Saunders

MANUAL OF

Nursing Care

Editor

JOAN LUCKMANN, MA, RN

Seattle, Washington

Medical Illustrations by

Kate Sweeney

W.B. SAUNDERS COMPANY
A Division of Harcourt Brace & Company
Philadelphia London Toronto Montreal Sydney Tokyo

W.B. SAUNDERS COMPANY
A Division of Harcourt Brace & Company

The Curtis Center
Independence Square West
Philadelphia, Pennsylvania 19106

Library of Congress Cataloging-in-Publication Data

Luckmann, Joan.
    Saunders manual of nursing care / Joan Luckmann; medical
artist, Kate Sweeney.—1st ed.
      p. cm.
    Includes indexes.
    ISBN 0–7216–5017–1
    1. Nursing—Handbooks, manuals, etc. I. Title. II. Title:
Manual of nursing care.
    [DNLM: 1. Nursing Process. WY 100 L941s 1997]
RT51.L83 1997
610.73—DC20
DNLM/DLC   95-50014

NOTICE

Nursing is an ever-changing field. Standard safety precautions must be followed, but as new research and clinical experience broaden our knowledge, changes in treatment and drug therapy become necessary or appropriate. Readers are advised to check the product information currently provided by the manufacturer of each drug to verify the recommended dose, the method and duration of administration, and contraindications. It is the responsibility of the treating physician, relying on experience and knowledge of the patient, to determine dosages and the best treatment for the patient. Neither the Publisher nor the editor assumes any responsibility for any injury and/or damage to persons or property.

THE PUBLISHER

To my loving children,
Karen and Chris;

my darling grandchildren,
Nicole and Michael;

my wonderful friends,
who have stood by me throughout my career in nursing;

and last but not least, my dog, **Peaches,**
who has been by my side every day as I've worked on the
Saunders Manual of Nursing Care.

Special Consultants

M. Linda Workman, PhD, RN, OCN, FAAN
Associate Professor
Frances Payne Bolton School of Nursing
Case Western Reserve University
Cleveland, Ohio

Elizabeth Crooks, MSN, RN, CCRN
Lecturer
Frances Payne Bolton School of Nursing
Case Western Reserve University
Cleveland, Ohio

Constance Visovsky, MS, RN,C
Instructor in Nursing
Frances Payne Bolton School of Nursing
Case Western Reserve University
Cleveland, Ohio

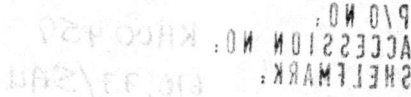

Contributors

Steve Alderfer, MSN, RN, CCRN
Instructor of Nursing, Eastern Mennonite University, Harrisonburg, Virginia
22 *Caring for People with Respiratory Disorders*

Kathleen Miller Baldwin, PhD, RN, CEN, CCRN
Assistant Professor, College of Nursing, University of Utah; Staff Nurse, Neuro Critical Care, University of Utah Medical Center, Salt Lake City, Utah
12 *Caring for People in Shock*

Cindy Bedell, MSN, RN, OCN
Breast Care Center, John Muir Medical Center, Walnut Creek, California
33 *Caring for People with Breast Disorders*

Carol Birch, MS, RN
Instructor, Medical-Surgical Nursing, College of Nursing, South Dakota State University, Rapid City, South Dakota
29 *Caring for People with Endocrine Disorders*

Karen M. Boyd-Sheehan, MSN, RN, OCN
Lincoln, California
32 *Caring for People with Sexually Transmitted Diseases*

Tess L. Briones, PhD(C), RN
Research Assistant, School of Nursing, University of Michigan, Ann Arbor, Michigan
28 *Caring for People with Hepatic, Biliary, and Pancreatic Disorders*

Barbara J. Burgel, MS, RN, NP, COHN
Clinical Professor, Occupational Health Nursing Graduate Program, University of California School of Nursing, University of California, San Francisco; Nurse Practitioner, Occupational Medical Clinic, The Medical Center at the University of California, San Francisco, San Francisco, California
38 *Caring for People with Environmentally and Occupationally Induced Disorders*

Gretchen J. Carrougher, MN, RN
Clinical Research Nurse, University of Washington Burn/Plastic Center, Harborview Medical Center, Seattle, Washington
36 *Caring for People with Burn Injuries*

Susan E. Chaney, EdD, RN, FNPC
Professor, College of Nursing, Texas Woman's University; Family Nurse Practitioner, Homeless Outreach Medical Services, Parkland Memorial Hospital, Dallas, Texas
7 *Caring for People with Disabilities*

Marilyn L. Conner, MS, RN, ONC, CCM
Clinical Nurse Specialist/Case Manager, Orthopaedics Department, Good Samaritan Hospital and Health Center, Dayton, Ohio
34 *Caring for People with Musculoskeletal Disorders*

Judi Davis, MS
Chief Dietitian, Home-Based Community Services, Torrant County Mental Health–Mental Retardation, Fort Worth, Texas
10 *Caring for People with Nutritional Disorders*

Lydia DeSantis, PhD, RN, FAAN
Professor of Nursing, School of Nursing, University of Miami, Coral Gables, Florida
2 *Providing Transcultural Nursing Care*

Pamela Duchene, DNS, RN, CRRN
New England Rehabilitation Hospital, Woburn, Massachusetts
16 *Caring for Older People*

Mary R. Dunbar, MN, MSW, RN
Coordinator, Chemical Dependency Program, Shoreline Community College; Creative Arts Therapist, Addiction Recovery Services, Swedish Medical Center, Seattle, Washington
40 *Caring for People with Tobacco, Alcohol, and Other Drug Addictions*

Linda Felver, PhD, RN
Department of Adult Health and Illness, School of Nursing, Oregon Health Sciences University, Portland, Oregon
9   Caring for People with Fluid, Electrolyte, and Acid-Base Imbalances

Sally K. Graham, MSN, RN
Adult/Geriatric Nurse Practitioner, Ever Care, Atlanta, Georgia
33   Caring for People with Breast Disorders

Mikel Gray, PhD, CUNP, CCCN, FAAN
Adjunct Professor of Nursing, Bellarmine College, Lansing School of Nursing, Louisville, Kentucky; Nurse Practitioner, Department of Urology, University of Virginia Medical Center, Charlottesville, Virginia
26   Caring for People with Urinary System Disorders

Oneida M. Hughes, PhD, RN
Professor, Nursing Education, College of Nursing, Texas Woman's University, Dallas, Texas
11   Caring for People in Pain

Barbara Innes, EdD, RN
Associate Professor, School of Nursing, Seattle Pacific University, Seattle, Washington
1   Problem Solving in Nursing

Susan Rowen James, MSN, RN
Assistant Professor, School of Nursing, Curry College, Milton, Massachusetts
15   Caring for Infants, Children, and Adolescents

Kathleen J. Jones, MS, RN, ANP
Adult Nurse Practitioner, Oncology Clinic, Walter Reed Army Medical Center, Washington, District of Columbia
30   Caring for Men with Sexual and Reproductive System Disorders

Annabelle M. Keene, MSN, RN
Associate Professor, Nursing Division, College of Saint Mary, Omaha, Nebraska
4   Obtaining the Basic Health History
5   Performing the Basic Physical Assessment
6   Performing the Basic Psychosocial Assessment

Suzanne Kier, PhD, RN
College of Nursing, Texas Woman's University, Dallas, Texas
25   Caring for People with Blood Disorders

Diane Klein, PhD, RN
Associate Professor of Medical-Surgical Nursing, Niehoff School of Nursing, Loyola University of Chicago, Maywood, Illinois
21   Caring for People with Immune and Autoimmune Disorders
8   Caring for People with Infections and Infectious Disorders

Kathryn K. Kremer, MSN, RN
Clinical Instructor, College of Nursing, Texas Woman's University; Staff Nurse, Parkland Memorial Hospital, Dallas, Texas
7   Caring for People with Disabilities

Marijo Letizia, PhD, RN,C
Assistant Professor of Medical-Surgical Nursing, Niehoff School of Nursing, Loyola University of Chicago, Maywood, Illinois
21   Caring for People with Immune and Autoimmune Disorders

Deitra Leonard Lowdermilk, PhD, RN,C
Clinical Professor, Department of Health of Women and Children, School of Nursing, University of North Carolina at Chapel Hill, Chapel Hill, North Carolina
31   Caring for Women with Sexual and Reproductive System Disorders

Laura E. Luecke, BSN, RN, CCRN
Nurse Internship Instructor, Parkland Memorial Hospital, Dallas, Texas
23   Caring for People with Cardiovascular Disorders

Mary E. Mancini, MSN, RN, CNA
Senior Vice President, Nursing Administration, Parkland Memorial Hospital, Dallas, Texas
23   Caring for People with Cardiovascular Disorders

Sue Ann McCann, MSN, RN
Dermatology Nurse Coordinator, University of Pittsburgh Medical Center, Pittsburgh, Pennsylvania
35   Caring for People with Integumentary Disorders

Ruth McCorkle, PhD, RN, FAAN
Professor of Oncology Nursing, School of Nursing, University of Pennsylvania, Philadelphia, Pennsylvania
43   Caring for People Who Are Dying and Their Families

Margaret M. McMahon, MN, RN, CEN
Clinical Instructor, Emergency Department, Atlantic City Medical Center, Atlantic City, New Jersey
37   Caring for People Experiencing Emergencies

Margaret Norton, MN, RN
Niehoff School of Nursing, Loyola University of Chicago, Maywood, Illinois
21   Caring for People with Immune and Autoimmune Disorders

Sally Olds, MSN, RN,C
Associate Professor and Chair, Department of Holistic Nursing, Beth-El College of Nursing and Health Sciences, Colorado Springs, Colorado
14   Caring for Women in the Childbearing Cycle

Judy Ozuna, MN, RN
Clinical Assistant Professor, Department of Biobehavioral Nursing and Health Systems, School of Nursing, University of Washington; Clinical Nurse Specialist in Neurology, Veterans Affairs Medical Center, Seattle, Washington
18   Caring for People with Neurologic Disorders

Ann Griswold Peirce, PhD, RN
School of Nursing, Columbia University, New York, New York
39 Caring for People Experiencing Life Crises

Rose Ann Peterson, MSN, RN
School of Nursing, Los Angeles County Medical Center, Los Angeles, California
3 Managing the Modern Clinical Environment

Mary Pickett, PhD, RN
Research Assistant Professor, School of Nursing, University of Pennsylvania, Philadelphia, Pennsylvania
43 Caring for People Who Are Dying and Their Families

Lana Ralston, MS, RN
School of Nursing, Texas Woman's University, Dallas, Texas
41 Caring for People with Mental Disorders

Nina A. Rauscher, BA, RN,C, ONC, CRRN
Nurse Clinician, Orthopaedics/Neuroscience/Rehabilitation, The North Shore Medical Center, Salem, Massachusetts
34 Caring for People with Musculoskeletal Disorders

Richard G. Rayome, BSN, RN, CCCN
Clinical Director, UroHealth of Kentucky, Inc., Louisville, Kentucky
26 Caring for People with Urinary System Disorders

Marian Williams Roman, MSN, RN, CS
Assistant Clinical Professor, Psychiatric-Mental Health Nursing, College of Nursing, Texas Woman's University; Consultant for Psychiatric Nursing/Clinical Nurse Specialist, Home Health Services of Dallas, Dallas, Texas
41 Caring for People with Mental Disorders

Linda Traxler Schuring, MSN, RN
Nursing Director of Balance Clinics, Warren Otologic Group, Warren, Ohio
20 Caring for People with Ear, Nose, Throat, Head, and Neck Disorders

Kim Sherer, MN, RN
Nursing Chair, Division of Nursing, Northern Oklahoma College, Tonkawa, Oklahoma
10 Caring for People with Nutritional Disorders

Susan W. Sheriff, PhD, RN
Assistant Professor, College of Nursing, Texas Woman's University, Dallas, Texas
13 Caring for People Undergoing Surgery

Barbara A. Sigler, MNEd, RN, CORLN
Adjunctive Instructor, School of Nursing, University of Pittsburgh; Clinical Nurse Specialist, Department of Otolaryngology, University of Pittsburgh Medical Center, Pittsburgh, Pennsylvania
20 Caring for People with Ear, Nose, Throat, Head, and Neck Disorders

JoAnne Turner, MN, RN
Clinical Nurse Specialist, Columbia Cardiology, Columbia, South Carolina
24 Caring for People with Peripheral Vascular and Lymphatic Disorders

Linda Anderson Vader, BS, RN, CRNO
Head Nurse, W. K. Kellogg Eye Center, University of Michigan, Ann Arbor, Michigan
19 Caring for People with Visual Disorders

Jeanette Baird Vaughan, MSN, RN, CCRN
School of Nursing, Texas Woman's University, Dallas, Texas
25 Caring for People with Blood Disorders

Kathleen Murphy White, PhD, RN
Assistant Professor, School of Nursing, University of Maryland at Baltimore, Baltimore, Maryland
27 Caring for People with Gastrointestinal Disorders

Marianne G. Zelewsky, MSN, RN,C
Assistant Professor, Community, Mental Health, and Administrative Nursing, Niehoff School of Nursing, Loyola University of Chicago; Consultant, HIV/AIDS Services, Catholic Charities, Chicago, Illinois
42 Caring for People with Human Immunodeficiency Virus Disease

Home Care Strategies were coordinated and edited by **Karen S. Martin**, MSN, RN, FAAN, Health Care Consultant, Omaha, Nebraska. Individual Home Care Strategies were written by the following people:
1. Alegent Health, Bergan Mercy Home Healthcare Services, Omaha, Nebraska. Contact person: Carolyn Geiger, BSN, RN, Director. Contributors: Karen Thomas, BSN, RN (Chapter 7); Bev Ordway, RN (Chapter 10); Joan Gilroy, BSN, RN, CRNH, and Lora Lea Brennan, BS, RN, CRNH (Chapter 11); Kathy Henely, RN (Chapter 13); Samantha Hoffman, OT, and Cathy Zimmerman, PT (Chapter 16); Barbara O'Malley, BS, RN (Chapter 17); Carolyn Geiger, BSN, RN (Chapter 22); Linda David, BSN, RN, Nancy Buras, AD, RN, and Ann Hovendick, AD, RN (Chapter 23); Christine Campbell, RN (Chapter 29); Peggy Kelley Curl, MSN, RN (Chapter 33); Bonnie Brown, BGS, RN, and Marcia Blum, CMSW, ACSW (Chapter 43).
2. Visiting Nurse Association of Cleveland, Cleveland, Ohio. Contact person: Barbara Kukla, MSN, RN, CNA, Vice President of Nursing Services. Contributors: Barbara M. Mundson, RN,C (Chapter 14); Kathryn J. Miller, BA, ADN (Chapter 15); Sandra Fogel, BSN (Chapter 18); Patricia M. Gracey, BSN, RN,C (Chapter 19); Elaine Ramos Pagan, RN (Chapter 20); Debra A. S. Passan, BSN, RN (Chapter 21); Penny King Paul, BA, RN (Chapter 24); Juliann Dobrozsi Seballos, RN (Chapter 25); Christine L. Schmitt, BSN, RN (Chapter 26); Patricia A. Gallagher, BSN, RN, CETN (Chapter 27); Peter Markovich, RN, BA, AD (Chapter 34); Deborah Spilker, BSN, RN,C (Chapter 35); Suzette Lusane, BSN, RN (Chapter 36); and Sallie Eddy, BSN, RN (Chapter 42).

Consultants

Barbara Brillhart, PhD, RN, CRRN
School of Nursing
University of Colorado Health Sciences Center
Denver, Colorado

Kathlyn Carlson, BSN, RN, MA, CPAN
Abbott Northwestern Hospital
Minneapolis, Minnesota

Linda Fletcher, MS, RN, CRRN
Crawford Health Care Management
Columbus, Georgia

Patricia J. Hughes, EdD, RN
Pacific Lutheran University
Tacoma, Washington

Judith Ann Kilpatrick, MSN, RN,C
Widener University
Chester, Pennsylvania

Doris Marshalek, MSN, CCRN
Community College of Allegheny County
Pittsburgh, Pennsylvania

Mary Patricia Norrell, BSN, RN,C
Ivy Tech State College
Columbus, Indiana

Mary E. Sampel, MSN, RN
St. Louis University
St. Louis, Missouri

Teresa Kelly Snyder, MN, RN, CS
Montana State University
Missoula, Montana

Janice M. Sylakowski, MS, RN
State University of New York at Buffalo
Buffalo, New York

Barbara Gayle Talik, BSN, MEd, RN
Northwest Technical Institute
Springdale, Arkansas

Reviewers

Mary Lou Altman, MSN, RN
University of Pittsburgh
Pittsburgh, Pennsylvania

Jill S. Anderson, MSN, RN, CS
University of Illinois at Chicago
Chicago, Illinois

Sarah Angermuller, MEd, MSN, CNRN, CCRN, CEN
Columbus College
Columbus, Georgia

Elizabeth Arnold, BSN, MEd, RN,C
Milton S. Hershey Medical Center
Pennsylvania State University
Hershey, Pennsylvania

Gretchen E. Bagley, MSN, MA
Pikes Peak Community College
Colorado Springs, Colorado

Linda Becker, MSN, RN,C
St. Clair County Community College
Port Huron, Michigan

Roxanne Bell, PhD, RN
College of West Virginia
Beckley, West Virginia

Margaret Bellak, MN, RN
Indiana University of Pennsylvania
Indiana, Pennsylvania

Nancy Berger, MSN, RN,C
Charles E. Gregory School of Nursing
Raritan Bay Medical Center
Perth Amboy, New Jersey

Wendy Blackburn, BAA, MNI, MAEd, RN, CNN
Fanshawe College
St. Michael's Hospital
London, Ontario, Canada

Kathleen Blade, MS, RN
St. Joseph Hospital School of Nursing
North Providence, Rhode Island

Donna Bosch, MSN, RN,C
University of Mary and Medcenter One
Bismarck, North Dakota

Carole Broxson, PhD, RN
Sinclair Community College
Dayton, Ohio

Bonita E. Broyles, BSN, MA, RN
Piedmont Community College
Roxboro, North Carolina

Roberta Bumann, MSN, RN
Department Of Nursing
Winona State University and St. Marys Hospital
of Rochester
Rochester, Minnesota

Janet E. Burton, BRE, MSN, RN
Bob Jones University
Greenville, South Carolina

Lee Anne Caffrey, MSN, RN, OCN
Memorial Sloan Kettering Cancer Center
New York, New York

Marissa Camanga-Reyes, MN, RN, CCRN
Harbor UCLA Medical Center
Torrance, California

Marcia Chorba, MSN, RN
Mercy Hospital School of Nursing
Pittsburgh, Pennsylvania

Bonnie L. Closson, MSN, RNCS, MRC, CRRN
Mayo Foundation, St. Mary's Hospital (MN)
Rochester, Minnesota

Diane G. Copenhaver, PhD, RN, CANP, CPNP
Coppin State University
Baltimore, Maryland

Judy K. Davidson, MN, RN, RN, CS
Columbus College
Columbus, Georgia

Paula Dawson, BSN, MEd, RN, CHES
Monroeville, Pennsylvania

Sharron K. Disbro, BSN, MA, RN, CNOR
University of Michigan
Ann Arbor, Michigan

Mary Rose Driggers, MSN, RN
Davidson County Community College
Lexington, North Carolina

Linda Fahey, MSN, ANP-C
California State University, Los Angeles
Los Angeles, California

Joyce Feldman, MSN, RN
Overlook Hospital
Summit, New Jersey

Diane M. Felser, MSN, RN
College of Nursing
University of Illinois
Chicago, Illinois

Vickie K. Fieler, MS, RN, OCN
University of Rochester Cancer Center
Rochester, New York

Patricia Finder-Stone, MS, RN
Northeast Wisconsin Technical College
Green Bay, Wisconsin

Cynthia Garrett, MSN, RN
University of North Carolina Hospitals
Chapel Hill, North Carolina

Mary Jo Gerlach, MSNEd, RN
School of Nursing
Medical College of Georgia
Athens, Georgia

Michele Gerwick, MSN, RN
Indiana University of Pennsylvania
Indiana, Pennsylvania

Debra S. Goodwin, BSN, MS, RN, ACLS
Belleair Surgical Center
Clearwater, Florida

Ann Smith Gregoire, MSN, RN, CRNP, CCRN
Thomas Jefferson University Hospital
Philadelphia, Pennsylvania

Gloria A. Hagopian, EdD, RN
College of Nursing
University of North Carolina, Charlotte
Charlotte, North Carolina

Lori Hendrickx, MSN, RN, CCRN
Montana State University
Bozeman, Montana

Shirley Hoeman, PhD, MPH, RN, CRRN, CNAA, CCM
Fairfield University
Fairfield, Connecticut

Nancy S. Hogan, PhD, RN, CS
University of Miami
Coral Gables, Florida

Holly Holden, BSN, RN, CEN
River District Hospital
and St. Clair County Community College
East China, Michigan

Cynthia L. Homan, MSN, RN,C
Good Samaritan Hospital
Downers Grove, Illinois

Charlotte L. Ingram, MS, RN, CS
Columbus College
Columbus, Georgia

Patricia Iyer, MSN, RN, CNA
Patricia Iyer Associates
Stockton, New Jersey

Anita Jackson, MS, RN,C
Ohio State Medical Center
Columbus, Ohio

Patricia Jakel, MN, RN, OCN
UCLA Medical Center
Los Angeles, California

Gwendolyn C. Jones, MSN, RN
North Carolina Central University
Durham, North Carolina

Linda Kocent, MSN, RN, CCRN
Thomas Jefferson University Hospital
Philadelphia, Pennsylvania

Eileen Mieras Kohlenberg, PhD, RN, CNAA
Adult Health Nursing
University of North Carolina at Greensboro
Greensboro, North Carolina

Mary Ann Krammin, PhD, RN
Oakland Community College
Waterford, Michigan

N. Robin Kubel, PhD, RN, PNP
Coppin State College
Baltimore, Maryland

Janet Kuhn, EdD, RN
Villanova University
Villanova, Pennsylvania

Nancy Kupper, MSN, RN
Tarrant County Junior College
Ft. Worth, Texas

Louise LaFramboise, MSN, RN
College of Nursing
University of Nebraska
Omaha, Nebraska

Janice G. Lanham, BSN, RN
TriCounty Technical College
Pendleton, South Carolina

Denise LeBlanc, BScN, RN
Humber College
and Scarborough General Hospital
Toronto, Ontario, Canada

J. Pierre Loebel, MA, MD
University of Washington
Seattle, Washington

Mary Ann Long, BSN, RN
Roswell Park Cancer Institute
Buffalo, New York

Denise Maguire, MS, RN,C
All Children's Hospital
St. Petersburg, Florida

Linda Nance Marks, EdD, RN, ANP
School of Nursing
University of Texas at Arlington
Arlington, Texas

Jean McLeod, MS, RN,C, CNA
Johns Hopkins Bayview Medical Center
Baltimore, Maryland

Mary Ellen McMorrow, EdD, RN, CCRN
College of Staten Island
Staten Island, New York

Ann F. Mead, MN, RN, GPN
Mississippi Gulf Coast Community College
Gulfport, Mississippi

Diane C. Meador, MSN, RN
University of Northern Colorado
Greeley, Colorado

Mary E. Mehok, MSN, RN, CCRN
Mercy Hospital
Pittsburgh, Pennsylvania

Mary Kemp Milsten, BSN, MS, RN
Saint Luke's College
Kansas City, Missouri

Terry R. Misener, PhD, RNCS, FAAN
College of Nursing
University of South Carolina
Columbia, South Carolina

Sharon Moran, MPH, RN,C
University of Hawaii
and Hawaii Community College
Hilo, Hawaii

Teri Morehouse, MS, RN
School of Nursing
University of Wyoming
Laramie, Wyoming

Sally W. Morgan, MS, RN, CS
Ohio State University Medical Center
Columbus, Ohio

Catherine Ann Myerholtz, MSN, RN
School of Nursing
Providence Hospital
Sandusky, Ohio

Carol J. Nelson, MSN, RN
Spokane Community College
Spokane, Washington

Sylvia E. Nissila, PhD, RN
College of St. Catherine
St. Paul, Minnesota

Netha O'Meara, MSN, RN
Wharton County Junior College
Wharton, Texas

Mary Frances Oneha, MN, RN
School of Nursing
University of Hawaii and Waianae Coast Comprehensive
Health Center
Honolulu Hawaii

Maureen O'Rourke, MS, RN, OCN
University of North Carolina at Chapel Hill
Chapel Hill, North Carolina

Brenda Owens, PhD, RN
Louisiana State University Medical Center
New Orleans, Louisiana

Linda J. Allan Pasto, MS, RN
Tompkins-Cortland Community College
Dryden, New York

Jennie S. Payne, MSN, RN
Edwards-Eve Clinic
Nashville, Tennessee

Sharon Ann Perrilliat-Stanley, MSN
Albuquerque Technical Vocational Institute
Community College
Albuquerque, New Mexico

Barbara Preib-Lannon, MS, RN,C
University of Illinois at Chicago
Chicago, Illinois

Shanti J. Pruitt, MN, RN, OCN
Indiana University Medical Center
Indianapolis, Indiana

Patti D. Quenzer, MSN, RN, RT
Southern West Virginia Community College
Williamsville, West Virginia

Rosemary Quinn-Cefaro, MS, RN, CDE, CNN, CNS
SUNY/HSC at Brooklyn Research Foundation
Brooklyn, New York

Rosemary Ann Roth, MSN, RN, CNOR, CNAA
The Genesee Hospital
Rochester, New York

Josephine R. Sears, BSN, MEd, RN
Springfield Technical Community College
Springfield, Massachusetts

Donna J. Seefeldt, MSN, RN, OCN
D'Youville College
Buffalo, New York

Lisa Anderson Shaw, MSN, MA, RN,C
College of Nursing
University of Illinois
University of Illinois Eye and Ear Infirmary
Chicago, Illinois

Joyce A. Shireman, BSN, PhD, RN
Coe College
Cedar Rapids, Iowa

Lois M. Short, MA, MN, RN, CNS-ARNP
Wichita State University
Wichita, Kansas

Linda A. Shortridge, MN, PhD, RN
Oregon Health Sciences University
Portland, Oregon

Gloria A. Smith, MS, RN
CM Health Care Resources
Deerfield, Illinois
and Baptist Hospital of Miami
Miami, Florida

Mary E. Soja, MSN, MA, RN
Indiana University School of Nursing
Indianapolis, Indiana

Lillian Sonnenschein, MSN, RN
St. Joseph Health Services
North Providence, Rhode Island

Patricia Soran, MS, RN
Boise State University
Boise, Idaho

Martha A. Spies, MSN, RN
Deaconess College of Nursing
St. Louis, Missouri

Karen J. Stanley, MSN, RN, OCN
Kaiser Permanente Hospital
Fontana, California

Louise Suit, EdD, RN
Harding University
Searcy, Arizona

Elizabeth D. Sullivan, MN, RN, OCN
City of Hope Medical Center
Duarte, California

Linda Tenenbaum, MSN, RN, OCN
Broward Community College
Ft. Lauderdale, Florida

Paula R. Timmerman, MSN, RN, OCN
Good Samaritan Hospital
Downers Grove, Illinois

Marilyn J. Vontz, MSN, PhD, RN
Bryan Memorial Hospital School of Nursing
Lincoln, Nebraska

Carole J. Petrosky Vozel, PhD, RN,C
School of Nursing
Western Pennsylvania Hospital
Pittsburgh, Pennsylvania

Penny J. Vukov-Zmora, MS, RN, CS
Good Samaritan Hospital
Downers Grove, Illinois

Margaret Washington, MN, RN
Charity School of Nursing
and Delgado Community College
New Orleans, Louisiana

Kathleen H. Werle, MSN, RN
Victor Valley College
Victorville, California
and California State University, Domingo Hills,
Carson, California

Nancy West, MN, RN, ACLS
Johnson County Community College
Overland Park, Kansas

Suzanne T. West, MSN, RN
Department of Nursing
Columbus College
Columbus, Georgia

Jeanne Whalen, BSN, RN, MICN, CEN
Carolinas Medical Center
Charlotte, North Carolina

Stuart L. Whitney, MS, RN, CS
School of Nursing
University of Vermont
Burlington, Vermont

Susan Karm Wieczorek, MSN, RN, CNS
Health Education Consulting Institute, Inc.
Columbus, Georgia

Sandra Lee Woods, MSN, RN, NP
University of Cincinnati Medical Center
Cincinnati, Ohio

◼ STUDENT REVIEWERS

Jill Bennett, RN
San Diego State University
San Diego, California

Rachel Winograd Bollenbecker, BA, BSN, RN
Olive View Medical Center
Sylmar, California

Kristin Cammack
Beth-El College of Nursing and Health Sciences
Colorado Springs, Colorado

Elaine Horton, SN
Beth-El College of Nursing and Health Sciences
Colorado Springs, Colorado

Rodger Jarabek, BA, ADN
Dakota Wesleyan University
Mitchell, South Dakota

Jeanne Lindner
California State University, Bakersfield
Bakersfield, California

Tina Rorick, BSN
California State University, Los Angeles
Acton, California

Preface

As the standard of education and requirements become of a higher character and the training more efficient, the trained nurse will draw nearer to science and its demands and take a greater share as a social factor in solving the world's needs.

Isabel Hampton Robb
NURSING ETHICS, 1901

Goal and Purposes

The 20th century was just beginning when Isabel Hampton Robb wrote her landmark textbook, *Nursing Ethics*. Over the decades, her predictions have come true. Nursing has grown into a respected profession, advanced in the sciences, and emerged into a powerful social force for "solving the world's needs." Now, on the brink of the 21st century, nurses face even greater challenges as they cope with new medical technologies, evolving health care policies, and social and cultural change. To provide nurses with the "cutting edge" information they must have to meet these challenges is the goal of the *Saunders Manual of Nursing Care*.

Specifically, we have structured the *Saunders Manual* to provide nurses with the following:

1. A review of the *broad principles* that underlie nursing practice such as (1) the 5 steps of the nursing process, (2) the principles of health care teaching, and (3) the legal and ethical aspects of nursing.

2. Strategies for *managing* the modern clinical area, coordinating patient care, directing the nursing staff, and identifying signs of stress and burnout in the nursing staff.

3. Methods for conducting a *holistic health assessment* that encompass both the physical examination and the psychosocial assessment.

4. Detailed and well-illustrated data concerning the assessment and care of people experiencing medical-surgical problems (e.g., fluid and electrolyte imbalances), medical-surgical disorders, and medical-surgical emergencies.

5. Realistic and practical solutions for overcoming the problems that continually arise in hospital, clinic, and home care situations.

6. Information on how to care for people with special developmental needs and problems, such as women in the childbearing cycle, infants, children, adolescents, and older people.

7. Specific guidelines for caring for people with special psychosocial needs and problems, such as people who are experiencing crises, people who are mentally ill, and people who are dying.

8. Sections that clearly address the important issue of cultural diversity and carefully tailor nursing care to the special needs of people from different racial, ethnic, and religious backgrounds.

Scope, Organization, and Content

The *Saunders Manual of Nursing Care* is both broad in scope and comprehensive in its coverage of important procedures, medical-surgical disorders, medical-surgical needs and problems, and emergencies. To cover the spectrum of professional nursing practice, the *Saunders Manual* is divided into 6 major units. The material in these units is in *outline format* for ease of use.

Unit I, "Challenges Facing Nurses in the 1990s and Beyond," focuses on the challenges that professional nurses must master to provide optimal nursing care and experience success and satisfaction in their careers. This unit addresses such important topics as the nursing process, problem solving, legal and ethical considerations, transcultural considerations, quality care, health care teaching, legal and ethical considerations, and the principles of nursing management.

Unit II, "Performing a Holistic Health Assessment," examines the process of performing basic physical and psychosocial assessments. This unit's 3 chapters describe interviewing techniques, methods for obtaining and recording a person's health history and current health status, physical examination techniques, and the essential components of the psychosocial assessment.

Unit III, "Caring for People with Special Medical-Surgical

Needs and Problems," contains separate chapters on caring for people with disabilities, infections and infectious disorders, nutritional disorders, fluid and electrolyte and acid-base imbalances, pain, and shock. In addition, Chapter 13 outlines the nursing care for people undergoing surgery. This unit describes such important interventions as physical rehabilitation techniques, intravenous therapy, diet therapy, and invasive and noninvasive pain and shock therapies.

Unit IV, "Caring for People with Special Developmental Needs and Problems," addresses the care of women in the childbearing cycle, infants, children, adolescents, and older people. The *Saunders Manual* does not attempt to present highly technical information about obstetric or neonatal care, nor does it describe all of the pediatric disorders in detail. Instead it focuses on those problems, conditions, and situations that the nurse who is in *general practice* frequently encounters—for example, women with unwanted pregnancies, mothers suffering from postpartum depression, children experiencing emergencies, and older people who are no longer able to care for themselves.

Unit V, "Caring for People with Medical-Surgical Disorders," is the heart of the *Saunders Manual*. This unit focuses on the major disorders that afflict each of the body systems. Detailed chapters cover these important topics clearly: cancer; neurologic disorders; visual disorders; ear, nose, throat, head, and neck disorders; immune and autoimmune disorders; respiratory disorders; cardiovascular disorders; peripheral vascular and lymphatic disorders; blood disorders; urinary system disorders; hepatic, biliary, and pancreatic disorders; endocrine disorders; sexual and reproductive system disorders of men and women; sexually transmitted disorders; breast disorders; musculoskeletal disorders; integumentary disorders; burn injuries; emergencies; and environmental and occupational disorders.

Unit VI, "Caring for People with Special Psychosocial Needs and Problems," describes the special needs and problems of people in crisis, people with drug addictions, people with AIDS, mentally ill people, and people who are dying; in other words, people who are found in all populations—hospital, clinic, and home. This unit guides nurses as they work with individuals who are trying to quit smoking or drinking, people who feel devastated by AIDS, and people who are anxious or depressed or experiencing a crisis such as domestic abuse.

The Appendix is composed of 4 sections. Appendix A focuses on the traditional health beliefs and practices of select cultures. Appendix B presents guidelines for obtaining specific laboratory cultures. Appendix C lists clinical laboratory values. Finally, Appendix D provides guidelines for isolation precautions in hospitals.

The *Saunders Manual* contains more than 750 illustrations, photographs, charts, and graphs. These illustrative materials act to clarify anatomy and physiology discussions, explain pathophysiology and symptoms, and demonstrate how to perform physical assessments and diagnostic tests. There is also an 8-page insert of 48 color illustrations of examples of dermatology, eye, and gastrointestinal disorders as well as AIDS-related disorders and burn injuries. In addition 82 formally prepared nursing procedures, many of which are illustrated, are presented in a step-by-step format with each step accompanied by a rationale.

Special Features

The *Saunders Manual of Nursing Care* has numerous excellent features that are integrated throughout the book and that serve to clarify and enliven the text.

- **Transcultural Considerations** boxes point out the traditional beliefs and customs of people from different cultures that affect their health, as well as the risk factors that may cause people from different cultures to be more vulnerable to certain disorders.
- **Nurse Advisory** boxes alert the nurse to the potential dangers and complications that may arise when caring for people with serious disorders and problems. These boxes emphasize the precautions that the nurse must observe to ensure safe care.
- **Elder Advisory** boxes remind the nurse of the special problems that older patients may experience—either as a result of disease or from iatrogenic causes.
- **Nursing Management** boxes are designed to help nursing managers make decisions concerning patients and staff and then take appropriate action.
- **Legal and Ethical Considerations** boxes increase the nurse's awareness of such vital issues as patient's rights, privileged communication, abortion, and euthanasia.
- **Clinical Controversy** boxes address controversial aspects of patient care such as the use of prophylactic antibiotics.
- **Learning/Teaching Guidelines** outline the health teaching information that patients and their families need to receive before going home. Seventy-six Learning/Teaching Guidelines provide nurses with clear and practical instructions for patients who are being discharged.
- **Home Care Strategies** are helpful tips on how to modify nursing techniques that are used in hospitals for the home. The *Saunders Manual* contains 25 Home Care Strategies; examples include "Infection Control in the Home," "Ostomy Care," "Care of the Surgical Incision," and "Home Chemotherapy."
- Large original illustrations combine artwork with textual material and consolidate and clarify vital information that is not duplicated elsewhere in the book.
- Extensive chapter bibliographies are broken down by subject matter (e.g., disorders, interventions, preventative measures). These bibliographies provide excellent reference material for the reader who wants to learn more about a particular problem or disorder.
- Lists of agencies that can be contacted for help end each chapter. Each list contains the names, addresses, and phone numbers of organizations that provide health care professionals, patients, and families with information and assistance (e.g., The American Heart Association, The National Cancer Institute, and The American Dietetic Association).

In summary, the reader will find that the *Saunders Manual of Nursing Care* provides nurses with the essential elements they need to practice their profession with competence and compassion. Within its pages, nurses will find clearly presented information, excellent illustrations, and clear guidelines for assessing, caring for, and teaching patients. We hope that the *Saunders Manual* will become a major source of knowledge and inspiration for nurses everywhere.

Acknowledgments

Researching, writing, editing, illustrating, and publishing a book as large and complex as the *Saunders Manual of Nursing Care* has involved the combined efforts of many talented and dedicated individuals. I am grateful to the following people:

Kate Sweeney, for her outstanding illustrations that make the *Saunders Manual* a useful and a beautiful book;

Linda Bedell, Developmental Editor, for her dedication to editing the manuscript and managing the length and for her constant encouragement;

Michael J. Brown, former Editor in Chief, Nursing Books, and **Darlene D. Pedersen**, former Senior Vice President and Editorial Director, Books Division, for giving me the opportunity to develop and edit the *Saunders Manual*;

Thomas Eoyang, Vice President and Editor in Chief, Nursing Books, for supporting the project;

Robin Levin Richman, Senior Developmental Editor, for her tremendous efforts to coordinate this huge project over the years;

Frank Polizzano, Production Manager, for expediting publication of this book;

Lee Ann Draud, Supervising Copy Editor, for her conscientious work on the manuscript;

Susan Blaker, Designer, for her elegant and efficient design;

David Kerprich, Marketing Manager, for developing a fine marketing campaign;

Lydia De Santis, PhD, RN, for the untold hours that she spent reviewing the manuscript for transcultural considerations and for bringing this vital information to light;

Margaret McMahon, MN, CEN, for her expert advice on the emergency conditions and procedures that are presented throughout the *Saunders Manual*;

Kelly Doran, MLS, for her library research and careful review of proof for the manuscript;

Charlie Smyth, for his valuable help with setting up the format for the *Saunders Manual*;

Lora Lee Wallace and **Dorene Johnson** for their secretarial support, and **Royale Landy** for the numerous telephone calls she made to health care agencies;

Debra Osnowitz, Developmental Editor, for her careful editing and her help with keeping the project on deadline;

I am grateful to the contributors and reviewers for the *Saunders Manual* who, over the years, gave so generously of their time, knowledge, and experience.

Once again, I want to thank all of you for your encouragement, support, and help and for your dedication to producing this outstanding book: *Saunders Manual of Nursing Care.*

JOAN LUCKMANN, MA, RN
Seattle, Washington

Contents

VI
Caring for People with Special Psychosocial Needs and Problems, 1833

Appendices

Color Figures

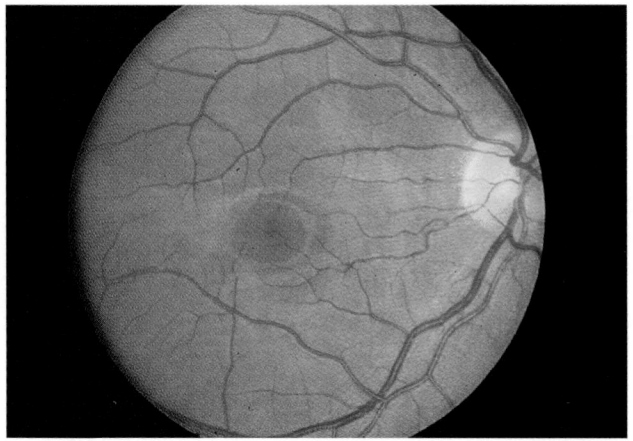

Color Figure 19–1. Normal fundus. (Courtesy of Ophthalmic Photography at the W.K. Kellogg Eye Center, University of Michigan, Ann Arbor, MI.)

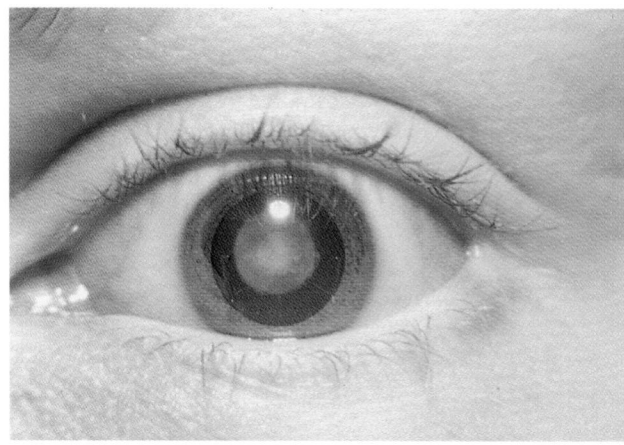

Color Figure 19–2. Congenital cataract. (Courtesy of Ophthalmic Photography at the W.K. Kellogg Eye Center, University of Michigan, Ann Arbor, MI.)

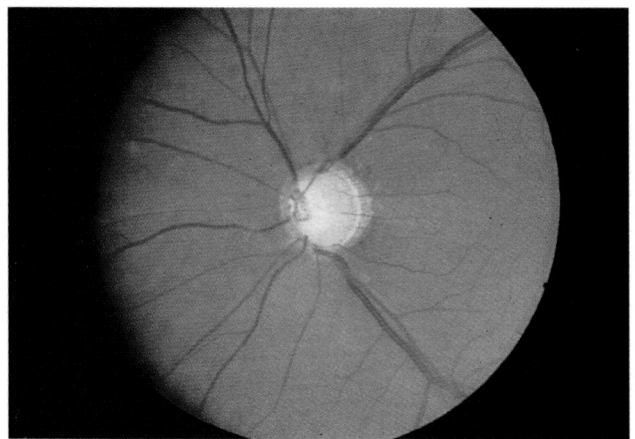

Color Figure 19–3. Cupped disk in glaucoma. (Courtesy of Ophthalmic Photography at the W.K. Kellogg Eye Center, University of Michigan, Ann Arbor, MI.)

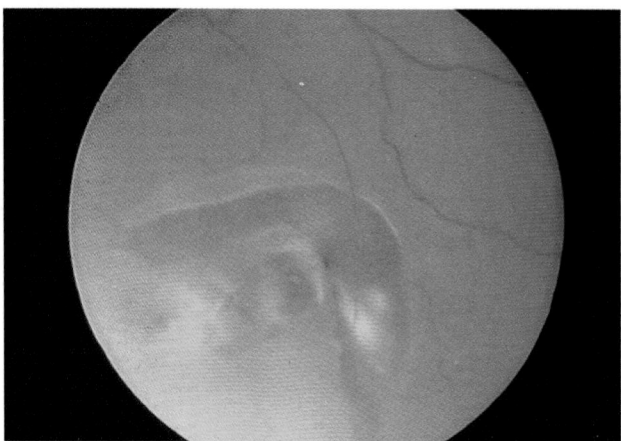

Color Figure 19–4. Rhegmatogenous retinal tear. (Courtesy of Ophthalmic Photography at the W.K. Kellogg Eye Center, University of Michigan, Ann Arbor, MI.)

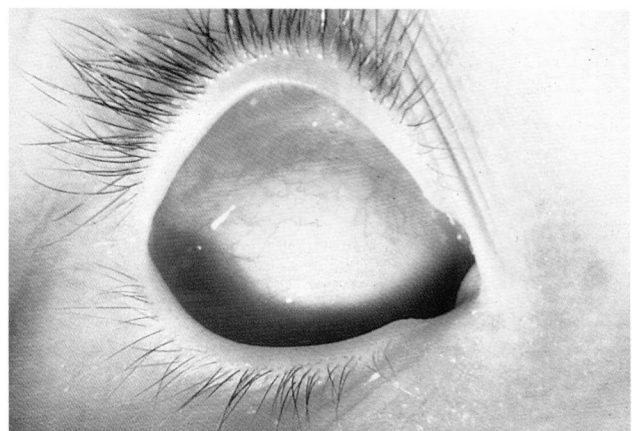

Color Figure 19–5. Healed socket after enucleation. (Courtesy of Ophthalmic Photography at the W.K. Kellogg Eye Center, University of Michigan, Ann Arbor, MI.)

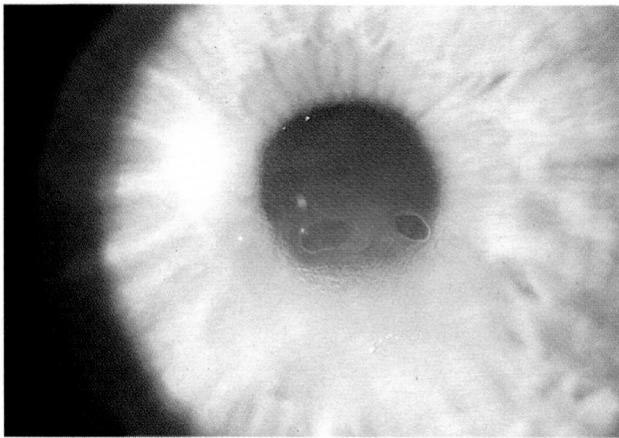

Color Figure 19–6. Fuchs' dystrophy. (Courtesy of Ophthalmic Photography at the W.K. Kellogg Eye Center, University of Michigan, Ann Arbor, MI.)

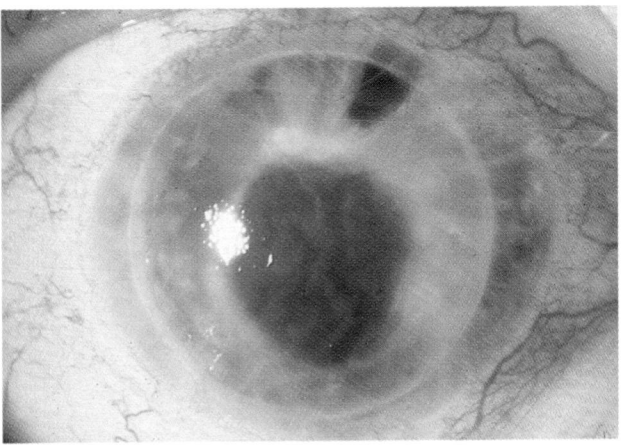

Color Figure 19–7. Corneal graft rejection. (Courtesy of Ophthalmic Photography at the W.K. Kellogg Eye Center, University of Michigan, Ann Arbor, MI.)

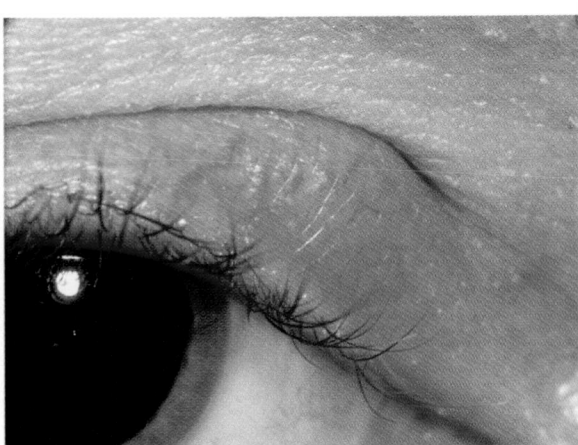

Color Figure 19–8. Chalazion. (Courtesy of Ophthalmic Photography at the W.K. Kellogg Eye Center, University of Michigan, Ann Arbor, MI.)

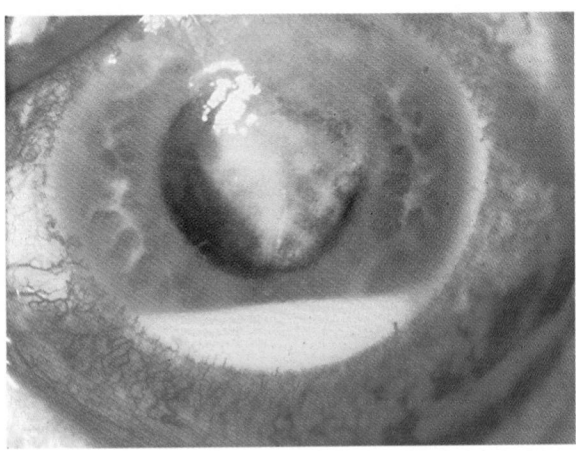

Color Figure 19–9. Corneal ulcer with hypopyon. (Courtesy of Ophthalmic Photography at the W.K. Kellogg Eye Center, University of Michigan, Ann Arbor, MI.)

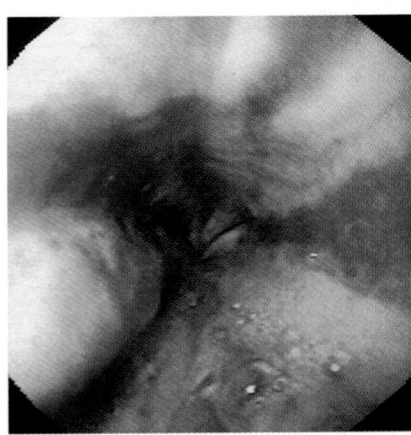

Color Figure 27–1. *Candida* esophagitis. (Courtesy of Surgical Endoscopy, University of Maryland Medical Center, Baltimore, MD.)

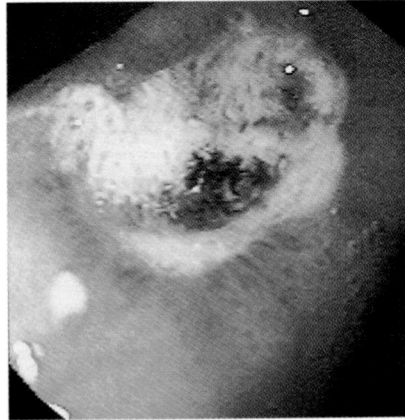

Color Figure 27–2. Gastric ulcer. (Courtesy of Surgical Endoscopy, University of Maryland Medical Center, Baltimore, MD.)

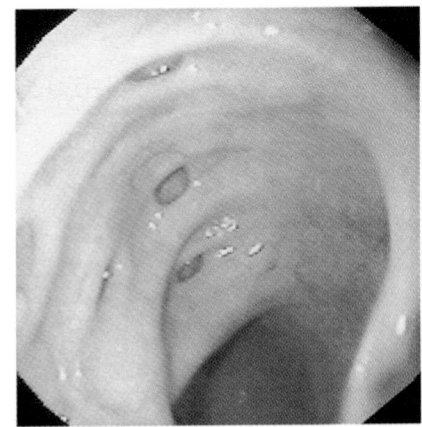

Color Figure 27–3. Diverticuli. (Courtesy of Surgical Endoscopy, University of Maryland Medical Center, Baltimore, MD.)

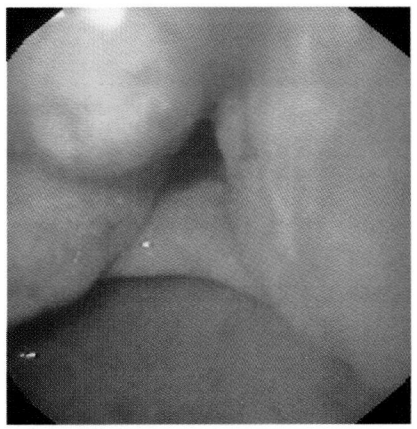

Color Figure 27–4. Gastric cancer. (Courtesy of Surgical Endoscopy, University of Maryland Medical Center, Baltimore, MD.)

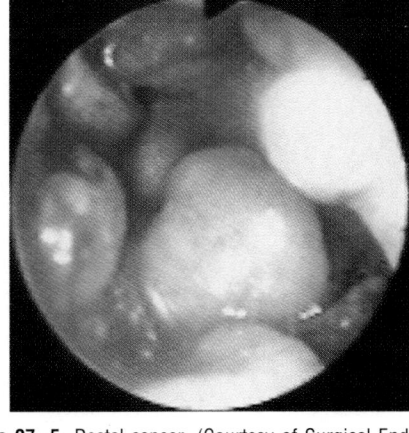

Color Figure 27–5. Rectal cancer. (Courtesy of Surgical Endoscopy, University of Maryland Medical Center, Baltimore, MD.)

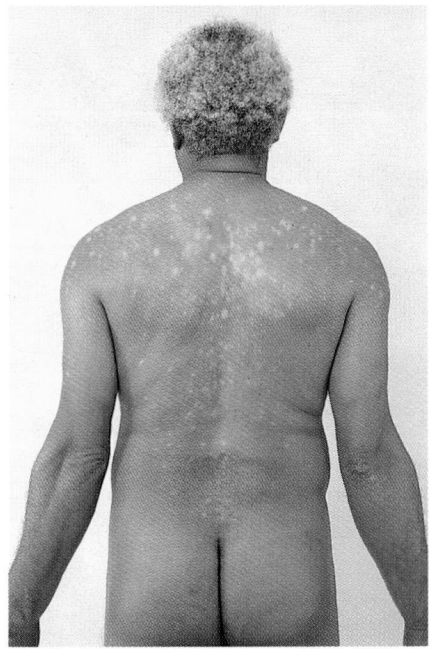

Color Figure 35–1. Arrangement of skin lesions. (Courtesy of Brian V. Jegasothy, MD.)

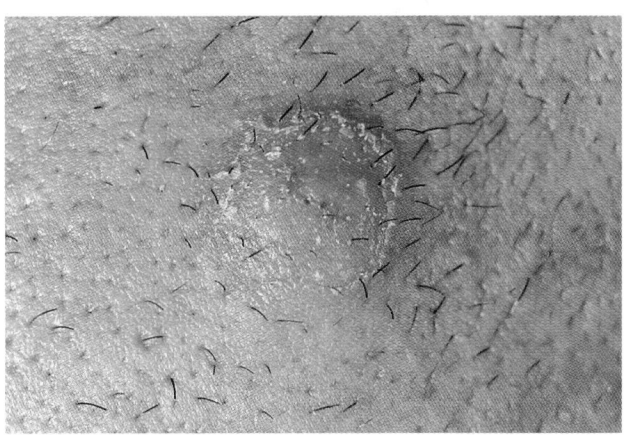

Color Figure 35–2. Folliculitis barbae. (Courtesy of Brian V. Jegasothy, MD.)

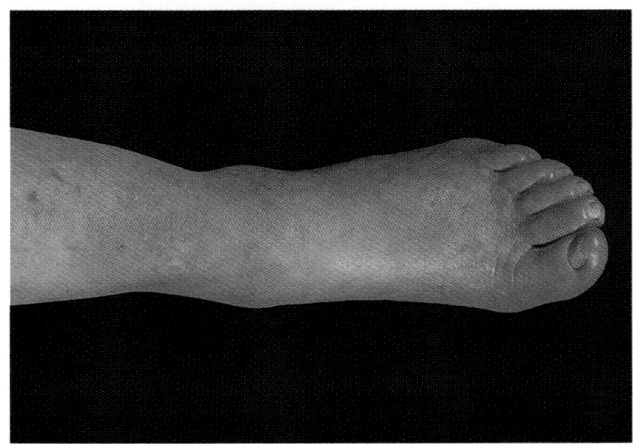

Color Figure 35–3. Cellulitis of foot. (Courtesy of Brian V. Jegasothy, MD.)

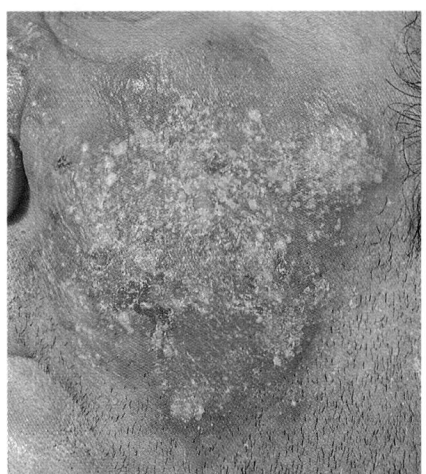

Color Figure 35–4. Erysipelas of face (left cheek, secondarily infected). (Courtesy of Brian V. Jegasothy, MD.)

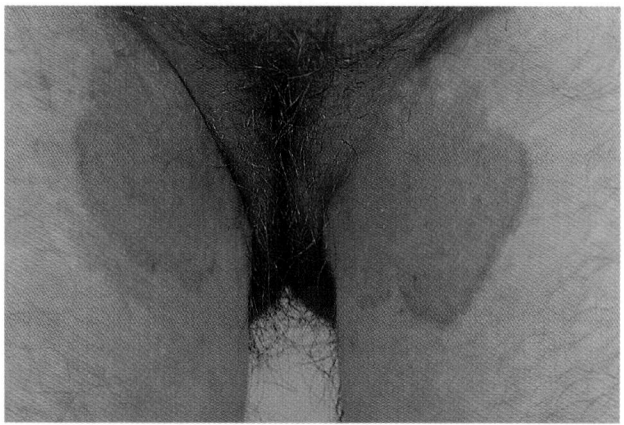

Color Figure 35-5. Tinea cruris. (Courtesy of Brian V. Jegasothy, MD.)

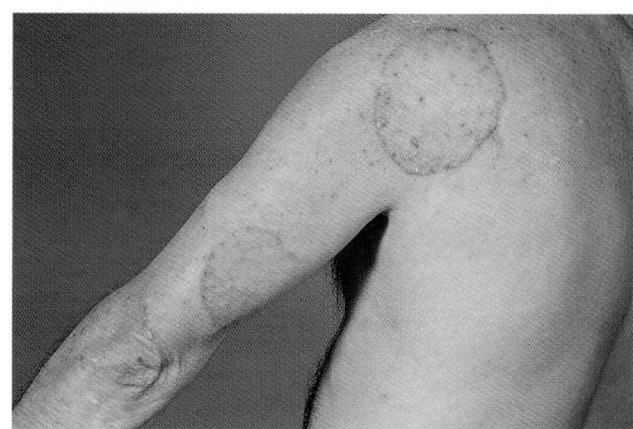

Color Figure 35-6. Tinea corporis. (Courtesy of Brian V. Jegasothy, MD.)

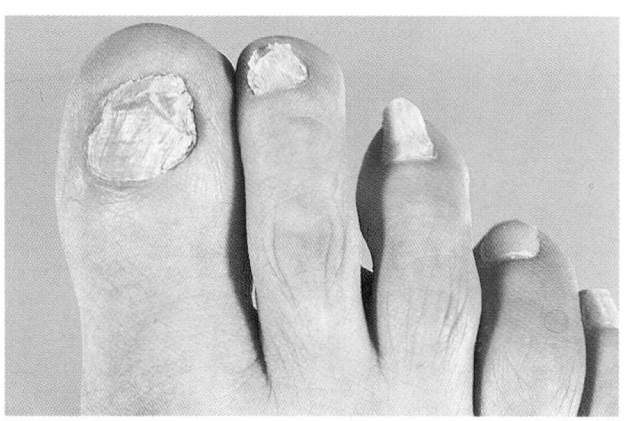

Color Figure 35-7. Onychomycosis. (Courtesy of Brian V. Jegasothy, MD.)

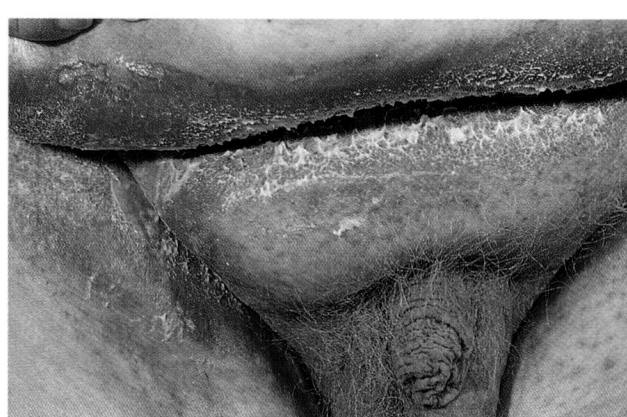

Color Figure 35-8. Intertrigo. (Courtesy of Brian V. Jegasothy, MD.)

Color Figure 35-9. Tinea versicolor. (Courtesy of Brian V. Jegasothy, MD.)

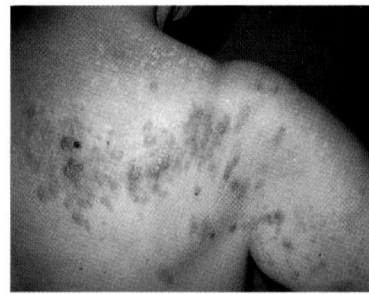

Color Figure 35-10. Herpes zoster. (From Lookingbill DP, and Marks JG Jr. *Principles of Dermatology.* 2nd ed. Philadelphia: WB Saunders, 1993, p 166.)

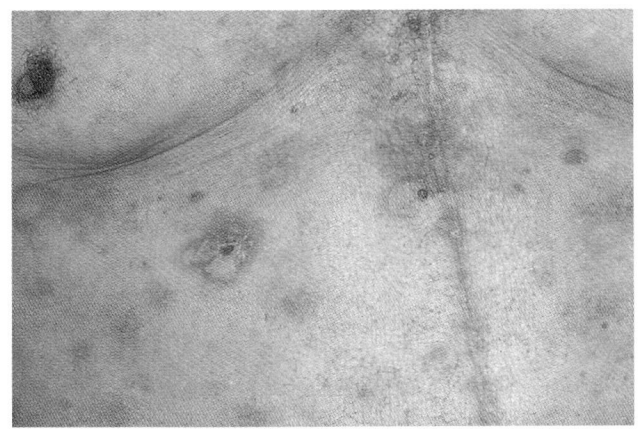

Color Figure 35-11. Pemphigus vulgaris. (Courtesy of Brian V. Jegasothy, MD.)

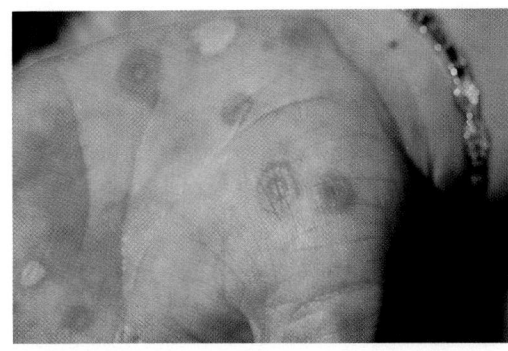

Color Figure 35-12. Erythema multiforme. (From Lookingbill DP, and Marks JG Jr. *Principles of Dermatology.* 2nd ed. Philadelphia: WB Saunders, 1993, p 243.)

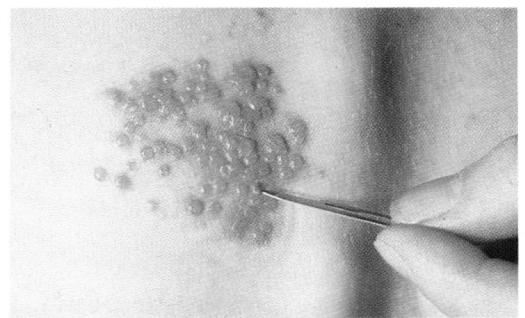

Color Figure 35-13. Herpes simplex. (From Lookingbill DP, and Marks JG Jr. *Principles of Dermatology.* 2nd ed. Philadelphia: WB Saunders, 1993, p 162.)

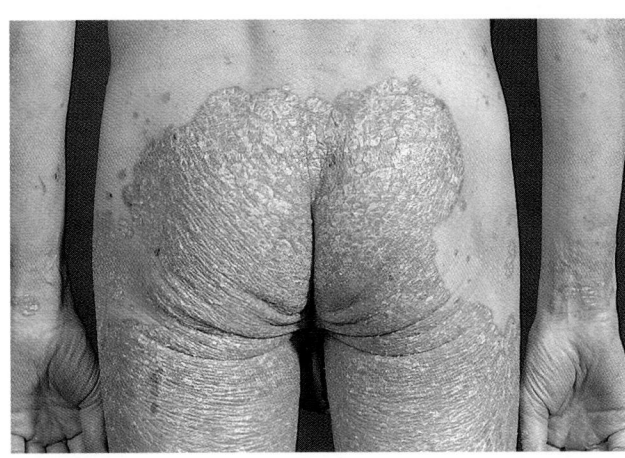

Color Figure 35-14. Psoriasis. (Courtesy of Brian V. Jegasothy, MD.)

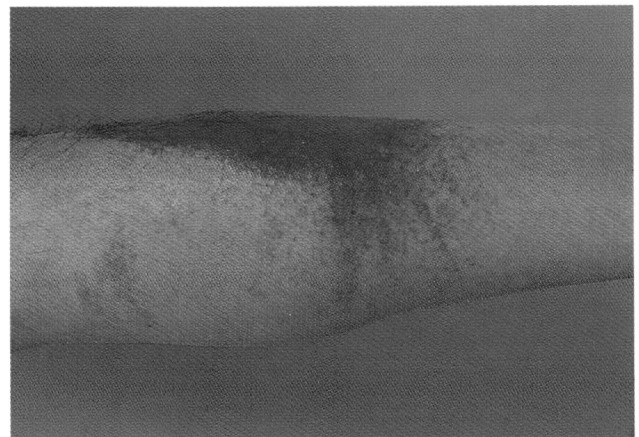

Color Figure 35-15. Contact dermatitis. (Courtesy of Brian V. Jegasothy, MD.)

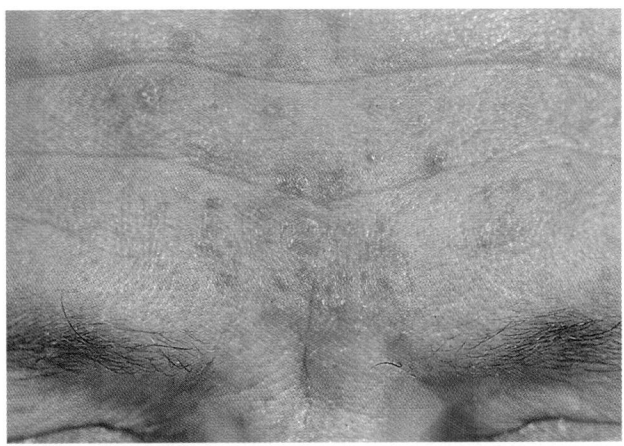

Color Figure 35-16. Acne rosacea. (Courtesy of Brian V. Jegasothy, MD.)

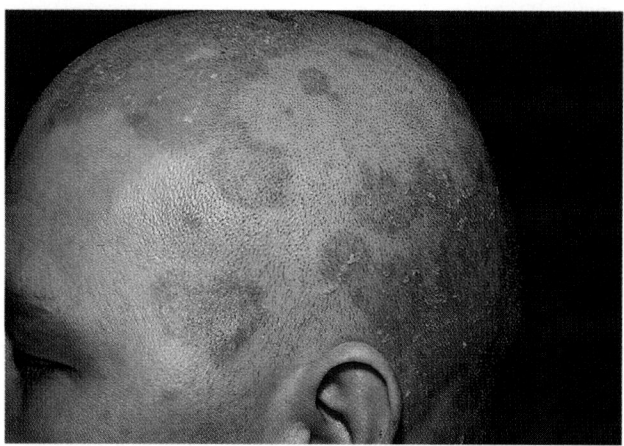

Color Figure 35–17. Seborrheic dermatitis. (From Callen JP, et al. *Dermatological Signs of Internal Disease.* 2nd ed. Philadelphia: WB Saunders, 1995, p 110.)

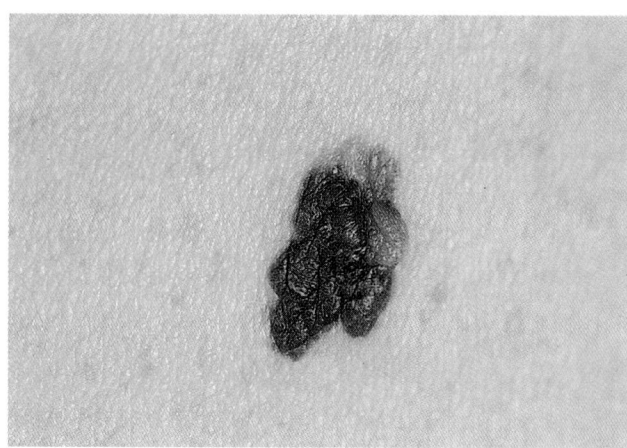

Color Figure 35–18. Superficial spreading melanoma. (Courtesy of Brian V. Jegasothy, MD.)

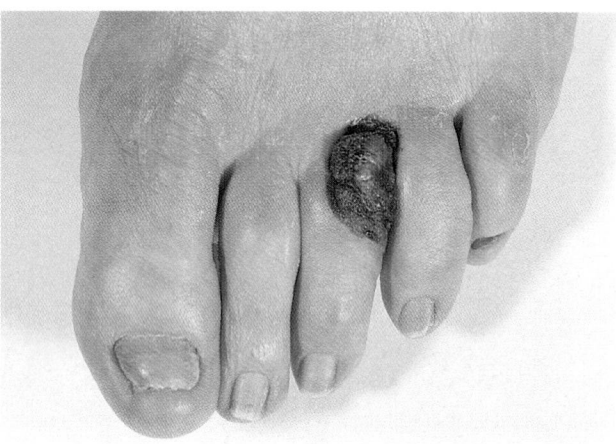

Color Figure 35–19. Nodular melanoma. (Courtesy of Brian V. Jegasothy, MD.)

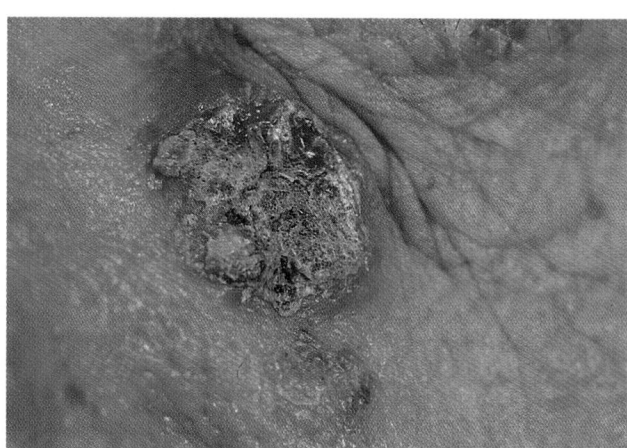

Color Figure 35–20. Basal cell carcinoma. (Courtesy of Brian V. Jegasothy, MD.)

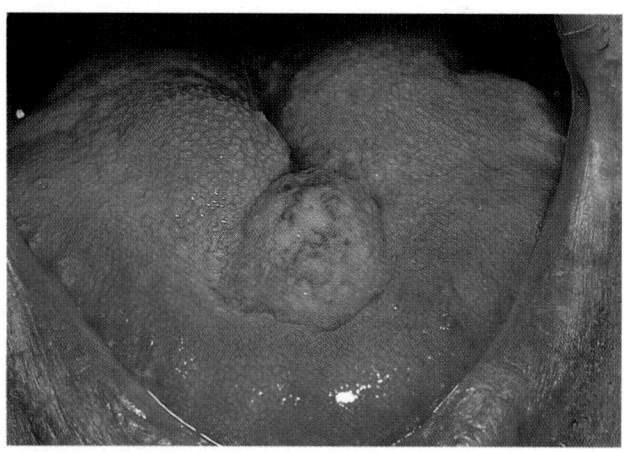

Color Figure 35–21. Squamous cell carcinoma. (Courtesy of Brian V. Jegasothy, MD.)

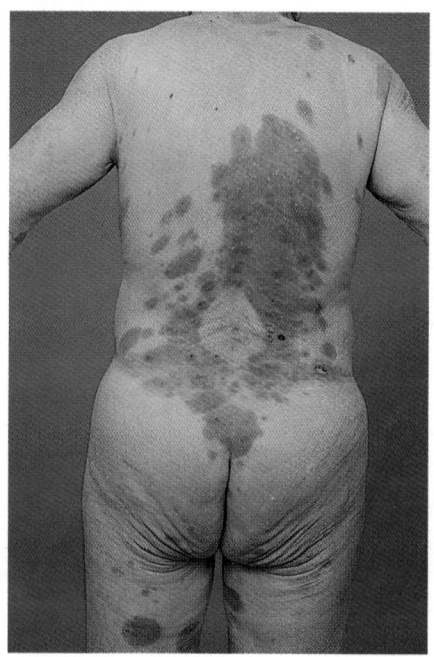

Color Figure 35–22. Ulcerated plaque stage of cutaneous T-cell lymphoma. (Courtesy of Brian V. Jegasothy, MD.)

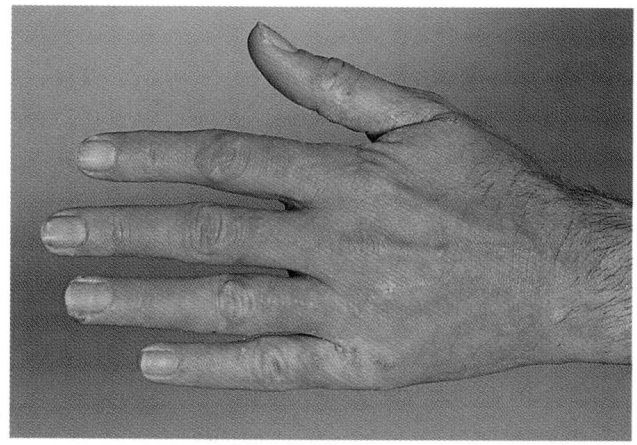

Color Figure 35–23. Scabies. (Courtesy of Brian V. Jegasothy, MD.)

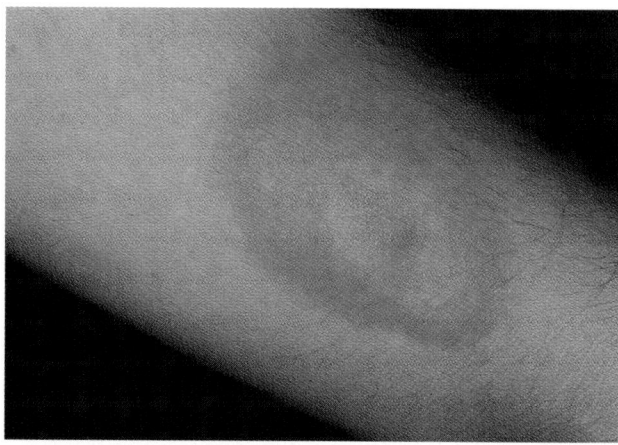

Color Figure 35–24. Erythema chronicum migrans of Lyme disease. (From Callen JP, et al. *Dermatological Signs of Internal Disease.* 2nd ed. Philadelphia: WB Saunders, 1995, p 261.)

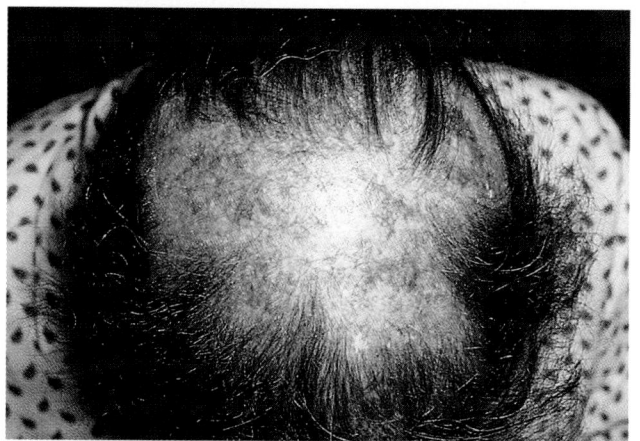

Color Figure 35–25. Scarring alopecia related to chronic graft-versus-host disease. (Courtesy of Brian V. Jegasothy, MD.)

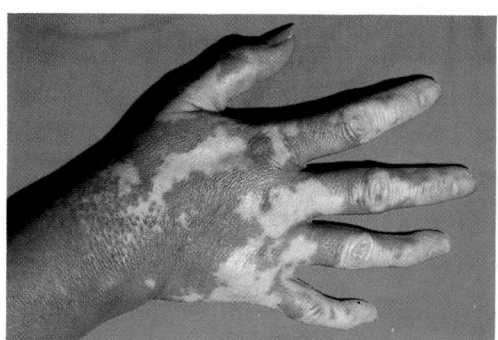

Color Figure 35–26. Vitiligo. (From Lookingbill DP, and Marks JG Jr. *Principles of Dermatology.* 2nd ed. Philadelphia: WB Saunders, 1993, p 208.)

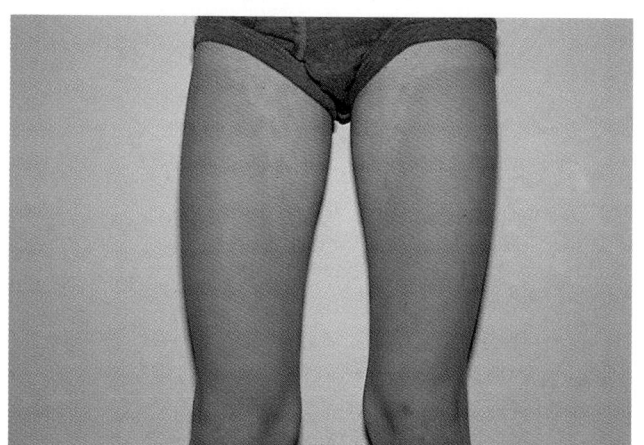

Color Figure 36–1. Superficial (1st-degree) burn injury. (Courtesy of the University of Washington Burn Center, Harborview Medical Center, Seattle, WA.)

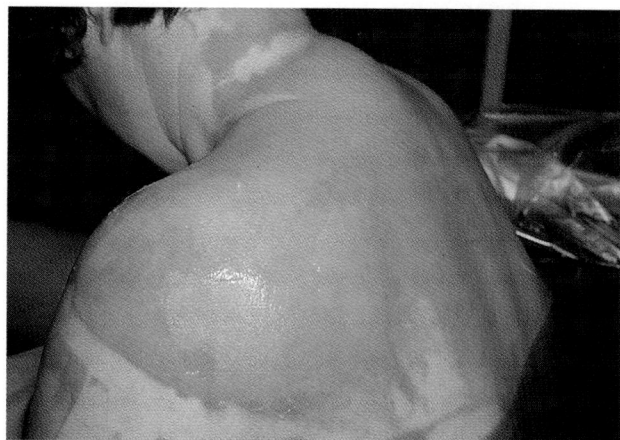

Color Figure 36–2. Partial-thickness (2nd-degree) burn injury. (Courtesy of the University of Washington Burn Center, Harborview Medical Center, Seattle, WA.)

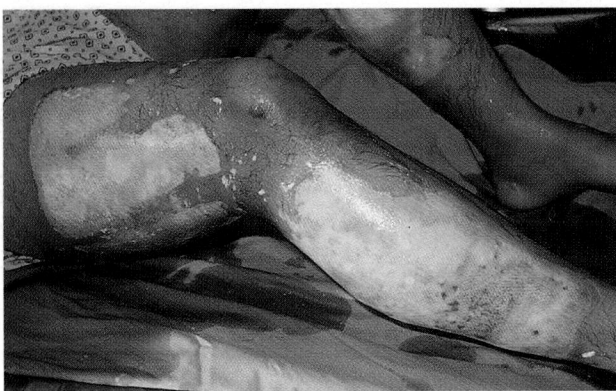

Color Figure 36–3. Full-thickness (3rd-degree) burn injury to lower leg. Thigh burn injury is a combination of deep, partial-thickness, and full-thickness burns. (Courtesy of the University of Washington Burn Center, Harborview Medical Center, Seattle, WA.)

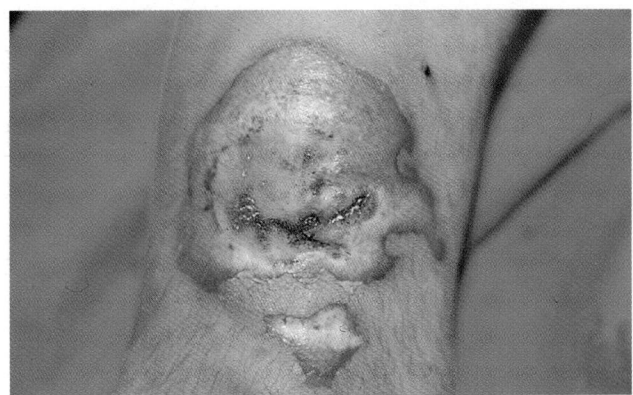

Color Figure 36–4. Full-thickness (4th-degree) burn injury at center of knee burn (blackened areas). (Courtesy of the University of Washington Burn Center, Harborview Medical Center, Seattle, WA.)

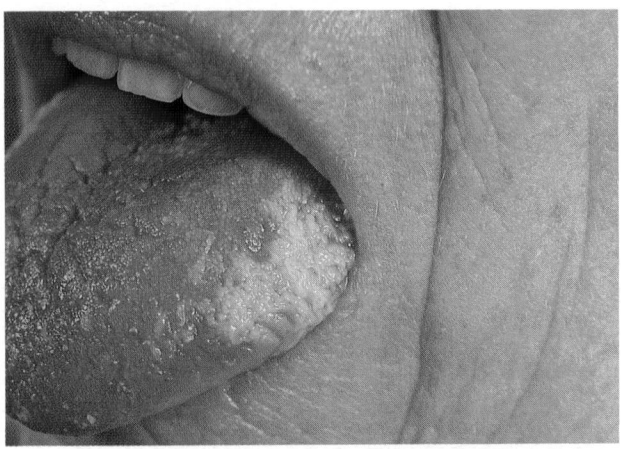

Color Figure 42–1. Hairy leukoplakia found in a woman who had received blood transfusions. (From Friedman-Kien AE, and Cockerell CJ. *Color Atlas of AIDS.* 2nd ed. Philadelphia: WB Saunders, 1996, p 89.)

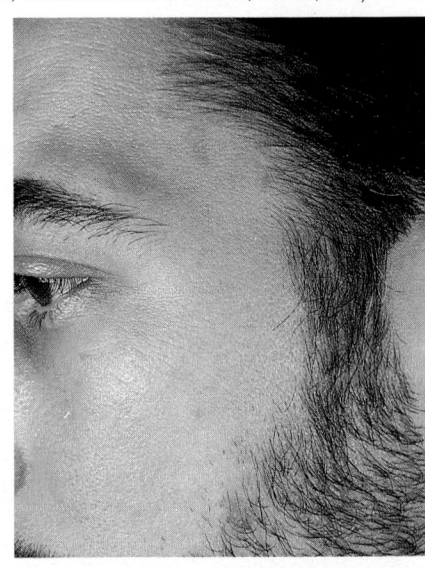

Color Figure 42–2. Epidemic Kaposi's sarcoma in the early stage (patch stage) of the disease. Lesions are slightly irregular in shape. (From Friedman-Kien AE, and Cockerell CJ. *Color Atlas of AIDS.* 2nd ed. Philadelphia: WB Saunders, 1996, p 48.)

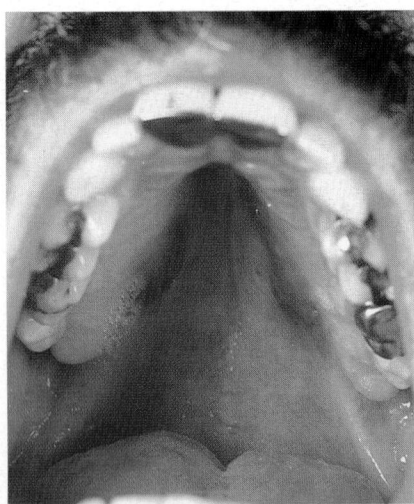

Color Figure 42–3. Epidemic Kaposi's sarcoma, plaque stage. These violet, symmetric plaques on the hard palate were among the earliest lesions to develop in this patient. (From Friedman-Kien AE, and Cockerell CJ. *Color Atlas of AIDS.* 2nd ed. Philadelphia: WB Saunders, 1996, p 59.)

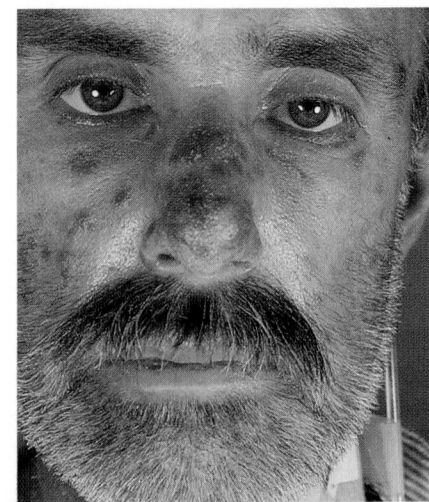

Color Figure 42–4. Epidemic Kaposi's sarcoma, advanced stage of the disease. (From Friedman-Kien AE, and Cockerell CJ. *Color Atlas of AIDS.* 2nd ed. Philadelphia: WB Saunders, 1996, p 58.)

Challenges Facing Nurses in the 1990s and Beyond

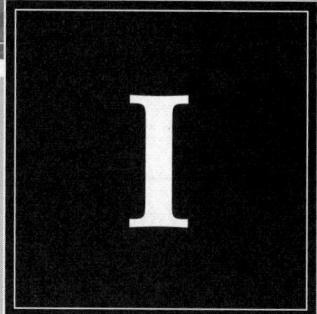

I

1
Problem Solving in Nursing

◼ OVERVIEW OF PROBLEM SOLVING IN NURSING

Approaches to Problem Solving

1. Unlearned problem solving: reflexive reaction to problems (e.g., lifting the foot off a sharp tack on the floor or pulling the finger back from a hot iron)
2. Trial-and-error approach: application of possible solutions, one after another, until the problem is solved; guesswork without systematic forethought or effective documentation of outcomes
3. Scientific method: systematic, logical method, using 7 steps to solve the problem
   a. Identification of general problem area
   b. Collection of relevant data from a variety of appropriate resources
   c. Analysis of data to formulate a hypothesis or theory
   d. Development of an action plan to test the hypothesis or theory
   e. Implementation of the action plan
   f. Evaluation of the outcomes, leading to acceptance or rejection of the hypothesis
   g. Modification of the action plan or termination of the process as appropriate

The Nursing Process: A Form of Problem Solving

1. The nursing process is an adaptation of the scientific method to make it specifically applicable to nursing care.
2. Historical perspective on the nursing process
   a. The term "nursing process" was first officially used in 1955. It represented early moves to differentiate nursing practice from medical practice and to establish a scientific basis for nursing.
   b. In 1973, the American Nurses Association (ANA) accepted the nursing process as a standard of practice.
   c. The ensuing years have been used to refine the steps of the nursing process further and to develop the skills needed to apply the process.
   d. A significant number of states use the nursing process as the foundation for their nurse practice acts.
3. Definitions of aspects of the nursing process
   a. **Process:** a series of actions intended to achieve specific outcomes. A process is also dynamic, always evolving.
   b. **Nursing process:** a deliberate, rational, systematic, goal-directed method of planning and providing nursing care. It is cyclic and *interactive*. Although the systematic sequence of steps is usually followed, the nurse often goes back to previous steps. For example, there are many returns to the assessment phase during the care of a patient (Fig. 1–1).
   (1) The nursing process consists of 5 steps: assessment, nursing diagnosis, planning, implementation, evaluation.
   (2) The nursing process can be used with individuals, families, groups, communities, and organizations. (This chapter emphasizes nursing process applied to individuals.)
   (3) Through consistent application, the nursing process becomes a natural way of thinking used throughout all aspects of nursing practice. As the nurse's expertise develops, so too does the depth and scope of application of the nursing process.

Critical Thinking and the Nursing Process

1. Critical thinking refers to thinking about a situation, problem, question, or phenomenon using information from a *wide* variety of sources. It means thinking in such a manner that more questions are generated, assumptions are identified and challenged, new connections are developed, and the scope of possible solutions is broadened (Box 1–1).
   a. Includes elements of reasoning: purpose, questions, concepts, information, points of view, assumptions, inferences, and consequences and implications
   b. Is a nonlinear way of thinking, not bound by sequential steps
   c. Requires attitudes of openness and inquisitiveness as well as facts and other empirical knowledge; involves reflective skepticism
   d. Uses cognitive skills of interpretation, analysis, inference, evaluation, explanation, justification, persuasion, and self-regulation; also uses intuition and hunches
   e. Examines the *environmental context* of the patient or event under consideration
   f. Involves thinking about *how* you are thinking in a way to improve your thinking skills
2. Many nurses believe that critical thinking includes the nursing process, and that the use of critical thinking throughout the nursing process is the foundation of holistic, creative, and effective patient care. Other nurses believe that critical thinking and the nursing process are contradictory, that the nursing process is too linear and

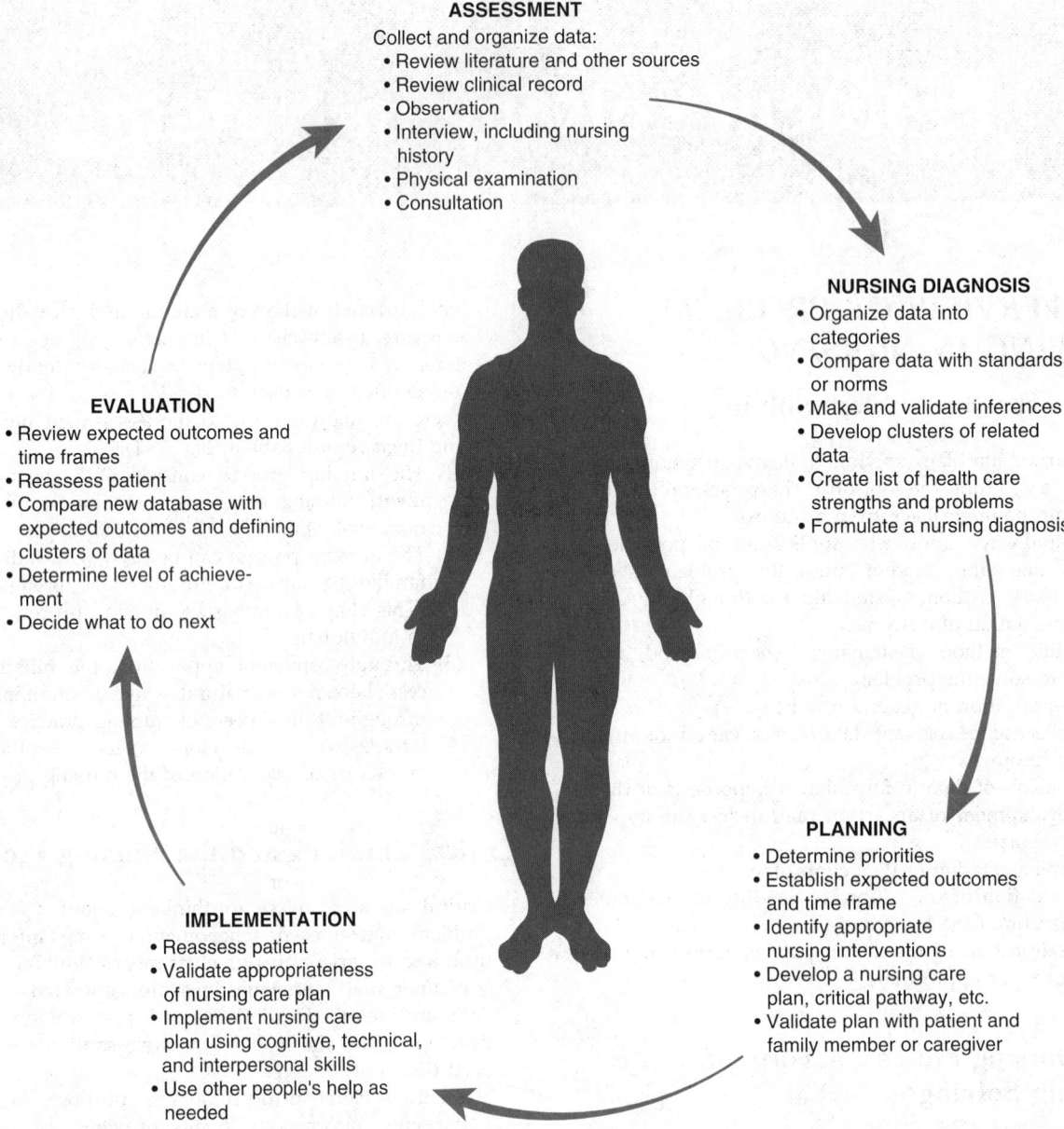

ASSESSMENT
Collect and organize data:
• Review literature and other sources
• Review clinical record
• Observation
• Interview, including nursing history
• Physical examination
• Consultation

NURSING DIAGNOSIS
• Organize data into categories
• Compare data with standards or norms
• Make and validate inferences
• Develop clusters of related data
• Create list of health care strengths and problems
• Formulate a nursing diagnosis

PLANNING
• Determine priorities
• Establish expected outcomes and time frame
• Identify appropriate nursing interventions
• Develop a nursing care plan, critical pathway, etc.
• Validate plan with patient and family member or caregiver

IMPLEMENTATION
• Reassess patient
• Validate appropriateness of nursing care plan
• Implement nursing care plan using cognitive, technical, and interpersonal skills
• Use other people's help as needed

EVALUATION
• Review expected outcomes and time frames
• Reassess patient
• Compare new database with expected outcomes and defining clusters of data
• Determine level of achievement
• Decide what to do next

Figure 1–1. Overview of the nursing process. (Modified from Bolander VB. *Sorensen and Luckmann's Basic Nursing.* 3rd ed. Philadelphia: WB Saunders, 1994.)

BOX 1–1. Fostering Critical Thinking

Examples of Questions Fostering Critical Thinking About a Situation, Problem, Question, or Phenomenon

After viewing a videotape of the interactions of a family in conflict, ask the following:

"What are you assuming in this situation?"
"What do you think is the main issue?"
"How did you come to that conclusion?"
"This patient just doesn't 'look' right; why do I think that?"
"Should I be looking at this from another point of view?"
"Can you justify this course of action?"
"What did you think the patient meant by his remark?"

---

has a strong potential for limiting a nurse's scope of thinking—for example, through the use of standardized nursing care plans.

◼ REVIEW: COMPONENTS OF THE NURSING PROCESS

Assessment

1. Assessment: the dynamic and continuous process of collecting, verifying, and organizing information about a person or other entity. Emphasis is on health status, environment, strengths, and concerns, as well as on the

person's cultural beliefs and practices. Assessment includes the formation and continual development of a database.

2. Sources of data
   a. Background nursing knowledge obtained from review of the literature and other sources, including multimedia programs; computer programs; and classes, workshops, and conferences. Knowledge gleaned from these sources helps the nurse do the following:
      (1) Know what information to seek in a given situation.
      (2) Differentiate between relevant and irrelevant data.
      (3) Prioritize data.
      (4) Recognize when data need to be verified or clarified.
      (5) Organize data into appropriate categories (e.g., nutritional status or patterns of bowel function).
      (6) Analyze data by providing a set of norms against which current information can be compared.
   b. Clinical record: medical history, current medical problems and interventions, laboratory values and results of other diagnostic tests, previous nursing assessments, nursing interventions and evaluation of outcomes, and information from other health care providers (e.g., social information regarding the support system at home and other information as appropriate to the patient)
   c. General observation of the patient and the environment. Information can be used to develop a general picture of the patient and guide an in-depth assessment.
   d. The interview, often considered the most important part of the assessment process, is usually completed before the physical examination. (Supplemental data may be obtained during the examination.)
      (1) Information guides further assessment, identifies expectations and concerns of the patient, gives the patient's perspective of the data and what this information means to the patient, and suggests how the patient may react to potential interventions. (See Chapter 2 for a discussion of the patient's "explanatory model.")
      (2) A formal part of the interview process is a health history (Fig. 1–2). This process seeks information about the patient that will help the nurse identify strengths and problems and guide the planning and implementation of *nursing* care. Typical components of a nursing history include descriptions of current health problems, past health history, current medications and treatments, allergies, personal and social history, cultural beliefs and practices related to health, review of physiologic systems with attention to activities of daily living, and advanced directives (existence and location of appropriate documents describing patient's desires about heroic resuscitation measures and organ donation).
   e. Physical examination uses psychomotor skills of inspection, palpation, percussion, and auscultation.
      (1) The patient may be asked to demonstrate certain activities (e.g., walking, bending, detection of noises and smells, and reading a visual acuity chart).
      (2) The physical examination also includes use of laboratory tests and other diagnostic examinations, such as radiographs, electrocardiograms, and pulmonary function tests.
   f. Consultations: Family and friends can often give important information about the patient's usual behavior patterns and coping mechanisms; recent changes in the patient's condition, including cognitive and behavior changes; resources available to the patient; and additional questions and concerns that the patient may not have been able to discuss. (See Chapter 2 for discussion of patient's "therapy management group.") Other health care providers who have been directly involved in the care of the patient (e.g., home health aides, physical therapists) may also be consulted.

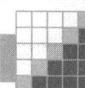 **LEGAL AND ETHICAL CONSIDERATIONS**

To protect the confidentiality of the patient, consultation with family members or friends requires permission by the patient. Many states have specific statutes identifying the need for permission, such as in the situation of an adolescent seeking assistance with birth control.

3. Domains to be assessed to develop a picture of a total person or group
   a. Physiologic: biologic and physical structure and functional characteristics
   b. Psychologic: emotional and cognitive characteristics
   c. Social: interactions with others or other systems (e.g., kinship roles, social status, social activities, social support system, financial resources)
   d. Cultural: primary language, shared beliefs, perceptions, and behaviors of groups (as well as individuals within groups) based on common heritage or ethnic or racial background
   e. Spiritual: beliefs and values that provide strength, hope, and meaning to life; religious beliefs
   f. Developmental: evolutionary process over time as a result of maturation, experience, or learning. Development is ultimately involved with each of the other 5 domains.

4. Types of data
   a. Subjective data: what the person *tells* you (e.g., description of pain, perceptions, feelings, or experiences, usually obtained during the interview)
   b. Objective data: what the nurse actually observes using the 5 senses (e.g., blood pressure reading, dryness of skin, redness of incision, yelling at spouse, musty odor of urine) and laboratory and radiograph results
   c. Correlation of subjective and objective data: Questions might include Does red, scaly skin also itch? Is the patient's reported shortness of breath supported by decreased lung sounds?

5. Health care needs to be identified
   a. Health promotion needs: activities directed toward improving or maintaining a person's health and well-

21514

ADMISSION DATE & TIME:		PRIMARY LANGUAGE IF NOT ENGLISH	ADMITTED FROM: ☐ HOME ☐ DIRECT _____ ☐ OTHER _____	☐ ED ☐ ECF	VITAL SIGNS			HT. IN.	WT. ☐ STANDING
ROOM NUMBER:		☐ SIGN LANGUAGE	MODE OF TRANSFER: ☐ BED ☐ GUERNEY	☐ W/C ☐ AMBULATED	T R /min	P /min BP	R /mmhg L	☐ STATED ☐ MEASURED	☐ ☐ BED CHAIR SCALE SCALE

COMMENTS:

Instruction of Routines and Services to Patient/Family

☐ Nurse call system
☐ Bed controls
☐ Side Rails
☐ Telephone/TV/Radio
☐ Intercom
☐ Visiting hours
☐ Smoking policy
☐ Identiband

SIGNATURE & TITLE

The valuables policy has been explained, and, I understand that Marian Medical Center does not assume responsibility for valuables (money, jewelry, or other personal effects) not secured in the Marian Medical Center safe.

_____ Signature
Patient or Responsible Person

La poliza tocante objectos de valor ha sido explicada, y yo entiendo que Marian Medical Center no asume responsibilidad for estos objectos (alhajas, dinero, etc.) o cualquier otra prenda personal que no sea asegurada en la caja fuerte de Marian Medical Center.

_____ Firma
Paciente o persona responsable por el paciente

ADMITTING DIAGNOSIS: _____

PATIENT STATEMENT/COMPLAINT: _____

CURRENT MEDICATIONS: (Prescribed and non prescribed.)

DISPOSITION OF MEDICATIONS: ☐ Home   ☐ To Pharmacy

PHARMACY

Medication	Dosage	Frequency	Last Dose	Medication	Dosage	Frequency	Last Dose

ALLERGIES

MEDICATIONS/FOODS	☐ NO KNOWN ALLERGIES	Type of Reaction

ADHESIVE TAPE: YES ☐ NO ☐	SIGNATURE OF R.N./L.V.N.
IODINE SKIN PREP: YES ☐ NO ☐	

PAGE I

PATIENT ADDRESSOGRAPH
STAMP PAGE I AND II

PATIENT ADMISSION ASSESSMENT
CHART

Figure 1–2. Sample admission nursing history. (From deWit SC. *Rambo's Nursing Skills for Clinical Practice.* 4th ed. Philadelphia: WB Saunders, 1994, p 398.)

21514

NEUROLOGICAL STATUS	

PUPIL SIZE CHART

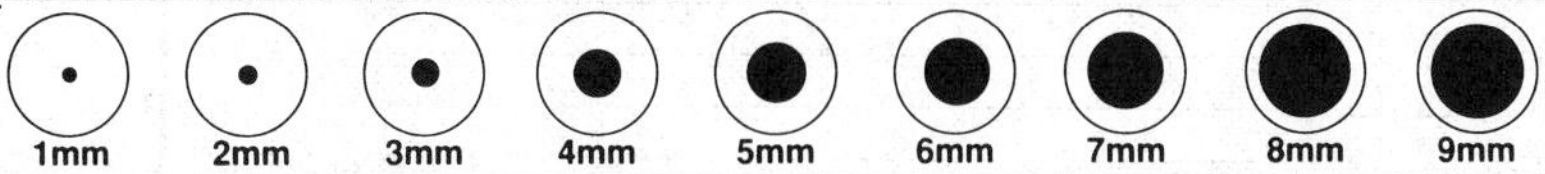

○ 1mm · ○ 2mm · ● 3mm ● 4mm ● 5mm ● 6mm ● 7mm ● 8mm ● 9mm

LEVEL OF CONSCIOUSNESS: ☐ ALERT ☐ ORIENTED
☐ Confused ☐ Slow to respond/Comprehend ☐ History of Seizures
☐ Disoriented ☐ Lethargic ☐ Vertigo ☐ Other
☐ Pupils: Right: _____ Left: _____

	If Pt. Uses	If with Patient

SENSORY LIMITATIONS: ☐ NONE NOTED
☐ Taste ☐ Speech ☐ Sight
☐ Touch ☐ Smell ☐ Hearing

Glasses ☐ ☐
Contact Lenses ☐ R ☐ L ☐ ☐
Hearing Aid ☐ R ☐ L ☐ ☐

COMMENTS:

DESCRIBE ABNORMAL FINDINGS

☐ Seizure precaution needed

FUNCTIONAL STATUS (LEVEL OF SELF CARE)

MOBILITY: ☐ NO LIMITATIONS
Limitations
☐ Walking
☐ Transfer
☐ Turning in bed
☐ Stairs
☐ Standing
☐ Generalized Weakness ☐ Other

DEVICES TO AID MOBILITY:

	If Pt. Uses	If with Patient

☐ None
Cane/Crutches/Walker ☐ ☐
Artificial Limbs ☐ R ☐ L ☐ ☐
Brace ☐ ☐

WEAKNESS/PARALYSIS:
☐ Upper Extremity ☐ R ☐ L   Lower Extremity ☐ R ☐ L

ASSISTANCE REQUIRED:
☐ Hygiene/Grooming ☐ Dressing ☐ Meals ☐ Other

CRITERIA FOR FALL PREVENTION
___ Age 65 or older
___ Altered mental status
___ History of falls
___ Impaired mobility/ balance
___ Ambulatory device cane / walker / w/c
___ Any of the following medications sedatives / narcotics diuretics muscle relaxants antihypertensives

PATIENTS WHO MEET TWO OR MORE CRITERIA ARE AT RISK

☐ **Patient instructed to ask for assistance when getting out of bed.**

RESPIRATORY

☐ Accessory Muscles ☐ Normal Limits (Rate) ☐ Nasal Flaring
☐ Dyspnea ☐ Secretions ☐ Tracheostomy
☐ Orthopnea ☐ Abnormal Breath Sounds ☐ Seasonal Breathing Difficulties
☐ Cough ☐ Oxygen ☐ Other

CARDIO VASCULAR

☐ REGULAR RHYTHM, RATE WITHIN NORMAL LIMITS
☐ Abnormal Pulses ☐ Abnormal Heart Sounds ☐ Pacemaker
Apical/Radial/Pedal ☐ Jugular Vein Distension ☐ Calf Tenderness
☐ Edema ☐ Other
☐ Vascular Access Device (type) _____

SKIN

☐ NORMAL TURGOR, TEMPERATURE & COLOR
☐ INTACT, MOIST MUCOUS MEMBRANES

☐ Edema ☐ Cyanotic
☐ Dry ☐ Flushed
☐ Diaphoretic ☐ Pale
☐ Jaundiced ☐ Rash
☐ Scaly ☐ Other

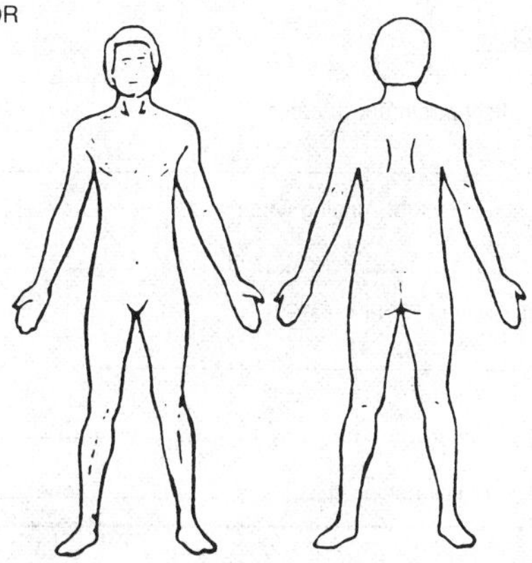

SKIN ASSESSMENT CODE
B - Bruises
D - Decubitus Grade I II III IV (circle)
L - Lacerations
S - Scar
R - Rash
A - Abrasions
Bu - Burn

POTENTIAL FOR SKIN BREAKDOWN:
☐ Poor General Health
☐ Decreased mental status
☐ Decreased oral/fluid intake
☐ Incontinence
☐ Decreased activity
☐ Immobility
☐ No problems

Patient who meet four or more criteria are "at risk for breakdown".

PAGE II   PATIENT ADDRESSOGRAPH

R.N. Signature _____

Date _____ Time _____

PATIENT ADMISSION ASSESSMENT
PHYSICAL ASSESSMENT

Figure 1–2. *Continued*

Illustration continued on following page

		YES NO	Any other Medical/Surgical Conditions:	COMMENTS:
MEDICAL HISTORY	Diabetes	☐ ☐	_____	
	Asthma	☐ ☐	_____	
	Epilepsy	☐ ☐	_____	
	Family Bleeding Tend.	☐ ☐	_____	
	Glaucoma	☐ ☐	_____	
	Cardiac	☐ ☐	_____	

ELIMINATION

BLADDER: ☐ DENIES PROBLEM   BOWEL: ☐ DENIES PROBLEM

☐ Nocturia   ☐ Other   Usual Bowel Pattern _____
☐ Burning   ☐ Catheter   Last BM _____
☐ Urgency   Date Placed _____ ☐ Laxative Use (List under medications)
☐ Urinary Incontinence   ☐ Other Aids _____
☐ Urinary Frequency   ☐ Ostomy, type _____
☐ Stress Incontinence

PERSONAL HABITS

DENIES USE   Type/Amount per day

Caffeine Beverages ☐   _____
Alcohol   ☐   _____
Tobacco   ☐   _____
Other   ☐   _____

NUTRITION

RECENT WEIGHT CHANGES _____   DENTURES YES ☐ NO ☐ PARTIAL ☐
RECENT DIETARY RESTRICTIONS _____ SWALLOWING DIFFICULTY YES ☐ NO ☐
FOOD ALLERGIES _____   OTHER CONCERNS: _____
FOOD INTOLERANCES _____

PEDIATRIC NUTRITION: Problems with eating _____
Special diet (baby - pureed or table food): _____   Special Formula: _____

Breast/bottle/cup _____   Special nipple: _____

PEDIATRICS

Are immunizations up to date? _____
Any exposure to communicable diseases: _____
    (When & Where)

Name child goes by: _____   Head Circumference: _____
Potty trained YES ☐ NO ☐

PSYCHOSOCIAL SPIRITUAL

DURABLE POWER OF ATTORNEY FOR HEALTH CARE _____ Yes   _____ No
    If yes, copy on chart _____
                         (date)

Religious or cultural beliefs which may affect treatment or care:
_____

Environmental concerns at home: (i.e. stairs, lack of running water):
_____

Concerns/worries of patient and/or family during hospitalization:
_____

Person to contact regarding: Name: _____
☐ Post hospital care/change
   in patient's condition   Relationship: _____ Phone: _____

SIGNATURE OF R.N./L.V.N. _____   DATE _____   TIME _____

PAGE III

Figure 1–2. *Continued*

being; common examples include improvements in diet, exercise, weight control, cessation of smoking, and stress management.

b. Health risk factors are conditions that increase the probability of developing certain illnesses or injuries.

(1) Nonmodifiable risk factors (e.g., family history, age, gender, race) cannot be influenced.

(2) Modifiable risk factors (e.g., obesity, sedentary lifestyle, smoking, high fat intake, overuse of alcohol, nonuse of safety helmet while bicycle riding,

anger management problems) can be reduced or eliminated.

c. Potential health problems: The presence of risk factors or existing health problems may predispose a person to illness or injury. For example, an overweight, sedentary person with a family history of heart disease who smokes is a high-risk candidate for a myocardial infarction. Also, a person with a fresh traumatic wound is at risk for the development of an infection.

d. Actual health problems: a situation or condition in which a person needs help to attain, maintain, or regain an optimal level of health. This may include helping the patient to attain a peaceful death.

6. Full versus focused assessment
   a. A full (complete) assessment is usually done when the person enters (is admitted to) a health care setting and is performed at individually determined intervals during a continuing patient–health care provider relationship.
   b. A focused (partial) assessment may be done in the following circumstances:
      (1) When the severity of the patient's condition precludes a full assessment (e.g., acute pain or breathing difficulties)
      (2) When a patient has sought health care for an episodic problem (e.g., sore throat, fractured arm, need for information about birth control measures)
      (3) To check on the progress of a specific potential or specific actual health problem
      (4) To evaluate the effectiveness of a nursing intervention (e.g., relief of pain by position change and medication)
      (5) When a nurse assumes care of a patient during an ongoing period of care (e.g., at the beginning of a shift in a hospital)
   c. A focused assessment is used more often than a full assessment.
7. Structures for organizing data
   a. These structures assist the nurse in the assessment process by doing the following:
      (1) Giving cues to pertinent data needed.
      (2) Pointing out gaps in the database.
      (3) Providing categories into which data can be placed for analysis.
      (4) Showing relationships between data and helping the nurse draw meaning from the database.
   b. Three models are commonly used.
      (1) Body systems approach (Box 1–2): easy-to-memorize categories but with a strong focus on physiologic assessment. This approach does not foster data collection from other domains.
      (2) Gordon's functional health pattern approach (Box 1–3) identifies patterns of behavior over time and facilitates recognition of functional and dysfunctional patterns.
      (3) The human response patterns approach (Box 1–4) facilitates development of nursing diagnoses.
      (4) Many health care settings have developed their own structure for organizing assessment data. They tend to have similar content but are organized differently.

(5) Functional health patterns and human response patterns approaches focus on nursing care. The body systems approach is a component of the medical model.

Diagnoses

1. Definitions (Table 1–1, p. 13)
   a. Diagnosis: statement about the nature of or conclusion regarding a condition or problem, following collection and analysis of relevant data.
   b. Nursing diagnosis: statement made by a nurse about an individual, a family, a group, or a community regarding potential or actual alterations in health status or life processes and responses to these alterations. Nursing diagnosis reflects identification and treatment of health concerns that are within the scope of nursing practice and includes the etiology of the diagnosis.
   c. Medical diagnosis: diagnosis formulated by a physician that reflects health concerns within the scope of medical practice. A medical diagnosis is usually focused on pathophysiology and disease or injury.
   d. Collaborative diagnosis: diagnosis that reflects health concerns requiring intervention within the domains of both nursing and medicine together. The physician usually has primary responsibility for the initial diagnosis, and the nurse monitors onset, change, and resolution of the problem and responds to changes with interventions prescribed by *both* nursing and medicine. Hypoglycemia is one example.
2. North American Nursing Diagnosis Association (NANDA)
   a. In the 1970s NANDA was formed to promote the development of and education about nursing diagnoses. Its primary activity has been to formulate a taxonomy of standardized nursing diagnoses to cover the scope of nursing practice (see Box 1–5).
   b. Approval of nursing diagnoses requires research to determine the significance and suitability of a proposed nursing diagnosis followed by testing in clinical practice and modification as needed.
3. Diagnostic process
   a. Organize assessment data into categories.
      (1) Categorizing is actually a bridge step between assessment and diagnosis; some definitions of assessment include categorization of data (see "Structures for Organizing Data" on this page for the beginning of this step).
      (2) Use a suitable framework to do this, e.g., Gordon's Functional Health Patterns or a health care institution's format.
      (3) Sometimes a piece of information fits into more than 1 category. Pick the most appropriate category and place it there. For example, getting up 4 times every night to go to the bathroom fits into at least 2 categories: elimination and sleep-rest; placement in either category should result in an appropriate nursing diagnosis.
   b. Compare data with standards and norms.
      (1) A standard or norm is a generally accepted value, model, or pattern. Examples include normal labo-

BOX 1–2. Body Systems Approach to Organizing Assessment

General Appearance

- *Observations*—age, sex, race, height, weight, nutritional status, development

Vital Signs

- Temperature
- Pulse (rate)
- Respirations
- *Blood pressure*—supine, sitting, right and left arms

Neurologic System

- Level of consciousness
- *Skull*—size, contour, symmetry, color, pain, tenderness, lesions, edema
- *Eyes*—acuity, visual loss, glasses, contacts, prosthesis, diplopia, photophobia, color vision, pain, burning, eyelid ptosis, edema, styes, exophthalmos, extraocular movement, position and alignment, strabismus, nystagmus, conjunctival color, discharge, vascular changes, corneal reflex, scleral color, vascularity, jaundice; pupils: size, shape, equality, reaction to light, accommodation
- *Neck*—symmetry, movement, range of motion, masses, scars, pain, stiffness; lymph nodes: size, shape, mobility, tenderness, enlargement
- *Reflexes*—Deep tendon reflexes, Babinski's sign, posturing

Musculoskeletal System

- *Activity level*—prescribed, actual, range of motion, gait
- *Extremities*—size, shape, symmetry, temperature, color, numbness, paresis, swelling, prosthesis, fracture
- *Joints*—symmetry, active and passive mobility, deformities, stiffness, fixation, masses, swelling, fluid, bogginess, crepitation, pain, tenderness
- *Muscles*—symmetry, size, shape, tone, weakness, cramps, spasms, rigidity, tremors
- *Back*—scars, sacral edema, spinal abnormalities, kyphosis, scoliosis, tenderness, pain

Respiratory System

- *Nose*—smell, nasal size, symmetry, flaring, sneezing, deformities, mucosal color, edema, exudate, bleeding, furuncles, pain, tenderness, sinus pain
- *Chest*—size, shape, symmetry, deformities, pain, tenderness, expansion, crepitation, tactile fremitus
- *Trachea*—deviation, scars
- *Breathing patterns*—rate, regularity, depth, effort, use of accessory muscles, cyanosis, clubbing, cough
- *Sounds*—normal, adventitious, intensity, pitch, quality, duration, equality, vocal resonance

Cardiovascular System

- *Cardiac patterns*—rate, rhythm, intensity, regularity, skipped or extra beats, point of maximal impulse, bruits, thrills, murmurs, rubs
- Precordial movements, neck veins, right and left cardiac borders, pacemaker, peripheral pulses

Gastrointestinal System

- *Mouth and throat*—odor, pain, ability to speak, bite, chew, swallow, taste; tongue: size, shape, protrusion, symmetry, color, hydration, markings, ulcers, burning, swelling, coating; gums: color, edema, bleeding, retraction, pain; teeth: number, absence, caries, caps, dentures, sensitivity to heat or cold; gag reflex, throat soreness, cough, sputum, hemoptysis
- *Abdomen*—size, color, contour, symmetry, fat, muscle tone, turgor, hair distribution, scars, umbilicus, striae, rashes, distention, abnormal pulsations; sounds: absent, hypoactive, hyperactive; tenderness, rigidity, free fluid, liver border, air bubble, splenic dullness, air rebound, muscle spasm, masses, guarding, pain
- *Rectum*—pigmentation, hemorrhoids, excoriation, rashes, abscess, pilonidal cyst, masses, lesions, tenderness, pain, itching, burning

Renal System

- *Urinary patterns*—amount, color, timing, odor, pH, sediment, frequency, urgency, hesitancy, burning, pain, dribbling, incontinence, hematuria, nocturia, oliguria, change in stream, enuresis, flank pain, polyuria, retention, stress incontinence, bladder distention

Reproductive System

- *Male*—*penis:* discharge, ulceration, pain, size, prepuce; *scrotum:* size, color, nodules, swelling, ulceration, tenderness, pain; *testes:* size, shape, swelling, masses, absence
- *Female*—*labia majora and minora, urethral and vaginal orifices:* discharge, swelling, ulcerations, nodules, masses, tenderness, pain, pruritus, Pap smear, menstrual flow, menopause
- *Breasts*—contour, symmetry, color, shape, size, inflammation, scars; masses: location, size, shape, mobility, tenderness, pain; dimpling, swelling; nipples: color, discharge, ulceration, bleeding, inversion, pain; axillae: nodes, enlargement, tenderness, rash inflammation

Integumentary System

- *Color*—pink, pale, red, jaundice, mottled, blanched, cyanotic

---

BOX 1–2. Body Systems Approach to Organizing Assessment *Continued*

- *Patterns*—pigmentation, vascularity, temperature, texture, turgor, lesions (type, color, size, shape, distribution), hematoma bruises, bleeding, scars, edema, dryness, ecchy-moses, masses (size, shape, location, mobility, tenderness), odors, petechiae, pruritus, edema, rash, ulcerations, drainage, necrosis

---

Modified from Bolander VB. *Sorensen and Luckmann's Basic Nursing.* 3rd ed. Philadelphia: WB Saunders, 1994, p 123; originally adapted from Iyer PW, et al. *Nursing Process and Nursing Diagnosis.* 2nd ed. Philadelphia: WB Saunders, 1991, p 276.

BOX 1–3. Gordon's Functional Health Patterns Approach to Assessment

Health Perception—Health Management

- Description of health (usual, current), preventive measures, previous hospitalizations and expectations of current hospitalization, description of illness (onset, cause), prior treatment (including compliance, anticipated self-care problems)

Nutritional-Metabolic

- Usual daily food and fluid intake, appetite, food restrictions or preferences, food supplements, recent weight change; swallowing, chewing, feeding problems

Elimination

- *Bowel*—usual time, frequency, color, consistency, assistive devices (laxatives, suppositories, enemas), constipation, diarrhea
- *Bladder*—usual frequency; problems with frequency, urgency, burning, retention, incontinence, dribbling, dysuria, polyuria; assistive devices
- *Skin*—condition, color, temperature, turgor, lesions, edema, pruritus

Activity-Exercise

- Usual daily or weekly activities, occupation, leisure-exercise patterns, limitations in ambulation, bathing, dressing, toileting, dyspnea, fatigue

Sleep-Rest

- *Usual sleep pattern*—bedtime, hours, sleep aids; problems falling asleep, staying asleep, feeling rested, naps

Cognitive-Perceptual

- *Sensory deficits*—hearing, sight, taste, smell, touch; problems with vertigo, heat or cold sensitivity, ability to read or write

Self-Perception

- Major concerns, health goals, self-description, effects of illness on self-perception; factors contributing to illness, recovery, health maintenance

Role-Relationship

- *Communication*—language; clear and relevant speech, expression, understanding
- *Relationships*—living arrangements, support system, family life, complaints (parenting, relatives, abuse, marital problems)

Sexuality-Reproductive

- Changes anticipated or experienced because of condition (fertility, libido, erection, pregnancy, contraception, menstruation), menopause

Coping—Stress Tolerance

- Decision making (independent, assisted), major life changes (past, future, desired), stress management (eat, sleep, take medication, seek help), comfort or security needs

Value-Belief

- Sources of strength, meaning, religion (importance, type, frequency of practice), recent changes in values, beliefs, needs during hospitalization

Physical Assessment

- General appearance, weight, and height
- Eyes: appearance, drainage, pupils, vision
- Mouth: mucous membranes, teeth
- Hearing: acuity, aids
- Pulses: rate, rhythm, volume
- Respirations: rate, quality, sounds
- Blood pressure
- Temperature
- Skin color, temperature, turgor, lesions, edema, pruritus
- Functional ability, dominant hand, use of arms, legs, hands, strength, grasp, range of motion, gait, use of aids, weight bearing, activities of daily living
- Mental status, orientation, long- and short-term memory, affect, eye contact

---

Modified from Bolander VB. *Sorensen and Luckmann's Basic Nursing.* 3rd ed. Philadelphia: WB Saunders, 1994, p 124; originally adapted from Iyer PW, et al. *Nursing Process and Nursing Diagnosis.* 2nd ed. Philadelphia: WB Saunders, 1991, pp 278–279.

BOX 1–4. Human Response Patterns Approach to Organizing Assessment Data

Exchanging

A human response pattern involving mutual giving and receiving

- *Cardiac*—apical rate, rhythm, point of maximal impulse, blood pressure (sitting, supine, standing, right and left)
- *Cerebral*—level of consciousness, pupils, eye opening, best verbal response, best motor response
- *Peripheral*—pulses, skin temperature, color, capillary refill, clubbing, edema
- *Skin integrity*—rashes, petechiae, abrasions, lesions, bruises, surgical incisions, other
- *Oxygenation*—respiratory rate, rhythm, depth, use of accessory muscles, dyspnea including precipitating factors, orthopnea, splinting, cough, sputum (color, amount, consistency), breath sounds, history of smoking
- *Physical regulation*—lymph nodes, temperature
- *Nutrition*—eating patterns, number of meals per day, special diet, food preferences and intolerances, food allergies, caffeine intake, appetite changes, nausea and vomiting, condition of mouth and throat, height, weight, ideal body weight, alcohol use
- *Elimination*—usual bowel habits, alterations from normal, constipation, diarrhea, incontinence; bowel sounds; usual urinary habits, alterations from normal, incontinence, retention, urine color, consistency, and odor
- *Safety*—risk for falls

Communicating

A human response pattern involving sending messages

- Read, write, and understand English; other languages; impaired speech; other forms of communication

Relating

A human response pattern involving establishing bonds

- *Relationships*—marital status, age and health of significant other, number of children, role in home, financial support, occupation, job satisfaction and concerns, physical and mental energy expenditures, sexual relationships, physical difficulties or effects of illness on sexuality
- *Socialization*—quality of relationships with others, patient's description, significant other's description, staff observations, verbalization of aloneness

Valuing

A human response pattern involving the assigning of relative worth

- Religious preference, important religious practices, spiritual concerns, cultural orientation, cultural practices

Choosing

A human response pattern involving the selection of alternatives

- Knowledge level
- *Coping*—patient's and significant other's usual problem-solving methods, patient's and significant other's method of managing stress, patient's affect, physical manifestations, available support systems
- *Participation*—compliance with past and current health care regimens, willingness to comply with future health care regimen
- *Judgment*—decision-making ability, patient's perspective, others' perspectives

Moving

A human response pattern involving the activity

- *Activity*—history of physical disability, limitations in daily activities, verbal reports of fatigue or weakness, exercise habits
- *Rest*—hours slept per night, feeling rested on awakening, sleeping aids, difficulty falling or remaining asleep
- *Recreation*—leisure activities, social activities
- *Environmental maintenance*—size and arrangement of home, stairs, and bathroom; safety needs, home responsibilities
- *Health maintenance*—health insurance, regular checkups, medications (prescription, availability)
- *Self-care*—client's ability to feed, bathe, dress, and toilet self
- *Meaningfulness*—verbalizes hopelessness, verbalizes or perceives loss of control
- *Sensory-perception*—history of restricted environment, impaired vision, glasses, impaired hearing, hearing aid, body position or motion, taste, touch, smell, reflexes

Perceiving

A human response pattern involving the reception of information

- *Self-concept*—patient's description of self, effects of illness or surgery on self-concept
- *Meaningfulness*—verbalizes hopelessness, verbalizes or perceives loss of control
- *Sensory perception*—history of restricted environment, vision impaired, glasses, contact lenses, prosthesis, auditory impaired, hearing aid, body position or motion, taste, touch, smell, reflexes

Knowing

A human response pattern involving meaning associated with information

- *Current health problems* (patient's and significant other's perception)
- *Health history*—previous illnesses, hospitalizations, or surgery; diseases of heart, peripheral vascular systems, lungs,

---

BOX 1–4. Human Response Patterns Approach to Organizing Assessment Data *Continued*

liver, kidneys; cerebrovascular disorders, rheumatic fever, thyroid, others
- *Current medications*—name, dosage, frequency, action
- *Risk factors*—hypertension, hyperlipidemia, smoking, obesity, diabetes, sedentary lifestyle, stress, alcohol use, oral contraceptives, family history
- *Readiness*—perception and knowledge of illness, tests, and surgery; expectations of therapy; misconceptions; readiness to learn; requests for information; educational level; learning barriers
- *Orientation*—level of alertness; orientation to person,

place, and time; appropriate behavior and communication
- *Memory*—intact, recent only, remote only

Feeling

A human response pattern involving the subjective awareness of information

- *Pain and discomfort*—onset, duration, location, quality, radiation; associated, aggravating, and alleviating factors
- *Emotional integrity-status*—recent stressful life events, fears, anxiety, grieving, source, physical manifestations

---

Modified from Bolander VB. *Sorensen and Luckmann's Basic Nursing*. 3rd ed. Philadelphia: WB Saunders, 1994, pp 125–126; originally modified from Iyer PW, et al. *Nursing Process and Nursing Diagnosis*. 2nd ed. Philadelphia: WB Saunders, 1991, pp 280–282.

ratory values, growth and development stages, normal vital signs boundaries, basic food groups, cultural norms for behavior, usual symptom patterns for a specific disease, and recommended immunization schedules.

NURSE ADVISORY

> Standards and norms are learned from literature and all other avenues of knowing, including personal experience.

(2) Determine which data match the standard or norm (are "within normal limits") and which data vary (are "abnormal").
(3) Compare data to what is normal for the patient. For instance, a blood pressure of 108/72 falls within normal limits according to published standards for a young adult. When the patient states that her normal blood pressure is 162/88, however, the blood pressure reading takes on a different meaning.

(4) Begin to determine which data are relevant and which are irrelevant. For example, the color of a person's hair is not usually relevant in making nursing diagnoses.
c. Make and validate inferences.
(1) Inferences are the process of assigning meaning to data.
(2) As soon as possible, inferences should be validated with the person (e.g., "Are you feeling nervous?").
d. Develop clusters of related data.
(1) The goal is to identify patterns.
(2) The inductive approach (reasoning from specific observations to general statements) is used to group data within a category and from different categories to form patterns.
(3) The ability to do this increases in direct proportion to the nurse's theoretical knowledge base, clinical experience, and general life experience.
(4) Identify and obtain missing data that may become known while trying to identify patterns.
(5) Identify inconsistent data as they relate to patterns formulated.

Table 1–1. Examples of Medical, Nursing, and Collaborative Diagnoses

Medical Diagnosis	Nursing Diagnosis	Collaborative Diagnosis
Formulated by physician; reflects health concern within the scope of medical practice	Made by a nurse; reflects health concern within the scope of nursing	Reflects health concern within the domains of both nursing and medicine. The physician makes the initial diagnosis, and the nurse monitors onset, change, and resolution and responds to changes.
Example: congestive heart failure	Example: high risk for impaired skin integrity related to edema and poor tissue perfusion	Example: peripheral edema (medical). Altered fluid balance: fluid volume excess (nursing). The physician would order diuretics, and the nurse would plan administration time of diuretics and monitor changes in weight and girth of extremities.

BOX 1–5. NANDA-Approved Nursing Diagnoses

Activity Intolerance
* Activity Intolerance, Risk for
† Adaptive Capacity: Intracranial, Decreased
Adjustment, Impaired
Airway Clearance, Ineffective
Anxiety
* Aspiration, Risk for
Body Image Disturbance
* Body Temperature, Risk for Altered
Breastfeeding, Effective
Breastfeeding, Ineffective
Breastfeeding, Interrupted
Breathing Pattern, Ineffective
Caregiver Role Strain
* Caregiver Role Strain, Risk for
Communication, Impaired Verbal
† Community Coping, Ineffective
† Community Coping, Potential for Enhanced
† Confusion, Acute
† Confusion, Chronic
Constipation
Constipation, Colonic
Constipation, Perceived
Decisional Conflict (Specify)
Decreased Cardiac Output
Defensive Coping
Denial, Ineffective
Diarrhea
* Disuse Syndrome, Risk for
Diversional Activity Deficit
* Dysfunctional Ventilatory Weaning Response
   (DVWR)
Dysreflexia
† Energy Field Disturbance
† Environmental Interpretation Syndrome, Impaired
Family Coping: Compromised, Ineffective
Family Coping: Disabling, Ineffective
Family Coping: Potential for Growth
Family Processes, Altered
† Family Processes: Alcoholism, Altered
Fatigue
Fear
Fluid Volume Deficit
* Fluid Volume Deficit, Risk for
Fluid Volume Excess
Gas Exchange, Impaired
Grieving, Anticipatory
Grieving, Dysfunctional
Growth and Development, Altered

Health Maintenance, Altered
Health Seeking Behaviors (Specify)
Home Maintenance Management, Impaired
Hopelessness
Hyperthermia
Hypothermia
Incontinence, Bowel
Incontinence, Functional
Incontinence, Reflex
Incontinence, Stress
Incontinence, Total
Incontinence, Urge
Individual Coping, Ineffective
† Infant Behavior, Disorganized
† Infant Behavior, Potential for Enhanced Organized
† Infant Behavior, Risk for Disorganized
Infant Feeding Pattern, Ineffective
* Infection, Risk for
* Injury, Risk for
Knowledge Deficit (Specify)
† Loneliness, Risk for
† Management of Therapeutic Regimen: Community, Ineffective
† Management of Therapeutic Regimen: Families, Ineffective
† Management of Therapeutic Regimen: Individual, Ineffective
† Management of Therapeutic Regimen: Ineffective
† Memory, Impaired
Noncompliance (Specify)
Nutrition: Less than Body Requirements, Altered
Nutrition: More than Body Requirements, Altered
Nutrition: Potential for More than Body Requirements, Altered
Oral Mucous Membrane, Altered
Pain
Pain, Chronic
Parental Role Conflict
† Parent/Infant/Child Attachment, Risk for Altered
Parenting, Altered
* Parenting, Risk for Altered
† Perioperative Positioning Injury, Risk for
* Peripheral Neurovascular Dysfunction, Risk for
Personal Identity Disturbance

Physical Mobility, Impaired
* Poisoning, Risk for
Post-Trauma Response
Powerlessness
Protection, Altered
Rape-Trauma Syndrome
Rape-Trauma Syndrome: Compound Reaction
Rape-Trauma Syndrome: Silent Reaction
Relocation Stress Syndrome
Role Performance, Altered
Self Care Deficit
   Bathing/Hygiene
   Dressing/Grooming
   Feeding
   Toileting
Self-Esteem, Chronic Low
Self-Esteem Disturbance
Self-Esteem, Situational Low
* Self-Mutilation, Risk for
Sensory/Perceptual Alterations (Specify)
   (Visual, Auditory, Kinesthetic, Gustatory, Tactile, Olfactory)
Sexual Dysfunction
Sexuality Patterns, Altered
Skin Integrity, Impaired
* Skin Integrity, Risk for Impaired
Sleep Pattern Disturbance
Social Interaction, Impaired
Social Isolation
Spiritual Distress (distress of the human spirit)
† Spiritual Well-Being, Potential for Enhanced
* Suffocation, Risk for
Sustained Spontaneous Ventilation, Inability to
Swallowing, Impaired
Thermoregulation, Ineffective
Thought Processes, Altered
Tissue Integrity, Impaired
Tissue Perfusion, Altered (Specify Type)
   (Renal, Cerebral, Cardiopulmonary, Gastrointestinal, Peripheral)
* Trauma, Risk for
Unilateral Neglect
Urinary Elimination, Altered
Urinary Retention
* Violence: Self-Directed or Directed at Others, Risk for

* Diagnoses with modified label terminology.
† New diagnoses added in 1994.
North American Nursing Diagnosis Association (1994). NANDA Nursing Diagnoses: Definitions and Classification 1995–1996. Philadelphia: NANDA.

e. Determine a list of health care strengths (e.g., a strong social support system) and problems (e.g., inadequate nutritional intake). These should flow logically from the clusters of related data.
4. Formulate a nursing diagnosis.
   a. Each nursing diagnosis must have a problem statement and an etiology. It may or may not include a defining cluster of data depending on the health care setting's policy or the norm of nursing practice.
      (1) The problem statement, sometimes called human response (e.g., impaired skin integrity), may be

selected from a list of NANDA-accepted nursing diagnoses or may, if necessary, be formulated for problems not represented on the list.
      (2) The etiology or primary factors contributing to the problem (e.g., related to (R/T) prolonged immobility) need to be something that a nurse can decrease, eliminate, or modify.
      (3) The defining cluster of data (e.g., as manifested or evidenced by open lesion on sacrum, serous drainage) must be related to the *nursing* diagnostic statement.

b. The desired characteristics of a nursing diagnosis include the following:
  (1) Clear and concise statement
  (2) Specificity
  (3) Patient-centered data
  (4) Accuracy
  (5) No inclusion of medical diagnosis
  (6) No inclusion of value judgments
  (7) Support by signs and symptoms within the database that reflect at least the major defining characteristics of that diagnosis
c. The nursing diagnosis should be validated with the patient.

Planning

1. Planning is a process of designing an action plan through which lifestyle behaviors can be supported or changed as appropriate and health problems can be prevented, reduced, or eliminated.
2. Determine priorities (Table 1–2).
  a. The setting, situation, and available resources often influence the priority assigned to a nursing diagnosis. For example, a nurse will give higher priority to teaching child safety in the home (high risk for injury) when working with a new parent than when working with a new postappendectomy patient. Available resources include people, cost, time, and equipment.
  b. Review the list of nursing diagnoses and assign priorities.
  c. Be sure to include the patient and family members or caregivers in the setting of priorities; congruency among the patient, caregivers, and nurse at this point will influence the outcome. Any differences should be mutually negotiated. (See Chapter 2 for therapy management group and cultural brokerage.)
  d. Priorities must be congruent with those of others on the health care team; incongruencies must be mutually negotiated. For example, if the physician wants the patient up walking for 30 minutes, but the nurse knows the patient gets short of breath after 5 minutes, these 2 health care providers need to collaborate.
  e. Priorities will change as the patient's condition and environment change over time.
3. Establish desired outcomes and time frame.

a. The desired outcome is a statement of the condition or behavior that indicates that the healthy lifestyle has been supported or that the health problem has been resolved. For example, if the health problem was poor oral hygiene, the desired outcome may be as follows: The patient will have improved oral hygiene as evidenced by no plaque with disclosing solution.
b. The desired outcome statement should be related to the health concern or human response stated in the nursing diagnosis. It should focus on patient outcomes and should be clear, concise, specific, realistic, measurable, and acceptable to patient, family members or caregivers, or both (mutually negotiated as necessary).
c. Set realistic, acceptable time frames that indicate when the health problem should be resolved. Note that potential health concerns may not have a specific time frame.
d. When health concerns require a major change or a long time to achieve, write interval short-term desired outcomes (e.g., progressive weight loss goals, exercise tolerance, learning about self-care by patient with diabetes). Interval outcomes provide the patient, family, and caregivers frequent benchmarks to celebrate; make a big task look more doable by breaking it into steps; and provide the nurse with predetermined intervals to evaluate progress.
4. Identify appropriate nursing interventions.
  a. Nursing interventions are actions or strategies within the scope of nursing practice aimed at achieving the desired outcomes within the appropriate time frame. They are sometimes called nursing orders.
  b. Nursing interventions relate directly to all parts of the nursing diagnosis and are therapeutically effective and safe. They provide specific instructions as to activity and times or frequencies of interventions. Interventions must be individualized and consistent with the medical care plan and those of other health care providers. They must be realistic and acceptable to the patient, family, and caregivers (and are mutually negotiated as necessary).
  c. Each nursing diagnosis has 1 to several nursing interventions, depending on the complexity of the health concern or human response (Table 1–3).
  d. Generating alternative nursing interventions or considering multiple options increases the chance of de-

Table 1–2. Planning by Determining Priorities

Priority Level	Characteristics
High	Life threatening or causing the patient so much distress that nothing else can be attended to (e.g., severe dyspnea, pain, or concern over safety of child)
Medium	Threat to health, actual or potential (e.g., smoking, poor family communication, low self-esteem, infected surgical incision, lack of knowledge about diabetes)
Low	Lifestyle behavior changes or health problems that the person can handle with minimal assistance (e.g., hygiene needs for elderly homebound person recovering from a fractured hip; helping new mother deal with moderate-level sibling rivalry of a 2 year old)

	Table 1–3. Sample Excerpt from Nursing Care Plan		
Nursing Diagnosis	**Expected Outcome(s)**	**Nursing Interventions**	**Evaluation**
Risk for impaired skin integrity R/T prolonged immobility (decreased circulation) and dry skin on extremities	Patient will have minimal impairment of skin integrity as evidenced by lack of redness, irritation, and skin breakdown by day of discharge	• Inspect skin, especially bony prominences, dependent areas, areas of edema, and extremities every 8 hr. • Change position every 2 hr. See posted schedule for position to be used each time. • Pad around bony prominences. • Keep heels off bed by using pillows. • Up in chair or ambulate as tolerated. • Use pull sheet and at least 2 people when moving patient. • Apply moisturizing lotion to dry skin.	2/1/96—no skin breakdown

veloping the most effective plan for the patient. Consider consequences, both positive and negative, of each option, and select the nursing interventions to be used with a particular patient.

5. Develop a nursing care plan, a critical pathway, or another plan format. Validate the entire plan with the patient and family or caregivers as appropriate; differences must be mutually negotiated.

  a. The nursing care plan is a written presentation of nursing diagnoses, desired outcomes and time frames, and nursing interventions.

    (1) It serves as a specific guide for individualized nursing care.

    (2) It provides for continuity of care through communication to all caregivers.

    (3) It serves as a guide for developing staff assignments.

  b. The format for nursing care plans varies among health care settings which often design a procedure or form to meet their needs or preference. Most nursing care plan formats have some similar characteristics.

    (1) Most have 4 categories: nursing diagnosis, desired outcome and time frame, nursing interventions, and the date the health concern resolved. If there is no actual category for resolution, there will be some other way to indicate this (e.g., highlighting or crossing out with single line).

    (2) Entries and changes must be dated and signed.

    (3) Most are written in ink; nursing care plans usually become a permanent part of the patient's medical record.

  c. Nursing care plans can be standardized. Preprinted plans list typical nursing diagnoses and interventions for a patient in a given situation. They are commercially prepared or developed by the health care setting. Standard plans give cues to the nurse and save time by avoiding the redundancy of writing the same diagnoses and interventions for different patients. These forms, however, must be individualized for the specific patient. Too often they are used as "cookbook recipes," so that patient-specific nursing diagnoses may not be included, nursing care plan and nursing interventions suggested do not fit with the patient's needs and resources, and transcultural perspectives are not reflected.

  d. Additional formats and adaptations to the nursing care plan are being developed constantly as nursing and health care changes. Some agencies do not use nursing care plans as such but instead use documentation processes to incorporate the nursing care process.

  e. Computer programs are being developed as a tool for nurses. Data input will prompt nurses regarding further assessment data needed, clusters of related data and nursing diagnoses, desired outcomes, and nursing interventions, and then will print the nursing care plans. A concern is that, as with standardized nursing care plans, the individual needs of the patient may not be addressed. Nurses must continue to use clinical judgment based on their theoretical knowledge base and experience.

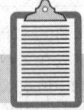

NURSING MANAGEMENT

When using computers for developing and documenting use of the nursing process, including the patient's database, review legal and ethical mandates about protecting the privacy of the patient.

6. Clinical pathways (also called critical care pathways and care maps) (see Chapter 3) are an adaptation of the nursing care plan, often combining the interdisciplinary care processes of nursing, medicine, and other related health care professionals, such as physical therapists (Fig. 1–3).
   a. Clinical pathways focus on desired outcomes, are usually short term, and prescribe interventions along a specific time line (e.g., Day 1, Day 2). They might, for example, spell out what the patient should have accomplished by each day following admission or surgery. If the patient does not achieve the expected outcomes for a specific day or days, the problem is called a *variance.* For example, a postsurgery patient might not move from parenteral to oral pain medications by the specified day or might develop a significantly elevated temperature.
   b. Clinical pathways serve as an effective guide to holistic nursing care for those patients following a typical course. (They also guide care given by other health care providers such as physicians or physical therapists.) The plan focuses attention on patients who have "fallen off" the clinical pathway—that is, have developed a variance. These patients can then receive intensified care if needed. Nursing staff resources can also be focused more appropriately.
      (1) Clinical pathways contribute to cost-effective health care by reducing length of episodic patient care needed and inappropriate use of resources.
      (2) They also provide data for analysis that can be used to improve the quality of care.
   c. The development of a clinical pathway is done preferably by a team of health care professionals who are actively involved in the care of patients in the selected population. Information is gathered from literature reviews, chart reviews, cost analyses for specific health problems, experiences of patients and care providers, and clinical practice guidelines published by professional organizations, legal bodies, and accreditation bodies.
      (1) Patterns of care, outcomes of care, priority problems, patient concerns, and costs are identified and analyzed.
      (2) Clinical outcomes are developed for each health problem, and the care process is mapped out with assigned time intervals; specified interventions are also placed on the time line. This process challenges the traditional aspects of care delivery and requires much discussion and negotiation among members of the interdisciplinary health care planning group.
      (3) Proposed clinical pathways are sent out to other health care professionals for review.
      (4) Clinical pathways become part of expected or standard practice.
      (5) Continued analysis of variances contributes to revision of a given clinical pathway as indicated.
   d. When a patient is admitted, the appropriate pathway is selected. The pathway is adapted to reflect the patient's needs, and the nurse must be careful not to use the clinical pathway as a cookbook recipe.
      (1) Nursing care is provided according to the clinical pathway.
      (2) Variances are noted and analyzed, and nursing interventions are modified to reduce or eliminate the variance and get the patient back onto the pathway. Variances must be documented. The information should be available to those who periodically review the clinical pathway so they can be up to date and effective.

Implementation

1. Implementation involves providing the patient care as determined by the previous steps in the nursing process.
2. Types of nursing interventions
   a. Independent nursing interventions are initiated by the nurse. They are based on theoretical knowledge and skills and are within the legal scope of nursing practice. They do not require an order from another health care professional. For example, changing a leaking colostomy bag, teaching a patient about the importance of balanced rest and exercise when recovering from surgery, and using moisturizing lotion for a patient with dry skin are all independent interventions.
   b. Dependent interventions must be initiated or ordered by another health care professional. Examples include prescription of medications, laboratory tests, and application of hot packs to an infected skin lesion.
   c. Collaborative, or interdependent, interventions are initiated in collaboration with another health care professional. Examples include planning *with* the physical therapist to develop an exercise program for a patient with an amputated leg, so that part of the program is performed by the nurse and part by the physical therapist. Continued collaboration facilitates effective progression and modification of the plan, as indicated.
3. Protocols and standing orders are standardized procedures that are instituted when a patient's condition indicates a need for their use.
   a. Protocols and standing orders do not require time-specific instructions from the health care professional (usually a physician) who has written them. The nurse can initiate them with reference to sound clinical judgment.
   b. Protocols and standing orders must be written into the patient's medical or nursing care plan, or both, and signed by the appropriate health care professional as soon as possible.
4. The implementation process reassesses the patient to allow health care providers to ascertain the patient's current condition and validate that the nursing care plan is still appropriate.
   a. Implement the plan using cognitive, technical, and interpersonal skills.
      (1) Cognitive (intellectual) skills include problem solving, decision making, clinical judgment, critical thinking, and creativity. For example, the nurse might use a knowledge of normal bowel function to determine what interventions to use to resolve a patient's constipation.

Clinical Pathway for Congestive Heart Failure

ICD-9 Code **428.0**   ELOS **5 days**

Nursing Diagnosis/ Collaborative Problem	Expected Outcome (The Patient Is Expected to...)	Met/ Not Met	Reason	Date/ Initials
Decreased cardiac output/fluid volume overload	Have a heart rate within baseline, no significant dependent edema, clear lungs, BP within baseline, and no neck vein distention			
Impaired gas exchange	Have ABGs WNL and respiratory rate within normal rate, rhythm, and depth with equal expansion and breath sounds			
Fatigue/activity intolerance	Perform ADLs without experiencing shortness of breath			
Potential for life-threatening dysrhythmias	Be free of life-threatening dysrhythmias; have normal sinus rhythm			

Aspect of Care	Date_____ Day 1	Date_____ Day 2	Date_____ Day 3	Date_____ Day 4	Date_____ Day 5
Assessment	Systems assessment; Code status/advance directives; Chest pain assessment with VS; VS q 1–4 h, as indicated; Mental status assessment QD; Breath sounds q 8 h	VS q 4 h; Chest pain assessment with VS; Breath sounds q 8 h; Teaching/learning ability assessment; assess barriers to learning	VS q 4–8 h, as indicated; Chest pain and mental status; Breath sounds q 8 h	VS q 8 h; Continue to monitor breath sounds q 8 h; Mental status assessment; Chest pain assessment	Same as Day 4
Teaching	Orient to hospital and unit; Review plan of care/clinical pathway with patient and family; Explain procedures and treatments carefully; Teach importance of reporting chest pain or unusual sensations	Review CHF diagnosis; Teach need for activity restriction/energy conservation	Begin teaching about cardiac meds, special diet, and wt monitoring	Continue with teaching/provide discharge instructions regarding: • Activity restrictions • Dietary/fluid restrictions • Meds (administration, side effects) • When to notify MD of significant changes such as swelling of hands and feet or sudden weight gain; Provide written materials from the American Heart Association	Review discharge instructions as listed on Day 4
Consults	Cardiologist, if needed; Dietician; Social worker	Cardiac rehab; OT for ADLs, if needed	N/A	N/A	N/A

Continued

Figure 1–3. Sample clinical pathway. (From Ignatavicius DD, and Hausman KA. *Clinical Pathways for Collaborative Practice.* Philadelphia: WB Saunders, 1995, pp 94–97.)

Aspect of Care (Cont'd)	Date_____ Day 1	Date_____ Day 2	Date_____ Day 3	Date_____ Day 4	Date_____ Day 5
Lab Tests	CBC, lytes, Mg^{+2} BUN, Cr, glucose (SMA-6 or 6/60) Cardiac enzymes q 8–12 h Digitalis level, if indicated ABGs, pulse ox, as ordered INR(PT)/APTT	Same as Day 1 Cardiac enzymes, if elevated INR(PT)/APTT QD if on anticoagulants	Same as Day 2	Repeat tests, as indicated Digtalis level	N/A
Other Tests	ECG Chest x-ray	ECG MUGA scan or echocardiogram	ECG	ECG, if indicated	N/A
Meds	Review med regimen before admission Digoxin Lasix (or other loop diuretic) IV push or PO as needed K^+ supplement, if low K^+ ACE inhibitor Anticoagulant, if clotting disorder or prophylactically Nitrates and/or inotropes (IV, PO, or topical)	Same as Day 1	Same as Day 2	Continue with meds PO	Same as Day 4
Treatments/ Interventions	Telemetry, if severe dysrhythmias O_2 via NC, as needed Daily wts (before breakfast) Strict I & O	Same as Day 1	Same as Day 2 Assess for transfer from telemetry	O_2 via NC, as needed Daily wts (before breakfast) Strict I & O	Same as Day 4
Nutrition	Fluid restriction Low sodium diet (NAS → 2 GM Na^+) per MD/dietician	Same as Day 1	Same as Day 2	Fluid restriction, if needed Low sodium diet	Same as Day 4
Lines/Tubes/ Monitors	Saline loc or IV fluids at KVO rate	Saline loc	Same as Day 2	Saline loc	D/C saline loc
Mobility/Self-Care	Bed rest Total care	Bed rest or BRPs/BSC with assistance, if no dyspnea May be up in chair for 10–15 min with assistance per MD Assist with ADLs as needed	May ambulate in room with assistance, if ambulatory Provide frequent rest periods Assist with ADLs as needed	Ambulate in room; may need assistance (walker or helper) Provide frequent rest periods	Same as Day 4
Discharge Planning	Assess home needs and family support/resources (focus on physical environment, e.g., stairs, location of bathroom)	Collaborate with social worker to determine disposition: home or NH	Same as Day 2	Assess need for referral to home health services (if discharged to home), including homemaker, nursing, OT/PT to increase activity tolerance	Arrange for follow-up appointment with MD per order

Figure 1–3. *Continued*

(2) Technical (psychomotor) skills involve doing "hands on" procedures, such as measurement of vital signs, parenteral medication administration, and bladder catheterization.

(3) Interpersonal skills involve verbal and nonverbal communication and are part of all nursing activities. Examples are holding the hand of a crying patient, convincing a patient to ambulate when the patient does not want to, teaching, counseling, and collaborating with a physician about a patient's needs.

b. Use other people resources as needed.

(1) Decide what the nurse will do, depending on knowledge and skill level, time available, and priorities.

(2) Identify other persons who have skills, time, motivation, expectation, and need for learning to provide some of the care. Examples include the patient, family, and other caregivers; licensed practical (or vocational) nurses; physical therapists; social workers; respiratory therapists; nursing assistants; home health aides; and volunteers. (See Chapter 2 for discussion of the patient's therapy management group.)

Evaluation

1. Evaluation is an ongoing process of appraisal done continually during the care process. This phase of the nursing process is used for making a clinical judgment about the following:

a. The continued relevance of the nursing diagnoses, desired outcomes and time frame, and nursing interventions.

b. The patient's level of achievement of desired outcomes, including appropriate progress toward them.

c. The effectiveness of nursing care.

2. The evaluation process reviews the desired outcomes and time frames in the nursing care plan. It includes a focused or full assessment as appropriate. Evaluation intervals will vary along a long continuum. Evaluation may occur every several minutes for a patient in an intensive care unit or every month for a school nurse monitoring the dental hygiene of a child.

a. Compare the new database with the desired outcomes and the defining cluster of data, if documented.

b. Determine the level of achievement of the expected outcomes: achieved fully, achieved partially, not achieved at all.

c. Determine additional nursing interventions.

(1) If the expected outcome is fully achieved, continue with the current nursing interventions or consider the health problem or human response resolved and remove it from the nursing care plan as appropriate. Then identify and reprioritize health care needed by the patient. Return to the assessment or diagnosis steps of the nursing process, or both.

(2) If the expected outcome is partially achieved or not achieved at all, reexamine the nursing diagnosis, expected outcomes, and time frame for relevance; validate the new database about the patient; and identify reasons for failure to achieve the expected outcomes fully (e.g., lack of effective communication, knowledge deficit, inadequate performance of nursing interventions, faulty equipment, or unrealistic expectations of the patient or family caregiver). Revise the nursing diagnosis, expected outcome, or time frame, or all of these, and modify the nursing interventions (e.g., adding interventions, deleting interventions, altering the way an intervention is performed, or changing its frequency).

d. Continue this process until the expected outcome has been fully achieved.

Documentation

1. It is essential that the steps of the nursing process be documented throughout the entire process. Documentation is important to achieve the purposes of the nursing care plan (see p. 16); to provide a legal record of professional nursing care given to a patient; to provide the information that will be used for research by accrediting bodies; and to refine nursing practice.

2. There are many methods and formats for documentation, often designed by individual health care settings (see Chapter 3).

◼ APPLYING THE NURSING PROCESS

Providing Direct Patient Care

1. Direct patient care is the most common application of the nursing process.

2. The process is a guide to the nursing interventions that will achieve health promotion, prevent potential health concerns, and lead to appropriate resolution of health problems or human responses.

Working with Other Health Care Personnel

1. The nursing process often involves assigning nursing care activities to someone else, then following up to make sure that the activities were done in an effective manner.

2. Part of the nurse's role is to delegate nursing interventions and to supervise the quality of their performance. This role is often included in states' Nurse Practice Acts.

3. The nurse must always remember that although some nursing activities may be delegated to others, clinical judgment based on the expected theoretical knowledge base and skills of the professional nurse cannot be delegated away.

4. Generally, this nursing responsibility is aimed at licensed practical or vocational nurses and nonlicensed assistive personnel such as nursing assistants, home health aides, patient care technicians, and nursing students, who are accountable to the nurse by law, job description, or policy of the health care setting. This responsibility may also involve the patient, family member, or friend.
5. Elements to be considered in decisions about delegation and supervision include the following:
   a. Assessment of the complexity of the patient's condition and nursing care needs.
   b. Determination of the stability of the patient's condition.
   c. Determination of the cognitive, technical, and interpersonal skills needed to provide the nursing care.
   d. Degree of supervision needed by the potential delegatee.
   e. Availability of the supervisor (see Chapter 3, "Principles of Delegation").

Quality Improvement

1. The nursing process provides a format for implementing a quality improvement program (see Chapter 3).
2. The process also provides data for measuring the outcomes of nursing care.

Nursing Research

1. The data about patients and the effectiveness of nursing interventions provide the basis for investigating research questions.
2. Of special interest are those studies aimed at improving the quality and cost effectiveness of health care in general and of nursing care in particular.

◼ PATIENT TEACHING AND THE NURSING PROCESS

Principles of Learning

1. Each person must be ready to learn physically, emotionally, and cognitively. The person must be free of moderate-to-severe pain, feel able to cope with the new information, and not be under the influence of anesthesia.
2. Readiness to learn also includes motivation or a sincere desire to learn. For instance, a person may not yet be ready to learn about ways to quit smoking or about the details regarding a new diagnosis of diabetes. Until motivated, the person will not "learn," no matter how much the nurse "teaches."
3. The environment must be conducive to learning. Consider the aesthetic, safety, comfort, and privacy elements in the environment. Also consider the general acceptance of and interest in the learner as demon-

strated by the nurse and others in the learning environment.
4. Content must be personally relevant to the learner. It is most easily learned if it can be connected with something that the learner already knows or has experienced. This connection requires that the nurse be continually validating relevance with the learner before and throughout the learning process.
5. A well-developed teaching plan generally moves from simple to complex, with each new concept evolving from what has already been learned. For example, a person with newly diagnosed diabetes may first need to learn about normal physiology of the pancreas and movement of glucose from the bloodstream into cells and *then* learn about what has happened to these normal processes before learning about blood glucose testing and dietary recommendations.
6. Active participation enhances learning by generating interest and encouraging the use of a variety of learning modes (e.g., visual, auditory, manual manipulation, problem solving).
7. Repetition of key facts and concepts reinforces learning. Repetition includes periodically helping the learner summarize the knowledge learned to validate accurate past learning and provide a bridge for new learning.
8. Putting new knowledge and skills into actual practice strengthens learning. Such practice needs to happen during or very soon after new learning has occurred, so as to prevent forgetting new material and help the learner make the transfer of knowledge into application in real life.
9. Learners need rewards to support their positive new behaviors. Examples of appropriate rewards include a smile and a compliment from the nurse, relief of pain and nausea, avoidance of complications from the disease process, and return to work.
10. Learners normally experience periodic learning plateaus and need to recognize and understand them. A learner needs to be supported by the nurse until readiness to learn new material returns.

Guidelines for Teaching

1. The nurse needs to determine the following:
   a. What to teach: Assess for knowledge deficits, interests, information, and skills needed to promote health or prevent and treat illness. Consult with patients to determine their perceived needs.
   b. When to teach: Include both formal, planned opportunities and informal, unplanned opportunities. When scheduling to meet the needs of the nurse and patient, consider what time of day the patient learns best.
   c. How to teach: Knowing the learning abilities, personality, and preferences of the client; the nature of the subject matter to be learned; and the teaching modes (e.g., demonstration, videotape, group discussion, reading material) that would be most appropriate in this situation.

2. In assessing the learner, the nurse must pay special attention to characteristics of the learner. These include age, gender, ethnic or racial background, religious beliefs, and visual and auditory acuity; level of education (including reading and comprehension ability); level of knowledge about the content to be learned; socioeconomic factors; and physiologic and psychologic factors that may influence the learning process.

Application of the Nursing Process to Patient Teaching

1. The nursing process provides a systematic approach that can be applied in a teaching-learning situation.

a. Assessment: establishing a database
b. Diagnosis: identifying learning needs or knowledge deficits
c. Planning: formulating learning objectives and intended outcomes; establishing a teaching plan to be used
d. Implementation: implementing the teaching plan
e. Evaluation: measuring patient's progress toward achievement of the learning outcomes and modifying the teaching plan as needed

2. Teaching-learning guidelines for many health problems are discussed in this book. They are meant to guide the nurse in teaching patients and present a short overview of the health problems and topics to include in the content of the teaching plan.

Bibliography

Books

Benner P. *From Novice to Expert*. Menlo Park, CA: Addison-Wesley Publishing Company, 1984.

Bolander VB. *Sorensen and Luckmann's Basic Nursing*. 3rd ed. Philadelphia: WB Saunders, 1994.

deWit SC. *Rambo's Nursing Skills for Clinical Practice*. 4th ed. Philadelphia: WB Saunders, 1994.

Flarey D. *Redesigning Nursing Care Delivery: Transforming our Future*. Philadelphia: JB Lippincott, 1995.

Ignatavicius DP, and Hausman KA. *Clinical Pathways for Collaborative Practice*. Philadelphia: WB Saunders, 1995.

Iyer PW, et al. *Nursing Process and Nursing Diagnosis*. 3rd ed. Philadelphia: WB Saunders, 1995.

North American Nursing Diagnosis Association. *NANDA Nursing Diagnoses: Definitions and Classification 1995–1996*. Philadelphia: NANDA, 1994.

Polit D, and Hungler B. *Nursing Research: Principles and Methods*. Philadelphia: JB Lippincott, 1995.

Schon D. *The Reflective Practitioner*. New York: Basic Books, 1983.

Vestal K. *Nursing Management: Concepts and Issues*. Philadelphia: JB Lippincott, 1995.

Journal Articles

Ford J, and Profetto-McGrath J. A model for critical thinking within the context of curriculum praxis. *J Nurs Educ* 33(8): 341–344, 1994.

Kataoka-Yahiro M, and Saylor C. A critical thinking model for nursing judgment. *J Nurs Educ* 33(8):351–356, 1994.

Koldjeski D. A restructured nursing process model. *Nurse Educator* 18(4):33–38, 1993.

Other Publications

Hall L. Quality of nursing care. *Public Health News*. Newark, NJ: State Department of Health, 1955.

2

Providing Transcultural Nursing Care

◼ *DEFINITIONS AND FOUNDATIONAL CONCEPTS*

Culture

Culture is an integrated system of learned values, beliefs, and practices that are characteristic of a society and that guide individual behavior—ways of thinking, feeling, and acting.

Transcultural Nursing

Transcultural nursing is the *integration* of the concept of *culture* into all aspects of nursing care (Box 2–1).

1. Transcultural nursing requires that you temporarily suspend or set aside your own cultural traditions (values, beliefs, practices) and role as nurse to perceive the situation as persons from another culture perceive it and act from a transcultural posture.
2. You must use aspects of each health culture under consideration to function as a "culture broker" and develop mutually acceptable and culturally appropriate nursing diagnoses and interventions.

Acculturation

Acculturation is the process of learning a different culture to adapt to a new or changing environment. The values, beliefs, and practices of the person's culture of origin may be retained without modification, replaced by those of the new culture, or modified to accommodate those of the new culture.

1. Physical-environmental acculturation: Adjustments to factors such as new housing; increased or decreased population density; and new climate, terrain, vegetation, and air and water quality.
2. Biologic acculturation: Adjustments to new factors such as diseases, genetic changes due to interbreeding, and increased or decreased nutritional status.
3. Cultural acculturation: Adjustments to factors such as religious, gender role, and institutional (economic, political, educational, and social) changes.
4. Psychologic acculturation: Adjustments such as mental

health alterations, psychosocial adjustments, and increased or decreased coping abilities.
5. The acculturation of an immigrant group into a new society usually occurs over 3 generations.
   a. The 1st generation (immigrants) generally seeks to preserve the cultural values of the group in the new society.
   b. The 2nd generation (children of immigrants) is educated in the institutions of the new society and becomes a subculture negotiating between the new society and the immigrant group.
   c. The 3rd generation (grandchildren of immigrants) is seen as a product of the new society.

Assimilation

Assimilation is the process of completely giving up or replacing one's values, beliefs, and practices with those of another culture.

Ethnic Group

An ethnic group is any group of individuals in a society that is culturally distinctive and has a unique identity based on shared traditions, national origin, physical and biologic characteristics (skin color, height, build), social markers (language, religion), and aesthetic markers (dress, music, dance, food).

Subculture

A subculture is a group that shares some of the characteristics of the larger population group of which it is a part but that is seen as a distinguishable subgroup (e.g., ethnic, gender, age, and occupational, or professional groups). The U.S. Census Bureau identifies 5 ethnic groups, which include multiple subcultural groups.

1. Hispanic: Peoples of Spanish origin, including persons of Cuban, Puerto Rican, Mexican, and South and Central American descent.
2. Black: Persons of African descent.
3. Asian or Pacific Islander: Persons of Chinese, Japanese, Filipino, Vietnamese, Korean, Samoan, Hawaiian, East Indian, Melanesian, and Guamian descent.

BOX 2-1. Relevance of Culture to Nursing

Culture largely determines human response to health and illness, because it defines concepts of health and illness, directs people's attempts to achieve health and treat illness, and influences communications with medical personnel (whether biomedical or ethnomedical).

As a nurse, you hold a particular view of health and illness that is based on your professional nursing education and individual experiences in nursing and nursing specialty. Your personal cultural beliefs and values and professional view of health and illness affect your interactions with patients and your ability to perceive the health care situation as they do. Differences in perceptions occur even if you are from the *same* cultural group or socioeconomic status as your patients. The same health care situation may be a separate reality for you and your patients. Recognize the discrepancies between your perception of reality and your patients' perceptions to avoid making nursing diagnoses and prescribing interventions that are socially and culturally unacceptable to patients.

Such unacceptable diagnoses and interventions have no meaning for patients, and they are unlikely to adhere to them. Patients are often mislabeled as "difficult," "uncooperative," "lacking knowledge," "unmotivated," or "noncompliant." Nurses are then often mislabeled by patients as "uncaring," "insensitive," "disrespectful," or "well-meaning but not especially knowledgeable."

To work successfully with patients of different cultures, nurses must suspend their cultural traditions. Suspending or setting aside your cultural tradition *does not mean* discarding your own cultural values, beliefs, or practices; considering them wrong; or adopting those of other people. It does mean remaining open and attempting to understand the patient's concept of health and illness and his or her explanatory model and considering the patient's perspective as important and integral to the development of culturally appropriate nursing diagnoses and interventions.

Take a culturally relativistic approach to patient care. Culture relativism means judging each culture on its own merits. It is based on the premise that patients have reasons for their health care decisions and responses. Cultural relativism has 4 interrelated propositions:

1. Each person's value system is learned in the course of everyday experiences.
2. Values people learn differ from society to society because of different learning experiences.
3. Values are relative to the society in which they occur.
4. Because values are not universal, the values of every culture in the world should be respected.

Remember that you cannot be totally accepting of every patient and that you cannot help every patient. Do not forget that you are a product of your own culture. There will be times when you cannot condone, promote, or accommodate your patients' cultural and health-culture values, beliefs, and practices. When you sense you are unable to help or accept the patient, your responsibility is to find another person who can assist the patient.

---

4. Native American: Persons of Eskimo and American Indian descent.
5. Non-Hispanic White: Persons of European or Anglo-Saxon descent (also referred to as Euro-American or Anglo-American).

Race

Race is a division of the human species that differs from other divisions based upon common hereditary traits that appear among members.

1. There are 3 broad racial divisions.

a. Black
b. White
c. Oriental–American Indian

2. Hereditary differences include variations in the following:
   a. Color: Skin, eyes, and mucus membranes
   b. Anatomic measurements: Body proportions; bone length and density; tooth size, shape, and density; pelvis and chest size; and soft tissue differences in blood vessels and muscles
   c. Growth and development: Height and growth rates; amount of body fat; skeletal and neurologic maturity; motor development; and age of onset of puberty and menopause
   d. Common clinical measurements: Temperature, pulse, respiration, hemoglobin and hematocrit; cholesterol, and APGAR scores
   e. Biochemical: Enzymatic (drug and alcohol metabolism, lactose intolerance) and malaria-related conditions (sickle cell hemoglobin, thalassemia, Duffy blood group, and G6PD deficiency)
3. Hereditary differences may lead to increased racial susceptibility to disease (see p. 47).
4. Racial characteristics cut across ethnic groups, because race is a biologic, not a social classification.

Biomedicine

(Western, modern, orthodox [official], scientific, or cosmopolitan medicine): A medical theory of disease and treatment practices based on manipulation of biochemical and physical processes that occur within the human body. The scientific world-view dominates Western medical thought. Nursing draws the majority of its medical content from biomedicine.

Ethnomedicine

Non-Western, traditional, or folk medicine: Cultural traditions, beliefs, and practices related to health and illness that are derived from other than biomedical theory.

Health-Seeking Behavior

Health-seeking behavior is the sequence of actions taken by an individual to prevent illness, maintain health, solve a health problem, and seek care for illness.

Ethnonursing

Ethnonursing is the study of nursing and nursing care values, beliefs, and practices as perceived by members of a cultural group.

Culture Competence

Culture competence is knowing, utilizing, and appreciating the effects of culture in resolving individual, family, or community problems. It requires both an awareness of your own cultural values, beliefs, and practices and the limitations ("blinders") they put on you and your reactions to others and an openness to, an understanding and acceptance of, and an adjustment to cultural differences between yourself and your patients.

Culture Brokerage

1. Culture brokerage: The process of translating cultural values, beliefs, and practices from 1 person or group to another and negotiating methods of resolving differences. The goal is to reduce conflict and promote cooperation.
2. Culture broker: A person who assumes the role, function, and responsibility of the culture brokerage process.

The Explanatory Model

1. Culture structures people's explanatory models (EMs) of health and illness.
   a. Explanatory model: A person's individual or cultural construct of reality, including health and illness.
   b. These models are based on life experiences with health and illness.
   c. A patient's EM may differ from the general beliefs about health and illness held by society or nurses.
2. Explanatory models of health and illness
   a. The concept of EMs applied to health maintenance and illness prevention will help you ascertain the person's beliefs and understanding regarding to health promotion.
      (1) How to prevent illness
      (2) How to maintain health
      (3) What self-care initiatives to take
      (4) How lifestyle affects health
      (5) How to avoid misfortune
   b. The concept of EMs applied to sickness will help you ascertain the person's beliefs and understanding of his or her illness.
      (1) What caused the illness (etiology)
      (2) When and how the illness began (mode of onset)
      (3) What the illness does and how it works (pathophysiology)
      (4) How bad the illness is and what its likely course will be (severity and prognosis)
      (5) What should be done about the illness (therapeutic regimen and nursing interventions)
      (6) Who should be consulted about it (therapy managers)
   c. The EMs of patients applied to sickness focus on *illness* rather than disease.
      (1) Disease: An alteration in the structure and function of the body. Disease is the focus of biomedicine. Pathophysiology is generally the same across cultures. Signs and symptoms are investigated via biologic and physiologic measurements.
      (2) Illness: A person's experience of being sick. It includes the following dimensions:
         • Physical-biologic (signs and symptoms)
         • Social-behavioral (roles, relationships, and actions)
         • Phenomenologic (feeling state)
         • Spiritual
   d. See page 28 for details on specific explanatory models.
3. Explanatory models of anatomy and physiology
   a. The majority of people in the world have developed explanatory models of anatomy and physiology indirectly.
      (1) Through making analogies with animals, such as buying animal parts in meat markets, slaughtering farm animals for food, sacrificing animals for religious purposes, observing animals give birth, and caring for injured or sick animals.
      (2) Through making practical observations about bodily sensations and conditions, such as, post hoc associations between an event and an onset of signs and symptoms; increased heart rate in response to various emotional states or exercise; occurrence of perspiration after exertion, exposure to heat, eating certain foods, and experiencing pain or fear; and feeling "bloated all over" before the onset of menstruation.
      (3) Through interpreting religious texts or dogma.
      (4) Through personal experience with illness.
      (5) Through media representations of the body, including advertisements of medications targeted for specific body parts; animation of the body in cartoons and advertisements; and technologic and science fiction representations of the body as a cyborg, mind as a computer, and organs as spare parts to be transplanted or replaced by machines.
      (6) Through information gained from other persons.
   b. Importance of body parts: Body parts may assume greater or lesser roles in explanatory models of anatomy and physiology because of the following:
      (1) Folklore and symbolism
         • The heart in traditional Chinese medicine is equated with the functions of an emperor.
         • The brain or head is often designated as the seat of ideas and intelligence.
         • The female breast is representative of sexual attractiveness.
         • The uterus symbolizes female fertility and femaleness.
         • Male genital organs symbolize virility and potency.
      (2) Their importance in biomedicine
         • United States: Brain death is used to establish physical death.
         • Japan: Brain death is but 1 element in establishing physical death according to burial rituals.
         • Germany: Heart functioning is considered central to general body functioning.
         • France: Liver functioning is considered central to health.
         • Britain: Colon functioning is considered central to health.

Table 2–1. World Views of Health and Illness

World View	Basic Premises	Health	Illness	Treatment
Biomedical (scientific)	1. Life is regulated by biochemical and physical processes. 2. Mechanism: Life processes can be determined by science and manipulated by humans through mechanical interventions. 3. Determinism: Natural phenomena are regulated by cause and effect relationships. 4. Objective materialism: that which is grounded in reality can be observed and measured. 5. Reductionism: Life processes can be reduced to their component parts. The whole can be determined by studying the unique characteristics of each of its parts.	Health is the absence of disease or of signs or symptoms of disease.	Disease is an alteration in the structure and function of the body. Disease has a specific cause, length of onset and course, and therapeutic regimen. Psychologic and physical disturbances can be understood through their underlying biochemical processes. Causation is attributed to trauma to body parts, pathogens, chemical imbalance, or degeneration or failure of body parts.	Treatment focuses on physical and chemical interventions.
Magicoreligious (supernatural)	1. Supernatural (SN) control: The world, nature, and all that exists within the world, including humans, are dependent on the actions of SN forces, which may be good or evil. These forces may take a number of forms: a supreme God, as in the Christian religion; a pantheon of gods, as in ancient Roman, Greek, or Egyptian religions or in more contemporary folk (indigenous) religions such as *santeria*, voodoo, and indigenous African religions; spirits that continue to exist in an afterlife: deceased ancestors, persons, or animals; emissaries of god(s): saints, spirits, and other ecclesiastic beings; psychic or ethereal forces or essences: magic, witchcraft, sorcery, or curses. 2. Personalistic: SN forces are directed at specific individuals, groups, or communities. 3. Punishment: SN forces are activated to seek retribution for unacceptable social behavior.	Health indicates the individual is blessed or favored by the SN.	Disease causation is mystical and not based on empiric (scientific) fact. A disease-causing foreign object or spirit intruder enters the body. Disease is a sign of punishment or possession by the SN.	Treatment is the removal of the foreign object or spirit intruder via prescribed rituals, countermagic, repentence, or subjecting oneself to the will of the SN.

Table 2–1. World Views of Health and Illness (Continued)

World View	Basic Premises	Health	Illness	Treatment
	4. Social control: Threat of SN punishment is used to prevent unacceptable behavior. 5. Mobilization: SN forces may be activated by a variety of means: a SN being, an individual who employs a sorcerer, or an individual who practices witchcraft, sorcery, or magic.			
Holistic	1. Everything in the universe is governed by the laws of nature, including human beings. 2. If the forces of nature are not kept in balance or harmony, disease and general chaos result. 3. Disturbances in environmental, sociocultural, and behavioral aspects of life upset the harmony in nature. 4. Fluctuations between harmony and disharmony are natural processes that occur throughout life. Individuals must change constantly to adapt to their ever-changing environment. The best adaptation to one's environment is achieved by living according to the social rules and engaging in self-care measures. 5. Emphasis is on prevention of illness and health maintenance.	Health is attained by achieving the best possible adaptation to a constantly changing environment. Perfect health is never possible because of the natural and continuous fluctuation between harmony and disharmony in the universe.	Disease is imbalance or lack of harmony between the human, metaphysical, and natural forces of the universe. 1. Disease prevention depends on maintaining a sense of harmony or balance between humans and the universe. 2. Disease extends beyond the body and includes disturbances in the person's sociocultural, physical, and metaphysical environments. Unemployment, crime, poverty, racial or religious discrimination, homelessness, famine, misfortune, and war are as much illness are as organic biomedical diseases.	Treatment is the restoration of harmony or balance within individuals; between individuals and their external physical, social, and metaphysical worlds; and within and between the forces of the universe.

Adapted from Herberg P. Theoretical foundations of transcultural nursing. *In* Andrews MM, and Boyle JS (eds). *Transcultural Concepts in Nursing Care.* Philadelphia: JB Lippincott, 1995.

(3) Their importance in ethnomedicine
- Haiti: The status of the blood is central to health.
- Jamaica: The functioning of the "belly" (abdominal cavity) is central to health.
- China, Saudi Arabia, and Mexico: The heart is central because of its role in the circulation of the vital life forces of *ch'i, ruh,* and *fuerza* respectively.

(4) Their replaceability. The more easily a body part or its function can be replaced, the less importance it may assume in terms of health maintenance and illness prevention measures.

c. Keep in mind that cultural constructs of anatomy and physiology change over time owing to factors such as the following:
(1) Exposure to health education
(2) Illness experience and disability
(3) Experience with various physiologic states such as pregnancy, weight gain, and weight loss
(4) One's emotional state
(5) The need for explanations of new illnesses, misfortune, and catastrophic events such as natural disasters
(6) Alteration in internal and external body image

◼ *MAJOR CULTURE BELIEFS AND PRACTICES ABOUT HEALTH*

Major World-Views of Health and Illness

1. See Table 2–1 for 3 perspectives on health illness and treatment.
2. Although Western medicine follows the biomedical view, most ethnomedical systems combine elements of the magicoreligious (supernatural) and holistic (naturalistic) world-views to explain illness causation and determine treatment.
   a. Supernatural causation is expressed or seen as a personalistic phenomenon.
      (1) The ill person is the victim, object of aggression, or receiver of punishment for specific reasons.
      (2) Causative agents may be human, nonhuman, or supernatural beings.
   b. Natural causation is expressed or seen as an impersonal phenomenon.
      (1) Illness comes from the forces of nature or conditions of the natural world such as wind or air, heat or cold, dampness or dryness, and imbalance of body elements (blood, bile, and phlegm).
      (2) The causative agent of the illness is the individual who puts himself or herself at risk by failing to avoid illness-producing situations or failing to take self-care measures such as adhering to the laws of nature, eating the correct diet, avoiding overexertion or becoming excessively tired, periodically cleansing the body of impurities that accumulate in the blood, leading a moderate lifestyle, and being respectful of others or conducting oneself in the culturally prescribed manner.
   c. Emotional illnesses may be attributed to chance or naturalistic causes rather than to the deliberate action of others.
3. The majority of ethnomedical systems focus on the effects of the social, physical, and supernatural environments on body structure and function.
   a. The physical (internal) functioning of the body is linked to the individual's spiritual and cognitive functioning.
      (1) The body, mind, and spirit are joined together and respond together in health and illness.
   b. Physical functioning is also linked to external events in the social, natural, and supernatural environments.

Sectors of Health Care

1. The 3 major sectors of health care found in most societies are the popular, folk, and professional (Table 2–2).
2. Each sector has its own way of explaining and treating illness, defining who should be the health care provider, and delineating how providers and patients should interact.
3. People may use any of the 3 sectors individually, in combination, or simultaneously.
4. The usual sequence of use is the following:
   a. Popular sector: Consulted initially to confirm illness or meaning of signs and symptoms and to determine appropriate self-care measures.
   b. Folk sector: Consulted if home remedies and self-care methods fail.
      (1) Consulted initially if causation is thought to be supernatural or a disharmony in the individual, society, or universe.
      (2) Consulted simultaneously with biomedicine to remove supernatural causation, restore harmony, and invoke supernatural and natural forces to enhance effectiveness of biomedicine.
   c. Professional sector: Consulted if home remedies and folk sector treatments are ineffective. May be consulted initially for illnesses or signs and symptoms for which it is considered best, such as acute trauma, surgery, or restoration of body parts.
5. Many newly arrived immigrant and refugee groups use the popular and folk sectors primarily. As they acculturate, they may begin to consult the professional sector more readily.
6. Use of the folk sector is not restricted to immigrants or specific cultural groups.
   a. Persons from all socioeconomic groups use the folk sector, including nurses and other health care professionals.
   b. Use of any sector is dependent on the causation attributed to the illness and access or availability of healers in other sectors.
7. If we understand why people are using multiple sectors of health care during their health-seeking behavior, we can do the following:
   a. Better explain the goals of the nursing intervention and biomedical treatment to patients.
   b. Be certain patients understand the advantages, disadvantages, and possible synergistic or incompatible effects of treatments from multiple sectors.
8. The use of multiple sectors provides patients with multiple therapy managers.

Ethnomedical Models of Anatomy and Physiology

1. One or more aspects of 4 basic models of anatomy and physiology appear in most ethnomedical systems. They are the following:
   a. Organ-machine model
   b. Plumbing model
   c. Balance models
   d. Blood status model
2. Organ-machine model
   a. Emphasis is placed on the role and function of organs and other body parts in health and illness.
   b. Certain organs are equated as body cavities regardless of other structures or organs present. For example, the thoracic cavity may be referred to as the chest, the lungs, or the heart.
   c. Organs vary as to their location, number, and function. For example, there may be 3 lungs—2 in the

Table 2–2. Sectors of Health Care

	Popular Sector	Folk Sector	Professional Sector
Alternative Terminology	Lay; nonprofessional, non–folk healer	Ethnomedical; traditional	Official; legally sanctioned; orthodox, e.g., biomedicine (U.S.); traditional Chinese medicine (China); ayurvedic medicine (India)
Role of Health Care Givers	Define and treat illness Determine if folk or professional care needed Seek advice and resources to manage condition, assess progress, and evaluate treatments from folk and professional sectors	Define and remove supernatural cause Restore balance Prevent illness and restore health	Define, treat, and prevent disease and illness

Activities	Illness recognized
	Self-care initiated
	No involvement of folk or professional healers
	Home remedies
	  Treatment of illness
	  Health maintenance
	  Illness prevention
	Consultation with:
	  Family, friends, clergy, neighbors, work groups, self-help groups, others who have had the same condition
	Take over-the-counter drugs
		Holistic care
		Treat illnesses due to
		  Supernatural forces
		  Imbalance in individual and physical, social, and metaphysical environments
		Treat illnesses not amenable to home remedies or professional medicine or professional medicine
		Treat culture-specific illnesses
		Rituals to prevent illness and misfortune
		Rituals to enhance the effect of biomedicine
			Question and examine patients
			Prescribe legally regulated treatments and drugs
			Admit patients to hospitals and other care facilities
			Perform highly technologic diagnostic procedures
			Confine patients against their will (e.g., psychotic or infectious diagnoses)
			Officially label patients as ill or well

Sequence	Initial diagnoses and treatment Seventy to 90% of health care is provided in this sector Self-limiting illnesses	Intermediary between popular and professional sectors May be initial or only source consulted depending on causation attributed to signs and symptoms	May be initial source or utilized simultaneously with folk and popular sectors Provides the least amount of health care of any sector
Source of Care	Family Self Friends Neighbors	Folk healers: secular, sacred, or combination of both	Legally sanctioned health care providers

Adapted from Hellman CG. *Culture, Health, and Illness*. Oxford: Butterworth-Heinemann, 1994.

region of the clavicles to give strength and motion to the upper extremities and 1 next to the heart to help it beat faster.

d. The prominence or importance of organs is related to their role in essential body functions. For example, the important organs are related to the 3 essential body functions in the Mexican explanatory model.

(1) Circulation: Heart, blood, and veins. **Fuerza,** the essential energy of life, is carried throughout the body in the blood. *Fuerza* fuels the body to accomplish one's work and maintain health.

(2) Temperature regulation: Heart, lungs, and stomach. Proper body function depends on a balance of hot and cold forces in the body. The heart generates heat during shivering for circulation throughout the body to raise its temperature. The lungs and stomach are seen as the repositories of cool air taken into the body for diffusion throughout. The lungs help the heart beat faster to dispense more heat.

(3) Digestion and nutrition: Heart, stomach, intestines, bladder, and veins. *Fuerza* is extracted from food in the stomach, concentrated as a juice, and passed into the intestine. The juice is absorbed from the intestines into the veins and circulated throughout the body.

e. Organs may be blamed for certain signs and symptoms when patients endow organs with physical and emotional properties. For example, weak lungs may be blamed for frequent colds, recurrent bronchitis and pneumonia, or shortness of breath.

f. Organs may be seen as parts of a machine.

g. Emphasis on body parts as causation of disease may lead to the concept of the body as a machine in which body parts that fail can be replaced or repaired. Also, the body needs ongoing sources of energy or fuel to continue functioning. Examples of the body as machine concept:

(1) African-American, Anglo-American, and Hispanic-

American beliefs that overuse of a body part will wear it out, causing pain and dysfunction.

(2) Hispanic-American concepts of needing to replenish or conserve *fuerza*.

h. Current biomedical practices have increasingly reinforced the ethnomedical concept of the body as machine.

(1) Biomedical health teaching uses explanations such as blockage of a blood vessel, the heart, intestine, or bladder; reaming out a vessel or tube; encouraging rest to "recharge one's batteries"; and flushing out the kidneys.

(2) Transplant surgery advances the idea of exchange of spare parts and, in conjunction with prolongation of life by external methods, has given rise to the "cyborg" image of the body.

(3) Computer modeling has advanced the concept of the body and mind as being controlled by circuits and programs located in the brain. Circuits can be reprogrammed to reenervate or infuse body parts. Deviant behavior, psychiatric illnesses, or personality disorders can be reprogrammed.

i. The body as machine has profound implications for health teaching and nursing care.

(1) Reinforces the responsibility of the individual in health maintenance and illness prevention.

(2) Stresses the effects of lifestyle on health and illness.

(3) Emphasizes the relationship of individual body parts to the functioning of the whole body.

(4) Uses the machine metaphor to make health education more relevant.

(5) Helps patients maintain realistic expectations about the effects of technology on body functioning, prolongation of life, and quality of life.

3. Plumbing model

a. The body is conceptualized as a series of hollow containers (cavities or chambers) connected to each other and body orifices by pipes or tubes (Box 2–2).

(1) The model is common in Western societies and among persons of middle and high socioeconomic status.

(2) Its origins stem from knowledge of the structure and physics of drainage systems.

b. As in the organ model, the containers are often referred to as single organs regardless of other structures they contain.

c. The connecting tubes or pipes are the intestine or "bowel"; blood vessels; esophagus; nerves, tendons, and ligaments; and "windpipe."

d. Substances that flow through the tubes include air or wind; energy or vital life forces; fluids; blood, urine, and menstrual blood; food; fecal matter; perspiration; and emotions.

e. Health is maintained by the continual and unimpeded flow of substances among cavities, body orifices, and the external body surface.

f. Illness results from blockage or severance of the connecting tube.

g. Common ethnomedical health maintenance and treatment measures associated with the plumbing model are the following:

BOX 2–2. The Plumbing Model of Anatomy and Physiology

The Jamaican ethnomedical concept of "belly" is an example of the plumbing model of anatomy and physiology. The belly is described as a large cavity or bag that extends from the end of the breast to the pelvis. The belly is packed full of other bags such as the "baby bag" (uterus) and bladder bag. The main tube of the body goes from the top of the body through the belly and ends at the bottom of the body.

Coming off the main tube are "tributary" bags and tubes. The tube and bag connections are not always tight. Substances passing along the main tube may slide off into the wrong tube, become stuck, and clog the system or fester and give rise to gas and other noxious impurities.

Most illness conditions originate in the belly because of its primary role in converting substances taken in into needed bodily elements while also expelling waste matter such as unused parts of food or drink, medicine, air, or impurities that have built up in the blood. Washouts of laxatives or purgatives of castor oil, epsom salts, or cathartic herbs should be done regularly to cut out "offending substances." The washouts also remove impurities in the blood. When the belly is said to be working, it is washing excess bad things down and out. Health is dependent on good belly functioning. The function of the belly can be aided through preventive measures such as drinking purifying teas and taking cleansing laxatives. Failure to observe such measures risks the purity of individuals, their blood, and system.

Adapted from Sobo EJ. "Unclean deeds": Menstrual taboos and binding "ties" in rural Jamaica. In Nichter M (ed). *Anthropological Approaches to the Study of Ethnomedicine*. Philadelphia: Gordon and Breach, 1992.

(1) Taking of laxatives or enemas to prevent blockage of the bowels.

(2) Avoiding the entrance of "evil air," gas, or other poisons into the body.

(3) Drinking large amounts of fluids to clean toxins and impurities out of the body; improve one's skin and complexion; and dilute the viscosity of body fluids to enhance their transport.

(4) Taking purgatives on a regular basis to cleanse the blood and organs of impurities.

(5) Taking measures to promote menstrual flow, expulsion of afterbirth, and postpartum fluids.

(6) Increasing activity to help the flow of body fluids.

(7) Using massage or digital manipulation of body parts or conducting pathways to dislodge blockages.

(8) Avoiding activities that will impede flow of body substances, such as the following:

- Slowing down blood flow by sleeping too much or not being active enough
- Causing a build up of pressure in body cavities by becoming emotionally upset
- Eating too much and clogging the system with excessive waste
- Exposing oneself to excessive or sudden cold that stops the menstrual flow

4. Balance models

a. These models are an ethnomedical adaptation of humoral and balance theories underlying the ancient medical systems of the world. Balance models are common in ethnic or racial groups adhering to the holistic world view.

b. Emphasis is placed on balance between internal and external forces or elements in the body.
  (1) External (cosmic) forces include food and fluid ingested; environmental elements such as climate, water, air, animals, seasons of the year, or time of day; position of celestial bodies; and supernatural entities.
  (2) Internal (body-mind-spirit) forces include emotions, genetic or inherited conditions; and fears and anxieties.
c. Health is maintaining harmonious or balanced relationships between individuals and their social, physical (natural), and supernatural environments.
d. Illness results from an imbalance or disharmony of elements within individuals or between individuals and aspects of their environment.
e. Treatment of illness involves measures to restore balance or harmony. The individual bears the major responsibility for health maintenance, illness prevention, and treatment success.

5. Hot-cold syndrome
a. The principle of hot and cold is the major balance concept from ancient medical systems adopted by many ethnomedical systems.
  (1) It is the central element of Latin-American and other Hispanic ethnomedical systems.
  (2) It is prominent in the ethnomedical systems of Caribbean, Asian and East Asian, Arab, and Mediterranean populations.
  (3) It has essentially disappeared from biomedicine.
b. Hot and cold are conceptualized as 2 opposite states of the body.
  (1) Health represents a balance between the 2 states.
  (2) Illness represents an imbalance between the 2 states.
  (3) Treatment is aimed at restoring the balance of hot and cold in the body.
c. Certain principles of the hot-cold syndrome are common to most ethnomedical systems. Hot and cold is a symbolic classification of the state of the body and has little to no relationship to the actual temperature or thermal state of the body.
  (1) Hispanic, Ancient Arab, and other ethnomedical systems drawing upon Hippocratic-Galenic humoral theory often relate hot-cold states to intrusion of hot or cold into the body from exposure to external elements, and intake of foods and medicine that may cause an imbalance in the production of body humors or affect the normal hot or cold state of the body or body part.
  (2) Going out of balance is a process of going from 1 state to another owing to internal or external factors.
    • External factors are such things as climate changes; activity level; excessive or prolonged exposure to elements such as heat or cold, dampness or dryness, wind, or darkness or brightness; and exposure to elements without proper dress or shelter.
    • Internal factors relate to the ingestion and metabolism of substances such as food, fluid, herbs, and medications.

(3) The hot-cold classification of internal factors relates to the symbolic power contained in or produced by substances rather than to their actual temperature. For example, chili peppers are hot to taste but may be classified as cold food owing to their cooling effect when the body is in a hot state. Chilled fruit juice is cold in temperature but may be classified as hot because of its warming effect when the body is in a cold state. Cold beer may be classified as hot because it contains alcohol, a hot substance.
(4) Medications and herbs may be classified as hot or cold because of the side effects they produce. For example, an antibiotic may be classified as hot because it can cause side effects that are considered to be hot illnesses, such as diarrhea, rash, or vomiting. Medications causing joint pain may be classified as cold because joint pain is a cold condition.
(5) Foods are usually dichotomized into parallel classifications of hot or cold. Some parallel food classifications contain intermediate or neutral food categories. See Table 2–3 for the parallel hot-cold food classification for Puerto Rican–Americans in New York City that contains an intermediate "cool" (fresco) category. See Table 2–4 for a Haitian hot-cold parallel food classification that contains a neutral category and variations on the hot-cold categories.
(6) There is great variation in the classification of ill-

Table 2–3. Puerto Rican–American Hot-Cold Classification of Foodstuffs, Medicines, and Herbs

Hot (caliente)	Cool (fresco)	Cold (frío)
Alcoholic drinks	Barley water	Avocado
Anise	Bicarbonate of soda	Bananas
Aspirin	Bottled milk	Coconut
Caster oil	Chicken	Lima beans
Chili peppers	Fruit	Sugar cane
Chocolate	Honey	White beans
Cinnamon	Magnesium carbonate	
Cod liver oil	Mannitol	
Coffee	Milk of magnesia	
Corn meal	Nightshade	
Evaporated milk	Orange flower water	
Garlic	Raisins	
Iron (Fe) tablets	Sage	
Kidney beans	Salt cod	
Onions	Watercress	
Peas		
Penicillin		
Tobacco		
Vitamins		

Note: Due to the idiosyncratic nature of hot-cold classifications of internal factors, there may be considerable variation in the above among Puerto Rican populations. Adapted from Harwood A. The hot-cold theory of disease: Implications for treatment of Puerto Rican patients. *JAMA* 216(7):1153–1158, 1971. Copyright 1971, American Medical Association.

nesses or internal factors such as hot or cold among ethnic and racial groups.

- Classification may be based on local, regional, cultural, or historical factors and are passed down by word of mouth.
- The hot-cold power of internal factors can be determined only by observing their effect on the body state or the illness classified as hot or cold.
- Individuals often reclassify internal factors based on their own idiosyncratic, practical experience with them.
- Introduction of new food items, medications, and over-the-counter drugs requires classification based on idiosyncratic, practical experience.
- New disease conditions incorporated into ethnomedical systems may have variable hot-cold properties attributed to them.
- Remedies may be given in improper amounts and prove ineffective despite their proper classification as hot or cold.

d. Treatment of illness due to hot-cold imbalance follows the law of opposites.
  (1) Hot illnesses are treated by ingestion of cold internal factors, reduction of exposure to hot external elements, or both.
  (2) Cold illnesses are treated by ingestion of hot internal factors, reduction of exposure to cold external elements, or both.

e. The hot-cold syndrome provides a basis for self-care and preventive care.

  (1) Health can be maintained by avoidance of extremes in behavior, intake of internal factors, and exposure to external elements.
  (2) Intake of internal factors and exposure to external factors can be tailored to certain life stages when hot or cold body states are known to prevail. For example, the very young and old may be considered to have naturally more cold body states. Therefore, warm or hot foods and exposure to warmer external factors would maintain health. Also, a warm body state may be believed to exist during pregnancy, so cold or cool foods and exposure to cooler external factors would promote a healthy pregnancy. A cold body state may be believed to exist during menstruation. Therefore, warm or hot internal factors and exposure to warm external factors would prevent clotting of blood or slowing or stopping the menstrual flow. Table 2–5 gives examples of conditions and expected behaviors of Puerto Rican–American patients adhering to hot-cold ethnomedical beliefs.

f. The hot-cold syndrome presents multiple challenges to the development of transcultural health care interventions.
  (1) The idiosyncratic and ever-changing nature of hot-cold classifications requires the ascertainment of the individual patient's explanatory model of illness and treatment.
  (2) Biomedical treatments and nursing interventions may be diametrically opposite of hot-cold principles.

Table 2–4. Haitian Hot-Cold Food Classification

Very Cold	Quite Cold	Cool	Warm	Very Hot
Avocado	Banana	Cane syrup	Eggs	Cinnamon
Cashew nuts	Grapefruit	Orange juice	Grapefruit juice	Clarin (raw rum)
Cassava bread	Lime	Tomato	Pigeon	Nutmeg
Coconut juice	Lime juice			Roasted coffee
Coconut meat	Okra			Rum
Mango	Orange			
Pineapple	Watermelon			

Neutral		
Banana juice	Eggplant	Pork
Beef	Goat meat	Pumpkin
Beets	Goat milk	River fish
Breadfruit	Kidney beans	Roasted peanuts
Brown rice	Lima beans	Sea fish
Carrot	Malanga	Spam
Cabbage	Milled corn	Sugar cane
Chicken	Noniced soft drinks	Sweet cassava
Coconut candy	Parsley	Sweet potato
Conch	Pigeon peas	White rice
Cow's milk	Plantain	Yam

Note: Due to the idiosyncratic nature of hot-cold classifications of internal factors, there may be considerable variation in the above among Haitian populations.
Adapted by permission of the Society for Applied Anthropology from Weiss HJC. Maternal nutrition and traditional food behavior in Haiti. *Hum Organ* 35:193–200, 1976.

Table 2–5. Behavior of Puerto Rican–Americans Related to Hot-Cold Conditions

Condition	Anticipated Behavior
Cold Conditions	
Arthritis	Refuses cold- or cool-classified internal factors
Common cold	Avoids exposure to cold
Painful joints	Accepts hot-classified internal factors
Postpartum	Avoids cold- or cold-classified internal factors
Menstruation	Avoids acidic foods and medicines
	Avoids exposure to cold
Hot Conditions	
Diarrhea	Refuses hot-classified internal factors
Rash	Accepts cold- or cool-classified internal factors
Ulcers	as therapy
Pregnancy	Avoids exposure to heat
Hot Substances	
Infant formula requiring evaporated milk	Infant formula will be made with whole milk to "refresh" or cool down the naturally warm stomach
	Infants given formula with evaporated milk will receive cool substances afterward to refresh or cool down the warm stomach
Penicillin required on an ongoing basis	Stops taking penicillin when experiences symptoms of side effects classified as hot conditions (e.g., rash, diarrhea, and constipation)
	Stops taking penicillin if experiences a hot illness

Adapted from Hardwood A. The hot-cold theory of disease: Implications for treatment of Puerto Rican patients. *JAMA* 216(7):1153–1158, 1971. Copyright 1971, American Medical Association.

- The biomedical belief in consumption of green, leafy, iron-containing vegetables during the postpartum period may be contraindicated by hot-cold beliefs. Postpartum is a cold body state and green-leafy foodstuffs are cold internal factors. Also, foods rich in potassium prescribed in conjunction with diuretics may be discontinued when a cold illness occurs because they are also commonly classified as cold foodstuffs.
- Most hot-cold classifications contain internal factors that are compatible with biomedical treatment regimens and nursing interventions. The biomedically preferred, recommended, and commonly prescribed foods, fluids, or medications usually have less common but equally effective alternatives within the acceptable hot-cold classification.
  (3) The principle of neutralization can be used to develop transcultural nursing interventions. Contraindicated foodstuffs, herbs, or medications can be administered with neutral foods or fluids. Contraindicated internal factors can be administered with a small quantity of the opposite classified food or drink. Hot classified biomedical food or medications needed for hot classified illnesses can be administered with cold classified foods or drink. Symptoms of side effects of medications may result in discontinuation of the medication. We should try to anticipate the occurrence of such symptoms and advise the intake of the appropriate hot-cold internal factor with their onset and during their course.

6. Blood status model
  a. The status and function of blood are central concepts in beliefs about health and illness in many ethnomedical systems. Blood beliefs are central concepts in the ethnomedical health cultures of African Americans, African Caribbeans, Anglos, Appalachian Americans, Asian Americans, and Arab Americans.
  b. Blood has both physiologic and social-psychologic meanings.
  c. Social-psychologic meanings generally center on the following:
    (1) Emotional states, as in blushing in embarrassment or humility, flushing with anger, and becoming pale with fright.
    (2) Social and kin relationships, as in "bad blood" between people, being "blood brothers" or sisters, "blood" kin, and "Blood is thicker than water."
    (3) Personality types, as in "Hot-blooded," "cold-blooded," and "sanguine" (even-tempered).
    (4) Gender qualities. Menstruation infers adulthood, womanhood, and fertility. Males are considered to have more and stronger blood than females.
    (5) Danger. Blood carries contaminants as in the human immunodeficiency virus or acquired immunodeficiency syndrome, the Ebola virus, malaria, and hepatitis B. Magical properties attributed to menstrual blood are considered dangerous to males and others in society. Menstruating women are subject to multiple social restrictions owing to the polluting power attributed to menstrual blood.
  d. Physiologic meanings center on beliefs about the characteristics of blood necessary to keep the person alive and well or normal. Table 2–6 illustrates African-Carribbean beliefs about blood and its relationship to health and illness.
  e. Cross-cultural principles about blood beliefs common to most ethnomedical systems
    (1) There is little to no differentiation or recognition of biomedical concepts related to blood components such as types of cells and fluids composing blood and electrolytes, minerals, and other elements contained in blood.
    (2) The heart is seen as the organ most responsible for circulating blood.
    (3) Imbalances in blood by most causes can be restored through medications and herbs; diet; purging; removal of blood (bloodletting) or avoidance of blood loss; modification of activity level; resolution of emotional, psychologic, and social conflict; or avoidance of prolonged exposure to extremes of climate and weather.
    (4) The status of blood is affected by gender and age. Older, younger, and female individuals are con-

Table 2–6. African-Caribbean Beliefs About Blood

Characteristics of Blood	Condition	Physiologic Basis	Ethnomedical Treatment
Quantity or volume	Stroke Headache Tachycardia Hemoptysis Difficulty breathing Visual disturbances	Too much blood High blood or blood rising to and accumulating in chest and head Effects of bad luck or negative emotions Eating too much rich food (red meat, red wine)	Medications Herbs Acid or astringent foods (lemon juice, vinegar, sour oranges, sauerkraut) Epsom salts Brine from pickles or olives
	Anemia Weakness (physical and mental) Fatigue Lassitude Pallor	Too little blood Low blood or falling blood Lack of rest and sleep Pregnancy Inadequate diet (eating too much astringent or acid foods)	Medications Herbs Red food and drink (beets, grape juice, liver, red wine, red meat)
Color	Yellow blood or jaundice Dark blood Pale or loss of reddish color Bright red or too red	Bile is entering blood Patient is moribund Weak blood Blood is too strong	Diet Medications Herbs
Viscosity	Anxiety Fear Hypertension Itching Urticaria	Thick blood Effects of environmental factors (stormy weather, waxing moon, high tide, changing seasons)	See treatment for too much or high blood
	Pallor Weakness Clotting Edema of lower extremities	Thin blood Weak blood Inactivity	See treatment for too little or low blood

Temperature	Rashes
	Urticaria
	Fever
	Nervousness
	Migraine headaches
		Hot blood
		  Sleeping
		  Physical exercise
		  Concentrating or thinking a good deal
		Hot body states: early weeks into pregnancy or after childbirth
		Ingestion of hot foods and medications
			Food and medications classified as cold or neutral
			Administer laxatives

	Quietness
	Malaria
	Excessive sleeping
		Cold blood
		Cold body states
		  Postpartum
		  Menstruation
		Ingestion of cold foods and medications
			Food and medications classified as hot or neutral

Purity	Urticaria
	Venereal disease
	Debilitating illnesses
	Infections
	Susceptibility to illness
	Migrating body pains
	Diarrhea
	Abdominal pain
	Dizziness, lightheadedness
	Numbness in extremities
	"Spoiled" breast milk
	Depression
		Bad blood
		Dirty blood
		Shock, fright, and stress
		Social conflict
			Medications
			Herbs
			  Catnip tea
			  Pokeweed leaves
			Purgatives
			Alleviation of stress and social conflict

Data from DeSantis L. Haitian immigrant concepts of health. *Health Values* 17(6):3–16, 1993; Farmer P. Bad blood, spoiled milk: Bodily fluids as moral barometers in rural Haiti. *Am Ethnol* 15(1):62–83, 1988; Laguerre MS. Haitian-Americans. In Harwood A (ed). *Ethnicity and Medical Care.* Cambridge: Harvard University Press, 1981; Laguerre M. *Afro-Caribbean Folk Medicine.* South Hadley, MA: Bergin and Garvey, 1987; and Scott CS. The theoretical significance of a sense of well-being for the delivery of gynecological care. In Bauwens EE (ed). *The Anthropology of Health.* St Louis: CV Mosby, 1978.

sidered to have less blood and weaker blood. They are affected by having more illnesses, less strength, and less energy.

(5) Persons receiving blood from another may take on the physical characteristics, personality traits, and illnesses of the donor.

(6) In cultures in which blood carries the essential life force or energy, loss of blood is equated with loss of the life force. Blood loss may not be regenerated, leaving the person in a permanently weakened state.

(7) Menstrual blood is often imbued with magical powers. Menstruating women are considered unclean and dangerously polluting. Excessive menstrual flow places women at risk for premature aging, infertility, lack of energy, and disease due to weak blood or lack of adequate blood.

(8) Decreased menstrual flow places a woman at risk for the following:
  • Disease due to impurities building up in the blood or "bad blood."
  • Excessive blood, leading to headaches, stroke, and heart problems.
  • Accumulation of blood in the uterus, causing cancer, sterility, or blood clotting.
  • Blood rising or backing up in the body, leading to quick tuberculosis (hemoptysis) or stroke.

(9) Menstrual blood and materials used to absorb it render menstruating women vulnerable to harm by others.

f. Challenges presented to developing transcultural nursing interventions by blood beliefs

(1) Foods and fluids used to adjust the volume or quality of blood may be contraindicated by biomedicine.

(2) Persons with blood beliefs may seek frequent biomedical assessments of their blood. Delay in reporting results will result in extreme apprehension. Telling them their blood is good or "okay" is often translated into a confirmation of good health. Telling them there is a problem with their blood may cause extreme apprehension unless translated into their explanatory model.

(3) Using negative or positive to describe blood tests may lead to misunderstanding. Saying a blood test result is negative may mean ethnomedically that the blood is bad or weak or that the person is moribund. Saying a blood test result is positive may mean ethnomedically that the blood is good, strong, or okay and that the person is healthy.

(4) Beliefs about blood may affect willingness to use or continued use of contraceptives due to side effects such as spotting between periods and decreased menstrual blood flow.

(5) Examples of questions to ascertain the patient's explanatory model about blood and menstruation are contained in Table 2–7.

Table 2–7. Clinical Questions to Ascertain Patients' Explanatory Models About Blood Beliefs

General Blood Beliefs

1. What does blood do in the body?
2. What kind of problems can people have with their blood? How can these problems be prevented or treated?
3. What happens when a person has too much blood? How can a person prevent having too much blood? How can it be treated?
4. What happens when a person has too little blood? How can a person prevent having too little blood? How can it be treated?
5. What problems have you had or are you having with your blood? What do you think caused them? What can be done to treat them?

Menstruation

1. Why do women menstruate? What causes menstruation? Why do menstrual periods start when they do? Why do menstrual periods stop when they do?
2. What is good about menstruation?
3. What is bad or not good about menstruation?
4. Where does menstrual blood come from?
5. If there is less flow or bleeding than usual, how does it affect your body and health?
6. If there is more flow or bleeding than usual, how does it affect your body and health?
7. Are there certain things you should not do when you are menstruating? Why?
8. Are there certain places you should not go when you are menstruating?

Data from Helman CG. *Culture, Health & Illness.* Oxford: Butterworth–Heinemann, 1994; Laguerre M. *Afro-Caribbean Folk Medicine.* South Hadley, MA: Bergin and Garvey, 1987; Scott CS. The theoretical significance of a sense of well-being for the delivery of gynecological care. In Bauwens EE (ed). *The Anthropology of Health.* St Louis: CV Mosby, 1978; and Snow LF, and Johnson SM. Modern day menstrual folklore. *JAMA* 237(25):2736–2739.

■ TRADITIONAL HEALTH CULTURES

Overview

1. People throughout the world have traditional ways in which they cope with the phenomena associated with the maintenance and promotion of health and well-being and the prevention and treatment of illness. They include cognitive and social dimensions.

a. Cognitive dimension: Values and beliefs that serve as blueprints for the health-seeking behavior of people.
  (1) Includes concepts of health maintenance, disease etiology, disease prevention, diagnosis, treatment, care, and cure
  (2) Develops from the world-view of individuals and their life experiences with health and illness
  (3) Based in most cases on the scientific, magicoreligious, or holistic world-view, or elements of several world views.

b. Social dimension: The organization of health care delivery and health-seeking behaviors.

(1) Includes concepts of health-related roles and behaviors of patients and their families, nurses, and others involved in health care.

(2) Patients may draw help and knowledge from the popular, folk, or professional health care sector or from combinations of sectors.

Traditional Healers

1. Traditional healers are people who specialize in forms of healing that are characteristic of ethnomedicine. They are not part of either the popular or the professional health care sectors. Traditional healers deal with forms of healing that are secular, sacred, or both.
   a. Secular healing: Use of organic and technical means of treating conditions due to natural causation. Types of secular healers include herbalists, bone setters, injectionists, granny midwives, and tooth extractors.
   b. Sacred healing: Use of nonorganic methods to treat conditions due to supernatural and natural causation.
      (1) Nonorganic methods of healing are semimystic and religious practices used to influence the mind and faith of the individual. Examples include amulets, chants, prayers, rituals, and information gained from reading omens and signs.
      (2) Types of sacred healers include sorcerers, shamans, spiritualists, mediums, voodoo priests and priestesses, and diviners.
      (3) Many traditional healers combine both sacred and secular healing methods.
2. The variety of traditional healers available in society depends on the number and type of competing health cultures.
   a. Cultural groups with a magicoreligious world-view require a large number of sacred healers.
   b. Cultural groups with a naturalistic world-view require a large number of secular healers.
   c. Cultural groups that have both magicoreligious and naturalistic views of health and illness require a large number of sacred and secular healers.
   d. Table 2–8 shows the variety, preparation, and areas of practice of traditional healers in several cultural groups.
3. Traditional healers have a holistic approach to healing.
   a. They deal with all aspects of the patient's relationships in the diagnoses and treatment of illness. Relationships include those with the social world, natural world or environment, and supernatural world.
   b. A disturbance in any aspect of the patient's life may cause physical or emotional signs or symptoms.
   c. Diagnosis often requires 2 steps.
      (1) Inquiry into the patient's recent social history and behavior.
      (2) Some form of divination to determine any underlying supernatural causation and direction for therapy.
   d. Therapy is directed at all aspects of the patient's life that are disrupted.
      (1) Resolving interpersonal conflicts
      (2) Prescribing medications, special diets, or activities for physical signs and symptoms

(3) Providing explanations and ritual treatments to relieve feelings of guilt, shame, anger, and depression
(4) Performing rituals to resolve problems between the patient and the supernatural
   e. Treatment sessions are often public and include all who are involved in or affected by the illness.
4. You will need to determine whether your patients are receiving treatment from a traditional healer.
   a. Questions 5 and 6 in Table 2–8 help determine whether traditional healers will be or have been consulted.
   b. You should inform the patient if the traditional and biomedical therapies are incompatible.
      (1) Your role as culture broker is important when therapies are incompatible (see p. 60).
      (2) You will need to include members of the patient's therapy management group in the culture brokerage process. They can assist in achieving a mutually acceptable intervention.
      (3) You or an intermediary from the patient's therapy management group may need to consult directly with the traditional healer. You, the traditional healer, and the therapy management group *all* have the *same goal*—helping the patient recover from the illness. Traditional healers often have alternative therapies they are able to use.
      (4) You may need to modify the preferred biomedical therapy or nursing intervention if no compromise is possible.
5. Patients often indirectly seek our approval to consult with a traditional healer when they indicate their illness has a nonbiomedical basis (supernatural or out-of-balance causation).
   a. Your responsibility is to do the following:
      (1) Clarify the patient's concern
      (2) Determine what the patient believes should be done and who should do it
      (3) Explain any concerns you may have about the patient's proposed plan
      (4) Respect the patient's right to consult with traditional healers
      (5) Work with the therapy management group to secure the needed traditional therapy

Ethnic and Racial Groups

1. The major ethnic and racial groups recognized by the U.S. Bureau of the Census have distinctive traditional (ethnomedical, folk) health-culture beliefs and practices.
2. The table in Appendix A uses representative subgroups to illustrate the traditional health-culture beliefs and practices for each broad ethnic and racial category. Bear in mind, however, that these examples are presented to show a range of possible responses and reactions and to provide a basis for comparing the explanatory model of health and illness held by each individual patient from the specified subcultural group or broad ethnic or racial category.
   a. They cannot be generalized to all members of the

Table 2–8. Traditional Healers, Preparation, and Area of Practice

	Healer	Preparation	Practice
African American (southern urban)	Family members, especially grandmother	Word of mouth Practical experience	*Secular:* Common, everyday self-limiting illnesses that respond to home remedies Illness prevention
	Wise woman ("old lady")	Practical experience of caring for and raising own children, grandchildren and other kin Develops reputation among family, friends, and neighbors of being knowledgeable about home remedies for common illnesses	*Secular:* Treatment and prevention of common, everyday illnesses Advice about child care and childrearing
	Herbalist	No formal training	*Secular:* Diagnose a variety of natural illnesses Dispense herbs to neutralize or eliminate harmful substances that impair the power of body to heal or protect itself
	Spiritualist	No formal training Power may be present at birth (twins) or given by God later in life Usually associated with fundamentalist Christian religion (Holy Ghost, Pentecostal)	*Sacred:* Cure illnesses sent by God as punishment Cure ailments beyond the power of biomedical practitioners (e.g., arthritis, hypertension, diabetes mellitus) Power of God is present in the body of the spiritualist and transferred to the ill person through laying on of hands Draws on the faith of the individual *Sacred or secular:* May combine laying on of hands with herbal therapy, massage, and life counseling
	Root doctor (root worker, conjure man or woman, voodoo priest or priestess)	Apprenticeship May be born with magical powers	*Sacred or secular:* Serves as intermediary between supernatural and natural worlds Enact or remove spells Counteract or protect against witchcraft or sorcery Combine magical powers with use of herbs Read omens and signs and prescribe therapy or preventive measures Counseling and magical powers with use of herbs
African Caribbean (Haitian)	Family members, primarily female	Word of mouth generation to generation Practical experience	*Secular:* Prevention and treatment of common, everyday illnesses
	Docture feuilles, bocars, dokte fe (leaf doctors, herbalists)	Apprenticeship training Hands-on experience Learn "formulas" for healing	*Secular:* Treats patients with herbs, roots, medicinal plants, and rituals Bone setting, burn treatments, and massage
	Droquistes	Apprenticeship	*Secular:* Make and sell potions to prevent or treat illnesses of natural causation
	Houngan (voodoo priest) Mambo (voodoo priestess)	Apprenticeship training in rituals Knowledge of prayers and herbal remedies from elders Long training in and study of mythology of spirits	*Sacred or secular:* Treatment of illnesses due to supernatural causation (angry voodoo spirits; dead ancestors; or magic, witchcraft, or sorcery) Treatment of illnesses that are long lasting or fail to respond to biomedicine
	Sages-femme, fam saj, matrone (lay midwife, wise woman)	Apprenticeship	*Secular:* Perform deliveries, prepartum and postpartum care, treats other "female" conditions related to reproduction

Table continued on following page

Table 2–8. Traditional Healers, Preparation, and Area of Practice (Continued)

	Healer	Preparation	Practice
			Uses herbs, massage, rituals, baths, and diet
	Piqurestes (injectionists)	Training in missions and other medical facilities	*Secular:* Give injections, change dressings
Hispanic (Puerto Rican)	Family member, especially oldest female	Word of mouth Practical experience	*Secular:* Common everyday illnesses that respond to home remedies
	Curandero or cuandera	Apprenticeship Gift from God	*Sacred or secular:* Knowledge of herbs, diet, massage, and ritual Commune with supernatural Conduct religious curing ceremonies
	Partera (lay midwife)	Apprenticeship training from older female relatives	*Secular:* Prepartum and postnatal care, herbal remedies, massage, treatment of natural illnesses affecting women
	Yerbero (herbalist)	No formal training	*Secular:* Preventive and curative care Treats both ethnomedical and biomedical illnesses
	Santiguadore (sabador)	Apprenticeship	*Secular:* Massage and manipulation of body for illnesses affecting the musculoskeletal and gastrointestinal systems Treats both ethnomedical and biomedical illnesses
	Spiritualist (espiritualualista, brujera, santero)	May be born with gift to foretell future Perfect skills through apprenticeship	*Sacred:* Prevention and diagnosis of illness due to magic, witchcraft, or sorcery; uses amulets, prayers, and other artifacts Some limited curative functions
Moslem (Iranian)	Family members, especially older women	Knowledge handed down generation to generation	*Secular:* Self-care measures such as bed rest, diet, herbs, home remedies, and childbirth assistance
	Dais (traditional midwife)	Apprenticeship Older women who have raised their own families	*Secular:* Prepartum and postpartum care Childbirth Newborn care Herbal therapies Massage
	Mullah (religious healer)	Religious training	*Sacred:* Prevention of illness via preparation of tawiz (amulet with verses from the Koran) Treat illnesses due to evil spirits Treat emotional problems, nervousness, excessive anxiety, and mental illness
	Injectionists	Self-taught	*Secular:* Administer medications prescribed by physicians Purchase and prescribe injectable medications on their own
	Hakimji (traditional healer)	Apprenticeship	*Sacred or secular:* Combine procedures and medicines from Urani and Greco-Arabic medical traditions
	Bonesetters	Apprenticeship	*Secular:* Sets broken bones Treats sprains, strains, dislocations, and generalized body pains
Native American (Navajo Indian)	Family members	Knowledge handed down from generation to generation	*Secular:* Common everyday illnesses of natural origin Prevention of illness

Table 2–8. Traditional Healers, Preparation, and Area of Practice (Continued)

Healer	Preparation	Practice
		Herbal remedies
Medicine man	Born with power to heal Acquire power to heal via vision or quest Apprenticeship with medicine man once power to heal is known	*Sacred or secular:* Diagnoses and treatment of supernatural or natural illness (meditation, trance state, divination, or star gazing) Use combination of herbs and curing ceremonies
Diagnostician	As per medicine man	*Sacred:* Diagnose underlying cause of illness via divination
Herbalists	Knowledge passed down generation to generation Apprenticeship	*Secular:* Diagnose and treat common illnesses of natural causation

subcultural group or to the broader ethnic or racial category.

b. Great variations in the health-culture beliefs and practices exist not only between but also among members of any given subcultural group. Examples of factors causing intragroup variation are the following:
   (1) Socioeconomic status
   (2) Race
   (3) Age
   (4) Gender
   (5) Educational level
   (6) Religious beliefs and practices, for example, level of religiosity; adherence to traditional or mainstream Christian, Islamic, or Jewish religions; or degree to which religion directs health-seeking behavior
   (7) Life experiences related to health and illness
   (8) Availability and access to biomedical and ethnomedical health care providers

3. Black (African American). The world-view is a combination of the magicoreligious and holistic world-views which forms the basis of health-culture beliefs and practices (see p. 28).
   a. Ideas about health and illness are drawn from the popular, ethnomedical, and biomedical health cultures and make little distinction between science and religion or mind and body. Everyday events affect all aspects of the person's life and his or her physical, social, and spiritual being. Good health is seen as an instance of good fortune as is job success and having a loving family. Illness is seen as an instance of personal misfortune as is poverty, lack of a job, and family discord. Things that cause misfortune in 1 area of life can result in misfortune in all areas of life.
   b. Illnesses are classified as natural and unnatural. The table in Appendix A lists natural and unnatural illnesses, their causation, and treatment. Natural illnesses are attributed to the person's failure to follow the 3 laws of nature (God's laws).
      (1) Human beings are bound by the same laws of nature as are the seasons, heavenly bodies, plants, and animals.
      (2) Human beings are to know, love, and serve God.
      (3) Human beings are to love each other. Unnatural illnesses are attributed to God withdrawing divine protection and making the person vulnerable to evil influences. The devil is in control. Evil influences are not responsive to biomedical treatment, self-care measures, help from family and friends, or the healing powers of prayer.
   c. Diagnosis of illness is dependent on the causation attributed to it and not necessarily to the presenting signs and symptoms.
      (1) The same signs and symptoms are interpreted differently in different situations and depend on the individual's assessment of risks he or she has been exposed to. For example, a stroke may be attributed to old age, divine punishment, excessive dietary intake of red meat, witchcraft by one's enemy, or abrupt stopping of the menses due to sudden exposure to cold.
      (2) Treatment of any illness cannot be separated from religious beliefs and practices. Healing of natural illnesses and restoration of divine protection occur within the context of religious ceremonies. One is dependent on God to send the "right" powerful healer when signs and symptoms continue despite trying biomedicine, prayer, or countermagic.
      (3) All illnesses are theoretically preventable if individuals take care in their relationships with God, nature, and other persons.
      (4) Certain persons are believed to be more vulnerable to natural illnesses.
         • Older people and children: Blood "thins" out and is unable to protect one against illness.
         • Women: Constitutionally weaker than men owing to menstruation, anatomic differences, and their reproductive function. They are most vulnerable when menstruating, during postpartum, and postabortion.
         • Unborn fetus: Well-being is totally dependent on maternal behavior during pregnancy.
   d. Family and friends are an integral part of the person's therapy management group regardless of illness causation or treatment prescribed from any sector of health care.

4. African-Caribbean (Haitian American). The world-view is a combination of magicoreligious and holistic, which forms the basis of health culture beliefs (see p. 28).
   a. In addition to belief in the healing power of the Christian God, there is often a concomitant belief system grounded in traditional (folk) religion such as voodoo and *santeria*.
      (1) Health maintenance and recovery from illness are dependent on faith in the power of the supernatural working in collaboration with traditional healers or biomedical health care providers.
      (2) African-Caribbean patients may respond to signs and symptoms initially with religious behavior rather than biomedical health-seeking behavior.
      (3) After appropriate rituals have been performed, it is not unusual for African-Caribbean patients to seek biomedical health care.
   b. Health is seen as the ability to work and to carry out one's activities of daily living. A healthy person is one who has a good appetite; looks well with shiny skin, bright eyes, and good color; is at peace; and moves without effort or pain.
   c. Illnesses are classified as supernatural or natural (see table in Appendix A).
      (1) Natural illnesses are the dominant illnesses in African-Caribbean health culture.
      (2) Supernatural illnesses are relatively rare. They are suspected when
         • A child becomes ill or dies.
         • Signs and symptoms do not respond to home remedies, biomedicine, or treatments from secular traditional healers.
         • Social conflict predates onset of signs and symptoms.
         • Onset is sudden and illness becomes life threatening.
         • Illness occurs in combination with other personal misfortunes, such as business failure, spousal infidelity, or family conflict.
         • Illness occurs after one gains power, wealth, or other good fortune that causes envy and anger in others.
   d. Implications for nursing care
      (1) African-Caribbeans will rely on family, kin, and friends for assistance in health and illness.
      (2) African-Caribbeans are not accustomed to being asked many questions during physical examinations. The nurse should keep questions to a minimum and explain the basis for the questions. Questions, especially those related to family history, are regarded with suspicion. Health care providers who ask many questions are seen as lacking competence.
      (3) Medications given via injection are more effective than those given orally.
      (4) Vitamin injections are an important method of maintaining or building up one's blood.
      (5) African-Caribbean patients are quite concerned about the status of their blood so you should make a point of explaining the reason for and result of all blood tests even if they are routine tests.
      (6) Purgatives with a castor oil base are commonly taken by adults and given to newborns, infants, and children. Pregnant women will take purgatives to cleanse the system of the fetus to remove impurities from its blood, produce a lighter-skinned child, and result in a more active newborn. Newborns are given purgatives to cleanse their systems of afterbirth and meconium, which is considered poisonous. Children and adults take purgatives regularly to remove impurities from the blood. You should be alert to signs and symptoms of dehydration in newborns and infants.
      (7) African-Caribbean patients have difficulty localizing symptoms of pain. You will need to be very precise in your physical assessment. Have them point to the affected part and locate the site of pain on the affected part. Let them describe the pain, as they are not usually accustomed to rating scales to determine pain intensity.
      (8) Family structure is usually extended. The grandmother, mother, or maternal aunt is responsible for health care in the home. Older siblings are given responsibility for child care of younger siblings.
5. White or Anglo American (lower and middle class Anglo American). The world-view is that science is the dominant basis of health-culture beliefs and practices (see p. 28).
   a. The scientific world-view does not mean that Whites use biomedical criteria to define health and illness or to direct their health-seeking behavior.
      (1) Whites incorporate a variety of self-care measures and home remedies into their health-seeking behavior.
      (2) A limited number of illness episodes are brought to biomedical health care providers.
   b. The scientific world-view does not exclude faith in God as a force in health and illness.
      (1) Whites do hold beliefs that faith in God will assist in protecting them from illness, aid in recovery from illness, or help cope with illness.
      (2) White groups do hold beliefs that suffering is a blessing from God.
      (3) White groups subscribing to fundamentalist Christian religious beliefs may consider illness as punishment from God.
   c. The scientific world-view does not mean that Whites totally exclude supernatural causation of illness.
      (1) Belief in the evil eye and curses exist as explanations for illness among such groups as Mediterranian Americans and Scandinavian Americans.
      (2) Belief in curses as an explanation for illness exists among such groups as Mediterranian Americans and German Americans.
   d. Health and illness are seen as multidimensional entities related primarily to physical functioning and feeling states.
      (1) Health is the absence of signs or symptoms of illness or conditions and the ability to function in a manner acceptable to oneself and one's group.
      (2) Illness interferes with the ability to function in a manner acceptable to one's group or oneself. Illness is indicated when pain occurs. Illness is indi-

cated when one experiences changes in bodily feeling states or functions without the presence of pain. Examples are the following:
  - Inability to see or interference with vision due to a cataract or detached retina
  - Glandular swelling without apparent infection or fever
  - Anemia without loss of blood or decrease in activity state

e. Most illness is due to natural causation. Table 3 in Appendix A details the dominant White concepts of illness causation.
  (1) The germ theory of illness is the dominant theory.
  (2) Social and physical environmental causation are achieving greater prominence as factors in illness causation.

f. Health maintenance measures are centered on diet and nutrition; taking vitamins, minerals, and tonics; exercising; maintaining regular bowel function through diet, laxatives, or enemas; living a moderate lifestyle; and obtaining adequate sleep and rest.

g. Implications for nursing care
  (1) There is wide variation in the experiencing and expression of signs and symptoms. Some White groups experience a large number of signs and symptoms and have difficulty localizing them during physical examinations. Examples are Italian Americans, Greek Americans, and French Americans. Also, some White groups do not readily or openly express signs and symptoms or pain. Examples are Irish Americans, German Americans, and Scandinavian Americans. Family structure is usually nuclear, and the spouse is generally the main health consultant. The mother or wife is the prime caregiver and diagnostician during illness.

6. Asian (Chinese American). The holistic world-view forms the primary basis for health-culture beliefs and practices.
  a. The oneness of all things and all people with nature, the universe, and the divine is the fundamental concept of all Chinese philosophic traditions, medicine, social life, and afterlife.
  b. Health results when the body works in a rhythmic and finely balanced manner, when the body adjusts to its external (physical) environment, and when functions and emotions are in a harmonious relationship.
  c. Illness is the opposite of health.
  d. Traditional Chinese medicine (TCM). Traditional Chinese medicine has always been a system of preventive medicine.
    (1) All things, people, and systems have a responsibility and place in the prevention and healing of illness.
    (2) The individual has the primary responsibility to prevent and heal illness.
    (3) Illness may have an external cause. All illnesses have an internal cause and involve a sickness of the spirit.
    (4) Knowledge of 6 interrelated components is helpful in understanding the conceptual framework of traditional Chinese medicine.
      - Tao
      - *Ch'i*
      - Yin and yang
      - Law of 5 elements
      - Meridians
      - Causative factors
    (5) Tao, *ch'i*, and yin and yang provide the philosophic basis of traditional Chinese medicine.
      - Tao: From the philosophic tradition of Taoism, it posits a way of life, a way of virtue, a way of heaven, and a way of death. Individuals, families, groups, and communities should flow with nature, avoid excesses or extremes, maintain a middle position, and practice moderation.
      - *Ch'i* (vitality): The "universal energy" or cosmic life force, *Ch'i* is the fundamental concept of the entire system of traditional Chinese medicine. *Ch'i* is the origin of all disease. Health is the balance or harmony in the flow of *ch'i;* illness results from an imbalance.
      - Yin and yang: These are cosmic forces representing the duality and unity of the universe and the tao. Illness occurs when yin and yang are out of balance.
    (6) Law of 5 elements (fire, earth, metal, water, and wood): This law provides a series of correspondences or associations between the external physical world and the internal milieu of the body.
    (7) Meridians and pulses: Meridians are invisible systems *(ching-lo)* or pathways that carry *ch'i* throughout the body. They regulate the organs, transport blood, and connect internal and external organs. Pulses are present in each organ. The rate, rhythm, and strength of the pulses taken together indicate the status of the organs and the balance or imbalance in the flow of *ch'i.* No difference among the pulses indicates perfect balance.
    (8) Causative factors: There are 7 internal and external factors that cause disease. Internal factors are excess or lack of emotions, constitution (hereditary), anxiety, and irregularity of food or drink. External factors are cold, heat, humidity, fire, dryness, dampness, and wind. Illness results from excess or deficiency of the internal or external causative factors, interruption of the flow of *ch'i*, loss of *ch'i*, imbalance of yin or yang, and failure to find or maintain "the way."
    (9) Diagnosis relies on the differentiation of signs or symptoms arising from somatic conditions and those from emotional disturbances. Somatization of signs and symptoms that arise from emotional distress is common in Chinese culture, and expression of physical signs and symptoms is more socially acceptable. The Chinese, however, are culturally reluctant to express emotion to others.
  e. Implications for nursing care
    (1) Expect the simultaneous use of multiple sectors of health care, and try to accommodate the use of alternate therapies.
    (2) Many self-care measures will be used, since traditional Chinese medicine and ethnomedicine place the major responsibility for prevention and treatment of illness on the individual. The role of the

health care practitioner is to support and encourage the patient.

(3) Collaborate with the patient and family in determining interventions. Loyalty to the family subjugates individual welfare to family welfare. Patients may be more concerned about the effect of their illness on the family than on themselves and may feel guilty and ashamed over letting down the family by becoming ill. Patients may also be reluctant to assert themselves.

(4) Be understanding about possible delays in seeking biomedical care. Because Chinese family cohesiveness and support result in a higher level of coping with and caring for ill members, care may be sought only after all other resources are exhausted. Delay is especially likely in emotional or psychiatric conditions.

(5) Remain alert to the tendency of patients to be submissive, quiet, and overly agreeable. Maintaining harmonious social relationships takes precedence even when the patient may disagree. Also, it is considered impolite and disrespectful to disagree with those in authority even when asked. Saying yes when one does not understand or agree prevents disruption in social harmony. Open expression of pain or the need to ask for assistance may be contraindicated or considered disrespectful.

(6) Avoid drawing large amounts of blood from patients, because blood contains *ch'i* and is the vital energy for adherents to traditional Chinese medicine and ethnomedicine.

(7) Try to limit excessive questioning or lengthy health teaching. "Talking" health care providers may confuse patients and convey incompetence. Instead, combine health teaching with demonstration and use more interactive techniques.

(8) Explore the context in which somatic signs and symptoms are manifested. Physical symptoms are a language of distress in Chinese culture, and should be put in the context of their onset and ongoing manifestations.

7. Hispanic (Puerto Rican–American). The world-view is the holistic world-view, which forms the primary basis of health-culture beliefs and practices (see p. 28).

a. Health and illness cannot be separated from interpersonal relationships, the forces of nature, God's will, and significant events. Mental and physical functioning cannot be separated. What affects the mind also affects the body and vice versa.

b. Health is seen as a gift from God, which the person must preserve by maintaining equilibrium in his or her life. Equilibrium is achieved by doing the following:
   • Maintaining an adequate and proper (balanced) diet
   • Avoiding interpersonal conflict by treating people kindly, fairly, and respectfully
   • Living a moderate lifestyle
   • Sharing whatever resources one has with others
   • Honoring God

c. Health is maintained through the following measures:
   • Praying to God
   • Taking herbs and spices to increase one's strength and resistance to illness
   • Wearing amulets
   • Keeping religious paraphernalia in the home

d. Illness causation is classified as natural and supernatural. The table in Appendix A summarizes the major natural and supernatural illnesses.

(1) Determination of causation is dependent on analysis of previous social and religious behavior.

(2) The same signs and symptoms may be interpreted differently depending on the circumstances surrounding their manifestation and response to treatment. Certain signs and symptoms may be attributed to natural causes 1 time and supernatural causes another time. Signs and symptoms that fail to respond to secular ethnomedical measures may then be reinterpreted as having a supernatural causation.

(3) **Spiritism** is the broad term used to describe illnesses of supernatural (spiritual) causation. Spiritism is the belief that spirits can enter the natural world and affect human behavior. Persons suffering from spiritism are not defined as sick or held responsible for their illnesses. The causation is external or from outside forces. The individual is a "passive" instrument of the treatment. The behavioral manifestations are seen as culturally appropriate and normal responses to the effect of spiritism.

(4) Failure of continued improvement in signs and symptoms with 1 therapy may indicate that the underlying causation has changed or that a new illness entity is occurring. Failure of signs and symptoms to respond to biomedical therapy may be taken as confirmation of supernatural causation.

(5) Emotional illnesses may have either natural or supernatural causation. Examples of such illnesses are *susto, mal aire, nervios,* and *locura* (see Table 3E in Appendix). Persons may be brought to biomedical health care providers to relieve signs and symptoms of aggressive behavior, agitation, and self-destructive actions. However, biomedical psychotherapy is not considered appropriate for illnesses with mental manifestations or ones caused by spiritism, for the following reasons:
   • Psychotherapy classifies the person as mentally ill or crazy, which carries great stigma in Puerto Rican society.
   • Psychotherapy considers the illness to be internal or the fault of the person.
   • Psychotherapy does not recognize the role of God or spirits in the illness.

e. Implications for nursing care. Keep 2 key cultural concepts in mind when caring for the Hispanic patient. They are *respecto* and *personalismo*.

(1) *Respecto* (respect): treating others and being treated with respect and dignity. This is achieved by dressing professionally, speaking with a correct

tone of voice, projecting a professional image, explaining all procedures, providing an explanation for all questions asked, and providing patients with an opportunity to express their opinions.

(2) *Personalismo:* treating each person as an individual. This can be achieved by building rapport before starting the history or physical; touching patients on the arm, shoulder, or back several times during the nurse-patient encounter; letting patients speak about their concerns even if they are seemingly unrelated to the condition as we perceive it; and learning a few words of Spanish or having the patient teach us some words.

(3) Hispanic patients usually expect a complete physical examination for any problem.

(4) Hispanic patients may perceive and express more symptoms than groups such as Whites, Asian Americans, and Native Americans. Do not mistake such behavior as an emotional problem or undue dramatization. What appears as dramatization is well within the cultural norm of Hispanic health culture. Hispanic patients have difficulty expressing degrees of pain or localizing pain.

(5) Hispanic patients may prefer to be treated by Hispanic health care providers because they generally speak the same language, and Hispanic patients believe they are more likely to understand and respect traditional health-culture beliefs and practices.

(6) The family plays a key role in all aspects of health care. Mothers of pregnant women are the key consultants in infant and child care, especially in infant feeding. The oldest female in the family is usually the family health consultant.

8. Native Americans (e.g., Navajo Indians)
   a. There is great cultural diversity among and within the approximately 500 Native-American tribes and nations in North America recognized by federal, state, or local governments.
   b. Cultural traditions shared by most Native-American tribes include the following:
      (1) An emphasis on cooperation rather than competition among individuals or groups
      (2) Sharing with and giving to others
      (3) Continual development of the self throughout life
      (4) The belief that nature is more powerful than human beings
      (5) Respect for elders
      (6) A present and seasonal (rhythmic) time orientation
      (7) Placing in importance the welfare and security of the extended family over individual success
      (8) Living in balance and harmony with nature
   c. World-view: The holistic world-view forms the primary basis of traditional Navajo health-culture beliefs and practices (see p. 28).
      (1) Health is achieved by living in harmony with the universe. The universe includes the individual, the family, the community and tribe, the environment (physical world), and the spirit world.
      (2) Individuals have both a physical and a spiritual dimension. These are considered 2 aspects of the

same reality. Each dimension is governed by different laws. Violation of the laws of 1 will affect the other. Living by the laws of both will results in a balanced, healthy, and happy life.

(3) The physical dimension requires that individuals treat their bodies and nature with respect. Earth and humans are seen as one. When individuals harm themselves, they harm the earth and vice versa.

(4) The spiritual dimension requires that individuals actively participate in developing their own potentialities through will or volition. The realities of existence can be learned through nonmaterial ways such as through dreams and visions, legends, spiritual teachings, traditions learned from sacred tribal myths and rituals, spirits and spirit protectors, and older people who act as guides and teachers of life. Individuals must develop the capacity to accept the realities of existence as a reflection of their unknown or unrealized potential. The newfound realities then become something more or different. There must be a balance between values individuals hold about themselves and about others. Lack of balance in values causes individuals and their families and communities to suffer illness and misfortune. The only source of failure in the process of self-development is the individual's failure to be guided by tribal traditions, which reveal the laws of the universe.

(5) The supernatural is ever present in Navajo life. The world is governed by supernatural powers and holy people, and failure to honor them through rituals results in lack of harmony between individuals and nature. All things of the Creator have a purpose and are to be respected. Being in harmony with the supernatural forces and the Creator is essential for health.

d. Illness occurs when there is disharmony in some aspect of the individual, environment, or supernatural.
   (1) The disharmony may result from actions of witches, disturbing the physical world, failure to observe proper ceremonies or improperly using a sacred ceremony, angering the spirit world (holy people), not taking care of the self, not observing the laws regulating the physical and spiritual dimensions of humans, failure to observe moderation and balance in all things, and not being respectful to others.
   (2) Navajo do not believe disease is caused by infections, communicable agents, or physiologic processes. The word "germ" does not exist in the Navajo language. The cause of a disease must be sought in individual actions that were counter to the laws of the universe.
   (3) Mental illnesses are also seen as due to disharmony.

e. All illnesses in Navajo health culture have a supernatural basis because all things surrounding humans in the environment and spirit world have supernatural power. Such power is regarded as benevolent if individuals live according to the laws that govern the universe. Illnesses resulting from failure to live by the laws of the universe are considered natural illnesses.

   (1) Some Navajo believe evil power exists in the form of witchcraft. Witchcraft is often given as an explanation of death, illness, prolonged hardship, and anxieties of life. The victim is held blameless. Spirits of the dead are often blamed for illness and misfortune.

   (2) Navajo have elaborate burial rituals and taboos surrounding contact with the dead, and violation of such taboos can result in illness.

   (3) Special ceremonies (sings or ways) are required to treat illnesses due to witchcraft and ghosts.

f. Navajo will seek treatment from both the biomedical and ethnomedical systems regardless of cause.

   (1) Biomedicine will be sought for treatment of signs and symptoms, but healing or restoring of harmony can only be achieved through ethnomedicine. Healing is based on a variety of concepts about life and not primarily on the actions of medicines, remedies, and treatments. Healing cannot be separated from Navajo religion and individual spirituality.

   (2) Chant ways or sings are the traditional healing ceremonies used to diagnose and restore balance. They are conducted by medicine men or singers.

g. Healing is achieved when the ill person becomes one with the holy people and comes into harmony with the universe.

   (1) Healing is done through medications, rest, diet, isolation, and sweat baths.

   (2) Herbs and plants compose the bulk of medications because they are natural products of the earth.

   (3) Medications must be solicited, prepared, and administered in accordance with the proper ceremonies to be effective.

h. Prevention of illness requires living by the laws of the physical and spiritual dimensions of human existence.

   (1) Amulets may be worn to ward off illness or witchcraft. Amulets are bags of herbs, fetishes, or other symbolic entities believed to have curative or protective powers.

   (2) Blessing ways are done at important life events to enhance good fortune, happiness, and health.

i. Implications for nursing care

   (1) You should endeavor to include family and community members in the care of Navajo patients. Navajo draw strength, spiritual comfort, and support from their family and community. You may need to suspend or alter agency rules limiting visitors.

   (2) You should work cooperatively with Navajo healers and facilitate their participation with hospitalized or institutionalized patients. You will need to know the essence of the healing ceremony so that you do not inadvertently invalidate it. Food, sacred objects, and other artifacts used in the ceremonies may need to remain near the patient for a period of time. You may need to intervene for patients and families with biomedical and

administrative personnel to permit needed referrals to Navajo healers.

   (3) The healing power of Navajo medicine is in the ceremony rather than in the actual medication or remedy.

   (4) Expect that there may be delay by Navajo patients in seeking biomedical care because diagnoses and cure may be attempted in the popular or ethnomedical system first.

   (5) Expect the individual Navajo to make his or her own decisions about treatment. The right of individuals to find their own way is a core Navajo cultural value and is extended to all Navajo, including children.

   (6) Familiarize yourself with the communication patterns of Navajo. Periods of silence and avoidance of eye contact convey respect. Nonverbal communication is a central feature of Navajo behavior. There is often no equivalent word in the Navajo language for an English word, necessitating use of greater descriptions in translation across languages.

■ THE TRANSCULTURAL NURSING PROCESS

Major Objectives

1. Avoid imposing one's cultural beliefs, practices, and concepts of health and illness on patients.
2. Respect (understand) patients' health-culture beliefs and practices.
3. Develop culturally appropriate nursing diagnoses and interventions that incorporate the patient's concept of clinical reality.
4. Avoid allowing cultural stereotypes to dictate interactions with individuals.
5. Consider patients as equal partners.
6. Advocate for the right of individuals to decide their health care options.

NURSE ADVISORY

Nurses are human beings with deeply held personal and professional values. You cannot be expected to fully accept every patient you encounter. If you feel unable to assist or accept patients with alternative health-culture beliefs and practices, you have an obligation to excuse yourself from the nurse-patient encounter and to find another person who can assume responsibility for patient care.

Transcultural Communication Techniques

1. Cross-cultural communication: Process by which persons from different ethnic or racial or subcultural groups send and interpret messages. The cycle of sending messages and responding to feedback is largely an unconscious process when done between persons of the same ethnic, racial, or subcultural group. It is also affected by the

Table 2–9. Factors That Commonly Affect the Communication Process

Factors	Examples
Personal characteristics of sender and receiver	Sociodemographic characteristics such as age, gender, income, and marital status. Past-life experiences, attitudes, and opinions
Cultural	Language and dialect, time or season of year, space and distance, dress, food digestion, good or bad manners, use and meaning of touch, meaning of gestures
Situational	Background noise, physical and emotional states of participants, climate (e.g., warm or cold room where interaction occurs), being interrupted by others, body odors of participants

Context in which the communication is sent and received	Inappropriate:
	  Proposing marriage at a funeral
	  Joking with dying patients that death is punishment for one's lifestyle
	Appropriate:
	  Teaching children dental care in school health class

factors shown in Table 2–9. Verbal and nonverbal communication processes of the major ethnic and racial groups in the United States are shown in Table 2–10.

NURSE ADVISORY

The ability to convey respect to patients is the key to any successful communication. All individuals and groups desire respect. In cross-cultural situations, you may be readily forgiven for inadvertently violating culturally prescribed communication behaviors if patients perceive you as sincere, empathetic, and trustworthy.

2. Barriers to cross-cultural communication are both verbal and nonverbal.
   a. Verbal barriers
      (1) Use of professional jargon (see Chapter 4)
      (2) Multiple dialects of the same language: Just as English can vary widely in how it is spoken and the words it uses (Black English, "The Queen's English," Appalachian English, West Indian English, Yankee English, and Southern English), so do other languages differ from dialect to dialect, complicating communication even between 2 "native" speakers.
      (3) Vocabulary differences between languages: Languages often do not have words for biomedical anatomic terms, names of illnesses, conditions, treatments, or feeling states (Table 2–11). For example, Haitian Creole has no word for "womb" or "virus," Mandarin Chinese has no equivalent term for "assessment"; Miccosukee Indians consider anxiety an illness and not a symptom related to another illness.

NURSE ADVISORY

To overcome medical terminology barriers, ask the patient to name or describe the entity, procedure, process, or feeling state in question, then use the patient's descriptions or terms in nurse-patient interactions.

      (4) Vocal intonation
      (5) Speed or rate of speech (see Table 2–9)
      (6) Speech punctuated by silence
   b. Nonverbal barriers (see also Chapter 4)
      (1) Space and spatial distance
      (2) Touch
      (3) Facial expressions
      (4) Eye contact

Table 2–10. Verbal and Nonverbal Communication Processes of Ethnic or Racial Groups*

Communication Process	Black	White	Asian (Chinese)	Hispanic (Mexican American)	Native American (Navajo)
Dominant language	English and Black English	English	Mandarin Chinese	Spanish	Navajo
Speech pattern	Rapid	Moderate	Slow with silences	Rapid	Slow with silences
Intonation	Loud	Moderate	Soft	Loud	Soft
Space	Close	Distant	Close	Close	Close
Time orientation	Present or future Polychronic† Flexible schedules	Future Monochronic‡ Clock regulated	Present or past Circular time	Present Polychronic Elastic time	Present or past Circular time
Express pain	Open or public	Closed or private	Closed or private	Open or public	Closed or private
Eye contact	Maintain but avoided for long periods	Maintain	Indicates rudeness	Maintain	Sign of disrespect

* Communication processes may change over time and may vary owing to sociodemographic factors and context (public or private).
† Polychronic time describes a period when several happenings occur and are tended to simultaneously.
‡ Monochronic time is linear and segmented so that the focus can be on one activity.
Data from Andrews MM, and Boyle JS (eds). *Transcultural Concepts in Nursing Care.* 2nd ed. Philadelphia: JB Lippincott, 1995; Hall ET. Proxemics: The study of man's spatial relations. *In* Gladstone I (ed). *Man's Image in Medicine and Anthropology.* New York: International University Press, 1963; Hall ET, and Hall MR. *Understanding Cultural Differences.* Yarmouth, ME: Intercultural Press, 1990; and Kluckhohn F. Dominant and variant value orientations. *In* Brink PJ (ed). *Transcultural Nursing: A Book of Readings.* Englewood Cliffs, NJ: Prentice-Hall, 1979.

Table 2–11. Variations in Meaning of Health Terminology

Biomedical Term	Sign or Symptom
Black (American)	
Anemia; low blood pressure	Low blood; tired blood; not enough blood
Constipation	Locked bowels; stopped up
Diabetes mellitus	Sugar; sweet blood
Diarrhea	Running off; grip
High blood pressure	High blood; too much blood
Hypertension	Being hyper and tense
Menstrual period	Red flag; the curse
Pain	Miseries; rheumatism
Syphilis	Bad blood; pox
Urinate	Pass water; tinkle; pee pee
Black (Caribbean, Virgin Islands)	
Anemia	Weak blood
Constipated	Can't go off
Delirium tremens	Harrows
Edematous	Gathering water
Epileptic seizure	Falling out
Hydrocephalic	Water head
Menstruating	Unwell; monthly; flowing; period
Nausea	Bad feeling
Strabismus	Cock-eye
Syphilis	Bad blood
Appalachian American	
Anemia; low blood pressure; lack of energy	Low blood
Diarrhea	Running off
Dizziness; light headedness	Blind staggers
Heavier than usual vaginal bleeding	Wasting
Hypertension	High blood
Hyperventilation	Drawing spell
Insomnia	Big eye
Mentally unbalanced	Tetched
Miscarriage	Bad luck
Nauseated	Deathly sick
Syncope	Deader than four o'clock
Tense; high strung	Hypertension
Tight and swollen	Strutted

Data from Burnum JF. Dialect is diagnostic. *Ann Intern Med* 100(6):899–901, 1984; Mitchell L. *101 Colloquial Expressions for Health Service Personnel.* Los Angeles: Mitsho, 1985; and Stokes LG. Delivering health services in a Black community. *In* Reinhardt AM, and Quinn MB (eds). *Current Practice in Family-Centered Community Nursing.* St. Louis: CV Mosby, 1977.

(5) Concepts of time
(6) Meaning of food

3. Overcoming cross-cultural communication problems
   a. Nurses need four areas of cross-cultural communication skills to overcome problems during the nurse-patient encounter.
      (1) Ability to perceive the health care problem or situation from the patient's perspective
      (2) Ability to recognize when the nurse or the patient is becoming resistant or defensive
      (3) Ability to reduce resistance and defensiveness
      (4) Ability to accept that cross-cultural communication errors will occur

   b. You can overcome cross-cultural communication problems by doing the following:
      (1) Assuming responsibility for learning about the cultural values, beliefs, practices, and behaviors of ethnic and racial groups we frequently encounter in the health care situation and adopting a patient-oriented learning style.
      (2) Performing a cultural assessment to ascertain the patient's concept of reality
      (3) Acting as a culture broker to further clarify the patient's perspective.
      (4) Considering what will happen if you impose biomedical or your own cultural beliefs, values, and practices on the patient and health care situation.
      (5) Acknowledging openly your concern or lack of understanding when a patient fails to respond or behave as you expect (e.g., suddenly breaking eye contact)
      (6) Sharing culturally appropriate personal information about yourself to personalize the nurse-patient encounter (e.g., talking about your family, home, or parenting experience)
      (7) Emulating the patient's verbal and nonverbal behavior
      (8) Using interpreters, when appropriate (see Chapter 4)

NURSE ADVISORY

Expect the nurse-patient encounter to be more time consuming when you do not speak the patient's language. If you organize the nurse-patient encounter so that the most important procedures or interactions are conducted first, you lessen the "fatigue factor" that can affect the patient, the interpreter, or yourself.

   c. Develop recovery skills to reestablish rapport with patients after the commission of cross-cultural communication errors.
      (1) Use patients as cultural informants. Realize that patients know more than you do about the situation, and seek their assistance in developing interventions.
      (2) Acknowledge your cultural limitations. Apologize and communicate your desire to learn how to avoid similar mistakes in the future. Use humor to alleviate the tension.
      (3) Consult cultural helpers or guides to contribute to understanding or mediation during sensitive encounters.
      (4) Refocus attention away from sensitive topics.
      (5) Allow patients to react to your mistakes without becoming defensive or angry.
      (6) Find another health care provider to take over if you cannot reestablish rapport.

Transcultural Nursing Assessment

1. Assessing the patient's concept of anatomy and physiology
   a. Health-seeking behavior is affected by concepts of the structure and function of the body.

b. Concepts of anatomy and physiology help patients to determine the significance of their signs and symptoms, decide whether to seek health care, choose among treatment options, and understand and adhere to health teaching.

2. Assessing the patient's EM: We can ascertain patients' EMs by doing a cultural assessment (cultural status examination).
   a. Table 2–12 gives examples of cultural assessment questions for illness.
      (1) Not all questions must be asked each time.
      (2) Questions should be open ended. Avoid yes-no responses. Allow patients to expand on their answers. Always try to ascertain the basis (why) of their responses.
      (3) Use questions to guide, not direct, the assessment process.

3. A different set of questions should be used to elicit EMs that are not illness based.
   a. Although the concept of EMs was developed for illness conditions, you can adapt it readily to health promotion; illness prevention; patient knowledge of anatomy, physiology, and signs and symptoms; and other aspects of patient care.
      (1) It is the *concept of EMs* that is critical to the transcultural nursing process.
      (2) The questions will vary according to what you wish to know.

4. When patients' EMs have been elicited, compare them with your EMs.
   a. Explain your EMs to patients.
   b. Ask your patients to explain their EMs to you.
   c. Discrepancies are noted between the EMs.
   d. Together with patients, negotiate or work out discrepancies between your EMs through the culture brokerage process (see p. 61).

5. The value of the EM approach to transcultural nursing
   a. Nurses become consciously aware of their EMs and their role in guiding interactions with patients.
   b. Nurses place themselves in the role of learners and patients in the role of teachers as we elicit their EMs.
   c. Nurses consider patients as equals in matters of health and illness.
   d. Nurses avoid the 5 fallacies of health-culture thinking.
      (1) Fallacy 1: All members of an ethnic or racial group hold identical values and beliefs about health and illness.
      (2) Fallacy 2: Nurses are guided in health care decision making by scientific reason, and patients are guided by ethnocentric beliefs.
      (3) Fallacy 3: Patients have no or limited knowledge about health and illness.
      (4) Fallacy 4: Health-culture beliefs and practices based on nonbiomedical premises are grounded in superstition and unrelated ideas.
      (5) Fallacy 5: Patients will change their health-culture beliefs and practices if nurses merely explain the underlying scientific rationale and logic of biomedicine.

6. Assessing risk factors
   a. Certain ethnic, racial, and population groups are at risk for specific disorders.
   b. Risk factors are usually an interplay between genetic composition and the following:
      (1) Ecology and environment
      (2) Culture and lifestyle
      (3) Socioeconomic factors
   c. Ecologic-environmental risk factors usually result from biologic adaptation that may be reversible, irreversible, or genetic.
      (1) Risk varies according to socioeconomic status, age, gender, and race.
      (2) Risk is usually related to climate, altitude, diet, and exposure to occupational and environmental hazards (see Chapter 38).
   d. Reversible biologic responses occur throughout life.
      (1) After a short-time exposure to ecologic conditions, the person is able to better tolerate them.
      (2) Examples are heat stress (excessive sweating), cold stress (vasoconstriction alternating with vasodilatation, shivering, and often an increased metabolic rate), and high altitude stress (shortness of breath, headache, and tachycardia).
   e. Irreversible biologic responses modify persons during their growth and development and cannot be reversed by adulthood.
      (1) Children exposed to heat during childhood are more slender, weigh less, and have more efficient sweat production due to greater body surface area by body weight.
      (2) Blacks, southwestern Native Americans, Asian Indians, and Australian Aborigines withstand heat better than Whites owing to more efficient sweat production.
      (3) Individuals raised in cold climates are less susceptible to cold injuries because of more efficient alternative sequences of vasoconstriction-vasodilation (hurting response) and increased metabolic rates.
         • Whites are less susceptible than Blacks to cold injuries.
         • Eskimos, Laplanders, and northern Native Americans have the least risk of cold injuries.
         • Populations with long-term exposure to high altitudes (3050 m or 10,000 ft) experience decreased fertility; decreased birth weight and increased placental weights (in an attempt to get more nutrients to the fetus); increased infant mortality rates; decreased skeletal size in response to decreased energy requirements; slower growth rates but longer growth periods; greater lung capacity and chest size; increased hematocrits, hemoglobin levels, red blood cell counts, and polycythemia due to hypoxic stress.
   f. Genetic responses to ecologic conditions do not require repeated childhood exposure. For example, population groups in tropical and subtropical regions have developed several hemoglobin and enzyme variants as a protective response against malaria, including sickle cell trait (in persons of African, Greek, Italian, Turkish, and Armenian ancestry) and α- and β-thalassemia (in persons from the Mediterranean,

Table 2–12. *Cultural Assessment Questions for Illness*

Questions	Reason for Asking
1. What do you think has caused your problem (condition)? *or* How would you describe the problem that has brought you to see me?	1. Allows patients to define the problem from their point of view, i.e., to describe their *illness* experience
2. Why do you think this has happened to you? Why did it happen now? Why has it affected *(name of body part)*? Why did it happen to you and not to someone else?	2. Permits patients to participate in the search for causality Determine patients' ideas of general and specific individual causality Determine if there is an underlying social causation factor, for example: Guilt over mistreatment of someone else Envy on the part of others Violation of a social taboo Failure to carry out obligations to others, ancestors, or supernatural entities Immoral behavior
3. How long have you had this problem? Why have you come for help now?	3. Gain information about patients' concept of time and severity of problem Are there unresolved issues from the past? Is there something that has just happened to trigger help seeking? Is there concern about the future?
4. What does your sickness do to you? *or* How does your sickness work?	4. Ascertain patient's concept of pathophysiology Valuable source of lay or folk etiologies Natural causation Out of balance Supernatural causation Lay interpretation of biomedical causation
5. What do you think should be done to help clear up (get rid of) your problem?	5. Learn patients' treatment plans or hidden agendas If specific tests, treatments, drugs, or diets are suggested, have patients describe how they will help Determine whether patients are using multiple medical systems Helps to bring popular, ethnomedical, and biomedical treatments together
6. Who else can help you get better?	6. Reassure patients all is being done to help resolve their illness Help ensure incorporating patients' therapy management group (healing network) into the plan or care Aids in determining alternative healing methods and care givers
7. What are the most important results you hope to receive from your care?	7. Determine patients' understanding of their prognosis
8. What are the problems your sickness has caused you? Who can or has helped you during your illness? *or* Are there other people who can help you with your problems?	8. Ascertain needs for health teaching and discharge planning Determine social support network and further define members of the therapy management group

Data from Kleinman A, Eisenberg L, and Good B. Culture, illness, and care: Clinical lessons from anthropological and cross-cultural research. *Ann Intern Med* 88(2):251–258, 1978; Molde S. Understanding patients' agendas. *Image* 18(4):145–147, 1986; and Pfifferling JH. A cultural prescription for medicocentrism. *In* Kleinman A, and Eisenberg L (eds). *The Relevance of Social Science for Medicine.* Boston: D Reidel, 1981.

Middle Eastern, and Southeast Asian regions). Genetic adaptation to ecologic conditions has resulted in increased incidence of disorders primarily due to race.

g. Risk factors due to culture and lifestyle
   (1) The interplay of culture and individual lifestyle with biologic and socioeconomic factors has resulted in an uneven distribution of disease conditions across ethnic and racial groups.
   (2) Cultural factors seldom act alone to cause illness conditions. They may contribute to their increased or decreased incidence.
   (3) Table 2–13 lists examples of the biocultural aspects of disease among selected ethnic racial groups. Cancer epidemiology is an example of how cultural factors and individual lifestyle affect the incidence of disease (Box 2–3).

h. Cultural practices may place certain members of ethnic or racial groups at risk when viewed from the biomedical perspective. Most of these practices have specific beneficial functions when viewed from the perspective of the culture where practiced. Examples of such practices are the following:
   (1) Haitian immigrant mothers giving newborns purgatives while keeping them on nothing by mouth: The purpose is to rid the body of poisonous afterbirth and meconium. The danger biomedically is dehydration, cachexia, and possible death. The danger culturally is the newborn's death due to retention of poisonous afterbirth. Failure to purge is considered a cultural sign of poor parenting.
   (2) The practice of coining, burning, cupping, or pinching by Southeast-Asian parents, certain Native-American groups, and Caribbean Blacks: The primary purpose is to treat various body pains but also to treat natural illnesses of a minor nature such as colds, fevers, nausea and vomiting, fainting and dizziness, coughing, and heat exhaustion. The function is to release the "wind" or noxious element causing the condition. The greater the bruise, burn mark, or raised erythema, the more effective the treatment. It is usually done on the chest, back, or abdomen; along the spine or trachea; or on the extremities. It may be done using herbs or other medications. From the biomedical

perspective, such measures are ineffective and border on physical abuse, especially when done on children.
   (3) Female circumcision
   (4) Fondling or kissing a child's genitals by Turkish adults: The purpose is to express admiration and celebration of the male child's virility and the female child's fertility. From the biomedical perspective, such practices could constitute sexual assault or psychologic seduction. In Turkey, such practices are a sign of parental affection and are necessary for normal psychosocial child development.
   (5) Physically punishing children by Haitian and Taiwanese parents: The purpose is to instill unquestioned obedience to and respect for parents, older adults, and those in authority. Artifacts (rods, sticks, and whips) to instill punishment along with hands-on methods and kneeling for long periods may be used. The biomedical perspective is that beating children constitutes physical child abuse.
   (6) When confronted with such practices, you will need to determine their purpose by exploring the patient's explanatory model, know the legal statutes relating to such practices to determine your legal accountability, attempt to find a culturally and legally sanctioned intervention by adopting the role of culture broker (see p. 61). Cultural accommodation or restructuring may be needed (see p. 61).

i. Risk factors due to socioeconomic status
   (1) It is extremely difficult to separate the effects of socioeconomic status from the effects of race, culture, and environment when determining risk factors. All are closely correlated with incidence and prevalence of disease.
   (2) Most of the major illnesses in the world today are caused by socioeconomic factors such as poverty; lack of access to potable water (which accounts for 80% of illnesses in the developing world), basic sanitation, education, and adequate housing; inadequate nutrition; maldistribution or lack of adequate health care personnel and facilities; low levels of immunization against preventable communicable diseases; environmental pollution due to poor regulation of industry; overpopulation; and accidents, especially vehicular, due to no safety regulations or limited enforcement of such.
   (3) Ethnic or racial differences in rates of illness are often reduced or eliminated when socioeconomic factors are controlled.

j. Culture-specific illnesses (CSIs): Clusters of symptoms, signs, and behaviors that are defined as illness by a cultural group but that are not considered illnesses by other cultural groups or medical systems.
   (1) Culture-specific illnesses are culturally derived explanations for physical (somatic) and psychologic signs or symptoms resulting from acute or chronic (unrelieved) psychosocial stress.
   (2) These illnesses cannot be understood or treated separately from the cultural, social, and environ-

---

BOX 2–3. Lifestyle and Incidence of Cancer

Rates of cervical cancer are lower in Jewish women with partners circumcised in accordance with Jewish religious practices; higher in Panamanian women who have multiple sex partners; and higher in Latin American women owing to high rates of prostitution, male penile cancer, and male promiscuity.

Nasopharyngeal cancer is highest in Hong Kong Chinese owing to childhood consumption of salted fish. Oral cancer is higher in western India and Malaysia because of betel nut chewing, higher in tobacco chewers, and higher in pipe smokers.

Lung cancer is lower in Mormons owing to religious prohibitions on tobacco use, lower in Jewish males because of decreased rates of smoking, and increasing in females in the United States because of increasing rates of cigarette smoking.

Table 2–13. Biocultural Aspects of Disease

Disease	Remarks
Alcoholism	Native Americans have double the rate of Whites; lower tolerance to alcohol among Chinese and Japanese Americans
Anemia	High incidence among Vietnamese due to presence of infestations among immigrants and low iron diets; low hemoglobin and malnutrition found among 18.2% of Native Americans, 32.7% of Blacks, 14.6% of Hispanics, and 10.4% of White children under 5 years of age
Arthritis	Increased incidence among Native Americans Blackfoot 1.4% Pima 1.8% Chippewa 6.8%
Asthma	Six times greater for Native American infants <1 yr; same as general population for Native Americans, ages 1–44 yr
Bronchitis	Six times greater for Native American infants <1 yr; same as general population for Native Americans, ages 1–44 yr
Cancer	Nasopharyngeal: High among Chinese Americans and Native Americans Esophageal: No. 2 cause of death for Black males aged 35–54 yr *Incidence:* White males 3.5/100,000 Black males 13.3/100,000 Liver: Highest among all ethnic groups are Filipino Hawaiians Stomach: Black males twice as likely as White males; low among Filipinos Cervical: 120% higher in Black females than in White females Uterine: 53% lower in Black females than White females Most prevalent cancer among Native Americans: biliary, nasopharyngeal, testicular, cervical, renal, and thyroid (females) cancer Lung cancer among Navajo uranium miners 85 times higher than among White miners Most prevalent cancer among Japanese Americans: esophageal, stomach, liver, and biliary cancer Among Chinese Americans, there is a higher incidence of nasopharyngeal and liver cancer than among the general population
Cholecystitis	*Incidence:* Whites 0.3% Puerto Ricans 2.1% Native Americans 2.2% Chinese 2.6%
Colitis	High incidence among Japanese Americans
Diabetes mellitus	Three times as prevalent among Filipino Americans as Whites; higher among Hispanics than Blacks or Whites Death rate is 3–4 times as high among Native Americans aged 25–34 yr, especially those in the West such as Utes, Pimas, and Papagos *Complications* Amputations: Twice as high among Native Americans as among the general U.S. population Renal failure: 20 times as high as general U.S. population, with tribal variation, e.g., Utes have 43 times higher incidence
G6PD	Present among 30% of Black males
Hepatitis	12% of Vietnamese refugees are hepatitis B surface antigen carriers
Influenza	Increased death rate among Native Americans age 45+
Ischemic heart disease	Responsible for 32% of heart-related causes of death among Native Americans
Lactose intolerance	Present among 66% of Hispanic women; increased incidence among Blacks and Chinese
Myocardial infarction	Leading cause of heart disease in Native Americans, accounting for 43% of death from heart disease; low incidence among Japanese Americans
Otitis media	7.9% incidence among school-aged Navajo children vs. 0.5% in Whites Up to ⅓ of Eskimo children <2 yr have chronic otitis media Increased incidence among bottle-fed Native Americans and Eskimo infants
Pneumonia	Increased death rate among Native Americans age 45+
Psoriasis	Affects 2–5% of Whites, but <1% of Blacks; high among Japanese Americans
Renal disease	Lower incidence among Japanese Americans

Table 2–13. Biocultural Aspects of Disease (Continued)

Disease	Remarks
Sickle cell anemia	Increased incidence among Blacks
Trachoma	Increased incidence among Native Americans and Eskimo children (3 to 8 times greater than general population)
Tuberculosis	Increased incidence among Native Americans
	Apache 2.0%
	Sioux 3.2%
	Navajo 4.6%
Ulcers	Decreased incidence among Japanese Americans

From Andrews MM. Transcultural nursing care. *In* Andrews MM, and Boyle JS (eds). *Transcultural Concepts in Nursing Care.* Philadelphia: JB Lippincott, 1995, pp 92–93. Originally data from Henderson G, Primeaux M. *Transcultural Health Care.* Menlo Park, CA: Addison-Wesley, 1981, Orque MS, Bloch B, and Monrroy LS. *Ethnic Nursing Care: A Multicultural Approach.* St. Louis: CV Mosby, 1983, and Overfield T. *Biologic Variation in Health and Illness: Race, Age, and Sex Differences.* Menlo Park, CA: Addison-Wesley, 1985.

mental contexts in which they are manifested and diagnosed. The physical signs and symptoms and behavior demonstrated by persons with a CSI are considered normal and appropriate responses by members of their ethnic or racial group.

(3) Culture-specific illnesses are often mislabeled (categorized) as psychosomatic or somatopsychic illnesses by biomedical health care providers.

(4) Examples of CSIs in Western societies that are not recognized as illness conditions in non-Western societies or outside of the biomedicine system are anorexia nervosa, bulimia, premenstrual syndrome, and agoraphobia.

(5) Table 2–14 is a representative listing of CSIs that are experienced by the major ethnic and racial groups in the United States and elsewhere but that are not recognized as illness conditions by biomedicine.

(6) Treatment of CSIs may include relieving the physical signs and symptoms through biomedicine and alleviating the underlying cultural, social, economic, political, and environmental stresses through ethnomedicine.

k. Knowledge of the relationship between risk factors and incidence and prevalence of disorders in ethnic and racial groups and populations can prevent needless surgeries, diagnostic studies, and misdiagnoses and can facilitate rapid diagnoses and culture-specific interventions. For example:

(1) Fever, abdominal pain, and leucocytosis may have different meanings in different ethnic or racial groups or populations.
- Northern European: Possible surgical conditions such as cholecystectomy or appendicitis
- Mediterranean groups: Familial Mediterranean fever in Greeks, Italians, and Turks
- Ashkenazic Jews: Familial Mediterranean fever
- Blacks: Sickle cell crisis

(2) Diarrhea, dehydration, and cachexia in newborns and infants may be any of the following:
- A side effect of newborn purging in Haitian infants

- An indication of early lactose intolerance in Native-American infants
- An indication of infectious disease in White infants

(3) Burn marks, bruises, or erythema on the chest, back, and extremities of children may be the result of any of the following:
- Spanking or whipping for disobedience in Haitian and Taiwanese children
- Curing rituals for pain or acute minor conditions in Native-American or Southeast-Asian children
- Physical abuse by parents of White children

(4) Flatulence, diarrhea, and associated gastrointestinal signs and symptoms in children may indicate any of the following:
- Sickle cell crises in Blacks
- Lactose intolerance in Asians and Native Americans
- Cystic fibrosis in Whites

(5) Stunted skeletal growth may indicate the following:
- Malnutrition in Haitian, Ethiopian, and rural African-American children in Alabama
- An irreversible response in children living at high altitudes in Peru, Papua New Guinea, Afghanistan, and Tibet.

l. *Caution:* We need to avoid attributing illness to or basing nursing care solely on race or culture. Such approaches erroneously and inadvertently promote the concept of racial, cultural, or gender superiority, inferiority, or determinism.

7. Assessing religious beliefs

a. Religion is a personal (individual) or institutionalized system of values, beliefs, and practices that defines the nature of reality, the meaning, origin, and destiny of life, and the myths and rituals that manifest them.

b. Religion is a symbolic expression of the models of the world used by people to explain the meaning of events and things.

c. Religion may or may not include belief in supernatural beings, events, or processes.

(1) Defining religion as a belief in supernatural beings or events is a distinction made mainly by those

Table 2–14. Culture-Specific Illnesses

Ethnic or Racial Group or Geographic Area	Culture-Specific Illness	Signs or Symptoms	Cultural Causation (Biomedical Classification)	Cultural Treatment
Black and African-Caribbean				
Southern Black Bahamian Haitian	Falling out (blacking out) Blacking out Indisposition	Sudden collapse, often without warning; seizure activity preceded by dizziness or "swimming" in the head; eyes open but unable to see or move; can hear and understand	*Natural:* Receipt of shocking news; extreme heat; witnessing or experiencing fear-arousing situations; excessive stress High blood—blood rises and accumulates in brain or back of neck, preventing adequate circulation Low blood—insufficient blood to nourish the brain *Supernatural:* Witchcraft; sorcery; punishment by God (Dissociative state)	*Natural:* Biomedical therapy for fainting or convulsions Food, diet, and herbal therapy to "cool" blood or bring blood down Food or tonics to build up quantity and quality of blood *Supernatural:* If natural therapy is ineffective: prayer; spiritual healing; root doctor to counteract witchcraft or sorcery
Haitian	Boufée delirante aigüe (spirit possession)	Sudden marked confusion; aggressive behavior; psychomotor excitement; may have visual and auditory hallucinations	Unwillingness to join voodoo church (Dissociative state)	Treated by traditional healer (houngan) who communes with loa (voodoo spirit) to determine treatment
Caribbean populations	Evil eye	See mal de ojo under Hispanic American		
Asian Pacific Islander				
East Indian	Shen-k'uei Dhat	Anxiety or panic state. Somatic complaints of fatigue, dizziness, general weakness, insomnia, back pain, frequent dreaming, graying of hair Sexual dysfunction: premature ejaculation; impotence Fear of loss of semen due to masturbation, nocturnal emissions, frequent intercourse, and white (milky) urine	Sexual excess (anxiety state)	Diet, herbs, rest
Japanese	Shinkei shitsu	Anxiety, hypochondriasis, fear of meeting people, feelings of inadequacy, obsessive-compulsive behavior Affects mainly young persons	Inability to meet expectations of society (Compulsive neurosis)	Morita therapy: Period of semi-isolation Period of simple labor to develop attitudes of self-acceptance
Chinese	Hsieh-ping (double sickness)	Trance state, disorientation, depression, anxiety, speaking in tongues, visual and auditory hallucinations, believes self to be possessed by dead relatives or friends to whom has been disrespectful	Lack of respect for dead, experiencing social conflict, punishment by supernatural (Dissociative state)	Traditional priest enters trance to commune with spirit world
Chinese (South China; Hong Kong and Malaysia) Malaysian Assam (Hindus)	Koro (genital retraction)	Male: Fear that penis will retract into body, causing death Female: Fear that vulva and breasts will disappear into	Sudden fright, exposure to cold, precipitated by real or imagined overindulgence in sex or masturbation (Anxiety state)	Assistance from same sex friends or kin Vigorous massage and pulling on body part until pain is alleviated

Table 2–14. *Culture-Specific Illnesses* (Continued)

Ethnic or Racial Group or Geographic Area	Culture-Specific Illness	Signs or Symptoms	Cultural Causation (Biomedical Classification)	Cultural Treatment
		body and cause death (much less prevalent than male Koro) Panic state: tachycardia, coldness and loss of sensation in extremities, pallor, sweating, stiffening of body, protrusion of eyes Pulling on penis, calling loudly for help; screaming with pain; may have loss of consciousness		Massage of extremities to restore feeling In extreme or chronic cases, the penis is secured to prevent retraction Medicinal potion to drink to keep penis erect
Chinese	Haak-tsan (soul loss)	See susto under Hispanic American		
Pacific Islands				
Indonesia Malaysia Burma Japan (Anui) Philippines Thailand	Latah (startle reflex) Yuan Imu Mali-mali Bahtschi	Trancelike dissociative behavior, depression, anxiety, hypersensitivity to sudden fright or startle, echolalia (repeating words of others), automatic obedience, coprolalia (speaking obscenities), pornolalia (vulgar sexual exclamations), reflexive, repetitive behavior Middle-aged females in subservient positions. Self-effacting individuals	Sudden, overwhelming stress; reaction to acute, traumatic experiences; reaction to objects or animals for which person has excessive fear (e.g., snakes, spiders, or worms) (Hysterical disorder)	Usually none unless person becomes homicidal
Indonesia Malaysia Papua New Guinea Highlands Polynesia	Amok (wild person behavior) Gila babi Gila mengamok Aha De Idize Be Cathard	Outbursts of violent and aggressive behavior bordering on rage directed at people, objects, or animals; experience amnesia, exhaustion, and return to consciousness at end of the episode; affects primarily males	Unbearable environmental stress, sleep deprivation, extreme heat, exhaustion, alcohol, depression, infection, fear and anger (Dissociative state)	Relieve stress Prevent harming others or self
Papua New Guinea Highlands Philippines	Mogo laya Lanti	See susto under Hispanic American See susto under Hispanic American		
Hispanic				
Mexican American Caribbean Central America	Caida de la mollera or mollera caida (fallen fontanel)	Vomiting, diarrhea, irritability, crying, depressed fontanel (Affects newborns and infants mainly)	Child has fallen and fontanel has become depressed, blow to head, rapid removal of nipple from mouth and fontanel is pulled into palate (Dehydration)	Put finger in child's mouth and press upward palate Apply soap-shaving poultice to fontanel Hold child upside down by the ankles with head touching a pan of warm water, hold for a few moments
Mexican American Caribbean Central American Latin American Mediterranean	Mal de ojo (evil eye)	Fever; restlessness; crying, vomiting; diarrhea (affects children mainly)	*Supernatural origin* Spell cast by a person envious of another person; spell is cast through envious glance or staring at the victim	*Prevention:* Admire and touch person while simultaneously saying "May God bless you" *Treatment:* By curandero or brujo

Table continued on following page

Table 2–14. Culture-Specific Illnesses (Continued)

Ethnic or Racial Group or Geographic Area	Culture-Specific Illness	Signs or Symptoms	Cultural Causation (Biomedical Classification)	Cultural Treatment
			Envious vision causes blood to heat, resulting in signs and symptoms (Phobic state)	Pass unbroken egg over body saying a prayer. Egg draws heat from body. Egg is broken, placed under bed overnight. If egg is "cooked by body's heat in the morning," person had mal de ojo
Hispanic populations	Empacho	Bolus of undigested food adheres to stomach or intestinal wall causing blockage; stomach pain; nausea and vomiting; diarrhea; anorexia	Eating too rapidly, too much or not enough; made to eat against one's will	Massage stomach or back firmly until a cracking or popping sound is heard. Administer laxative
Guatemalan	Colerina	See amok		
Peru	Colerina			
Puerto Rican	Mal de pelea			
Hispanic populations	Susto, espanto (soul loss)	Restless sleep, anxiety, irritability, insomnia, anorexia, vomiting, diarrhea, trembling, sweating, tachycardia, depression, phobic behavior, loss of interest in personal appearance	Sudden fright, causing the soul to leave the body	Curandero, espiritualista, or santero
Central and Latin American			Dreaming and awakening before one's soul has reentered the body	Religious ceremony
Andean groups			Witchcraft or sorcery (Anxiety state)	Seance to locate wandering soul and entice it into body
Cuban	Espirituamento de susto			Counseling by family and traditional healer
Chile	Saladera			Countermagic to remove witchcraft or sorcery
Peru		Prevalent in females, young children, and persons unable to fulfill their social roles		
Native American				
Eskimo	Pibloktog (Arctic hysteria)	Brooding, depression, tremors, anxiety, screaming and crying, running and jumping in fire or water, violent aggressive behavior, tear clothes off, speak in tongues, alterations in consciousness, fatigue, confusion, amnesia	Sudden fright; shame; acute stress and worry; frustration; response to harsh climate, threat of starvation, or accidents (Anxiety state)	Prevention of harm to self or others. Relief of stress
Kiowa Apache	Ghost sickness	Terror state: becomes hypersensitive to touch and sound believed to be from ghost of dead ancestor, fear of body palsy if looks at ghost, eating disorders	Mourning loss of significant person. Possession by ancestor's ghost (Dissociative state)	Medicine man to commune with spirit world
Navajo	Ghost sickness	Generalized weakness, nightmares, feelings of danger, anoxeria, dizziness and syncope, fearfulness, inability to breathe freely, may have hallucinations	Witchcraft (Dissociative state)	Medicine man to counteract witchcraft
Yaqui	Womita	See susto under Hispanic		

Data from Andrews MM, and Boyle JS (eds). *Transcultural Concepts in Nursing Care*. 2nd ed. Philadelphia: JB Lippincott, 1995; Kiev A. *Transcultural Psychiatry*. New York: The Free Press, 1972; Simons RC, and Hughes CC (eds). *The Culture-Bound Syndromes*. Boston: D Reidel 1985; and Yap PM. The culture-bound syndromes. *In* Landy D (ed). *Culture, Disease and Healing*. New York: Macmillan, 1977.

holding a Western, scientific world-view. Christianity, Islam, some forms of Hinduism, and most tribal religions have beliefs in supernatural beings. Scientism, other forms of Hinduism, and some forms of Buddhism do not.

d. Functions of religion
 (1) Explanatory: Answers existential questions essential to give meaning to dimensions of human existence (e.g., how the world was created).
 (2) Validation and control of social behavior: Posits rules and relationships of a celestial order that sustain the moral and social order of a society.
 (3) Enhances the human ability to cope: Provides psychologic reinforcement during times of tragedy, crisis, and anxiety.
 (4) Gives security and meaning to events in a natural world that is seen as capricious and unpredictable. Such events include illness, death, failure and misfortune, natural and human-made disaster.

e. Religion is closely related to health, illness, and healing in all societies.
 (1) Religion provides an explanation for causation of illness and misfortune.
 (2) Religion provides an explanation for prevention of illness and misfortune.
 (3) Religion provides a basis for therapy decisions and healing strategies. Many religious beliefs and practices related to the etiology and prevention of illness and misfortune also form the basis of their treatment or reversal. Table 2–15 summarizes the health-culture beliefs and practices of major religions found in North America. Individuals may combine beliefs and practices from the major world religions listed in the table with those of traditional or folk religions. Examples:
 • The combination of African traditional religions with beliefs in magic and spirits and Catholicism: Cuban *santeria*, Haitian voodoo, and Jamaican *obeah*
 • The merging of Chinese traditional religion with beliefs in magic, spirits, and pantheons of gods with the guiding principles for morality, behavior, and science from Buddhism, Confucianism, and Taoism.

f. Examples of general protective measures are the following:
 (1) Wearing amulets (charms, good luck symbols, or sayings), clothing, or jewelry
 (2) Carrying or hanging a talisman (object imbued with supernatural powers) nearby
 (3) Making noise to scare or ward off evil entities (e.g., jewelry that tinkles when the person moves)
 (4) Drinking or ingesting potions, tonics, herbs, or foods
 (5) Avoiding certain activities at specific times (e.g., pregnant women or young children not attending funerals so that the illness or entity causing death does not enter or affect them)
 (6) Carrying out proper disposal or care of things that have come into contact with or been part of a person's body, such as umbilical cords or placentas

 (7) Performing religious ceremonies or otherwise demonstrating one's faith in the supernatural (e.g., baptizing newborns and children)
 (8) Avoiding behaviors that disrupt relationships (e.g., failing to share wealth or resources with others in need)
 (9) Avoiding behaviors that are not socially sanctioned, such as adultery

g. Nurses should attempt to facilitate such protective measures as much as possible to avoid causing or exacerbating an illness or misfortune.
 (1) Most protective measures are neutral or adaptive from the biomedical perspective.
 (2) See page 61 regarding cultural maintenance and cultural accommodation of health-culture beliefs and practices.

h. Religious beliefs and practices may also contribute to illness problems by causing feelings of guilt or remorse, delay in seeking care, or failure to institute treatments.
 (1) Patients may delay seeking or instituting biomedical care by turning to the religious system first for diagnoses and initial treatment, seeking religious sanction to obtain biomedical care, and validating biomedical treatments prescribed before instituting them.

i. You can alleviate such problems by doing the following:
 (1) Demonstrating a patient-oriented learning style.
 (2) Asking patients the reasons for their feelings or questions to clarify the problem.
 (3) Seeking assistance from persons knowledgeable about patients' religious practices. Sources may include ordained or lay clergy, traditional healers, religious scholars, other adherents of the religion, and family and kin.
 (4) Being respectful of and sensitive to patients' viewpoints.
 (5) Assuming the role of culture broker to institute religiously appropriate interventions.

j. Basing nursing care on religious beliefs does not necessarily meet the spiritual needs of patients. Meeting spiritual needs involve helping patients to do the following:
 (1) Mobilize their inner resources to cope with and find meaning in illness, life crises, or social deprivation
 (2) Restore their self-dignity and preserve their self-worth when faced with dehumanizing events and overwhelming adversity
 (3) Find God or some unifying truth of a personal nature
 (4) Find strength in and peace and satisfaction with one's life

k. When attempting to give spiritual care, you must be careful not to do the following:
 (1) Impose your own religious beliefs on patients
 (2) Conclude that "finding religion" will make a person "spiritually richer" or spiritually stronger

8. Assessing dietary restrictions (see Chapter 4 for details)

Table 2–15. Selected Religion's Responses to Health Events

Event	Reaction	Event	Reaction
Baha'i: "All healing comes from God."		Birth control	Individual judgment
Abortion	Forbidden	Blood and blood products	Ordinarily not used by members
Artificial insemination	No specific rule	Diet	No restrictions
Autopsy	Acceptable with medical or legal need		Abstain from alcohol and tobacco, some from tea and coffee
Birth control	Can choose family planning method	Euthanasia	Contrary to teachings
Blood and blood products	No restrictions for use	Healing beliefs	Accepts physical and moral healing
Diet	Alcohol and drugs forbidden	Healing practices	Full-time healing ministers
Euthanasia	No destruction of life		Spiritual healing practiced
Healing beliefs	Harmony between religion and science	Medications	None
Healing practices	Pray		Immunizations or vaccines to comply with law
Medications	Narcotics with prescription		
	No restriction for vaccines	Organ donations	Individual decides
Organ donations	Permitted	Right to die issues	Unlikely to seek medical help to prolong life
Right to die issues	Life is unique and precious—do not destroy	Surgical procedures	No medical ones practiced
Surgical procedures	No restrictions	Visitors	Family, friends, and members of the Christian Science community and healers, Christian Science nurses
Visitors	Community members assist and support		
Buddhist Churches of America: "To keep the body in good health is a duty—otherwise we shall not be able to keep our mind strong and clear."			
		Church of Jesus Christ of Latter Day Saints	
Abortion	Patient's condition determines	Abortion	Forbidden
Artificial insemination	Acceptable	Artificial insemination	Acceptable between husband and wife
Autopsy	Matter of individual practice	Autopsy	Permitted with consent of next of kin
Birth control	Acceptable	Birth control	Contrary to Mormon belief
Blood and blood products	No restrictions	Blood and blood products	No restrictions
Diet	Restricted food combinations	Diet	Alcohol, tea (except herbal teas), coffee, and tobacco are forbidden
	Extremes must be avoided		
Euthanasia	May permit		Fasting (24 hr without food and drink) is required once a month
Healing beliefs	Do believe in healing through faith		
Healing practices	No restrictions	Euthanasia	Humans must not interfere in God's plan
Medications	No restrictions	Healing beliefs	Power of God can bring healing
Organ donations	Considered act of mercy; if hope for recovery, all means may be taken	Healing practices	Anointing with oil, sealing, prayer, laying on of hands
Right to die issues	With hope, all means encouraged	Medications	No restrictions; may use herbal folk remedies
Surgical procedures	Permitted, with extremes avoided		
Visitors	Family, community	Organ donations	Permitted
		Right to die issues	If death inevitable, promote a peaceful and dignified death
Roman Catholic: "The prayer of faith shall heal the sick, and the Lord shall raise him up."			
		Surgical procedures	Matter of individual choice
Abortion	Prohibited	Visitors	Church members (elder and sister) family and friends
Artificial insemination	Illicit, even between husband and wife		
Autopsy	Permissible		
Birth control	Natural means only	**Hinduism: "Enricher, Healer of disease, be a good friend to us."**	
Blood and blood products	Permissible		
Diet	Use foods in moderation	Abortion	No policy exists
Euthanasia	Direct life-ending procedures forbidden	Artificial insemination	No restrictions exist but not often practiced
Healing beliefs	Many within religious belief system		
Healing practices	Sacrament of sick, candles, laying-on-of-hands	Autopsy	Acceptable
		Birth control	All types acceptable
Medications	May take if benefits outweigh risks	Blood and blood products	Acceptable
Organ donations	Justifiable	Diet	Eating of beef is forbidden
Right to die issues	Obligated to take ordinary, not extraordinary, means to prolong life	Euthanasia	Not practiced
		Healing beliefs	Some believe in faith healing
Surgical procedures	Most are permissible except abortion and sterilization	Healing practices	Traditional faith healing system
		Medications	Acceptable
Visitors	Family, friends, priest	Organ donations	Acceptable
	Many outreach programs through church to reach the sick	Right to die issues	No restrictions
			Death seen as "one more step to nirvana"
Christian Science		Surgical procedures	With an amputation, the loss of limb seen as due to "sins in a previous life"
Abortion	Incompatible with faith		
Artificial insemination	Unusual	Visitors	Members of family, community, and priest support
Autopsy	Not usual; individual or family decide		

Table 2–15. Selected Religion's Responses to Health Events (Continued)

Event	Reaction	Event	Reaction
Islam: "The Lord of the world created me—and when I am sick, He healeth me."			If death inevitable, no new procedures need to be undertaken, but those ongoing must continue
Abortion	Accepted	Surgical procedures	Most allowed
Artificial insemination	Permitted husband to wife	Visitors	Family, friends, rabbi, many community services
Autopsy	Permitted for medical and legal purposes		
Birth control	Acceptable	**Mennonite**	
Blood and blood products	No restrictions	Abortion	Therapeutic acceptable
Diet	Pork and alcohol prohibited	Artificial insemination	Individual conscience; husband to wife
Euthanasia	Not acceptable	Autopsy	Acceptable
Healing beliefs	Faith healing generally not acceptable	Birth control	Acceptable
Healing practices	Some use of herbal remedies and faith healing	Blood and blood products	Acceptable
Medications	No restrictions	Diet	No specific restrictions
Organ donations	Acceptable	Euthanasia	Not condoned
Right to die issues	Attempts to shorten life prohibited	Healing beliefs	Part of God's work
Surgical procedures	Most permitted	Healing practices	Prayer and anointing with oil
Visitors	Family and friends provide support	Medications	No restrictions
		Organ donations	Acceptable
Jehovah's Witnesses		Right to die issues	Do not believe life must be continued at all cost
Abortion	Forbidden	Surgical procedures	No restrictions
Artificial insemination	Forbidden	Visitors	Family, community
Autopsy	Acceptable if required by law		
Birth control	Sterilization forbidden; Other methods individual choice	**Seventh-Day Adventist**	
		Abortion	Therapeutic acceptable
Blood and blood products	Forbidden	Artificial insemination	Between husband and wife
Diet	Abstain from tobacco, moderate use of alcohol	Autopsy	Acceptable
Euthanasia	Forbidden	Birth control	Individual choice
Healing beliefs	Faith healing forbidden	Blood and blood products	No restrictions
Healing practices	Reading scriptures can comfort the individual and lead to mental and spiritual healing	Diet	Encourage vegetarian diet
		Euthanasia	Not practiced
Medications	Accepted except if derived from blood products	Healing beliefs	Divine healing
		Healing practices	Anointing with oil and prayer
Organ donations	Forbidden	Medications	No restrictions; Vaccines acceptable
Right to die issues	Use of extraordinary means an individual's choice	Organ donations	Acceptable
		Right to die issues	Follow the ethic of prolonging life
Surgical procedures	Not opposed, but administration of blood during surgery is strictly prohibited	Surgical procedures	No restrictions; Oppose use of hypnotism
Visitors	Members of congregation and elders pray for the sick person	Visitors	Pastor and elders pray and anoint sick person; Worldwide health system includes hospitals and clinics
Judaism: "O Lord, my God, I cried to Thee for help and Thou has healed me."		**Unitarian-Universalist Church**	
Abortion	Therapeutic permitted; some groups accept abortion on demand	Abortion	Acceptable, therapeutic and on demand
Artificial insemination	Permitted	Artificial insemination	Acceptable
Autopsy	Permitted under certain circumstances; All body parts must be buried together	Autopsy	Recommended
Birth control	Permissible, except with Orthodox Jews	Birth control	All types acceptable
Blood and blood products	Acceptable	Blood and blood products	No restrictions
Diet	Strict dietary laws—milk and meat not mixed; predatory fowl, shellfish, and pork products forbidden; kosher products only may be requested	Diet	No restrictions
		Euthanasia	Favor nonaction; May withdraw therapies if death imminent
Euthanasia	Prohibited	Healing beliefs	Faith healing: seen as "superstitious"
Healing beliefs	Medical care expected	Healing practices	Use of science to facilitate healing
Healing practices	Prayers for the sick	Medications	No restrictions
Medications	No restrictions	Organ donations	Acceptable
Organ donations	Complex issue; some practiced	Right to die issues	Favor the right to die with dignity
Right to die issues	Right to die with dignity	Surgical procedures	No restrictions
		Visitors	Family, friends, church members

From Spector RE. *Cultural Diversity in Health and Illness.* Norwalk, CT: Appleton & Lange, 1991, pp 137–142. Originally adapted from Andrews MM, and Hanson PA. Religious beliefs: Implications for nursing practice. In Boyle JS, and Andrews MM (eds). *Transcultural Concepts in Nursing Care.* Glenview, IL: Scott, Foresman & Co/Little, Brown College Division, 1989, pp 377–416. Selected statements from *Health and Healing in the World's Great Religions*, a poster from the Fellowship for Spiritual Understanding, Palo Verdes, CA, 1972.

9. Assessing the patient's family and social support system
   a. Assess the family from 2 perspectives because of the role it plays in the health and welfare of its members.
      (1) As an environment in which individual family members are nurtured and developed throughout life, it provides for members' basic physical and psychosocial needs as well as material needs.
      (2) As the patient when it is unable to provide the healthy environment needed by its members. The family as a whole or its individual members may need assistance when illness occurs. Examples:
         • Caregivers of older or chronically ill members who become isolated and emotionally distraught due to the constancy of care needed
         • Parents who become anxious or fearful when children are ill
         • Children who need reassurance to cope with fears of death when parents are ill
         • The family as a whole when the mother-wife or father-husband becomes ill, because of the need to deal with loss of financial income, maintaining household functioning, and loss of spouse or parent relationships
         • The family as a whole when crises occur
         • The family as a whole when general lifestyle changes must be implemented as part of the therapy regimen of ill members
   b. The family is essential to health care decision making about ill members.
      (1) Nursing interventions cannot be based on the nuclear family structure that has long dominated biomedical health care thinking and program models because it represents the family structure in only 6 percent of known societies.
      (2) Extended family members are integral to health care decision making and caregiving in the vast majority of known societies. Do not consider others who accompany the patient as outsiders or disruptive to decision-making processes. Instead, consult and include them in interventions and health teaching. Such members constitute the family as environment and patient. Table 2–16 summarizes information related to family structure and health culture of major ethnic and racial groups.

(3) Do not assume that the ill adult or legal next of kin are the primary decision makers for ill family members. Parents may need to consult with older family members in elder-dominated societies. Heads of households may be responsible for deciding who gets care, when it is given, and who gives it. Husbands may need to be consulted in all decisions about wives in gender-differentiated societies. Same-sex partners in gay and lesbian families may be the preferred caregivers and decision makers.
   c. The variety of family structures and roles and relationships makes it imperative that you know the cultural and health-culture values, beliefs, and practices affecting family functioning during health and illness.
   d. It is important to remember that families modify and are modified by the cultural and health-culture values, beliefs, and practices of the society of which they are a part.
      (1) Modification may occur due to relocation, as in immigration, migration, or refugeeism; changes in educational or socioeconomic status; exposure to new ideas, inventions, or persons from other ethnic or racial or socioeconomic groups; accessibility to new forms of health care; natural disasters or upheavals; and the acculturation process.
      (2) Family modification of culture and cultural modification of the family require that we assess each family on an individual basis.

NURSE ADVISORY

Although it is important to know the basic family structure of your patients' ethnic, racial, or subcultural groups, it is *more important* to view your patients within their family environment. Families modify the culture of the larger social group in many ways. Not all roles and relationships in individual families reflect those commonly attributed to a culture or family type.

   e. Immigrant and refugee families are particularly vulnerable to illness due to changes in their structures and functions.

Table 2–16. Family Structure and Health Culture of Major Ethnic and Racial Groups

Characteristics*	Black	White	Hispanic (Puerto Rican American)	Asian (Chinese American)	Native American (Navajo)
Dominant family structure	Nuclear or extended	Nuclear	Extended or nuclear	Extended or nuclear	Extended
Residence pattern	Matrilocal	Neolocal†	Patrilocal	Patrilocal	Matrilocal
Dominant relationship	Network of kin	Husband-wife	Mother-child	Parent-child	Network of kin
Dominant world-view	Magico religious	Scientific	Holistic	Holistic	Holistic
Primary caregiver in illlness	Female kin	Mother-wife	Mother-wife	Female kin	Family and kin network
Child caregiver	Network of kin	Parents	Mother-wife and female kin	Female kin	Family and kin network
Dominant religion	Black churches	Protestant	Catholic	Christianity and Buddhism	Native American

* There will be considerable intragroup variation due to factors such as sociodemographic variables, degree of acculturation, and the immigration process.
† Neolocal indicates the married couple sets up their own independent residence.

(1) Separation from members of the family unit in the country of origin

(2) Loss of extended family support

(3) Loss of social status

(4) Existence at a poverty level

(5) Changes in roles and relationships related to gender (female-male), spouse (husband-wife), parenting (parent-child), and generation (ancestor-parents–descendants-children)

(6) Questioning of traditional cultural values, beliefs, and practices due to the acculturation process

(7) Need for new language, job skills, or both

Transcultural Nursing Diagnoses

1. North American Nursing Diagnostic Association (NANDA) nursing diagnoses may inadvertently cause us to impose our health-culture beliefs and practices on patients.
   a. The NANDA nursing diagnoses, which are based in the scientific world-view of health and illness, represent problems *nurses* perceive patients to have.
   b. Applying NANDA nursing diagnoses to patients holding other world-views places them at risk for being labeled abnormal.
      (1) Patient health-seeking behaviors may be quite normal and consistent with their world-view and health culture.
      (2) Do not apply NANDA nursing diagnoses before you determine the patient's explanatory model.
      (3) Do not formulate nursing interventions based on NANDA nursing diagnoses independent of the culture brokerage process (see p. 61) (Box 2–4).
2. The NANDA nursing diagnoses focus exclusively on the patient. This patient-centered focus leads nurses inadvertently to do the following:
   a. Assume the patient is at fault, lacking in some way, or needing to change
   b. Deny the reality of cultural and health-culture values, beliefs, and practices other than our own
   c. Absolve ourselves and the health care system of the need to change to accommodate patients' health-culture beliefs and practices

---

BOX 2–4. Nursing Diagnoses and Cultural Accommodation

It would be improper to label a Black woman as noncompliant because she insists on drinking aloe water to treat her diabetes mellitus instead of modifying her diet in accordance with dietary teaching. Aloe water is quite bitter and is commonly believed to "bitter-up" blood that is "sweet" or has too much "sugar." Sugar in the blood is a common explanation for diabetes mellitus in the Black health culture. The treatment is to dilute the sugar via intake of fluids and food that have a bitter taste.

Rather than to label her noncompliant, you can take a more fruitful course of action by seeking some type of cultural accommodation intervention—allowing her to continue to drink the aloe water. At the same time, you should do 4 things: (1) Learn from her what else she believes is effective against diabetes, (2) determine what she can realistically include in her diet and activities from the biomedical model of diabetes care, (3) seek common ground between her beliefs and yours, and (4) set up a new plan of care that sets new priorities and goals acceptable to both her and you.

---

d. Focus our nursing interventions and health teaching on changing the patient

3. The NANDA nursing diagnoses that are especially problematic when applied from a transcultural perspective are those related to the following:
   a. Knowledge deficit: Patients adhering to health-culture beliefs and practices from the popular or ethnomedical systems do not have a knowledge deficit. Their decision-making and health-seeking behavior are being directed by a different system of thought.
      (1) It is ethnocentric to say that patients have a knowledge deficit because they do adhere to your health-cultural beliefs and practices.
      (2) You also have a knowledge deficit if you base your decision making and nursing interventions solely on your health-culture beliefs and practices.
   b. Impaired functioning: You and the patient are both impaired when guided by different health-culture beliefs and practices. The patient's inability to function in your health culture may be related to your inability to be transcultural.
   c. Impaired verbal communication: The problem may be based in *barriers* to communication and not in an inability to communicate verbally.
      (1) When you and the patient speak different languages, the problem is your mutual inability to understand each other.
      (2) Speech patterns in one culture may mimic pathophysiologic speech patterns in another culture.
         • Aphasia in a trance state entered into for a curing ceremony in Polynesia
         • Glossolalia (speaking in tongues) during religious ceremonies in Pentecostal religion
         • Talking slowly, deliberately punctuating each word, and pausing between words as in Appalachian and Native-American groups
         • Mumbling by Asian patients as a sign of deference to authority
      (3) Speech patterns may be affected by the stress of the sociocultural setting. Patients may *seem* unable to speak normally when they attempt to express themselves in another language.
      (4) Nonverbal communication between the nurse and the patient may interfere with verbal communication. Your eye contact, body language, and facial expression may convey to patients that you expect no response.
   d. Noncompliance: Patients who make decisions based on health-culture beliefs different from yours are not noncompliant. They are adhering to an alternative health-culture and explanatory model. When we label them noncompliant, we are being ethnocentric and assuming that our health-culture beliefs and practices are superior. Patients have the *right to decide* what they will or will not do. Patients may choose not to adhere to nursing interventions for many reasons.
      (1) Concepts of time may delay implementation.
      (2) Religious beliefs may prohibit adhering to the recommended treatment regimens.
      (3) Therapy management groups may counsel against your recommendations.

(4) Nursing interventions may not be meaningful to patients.

(5) Symptom relief may be interpreted as indicating the illness is over.

(6) Nursing interventions may be directed at relieving signs or symptoms that patients do not consider important.

4. To lessen the cultural limitations of NANDA nursing diagnoses, nurses must evaluate patient behavior from the perspective of the patient's health culture.

5. Transcultural nursing focuses nursing interventions on nurses and the system as well as on the patient.

a. Change may be required on the part of nurses or the health care system to accommodate, maintain, or reinforce patients' health-culture beliefs and practices.

b. To make nursing interventions meaningful and acceptable to patients, we may need to do the following:

(1) Reprioritize nursing goals

(2) Change procedures

(3) Negotiate a compromise between nurses' health-culture beliefs and practices and those of patients

NURSE ADVISORY

There is no easy or standard method for negotiating mutually acceptable and culturally appropriate nursing interventions because the method depends on where the differences exist in the nurse's and patient's explanatory models, if the interventions affect care, and the context in which the interventions are to be implemented.

(4) Accommodate patient health-culture beliefs and practices

Planning Transcultural Care with the Therapy Management Group

1. Biomedical treatment usually focuses on the individual and changing his or her beliefs, practices, and attitudes, whereas ethnomedical treatment often requires the active participation of others involved in circumstances causing the illness (immediate family or other relatives, friends, neighbors, or business associates).

2. Nursing interventions for patients who believe in social and supernatural causation may need to be community based as well as directed at the individual.

a. Intervention is directed at relieving underlying social or supernatural causation.

b. Intervention may require working with appropriate ethnomedical healers or ordained or nonordained clergy.

c. Intervention may require collaboration with the person's therapy management group.

Therapy Management Groups and Specific Approaches to Health Care

1. Therapy management groups: Networks of individuals who people rely on to help with matters of health and illness.

a. Members may include the following:

(1) Family and kin (Box 2–5)

(2) Friends

(3) Neighbors

(4) Ordained clergy and nonordained spiritual healers

(5) Traditional healers (see p. 36)

(6) Persons who have experienced the same signs or symptoms

(7) Nurses and other biomedical health care providers

b. Functions may include the following:

(1) Making the diagnosis

(2) Arranging for therapeutic consultations across all 3 sectors of health care (see p. 28)

(3) Selecting treatment modalities across all 3 sectors of health care

(4) Evaluating biomedical, ethnomedical, and nursing (caring) interventions

(5) Doing health teaching

(6) Providing support and care

(7) Assessing the patient's progress

(8) Determining the patient's prognosis

2. The therapy management group is usually consulted before people seek biomedical and nursing care.

3. The therapy management group will be consulted after biomedical and nursing care is received to verify its correctness and effectiveness.

4. The composition of the therapy management group varies depending on the patient's age, gender, marital status, socioeconomic level, religion, and ethnicity or race.

a. Immigrants and refugees may have a limited number of persons in their therapy management group owing to the nature and timing of the immigration process.

(1) A new therapy management group may need to be formed to replace members remaining in their country of origin.

(2) The absence of their normal support group may add additional stress to their illness episode.

b. Cultural assessment questions 6 and 8 in Table 2–10 can help determine who should be members of the person's therapy management group. In addition, consider questions such as the following:

• Who else can help me learn more about your condition?

• Who else can help me understand why this has happened?

5. You need to include members of the therapy management group when you do the following:

a. Attempt to understand the patient's explanatory model

b. Do health teaching

c. Negotiate nursing interventions that are mutually acceptable to you and the patient

<table>
</table>

> ## BOX 2–5. Who Is "Family"?
>
> The family is the primary social unit in human societies. The majority of families are based on some form of kinship through 2 basic dyadic relationships: marriage (legal or consensual) between husband and wife, which socially sanctions and regulates mating and reproduction; and biologic descent of children from parents, which provides bases for childrearing and enculturation of children into society. Adoption of members is an extension of biologic descent.
>
> The functions of families vary cross-culturally but generally include the following:
> - Biologic: unit of reproduction
> - Sociologic: defines roles and relationships within the family unit and between the family and the wider society
> - Cultural: passes on values, beliefs, and practices of society from generation to generation
> - Economic: basic unit of production, consumption, and for meeting each member's material needs
> - Psychologic: provides a nurturing environment that promotes a sense of safety, self-worth, and self-esteem within members
>
> The types of families are the following:
> - Orientation: family into which one was born or adopted
> - Procreation: family one creates through marriage and reproduction of children
> - Nuclear: two generations consisting of husband, wife, and biologic or adopted children
> - Blended (reconstituted): two generations consisting of husband, wife, and children from previous parental relationships
> - Nuclear-dyad: one generation consisting of a married couple without children
> - Single-parent: two generations consisting of 1 parent and 1 or more children by biologic descent or adoption
> - Extended: multigenerational kinship grouping that includes the nuclear family and kin by adoption and marriage
> - Alternative: consists of 2 or more unmarried adults who live together with or without children; includes gay or lesbian families; communes; and religious or cult organizations
>
> In gay or lesbian families, children may be present via adoption or custody after divorce. Gay or lesbian couples often are stigmatized by society and their own families of orientation and procreation. You will need to know the laws of your state regarding marriage, adoption of children, and next of kin issues when working with these families, because you may need to broker between the same-sex partner as caregiver and the desires and legal rights of the families of orientation and procreation. The wishes of the gay and lesbian partners should be respected as much as possible within the bounds of legal statutes governing such relationships.
>
> Multigenerational families have emerged in the United States resulting in the "sandwich generation." Adult couples have older parents and children with grandchildren who return to live with them.
>
> Many societies may add persons to families who are not related by marriage, descent, or adoption:
> - Godparents in Roman Catholic populations
> - African societies may extend the title of "brother" or "sister" to others residing in small communities or surrounding neighborhoods.
> - "Patrons" are adopted from families of higher socioeconomic status in Latin American, Central American, and Mediterranean countries.
>
> Such persons are turned to for assistance throughout the family life cycle. They become part of family members' therapy management groups and provide sources of financial, social, and material support. They become role models and mentors, and are consultants in major family decisions. They assist with childrearing and child care.
>
> Extended family structures have advantages over nuclear family structures in health and illness situations. Multiple caregivers for children are available when parents are ill, incapacitated, dead, or absent for periods of time. They provide a safety valve for prevention of child abuse by parents and spousal abuse. They provide economic and social support in times of crises, cultural or social change, and life-stage transitions.

6. To include members of the therapy management group in nursing care, you should do the following:
   a. Look beyond the nurse-patient dyad or nurse-patient-family triad when assessing patients and developing nursing interventions.
   b. Consider yourself as *part* of the patient's therapy management network and not as *the* therapy manager.
7. Failure to include members of the therapy management group in planning nursing interventions will likely result in the following:
   a. Inability to develop interventions that are meaningful to the patient
   b. Patients who do not adhere to biomedical therapy and nursing interventions

Transcultural Nursing Interventions

1. Nurse-patient negotiation: A nurse-patient *negotiation model* is inherent in transcultural nursing. The negotiation model is based on the following basic premises.
   a. Discrepancies are likely to exist between the EMs of nurses and patients.
      (1) Nurses and patients learn about health and illness through different life experiences.
      (2) Nurses and patients may have different concepts about what is wrong, what should be done, who should do it, and how nurses and patients should interact in the health care situation.
   b. People do not necessarily conform to cultural stereotypes or adhere to treatments advocated by biomedicine and nursing. Knowledge of the health culture of a patient's ethnic or racial group is important. However, such knowledge *in and of itself* cannot predict whether patients' EMs of their health condition will be reflected in their health-seeking behavior. The nurse's role in any nurse-patient encounter is to determine the patient's EM of the health condition.

> ### NURSE ADVISORY
>
> There is no recipe approach to patient care. Patients do not automatically respond to health and illness based on their cultural heritage, socioeconomic status, gender, sexual identity, religious denomination, occupation, or other defining sociodemographic characteristics.

2. Cultural brokerage as intervention
   a. Nurses act as cultural brokers in 2 ways.
      (1) Interpreting messages, instructions, health-culture beliefs and practices, and nonverbal behaviors from one individual or group to another
      (2) Negotiating interventions to address differences that may occur between individuals and groups in the health care encounter.

NURSE ADVISORY

The cultural brokerage process often requires compromise and change on the part of *both* the nurse and the patient.

b. As a nursing intervention, cultural brokerage is based on the strategies of therapeutic use of time, power equalization, and viewing cultural assessment as a process.

   (1) Therapeutic use of time: At each step of the brokerage process, both the nurse and the patient require time to obtain and process the necessary information to make informed decisions. Interactions with patients require more time if the nurse and the patient are from different ethnic or racial groups. Patients expect nurses to listen quietly, politely, and patiently to their explanations and descriptions of illnesses. Patients may require the presence of other members of their therapy management group throughout the brokerage process.

   (2) Power equalization: Patients and their families must be given the opportunity to participate fully in the health care decision-making process.

   (3) Cultural assessment as process: The patient's perspective or EM is elicited at every step of the culture brokerage process.

c. The results of cultural brokerage are cultural maintenance, accommodation, or restructuring.

d. Cultural maintenance (preservation): Inclusion of neutral or helpful health culture beliefs and practices from the patient's EM. Examples:

   (1) Allowing patients to wear amulets (charms, metals, beads, pendants, or feathers) to prevent harm.

   (2) Repositioning rather than removing religious clothing during treatment or surgery.

   (3) Permitting Hindu family members to care for the body immediately after death.

e. Cultural accommodation (negotiation or translation across cultures): Inclusion of both the patient's and the nurse's needs and points of view in nursing interventions. Examples:

   (1) Giving a medication in liquid rather than pill form when patients believe liquids are more effective.

   (2) Allowing postpartum women to take sponge baths or to apply warm soaks to episiotomies rather than to take sitz baths, showers, or baths. It is a common ethnomedical belief that water or air will enter the body via the vagina and cause illness or pain until the womb (uterus) closes (returns to its normal state and position).

   (3) Allowing designated family members to make decisions regarding therapies in patients with terminal illnesses. For example, in certain Hispanic and Asian cultural groups, it is the family's responsibility and obligation to relieve patients of worry or concern to make the remainder of their life as long, happy, and carefree as possible. You can help families meet this cultural obligation by working closely with legal counsel to draft proper procedures to ensure the family is authorized to do so.

   (4) Explaining to surgical staff that shaving of body hair is not permitted by many ethnic and racial groups for reasons such as altered body image or self-concept, religion, or health maintenance. Options to shaving hair are the following:
      • The area needing shaving should be limited in scope and negotiated with the patient.
      • The procedure may be done without shaving.
      • The patient can be allowed to use culturally prescribed methods to counteract the potential harm done by shaving or cutting hair.

f. Cultural restructuring (promoting adaptation or teaching new skills): Modification of health-culture beliefs and practices and general lifeways to assist patients to adapt to new or changing sociocultural environments.

   (1) Cultural restructuring or behavior change is usually needed when beliefs and practices are considered illegal, abusive, or neglectful by society, including spousal violence, excessive physical punishment of children, inadequate parenting, and withdrawal from or failure to enroll children in school.

   (2) Examples of cultural restructuring are:
      • Explaining to health care providers and legal authorities that circumscribed, cigarette-like or coinlike burns on a child's body may signify coining or burning—a Southeast Asian healing practice. In addition, immigrant parents must be told that such acts are regarded as abusive by the new society and will likely result in legal prosecution if continued. Nurses should negotiate alternative means of treatment with parents so that they are assured their child will recover from the illness without coining or burning.
      • Explaining to immigrant and refugee parents that adolescent children should not be kept out of school to care for younger siblings. Refugeeism often prevents extended family or kin migration. Child care responsibilities then fall totally to parents and older children. Nurses need to help immigrant parents find alternative child care assistance and promote the value of educating children.
      • Assisting spouses, who have been physically and mentally abused by their mates, to remove themselves from the abusive relationship. When such abuse occurs among immigrants and refugees, it may signify acculturation stress—inability to fulfill the cultural role of husband or wife, parent, or family member in the new society.

   (3) Cultural restructuring may pose significant ethical,

moral, and legal problems when you act as a culture broker because nurses are expected to respect individual rights, be sensitive to health-culture beliefs and practices, protect vulnerable individuals (children, elderly, ill, and refugees) from harm and abuse, and adhere to legal codes.

(4) Before taking action against unsafe cultural practices in nonemergency situations, be certain to explore all possible methods of change, understand the benefits and risks of the practice, and apprise all individuals concerned of the consequences of continuing the practice.

NURSE ADVISORY

When cultural beliefs and folk healing practices put vulnerable individuals at physical risk, your primary responsibility is to prevent physical injury.

g. Benefits of cultural brokerage in the clinical setting are the following:
(1) Patients will have a higher level of satisfaction with nursing interventions and biomedical treatments.
(2) Nurses will experience less frustration when caring for culturally diverse patients.
(3) Patients will have a greater understanding of nursing interventions and adhere more readily to them.
(4) Nurses will gain a greater understanding of their patients and more readily develop realistic and holistic nursing care plans.
(5) Nurses will have an increased understanding of the patients' *illness* experience and place less emphasis on the treatment of *disease.*
(6) Nurses will be able to develop more practical and meaningful health teaching and education programs for patients.

3. Steps in the cultural brokerage process
a. Determine how the patient, family, or members of the patient's therapy management group conceptualize the problem. What is their EM?
b. Compare the patient's perspective (EM) with your own.
c. Explain your EM to the patient.
(1) Give your explanation at the patient's level of understanding.
(2) Use the same words and concepts the patient uses to describe his or her EM. Make certain that you understand the frame of reference the patient is using when describing his or her EM.
d. Develop a mutually acceptable nursing intervention or "working alliance" with the patient. This can be done rapidly under the following circumstances:
(1) You and the patient hold similar health-culture perspectives on the same problem.
(2) Your expectations shift toward the patient's expectations.

(3) The patient's expectations shift toward yours.
e. Clarify areas of conflict when you and the patient are unable to agree on mutually acceptable nursing interventions.
f. Attempt to reach a compromise with the patient when neither you nor the patient are able to accept the other's perspective. The compromise should do the following:
(1) Meet ethical standards of care
(2) Ensure the patient's rights
(3) Include appropriate knowledge from your point of view and that of the patient
g. When compromise is reached, you *and* the patient must do the following:
(1) Abide by it
(2) Monitor the implementation progress
(3) Seek renegotiation and clarification when problems arise
h. If no compromise is possible, you must do the following:
(1) Be certain you have presented your view as clearly as possible
(2) Be certain you have sought to understand the patient's perspective as much as possible
(3) Be willing to recognize the patient's right to decide what health care measures to take
(4) Refer the patient to another health care provider who can assist
(5) Understand the patient has the right to seek assistance from other health care providers if he or she chooses

Transcultural Nursing Evaluation

1. Do not feel the cultural brokerage process has failed if patients do not agree to try or do not adhere to nursing interventions. Patients have the right to determine their own health care options.
2. Successful interventions in transcultural nursing may include the following:
a. Cultural maintenance
b. Cultural accommodation
c. Cultural restructuring
d. Greater mutual understanding and trust between nurses and patients with or without a mutually agreed on intervention
e. Greater adherence on the part of patients to nursing interventions and treatment regimens
f. Increased willingness on the part of nurses and patients to compromise and accommodate each other
g. Increased awareness on the part of nurses and their health care colleagues of the effect of patients' EMs on their health-seeking behavior
h. Development of practical and meaningful approaches to health teaching and health education programs
i. Greater emphasis placed on interventions related to the patient's illness experience and less emphasis placed on the treatment of disease.

Bibliography

Books

Andrews MM, and Boyle JS (eds). *Transcultural Concepts in Nursing Care.* 2nd ed. Philadelphia: JB Lippincott, 1995.

Bailey EJ. *Urban African American Health Care.* Lanham, MD: University Press of America, 1991.

Bannerman RH, Burton J, and Ch'en WC (eds). *Traditional Medicine and Health Care Coverage.* Geneva, Switzerland: World Health Organization, 1983.

Bopp J, and Bopp M. *The Sacred Tree.* Wilmont, WI: Lotus Light, 1984.

Buckley T, and Gottlieb A (eds). *Blood Magic: The Anthropology of Menstruation.* Berkeley, CA: University of California Press, 1989.

Camino LA, and Krulfeld RM (eds). *Reconstructing Lives, Recapturing Meaning: Refugee Identity, Gender, and Culture Change.* Basel, Switzerland: Gordon Breach, 1994.

Clark M. *Health in the Mexican American Culture.* Berkeley, CA: University of California Press, 1959.

Comas-Diaz L, and Griffith EEH (eds). *Clinical Guidelines in Cross-Cultural Mental Health.* New York: John Wiley & Sons, 1988.

Cruickshank JK, and Beevers DG. *Ethnic Factors in Health and Disease.* London: Wright, 1989.

Freund PF, and McGuire MB. *Health, Illness, and the Social Body.* Englewood Cliffs, NJ: Prentice-Hall, 1995.

Galanti GA. *Caring for Patients from Different Cultures.* Philadelphia: University of Pennsylvania Press, 1991.

Gaw A (ed.). *Cross-Cultural Psychiatry.* London: Wright, 1982.

Good CM. *Ethnomedical Systems in Africa.* New York: Guilford, 1987.

Hall ET, and Hall MR. *Understanding Cultural Differences.* Yarmouth, ME: Intercultural Press, 1990.

Hammerschlag CA. *The Dancing Healers: A Doctor's Journey of Healing with Native Americans.* San Francisco: Harper & Row, 1988.

Harwood A (ed). *Ethnicity and Medical Care.* Cambridge: Harvard University Press, 1981.

Helman CG. *Culture, Health and Illness.* Oxford: Butterworth-Heinemann, 1994.

Kavanagh KH, and Kennedy PH. *Promoting Cultural Diversity: Strategies for Health Care Professionals.* Newbury Park, CA: Sage, 1992.

Kiev A. *Transcultural Psychiatry.* New York: The Free Press, 1972.

Kleinman A. *Patients and Healers in the Context of Culture.* Berkeley, CA: University of California Press, 1980.

Kleinman A. *The Illness Narratives.* New York: Basic Books, 1988.

Kleinman A, and Good B (eds). *Culture and Depression: Studies in Anthropology and Cross-Cultural Psychiatry of Affect and Disorder.* Berkeley, CA: University of California Press, 1985.

Laguerre M. *Afro-Caribbean Folk Medicine.* South Hadley, MA: Bergin and Garvey, 1987.

Lefley HP, and Pederson PB. (eds). *Cross-Cultural Training for Mental Health Professionals.* Springfield, IL: Charles C Thomas, 1986.

Leininger MM (ed). *Culture Care Diversity and Universality: A Theory of Nursing.* New York: National League for Nursing, 1991.

Leslie C (ed). *Asian Medical Systems: A Comparative Study.* Berkeley, CA: University of California Press, 1976.

Maloney C (ed). *The Evil Eye.* New York: Columbia University Press, 1976.

Marsella AJ, and White GM. *Cultural Conceptions of Mental Health and Therapy.* Boston: D Reidel, 1984.

Martinez RA. *Hispanic Culture and Health Care.* St. Louis: CV Mosby, 1978.

McElroy A, and Townsend PK. *Medical Anthropology in Ecologial Perspective.* Boulder, CO: Westview, 1985.

Mitchell L. *101 Colloquial Expressions for Health Service Personnel.* Los Angeles: Mit-sho, 1985.

Moran EF. *Human Adaptability: An Introduction to Ecological Anthropology.* Boulder, CO: Westview, 1982.

Orque M, Block OB, and Monrroy L (eds). *Ethnic Nursing Care.* St. Louis: CV Mosby, 1971.

Overfield T. *Biologic Variation in Health and Illness.* New York: CRC Press, 1995.

Parkes AS. *Backlash.* Cambridge, England: Parkes Foundation, 1993.

Payer L. *Medicine and Culture.* New York: Henry Holt, 1988.

Polednak AP. *Host Factors in Disease: Age, Sex, Racial and Ethnic Group, and Body Build.* Springfield, IL: Charles C Thomas, 1987.

Rathwell T, and Phillips D (eds). *Health, Race and Ethnicity.* London: Croom Helm, 1986.

Scheper-Hughes N (ed). *Child Survival.* Boston: Reidel, 1987.

Sheikh AA, and Sheikh KS (eds). *Eastern and Western Approaches to Healing: Ancient Wisdom and Modern Knowledge.* New York: John Wiley & Sons, 1989.

Simmons M. *Witchcraft in the Southwest.* Lincoln, NB: University of Nebraska Press, 1974.

Simons RC, and Hughes CC (eds). *The Culture-Bound Syndromes.* Boston: D Reidel, 1985.

Snow LF. *Walkin' Over Medicine.* Boulder, CO: Westview, 1993.

Spector RE. *Cultural Diversity in Health and Illness.* Norwalk, CT: Appleton & Lange, 1991.

Spicer EH (ed). *Ethnic Medicine in the Southwest.* Tucson, AZ: University of Arizona Press, 1977.

Spradley J, and McCurdy J. *Conformity and Conflict.* Boston: Little, Brown & Co, 1977.

Waxler-Morrison N, Anderson JM, and Richardson E (eds). *Cross-Cultural Caring: A Handbook for Health Professionals in Western Canada.* Vancouver, BC: University of British Columbia Press, 1990.

Weiss KA. *Genetic Variation and Human Disease.* New York: Cambridge University Press, 1993.

Winthrop RH. *Dictionary of Concepts in Cultural Anthropology.* New York: Greenwood, 1991.

Young JC. *Medical Choice in a Mexican Village.* New Brunswick, NJ: Rutgers University Press, 1981.

Chapters in Books

Ahern EM. The power and pollution of Chinese women. *In* Wolf AP (ed). *Studies in Chinese Society.* Stanford, CA: Stanford University Press, 1978.

Berry JW, and Kim U. Acculturation and mental health. *In* Dasen PR, Berry JW, and Sartorius N (eds). *Health and Cross-Cultural Psychology: Toward Application.* Newbury Park, CA: Sage, 1988.

Blumhagen D. The meaning of hypertension. *In* Chrisman NJ, and Maretzki TW (eds). *Clinically Applied Anthropology. Anthropologists in Health Science Settings.* Boston: D Reidel, 1982.

Chung K. Chinese Americans. *In* Giger JN, and Davidhizar RE (eds). *Transcultural Nursing: Assessment and Intervention.* St. Louis: Mosby–Year Book, 1991.

Fife AE. Birthmarks and psychic imprinting of babies of Utah folk medicine. *In* Hand WD (ed). *American Folk Medicine.* Berkeley, CA: University of California Press, 1976.

Frazer JG. Sympathetic magic. *In* Lessa WA, and Vogt EZ (eds). *Reader in Comparative Religions: An Anthropological Approach.* New York: Harper & Row, 1979.

Good BJ, and DelVecchio-Good MJ. The meaning of symptoms: A cultural hermeneutic model for clinical practice. *In* Kleinman A, and Eisenberg L (eds). *The Relevance of Social Science for Medicine.* Boston: D Reidel, 1981.

Hall ET. Proxemics: The study of man's spatial relations. *In* Galdston I (ed). *Man's Image in Medicine and Anthropology.* New York: International Universities Press, 1963.

Hanley CE. Navajo Indians. *In* Giger JN, and Davidhizar RE (eds). *Transcultural Nursing.* St. Louis: Mosby–Year Book, 1991.

Kluckhohn F. Dominant and variant value orientations. *In* Brink PJ (ed). *Transcultural Nursing: A Book of Readings.* Englewood Cliffs, NJ: Prentice-Hall, 1979.

Olson EM. Socioeconomic and psychocultural contexts of child abuse and neglect in Turkey. *In* Korbin JE (ed). *Child Abuse and Neglect: Cross-Cultural Perspectives.* Berkeley, CA: University of California Press, 1981.

Pederson P. The three stages of multicultural development: Awareness, knowledge, and skill. *In* Pederson P (ed). *A*

Handbook for Developing Multicultural Awareness. Alexandria, VA: American Association for Counseling and Development, 1988.

Pfifferling JH. A cultural prescription for medicocentrism. *In* Kleinman A, and Eisenberg L (eds). *The Relevance of Social Science for Medicine*. Boston: D Reidel, 1981.

Potter JM. Cantonese shamanism. *In* Wolf AP (ed). *Studies in Chinese Society*. Stanford, CA: Stanford University Press, 1978.

Scott CS. The theoretical significance of a sense of well-being for the delivery of gynecological health care. *In* Bauwens EE (ed). *The Anthropology of Health*. St. Louis: CV Mosby, 1978.

Sobo EJ. "Unclean deeds": Menstrual taboos and binding "ties" in rural Jamaica. *In* Nichter M (ed). *Anthropological Approaches to the Study of Ethnomedicine*. Philadelphia: Gordon and Breach, 1992.

Stokes LG. Delivering health services in a Black community. *In* Reinhardt AM, and Quinn MB (eds). *Current Practice in Family-Centered Community Nursing*. St. Louis: CV Mosby, 1977.

Tripp-Reimer T, and Brink PJ. Culture brokerage. *In* Bulecheck GM, and McCloskey JC (eds). *Nursing Interventions*. Philadelphia: WB Saunders, 1985.

Wolf AP. Gods, ghosts, and ancestors. *In* Wolf AP (ed). *Studies in Chinese Society*. Stanford, CA: Stanford University Press, 1978.

Wu DYH. Child abuse in Taiwan. *In* Korbin JE (ed). *Child Abuse and Neglect: Cross-Cultural Perspectives*. Berkeley, CA: University of California Press, 1981.

Yap PM. The culture-bound syndromes. *In* Landy D (ed). *Culture, Disease, and Healing*. New York: Macmillan, 1977.

Journal Articles

Anderson JM. Health care across cultures. *Nurs Outlook* 38(3):136–139, 1990.

Bailey EJ. Hypertension: An analysis of Detroit African American health care treatment patterns. *Hum Org* 50(3):287–296, 1991.

Burnum JF. Dialect is diagnostic. *Ann Intern Med* 100(6):899–901, 1984.

Charonko CV. Cultural influences in "noncompliant" behavior and decision making. *Holistic Nurs Pract* 6(3):73–78, 1992.

Chrisman NJ. The health seeking process: An approach to the natural history of illness. *Culture Med Psychiatry* 1(4):351–371, 1977.

Currier RL. The hot-cold syndrome and symbolic balance in Mexican and Spanish-American folk medicine. *Ethnology* 5(3):251–263, 1966.

DelVecchio-Good MJ. Of blood and babies: The relationship of popular Islamic physiology on fertility. *Soc Sci Med* 14B(3):147–156, 1980.

DeSantis L. Cultural factors affecting newborn and infant diarrhea. *J Pediatr Nurs* 3(6):391–398, 1988.

DeSantis L. Haitian immigrant concepts of health. *Health Values* 17(6):3–16, 1993.

DeSantis L. Making anthropology clinically relevant to nursing care. *J Adv Nurs* 20:707–715, 1994.

DeSantis L, and Halberstein R. The effects of immigration on the health care system of South Florida. *Hum Org* 51(3):223–234, 1992.

DeSantis L, and Thomas JT. Health education and the immigrant Haitian mother: Cultural insights for community health nurses. *J Public Health Nurs* 9(2):87–96, 1992.

Diaz-Duque OF. Overcoming the language barrier: Advice from an interpreter. *Am J Nurs* 82(9):1380–1382, 1982.

Fabrega H. The study of disease in relation to culture. *Behav Sci* 17(2):183–203, 1972.

Fabrega H. The need for an ethnomedical science. *Science* 189:969–975, 1975.

Farmer P. Bad blood, spoiled milk: Bodily fluids as moral barometers in rural Haiti. *Am Ethnol* 15(1):62–83, 1988.

Farmer P. Sending sickness: Sorcery, politics, and changing concepts of AIDS in rural Haiti. *Med Anthropol Q* 4(1):6–27, 1990.

Fong CM. Ethnicity and nursing practice. *Top Clin Nurs* 7(3):1–10, 1985.

Foreman JT. Susto and the health needs of the Cuban refugee population. *Top Clin Nurs* 7(3):40–47, 1985.

Foster GM. Disease etiologies in non-western medical systems. *Am Anthropol* 78(4):773–782, 1976.

Friedl J. Explanatory model of black lung: Understanding the health-related behavior of Appalachian coal miners. *Culture Med Psychiatry* 6(1):3–6, 1982.

Geissler EM. Nursing diagnoses of culturally diverse patients. *Internat Nurs Rev* 38(5):150–152, 1991.

Geissler EM. Transcultural nursing and nursing diagnoses. *Nurs Health Care* 12(4):190–192, 203, 1991.

Germain CP. Cultural care: A bridge between sickness, illness, and disease. *Holistic Nurs Pract* 6(3):1–9, 1992.

Good BJ. The heart of what's the matter: The semantics of illness in Iran. *Culture Med Psychiatry* 1:25–58, 1977.

Grasska MA, and McFarland T. Overcoming the language barrier: Problems and solutions. *Am J Nurs* 82(9):1376–1379, 1982.

Groce NE, and Zola IK. Multiculturalism, chronic illness and disability. *Pediatrics* 19(5):1048–1055, 1993.

Hartman MA, and Harrison JK. Health beliefs and practices in a middle-income Anglo-American neighborhood. *Adv Nurs Sci* 4(1):49–64, 1982.

Harwood A. The hot-cold theory of disease: Implications for treatment of Puerto Rican patients. *JAMA* 216(7):1153–1158, 1971.

Hautman MA. Self-care responses to respiratory illness among Vietnamese. *West J Nurs Res* 9(2):223–243, 1987.

Hoeman SP. Cultural assessment in rehabilitation nursing practice. *Nurs Clin North Am* 24(1):277–289, 1989.

Janzen JM. Therapy management: Concept, reality, process. *Med Anthropol Q* 1(1):69–84, 1987.

Jezewski MA. Culture brokerage in migrant farmworker health care. *West J Nurs Res* 12(4):497–513, 1990.

Johnson KE, and Rodgers S. When cultural practices are health risks: The dilemma of female circumcision. *Holistic Nurs Pract* 8(2):70–78, 1994.

Johnson TM. Premenstrual syndrome as a western culture-specific disorder. *Culture Med Psychiatry* 11:337–356, 1987.

Kavanagh KH. Transcultural nursing: Facing the challenges of advocacy and diversity/universality. *J Transcult Nurs* 5(1):4–13, 1993.

Kelley J, and Frisch NC. Use of selected nursing diagnoses: A transcultural comparison between Mexican and American nurses. *J Transcult Nurs* 2(1):16–22, 1990.

Kleinman A, Eisenberg L, and Good, B. Culture, illness and care: Clinical lessons from anthropological and cross-cultural research. *Ann Intern Med* 88(2):251–258, 1978.

Kleinman A, and Sung LH. Why do indigenous practitioners successfully heal? *Soc Sci Med* 13B(1):7–26, 1979.

Kosko DA, and Flaskerud JH. Mexican American, nurse practitioner, and lay control group beliefs about cause and treatment of chest pain. *Nurs Res* 36(4):226–230, 1987.

LaFargue JP. Mediating between two views of illness. *Top Clin Nurs* 7(3):70–75, 1985.

Leininger M. Issues, questions, and concerns related to the nursing diagnoses cultural movement from a transcultural nursing perspective. *J Transcult Nurs* 2(1):23–32, 1990.

Leininger M. Becoming aware of types of health practitioners and cultural imposition. *J Transcult Nurs* 2(2):32–39, 1991.

Lipson JG, and Meleis AI. Culturally appropriate care: The case of immigrants. *Top Clin Nurs* 7(3):48–56, 1985.

Littlewood J. A model for nursing using anthropological literature. *Soc Sci Med* 26(3):221–228, 1989.

Low SM. Culturally interpreted symptoms or culture-bound syndrome: A cross-cultural review of nerves. *Soc Sci Med* 21(2):187–196, 1985.

Lynough SE, and Bates B. The two languages of nursing and medicine. *Am J Nurs* 73:66–69, 1973.

Maduro R. Curanderismo and Latino views of disease and caring. *West J Med* 139:868–874, 1983.

Minami H. East meets West: Some ethical considerations. *Int J Nurs Stud* 22(4):311–318, 1985.

Molde S. Understanding patients' agendas. *Image* 18(4):145–147, 1986.

Muecke M. Caring for Southeast Asian refugee patients in the U.S.A. *Am J Public Health* 73(4):431–438, 1983.

Opler ME. The cultural definition of illness in village India. *Hum Organ* 22(1):32–35, 1963.

Philippe J, and Romain JB. Indisposition in Haiti. *Soc Sci Med* 13B(2):129–133, 1979.

Plawecki HM, Sanchez TR, and Plawecki JA. Cultural aspects of caring for Navajo Indian clients. *J Holistic Nurs* 12(3):291–306, 1994.

Prince R. The concept of culture-bound syndromes: Anorexia nervosa and brain-fag. *Soc Sci Med* 21(2):197–203, 1985.

Putsch RW. Cross-cultural communication: The special case of interpreters in health care. *JAMA* 254(23):3344–3348, 1985.

Roberson MHB. The influence of religious beliefs on health choices of Afro-Americans. *Top Clin Nurs* 7(3):57–63, 1985.

Roberson MHB. The meaning of compliance: Patient perspectives. *Qual Health Res* 2(1):7–26, 1992.

Scott CS, et al. Hispanic and Black American adolescents' beliefs relating to sexuality and contraception. *Adolescence* 23(91):667–688, 1988.

Sherblom S, Shipps TB, and Sherblom JC. Justice, care and integrated concerns in the ethical decision making of nurses. *Qual Health Res* 3(4):442–464, 1993.

Simmons SJ. Health: A concept analysis. *Int J Nurs Stud* 26(2):155–161, 1989.

Snow LF. Sorcerers, saints and charlatans: Black folk healers in urban America. *Culture Med Psychiatry* 2:69–106, 1978.

Snow LF, and Johnson SM. Modern day menstrual folklore. *JAMA* 237(25):2736–2739, 1977.

Thorne SE. Constructive noncompliance in chronic illness. *Holistic Nurs Pract* 5(1):62–69, 1990.

Tripp-Reimer T. Retention of a folk-healing practice (matiasma) among four generations of urban Greek immigrants. *Nurs Res* 32(2):97–101, 1983.

Tripp-Reimer T, Brink, PJ, and Saunders JM. Cultural assessment: Content and process. *Nurs Outlook* 32(2):78–82, 1984.

Weidman HH. Falling-out: A diagnostic and treatment problem viewed from a transcultural perspective. *Soc Sci Med* 13B(2):95–112, 1979.

Weidman HH. The transcultural view: Prerequisite to interethnic (intercultural) communication in medicine. *Soc Sci Med* 13B(2):85–87, 1979.

Weise HJC. Maternal nutrition and traditional food behavior in Haiti. *Hum Org* 35:193–200, 1976.

Weiss MG. Cultural models of diarrheal illness: Conceptual framework and review. *Soc Sci Med* 27(1):5–16, 1988.

Wenger AFZ. Cultural meaning of symptoms. *Holistic Nurs Pract* 7(2):22–35, 1993.

Zola IK. Culture and symptoms: An analysis of patients' presenting complaints. *Am Soc Rev* 31:615–630, 1966.

3

Managing the Modern Clinical Environment

◼ NURSES AS MANAGERS

Roles of the Nurse as Manager

1. Leader
   a. A manager encourages others to follow by using personal characteristics such as charisma, knowledge, trust, and enthusiasm.

A leader
- has a mission that matters
- is a big thinker
- has high ethics
- masters change
- is sensitive
- is a risk taker
- is a decision maker
- uses power wisely
- communicates effectively
- is courageous
- is a team member
- is committed

Reprinted by permission of The Putnam Publishing Group from Bethel SM. *Making a Difference: 12 Qualities That Make You a Leader.* New York: GP Putnam's Sons, 1990. Copyright © 1990 by Sheila Murray Bethel.

2. Educator
   a. Managers have a responsibility to develop the skills of the nursing staff through presentations by experts such as clinical specialists.
   b. Most education occurs informally between manager and staff through role modeling. Remember: Your behavior is *always* noticed by staff. (See also "Researcher" and "Facilitator.")
3. Administrator
   a. Administration includes developing, executing, and evaluating policies and standards.
   b. Administrators must balance budgetary limitations with the need to provide sufficient resources (staff, equipment, supplies) for job accomplishment and to ensure quality of care.
4. Problem solver
   a. Managers of nursing staff are responsible for solving a wide range of problems.
   b. The steps in problem solving are as follows:
      (1) Assess the situation.

(2) Define the problem requiring a solution.
(3) List several possible solutions.
(4) Determine short-term and long-term goals.
(5) Analyze and select 1 solution.
(6) Implement the solution.
(7) Evaluate the effectiveness of the solution.
   c. Involve staff early on in problem solving to engage them in shared decision making, thus promoting their support of the solution.
5. Coordinator
   a. The coordinator role is one in which the manager facilitates the group's efforts toward goal achievement.
   b. The manager must do the following:
      (1) Help staff to identify the priority needs of the patient and initiate a plan of care.
      (2) Obtain support from other departments and disciplines.
      (3) Monitor supplies and equipment maintenance.
      (4) Motivate staff as needed.
      (5) Ensure follow-through on all problem-solving efforts.
6. Advocate
   a. Advocacy is the act of pleading a cause for someone who is unable to do so.
   b. Just as a nurse's advocacy helps patients to become more informed decision makers, so does the manager's advocacy toward staff help them to do the following:
      (1) Make more informed decisions.
      (2) Become willing to take risks.
      (3) Feel supported.
      (4) Become better patient advocates.
7. Counselor
   a. A counselor is one who gives expert advice.
   b. Managers need to advise and counsel staff members
      (1) On their educational and career pursuits.
      (2) On their current performance—positive or negative—noting strengths and areas needing improvement.
      (3) On how they can best contribute to the functioning of the unit.
8. Researcher
   a. Involvement in research may include identification of clinical problems for study, participation on research review committees, implementation of research pro-

tocols, and evaluation of research reports for application to nursing practice.

    b. Managers need to motivate their staff to expand their knowledge of relevant research findings.

9. Facilitator

    a. Facilitators help make any action easier to achieve.

    b. Facilitators identify barriers to goal achievement and plan strategies to overcome them.

10. Case manager in hospital settings

    a. The case manager is responsible for the following:

       (1) Planning nursing treatment modalities.

       (2) Facilitating communication among workers in all disciplines.

       (3) Teaching less experienced nurses the concept of case management.

       (4) Supervising care to ensure its appropriateness.

11. Managers in nonhospital settings

    a. Clinic manager or supervisor

       (1) Interviews and recommends nurses for employment.

       (2) Assigns nurses to specific clinics.

       (3) Interacts with patients and families for problem solving.

       (4) Collaborates with physicians and those in other disciplines to provide for the smooth transfer of patients from one clinic to another.

       (5) Provides for adequate supplies and equipment.

       (6) Counsels staff regarding performance.

       (7) Reviews records for quality of documentation and appropriateness of care.

       (8) Participates in the development of the budget.

    b. Long-term care manager or director

       (1) Interviews and hires prospective employees and staffs the facility according to organization policy and state and federal requirements.

       (2) Counsels staff regarding performance.

       (3) Arranges in-service education for a largely nonlicensed staff.

       (4) Collaborates with the medical director and attending physicians to review patients and their progress.

       (5) Meets regularly with members of other relevant disciplines to discuss the patients' care plans.

       (6) Defines nursing policy and sets standards of care.

       (7) Prepares the nursing budget.

       (8) Participates in quality of care reviews.

    c. Home care manager or supervisor

       (1) Interviews and recommends nurses for hire.

       (2) Assigns nurses their case loads.

       (3) Obtains authorization for care from payment source.

       (4) Ensures quality through chart audits.

       (5) Obtains physicians' signatures for treatment orders.

       (6) Ensures that patients are getting the appropriate level of service.

Traditional Types of Nurse Management

1. Vice president

    a. Is responsible for the management of all nursing services and policy development within the department of nursing, including the system of patient care delivery.

    b. Has responsibility that may extend to other departments that have patient contact such as physical therapy, pharmacy, and radiology.

    c. Can also be titled assistant administrator or director of nursing services.

    d. Reports to the chief executive officer (hospital administrator or president).

2. Supervisor

    a. Has selected administrative management responsibilities for a limited area (e.g., emergency department, operating suite, or a shift such as 3:00 P.M. to 11:00 P.M. or 11:00 P.M. to 7:00 A.M.).

    b. Is used in traditional nursing organizations.

    c. Reports to the director or assistant director of nursing.

3. Nurse manager (head nurse)

    a. Is a pivotal and powerful position when used appropriately.

    b. Has full management responsibility for 1 or more patient care units over a 24-hour period.

    c. Develops standards and coordinates care specific to assigned areas.

    d. Reports to the director or vice president of nursing.

4. Charge nurse

    a. Has responsibility for the care being delivered on an assigned unit during 1 shift.

    b. Is used in traditional nursing organizations.

    c. Can be a permanent position or rotated among various nurses on the unit.

    d. Reports to the nurse manager.

5. Team leader

    a. Is responsible for leading a "team" of RNs and ancillary personnel in caring for a group of patients on a given patient care unit for 1 shift.

    b. Is usually used in traditional nursing organizations.

    c. Coordinates care given by team members for the purpose of meeting team goals.

6. Case manager

    a. Responsible for coordinating the care of a case load of patients from preadmission to postdischarge in a case management or managed care system (discussed later in this chapter).

    b. Works collaboratively with other nurses (and in some situations with persons in other disciplines) to move the patient through a hospital stay efficiently.

    c. Requires advanced nursing skills or advanced managerial and communication skills, usually at the master's degree level.

    d. Reports to the nurse manager or chief nursing officer, depending on the type of nursing organization.

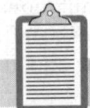

NURSING MANAGEMENT

Visibility is a key nursing management behavior. Show your nurses you care by regularly being in the patient care areas. Walking around lets you observe concern for quality, interact with persons from other disciplines, and get a better feel for staffing.

◼ *PROMOTING COMMUNICATION*

As managers, nurses must relate to one another, to patients and families, and to persons in other disciplines to be effective. Information about assignments, about how to operate special equipment, about the quality of a nurse's performance, and about the patient's response to treatment are all vital to the functioning of the health care team and the organization. Communication, then, is the process that links people together in their efforts to meet patient needs.

Principles of Effective Communication

1. Elements (Fig. 3–1)
   a. **Sender**—the person with something to say
   b. **Message**—what the sender wants to say
   c. **Receiver**—the person to whom something is being said
2. Basic principles
   a. **Knowledge and credibility.** Review subject matter before providing others with important information. Being knowledgeable helps to establish your credibility and fosters trusting relationships.
   b. **Caring.** Show interest and compassion when interacting with other people. Remain objective. Try to be positive and nonjudgmental.
   c. **Listening.** Take the time to listen actively to another person's questions and concerns. Avoid planning a response until the person has finished speaking.
   d. **Clarity.** Use simple words and explanations. Speak slowly and clearly. Identify and clarify misunderstandings.
   e. **Validation.** Verify that the person understands what you are saying. Ask the person to rephrase what you have said in his or her own words.
   f. **Humor.** Laughing at oneself or at a particular situation can be therapeutic and can add levity during a time that might otherwise be too serious.
   g. **Nonverbal cues.** Compare nonverbal behaviors with the stated message when trying to determine the intended message. Because appearance is also a nonverbal cue, be sure your clothing says what you wish.
3. Shared decision making
   a. Nurses make decisions based on their personal values, life experiences, perceptions, education, and knowledge.
   b. Working together as a group helps nurses feel more committed to one another and to the decision. Group members can also pool their ideas and arrive at creative alternatives to primary decisions.
   c. The effectiveness of a decision usually depends on the dynamics of the group.

COMMUNICATION = GETTING THROUGH

Sender ⟶ Intended message ⟶ Receiver

Figure 3–1. Effective communication.

   d. Decisions may be unanimous, by consensus, or by majority rule.
4. Conflict resolution
   a. Conflict occurs when 2 people or groups differ greatly in their ideas, roles, or actions. One or both may perceive a threat.
   b. Conflict in a dynamic organization is inevitable.
   c. Conflict is most commonly handled by withdrawal. Conflict is also resolved by using force, conciliation, smoothing over, compromise, or confrontation.
   d. Nurses trained in communication skills learn that each of the aforementioned styles can be employed under specific circumstances as long as a few basic rules are followed.
      (1) Clearly identify the issue through active listening.
      (2) Confront only the issue, not the person.
      (3) Discuss privately, away from patients and the central nursing area.
      (4) Focus on solving the problem.
      (5) Include a neutral party (such as the manager) to medate if the principals are unable to resolve the conflict.

Communicating with the Nursing Staff

1. Communicating with individual nurses
   a. To establish positive interpersonal communication, the manager first needs to become acquainted with the nursing team.
      (1) In a one-to-one meeting with each member of the staff, the manager should do the following:
         • Actively listen and allow the nurse to do most of the talking.
         • Briefly discuss the nurse's professional goals, along with any concerns the nurse might have.
      (2) Exhibit warmth, caring, and honesty—the cornerstones on which to build a trusting relationship with staff.
   b. Communication also includes making nurses aware of the quality of their performance.
      (1) Observe the staff delivering care.
      (2) Praise professional behavior (within earshot of peers, if culturally acceptable).
      (3) Deal with negative behavior promptly and in private. Address negative behavior immediately or within a few hours. (Sometimes you may need to prepare ahead for the counseling session and get your own emotions under control.)
         • Meet with the nurse in an office or other private place.
         • Inform the nurse of observed unacceptable behavior.
         • Allow the nurse an opportunity to respond.
         • Delineate expectations clearly and concisely.
         • Avoid long, drawn-out discussions, which tend to undermine the seriousness of the problem.
         • Arrange a time to review progress.
      (4) Document both positive and negative behavior as well as feedback, and keep the documentation in the nurse's file. These records help the manager to

- Review performance at annual evaluation.
- Keep track of patterns of behavior.
- Note responses to constructive criticism.
2. Communicating with groups of nurses
  a. Schedule an initial meeting with groups of staff to determine the staff-to-staff and staff-to-manager dynamics.
    (1) Distribute an agenda that states meeting objectives.
    (2) Set clear expectations regarding standards of care, problem solving, scheduling, and other issues pertinent to unit operations.
    (3) Allow ample time for the nursing staff to react, clarify, and respond.
    (4) If response is minimal, ask for feedback to ensure that the message was received.
    (5) Encourage questions.
  b. Establish routines to make information exchange an ongoing process.
    (1) Keep flexible work hours to allow direct access by nurses on all shifts.
    (2) Make rounds regularly with key staff members to review issues involving patients, and then discuss issues of importance to staff.
    (3) Remain sensitive to the changing needs of patients and staff.
    (4) Promote a nurturing environment through active listening and appreciation for the other person.
  c. When trying to reach a large staff (and possibly members of other disciplines), written memorandums are an effective communication tool.
    (1) Keep memos brief and clear.
    (2) Have a reliable staff member read and critique memos before circulating them.
    (3) Have staff members initial the memo after they have read it (to promote accountability).
    (4) Avoid sending notes to individuals about specific problems. This tends to annoy staff rather than to change behavior.
    (5) Avoid using a "communication book," which often becomes a person-to-person or shift-to-shift complaint log and leads to polarization of staff.
    (6) With staff input, develop a system for getting information to part-time or vacationing staff.
  d. Group meetings
    (1) Individuals behave differently when communicating in groups because they are aware of being observed by others.
    (2) Group size and composition affect how individuals communicate.
    (3) Members of the group usually perceive information differently, based on past experiences and individual preferences.
    (4) Group members may take on different roles depending on what they feel needs to be done.
      - Task roles such as coordinator or energizer may be taken on by a member or the leader, and one person may perform several roles.
      - Group building and maintenance roles such as harmonizer or gatekeeper serve to keep the group working toward its goal and can be taken on by members or by the leader.

- Individual roles are used by members to meet their own needs and may include roles such as aggressor, recognition seeker, or special interest pleader.
    (5) Knowing which roles group members usually assume helps the nurse manager or group leader to put together productive task groups and committees.
    (6) Group training for the nurses helps them become aware of their roles and learn how their behaviors influence outcomes.

Helping Nurses Communicate with One Another

1. Emphasize to nurses that they have certain responsibilities toward one another. They must
  a. Be open and direct with information and concerns.
  b. Be clear and concise with instructions, verbal or written.
  c. Be courteous at all times, even when under pressure.
  d. Trust one another's ability, even when communication styles differ.
  e. Nurture one another.
2. Encourage nurses who work together to develop mutual understanding by
  a. Learning about one another's values and beliefs.
  b. Learning about and respecting any cultural differences (see "Communicating with Nurses, Physicians, Staff, and Patients of Different Cultures").
  c. Being genuine and sensitive to one another's needs.
  d. Praising one another for a job well done (peers and leaders alike).
  e. Agreeing to manage any conflict that might occur.
3. Develop change-of-shift reporting procedures.
  a. Types of reporting methods for change of shift are as follows (nos. 1–3 usually require a report form for organization of data, including types and times for tasks to be done):
    (1) Face-to-face reporting between two nurses or between off-going nurse and on-coming shift or team.
    (2) Taped reporting from off-going nurse to on-coming shift or team.
    (3) Walking rounds by off-going nurse and on-coming nurse. This face-to-face method includes viewing the patient, performing a mini-assessment, or both.
    (4) Computer-generated reporting, which includes input data from off-going nurses, the laboratory, and other departments performing diagnostic tests and physicians' progress notes.
  b. Face-to-face reports are more effective than taped reports because of the following:
    (1) Anything misunderstood can be clarified immediately.
    (2) Last-minute changes can be managed.
  c. Changes in patient condition must be reflected on the care plan or Kardex (if used).
  d. Use of the care plan in reporting helps the nurse determine whether the patient has met his or her goals.

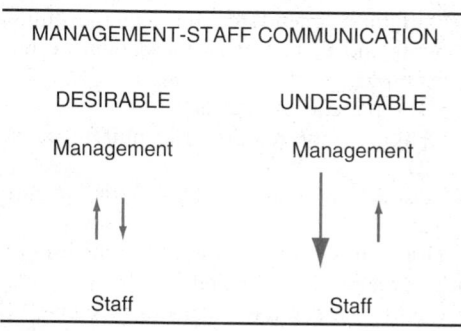

Figure 3–2. Management-staff communication.

e. Form and style of report may vary with pattern of nursing care delivery, agency policies, and group preferences.
4. Hold regular staff meetings.
   a. Plan an agenda for your meeting. Agendas do the following:
     (1) Help staff members prepare for the meeting.
     (2) Help keep the staff focused on specific issues.
     (3) Help prevent disgruntled staff members from disrupting a meeting with complaints and gripes.
   b. Share and discuss ongoing plans, programs, and concerns.
     (1) Replace rumors with facts.
     (2) Discuss concerns regarding other units or departments.
     (3) Take issues requiring upper management involvement to the appropriate person and convey management response (follow-through) at next meeting or sooner (Fig. 3–2). (This upward communication also keeps management in touch with how the nursing staff feel about new or changed programs and practices.)

Communicating with Physicians

1. Establish a foundation of trust and communication.
   a. Get to know each physician—*before* a problem arises.
   b. Arrange meetings with individuals or specialty groups of physicians to discuss needs and services.
   c. Review protocol for such items as use of conference rooms, rounds, and orders, as well as problems or perceived problems with nursing care.
     (1) Have physicians agree to seek out the primary nurse or case manager.
     (2) Have the case manager, primary nurse, or designee make rounds with physicians.
   d. Stress the importance of open communication between physician and nurse in providing patient care.
     (1) Make sure the nurse shares with the physician any information about patient needs and response to treatment.
     (2) Make sure the physician shares with the nurse plans for care, including new treatment or further diagnostic tests.
     (3) Have physicians discuss plans for discharge with nurses, including any home care or clinic follow-up that the patient may require.

2. Physicians and nurses must agree to respect one another, their positions, and their educational qualifications.
   a. Nurses and physicians should ask and answer questions politely and informatively.
   b. *Nurses* should have all facts together before phoning physicians, especially if treatment changes are needed.
   c. *Physicians* should respond quickly when phoned at any hour.
   d. Both groups must agree to avoid outbursts in front of patients and staff.
   e. Nurses and physicians should meet privately to discuss disagreements about the care being provided by either group.

When telephoning physicians about a change in patient condition, do the following:

1. Identify yourself, the hospital, and the hospital unit or ward.
2. Do not apologize for calling.
3. Identify the patient and diagnoses.
4. State the problem and include:
   - vital signs and level of consciousness
   - appearance of the patient, the wound, or both
   - response to interventions
   - any other pertinent data
5. Ask for orders or physician presence, if indicated.
6. If you encounter rude behavior, remain calm but assertive.
7. Document that the call was made.

Communicating with the Health Care Team, Patients, and Family

1. The health care team
   a. Encourage one-to-one problem solving as problems arise.
   b. Arrange regular interdisciplinary meetings to plan patient care improvement collaboratively.
   c. Keep the group on friendly terms. Inject humor to reduce tension when appropriate.
   d. Agree to try new approaches and give feedback.
   e. If feedback includes negative comments, include some positive findings (an idea cannot be *all* bad).
   f. Rotate the nurses responsible for attending these meetings to improve accountability and verbal communication skills.
   g. Recognize that being "very busy" does not mean we must avoid dealing with persons from other disciplines.
     (1) Taking a moment to respond to questions about the patient or the care provided can result in overall improvement of that care or treatment.
     (2) A friendly and professional exchange can improve relationships between individuals from different disciplines, laying the groundwork for good communication under more difficult circumstances.
2. Patients and family
   a. Begin patient rounds early in the shift to make quick assessments and to assure patients of your availability.

b. Listen to what patients have to say about their condition, their care, and their feelings.
c. Ensure that nurses keep patients informed of all treatment plans. Involve patients and their families in developing the plans when possible.
d. Always speak in simple language, without being condescending.
e. Make time to talk to family members. Time given early on can save time later.
f. Smile—softly and frequently.

Communicating with Nurses, Physicians, Staff, and Patients of Different Cultures

1. Nurses must try to understand the customs and beliefs of persons of different cultures. To accomplish this with their peers they can do the following:
   a. Develop one-to-one relationships.
   b. Meet regularly (monthly or biweekly) to discuss the meaning of verbal and nonverbal expressions that may unknowingly be hurtful.
   c. Agree to talk immediately when cultural miscommunications occur to avoid future embarrassment.
2. Together with physicians and staff, develop a plan for communicating with patients who have limited English proficiency.
   a. Purchase or make flash cards in the languages common to the area.
   b. Use prepared lists of frequently asked questions and answers in these and several other languages (be sure to include phonetic pronunciations).
   c. Develop a plan with a family member for calls to be made at certain times of the day by nurses or physicians to clarify or discuss significant communication problems regarding the patient or the patient's progress. Include the following:
      • Who will act as an interpreter
      • What times the interpreter will be available
      • How to contact the interpreter
   d. Know the name of a staff member who can interpret for the patient if necessary (keep a hospital-wide interpreter list available on the unit).
   e. Recognize the need to be flexible with visiting policies for people of different cultures.

◼ OVERCOMING STAFFING AND SCHEDULING PROBLEMS

Staffing and Scheduling Considerations

1. Staffing and scheduling techniques
   a. Plan for the number and types of nurses needed to deliver care to a specific patient population.
      (1) Develop the plan in conjunction with nursing administration.
      (2) Make changes if the patient population changes (usually at the time the annual budget is prepared).
      (3) Staff mix depends on the average number of patients and the acuity of the patient population. For example:
         • The patient number is 20.
         • High acuity requires the unit to be staffed for 24.
         • An RN is substituted for 1 of the nurse assistants.
   b. Develop a monthly or bimonthly schedule of how the staffing plan will be implemented.
      (1) Identify each nurse according to name, title, hours, and days to be worked.
      (2) Cover the 7-day week, 24-hour day with the number and mix of nurses necessary to provide care, using shifts such as the following:
         • 8-hour shifts, 5 days per week
         • 10-hour shifts, 4 days per week
         • 12-hour shifts, 3 to 4 days per week
         • 12-hour shifts, 7 days on and 7 off
         • Part-time, less than 8 hours per day or 40 hours per week
         • Job sharing, 2 people share 1 full-time position
   c. Avoid problems by keeping these things in mind:
      (1) Match patient needs to nurse skill level.
      (2) Reassign nurses after 4 or 5 days of caring for patients with intense needs.
      (3) Be flexible in trying new approaches to staffing and scheduling; for example, partial shifts allow experienced nurses to help out when home responsibilities might otherwise keep them out of the work force, and can also help keep costs under control.
      (4) Whenever possible, involve staff members in planning the work schedule and encourage them to hold one another accountable.
   d. To avoid staffing problems because of last-minute requests, limit any changes once schedule is posted to those made by nurses who find their own replacements from regular staff (at no additional cost to the unit), with your approval.
2. Reducing turnover by increasing job satisfaction
   a. Turnover usually occurs when roles are not well defined and when workers feel they have no say in the day-to-day practice of their profession.
   b. Autonomy in decision making not only increases accountability but also raises self-esteem, leading to improved role performance.
   c. Improved performance leads to recognition and an even higher level of self-esteem, self-actualization, and satisfaction in the work place.
   d. Work satisfaction is also enhanced by flexible and versatile staffing schedules.
3. Coping with changing staffing needs
   a. Short staffing of RNs
      (1) When short staffing occurs, nurses who are cross-trained in several areas or departments can increase the pool of nurses who can be called on, and thus prevent the need for using a nurse totally unfamiliar with the unit.
      (2) Cross-training also works when nurse numbers seem high, allowing nurses to be used in other

nursing areas or departments rather than in a particular unit.
- Downsizing is an option, but sacrificed positions may never again be approved and obtained.
- The versatile RN is valuable to the organization that is trying to streamline operations.
- RN staffs are associated with improved patient outcomes.

Building a Professional Staff

1. Evaluating staff performance and validating staff competency
   a. Annual performance evaluations are integral to the staff's professional development because they identify employee strengths and weaknesses and clarify employee and organizational goals. They are also used to promote job satisfaction; guide promotion, transfer, and separation decisions; and ensure competent nursing practice.
   b. Effective performance evaluations share the following characteristics:
      (1) Performance measures are based on a job description in which primary duties and the employee's characteristics and qualifications for adequate job performance are clearly stated.
      (2) Multiple observations and raters are used to increase evaluation reliability. Improved performance is more likely to occur when the employee, manager, and professional peers contribute to the evaluation process.
      (3) Performance appraisal tools are standardized and include detailed instructions and definitions of performance dimensions.
      (4) Evaluators have formal training in performance appraisal.
      (5) Performance evaluations are tied to a system of rewards and sanctions.
   c. Performance evaluation reliability may be compromised by the following:
      (1) Inadequate definition of performance.
      (2) Environmental problems, time constraints, and other situational factors that intrude on and distort the evaluator's judgment.
      (3) Temporary individual changes such as fatigue, illness, and mood of the employee or rater that influence the evaluation and lead to an inaccurate picture of actual performance.
      (4) Rater objectivity that is impaired by first impressions, stereotypic thinking, or personal relationships.
2. Developing staff strengths
   a. The nurse manager begins this process by hiring the right people who have the following characteristics:
      (1) Integrity, compassion, and enthusiasm along with a sense of humor, good communication skills, and an ability to get along well with coworkers.
      (2) An ability to clearly state what their previous job included and what they liked best and least about it.
      (3) References that describe the nurse as dependable, trustworthy, and possessing a good grasp of the knowledge required of the role.
   b. Once the nurse is hired, have him or her share expertise with peers in either a classroom or an informal setting.
   c. Give praise for a job well done.
   d. Encourage participation in programs that educate the whole person.
      (1) Post available programs, both internal and external. Arrange time for attendance.
      (2) Stress the need for development in areas beyond the nurse's specialty, such as human relations, legal and ethical issues, and management.
   e. Promote involvement in professional organizations to broaden knowledge of issues that affect the profession as a whole. Make literature, journals, and applications to professional organizations available.
   f. Support and encourage nurses' efforts to advance their education at local colleges and universities by allowing flexible work schedules.
3. Providing in-service education
   a. The purpose of in-service education is to maintain competent nursing practice.
   b. It usually includes programs about new procedures, operation of new equipment, or changes in policy.
   c. In-service training is generally a part of a larger department of staff development.
   d. Such training may be centralized (a pool of instructors teaches a core of more general topics and information) or decentralized (specialty instructors teach selected content to staff who work in specialized areas).

Managing Stress and Burnout Among the Nursing Staff

1. Identifying causes of stress and burnout
   a. Stress that lasts over long periods usually has undesirable effects on body systems or behavior.
   b. Causes of stress include role conflicts, emotional responses to patient suffering, skill inadequacy, disrespect among nurses, understaffing, highly structured nurse leaders, and low morale.
   c. Symptoms of stress include headache, fatigue, irritability, insomnia, and increased feeling of pessimism, all of which lead to absenteeism.
   d. A stress condition common among those who care for people in need is "compassion fatigue," a result of always putting someone else's needs before your own.
2. Counseling and educating the nursing staff
   a. Like patients, nurses may need help in coping with stress.
      (1) Observe staff for changes in work behaviors that may indicate high stress.
      (2) Schedule monthly support groups for nurses in high-stress patient care areas.
      (3) If your hospital has a staff psychologist, evidence of high stress is a good reason to engage his or her services (call directly or have upper-level

DECLARE WAR ON BURNOUT: 12 Tips for Professional Self-Care

1. Practice what we preach. Concentrate on good health habits.
2. Believe in what you do; value it and have respect for the demands it places on you.
3. *Just say no* to unsafe assignments and unrealistic expectations.
4. Look for the opportunity in the problem.
5. Develop and maintain professional liaisons both from within and outside your work setting.
6. Choose when to stand firm and when to let go.
7. Explore your options and focus on solutions.
8. Educate yourself, the consumer, your colleagues, and others about the scope and boundaries of your role.
9. Keep informed of nursing issues and strategies—not only in your specialty, but in your profession.
10. Stay calm and professional. There are no points for frenzy.
11. Work from within to make changes and leave if you have to. There is honor in knowing your limits.
12. Laugh! Let your light shine!

From Billings C. Declare war on burnout: 12 Tips for professional self-care. *Am Nurse*, November/December 1992.

nursing management make arrangements for regularly scheduled group sessions).
  b. Emphasize to your staff the need to guard their physical and mental health by taking assigned breaks and seeking support from peers.
  c. Teach staff to recognize that they cannot solve every problem. Some problems must be handled within another discipline or at a higher level of management.
  d. Encourage staff to care for one another.
    (1) Recognize when a peer is in need and when offering support *can* make a difference.
    (2) An environment in which nurses nurture one another promotes cohesiveness and reduces turnover.

Promoting a Nurturing Work Environment

1. A nurturing work environment nurtures the staff as well as the patients and their families.
  a. Nurses are respected for their input in problem solving even when 2 caregivers disagree about the solution.
  b. Nurses are valued as whole individuals, not just as clinical experts.
  c. The focus of care is the patient and family.
2. The nurse manager and other clinical leaders set the tone for a nurturing environment through calm and efficient problem solving, even during periods of chaos.
3. The physical setting should allow adequate work space for nurses to prepare medications, complete documentation, or conduct conferences without interruption.
4. Mutual respect and frequent praise motivates staff to be productive and sensitive in their care delivery and supportive of one another in the day-to-day work environment.

Working with the Physically Impaired Nurse

1. Recognize that such nurses are aware of their physical limitations.
2. Know and be alert to the performance expectations as defined in the employment agreement.
3. The type of physical impairment determines the extent of physical work a nurse can do; some may be limited to skills requiring evaluation or supportive interaction.
4. Do not patronize—treat the nurse as you do other employees or coworkers.
5. Learn from the nurse's expertise and share your knowledge with them.

Working with the Chemically Dependent Nurse

1. The American Nurses Association estimates that 6 to 8 percent of nurses impair their performance through the use of drugs or alcohol.
2. A number of hospitals and facilities have their own intervention teams, whose members are experienced at confronting, supporting, and monitoring the impaired employee.
3. Because denial is a common behavior in addicted persons, confrontation initiated by inexperienced coworkers may be unsuccessful and create hostility.
4. Review your organization policies for guidance.
5. If you suspect that a nurse has this problem, *do not* ignore it.
6. Your duty to your patients takes precedence over loyalty to a coworker.
7. Keep a record of subtle changes in behavior to help recognize if a pattern exists, noting any unexplained absences from the unit.
8. Immediately report the following signs to your supervisor:
  a. Alcohol on the breath
  b. Slurred speech
  c. Tremors or shaking
9. Do not discuss the nurse's problem with coworkers.
10. Remember: Reporting a colleague may save his or her license and life!

◼ PRINCIPLES OF TOTAL QUALITY MANAGEMENT

Total quality management (TQM) is a concept that guides all members of an organization and promotes high-level performance to complete a task or project. In a health care environment, the primary goal is a satisfied patient.

Basic Quality Management Principles

1. The patient is satisfied when care is personalized.
2. Staff can personalize care when empowered to make decisions about patient care.

3. Nonnursing caregivers (other professionals) deliver care at the patient's bedside whenever possible.
4. Good decisions are developed with cross-training.
5. Teamwork is the prevailing spirit.

Techniques of Quality Management

1. A program to ensure quality is based on a patient-centered organizational philosophy.
2. All staff, rather than a specific group or department, are involved in ensuring quality.
3. Cross-training and development are ongoing.
4. Care is measured against standards developed by staff and based on a business technique known as "bench-marking."

Benchmarking is the process in which a company finds and implements the best practices of other companies to improve its own products or services.

1. Do a critical review of competitors to determine the best products or services.
2. Determine where improvement would result in better care.
3. Use benchmarks to provide realistic targets for quality management.

---

5. Standards are reviewed and updated as necessary.
6. Staff members are recognized and valued for their contributions.
7. A commitment exists to continuously improve patient care services.
8. "Quality circles" are organized to engage employees in improving the work process and removing communication barriers between workers and management.

Quality circles is a participative management technique initiated in Japan after World War II based on the techniques of an American, Dr. Edward Deming.

• Representative groups of 5 to 10 people meet regularly, approximately 1 hour per week, to share common interests and solve problems.
• Groups manage themselves with the assistance of managers who are peer group members.
• Group mix is multidepartmental and multilevel to promote communication.
• Each group must reach consensus before decisions or recommendations are made.
• Overall morale and accountability improve with a resulting increase in productivity.

Decentralized Nursing Organizations

1. Decision making and policy formation move from the chief nursing officer to the nurse manager or the RN, or both, in charge of bedside care.
2. Responsibility and accountability are increased.

3. Fewer levels of management exist between the bedside nurse and the chief nursing officer.
4. Self-directed nurses have the autonomy they need to perform to the best of their ability.

◼ ENSURING QUALITY CARE IN A COST-SENSITIVE ENVIRONMENT

Restructuring Nursing Care Delivery

1. Primary nursing care delivery systems, developed in the 1970s and 1980s, rely on the registered nurse to assume responsibility for most aspects of patient care.
2. The socioeconomic influences of an aging American population that consumes ever greater health care resources and the advent of prospective and capitated reimbursement systems demands more efficient and less costly nursing care delivery.
3. Work redesign is the development of a nursing care delivery system based on the following:
   a. *Re-engineering* that determines nursing task and job viability in the clinical environment based on expected outcomes
   b. *Process improvement* that simplifies tasks and eliminates waste and work duplication
   c. *Skill mix analysis* that determines the appropriate skill level for task completion
4. Registered nurses practice in expanded professional roles in which they plan and coordinate patient care.
5. Basic nursing and support tasks are delegated by the registered nurse to nonprofessional staff such as licensed practical nurses or multiskilled unlicensed assistive personnel.
6. Quality patient care is ensured when unlicensed assistive personnel have the following:
   a. A minimum educational requirement for hire
   b. Proper training in basic nursing care delivery
   c. Validation of fundamental care skills
   d. Clearly defined roles within a written job description
   e. Properly delegated and adequately supervised assignments
   f. The ability to communicate effectively with patients, families, and professional staff
   g. Values that embrace the essentials of caring

Principles of Delegation

1. Delegation is giving another person the responsibility for meeting an identified outcome.
2. Delegation occurs from the top of the chain of command downward. Registered nurses delegate tasks to licensed practical nurses, unlicensed assistive personnel, and other support staff.
3. The registered nurse must know the individual's scope of practice, educational preparation, and competence before delegation.
4. The following factors influence whether an activity can be delegated:
   a. Potential for harm—the greater the risk for harm, the

less likely the activity is delegated to a nonprofessional.

b. Complexity of task—complex tasks require extensive training and assurance of competency.

c. Predictability of outcome and required problem solving—routine, stable, controllable tasks with predictable outcomes are most appropriate for delegation.

d. Need for assessment and nursing judgment—nursing assessment and judgment is the sole responsibility of the professional nurse and may not be delegated.

e. Regulatory mandates—Nurse Practice Acts vary from state to state and dictate the standard of professional and vocational nursing practice within that state. Delegation may not occur outside of state regulations.

Promoting a Therapeutic Environment

1. Patients generally recuperate faster in a safe and therapeutic environment where the nurses are caring and well informed.

2. Promoting safety

   a. Ensure staff awareness of current isolation techniques for the handling of specific organisms, whether brought in by patients or acquired in the hospital (nosocomial). Support the staff in their efforts to report breaks in technique by physicians, nurses, and other health care providers (see Chapter 8 for details).

   b. Regularly review procedures designed to minimize staff injuries such as transfer techniques (see Chapter 7 for details).

   c. Develop a maintenance program that keeps equipment in good working order, thus preventing injuries to staff and patients.

      (1) Involve staff in keeping equipment clean and in reporting minor malfunctions that can be repaired before equipment fails.

      (2) Work with the environmental services and maintenance departments to develop a preventive maintenance program.

   d. Monitor work areas for obstructions to safety occurring during patient care delivery, such as spilled bath water or linens or needle caps on the floor, all of which can cause falls and injuries.

   e. Emphasize to staff that hurrying or running usually impairs rather than improves speed and frequently brings about an undesirable sense of tension throughout the unit.

3. Promoting comfort

   a. Patients are usually most comfortable when they

      (1) Have confidence in their nurses and doctors as competent professionals.

      (2) Are free of pain.

      (3) Are informed of what they will encounter.

      (4) Receive hot food and cold water.

      (5) Have family or significant friends present.

   b. Staff members usually are most comfortable when they

      (1) Have adequate knowledge to provide safe, competent care.

      (2) Have sufficient staffing, supplies, and equipment to meet the care needs of their patients.

Enforcing Institutional Policies, Procedures, and Legal Safeguards

1. Identifying and controlling potential areas of legal liability

   a. Review with your staff areas in which problems have been identified by the facility's risk management and quality management programs.

   b. Discuss the areas most commonly brought to litigation. For example:

      (1) The patient's failure to be informed before consenting to a treatment.

      (2) Patient falls.

      (3) Medication and treatment errors, especially those related to improper identification.

   c. Take steps to correct existing problems.

      (1) Seek the help of a clinical or management specialist for problems requiring expertise.

      (2) Review with staff any patient care issues that might develop into legal problems.

         • Early discharges may lead to heavy burdens on families and result in inadequate and potentially unsafe care and complications. Suggest or arrange home care for patients requiring further nursing intervention and follow up periodically with a phone call for the more complicated cases (not uncommon in case-managed environments).

         • Do not breach the patient's right to informed consent. A breach could be interpreted as "assault" or "battery," legal terms meaning that the person's body was invaded without an understanding of what was to be done. Although the physician is the person legally responsible for obtaining the consent, the nurse plays a key role in determining whether there is any confusion or lack of awareness on the part of the patient about to receive treatment.

         • Familiarize yourself with equipment you use. Improper use of equipment such as monitors and infusion pumps can expose you to litigation, even though it is the hospital's responsibility to provide information about equipment and to maintain the equipment in proper working order. Nurses are responsible for accessing the education offered by the hospital and for checking equipment to ensure its readiness for use.

         • Document clearly and accurately. Although many nurses have learned the common legal dictate "if it wasn't documented then it wasn't done," other aspects of documentation such as the legibility of the writing or the procedure for error correction (e.g., erasing, scribbling over, use of correction fluid) are frequently called into question. Facility policies usually address the expected behavior for handling errors, such as a single-line-only through an error along with the nurse's initials, the date, and the time the late entry was made to correct the error. All of them say absolutely *no* erasures or use of correction fluid or tape.

(3) Remind staff that their caring and apologetic behavior in the event of error goes a long way toward *preventing* litigation.

2. Enforcing reporting and recording requirements
   a. Advise staff to report any suspected problem of negligence or malpractice.
      (1) Respond immediately with an appropriate investigation.
      (2) Involve upper management.
   b. Monitor staff awareness of, and adherence to, documentation policies.
   c. Key items to document are the following:
      (1) Nursing care that is pertinent, precise, and reflects the patient's status.
      (2) The patient's needs, problems, capabilities, and limitations.
      (3) Nursing interventions and patient response.
   d. Follow up with counseling and education to correct any documentation problem.
   e. Reevaluate key documentation items periodically to ensure accuracy and consistency.
   f. Encourage nurses to evaluate each others' documentation (for some, documentation is much easier than for others).
3. Protecting the ethical and legal rights of patients and staff

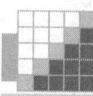

LEGAL AND ETHICAL CONSIDERATIONS

American Hospital Association Patients' Bill of Rights

Every patient has the right to

1. Considerate and respectful care.
2. Relevant, current, and understandable information concerning diagnosis, treatment, and prognosis.
3. Informed consent to or refusal of care.
4. Advance directive, e.g., living will, health care proxy, or durable power of attorney for health care.
5. Privacy.
6. Confidentiality.
7. Access to own medical records, except when restricted by law.
8. Reasonable response by hospital to patient request for care or transfer to another facility.
9. Information on potential business conflicts of interest among health care providers, which might affect patient's care.
10. Information on research studies or human experimentation affecting care and treatment or requiring direct patient involvement and the right of patient to refuse participation in same.
11. Reasonable continuity of care.
12. Information on hospital policies and practices that relate to patient care.

Adapted with permission from the American Hospital Association. Copyright 1992.

a. Make staff aware of the Nurse Practice Act, and give everyone a copy.
   (1) Note that the provisions of the Nurse Practice Act vary somewhat from state to state.

(2) Provisions common to many states include definitions of registered nursing and vocational or practical nursing, authority given to the state board regarding educational requirements and state regulations, and punishable violations of the practice act.
(3) Hold a conference to discuss application to the general or extended-role practitioner.

b. Get staff involved in the hospital's risk management program beyond the minimal participation of occasionally completing an incident report form.
c. Keep staff updated on changes or new policies and involve them, when possible, in making changes or developing new standards.
d. Have new staff review the policies and procedures and be sure to verify their understanding (rotate staff through the responsibility of being the "new policy" or "new equipment" informant of the month).

Diagnosis-Related Groups and Length of Stay

1. Using diagnosis-related groups (DRGs)
   a. The DRGs are a system of reimbursement standards utilized by the federal government to pay for care received by all Medicare patients.
      (1) The payment schedule is predetermined, based on the average number of hospitalization days (also called average length of stay) needed for a specific diagnosis.
      (2) Costs beyond the days specified are absorbed by the hospital or other facility, and special consideration may be given in a few circumstances with a written request by the hospital.
      (3) Any profits from keeping costs below the average are retained by the hospital or other care facility.
      (4) To keep costs down, health care facilities are reducing length of stay, leading to increasing numbers of higher acuity patients.
2. Nursing responsibilities associated with DRGs
   a. Every effort must be made to assist the patient in moving toward goal achievement as rapidly as possible.
   b. Highly skilled assessments allow the nurse to note patient progress and to intervene (with members of other disciplines if necessary), to alter intervention as needed, and to improve patient outcome.
   c. Teaching the patient the reasons for therapy and how to provide self-care not only makes the patient a more informed participant in the care team but increases the opportunity for an early or scheduled discharge date.
   d. Expertise in developing and using "critical pathways" (explained later in this section) will assist nurses in meeting length of stay parameters.

Instituting Case Management and Critical Pathways

1. Joint Commission on Accreditation of Healthcare Organizations (JCAHO) Standards

a. In 1975 the JCAHO urged the use of outcome criteria to evaluate nursing.
b. Today the JCAHO continues to recommend the use of outcome criteria using a collaborative approach to patient-focused care.
c. This collaborative effort by the interdisciplinary work group begins before admission and continues until discharge.

2. Case management
a. Preadmission planning and evaluation can begin in the physician's office, where a nurse case manager may be contacted by a physician.
    (1) The nurse can arrange to meet the patient at the hospital several days in advance of a scheduled procedure.
    (2) Patient and family teaching may begin at this time, along with some preprocedure diagnostic tests.
b. Collaborative inpatient planning and evaluation begins on admission with a nursing assessment and evaluation by other members of the patient-focused team.
    (1) An interdisciplinary plan for the patient's care based on expected outcomes, also known as a care map or clinical path, is then initiated.
    (2) In some organizations one professional is assigned the case manager position and assumes accountability for the coordination and delivery of diverse elements of care, whereas in others the responsibility may be assigned to an interdisciplinary team.
    (3) Goals are developed in concert with the patient and family who agree on the plan.
    (4) The team evaluates patient progress daily and collaborates to resolve any patient problems.
c. Collaborative discharge planning and evaluation begin early in the hospital stay.
    (1) The plan of care includes what the patient will need, from any discipline or specialty when discharged.
    (2) Contacts are made and contracts developed with home service providers to ease the transition from hospital to home.
    (3) A network of family and friends can also be established for helping out at home.
d. Collaborative home care planning and evaluation occur among the patient, family, and home care professionals.
    (1) Visits are made to administer care, evaluate progress, and reinforce the care efforts of family and friends.
    (2) Physicians are contacted regarding progress and any need for change in therapy by the field case manager.
    (3) Records are reviewed by all members of the team, and contacts are made to clarify or resolve concerns with the purpose of keeping the care focus on the patient's achievement of goals.

3. Critical pathways (see Chapter 1)

■ THE FUTURE OF NURSING MANAGEMENT

Nursing Informatics

1. Involves all aspects of technology related to nursing care delivery and includes but is not limited to:
a. Financial reports about productivity and expenditures.
b. Laboratory and other diagnostic data reporting.
c. Care plans and patient summaries.
d. Quality management tools.
e. Patient databases used for patient follow-up and research.
2. Future technology in computers will include the following:
a. Voice technology to ease the process of data entry.
b. Point-of-care systems at the patient's bedside or portable units small enough to move about from bed to bed.
c. Regional, national, and global information networks.
d. Electronic networks that link patients at home to medical, nursing, and support services.

Nursing Research

1. More nurses will be involved in research under the direction of a doctorally prepared nurse researcher.
2. Nursing research will continue to focus on validation of nursing practice through empiric data.
3. Research will include such topics as the following:
a. The most cost-effective staff mix for the best possible outcomes.
    (1) Staffing will be determined by nurse researchers.
    (2) Nurses will be more responsive to the results than when staffing determinations were made based on data collected by industrial engineers.
b. Effective models of managed care.
c. Effects of continuous quality improvement processes, which are data based.

Nursing Management in the Twenty-First Century

1. Nursing practice will be driven by 2 major forces: the global economy and computer technology.
2. The nursing work force
a. Expect the nursing work force to become more culturally diverse with a greater number of men choosing nursing careers.
b. Competition for nursing positions will increase. Nurses will be required to be flexible and multiskilled to remain employable.
c. Schools of nursing will admit more 2nd-career students.
3. Education

a. Advanced education will be important to gain the expertise needed to care for the increasing numbers of critically ill patients.

b. Education will also be needed for nurses to become more expert at health promotion as the focus of health care shifts from managing illness to maintaining wellness.

c. Management skills and leadership development will be necessary to prepare registered nurses to lead interdisciplinary teams.

Bibliography

Books

Bethel JM. *Making a Difference: 12 Qualities That Make You a Leader*. New York: GP Putnam's Sons, 1990.

Black JM, and Matassarin-Jacobs E [eds]. *Luckmann and Sorensen's Medical-Surgical Nursing: A Psychophysiologic Approach*. 4th ed. Philadelphia: WB Saunders, 1992.

Bolander VB. *Sorensen and Luckmann's Basic Nursing: A Psychophysiologic Approach*. 3rd ed. Philadelphia: WB Saunders, 1994.

Bullough B, and Bullough V. *Nursing Issues for the Nineties and Beyond*. New York: Springer Publishing Co, 1994.

Deloughery GL. *Issues and Trends in Nursing*. St. Louis: Mosby–Year Book, 1990.

Douglas LM. *The Effective Nurse, Leader and Manager*. St. Louis: Mosby–Year Book, 1992.

Gillies DA. *Nursing Management, a Systems Approach*. 3rd ed. Philadelphia: WB Saunders, 1994.

Griffin RW, and Ebert R. *Business*. 3rd ed. Englewood Cliffs, NJ: Prentice-Hall, 1992.

Grohar-Murray ME, and Di Croce HR. *Leadership and Management in Nursing*. Norwalk, CT: Appleton & Lange, 1992.

Hamilton PM. *Realities of Contemporary Nursing*. Redding, MA: Addison-Wesley, 1992.

Marquis BL, and Husten CJ. *Management Decision Making for Nurses*. 2nd ed. Philadelphia: JB Lippincott, 1994.

Mitchell PR, and Grippando GM. *Nursing Perspectives and Issues*. 5th ed. Albany, NY: Delmar Publishers, Inc, 1993.

Swansburg C. *Management and Leadership for Nurse Managers*. Boston: Jones and Bartlett Publishers, 1990.

Wywialowski E. *Managing Client Care*. St. Louis: Mosby–Year Book, 1993.

Zerwekh J, and Claborn JC. *Nursing Today: Transition and Trends*. Philadelphia: WB Saunders, 1994.

Chapters in Books and Journal Articles

Barden RM. Evaluating critical care staff. *In* Cardin S, and Ward CR (eds). *Personnel Management in Critical Care Nursing*. Baltimore: Williams & Wilkins, 1989.

Barkauskas VH. Case management within home care. *Home Healthc Nurse* 12(1):8, 1994.

Barter M, and Furmidge ML. Nursing's new frontier: Reinventing our practice in a restructured health care system. *Semin Nurse Managers* 3(4):166–174, 1995.

Brandt MA. Caring leadership: Secret and path to success. *Nurs Manage* 25(8):68–72, 1994.

Brider P. The move to patient-focused care. *Am J Nurs* 92(9):26–33, 1992.

Brown KC. Written communication. A key management skill. *AAOHN J* 38(9):455–456, 1990.

Bushardt SC, and Fowler AR. Performance evaluation alternatives. *JONA* 18(10):40–44, 1988.

Chu S, and Thom J. Information technology as a practice strategic weapon in health care. *J Nurs Adm* 24(4):5–9, 1994.

Duffield C. Nursing unit managers. Defining a role. *Nurs Manage* 25(4):63–67, 1994.

Everson-Bates S. First-line nurse managers in the expanded role, an ethnographic analysis. *J Nurs Adm* 22(2):32–37, 1992.

Fiesta J. Criminal liability for the nurse. *Nurs Manage* 23(5):16–17, 1992.

Fondiller S. The new look in nursing documentation. *Am J Nurs* 91(9):65–75, 1991.

Fowler A, et al. Retaining nurses through conflict resolution. *Health Prog* 25–29, 1993.

Fraser LE, et al. Patient care plans for intershift report. *J Pediatr Nurs* 6(5):310–316, 1991.

Harrell MS. Practical strategies for delegation and team building in a redesigned environment. *Semin Nurse Managers* 3(4):180–184, 1995.

Hughes TL, and Smith LL. Is your colleague chemically dependent? *Am J Nurs* 94(9):31–35, 1994.

Hurley ML. Focusing on outcomes. *RN* 57(5):57–60, 1994.

Hurley ML. Where will you work tomorrow? *RN* 57(8):31–35, 1994.

Roberts-DeGennaro M. Generalist model of case management practice. *J Case Manage* 2(3):106–111, 1993.

Russ AM. Downsizing: A survival kit for employees. *Nurs Manage* 25(6):66–67, 1994.

Simpson RL. How technology enhances total quality improvement. *Nurs Manage* 25(6):40–41, 1994.

Smith LL. Coping with disability: Nurse administrators' obligations under the Americans with Disabilities Act. *J Nurs Adm* 22(3):29–31, 1992.

Tahan H. The nurse case manager in acute care settings: Job descriptions and function. *J Nurs Adm* 23(2):53–60, 1993.

Tonges MC, and Lawrenz E. Reengineering: The work design-technology link. *J Nurs Adm* 23(10):15–22, 1993.

Townsend MB. Twenty-four hour care terms. *Nurs Manage* 25(6):62–64, 1994.

Performing a Holistic Health Assessment

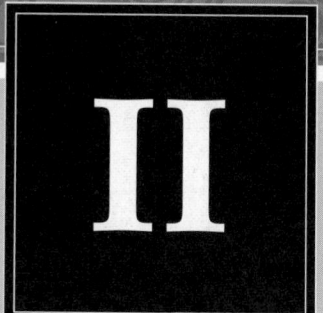

II

4

Obtaining the Basic
Health History

◼ OVERVIEW

Definition

1. A basic health history is an accurate and complete account of a person's past and current health.
   a. It describes the person as a whole, and how he or she interacts with the environment.
   b. It includes information about the person's strengths, problems, beliefs, values, health practices, and needs.
   c. It may be taken when the person enters the health care system (the extent and depth may vary as time and the person's condition permit). Or portions of the history may be taken over time, depending on the person's health needs.
2. The health history is the first step in health assessment, which is the first step in the nursing process.

Purposes

> The overall goal in taking a basic health history is to evaluate the status of the person's well-being.

1. To collect *subjective* data about a patient.
2. To create a patient database by combining this subjective history with *objective* data from a physical examination and laboratory studies.
3. To help you establish a trusting relationship with a patient.

Uses

1. To screen people for health problems and abnormal symptoms.
2. To assess lifestyles of the healthy to evaluate their usual health promotion and health maintenance behaviors and the effectiveness of these behaviors.
3. To assess health problems of the ill and their reaction to these problems.
4. To make nursing judgments and develop nursing diagnoses.

5. To identify realistic goals and outcomes to help people manage their responses to health problems.
6. To explore the effectiveness of a person's efforts to manage health problems through self-care.
7. To initiate discharge or follow-up planning by identifying potential future needs of the person.

Legal and Ethical Issues

1. History taking involves an unwritten (verbal) contract between you and the person.
2. Defining the terms of the contract early in the process reduces interpersonal stress and helps the nurse and patient set mutual goals and establish an atmosphere of trust.
3. The "contract" describes your role and the patient's role.
   a. It establishes a basis for shared management of the person's health problem.
   b. It clarifies expectations about what you can accomplish and what is expected of the patient.
4. Terms for the verbal contract might include the following:
   a. Time and place for the interview and any additional sessions, such as the physical examination.
   b. Length of the interview.
   c. Number of sessions needed for completion.
   d. Purpose of the interview.
   e. Your stated expectation that the person will actively participate throughout the assessment process.

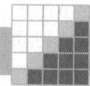 **LEGAL AND ETHICAL CONSIDERATIONS**

The patient has the right to every consideration of privacy. Case discussion, consultation, examination, and treatment should be conducted so as to protect each patient's privacy.

The patient has the right to expect that all communications and records pertaining to his/her care will be treated as confidential by the hospital, except in cases such as suspected abuse and public health hazards when reporting is permitted or required by law. The patient has the right to expect that the hospital will emphasize the confidentiality of this information when it releases it to any other parties entitled to review information in these records.

Reprinted with permission from the American Hospital Association's Patient's Bill of Rights. Copyright 1992.

f. Mutual agreement about the presence or participation of other people during the assessment process (e.g., spouse, family members or friends, interpreters, other health professionals).

g. Your responsibilities regarding confidentiality of information divulged by the person.

(1) Patients have a right to know who will have access to the information they give you. This information should be shared only with nursing staff, physicians, and other health team members who *need* access to the information.

NURSE ADVISORY

Do *not* discuss the person's health history with nonmedical personnel or the person's family or friends without the person's permission.

---

(2) Assure patients that information is kept confidential unless it puts you or others under a legal obligation. For example, you must report the following:

• Physical abuse of a child or an elderly person.

• Gunshot wounds.

• Certain infectious diseases, such as tuberculosis, syphilis, cholera, typhus, and malaria. Infection with the human immunodeficiency virus does not have to be reported to the Centers for Disease Control and Prevention (CDC), but some states require that it be reported. Acquired immunodeficiency syndrome must be reported to the CDC when accompanied by opportunistic disorders (see Chapter 42).

(3) If you are required to report a problem you suspect exists, explain this requirement. If this explanation leads the person to attempt to leave the interview, explain the dangers of *not* continuing with assessment and treatment so that the person can make an informed decision.

h. Any fees or costs, if applicable.

5. If the person cannot speak or understand English (or the language in which you conduct the interview), you have an ethical (and in some cases legal) obligation to arrange for an interpreter (see no. 6 under "Obtaining the Health History").

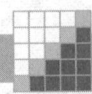

LEGAL AND ETHICAL CONSIDERATIONS

Under U.S. federal laws, any health care facility that receives federal funds from the Department of Health and Human Services *cannot* deny an interpreter to anyone seeking or receiving treatment. Moreover, under Title 45 Code of Federal Regulations, part 80, "such aids must be provided without additional charge to persons needing them in order to benefit equally from any service, program, or activity."

■ OBTAINING THE HEALTH HISTORY

Preparing and Planning for the Interview

1. Arrange the environment to promote accurate communication, rapport, and development of trust.

2. Maintain privacy.
   a. If possible, go to a vacant room and close the door.
   b. In a multibed room, close the cubicle curtains, and give your undivided attention to the person. Try to keep your voice low so that you will not be overheard.

3. Reduce interruptions. Inform colleagues that you have scheduled an interview, and refuse calls except for emergencies.

4. Create a favorable physical environment.
   a. Adjust the room temperature to a comfortable level.
   b. Control the lighting to avoid glare on your writing surface or a bright light shining into the patient's face.
   c. Reduce the noise level by turning off the radio, television, or unnecessary equipment.
   d. Remove distracting objects such as clutter, mail, or extra equipment.
   e. Arrange chairs to face each other at a slight angle, 2 to 4 feet apart, so that you are at eye level with the person.
   f. Allow the person to remain in street clothes, if possible.

5. Avoid long interviews that may tire the person. Schedule more than one session if needed.

6. If the patient does not speak fluent English, arrange for an interpreter.
   a. Choose an interpreter (if needed) carefully, to protect the person's privacy and to ensure accuracy.
   b. Ask if there are people who should *not* be asked to interpret, such as a young man to interpret for an older woman.
   c. If possible, meet with the interpreter *before* meeting with the patient and advise the individual of the nature of the questions you will be asking.

TRANSCULTURAL CONSIDERATIONS

Obtaining a complete health history means asking many technical questions—and often getting technical answers. Such communication is impossible with someone who does not speak your language unless an interpreter is brought in to bridge the language gap.

Although you may be forced to use a family member to interpret during an emergency, use a professional interpreter whenever possible. A patient may be more willing to give certain types of information—especially about sexual matters—to a stranger he or she will never see again than to a family member who must be faced daily in the years to come. Moreover, embarrassment or shame are unlikely to keep the professional from omitting such information from a translation. In addition, an experienced interpreter will follow up on a patient's vague answer to obtain more specific information or to clarify his or her meaning.

Conducting the Interview

1. Conducting the interview involves introducing new topics, developing and exploring topics, and assisting the person to respond to a series of questions.
2. Opening the interview
   a. Always introduce yourself and state how you want to be addressed. Address the person by surname, then ask the person's preference in address.
   b. Help the person to become comfortable. Offer a chair, a glass of water, or time to prepare for the interview.
   c. Explain the purpose of the interview and how long it will last.
   d. Establish the terms of the verbal contract (see "Legal and Ethical Issues"). Encourage the person to ask questions.
   e. Explain that you will be taking notes on the person's responses to your questions.
      (1) Take notes sparingly, as extensive note taking may interfere with active listening and rapport.
      (2) Use a pocket-sized outline or agency-approved form.

NURSE ADVISORY

Give the person your undivided attention.

3. Use verbal techniques to promote rapport by helping the person feel comfortable, relaxed, and respected. Building trust and rapport results in more accurate data.
   a. Describe what will be done during the interview and what to expect.
   b. Explain why you are asking for certain information even if it does not seem related to the immediate situation. Include the following reasons in your explanation:
      (1) To identify actual or possible problems.
      (2) To determine the resources available to and barriers faced by the person in resolving health care problems.
      (3) To assess whether the person is adapting to the effects of a condition. For example, you might ask a person with arthritis about the preferred method of bathing (tub bath or shower), the ability to negotiate stairs in the home, and whether there have been changes in the frequency or positions assumed for sexual intercourse.
   c. Ask *closed* or *directed* questions only for specific information. Direct questions usually receive short, limited answers. This method may limit rapport.
   d. Ask *open-ended* questions to introduce a topic and to obtain detailed information on topics. Such questions allow the person to answer freely, using longer phrases and sentences to express feelings and opinions.
   e. Try to allow for some flexibility in the interview to accommodate the nature of the person's problems, his or her answers, and any areas of hesitancy in response.

f. Use prompts such as "Go on" to encourage a person to keep talking.
g. Include transition statements to signal movement from one topic to another, and give the person a chance to finish discussing each topic before moving on. For example, "I have no more questions about _____. Is there anything else you want to add?"
h. Use *reflection*.
   (1) Repeat the person's words to encourage explanation or description of a problem.
   (2) Focus on an expressed feeling to help clarify what the person means. For example, "You feel anxious when the pain starts?"
i. Use *empathy* to acknowledge the person's feelings before he or she mentions them. For example, if the person says "I'm not used to being in bed all day with nothing to do," you might respond, "It must be hard when you're used to being busy at work and at home."
j. Use the following methods to clarify vague, ambiguous, conflicting, or confusing information:
   (1) Restate what the person has said in more specific words. For example, "Do you mean . . . ?"
   (2) State what you think the person is implying. For example, "The pain was in your chest; were you afraid that it was something serious?"
   (3) Define time limits by placing an event in sequence. For example, "What were you doing when the pain began?"
   (4) Seek validation of specific symptoms or concerns. For example, "Did the pain last longer than a minute?"
k. Explore observed actions, feelings, or statements to clarify inconsistencies between verbal and nonverbal behavior or to amplify the person's story.
   (1) Mention your observations to help a person modify or explain inconsistencies. For example, "You say you are relaxed, but your fists are clenched."
   (2) Make observations to help you understand nonverbal behavior and to encourage the person to reveal other concerns. For example, "I see that you rub your arm when we talk about your chest pain. Does the pain travel to your arm?"
l. Interpret the person's answers by sorting the data and drawing conclusions.
m. Share facts, observations, and your interpretations with the person and get him or her to validate, refute, or reinterpret the conclusions. Encourage the person to be an active member of the health care team.
n. Summarize the perceived health problems for the person's review and to signal the end of the interview or a transition to another topic.
o. Use active listening techniques.
   (1) Active listening requires your full attention. Focus on the person and on what he or she is saying (or not saying).
   (2) Avoid thinking about what you will say next.
   (3) Look at the person, lean forward slightly, keep your arms relaxed, and maintain a comfortable level of eye contact.

p. Use silence as a technique.
   (1) Silence allows you and the person to think about and organize what you both want to say.
   (2) Following a question, give the person time to answer while you observe his or her reactions, including nonverbal behavior.

NURSE ADVISORY

Silence encourages the person to continue. Avoid the urge to fill the quiet with dialogue.

   (3) *Transcultural considerations:* Recognize that the communication style of some ethnic groups (e.g., Asians and Native Americans) includes prolonged silences to indicate reflection and consideration of a subject. Allow extra time for responses on the part of such persons.
4. Use nonverbal techniques to enhance your relationship with the person and to obtain unspoken information about him or her.
   a. Forms of nonverbal communication include physical appearance, posture and body language, facial expression, eye movement, voice, and touch (Table 4–1).

NURSE ADVISORY

Use touch judiciously, especially in taking the health history. Touch can be a source of comfort to a patient in distress, but it can also be subject to misinterpretation.

   b. Your nonverbal actions convey messages to the person and may help him or her respond to your questions.
   c. The person's nonverbal behavior can reveal how he or she feels about your questions and the health issues under discussion.
      (1) If a topic is uncomfortable to discuss, the person may stiffen, shift in the chair, or pull away from you slightly and block further discussion.
      (2) The person may become more animated, lean forward, and make eye contact if the topic is important.
   d. Be sure your verbal and nonverbal messages agree and convey friendliness, sincerity, and patience. For example, do not say "Take your time" and then shift in your chair, tap your foot, glance at your watch, or shuffle your notes, which the person may interpret as impatience or annoyance.
5. Techniques to avoid
   a. Verbal and nonverbal techniques that restrict the person's responses or make them unclear.
      (1) Leading or biased questions suggest to the person that there is a "correct" or most acceptable answer. For example, "You don't smoke, do you?"
      (2) Complex questions confuse both parties, because

an answer may apply to only one part of the question. For example, does the answer "yes" to the question "Do you ever have blurred vision, headaches, or dizziness?" mean the person has all three, two, or only one symptom? Do the symptoms occur together or at different times?
      (3) Persistent questions in one area can make the person uncomfortable, defensive, and reluctant to continue the interview. If the person indicates a particular topic is painful to discuss, drop the subject, at least temporarily. If the information is important, bring the topic up again later in the interview, when the person may be more comfortable with you. If information is crucial because emergency treatment may depend on it, explain this to the person and attempt to elicit the information.
   b. "Why" or "how" questions, which may put people on the defensive if they think you are blaming or condemning them or if they feel you expect an answer they cannot supply.
   c. False reassurances and platitudes, which may relieve your anxiety but devalue the person's feelings. For example, "It will be all right" does not allow the person to express fears or other feelings.
   d. Deference to the physician's authority, which implies lack of respect for the patient and suggests inferiority or dependency. For example, "The doctor will decide what to do."
   e. Unfamiliar jargon or inappropriate terms, which may be confusing or frightening. The person may believe you are withholding information or may be too embarrassed to ask for clarification.
   f. Cliches and stereotyped responses, which deny the person's individuality and discourage discussion of feelings. For example, "Pain is common in this problem."
   g. *Distancing*—using depersonalizing language—which deprives the person of identity, is impersonal, and implies disinterest in the person's uniqueness. For example, "We'll need to check the leg" (instead of "your leg").
   h. Excessive talking, which interferes with the person's ability to express his or her needs and concerns.
   i. Changing the subject or interrupting, which disrupts the person's thoughts and conveys boredom, lack of empathy, or impatience. You may also confuse or distract the person.
   j. Signaling that a response is "good," which implies that a different response is "not good" and may inhibit the person from supplying additional information.
   k. Jumping to conclusions and premature interpretation of data, which may be incorrect and may stifle further revelations, especially if the person perceives disapproval.
   l. Responding defensively to verbal attack against "the system," which may further antagonize the person and inhibit his or her expression.
6. If problems arise in taking the health history, look for

Table 4–1. Nonverbal Behaviors and the Health History

Nonverbal Behavior	Patient Behaviors	Transcultural Considerations	Nurse Behaviors
Physical appearance (dress and grooming)	Reflects socioeconomic status, role image (businessperson, shop clerk, student), attitude (fastidious, casual, provocative), physical and mental function, ability to maintain appearance (physical or emotional self-care ability, self-regard), general health or illness	May be culturally determined (Amish people wear 19th-century clothing; Indian women wear saris; Arab men wear long robes, beards, and head coverings)	Be aware of your own values regarding dress, grooming, and attractiveness. Do not let them interfere with your ability to help people whose values differ from yours. Neat grooming and professional attire enhance your own credibility.
Posture and body language (position, gestures, muscle tension)	May convey thoughts and feelings. Open position (large muscles extended) suggests relaxation, comfort, willingness to divulge information. Closed position (limbs crossed or close to body) suggests anxiety or defensiveness. Changing position (from open to closed) or tensing muscles suggests discomfort with current topic. Revealing gestures include head nodding (agreement/acceptance or disagreement), hand wringing (anxiety), finger pointing (anger, locating a symptom), and fist clenching (anxiety, discomfort, or anger).	Differs among cultures (bowing one's head in the presence of a superior is traditional in many Asian cultures; pointing is unacceptable to Navajos; waving to attract attention and pointing the toes out from the body are not acceptable to Vietnamese)	Remain calm, relaxed, and seated to show your interest in the person.
Facial expression (e.g., smiling, frowning, yawning)	Can indicate alertness, interest, relaxation, anxiety, fear, anger, pain, or suspicion	Members of some cultures, especially Asians, may view open expressions of emotion as inappropriate.	Look attentive, sincere, and interested. Avoid expressions of boredom, disgust, or disbelief.
Eye contact and movement (steady, direct gaze; averted eyes; darting eyes; blinking)	Can reflect level of attention and interest. Lack of eye contact may be seen as shyness, guilt, confusion, boredom, apathy, withdrawal, or depression. Pupil size can indicate anxiety, tension, fright (dilation), or relaxation (contraction).	Depending on culture, eye contact may be seen as disrespectful (Navajo), rude (Chinese), or an act of aggression (Vietnamese).	Maintain eye contact with periodic breaks. Avoid staring.
Voice (tone, intensity, rapidity, pitch, pauses)	Loud, rapid speech often accompanies anxiety. Slow, monotonous speech with frequent pauses can signal depression.	In many cultures (Appalachian, Native American, Asian) soft speech and multiple pauses are normal voice patterns.	Keep your voice even and low. Adjust the volume to the hearing ability of the person. Use pauses to signal subject transitions and allow time for person to respond.
Touch	Age, sex, experience, and current circumstances affect how the person interprets touch (touching a person's arm may be viewed as an invasion of personal space or as an attempt to comfort).	Cultural norms regarding touch vary widely. Members of some cultures freely touch one another (Italian, Spanish). Other cultures limit touch severely (English, Asian). Touching between genders may be highly unacceptable or forbidden.	As a rule, avoid touching during the interview.

Table 4–2. Guide to Basic Health History Assessment

Interview date (included as a baseline for later reference)

Biographic and Demographic Data

Full name (include nicknames, aliases, and other alternative forms, if applicable)
Age
Sex
Race
Nationality or ethnic background
Primary language
Date and place of birth
Significant others (family or friends) and relationship to person
Home address (and alternate contact address, if applicable)
Phone number(s)
Occupation (usual and current)

Social Security number
Religion
Emergency contact
Legal guardian (if necessary)
Source of information and reliability as a historian (note use of an interpreter, if needed)
Source of referral to agency and/or usual primary caregiver
Health insurance information
Advance directive and/or living will information

Current Symptoms

Reason for Seeking Health Care (in person's own words)

Symptom Analysis (in-depth analysis of up to 3 symptoms):

- Last time person was well (discriminate between onset of symptom and when person became concerned about it)
- Date and time of onset, including time period over which symptom evolved (slow? abrupt?)
- Setting (what was person doing and where was person when symptom began?)
- How was person feeling before problem's onset?
- Location of symptom (localized? diffuse? radiating?)
- Quality (description) of symptom's characteristics (burning? piercing? stabbing? dull? aching? throbbing?)
- Quantity or severity rated by person using an analogue scale (e.g., 1 to 10, with 1 as the least and 10 as the most or worst)
- Duration or how long symptom lasts (intermittent? constant? goes away completely?)
- Frequency or how often symptom occurs (daily? weekly? monthly?)
- Factors that seem to bring on the symptom
- Factors that seem to aggravate the symptom (activity? weather? eating? medication? position? fatigue? time of year or day?)
- Factors that relieve symptoms (rest? sleep? medication? heat? cold?)
- Associated factors or symptoms in other body systems that seem concurrent. Review the associated body system at this time instead of later.
- Does symptom interfere with person's usual activities? Do interferences cause problems (what types) for the person?

Past Health History

Developmental (may not be appropriate for adults)

- Any known problems with growth and development, including prenatal or birth history (e.g., premature delivery or low birth weight) or delay in language, speech, motor skills?

Immunizations

- Childhood immunizations (tetanus, diphtheria, pertussis, measles, mumps, rubella, polio, *Haemophilus b* conjugate, hepatitis B) given when? Kept up to date?
- Last dates of tetanus booster and influenza vaccination?
- If age 65 or older, has received pneumococcal vaccination?

Past Illnesses (childhood and adulthood)

- Ever had measles (rubeola), mumps, rubella, chicken pox, whooping cough (pertussis), scarlet fever, strep throat, rheumatic fever, poliomyelitis, asthma, tuberculosis, pneumonia?
- Presence of diabetes mellitus, heart disease, hypertension, kidney problems, ulcers, thyroid problems, migraine headaches, seizure disorders, stroke (cerebral vascular accident), arthritis, Lyme disease, cancer, anemia, sickle cell anemia, bleeding tendencies, or human immunodeficiency virus infection?

Hospitalizations

- Date and reason for each admission
- Summary of treatment, length of hospitalization
- Name of primary care physician(s)
- Outcomes and person's reaction to hospitalizations

Table 4–2. Guide to Basic Health History Assessment
(Continued)

Past Health History

Surgeries

- Date and type of procedures performed
- Name of surgeon(s)
- Performed as inpatient or outpatient?
- Outcomes and person's reaction to surgeries

Obstetric History (if applicable)

- For completed pregnancies: Number; course of each pregnancy, labor, delivery, and postpartum period; delivery date; birth weight, sex, and infant's health
- For incomplete pregnancies: Number; duration of pregnancy; date and circumstances of termination (spontaneous or induced abortion, stillbirth)
- Complications

Last Visit(s) to Health Care Providers

- Most recent dates for dental, physical, vision, and hearing examinations
- Results of screening or diagnostic tests performed, such as electrocardiogram, radiology studies, Papanicolaou (Pap) smear, purified protein derivative (PPD) or tuberculosis tine test

Allergies

- Known allergens: Medications (true allergic reactions only and not side effects), food, contact agents (fabric, nickel), and environmental agents (dust, dander, pollens, cigarette smoke)
- Allergic reactions (rash, pruritus, watery eyes, nasal congestion, running nose, breathing difficulty)

Medications

- What is currently taken: Prescription (including birth control pills), nonprescription over-the-counter (aspirin, vitamins, antacids, cold and allergy preparations, topical creams and lotions—ask about by name, as many people do not think of these as medications), recreational drugs?
- For all medications: Name; dose; route; frequency and time of day taken; reason for taking; any problems with taking; who prescribed each drug and when?

Family Health History

- Members' ages, cause of death, and age at death
- Does/did any family member have heart disease, hypertension (high blood pressure), cerebral vascular accidents (stroke), epilepsy (seizures), migraines or headaches, mental illness, Alzheimer's disease, Huntington's chorea, alcoholism, tuberculosis, asthma, allergies, diabetes mellitus, thyroid problems, eating disorders (overeating, undereating, self-induced vomiting), obesity, kidney disease, arthritis, cancer (type), sickle cell anemia, anemia, hemophilia, human immunodeficiency virus infection, developmental delay?

possible barriers to communication and apply special techniques to overcome these barriers.

a. Barriers to communication include semantic, transcultural, socioeconomic, age, and gender differences as well as physical and mental impairments.

b. *Semantic (word-based) barriers* are related to the meanings in language. Use easily understood words and avoid medical or technical terms unless you explain their meaning.

c. *Transcultural barriers* are related to cultural differences between you and the patient (see Chapter 2). To overcome the tendency toward **ethnocentrism** (the tendency to view your own culture as superior to any other), follow these guidelines:

(1) Avoid cultural stereotyping. Both your cultural background and that of the patient may affect the interview process and how you perceive each other. However, do not *assume* that a person will-hold certain values because he or she is a member of a particular cultural group; inquire about the individual's values.

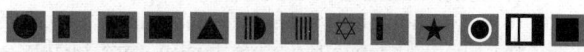

TRANSCULTURAL CONSIDERATIONS

Cultural stereotyping can seriously interfere with your relationshi with a patient. The patient may become angry and withhold infor mation, thus jeopardizing your ability to make accurate nursin diagnoses.

Similarities among people allow for grouping, which can be use ful in establishing a starting point. However, each member of a group is an individual with unique differences. Avoid the tendency to generalize from a group's similar characteristics and apply them rigidly to a specific person (stereotyping). Stereotyping can lead to missed diagnoses if you attempt to make the information from the person fit a stereotyped image.

(2) Become familiar with culture-related behavi demonstrated by persons from cultures wi which you commonly interact (e.g., aggressiv quiet, passive) to help you understand them.

(3) Recognize the person's preferred personal spatial distance and do not cross these boundaries without permission.

(4) Consider nonverbal communication in its cultural context, especially eye contact, body language, touch, and use of silence (see Table 4–1).

(5) Identify cultural norms governing male-female relationships at the beginning of the interview. For example, "Is there anything I should know about how men and women in your culture act with each other so that I do not offend you?" Whenever possible, try to adhere to these norms to avoid creating uncomfortable or forbidden situations.

(6) Be aware that some cultures restrict discussion of certain topics (e.g., deceased people). If you ask about a restricted topic inadvertently, apologize for making the person uncomfortable. If the information is vital, explain why it is necessary. Respect that the person may refuse or be unable to discuss the topic.

(7) Throughout the interview, keep in mind that different cultural values may affect all aspects of health and health care, including (but not limited to) beliefs, values, nutritional practices, religion, and spirituality (see also Chapter 6).

d. *Socioeconomic barriers* are related to the person's social support network, educational background, or economic status. Use the following information to help overcome these blocks:

(1) Ask about the person's social support network—those people most important in the person's life in matters of health and illness. The network may include family members, peers, friends, spiritual advisers, or alternative health care practitioners (see Chapter 6 for more detail).

 • Determine whether social support network members are available to assist the person in answering health questions. You may need to help the person contact people or to arrange for a social worker to do so.

 • A patient without an obvious support network (e.g., a homeless person) may have sought treatment in an alternative health care facility, such as a freestanding clinic. If the patient can remember the name of the clinic, call the clinic personnel and ask for additional health history information.

 • The presence of too many family members or friends is distracting and interferes with the interview. Limit the number of people present to those whose presence is essential.

(2) Educational issues include language ability, literacy, and learning style. Ask about the highest level of education the person has attained. This knowledge may help you choose your words. Determine whether the person can read and write in English or in another language. You may need to adapt written materials for the person to understand. Ask about the person's preferred learning style: written material, verbal explanation, visual demonstration, or a combination of techniques.

(3) Economic status can be a block if the person is worried about the cost of health care, including your services.

 • Ask whether the person's health care insurance is adequate to meet the anticipated needs. Make arrangements for assistance (e.g., enrollment in Medicare or Medicaid) if necessary.

 • Ask whether the person has other pressing financial concerns that may compete with paying for health care. The person may feel that a temporary "fix the problem" approach is all that is necessary for now and seek to hurry the interview.

 • If appropriate, refer the person to a social worker or other counseling service of the person's choice.

e. Age and gender barriers

(1) Older people may require more time because of physical impairments (e.g., deafness or other physical disabilities; see later discussion), because they have longer health histories to review than younger persons (see also Chapter 16), or because of both.

(2) Whenever possible, interview minor children in the presence of their parents or guardians. Very young children especially may be unable to supply health history information on their own (see also Chapter 15).

(3) Communication styles of men and women may differ, which may affect the interview process between you and a patient of the opposite sex. Men may attempt to dominate the interview and may have difficulty expressing their thoughts and feelings. Women may express their emotions and feelings more freely, especially to another woman.

7. Communicating with persons with a physical or mental impairment can be challenging. The following suggestions may be helpful.

a. Hearing-impaired people

(1) For persons with a slight to moderate impairment, ask if they prefer lip reading, signing, or writing (see Chapter 20).

 • Speak naturally and distinctly. Do not shout; it distorts sounds. Slow speech and exaggerated mouthing of words are harder to understand.

 • Face the person so that your face is illuminated and easier for the person to see. If you have a beard or a mustache or speak with a foreign accent, arrange for another nurse to perform the assessment, as these traits may interfere with the deaf person's ability to read your lips.

 • Ask if the person has a "good" ear and, if so, speak in that direction.

 • Attract the person's attention before beginning to speak. Supplement your words with pantomime.

 • Use written forms for parts of the history such as the past health history and review of systems.

(2) For the person who is completely deaf, ask if the

person knows sign language and would like an interpreter. Allow time for signing.

b. Visually impaired people do not need modification of the health history interview unless they have other problems that interfere with communication. Use a normal tone of voice; remember that your nonverbal communication will not be seen by the person, but sounds and movements will be heard (see Chapter 19).

c. Physically impaired people may not require modification of the health history format unless they are unable to tolerate the length of a complete interview or have speech problems (e.g., from cerebral palsy). Schedule several sessions or arrange for a family member to assist in the interview if necessary.

d. The abilities of intellectually impaired people to participate in the health history interview vary greatly.

(1) Determine whether the individual is legally competent. If not, be sure to obtain the consent and assistance of the person's legal guardian.

(2) For the mildly or moderately impaired person, use simple phrases. Schedule several brief sessions to accommodate a shortened attention span.

(3) For the severely impaired person, ask a family member or friend to provide information.

e. People under the influence of mind-altering substances may perceive your questions and actions as threatening (see also Chapter 40).

(1) Remain calm and ask simple, direct questions. Do not scold or show disgust.

(2) Complete only those portions of the history interview that are necessary for the person's immediate care needs. Plan to return after the person is no longer under the influence of a substance.

f. Emotionally disturbed people may have difficulty participating in an interview, depending on the nature of their problem (see also Chapter 41).

(1) Remain calm and ask simple, direct questions.

(2) You may need to reschedule the interview, complete portions over several sessions, or ask a family member or friend to supply information.

Closing the Interview

1. Give the person the initiative by saying that you have completed your questions. Ask if there is anything else he or she would like to discuss.

2. Summarize your findings and conclusions about the person's health status, and ask the person to confirm or amend them.

3. Explain what will happen next, such as follow-up plans or preparations for the physical examination.

4. Do not end abruptly or awkwardly, as doing so may damage your therapeutic relationship with the person. For example, you might say, "Our interview is almost finished. Thank you for talking with me and helping me to understand you better."

■ RECORDING THE BASIC HEALTH HISTORY

A Note on Data Collection

1. A suggested sequence for data collection follows.

2. Note that the sequence—and the depth of questioning—depends on the agency's form, the person's specific situation, and time constraints.

Biographic and Demographic Data

1. These data (Table 4–2) identify the individual.

2. They provide sociocultural information that can serve as clues for personal health risk (see "Health Risk Appraisal" in Table 4–3).

Current Symptoms

1. Also called chief complaint (CC) and history of present illness (HPI) (see Table 4–2).

2. Use the person's own words to describe the reason for the visit. This is *not* a medical diagnosis.

3. Explore each symptom with a symptom analysis.

Past Health History

1. Explore the individual's perceptions of past health events, how he or she responded to illness episodes, and the significance of these illnesses to the person (see Table 4–2).

2. Past health and illness events can have lingering effects on current health status

Family Health History

1. Information on the patient's family members can help identify risk factors that are genetic or familial in origin (see Table 4–2).

2. Family members include the person's blood relatives (grandparents, parents, aunts, uncles, sisters, brothers, and children) as well as the spouse.

3. Many diseases have a strong genetic link (e.g., diabetes mellitus, polycystic kidney disease). Other health problems occur in family groups because of an increased risk of exposure, rather than a known genetic factor (e.g., tuberculosis, hepatitis).

4. Family history information should include the ages of living members and the ages at death and causes of death of deceased members. A family tree similar to that shown in Figure 4–1 may be useful in recording such information.

Text continued on page 99

Table 4–3. Health Risk Appraisal

Risk Factors*	Examples of Potential Health Problems	Key Questions and Issues to Include
Genetic or Family Related		
Heart disease (onset before age 50)	Cardiovascular disease; hypercholesterolemia; hyperlipidemia	Is there any history of heart problems in your family (describe)? Have you ever had your blood cholesterol measured? Do you know your cholesterol level? Do you smoke or did you ever smoke (what? how much? how long?)? Does anyone smoke in your home? Do you exercise regularly (type? frequency? duration?)? What type of diet do you eat (describe)? Do you take any medicine for heart problems?
Hypertension	Cardiovascular disease; stroke	Do you or anyone in your family have a history of high blood pressure or stroke? Do you know what your blood pressure is? Do you take your own blood pressure or have it taken? Do you take any medicine for high blood pressure? How much salt do you use in cooking and on your food? Are you overweight or have you been told you should lose weight? (Also ask about exercise and activity patterns.)
Alcoholism	Alcohol abuse and related problems (e.g., cirrhosis, pancreatitis, accidents)	Is there a history of alcohol abuse in your family (who?)? How much alcohol do you drink in a week (beer, wine, wine coolers, mixed drinks, hard liquor)? Do you ever go on a binge (how often? how much alcohol?)? Did you drink a lot of alcohol in the past? If so, when did you stop? Have you ever gotten sick because of drinking too much? Have you ever tried to get help for a drinking problem? Are you interested in trying to stop drinking?
Diabetes	Diabetes, glucose intolerance, hyperglycemia	Does anyone in your family have diabetes (high blood sugar)? Who? How old were they when they got it? Did they need to take insulin or pills for it? Are you always hungry or thirsty? Do you have to urinate a lot (describe)? Do sores and cuts take a long time to heal? Do you take medicine for diabetes (what? how much? how often?)? Do you follow a special diet for high or low blood sugar (describe)? Do you measure your blood sugar (how often? with what?)? Do you have enough supplies to measure your blood sugar?
Obesity	Obesity-related problems (e.g., heart disease, hypertension, diabetes, muscle and joint injury)	Is anyone in your family overweight (who?)? Have you ever had a weight problem (describe)? Can you lose weight and keep it off? Do you try to diet? What kind(s) of diet(s) have you tried in the past? Did they work? Have you tried using a support group (e.g., Weight Watchers, TOPS) to help (did it help?)?
Breast cancer (in mother, sisters, daughters)	Breast cancer	Has anyone in your family had breast cancer (who)? How old were they when diagnosed? Do you practice breast self-examination (how often? when in relation to the menstrual cycle or when in month if past menopause?)? Have you ever had a mammogram (when last? results?)? How often do you have mammograms? Do you have problems with breast lumps? Have you ever had surgery on your breasts (when?)?
Fair skin tones	Skin cancer	Have you or a family member ever had skin cancer? Do you use a sunscreen and wear protective clothing when out in the sun? Do you do a head-to-toe skin self-inspection monthly? Have you ever had a skin growth removed (when?)? Have you ever had a severe sunburn?
Hypersensitivity reactions (describe)	Allergic reactions (e.g., bronchospasm, asthma, rhinitis, eczema, atopic dermatitis)	Do you or a family member have allergies (describe)? Do you know what triggers your allergy symptoms? Have you ever been tested for what triggers your symptoms? Do you take medicine for symptoms (what? how much? when?) or allergy shots to make you less sensitive?
Personal Habits		
Nutrition (e.g., consumption of calcium, fiber, caffeine, sodium, alcohol, fat)	Obesity, underweight, heart disease, hypertension, irritability, cancer of colon, osteoporosis	Describe your typical 24-hour diet. (Compare the person's recent diet pattern to the typical diet.) Have there been recent changes (appetite increase or decrease)? Do you have any medical dietary restrictions? Do you have problems with this diet? Do you have any cultural, ethnic, religious, or self-imposed restrictions on your diet or how food is prepared? Describe your food likes and dislikes. Do you take vitamins, minerals, or other types of diet supplements? Have you ever had anorexia or bulimia? What is your usual weight range? Is your weight stable? Have you gained or lost weight within the past 6 months? Who usually does the food shopping (the cooking?) for your family? Is there enough money to buy food for you and your family? Are you able to get to the grocery store? Do you have problems walking that make it difficult for you to do your shopping? Do you have problems chewing or swallowing?

	Table 4–3. Health Risk Appraisal (Continued)	
Risk Factors*	**Examples of Potential Health Problems**	**Key Questions and Issues to Include**
Elimination	Constipation, diarrhea, colon cancer, bladder cancer, incontinence	How often do you have a bowel movement? How often do you urinate? Has there been a change in the appearance of your urine or bowel movements or in how often you go? Do you use laxatives, suppositories, or enemas? (Consider the amount of fiber in the person's diet.) How much liquid do you drink during the day? Do you limit how much or when you drink? Why?
Tobacco use (smoked and smokeless)	Cancer of the mouth or lung, cardiovascular disease, respiratory disease	Do you smoke or have you ever smoked (type of tobacco product used, how much per day or week, for how long?)? Do you or have you ever chewed tobacco or snuff? Has your use of tobacco products changed (increased or decreased) over time? Do you smoke more if you feel stressed? Have you ever tried to stop (did you succeed?)? Do you want to stop? Do you have persistent cough, sore in mouth that does not heal, chronic hoarseness, or spitting up blood?
Alcohol consumption		(See previous discussion under "Alcoholism" in "Genetic or Family Related" risk factors section.)
Recreational drug use	Addiction; overdose; hepatitis; harmful side effects, including death	Do you take unprescribed drugs, medicines, or other psychoactive substances (e.g., street drugs; inhalants such as glue, paint thinner, or cleaning fluids)? Why? How much do you use in one day or week? How long have you used these substances? Has your pattern of using them changed with time (do you use them more or less?)? Are there times when you use them more often (e.g., when you feel stressed?)? Have you ever had a "bad time" after taking them (describe)? Do you want to quit? Do you need help to quit?
Safety awareness	Unintentional injury or death	Do you wear seatbelts when in a car or other vehicle? Do you drive after drinking alcohol? When you play a sport or do yard work or repair jobs, do you wear protective gear such as goggles, gloves, mask, ear plugs, body pads, or similar items? Do you operate heavy machinery? Do you know how to swim?
Sleep and rest patterns	Fatigue, lowered resistance to illness, increased risk of accidental injury	How many hours of sleep do you get every day? Do you find it is enough for you to feel rested? Do you get most of your sleep during the night or do you have a different schedule? Do you have problems falling asleep or staying asleep? Do you awaken at night gasping for air? Has anyone ever complained that you snore? Do you use anything to help you get to sleep (e.g., food, beverage, medication, reading)? Do you take naps? Do you get drowsy during the day?
Activity and exercise patterns	Strains, sprains, fractures; unintentional injury; obesity; cardiovascular disease	Describe your usual daily activities. Does this schedule change when you have time off from work (describe)? Do you follow an exercise plan? How often do you exercise? For how long at a time? Do you do warm-up and cool-down exercises? Have you ever had a problem from exercising (e.g., pain, dizziness)?
Recreation and relaxation patterns	Unrelieved stress or tension, irritability, unintentional injury, fatigue	What kinds of things do you enjoy doing to help you relax and have fun (include hobbies)? Do you get to spend as much time doing fun things as you would like? Do you like to do things with friends or family or do you prefer to be alone?
Lifestyle		
Lack of regular exercise		(See previous discussion under "Activity and Exercise Patterns" in "Personal Habits" risk factors section.)
Stress and coping ability (see also text discussion of stress assessment)	Fatigue, irritability, frequent illness, unintentional injury	Describe what you find stressful in your life at this time. Are you able to manage your stress level? What have you done to help yourself cope? Do you need help managing your stress level?
Lack of self-care activities to promote health	Numerous health problems	Do you get regular checkups to screen for health problems (e.g., blood pressure; vision; hearing; dental; pelvic; breast)? Do you remember when you got your last tetanus immunization? (Also ask about other immunizations.) Do you do any type of self-examination for health problems (e.g., breast self-examination)? (If the person has a chronic disease such as arthritis or hypertension, ask how he or she manages the effects of the disease, including diet and medications.)

Table continued on following page

Table 4–3. Health Risk Appraisal (Continued)

Risk Factors*	Examples of Potential Health Problems	Key Questions and Issues to Include
High-risk sexual activity	Unplanned pregnancy, sexually transmitted diseases (STDs), cervical cancer	How many sexual partners have you had in the past? Do you currently have intercourse with more than one person? Are you in a stable relationship at this time? Have you always used protection (e.g., a condom) when you had intercourse? Have you ever been treated for an STD (which? with what? were there any problems?)? Do you know about "safe" sexual practices? Would you like information on them?
Travel abroad	Diseases found in locale visited (e.g., parasites, malaria, cholera)	Did you get any immunizations before traveling? Did you eat any fresh fruit or vegetables (washed or unwashed) while there? Did you use ice or drink the local water without boiling or chemically treating it? Did you go swimming?
Environmental and Occupational		
Home environment	Unintentional injury, poisoning, strained interpersonal relationships	Describe your home. How old is it? Is there enough living space for your household members? How many people live in your home? Is there a private place for you to go when you need it? Does your home have enough light and ventilation (e.g., heating and cooling) for your needs? Where do you store cleaning solutions, chemicals, paint, tools, electrical equipment? Do you have smoke alarms (where?)? How often do you check them (change batteries?)? Do you have a plan to get everyone out of the home in case of fire? Does everyone know the plan? Do you know how to call for emergency help (e.g., 911)? Do you have easy access to a health care facility? Do you have a way to get there? Do you know of any environmental safety problems (e.g., air or water pollution, toxic waste disposal, radon gas) in your neighborhood or community?
Work environment	Symptoms related to stress response, job-related injuries (e.g., back strain, eye strain, "sick building" syndrome)	What types of jobs have you had in the past? Describe your current job. How many hours per day or week do you work? Are you satisfied with your job? How far do you commute to work? Do you get time for breaks and meals during work hours? Is your workplace well ventilated? Is there enough light to work without eye strain? Does your job involve heavy lifting or moving heavy objects? Do you operate machinery or heavy equipment? Do you wear safety gear (e.g., goggles, ear plugs, hard hat, work boots, insulated gloves) if your job is hazardous?
Noise level exposure	Hearing deficit	How noisy is your home? Your workplace? How much traffic is there on the street where you live? Do you live or work near an airport or a major highway? Do you operate any power tools, machinery, or heavy equipment? Have you ever had ear or hearing problems after listening to loud noises (describe, e.g., buzzing or ringing in the ears, diminished ability to hear)? Do you have a noisy hobby (e.g., woodworking, target shooting, hunting, playing in a band)?
Chemical fume or particle exposure	Toxic symptoms, pulmonary or skin problems	Do you work with pesticides, inhalants, or heavy metals (e.g., lead or mercury)? Do you wear a mask or respirator when using chemicals that can become airborne (e.g., paints, cleaning solutions, aerosols)? What other type of protective gear or clothing do you wear when you work with chemicals? Where do you store these clothes, and how do you clean them after use?
Socioeconomic		
Lack of health and dental insurance	Delayed or postponed treatment of health problems, undetected health problems	What kind of health and dental insurance do you have? Does it cover your health and illness care needs? Do you ever wait to get medical help because you worry about how you will pay for it? Do you want to talk to someone about getting help to pay for your care? Do you have enough money for other expenses of your family (e.g., rent, utilities)?
Recent immigration	Diseases or health problems common to the area of origin	What immunizations have you ever received (see Table 4–2)? What diseases and health problems are common in the country you come from because of the climate, living conditions, water supply, and the like? Have you ever had any of these diseases or health problems (describe)?

* Risk factors are representative and not inclusive.

Table 4–4. Review of Systems

Body Systems	Examples of Information and Questions to Cover
General	Any fever, chills, sweats, night sweats, weakness, weight loss or gain (in past 6 months), fatigue, malaise, nausea or vomiting, headaches, mood changes?
Integument Skin	Any past skin problems (e.g., scars, birthmarks, moles)? Ever had any skin lesions removed (describe)? Any current problems with dryness, psoriasis, eczema, pruritus (itching), rashes or other skin eruptions, odor, sore that does not heal, or change in skin lesion or growth? Do you bruise easily? Describe your skin care habits (e.g., use of soap, lotions, skin oils).
Hair	Any alopecia (hair loss), dryness, dandruff, or brittleness? Do you use hair dye or have a permanent wave? Describe your hair care habits (e.g., frequency of shampooing, use of conditioner, combing vs. brushing).
Nails	Any brittleness, cracking, splitting? Change in nail texture? Do you bite your nails? Wear nail polish? Have artificial nails?
Hematopoietic	Any problems with fatigue, unusual bleeding, easy bruising, anemia, or leukemia? Ever had a transfusion of blood or a blood product (were there any problems?)? Ever been exposed to radiation or toxic agents (describe)? Do you know your blood type (if Rh negative and you have been pregnant, do you recall receiving RhoGAM?)? Do you know if you have any unusual type of antibodies (describe)?
Endocrine	Any history of diabetes, goiter, thyroid, or abnormal growth or development? Ever been treated with hormones (describe) or had neck surgery (describe)? Any current problem with heat or cold intolerance, weakness, tremors, nervousness, dry skin or hair, excessive sweating, change in hair distribution, excess hair growth in unusual places (hirsutism), impotence, change in sexual activity or libido, increased thirst (polydipsia), increased urination (polyuria), or increased hunger (polyphagia)?
Head	Ever had a blow, trauma, or injury to the head? Any current problems with headaches (unusual or severe), lightheadedness or dizziness, syncope (fainting or loss of consciousness), vertigo (sense of spinning or moving in space [subjective], sense of objects moving around in space [objective]), seizures?
Eyes	Any history of eye infections (pink eye or conjunctivitis), eyelid cyst (chalazion), stye (hordeolum), glaucoma, cataracts, "lazy eye" (amblyopia), strabismus, detached retina? Ever received a blow to the eye or had eye surgery (describe)? Any current problems with change in vision (either in general or in part of the visual field or in night vision), failing vision or blindness, blurred vision, double vision (diplopia), spots or floaters, redness, pain, itching, excess tearing (lacrimation), dryness, discharge or drainage, swelling around the eyes, unusual sensations or twitching, light sensitivity (photophobia), reading, seeing distant objects? Do vision problems interfere with daily activities? Do you wear eye glasses or contact lenses (when was the last prescription change?)? When was the last eye examination (results?)? Last glaucoma check (results?)? Do you wear an eye prosthesis (how do you care for it?)?
Ears	Any history of ear infections or earaches, diminished hearing or loss of hearing? Any current problems with diminished hearing; deafness; increased sensitivity to sound; feeling of fullness in the ear; ear pain; discharge or drainage (describe); vertigo; or ringing (tinnitus), crackling, buzzing, or other sounds in the ears? Any problems with excess ear wax? How do you clean your ears (use cotton-tipped swabs, hair pins, or other sharp, foreign objects?)? Do you wear a hearing aid? When was last ear or hearing examination (results?)?

Table continued on following page

Table 4–4. *Review of Systems* (Continued)

Body Systems	Examples of Information and Questions to Cover
Nose and Sinuses	Any history of frequent colds, sinus infections, nasal stuffiness, allergies, hay fever, or nasal trauma or fracture? Any current problems with sneezing, postnasal drip, runny nose (rhinitis), difficulty breathing through the nose, pain over the sinuses, or nosebleed (epistaxis)? Any change in the sense of smell? Do you use nasal sprays or other cold, allergy, or sinus medications (type? amount? frequency?)?
Mouth and Pharynx	Any history of sore throat or oral infections such as strep throat, cold sores (herpes), or thrush (*Candida*)? Ever had oral or dental surgery (describe)? Any current problems with mouth or tongue lesions (sore, abscess, ulcer), bleeding gums, increased saliva, dry mouth, mouth pain, sore throat, hoarseness, voice change, difficulty chewing or swallowing, halitosis, change in taste? Do you use tobacco products (type? amount? frequency? current use patterns?)? Do you wear dentures or bridges (do they fit well? do you wear them most of the time?)? Describe your dental hygiene practices (brushing, flossing, use of fluoride toothpaste). When was last dental examination (results?)? Were radiographs taken?
Neck	Any history of neck injury, goiter, pain, limited movement, or swollen glands? Any current problem with stiffness, tenderness, pain, swelling, or lumps in the neck?
Breasts and Axillae	Any personal or family history of fibrocystic breast disease, cancer of the breast, or breast surgery? Any current problems with enlargement (gynecomastia), itching (pruritus), nipple discharge, breast lumps, dimpling or change in breast skin texture or color, change in appearance of the nipples, breast pain, tenderness, or swelling? Do you take corticosteroid medications (describe)? Do you perform breast self-examination (if so, when and using what technique?)? *If patient is female:* Do you take any estrogen (e.g., birth control pills)? Did you ever breast-feed a child? Have you had mammograms (when? how often? results?)?
Respiratory	Any past history of breathing problems such as asthma, emphysema, wheezing, pleurisy, pneumonia, bronchitis, tuberculosis (describe any treatment received), or whooping cough? Ever smoked or used tobacco products (type? amount? length of time used? attempts to stop?)? If a former smoker, how long ago did you quit? Any current problems with chronic cough, sputum production (describe), blood in sputum (hemoptysis), night sweats, shortness of breath with or without exertion (dyspnea), ability to tolerate exercise or activity of daily living without becoming short of breath, difficulty breathing without elevating the head when supine (orthopnea), pain with breathing, blue-tinged nail beds or tips (cyanosis)? Ever had a chest radiograph (results?) or a skin test for tuberculosis (results?)?
Cardiovascular	Any history of congenital heart problems, rheumatic fever, heart murmur, myocardial infarction (MI), coronary artery disease, cardiac surgery, hypertension, or thyroid problems? Any family history of hypertension or MI before age 50? Any current problems with chest discomfort or pain, syncope, vertigo, palpitations, sudden awakening at night with difficulty breathing (paroxysmal nocturnal dyspnea), dyspnea on exertion, orthopnea, sudden weight gain, edema of hands or feet, hyperlipidemia or hypercholesterolemia? Ever had any cardiac tests: electrocardiogram (ECG), stress ECG, coronary angiogram, echocardiogram, electrophysiologic studies?
Peripheral Vascular	Any history of varicose veins, diabetes, hypertension, pain in the extremities, injury to an extremity (describe), or edema of the hands or feet? Any current problems with lymph node swelling or tenderness; pain in the legs with walking that is relieved by resting (claudication resting), numbness or coldness of an extremity, discoloration or ulceration on extremities (especially feet and ankles), hair loss on an extremity, nail changes? Ever had any vascular tests such as Doppler studies? Do

Table 4–4. Review of Systems (Continued)

Body Systems	Examples of Information and Questions to Cover
	you spend prolonged periods of time standing? *If patient is female:* What type of hose (e.g., support hose) do you wear? Do you use garters or other means of securing the hose?
Gastrointestinal	Any history of indigestion, heartburn, ulcers, hernia, liver disease, hepatitis (type?), gallbladder disease, pancreatic disease, appendicitis, or abuse of alcohol? Any family history of alcohol abuse or cancer of the stomach, liver, pancreas, intestines, or colorectal area? Any current problems with weight loss or gain, change in appetite or taste, food intolerance, belching, nausea or vomiting, blood in emesis (hematemesis), pain or indigestion with eating, difficulty swallowing, diarrhea, constipation, bowel incontinence, flatulence, changes in bowel habits or stool characteristics (e.g., clay colored or blood in stool, ribbon-like stools), hemorrhoids (any pain or bleeding, especially with defecation?), rectal pain or itching, pain or swelling (ascites) in the abdomen, or jaundice? Do you use digestive aids, laxatives, enemas, or suppositories (describe)? Ever had tests of the gastrointestinal (GI) system (barium swallow, upper GI series, barium enema, sigmoidoscopy, colonoscopy, Hemoccult test, gallbladder radiographs or ultrasound, liver scan)? Results?
Urinary	Any history of bladder infection, kidney problems, urinary tract stones, sexually transmitted diseases? Any family history of renal disease? Any current problems with change in urinary patterns, weak stream, hesitancy, urgency, frequency, increased or decreased amount of urine (polyuria or oliguria), change in color of urine, foaming in the urine (proteinuria), pus in the urine (pyuria), dribbling or incontinence, nocturia, pain urinating (dysuria), flank or low back pain, or discharge from the urethra? Ever had tests of the urinary system (urinalysis, cystoscopy, intravenous pyelogram)? Results?
Genitoreproductive	
General	Any history of sexually transmitted diseases (STDs); infertility; problems with sexual performance; urethral discharge; odor; pain; burning; itching; or genital lesions, sores, or ulcers? Ever had surgery on the genitoreproductive system (describe)? Do you use any contraceptives (type?)? Are you satisfied with the type used or do you want to change? Do you know how to avoid STDs or want information on the topic?
Female	Any history of pelvic inflammatory disease, endometriosis, abnormal Papanicolaou (Pap) test results? Any personal or family history of reproductive cancer (cervix, uterus, ovary, breast)? Any current problems with premenstrual issues (bloating, weight gain, fatigue, mood changes), irregular menstrual periods, excessive menses (dysmenorrhea), painful menses, absence of menses (amenorrhea), bleeding other than with menses (metrorrhagia), painful intercourse (dyspareunia), postcoital pain or bleeding? (Review the menstrual cycle history for age at menarche and menopause, if applicable, the duration and amount of menstrual flow, and the last menstrual period.) When was your last pelvic examination and Pap test (results?)?
Male	Any history of inguinal hernia, prostate problems, impotence? Any family history of reproductive cancer (prostate, penis, testes)? Any current problems with testicular pain or mass or blood in the ejaculate? When was your last physical examination that included checking the prostate and for hernia (results?)? Do you know how to perform testicular self-examination (how often do you do it?)?
Musculoskeletal	Any history of sprains, strains, fractures, dislocations, arthritis, gout, backache, bursitis, osteomyelitis, scoliosis, or flat feet? Any family history of arthritis, gout, or muscular dystrophy? Any current problems with muscle twitches, cramps, or spasms; involuntary movements, pain, or weakness; muscle atrophy; joint pain, stiffness, swelling, redness, deformity, or limited movement; noise or grating with joint movement (crepitation); backache; spinal deformity; limitation in

Table continued on following page

Body Systems	Examples of Information and Questions to Cover
	walking, gait, running, sports activities, or activities of daily living? Ever had tests of the musculoskeletal system (skeletal radiographs or electromyography)?
Neurologic	Any history of loss of consciousness, fainting, seizures, paralysis, numbness or tingling (paresthesia), trauma to the nervous system, or stroke? Any family history of stroke, seizures, or neurologic disease such as Huntington's chorea? Any current problems with vertigo, syncope, paresthesia, paralysis, headache, loss of balance, seizures, uncoordinated or involuntary movements (tics, tremors, clumsiness), speech problems, or memory (short- or long-term) problems? Are neurologic problems interfering with activities of daily living (describe)? Ever had neurologic tests (electroencephalography, lumbar puncture, computed tomography of the head)? Results?
Psychiatric	Any history of depression, bipolar disorder, schizophrenia, obsessive-compulsive tendency (does it interfere with your activities of daily living?)? Any sleeping problems, memory problems, anxiety attacks, eating disorders (e.g., anorexia or bulimia nervosa)? Any family history of depression, bipolar disorder, or schizophrenia? Ever been treated for mental or emotional health problems or taken psychotropic medications (describe)? Any current problems with mood swings, sleeping problems, anxiety (especially if it interferes with activities of daily living), nervousness, increased or decreased appetite, memory lapses, inability to concentrate, change in energy level or inability to complete tasks, phobias, delusions, or hallucinations? Any recent change in relationships with family members or friends?

Table 4–4. Review of Systems (Continued)

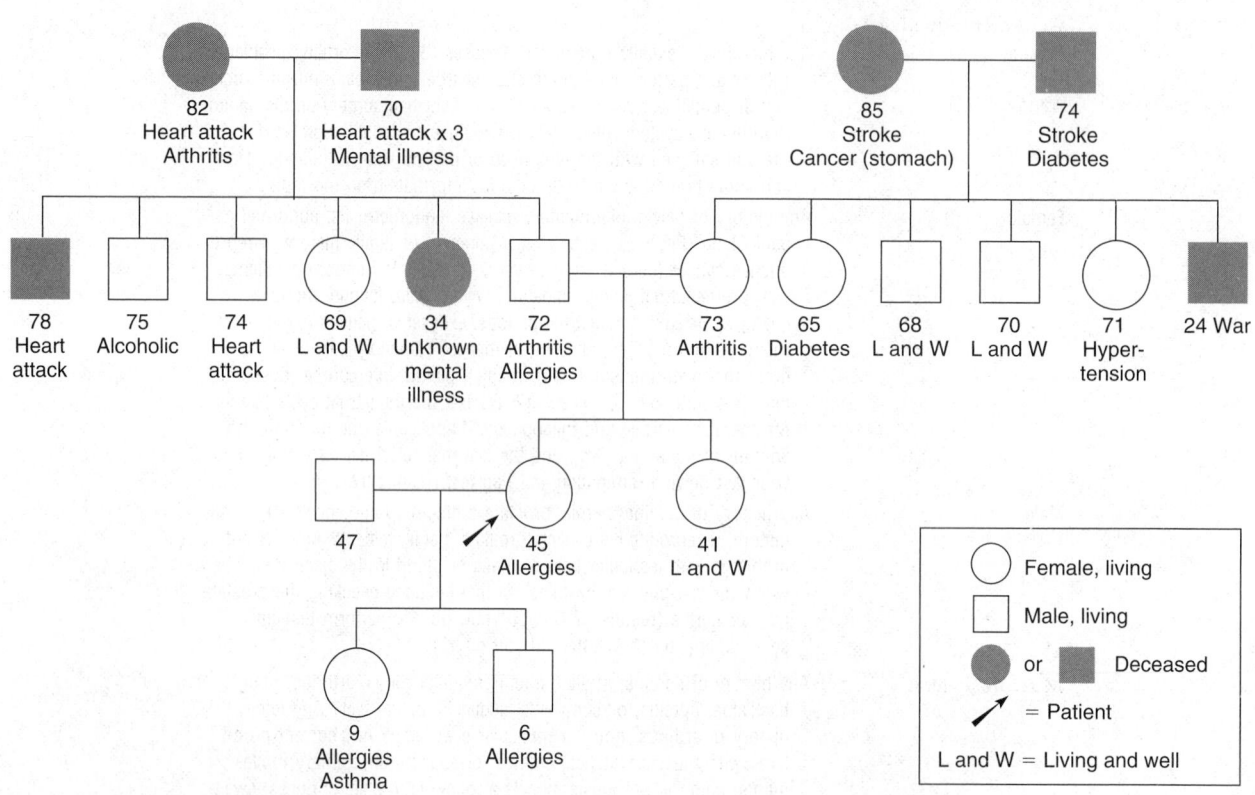

Figure 4–1. Diagram of a family history. (From Black JM, and Matassarin-Jacobs E [eds]. *Luckmann and Sorensen's Medical-Surgical Nursing: A Psychophysiologic Approach.* 4th ed. Philadelphia: WB Saunders, 1993, p 166.)

Psychosocial History

1. To complete a basic health history, you must also consider a patient's psychosocial history.
2. See Chapter 6 for details on obtaining a psychosocial history.

Health Risk Appraisal

1. Health risk appraisal is the analysis of all known factors about a person's life situation, habits, and health-related activities (or lack thereof).
2. Purposes of health risk appraisal
   a. To examine factors affecting the person's potential for developing health problems
   b. To identify people at risk who may benefit from preventive intervention
   c. To recommend screening and preventive measures based on current guidelines, such as those published by the American Cancer Society and the American Heart Association.

3. Table 4–3 identifies potential questions regarding various categories of health risk factors.
   a. Discriminate between changeable (e.g., diet, exercise) and nonchangeable (e.g., age, gender) risk factors.
   b. Assess the person's motivation to modify or reduce personal risk factors.
4. Evaluate the person's resources for and barriers against modifying or reducing personal risk factors.

Review of Systems

1. Proceed in head-to-toe fashion, and phrase questions and terms in simple language (Table 4–4). Avoid medical terms or jargon.
2. Survey past and current health status of each body system by reviewing common symptoms.
3. Explore symptoms confirmed by the person with a symptom analysis.
4. Be alert for signs of health problems mentioned.

Bibliography

Books

Alfaro R. *Applying Nursing Diagnosis and Nursing Process: A Step-by-Step Guide.* 2nd ed. Philadelphia: JB Lippincott, 1990.

American Academy of Pediatrics. *Guidelines for Health Supervision: II.* 2nd ed. Elk Grove Village, IL: Author, 1988.

American Nurses Association. *Clinician's Handbook of Preventive Services: Put Prevention into Practice.* Waldorf, MD: Author, 1994.

American Nurses Association. *Position Statement on Cultural Diversity in Nursing Practice.* Kansas City, MO: Author, 1991.

Bernstein L, and Bernstein RS. *Interviewing — A Guide for Health Professionals.* 4th ed. Norwalk, CT: Appleton-Century-Crofts, 1985.

Bowers AC, and Thompson JM. *Clinical Manual of Health Assessment.* St. Louis: CV Mosby, 1992.

Clark CC. *Wellness Nursing: Concepts, Theory, Research, and Practice.* New York: Springer Publishing Co, 1986.

Doenges ME, and Moorhouse MF. *Application of Nursing Process and Nursing Diagnosis: An Interactive Text.* Philadelphia: FA Davis, 1992.

Gordon M. *Nursing Diagnosis: Process and Application.* 2nd ed. New York: McGraw-Hill, 1987.

Hill LH, and Smith N. *Self-Care Nursing: Promotion of Health.* 2nd ed. Norwalk, CT: Appleton & Lange, 1990.

Jarvis C. *Physical Examination and Health Assessment.* Philadelphia: WB Saunders, 1992.

Malasanos L, Barkauskas V, and Stoltenberg-Allen K. *Health Assessment.* 4th ed. St. Louis: CV Mosby, 1990.

Morton PG. *Health Assessment in Nursing.* 2nd ed. Springhouse, PA: Springhouse, 1993.

Murray RB, and Zentner JP. *Nursing Assessment and Health Promotion: Strategies Through the Life Span.* 5th ed. Norwalk, CT: Appleton & Lange, 1993.

Pender NJ. *Health Promotion in Nursing Practice.* 2nd ed. Norwalk, CT: Appleton & Lange, 1987.

Stanhope M, and Lancaster J. *Community Health Nursing: Process and Practice for Promoting Health.* 3rd ed. St. Louis: CV Mosby, 1992.

Thomas CL (ed). *Taber's Cyclopedic Medical Dictionary.* 16th ed. Philadelphia: FA Davis, 1989.

U.S. Preventive Services Task Force. *Guide to Clinical Preventive Services: An Assessment of the Effectiveness of 169 Interventions.* Baltimore: Williams & Wilkins, 1989.

Varcarolis EM. *Foundations of Psychiatric Mental Health Nursing.* Philadelphia: WB Saunders, 1990.

Chapters in Books

Keene A. Health assessment. *In* Black JM, and Matassarian-Jacobs E (eds). *Luckmann and Sorensen's Medical-Surgical Nursing: A Psychophysiologic Approach.* 4th ed. Philadelphia: WB Saunders, 1993.

Title 45 Code of Federal Regulations, part 80—Nondiscrimination under programs receiving Federal assistance through the Department of Health and Human Services, effect of Title 6 of the Civil Rights Act of 1964. Department of Health and Human Services, 45 CFR A(10-1-94 edition), 292–293.

Journal Articles

American Medical Association. Medical evaluations of healthy persons (Report of the Council on Scientific Affairs). *JAMA* 249:1626–1633, 1983.

Bamberg R, et al. The effect of risk assessment in conjunction with health promotion education on compliance with preventive behaviors. *J Allied Health* 18(3):271–280, 1989.

Bonheur B, and Young S. Exercise as a health-promoting lifestyle choice. *Appl Nurs Res* 4:2–6, 1991.

Braverman BG. Eliciting assessment data from the patient who is difficult to interview. *Nurs Clin North Am* 25:743–750, 1990.

Breslow L, and Somer A. The lifetime health monitoring program. *N Engl J Med* 296:601–608, 1977.

Burnard P. Discussing spiritual issues with clients. *Health Vision* 61(12):371–372, 1988.

Cameron CT, and McNeil EL: The importance of history. *J Emerg Nurs* 2(3):21–22, 1976.

Diaz-Duque OF. Advice from an interpreter. *Am J Nurs* 82(9):1380–1382, 1982.

Dirckx JH. Talking with patients, the art of history taking. *Clin Nurs Pract* 3:13–14, 1985.

Grasska MA, and McFarland T. Overcoming the language barrier: Problems and solutions. *Am J Nurs* 82(9):1376–1379, 1982.

Pulsch RW. Cross-cultural interpreters in health care. *JAMA* 254(23):3344–3348, 1985.

Schneiderman H. The review of systems, an important part of comprehensive examination. *Postgrad Med* 71:151–158, 1982.

Selleck KJ. Nurses' interpersonal behavior and the development of helping skills. *Int J Nurs Stud* 28(1):3–11, 1991.

Spillane RK. Assessment: Getting the patient's point of view—early. *Nurs Manage* 18(5):20–28, 1987.

Tom CK. Nursing assessment of biological rhythms. *Nurs Clin North Am* 11:621–630, 1976.

Topf M. Verbal interpersonal responsiveness. *J Psychosoc Nurs* 26(7):8–16, 1988.

Agencies

Nutrition Screening Initiative
1010 Wisconsin Avenue, NW
Suite 800
Washington, DC 20007

AT&T Language Line
(a 24-hour service providing interpreters in approximately 140 languages)
(408) 648–7541

5
Performing the Basic Physical Assessment

■ PURPOSES OF THE PHYSICAL ASSESSMENT

The purposes of the physical assessment are to assess the patient's current physical health status, interpret the physical health data, and make clinical decisions on the basis of the data.

Assess Current Physical Health Status

1. Collect *objective* physical health data to establish a current baseline for the patient against which to compare the findings of previous and subsequent assessments.
2. Supplement and validate the patient's subjective data about his or her physical health status.

Interpret the Physical Health Data

1. Differentiate normal from abnormal physical findings by comparing the patient's data against known standards.
2. Compare the patient's current physical health status with his or her previous status.

Make Clinical Decisions

1. Review and compare the physical examination data for defining characteristics that will help you formulate nursing diagnoses.
2. Monitor the patient's physical health status (e.g., take vital signs) to assess the effectiveness of nursing and medical interventions and note any changes.
3. Evaluate expected patient outcomes to determine whether they have been accomplished.

■ PREPARING FOR THE PHYSICAL ASSESSMENT

Assemble Equipment

1. Gather all necessary equipment before beginning the physical examination.
   a. Arrange the equipment to be within your reach in the order in which you will use it during the examination.

   b. Become familiar with the equipment. Make sure you know how to assemble and use each piece.
   c. Check that all equipment functions properly. Replace bulbs, charge or change batteries, and refill containers.
2. Figure 5–1 shows equipment commonly used in the physical examination.

Prepare the Environment

1. The setting can be anywhere: an office, a clinic cubicle, the home, or a screened bedside, for example.
2. Provide privacy to promote comfort and rapport.
3. Reduce or eliminate extraneous noise so that you and the patient can concentrate on the examination. Some assessments, such as auscultating the heart and lungs, require a quiet environment.
4. Make sure the room is neither too warm nor too cool; the patient may be wearing only a gown or examination wrap.
5. Provide sufficient overhead light. Supplement this with a flashlight, penlight, or oto-ophthalmoscope.

Plan and Organize the Approach

1. Develop a thorough and systematic approach and use it routinely to avoid missing parts of the examination.
   a. A head-to-toe approach is commonly used to organize the examination. You can integrate assessments of body regions (e.g., the head and neck) and body systems (e.g., the neurologic or integumentary system).
   b. Table 5–1 presents an example of an integrated head-to-toe sequence for an adult physical examination. The specifics on each area to be examined are presented later in this chapter.
2. Be flexible, allowing for the patient's needs. For example, if the patient is nervous about being examined, begin with a general assessment of the neurologic or musculoskeletal system before examining areas that expose the body, such as the anterior thorax.
3. Be efficient. Do not waste time and energy.
   a. Keep position changes to a minimum to keep from fatiguing the patient.
   b. When possible, use a piece of equipment to examine an entire body region or body system before returning it to the equipment tray. For example, use the reflex

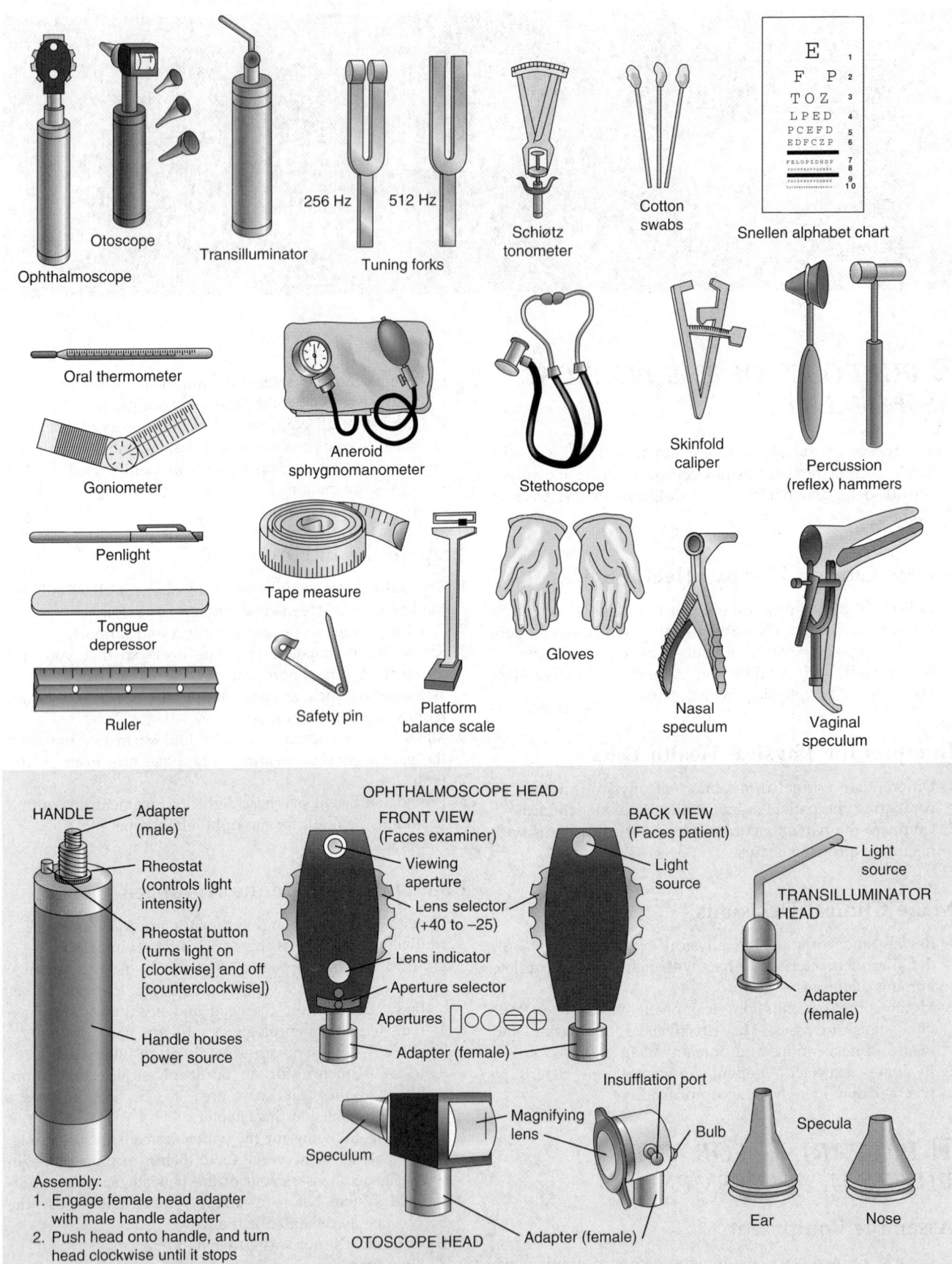

Figure 5–1. Equipment commonly used in a physical examination. The various stages of the physical examination can require a variety of equipment. Major instruments are illustrated. In addition, examination equipment may include any or all of the following: cotton balls, cotton-tipped applicators, examination gloves, flashlight or floor lamp, gauze sponges, glass of water, water-soluble lubricant, penlight, ruler, safety pins, supplies for tests and specimens (e.g., Papanicolaou, guaiac), tape measure, tongue blades, watch with second hand. (Redrawn from Black JM, and Matassarin-Jacobs E [eds]. *Luckmann and Sorensen's Medical-Surgical Nursing: A Psychophysiologic Approach.* 4th ed. Philadelphia: WB Saunders, 1993, p 218.)

Table 5–1. Sequence for Integrated Head-to-Toe Assessment	
Body Region/System	**Subregions/Systems**
General survey	Vital signs
	Appearance
	Behavior
Head and neck	Head
	Face
	Eyes
	Ears
	Nose
	Sinuses
	Mouth
	Pharynx
	Neck
Upper extremities	Upper extremities (including integumentary and peripheral vascular systems)
	Spine (reflexes)
	Musculoskeletal system
	Neurologic system
Posterior thorax	Spine
	Ribs
	Muscles
	Lungs
	Kidneys
Anterior thorax	Thorax
	Lungs
	Heart
	Carotid arteries
	Jugular veins
	Breasts and axillae
Abdomen	General examination
	Liver
	Spleen
	Kidneys
	Aorta
	Inguinal areas
Lower extremities	Lower extremities (including integumentary and peripheral vascular systems)
	Spine (reflexes)
	Musculoskeletal system
	Neurologic system
General neurologic and spine	Sensory function
	Gross motor function and balance
	Spine profile
Genitalia	External
	Internal
Anus and rectum	Anus
	Rectum

hammer to assess all the deep tendon reflexes and the plantar reflex in quick succession.
c. If you examine a body region or system that requires several position changes (e.g., the heart) assess whether the patient can tolerate it. You may need to adapt the sequence to accommodate the patient.
4. Identify anatomic landmarks and discriminate abnormal findings. Use these landmarks to locate areas to examine and as reference points when recording findings.

Prepare the Patient

1. Prepare the patient psychologically.
   a. Try to alleviate the patient's anxiety about being examined.
      (1) Approach the patient calmly and professionally.
      (2) Use a relaxed tone of voice and facial expression to put the patient at ease and promote trust.
   b. Describe the examination process to the patient using words he or she can understand.
      (1) Explain what you will do before starting so the patient knows what to expect and can cooperate.
      (2) Give further explanations and instructions as you proceed.
      (3) Tell the patient ahead of time if you plan to collect specimens during the examination (e.g., a throat culture or Papanicolaou [Pap] smear).
   c. Encourage the patient to express discomfort or other concerns as the examination proceeds.
      (1) Watch the patient's facial expressions and body language throughout the examination for nonverbal cues of anxiety or fear (see Chapter 4). Examples are draping pulled close around a body part and tense or contracted muscles.
      (2) Never force the patient to continue if he or she wishes to stop. Try to avoid misunderstandings by explaining what you are doing and why.
2. Prepare the patient physically.
   a. Ask the patient to empty the bladder before you begin the physical examination.
      (1) An empty bladder facilitates a more comfortable examination of the abdomen, genitalia, and rectum.
      (2) If a urinalysis is part of the examination, instruct the patient on how to collect a specimen (see Chapter 26).
   b. Arrange draping.
      (1) Provide the patient with a gown or paper drape that will preserve the patient's privacy while allowing access for examination.
      (2) Uncover only the area you are examining. Keep the rest covered to prevent unnecessary exposure.
   c. Position the patient.
      (1) Help the patient assume and change positions (Fig. 5–2).
      (2) Adapt positioning when the patient has a disability or limitation, such as arthritis, back pain, joint deformity, or weakness.
      (3) Keep the patient in an uncomfortable or embarrassing position only as long as needed.

◼ PHYSICAL ASSESSMENT TECHNIQUES

General Principles of Physical Assessment

1. Use the patient as a self-standard or "control."
   a. The body is almost symmetric, and each person has unique similarities in structure and appearance.
   b. Compare the findings for one side of the body with those for the other side.

POSITION	AREAS EXAMINED	RATIONALE	CONTRAINDICATIONS
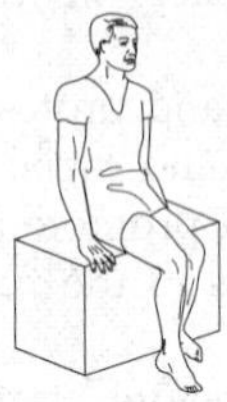 Sitting	Vital signs, head and neck, back, posterior and anterior thorax and lungs, breasts, axillae, heart, upper and lower extremities, reflexes	Sitting upright allows for full lung expansion and better visualization of upper body symmetry.	Elderly and weak people may be unable to sit without support. Alternate position is supine with head of bed elevated.
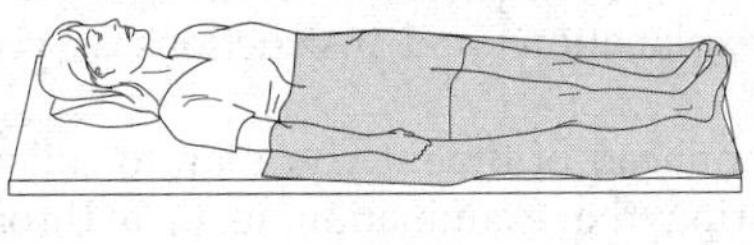 Supine	Vital signs, head and neck, anterior thorax and lungs, breasts, axillae, heart, abdomen, extremities, peripheral pulses	This is a relaxed position for most people. It provides access to pulse sites and prevents contracture of abdominal muscles, especially if a small pillow is placed under the knees.	Patients with cardiovascular and respiratory problems may be unable to lie flat without becoming short of breath. Alternate position is to raise head of bed. Patients with low back pain may be unable to lie flat without flexing the knees.
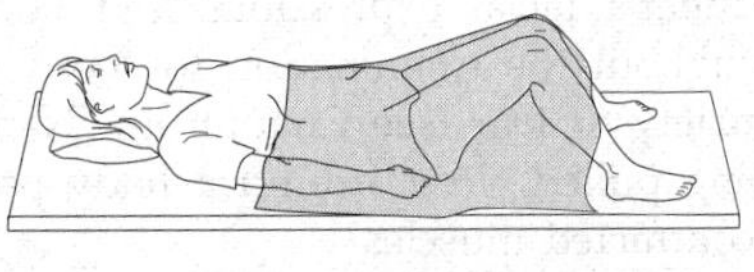 Dorsal recumbent	Vital signs, head and neck, anterior thorax and lungs, breasts, axillae, heart, abdomen, extremities, peripheral pulses, vagina	Flexed knees reduce tension on lower back and abdominal muscles and increase comfort.	Same as for supine. The person should not raise the arms over the head or clasp the hands behind the head, as this increases contraction of abdominal muscles.
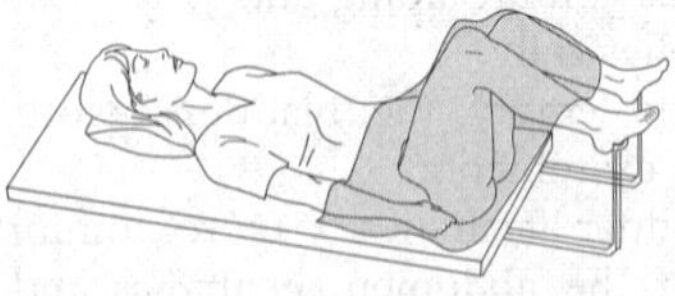 Lithotomy	Female genitalia, reproductive tract, and rectum	This position maximally exposes the genitalia and facilitates the insertion of a vaginal speculum.	This position is assumed immediately before it is needed as it is embarrassing and uncomfortable. The person is kept draped. People with arthritis or joint deformity may be unable to assume this position. Alternate positions are dorsal recumbent or Sims.
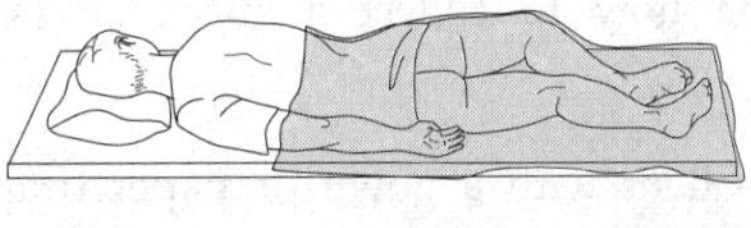 Sims (posterior view)	Rectum, vagina	Flexion of the upper hip and knee improves exposure of the rectal area.	People with deformities of the hip or knee may be unable to assume this position. Older people and obese patients may be uncomfortable.
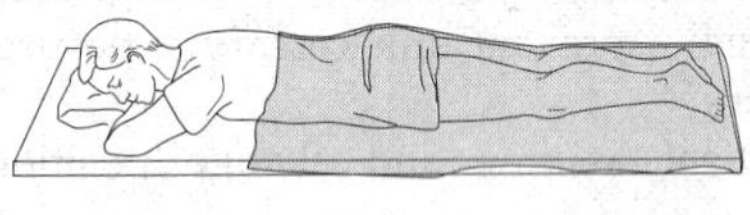 Prone	Posterior thorax, hip movement, popliteal pulses	This position is used to assess hip extension. Sometimes popliteal pulse palpation is facilitated in this position.	This position is not well tolerated by older people or patients with cardiovascular or respiratory problems.
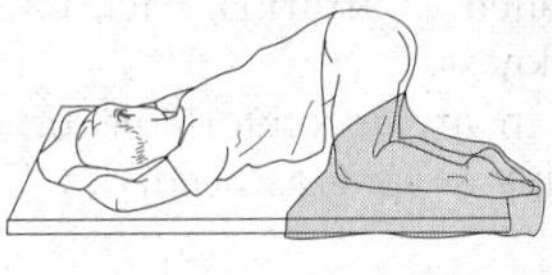 Knee-chest	Rectum, prostate	This position provides maximal exposure of the anal and rectal areas and facilitates insertion of instruments into the rectum.	Poorly tolerated by people with cardiovascular or respiratory problems. Persons with difficulty flexing hips or knees may be unable to assume this position. Alternate position is Sims or standing, bent over examining table.
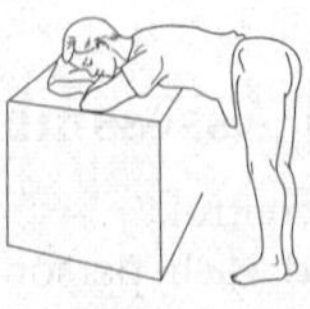 Standing, bent over examining table	Rectum, prostate	This is a more comfortable position than knee-chest and allows for palpation of the prostate gland.	This position is assumed immediately before it is needed as it is embarrassing. Persons with back problems may need assistance.

Figure 5–2. Common physical examination positions and their applications. (Redrawn from Black JM, and Matassarin-Jacobs E [eds]. *Luckmann and Sorensen's Medical-Surgical Nursing: A Psychophysiologic Approach.* 4th ed. Philadelphia: WB Saunders, 1993, p 224.)

2. Compare your findings with known parameters of what is "normal" for the patient's age, sex, and ethnic background. For example, baldness is a normal finding for a middle-aged man but not for a teenager, and men generally have more muscle mass than women do.
3. Examine known or suspected problem areas carefully.
   a. Include areas identified by the patient and areas you suspect may be at increased risk on the basis of the patient's history and risk profile.
   b. To avoid causing the patient unnecessary anxiety, explain why you are examining an area thoroughly.

NURSE ADVISORY

> During the examination, watch for such reactions as tensing or flinching, which often indicate a potential problem area that needs in-depth assessment.

4. Be alert for health teaching opportunities. Provide accurate health information and correct misconceptions. Reinforce health promotion practices such as regular dental hygiene, eye examinations, and breast self-examination.

Inspection

1. **Inspection** is systematic, deliberate visual examination. It reveals information about size, shape, color, texture, symmetry, position, and deformity.
2. Inspection is the 1st technique of physical assessment.
   a. It begins the moment you meet the patient, even before the health history interview. Inspection continues throughout the physical examination.
   b. Perform an initial inspection before you perform the hands-on techniques palpation, percussion, and auscultation. These other techniques can alter subsequent findings.
3. Show concern for the patient during the inspection.
   a. Explain the process as you perform your inspection, saying, for example, "I'm just going to look at your face and neck for anything unusual."
   b. Expose each area you examine to good light to allow complete visualization. Remember to keep the rest of the body draped.
4. Use special equipment to enhance inspection.
   a. Specula (nasal, ear, and vaginal) combined with supplemental light permit visual access to body cavities and orifices.
   b. Other equipment includes tongue depressors, a marking pen, a tape measure, skinfold calipers, eye charts, and a goniometer (see Fig. 5–1).

Palpation

1. **Palpation** is the use of touch to examine an area. It reveals information about masses (position, size, shape, consistency, and mobility), pulsation, organ size, tenderness or pain, swelling, tissue firmness and elasticity, vibration, crepitus, temperature, variation in texture, and moisture.

2. Palpation is the 2nd technique of physical assessment.
   a. It usually follows inspection to confirm what you saw during inspection.
   b. In assessment of the abdomen, however, palpation comes last (after inspection, auscultation, and percussion), because it may interfere with accurate assessment of abdominal organs if it precedes other techniques.
3. Encourage the patient to relax before and during palpation to facilitate examination.
   a. Position the patient comfortably to minimize muscle tension, which will feel like muscle rigidity.
   b. Encourage the patient to breathe regularly and slowly and not to hold his or her breath.
   c. Ask the patient to point out any tender areas before you start. Palpate these areas last while you observe for signs of discomfort or pain. Be prepared to stop if the patient is too uncomfortable.
   d. Warm your hands, either by rubbing them together lightly or by running them under warm water.
   e. Keep your fingernails short and smooth.
   f. People tend to stiffen when suddenly touched. Approach slowly and proceed systematically, explaining as you go.
   g. Avoid applying prolonged pressure in one area. It is uncomfortable for the patient, and your ability to perceive structures diminishes with prolonged palpation.
4. Use the most sensitive parts of your hands and fingers to palpate specific characteristics as follows.
   a. Use your **fingertips or finger pads** for fine touch (e.g., to palpate pulses, lymph nodes, and breast tissue).
   b. Use the **dorsum of your fingers or hand** to discriminate skin temperature.
   c. Use the **palmar surface** of your hand over the metacarpophalangeal joints and the **ulnar aspect** of your hand on the chest wall to assess lung vibration with vocalization (tactile fremitus).
   d. Grasp the tissue lightly with your **index finger and thumb** to assess position, consistency, mobility, size, shape, and turgor.
5. Proceed gradually from light to deep palpation to help the patient adjust to varying pressures (Fig. 5–3).
   a. Begin the **light palpation** to assess superficial structures such as skin lesions or lymph nodes. Depress the underlying tissue approximately 1 to 2 cm (1/2–3/4 of an inch).
   b. Use **deep palpation** to determine the size and condition of underlying organs or structures. Depress the underlying tissue approximately 4 to 5 cm (1 1/2–2 inches).
      (1) Proceed slowly to avoid injuring internal organs with sudden or forceful pressure.
      (2) Use 1 hand or both hands.
   c. In **bimanual palpation,** use both hands for deep palpation or to trap a movable structure, such as a kidney.
      (1) In deep palpation, place your sensing hand lightly on the patient's skin over the structure you wish to palpate. Position your active hand over the sensing hand to apply pressure.

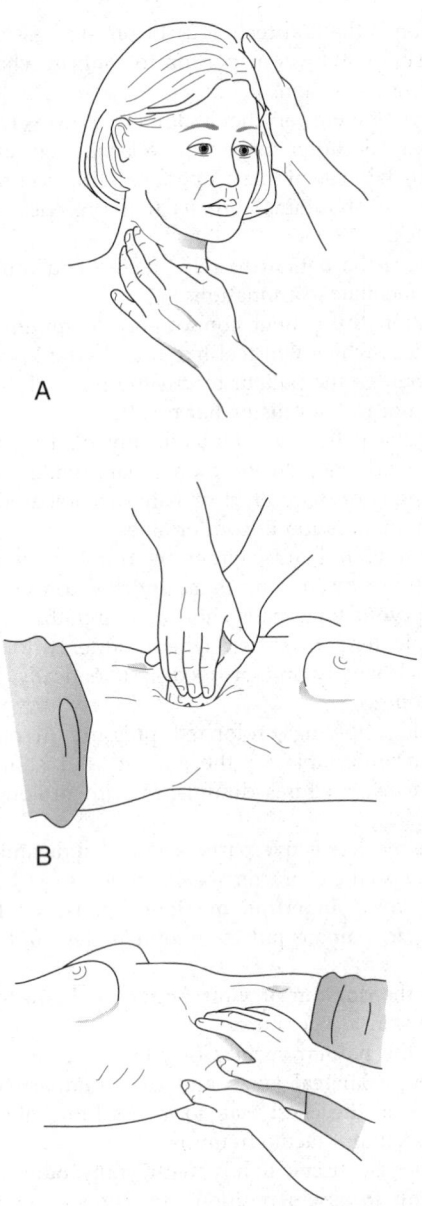

Figure 5–3. Hand positions used in palpation. *A*, Light palpation employs the lightest pressure possible to assess structures under the skin's surface, such as lymph nodes. *B*, Deep palpation is used to assess the condition of underlying organs such as in the abdomen using 1 or both hands. *C*, Bimanual palpation is used to trap and assess hard-to-palpate organs (e.g., kidney or spleen) or to stabilize an organ with 1 hand while the other hand palpates (e.g., liver). (Redrawn from Black JM, and Matassarin-Jacobs E [eds]. *Luckmann and Sorensen's Medical-Surgical Nursing: A Psychophysiologic Approach.* 4th ed. Philadelphia: WB Saunders, 1993, p 219.)

    (2) To trap a movable structure, place 1 hand under or behind the structure to stabilize it while you palpate with your dominant hand.

NURSE ADVISORY

Do not apply direct pressure with the sensing hand in bimanual deep palpation. Allow the hand to remain sensitive to underlying structure characteristics.

---

    d. **Ballottement** is a palpation technique that is used to assess a floating object such as the kidney or a fetus. Push fluid-filled tissue toward the palpating hand so that the object floats against the fingertips. Ballottement is also used to assess for free fluid in tissue spaces where it is not usually found, for example, edema around the knee.

6. Take precautions when palpating:
    a. Do not obstruct an artery's blood flow by palpating too firmly or continuously.
    b. Never palpate both carotid arteries at the same time.

Percussion

1. **Percussion** is the production of sound and vibration by striking (tapping or thumping) the skin. It reveals information about location, size, and density of superficial abnormal masses and pain in underlying areas up to a depth of 3 to 5 cm (1–2 inches).
2. Percussion is the 3rd technique of physical assessment.
    a. In most assessments, perform percussion after inspection and palpation and before auscultation. In abdominal assessment, however, perform percussion after inspection and auscultation and before palpation.
    b. Percussion helps confirm suspected abnormal findings from palpation and auscultation (e.g., a mass or consolidation).
3. Encourage the patient to relax during percussion to facilitate the examination.
    a. Position the patient comfortably.
    b. Encourage the patient to breathe regularly unless instructed otherwise. For example, when you percuss to determine the extent of organ (e.g., lungs, liver, or spleen) movement with respiration, instruct the patient to inhale or exhale deeply.
    c. Percuss tender areas gently. Be prepared to stop if the patient is uncomfortable.
    d. Explain what you will do before you touch the patient to avoid startling him or her.
    e. Avoid percussing the patient's skin with your fingernail to prevent scratching (as in direct finger percussion).
4. There are 2 primary methods and 1 secondary method of percussion (Fig. 5–4).
    a. **Direct percussion** involves striking the body surface with 1 or 2 fingers (over the sinuses) or the fist (blunt percussion over the kidneys). Use these maneuvers to assess tenderness.
    b. **Indirect percussion** involves striking the body surface through an intermediary finger (over the lungs) or hand (over the liver or spleen to assess tenderness) placed firmly on the skin.
        (1) Indirect percussion requires dexterity, patience, practice, and a short nail on the percussing finger.
        (2) Common errors in technique are discussed in the legend to Figure 5–4.
    c. **Blunt percussion** with a reflex hammer helps you assess deep tendon reflexes.
5. Evaluate the sounds produced in relation to the location of underlying structures. Tissue density determines the sound produced (Table 5–2):

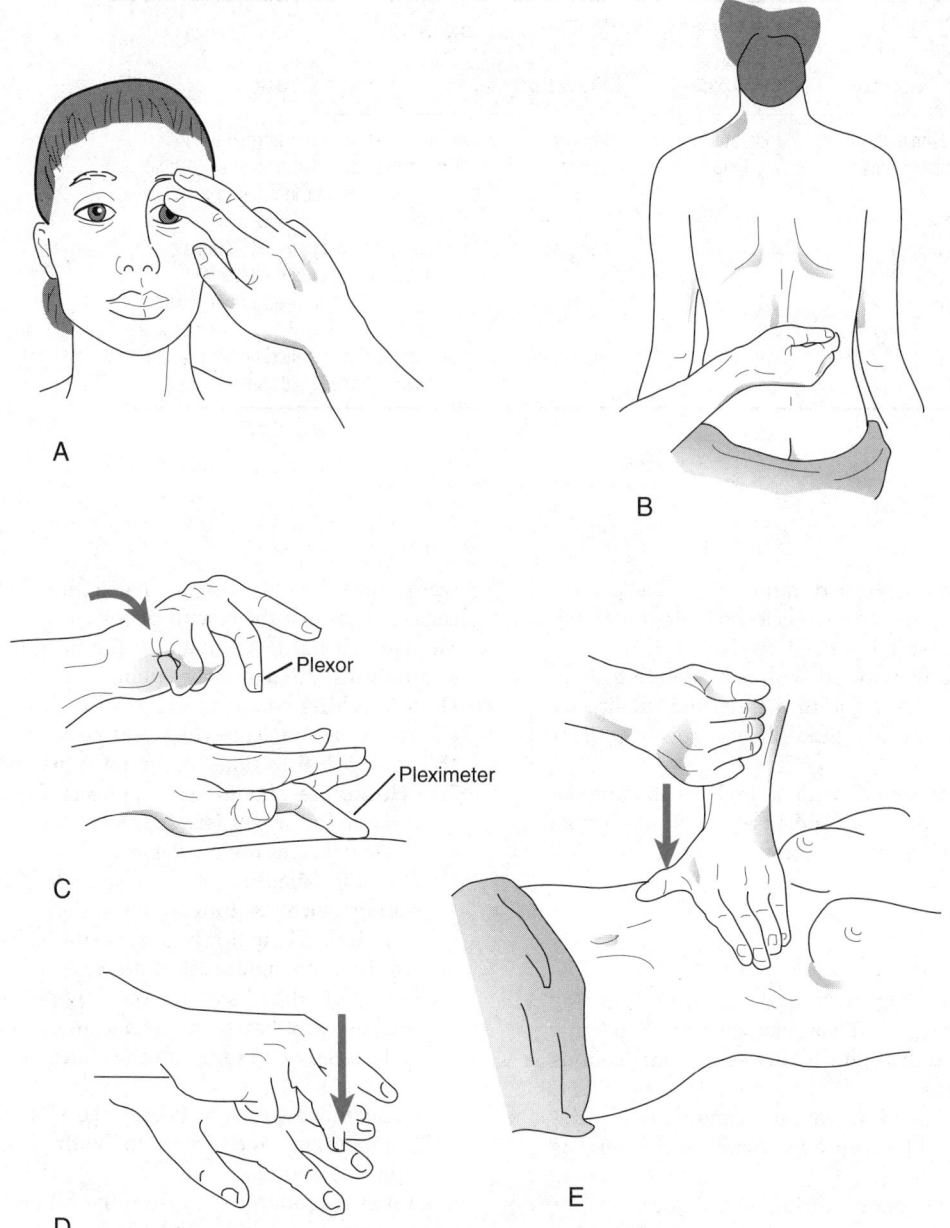

Figure 5-4. Percussion. *Direct percussion. A*, One or 2 fingers are used to percuss directly against the body's surface, such as an adult's sinuses to elicit tenderness or a child's thorax to assess sounds. *B*, The ulnar surface of the fist is used to gently strike the body's surface over an underlying organ such as at the costovertebral junction to assess for kidney tenderness. *Indirect percussion. C*, The pleximeter (distal phalanx of nondominant hand's middle finger) is placed firmly on the patient's skin surface over soft tissue. The remaining fingers are hyperextended so that only the single joint is in contact with the skin. Failure to do this dampens (i.e., diminishes) the sound. The middle finger of the dominant hand is bent at its distal interphalangeal joint to create a hammer (i.e., plexor). *D*, The plexor moves in an arc to strike the pleximeter sharply and quickly at a perpendicular angle over the joint. The wrist remains relaxed and the forearm stationary to ensure a sharp blow. Resting the palm of the nondominant hand on the body surface, loose contact of the pleximeter with the skin surface, and delivering a weak blow with the plexor dampen the sound. The same amount of force is delivered with each blow for accurate comparison of sounds. A light, quick blow produces the clearest sound. The blows may be repeated rapidly 3 or 4 times to assess the sound. *E*, The palm of the left hand is placed over the area to be percussed, and the ulnar surface of the right fist is used to gently strike the left hand. (Redrawn from Black JM, and Matassarin-Jacobs E [eds]. *Luckmann and Sorensen's Medical-Surgical Nursing: A Psychophysiologic Approach.* 4th ed. Philadelphia: WB Saunders, 1993, p 220.)

a. **Resonance:** A moderate to loud sound with a low pitch and moderate duration results from air-filled tissue found in the normal lung. Resonance has a clear, hollow quality.
b. **Hyperresonance:** A loud, booming sound with a low

pitch and longer duration than resonance results from overinflated, air-filled tissue (e.g., pulmonary emphysema) in adults. Hyperresonance is normal in a child because of the thin chest wall.
c. **Tympany:** A loud, drumlike or musical sound with a

Table 5–2. Percussion Sounds

Sound	Loudness	Duration	Cause
Resonance	Moderate to loud	Moderate	Air-filled tissue in the normal lung
Hyperresonance	Very loud	Longer	Overinflated, air-filled tissue, as in pulmonary emphysema; normal in a child's lung
Tympany	Loud	Longest	Enclosed, air-containing structures (stomach's gastric bubble, intestine)
Dull	Soft	Short	Dense, mostly fluid-filled organ (liver, spleen)
Flat	Very soft	Very short	Very dense tissue, when no air present (muscle, bone, solid tumor)

high pitch and the longest duration of all the percussion sounds results from enclosed, air-containing structures (e.g., gastric bubble, bowel).

d. **Dull:** A soft, muffled sound with a moderate to high pitch and short duration with a thudding quality results from dense, mostly fluid-filled tissue (e.g., liver or spleen).

e. **Flat:** A very soft sound with a high pitch and the shortest duration of all the percussion sounds results from very dense tissue (e.g., muscle, bone, or solid tumor).

Auscultation

1. **Auscultation** is listening to sounds produced in the heart, lungs, abdomen, and vascular system. You must practice to be able to distinguish between normal sounds and abnormal sounds.

2. Auscultation is the last examination technique in a physical assessment, except in an abdominal assessment, as discussed earlier.

3. Show concern for the patient during auscultation.
   a. Keep the person warm to prevent shivering. Shivering can produce sounds that interfere with what you are trying to hear.
      (1) Use drapes and adjust the room temperature.
      (2) Warm the chestpiece of the stethoscope in your hand before you place it on the patient's skin.
   b. To allay anxiety, explain to the patient what you will do while you listen over 1 area for what may seem like a long time. For example, cardiac auscultation requires concentrated (focused) listening over each auscultation point for several cardiac cycles.

4. A **stethoscope** enhances your ability to hear but amplifies sound only if it has an amplifier attachment. Select a stethoscope to fit you and suit your needs.
   a. The **earpieces** of a stethoscope may be plastic or rubber. They should fit your ear canal snugly, to block extraneous sounds, but should not hurt. Experiment to find the most comfortable fit.
   b. The **binaurals** (curved, metal tubes) should slope for-

ward toward your nose to match the slope of your ear canal. Adjust them with pliers.
   c. The **tension bar** lets you adjust the fit of the earpieces and reduces kinking of the tubing.
   d. **Double tubing** conducts sound to both ears from the chestpiece. It should be thick and no longer than 12 to 15 inches for distortion-free sound transmission.
   e. The **chestpiece** should have at least 2 endpieces, a diaphragm and a bell (see Fig. 5–1). Adult, pediatric, and neonatal sizes are available.
      (1) Use the **diaphragm** to listen to high-pitched sounds such as lung, bowel, and normal heart sounds. Hold it firmly against the skin to form a seal tight enough to leave a ring.
      (2) Use the **bell** to listen to soft, low-pitched sounds, such as extra heart sounds and murmurs.
         • Place the bell lightly on the skin's surface to just form a seal.
         • Too much pressure causes the skin to mimic a diaphragm and interfere with hearing low-pitched sounds.

5. Successful auscultation depends on the following:
   a. Listen over bare skin only. Clothing, a gown, or a sheet prevents sound transmission and may distort your findings.
   b. If an area of skin is particularly hairy, friction on the chestpiece will sound like crackling.
      (1) Over the lungs, you may mistake this crackling for the abnormal sound of crackles.
      (2) Wet the hair first to prevent crackling. Do not shave the hair to prevent crackling.
   c. Prevent the binaurals from rubbing together or striking other objects, causing a misleading clunking sound.
   d. Reduce room noise as much as possible (e.g., turn off the television and close the door). Background noise produces a roar that affects your ability to hear.
   e. Concentrate on the sound you wish to hear and tune out other sounds. This is important when listening to heart and lung sounds, which may be heard simultaneously.

Olfaction

1. **Olfaction** involves using the sense of smell to detect body odors. Perform this technique throughout the physical assessment.
2. Be alert for unusual odors, which may indicate health problems. For example, an ammonia odor in urine suggests a urinary tract infection; halitosis could mean poor oral hygiene or an oral or sinus infection.

◼ PERFORMING THE ADULT PHYSICAL EXAMINATION

General Survey

1. The general survey begins the physical examination.
2. Note the patient's general appearance and behavior. Begin when you first greet the patient and continue throughout the history interview.
   a. Relate your observations to the patient's cultural, educational, and socioeconomic backgrounds, as well as to his or her current health or illness status.
   b. Let signs of problems or abnormalities guide your examination. For example, if the patient is unkempt and has a noticeable body odor, examine the hair, skin, and nails to assess hygiene.
3. Survey the specific aspects of appearance and behavior.
   a. Apparent age: Does the patient look his or her stated age? Or does the patient look older or younger than his or her age?
      (1) Chronic illness may make a person appear prematurely aged.
      (2) Transcultural considerations:
         • Members of certain ethnic groups exposed to excessive sun (e.g., Hispanic migrant workers) appear older than their age.
         • Members of cultures with shorter life spans also may appear older than their age.
      (3) When aging appears premature, assess body systems for other signs of aging (e.g., loss of subcutaneous tissue and muscle mass).
      (4) When the patient appears youthful for his or her stated age, assess body systems for signs of age (e.g., skin tone and elasticity, joint flexibility, and range of motion).
   b. Sex: Is the patient's sexual development appropriate for his or her gender and age? Deviations from normal include signs of precocious or delayed puberty in a child, gynecomastia in a man, and micromastia or hirsutism in a woman.
   c. Racial and ethnic group: Is the patient's physical appearance consistent with that of a recognized racial or ethnic group?
   d. Apparent state of health: Determine whether the patient looks healthy, frail, or ill, and note any deformities or absent body parts. This will help you organize and prioritize your approach to the examination.
   e. Signs of distress or discomfort: Ideally, the patient is relaxed and comfortable. If not, determine why.
      (1) If the patient is in pain (wincing), anxious (darting or downcast eyes), gasping for air, or has some other problem, you may have to adapt the examination.
      (2) Transcultural considerations: Is the patient's discomfort related to cultural differences between the two of you? For example, does the patient fear exposure of body parts that are usually kept covered from strangers?
   f. Body build, height, and weight: Is the patient's body proportionate in weight and height? Note excessive shortness, tallness, obesity, thinness, or unusual distribution of or lack of body fat versus the normal ranges for age, sex, and racial and ethnic background. (You will take precise measurements later in the examination.)
      (1) Body build can reflect the degree of physical fitness (e.g., weight training versus no exercise).
      (2) Biocultural differences: Norms differ for various racial and ethnic groups.
         • In general, White men are slightly taller than Black men, whereas Black and White women are about the same height.
         • Blacks have longer legs and arms and shorter trunks than Whites. White men look somewhat heavier than Black men because of weight distribution in the trunk. Black women often weigh more than White women of the same height.
         • Asians are lighter and shorter and have smaller body frames than either Blacks or Whites, on average.
         • Asians and Native Americans often have longer trunks and shorter limbs than Whites.
         • Second- and 3rd-generation immigrants (i.e., children and grandchildren of immigrants) are taller and heavier than 1st-generation immigrants of the same age and gender.
         • Members of lower socioeconomic groups have a greater tendency to be obese than do members of the middle class, and members of upper socioeconomic groups are the least likely to be obese.
   g. Posture: Posture reflects mood as well as physical status. Observe the patient's posture throughout the examination.
      (1) Standing posture should be erect, with shoulders, hips, and knees aligned over the ankles and weight equally distributed on both feet.
      (2) In the sitting position, the back should be straight, the arms relaxed, and the shoulders slightly rounded.
   h. Gait: Observe the patient walking.
      (1) Gait should be smooth and coordinated, the arms swinging freely opposite to leg movement.
      (2) Note any abnormal gait (e.g., shuffle, limp, stagger, foot drag) or use of mobility aids (e.g., a cane).
   i. Movements: Watch the patient's body movements throughout the examination.
      (1) Movements should be purposeful and controlled and absent of tremors, rigidity, tics, spasticity,

immobility, or fasciculations (small contractions of muscles under the skin).

  (2) Range of motion should be full and symmetric.

  j. Dress: Note whether the patient's clothing is suitable for the climate, weather, and season and for age, cultural background (e.g., saris or veils), socioeconomic status, and current condition. Clothing may provide clues to the patient's mental and physical health.

    (1) A depressed person may wear drab, dirty, or disheveled clothing, suggesting lack of energy for self-care.

    (2) Dirty or disheveled clothing may also reflect physical problems with self-care.

  k. Hygiene and grooming: Are the patient's hair, nails, and skin clean and neat? Age, sex, socioeconomic status, and occupational factors may influence the patient's appearance.

    (1) Someone who does manual labor for a living may have rough, stained hands and broken nails.

    (2) Transcultural considerations: What is considered normal grooming varies with culture and racial and ethnic group.

      • Native American men have little facial hair and do not shave. Muslim men often have beards.

      • Some orthodox religions have rules regarding grooming by both men and women, including rules for hair length and style and use of makeup, that differ from mainstream American conventions.

      • Some Islamic women shave their perineum.

  l. Body and breath odor: Note body or breath odor relative to the patient's activity level, food choices, hygiene, and health status. Examples are perfume, perspiration, cigarette smoke, alcohol, acetone, blood, and decaying tissue.

    (1) Some foods (e.g., garlic and curry) result in breath odors as they are metabolized.

    (2) Infected skin lesions can have strong odors; a bowel obstruction may result in a fecal breath odor.

    (3) Transcultural considerations

      • In many cultures people do not use deodorants.

      • Asians and Native Americans have a milder body odor than do Whites and Blacks, because they have fewer apocrine sweat glands.

  m. Mental status: Assess mental status—including level of consciousness, orientation, mood, affect, speech, and thought processes—during the health history interview and each time you interact with the patient. (See Chapter 6 for details on performing a complete mental status examination when you suspect a serious problem.)

    (1) Level of consciousness: Normal findings are alertness and responsiveness to questions. Abnormal findings include confusion, drowsiness, lethargy, and inattentiveness.

    (2) Orientation: The patient should be oriented to time, place, person, and situation and demonstrate appropriate facial expression, eye contact, and body language.

    (3) Mood and affect: Mood and affect should match and be consistent with the patient's situation.

      • The patient should be comfortable and cooperative.

      • Abnormal findings include hostility, anger, and suspicious or challenging behavior.

    (4) Speech: The patient should speak clearly, fluently, and evenly, without hesitancy or difficulty of expression.

    (5) Thought processes: The patient's thought processes should be logical, coherent, and relevant. The patient's vocabulary should match his or her educational and cultural background.

    (6) Transcultural considerations: Members of cultures that value silence (e.g., Appalachians and Native Americans) often speak slowly and seem to meditate on each word, which may give them the appearance of hesitancy and disjointedness.

  n. Level of cooperation: Assess the patient's cooperation with the examination.

    (1) Does the patient willingly discuss information, or is he or she distant, silent, withdrawn, angry, hostile, or suspicious?

    (2) Note how much eye contact the patient makes and signs of anxiety, such as tense, closed body language.

4. Note skin color.

  a. Assess overall skin color as you interview the patient. Observe the face and visible skin surfaces.

  b. Skin color varies with genetic background, but normally it is even and free from lesions. Abnormal findings include pallor, flushing, ruddiness, cyanosis (a blue tinge), jaundice, and irregular pigmentation.

  c. Examine remaining skin surfaces as you inspect each body region. Look for moles, skin tags, scars, bruises, or other variations in color that may indicate a health problem.

  d. Transcultural considerations

    (1) Overall skin tone varies greatly among individuals, depending on the amount of melanin deposits they have. Lighter skin tones contain less melanin and are thus at greater risk for skin cancer from exposure to ultraviolet rays.

    (2) The palms and soles of darker-pigmented people may look pink compared with the rest of their skin, because there are few melanin deposits in these areas.

5. Take vital signs.

  a. Temperature: Take the patient's temperature orally, rectally, axillarily, or tympanically.

    (1) Normal oral range is 36 to 37.5 degrees Celsius (96.8–99.5 degrees Fahrenheit) with an average of 37 degrees Celsius (98.6 degrees Fahrenheit).

    (2) Rectal temperature is usually 1 degree Fahrenheit higher than oral temperature.

    (3) Axillary temperature is usually 1 degree Fahrenheit lower than oral temperature.

    (4) Tympanic temperature is considered comparable to the oral temperature.

    (5) Note time of day to allow for the circadian rise in

Table 5-3. Vital Signs Across the Life Span

Vital Sign	Newborn	Adult	Older Adult
Temperature			
°Fahrenheit	98.6–99.8	96.8–99.5	96.5–97.5
°Celsius	37–37.7	36–37.5	35.8–36.4
Pulse rate (beats per minute)	70–190	60–100	60–100
Respiratory rate (breaths per minute)	30–80	12–20	15–25
Blood pressure			
Systolic	50–52	95–140	140–160
Diastolic	25–30	60–85	70–90

temperature during the late afternoon and early evening.

(6) Body temperature increases after vigorous exercise, with psychologic and physiologic stress, and in response to increased circulating levels of thyroid and growth hormone.

(7) Older adults often have a lower baseline temperature (Table 5–3).

b. Pulse: Palpate the radial pulse (Fig. 5–5) for 15 seconds and multiply by 4 (if it is regular) or for 1 full minute (if irregular) for accurate results. Note rate, rhythm, amplitude (force), and elasticity.

(1) Rate: Resting adult pulse rate ranges from 60 to 100 beats per minute. Bradycardia is a rate below 60, and tachycardia is a rate above 100.

  • Heart rate varies slightly with respiration, speeding up with inspiration and slowing during expiration.

  • Pulse rate increases with an increase in body temperature.

  • Physically fit, conditioned people have a lower resting baseline pulse rate than do people who are not in shape.

  • Men usually have lower pulse rates than do women.

  • Resting baseline pulse rates are often higher in older people than in young and middle-aged people.

(2) Rhythm: Resting heart rate is normally even and regular, with pulsations at equal intervals and of similar strength or amplitude.

  • Describe irregular rhythms or patterns if you note them.

  • Auscultate the apical pulse while you palpate the radial pulse. For every cardiac systole, you should feel a pulsation.

(3) Amplitude: The amplitude of the pulse indicates the heart's stroke volume. It is commonly recorded using a 3- or 4-point scale (Box 5–1).

(4) Elasticity: The resiliency of an arterial wall is a measure of its elasticity. Arterial pulses should feel springy directly against your fingers.

c. Respiration: Count the patient's respirations for 30 seconds and multiply that number by 2 if respirations are regular or count for 1 full minute if respira-

---

BOX 5–1. Rating and Recording Pulse Amplitude

Rate and record the pulse amplitude using a standard system for clear communication among health professionals. The following scale is common. (A variation is a 4-point scale in which 3+ is considered an increased amplitude but within normal limits and 4+ is considered bounding. Use the scale approved by your agency.) Note that the 2+ rating is expected for the particular pulse being examined. A 2+ rating for a pedal pulse feels different from a 2+ rating for a carotid pulse because of the different size of vessel lumens and distance from the heart. Express the pulse amplitude in relationship to the rating scale norm. For example, the notation 2+/3+ indicates that the pulse was rated 2+ on a 3-point rating scale in which 2+ is normal.

0   **Absent.** Pulse is indiscernible to palpation.

1+ **Weak, thready.** Pulse is difficult to palpate and easily obliterated by slight pressure.

2+ **Normal.** Pulse is readily palpable and can be obliterated only with strong pressure.

3+ **Bounding.** Pulse is easily palpable, forceful, and not easily obliterated by pressure.

---

tions are irregular. (See Chapter 22 for details on the respiratory system.) Note whether respiration is labored or unlabored and the rate, rhythm (pattern), and depth of respirations.

(1) Labored versus unlabored respiration: Labored respiration (dyspnea) is difficult breathing that involves active use of accessory inspiratory and expiratory muscles. Unlabored respiration (eupnea) is quiet, relaxed, normal breathing.

(2) Rate: The resting adult respiratory rate ranges from 12 to 20 breaths per minute. Respiratory rate is approximately a 1:4 ratio with the pulse rate. It increases in response to activity, anxiety, and increased temperature.

(3) Pattern: Respirations normally are regular, even, quiet, and effortless; note sighing, pursed-lip breathing, or abnormal inspiration or expiration. See Chapter 22 for examples of respiratory patterns.

(4) Depth: Resting respirations should be of even depth except for the occasional sigh. The depth is an indication of the tidal volume, that is, the amount of air inhaled with each breath.

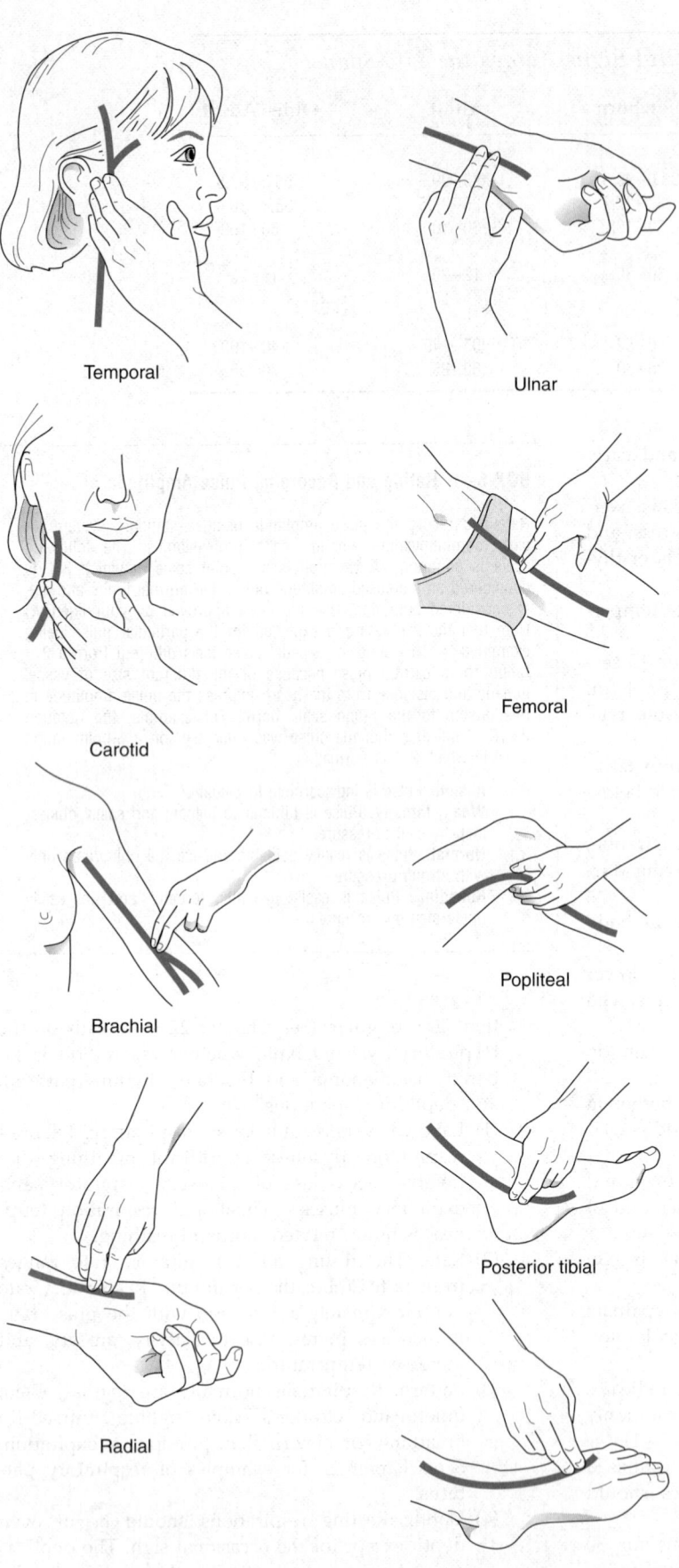

Temporal

Ulnar

Carotid

Femoral

Brachial

Popliteal

Radial

Posterior tibial

Dorsalis pedis

Figure 5–5. Assess peripheral pulses bilaterally, and note pulse amplitude, rhythm, and symmetry. (Redrawn from Black JM, and Matassarin-Jacobs E [eds]. *Luckmann and Sorensen's Medical-Surgical Nursing: A Psychophysiologic Approach.* 4th ed. Philadelphia: WB Saunders, 1993, p 1263.)

d. Blood pressure: Auscultate the patient's blood pressure in both arms and compare the 2 readings (see Chapter 23 for details on blood pressure taking). A difference of 5 to 10 mm Hg between the 2 arms is normal; report larger differences.

(1) Normal systolic pressure ranges from 95 to 140 mm Hg; normal diastolic pressure ranges from 60 to 85 mm Hg. Evaluate the patient's blood pressure in light of current circumstances and previous readings. Report changes of more than 5 to 10 mm Hg between readings or a trend of either increasing or decreasing systolic or diastolic pressures. (See Chapter 23 for a discussion of the diagnosis and treatment of individuals with a diastolic pressure consistently over 85.)

(2) An auscultatory gap, an audible pause of 10 to 15 mm Hg in Korotkoff sounds as the cuff is deflated, may be noted in some individuals with high diastolic readings. It may cause inaccurate systolic readings if you do not initially inflate the cuff above the true systolic pressure.

(3) Pulse pressure is the difference between the systolic and diastolic pressures. It usually is 30 to 40 mm Hg. Report differences greater than 40 mm Hg.

(4) Blood pressure increases with exercise, stress response, strong emotional response, and obesity. Blood pressure also has a diurnal rhythm, similar to that of body temperature.

(5) Transcultural considerations
  • African Americans, particularly women, have higher than normal baseline blood pressures.
  • The incidence of hypertension is higher in Blacks than in Whites in the United States and is extremely high among Caribbean Blacks.

6. Measure height, weight, and body frame.
  a. Measure height and weight while the patient stands on a balance scale equipped with a measuring ruler. If the patient cannot stand, use an alternative, such as a chair scale.
  b. Compare results to a standard table such as the one presented in Chapter 10. Weight should be within range for the patient's sex, height, body frame, and racial or ethnic group.
  c. Use the guidelines presented in Table 5–4 to calculate the patient's ideal body weight. Weight 20 percent above or 10 percent below a person's ideal body weight increases the risk of nutritional problems.
  d. How to measure a patient's body frame accurately is discussed in Chapter 10.

7. Assess balance.
  a. Observe the patient's ability to balance and maintain an upright posture.
  b. If the patient cannot stand or sit without assistance, take safety precautions or alter the sequence of the physical examination and positioning of the patient.
  c. Additional assessment techniques for balance are included in the discussion of neurologic assessment in Chapter 18.

8. Check nutritional status.
  a. Nutritional indices include height, weight, ideal body weight, triceps skinfold thickness, midarm circumference, and the midarm muscle circumference.
  b. The midarm muscle circumference is calculated from the triceps skinfold thickness and midarm circumference (Fig. 5–6) and indicates a person's reserves of protein and calories.
  c. Transcultural considerations
    (1) American nutritional indices are based on data collected from the U.S. population. These stan-

Table 5–4. Calculating Ideal Body Weight

Adult Male*	Adult Female*
Take 106 lb for the first 5 ft of height; add 6 lb/inch for each additional inch over 5 ft	Take 100 lb for the first 5 ft of height; add 5 lb/inch for each additional inch over 5 ft

Small frame — Calculate 10% of the amount for medium frame and subtract it from the first amount (i.e., ideal body weight [IBW] is 10% less for individuals with small frames)

Large frame — Calculate 10% of the amount for medium frame and add it to the first amount (i.e., IBW is 10% more for individuals with large frames)

Example — An adult male is 6'1" tall with a large body frame. His IBW is calculated as follows:
6'1" = 5 ft plus 13 in
First 5 ft of height = 106 lb
Additional height over 5 ft = (13) × (6) = 78 lb
Medium frame IBW = 106 + 78 = 184 lb
Allowance for large frame = (10% × 184 = 18.4 lb
Large frame IBW = 184 + 18.4 = 202.4 lb

* These formulas are for adults with a medium body frame. Adjust formulas for people with small or large frames. Adjustment is the same formula for both sexes.
Data are from the American Dietetic Association. *Handbook of Clinical Dietetics.* New Haven, CT: Yale University Press, 1981. From Keene A. Physical examination. *In* Black J, and Matassarian-Jacobs E. (eds). *Luckmann and Sorensen's Medical-Surgical Nursing: A Psychophysiologic Approach.* 4th ed. Philadelphia: WB Saunders, 1993, p 235.

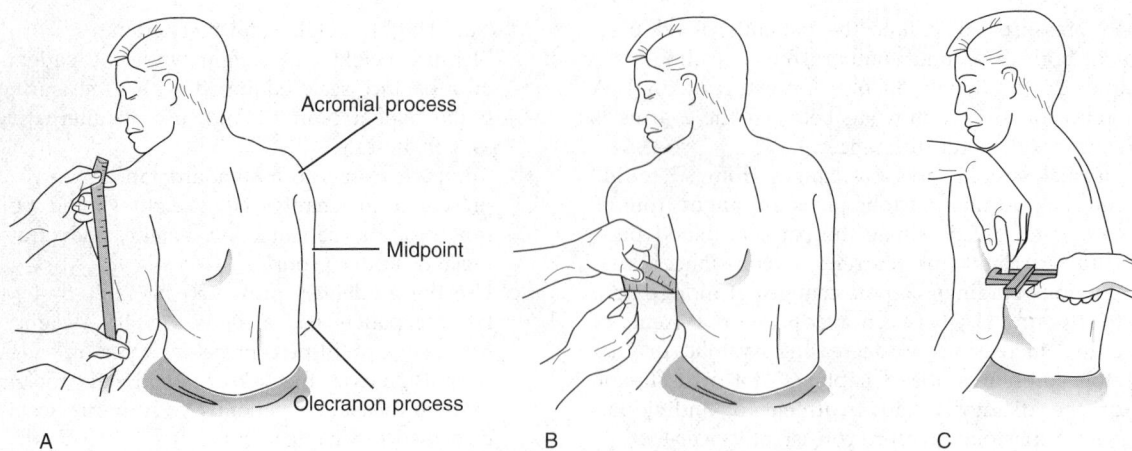

Acromial process

Midpoint

Olecranon process

A   B   C

Figure 5–6. Measuring adipose and skeletal muscular tissue to estimate the person's reserves of protein and calories. *A*, Locate the *midpoint* of the person's relaxed, nondominant upper arm by palpating the acromial and olecranon processes and measuring the distance between the 2 points with a tape measure. Mark the posterior aspect of the arm at the midpoint with a pen. *B*, Measure *midarm circumference (MAC)* at the midpoint, keeping the tape measure level. *C*, Just above the midpoint at the posterior aspect of the arm, grasp the person's skin and subcutaneous tissue between thumb and index finger, freeing it from the underlying muscle mass. Place the calipers at the midpoint just below the fold of grasped tissue. Squeeze the calipers until they equilibrate at the "measure" markings. Read the measurement to the nearest mm. Repeat the readings 2 more times, allowing a rest period of 3 seconds between readings. Calculate the average of the 3 readings for the *triceps skin fold thickness (TSF)*. *D*, Compare the person's values for MAC, TSF, and MAMC to the following standards to determine nutritional risk status. *Undernutrition* is indicated by a measurement below 90% of the standard. *Protein-calorie malnutrition* is indicated by a measurement of less than 60% of the standard, especially for the MAMC. *Obesity* is indicated by a TSF measurement 120% or more above the standard. (Redrawn from Black JM, and Matassarin-Jacobs E [eds]. *Luckmann and Sorensen's Medical-Surgical Nursing: A Psychophysiologic Approach.* 4th ed. Philadelphia: WB Saunders, 1993, p 239.)

dards may or may not be valid for recent immigrants.

(2) Recent immigrants may be at risk for nutritional problems developed earlier. Also, they may have trouble finding familiar foods or adapting to new foods in the United States.

(3) Recent immigrants may also develop nutritional problems if they decrease their activity level.

Screening Body Systems

1. Examine the following body regions carefully. (See the "Assessment" section in each chapter in Unit V for additional information about assessing each body system.) Table 5–5 presents an example of a complete written physical examination.

2. **Integument:** Assess the patient's integument as you examine each body region. You may report significant or abnormal findings as part of each regional assessment or separately.

   a. Skin
      (1) Equipment: You need good lighting for complete visualization. Wear gloves if open areas or draining lesions are present.
      (2) Anatomic landmarks provide reference points for making and recording observations.
      (3) Inspection
         • The skin should be warm, smooth, slightly moist, and of the same general tone throughout. Areas that are regularly exposed will be darker.

• Note skin color (see p. 110). Skin that is protected from the sun and exposure by clothing is lighter in color, especially in light-skinned patients.

• Skin tones range from light ivory to deep brown, yellow to olive, or light pink to dark, ruddy pink.

• Less pigmented areas reveal abnormal findings more readily than heavier pigmented surfaces do. For example, **pallor** is best seen in the buccal mucosa or conjunctivae, particularly in dark-skinned patients. **Cyanosis** is best seen in the nail beds, conjunctivae, and oral mucosa. **Jaundice** can be seen in the sclerae (near the limbus), at the junction of the hard and soft palates, and over the palms.

• **Hyperpigmented** (increased) and **hypopigmented** (decreased) areas may result from variation in melanin deposits or blood flow. Palpate for skin temperature and for tissue edema over these areas to assess circulation.

• **Superficial venous vascular patterns** are usually symmetric. Look for areas of increased vascularity (e.g., hemangioma or telangiectasia), which often are normal findings. Prominent veins are normal in a muscularly developed person who lifts weights or performs hard physical labor; in a less muscular person, they may indicate an underlying health problem, such as a vascular obstruction (e.g., varicose veins).

Table 5–5. Example of a Recorded Physical Examination

Data*	Example†
Date of examination	July 14, 1993
Name	John Jones
General survey	Well-nourished, well-developed White male in no apparent distress; appears stated age of 37. Posture, erect, gait smooth and even, no deformity. Neatly groomed; no breath or body odors. Alert, cooperative. Pleasant affect; smiles occasionally. Speech clear, even. Responds to questions thoughtfully with intermittent eye contact. Memory intact; oriented to time, place, and person; reliable historian
Vital signs	T = 98.5 F; P = 76, regular; R = 14, even; BP = 140/86, left arm (sitting); BP = 138/88, right arm (sitting); no auscultatory gap
Nutritional status	Height = 6'0"; weight = 220 lb; body frame = large; IBW = 195.8 lb; percent IBW = 110.6%; MAC = 28.2 cm (96.2% standard); TSF = 12.3 mm (98.4% standard); MAMC = 24.3 cm (96.0% standard). Sedentary lifestyle with occasional periods of moderate to intense activity
Mental status	Thought process clear, logical. Evidence of active problem-solving behavior (e.g., recent job transfer for a promotion and home purchase). Articulate. No difficulty in recalling recent or past events. Serial 7s deferred
Integument	
Skin	Skin tones light to medium tan over arms and legs, pale over abdomen and back; even, except for irregular light patches over nape of neck, anterior torso, and medial arms. Warm, smooth, supple, dry patches on elbows, knees, and feet. Turgor immediate. Scars: left lateral knee (6 cm), left medial knee (5 cm), and RLQ (4 cm)
Hair	Dark brown, thick, wavy hair; no dandruff or nits; no alopecia. Coarse body hair, with usual male distribution
Nails	Short, groomed, rounded without cracking or peeling; cuticles intact; beds pink; immediate capillary refill upon blanching; no lesions; angle <160°
Head	Normocephalic; no lesions or tenderness; face symmetric at rest and with movements; TMJ: no crepitus, full mobility; CN II–XII intact, CN I not tested; temporal artery 2+/3+ bilaterally, soft
Eyes	Acuity per Snellen chart (unaided): OD = 20/25, OS = 20/20, OU = 20/20. Full visual fields to confrontation. EOMs intact, no nystagmus; PERRLA, direct and consensual; cover/uncover test = no eye movement; corneal light reflections equal (Hirschberg's). Eyebrows symmetric, full, groomed; lashes full, with outward curve. Lids approximated when closed and rest at limbus borders when open; palpebral fissures equal; no lesions. Lacrimal apparatus functioning. Sclerae white; palpebral conjunctivae pink; bulbar conjunctivae clear; corneas and anterior chambers clear; globes firm; lenses clear. Disk margins sharp with nasal blurring; bilateral cup-to-disk ratio 1:3, cups symetric. No A-V nicking; ratio 2:3. Fovea not visualized
Ears	Auricles symmetric; no lesions or tenderness over tragus. Canals lined with soft cerumen; no tenderness or discharge. TMs grey, cone of light at 4:00, right ear; at 7:00 left ear; no retraction; landmarks visualized. No lateralization; AC > BC, bilaterally; whisper heard at 3 ft
Nose and sinuses	Nose angled to right; no nasal flaring, lesions, discharge, or tenderness; patent bilaterally (better on right); septum deviated from midline to the right; mucosa pink, moist. Inferior, middle turbinates pink; clear discharge present; frontal and maxillary sinuses nontender, transilluminate
Mouth and pharynx	Lips pink, symmetric, smooth, moist, and without lesions. Gingivae pink, intact; 28 teeth present, 3rd molars absent, rest without caries; fillings in all 1st and 2nd molars; no malocclusion. Mucosa pink, smooth; no lesions; Stensens's ducts visualized bilaterally. Tongue midline, with full mobility and strength; no lesions or fasciculation; papillae present, light white coating. Saliva pool in floor of mouth. Palates intact, smooth, symmetric, and pink; palates and uvula rise in midline with phonation. Pillars pink, tonsils 1+. Pharynx pink, no drainage; gag reflex intact. Voice clear, strong; swallows without difficulty; taste perception deferred
Neck	Symmetric; no masses or swelling; full ROM of cervical spine. Trapezius muscles tender with movement; no masses or stiffness. Occipital, postauricular, postcervical, supraclavicular, superficial and deep cervical, preauricular, and submental nodes nonpalpable. Tonsillar and submandibular nodes felt bilaterally: 0.5 cm, soft, round, mobile, and nontender. Trachea midline, mobile, and nontender. Thyroid isthmus soft; rest of gland not palpable; no bruit. JVD absent sitting upright and in lower 3rd of neck above sternal notch when supine; carotids 2+/3+ bilaterally, no bruit
Thorax and lungs	AP:lateral diameter 1:2. Breathing quiet, unlabored, without use of ancillary muscles or retractions; rate 14, regular. Thorax symmetric; no tenderness or masses; tactile fremitus symmetric; resonant throughout; thoracic expansion equal; diaphragmatic excursion equal, 3 cm. Breath sounds vesicular in periphery; no crackles or wheezes. No CVA tenderness bilaterally
Heart	Precordium without lifts, heaves, or thrills. Apical impulse at 5th ICS, 1 cm right of LMCL; diameter: 1.5 cm. No pulsations in epigastrium. Regular rhythm with apical rate of 74. S-1 and S-2 regular; no splitting, gallops, murmurs, or rubs. No changes in sounds with position changes

Table 5–5. *Example of a Recorded Physical Examination* (Continued)

Data*	Example†
Peripheral vascular system	Brachial, radial, femoral, and posterior tibial pulses 2+/3+ bilaterally. Ulnar, popliteal, and dorsalis pedis pulses 1+/3+ bilaterally. Epitrochlear, vertical inguinal, and popliteal nodes nonpalpable. Horizontal inguinal nodes palpable (2 in right groin, 3 in left groin), 1 cm, round, mobile, and nontender; no edema. Homans' sign negative bilaterally. Calves nontender; varicosities absent
Breasts and axillae	Breasts rounded and symmetric in all positions; skin smooth, with even contour and no lesions. Vascular pattern not evident. Areola and nipple symmetric bilaterally, no puckering or inversion. Soft, no masses or discharge, and nontender. Axillae hair thick. No rashes, lesions, or hyperpigmentation; nodes nonpalpable and nontender
Abdomen	Symmetric, flat. Visible pulsations or peristalsis absent. Umbilicus midline, inverted. Rectus muscles intact at rest and with straining. No striae. Scar in RLQ, 4 cm (appendectomy). Bowel sounds active all quadrants. No vascular bruits, venous hum, or friction rubs. Abdominal aortic pulsation in epigastrium palpable, thrusting, and nonradiating. Abdomen nontender; no guarding or rigidity; tympany throughout. Liver span: 10 cm at RMCL and 5 cm at MSL. Palpable 1 cm below right costal margin at RMCL, smooth. Splenic dullness at LAAL, 6th ICS. Kidneys nonpalpable; no rebound tenderness. Inguinal areas without bulging
Neurologic system	Gross and fine motor coordination intact; Romberg's test negative; no arm drift or pronation; see Head for CNs. Performs rapid alternating movements and point-to-point maneuvers without difficulty. Gait steady; maintains balance on toes and heels. Sensation to light touch, pain, and vibration intact distally, over trunk, neck, and face. Position sense of fingers and toes intact; stereognosis and graphesthesia present bilaterally. Two-point discrimination: 2 mm on index fingers bilaterally. See diagram for DTRs and plantar reflex

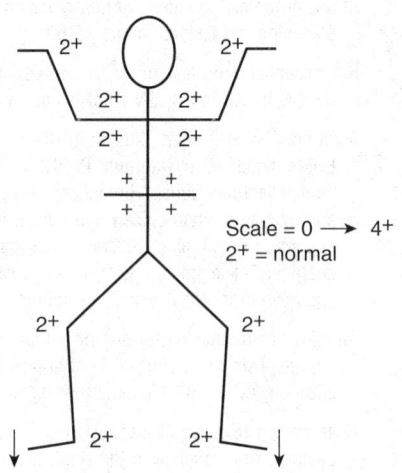

Musculoskeletal system	Muscle masses smooth, firm, nontender, and without fasciculations or lesions. Strength equal at 5/5 bilaterally for all major muscle groups: neck, deltoids, triceps, wrists, fingers, grip strength, hips, hamstrings, quadriceps, ankles, and feet. ROM is WNL for all joints. Palpable coarse crepitus in left knee and fine crepitus in shoulders. Extremities symmetric, without deformity; spine straight; no kyphosis, lordosis, or scoliosis. Para-vertebral muscles nontender and soft; joints symmetric and nontender except for left knee; no edema or nodules
Genitalia	Mature, circumcised male external genitalia. Pubic hair clean; skin without lesions or parasites. Glans smooth; no lesions. No discharge or foul odor from meatus; meatus positioned centrally. Penile shaft smooth, semifirm, and nontender. Scrotum: testes descended, symmetric, firm, movable, and nontender; no masses; epididymis smooth and nontender bilaterally; spermatic cords smooth and nontender. No bulge in inguinal areas at rest or with Valsalva maneuver. Unable to palpate inguinal canal
Rectum	Perianal area: no rashes, lesions, or hemorrhoids at rest or with Valsalva maneuver; sphincter intact. Rectal wall smooth, without tenderness or masses; prostate smooth, firm, movable, and nontender. Stool brown and negative for occult blood
Summary	Generally healthy. Possible borderline hypertension. Deviated nasal septum, nonproblematic. Muscle tension in neck. Increasing left knee tenderness and crepitus following knee anthrotomy. Does not practice TSE
Nursing diagnoses	Review the nursing diagnoses you tentatively formulated after the health history interview in light of the present physical examination data. Validate, revise, add, or discard diagnoses after careful evaluation. The following diagnoses are not listed in order of priority for Mr. Jones:

Table 5–5. Example of a Recorded Physical Examination (Continued)

Data*	Example†
	Altered health maintenance R/T positive family history of hypertension in both maternal and paternal lines, amount of salt consumption per diet history, borderline high systolic and diastolic BP readings, sedentary lifestyle, erratic exercise regimen, being 10% over IBW, perceived stressors of recent job promotion, new home with a large mortgage, increasing frequency of tension headaches, lack of an outlet to "let off steam," lack of knowledge about TSE.
	Impaired physical mobility R/T changes in left knee integrity and function and lack of knowledge about a medical resource since recent move to the community.
Nursing interventions	1. Discuss with Mr. Jones and his wife a referral to the dietitian for counseling regarding a low-salt, low-fat diet.
	2. Review with Mr. Jones the need for regular TSE and the technique. Encourage him to practice and perform TSE monthly.
	3. Encourage Mr. Jones to build into his schedule "personal time," that is, time to relax. Ask him to identify what works for him and has been successful in the past.
	4. Explore options for a regular aerobic exercise regimen with Mr. Jones to help with weight control and relief of tension.
	5. Discuss with Mr. Jones whether he wishes a referral to an orthopedic surgeon for further evaluation of his knee.
	6. Discuss with Mr. Jones his risk profile for hypertension. Explain how other recommendations in this plan may help him regulate his BP. Recommend regular monitoring of his BP and help him schedule appointments if he opts to do this.

* See text for data to collect.
† Patient's history is not included.
IBW, Ideal body weight; MAC, midarm circumference; TSF, triceps skinfold thickness; MAMC, midarm muscle circumference; RLQ, right lower quadrant; TMJ, temporomandibular joint; CN, cranial nerve; OD, right eye; OS, left eye; OU, both eyes; EOMs, extraocular muscles; PERRLA, pupils equal, round, reactive to light and accommodation; A-V, arteriovenous; TMs, tympanic membranes; AC, air conduction; BC, bone conduction; ROM, range of motion; JVD, jugular venous distention; AP, anteroposterior; CVA, costovertebral angle; LMCL, left midclavicular line; RMCL, right midclavicular line; MSL, midsternal line; LAAL, left anterior axillary line; ICS, intercostal space; DTRs, deep tendon reflexes; WNL, within normal limits; TSE, testicular self-examination.

- Examine **scars and bruises** for location, color, length, and width. Correlate their presence with the patient's health history.
- Note excess **moisture,** such as perspiration, which may indicate fever, anxiety, or a warm room.
- Look for **edema** (swelling), especially in the extremities, over the sacrum, and around the eyes. Edema may result from a number of health problems, such as cardiac enlargement, renal failure, or allergic reactions.
- **Lesions** can occur anywhere. Describe their type, color, location, size, distribution, and configuration. Use palpation to examine lesions completely. Normal lesions are freckles; most moles (pigmented nevi) and birthmarks; and age-related changes such as lentigines, skin tags, or seborrheic keratoses; other lesions may be abnormal. See Chapter 35 for a description of the types of skin lesions.
- Transcultural considerations: Skin areas influenced by hormones (e.g., the nipples, areola, labia majora, and scrotum) are darker than the rest of the skin, especially in Blacks and Asians.
- (4) Palpation: Palpate the skin to assess moisture, temperature, texture, turgor and elasticity, edema, tenderness, and lesions.
  - **Moisture** is the skin's state of hydration for both wetness and oiliness. Skin is normally slightly moist, with increased moisture in intertriginous areas such as the axillae and groin. Wet, cool (i.e., clammy) skin is abnormal.
  - Assess **temperature** with the dorsum of your hand. The skin should feel uniformly warm as a reflection of circulation. Compare areas that feel hypothermic or hyperthermic with these same areas on the opposite side of the body and look for accompanying color changes.
  - Palpate for **texture** by touching the skin lightly with your fingertips. The skin should feel smooth, soft, and resilient without lumps or areas of thickening or thinning (atrophy). Skin is uniformly thin over most of the body, except for the palms and soles.
  - **Turgor and elasticity** reflect the skin's resiliency and hydration status. With your thumb and index finger, lightly pinch a skinfold over the forearm and then release it. When turgor is normal, the skin returns to its baseline contour within 3 seconds. If the skin remains elevated (i.e., tented) longer than 3 seconds, turgor is decreased. Turgor decreases with age as the skin loses elasticity. An alternate location to assess turgor is over the sternum.
  - **Edema** is a collection of fluid that separates the surface of the skin from the pigmented and vascular layers of the skin, resulting in a blanched appearance and a change in surface

contour. Palpate edematous areas for consistency, temperature, shape or extent, tenderness, and mobility. Press 1 or 2 fingers firmly against the edematous area for 5 seconds to assess for **pitting edema.** Pitting is a residual indentation left by the finger's pressure when fluid is displaced from the underlying tissue. Express the depth of pitting in millimeters or centimeters (see Chapter 24).

- For the patient to verbalize that the area is **tender** when you palpate is not normal. Look also for guarding, wincing, or other reactions. Although expressed tenderness is subjective, record it as an objective finding.
- Palpate **lesions** to determine their contour (e.g., flat, raised, or depressed), size, consistency (e.g., firm or soft), mobility (e.g., mobile, immobile, or fixed to underlying tissue), and tenderness. Press or stretch lesions and observe for blanching.

NURSE ADVISORY

Wear gloves to palpate mucous membranes and open or draining lesions or when discharge is present.

(5) Olfaction: The skin should be free of pungent odors. Pungent odors may be related to the presence of bacteria on the skin, inadequate hygiene, or draining lesions.

(6) Other tests performed on skin lesions include examination under a Wood's light and potassium hydroxide preparation. These tests are discussed in Chapter 35.

b. Hair

(1) Use good lighting when examining body hair and wear gloves if infestation or lesions are present. Before examining the hair, explain to the patient that you will be touching his or her hair as you examine it.

(2) Distribution and quantity of body hair vary greatly among individuals and are affected by racial, ethnic, and genetic factors.

- Fine hair covers most of the body and is the same color as scalp hair. **Hirsutism** is an excess of body hair. **Alopecia** is hair loss or thinning of the hair and may result from a genetic predisposition to baldness or an underlying health problem or its treatment (e.g., recent chemotherapy).
- The eyebrows, eyelashes, and scalp hair are coarse terminal hairs. Hair distribution is thickest on the scalp and in the axillae and pubic area in adults. Puberty initiates changes in pubic, axillary, and facial hair. In women, the pubic hair pattern is an inverted triangle; in men it is an upright triangle.

(3) Inspect hair for distribution (discussed above), color, texture, lubrication, and signs of infestation.

- Hair **color** may vary from pale blond to black. With aging, color turns to gray or white as melanin production declines. Genetic factors affect the onset of graying. Ask the patient if he or she uses hair dyes or color rinses.
- The **texture** of individual hair shafts may range from thin and fine to thick and coarse. Hair may be straight, curly, or wavy and is affected by shampoos, curling irons, hair dryers, dyes, and permanent waving.
- **Lubrication** is affected by the type of hair care products used as well as dietary protein intake and febrile illness. Insufficient protein intake and illness may leave the hair dry and brittle.
- **Infestation** of scalp hair (with *Pediculus capitis,* or head louse) or pubic hair (with *Pediculus pubis,* or pubic louse) may be seen. Eyebrows, eyelashes, axillary hair, beards, and other body hair may also be infested. Examine hair for nits (eggs), which are white, oval patches adhered to the shafts, particularly behind the ears and along the back of the neck (see Chapter 35).

(4) Palpate scalp hair by rolling it between your fingers to assess texture and lubrication further.

(5) Hair odors may reflect the patient's hygiene, hair care products, or recent activity (e.g., exercising or smoking).

c. Nails

(1) Examine the patient's fingernails and toenails. They reflect the patient's overall health and provide clues to the patient's nutritional and respiratory status.

(2) Inspect the nails for color, shape and contour, texture, thickness, and integrity.

- The **color** of the nail plate is clear, allowing you to see the underlying vascular bed, which is pink in patients with light skin and darker pink in patients with dark skin. Pallor may signal anemia or a low hemoglobin level. Cyanosis may accompany decreased arterial circulation and oxygenation (see Chapter 22 and 23).
- In terms of **shape and contour,** the nail is normally slightly curved or flat, with a convex profile. Inspect the angle of the nail base where it joins the cuticle. It should be 160 degrees or less.
- **Clubbing** of nails results from prolonged oxygen deficiency, such as occurs in emphysema, chronic bronchitis, or cardiac failure. The nail bed angle flattens to 180 degrees in early clubbing and then increases in late clubbing from the chronic hypoxemia (see Chapter 22). The distal phalanx may look splayed (i.e., rounder and wider).
- Nail **texture** is smooth and regular. Pits, splitting, grooves, or lines may indicate a nutri-

tional deficiency or interrupted nail growth (as occurs in acute illness).
- Nail **thickness** is uniform. Thick, ridged nails accompany chronic arterial insufficiency.
- The **integrity** of the nails refers to the condition of the edges and cuticles. They should be clean and smooth, without redness or swelling. Dirty, broken nails and rough, dry, or cracked cuticles may reflect hygiene or the patient's occupation. Jagged nails, nails bitten to the quick, or inflamed cuticles may indicate nervousness.
- Transcultural considerations: Areas of brown or black pigment and linear bands or streaks on the nail plate may be seen in dark-skinned patients.

(3) Palpate nail bases for firmness, and check blanching of fingernails and toenails. Spongy nail beds accompany clubbing. Press firmly over the nail bed to blanch them and then release the pressure. Note how long it takes for the color of the nail bed to return to baseline, indicating peripheral circulation. Normal response time is immediate; longer than 3 seconds is considered a delayed response.

3. **Head and neck:** The head and neck include parts of multiple body systems that, although examined simultaneously, often are reported separately in the findings.
  a. Head
   (1) Equipment: Wear gloves if lesions are present. If the temporal arteries are hard or tender (see below), use a stethoscope to assess them further.
   (2) Anatomic landmarks are the top of the ears in relation to the lateral corner of the eyes and the breadth of the forehead.
   (3) Perform inspection and palpation of the head simultaneously, with the person sitting on the edge of the examining table.
   (4) Inspect for size, shape, contour, and symmetry.
   - The **size** of the head should be in proportion to the patient's body and be approximately 12 percent of the total body size (normocephalic).
   - The **shape** is round, with bony prominences anteriorly (frontal area) and posteriorly (occiput).
   - The **contour** is smooth without bumps, lumps, or depressions.
   - The head and its structures are generally **symmetric.**
   (5) Palpate lightly for nodules, masses, or tenderness. The skull should feel smooth and hard as your fingertips rotate along the midline and over the sides.
   (6) Palpate the temporal arteries (see Fig. 5–5), which should feel soft, and rate the pulse amplitude (see Box 5–1).
   (7) If the temporal arteries feel hard or are tender, auscultate with the bell of the stethoscope for a **bruit** (a turbulence in the vessel that sounds

like a muffling or blunting of the pulse beat) (see Chapter 23).
  b. Face
   (1) Equipment: Cotton wisp and a sharp object such as a sterile needle or safety pin or the pointed end of a pen's cap are needed for the neurologic assessment.
   (2) Inspect the face for symmetry, skin color, hair distribution, and facial movements. (This is easily done during the health history interview and general survey.)
   - The face should be **symmetric** at rest, while the patient talks, and when you ask the patient to perform specific maneuvers to assess cranial nerve function (see Chapter 18).
   - **Skin color** should be distributed evenly.
   - Regarding **hair distribution,** in Whites fine hair covers the cheeks and upper lip in women and coarser, dark hair over the cheeks, upper lip, and chin is common in men; many Blacks and Native Americans have sparse facial hair.
   - Assess cranial nerve VII (facial) by asking the patient to raise the eyebrows, frown, close the eyelids tightly while you try to open them, smile, and puff out the cheeks.
   - Assess cranial nerve V (trigeminal) by asking the patient to clench the jaws together while you try to open his or her mouth against the resistance.
   (3) Palpate the temporal and masseter muscles for symmetry (cranial nerve V) while the patient clenches his or her jaws together.
   (4) Ask the patient to open and close his or her mouth slowly while you palpate the temporomandibular joints. Movement should be smooth and without crepitus (a clicking or grinding sensation) or tenderness, which are abnormal.
   (5) Test facial sensation of cranial nerve V by randomly touching the patient's face with a cotton wisp and a sharp object while his or her eyes are closed. Cue the patient about what the light touch and sharp touch will feel like before beginning. Lightly stroke with the wisp or press the sharp point over the patient's forehead, cheeks, and chin on both sides of midline. The patient should be able to discriminate light from sharp touch and the location on both sides.

4. **Eyes**
  a. Equipment: A Snellen wall chart or hand-held card, an opaque eye cover (e.g., an index card), a penlight and pen, and an ophthalmoscope are needed.
  b. The external anatomic landmarks of each eye include the eyebrow, eyelashes, globe, palpebral fissures, lid margins, conjunctivae (bulbar and palpebral), sclera, limbus, cornea, pupil, and iris. Internal landmarks are the lens, anterior chamber, retina, optic disk, macula, and retinal blood vessels (see Chapter 19).

c. Inspect the **external eye** structures and functions while the patient sits with his or her eyes at your eye level. The eyes should be aligned symmetrically, without protruding or appearing sunken.

(1) The **eyebrows** should be symmetric, with the hair distributed evenly. Hair loss at the lateral aspects may occur with aging. The skin may be dry and flaking (dandruff), which is abnormal. The eyebrows should move smoothly under control of cranial nerve VII (facial).

(2) The **eyelashes** should be evenly distributed and curve outward, away from the globe. Lashes that curve inward because of eyelid inversion are abnormal and may irritate and damage the cornea.

(3) Note the **eyelids'** position, skin quality and characteristics, blinking, and frequency of blinking.

- The lids should not sag, droop, invert, or evert. When open, the upper lid rests at the top of the iris and the lower lid at the bottom, so that the sclera is not visible above or below the iris. Sagging of the upper lid to the extent that it covers the pupil is called **ptosis.** Ptosis may occur with aging, edema, 3rd cranial nerve dysfunction, or neuromuscular disorders.

- Ask the patient to close his or her eyelids while you inspect them. The lids should close enough to cover the globe. Note skin color. Elevate the eybrows gently with your fingers to inspect for lesions on the upper lid. Ask the patient to open the eyes while you look for lesions on the lower lid.

- Note the patient's ability to blink, approximately 20 times a minute. Rapid, infrequent, or asymmetric blinking is abnormal.

(4) Inspect the conjunctivae and sclerae for color, texture, lesions, and foreign bodies.

- The **bulbar conjunctivae** are colorless, transparent, and smooth, allowing you to see small blood vessels on the sclerae.

- You may wish to wear gloves to inspect the **palpebral conjunctivae.** Wash your hands before and after touching the conjunctivae. Retract each lower lid by pushing it down against the bony orbit while the patient looks up. Note whether the lid lining is pink to light red. A bright red or pale color is abnormal. If the lower palpebral conjunctivae are normal, you need not examine the upper conjunctivae.

- Evert each upper eyelid by gently pulling the lid down while the patient looks down. Place a cotton-tipped applicator just above the upper lid margin and push down on the lid, turning it inside out over the applicator. After inspecting the conjunctiva, return the lid to its normal position by pulling the eyelashes forward while the patient looks up.

- Transcultural considerations: Blacks may have yellow, fatty deposits on the undersurface of their lids, away from the cornea. The sclerae are white in Whites and may be gray-blue in Blacks. Dark-skinned patients may have brown flecks on the sclerae.

(5) Inspect the **lacrimal apparatus** in the upper outer wall of the anterior orbit and the area between the lower lid and nose for edema or redness. Look for a moist globe free of excess tearing.

(6) Palpate the **lacrimal sac** inside the orbit rim near the inner canthus. There should be no regurgitation of fluid from the sac or puncta.

(7) After asking the patient to close the eyes and look down, palpate the **globes** gently for firmness. With your thumbs, apply slight pressure on the upper eyelids, over the sclerae. The globes should feel equally firm yet yielding (see Chapter 18).

(8) Examine the cornea. Shine a penlight through the **cornea** from an oblique angle while from the opposite side you inspect the cornea for transparency; color; and smooth, convex curvature.

- There should be no corneal surface irregularity or cloudiness or opacity in the **anterior chamber.** Note the depth of the chamber between the cornea and the iris. It normally is approximately 3 mm. If chambers are shallower or deeper, refer the patient to an ophthalmologist for further examination.

- A thin white ring around the edge of the cornea in older patients (arcus senilis) is normal.

- The **iris** should be even in color and should not bulge. Note whether the iris constricts with the light, making the pupil smaller.

(9) Inspect the **pupils** for size, shape, equality, and reactivity to light and accommodation (under control of cranial nerves III, IV, and VI).

- Pupils normally are black and round, have smooth borders, and are equal in size.

- To test **direct response** to light, dim the lights, which will dilate the pupils, and ask the patient to look straight ahead. Bring the penlight toward the pupil from the side to shine directly on the pupil. The pupil should constrict briskly and evenly. Repeat the maneuver on the opposite pupil; the response should be the same.

- To test **consensual response** to light, shine the penlight on 1 pupil while you observe the opposite pupil for constriction. Repeat for the other eye. The responses of both pupils should be the same.

- Test **accommodation** by holding the penlight 10 to 15 cm (4–6 inches) away from the patient's nose. Instruct the patient to look first at the penlight, then straight ahead toward the distant wall, and then back at the penlight. Observe whether the pupils dilate with distance and constrict with near vision.

- Move the penlight toward the bridge of the patient's nose and observe for the pupils to converge and constrict.
- Record normal pupil reaction as *PERRLA*—*p*upils *e*qual, *r*ound, *r*eactive to *l*ight and *ac*commodation. Abnormal results include light intolerance (photophobia), irregular or unequal pupils, and pupils that do not react to light or accommodation.

(10) Test **extraocular movement** through 6 cardinal positions of gaze using the penlight or your finger held 30 cm (12 inches) in front of the patient's eyes. This maneuver tests the function of the 6 muscles that control conjugate eye movement (cranial nerves III, IV, and VI).
- Instruct the patient to look straight ahead and keep his or her head still while your finger moves slowly in a wide, extended H pattern (see Chapter 19). Do not go beyond the patient's field of vision. Move your finger from the center outward along each of the 6 directions. Pause briefly at the endpoint of each direction to observe for **nystagmus,** an abnormal, involuntary, rapid, oscillating movement of the globe. Nystagmus, in the positions of extreme lateral gaze is normal and is called endpoint nystagmus. Return to the center.
- Lack of conjugate eye movement and the covering of more than a small portion of the iris with the upper eyelid also are abnormal findings.

(11) While the patient continues to look straight ahead, shine the penlight at the bridge of the nose from a distance of 30 to 38 cm (12–15 inches). Look for the **corneal light reflection** (Hirschberg's test) of the penlight. The light's reflection should be at the same position on each cornea. Asymmetric reflection may indicate **strabismus** or a lack of conjugate eye movement toward an object. You will observe for strabismus further with the cover-uncover test.

(12) Elicit the **corneal reflex** to test cranial nerves V and VII. While the patient stares straight ahead, move your hand quickly from down and behind the patient in toward 1 eye, stopping short of touching it. The patient should blink the eye and possibly tear. Test both eyes.
- Alternative maneuvers include using a sterile cotton wisp to lightly touch each cornea and directing a puff of air across the cornea with a syringe or insufflation bulb from an otoscope.
- Because of decreased sensitivity to the stimulus, patients who wear contact lenses may not respond to the same degree as people who do not wear lenses.

(13) Perform the **cover test** for both eyes to assess eye muscle function and alignment. Ask the patient to stare straight ahead at a fixed point while you cover 1 eye with an index card and observe the uncovered eye for a steady, fixed gaze. Remove the eye cover and observe for movement in that eye. The gaze should remain steady. If either eye moves during the cover-uncover process, the eyes are out of alignment.

(14) Test the patient's **visual fields** (peripheral vision) by the confrontation method. This maneuver assumes that you have normal peripheral vision, which is 50 degrees superiorly, 90 degrees temporally, 70 degrees inferiorly, and 60 degrees nasally.
- Sit at eye level with the patient about 60 cm (2 ft) away. Both of you cover 1 eye, directly opposite each other (e.g., your left eye, the patient's right eye). Hold a penlight or your finger midway between the two of you at the periphery of your visual fields.
- Start with your finger in the superior field and proceed clockwise. Move your finger in toward midline until the patient states he or she can see it. You should be able to see your finger about the same time.
- For the temporal fields, start with your finger in a position slightly behind the patient's visual field.

d. Check **visual acuity** with the eye chart to assess cranial nerve II (optic). Test each eye separately by covering 1 eye with the eye cover and then test both eyes together. If the patient wears eyeglasses or contact lenses, test acuity with and without the lenses.
- The patient stands or sits 20 feet from the wall chart or holds the hand card 30 to 36 cm (12–14 inches) away from the face. Point to the line you wish the patient to read.
- Credit the patient for the smallest line of print he or she is able to read with 50 percent or greater accuracy. Use the standardized numbers printed in the margins of the eye chart to record results.
- **Normal vision** is 20/20; that is, the patient is able to read at 20 feet what a person with normal vision can read at 20 feet.
- **Myopia** (nearsightedness) is visual acuity of 20/30 or greater; that is, the patient reads at 20 feet what a person with normal vision can read at 30 feet.
- **Hyperopia** (farsightedness) is visual acuity of 20/15 or less; that is, the patient reads at 20 feet what a person with normal vision can read at 15 feet. Refer the patient whose visual acuity is 20/30 or greater to a specialist for further examination.
- Test **near vision** with the fine print on the hand-held card, or a newspaper, held 30 to 36 cm (12–14 inches) away. The patient may wear corrective lenses.
- The patient should be able to read the material clearly (no blurring) without moving the card. If this is not the case, refer the patient to a specialist.

e. Use the ophthalmoscope to inspect the structures posterior to the iris (see Chapter 19).
- Hold the ophthalmoscope in your right hand to examine the patient's right eye with your right

eye. Use your left hand and left eye to examine the patient's left eye.

- Hold the ophthalmoscope with your thumb, middle finger, and 4th finger. Your index finger will manipulate the diopter setting. Your 5th finger should rest on the patient's cheek to steady your hand and avoid bumping the patient's face with the instrument, and to anticipate any sudden head movement. Place your other hand toward the top of the head, with your thumb over the patient's eyebrow and fingers, to steady head movement.
- Dim the lights to promote pupil dilation. You will see only limited portions of the fundus at any 1 time unless the patient has received mydriatic eye drops.
- Turn on the ophthalmoscope light. Use the large, round aperture with white light for routine examination and the small, round aperture with white light for small pupils. Hold the ophthalmoscope up to your eye. Instruct the patient to stare at a point over your shoulder and to remain steady.
- Start from 30 cm (12 inches) away at a 15-degree lateral angle from the patient's eye. Set the diopter dial to +8 or +10 (black numbers). If you wear glasses, keep them on. The ophthalmoscope does not correct for astigmatism.
- Aim the light on the patient's pupil and look for the **red reflex,** a red glow from the light reflecting off the retina. Follow the red glow as you move the ophthalmoscope toward the patient and change the diopter setting to +6. If you lose sight of the red glow, you are not looking at the pupil. Adjust your angle accordingly. If the patient blinks, you will see a moving shadow and lose the red reflex. Maintain your position until the patient stops blinking.
- Note whether any dark shadows or black dots interrupt the red reflex. There should be none. Check the cornea and lens for transparency.
- Continue until your forehead is almost touching the patient's. Adjust the diopter setting until the **fundus** is in focus. If both you and the patient have normal vision, the diopter setting will be at 0 (zero). Use one of the negative diopter settings (red numbers) if the patient is nearsighted. Use one of the positive diopter settings (black numbers) if the patient is farsighted.
- Check the **retina** for color, pigmentation, hemorrhage, or exudate. Color can range from light red to dark red-brown, depending on skin color. Pigment is more noticeable in dark-skinned people and older people. There should be no signs of hemorrhage or exudate.
- Find the **optic disk** by following a blood vessel as it becomes larger, leading to the disk on the nasal side of the retina. Examine the disk for color, shape, sharpness of margins, pigmentation, and presence of the physiologic cup. Color ranges from creamy yellow to pink. The shape is round or oval. Disk margins should be sharp, although blurring at the nasal margin is normal. Pigmenta-

tion may vary. The cup may or may not be distinct in the middle of the disk as a brighter yellow or white. It should be no wider than half the diameter of the disk. Use the disk diameter to measure distances and other fundus structures, comparing their location with the hours on a clockface.

- Follow the **retinal vessels** out from the disk into 4 quadrants. Note their number, color, ratio of arterial to venous width, caliber, characteristics of arteriovenous crossings, tortuosity, and pulsations. Each quadrant has a paired artery and vein, which may appear straighter on the nasal side than in the lateral superior temporal or lateral inferior directions. Arteries are brighter red than veins and may look shiny as they reflect the light. Retinal arteries vary in width but are narrower than veins (e.g., two thirds or four fifths the width of veins). Both arteries and veins should narrow as they extend away from the optic disk. Look for interruptions, pinching, or displacement where arteries and veins cross. Mild tortuosity of vessels and slight pulsation in the veins near the disk are normal.
- Last, look for the **macula** on the temporal side of the optic disk at a distance of 2 disk diameters. It is the same size as the disk and is darker than the rest of the fundus. Signs of clumped pigment may occur with aging or may be abnormal. The patient's eyes will water and be uncomfortable while the light is shining on the macula, so be quick. Try to visualize the **fovea** in the middle of the macula, which may be seen as a white dot before the patient blinks and looks away.

f. Other tests that may be performed on the eyes are refraction, complete visual fields, color vision, and tonometry (see Chapter 19).

5. **Ears**
   a. Equipment: An otoscope and a tuning fork (512 Hz) are needed.
   b. External anatomic landmarks are the pinna, tragus, mastoid process, and external ear canal. Internal anatomic landmarks are the tympanic membrane, cone of light, umbo, handle and short process of the malleus, pars flaccida, and pars tensa.
   c. Examine the external ear.
      (1) Inspect the **pinnae** for placement, color, size, symmetry, lesions or masses.
         - Each pinna should be of equal size and symmetrically located with the upper point of attachment in line with the outer canthus. The vertical axis of each pinna should deviate no more than 10 degrees.
         - Each pinna should be the same color as the facial skin, without redness, pallor, or cyanosis. The skin should be smooth and free of flaking, scaling, and cysts or other lesions.
         - Assess the mobility of each pinna by gently moving it up, down, and back and folding it forward. It should be elastic and recoil without tenderness or pain.

• Palpate the cartilage of the pinna for firmness, tenderness, and swelling.

(2) Palpate over the **tragus** and behind the ear over the mastoid for tenderness, which is abnormal.

(3) Inspect the **external ear canal** for size (to determine which speculum to use in the otoscopic examination), redness, swelling, discharge, or foreign bodies, all of which should be absent. A small amount of **cerumen** is normal.

d. Perform the otoscopic examination (Fig. 5–7).

(1) Select the largest speculum that will fit into the patient's ear canal comfortably. Turn on the light. Hold the otoscope in your right hand to examine the patient's right ear and in your left hand for the left ear. You may hold the otoscope either upright or upside down.

(2) Brace the back of your hand and fingers lightly on the patient's cheek. This steadies the instrument and allows you to anticipate sudden movements of the patient's head.

(3) Tilt the patient's head away from you and toward his or her opposite shoulder. Grasp the top of the pinna firmly with your free hand and pull it up and back (adult or older child) or down (child under age 3) to straighten the ear canal. Retract the pinna firmly throughout the examination until you remove the otoscope from the ear canal.

(4) Watch as you insert the speculum slowly and gently into the canal, following its slope down and toward the nose. Then look through the lens. Avoid touching the inner lining of the canal, which is sensitive to pain. Reposition the otoscope or the patient's head as necessary to see structures.

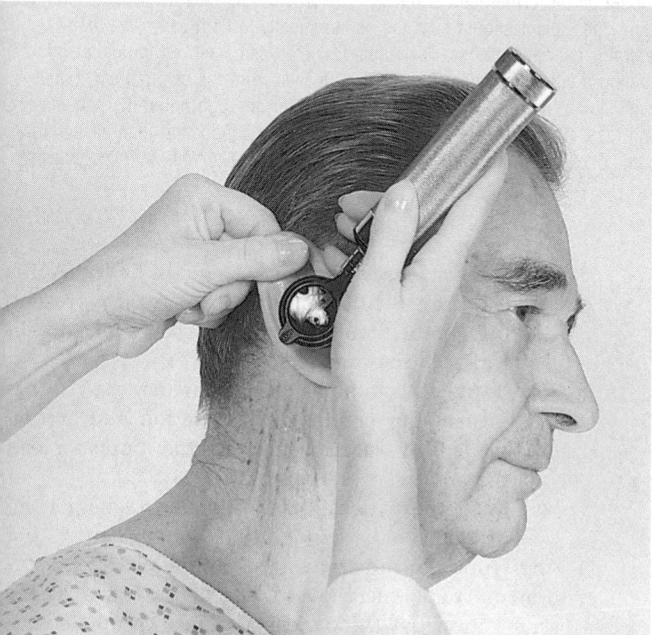

Figure 5–7. Otoscopic examination of the ear. (From Jarvis C. *Physical Examination and Health Assessment.* 2nd ed. Philadelphia: WB Saunders, 1996, p 362.)

(5) Inspect the ear canal for cerumen, color, lesions, foreign bodies, or discharge. If cerumen obstructs the canal, it must be removed for successful visualization of the tympanic membrane and accurate testing of hearing. Follow your institution's protocol for removing cerumen. (*Note:* Clean any discharge from the speculum before using it on the opposite ear.)

(6) Look for the **tympanic membrane** as a shiny reflection. You can see only portions of the membrane at one time and must reposition the otoscope carefully to see all the landmarks. The membrane should be shiny and a translucent pearl-gray.

(7) Locate the **cone of light** at the 5:00 position in the right ear and the 7:00 position in the left ear. Abnormalities of the tympanic membrane or in the middle ear may alter its location and appearance.

(8) Examine the tympanic membrane for scars (white patches) or perforations (round or oval darker areas).

(9) The tympanic membrane is flat and slightly concave at its center. It moves if the patient performs the Valsalva maneuver. Abnormal findings include retraction, bulging, or immobility with insufflation.

(10) Visualize the **annulus** (which surrounds the entire membrane), the **pars flaccida** (at the superior border), the **pars tensa** (lower two thirds of the membrane), the **umbo** in the center, the **long process of the malleus** (behind the umbo and angling upwards), and the **short process of the malleus** (at the upper end of the malleus just under the pars flaccida).

e. Test each ear for **hearing** continuously as you talk to the patient throughout the physical examination. Observe whether the patient cups 1 ear to hear better, turns his or her head, or leans toward you while listening.

f. The **voice test** assesses gross hearing acuity (auditory portion of cranial nerve VIII). Ask the patient to occlude 1 ear with a finger. Stand 30 to 60 cm (1–2 ft) away from the uncovered ear, so that the patient cannot see your lips. Slowly whisper several unrelated words, pausing for the patient to repeat them. If the patient cannot hear the words repeat the process while speaking more loudly. Repeat for the opposite ear. If results are abnormal, proceed to the Weber and Rinne tests.

g. The **Weber test** (Fig. 5–8) assesses bone conduction (BC) of sound with a tuning fork. Hold the tuning fork at the base of its handle and not by its prongs (to avoid dampening the sound). Strike the prongs softly against the heel of your hand, setting them into vibration. Do not strike the prongs on the edge of the table or another object.

(1) Quickly place the handle on the patient's skull at midline. Ask the patient whether he or she hears the sound equally in both ears (normal) or the sound is louder in 1 ear than the other

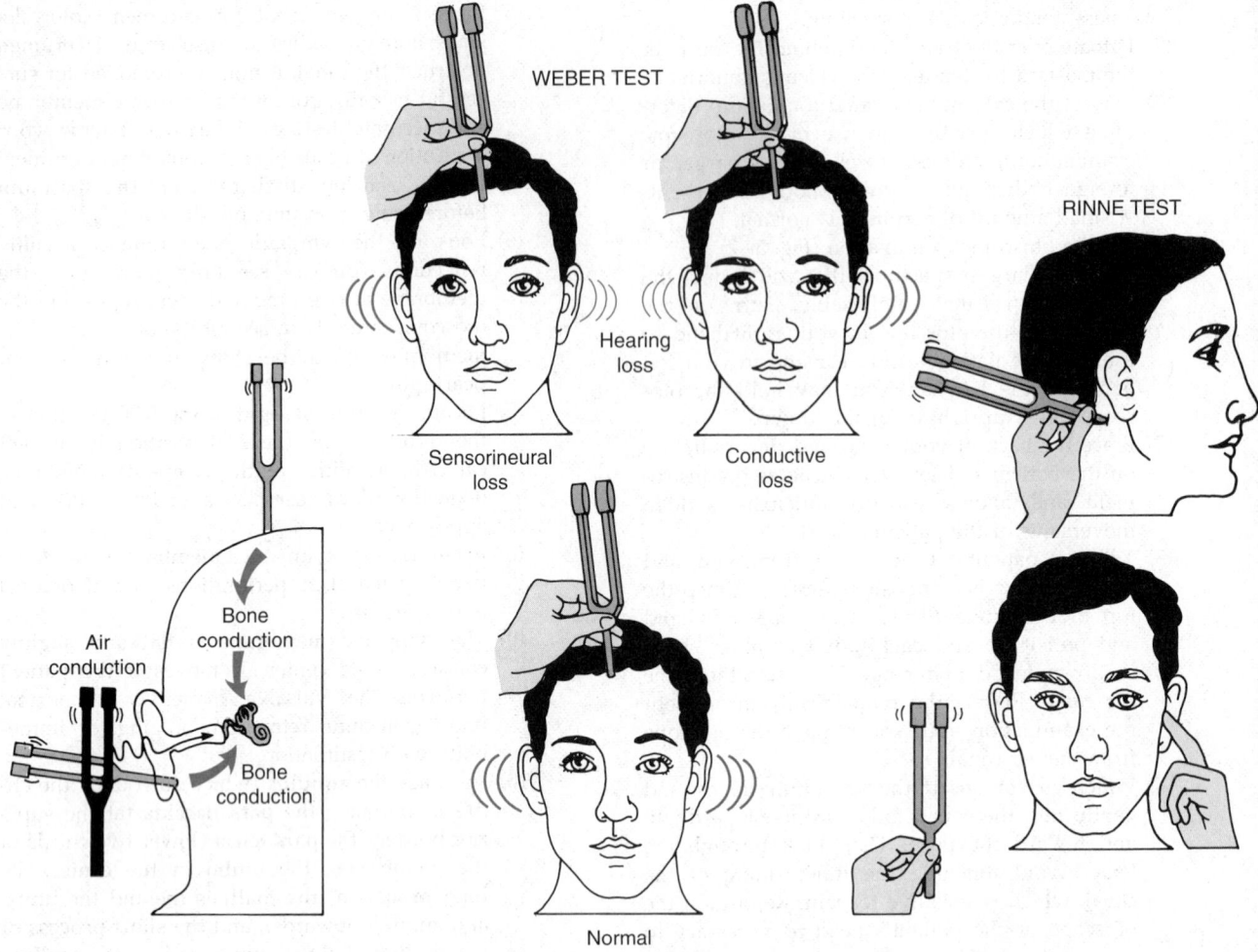

Figure 5-8. The Weber and Rinne tests for hearing loss. The Weber test is used to detect lateralization of hearing damage; the Rinne test distinguishes between conductive hearing loss and sensorineural hearing loss. The 2 tests should be performed consecutively. The Weber test uses a vibrating tuning fork placed on the patient's head or nose to produce a centrally located stimulus. The patient should hear the sound equally in both ears. The tone is louder in an ear with unilateral conductive loss and quieter in an ear with unilateral sensorineural loss. The Rinne test then characterizes the unilateral hearing loss as conductive or sensorineural. The Rinne test is performed by holding a vibrating tuning fork about 2 inches from the external ear. When the patient cannot hear the sound, the tuning fork is placed on the mastoid bone. When the tone is louder through air than through bone, the patient has a positive Rinne finding, which indicates normal hearing or sensorineural hearing loss. A negative Rinne finding (louder bone conduction than air conduction) indicates a conductive loss. (From Black JM, and Matassarin-Jacobs E [eds]. *Luckmann and Sorensen's Medical-Surgical Nursing: A Psychophysiologic Approach.* 4th ed. Philadelphia: WB Saunders, 1993, p 875.)

(lateralization). Note to which ear the sound lateralizes.

(2) Lateralization may indicate either a conduction or a sensorineural loss, depending on the underlying problem. Continue with the Rinne test.

h. The **Rinne test** (see Fig. 5–8) compares bone conduction (BC) with air conduction (AC) (see Fig. 5–8*B* and *C*).

(1) Set the tuning fork into vibration. Place it 1st on the mastoid process (BC) and ask the patient to tell you when he or she no longer hears the sound. Quickly move the tuning fork to position the prongs in front of the patient's ear canal (AC). The patient should still be able to hear the sound. Ask the patient to tell you when the sound is gone.

(2) The normal response is AC is greater than BC by a ratio of 2:1 (positive Rinne test).

(3) Abnormal results are AC equals BC or AC is less than BC (a negative Rinne test), representing conduction loss in the presence of lateralization to the same ear.

(4) If the 2:1 ratio of AC is greater than BC is present but shortened in duration and accompanied by lateralization to the opposite ear, there is a sensorineural loss.

(5) Refer the patient for additional screening if indicated.

i. The vestibular apparatus (the vestibulocochlear portion of cranial nerve VIII) is usually tested at the time you assess the patient's balance during neurologic assessment.

6. **Nose and sinuses**

a. Equipment. A penlight and a nasal speculum, or an otoscope fitted with a nasal speculum and a transilluminator (see Fig. 5–1), are needed. If you plan to test olfaction, you also need a supply of various substances for the patient to smell (e.g., coffee grounds, cinnamon, cloves, peppermint).

  b. External anatomic landmarks are the external nose, including the nares. Internal landmarks are the vestibule, nasal mucosa, septum, turbinates, nasal canals, and sinuses.

  c. Examine the **external nose.**

    (1) Inspect the external nose for alignment, symmetry, color, discharge, nasal flaring, and lesions. The nose should be straight, without deviation from midline, and it should be the same color as the facial skin. The presence of a discharge, nasal flaring with breathing, and lesions are abnormal findings.

    (2) Palpate the nose for alignment, lesions, tenderness, and patency. There should be no masses, lesions, or tenderness. Ask the patient to occlude one naris with a finger and breathe through the open naris with the mouth closed. Repeat for the opposite naris. The patient should be able to breathe easily through both nares.

    (3) Ask the patient to tip his or her head back while you inspect the outer nares for crusting, bleeding, or dryness, which should be absent. Note whether the **septum** is at midline.

    (4) Use a penlight to inspect the **vestibules.** Coarse hair is normal. You may be able to see the inferior nasal mucosa, which should be moist and pink. Further examination is conducted with a nasal speculum and light source.

  d. Examine the internal nose with the nasal speculum attached to the otoscope head or use a metal nasal speculum and penlight (Fig. 5–9). Ask the patient to tip his or her head back. With your free hand, lightly push the tip of the nose up and insert the speculum gently into 1 naris. Do not scrape the mucosa.

    (1) Inspect the **mucosa** for color, moisture, and discharge. The mucosa should be dark pink

and moist, without signs of discharge, inflammation, pallor, or cyanosis.

    (2) Note the septum's midline position and look for masses, perforation, or exudate, which should be absent.

    (3) Inspect the **turbinates** (only the inferior turbinate and part of the middle turbinate are visible; the superior turbinate is not). They should be of the same color as the mucosa and free of exudate, swelling, or inflammation.

  e. Assess the **sinuses** using palpation and percussion. If they are tender, transilluminate them.

    (1) Palpate the **frontal sinuses** simultaneously, using your thumbs (Fig. 5–10). Press gently above the eyes, just under the bony ridge of the orbits. The frontal sinuses should be free of tenderness, swelling, or bogginess.

    (2) Palpate the **maxillary sinuses** with either your index and middle fingers or your thumbs. Gently press on each side of the nose just under the zygomatic bones.

    (3) Use direct finger percussion over the eyebrows (frontal sinuses) and under the eyes at their midpoint (maxillary sinuses) to assess further for tenderness.

    (4) If tenderness is present, attempt to transilluminate the sinuses to assess for congestion (see Chapter 20). Use a penlight or the transilluminator head and darken the room.

    (5) Place the light source against the orbital bone immediately below the eyebrow and shield the light with your free hand. Normally, a red glow appears over the frontal sinus area. If the sinus is congested, the area will remain dark.

    (6) Repeat this test for the maxillary sinus by placing the light beneath the center of the eye and the zygomatic bone. Direct the light down and in toward the roof of the mouth. Ask the patient to open his or her mouth while you look for the red glow on the hard palate on the illuminated side.

  f. If you plan to test the patient's sense of smell (cranial nerve I), ask the patient to close his or her eyes and occlude 1 naris with a finger. Test each side separately and randomly. Hold the test substance under the naris and ask the patient to sniff and identify the separate odors.

7. **Mouth and pharynx**

  a. Equipment: You need gloves, a tongue depressor, a penlight, gauze pads, and substances to assess taste sensation (cranial nerves VII and IX) if the patient reports any problems in this area.

  b. Anatomic landmarks are the lips, teeth, gingivae, oral mucosa, Stensen's ducts, Wharton's ducts, tongue, hard and soft palates, uvula, anterior and posterior pillars, tonsils, and posterior oropharynx. (see Chapter 27).

  c. Inspect the patient's **lips** for color, texture, contour, hydration, and lesions. The lips should be pink, smooth, moist, and without lesions, fissures, crusts, or cyanosis. The color may be darker pink in dark-skinned patients.

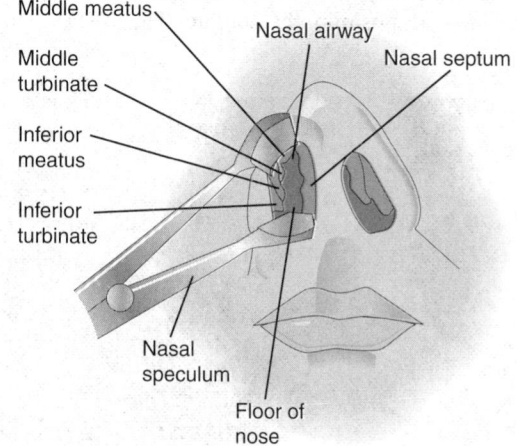

Figure 5–9. Insertion of a nasal speculum, showing the visible portions of internal structures. (Redrawn from Black JM, and Matassarin-Jacobs E [eds]. *Luckmann and Sorensen's Medical-Surgical Nursing: A Psychophysiologic Approach.* 4th ed. Philadelphia: WB Saunders, 1993, p 926.)

Middle meatus

Middle turbinate

Inferior meatus

Inferior turbinate

Nasal airway

Nasal septum

Nasal speculum

Floor of nose

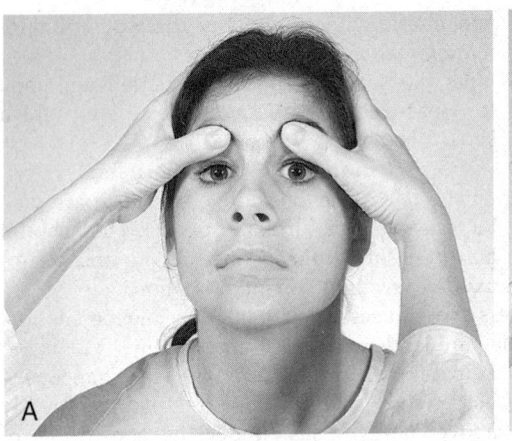
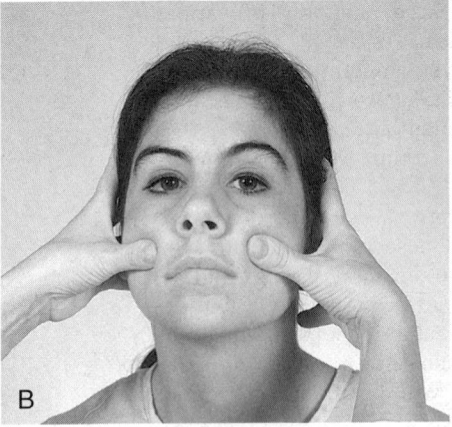

Figure 5–10. Palpation of the maxillary and frontal sinuses. (From Jarvis C. *Physical Examination and Health Assessment*. 2nd ed. Philadelphia: WB Saunders, 1996, p 398.)

d. Inspect the **oral mucosa** using the penlight and tongue depressor. Ask the patient to remove any dentures before you begin. Wear gloves.

  (1) Retract the lips from the gums using your fingers or a tongue depressor. Use a penlight to inspect the mucosa lining the lips and gums. Retract the buccal mucosa and inspect the lining of the cheeks. Look for masses, lesions, and discoloration. Note hydration.

  (2) The mucosa should be glistening and moist, pink, and smooth. Dark-skinned patients may have pigmented areas on the mucosa and gums. There should be no masses, lesions, vesicles, or ulcers.

  (3) Note the openings of **Stensen's ducts** on the buccal mucosa, opposite the upper 2nd molars. They look like dimples and should be without swelling or redness.

e. Inspect the **gingivae and teeth** while you inspect the mucosa. Note the color of the gingivae and look for edema, bleeding, retraction (pulling away from the teeth), and lesions.

  (1) The gingivae should be pink (dark patches in dark-skinned patients are normal). There should be no bleeding, swelling, retraction, inflammation, drainage, or lesions.

  (2) Note the number of teeth present, their color, and their condition. Adults with no history of extractions usually have 32 teeth that are light yellow to white, and shiny. Note missing or loose teeth, areas of chalky white or dark discoloration on the enamel, or plaque, all of which are abnormal findings. Ask if the patient has bridges or fillings.

  (3) Ask the patient to open and close his or her mouth while you inspect the alignment of the teeth. The upper and lower molars should line up, and the upper teeth should override the lower teeth slightly.

  (4) If the patient wears dentures, inspect them for broken or worn areas that may irritate the underlying tissues. Inspect those tissues for redness or ulceration.

  (5) Palpate the gingivae. They should feel firm and smooth and should not bleed or feel boggy (soft).

f. Inspect the **tongue and floor of the mouth** by asking the patient to stick out his or her tongue. Note the tongue's position, symmetry, color, size, texture, and mobility and the presence of a coating, lesions, or fasciculations.

  (1) The tongue should protrude at midline without deviation or tremor (cranial nerve XII). It should be symmetric and lie in the floor of the mouth behind the lower teeth when at rest. Its color is dark pink. Its texture is rough on the dorsal surface (from the papillae, or taste buds) and smooth on the lateral margins. The surface should be moist and may have a light white coating.

  (2) Ask the patient to lift the tongue to the roof of the mouth; curl it down toward the chin; move it back and forth rapidly; and push it against the tongue depressor, first to the left and then to the right. These movements test the function of cranial nerves IX and XII. The tongue should be freely mobile and equally strong from side to side.

  (3) Inspect the underside of the tongue and the floor of the mouth. Use the penlight and either the tongue depressor or gauze sponge to grasp and position the tongue (Fig. 5–11). The area

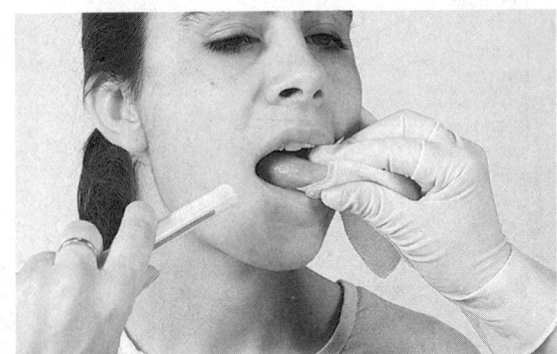

Figure 5–11. Inspection and palpation of the mouth and gums. (From Jarvis C. *Physical Examination and Health Assessment*. 2nd ed. Philadelphia: WB Saunders, 1996, p 401.)

should be moist, and pooling of saliva is normal. Look for the openings of **Wharton's ducts** at the base of the tongue on either side of the frenulum. There should be no lesions, red plaque, or leukoplakia.

(4) Palpate the entire tongue, including its base, and the floor of the mouth for lesions, cysts, or nodules, which should be absent.

g. Ask the patient to tip back his or her head. Inspect the roof of the mouth, palates, and uvula using the penlight.

(1) Inspect the **hard and soft palates** for color, shape, texture, and presence of bony deformity. The palates should be light pink and symmetric. Rough ridges on the hard palate are normal; the soft palate should be smooth. Bony growths (exostoses) may normally be present on the hard palate.

(2) Inspect the **uvula** by placing the tongue depressor on the middle 3rd of the tongue and depressing it lightly. Ask the patient to say ''Ah'' while you look to see that the uvula and soft palate rise in the midline without deviation (cranial nerve X).

h. Keep the tongue depressor in place and inspect the **tonsils**, which are located between the anterior and posterior pillars. The pillars are normally pink and smooth. The tonsils, if present, are normally oval, pink, smooth, and symmetric. Their size may vary, but the tonsilar tissue should lie behind the anterior pillar and not extend into the midline. Folds on the surface of the tonsils are normal but should be free of exudate or white spots. If the tonsils are enlarged, grade them according to the following scale:
- Grade 1 = Tonsils are behind the pillars
- Grade 2 = Tonsils are between the pillars and uvula
- Grade 3 = Tonsils touch the uvula
- Grade 4 = Tonsils extend the midline of the oropharynx

i. Inspect the **pharynx** for color and the presence of drainage on the posterior wall. The pharynx is normally pink and smooth and without edema, ulcers, inflammation, or exudate.
- Clear drainage along the posterior pharynx may indicate allergic rhinitis; yellow or green exudate may signal sinus infection. The patient should be referred for follow-up in either case.
- Assess the functioning of cranial nerves IX and X by eliciting the **gag reflex** with the tongue depressor. Gently touch 1 side of the posterior pharynx and observe the patient's reaction. Be sure to test both sides.

j. Assess the patient's **voice** throughout your interactions. Note pitch, volume, and clarity. Ask the patient to **swallow** and note the level of ease with which this is done. These actions test cranial nerves IX and X. Hoarseness, rasping, uneven pitch, fluctuating volume, and difficulty swallowing are abnormal.

k. Note whether the patient's **breath** has an unusual odor, which may indicate an underlying problem. Examples are poor dental hygiene, sinus infection, alcohol ingestion, diabetes mellitus, and uremia.

l. The sense of **taste** (cranial nerves VII and IX) is usually not assessed unless the patient reports a problem. If you tested the patient's sense of smell, test his or her sense of taste as well. The two are closely linked.

(1) Ask the patient to close the eyes and stick out the tongue. Test each side of the anterior and posterior aspects of the tongue with 4 substances: salt (salt), sugar (sweet), vinegar or lemon juice (acid), and bitters or quinine (bitter).

(2) Apply the substances with a dropper or cotton applicator in a random pattern. Instruct the patient to rinse his or her mouth with water between each taste. The patient should be able to discern each taste.

8. **Neck**

a. Equipment: A stethoscope, glass of water, and straw are needed.

b. Anatomic landmarks include the neck muscles (trapezius and sternocleidomastoid), cervical spine, salivary glands (parotid, sublingual, and submaxillary), cervical lymph nodes (occipital, postauricular, postcervical, supraclavicular, superficial and deep cervical, tonsillar, submandibular, submental, and preauricular), trachea, thyroid gland, and neck vessels (carotid arteries and jugular veins).

c. The patient is sitting except when you inspect the jugular veins. Inspect the patient's neck for symmetry, swelling, and masses. There should be no swelling or masses.

d. Ask the patient to flex his or her head laterally by trying to touch each ear to the shoulders, turning the head to the right and to the left in lateral rotation; and tipping the head back and then bringing the chin forward to the chest. These maneuvers test neck muscle flexibility and **cervical spine** range of motion. There should be no stiffness, pain, or tenderness.

e. Ask the patient to turn his or her head to the right and to the left and then turn it back to the center while you apply resistance with your hand against the side of the head. Also ask the patient to shrug his or her shoulders upward while you apply resistance to them. The patient should be able to push his or her shoulders firmly against your hands with equal strength on both sides. These 2 maneuvers test the functioning of cranial nerve XI.

f. Inspect and palpate the areas over the parotid, sublingual, and submandibular **salivary glands** for swelling and tenderness, which should be absent.

g. Inspect the surface overlying the **cervical nodes** for masses or scars. Compare with the contralateral side.

h. Palpate all cervical nodes for size, shape, consistency, discreteness, mobility, and tenderness. Palpate with the pads of your 1st 3 fingers, making a gentle, circular motion. Keep your fingertips in contact with the skin and slide the skin over the underlying nodes. Be careful not the use too much pressure, because it obliterates small, palpable nodes. Use a methodic, thorough approach.

    (1) Lymph nodes are not normally palpable, but it is common to find small (1 cm or less), round, soft, single, mobile, nontender nodes in the cervical area.

    (2) Nodes that are large (greater than 1 cm in diameter), hard, tender, matted together, or fixed to underlying structures are abnormal.

i. Inspect and palpate the **trachea** for symmetry and location.

    (1) Locate the suprasternal notch over the manubrium and slide your thumb and index finger apart laterally so that the trachea is between your fingers.

    (2) The spaces formed by the clavicles, the anterior aspect of the sternocleidomastoids, and the trachea should be symmetric, without lateral deviation. The trachea should be slightly mobile from side to side.

j. Examine the **thyroid gland** using inspection, palpation, and auscultation.

    (1) Stand in front of the patient and inspect the lower neck for symmetry and visible masses. Ask the patient to hyperextend the neck and swallow (offer the patient a glass of water, if needed) while you observe the thyroid and cricoid cartilage move upward with the swallowing action. There should be no bulging over the gland, because the thyroid is usually not visible.

    (2) Palpate the gland using either an anterior or a posterior approach (Fig. 5–12).

      • In the **anterior approach,** slide your finger down the anterior neck, locating the thyroid and cricoid cartilages and the thyroid isthmus. The isthmus feels soft and compressible compared with the firmer cartilage ring just superior to it. Ask the patient to swallow while you palpate the isthmus. The isthmus should rise in the neck and should not be enlarged. Palpate the lobes of the gland by flexing the patient's head toward the side of the lobe you want to palpate to relax the neck muscles. Use your right hand to displace the thyroid gently toward the patient's right while the head is flexed to the right. Palpate the right lobe with your left fingers while the patient swallows and the gland rises. Use your left hand to displace the thyroid toward the patient's left while the head is flexed to the left. Palpate the left lobe with your right fingers. The thyroid gland is usually not palpable. If it is, note the texture. The gland should be smooth, without lumps or roughness.

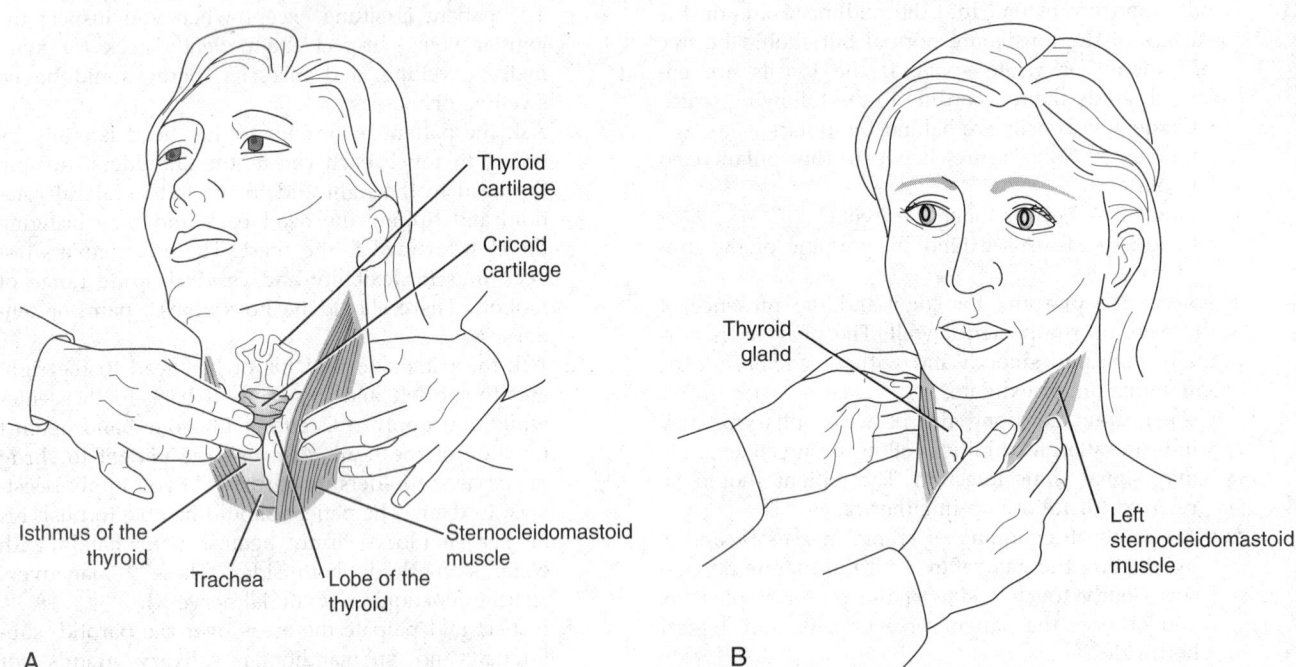

A

B

Figure 5–12. Palpation of the thyroid. *A,* Posterior approach for thyroid palpation. The examiner stands behind the patient. The patient is asked to lower the chin to relax the neck muscles and turn the head slightly to the right. To examine the right lobe of the thyroid, the examiner uses the finger of the left hand to displace the trachea slightly to the right. This moves the thyroid laterally. The lobes can then be palpated by the fingers of the right hand. Projection of the thyroid can be assisted by having the patient drink water. *B,* Anterior approach to thyroid palpation. The examiner stands in front of the patient. To examine the right lobe of the thyroid, the examiner uses the fingers of the left hand to displace the trachea slightly to the right. With the fingers of the left hand, the thyroid is palpated. The patient is asked to swallow and flex the head slightly and turn. Thyroid enlargement can also be assessed for by palpating deep on each side of the sternocleidomastoid muscle. (Redrawn from Black JM, and Matassarin-Jacobs E [eds]. *Luckmann and Sorensen's Medical-Surgical Nursing: A Psychophysiologic Approach.* 4th ed. Philadelphia: WB Saunders, 1993, p 1770.)

- In the **posterior approach,** stand behind the patient and reach your hands around his or her neck to locate the isthmus with your fingers. The remainder of the maneuver is similar to that used in the anterior approach.
      (3) If the thyroid gland is enlarged, auscultate the lobes with the bell of the stethoscope. Enlargement results in increased blood flow through the gland, which may be heard as a bruit.
  k. Assess the **neck vessels** while the patient is sitting and later during the anterior thorax examination, when he or she is supine or in the semi-Fowler's position.
      (1) Inspect the area over the **carotid arteries** for visible pulsations. Sometimes a pulse wave may be seen just below the angle of the jaw.
      (2) Palpate each artery individually. Do not massage the area or press too firmly over the carotid sinus near the angle of the jaw. This may stimulate a vagal response, causing bradycardia and syncope.
      (3) Locate the artery by sliding your fingers from the trachea to the medial side of the sternocleidomastoid muscle while the patient turns his or her head to that same side. Note the pulse amplitude. The pulse should thrust against your fingers, and the artery walls should feel elastic and smooth.
      (4) Auscultate each carotid artery with the bell of the stethoscope to assess for bruits. Ask the patient to hold his or her breath momentarily while you listen. There should be no vascular sounds. If you hear a bruit, palpate the artery again to assess for a **thrill** (a vibrating sensation that feels like a purring cat), which indicates turbulent blood flow related to narrowing of the vessel lumen.
      (5) Inspect the areas over the **jugular veins** for distention. When the patient is sitting, the jugular veins should be flat. Bilateral distention indicates increased venous system blood volume and right heart overload. Unilateral distention indicates vessel obstruction on that side. Examine the jugular veins further when you assess the anterior thorax.

9. **Upper extremities**
  a. The upper extremities include parts of multiple body systems that may be examined in an integrated manner but are reported separately in the findings. These systems include the integumentary (see earlier section), peripheral vascular, musculoskeletal, and neurologic systems. Some practitioners perform this part of the physical examination before they examine the head and neck. Others examine both the upper and lower extremities toward the end of the examination. Be consistent and thorough in your approach.
  b. Peripheral vascular system
      (1) The patient is still seated.
        - Palpate the **peripheral pulses** (radial, ulnar, and brachial). Assess rhythm and amplitude

(see p. 111 and Fig. 5–5) by palpating each pair of pulses simultaneously. Use your right hand to palpate the patient's left pulses and your left hand to palpate the right pulses. The same right and left pulses (e.g., right and left radial) should have the same pulse amplitude and rhythm.
      (2) Palpate the **epitrochlear lymph nodes,** located proximal to the medial epicondyle of the humerus between the biceps and triceps muscles. (See p. 105 for a discussion of lymph node palpation.) They should be nonpalpable.
      (3) Note whether there is **edema** in the extremities.
  c. Musculoskeletal system
      (1) Equipment: A tape measure and goniometer are needed if there are abnormal findings.
      (2) Inspect the arms for symmetry, alignment, and proportion relative to the trunk of the body.
      (3) Inspect and palpate muscle groups for size, symmetry, and **tone** (the state of tension in a muscle at rest, felt as firmness). Note involuntary movements. Begin proximally at the shoulders and work distally to the fingers, or vice versa. The muscles should be nontender; firm; equal in size bilaterally; and without fasciculations, lumps, or bulges. If muscle groups look unequal, measure them with a tape measure and compare measurements. In the dominant arm, slight **hypertrophy** (increased muscle mass) is a normal finding and **atrophy** (decreased mass) is abnormal.
      (4) Assess **muscle strength** in the major muscle groups of the upper arms, forearms, wrists, and fingers by applying resistance to the patient's movements with your hands.
        - Test muscle group extensors and flexors in pairs for greatest efficiency. For example, ask the patient to first extend and then flex the elbow while you attempt to prevent these movements.
        - Rate muscle strength using the scale shown in Chapter 18 (see Fig. 18–13).
      (5) Inspect and palpate each **joint and bone** for symmetry, swelling, tenderness, crepitus, or deformity.
        - Palpate the joints as they move for **crepitus** (a grating sound or sensation). The joints should feel smooth as they move and should be free of nodules.
        - Ask the patient to put each joint (shoulder, elbow, wrist, and finger) through active range of motion. (See Chapter 7.) If you observe a limitation, use a goniometer to measure the angle of joint movement.
  d. Neurologic system
      (1) You may elect to complete parts of the assessment of the neurologic system at this time or complete the entire neurologic assessment toward the end of the physical examination. The parts often performed at this time are assessments of motor function, deep tendon re-

flexes (DTRs), and cerebellar function. Sensory function is best assessed for the entire body at one time. You have already assessed motor function as part of the musculoskeletal examination when you assessed muscle tone, strength, and movement. If you test **DTRs** for the upper extremities, be efficient and test the lower extremity DTRs and plantar reflex also.

(2) Equipment: You will need a reflex hammer to test DTRs. The patient may be seated or lying.

(3) Anatomic landmarks are the biceps, triceps, and brachioradialis muscles and their attached tendons in the upper extremities and the quadriceps and gastrocnemius muscles and their attached tendons (including the Achilles tendon) in the lower extremities.

(4) Testing of the DTR arcs assesses the integrity of both sensory and motor pathways, as well as their associated spinal cord segments (see Fig. 18–17).

(5) Use the following guidelines:
- All DTRs may be assessed with the patient either sitting or lying.
- Support the joint where the tendon is being tested so that the attached muscle is relaxed.
- Use the pointed end of the triangular reflex hammer to strike small areas (e.g., place your thumb over the biceps tendon and strike your thumb). Use the flat end of the hammer to strike larger areas, such as the Achilles tendon.
- Hold the reflex hammer loosely between your thumb and fingers so that it can swing in an arc. Swing the reflex hammer by moving only your wrist, not your elbow or arm. Tap the tendon briskly. Note the speed, force, and amplitude of the reflex response.
- Compare reflex responses bilaterally. Grade reflexes on a 0 to 4+ scale. Consider the strength of the reflex in relation to the bulk of the muscle mass. Repeat testing of reflexes that are graded 0 or 1+ by using reinforcement at the same time you strike the tendon. Note in the recording that reinforcement was used.

(6) Grade DTRs as follows:
- 0 = Response absent
- 1+ = Response diminished
- 2+ = Response normal
- 3+ = Response brisker than expected (may or may not be abnormal)
- 4+ = Response very brisk, hyperactive, or clonic (i.e., alternating involuntary contraction and relaxation of skeletal muscles); often associated with spinal cord disorders

(7) **Reinforcement** increases the general reflex response when the patient isometrically contracts other muscle groups. For example, for upper extremity DTRs ask the patient either to clench the teeth together or contract the quadriceps muscles by pushing the thighs against the table. For lower extremity DTRs, ask the patient to lock the fingers together and then try to pull them apart.

(8) Assess **cerebellar function** by observing the patient's coordination as he or she performs specific rapid alternating movements and point-to-point touching.
- Ask the patient to alternately pronate and supinate both hands on his or her thighs as quickly as possible. An alternative maneuver is to have the patient touch each finger to the thumb (opposition) quickly. These movements should be performed rapidly and smoothly.
- Ask the patient touch his or her nose with an index finger, first with eyes open and then with eyes closed, for several repetitions. Then ask the patient to touch his or her nose alternating with touching your index finger, which you hold out at arm's length from the patient. Repeat several times while you move your finger in different directions. The patient should be able to perform accurately.
- Maneuvers for assessing cerebellar function in the lower extremities are discussed on p. 142.

10. **Posterior thorax**

a. Assessment of the posterior thorax includes parts of the integumentary, musculoskeletal, respiratory, and urinary systems.

b. The patient should be sitting, especially for the lung assessment. If the patient cannot sit either unaided or with assistance, you may examine first 1 side and then the other by turning the patient from side to side. The entire posterior thorax should be undraped for the examination.

c. Integumentary system: Inspect the skin as you inspect the thorax.

d. Musculoskeletal system
(1) Inspect the **spine** for alignment; it should be straight and without lateral deviation.
(2) Palpate the **spinous processes** for tenderness and lateral curvature, which should be absent.
(3) Inspect the **rib cage and scapulae** for symmetry, shape, and movement with respiration.
- Each hemithorax should move in and out equally with respirations. The ribs slope obliquely downward so that the **costovertebral angles** (formed by the ribs joining the spine) are approximately 45 degrees.
- Compare the ratio of the anteroposterior diameter to the transverse diameter, i.e., the **anteroposterior to lateral diameter,** at the level of the lower sternum. The anteroposterior to lateral diameter normally ranges from 1:2 to 5:7 in adults.
- The **scapulae** lie close against the thoracic wall and are symmetric.
- Abnormal findings include asymmetry, increased costovertebral angles, and an anteroposterior to lateral diameter approaching 1:1 (barrel chest).
(4) Inspect the thoracic **musculature** and intercostal

spaces for signs of bulging or retraction with respirations, which should be absent. Contour is symmetric.

(5) Lightly palpate over the **paravertebral muscles** for tenderness and spasm. They should feel smooth.

(6) Palpate lightly over the entire posterior and lateral thorax for masses and tenderness, which should be absent. Avoid deep palpation if areas of pain or tenderness are found; you may inadvertently displace a rib segment against an underlying organ.

(7) Place the palms of your hands on the lower borders of the thorax to assess **thoracic excursion** (respiratory excursion). Your thumbs should be approximately 5 cm (2 inches) apart and level with the 10th ribs, pointing toward the spine. Spread the rest of your fingers laterally over the thorax. Push your thumbs together slightly so that a small fold of skin arises between them.
  • Ask the patient to take a deep breath while you observe and feel the chest movement.
  • Your thumbs should move apart equally and simultaneously, approximately 3 to 5 cm (1.5–2.0 inches), during excursion. Asymmetry and hesitancy in taking a deep breath (splinting or guarding) are abnormal findings.

e. Lungs

(1) Equipment: You will need a stethoscope, ruler, and pen for this portion of the thoracic assessment.

(2) Posterior thorax anatomic landmarks are the cervical and thoracic vertebrae, scapulae, ribs, vertical anatomic reference lines (midline, midscapular, posterior axillary, and midaxillary), location of the underlying lung lobes and fissures, and level of the diaphragm.

(3) Observe **respirations** in more detail, noting rate, depth, pattern, and how much effort the patient has to make to breathe.

(4) Palpate **tactile fremitus** (vocal fremitus) over the posterior lung fields. Fremitus is the vibration produced in the airways when the patient vocalizes sounds.
  • Ask the patient to cross his or her arms over the chest to spread the scapulae apart, increasing the area of accessible lung tissue. Instruct the patient to say "99" each time your hands touch his or her back.
  • Palpate with either the ball or ulnar aspect of your hands. Assess the right and left sides at the same time for comparison. Begin over the lung apices, move to the area over the tracheal bifurcation, and then proceed down either side of the spine. Continue over the lung bases posteriorly and laterally.
  • Vibrations are usually most strong at the lung apices and over the tracheal bifurcation and diminish toward the bases. If the vibrations

are faint, ask the patient to speak louder using a deeper voice.
  • If tactile fremitus is increased, decreased, or asymmetric, auscultate the vocal sounds for bronchophony, egophony, and whispered pectoriloquy (see Chapter 21).

(5) Use indirect finger percussion over the interspaces to assess for fluid or consolidation in underlying lung tissue, as well as diaphragmatic excursion (Fig. 5–13).

(6) Ask the patient to cross his or her arms over the chest to spread the scapulae. The patient can also raise his or her arms straight overhead. Follow the same sequence as for tactile fremitus palpation.
  • Percuss only over the apices and between the interspaces, parallel to the ribs and between the spine and scapulae, to the level of the 10th ribs.
  • Continue over the bases laterally to the midaxillary lines and then from the axillae to the 8th ribs.
  • The sound should be resonant throughout the lung fields and dull over the diaphragm.

(7) Determine **diaphragmatic excursion** as the diaphragm moves during maximal inspiration and expiration (Fig. 5–14).
  • Ask the patient to take a deep breath and hold it while you percuss down one midscapular line from the area of resonance to dullness. Mark the level with a pen where the

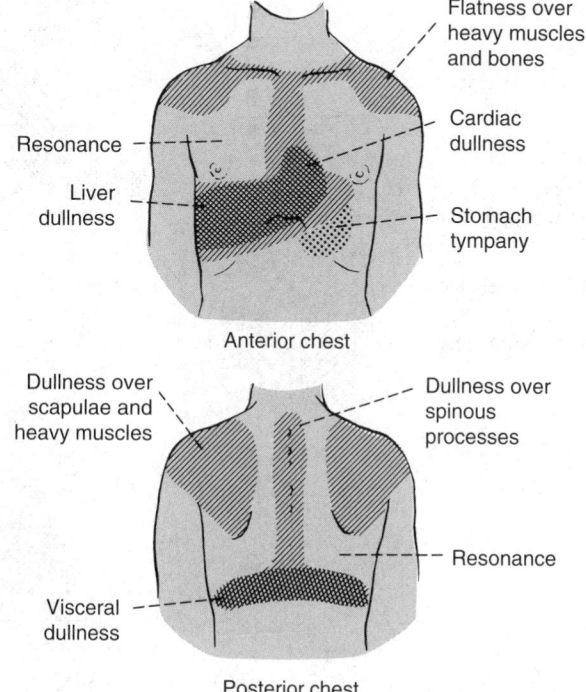

Figure 5–13. Location of thoracic percussion tones and their associated structures. (From Black JM, and Matassarin-Jacobs E [eds]. *Luckmann and Sorensen's Medical-Surgical Nursing: A Psychophysiologic Approach.* 4th ed. Philadelphia: WB Saunders, 1993, p 921.)

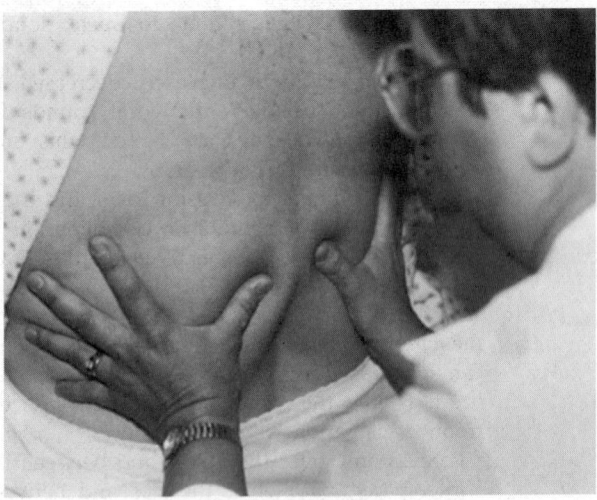

Figure 5-14. Thoracic excursion assesses the degree and symmetry of chest movement. (From Black JM, and Matassarin-Jacobs E [eds]. *Luckmann and Sorensen's Medical-Surgical Nursing: A Psychophysiologic Approach.* 4th ed. Philadelphia: WB Saunders, 1993, p 920.)

sound changes. Repeat this maneuver on the other side.

- Allow the patient to rest a moment and then ask him or her to exhale deeply and hold it

while you percuss up the midscapular line from the pen mark (dullness) to where the sound changes to resonance. Mark this level with the pen. Repeat for the other side.

- Measure the vertical distance between each set of pen marks; this is the diaphragmatic excursion. The distance is approximately 5 to 7 cm (2.0–2.5 inches) in men and 3 to 5 cm (1–2 inches) in women. The lines on the patient's right side may be slightly higher than those on the left because of the presence of the liver.

(8) Auscultate the posterior lung fields using the same sequence you used for palpation of fremitus and percussion (Fig. 5–15).

- Place the diaphragm of the stethoscope over the apices and intercostal spaces to listen for the sounds created by air moving through the tracheobronchial tree.
- Be familiar with the characteristics of normal breath sounds and their location. (See Chapter 22.)
- Ask the patient to breathe through the mouth, taking a slow, deep breath each time you place the stethoscope on his or her back.
- Listen at each point for a complete respira-

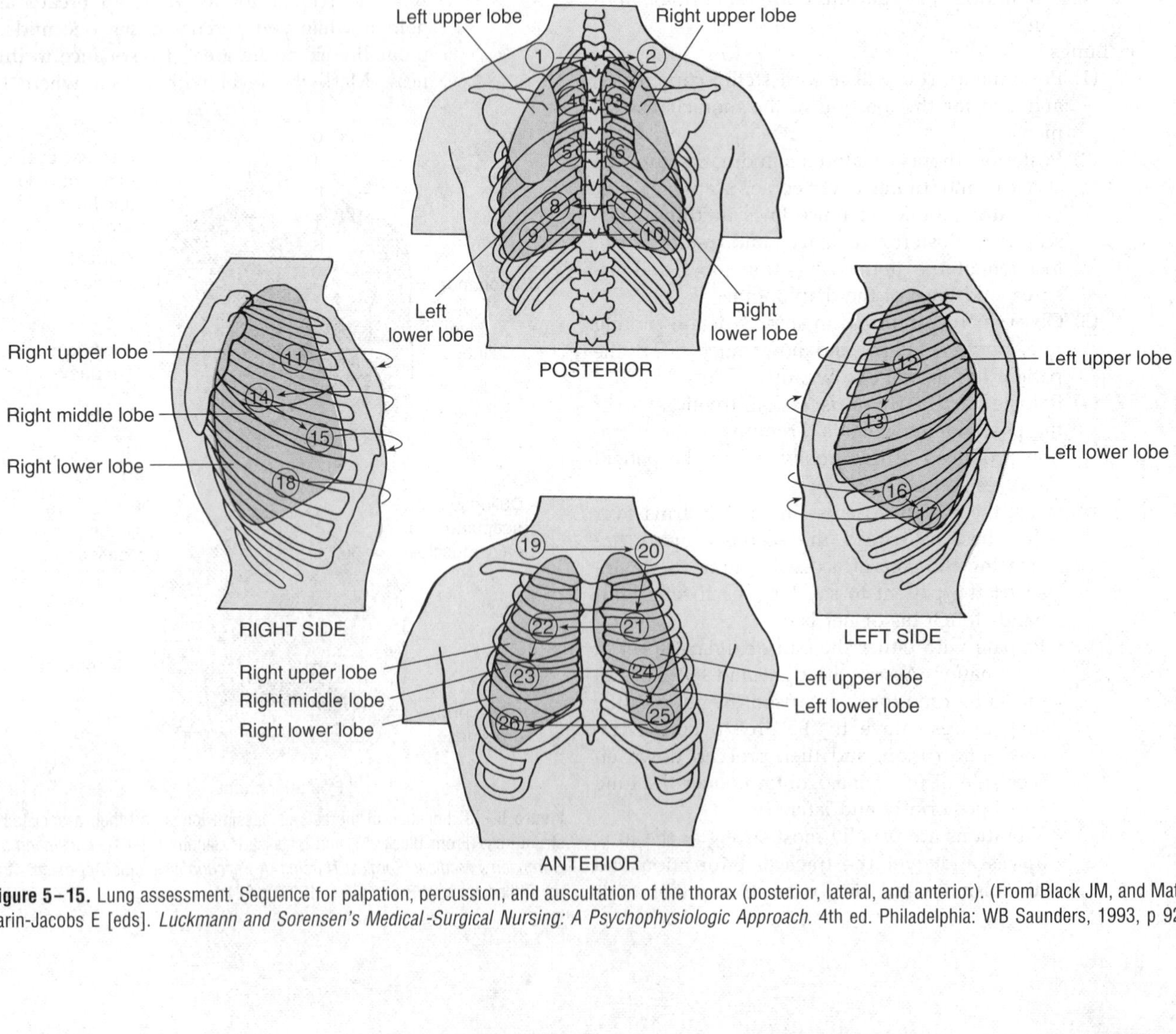

Left upper lobe   Right upper lobe

Left lower lobe   Right lower lobe

POSTERIOR

Right upper lobe
Right middle lobe
Right lower lobe

RIGHT SIDE

Left upper lobe

Left lower lobe

LEFT SIDE

Right upper lobe
Right middle lobe
Right lower lobe

Left upper lobe
Left lower lobe

ANTERIOR

Figure 5-15. Lung assessment. Sequence for palpation, percussion, and auscultation of the thorax (posterior, lateral, and anterior). (From Black JM, and Matassarin-Jacobs E [eds]. *Luckmann and Sorensen's Medical-Surgical Nursing: A Psychophysiologic Approach.* 4th ed. Philadelphia: WB Saunders, 1993, p 921.

tory cycle. If breath sounds are faint, ask the patient to breathe more deeply. Do not let the patient hyperventilate or fatigue him or her.

- The sounds heard over the posterior and lateral thorax are usually **vesicular** and those heard between the scapulae over the tracheal bifurcation **bronchovesicular.**
- Abnormal sounds result from air flow obstruction related to airway narrowing. Airway narrowing may be caused by fluid, mucus, inflammatory edema, rapid changes in the diameter of the airway lumen, or inflammation of the pleural lining, resulting in abnormal breath sounds called **adventitious sounds.** Absent breath sounds may be found in patients whose lung lobes have collapsed or have been removed surgically. Abnormal breath sounds are discussed in detail in Chapter 22.

f. Kidneys
(1) The kidney may be assessed during the posterior thorax examination because of its retroperitoneal location.
(2) Use blunt percussion (first percussion) over the lower costovertebral angles to assess for kidney tenderness (Fig. 5–16). Gentle blunt percussion normally yields no tenderness or discomfort for the patient.

11. **Anterior thorax**
a. Assessment of the anterior thorax includes assessment of parts of the integumentary, musculoskeletal,

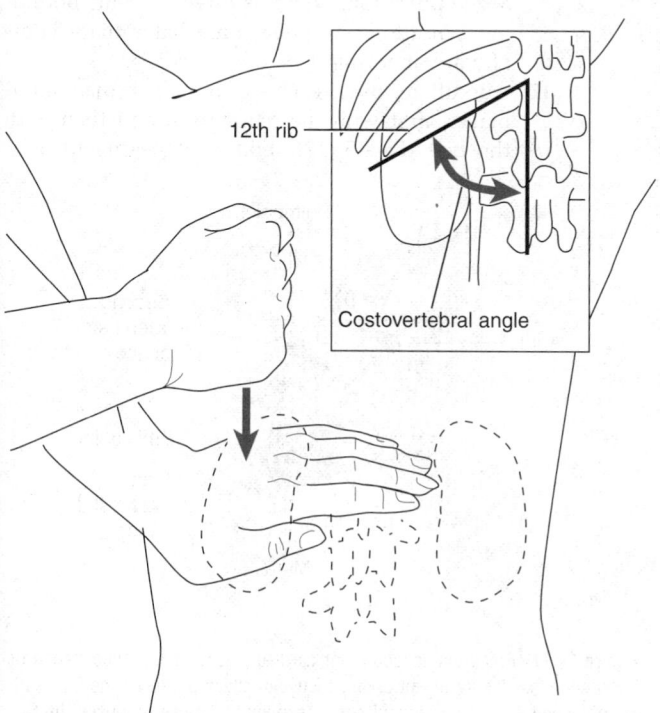

Figure 5–16. Percussion over the costovertebral angle. (Redrawn from Black JM, and Matassarin-Jacobs E [eds]. *Luckmann and Sorensen's Medical-Surgical Nursing: A Psychophysiologic Approach.* 4th ed. Philadelphia: WB Saunders, 1993, p 1420.)

respiratory, cardiovascular, and reproductive systems.

b. Stand at the patient's right side while he or she sits for the beginning of this examination of the lungs and thorax, heart and great vessels, and breasts and axillae. Continue the examination of these structures after you assist the patient to a supine position, which you may modify depending on the patient's status.

c. Equipment: You will need a stethoscope to examine the lungs and heart. If the jugular veins are distended, you may measure the extent of distention with a ruler and a straight edge.

d. Musculoskeletal: Inspect the rib cage for symmetry, shape, and movement. Note the **costal angle** where the ribs meet the sternum. It is usually about 90 degrees or less.

e. Lungs
(1) Anatomic landmarks for the lungs in the anterior thorax are the clavicles, sternum (including the sternal notch, manubrium, sternal angle or angle of Louis, body of the sternum, and xiphoid process), ribs and interspaces, and vertical anatomic reference lines (midsternal, midclavicular, anterior axillary, and midaxillary).
(2) Inspect the skin.
(3) Observe the patient's respiratory pattern, looking for intercostal bulges or retractions and use of the accessory muscles of breathing, such as the sternocleidomastoids, trapezius, or abdominal muscles.
- Men tend to breathe diaphragmatically, whereas women tend to use their costal muscles to breathe.
- Consciousness that you are observing may make the patient alter his or her rate and depth of respirations.
(4) Palpate for **tactile fremitus** using the same technique you used for the posterior thorax. Begin over the lung apices above the clavicles and proceed down the chest on either side of the sternum of the level of the 6th ribs; then move laterally toward the midaxillary line. Displace breast tissue gently, if necessary, for optimal palpation. Vibrations are strongest at the apices and diminish toward the bases and sides.
(5) Palpate **respiratory excursion** using the same technique you used for the posterior thorax.
- Place your hands on the lower anterior rib cage with your fingers extended laterally along the costal margins and your thumbs pushing up a skin fold.
- Ask the patient to take a deep breath while you observe the chest expansion.
(6) Percuss the anterior thorax over the lungs systematically. Use indirect finger percussion. Begin just above the clavicles and proceed down either side of the sternum, percussing over the interspaces.
- Percussion may be done with the patient sitting, but it may be easier if he or she is supine.

- Know which organs underlie the lungs and thorax and be familiar with the percussion sounds produced over the liver, heart, and stomach. The lung fields should be resonant throughout, with dullness over the liver and heart and tympany over the gastric bubble. Percussing a rib yields a flat sound.
- Displace breast tissue laterally to percuss from the 4th to 6th ribs to produce the best results.

(7) Auscultate the lung fields with the diaphragm of the stethoscope, following the same pattern you used for palpation and percussion.
- Having the patient in a sitting position enhances chest expansion and allows you to assess the lower lobes with more accuracy.
- Instruct the patient to breathe as for auscultation of the posterior thorax. Breath sounds are normally vesicular over the peripheral lung fields, bronchovesicular over the mainstem bronchi, and bronchial (tubular) over the lower trachea. Note the presence and characteristics of any adventitious sounds.
- Auscultate voice sounds if tactile fremitus is abnormal (see Chapter 22).

g. Heart
(1) Physical examination of the **heart** includes inspection, palpation, and auscultation. Percussion is rarely performed clinically and is not discussed here. A quiet room and a good stethoscope are essential for accurate cardiac auscultation.
(2) You must be able to visualize cardiac anatomy in relation to thoracic landmarks and cardiac cycle events in relation to the heart sounds. Repeated, diligent practice will help you learn these.
- Locate the cardiac landmarks before you begin.
- Palpate **Louis' angle** at the manubrialsternal junction. The 2nd ribs are attached to the sternum at this level. Slide your fingers over the 2nd ribs then inferiorly into the 2nd intercostal spaces. The 2nd intercostal spaces at the right and left sternal borders are the **aortic and pulmonic areas,** respectively.
- Continue down the left sternal border to the 3rd interspace (sometimes known as **Erb's point**). Proceed to the 4th or 5th interspace at the sternal border, which is the **tricuspid area.**
- The **mitral area** is in the 5th intercostal space toward the left midclavicular line, approximately 5 to 7 cm (2–3 inches) from the sternal border. This area is also known as the **apical area.**

(3) Inspect the **precordium** (the area overlying the heart) while the patient is seated. Stand at the patient's right side and look across the chest tangentially. This enhances detection of pulsations, bulging, heaving, or thrusting.

- There should be no signs of movement over the sternal borders. Thrusting movements, caused by enlarged ventricles pushing against the chest wall, are abnormal. These are called **lifts or heaves.**
- You may observe a slight pulsation over the apical area where the apex of the left ventricle is closest to the chest wall. This is called the **point of maximal impulse** or **apical impulse.** It is visible in approximately half the population and difficult to see in women because of the overlying breast tissue.

(4) Inspect over the **epigastrium,** just distal to the xiphoid process, for aortic pulsations. These pulsations may be seen in people with thin chest walls.

(5) Palpate over each of the 5 cardiac landmarks using the ball of your hand to detect lifts or thrills.
- A lift or heave will push against your hand, lifting it from the chest wall. A thrill feels like a cat purring and is caused by the vibration from valvular murmurs.
- If you feel pulsations or thrills, auscultate simultaneously to help time their occurrence in relation to the cardiac cycle.
- The apical impulse may be felt in many patients and should be no longer than the width of the interspace, or 1 to 2 cm (1/2 inch) in diameter. The impulse may be more readily palpable with the patient in a left lateral recumbent position, which moves the left ventricle closer to the chest wall.

(6) Palpate over the epigastrium for an abdominal aortic pulsation, which is often present. Bounding pulsations or pulsations that radiate laterally are abnormal.

(7) Auscultate over each of the 5 cardiac landmarks, first with the diaphragm and then with the bell (Fig. 5–17). You may begin either at

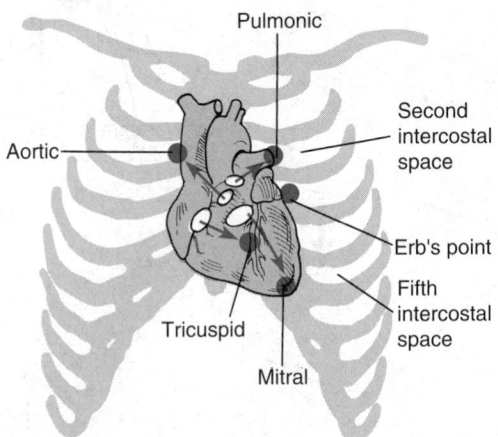

Figure 5–17. Precordial locations for cardiac palpation and auscultation of heart sounds. Closure of mitral and tricuspid valves produces the S1 heart sound; closure of pulmonic and aortic (semilunar) valves produces the S2 heart sound. (Redrawn from Black JM, and Matassarin-Jacobs E [eds]. *Luckmann and Sorensen's Medical-Surgical Nursing: A Psychophysiologic Approach.* 4th ed. Philadelphia: WB Saunders, 1993, p 1114.)

the base (over the aortic area) or at the apex (over the mitral area), but be consistent in your approach and listen over all areas. For a complete examination, listen while the patient is sitting and again while he or she is supine with the head elevated 30 to 45 degrees.

(8) Listen for **S-1** and **S-2**, the first 2 heart sounds. Each pair of S-1 and S-2 sounds is 1 cardiac cycle. Allow several cardiac cycles to occur at each location so that you clearly discern the sounds and their meaning.

- S-2 (the "dub" in "lub dub") is loudest at the aortic and pulmonic areas and is thought to be caused by the closure of the aortic and pulmonic values. Once you have identified S-2, use it as a guide when listening in the other areas. S-2 occurs at the end of systole and just before diastole.
- S-1 ("lub") is loudest at the tricuspid and mitral areas and is thought to be caused by the closure of these valves, just before systole and after diastole.
- You may hear a slight splitting of S-2 over the pulmonic area and Erb's point, in which the aortic and pulmonic components of the sound are heard separately rather than as one sound. Normal physiologic splitting is more noticeable during inspiration and disappears with expiration. To hear a split S-2 more clearly, ask the patient to breathe deeply through the nose and lean forward, bringing the base of the heart closer to the chest wall.
- Once you have distinguished the heart sounds, count the **apical rate** and note the **rhythm.** If the rhythm is irregular, auscultate the apical pulse while you simultaneously palpate the radial pulse for a **pulse deficit.**
- Use the bell to listen for extra heart sounds (S-3 and S-4) and murmurs. See Chapter 22 for a more complete discussion of these abnormal sounds.

(9) Help the patient to the supine position, and repeat the inspection, palpation, and auscultation over the cardiac landmarks.

- The point of maximal impulse may be palpable with the patient in this position if it was not previously.
- Ask the patient to turn to the left lateral recumbent position to move the apex of the heart closer to the chest wall. This position enhances auscultation of a suspected S-3 or S-4, both of which are considered abnormal in adults older than age 30.

(10) Describe any abnormal sounds in relation to the cardiac cycle. Refer the patient to the physician for further evaluation.

h. Carotid arteries

(1) The **carotid arteries** may be assessed as part of the head and neck examination or cardiac examination.

(2) Rate the pulse amplitude and auscultate for bruits.

i. Jugular veins

(1) Inspect the jugular veins for distention while the patient is supine with the head elevated 30 to 45 degrees (Fig. 15–18). The vessels should be flat. If you observe venous distention, measure its level above the right atrium (in centimeters) by using the jugular vein pulsations as a landmark. This is a rough estimate of the pressure in the right atrium.

(2) The vessels should not bulge, feel hard, or be distended to the level of the jaw. Unilateral distention is abnormal and may reflect serious underlying pathology.

(3) When the patient is lying flat, it is normal to observe vessel distention from the clavicle to the jaw angle.

j. Breasts and axillae

(1) You may sequence examination of the breasts before or after assessment of the lungs and heart. Some practitioners prefer to integrate the assessments of lungs, heart, breasts, and axillae so that all those portions performed while the patient is sitting are completed before the patient assumes a supine position.

(2) Examine the breasts and axillae of both men and women. Men have a small amount of glandular tissue beneath each nipple that may give rise to neoplastic growths.

(3) Ask women about their last menstrual period. Breasts are usually the most tender the week before the onset of menses and the least tender the following week. If the patient reports that 1 breast is tender, begin palpation with the opposite breast.

(4) Both breasts should be exposed for accurate comparison. Begin with the patient seated.

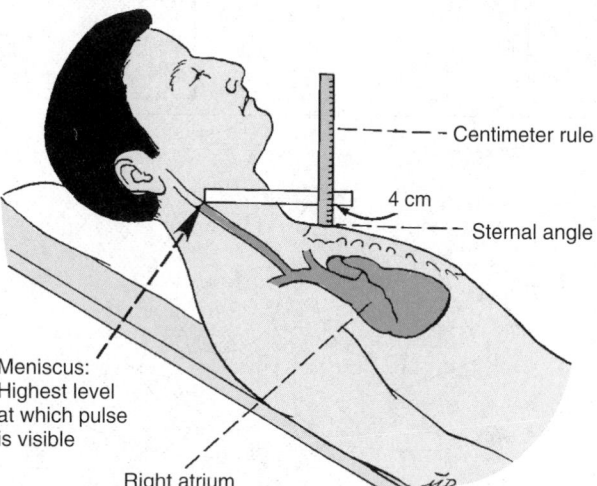

Figure 5–18. Estimation of jugular vein measurement to assess central venous pressure. (From Black JM, and Matassarin-Jacobs E [eds]. *Luckmann and Sorensen's Medical-Surgical Nursing: A Psychophysiologic Approach.* 4th ed. Philadelphia: WB Saunders, 1993, p 1113.)

(5) Inspect the breasts while the patient sits quietly with arms at the sides, then with the arms raised overhead, and finally with the hands pressed firmly on the hips. If a woman has large or pendulous breasts, ask her to lean over so that the breasts hang free and inspect their contour.

- Inspect the breasts for symmetry, size, shape, contour, skin characteristics, vascular pattern, and nipple and areola characteristics in all positions (Fig. 5–19).
- The breasts should be symmetric. It is normal for 1 breast to be slightly larger than the other, however. They should point laterally and hang evenly between the 3rd and 4th ribs with the nipples approximately level with the 4th intercostal space when the patient sits with the arms at the sides. The breasts hang lower in older women because of the loss of tissue elasticity. Older and obese men may have **gynecomastia** (breast enlargement), but unilateral enlargement is unusual.
- Contour should be even; there should be no dimpling (retraction), masses, or surface flattening. The color should be the same as the abdomen. **Striae** (stretch marks) may be noted in women. They are reddish if they developed recently and become pale with

age. If venous patterns are noticeable, they should be symmetric. There should be no signs of hyperpigmentation or edema.
- Ask the patient to raise the arms overhead while you examine the lateral surface and undersurface of each breast. Contraction of the pectoral muscles will emphasize any signs of retraction or skin flattening. In women, especially those with large breasts, you may note redness or excoriation from brassiere rubbing.
- The breasts should elevate evenly so that the areolae remain at the same level.
- Ask the patient to put the hands on the hips and press inward firmly while you continue to inspect for masses, retraction, or skin flattening, all of which are abnormal findings.

(6) Inspect the areolae and nipples for size, shape and contour, symmetry, surface characteristics, masses, and lesions.

- The **areolae** are pink in Whites and darker pink in dark-skinned patients. Slight asymmetry is common, although the nipples should point in symmetric directions. Shape is round or oval. Masses or lesions are abnormal.
- You may observe prominent **Montgomery's tubercles** around the nipple. The **nipples** are round, equal in size, soft, smooth, and of the same color.

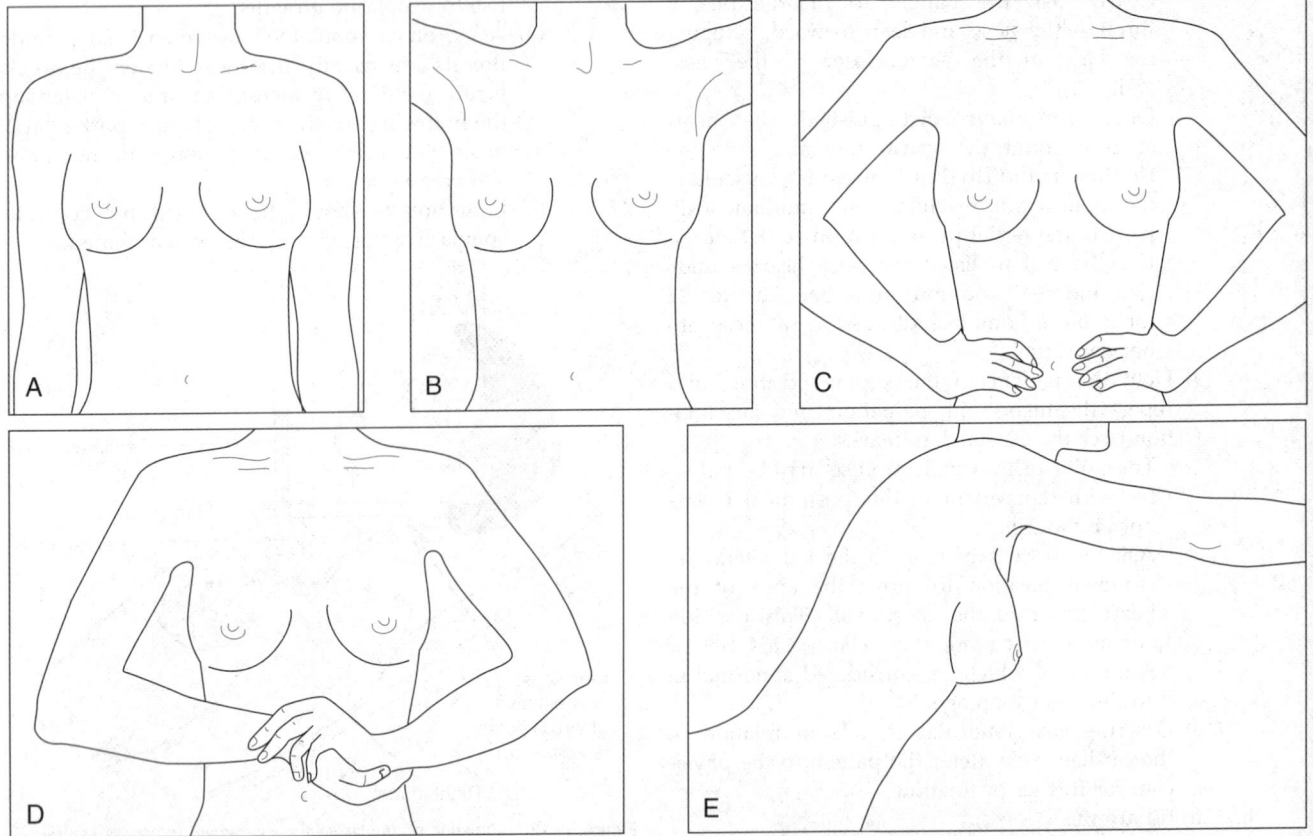

Figure 5–19. Positions for breast examination. *A*, Arms at sides. *B*, Hands raised overhead. For tightening pectoral muscles, the examiner asks the patient to press hands firmly on hips *(C)* or to press hands together *(D)*. *E*, Breasts may also be examined with the woman leaning forward at the waist, allowing the breasts to hang down. (Redrawn from Black JM, and Matassarin-Jacobs E [eds]. *Luckmann and Sorensen's Medical-Surgical Nursing: A Psychophysiologic Approach.* 4th ed. Philadelphia: WB Saunders, 1993, p 2059.)

- If 1 or both nipples are inverted, ask the patient whether this is a recent occurrence. Nipple inversion that has been present since puberty is often normal, but recent inversion is not.
- There should be no rashes, crusts, cracks, ulcers, or discharge from the nipples unless the patient is in the late stages of pregnancy, when colostrum may leak from the nipples.

(7) Ask the patient to raise the arms again for you to inspect the axillae for rashes, masses, and areas of unusual pigmentation. Axillary hair may be present unless the patient shaves it or uses a depilatory.

(8) Palpate the axillae while the patient is still sitting. You may also palpate the breasts at this time, but you may find it easier to do so with the patient supine. Patients who have large, pendulous breasts; a history of breast masses or cancer; or a high risk of breast cancer should have their breasts palpated in both positions.

- Palpate the axillae of both men and women. Help the patient relax the arm, shoulder, and chest muscles on the side you are palpating by supporting the arm.
- Palpate the 5 chains of accessible lymph nodes (pectoral or anterior, midaxillary or central, subscapular or posterior, brachial or lateral, and infraclavicular) associated with breast lymphatic drainage (Fig. 5–20).
- Palpate the edge of the pectoralis major muscle along the anterior axillary line, using both hands if necessary, to examine the pectoral nodes.
- Reach high up into the axilla at the midaxillary line to palpate the midaxillary nodes against the ribs and serratus anterior.
- Palpate the subscapular nodes along the posterior axillary fold along the anterior edge of the latissimus dorsi.
- Palpate the brachial nodes along the upper inner arm along the humerus.
- Palpate under the midclavicular area for the infraclavicular nodes. You already palpated the supraclavicular nodes, which also receive breast lymphatic drainage, when you palpated the cervical nodes.
- All nodes should be nonpalpable. The existence of 1 or 2 small, nontender, mobile central nodes may be normal. Abnormal findings include firm, fixed nodes that may or may not be tender. Note the number of nodes felt and their location, size, shape, mobility, tenderness, and consistency.

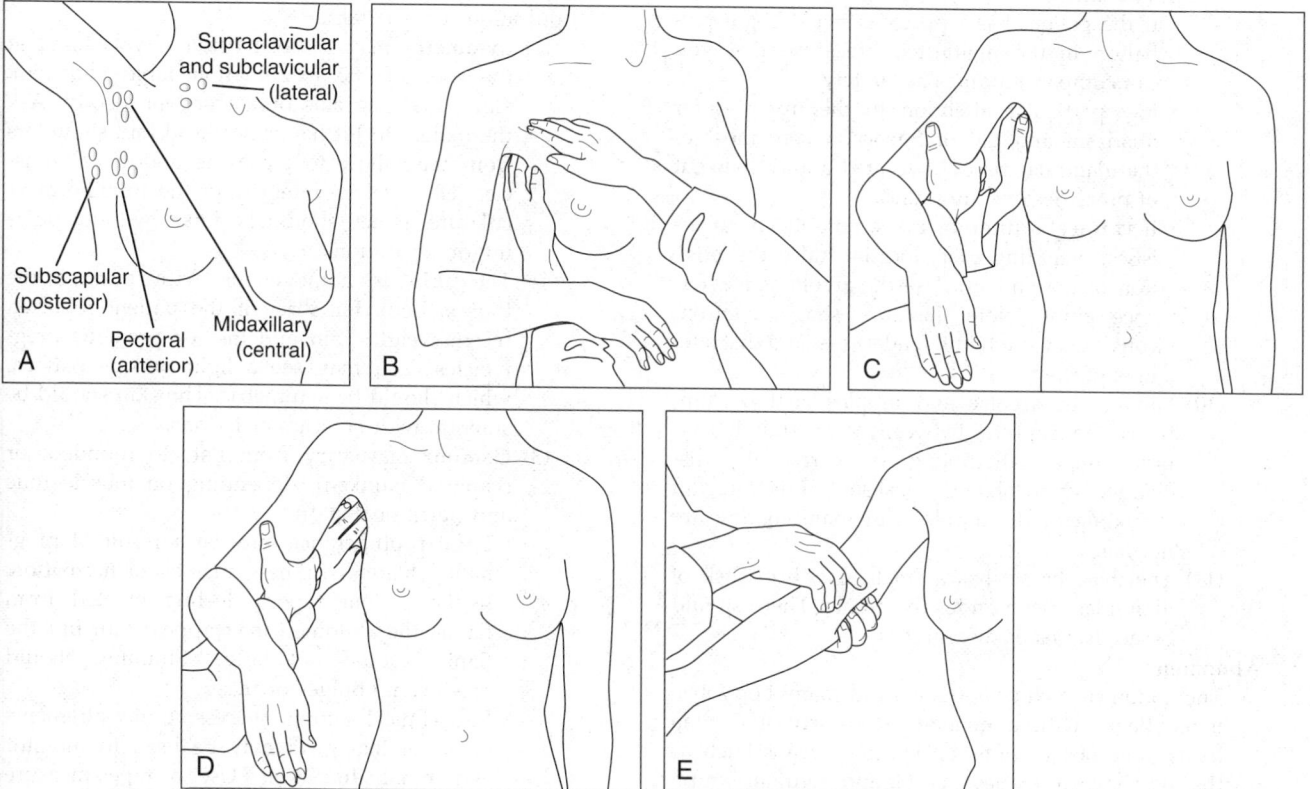

Figure 5–20. Assessment of axillary lymph nodes. *A*, Location of the groups of nodes to be examined. *B*, Pectoral (anterior) nodes. *C*, Midaxillary (central) nodes. *D*, Subscapular (posterior) nodes. *E*, Brachial (lateral) nodes. Axillary nodes are also palpated for male patients. (Redrawn from Black JM, and Matassarin-Jacobs E [eds]. *Luckmann and Sorensen's Medical-Surgical Nursing: A Psychophysiologic Approach.* 4th ed. Philadelphia: WB Saunders, 1993, p 2060.)

(9) Palpate breast tissue systematically so that you examine all areas, including the tail of Spence in the upper outer quadrant. Any one of several approaches is acceptable, as long as you include each of the 4 quadrants, the areolae, and the nipples.

- Palpation variations include moving in widening concentric circles, using a wheel-and-spokes pattern, or going back and forth across the breast from the superior to the inferior aspects. A bimanual technique may be used when the breasts are large and the patient is sitting.
- When the patient is supine, place a small folded towel under the shoulder on the same side you are palpating. This helps distribute the breast tissue more evenly over the chest wall. Ask the patient to place the arm on that side behind the head.
- Slide your fingers along the breast using a rotary motion to press the tissue against the chest wall. Keep your fingers in contact with the skin. You may feel a firm, curved ridge along the inferior breast; this is the **inframammary ridge.**
- Breast consistency varies from firm, homogeneous, and elastic in young women to stringy and nodular in older women. Consistency also varies with the menstrual cycle. Before menstruation, the breasts are more nodular and fuller.
- If the patient has reported a mass, begin palpation in the unaffected breast so that you can compare findings accurately.
- Pay particular attention to the upper outer quadrant and tail of Spence, where most of the glandular tissue is located and 50 percent of breast lesions are found.
- If you feel a lump or mass, note its characteristics, including exact location (also the position of the patient). Use the areola as a reference point. Note the size, shape, contour, consistency, mobility, tenderness, and discreteness of the mass.

(10) Palpate the areolae and nipples gently. Compress the nipples between your thumb and index finger, attempting to express any discharge, which should be absent. Erection and wrinkling of the nipple with manipulation are normal.

(11) The male breast has a small, flat, firm disk of glandular tissue under the areola. There should be no masses or discharge.

12. **Abdomen**
    a. The abdomen includes organs from many body systems. Begin with a general assessment and then focus your observations on specific organs such as the liver, spleen, kidneys, aorta, and inguinal lymph nodes (see Chapter 27).
    b. The patient should be supine with a small pillow under the head, arms relaxed at the sides, and the abdomen relaxed. Flexing the knees slightly helps the patient to relax the abdominal muscles as well as relieve any lower back discomfort. Stand at the patient's right side throughout the abdominal examination, except where noted in the following discussion.
    c. Ask the patient whether he or she needs to empty the bladder before you begin. Percussion and palpation over a full bladder are uncomfortable.
    d. Expose the abdomen from the xiphoid process to the symphysis pubis for complete visualization and examination. If the patient is a woman, keep her breasts covered and a drape over the pubic area and lower extremities. Use tangential lighting to enhance inspection.
    e. Remember that the sequence for abdominal assessment varies from the usual. Inspection and auscultation, the nonmanipulative techniques, come first, before percussion and palpation.
    f. Equipment: You will need a stethoscope, ruler, pen, and tongue depressor.
    g. Be familiar with the underlying organs of the abdomen. Use a standard reference for abdominal mapping, such as the 4 quadrants or the 9 regions (see Fig. 27–7). Both methods of reference are often used interchangeably when reporting findings.
    h. Inspect the abdomen using tangential lighting. Look across the abdomen from a standing position and then stoop to look across the abdomen at eye level. Observe the skin. Look for symmetry, contour, the umbilicus's placement, and movements related to pulsations or peristalsis.
       (1) **Symmetry** may be seen better if you stand at the foot of the examination table and look along the long axis of the patient's body. Ask the patient to lift his or her head and shoulders from the pillow to tense the abdominal muscles. Observe the integrity of the midline musculature, which should be intact without bulging or separation.
       (2) The **skin** is homogenous with that of the thorax. Look for striae if the patient reported recent weight gain and loss or previous pregnancies. You may see a light venous pattern, which should be symmetric. The skin should be smooth, with no scars or lesions.
       (3) **Contour** may vary from flat, to rounded, or scaphoid (sunken), depending on muscle tone and nutritional status.
          - Local protuberance may be a result of pregnancy, bladder fullness, masses, or herniation. If the patient reports feeling bloated from flatus, the abdomen may appear taut but the flanks should not bulge. Straining should produce no bulges or masses.
          - In a clinical setting, successive measurements of abdominal girth may be used to monitor abdominal distention. Use a tape measure placed at the level of the umbilicus and mark the level with a pen.
       (4) The **umbilicus** is at midline, inverted, and

round. There should be no bulges, discharge, or sign of inflammation. Straining or deep inspiration should produce no bulges or hernias.

(5) Visible **pulsations and peristaltic waves** are usually not seen. You may see a slight aortic pulsation over the epigastrium in thin patients. Observe whether the patient restricts respiration because of abdominal pain or discomfort.

i. Auscultate bowel sounds, vascular sounds, and friction rubs. Ask the patient to breathe quietly as you listen. Also ask the patient when he or she last ate, because bowel sounds increase shortly after eating and several hours after a meal. If a meal is long overdue, the bowel sounds may be loud.

(1) Listen over each quadrant with the diaphragm of the stethoscope.

(2) Place the diaphragm over each quadrant in a systematic manner. Many nurses begin in the right lower quadrant midway between the symphysis pubis and the anterior iliac spine, over the ileocecal valve.

(3) **Bowel sounds** are high-pitched gurgles that occur every 5 to 20 seconds. Describe bowel sounds as **audible** (present), **hypoactive** (soft and infrequent; fewer than 3 per minute), **hyperactive** (loud and increased in frequency), or **silent** (absent). If you believe bowel sounds are silent, listen over each quadrant at least 3 to 5 minutes to confirm that bowel motility has stopped.

(4) Place the bell of the stethoscope over the aorta, renal, iliac, and femoral arteries to assess for bruits, which should be absent (Fig. 5-21). Auscultate the aorta at midline, superior to the umbilicus and inferior to the xiphoid.
  • Locate the renal arteries at or just lateral to the upper abdominal midline toward the flanks.
  • Locate the iliac arteries just lateral to the midline below the umbilicus.

• Auscultate the femoral arteries in each groin midway between the pubic bone and the femur head.

(5) You may hear a **venous hum** when you listen over the epigastrium. It indicates increased collateral circulation between the portal and systemic venous systems, such as is found in hepatic cirrhosis.

(6) Listen for **peritoneal friction rubs** over the lower borders of the liver (right lower thorax) and spleen (left lower thorax) at the anterior axillary lines (see Chapter 28). Ask the patient to inhale deeply while you listen for a grating sound that varies with respirations. These sounds indicate inflammation of the organ's peritoneal surface.

j. Percuss lightly and methodically over all abdominal quadrants to assess for air, fluid, and masses (see Fig. 27-7). Also percuss over major organs to assess their size.

(1) Tympany is the predominant sound over all quadrants, except over the liver and spleen, which sound dull. Note the presence of the gastric air bubble in the left upper quadrant near the midclavicular line over the lower border of the ribs.

(2) Dullness superior to the symphysis pubis is usually from a distended bladder. Note the level of distention as the distance from the border of dullness to the umbilicus.

(3) Other areas of dullness may be caused by the presence of solid masses (e.g., an enlarged liver or spleen, stool in the colon, or a tumor) or fluid (ascites). If you find unexpected areas of dullness, alternate between percussion and palpation to determine the nature of the abnormality. If the patient reports abdominal tenderness, percuss this area last to avoid increasing the patient's discomfort and prevent him or her from tensing (guarding) the abdominal muscles.

(4) Use percussion to determine liver size for later palpation. Percuss the span of the liver in the right midclavicular line and the midsternal line. Liver size varies with body size.
  • Begin by percussing in the right midclavicular line either superior or inferior to the estimated borders of the liver. Superiorly, begin at the 3rd intercostal space over lung resonance and percuss down the thorax until the sound changes to dull. Mark this level with a pen.
  • Inferiorly, begin over abdominal tympany and percuss upward until the sound changes to dull. Mark the level with a pen.
  • At the midsternal line, percuss upward from above the umbilicus from tympany to dull and mark the level. Superiorly, percuss down the sternum (it will be flat) until the sound of the percussion note changes (it will be flat or dull). Mark the level.

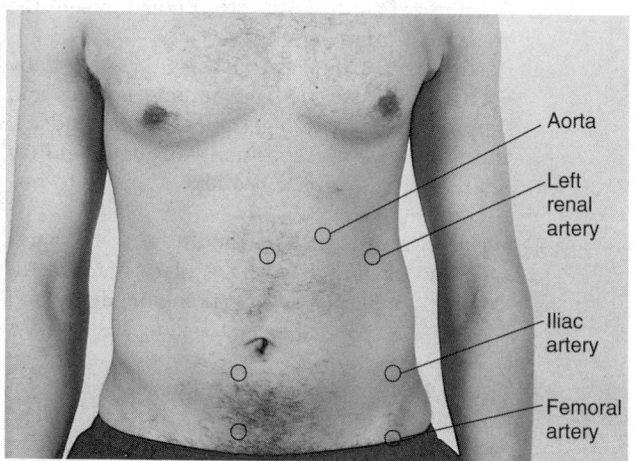

Figure 5-21. Auscultate the abdomen (aorta, renal arteries, iliac and femoral arteries) for vascular sounds or *bruits*. (From Jarvis C. *Physical Examination and Health Assessment*. 2nd ed. Philadelphia: WB Saunders, 1996, p 614.)

- Measure the distance between each set of marks, at the right midclavicular line and midsternal line. Liver span ranges from 6 to 12 cm (2.5–5.0 inches) at the right midclavicular line and from 4 to 8 cm (1.5–3.0 inches) at the midsternal line. The lower border of the liver in the right midclavicular line is usually at the right costal margin, and the upper border is between the 5th and 7th intercostal spaces. Measurements larger than the norms indicate liver enlargement.
- Ask the patient to take a deep breath and hold it at maximum inspiration while you percuss the lower liver border again. Deep inspiration causes the diaphragm to push the liver into the abdomen. Mark and note the distance of **liver descent,** which usually is 2 to 3 cm (about 1 inch). You will use this lower mark as a guide to palpate the liver.

(5) Percuss to determine spleen size. The spleen is noted as a small area of dullness just posterior to the left midaxillary line between the 6th and 10th ribs. It normally has a span of approximately 7 cm (2.5–3.0 inches). If the spleen enlarges, the area of dullness shifts to below the 10th rib, toward or beyond the left anterior axillary line.

(6) After all other assessments have been completed, perform blunt (fist) percussion to assess for liver tenderness. This maneuver may be uncomfortable for the patient if liver tenderness exists. Tell the patient before you percuss to avoid a surprised reaction that you may interpret as an expression that the area is tender. Note the patient's reaction to the blows. To avoid traumatizing the liver, use only indirect fist percussion over the costal margin at the right midclavicular line. This maneuver is also known as the "liver tap." For comparison, also perform indirect fist percussion over the left costal margin at the midclavicular line.

(7) Blunt percussion over the kidneys is discussed in the section on the posterior thorax examination.

k. Palpate all abdominal quadrants to detect areas of tenderness, masses, hernias, distention, bladder distention, aortic and femoral pulses, inguinal lymph nodes, and organ size.

(1) Perform **light palpation** systematically in all quadrants. If the patient is ticklish, begin with a variation of bimanual palpation in which you place the patient's hand on top of yours until he or she becomes accustomed to the touch.

(2) Palpate tender areas last.

(3) The abdomen should feel smooth, soft, relaxed, and nontender. The bladder is nonpalpable when it is empty. If the bladder is distended, it is felt midline, superior to the symphysis pubis and inferior to the umbilicus, as a rounded, smooth, tense mass.

(4) Perform **deep palpation** to assess for masses and organ size. If you feel a mass, try to determine its size, location, shape, consistency, tenderness, mobility (especially with respiration), and pulsatility. Avoid aggressive deep palpation over masses that are tender or pulsating and over recent surgical incisions. Abdominal structures that you may mistake for masses are the aorta; portions of the ascending, descending, or sigmoid colon that are filled with feces; the uterus; the lateral borders of the rectus abdominis muscles; the common iliac arteries; and the sacral prominence (in very thin patients). Tenderness may be a normal variation over the xiphoid, cecum, and sigmoid colon. Feces in the ascending and descending colon may feel soft and moveable.

(5) Palpation of the aorta is discussed in the section on the anterior thorax examination.

(6) Locate and palpate the **femoral pulses.** Note and rate the pulse amplitude.

(7) Palpate the inguinal and femoral areas for the **inguinal lymph nodes.** The superior (horizontal) and inferior (vertical) chains are usually nonpalpable, although small, soft, mobile, nontender nodes are common. The inguinal area should be free of bulges or masses.

l. Palpate for **rebound tenderness** in the lower quadrants, which indicates inflammation of the underlying peritoneum. Press your fingers into the abdominal wall slowly and deeply. Release the pressure quickly. If the patient reports pain or increased tenderness with the release of pressure (rebound), the test is positive.

m. Palpate the liver for size, masses, and nodules.

(1) Place your left hand under the patient's right posterior thorax over the 11th and 12th ribs. Push the thorax upward. Place your right hand below the right costal margin at the lowest pen mark where you percussed the liver's descent with maximum inspiration. Your fingers should point upward toward the costal margin.

(2) Ask the patient to take a deep breath, using the abdominal muscles.

(3) As the patient inhales, push gently up and in. Feel for the liver's edge bumping against and slipping over your fingertips as it descends. If you do not feel it, reposition your hand and try again after the patient has had a chance to rest a moment.

(4) The liver's edge, if felt, should be firm, sharp, and smooth and have a regular contour. Attempt to palpate at several points medially and laterally to assess the edge along its inferior border.

(5) An alternate palpation technique is to use bimanual palpation with the left hand placed over the right. Place your hands below the right costal margin and proceed as just described.

(6) The liver is difficult to palpate in patients who are obese or tense or have taut abdominal muscles.

(7) Abnormal findings include the liver's feeling hard, nodular, or tender.

n. Perform spleen palpation on the left side of the abdomen below the costal margin. Use a technique similar to the one you used for liver palpation. If spleen percussion shows the spleen to be enlarged, do not attempt to palpate, because you may rupture it.

(1) Ask the patient to turn onto his or her right side to allow gravity to bring the spleen forward and down, closer to the abdominal wall.

(2) Place your left hand behind the patient's left posterior rib cage and push forward while palpating with the right hand. Help the patient return to the supine position when you are done.

(3) The spleen usually is nonpalpable.

o. Palpate the kidneys using a bimanual technique. The right kidney is more accessible to palpation, because it lies lower in the retroperitoneal space.

(1) Place your left hand under the patient's right flank to push and elevate the right kidney anteriorly. Place your right hand on the abdominal wall at the right midclavicular line inferior to the costal margin. Because the kidney moves downward with inspiration, the lower pole may be felt.

(2) Ask the patient to take a deep breath and hold it. At that point, push your hands together in an attempt to capture the kidney between your fingers.

(3) If it is palpable, the kidney feels smooth and firm without hardness, tenderness, or nodularity.

(4) Repeat the maneuver on the patient's left side, placing your left hand under the left flank and palpating with your right hand. The left kidney usually is nonpalpable.

p. Attempt to elicit the **abdominal reflexes,** which are superficial cutaneous neurologic reflexes.

(1) Use the tongue depressor to stroke each quadrant horizontally from the lateral aspect toward the umbilicus. Use light, quick strokes.

(2) If the reflexes are present, the abdominal muscles contract so that the umbilicus deviates toward the direction of the stimulus. The reflex may be absent in obese patients and patients who have had abdominal incisions in the area being tested.

13. **Lower extremities**

a. Assessment of the lower extremities is similar to that of the upper extremities. You may perform this part of the physical examination after you assess the upper extremities or toward the end of the examination, when you perform the general neurologic assessment.

b. Many of the assessments may be made while the patient is supine, after the abdominal examination. Several observations require the patient to stand or sit on the edge of the examination table.

c. Integument

(1) The **skin** over the lower extremities should be warm, smooth, slightly moist, and of the same tone as the skin over the rest of the body, except areas exposed to the sun. Palpate with the dorsum of your hands over the lower legs to detect local areas of increased temperature, which should be absent.

(2) There should be no lesions or masses, and turgor should be immediate.

(3) Examine the toenails for grooming. They should be trimmed straight across, without sign of inflammation. Blanch the nail beds and observe for capillary refill. Note the presence of corns, calluses, or deformities.

(4) Examine the **hair distribution;** it should be even. Hair becomes sparse over the lower legs and feet with age or decreased circulation. In men, the level of hair loss may correspond to the type of socks worn and should not be confused with vascular deficiency.

d. Peripheral vascular system

(1) Palpate the **peripheral pulses** (popliteal, posterior tibial, and dorsalis pedis). Assess the rhythm and rate the pulse amplitude. If you did not palpate the femoral arteries when you assessed the abdomen, do so now.

(2) Popliteal pulses often are nonpalpable. If you have difficulty finding them, help the patient turn prone and flex the knees. Palpate deeply into the popliteal fossae, one at a time.

(3) Dorsalis pedis pulses may be nonpalpable in otherwise healthy patients. Look for other signs of peripheral circulation, such as blanching of the distal toes and warm skin temperature.

(4) Palpate the **popliteal lymph nodes** in the lateral aspects of the popliteal fossae. They usually are nonpalpable.

(5) Assess for **edema** by palpating with your thumbs over the dorsum of the feet and lower shins. Note any residual depression in the skin.

(6) Assess for **phlebitis** by gently squeezing the calf muscles against the tibia. There should be no tenderness.

• Observe for **Homans' sign,** a test for thrombophlebitis. Extend the patient's leg, place your left hand on the knee, and place your right hand across the sole of the foot. Sharply dorsiflex the foot. The patient should not report pain in the calf. The presence or absence of Homans' sign is not conclusive, however; there may be false-positive as well as false-negative results.

• Inspect the legs for varicose veins, which appear as knotted or hardened cordlike bulges under the skin. Further examination is best done when the patient stands and you can see distended vessels more easily.

• If either the calves or thighs look enlarged or swollen, measure their circumference with a tape measure at the same level on each leg.

Compare results. The measurements should be within 1 cm (1/2 inch).

e. Musculoskeletal system

(1) Observe the lower extremities for symmetry, alignment, and proportion to the rest of the body.

(2) Inspect and palpate muscle groups for size, symmetry, and tone. Note involuntary movements. Begin either proximally at the hip or distally at the feet. There should be no tenderness, fasciculations, lumps, or bulges. If muscle groups look uneven, measure them with the tape measure.

(3) Assess **muscle strength** in the major muscle groups of the hips, hamstrings, quadriceps, ankles, and feet. See the discussion of rating muscle strength on p. 129.

(4) Inspect and palpate each **joint** and **bone** for symmetry, swelling, tenderness, crepitus, and deformity.

(5) Ask the patient to put each joint (hips, knees, ankles, and feet) through its range of motion. Each joint may be assessed with the patient supine except for hip hyperextension, which is observed while the patient stands or is prone. If you observe a limitation, measure the angle of joint movement with a goniometer.

f. Neurologic system

(1) If you did not do so earlier when you assessed the upper extremities, assess the lower extremity DTRs (patellar and Achilles reflexes) now. See pp. 129–130 for a discussion of testing and rating these reflexes.

(2) Assess the **plantar reflex,** a superficial cutaneous reflex. Use the pointed handle of the reflex hammer to stroke firmly along the lateral aspect of the sole from the heel and across the ball of the foot in 1 continuous motion. This normally produces plantar flexion of the great toe (i.e., a negative Babinski's sign). Abnormal results are for the great toe to dorsiflex and the remaining toes to fan. Note this as a positive Babinski's sign (see Chapter 18).

(3) Assess **cerebellar function** as the patient performs specific rapid alternating movements and point-to-point touching. Ask the patient to alternate tapping the balls of his or her feet against your hands as quickly as possible. The movements should be smooth and coordinated. Ask the patient to place the heel of 1 foot on the opposite knee and slide the heel down the shin toward the foot. The movement should be smooth, with the heel remaining on the shin without wobbling or sliding off. Repeat for the opposite leg.

14. **General neurologic and spine**

a. There are 6 components in the general neurologic assessment. Many of these assessments are integrated throughout the physical examination but are recorded so that significant findings can be evaluated in a meaningful way. The general neurologic assessment includes mental status (cerebral function), cranial nerve function, cerebellar function, motor function, sensory function, and DTRs. The examination is conducted with the patient either sitting or supine, except where noted.

b. **Mental status** assessment is discussed in detail in Chapter 4 as part of the health history and in Chapter 6.

c. Assessment of **cranial nerve function** is discussed in "Head and Neck." See Chapter 18 for additional information.

d. Assessment of **cerebellar function** includes examination of posture, gait, and the ability to move with coordination and balance.

(1) Observe the patient's posture and gait as discussed in "General Survey."

(2) Ask the patient to walk in a straight line, first forwards and then backwards. The patient should be able to do this without weaving, stumbling, or widening his or her stance to maintain balance. Ask the patient to stand quietly with the feet together, first with the eyes open and then with the eyes closed. The patient should be able to maintain balance with only slight swaying for at least 5 seconds. The nurse should remain nearby to prevent a fall or an injury to the patient, should he or she lose balance.

(3) Assess the patient's ability to perform rapid alternating movements and point-to-point maneuvers. (See "Upper Extremities" and "Lower Extremities.")

e. Assess **motor function** continuously as you examine the skeletal system, because bony deformities affect motor function. Assess muscle mass, tone, and strength and abnormal movements such as tics, fasciculations, or twitches.

(1) Observe **muscle mass** for symmetry and distribution. Consider the patient's sex, body build, and usual types of activity and exercise.

(2) Assess **tone** when you test muscle strength and resistance (see p. 129) during passive motion of the extremities and other body parts.

(3) Assess the strength of the major muscle groups of the upper and lower extremities (see pp. 129 and this page for discussions). Also ask the patient to perform the following maneuvers to further evaluate gross motor function and balance.

• Observe the patient while he or she walks first on the toes and then on the heels. Ask the patient to hop first on 1 foot and then the other.

• Ask the patient to extend his or her arms and perform several shallow knee bends.

(4) The patient should be able to perform the maneuvers without difficulty. There should be no unusual muscle movements or tremors.

f. Assess **sensory function** over the entire body. You may complete a portion of this assessment when you test cranial nerve function as part of the head and neck examination.

(1) Sensory functions include the perception of light touch, pain, pressure, temperature, vibration, proprioception (position sense), tactile localization, and discrimination (i.e., 2-point discrimination, stereognosis, graphesthesia, and point localization), as well as seeing, hearing, smelling, and tasting (Table 5–6).

(2) Temperature perception usually is not tested if the patient's perception of pain is intact.

(3) If the patient's perception of pain, light touch, and vibration are intact, you do not need to test the remaining portions of the sensory examination.

(4) If the patient's perception of a stimulus is intact distally, it generally is intact proximally also, and you need not test any further. If the patient cannot perceive a stimulus distally, proceed proximally until he or she can distinguish the stimulus.

(5) Apply the stimuli randomly so that the patient cannot anticipate where or when you will touch him or her next.

(6) Always test the patient with his or her eyes closed. Cue the patient to what the stimuli are and how they feel before you begin each portion of the sensory examination.

(7) Always compare findings from side to side and from distal to proximal.

g. **Deep tendon reflexes** are discussed in detail in "Upper Extremities" and "Lower Extremities."

h. Portions of the **spine** assessment are completed in the examinations of the head and neck and the posterior thorax. In addition to inspecting and palpating the spine and paravertebral muscles, assess spine alignment and range of motion.

(1) Inspect **spine alignment** from the anterior, lateral, and posterior aspects by examining the patient's posture. The spine should be straight, without lateral deviation (scoliosis). Look for the normal curvature of the cervical, thoracic, and lumbar areas. There should be no signs of kyphosis (exaggerated thoracic curvature, or humpback) or lordosis (exaggerated lumbar curvature, or swayback). The shoulders and hips should be even; the arms should hang evenly; and there should be no protuberance of 1 scapula, hemithorax, or hip.

(2) Assess the spine for **range of motion.**

15. **Genitalia**

a. Examination of the genitalia includes external and internal structures. Portions of the internal examination are accessed through the rectum and are discussed in "Anus and Rectum." Assessment of the genitalia provides information about the patient's reproductive and urinary systems.

b. Assessment of the genitalia may be embarrassing, uncomfortable, or anxiety producing for the patient. Make the patient comfortable by being nonjudgmental, relaxed, and confident.

(1) Explain what you will do before proceeding. Avoid quick movements, because they may cause the patient to become tense, increasing his or her discomfort.

(2) Provide privacy. Warm your hands and any instruments you use under warm running water. Wear gloves. Use a water-soluble lubricant to ease insertion of instruments or your fingers.

(3) Be professional. Avoid actions or remarks that the patient may misconstrue as unintentionally judgmental or sexually provocative. A male patient may fear that he will have an erection during the examination and that it will be misinterpreted by you. Use a firm, deliberate touch rather than a gentle stroke. If a man has an erection during the examination, do not stop the examination. Reassure him that this is a normal physiologic response to being touched. Continue with the examination.

(4) Some agencies require that an examiner be accompanied by an assistant of the same sex as the patient if the examiner and the patient are of opposite sexes or if the patient is extremely anxious or has previously exhibited unpredictable behavior.

c. Ask the patient whether he or she needs to empty the bladder before you begin.

d. Assess secondary sexual characteristics (pubic hair distribution and genitalia developmental stage) as you examine the external genitalia.

e. Male genitalia (see Chapter 30)

(1) Examine the skin and hair of the pubic area, the penis and scrotum, and the inguinal areas.

(2) The man may be supine for all of the examination, except when you check the inguinal areas for hernias, when he should stand. Alternatively, he may stand for the entire examination while you are seated.

(3) Equipment: You will need gloves, a transilluminator or a flashlight, culture-obtaining materials, and culture media, as needed.

(4) Inspect the external genitalia and perineum and observe the **pubic hair and skin**. Pubic hair distribution in the adult is triangular, with hair covering the symphysis pubis, the base of the penis, and the inner aspects of the thighs. Distribution also may spread toward the umbilicus in a diamond pattern. Inspect the hair for nits and the skin for parasites, rashes, excoriation, and lesions. Masses, lesions, edema, and offensive odors should be absent. **Scrotal skin** is darker than other skin surfaces and is loose and wrinkled. **Penile skin** in the flaccid penis is wrinkled with rugae.

(5) Inspect and palpate the **penis** for lesions, nodules, swelling, inflammation, and discharge.

• The **foreskin** covers the glans unless it has been circumcised. Ask the patient to retract the foreskin to expose the **glans,** which should be easy to do unless there is scarring or adhesions. You may note a small amount of thick, white **smegma** between the glans

Table 5–6. Assessing Sensory Neurologic Function

Function	Equipment	Technique	Comments
Light touch	Cotton wisp	Lightly touch the patient's skin with cotton wisp over the forehead, cheek, neck, dorsum of the hand, lower arm, abdomen, foot, and lower leg. Alternately touch the right side and then the left side for comparison of symmetric dermatomes.	Ask the patient to say "now" or a similar response when he or she feels the stimulus. Test areas where skin is thin and more sensitive.
Point localization	Cotton wisp or finger	Proceed as in technique for light touch.	Ask the patient to state where the skin has been touched or to point to the place. This may be done instead of having the patient say "now."
Pain	Sterile safety pin or needle	Alternately touch the sharp and dull ends of the safety pin or needle to the skin's surface. Present stimuli no sooner than 2 sec apart to avoid a summation effect. If sensory loss exists, test proximally every 2.5 cm (1 inch) until the boundary of normal sensation is mapped.	Ask the patient to state whether he or she feels "sharp" or "dull" pain when the stimulus is applied. Avoid areas of thickened skin, which are less sensitive to pain. Older patients are less sensitive to pain bilaterally.
Deep pressure	None	Gently squeeze the patient's Achilles tendons, calf muscles, and forearm.	Ask the patient to state whether there is discomfort. Note whether patient withdraws an extremity.
Temperature	Two test tubes: one filled with hot water and one with cold water	Alternately touch the patient's skin with the hot test tube and cold test tube. Retest areas where pain sensation is abnormal.	Omit this test if pain sensation is normal. If test is given, ask the patient to say "hot" or "cold" when the stimulus is applied.
Vibration	Large 128-Hz tuning fork	Touch handle of vibrating tuning fork to the distal interphalangeal joints of fingers and great toes. If the patient shows no perception of vibration, continue proximally to the wrists and ankles, and elbows and knees, and the acromion processes and anterior iliac spines until you determine where the patient can feel vibrations. Periodically stop vibrations while tuning fork is still on the bone to determine whether the patient can distinguish when vibrations cease. Alternatively, place handle of nonvibrating tuning fork on the patient's bones.	Ask the patient to say "yes" or "now" when vibrations are felt. Ask the patient to say "no" or "gone" when vibrations are no longer felt.
Position or proprioception	None	Test the patient's middle fingers and great toes by moving the distal phalanges up and down. Hold the distal phalanx by the lateral aspects (while the rest of the hand or foot is supported) between your thumb and index finger. Grasp the finger or toe with your free thumb and index finger and move the distal portion of the digit alternately up, down, and to a neutral position.	Ask the patient to say "up," "down," or "neutral" to identify the final position of the digit. Avoid touching or rubbing adjacent digits when moving the distal phalanx.
Tactile localization (double simultaneous stimulation)	None	Touch the patient on both sides of the body at the same time in symmetric areas, alternating with nonsymmetric areas (e.g., right forearm and left trunk).	Ask the patient to state where skin has been touched. The patient should be able to feel and identify both stimuli. If point localization is normal but double stimulation is abnormal and only 1 touch is felt, **extinction** exists.
Two-point discrimination	Two sterile safety pins or needles	Lightly touch the points of 2 safety pins or needles simultaneously to the patient's skin. Hold the needle tips 2–3 mm apart to test the fingertips. Repeat with the tips together and with just 1 needle. Test other areas, such as the palms of the hands, forearms, back, toes, and upper thighs.	Ask the patient to identify whether 1 or 2 pin pricks are felt. Normally a patient can distinguish 1 from 2 needle pricks on the fingertips at 2 mm apart; on the palms of the hands at 8–12 mm apart; on the forearms at 40 mm apart, on the back 40–60 mm apart; on the toes 3–8 mm apart; and on the upper thighs at 70 mm apart.
Stereognosis	Small, common objects (e.g., a key, coin, and paper clip)	Place an object in the patient's hand and ask him or her to identify it by name. Repeat for the opposite hand.	Use commonly recognized objects. If the patient has a motor impairment and cannot manipulate the objects, test for graphesthesia.
Graphesthesia	Blunt end of pen or pencil	Use the blunt end of the pen or pencil to "write" a single-digit number on the patient's palm. Make sure the direction of the number faces patient so it is right-side up from his or her perspective. Repeat for the opposite hand.	Ask the patient to identify the number.

144

and the foreskin, which is normal. Other discharges are abnormal and should be cultured.

- The area should be free of lesions. If you note any, palpate them for tenderness, size, shape, and consistency.
- Inspect the **penile shaft** and **urethral meatus.** The dorsal vein may be prominent on the shaft. The meatus should be located as a slit at the tip of the penis. It should be pink, without ulcers, scars, inflammation, or discharge. A meatus that is located on the underside of the penile shaft is a **hypospadias;** one located on the upper side is an **epispadias.** Both are congenital malpositions of the meatus.
- Compress the glans between thumb and index finger to open the meatus and inspect for discharge. If the patient reports a urethral discharge, ask him to compress the penile urethra from base to tip between his thumb and fingers in an attempt to express a discharge, which you should obtain for a culture.
- Palpate the penile shaft gently between your thumb and 1st 2 fingers. It should feel smooth and semifirm, allowing the skin to move easily over underlying structures. There should be no nodules, thickened or hard areas, or tenderness.

(6) Inspect and palpate the **scrotum** for symmetry, size, shape, and swelling. Each half of the scrotum should contain a testis, epididymis, and vas deferens. The left testis usually hangs lower than the right testis.

- Scrotal size varies with ambient temperature: Cold results in contraction towards the body and heat results in relaxation.
- Ask the patient to hold his penis first to 1 side and then to the other and to lift his scrotum while you inspect the scrotum. The skin should be loose, without tenseness.
- The **testes** are oval; are approximately 2×4 cm ($4/5 \times 1\ 3/5$ inches); and should feel firm and rubbery, without nodules or masses. An elderly man will have smaller, less firm testes. In a young adolescent, note whether the testes are present in the scrotum. If not, palpate along the inguinal canals to determine their presence. Refer the patient with an undescended testis or palpable lump to a physician.
- Palpate each **epididymis** between your thumb and index finger. The epididymides are located on the superior aspects of the testes and extend down the posterior surfaces. Each epididymis should feel soft and resilient, and the patient may report tenderness upon palpation. Swelling and hardness are abnormal.
- Palpate each **vas deferens** (spermatic cord) along its length from the superior lateral aspect of the testis toward the inguinal canal. Differentiate the vas deferens from the epididymis by its firmer, tubular characteristics. There should be no thickening or asymmetry.

- If you find swelling, nodules, or other abnormalities during the scrotal examination, transilluminate the scrotum. Darken the room and use a transilluminator or flashlight. Shine the light through the scrotum from behind and look for the outline of the testes. Serous fluid in the scrotum transilluminates as a red glow; solid lesions, such as a hematoma or mass, do not transilluminate and cast a dark shadow. Describe the characteristics of any abnormality.

(7) Ask the patient to stand while you examine the **inguinal areas** for a hernia (a prolapse or protrusion of a loop of intestine through the inguinal wall or canal).

- A **direct inguinal hernia** enters the inguinal canal behind the external ring because of a weakened abdominal wall; it does not pass through the inguinal canal. An **indirect inguinal hernia** enters the inguinal canal through the internal ring and can remain in the canal or pass down through the external ring into the scrotum.
- To examine the right inguinal area, ask the patient to shift his weight to the left leg; for the left canal, ask the patient to shift his weight to the right leg.
- Inspect the inguinal areas for bulges while the patient stands quietly and again as he performs the Valsalva maneuver. There should be no bulges.
- Assess for a hernia by gently inserting your index finger into the loose scrotal skin, invaginating it, and following the vas deferens to the external inguinal ring. The ring feels like a triangular slitlike opening. Ask the patient to bear down while you feel for a bulge, which should be absent.
- Next, gently attempt to insert your finger through the external ring into the inguinal canal. (Asking the patient to flex the knee on that same side may help relax the muscles, which may make insertion easier.) Advance your finger into the canal and ask the patient to bear down. Feel for a mass that touches your fingertip and retreats back up the canal when the patient relaxes.
- Complete the examination of the internal genitalia when you assess the rectum.

f. Female genitalia (see Chapter 31)

(1) Examine the skin and hair of the pubic area, the perineum, the external genitalia (the labia majora and minora, clitoris, vestibule, and introitus), and the internal genitalia (vagina, cervix, uterus, and adnexae).

(2) Help the patient assume a lithotomy position and keep her draped until you begin the examination. If you plan to examine only the external genitalia, the patient does not have to place her feet into stirrups.

- Help the patient flex and abduct her hips and knees. Her arms should be at her sides or crossed over the chest; her head may be elevated on a pillow. If the patient has lower back pain or cannot assume this position, she may assume Sim's position. An assistant may need to help the patient abduct 1 or both legs. Sit at the end of the examining table.

- Equipment: If you plan to perform a complete pelvic examination, you will need lubricant, a vaginal speculum of appropriate size, and an adjustable source of direct light. To collect specimens, including a Pap smear, you will need a cervical scraper, glass slides, long cotton-tipped applicators, and fixative.

(3) Inspect and palpate the external genitalia and perineum and observe the mons pubis, perineum, and vulva. Before touching the perineum or vulva, place your hand on the patient's thigh to avoid startling her.

- The **mons pubis,** superior to the labia, is usually covered by pubic hair that is distributed in an inverse triangular pattern over the mons, anterior vulva, and medial aspects of the upper thighs. Inspect the hair for nits and the skin for parasites, irritation, inflammation, edema, and lesions. There should be no offensive odor. The perineal skin is slightly darker than the rest of the body.
- The **labia majora** are symmetric, rounded, and full and free of edema, inflammation, or lesions. They tend to gape in women who have had a vaginal delivery, allowing the labia minora to show. After menopause, the labia majora atrophy slowly.
- The **labia minora** are thinner than the labia majora and 1 may be larger than the other. Gently separate the labia majora and labia minora to examine the **vulva** and remaining external structures.
- Place the thumb and index finger of your nondominant hand inside the labia minora and retract the tissue laterally. A firm hold is needed to avoid unnecessary manipulation of sensitive tissues. Inspect the clitoris, urethral meatus, hymen (if present), and vaginal orifice (introitus) for discharge, inflammation, edema, or lesions, which should be absent.
- The **clitoris** is approximately 1 cm wide and 2 cm long and of the same color as the rest of the vulva.
- When you examine the **introitus,** also inspect the **hymen**, which is just inside the introitus. The hymen may be prominent and restrict the vaginal opening in a virgin, or it may be mostly absent, as in a sexually active patient.
- Palpate the posterior labia majora between your thumb and index finger (just inside the vagina) to assess **Bartholin's glands** (see Procedure 31–1). These glands usually are not obvious or palpable. If you express a discharge from the glands, obtain a specimen for culture and change gloves before proceeding with the rest of the examination.

- Inspect the **urethral meatus** between the clitoris and introitus. The meatus should be midline, should look like a slit or dimple, and should be the same color as the vulva. It should be free of discharge, swelling, and inflammation.
- Palpate **Skene's glands** (paraurethral glands), which are on either side of the urethral meatus. Insert your index finger into the vagina and gently press up and out to milk the urethra. There should be no discharge or pain. If a discharge is present, culture it and change gloves before you continue the examination.
- Assess the integrity of the **pelvic floor** musculature. Palpate the perineum. It should feel thick and smooth in a nulliparous woman and thin in a multiparous woman.
- Insert your index and middle fingers into the vagina and ask the patient to contract her pelvic floor muscles as if trying to stop the flow of urine. The tone and strength of muscle contracture vary with parity. Ask the patient to bear down (the Valsalva maneuver) while you feel for any bulges in the vaginal wall that press against the introitus. There should be no bulges or urine leakage. An anterior wall bulge may indicate a **cystocele** (urinary bladder prolapse) and a posterior bulge a **rectocele** (rectal wall prolapse).
- Palpate the vagina for length to determine which size of vaginal speculum to use.

(4) Inspect and palpate the internal genitalia during the speculum examination and bimanual examination.

- Select the appropriate-size vaginal speculum for the patient and warm and lubricate it under warm running water. Do not use any other lubricant, because it may distort the results of any cytology specimens.
- Hold the speculum, blades closed, in your right hand with your index and middle fingers around the blades and your thumb under the thumbscrew. This prevents accidental opening of the blades as you insert them into the vagina.
- Push the introitus down posteriorly with your left index and middle fingers, opening it for insertion of the speculum.
- Hold the speculum blades obliquely to the introitus and insert the speculum over your left fingers while the woman bears down. Do not apply pressure anteriorly against the urethra. The perineal muscles will relax and allow the introitus to open. Remove your left fingers once the speculum blades are in the vagina and rotate the blades horizontally. Gently continue to insert the speculum downward toward the sacrum, following the vaginal slope. When the speculum is inserted

completely, open the blades by squeezing the handles together.

- Look for the **cervix**. If you do not see it, close the blades, withdraw them slightly, and reinsert with a more posterior slant. Once you see the cervix, lock the blades of the speculum in the open position with the thumbscrew.
- Inspect the cervix for color (pink and even), position (midline, projecting 1–3 cm into the vagina), shape (round), size (2.5 cm in diameter), os (round in nulliparous women and horizontal and slitlike in parous women), and surface characteristics (smooth, without erosion or lesions). Note any secretions.
- Obtain specimens if indicated (e.g., endocervical swab, cervical scrape, vaginal pool, saline mount, KOH preparation, and gonorrhea culture).
- Inspect the vaginal wall as you remove the speculum. Loosen the thumbscrew and hold the blades open. Slowly withdraw and rotate the speculum as you inspect. The wall should be pink, moist, and smooth and have deep rugae. There should be no inflammation or lesions, and any discharge should be odorless and thin and clear or opaque and stringy. As the blades near the introitus, close them without pinching the mucosa or pulling any pubic hair. Turn the blades obliquely to remove them from the vagina.

(5) Palpate the internal genitalia bimanually for location, size, mobility, masses, or tenderness. Stand and place 1 hand on the patient's abdomen over the symphysis pubis. Lubricate and insert 2 fingers of the other hand (usually your dominant hand) into the vagina.

- Keep your index and middle fingers extended, your thumb abducted, and your 4th and 5th fingers flexed onto your palm (obstetric position). Insert your fingers, applying any pressure posteriorly. Wait until the vaginal wall relaxes before inserting your fingers fully. Palpate the vaginal wall. It should feel smooth, without nodules or tenderness.
- Feel the cervix at midline with the palmar surface of your fingers. Note its consistency (smooth and firm, like the cartilage of the nose), shape (round), and mobility (moveable from side to side without pain).
- Palpate the anterior, posterior, and lateral fornices, all of which should feel smooth. Place your fingers in the posterior fornix and your other hand midway between the symphysis pubis and umbilicus. Push your hands together to palpate the uterus. Note its size, shape, consistency, position, mobility, and tenderness or pain. It should feel firm, smooth, rounded, mobile, and nontender. Move your fingers into the lateral fornix and

position your other hand in the lower quadrant just inside the anterior iliac spine (to the right to palpate the patient's left adnexa and to the left to palpate the patient's right adnexa). Push your abdominal hand in and down to try and capture the ovary. It often is nonpalpable, but if you feel it, it should be smooth, firm, oval, and movable. The patient may say she feels "something move" but should not feel pain.

- Withdraw your fingers from the patient's vagina and note any secretions on your glove.

(6) Palpate using a rectovaginal approach to assess the rectovaginal septum, posterior uterine wall, cul-de-sac, and rectum. Change gloves to prevent spreading any organisms and lubricate your first 2 fingers.

- Tell the patient that this part of the examination may give her an uncomfortable feeling, similar to the urge to move the bowels. Ask her to bear down as you insert your index finger into the vagina to the cervix and your middle finger into the rectum. Push down with your abdominal hand while you palpate.
- The rectovaginal septum should feel smooth, thin, firm, and resilient. The cul-de-sac usually is not felt. The uterine wall should be firm and smooth.
- Rotate the finger in the rectum to palpate the rectal wall and sphincter tone. (See "Anus and rectum.") As you remove your finger from the patient's rectum, note the presence of stool and test it for occult blood.

16. **Anus and rectum**
   a. Examination of the anus and rectum provides information about the gastrointestinal and reproductive systems.
   b. Examination of the anus and rectum may be embarrassing and uncomfortable for the patient. Use a matter-of-fact approach and manipulate tissues slowly and gently to avoid causing the patient unnecessary discomfort.
   c. Review the anatomies of the anus and rectum so that you are familiar with their structures.
   d. Equipment: Wear gloves and lubricate your palpating finger generously with water-soluble lubricant. If you plan to collect a stool sample for occult blood (guaiac), have a hemoccult slide ready.
   e. Positioning of the patient for rectal examination depends on the circumstances of the preceding physical examination.
      (1) If the rectal examination follows a vaginal examination, examine the woman in the lithotomy position immediately after examining the internal genitalia. Use a bimanual approach (described above) with your index finger in the vagina and your middle finger in the rectum. If you are examining only the anus and rectum in

a woman, without peforming an intravaginal examination, help the patient assume the Sim's or dorsal recumbent position.

    (2) The Sim's position should also be assumed by a man if you are examining only the anus and rectum. If you are examining a man's internal genitalia as well as the anus and rectum, ask the patient to stand and lean over the examining table. This position facilitates palpation of the prostate gland.

  f. Drape the patient to prevent unnecessary and embarrassing exposure.

  g. Inspection of the anus. Spread the buttocks apart with your nondominant hand. Examine the perianal skin and anus.

    (1) The **perianal skin** is darker than that of the surrounding buttocks and should be intact. The **anal area** has coarse, moist, hairless skin.

    (2) Note whether the anus is closed and without signs of rectal prolapse or hemorrhoids. A **rectal prolapse** is a protrusion of rectal mucous membrane through the anus. **Hemorrhoids** are dilated veins that appear as reddened skin protrusions. The perianal area should be without fissures (cracks), excoriation, rashes, inflammation, ulceration, abscesses, lumps, or fistula openings.

    (3) Ask the patient to bear down while you inspect for rectal prolapse, protruding internal hemorrhoids, polyps, and fissures. The increased intra-abdominal pressure may cause an abnormality to become more prominent.

    (4) Lubricate the index finger of your dominant hand and place it over the anus.

    (5) Ask the patient to bear down, which relaxes the anal sphincter. As the sphincter relaxes, insert your index finger slowly and gently into the anal canal, pointing toward the patient's umbilicus. Tell the patient that it is normal to feel as though he or she will have a bowel movement. If it is difficult to insert your finger or you meet resistance or rectal bleeding, stop and remove your finger.

    (6) The **anal canal** extends toward the umbilicus approximately 3 cm (1.0–1.5 inches), where it joins the rectum at the anorectal junction. Ask the patient to tighten the anal muscles around your finger while you assess the **anal sphincter** tone. It should be strong.

    (7) Rotate your finger around the **anal wall** to assess for nodules, masses, or tenderness, which should be absent. Advance your finger slowly to the anorectal junction, where the rectum widens and turns posteriorly along the coccyx and sacrum.

  h. Palpation of the rectum

    (1) Palpate around the **rectal wall** and along the curve of the coccyx, which is mobile. Advance your finger to its fullest extent, approximately 6 to 10 cm (2–4 inches) into the rectum, and palpate for tenderness or masses. The rectal wall should be smooth and nontender. If you palpate an abnormality, document its location (e.g., "left lateral wall 1 cm proximal to internal anal sphincter") and characteristics.

    (2) Once your finger is inserted fully, ask the patient to bear down again while you feel for a descending mass pushing against your finger. There should be none.

    (3) In a man, palpate the **prostate gland** through the anterior rectal wall. The prostate gland feels like a rounded, heart-shaped structure approximately 2.5 to 4 cm (1.0–1.5 inches) in diameter. Its borders are discrete. Feel for the **median sulcus** (groove), which separates the posterior prostate into 2 lateral lobes. The gland is firm, rubbery, nontender, and movable. Enlargement, bogginess, nodules, hardness, and tenderness are abnormal findings.

    (4) In a woman, palpate the **cervix** through the **rectovaginal wall** along the anterior rectum. The rectovaginal wall is firm, smooth, and resilient. The cervix feels round, smooth, firm, and movable without tenderness. Do not mistake the cervix or a vaginal tampon for a rectal mass.

    (5) As you withdraw your finger from the rectum, observe for the presence of stool on your glove. Feces, if present, is usually brown. Mucus, blood, and black and tarry or light tan or gray stool are abnormal findings. Test a sample of stool from your glove for occult blood, which should be negative. If you suspect that the patient has a sexually transmitted disease, you may wish to obtain a rectal culture.

    (6) Wipe the patient's perianal area with a tissue. Inform the patient that the examination is over.

17. Ending the examination

  a. Help the patient assume a comfortable position. Close the gown or wrap and provide wipes or tissues if needed.

  b. Dispose of used equipment and supplies that cannot be sterilized or cleaned. Clean nondisposable equipment and restock the equipment tray for future use.

◘ USING THE FINDINGS OF THE PHYSICAL ASSESSMENT

Recording the Findings

1. Use forms and formats approved by your agency.
2. Record both normal and abnormal findings as soon as possible after completing the examination. Be objective. Use clear, concise, descriptive terms. Avoid vague descriptors such as "good," "poor," "fair," "normal," "moderate," and the like.

Analyzing the Data

1. The complete results of the physical examination, together with the health history, should form a substantial database.
2. Review all data, summarize the patient's strengths, and determine his or her health risk profile.
3. Validate, revise, or discard any tentative nursing diagnoses you formulated after completing the patient's health history. Add new nursing diagnoses that are supported by the physical examination findings.
4. Discuss your findings and nursing diagnoses with the patient. Formulate an action plan together. The plan should include referring the person to a physician for further assessment if there is a serious abnormality.

Preparing a Summary and Making Recommendations

1. Summarize the patient's problem areas and the action plan. Determine which health problems are nursing diagnoses that you can manage either independently or in collaboration with colleagues.
2. If necessary, refer the patient to appropriate health care professionals for additional care or follow-up.

Bibliography

Books

American Dietetic Association. *Handbook of Clinical Dietetics.* New Haven, CT: Yale University Press, 1981.

Bates B. *A Guide to Physical Examination.* 5th ed. Philadelphia: JB Lippincott, 1991.

Doenges ME, and Moorhouse MF. *Application of Nursing Process and Nursing Diagnosis: An Interactive Text.* Philadelphia: FA Davis, 1992.

Giger JN, and Davidhizer RE. *Transcultural Nursing: Assessment and Intervention.* St. Louis: Mosby–Year Book, 1991.

Jarvis C. *Physical Examination and Health Assessment.* 2d ed. Philadelphia: WB Saunders, 1996.

Malasanos L, Barkauskas V, and Stoltenberg-Allen K. *Health Assessment.* 4th ed. St. Louis: CV Mosby, 1990.

Morton PG. *Health Assessment in Nursing.* 2nd ed. Springhouse, PA: Springhouse, 1993.

Polednak AP. *Host Factors in Diseases: Age, Sex, Racial, and Ethnic Group, and Body Build.* Springfield, IL: Charles C. Thomas, 1987.

Seidel HM, et al. *Mosby's Guide to Physical Examination.* 2nd ed. St. Louis: CV Mosby, 1991.

Swartz MH. *Textbook of Physical Diagnosis.* Philadelphia: WB Saunders, 1989.

Chapters in Books

Keene A. Physical examination. *In* Black JM, and Matassarian-Jacobs E (eds). *Luckmann and Sorensen's Medical-Surgical Nursing: A Psychophysiologic Approach.* 4th ed. Philadelphia: WB Saunders, 1993, pp. 215–244.

Articles

Curtas S, et al. Evaluation of nutritional status. *Nurs Clin North Am* 24:301–313, 1989.

Erickson RS, and Yount ST. Comparison of tympanic and oral temperatures in surgical patients. *Nurs Res* 40:90–93, 1991.

Fraden J, and Lackey RP. Estimation of body sites temperatures from tympanic measurements. *Clin Pediatr* 30: (Suppl 4): 65–70, 1991.

Grant JP, et al. Current techniques of nutritional assessment. *Surg Clin North Am* 61:437–463, 1981.

Joint National Committee on Detection, Evaluation, and Treatment of High Blood Pressure. 1988 report. *Arch Intern Med* 148:1023–1038, 1988.

Shinozaki T, et al. Infrared tympanic thermometer. Evaluation of a new clinical thermometer. *Crit Care Med* 16:148–150, 1988.

6

Performing the Basic Psychosocial Assessment

■ OVERVIEW

Definition

1. Psychosocial assessment includes collecting information about a patient's psychologic patterns, sociologic experiences, and environmental influences.
   a. **Psychologic patterns** are the person's unique thoughts, feelings, emotions, motivations, mental status, strengths, and shortcomings.
   b. **Sociologic experiences** are those parts of a person's life that are affected by or dependent on others, including his or her roles and relationships within the family, in groups, and in society. A person's experiences are influenced by cultural and spiritual factors that originate both internally and externally.
   c. **Psychosocial considerations** are a mixture of the psychologic and sociologic dimensions. It is impossible to separate a person's psychologic and sociologic influences, the interactions between these dimensions, and their effect on the physiologic dimension.
   d. **Environmental influences** include factors such as the community and neighborhood in which a person lives and conditions (safe or unsafe) within the person's workplace or school.

Purposes

1. To assess the total person, including the effects of physical, emotional, social, spiritual, intellectual, and cultural stresses on the person.
2. To integrate psychosocial assessment into the nursing history interview and physical assessment (see Chapters 4 and 5).
3. To identify actual, potential, or possible problem areas that may affect the person's ability to function in the family and in society or that may interfere with recovery from an illness or injury.
4. To gain insight into the person and the person's interac-

tions with friends and family members, the community, and other sources of influence.

Benefits

1. Promoting comprehensive nursing care
   a. Psychosocial assessment helps you to establish a comprehensive database to use in formulating relevant nursing diagnoses based on identified needs or problems.
   b. Psychosocial assessment is essential to a holistic approach to nursing. More than half the disorders that nurses diagnose and treat independently are psychosocial.

2. Building therapeutic relationships
   a. Psychosocial assessment helps you view each patient as unique.
   b. Successful nurse-patient communication helps promote rapport and establish trust.
   c. Rapport helps patients feel comfortable about revealing personal information that may affect their health status or ability to cope with a health problem. Trust enables patients to feel that you are as interested in their well-being as they are.
   d. Planning effective, therapeutic interventions depends on assessing accurately how the patient and the patient's significant others will respond to the patient's health needs and problems.

◻ PERFORMING THE PSYCHOSOCIAL ASSESSMENT

General Guidelines

1. The person must be conscious, alert, and cooperative for you to perform a psychosocial assessment (Table 6–1).
2. Provide privacy for the interview, and select a time when the person is free from distractions.
3. Employ communication skills and therapeutic use of self (see Chapter 4). Use open-ended questions to avoid receiving answers the patient thinks you want to hear.
4. Be tactful and nonjudgmental. Many topics are personal and sensitive or difficult for a person to discuss.
5. Avoid pressuring the person to discuss topics that seem to cause discomfort. Revisit them after trust has been established.

Table 6–1. Guide to Psychosocial Assessment

1. Explore history of psychosocial problems
   - Personal history
   - Family history
2. Assess psychologic components
   - General appearance
     Dress
     Hygiene and grooming
     Posture
     Motor activity
     Facial expression
   - Recent level of stress
     Current perceived level of stress
     Adjustment to past stressors
     Signs of response to stress
     Usual coping pattern
   - Mental status and level of understanding
     Level of consciousness (LOC)
     Orientation
     Mood and affect
     Speech and communication (language)
     Thought process and content
     Attention span
     Memory
     General fund of knowledge
     Calculation ability
     Ability to reason and think abstractly
     Perception
     Judgment
   - Behavior
     Verbal
     Nonverbal
     Reaction to interview
   - Personality style
   - Motivation
   - Personal strengths
   - Values and beliefs
     Self-concept, self-esteem
     Body image
     Locus of control
   - Spirituality
   - Psychosocial risk factors
3. Assess sociologic components
   - Psychosocial level of development
   - Social network
     Support systems
   - Socioeconomic status
   - Lifestyle
   - Sexuality
4. Assess transcultural components

NURSE ADVISORY

Psychosocial assessment requires a trusting relationship between interviewer and patient. If you are unable to build such a relationship with a particular patient, you may need to request that another nurse perform the assessment.

---

6. Be aware of your own feelings and reactions to the person and his or her situation. Your anxiety level, values, and personal biases can affect the nurse-patient relationship and its outcome.
7. Be aware of cultural biases, and avoid labeling a person's beliefs or behavior in the context of your own cultural beliefs.
8. Do not assume there is one "correct" reaction for every person in a given situation.

Explore the History of Psychosocial Problems

1. Inquire about experiences with psychosocial problems, including hospitalizations or other psychotherapy.
   a. The patient may continue to be affected by emotional or mental health problems or may fear a recurrence of a problem, especially if his or her health status is compromised.
   b. Ask about past or current use of psychotropic medications or drugs and whether the patient experienced any side effects.
   c. *Transcultural considerations:* Some ethnic groups (e.g., Asian, Hispanic) require lower doses of various psychotropic medications, and experience side effects at lower doses than do Whites.
2. Ask whether there is a history of psychosocial problems in the patient's family.
   a. Some mental health problems (e.g., depression, schizophrenia) have been linked to biologic and possibly genetic causes.
   b. The patient may have concerns about developing an emotional or mental health problem because of a family tendency toward such problems.
   c. *Transcultural considerations:* Some ethnic groups (e.g., Asian Americans) view mental illness as a stigma and may be reluctant to discuss this topic. Psychosocial problems may be expressed as somatic complaints, for example, headaches, stomach aches, weakness, or dizziness.

Assess Psychologic Components

1. Assess general appearance. Dress, hygiene, posture, motor activity, and facial expression can all provide clues to psychosocial status (see Chapter 5).
   a. *Dress:* Dress is an indicator of self-esteem, body image, mood, socioeconomic status, and self-care ability.
      (1) Clothing can be neat, in good repair, clean, disheveled, torn, or soiled.
      (2) Bright clothes may hint at a cheerful disposition, and drab, dull colors may signal depression.
   b. *Hygiene and grooming:* Grooming and hygiene reflect mood, self-esteem, body image, socioeconomic status, and self-care ability. A person can be neat, clean, unkempt, or unwashed or have body odor. Attention to appearance takes physical and emotional energy.
   c. *Posture:* Posture reflects mood, self-esteem, body image, and level of anxiety.
      (1) A person's posture may be tall and erect, relaxed, hunched, stooped, or tense.
      (2) A person's posture may change when someone else is present, depending on the relationship between the 2 persons (e.g., dominant-submissive, aggressor-victim, protector-ward).
   d. *Motor activity:* Motor activity can indicate level of anxiety, underlying physical conditions, or side effects of medication.
      (1) Movements may be calm, quiet, controlled, agitated, restless, or erratic.
      (2) Unusual movements include tics, tremors, repetitive gestures, handwringing, foot tapping, swaying, and persistent touching, rubbing, or other handling of objects.
      (3) A person may react to increased levels of anxiety with increased motor activity, or he or she may withdraw and become still.
   e. *Facial expression:* Facial expression often mirrors mood and emotional state.
      (1) A change in facial skin color, such as a sudden reddening flush or pallor, may indicate increased anxiety.
      (2) A change in affect (mood) during the interview may provide clues to underlying conflicts. Also note whether the patient displays an appropriate *range* of affect.
   f. *Transcultural considerations:* Evaluate all psychosocial data in their sociocultural context. For example, Native Americans and Asians may not readily reveal their feelings and emotions through their body language and facial expressions.
2. Assess recent level of stress.
   a. Assess the person's current perceived level of stress.
      (1) Recent stressors, both major and minor, affect a person's ability to function and cope with additional stressors.
      (2) Recent stressors also may reactivate unresolved past stressors (e.g., the death of a sibling may reactivate unresolved grief from earlier losses).
   b. Assess stress from major stressors.
      (1) Changes and losses in a person's life, including

health, work, home and family; and personal, social, and financial status.

- Change and loss are inevitable in everyone's life.
- Changes and losses range from minor to major.
- Categorizing a change or loss as minor or major can be done only by the person affected by the event.
- Minor change or loss is perceived by the person as manageable and nonthreatening.
- Major change or loss is perceived by the person as potentially overwhelming and possibly life threatening.
- Reactions to change or loss may be positive (or desirable), negative (undesirable), or neutral (having no effect). The person's perception of or reaction to a specific event can change over time, becoming more or less positive or negative.
- Reaction to a specific event depends on how the person learned to cope with change and loss, the significance of the event, the person's physical and emotional state at the time the event occurred, the person's perceived control over the event's occurrence, the accumulation of changes and losses throughout the person's lifetime, and how the person has resolved the effects of these previous events.
- A large number of recent changes or losses, especially those rated as having negative or undesirable effects, may lead to health problems.

---

   (2) Normal responses to loss proceed through a series of stages, the timing of which varies from person to person and situation to situation (Table 6–2).
   c. *Transcultural considerations:* Try to evaluate the effect of change or loss from the patient's sociocultural perspective. All cultures do not view the same event in the same way (e.g., death of a parent). Failure to come to terms with loss leaves a person less able to cope with future losses and at risk for extreme reactions such as attempts at suicide.

NURSE ADVISORY

Do not ignore *any* comment that indicates a patient is considering suicide. Such individuals may well attempt to kill themselves. Bring your findings to psychiatric professionals *immediately.*

   d. Ask the person about changes, losses, and other stressors that have occurred during the past 6 months to 1 year. Table 6–3 lists possible stressors and rates their impact on a person's well-being.
      (1) Place the stressors in a time line. Try to rank them from least to most severe.
   e. Ask the person whether he or she has adjusted well to personal stressors in the past.
      (1) Has the person resolved the effects of loss or change? Has he or she been able to move on and continue to function in daily life?
      (2) Does the person remain affected and influenced by unresolved stress? For example, is the person angry and aggressive or withdrawn and passive?

Table 6–2. Stages of Recovery in Response to Stressful Loss		
Stage*	**Description**	**Example**
Shock and denial	Initial disbelief that the loss occurred. Person may be unable to function physically or psychologically.	"This is happening to someone else, not me!" "These tests are wrong!"
Anger and depression	Reactions occurring after the person realizes that the loss has actually happened. *Anger* can take form as verbal lashing out, blaming others for the loss, or criticizing. (Health care professionals are often targets of anger during this stage.) *Depression* may be displayed as sadness, guilt, crying, or self-directed violence. The person may feel helpless, hopeless, fearful, lonely, guilty, or desperate.	"This wouldn't have happened if you had been there!" "I should have insisted that my husband see the doctor sooner."
Understanding and acceptance	The person experiences an inner peace and calm as the loss is put into perspective. (*Note:* If another loss or stressful event occurs before the person completes this stage, he or she may regress and need to rework feelings and emotions related to the previous loss.)	"It's been hard but I need to go on." "My mother was so ill and suffered so much that her death was a blessing."

* The length, intensity, and scope of the stages vary with the person's perception of the event and the type of loss.

TRANSCULTURAL CONSIDERATIONS

When dealing with members of refugee groups, you may need to explore the circumstances of their move, feelings about leaving their country of origin, responsibilities to those left behind, and acceptance of the new host society and culture.

f. Assess for signs of the stress response. The stress response is a normal physical reaction to both physical and psychologic stressors (Fig. 6–1).
  (1) Levels of neurotransmitters, such as norepinephrine and serotonin, change during the stress response.
  (2) Altered levels of neurotransmitters affect the function of the sympathetic and parasympathetic nervous systems and result in physical signs such as increased heart rate, blood pressure, and rate and depth of respiration; increased alertness; dilated pupils; muscle tenseness; and cool, pale skin.
  (3) Physical reactions to stress include disruptions in the person's usual rest, eating, elimination, and activity patterns, including sexual activity.
g. Ask about the patient's pattern of coping wth stress.

NURSE ADVISORY

Avoid asking leading questions about physical activity patterns. That is, instead of asking, "Have you been sleeping less?" say, "How have you been sleeping . . . Is that your usual pattern?"

  (1) **Coping** is the process (conscious and unconscious) of adapting to or managing the effects of stress.
  (2) A **coping pattern** (or style) is what a person usually does in response to difficult times or perceived stress. Examples of coping styles include the following:
  • Confrontive: Facing the problem
  • Evasive: Engaging in avoidance behavior
  • Optimistic: Using positive thinking
  • Fatalistic: Feeling hopeless
  • Emotive: Expressing emotions openly
  • Palliative: Making oneself feel better
  • Supportant: Using support systems
  • Self-reliant: Depending on oneself
  (3) **Coping strategies,** unlike **defense mechanisms,** which are unconscious, are specific skills or actions that are consciously selected by a person to help manage the effects of stress (see Chapter 41).

Table 6–3. Stress Ratings of Various Life Events

Events	Scale of Impact
Death of spouse	100
Divorce	73
Marital separation	65
Jail term	63
Death of close family member	63
Personal injury or illness	53
Marriage	50
Fired at work	47
Marital reconciliation	45
Retirement	45
Change in health of family member	44
Pregnancy	40
Sex difficulties	39
Gain of a new family member	39
Business readjustment	39
Change in financial state	38
Death of close friend	37
Change to different line of work	36
Change in number of arguments with spouse	35
Mortgage over $10,000	31
Foreclosure of mortgage or loan	30
Change in responsibilities at work	29
Son or daughter leaving home	29
Trouble with in-laws	29
Outstanding personal achievement	28
Wife begins or stops work	26
Begin or end school	26
Change in living conditions	25
Revision of personal habits	24
Trouble with boss	23
Change in work hours or conditions	20
Change in residence	20
Change in schools	20
Change in recreation	19
Change in church activities	19
Change in social activities	18
Mortgage or loan less than $10,000	17
Change in sleeping habits	16
Change in number of family get-togethers	15
Change in eating habits	15
Vacation	13
Christmas	12
Minor violations of the law	11

Adapted by permission of the publisher from Holmes TS, and Holmes TH. Short-term intrusions into life-style routine. *J Psychosom Res* 14:121–132, 1970. Copyright 1970 by Elsevier Science, Inc.

Examples of positive coping strategies include the following:

- Maintaining an established routine
- Limiting or avoiding changes
- Setting a period of time aside to focus on and adapt to stressors
- Using one's time efficiently
- Modifying the environment to reduce stressful situations
- Engaging in regular exercise
- Using humor

- Eating a sound diet
- Obtaining sufficient rest and sleep
- Learning and practicing relaxation techniques
- Building a support system
- Enhancing self-esteem
- Praying

(4) Ask what helps the person manage the effects of stress. When patients have difficulty answering, ask them to describe the worst period in their lives and how they got through it.

(5) Ask how long it took the person to resolve or get over the effects of the stressful event. In assessing the person's coping skills, bear in mind that major losses usually take longer to resolve than minor annoyances.

(6) Assess whether the person's usual coping strategies are adequate to deal with current stressors. Ask the person what was done in previous, similar situations that was helpful. Also ask what was not helpful. The person may need guidance in developing new coping strategies if the usual ones are likely to be ineffective or unworkable. For example, a person who uses physical activity (e.g., walking or working out) to relieve the effects of stress may need help if faced with a health problem that restricts mobility or activity.

(7) *Transcultural considerations:* Some cultures use rituals to resolve events. The timing of such rituals may not seem appropriate to you. For example, many Asian cultures observe 2- to 5-year mourning periods. Also, in dislocated groups, any assistance offered may need to be group or community based rather than individually based.

3. Assess mental status and level of understanding.

  a. **Mental status** refers to the person's current level of functioning emotionally, intellectually (cognitively), and perceptually, and to his or her level of understanding. Mental status is reflected in general appearance and behavior (see also "Assess Psychologic Components" in this chapter and Chapters 4 and 5).

  (1) If you note a dysfunction in any of these areas, try to describe—not label—the person's behavior. For example, say, "The person is quiet, turns away, and does not interact with others when addressed" rather than "The person is depressed."

  (2) *Transcultural considerations:* Note that changes in level of awareness, withdrawal, or trancelike states are normal coping behaviors in some cultural groups, especially Asians, Pacific Islanders, and Native Americans.

  b. To assess level of understanding, determine the person's perception of his or her current situation and its present and future significance.

  (1) This assessment is directed to the person who has a health problem or is at risk for developing one.

  (2) The goal is to determine whether the person is able to foresee the effects a current health problem will continue to have on life.

  (3) Patients with understanding deficits may require

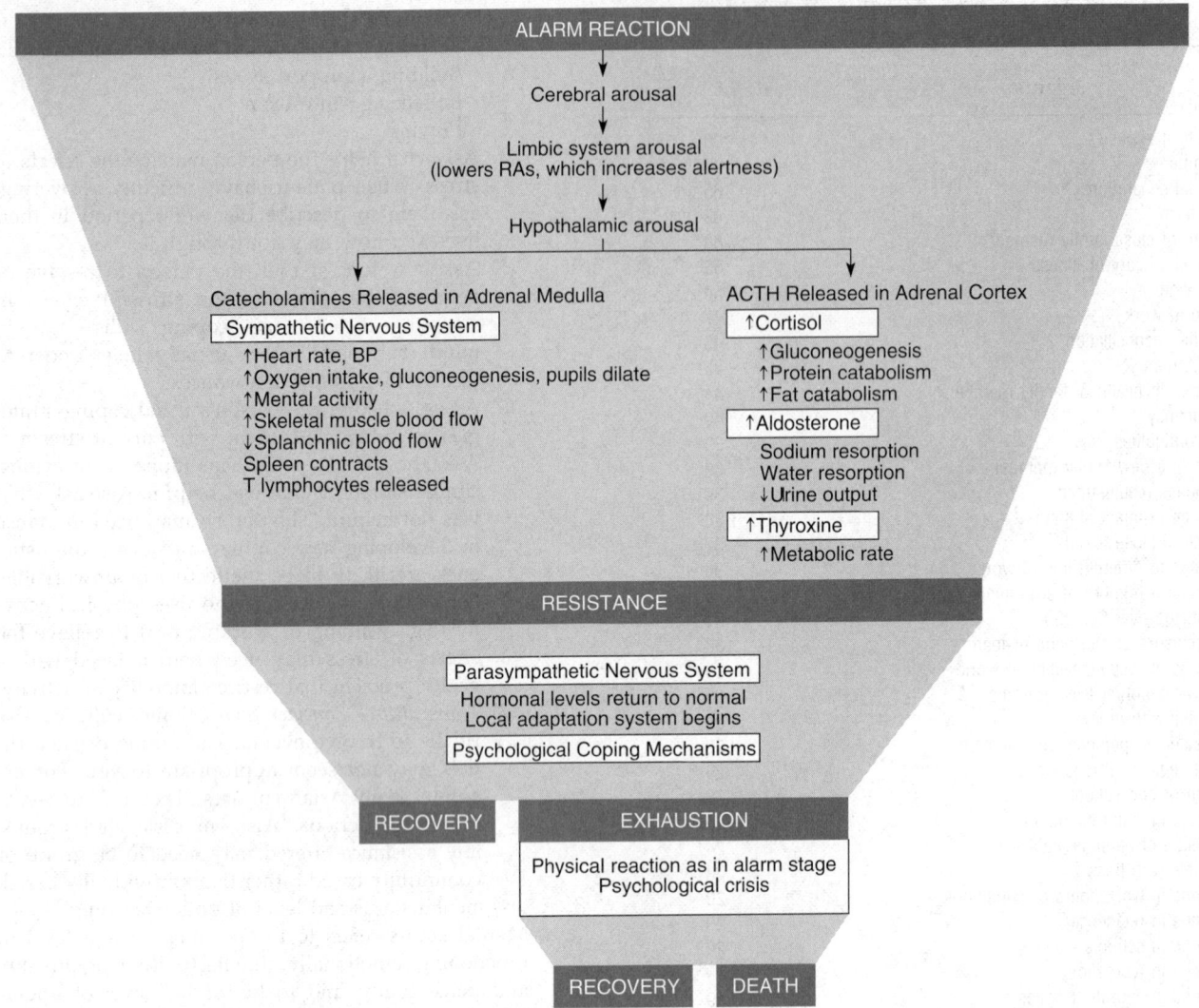

Figure 6–1. The general adaptation syndrome ("fight or flight") occurs in response to physical or physiologic stressors. (*From* Black JM, and Matassarin-Jacobs E [eds]. *Luckmann and Sorensen's Medical-Surgical Nursing: A Psychophysiologic Approach.* 4th ed. Philadelphia: WB Saunders, 1993, p 46.)

frequent assessment of their health status and teaching and learning reinforcement to maintain a healthy state.

(4) In conducting the assessment, make allowances for whether the patient has had time to consider the problem and its ramifications thoroughly. Victims of acute onset problems may need time to prepare psychologically.

(5) Ask open-ended questions such as the following:

- "What brings you here today?"
- "When did you first notice the problem?"
- "How do you think the health care team can help you?"
- "Do you foresee any problems when you go home?"
- "How are members of your family (or close friends) reacting to your problem?" (See explanatory model questions under cultural assessment in Chapter 2.)

c. A complete, detailed mental status assessment includes observing the patient's general appearance (see earlier discussion), as well as the following areas:

(1) **Level of consciousness** (LOC) is the person's state of awareness and orientation. Awareness ranges on a continuum from unconscious to manic (Fig. 6–2).

(2) **Orientation** is the person's ability to identify *person* (self), *place* (present location), *time* (date), and *situation* (present circumstances). Orientation ranges on a continuum from comatose to completely oriented (Fig. 6–3). Ask the following questions: "What is your name?", "Where are you now?", "What year (month, day) is it?", and "What is happening to you?" or "What brought you here?"

(3) **Mood** consists of the subjective feelings that color one's outlook; its visible display is called **affect.** Assess mood by asking the patient to

Alert
Comatose
Stuporous
Hypersomnolent
Drowsy
Hyperalert
Suspicious
Paranoid
Manic

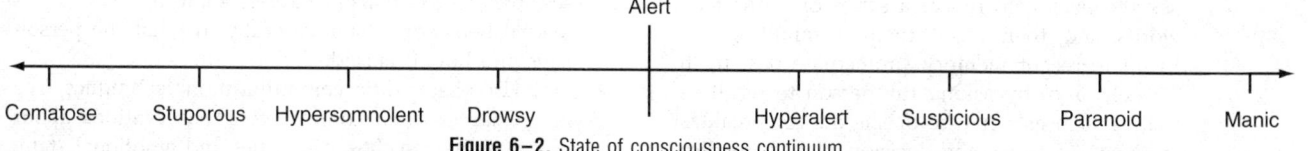

Figure 6–2. State of consciousness continuum.

NURSE ADVISORY

Subtle changes in level of consciousness and orientation are significant indicators of a person's neurologic and psychologic status. Report changes in level of consciousness immediately.

describe how he or she feels. Be especially alert for abnormalities such as depression or suicidal thoughts. Mood and affect should agree. For example, "The woman cried when she learned of her husband's serious accident." Inappropriate affect refers to a response that is unusual in a given situation. For example, "The patient smiled when informed that a tumor had spread." Blunted or flat affect means that the usual range of emotions is lacking. The person tends to respond with an understated response or none at all.

NURSE ADVISORY

Be aware that depression and suicidal thoughts are not limited to people with a history of psychiatric disorders. They may be present in people with medical-surgical problems.

Transcultural considerations: Cultural differences in language and mannerisms may result in an inaccurate assessment of mood and affect. For example, Latin Americans and Asians may display somatic problems (fatigue, weight loss, sleep disturbance) rather than cognitive or affective signs of stress or depression. Native Americans tend to keep their thoughts private and not to display emotions.

(4) **Speech and communication (language).** Assess speech and language by focusing on the form, not the content, of the person's speech. Describe rate of speech, volume, voice modulation, pitch, spontaneity, articulation, coherence, length of responses to questions, pauses, and hesitancy before replying to questions. Also note changes in the person's tone of voice brought on by discussing a particular topic, and be alert to abrupt changes of subject.

Transcultural considerations: Members of some cultures, such as persons from Appalachia, often speak slowly and deliberately and so may appear to be mentally slow. In contrast, members of some Asian cultures may speak rapidly and nonstop and so may appear unduly agitated.

(5) **Thought process,** called cognitive style, reflects the way a person functions intellectually. It includes reasoning ability, association of ideas, and organization of thoughts. Note the progression of speech. Does it proceed spontaneously, logically, coherently, and relevantly toward a goal-directed conclusion? Examples of thought disorders include loose association or flight of ideas, blocking, preoccupation, delusions, obsessions, phobias, and impaired memory.

Transcultural considerations: Note that what may seem to be a thought disorder may simply reflect a cultural norm with which you are unfamiliar.

(6) **Content** is reflected in what the person decides to talk about. Is the person's speech related to the topic under discussion? Is it consistent and logical?

(7) **Attention span** is the ability to focus or concentrate consciously on a task or activity over time. Assess attention span with a digit-span test or a serial-7s or -3s test. Digit span tests the patient's ability to repeat a series of numbers you create. Use 5 to 7 numbers forward and up to 5 numbers backward. Serial 7s and 3s also test calculation ability and memory. Ask the person to count backward from 100 by subtracting 7 (or 3) repeatedly until he or she is unable to continue.

Transcultural considerations: Some cultural groups are not oriented toward numbers or retention of numbers. They do better with concrete events and names.

(8) **Memory** is the ability to retain and recall information and experiences. Assess immediate memory with a digit-span or serial-7s test, or

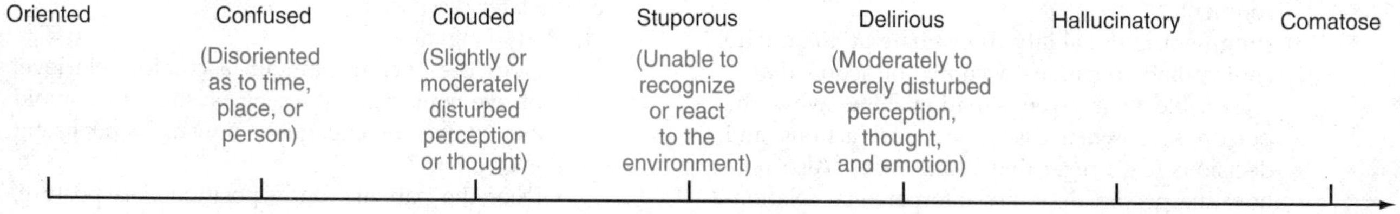

Oriented
Confused
(Disoriented as to time, place, or person)
Clouded
(Slightly or moderately disturbed perception or thought)
Stuporous
(Unable to recognize or react to the environment)
Delirious
(Moderately to severely disturbed perception, thought, and emotion)
Hallucinatory
Comatose

Figure 6–3. Orientation continuum.

ask the person to repeat a series of 3 unrelated words and then recall them 5 minutes later. Evaluate recent memory (immediate past up to 2 weeks ago) by asking the person to recall activities such as what he or she ate for breakfast or what led up to the decision to seek medical help. Test long-term memory by asking the person to relate information about his or her childhood. You should have a way of verifying the information, by consulting either health records or a family member.

(9) **General fund of knowledge** is a general evaluation of intelligence. Ask the person to identify commonly known people, places, events, or facts that you can verify. Examples are famous people, large cities, and major holidays.

Transcultural considerations: Questions must be culturally relevant. Immigrants, for example, may have little knowledge of the host culture.

(10) **Calculation ability** is a function of intelligence, memory, attention span, logical thinking, and educational level. Ask the person to perform simple addition, subtraction, multiplication, and division without pencil and paper.

Transcultural considerations: As with literacy and cultural knowledge, lack of arithmetic proficiency among immigrants may not reflect lack of intelligence.

(11) **Abstract thinking or reasoning** is the ability to consider words and ideas beyond their concrete and literal meanings. Assess abstract reasoning ability by asking the person to describe similarities between two objects (e.g., ''How are a tree and a bush alike?''). Avoid asking the person to interpret the meaning of a proverb or fable unless it is culturally meaningful.

Transcultural considerations: Present-oriented cultural groups often think in a concrete rather than an abstract manner. The level of formal education may also affect a person's ability to think abstractly versus concretely.

(12) **Perception** is the ability to recognize and understand the self, the environment, and relationships with others. It is a function of the senses of vision, hearing, touch, and smell and of interpretation of sensory stimuli, which may be culturally influenced. Perceptual distortion is the misinterpretation of stimuli. Examples of perceptual distortion are hallucinations (visual, tactile, and auditory) and illusions. Assess for perceptual distortion by observing whether the person's verbal and nonverbal behavior is related to what is happening in the current environment.

(13) **Judgment** is the ability to evaluate and compare choices and to pursue a course of action that is reasonable in a given situation. Note what the person says when discussing past actions and decisions (e.g., regarding health care). Also note how the person describes interpersonal relationships and responsibilities related to family, job, or financial obligations.

4. Assess behavior (see also Chapters 4 and 5).
   a. Verbal behavior: Listen carefully to what the person says and how it is said.
      (1) Use therapeutic communication techniques (see Chapter 4) to confirm your observations about possible psychosocial issues and emotional state.
      (2) Pay attention to what is *not* said. The person may be unable to verbalize concerns without help and reassurance.
   b. Nonverbal behavior: Observe the person's nonverbal behavior, such as manner of dress, posture, movements, facial expression, and other body language.
      (1) Look for signs of anxiety (tensed muscles, increased or decreased activity, nervous mannerisms, hyperventilation), which may need to be dissipated before you can continue the interview.
      (2) Note whether the person's nonverbal behavior matches what he or she is saying.
   c. Reaction to the interview: Verbal and nonverbal reactions to the interview reveal information about emotional state, ability to trust, and ability to relate to others. Reactions include friendly, suspicious, hostile, indifferent, and flirtatious behavior.

NURSE ADVISORY

When describing a patient's verbal and nonverbal behavior during an interview, *avoid labeling.* Instead, describe the behavior without interpreting it. For example, "The patient hesitates before answering questions" is an observed fact. "The patient is evasive" is judgmental and possibly incorrect.

   d. Validate your observations with the person. All behavior has meaning, but the meaning may not be clear to others, including the nurse conducting the interview.
5. Assess personality style.
   a. Personality style is the way a person usually interacts with others socially.
      (1) Personality style can interfere with a person's ability to adapt to a health problem if it creates communication difficulties with caregivers or family or friends.
      (2) Examples of personality styles are dependent, independent, controlled (orderly), relaxed, dramatic, suspicious (guarded), accepting, self-sacrificing, superior, inferior, and aloof (detached).
   b. As you talk to the person, pay attention to the way he or she interacts with you. Note the following clues, remembering to consider transcultural variations (some of these are discussed in Chapter 4; also see the later discussion).
      (1) Body language
         • Does the person maintain a comfortable level of eye contact, or does he or she either avoid eye contact or engage in unusually persistent eye contact?
         • Does the patient's body position (i.e., posture, position of arms and legs) indicate withdrawal, relaxation, tension, or aggression?

(2) Descriptions of feelings
- Does the person avoid discussing feelings, certain topics, or both? Does the person express feelings freely or even dramatically?
- Does he or she describe intellectual reactions to situations without also expressing feelings about what happened?
- Does the person dwell on his or her reaction to a situation, expressing guilt?

(3) Descriptions of relationships
- Does the patient freely describe his or her relationships with family members and friends or avoid such discussions?
- Does the person demonstrate emotional reactions when discussing his or her health problem and its effects on family and close friends?

(4) Interactions with others: Does the person initiate discussion or avoid conversation unless directly addressed?

6. Assess motivation.
   a. Motivation is what drives a person to action or thought. Its stimulus is either internal (e.g., personal needs or desires) or external (e.g., a threat to one's health).
   b. When you know what motivates your patient, you will be able to help the patient make important health care decisions, such as starting an exercise program or adhering to a therapeutic diet.
   c. Helping the person to identify strengths, values and beliefs, and feelings about self enables him or her to make more informed decisions.

7. Assess personal strengths (see also Chapter 4).
   a. Personal strengths are internal and external factors that help a person adapt to and cope with stressors.
   b. Internal factors are physiologic or psychologic.
      (1) Physiologic factors are the immune system, nutritional status, physiologic defense systems, genetic predisposition to health, and current status of each body system.
      (2) Psychologic factors include defense mechanisms (see Chapter 41), usual coping ability, current coping ability, interpersonal style, and spiritual state (such as hopefulness).
   c. External factors include the social environment (usual coping style of family and friends; social support systems; the assessment by the health care team); and the physical, economic, and cultural environments.

8. Assess values and beliefs (see also Chapter 4 and Table 6–4).
   a. Values are the principles, standards, and qualities that a person (or cultural group) cherishes and holds dear.
   b. Beliefs are a person's (or group's) ideas, expectations, attitudes, and opinions.
      (1) Values and beliefs are acquired as the person grows and interacts with the environment. They influence a person's perspectives on health, wellness, illness, and whether health care is worthwhile.
      (2) Awareness of the person's values and beliefs gives you insight into his or her behavior.

Table 6–4. Guide for Assessing Values, Beliefs, and Spirituality

Key Questions or Issues

Values and Beliefs
- What things in your life help you want to live each day (e.g., health, respect of others, happiness, loving relationships with family, time to spend with loved ones, friendships, religious beliefs, financial security, having a job or work to do)?
- How important is your health to you? To your family or friends? (Ask person to rate importance on a scale of 1 to 10, where 10 is of most importance and 1 is the least.)
- What do you hope to accomplish in your lifetime (e.g., rear children successfully, become rich or famous, have a satisfying job or career)?
- Have you accomplished what you set out to do in your life? Are you satisfied or dissatisfied? If you were to come into a lot of money (win a lottery, inheritance), what would you do with it?
- Are there specific factors that influence you when you have to make important decisions (e.g., being fair or honest, getting a fair deal, examining all sides of the issue)?
- Have you had any of your beliefs or values challenged recently? Have such challenges made you uncomfortable?
- Have you changed any of your values or beliefs recently? Has this change put a strain on your relationship with family or friends? Are you comfortable with the change?

Self-Concept, Self-Esteem, Body Image
- Describe yourself as you believe others see you and as you see yourself (e.g., emotional health, usual mood and what affects it, ability to cope with daily stressors, physical appearance, stamina, intelligence).
- What do you like about yourself? What do you wish you could change about yourself?
- Has anything happened recently to change your feelings about yourself (e.g., change in health status or physical agility, a loss of some kind, a role change)? Do you feel more positive or negative about yourself because of this change?
- Describe how you feel when you become ill or in some way incapacitated and are unable to carry on your daily activities.

Locus of Control
- Do you feel that you can control or manage factors that affect your health (e.g., whether you smoke or exercise, what you do and do not eat, getting regular checkups)?
- Do you feel that you can control or manage factors that affect your life (e.g., your job, where you live, who your friends are)?
- Is there anybody or anything that you believe is responsible for what happens to you in your life (e.g., a supreme being, fate, luck)?

Spirituality
- Do you have a preferred religion or religious beliefs?
- Is your religion an important influence in your life? Does it give you guidance in your daily life?
- How often do you attend worship services? Does it bother you if you are ill or unable to attend worship services? What do you do if you cannot attend services?
- Are there other things besides religion that are important to you as you go about your daily life?
- Is there someone you consider to be your spiritual adviser? Describe how this person makes you feel better. Do you need to talk to this person?
- Is there anything special that you do when you feel a need for spiritual support? Do you need help to practice your beliefs at this time?
- Do you have any religious or spiritual beliefs about health and illness (e.g., illness as a punishment, certain foods to eat or avoid, or practices that should be done or avoided) that the health care team should be aware of?
- Can the health care team be of spiritual help to you?

c. Self-concept is a set of beliefs about self that affects what a person thinks, says, and does; its expression is called self-esteem or self-worth.

   (1) Self-concept includes the person's perception of his or her identity, worth, capabilities, and limitations and of the way he or she fits into the environment.

   (2) A person's self-concept influences the way other people view and act toward the person.

   (3) Body image is a person's perception of his or her own body (i.e., how one thinks one looks). Body image influences self-concept and self-esteem. Body image is influenced by feedback from other people and can change, becoming more positive or more negative.

   (4) Locus of control refers to a person's sense of mastery or influence over events, including health status. People with an internal locus of control are apt to engage in health promotion behaviors, believing that they can ward off or abate the effects of illness. People with an external locus of control may believe that their health status is a result of fate. They may be less able to participate actively in the management of their health or illness without encouragement from others.

9. Assess spirituality (see Table 6–4).

   a. Spirituality involves finding meaning and purpose in life. Although it may include religious beliefs, spirituality goes beyond such beliefs to encompass the individual's interpretations of such mysteries as life and death, good and evil, pain and suffering.

      (1) These interpretations arise from the interaction among a person's family and cultural background; education; and unique feelings, thoughts, and goals.

      (2) A person's spiritual beliefs and values affect all aspects of his or her life, including relationships with others, sense of right and wrong, locus of control, and beliefs about health and health care.

   b. Holistic nursing care includes the spiritual dimension of the person as well as the physiologic and psychologic dimensions.

      (1) Maintaining optimal health and wellness requires a balance among physiologic, psychologic, and spiritual dimensions.

      (2) Disturbances in one of a person's dimensions can precipitate a problem in one or both of the other dimensions. For example, a loss of physical health may precipitate mental problems (depression, anger) and spiritual distress (a sense of abandonment or hopelessness).

      (3) Conflicts among a person's beliefs, values, and goals can produce spiritual distress, which may manifest itself as physical or psychologic problems.

   c. Assess spirituality *after* you have established a trusting relationship with the patient.

      (1) Acknowledge the person's feelings and need for privacy.

      (2) Offer to discuss spirituality and the person's needs when he or she is ready. Ask if there is someone else who can assist the person with spiritual support, if needed.

      (3) Be aware of your own spirituality and beliefs as you assist the person. Do not let these beliefs interfere with the therapeutic relationship.

      (4) Because of its personal nature, some people may be reluctant to discuss their spiritual beliefs. If the person declines to discuss the topic, do not persist.

   d. Observe the person's verbal and nonverbal behavior and affect. Note signs of anxiety, anger, sadness, or agitation, which may indicate spiritual distress.

10. Assess for psychosocial risk factors that increase the chances of illness or disease. Such risk factors include the following:

    a. High stress levels, poor coping skills, or both

    b. Risk-taking behaviors (e.g., avoiding safety precautions, sexual promiscuity)

    c. External locus of control

    d. Loss of or change in beliefs or values

    e. Spiritual distress

    f. Nutritional, sleep, exercise, or recreation deficits

    g. Financial problems

    h. Lack of social support (see "Assess the person's social network" in the following section).

Assess Sociologic Components

1. Assess psychosocial level of development.

   a. Understanding the person's level of psychosocial development gives you insight into his or her life situation and its effect on health status.

   b. Psychosocial development occurs throughout a person's life and includes physical, emotional, psychologic, social, and cognitive growth and maturation (see also Chapter 15).

   c. Some developmental changes occur slowly and others rapidly.

   d. Although grouping of changes into stages or tasks is a useful way to organize such changes, stages and tasks are not actually totally distinct or exclusive.

   e. A person may grow and change in certain developmental areas more quickly than in other areas. These changes are affected by age, individual considerations, and environmental factors.

   f. *Transcultural considerations:* Most models of psychosocial development are based in Western cultural beliefs and values and so may be irrelevant for people from other cultures.

2. Assess the person's social network (Table 6–5).

   a. A social network comprises all the people who are connected to and interact with a person.

   b. Network members include family members; neighbors; friends; employers; coworkers; teachers; classmates; and members of any groups, clubs, or organizations to which a person belongs. Cultural background and socioeconomic status influence the composition and extent of a person's social network.

Table 6–5. Guide for Assessing Social Network and Support Systems

Family

- Describe your family: Who are its members and what are their relationships to you?
- What roles do you and your family members have (e.g., parent, child, spouse, sibling, other relative, teacher, provider, role model, best friend, authority figure, peacemaker)?
- Who in your family do you feel closest to? Are there other people not related to you whom you consider important (i.e., significant others)?
- Do you and your family members (or significant others) get along with one another?
- Are there any problems within your family or with significant others that have strained your relationships with one another (e.g., change in living space, marital problems, arguments)?

Friends

- Are friendships important to you?
- Are you satisfied with the friendships that you have now?
- Who would you identify as your best friend?
- Are your friends accepted by your family and significant others?
- Describe your relationships with your friends.

Other Sources of Support

- Describe your relationships with coworkers.
- Is there someone at work in whom you confide?
- What types of groups, clubs, or organizations do you belong to? How important are they to you? Do you view them as sources of support?
- If you had a problem or were in a crisis, who would you turn to for help? Is this person available?
- Are there other things that help you when you need support during stressful times (e.g., a pet or inanimate object)?
- Do you have a pet or animals that are important to you? Is there someone who will take care of them for you if you are unable to do so?

(1) Health care professionals may become part of a person's social network when a need for health care arises.

c. The social network helps define a person's self-image and sense of belonging. It is a source of support, approval, rewards, and love and a framework for sharing values, beliefs, attitudes, and norms.

d. Consider the person's psychosocial level of development (Table 6–6) when assessing his or her social network. Awareness of the person's developmental stage and tasks is crucial when planning to enlist social network members as resources in a patient's care.

4. Assess socioeconomic status (see also Chapter 4).
   a. Socioeconomic status refers to one's financial and social positions within society.
      (1) Socioeconomic status influences the way a person is perceived as well as the way he or she perceives others.
      (2) It affects physical and psychologic well-being by influencing how much money and time are available to attend to health care needs, by defining who has access to the health care system, and by controlling what services are available.
   b. Ask about the patient's occupation, current employment status, work-related concerns, financial worries, ability to work, health insurance coverage, ability to afford health care services, educational background, and hopes and goals.

5. Assess lifestyle (see also Chapter 4).
   a. Lifestyle reflects a person's psychologic and sociologic influences, including socioeconomic status and interpersonal relationships. It is reflected in daily patterns of living, such as habits, routines, and other typical activities.
   b. Lifestyle choices are often made consciously and help the person maintain control over and function in his or her environment.
   c. Ask about health habits (use of alcohol, medications, recreational drugs, nicotine, safety practices), sleep and rest patterns, work and study routines, recreational and leisure activities, diet and nutrition, stress level, methods used to reduce stress, interpersonal relationships, home setting, and access to reliable transportation.
   d. *Transcultural considerations:* Remember to consider transcultural influences as the person describes his or her lifestyle, especially in relation to gender and life stage, religious beliefs and practices, family and community roles and responsibilities, and socioeconomic status.

6. Assess sexuality.
   a. Sexuality is the behavioral expression of a person's sexual identity. It encompasses sexual relationships between people as well as one's self-concept about being male or female.
   b. Assess areas such as physical health problems that have implications for sexuality and its expression, concerns with sexual role performance, issues of sexual role function, and the effect of environmental restrictions on sexual expression (see also Chapters 30 and 31).
      (1) Examples of physical health problems are disorders involving sexual organs, such as cancer or sexually transmitted diseases, and disorders that affect physical appearance and attractiveness, such as skin lesions, physical deformities, paralysis, or colostomy. (See also Chapters 7, 17, 18, 27, and 35 for more on these topics.)
      (2) Concerns with sexual role performance include infertility, frigidity, impotence, premature ejaculation, inability to achieve orgasm, and pain with intercourse.
      (3) Issues of sexual role function include homosexuality, bisexuality, sexual ambiguity, transsexual surgery, and transvestism.
      (4) Environmental restrictions on sexual expression include lack of privacy from hospitalization or residency in a long-term care facility.
   c. Remember that sexuality and sexual behavior are sensitive topics for many people, especially those who are not from middle-class American backgrounds. Some people are embarrassed to discuss their concerns and do not volunteer information but are relieved when you bring up the subject in a nonthreatening way.
   d. Do not allow personal beliefs and values to interfere with your ability to help the person express concerns.
      (1) Be nonjudgmental and neutral in your behavior.
      (2) If the person is uncomfortable, acknowledge his or

Level of Development	Approximate Age Range	Developmental Tasks
Table 6–6. Psychosocial Developmental Tasks: Adolescence Through Adulthood		
Adolescence	12–20 years	Achieve a stable identity Establish independence Assume an adult sex role Select a vocation or career
Early adulthood	18–25 years	Begin an occupation Select a mate and establish a relationship Start a family Raise children Manage a home
Middle adulthood	25–65 years	Accept the physiologic changes of midlife Develop or rediscover a satisfying personal relationship with one's spouse or significant other Assist children to become happy, responsible, independent adults Develop new roles with aging parents, emotionally preparing for their deaths Obtain satisfaction with one's career and prepare for retirement Develop leisure time activities Achieve social and civic responsibilities
Late adulthood	65+ years	Adjust to decreases in physical strength and health Adjust to retirement and reduced income Adjust to death of spouse and other loved ones Establish an explicit affiliation with one's own age group Adjust and adapt to social roles in a flexible way Establish satisfactory living arrangements

her feelings and move on to another topic. Offer to return to the subject of sexuality later, when the person is more comfortable discussing it.

(3) Some people are never comfortable discussing their sexuality even if they perceive a problem in this area. If there is a specific need for such information, explain it to the patient and ask about only what is necessary to assess the person's needs.

e. In addition to questions about sexual reproduction and health (see Chapter 4), ask questions such as the following:

(1) Are you satisfied with being a man (or a woman)? Have you ever wished you were of the opposite sex?

(2) Are you satisfied in your sexual relationships with your sexual partner or partners (e.g., frequency and quality of interactions)?

(3) Has there been a change in your sexual function? If so, how has it changed and how long has it been this way? Is this change for the better or worse?

Assess Transcultural Components

1. A person's culture *influences*—though it does not control absolutely—every aspect of living: how he or she thinks, behaves, and feels.
2. Culture affects psychosocial development because as children grow up, they learn the standards and values of the group into which they are born. Cultural norms may be written or unwritten.
3. Psychosocial assessment must occur within the context of the person's cultural orientation if subsequent evaluations of behavior are to be valid.
4. Use the following guidelines to assess the person who is culturally different from you.
   a. Be as aware as you can of your own cultural background and the ways it influences you.
   b. Avoid ethnocentrism, the belief that one's own culture is superior to all others.
   c. Remember that although your previous experiences in transcultural relationships may be helpful when assessing a person, stereotyping all people of similar cultural backgrounds is dangerous and counterproductive (see Chapter 4). People are individuals, not just members of certain groups.
5. To assess transcultural considerations, ask questions such as those in Table 6–7.

◼ UTILIZING PSYCHOSOCIAL FINDINGS

Record Findings

1. Use forms and formats approved by your agency.
2. Record your findings as soon as possible after the interview has been completed.

Table 6–7. Guide to Assessing Transcultural Components

Identification with a Cultural Group

- How do you identify yourself to others when you are asked what nationality or what ethnic group you belong to?
- Describe how strongly you feel about your ethnic roots. Do you see yourself as a member of your ethnic group first, or do you think of yourself as a/an _____ (American, Canadian, or other) first?
- How do you identify yourself when you are asked about your racial background (e.g., Black, African American, Native American, Hispanic, Asian)?
- Where were you born? Your parents? What countries (or regions of this country) have you lived in and when?

Communication

- What language do you speak at home? Do you speak or read other languages? Do you prefer to speak in a language other than English?
- Do you want to have an interpreter? Is there someone (e.g., friend, relative) whom you want to interpret for you? Is there anyone (e.g., someone of the opposite sex, a person who is older or younger than you, a person you see as a rival or enemy) who should not interpret?
- Who do you prefer to take care of you when you need health care (e.g., a person of the same cultural background/same sex/same age as you)?

Values, Beliefs, and Attitudes

- Can you identify any special beliefs or practices you have that are influenced by your ethnic or cultural background? For example, are there things that you or your relatives do when a baby is born? When someone dies? When you or your family members are ill?
- Is there anything special that you or your family do to stay healthy that is culturally or ethnically based (e.g., eat or avoid certain foods, use herbs, call in someone who has special powers or gifts to help you stay well or get well)?

Cultural Sanctions and Restrictions

- Is there anything in your cultural beliefs that the health care team should know about when taking care of you? For example, do you need to keep parts of your body covered to prevent others from seeing them?
- Are there certain types of procedures that your culture forbids you to have done (e.g., hysterectomy, vasectomy)?
- If you had a serious operation in which part of your body had to be removed (amputation) or cut out (excision), how should this body part be handled (e.g., preserved, buried, cremated, no special treatment)?
- Are there any topics or subjects that you do not wish to talk about because it is not allowed by your beliefs (e.g., discussing people who have died)?

Health-Related Beliefs and Practices

- Is there anything in your beliefs that you feel helps you to be (or stay) healthy (e.g., do you believe certain foods, beverages, potions, or herbs are good for you)?
- Is there anything special that you traditionally do or wear to help you stay healthy or bring you luck (e.g., amulet; prayers to ancestors, saint, supreme being, or other being; certain rituals)?
- Do you believe in or use nonmedical people to help you get better or heal you when you are sick (e.g., curandero, shaman, imam, monk, elder, minister, or other spiritual adviser)? How do you know when to contact this person?
- Is there anything that you believe is not good for your health or that causes illness or sickness (e.g., illness is a punishment for doing something "wrong," you are under a spell or curse, your body is not in harmony or balance with nature, there is an imbalance between good and bad [positive and negative] forces within your body such as yin/yang or hot/cold)?
- Are there any types of healing practices or beliefs that you have or feel you need (e.g., use of herbal remedies or potions, eating special foods, massage or other type of special touch, wearing a special charm or talisman to ward off evil spirits, special prayers or incantations, specific healing practices or ceremonies)?
- When you are ill or sick, do your family and significant others expect you to act in a certain way (e.g., to play a particular "sick role")?
- Who decides when you are sick or when you are no longer sick?
- Who usually helps take care of you when you are sick?

Nutritional Beliefs and Practices

- Identify foods that you believe are healthy for you to eat and foods that you believe you should avoid because they are unhealthy.
- Describe how food is prepared in your home (e.g., frying, steaming, use of cooking oils [type], how long foods are cooked, what types of seasonings are used or avoided, what foods may or may not be served together at the same meal, use of special cookware or dishes to serve food).
- Do you have certain religious beliefs that control the type of foods you eat and should not eat (e.g., kosher diet) or how food is prepared? (Also see previous question.)
- Do you fast or abstain from specific foods at certain times during the week or year because of religious beliefs?
- If you believe in "fasting" for religious reasons, describe what this means to you. Do you avoid certain foods or beverages? Do you eat only at specified times during the day?
- Are you ever allowed to break your religious rules of diet or fasting if you are ill? Who makes this decision and who would tell you that it is all right to break a dietary rule?

Socioeconomic Issues

- Is there anyone in your circle of family, friends, or spiritual advisers (i.e., social network) whom you feel influences your health or illness status?
- Are there special things that the members of your social network and support system do to help you when you are sick or to help you get better? Describe how these people would help take care of you if you were ill (e.g., stay by your side continuously, do things for you or your family, help your family).
- Describe the roles that your family members play when one of the members is ill.
- Do you expect your family members to help take care of you when you are sick? Describe what types of activities they might participate in (e.g., give you a bath, prepare your food, help to feed you, be there with you).
- Will your illness put a financial strain on your family? Who is the main wage earner in the family? Does anyone else help contribute to the family's income? Are there other sources for the family for financial income?

Educational Background

- Can you read and write English, or do you feel more comfortable with another language?
- How much schooling have you had?
- When you learn about new things, is there a special way that you prefer to learn? For example, do you like to read information first, or do you like to watch someone perform a new skill and then try to repeat it? Does it help for you to talk to someone and ask questions?

---

a. Be descriptive (objective), clear, and concise.
b. Use the person's subjective statements to illustrate or amplify the descriptions as necessary.
c. *Transcultural considerations:* Note whether the person indicates that certain data have cultural significance. Also note whether an interpreter has assisted with the interview or has elaborated about the cultural importance of certain data.

Analyze the Data

1. Psychosocial data, along with the data from the person's history and physical examination, should provide a comprehensive database.
   a. Remember that the physiologic, psychologic, and spiritual dimensions of a person are closely linked. A problem in 1 dimension also may be reflected in 1 or both of the other dimensions.
2. Review all the data, and summarize the person's strengths and problem areas.
3. After considering the psychosocial data, validate, revise,

or discard any tentative nursing diagnoses that had been formulated previously and were based only on data from the patient's history and physical examination.

4. If appropriate, formulate new nursing diagnoses that address psychosocial problems evidenced by the data.
5. Discuss your findings and nursing diagnoses with the patient. Formulate an action plan *together*.
   a. If a psychosocial problem exists, the plan should include a referral to a specialist in psychiatric and mental health care or social services.
   b. *Transcultural considerations:* Consult a cultural nurse specialist, nurse anthropologist, or other expert in the person's culture if you suspect a problem in the cultural dimension of psychosocial mental health. Some "problems" may not be problems at all but culturally acceptable ways of coping or other behavior.

Prepare Summary and Make Recommendations and Referrals

1. Summarize the patient's problem areas and the action plan. Determine which problems are nursing diagnoses that you can manage either independently or in collaboration with colleagues.
2. If necessary, refer the patient to appropriate health care professionals for additional care or follow-up.
3. *Transcultural considerations:*
   a. Consider referral to traditional (folk) practitioners as indicated.
   b. Some groups (Hispanic) are more likely to participate in a therapeutic plan if it is located in the local community and the services are available during weekend and evening hours.

Bibliography

Books

Barry PD. *Psychosocial Nursing Assessment and Intervention: Care of the Physically Ill Person.* 2nd ed. Philadelphia: JB Lippincott, 1989.

Bolander VR. *Sorensen and Luckmann's Basic Nursing: A Psychophysiologic Approach.* 3rd ed. Philadelphia: WB Saunders, 1994.

Carpenito LJ. *Nursing Diagnosis: Application to Clinical Practice.* 4th ed. Philadelphia: JB Lippincott, 1992.

Carson VB. *Spiritual Dimensions of Nursing Practice.* Philadelphia: WB Saunders, 1989.

Clark CC. *Wellness Nursing: Concepts, Theory, Research, and Practice.* New York: Springer Publishing Co, 1986.

Cook JS, and Fontaine KL. *Essentials of Mental Health Nursing.* 2nd ed. Redwood City, CA: Addison-Wesley, 1991.

Cox HC, et al. *Clinical Applications of Nursing Diagnosis: Adult, Child, Women's, Psychiatric, Gerontic and Home Health Considerations.* 2nd ed. Philadelphia: FA Davis, 1993.

Fawcett CS. *Family Psychiatric Nursing.* St. Louis: CV Mosby, 1993.

Helman C. *Culture, Health and Illness.* Boston: Wright, 1990.

Hill LH, and Smith N. *Self-Care Nursing: Promotion of Health.* 2nd ed. Norwalk, CT: Appleton & Lange, 1990.

Hymovich DP, and Hagopian GA. *Chronic Illness in Children and Adults: A Psychosocial Approach.* Philadelphia: WB Saunders, 1992.

Jarvis C. *Physical Examination and Health Assessment.* 2nd ed. Philadelphia: WB Saunders, 1996.

Longo DC, and Williams RA. *Clinical Practice in Psychosocial Nursing: Assessment and Intervention.* 2nd ed. Norwalk, CT: Appleton-Century-Crofts, 1986.

Malasanos L, Barkauskas V, and Stoltenberg-Allen K. *Health Assessment.* 4th ed. St. Louis: CV Mosby, 1990.

Pender NJ. *Health Promotion in Nursing.* 2nd ed. Norwalk, CT: Appleton & Lange, 1987.

Wilson HS, and Kneisl CR. *Psychiatric Nursing.* 4th ed. Redwood City, CA: Addison-Wesley, 1992.

Chapters in Books

Balzer JW. The nursing process applied to family health promotion. *In* Stanhope M, and Lancaster J (eds). *Community Health Nursing: Process and Practice for Promoting Health.* 3rd ed. St. Louis: CV Mosby, 1992.

Flaskerud JH. Transcultural concepts in mental health nursing. *In* Boyle JC, and Andrews MM (eds). *Transcultural Concepts in Nursing.* Glenview, IL: Scott, Foresman, 1989.

Hutchinson SA. Cultural considerations. *In* Wilson HS, and Kneisl CR (eds). *Psychiatric Nursing.* 4th ed. Redwood City, CA: Addison-Wesley, 1992.

Leveck PG. The role of culture in mental health and illness. *In* Cook JS, and Fontaine KL (eds). *Essentials of Mental Health Nursing.* 2nd ed. Redwood City, CA: Addison-Wesley, 1991.

Rahe RH. Life changes and near-future illness reports. *In* Levi L (ed). *Emotions: Their Parameters and Measurement.* New York: Raven Press, 1975.

Werner JS, and O'Neill SE. Nursing assessment and role in stress management. *In* Lewis SM, and Collier IC (eds). *Medical-Surgical Nursing: Assessment and Management of Clinical Problems.* 3rd ed. St. Louis: CV Mosby, 1992.

Journal Articles

Brink P. Value orientations as an assessment tool in cultural diversity. *Nurs Res* 35:198, 1984.

Brink PJ. Cultural aspects of sexuality. *Holistic Nurs Pract* 1:12–20, 1987.

Dirckx JH. Talking with patients: The art of history taking. *Clin Nurs Pract* 3:13–14, 1985.

Grossman D. Enhancing your "cultural competence." *Am J Nurs* 94(7):58–62, 1994.

Hays A. The set test to screen mental status quickly. *Geriatr Nurs* 5:96–97, 1984.

Lipson J, and Melies A. Culturally appropriate care: The case of immigrants. *Top Clin Nurs* 7(3):48–56, 1985.

Martocchio BC. Grief and bereavement: Health through hurt. *Nurs Clin North Am* 20(2):327–341, 1985.

Rahe RH. Epidemiological studies of life change and illness. *Int J Psych Med* 6 (1–2):133–146, 1975.

Rawnsley M. Toward a conceptual base for affective nursing. *Nurs Outlook* 28:244, 1980.

Sarason IG, Johnson JH, and Siegal JM. Assessing the impact of life changes: Development of life experiences survey. *J Consult Clin Psychol* 46(5):932–946, 1978.

Utz S. Motivating self-care: A nursing approach. *Holistic Nurs Pract* 4(2):13–21, 1990.

Agencies

American Psychiatric Nurses
   Association
1200 19th Street, NW
Suite 300
Washington, DC 20036
(202) 857-1133

Transcultural Nursing Society
College of Nursing and Health
Madonna University
36600 Schoolcraft Road
Livonia, MI 48150
(313) 591-8320

Mental Health Counselors Association
5999 Stevenson Avenue
Alexandria, VA 22304
(800) 326-2642

Caring for People with Special Medical-Surgical Needs and Problems

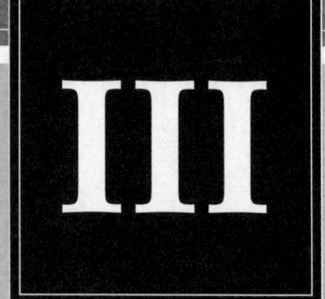

III

7
Caring for People with Disabilities

◼ DEFINITIONS AND INCIDENCE

Definitions

1. **Impairment** is any physiologic or mental condition that limits major life activities, according to the Americans with Disabilities Act (ADA) of 1990.
   a. Major life activities include walking, learning, caring for oneself, performing manual tasks, seeing, hearing, breathing, or working.
   b. Examples of impairments include heart disease, cancer, epilepsy, diabetes, learning disorders, psychosis, mental retardation, alcoholism, infection with the human immunodeficiency virus, and conditions requiring wheelchairs (e.g., spinal cord injury).
   c. Impairments may be inherited or may result from trauma or a disease process (such as arthritis).
   d. Impairments may be temporary or permanent and may or may not be associated with an active pathologic condition.

> **NURSE ADVISORY**
>
> Care for each disabled person as a whole person, rather than a person with a specific illness or disability.

2. **Disability** is a limited functional ability resulting from an impairment; it is the term preferred over "handicap." Disability exists when a physical impairment prevents a person from performing major activities such as self-care, communication, mobility, or working.
3. **Functional ability** is a person's ability to perform the activities of daily living independently and to perform expected roles.
4. **Activities of daily living** include hygiene (practices that promote cleanliness and health), cooking, driving or using public transportation, and managing money.
5. **Self-care** is the practice of activities that maintain life, health, and well-being.
   a. This behavior acts to restore equilibrium. When self-care is not maintained, illness, disease, or death occurs. Self-care is integral to rehabilitation.
   b. Self-care has 2 phases: decision making, when the person has input regarding activity, and production, when the person performs activity.
6. **Rehabilitation** is the process of maximizing the use of a

person's capabilities to achieve optimal growth and functioning.
   a. The major goal of rehabilitation is to enable a person to achieve the highest level of function.
   b. Secondary goals include preventing complications, modifying effects of disability, and improving quality of life for persons with chronic illness.
7. Chronic illness includes all impairments or pathologic deviations characterized by 1 or more of the following features:
   a. Illness duration of longer than 6 months
   b. Residual disability
   c. Nonreversible pathologic alteration as a cause of illness
   d. Need for special training
   e. Expectation of a long period of supervision, observation, or care

Incidence and Socioeconomic Impact

1. Approximately 50 percent of Americans have 1 or more chronic diseases, such as coronary artery disease, cancer, and arthritis, that cause varying degrees of disability.
2. Approximately 43 million Americans have 1 or more physical or mental disabilities.
   a. Approximately 1 million persons are blind or visually impaired, and 13 million are deaf or hearing impaired (see Chapters 19 and 20).
   b. Approximately 7,959,000 persons have limited mobility.
   c. Approximately 500,000 persons use a wheelchair.
   d. Approximately 10,000 people (primarily males under the age of 40) sustain a spinal cord injury every year, and around 200,000 people with spinal cord injuries are currently living in the United States.

◼ TRANSCULTURAL CONSIDERATIONS

Transcultural Attitudes Toward Disability

1. Some cultures view illness as a punishment, believing that sick people have offended the supreme being or broken a divine law (taboo).
2. A belief in curses and evil spirits as a cause for illness is particularly strong among African, Caribbean, Native American, and Pacific Basin societies.

a. Persons in these societies may look on a sick person as a victim. Friends and family fear being close to the person because they believe that the spell may affect them. Furthermore, the family of the sick person may also be considered cursed.

b. Members of these cultures sometimes believe that illness is passed along for generations through the blood. They may view genetically transmitted diseases, especially in cases of insanity or mental retardation, as the result of incest or the marriage of close relatives.

3. People in cultures that hold a widespread belief in reincarnation (especially East Asian populations) tend to view illness as the result of misconduct in past lives. They sometimes believe that acceptance of suffering is a virtue that will either pay for past sins or help the soul attain purity sooner. They may perceive those who help a suffering person as interfering with the person's "karma" or destiny.

4. In some other cultures, people believe that illness is the responsibility of the sick person.

a. Illness may result from an imbalance between hot and cold or yin and yang. To correct the imbalance, the sick person must take appropriate action.

b. In some cases, a person with a permanent disability is viewed as continually impure and thus responsible for the disability.

5. In still other cultures, people view illness as God's will.

a. Some Roman Catholic Hispanics regard illness as an opportunity to grow closer to God.

b. Parents with a disabled child may believe that they have been singled out by God because they showed kindness to disabled persons in the past.

c. Some people believe that disabled people exist as a part of God's plan.

Transcultural Attitudes Toward Self-Care

1. Many non-Western cultures, such as Native American, African, Caribbean, and Pacific Basin societies, value interdependence, interconnectedness, companionship, and responsibility for others as opposed to the Western values of independence, individualism, autonomy, self-reliance, self-control, and self-management.

2. Promoting self-care in a person with non-Western values is not likely to be effective because the frame of reference does not include Western ideas and values.

Transcultural Attitudes Toward Rehabilitation

1. Attitudes of various cultural groups toward rehabilitation vary according to the perceived causes of the disability.

a. If the disability is perceived to be shameful, the person or family may believe that they are unworthy to receive help.

b. In some cases, the disabled person may be abandoned or locked away from society.

2. Some groups, particularly East Asians, do not encourage the use of a prosthesis because it does not cure the problem. If the disability keeps the person from living a "normal" life, the family may choose not to spend its resources on medical care.

3. In cultures that value male children over female children, especially Chinese or other Asian cultures, some families may do everything possible for a disabled son but pay less attention to a disabled daughter.

◾ IMPACT OF BEING PHYSICALLY DISABLED

Physical Impact

1. Disabled persons may have problems with self-care activities such as feeding, bathing, hygiene (e.g., applying deodorant or cosmetics), dressing, toileting, and ambulation.

2. Disabled persons may experience alterations in patterns of urinary elimination, impairment of skin integrity, or alterations in bowel elimination, depending on the type of motor impairment.

3. Disabled persons may need physical aids such as wheelchairs, crutches, hearing aids, or visual aids.

a. Physical mobility has 4 areas of aids that concern nurses: bed, transfers, wheelchair, and ambulation.

(1) Bed mobility aids include side rails, overhead frame, and trapeze to aid the patient.

(2) Transfers aids include mechanical lift devices, bath bench, shower chair, and sliding boards.

(3) Wheelchairs can be the major mode of locomotion or can be used in addition to ambulation to conserve the patient's energy.

- Prescriptions for wheelchair types are based on patient needs, cosmetic factors, and occupational factors.
- Wheelchairs are electrically or manually powered.
- Electric wheelchairs have rechargeable batteries. Control systems for electric wheelchairs include joysticks, pneumatic switches, and voice-activated controls.

(4) Ambulation may require assistive devices such as canes, crutches, walkers, orthoses, and prostheses.

b. Sensory aids for the visually impaired include large-print books, talking books, a path sounder (a boxlike device used to aid travel), a laser cane (which sends out beams), the Optacon reading machine (which converts printed characters into sounds), and the Kurzweil Reading Machine (which uses a computer-controlled camera that scans a printed page and transcribes it into synthetic speech).

c. Hearing-impaired patients with conductive hearing loss use hearing aids as assistive devices for simple amplification. Other assistive devices for the hearing impaired include a telephone amplifier or a teletypewriter.

4. Physical barriers encountered by the disabled person include many physical and structural restrictions.
   a. Homes, schools, and buildings are often without ramps, elevators, or restrooms that are accessible to the physically disabled. Elevators are often too small to accommodate wheelchairs.
   b. Steps and curbs also cause problems for persons in wheelchairs. Often, able-bodied members of society use parking spaces that are set aside for the disabled. Public transportation may not be available to the physically disabled, or, if available, may involve long waiting times.
   c. External barriers for disabled people include limited accessibility to services and housing.
   d. In recent years, Americans with Disabilities Act has sought to minimize these problems by prohibiting discrimination against the physically disabled in the areas of public services, transportation, and accessibility to many privately owned businesses such as hotels, stores, restaurants, and office buildings.
      (1) Public transportation must accommodate the disabled, and ramps and elevators must be installed.
      (2) Existing buildings must be modified by adding ramps, widening doorways, adapting restrooms, and clearing entrances and halls of obstructions.

Psychologic Impact

1. Physical disability affects persons whether they are born disabled or become disabled. Factors influencing adaptation to physical disability include the person's age at onset of the physical disability, body image, nature of the disability and meaning to the person, cultural beliefs, and psychologic support from the family and nurse.
   a. Persons who are born disabled have the disability as part of their identity from birth.
      (1) In certain aspects, it may be easier for a child to adjust to functional limitations than for a person who becomes disabled in later life. A child learns to adapt to tasks and loss of function early in life. The presence of disability may influence an infant's sense of trust owing to frequent hospitalizations and separation from parents.
      (2) Children who are born disabled may not be expected to survive. If they do survive, the vulnerable child syndrome may develop in which the child exhibits separation, sleep, and feeding problems. When they reach school age, these children exhibit school phobia, poor academic performance, and hypochondria.
   b. Persons who become disabled (e.g., from a spinal cord injury) generally pass through a series of psychologic responses to their condition:
      (1) Grief or anger is expressed over the loss of certain abilities. This is especially true when a disability is acquired after early childhood.
      (2) The person denies that change has occurred and insists on maintaining the old body image.
      (3) Depression or anxiety may develop as the person finally acknowledges that the disability is permanent.
      (4) The person gradually accepts and adapts to the new body structure. Adaptation depends on the following:
         • The nature of the person's prior concept of body image, that is, the person's subjective attitude toward one's own body
         • The meaning of the investment in the care of the body and attractiveness to the person
         • The person's coping abilities
         • Responses from family and friends
         • Society's perception of beauty and wholeness
         • The nature of the physical limitation (e.g., a long-distance runner would have more difficulty coping with paraplegia than a nonathletic person)
         • Resources (e.g., support from family, friends, health professionals, support groups, and community agencies)

2. Nursing management for initial psychologic responses is to evaluate the person's assets, promote positive self-statements, teach coping strategies, modify role, and help set realistic goals for adaptation, especially if the patient has a permanent disability.

3. Powerlessness
   a. Individuals with physical disabilities, whether the disabilities are lifelong or of recent origin, often experience profound feelings of powerlessness.
   b. Feelings of powerlessness may arise if persons with disabilities think that there is nothing they can do to change their disability.
   c. Individuals are most likely to feel powerless if they think they cannot achieve self-care.

4. Coping challenges and difficulties
   a. The person with a disability faces many coping tasks, such as maintaining a sense of normality, modifying daily routines, maintaining self-concept, dealing with role changes, managing stress, and complying with prescribed regimens.
   b. The more coping tasks confronting a disabled person, the greater the chance that the individual will feel powerless.

Socioeconomic Impact

1. Impact of social isolation—interpersonal interaction less than that desired for personal integrity
   a. The person with a physical disability indicates a desire for increased human interaction, feels rejected, and expresses feelings of being different from others. Owing to fear of rejection, physically disabled persons may avoid social interactions or gatherings.
   b. Self-concept is a product of social interaction. Physically disabled individuals who perceive more social support from friends and family exhibit more positive body images, more self-esteem, and less depression than others.

2. Impact on social life. Physical disability affects all areas of the person's social life including family life, interac-

tion with friends, education, economic status, and vocation. A stigma is attached to being disabled. Some disabilities are viewed as being more disabling than others, so the amount of stigmatization varies accordingly. The least ambivalence is felt toward blind persons, and the next least toward deaf persons. Persons with paralyzed limbs (e.g., people with paraplegia) are viewed more positively than those with face, head, or trunk disabilities.

   a. Able-bodied members of society tend to reject disabled people because they are reminded of their own vulnerability and mortality. Disabled people are devalued and stereotyped. Some able-bodied people avoid interacting with the disabled person because disabilities are unsettling.

   b. Societal expectations of nondisabled people, such as gaining accomplishments and possessions, may not be reasonable for those with physical disabilities, increasing the likelihood that society will treat those with disabilities as outsiders.

   c. Disabilities, both new and lifelong, can disrupt or limit normal relationships with friends. Some people tend to pity the disabled and try to help them when they do not want help. Therefore, it is sometimes difficult to form friendships. In addition, the disabled person may become increasingly dependent on others.

   d. Fear of embarrassment may prevent the physically disabled person from developing close personal relationships. For example, persons with spinal cord injury may fear having accidental bowel movements in public or may fear falling out of a wheelchair.

3. Impact on education
   a. Children born with physical disabilities, such as cerebral palsy and muscular dystrophy, are often still placed in special educational facilities. Many people believe that the physically disabled are mentally retarded as well.
   b. In college, students with physical disabilities are often counseled out of professional programs. For example, medical and dental schools often deny admission to young adults treated for cancer.

4. Impact on vocation
   a. Limited job prospects may exist for persons who are born disabled or are disabled at an early age. The disabled who are hired are often given lower level clerical positions because employers may think they do not have the stamina for physical work. For example, a person with cystic fibrosis may need chest percussion several times a day, which would require time taken from work.
   b. Becoming disabled may cause a person to lose a job or force a person to change jobs. For example, a police officer with a spinal cord injury may have to seek a more sedentary job.

5. Impact on economic status
   a. Persons who become disabled may lose income, either temporarily (loss of salary while recuperating) or permanently (loss of job). Workers' compensation and other disability insurance programs often provide only poverty-level payments. If the disability strikes during midlife or middle age, the person's capacity for vocational development is often disrupted. The person may be forced to retire.
   b. Disabled individuals often have high "out-of-pocket" health care costs, because private insurance and Medicare limit coverage for many problems.
   c. The annual cost of disabilities ranges from $10 billion to $100 billion and is more than 7 percent of the gross national product in the United States. Because approximately 25 percent of any population consists of disabled persons, these cost estimates include prescribed treatment and rehabilitation programs. For example, it is estimated that the lifetime care costs for a paraplegic are $180,000 to $225,000. In addition, some insurance companies do not cover disability expenses or adaptive equipment.

6. Impact on family
   a. In addition to bearing the costs of the disabled person's illness, family members may have to stop working to care for the disabled person. Overall, the decrease in family income may exceed 40 percent.
   b. Family members may be forced into new roles when a formerly independent person becomes dependent as the result of a disability.
   c. The family may experience increasing feelings of powerlessness or resentment.

ASSESSING PEOPLE WITH DISABILITIES

Health History

1. Collect information on the history of the disability, pain, and sensory changes (e.g., tingling, burning).
2. Inquire about current medications, rehabilitation programs, and other treatment programs, including physical and occupational therapy.

TRANSCULTURAL CONSIDERATIONS

Persons belonging to a non-Western cultural group may use traditional or alternative health practices as well as Western medicine. Some herbal remedies may cause drug interactions or symptoms that are difficult to differentiate from the symptoms of the disease process. Traditional Chinese medicine uses practices such as moxibustion and scraping, which may appear as bruises or burns and have often been confused with marks caused by child abuse.

3. Note the use of aids, such as wheelchairs, crutches, canes, braces, glasses, and hearing aids.
4. Activities of daily living may be altered by disabilities affecting the musculoskeletal system. Activities of daily living that rely on musculoskeletal system activity include dressing, grooming, bathing, toileting, feeding, mobility (e.g., moving from bed to chair), and verbally communicating.

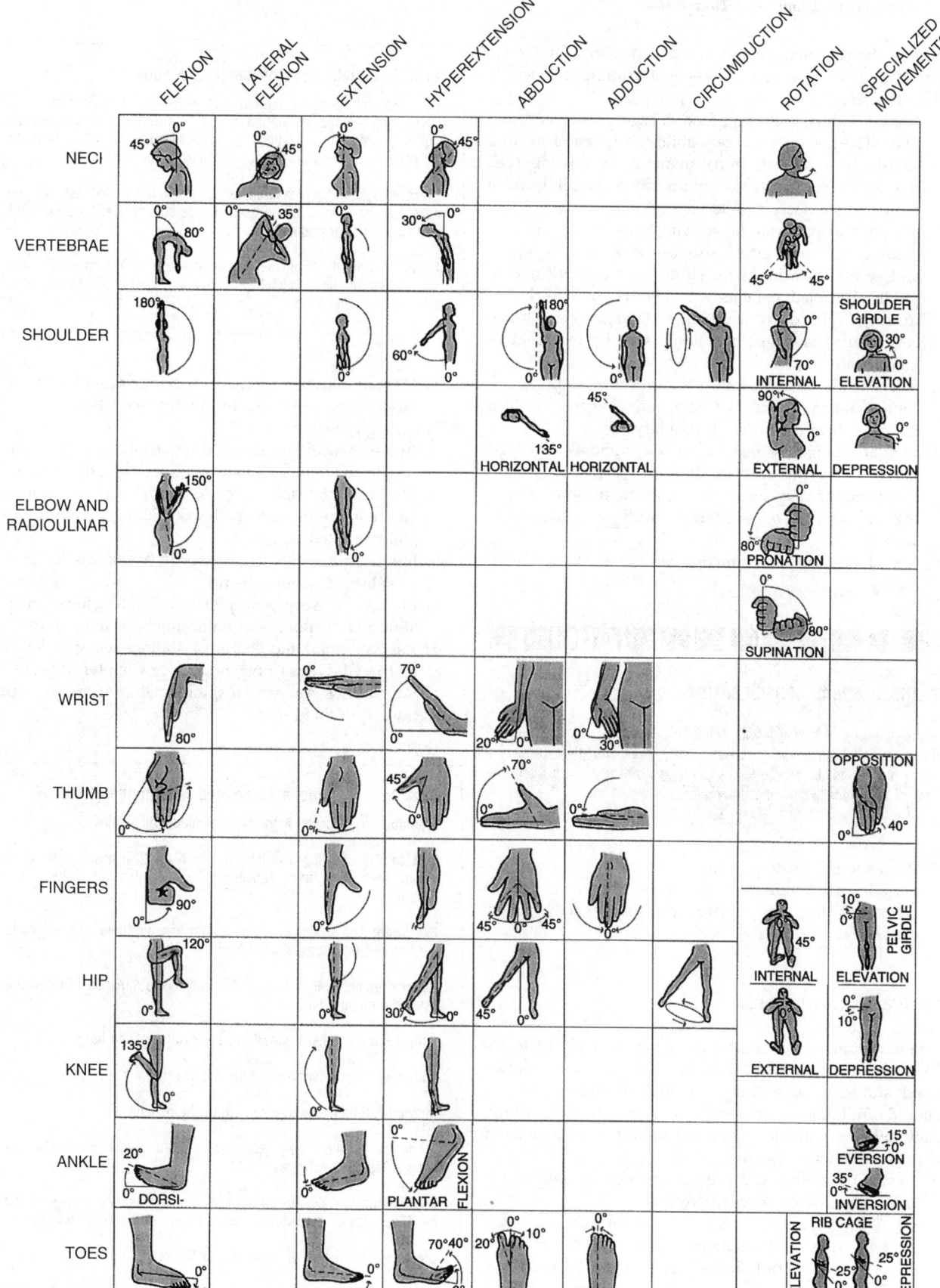

Figure 7–1. Assessing joint range of motion (ROM). All joints are at 0 degrees when in anatomic position. ROM begins at 0 degrees, as shown by solid lines. Attainment of the average normal ROM is shown by dotted lines and the number of degrees in the angle formed by the 2 lines. Shoulder flexion and abduction to 180 degrees include scapular motions. Hip flexion to 120 degrees is with the knee flexed. (From Black JM, and Matassarin-Jacobs E [eds]. *Luckmann and Sorensen's Medical-Surgical Nursing: A Psychophysiologic Approach.* 4th ed. Philadelphia: WB Saunders, 1993, p 1877.)

5. Assess the disabled person and the person's family for habits and life patterns. Assessment parameters include the following:
   a. Dietary habits, including food allergies, likes, and dislikes. The person's self-care ability in terms of feeding should be included. Impairment of swallowing (i.e., the decreased ability to voluntarily pass solids from mouth to stomach) should be assessed.
   b. Elimination patterns, bowel and bladder function, including use of enemas, suppositories, and laxatives, and access to facilities for elimination at work and in public. Disabled persons with bladder or bowel dysfunction related to neurologic damage (e.g., spinal cord injury) are most commonly seen by the rehabilitation team.
   c. Sleep habits, including numbers of hours slept, medications taken before bedtime, and changes in sleep patterns since the onset of disability.
   d. Weight changes, especially in the immobile disabled person, since the onset of disability. Increased weight (overweight) may affect the disabled person's ability to use supportive equipment such as crutches or walkers.
   e. Sexual patterns and function since the onset of disability.

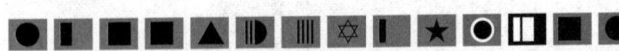

TRANSCULTURAL CONSIDERATIONS

Address issues of sexuality with sensitivity. Members of many cultures do not discuss such subjects openly, even with their peers. Some may be totally unable to discuss sexual practices with members of the opposite sex other than their sexual partners.

   f. Recreational patterns and exercise. For example, various neuromuscular disorders result in muscle weakness that may impair recreational activities or exercise ability.

Physical Examination

1. Limited mobility can affect virtually every body system.
2. Musculoskeletal system: Whether the deformity developed suddenly or gradually should be determined, as should limitation of movement and its link to activity. Immobility is variable in certain conditions, such as from degenerative joint disease.
   a. Assess premorbia and present function as well as active and passive ranges of motion.
      (1) A specific range (extent) of motion exists for each joint (Fig. 7–1). Range of joint motion may be described as full, limited, or severely limited (Box 7–1). Definitions associated with range of motion are listed in Box 7–2.
      (2) Range of joint motion is measured by an instrument called a goniometer, which resembles a protractor (Fig. 7–2).

BOX 7–1. Definitions of Range of Motion

Full: Normal range of motion that a healthy joint is capable of performing. Range of motion is full if movement occurs without stiffness, pain, or crepitation. The value of range of motion is within 10 percent to 20 percent of the predicted value for that joint.

Limited: When the measured range of motion is between 50 percent and 80 percent of normal. The person may experience some stiffness, pain, or crepitation.

Severely limited: When the measured range of motion is less than 50 percent of the predicted. The person experiences severe pain, stiffness, or crepitation.

---

   b. Manual muscle testing is used to describe range of motion and resistance to gravity (see Chapter 5).
3. Neurologic system
   a. Assess neurologic functioning before injury or illness problems (e.g., limited motion, spastic paralysis), physical condition, reflexes, cranial nerve functioning, and communication patterns. Changes in functional ability should be noted.
   b. Identify the existence of paresis (weakness) or paralysis (absence of movement).
   c. Identify sensory and perceptual alterations, such as abnormal responses to pain, touch, or temperature.
   d. Assess mental and cognitive abilities using scales such as the Glasgow Coma Scale (see Chapter 18) and the Rancho Los Amigos Hospital Scale of Cognitive Functioning (Table 7–1).

BOX 7–2. Definitions Associated with Range of Motion

Median: Pertaining to or toward the middle or midline

Flexion: The bending of a joint in which the 2 adjacent parts move toward each other, thus reducing the angle at the joint between the 2 parts

Extension: The straightening of a joint in which two adjacent parts are brought into straight alignment

Hyperextension: Movement of the joint in the direction of extension beyond a straight line

Abduction: Movement away from the midline of the body

Adduction: Movement toward the midline of the body

Internal rotation: Turning away from the midline

Pronation: Turning the forearm so that the palmar surface of the hand is facing downward

Supination: Turning the forearm so that the palmar surface of the hand is facing upward (also referred to as radioulnar articulation)

Deviation: Abduction or adduction of the wrist

Opposition: Placement of the palmar surface of the thumb so that it touches the base of the fingers

From Rehabilitation Institute of Chicago Division of Nursing. *Rehabilitation Nursing Procedures Manual.* Rockville, MD: Aspen, 1990.

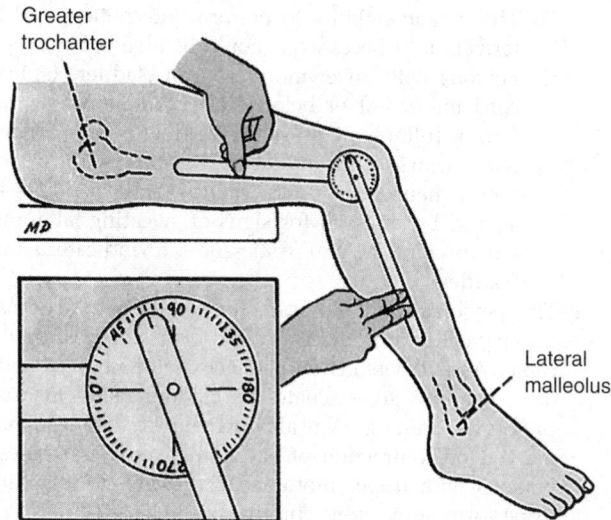

Greater trochanter

Lateral malleolus

Figure 7–2. Using a goniometer. (From Black JM, and Matassarin-Jacobs E [eds]. *Luckmann and Sorensen's Medical-Surgical Nursing: A Psychophysiologic Approach.* 4th ed. Philadelphia: WB Saunders, 1993, p 1876.)

4. Gastrointestinal system
   a. Assess the disabled person's nutritional pattern. Swallowing disorders may be associated with neurologic conditions such as stroke, head trauma, multiple sclerosis, or cerebral palsy. Assess facial asymmetry, drooling, oral muscle weakness, chewing ability, dentition, weight pattern, and level of consciousness.
   b. Note the presence of nausea, vomiting, anorexia, constipation, diarrhea, and weight gain or loss.
   c. If indicated, check the person's blood glucose, hemoglobin, or serum albumin level.
   d. If the person is experiencing elimination problems, a change in activity, diet, or medication may be the cause.
   e. Neurogenic bowel may occur as a result of central nervous system vascular disorders (e.g., stroke), traumatic injury (e.g., spinal cord injury), or neurologic disease (e.g., multiple sclerosis).
      (1) These conditions result in loss of gastrointestinal tract innervation, with resulting constipation or incontinence.
      (2) Alterations in diet and activity may lead to neurogenic bowel.
   f. Identify the type of neurogenic bowel exhibited by the person.
      (1) Uninhibited neurogenic bowel from damage to upper motor neurons (from stroke, trauma, or multiple sclerosis) results in involuntary and sudden defecation.
      (2) Reflex neurogenic bowel (from incomplete or complete spinal cord trauma) results in purely reflexive defecation.

Table 7–1. Rancho Los Amigos Hospital: Scale of Cognitive Functioning	
Level of Response	**Behavior**
I None	Unresponsive to auditory, visual, or tactile stimuli
II Generalized	Reacts inconsistently and nonpurposively to stimuli. Delayed and limited responses
III Localized	Reacts specifically but inconsistently to stimuli. Responses are related to type of stimuli presented, such as visually focusing on an object or responding to sounds
IV Confused-agitated	Extremely agitated and in a high state of confusion. Nonpurposeful and aggressive behavior. Unable to fully cooperate with treatments owing to short attention span. Requires maximal assistance with self-care
V Confused-inappropriate, nonagitated	Alert and can respond to simple commands on a more consistent basis. Highly distractible. Needs constant cueing to attend to an activity. Memory is impaired, with confusion regarding past and present. Can perform self-care activities with assistance. May wander and needs to be watched carefully
VI Confused-appropriate	Shows goal-directed behavior, but still needs direction. Follows simple tasks consistently, and shows carry-over for relearned tasks. More aware of his or her deficits, and has increased awareness of self, family, and basic needs
VII Automatic-appropriate	Appears oriented in home and hospital, and goes through daily routine automatically. Shows carry-over for new learning, but still requires structure and supervision to ensure safety and good judgment. Able to initiate tasks in which he or she has an interest
VIII Purposeful-appropriate	Totally alert, oriented, and shows good recall of past and recent events. Independent in the home and community

From Black JM, and Matassarin-Jacobs E (eds). *Luckmann and Sorensen's Medical-Surgical Nursing: A Psychophysiologic Approach.* 4th ed. Philadelphia: WB Saunders, 1993, p 140.

(3) Areflexia neurogenic bowel results from a complete or incomplete lower motor neuron system pathologic condition below or at T12 that is characterized by partial or total sensory loss in both the perineum and rectum and in loss of external sphincter control.

g. Examine the abdomen for decreased or increased bowel sounds and distention.

h. Perform a rectal examination for fecal impaction, sphincter tone, and anal reflex.

i. Assess person's self-care ability for bowel training programs.

5. Urologic system

a. Assess the type of urinary incontinence that the disabled person exhibits: urge, stress, overflow, or functional loss related to neurologic damage.

b. Assess the person's regular urinary pattern, including number of times per day that the person usually voids and whether the person wakes up at night to void.

c. Determine the effect of any medications on urinary status. Medications that influence urinary continence include diuretics, anticholinergics, β-blockers, and antidepressants.

d. Assess the person's past and present problems, such as incontinence, retention, or impaired bladder function (e.g., neurogenic bladder or history of urinary tract infections).

e. Physical assessment data include color, amount, cloudiness, and blood in the urine, presence of bladder distention, condition of external genitalia, and urinary meatus. Measure the amount of voiding over 24 hours.

f. Monitor laboratory reports of urinalysis, blood urea nitrogen, culture, and serum creatinine levels.

g. Determine the classification of neurogenic bladder and type of voiding problem.

(1) Persons with uninhibited neurogenic bladder (persons with lesions of the brain) may exhibit frequency, urgency, and nocturia, resulting in urge incontinence.

(2) Persons with reflex neurogenic bladder (spinal cord lesions above T12–L1) exhibit decreased bladder capacity, increased resistance to urine outflow, and high urine residuals.

(3) Persons with areflexia neurogenic bladder (e.g., patients with spinal cord injuries who have lesions at or below T12–L1) exhibit decreased sensation of fullness, increased bladder capacity, and high residual urine.

(4) Persons with motor paralytic neurogenic bladder (such as that caused by trauma or poliomyelitis) may exhibit overflow incontinence.

(5) Persons with sensory paralytic neurogenic bladder (as in multiple sclerosis) may exhibit decreased sensation of bladder fullness or infrequent voiding with large output.

h. Because nursing management depends on nursing assessment, the level of bladder retraining the person has attained should be assessed.

(1) Immobile persons may have continuous bladder irrigation or drainage via an indwelling catheter.

(2) The person's ability to perform intermittent catheterization, if necessary, should be assessed.

(3) Persons with lower motor neuron bladders (spinal cord injuries at or below T12–L1) have no sensation of fullness or pressure. Voiding is involuntary and occurs with overflow. Persons with upper motor neuron bladders (injuries above T12–L1) should be assessed for signs of sweating, abdominal discomfort, and restlessness to indicate a full bladder.

i. The person's ability to care for catheters or external urinary collection devices should be assessed, if applicable. Assess persons with lower motor neuron bladder for ability to evacuate the bladder using manual pressure straining (Valsalva maneuver, Credé's maneuver, or contraction of abdominal muscles). Assess persons with upper motor neuron bladder for ability to perform suprapubic stimulation.

j. Assess for signs of urinary tract infection in patients with a spinal cord injury (e.g., burning; low back, suprapubic, abdominal or flank pain; chills and fever; positive urine cultures).

6. Cardiovascular system

a. Check for symptoms of decreased cardiac output, such as chest pain, diaphoresis, or decrease in systolic blood pressure of more than 10 mm Hg from the person's normal level. These symptoms may indicate activity intolerance. Other causes of activity intolerance include depression, chronic illness with disability, and prolonged immobility.

b. Inquire about fatigue, especially with activity. Fatigue, weakness, or vertigo may be associated with activity intolerance.

c. The following guidelines are used to assess the person:

(1) Adequacy of basic physiologic energy resources (such as oxygen and rest)

(2) Changes linked to the disability resulting in reallocation of energy expenditure, such as increased energy to daily activities, self-care, or maintenance of physical integrity

(3) Adequacy of nutritional intake for energy expenditure

7. Respiratory system

a. Respiratory impairment is exhibited by disabled persons with neurologic injury, neuromuscular diseases, or premorbid chronic respiratory disease.

b. The disabled person may have a neurologic impairment that affects the respiratory system.

c. The level of activity that the person can tolerate before experiencing shortness of breath should be established.

d. The nurse should assess the person's ability to perform self-care activities, such as conserving energy with performing activities of daily living, pulmonary toilet, and maintenance of specialized pulmonary equipment such as ventilators.

e. If there are symptoms of cough, dyspnea, hemoptysis, or chest pain, the person should be referred for medical treatment.

f. The person should be checked for fatigue.

8. Integumentary system
    a. Collect information regarding the patient's ability for self-care of skin and skin alterations.
    b. Inspect the color, dryness, lesions, and turgor of the skin.
    c. Note actual and potential skin interruptions.
    d. Any pressure ulcers should be described in terms of depth and diameter (in centimeters), stage (Fig. 7–3), location, color of wound bed, drainage (color, odor, consistency), presence of undermining sinus tract (may be associated with stage 4 pressure ulcers), pressure-relieving devices in use (see p. 192), and heat or edema (possible presence of infection).
    e. Assess the person's physical condition, mental state, and continence. Impaired ability of bed- or chair-bound persons to reposition self increases the risk of pressure ulcer development.

9. Reproductive system
    a. Assess the disabled person's reproductive patterns and specific factors related to physical disability.
    b. Determine premorbid and current sexual patterns and level of activity.
    c. Assess substance use that may alter sexual function, such as use of antidepressants, antihypertensives, diuretics, tranquilizers, opiates, or marijuana.
    d. Examine sensorimotor testing: motor function of the lower extremities, tactile sensation of the genital area, and rectal and urinary strength and tone.
    e. Assess for altered sexuality patterns related to physical disability (Table 7–2).

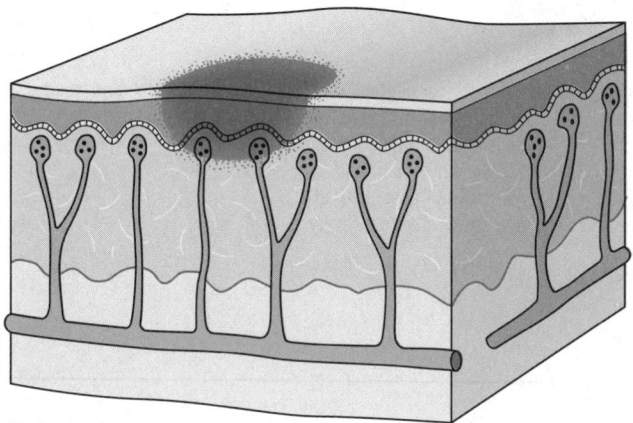

Stage I

Soft tissue swelling or ulceration lasting 24 hours or longer. Nonblanchable erythema of intact skin, heralding lesion of skin ulceration.

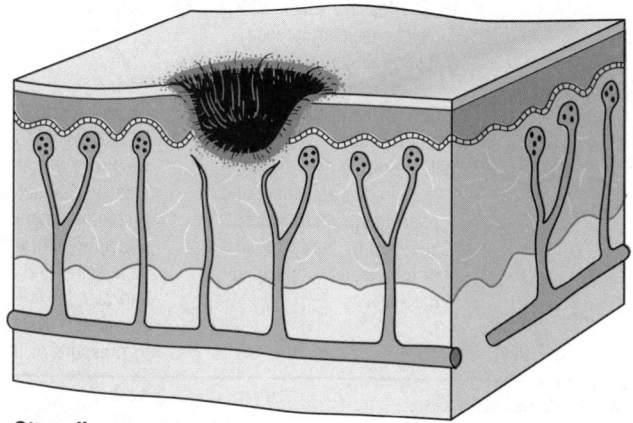

Stage II

Full-thickness ulcers penetrating the dermis. Subcutaneous tissue remains intact. Ulcer is superficial and appears clinically as an abrasion, blister, or shallow crater.

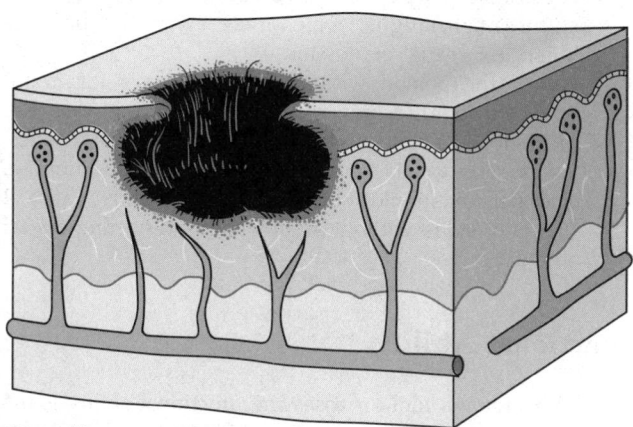

Stage III

Full-thickness skin loss involving damage of subcutaneous tissue that may extend down to, but not through, underlying fascia. Ulcer appears as a deep crater with or without undermining of adjacent tissue.

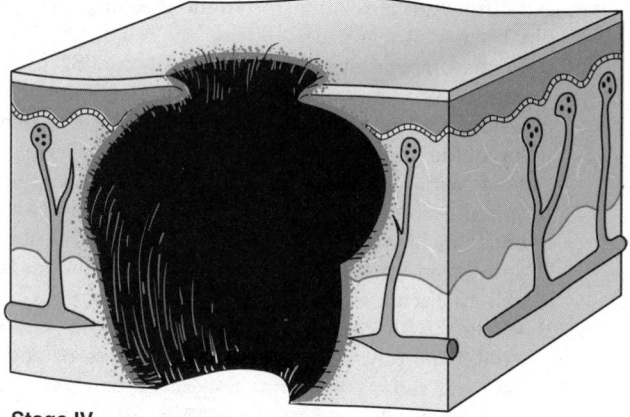

Stage IV

Full-thickness skin loss with extensive destruction, tissue necrosis, or involvement of muscle, bone, or supporting structures. Bone might be exposed.

Figure 7–3. Stages of pressure ulcers. (Redrawn and modified from Black JM, and Matassarin-Jacobs E [eds]. *Luckmann and Sorensen's Medical-Surgical Nursing: A Psychophysiologic Approach.* 4th ed. Philadelphia: WB Saunders, 1993, p 394.)

Table 7–2. Reproductive Capabilities After Disability

Diagnosis	Fertility	Pregnancy	Childbirth	Parenting
Arthritis (includes hip and knee disease)	Unchanged	Increased pressure on joints due to weight gain	Potential need for cesarean section depending on joint involvement	Increased energy needs and pressure on joints required in child care
Brain injury	Males: Possible premature ejaculation due to decreased attention span Males and females: Poor libido and behavioral changes and social inappropriateness may interfere with sexual relationships	Cognitive deficits possibly requiring assistance to ensure good prenatal care	Spasticity and sensory deficits may necessitate planned labor induction or a cesarean section	Cognitive, temper control, memory, safety awareness, activities of daily living, or mobility deficits possibly requiring client to obtain assistance
Stroke	Females: Unchanged (see Brain injury) Males: Possible vascular or psychogenic impotence (see Brain injury)	Plan around fully stabilized CVA, especially hemorrhagic CVA, if possible	(see Brain injury)	(see Brain injury)
Spinal cord injury	Females: Temporary disruption of the menstrual cycle and ovulation Males: Erectile dysfunction, retrograde ejaculation, and poor spermatozoa count and quality due to the loss of temperature-regulating mechanisms	Need for close medical supervision, possible increase in spasms due to the weight of the fetus, increased fatigue, circulation problems, edema, more difficulty with activities of daily living and transfers, and bladder infections or autonomic dysreflexia due to pressure of the fetus	Inability to feel contractions in injuries at or above T10, possibility of induction of a cesarean section and vaginal delivery, possibility of dysreflexia during delivery	Need for home and equipment modifications

CVA, Cerebrovascular accident.
Reprinted from Mumma C. *The Specialty Practice of Rehabilitation Nursing—A Core Curriculum.* 3rd ed. Skokie, IL: Rehabilitation Nursing Foundation, 1993, p. 163, with permission of the Rehabilitation Nursing Foundation, 5700 Old Orchard Road, First Floor, Skokie, IL 60077–1057. Copyright © 1993. Rehabilitation Nursing Foundation.

(1) Physical limitations in preferred sexual positions may be present.
(2) Reproductive capabilities may be impaired (see Table 7–2)

f. In patients with spinal cord injury, assess the person's sexual function in relationship to the level and type of spinal injury (Table 7–3).

(1) In men, spinal segments T11 to L1 and S2 to S4 control erection and ejaculation. The higher the lesion, the more likely it is that the person may have the ability to attain an erection. Disabled men with upper motor neuron and incomplete spinal lesions are more likely to be able to have an erection. Men with low or incomplete cord lesions and lower motor injuries are more likely to be able to ejaculate.

(2) Women with complete spinal cord lesions rarely exhibit the physiologic orgasmic response of vaginal contractions. In women with spinal cord injury, assess for menstrual status. Some women may experience amenorrhea up to 1 year after injury. Fertility is rarely impaired in women with spinal cord injury.

g. Determine self-care ability for sexual positioning in the person with cerebral palsy. Limited mobility, tremors, and muscle spasms may affect sexual functioning in these individuals.

h. Stroke may result in limitations of movement on the affected side. Although sexual ability is not affected by stroke, the disabled person may require footboards or hand levers for support if weakness exists.

i. Assess the person with rheumatoid arthritis for pain, stiffness, or fatigue, which may affect the person's ability for sexual expression.

j. Assess the person with multiple sclerosis for impotence (in men), achievement of orgasm, and decrease of libido, which occurs progressively with the disease.

k. Assess the cardiac patient for aerobic conditioning. The person should be able to comfortably climb 2 flights of stairs without angina before resuming sexual activity.

Functional Ability

1. The best-known tool for assessing functional ability is the Katz Index of Activities of Daily Living (Fig. 7–4). It includes 6 functional areas of bathing, dressing, toileting, transfer, continence, and feeding; the order of items reflects increased progression in loss and acquisition of function.
2. Assess the person's physical ability to return to a former occupation.
   a. Collect data on the patient's employment background and education.

Table 7–3. Sexual Function in Patients with Spinal Cord Injury

Sexuality	Reproductive Functioning	Special Considerations for Contraceptive Methods
Females		
Lesions at C1–C3: Reflex lubrication is probable. Erogenous areas may develop above injury. Libido is intact. Lesions at C4–C6: Psychogenic lubrication is unlikely. Nongenital orgasm may be experienced. Lesions at C7: Able to use hands for holding and caressing. Lesions at T12–L5: Psychogenic stimulation of the clitoris, lubrication, labial swelling, and skin flush are possible but unlikely.	Menstruation and fertility unaffected. Pregnancy is not affected. Incidence of bladder infection during pregnancy increases. Risk of autonomic hyperreflexia during delivery and labor increases.	Birth control pills are contraindicated when circulatory problems are present; thrombophlebitis could go undetected owing to lack of sensation in extremities. Intrauterine device may be contraindicated because pelvic inflammatory disease and other problems could remain undetected owing to lack of sensation. Patient must be able to assess for vaginal bleeding.
Males		
Lesions at C1–C3: Reflex erection is caused by genital stimulation. Psychogenic erection is not possible. Erogenous areas above injury site may develop. Libido is intact. Lesions at C4–C6: Reflex erection is possible. Nongenital orgasm may be experienced; no ejaculation. Oral sex is possible. Libido is intact. Lesions at C7: Holding and caressing with hands are possible. Lesions at T12–L5: Psychogenic stimulation and erection are possible; no reflex erection. Lesions at S2–S4: Reflex erection is possible. Ejaculation is possible but may be retrograde.	Semen can be obtained from the bladder of patients who have retrograde ejaculation. For patients who cannot ejaculate, semen can be obtained through glandular vibratory stimulation. In general, semen quality is impaired, with poor motility the most common abnormality. Some patients are candidates for penile prosthesis.	Patient or partner may apply condom.

Modified from Black JM, and Matassarin-Jacobs E (eds). *Luckmann and Sorensen's Medical-Surgical Nursing: A Psychophysiologic Approach.* 4th ed. Philadelphia: WB Saunders, 1993, p 810.

b. Identify the manual and cognitive demands of the job held before the onset of the disability.
   (1) Physical demand of jobs ranges from light (0 to 10 pounds lifted frequently) to heavy (more than 100 pounds lifted frequently).
   (2) Cognitive demands of the job are the mental activities that the job requires. The nurse assesses these demands if the person desires to return to a former job. These demands are ascertained from the job description.
   (3) The nurse additionally assesses the person's educational level; cognitive abilities from past jobs; and statements about job interests, training, and aspirations. The nurse assesses the person's recent attention span, short- and long-term memory, and thought processes.
3. Assess functional ability and whether the person requires assistance or can be independent in bowel elimination. If assistance is needed, assess the ability of family to help.

Psychosocial History

1. Assess the patient's feeling of powerlessness, using a tool such as that shown in Figure 7–5.

2. Determine the person's self-esteem and body image through direct questions and through observations.
   a. Questions to ask the patient include the following:
      (1) How comfortable are you with initiating interactions with other people?
      (2) What opportunities do you have for socialization?
      (3) Who are the important persons in your life?
      (4) How do you feel about your attractiveness to potential sexual partners?
      (5) How do you feel about your worth or value compared with that of other people?
      (6) How do you take care of your personal hygiene and dress?
      (7) Have you altered your sexuality patterns since the onset of your physical disability? If so, how?
      (8) Since the onset of your physical disability, has there been a change in social interaction? If so, what has it been?
      (9) How do you think your disability has affected your work?
   b. Observations include the following:
      (1) Visibility of disability (e.g., loss of limb, paralysis, disfigurement)
      (2) Visibility of equipment or other aids necessitated by the disability
      (3) Presence of pain

Name_____   Date_____

For each area of functioning listed below check description that applies. (The word "assistance" means supervision, direction of personal assistance.)

Bathing—sponge bath, tub bath, or shower

_____   _____   _____

Receives no assistance (gets in and out of tub by self if tub is usual means of bathing)	Receives assistance in bathing only one part of body (such as back or a leg)	Receives assistance bathing more than one part of body (or does not bathe self)

Dressing—gets clothes from drawers; puts on clothes, including underclothes, outer garments; manages fasteners (including braces, if worn)

_____   _____   _____

Gets clothes and gets completely dressed without assistance	Gets clothes and gets dressed without assistance except for tying shoes	Receives assistance in getting clothes or in getting dressed or stays partly or completely undressed

Toileting—going to the "toilet room" for bowel and urine elimination; cleaning self after elimination and arranging clothes

_____   _____   _____

Goes to "toilet room," cleans self, and arranges clothes (may use object for support such as cane, walker, or wheelchair and may manage night bedpan or commode, emptying same in morning)	Receives assistance in going to "toilet room" or in cleaning self or in arranging clothes after elimination or in use of night bedpan or commode	Does not go to room termed "toilet" for the elimination process

Transfer

_____   _____   _____

Moves in and out of bed and in and out of chair without assistance (may use objects for support such as cane or walker)	Moves in or out of bed with assistance	Does not get out of bed

Continence

_____   _____   _____

Controls urination and bowel movement completely by self	Has occasional "accidents"	Supervision helps keep urine or bowel control; catheter is used or is incontinent

Feeding

_____   _____   _____

Feeds self without assistance	Feeds self except for getting assistance in cutting meat or buttering bread	Receives assistance or is fed partly or completely by tubes or intravenous fluids

Figure 7–4. Katz index of activities of daily living evaluation form. (From Katz S, et al. Studies of illness in the aged. The index of ADL: A standardized measure of biological and psychological function. *JAMA* 185:94, 1963. Copyright 1963, American Medical Association.)

3. Assess the patient's coping ability, including the ability to manage stress, to modify daily routines, and to comply with regimens.
4. Assess the person's social support system

a. Family members or other persons may be able to assist the disabled person in ambulating around the home and with transportation in the community.

Directions:

Check _____ the verbal expression and behaviors that are applicable to the patient. The defining characteristics are keyed (L) low, (M) moderate, and (S) severe. Low- or moderate-defining characteristics are important cues. Indicators ranked as severe could be termed "critical indicators" of the nursing diagnosis of powerlessness. If any of these indicators is present, the patient may be experiencing powerlessness.

Verbal Indicators:

_____ Uncertainty about fluctuating energy level (L)
_____ Dissatisfaction and frustration over inability to perform previous tasks or activities (M)
_____ Uncertainty about treatment outcome (M)
_____ Doubt regarding role performance (M)
_____ Reluctance to express true feelings, fearing alienation of self from care givers (M)
_____ Expression of having no control or influence over situations (S)
_____ Expression of having no control or influence over self-care (S)
_____ Expression of having no control or influence over outcomes (S)

Behavioral Indicators:

_____ Apathy (M)
_____ Nonparticipation in care or decision making when opportunities are provided (M)
_____ Dependence on others that may result in irritability, resentment, anger, and guilt (M)
_____ Inability to monitor progress (M)
_____ Does not defend self-care practice when challenged (M)
_____ Inability to seek information regarding self-care (M)
_____ Hesitant to plan for future, set goals (M)
_____ Depression over physical deterioration that occurs despite patient compliance with regimens (S)
_____ Passivity (S)

Figure 7–5. Assessment tool for powerlessness. (From Miller JF. *Coping with Chronic Illness: Overcoming Powerlessness.* Philadelphia: FA Davis, 1992.)

b. The patient's home environment may contain physical barriers to mobility; family members may be aware of such problems and have plans to overcome them.

c. The nurse should assess the disabled person's sexual partner's response to the recent disability in terms of economic resources and sexuality. Assessment of the disabled person and partner includes identifying changes in each person's sexual response, identifying alternate types of acceptable sexual expression, and helping the couple to adapt to alterations in sexual performance.

d. If the patient is newly disabled, the nurse should determine whether family or friends can help with the patient's self-care in both the short and the long term.

e. The nurse should assess any person who is or will be engaged in caring for the patient's housework or functional activities of daily living. To assess the disabled person's safety and level of independence, the nurse should have the disabled person demonstrate activities of daily living in the home and community while using assistive devices.

◼ REHABILITATION

Overall Goal

1. The main goal of rehabilitation is to restore maximal functional abilities and self-care skills consistent with the individual's disability.
2. Desired goals of rehabilitation include achieving and maintaining an acceptable quality of life for the disabled person.

3. The person should be enabled to return to successful function within the community.

Rehabilitation Team

1. Successful rehabilitation depends on coordinated efforts by members of different disciplines to maximize opportunities for educating and otherwise assisting the disabled person to return to maximal functioning in all regards—physical, mental, and spiritual. This comprehensive approach fosters optimal patient outcomes.

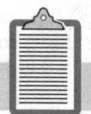

NURSING MANAGEMENT

The function of cooperative practice is to provide high-quality care for disabled patients and to improve patient satisfaction with that care.

The purpose of team collaboration is to integrate each discipline's care regimen into a single comprehensive approach to the patient's need.

Collaboration develops when team members—including the patient and the patient's family—communicate and provide feedback on the overall plan. The goals of collaborative practice are to
- Assess the needs and functional ability of the patient
- Develop and document an interdisciplinary management plan based on patient and team goals
- Provide continuity of care in implementation of a management plan
- Evaluate the extent of goal achievement by the patient
- Plan the discharge of the patient

2. Team members include nurses, physicians, physical therapists, occupational therapists, speech pathologists, recreational therapists, aides, social workers, vocational counselors, psychologists, nutritionists, transcultural nurse specialists, the disabled person, and the disabled person's family members (Table 7–4).
   a. The size and composition of the team depend on the size, type, and financial resources of the rehabilitation setting.
   b. The team is actively involved in planning for the patient's discharge from the rehabilitation facility. Team members assess the patient's ability to provide self-care at home. Team members also determine what equipment and supplies the patient will need at home, and they refer the patient to sources where such items are sold, rented, or donated.
   c. The disabled person generally has the final authority regarding treatment plans and interventions.
3. Nursing role
   a. The nurse may serve as team leader and coordinator.
   b. The nurse performs activities that maintain and re-

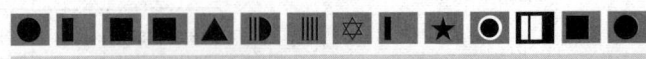

TRANSCULTURAL CONSIDERATIONS

In some elder-centered cultures (e.g., Hispanic, Appalachian, East Indian, Native American), the head of the family may make health care decisions for all members of the family.

store function and prevent complications or further loss of function.
   c. The nurse provides direct care to the disabled person while the person develops maximal self-care independence.
   d. In rehabilitation facilities, the nurse develops nursing care plans directed toward such rehabilitation goals as improved mobility and bowel, bladder, and skin self-management.
   e. The nurse may assume an independent role in coordinating services such as education, discharge planning, and referrals.

Table 7–4. Members of the Rehabilitation Team and Their Roles

Team Member	Role
Rehabilitation nurse	Provides direct or indirect patient care to rehabilitation clients. Direct patient care involves client assessment, personal hygiene, nursing procedures, counseling, administering medications, and patient education. Indirect patient care involves giving and receiving shift report, making rounds, noting physician orders, supervising nonlicensed personnel, and charting.
Physical therapist	Evaluates and manages mobility needs of patients, such as moving with crutches.
Occupational therapist	Helps the disabled person reestablish fine-motor skills used in hygiene or other activities of daily living.
Speech-language pathologist	Retrains persons with language or feeding (chewing and swallowing) problems. Evaluates and treats communication and eating disorders.
Recreational therapist	Develops leisure activities that will assist the disabled person with reentry into society.
Aides	Work under the direction of registered nurses in the physical care of the disabled person.
Social worker	Works with disabled persons to identify community or support resources including income, housing, transportation, and recreational resources. Provides information related to support groups and organizations for specific disabilities.
Vocational counselor	Assesses disabled persons' job-related skills and abilities and helps them obtain retraining, education, and jobs.
Psychologist	Counsels disabled persons and their families in dealing with psychologic or other coping problems.
Nutritionist	Evaluates and provides for the nutritional needs of disabled persons, including monitoring of weight.
Transcultural nurse specialist	Assesses cultural responses to disability and rehabilitation on the part of disabled persons and their families.
Rehabilitation engineer	Designs adaptive equipment for severely disabled to maintain some level of functioning.

Table 7–5. Functional Goals in Spinal Cord Injury

Spinal Cord Level	Muscle Function	Functional Goals
C1–C2	Has no phrenic nerve function	Respirations managed with phrenic pacemaker
C3–C4	Neck control Scapular elevators Diaphragm function may be weak or absent	Manipulate electric wheelchair with breath control, chin control, or voice activation Limited self-feeding with ball-bearing feeders Operate environmental control units
C5	Fair-to-good shoulder control Functional deltoids, biceps, or both Elbow flexion	Dress upper trunk Turn self in bed with or without arm slings Propel wheelchair with or without friction-surface handrims Self-feeding with handsplints or following tenodesis Assist getting to and from bed May learn to write or type
C6	Good shoulder control Wrist extension Supinators	Dress upper trunk, sometimes dress lower trunk Turn self in bed with arm slings Propel wheelchair with handrim projections Self-feeding with handsplints Transfer from wheelchair to bed with or without minimal assistance (e.g., sliding board) Assist getting to and from commode chair Self-catheterization
C7	May have weak shoulder depression Weak elbow extension Some hand function Triceps	Independent in transfer to bed, car, and toilet Total dressing independence Wheelchair without handrim projections Self-feeding with no assistive devices
T1–T4	Good-to-normal upper extremity muscle function Intrinsic muscles of the hand No trunk control	Independent in transfer to bed, car, and toilet Total dressing independence Wheelchair with standard handrims Self-feeding with no assistive devices Transfer from wheelchair to floor and return Wheelchair up and down curb Transfer from wheelchair to tub and return
T5–L2	Partial-to-good trunk stability	Total wheelchair independence Limited ambulation with bilateral long leg braces and crutches (injury at T12 or below)
L3–L4	All trunk-pelvic stabilizers intact Hip flexors Adductors Quadriceps	Ambulation with short leg braces with or without crutches, depending on level
L5–S3	Hip extensors Abductors, knee flexors, ankle control	No equipment needed if plantar flexion is strong enough for push off at end of stance

Modified from Rancho Los Amigos Hospital, Physical Therapy Department, Downey, CA. From Black JM, and Matassarin-Jacobs E (eds). *Luckmann and Sorensen's Medical-Surgical Nursing: A Psychophysiologic Approach.* 4th ed. Philadelphia: WB Saunders, 1993, p 801.

Setting Specific Goals

1. Prevention of injury
   a. Maintain activity levels to avoid deterioration of an unaffected part.
   b. Eliminate factors that may contribute to further injury, for example, removing heating pads, wrinkled linens, or frayed electrical cords and picking up from cluttered floors.
2. Restoration of function
   a. Restore as much function as possible to the affected part.
   b. Increase functional ability to the highest level, contributing to improved quality of life. Table 7–5 provides an example of functional goals in spinal cord injury.
   c. Promote a sense of well-being.
3. Increase the patient's knowledge about and acceptance of the limitations imposed by the disability.
4. Improve the coping skills of the disabled person and that person's family. Engel categorized the 4 phases of coping behavior associated with the grief brought about by chronic illness as shock and disbelief, developing awareness, restitution, and resolution. The response of each person or family member varies, however, and adjustment is highly individualized. Nursing interventions should be designed according to the behavioral responses observed and should build on the person's past coping abilities or styles.

Overcoming Barriers

1. Barriers to rehabilitation may be physical, psychologic, or sociologic (see pp. 168–170).
2. Ability to overcome barriers depends on the following:
   a. Visibility of disability
   b. Knowledge about the disability and rehabilitation
   c. Availability of rehabilitation services
   d. Individual and family coping skills
3. To help disabled persons overcome these barriers, the rehabilitation team must do the following:
   a. Accurately assess each patient's disability—and abilities—and help patients come to terms with the extent and nature of any new limitations.
   b. Work with disabled persons to develop a rehabilitation plan to restore maximal functioning.
   c. Provide necessary physical, emotional, and social rehabilitation services, including giving referrals outside the institution, such as to help arrange for a permanent assistant for those who cannot care for themselves.
4. To provide strategies for assisting the patient to adapt to a disability, the rehabilitation team must do the following:
   a. Tailor interventions that are congruent with the person's stage of grief.
   b. Encourage the patient to express feelings.
   c. If assessment indicates that the patient lingers in a stage of denial, anger, or depression, refer the patient to the team psychologist or social worker.
   d. Assist the patient to identify prior successful coping strategies, support systems, or individual strengths such as motivation, beliefs, or sense of humor.
5. Strategies for modifying an environment for a person with disabilities include the following:
   a. Providing adaptive devices to help the client perform activities of daily living
   b. Before discharge, assessing the client's house or apartment for accessibility is usually the responsibility of the occupational therapist
   c. Assessing the need for ramps or safety features such as guard rails and smoke alarms
6. Providing information on community resources for persons with disabilities:
   a. Resources include educational materials, support groups, financial assistance, religious organizations, self-help groups, and mental health services.
   b. The disabled person's physical and psychologic strengths can be enhanced by teaching self-care skills and by identifying supportive resources within the family.

Promoting Function in the Activities of Daily Living

1. Therapeutic exercise
   a. Regular movement is important for the disabled person to prevent cardiovascular complications (e.g., orthostatic hypotension, thrombus formation) resulting from immobility.
   b. Range of joint motion exercises take 4 forms:
      (1) Passive exercises are performed for immobilized patients to the extent that they are unable to do the work involved in exercising 1 or more of their joints. The caregiver doing the exercises supports the dependent part while putting an immobilized joint through the full range of motion. Procedure 7–1 illustrates passive range-of-motion exercises.
      (2) Active-assisted exercises are used for patients who can partially move at an affected joint, and the nurse encourages the disabled person to do as much of each exercise as possible. When the disabled person can move the joint no farther, the nurse supports the dependent body part and completes the exercise by passive range of motion. The exercise is repeated 3 times before the next activity.
      (3) Active exercise is performed by the disabled person independently by exercising 1 or more joints through complete range of motion several times a day. The nurse teaches the disabled person the proper techniques.
      (4) Resistive exercises are similar to the active exercises except that some force is exerted during each movement to prevent easy movement of the limb. For example, ankle weights may be added to increase resistance during knee or hip exercises.
   c. Isometric and isotonic exercises build both mass and strength (Table 7–6).

Procedure 7–1
Performing Passive Range-of-Motion Exercises

Definitions/Purposes	Range-of-motion exercises are isotonic exercises that move a joint through its predicted full range. The nurse, physical therapist, or family member does passive range of motion when the client is unable to move the joint without assistance. These exercises are usually done at least 3 or 4 times a day, with 3 to 5 repetitions of each movement. The main reason for doing these exercises is to prevent the development of contractures, which interfere with the activities of daily living.
Contraindications/Cautions	Do not perform range of motion on inflamed or hot joints. Do not perform range of motion past the point of pain or beyond predicted joint limits. Movements should be smooth and slow. If the muscle spasms, back off the pressure slightly and maintain a functional position until the spasm eases. Support the joints with your hands. Stop the exercises if the patient becomes fatigued. In cases of orthopedic trauma, consult with a physician to determine when exercises should begin, what types are appropriate, and which joints should be included. Other contraindications include exercising an extremity when there is deep vein thrombosis, arterial lines or intravenous access devices in or near the joint, acute joint bleed in a hemophiliac, or immediately postoperatively after a skin graft or flap procedure.
Learning/Teaching Activities	Teach the patient and family the correct movements and terms for each exercise (Box 7–1 and 7–2). Teach the patient to do range of motion actively as soon as possible, to report pain or other problems to the nurse, and to follow an individualized plan that specifies the joint range and number of repetitions. Teach correct posture and body alignment. Teach the patient to breathe deeply and to hold each movement for several counts. Provide the patient and family with written guidelines and instructions for reinforcement.

Preliminary Activities

Assessment/Planning	• Review the chart for contraindications. • Know the baseline level of activity for this disabled person. • Make decisions regarding type and frequency of range-of-motion exercises in conjunction with physician orders and in collaboration with the physical therapist. • Record the program on the nursing care plan. • Schedule range-of-motion activities to coincide with routine care, if possible.
Equipment	• Bed with firm mattress or padded table • Nonrestrictive clothing for the patient • Bath blanket, if required, for drape
Preparation	• Explain what will be done and why. • Provide for privacy. • Raise bed to working height, lock wheels. • Help patient don exercise clothing. Maintain modesty with bath blanket if only a hospital gown is available. The patient's feet should be bare. • Position the person flat in bed (unless contraindicated), supine and without a pillow. • Remind the patient to report changes in joints or the presence of pain.

Procedure

Action	Rationale/Discussion
1. Facing the patient's head, lower the side rail nearest you.	1. Facing the direction of movement avoids twisting the spine.
2. Shift the patient close to you on the edge of the bed.	2. Avoid back strain by keeping the patient's weight close to your center of gravity.
3. Check the patient's body alignment.	3. Proper alignment helps the body parts move correctly during the exercises.
4. While supporting the patient's head and neck, slowly move the joint through its range of motion, repeating each movement 3 to 5 times.	4. Slow movements of the head help to prevent dizziness.
5. Flex the spine by raising the head of the bed as high as it will go and allow the patient's head to droop forward. Move the head back to the mattress and lower the bed flat. Repeat.	5. Spinal exercises may or may not be included in the routine range-of-motion exercises. There is some degree of spinal flexion and extension every time the head of the bed is raised and lowered.
6. Beginning with the arm nearest you, support the elbow and wrist and put the shoulder through its range of motion.	6. Flexing the elbow helps keep the patient's arm from hitting the wall or head of the bed.

(continued)

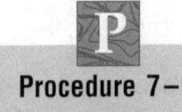

Procedure 7–1

(continued)

Action	Rationale/Discussion
7. Pronate and supinate the elbow, using a handshake position.	7. This position keeps you from rotating too far.
8. Flex and extend the wrist, then laterally and medially flex it.	8. Lace your finger with the patient's so that you do not exceed normal range.
9. Abduct and adduct the fingers, make a fist and extend the fingers, flex the thumb to touch each finger.	9. These motions are important for the full use of the hand in activities of daily living.
10. Move to the hip. Support the knee and ankle during these maneuvers. Flex and extend both hip and knee at the same time unless contraindicated. Abduct and adduct the hip, holding the leg close to your body. Internally and externally rotate the hip. Circumduct the hip as widely as possible.	10. As the knee approaches the hip, move your hand to the lateral side to prevent external rotation of the hip. As it returns to the bed, place your hand under the knee again to prevent hyperextension. Holding the weight close to you helps prevent back strain.
11. Plantar flex and dorsiflex the ankle, then invert and evert it.	11. If foot drop is developing in the patient, concentrate on dorsiflexion.
12. Invert and evert the metatarsals; flex and extend the toes; abduct and adduct the toes.	12. While inverting and everting, the heel is stable and the ball of the foot moves. All the toes may be exercised together.
13. Raise the side rail and move to the other side. Repeat the extremity movements beginning with the shoulder.	13. The neck and spine have already been exercised sufficiently.
14. When the joints on the second side are completed, turn the patient into a prone position if possible.	14. Turning allows completion of exercises for shoulder, spine, and hip.
15. Supporting the wrist and elbow, hyperextend the shoulder and lower it again.	15. The average person can hyperextend 45 degrees to 60 degrees.
16. Raise the head of the bed to hyperextend the spine, then lower it. Repeat.	16. This allows the bed to do the work, saving back strain.
17. Supporting the knee and ankle, hyperextend the hip.	17. Because hip flexion contractures develop in bed-ridden patients, this may not be possible.
18. Raise the side rail and repeat on the other side.	18. This completes the required exercises.
19. Place the patient in an aligned position for comfort.	19. This allows the patient to rest.

Final Activities

Replace the covers, check vital signs, raise side rails, place call bell within reach. Chart any deviations from previous findings in range of motion, presence of pain, stiffness, spasms, or other untoward effects. Note the number of repetitions and the joints involved. Record vital signs and state how the person tolerated the procedure.

Adapted from Bolander VB (ed). *Sorensen and Luckmann's Basic Nursing: A Psychophysiologic Approach.* 3rd ed. Philadelphia: WB Saunders, 1994.

(1) In isotonic exercises, muscle tension remains constant while muscles shorten (contract) to do work. Such exercises increase the mass and strength of the muscles worked.

(2) In isometric exercises, muscle tension increases while muscle length remains constant. Although such exercises do no work, they do use energy and increase the mass and strength of the muscles involved.

d. The process for teaching any type of exercise is the following:

(1) The nurse demonstrates the exercise.

(2) The patient performs the exercise.

(3) As patients near discharge, they (or a family member) become increasingly responsible for performing the exercise regularly.

2. Assisted ambulation devices (see Chapter 34)

Table 7–6. Comparison of Isometric and Isotonic Exercises

Isometric Exercises	Isotonic Exercises
Pushing or pulling against an immovable object	Active range of motion
Hold muscle contractions for a minimum of 6 seconds, extending to 10 to 15 seconds as strength improves	Weight lifting
Immobilized clients push their feet against an immovable footboard	Calisthenics
	Bed exercises: the patient flexes and extends fingers and thumbs, as in squeezing a rubber ball, and flexes and extends elbows, knees, or hips
Muscle-setting exercises	Bed pushups

a. The type of assisted ambulation device depends on the disabled person's limitations.

b. Crutches are used for persons with limitations of lower extremity function but who have full use of upper extremities.

c. Tripod, quad, or broad-based canes are appropriate for persons with paralysis or weakness on 1 side of the body.

d. Walkers are for persons who have weakness in both upper and lower extremities or for older persons with hip problems, arthritis, or neuromuscular disease.

e. Wheelchairs may provide the only source of mobility for patients with spinal cord injuries. The wheelchair should be designed for good back support and should allow the patient to propel the chair.

3. Resumption of activities of daily living while in hospital
   a. The rehabilitation team encourages the person to perform self-care activities as soon as medically possible.
   b. The team helps the person become mobile and independent through teaching safe transfer and ambulation methods.
   c. The person is placed in an upright position if possible.
   d. The person should be placed in a sitting or squatting position, if possible, for defecation.
   e. If the person's urinary function must be managed through a bladder program, the nurse teaches this self-care method.
   f. Assistive devices are provided for self-care skills and ambulation.

Preventing and Treating Complications and Deformities

1. Positioning
   a. Prevent complications such as skin breakdown and contracture by proper and frequent changes of position. Patients who cannot turn themselves should be turned every 2 hours. Disabled persons confined to wheelchairs should be taught to raise their buttocks from the chair for 10 to 15 seconds every 15 minutes; this is very important for patients with spinal cord injuries.

NURSE ADVISORY

Generally, nurses should not lift more than 35 percent of their body weight without assistance. For example, a 60-kg (132-pound) nurse should not lift greater than 21 kg (46 pounds) alone.

   b. Position changes stimulate circulation and lung expansion and alleviate pressure. Procedure 7–2 illustrates recommended procedures for safely lifting and positioning immobile patients.
   c. Check correct body alignment from head to toe by drawing an imaginary line from the chin to the sym-

physis pubis. If the line is straight, the patient is in correct alignment.

   d. Special equipment is used to foster correct positioning and maintain correct body alignment (Procedure 7–3).
      (1) Positioning aids may be developed from supplies on the nursing unit or from the person's home.
      (2) Aids such as splints may be ordered by the physiatrist and fitted by the occupational therapist. For the patient with a lumbar spinal injury, a back brace may be prescribed to help stabilize the spine while it heals.
      (3) Pillows are used by the nurse to position, stabilize, or support a pressure area. A folded towel or bath blankets may be substituted.
      (4) The nurse can make a trochanter roll from a bath blanket or flannel sheet. The roll is used to prevent outward rotation of the hip when the client is supine. The nurse should place trochanter rolls under the patient's hip and thighs to form a roll along the outer aspect of the thighs.
      (5) Foot supports include blanket-covered boxes, resting leg splints, or high-top sneakers. These supports serve as alternatives to a footboard.
      (6) Hand rolls can be devised by the nurse from soft rubber balls. Hand rolls are used to position the hand in a slightly flexed position.
      (7) Splints may be used to support wrists, thumbs, and fingers, especially for those persons who have moderate or severe spasticity.
      (8) Mechanical beds and turning frames facilitate the turning of disabled persons and changing their position. Examples include Stryker Wedge Frames, Stryker CircOlectric beds, ROTO REST oscillating beds, and Air-fluidized beds.

NURSE ADVISORY

When working with obese patients, the following equipment may be used.
- Extra large, or thigh, blood pressure cuff
- "Big Boy" bed
- Heavy duty wheelchair
- Extra large hospital gown
- Hoyer lift
- Scales—clients weighing more than 350 pounds probably have to be weighed on commercial or loading dock scales.

2. Preventing external hip rotation
   a. External hip rotation is a complication of bed rest in which the hip rotates outward while patients are on their back.
   b. A trochanter roll is placed from the crest of the ileum to the midthigh area and a footboard is placed while the patient is in a dorsal position.
3. Preventing foot drop (plantar flexion)
   a. Foot drop results from muscular contractures in the Achilles tendon and maintenance of the foot in this position as a result of muscle spasticity (excess tonus), paralysis with flaccidity (decreased tonus), or me-

Procedure 7–2
Lifting Immobilized Patients from Bed

Definitions/Purposes	One or more nurses or helpers move a patient out of bed to a wheelchair or gurney. Proper lifting reduces the amount of work required and helps ensure safe body mechanics for the patient and nurse during the transfer.
Contraindications/Cautions	When using mechanical devices, become familiar with the manufacturer's recommendations for safe use and practice under supervision until you are comfortable with the procedure. Prior to transfer, make sure wheels are locked and prevent rolling by bracing the chair or bed against a wall. Avoid tension on any tubes during the transfer. If the patient is very heavy, obtain additional help.
Learning/Teaching Guidelines	Encourage the patient to do as much as possible to assist. Teach correct body alignment and body mechanics to avoid future injury.

Preliminary Activities

Assessment/Planning	• Review chart for diagnosis and activity orders, presence of skin lesions, bone disorders, and so on. • Plan type and method of move. • Determine the number of helpers needed. • Clear the area of clutter to provide working space. • Make sure equipment works before using it.
Equipment	• High-low bed, if available • Bath blanket • Hoyer lift • Wheelchair or gurney
Preparation	• Review equipment and plan the move. • Fan-fold linen to the foot of the bed. • Unhook urinary drainage bags, clamp nasogastric tubes and move intravenous bags so that they will not be pulled during the transfer.
Procedure	Using a Hoyer lift for transfer

Action	Rationale/Discussion
1. Center the sling under the patient by rolling the patient side to side.	1. Assess sling placement under the patient for (a) equal distance from side to side and (b) support of the person's weight.
2. Widen base-adjusting lever and lock the lever.	2. A wide base of support gives greater stability.
3. Position lift base under the bed with the boom centered over the sling.	3. Weight balanced over the center of gravity is more stable.
4. While holding onto the boom, open the release valve and lower the boom enough to attach the sling.	4. The boom is kept from swinging and hitting the patient.
5. Attach the boom to the sling with straps or chains using an S hook. The shorter arm of the strap goes closer to the client's back.	5. The S hook faces away from the patient to avoid scratching injuries. The sling forms a bucket seat. Make sure attachments are secure and the patient is centered in the sling.
6. Direct the patient to cross arms over chest or grasp straps.	6. This position provides a sense of security and keeps hands from being injured during the lift.
7. Close the release valve; pump up the level enough for the sling to clear the bed.	7. Assess the patient's balance in the sling. Lower and readjust if necessary.
8. The first helper guides the lift parallel with the bed, using steering bars while the second helper lifts the patient's legs off the bed and steadies the sling.	8. Use of 2 helpers increases safety. Heels may rub on sheets if they are not supported.
9. Move the wheelchair between the base support legs and lock wheels.	9. Minimize the distance that the patient must be transported in the sling.
10. The first helper slowly releases the valve to lower the boom while the second helper guides the patient into the chair.	10. Release pressure slowly. The patient may be startled if the boom lowers too quickly.

P

Procedure 7–2

(continued)

Three-Person Carry from Bed to Stretcher

Action	Rationale/Discussion
1. Position the stretcher at a right angle to the head or foot of the bed.	1. Such positioning allows for carrying the patient the least possible distance.
2. Raise the bed to match gurney height and lock wheels on the bed and stretcher.	2. Equalizing height minimizes bending to move the patient. Locking wheels prevents accidental shifts and maximizes safety.
3. Three persons work together to shift the patient to the side of bed.	3. Shared work minimizes strain. The patient's arms are crossed to prevent dragging.
4. Three persons arrange themselves alongside of the patient to support the head and shoulders and the hips and legs.	4. The strongest person holds a male patient's head or a female patient's hips.
5. Helpers slide their arms under the patient and, on an agreed signal, roll the patient toward their chests on their arms, keeping elbows on bed.	5. Weight is brought close to the center of gravity and elbows are used as a fulcrum.
6. Helpers step backward as a unit, pivot toward the gurney, and move to the stretcher.	6. Moving as a unit maintains the patient's body alignment and prevents injury.
7. Helpers place elbows on the gurney's edge and slowly lower their forearms to place the patient on the center of it.	7. Weight is kept in the center of the support, and movement of the patient's weight is controlled.

Final Activities

Cover the patient with a bath blanket for warmth and modesty. Raise the side rails of the gurney. Remind the patient to keep arms inside the gurney or wheelchair while it is moving.

chanical (positional) restriction of motion. Mechanical restriction of motion can result when immobilized patients lie supine for a long period of time with the weight of bed covers on their feet forcing the toes down and the ankles into a position of plantar flexion.

   b. Foot drop is most common among immobile patients.

   c. Patients who wear high-top tennis shoes can keep their feet at right angles to the legs in bed.

   d. Trochanter rolls are applied to keep the legs in neutral position.

   e. The patient should perform flexion and extension exercises frequently.

4. Preventing skin breakdown and pressure sore formation

   a. Skin breakdown is a serious threat to disabled persons who have had a sudden change of health status, altered mobility, or a major change in nutritional status.

   b. The patient should be continually assessed for general physical condition, mobility, sensory perception, diaphoresis, nutrition, and existing skin breakdown.

   c. To maintain skin integrity, friction, shearing, and undue pressure over bony prominences should be avoided.

      (1) Friction is damage caused by skin rubbing against a surface.

      (2) Shearing is damage caused by tissue layers sliding against each other under the pressure of gravity

(Fig. 7–6). It is a common problem for wheelchair-bound patients and patients slumped in bed.

      (3) Pressure is force exerted on an area. Pressure causes ischemia (deficiency of blood flow to an area due to constriction or obstruction of a blood

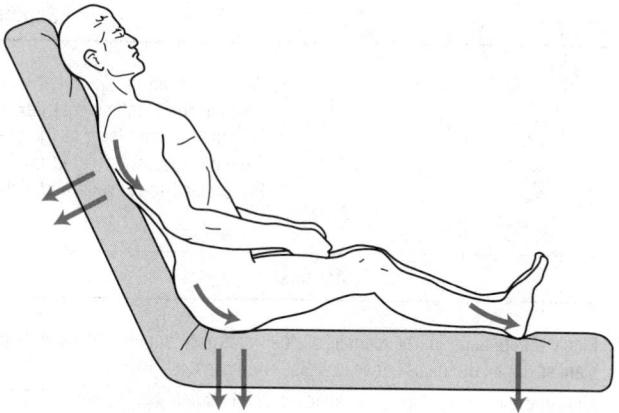

Figure 7–6. Shearing forces pull tissue layers apart when tissues nearer the bone slide downward and forward, whereas tissue layers nearer the skin tend to be held in place by friction between skin and sheets. (Redrawn from Bolander VB [ed]. *Sorensen and Luckmann's Basic Nursing*. 3rd ed. Philadelphia: WB Saunders, 1994, p 742.)

Procedure 7–3
Positioning Immobilized Patients in Bed

Definitions/Purposes — A person is placed in a safe position with correct body alignment to prevent or minimize the complications of immobility.

Contraindications/Cautions — Patients need to move at least every 2 hours to prevent skin breakdown and contractures. Use mechanical assist devices as needed or obtain help if the patient is very heavy. Two or more persons are needed to move patients with spinal injuries because the spine must be aligned at all times. Sheets must be clean, dry, and wrinkle-free. Be careful not to dislodge tubes or intravenous lines when moving the patient.

Learning/Teaching Guidelines — Have the patient help as much as possible to increase muscle strength. Explain what will be done and how, even if the patient is unconscious. If the patient is likely to be bedridden for a prolonged period, teach family members as well as the patient the principles of preventing complications of immobility. Encourage the patient to report any discomfort or difficulty breathing.

Preliminary Activities

Assessment/Planning
- Review diagnosis and activity orders.
- Assess mobility level and limitations of movement.
- Assess level of consciousness and ability to cooperate.
- Decide what position the patient should assume, based on turning schedule (see Fig. 7–8).
- Obtain helpers and equipment if required.

Equipment
- Clean, dry linens and gown
- Turning sheet
- Side rails
- Pillows of various sizes
- Bath blanket
- Incontinence pad, if necessary
- Clean, high-top shoes for supine positioning

Preparation of the Patient
- Discuss with the patient and helpers how the move will be done.
- Provide privacy, avoid drafts, preserve the patient's modesty.
- Adjust the bed to working height and lock wheels.
- Cover the patient with the bath blanket and fan-fold the top sheet.
- Lower the head of the bed to a flat position if the patient is able to tolerate it.
- Clear the bed of positioning devices and change soiled linens if required. Place the turning sheet under the patient if needed.

Supine Position

1. Keep the head in alignment with the spine.
2. Position the trunk so that flexion of the hips is minimal.
3. Flex the person's arm at the elbow with hands resting on the abdomen.
4. Patient's toes are pointed up.
5. Place small towel rolls under the greater trochanters in the hip joints.

Actions	Rationale/Discussion
1. Place the patient in the center of the mattress, supine. Place a bath blanket under the hips, between waist and knees.	1. Placement of linens and pad should be done first to avoid moving the patient later.
2. Align the shoulders, hips, and knees on both sides.	2. Proper alignment reduces muscle strain.
3. Roll the ends of the folded bath blanket under and wedge them under the thighs to maintain hip extension with a slight separation of the legs.	3. This trochanter roll prevents external rotation of the hips. Separating the legs keeps the skin surfaces from chafing against each other.
4. Place a pillow under the patient's head, neck, and shoulders.	4. The pillow should support the cervical curvature without causing flexion of the neck.
5. Place the patient's upper arms on a small pillow or rolled towel and the lower arms on a larger pillow.	5. Venous drainage of the hands is promoted and rubbing of elbows on the sheets is prevented.

Procedure 7–3

(continued)

Actions	Rationale/Discussion
6. Place splints on wrists and hands if needed.	6. Wrists and hands are kept in functional position.
7. Apply high-top shoes and lace firmly. Place a pillow under the patient's ankles and lower legs.	7. Functional position of the feet is maintained. Heels are kept off the bed and venous drainage is promoted.

Side-Lying Position

1. Keep the head in alignment with the spine.
2. Keep the body in alignment and do not twist it.
3. Place the upper hip joint slightly forward and support it with a pillow in a position of slight abduction.
4. Support the flexed arm with a pillow.

Actions	Rationale/Discussion
1. Remove positioning devices and assess skin.	1. When the patient lies on one side, some skin is not visible.
2. Lower the side rail and move the patient toward the near side of the bed. The patient will turn toward the far side.	2. Moving the patient to the side of the bed allows the patient to be centered on the mattress when turned.
3. Raise the rail and go to the other side. Abduct the near shoulder approximately 90 degrees and flex the elbow.	3. The patient does not roll onto the arm during the turn.
4. Gently grasp the patient's shoulder and the thigh just above the knee, pulling the patient toward you.	4. Pulling is easier than pushing.
5. Adjust the head pillow. Place a pillow between the patient's arms and another under the upper knee.	5. Pillow placement allows chest expansion and prevents internal rotation of the shoulder. Bony knees do not rub together and cross-adduction of the hip is prevented.

Prone Position

1. Turn the patient's head laterally and place it in alignment with the rest of the body.
2. Arms are abducted and externally rotated at the shoulder joint; flex the elbows.
3. Place a small, flat support under the pelvis.
4. Lower extremities remain neutral.
5. Suspend the toes over the edge of the mattress.

Actions	Rationale/Discussion
1. Assemble at least 3 persons: 1 on each side of the bed and 1 to support the neck and head. Lower the side rails. Remove pillows and positioning devices. Grasp the lift sheet firmly next to the patient's body and move the patient down to the foot of the bed.	1. Using more helpers and a lift sheet helps prevent shearing injury to the skin.
2. Move the patient to the side of the bed opposite the planned turn.	2. There is more room for the patient to turn safely.
3. Place pillows next to the patient in the following places: (a) the lower chest and abdomen for women, waist to pubis for men, (b) thighs below the hips, (c) lower legs above the ankles. Use 2 pillows if the feet cannot hang off the end of the bed.	3. Pillows maintain alignment and support weight. (a) Breasts and scrotum are protected from pressure while the lumbar curve is minimized. (b) Knees are kept off sheets. (c) Knees and spine are kept from hyperextension.
4. Place arms along the patient's sides with palms next to thighs.	4. Arm injuries are prevented during the turn.
5. Stand on side toward which the patient will turn. Bring the patient's far leg over the near leg.	5. This position allows for good body mechanics and easier turning.
6. Gently grasp the patient's shoulder and hip. On the count of 3, pull the patient toward you, over the arm and face down as assistants control the patient's head and neck during the turn.	6. Pulling is easier than pushing. Grasping the body gives more control during the turn. Moving as a unit keeps the body in alignment.

(continued)

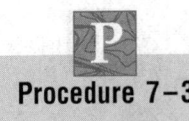

Procedure 7–3

(continued)

Actions	Rationale/Discussion
7. Check that the patient is breathing. Position a small pillow under the head. Turn the head to the side if necessary.	7. Ensure that the mattress is not occluding airway. This positioning allows for drainage of secretions and cushioning of the face.
8. Abduct both shoulders 90 degrees. Place small rolls under the shoulders and axillae. Apply wrist or hand splints if needed.	8. Joint motion is maintained by preventing adduction. Hands and wrists are kept in functional position.
9. Check body alignment. Feet should hang over the end of the mattress or be supported by pillows to allow a 90-degree flexion at the ankle.	9. Correct alignment promotes comfort and reduced muscle strain, and prevents foot drop.
10. Rearrange the patient's shoulder and arm position periodically.	10. Range of joint motion is increased, and the patient is more comfortable.
11. Frequently check on the patient in this position.	11. Some patients find this position uncomfortable for longer than a short time and dyspnea may develop.

Final Activities

Check for correct body alignment. Make sure any tubes are not occluded. Check linens for wrinkles and straighten if necessary. Assess exposed skin. Ascertain the patient's level of comfort. Place the call bell within reach. Raise the side rails. Discard any soiled linens. Document assessment data.

vessel) if it exceeds the maximum capillary pressure in the skin (approximately 35 mm Hg) for a prolonged period of time.

   d. To prevent new pressure sores, promote healing of existing ones and avert necrosis of deeper structures.

     (1) Examine skin surfaces, especially bony prominences and other areas at risk of breakdown (Fig. 7–7). Skin surfaces should be examined at least every 2 hours when the patient must be repositioned or turned.

     (2) Continuously monitor the patient's position using a device such as that shown in Figure 7–8.

     (3) Change bed linen as often as necessary to keep it dry and free of wrinkles and foreign objects that may injure the skin.

     (4) Elevate the feet with pillows under the calves to avoid putting pressure on the heels.

     (5) Use incontinence measures for any patient who is incontinent of stool or urine.

     (6) See Table 7–7 for techniques of pressure ulcer management related to the stage of the ulcer.

     (7) Keep records of all sores and their treatment.

5. Bowel and bladder management

   a. Patients with physical disabilities such as spinal cord injury may experience bowel incontinence, bladder incontinence, or both.

   b. Urinary tract problems can lead to life-threatening situations in the disabled person such as sepsis, urinary retention, or shock.

   c. Persons who do not manage bowel care may experience constipation or incontinence.

   d. Bowel management includes fluid and diet management, rectal digital stimulation, and use of supposi-

tories. Basic components common to all bowel programs include a "clear" bowel to start, timing, appropriate diet and fluid intake, exercise, privacy, and positioning.

   e. For the disabled person with diarrhea, the nurse should first check the patient for an impaction. If the person is impacted, the basic components of bowel management should be initiated. If impaction is not the cause, other causes should be investigated, such as disease or medication. If the person experiences bowel incontinence, the nurse offers emotional support. The person may be embarrassed or anxious (see Chapter 27).

   f. Bladder management includes fluid management, a bladder training program, intermittent catheterizations, and use of indwelling catheters (see Chapter 26). Special equipment needed by disabled persons for bowel or bladder elimination includes hand bars, raised toilets, and other supplies such as catheters.

Applying the Nursing Process

NURSING DIAGNOSIS: Ineffective individual coping R/T powerlessness

1. *Expected outcomes:* Within a specified period of time, the person should be able to do the following:

   a. Participate in self-care (see Learning/Teaching Guidelines for Self-Care in Disability)

   b. Participate in long-term and short-term goal setting

  c. Make some personal decisions
  d. Evaluate self for strengths and assets
  e. Evaluate past successful coping strategies
2. *Nursing interventions*
  a. Provide an environment conducive to independence (e.g., place items within reach and encourage the person in self-care activities).
  b. Establish rapport with the patient.
  c. Help the patient identify past successful coping strategies.

SUPINE

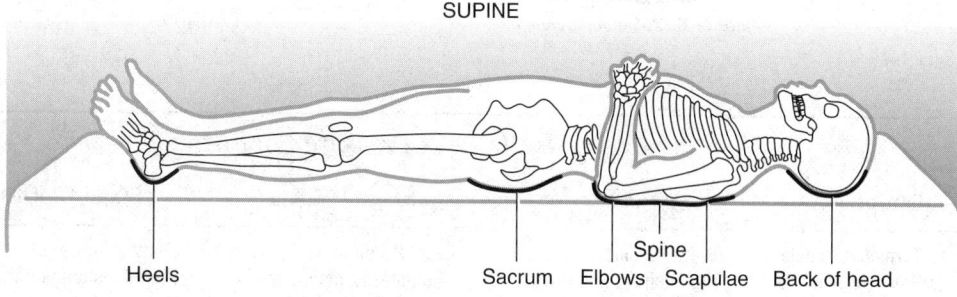

SIDE-LYING

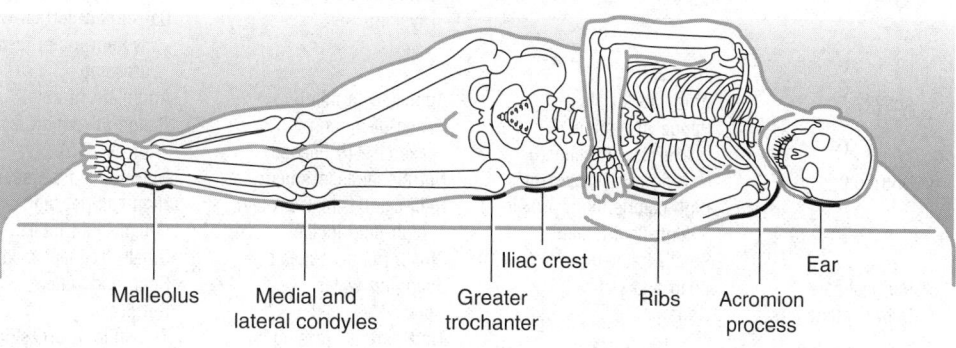

Figure 7–7. Common pressure ulcer sites (supine, side-lying, and prone). (From Bolander VB [ed]. *Sorensen and Luckmann's Basic Nursing.* 3rd ed. Philadelphia: WB Saunders, 1994, p 742.)

PRONE

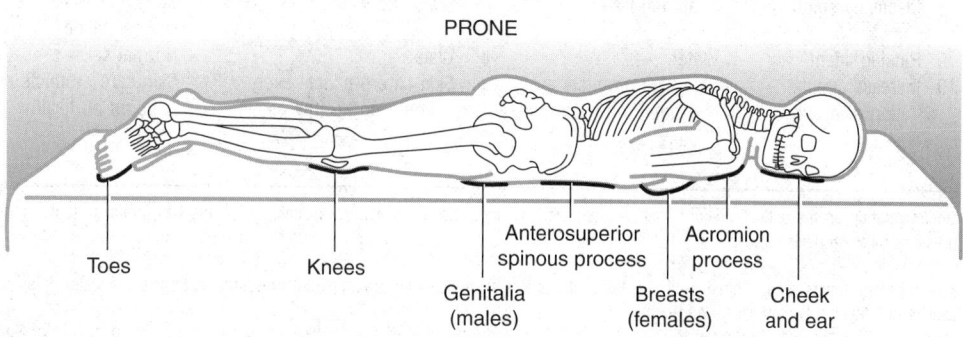

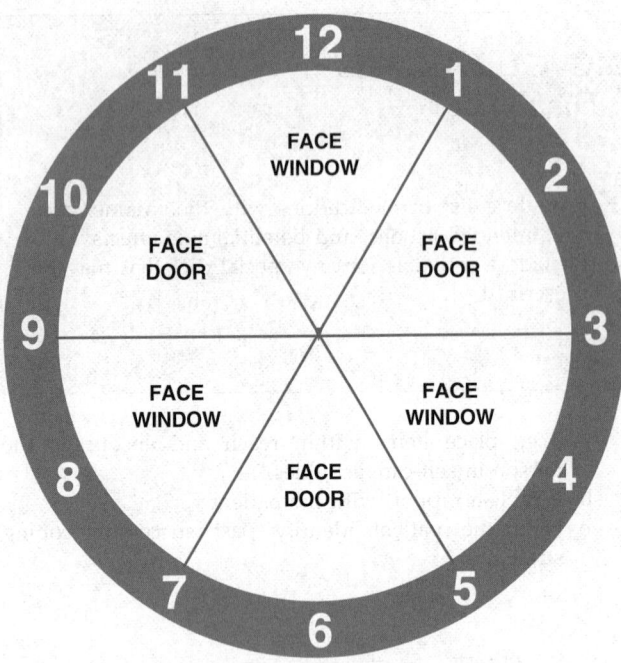

Figure 7–8. Positioning clock.

d. Facilitate the person's self-assessment of strengths and weaknesses.
e. Assist the person in identifying realistic long- and short-term goals.
f. Focus on areas where the patient has control of outcomes.

NURSING DIAGNOSIS: Body image disturbance R/T change in appearance or function of the person

3. *Expected outcomes:* After counseling, the person should do the following:
   a. Verbalize acceptance of appearance
   b. Implement new coping patterns
   c. Demonstrate willingness and ability to assume self-care responsibilities
   d. Initiate new or reestablish existing support systems
4. *Nursing interventions*
   a. Establish a trusting relationship with the patient.
   b. Promote social interaction.
   c. Assess the meaning of the loss for the patient and family.

Table 7–7. Pressure Sore Management

Plan of Action	Stage I Ulcer	Stage II Ulcer	Stage III Ulcer	Stage IV Ulcer
1. Turning schedule	Every 2 hours	Every 2 hours	Every 2 hours	Every 2 hours
2. Pressure relief devices	High-density foam mattress	High-density foam mattress, Roho mattress	High-density foam mattress, Roho mattress	Air-fluidized bed, Roho mattress
3. Dressing treatment	Occlusive dressing Transparent dressing	Transparent dressing Occlusive wafer dressing Carrington dermal wound system	Transparent dressing Occlusive wafer dressing Wet to dry dressing Carrington dermal wound system moist-to-moist dressing	Wet to dry dressing Transparent dressing Surgical flap/Carrington dermal wound system moist-to-moist dressing
4. Activity	Ambulate (if able) Range-of-motion exercise (if needed)	Ambulate (if able) Range-of-motion exercise (if needed)	Ambulate (if able) Range-of-motion exercise (if needed)	Ambulate (if able) Range-of-motion exercise (if needed)
5. Nutrition	Nutritional assessment High-calorie, high-protein, high-fluid intake Small, frequent meals	Nutritional assessment High-calorie, high-protein, high-fluid intake Small, frequent meals	Nutritional assessment High-calorie, high-protein, high-fluid intake Small, frequent meals	Nutritional assessment High-calorie, high-protein, high-fluid intake Small, frequent meals
6. Perineal care	Soap and water	Soap and water	Soap and water	Soap and water
7. Débridement	None	None Transparent dressing*† Mechanical*† Occlusive wafer dressing*†	Surgical Transparent dressing*† Mechanical/chemical*† Occlusive wafer dressing*†	Surgical Transparent dressing*† Mechanical/chemical*†
8. Cleansing solution	Soap and water	Soap and water	Soap and water Normal saline	Soap and water Normal saline
9. Rinsing agent	Water	Water	Normal saline	Normal saline
10. Increase circulation of healthy skin	Skin care products every 2 hours on healthy tissue	Skin care products every 2 hours on healthy tissue	Skin care products every 2 hours on healthy tissue	Skin care products every 2 hours on healthy tissue Consider silver sulfadiazine in the wound

Documentation on the patient's record shall include location, stage, size (in centimeters), color of wound bed, drainage (color/odor/consistency), presence of sinus tract, and pressure-relieving device in use.
* Not available.
† Skin care products—i.e., United, Hollister, Bard, etc. (cleanser, moisturizer). Transparent dressings and occlusive wafer dressings provide a moist wound environment that assists in softening wound eschar and debris.
From Dallas County Hospital District Nursing Service. *Policy and Procedure Manual.* Dallas, TX: Dallas County Hospital District Nursing Service, 1993.

d. Facilitate the grieving process.

e. Encourage family members to share feelings about the loss with the person.

f. Encourage the person to obtain a prosthesis as soon as possible.

g. Encourage the person to look at, touch, and care for the operative site.

NURSING DIAGNOSIS: Knowledge deficit R/T medical treatment regimen

5. *Expected outcomes:* By the time of discharge, the patient should be able to do the following:

a. Demonstrate proper use of medications by stating the names, doses, and purposes of each medication, and by stating the side effects that necessitate medical attention

b. State signs and symptoms of infection or complications that require medical follow-up

c. Demonstrate understanding of diet by choosing appropriate foods from a list

d. Demonstrate beginning competence at prescribed exercise program

e. Demonstrate care of prosthesis or operative site

f. Demonstrate skills involved in the treatment regimen such as self-catheterization, suctioning, and transfer from bed to wheelchair

g. State the frequency of follow-up visits

6. *Nursing interventions*

a. Provide the patient with a list of medications, doses, purposes, and side effects.

b. Review the medications with the patient each time they are given.

c. Assist the person with menu choices.

d. Assist the person with the exercise program as appropriate.

e. Demonstrate care of the prosthesis or operative site, then ask for a return demonstration.

NURSING DIAGNOSIS: Risk for disuse syndrome R/T loss of function in the affected part

7. *Expected outcomes:* By the time of discharge, the patient should be able to demonstrate the following:

a. Intact skin and tissue integrity

b. Adequate or maximal pulmonary function

c. Maximal peripheral blood flow

d. Full range of motion

e. Bowel, bladder, and renal function within normal limits

f. Use of social contacts and activities when possible

8. *Nursing interventions*

a. Identify causative agent for disuse.

b. Promote optimal respiratory function.

c. Assist the patient in maintaining usual bowel patterns.

d. Prevent pressure ulcers.

e. Promote venous return.

f. Maintain limb mobility and prevent contractures.

g. Prevent urinary stasis and calculi formation.

h. Reduce and monitor bone demineralization.

i. Encourage sharing of feelings regarding prolonged immobility.

j. Encourage the person to make as many independent decisions as possible.

k. Encourage the person to make use of support systems.

NURSING DIAGNOSIS: Self-care deficit R/T impaired physical mobility

9. *Expected outcomes:* Before discharge, the person should be able to do the following:

a. Identify preferences in self-care activities (time, products, location)

b. Demonstrate optimal hygiene after assistance

c. Participate physically or verbally in feeding, dressing, toileting, and bathing activities

10. *Nursing interventions*

a. Assess the patient for causative or contributing factors.

b. Promote optimal participation.

c. Promote self-esteem and independence.

d. Evaluate the patient's ability to participate in each self-care activity.

NURSING DIAGNOSIS: Altered family processes R/T long-term change in health status of a family member

11. *Expected outcomes:* By the time of discharge, the family members should be able to do the following:

a. Verbalize feelings frequently to health care providers and each other

b. Participate in the care of the ill family member

c. Facilitate the return of the ill family member from having a sick role to a well role

d. Maintain a system of mutual support for each family member

e. Identify available appropriate resources

12. *Nursing interventions*

a. Assess the situation for causative and contributing factors.

b. Create a supportive environment for patients and family members.

c. Facilitate family strengths.

d. Promote cohesiveness.

e. Encourage sharing of feelings between the family members and the patient.

f. Assist the family with appraisal of the situation.

g. Provide the family with anticipatory guidance as the illness progresses.

h. Discuss implications of long-term care for the person and the family.

NURSING DIAGNOSIS: Altered skin integrity R/T pressure ulcer on the sacrum

13. *Expected outcomes:* After intervention, the person should have the following:
    a. An acceptable level of comfort
    b. A decrease in pressure ulcer size with formation of a scar before discharge
14. *Nursing interventions*
    a. Keep patients off their back as much as possible.
    b. Keep patients clean and dry.
    c. Follow pressure ulcer protocol for wound care procedures.
    d. Culture the wound and administer antibiotics as ordered.

◼ DISCHARGE PLANNING AND TEACHING

Fitting the Plan to the Person

1. At the time of discharge from an acute care facility, disabled persons fall into the following categories:
   a. Discharged directly to home with extensive home health care resources required
   b. Admitted to a rehabilitation center
   c. Admitted to an extended care facility
2. At the time of discharge from a rehabilitation facility, disabled persons fall into the following categories:
   a. Discharged directly to home with little support needed
   b. Discharged to home with some kind of community or family support needed
   c. Discharged to some type of residential home

Developing the Plan

1. Discharge planning begins the moment a patient is admitted to a care facility, and it continues throughout the patient's stay.
2. Discharge planning should be a collaborative effort by the rehabilitation team.
   a. Nurses must be aware of options available for the patient after discharge and must communicate these to the person.
   b. The social worker is often the coordinator of social services. Social services include those offered by rehabilitation agencies to assist the person and family with financial problems, income replacement, medical coverage for rehabilitation and equipment needs, home structural modifications, transportation, extended care placement, and recreational needs.
   c. Nurses coordinate community referrals to community nursing agencies to ensure that nursing services are not interrupted when the patient is discharged back to the community. This follow-up care may include private physicians, public health departments, or home health agencies that provide nursing care, physical therapy, or other services needed for physical care.
3. The 1st step in discharge planning is to gather data on the disabled person's
   a. Mental status

b. Coping abilities, especially regarding new situations such as use of canes or braces
c. Physical status, including physical assessment data, review of systems, physical examination findings, and activity level
d. Functional status, including self-care ability and management of activities of daily living, and assistive devices required
e. Family for their ability and willingness to participate in the rehabilitation program and self-care programs
f. Medical treatment plan, including medications, diet, bladder and bowel programs, and skin care protocols

HOME CARE STRATEGIES

Prevention of Pressure Ulcers

A pressure ulcer is caused when part of the body is pressed continuously against a hard surface, such as a mattress or chair. Prevention is the key to eliminating multiple problems resulting from the development of skin breakdown. The following risk factors increase the development of skin breakdown, especially in the home setting.
- Bed or chair confinement
- Inability to move
- Loss of bowel or bladder control
- Poor nutrition
- Lowered mental awareness
- Absent, inconsistent, or uninformed primary caregiver

The presence of a knowledgeable caregiver or family member to assist with a program for the prevention of skin breakdown is critical. A caregiver can be instructed about the techniques for preventing pressure and about the protocols to care for the specific skin problems of the patient. The team approach, involving the patient and caregiver along with the professional home care staff, can make a dramatic difference in achieving positive outcomes.

1. For those confined to a bed or chair, there are special mattresses and chair cushions that contain foam, air, gel, or water to assist with pressure relief.
2. Teach patients to reposition using a schedule that will fit into their daily routine. Show family members how to maintain a desired position for a specified amount of time and keep instructions simple and specific.
3. Teach the patient and family about the use of elbow and heel protectors and the correct way to apply them.
4. Use a protective dressing (e.g., hydrocolloid gel or transparent dressing) when needed, for specific areas prone to breaking down or areas of previous difficulty.

Although there are many factors that prevent skin breakdown, pressure relief is one of the most critical. It should be the primary focus of home health care nurses' instructions as they teach patients and families to take an active role in their own care.

4. Discharge planning is part of early goal setting in the rehabilitation process; it promotes continuity of care and is critical to the success of controlling inpatient length of stay.
5. Team members communicate the patient's discharge needs and convey that information to the team member who is coordinating the discharge.
6. One team member coordinates transfer to an extended care facility or discharge to home.
7. The team makes referrals to appropriate and available resources.

LEARNING/TEACHING GUIDELINES
for Patients with Spinal Cord Injury Who Are Being Discharged Home

General Overview

1. Include the family when teaching the patient about spinal cord injury and self-care. Explain the rationale for all treatments and medications, and emphasize the potential consequences of noncompliance.
2. Consult with social services, and supply the patient with a list of available community resources and services that provide equipment for home use as well as home care nursing and housekeeping services.
3. Refer the patient to physical therapy for assistive devices designed to help the person maintain as much function as possible. Encourage the patient to continue in an exercise program and to perform weight-bearing activities after discharge home.
4. Arrange for a follow-up visit with the physician. Let the physician know if you have assessed that the patient is severely depressed about the spinal cord injury and needs psychiatric or sexual counseling.
5. Provide the patient and family with a telephone number to call if they have questions or concerns.

Instructions for Home Care

1. Encourage the patient to maintain an established elimination schedule. Remind the person that it is important to continue to follow the bowel retraining program and the bladder retraining program that was instituted during hospitalization.
2. Have a dietitian talk with the patient and family about the importance of drinking fluids (at least 8 glasses of fluid a day) and eating a diet high in bulk and roughage. These measures act to reduce constipation and impaction. Forcing fluids up to 2000 to 3000 ml helps to prevent kidney stones and urinary tract infections.

3. Urge the patient to avoid prolonged pressure on areas of the body that are prone to skin breakdown. Remind the patient and family to inspect pressure areas daily, to use repositioning techniques, to shift body weight when sitting in a wheelchair to prevent the shearing force, and to keep the skin clean and free from excessive moisture.
4. Instruct the patient in important safety measures. Because spinal cord injury results in sensory loss, the patient needs to avoid wearing ill-fitting shoes. Also, because of loss of sensation in the feet, the patient needs to receive regular foot and nail assessment and care.

    To prevent scalds from very hot shower or bath water, the temperature setting for the water heater at home needs to be lowered to around 41 to 46 degrees Celsius (105.8–114.8 degrees Fahrenheit). Also warn the person that hot water bottles and heating pads can severely burn individuals who suffer from sensory loss.
5. Remind the patient to avoid situations that can precipitate muscle spasms, for example, prolonged sitting, cold temperatures, and emotional upsets. Also touching the patient during position changes or treatments can cause spasms.
6. Review the signs of autonomic dysreflexia with the patient and family (see Chapter 37). Autonomic dysreflexia, which must be immediately treated as an acute medical emergency, can occur at any time, but is most common within 1 to 2 years after injury. The most common cause of autonomic dysreflexia is a distended bladder.
7. Teach the patient how to assess for and prevent deep vein thrombosis. Encourage the family or other home care providers to perform passive range-of-motion exercises on the limbs at least daily. The use of antiembolic socks also helps to prevent this complication.

8. The team communicates both verbally and in writing to referral agencies regarding the patient's status and needs.
9. The team disengages from patients and their families to promote their independence and transition back into the community.
10. For an example of discharge teaching for disabled people, see Learning/Teaching Guidelines for Patients with Spinal Cord Injury Who Are Being Discharged Home.

◼ *PUBLIC HEALTH CONSIDERATIONS*

Preventing Accidents

1. Nurses can provide and support educational programs that address alcohol and drug abuse, use of adult and child passenger restraint systems, safe handling of firearms, and prevention of falls and diving accidents.
2. As an educator, the nurse can assist in preventing traumatic and, perhaps, permanent disabilities.

Educating the Public

1. Practice is guided by the *Code for Nurses with Interpretive Statements* (Box 7–3).
2. Nurses can provide public education programs about a variety of disabilities.
3. Nurses can incorporate the disabled into these programs to give the public an opportunity to interact with the disabled.
4. Nurses can speak at service club meetings.
5. Nurses can educate the public on accident prevention.

BOX 7–3. American Nurses Association Code for Nurses

1. The nurse provides services with respect for human dignity and the uniqueness of the client, unrestricted by considerations of social or economic status, personal attributes, or the nature of health problems.
2. The nurse safeguards the client's right to privacy by judiciously protecting information of a confidential nature.
3. The nurse acts to safeguard the client and the public when health care and safety are affected by the incompetent, unethical, or illegal practice of any person.
4. The nurse assumes responsibility and accountability for individual nursing judgments and actions.
5. The nurse maintains competence in nursing.
6. The nurse exercises informed judgment and uses individual competence and qualifications as criteria in seeking consultation, accepting responsibilities, and delegating nursing activities to others.
7. The nurse participates in activities that contribute to the ongoing development of the profession's body of knowledge.
8. The nurse participates in the profession's efforts to implement and improve standards of nursing.
9. The nurse participates in the profession's efforts to establish and maintain conditions of employment conducive to high quality nursing care.
10. The nurse participates in the profession's effort to protect the public from misinformation and misrepresentation and to maintain the integrity of nursing.
11. The nurse collaborates with members of the health professions and other citizens in promoting community and national efforts to meet the health needs of the public.

From American Nurses Association. *Code for Nurses with Interpretive Statements*. Washington, DC: Author, 1985, p 1.

6. Nurses can actively participate in professional organizations.
7. Nurses can act as a community advocate to promote increased environmental accessibility and decreased architectural barriers for disabled persons.
8. Nurses can attend public hearings regarding issues affecting people with disabilities and serve on committees when possible.

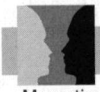 **CLINICAL CONTROVERSIES**

Many times a physician will write a do not resuscitate (DNR) order for a person who is terminally ill or has suffered a critical injury. Do not resuscitate means that if the person goes into cardiac or respiratory arrest, resuscitation should not be initiated. This order prevents the staff from performing cardiopulmonary resuscitation on a patient for whom resuscitation would only prolong death. Policies vary among institutions regarding the frequency with which these orders must be renewed and how they should be documented. In some states, the physician is not legally required to get permission from the patient or the family to write such an order. Ethically, it is best for such a decision to be made with the full cooperation of all parties.

Sometimes the physician cannot get the person or family to agree to a DNR order, even though such an order is medically sound. In such cases, the doctor may tell the nursing staff to do a "Code Gray" or "Slow Code." This means that when the person experiences cardiac arrest, the staff is to wait for some prolonged time before notifying the code team. The intended result is that the patient will be unable to be resuscitated. There are ethical problems with this approach. First, the doctor is asking the nurses to conspire in keeping the family ignorant of what is planned. Second, the nurses may be put in jeopardy for failing to perform cardiopulmonary resuscitation in a timely fashion when the patient has no legal DNR order. Third, the family will be paying for a resuscitation attempt that was not made in good faith.

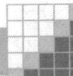 **LEGAL AND ETHICAL CONSIDERATIONS**

The following is a brief history of statutes effected to help disabled persons.

1. Economic Opportunity Acts (1964 and 1974)
   a. Initiated the Head Start program
   b. Included children with disabilities in 1974
2. Rehabilitation Act (1973 and 1978)
   a. Provided funding for vocational rehabilitation
   b. Provided funding for affirmative action efforts to employ qualified disabled persons
   c. Provided funding for independent living programs
3. Americans with Disabilities Act (1990)
   a. Mandated nondiscrimination in the employment of persons with disabilities
   b. Mandated barrier-free transportation in systems and buildings

9. Nurses can contact legislators to support such funding programs as those for transferring disabled persons to independent living centers or those that supplement income for persons with disabilities that inhibit work performance.

Legal Rights

1. A number of federal laws protect the rights of disabled persons in the United States.
2. Main rights of the disabled persons invoke several legal considerations and patient rights (Box 7–4).
3. Despite laws, disabled people still encounter job discrimination and access problems.
4. Nurses' guidelines for conduct to help the disabled obtain their rights include the following:
   a. Practice according to the *Code for Nurses with Interpretive Statements*
   b. Maintain patient confidentiality
   c. Act as a patient advocate
   d. Deliver care in a nondiscriminatory manner
   e. Preserve the disabled client's autonomy, dignity, and rights
   f. Ensure compliance with state laws
   g. Encourage the formation of ethics committees in rehabilitation settings

BOX 7–4. Main Rights of Disabled Persons

Right	Description
Informed consent	Consent is obtained from a patient after the person has been fully informed about the risks of either agreeing to or refusing to submit to an operation or procedure.
Living will	Living wills are recognized legal documents in 40 states and the District of Columbia. They allow persons to make their wishes known before hospitalization regarding medical treatment or conditions that may result in some incompetency.
Right to receive or refuse treatment	Those deemed competent have a constitutional right to refuse treatment. Their decision may be overruled in life-threatening situations.
Autonomy	Not being controlled by others.
Guardianship	A surrogate exercises rights for a minor or an incompetent adult.

Bibliography

Books

Andrews M, and Boyle JS (eds). *Transcultural Concepts in Nursing Care*. Philadelphia: JB Lippincott, 1995.

Black JM, and Matassarin-Jacobs E (eds). *Luckmann and Sorensen's Medical-Surgical Nursing: A Psychophysiologic Approach*. 4th ed. Philadelphia: WB Saunders, 1993.

Bolander VB (ed). *Sorensen and Luckmann's Basic Nursing: A Psychophysiologic Approach*. 3rd ed. Philadelphia: WB Saunders, 1994.

Brink PJ (ed). *Transcultural Nursing: A Book of Readings*. Englewood Cliffs, NJ: Prentice-Hall, 1979.

Carpenito LJ. *Nursing Diagnosis: Application to Clinical Practice*. Philadelphia: JB Lippincott, 1993.

Castiglia PT, and Harbin RE. *Child Health Care Process and Practice*. Philadelphia: JB Lippincott, 1992.

Charmaz K. *Good Days and Bad Days: The Self in Chronic Illness*. Newark, NJ: Rutgers University Press, 1993.

Dallas County Hospital District. *Physical Therapy Policy Manual*. Dallas, TX: Parkland Memorial Hospital, 1989.

Dallas County Hospital District Nursing Service. *Policy and Procedure Manual*. Dallas: Parkland Memorial Hospital, 1993.

Dittmar S. *Rehabilitation Nursing*. St. Louis: CV Mosby, 1989.

Dobson S. *Transcultural Nursing*. London: Scutari Press, 1991.

Ebersole P, and Hess P. *Toward Healthy Aging*. St. Louis: CV Mosby, 1994.

England DA. *Collaboration in Nursing*. Rockville, MD: Aspen, 1985.

Fraley AM. *Nursing and the Disabled*. Boston: Jones & Bartlett, 1992.

Fuller J, and Schaller-Ayers J. *Health Assessment*. Philadelphia: JB Lippincott, 1994.

Giger JN, and Davidhizar RE. *Transcultural Nursing Assessment and Intervention*. St. Louis: CV Mosby, 1991.

Hickey JV. *The Clinical Practice of Neurological and Neurosurgical Nursing*. Philadelphia: JB Lippincott, 1992.

Kozier B, Erb G, and Olivieri R. *Fundamentals of Nursing*. Redwood City, CA: Addison-Wesley, 1991.

Leininger MM. *Transcultural Nursing: Concepts, Theories and Practices*. New York: John Wiley & Sons, 1978.

Leininger MM (ed). *Culture Care Diversity and Universality: A Theory of Nursing*. New York: National League for Nursing Press, 1991.

Marinelli RP, Dell O, and Arthur E (eds). *The Psychological and Social Impact of Disability*. New York: Springer, 1991.

McCourt AE (ed). *The Specialty Practice of Rehabilitation Nursing: A Core Curriculum*. Skokie, IL: Rehabilitation Nursing Foundation, 1993.

Miller JF. *Coping with Chronic Illness*. Philadelphia: FA Davis, 1992.

Perry G, and Potter PA. *Clinical Nursing Skills and Techniques*. St. Louis: CV Mosby, 1990.

Rehabilitation Institute of Chicago Division of Nursing. *Rehabilitation Nursing Procedures Manual*. Rockville, MD: Aspen, 1990.

Samovar L, and Porter R. *Intercultural Communication*. Belmont, CA: Wadsworth, 1991.

Seidel HM, et al. *Mosby's Guide to Physical Examination*. St. Louis: Mosby-Year Book, 1995.

Sparks SM, and Taylor CM. *Nursing Diagnosis Reference Manual*. Springhouse, PA: Springhouse, 1991.

Spector RE. *Cultural Diversity in Health and Illness*. Norwalk, CT: Appleton & Lange, 1991.

Stanley M, and Beare PG. *Gerontological Nursing*. Philadelphia: FA Davis, 1995.

Suddarth DS. *Manual of Nursing Practice*. Philadelphia: JB Lippincott, 1991.

US Bureau of the Census. *Statistical Abstracts of the U.S.* 10th ed. Washington, DC: US Department of Commerce, 1988.

Wright LM, and Leahey M. *Families and Chronic Illness*. Springhouse, PA: Springhouse, 1987.

Chapters in Books and Journal Articles

Definitions and Incidence

Watson PG. The Americans with Disability Act: More rights for people with disabilities. *Rehabil Nurs* 15(6):325–328, 1990.

Transcultural Attitudes Toward Disability

Adams R, Briones E, and Rentfro A. Cultural consideration: Developing a nursing care delivery system for a Hispanic community. *Nurs Clin North Am* 27(1):107–117, 1992.

Barkauskas VH, et al. Cultural considerations in health assessment. *In* Stoltenberg-Allen K, Bauman L, and Darling-Fisher C. *Health and Physical Assessment*. St. Louis: CV Mosby, 1994.

Gellman W. Roots of prejudice against the handicapped. *J Rehabil* 25:4–6, 25, 1959.

Hammond DC. Cross cultural rehabilitation. *J Rehabil* 37:34–36, 44, 1971.

Hoeman SP. Cultural assessment in rehabilitation nursing practice. *Nurs Clin North Am* 24(1):277–289, 1989.

Kleinman A, Eisenberg L, and Good B. Culture, illness and care: Clinical lessons. Anthropologic and cross-cultural research. *Ann Intern Med* 88:251–258, 1978.

Morse JM. Transcultural nursing: Its substance and issues in research and knowledge. *Recent Adv Nurs Sci* 18:129–141, 1990.

Weller B. Nursing in a multicultural world. *Nurs Stand* 5(30):31–32, 1991.

Wenger A. Transcultural nursing and health care issues in urban and rural contexts. *J Transcult Nurs* 3(2):4–10, 1992.

Impact of Being Physically Disabled

Engel GL. Grief and grieving. *Am J Nurs* 64(9):93–98, 1964.

Assessing People with Disabilities

French GT, and Ledwell-Sifner K. A method for consistent documentation of pressure sores. *Rehabil Nursing* 16(4):204–207, 1991.

Juarez VJ. Interrator reliability of the Glasgow Coma Scale. *J Neurosci Nurs* 27(5):283–286, 1995.

Katz S, et al. Studies of illness in the aged. *JAMA* 185(12):914–919, 1963.

McCloskey JC. How to make the most of body image theory in nursing practice. *Nursing* 6(5):68–72, 1976.

Piper B, et al. The development of an instrument to measure the subjective dimension of fatigue. *In* Funk E, et al (eds). *Key Aspects of Comfort: Management of Pain, Fatigue and Nausea*. New York: Springer, 1989.

Ryden MB. Energy: A crucial consideration in the nursing process. *Nurs Forum* 16(1):71–80, 1977.

Venn MR, et al. The influence of timing and suppository use on efficiency and effectiveness of bowel training after a stroke. *Rehabil Nurs* 17(3):116–120, 1992.

Rehabilitation

Ackerman LL. Intervention related to neurologic care. *Nurs Clin North Am* 27(2):325–346, 1992.

Alywahby NF. Principles of teaching for individual learning of older adults. *Rehabil Nurs* 14(6):330–333, 1989.

Brillhart B, and Sills FB. Analysis of the roles and responsibilities of rehabilitation nursing staff. *Rehabil Nurs* 19(3):145–150, 1994.

Buchanan LC. A rehabilitation clinical nurse specialist: Evolution of the role in a home health setting. *Holistic Nurs Pract* 6(2):42–50, 1992.

Buckwalter KC, et al. Increasing communication ability of aphasic/dysarthric patients. *West J Nursing Res* 11(6):736–747, 1989.

Camara T. Community-based rehabilitation. *World Health* 48(5):4–5, 1995.

Gadow S. Existential advocacy: Philosophical foundations of nursing in ethical problems. *In* Murphy CP, and Hunter H (eds). *Ethical Problems in the Nurse-Patient Relationship*. Boston: Allyn & Bacon, 1983.

Goerdt A. Disability prevention and rehabilitation. *World Health* 48(5):4–5, 1995.

Harrison MB, et al. Practice guidelines for the prediction and prevention of pressure ulcers: Evaluating the evidence. *Appl Nurs Res* 9(1):9–17, 1996.

Hegeman KM. A care pattern for the family of a brain trauma client. *Rehabil Nurs* 13(5):254–262, 1988.

Janowski MJ. A road map for stroke recovery. *RN* 59(3):26–30, 1996.

Johnson BP. One family's experience with head injury: A phenomenological study. *J Neurosci Nurs* 27(2):113–118, 1995.

Kohnke MF. The nurse as advocate. *Am J Nurs* 80(11):2038–2040, 1980.

Palmer M, and Wyness MA. Positioning and handling: Important considerations in the care of the severely head-injured patient. *J Neurosci Nurs* 20(1):42–49, 1988.

Richmond TS, Metcalf J, and Daly, M. Requirements for nursing care services and associated costs in acute spinal cord injury. *J Neurosci Nurs* 27(1):47–51, 1996.

Rintala DH, et al. Family relationships and adaptation to spinal cord injury: A qualitative study. *Rehabil Nurs* 21(2):67–74, 1996.

Robinson-Smith G, and Mahoney C. Coping and marital equilibrium after stroke. *J Neurosci Nurs* 27(2):83–89, 1995.

Sisson RA. Cognitive status as a predictor of right hemisphere stroke outcomes. *J Neurosci Nurs* 27(3):152–156, 1995.

Spica MM. Sexual counseling standards for the spinal cord-injured. *J Neurosci Nurs* 21(1):56–60, 1989.

Swarczinski C, and Graham P. From ICU to rehabilitation: A checklist to ease the transition for the spinal cord injured. *J Neurosci Nurs* 22(2):89–91, 1990.

Discharge Planning and Teaching

Diehl LN. Client and family learning in the rehabilitation setting. *Nurs Clin North Am* 24(1):257–264, 1989.

Public Health Considerations

American Nurses Association. *Code for Nurses with Interpretive Statements.* Washington, DC: Author, 1985.

Americans with Disabilities Act of 1990, PL 101-336. U.S.C. 1990.

Suter-Gut D, et al. Post-discharge care planning and rehabilitation of the elderly surgical patient. *Clin Geriatr Med* 6(3):669–683, 1990.

White MJ, and Holloway M. Patient concerns after discharge from rehabilitation. *Rehabil Nurs* 15(6):316–318, 1990.

Agencies and Resources

Agencies

Alzheimer's Disease

Alzheimer's Association
919 North Michigan Avenue, Suite 1000
Chicago, IL 60611

Alzheimer's Information Referral Line
(800) 272–3900

Amyotrophic Lateral Sclerosis

The ALS Association—Greater New York Chapter
40 Wall Street, Suite 2111
New York, NY 10005
(212) 248–9000

Amyotrophic Lateral Sclerosis Society of America
21021 Ventura Boulevard, Suite 321
Woodland Hills, CA 91364
(800) 782–4747

Arthritis

Arthritis Foundation—New York Chapter
67 Irving Place
New York, NY 10003
(212) 477–8700
(800) 283–7800 (to locate nearest chapter in your city)

Arthritis Foundation—Virginia Chapter
3805 Cutshaw Avenue, Suite 200
Richmond, VA 23230
(804) 359–1700

Blind

American Foundation for the Blind (AFB)
11 Penn Plaza, Suite 300
New York, NY 10001
(212) 502–7600
(800) 232–5463 Information line

Association of Radio Reading Services
c/o Radio Information Services
2100 Wharton Street, Suite 140
Pittsburgh, PA 15203
(412) 488–3944

Guide Dogs for the Blind
P.O. Box 151200
San Rafael, CA 94915
(800) 295–4050

National Association for the Visually Handicapped
22 West 21st Street
New York, NY 10010
(212) 889–3141

National Library Service for the Blind and Physically Handicapped
Library of Congress
Washington, DC 20542
(800) 424–8567

Burns

American Burn Association
University of Utah Medical Center
50 North Medical Drive
Salt Lake City, UT 84132
(800) 548–2876

National Burn Victim Foundation
32–34 Scotland Road
Orange, NJ 07050
(800) 803–5879

Cancer

American Cancer Society (National Office)
1599 Clifton Road, N.E.
Atlanta, GA 30329
(404) 320–3333
(800) ACS-2345 To locate nearest office in your city

Cancer Information Service
(800) 4-CANCER

The Connecticut Hospice, Inc.
61 Burban Drive
Branford, CT 06405
(203) 481–6231
(800) 8-HOSPICE

Deaf

American Deafness and Rehabilitation Association
P.O. Box 251554
Little Rock, AR 72225
(501) 868–8850

Deafness Research Foundation
15 West 39th Street, 6th Floor
New York, NY 10018
(212) 768–1181
(800) 535–3323

National Association of the Deaf
814 Thayer Avenue
Silver Springs, MD 20910
(301) 587–1788
(800) 237–6213 Captioned films and video program

Disabilities

Consortium for Citizens with Disabilities
1730 K Street N.W., Suite 1212
Washington, DC 20006
(202) 785–3388

Disability Rights, Education, & Defense Fund
1633 Q Street, N.W., Suite 220
Washington, DC 20009
(202) 986–0375

Dystonia Medical Research Foundation
1 East Wacker Drive, Suite 2430
Chicago, IL 60601–2001
(312) 755–0198
(800) 377–DYST

Independent Living-Housing (ILH)
1301 Belmont Street, N.W.
Washington, DC 20009
(202) 797–9803

Massachusetts Office on Disability
1 Ashburton Place, Room 1305
Boston, MA 02108
(617) 727–7740
(800) 322–2020

National Organization on Disability
910 16th Street N.W., Suite 600
Washington, DC 20006
(202) 293–5960

Epilepsy

Epilepsy Foundation of America (National
  Headquarters)
4351 Garden City Drive, Suite 406
Landover, MD 20785
(800) 332–1000

Home Health

American Federation of Home Health
  Agencies
1320 Fenwick Lane, Suite 100
Silver Springs, MD 20910
(301) 588–1454

National Association for Home Care
228 7th Street, S.E.
Washington, DC 20003
(202) 547–7424

Multiple Sclerosis

National Multiple Sclerosis Society
733 3rd Avenue, 6th Floor
New York, NY 10017
(212) 986–3240
(800) FIGHT-MS

Nursing Homes

American Association of Homes &
  Services for the Aging
AAHSA Publications, Department 5119
Washington, DC 20061–5119
(800) 508–9442

Nursing Home Information Service
c/o National Council of Senior Citizens
1331 F Street, N.W.
Washington, DC 20004
(202) 347–8800

Parkinson's Disease

American Parkinson's Disease Association
1250 Highland Boulevard
Staten Island, NY 10305
(800) 223–2732

National Parkinson's Disease Foundation
  (NPF)
1501 N.W. Ninth Avenue
Miami, FL 33136
(800) 327–4545

Parkinson's Disease Support Groups of
  America
11376 Cherry Hill Road, No. 204
Beltsville, MD 20705
(301) 937–1545

Rehabilitation

National Hospital Medical Center
2455 Army Navy Drive
Arlington, VA 22206
(703) 920–6700

National Rehabilitation Hospital
102 Irving Street, N.W.
Washington, D.C. 20010
(202) 877–1707

Spinal Cord Injury

American Paralysis Association
500 Morris Avenue
Springfield, NJ 07081
(800) 225–0292

National Paralysis Foundation
16415 Addison Road
Dallas, TX 75248
(800) 925–CURE

National Spinal Cord Injury Association
  Hotline
545 Concord Avenue, Suite 29
Cambridge, MA 02138
(800) 962–9629

National Spinal Cord Injury Hotline
2200 North Forest Park Avenue
Baltimore, MD 21207
(800) 526–3456

Stroke

The National Stroke Association
96 Inverness Drive East, Suite I
Englewood, CO 80112–5112
(303) 771–1700
(800) STROKES

Resources

Adaptive Devices
Enrichments Catalogue
(800) 323–5547
Assistive devices catalogue for the
  disabled

Comfort House
(800) 359–7701
Products source for the disabled

Ostomy Association, Inc.
1111 Wilshire Boulevard
Los Angeles, CA 90017
(213) 255–4681
Information calls on Tuesdays only

Sears Home Health Care Catalogue
(800) 948–8800
Catalogue request department

8

Caring for People with Infections and Infectious Disorders

OVERVIEW OF INFECTIOUS PROCESSES

Definitions

1. **Infection** is the invasion of normally sterile body tissue by infectious organisms that multiply, producing tissue injury and a local inflammatory response that *may* progress to systemic manifestations.
   a. **Infectious organisms** are parasites that survive at the expense of the host they invade.
   b. Infection occurs when a tissue is exposed to contamination by a pathogen that successfully colonizes.
2. **Infectious disease** is an illness produced by an infection that causes clinically manifested signs and symptoms.
3. **Communicable disease** is an illness caused by infectious organisms or their toxins that can be transmitted, either directly or indirectly, from 1 person to another.
4. The **communicable period** is the time during which the infectious organism is present in sufficient amounts in body fluids or tissues to be transmitted, directly or indirectly, to another person. The communicable period varies with each infectious disease.
5. **Contamination** is the presence of an infectious organism on a body surface or an inanimate object.
   a. Contaminated individuals, animals, or objects can transmit certain infectious organisms to other individuals, animals, or objects.
   b. Breaks in the skin or in mucous membranes allow infectious organisms to invade body tissues.
6. **Colonization** is the establishment of replicating organisms on or in the body. Colonization results in infection *only* if the organisms are pathogenic and host defenses are inadequate to prevent spread of the organism. Examples of colonization include *Staphylococcus aureus* on the skin, which can lead to a wound infection, and *Escherichia coli* in the trachea, which can cause pneumonia.
7. A **nosocomial infection** is one that develops while in a hospital or another health care facility and that was neither present nor incubating at the time of admission.
   a. Nosocomial infections contribute significantly to the morbidity and mortality of hospitalized persons.
   b. They increase the length of hospitalization and increase the cost of health care in the United States by approximately $1 billion annually.
   c. Nosocomial infections currently occur in 5% of hospitalized persons, or approximately 2 million nosocomial infections per year in the United States. The highest rates of nosocomial infections occur in care units where immunosuppressed persons are housed and where invasive devices are frequently used (e.g., in medical and surgical critical care, burn, and transplant units).

Frequency Patterns of Infectious Diseases

1. **Sporadic:** A disease that occurs occasionally and irregularly in a particular geographic area or population over a specified period.
2. **Endemic:** A disease that occurs continuously in a particular geographic area over a specified period.
3. **Epidemic:** A significant increase in the frequency of a disease above its usual occurrence in a particular geographic area or population.
4. **Pandemic:** A disease that affects a large number of people in a large geographic area. A pandemic also refers to an epidemic occurring at the same time in many areas of the world.

Stages of Infectious Disease

1. The progression of an infection from initial exposure to a pathogen to an active infectious disease occurs in stages whose length and outcome depend both on the characteristics of the pathogen and the host resistance factors.
2. The stages of infection are incubation, active disease, and latency.
   a. **Incubation.** Begins when a pathogen invades host tissue. The pathogen multiplies and may spread to other tissues. Clinically obvious signs and symptoms are not present in this stage, which varies with each pathogen. However, the person may experience general weakness, fatigue, lack of appetite, headache, and muscle aches.
   b. **Active disease.** May be asymptomatic or symptomatic.
      (1) Asymptomatic disease. An inapparent, subclinical, mild infection without obvious signs or symp-

toms, which can involve an immune response against the pathogen. If the pathogen is not destroyed, the person can become an asymptomatic reservoir (carrier) of the pathogen.

(2) Symptomatic disease. Clinically obvious disease in which the person feels ill. Possible outcomes are death; full recovery, with or without subsequent immunity to reinfection; or conversion of the acute infection to a chronic disease if the pathogen is not destroyed.

c. **Latency.** Time between episodes of active disease. Pathogen remains dormant or replicates but is quickly eliminated by the immune system and does not produce clinical signs or symptoms. Proliferation of the pathogen can be reactivated by stress, exposure to certain chemicals, and other infections, and a new active stage follows. Examples of pathogens producing infections with latent stages are herpesvirus and human immunodeficiency virus (HIV).

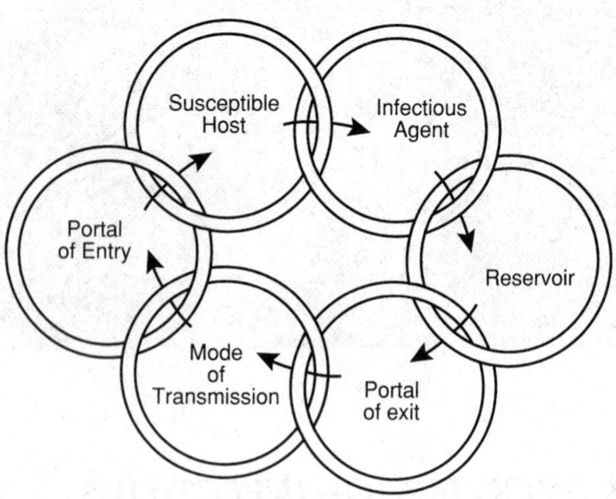

Figure 8–1. The chain of infection. (From Bolander V. *Sorensen and Luckmann's Basic Nursing: A Psychophysiologic Approach.* 3rd ed. Philadelphia: WB Saunders, 1994, p 507.)

Psychosocial Considerations

1. Stigmas can be associated with some infections.
   a. Certain infections may be viewed as punishment for aspects of the person's lifestyle, such as sexual or hygienic practices, or as punishment sent by God for some misdeed.
   b. People with some infections, such as HIV or tuberculosis, may be stigmatized because of fear of contracting the infection.
   c. Stigmas associated with infections can lead to social isolation, loneliness, and inability to find or maintain employment.
2. Problems of living with a chronic infection can include the following:
   a. Economic strain caused by the costs of treatment, complications from the disease, impaired ability to work, or a combination of these.
   b. Loss of self-esteem associated with impaired image as a productive member of the family or community.
   c. Loss of independence as a result of continued dependence on health care providers, family, or both.
   d. Grief or depression associated with a chronic, and in some cases a terminal, infectious disease.
   e. Chronic pain.
   f. Guilt regarding lifestyle choices that increased the risk for infection.
   g. Conflict in interpersonal relationships, and potential for transmitting the infection to others.
   h. Suicidal ideation resulting from any of these factors.

◼ THE CHAIN OF INFECTION

Elements in the Chain

1. The chain of events in the development of an infectious disease depends on several factors (Fig. 8–1):
   a. A pathogenic organism (infectious agent)
   b. A reservoir where the infectious agent resides.

c. A mode of escape from the reservoir
d. A mode of transmission to the human host
e. A portal of entry for the organism
2. Disease transmission can be interrupted by breaking the chain at any point, but the mode of transmission is the weakest link in the chain.
3. Whether an infectious disease develops in a person exposed to an infectious organism is determined by characteristics of the infectious organism and susceptibility of the host.

Human Infectious Agents

1. **Viruses** are the smallest pathogens (Table 8–1).
   a. Life cycle of a virus (Fig. 8–2)
      (1) The virus attaches to the host cell.
      (2) The virus penetrates the host cell.
      (3) The virus loses its cell coat, exposing its core genetic material in the host cell's cytoplasm.
      (4) The virus replicates.
      (5) The virus exits the host cell.
   b. Structure of a virus
      (1) Viruses contain a central core of single- or double-stranded DNA or RNA that contains their genetic information.
      (2) A protective protein coat (capsid) surrounds the nucleic acid core and helps the virus attach to host cells.
      (3) Some viruses also contain an outer envelope composed of lipid and glycoprotein that surrounds the capsid. The envelope is mainly derived from host cell membranes as the virus exits from the cell.
   c. Mechanisms by which viruses cause cell injury:
      (1) Rupture of the host cell as the virus exits
      (2) Fusion of many virus-infected cells, causing cell dysfunction and death
      (3) Stimulation of excessive or abnormal host cell division, leading to cancer

Table 8–1. Selected Organisms That Cause Disease in Humans

Organism	Disease
Viruses	
DNA Viruses	
Adenovirus	Pharyngitis, conjunctivitis, pneumonia
Cytomegalovirus	Mononucleosis-like syndrome, pneumonia, retinitis
Epstein-Barr virus	Mononucleosis, chronic fatigue syndrome, Burkitt's lymphoma (possibly)
Hepatitis B virus	Hepatitis
Herpes simplex virus	Fever blisters, genital herpes
Herpes zoster virus	Shingles
Human papilloma virus	Warts, associated with cervical and penile cancers
Parvovirus	Gastroenteritis
Varicella-zoster virus	Chickenpox, shingles
RNA Viruses	
Coxsackie virus	Myocarditis, cardiomyopathy, gastroenteritis, upper respiratory tract infection
Hantavirus	Hemorrhagic fever with renal syndrome
Hepatitis A, C, and delta viruses	Hepatitis
Human immunodeficiency virus (HIV)	HIV infection and acquired immunodeficiency syndrome (AIDS)
Influenza virus	Upper respiratory tract infection, pneumonia
Mumps virus	Parotitis, orchitis
Respiratory syncytial virus	Upper respiratory tract infection, bronchiolitis, pneumonia
Rhabdovirus	Rabies
Rhinovirus	Common cold, pneumonia
Rubella virus	German measles
Rubeola virus	Rubeola (measles)
Mycoplasma	
Mycoplasma orale	Oropharyngeal infections
Mycoplasma pneumoniae	Atypical pneumonia
Ureaplasma urealyticum	Genitourinary tract infection
Chlamydiae	
Chlamydia trachomatis	Cervicitis, conjunctivitis, epididymitis, urethritis
Chlamydia pneumoniae	Pneumonia, bronchitis, pharyngitis
Rickettsiae	
Rickettsia akari	Rickettsial pox
Rickettsia burnetii	Q fever
Rickettsia quintana	Trench fever
Rickettsia rickettsii	Rocky mountain spotted fever
Rickettsia typhi	Endemic typhus
Bacteria	
Gram-Negative Bacteria	
Bacteroides	Brain and lung abscess, peritonitis
Bordetella pertussis	Whooping cough
Enterobacter	Urinary and biliary tract infections, peritonitis
Escherichia coli	Urinary tract infections, peritonitis, diarrhea
Haemophilus influenzae	Nasopharyngitis, pleuritis, pneumonia, meningitis
Helicobacter pylori	Gastritis and gastrointestinal ulcers
Klebsiella pneumoniae	Pneumonia, lung abscess
Legionella pneumophila	Legionnaire's disease (pneumonia)
Neisseria gonnorrhoeae	Gonorrhea
Neisseria meningitidis (meningococcus)	Meningitis
Proteus species	Peritonitis, pneumonia, urinary tract infection

Table continued on following page

Table 8–1. Selected Organisms That Cause Disease in Humans (Continued)

Organism	Disease
Pseudomonas aeruginosa	Urinary tract, middle ear, and wound infections, pneumonia
Salmonella typhi	Typhoid fever
Other *Salmonella* species	Food poisoning (gastroenteritis)
Shigella species	Shigellosis (diarrhea, abdominal pain)
Gram-Positive Bacteria	
Clostridium botulinum	Food poisoning causing muscle paralysis
Clostridium difficile	Deep wound infections, diarrhea
Clostridium tetani	Tetanus
Clostridium perfringens	Gas gangrene
Corynebacterium diphtheriae	Diphtheria
Enterococcus	Enterocolitis, endocarditis
Listeria monocytogenes	Listeriosis (meningoencephalitis, septicemia)
Mycobacterium leprae	Leprosy
Mycobacterium tuberculosis	Tuberculosis
Staphylococcus aureus (coagulase positive)	Skin, wound, middle ear, and urinary tract infections; pneumonia; food poisoning; osteomyelitis; endocarditis; toxic shock syndrome; conjunctivitis
Staphylococcus epidermidis (coagulase negative)	Urinary tract infections, endocarditis
Streptococcus pneumoniae	Pneumonia
Streptococcus pyogenes (group A β-hemolytic)	Rheumatic fever, pharyngitis, endocarditis, cellulitis, glomerulonephritis
Streptococcus viridans	Dental caries, endocarditis
Treponema pallidum	Syphilis
Vibrio parahaemolyticus	Watery diarrhea and abdominal cramps
Fungi	
Aspergillus	Aspergillosis (pulmonary or systemic infection)
Blastomyces dermatitidis	Blastomycosis (cutaneous or pulmonary)
Candida albicans	Candidiasis (mucocutaneous or visceral)
Coccidioides immitis	Coccidioidomycosis (pulmonary, meningeal, or systemic infection)
Cryptococcus neoformans	Cryptococcosis (pulmonary or meningeal)
Histoplasma capsulatum	Histoplasmosis (pulmonary or systemic)
Pneumocystis carinii	Opportunistic pneumonia
Protozoa	
Cryptosporidium	Gastroenteritis
Entamoeba histolytica	Amebiasis (gastroenteritis, liver abscess)
Giardia lamblia	Giardiasis (diarrhea, malabsorption)
Leishmania species	Mucocutaneous visceral infection
Plasmodium species	Malaria
Toxoplasma gondii	Toxoplasmosis (central nervous system, eye, muscle infections)
Trypanosoma species	Trypanosomiasis (sleeping sickness)
Helminths	
Cestodes (Tapeworms)	
Diphyllobothrium latum (fish tapeworm)	Intestinal infection
Echinococcus granulosus	Lung, liver, and intestinal infections
Taenia saginata (beef tapeworm)	Intestinal infection
Taenia solium (pork tapeworm)	Muscle, brain, eye, and intestinal infections
Nematodes	
Ascaris lumbricoides (roundworm)	Intestinal and pulmonary infections
Enterobius vermicularis (pinworm)	Cecum, colon, and perianal infections
Necator americanus (hookworm)	Intestinal and pulmonary infections
Strongyloides stercoralis	Intestinal systemic infections and immunodeficiency disorders

Table 8–1. Selected Organisms That Cause Disease in Humans (Continued)

Organism	Disease
Trichinella spiralis	Skeletal muscle infections
Trichuris trichiura (whipworm)	Cecum and colon infections
Trematodes (Flukes)	
Clonorchis sinensis	Liver infection
Fasciola hepatica	Liver infection
Fasciolopsis buski	Intestinal infection
Heterophyes	Intestinal infection
Metagonimus yokogawai	Intestinal infection
Schistosoma mansoni, japonicum, and *haematobium*	Kidney and liver infections

(4) Inhibition of cell protein or nucleic acid synthesis, leading to cell death

(5) Invasion of white blood cells, impairing immune defenses and leading to secondary infections

(6) Inflammation

(7) Destruction of host cells by the immune system, which recognize the viral-infected cell as foreign (non-self), because it contains viral antigens on its cell membrane

(8) Persistent infection and inflammation, causing progressive organ dysfunction (often as a result of

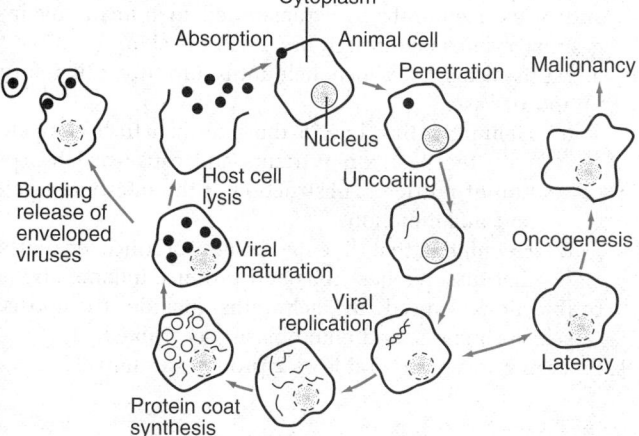

Figure 8–2. A generalized viral cycle. The viral particle binds, by its receptors, to a host cell (1). It then penetrates the cell and becomes uncoated (2 and 3). Some viruses replicate their components, which then assemble in the host cell (4) and are released by budding from the cell membrane (5). The virus can also spread by cell-to-cell contact (6) without being released. In addition, it can remain dormant within cells, to be reactivated at a later date (7). Some viruses can insert their genetic material into the host cell genome, where they remain latent (8). Their proteins may be expressed on the surface of the cell. Subsequently, the cell may become productive (4) or undergo neoplastic transformation (9). Some viral infections may be abortive (10), either because the host cell is nonpermissive for infection or because the virus is defective. Abortive infections (like productive infections) can lead to cell death (11). (Redrawn from Porth CM. *Pathophysiology.* 4th ed. Philadelphia: JB Lippincott, 1994, Fig. 12–2.)

an autoimmune response, as occurs in insulin-dependent diabetes mellitus)

d. Infections caused by viruses include the common cold, hepatitis, encephalitis, meningitis, myocarditis, varicella, mumps, and rubella.

2. **Mycoplasma** are extracellular organisms. Only a few species cause disease in humans (see Table 8–1).

a. Mechanisms by which mycoplasma cause cell injury and disease:

(1) Inflammation

(2) Epithelial cell injury

(3) Superinfection with other organisms

b. Infections caused by mycoplasma include *Mycoplasma* (atypical) pneumonia, urethritis, and pelvic inflammatory disease.

3. **Chlamydiae** are intracellular organisms that contain both RNA and DNA, but cannot synthesize their own adenosine triphosphate for energy. They are very resistant to attack by phagocytic cells.

a. Life cycle

(1) Chlamydiae are passively taken up into host cells.

(2) They replicate inside of cells using their own genetic material, not the host cell's genetic material as do viruses.

b. Mechanisms by which chlamydiae produce tissue injury and disease include both acute and chronic inflammation. Most of the damage done to humans by chlamydia is the result of infection by *Chlamydia trachomatis.*

c. Infections caused by chlamydiae include conjunctivitis, urethritis, pneumonia, and cervicitis (see Table 8–1).

4. **Rickettsiae** are structurally similar to gram-negative bacteria. They can multiply only within host cells.

a. Life cycle

(1) Rickettsiae are transmitted to humans through the bite of ticks, fleas, mites, or lice.

(2) Rickettsiae enter and multiply primarily in vascular endothelial cells.

(3) They are then expelled by the host cell or rupture the host cell as they exit.

b. Mechanisms by which rickettsiae produce cell injury and disease:
   (1) Damage to vascular endothelial cells, triggering the inflammatory response and leading to cell necrosis and a rash.
   (2) Accumulation of phagocytic cells and platelets at the site of infection, forming microthrombi, which decrease blood flow.
c. Infections caused by rickettsiae include Rocky Mountain spotted fever, typhus, and Q fever (see Table 8–1).

5. **Bacteria:** Most bacteria are extracellular organisms. Bacteria differ in shape, their reaction to a Gram stain, and their reaction to oxygen.
   a. Shape: Bacteria may be round (cocci, diplococci, streptococci, and staphylococci), or spiral shaped (spirochetes), or rod shaped (bacilli).
   b. Gram stain (see "Special Diagnostic Tests" under "Assessing People with Infections"): Gram-positive bacteria have cell walls with a thick proteoglycan layer, allowing the walls to retain the Gram stain dye. Gram-negative bacteria have less proteoglycan in their cell walls, causing a loss of dye and greater alcohol decolorization.
   c. Oxygen dependence
      (1) Aerobic bacteria survive in the presence of oxygen.
      (2) Anaerobic bacteria survive without oxygen.
      (3) Facultative anaerobic bacteria can survive with or without oxygen.
   d. Mechanisms by which bacteria cause cell injury and disease:
      (1) Destructive proteins are synthesized and secreted primarily by gram-positive bacteria. Cytolytic toxins cause disruption of cell membranes resulting in cell lysis. Enterotoxins cause vomiting and diarrhea. Epidermolytic toxins cause skin exfoliation. Neurotoxins block nerve transmission.
      (2) Disruption is caused by endotoxins, which are fragments of outer cell walls of gram-negative bacteria. Endotoxins are either shed from live bacteria or released when the bacteria are killed by host defenses or antibiotics. They are potent stimulators of host defense systems and can cause serious alterations in metabolism and coagulation and in pulmonary, cardiovascular, and neurologic functions, which can lead to shock.

NURSE ADVISORY

> Under the right conditions, any bacterium may become a pathogen.

---

   e. Infections caused by bacteria include pneumonia, cellulitis, urethritis, cervicitis, pharyngitis, otitis media, osteomyelitis, meningitis, and skin and wound infections (see Table 8–1).
6. **Fungi** are mainly extracellular organisms that resemble plants because they grow as branching filaments. Although fungi can infect any area of the body, they are most common in areas that have a direct link to the outside world.
   a. Mechanisms by which fungi cause cell injury and disease:
      (1) Induction of hypersensitivity reactions (see Chapter 21).
      (2) Acute or chronic inflammation.
      (3) Thrombosis or hemorrhage of blood vessels.
      (4) Abscess formation.
   b. Examples of infections caused by fungi include tinea corporis, tinea pedis, vaginal or systemic candidiasis, and coccidioidomycoses (see Table 8–1).
7. **Protozoa** are intracellular parasites that can move easily from place to place. They include *Sarcodina*, ciliates, flagellates, and sporidia. Protozoa differ in their location of reproduction in the body and in their structural and functional characteristics.
   a. Mechanisms by which protozoa cause cell injury and disease:
      (1) Multiplication inside cells, causing interference with cell metabolism.
      (2) Formation of pores in host cell membranes, causing the cell to rupture.
      (3) Formation of cysts.
      (4) Induction of inflammation.
   b. Examples of infections caused by protozoa include amebiasis, malaria, pneumonia, and toxoplasmosis (see Table 8–1).
8. **Helminths** are multicellular organisms shaped like pathogenic worms. They are large enough to be seen without a microscope. The development of helminths takes place in several hosts, including fish, animals, and humans. The offspring (*larvae*) of helminths are excreted in urine and feces. Helminths are transmitted to humans by ingestion or bites or through breaks in the skin.
   a. Mechanisms by which helminths produce cell injury and disease:
      (1) Helminths that live in the intestinal tract compete with the host for nutrients and cause malabsorption of nutrients, obstruction of the intestinal tract, and inflammation.
      (2) Helminths that live in tissues produce enzymes that dissolve host cells and produce inflammation.
   b. Infections caused by helminths include trichinosis, schistosomiasis, and enterobiasis (see Table 8–1).
9. Emerging infections. Table 8–2 provides examples.

Reservoirs of Infectious Agents

1. A **reservoir** is a place where infectious agents live and multiply. It serves as a source for transmission of infection to susceptible hosts.
2. Living reservoirs
   a. Human reservoirs: Persons with an infection in any stage: incubation, active, or latency. Persons who are *carriers* of an infectious organism—that is, persons who harbor an infectious organism in the absence of overt clinical disease. The carrier state may be temporary or chronic.
   b. Animal reservoirs: *Zoonotic* infections are those trans-

Table 8–2. Selected Examples of Emerging Infections

Infection	Pathogen	Mode of Transmission	Clinical Manifestations	Medical Management
Ebola hemorrhagic fever	Ebola virus	Contact with body fluids and airborne transmission from infected animals or humans	Fever, hemorrhagic disease, shock, with high lethality	Supportive therapy
Escherichia coli hemolytic uremic syndrome	*Escherichia coli* strain 0157:H7	Ingestion of contaminated ground meat	Hemorrhagic colitis with bloody diarrhea, thrombocytopenia, renal failure, hemolytic anemia with high lethality	Antibiotics and supportive therapy
Hantavirus pulmonary syndrome	Hantavirus (Muerto Canyon virus)	Inhalation of particles from saliva, urine, or feces of infected deer mice	Fever, myalgia, rapidly progressive noncardiogenic pulmonary edema, thrombocytopenia, hypotension, shock with high mortality	Ribavirin (Virazole), which is effective if administered early Circulatory and ventilatory support
Human granulocytic ehrlichiosis	Genetic variant of *Ehrlichia phagocytophilia* and *Ehrlichia equi*	Bite of the deer tick	Fever, chills, severe headache, leukopenia, anemia, thrombocytopenia, renal failure, pulmonary failure, lethal without appropriate treatment	Tetracycline or doxycycline: responds quickly to treatment with full recovery

Emerging infections are those that have recently appeared in humans or are expanding in the geographic areas affected. They are caused by new genetic variations of microorganisms or by preexisting microorganisms that have recently gained access to the human population. Changing environmental conditions and lifestyles provide new opportunities for microorganisms to cross species from animals to humans.

mitted from an animal reservoir. Infection derived from an animal reservoir may be more serious (e.g., rabies) or less serious (e.g., cowpox) for humans than for the animal acting as the reservoir.

   c. Arthropod reservoirs: Some arthropod reservoirs act only in a mechanical manner to carry infectious agents from one place to another. Other arthropod reservoirs act in a biologic manner as a necessary step in the life cycle of certain infectious agents.

3. Inanimate reservoirs
   a. Soil: Many organisms living in soil are pathogenic only to immunosuppressed individuals. Soil is a reservoir for some pathogenic bacteria (e.g., *Clostridium tetani*) and fungi.
   b. Food: Food may be contaminated by equipment or by humans during handling. Contamination may come from infected animals or their products (e.g., *Salmonella* infection from poultry or eggs). Storage of food at higher than optimal temperatures favors the growth of microorganisms.
   c. Water: Most microorganisms found in public water supplies are not pathogenic. Water provides a favorable environment for the proliferation of some pathogenic organisms (e.g., *Legionella* in shower heads and cooling systems, and *Pseudomonas* in the water of respiratory therapy equipment). Water supplies polluted with sewage act as a reservoir for many types of bacteria, viruses, and protozoa.
   d. Fomites: **Fomites** are contaminated inanimate articles such as clothing, bed linens, eating utensils, respiratory therapy equipment, needles, and surgical instruments.

Portals of Exit

1. The portal of exit of an infectious agent from its reservoir determines its mode of transmission. There may be more than 1 portal of exit for an infectious agent.
2. Portals of exit from human reservoirs and associated infectious materials include the following:
   a. Respiratory tract (secretions and sputum)
   b. Oral cavity (saliva and secretions)
   c. Gastrointestinal tract (feces)
   d. Genitourinary tract (urine, secretions, semen)
   e. Body surface (skin cells, hair, exudates)
   f. Skin lesions (blood)
   g. Eyes (tears, exudates)
   h. Placenta (transplacental transmission)

Modes of Transmission

1. Once an infectious agent has escaped from its reservoir, it can be transmitted to a host through either direct or indirect contact.
2. Direct contact requires close physical contact between a live source of infection (person or animal) and the recipient of the infection. Examples include touching, kissing, sexual contact, bites, and in-utero transmission.

3. Indirect transmission of infection takes place through an intermediate such as a vector or an inanimate vehicle. Indirect transmission requires that the infectious agent be able to survive outside the human host.
   a. **Vectors** are living intermediates, such as insects and arachnids.
   b. Inanimate vehicles include food, water, soil, fomites, biologic materials (e.g., blood products), invasive medical equipment (e.g., needles, tubing, and catheters), and airborne particles that are inhaled (e.g., small droplet nuclei or dust particles).

Conditions Favoring Infectious Agents

1. The ability of any type of organism to produce an infectious disease and the seriousness of that disease are determined by the organism's pathogenicity, virulence, toxigenicity, and antigenicity and by the ability (or inability) of the host's immune system to counter the attack.
2. **Pathogenicity:** The ability to produce disease in a normal host as determined by the following:
   a. Rate of multiplication of the pathogen
   b. Production of a toxin
   c. Resistance to destruction by host defense mechanisms
   d. Stimulation of host defense mechanisms that result in tissue damage
   e. Virulence
3. **Virulence:** Potency or ability of a pathogen to produce serious disease.
   a. Measured by the number of microorganisms needed to kill a host.
   b. Range of virulence
      (1) Low virulence (e.g., the rhinovirus causing the common cold)
      (2) Intermediate virulence (e.g., poliomyelitis virus)
      (3) High virulence (e.g., rabies virus)
4. **Toxigenicity:** The ability to produce tissue injury by production of exotoxins or endotoxins (primarily found in bacteria).
5. **Antigenicity:** Ability of a pathogen to stimulate an immune response in the host.
   a. Some pathogens trigger B lymphocytes to produce antibodies, and other pathogens activate T lymphocytes (see Chapter 21).
   b. The result can be destruction of the pathogen, further tissue damage, or both.

Host Susceptibility to Infectious Agents

1. Whether the transmission of an infectious agent to a host actually results in an infection depends to a large extent on the susceptibility of the host. Host susceptibility is increased by host-related and treatment-related factors that decrease either the effectiveness of immune defenses or the body's protective barriers.
2. Host-related risk factors
   a. Age: Risk for infection is higher in the very young and the very old because of deficiencies in the immune system.

   (1) The immune system is immature at birth; B lymphocytes have a limited ability to produce antibodies, and T lymphocytes, neutrophils, and macrophages have a limited ability to destroy infectious agents.
   (2) The immune system becomes less effective with advancing age, resulting in a decreased ability of B lymphocytes to produce certain antibodies and a decreased ability of T lymphocytes to proliferate in response to infectious agents.
   b. Malnutrition: Nutritional deficiencies of protein, vitamins, or minerals decrease host defenses and increase susceptibility to infection.
   c. Immunodeficiency syndromes: Primary and secondary immunodeficiency syndromes increase susceptibility to infection.
      (1) Primary immunodeficiency syndromes are caused by genetic or developmental disorders (see Chapter 21).
      (2) Secondary immunodeficiency syndromes are caused by a reaction to treatments such as chemotherapy and radiotherapy or by an underlying disease process that can be acquired at any time throughout life. Examples include HIV (see Chapter 42) and leukemia (see Chapter 25), cancer (see Chapter 17), severe burns (see Chapter 36), or trauma (see Chapter 37).
   d. Loss of skin or mucous membrane integrity: Microorganisms gain easy entrance into body tissues.
   e. Alcohol abuse: Increased susceptibility to infection occurs by impairing a variety of host defense mechanisms (see Chapter 40).
   f. Intravenous drug abuse: Increased susceptibility occurs by impairing a variety of host defense mechanisms. Drug abuse also increases risk of exposure to pathogens if needles are shared with others (see Chapter 40).
   g. Acute or chronic illness: Structural or functional alterations favor invasion by microorganisms or decrease immune effectiveness, or both (e.g., diabetes).
3. Treatment-related risk factors
   a. Prolonged hospitalization: Chance of exposure to microorganisms in the environment from other infected patients, contaminated objects, or hospital personnel increases.
   b. Medication-induced immunosuppression.
   c. Invasive procedures: Technologic advances have increased the use of invasive procedures and devices for the diagnosis, monitoring, and treatment of disease and thus the opportunities for infection.
      (1) Invasive procedures and devices include surgery, catheters, tubes, and intravenous, intra-arterial, and intracranial lines.
      (2) Associated mechanisms responsible for increased risk for infection include breakdown in integrity of skin or mucous membranes as a physical barrier against infection, and devices implanted in the body. Implants often cause inflammation and subsequent formation of a *biofilm* made of proteins such as fibrin and fibronectin. Bacteria (which may enter during placement of the device or dur-

ing an episode of bacteremia) adhere to the biofilm and multiply. These bacteria are inaccessible to immune defenses.

d. Splenectomy: Decreased ability to clear infectious agents from the body occurs because the spleen, an important lymphoid organ, contains macrophages and T and B lymphocytes.

Nosocomial Infections

1. Types of pathogens causing nosocomial infections
   a. Bacteria cause approximately 85 percent of nosocomial infections. Aerobic gram-negative bacilli are the most frequent cause, followed by staphylococci and then streptococci.
   b. Viruses cause only about 5 percent of nosocomial infections and include hepatitis B, hepatitis C, herpes simplex, cytomegalovirus, varicella zoster, and Epstein-Barr viruses.
   c. Fungi that most often cause nosocomial infections include *Candida* and *Aspergillus*.
   d. The protozoans *Plasmodium* and *Toxoplasma* are rare causes of nosocomial infections.
2. Sources of nosocomial pathogens
   a. Endogenous pathogens, which are part of the person's normal flora, are flora that has been altered by the antimicrobial therapy, the underlying disease process, or the hospital environment.
      (1) Some endogenous microorganisms are not normally pathogenic, but in an immunosuppressed person they can become pathogenic, opportunistic organisms.
      (2) Microorganisms and their toxins can migrate from the gastrointestinal tract into lymphatic and blood vessels when intestinal permeability is increased, as in states of hypoperfusion, inflammation, and reperfusion injury. Reperfusion injury occurs when blood flow returns after a period of ischemia.

NURSE ADVISORY

Early enteral feeding, within a day or two of serious illness or injury, helps maintain the integrity of the gastrointestinal mucosa and helps prevent the translocation of microorganisms out of the intestinal tract and into the blood.

---

      (3) Colonization of microorganisms in the oropharyngeal area occurs in approximately 50 percent of patients within a few days of hospital admission. Aspiration of the microorganisms from the colonized oral pharynx into the lower respiratory tract may cause pneumonia. Aspiration is most likely to occur in persons with a decreased level of consciousness, an impaired gag reflex, or impaired airway mucociliary clearance.
      (4) *Staphylococcus aureus, Staphylococcus epidermidis,* and gram-negative bacilli frequently colonize the skin of all persons. These organisms can then enter body tissues when skin breaks down or invasive procedures are performed.
   b. Exogenous pathogens originate from one or more reservoirs in the hospital. Identification of the reservoir is crucial for controlling nosocomial infections.
      (1) Equipment and supplies: Common sources of nosocomial infections include respiratory therapy equipment, intravenous tubing, needles, urinary catheters, central venous catheters, and cystoscopes.
      (2) Other people: Hospitalized persons, visitors, or hospital personnel often directly or indirectly transmit infections.

■ ASSESSING PEOPLE WITH INFECTIONS

Key Symptoms and Their Pathophysiologic Bases

1. The exact signs and symptoms of localized and systemic infections depend on the causative organisms, the tissue or tissues affected, and the stage of the disease.
2. The clinical manifestations of an infection result from the direct effects of the microorganism or its toxins, the inflammatory response (see Chapter 21), and the resultant cell damage. Some general clinical manifestations (Table 8–3) should alert you to the possibility of an infection.

The development of a fever requires a functioning immune system. Newborns, infants, older adults, and immunocompromised persons have a poorer prognosis if they are unable to produce a fever in the presence of an infection.

---

3. Fever may result if endogenous pyrogens (polypeptides produced by the body cells, especially monocytes and macrophages, that raise body temperature) reset the hypothalamic temperature center to a higher level. Body temperature rarely rises above 41 degrees Celsius (105.8 degrees Fahrenheit) because of an infection (Fig. 8–3). Temperatures above this level are usually the result of another mechanism, such as hyperthermia secondary to high environmental temperatures or injury to the hypothalamic heat control center.
   a. Fever progresses in 3 stages (Fig. 8–4).
      (1) Stage I (cold stage). Begins when the hypothalamic heat regulatory center is reset to a higher level, which activates heat-producing (increased metabolic rate and shivering) and heat-conserving (peripheral vasoconstriction) mechanisms and causes the temperature to rise. The person complains of feeling cold and has gooseflesh (piloerection).
      (2) Stage II (heat maintenance stage). Begins when the temperature has increased to that level directed by the reset hypothalamus. The person complains of

Table 8–3. Key Signs and Symptoms of Infection in Various Organ Systems

System	Signs and Symptoms Suggestive of Infection
Generalized	Fever, chills, malaise, fatigue, anorexia, light-headedness, inability to concentrate, apathy, aching muscles
Skin	Inflammation, rash, pruritus
Immune system	Lymphadenopathy, altered differential white blood cell count (see Chapter 21)
Gastrointestinal and hepatobiliary systems	Nausea and vomiting, anorexia, diarrhea, weight loss, abdominal cramps or pain, jaundice
Respiratory system	Sore or inflamed throat; cough; green, yellow, rust-colored, or foul-smelling sputum; sneezing; dyspnea; nasal discharge; congestion; abnormal lung sounds such as rales, rhonchi, or a pleural friction rub; increased respiratory rate.
Cardiovascular system	Heart murmurs, decreased cardiac output, vasculitis, tachycardia
Genitourinary system	Urgency, frequency, or discomfort on urination; oliguria or polyuria; hematuria; pyuria; foul-smelling urine; pelvic or flank pain; vaginal or urethral discharge
Musculoskeletal system	Muscle weakness, decreased range of motion, tenderness, swelling, or redness of the joints
Nervous system	Weakness, abnormal sensations, confusion, headache, seizures, nuchal rigidity
Auditory system	Inflammation, pain, or drainage in the auditory canal; change in hearing acuity
Visual system	Conjunctivitis, scleritis, iritis, increased lacrimation, itching, decreased visual acuity

feeling hot, appears flushed, and the skin feels warm.

(3) Stage III (defervescent or heat dissipating stage). Begins when hypothalamic setpoint returns to normal and heat loss mechanisms, such as sweating and peripheral vasodilation, are activated.

NURSE ADVISORY

Identifying the patient's fever pattern can help you determine the cause of the infection.

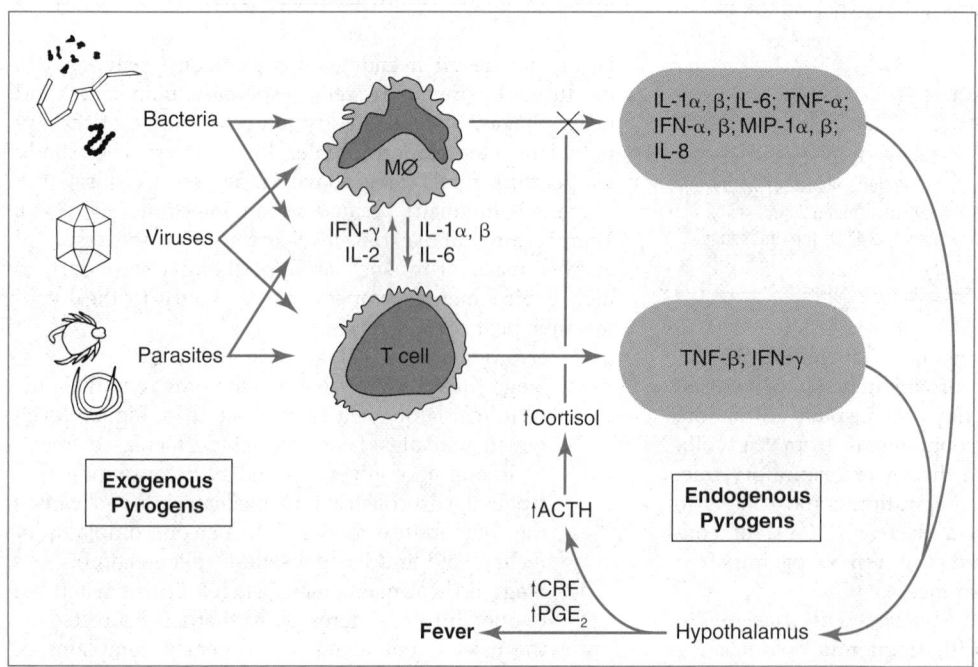

Figure 8–3. Mechanisms of fever production. ACTH, Adrenocorticotropic hormone; CRF, corticotropin-releasing factor; PGE$_2$, prostaglandin E$_2$; MØ, macrophage; INF, interferon; IL, interleukin; TNF, tumor necrosis factor; MIP, macrophage inflammatory protein. (From Wyngaarden JB, Smith LH Jr, and Bennett JC [eds]. *Cecil Textbook of Medicine.* 19th ed. Philadelphia: WB Saunders, 1992, p 157.)

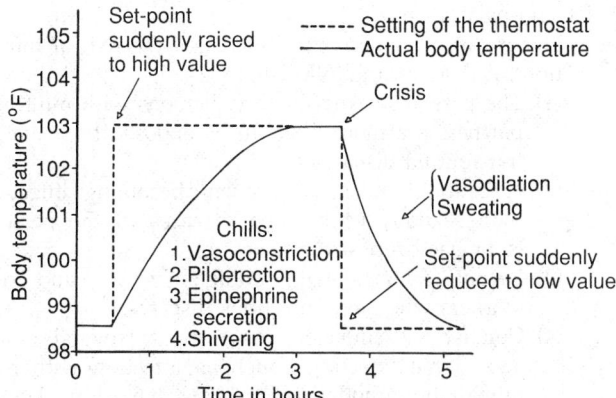

Figure 8–4. Stages of fever. (From Guyton AC, and Hall JE. *Textbook of Medical Physiology.* 9th ed. Philadelphia: WB Saunders, 1996, p 920.)

b. Fever can take 4 patterns.
(1) **Constant fever** is a persistent temperature elevation varying less than 1 degree Celsius throughout the infectious disease. Constant fever often occurs in typhoid fever, gram-negative bacterial pneumonia, and rickettsial infections.
(2) **Remittent fever** is a pattern of elevations and falls in temperature greater than 2 degrees Celsius (without returning to normal) over a 24-hour period. Remittent fever often occurs in salmonella infections.
(3) **Intermittent fever** is a cycle of temperature elevations and returns to normal over a 24-hour period. Intermittent fever often occurs in miliary tuberculosis, intermittent bacteremias, and bacterial endocarditis.
(4) **Relapsing fever** is a recurrence of fever after return to normal temperature and apparent recovery. Relapsing fever often occurs in infections transmitted by ticks and rodents.
c. The beneficial effects of fever include the following:
(1) Release of endogenous pyrogens, which increase the production of T and B lymphocytes and interferon, important antipathogenic agents.
(2) Enhanced phagocytosis and killing of some microorganisms.
(3) Drowsiness, leading persons to apply energy normally used for everyday living to fight the infection instead.
d. The harmful effects of fever include the following:
(1) Discomfort and restlessness.
(2) Increased oxygen consumption. For each 1 degree Celsius increase in temperature, there is a 13 percent increase in oxygen consumption as a result of the increased metabolic rate.
(3) Increased caloric requirements. Metabolic changes can lead to protein catabolism and negative nitrogen balance.
(4) Dehydration. Sweating and loss of water vapor from increased respiratory rate can cause dehydration.
e. Neurologic effects. Temperatures greater than 40 degrees Celsius (104 degrees Fahrenheit) can cause delir-

ium and seizures, further increasing oxygen consumption.
f. Respiratory effects. Temperatures greater than 41.1 degrees Celsius (106 degrees Fahrenheit) can damage the heat regulatory center and cause widespread cell damage (Box 8–1).
4. Changes occur in heart rate, respiratory rate, and blood pressure.
a. Tachycardia usually occurs with infections because the accompanying fever increases oxygen demands,

---

BOX 8–1. Fever of Unknown Origin

Definitions

- Fever of unknown origin (FUO) must meet the following three criteria first described by Petersdorf and Beeson in 1961 and modified by Durack and Street in 1991:
 1. Duration of at least 3 weeks
 2. Temperature greater than 38.3°C (101°F) on several occasions
 3. Undetermined cause after assessment in 3 outpatient visits or 3 days in the hospital
- Nosocomial FUO: fever in a hospitalized person in whom infection was not present or incubating at admission that is caused, for example, by infected intravascular lines, drug fever, sinusitis secondary to intubation, or *Clostridium difficile* colitis.
- Neutropenic FUO: fever in a person with fewer than 500 neutrophils per mm³ caused, for example, by focal fungal, bacterial, herpes simplex, or cytomegalovirus infections.
- HIV-associated FUO: fever in person who tests positive for the human immunodeficiency virus that is caused, for example, by *Pneumocystis carinii*, tuberculosis, toxoplasmosis, histoplasmosis, or non-Hodgkins lymphoma.
- Classic FUO: fever in persons not fitting the previous 3 categories.

Causes

- Infections such as extrapulmonary tuberculosis, abscesses, endocarditis, histoplasmosis, and unusual infections acquired outside the United States.
- Neoplasms such as lymphoma, myeloma, leukemia, and metastatic cancers.
- Multisystem inflammatory diseases such as giant cell arteritis and adult-onset Still's disease.
- Factitious fever: Persons pretending to have a fever as a result of an emotional disorder or for the purpose of malingering.

Medical Diagnosis

- Laboratory tests include multiple blood cultures, erythrocyte sedimentation rate, serologic tests for infectious agents and antibodies, serum enzyme and blood chemistries, skin tests for tuberculosis and to detect anergy, and spinal fluid examination.
- Radiologic studies include ultrasonography, computed tomography, magnetic resonance imaging (MRI), radionuclide scans, and upper and lower gastrointestinal scans.
- Tissue biopsy to detect infection, inflammation, or connective tissue disorders.
- Exploratory laparotomy if other tests suggest an intra-abdominal or retroperitoneal source of fever.

Medical Management

- A course of antibiotics guided by suspicion as to the underlying infectious agent.
- Nonsteroidal anti-inflammatory drugs.
- No treatment and reevaluation after several weeks or months for persons with FUO that is not progressive or associated with other manifestations and without clues as to the cause.

and the heart beats faster to improve oxygen delivery to tissues. For each 1 degree Celsius increase in temperature in an adult, heart rate increases by approximately 20 beats per minute.

  b. Tachypnea, an increased respiratory rate, usually occurs with infection as a result of fever and increased oxygen demands. For each 1 degree Celsius increase in temperature, respiratory rate increases by approximately 7 breaths per minute.

  c. Tachypnea can also result from a reflex response to hypoxemia occurring in pulmonary infections or in severe sepsis.

  d. Blood pressure can increase due to vasoconstriction during development of a fever with an infection. Blood pressure can decrease during an infection due to impaired cardiac function or the development of septic shock.

5. Inflammation is the body's normal response to the invasion of pathogens (see also Chapter 21). Inflammation is characterized by pain, redness, swelling, and heat at the site. If successful in walling off and destroying or neutralizing pathogens, inflammation will remain localized; if not, inflammation can spread systemically.

History of Exposure and Risk of Susceptibility

1. Travel history. Fast and economical air travel allows millions of people to encounter infectious diseases to which they do not have immunity. Travel also allows infected persons and vectors to be transported from areas in which an infectious disease is endemic, to areas in which it is rare or nonexistent. When pathogens are brought into countries where they are rare and an unlikely cause of infection, delays in diagnosis and treatment often occur and a poor outcome results. If a patient is a recent immigrant, inquire about the country of origin and the length of time since leaving that country. Ask all travelers about the following:

  a. Where and when a person has traveled and the length of stay.

  b. Whether travel included rural or remote areas in which sanitation facilities may have been lacking.

  c. Whether raw fruits or vegetables were consumed during the trip.

  d. Whether precautions, such as vaccinations or prophylactic antibiotics, were taken when traveling to areas with endemic or epidemic infectious diseases.

Living and working conditions can put a person at greater risk of infection, because close contact with others in crowded city and office environments increases exposure to pathogens. In addition, poor sanitation, either in impoverished areas or in the aftermath of natural disasters such as floods, increases risk of exposure to infectious agents. Finally, the inability to cope with high-stress lifestyles is linked to immunosuppression and increased susceptibility to infections.

---

2. Psychosocial history

  a. History of human contact (increases the risk of infection). Ask about the following:

    (1) The person's sexual history. Persons with multiple partners are more likely to be exposed to sexually transmitted diseases.

    (2) Precautions taken to prevent becoming infected with sexually transmitted diseases (if the person is, or has been, sexually active).

    (3) Recent contacts with family, friends, and co-workers who have infectious diseases.

    (4) Contact with infected people up to several years ago. Some infections, such as infection with the human immunodeficiency virus, have long latent or incubation periods.

  b. Recent stress level.

3. History of arthropod and animal contact (increases risk of infection). Ask about the following:

  a. Whether the person has had any recent contact with pets or wild animals, including birds.

  b. Whether the person was bitten by an insect or tick within the past month.

  c. Whether the person's residence or place of work is infested with insects or rodents.

  d. Whether the person handles dead animals or is exposed to animal excrement.

4. Diet history. Ask about the following:

  a. Whether the person drinks unpasteurized milk or eats unpasteurized milk products.

  b. Whether the person eats raw or undercooked meat, fish, chicken, or eggs.

  c. Whether the person has recently eaten canned foods that could have been contaminated by botulin.

  d. Whether the person's water supply could have been contaminated (e.g., by flooding).

TRANSCULTURAL CONSIDERATIONS

In some cultures, sharing of food or drink is a common practice. Because this practice can increase the risk of exposure to many pathogens, be sure to ask about it.

5. Transplantation and transfusion history. Ask about the following:

  a. Whether the person has had any organ or tissue transplants and when these procedures were performed. Transplanted tissue can transmit microorganisms, such as cytomegalovirus, from the donor.

  b. Whether the person has had a transfusion with blood or blood products. Blood is not screened for all infectious agents and may have been taken from a donor before clinical manifestations of illness became evident. Also, because some screening tests, such as those for human immunodeficiency virus infection, are based on the detection of antibodies, blood can be donated before the body has been able to produce a detectable level of antibodies.

6. History of recurrent infections
   a. Determine whether the person has had any infectious disease that recurs and, if so, how often it recurs.
   b. Microorganisms that can cause recurrent infections include herpes simplex, *Chlamydia trachomatis*, cytomegalovirus, hepatitis B or C virus, and *Candida*.
7. History of childhood communicable diseases
   a. Ask whether the person has had childhood communicable diseases such as mumps, measles, chickenpox, and rheumatic fever.
   b. Record the types and dates of all vaccinations.
8. History of host susceptibility. Ask about the following:
   a. Whether the person has a chronic disease or condition associated with immune suppression or decreased healing such as diabetes mellitus, renal failure, or liver disfunction. Has the person had a splenectomy?
   b. Whether a woman is pregnant. Hormonal changes during pregnancy cause a degree of immune suppression.
   c. Whether the person is receiving a therapy that causes immune suppression, such as corticosteroids, cancer chemotherapy, radiation, or drugs to suppress rejection of transplanted organs.
   d. Whether the person is taking any anti-inflammatory drugs such as aspirin, ibuprofen, or indomethacin.

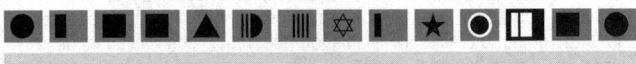

TRANSCULTURAL CONSIDERATIONS

To determine a patient's explanatory model for an infection (the patient's reasons for why an infection developed), you will need to perform a cultural assessment (see Chapter 2).

Physical Examination

1. Vital signs (see Table 8–3)
2. Skin and mucous membranes
   a. Inspect for breaks in integrity that allow pathogens to enter the body.
   b. Inspect for signs of inflammation.
   c. Inspect for bites or scratches from an insect or animal or from another human being.
   d. Inspect for signs of dehydration such as decreased skin turgor; dry, fissured mucous membranes; weak, thready pulse; hypotension; and decreased urine output. Dehydration can be caused by fever, diarrhea, or vomiting associated with an infection.
   e. Closely inspect body surfaces, including the fingernails and toenails, areas between the fingers and toes, and areas under the breasts and scrotum; mucous membranes in the mouth, throat, nasal cavity, and vagina; and eyes and ears.
   f. During inspection, note any change in skin color or temperature; macular, papular, or vesicular eruptions; ulcers; and color, consistency, and odor of any drainage, especially purulent drainage.
3. Lymph node palpation: Lymph nodes usually change in the area of infection because of proliferation of B and T lymphocytes inside. Palpate all superficial lymph nodes, noting lymph node diameter greater than 2 cm, hardness, tenderness, and immobile nodes (see Chapter 21).
4. Listen to lungs for diminished or absent breath sounds and abnormal breath sounds such as rales (crackles) or rhonchi.

Special Diagnostic Tests

1. Staining of specimens for microorganisms identifies the general type of microorganism, but confirmation of the specific species causing an infection usually requires culturing.
   a. The Gram stain differentiates bacteria into 2 major categories.
      (1) Gram-positive bacteria have cell walls that retain the stain. Gram-positive bacteria include *Streptococcus pneumoniae*, β-hemolytic streptococcus, and *Staphylococcus aureus*.
      (2) Gram-negative bacteria have cell walls that do not retain the gram stain. Gram-negative bacteria include *Escherichia coli*, *Pseudomonas*, *Salmonella*, *Bacterioides*, and *Neisseria gonorrhoeae*.
   b. The acid-fast stain identifies bacteria such as *Mycobacterium tuberculosis*, *Nocardia*, and *Actinomyces* that retain carbolfuchsin stain after treatment with acid.
   c. Immunofluorescent stains consist of antibodies linked to a compound that fluoresces when exposed to ultraviolet light. These antibodies bind to antigens on certain microorganisms. Immunofluorescent stains are used to identify cells infected with certain viruses, such as cytomegalovirus and herpes simplex, and to identify bacteria that are difficult to grow in culture, such as *Legionella*.
2. Culture and sensitivity tests
   a. Culture media provide environments in which pathogens can multiply, thus providing a sufficient number for staining, microscopic examination, and other identification procedures. Culture results take a minimum of 2 days and can take up to several weeks for some slow-growing organisms such as *M. tuberculosis*.
   b. Sensitivity tests determine which antibiotics are capable of killing the bacteria cultured.
   c. Types of pathogens that can be cultured include bacteria, fungi, viruses, and mycoplasma.
   d. Substances cultured include all body fluids: exudates, aspirates, and urine. Stool, biopsied tissue, and intravascular catheter tips are also frequently cultured.
   e. Follow the general guidelines for collecting culture specimens to ensure prompt and accurate organism identification.
      (1) Explain the procedure and its purpose to the patient (Box 8–2).
      (2) Collect specimens before administering antimicrobial agents, which can alter the growth of pathogens and result in misleading culture results. If the person is already receiving antimicrobial therapy, record the information on the laboratory requisition form.
      (3) Aseptically prepare the body site for specimen collection to avoid contamination with normal flora.

BOX 8-2. Guidelines for Collection of Specimens for Culture

Blood Culture

Patient Preparation: Cleanse the area over the venipuncture site with alcohol, then with an iodine solution. Allow the iodine solution to remain on the skin for 1 minute before removal with an alcohol swab. Wear sterile gloves if palpating the venipuncture site after it is cleansed.

Procedure: Perform a venipuncture and withdraw at least 10 ml of blood. Place half the blood into a culture tube for aerobic organisms and half the sample into a culture tube for anaerobic organisms. Blood cultures are usually drawn on at least 2 consecutive days.

Results: Normally blood is sterile. If pathogens are present, most can be detected in blood after 72 hours of culture. Bacteria that may be found in a blood culture include *Streptococcus* species, *Escherichia coli*, *Staphylococcus aureus*, *Bacteroides*, and *Neisseria meningitidis*. Viruses and fungi can also be detected.

Sputum Culture

Patient Preparation: Teach the patient to expectorate sputum by first taking a few deep breaths and then coughing deeply. It is important to obtain a sputum and not a saliva sample. The patient may require increased fluid intake, tracheal suctioning, or postural drainage to obtain sputum.

Procedure: Wear a mask during the procedure. Use a sterile sputum cup or a sputum trap if tracheal suctioning is used. Send the specimen to the laboratory immediately.

Results: Sputum culture results are often difficult to interpret because the specimen is contaminated with flora in the oral cavity and trachea. Pathogens that may be found include *Streptococcus pneumoniae*, *Mycobacterium tuberculosis*, *Enterobacter*, *Haemophilus influenzae*, *Pseudomonas aeruginosa*, and *Staphylococcus aureus*.

Throat Culture

Patient Preparation: Inform the patient that swabbing of the throat may cause a gag reflex.

Procedure: Use a tongue depressor to avoid contact with structures in the oral cavity. Visualize the throat with a flashlight. With a sterile swab, wipe the posterior pharynx including areas of suspected infection, such as areas of inflammation, ulceration, or vesicles. Place the swab in a sterile collection tube and send to the laboratory immediately.

Results: Pathogens that may be cultured include group A β-hemolytic streptococcus, *S. pneumoniae*, *Corynebacterium diphtheriae*, *Bordetella pertussis*, *H. influenzae*, and *Candida albicans*.

Nasopharyngeal Culture

Patient Preparation: Explain to the patient that a specimen will be obtained from the back of the throat and that the procedure may cause some discomfort or trigger a gag reflex.

Procedure: Use a cotton swab attached to a flexible tube to collect the specimen. Tilt the patient's head back and gently pass the swab through the nose into the nasopharynx. Rotate the swab before removing it. Either streak the swab onto a culture plate immediately or send the swab in a tube with transport medium to the laboratory.

Results: Pathogens that may be cultured include *B. pertussis*, *H. influenzae*, *N. meningitidis*, *C. diphtheriae*, group A β-hemolytic streptococcus, and *C. albicans*.

Wound Culture

Patient Preparation: Cleanse the skin around the wound to avoid contamination of the specimen with skin flora.

Procedure: Collect specimens using a sterile swab, gently rotating it before removal. A sterile syringe can be used to aspirate wound exudates. A minimum of 0.5 ml is required. Collect samples from several wound sites, including superficial and deep areas, using a different swab or syringe for each site. Place 1 sample into a culture tube for aerobic organisms and another sample into a culture tube for anaerobic organisms, being careful not to allow contact with air, which can kill anaerobic organisms. Send the specimens to the laboratory immediately.

Results: Organisms most frequently causing a wound infection include *S. aureus*, *E. coli*, *Pseudomonas*, *Proteus*, streptococci, *Bacteroides*, *Clostridium*, and fungi.

Urine Culture

Patient Preparation: Instruct the patient how to collect a clean voided midstream urine specimen to avoid contamination of the specimen with flora in the perineal area. If catheterization or suprapubic aspiration will be used to obtain the specimen, explain the procedure.

Procedure: Collect the urine specimen as ordered. Collect at least 1 ml but do not fill more than half of the container. If collecting the specimen from an indwelling catheter, withdraw urine from a port in the tubing, after wiping it with alcohol, using a sterile syringe. Do not take urine from the drainage bag. Send the specimen to the laboratory immediately. If transport to the laboratory is delayed longer than 30 minutes, refrigerate the specimen at 4 degrees Celsius. If the patient is undergoing diuresis, note this on the requisition because dilute urine can lower bacterial counts.

Results: Bacterial counts of 100,000 or more per ml of urine are a definite indication of a urinary tract infection. Bacterial counts of 10,000 to 100,000 per ml indicate a probable infection, especially if the specimen was obtained by bladder catheterization. Bacterial counts of less than 10,000 per ml usually indicate a contaminated specimen; however, they could indicate an infection in a patient who is also symptomatic. The most common organism causing a urinary tract infection is *E. coli*. An acid-fast stain can be requested to detect *M. tuberculosis* in the urinary tract.

Stool Culture

Patient Preparation: If the patient is to collect the specimen at home, provide instruction on the proper collection technique as discussed below.

Procedure: Collect the stool specimen directly into a plastic-coated container or a clean, dry bedpan, and transfer the specimen to the container with a tongue blade. Avoid contact of the stool with urine. If blood or mucus is present in the stool, include it with the specimen. One gm of solid stool or 15 ml of liquid stool is adequate. If using a sterile swab to obtain the specimen, insert it past the anal sphincter and rotate it several times before removal. Either inoculate a culture plate with the swab immediately or place the swab into a tube with buffered transport medium. If protozoa are suspected to be present, collect specimens over several days, which will increase the chance of sampling the protozoa that have cyclic life cycles. Use cellophane tape pressed over the perineal area to collect pinworms if a specimen cannot be sent to the laboratory immediately because some fecal organisms die with a fall in temperature.

Results: Pathogenic organisms that can be cultured in stool include *Clostridium difficile*, *Clostridium botulinum*, *Clostridium perfringens*, *Salmonella*, *Shigella*, *S. aureus*, *Campylobacter jejuni*, *Vibrio cholerae*, helminths, and protozoa.

(4) Protect yourself and others from contamination during collection and handling of the specimen by wearing gloves and not contaminating the outside of the specimen container.

(5) Label the specimen with the patient's and the physician's names, room number, date, time, and method of collection, and the test or tests to be performed.

(6) Transport in a timely manner.

3. Hematologic tests (see also Chapter 25)
   a. Differential white blood cell (WBC) count: A change in the number of certain WBC types is characteristic of certain infectious diseases (see Chapter 21). In *most* serious infections, the total WBC count increases above 10,000 per mm³, as the bone marrow increases production of these cells to combat the infection. In some infectious diseases, however, the total WBC count decreases.
      (1) **Neutropenia** (decreased number of neutrophils, which are polymorphonuclear leukocytes and which function in phagocytosis of microorganisms) occurs in many viral infections, in overwhelming bacterial infections, and in some infections with rickettsiae and protozoa.
      (2) **Neutrophilia** (increased neutrophil count) occurs in acute infections caused mainly by bacteria and rickettsiae and a few viruses and protozoa.
      (3) **Eosinopenia** (decreased number of eosinophils, which are leukocytes that help regulate inflammation and protect against infections with helminths) occurs in infectious mononucleosis and in conditions in which corticosteroid levels are increased. For example eosinopenia occurs during stress, as a result of therapy with a corticosteroid drug, or in states of excess adrenal secretion of corticosteroids.
      (4) **Eosinophilia** (increased eosinophil count) occurs in infections caused by helminths and some other parasites.
      (5) **Lymphopenia** (decreased lymphocyte count) occurs in human immunodeficiency virus infection and in the presence of immunosuppressive drugs.
      (6) **Lymphocytosis** (increased lymphocyte count) occurs in most viral infections and chronic bacterial infections such as tuberculosis.
      (7) **Monocytosis** (increased number of monocytes, which are large mononuclear leukocytes and function in phagocytosis of microorganisms) occurs in some viral, rickettsial, and protozoan infections and in the recovery phase of acute bacterial infections.
   b. Erythrocyte sedimentation rate (ESR): This nonspecific test detects an inflammatory process but does not indicate whether an infection (or what type of infection) is causing it.
      (1) The ESR measures, in millimeters per hour, the rate at which erythrocytes fall to the bottom of a test tube.
      (2) The ESR increases in the presence of increased proteins (e.g., immunoglobulins) in the blood because the proteins cause the cells to stick together (rouleaux formation), so that they are heavier and fall faster.
      (3) The blood sample can undergo centrifugation to speed up the test.
   c. C-reactive protein (CRP): C-reactive protein is synthesized by the liver and normally is present in the blood in only trace amounts. It functions in activation of the complement system (a group of plasma proteins involved in the immune response). Levels of CRP increase in the blood during an inflammatory response.

4. Urinalysis: The following information obtained from a routine urinalysis provides clues regarding the presence of a urinary tract infection: urine color, odor, clarity, pH, specific gravity, presence of nitrites, bacteria, or yeast (see Box 8–2 for information on urine cultures).
5. Immunologic tests (see Chapter 21)
6. Molecular methods: The newest methods of identifying microorganisms are based on indirect analysis of their gene products (phenotyping) or direct analysis of their genes (plasmid fingerprinting, genomic fingerprinting, and DNA amplification). These methods have greatly improved the ability to pinpoint the source and mode of transmission of outbreaks of infectious diseases and the diagnosis of individual infections.
7. Scans: Body scans are used to locate many types of masses, including abscesses or inflammatory lesions.
   a. *Computed axial tomography (CT) scans*, or multiple x-ray beams, provide a high-resolution anatomic image of masses such as an abscess in the brain or abdomen.
   b. In a gallium scan, radioactive gallium is injected and taken up by cells in an abscess or an area of inflammation. The area of radioactivity is located by a scanner.
   c. Using indium-111—WBC inflammatory imagery—a sample of WBCs is removed, tagged with radioactive indium, and then reinjected. Labeled WBCs travel to an area of infection and can be located by a scanner.

◼ INTERVENTIONS TO TREAT INFECTIONS

Avoiding Spread of Infection

1. The spread of infection can be stopped at any point in the chain of infection.
2. Figure 8–5 shows barriers to the transmission of disease.

Helping Patients Cope with Psychosocial Concerns

1. Question the person and listen with a nonjudgmental attitude regarding the psychosocial implications of the infection.
2. Determine how the person was able to cope effectively with adverse events in the past, and facilitate this coping pattern.
3. Help the person cope by making referrals to social services, clergy, and community support groups.
4. Educate the person with the infection and the person's family, friends, and community (possibly with the assistance of a school nurse or occupational health nurse) to prevent transmission and social isolation.

Reducing Fever

1. Situations requiring fever reduction
   a. Because fevers have beneficial effects, temperatures lower than 38.9 degrees Celsius (102 degrees Fahren-

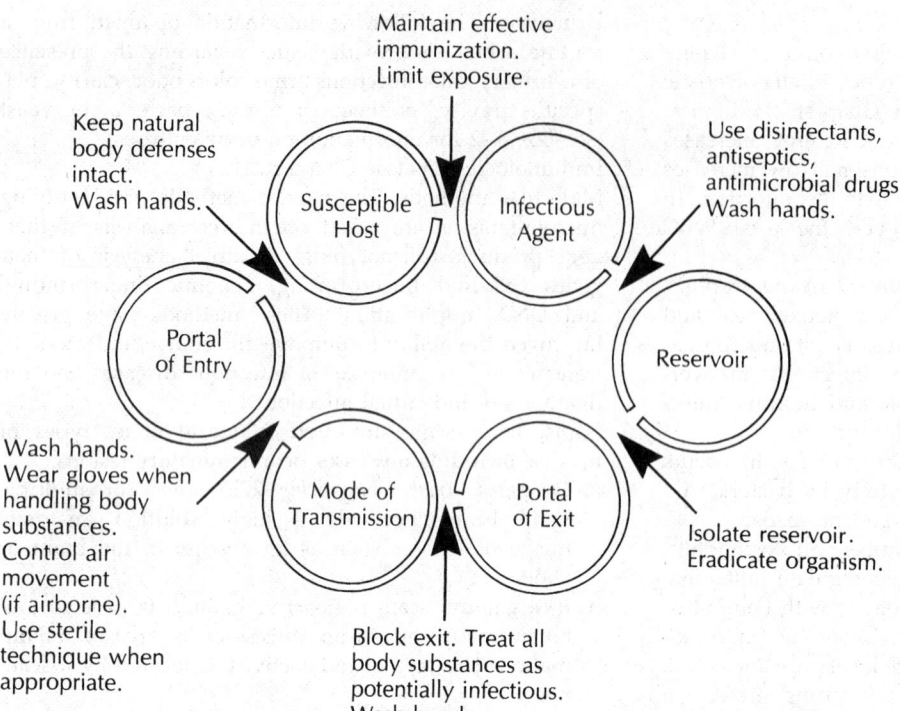

Keep natural body defenses intact. Wash hands.

Maintain effective immunization. Limit exposure.

Use disinfectants, antiseptics, antimicrobial drugs. Wash hands.

Figure 8–5. Breaking the chain of infection. Note the actions (arrows) that can create barriers to transmission of disease. (From Bolander V. *Sorensen and Luckmann's Basic Nursing: A Psychophysiologic Approach.* 3rd ed. Philadelphia: WB Saunders, 1994, p 512.)

Wash hands. Wear gloves when handling body substances. Control air movement (if airborne). Use sterile technique when appropriate.

Isolate reservoir. Eradicate organism.

Block exit. Treat all body substances as potentially infectious. Wash hands.

heit) generally should not be reduced in persons who are able to tolerate the increased metabolic demands associated with the fever.

b. Temperatures between 40 degrees Celsius (104 degrees Fahrenheit) and 41.1 degrees Celsius (106 degrees Fahrenheit) should be reduced with antipyretics and tepid sponge baths.

c. Temperatures greater than 41.1 degrees Celsius (106 degrees Fahrenheit) are life threatening and must be lowered immediately with antipyretics and physical cooling.

d. Any degree of fever should be reduced in a person who is very uncomfortable or unable to tolerate the associated increased metabolic and oxygen demands (e.g., because of cardiac or pulmonary disease or a predisposition to seizures).

2. Methods of fever reduction
   a. Pharmacologic interventions for reducing fevers
      (1) Aspirin. Aspirin inhibits prostaglandin synthesis in the hypothalamic heat regulatory center, which decreases the temperature setpoint and triggers heat loss mechanisms such as vasodilation and sweating. Aspirin is a potent inhibitor of platelet aggregation and prolongs bleeding time. *Avoid giving aspirin to children who have viral diseases.*

 DRUG ADVISORY

Because aspirin is a common allergen and can cause anaphylaxis, determine whether the patient is allergic to it *before* administration.

   (2) Acetaminophen. The antipyretic action of acetaminophen is similar to that of aspirin. Acetamino-

phen, however, does not decrease platelet aggregation or prolong bleeding. In high doses, acetaminophen has hepatotoxic effects.

   b. Nonpharmacologic methods for reducing fever

NURSE ADVISORY

Do not attempt to lower body temperature with external cooling (e.g., sponging with cold water or alcohol rubs), because skin temperature will fall below core temperature and trigger heat gain mechanisms such as shivering; which will increase body temperature and oxygen demands.

   (1) Extreme external cooling with ice water baths or a cooling mattress is usually contraindicated because these measures do not treat the cause of the fever—that is, the resetting of the hypothalamus.

   (2) Sponging with *tepid* water cools the body surface as the water evaporates and can help to reduce a fever. Sponging should not be performed until 30 minutes after the administration of an antipyretic so that the hypothalamic temperature set point will be lowered. Otherwise, the body will resist the cooling attempt, and shivering can occur.

Maintaining Nutrition and Fluid and Electrolyte Balance

1. Consult with the nutrition team to ensure that the patient has an adequate nutritional intake to meet the increased energy requirements associated with a fever, the

immune response, and tissue healing from an infection (see Chapter 10).

2. Observe for signs of a fluid deficit, which can be caused by diaphoresis, increased respiratory rate, vomiting, or diarrhea caused by an infection. Provide for adequate fluid intake (see Chapter 9).

3. Monitor electrolyte levels and watch for manifestations of an electrolyte imbalance.

Eliminating Infection: Antimicrobial Therapy

1. General principles and nursing implications
   a. To reduce morbidity and mortality in a patient with a potentially life-threatening infection, the physician may initiate empiric antimicrobial therapy as soon as there are clinical manifestations of infection and before culture results are available.
   b. The physician needs to base the agent, dose, and route of administration on these clues to the identity and characteristics of the etiologic pathogen:
      (1) Clinical manifestations and the suspected site of infection.
      (2) Whether the infection is community or hospital acquired (nosocomial).
      (3) Usual antimicrobial susceptibility of the suspected pathogen.

DRUG ADVISORY

Before starting antimicrobial therapy, obtain the person's history of drug allergies. Many antimicrobial agents have structural similarities, and a person with an allergy to one agent may be allergic to another agent in the same class.

   c. After culture results have identified the etiologic pathogen, the physician narrows the antibiotic spectrum to attack the specific pathogen and to decrease the risk of antibiotic toxicity, resistance, or superinfection.
   d. For people with moderate to severe renal impairment, the physician must adjust the dosage for agents excreted primarily by the kidneys.
   e. Once antimicrobial therapy begins, the nurse must do the following:
      (1) Help maintain effective blood levels that are above the **minimum inhibitory concentration**—the lowest concentration of the drug known to inhibit multiplication of the pathogen—by administering the antimicrobial agent at the correct time, dose, and route.
      (2) Monitor the patient's response and the changes in signs and symptoms of infection to see if the antimicrobial agent is effective.
      (3) Monitor the patient for adverse reactions.
      (4) Check the patient's entire drug regimen for drug or nutrient interactions.

DRUG ADVISORY

Instruct patients to complete the prescribed course of antimicrobial therapy. Warn them not to stop taking the medication when they start feeling better.

2. Antibiotics (see Clinical Controversies below)

CLINICAL CONTROVERSIES

The emergence of antibiotic resistance is one important reason why antibiotic therapy for bacterial infections may fail. Increasingly, bacteria are becoming resistant, in large part because of the widespread or inappropriate use of antibiotics, which leads to the killing of susceptible bacteria and allows more resistant strains to proliferate. The widespread use of antibiotics in farm animals has increased the number of resistant bacteria ingested in meat and milk.

Inappropriate uses of antibiotics include treatment for viral infections or for fevers without other indications of infection, failure to complete a prescribed course of antibiotics, or ingestion of antibiotics prescribed for another person.

The prophylactic use of antibiotics is controversial because of the risk of adverse reactions and the development of resistant bacteria. Antibiotic prophylaxis is usually required prior to invasive procedures such as tooth extraction or invasive diagnostic tests, especially if the patient has prosthetic heart valves or has a history of (a) bacterial endocarditis, (b) mitral valve prolapse, or (c) certain congenital heart malformations. Patients with orthopedic prostheses receive prophylactic antibiotics only if other risk factors for infection are also present.

Examples of bacterial resistance to antibiotics include *Staphylococcus aureus* resistance to all antibiotics except vancomycin; *Mycobacterium tuberculosis* resistance to isoniazid and rifampin; *Enterococcus* resistance to penicillins, cephalosporins, vancomycin, aminoglycosides, and tetracycline; *Streptococcus pneumoniae* resistance to penicillins and cephalosporins; *Neisseria gonorrhoeae* resistance to penicillin and tetracycline; and *Haemophilus influenzae* resistance to penicillins, tetracycline, and trimethoprim-sulfamethoxazole.

   a. Beta-lactam antibiotics
      (1) Beta-lactam antibiotics all contain a β-lactam ring, which is necessary for antibacterial activity.
      (2) Beta-lactam antibiotics include cephalosporins, penicillins, carbapenems, and monobactams (Table 8–4).
      (3) Beta-lactam antibiotics inhibit a bacterial enzyme known as penicillin-binding protein, which completes bacterial cell wall synthesis. When this enzyme is inhibited by antibiotics, the cell wall weakens, and the bacteria rupture.
   b. Aminoglycosides
      (1) The aminoglycosides are used to treat serious infections caused by certain gram-negative bacteria. They destroy bacteria by binding to bacterial ribosomes and inhibiting protein synthesis.
      (2) Commonly used aminoglycosides are gentamicin, tobramycin, amikacin, netilmicin, streptomycin, and kanamycin.

Table 8–4. Antibiotics

Actions and Uses	Adverse Reactions/ Contraindications	Drug Interactions	Nursing Implications

Aminoglycosides: Amikacin, gentamicin, kanamycin, neomycin, netilmicin, streptomycin, tobramycin

Actions and Uses	Adverse Reactions/ Contraindications	Drug Interactions	Nursing Implications
Bactericidal activity through binding to bacterial ribosomes, thus inhibiting synthesis of proteins required for replication Effective against most gram-negative bacteria except anaerobes Reserved for treatment of serious infections (because of toxicity) Does not penetrate bone or central nervous system	Nephrotoxicity and ototoxicity (with possible irreversible hearing loss) Neuromuscular depression due to decreased acetylcholine release most likely in people with neuromuscular disease or those receiving neuromuscular blocking agents Contraindicated during pregnancy because of risk of eighth cranial nerve damage and possible deafness of the fetus	Increased potential for nephrotoxicity and ototoxicity when used with other drugs having the same adverse effects Can produce skeletal muscle paralysis when used with neuromuscular blocking agents Synergistic with penicillin, which increases bacterial permeability	Because of toxicity, carefully monitor serum levels and adjust the dosage as ordered Monitor renal function and hearing (use audiometry for best determination of early hearing loss in those at high risk)

Beta-lactam antibiotics: Penicillins (amoxicillin, ampicillin, bacampicillin, carbenicillin, cloxacillin, dicloxacillin, methicillin, mezlocillin, nafcillin, oxacillin, penicillin G, penicillin V, piperacillin, ticarcillin)

Actions and Uses	Adverse Reactions/ Contraindications	Drug Interactions	Nursing Implications
Bactericidal activity Inhibition of cell wall synthesis, causing lysis Effective against gram-positive and gram-negative bacteria Susceptibility varies Effectiveness limited by bacterial β-lactamase, which destroys the β-lactam ring Some semisynthetic penicillinase-resistant agents available	Allergic reactions, hypernatremia or hyperkalemia (due to sodium or potassium in the penicillin preparation), thrombophlebitis, anemia, leukopenia, impaired platelet aggregation, seizures, nephritis Contraindicated if the person has a history of hypersensitivity to any penicillin preparation	Effectiveness decreased by bacteriostatic antibiotics such as tetracyclines and erythromycin Probenecid decreases renal clearance of penicillins and prolongs their action Acidifying agents, such as ammonium chloride, ascorbic acid, orange juice, and cranberry juice, destroy penicillin Ampicillin can interfere with oral contraceptives	Obtain a thorough history of allergic reactions Have emergency drugs and equipment available for cases of anaphylactic shock Monitor electrolyte levels Tell outpatients to notify nurse or physician of rash or decreased urination Tell outpatients to go immediately to an emergency department if they develop shortness of breath

Carbapenems (imipenem-cilastin)

Actions and Uses	Adverse Reactions/ Contraindications	Drug Interactions	Nursing Implications
Imipenem in combination with cilastin decreases drug inactivation by the kidneys Imipenem is a β-lactam antibiotic structurally different from the penicillins and cephalosporins but with a similar mechanism of action Effective against a wide range of gram-positive, gram-negative, and anaerobic bacteria Used to treat serious infections caused by antiobiotic-resistant bacteria	Nausea, vomiting, diarrhea, colitis, thrombophlebitis, fever, pruritus, urticaria, dyspnea, hyperventilation, fatigue, confusion, dizziness, somnolence, seizures, tachycardia, hypotension, oliguria, transient hearing loss	Similar to interactions with penicillin Concurrent use with ganciclovir can cause seizures; use with probenecid results in increased serum concentration and possible toxicity	Use seizure precautions for persons with head injury, intracranial neoplasms, renal insufficiency, or history of seizures Carefully monitor for allergic reactions in persons with history of allergy to penicillins, because cross-reactivity to imipenem is possible

Cephalosporins: First generation: cefadroxil, cefazolin, cephalexin, cephalothin, cephapirin, cephradine; second generation: cefaclor, cefamandole, cefmetazole, cefonicid, ceforanide, cefotetan, cefoxitin, cefprozil, cefuroxime; third generation: cefixime, cefoperazone, cefotaxime, cefpodoxime, ceftazidime, ceftizoxime, ceftriaxone

Actions and Uses	Adverse Reactions/ Contraindications	Drug Interactions	Nursing Implications
Bactericidal, with mechanism of action similar to penicillins From first to third generations, activity increases against gram-negative organisms and	Allergic reactions, nephrotoxicity, thrombophlebitis, nausea, vomiting, diarrhea Cephalosporins with a methylthiotetrazole group (especially cefa-	Nephrotoxicity potentiated by loop diuretics and aminoglycosides Probenecid decreases renal excretion and prolongs action Tetracyclines decrease effectiveness	Obtain thorough history of allergic reactions to any penicillin or cephalosporin Monitor renal function Tell the person to report severe

Table 8–4. Antibiotics (Continued)

Actions and Uses	Adverse Reactions/ Contraindications	Drug Interactions	Nursing Implications
decreases against gram-positive organisms Second and third generations more resistant to destruction by bacterial β-lactamase enzymes Third generation active against some first-generation–resistant bacteria	mandole and cefoperazone) impair prothrombin synthesis and can lead to bleeding Some agents cause false-positive glucose reaction in urine Disulfiram-like reaction with alcohol for cefamandole or cefoperazone		diarrhea, especially with blood or mucus; explain risk of drug-induced pseudomembranous colitis Advise the person not to ingest alcohol during treatment Do not give with tetracyclines

Monobactams (aztreonam)

Bacterial lysis by inhibition of cell wall synthesis Resistant to destruction by most bacterial β-lactamase enzymes Effective against gram-negative bacilli without the toxicity of the aminoglycosides Ineffective against gram-positive and anaerobic bacteria Can be used for persons allergic to other β-lactam antibiotics because of low cross-reactivity with these drugs	Gastrointestinal disturbances, including nausea, vomiting, and diarrhea Headache, weakness, paresthesia, altered taste, jaundice, elevated liver enzymes, blood dyscrasia Use with caution for persons with liver or renal dysfunction	Effectiveness decreased against β-lactamase–secreting gram-negative bacteria when aztreonam is used with cefoxitin and imipenem	Monitor liver and renal function and complete blood count

Macrolides: Azithromycin, clarithromycin, erythromycin

Bacteriostatic or bactericidal depending on concentration and bacterial susceptibility Binding to a subunit on the bacterial ribosome interferes with protein synthesis Effective against most gram-positive bacteria but have limited activity against gram-negative bacteria Very effective against *Campylobacter jejuni, Chlamydia trachomatis, Legionella pneumophila, Mycoplasma pneumoniae,* and *Treponema pallidum* Can be used for people allergic to penicillin	Relatively low toxicity but can cause nausea, vomiting, diarrhea, transient hearing loss, phlebitis at the infusion site, and allergic reactions Some forms can be hepatotoxic	Inhibits hepatic metabolism and increases serum concentration and potential for toxicity of many drugs, including cyclosporine, theophylline, and warfarin Can increase absorption of oral digoxin because they kill digoxin-metabolizing bacteria in the intestine Should not be administered with the antihistamines terfenadine or astemizole because of increased risk of inducing ventricular dysrhythmias	Monitor liver function and use with caution for people with liver dysfunction For people on theophylline who require erythromycin, monitor serum levels of theophylline

Quinolones: Cinoxacin, ciprofloxacin, enoxacin, lomefloxacin, nalidixic acid, norfloxacin, ofloxacin

Bactericidal activity Inhibition of a bacterial enzyme necessary for DNA replication and repair Effective against a variety of gram-negative aerobic bacteria Specific indications vary with different agents	Usually well tolerated and only occasionally cause nausea, vomiting, diarrhea, allergic reactions, nephritis, or central nervous system toxicity (headache, dizziness, drowsiness, confusion, visual disturbances, seizures) Contraindicated during pregnancy and lactation and for children younger than 16 years of age because of impairment of cartilage development	Decreased absorption with aluminum-, calcium-, or magnesium-containing compounds (e.g., antacids) and with iron or zinc Ciprofloxacin, enoxacin, norfloxacin, and ofloxacin can inhibit hepatic enzymes, which metabolize theophylline, resulting in increased theophylline levels and toxicity	Ensure that the person has adequate fluid intake to prevent the formation of drug crystals in the urinary tract Separate administration of quinolones and calcium-, magnesium-, aluminum-, iron-, or zinc-containing compounds by at least 2 hr

Table continued on following page

Table 8–4. Antibiotics (Continued)

Actions and Uses	Adverse Reactions/ Contraindications	Drug Interactions	Nursing Implications
Sulfonamides: Sulfacetamide, sulfacytine, sulfadiazine, sulfamethizole, sulfamethoxazole, sulfapyridine, sulfasalazine, sulfisoxazole, trimethoprim-sulfamethoxazole			
Bacteriostatic or bactericidal activity, depending on concentration Impairs synthesis of folic acid, an essential nutrient synthesized by bacteria, which cannot absorb it (trimethoprim further blocks folic acid synthesis) Effective against some gram-positive cocci and gram-negative bacilli, but many bacteria are resistant Used to treat urinary tract infection because effective concentrations do not cause renal damage	Allergic reactions due to sulfa component Can cause anemia, leukopenia, thrombocytopenia, gastrointestinal upset, headache, dizziness, seizures, hallucinations, fatigue, and insomnia Contraindicated for pregnant women near term and for newborns because agents displace bilirubin from protein-binding sites, resulting in jaundice and kernicterus	Because of competition for protein-binding sites, sulfonamides can displace or be displaced by other drugs that bind to plasma proteins: warfarin, oral hypoglycemics, and phenytoin. The result is increased concentration of active drug.	Monitor for allergic reactions, liver and renal function, and complete blood count
Tetracyclines: Chlortetracycline, demeclocycline, doxycycline, meclocycline, minocycline, oxytetracycline, tetracycline			
Bacteriostatic activity with broad-spectrum activity against gram-positive and gram-negative bacteria, rickettsiae, and mycoplasma Impair protein synthesis by binding to a ribosomal subunit Many bacterial strains have developed resistance	Impaired bone growth and discoloration of teeth because of calcium binding, especially during active periods of mineralization (up to 7 years of age) Photosensitivity, hepatic necrosis, renal failure, and diarrhea Contraindicated during pregnancy and lactation Contraindicated for children younger than 8 years All agents except doxycycline and minocycline contraindicated in the presence of renal insufficiency	Tetracyclines decrease the effectiveness of penicillins and cephalosporins and should not be administered concurrently Aluminum-, calcium-, and magnesium-containing compounds combine with oral tetracyclines and decrease their absorption Food in the intestinal tract also decreases their absorption	Obtain drug history, noting especially hypersensitivity to lidocaine or procaine, which may react adversely to the lidocaine in oxytetracycline or the procaine in the intramuscular preparation of tetracycline High risk for secondary infections because of broad-spectrum activity that upsets the balance of normal flora Observe for signs of secondary infections, especially *Candida,* and provide good preventive hygiene
Vancomycin			
Structure different from other antibiotics Drug of choice for treating methicillin-resistant *Staphylococcus aureus* and methicillin-resistant *Staphylococcus epidermidis* Inhibits bacterial cell wall synthesis Bactericidal for some microorganisms and bacteriostatic for others Used for intestinal infections caused by susceptible organisms	Anaphylactoid reactions, phlebitis at the infusion site, ototoxicity, nephrotoxicity, leukopenia, and thrombocytopenia Rapid intravenous infusion causes histamine release and red neck syndrome, characterized by erythema of the neck and upper torso, pruritus, and hypotension	Additive nephrotoxicity and ototoxicity when used with other agents with these same adverse effects	Infuse slowly (1 gm over 60 min) to decrease incidence of red neck syndrome Assess for hearing loss Monitor renal function Dosage reduction required for people with renal insufficiency

(3) The aminoglycosides are highly toxic. Adverse reactions include ototoxicity, resulting in reversible or irreversible hearing loss, and nephrotoxicity. Because aminoglycosides are excreted primarily by the kidneys, be sure that a dosage adjustment is made for people with renal insufficiency.

c. Macrolides

(1) Macrolides are used primarily to treat skin and upper respiratory infections. They can be used for persons allergic to penicillin. They are effective against most streptococci, *Legionella,* and *Mycoplasma pneumoniae* bacteria.

(2) Most macrolides are bacteriostatic and stop bacterial growth by interfering with protein synthesis.

(3) Macrolides include erythromycin, clarithromycin, roxithromycin, azithromycin, and dirithromycin.

(4) Macrolides are among the safest antibiotics, but they do have some adverse effects. Watch for phlebitis at the intravenous infusion site, fever, and rash.

d. Quinolones

(1) Quinolones are effective against most gram-negative bacilli. They can enter certain host cells and are therefore effective against some intracellular bacteria.

(2) They inhibit a bacterial enzyme that is necessary for the replication and repair of DNA.

(3) The quinolone class includes norfloxacin, ciprofloxacin, nalidixic acid, and clinafloxacin.

(4) Quinolones are usually well tolerated and only occasionally cause nausea or vomiting or central nervous system toxicity at high doses. The use of quinolones is contraindicated in children.

e. Tetracyclines

(1) Tetracyclines are among the oldest antibiotics, and because of their long-term use, many bacteria have developed resistance to them. They are effective against some gram-positive and gram-negative bacteria and rickettsiae. The tetracyclines inhibit bacterial protein synthesis and are bacteriostatic.

(2) This group includes tetracycline, oxytetracycline, chlortetracycline, demeclocycline, methacycline, doxycycline, and minocycline.

(3) Adverse effects of the tetracyclines include a rash on sun exposure, brown discoloration of the teeth, and retardation of bone growth in children and developing fetuses.

f. Sulfonamides

(1) Sulfonamides have also been used for a long time, and many bacteria have become resistant to them. They are effective against most gram-negative bacilli and some gram-positive cocci. They are bacteriostatic and are used to treat certain urinary tract infections and gastroenteritis.

(2) This group includes trimethoprin-sulfadiazine, sulfisoxazole, sulfadiazine, and sulfamethoxazole.

(3) Adverse reactions, mainly due to the sulfa component in these drugs, include rash and anaphylaxis. On rare occasions, hemolysis, thrombocytopenia, and leukopenia have occurred.

g. Vancomycin

(1) Vancomycin is a glycopeptide and is structurally unlike the other antibiotic classes. It is used mainly to treat infections with staphylococci or streptococci that are resistant to beta-lactam antibiotics or to treat persons allergic to the beta-lactams.

(2) It inhibits bacterial cell wall synthesis and is bacteriocidal.

(3) At high blood levels, vancomycin can cause nephrotoxicity and ototoxicity.

 DRUG ADVISORY

Infuse vancomycin slowly. Rapid infusion can produce red neck syndrome with erythema of the neck and upper torso, tingling, and hypotension caused by histamine release.

3. Antiviral agents: Currently available antiviral agents include drugs that inhibit various steps in the viral life cycle (Table 8–5).

4. Antifungal agents: Agents used most often for the treatment of systemic fungal infections are amphotericin B, fluconazole, flucytosine, and ketoconazole (Table 8–6).

Eliminating Infection: Medical-Surgical Interventions

1. Hyperbaric oxygen therapy

a. Breathing 100 percent oxygen at higher-than-atmospheric (barometric) pressure in a closed chamber increases the amount of dissolved oxygen transported in plasma, and can increase the PaO_2 to as high as 2000 mm Hg (normal PaO_2 = 80–100 mm Hg).

b. The oxygen-rich environment improves leukocyte phagocytic activity and kills anaerobic bacteria, such as *Clostridium perfringens* (the cause of gas gangrene).

NURSE ADVISORY

Take the following precautions for persons undergoing hyperbaric oxygen (HBO) therapy: (1) Warn the person against smoking for several hours before and after treatment to decrease lung irritation from breathing high oxygen levels; (2) teach the person to prevent pressure buildup in the ears (e.g., by swallowing); and (3) be sure that everyone in the HBO chamber wears 100 percent cotton clothing to prevent static electricity and sparks that could cause a fire.

c. Monitor the person for the following complications during hyperbaric oxygen therapy:

(1) Ear or sinus pain (from pressure buildup)

(2) Respiratory difficulty (a pulmonary manifestation of oxygen toxicity)

(3) Seizures (a central nervous system manifestation of oxygen toxicity)

(4) Bradycardia (a reflex response to hyperoxia)

2. Surgery: Surgery may be necessary to remove a source of infection that is unresponsive to antimicrobial therapy.

a. An abscess contains living organisms that can escape and travel to other tissues and cause infections at multiple sites. As the abscess grows, it exerts pressure on adjacent tissue, causing atrophy and pain. Rupture of an abscess causes severe sepsis and shock.

b. Surgery provides direct examination of all abscesses in the area and direct access for abscess drainage. Surgery also allows simultaneous correction of underlying cause of the abscess (e.g., a perforated bowel).

c. Removal of foreign materials may be necessary. Infections at a site of foreign material (e.g., orthopedic

Table 8–5. Antiviral Agents

Actions and Uses	Adverse Reactions/ Contraindications	Drug Interactions	Nursing Implications
Acyclovir (Zovirax)			
A nucleoside analogue activated by the viral enzyme thymidine kinase Inhibits viral DNA synthesis Effective against herpes simplex and varicella-zoster but less effective against Epstein-Barr virus and cytomegalovirus Penetrates the central nervous system (CNS) and therefore is used to treat herpes encephalitis Does not eradicate latent herpes infection	Adverse reactions uncommon but include renal dysfunction, allergy, hypotension, headache, seizures, drowsiness, lethargy, confusion, tremors, fever, nausea, vomiting, diarrhea, and phlebitis at the infusion site	Concurrent use of other nephrotoxic agents increases risk of adverse effects Probenecid decreases the elimination of acyclovir Use with zidovudine can increase drowsiness and lethargy	Monitor renal function Keep the person adequately hydrated during intravenous infusion to maintain urine flow and prevent precipitation of acyclovir in the renal tubules Inform the person that acyclovir does not eliminate latent herpes infections
Amantidine (Symmetrel)			
Prevents influenza A virus from uncoating in respiratory epithelial cells, thus inhibiting viral replication Used for the prevention and treatment of influenza A infections	Anorexia, nausea, vomiting, constipation, dry mouth and throat, anxiety, insomnia, impaired concentration, hallucinations, visual disturbances, weakness, headaches, rash, hypotension, palpations, ankle edema	Alcohol use increases the risk for CNS depression Increased anticholinergic effects (dry mouth, blurred vision, confusion, hallucinations) when used with an anticholinergic agent Increased CNS stimulation (insomnia, nervousness, dysrhythmias) when used with a CNS stimulant	Monitor older adults for confusion and difficulty with urination Monitor blood pressure Use cautiously in persons with epilepsy because the drug can increase incidence of seizures Caution the person to avoid alcohol ingestion during therapy Advise the person to report insomnia, confusion, or hallucinations to the physician because these are signs of CNS toxicity
Didanosine (ddI, Videx)			
A nucleoside analogue that competes with viral nucleosides, thus blocking viral DNA synthesis Used to treat immunodeficiency virus infections	Peripheral neuropathy (aching, burning, or tingling sensations), pancreatitis (which can be fatal), nausea, vomiting, diarrhea, abdominal pain, headache, insomnia, rash, pruritus, hyperuricemia, leukopenia	Increased risk of serious pancreatitis if used with other agents toxic to the pancreas, such as pentamidine Contains a buffer and can decrease absorption of drugs that require an acid medium for absorption, such as ketoconazole, quinolones, and tetracyclines	Administer on an empty stomach Administer drugs requiring an acid medium for absorption at least 2 hr before didanosine
Foscarnet (Foscavir)			
A pyrophosphate analogue that inhibits the viral enzyme DNA polymerase, thus blocking DNA synthesis Effective against herpesviruses, including cytomegalovirus and acyclovir-resistant herpes simplex and herpes zoster	Nephrotoxicity, anemia, hypotension, confusion, seizures, fever, nausea, vomiting, anorexia, and chelation, which lowers serum levels of calcium, magnesium, and potassium	Increased risk of nephrotoxicity when used concurrently with other nephrotoxic agents Concurrent use with pentamidine can cause severe hypocalcemia, hypomagnesemia, and nephrotoxicity	Monitor renal function Monitor serum levels of calcium, magnesium, and potassium
Ganciclovir (Cytovene, DHPG)			
A nucleoside analogue structurally similar to acyclovir but with inhibition of viral DNA synthesis Effective against herpesviruses including cytomegalovirus,	Fever, rash, nausea, vomiting, phlebitis at the infusion site, anemia, neutropenia, thrombocytopenia, malaise, headache, drowsiness, ataxia, confusion,	Bone marrow suppression potentiated by concurrent bone marrow–suppressing agents Severe hematologic toxicity possible when used with zidovudine	Monitor renal and liver function and complete blood count

Table 8–5. Antiviral Agents (Continued)

Actions and Uses	Adverse Reactions/ Contraindications	Drug Interactions	Nursing Implications
herpes simplex, and herpes zoster Most often used to treat retinitis, esophagitis, pneumonia, and colitis caused by cytomegalovirus infections	and serious renal and liver dysfunction Contraindicated for those with hypersensitivity to ganciclovir or acyclovir	Probenecid increases the potential for toxicity Can cause seizures when used with imipenem	

Ribavirin (Virazole)

A nucleoside analogue that inhibits viral DNA and RNA synthesis Used mainly in aerosol form to treat bronchitis and pneumonia caused by respiratory syncytial virus in infants and children Effectiveness in adults is questionable	Bronchospasm, dyspnea, rash, anemia, conjunctivitis, weakness, hypotension, cardiac arrest Contraindicated during pregnancy because of teratogenic potential	No significant interactions known	Health care personnel and visitors, especially pregnant women, should avoid exposure to aerosolized ribavirin at the patient's bedside Prevent accumulation of the aerosolized drug on valves or in tubing of mechanical ventilators because it can cause ventilator malfunction

Vidarabine (adenine arabinoside, ara-A, Vira-A)

An inhibitor of viral DNA polymerase, thus inhibiting viral DNA synthesis Effective against DNA viruses including herpes simplex, varicella-zoster, and cytomegalovirus Penetrates the blood-brain barrier and used to treat herpes encephalitis	Tremors and ataxia, anemia, photosensitivity, Parkinson-like reaction, encephalopathy (more likely to occur in those with renal or liver dysfunction)	Allopurinol can interfere with metabolism of vidarabine	Monitor the person's neurologic and hematologic status

Zalcitabine (dideoxycytidine, ddC)

A nucleoside analogue that inhibits the reverse transcriptase enzyme and thus inhibits viral replication Used in combination with zidovudine to treat advanced infection with the human immunodeficiency virus	Pancreatitis, hepatitis, stomatitis, peripheral neuropathy, nausea, vomiting, dysphagia, abnormal taste sensations, ototoxicity, headache, dizziness, fatigue, myalgia, arthralgia, anemia, leukopenia	Additive peripheral neuropathy when used with didanosine	Monitor the person's complete blood count, serum amylase, and signs of adverse reactions

Zidovudine (azidothymidine, AZT, Retrovir)

A nucleoside analogue that inhibits the reverse transcriptase enzyme and thus inhibits viral replication Used to treat human immunodeficiency virus infection	Anorexia; nausea; vomiting; abdominal pain; hematologic toxicity, including serious anemia and neutropenia; headache; seizures; rash; nail discoloration	Can cause incapacitating lethargy and drowsiness when used with acyclovir Acetaminophen, probenecid, and sulfonamides decrease clearance of zidovudine and thereby increase risk of toxicity	Administer on an empty stomach Monitor complete blood count

prostheses or artificial heart valves) are often unresponsive to antibiotic therapy because the foreign materials shield the pathogens from host immune defenses and antibiotics.

  d. Removal of necrotic tissue may be the only way to eliminate infecting organisms and clean up the area to allow healing to take place. Dead tissue is a good environment for growth of some organisms such as anaerobic bacteria. Antimicrobial agents may be ineffective in eliminating infection at the site of dead,

Table 8–6. Antifungal Agents

Actions and Uses	Adverse Reactions/ Contraindications	Drug Interactions	Nursing Implications
Amphotericin B (Fungizone)			
Fungistatic or fungicidal depending on concentration and fungal sensitivity Binds to fungus cell membrane causing increased permeability and loss of intracellular contents Has a wide spectrum of antifungal activity and is used for localized and systemic fungal infections Poorly distributed to the central nervous system	Chills, fever, anorexia, headache, nausea, vomiting, diarrhea, bone marrow suppression, ototoxicity, nephrotoxicity, hypersensitivity reaction, hypokalemia, hypomagnesemia, thrombophlebitis at the intravenous infusion site	Additive nephrotoxicity with other nephrotoxic agents such as aminoglycosides, cisplatin, cyclosporine, furosemide, and vancomycin Amphotericin-induced hypokalemia increases risk of digitalis toxicity Concurrent use of glucocorticoids or mineralocorticoids increases risk for severe hypokalemia	Monitor renal function, serum potassium and magnesium, and complete blood count Assess for hearing loss, vertigo, and tinnitus Check intravenous infusion site for extravasation and thrombophlebitis
Fluconazole (Diflucan)			
Inhibits fungal metabolism Used to treat mucocutaneous *Candida* infections and cryptococcal meningitis	Nausea, vomiting, rash, headache, hepatotoxicity	Can prolong warfarin activity and increase risk of bleeding Rifampin can increase metabolism of fluconozole so that the drug may need an upward dosage adjustment Can increase serum levels of phenytoin Can increase serum concentration of oral hypoglycemic agents, resulting in hypoglycemia	Monitor liver function tests
Flucytosine (Ancobon)			
Fungistatic or fungicidal (at higher dosages) Converted to fluorouracil inside fungal cells and so interferes with nucleic acid synthesis, resulting in fungal cell death Effective against some *Candida* species, *Cryptococcus neoformans,* and some isolates of other fungal species Rarely used as a single antifungal agent because resistance often develops during therapy	Bone marrow suppression, nausea, vomiting, diarrhea, renal and liver impairment, headache, drowsiness, confusion, dizziness Avoid concurrent use with other hepatotoxic or nephrotoxic drugs Contraindicated in pregnancy	Toxicity increases if used concurrently with other bone marrow depressants	Monitor renal and liver function tests and white blood cell and platelet counts Caution the person to avoid driving and other activities requiring alertness until the response to the medication is known Advise the person to notify the physician if a rash, excessive bleeding, bruising, or weakness develops
Griseofulvin (Grifulvin V, Grisactin, Fulvicin P/G, Gris-PEG)			
Fungistatic agent used for infections of the skin and nails Deposits in precursor skin and nail cells, making them resistant to fungal infection Exfoliation of previously infected cells occurs, and remaining cells are resistant to fungal infection	Headache, dizziness, blurred vision, hearing loss, nausea, vomiting, diarrhea, dry mouth, sore throat, black furry tongue, urticaria, fever, photosensitivity, proteinuria, leukopenia Risk of cross-sensitivity in people allergic to penicillin Contraindicated for those with severe liver disease	Can decrease effectiveness of oral anticoagulants and oral contraceptives Can increase the central nervous system depressant effect of alcohol Barbiturates decrease blood level and effectiveness of the drug	Explain why long-term therapy (weeks to months) is required to eradicate infection Caution the person to avoid alcohol during therapy Warn about possible photosensitivity
Ketoconazole (Nizoral)			
Broad-spectrum fungistatic and fungicidal activity	Nausea, vomiting, diarrhea, fever, dizziness, headache, hepatotox-	Additive hepatotoxicity with other hepatotoxic agents	Monitor liver function tests Note that at least 2 hours should

Table 8–6. Antifungal Agents (Continued)

Actions and Uses	Adverse Reactions/ Contraindications	Drug Interactions	Nursing Implications
Impairs fungal cell membrane synthesis, causing leakage of cell contents Used to treat candidiasis and systemic fungal infections Not recommended for central nervous system infections because of poor penetration across the blood-brain barrier	icity, pruritus, photophobia, gynecomastia, impotence	Can increase activity of oral anticoagulants and cyclosporine Antacids, anticholinergics, histamine$_2$ blockers, and didanosine increase gastrointestinal pH and decrease absorption	separate ingestion of agents that increase gastric pH and ketoconazole Caution person to avoid prolonged exposure to bright light and to wear sunglasses outdoors to decrease photophobia Also caution against concurrent alcohol ingestion
Nystatin (Mycostatin, Nilstat, Nystex)			
Fungistatic and fungicidal activity Binds to fungal cell membrane, causing increased permeability and loss of cell contents Used to treat localized *Candida* infections of the skin, mucous membranes, vagina, and intestines	Nausea, vomiting, diarrhea, stomach pain Contraindicated for those with hypersensitivity to nystatin or additives found in some preparations such as alcohol, povidone, and propylene glycol	No significant interactions known	Instruct person about proper ingestion of oral suspension or topical or vaginal application

underperfused tissue because they do not reach the microorganisms.

Preventing Nosocomial Infections

1. Urinary tract infections
   a. The urinary tract is the most common site of nosocomial infections. Urinary tract infections are characterized by pyuria (greater than 10 white blood cells per high-power microscopic field, or greater than 100,000 bacteria per ml of urine collected from a clean-catch specimen, or between 10,000 to 100,000 bacteria per ml if the specimen was collected by bladder catheterization).

NURSE ADVISORY

An indwelling Foley catheter is the most common cause of nosocomial infections of the urinary tract.

   b. Preventive measures
      (1) Catheterize the bladder only when absolutely necessary.
      (2) Insert catheters with strict adherence to aseptic technique.
      (3) Clean the urinary meatus-catheter junction at least once daily.
      (4) Empty the urine bag before it is full so that the outflow of urine is not obstructed.
      (5) Keep the tubing and bag below the level of the bladder to prevent the backflow of urine into the bladder.
      (6) Keep the bag off the floor.
      (7) Clean ports before and after emptying urine or taking samples.
      (8) Wash and dry perineal and rectal areas frequently, especially if the patient is incontinent of stool.
      (9) Remove the catheter as soon as possible.
2. Wound infections (see also Chapter 13 and Chapter 37).
   a. The incidence of wound infections is partly related to the degree of contamination of the wound during surgery. Wound infections are characterized by purulent drainage and positive results on wound cultures.
   b. Preventive measures
      (1) Thoroughly cleanse the skin with an antiseptic soap preoperatively.
      (2) Use aseptic technique during surgery and dressing changes.
      (3) Use appropriate ventilation systems in the operating rooms to decrease the spread of airbone pathogens.
      (4) Administer prophylactic antibiotics before bowel surgery.
3. Nosocomial pneumonia
   a. The major risk factors for nosocomial pneumonia are intubation, upper abdominal or thoracic surgery, ineffective cough reflex, and increased gastric pH (caused, for example, by use of antacids or histamine blockers, which facilitate the growth of intestinal flora).
   b. Preventive measures
      (1) Encourage deep breathing and coughing.
      (2) Encourage early ambulation.
      (3) Properly sterilize all respiratory therapy equipment.

(4) Use aseptic technique for intubation and endotracheal suctioning.

(5) Maintain good oral hygiene to decrease colonization of the oropharyngeal tract.

(6) Administer medication. Some research documents the effectiveness of sucralfate (a drug that coats the stomach but does not increase gastric pH) in preventing stress ulcers without increasing the risk of pneumonia.

4. Cutaneous infections
   a. Major risk factors for skin infections include burns and pressure ulcers (see Chapters 7 and 36). Cutaneous infections are characterized by purulent drainage or positive cultures.
   b. Preventive measures
      (1) Turn the person every hour or use an automatic rotating bed.
      (2) Massage the skin to improve circulation.
      (3) Promote good nutrition to maintain skin integrity.
      (4) Keep skin clean and dry.

5. Bacteremias
   a. Bacteremias develop from infections elsewhere in the body (e.g., wound or pulmonary infections); from contaminated blood, fluids, and intravascular devices; or from contamination during injection of medications into vascular lines.
   b. Preventive measures
      (1) Insert and manage vascular lines using aseptic technique.
      (2) Use aseptic technique when cleaning intravascular insertion sites.
      (3) Before use, check intravenous tubing and bags for cracks.
      (4) Change intravenous tubing, following institutional policy.
      (5) Check intravenous solutions for discoloration and clarity (cloudy solutions may indicate contamination).
      (6) Whenever possible, have the pharmacy mix intravenous solutions.
      (7) Use aseptic technique when adding medications to intravenous bags or ports.
      (8) Use measures to prevent other infections that can lead to bacteremia.

General Preventive Measures

1. Hand washing
   a. The spread of microorganisms that either have colonized the hands or are transient residents on the hands is a common cause of nosocomial infections (Box 8–3).
   b. Hand washing is necessary even if gloves are worn, because the hands can become contaminated through a tear in the glove or during the removal of gloves. See Procedure 8–1 for general principles and agents for hand washing.
2. Sterile technique: See Table 8–7 for principles and nursing interventions related to maintaining a sterile field (see also Chapter 13).

BOX 8–3. Nursing Management for Infection Control

The prevention, monitoring, and reporting of infections of both patients and staff is an important responsibility of the nurse manager. To train new staff and to review procedures for continuing staff, you should conduct in-service programs on topics related to infection control and reporting, such as hand washing procedure, aseptic technique, body substance isolation, and universal precautions.

Communication and collaboration of the nurse manager with the following departments is also important for infection control:

- The infection control service is a resource for staff in-service programs and the latest information related to the treatment and reporting of infections. Collaborate with this team in identifying and reporting infections and enforcing their infection control policies. Also be aware of procedures to follow in cases of an epidemic.
- The occupational health department is charged with protecting personnel from infection while on duty and preventing infected staff from transmitting their infection to patients. Be aware of and enforce your institution's policy regarding the follow-up of staff who have been exposed while on duty to such infections as human immunodeficiency virus, hepatitis, and tuberculosis. Also make your staff aware of the preventive measures available through the occupational health department (e.g., hepatitis B and other vaccines). Enforce work restrictions that are set by the occupational health department for staff with communicable diseases.
- The housekeeping department is responsible for the cleanliness of the environment and the disposal of medical waste according to local regulations. Enforce your institution's policy regarding decontamination of objects following contamination with body fluids. Use a disinfectant approved by the Environmental Protection Agency. Also keep clean supplies separate from used or soiled items.

---

3. Isolation procedures
   a. Body substance isolation (precautions) is based on the principle that any person is potentially a carrier of a pathogen, even in the absence of a positive culture or clinical manifestations of infection.
   b. Body substance isolation protects against contact with a patient's solid or fluid substances, such as blood, urine, feces, saliva, cerebrospinal fluid, and wound drainage.
   c. Body substance isolation has been shown to be better at protecting both the patient and the staff from infection than the older, category-specific method of isolation based on the patient's diagnosis.
   d. Guidelines for observing body substance isolation precautions, which have been adapted from the work of Lynch and associates, are as follows:
      (1) Wear clean gloves for anticipated contact with blood, mucous membranes, secretions, excretions, tissue samples, nonintact skin, and moist body substances. Change gloves between patient contacts and between activities related to the same patient (to prevent cross-contamination from one area of the patient to another).
      (2) Wash your hands (see Procedure 8–1) before each new patient contact and whenever your hands become soiled.
      (3) Use additional barriers, such as masks, goggles, hair or shoe covers, or plastic aprons, when blood or other body substances could splash

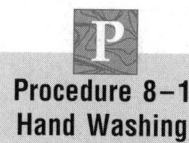

Procedure 8–1
Hand Washing

Equipment	• Soap (liquid, leaflet, powder) or antimicrobial soap solution • Running water • Paper towels • Nail cleaner, if necessary
Definition/Purpose	To remove transient microorganisms from the skin of the hands. Chemical forces include antimicrobial soap solutions and bar, leaflet, powder, or liquid soaps. Mechanical forces include friction during the washing and flushing away during the rinsing. Hand washing helps control infectious disease by decreasing the possibility of cross-contamination. Hand washing is the single most effective means of promoting good medical asepsis.
Contraindications/Cautions	Health care workers must wash their hands so frequently that the skin can break down. It is important to wash the hands for a sufficient time to remove microbes, but not to prolong the procedure unnecessarily. Likewise, cleaning under the fingernails with sharp instruments such as nail files or plastic fingernail cleaners can damage delicate tissues. Use such instruments only when visible soil has accumulated and cannot be removed otherwise. Keep fingernails short to reduce the area where microbes may harbor and thus reduce the total number of microbes on the hands. Report to your supervisor any lesions on your hands, such as broken skin, a rash, or one or more vesicles. Such lesions are capable of harboring microbes, are potential portals of entry for pathogens, and may be made worse by hand washing.
Learning/Teaching Guidelines	Patients may be frightened of acquiring an infectious disease from health care workers. Telling them that you are going to wash your hands or, if facilities allow, actually washing your hands in their presence can reassure them. Teaching patients and family members how to wash their own hands effectively may be an important part of teaching them self-care.

Preliminary Activities

	Long sleeves are inconvenient in the clinical area. The distal portion of the sleeves can easily be soiled during work and can get wet during hand washing. It is easier not to wear long sleeves at all, but, if worn, the sleeves must be rolled up or pushed up before each hand washing. Likewise, your wristwatch should either be worn 2.5 to 5 cm (1 to 2 in.) above the wrist at all times, or it will have to be moved up on the arm before each hand washing.
Assessment/Planning	Plan to wash your hands at least • at the beginning of the work day • before giving any nursing care • after giving any nursing care • after using the toilet • before eating or handling food Also wash your hands when providing nursing care whenever there is a chance of transmitting pathogenic microorganisms from a potentially contaminated area to a cleaner area; for example, • before assisting the patient with eating • before contact with mucous membranes or nonintact skin (e.g., before any invasive procedure or contact with a wound) • after soilage of the hands with most body substances (e.g., after contact with any blood or body fluid when assisting with client toileting, wound care, or invasive procedures, even if gloves are worn) When not caring for patients, plan to wash your hands whenever necessary; for example, • before eating • after contaminating your hands by touching your hair, wiping your nose, or using the toilet
Procedure	

Actions	Rationale/Discussion
1. Standing well back from the sink, turn on the water and adjust the flow to a comfortable temperature: 105°F to 110°F (40.5°C to 43.3°C).	1. Standing close to running water exposes the uniform to splashing. Having to adjust water temperature that is too hot or too cold later (before rinsing) may require touching faucets that are considered contaminated with hands that have just been cleaned.
2. Wet hands well with water before soaping them with liquid soap, a soap leaflet, powdered soap, or an antimicrobial soap solution.	2. The addition of water to soap promotes the formation of suds that help to emulsify body secretions, oils, or greases that may be present on the hands and that tend to protect microbes. With some antimicrobial soaps, the addition of water reduces skin irritation.

(continued)

P

Procedure 8–1

(continued)

Actions	Rationale/Discussion
If a bar soap is used, rinse it to flush away surface dirt before lathering with it, and again before replacing it in the soap dish.	Although soap can serve as a medium for the growth of bacteria, there is no evidence that rinsing the bar is effective in reducing bacterial growth. Rather, the rinsed bar is more esthetically pleasing.
3. If it is the first hand wash of the day or if hands are grossly soiled, clean under fingernails with file or plastic fingernail cleaner, as necessary. Otherwise, clean under each fingernail with a fingernail from the opposite hand.	3. Fingernails can harbor microbes. Cleaning helps remove subungual microbes and thus decreases microbe proliferation. Sharp instruments can damage delicate subungual tissues and should be used with care and only when necessary.
4. Rub palms and fingers together using friction. Pay particular attention to places where microbes can hide (e.g., under and around fingernails and in the knuckle creases). Also give attention to the thumbs and to the lateral aspects of the hand and fifth fingers. If a ring is worn, move it enough to clean the finger under it and wash the ring with friction as well as the fingers.	4. Friction helps to loosen microbes so they can be removed. These areas are often overlooked during hand washing.
5. Continue washing for at least 10 seconds.	5. Ten seconds is the minimum acceptable time established for hand washing, but more time may be taken if required.
6. With fingernails lower than wrists, rinse hands well under running water.	6. Rinse water will flush loosened microbes away from the cleanest part of the hands (the wrists) toward the least clean part (the fingernails). Thorough rinsing removes residual soap solution that can dry the skin of the hands.
7. Thoroughly dry hands with paper towel.	7. Paper towels are disposable and are used only once, so they do not contribute to cross-contamination. Hands that are not thoroughly dried are prone to maceration.
8. Unless foot or knee controls are being used, use a paper towel to turn off water faucet.	8. The towel serves as a barrier between clean fingers and contaminated faucet handles.
9. Carefully discard paper towel.	9. Touching the waste container contaminates clean fingers. Having to pick up a paper towel from the floor can contaminate clean hands and is a waste of time and energy.

Final Activities

Use extra paper toweling as a barrier to protect your clean hands as you wipe up splashed water and suds as necessary to keep the work area clean and dry.

Adapted from Bolander V (ed). *Sorensen and Luckmann's Basic Nursing: A Psychophysiologic Approach*. 3rd ed. Philadelphia: WB Saunders, 1994.

onto your face, mucous membranes, skin, or clothing.

(4) Transport soiled, reusable articles and trash in plastic bags or rigid containers to prevent leaking.

(5) Place sharp instruments and unrecapped needles in puncture-resistant rigid containers. For reusable needles use a recapping device.

(6) Provide a private room for patients with diseases transmitted by the airborne route (e.g., pulmonary tuberculosis). Wear a mask. Place a large sign on the door to the room of such patients instructing all persons to check with the nurse before entering. Also provide a private room for patients who soil articles in the environment with body secretions.

(7) When contacting patients with diseases such as measles, rubella, mumps, or chickenpox, health care workers immune to these infections are not

required to take extra barrier precautions. Susceptible personnel should not care for patients with these diseases.

e. Box 8–4 lists universal blood and body fluid precautions that were initially developed to protect health care professionals from infection with the human immunodeficiency virus.

◼ COMPLICATIONS OF INFECTION

Sepsis

1. **Sepsis** is the systemic host response to an infection that has progressed to the systemic level. Sepsis exists when two or more of the following criteria are present:

Table 8–7. Selected Scientific Principles and Related Nursing Interventions for Maintaining a Sterile Field

Principle	Nursing Interventions
Sterile objects that are out of the line of vision are considered questionable or their sterility cannot be guaranteed. Waist level and table level are considered margins of safety that can be uniformly enforced and that promote maximum visibility of the sterile objects.	Always face the sterile field. Do not turn your back or side on a sterile field. Keep sterile equipment above your waist level or above table level.
Microorganisms from the oral cavity are spread into the air when a person speaks or coughs and the organisms may drop onto the sterile field.	Do not speak, cough, sneeze, or laugh over a sterile field. If it is necessary to do any of these, turn your head away from the sterile field.
When a nonsterile object is held above a sterile object, gravity causes microorganisms to fall onto the sterile object.	Never reach across the sterile field. Instead (1) move yourself around the field (while continuing to face the field), (2) reach around the edges of the sterile field, or (3) cautiously turn the entire sterile field either by touching the edges of the bottom wrapper or by reaching underneath the bottom wrapper.
A sterile object becomes contaminated when touched by a nonsterile object. A sterile field cannot be contaminated by a sterile object.	Never touch a sterile field with any object that is not sterile. Sterile objects (or hands covered with sterile gloves) may safely touch or pass over a sterile field.
A general rule is that there is a 2.5-cm (1-inch) margin of safety around the outside edge of a sterile field. This 2.5-cm (1-inch) border is considered contaminated. Microorganisms are present in, and travel on, air currents.	The unsterile hand may touch the edge of the sterile field if necessary to make a small adjustment. Prevent excessive air currents around the sterile field (e.g., close the door before opening the sterile field, move slowly, minimize flapping of clothing and drapes).
Sterilization indicators are used to demonstrate whether an object has been exposed to the sterilization process. Sterility expiration date indicates the last possible date on which the contents of the package can be assumed to be sterile. Only intact wrappings protect sterile objects from contamination.	Never assume that an object is sterile. Always check the sterilization indicators on or inside of wrappers of sterile objects. Always check the sterility expiration date, which is clearly stated on the package. Always check to be sure the sterile package is intact. Look for holes, tears, watermarks, or other signs that might indicate contamination.
Any object is considered contaminated if its sterility is in question. When a liquid connects a nonsterile surface to a sterile one, microorganisms may be transferred from the unsterile to the sterile area. Consequently, the sterile area becomes contaminated by capillary attraction.	If the sterility of an object is in doubt, do not use it. Handle liquids cautiously near the sterile field to prevent drapes or wrappers from becoming wet. Do not allow splashing to occur.
Microorganisms do not pass easily through a dry surface; rather, they tend to move slowly along the surface. That which is sterile remains sterile unless contaminated, but one part of an instrument may be sterile and another part contaminated as long as it is clear what is sterile and what is not.	Dry sterile objects (e.g., sterile towel) may have one surface that is contaminated and one surface that is sterile. A sterile object (e.g., a pair of scissors) may be picked up from a sterile field with a sterile instrument (e.g., a forceps) and touched with bare hands on parts of the object that can be contaminated (e.g., touched handles become contaminated). The tips, however, may still be considered sterile if they touch only that which is sterile (e.g., the tips may be placed within the sterile field's 2.5-cm [1-inch] border while the contaminated handles stay outside of the 2.5-cm [1-inch] border).
Fluid flows downward by gravity. Fluid that flows into a contaminated area becomes contaminated. Fluid that is contaminated can flow back into a sterile area and contaminate it.	When working with liquids on a sterile field by using forceps with contaminated handles, always be certain to keep the tips of the forceps pointed downward.

From Bolander V (ed). *Sorensen and Luckmann's Basic Nursing: A Psychophysiologic Approach.* 3rd ed. Philadelphia: WB Saunders, 1994.

a. Rectal temperature greater than 38 degrees Celsius or less than 36 degrees Celsius

b. Heart rate greater than 90 beats per minute

c. Respiratory rate greater than 20 breaths per minute or $Paco_2$ less than 32 mm Hg (a result of hyperventilation)

d. White blood cell count greater than 12,000 per mm^3 or less than 4000 per mm^3 or more than 10 percent of the total white blood cell count as immature cells.

Severe Sepsis

1. Severe sepsis is accompanied by organ dysfunction, decreased tissue perfusion, or hypotension (systolic blood

BOX 8-4. Universal Precautions

Universal precautions are intended to prevent parenteral, mucous membrane, and nonintact skin exposures of health care workers to blood-borne pathogens. Universal precautions apply to blood and to other body fluids containing visible blood, semen, vaginal secretions, cerebrospinal fluid, synovial fluid, pleural fluid, peritoneal fluid, pericardial fluid, and amniotic fluid. Universal precautions do not apply to feces, nasal secretions, sputum, sweat, tears, urine, and vomitus unless they contain visible blood.

Barrier Guidelines

1. Disposable gloves (vinyl, latex) should be worn when in contact or when there is potential for contact with blood, body fluids, or other fluids that may contain human immunodeficiency virus (HIV) or other blood-borne pathogens. Gloves should be removed after each client contact. Rubber gloves can be used for equipment cleaning.
2. Hands should be washed between clients, after any exposure, and after removal of gloves.
3. Protective eyewear, face shields, and/or masks should be worn during procedures that may aerosolize blood.
4. Impervious gowns should be worn when there is potential for exposure to large quantities of blood, such as in the labor and delivery area or emergency room.

Needle Precautions

1. Needles should never be recapped after use; keep in mind that most needlesticks are the result of missed needle recapping.
2. Do not cut, break, or bend needles after use; this may release aerosolized blood from the needle shaft.
3. Do not leave used needles lying around.
4. Do not dispose of needles in ordinary receptacles; instead, use appropriately labeled, impermeable needle containers.

From Bolander V (ed). *Sorensen and Luckmann's Basic Nursing: A Psychophysiologic Approach.* 3rd ed. Philadelphia: WB Saunders, 1994.
Adapted from the Centers for Disease Control. Update: Universal precautions for prevention of transmission of human immunodeficiency virus, hepatitis B virus, and other bloodborne pathogens in health-care setting. *MMWR 37*(3): 377–388, 1988.

pressure less than 90 mm Hg, or a decrease of more than 40 mm Hg from the person's baseline value in the absence of other causes of hypotension).
2. Clinical manifestations of decreased tissue perfusion include the following:
   a. Lactic acidosis: Plasma lactate greater than 1.8 mEq/L in arterial blood or 2.2 mEq/L in venous blood
   b. Oliguria: Urine output less than 0.5 ml per kg per hour
   c. Acute alteration in mental status

Septic Shock

1. **Septic shock** is the end stage of an overwhelming systemic infection in which perfusion is inadequate to meet the metabolic demands of tissues (see Chapter 12).
2. The criteria for septic shock are evidence of sepsis-induced hypotension that persists despite adequate fluid replacement and evidence of decreased tissue perfusion.

Experimental Agents for the Treatment of Sepsis

1. Many people develop septic shock and die of severe infections because of tissue damage caused by overstimulation of host defense systems, and not because of the direct effects of the pathogen.
2. Therapies for sepsis currently under investigation are directed at blocking the harmful effects caused by host responses to infection and the action of endotoxin, a component of the cell wall of gram-negative bacteria, which activates host defenses.

◼ APPLYING THE NURSING PROCESS

NURSING DIAGNOSIS: Risk for infection R/T increased host susceptibility due to malnutrition, immunodeficiency, invasive monitoring, a wound, or nonintact skin

1. *Expected outcomes*
   a. The person will remain free of infection.
   b. Immune function will be maintained as optimally as possible.
   c. Infection will be recognized early, to allow for prompt treatment.
2. *Nursing interventions*
   a. Determine the person's risk for infection, including host-related and treatment-related risk factors.
   b. Adhere strictly to policy on hand washing, use of gloves, and aseptic technique.
   c. Mobilize respiratory secretions with adequate hydration, coughing and deep breathing, incentive spirometry, and position changes.
   d. Maintain skin integrity by keeping skin lubricated and dry and by changing position at least every 2 hours.
   e. Decrease risk of urinary tract infection by maintaining perineal hygiene and preventing urinary stasis.
   f. Avoid placing the person in the same room with someone who has an infection.
   g. Help the person decrease stress, which causes increased secretion of immunosuppressant glucocorticoid hormones.
   h. Monitor for signs and symptoms of infection (see Table 8–3).
   i. Obtain specimens for cultures as ordered (see Box 8–2).

NURSING DIAGNOSIS: Risk for altered body temperature R/T infectious process

1. *Expected outcomes*
   a. The person will be able to tolerate the increased metabolic demands associated with an elevated body temperature.
   b. Comfort will be maintained.

c. Body temperature will return to normal in response to treatment of the infection.

2. *Nursing interventions*
   a. Monitor body temperature at least every 4 hours, by the same route, and at the same times of the day.
   b. Monitor cardiovascular and respiratory status to determine ability to meet the increased oxygen demands associated with a fever.
   c. Maintain comfort by positioning and providing clean and dry bed clothing.
   d. Report onset of chills because blood cultures obtained at that time are more likely to detect intermittent bacteremias.
   e. Administer antimicrobial therapy as ordered.
   f. Administer antipyretics as ordered.

NURSING DIAGNOSIS: Risk for fluid volume deficit R/T diaphoresis due to fever, gastrointestinal fluid loss secondary to vomiting or diarrhea, and water vapor loss secondary to increased respiratory rate

1. *Expected outcomes:* Fluid balance will be maintained.
2. *Nursing interventions*
   a. Monitor intake and output and daily weights.
   b. Watch for signs and symptoms of fluid volume deficit including complaints of thirst, decreased skin turgor, orthostatic hypotension, tachycardia, weak pulse, oliguria, concentrated urine, and decreased tissue perfusion (see Chapter 9).
   c. Force fluids, unless contraindicated, to balance fluid losses.
   d. Monitor laboratory tests that would reflect hemoconcentration, such as hematocrit and blood urea nitrogen (BUN).

NURSING DIAGNOSIS: Impaired social interactions R/T isolation for airborne infection

1. *Expected outcomes*
   a. The person verbalizes feelings related to isolation.
   b. The person will have interpersonal contacts without transmission of infection to others.
   c. The person will have a realistic and positive self-image.
2. *Nursing interventions*
   a. Discuss with the person the impact of the infectious disease on self-image and social interactions.
   b. Determine the effect of the person's culture on the perception of having an infectious disease.
   c. Provide frequent contacts with the person, maintaining appropriate isolation procedure.
   d. Provide stimuli in the person's environment such as reading materials, radio, and television.
   e. Explain how the person can maintain social contacts during hospitalization and at home (if long-term precautions are required) without transmitting the infection to others.

■ DISCHARGE PLANNING AND TEACHING

1. Assess the person's understanding of the infectious disease process and its treatment.
2. Provide a comfortable environment conducive to learning.
3. Teach patient and family members about the mode of transmission and preventive measures specific to their infection and infections in general.
4. Explain the importance of completing the full course of antimicrobial therapy.
5. Explain the danger of using antimicrobial medications prescribed for others or for a previous infection.
6. Explain the role of good nutrition in maintenance of resistance to infection.
7. Teach the person the signs and symptoms of infection and the time to report to the physician or nurse.
8. Teach the person—with a return demonstration—required self-care procedures such as intravascular line care, bladder catheterization, or dressing changes.
9. Identify home care needs, and make referrals for additional support as necessary.

■ PUBLIC HEALTH CONSIDERATIONS

Reporting and Control

1. Successful eradication of infectious diseases requires accurate reporting so that appropriate therapy and preventive measures can be initiated.
2. Physicians *must* report certain communicable diseases to state health departments. State laws vary as to which diseases must be reported. Information regarding mandatory reporting and the appropriate level (local, state, national, or international) can be found in the latest report of the American Public Health Association's *Control of Infectious Diseases in Man*.
3. In addition to individual case reports of infectious disease, any unusual occurrence, such as an increase in incidence that could represent an epidemic, must be reported to the local health authority. Throughout history infectious diseases have been a leading cause of disability and death, prompting nations to cooperate in efforts to eradicate them. The World Health Organization (WHO), a division of the United Nations, is responsible for the prevention, control, and monitoring of infectious diseases on a worldwide basis. Worldwide eradication of infectious diseases includes smallpox, which has been eradicated by vaccinations, and rubella, rubeola, and poliomyelitis, which the World Health Organization hopes to eradicate by the end of the 20th century through vaccinations. The Centers for Disease Control and Prevention (CDC), in Atlanta, Georgia, is responsible for controlling communicable diseases in the United States.
4. Home health nurses participate in the control of communicable diseases in the community by reporting, assessing the home environment, and providing instruction on

proper hygiene; handling of contaminated objects; use of gowns, gloves, and masks; safe food preparation; and using uncontaminated water supplies.

Factors Hindering Eradication of Infectious Diseases

1. Difficulty in developing safe and effective vaccines when faced with constantly mutating pathogens.
2. Tendency of arthropod vectors to develop immunity to antimicrobial agents and insecticides.
3. Lack of adequate delivery to and compliance by people in need of vaccinations or antimicrobial therapy.
4. Cost of vaccines and implementation of sanitation technology.
5. Unwillingness of individuals to take preventive measures (e.g., to use "safer sex" practices to prevent spread of the human immunodeficiency virus).

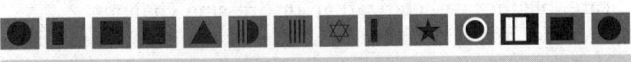

TRANSCULTURAL CONSIDERATIONS

Some cultures have serious taboos against the use of vaccines and other preventive measures that make it difficult, or even impossible, to lower the rates of certain infections.

Immunizations to Alter Host Resistance

1. Immunizations can induce either active or passive immunity (see Chapter 21).
   a. **Active artificial immunity** is acquired by injection or ingestion of microorganisms or their toxins that have been altered so that they stimulate an immune response without actually causing the disease. Microorganisms used in immunizations are either killed or attenuated (living but weakened). Immunization protocols are recommended by the Committee on Infectious Diseases of the American Academy of Pediatrics and by the United States Public Health Service Advisory Committee on Immunization Practices (see Chapter 15).

NURSE ADVISORY

Inform patients or their parents or another family member regarding the need for immunizations and keeping accurate records about possible adverse effects and the action to take.

   (1) Contraindications to active immunizations include the following:

- Do not administer immunizations prepared in chicken or duck eggs to persons allergic to eggs.
- Check the package insert for other ingredients, and do not administer the immunization to persons allergic to those ingredients.
- Because of risk to the fetus, do not administer live, attenuated viral immunizations to pregnant women or to those who are likely to become pregnant within 3 months after being immunized.
- Do not administer live, attenuated immunizations to immunosuppressed persons because the microorganisms may be able to replicate uncontrolled, and cause a full-blown case of the disorder.
   (2) Adverse reactions to active immunizations include a local inflammatory reaction at the site of injection and, occasionally, a mild to moderate systemic reaction, including fever, headache, and muscle aches. A few severe reactions, including deaths, have been caused by reactions to immunizations.
   b. **Passive artificial immunization** provides rapid induction of immunity by the injection of antibodies produced by another person or animal. Antibodies bind and inactivate viruses, bacteria, or their toxins. Passive artificial immunity lasts only a few weeks.
   (1) Passive immunization is indicated when there is an urgent need to protect a person already exposed to an infectious disease without waiting for immunity to develop after active immunization. Passive immunization is also used to treat infectious diseases for which active immunization is unavailable.
   (2) Passive immunization, in the form of human immune serum, is available for hepatitis A, hepatitis B, measles, mumps, pertussis, poliomyelitis, rabies, and tetanus.
   (3) Antitoxin is available for botulism, gas gangrene, tetanus, and snake venom.

DRUG ADVISORY

Closely monitor people for an hour after administration of antiserum or antitoxin for signs of an anaphylactic reaction.

2. Immunizations for high risk groups: In addition to routine immunizations, additional immunizations are recommended for those at high risk for exposure to or for serious complications from infectious diseases.
   a. Annual influenza immunizations are recommended for persons older than 60 years of age and for those with chronic pulmonary or cardiac disorders.
   b. A pneumococcal polysaccharide vaccine is recommended for children and adults with chronic illness and for those older than 65 years of age.

Bibliography

Books

Benenson AS (ed). *Control of Communicable Diseases Manual.* Washington, DC: American Public Health Association, 1995.

Ellner PD, and Neu HC. *Understanding Infectious Disease.* St. Louis: Mosby–Year Book, 1992.

Feigin RD, and Cherry JD. *Textbook of Pediatric Infectious Diseases.* Philadelphia: WB Saunders, 1993.

Gorbach SL, Bartlett JG, and Blacklow NR (eds). *Infectious Diseases.* Philadelphia: WB Saunders, 1992.

Mandell GL, Douglas RG, and Bennent JE. *Principles and Practices of Infectious Disease.* New York: Churchill Livingston, 1990.

Chapters in Books and Journal Articles

Overview of Infectious Diseases

Ackerman MH. The systemic inflammatory response, sepsis, and multiple organ dysfunction: New definitions for an old problem. *Crit Care Nurs Clin North Am* 6(2):243–250, 1994.

Bone RC, et al. Definitions for sepsis and organ failure and guidelines for the use of innovative therapies in sepsis. *Chest* 101(6):1644–1655, 1991.

Paul WE. Infectious disease and the immune system. *Sci Am* 269(3):91–97, 1993.

Stengle J, and Dries D. Sepsis in the elderly. *Crit Care Nurs Clin North Am* 6(2):421–427, 1994.

Assessment of People with Infections

Bruce JL, and Grove SK. Fever: Pathology and treatment. *Crit Care Nurse* 12(1):40–49, 1992.

Corbett JV. Hematological tests. *In* Corbett JV (ed). *Laboratory Tests and Diagnostic Procedures with Nursing Diagnoses.* 2nd ed. Norwalk, CT: Appleton & Lange, 1987.

Letizia M, and Janusek L. The self-defense mechanism of fever. *MedSurg Nurs* 3(5):373–377, 1994.

Tomkins LS. The use of molecular methods in infectious diseases. *N Engl J Med* 327(18):1290–1297, 1992.

Treatment of Infection

Beam TR. Anti-infective drugs in the prevention and treatment of sepsis syndrome. *Crit Care Nurs Clin North Am* 6(2):275–293, 1994.

Colletti RC, Dew RB, and Goulart AE. Antiendotoxin therapy in sepsis. *Crit Care Nurs Clin North Am* 5(2):345–353, 1993.

Ezzell C. Anti-septic strategies: New drugs hold promise for treating life-threatening bacterial infections. *Science News* 142:140–142, 1992.

Fink MP. Adoptive immunotherapy of gram-negative sepsis: Use of monoclonal antibodies to lipopolysaccharide. *Crit Care Med* 21(2):532–539, 1993.

Klein D, and Witek-Janusek L. Advances in immunotherapy of sepsis. *Dimens Crit Care Nurs* 11(2):75–89, 1992.

Lanifield M, and Conill AM. Antibiotic prophylaxis. *Hosp Pract* 27(3A):126–129, 1992.

Lynch P, et al. Implementing and evaluating a system of generic infection precautions: Body substance isolation. *Am J Infect Control* 18:1–12, 1990.

Sanford JP. Drug interactions to watch for during antibiotic therapy. *J Crit Illness* 7(3):450–459, 1992.

Walsh ML, and Johnson CC. Update on antimicrobial agents. *Nurs Clin North Am* 26(2):341–360, 1991.

Nosocomial Infections

Duncan I, and Batchelor C. Assessment of the effectiveness of body substance precautions as the infection control system of a large teaching hospital. *Am J Infect Control* 21:302–309, 1993.

Goldman D, and Larson E. Handwashing and nosocomial infections. *N Engl J Med* 327(2):120–122, 1992.

Jarris W, et al. Nosocomial infection rates in adult and pediatric intensive care units in the United States. *Am J Med* 91(suppl 3B):1855–1915, 1991.

Lee B, Chang RW, and Jacobs S. Intermittent nasogastric feeding: A simple and effective method to reduce pneumonia among ventilated ICU patients. *Clin Intens Care* 1:100–102, 1990.

Leu HS, et al. Hospital acquired pneumonia: Attributable mortality and morbidity. *Am J Epidemiol* 129:1258–1267, 1989.

Lynch P, et al. Rethinking the role of isolation precautions in the prevention of nosocomial infections. *Ann Intern Med* 107(2):243–246, 1987.

Torres A, et al. Incidence, risk, and prognosis factors of nosocomial pneumonia in mechanically ventilated patients. *Am Rev Respir Dis* 142:523–528, 1990.

Yannelli B, and Gurevich I. Infection control in critical care. *Heart Lung* 17(6):596–601, 1988.

Public Health Considerations

Centers for Disease Control. Recommendations of the Immunization Practices Advisory Committee: Diptheria, tetanus, and pertussis—recommendations for vaccine use and other preventive measures. *MMWR* 40(RR-10):1–28, 1991.

Centers for Disease Control. Recommendations of the Immunization Practices Advisory Committee: *Haemophilus* b conjugate vaccines for prevention of *Haemophilus influenzae* type b disease among infants and children two months of age and older. *MMWR* 40(RR-1): 1–7, 1991.

Centers for Disease Control. Recommendations of the Immunization Practices Advisory Committee: Measles prevention. *MMWR* 38(S-9): 5–18, 1989.

Centers for Disease Control. Recommendations of the Immunization Practices Advisory Committee: Protection against viral hepatitis. *MMWR* 39(RR-2):1–26, 1990.

Centers for Disease Control. Vaccine adverse event reporting system—United States. *MMWR* 39(41):730–733, 1990.

Centers for Disease Control and Prevention. Recommendations of the Immunization Practices Advisory Committee: Prevention and control of influenza: Part 1, vaccines. *MMWR* 42(RR-6):1–14, 1993.

9

Caring for People with Fluid, Electrolyte, and Acid-Base Imbalances

◼ NORMAL FLUID, ELECTROLYTE, AND ACID-BASE BALANCE

Fluid Balance

1. Overview
   a. The percentage of fluid in the body depends on the person's age. Infants have the highest proportion of body fluid by weight (70–75%), adults are typically 60 percent fluid, and older people have the lowest proportion of fluid by weight (45–50%).
   b. Women have a greater proportion of body fat, and therefore less fluid by weight, than men. Obese persons have relatively less fluid than lean persons.
   c. Fluid balance is a dynamic process that has 3 normal components (*intake*, *distribution*, and *excretion*) and an additional component (*loss through abnormal routes*) that occurs in many persons.
      (1) Fluid intake. Routes of fluid intake include the gastrointestinal tract (oral, through tubes, or rectal), parenteral (intravenous, into bone marrow), pulmonary (near drowning, ultrasonic nebulizers), and other routes (e.g., irrigation of body cavities). For normal fluid balance, fluid intake must match fluid excretion and loss of fluid through abnormal routes.
      (2) Fluid distribution. The 2 major fluid compartments are extracellular (outside the cells) and intracellular (inside the cells). In a child or an adult, approximately one third of body water is in the extracellular fluid compartment. The other approximately two thirds of body water is inside the cells (intracellular fluid). An infant has more extracellular fluid than intracellular fluid. The distribution of fluid between the extracellular and intracellular compartments depends on the process of osmosis.
      The extracellular fluid compartment has 2 subcompartments: vascular and interstitial. The vascular fluid (inside blood vessels) is approximately one third of extracellular fluid. The interstitial fluid (fluid between the cells) is approximately

two thirds of extracellular fluid. The distribution of extracellular fluid between the vascular and interstitial subcompartments depends on the process of capillary filtration.
      Transcellular fluids may be viewed as a minor fluid compartment. Transcellular fluids are fluids such as cerebrospinal, synovial, and intestinal that are secreted by epithelial cells.
      (3) Fluid excretion. The normal routes of fluid excretion are kidneys, gastrointestinal tract, skin, and lungs. With normal renal and hormonal function, a fluid intake above body requirements results in an increased urine output; decreased fluid intake, increased fluid excretion through feces or sweat, or loss of fluid through abnormal routes causes decreased urine output. Abnormal increases or decreases in urine volume produce increased or decreased fluid excretion that must be balanced by changes in fluid intake to maintain fluid balance. Diarrhea causes increased fluid excretion through the gastrointestinal tract. Fluid is excreted through the skin as insensible perspiration (not visible to the eye) and as visible sweat. Fluid is excreted through the lungs as water vapor during exhalation. Fever increases fluid excretion through the skin via insensible perspiration and through the lungs.
      (4) Fluid loss through abnormal routes. Abnormal routes of fluid loss include emesis, fistulas, secretions through drainage or suction tubes, hemorrhage, dialysis, wound exudate, evaporation from body during surgery, and paracentesis and similar procedures. Fluid loss through abnormal routes must be balanced by increased fluid intake to maintain fluid balance.
   c. For normal fluid balance, both the *volume* and the *concentration* (osmolality) of body fluid must be within normal limits. Normal osmolality is 280 to 300 mOsm per kg (Table 9–1).
2. Extracellular fluid volume balance: The volume of the extracellular fluid is regulated in large part by the hormone aldosterone (Fig. 9–1).
3. Serum sodium (osmolality) balance: The concentration

235

Table 9–1. Normal Osmolality, Electrolyte, and Acid-Base Values for Adults

Serum

Bicarbonate (HCO_3^-)	22–26 mEq/L
Calcium (Ca^{++})	9–11 mg/dl (4.5–5.5 mEq/L)
Chloride (Cl^-)	95–108 mEq/L
Magnesium (Mg^{++})	1.5–2.5 mEq/L (1.8–3.0 mg/dl)
Osmolality	280–300 mOsm/kg
Phosphate (Pi)	2.5–4.5 mg/dl
Potassium (K^+)	3.5–5.0 mEq/L
Sodium (Na^+)	135–145 mEq/L

Arterial Blood

PaCO_2	36–44 mm Hg
pH	7.35–7.45

(osmolality) of body fluid is regulated in large part by antidiuretic hormone (ADH). (Fig. 9–2)

Electrolyte Balance

1. Overview
   a. Electrolyte balance is a dynamic process that has 3 normal components:
      (1) Electrolyte intake and absorption
      (2) Electrolyte distribution
      (3) Electrolyte excretion
   b. A 4th component, loss of electrolytes through abnormal routes, also occurs in many instances.
   c. When a person has normal electrolyte balance, electrolyte excretion and loss through abnormal routes are balanced by electrolyte intake and absorption, so that the total amount of the electrolytes in the body does not change. In addition, the distribution of electrolytes between body compartments is appropriate.
2. Electrolyte intake and absorption
   a. The normal route of electrolyte intake is oral.
   b. Additional routes of electrolyte intake include intravenous, rectal (phosphate or magnesium from enemas), pulmonary (magnesium from near drowning in salt water), and via tubes or irrigation of body cavities.
   c. Many factors can decrease oral electrolyte intake.
      (1) Anorexia, weakness, dyspnea, nausea, fad diets
      (2) Low income and lack of transportation, cooking facilities, refrigeration, language skills, and knowledge
   c. Electrolyte absorption from the gastrointestinal tract varies, depending on the type of electrolyte.
      (1) Potassium is absorbed easily when there is a greater concentration of potassium in the intestines than in the blood.
      (2) Calcium is absorbed best from the duodenum by a process that requires vitamin D.
      (3) Magnesium is absorbed primarily from the terminal ileum.
      (4) Phosphate is absorbed from the small intestine.

EXTRACELLULAR FLUID VOLUME BALANCE

Hypovolemia or any other cause of decreased blood flow through the renal arteries causes an increase in renin, which increases the secretion of aldosterone through the renin-angiotensin-aldosterone system. The renal action of aldosterone then increases extracellular fluid volume. Aldosterone is secreted by the adrenal cortex, circulates in the blood, and causes the kidneys to retain sodium and water in the same concentration as normal body fluids (isotonic), which in turn expands the extracellular fluid volume without changing its concentration.

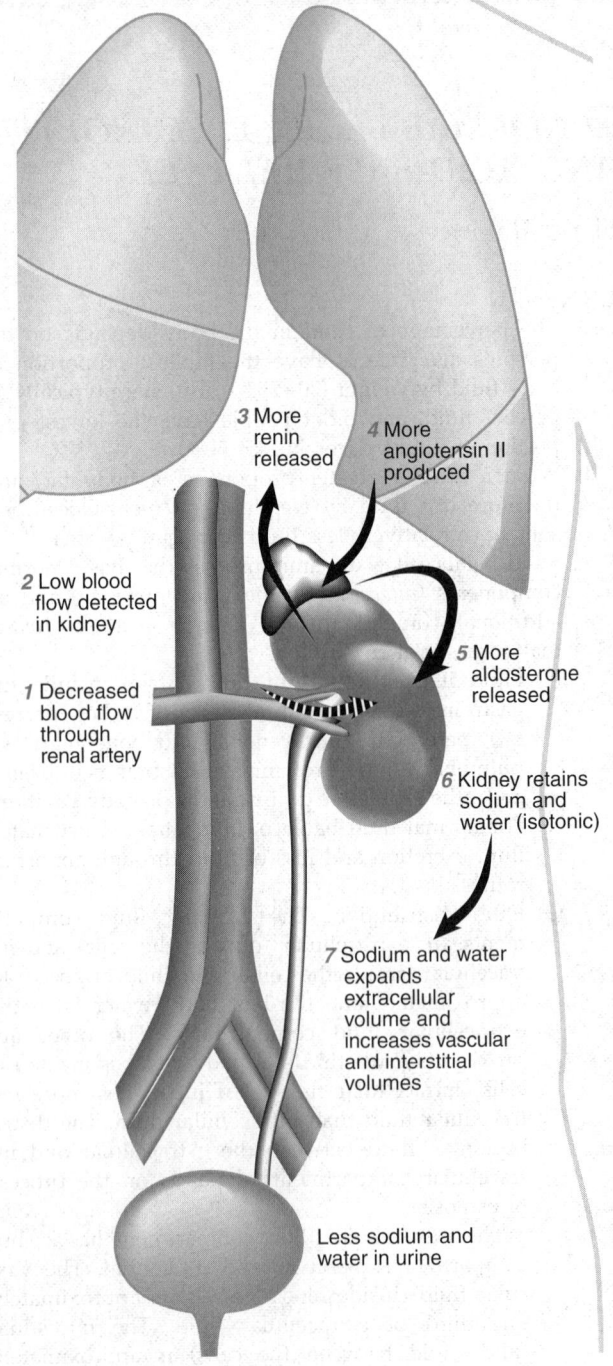

3 More renin released

4 More angiotensin II produced

2 Low blood flow detected in kidney

5 More aldosterone released

1 Decreased blood flow through renal artery

6 Kidney retains sodium and water (isotonic)

7 Sodium and water expands extracellular volume and increases vascular and interstitial volumes

Less sodium and water in urine

Figure 9–1.

OSMOLALITY: SERUM SODIUM BALANCE

The concentration (osmolality) of body fluid is regulated in large part by antidiuretic hormone (ADH), which is synthesized in the hypothalamus but is released from the posterior pituitary gland. ADH circulates in the blood and causes the kidneys to retain water, which dilutes body fluids. When the osmolality of body fluid increases, more ADH is released. The renal action of ADH then dilutes body fluids so that homeostasis is restored. When the osmolality of body fluid decreases, less ADH is released. Lack of the renal action of ADH then allows more water to be excreted in the urine and concentrates body fluids so that homeostasis is restored.

Serum sodium concentration reflects the osmolality of the blood but does not indicate sodium level in the body. Changes in the serum sodium concentration alter the amount of fluid in the intracellular compartment. The sodium-potassium pump in cell membranes keeps sodium ions from entering cells. When the serum sodium concentration increases, water leaves cells by the process of osmosis to equalize the osmolality. When the serum sodium concentration decreases, water enters the cells by the process of osmosis to equalize the osmolality.

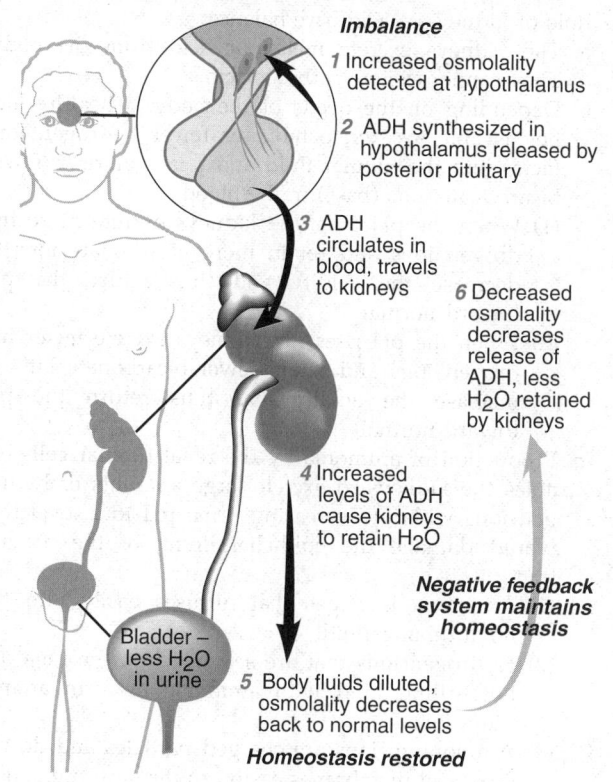

Imbalance

1 Increased osmolality detected at hypothalamus

2 ADH synthesized in hypothalamus released by posterior pituitary

3 ADH circulates in blood, travels to kidneys

4 Increased levels of ADH cause kidneys to retain H₂O

5 Body fluids diluted, osmolality decreases back to normal levels

6 Decreased osmolality decreases release of ADH, less H₂O retained by kidneys

Negative feedback system maintains homeostasis

Bladder – less H₂O in urine

Homeostasis restored

Figure 9-2.

d. Many factors can impair electrolyte absorption, so that electrolytes are eliminated in the feces and do not enter the blood.
  (1) Diarrhea (including laxative abuse)
  (2) Malabsorption syndromes

  (3) Undigested fat (binds calcium and magnesium)
  (4) Dietary substances, such as phytates, that bind calcium and magnesium.
3. Electrolyte distribution
  a. Electrolytes are distributed among the extracellular fluid and intracellular fluid and other body compartments, such as bone.
  b. The extracellular fluid has high concentrations of sodium and chloride but low concentrations of potassium, calcium, magnesium, and phosphate.
  c. The intracellular fluid has high concentrations of potassium, magnesium, and phosphate but low concentrations of sodium and chloride. The concentration of calcium in intracellular fluid is low, but it is higher than in the extracellular fluid.
  d. Bones have large amounts of calcium, magnesium, and phosphate.
  e. Several hormones are important in normal electrolyte distribution.
    (1) Insulin and epinephrine cause potassium and phosphate to move from the extracellular fluid into cells.
    (2) Parathyroid hormone causes calcium and phosphate to move from bones into the extracellular fluid. Calcitonin moves calcium into bones.
  f. Electrolytes can also be distributed among different chemical forms in the extracellular fluid, some of which are physiologically inactive.
    (1) Calcium and magnesium in the blood exist in 3 forms:
      • Bound to plasma proteins, a physiologically inactive form of electrolyte
      • Bound to citrate and other small ions, also a physiologically inactive form of electrolyte
      • Free ionized form, the physiologically active form of electrolyte
    (2) Increased pH (blood more alkaline) causes more calcium and magnesium to bind to plasma proteins and thus decreases the concentration of physiologically active electrolyte.
4. Electrolyte excretion
  a. Normal routes of electrolyte excretion are urine, feces, and sweat.
  b. Several hormones are important in normal electrolyte excretion.
    (1) Aldosterone and cortisol facilitate the excretion of potassium in the urine.
    (2) Parathyroid hormone increases urine excretion of phosphate and decreases urine excretion of calcium.
  c. Impaired renal function causes electrolytes to accumulate in the blood unless their intake is reduced.
  d. Increased fecal excretion of electrolytes occurs with diarrhea.
5. Loss of electrolytes through abnormal routes
  a. Abnormal routes of electrolyte loss include vomiting, nasogastric or intestinal suction, wound or fistula drainage, paracentesis, and electrolytes lost in removal of irrigation fluid.
  b. To maintain electrolyte balance, electrolytes lost through abnormal routes must be replaced by increasing electrolyte intake above the amount excreted normally through urine, feces, and sweat.

Acid-Base Balance

1. Overview
   a. The degree of acidity of body fluids is measured by their pH.
      (1) The pH is the negative logarithm of the hydrogen ion concentration. Hydrogen ions are acid. Bicarbonate ions are base (alkaline).
      (2) The normal pH range of the arterial blood is 7.35 to 7.45 except at birth, when it is 7.11 to 7.36.
      (3) A decrease in pH indicates more acidity.
      (4) An increase in pH indicates more alkalinity.
   b. Cellular metabolism creates 2 kinds of acids that must be excreted from the body or they will accumulate to dangerous levels.
      (1) Carbonic acid (carbon dioxide and water)
      (2) Metabolic acids such as sulfuric acid and lactic acid
   c. The body deals with the acids it produces by buffering them in the body fluids and by excreting them through the lungs and the kidneys.
2. Role of buffers in acid-base balance
   a. Buffers are chemicals that take up or liberate hydrogen ions to prevent large changes in pH.
   b. Every body fluid has buffers (Table 9–2).
   c. Metabolic acids are buffered extensively by the bicarbonate buffer system. Therefore, a change in the amount of metabolic acid is detected clinically as a change in the serum bicarbonate concentration.
      (1) If too much metabolic acid is present, the bicarbonate concentration decreases because bicarbonate is used in buffering.
      (2) If not enough metabolic acid is present, the bicarbonate concentration increases because bicarbonate is not being used in buffering.
   d. Carbonic acid is not buffered by the bicarbonate buffer system but by other buffer systems. It is transported in the blood primarily as carbon dioxide. Therefore, a change in the amount of carbonic acid is detected clinically as a change in the Pa_{CO_2}.
      (1) An increase in carbonic acid is detected clinically as an increased Pa_{CO_2}.
      (2) A decrease in carbonic acid is detected clinically as a decreased Pa_{CO_2}.
   e. Buffering occurs immediately when acid or base is added to the blood.
3. Role of lungs in acid-base balance
   a. The lungs excrete carbonic acid from the body in the form of carbon dioxide and water. They cannot excrete metabolic acids.
   b. The rate and depth of respirations determine how much carbonic acid is excreted.
      (1) A decrease in the rate and depth of respirations (hypoventilation) decreases the amount of carbonic acid excreted and allows more carbon dioxide to accumulate in the blood, thus decreasing the pH.
      (2) An increase in the rate and depth of respirations (hyperventilation) increases the amount of carbonic acid excreted and removes more carbon dioxide from the blood, thus increasing the pH.
   c. The rate and depth of respirations are modified by input from the chemoreceptors that monitor the pH, Pa_{CO_2}, and Pa_{O_2} of arterial blood.
      (1) If the pH decreases or the Pa_{CO_2} rises, rate and depth of respirations increase to remove excess carbon dioxide (carbonic acid) and thus return the pH toward normal.
      (2) If the pH increases or the Pa_{CO_2} falls, rate and depth of respirations decrease to accumulate more carbon dioxide (carbonic acid) and thus return the pH toward normal.
   d. Adjustment of blood pH by the lungs is normally rapid and occurs within minutes.
4. Role of kidneys in acid-base balance
   a. The kidneys excrete metabolic acid from the body. They cannot excrete carbonic acid.
   b. Depending on the needs of the body, a healthy kidney is able to excrete more or fewer hydrogen ions (acid) into the tubular fluid and retain more or fewer bicarbonate ions (base) in the blood.
      (1) When the pH falls, the kidneys excrete more hydrogen ions and retain more bicarbonate ions to decrease the acidity and thus return the pH toward normal.
      (2) When the pH rises, the kidneys excrete fewer hydrogen ions and retain fewer bicarbonate ions to increase the acidity and thus return the pH toward normal.
   c. Production of ammonia by the renal tubular cells enables the kidneys to excrete large amounts of hydrogen ions without decreasing urine pH to a level that would damage the epithelial lining of the urinary tract.
      (1) Ammonia is a gas that diffuses easily into the renal tubular fluid.
      (2) Hydrogen ions that are secreted into the renal tubular fluid bind with ammonia to form ammonium ions.
      (3) Ammonium ions are charged particles and do not cross cell membranes easily, so they are trapped in the renal tubular fluid and are excreted in the urine.
      (4) When the pH of the blood falls, the kidneys make more ammonia to help excrete more hydrogen ions.
   d. The kidneys normally respond to changes in blood pH more slowly than the lungs and may take several days to adjust the pH if the change has been large.

Table 9–2. Important Buffers in Body Fluids

Buffer	Major Sites
Bicarbonate	Extracellular fluid (plasma and interstitial)
Phosphate	Intracellular fluid; urine
Hemoglobin	Inside red blood cells
Protein	Plasma; intracellular fluid

◼ *FLUID, ELECTROLYTE, AND ACID-BASE IMBALANCES*

Fluid Imbalances

1. Types of fluid imbalances
   a. Extracellular fluid volume imbalances
      (1) Extracellular fluid volume imbalances are *volume* disorders. The concentration of the fluid is normal (except with combined imbalances); there is just too much or too little of it.
      (2) Extracellular fluid volume deficit is a decreased volume of fluid in the vascular and interstitial compartments.
      (3) Extracellular fluid volume excess is an increased volume of fluid in the vascular and interstitial compartments.
   b. Serum sodium (osmolality) imbalances
      (1) Serum sodium (osmolality) imbalances are *concentration* disorders and cause changes in intracellular fluid volume. The extracellular volume of fluid is normal (except with combined imbalances); however, it is too concentrated or too dilute.
      (2) Hyponatremia is a decreased concentration of sodium in the extracellular fluid; the extracellular fluid is too dilute, and the cells are swollen (increased intracellular volume).
      (3) Hypernatremia is an increased concentration of sodium in the extracellular fluid; the extracellular fluid is too concentrated, and the cells are shriveled (decreased intracellular volume).
2. General causes of fluid imbalances
   a. Causes of extracellular fluid volume imbalances
      (1) Conditions that produce losses or gains of isotonic saline cause extracellular fluid volume imbalances. Extracellular fluid volume deficit is caused by loss of isotonic saline from the body or into an inaccessible 3rd space. **Examples:** hemorrhage, diarrhea and emesis with replacement of water but not saline. Extracellular fluid volume excess is caused by gain of isotonic saline in the body. **Examples:** chronic congestive heart failure, hyperaldosteronism.
   b. Causes of serum sodium (osmolality) imbalances (see Fig. 9–2)
      (1) Conditions that change the relative proportion of water to sodium in the body fluids cause serum sodium imbalances. **Hyponatremia** is caused by a gain of relatively more water than sodium or by a loss of relatively more sodium than water. **Examples:** excessive infusion of 5 percent dextrose in water (D5W), increased antidiuretic hormone (ADH) secretion. **Hypernatremia** is caused by loss of relatively more water than sodium or by gain of relatively more sodium than water. **Examples:** diarrhea and emesis with no fluid replacement, tube feedings without extra water, decreased ADH (diabetes insipidus).
3. People at risk for fluid imbalances (Table 9–3)

Electrolyte Imbalances

1. Overview
   a. Because electrolytes are frequently shifted between the extracellular fluid and the intracellular or bone electrolyte pools, the plasma concentration of an electrolyte does not necessarily indicate the whole body electrolyte content.
   b. Blood is the most available body tissue for the measurement of electrolyte concentration.
2. Types of electrolyte imbalances

Table 9–3. People at Risk for Fluid Imbalances	
Risk Factor	**Explanation**
Vomiting	Fluid loss through abnormal route
Diarrhea	Increased fluid excretion through normal route
Gastrointestinal suctioning	Fluid loss through abnormal route
Large amounts of wound drainage	Fluid loss through abnormal route
Burns	Fluid loss through abnormal route, altered fluid distribution, increased fluid excretion through normal route
Large diaphoresis	Increased fluid excretion through normal route
Tube feedings	Highly concentrated particle intake causes renal water loss
Too much or too little aldosterone or cortisol	Decreased or increased excretion of saline (sodium and water)
Congestive heart failure, cirrhosis, or nephrotic syndrome	Pathophysiologic conditions accompanied by increased aldosterone
Too much or too little antidiuretic hormone	Decreased or increased excretion of water
Newborns	Very high percentage of body weight is water; immature kidneys
Older people	Small percentage of body weight is water; diminished thirst; decreased renal concentrating ability

Table 9-4. People at Risk for Electrolyte Imbalances

Risk Factor	Explanation
Poor nutritional intake	Decreased intake of K^+, Ca^{++}, Mg^{++}
Chronic diarrhea	Decreased absorption of Ca^{++}, Mg^{++}; increased fecal excretion of K^+
Repeated vomiting or nasogastric suction	Decreased intake of K^+, Ca^{++}, Mg^{++}; loss through abnormal route; increased renal excretion of K^+
Too much or too little aldosterone	Altered excretion of K^+, Mg^{++}
Too much or too little cortisol	Altered excretion of K^+, Mg^{++}
Too much or too little insulin	Altered distribution of K^+
Too much or too little parathyroid hormone	Altered absorption, distribution, and excretion of Ca^{++}
Diuretic therapy	Increased excretion of K^+, Mg^{++}, Pi, Na^+
Oliguric renal failure	Decreased excretion of K^+, Mg^{++}, Pi; decreased Ca^{++} absorption, altered Ca^{++} distribution
Alcohol abuse	Decreased intake of K^+, Ca^{++}, Mg^{++}; decreased absorption of Ca^{++}, Mg^{++}; altered distribution of Ca^{++}, Mg^{++}, Pi; increased excretion of K^+, Ca^{++}, Mg^{++}; loss of K^+, Mg^{++} through abnormal routes
Massive blood transfusion	Increased K^+ intake, altered distribution of Ca^{++}, Mg^{++} (citrate binding)

a. Plasma electrolyte deficits
   (1) A plasma electrolyte deficit is a plasma concentration of an electrolyte below the lower limit of the normal range.
   (2) Plasma electrolyte deficits cause signs and symptoms even if whole body electrolyte content is normal because the electrolyte is distributed abnormally.
b. Plasma electrolyte excesses
   (1) A plasma electrolyte excess is a plasma concentration of an electrolyte above the upper limit of the normal range.
   (2) Plasma electrolyte excesses cause signs and symptoms even if whole body electrolyte content is normal because the electrolyte is distributed abnormally.
3. General causes of electrolyte imbalances
   a. Causes of plasma electrolyte deficits
      (1) Decreased electrolyte intake or absorption. **Examples:** hypokalemia from fad diet low in potassium; hypomagnesemia from chronic diarrhea or ileal resection.
      (2) Shift of electrolyte from extracellular fluid into cells or into a physiologically unavailable form in the plasma. **Examples:** hypokalemia due to hypothermia or insulin excess; ionized hypocalcemia due to alkalosis and binding of calcium to free fatty acids in the blood.
      (3) Increased electrolyte excretion through normal routes. **Examples:** hypokalemia and hypomagnesemia from diarrhea or diuretic therapy.
      (4) Electrolyte loss through abnormal routes. **Examples:** hypokalemia and hypomagnesemia from repeated emesis, prolonged nasogastric suction, or fistula drainage.
   b. Causes of plasma electrolyte excesses
      (1) Increased electrolyte intake or absorption. **Exam-**

ples: hyperkalemia from massive blood transfusion; hypercalcemia from overdose of vitamin D.
   (2) Shift of electrolyte from electrolyte pools into the extracellular fluid. **Examples:** hypercalcemia from bone resorption due to circulating factors produced by malignant tumor; hyperkalemia and hyperphosphatemia from massive cell death due to crushing injury.
   (3) Decreased electrolyte excretion through normal routes. **Examples:** hyperkalemia, hypermagnesemia, and hyperphosphatemia from acute or chronic oliguric renal failure.
4. People at risk for electrolyte imbalances (Table 9-4)

Acid-Base Imbalances

1. Overview
   a. Acidosis is a condition that tends to decrease the pH of the blood. If the blood pH actually decreases, the acidosis has caused acidemia (decreased blood pH).
   b. Alkalosis is a condition that tends to increase the pH of the blood. If the blood pH actually increases, the alkalosis has caused alkalemia (increased blood pH).
   c. Acid-base imbalances are categorized according to the kind of acid that is out of balance.
2. Types of acid-base imbalances
   a. Respiratory acid-base imbalances
      (1) Respiratory acid-base imbalances are disorders of carbonic acid.
      (2) Respiratory acidosis is a condition in which there is too much carbonic acid (carbon dioxide) in the blood.
      (3) Respiratory alkalosis is a condition in which there is too little carbonic acid (carbon dioxide) in the blood.
   b. Metabolic acid-base imbalances

(1) Metabolic acid-base imbalances are disorders of metabolic acid.

(2) Metabolic acidosis is a condition in which there is relatively too much metabolic acid in the blood.

(3) Metabolic alkalosis is a condition in which there is relatively too little metabolic acid in the blood.

c. Compensatory mechanisms for acid-base imbalances

(1) If the pH of the blood rises too high or falls too low, the person will die.

(2) The body has compensatory mechanisms for acid-base imbalances that operate to return the pH to normal levels even though the imbalance still exists.

(3) Compensation for respiratory acid-base imbalances (respiratory acidosis and respiratory alkalosis) is performed by the kidneys over several days (Fig. 9–3).

(4) Compensation for metabolic acid-base imbalances (metabolic acidosis and metabolic alkalosis) (Fig. 9–4) is performed by the lungs over several hours.

3. General causes of acid-base imbalances

a. Causes of respiratory acid-base imbalances: Conditions that change the excretion of carbonic acid by the lungs cause respiratory acid-base imbalances. Respiratory acidosis is caused by decreased excretion of carbonic acid as a result of decreased alveolar ventila-

---

RESPIRATORY ACIDOSIS AND RESPIRATORY ALKALOSIS

Respiratory Acidosis

Respiratory acidosis is caused by accumulation of carbonic acid. During respiratory acidosis, the kidneys excrete more metabolic acids and retain more bicarbonate than usual. Renal compensation for respiratory acidosis produces a compensatory metabolic alkalosis, which helps to keep pH from falling too low although it does not correct the original carbonic acid excess. Renal compensation for a respiratory acid–base imbalance takes several days.

Respiratory Alkalosis

Respiratory alkalosis is caused by a deficiency of carbonic acid. During respiratory alkalosis, the kidneys excrete fewer metabolic acids and retain less bicarbonate than usual. Renal compensation for respiratory alkalosis produces a compensatory metabolic acidosis by retaining more acids in the body and, thus, helps to keep pH from rising too high. Renal compensation does not, however, correct the original carbonic acid deficit.

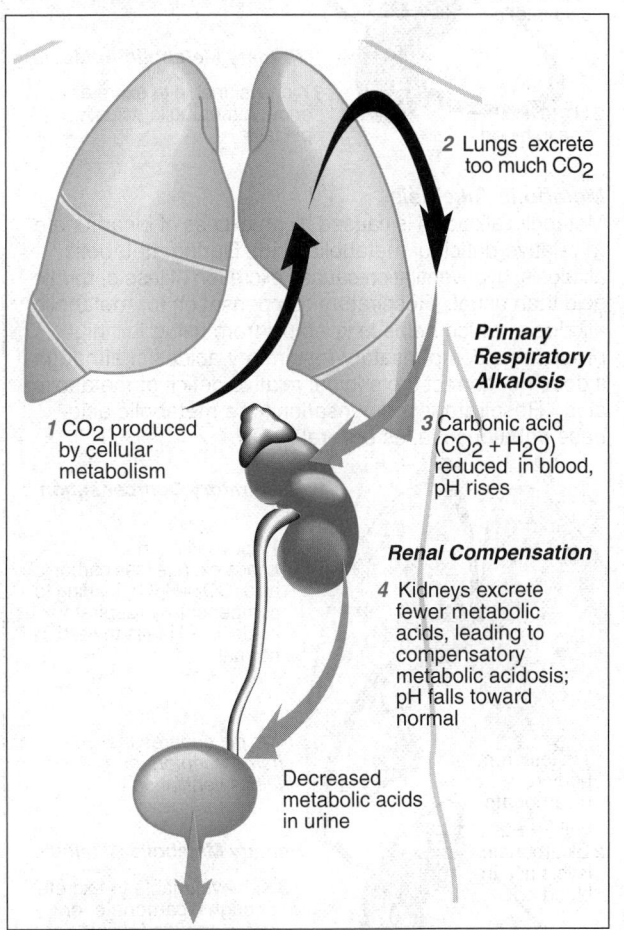

2 Lungs cannot excrete enough CO_2

Primary Respiratory Acidosis

1 CO_2 produced by cellular metabolism

3 Carbonic acid ($CO_2 + H_2O$) builds up in blood and pH falls

Renal Compensation

4 Kidneys excrete more metabolic acids, leading to compensatory metabolic alkalosis; pH rises toward normal

Increased metabolic acids in urine

2 Lungs excrete too much CO_2

Primary Respiratory Alkalosis

1 CO_2 produced by cellular metabolism

3 Carbonic acid ($CO_2 + H_2O$) reduced in blood, pH rises

Renal Compensation

4 Kidneys excrete fewer metabolic acids, leading to compensatory metabolic acidosis; pH falls toward normal

Decreased metabolic acids in urine

Figure 9–3.

METABOLIC ACIDOSIS AND ALKALOSIS

Metabolic Acidosis

Metabolic acidosis is caused by a relative excess of metabolic acid. During metabolic acidosis, hyperventilation causes excretion of more carbonic acid than usual. Respiratory compensation for metabolic acidosis, which helps to keep pH from falling too low by removing more acid from the body, produces a compensatory respiratory alkalosis, although it does not correct the original relative excess of metabolic acid.

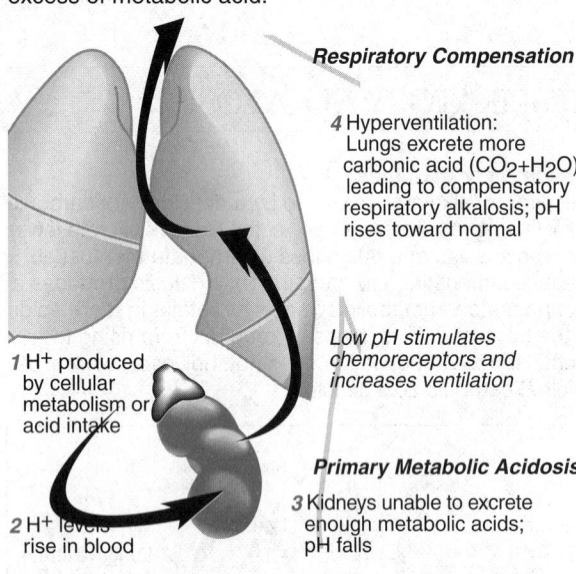

Respiratory Compensation

4 Hyperventilation: Lungs excrete more carbonic acid ($CO_2 + H_2O$) leading to compensatory respiratory alkalosis; pH rises toward normal

Low pH stimulates chemoreceptors and increases ventilation

1 H^+ produced by cellular metabolism or acid intake

2 H^+ levels rise in blood

Primary Metabolic Acidosis

3 Kidneys unable to excrete enough metabolic acids; pH falls

Metabolic Alkalosis

Metabolic alkalosis is caused by an excess of bicarbonate (a relative deficit of metabolic acid). During metabolic alkalosis, hypoventilation causes excretion of less carbonic acid than usual. Respiratory compensation for metabolic alkalosis, which helps to keep pH from rising too high, produces a compensatory respiratory acidosis, although it does not correct the original relative deficit of metabolic acid. Respiratory compensation for a metabolic acid-base imbalance takes several hours.

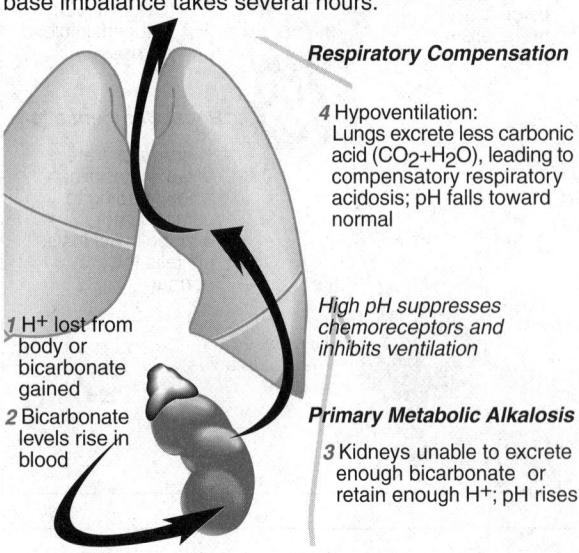

Respiratory Compensation

4 Hypoventilation: Lungs excrete less carbonic acid ($CO_2 + H_2O$), leading to compensatory respiratory acidosis; pH falls toward normal

High pH suppresses chemoreceptors and inhibits ventilation

1 H^+ lost from body or bicarbonate gained

2 Bicarbonate levels rise in blood

Primary Metabolic Alkalosis

3 Kidneys unable to excrete enough bicarbonate or retain enough H^+; pH rises

Figure 9–4.

---

tion. Respiratory alkalosis is caused by increased excretion of carbonic acid as a result of hyperventilation.

b. Causes of metabolic acid-base imbalances: Conditions that cause a relative excess or deficit of metabolic acids cause metabolic acid-base imbalances. Metabolic acidosis is caused by accumulation of metabolic acids or loss of bicarbonate. Metabolic alkalosis is caused by accumulation of bicarbonate or loss of metabolic acids.

4. People at risk for acid-base imbalances (Table 9–5)

◾ *ASSESSING PEOPLE WITH FLUID, ELECTROLYTE, AND ACID-BASE IMBALANCES*

Key Symptoms and Their Pathophysiologic Bases

1. Signs and symptoms of fluid imbalances
   a. Extracellular volume imbalances: sudden changes in body weight (1 L of fluid weighs 1 kg or 2.2 lb), signs and symptoms due to increased or decreased vascular volume (degree of jugular vein distention, character of pulse), signs due to changes in interstitial volume (decreased skin turgor or edema).
   b. Serum sodium imbalances (intracellular fluid volume imbalances): decreased level of consciousness (brain cells swell or shrivel due to osmotic changes). The severity of the clinical manifestations depends on how fast the serum sodium concentration changes.
2. Signs and symptoms of electrolyte imbalances
   a. Decreased muscle strength, increased or decreased neuromuscular excitability, constipation or diarrhea, cardiac dysrhythmias, and electrocardiogram changes.
   b. Electrolyte imbalances alter resting membrane potentials (potassium and sodium imbalances), threshold potentials (calcium imbalances), release of acetylcholine (magnesium imbalances), or intracellular metabolism and availability of adenosine triphosphate (phosphate imbalances).
3. Signs and symptoms of acid-base imbalances
   a. Altered level of consciousness, cardiac dysrhythmias, increased or decreased rate and depth of respirations.
   b. Altered intracellular pH impairs function of brain cells and cardiac cells; chemoreceptors cause altered rate and depth of respirations in compensation for metabolic acid-base imbalances.

Health History

1. Intake of fluid, electrolytes, and bicarbonate
   a. Appetite, nausea, dietary restrictions, dietary supplements, special diets (including weight loss diets), use of salt, intake of fruits (potassium), green vegetables (magnesium), dairy products (calcium), use of antacids (calcium, magnesium, sodium bicarbonate)
   b. Ability to swallow liquids, daily fluid intake, thirst, fluid and nutrient intake by routes such as tube feedings or intravenously
2. Excretion of fluid, electrolytes, and bicarbonate

Table 9–5. People at Risk for Acid-Base Imbalances	
Risk Factor	**Explanation**
Pathophysiology of lungs or chest wall	Decreased ability to excrete carbonic acid
Renal pathophysiology	Decreased ability to excrete metabolic acids if oliguric; may have altered excretion of bicarbonate
Diabetes mellitus	Accumulation of metabolic acids
Other endocrine pathophysiology	Depends on the pathophysiology; may accumulate metabolic acids or bicarbonate
Prolonged vomiting or gastric suction	Loss of acid
Prolonged diarrhea	Increased excretion of bicarbonate
Newborns	Immature kidneys
Older people	Decreased ability to excrete an acid load

a. Amount and color of urine output, history of renal disease, use of diuretics or corticosteroids
b. Changes in bowel patterns, diarrhea, constipation, use of laxatives or enemas

3. Abnormal losses of fluid, electrolytes, and acid or bicarbonate: Vomiting, tubes to suction, wound or fistula drainages

4. History of hormone imbalances or disease processes that commonly cause fluid, electrolyte, or acid-base imbalances: Diabetes mellitus, hyperaldosteronism, congestive heart failure, cirrhosis, adrenal insufficiency, Cushing's syndrome, diabetes insipidus, syndrome of inappropriate antidiuretic hormone secretion (SIADH), respiratory disorders, hyperthyroidism, chronic alcohol abuse

5. Symptoms: Fatigue, lightheadedness on standing, dyspnea, muscle weakness, muscle cramping, tingling, tightness of shoes or rings (edema)

Physical Examination

1. Level of consciousness: Decreased level of consciousness may occur with hypernatremia, clinical dehydration, hyponatremia, and acid-base imbalances.
2. Cardiac rate and rhythm
   a. Character of pulse
      (1) Thready, rapid pulse occurs with extracellular fluid volume deficit and clinical dehydration.
      (2) Bounding pulse occurs with extracellular fluid volume excess.
   b. Rate and regularity of pulse
      (1) Cardiac dysrhythmias may occur with electrolyte and acid-base imbalances.
      (2) Tachycardia occurs with respiratory acidosis and metabolic acidosis; tachycardia with thready pulse occurs with extracellular fluid volume deficit and clinical dehydration.
      (3) Bradycardia occurs with hypermagnesemia and severe metabolic acidosis.
   c. Electrocardiogram changes: These changes occur with electrolyte imbalances.
3. Respiratory rate, depth, and lung sounds in dependent portions of the lungs
   a. Increased rate and depth may be the cause of respiratory alkalosis or compensation for metabolic acidosis.
   b. Decreased rate and depth may be the cause of respiratory acidosis or compensation for metabolic alkalosis.
   c. Decreased depth may be due to muscle weakness from hypokalemia, hyperkalemia, or severe hypophosphatemia.
   d. Crackles in dependent portions may occur with extracellular fluid volume excess; assess lung bases if the person is upright and posterior portion if the person is supine.
4. Postural blood pressure measurement (adults and adolescents)
   a. First measure blood pressure and heart rate with the person supine.
   b. Then measure blood pressure and heart rate with the person standing or sitting with the legs dependent (not sitting with legs stretched out horizontally).
   c. Postural blood pressure drop occurs with extracellular fluid volume deficit and clinical dehydration.
      (1) Criteria for postural blood pressure drop: systolic pressure decreases more than 15 mm Hg, diastolic pressure decreases 10 mm Hg or more, and heart rate increases.
      (2) If the blood pressure decreases but the heart rate does not increase, the patient may have autonomic neuropathy rather than an extracellular fluid volume deficit. (With autonomic neuropathy, the autonomic baroreceptor reflexes that normally adjust blood pressure do not work effectively.)
      (3) Persons who have a transplanted heart may not have the heart rate increase even if they do have an extracellular fluid volume deficit.
   d. Look for other signs of decreased vascular volume first in infants and children, because their blood pressure compensates well for reduced vascular volume until it is very severe.
5. Other assessments of vascular volume
   a. Fullness of anterior fontanel (infants)
   b. Small vein filling time (see p. 261)
   c. Capillary refill time
   d. Neck vein filling
   e. Central venous pressure (see Chapter 23)
   f. Dryness of mucous membranes
   g. Presence or absence of tears and sweat
   h. Urine output

6. Bowel sounds: Decreased or absent with hypokalemia and hypercalcemia
7. Assessments of interstitial volume
   a. Skin turgor
      (1) Pinch up the skin over the sternum (all ages) or over the ribcage (infants) and release it.
      (2) If the skin stays pinched up (tented), this indicates extracellular fluid volume deficit or clinical dehydration, rapid recent loss of body mass, or changes due to normal aging in the skin.

ELDER ADVISORY

Skin turgor is not an accurate assessment of extracellular fluid volume deficit in older people. Physiologic changes of normal aging cause the skin to stay pinched up even when extracellular fluid volume is normal. Use other assessments for evaluating older people.

---

(3) Do not test skin turgor on the arm in adults (sun exposure and weathering may give false results) or over the abdomen in infants (may give false results if abdomen is distended or infant is chubby).
      (4) Skin turgor may also be tested over the forehead, but over the sternum is preferred because many persons are sensitive to the pinching sensation.
   b. Edema occurs with extracellular fluid volume excess. Look for edema in the dependent portions of the body: ankles if upright or seated, sacrum if supine, around eyes if prone.
8. Muscle strength
   a. Muscle weakness or flaccid paralysis, initially most obvious in thighs, occurs with both hypokalemia and hyperkalemia.
   b. General muscle weakness occurs with hypercalcemia.
9. Neuromuscular excitability
   a. Deep tendon reflexes: decreased with hypercalcemia and hypermagnesemia; increased with hypocalcemia and hypomagnesemia
   b. Chvostek's sign and Trousseau's sign (described under hypocalcemia): positive, indicating increased neuromuscular excitability with hypocalcemia and hypomagnesemia
10. Body weight
    a. Compare body weight with previous day's weight if available or measure as baseline for future comparison.
    b. Have person empty bladder; empty drainage bags; use same scale, same amount of clothing, same amount of bed linens; if cast or bulky dressings are added or removed, weigh them and adjust comparison weight accordingly; weigh at the same time each day if possible.
    c. Sudden (overnight) increase occurs with extracellular fluid volume excess.
    d. Sudden (overnight) decrease occurs with extracellular fluid volume deficit and clinical dehydration.

Special Diagnostic Studies

1. Extracellular fluid volume imbalances are diagnosed from results of the history and physical examination.
2. Serum sodium imbalances (intracellular volume imbalances) and electrolyte imbalances are diagnosed from laboratory tests on some form of blood (plasma, serum, capillary) (see Table 9–1).
3. Acid-base imbalances are diagnosed from arterial blood gas measurements or occasionally from venous blood measurements (see Table 9–1).

◼ INTRAVENOUS FLUID THERAPY

Purpose of Intravenous Therapy

1. Provide water, electrolytes, and nutrients when people cannot ingest enough orally.
   a. *Maintenance* intravenous therapy matches daily fluid and electrolyte excretion and thus prevents the person from developing an imbalance.
   b. *Replacement* intravenous therapy replenishes fluid and electrolytes that are depleted and thus corrects imbalances that have already developed.
2. Provide vascular access for infusion of medications or blood components.
3. Allow vascular access for monitoring devices.

Benefits and Drawbacks of Intravenous Therapy

1. Benefits
   a. Provides immediate access to the vasculature for rapid delivery of specific amounts of fluids, electrolytes, nutrients, and medications without time required for absorption from gastrointestinal tract or tissues.
   b. Allows delivery of blood and other agents that would be destroyed in the gastrointestinal tract.
   c. Provides a route for delivery of fluids, electrolytes, nutrients, and medications to persons who cannot take adequate amounts orally due to decreased level of consciousness, inability to swallow, gastrointestinal pathophysiology, or therapeutic restrictions (NPO orders).
   d. Enables administration of accurate doses of medication and rapid measurement and titration of medications.
2. Drawbacks
   a. Venipuncture causes initial pain and is distressing to many persons.
   b. Intravenous therapy provides a potential route of entry for microorganisms into the body.
   c. Adverse reactions or hypersensitivity reactions to medications may occur very rapidly, because medications enter the blood immediately.
   d. Excessive or too rapid infusion of solution may cause fluid overload or electrolyte imbalance.

e. Incompatibilities occur when certain solutions and medications are mixed.

f. The nurse may be exposed to another person's blood, which may transmit disease.

g. Complications of intravenous therapy include fluid and electrolyte overload, infiltration, inflammation (phlebitis), infection, hematoma, and air embolism (discussed later in this chapter).

Intravenous Solutions

1. Types of intravenous fluids
   a. *Isotonic fluids* are solutions with the same osmolality as the body fluids.
      (1) Isotonic sodium-containing fluids are used to expand the extracellular fluid compartment. Approximately one third of the isotonic fluid infused stays in the vasculature. Approximately two thirds of the isotonic fluid infused distributes into the interstitial fluid compartment. Isotonic fluids do not enter the cells because there is no osmotic force to shift them.
      (2) Examples of isotonic fluids are normal saline (0.9% NaCl), Ringer's solution, lactated Ringer's solution, and replacement electrolyte solutions (e.g., Normosol-R).
      (3) Isotonic fluids are used clinically to treat hemorrhage, hypovolemia, extracellular fluid volume deficit, or as an initial treatment of clinical dehydration.
   b. *Hypotonic fluids* are solutions that are more dilute (have lower osmolality) than body fluids.
      (1) Hypotonic fluids are used to expand the intracellular fluid compartment. Hypotonic fluids that contain sodium are used to expand both extracellular and intracellular compartments.
      (2) Hypotonic fluids dilute extracellular fluid and cause movement of water into cells by osmosis.
      (3) How much of the hypotonic fluid enters the cells depends on whether the solution contains sodium. If a hypotonic solution does not contain sodium (i.e., D5W), approximately two thirds of the fluid infused enters the cells. The remaining one third of the hypotonic fluid infused stays in the extracellular compartment (vascular and interstitial). If a hypotonic solution contains sodium, its distribution can best be understood by considering it to be normal saline with extra water added. The saline portion of the fluid distributes into the extracellular compartment; approximately two thirds of the extra water enters the cells.
      (4) Examples of hypotonic fluids are D5W, half-normal saline (0.45% NaCl), quarter-normal saline (0.225% NaCl), and maintenance electrolyte solutions (e.g., Normosol-M in D5W).
      (5) Hypotonic fluids are used to maintain open vascular access, replace water excreted in breathing, replace hypotonic sodium-containing body fluids (sweat, emesis, urine), and maintain daily fluid balance.
   c. *Hypertonic fluids* are solutions that are more concentrated (have higher osmolality) than the body fluids.
      (1) Hypertonic fluids are used to shrink the intracellular fluid compartment.
      (2) Hypertonic fluids concentrate extracellular fluid and cause movement of water from cells into extracellular fluid by osmosis.
      (3) A clinical example of hypertonic fluid use is infusion of 3 percent saline for emergency treatment of seizures from hyponatremia.
   d. *Plasma expanders* are solutions containing large particles that remain in the vasculature and do not enter the interstitial fluid.
      (1) Plasma expanders are used to increase the vascular volume rapidly.
      (2) Plasma expanders increase blood colloid osmotic pressure and thus draw fluid into the blood vessels.
      (3) Examples of plasma expanders are albumin, plasma protein fraction (Plasmanate), dextran, and hetastarch (Hespan).
      (4) Plasma expanders are used during hemorrhage and severe hypovolemia.

2. Composition of intravenous fluids and precautions for their use (Table 9–6)

Intravenous Therapy Equipment

1. Vascular access
   a. Choice of type of device depends on expected infusion time and potential complications.
      (1) Steel needles may be used in peripheral veins when the infusion time will be short. Steel needles cause less trauma than catheters on insertion and are less likely to cause hypersensitivity reactions. Infiltration is more common with steel needles.
      (2) Plastic catheters are used in peripheral veins when longer infusion times are expected. Plastic catheters may cause catheter embolism if the tip breaks.
      (3) Vascular access ports, implanted surgically under the skin, are used for long-term conditions that require repeated intravenous therapy. Use of vascular access ports requires palpation to locate the port, which may be difficult in obese persons. Sterile technique is used to inject through the skin into the self-sealing portal; may be poorly accepted by persons who fear needles.
      (4) Central venous catheters, inserted by physicians or advanced practice nurses, are used for long-term therapies with multiple drugs or highly concentrated or potentially-irritating agents. Air embolism is a serious complication of central venous catheters. With a multiple-lumen catheter, marking the lumen used for medications and flushing before and after use will help keep the lumen patent.
      (5) Peripherally inserted central catheters (PICC) lines, inserted by physicians or advanced practice

Table 9–6. Composition of Common Intravenous Fluids and Precautions for Their Use

Fluid	Tonicity	Sugar (gm/L)	Na⁺	Cl⁻	K⁺	Ca⁺⁺	Mg⁺⁺	HCO₃⁻	Other	Precautions
				(Values are mEq/L)						
D5W (5% dextrose in water)	Hypotonic effect in body after sugar enters cells; isotonic before administration	50	—	—	—	—	—	—	—	Excess causes hyponatremia; contains no electrolytes, so person needs a source of K^+, Ca^{++}, and Mg^{++} to prevent electrolyte deficits; does not provide enough calories for daily needs; will not correct hypovolemia (has no Na^+)
D10W (10% dextrose in water)	Hypotonic effect in body after sugar enters cells; hypertonic before administration	100	—	—	—	—	—	—	—	High osmolality irritates veins; administer slowly to allow sugar metabolism; contains no electrolytes, so person needs source of K^+, Ca^{++}, and Mg^{++} to prevent electrolyte deficits; will not correct hypovolemia (has no Na^+)
0.9% NaCl (normal saline [NS])	Isotonic	—	154	154	—	—	—	—	—	Excess causes ECV overload; monitor for pulmonary edema; person needs source of K^+, Ca^{++}, and Mg^{++}; use caution with CHF, renal failure, or liver disease
0.45% NaCl (half NS)	Hypotonic	—	77	77	—	—	—	—	—	Excess causes ECV overload plus hyponatremia; person needs source of K^+, Ca^{++}, and Mg^{++}
0.33% NaCl (one third NS)	Hypotonic	—	56	56	—	—	—	—	—	Excess causes hyponatremia plus possible ECV overload; person needs source of K^+, Ca^{++}, and Mg^{++}
3% saline	Hypertonic	—	513	513	—	—	—	—	—	Excess causes dangerous hypernatremia; administer slowly, with caution; monitor serum Na^+ and level of consciousness closely

Solution	Tonicity	Dextrose	Na^+	Cl^-	K^+	Ca^{++}	Mg^{++}		Other components	Comments
5% saline	Hypertonic	—	855	855	—	—	—	—	—	Excess causes dangerous hypernatremia; administer slowly, with extreme caution; monitor serum Na^+ and level of consciousness closely
D5 one half NS	Hypotonic effect in body after sugar enters cells	50	77	77	—	—	—	—	—	Excess causes ECV overload plus hyponatremia; person needs source of K^+, Ca^{++}, and Mg^{++}
D5 one quarter NS	Hypotonic effect in body after sugar enters cells	50	38.5	38.5	—	—	—	—	—	Excess causes hyponatremia plus possible ECV overload; person needs source of K^+, Ca^{++}, and Mg^{++}
Ringer's solution	Isotonic	—	147	156	4	4	—	—	—	Excess causes ECV overload; monitor for pulmonary edema; use with caution with CHF, renal failure, or liver disease
Lactated Ringer's solution	Isotonic	—	130	109	4	3	—	—	Lactate (source of HCO_3^-)	Excess causes ECV overload and metabolic alkalosis; monitor pH and s/s pulmonary edema; use with caution with CHF or renal failure; avoid with liver disease
Replacement electrolyte solutions (e.g., Isolyte S, Normosol-R, Plasma-Lyte 148)	Isotonic	—	140	98	5	—	3	—	Acetate, gluconate (sources of HCO_3^-)	Excess causes ECV overload and possible metabolic alkalosis; monitor s/s pulmonary edema; use with caution with CHF, renal failure, or liver disease
Replacement electrolyte solutions containing calcium (e.g., Isolyte E, Plasma-Lyte R)	Isotonic	—	140	103	10	5	3	—	Acetate and other sources of HCO_3^-	Excess causes ECV overload and metabolic alkalosis; monitor s/s pulmonary edema; watch for adequate urine output to prevent hyperkalemia
Maintenance hypotonic electrolyte solutions (e.g., Normosol-M, Plasma-Lyte 56)	Hypotonic	—	40	40	13	—	3	—	Acetate (source of HCO_3^-)	Excess causes hyponatremia plus possible ECV overload and metabolic alkalosis; watch for adequate urine output to prevent hyperkalemia

ECV, Extracellular volume; CHF, congestive heart failure; s/s, signs and symptoms.

247

nurses, are also used for long-term therapies that require repeated venous access. They are often used in home care because they are easier to insert than traditional central lines. A small amount of bleeding may occur at the insertion site for 24 hours; bleeding after that time is not expected. The most common complication is phlebitis; air embolism is possible but less common than with traditional central lines because the insertion site for PICC lines is below the heart level.

b. Choose the size of the peripheral catheter or needle depending on the solution to be infused and the diameter of the available vein.

(1) For rapid emergency fluid administration, blood products, or anesthetics, use large-bore devices (small gauge numbers) such as 14-, 16-, or 18-gauge catheters or 19-gauge needles.

(2) For peripheral fat infusions, use 20-gauge catheters or 21-gauge needles.

(3) For standard intravenous fluids and clear liquid medications, use 22-gauge catheters or 23-gauge needles.

(4) If the person has very small veins, use 24-gauge catheters or 25-gauge needles.

c. Attach an intravenous lock (saline lock) for intermittent infusion through peripheral lines.

d. Attach tubing (see below) for continuous infusion through peripheral lines.

2. Fluid containers

a. Flexible plastic bags

(1) Squeeze the bag to check for small punctures before hanging it.

(2) Never write directly on a plastic intravenous bag with a marking pen because it may be absorbed into the solution; use a ballpoint pen to write on a label or tape before placing it on the bag.

(3) After adding potassium chloride (KCl) or other agents to bags, mix the container end to end several times before hanging it to prevent infusion of a bolus.

b. Rigid plastic and glass bottles

(1) Examine the bottle for cracks before hanging it.

(2) Some medications (e.g., nitroglycerine) absorb into soft plastic and should be mixed only in glass bottles.

3. Pumps and infusion control devices

a. Infusion pumps and controllers are electronic devices that allow accurate infusion of fluid and have alarms to indicate various problems.

(1) Controllers depend on gravity, whereas pumps exert pressure to cause the fluid to flow.

(2) These devices are used for continuous or intermittent infusion of fluid and solutions of medications; most are not acceptable for infusion of blood products.

(3) Most pumps and controllers are attached to the intravenous line setup beneath the fluid container and drip chamber.

(4) Syringe pumps are attached to prefilled syringes of medication and use microbore tubing, which attaches to an injection port of a continuous intravenous line or to an intravenous lock.

(5) Read the directions carefully, understand how to operate and troubleshoot the device, and demonstrate competency before using it.

(6) Double-check the settings on a pump or controller because it is designed to deliver whatever is programmed into it.

(7) Explain the purpose of the device to the patient to reduce the anxiety of being attached to a machine.

b. Volume control sets are fluid chambers with gradations marked on them that can be inserted into an intravenous line setup to control maximum fluid infusion for persons who could easily become fluid overloaded (e.g., small children).

4. Tubing

a. Vents. A vent allows air to enter the intravenous fluid container as the fluid leaves. A vented adapter can be used to add a vent to a nonvented tubing system.

(1) Look at the fluid container to determine whether vented tubing is needed.

(2) Use nonvented tubing for flexible bags because they collapse as the fluid leaves. Vented tubing may be used with flexible containers, but it is not necessary.

(3) Use vented tubing for glass or rigid plastic containers to allow air to enter and displace the fluid as it leaves. Fluid will not flow from a rigid intravenous container unless it is vented.

b. Drip chambers (macrodrip and microdrip). Where the drop enters the drip chamber differentiates one type from the other; microdrip chambers have a short vertical metal piece where the drop forms. The packaging indicates how many drops per milliliter (gtt/ml) are delivered (the drop factor).

(1) Choose the drip chamber based on the projected infusion rate and type of solution.

(2) Use a microdrip chamber (delivers 60 drops/ml) if fluid will be infused at a slow rate (less than 50 ml/hr), if the solution contains potent medications that need to be titrated (as in critical care settings), and in many pediatric settings.

(3) Use a macrodrip chamber (delivers 10, 15, or 20 drops/ml) if the solution is thick or will be infused rapidly.

c. Filters

(1) Filters are used in intravenous lines to trap small particles, such as undissolved antibiotics or salts or medications that have precipitated from solution. They provide protection by preventing particles from entering the person's veins.

(2) Follow your institutional policy regarding the use of filters. Use a 0.22-micron filter for most solutions, a 1.2-micron filter for solutions containing lipids or albumin, and a special blood filter for blood components.

(3) Change filters every 24 to 72 hours, according to institutional policy, to prevent bacterial growth and release of endotoxin.

d. Other tubing considerations

(1) If a needleless system is being used, use the appropriate tubing that has resealable ports or one-way valves. A plastic cannula is used for resealable injection ports without caps. A white ring

identifies a resealable port. Injection ports with caps are one-way valves designed to fit a syringe tip. Use a new replacement cap after each procedure to keep the port sterile. Do not administer total parenteral nutrition or blood products through a one-way valve.

(2) If a pump or controller will be used, use the special tubing for the specific device.

(3) Add extension tubing for children, restless persons, or those with special mobility needs.

(4) Choose shorter (secondary) tubing for "piggyback" solutions, connecting them to the injection site nearest to the drip chamber.

(5) Use special tubing for nitroglycerine and other medications that absorb into soft plastic.

Intravenous Therapy Procedures

1. Calculating intravenous fluid flow rates (Procedure 9–1)
2. Venipuncture and starting an intravenous infusion (Procedure 9–2)

 CLINICAL CONTROVERSIES

Transparent dressings are used widely for covering intravenous sites and are replacing the more traditional sterile gauze dressings.

Several researchers have studied infection rates with transparent dressings and those with gauze dressings. One meta-analysis (statistical procedure to synthesize results of many research studies) concluded that transparent dressings are associated with increased risk of catheter infection.

Nevertheless, ease of use, ability to assess the intravenous site visually, and reduced frequency of dressing changes are the key factors that influence clinicians to choose transparent dressings for intravenous sites. The infection risk remains a source of controversy.

3. Connecting piggyback infusions (Procedure 9–3)
4. Discontinuing an intravenous infusion (Procedure 9–4)
5. Administering an "IV push" medication (Procedure 9–5)

Complications of Intravenous Therapy

1. Fluid and electrolyte overload
   a. Causes: Too rapid, excessive, or inappropriate infusion of intravenous fluid leads to fluid, electrolyte, or acid-base imbalance, depending on the type of solution infused.
   b. Prevention
      (1) Read the label carefully to verify correct solution.
      (2) Calculate drip rate accurately.
      (3) Use an infusion control device.
      (4) Use colored stickers to mark solutions containing potassium or other electrolytes.
      (5) Add a time strip to the intravenous bag or bottle.
      (6) Check the drip rate or pump settings frequently to verify that they are correct; sometimes patients, visitors, or other health care providers alter the rate. Also, the flow at some intravenous sites may vary with the patient's position.

(7) If the pump or controller has a lockout button, activate it after setting the infusion rate.

   c. Nursing assessment
      (1) Review the signs and symptoms of excess of the solutions being infused. Signs and symptoms and specific assessments for extracellular fluid volume (saline) excess, hyponatremia (water excess), hyperkalemia, hypercalcemia, hypermagnesemia, hyperphosphatemia, metabolic acidosis, and metabolic alkalosis are presented later in this chapter.
      (2) Perform the appropriate assessments frequently.
   d. Nursing intervention if complication occurs
      (1) Decrease drip rate to minimum level ("keep-open" rate).
      (2) Notify physician immediately.
      (3) Use independent nursing actions specific to the imbalance that has developed. These are outlined with each imbalance later in this chapter.

2. Infiltration (extravasation)
   a. Causes: Infusion of solution into subcutaneous tissue when the intravenous needle or catheter slips out of the vein or is pushed through the posterior wall of the vein, or when vein back pressure increases due to venospasm or clot.

ELDER ADVISORY

Older adults are at greatly increased risk for infiltration because they have fragile veins.

   b. Prevention
      (1) Avoid venipuncture over an area of flexion.
      (2) Anchor the venipuncture cannula and a loop of tubing securely.
      (3) Use an armboard or a splint for an active or a restless person.
   c. Nursing assessment
      (1) Inspect the site for edema and coolness; compare with opposite extremity to note small amounts of swelling.

ELDER ADVISORY

Because older people have less subcutaneous fat, a considerable amount of fluid can accumulate in their tissues before swelling becomes evident.

      (2) Watch for substantially decreased or stopped infusion rate.
      (3) While watching the drip rate, occlude the vein a few inches above the area where the cannula or needle tip should be. If the tip is in the tissues, the infusion will continue to flow; if the tip is still in the vein, the flow will stop.
      (4) Alternatively, lower the intravenous fluid con-

Text continued on page 259

Procedure 9–1
Calculating Intravenous Fluid Flow Rates

Definition/Purpose	To determine the rate at which to infuse an intravenous fluid so that it flows during the prescribed time interval. Drip rates set visually are calculated in gtt per min. If an infusion pump or controller is used, the setting may be in ml per min or ml per hr.
Contraindications/Cautions	Inaccurate flow rates can jeopardize the patient. If the flow rate is too fast, the person may develop phlebitis from vein irritation by the solution, extracellular fluid volume excess, hyponatremia, plasma electrolyte excesses, metabolic acid-base imbalances, or drug overdose, depending on the content of the infusion. If the flow rate is too slow, the person will not receive the therapeutic effects of the fluid, electrolytes, or medication in the solution. If you are tired, distracted, hurried, or tend to make arithmetic errors, use a calculator for accuracy.
Learning/Teaching Activities	Provide the following information: (1) explain that you have set the rate so that it will flow at the right speed; (2) indicate that you will check it frequently to make sure it runs correctly; and (3) ask the person and any visitors not to adjust it.

Preliminary Activities

Equipment	• Fluid infusion order • Pencil and paper • Calculator (optional)
Assessment/Planning	• Decide whether you will use an infusion pump or controller or count drip rates visually. • If counting drip rates visually, look at the packaging to determine the gtt per ml (drop factor) delivered by the tubing you will be using. • If using an infusion pump or controller, look at the control panel to determine what units are needed to set the flow rate (e.g., ml/min; ml/hr).

Procedure

Actions	Rationale/Discussion
1. Decide in what units you need the flow rate.	1. If counting visually, gtt/min. If pump or controller, use the rate requested on the control panel (ml/min, ml/hr).
2. If fluid order is written in liters, convert liters to ml by multiplying by 1000.	2. Volume may be written in liters or ml. 1 liter = 1000 ml. *Example:* Fluid order: 2 liters D5W. Calculation: 2 liters × 1000 ml/liter = 2000 ml.
3. Read the fluid order to determine the volume of solution (in ml) to be infused in 1 hr. If the order indicates a volume for several hours, divide the total volume by the total number of hours to determine the volume for 1 hr.	3. *Example:* Fluid order: 2 liters D5W over 8 hr. Calculation: 2000 ml ÷ 8 hr = 250 ml/hr.
4. If the control panel requests ml per hr, you have finished calculating the flow rate. If you need flow rate in ml per min or gtt per min, continue calculating.	4. The units you need to set the rate for the equipment you are using will determine what you need to calculate.
5. Divide the rate in ml per hr by 60 to determine ml per min. If control panel requests ml per min, you have finished calculating the flow rate. If you need flow rate in gtt per min, continue calculating.	5. 1 hr = 60 min. *Example:* 250 ml/hr ÷ 60 min/hr = 4 ml/min.
6. Multiply the ml per min by the gtt per ml (drop factor) from the tubing package to determine the flow rate in gtt per min.	6. Different drip chambers deliver drops of different sizes. *Example:* package indicates 15 gtt/ml. Calculation: 4 ml/min × 15 gtt/ml = 60 gtt/min.
7. The above steps are equivalent to using the following formula:	

$$\frac{\text{total volume of solution (ml)} \times \text{gtt/ml delivered by drip chamber}}{\text{number of hours ordered to infuse} \times 60 \text{ min/hr}} = \text{flow rate (gtt/min)}$$

Final Activities

Recheck your calculations to ensure accuracy. Write down the calculated flow rate and carry it with you to adjust the infusion so that you do not forget it or confuse flow rates for two different persons. Document flow rate according to institutional policy. *Note:* to help prevent medication errors, always recalculate the flow rate at the beginning of each shift.

Procedure 9–2
Venipuncture and Starting an Intravenous Infusion

Definition/Purpose	To insert a needle or cannula into a vein to allow infusion of fluids or medications. Tubing is attached to provide continuous fluid infusion. For intermittent infusion, an intravenous (IV) lock (saline lock; heparin lock) is attached.
Contraindications/Cautions	Read the label on the IV fluid container carefully to ensure that you have the correct solution. Do not start an IV infusion in an arm that has a dialysis access, is edematous, is affected by a cardiovascular accident, or is on the same side as a mastectomy. When choosing site, consider the solution to be infused; use larger veins for irritating solutions.
Learning/Teaching Activities	Provide the following information: (1) explain the purpose of the procedure; (2) describe the procedure regardless of the person's level of consciousness.

Preliminary Activities

Equipment	• Disposable gloves
	• Intravenous needle or catheter (see text)
	• Tourniquet
	• Alcohol swabs or sterile gauze and antiseptic (according to institutional policy)
	• Transparent intravenous dressing or other dressing (according to institutional policy)
	• Tape
	• Armboard (optional)
	• If starting continuous infusion:
	  • Intravenous fluid container
	  • Sterile tubing
	  • Filter, if institutional policy
	  • Infusion pump or controller, if desired or indicated
	• If inserting IV lock for intermittent infusion:
	  • Intravenous lock
	  • Sterile syringe with 2 or 3 ml normal saline and 25-gauge needle or needleless connector, as appropriate for the IV lock
	  • If institutional policy indicates, sterile syringe containing 0.5 to 1.0 ml heparin flush solution (100 units/ml) with needle or needleless connector, as appropriate for the IV lock

Assessment/Planning	• Read the order and calculate the desired infusion flow rate (see Procedure 9–1). • If the IV fluid contains potassium or magnesium, be sure that the person has adequate renal function. • Select appropriate tubing for the fluid container (see tubing discussion in text). • If inserting an IV lock, determine whether a needle is needed to connect the IV infusion or a needleless system is in use. • If inserting an IV lock, determine the institutional policy regarding heparin or saline flush. • Determine whether the person is right- or left-handed, has a dialysis access, has an extremity that is edematous, or is affected by a cardiovascular accident or lymph node dissection (e.g., mastectomy).
Preparation of Person	• Be sure that you have identified the right person. • Explain the procedure and the purpose of infusion to the person. • Ask if the person has had an IV infusion started previously, and assess anxiety level. • The individual should be in a stable sitting or lying position. • If appropriate, discuss placement (right or left arm) with the person.

Procedure

Actions	Rationale/Discussion
1. Wash your hands.	1. Maintain asepsis.
2. Verify that the fluid container is not cracked or leaking and that the solution is clear and does not contain crystals.	2. Holding container up to the light facilitates checking for cracks, cloudiness, and crystals. Squeeze the plastic bag gently to check for leaks. Detection of possible contamination or decomposition of solution protects the patient.
3. Attach tubing to fluid container, hang it, and prime the tubing while maintaining sterility. If using pump or controller, follow manufacturer's directions for setup and priming.	3. Priming removes air from the system. Sterility is necessary to prevent infection.

(continued)

Procedure 9-2

(continued)

Actions	Rationale/Discussion
4. Select the most distal insertion site above digital veins. For adults, use metacarpal (back of hand), basilic, or cephalic (inner forearm) veins. For elders, avoid metacarpal veins. For infants, use scalp, hand, or foot veins. Be sure that you have enough straight vein above the insertion site for the length of needle or catheter. Apply tourniquet briefly if needed to visualize veins.	4. Use of most distal site saves more proximal sites for later use. Avoid areas over joints and scarred or inflamed veins. Save veins in antecubital fossa for laboratory or emergency use if possible. In adults, veins in lower extremities are used only if absolutely necessary due to potential for thrombophlebitis. In older people, metacarpal veins are often fragile.
5. Position yourself for easy access with adequate lighting.	5. Facilitate successful venipuncture.
6. Open equipment package, maintaining sterility.	6. Prevent infection.
7. Apply tourniquet about 10 to 15 cm (4–6 in) above chosen insertion site. Ensure that distal pulse is still palpable.	7. Properly applied tourniquet reduces venous return so that superficial veins are distended but does not impede arterial blood flow. Do not leave tourniquet applied for more than 2 min; loosen and reapply if necessary.
8. Put on gloves.	8. Universal precautions.
9. If vein is not clearly distended, have person open and close fist a few times.	9. Other techniques to increase venous distention include keeping vein below heart level, tapping very lightly over the site with the flats of your fingers, and wrapping the arm with a warm, moist towel before applying the tourniquet.
10. Cleanse the insertion site using firm pressure in concentric circles from the center outward. Allow to air dry or blot center with a sterile gauze.	10. Reduce potential for infection. Follow institutional policy for cleansing agent. If choice is available, avoid using alcohol for older people (unless sensitive to iodine) because it dries the skin.
11. Remove needle guard, maintaining sterility.	11. Prevent infection.
12. Stabilize the vein by grasping the person's arm or hand with your nondominant hand so that your thumb is beside the vein and about 5 cm (2 in) distal to the insertion site. Use your thumb to apply gentle traction on the skin toward the person's hand or fingers.	12. Facilitate piercing the vein by keeping it from rolling away from the needle. Decreased subcutaneous fat in elders allows veins to roll more easily, so stabilization is especially important.

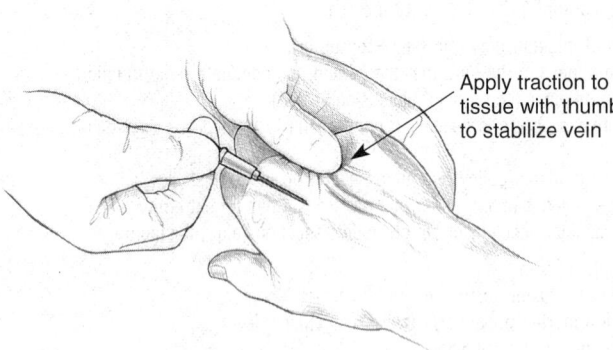

Apply traction to tissue with thumb to stabilize vein

Actions	Rationale/Discussion
13. Assess the person's anxiety level and provide reassurance or verbal distraction while you proceed, if possible.	13. Increase patient comfort.
14. Hold the needle bevel up, and insert it at a 45-degree angle using a smooth motion. You will feel a slight "give" when the needle enters the vein.	14. Small, sharp portion of needle should enter vein first. Sudden decrease in resistance is due to needle entering vein from denser tissue.
15. Check the flashback chamber for blood return.	15. Confirm placement in vein.
16. Lower the hub toward the skin (more parallel to the course of the vein), and advance a little into the vein.	16. Change of angle prevents puncturing opposite wall of vein. If inserting catheter, advance enough so that catheter tip as well as needle tip is within the vein.
17. If inserting catheter, separate needle from catheter by pulling back on needle hub slightly and then holding it steady while advancing catheter	17. Allow needle to strengthen catheter without puncturing opposite wall of vein. To avoid shearing off the catheter tip, do not advance the needle

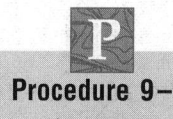

Procedure 9–2

(continued)

Actions	Rationale/Discussion
the remaining distance. Allowing 1 or 2 drops of IV fluid to infuse before advancing catheter may ease catheter entry.	once it has been pulled back from the catheter. A few drops of fluid dilate vein, allowing catheter to enter more easily.

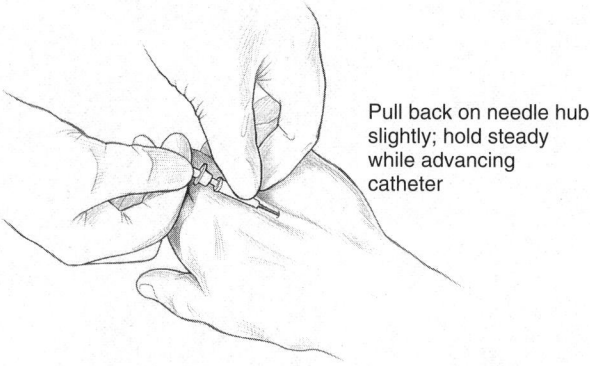

Pull back on needle hub slightly; hold steady while advancing catheter

Actions	Rationale/Discussion
18. Release tourniquet.	18. Release venous congestion to reduce blood leakage.
19. If inserting catheter, remove needle, holding catheter in place.	19. Prevent dislodging catheter.
20. Insert primed IV tubing, being careful to stabilize the hub. Turn on infusion at slow rate. If using IV lock, flush it according to institutional policy.	20. Start fluid flow as soon as possible to prevent clot formation at tip of catheter or needle. Watch for infiltration or hematoma. Adjust final rate later if necessary, after site is stabilized by taping.
21. Secure the site with a tape chevron: place the center of a 10 cm (4 in) strip of tape, sticky side up, under the hub; cross each end over to secure to skin without taping over the puncture site. If a butterfly (winged) needle was used, tape the wings flat using a crosswise strip of tape, in addition to a chevron. If a sterile transparent occlusive dressing will be used, the catheter hub may be taped with two crosswise pieces of tape and the chevron omitted.	21. Prevent dislodging of IV access. Protect skin from irritation by placing tape between hub and person's skin. Keeping tape off puncture site reduces potential for infection and allows visual inspection. Choose appropriate tape for elders and other persons with fragile skin. Transparent dressings facilitate visual inspection of the site but may have increased risk of infection.

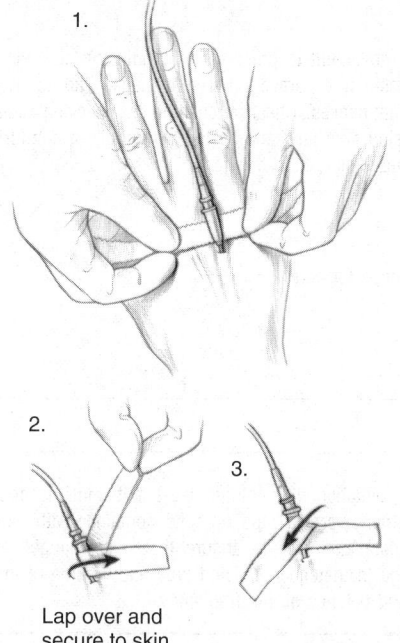

Lap over and secure to skin

(continued)

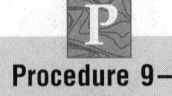

Procedure 9–2

(continued)

Actions	Rationale/Discussion
22. Apply transparent or other dressing over puncture site as indicated by institutional policy.	22. Institutional policy varies regarding use of antimicrobial ointment or dressing.
23. Make a loop of tubing, being careful not to kink it, and tape it to the person's arm or hand.	23. Prevent dislodging if tubing is pulled.

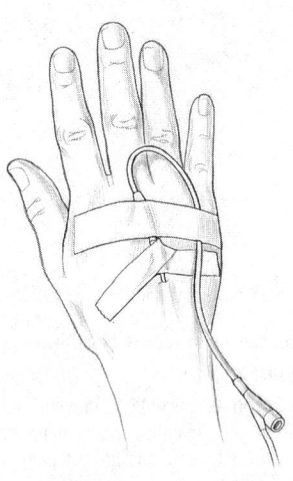

24. Adjust infusion flow rate to level calculated previously.	24. Deliver fluid as ordered.
25. Apply a tape label on which you have written date, gauge, catheter length, and your initials. Do not write on tape over the vein.	25. Document according to institutional policy to provide accessible information to guide use and replacement of intravenous access. Writing over vein may cause puncture or damage.
26. Remove gloves and wash your hands. You may remove gloves earlier to facilitate working with tape as long as no blood leakage has occurred.	26. Maintain universal precautions and asepsis.
27. If the intravenous site is near a joint or is unstable, or if person is not alert and may dislodge the system, use an armboard: place armboard under the arm or hand, allowing fingers to curl over the end in functional position; pad it at the wrist joint; tape armboard to the extremity, being careful not to impede circulation. For small children, you may need to pin the armboard to the sheet or tape a paper cup over the insertion site; cut a hole in the bottom of the paper cup before taping it to allow visualization of site.	27. Prevent movement to preserve intact infusion site. Place hand in functional position to prevent nerve damage. Pad to avoid pressure on bony prominences. Check circulation by checking radial pulse, watching infusion flow rate, and asking person about comfort. Ensure stabilization and visualization of site.
28. Check to see how person tolerated procedure.	28. Assess need for care.

Final Activities

Ask if the person has any questions. Label fluid container with colored label if it contains potassium or other additives, including medications. Add time strip (mark vertical tape on fluid container with expected times) to assist monitoring of infusion. Label tubing with date and time to ensure that it is changed as prescribed by institutional policy. Document location of site, gauge, catheter length, and type and volume of infusion according to institutional policy. Check progress of infusion and patency of site frequently.

Procedure 9–3
Connecting Piggyback Infusions

Definition/Purpose	To infuse an intravenous solution of medication using a preestablished intravenous line. The fluid container with the preestablished intravenous line is the primary infusion; the medication in solution is the secondary (piggyback) infusion. After the secondary infusion is complete, it is removed, leaving the primary infusion in place.
Contraindications/Cautions	Mixing solutions in intravenous lines may cause them to precipitate in the line if they are not compatible. Always check for incompatibility. Use a compatibility chart found in the medication preparation area, look in a reference book, or ask a pharmacist.
Learning/Teaching Activities	Provide the following information: (1) describe procedure regardless of person's level of consciousness; (2) explain that the existing intravenous line will be used and that the person will not have an additional needle stick.

Preliminary Activities

Equipment	• Intravenous fluid container with secondary (piggyback) solution • Sterile tubing for secondary (piggyback) container • Sterile 19- or 20-gauge needle or needleless connector, as appropriate • Sterile syringe with 2 or 3 ml normal saline and needle or needleless connector if the 2 solutions are not compatible • Alcohol swabs or sterile gauze and antiseptic (according to institutional policy)
Assessment/Planning	• Read the order for the medication in the secondary (piggyback) infusion, look at the container to determine the volume to be infused, and calculate the infusion flow rate (see Procedure 9–1). Typically, the solution is 50 to 100 ml and is infused over 30 to 60 min. Check with a pharmacist if infusion duration is not clear. • Select appropriate tubing for the secondary (piggyback) container (see tubing discussion in text). Determine whether a needle is needed to connect to the infusion port on the primary line or a needleless system is in use. • Check compatibility of the medication with the solution infusing through the primary intravenous line. • Check the medical records for any allergy to the medication.
Preparation of Person	• Be sure that you have identified the right person. • Ask regarding medication allergies. • Explain the procedure and the purpose of the infusion to the person. • The individual should be in a stable sitting or lying position so that the intravenous line does not move.

Procedure

Actions	Rationale/Discussion
1. Wash your hands.	1. Maintain asepsis.
2. Check patency of primary infusion: determine that primary infusion is flowing by watching drip chamber or control panel of infusion pump or controller; look for signs of infection or infiltration (see discussion in text).	2. Primary line must be operative to infuse secondary fluid into it; prevent infusing medication into tissues instead of vein.
3. Attach tubing to secondary container, hang it, attach needle or connector (if needed) to other end of tubing, and prime the tubing while maintaining sterility.	3. Priming removes air from the system. Sterility is necessary to prevent infection.
4. What you do next depends on whether the two solutions are compatible and exactly what type of tubing is supplied.	4. The directions on the secondary tubing package will clarify exact procedure.
5. *If the primary and secondary solutions are not compatible* and no alternate site for administration is feasible, clamp the primary infusion, clean an injection port on the primary line that is below the clamp, flush the line with normal saline using a syringe, and then attach the secondary (piggyback) tubing to the injection port.	5. Clears the primary solution from the tubing and fills it with saline. This procedure prevents precipitation of incompatible solutions in the intravenous line.
6. *If the primary and secondary solutions are compatible,* clean an injection port on the primary tubing above the clamp, flush the port with normal saline, and attach the secondary (piggyback) tubing to the injection port.	6. Mixing of compatible solutions in the primary tubing will not cause a problem.
7. Lower the primary fluid container by hanging it on an extension hook.	7. Fluid will flow faster from the container that is higher, so the secondary fluid container will empty first. If the primary tubing has a "backcheck" valve, the primary infusion will stop until the secondary infusion is complete and then resume.

(continued)

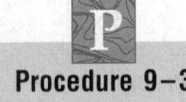

Procedure 9–3
(continued)

Actions	Rationale/Discussion
8. Adjust flow rate of secondary (piggyback) infusion. With the incompatible solutions setup, use the clamp on the secondary tubing to adjust the rate. With the compatible solutions setup, open the secondary tubing clamp fully and use the primary tubing clamp to adjust the rate.	8. Ensure that it will be delivered as ordered. Use the clamp on the tubing that is closest to the venipuncture site to adjust the rate.
9. Note the time.	9. Determine when the secondary infusion should be finishing so you can organize your care to be available.

Final Activities

Ask if person has any questions. Document type and volume of fluid, type and volume of flush solution, and dose of medication infused according to institutional policy. Check progress of infusion frequently. After secondary (piggyback) infusion is complete, remove secondary tubing from injection port, raise primary fluid container, and readjust primary infusion rate. If the 2 solutions were incompatible, flush the primary tubing with normal saline after removing the secondary tubing.

Procedure 9–4
Discontinuing an Intravenous Infusion

Definition/Purpose	To remove an intravenous needle or a cannula from the infusion site.
Contraindications/Cautions	If the person is hypovolemic with a decreased level of consciousness, be sure that another intravenous infusion site is already in place before discontinuing the 1st infusion site.
Learning/Teaching Activities	Provide the following information: (1) describe procedure regardless of person's level of consciousness; (2) explain that you will apply pressure after removing the needle or cannula to prevent bleeding.

Preliminary Activities

Equipment	• Disposable gloves • 2 × 2 sterile gauze sponge • Adhesive bandage
Assessment/Planning	• Find out if the person has a bleeding disorder or is receiving anticoagulants. • Find out the reason for discontinuing the intravenous infusion (e.g., phlebitis, routine rotating of sites to prevent phlebitis, person no longer needs intravenous therapy). • Find out if venipuncture for another intravenous site will be needed. • If a cannula is to be removed, find out its length.
Preparation of Person	• Explain the procedure to the person. Ask if the person has had an intravenous infusion discontinued previously, and assess anxiety level. • The individual should be in a stable sitting or lying position.
Procedure	

Actions	Rationale/Discussion
1. Wash your hands.	1. Maintain asepsis.
2. Put on gloves.	2. Universal precautions.

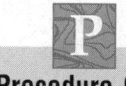

Procedure 9–4
(continued)

Actions	Rationale/Discussion
3. Turn off intravenous infusion.	3. Prevent leakage.
4. Remove any dressing; untape tubing and needle hub from patient, being careful to stabilize the hub.	4. Allow access while preventing damage to vein.
5. Place 2 × 2 gauze sponge over infusion site, and withdraw the needle or cannula without putting any pressure on it.	5. Have gauze in place to apply pressure rapidly after removal; no pressure during removal protects vein from damage.
6. Immediately put pressure on the infusion site with the gauze until there is no bleeding (at least 1 min); elevate site if practical.	6. Promote hemostasis with pressure and elevation. Person with bleeding disorder or anticoagulant therapy will need pressure for longer time (5–10 min).
7. Inspect site.	7. Detect redness or swelling.
8. Apply adhesive bandage to the site.	8. Protect from contamination or trauma.
9. If a cannula was removed, inspect the end and measure it to ensure that the full length was removed.	9. Detect cannula embolism from broken cannula.
10. Dispose of equipment safely.	10. Universal precautions.
11. Remove gloves. Wash hands.	11. Maintain asepsis.

Final Activities

If venipuncture for another intravenous infusion is not planned and no other infusion site is already in place, discuss with person the need for adequate oral fluid intake and help plan practical ways to make that possible. Ask if person has any questions. Document removal of intravenous infusion site according to institutional policy.

Procedure 9–5
Administering an "IV Push" Medication

Definition/Purpose

To administer a medication from a syringe directly into a vein through a preexisting intravenous (IV) lock (saline lock; heparin lock) or infusing IV line. Intravenous push medications may also be given through direct venipuncture. Venipuncture is described in Procedure 9–2.

Contraindications/Cautions

Adverse reactions may occur rapidly because the medication is given intravenously. Giving the medication too rapidly is likely to cause serious adverse effects. Careful dilution is necessary to prevent irritation of the vein.

Learning/Teaching Activities

Provide the following information: (1) explain the purpose of the procedure; (2) describe the procedure regardless of the person's level of consciousness.

Preliminary Activities

Equipment

- Disposable gloves
- Alcohol swabs
- Medication in proper dose and dilution in syringe with needle or needleless connector, as appropriate for the system.
- Two sterile syringes, each with 2 or 3 ml normal saline (or 1 syringe with 4 or 6 ml saline) and 25-gauge needle or needleless connector, as appropriate for the system.
- If institutional policy indicates using an IV lock, sterile syringe containing 0.5- to 1.0-ml heparin flush solution (100 units/ml) with needle or needleless connector, as appropriate for the IV lock.

Assessment/Planning

- Compare the medication order and the label on the medication container to determine that they match.
- Determine the necessary dilution for IV push administration by consulting a reference book, computerized database, or pharmacist. Double-check the dose, and dilute it carefully.

(continued)

Procedure 9-5
(continued)

- Determine how rapidly the medication is to be given by consulting a reference book, computerized database, or pharmacist. Times may vary from 1 to 30 min.
- Determine desired therapeutic actions and common adverse reactions of the medication, and decide which assessments are the most appropriate.
- If giving medication through an IV lock or existing IV line, determine whether a needle is needed or a needleless system is in use.
- If giving medication through an IV lock, determine the institutional policy regarding heparin or saline flush.
- If giving medication through an existing IV line, determine the compatibility of the medication with the IV fluid that is infusing.

Preparation of Person
- Be sure that you have identified the right person.
- Explain the procedure and the purpose of the medication to the person.
- The individual should be in a stable sitting or lying position.

Procedure

Actions	Rationale/Discussion
1. Wash your hands.	1. Maintain asepsis.
2. Position yourself for easy access with adequate lighting. For injection times over 1 min, sitting is recommended.	2. Facilitate successful procedure.
3. Put on gloves.	3. Universal precautions. If injecting into an IV line, gloves may not be needed but should be at hand in case manipulation of the IV site becomes necessary.
4. Determine that the IV site is patent.	4. Prevent injection into tissues rather than vein.
5. Cleanse the IV lock or injection port with an alcohol swab. With an IV line, use the distal port (closest to the person). Allow to air dry or blot center with a sterile gauze.	5. Prevent infection.
6. Remove needle guard or protective cap of needleless system, maintaining sterility.	6. Prevent infection.
7. Flush with 2 or 3 ml of normal saline. If the medication is incompatible with the IV solution, turn off the infusion before flushing the line. If the solutions are compatible, leave the infusion running.	7. Ensure patency; prevent clotting and possible incompatibilities by clearing aspirated blood and any heparin from the IV lock reservoir or the infusing IV solution from the IV line. Injection while an IV infusion is running dilutes the medication further and helps avoid vein irritation.
8. Insert syringe and inject the medication slowly over the required time interval, assessing the person closely for changes in condition that may indicate adverse reaction	8. Prevent adverse reactions from too rapid administration. Detect adverse reactions early, should they occur.
9. If an adverse reaction does occur, stop administering the medication, remove the syringe, flush (see step 11), and consult the physician or nurse practitioner.	9. Seek appropriate care.
10. Assess the person's anxiety level and provide reassurance or verbal distraction while you proceed.	10. Increase the person's comfort.
11. After administering the medication, remove the syringe and flush with 2 or 3 ml of normal saline. With an IV lock, if institutional policy indicates, finish with a heparin flush.	11. Promote patency of the device and prevent incompatibilities.
12. With an existing IV line, turn on the flow if you stopped it previously; check the infusion flow rate.	12. Maintain delivery of fluid as ordered.
13. Check to see how person tolerated procedure.	13. Assess need for care.
14. Remove gloves and wash hands.	14. Universal precautions and maintain asepsis.

Final Activities

Ask if person has any questions. Dispose of equipment safely. Document medication, dose, time, flushes, and person's condition according to institutional policy.

tainer while watching the tubing near the intravenous site; if the cannula or needle is still in the vein, a "flashback" of blood will appear in the tubing.

d. Nursing actions if complication occurs
(1) Discontinue infusion site immediately.
(2) If a vasoconstrictor or irritating agent has been infused, apply emergency local therapy as ordered, to prevent tissue sloughing.
(3) With less irritating agents, elevate the extremity and apply compress according to institutional policy or the person's preference.

CLINICAL CONTROVERSIES

Traditionally, nurses apply a warm, moist compress to the site and elevate the extremity following discontinuation of an infiltrated intravenous line. Sometimes a cold moist compress is applied.

Some studies on infiltrated saline solutions have shown that application of warmth caused significantly faster reabsorption of the infiltrate than application of cold. There was no difference in amount of pain reported by patients. Elevation did not speed reabsorption. Statistical comparison indicated no difference between application of moist heat and no treatment at all.

Elevation of the extremity and use of warm moist compresses are still controversial. The above studies examined small infiltrations of various saline solutions; they did not study D5W or solutions containing caustic medications. At least in the case of saline, current research indicates that patient preference may be the treatment of choice.

3. Phlebitis
a. Causes
(1) Inflammation of a vein caused by chemical irritation from the intravenous solution or medications, mechanical irritation from the needle or cannula, or accompanying local infection.
(2) Development of a clot (thrombophlebitis) may occur.
b. Prevention
(1) To reduce mechanical irritation, choose cannula or needle smaller than the vein, avoid areas of flexion, and anchor securely, using armboard or splint for restless or very active person.
(2) Avoid very small veins for infusion of irritating solutions.
(3) Avoid infusing into lower extremities in adults or children of walking age.
(4) Change venipuncture site every 48 to 72 hours, according to institutional policy.
c. Nursing assessment
(1) Inspect vein near site frequently for heat, redness, tenderness, and swelling along the course of the vein.
(2) Vein may feel hard or cordlike with thrombophlebitis.
d. Nursing actions if complication occurs
(1) Discontinue infusion site.
(2) Apply warm, moist compress.
(3) Provide teaching and reassurance.

4. Infection
a. Causes: Local or systemic growth of microorganisms that gained entry to the body through the venipuncture site.
b. Prevention
(1) Use careful aseptic technique in assembling intravenous lines and fluid containers.
(2) Check fluid containers for cracks, leaks, cloudiness (if solution should be clear), or other evidence of contamination.
(3) Wash hands before gloving and prepare venipuncture site according to institutional policy before venipuncture.
(4) Change tubing and site dressings every 24 to 72 hours, according to institutional policy; use antimicrobial ointment at site (after checking for allergies) if included in protocol. Label the tubing with date and time to ensure that it is changed as prescribed by institutional policy.
(5) Write date and time on fluid containers, and be sure the solution is not infused for more than 24 hours.
c. Nursing assessment
(1) Local infection: inflammation at site (see previous discussion) plus exudate
(2) Systemic (sepsis): malaise, chills and fever, nausea, vomiting, headache, backache, tachycardia, septic shock, positive blood culture
d. Nursing actions if complication occurs
(1) Discontinue infusion site, place sterile cap on venipuncture device, and save the entire setup for possible culture.
(2) Monitor vital signs carefully, and notify physician.
(3) With sepsis, obtain blood samples as ordered for culture. Use the other arm to differentiate sepsis from local infection at the intravenous site.
5. Hematoma
a. Causes: Collection of blood into the tissues during unsuccessful venipuncture or after venipuncture site is discontinued.
b. Prevention
(1) Avoid piercing posterior wall of vein during venipuncture.
(2) Do not apply a tourniquet to an extremity immediately after an unsuccessful venipuncture.
(3) When discontinuing an infusion site, apply pressure to the site for at least 1 minute immediately after the device is removed and elevate the extremity; apply pressure longer (5–10 min) for persons who take anticoagulants or have bleeding disorders.
c. Nursing assessment: Observe for hard, painful lump at site.
d. Nursing actions if complication occurs
(1) Apply ice immediately.
(2) Apply pressure and elevate.
6. Air embolism
a. Causes: Bolus of air enters the veins through an inadequately primed intravenous line or a loose connection or during central venous line insertion, tubing change, or removal.

LEARNING/TEACHING GUIDELINES
for People Receiving Intravenous Therapy at Home

1. Explain the purpose of the therapy, and give an overview of the procedures. Remember to include the family or any caregivers in the teaching session as well as the person receiving the intravenous (IV) therapy.
2. Teach the importance of hand washing and how to do it properly.
   a. If the home does not have running water, help the person set up a basin and pitcher or other arrangement in a convenient location.
   b. With this and all psychomotor procedures, demonstrate first and have the person return the demonstration.
3. Define sterile, explain the importance of sterile technique, and teach the person how to establish and maintain sterility during the required procedures.
4. Demonstrate the equipment and how it works.
   a. Provide a diagram of the equipment setup for the person to follow while you demonstrate.
   b. Demonstrate changing an IV bag, hanging medi-

cations, or other procedures pertinent to the person's situation.
   c. Show how to set and monitor the drip rate and operate the controls on the pump or controller, if used.
   d. Provide basic equipment troubleshooting information.
5. Explain how to monitor the site for infiltration and inflammation and what to do if these occur.
6. Explain the infusion schedule, and help the person plan ways to incorporate it into daily life.
   a. Discuss the person's schedule, and do joint problem solving about potential difficulties.
   b. Demonstrate how to wrap the IV site so the person can take a shower, if pertinent.
7. Provide written instructions to reinforce the teaching.
8. Give the name and telephone number of the person to contact when questions arise. Explain when the nurse will visit again. If the home does not have a telephone, establish a mechanism by which the person can make contact if questions arise.

---

b. Prevention
   (1) Peripheral lines: Prime tubing with fluid before use and inspect for air bubbles, which may alarm patient and family members; remove any visible bubbles; secure all connections; replace fluid containers before they are completely dry; adjust any stopcocks correctly; use pump or controller with an air sensor.
   (2) Central lines: As above; for central line insertion, tubing changes, and line removal, place person in Trendelenburg position and teach him or her to perform the Valsalva maneuver to increase pressure in central veins while system is open.
c. Nursing assessment: Be alert for sudden onset of tachycardia, dyspnea, cyanosis, hypotension, decreased level of consciousness, and possible mill wheel murmur (continuous loud "turning" sound over the precordium due to air in right ventricle).
d. Nursing actions if complication occurs
   (1) Clamp tubing.
   (2) Immediately turn person on left side, with head of bed lowered, to trap air in the right atrium.
   (3) Monitor vital signs, and notify physician.
   (4) Administer oxygen if needed.
   (5) Provide emotional support.

Home Intravenous Therapy

1. When intravenous therapy is performed at home, teaching the person and family or caregivers becomes very important.
   a. After explaining and demonstrating, have the person

perform the procedures (return demonstration) under supervision.
   b. Remember that people learn less effectively when they are anxious or in pain.
   c. Expect the person to have questions; allow opportunity for questions and provide a telephone number or other source to contact for questions that will arise.
   d. Provide information in several ways (verbal, diagrams, written instructions) that are appropriate to the person's learning style, literacy level, and language (Learning/Teaching Guidelines for People Receiving Intravenous Therapy at Home).

◼ EXTRACELLULAR FLUID VOLUME DEFICIT

Definition

1. Extracellular fluid volume deficit is too little isotonic fluid in the extracellular fluid compartment. Both vascular and interstitial compartments are contracted.
2. Extracellular fluid volume deficit may occur singly or together with hypernatremia (water deficit). The combination of extracellular fluid volume deficit and hypernatremia is *clinical dehydration*.

Incidence and Etiology

1. Loss of sodium-containing body fluids
   a. Gastrointestinal fluids. **Examples:** vomiting, diarrhea, nasogastric or intestinal suction, fistula drainage.

b. Urine. **Examples:** Adrenal insufficiency (decreased aldosterone), salt-wasting renal disorders, excessive diuretic therapy, prolonged bed rest.
  c. Other body fluids. **Examples:** wound exudate, burns, hemorrhage, 3rd space fluid accumulation (e.g., ascites).
2. Many body fluids are hypotonic sodium-containing fluids (e.g., most gastrointestinal fluids, sweat). They are like isotonic saline with additional water added. The loss of the isotonic saline portion of these fluids causes extracellular fluid volume deficit.

Clinical Manifestations and Pathophysiology (Table 9–7)

Diagnostics

1. Assessment
  a. Measure weight daily.
    (1) If extracellular fluid volume deficit is due to 3rd space fluid accumulation (e.g., ascites), weight will

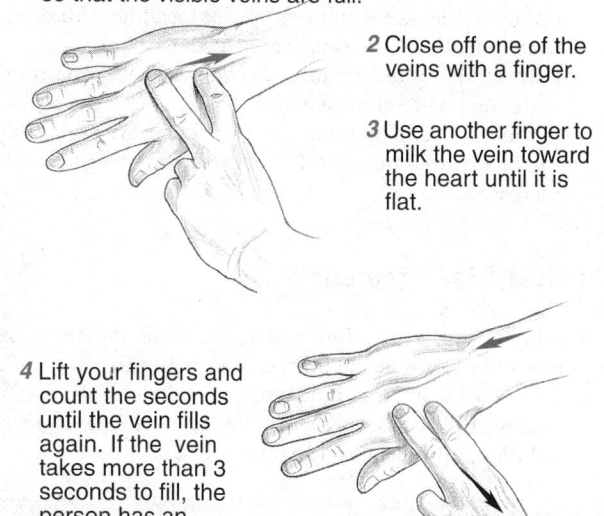

ASSESSING SMALL VEIN FILLING TIME

1 Place the person's hand below the level of the heart, so that the visible veins are full.

2 Close off one of the veins with a finger.

3 Use another finger to milk the vein toward the heart until it is flat.

4 Lift your fingers and count the seconds until the vein fills again. If the vein takes more than 3 seconds to fill, the person has an extracellular fluid volume deficit, unless arterial disease is present.

Figure 9–5.

Table 9–7. Clinical Manifestations of Extracellular Fluid Volume Deficit and Excess with Their Pathophysiologic Bases

Clinical Manifestation	Pathophysiologic Basis
Extracellular Fluid Volume Deficit	
Sudden loss of weight (unless 3rd space fluid accumulation)	A liter of fluid weighs 1 kg
Postural blood pressure drop	Inadequate vascular volume
Flat neck veins when supine	Inadequate vascular volume
Rapid thready pulse	Inadequate vascular volume; cardiac response to baroreceptor reflex
Increased small vein filling time	Inadequate vascular volume
Sunken fontanel (infants)	Inadequate vascular volume
Dryness of opposing mucous membranes	Inadequate vascular volume
Absence of tears and sweat	Inadequate vascular volume
Decreased skin turgor	Inadequate interstitial volume
Longitudinal furrows in the tongue	Inadequate interstitial volume
Soft, sunken eyeballs	Inadequate interstitial volume
Lightheadedness, syncope	Decreased perfusion of brain
Decreased capillary refill time	Decreased tissue perfusion
Oliguria	Decreased renal perfusion
Signs of hypovolemic shock	Inadequate vascular volume
Extracellular Fluid Volume Excess	
Sudden gain of weight	A liter of fluid weighs 1 kg
Full neck veins when upright	Excessive vascular volume
Bounding pulse	Excessive vascular volume
Tense or bulging fontanel (infants)	Excessive vascular volume
Edema in ankles or other dependent area	Excessive interstitial volume
Crackles in dependent portions of lungs	Pulmonary edema from excessive vascular volume
Dyspnea or orthopnea	Pulmonary edema
Pink frothy sputum	Pulmonary edema

not decrease because the fluid is still in the body, although it is not available to the normal extracellular fluid compartments.
  b. Take postural blood pressure measurements in adults or adolescents, as described in the Physical Examination section of this chapter; assess pulse rate and character.
  c. Assess neck vein filling. Before neck veins are totally flat, they may be seen collapsing with inspiration.
  d. Assess small vein filling time (Fig. 9–5).
    (1) Small vein filling time may be assessed using the hand or the foot.
    (2) Small vein filling time is not a useful assessment in persons who have severe peripheral arterial disease.
  e. Check skin turgor, as described in the Physical Examination section of this chapter.
  f. Watch for longitudinal furrows in the tongue, sunken eyeballs, or absence of tears and sweat.
  g. Assess dryness of opposing mucous membranes (e.g., between cheek and gum).
  h. In infants, check for sunken anterior fontanel.
  i. Watch for signs of decreased organ and tissue perfusion.
    (1) Light-headedness, syncope
    (2) Oliguria
    (3) Decreased capillary refill time
    (3) Hypovolemic shock, the very last manifestation (see Chapter 12)

2. Medical diagnosis
   a. Extracellular fluid volume deficit is diagnosed by combining patient history with clinical manifestations.
   b. The serum sodium concentration does not change with an isolated extracellular fluid volume deficit. A serum sodium imbalance (osmolality imbalance) may occur at the same time as an extracellular fluid volume deficit but is a separate disorder.
   c. Extracellular fluid volume deficit with hypernatremia is defined as clinical dehydration.
   d. If the extracellular fluid volume deficit arises rapidly, the blood urea nitrogen (BUN) and hematocrit may be increased.

Clinical Management

1. Treatment for extracellular fluid volume deficit is replacement of isotonic sodium-containing fluid.
   a. The most common intravenous isotonic sodium-containing fluids are normal saline (0.9% NaCl), Ringer's solution, and lactated Ringer's solution.

NURSE ADVISORY

> To detect rebound extracellular fluid volume excess, listen to the dependent portions of the lung for crackles during infusion of intravenous isotonic fluid.

   b. Oral replacement may also be accomplished by giving fluids that contain sodium (such as salty broth), by providing salty foods along with liquid, or by using commercial pediatric oral rehydration fluids.
   c. If the person has clinical dehydration (combined extracellular fluid volume deficit and hypernatremia), intravenous isotonic sodium-containing fluid will be followed by more dilute sodium-containing fluids such as one half normal or one quarter normal saline. This therapy provides replacement of both the extracellular volume (isotonic) and the extra water needed to dilute the body fluids back to their normal concentration.

Applying the Nursing Process

NURSING DIAGNOSIS: Fluid volume deficit R/T excessive loss or inadequate intake of sodium-containing fluid

1. *Expected outcomes:* Following intervention, the person's extracellular fluid volume should return to normal, as evidenced by disappearance of signs and symptoms and normal results on assessment of vascular and interstitial volume.
2. *Nursing interventions*
   a. Initiate intake and output recording and daily weights.
   b. Manage the replacement of isotonic sodium-containing fluid. Replacement fluid must contain sodium to hold the fluid in the extracellular fluid compartments.

NURSING DIAGNOSIS: Risk for injury R/T postural hypotension or syncope

1. *Expected outcomes:* Following instruction, the person will remain free of injury from falls.
2. *Nursing interventions*
   a. Teach the person to get up slowly and have something sturdy to hold onto in case of light-headedness.
   b. Encourage the person to be as active as possible within the limits of safety.

Discharge Planning and Teaching

1. Before hospital discharge, people need to learn the following:
   a. About extracellular fluid volume deficit and its treatment, including its specific cause in each person's case.
   b. How to prevent extracellular fluid volume deficit in the future.
   c. How to detect early signs of extracellular fluid volume deficit in case it recurs.
2. Learning/Teaching Guidelines for People with Clinical Dehydration are outlined on page 267.

■ EXTRACELLULAR FLUID VOLUME EXCESS (SALINE EXCESS)

Definition

Extracellular fluid volume excess is too much isotonic fluid in the extracellular fluid compartment. Both vascular and interstitial compartments are expanded.

Incidence and Etiology

1. Gain of excessive isotonic saline
   a. Intravenous. **Examples:** excessive infusion of isotonic normal saline, Ringer's solution, or Ringer's lactate.
   b. Renal. **Examples:** glucocorticoid therapy, excessive aldosterone. Excessive aldosterone is produced by aldosterone-secreting tumors and, more commonly, as a compensatory mechanism in congestive heart failure, cirrhosis, and nephrotic syndrome.
   c. Oral. **Example:** dietary intake of salty foods and water. Temporary excess unless combined with renal mechanism.

Clinical Manifestations and Pathophysiology (see Table 9–7)

Diagnostics

1. Assessment
   a. Measure weight daily.

b. Assess neck vein filling. Neck veins that are full when the person is upright or sitting with the backrest at greater than a 45-degree angle indicate extracellular fluid volume excess.

c. Note character of the pulse.

d. Assess dependent portions of the body for edema.
   (1) Measure circumference of ankles to detect changes in amount of edema.
   (2) Ask the person for permission to mark a spot on the skin to locate the measurement point so that measurements can be taken in the same place each time. Measurement location can also be recorded by distance above a particular bony landmark.

e. Keep a close watch for indications of pulmonary edema.
   (1) Crackles, initially in the dependent portions of the person's lungs
   (2) Dyspnea or orthopnea
   (3) Pink frothy sputum

f. In infants, check for a tense or bulging anterior fontanel.

2. Medical diagnosis
   a. Extracellular fluid volume excess is diagnosed from history and clinical findings.
   b. The serum sodium concentration does not change with an uncomplicated extracellular fluid volume excess.
   c. If extracellular fluid volume excess arises rapidly, the hematocrit may be decreased.

Clinical Management

1. Treatment for extracellular fluid volume excess usually involves diuretic therapy to remove excess saline.

NURSE ADVISORY

When diuretics are used to treat extracellular fluid volume excess, monitor the person's postural blood pressure because diuretic therapy may cause rebound extracellular fluid volume deficit.

2. If the person has a disease process that causes extracellular fluid volume excess, such as congestive heart failure, sodium restriction is usually prescribed.

Applying the Nursing Process

NURSING DIAGNOSIS: Fluid volume excess R/T excessive intake or inadequate excretion of sodium-containing fluid

1. *Expected outcomes:* Following intervention, the person's extracellular fluid volume should decrease toward normal.
2. *Nursing interventions*

a. Initiate intake and output recording and daily weights.
b. Manage the prescribed sodium restriction.

NURSING DIAGNOSIS: Risk for impaired gas exchange R/T fluid in alveoli

1. *Expected outcomes:* Following intervention, the person should be well-oxygenated, as evidenced by normal Pao$_2$, absence of crackles, dyspnea, cough, or pink frothy sputum.
2. *Nursing interventions*
   a. Monitor carefully for pulmonary edema (see earlier discussion).
   b. Position in semi-Fowler's to high Fowler's position.
   c. If pulmonary edema occurs, help the person deal with anxiety caused by dyspnea while providing appropriate therapy (see Chapter 22).

NURSING DIAGNOSIS: Risk for impaired skin integrity R/T edema

1. *Expected outcomes:* Following intervention, the person's skin integrity should be maintained, as evidenced by absence of reddened areas or breaks in skin.
2. *Nursing interventions*
   a. Provide careful skin care for edematous areas, keeping them clean and dry.
   b. Position the person carefully to avoid friction or pressure on edematous tissue; elevate edematous parts if possible.

NURSING DIAGNOSIS: Risk for altered body image R/T edema

1. *Expected outcomes:* Following discussion, the person should not avoid interpersonal contacts from embarrassment about appearance.
2. *Nursing interventions*
   a. Provide opportunities for the person to talk about feelings about presence of edema.
   b. Give permission to voice feelings by indicating that sometimes people feel uncomfortable about their appearance when they have swollen ankles or legs and ask how the person feels.

Discharge Planning and Teaching

1. Before hospital discharge, people need to learn the following:
   a. About extracellular fluid volume excess and its treatment, including its specific cause in each person's case.
   b. How to manage a prescribed sodium restriction.
   c. Which foods are rich in sodium.

LEARNING/TEACHING GUIDELINES
for People with Extracellular Fluid Volume Excess

1. Describe the processes that cause extracellular fluid volume excess, and explain how the person's signs and symptoms result from too much salt water in the blood vessels and between the cells.
2. Explain the prescribed therapy, and help the person plan ways to incorporate it into daily life.
   a. If a potassium-wasting diuretic is prescribed, include teaching about hypokalemia (see Learning/Teaching Guidelines for People with Hypokalemia) as well as about the medication itself (see Chapter 23).
   b. If a low-sodium diet is prescribed, ask the person what types of foods he or she usually eats (to assess cultural preferences), identify foods that are high in sodium, and plan low-sodium alternatives (see Learning/Teaching Guidelines for management of low-sodium diet in Chapter 23).
3. Discuss symptom assessment and management.
   a. Explain that reduction of the signs and symptoms indicates that therapy is working well and that therapy may need to be continued to keep signs and symptoms under control.
   b. Teach how to monitor daily weights, and help the person prepare a chart for recording date and weight.
   c. Demonstrate how to measure ankle circumference to assess edema, if appropriate.
   d. Explain that edematous tissue is fragile and needs special care to keep it clean, dry, and free from pressure or scratching.
   e. Indicate that the person should contact the health care provider if symptoms worsen (e.g., shortness of breath when not exercising) or reappear after they have gone away, or if lightheadedness occurs (potential need for adjustment of therapy).

d. How to detect signs of extracellular fluid volume excess in case it recurs or worsens.
e. How to weigh daily and what to do with the information. (Learning/Teaching Guidelines for People with Extracellular Fluid Volume Excess).

▣ HYPONATREMIA (INTRACELLULAR FLUID VOLUME EXCESS)

Definition

Hyponatremia is a plasma sodium concentration below normal. It indicates that the body fluids are too dilute (Table 9–8).

Table 9–8. Clinical Manifestations of Hyponatremia and Hypernatremia with Their Pathophysiologic Bases

Clinical Manifestation	Pathophysiologic Basis
Hyponatremia	
Confusion, lethargy, coma	As plasma sodium concentration falls, water enters brain cells by osmosis; cerebral cell swelling causes decreased level of consciousness.
Seizures	Rapid changes in cerebral cell size
Hypernatremia	
Confusion, lethargy, coma	As plasma sodium concentration rises, water leaves brain cells by osmosis; cerebral cell shrinking causes decreased level of consciousness.
Thirst	Osmosensitive cells in hypothalamus trigger thirst
Seizures	Rapid changes in cerebral cell size

Incidence and Etiology

1. Gain of relatively more water than sodium
   a. **Examples:** excessive infusion of D5W, excessive tap water enemas, distilled water used to irrigate body cavities, near-drowning in fresh water, giving infants water instead of milk in low-income situations, excessive ADH.
      (1) Secretion of ADH is increased by pain, nausea, trauma, anesthesia and surgery, physiologic stressors, and psychologic stressors.
      (2) Increased ADH is also caused by some head injuries, ectopic ADH secreted by certain malignant tumors, and by the syndrome of inappropriate ADH (SIADH).
2. Loss of relatively more sodium than water. **Examples:** vomiting, diarrhea, diaphoresis with tap water (and no salt) replacement, distilled water used to irrigate body cavities

ELDER ADVISORY

In some older people, thiazide diuretics cause hyponatremia through loss of relatively more salt than water in the urine.

Clinical Manifestations and Pathophysiology (see Table 9–8)

Diagnostics

1. Assessment
   a. Assess level of consciousness and neurologic status.
   b. Watch for seizures. Seizures occur more commonly when the plasma sodium concentration falls rapidly.

2. Medical diagnosis: Serum sodium concentration below 130 mEq/L. Although the lower limit of the normal range of serum sodium is 135 mEq/L, hyponatremia is not usually diagnosed until the serum sodium concentration has fallen to 130 mEq/L.

Clinical Management

1. The usual therapy for hyponatremia is water restriction. The restricted intake allows the kidneys to excrete the excess water and return the plasma sodium concentration to normal.
2. If the person has seizures or major neurologic changes, hypertonic saline (5% NaCl) may be given intravenously to raise the plasma sodium concentration above the danger level (but not back to normal). The serum sodium concentration is then allowed to return to normal slowly, often over 24 hours or more.
3. Medications (e.g., demeclocycline) that make the kidneys less responsive to ADH may be used.

DRUG ADVISORY

Hypertonic saline infusions can be dangerous. They may cause rapid osmotic fluid shifts in the brain, with severe neurologic consequences. Infuse hypertonic saline slowly, using a controller or infusion pump if possible. Monitor serum sodium and neurologic status closely.

Applying the Nursing Process

NURSING DIAGNOSIS: Risk for injury R/T decreased level of consciousness

1. *Expected outcomes:* Following intervention, the person should remain free of injury.
2. *Nursing interventions*
   a. Provide safety measures appropriate to the person's level of consciousness.
   b. Provide frequent position changes and skin care to prevent development of pressure ulcers.

NURSING DIAGNOSIS: Self-care deficit R/T decreased level of consciousness

1. *Expected outcomes:* Following intervention, the person's hygiene should be maintained at a culturally acceptable level.
2. *Nursing interventions*: Provide assistance, while encouraging as much independence as possible and adhering to the person's preferences and cultural values.

NURSING DIAGNOSIS: Discomfort and anxiety R/T thirst and fluid restriction

1. *Expected outcomes:* Following instruction, the person should comply with prescribed fluid restriction.
2. *Nursing interventions*
   a. Explain the reason for the fluid restriction to the patient and family members.
   b. Provide opportunities for the person to express feelings about fluid restriction.
   c. Give frequent oral care to keep mucous membranes moist, which decreases thirst.
   d. Remove extra liquids from meal trays before the person sees them.
   e. Allow the person as much control as possible regarding the fluid restriction, depending on level of consciousness.
      (1) Plan the timing of fluid intake with the person.
      (2) Let the person choose what type of fluids to drink when allowed.
      (3) Have the person keep a fluid intake record.
      (4) Tell the person to swish allowed fluid around the mouth to moisten mucous membranes before swallowing.
      (5) Teach sham drinking (swish water around the mouth and spit it out without swallowing any) to relieve thirst.
   f. Consolidate intravenous medications as much as possible, within the limits of compatibilities, to reduce intravenous fluids and increase oral fluids.

Discharge Planning and Teaching

1. Before hospital discharge, people need to learn the following:
   a. About hyponatremia and its treatment, including its specific cause in each person's case.
   b. How to manage fluid restriction.
   c. How to prevent hyponatremia in the future.
   d. How to detect early signs of hyponatremia in case it recurs (Learning/Teaching Guidelines for People with Hyponatremia).

■ *HYPERNATREMIA (INTRACELLULAR FLUID VOLUME DEFICIT)*

Definition

1. Hypernatremia is a plasma sodium concentration above normal. It indicates that body fluids are too concentrated (see Table 9–8).
2. Hypernatremia may occur singly or together with extracellular fluid volume deficit. The combination of hypernatremia and extracellular fluid volume deficit is *clinical dehydration*.

Incidence and Etiology

1. Loss of relatively more water than sodium. **Examples:** emesis, diarrhea, diaphoresis without fluid replacement or with isotonic replacement, insufficient ADH. Secretion

---

LEARNING/TEACHING GUIDELINES
for People with Hyponatremia

1. Describe the processes that cause hyponatremia, and explain how the person's signs and symptoms result from body fluids being too dilute.
2. Explain the prescribed fluid restriction, and help the person and family plan ways to manage it, if appropriate.
   a. Help the person make a chart to keep track of fluid intake.
   b. Work with the person to make a plan regarding how to space out fluids for maximum comfort.
   c. Explain that keeping the inside of the mouth moist by swishing water around and then spitting it out (sham drinking) will decrease thirst.
   d. Indicate that cold or hot liquids often satisfy thirst better than lukewarm ones.
3. If the hyponatremia is preventable (e.g., excessive use of tap water enemas or replacement of emesis with tap water), discuss ways to change the practices that caused it.

---

of ADH is decreased by ethanol, some head injuries, and diabetes insipidus.

2. Gain of relatively more sodium than water. **Examples:** limited access to water, self-limited water intake, inability to respond to thirst, decreased thirst sensation, difficulty swallowing liquids, tube feedings without adequate water intake, infusion of hypertonic saline.
   a. Persons who are unable to respond to thirst include those who are confused, weak, aphasic, paralyzed, developmentally delayed, or comatose.
   b. The high concentration of tube feedings (even isotonic ones) provides insufficient water for daily maintenance. In addition, it causes the kidneys to excrete water while excreting the high particle load from tube feedings.

ELDER ADVISORY

Hypernatremia from tube feedings is more common in older adults than in middle-aged or young adults. Be sure to supply extra water between tube feedings.

c. The thirst sensation is diminished with normal aging, which places elders at high risk for hypernatremia.

Clinical Manifestations and Pathophysiology (see Table 9–8)

Diagnostics

1. Assessment
   a. Assess level of consciousness.
   b. Ask the person regarding thirst.

ELDER ADVISORY

Thirst is not a reliable indicator of hypernatremia in older people because their thirst response to increased osmolality is blunted.

c. Watch for seizures. Seizures occur more commonly when the plasma sodium concentration rises rapidly.
2. Medical diagnosis: Serum sodium concentration above 145 mEq/L in adults and children and 162 mEq/L in newborns.

Clinical Management

1. Treatment for hypernatremia is replacement of water until the serum sodium concentration returns to normal.
   a. Water replacement may be intravenous (e.g., D5W) or oral.

NURSE ADVISORY

Intravenous replacement of water in hypernatremia must be performed slowly. Too rapid replacement will cause osmotic fluid shifts in the brain and may cause cerebral edema or intracranial hemorrhage, especially in infants. Monitor serum sodium and neurologic status frequently.

   b. If the person is clinically dehydrated (combined extracellular fluid volume deficit and hypernatremia), intravenous isotonic sodium-containing fluid will be followed by more dilute sodium-containing fluids such as one half normal or one quarter normal saline. This therapy provides replacement of both the extracellular volume (isotonic) and the extra water needed to dilute the body fluids back to their normal concentration.

Applying the Nursing Process

NURSING DIAGNOSIS: Risk for injury R/T decreased level of consciousness

1. *Expected outcomes:* Following intervention, the person should remain free of injury.

LEARNING/TEACHING GUIDELINES
for People with Clinical Dehydration

1. Describe the processes that cause clinical dehydration, and explain that the person's signs and symptoms result from not enough fluid in the body.
2. Explain the need to replace fluid with liquids that contain salt, and help the person plan ways to manage this therapy.
   a. Explain that although usually we recommend that people decrease the salt in their diet, some salt is necessary when a person has clinical dehydration because sodium holds the water in the body.
   b. For replacement fluids, recommend using bouillon, juice and salty crackers, or commercial oral rehydration fluids and avoiding fluid labeled low sodium.
   c. Indicate that sugar helps sodium be absorbed from the intestines into the blood, so diet drinks are not as useful as sugar-containing ones when replacing body fluid losses.
   d. If the person is vomiting, small amounts (e.g., 1 or 2 tablespoons) of fluid should be taken every 15 to 30 minutes.
3. Discuss symptom assessment and management.
   a. Indicate that people often get lightheaded when they do not have enough body fluids, so safety precautions should be taken.
   b. Explain that reduction of the signs and symptoms indicates that fluid therapy is working well and should be continued until the health care provider indicates it is safe to stop.
   c. Indicate that the person should contact the health care provider if symptoms get worse, do not go away, or reappear after they have gone away.
4. Describe how to prevent clinical dehydration by increasing fluid intake to match fluid excretion and loss.
   a. Discuss the importance of replacing body fluid losses immediately with sodium-containing fluids (not tap water) to prevent clinical dehydration in the future.
   b. Review the signs and symptoms of clinical dehydration, and explain how to recognize it early so that the person can seek health care if home rehydration is not successful.

2. *Nursing interventions*
   a. Provide safety measures appropriate to the person's level of consciousness.
   b. Provide frequent position changes and skin care to prevent development of pressure ulcers.

NURSING DIAGNOSIS: Self-care deficit R/T decreased level of consciousness

1. *Expected outcomes:* Following intervention, the person's hygiene should be maintained at a culturally acceptable level.
2. *Nursing interventions*: Provide assistance, while encouraging as much independence as possible and adhering to the person's preferences and cultural values.

Discharge Planning and Teaching

1. Before hospital discharge, people need to learn the following:
   a. About hypernatremia and its treatment, including its specific cause in each person's case.
   b. How to manage replacement of water.
   c. How to detect early signs of hypernatremia in case it recurs (Learning/Teaching Guidelines for People with Clinical Dehydration).

☐ HYPOKALEMIA

Definition

Hypokalemia is a plasma potassium concentration below normal. Intracellular potassium may be low, normal, or even high when the plasma potassium concentration is low (Table 9–9).

Incidence and Etiology

1. Decreased potassium intake. **Examples:** anorexia, NPO orders, fad diets
2. Shift of potassium from the extracellular fluid into cells. **Examples:** excessive insulin, hyperalimentation, alkalosis, hypothermia, excessive epinephrine or β_2-adrenergic medications.
3. Increased potassium excretion. **Examples:** diarrhea, laxative abuse, potassium-wasting diuretics, osmotic diuresis, hypomagnesemia, excessive aldosterone, glucocorticoid excess.
4. Loss of potassium through abnormal routes. **Examples:** vomiting, gastric or intestinal suction

Clinical Manifestations and Pathophysiology (see Table 9–9)

Diagnostics

1. Assessment
   a. Check for muscle weakness or flaccid paralysis.
      (1) Muscle weakness usually starts in the legs and is bilateral and ascending.
      (2) Ask about difficulty climbing stairs or rising from low or overstuffed chairs.
   b. Assess depth of respirations.

Table 9–9. Clinical Manifestations of Hypokalemia and Hyperkalemia with Their Pathophysiologic Bases

Clinical Manifestation	Pathophysiologic Basis
Hypokalemia	
Skeletal muscle weakness, flaccid paralysis	Muscles are hyperpolarized and thus unresponsive to stimuli
Shallow respirations	Weakness of respiratory muscles
Cardiac dysrhythmias	Altered cardiac cell resting membrane potential, more rapid diastolic depolarization, decreased conduction velocity, changes in refractory period
ST depression, decreased amplitude or inverted T waves, presence of U waves, PR and QT prolongation on electrocardiogram	See above
Constipation, abdominal distention, decreased or absent bowel tones, paralytic ileus	Unresponsiveness of hyperpolarized gastrointestinal smooth muscle
Postural hypotension	Unresponsiveness of hyperpolarized vascular smooth muscle
Polyuria, nocturia	Renal unresponsiveness to antidiuretic hormone causes larger volume of more dilute urine
Hyperkalemia	
Skeletal muscle weakness or flaccid paralysis	Muscles are hypopolarized but become unresponsive to stimuli because they cannot repolarize after an action potential
Cardiac dysrhythmias	Altered cardiac cell resting membrane potential, shorter action potentials, more rapid repolarization, decreased conduction velocity
Peaked narrow T waves, ST depression, wide QRS, sine wave on electrocardiogram	See above
Cardiac arrest	Asystole; see above
Abdominal cramping, diarrhea, increased bowel tones	Hypopolarized gastrointestinal smooth muscle becomes hyperactive and increases peristalsis

c. Monitor heart rate and rhythm.
d. Assess for constipation or paralytic ileus.
 (1) Listen for bowel tones in all 4 quadrants.
 (2) Watch for abdominal distention.
 (3) Ask about bowel pattern.
e. Assess for postural hypotension.
 (1) Measure postural blood pressure.
 (2) Ask person about lightheadedness on standing.
f. Measure urine output.
2. Medical diagnosis: Plasma potassium concentration below 3.5 mEq/L in adults and children or below 3.9 mEq/L in newborns.

Clinical Management

1. Give oral or intravenous potassium as ordered until the plasma potassium concentration returns to normal.
 a. Potassium chloride (KCl) is the most common oral and intravenous form.
 b. Potassium phosphate is used for potassium replacement in diabetic ketoacidosis.
2. Treat the cause of the hypokalemia.

℞ DRUG ADVISORY

Potassium salts are irritating to tissues in high concentrations. Watch for gastrointestinal distress with oral potassium. Give oral potassium with food to decrease mucosal irritation.

Watch for heat and redness at the infusion site for intravenous potassium. Dilute intravenous potassium carefully and infuse it slowly to avoid giving a potassium bolus, which may cause ventricular fibrillation or cardiac arrest. Use a controller or infusion pump if possible to maintain the correct intravenous flow rate.

3. If the person is receiving digitalis, monitor for digitalis toxicity.

NURSE ADVISORY

If a person who is receiving digitalis develops hypokalemia, digitalis toxicity may occur. Monitor for digitalis toxicity (anorexia, nausea, emesis, cardiac arrhythmias, bradycardia) and administer potassium replacement as prescribed before administering digitalis.

LEARNING/TEACHING GUIDELINES
for People with Hypokalemia

1. Describe the processes that cause hypokalemia, and explain how the person's signs and symptoms result from not enough potassium in the blood.
2. Explain the need for increased potassium intake and help the person plan ways to incorporate it into daily life.
   a. If potassium supplements are prescribed, explain the importance of taking them regularly.
   b. Demonstrate how to mix powdered potassium chloride with cold juice or sherbet to make it taste better.
   c. Ask the person what types of foods he or she usually eats (to assess cultural preferences), and identify foods that are high in potassium.
   d. Help make menu plans to increase intake of potassium-rich foods such as oranges, bananas, peaches, prunes, raisins, dates, dried apricots, strawberries, cantaloupe, almonds, and potatoes.
3. Discuss symptom assessment and management.
   a. Explain that reduction of the signs and symptoms indicates that therapy is working well and that increased potassium intake may need to be maintained to keep blood potassium normal.
   b. Indicate that the person should contact the health care provider if symptoms worsen (e.g., legs too weak to climb stairs) or reappear after they have gone away, or if severe gastrointestinal distress occurs, or urine becomes dark yellow and scant (potential need for adjustment of therapy).
4. If the hypokalemia is preventable (e.g., laxative abuse), discuss ways to change the practices that caused it.

Applying the Nursing Process

NURSING DIAGNOSIS: Risk for injury R/T muscle weakness and postural hypotension

1. *Expected outcomes:* Following intervention, the person should remain free from injury.
2. *Nursing interventions*
   a. Provide safety measures appropriate to the person's degree of muscle weakness.
      (1) Raised bedrails
      (2) Bedpan or bedside commode
      (3) Sturdy stool for climbing into and out of bed
      (4) Straight chair instead of overstuffed or low chair
   b. Instruct person with postural hypotension to rise slowly and to hold onto something while rising to avoid falling.

NURSING DIAGNOSIS: Impaired gas exchange R/T cardiac dysrhythmias or respiratory muscle weakness

1. *Expected outcomes:* Following intervention, the person should remain well oxygenated, as evidenced by normal PaO_2, cardiac output, and capillary filling and lack of cyanosis.
2. *Nursing interventions*
   a. Apply cardiac monitor if apical pulse is irregular.
   b. Monitor for signs and symptoms of decreased cardiac output.
   c. If respirations are becoming more shallow, be ready to institute mechanical ventilation if necessary.

NURSING DIAGNOSIS: Constipation R/T unresponsive, gastrointestinal smooth muscle

1. *Expected outcomes:* Following intervention, the person should regain customary bowel pattern.
2. *Nursing interventions*
   a. Explain reason for constipation to the person.
   b. Encourage fluids, provide privacy at the person's usual elimination time.

NURSING DIAGNOSIS: Self-care deficit R/T muscle weakness

1. *Expected outcomes.* Following intervention,
   a. The person's hygiene should be maintained within culturally acceptable levels.
   b. The person should state satisfaction with degree to which other activities of daily living are performed.
2. *Nursing interventions*
   a. Discuss activities of daily living and determine what assistance is needed.
   b. Provide assistance, while encouraging as much independence as possible and adhering to the person's preferences and cultural values.

Discharge Planning and Teaching

1. Before hospital discharge, people need to learn the following:
   a. About hypokalemia and its treatment, including its specific cause in each person's case.
   b. How to manage their specific potassium supplements.
   c. Which foods are rich in potassium.
   d. How to detect early signs of hypokalemia in case it recurs.
2. People who take digitalis need to know that hypokalemia can cause therapeutic levels of digitalis to be toxic (Learning/Teaching Guidelines for People with Hypokalemia).

◼ *HYPERKALEMIA*

Definition

Hyperkalemia is a plasma potassium concentration above normal. Intracellular potassium may be high, normal, or even low even when the plasma potassium concentration is high (see Table 9–9).

Incidence and Etiology

1. Increased potassium intake
   a. **Examples:** excessive infusion of intravenous potassium, insufficient mixing of potassium salts added to intravenous containers, multiple blood transfusions, and children who eat huge quantities of potassium-containing salt substitute.
   b. If renal function is normal, excessive oral intake of potassium does not usually cause hyperkalemia because the kidneys excrete the excess. If renal function is decreased, oral potassium intake may result in hyperkalemia.
2. Shift of potassium from cells to the extracellular fluid. **Examples:** lack of insulin, metabolic acidosis due to relative excess of mineral acids (e.g., diarrhea), crushing injuries, sickle cell crisis, tumor lysis syndrome.
3. Decreased potassium excretion. **Examples:** oliguria from any cause, including acute or chronic renal failure, severe hypovolemia, adrenal insufficiency, potassium-sparing diuretics, angiotensin-converting enzyme inhibitors.

NURSE ADVISORY

To prevent hyperkalemia, always check renal function to see that it is adequate (i.e., at least 30 ml/hr in adults) before giving potassium supplements.

Clinical Manifestations and Pathophysiology (see Table 9–9)

Diagnostics

1. Assessment
   a. Check for muscle weakness or flaccid paralysis.
      (1) Muscle weakness usually starts in the legs and is bilateral and ascending. Hyperkalemic persons may have "heavy legs" and difficulty climbing stairs.
      (2) Hyperkalemic infants have more flaccid muscles and kick less vigorously than usual.
   b. Assess depth of respirations. Although it is uncommon, hyperkalemia may cause weak respiratory muscles.
   c. Monitor heart rate and rhythm.
   d. Assess for abdominal cramping or diarrhea.

2. Medical Diagnosis: Serum potassium concentration above 5.0 mEq/L in adults and children or above 5.9 mEq/L in newborns.

Clinical Management

1. Give medical therapy as ordered until the serum potassium concentration returns to normal.
   a. Kayexalate (sodium polystyrene sulfonate) may be given orally or as a retention enema. It binds potassium ions and carries them out in the feces.

NURSE ADVISORY

To prevent constipation, be sure that sorbitol is given with sodium polystyrene sulfonate.

   b. Intravenous insulin and glucose drives extracellular potassium into cells. Glucose in the solution prevents hypoglycemia. Intravenous bicarbonate also drives extracellular potassium into cells.
   c. Intravenous calcium reduces the cardiac effects.
   d. Potassium-wasting diuretics may be used to increase potassium excretion.
   e. Dialysis may be necessary.
2. Treat the cause of the hyperkalemia.

Applying the Nursing Process

NURSING DIAGNOSIS: Risk for injury R/T muscle weakness

1. *Expected outcomes:* Following intervention, the person should remain free from injury.
2. *Nursing interventions*
   a. Provide safety measures appropriate to the person's degree of muscle weakness.
      (1) Raised bedrails
      (2) Bedpan or bedside commode
      (3) Sturdy stool for climbing into and out of bed
      (4) Straight chair instead of overstuffed or low chair

NURSING DIAGNOSIS: Risk for decreased cardiac output R/T cardiac dysrhythmias or cardiac arrest

1. *Expected outcomes:* Following intervention, the person should maintain normal cardiac output, as evidenced by adequate urine output, normal capillary filling, normal PaO_2, and lack of cyanosis.
2. *Nursing interventions*
   a. Apply cardiac monitor if apical pulse is irregular.
   b. Apply monitor if blood is being transfused rapidly or multiple units are administered.

c. Monitor for signs and symptoms of decreased cardiac output.

NURSING DIAGNOSIS: Self-care deficit R/T muscle weakness

---

1. *Expected outcomes:* Following instruction,
   a. The person's hygiene will be maintained within culturally acceptable levels.
   b. The person will state satisfaction with degree to which other activities of daily living are performed.
2. *Nursing interventions*
   a. Discuss activities of daily living and determine what assistance is needed.
   b. Provide assistance, while encouraging as much independence as possible and adhering to the person's preferences and cultural values.

Discharge Planning and Teaching

1. Before hospital discharge, people need to learn the following:
   a. About hyperkalemia and its treatment, including its specific cause in each person's case.
   b. How to prevent hyperkalemia from recurring, if possible.
   c. How to detect early signs and symptoms of hyperkalemia, in case it recurs (Learning/Teaching Guidelines for People with Hyperkalemia).

◼ HYPOCALCEMIA

Definition

Hypocalcemia is a plasma calcium concentration below normal. Whole body calcium content may be low, normal, or even high when the plasma calcium concentration is low (Table 9–10).

Incidence and Etiology

1. Decreased calcium intake or absorption
   a. **Examples:** diet poor in dairy products and other calcium sources, chronic diarrhea, laxative abuse, steatorrhea, vitamin D deficiency
   b. Vitamin D deficiency causes hypocalcemia by interfering with calcium absorption. **Examples:** lack of access to sunlight, uremic syndrome, overuse of oral mineral oil.
2. Shift of calcium from the extracellular fluid into the bones or into a physiologically unavailable form
   a. **Examples:** hypoparathyroidism, hypomagnesemia, hyperphosphatemia, alkalosis, citrate from blood transfusions, liver transplant (citrate toxicity)
   b. When calcium in the plasma binds to plasma proteins or small ions such as citrate, it becomes physiologically unavailable and the ionized calcium concentration decreases.
3. Increased calcium excretion. **Examples:** steatorrhea, medications that cause renal calcium wasting (e.g., antineoplastics)
4. Loss of calcium through abnormal routes. **Examples:** acute pancreatitis, fistula or wound drainage

Clinical Manifestations and Pathophysiology (see Table 9–10)

Diagnostics

1. Assessment
   a. Check for increased neuromuscular excitability.
      (1) In adults or children, check Chvostek's sign (Fig. 9–6) or Trousseau's sign (Fig. 9–7).
      (2) In adults and children, watch for muscle twitching, grimacing, carpal spasm, pedal spasm, laryngospasm, seizures.
      (3) Ask about muscle cramping and any tingling around the mouth or in the fingers.

Table 9–10. Clinical Manifestations of Hypocalcemia and Hypercalcemia with Their Pathophysiologic Bases

Clinical Manifestation	Pathophysiologic Basis
Hypocalcemia	
Positive Chvostek's sign, Trousseau's sign, muscle cramping, tingling around mouth or in fingers, muscle twitching, grimacing, hyperactive reflexes, carpal spasm, pedal spasm, laryngospasm, seizures	Increased neuromuscular excitability
Cardiac dysrhythmias	Prolonged plateau phase of cardiac cell action potentials, decreased conduction velocity
Prolonged QT interval on electrocardiogram	See above
Crackles in dependent portions of lungs	Congestive heart failure due to impaired myocardial contractility
Hypotension (acute hypocalcemia only)	Decreased peripheral vascular resistance and impaired cardiac function
Hypercalcemia	
Fatigue, skeletal muscle weakness, decreased reflexes	Decreased neuromuscular excitability
Confusion, lethargy, coma	Decreased neural excitability
Personality change, psychosis	Altered function of central nervous system
Constipation, anorexia, nausea	Decreased excitability of gastrointestinal smooth muscle
Cardiac dysrhythmias	Shortened plateau phase of cardiac cell action potentials, faster diastolic depolarization in sinus node, delayed atrioventricular conduction
Short QT interval on electrocardiogram, J wave if severe	See above
Polyuria	Renal unresponsiveness to antidiuretic hormone causes larger volume of more dilute urine
Pain of renal colic, calculi in urine	Urinary calculi from high concentration of urine calcium
High blood pressure (acute hypercalcemia only)	Increased peripheral vascular resistance

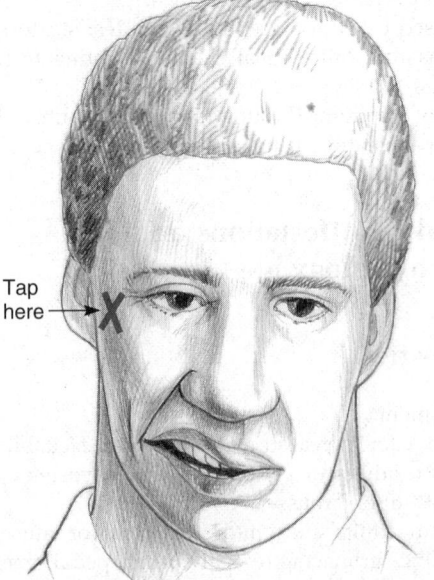

Figure 9–6. Assessing Chvostek's sign. Tap the side of the face in front of the ear and watch the cheek and corner of the mouth. If obvious muscle contraction draws up the cheek and mouth, this is a positive Chvostek's sign, which indicates increased neuromuscular excitability.

(4) In infants, watch for tremors, muscle twitching, and transient tonic-clonic seizures. A positive Chvostek's sign is normal in a newborn.

(5) Assess reflexes.

b. Monitor heart rate and rhythm and blood pressure.

c. Listen for crackles in the dependent portions of the lungs.

2. Medical diagnosis: Serum calcium concentration below 9 mg/dl (4.5 mEq/L) or ionized calcium below 1.14 mM/L.

Clinical Management

1. Give oral or intravenous calcium as ordered until the serum calcium concentration returns to normal.

 DRUG ADVISORY

Do not mix calcium with intravenous solutions containing bicarbonate or phosphate because crystals will form in the tubing. Watch carefully to avoid infiltration of intravenous calcium because calcium solutions cause severe tissue damage. Using an intravenous infusion pump, give calcium infusions slowly to prevent bradycardia or heart block.

2. Treat the cause of the hypocalcemia.

LEARNING/TEACHING GUIDELINES
for People with Hypocalcemia

1. Describe the processes that cause hypocalcemia, and explain how the person's signs and symptoms result from not enough calcium in the blood.
2. Explain the need for increased calcium intake, and help the person plan ways to incorporate it into daily life.
   a. If calcium supplements are prescribed, explain the importance of taking them regularly.
   b. Ask the person what types of foods he or she usually eats (to assess cultural preferences), inquire about tolerance and acceptability of dairy products, and identify foods that are high in calcium.
   c. Help make menu plans to increase intake of calcium-rich foods such as dairy products (if acceptable), oranges, broccoli, canned salmon, sardines, and tofu.
3. Discuss symptom assessment and management.

   a. Explain that reduction of the signs and symptoms indicates that therapy is working well and that increased calcium intake may need to be maintained to keep blood calcium normal.
   b. Describe how to control neuromuscular and environmental stimuli to provide safety and comfort until increased neuromuscular excitability is resolved.
   c. Indicate that the person should contact the health care provider if symptoms worsen (e.g., spontaneous muscle twitching) or reappear after they have gone away, if muscles become weak and heavy, or if constipation suddenly occurs (potential need for adjustment of therapy).
4. If the hypocalcemia is preventable (e.g., laxative abuse), discuss ways to change the practices that caused it.

Applying the Nursing Process

NURSING DIAGNOSIS: Risk for impaired gas exchange R/T potential laryngospasm

1. *Expected outcomes:* Following intervention, the person should maintain oxygenation, as evidenced by normal PaO_2, regular respirations, and lack of use of accessory respiratory muscles.
2. *Nursing interventions*
   a. Monitor for crowing respirations that could indicate laryngospasm.
   b. Find out where the 10 percent calcium gluconate solution is kept for emergency infusion in case of laryngospasm.

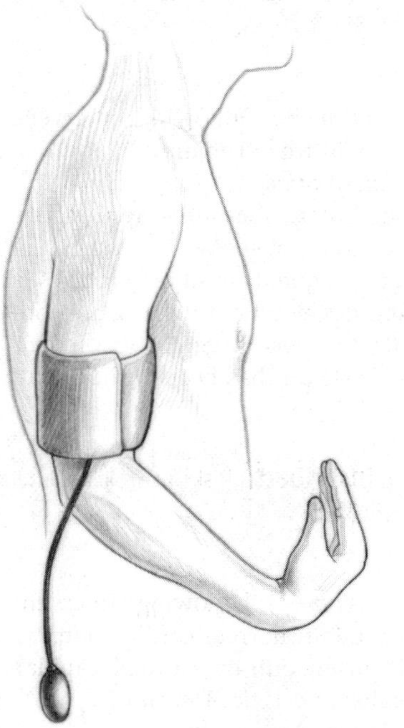

NURSING DIAGNOSIS: Risk for decreased cardiac output R/T cardiac dysrhythmias

1. *Expected outcomes:* Following intervention, the person should maintain normal cardiac output, as evidenced by adequate urine output, normal capillary filling, normal PaO_2, and lack of cyanosis.
2. *Nursing interventions*
   a. Apply cardiac monitor if apical pulse is irregular.
   b. Apply monitor if blood is being transfused rapidly or multiple units are administered.
   c. Monitor for signs and symptoms of decreased cardiac output.

NURSING DIAGNOSIS: Risk for injury R/T seizures

1. *Expected outcomes:* Following intervention, the person should not be injured if a seizure occurs.
2. *Nursing interventions*: Institute seizure precautions if appropriate.
   a. Raised and padded bedrails
   b. Reduced environmental stimuli

Figure 9–7. Assessing Trousseau's sign. Place a blood pressure cuff around the upper arm, inflate it, and watch the patient's hand. If the fingers extend while the wrist flexes (carpal spasm), this is a positive Trousseau's sign, which indicates increased neuromuscular excitability.

NURSING DIAGNOSIS: Anxiety R/T paresthesias and muscle twitching

1. *Expected outcomes:* Following instruction, the person's verbal and behavioral manifestations of anxiety (interpreted according to the person's culture) will be reduced.
2. *Nursing interventions*
   a. Explain cause of paresthesias and twitching.
   b. Provide anxiety-relieving interventions appropriate to the person's developmental level and cultural values.

Discharge Planning and Teaching

1. Before hospital discharge, people need to learn the following:
   a. About hypocalcemia and its treatment, including its specific cause in each person's case.
   b. How to prevent hypocalcemia from recurring, if possible.
   c. How to detect early signs and symptoms of hypocalcemia, in case it recurs (Learning/Teaching Guidelines for People with Hypocalcemia).

◼ HYPERCALCEMIA

Definition

Hypercalcemia is a plasma calcium concentration above normal. Whole body calcium may be high, normal, or even low even when the plasma calcium concentration is high (see Table 9–10).

Incidence and Etiology

1. Increased calcium intake or absorption. **Examples:** ingestion of large amounts of calcium-rich foods concurrently with large doses of antacids (milk-alkali syndrome) or megadoses of vitamin D or vitamin A, excessive infusion of intravenous calcium
2. Shift of calcium from bones to the extracellular fluid. **Examples:** hyperparathyroidism, prolonged immobilization (especially adolescent males with spinal cord injuries), bone tumors, cancers that produce bone-resorbing factors that circulate in the blood
3. Decreased calcium excretion. **Example:** thiazide diuretics

Clinical Manifestations and Pathophysiology (see Table 9–10)

Diagnostics

1. Assessment
   a. Check for fatigue and skeletal muscle weakness; assess reflexes.
   b. Assess level of consciousness.
   c. Monitor heart rate and rhythm and blood pressure.
   d. Measure urine output, strain urine for calculi.
   e. Assess for constipation, anorexia, nausea.
2. Medical diagnosis: Plasma calcium concentration above 11 mg/dl (5.5 mEq/L)

Clinical Management

1. Give medical therapy as ordered until the plasma calcium concentration returns to normal.
   a. Oral fluids, intravenous saline, or the diuretic furosemide may be used to increase urine excretion of calcium.

 DRUG ADVISORY

If phosphate salts are ordered for a person who has hypercalcemia, they should be given very cautiously because calcium phosphate salts may precipitate in the body and cause tissue damage.

b. Glucocorticoids or calcitonin may be ordered to decrease bone resorption.
   c. Dialysis may be used.
2. Treat the cause of the hypercalcemia.

Applying the Nursing Process

NURSING DIAGNOSIS: Risk for injury R/T decreased level of consciousness

1. *Expected outcomes:* Following intervention, the person should remain free of injury.
2. *Nursing interventions*
   a. Provide safety measures appropriate to the person's level of consciousness.
   b. Provide frequent position changes and skin care to prevent development of pressure sores.
   c. Handle the person gently to prevent pathologic fractures if calcium has been withdrawn from bones.

NURSING DIAGNOSIS: Risk for decreased cardiac output R/T cardiac dysrhythmias.

1. *Expected outcomes:* Following intervention, the person should maintain normal cardiac output, as evidenced by adequate urine output, normal capillary filling, normal PaO₂ results, and lack of cyanosis.
2. *Nursing interventions*
   a. Apply cardiac monitor if apical pulse is irregular.
   b. Monitor for signs and symptoms of decreased cardiac output.

LEARNING/TEACHING GUIDELINES
for People with Hypercalcemia

1. Describe the processes that cause hypercalcemia, and explain how the person's signs and symptoms result from too much calcium in the blood.
2. Explain the need for decreased calcium intake and increased fluid intake, and help the person plan ways to incorporate these into daily life.
   a. Ask the person what types of foods he or she usually eats (to assess cultural preferences), identify foods that are high in calcium (e.g., milk, cheese, ice cream, oranges), and plan low-calcium alternatives.
   b. Work with the person to set up a schedule for regular fluid intake throughout the day, setting a goal and a way to keep track of fluid intake.
3. Discuss symptom assessment and management.
   a. Explain that reduction of the signs and symptoms indicates that therapy is working well.
   b. Indicate that the person should contact the health care provider if symptoms worsen (e.g., lethargy) or reappear after they have gone away.
4. If the hypercalcemia is preventable (e.g., megadoses of vitamin D), discuss ways to change the practices that caused it.

NURSING DIAGNOSIS: Risk for injury R/T calcium precipitation in urinary tract

1. *Expected outcomes:* Following intervention, the person should not develop calcium precipitation or urinary calculi, as evidenced by unobstructed flow of urine, absence of stones in urine, and lack of acute pain consistent with calculus in ureter.
2. *Nursing interventions*
   a. Supply enough fluids (3–4 L daily for an adult) to keep the urine dilute.
   b. Keep the urine acidic by preventing urinary tract infections and by increasing intake of prune and cranberry juices and acid-ash diet.

NURSING DIAGNOSIS: Self-care deficit R/T muscle weakness or decreased level of consciousness

1. *Expected outcomes:* Following intervention,
   a. The person's hygiene should be maintained within culturally acceptable levels.
   b. The person should state satisfaction with degree to which other activities of daily living are performed.
2. *Nursing interventions*
   a. Discuss activities of daily living and determine what assistance is needed.
   b. Provide assistance, while encouraging as much independence as possible and adhering to the person's preferences and cultural values.

NURSING DIAGNOSIS: Constipation R/T decreased gastrointestinal smooth muscle excitability and motility

1. *Expected outcomes:* Following intervention, the person should regain customary bowel pattern.

2. *Nursing interventions*
   a. Explain reason for constipation to the person.
   b. Encourage fluids, provide privacy at the person's usual elimination time.

Discharge Planning and Teaching

1. Before hospital discharge, people need to learn the following:
   a. About hypercalcemia and its treatment, including its specific cause in each person's case.
   b. How to prevent hypercalcemia from recurring, if possible.
   c. How to detect early signs and symptoms of hypercalcemia, in case it recurs (Learning/Teaching Guidelines for People with Hypercalcemia).

◻ *HYPOMAGNESEMIA*

Definition

Hypomagnesemia is a plasma magnesium concentration below normal. Intracellular magnesium may be low, normal, or even high when the plasma magnesium concentration is low (Table 9–11).

Incidence and Etiology

1. Decreased magnesium intake or absorption. **Examples:** chronic malnutrition, chronic alcoholism, chronic diarrhea, laxative abuse, malabsorption syndromes, ileal resection, steatorrhea
2. Shift of magnesium from the extracellular fluid into cells or bone or into physiologically unavailable form. **Examples:** alcohol withdrawal, citrate from blood transfusions, liver transplant (citrate toxicity)
3. Increased magnesium excretion. **Examples:** steatorrhea,

Table 9–11. Clinical Manifestations of Hypomagnesemia and Hypermagnesemia with Their Pathophysiologic Bases

Clinical Manifestation	Pathophysiologic Basis
Hypomagnesemia	
Positive Chvostek's sign, Trousseau's sign, muscle twitching, grimacing, muscle cramping, tingling around mouth or in fingers, carpal spasm, pedal spasm, hyperactive deep tendon reflexes, nystagmus, tremors, seizures	Increased neuromuscular excitability
Dysphagia	Incoordination of swallowing muscles
Cardiac dysrhythmias	Decreased activity of Na$^+$, K$^+$-ATPase causes increased Na$^+$ and decreased K$^+$ in cardiac cells, sinus node fires more rapidly, decreased duration of cardiac action potentials, changes in refractory period
Abnormal ST and T waves on electrocardiogram	See above
Hypertension	Increased peripheral vascular resistance
Hypermagnesemia	
Weak or absent deep tendon reflexes, muscle weakness, flaccid paralysis	Decreased neuromuscular excitability
Drowsiness, lethargy, coma	Decreased neural function
Hypotension	Decreased peripheral vascular resistance
Bradycardia	Decreased cardiac conduction
Cardiac dysrhythmias	Decreased conduction velocity, longer refractory period, altered neurotransmitter release
Increased amplitude of T waves, prolonged PR and QRS on electrocardiogram	See above
Cardiac arrest	Asystole; see above
Respiratory arrest	Neural dysfunction

hyperaldosteronism, chronic alcoholism, diabetic ketoacidosis, diuretic therapy, medications that cause renal magnesium wasting (e.g., antineoplastics)
4. Loss of magnesium through abnormal routes. **Examples:** vomiting, nasogastric or intestinal suction, acute pancreatitis

Clinical Manifestations and Pathophysiology (see Table 9–11)

Diagnostics

1. Assessment
   a. Check for increased neuromuscular excitability.
      (1) In adults or children, check Chvostek's sign or Trousseau's sign (see Figs. 9–6 and 9–7).
      (2) Watch for muscle twitching, grimacing, carpal spasm, pedal spasm, dysphagia, nystagmus, tremors, and seizures.
      (3) Ask about muscle cramping and any tingling around the mouth or in the fingers.
      (4) Test deep tendon reflexes.
   b. Monitor heart rate and rhythm and blood pressure.
2. Medical diagnosis: Plasma magnesium concentration below 1.5 mEq/L (1.8 mg/dl)

Clinical Management

1. Give magnesium replacement as ordered until the plasma magnesium concentration returns to normal. Magnesium sulfate may be given orally, intramuscularly, or intravenously.

 DRUG ADVISORY

Watch for diarrhea if giving oral magnesium sulfate. Turn down the rate if flushing occurs or if the person suddenly feels very warm when administering intravenous magnesium salts. Monitor deep tendon reflexes during intravenous magnesium infusion to check for rebound hypermagnesemia.

2. Treat the cause of the hypomagnesemia.

Applying the Nursing Process

NURSING DIAGNOSIS: Risk for decreased cardiac output R/T cardiac dysrhythmias or cardiac arrest

1. *Expected outcomes:* Following intervention, the person should maintain normal cardiac output, as evidenced by

---

LEARNING/TEACHING GUIDELINES
for People with Hypomagnesemia

1. Describe the processes that cause hypomagnesemia, and explain how the person's signs and symptoms result from not enough magnesium in the blood.
2. If the cause of hypomagnesemia is not identified, assess for bulimia or alcohol abuse; explain the effects of these behaviors, and discuss entry into treatment if appropriate.
3. Explain the need for increased magnesium intake, and help the person plan ways to incorporate it into daily life.
   a. If magnesium supplements are prescribed, explain the importance of taking them regularly.
   b. Ask the person what types of foods he or she usually eats (to assess cultural preferences), and identify foods that are high in magnesium.
   c. Help make menu plans to increase intake of magnesium-rich foods such as dark green vegetables, whole grains, nuts, soybeans, and almonds.
4. Discuss symptom assessment and management.
   a. Explain that reduction of the signs and symptoms indicates that therapy is working well and that increased magnesium intake may need to be maintained to keep blood magnesium normal.
   b. Describe how to control neuromuscular and environmental stimuli to provide safety and comfort until increased neuromuscular excitability is resolved.
   c. Indicate that the person should contact the health care provider if symptoms worsen (e.g., spontaneous muscle twitching) or reappear after they have gone away, or if diarrhea occurs or muscles become heavy and unresponsive (potential need for adjustment of therapy).
5. If the hypomagnesemia is preventable (e.g., laxative abuse), discuss ways to change the practices that caused it.

---

adequate urine output, normal capillary filling, normal PaO_2 results, and lack of cyanosis.
2. *Nursing interventions*
   a. Apply cardiac monitor if apical pulse is irregular.
   b. Apply monitor if blood is being transfused rapidly or multiple units are administered.
   c. Monitor for signs and symptoms of decreased cardiac output.

NURSING DIAGNOSIS: Risk for injury R/T seizures

---

1. *Expected outcomes:* Following intervention, the person should not be injured if seizure occurs.
2. *Nursing interventions*: Institute seizure precautions if appropriate.
   a. Raised and padded bedrails
   b. Reduced environmental stimuli

NURSING DIAGNOSIS: Anxiety R/T paresthesias and muscle twitching

---

1. *Expected outcomes:* Following intervention, the person's verbal and behavioral manifestations of anxiety (interpreted according to the person's culture) should be reduced.
2. *Nursing interventions*
   a. Explain cause of paresthesias and twitching.
   b. Provide anxiety-relieving interventions appropriate to the person's developmental level and cultural values.

Discharge Planning and Teaching

1. Before hospital discharge, people need to learn the following:
   a. About hypomagnesemia and its treatment, including its specific cause in each person's case.
   b. How to prevent hypomagnesemia from recurring, if possible.
   c. How to detect early signs and symptoms of hypomagnesemia, in case it recurs (see Learning/Teaching Guidelines for People with Hypomagnesemia).

◼ HYPERMAGNESEMIA

Definition

Hypermagnesemia is a plasma magnesium concentration above normal. Intracellular magnesium may be high, normal, or even low when the plasma magnesium concentration is high (see Table 9–11).

Incidence and Etiology

1. Increased magnesium intake
   a. **Examples:** excessive intake of magnesium-containing medications (antacids, cathartics, enemas), excessive infusion of intravenous magnesium, near drowning in sea water
   b. Administration of magnesium sulfate to the mother for treatment of preeclampsia can cause hypermagnesemia in the newborn.

LEARNING/TEACHING GUIDELINES
for People with Hypermagnesemia

1. Describe the processes that cause hypermagnesemia, and explain how the person's signs and symptoms result from too much magnesium in the blood.
2. Explain the need for decreased magnesium intake, and help the person plan ways to incorporate it into daily life.
   a. Ask the person what types of foods he or she usually eats (to assess cultural preferences), identify foods that are high in magnesium (e.g., nuts, dark green vegetables), and plan low-magnesium alternatives.
   b. Identify antacids and laxatives that contain magnesium and help the person plan magnesium-free alternatives.
3. Discuss symptom assessment and management.
   a. Explain that reduction of the signs and symptoms indicates that therapy is working well and that decreased magnesium intake may need to be maintained to keep blood magnesium normal.
   b. Indicate that the person should contact the health care provider if symptoms worsen (e.g., drowsiness and weak muscles) or reappear after they have gone away.
4. If the hypermagnesemia is preventable (e.g., person with chronic renal failure using magnesium antacids), discuss ways to change the practices that caused it.

---

2. Shift of magnesium from cells or bone to the extracellular fluid. **Example:** hyperparathyroidism
3. Decreased magnesium excretion. **Examples:** adrenal insufficiency; oliguria from any cause, including acute or chronic renal failure; severe hypovolemia

Clinical Manifestations and Pathophysiology (see Table 9–11)

Diagnostics

1. Assessment
   a. Check for decreased neuromuscular irritability.
      (1) Monitor deep tendon reflexes, assess for muscle weakness or flaccid paralysis.
      (2) Hypermagnesemic newborns have flaccid muscles and lie in an extended posture.
   b. Monitor rate and depth of respirations.
   c. Assess level of consciousness.
   d. Measure blood pressure.
2. Medical diagnosis: Plasma magnesium concentration above 2.5 mEq/L (3 mg/dl)

Clinical Management

1. Give medical therapy as ordered until the plasma magnesium concentration returns to normal.
   a. Oral fluids, intravenous saline, or diuretics may be used to increase urine excretion of magnesium.
   b. Dialysis may be necessary.
2. Treat the cause of the hypermagnesemia.

Applying the Nursing Process

NURSING DIAGNOSIS: Risk for injury R/T decreased level of consciousness

1. *Expected outcomes:* Following intervention, the person should remain free of injury.
2. *Nursing interventions*
   a. Provide safety measures appropriate to the person's level of consciousness and degree of muscle weakness.
   b. Provide frequent position changes and skin care to prevent development of pressure sores.

NURSING DIAGNOSIS: Risk for impaired gas exchange R/T cardiac dysrhythmias, cardiac arrest, or respiratory arrest

1. *Expected outcomes:* Following intervention, the person should maintain normal oxygenation, as evidenced by normal PaO_2, cardiac output, capillary filling, and respiratory rate and depth, and lack of cyanosis.
2. *Nursing interventions*
   a. Apply cardiac monitor if apical pulse is irregular.
   b. If respiratory rate is decreasing, be ready to institute mechanical ventilation if necessary.

NURSING DIAGNOSIS: Self-care deficit R/T muscle weakness and decreased level of consciousness

1. *Expected outcomes:* Following intervention, the person's hygiene should be maintained within culturally acceptable levels.

2. *Nursing interventions*: Provide assistance, while encouraging as much independence as possible and adhering to the person's preferences and cultural values.

Discharge Planning and Teaching

1. Before hospital discharge, people need to learn the following:
   a. About hypermagnesemia and its treatment, including its specific cause in each person's case.
   b. How to prevent hypermagnesemia from recurring, if possible.
   c. How to detect early signs and symptoms of hypermagnesemia, in case it recurs (Learning/Teaching Guidelines for People with Hypermagnesemia).

◼ *HYPOPHOSPHATEMIA*

Definition

Hypophosphatemia is a plasma phosphate concentration below normal. Intracellular phosphate may be low, normal, or even high when the plasma phosphate concentration is low (Table 9–12).

Incidence and Etiology

1. Decreased phosphate intake or absorption. **Examples:** malabsorption syndromes, chronic diarrhea, excessive or prolonged use of antacids
2. Shift of phosphate from the extracellular fluid to the cells or bone. **Examples:** excessive insulin, hyperalimentation, refeeding after starvation or malnutrition, hyperventilation (respiratory alkalosis)
3. Increased phosphate excretion. **Examples:** diabetic ketoacidosis, alcohol withdrawal, diuretic phase after burns, diuretic therapy, hyperparathyroidism
4. Loss of phosphate through abnormal routes. **Examples:** vomiting, hemodialysis

Clinical Manifestations and Pathophysiology (see Table 9–12)

Diagnostics

1. Assessment
   a. Check for muscle weakness and decreased reflexes.
      (1) With severe symptomatic hypophosphatemia, muscle weakness may progress rapidly until the person is unable even to turn over when in bed.

Table 9–12. Clinical Manifestations of Hypophosphatemia and Hyperphosphatemia with Their Pathophysiologic Bases

Clinical Manifestation	Pathophysiologic Basis
Hypophosphatemia	
Muscle weakness, decreased reflexes	Impaired cellular metabolism from lack of phosphate compounds such as ATP; impaired oxygenation from decreased 2,3-DPG in erythrocytes
Shallow respirations	Respiratory muscle weakness
Muscle aching, paresthesias	Altered cellular metabolism
Anorexia, nausea	Decreased function of gastrointestinal smooth muscle
Malaise, irritability, apprehension	Impaired cerebral oxygenation and cellular metabolism
Confusion, stupor, coma	Decreased level of consciousness, due in part to lack of ATP and impaired oxygenation from decreased 2,3-DPG
Crackles in dependent portions of lungs (if severe)	Congestive cardiomyopathy from lack of ATP and other phosphate compounds
Hyperphosphatemia	
Persons who do not have renal failure:	
Manifestations of hypocalcemia (See Table 9–10)	The plasma calcium concentration falls as the plasma phosphate concentration rises.
Persons who have chronic renal failure:	
Pruritus	Both plasma calcium and phosphate concentrations are high. Calcium phosphate salts precipitate in soft tissues
Eye discomfort, conjunctival redness	Precipitation of calcium phosphate salts in eye
Joint pain	Precipitation of calcium phosphate salts in joints
Worsening oliguria	Precipitation of calcium phosphate salts in kidney

ATP, Adenosine triphosphate; 2,3-DPG, 2,3-diphosphoglycerate.

LEARNING/TEACHING GUIDELINES
for People with Hypophosphatemia

1. Describe the processes that cause hypophosphatemia, and explain how the person's signs and symptoms result from not enough phosphate in the blood.
2. Explain the need for increased dietary intake (if malnutrition related) or ways to increase phosphate absorption (less use of antacids and laxatives), and help the person plan ways to incorporate this into daily life.
   a. If phosphate supplements are prescribed, explain the importance of taking them regularly, and remind the patient that chilling them makes them more palatable.
   b. Explain that phosphate is abundant in many foods (milk, meat, fish, poultry, processed foods) and that using a lot of antacids and laxatives keeps it from being absorbed from the intestines so that the body can use it.
   c. Assess dietary intake, and use those data as a basis for planning with the person how to increase the consumption of phosphate, if needed.
3. Discuss symptom assessment and management.
   a. Explain that reduction of the signs and symptoms indicates that therapy is working well and that increased dietary intake or specific ways to increase phosphate absorption may need to be maintained to keep blood phosphate normal.
   b. Indicate that the person should contact the health care provider if symptoms worsen (e.g., increased muscle weakness) or reappear after they have gone away, or if tingling or muscle cramping occurs (need to decrease oral phosphate replacement).
4. If the hypophosphatemia is preventable (e.g., prolonged overuse of magnesium-aluminum antacids or laxative abuse), discuss ways to change the practices that caused it.

---

(2) Monitor depth of respirations.
   b. Inquire about anorexia, nausea, muscle aching, bruising, malaise, irritability, apprehension, paresthesias.
   c. Monitor level of consciousness.
   d. If severe, listen for crackles in dependent areas of lungs.
2. Medical diagnosis
   a. Serum phosphate concentration below 2.5 mg/dl in adults, below 4.5 mg/dl in children, or below 4.3 mg/dl in newborns. Mild hypophosphatemia may not cause symptoms.
   b. Severe symptomatic hypophosphatemia occurs when the serum phosphate concentration falls below 1.0 mg/dl in adults and children.

Clinical Management

1. Give phosphate replacement as ordered until the plasma phosphate concentration returns to normal.
   a. For mild hypophosphatemia, oral phosphates may be ordered.
   b. For severe symptomatic hypophosphatemia, intravenous phosphate is used initially.

DRUG ADVISORY

Intravenous phosphate may cause hypocalcemia. When infusing it, monitor for paresthesias and increased neuromuscular excitability. Check that urine output is adequate to limit the risk of hyperphosphatemia.

2. Treat the cause of the hypophosphatemia.

Applying the Nursing Process

NURSING DIAGNOSIS: Risk for injury R/T muscle weakness and decreased level of consciousness

1. *Expected outcomes:* Following intervention, the person should remain free of injury.
2. *Nursing interventions*
   a. Provide safety measures appropriate to the person's degree of muscle weakness and level of consciousness.
   b. Turn the person on a regular schedule if muscle weakness is extreme.
   c. Provide careful skin care if muscle weakness impairs mobility.

NURSING DIAGNOSIS: Risk for impaired gas exchange R/T respiratory muscle weakness

1. *Expected outcomes:* Following intervention, the person should be well oxygenated, as evidenced by normal respiratory rate and depth and Pao_2.
2. *Nursing interventions*
   a. Position to facilitate chest expansion.
   b. Monitor for hypoventilation.

NURSING DIAGNOSIS: Risk for injury R/T seizures

1. *Expected outcomes:* Following intervention, the person should not be injured if seizure occurs.
2. *Nursing interventions:* Institute seizure precautions if appropriate.
   a. Raised and padded bedrails
   b. Reduced environmental stimuli

NURSING DIAGNOSIS: Anxiety R/T paresthesias and muscle weakness

1. *Expected outcomes:* Following intervention, the person's verbal and behavioral manifestations of anxiety (interpreted according to the person's culture) should be reduced.
2. *Nursing interventions*
   a. Explain cause of paresthesias and muscle weakness.
   b. Provide anxiety-relieving interventions appropriate to the person's developmental level and cultural values.

NURSING DIAGNOSIS: Self-care deficit R/T muscle weakness and decreased level of consciousness

1. *Expected outcomes:* Following intervention, the person's hygiene should be maintained within culturally acceptable levels.
2. *Nursing interventions:* Provide assistance, while encouraging as much independence as possible and adhering to the person's preferences and cultural values.

Discharge Planning and Teaching

1. Before hospital discharge, people need to learn the following:
   a. About hypophosphatemia and its treatment, including its specific cause in each person's case.
   b. How to prevent hypophosphatemia from recurring, if possible.
   c. How to detect early signs and symptoms of hypophosphatemia, in case it recurs (Learning/Teaching Guidelines for People with Hypophosphatemia).

◼ *HYPERPHOSPHATEMIA*

Definition

Hyperphosphatemia is a plasma phosphate concentration above normal levels. Intracellular phosphate may be high, normal, or even low when the plasma phosphate concentration is high (see Table 9–12).

Incidence and Etiology

1. Increased phosphate intake. **Examples:** overuse of phosphate-containing enemas and cathartics, excess phosphate therapy
2. Shift of phosphate from cells to the extracellular fluid. **Examples:** tumor lysis syndrome, crush injuries, rhabdomyolysis
3. Decreased phosphate excretion. **Examples:** hypoparathyroidism, oliguria from any cause, including acute and chronic renal failure

Clinical Manifestations and Pathophysiology (see Table 9–12)

Diagnostics

1. Assessment
   a. Check for the increased neuromuscular excitability of hypocalcemia, as outlined previously in this chapter.
   b. Monitor for the effects of precipitation of calcium phosphate salts in soft tissues.
      (1) Ask regarding pruritus, eye discomfort, or joint pain.
      (2) Assess for conjunctival redness.
      (3) Monitor urine output.
2. Medical diagnosis: Plasma phosphate concentration above 4.5 mg/dl in adults, above 6.5 mg/dl in children, or above 9.3 mg/dl in newborns.

Clinical Management

1. Give medical therapy as ordered (depends on specific cause) until the plasma phosphate concentration returns to normal.
   a. With normal renal and cardiac function, fluid intake is increased to promote renal excretion of phosphate.
   b. Persons who have renal failure are prescribed phosphate binders to ingest during meals to bind phosphate in the gastrointestinal tract and remove it in the feces.
   c. Dialysis may be necessary.
2. Treat the cause of the hyperphosphatemia.

Applying the Nursing Process

See nursing diagnoses for hypocalcemia, listed previously in this chapter.

NURSING DIAGNOSIS: Risk for injury R/T calcium phosphate precipitation

1. *Expected outcomes:* Following intervention, the person should remain free of injury.

LEARNING/TEACHING GUIDELINES
for People with Hyperphosphatemia

1. Describe the processes that cause hyperphosphatemia, and explain how the person's signs and symptoms result from too much phosphate in the blood.
2. Explain the need for decreased phosphate intake, and help the person plan ways to incorporate it into daily life.
   a. Explain that phosphate is abundant in many foods and that phosphate binders (aluminum antacids) need to be taken during meals to keep phosphate from being absorbed from the intestines.
   b. Ask the person what types of foods he or she usually eats (to assess cultural preferences), identify foods that are extremely high in phosphate (e.g., cola drinks, ready-made frozen foods), and plan lower-phosphate alternatives.
3. Discuss symptom assessment and management.
   a. Explain that reduction of the signs and symptoms indicates that therapy is working well and that decreased phosphate intake and phosphate binder therapy may need to be maintained to keep blood phosphate normal.
   b. Indicate that the person should contact the health care provider if symptoms worsen (e.g., itching) or reappear after they have gone away.
4. If the hyperphosphatemia is preventable (e.g., person with chronic renal failure noncompliant with phosphate binder therapy), discuss ways to change the practices that caused it.

2. *Nursing interventions*
   a. Increase fluid intake to keep urine dilute (unless contraindicated by oliguria).
   b. If person develops pruritus, manicure fingernails smoothly to prevent excoriation of skin; use interventions to reduce itching; supply distraction.

Discharge Planning and Teaching

1. Before hospital discharge, people need to learn the following:
   a. About hyperphosphatemia and its treatment, including its specific cause in each person's case.
   b. How to prevent hyperphosphatemia from recurring, if possible.
   c. How to detect early signs and symptoms of hyperphosphatemia, in case it recurs (Learning/Teaching Guidelines for People with Hyperphosphatemia).

◼ RESPIRATORY ACIDOSIS

Definition

1. Respiratory acidosis is an excess of carbonic acid in the blood, which is seen clinically as an elevated partial pressure of carbon dioxide in the blood.
2. Respiratory acidosis decreases the pH of the blood. However, if full renal compensation has occurred, then the pH will be in the low normal range.
3. Respiratory acidosis may be primary or compensatory.

Incidence and Etiology

1. Primary respiratory acidosis is caused by pathophysiologic processes that interfere with gas exchange, neuromuscular function of the chest, or regulation of respiration by the central nervous system (Table 9–13).

2. Compensatory respiratory acidosis is a response to metabolic alkalosis.
   a. Compensatory respiratory acidosis occurs when increased blood pH from metabolic alkalosis suppresses the chemoreceptors and causes hypoventilation; hypoventilation causes carbon dioxide (carbonic acid) to accumulate.
   b. Increased carbonic acid from compensatory respiratory acidosis helps neutralize the excess bicarbonate of metabolic alkalosis, bringing pH toward the normal range.

Clinical Manifestations and Pathophysiology (Table 9–14)

Diagnostics

1. Assessment
   a. Assess level of consciousness.

Table 9–13. Etiology of Respiratory Acidosis

General Causes	Examples
Impaired gas exchange	Emphysema, severe asthma, bronchiectasis, airway obstruction, pneumonia, atelectasis, pulmonary edema, obstructive sleep apnea
Impaired neuromuscular function of chest	Chest injury, recent chest surgery, respiratory muscle fatigue, hypokalemic muscle weakness, Guillain-Barré syndrome, myasthenia gravis, severe kyphoscoliosis
Impaired central regulation of respiration	Suppression of respiration by medications (e.g., narcotics, barbiturates), central sleep apnea
Compensation for metabolic alkalosis	See explanation in text

Table 9–14. Clinical Manifestations of Respiratory Acidosis with Their Pathophysiologic Bases

Clinical Manifestation	Pathophysiologic Basis
Decreased level of consciousness (disorientation, lethargy, somnolence)	Decreased pH in central nervous system
Tachycardia	Catecholamine release from adrenal medulla
Cardiac dysrhythmias	Decreased pH in cardiac cells, altered response to catecholamines
Headache	Cerebral vasodilation
Blurred vision	Increased intracranial pressure from cerebral vasodilation
Hypoventilation	The cause, rather than the result, of respiratory acidosis

b. Monitor heart rate and rhythm.
c. Ask about presence of headache or blurred vision.
d. Monitor respiratory rate and depth.

2. Medical diagnosis: Partial pressure of carbon dioxide ($PaCO_2$) above 44 mm Hg in adults and children or above 34 mm Hg in infants (Table 9–15).

Clinical Management

1. Give medical therapy as ordered until the $PaCO_2$ returns to normal or baseline. The major focus of medical therapy is increasing alveolar ventilation by treating the underlying condition. Successful treatment of the underlying condition increases alveolar ventilation and thus resolves respiratory acidosis or improves the condition (underlying irreversible lung disease may cause chronic respiratory acidosis). Interventions to increase alveolar ventilation are presented in Chapter 22.

Applying the Nursing Process

NURSING DIAGNOSIS: Risk for injury R/T decreased level of consciusness

1. *Expected outcomes:* Following intervention, the person should remain free of injury.
2. *Nursing interventions*
   a. Provide safety measures appropriate to the person's level of consciousness.
   b. Provide frequent position changes and skin care to prevent development of pressure ulcers.

NURSING DIAGNOSIS: Decreased cardiac output R/T cardiac dysrhythmias

1. *Expected outcomes:* Following intervention, the person should maintain normal cardiac output, as evidenced by adequate urine output, normal capillary filling, normal PaO_2 levels, and lack of cyanosis.
2. *Nursing interventions*
   a. Apply cardiac monitor if apical pulse is irregular.
   b. Monitor for signs and symptoms of decreased cardiac output.

NURSING DIAGNOSIS: Ineffective breathing pattern (hypoventilation) R/T impaired gas exchange, impaired neuromuscular chest function, and/or impaired central regulation of respiration

1. *Expected outcomes:* Following intervention, the person should regain normal respiratory rate and depth.
2. *Nursing interventions:* Institute measures to increase alveolar ventilation. See Chapter 22.

NURSING DIAGNOSIS: Headache R/T cerebral vasodilation from elevated $PaCO_2$

1. *Expected outcomes:* Following intervention, the person should evidence verbal and nonverbal behaviors (interpreted within the person's culture) of decreased pain.
2. *Nursing interventions*
   a. Explain cause of pain.
   b. Provide nonnarcotic and nonpharmacologic pain relief.

Table 9–15. Laboratory Values in Respiratory Acidosis

Laboratory Measure	Uncompensated (Acute) Respiratory Acidosis	Partially Compensated Respiratory Acidosis	Fully Compensated Respiratory Acidosis
$PaCO_2$ (marker of the problem)	Above normal	Above normal	Above normal
HCO_3^- (marker of renal compensation)	Normal range	Slightly above normal	More above normal
pH (end result of problem and any compensation)	Below normal	Below normal but moving toward it	Low normal range (< 7.40)

LEARNING/TEACHING GUIDELINES
for People with Respiratory Acidosis

1. Describe the processes that cause respiratory acidosis, and explain that the person's signs and symptoms result from too much carbon dioxide (carbonic acid) in the blood.
2. Explain the need to improve respiratory function, and help the person plan ways to incorporate necessary therapy into daily life (see Chapter 22).
3. Discuss symptom assessment and management.
   a. Point out that the signs and symptoms the person is experiencing are due both to respiratory acidosis and to the underlying condition that caused it.
   b. Explain that reduction of the signs and symptoms indicates that therapy is working well and should be continued until the health care provider indicates it is safe to stop.
   c. Indicate that the person should contact the health care provider if symptoms worsen or reappear after they have gone away.
   d. Review the signs and symptoms of the underlying condition, and explain how to recognize it so that the person can seek health care before it leads to respiratory acidosis in the future.
4. If the respiratory acidosis is potentially preventable (e.g., acute respiratory infection in person with chronic obstructive pulmonary disease), discuss ways to change the practices that contributed to it.

NURSE ADVISORY

Narcotic analgesics are inappropriate for persons who have respiratory acidosis because narcotics may depress respirations and worsen the acidosis.

Discharge Planning and Teaching

1. Before hospital discharge, people need to learn the following:
   a. About respiratory acidosis and its treatment, including its specific cause in each person's case.
   b. How to prevent the underlying condition that caused respiratory acidosis from recurring, if possible.
   c. How to detect early signs and symptoms of the underlying condition and of respiratory acidosis, in case they recur (Learning/Teaching Guidelines for People with Respiratory Acidosis).

▣ METABOLIC ACIDOSIS

Definition

1. Metabolic acidosis is a relative increase of metabolic acids (any acid except carbonic acid) in the blood, which is seen clinically as a decreased bicarbonate concentration.
2. Metabolic acidosis decreases the pH of the blood. However, if full respiratory compensation (hyperventilation) has occurred, then the pH will be in the low normal range. Respiratory compensation may be limited by respiratory muscle fatigue.
3. Metabolic acidosis may be primary or compensatory.

Incidence and Etiology

1. Primary metabolic acidosis is caused by pathophysiologic processes that cause accumulation of metabolic acid or loss of bicarbonate (Table 9–16).
2. Compensatory metabolic acidosis is a response to prolonged respiratory alkalosis.
   a. Compensatory metabolic acidosis occurs when increased blood pH from prolonged respiratory alkalosis causes the kidneys to retain metabolic acid and excrete more bicarbonate.
   b. Increased metabolic acid from compensatory metabolic acidosis helps balance the carbonic acid deficiency of respiratory alkalosis and brings the pH back toward normal.

Table 9–16. Etiology of Metabolic Acidosis

General Causes	Examples
Accumulation of metabolic acids	
• Ingestion of acid or substances that are converted to acid	Aspirin, methanol, antifreeze (ethylene glycol), boric acid, ammonium chloride
• Increased production of metabolic acid	Hyperthyroidism, hypermetabolic states, lactic acidosis, shock, diabetic ketoacidosis, starvation, alcoholic ketoacidosis
• Decreased excretion of metabolic acid	Oliguric acute or chronic renal failure, severe hypovolemia, shock, hypoaldosteronism, type 1 renal tubular acidosis
Loss of bicarbonate	Prolonged diarrhea, intestinal decompression, fistula drainage, vomiting of intestinal contents, type 2 renal tubular acidosis
Compensation for respiratory alkalosis	See explanation in text

Table 9–17. Clinical Manifestations of Metabolic Acidosis with Their Pathophysiologic Bases

Clinical Manifestation	Pathophysiologic Basis
Decreased level of consciousness (confusion, drowsiness, lethargy, stupor, coma)	Decreased pH in central nervous system
Tachycardia (initially)	Catecholamine release from adrenal medulla
Bradycardia (if severe)	Decreased cardiac conduction
Cardiac dysrhythmias	Decreased pH in cardiac cells, decreased contractility, decreased conduction
Headache	Poorly understood mechanisms
Abdominal pain	Poorly understood mechanisms
Hyperventilation	Compensatory mechanism for metabolic acidosis

Clinical Manifestations and Pathophysiology (Table 9–17)

Diagnostics

1. Assessment
   a. Assess level of consciousness.
   b. Monitor heart rate and rhythm.
   c. Ask about presence of headache or abdominal pain.
   d. Monitor respiratory rate and depth.
2. Medical diagnosis: Serum bicarbonate concentration below 22 mEq/L in adults and children or below 19 mEq/L in infants (Table 9–18).

Clinical Management

1. Give medical therapy as ordered until the plasma bicarbonate concentration returns to normal.
   a. The major focus of medical therapy is treating the cause of the metabolic acidosis and supporting renal function.
   b. If the pH is extremely low, intravenous sodium bicarbonate may be administered to increase the pH.
   c. Lactate, citrate, and acetate are metabolized by the

 DRUG ADVISORY

Monitor for complications of sodium bicarbonate therapy: rebound metabolic alkalosis (paresthesias, decreasing level of consciousness), hypocalcemia (paresthesias, tetany), hypokalemia (muscle weakness, cardiac arrhythmias), extracellular fluid volume excess (crackles, distended neck veins), hypernatremia (with ampules of sodium bicarbonate; increasing confusion and lethargy).

liver to bicarbonate and are alternate forms of bicarbonate therapy.
   d. Dichloroacetate increases metabolism of lactate and may be used to treat lactic acidosis.

Applying the Nursing Process

NURSING DIAGNOSIS: Risk for injury R/T decreased level of consciousness

1. *Expected outcomes:* Following intervention, the person should remain free of injury.
2. *Nursing interventions*
   a. Provide safety measures appropriate to the person's level of consciousness.
   b. Provide frequent position changes and skin care to prevent development of pressure ulcers.

NURSING DIAGNOSIS: Risk for decreased cardiac output R/T cardiac dysrhythmias

1. *Expected outcomes:* Following intervention, the person should maintain normal cardiac output, as evidenced by adequate urine ouput, normal capillary filling, normal PaO2 levels, and lack of cyanosis.
2. *Nursing interventions*
   a. Apply cardiac monitor if apical pulse is irregular.
   b. Monitor for signs and symptoms of decreased cardiac output.

NURSING DIAGNOSIS: Risk for injury R/T dry oral mucous membranes from hyperventilation

Table 9–18. Laboratory Values in Metabolic Acidosis

Laboratory Measure	Uncompensated (Acute) Metabolic Acidosis	Partially Compensated Metabolic Acidosis	Fully Compensated Metabolic Acidosis
$PaCO_2$ (marker of respiratory compensation)	Normal range	Below normal	More below normal
HCO_3^- (marker of the problem)	Below normal	Below normal	Below normal
pH (end result of problem and any compensation)	Below normal	Below normal but moving toward it	Low normal range (< 7.40)

LEARNING/TEACHING GUIDELINES
for People with Metabolic Acidosis

1. Describe the processes that cause metabolic acidosis, and explain that the person's signs and symptoms result from too much acid in the blood.
2. Explain how the prescribed therapy will decrease the acid in the blood.
3. Discuss symptom assessment and management.
   a. Explain that rapid deep breathing is the body's way of compensating for metabolic acidosis and is a helpful process that will disappear when the extra acid is removed by the kidneys.
   b. Explain that reduction of the signs and symptoms indicates that therapy is working well.
   c. Indicate that the person should contact the health care provider if symptoms worsen or reappear after they have gone away.
4. If the metabolic acidosis is potentially preventable (e.g., starvation ketoacidosis due to fasting to lose weight; diabetic ketoacidosis), discuss ways to change the practices that contributed to it.

---

1. *Expected outcomes:* Following intervention, the person should have moist mucous membranes with no evidence of flaking or cracks.
2. *Nursing interventions*
   a. Provide frequent oral care.
   b. Position to facilitate chest expansion. Hyperventilation is a useful compensatory mechanism for metabolic acidosis.

NURSING DIAGNOSIS: Headache R/T poorly understood mechanisms

1. *Expected outcomes:* Following intervention, the person should evidence verbal and nonverbal behaviors (interpreted within the person's culture) of decreased headache.
2. *Nursing interventions*
   a. Explain that headache is due to metabolic acidosis.
   b. Provide nonnarcotic and nonpharmacologic pain relief. Avoid suppressing respiratory compensation with narcotics.

NURSING DIAGNOSIS: Abdominal pain R/T poorly understood mechanisms

1. *Expected outcomes:* Following intervention, the person should evidence verbal and nonverbal behaviors (interpreted within the person's culture) of decreased abdominal pain.
2. *Nursing interventions*
   a. Explain that the abdominal pain is due to metabolic acidosis and that it will decrease following treatment.
   b. Provide nonnarcotic and nonpharmacologic pain relief. Avoid suppressing respiratory compensation with narcotics.

NURSING DIAGNOSIS: Self-care deficit R/T decreased level of consciousness

1. *Expected outcomes:* Following intervention, the person should maintain hygiene at culturally acceptable level.
2. *Nursing interventions:* Provide assistance, while encouraging as much independence as possible and adhering to the person's preferences and cultural values.

Discharge Planning and Teaching

1. Before hospital discharge, people need to learn the following:
   a. About metabolic acidosis and its treatment, including its specific cause in each person's case.
   b. How to prevent metabolic acidosis from recurring, if possible.
   c. How to detect early signs and symptoms of metabolic acidosis, in case it recurs (Learning/Teaching Guidelines for People with Metabolic Acidosis).

■ RESPIRATORY ALKALOSIS

Definition

1. Respiratory alkalosis is a deficit of carbonic acid in the blood, which is seen clinically as a decreased partial pressure of carbon dioxide in the blood.
2. Respiratory alkalosis increases the pH of the blood. However, if full renal compensation has occurred, the pH will be in the high normal range.
3. Respiratory alkalosis may be primary or compensatory.

Incidence and Etiology

1. Primary respiratory alkalosis is caused by pathophysiologic processes or emotional circumstances that lead to hyperventilation (Table 9–19).
2. Compensatory respiratory alkalosis is a response to metabolic acidosis (see Figure 9–3).
   a. Compensatory respiratory alkalosis occurs when decreased blood pH from metabolic acidosis stimulates

Table 9–19. Etiology of Respiratory Alkalosis

General Causes	Examples
Hyperventilation	Hypoxemia, pain, anxiety, prolonged gasping-type crying, mechanical overventilation, stimulation of central regulatory mechanisms by fever or infection
Compensation for metabolic acidosis	See explanation in text

the chemoreceptors and causes hyperventilation; hyperventilation removes carbon dioxide (carbonic acid) from the body.

b. Decreased carbonic acid from compensatory respiratory alkalosis helps balance the decreased bicarbonate of metabolic acidosis and brings pH back toward normal.

Clinical Manifestations and Pathophysiology (Table 9–20)

Diagnostics

1. Assessment
   a. Ask about presence of lightheadedness and watch for syncope.
   b. Watch for diaphoresis.
   c. Monitor heart rate and rhythm.
   d. Assess for increased neuromuscular excitability.
      (1) Ask about muscle cramps or tingling of fingers, toes, or area around mouth.
      (2) Test Chvostek's sign (not useful for infants).
      (3) Watch for grimacing, carpal spasm, pedal spasm, tetany.
   e. Monitor respiratory rate and depth.
   f. Measure Pa_{O_2}. Because decreased Pa_{O_2} may be the cause of hyperventilation, it is crucial to assess Pa_{O_2} to determine the appropriate therapy for respiratory alkalosis.
2. Medical diagnosis: Partial pressure of carbon dioxide (Pa_{CO_2}) below 36 mm Hg in adults and children or below 30 mm Hg in infants (Table 9–21).

Table 9–20. Clinical Manifestations of Respiratory Alkalosis with Their Pathophysiologic Bases

Clinical Manifestation	Pathophysiologic Basis
Lightheadedness, syncope	Cerebral vasoconstriction, lack of oxygen, increased pH inside brain cells
Diaphoresis	Unclear
Cardiac dysrhythmias	Increased pH inside cardiac cells
Muscle cramps; tingling of fingers, toes, or around mouth; positive Chvostek's sign; grimacing; carpal spasm; pedal spasm; tetany	Increased neuromuscular excitability; more plasma calcium binds to plasma proteins, decreasing the physiologically available ionized calcium
Hyperventilation	The cause, rather than the result, of respiratory alkalosis

Clinical Management

1. The focus of medical therapy depends on the cause of respiratory alkalosis.
   a. Treat the original cause.
      (1) If due to decreased Pa_{O_2}, increase the person's oxygenation. Hyperventilation is a beneficial physiologic response if Pa_{O_2} is low.
      (2) If hyperventilation is a response to metabolic acidosis, treat the metabolic acidosis and monitor for respiratory muscle fatigue. Hyperventilation is a helpful compensatory response to metabolic acidosis.
      (3) If due to pain, fever or infection, treat these.
      (4) If due to anxiety, use supportive listening and direct attention to decreasing the respiratory rate. Count aloud slowly and ask the patient to match breathing rate to the counting rate. Have the patient rebreathe expired air by breathing into a paper bag.

NURSE ADVISORY

Always check the person's Pa_{O_2} before using interventions to decrease respiratory rate. It is dangerous to slow the respiratory rate in a person who is hypoxemic.

Table 9–21. Laboratory Values in Respiratory Alkalosis

Laboratory Measure	Uncompensated (Acute) Respiratory Alkalosis	Partially Compensated Respiratory Alkalosis	Fully Compensated Respiratory Alkalosis
Pa_{CO_2} (marker of the problem)	Below normal	Below normal	Below normal
HCO_3^- (marker of renal compensation)	Normal range	Slightly below normal	More below normal
pH (end result of problem and any compensation)	Above normal	Above normal but moving toward it	High normal range (>7.40)

b. Respiratory alkalosis may be induced deliberately by mechanical overventilation to reduce intracranial pressure in head injuries.

Applying the Nursing Process

NURSING DIAGNOSIS: Risk for injury R/T syncope

1. *Expected outcomes:* Following intervention, the person should remain free of injury.
2. *Nursing interventions:* Provide appropriate safety measures.

NURSING DIAGNOSIS: Risk for decreased cardiac output R/T cardiac dysrhythmias

1. *Expected outcomes:* Following intervention, the person should maintain normal cardiac output, as evidenced by adequate urine output, normal capillary filling, normal PaO_2 levels, and lack of cyanosis.
2. *Nursing interventions*
   a. Apply cardiac monitor if apical pulse is irregular.
   b. Monitor for signs and symptoms of decreased cardiac output.

NURSING DIAGNOSIS: Anxiety R/T lightheadedness, paresthesias, and muscle cramps

1. *Expected outcomes:* Following instruction, the person should show verbal and nonverbal behaviors (interpreted within the person's culture) of decreased anxiety.
2. *Nursing interventions*
   a. Recognize that whether anxiety caused the initial hyperventilation, the symptoms of respiratory alkalosis often provoke anxiety.
   b. Listen to and reflect the patient's feelings.
   c. Explain the reason for these sensations, and reassure that they are temporary.
   d. Tell the person to avoid crossing the legs, which may worsen cramps and tingling in the feet.
   e. Teach muscle relaxation or other anxiety-reduction techniques.

Discharge Planning and Teaching

1. Before hospital discharge, people need to learn the following:
   a. About respiratory alkalosis and its treatment, including its specific cause in each person's case.
   b. How to reduce anxiety and control breathing rate if hyperventilation was anxiety related.

■ METABOLIC ALKALOSIS

Definition

1. Metabolic alkalosis is a relative deficit of metabolic acid in the blood, which is seen clinically as an increased bicarbonate concentration.
2. Metabolic alkalosis increases the pH of the blood. Partial respiratory compensation (hypoventilation) occurs but is limited by the need for oxygen.
3. Metabolic alkalosis may be primary or compensatory.

Incidence and Etiology

1. Primary metabolic alkalosis is caused by pathophysiologic processes that cause a gain of bicarbonate or a loss of metabolic acids (Table 9–22).
2. Compensatory metabolic alkalosis is a response to prolonged respiratory acidosis (see Fig. 9–3).
   a. Compensatory metabolic alkalosis occurs when decreased blood pH from prolonged respiratory acidosis causes the kidneys to retain bicarbonate and excrete more metabolic acid.
   b. Decreased metabolic acid from compensatory metabolic alkalosis helps balance the carbonic acid deficiency of respiratory acidosis and brings pH back toward normal.

Clinical Manifestations and Pathophysiology (Table 9–23)

Diagnostics

1. Assessment
   a. Assess level of consciousness.
   b. Assess for increased neuromuscular excitability initially.
      (1) Ask about muscle cramps or tingling of fingers, toes, or area around mouth.

Table 9–22. Etiology of Metabolic Alkalosis

General Causes	Examples
Gain of bicarbonate	Overuse of baking soda as an antacid, excess infusion of intravenous bicarbonate, massive blood transfusion, hypovolemia
Loss of metabolic acid	Vomiting, gastric suction, hypokalemia, hyperaldosteronism, excessive glucocorticoids, hypovolemia
Compensation for respiratory acidosis	See explanation in text

Table 9–23. Clinical Manifestations of Metabolic Alkalosis with Their Pathophysiologic Bases

Clinical Manifestation	Pathophysiologic Basis
Initially:	
Belligerence	Central nervous system excitation
Muscle cramps; tingling of fingers, toes, or around mouth; grimacing; carpal spasm; pedal spasm; tetany; seizures	Increased neuromuscular excitability
Later:	
Decreased level of consciousness (confusion, lethargy, coma)	Central nervous system depression
Cardiac dysrhythmias	Increased pH inside cardiac cells; hypokalemia
Nausea, vomiting	Unclear
Hypoventilation	Compensatory mechanism for metabolic alkalosis

(2) Watch for grimacing, carpal spasm, pedal spasm, tetany, seizures.

c. Monitor heart rate and rhythm.

d. Ask about presence of nausea or vomiting.

e. Monitor respiratory rate and depth.

2. Medical diagnosis: Serum bicarbonate concentration above 26 mEq/L in adults and children or above 23 mEq/L in infants (Table 9–24).

Clinical Management

1. Give medical therapy as ordered until the plasma bicarbonate concentration returns to normal.

   a. The major focus of medical therapy is treating the cause of the metabolic alkalosis and supporting renal function.

      (1) Intravenous saline is used to increase renal excretion of bicarbonate.

      (2) Potassium salts are usually given to correct the hypokalemia.

   b. If the pH is extremely high, or if saline and potassium therapy are not effective, intravenous hydrochloric acid or ammonium chloride may be administered to decrease the pH.

DRUG ADVISORY

Monitor intravenous hydrochloric acid carefully. It is irritating to veins (redness, pain at infusion site) and may cause rebound metabolic acidosis (decreasing level of consciousness, cardiac arrhythmias, increased rate and depth of respirations).

   c. Dialysis may be used.

Applying the Nursing Process

NURSING DIAGNOSIS: Risk for injury R/T altered level of consciousness and potential for seizures

1. *Expected outcomes:* Following intervention, the person should remain free of injury.

2. *Nursing interventions*

   a. Provide safety measures appropriate to the person's level of consciousness, recognizing that safety needs differ as excitation changes to central nervous system depression.

   b. Institute seizure precautions if appropriate in the initial stage.

   c. Provide frequent position changes and skin care to prevent development of pressure ulcers if level of consciousness is decreased.

NURSING DIAGNOSIS: Risk for decreased cardiac output R/T cardiac dysrhythmias

1. *Expected outcomes:* Following intervention, the person should maintain normal cardiac output, as evidenced by adequate urine output, normal capillary filling, normal PaO_2 levels, and lack of cyanosis.

2. *Nursing interventions*

   a. Apply cardiac monitor if apical pulse is irregular.

Table 9–24. Laboratory Values in Metabolic Alkalosis

Laboratory Measure	Uncompensated (Acute) Metabolic Alkalosis	Partially Compensated Metabolic Alkalosis	Fully Compensated Metabolic Alkalosis
$PaCO_2$ (marker of respiratory compensation)	Normal range	Above normal	Does not usually occur, because respiratory compensation (hypoventilation) is limited by the need for oxygen.
HCO_3^- (marker of the problem)	Above normal	Above normal	
pH (end result of problem and any compensation)	Above normal	Above normal but moving toward it	

b. Monitor for signs and symptoms of decreased cardiac output.

NURSING DIAGNOSIS: Risk for injury R/T potential aspiration of vomitus

1. *Expected outcomes:* Following intervention, the person should not aspirate if emesis occurs.
2. *Nursing interventions:* Position person on side if nauseated.

NURSING DIAGNOSIS: Self-care deficit R/T decreased level of consciousness

1. *Expected outcomes:* Following intervention, the person should maintain hygiene at culturally acceptable level.
2. *Nursing interventions:* Provide assistance, while encouraging as much independence as possible and adhering to the person's preferences and cultural values.

Discharge Planning and Teaching

1. Before hospital discharge, people need to learn the following:
   a. About metabolic alkalosis and its treatment, including its specific cause in each person's case.
   b. How to prevent metabolic alkalosis from recurring, if possible.

Bibliography

Books

Kokko JP, and Tannen RL. *Fluids and Electrolytes.* 2nd ed. Philadelphia: WB Saunders, 1990.

Metheny NM. *Fluid and Electrolyte Balance: Nursing Considerations.* 3rd ed. Philadelphia: JB Lippincott, 1996.

Rose BD. *Clinical Physiology of Acid-Base and Electrolyte Disorders.* 4th ed. New York: McGraw-Hill, 1994.

Chapters in Books and Journal Articles

Fluid and Electrolyte Imbalances

Balistreri WF. Oral rehydration in acute infantile diarrhea. *Am J Med* 88(S6A): 30S–33S, 1990.

Bove LA. Restoring electrolyte balance: Sodium and chloride. *RN* 59(1):25–29, 1996.

Cirolia B. Understanding edema: When fluid balance fails. *Nurs 96* 26(2):66–70, 1996.

Cullen L. Interventions related to fluid and electrolyte balance. *Nurs Clin North Am* 27:569–597, 1992.

DeAngelis R. Hypokalemia. *Crit Care Nurs* 11(7):71–75, 1991.

Felver L. Fluid and electrolyte balance and imbalances. *In* Patrick ML, et al (eds). *Medical-Surgical Nursing: Pathophysiological Concepts.* 2nd ed. Philadelphia: JB Lippincott, 1991.

Felver L. Fluid and electrolyte balance and imbalances. *In* Woods SL, et al (eds).

Cardiac Nursing. 3rd ed. Philadelphia: JB Lippincott, 1995.

Kaplan M. Hypercalcemia of malignancy: A review of advances in pathophysiology. *Oncol Nurs Forum* 21(6):1039–1046, 1994.

Kositzke JA. A question of balance: Dehydration in the elderly. *J Gerontol Nurs* 16(5):4–11, 1990.

Perez A. Electrolytes: Restoring the balance. Hyperkalemia. *RN* 58(11):32–37, 1995.

Perez A. Restoring electrolyte balance: Hypokalemia. *RN* 58(12):33–35, 1995.

Squire DL. Fluid and electrolyte issues for pediatric and adolescent athletes. *Pediatr Clin North Am* 37:1085–1101, 1990.

Woodtli A. Thirst: A critical care nursing challenge. *Dimens Crit Care Nurs* 9(1):6–15, 1990.

Yarnell RP, and Craig MP. Detecting hypomagnesemia: The most overlooked electrolyte imbalance. *Nursing* 21(7):55–57, 1991.

Zaloga G. Hypocalcemic crisis. *Crit Care Clin* 7:191–199, 1991.

Acid-Base Imbalances

Brenner M, and Welliver J. Pulmonary and acid-base assessment. *Nurs Clin North Am* 25:761–770, 1990.

Felver L. Acid-base balance and imbalances. *In* Patrick ML, et al (eds). *Medical-Surgical Nursing: Pathophysiological Concepts.* 2nd ed. Philadelphia: JB Lippincott, 1991.

Felver L. Acid-base balance and imbalances. *In* Woods SL, et al (eds): *Cardiac*

Nursing. 3rd ed. Philadelphia: JB Lippincott, 1995.

Janusek LW. Metabolic acidosis. *Nursing 90* 20(7):52–53, 1990.

Taylor L, and Stephens D. Arterial blood gases: Clinical application. *J Post Anesth Nurs* 5:264–272, 1990.

Intravenous Fluid Therapy

Dibble SL, Bostrom-Ezrati J, and Rizzuto C. Clinical predictors of intravenous site symptoms. *Res Nurs Health* 14:413–420, 1991.

Hadaway LC. IV tips. *Geriatric Nurs* 12:78–81, 1991.

Hastings-Tolsma MT, et al. Effect of warm and cold applications on the resolution of IV infiltrations. *Res Nurs Health* 16:171–178, 1993.

Hoffman KK. Transparent polyurethane films as an intravenous catheter dressing: Meta-analysis of the infection risks. *JAMA* 268:2072–2076, 1992.

Holliman CJ, and Wuerz RC. Proper usage of intravenous fluids. *Resident Staff Physician* 38:23–27, 1992.

Kamitomo V, and Olson K. Using normal saline to lock peripheral intravenous catheters in ambulatory cancer patients. *J Intravenous Nurs* 19:75–78, 1996.

Yucha CB, and Hastings-Tolsma M. IV infiltration—no clear signs, no clear treatment? *RN* 57(12):34–38, 1994.

Yucha CB, Hastings-Tolsma M, and Szeverenyi N. Effect of elevation on intravenous extravasations. *J Intravenous Nurs* 17:231–234, 1994.

Agencies and Resources

Intravenous Nurses Society, Inc.
Fresh Pond Square
10 Fawcett Street
Cambridge, MA 02138
(617) 441–3008

10
Caring for People with Nutritional Disorders

◼ BASICS OF NUTRITION

Principles of Nutrition

1. Basic concepts
   a. Nutrition involves eating, digesting, and absorbing foods to furnish the body with nutrients, substances the body cannot produce.
   b. No single food provides all the nutrients needed by the body.
2. Nutrients
   a. Nutrients are necessary for life, growth, and health.
   b. Nutrients also are required to promote repair and maintenance of the body.
   c. Our bodies need the same kinds of nutrients throughout life; only the *amounts* change. Requirements change according to the following:
      (1) How efficiently the body uses foods
      (2) Stage of growth and development
      (3) Gender, body size, weight, physical activity, and state of health
   d. The body can convert some nutrients into other nutrients to meet its physiologic needs.
   e. The nutritive value of any specific food is dependent on several factors:
      (1) Content and amount of nutrients in a specific food that the body can use
      (2) Content and bioavailability of nutrients in other foods in the person's diet
      (3) Nutrient requirements for that person
   f. Food processing, storage, and preparation affect the amounts of nutrients in food.
   g. A nutritious diet provides the required nutrient levels in the required balance.
   h. Increasing the variety of foods consumed is beneficial. Variety reduces the probability of the person developing the following:
      (1) Isolated nutrient deficiencies (e.g., a potassium deficiency)
      (2) Isolated nutrient excesses (e.g., vitamin A toxicity)
      (3) Toxicity due to nonnutritive components or contaminants in any particular food
   i. If a person's intake of any single nutrient changes, the amounts of other nutrients in the diet also change as a result of different food choices. (For instance, when cholesterol intake is decreased, calcium and iron intake are usually lower because of different foods chosen.)

Elements of Basic Nutrition

1. Calories (cal): kilocalorie (usually called a calorie) is the basic measure of nutritional energy. It is the amount of heat (energy) required to raise the temperature of 1 kg of water 1 degree Celsius.
2. Energy-producing nutrients
   a. Aside from water, the body's greatest nutritional need is for energy. Carbohydrates, proteins, and fats in food provide energy. Limited quantities of fat stores in the body can also supply energy.
   b. Carbohydrates consist of monosaccharides, disaccharides, and polysaccharides (soluble and insoluble fiber).
      (1) Monosaccharides and disaccharides constitute simple carbohydrates, which include naturally occurring sugars (fruits and milk) and concentrated sweets (honey and table sugar).
      (2) Polysaccharides are commonly called complex carbohydrates and contain numerous sugar molecules. Grains, breads, pastas, vegetables, beans, and peas are sources of complex carbohydrates.
      (3) Soluble fiber is almost totally digested and performs several functions: lowers cholesterol, keeps blood sugar levels stable, delays gastric emptying, binds bile acids, and reduces fat absorption. Conversely, insoluble fiber is largely undigested. Functions include absorbing water, increasing stool bulk, and promoting gastrointestinal muscle tone, thereby preventing or relieving constipation. High-fiber foods are not high in calories. Table 10–1 lists sources of soluble and insoluble fiber.
      (4) Functions of carbohydrates include (a) providing energy; (b) producing nonessential amino acids; (c) facilitating normal metabolism of fats; (d) promoting gastrointestinal (GI) health (fiber); and (e) providing good sources of protein, minerals, and B vitamins (complex carbohydrates).
      (5) Energy value, sources, and recommended amounts of carbohydrate intake are listed in Table 10–1.
   c. Proteins are made of 22 amino acids, essential compounds that contain nitrogen. Amino acids are the

Table 10–1. Energy-Containing Nutrients

Nutrient	Energy Value	Recommended Amounts	Sources	Hyper- or Hypo- States
Carbohydrate	4 cal/gm	55–58%*	Milk, grain products, fruits and vegetables; sugars, syrups, jellies, honey, candies, many desserts	*Hyper:* Caries; too many concentrated sweets consumed can decrease intake of vital nutrients and increase risk for obesity *Hypo:* Rarely occurs
Fiber		20–30 gm/day	*Insoluble fiber:* Brans, whole wheat products, whole grain oats, brown rice, nuts, dried beans and peas, bananas, apples, fruits with edible seeds; cauliflower, potatoes, green beans and peas, broccoli, carrots *Soluble fiber:* Oat products, barley, dried beans and peas, apples, potatoes, citrus fruits, broccoli, carrots, psyllium, pectin	*Hyper:* Bloating; flatulence *Hypo:* Constipation; hemorrhoids
Protein	4 cal/gm	12%*; 0.8 gm/kg body weight for adults	Meats: Chicken, beef, pork, fish; milk; cheese; eggs; nuts; dried beans and peas; bread and cereal products	*Hyper:* May result in dehydration, especially in infants; excess protein intake will be stored as adipose fat, not muscle *Hypo:* Protein-energy malnutrition; kwashiorkor; marasmus; dry, flaky skin; slow healing time; prone to infections; dull, dry, brittle hair
Fat	9 cal/gm	30%* or less	*Saturated:* Beef, lamb, luncheon meats, pork, hard yellow cheese, cream, butter, lard, coconut oil, palm oil, hydrogenated vegetable oils, regular margarine *Monounsaturated:* Duck, goose, eggs, chicken, turkey, olive and peanut oil *Polyunsaturated:* Fish, shellfish, salmon, tuna. Oils: safflower, corn, cottonseed, sesame, soybean, sunflower; special margarines listing liquid oil first	*Hyper:* Obesity; elevated blood lipid levels; cancer; cardiovascular disease *Hypo:* Dry skin; dull hair; sensitivity to cold temperatures

* Percentage of total calories of the diet.

building blocks for body proteins (hair, bones, muscles).

(1) Eight amino acids must be obtained from protein-containing foods because the body cannot manufacture them; these amino acids are termed essential amino acids. All of the other amino acids can be synthesized in the body and are called nonessential amino acids.

(2) Functions of protein include building new body tissues and replacing body tissues that are constantly being catabolized or broken down, producing regulatory enzymes and hormones, helping to regulate fluid balance, assisting in acid-base balance, providing resistance to disease (antibodies or immunoglobulins), transporting insoluble lipids through the blood, and serving as a source of energy (see Table 10–1).

d. Fats or Lipids

(1) Fats consist of triglycerides (fatty acids) and glycerol (alcohol portion to which fatty acids attach). Fats also supply cholesterol, a fatlike substance.

(2) Triglycerides can vary greatly. Saturated fatty acids have all the hydrogen bonds they can hold; lower intake of these in the American diet is desirable. Monounsaturated fatty acids have 1 double bond; increased intake is recommended. Polyunsaturated fatty acids have 2 or more double bonds; excessive amounts may promote carcinogenesis. Short-chain and medium-chain triglycerides are more readily digested and absorbed. Long-chain fatty acids are prevalent in vegetable oils.

(3) Functions of fats include providing a concentrated source of energy, providing a high satiety value, improving the palatability of the diet, providing essential fatty acids, promoting absorption of fat-soluble vitamins, and protecting vital organs and providing insulation.

e. Energy value, requirements, sources, and diseases or conditions associated with carbohydrate, protein, and fat intake are listed in Table 10–1.

3. Vitamins

a. Vitamins catalyze all reactions using proteins, fats, and carbohydrates.

b. The body requires very small amounts of vitamins.

c. Vitamins do not provide energy or building material for the body.

d. Most vitamins perform several tasks.

e. Vitamins can be fat soluble or water soluble.
  (1) Fat-soluble vitamins include vitamins A, D, E, and K. They can be stored in the body, predisposing to toxicities. Fat-soluble vitamins are fairly stable to heat, as in cooking. Fat-soluble vitamins are absorbed in the intestine along with fats and lipids in foods. They require bile for absorption.
  (2) Water-soluble vitamins include all the B vitamins and vitamin C. The B vitamins contain nitrogen. Water-soluble vitamins are necessary for almost every cellular reaction in the body. The body needs a daily source to prevent deficiencies. Deficiencies generally take 1 to 2 months to develop. Most water-soluble vitamins are readily absorbed from the jejunum.
f. Table 10–2 lists sources, recommended allowances, deficiency and toxicity symptoms of all vitamins.
4. Minerals
  a. Minerals are essential for proper physiologic functioning of the body. Table 10–3 lists a summary of minerals and their sources and effects of deficiency and toxicity.
  b. Functions of minerals
    (1) Regulate the activity of many enzymes
    (2) Help membrane transfer of essential compounds
    (3) Maintain nerve and muscular irritability
    (4) Are structural components of body tissues
    (5) Contribute indirectly to the growth process
    (6) Are important antioxidants, substances that help protect the body against certain diseases, especially cancer (e.g., zinc, copper, selenium, manganese)
5. Fluids and electrolytes
  a. Because body cells live in a fluid medium, water is required for survival.
  b. Electrolytes are important for both water balance and acid-base balance (see Chapter 9 for a discussion of fluids and electrolytes).

Nutritional Guidelines for Healthy Adults

1. Recommended daily allowances (RDAs)
  a. The RDAs identify specific amounts of essential nutrients that meet the known nutrient needs of practically all healthy people at various stages of life.
  b. The U.S. government publishes the RDAs based on the recommendations of reputable scientists and scientific research studies.
  c. The RDAs are guidelines for large groups of healthy people; comparing nutrients in menus or in diets with the RDAs is a tedious, time-consuming task. People need information in terms of foods they eat, not nutrient amounts.
  d. Generally a diet that provides two thirds of the RDA is considered adequate.
2. Dietary guidelines for Americans
  a. The dietary guidelines are intended for healthy Americans and people at risk of developing chronic diseases (family history of obesity, high blood pressure, or elevated cholesterol levels) who want to avoid nu-

tritional deficiencies and reduce the risk of acquiring some of these diseases.
  b. These 7 guidelines address problems of overconsumption of food rather than those of inadequate nutrients or intake because deficiency diseases occur less frequently in the United States. The guidelines are as follows:
    (1) Eat a variety of foods.
    (2) Balance the food you eat with physical activity. Maintain or improve your weight.
    (3) Choose a diet with plenty of grain products, vegetables, and fruits.
    (4) Choose a diet low in fat (no more than 30% of total calories), saturated fat, and cholesterol (no more than 300 mg per day).
    (5) Choose a diet moderate in sugars.
    (6) Choose a diet moderate in salt and sodium.
    (7) If you drink alcoholic beverages, do so in moderation.
3. Food pyramid. This tool replaces the basic 4 food groups to help people implement the dietary guidelines (Fig. 10–1; Box 10–1).
4. Nutrition labels. The nutrition labels on product packaging promote awareness of nutrients in a food and comparison of nutritional values for various products (Fig. 10–2).
5. Energy requirements
  a. People at their desirable weight or moderately active persons should multiply 15 times their ideal body weight (IBW) in pounds. The IBW denotes a weight for height considered to be healthy for a person.
  b. To estimate caloric requirements of obese or inactive adults, multiply 10 times their IBW.
  c. For thin or very active adults, multiply 20 times the IBW.
  d. For people older than age 55 or for sedentary people, multiply 13 times their IBW.
  e. For adults who want to lose weight, follow the above multiplication factor guidelines and subtract 500 calories from the total number.

Transcultural Food Patterns and Nutrition-Related Health Problems

1. Besides physiologic needs, food meets a person's personal, social, and cultural needs. Nurses should consider several facts about food patterns when working with people of various cultures.
2. Asian practices
  a. Asian people have maintained strong ties to their native foods.
  b. Nourishment of the body is important; Asians believe health is balanced by a harmonious mixture of foods.
  c. Many Asians are lactose intolerant.
  d. Nutritionally helpful practices
    (1) The yin-yang concept has been beneficial, creating dietary variety and balancing animal protein, grain, and vegetable consumption.
    (2) Moderation is important; Asians often reject extremely unbalanced diets.

Text continued on page 301

Table 10–2. Summary of Vitamins and Management of Hyper- and Hypo- States

Vitamins and Adult RDAs, IV Dosage, Diagnostic Tests	Sources	Causes of Hyper- or Hypo- States	Manifestations	Nursing Interventions
Vitamin A (retinol, carotene) *Diagnostic Tests:* Serum tocopherol/carotene level; retinol-binding protein	Liver and other organ meats; egg yolk; green, yellow, or orange vegetables and fruits; tomatoes; whole milk and cheese; cream; fortified margarine; fatty fish, fish oils	*Hyper:* Too much vitamin A supplement *Hypo:* Inadequate intake; chronic fat malabsorption; alcoholism; hepatic disease; chronic use of mineral oil, neomycin, cholestyramine	*Hyper:* Bulging of the fontanelle, headache, vomiting, diplopia, alopecia, dry mucous membranes, liver damage *Hypo:* Night blindness, xerophthalmia, Bitot's spots, keratinization of epithelium, follicular hyperkeratosis, growth retardation, skin and mucous membrane infections, blindness	Explain that vitamin prescriptions should be followed explicitly and should never be shared with friends. Recommend storing vitamins in a cool, dark place. Encourage intake of vitamin A–rich foods. Provide oral or IV supplements as prescribed; a water-miscible form may be necessary for fat malabsorption. Inform people that Vitamin A acts as an antioxidant to protect against lung, breast, oral mucosa, esophageal, and bladder cancers.
Vitamin D: 5 μg; 5 μg IV *Diagnostic Tests:* Serum calcium, alkaline phosphatase; serum 25-(OH vitamin D) or 1,25-(OH$_2$ vitamin D)	Fortified milk, fortified margarine; fish oil; liver; butter; egg yolk. Synthesized in skin by ultraviolet light	*Hyper:* Giving incorrect amounts of a concentrated calciferol preparation Excessive intake of fortified foods (especially infants) *Hypo:* Inadequate exposure to sunshine; hepatic or renal disease; malabsorption; abnormalities in calcium balance and bone metabolism caused by malfunctioning parathyroid gland; cholestyramine, glucocorticoids, phenobarbital; diphenylhydantoin, mineral oil	*Hyper:* Early symptoms—anorexia; nausea; vomiting; diarrhea; bloody stools; polyuria, muscular weakness; lassitude, headache; hypercalcemia, increased phosphorus More serious symptoms—renal failure and calcification *Hypo:* Children—rickets, enlarged joints, bowed legs, deformities of the chest, spine, and pelvis Infants—tetany Adults—osteomalacia	Provide supplemental amounts for rickets and osteomalacia, as ordered. When supplements are prescribed, monitor color of urine (cloudiness or a red color may indicate toxicity) and calcium phosphate and urea levels. If overdose occurs, induce emesis or gastric lavage, or administer mineral oil to increase fecal excretion. Explain the importance of taking or giving the exact prescribed dose to avoid toxicity. Closely monitor persons taking digitalis preparations and vitamin D supplements concurrently; elevated calcium levels may cause dysrhythmias. Advise persons with chronic renal failure to avoid magnesium-containing antacids or laxatives if they are taking vitamin D supplements (causes magnesium toxicity).
Vitamin E (tocopherol) *Diagnostic Tests:* Serum tocopherol esters, vitamin E	Vegetable oils and margarines; whole grains; wheat germ; green leafy vegetables; nuts; liver	*Hyper:* Rarely seen *Hypo:* In newborns, poor placental transfer of vitamin K and inadequate production; malabsorption; polyunsaturated fat increases requirement	*Hyper:* None known *Hypo:* Red blood cell (RBC) hemolysis and abnormal fat deposits; reticulocytosis; thrombocytosis. Deficiency unlikely except in premature infants who may develop hemolytic anemia. Adults with malabsorption—neuropathy and myopathy with creatinuria	Vitamin E may help the immune system function better, so encourage intake of vitamin E–rich foods by hospitalized persons. Also acts as an antioxidant and prevents breakdown of RBCs. Give high levels of vitamin E supplementation only with proper medical supervision. Teach persons taking anticoagulant therapy to avoid vitamin E supplements. If iron supplements are needed, advise discontinuation of vitamin E supplements until improvement is observed in iron status.

294

Vitamin (Diagnostic Test)	Food Sources	Hyper/Hypo Conditions	Hyper/Hypo Clinical Signs	Nursing Considerations
Vitamin K menadione, phylloquinone *Diagnostic Test:* Prothrombin time	Green leafy vegetables; kale; cauliflower; cabbage; egg yolk; soybean oil; liver; manufactured by GI microflora	*Hyper:* None documented from oral intake of vitamin K; synthetic menadione may cause hemolytic anemia, hyperbilirubinemia, and jaundice in the newborn. *Hypo:* Prolonged courses of antibiotics; malabsorption syndromes; cholestyramine; coumarin; anticoagulants	*Hyper:* Kernicterus, jaundice *Hypo:* Low serum prothrombin and prolonged blood clotting times; hemorrhagic disease of the newborn; hemorrhages	Double-check dosage of menadione given to infants because overdose may cause irreversible brain damage. Store injectable or colloidal solutions in a cool dark place. If administration is IV, monitor for severe or even fatal reactions, including transient facial flushing, sweating, a sense of constriction in the chest, weakness; more serious effects include shock or even cardiac and respiratory failure. Suggest water-soluble forms of vitamins K_1 and K_2 for persons with fat malabsorption. Discourage vitamins A and E supplements if person is prone to vitamin K deficiencies. Teach persons on dicumarol or warfarin therapy that large amounts of vitamin K–rich foods are contraindicated.
Vitamin C (ascorbic acid) *Diagnostic Tests:* Serum ascorbate; urinary ascorbic acid concentration	Citrus fruits; strawberries; cantaloupe, tomatoes, sweet peppers; cabbage; potatoes; turnip greens; broccoli; mango; fresh peaches	*Hyper:* Supplemental doses promoted as increasing resistance to colds and other respiratory diseases *Hypo:* Avoidance of acidic foods to control esophageal reflux; peritoneal dialysis or hemodialysis; increased requirement during physiologic stress; smoking; drug abusers, anorectic medications; alcohol; anticonvulsants; oral contraceptives; tetracycline; aspirin	*Hyper:* Diarrhea, hypoglycemia, oxaluria, dependency or rebound effect; large amounts interfere with vitamin B_{12} absorption *Hypo:* Delayed wound healing; bruise and hemorrhage easily; gingivitis; anemia; scurvy	Monitor for subclinical deficiency symptoms—anorexia, increasing debilitation, sensitivity to touch, easily bruised. Avoid rapid administration IV, especially in persons with renal insufficiency. Teach persons that vitamin C acts as an antioxidant to reduce risk of stomach cancer. Avoid regular IV fluids containing 3 gm of ascorbic acid in iron-overloaded persons. Teach persons who form kidney stones to avoid high doses of vitamin C. Warn persons taking large amounts of vitamin C to gradually reduce doses to avoid scurvy. Inform people that chewable vitamin C tablets may lead to erosion of dental enamel.
Thiamin (vitamin B_1) *Diagnostic Tests:* Urinary thiamin; RBC transketolase; RBC thiamin	Pork; liver; chicken; beef; whole grains; enriched cereals; legumes	*Hyper:* None known *Hypo:* Alcoholism; ingestion of raw fish; chronic febrile states; total parenteral nutrition; thyrotoxicosis; malabsorption	*Hyper:* Rarely occurs *Hypo:* Early signs—depression, irritability, poor appetite, fatigue, apathy, vasodilation (ruddy skin) Wet beriberi—dependent edema, dyspnea, palpitations; cardiac failure Dry beriberi—peripheral polyneuritis. Alcoholic polyneuropathy—myelopathy, cerebellar signs, anorexia, hypothermia Wernicke-Korsakoff syndrome—confabulation, disorientation	If deficiency is suspected or diagnosed, observe for symptoms of other vitamin B deficiencies. Advise persons with beriberi to decrease physical activity and rest frequently. Advise persons to keep the vitamin in an air-tight, light-resistant, nonmetallic container. Remember that clinical response to thiamin therapy is often dramatic, but ultimate recovery may be incomplete; relapses may occur. Recovery is extremely slow after prolonged paralysis. Offer emotional support to prevent depression or hopelessness. If lactic acidosis is occurring for an unknown reason, suspect thiamin deficiency. Only give IV push in life-threatening wet beriberi. When administering large doses, test for hypersensitivity.

Table continued on following page

Table 10–2. Summary of Vitamins and Management of Hyper- and Hypo- States (Continued)

Vitamins and Adult RDAs, IV Dosage, Diagnostic Tests	Sources	Causes of Hyper- or Hypo- States	Manifestations	Nursing Interventions
Riboflavin (vitamin B$_2$) *Diagnostic Tests:* Urine riboflavin; RBC glutathione reductase activity coefficient (high level indicates deficiency)	Milk; liver; meat; fish; enriched cereal products; yeast	*Hyper:* None known *Hypo:* Uncommon; encountered in persons with multiple nutrient deficiencies related to poor nutrient absorption or utilization; hyperthyroidism; hypothyroidism; chronic alcoholism; phenothiazines; antibiotics	*Hyper:* None known *Hypo:* Dermatitis, especially in the scrotal or vulval area; glossitis; depapillation of tongue; cheilosis; tearing, burning, and itching of eyes	Protect vitamin from light. Closely monitor persons with increased nitrogen losses due to catabolism for possible riboflavin deficiency. Teach people that enriched products provide more riboflavin than their whole grain counterparts. Warn persons that riboflavin supplements will make the urine an intense yellow color. Inform persons that a mixed diet that contains 2 cups of milk and 4 to 6 ounces of meat daily ensures an adequate riboflavin supply.
Niacin (nicotinamide, nicotinic acid) *Diagnostic Test:* N' methylnicotinamide	Liver; poultry; beef; fish; eggs; whole grain and enriched cereals; legumes; seeds; nuts; yeast	*Hyper:* Supplemental doses of nicotinic acid taken to lower serum lipids *Hypo:* Alcohol; cytotoxic drugs; antituberculous drugs; tryptophan intake	*Hyper:* Nicotinic acid may cause flushing, nausea, itching, tachycardia, fainting, blurred vision, abnormal liver function, and gout *Hypo:* Pellagra—diarrhea, dermatitis, depression or dementia; scarlet, raw depapillated, and fissured tongue Hartnup's disease—aminoaciduria, pellagra-like rash, cerebellar ataxia	Teach persons the following: Nicotinamide is a form of niacin but does not lower serum lipids. Flushing, while uncomfortable, is harmless; timed release of nicotinic acid, aspirin, or both may lessen this response. Nicotinamide is not a vasodilator and does not cause adverse effects associated with nicotinic acid. Persons with diabetes mellitus should not take niacin supplements unless prescribed by the physician (elevates glucose levels). Warn persons receiving niacin therapy to avoid alcohol, report dark-colored urine, light-colored stools or jaundice to the physician; if skin reactions appear, stay out of the sun. Assess for riboflavin deficiency because these often occur together; supplemental riboflavin should accompany niacin treatment. Provide vitamin supplements with meals to avoid adverse GI effects.
Folate (folic acid, folacin) *Diagnostic Tests:* Serum and RBC folate levels	Green leafy vegetables; liver; beef; fish; whole grains; legumes; lima beans; grapefruit; oranges	*Hyper:* None known *Hypo:* Increased requirements, as during pregnancy, chemotherapy; vitamin B$_{12}$ deficiency; alcohol; anticonvulsants; oral contraceptives; pyrimethamine; triamterene; analgesics; salicylates; cytotoxic agents; anti-inflammatory agents; H$_2$ receptor blockers; antacids	*Hyper:* None known *Hypo:* Megaloblastic anemia; stomatitis; glossitis; diarrhea; stunted growth; frequent infections; depression; mental confusion; neural tube defects in infants born to folate deficient mothers	Especially assess persons with conditions that increase metabolic rate (infection, hyperthyroidism, increased cell turnover, rapid tissue growth, malignant tumor) for folate deficiency (megaloblastic anemia). Remember that folate supplementation in pernicious anemia results in remission of hematologic abnormalities but not the neurologic deficits; a correct diagnosis is imperative before initiating corrective treatment. Inform persons that high folate supplementation for persons taking phenytoin can decrease effectiveness of the medication. Teach people that folate is easily destroyed by food processing or heat; raw vegetables provide more folate than cooked ones.

Nutrient / Diagnostic Tests	Food Sources	Causes (Hyper/Hypo)	Signs and Symptoms (Hyper/Hypo)	Nursing Implications*
Pyridoxine (vitamin B_6, pyridoxal) *Diagnostic Test:* RBC aspartate amino transferase activity coefficient (high level indicates deficiency)	Meats; fish; corn; legumes; seeds; grains; potatoes; green leafy vegetables; green beans; bananas	*Hyper:* Supplemental doses given for coronary heart disease, cancer, premenstrual syndrome *Hypo:* Deficiency rarely occurs alone, usually accompanied by other B vitamin deficiencies; excessive protein intake; oral contraceptive agents, isoniazid, levodopa, cycloserine, penicillamine therapy	*Hyper:* Ataxia; severe sensory neuropathy; bone pain and muscle weakness; hypotonia in neonates *Hypo:* Nervous irritability; seborrhea-like skin lesions with cheilosis and glossitis; weakness; anemias (hypochromic, microcytic, and of pregnancy); impaired immune responses; convulsions (in infants)	Teach persons not to take vitamin B_6 unless ordered by a physician. Vitamin B_6 supplements may be recommended for women taking oral contraceptive agents, especially if anticipating a pregnancy in the near future. Remember that serum levels are low in persons with chronic renal failure, but supplementation may not be warranted. Inform person that excessive pyridoxine can reduce clinical benefits of levodopa therapy in Parkinson's disease; encourage limited intake of foods fortified with vitamin B_6. If person is on isoniazid and rifampin for tuberculosis, supplements of pyridoxine are necessary if the ordered antitubercular medication does not contain pyridoxine.
Vitamin B_{12} (cyanocobalamin) *Diagnostic Tests:* Serum vitamin B_{12} level, Schilling test	Only in animal foods: liver, meats, salt-water fish, oysters, milk, eggs; synthesized by microorganisms in the GI tract	*Hyper:* None known *Hypo:* Strict vegetarians and breast-fed babies of strict vegetarians; gastrectomy or lack of intrinsic factor; bacterial overgrowth; megadoses of vitamin C; terminal ileal disease or resection; cholestyramine	*Hyper:* None known *Hypo:* Pernicious or megaloblastic anemia; peripheral neuropathy; stomatitis, glossitis, bright red tongue; weakness; personality changes	Teach strict vegetarians that a daily supplement of vitamin B_{12} may be required. Be sure persons who have had permanent gastric surgery or ileal damage are aware of lifelong requirements for monthly vitamin B_{12} injections. Inform person that concomitant ingestion of megadoses of ascorbic acid (foods or tablets) can destroy substantial amounts of vitamin B_{12} and produce deficiency. Provide oral doses with meals when intrinsic factor secretion is elevated.
Pantothenic acid *Diagnostic Tests:* Urine and whole blood pantothenic acid levels	Present in all plant and animal foods; meats; legumes; whole grains	*Hyper:* High dosage of supplements *Hypo:* Only documented in persons using a metabolic antagonist or semisynthetic diet devoid of pantothenic acid	*Hyper:* Occasional diarrhea *Hypo:* Postural hypotension, rapid heart rate on exertion; abdominal distress—anorexia, constipation, flatulence; numbness and tingling of the extremities	Teach people that diets including whole grain unprocessed foods contain more pantothenic acid.
Biotin *Diagnostic Tests:* Whole blood and urine biotin levels	Liver, meat, egg yolk, cereals, yeast, milk; synthesized by microorganisms in GI tract	*Hyper:* None reported in humans *Hypo:* Suppression of colonic bacterial production as a result of long-term antibiotic therapy; prolonged IV therapy; gastrointestinal fistulas; high levels of zinc supplementation	*Hyper:* None known *Hypo:* Depression and anorexia; glossitis; dermatitis; alopecia and loss of hair color; lethargy; paresthesias; seborrheic dermatitis in infants under 6 months of age	Teach persons to cook eggs to decrease avidin's binding capacity and minimize danger of *Salmonella* poisoning. Explain that a balanced diet that includes a variety of foods contains adequate amounts of biotin, so supplements are unnecessary.

*In all cases, nurses should assess persons for deficiency or toxicity symptoms. A diet history helps determine causes. Encourage persons to increase or decrease dietary intake of foods high in that nutrient, as appropriate. Explain how to consume adequate amounts of nutrients by eating a well-balanced diet using a variety of foods.

Table 10–3. Summary of Minerals and Management of Hyper- and Hypo- States

Minerals and Adult RDAs, IV Dosage, Diagnostic Tests	Sources	Causes of Hyper- or Hypo- States	Manifestations	Nursing Interventions
Calcium *Diagnostic Tests:* Serum and urine calcium levels	Milk and other dairy products, dark green leafy vegetables, salmon, sardines, fortified fruit beverages	*Hyper:* Overdoses of cholecalciferol or vitamin D preparations, hyperparathyroidism, certain types of bone disease, sarcoidosis, cancer *Hypo:* Hypoparathyroidism, some bone diseases, certain kidney diseases, low serum protein levels; anticonvulsants, corticosteroids, diphosphonates, diuretics, laxatives	*Hyper:* Constipation, renal calculi, calcification of soft tissues; inhibits absorption of iron and zinc *Hypo:* Rickets, osteoporosis, osteomalacia, paresthesias, tetany, convulsions; may contribute to hypertension	When calcium levels are abnormal, correction of the primary problem is usually necessary rather than dietary calcium adjustments. Check the serum protein and albumin and parathyroid hormone levels before becoming concerned over the calcium level. For persons with hypercalcemia, limit high-calcium foods and encourage fluid intake. Monitor electrocardiogram when giving calcium IV. Give calcium supplements with some form of sugar and vitamin D to enhance absorption. If usual intake is low, encourage increased consumption of dairy products if tolerated. If the person dislikes milk products, powdered milk can be added to many items.
Phosphorus *Diagnostic Tests:* Serum and urine phosphorus levels	Milk and dairy products, meats, whole grains, legumes, nuts	*Hyper:* Hypoparathyroidism or renal insufficiency *Hypo:* Increased calcium excretion; bone loss; long-term ingestion of aluminum hydroxide antacids; malabsorption syndromes, such as sprue and celiac disease; renal tubular disease; total parenteral nutrition; alcohol withdrawal; diuretics; antacids	*Hyper:* Tetany, convulsions *Hypo:* Muscle weakness, increased calcium excretion, bone loss, cardiac and respiratory failure, glucose intolerance, diminished RBC, growth retardation in children	Teach person that oral supplements are poorly tolerated, usually causing diarrhea; milk is a good source of phosphate.
Magnesium *Diagnostic Tests:* Serum and urine magnesium levels	Whole-grain products, nuts, beans, green leafy vegetables, bananas	*Hyper:* Kidney failure *Hypo:* Gastrointestinal abnormalities with diarrhea, renal disease, general malnutrition, alcoholism, diuretics, infants of diabetic mothers, alcohol, amphotericin B, diuretics, gentamicin, platinum-containing chemotherapeutic agents	*Hyper:* Weakness, drowsiness, vasodilation, decreased respiration, diarrhea *Hypo:* Personality changes: vomiting; neuromuscular dysfunction, muscle spasm, convulsions, hyperexcitability, tremors; cardiac dysrhythmias; anorexia; apathy; coma	Remember chronic alcoholics may require magnesium therapy after an acute attack of delirium tremens because of high urinary losses of magnesium. Explain that unrefined grains and vegetables provide more magnesium than refined processed foods. If persons on dialysis need antacids, emphasize the use of aluminum- or calcium-based antacids or laxatives rather than magnesium hydroxide.

Mineral / Diagnostic Tests	Food Sources	Conditions	Nursing Considerations
Iron *Diagnostic Tests:* Serum iron, total iron-binding capacity, hemoglobin, hematocrit, serum ferritin	Liver, meats, egg yolk, dark green vegetables, enriched breads and cereals	*Hyper:* Hemochromatosis; hemosiderosis—excessive iron intake, multiple blood transfusions, failure to regulate absorption *Hypo:* Dietary deficiency, increased requirements for growth; increased iron losses; inadequate absorption secondary to diarrhea; decreased acid secretion; antacid therapy; duodenal or jejunal disease or resection; antacids, cholestyramine, coumarin, heparin, isoniazid, chloramphenicol, acetyl-salicylic acid	Do not encourage iron supplements without laboratory testing that indicates a deficiency. Closely monitor alcoholics and persons who receive numerous blood transfusions for iron toxicity. Absorption is improved by giving on an empty stomach, but this may cause a stomach upset. Inform person that a vitamin C–rich food with supplements or with meals increases absorption of iron, especially nonheme iron. Avoid giving iron supplements with milk because calcium in milk interferes with iron absorption. Avoid giving iron supplements with coffee and tea because this decreases iron absorption, but these beverages can be drunk 1 hr before the meal. Teach person that iron supplements cause stools to turn black. Give elixir iron preparations with straw to avoid staining teeth.
Zinc *Diagnostic Tests:* Plasma and 24-hour urine zinc	Meats, eggs, crustaceans, leafy and root vegetables	*Hyper:* Vomiting, diarrhea, epigastric pain, lethargy, fatigue; renal damage, pancreatitis, death *Hypo:* Dietary deficiency, decreased absorption (high fiber, phytate, calcium, phosphate, copper or iron intake), pica, malabsorption syndromes, pancreatic insufficiency, alcoholism, chronic renal disease, sickle cell disease, thalassemia; thiazide diuretics, oral penicillamine therapy, corticosteroids, oral contraceptives	Teach person that chronic consumption of 15-mg zinc supplements may cause toxicity symptoms. Because of detrimental effects of too much zinc, advise persons to take zinc supplements only if ordered by the physician. Zinc supplements are rarely needed if a well-balanced diet is consumed; give zinc supplements only to persons who will benefit. Persons with taste abnormalities secondary to zinc deficiency may respond to supplementation, but additional zinc is not effective in restoring normal taste acuity associated with other conditions. Teach persons that zinc supplementation interferes with use of iron and copper and adversely affects high-density lipoproteins. Give between meals without food to enhance absorption, but this may cause gastric distress. Do not give milk with zinc supplements because calcium in the milk interferes with zinc absorption. Teach persons that meats are the preferred source of zinc. Small amounts of animal protein can significantly improve absorption of zinc from a legume-based meal.
Iodine *Diagnostic Tests:* Thyroid-stimulating hormone level, thyroxine and triiodothyronine levels, 24-hr urine iodine levels, serum protein-bound iodine	Iodized salt, saltwater fish	*Hyper:* Parotitis, headache, goiter, Graves' disease *Hypo:* Goiter, myxedema, stillbirths, abortions, congenital anomalies, mental retardation, deaf mutism, cretinism, hypothyroidism, mild depression of mental functions	Inform person that iodine supplements (saturated solution of potassium iodide) may cause gastric irritation and have a metallic taste. Advise the person to take through a straw to prevent staining teeth.

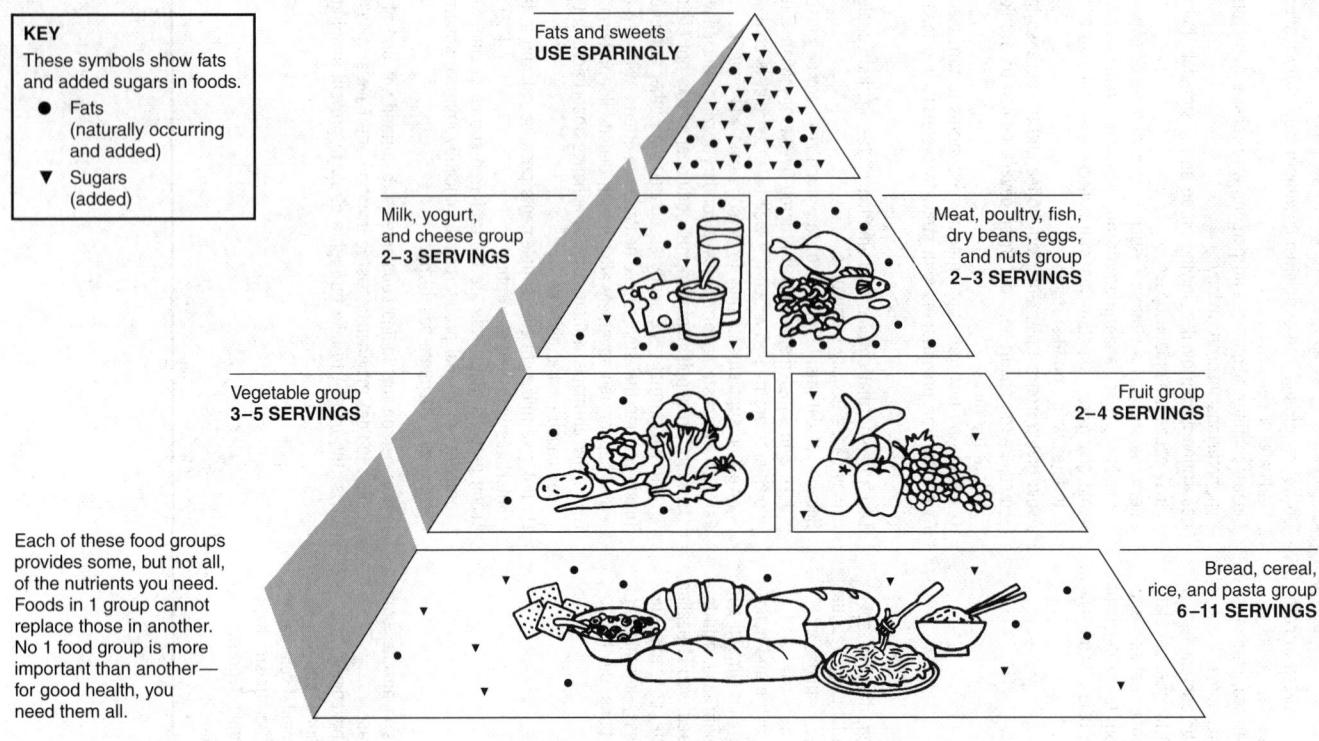

KEY

These symbols show fats and added sugars in foods.

● Fats (naturally occurring and added)

▼ Sugars (added)

Fats and sweets **USE SPARINGLY**

Milk, yogurt, and cheese group **2–3 SERVINGS**

Meat, poultry, fish, dry beans, eggs, and nuts group **2–3 SERVINGS**

Vegetable group **3–5 SERVINGS**

Fruit group **2–4 SERVINGS**

Bread, cereal, rice, and pasta group **6–11 SERVINGS**

Each of these food groups provides some, but not all, of the nutrients you need. Foods in 1 group cannot replace those in another. No 1 food group is more important than another—for good health, you need them all.

What Counts as 1 Serving?

▶ The amount you eat may be more than 1 serving. For example, a dinner portion of spaghetti would count as 2 or 3 servings.

Bread, Cereal, Rice, and Pasta Group

1 slice of bread
½ cup of cooked rice or pasta
½ cup of cooked cereal
1 ounce of ready-to-eat cereal

Vegetable Group

½ cup of chopped raw or cooked vegetables
1 cup of leafy raw vegetables

Fruit Group

1 piece of fruit or melon wedge
¾ cup of juice
½ cup of canned fruit
¼ cup of dried fruit

Milk, Yogurt, and Cheese Group

1 cup of milk or yogurt
1½ ounces of natural cheese
2 ounces of process cheese

Meat, Poultry, Fish, Dry Beans, Eggs, and Nuts Group

2½ to 3 ounces of cooked lean meat, poultry, or fish
Count ½ cup of cooked beans, or 1 egg, or 2 tablespoons of peanut butter as 1 ounce of lean meat

Fats and Sweets

LIMIT CALORIES FROM THESE especially if you need to lose weight

How Many Servings Do You Need Each Day?

	Women and Some Older Adults	Children, Teen Girls, Active Women, Most Men	Teen Boys and Active Men
Calorie level*	About 1600	About 2200	About 2800
Bread Group	6	9	11
Vegetable Group	3	4	5
Fruit Group	2	3	4
Milk Group	2–3†	2–3†	2–3†
Meat Group	2 for a total of 5 ounces	2 for a total of 6 ounces	3 for a total of 7 ounces

*These are the calorie levels if you choose low-fat, lean foods from the 5 major food groups and use foods from the fats and sweets group sparingly.

†Women who are pregnant or breast-feeding, teenagers, and young adults to age 24 need 3 servings.

Figure 10–1. The pyramid depicts 3 essential elements of a healthy diet for adults: proportions, variety, and moderation. It is not a rigid prescription but a general guide for choosing a variety of foods to obtain the needed nutrients and the correct amounts of calories to maintain a healthy weight. (From the U.S. Department of Agriculture, Human Nutrition Information Service, and the Food Marketing Institute.)

Nutrition information
provided for 1 serving

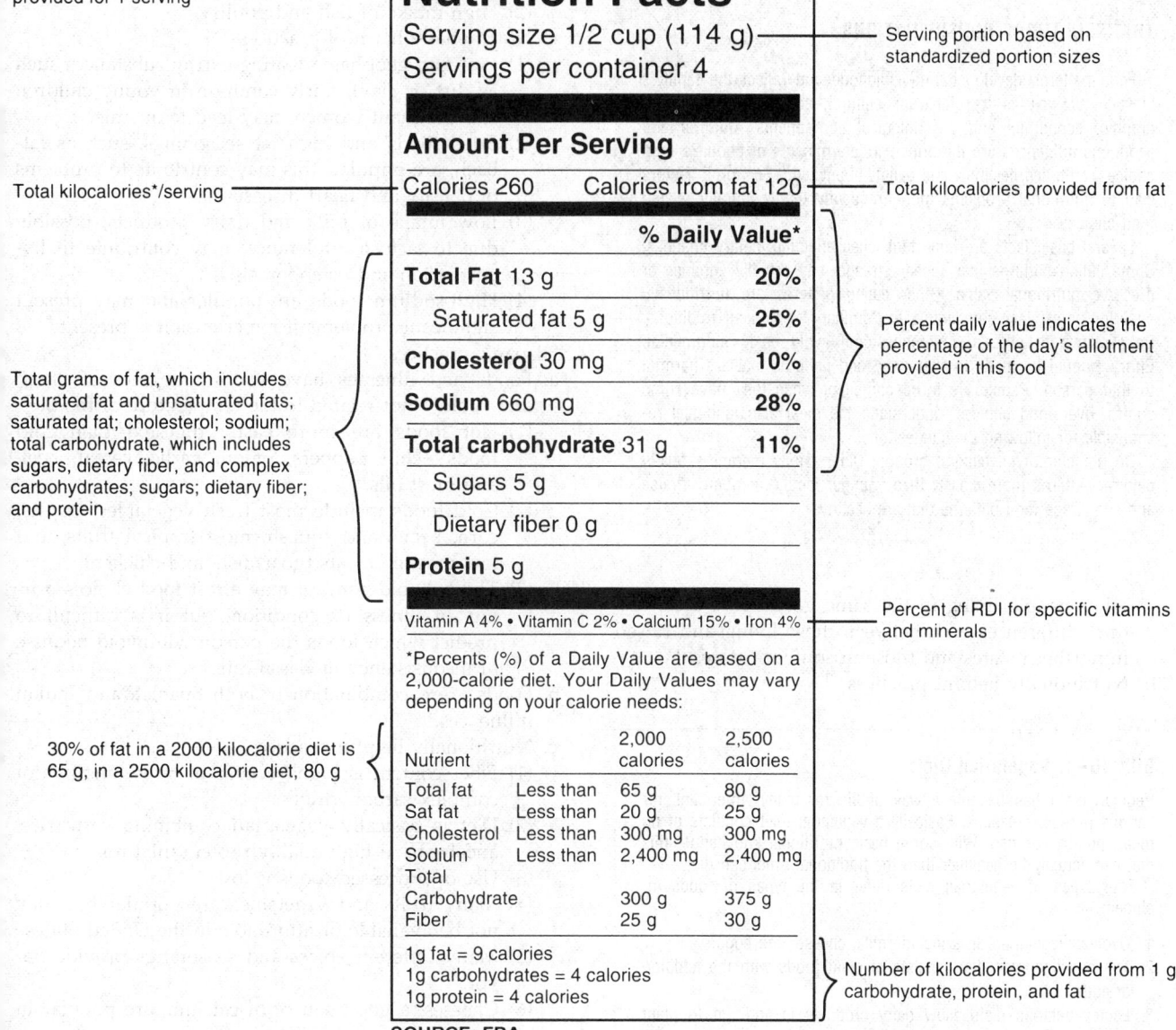

Serving portion based on
standardized portion sizes

Total kilocalories*/serving

Total kilocalories provided from fat

Total grams of fat, which includes
saturated fat and unsaturated fats;
saturated fat; cholesterol; sodium;
total carbohydrate, which includes
sugars, dietary fiber, and complex
carbohydrates; sugars; dietary fiber;
and protein

Percent daily value indicates the
percentage of the day's allotment
provided in this food

Percent of RDI for specific vitamins
and minerals

30% of fat in a 2000 kilocalorie diet is
65 g, in a 2500 kilocalorie diet, 80 g

Number of kilocalories provided from 1 g
carbohydrate, protein, and fat

Nutrition Facts

Serving size 1/2 cup (114 g)
Servings per container 4

Amount Per Serving

Calories 260   Calories from fat 120

% Daily Value*

Total Fat 13 g	**20%**
Saturated fat 5 g	**25%**
Cholesterol 30 mg	**10%**
Sodium 660 mg	**28%**
Total carbohydrate 31 g	**11%**
Sugars 5 g	
Dietary fiber 0 g	
Protein 5 g	

Vitamin A 4% • Vitamin C 2% • Calcium 15% • Iron 4%

*Percents (%) of a Daily Value are based on a
2,000-calorie diet. Your Daily Values may vary
depending on your calorie needs:

Nutrient		2,000 calories	2,500 calories
Total fat	Less than	65 g	80 g
Sat fat	Less than	20 g	25 g
Cholesterol	Less than	300 mg	300 mg
Sodium	Less than	2,400 mg	2,400 mg
Total Carbohydrate		300 g	375 g
Fiber		25 g	30 g

1g fat = 9 calories
1g carbohydrates = 4 calories
1g protein = 4 calories

SOURCE: FDA

Figure 10–2. Explanation of the latest nutrition food label. The term "daily value" used on the label reflects 2 new sets of dietary standards: (1) Reference daily intakes (RDIs), a new term for the U.S. recommended dietary allowances (RDAs), are based on a population-adjusted average of all the age and sex groups of RDA values, excluding those for pregnant and lactating women; (2) daily reference values (DRVs) are based on desirable levels of nutrients that are considered important for health: total fat, saturated fatty acids, protein, cholesterol, carbohydrate, fiber, and sodium. (From the U.S. Department of Health and Human Services, Food and Drug Administration, Washington, D.C., 1991.)

(3) Overeating is not prevalent.
(4) Food intake consists primarily of carbohydrate foods (rice) with small amounts of meat and fruit for dessert.
(5) Vegetables are minimally cooked.
(6) Tofu, a popular soybean product, can be a good source of calcium if calcium salts are used in making it.
e. Nutritionally harmful practices
(1) Condiments (soy sauce, pickles, nuoc mam, and kimchi) contain large amounts of sodium.

(2) Raw fish carry a risk of infestation with fish tapeworms and may cause stomach cancer and gastroenteritis.
(3) Rinsing rice decreases nutrient value.
(4) Long-term abuse of ginseng (used as an aphrodisiac by Koreans) may lead to hypertension. Other adverse reactions include nervousness, sleeplessness, skin eruptions, morning diarrhea, edema, and irregularities in blood glucose level.
3. Practices of Blacks
a. Patterns are relatively consistent with food patterns of

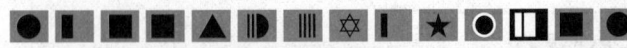

TRANSCULTURAL CONSIDERATIONS

Food patterns develop during childhood and reflect the family's lifestyle as well as its ethnic or cultural, social, religious, geographic, economic, and psychological components. Cultural and economic influences are the principal determinants of people's food choices, attitudes, feelings, and beliefs about food. Economic factors lead to nutritional problems more frequently than culturally related food choices.

Several basic facts are important when effecting dietary changes. Some eating patterns that appear strange may actually enhance or preserve nutritional value. Other eating patterns are nutritionally superior or at least comparable to "ordinary" American traditions. Be sensitive to other's preferences and avoid being judgmental. Efforts should be made to alter only food patterns that are harmful to that person. People are more compliant when they have some control over food choices, understand the meal plan, and feel responsible for following the suggestions.

Do not stereotype cultural groups. Older family members follow cultural patterns more closely than younger family members. Praise and encourage food patterns that are healthy.

other people living in the same geographic area; distinct differences exist between those living and raised in northern states and those living in southern states.
b. Nutritionally helpful practices

BOX 10–1. Vegetarian Diets

Vegetarianism has become a way of life for many Americans for various personal reasons. Basically a vegetarian diet consists of no meat, poultry, or fish. With some basic nutritional knowledge, this diet can actually be healthier than the traditional American diet.

Four types of vegetarian diets differ in the types of foods included:

1. Ovolactovegetarian diets include milk, cheese, and eggs.
2. The ovovegetarian diet consists of plant foods with the addition of eggs.
3. Lactovegetarian diets allow dairy products in addition to plant foods.
4. Vegan or strict vegetarian diets contain only food from plants, including vegetables, fruits, and grains.

The Food Guide Pyramid can still be used for planning well-balanced menus, using various combinations of protein-containing foods to complement one another. The major difference is the protein source. In general, dried beans and peas, nuts, nut butters, and seeds are the principal source of protein for vegans. For the other vegetarians, adequate amounts of protein are furnished from eggs, cheese, nuts, and dried beans and peas. A mixture of protein-containing foods throughout the day will provide enough essential amino acids. Some groups, especially Seventh-Day Adventists, supplement protein intake with many textured vegetable protein products.

There is no reason why an adequate diet cannot be obtained. The limitations of the vegetarian diet should be recognized during periods of growth or during periods of increased catabolism (such as stress, surgery, and illness) in which protein requirements are increased. If no meat products are eaten, as in the vegan diet, vitamin B_{12} may be of concern. Brewer's yeast, tempeh (fermented soy), or fortified breakfast cereals or vitamin supplements can be a source of vitamin B_{12} for vegans.

---

    (1) High intake of yellow and dark green leafy vegetables.
    (2) High intake of fish and poultry.
  c. Nutritionally harmful practices
    (1) Pica and geophagia (eating earthy substances such as dirt or clay), fairly common in young children and pregnant women, may lead to anemia.
    (2) Fried foods and high fat seasonings, such as fatback, are popular; this may contribute to problems of obesity and heart disease.
    (3) Low intake of milk and dairy products, possibly due to lactose intolerance, may contribute to hypertension and osteoporosis.
    (4) High-sodium foods are popular and may present significant problems if hypertension is present.
4. Hispanic practices
  a. Foods and illnesses have varying degrees of "hot" and "cold" (not related to the temperature of food).
    (1) Hot foods are more easily digested than cold foods—chili peppers, onion, garlic, cereal, beef, and most oils.
    (2) Cold foods include most fresh vegetables, staples, corn, beans and squash, most tropical fruits, and low-prestige meats (goat, fish, and chicken).
    (3) The hot-cold concept may affect food choices during an illness or condition, but it is difficult to predict which foods the person will avoid because of inconsistency in classifications.
  b. Foods are a combination of both Spanish and Indian influences.
  c. Nutritionally helpful practices
    (1) Fiber content is high because of large amounts of complex carbohydrates.
    (2) Diet is basically vegetarian combining corn, rice, and beans, a high-quality protein mixture.
    (3) Use of processed foods is low.
    (4) Many fruits and vegetables are popular but may not be available or affordable in the United States.
    (5) Many different spices and seasonings provide flavor.
    (6) Cheeses, a good source of calcium, are popular in meal preparation.
  d. Nutritionally harmful practices
    (1) With acculturation, animal protein intake is increasing.
    (2) Long cooking periods for vegetables cause heavy nutrient losses.
    (3) Most cooking procedures rely heavily on added saturated fats, especially lard, salt pork, and bacon fat.
    (4) Adults consume limited amounts of milk.
5. Italian practices
  a. Warmth and fellowship permeate leisurely mealtimes.
  b. Cultural foods are an integral component of family and social gatherings.
  c. Typical mealtimes include a light breakfast, larger lunch, and small evening meal.
  d. Nutritionally helpful practices
    (1) Complex carbohydrates (pastas and bread) are used extensively.
    (2) Foods are seasoned with olive oil, garlic, tomato puree, and a mixture of herbs.

(3) Consumption of greens and vegetables is high.
e. Nutritionally harmful practices
(1) Milk consumption is low.
(2) Breads may not be enriched and do not contain milk.
6. Native American practices
a. Food has great religious and social significance.
b. Traditional foods vary among tribes, but the basic diet consists of corn, beans, and squashes.
c. Diets on some reservations are poor, usually because of food availability and cost; some commodity foods may be available.
d. Poor nutrition is directly related to several leading causes of death: heart disease, cirrhosis of the liver, obesity, and obesity-related diabetes.
e. Nutritionally helpful practices
(1) Diets are high in carbohydrates.
f. Nutritionally harmful practices
(1) Diets are high in calories, saturated fat, sodium, and sugar.
(2) Fresh fruits and vegetables may not be available or are too expensive.
(3) The diet lacks variety.
7. Religious group influences on dietary practices
a. Jewish: All Orthodox and many Conservative Jews adhere to a kosher diet. Reform Jews do not usually follow kosher dietary laws. Intricate, complex guidelines for food preparation are required for a kosher diet. Pork, shellfish, and combining meat with milk products are prohibited. A dietary consult is highly recommended so appropriate changes can be made to increase compliance.
b. Muslim: Pork, pork products, foods made with pork, animal fat shortening, and alcoholic products or beverages are prohibited. Kosher meats are acceptable. Fasting is a common practice.
c. Seventh-Day Adventists: No alcoholic or caffeine-containing beverages are allowed. Between meal snacks are discouraged. A vegetarian diet may be followed. Meats, especially pork and shellfish, may be eliminated from the diet.

■ ASSESSING NUTRITIONAL STATUS

Purpose of Nutritional Screening

1. Nutritional screening is the gathering of subjective and objective data from the person, family members, and the

---

BOX 10–2. Diet History

I. Fluids
  A. Usual fluid intake amount
  B. Recent changes in amount (increased, decreased, or unchanged)
  C. Beverage preferences
  D. Frequency of intake
  E. Beverages not tolerated
II. Nutrition
  A. Recent weight changes
  B. Appetite and food preferences
    1. Recent appetite changes (increased, decreased, or unchanged)
    2. Amount of food eaten
    3. Favorite foods
    4. Foods disliked
    5. Foods not tolerated and why
    6. Food allergies
    7. Where meals are taken
    8. Duration of meals
    9. Who purchases and prepares the food
    10. Snacking habits
    11. Number of feedings daily
    12. Vitamin or mineral or other dietary supplements
    13. Budgeting problems
    14. Substance intake (type, including alcohol and drugs, and amount)
    15. Personal or religious restrictions (e.g., kosher or vegetarian)
  C. Diet
    1. Type of special diet
    2. Problems and concerns or successes with diet
    3. Nutrient adequacy*
      a. Dietary recall is a recollection of all foods and amounts eaten by the person on the previous day.
      b. Food diary is maintained by the person for 3 to 7 days

and consists of a record of foods eaten, the amounts, the method of preparation, where the food is eaten, and the time of intake.
      c. Food frequency form is a food checklist to ascertain the number of times per day, week, or month that specific foods or categories of food are eaten.
III. Current and previous medical-surgical problems involving nutrition
  A. Teeth and mouth
    1. Condition of teeth
    2. Dentures
    3. Difficulties in chewing
    4. Soreness in mouth
    5. Difficulty swallowing
    6. Problems with choking
    7. Recent changes in taste
  B. Gastrointestinal problems
    1. Excessive belching or heartburn
    2. Indigestion
    3. Nausea
    4. Vomiting
    5. Gastrointestinal surgeries
  C. Elimination problems
    1. Bowels
      a. Constipation or diarrhea
      b. Recent changes in bowel movements
      c. Frequency of bowel movements
      d. Use of laxatives or enemas, or other practices
    2. Difficulty urinating
      a. Recent changes (increased, decreased, or unchanged)
    3. Other physical or medical problems
    4. Current medications
  D. Physical assessment
    1. Anthropometric measures
    2. Laboratory test results

---

* These techniques for determining actual and habitual dietary intake provide a rough estimate of actual nutrient intake that can be compared with standards (RDA, Food Guide Pyramid, Dietary Guidelines for Americans).
From Davis JR, and Sherer K. *Applied Nutrition and Diet Therapy for Nurses.* 2nd ed. Philadelphia: WB Saunders, 1994, p 287.

Table 10–4. *Nutrient Antagonist Medications and Nutritional Interventions*

Medication	Nutrients Affected	Nursing Interventions
Antiacne		
Isotretinoin	Vitamin A	Avoid vitamin A supplements to prevent additive toxic effects. Monitor for skeletal changes with bony spurs.
Anticonvulsants		
Phenytoin, primidone	Vitamins D, K, B_{12}, and folic acid	Monitor for symptoms of deficiency, especially megaloblastic anemia. Supplement folate (< 5 mg/day), if ordered. Encourage some daily exposure to sunshine. Encourage intake of foods to provide needed vitamins. Provide supplements if needed.
Anti-inflammatory Drugs		
Aspirin	Vitamin C, folic acid, and iron	Monitor for hypoprothrombinemia and anemia. Provide vitamin C and folate supplements if needed. Advise person to take with meals, milk, or antacids and to avoid alcohol.
Sulfasalazine	Folic acid	Monitor for anemia (uncommon). Advise intake of good food sources.
Antimicrobials		
Moxalactam	Vitamin K	Monitor for bleeding problems. Encourage vitamin K–rich foods.
Neomycin	Vitamins A, D, K, B_{12}, and folic acid	Monitor nutrient levels, red blood count indices, and for diarrhea. Encourage well-balanced diet.
Pyrimethamine	Folic acid	Monitor for megaloblastic anemia. Treat with folate, > 25 mg/week, or supplement with folinic acid.
Trimethoprim	Folic acid	Monitor for megaloblastic anemia. Encourage intake of foods rich in folic acid.
Tetracycline	Folic acid, vitamins C and K, and calcium	Take medication 1 hr before meals or 2 hr after meals, not with milk formulas, dairy products, or iron supplements.
Antineoplastic		
Methotrexate	Folic acid, vitamin B_{12}	Monitor folate and vitamin B_{12} status and weight. Low serum folate levels predispose persons to toxic drug effects, but folate preparations alter drug responses. Be sure person is eating well and avoids alcohol. Suggest nutritional supplements if intake is poor.
Antiparkinsonian		
Levodopa	Vitamin B_6	Monitor for serum levels and physical signs of deficiency. Avoid vitamin supplements with high levels of pyridoxine. Take with carbohydrate foods to avoid gastrointestinal irritation but not with any high protein foods, which impair drug absorption.
Antipsychotic		
Chlorpromazine, thioridazine, fluphenazine, thiothixene	Riboflavin	Assist person in choosing low-calorie foods to help satiate the increased appetite. Monitor for riboflavin depletion. Avoid alcohol.
Antitubercular Drugs		
Isoniazid	Vitamin B_6, niacin, and vitamin D	Monitor for peripheral neuropathy, anemia, convulsions (infants). Give on empty stomach for optimal absorption, not with high-carbohydrate foods. Pyridoxine supplement recommended. Because some preparations already contain pyridoxine, check before giving the supplement.
Cardiovascular Drugs		
Cholestyramine or colestipol	Vitamins A, D, K, and folic acid; iron	Monitor vitamins B_{12} and A and red blood cell status. Encourage well-balanced low-fat diet. Provide supplements as needed.
Digitalis	Thiamin, potassium, magnesium	Monitor weight and appetite, potassium levels, and observe for unusual muscle weakness. Encourage high-potassium foods, low-sodium diet, and adequate intake of magnesium, calcium, and calories.
Hydralazine	Vitamins B_6 and D, niacin	Monitor for peripheral neuropathy and anemia. Pyridoxine supplement may be needed. Limit alcohol intake.
Thiazides	Potassium, glucose and lipid levels; magnesium, zinc	Monitor for laxative abuse, potassium levels, and blood glucose and lipid levels. Encourage increased potassium intake or supplements; encourage adequate magnesium and zinc intake.
Triamterene	Folic acid, potassium	Monitor folate levels. Avoid potassium-containing salt substitutes and large amounts of high-potassium foods. Encourage folate-rich foods.
Warfarin	Vitamin K	Encourage balanced diet with consistent intake of vitamin K. Check multivitamin preparations for vitamin K content. Monitor vegetarian diets. Avoid alcohol and vitamin E supplements.

Table 10–4. *Nutrient Antagonist Medications and Nutritional Interventions* (Continued)

Medication	Nutrients Affected	Nursing Interventions
Gastrointestinal Drugs		
Emollients	Vitamins A and D	Do not give with meals or when fat-soluble vitamins are eaten. Fat-soluble vitamin supplement may be needed.
Musculoskeletal Drugs		
Penicillamine	Vitamins B_6 and D, niacin, zinc, copper	Monitor pyridoxine level; for peripheral neuropathy, mineral depletion, and weight loss. Encourage well-balanced diet. Routine supplementation of pyridoxine is recommended for long-term therapy. Zinc deficiency may result in taste changes and decreased intake.
Oral Contraceptives		
Estrogen-progestin combinations	Vitamin B_6 and C, folic acid	Monitor folate levels; for megaloblastic anemia. Encourage foods high in folic acid and pyridoxine, but routine supplements are not necessary. Megadoses of vitamin C increase estrogen levels.

medical record to help determine nutritional status and identify people who may benefit from nutritional intervention.

2. For optimal effectiveness, nutritional screening includes consideration of physical, biochemical, and anthropometric parameters and a thorough dietary history.

History

1. Assess the intake of foods and the interrelationships among diet, medications, lifestyle, and physiologic-psychologic conditions to recognize actual or high-risk nutritional problems (Box 10–2).
2. Assess for any caloric excess or deficit in relationship to the person's gender, height, weight, and age.
3. Determine what, when, and how often the person is eating and why specific foods are eaten (likes, dislikes, intolerances, supplements, special diets).
4. Consider current and previous health problems (surgeries, disease processes) that may affect nutritional status.
5. Explore nutrient-drug interactions that may affect nutrition. Both prescription and over-the-counter drugs may lead to nutrient deficiencies secondary to decreased food intake or increased nutrient requirements because of altered nutrient absorption, metabolism, or excretion.
   a. Nutrient depletions occur gradually with regular drug use for long periods.
   b. Deficiencies most frequently occur in persons with multiple drug regimens; marginal nutritional status because of a poor diet, chronic disease, drug abuse, or physiologic stress; or impaired metabolic or excretory functions.

ELDER ADVISORY

Older people are particularly at risk for nutrient deficiencies because of their need for many drugs combined with poor eating habits and a slow rate of drug metabolism.

c. Medications that are particularly known for their antinutrient effects or are affected by large amounts of specific nutrients are listed in Table 10–4.
d. The nursing assessment should list all the drugs a person is taking—prescription, over the counter, and any home remedies, such as sodium bicarbonate or herbal teas.
e. When an expected response to a planned therapeutic program does not occur, consider the possibility of interactions among the disease state, drugs, and food.
f. Unless contraindicated, dietary modifications to include foods rich in the affected vitamins and minerals are preferable to taking supplements.
g. Advise against drastic modification of the diet or food "binges" without consulting the physician or pharmacist.
h. Teach the person about the purpose of the drug and the proper time to take it.

6. History of weight loss (see Box 10–2)
   a. Weight loss indicates the use of lean body mass (muscle and organ tissue), fat stores, or both for energy.
   b. If fluid loss is not significant, weight loss is a good indicator of current nutritional status.

NURSE ADVISORY

People, especially obese ones, with protein-energy malnutrition may maintain weight because water and collagen replace the fat and muscle tissue being catabolized.

c. The significance of involuntary weight loss is shown in Figure 10–3.

Physical Assessment

1. Physical assessment can reveal existing nutritional deficiencies and must correlate with other assessment parameters (laboratory data and dietary history).

Body Weight

Desirable Body Weight (Hamwi Method)

a. Males: 106 lb for the first 5 ft;
             6 lb for each inch over 5 ft.
b. Females: 100 lb for the first 5 ft;
             5 lb for each inch over 5 ft.
c. Frame: Add 10% for large frame.
             Subtract 10% for small frame.

Frame Size

1. Measure the client's right wrist (in centimeters) at the point of smallest circumference, just distal to the styloid process of the radius and ulna.

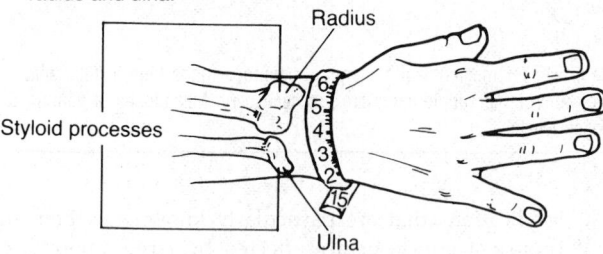

2. Obtain the client's height (in centimeters) without shoes.

3. Divide the client's wrist circumference into the height to obtain the "r" value:

$$r = \frac{\text{height (in cm)}}{\text{wrist circumference (in cm)}}$$

4. Use the chart shown to determine the client's body frame size based on the calculated "r" value and sex:

	Adult Males	Adult Females
Small frame	r>10.4	r>10.9
Medium frame	r = 9.6 – 10.4	r = 9.9 – 10.9
Large frame	r<9.6	r<9.9

(Adapted from Grant JP, et al. Current techniques of nutritional assessment. *Surg Clin North Am* 61: 437–463, 1981.)

Classification of Weight (based on deviations from ideal body weight [IBW])

$$\% \text{ IBW} = \frac{\text{Actual weight}}{\text{Usual body weight}} \times 100$$

% IBW	Indication
>120	Obesity
110–120	Moderately overweight
80–90	Moderate depletion
<70	Severe depletion

Weight Changes

$$\text{Percent weight change} = \frac{(\text{Usual weight} - \text{actual weight})}{\text{Usual weight}} \times 100$$

Time	Significant weight loss	Severe weight loss
1 month	5%	>5%
3 months	7.5%	>7.5%
6 months	10%	>10%

Body Fat

Classification	Men	Women
Desirable	15–18%	20–25%
Minimal	2–3%	12%
Obesity	25%	30%

Body Mass Index

Body mass index can be determined by using the formula:

$$\text{Body mass index (BMI)} = \frac{\text{Weight (kg)}}{\text{Height}^2 \text{ (m}^2)}$$

Or by using the nomogram below: After measuring height to the nearest inch and weight to the nearest pound, mark the values on the nomogram. Use a straight edge to connect the 2 points and circle the spot where this straight line crosses the center line (body mass index).

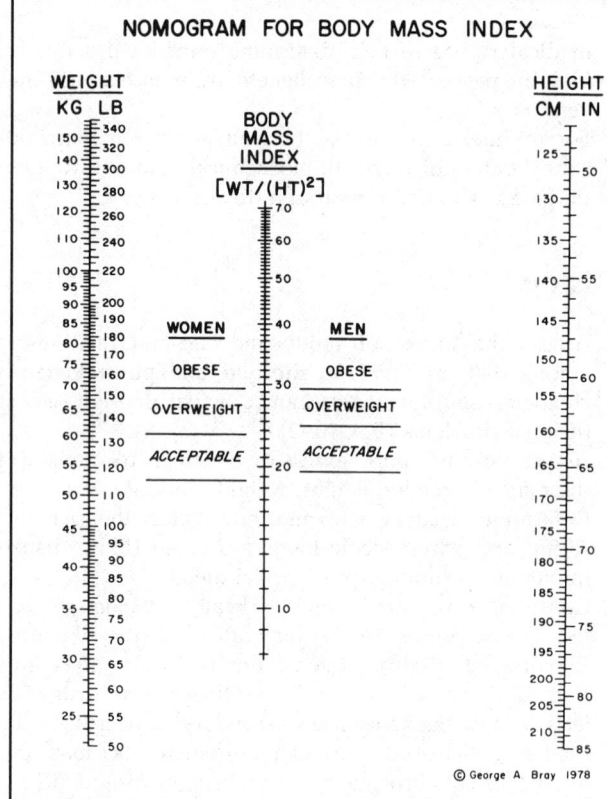

Classification of BMI	Kg/m²
Underweight	<20 for men
	<19 for women
Acceptable	20–25
Obesity (low risk for health problems)	25–30
High risk	35–40
Very high risk	>40

Figure 10–3. Anthropometric assessment tools. Nomogram © George A. Bray, M.D., 1978.

2. Table 10-5 lists clinical findings that are associated with specific nutrient deficiencies.

Anthropometric Measurements

1. Height
   a. Information provided by the person or a family member is usually inaccurate.
   b. Obtain a baseline height without shoes, noting any spinal curvature.
2. Body frame
   a. Bone structure determines body frame size.
   b. Determine frame size by wrist measurement (see Fig. 10-3).
   c. Body frame helps determine appropriate weight.
3. Weight
   a. An accurate body weight is the cornerstone of a good nutritional assessment and a baseline for future reference.
   b. Weight is a nonspecific measure of all body components, including fat, protein, and water.
   c. Desirable body weight, or IBW, is a weight for height that is considered healthy for a person.
      (1) Use the formula shown in Figure 10-3 to estimate IBW.
      (2) The Metropolitan Life Insurance Table is another standard for determining desirable weight (Table 10-6)
      (3) Weight can be classified based on deviations from IBW (see Fig. 10-3).
   d. Compare accurate weights with standards to determine whether the person is overweight, at IBW, or underweight.
   e. In the hospital, weigh persons daily or as ordered, at the same time of day with approximately the same amount of clothing.
   f. Weight is frequently used to assess nutritional status, but body fat is the main health concern.
   g. Usual body weight is more useful than IBW when working with ill persons.
4. Body fat
   a. Fat and weight distribution
      (1) Location of fat stores is classified as android or gynoid obesity.
      (2) **Android obesity** (apple-shaped bodies) indicates excessive fat stores in the abdominal area; is characteristic of men; and is associated with increased risk of coronary heart disease, hypertension, and certain cancers (especially breast and endometrial).
      (3) **Gynoid obesity** (pear-shaped bodies) indicates fat stores in the hips or femoral area; it is typical of women and relatively benign. Those with gynoid obesity have more difficulty losing weight and maintaining IBW.
      (4) More information on body fat is in Figure 10-3.
   b. Body mass index
      (1) Body mass index estimates total body mass but shows the highest correlation with actual body fat.
      (2) Determine body mass index and classifications using the information provided in Figure 10-3.
   c. Skinfold measurements
      (1) Skinfold measurements indirectly measure body fat, reflecting subcutaneous fat stores.
      (2) Special skinfold calipers are used.
      (3) Triceps skinfold measurements are determined most frequently. Because they require practice to ensure both precision and accuracy, dietitians usually perform this assessment.
   d. Underwater weighing
      (1) Many sports and fitness centers determine body fat by weighing the body under water.
      (2) This relatively simple technique is the most reliable method of determining body fat and fat-free mass.
      (3) The weight of a submerged body is compared with its out-of-water weight to estimate body density.
   e. Electrical impedance measurements
      (1) Total body electrical conductivity estimates body fat and lean tissue based on differences in electromagnetic waves.
      (2) Electrodes placed on the body measure the impedance or resistance.
      (3) Results are very reliable compared with those of underwater weighing.
5. Midarm circumference
   a. This test, usually conducted by a registered dietitian, is an index of the arm's total area and reflects caloric adequacy.
   b. Using an equation, the amount of subcutaneous fat (measured by skinfold thickness) is subtracted from the midarm circumference to estimate lean tissue in the arm.
   c. Midarm circumference indirectly measures body proteins.

Psychosocial Assessment

1. Emotions, feelings, and attitudes can alter food intake.
   a. Depression and suicidal tendencies usually cause a person to decrease food intake.
   b. Anxiety may lead to increased food intake.
   c. Food intake may decrease if a person is angry or afraid.
   d. Fear of becoming fat can decrease intake severely.
      (1) Some mental illnesses can result in physical signs and symptoms that affect nutritional status, such as binging and purging or self-inflicted starvation.
2. Economic and social factors can also affect nutritional status.
   a. Funds available for food purchases.
   b. Types of transportation and facilities available for purchasing, preparing, and storing foods.
   c. People experiencing loneliness or living alone generally do not eat as much as people who eat with others.

Laboratory Tests

1. Protein levels. Serum proteins (albumin, transferrin, and prealbumin levels) and 24-hour urine urea nitrogen excretion reflect visceral protein stores (Table 10-7).

Table 10–5. Clinical Findings Associated with Specific Nutrient Deficiencies

	Physical Findings	Possible Nutrient Deficiency
Hair	Alopecia (loss of hair)	Protein, biotin, zinc
	Dyspigmentation	Protein, biotin
	Flag sign	Protein
	Easily plucked hair	Protein
Nails	Transverse ridging	Protein
	Koilonychia (spoon shaped)	Iron
Skin	Dryness	Vitamin A, essential fatty acids, zinc
	Follicular hyperkeratosis (resembles goose flesh on buttocks and arms)	Vitamins A and C, essential fatty acids
	Petechiae	Vitamin C
	Purpura	Vitamins C and K
	Dermatitis	Niacin
	Nasolabial seborrhea	Niacin, riboflavin, vitamin B_6
	Pigmentation, desquamation of sun-exposed areas	Niacin
Eyes	Night blindness, Bitot's spots, xerophthalmia (dry, thickened conjunctiva and cornea)	Vitamin A
	Angular blepharitis	Riboflavin
Perioral	Cheilosis (cracks at the corner of the lips)	Vitamin B_6, riboflavin, niacin
	Angular stomatitis (inflamed oral mucous membranes)	Riboflavin, niacin, vitamin B_6
Oral	Bleeding, swollen gums	Vitamin C
	Magenta tongue	Riboflavin
	Atrophic papillae	Iron, niacin, folate, vitamins B_{12} and E
	Glossitis (beefy, red, swollen tongue)	Riboflavin, niacin, folate, iron, vitamins B_6 and B_{12}
	Hypogeusia	Zinc
Subcutaneous tissue	Edema	Protein, thiamin
	Wasted	Energy
Musculoskeletal system	Muscle wasting	Protein
	Bowlegs	Vitamin D, calcium
	Beading of ribs	Vitamin D, protein
	Tenderness	Vitamin C
Neurologic	Dementia	Niacin, vitamin B_{12}
	Confabulation, disorientation	Thiamin
	Peripheral neuropathy	Thiamin, vitamins B_6 and B_{12}
	Tetany	Calcium, magnesium
Other	Parotid enlargement	Protein
	Heart failure	Thiamin, phosphorus
	Poor wound healing, decubitus ulcers	Protein, vitamin C, zinc
	Hepatomegaly	Protein

NURSE ADVISORY

Although protein levels do not always indicate malnutrition, they do indicate an increased *risk* of malnutrition and a critical need for adequate nutrition.

a. Albumin provides 70 percent of colloid osmotic pressure of plasma.

(1) Levels indicate rate of synthesis by the liver, catabolism, loss into interstitial fluids, or abnormal external losses.
(2) Albumin levels are good indicators of long-term nutritional status if no current illness or condition is present.
(3) Decreased albumin results in peripheral edema, decreased nutrient absorption, and less transport of small molecules (medications, hormones, and vitamins).

Table 10–6. Metropolitan Life Height and Weight Tables

Men					Women				
Height		Small Frame	Medium Frame	Large Frame	Height		Small Frame	Medium Frame	Large Frame
Feet	*Inches*				*Feet*	*Inches*			
5	2	128–134	131–141	138–150	4	10	102–111	109–121	118–131
5	3	130–136	133–143	140–153	4	11	103–113	111–123	120–134
5	4	132–138	135–145	152–156	5	0	104–115	113–126	122–137
5	5	134–140	137–148	144–160	5	1	106–118	115–129	125–140
5	6	136–142	139–151	146–164	5	2	108–121	118–132	128–143
5	7	138–145	142–154	149–168	5	3	111–124	121–135	131–147
5	8	140–148	145–157	152–172	5	4	114–127	124–138	134–151
5	9	142–151	148–160	155–176	5	5	117–130	127–141	137–155
5	10	144–154	151–163	158–180	5	6	120–133	130–144	140–159
5	11	146–157	154–166	161–184	5	7	123–136	133–147	143–163
6	0	149–160	157–170	164–188	5	8	126–139	136–150	146–167
6	1	152–164	160–174	168–192	5	9	129–142	139–153	149–170
6	2	155–168	164–178	172–197	5	10	132–145	142–156	152–173
6	3	158–172	167–182	176–202	5	11	135–148	145–159	155–176
6	4	162–176	171–187	181–207	6	0	138–151	148–162	158–179

Weights at ages 25–59 based on lowest mortality. Weight in pounds according to frame (in indoor clothing weighing 5 lbs, shoes with 1-inch heels).

Courtesy of the Metropolitan Life Insurance Co., New York, *Statistical Bulletin.*

Weights at ages 25–59 based on lowest mortality. Weight in pounds according to frame (in indoor clothing weighing 3 lbs, shoes with 1-inch heels).

b. Transferrin is an iron-carrying protein.
   (1) Transferrin reflects short-term changes in visceral proteins and is more sensitive regarding current nutritional status.
   (2) It is unreliable as a nutritional marker when hydration status is abnormal (fluid volume excess or fluid volume deficit).
   (3) Low levels indicate higher risk for anergy, sepsis, and mortality.
c. Thyroxine-binding prealbumin is a carrier protein for retinol-binding protein.
   (1) It correlates better with nitrogen balance than albumin or transferrin.
   (2) Prealbumin levels drop rapidly with sudden demands for protein synthesis, which occur with infection and trauma.
d. A 24-hour urinary nitrogen excretion determines the extent of protein breakdown and adequacy of protein intake.

   (1) Ammonia, a toxic substance, is changed to urea in the liver and excreted in the urine.
   (2) Negative nitrogen balance occurs when protein breakdown is higher than rates of synthesis.
   (3) To determine balance, food intake records and urine samples are collected concurrently.
   • Nurses record the type and amount of all foods and fluids consumed.
   • Nurses collect all urine excreted during the 24-hour period, as ordered.
   • Nurses maintain an accurate 24-hour stool collection, if ordered.
   • Dietitians determine the amount of nitrogen consumed from records maintained by the nurse.
   • Laboratory determines the amount of nitrogen in urine and stool.
   • Dietitians or the physician calculate whether the person is in nitrogen balance.

Table 10–7. Assessment of Visceral Proteins

Protein	Function	Normal	Degree of Malnutrition		
			Mild	*Moderate*	*Severe*
Albumin (g/dl)	Carrier protein; maintains colloid osmotic pressure	>3.5	3.0–3.5	2.5–3.0	<2.5
Transferrin (mg/dl)	Transports iron	>200	180–200	160–180	<160
Prealbumin (mg/dl)	Transports thyroxin and retinol-binding protein	>15	10–15	5–10	<5
Total lymphocyte count (mm³)	Reflects immune and protein status	>1500	1200–1500	800–1200	<800

From Davis JR, and Sherer K. *Applied Nutrition and Diet Therapy for Nurses.* 2nd ed. Philadelphia: WB Saunders, 1994.

2. Total lymphocyte count (TLC) reflects immune status and may indicate the severity of protein malnutrition because proteins are necessary to produce antibodies (see Table 10–7). Calculate the TLC from the complete white blood count (WBC) and percentage of lymphocytes using this formula:

$$TLC = \text{percent of lymphocyte (use decimal)} \times WBC$$

3. Lipid levels. Cholesterol, low-density lipoprotein, and high-density lipoprotein levels reflect dietary intake of fat and are indicators for risk of cardiovascular disease. If cholesterol and low-density lipoprotein levels are high, the person is at increased risk of heart disease and generally has a high fat intake, especially of saturated fat.
4. Blood glucose levels. The body's cells prefer glucose for energy. A consistent blood glucose level is necessary for normal body functioning. If the level is too low, hypoglycemia results; if the level is too high, hyperglycemia can occur.
5. Urinalysis
   a. Recent nutrient intake rather than usual intake is reflected in urine findings.
   b. Two findings are important when assessing nutrient intake.
      (1) Urine protein levels—usually negative. If positive, the person is losing protein, which reduces building and repairing of the body.
      (2) Urine ketones levels—normally negative. If positive, the person is using fat for energy rather than carbohydrates, indicating the person is not receiving enough carbohydrate intake or carbohydrates are not being utilized properly by the body.

◼ DIETARY INTERVENTIONS

Therapeutic Diets

There are many different diets used as part of therapy for various disorders including hospital, dysphagia, low-fat, low-residue, low-sodium, and soft diets. Only the more commonly used diets are discussed.

1. Hospital diets. See Table 10–8 for the various hospital diets
2. Dysphagia diets
   a. Purpose: A dysphagia diet decreases the risk of aspiration in persons who are unable to swallow safely because of neurologic deficits.

NURSE ADVISORY

Be careful not to confuse a texture-modified diet for persons with chewing problems and a texture-modified diet for persons with swallowing problems. Texture modifications for chewing problems are usually individualized according to the person's tolerance and acceptance (chopped, ground, or pureed). Dysphagia diets specify the texture of the food and the type of liquid tolerated.

   b. Dysphagia should be suspected if a person has weak facial (drooping mouth), oral, neck, or tongue muscles or if a person coughs or chokes frequently when taking foods or fluids.
   c. Assessment includes evaluating the medical history and diet history, performing physical and neurologic examinations, and videotaping a barium swallow.
   d. Special considerations
      (1) Usually the speech-language pathologist provides training and recommends specific techniques to facilitate a safe swallow. These guidelines are followed for anything provided orally (medications, fluids) (Box 10–3).
      (2) People with dysphagia are sometimes allowed nothing by mouth and receive nutriment via tube feedings while receiving oral-pharyngeal muscle therapy when relearning to swallow safely.
      (3) If the person can swallow some foods safely, the diet order specifies consistency or texture of foods (pureed, pureed with texture, finely chopped, chopped foods) and thickness of liquids (thin, medium thick, or spoon thick).
      (4) Unless recommended by a speech-language pathologist, avoid pureed foods because their lack of texture fails to stimulate a swallow reflex, thereby increasing aspiration risk.
      (5) Normal diet texture progression is from thick pureed foods (semisolid consistency) to foods requiring little chewing (ground) to chewable foods in bite-sized pieces (sugar cube size).
3. Low-fat diets
   a. Purpose: Low-fat diets are appropriate to prevent and treat chronic health problems (e.g., obesity, heart disease, cancer).
      (1) They may also be ordered to relieve symptoms associated with specific health problems in which the body is unable to digest or absorb fats—diarrhea and steatorrhea.
      (2) Low-fat diets are used for **maldigestion** (chronic pancreatitis, cystic fibrosis, postgastrectomy dumping syndrome, pernicious anemia, biliary obstruction, cholestyramine) and for **malabsorption** (various abnormalities in the small bowel such as Crohn's disease, small bowel resection, tropical sprue, celiac disease).
   b. Special considerations
      (1) Explain to the person why food choices should be altered.
      (2) Teach the person which foods to eliminate from the diet and alternatives for maintaining adequate nutrient intake (Table 10–9).
      (3) Explain how much fat is allowed and how to determine fat content of food by reading nutrition labels. (Labels show gm of fat and percentage of fat for a 2000-calorie diet.) Malabsorption disorders are usually controlled by limiting fat to 50 gm daily. Diets to prevent chronic diseases, to encourage weight loss, and to prevent heart disease usually limit fat to less than 30 percent of the total caloric intake. To determine the percentage of fat a specific food provides for a given caloric

Table 10–8. Types of Hospital Diets

	Clear Liquid Diet	Full Liquid Diet	Soft Diet*	Regular—House General—Full
Description	Temporary diet consisting of clear liquids without residue; nonstimulating, non–gas-forming, nonirritating	Diet liquid at room temperature or liquefied at body temperature	Normal diet modified in consistency to have no roughage Liquids and semisolid food; easily digested	Practically all foods; simple, easy-to-digest foods, simply prepared, palatably seasoned
Adequacy	Inadequate: lacking in protein, minerals, vitamins, and calories	Can be adequate with careful planning: adequacy depends on liquids consumed	Entirely adequate liberal diet	Adequate and well balanced
Uses	Acute illness and infections Postoperatively Temporary food intolerance To relieve thirst Reduce colonic fecal matter 1- to 2-hr feeding intervals	Between clear liquid and soft diets Postoperatively Acute gastritis and infections Febrile disorders Intolerance for solid food 2- to 4-hr feeding intervals	Between full liquid and light or regular diet Between acute illness and convalescence Acute infections Chewing difficulties Gastrointestinal disorders 3 meals with or without between-meal feedings	For uniformity and convenience in serving hospital patients Ambulatory people Immobilized people not requiring therapeutic diets
Foods Allowed	Water, tea, coffee, coffee substitutes Fat-free broth Carbonated beverages Synthetic fruit juices Ginger ale Plain gelatin Sugar	All liquids on clear liquid diet plus: All forms of milk Strained soups Fruit and vegetable juices Eggnog Plain ice cream and sherbet Plain gelatin dishes Soft custard Cereal gruels	All liquids Fine and strained cereals Cooked tender or puréed vegetables Cooked fruits without skins and seeds Ripe bananas Ground or minced meat, fish, poultry Eggs and mild cheeses Plain cake and puddings Moderately seasoned foods	All types of foods
Modifications	Liberal clear liquid diet: add fruit juices, egg white, whole egg, thin gruels	Consistency for tube feedings: foods that will pass through tube easily	Low residue—no fiber Bland—no chemical, thermal, physical stimulants Cold soft—tonsillectomy Mechanical soft—requiring no mastication Light diet—intermediate between soft and regular	For a light or convalescent diet: fried foods, rich pastries, fat-rich foods, coarse vegetables, raw fruits may be omitted

*Because of trend toward more liberal interpretation of diets and foods, soft diet may be combined with light diet in some hospitals.
Modified from Keane CB. *Saunders Review for Practical Nurses.* 4th ed. Philadelphia: WB Saunders, 1982.

level, use the following equation:

$$\text{Gm of fat in a food} \times 9 = \text{total calories provided by fat}$$

$$\frac{\text{Total fat calories}}{\text{Total calories required}} \times 100 = \text{\% total calories from fat}$$

If a food contains less than 30 percent fat, it is generally a wise choice, but some fats and oils that are 100 percent fat are necessary to provide adequate fat-soluble vitamins and essential fatty acids; therefore, food items are averaged together to determine whether an item that exceeds 30 percent fat would cause the day's or week's intake to exceed the overall 30 percent desired fat level.

(4) Emphasize that if weight maintenance is the goal, the person will need to eat significantly more food.

(5) Fruits and vegetables (except avocado, olives, and coconut) contain minimal amounts of fat; liberal use of these is desirable.

4. Low-residue diets

a. Purpose: Low-residue (low-fiber) diets place less strain on intestines because this type of diet is easier to digest.

b. This diet is usually used for ulcerative colitis, diverticulitis, and irritable bowel syndrome.

c. Special considerations

(1) Limit milk and milk products to 2 cups per day.

BOX 10-3. Nursing Interventions for People with Dysphagia

Safety Tips for Preventing Aspiration

1. If the person experiences difficulty with foods or liquids or coughs and chokes, discontinue the feeding. Note any particular types of food or textures that cause problems and report to physician, speech language pathologist, or dietitian.
2. Be sure suction equipment is within reach when providing anything orally.
3. Do not allow individual to self-feed unless the person will be safe and alert throughout the meal. The person's safety is paramount.
4. Position person in an upright sitting position with 90-degree flexion at the hips during eating to prevent aspiration. A semiupright position (30–45 degrees) is maintained for at least 30 minutes following feedings.
5. Sufficient time for eating must be allowed. However, after eating for about 30 minutes, the person may tire which will increase risks of a dysfunctional swallow; small, frequent (4–6) feedings promote adequate nutrition without tiring.
6. Make sure the person is well rested before feeding, and remove distractions during feeding to allow concentration on chewing and swallowing.
7. If one side of the face is weak or paralyzed, head rotation toward the weaker side will improve swallowing. Neck flexion during swallowing facilitates glottis closure and enhances swallowing.
8. Place food on stronger side of mouth if individual has had a stroke affecting 1 side of the body.
9. Check the person's mouth after meals and remove any pocketed food with a toothette (a spongy tip on a stick used to cleanse the oral cavity) to decrease chances of inadvertent aspiration of food retained in the mouth.

Tips for Feeding the Person

1. If the person must be fed, begin by offering a quarter teaspoonful of food. Never give more than one half a heaping teaspoon; too much food may cause the patient to aspirate.
2. Apply slight downward pressure on the tongue when removing a spoon from the mouth.
3. Watch the thyroid cartilage (Adam's apple) to determine whether the person has swallowed before giving more food or drink.
4. Allow the person to indicate readiness for the next mouthful.
5. Converse only as needed. Communication may be distracting for people who are relearning the swallowing process, but verbal direction for eating may be necessary.

Tips About Foods, Aromas, and Temperature

1. If excessive drooling or salivation occurs or if excessively thick phlegm is produced, avoid uncooked milk products (milk and ice cream). Cream soups and puddings are acceptable. Some juices, such as cranberry, pineapple, and grapefruit (thicken if needed), or papain may help cut mucus.
2. Slippery foods are easier to swallow but more difficult to control in the mouth during mastication (e.g., toast is tolerated better than bread, a boiled potato instead of mashed potatoes).

3. Moistened foods can be manipulated easier in the mouth; use gravies, sauces, mayonnaise, or catsup to moisten foods.
4. Foods that fall apart easily, such as corn kernels or peas, plain ground meat, rice, and dry cottage cheese, can be aspirated easily.
5. Sticky foods such as peanut butter or soft bread with a hard crust should be avoided.
6. Foods with a combination of textures, such as soups, are very difficult to control orally until a swallow is initiated.
7. Mildly sweetened and salted foods are generally favored because flavor initiates a better swallow by increasing saliva production.
8. Temperature guidelines provided by the speech language pathologist are important because food temperatures (hot or cold) may be necessary to stimulate the swallow reflex. When nerve function is impaired, cold temperatures stimulate swallowing.
9. Thin beverages are the most difficult to manipulate; thickened beverages are easier for the tongue to manipulate and will help initiate the oral phase of swallowing. Beverages may be thickened to nectar, honey, or pudding consistency using a modified food starch, such as Thick-it (Milani), or Thick and Easy (American Institutional Products).

Adaptive Equipment

1. Utilize adaptive equipment per speech language pathologist's recommendation.
2. If the person tends to put too much food into the mouth too rapidly, place a single food item in front of the person and provide a spoon with a small bowl to limit bite size.
3. For individuals who can close lips but have a weak or delayed swallow reflex, offer fluids in a glass that is three quarters full to prevent tilting the head too far back.
4. Use cutout nose glass if recommended by the speech language pathologist. For people who have difficulty propelling liquids back into the mouth but have a functional swallow reflex, offer fluids in a glass that is one third or less full to promote tilting the head back so fluid flows further back into the throat.

Monitoring

1. Hydration status is frequently overlooked. Because thickened beverages are not well accepted, the person may consume less fluid. Plain or flavored gelatin, thick sauces, creamed soups, and pureed fruits and vegetables in an appropriate consistency can increase fluid intake.
2. Monitor for deterioration of nutritional status, as food intake frequently decreases because of decreased palatability, apathy, poor endurance, or depression; note and report intake and weight loss to a dietitian or physician. Nutritional supplements (thickened or puddings) can provide complete nutrition in a concentrated form when appetite is poor.
3. If person is taking an anticholinergic drug, monitor swallowing. Anticholinergic medications decrease saliva and make swallowing more difficult.

---

(2) Fruits and vegetables without skins are allowed. Fruit (except prune) and vegetable juices are also desirable. Canned fruit and cooked tender vegetables such as asparagus, green beans, tomato sauce, and eggplant can be included.

(3) White or refined breads and cereals are encouraged.

(4) All types of lean tender meats without grease are allowed.

5. Low-sodium diets

a. Purpose: Low-sodium diets are appropriate to treat chronic cardiovascular heart problems (hypertension, heart disease, congestive heart failure) and diseases causing fluid retention (cirrhosis).

Table 10–9. Guidelines for Low-Fat Diets

Frequently Consumed High-Fat Foods	Alternative Foods
Fried foods	Roast, bake, grill, stir-fry, or broil foods when possible. Baste meats with broth or stock. Use nonstick cookware and an aerosol cooking spray.
Fatty meats (bacon, sausage, choice grade meats, frankfurters, luncheon meats)	Choose 2 or 3 servings of meat, poultry, or fish with a daily total of about 6 oz. Choose a vegetarian entree (dry beans and peas) at least once a week. Trim visible fat from meat; remove skin from poultry before eating. Choose beef grade "select" because it contains less fat marbling. Leaner cuts of meat include flank, sirloin, or tenderloin, loin pork chops. Marinate leaner cuts of meat in lemon juice, flavored vinegars, or fruit juices.
Cheese (aged cheese and cream cheese)	Choose cheese with 6 gm or less of fat/oz such as farmer's cheese.
High-fat snacks (potato chips, some crackers, dips)	Substitute pretzels, fat-free chips, regular crackers.
Salad dressing, mayonnaise, sour cream	Use fat-free or reduced-fat salad dressings and sour cream. Substitute plain low-fat yogurt for mayonnaise or sour cream. Rely on mustard and salad greens to add moisture to sandwiches rather than high-fat spreads.
Gravies	Use the paste method for making gravy or sauces (add flour or cornstarch to cold liquids slowly and blend well).
Homogenized whole milk products	Use skim milk, buttermilk, low-fat yogurt, and cottage cheese.
Margarine and seasonings such as lard, bacon, or ham	Use jam, jelly, or marmalade spread instead of butter or margarine. Season with herbs, lemon juice, or stock rather than lard, bacon, or ham.

b. Special considerations
   (1) Explain to the person why food choices must be altered. Almost all foods and beverages, including water, contain sodium.
   (2) Teach the person which foods to eliminate or decrease in the diet.
   (3) Explain how much sodium is allowed and how to determine sodium content of food by reading nutrition labels. Any listing of "sodium," "Na+," "NaCl," or "MSG" indicates sources of sodium. If the food product contains less than 140 mg per serving and per 100 gm of food, it can be labeled low sodium. One gm of salt contains 388 mg of sodium. Processed foods, including canned, boxed, and some frozen foods (excluding fruits and vegetables), are high in sodium. Baking powder, baking soda, meat tenderizer, and soy sauce contain large amounts of sodium.
   c. Several levels of dietary sodium restriction can be ordered:
      (1) **No added salt:** Consists of 4 to 5 gm per day. Avoid salty and high-sodium processed foods. Avoid adding salt to food at the table. Small amounts may be used in cooking.
      (2) **Mild restriction:** Consists of 2 to 3 gm per day. Foods can be lightly salted during cooking, but salt is not allowed at the table. Pickles, olives, bacon, ham, chips, canned soups, salted nuts, and crackers are omitted.
      (3) **Moderate and severe restriction:** Generally not used for long periods of time because of noncompliance. These diets are useful in treating edema or severe congestive heart failure or cirrhosis with massive edema. Moderate restriction consists of 1 gm of sodium per day; severe is 0.5 gm per day.
      (4) Medications, especially some antacids, cough medicines, and laxatives, are high in sodium. Intake of these medications is monitored and in some cases discontinued.
6. Soft diet. See Table 10–8.

NURSE ADVISORY

When a strict sodium restriction is imposed, monitor food intake because some people, especially older people, have difficulty adjusting to these dietary changes. If food intake is severely curtailed as a result of the diet, consult a registered dietitian or the physician for possible alternatives.

Nutritional Support

1. Goals
   a. Replete body stores or prevent nutritional deficiencies when oral intake is inadequate to meet nutritional requirements.
   b. Different methods of providing increased nutritional support are employed when appetite is poor, early satiety occurs, nausea and vomiting are present, oral feedings are hazardous, or the GI tract is not functioning.
      (1) The preferred method is to provide oral feedings using frequent feedings of regular foods or foods modified in texture, flavor, or both.
      (2) If the person is unable to consume adequate amounts of regular foods, oral supplements of nutritionally complete formulas can be an adjunct to the normal diet.
      (3) Alternative methods of nutriment (enteral or parenteral nutrition) can maintain nutritional status if oral feedings are inadequate.
2. Controlling anorexia
   a. Controlling physical conditions that help make eating more pleasant can increase nutrient intake.

(1) Keep the environment clean and attractive.

(2) Protect the person from unpleasant odors and sights.

(3) Make sure the person is well rested before meals by scheduling unpleasant or painful procedures or treatments at least 1 hour before meals.

(4) Provide personal hygiene before meals.

(5) Provide comfort measure (back massage or linen change) before meals.

(6) If needed allow person to go to the bathroom before meals.

(7) Depending on medical condition, place person in a comfortable eating position.

(8) Assist person with preparing (opening cartons, cutting meat, buttering bread) and eating food as needed.

3. Antinausea and vomiting interventions

a. Withhold liquids and foods until vomiting is arrested; then begin with clear liquids or crushed ice.

b. Initially offer apple juice, iced tea, dry crackers or dry toast, and gelatin. Then proceed with other clear, cold beverages or juices followed by small quantities of easily digested foods, as tolerated.

c. Limit fluids during mealtimes, including soups. Liquids may be better tolerated before or after the meal.

d. Encourage soft, bland foods such as rice, soft-cooked eggs, custards, nectars, cottage cheese, applesauce, and vanilla ice cream.

e. Avoid offering highly spiced and acidic foods because these may be poorly tolerated.

f. Avoid fried, greasy, or fatty foods.

g. Offer cold foods or foods at room temperature rather than hot foods because cold foods are better tolerated.

h. Provide small, frequent feedings to avoid an empty stomach and increase food intake. Always have snacks available; waiting even for a few minutes may lessen the desire to eat.

i. Encourage the person to eat slowly, take small bites, and chew foods thoroughly.

j. Suggest avoiding cooking foods or being in areas during food preparation, as aromas from hot foods may aggravate nausea.

k. Alter mealtimes to coincide with the person's appetite.

l. Provide antiemetic medications 30 minutes before meals, if ordered.

m. Avoid favorite foods when the stomach is upset to prevent learned aversions.

n. Encourage family members to suggest and provide favorite foods when the person is feeling well.

o. Encourage the person to rest for approximately 1 hour after food intake. If reclining, have head 4 inches above the feet.

4. Interventions to avoid early satiety

a. Keep a diet diary to determine how much is being eaten.

b. Encourage foods high in carbohydrates because these foods are digested faster, which prevents early satiety and improves the ability to eat more often.

c. Provide small, frequent feedings.

d. Frequently offer small amounts of easily digestible foods.

e. Provide snacks.

5. Interventions to increase nutrient intake

a. Suggest alternative foods for restricted foods that retain the cultural, social, and personal habits of the person.

b. Educate and plan with the person to reconstruct eating habits so that more nutritious foods are chosen.

(1) Explain how the diet enhances health and minimizes discomforts of the disease.

(2) Use "teachable moments" to stress good nutrition, for example, when watching food commercials, when completing the food menu, and when eating meals.

(3) Plan methods to implement the diet at home by exploring the specific needs of the person and the workability of the diet.

c. Include high-calorie, nutrient-dense snacks or nutrition supplements rather than foods that are low in calories or contain minimal nutrients (e.g., salads, broth-type soups, carbonated beverages).

d. Maintain an inventory of easy-to-prepare foods such as frozen dinners, eggs, and nutrition supplements.

e. Offer high-calorie, high-protein milk shakes that can be prepared in advance, frozen in individual portions, and slightly thawed in the microwave when needed.

f. If tolerated, add skim milk powder or evaporated milk to dishes such as casseroles, hot cereals, and mashed potatoes.

g. Encourage snacks such as ice cream, puddings, cheese, and dried fruit.

h. Use evaporated milk, half-and-half, or cream rather than milk in drinks or food preparation.

i. Add cheese to casserole-type dishes, sandwiches, vegetables, and eggs.

j. Add fats, such as gravies, butter, cream, creamed soups, and whole milk, to provide a concentrated source of calories and reduce the volume of food needed.

k. Provide high-fat breads such as muffins, biscuits, and croissants.

l. Avoid artificial sweeteners; instead use sugar, honey, or corn syrup.

m. Encourage minimal amounts of liquids at mealtime.

n. Provide small, frequent feedings.

o. Serve a larger meal when the person's appetite is best.

p. Suggest liquid (or pudding) nutritional supplements because these products are more nutrient dense than most foods and provide protein, vitamins, and minerals that enhance oral intake. If several nutritional supplements are available, allow the person to choose preferred formulas to ensure compliance. Very cold supplements are more palatable. Persons will usually consume more supplement if it is left in an ice bucket in the room.

q. Suggest glucose polymers, such as Polycose (Ross) or Moducal (Mead Johnson), to provide needed calories and spare protein. Their mild sweetening effect only slightly alters the taste of foods.

r. Suggest the use of a fat supplement, such as Microlipid (Sherwood Medical), to provide a concentrated form of calories.

Enteral Nutrition

1. Advantages
   a. Tube feedings are physiologically more natural, less expensive, and nutritionally more complete than routine intravenous solutions for persons who are unable to consume adequate calories orally but who have a functional GI tract.
   b. The gut uses nutrients more efficiently, and fewer metabolic upsets occur.
   c. Use of the GI tract helps maintain intestinal integrity by promoting anatomic or immune functions.
   d. Early initiation of enteral feedings establishes and maintains positive nitrogen balance sooner, lessens hypermetabolic response, prevents paralytic ileus, and reduces costs.
2. Disadvantages
   a. Tube feedings deprive the patient of the psychologic and social pleasures of eating.
   b. By bypassing the oral cavity, tube feedings prevent the patient from enjoying the taste of food and the pleasure of chewing it.
3. Types of formulas: Formulas or "medical foods" are designed to be consumed or administered enterally under the supervision of a physician to treat a disease or condition for which distinctive nutritional requirements are established by medical evaluation. The most commonly used formulas are polymeric formulas and elemental formulas.
   a. Polymeric formulas
      (1) Contain intact nutrients and require a normally functioning GI tract.
      (2) Most contain 1 calorie per ml, but they may contain up to 2 calories per ml.
      (3) Are convenient, microbiologically safe, and consistent in their nutrient content and osmolality.
      (4) Those intended as oral supplements are flavored.
   b. Elemental formulas
      (1) Are appropriate when the GI tract is not wholly functional or when minimal fecal residue is necessary.
      (2) Protein in the form of short-chain peptides or pure amino acids requires little or no digestion for absorption.
      (3) Some formulas contain very little fat, but several newer products use a large percentage of medium-chain triglyceride oils.
      (4) Contain electrolytes, minerals, and trace elements.
4. Indications for use: anytime the person is unable to consume adequate nutrition orally but has a functioning GI tract
   a. Hypermetabolic conditions—major trauma, burns, sepsis
   b. Neurologic impairments—stroke, coma
   c. Pre- and postoperatively—intestinal, head and neck, or esophageal surgery
   d. During certain therapies—chemotherapy
   e. Oral-esophageal problems—acquired immunodeficiency syndrome (AIDS)
   f. Specific organ dysfunction—liver, renal, pancreatic, respiratory
   g. Intestinal dysfunction—Crohn's disease, short-bowel syndrome, AIDS
5. Routes for administration: depend on anticipated duration of feeding, condition of the GI tract, and potential for aspiration
   a. Nasogastric (nose to stomach)
      (1) Advantages: well tolerated, uses digestive and absorptive functions fully, reduced risk of hyperosmolar solution causing gastric distention, nausea, and vomiting
      (2) Disadvantages: increased risk of aspiration, reflux esophagitis
   b. Nasoduodenal-nasojejunal (nose to duodenum or jejunum)
      (1) Advantages: less likely to be aspirated; can use intact nutrient formulas if delivered slowly
      (2) Disadvantages: mercury-weighted or tungsten-weighted tubes must be radiographed for placement; may cause "dumping syndrome"
   c. Gastrostomy (surgical opening into stomach)
      (1) Advantages: can be performed at the bedside with minimal sedation; rarely pulled out inadvertently; well tolerated because the stomach is utilized; polymeric formulas are well tolerated.
      (2) Disadvantages: some risk of aspiration; ostomy site may become irritated and infected.
   d. Jejunostomy (surgical opening into jejunum)
      (1) Advantages: less risk of aspiration; uses absorptive function of GI tract.
      (2) Disadvantages: administration must be slow, delivered by continuous drip by pump; elemental formulas may be necessary.
6. Methods of delivery
   a. Bolus feedings deliver 300 to 400 ml of formula intermittently every 3 to 6 hours over a 30- to 60-minute period.
   b. Continuous feedings infuse all the person's nutritional requirements over a 24-hour period using a mechanical pump.
   c. Cyclic feedings infuse over an 8- to 16-hour period either during the day or night. Nighttime feedings allow oral feedings during the day and are less likely to interfere with appetite; daytime feedings are best when risk of aspiration or tube dislodgment is high.
7. Nursing care
   a. Refer to Chapter 27 for information on insertion, irrigation, and removal of tubes.
   b. Do not administer any formula if bowel sounds are absent.
   c. Always confirm tube placement before initiating a feeding.

d. Check residuals, as ordered, especially if the method of feeding is bolus. Always replace gastric residuals.

e. For intermittent feedings, raise the head of the bed to 30 to 45 degrees during feedings and for 30 minutes to 1 hour after feeding to decrease the risk of aspiration. For continuous feedings, elevate the head of the bed 30 degrees at all times.

f. When nourishment has been withheld longer than 7 days and the formula is hyperosmolar, initiate the feeding at a slower rate of 35 to 50 ml per hour, advancing by 15 to 25 ml per hour every 8 to 12 hours until reaching the optimal caloric goal.

g. Even if feeding falls behind schedule, do not increase the rate.

h. Use aseptic technique and basic principles of good hand washing to prevent bacterial contamination.

i. Change feeding container and tubing daily.

j. Provide formulas in a closed system container, if available, to prevent bacterial contamination.

k. If closed system container is not available, do not hang more than will infuse in an 8-hour period.

l. Check expiration date on the formula; do not use a formula that has expired.

m. Shake formula to make sure particles are in suspension.

n. Chart volume of formula administered separately from that of water given.

o. Provide adequate fluids (1500 to 2000 ml) to prevent hypernatremia and fluid volume deficit and to maintain a satisfactory urinary output. Monitor fluid intake and output, physical signs, and laboratory data, such as blood urea nitrogen and sodium levels. Provide additional fluids, if needed, based on the person's fluctuating status (e.g., fever, vomiting, diarrhea).

p. Provide routine oral hygiene for the person—brush the teeth and gums to moisten the lips and oral mucous membranes.

q. Monitor or chart the patient's physical tolerance (constipation, diarrhea, distention) and psychosocial tolerance for feedings.

8. Complications

a. Serious complications may occur from enteral feedings; correct formula selection and proper administration techniques prevent most complications.

b. The most frequent complications are diarrhea, aspiration, and obstructed tube. Causes and treatment for many problems associated with tube feedings are outlined in Figure 10–4.

9. Transitional feedings: A transitional or weaning period maintains nutritional status while making the transition from tube to oral feedings. Despite the person's desire to enjoy oral feedings, the stomach has atrophied, and early satiety is common.

a. Gradually decrease the amount of formula to promote appetite.

b. Provide 5 to 6 small feedings daily using nutrient-dense foods.

c. Maintain accurate records of person's intake so the dietitian can evaluate for adequacy of intake.

10. Home enteral nutrition

HOME CARE STRATEGIES

Enteral Feedings
You need to carefully evaluate patient needs and response to therapy. Safe delivery of care and quality of life are primary goals.
During a nutritional assessment in the home, keep the following in mind:

- Nasogastric access is acceptable in short-term therapy only and is less common than direct access to stomach or small intestine.
- When selecting a pump and supplies, consider the following: reimbursement, backup pumps for isolated areas, portable pumps for the ambulatory patient, and battery backup.
- Consult the dietitian about the appropriate formula for the patient's individual caloric and nutritional needs.
- Assess the correct placement of the tube: aspiration of stomach contents, auscultation of air movement into stomach.
- Elevate the head of the bed when administering feeding and 30 minutes after feedings.
- Maintain tube patency through plentiful irrigation of water. Flush the feeding tube with 50 ml of water before and after feeding and with each administration of medication. To declot feeding tubes, cola, meat tenderizer, and tea are effective.
- Feeding containers should be cleaned with warm water, air dried, and stored in a covered, dry area. Supplies should be changed at regular intervals appropriate for the patient's delivery system.
- Nighttime infusion increases the patient's independence during the day.
- Cleanse the healed insertion site with soap and water daily.
- Consult the pharmacist about available elixirs and potential problems if crushing pills.
- Monitor bowel response to therapy, and instruct the patient on interventions: rate change, medication for diarrhea or constipation, increase or decrease in water amounts.
- Assess caregiver and patient competence and comfort with the procedure by direct observation of technique and evaluation of problem-solving ability.
- Commonly ordered laboratory tests are chemistry profile, albumin, prealbumin, and transferrin levels.
- Provide open discussion and instruction concerning lifestyle activities (e.g., mealtime, physical, sexual, work).
- Instruct on proper oral care: twice a day brushing, frequent rinses, use of mints and chewing gum.
- Instruct on purchasing supplies, such as tube feeding formula.

Patient teaching materials are available through nutritional support companies such as Ross Nutritional System and Clintec Nutrition Company.

a. Work closely with other team members to ensure person and family members are knowledgeable about how to deliver the formula and problems that may occur.

b. Allow person and family members to observe and demonstrate the steps in administering the feeding.

c. Techniques persons and family members should know before discharge are provided in Learning/ Teaching Guidelines for Self-Care in Enteral Feedings.

Parenteral Nutrition

1. Indications for use

a. Parenteral nutrition provides required nutrients when the GI tract is dysfunctional.

b. Veins are used to provide nourishment in contrast to

LEARNING/TEACHING GUIDELINES
for Self-Care in Enteral Feedings

1. Assure the person and family members that nutritional requirements can be provided adequately with enteral feedings.
2. Demonstrate and have the person and family members demonstrate their ability to prepare and administer the formula, including the following:
   a. Clean technique for tube and site care
   b. Preparation and storage of formula
   c. Ability to utilize equipment and infuse formula
   d. Recognition and appropriate response to complications, equipment maintenance, and malfunctions
3. Stress the importance of providing additional fluids (specify amount) to flush tube and for adequate hydration.
4. Explain procedures for administering medications through the tube.
5. Provide written instructions.
6. Explain the importance of maintaining accurate records: document weight, formula, and water provided, bowel patterns and flatulence; emesis and gastric residual, which is the amount left in the stomach after a period of time following a feeding.
7. Explain follow-up arrangements (in-home visits by home health nurses), who to contact regarding any problems, and return appointments to the physician.

---

standard intravenous therapy that provides only glucose, electrolytes, and fluid.

NURSE ADVISORY

Standard dextrose IV solutions, although delivered through the veins, are not considered a form of nutrition support; a liter of D5W provides only 170 calories. Dextrose solutions prevent or correct more imminent problems of fluid and electrolyte balance.

c. Persons unable to tolerate enteral feedings within 7 to 10 days should receive parenteral nutrition to prevent subcutaneous fat and muscle protein from being used for energy.
   (1) Peripheral parenteral nutrition uses small peripheral veins to infuse isotonic or hypotonic or slightly hypertonic (20%) solutions to preserve lean body mass, and its use is anticipated for only 5 to 7 days.
   (2) Total parenteral nutrition (TPN), also called central parenteral nutrition, uses a central vein to infuse hypertonic solutions and is appropriate for persons with high energy requirements to promote cell growth and repletion for more than 7 days.
2. Composition of parenteral solutions
   a. Energy
      (1) Various combinations of dextrose, fat emulsions, or both provide calories.
      (2) Excessive amounts of energy may produce undesirable metabolic complications (see page 331).
      (3) Energy requirements can best be determined using a metabolic cart.
      (4) Most adults require approximately 1500 calories per day postoperatively to prevent catabolism of body protein, but persons with a hypermetabolic condition require more than 2000 calories.
   b. Dextrose
      (1) Dextrose solutions range from 10 to 70 percent.
      (2) Hypertonic dextrose solutions used in TPN may necessitate the use of insulin to prevent hyperglycemia.
   c. Lipid emulsions
      (1) Lipid emulsions are isotonic and contain 10 or 20 percent safflower or soybean oil, egg yolk phospholipids (as emulsifiers), and glycerin.
      (2) Fat emulsions are "piggybacked" with amino acid and dextrose solutions, or all 3 can be mixed in the same bag (called total nutrient admixture).
      (3) When TPN continues for more than 2 to 3 weeks, lipid emulsions are necessary to prevent essential fatty acid deficiency.
      (4) Using both dextrose and lipids has many advantages; for example, they are physiologically more natural, enhance protein repletion, and avoid overloading metabolic pathways (improved glucose tolerance and less fluid retention).
      (5) Refrigerate lipid emulsions to prevent aggregation of fat particles.
      (6) Do not use lipid emulsions if oil globules appear or if a "ring" is present in 3-in-1 mixtures.
   d. Protein
      (1) Protein infusions contain both essential and nonessential amino acids.
      (2) They are used principally for protein repletion and are not relied on for calories.
      (3) Amino acids are commercially available in 3 to 15 percent concentrations.
   e. Vitamins and minerals
      (1) During TPN therapy, the RDAs for vitamin or mineral requirements are not appropriate because the GI tract is bypassed.
      (2) Intravenous multivitamin and mineral preparations, recommended by the American Medical As-

**TROUBLE SHOOTING GUIDE
FOR TUBE FEEDING**

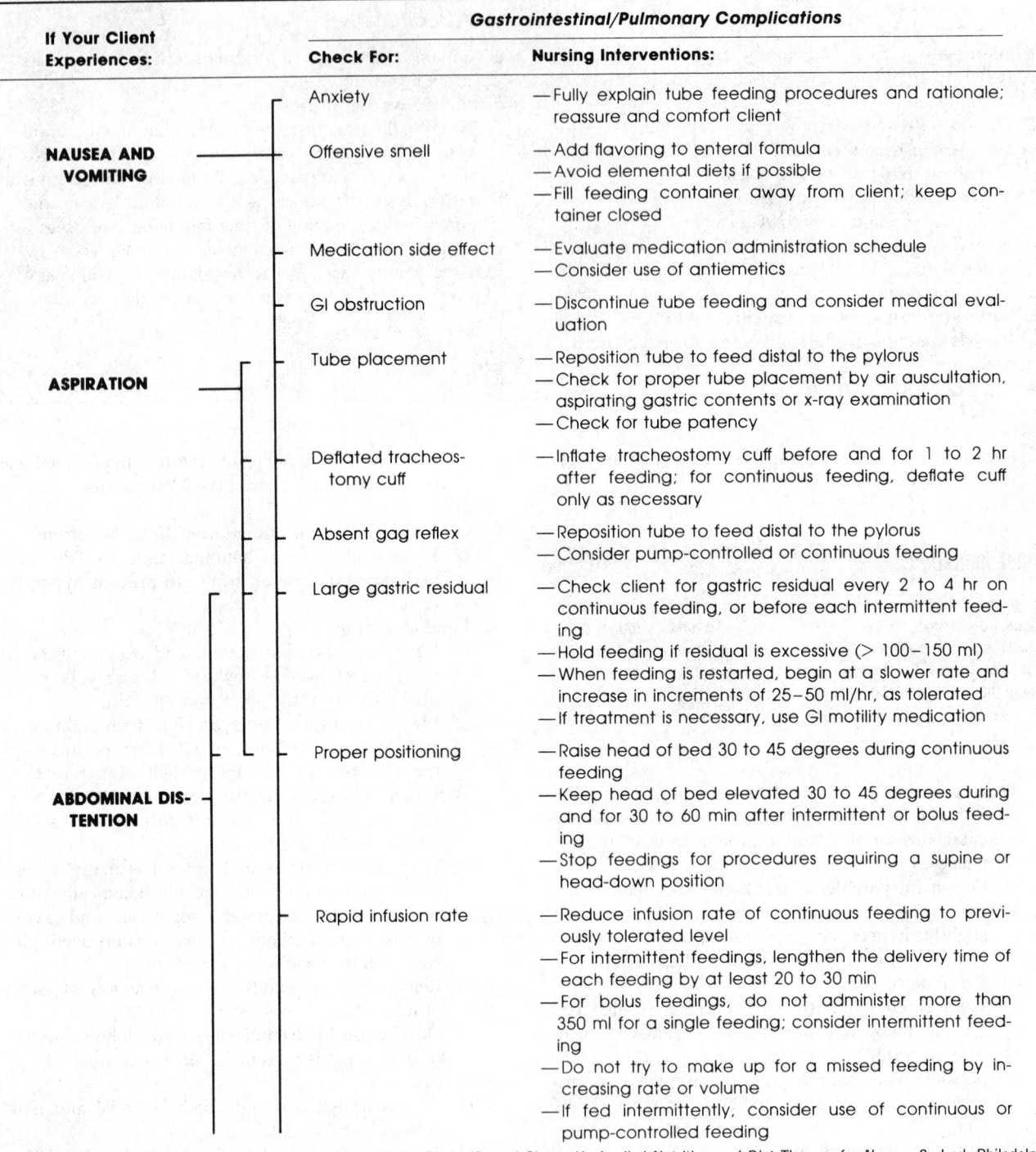

If Your Client Experiences:	Gastrointestinal/Pulmonary Complications	
	Check For:	Nursing Interventions:
NAUSEA AND VOMITING	Anxiety	—Fully explain tube feeding procedures and rationale; reassure and comfort client
	Offensive smell	—Add flavoring to enteral formula —Avoid elemental diets if possible —Fill feeding container away from client; keep container closed
	Medication side effect	—Evaluate medication administration schedule —Consider use of antiemetics
	GI obstruction	—Discontinue tube feeding and consider medical evaluation
ASPIRATION	Tube placement	—Reposition tube to feed distal to the pylorus —Check for proper tube placement by air auscultation, aspirating gastric contents or x-ray examination —Check for tube patency
	Deflated tracheostomy cuff	—Inflate tracheostomy cuff before and for 1 to 2 hr after feeding; for continuous feeding, deflate cuff only as necessary
	Absent gag reflex	—Reposition tube to feed distal to the pylorus —Consider pump-controlled or continuous feeding
	Large gastric residual	—Check client for gastric residual every 2 to 4 hr on continuous feeding, or before each intermittent feeding —Hold feeding if residual is excessive (> 100–150 ml) —When feeding is restarted, begin at a slower rate and increase in increments of 25–50 ml/hr, as tolerated —If treatment is necessary, use GI motility medication
ABDOMINAL DISTENTION	Proper positioning	—Raise head of bed 30 to 45 degrees during continuous feeding —Keep head of bed elevated 30 to 45 degrees during and for 30 to 60 min after intermittent or bolus feeding —Stop feedings for procedures requiring a supine or head-down position
	Rapid infusion rate	—Reduce infusion rate of continuous feeding to previously tolerated level —For intermittent feedings, lengthen the delivery time of each feeding by at least 20 to 30 min —For bolus feedings, do not administer more than 350 ml for a single feeding; consider intermittent feeding —Do not try to make up for a missed feeding by increasing rate or volume —If fed intermittently, consider use of continuous or pump-controlled feeding

Figure 10–4. Troubleshooting guide for tube feeding. (From Davis JR, and Sherer K. *Applied Nutrition and Diet Therapy for Nurses.* 2nd ed. Philadelphia: WB Saunders, 1994, pp 362–365. Original source: Sandoz Nutrition, Clinical Products Division, Minneapolis, MN.)

sociation (listed in Tables 10–2 and 10–3), are available; these are usually added to the bag just before its infusion.

    (3) Provide vitamin K intramuscularly once a week as ordered.

3. Nursing interventions

    a. Monitor the pump flow rate every hour. The infusion must be constant and uninterrupted to prevent hyper-

glycemia and osmotic diuresis and provide the whole solution in the allotted amount of time.

    b. "Catch up" is not allowed unless specified by the physician.

    c. Perform central line or venous access device assessments.

    d. Monitor laboratory data according to the following schedules:

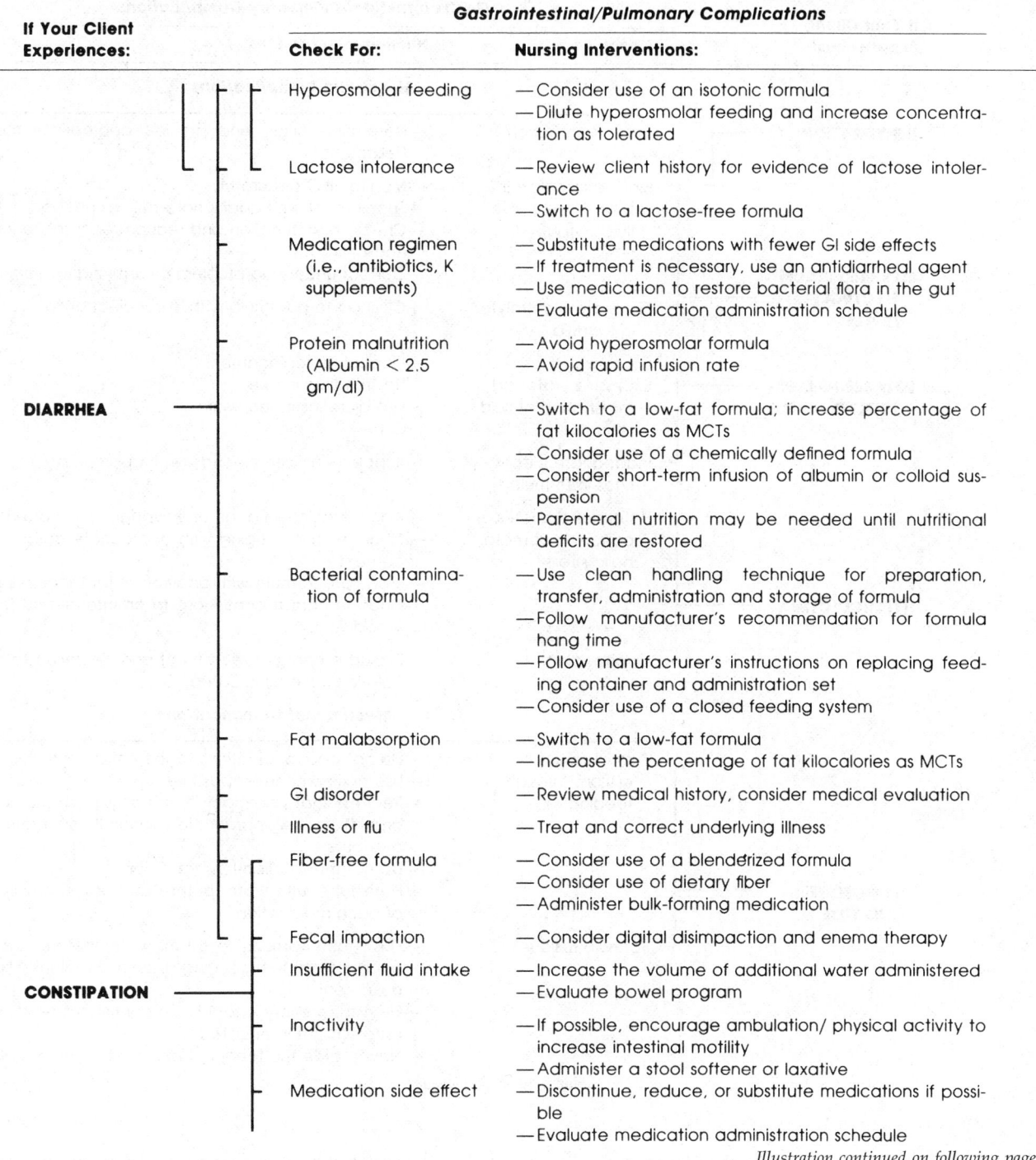

Gastrointestinal/Pulmonary Complications

If Your Client Experiences:	Check For:	Nursing Interventions:
DIARRHEA	Hyperosmolar feeding	—Consider use of an isotonic formula —Dilute hyperosmolar feeding and increase concentration as tolerated
	Lactose intolerance	—Review client history for evidence of lactose intolerance —Switch to a lactose-free formula
	Medication regimen (i.e., antibiotics, K supplements)	—Substitute medications with fewer GI side effects —If treatment is necessary, use an antidiarrheal agent —Use medication to restore bacterial flora in the gut —Evaluate medication administration schedule
	Protein malnutrition (Albumin < 2.5 gm/dl)	—Avoid hyperosmolar formula —Avoid rapid infusion rate —Switch to a low-fat formula; increase percentage of fat kilocalories as MCTs —Consider use of a chemically defined formula —Consider short-term infusion of albumin or colloid suspension —Parenteral nutrition may be needed until nutritional deficits are restored
	Bacterial contamination of formula	—Use clean handling technique for preparation, transfer, administration and storage of formula —Follow manufacturer's recommendation for formula hang time —Follow manufacturer's instructions on replacing feeding container and administration set —Consider use of a closed feeding system
	Fat malabsorption	—Switch to a low-fat formula —Increase the percentage of fat kilocalories as MCTs
	GI disorder	—Review medical history, consider medical evaluation
	Illness or flu	—Treat and correct underlying illness
CONSTIPATION	Fiber-free formula	—Consider use of a blenderized formula —Consider use of dietary fiber —Administer bulk-forming medication
	Fecal impaction	—Consider digital disimpaction and enema therapy
	Insufficient fluid intake	—Increase the volume of additional water administered —Evaluate bowel program
	Inactivity	—If possible, encourage ambulation/ physical activity to increase intestinal motility —Administer a stool softener or laxative
	Medication side effect	—Discontinue, reduce, or substitute medications if possible —Evaluate medication administration schedule

Illustration continued on following page

Figure 10–4 *Continued*

(1) Measure daily until stable, then 2 to 3 times weekly: electrolytes (sodium, potassium, chloride, carbon dioxide), glucose, phosphorus, blood urea nitrogen, creatinine, triglycerides (if fat emulsion prescribed).

(2) Measure 1 to 2 times weekly: complete blood count, calcium, magnesium, liver function tests, albumin, prealbumin-transferrin, prothrombin time.

4. Complications: Parenteral feedings can cause many complications; nursing interventions for more prevalent complications are presented.

a. Sepsis

(1) Monitor for sudden elevation of glucose.

(2) Use aseptic technique when hanging solution and preparing tubing to prevent bacterial contamination.

**TROUBLE SHOOTING GUIDE FOR
TUBE FEEDING** *Continued*

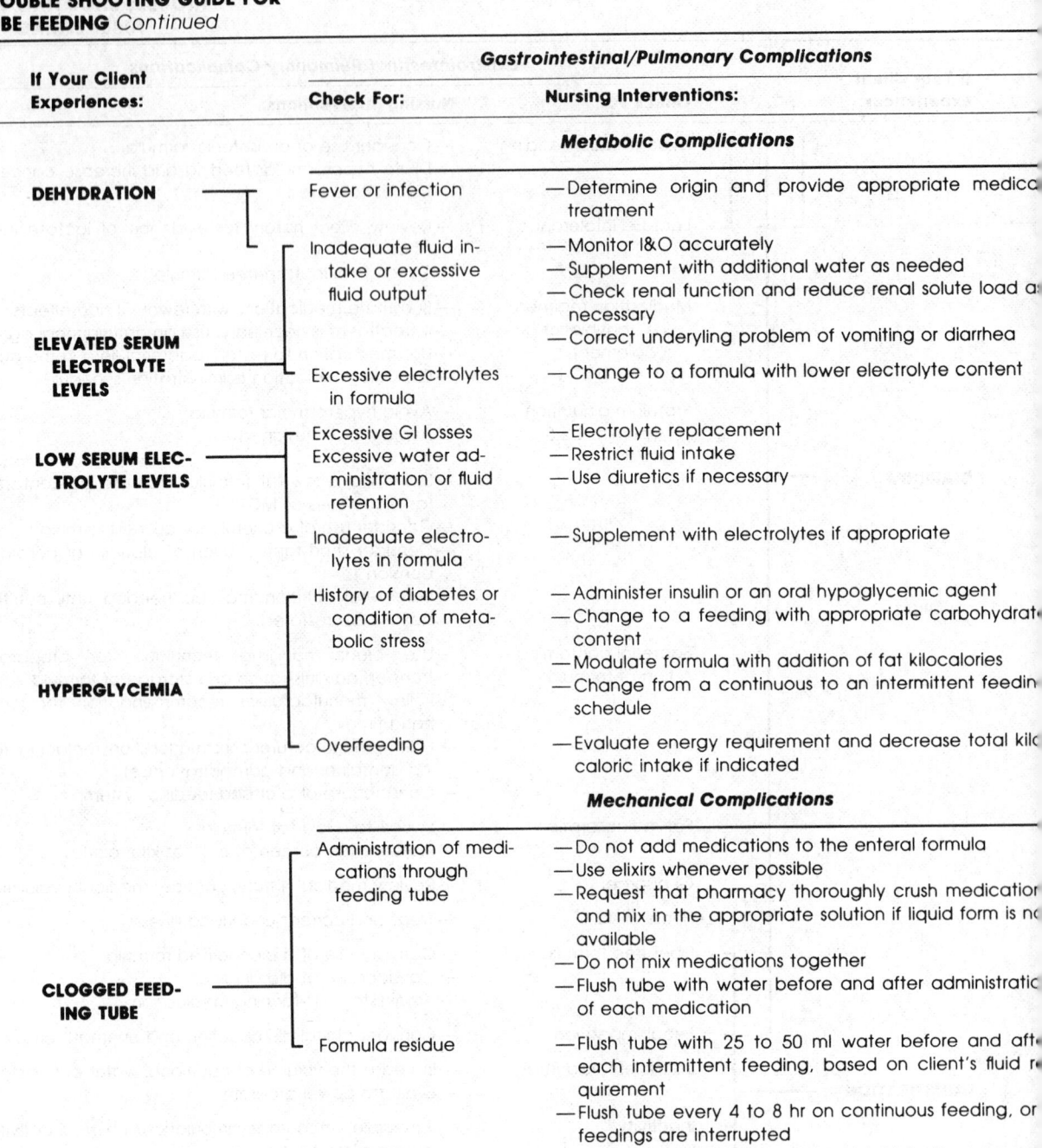

If Your Client Experiences:	Check For:	Nursing Interventions:
		Metabolic Complications
DEHYDRATION	Fever or infection	—Determine origin and provide appropriate medica treatment
ELEVATED SERUM ELECTROLYTE LEVELS	Inadequate fluid intake or excessive fluid output	—Monitor I&O accurately —Supplement with additional water as needed —Check renal function and reduce renal solute load a necessary —Correct underlying problem of vomiting or diarrhea
	Excessive electrolytes in formula	—Change to a formula with lower electrolyte content
LOW SERUM ELECTROLYTE LEVELS	Excessive GI losses Excessive water administration or fluid retention	—Electrolyte replacement —Restrict fluid intake —Use diuretics if necessary
	Inadequate electrolytes in formula	—Supplement with electrolytes if appropriate
HYPERGLYCEMIA	History of diabetes or condition of metabolic stress	—Administer insulin or an oral hypoglycemic agent —Change to a feeding with appropriate carbohydrat content —Modulate formula with addition of fat kilocalories —Change from a continuous to an intermittent feedin schedule
	Overfeeding	—Evaluate energy requirement and decrease total kilc caloric intake if indicated
		Mechanical Complications
CLOGGED FEEDING TUBE	Administration of medications through feeding tube	—Do not add medications to the enteral formula —Use elixirs whenever possible —Request that pharmacy thoroughly crush medicatior and mix in the appropriate solution if liquid form is nc available —Do not mix medications together —Flush tube with water before and after administratic of each medication
	Formula residue	—Flush tube with 25 to 50 ml water before and aft each intermittent feeding, based on client's fluid re quirement —Flush tube every 4 to 8 hr on continuous feeding, or feedings are interrupted —Never force the feeding tube stylet into the tube

Figure 10–4 *Continued*

(3) If infection occurs, notify the physician.
b. Hyperglycemia and hypoglycemia
(1) Monitor flow rate hourly.
(2) Identify and monitor closely blood glucose levels of persons at risk of developing blood glucose problems (early phase injury; diabetes mellitus; pancreatic disease; hormonal abnormalities; liver disease; sepsis; surgery; use of β-blockers, phenytoin, steroids, epinephrine, thiazide diuretics).

(3) Explain why hyperglycemia is occurring to clarify any confusion or concern about diabetes.
c. Lipid overload
(1) Give initial fat solution slowly, following facility guidelines.
(2) Notify the physician if an acute reaction or a fat overload occurs (hyperlipidemia, fever, focal seizures, pruritic urticaria, leukocytosis, hepatosplenomegaly).
d. Nutrient deficiencies

(1) Monitor physical status for possible nutrient excesses or deficiencies.
5. Transitional feedings
a. Because the GI tract has not been utilized, this transition can be surprisingly difficult for many people.
(1) The secretion of many intestinal enzymes may be low, causing an intolerance to lactose, gluten, hyperosmolar clear liquids, and large amounts of fats.
(2) People may not feel hungry and may experience early satiety.
b. If making a transition from TPN to tube feedings, begin with an isotonic formula at a reduced rate (25–50 ml/hr). Occasionally people need elemental formulas.
c. If transitioning from TPN to oral feedings, be sure that swallowing function is consistent and normal.
(1) Encourage easily digested liquids, using 30 to 60 ml of clear liquids with a low osmolality at 20- to 30-minute intervals.
(2) After 24 hours, initiate small amounts of full liquids. Most polymeric formulas are appropriate because they do not contain lactose.
(3) Introduce solid foods the next day and decrease TPN by 50 percent.
6. Home parenteral nutrition
a. Training for home therapy
(1) Training for home parenteral feedings is similar to that provided for home enteral feedings; it may take from 2 to 3 weeks to teach the principles of asepsis, catheter care, care of parenteral nutrient solutions and pump, parameters to monitor, and problem solving.
(2) Involve the person and family members.
(3) Inform the person and family members of home health care facilities, social workers, Medicare, support groups, and suppliers of equipment and parenteral infusion.
b. Home health care
(1) Home health care is vital to monitor for potential problems, especially catheter care to prevent sepsis.
(2) Laboratory values should be monitored by the physician every 2 weeks for at least the first 6 weeks. As these results improve and normalize, testing can be less frequent.

◼ NUTRITIONAL DISORDERS AND ALTERATIONS

Obesity

1. Definition
a. Overweight, defined as excess weight for height, is a 10 to 20 percent increase over IBW.
b. Obesity, or a 20 percent increase over IBW, is an excess accumulation of body fat.
c. Morbid obesity is 100 pounds over IBW.
2. Incidence and socioeconomic impact

a. Energy balance is difficult to achieve with today's sedentary lifestyles and jobs, which are low in energy expenditure and include readily available high-calorie foods.
b. Obesity is on the rise. More than 26 percent of the U.S. population are overweight. More women are overweight than men.
c. Being overweight can decrease the quality and quantity of life as well as the individual's productivity.
3. Risk factors
a. Sedentary lifestyle
b. Family history of obesity
c. Presence of or family history of hypertension, coronary heart disease, diabetes mellitus, endocrine diseases
d. Fat distribution
e. High fat intake
f. Taking drugs associated with hyperphagia (glucocorticoids, amitriptyline, lithium, cyproheptadine, phenothiazines, birth control pills)
4. Etiology
a. Obesity is the result of a consistent overconsumption of calories in relation to expenditure of energy.
b. Many factors regulate and influence control of food intake. Precise causes of obesity are not well understood, but many factors are involved.
c. Heredity
(1) Genetic factors contribute to obesity, especially regarding fat distribution (hips, thighs, waist).
(2) Children with one or both obese parents are at high risk of becoming obese.
d. Hypothyroidism
(1) In hypothyroidism, basal metabolic rate is lower because of a deficiency in thyroid secretion that results in less caloric expenditure.
(2) Obesity related to this metabolic disorder accounts for less than 1 percent of overweight people.
5. Pathophysiology
a. Increased numbers of fat cells—hyperplastic obesity
(1) Cell multiplication occurs during peak growth periods: late infancy, early childhood up to 6 years of age, adolescence, and pregnancy.
(2) The total number of fat cells increases when obesity develops during these periods, but obese infants do not necessarily become obese children.
(3) Persons with hyperplastic obesity have trouble losing weight and regain the weight more rapidly following weight loss.
b. Increased fat cell size—hypertrophy obesity
(1) Expansion of fat cells increases body weight.
(2) This type of obesity occurs primarily after puberty and usually correlates with android distribution.
(3) Persons who are 75 percent above ideal body weight usually have hypertrophic obesity.
6. Clinical manifestations
a. Obesity is manifested under the following conditions:
(1) A greater than 20 percent increase of IBW

(2) A greater than 25 percent body fat (men); greater than 30 percent body fat (women)

(3) A basal metabolic rate above 30 kg/m²

b. Morbid obesity is characterized by:

(1) A body weight of 100 pounds over IBW

(2) A more than 30 percent increase over IBW

(3) A basal metabolic index of more than 40

7. Diagnostics

a. Determine whether it is in the person's best interest to lose weight.

(1) Is the person's health in sufficient jeopardy to warrant weight reduction?

(2) How much weight should be lost?

(3) How does the person feel about his or her current weight?

(4) Is the person motivated to make changes for internal or external reasons? (Internally motivated people are more likely to succeed.)

(5) Are objectives realistic?

(6) How stable is the person's weight?

(7) How will weight loss affect the person's relationships with family and friends?

b. Physical examination: check weight for height, with consideration of frame size, using Figure 10–3, or Metropolitan Life Insurance Tables; evaluate fat using basal metabolic index, triceps skin fold measurements, underwater weighing, or impedance measurements; assess risk factors, age of onset of obesity, frequency and level of physical activity.

c. Dietary: ask about fat intake, total volume and frequency of eating, special or fad diets used.

d. Diagnosis is based on deviations from IBW using the formula presented previously in Figure 10–3.

8. Clinical management

a. Goal of clinical management

(1) To lose 1 to 2 pounds per week until desired body weight is reached

b. Nonpharmacologic interventions

(1) Decreasing caloric intake. Lower caloric intake to 1200 calories for women and 1500 calories for men. Limit fat intake to 45 to 65 gm per day. Very low calorie diets containing fewer than 800 calories per day may be recommended for severely or morbidly obese adults.

(2) Increasing exercise. Helps maintain muscle mass and increases caloric expenditure.

(3) Nutritional counseling. A registered dietitian can help people understand their eating habits and obtain a diet plan tailored for their lifestyle and food preferences.

(4) Mental health counseling. Behavior modification and other mental health techniques are beneficial in any weight control program because people learn new ways of dealing with old habits. Refer to Chapter 41.

c. Pharmacologic interventions

(1) Drugs are not used routinely, but some prescriptions help suppress appetite. The most commonly used medications include amphetamines and bulking agents.

d. Special medical-surgical procedures

(1) Gastrointestinal surgery may be recommended for morbid obesity. The preferred surgery is vertical banded gastroplasty, which limits stomach capacity.

(2) Liposuction and lipectomy

(3) Intragastric balloon

(4) Jaw wiring

9. Complications

a. Premature death

b. Increased risk for the following:

(1) Non–insulin-dependent diabetes mellitus

(2) Hypertension

(3) Cardiovascular disease

(4) Gallbladder disease

(5) Colon and postmenopausal breast cancer

(6) Wound infections

c. Decreased fertility

d. Slowed recovery from surgery with possible complications such as pneumonia and thrombophlebitis

e. Increased problems with sleep apnea, gout, and arthritis

10. Prognosis

a. Eighty to 100 percent of those who lose significant amounts of weight regain it.

b. To maintain weight loss, people must realize changes in eating and exercising habits are lifelong processes.

11. Applying the nursing process

NURSING DIAGNOSIS: Altered nutrition, more than body requirements, R/T imbalance of food intake versus activity expenditure

a. *Expected outcomes:* Following instruction, the person should be able to do the following:

(1) Lose 1 to 2 pounds per week until desired weight is achieved.

(2) State the importance of decreasing intake and increasing exercise.

b. *Nursing interventions*

(1) Correct knowledge deficits concerning the cause and complications of obesity and the importance of exercise, reducing caloric intake, and changing eating patterns for life.

(2) Help the person and family members comply with the interventions and eat in normal settings with some adjustments in food choices.

(3) Help the person and family members make changes in lifestyle to increase energy expenditure.

(4) Implement nonpharmacologic interventions mentioned previously.

NURSING DIAGNOSIS: Noncompliance R/T lack of motivation to adhere to the therapeutic regimen

a. *Expected outcomes:* Following instruction, the person should adhere to ordered diet, eat at least 75 percent of meals ordered and be able to plan a low-calorie diet.

LEARNING/TEACHING GUIDELINES
for Losing Weight

General Overview

1. Explain that weight loss is associated with a decrease in serum glucose, cholesterol, systolic blood pressure, and uric acid. Other physical conditions that can be expected to improve with weight loss include shortness of breath, ease of tiring, fluid retention, gastric disorders, headaches, decline in energy level, lack of interest in sex, joint pains, muscle cramps, low pulse rate, restless sleep, urinary infections, and varicose veins.
2. Explain that any treatment for weight loss should always be a serious undertaking with a high level of motivation and long-term commitment. This approach increases the chances that the plan will be followed until weight is lost and that weight loss will be maintained.
3. The recommended amount of weight loss is 1 to 2 pounds per week.
4. To lose 1 pound, there must be a deficit of 3500 calories, which may be achieved by decreasing energy intake by 500 calories per day and increasing energy expenditure equally.
5. Explain the difficulties in maintaining weight loss. Fatty tissues are conducive for refilling. Therefore, overweight individuals must change their eating patterns and learn skills to maintain weight loss.
6. Individuals should monitor their weight weekly, even after their target weight has been reached.
7. Help the person locate a local weight control program that incorporates behavior modification, diet, and exercise.
8. If medication has been prescribed, explain the dosage, when it is taken, potential side effects, and measures to minimize side effects.

Calorically Reduced Diets

1. Explain the importance of a well-balanced diet that contains adequate amounts of nutrients but is low in calories.
2. Point out these facts about reduction diets:
   a. Foods from each food group are needed to meet all nutrient needs except energy.
   b. It is very important that the total amount of food is divided into 3 or more feedings to lessen deprivation syndrome and eliminate excessive food intake. (Breakfast is very important.)
   c. The diet must be appealing, flexible, and affordable because the person should be able to live with these changes for life.
   d. Fat is reduced to less than 30 percent of total calories because fats are the most concentrated source of energy.
   e. A minimum of 20 percent of caloric intake from fat is needed to increase satiety and provide fat-soluble vitamins and essential fatty acids.
   f. See Table 10–9 for suggestions for lowering dietary fat.
   g. The diet should provide 50 to 60 gm of protein.
   h. Moderate amounts of complex carbohydrates are allowed, but minimal amounts of sugar and other sweeteners are used.
   i. Encourage high-fiber foods such as raw vegetables and other "fillers" such as bouillon or broth-type soups.
   j. Encourage the person to weigh out or measure the food.
3. Help the person change some patterns that contribute to overeating:
   a. Encourage the person to maintain a diary that records what was eaten, how much, when, and why; this helps reveal antecedents for food intake.
   b. Eat regularly in the same place.
   c. Sit down to eat.
   d. Put down the utensils between each bite.
   e. Do not watch television or read while eating.
   f. Take at least 20 minutes to eat each meal.
   g. Arrange an attractive meal on a small plate.
   h. Leave a small amount of food on the plate (1 or 2 bites).
   i. Store (or freeze) leftover food immediately to avoid returning for 2nd helpings.
   j. Buy only appropriate food to have available.
   k. Do not taste while preparing; an alternative is to chew gum or brush teeth to help resist temptations.
4. If a very low calorie diet is being used:
   a. Discuss the program regimen.
   b. Explain that close medical supervision is essential while on the diet.
   c. A maintenance program for at least 12 months is vital. (Maintenance of weight loss is 36 percent for women and 39 percent for men after 42 months.)
5. Even if the person has had surgery to help with weight loss, dietary changes are necessary to effect this weight loss and prevent other complications.
6. If surgical procedures are appropriate or have been done, explain the plan and dietary problems that may occur. These precautions are more important following vertical banded gastroplasty:
   a. Initially following surgery, the diet is restricted to liquids, 10 to 30 ml taken over a 30-minute period.
   b. Soft, high-calorie dense liquids and foods (ice cream, cheese, milk shakes) and easily dissolvable foods (cake and cookies) are avoided.

(continued)

c. Red meat, soft bread, pasta, and citrus membranes may result in obstruction.

d. Adequate chewing is important.

e. Foods should not be "flushed" down with liquids.

Exercise

1. Recommend a consultation with the physician before starting any weight loss program, especially with regard to the safety of exercise.

2. Discuss ways the person can become involved in an exercise program or increase energy expenditure.

3. Point out the benefits of exercise:
   a. Exercise reduces loss of muscle mass and burns calories.
   b. Energy expenditure declines when energy intake is reduced, possibly because of loss of lean body mass, decreased cost of physical activity as a result of lower body weight, and lower thermogenic effect of food related to decreased intake.
   c. Exercise is an alternative behavior for eating and prevents boredom.

4. Explain that the ideal goal is an exercise of adequate intensity for at least 20 minutes 3 times a week, but any exercise activity, even though it is below ideal level, still offers physiologic and metabolic benefits. Energy saved by parking the car closer to walk less or watching television an extra 30 minutes instead of a more active pursuit can easily cause a weight gain of 10 to 20 pounds per year.

5. Discuss which types of exercise the person prefers because any exercise program will last only if the person enjoys that activity.

---

    b. *Nursing interventions*

      (1) To help the person comply, explain the causes of obesity and discuss the health and social benefits of weight loss.

      (2) Encourage family and friends to provide support, understanding, and praise.

      (3) Encourage participation in a weight control group (local chapters of Weight Watchers International, Thin Within, Dieters Workshop, TOPS, and other weight reduction groups).

12. Discharge planning and teaching
    a. Overweight people need to understand the risks of obesity, the ways to decrease caloric intake, the importance of an exercise program, the reasons for changes in food patterns, and the requirement that these changes be permanent.
    b. Learning/Teaching Guidelines for Losing Weight are outlined above.

Anorexia Nervosa

1. Definition
   a. Deliberate weight loss leading to maintenance of body weight 15 percent below that expected.
   b. Intense fear held by an underweight individual of gaining weight or becoming fat.
   c. Disturbance in the way in which an individual perceives body weight, size, or shape.

2. Incidence and socioeconomic impact
   a. Incidence is rising (more than previously expected) among those in the late teens and early twenties.
   b. Occurs primarily in adolescent girls, but adolescent boys and middle-aged men and women can be affected.
   c. Ten percent of those affected are male.
   d. People in sports and professions that require a low weight (wrestlers, ballet dancers, models) are being diagnosed more frequently with this eating disorder.

3. Risk factors
   a. Overachieving, close-knit families
   b. Family history of eating disorders or alcohol abuse
   c. Upper-class or middle-class background
   d. Previous GI disorders in infancy and childhood
   e. Slow gastric emptying

4. Etiology
   a. There is no one known, accepted theory for the cause of anorexia nervosa.
   b. Most professionals believe multifaceted psychologic problems correlate with family relationships and possibly some biologic factors.

5. Pathophysiology: A severe decrease in nutrient and caloric intake literally places the person in a state of starvation. The person's body is "eating itself up" to obtain the needed nutrients to survive.

6. Clinical manifestations
   a. Extreme weight loss, "skin and bones" appearance
   b. Self-imposed dieting
   c. Excessive physical activity
   d. Preoccupation with caloric content of foods
   e. Wearing oversized clothing; person feels fat
   f. Weighing oneself numerous times a day (may be up to 20 times)
   g. Wanting to break the 100 pound mark, that is, weigh less than 100 pounds
   h. Hypothermia
   i. Bradycardia
   j. Amenorrhea

7. Diagnostics
   a. History: family relationships, family attitudes about

weight, exercise habits, menses history, relevant medical history, self-medication

b. Physical examination: body image, former weight, present weight, IBW, percentage weight changes, triceps skinfold fat

c. Dietary: food preferences, detailed diet history (number and content of meals and snacks), appetite; dieting practices; knowledge of nutritional and caloric values of food; perception of excessive intake; person's or family members' beliefs about food intake

d. Laboratory tests: low white blood cell count, decreased hemoglobin if patient is anemic, elevated hematocrit if patient is dehydrated, hypokalemia, hypocalcemia, elevated blood urea nitrogen; depressed albumin; elevated cholesterol

e. Three major features are required for a diagnosis of anorexia nervosa:

(1) Self-inflicted weight loss (15% below expected or original body weight) by avoiding foods considered fattening

(2) Amenorrhea in a woman and less sexual interest and activity in a man

(3) A psychologic fear of being unable to control eating and being too fat (distorted body image)

8. Clinical management

a. Goals of clinical management: The person must be physiologically and psychologically stable before any nutritional goals can be effective.

(1) Refeeding for weight gain

(2) Normalizing eating habits

b. Nonpharmacologic interventions

(1) Promoting intake: Options for repletion of nutritional status include a regular diet, the use of nutritional supplements (alone or in combination with food intake), a total fluid diet, tube feedings (for persons whose weight is 40% below their IBW), or TPN (only for a metabolically unstable person).

• Initially provide easily digested foods with 4 or 5 feedings daily.

• Maintain accurate records of food intake, if ordered. (Be sure person actually eats the food.)

• Allow person to be in control of food eaten and subsequent weight gain.

• Gradually increase the number of calories provided. These increases should be noticeable to the person but not overwhelming.

• Encourage calorie-dense foods to reduce the bulk of meals.

• Gradually introduce foods the person previously avoided.

• Limit mealtime to 30 minutes.

(2) Nutritional counseling: All team members, including the psychologist, dietitian, and nurse, provide nutritional counseling because anorexia nervosa patients have many inaccurate beliefs about food and an inability to differentiate food and nutrition truths from myths. Do not have prolonged discussions about food or make food an issue. Allow the person to make choices. Do not force-feed; food rejection is part of this illness.

(3) Mental health counseling: It is necessary for the treatment of this disorder to help the person make positive statements about self and get in touch with own body image; see Chapter 41.

c. Pharmacologic interventions

(1) Tricyclic antidepressants and monoamine oxidase inhibitors may promote weight gain.

(2) Metoclopramide increases gastric emptying rate, which negates the delayed gastric emptying time most persons with anorexia nervosa experience.

(3) Clomiphene citrate may be prescribed to restore menses.

(4) Antianxiety medications may be ordered to decrease anxiety before meals.

d. Special medical-surgical procedures: Enteral and total parenteral feedings may be required.

9. Complications

a. Cardiac dysrhythmias

b. Dehydration

c. Superior mesenteric artery syndrome, which causes vascular compression of the distal duodenum

d. Decreased bone mineral density, possibly leading to osteoporosis

e. Tetany

f. Seizures

10. Prognosis

a. Changing and maintaining eating habits is extremely difficult for anorexia nervosa patients; it usually takes years for these changes to become ingrained.

b. Prognosis is poor if the following factors are present:

(1) Duration of illness is long.

(2) Weight is extremely low when treatment is initiated.

(3) Social interactions are difficult.

(4) Relationship with family is disturbed.

(5) Prior treatments have been tried.

11. Applying the nursing process

> **NURSING DIAGNOSIS:** Altered nutrition: less than body requirement R/T inadequate food intake

a. *Expected outcomes:* Following instruction, the person should gain 1 pound per week until desired body weight is achieved.

b. *Nursing interventions*

(1) Explain that poor eating habits lead to health problems such as osteoporosis and increased infectious illnesses.

(2) Correct knowledge deficits concerning the relationship between energy intake–expenditure and weight and that between nutrition and health.

(3) Initially encourage the person to stop losing weight and to improve the nutritional status; then encourage gradual weight gain through self-feeding.

(4) Refrain from providing too much food. Because of a low basal metabolic rate and low weight, small quantities will maintain weight.

LEARNING/TEACHING GUIDELINES
for People with Anorexia Nervosa

General Overview

1. Describe the ramifications and the dangers of anorexia nervosa.
2. Explain that inadequate dietary intake and malnutrition are serious consequences of the problem but that the condition is psychologic in nature.
3. If the person is extremely malnourished, explain that the first concern is to reestablish physiologic stability.
4. Point out that it is very important to eat at least 4 times a day.
5. Discuss the person's goal for weight gain; an increase of 1 pound weekly is ideal.
6. Explain how emotions and physical aspects relate to food intake and weight changes.
7. Work with the person to establish a specific set of dietary guidelines (contracts) so the individual will maintain a feeling of control.
8. Encourage the individual to maintain a journal, recording time and quantity of specific food eaten, feelings, and thoughts.

Weight Gain

Point out these important facts about health and weight:

1. Regular eating patterns are important to maintain one's health.
2. Discuss the necessity of a proper balance of caloric and nutrient intake with energy expenditure for health.
3. Explain that emotions and physical well-being are related to food intake and weight changes.

4. Try to counter false beliefs about food with factual information. If answers cannot be provided, inform the dietitian so factual information can be provided.
5. Explain that the discomfort felt after eating is because the stomach has atrophied (shrunk); eating will become more comfortable as the capacity increases.
6. Explain that rapid weight gain will occur with early refeeding as the body retains water and increases liver and muscle glycogen stores. Assure the person that this state will resolve if a well-balanced diet is eaten.
7. Emphasize that once goal weight is reached, a maintenance diet plan will be provided to prevent further weight gain.

Pharmacologic

1. Tell persons who are taking prescribed medications the name of the drug and its desired effect. Also describe dosage, timing of medication, potential side effects, and measures to minimize side effects.
2. If a monoamine oxidase inhibitor is prescribed, advise the person to avoid cheese (except cottage and cream cheese), smoked or pickled fish, liver, Italian green beans, meats and yeast extracts, dry sausage, sauerkraut, beer, ale, chianti wine, and vermouth. Consume avocados, bananas, soy sauce, sour cream, and yogurt in moderation.
3. If prescribed, explain that clomiphene stimulates ovulation, but this drug may not be effective until fat stores are replenished.

---

(5) Implement strategies listed under nonpharmacologic interventions.

NURSING DIAGNOSIS: Anxiety R/T increased food intake and subsequent weight gain

a. *Expected outcomes:* Following instruction, the person should state that anxiety has decreased.
b. *Nursing interventions*
   (1) Assist the person to adopt a healthy lifestyle in which she or he is in control; let the person make some choices, but these choices cannot center around whether to eat. Use a matter of fact manner to indicate eating is expected.
   (2) Help the person gain confidence in ability to eat spontaneously and still maintain an appropriate weight.

NURSING DIAGNOSIS: Risk for noncompliance R/T food refusal or overexercising

a. *Expected outcomes:* Following instruction, the person should adhere to ordered diet, eat at least 75 percent of meals ordered, and be able to plan a well-balanced, nutrient-adequate diet.
b. *Nursing interventions*
   (1) Assist the person to comply with the nutritional, medical, and psychologic interventions.
   (2) Explain that by eating, the person will still be in control of life and actually will be in more control because of improvements in health and well-being.
   (3) Set limits on exercising.

NURSING DIAGNOSIS: Risk for fluid volume excess R/T retaining fluid during refeeding

a. *Expected outcomes:* Following interventions, the person should not experience edema in the extremities or face.
b. *Nursing interventions*
    (1) Offer a low-salt diet.
    (2) Limit fluids to 1000 to 1500 ml per day.
    (3) Monitor intake and output.
    (4) Elevate feet as needed.
    (5) Do not give diuretics for this edema unless cardiac problems develop.
12. Discharge planning and teaching
    a. Before discharge, the person and family members need to learn about anorexia and understand the psychologic problems causing it, diet and weight balance, and appropriate quantities of food necessary for weight maintenance (Learning/Teaching Guidelines for Persons with Anorexia Nervosa).
    b. Provide handouts, booklets, articles, and other written information about nutrition to allow the person to control which information is accepted.
    c. Refer to the American Anorexia and Bulimia Association, Anorexia and Related Eating Disorders, or Anorexia Nervosa and Associated Disorders organizations.

Bulimia

1. Definition
    a. Periodic episodes of binge eating
    b. Feelings that eating behaviors are out of control during the eating binges
    c. Routine practice of self-induced vomiting, use of laxatives or diuretics, adherence to strict dieting or fasting, or practice of vigorous exercise to prevent weight gain
    d. Persistent overconcern about body shape and weight
2. Incidence and socioeconomic impact
    a. Occurs more frequently than anorexia nervosa.
    b. Affects mainly women in their twenties.
    c. Twenty percent of the people affected are male.
3. Risk factors
    a. History of alcohol, sexual, and physical abuse
    b. Emotional problems such as depression, loneliness, boredom, anger, anxiety
    c. Frequent mood swings
    d. Conflicts in relationships, work situation, or both
    e. History of being slightly overweight
4. Etiology
    a. Causes of individuals being fearful of becoming fat are poorly understood.
5. Pathophysiology
    a. An intense fear of becoming fat leads the person to control this fear by repeatedly restraining eating. However, this does not work, and binging and purging occur.
    b. Binging can result from emotional or physical needs. After binging, the person feels depressed and self-critical. In an effort to regain control and rid the body of excessive calories, the person purges.
6. Clinical manifestations

a. Normal weight or slightly under or overweight
b. Ten-pound weight fluctuations
c. Preoccupation with appearance
d. Knowledge that eating habits are abnormal
e. Enlarged parotid glands
f. Teeth brown with loss of enamel; caries present
g. Abuse of laxatives or diuretics, vomiting, or both
h. Calluses or cuts on knuckles and fingers
i. Compulsive stealing of food and money
7. Diagnostics
    a. History: type of purging used (vomiting, laxative, diuretic abuse)
    b. Physical examination: weakness, lethargy, hoarseness, esophagitis, oral lesions, dehydration, irregular menses, constipation, height, weight/weight changes, IBW
    c. Psychologic: low self-esteem, worthlessness, guilt, shame
    d. Dietary: frequency of binging and purging, list of forbidden foods, alcohol intake
    e. Laboratory tests: elevated amylase levels; metabolic alkalosis; hypokalemia; hypochloremia; calcium, magnesium, and sodium levels; hemoglobin; folate
    f. Medical diagnosis of bulimia includes a minimal average of 2 binge eating episodes a week for at least 3 months; fear of inability to stop eating voluntarily; self-induced vomiting, use of laxatives or diuretics, fasting, or vigorous exercise to prevent weight gain; and persistent overconcern with body shape and weight.
8. Clinical management
    a. Goals of clinical management
        (1) Normalize eating habits
        (2) Correct nutritional deficiencies
        (3) Reduce binge-and-purge cycles
    b. Nonpharmacologic interventions
        (1) Promoting intake: Physiologic and psychologic stabilization must occur before persons can control their eating behaviors. Following feedings, involve the person in a social setting for up to 1 hour to reduce opportunities for purging. Exclude high-risk binge foods initially, then slowly reintroduce them. Use a firm, direct approach for promoting normal eating patterns.
        (2) Nutritional counseling: Help the person understand the importance of nutrition for health and the use of the Food Guide Pyramid to maintain health. Make a contract with the person not to binge or purge. Help the person understand that once weight is stable and problem behaviors are under control, the need for a gradual weight loss program can be reassessed. Help them understand food, eating, and self-image so they can approach the problem in another way. Refer to a dietitian.
        (3) Mental health counseling: Counseling is necessary for bulimics to cope effectively because there is a strong resistance to changing their behaviors (see Chapter 41).
    c. Pharmacologic interventions: Antidepressants may help control binge behaviors.

LEARNING/TEACHING GUIDELINES
for People with Bulimia

General Overview

1. Discuss the health consequences of these behaviors (e.g., electrolyte imbalances, muscle spasm, kidney problems, and cardiac arrest).
2. Assist the person in maintaining a journal recording time of binging and purging, behavior before and after, thoughts before and after, and money spent on food.
3. Help the person understand that purging does not negate the effects of foods consumed.
4. When the cause of binging is determined, collaborate about alternate methods of dealing with stress, for example, writing, talking, or painting.
5. Encourage exercise so the person can consume more calories.

Maintaining Healthy Weight

1. Help the person plan well-balanced meals that are low in calories. Specify appropriate quantities of food that will help to maintain weight (approximately 1200 cal/day).
2. Explain that 3 meals a day plus 1 snack will avoid food deprivation syndrome and impulsive snacking.
3. Explain that when food is eaten out of the original container rather than on a serving dish, the temptation to overeat is greater. The risk of overeating may be decreased by eating only at the dining table.
4. Suggest persons increase fiber and fluid intake rather than using laxatives.
   a. Increased consumption of fruits (2 to 4 servings) and vegetables (3 to 5 servings) help provide fiber and foods that are relatively low in calories. These can be used in sandwiches, brown bag lunches, or as snacks.
   b. Choose cereals with at least 2 gm of fiber but no more than 2 gm of fat per serving.
   c. Use breads and cereals in which the first item in the ingredient list is "whole wheat" or "whole grain."
   d. Prepare raw vegetables to eat with a low-fat dip as appetizers or snacks.
   e. Add a little bran or wheat germ to recipes, even casseroles, main dishes, pancakes, and cooked cereal.
   f. Drink tomato juice.

- Tricyclics (nortriptyline hydrochloride and desipramine hydrochloride)
- Monoamine oxidase inhibitors (phenelzine sulfate, tranylcypromine sulfate)
- Serotonergic agonists (fluoxetine and sertraline hydrochloride)

9. Complications
   a. Hypokalemia
   b. Metabolic alkalosis
   c. Gastric dilation and possible rupture
   d. Reflex constipation from overuse of laxatives
   e. Fluid volume deficit
   f. Heart dysrhythmias
   g. Kidney problems
   h. Tetany
   i. Esophagitis, esophageal perforation, and rupture
10. Prognosis: Bulimics have a less favorable prognosis than anorectics. Frequently bulimics do not want to change because their behavior helps them feel in control and powerful.
11. Applying the nursing process

NURSING DIAGNOSIS: Altered nutrition: Risk for more than body requirements R/T increased food intake secondary to binging

a. *Expected outcomes:* Following instruction, the person should do the following:
   (1) Maintain weight for height or lose 1 to 2 pounds per week until desired body weight is achieved.
   (2) Identify critical variables in the binge-and-purge cycle, consume "forbidden foods" without guilt, and develop new coping strategies.
b. *Nursing interventions*
   (1) Correct knowledge deficits concerning the complications of the disorder and how to balance caloric intake with expenditure.
   (2) Help the person comply with the therapeutic regimen and develop a healthy lifestyle.
   (3) Offer well-balanced meals that are low in calories, and slowly reintroduce "forbidden foods."
   (4) Enable the person to employ different coping mechanisms other than binging and purging.
   (5) Help the person express negative feelings, such as anger, frustration, and anxiety.
   (6) Implement suggestions previously listed in nonpharmacologic interventions.

NURSING DIAGNOSIS: Risk for fluid volume deficit R/T purging cycles

a. *Expected outcomes:* Following instruction, the person should demonstrate adequate urine output, good skin turgor, moist mucous membranes, and other parameters that reflect normal fluid balance.

b. *Nursing interventions*
(1) Monitor intake and output.
(2) Offer fluids as needed.
(3) If person used vomiting, laxatives, or diuretics to purge, monitor not only fluids but also potassium, as severe cardiac problems can result from potassium deficits.
12. Discharge planning and teaching
a. Teach the person to control weight by decreasing caloric intake, choosing a variety of foods from the Food Guide Pyramid, and eating at least 3 times a day (Learning/Teaching Guidelines for Persons with Bulimia).
b. Provide handouts and pamphlets about food and its relationship to health.
c. Refer to the American Anorexia and Bulimia Association and the Anorexia Nervosa and Bulimia Resource Center for valuable information.

Protein-Energy Malnutrition

1. Definition: A deficiency in protein, calories, or both.
a. Classifications
(1) **Marasmus** is a deficiency of both calories (energy) and protein.
(2) **Kwashiorkor** is a protein deficiency only and appears in the United States when nutrient requirements are high but intake is curtailed.
2. Incidence and socioeconomic impact
a. Protein-energy malnutrition is becoming more prevalent because the number of homeless people and migrant workers is increasing.
b. It is estimated that approximately 50 percent of all hospital admissions have some form of protein-energy malnutrition.
c. Protein-energy malnutrition can result in increased absenteeism from work and school.
d. When protein-energy malnutrition is present, learning is affected adversely.
e. The ability to become fully productive adults is diminished in persons who have protein-energy malnutrition.
3. Risk factors
a. Homelessness
b. Immigrant status
c. Financial difficulties or poverty
d. Age, particularly older people
e. Multiple medications regimen
f. Chronic diseases
g. Stress and trauma
4. Etiology
a. Decreased nutrient intake: refusal to eat foods provided, difficulty in purchasing and preparing food, financial constraints, or poor cooking facilities can all contribute to decreased nutrient intake. People with cancer, AIDS, GI disorders, chronic obstructive pulmonary disease, and problems of substance abuse are also included in this category.
b. Increased nutritional requirements: Illness, stress, and trauma have catabolic effects that increase nutri-

tional requirements when oral intake is poor. Typical cases are persons under acute stress who have been on standard intravenous dextrose solutions for an extended period (2 weeks or more).
c. Increased nutrient losses: Prolonged diarrhea, vomiting, or both or an inability to absorb or digest nutrients causes an increase in nutrient losses.
d. Usually takes 2 weeks to develop.
5. Pathophysiology
a. With decreased nutrient intake the body starts to "feed" on itself. After glycogen stores are depleted (12–24 hr) protein tissues are catabolized for glucose. This leads to a decreased basal metabolic rate, which results in energy needs being decreased and body proteins being conserved. Also, fat is broken down for energy, leading to ketone production.
6. Clinical manifestations
a. Marasmus
(1) Extremely underweight, emaciated
(2) Normal hair
(3) Wasted, drawn appearance
(4) Decreased muscle mass
(5) Fat loss
(6) No edema
b. Kwashiorkor
(1) Well-nourished appearance
(2) Easily pluckable hair
(3) Round, moon face
(4) Decreased muscle mass
(5) Fat loss minimal
(6) Edema
7. Diagnostics
a. History: risk factors, knowledge, ability to care for self, purchase and prepare food; length of time on dextrose intravenous solutions
b. Physical examination: body weight, weight gain or loss, percent weight loss, triceps skinfold fat, midarm muscle circumference; diarrhea, anorexia
c. Dietary: appetite, food intake, taste or smell alterations, unpalatable modified diets, chewing or swallowing disorders
d. Laboratory tests: albumin, transferrin, prealbumin; glucose, total lymphocyte count; cholesterol, triglycerides
e. Marasmus is a chronic illness with gradual wasting leading to severe cachexia. Diagnosis is principally based on anthropometric findings: weight less than 80 percent of standard for height, triceps skinfold less than 3 mm, midarm muscle circumference less than 15 cm.
f. Trauma or a life-threatening illness results in a hypermetabolic state; kwashiorkor may develop if nutrient intake is inadequate. Diagnosis is based primarily on laboratory findings: serum albumin less than 2.8 gm per dl, total iron binding capacity less than 200 μg per dl, lymphocytes fewer than 1500/mm^3.
8. Clinical management
a. Goals of clinical management
(1) Correct the nutritional deficiencies
(2) Reverse the downward trend

b. Nonpharmacologic interventions
  (1) Marasmus: Increase calories and protein gradually to allow for readaptation of metabolic and intestinal functions. Monitor closely for metabolic imbalances such as hypophosphatemia and cardiorespiratory failure. Monitor intake and report any problems to the dietitian or physician or both. Weigh the person twice a week, or as ordered.
  (2) Kwashiorkor: Implement aggressive nutritional support to provide the high caloric and protein requirements.
c. Pharmacologic interventions
  (1) Marasmus: If the person is unable to consume adequate amounts, nutritional support with liquid nutritional supplements, tube feeding, or TPN may be initiated at a slow rate with gradual increases.
  (2) Kwashiorkor: Enteral or parenteral feedings are usually necessary to provide adequate nutrients; if the person can eat, liquid nutritional supplements, enteral, or parenteral feedings may supplement oral intake.
d. Special medical-surgical procedures: Enteral and parenteral feedings are usually required.
9. Complications
  a. Increased chance of infection
  b. Poor healing of wounds
  c. Mental lassitude
  d. Diminished cardiac output
  e. Reduced vital capacity
  f. Increased morbidity and mortality
10. Prognosis
  a. Marasmus: Usually is not life threatening, but response and cure are lengthy, slow processes.
  b. Kwashiorkor: Aggressive nutritional support is required to prevent the high mortality rate.
11. Applying the nursing process

NURSING DIAGNOSIS: Nutrition: Less than body requirements R/T increased metabolic requirements and/or decreased intake secondary to financial problems, anorexia, knowledge deficit, and the like

a. *Expected outcomes:* Following instruction, the person should gain 1 to 2 pounds per week until desired body weight is obtained, consume 85 percent of ordered diet, and plan a nutrient-dense, well-balanced, high-calorie, high-protein diet.
b. *Nursing interventions*
  (1) If adequate nutrient intake via oral intake of regular foods is not feasible, follow nutritional support orders, for example, nutritional supplements, enteral feedings, or TPN, or a combination thereof. Explain the type of intervention and the rationale for its use. Explain the plan for resuming normal food intake.
  (2) Discuss the problems associated with inadequate food intake, and try to determine why it has occurred.
  (3) Refer to nonpharmacologic interventions for more information, depending on the type of mal-

nutrition (protein-energy malnutrition, marasmus, or kwashiorkor).
12. Discharge planning and teaching
  a. Before discharge, people need to understand that an adequate diet is essential to prevent health problems and how to obtain adequate nutrients.
  b. If indicated, refer to a social worker for government programs (food stamps, Meals on Wheels) and other community resources available.
  c. If oral intake is not adequate before discharge, teach individuals how to maintain the method of nutritional support currently being used (tube feeding, TPN) or tell the person where nutritional supplements can be purchased.

BOX 10–4. Drugs That May Decrease Food Intake

Suppress the Appetite Center
Anorexiants
Chlorphentermine
Haloperidol

Nausea-Producing
Antimicrobials
Antineoplastics
Cardiac glycosides
Iron preparations
Nonsteroidal anti-inflammatory drugs

Inflamed Mouth
Antineoplastics

Elevated Blood Glucose
Glucagon
Sympathomimetics

Delayed Gastric Emptying
Beta-adrenergic stimulants, such as salbutamol
Bulk-forming laxatives
Levodopa

Anorexia
Alcohol
Amphetamines
Antineoplastics

Altered Sensitivity to Taste or Smell
Allopurinol
Amphetamines
Antidiabetics
Antilipemics
Antimicrobials
Antineoplastics
Captopril
Carbamazepine
Disulfiram
Furosemide
Levodopa
Lithium carbonate
Methimazole
Penicillamine
Phenytoin
Potassium iodide
Tricyclic antidepressants

Other Nutritional Disorders and Alterations

1. General effects of illness
   a. Decreased appetite is prevalent during many illnesses because of the following:
      (1) Apathy
      (2) Anorexia
      (3) Drugs that directly suppress the appetite center (Box 10–4), (b) decrease ability to smell or taste, (c) alter taste, (d) cause nausea and vomiting, (e) delay gastric emptying, and (f) cause mouth soreness.
      (4) Pain
      (5) Inactivity
      (6) Modified diets
   b. Nutrient requirements usually increase during illness because of the following:
      (1) Decreased absorption of nutrients
      (2) Increased losses of electrolytes and nitrogen
      (3) Increased metabolic rate
   c. Psychosocial needs
      (1) Psychologic stress accompanies most health problems.
      (2) Hospitalization causes psychologic stress because of unfamiliar surroundings, routines, and meals; apprehension about what is going to happen, and dependence on others for care, meals, and all other needs.
      (3) Stress can be both the cause and the consequence of poor intake.

2. Hypermetabolic conditions
   a. Hypermetabolism indicates an increased expenditure of resting energy and oxygen utilization that occurs in direct proportion to the extent and severity of an injury or infection.
   b. Hypercatabolism, or marked loss of protein and fat, accompanies hypermetabolism.
   c. Physiologic stress can lead to a hypermetabolic response:
      (1) Injury—trauma, spinal cord, head, burns
      (2) Surgery
      (3) Infection, especially sepsis
   d. Nutritional concerns for a hypermetabolic person
      (1) The primary goals include preventing weight loss that results from depleted muscle mass and fluid losses and restoring anabolism by furnishing nutrients to meet increased demands and replace lost tissue protein.
      (2) Implement aggressive nutritional support when the blood glucose level decreases.
      (3) Provide nutrients in whatever form the person can handle (oral feedings plus nutritional supplements, tube feedings, or TPN).
      (4) The amount of calories provided are crucial.
         • The amount required is secondary to the type of insult but is generally around 1.2 to 1.5 times the basal energy expenditure or 35 to 45 calories per kg daily.
         • Normally 2000 to 3000 calories per day meet these requirements; however, with burns this amount can increase to 4000 to 7000 calories per day.

Table 10–10. Referral Chart for Community Nutrition Resources

Population Group	Risk Factor	Referral Source*	Contact
Pregnant and lactating women	Low income	Food stamps	Welfare office
	Anemia, inadequate weight gain, age-related risk factor, inadequate diet, adolescent pregnancy, inadequate health care, or lack of food and nutrition information	WIC Program Maternity and Infant Care Project EFNEP Prenatal education	City, county, or state health department State health department Land-grant universities Prenatal clinic or private health care team
Infants	Low birth weight, failure to thrive, or poor growth patterns	WIC Program	City, county, or state health department
	Inadequate health care	Children and Youth Project	State health department
Children	Poor growth patterns, inadequate diet, or anemia	WIC Program (up to 5 years of age) Children and Youth Project (up to 18 years of age)	City, county, or state health department State health department
	Low income	Headstart (preschool) School lunch School breakfast	Local community action project Board of education Local community action project
Elderly	Low income	Food stamps Congregate meal sites	Welfare office Social service agency
	Homebound	Meals on Wheels	Social service agency
	Diabetes	American Diabetes Association	Local chapter
	Obesity	Weight reduction groups	(See adult section)
	Cardiovascular disease	American Heart Association	Local chapter

*This is only a partial listing. Program may vary in different parts of the United States. Also see list of Agencies and Resources (p 337).
Adapted from Finkelhor S. Nutrition resources. *Med Clin North Am* 63(5):1117–1123, 1979.

Table 10–11. Nutritional Impact of and Nursing Interventions for Miscellaneous Other Disorders

Potential Nutritional Impact	Recommended Dietary Changes or Interventions
Gastrointestinal Disorders	
Because the gastrointestinal tract is the only natural way of providing nutriment to the body, these disorders can be particularly devastating to nutritional status. With altered GI functions, digestion, absorption, or both are usually compromised.	Offer small, frequent feedings to minimize irritation while maintaining nutritional status. Reduce stress, anxiety, and frustration, as this may be as important as providing adequate nutrition. Limiting fat intake is recommended for the following: obesity, gallbladder disease, malabsorption syndromes. Increasing fiber intake may lessen risk of various GI diseases. Increased fiber intake is suggested for constipation, irritable bowel disease, diverticulosis. Increasing intake of soluble fiber is recommended for obesity and diarrhea. However, fiber restriction may be warranted during acute phases of ulcerative colitis, Crohn's disease, and diverticulitis.

Lactose Intolerance

Congenital Lactase Deficiency: A rare condition, which may be present at birth because of an inborn error of metabolism.
Lactase Deficiency: The most common condition. A developmental age-related decrease in lactase activity.
Secondary Lactase Deficiency: Low lactase activity. Usually temporary secondary to GI disease or intestinal mucosa damage, such as bacterial infections.
  Lactase deficiency occurs in about 92% of Asians, 79% of Native Americans, 75% of Blacks, 51% of Hispanics, and 21% of whites.

Because of insufficient amounts of lactase enzyme, malabsorption of the disaccharide lactose leads to diarrhea, abdominal cramps, and flatulence. Because milk and milk products provide the most readily available source of calcium to the body, people with malabsorption disorders are prone to osteoporosis. When lactose-containing products are avoided, measures should be taken to provide adequate amounts of calcium. Milk and milk products are also good sources of protein, riboflavin, potassium, and magnesium. Because of different tolerance levels, each person needs to experiment to determine which method is most effective for providing necessary nutrients without discomfort. Usually the amount of lactose tolerated is cumulative: for example, a person may be able to tolerate cheese on an English muffin or crackers (made without milk) but may not be able to tolerate cheese on regular bread that contains milk.	Reduce lactose-containing foods, but because of the nutritional significance of milk and other milk-containing products, total elimination is not advisable. Lower the amount of dairy products to the person's tolerance level because lactose digestion is not an all-or-nothing phenomenon. Whole milk is tolerated better than skim milk, especially if taken with a meal and limited to 4 oz at a time. Fermented dairy products—especially unflavored yogurt, but also buttermilk, aged cheese (Swiss, Colby, longhorn), soft cheese (cream cheese, Neufchatel, cottage cheese, farmer's, ricotta), and sour cream—are well tolerated. Suggest commercially available lactase, available in tablet or liquid form to hydrolyze the lactose in milk products or use lactose-hydrolyzed commercially available milk. Follow the instructions carefully when using lactase enzymes. Suggest increasing intake of other calcium-containing foods: salmon and sardines canned with bones, spinach, kale, broccoli, turnip and beet greens, molasses, tofu, almonds, orange, eggs, and shrimp. Consider using commercially available nutrition supplements such as Ensure (Ross) or Resource (Sandoz) that are lactose free. If the above suggestions are not feasible to maintain an adequate intake of at least 600 mg calcium, consult a physician or registered dietitian for calcium supplements that are well absorbed. These supplements may also need to include vitamin D.

Endocrine Disorders

Diabetes mellitus (main metabolic disorder treated by diet)

Despite the use of insulin that helps normalize blood glucose levels, disturbances in lipid and protein occur. Electrolyte imbalances are also prevalent. Goals of the diabetic diet, discussed in Chapter 28, are to maintain good control of the diabetes, to prevent long-term complications associated with diabetes, and to promote near normal blood glucose and lipid levels.	Amount of dietary fat is limited for persons with diabetes. In diabetes, carbohydrate is increased to 60% using principally complex carbohydrates and limited amount of simple sugars. Increased intake of soluble fiber is recommended for diabetics.

Adrenal, Thyroid, and Parathyroid Dysfunction

Imbalances of hormones secreted by these glands directly affect how the body handles nutrients.	For adrenal problems a high-protein, moderate-carbohydrate diet is recommended; concentrated sugars are avoided; vitamin C is encouraged.

Table 10–11. Nutritional Impact of and Nursing Interventions for Miscellaneous Other Disorders (Continued)

Potential Nutritional Impact	Recommended Dietary Changes or Interventions
Glucocorticoids, secreted by the adrenal glands, affect carbohydrate, protein, and lipid metabolism. Thyroid hormones control the rate of biochemical processes, the metabolism of carbohydrates, fats, and proteins, and basal metabolic rate. The body needs iodine from the diet to synthesize these hormones. The parathyroid hormones help maintain a constant serum calcium level. With modern technology, the most effective treatment is hormonal replacement.	For hypothyroidism: Limit calories as needed; encourage fluids and high-fiber foods to prevent constipation; recommend iodized salt consumption. For hyperthyroidism: Encourage a high-calorie (3000 cal), high-protein (1–2 gm/kg), nutrient-dense diet; offer snacks frequently; encourage 3–4 L/day of fluids; limit high-fiber foods; follow suggestions for lactose intolerance as persons with hyperthyroidism are prone to lactose intolerance. For parathyroid dysfunctions: In hypo states: Offer a high-calcium and high–vitamin D diet; calcium supplements are usually required because diet alone cannot supply the necessary amounts. In hyper states: Offer a low-calcium and low–vitamin D diet; encourage 2–3 L/day of fluids to prevent kidney stones and constipation.

Hypertension

Dietary modifications lower blood pressure for many persons with mild to moderate hypertension. The following nutritional factors are associated with high blood pressure: obesity, high sodium intake, and >1–2 oz daily of alcohol intake. However, the following are correlated with low blood pressure: high potassium and calcium intake.	Encourage weight loss, a low-calorie diet, and increased exercise, as these are the the most effective nonpharmacological interventions for reducing blood pressure in persons with mildly elevated diastolic blood pressure. Suggest a well-balanced diet to provide adequate amounts of calcium, potassium, and magnesium. Low-sodium diets can enhance antihypertensive effects of medications. Refer to Chapter 23 for more information on hypertension.

Coronary Heart Disease

Nutritional aspects can be manipulated to alter several risk factors for coronary heart disease: increased weight, serum low-density lipoproteins, serum cholesterol, and blood pressure. To make these changes realistic, the National Cholesterol Education Program has outlined a 2-step approach to diet therapy to reduce total intake of fat, saturated fatty acids, and cholesterol, and to promote weight loss in overweight persons.	Encourage the Step 1 diet: Total fat intake is 30% of total caloric intake, saturated fat is <10% of total caloric intake, and cholesterol intake is <300 mg. (This is the recommended diet in the 7 guidelines for Americans.) If the Step-1 diet is not effective in lowering serum cholesterol, a registered dietitian should help the person in adopting the Step-2 diet: Fat intake <30% of total caloric intake; saturated fat is decreased to <7% of calories; cholesterol intake <200 mg. Provide support and praise for these people; this diet should become a lifelong habit. Encourage intake of soluble fiber, as this can decrease cholesterol serum levels.

Renal Disorders

Parts of the kidney (nephrons, tubules, glomerulus) eliminate or retain various nutrients depending on the body's needs. Dietary modifications depend on which part of the kidney is diseased. Nutrients that may be of concern: protein, calcium, potassium, sodium, phosphorus, fluid. Calories (energy) intake become a major concern because of the poor appetite these people experience. Foods that produce or contain too much "waste" are limited to prevent accumulation. The following nutritional complications can occur: protein losses; fluid and electrolyte imbalances; acidosis, calcium and phosphorus imbalances; lipid alterations; anemia; mineral and vitamin alterations; and weight loss.	Depending on the disorder, limit intake of the nutrients previously listed. Follow the renal exchange lists, similar to diabetic exchange lists, to help people choose appropriate foods in correct amounts. Because of the complexities of this diet, refer persons to a registered dietitian to be sure adequate nutrients are provided with the many restrictions imposed. Monitor sodium and potassium intake. Implement measures to control edema.

Immune Disorders (Cancer, AIDS, Allergies)

A majority of the immune disorders cause an increase in metabolism that affects carbohydrate, fat, and protein utilization. Anorexia, diarrhea, malabsorption, nausea, vomiting, early satiety, and distorted sense of taste occur, especially in cancers and in AIDS. From these effects almost every nutrient is adversely affected either during ingestion, digestion, absorption, metabolism, or utilization.	*Cancer:* Increasing intake of cruciferous vegetables, high-fiber food, vitamins A and C and maintaining ideal body weight are suggestions to reduce the risk of cancer. Increase nutrient and caloric intake to prevent "stealing" of nutrient by the tumor itself. This is very difficult and takes creativity because the person is usually anorectic. Encourage a high-protein (1.3 gm/kg) and high-calorie (35–42 cal/kg) diet.

Table continued on following page

Table 10–11. Nutritional Impact of and Nursing Interventions for Miscellaneous Other Disorders (Continued)

Potential Nutritional Impact	Recommended Dietary Changes or Interventions
Food allergies often cause a person to eliminate an entire food group, increasing the occurrence of serious nutrient deficiencies. Allergies can result from the food itself or from the additives or components in foods. Typical food sources include milk, wheat, beef, pork, corn, soy, nut, egg, and fish. Food additives are usually sulfites, monosodium glutamate, nitrates, and tartrazine. Generally, the components that cause the most problems are histamine, monoamines, salicylate, and methylxanthines.	Implement nutritional interventions previously discussed in this chapter for nausea, vomiting, early satiety, and anorexia. Avoid acidic beverages and food temperature extremes if oral lesions are present. Parenteral and enteral feedings may be necessary. *AIDS:* Only the difference from cancer will be discussed. Encourage a high-protein (2.5 gm/kg) and high-calorie (35–40 cal/kg) diet in small, frequent feedings. Instruct the person to eat meats that are well done; never to eat raw foods such as eggs, fruits, vegetables, fish, or meats, as in sushi or steak tartare; not to mix cooked foods with raw meats or vegetables; and to avoid unpasteurized milk or cheeses, cold cuts, and tofu. *Allergies:* Encourage elimination or rotation diets. Teach the person how to replace the eliminated food with those of similar nutrient value. For most allergies, consult a registered dietitian to enhance compliance with diet and nutritional adequacy of the diet. Teach people how to read food labels for offending food. Refer to Food Allergy Center and the Food Allergy Network.

Alcoholism and Other Drug Addictions

Chemical dependency frequently leads to malnutrition. Nutritional problems are encountered because (1) vitamins needed to metabolize energy are inactivated; (2) the damaged liver is unable to store adequate amounts of nutrients; (3) nutrient utilization is poor; (4) nutrients help detoxify and metabolize drugs; (5) food intake is usually poor (except with marijuana users); and (6) even when caloric intake is adequate (as with marijuana users), food choices are poor, with large amounts of high-fat foods and few fruits and vegetables.	Provide palatable, nourishing meals and supplements. Encourage normal eating patterns. Provide nutritional education and counseling to the user and family members. Help persons and family in development of an eating plan supportive of stable recovery. Offer 2000 ml fluid daily. Encourage a diet high in complex carbohydrates with moderate amounts of protein and low fat intake. Explain to alcoholics that a diet high in proteins and fat can lead to drinking binges. Refer to Alcoholics Anonymous, Narcotics Anonymous, Cocaine Anonymous, Al-Anon, Alateen, Women for Sobriety, or National Council on Alcoholism and Drug Dependence.

- Using a portable metabolic cart (a machine that is programmed to calculate the exact caloric requirements or resting energy expenditure of patients), caloric requirements for these patients should be determined to prevent the problems that may occur when the patient receives too many calories, for example hyperglycemia, hepatic abnormalities, fatty liver, infiltration, and ventilator dependence.
  - e. Protein and fluid losses are increased not only from increased resting metabolic rate but also from exudate, discharge, hemorrhage, vomiting, fever, or diuresis.
    - (1) Protein requirements can range from 1.0 to 2.5 gm per kg body weight depending on the severity of the stress; for the burned person 20 to 25 percent of the total caloric requirements should be protein.
    - (2) Fluid levels must be replaced, but extreme care must be taken not to overload the person because

hypermetabolism can lead to renal shutdown; thus, monitoring intake and output is crucial. Usually 2 to 4 liters are required, unless there is a preexisting cardiac disease.
  - f. Foods high in vitamin A, vitamin C, and zinc should be offered, as these nutrients enhance healing.
  - g. To ensure goals are being met, the person is weighed every other day until weight is stable; then weighing takes place weekly.
3. Pregnancy and lactation
  - a. Most nutrient requirements increase to some extent because of increased growth and metabolism.
    - (1) Pregnancy
      - **Calories**—An additional 300 calories per day are required during the 2nd and 3rd trimester. No extra calories are needed during the 1st trimester unless the woman is severely underweight.

- **Protein**—An extra 10 to 14 gm per day are suggested.
  - (2) Lactation
    - **Fluid**—1000 ml per day extra
    - **Calories**—an additional 500 calories per day; total 2000 to 2500 calories per day
  b. Appropriate weight gain reflects the adequacy of energy intake.
    - (1) First trimester: 2 to 4 pounds
    - (2) Second and 3rd trimester: 1 pound per week
    - (3) Overall weight gain: 25 to 35 pounds
  c. Although the mother must provide nutrients for 2, energy requirements are not doubled and foods must be chosen wisely, using mostly nutrient-dense low-calorie foods.
  d. Lack of funds and knowledge can affect the outcomes of pregnancy and lactation adversely; resources are available, so refer as needed (Table 10–10).
  e. Specific nutritional problems for pregnancy and lactation are discussed in Chapter 14.
4. Geriatric influences

a. Energy requirements are lower as a result of lower body metabolism and decreased activity levels.
b. Most other nutrient requirements are the same as those for younger adults, or they may increase because of functional decline of many body organs, affecting absorption, transportation, metabolism, or excretion of nutrients.
c. Older people differ from one another more than any other group. For instance, one 85-year-old person may be very active and healthy, whereas another may be confined to a wheelchair and disoriented. By contrast, we expect all infants to sit and walk at approximately the same age.
d. Nutritional problems are frequently a result of socioeconomic and psychologic factors. Some of the socioeconomic factors can be minimized by using the community resources listed in Table 10–11.
e. Malnutrition usually occurs gradually and is frequently unrecognized until full-blown medical problems develop.

BOX 10–5. Healthy People 2000

Healthy People 2000: Nutrition Priority Areas

1. Reduce coronary heart disease deaths to no more than 100 per 100,000 people.
2. Reverse the rise in cancer deaths to achieve a rate of no more than 130 per 100,000 people.
3. Reduce overweight to a prevalence of no more than 20 percent among people ages 20 and older and no more than 15 percent among adolescents ages 12 through 19.
4. Reduce growth retardation among low-income children ages 5 and younger to less than 10 percent.
5. Reduce dietary fat intake to an average of 30 percent of calories or less, and average saturated fat intake to less than 10 percent of calories among people ages 2 and older.
6. Increase complex carbohydrates and fiber-containing foods on the diets of adults to 5 or more daily servings for vegetables and fruits and to 6 or more daily servings for grain products.
7. Increase to at least 50 percent the proportion of overweight people ages 12 and older who have adopted sound dietary practices combined with regular physical activity to attain an appropriate body weight.
8. Increase calcium intake so at least 50 percent of youth ages 12 through 24 and 50 percent of pregnant and lactating women consume 3 or more servings daily of foods rich in calcium, and at least 50 percent of people ages 25 and older consume 2 or more servings daily.
9. Decrease salt and sodium intake so at least 65 percent of home meals are prepared without adding salt, at least 80 percent of people avoid using salt at the table, and at least 40 percent of adults regularly purchase foods modified or lower in sodium.
10. Reduce iron deficiency to less than 3 percent among children ages 1 through 4 and among women of childbearing age.
11. Increase to at least 75 percent the proportion of mothers who breast-feed their babies in early postpartum period and to at least 50 percent the proportion who continue breast-feeding until their babies are 5 to 6 months old.
12. Increase to at least 75 percent the proportion of parents and caregivers who use feeding practices that prevent baby bottle tooth decay.
13. Increase to at least 85 percent the proportion of people ages 18 and older who use food labels to make nutritious food selections.
14. Achieve useful and informative labeling for virtually all processed food and at least 40 percent of fresh meats, poultry, fish, fruits, vegetables, baked goods, and ready-to-eat carryout foods.
15. Increase to at least 5000 brand names the availability of processed food products that are reduced in fat and saturated fat.
16. Increase to at least 90 percent the proportion of restaurants and institutional food service operations that offer identifiable low-fat, low-calorie food choices, consistent with the *Dietary Guidelines for Americans.*
17. Increase to at least 90 percent the proportion of school lunch and breakfast services and child care food services with menus that are consistent with the nutrition principles in the *Dietary Guidelines for Americans.*
18. Increase to at least 80 percent the receipt of home food services by people ages 65 and older who have difficulty in preparing their own meals or are otherwise in need of home-delivered meals.
19. Increase to at least 75 percent the proportion of the nation's schools that provide nutrition education from preschool through 12th grade.
20. Increase to at least 50 percent the proportion of worksites with 50 or more employees that offer nutrition education and/or weight management programs for employees.
21. Increase to at least 75 percent the proportion of primary care providers who provide nutrition assessment and counseling and/or referral to qualified nutritionists or dietitians.

From U.S. Dept. of Health and Human Services, Public Health Service. *Healthy People 2000: National Health Promotion and Disease Prevention Objectives.* Washington, DC: U.S. Government Printing Office, 1990.

f. Nutritional challenges of older persons are addressed in Chapter 16.

5. Other disorders (see Table 10–11)

◼ PUBLIC HEALTH CONSIDERATIONS

Healthy People 2000

1. In 1990, the U.S. Department of Health and Human Services released the document, *Healthy People 2000,* to increase the healthy lifespan, reduce health disparities, and achieve access to preventive services for all Americans.
2. To help meet these goals, specific objectives were identified in 21 different priority areas, involving nutrition (Box 10–5).
3. Based on a progress review in 1992, objectives showing positive results were improved death rate from coronary heart disease, increased numbers of people using nutrition labels to make food choices, and increased numbers of restaurants offering low-fat, low-calorie menu choices.

Nutrition Screening Initiative

1. Because of health concerns of the older population, the American Dietetic Association, the American Academy of Family Physicians, and the National Council on Aging developed a Nutrition Screening Initiative. The purpose is to identify older people at nutritional risk before serious health problems occur.
2. The goal is to identify risk factors and implement preventive interventions before the situation becomes severe by following these procedures:
   a. A person or caregiver completes the checklist that identifies factors that can increase the risk for poor nutritional status (poor eating habits, financial difficulties, unintentional weight gain or loss, multiple drug use). The higher the score, the more the person is at risk. Depending on the score, the person continues with previous eating habits, needs to be rechecked in 3 months, or is referred to a professional to determine the severity of the problem and the measures to be initiated. Sometimes the measures are implemented easily (transportation needs, economic assistance, assistance with shopping), whereas in other cases more extensive involvement is required (e.g., medical intervention and possibly hospitalization).

Bibliography

Books

Davis JR, and Sherer K. *Applied Nutrition and Diet Therapy for Nurses.* 2nd ed. Philadelphia: WB Saunders, 1994.

Mahan LK, and Escott-Stump S. *Krause's Food Nutrition & Diet Therapy.* 9th ed. Philadelphia: WB Saunders, 1996.

Williamson D. *Assessment and Diagnosis of Eating Disorders: Obesity, Anorexia, and Bulimia Nervosa.* New York: Pergamon Press, 1990.

Chapters in Books and Journal Articles

Anorexia Nervosa and Bulimia

Edelstein C, et al. Early clues to anorexia and bulimia. *Patient Care* 23(13):155–175, 1989.

Kent A. Advances in bulimia nervosa. *Practitioner* 235(1502):396–399, 1991.

McKenna M. Assessment of the eating disordered patient. *Psych Ann* 19(9):467–472, 1989.

Meades S. Suggested community psychiatric nursing interventions with clients suffering from anorexia nervosa and bulimia nervosa. *J Adv Nurs* 18(3):364–370, 1993.

Plehn K. Anorexia nervosa and bulimia: Incidence and diagnosis. *Nurs Pract* 15(4):22–31, 1990.

Yen JL. General overview and treatment considerations of anorexia and bulimia. *Compr Ther* 18(1):26–28, 1992.

Hypertension

Kushiro T, et al. Role of sympathetic activity in blood pressure reduction with low calorie regimen. *Hypertension* 17(6, pt 2):965–968, 1991.

Schmid TL, et al. Demographic, knowledge, physiological, and behavioral variables as predictors of compliance with dietary treatment goals in hypertension. *Addict Behav* 16(3–4):151–160, 1991.

Stevens VJ, et al. Weight loss intervention in phase 1 of the Trials of Hypertension Prevention. The TOHP Collaborative Research Group. *Arch Intern Med* 153(7):849–858, 1993.

The treatment of mild hypertension study. A randomized, placebo-controlled trial of a nutritional-hygienic regimen along with various drug monotherapies. The Treatment of Mild Hypertension Research Group. *Arch Intern Med* 151(7):1413–1423, 1991.

Transcultural Food Patterns

Cerrato PM. Suggest diets with a difference. *RN* 56(2):67–72, 1993.

Female Nutrition

Cerrato PM. Teens can shape their postmenopausal years. *RN* 55(3):65–66, 68, 1992.

Freed GL, et al. A practical guide to successful breast-feeding management. *Am J Dis Child* 145(8):917–921, 1991.

Gizis FC. Nutrition in women across the life span. *Nurs Clin North Am* 27(4):971–982, 1992.

Suitor CW, et al. Nutrition care during pregnancy and lactation: New guidelines from the Institute of Medicine. *J Am Diet Assoc* 93(4):478–479, 1993.

Obesity

Atkinson RL, et al. Combination of very-low-calorie diet and behavior modification in the treatment of obesity. *Am J Clin Nutr* 56(1 suppl):199S–202S, 1992.

Bowyer CA. Dietary aspects of treatment. *Int J Obes* 16(suppl 2):S47–S48, 1992.

Gabel LL, et al. Dietary prevention and treatment of disease. *Am Fam Physician* 46(5 suppl):41S–48S, 1992.

Goldstein DJ. Beneficial health effects of modest weight loss. *Int J Obes* 16(6):397–415, 1992.

Pi-Sunyer FX. The role of very-low-calorie diets in obesity. *Am J Clin Nutr* 56(1 suppl):240S–243S, 1992.

Schlundt DG, et al. The role of breakfast in the treatment of obesity: A randomized clinical trial. *Am J Clin Nutr* 55(3):645–651, 1992.

Targeting weight-reduction programs. *Nutr Rev* 48(11):414–416, 1990.

AIDS

Cerrato PL. What diet can do to combat HIV infection. *RN* 56(6):71–72, 1993.

Keithley JK, et al. Nutritional alterations in persons with HIV infections. *Image J Nurs Sch* 24(3):183–189, 1992.

Singer P, et al. Risks and benefits of home parenteral nutrition in the acquired immunodeficiency syndrome. *JPEN* 15(1):75–79, 1991.

Malabsorption

Cerrato PL. The patient's eating—why is he losing weight? *RN* 55(4):77–80, 1992.

Nutrition Support

Bell SJ, et al. Generic enteral formulas: A new idea for the 1990s. *Nutr Clin Pract* 10(6):237–241, 1995.

Bockus S. Troubleshooting your tube feedings. *Am J Nurs* 91(5):24–28, 1991.

Clevenger FW, and Rodriquez DJ. Decision-making for enteral feeding administration: The why behind where and how. *Nutr Clin Pract* 10(3):104–113, 1995.

Faller N, and Lawrence KG. Comparing low profile gastrostomy tubes. *Nursing 93* 23(12):46–48, 1993.

Friend B. Hospital at home. Self-service. *Nurs Times* 88(44):26–28, 1992.

Gionino S, et al. The ABCs of TPN. *RN* 59(2):42–47, 1996.

Heather DJ, et al. Effect of a bulk-forming cathartic on diarrhea in tube-fed patients. *Heart Lung* 20(4):409–413, 1991.

Kapadia SA, et al. Influence of three different fiber-supplemented enteral diets on bowel function and short-chain fatty acid production. *JPEN* 19(1):63–68, 1995.

Kudsk KA, et al. Visceral protein response to enteral versus parenteral nutrition and sepsis in patients with trauma. *Surgery* 116:516–523, 1994.

Murphy LM, and Conforti CG. Nutritional support of the cardiopulmonary patient. *Crit Care Nurs Clin North Am* 5(1):57–64 1993.

Pitts DM, et al. Nutritional support for the patient with diabetes. *Crit Care Nurs Clin North Am* 5(1):47–56, 1993.

Welch SK. Certification of staff nurses to insert enteral feeding tubes using a research-based procedure. *Nutr Clin Pract* 11(1):21–27, 1996.

Nutrition Assessment

Charney P. Nutrition assessment in the 1990s: Where are we now? *Nutr Clin Pract* 10(4):131–139, 1995.

Dwyer JT, et al. Assessing nutritional status in elderly patients. *Am Fam Physician* 47(3):613–620, 1993.

Gianino S, and St. John RE. Nutritional assessment of the patient in the intensive care unit. *Crit Care Nurs Clin North Am* 5(1):1–16, 1993.

Ham RJ. Indicators of poor nutritional status in older Americans. *Am Fam Physician* 45(1):219–228, 1992.

Natarajan VS, et al. Assessment of nutrient intake and associated factors in an Indian elderly population. *Age Ageing* 22(2):103–108, 1993.

Posner BM, et al. Nutrition and health risks in the elderly: The nutrition screening initiative. *Am J Public Health* 83(7):972–978, 1993.

Sidenvall B, and Ek AC. Long-term care patients and their dietary intake related to eating ability and nutritional needs: Nursing staff interventions. *J Adv Nurs* 18(4):565–573, 1993.

Protein-Energy Malnutrition

Constans T, et al. Protein-energy malnutrition in elderly medical patients. *J Am Geriatr Soc* 40(3):263–268, 1992.

Norris MK. Assessing albumin values. *Nursing* 22(1):84, 1992.

Heart Disease

Hinders S. Calcium and cholesterol: A balancing act. *Am J Nurs* 91(12):35, 1991.

Unosson M, et al. Demographical, sociomedical and physical characteristics in relation to malnutrition in geriatric patients. *J Adv Nurs* 16(12):1406–1412, 1991.

Agencies and Resources

AIDS

Task Force on Nutrition Support in AIDS
Wang Associates, Inc.
19 West 21st Street
New York, NY 10010

Anorexia Nervosa and Bulimia

American Anorexia and Bulimia Association
418 East 76th Street
New York, NY 10021

Anorexia Nervosa and Related Eating Disorders
P.O. Box 5102
Eugene, OR 97405

National Association of Anorexia Nervosa and Associated Disorders
P.O. Box 7
Highland Park, IL 60035

General

American Dietetic Association
216 West Jackson Boulevard, Suite 800
Chicago, IL 60606–6995
(800) 366–1655 (consumer hotline)

Food Research and Action Center (FRAC)
2011 I Street, N.W.
Washington, DC 20006

National Dairy Council
11 North Canal Street
Chicago, IL 60606

Nutrition Foundation
888 17th Street, N.W.
Washington, DC 20006

Society for Nutrition Education
1700 Broadway, Suite 300
Oakland, CA 94612

11
Caring for People in Pain

□ *PAIN*

Definition

1. Pain is a subjective sensation caused by noxious stimuli that signal actual or potential tissue damage.
   a. Pain can be perceived only by the person experiencing it.
   b. The interpretation of and response to pain is influenced by psychologic and cultural factors, such as values, beliefs, religion, norms, and customs. These factors also help determine the significance and meaning that pain holds for each person.

Neurophysiologic Mechanism of the Pain Experience

1. **Reception** refers to the neurophysiologic basis of the pain process.
   a. Noxious stimuli that cause pain are thermal, chemical, mechanical, or electrical.
   b. When peripheral tissues are damaged, chemical substances known as prostaglandins are secreted, which stimulate free nerve endings (nociceptors) in the tissues and convert pain stimuli into electrical impulses.
   c. Free nerve endings, or nociceptors, are located in various tissues throughout the body. However, other receptors in the body may also be activated by any type of intense stimulation and they may convert pain stimuli into electrical impulses.
   d. The nerve impulses travel along peripheral afferent nerve fibers (1st-order neurons) to the spinal cord, where neurotransmitter substances are secreted. These chemical substances (e.g., serotonin, dopamine, glycene, gamma-aminobutyric acid) either excite or inhibit the transmission of pain impulses across the synaptic cleft.
   e. Two types of peripheral afferent nerve fibers transmit stimuli: myelinated A fibers, which are large in diameter, transmit impulses rapidly, but generally do not transmit pain stimuli; and unmyelinated C fibers, which are small in diameter, slower, and responsible for transmitting pain stimuli.
   f. Both myelinated A fibers and unmyelinated C fibers enter the spinal cord through the dorsal roots of the spinal nerves (2nd-order neurons) and synapse with longer afferent nerve fibers in the dorsal column and spinothalamic tract.

   g. The pain impulses travel up the dorsal column and the spinothalamic tract (3rd-order neurons) and transmit pain information to the higher centers in the brain, including the reticular formation, limbic system, thalamus, and cerebral cortex.
   h. Melzack and Wall's **gate control theory of pain** (1965) suggests that a neural system composed of a specialized body of cells known as the substantia gelatinosa, located in lamina II and III of the dorsal horn of the spinal cord, acts as a gating mechanism and can decrease or block the transmission of pain stimuli.
      (1) When the intensity of stimuli transmitted by large-diameter myelinated A fibers exceeds the intensity of pain stimuli transmitted by small-diameter unmyelinated C fibers, it closes the gate to the pain stimuli.
      (2) In addition, sensory stimuli from the higher brain centers (e.g., auditory, visual) and selective brain processes (e.g., emotions, cognition) are capable of transmitting impulses by efferent neurons that activate the transmission T cells in the dorsal horn of the spinal cord and close the gate to incoming pain stimuli (Fig. 11–1).
   i. The body manufactures endogenous substances or endorphins that have analgesic properties. These substances are located within the central nervous system.
      (1) These endogenous chemicals bind with opiate receptors on afferent neurons at the synaptic cleft and inhibit the secretion of neurotransmitter substances, which in turn block the transmission of pain stimuli (Fig. 11–2).
2. **Perception** is the point at which the sensation of pain is experienced. The perception of pain is influenced by 3 interacting systems: the sensory-discriminative system, the motivational-affective system, and the cognitive-evaluative system.
   a. The sensory-discriminative system is located in the thalamus and cerebral cortex. It influences perception of the location, intensity, and character of the pain.
   b. The motivational-affective system is located in the limbic system and reticular formation of the brain stem. It influences protective or avoidance reactions and emotional responses to pain.
   c. The cognitive-evaluative activities occur in the higher cortical centers. They are influenced by a person's cultural background, experiences with pain, and the meaning of the pain.
      (1) The cognitive-evaluative system may influence both the sensory-discriminative and motivational-

GATE CONTROL THEORY OF PAIN

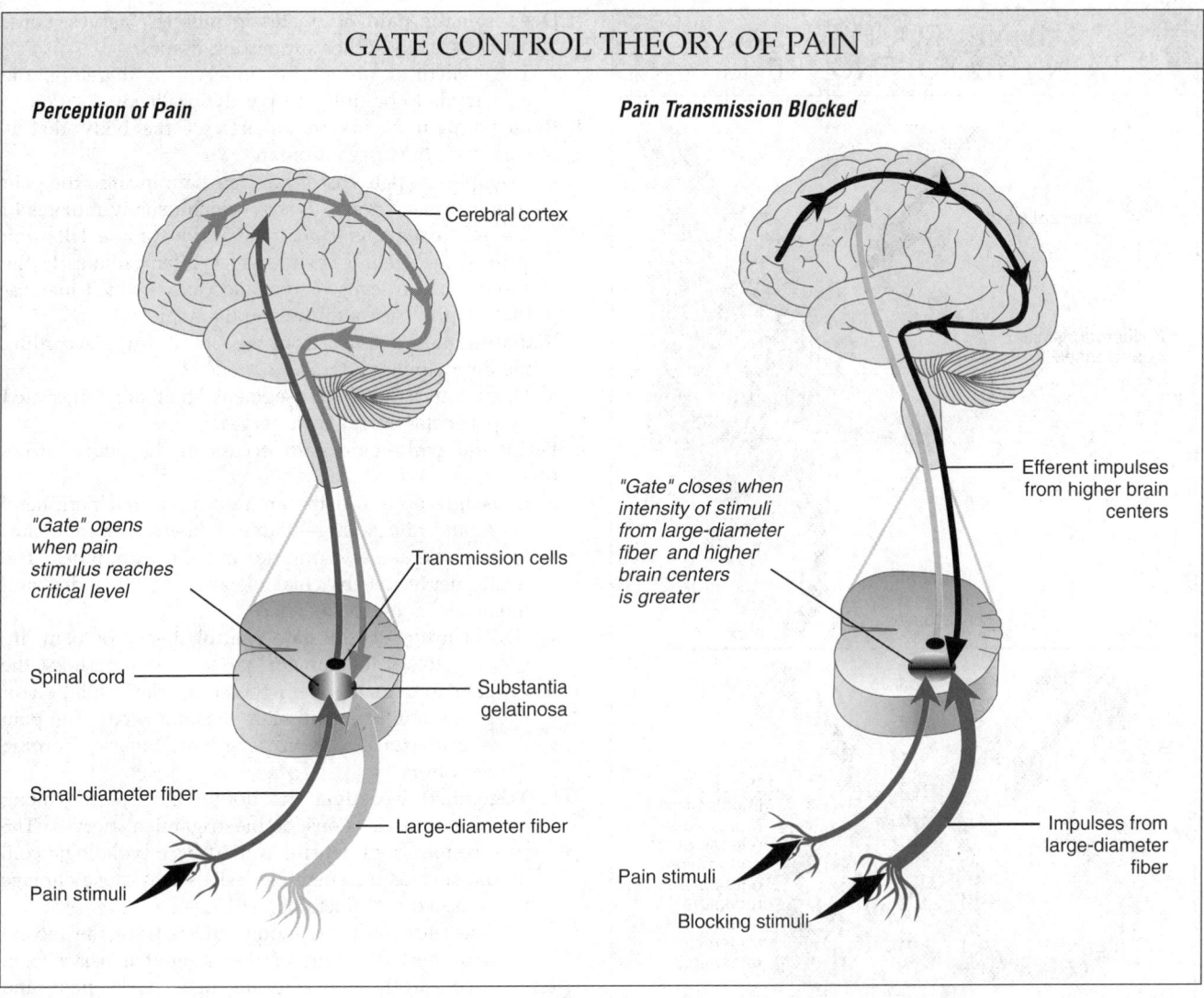

Perception of Pain

Cerebral cortex

"Gate" opens when pain stimulus reaches critical level

Transmission cells

Spinal cord

Substantia gelatinosa

Small-diameter fiber

Large-diameter fiber

Pain stimuli

Pain Transmission Blocked

"Gate" closes when intensity of stimuli from large-diameter fiber and higher brain centers is greater

Efferent impulses from higher brain centers

Impulses from large-diameter fiber

Pain stimuli

Blocking stimuli

Figure 11–1.

affective components of pain perception, and it accounts for the psychologic responses to pain perception.
3. **Reaction** refers to the physical and psychologic responses to pain perception.
4. **Tolerance** refers to the maximum level of pain tolerated.

◼ *TYPES OF PAIN*

Duration

1. **Acute pain** is generally caused by tissue damage. Its duration is relatively short, less than 6 months. The pain subsides with the appropriate interventions and as resolution of tissue damage occurs.
2. **Chronic pain** is of prolonged duration, lasting at least 6 months. Based on certain distinguishing characteristics, chronic pain may be classified as recurring acute pain, ongoing time-limited pain, and chronic benign pain.
   a. **Recurring acute pain** is characterized by recurring

episodes of pain that may continue over a lifetime. Examples include migraine headaches and sickle cell crises.
   b. **Ongoing time-limited pain** is characterized by a prolonged period of pain. The pain has a high probability of ending with appropriate interventions. Examples include burn pain and cancer pain.
   c. **Chronic benign pain** is generally due to non–life-threatening causes. It may not be responsive to many commonly used interventions and may continue for the remainder of the person's life. Examples include pain caused by rheumatoid arthritis, peripheral neuropathy, and Raynaud's disease.

Location

1. **Superficial or cutaneous pain** is localized on the skin or the body surface.
   a. The intensity of the pain usually correlates with the intensity of the stimulus; for example, pain can have a throbbing quality resulting from inflammation of the

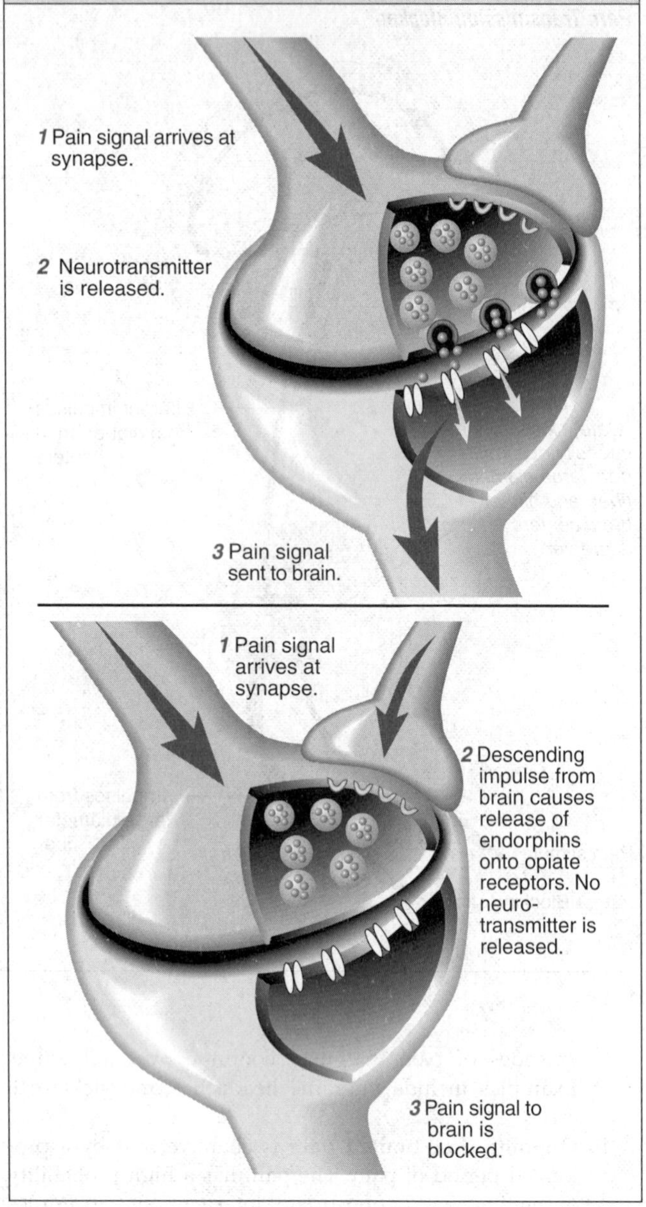

THE NEUROCHEMICAL PAIN THEORY: ENDORPHINS

1 Pain signal arrives at synapse.

2 Neurotransmitter is released.

3 Pain signal sent to brain.

1 Pain signal arrives at synapse.

2 Descending impulse from brain causes release of endorphins onto opiate receptors. No neurotransmitter is released.

3 Pain signal to brain is blocked.

Figure 11–2.

tissues, a sharp quality resulting from a pin stick, or a stinging quality resulting from an insect bite.

2. **Deep visceral pain** occurs in the internal organs.
   a. The pain tends to be diffused but may become localized if it continues. It may be constant or intermittent.
   b. The quality of the pain is influenced by the stimulus and may be characterized as burning, dull, aching, or sharp.
   c. Visceral pain may be accompanied by pain referred to superficial body locations, either adjacent to or remote from the affected organ. Visceral referred pain usually occurs in body areas that are innervated by a particular spinal cord segment or nerve endings.

3. **Deep somatic pain** originates in muscles, nerves, bone, blood vessels, and other supporting tissues.
   a. The structures are poorly innervated; therefore, the pain tends to be dull and poorly localized.
4. **Referred pain** occurs in an area of the body that is remote from the affected organ.
   a. Examples of patterns of referred pain include the pain from coronary heart disease, which usually radiates to the left axilla and down the inside of the left arm; pain in the pleural cavity, which often radiates to the shoulder; pain caused by cholecystitis, which may radiate to the back and the scapula angle.
5. **Radiating pain** extends from the site of origin according to the dermatome patterns.
   a. Dermatomes are body segments that are innervated by particular spinal cord nerves.
6. **Peripheral pathologic pain** occurs in the neural structures.
   a. **Causalgia** occurs in the area of an injured peripheral nerve and affects large-diameter fibers. Common sites for peripheral nerve injuries are the extremities. The sciatic nerve, the brachial plexus, and the radial and ulnar nerves can be affected.
      (1) According to the gate control theory of pain, injury to large-diameter nerve fibers permits the gate to remain open; therefore, the inhibition of pain stimuli transmission does not occur. The pain is characterized by a persistent, intense, burning sensation.
   b. **Trigeminal neuralgia** (tic douloureux) occurs along one or more divisions of the trigeminal nerves. The pain results from neuritis caused by a pathologic condition, such as degenerative lesions that cause damage to the nerve root fibers.
      (1) The sites most commonly affected are the second and third divisions of the trigeminal nerve; pain occurs in the mouth, gums, lips, cheeks, nose, and surface of the head.
      (2) The pain may be characterized by episodes of severe pain that last for a short period, or it may be ongoing. The pain may be precipitated by mechanical stimulation of the affected area, or it may occur spontaneously.
   c. **Postherpetic neuralgia** occurs following infection of the dorsal root ganglia. The infection is caused by the varicella-zoster (herpes zoster) virus.
      (1) Infection caused by the varicella-zoster virus destroys large-diameter nerve fibers of the dorsal root ganglia of the affected nerves. This process in turn destroys or decreases the capacity to close the gate to incoming pain stimuli, resulting in spontaneous pain.
      (2) Pain, along with vesicular eruptions caused by the infection, occurs along the distribution of the peripheral nerves arising from the affected dorsal root ganglia. Because of the patterns of the peripheral nerve distribution, the pain and vesicular eruptions may encircle body areas completely, such as the cervical, thoracic, lumbar, and sacral areas.
      (3) The pain is characterized by burning, dull, or

sharp sensations, varying in intensity from mild to severe. The pain may subside after the vesicular lesions heal; however, some patients may experience residual chronic pain indefinitely.

d. **Phantom pain** is perceived as occurring in a nonexistent body part, such as an amputated limb or breast.

(1) The mechanism of the pain perception is not clear. A variety of hypotheses have been proposed, including chronic low-level sensory input, abnormal neural activity in the dorsal horn of the spinal cord, and emotional factors. One hypothesis suggests that all of these factors may contribute to phantom pain.

e. **Headache** occurs in pain-sensitive structures in the head. Pain-sensitive structures include the blood vessels; the venous sinuses; the tentorium; the first 3 cervical nerves; the cranial nerves; the cranial periosteum; and the skin and tissues covering the cranium, muscles, and dura at the base of the brain.

(1) Types of headaches include muscle contraction/ tension, migraine, cluster, and headaches secondary to disease. See Chapter 18.

f. **Cancer pain** may be either acute or chronic in nature.

(1) Acute pain may occur as an early symptom of the underlying pathologic condition. It may also be induced by diagnostic procedures, surgery, or chemotherapy. Acute pain is usually time limited and often responds to a short course of analgesics.

(2) Chronic pain may occur as the cancer progresses or metastasizes to soft tissues, bone, and nerves. It also may be associated with ongoing cancer therapy (see Chapter 17).

g. **Psychologic pain** refers to pain for which there is no detectable physiologic or organic origin. The pain is believed to arise from mental or emotional factors. All pain has a psychologic component; however, the occurrence of pure psychologic pain is probably rare.

(1) It is important to remember that pain is a subjective experience. All pain is meaningful for the patient. The caregiver must never assume that the pain is imagined.

(2) Careful assessment and planning are significant. The assessment should include the patient's perception of the pain, its source, and meaning; the patient's attitude toward the pain and motivation; the expectation of the caregiver; and related factors. Emotions such as anxiety, depression, and hostility may be reactions to the pain. They frequently accompany psychologic pain.

(3) The nurse should appreciate the reality of the pain experience and, based on the assessment, develop a plan to provide pain relief, if possible.

▣ PHYSICAL RESPONSES TO PAIN

Physiologic Responses

1. Perception of pain activates the autonomic nervous system as part of the body's stress response.
   a. Low-intensity to moderate-intensity pain stimulates the sympathetic nervous system, resulting in physiologic responses. These responses include increased oxygen consumption, increased respiratory rate, increased rate and force of heart beat, increased blood pressure, decreased urinary output, increased muscle tension, and increased levels of blood glucose and epinephrine.
   b. When the pain is of high intensity, a parasympathetic response occurs as a compensatory reflex, resulting in a decrease in heart rate and blood pressure. If the pain continues, the body gradually adapts and the sympathetic responses subside.

Behavioral Responses

1. Behavioral responses to pain are mediated by the sensory-discriminative system. These responses are influenced by a variety of factors, such as pain tolerance level, cultural beliefs and values, prior experiences with pain, meaning of the pain, intensity of the pain, and situational factors, such as the caregiver's attitude.
   a. Behavioral responses include crying, moaning, quietness, restlessness, irritability, facial grimaces, clenching hands, muscle tension, perspiring, protective body posturing, and verbal reports of pain.
   b. When the pain is chronic in nature and the adaptive process has occurred, pain behavior may change. The "acute model" of moaning, grimacing, and the like may disappear and be replaced by a quieter demeanor, depression, lack of attention to personal appearance, loss of appetite, and withdrawal from social interaction.

▣ PSYCHOSOCIAL RESPONSES TO PAIN

Cognitive-Evaluative Component

1. The psychologic responses to pain are mediated by the cognitive-evaluative component of pain perception. These responses are influenced by a variety of factors, such as knowledge related to the cause of the pain, cultural beliefs and attitudes toward pain, past experiences with pain, and a sense of control over the pain or a sense of powerlessness to alter the pain.
2. Cultural beliefs and values, prior experiences with pain, knowledge regarding pain, and the like are subserved, at least in part, in memory stores by the cortical processes.
   a. The cognitive processes analyze the incoming sensory stimuli and their physical properties and evaluate them in terms of cultural beliefs and values, attitude, prior pain experiences, their meaning, and so forth.
   b. This analysis may affect the sensory-discriminative system and the motivational-affective system.
   c. These psychologic processes significantly influence one's perception of the quality and intensity of pain.
   d. Common psychologic responses to pain include fear, anxiety, anger, stoicism, denial, depression, and withdrawal.

Religious Beliefs

1. Religious beliefs and values strongly influence the way many people interpret health and illness and respond to the symptoms of illness, including pain. The religious beliefs and values of some cultural groups or subgroups may conflict with some conventional biomedical health care practices, such as the beliefs and values of Jehovah's Witnesses regarding the use of blood.
2. Religious beliefs may serve as a source of comfort for some people and increase their ability to cope with illness. However, religious beliefs may also affect a person's willingness to seek conventional medical treatment, as such action may be interpreted as showing a lack of faith in God and the healing power of prayer.

Socioeconomic Status

1. Socioeconomic status affects one's ability to secure health care and the nature of the care obtained. For example, persons of low socioeconomic status often tolerate pain for a long time before seeking relief because they lack health insurance or accessible health care services.
2. A prevailing premise in the United States is that health care is a commodity to be purchased. The higher the socioeconomic status, the more likely the person is to seek pain relief earlier.

Occupation

1. Occupation also affects the decision to seek care.
2. Persons with jobs requiring a great deal of physical exertion often do not seek help for pain because pain is considered normal, that is, a natural result of exertion on the job. Unless the pain interferes with their ability to function, it may not be considered significant.

Educational Background

1. The educational background of the person may influence his or her understanding of the cause and effect relationship of pain.
2. The higher the level of understanding about the cause of the pain and the ways it may be controlled, the lower the level of anxiety and the more likely the person is to seek biomedical assistance and to adhere to therapy.

◼ TRANSCULTURAL ATTITUDES TOWARD PAIN

The Patient's Attitude Toward Pain

1. An individual's definition of pain, like that of health and illness, is culturally determined. Pain is a highly personal experience influenced by cultural learning, the meaning of the situation, and other factors unique to the individual.

2. A patient's reaction to pain is influenced by the perception of the pain sensation and the motivational-affective system. Expressions of pain may vary considerably. To adequately interpret patients' responses to pain, you must view them within an ethnic cultural framework.
   a. Mexican Americans tend to view pain as a necessary part of life and as an indicator of the seriousness of an illness. Men often tolerate pain until it becomes unbearable.
   b. Puerto Rican patients often deny or avoid dealing with pain but may exhibit a high anxiety level.
   c. Black patients also may deny or avoid dealing with pain. Black patients often tolerate pain until it becomes unbearable, and they must seek emergency care. Both Black and Puerto Rican patients may perceive an overt reaction to pain as a threat to their self-esteem and view denial and avoidance behavior as more acceptable to the caregiver.
   d. Native Americans traditionally exhibit a stoic attitude and tolerate a high level of pain. Some patients may not seek pain relief and may tolerate pain until they are physically disabled.
   e. Asians
      (1) In many Asian cultures, pain is regarded as a serious symptom of illness for which biomedical care is sought. Acupuncture is a popular treatment for many health problems, including pain.
      (2) Japanese Americans regard pain as an integral part of illness and traditionally exhibit a stoic attitude toward it. Some Japanese Americans feel that it is disgraceful to express pain verbally, even when pain perception is intense. Patients may refuse pain medication when it is offered.
   f. Whites
      (1) Pain is regarded as a symptom of illness or injury. Evidence suggests that Whites exhibit a moderate level of pain tolerance and that they express pain behavior more readily than Blacks and are more likely to seek pain relief.
      (2) The majority of Whites seek biomedical care when they consider their symptoms to be serious.

The Nurse's Attitude Toward Pain

1. Because the United States is a culturally diverse society, nurses come in contact with patients from a variety of cultural backgrounds. The nurse's understanding of cultural influences is crucial in the management of pain.
2. Perhaps without conscious awareness, nurses often project their values onto patients from different cultures and with different beliefs and values. When the patient's behavior does not conform to expectations, the nurse may deny observing pain indicators and leave the patient to deal with the pain.
   a. Research suggests that some nurses prefer silence and self-control as responses to pain. Many nurses in the United States, most of whom are White, middle-class women, have been socialized to value self-control and a degree of stoicism in response to pain, as opposed to overt expressions of strong feelings.

b. Some nurses think that "good" patients should not complain, that they should control their pain in a stoic manner. Because of this stoicism, it is imperative that the nurse be especially attuned to nonverbal expressions of pain. Body tension is one of the cues that may signal the need for medication for pain relief.

3. Value clarification is an important process that enhances the nurse's understanding and awareness of personal values. An understanding of one's own values is crucial to dealing effectively with patients whose values and attitudes may be strikingly different from your own.

4. Cultural diversity exists in all health care delivery settings. By incorporating knowledge of cultural influences and patients' values into a framework for nursing practice, pain management is likely to be more effective.

TRANSCULTURAL CONSIDERATIONS

1. Pain is a complex phenomenon that is perceived differently by each individual.
2. The definition of pain, like that of health and illness, is culturally determined.
3. Pain expressions vary among patients of the same cultural background and vary even in the same patient in different situations.
4. The patient's behavior in response to pain is influenced by cultural definitions of how he or she should act and the meaning of the pain.
   a. The personal significance of the pain is influenced by one's cultural heritage.
   b. Exhibiting a helpful attitude and seeking reasons for behavior should promote the nurse's understanding of the situation and prevent labeling and stereotyping patients.
5. Knowledge of other cultures aids the nurse in examining her or his own cultural background, values, and beliefs, which promotes increased understanding of self.
6. A patient's nonverbal response to pain may not be due to cultural influences but rather to situational circumstances.
7. As much consideration and sensitivity should be shown for patients' non-Western values and practices as is shown for patients' Western values and practices in the management of pain.
   a. For example, patients experiencing pain should be allowed to incorporate their religious rituals and practices, as well as other alternative measures, such as herbal remedies, to aid in pain relief.
8. Patients of all cultures deserve competent care, including pain relief, clear explanations, and a helpful attitude from the caregivers.
9. The principle of justice is inherent in nursing practice when the efforts to relieve pain are extended to all patients.

◼ ASSESSING PEOPLE IN PAIN

Symptoms

1. The McGill-Melzack Pain Questionnaire is designed to measure the patient's pain symptoms. The questionnaire contains 5 basic components.

   a. *Pain Rating Index* (PRI): Twenty descriptive words or adjectives are used to describe the pain quality. These words are divided into 4 major groups of adjectives suggested by patients who helped to test the questionnaire in its research stage: 1–10 sensory, 11–15 affective, 16 evaluative, and 17–20 miscellaneous.
   b. *Number of words chosen* (NWC): This indicates the number of words chosen from the total of 20 in the group.
   c. *Present Pain Intensity* (PPI): The patient selects the word that most accurately describes the pain intensity.
   d. *Line Drawing of the Body:* The patient can describe the location of the pain and indicate whether it is internal or external and whether it is constant, periodic, or brief.
   e. *List of Symptoms:* The patient can describe the symptoms experienced.
   f. Space is provided to solicit information regarding the patient's sleep pattern, food intake, and activity pattern.

2. If thorough instructions are given and if the patient is able, the questionnaire may be completed by the patient; otherwise, to ensure accuracy, it may be completed by the nurse.
   a. Explain to the patient that he or she will read several groups of words, some of which may describe the patient's pain at this time. If so, the patient should select 1 word from each group; however, the patient is not required to select a word from every group—only the words that describe the pain.
   b. Next, ask the patient to pinpoint the location of the pain on the body line drawings and indicate the frequency of the pain. Ask the patient to describe his or her sleep pattern, food intake, and activity level.

3. To calculate the results of the assessment, do the following:
   a. Rank each word in each group of words and assign it the number value corresponding to its order in the group. For example, in the 1st (sensory, 1–10) group, "flickering" = 1, "quivering" = 2, "pulsing" = 3, and so on.
   b. Start again with each new group and assign a number value.
   c. Add up the number value the patient chose for each group of words (sensory, affective, evaluative, and miscellaneous) and mark these 4 totals in the spaces provided on the questionnaire. Mark the number of words chosen (NWC) and the present pain intensity (PPI) in the spaces provided.
   d. Write the patient's name, diagnosis, pain medication schedule, date and time of assessment, and your comments on the questionnaire.

4. This assessment should provide the caregiver with significant information regarding the patient's pain and should be used as a basis for pain treatment. After treatment and after the pain medication should have taken effect, reassessment should reflect the changes (or lack of them) in the PRI totals. This information should be used in planning more effective pain relief (Fig. 11–3).

McGill - Melzack Pain Questionnaire

Person's Name_____ Date _____ Time _____ am/pm
Analgesic(s)_____ Dosage_____ Time Given_____ am/pm
_____ Dosage_____ Time Given_____ am/pm
Analgesic Time Difference (hours):   +4   +1   +2   +3

PRI: S _____ A _____ E _____ M(S) _____ M(AE) _____ M(T) _____ PRI(T) _____
(1-10)   (11-15)   (16)   (17-19)   (20)   (17-20)   (1-20)

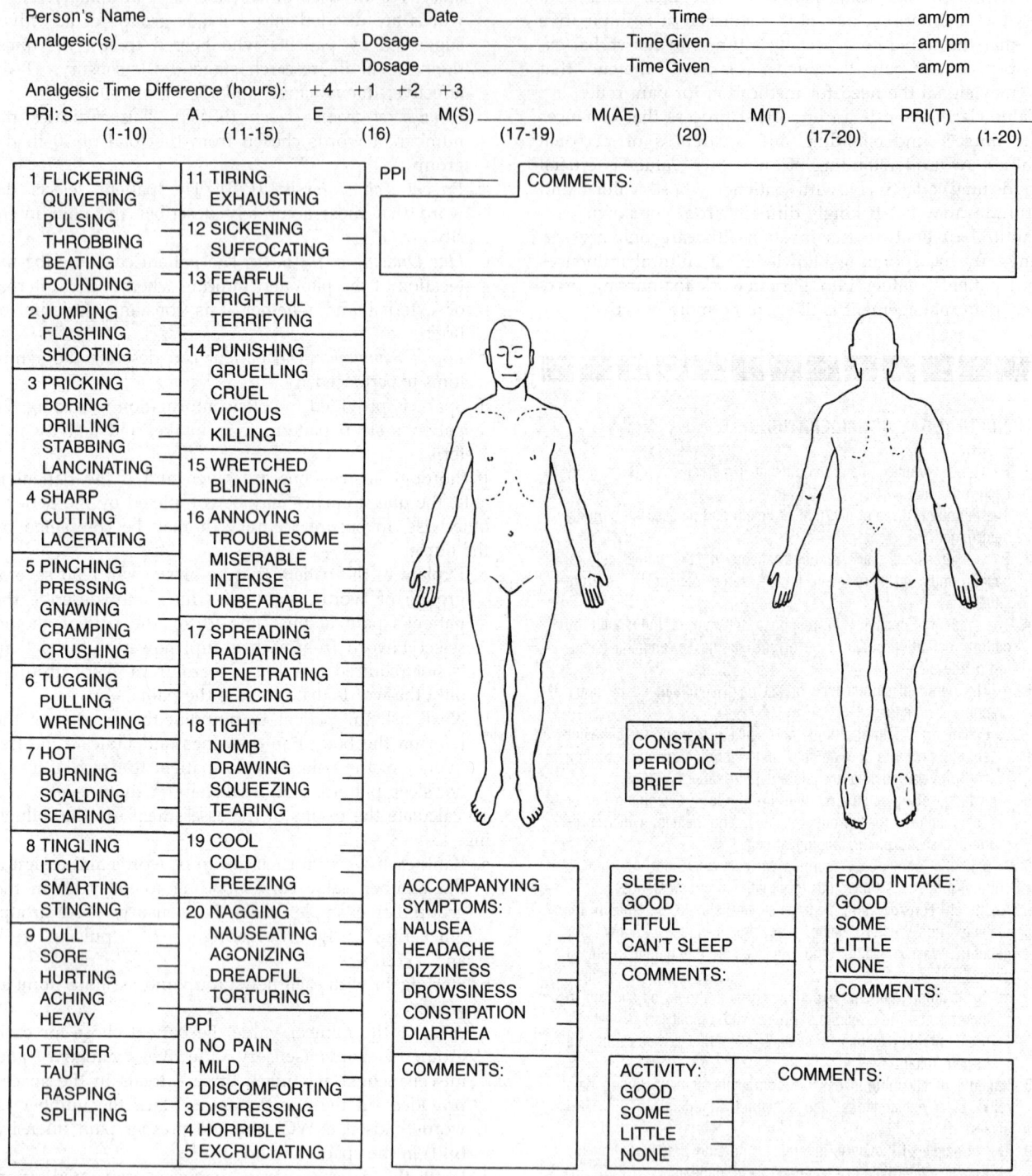

1 FLICKERING QUIVERING PULSING THROBBING BEATING POUNDING	11 TIRING EXHAUSTING
2 JUMPING FLASHING SHOOTING	12 SICKENING SUFFOCATING
3 PRICKING BORING DRILLING STABBING LANCINATING	13 FEARFUL FRIGHTFUL TERRIFYING
4 SHARP CUTTING LACERATING	14 PUNISHING GRUELLING CRUEL VICIOUS KILLING
5 PINCHING PRESSING GNAWING CRAMPING CRUSHING	15 WRETCHED BLINDING
6 TUGGING PULLING WRENCHING	16 ANNOYING TROUBLESOME MISERABLE INTENSE UNBEARABLE
7 HOT BURNING SCALDING SEARING	17 SPREADING RADIATING PENETRATING PIERCING
8 TINGLING ITCHY SMARTING STINGING	18 TIGHT NUMB DRAWING SQUEEZING TEARING
9 DULL SORE HURTING ACHING HEAVY	19 COOL COLD FREEZING
10 TENDER TAUT RASPING SPLITTING	20 NAGGING NAUSEATING AGONIZING DREADFUL TORTURING

PPI _____

COMMENTS:

CONSTANT
PERIODIC
BRIEF

ACCOMPANYING SYMPTOMS:
NAUSEA
HEADACHE
DIZZINESS
DROWSINESS
CONSTIPATION
DIARRHEA

COMMENTS:

SLEEP:
GOOD
FITFUL
CAN'T SLEEP
COMMENTS:

FOOD INTAKE:
GOOD
SOME
LITTLE
NONE
COMMENTS:

ACTIVITY:
GOOD
SOME
LITTLE
NONE

COMMENTS:

PPI
0 NO PAIN
1 MILD
2 DISCOMFORTING
3 DISTRESSING
4 HORRIBLE
5 EXCRUCIATING

Figure 11–3. McGill-Melzack Pain Questionnaire. (From Ronald Melzack, PhD, McGill University, Montreal, Canada, 1975. Reprinted with permission.)

History

1. The patient's pain history provides essential information about the pain experience. It should provide a chronology of events, including factors that are relevant to the pain location, onset, duration, intensity, quality, and precipitating and alleviating factors.

a. **Location.** To assess pain location, ask the patient to identify on the body line drawings the area or areas of pain or discomfort. Ask specific questions about the pain. Examples of questions include the following:
• Is the pain localized or diffused?
• Does it involve a large body area?
• Is the pain superficial or deep? Does it move?

- Is the pain on 1 side of the body or on both sides?
- Identify all areas of the pain on the body figures.
  b. **Onset.** To assess the onset of pain, ask specific questions. Examples of questions include the following:
- When did the pain begin?
- Was the onset sudden or gradual?
- What were you doing at the time the pain began?
- Did any specific thing trigger the pain?
- Is the pain constant or intermittent?
- Have you experienced this type of pain before? If so, what caused its onset?
  c. **Duration.** Duration refers to the length of time the pain is felt. To assess pain duration, the nurse should ask questions, such as the following:
- How long does the pain last with each occurrence?
- When did you last experience the pain?
- How frequently does it occur?
  d. **Intensity**
  (1) Pain intensity is the most subjective characteristic of the pain experience.
  (2) Assess pain intensity with the use of a scale designed to quantify the intensity of pain.
  (3) The numeric pain scale is a 10-point scale consisting of a line divided by numbered points from 0 to 9, which indicate pain intensities. Zero indicates no pain, and 9 indicates severe pain.

SIMPLE DESCRIPTIVE PAIN INTENSITY SCALE*

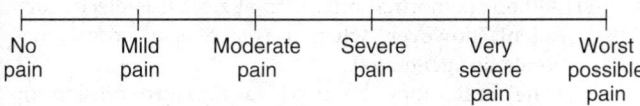

0 – 10 NUMERIC PAIN INTENSITY SCALE*

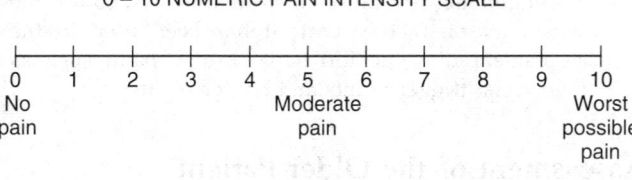

VISUAL ANALOG SCALE (VAS)†

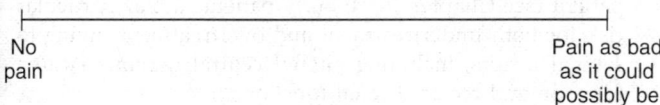

*If used as a graphic rating scale, a 10-cm baseline is recommended.
†A 10-cm baseline is recommended for VAS scales.

Figure 11–4. Pain intensity scales. (From U.S. Department of Health and Human Services Public Health Service. *Clinical Practice Guideline. Acute Pain Management: Operative and Medical Procedures and Trauma.* Publication 92-0032. Rockville, MD: Agency for Health Care Policy and Research, 1992.)

(4) A descriptive pain scale consists of a line that reflects points of increasing levels of pain intensity; for example, no pain, mild pain, moderate pain, severe pain, and unbearable pain.
(5) A visual analogue scale is a line on which 1 end represents no pain and the other end represents severe or worst pain (Fig. 11–4).
(6) Ask the patient to identify a point on the scale that corresponds to the perception of the pain intensity at the time of the assessment.
(7) The pain scale is also useful in evaluating changes in pain intensity after treatment.
  e. **Quality.** Pain quality refers to another subjective characteristic of pain.
  (1) The quality of pain may be assessed by asking certain questions or by using an assessment tool designed to assess pain quality. Ask the patient to "describe what your pain feels like." Words such as sharp, dull, stabbing, crushing, burning, throbbing, and aching are examples of descriptive terms that are often used.
  (2) The McGill-Melzack Pain Questionnaire (discussed earlier) contains 20 descriptive terms designed to assess the quality of pain.
  f. **Factors that precipitate and alleviate pain.** Pain may be precipitated or aggravated by certain factors. Likewise, it may be alleviated or ameliorated by certain factors. It is important to assess the patient's perception regarding factors or events that precipitate and alleviate the pain.

NURSE ADVISORY

Pain Precipitating Factors	Pain Alleviating Factors
Sudden movements or jarring	Analgesics
Emotional stress	Position change
Muscle tension	Relaxation
Exercise or stretching	Rest
Physical exertion	Sleep
Lifting objects	Massage
Exposure to cold temperature	Heating pad
Coughing	Ice bag
Eating large meals	Music therapy
Eating certain foods	Therapeutic touch
Constipation	Guided imagery

  g. **Associated factors.** It is important to assess the effects of pain on activities of daily living. Ask questions regarding the patient's ability to participate in self-care and daily activities. Examples of questions include the following:
- How has the pain interfered with your lifestyle and routine activities?
- Are you able to perform routine hygiene measures?
- Are you able to work and function in your regular job?
- Does the pain interfere with your normal exercise routine?

- Does the pain interfere with your sleep? Eating patterns?
- How does the pain affect family members?
- What factors are used to cope with pain of varying intensities?
- What do you usually do during an episode of pain?

Physical Examination

1. The physical examination includes the following observations of the overt physiologic responses and motor and body movements.
   a. The patient's overall appearance: facial expression, posture, gait, and motor activity.
   b. Autonomic nervous system responses, such as increased blood pressure, increased respiratory rate, increased rate and force of heart beat, increased muscle tension, decreased urinary output, and dilated pupils.
   c. Parasympathetic reflex responses, such as decreased heart rate, decreased blood pressure, decreased gastrointestinal motility, and nausea and vomiting.
   d. Body area of pain and discomfort
      - Inspect and palpate the painful body area.
      - Palpate or press carefully and systematically throughout the painful area and at locations away from the pain area.
      - Observe the patient's responses.
      - Identify pain trigger points.
      - Test the range of motion of affected joints.
      - Assess for decreased sensation or increased hypersensitivity.

Psychosocial Assessment

1. The psychosocial assessment includes observations of the patient's behavioral responses, social interaction, knowledge and understanding about the pain, and psychologic response.
   a. Behavioral response to pain may include crying, irritability, moaning, quietness, grimacing, tense facial muscles, body posturing, and verbal reports of pain.
   b. Social interaction in relation to pain may include such behaviors as avoidance of conversation, social withdrawal, isolation, preoccupation with the pain experience, and preoccupation with pain relief.
   c. The level of knowledge and understanding about the pain may be assessed by the use of open-ended questions, such as the following:
      - Tell me about your pain.
      - What is the source of the pain?
      - Tell me what you have been told about the pain.
      - Tell me what the pain means to you.
      - What are your expectations regarding the pain?
   d. Psychologic response to pain may be assessed through careful observations while interacting with the patient, and the use of open-ended questions. Examples of psychologic responses include fear, anxiety, frustration, despair, hopelessness, powerlessness, anger, denial, and stoicism.

Special Diagnostic Tools

1. The Hughes pain assessment tool is designed to assess relevant information about the patient's pain, including the onset, location, frequency of occurrence, duration, intensity, and quality.
   a. It assesses the patient's perception of the cause of the pain, the precipitating and alleviating factors, and the coping strategies used.
   b. It assesses the patient's sleep pattern, dietary pattern, and factors that interfere with these patterns.
   c. It assesses the patient's medication schedule, including nonprescription and allergy medications.
   d. In addition, it contains space for the patient's name and relevant demographic information, diagnosis, primary language, religious preference, physician's name, and vital signs. Space is provided for the patient to include comments or special concerns relevant to the treatment.
   e. You should perform the assessment and complete the tool as the patient responds to the questions (Fig. 11–5).
2. Physical measures of pain
   a. The **thymometer** is a toning instrument that is used to measure pain by having the patient manipulate the intensity of the tone to match the intensity of pain.
   b. The **electromyograph** (EMG) is an instrument that is used to measure the intrinsic electrical properties of skeletal muscles.
      (1) When the normal muscle is at rest, it is electrically silent; however, when it is active, electrical currents are generated.
      (2) The EMG may be used to measure tension of frontalis or temporal muscle groups. The muscle activity can be measured and recorded by use of a biofeedback monitor.
   c. The **algometer** is an instrument that is used to test the sensitivity of a body part. It has been used in the assessment of some forms of chronic pain, such as myofascial trigger points and tender points.

Assessment of the Older Patient

1. Individualized assessment and planning are important for safe and effective pain management in the elderly patient (see Chapter 16). Elderly patients are at particular risk for both undertreatment and overtreatment owing to several factors, including altered central nervous system function and reduced renal function.
2. The elderly tend to have increased fat-to-lean body mass ratios and reduced glomerular filtration rates.
   a. They are more sensitive to the analgesic effects of opioid analgesics, as they experience a higher peak and longer duration of pain relief than younger patients. Narcotic analgesics tend to produce a longer duration of pain relief in older patients because these drugs are excreted at a slower rate.
   b. They also are more sensitive to sedation and respiratory depression, probably owing to altered distribution and excretion of the drugs.

HUGHES' PAIN ASSESSMENT TOOL

Name _____ Age _____ Sex: M _____ F _____

Education _____ Primary Language _____

Occupation _____ Religious Preference _____

Diagnosis _____ Physician _____

Wt. _____ Ht. _____ B/P _____ Pulse _____ T. _____ R. _____

Onset of pain: Date _____ Sudden onset _____ Gradual onset _____

Location of pain: Localized in _____

                  Diffused over _____

Nature of occurrence: Constant _____ Intermittent _____

Intensity of pain: 0   1   2   3   4   5   6   7   8   9   10

                 No   Mild   Moderate   Severe   Overwhelming

                 pain   pain   pain   pain   pain

Quality of the pain: Burning _____, Sharp _____, Throbbing _____, Aching _____,

    (Other: please describe): _____

What time of day does the pain occur? _____

How often does it occur? _____

How long do the pain episodes last? _____

What do you think has caused the pain? _____

What makes the pain worse? _____

What has been helpful in relieving (or controlling) the pain in the past? _____

_____

How do you usually deal with stressful situations? _____

Do you have family support? Yes _____ No _____

    If yes, are they available to assist you, if needed? Yes _____ No _____

Usual sleep pattern: When _____ Number of hours _____

    Quality of sleep _____ Sedatives: Yes _____ No _____

Current dietary pattern _____

    Are you on a special diet? Yes _____ No _____

    If yes, please describe _____

Do any foods or medications upset your stomach? Yes _____ No _____

    If yes, please describe _____

Do any foods or medications interfere with your sleep pattern? Yes _____ No _____

    If yes, please describe _____

Medications: Please list all prescription medications and nonprescription medications that you take, including vitamins, laxatives, and occasional medications. Please include home remedies, if used. (Use the back of this page, if necessary.)

Name of Medication: **Schedule when taken:**

_____

_____

_____

_____

_____

_____

_____

Figure 11–5.

Illustration continued on following page

Allergies: *Medications?* If yes, please describe _____

_____

Foods? If yes, please describe _____

_____

Seasonal? If yes, please describe _____

_____

Do you have any beliefs or concerns related to your religious, spiritual, dietary practices, etc., that may be affected adversely by routine or conventional health care practices? If so, please describe them:

_____

_____

_____

Figure 11-5 *Continued*

3. Age-related changes in pharmacokinetics and pharmacodynamics contribute to a variety of adverse drug effects that have been reported in the elderly.
   a. The risks for gastric and renal toxicity from nonsteroidal anti-inflammatory drugs (NSAIDs) are increased among elderly patients.
   b. Common drug reactions include cognitive impairment, constipation, and headaches.
4. Some barriers to pain assessment in the elderly include cognitive impairment and dementia. Diminished vision and hearing may interfere with the use of some pain assessment scales. However, as with most patients, the nurse should be able to obtain an accurate self-report of pain from the elderly patient.
5. When it is not possible to obtain the patient's self-report, the nurse should monitor the patient more closely for behavioral cues for pain, such as restlessness or agitation. The absence of pain behavior does not negate the presence of pain.

DRUG ADVISORY

Older people often suffer from chronic diseases or have multiple sources of pain for which they may be receiving more than one medication. Special attention and teaching are required to detect early signs of drug interactions or drug toxicity related to reduced excretory capacity and altered drug sensitivity.

Assessment of Children

1. Children vary greatly in their cognitive and emotional development. Pain assessment strategies should be tai-

lored to the child's developmental level and physical abilities and to the situation.

2. The numeric rating scale that ranges from 0 (no pain) to 10 (worst pain) or the horizontal word-graphic rating scale with words to describe how much pain the patient has (no pain, little pain, medium pain, large pain, worst possible pain) may be used successfully to assess pain in children aged 4 and older or in those who understand the concepts of order, numbers, and words.
   a. Pain assessment in children younger than 7 requires different assessment strategies and tools because the ability of younger children to conceptualize is limited.
      (1) Several pain assessment tools are available for young children, such as the Wong-Baker FACES Pain Rating Scale that contains 6 faces expressing increasing levels of discomfort or distress from "smiling" to "crying."
      (2) Pain assessment must be accompanied by explanation (Figs. 11-6 and 11-7).
   b. Behavioral observation is necessary to assess pain in babies, very young children, and adults who cannot communicate. Behaviors may include a decrease in activity, failure to move an extremity, crying or grimacing with movement, irritability, and apathy.
3. Children and their parents should be actively involved in pain assessment and management. Use the parents' report of pain and information provided through inter-

No pain	Little pain	Medium pain	Large pain	Worst possible pain

Figure 11-6. The word-graphic rating scale. (From the Adolescent pediatric pain tool. *In* Savedra MC, et al. *Adolescent Pediatric Pain Tool [APPT] Preliminary User's Manual.* San Francisco, CA: University of California, 1989.)

Table 11-1. Pain Interview of Children

Child Form	Parent Form
Tell me about the hurt you're having now.	Tell me about the pain your child is having now.
Elicit descriptors, location, and cause.	Elicit descriptors, location, and cause.
What would you like me to do for you?	What would you like me to do for your child?

From U.S. Department of Health and Human Services. *Clinical Practice Guideline: Quick Reference Guide for Clinicians. Acute Pain Management in Infants, Children, and Adolescents: Operative and Medical Procedures.* AHCPR Publication No. 92-0020, 1993. Adapted with permission from Hester NO, and Barcus CS. Assessment and management of pain in children. *Pediatrics: Nursing Update* 1:2-8, 1986, published by CPEC, Inc.

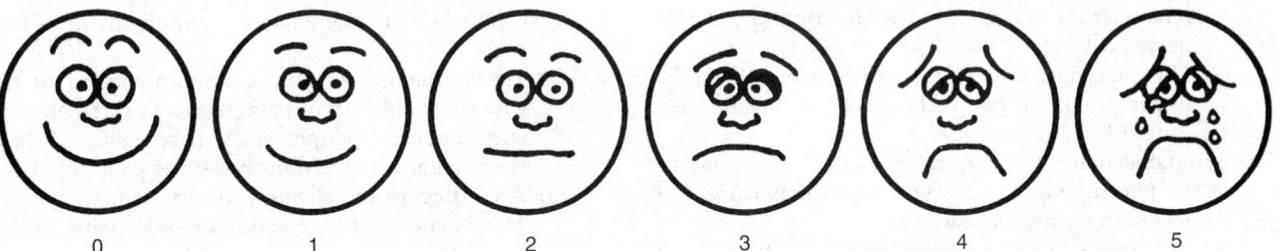

Explain to the person that each face is for a person who feels happy because he has no pain (hurt) or sad because he has some or a lot of pain. **Face 0** is very happy because he doesn't hurt at all. **Face 1** hurts just a little bit. **Face 2** hurts a little more. **Face 3** hurts even more. **Face 4** hurts a whole lot. **Face 5** hurts as much as you can imagine, although you don't have to be crying to feel this bad. Ask the person to choose the face that best describes how he or she is feeling.

Figure 11–7. Wong-Baker FACES Pain Rating Scale. (From Whaley L, and Wong D. *Essentials of Pediatric Nursing.* 4th ed. St. Louis: Mosby–Year Book, 1993, p 597.)

view when the child is unwilling or unable to give a self-report.

◼ INTERVENTIONS USED TO TREAT PAIN

Invasive Interventions

1. Intravenous administration is the parenteral route that may be used for bolus administration and continuous infusion of opioid analgesics.
2. Intraspinal infusion of narcotic analgesics may be administered by the epidural or intrathecal routes.
   a. **Epidural infusions** are administered next to the spinal cord, and they diffuse across the dura, a lipid membrane. Highly lipid-soluble narcotics, such as fentanyl citrate, have a rapid onset and prolonged duration; narcotics with low lipid solubility, such as morphine, have a slow onset of action.
   b. **Intrathecal infusions** are given into the subarachnoid space and do not cross the dura. Water-soluble narcotics, such as morphine, will diffuse more rapidly when given intrathecally rather than epidurally.
   c. Narcotic analgesics administered by **intraspinal infusion** are thought to control pain by stimulating the opiate receptors in the substantia gelatinosa, which inhibits the release of neurotransmitter substances.
3. **Implantable infusion pump** is an intraspinal route for administering narcotic analgesics.
   a. The infusion pump reservoir is usually placed subcutaneously in the lateral lower abdominal quadrant. A catheter leading from the pump reservoir is inserted, either into the thoracic or the lumbar region.
   b. The narcotic analgesic, usually preservative-free morphine, is placed in the reservoir and delivered at a slow, preset dosage and rate.
   c. The pump is refilled at regular intervals and the dosage adjusted.
   d. This method may be used for terminal cancer patients or those with intractable pain who have not received adequate pain control by other means.
4. **Local neural blockade** involves the use of local anesthetic or cryoprobe to block the intercostal nerves. The cryoprobe method includes infusion of local anesthetics

through an interpleural catheter. The nerve blockade may be continuous or intermittent.

5. **Implantable electrical stimulation systems**
   a. Percutaneous epidural dorsal column stimulation is a pain control measure that requires permanently implanting electrodes in the epidural space in the spinal cord, with an external power source. Dorsal column nerve stimulation is controlled by the patient.
   b. Extrapolating from the gate control theory of pain, large-diameter myelinated afferent nerve fibers in the posterior column of the spinal cord are stimulated, which closes the gate to pain stimuli below the dorsal column stimulation area.
   c. Dorsal column electrical stimulation may be used for pain control in patients experiencing chronic intractable pathologic pain, in which more conventional methods have not been successful.
   d. Peripheral nerve implant stimulation is a pain control measure that consists of permanently implanting electrodes around a peripheral nerve that innervates the painful area or body part. The power source is external, and nerve stimulation is controlled by the patient.
   e. The mechanism of pain control is produced by the stimulation of large-diameter myelinated A nerve fibers that close the gate to the transmission of pain stimuli.
   f. Peripheral nerve implant stimulation may be used selectively for pain control for intractable pain caused by such conditions as sciatic nerve injury, femoral nerve injury, and herpes zoster infection of the ophthalmic nerve.
6. Neurosurgical interventions
   a. **Neurectomy** is a surgical procedure in which the peripheral nerve fibers are severed from the spinal cord, blocking the transmission of pain stimuli.
      (1) The procedure is done to control severe pain in a well-defined localized area of the body that is innervated by the nerve that is severed.
      (2) This surgical measure is most often used to control the pain resulting from trigeminal neuralgia, in which case the 5th cranial nerve is resected.
   b. **Rhizotomy** is a surgical procedure that requires resection of a posterior nerve root at the point just before it enters the spinal cord.
      (1) Sensory nerve impulses enter the spinal cord by the posterior nerve roots. Resection of a nerve root

relieves pain arising from the distribution of that nerve root.

    (2) This procedure may be used to control pain in the upper trunk of the body, such as severe pain caused by lung cancer.

c. **Sympathectomy** is a surgical procedure that consists of the interruption of afferent visceral nerve fibers of the sympathetic nervous system.

    (1) This procedure may be used to control the pain of causalgia and post-traumatic sympathetic dystrophy.

d. **Tractotomy** is a surgical procedure in which the second-order neurons are severed in the spinothalamic tract. This procedure may be employed to control pain in the face, neck, and upper arm that results from such conditions as head and neck cancer.

e. **Cordotomy** is the most common neurosurgical procedure for pain relief. Cordotomy is a surgical procedure that accomplishes either unilateral or bilateral interruption of the pain pathways in the anterolateral spinothalamic tract.

    (1) This procedure may be used to control intractable lower body (below the arms) pain in patients with a short life expectancy, such as patients who have pain resulting from extensive cancer in the pelvic area.

    (2) Percutaneous cordotomy does not require a skin incision and can be performed under local anesthesia. Evidence indicates that this procedure can provide analgesia for up to 2 years.

f. **Hypophysectomy** is a surgical procedure that removes the pituitary gland. This procedure may be used to control intractable pain resulting from metastatic breast cancer, prostate cancer, and bone cancer.

7. Acupuncture

a. Acupuncture is a common treatment method in traditional Chinese medicine. It is a pain control technique that requires the insertion of sharp needles into specific points of the body, which produces mechanical stimulation of the large-diameter A nerve fibers that close the gate to pain stimuli.

b. Acupuncture is based on the energy theory. The needles are inserted along the meridians or energy pathways of the body that affect organs and bodily functions.

c. The analgesic affects of acupuncture are also attributed to the stimulation of endorphins in the nervous system, which alter or modulate the transmission of pain impulses.

Noninvasive Interventions

1. Cutaneous stimulation

a. **Transcutaneous electrical nerve stimulation (TENS)** provides stimulation by the use of a battery-powered current generator with electrodes that are applied to the skin. The electrodes may be applied directly over the nerve that innervates the painful area or directly over the painful area itself.

    (1) TENS produces stimulating pulses transcutaneously to nerve fibers, which interfere with the conduction of afferent pain stimuli to the spinal cord.

    (2) The mechanism of pain control, according to the gate control theory of pain, relates to stimulation of large-diameter peripheral A nerve fibers, which close the gate to the transmission of pain impulses.

    (3) According to the chemical theory of pain control, TENS activates the secretion of endorphins, which bind with opiate receptors in the dorsal horn of the spinal cord and inhibit the release of neurotransmitter substances, which alters the perception of pain. According to the gate control theory of pain, large fibers are activated and close the gate to central pain perception.

b. **Heat therapy** consists of the application of moist or dry heat to the skin. Heat therapy may be in the form of superficial heat or deep heat.

    (1) Dry superficial heat application may be accomplished by the use of a covered electrical heating pad, heat lamps, or covered hot water bottles.

    (2) Moist superficial heat application may be accomplished by the use of moist hot compresses, baths, sitz baths, soaks, electrical heating pads designed for moist heat application, or whirlpool.

    (3) Deep heat therapy involves the use of diathermy or ultrasound applied with special equipment, usually by a physical therapist or a person trained in the technique.

    (4) Heat therapy generally requires intermittent applications, with the heat applied for 15 to 30 minutes, or as ordered by a physician. Precautions must be taken to prevent burns.

    (5) According to the gate control theory of pain, heat stimulates large-diameter myelinated A nerve fibers, which close the gate to the transmission of pain stimuli to higher brain centers.

    (6) In addition, heat produces dilation of blood vessels, increases local blood flow, and promotes muscle relaxation, which reduces tension.

    (7) Superficial heat therapy is often used to relieve local superficial pain, such as sprains and bruises, muscle spasms, arthritis, perineal pain, and some forms of chronic pain.

    (8) Heat should not be used immediately following a traumatic injury when inflammation and swelling are present. Cold therapy may be more appropriate.

c. **Cold therapy** for pain relief requires the application of moist or dry cold to the skin. Dry cold may be applied by using an ice bag. Moist cold may be applied with cold moist compresses, chemical cold packs, or cold soaks and baths.

    (1) The mechanism of pain relief through cold application involves slowing the transmission of first-order neurons, thereby decreasing the transmission of pain stimuli. The perception of pain is decreased further by the sensation of cold.

    (2) In addition, cold causes constriction of the peripheral blood vessels, which decreases the local release of pain-producing substances (e.g., histamine, serotonin, bradykinin), which in turn reduces inflammation and swelling.

(3) Cold therapy may be used to relieve pain caused by a variety of conditions, including postoperative pain, burns, soft tissue injuries, muscle spasms, sprains and traumatic injuries, and some chronic pain syndromes. Precautions must be taken to prevent tissue injury from the cold, such as frostbite.

d. **Therapeutic touch** is an experimental therapy based on the assumption that the human body is an energy field that has inherent pattern and organization. The theory is that the body and the environment are open systems and constantly exchange energy and matter. A disruption in the pattern and organization of the energy field is thought by some practitioners to result in illness, including pain.

(1) Therapeutic touch is thought to be a process of mental concentration and focusing. The hands are used to locate and transmit energy to restore the body's energy field to organization and pattern. The effective use of therapeutic touch requires special training.

(2) The mechanism of pain relief from therapeutic touch is not fully understood. One hypothesis suggests that therapeutic touch may cause activation of the endorphins in the central nervous system and inhibit or modulate the transmission of pain stimuli.

(3) In addition, the cognitive-evaluative component of pain perception may be activated by the caring, compassion, and empathy conveyed during therapeutic touch. This process may promote the patient's emotional sense of well-being, which may contribute to decreased pain perception.

(4) Therapeutic touch for pain relief has been employed for a variety of problems, including postoperative pain, tension headaches, migraine headaches, and acute low back pain. It may be used in conjunction with other treatment measures in the management of chronic nonmalignant pain and other types of pain.

e. **Massage** for pain relief involves superficial stimulation of the body by applying light to deep pressure to the skin in a smooth and patterned fashion using rubbing, stroking, kneading, or chopping motions.

(1) The 4 basic techniques of massage are tapotement, kneading, petrissage, and effleurage (Box 11–1). Tapotement and petrissage have a stimulating effect; kneading and effleurage have a relaxing effect.

(2) Extrapolating from the gate control theory of pain, massage stimulates the large-diameter A nerve fibers, which closes the gate to the transmission of pain stimuli. In addition, massage produces relaxation and relief of muscle tension, which contributes to pain relief.

(3) Massage is often used to relieve the pain of aching muscles, back pain, and neck and shoulder pain.

f. **Vibration** is a form of cutaneous stimulation. Manual, battery-powered, or electrical vibrating devices are used.

(1) Vibration produces stimulation of the large-diameter A nerve fibers, which closes the gate to the transmission of pain stimuli.

BOX 11-1
EFFLEURAGE MASSAGE

1 In the prone or semiprone position, drape the patient so that the back, shoulders, and upper buttocks are exposed.

2 Wash hands. Pour a moderate amount of lotion into the palm of your hand and warm by rubbing your hands together. Tell the patient when you are ready to begin.

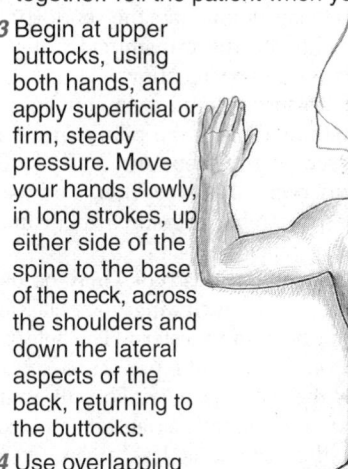

3 Begin at upper buttocks, using both hands, and apply superficial or firm, steady pressure. Move your hands slowly, in long strokes, up either side of the spine to the base of the neck, across the shoulders and down the lateral aspects of the back, returning to the buttocks.

4 Use overlapping strokes to cover the entire area.

5 Repeat several times, using additional lotion as needed to reduce friction between your hands and the patient's skin.

6 Next, using a kneading motion, gently rub your hands over the upper shoulders and scapula areas and work downward to the sacrum and iliac spine. Use additional lotion as needed.

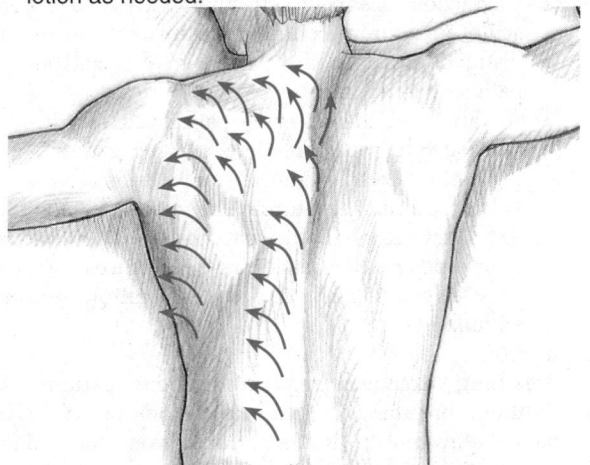

7 Repeat steps 3-6 for 6-10 minutes.

8 Observe for nonverbal cues indicating the patient's level of comfort. The time required to promote patient comfort and achieve a relaxed state will vary.

(2) Vibration is often applied to the shoulder and neck areas but also may be applied to any body part for relief of muscle tension and pain.

2. Auditory stimulation
   a. **Music therapy** consists of using selected musical compositions to produce distinct sensory stimuli for varied periods of time.
      (1) The mechanism of pain relief from the sensory stimuli of music is not clear. One hypothesis suggests that the effects of music on the affective component (improved mood and sense of well-being) and the cognitive component (increased control, distraction) may stimulate the endorphins that inhibit or modulate the transmission of pain stimuli and decrease pain perception.
      (2) In addition, the sensory stimuli from music may produce counterstimulation to the pain stimuli, resulting in decreased pain perception.
      (3) Music therapy has been employed alone and as an adjunct to other pain relief measures to promote relaxation and pain relief.
      (4) Easy listening music of various types may be used for its therapeutic effects, including jazz, classical, rock, folk, and country and western. The selection should be based on the patient's preference.
   b. **Distraction** involves the use of sensory stimuli, which become the focus of the patient's attention and concentration; in turn, the patient is less aware of the pain sensation.
      (1) The exact mechanism of pain relief from distraction is not clear. One premise is that the dominance of sensory stimuli provided by the distraction measure may produce counterstimulation to the pain stimuli, activating the secretion of endorphins, which inhibit or modulate the transmission of pain stimuli.
      (2) Distraction has been effective in relieving both acute and chronic pain. Unfortunately, when the distraction ceases, the patient may focus on the pain sensation again.
      (3) A variety of measures are employed for distraction, such as music, reading, playing games, visiting with family members, and various types of hobbies, including needlepoint, painting, and the like. Distractors should be chosen using the patient's perspective, including preferences and energy level and should produce multiple sensory stimulation.
3. Relaxation
   a. **Breathing exercises** require different patterns of rhythmic breathing for varying periods of time. The patient's awareness and concentration are focused on the breathing.
      (1) Deep rhythmic inhalations and exhalations performed in a steady pattern maintain an even flow in breathing and produce total body relaxation. The breathing cycle should be repeated 8 to 10 times.
      (2) Breathing exercises may be used to promote relaxation and are a form of distraction.
   b. **Relaxation response** is a relaxed state that may be elicited voluntarily and results in decreased sympathetic nervous system activity and increased parasympathetic nervous system activity. These changes, in turn, cause a series of physiologic and psychologic changes, such as decreased oxygen consumption, decreased muscle tension, decreased heart rate, decreased systolic and diastolic blood pressure, decreased respiratory rate, and reduced anxiety level.
      (1) The mechanism of pain relief involves the decrease in muscle tension and peripheral blood flow, which results in a decreased transmission of pain stimuli in the 1st-order neuron. Decreased sympathetic nervous system activity results in decreased levels of neurotransmitter substances, such as epinephrine, causing a decrease in the transmission of pain stimuli in 2nd-order neurons. The lowered anxiety level and calm emotions also contribute to pain relief.
      (2) Eliciting the relaxation response requires 4 essential elements: (1) a quiet environment; (2) a comfortable position, either sitting or lying; (3) a mental device, such as a word or phrase on which to focus concentration; and (4) a passive attitude, allowing oneself to relax.
      (3) The relaxation reponse, as well as other types of relaxation such as progressive relaxation, has been effective in relieving both acute and chronic pain. It may also be used as an adjunct to other pain relief measures.
   c. **Progressive relaxation training (PRT)** emphasizes the relaxation of voluntary skeletal muscles. The patient is encouraged to "tense" and then "relax" successive muscle groups. Attention is focused on discriminating between the feelings experienced when the muscles are relaxed and those experienced when they are tensed.
      (1) When teaching a patient to do progressive muscle relaxation, the muscles should initially be grouped into 16 groups and tensed and relaxed in sequential order. After mastery of the 16 groups, the muscles may be grouped into fewer groups, such as 7, and then into 4 muscle groups.

Progressive Relaxation Training (PRT)
Muscle groups relaxed in sequential order

1. Dominant hand and forearm
2. Dominant biceps
3. Nondominant hand and forearm
4. Nondominant biceps
5. Forehead
6. Upper cheeks and nose
7. Lower cheeks and jaw
8. Neck and throat
9. Chest, shoulders, and upper back
10. Lower back, buttocks, and pelvic region
11. Dominant thigh
12. Dominant calf
13. Dominant foot
14. Nondominant thigh
15. Nondominant calf
16. Nondominant foot

(2) The basic procedure for teaching progressive relaxation:
  - Focus attention on muscle group.
  - Instruct patient to tense a muscle group at a predetermined signal (e.g., "When I say 'now,' tense").
  - Maintain muscle tension for 5 to 7 seconds, using a shorter duration for foot muscles.
  - Release tension at a predetermined signal (e.g., "Relax").
  - Guide or coach the patient in tensing and relaxing muscle groups in sequential order, progressing through the 16 groups.
  - Instruct the patient to concentrate on the relaxed muscles, and to discriminate differences in sensations between relaxed and tensed muscles.
  - Guide the patient in using the technique in each muscle group twice.

(3) The patient should be assisted and encouraged to practice the relaxation response or progressive relaxation technique at least twice a day until it can be performed successfully.

(4) Some precautions for the use of relaxation have been reported. These precautions include the following:
  - When performing progressive relaxation, cardiac patients should be given special instructions not to tense muscles tightly.
  - The physiologic response generated by relaxation can intensify the effects of some medications, for example, hypotensive agents.
  - In persons who are depressed, relaxation may precipitate further withdrawal.

d. **Guided imagery** uses the patient's imagination to create images that focus attention away from the pain sensation.

(1) The patient selects a sensory image, such as a scene or an experience, that is particularly pleasant and relaxing. The patient engages all of the senses in the experience and focuses on the sensations provoked by the scene or experience. The patient is assisted by a coach or a therapist or uses a taped recording. A session may be 15 to 20 minutes in duration.

(2) Guided imagery is a form of distraction. The mechanism of pain relief involves focusing attention and awareness away from the pain sensation. The dominance of incoming sensory stimuli produced by the pleasant scene or experience may cause counterstimulation of the pain stimuli, resulting in decreased pain perception.

e. **Biofeedback** requires the control of automatically regulated body functions to alter the body's responses in more healthful ways.

(1) The patient learns about the body's biologic functions and learns to alter these responses to specific or desired levels. The process of learning biofeedback is facilitated by the use of a physiologic monitor, which displays feedback produced by physiologic changes.

(2) Feedback is based on physiologic changes that reflect relaxation. The physiologic responses to be altered usually include muscle tension, blood pressure, heart rate, and hand temperature. Body sensations such as pain may also be altered.

(3) Biofeedback has been effective in relieving pain resulting from muscle tension and stress, muscle spasms, lower back pain, headaches, hypertension, and stress-related syndromes.

4. **Rest and sleep**

a. Rest is a period of inactivity of the body that allows both physical and mental relaxation.

b. Mental relaxation is accompanied by calmness of the mind and mental processes, reduced anxiety and irritability, and improved sense of well-being.

c. Physical relaxation is accompanied by decreased demands on the body, including decreased oxygen requirements; decreased basic metabolic rate; decreased blood pressure, heart rate, and cardiac output; and decreased musculoskeletal activity, all of which result in decreased stimulation of injured tissues.

d. Sleep is a state of altered consciousness that is accompanied by decreased bodily functions. These changes in bodily functions include reduced demands on the body and reduced energy output, suspended musculoskeletal activity, and decreased oxygen consumption, metabolic rate, cardiac output, heart rate, and respiratory rate.

e. Sleep is associated with nerve cell activity and neurotransmitters, such as serotonin, acetylcholine, and norepinephrine, which play an intimate role in mood and pain perception.

f. Rest and sleep are basic physiologic and psychologic needs and are major energy sources. The reduced stress and tension promote rejuvenation of the body, restore body energy, and promote an improved sense of well-being. Pain perception is reduced, and the ability to cope is improved.

g. Rest and sleep deprivation results in fatigue, irritability, restlessness, and exhaustion, which can influence the perception of pain and decrease coping ability and sense of well-being.

h. Adequate rest and sleep promote physical and mental well-being, reduce pain perception, and enhance coping ability in both acute and chronic pain.

5. **Hypnosis**

a. Hypnosis refers to an altered state of consciousness in which the patient's concentration is sharply focused. It is accompanied by a feeling of relaxation. An awareness of the peripheral environment is maintained but at a decreased level.

b. In the altered conscious state, the patient is more receptive to suggestions of a positive and comforting nature, such as blocking pain sensations, minimizing fear and anxiety, and maintaining a sense of control. The patient's behavior remains within the limits of his or her moral code.

c. The mechanism of pain control is not clear. One hypothesis suggests that pain information is processed in the higher brain centers at an unconscious level and pain perception does not occur.

d. Suggestions for hypnotic pain control include the following:
  (1) Altering the perception of pain by blocking pain sensations.
  (2) Altering the sense of powerlessness and potentiating the patient's inner strength and sense of control.
  (3) Decreasing the patient's fear and anxiety and enhancing the sense of well-being.
  (4) Moving the pain to a less important area of the body as perceived by the patient.
  (5) Minimizing the time that pain is experienced and maximizing the time the patient is pain free.
  (6) Substituting pain sensations with pleasant sensations, such as coolness, warmth, or pressure.
e. Hypnosis has been used effectively to promote comfort and relieve both acute and chronic pain.

Pharmacologic Interventions

1. Principles of analgesic administration
  a. **Assessment.** The patient should be assessed before and after an analgesic is administered to maximize safety and ensure adequate pain relief. Important factors to be assessed before an analgesic is administered include drug allergies or sensitivity, other medications being taken, body weight, the person's pain experience, and body systems.
  b. **Drug allergies or sensitivities.** Before administering analgesics such as aspirin or morphine, ensure that the patient does not have a history of untoward reactions to the medications. When possible, ask the patient or family members about drug allergies or sensitivities.
  c. **Other medications.** Some drugs are contraindicated when certain drugs are being taken or when certain conditions exist. For example, meperidine (Demerol) is contraindicated for patients receiving monoamine oxidase (MAO) inhibitors and for patients with impaired renal function.
  d. **Body weight.** Ten mg of morphine per 70 kg of body weight is considered standard. The analgesic effect is dose related, and some patients may require higher or lower doses. Ascertain the patient's body weight by actually weighing the patient or by asking the patient or family members.
  e. **Individual pain experience.** Because pain is experienced by each person differently, there is no way to know for certain how much pain a patient is experiencing from a particular health problem or procedure, such as surgery. Likewise, it is difficult to know for certain what dosage of analgesic is needed to control a patient's pain.
    (1) One method of treating postoperative pain is to administer a standard dosage of analgesic following a particular surgical procedure and then increase or decrease the potency of subsequent doses on the basis of an evaluation of the patient's response to the initial dose. This method of titrating the amount and kind of analgesic needed should be based on the patient's response to the medication, including any side effects.

f. **Body systems.** Because all analgesics have the potential to produce mild to severe side effects, it is important to assess the patient's body systems, including hepatic function and status of cardiac, respiratory, renal, and nervous systems before and after administering analgesics.
  (1) Most analgesics are metabolized by the liver or kidney. Renal excretion is a major route of elimination of pharmacologically active opioid metabolites. Any impairment of function in these organs influences the pharmacokinetics of the analgesic and can result in drug accumulation. Nonopioid analgesics are often contraindicated in patients with impaired hepatic and renal function.
  (2) Opioid analgesics are contraindicated when respiratory depression (less than 10 breaths per minute) is present. Patients with respiratory insufficiency are usually those with chronic obstructive pulmonary disease, cystic fibrosis, or neuromuscular disorders affecting respiratory effort. These patients are vulnerable to the respiratory depressant of opioid analgesics because their respiratory drive is already compromised.
  (3) Opioid analgesics are contraindicated in patients with head injuries. The decreased respirations increase carbon dioxide retention, and carbon dioxide causes dilation of intracranial blood vessels.
g. **Planning.** Careful planning is required to provide effective and safe pain relief. Assessment and reassessment on an ongoing basis are essential.
h. **Ethical considerations** are also important in the management of pain.
2. Nonsteroidal anti-inflammatory drugs

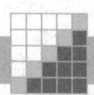

LEGAL AND ETHICAL CONSIDERATIONS

1. The nurse should respect patients' autonomy by allowing them to determine when they need pain relief.
2. The patient's self-report is the single most important and reliable source regarding the pain experience.
3. The patient's report of pain might be enhanced or hampered by the nurse's attitude and mannerisms.
4. The nurse should avoid cultural imposition, that is, dictating to patients what effect the pain should have on them and how they should behave.
5. The nurse should avoid stereotyping patients because they are members of a particular culture.
6. Nurses should clarify and be aware of their values and acknowledge that the values of patients may be different from their own.
7. Cultural sensitivity is fundamental to pain assessment and management.
8. Active kindness is inherent in the nurse's authentic efforts to relieve patient's pain.
9. Nurses should not prejudge a patient's pain using their own standards and values.
10. Placebos should not be administered as a test for pain.
11. One of the goals of nursing is to relieve suffering. Rationing pain control is not considered ethically defensible.
12. Nonmaleficence is inherent in efforts to prevent the devastating and dehumanizing effects of pain on the patient.
13. Patients have the right to have their pain relieved.

a. **Definition and use.** Nonsteroidal anti-inflammatory drugs are commonly used in the management of mild to moderate pain. This class encompasses a group of drugs that produces similar effects in the body. They vary in chemical structure, onset of action, and duration of action. These drugs have analgesic, anti-inflammatory, and antipyretic properties. They are absorbed in the gastrointestinal tract, and most of them are metabolized in the liver and excreted primarily by the kidneys.

b. **Mechanism of action.** The primary mechanism of the analgesic and anti-inflammatory actions is believed to be the inhibition of prostaglandin synthesis and formation and the inhibition of leukocyte migration and release of lysosomal enzymes. The antipyretic effect is mediated by the hypothalamus in the higher brain center and may inhibit the action of the endogenous pyrogens on the heat-regulating center, producing vasodilation and increased heat dissipation.

c. **Types of NSAIDs.** A wide variety of drugs are included in the NSAID category. Representative drugs in the NSAID category are shown in Table 11–2.

d. **Adverse effects.** At least many of the adverse effects of NSAIDs may be related to the analgesic and anti-inflammatory effects of the drugs on prostaglandins. NSAIDs reduce inflammation and pain by inhibiting the synthesis and formation of prostaglandins.

 (1) Prostaglandins are found throughout the body in most body tissues and fluids. They play significant roles in the biologic functioning of the body.

 (2) In the gastrointestinal tract, prostaglandins reduce the production of gastric acid and increase the secretion of mucus. When they are blocked or inhibited by the use of a NSAID, an increase in gastric acid and a decrease in gastric mucus result. This reaction may lead to a variety of gastric symptoms or adverse effects.

 (3) Gastrointestinal tract disturbances are the most common adverse effects caused by NSAIDs. These include gastric irritation, nausea, dyspepsia, abdominal pain, ulceration, bleeding, diarrhea, anemia, and hepatotoxicity.

 (4) Central nervous system adverse effects may include headaches, dizziness, tinnitus, vertigo, drowsiness, decreased attention span, and mental confusion.

 (5) Renal system adverse effects may include cystitis, urinary retention, hematuria, kidney necrosis, nephrotic syndrome, and renal insufficiency.

 (6) The eyes are occasionally affected by the use of NSAIDs. The adverse effects may include blurred vision and decreased acuity.

e. **Nursing implications.** Before administering an analgesic, assess the patient's medication history, including allergies and sensitivities. A common assumption is that patients who are allergic to aspirin are most likely allergic to NSAIDs. Usually NSAIDs are contraindicated in patients with asthma.

 (1) Patient teaching should emphasize the prevention of drug-drug interactions as well as drug-alcohol interactions. Teach the patient to recognize adverse signs and symptoms and to report them promptly.

 (2) Teaching should include the use of measures to prevent or minimize gastrointestinal disturbances caused by an oral NSAID, such as taking it with food or an antacid and avoiding lying down immediately after an oral dose.

 (3) Subjective and objective data, including laboratory results that are likely to be affected by the drug therapy, should be monitored at regular intervals. Teach the patient the importance of returning for regular checkups after discharge.

3. Narcotics-opioids

a. **Definition and use.** Narcotic analgesics are used to relieve moderate to severe pain. Narcotic analgesics are classified as agonists, agonists-antagonists, and antagonists based on their pharmacotherapeutic properties.

b. **Mechanism of action.** *Narcotic agonists* act by binding to opiate receptors in the peripheral and central nervous system, producing analgesic effects. Morphine serves as the standard against which the effectiveness of other narcotics are measured. *Narcotic agonists-antagonists* are drugs that have mixed properties. The agonist properties relieve pain, and the antagonist properties decrease the risks of adverse effects and toxicity. *Narcotic antagonists* are drugs that act by blocking the effects of narcotic agonist drugs, including pain relief and adverse effects. They attach to the opiate receptors and prevent narcotic agonists and the endorphins from producing their effects.

c. **Types of narcotics.** Representative drugs from the agonist, agonist-antagonist, and antagonist categories are included in Table 11–3.

d. **Adverse effects of narcotic agonists.** Narcotic agonists produce a variety of adverse reactions that affect most systems in the body.

 (1) Central nervous system adverse effects may include headaches, confusion, dizziness, drowsiness, sedation, insomnia, agitation, dysphoria, euphoria, and psychic dependence.

 (2) Cardiopulmonary adverse effects may include hypertension, hypotension, syncope, tachycardia, bradycardia, palpitations, apnea, respiratory depression, and cardiopulmonary arrest.

 (3) Gastrointestinal adverse effects may include nausea, vomiting, dry mouth, anorexia, and constipation.

 (4) Genitourinary adverse effects may include urinary hesitancy and urinary retention.

 (5) Itching, nausea and vomiting, sedation, and respiratory depression are the most common adverse effects.

e. **Adverse effects of narcotic agonists-antagonists.** Narcotic agonist-antagonist adverse reactions include lethargy, lightheadedness, sedation, headaches, blurred vision, dizziness, agitation, and euphoria.

 (1) In addition, symptoms such as hypertension, hypotension, palpitations, nausea, vomiting, dry mouth, and respiratory depression may occur.

 (2) Narcotic agonist-antagonist adverse reactions tend

Table 11–2. Nonsteroidal Anti-inflammatory Drugs

NSAIDs	Potential Adverse Effects	Precautions
Aspirin (acetylsalicylic acid)	Gastric irritation, dyspepsia, bleeding, nausea, vomiting, tinnitus, deafness, hypersensitive reaction; inhibits platelet aggregation	Administer with food, milk, or antacids to minimize gastric effects. Monitor for signs of gastrointestinal bleeding, such as tarry stools. Monitor for signs of hypersensitivity.
Acetaminophen (Tylenol)	May cause liver toxicity after prolonged use	Lacks anti-inflammatory effects
Ibuprofen (Motrin, Advil, Nuprin)	Gastric irritation, fluid retention, edema	Administer with food to minimize the gastric effects. Monitor for signs of fluid retention; monitor weight periodically.
Naproxen (Naprosyn)	Gastric irritation	Administer with food to minimize the gastric effects.
Indomethacin (Indocin)	Gastric irritation, nausea and vomiting, abdominal pain, headache, confusion, dizziness, syncope, fluid retention, edema	Administer with food or antacids to minimize gastric effects. Assess for edema; monitor weight periodically. Monitor blood count, ophthalmic effects. Assess baseline liver and kidney function test results before beginning long-term therapy.
Sulindac (Clinoril)	Abdominal pain, nausea, diarrhea, and constipation	Administer with food to decrease gastrointestinal effects.
Choline magnesium trisalicylate (Trilisate)	Gastric irritation, tinnitus	Administer with food to minimize gastric effects.
Tolmetin (Tolectin)	Gastric irritation, elevated blood pressure, headaches, abdominal pain, diarrhea	Administer with milk, food, or antacids to minimize gastric effects. Weigh weekly; observe for signs of edema. Monitor blood pressure regularly. Monitor for nose bleed and tarry stools.
Fenoprofen (Nalfon)	Gastric pain, dyspepsia, nausea, constipation, renal toxicity	Administer with meals to decrease gastric effects. Monitor kidney function test results.
Diflunisal (Dolobid)	Has a lower incidence of the same adverse effects as aspirin	Administer with food or antacid to decrease gastric effects.
Mefenamic acid (Ponstel)	Gastric irritation	Administer with meals to avoid gastric effects. Monitor for signs of bleeding, such as tarry stools and easy bruising.
Piroxicam (Feldene)	Gastric symptoms similar to aspirin. Inhibits renal excretion of lithium, resulting in toxicity.	Administer with food or antacid to prevent gastric symptoms. Observe for tremors. Monitor for lithium blood levels.
Phenylbutazone (Butazolidin)	Gastric irritation, nausea, vomiting, renal toxicity, hepatic toxicity, thrombocytopenia, sodium retention, increased hypoglycemic effects	Administer with meals to decrease gastric effects. Observe for signs and symptoms of hypoglycemia, such as tremors, lightheadedness, and diaphoresis.

Table 11–3. Narcotics-Opioids		
Narcotics-Opioids	**Comments**	**Precautions**
Narcotic Agonists		
Morphine	Used as the standard of comparison for other narcotic analgesics.	Monitor respiratory rate; if less than 10 breaths per minute, withhold drug. Use with caution in patients with impaired ventilation, bronchial asthma, liver failure, increased intracranial pressure, and elderly patients.
Meperidine (Demerol)	Duration of action is slightly shorter than morphine.	Monitor respiratory rate, depth, and rhythm. Monitor blood pressure and pulse rate. Do not use in patients with impaired renal function. Effects tend to accumulate with prolonged use, causing central nervous system symptoms, such as hyperirritability.
Hydromorphone (Dilaudid)	Duration of action is slightly shorter than that of morphine.	Precautions required are the same as those for morphine.
Methadone (Dolophine)	In addition to its analgesic effects, it is used in oral form for detoxification and maintenance programs for opiate addiction.	Monitor vital signs before and regularly after administration. May accumulate with prolonged use, causing excessive sedation. Use with caution in elderly and debilitated patients.
Codeine	Often used in combination with nonnarcotic analgesics.	Use with caution in patients with impaired ventilation.
Narcotic Agonists-Antagonists		
Pentazocine (Talwin)	Abuse of is greater than that of morphine.	May cause psychotomimetic effects. May precipitate withdrawal symptoms in physically dependent patients.
Nalbuphine (Nubain)	Incidence of psychotomimetic effects lower than that with pentazocine.	May precipitate withdrawal symptoms in narcotic-dependent patients.
Butorphanol (Stadol)	Less likelihood of abuse.	May precipitate withdrawal symptoms.
Narcotic Antagonists		
Naloxone hydrochloride (Narcan)	Used to reverse respiratory depression from narcotic overdose.	Monitor patient's vital signs before and after administration. Have emergency equipment available, including oxygen, ventilation equipment, and intravenous fluids.
Naltrexone (Trexan)	Often used as adjunctive therapy for drug rehabilitation from opioids. Potential adverse effects include abdominal pain and cramps, nausea, vomiting, headaches, muscle and joint pain, irritability.	Administer with food or milk to reduce gastric symptoms. Use with caution in cardiovascular disease. Monitor liver function studies baseline and regularly thereafter.

to occur less frequently than reactions to narcotic agonists.

f. **Adverse effects of narcotic antagonists.** Narcotic antagonist adverse reactions include nausea, vomiting, anorexia, headaches, hypertension, palpitations, anxiety, nervousness, depression, disorientation, blurred vision, and tinnitus.

g. **Nursing implications.** Nurses must have a sound knowledge base of commonly used narcotic analgesics. You should be knowledgeable about drug dosage, frequency of administration, route of administration, onset of action, duration of action, potential adverse effects, and drug-drug interactions.

(1) It is imperative that you know the federal, state, and institutional regulations regarding narcotics and controlled substances.

(2) A thorough patient assessment, including a drug history, is critically important. Review the patient's problems, such as allergies, hypertension, gastric problems, and previous experience with pain medication. Obtain and record baseline data.

(3) Collaborate with patient, family, and health team members regarding the goals of therapy, interventions to achieve them, and evaluation of outcomes. Review with the patient and family the anticipated benefits and possible adverse effects of the therapy. Implement measures to maximize the benefits and minimize the adverse effects.

(4) Reassess the patient at frequent intervals to determine the effectiveness of therapy, as well as the adverse effects.

(5) Emphasize the importance of the patient's participation in controlling the pain by promptly reporting pain perception and pain relief through the use of drug therapy and nonpharmacologic measures.

(6) Assess the patient's pain before administering each dose of analgesic medication, including perception of pain onset, duration, location, intensity, and quality. Assess for adverse effects. Record the patient's response to pain and response to the analgesic drug therapy.

4. Analgesic adjuvants
a. **Definition and use.** Analgesic adjuvants are drugs that are used in combination with narcotic analgesics and NSAIDs to potentiate their actions or to counteract the adverse effects caused by them or to do both.

b. **Types of analgesic adjuvants and their mechanisms of action.** A variety of drugs in a number of different categories have been used as analgesic adjuvants. These categories include central nervous system stimulants, tricyclic antidepressants, antihistamines, anticonvulsants, antipsychotics, and benzodiazepines.

(1) *Central nervous system stimulants* such as dextroamphetamine may be used to counteract the sedative effect, which may be caused by the use of narcotic analgesics. The use of dextroamphetamine, for example, has been reported to effectively reverse the sedating effects of morphine and potentiate its analgesic effects.

(2) *Tricyclic antidepressants* such as amitriptyline hydrochloride are believed to increase the neurotransmitter substances serotonin and norepinephrine, normalizing the receptor site associated with depression. These drugs are also effective in relieving pain related to neuropathy and postherpetic neuralgia. They may be used as analgesics independent of their antidepressant effect.

(3) *Antihistamines* such as hydroxyzine (Vistaril, Atarax) are used in combination with narcotic analgesics, primarily to counteract the adverse effects of nausea and vomiting. Antihistamine antiemetics may prevent nausea and vomiting by inhibiting cholinergic stimulation of the chemoreceptor target zone and vomiting center in the vestibular nuclei.

(4) *Anticonvulsants* such as carbamazepine (Tegretol) stabilize nerve cell activity against hyperexcitability by inhibiting the spread of seizure activity or neuromuscular transmission in general. The effects include muscle relaxation, sedation, and the relief of pain caused by trigeminal neuralgia, postherpetic neuralgia, post-traumatic neuralgia, and glossopharyngeal neuralgia.

(5) *Antipsychotics* such as chlorpromazine hydrochloride (Thorazine) may act by depressing the reticular activating system, the hypothalamus, and the chemoreceptor trigger zone and by affecting the vomiting center. These drugs are often used for their tranquilizing effects to calm agitated patients.

(6) *Benzodiazepines* such as diazepam (Valium) potentiate the action of the neurochemical γ-aminobutyric acid (GABA), decreasing excitatory stimulation of the limbic system to help control emotions. Diazepam may be used in combination with narcotic analgesics for its antianxiety muscle relaxant effects.

(7) Representative adjuvant agents, comments, and precautions to take when administering them are shown in Table 11–4.

6. Patient-controlled analgesia
a. Patient-controlled analgesia (PCA) refers to a method that allows the patient to control pain by using an intravenous drug delivery system (Fig. 11–8).

(1) This method allows a prescribed narcotic analgesic to be self-administered in controlled doses at a frequency necessary to manage the pain effectively.

b. A variety of commercial PCA delivery systems are available, including computerized systems. An essential feature of the PCA generally is that it can be programmed to deliver a dose of the prescribed analgesic directly into the intravenous line when the patient pushes a button. Another essential feature controls the intravenous dosages by using an adjustable lockout mechanism. This measure helps to safeguard the patient by preventing overmedication.

c. Many of the devices are designed to record each time the patient pushes the button, that is, attempts to administer a dose of medication, as well as each time a dose is actually administered.

Table 11-4. Analgesic Adjuvants

Analgesic Adjuvants	Comments	Precautions
CNS Stimulant		
Dextroamphetamine	May be habit forming.	Avoid the use of caffeine. Monitor blood pressure and for excessive stimulation.
Tricyclic Antidepressant		
Amitriptyline (Elavil)	Interacts with MAO inhibitors. Potential adverse effects include sedation and respiratory depression.	Monitor blood pressure, level of consciousness; monitor for urinary retention.
Antihistamine		
Hydroxyzine (Vistaril, Atarax)	Produces synergistic analgesic effects. Potential adverse effects include sedation and respiratory depression.	Monitor for dry mouth, visual disturbances, urinary retention, and constipation. Monitor respiratory status at frequent intervals.
Anticonvulsant		
Carbamazepine (Tegretol)	Potential adverse effects are hematopoietic toxicity, sour mouth and throat, fever, fatigue, dizziness, and ataxia.	Monitor complete blood count. Monitor for sour mouth and throat, fever, fatigue, pulse rate, dizziness. Exercise caution when ambulating.
Benzodiazepine		
Diazepam (Valium)	Potential adverse effects include drowsiness, lightheadedness, dizziness, ataxia, slurred speech, headache, dry mouth, and anorexia.	Monitor for excessive sedation and CNS symptoms.
Antipsychotics		
Chlorpromazine (Thorazine)	Potential adverse effects include sedation, dizziness, and hypotension.	Monitor blood pressure for orthostatic hypotension and excessive sedation.

CNS, Central nervous system; MAO, monoamine oxidase.

d. The use of PCA is based on the premise that pain is an individual subjective experience and the patient can best determine the amount of analgesic needed for pain relief.

e. Certain criteria for patient selection have been identified. These criteria include the following:
   (1) The patient is experiencing or is expected to experience moderate to severe pain, such as postoperative pain.
   (2) The patient is mentally competent.
   (3) The patient is physically capable of activating or pushing the button.
   (4) The patient has no history of sensitivity to morphine or to other opiates.
   (5) The patient has no history of significant hepatic or renal disease.
   (6) The patient has no recent history of substance abuse.

f. Commonly used narcotic analgesics for PCA therapy include morphine, meperidine, and hydromorphone.
   (1) Potential adverse effects include nausea, vomiting, anxiety, allergic reactions, itching, sedation, constipation, urinary retention, and respiratory depression.

g. The overall advantages and benefits of the PCA method of pain management include the following:
   • Increased patient satisfaction
   • Decreased anxiety level
   • Improved pain relief
   • Reduced sedation and increased alertness
   • Decreased narcotic usage
   • Enhanced sense of control
   • Increased sense of well-being

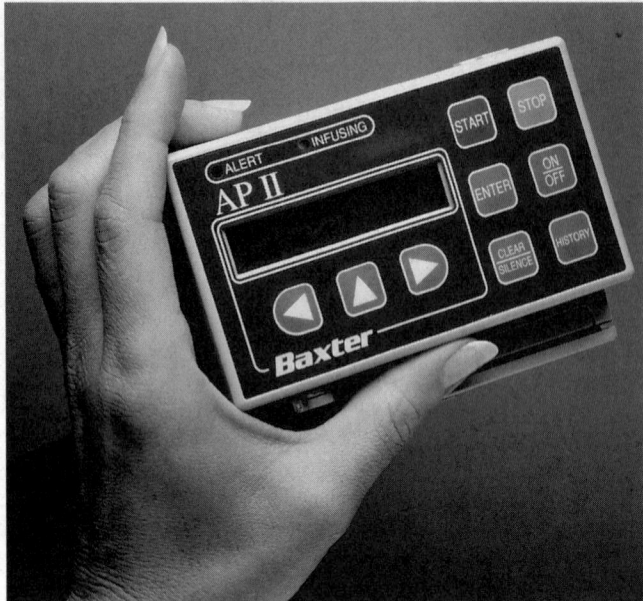

Figure 11-8. Patient-controlled analgesia pump. (Courtesy of Bard MedSystems Division, Baxter Healthcare Corp.)

h. In addition, postoperative patients tend to have better pain control and are less hesitant and more willing to engage in activities such as turning, coughing and deep breathing, ambulating, and self-care activities. A relationship between use of PCA and reduced length of hospital stay has been reported.

Multidisciplinary Approach to Pain Control

1. **Nurse.** A pain management plan may be developed by the health team in collaboration with the patient. The nurse is in an ideal position to coordinate the efforts of the health team members to obtain maximum pain relief for the patient. The nurse can work with the team members and the patient to plan the most appropriate therapies for the patient. She or he retains the responsibility for monitoring and evaluating the patient's overall response to therapy.
2. **Physical therapist.** The physical therapist determines the exercises and treatments that are appropriate for the patient. Treatments may include the use of heat or cold therapy, TENS, or ultrasound or muscle stimulator to decrease pain from muscle spasms. Daily walks and hydrotherapy may be used to help exercise and relax muscle groups.
3. **Occupational therapist.** The occupational therapist assesses the patient's capacity for self-care or level of needed assistance with activities of daily living and assists the patient in learning methods to control and reduce pain and resume a functional lifestyle.
4. **Clinical psychologist.** The clinical psychologist helps the patient learn cognitive and behavioral strategies to relieve pain and develop coping strategies and provides

emotional support. In addition, he or she helps family members to understand the patient's behavior and maintain adequate family dynamics.

5. **Social worker.** The social worker assists in the investigation of problems and their resolution, for example, insurance-related problems, preparation for home care, and mobilization of needed family and community resources to provide continuity of care. The social worker can usually direct the patient and family to helpful resources, such as pain clinics, support groups, transportation for follow-up appointments, and assistive devices.
6. **Spiritual or religious counselors.** Spiritual or religious counselors should be available to the patient who indicates such a desire. Many patients derive benefits from their religious beliefs. Religious or spiritual values and practices may be a positive influence in an individual's ability to cope with pain.
7. **Dietitian.** The dietitian can contribute to the pain relief program by designing a diet that increases the serotonin level in the brain, achieves or maintains ideal body weight, and provides the needed nutrients. Serotonin is a neurotransmitter that affects pain perception. The diet is designed to encourage the body to use its own natural pain relievers. Maintaining or achieving ideal body weight also is important because excess weight places stress on joints and muscles and can therefore contribute to pain.

■ APPLYING THE NURSING PROCESS

NURSING DIAGNOSIS: Knowledge deficit R/T pain management, including alternative therapies to control pain

1. *Expected outcomes:* Following instructions, the patient should be able to do the following:
   a. Demonstrate an understanding of alternative pain control measures. Successfully elicit the relaxation response.
   b. Engage in diversional activities: reading, watching television, listening to music.
   c. Report more effective pain relief and enhanced sense of well-being.
2. *Nursing interventions*
   a. Teach the patient and family about alternative measures to aid in controlling pain, such as relaxation, breathing exercises, the use of TENS, the use of heat and cold applications, and music therapy.
   b. Assess the patient's willingness to use alternative pain control measures in addition to the pharmacologic therapy.
   c. Teach the patient how to elicit the relaxation response. Encourage the patient to practice at specified times during the day. Provide a quiet environment, coaching, and assistance as needed.

d. Assess the patient's preferences for reading materials and music and make these available for use.

NURSING DIAGNOSIS: Pain R/T movement of abdominal incision and skin irritation

1. *Expected outcomes:* Following instructions and therapy, the patient should be able to do the following:
   a. Splint the incisional area with a pillow or hands when coughing or moving about.
   b. Remain mobile and report minimum pulling, pain, or both around the incisional area with movement or coughing.
   c. Acknowledge the role of splinting in lessening pain from a dressing change.
2. *Nursing interventions*
   a. Teach the patient how to splint the incisional area with a pillow when turning and coughing and moving about.
   b. Provide music therapy (patient's preference) 30 minutes before each dressing change.
   c. Administer narcotic or nonnarcotic analgesic, or both, 30 minutes before dressing change.
   d. Cleanse skin around abdominal incision with mild soap and water to remove antibiotic solution.
   e. Continue music therapy for at least 30 minutes after completion of dressing change.

Additional Nursing Diagnoses

- Activity intolerance
- Altered role performance
- Altered thought processes
- Anxiety
- Chronic pain
- Fear
- Impaired physical mobility
- Self-care deficit
  a. Bathing-hygiene, dressing-grooming
  b. Feeding
- Sleep pattern disturbance
- Social isolation

◼ *DISCHARGE PLANNING AND TEACHING*

1. Discharge planning and teaching should begin following the admission assessment and diagnosis and continue throughout the patient's hospitalization and in some instances after discharge. Teaching should be designed to help the patient develop a combination of cognitive, affective, and psychomotor skills for controlling the pain. Successful patient teaching also helps patients accept health-related information, become partners in their pain management regimen, and incorporate health information into daily routines.

HOME CARE STRATEGIES

Pain Management

Pain management in the home setting has a unique set of challenges. Remember the following:

- **Drug availability**—Know the state pharmacy regulations relating to dispensing controlled drugs. Will a signed prescription form be necessary? How will the patient obtain the prescription from the physician? How will the patient obtain the drug?
- **Cost**—Know the cost of medications to assist with recommendations to the physician. Check with the pharmacist regarding special programs through pharmaceutical companies for financial assistance.
- **Schedule of medication administration**—Compliance is more difficult if the patient or caregiver needs to be awakened for scheduled medications during the nighttime hours. The use of long-acting products with breakthrough dosing available will help the patient and family to establish a manageable schedule.
- **Reporting of pain**—Encourage the patient and family to utilize a pain diary that includes a pain rating and the use of scheduled and as needed medications. Write special instructions for the patient and family in the diary for easy reference.
- **Caregiver's perception of pain**—Instruct the patient and caregiver regarding the pain management plan. Participation is crucial to effective pain management. Dispel myths about pain and use of narcotics.
- **Uncontrolled pain**—Instruct the patient and caregiver regarding the procedure to follow if pain is not controlled. Make the on-call staff aware of current orders and dose ranges of prescribed medications. Persistent pain becomes a family crisis, which usually results in a hospital admission. This could be prevented with a well-established pain management plan.
- **Maintaining pain control**—As pain decreases with effective management, instruct the patient and caregiver to continue using regularly scheduled medications to maintain control. Misinformed patients may assume that pain that is managed no longer needs to be treated.
- **Safety and storage**—Assess the home setting for special concerns related to vulnerable adults, children, and pets. Monitor the supply of medications during regularly scheduled visits to maintain an adequate supply.

2. The discharge plan should be developed with the health care team in collaboration with the patient and the patient's family. The patient and family should be provided with a written pain management plan and relevant related information regarding the following:
   a. The pain, its source, and the expected outcome of therapy.
   b. The prescribed analgesic or analgesics, dosage, and frequency of administration.
   c. The potential side effects and measures to prevent or minimize these and how to report untoward symptoms promptly should they occur. Provide the patient with written information, including the names of the persons to contact about pain or medication problems.
   d. Potential drug interactions and specific precautions to follow when taking the medications.
3. Teach the patient and family about alternative pain management measures, such as breathing exercises, relaxation, the use of TENS, heat and cold applications, biofeedback, and the use of music therapy.
   a. Teach the patient how to elicit the relaxation response and schedule practice sessions before discharge.

4. Make a referral for home care physical therapy, if necessary, to assist with the use of TENS, massage, or heat or cold treatments.

5. Make a referral for visiting nurse home care if it is anticipated that the patient will require assistance or supervision with the pain relief regimen after discharge.

6. Promote the patient's autonomy and sense of control in managing the pain.

7. Emphasize the importance of keeping appointments for follow-up care.

8. Evaluate teaching and learning to determine whether the patient has acquired the knowledge and skills taught. Assessment and evaluation are ongoing and influence adjustment or changes in the teaching strategies or other components of the plan.

Bibliography

Books or Pamphlets

American Pain Society. *Principles of Analgesic Use in the Treatment of Acute Pain and Chronic Pain*. 3rd ed. Skokie, IL: American Pain Society, 1993.

Benson H. *The Relaxation Response*. New York: William Morrow, 1975.

Black JM, and Matassarin-Jacobs E. *Luckmann and Sorensen's Medical-Surgical Nursing: A Psychophysiologic Approach*. 4th ed. Philadelphia: WB Saunders, 1993.

Bulechek GG, and McCloskey JC. *Nursing Interventions: Essential Nursing Treatments*. 2nd ed. Philadelphia: WB Saunders, 1992.

Clark JB, Queener SF, and Karb VB. *Pharmacological Basis of Nursing Practice*. 3rd ed. St. Louis: CV Mosby, 1990.

Eliopoulos C. *Caring for the Elderly in Diverse Care Settings*. Philadelphia: JB Lippincott, 1990.

Ferri RS. *Care Planning for the Older Adult: Nursing Diagnosis in Long-Term Care*. Philadelphia: WB Saunders, 1994.

Giger JN, and Davidhizar RE. *Transcultural Nursing*. St. Louis: CV Mosby, 1991.

Hanson RW, and Gerber KE. *Coping with Chronic Pain*. New York: The Guilford Press, 1990.

Ignatavicius DD, and Bayne MV. *Medical-Surgical Nursing: A Nursing Process Approach*. Philadelphia: WB Saunders, 1991.

Lance JW. *Mechanism and Management of Headache*. 5th ed. Boston: Butterworth-Heinemann, 1993.

McCaffery M. *Nursing Management of the Patient with Pain*. 2nd ed. Philadelphia: JB Lippincott, 1979.

Melzack R. *The Puzzle of Pain*. New York: Basic Books, 1973.

Specter RE. *Cultural Diversity in Health and Illness*. 3rd ed. Norwalk, CT: Appleton & Lange, 1991.

U.S. Department of Health and Human Services. *Clinical Practice Guidelines. Acute Pain Management: Operative or Medical Procedures and Trauma*. Rockville, MD: Agency for Health Care Policy and Research, Public Health Services. Publication 92-0032. February 1992.

U.S. Department of Health and Human Services. *Management of Cancer Pain: Adults—Quick Reference Guide #9*. Rockville, MD: Agency for Health Care Policy and Research, Public Health Services. Publication No. 94-0593.

U.S. Department of Health and Human Services. *Management of Cancer Pain: Clinical Practice Guideline #9*. Rockville, MD: Agency for Health Care Policy and Research, Public Health Services. Publication No. 94-0592.

U.S. Department of Health and Human Services. *Managing Cancer Pain: Patient Guide*. Rockville, MD: Agency for Health Care Policy and Research, Public Health Services. Publication No. 94-0595.

U.S. Department of Health and Human Services. *Pain Control After Surgery—A Patient's Guide*. Rockville, MD: Agency for Health Care Policy and Research, Public Health Services. Publication No. 92-0021.

Watt-Watson JH, and Donovan MI. *Pain Management: Nursing Perspective*. St. Louis: Mosby–Year Book, 1992.

Williams BR, and Baer CL. *Essentials of Clinical Pharmacology in Nursing*. Springhouse, PA: Springhouse Corporation, 1990.

World Health Organization. *Cancer Pain Relief*. Albany, NY: Author, 1986.

World Health Organization. *Cancer Pain Relief and Palliative Care*. Albany, NY: Author, 1990.

World Health Organization. *Palliative Cancer Care: Pain Relief and Management*. Albany, NY: Author, 1993.

Journal Articles

American Health Consultants. The ethics of rationing pain control. *Medical Ethics Advisor* 9(9):110–111, 1993.

Anderson JM. Health care across cultures. *Nurs Outlook* 83(3):136–139, 1990.

Beck SL. The therapeutic use of music for cancer related pain. *Oncol Nurs Forum* 18(8):1327–1336, 1991.

Collier M. Controlling postoperative pain with patient-controlled analgesia. *Prof Nurs* 6(2):121–126, 1990.

Dalessio DJ. Diagnosis and treatment of cranial neuralgias. *Med Clin North Am* 75(3):605–615, 1991.

Diamond S. Migraine headaches. *Med Clin North Am* 75(3):545–565, 1991.

Ferrell BR, McCaffery M, and Ropchan R. Pain management as a clinical challenge for nursing administration. *Nurs Outlook* 40(6):263–268, 1992.

Ferrell BR, et al. Impact of cancer pain on family caregivers. *Oncol Nurs Forum* 18(8):1303–1308, 1991.

Greipp ME. Undermedication for pain: An ethical model. *Adv Nurs Sci* 15(1):44–53, 1992.

Harrison A. Assessing patient's pain: Identifying reasons for error. *J Adv Nurs* 16(1):1018–1025, 1991.

Henkle JO, and Kennerly SM. Cultural diversity: A resource for planning and implementing nursing care. *Public Health Nurs* 7(3):145–149, 1990.

Jacox A. A guideline for the nation: Managing acute pain. *Am J Nurs* 92(5):49–55, 1992.

Kachoyeanos MK, and Friedhoff M. Cognitive and behavioral strategies to reduce children's pain. *MCN* 18(1):14–19, 1993.

Kawamura J, and Meyer JS. Headaches due to cerebrovascular disease. *Med Clin North Am* 75(3):617–625, 1991.

Kudrow L. Diagnosis and treatment of cluster headache. *Med Clin North Am* 75(3):579–593, 1991.

Kunkel RS. Diagnosis and treatment of muscle contraction (tension-type) headache. *Med Clin North Am* 75(3):595–603, 1991.

McGuire L. The nurse's role in pain relief. *MedSurg Nurs* 3(2):94–98, 1994.

Melzack R, and Wall PD. Pain mechanism: A new theory. *Science* 150(36):971–972, 1965.

Miaskowski C. Current concepts and management of acute pain. *MedSurg Nurs* 2(9):28–32, 1993.

Miaskowski C. Current concepts in the assessment and management of cancer-related pain. *MedSurg Nurs* 2(2):113–118, 1993.

Mondell BE. Evaluation of the patient presenting with headache. *Med Clin North Am* 75(3):521–539, 1991.

Snelling J. The effect of chronic pain on the family unit. *J Adv Nurs* 19(3):543–551, 1994.

Thomas VJ, and Rose FD. Patient controlled analgesia: A new method for old. *J Adv Nurs* 18(11):1719–1720, 1993.

Villarruel AM, and deMontellano BO. Culture and pain: A Mesoamerican perspective. *Adv Nurs Sci* 15(1):21–32, 1992.

Walding MF. Pain, anxiety, and powerlessness. *J Adv Nurs* 16(4):388–397, 1991.

Weinrich SP, and Weinrich MC. The effects of massage on pain in cancer patients. *Appl Nurs Res* 3(4):140–145, 1990.

Agencies

Pain Management Resources

American Pain Society
P.O. Box 468
Des Plaines, IL 60016–0468
(708) 966–5595

American Society of Pain Management
  Nurses
P.O. Box 6604
Denver, CO 80206–0604
(303) 494–4215 (phone/fax)

U.S. Department of Health and
  Human Services
Public Health Service
Agency for Health Care Policy and
  Research
AHCPR, Publications
  Clearinghouse
P.O. Box 8547
Silver Springs, MD 20907
(800) 358–9295

World Health Organization
WHO Publication Center
49 Sheridan Avenue
Albany, NY 12210
(518) 436–9686

12
Caring for People in Shock

■ DEFINITION OF SHOCK AND PATHOPHYSIOLOGIC OVERVIEW

Definition of Shock

1. Shock is a pathologic condition characterized by inadequate tissue perfusion. It is a multicausal, progressive syndrome that results in cellular dysfunction and cellular death and may result in the patient's death.
2. Shock occurs when 1 of the following 2 things happens.
   a. The cardiovascular system fails to deliver adequate amounts of oxygen and glucose to the cells.
   b. The cells are unable to use the available amounts of oxygen and nutrients.

Pathophysiologic Overview

1. Regardless of cause, all types of shock result in the *same* pathophysiology and produce the *same* signs and symptoms.
2. All types of shock impair cellular metabolism of oxygen and glucose. Cells use oxygen and glucose to aerobically synthesize adenosine triphosphate (ATP), the energy source for cell functions.
3. Without oxygen and glucose, cells revert to anaerobic metabolism to produce ATP, resulting in inadequate production of ATP and production of lactic acid. When ATP is insufficient, the following occur:
   a. Metabolic acidosis
   b. Cellular dysfunction and cellular death (Fig. 12–1)
4. As cellular dysfunction and cellular death increase, organ systems begin to fail. When 3 or more vital organ systems fail, the person's death is imminent.

■ SHOCK: CLASSIFICATIONS, CAUSES, AND RISK FACTORS

Hypovolemic Shock

1. Hypovolemic shock results from loss of circulating fluid volume, which leads to inadequate intravascular volume. It is caused by external fluid losses, internal fluid losses, or both.

2. External fluid losses include the following (see Chapter 9):
   a. Hemorrhage
   b. Severe vomiting
   c. Severe diarrhea
   d. Excessive diuresis
   e. Inadequate fluid intake
   f. Temperature elevation
   g. Severe dehydration
3. Internal fluid losses: Fluids shift from the vasculature into organs or intracellular spaces. Conditions or examples of pathology incorporating fluid loss or shifts are as follows:
   a. Ileus
   b. Intestinal obstruction
   c. Burns (see Chapter 36)
   d. Peritonitis
   e. Ascites
   f. Pancreatitis
4. Risk factors
   a. Traumatic injury
   b. Alcoholism
   c. Severe diarrhea, vomiting, or both

Cardiogenic Shock

1. Cardiogenic shock results from major left ventricular dysfunction, leading to heart failure, ineffective pumping of blood, inadequate cardiac output, and decreased tissue perfusion.
2. Causes (see Chapter 23)
   a. Myocardial infarction—especially anterior-wall myocardial infarction
   b. Heart failure
   c. Cardiomyopathy
   d. Acute arrhythmias
   e. Acute pericardial tamponade
   f. Severe heart valve malfunction
   g. Massive pulmonary embolism
   h. Tension pneumothorax
   i. Myocarditis
   j. Dissecting abdominal aortic aneurysms
3. Risk factors
   a. Cardiovascular stress with previous myocardial damage
   b. Acute myocardial infarction involving more than 40 percent of the left ventricle

CELL DEATH

Normal Cell
- Cell membrane intact
- Normal aerobic metabolism
- Fluids in balance
- Electrolytes in balance
- Wastes removed

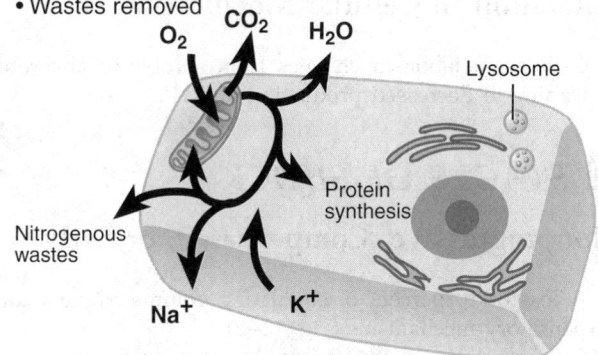

Cell in Early Shock
- Hypoxia leads to inadequate tissue perfusion
- Cell swells, membrane permeability increases
- Anaerobic metabolism
- Cell pH rises

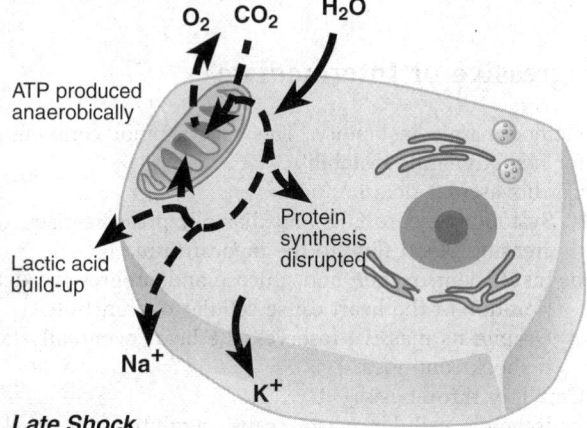

Late Shock
- Cell death
- Cell membrane destroyed
- Anaerobic metabolism continues
- Increasing pH
- Increased capillary pressure drives fluids into cell

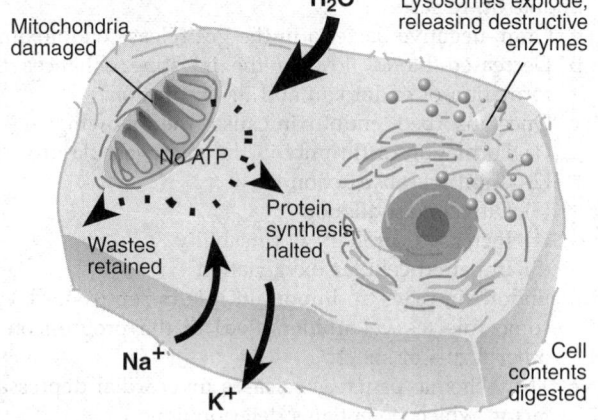

Figure 12–1. Normal cell versus cell in shock. ATP, Adenosine triphosphate.

---

   c. Dysrhythmias
   d. Obstructed left ventricular function

Distributive (or Vasogenic) Shock

1. Neurogenic shock
   a. Neurogenic shock results from generalized vasodilation and loss of vasomotor tone, causing the following:
      (1) A massive increase in vascular capacity
      (2) Pooling of blood in the periphery
      (3) Decreased venous return to the heart
   b. Causes (see Chapter 18)
      (1) Spinal cord injuries
      (2) Anesthetic paralysis
      (3) Reflex vasodilation (vasovagal response)
      (4) Head trauma
      (5) Extreme pain
   c. Risk factors
      (1) Traumatic injury
      (2) Diseases of the spinal cord
      (3) Spinal or deep general anesthesia
      (4) Drugs that cause vasomotor center depression
      (5) Snake venom
2. Anaphylactic shock
   a. Anaphylactic shock results from an antigen-antibody reaction, which releases histamine or histamine-like substances, causing the following:
      (1) Pooling of blood in the periphery from vasodilation
      (2) Fluid and protein shifts from leaking capillaries
      (3) Decreased venous return to the heart
   b. Causes (see Chapter 21)
      (1) Adverse drug reactions
      (2) Food intolerances
      (3) Pollen hypersensitivity
      (4) Hypersensitivity to insect stings
      (5) Hypersensitivity to foreign proteins in the serum (transfusion reaction)
   c. Risk factors
      (1) Unrecognized allergy
      (2) Accidental exposure to a known allergen
3. Septic shock
   a. Septic shock is a syndrome marked by altered hemodynamics, decreased tissue perfusion, and loss of cellular energy.
   b. It develops because of the body's immune and inflammatory responses to endotoxin following bacteremia, usually caused by gram-negative bacteria (> two thirds of cases), and produces the following:
      (1) Fever
      (2) Cellular dysfunction
      (3) Marked vasodilation
      (4) Peripheral pooling of blood
      (5) Decreased systemic vascular resistance
   c. Causes (see Chapter 8)
      (1) Gram-negative bacteria endotoxins—most common causative factor
      (2) Gram-positive bacteria—most common cause of toxic shock

(3) Fungi
(4) Viruses
(5) Rickettsiae
d. Risk factors
(1) Immunosuppression from either disease or drugs
(2) Extremes of age—being very old or very young

☐ THE BODY'S REACTION TO SHOCK

Activation of Compensatory Mechanisms

1. Activation of the central nervous system ischemic response
    a. The central nervous system ischemic response is activated when the following occur:
        (1) Carotid and aortic baroreceptors, responding to a decrease in blood pressure and a drop in intravascular fluid volume, slow discharges that inhibit the vasomotor center.
        (2) Changes in pH and P_{CO_2} stimulate the carotid body chemoreceptors.
    b. These changes stimulate the vasomotor center, activating the sympathetic nervous system.
2. Activation of the sympathetic nervous system
    a. Changes in the ratio of fluid volume to intravascular space activate the sympathetic nervous system.
    b. Alpha-adrenergic effects result from stimulation of the sympathetic nervous system receptors in the smooth muscle (α-$_1$) and the presynaptic neuron (α-$_2$). Effects include the following:
        (1) Vasoconstriction, which maintains systolic blood pressure and elevates diastolic blood pressure, produces a narrowed pulse pressure.
        (2) Circulation to the brain is improved, but circulation decreases to other organs.
    c. Beta-adrenergic effects result from stimulation of the sympathetic nervous system receptors in the myocardium and adipose tissue (β-$_1$) and the bronchial smooth muscle and vessel walls (β-$_2$). Effects include the following:
        (1) Increased heart rate, increased contractility, and increased stroke volume boost cardiac output.
        (2) Myocardial oxygen demand increases.
        (3) Bronchodilation and vasodilation occur.
3. Activation of the renin-angiotensin-aldosterone system
    a. Activation of the renin-angiotensin-aldosterone system results from decreased kidney perfusion caused by constriction of the renal artery.
    b. Renin released from the juxtaglomerular cells combines with angiotensin from the liver. This combination produces angiotensin I, which is converted to angiotensin II, a potent vasoconstrictor.
    c. Angiotensin II causes increased secretion of aldosterone from the adrenal cortex, which decreases sodium and water excretion from the kidneys.
    d. Angiotensin III, another product of this system, causes the following:
        (1) Increased sympathetic nervous system activity

(2) Increased release of antidiuretic hormone
(3) Increased reabsorption of water in the kidneys
(4) Thirst
e. The main result of the activation of the renin-angiotensin-aldosterone system is an increase in circulating volume.

Alteration in Cellular Metabolism

1. Cellular metabolism changes from aerobic to anaerobic, leading to decreased production of ATP.

☐ STAGES OF SHOCK

Nonprogressive, Compensated, or Early

1. A loss of 10 percent of circulating volume triggers compensatory mechanisms (Fig. 12–2).
2. Sympathetic nervous system responses and renin-angiotensin-aldosterone response compensate and prevent further deterioration.
3. Cardiac output and blood pressure remain normal.
4. The person recovers if shock does not enter the more severe progressive phase.

Progressive or Intermediate

1. Hemodynamic instability. The body cannot compensate for hemodynamic instability.
2. Cardiovascular deterioration
    a. Systolic pressure falls and diastolic pressure rises, decreasing blood flow to the myocardium.
    b. Insufficient oxygen and glucose and progressive deterioration of the heart cause cellular dysfunction.
    c. Despite its massive reserves, the heart eventually fails if shock continues.
3. Capillary thrombosis
    a. Ischemic cellular wastes cause agglutination or clotting in the small vessels.
    b. Sluggish blood flow in the microvasculature decreases the flow of oxygen and glucose to the cells.
4. Capillary permeability. Capillary hypoxia and lack of glucose increase capillary permeability.
5. Endotoxin release
    a. Gram-negative bacteria in the gut release endotoxin.
    b. Decreased blood flow to the intestine enhances the formation of endotoxin and its absorption.
    c. Once absorbed, endotoxin causes the following:
        (1) Formation of thrombi in the microvasculature
        (2) Capillary obstruction
        (3) Diffuse vasodilation
        (4) Increased capillary permeability
        (5) Impaired cellular oxygenation
    d. Endotoxin plays an important role in septic shock and some role (as yet unidentified) in the progression of other forms of shock.
    e. The ischemic pancreas releases myocardial depressant factor, which potentiates deterioration.

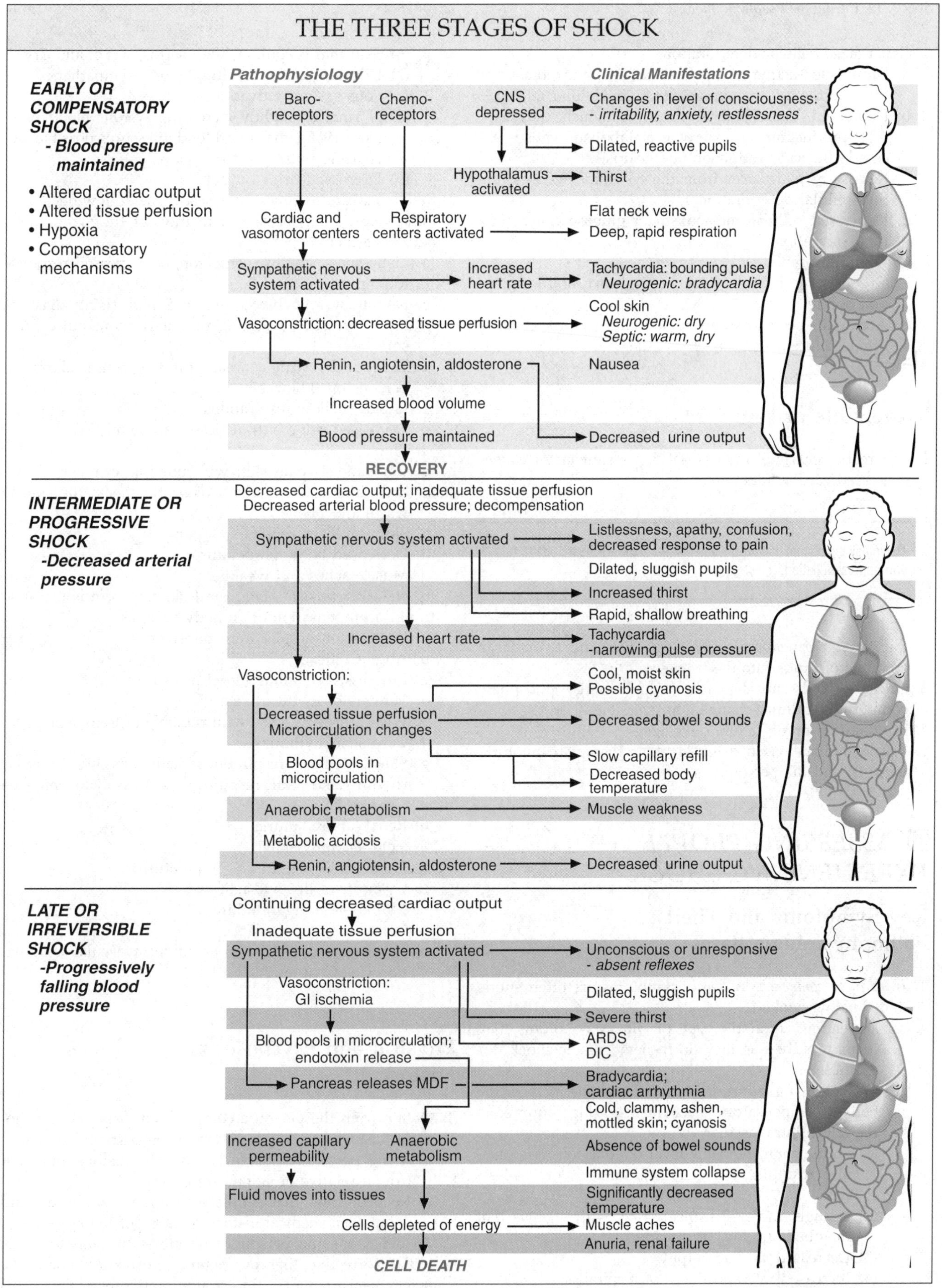

THE THREE STAGES OF SHOCK

Pathophysiology   **Clinical Manifestations**

EARLY OR COMPENSATORY SHOCK
- Blood pressure maintained

- Altered cardiac output
- Altered tissue perfusion
- Hypoxia
- Compensatory mechanisms

Baro-receptors   Chemo-receptors   CNS depressed → Changes in level of consciousness: - *irritability, anxiety, restlessness*

→ Dilated, reactive pupils

Hypothalamus activated → Thirst

Cardiac and vasomotor centers   Respiratory centers activated → Flat neck veins
Deep, rapid respiration

Sympathetic nervous system activated → Increased heart rate → Tachycardia: bounding pulse
Neurogenic: bradycardia

Vasoconstriction: decreased tissue perfusion → Cool skin
Neurogenic: dry
Septic: warm, dry

→ Renin, angiotensin, aldosterone → Nausea

Increased blood volume

Blood pressure maintained → Decreased urine output

RECOVERY

INTERMEDIATE OR PROGRESSIVE SHOCK
-Decreased arterial pressure

Decreased cardiac output; inadequate tissue perfusion
Decreased arterial blood pressure; decompensation

Sympathetic nervous system activated → Listlessness, apathy, confusion, decreased response to pain

→ Dilated, sluggish pupils

→ Increased thirst

→ Rapid, shallow breathing

Increased heart rate → Tachycardia -narrowing pulse pressure

Vasoconstriction: → Cool, moist skin
Possible cyanosis

Decreased tissue perfusion
Microcirculation changes → Decreased bowel sounds

Blood pools in microcirculation → Slow capillary refill
Decreased body temperature

Anaerobic metabolism → Muscle weakness

Metabolic acidosis

→ Renin, angiotensin, aldosterone → Decreased urine output

LATE OR IRREVERSIBLE SHOCK
-Progressively falling blood pressure

Continuing decreased cardiac output
Inadequate tissue perfusion
Sympathetic nervous system activated → Unconscious or unresponsive - *absent reflexes*

Vasoconstriction: GI ischemia → Dilated, sluggish pupils

→ Severe thirst

Blood pools in microcirculation; endotoxin release → ARDS
DIC

→ Pancreas releases MDF → Bradycardia; cardiac arrhythmia

Cold, clammy, ashen, mottled skin; cyanosis

Increased capillary permeability   Anaerobic metabolism → Absence of bowel sounds

→ Immune system collapse

Fluid moves into tissues → Significantly decreased temperature

Cells depleted of energy → Muscle aches

→ Anuria, renal failure

CELL DEATH

Figure 12–2. Stages of shock and signs and symptoms of shock and their pathophysiologic bases. CNS, Central nervous system; MDF, myocardial depressant factor; ARDS, adult respiratory distress syndrome; DIC, disseminated intravascular coagulation.

6. Generalized cellular deterioration
   a. Diminished active transport of sodium and potassium through the cell membrane results in cellular edema.
   b. Depressed mitochondrial function, which decreases ATP production by anaerobic metabolism, causes excess lactic acid production and acidosis.
   c. Release of hydrolases from the lysosomes causes further cellular deterioration.
   d. Depressed cellular metabolism of glucose causes cellular starvation.
7. Organ deterioration
   a. Organs, especially the liver, lungs, heart, and kidneys, deteriorate.
   b. Areas of necrosis develop within organs, causing organ failure.

Irreversible or Late

1. Pancreatic release of myocardial depressant factor causes decreased cardiac function.

> The most significant factors in late-stage shock are heart deterioration and vasodilation.

2. Capillary permeability results in movement of large amounts of fluids into the tissues.
3. Once the cells are depleted of high-energy phosphate compounds, cellular change is irreversible.
4. Multisystem organ failure develops.
5. Tissue damage is so extensive that therapy cannot reverse it, and the person dies.

■ ASSESSING PEOPLE EXPERIENCING SHOCK

Key Symptoms and Their Pathophysiologic Bases

1. In *early or compensatory shock*, symptoms are often subtle and thus overlooked.
   a. Depending upon the type of shock, symptoms may occur rapidly—as they do in hemorrhagic shock, for example.
   b. The following symptoms result from activation of the body's compensatory mechanisms, which counteract the fall in intravascular volume.
      (1) Subtle changes in the level of consciousness, usually resulting in irritability, anxiety, or restlessness
      (2) A slight increase in heart rate, with a pulse that may be bounding or thready
      (3) Decreased cardiac output
      (4) Increased rate and depth of respiration
      (5) Thirst

(6) Skin that is cool, or, with sepsis, warm and dry
(7) Dilated pupils resulting from sympathetic nervous system activation
(8) Normal or slightly increasing systolic blood pressure; rising diastolic blood pressure; possible decreasing pulse pressure
(9) Decreased urine output

2. In *intermediate or progressive shock*, the following symptoms result from massive activation of the sympathetic nervous system.
   a. Listlessness, apathy, confusion, or decreased response to pain
   b. Falling systolic blood pressure and rising diastolic blood pressure, resulting in a narrowing pulse pressure
   c. Tachycardia with a weak, thready pulse, except in persons on β-blockers
   d. Rapid, shallow respirations
   e. Decreased urine output (less than 30 ml/hr)
   f. Thirst
   g. Cool, moist, pale skin with possible cyanosis. However, in the warm phase of septic shock, the skin is warm and flushed.
   h. Slow capillary refill
   i. Decreased body temperature
   j. Muscle aches and weakness
3. In *late or irreversible shock*, the following symptoms arise from decompensation of all body systems.
   a. Unconsciousness or unresponsiveness
   b. Absent reflexes
   c. Progressively falling blood pressure
   d. Slowing of the heart rate
   e. Weak, thready pulse with possible pulse deficit
   f. Cardiac arrhythmias
   g. Slow, shallow respirations with possible irregular rhythms and adult respiratory distress syndrome (see Chapter 22)
   h. Renal failure, anuria
   i. Cold, clammy skin
   j. Significantly decreased temperature
   k. Cyanosis of lips and nail beds
   l. Multisystem organ failure
   m. Immune system collapse
   n. Development of disseminated intravascular coagulation (see Chapter 25)

Physical and Psychosocial History

1. Obtain from the person a complete physical and psychosocial history and a description of the current problem.
   a. If the person is unable to give the history, obtain it from a relative or significant other.
   b. Keep in mind that people may not always be truthful about their medical history or cause of injury.
2. To determine the person's baseline status and to guide initial corrective therapy, obtain information about the mechanism of injury, time frame, and prehospital treatment.

Physical Examination

1. Conduct a head-to-toe, front-to-back physical examination of the person for signs and symptoms of shock.
2. Identify areas of injury that may be responsible for shock. Findings vary with the stage of shock.
   a. A fractured femur or fractured pelvis may produce symptoms of hypovolemic shock in the absence of other injuries.
   b. Injury to the kidneys may produce profound shock in the absence of outward findings. Test urine for the presence of blood.
3. Assess neurologic status
   a. As shock progresses, the person's level of consciousness ranges from (1) to (2) to (3) as follows.
      (1) Inability to concentrate, restlessness, agitation, anxiety or confusion or both
      (2) Bizarre behavior, lethargy or apathy or both
      (3) Unconsciousness and unresponsiveness
   b. Pupils progress from normal and reactive to dilated and reactive to dilated and sluggish reaction (Fig. 12–3).
4. Assess cardiovascular status

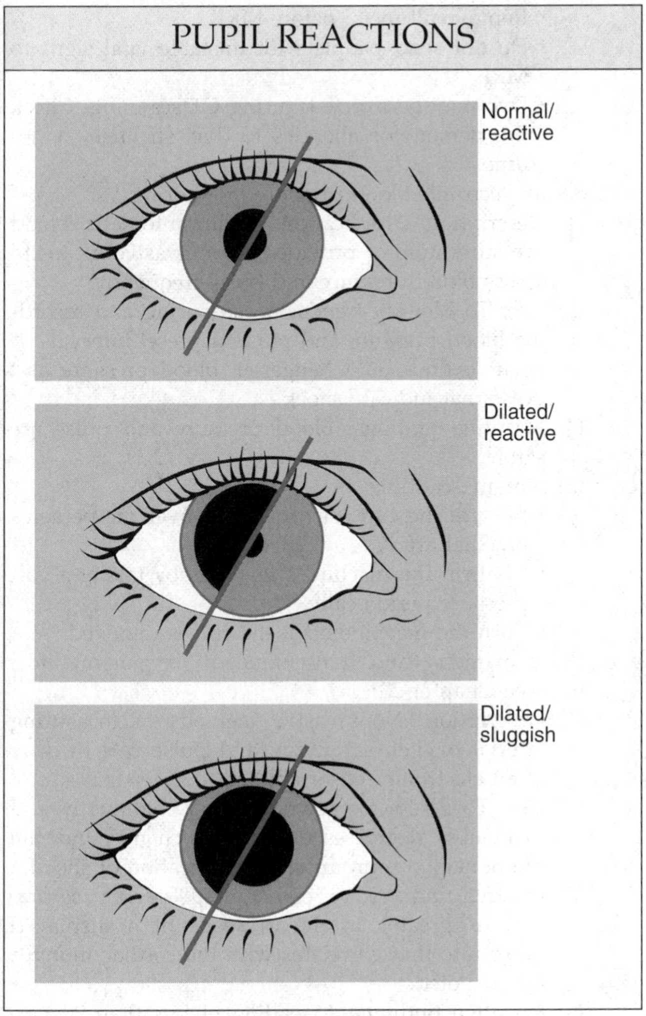

PUPIL REACTIONS

Figure 12–3.

BLOOD PRESSURE CHANGES IN SHOCK

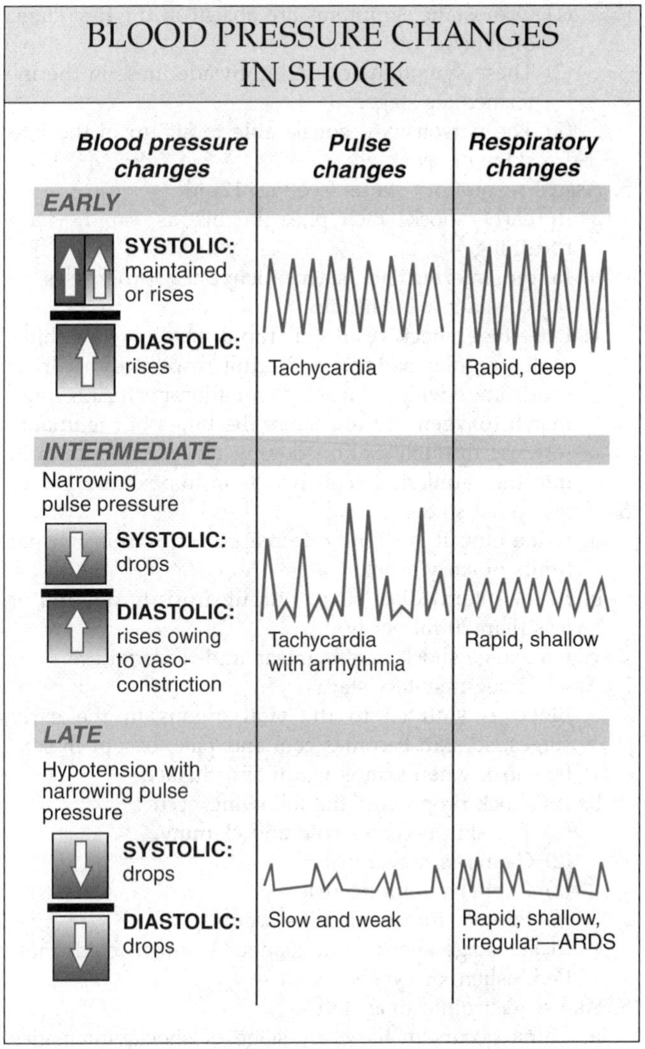

Figure 12–4. Blood pressure, pulse, and respiratory changes. ARDS, Adult respiratory distress syndrome.

a. Blood pressure varies with the stage of shock (Fig. 12–4).
   (1) Initially, systolic blood pressure is maintained or rises, and diastolic blood pressure rises. A decreased pulse pressure may result.
   (2) Systolic blood pressure drops as shock progresses, but vasoconstriction raises diastolic pressure, resulting in a narrowing pulse pressure.
   (3) Further progression results in frank hypotension with a widening pulse pressure.
   (4) If shock is untreated, cardiovascular collapse with no blood pressure results.
b. Pulse (see Fig. 12–4)
   (1) You may see initial tachycardia from sympathetic stimulation.
   (2) As shock worsens, this progresses to tachycardia with arrhythmias and weak, rapid, thready peripheral pulses.
   (3) In late-stage shock, you may see an extremely slow and weak or absent pulse.
c. Orthostatic symptoms

(1) Orthostatic symptoms are absent in the first stage of shock.

(2) These symptoms cause lightheadedness in the intermediate stage.

(3) The person may not be able to sit up in the late stage of shock.

5. Assess respiratory status (see Fig. 12–4)

a. In early shock, tachypnea begins as rapid, deep breathing.

b. In the intermediate stage, tachypnea progresses to rapid, shallow breathing.

c. Late-stage shock results in rapid, shallow breathing with irregular patterns and adult respiratory distress syndrome, which causes ventilation-perfusion mismatch (oxygen-rich air enters the lungs but is unable to cross through malfunctioning alveolar membranes into the capillaries). This results in hypoxemia.

6. Assess renal status

a. Urine output is slightly decreased but within normal limits in early shock.

b. In the intermediate stage, output drops to oliguria of less than 20 ml per hour.

c. Late-stage shock causes anuria and renal failure.

7. Assess integumentary status

a. Blood is shunted to the vital organs in the early stages, so skin becomes cool and pale, except in septic shock when skin is warm and flushed.

b. As shock progresses, the following occur:

(1) The skin becomes cold and clammy.

(2) Cyanosis may appear.

(3) Capillary refill decreases.

(4) Edema from fluid shifts occurs.

c. In late-stage shock, skin changes result in cold, mottled, ashen, or cyanotic skin.

8. Assess gastrointestinal status

a. Thirst occurs in the early stage of shock, intensifies in the intermediate stage, and is severe in late shock.

b. Bowel sounds become hypoactive as blood is shunted to other organs. This progresses to absence of bowel sounds (paralytic ileus) and formation of a stress ulcer.

9. Assess musculoskeletal status

a. Muscles weaken as blood is shunted to more vital organs

b. Muscles ache as lactic acid production increases in ischemic muscles.

10. Assess metabolic status

a. Except in the warm phase of septic shock, core temperature falls in all types of shock when the body is exposed to cold. In septic shock, core temperature rises.

b. Aerobic metabolism of nutrients converts to anaerobic metabolism, which produces lactic acid and other acids, resulting in acidosis.

Diagnostic Studies

1. Noninvasive assessment techniques

a. Noninvasive cardiology studies

(1) Description: Electrocardiogram, echocardiogram, and multiple-gated acquisition (MUGA) scanning provide information about cardiac function.

(2) Use: To assess damage to the left ventricle and structures within the heart in cardiogenic shock.

(3) Positive findings: Areas of damage are identified.

(4) Negative findings: No damage is identified.

(5) Nursing cautions: Dye is injected intravenously during a MUGA scan. An allergic reaction can occur. Check the person for allergies to dye, shellfish, or iodine.

b. Radiographic studies

(1) Description: The following radiographic studies are used in hypovolemic, neurogenic, and cardiogenic shock.

• Simple radiographs

• Computed tomography (CT) scans

• Magnetic resonance imaging (MRI)

• Positron-emitted tomography (PET)

(2) Use: To determine areas of injury responsible for the shock state.

(3) Positive findings: Areas of injury are seen.

(4) Negative findings: No injury is seen.

(5) Nursing cautions

• The person may need sedation to lie still for the procedure.

• Remove all metal before MRI.

• Do not send people with unstable vital signs to MRI.

• Dye may be injected during CT scanning. Check the person for allergies to dye, shellfish, or iodine.

c. Serial electronic blood pressure monitoring

(1) Description: Application of an automatic blood pressure monitor provides a noninvasive means to assess blood pressure and pulse frequently.

(2) Use: To identify trends by measuring and recording blood pressure and pulse at preset intervals.

(3) Positive findings: Changes in blood pressure and pulse that indicate shock.

(4) Negative findings: Blood pressure and pulse are stable.

(5) Nursing cautions

• Be sure the cuff microphone is over the person's brachial artery.

• Confirm the machine's readings by taking a cuff pressure periodically.

• Turn the machine off if the cuff is removed.

d. Pulse oximetry and transcutaneous oxygen monitoring (see Chapter 23)

(1) Description: Noninvasive methods of measuring arterial oxygen saturation and pulse rate by way of an electronic sensor applied to the skin.

(2) Use: To assess oxygen saturation continually and to identify decreases rapidly, which may indicate pulmonary compromise, a complication of shock.

(3) Positive findings: A reading of 90 percent saturation or greater in the presence of a displayed pulse rate that correlates with the cardiac monitor rate is noted.

(4) Negative findings: A reading of less than 90 percent saturation in the presence of a displayed

pulse rate that correlates with the cardiac monitor rate is recorded.
(5) Nursing cautions
- If the displayed pulse does not correlate with the cardiac monitor rate, you cannot consider the oxygen saturation accurate.
- Oxygen saturation does not reflect arterial oxygen content. Arterial blood gases must also be measured to determine this parameter.

e. Serial neurologic checks (see Chapter 18)
(1) Description: Tests performed every 1 to 4 hours to assess pupil size and reactivity, orientation, level of consciousness, sensation, and movement.
(2) Use: To detect changes that may signify worsening of shock.
(3) Positive findings: Nonreactive pinpoint or completely dilated (blown) pupils, unequal pupils in both size and reactivity; restlessness, confusion, lethargy, stupor, coma; inability to feel painful stimuli; inability to move extremities or to overcome gravity or resistance with any or all extremities are noted.
(4) Negative findings: Pupils are equal and round, and react to light and accommodation; the person is oriented to time, place, other people, and the past; the person responds appropriately to light pain; he or she can overcome gravity and resistance by moving extremities.
(5) Nursing cautions
- Persons with cataracts have unequal and often nonreactive pupils.
- Neurologic findings may not improve or decline steadily during shock. One examination result that shows improved or declining findings is not definitive. Look at the trends, not single examination findings.

f. Core temperature measurement
(1) Description: Measure the temperature of the head and trunk intermittently via a temperature probe inserted into the ear; or measure the temperature continuously via a temperature probe inserted into the rectum, into the bladder as part of an indwelling catheter, or into the stomach as part of a nasogastric tube.
(2) Use: To monitor core temperature intermittently or continuously.
(3) Positive findings: Hypothermia or hyperthermia unresponsive to treatment is noted.
(4) Negative findings: No uncontrollable temperature variations are found.
(5) Nursing cautions
- Be sure the ear probe fits snugly into the ear canal before you take a reading.
- Indwelling rectal probes are easily dislodged.

2. Invasive assessment techniques
a. Laboratory studies (see Chapter 25)
(1) Description: Laboratory studies frequently done in shock include complete blood count, serum glucose, serum electrolytes, serum creatinine, blood urea nitrogen, serum enzymes, arterial blood gases, urinalysis, and urine osmolality.

(2) Use: To assess the amount of injury done to the body by the shock state and to evaluate interventions used to treat the shock state.
(3) Positive findings
- In nonhemorrhagic hypovolemic shock, elevated hematocrit, hemoglobin, and red blood cell count (reflecting hemoconcentration) before intravenous fluid resuscitation; decreased hematocrit, hemoglobin, and red blood cell count follow fluid replacement
- Elevated serum creatinine, blood urea nitrogen, and cardiac enzymes in cardiogenic shock; elevated liver and pancreatic enzymes in shock following abdominal trauma
- Alkalosis in early shock, progressing to acidosis with a decreased bicarbonate level in late shock; decreased arterial carbon dioxide level in early shock secondary to hyperventilation, progressing to increased levels in late shock
- Decreased arterial oxygen concentration and elevated urine specific gravity and osmolality in early shock, falling to below normal as shock progresses
(4) Negative findings: No abnormalities are noted in laboratory test results.
(5) Nursing cautions: Serial laboratory tests should be done to determine trends in the person with shock. The dynamic, rapidly changing nature of the shock state makes results of single tests unreliable.

b. Urinary output assessment via catheter
(1) Description: Insertion of an indwelling catheter, and measurement of urine every hour.
(2) Use: To determine hydration and to assess the adequacy of fluid replacement.
(3) Positive findings: Urinary output is greater than 30 ml per hour or 240 ml per 8 hours.
(4) Negative findings: Urinary output is less than 30 ml per hour or 240 ml per 8 hours.

Acute renal failure is one of the major complications of shock.

---

c. Hemodynamic monitoring with central venous pressure or pulmonary artery catheter (see Chapter 23)
(1) Description: A central catheter is inserted to perform invasive monitoring of changes in the cardiovascular system secondary to the shock state.
(2) Use: To measure central venous pressure, pulmonary artery pressure, pulmonary capillary wedge pressure, cardiac output, cardiac index, and systemic vascular resistance in the person with shock.
(3) Positive findings:
- *Cardiogenic shock:* Elevated pulmonary artery pressure, pulmonary capillary wedge pressure, and systemic vascular resistance; decreased cardiac output and cardiac index
- *Septic shock:* Elevated cardiac output and cardiac

index in the early stage, which decrease as shock progresses; and decreased pulmonary artery pressure, pulmonary capillary wedge pressure, and systemic vascular resistance, which elevate as shock progresses
- *Hypovolemic shock, anaphylactic shock, neurogenic shock:* Decreased pulmonary artery pressure, pulmonary capillary wedge pressure, cardiac output, cardiac index, and systemic vascular resistance

(4) Negative findings: Normal values are noted for the tested parameters.

(5) Nursing cautions: Serial tests should be done to determine trends in the person with shock. The dynamic, rapidly changing nature of the shock state makes the results of single tests unreliable.

d. Continuous monitoring of mean arterial pressure (see Chapter 23)

(1) Description: Insertion of a peripheral arterial catheter and attachment to a device that monitors blood pressure.

(2) Use: To monitor blood pressure continuously during the shock state, so that trends may be identified accurately and quickly.

(3) Positive findings: Hypotension responsive or unresponsive to treatment is noted.

(4) Negative findings: Blood pressure is within normal limits.

(5) Nursing cautions: Confirm that the continuous readings correlate with a manual cuff pressure every 4 hours and as needed. Be sure the waveform is crisp, and do not trust pressures when the waveform is dampened.

e. Peritoneal lavage (see Chapter 27)

(1) Description
- Insert a cannula, through a small stab wound, into the peritoneal cavity.
- Instill 1 liter of Ringer's lactate through intravenous tubing connected to the cannula.
- After gravity drainage removes the fluid from the peritoneum, send it to the laboratory for analysis.

(2) Use: To determine the presence of free blood in the peritoneal cavity.

(3) Positive findings: A spontaneous return of bright red blood, or a red blood cell count of greater than 100,000 per mm³ after blunt trauma, or a red blood cell count of greater than 50,000 per mm³ after penetrating trauma is noted.

(4) Negative findings: No blood, or red blood cells counts lower than the previously noted parameters are measured.

(5) Nursing cautions
- Use 1 or 2 sutures to close the wound.
- Apply a dry, sterile dressing, and check it frequently for bleeding.
- Positive results require immediate surgery. Prepare to administer preoperative care.

f. Endoscopy

(1) Description: Insertion of a flexible, fiberoptic scope through the mouth or anus.

(2) Use: To identify and repair sources of hemorrhage within the gastrointestinal tract, thus arresting and reversing shock.

(3) Positive findings: Frank bleeding from areas within the gastrointestinal tract is noted.

(4) Negative findings: No bleeding or areas of potential bleeding are found.

(5) Nursing cautions
- Withhold oral fluid and food before the procedure.
- Sedation may be necessary.
- After the procedure, observe emesis and feces for blood.

g. Angiography

(1) Description: Injection of dye into arteries or veins, followed by radiographs of the area

(2) Use: To determine vessel tears and extravasation of blood.

(3) Positive findings: Extravasation of dye is noted.

(4) Negative findings: Vessels are intact.

(5) Nursing cautions: Check to see if the person is allergic to the dye, iodine, or shellfish. Allergic reaction to the dye can occur with or without these allergies.

h. Exploratory surgery (see Chapter 13)

(1) Description: Surgery is performed to explore the abdominal or chest cavity.

(2) Use: To identify and repair injuries and sources of hemorrhage, thus arresting and reversing shock.

(3) Positive findings: Vessel, tissue, or organ injury is noted.

(4) Negative findings: No injury is found.

(5) Nursing cautions
- Withhold oral fluids and food until surgery is deemed unnecessary.
- The surgeon should examine the person before he or she is given pain medication. Medications for pain relief may mask important signs and symptoms.

i. Monitoring of serial laboratory results throughout the assessment and intervention phases.

(1) Description
- Monitoring of complete blood cell count, blood chemistries, and urinalysis in all types of shock.
- Monitoring of cardiac enzymes in cardiogenic shock.
- Monitoring of blood culture results in septic shock.

(2) Use: Trends over time in laboratory test results show response to therapy for shock.

(3) Positive findings: Abnormal findings consistent with shock are seen.

(4) Negative findings: Normal findings are noted in laboratory test results.

(5) Nursing cautions
- Hemoconcentration before fluid replacement may make hemoglobin and hematocrit results appear normal or high.
- Elevation in serum glucose level is a stress response to the shock state, and does not necessarily indicate diabetes mellitus.

• Potassium migrates to the intracellular spaces and is reflected in a low serum potassium level, which requires intravenous replacement. Monitor serum potassium findings closely. The person may become hyperkalemic as shock improves with intervention.

◙ DIAGNOSING PEOPLE WITH SHOCK

Indicators of Shock

1. A downward trend in the level of consciousness, beginning with anxiety or restlessness and progressing to coma
2. A blood pressure that is initially normal and then decreases, requiring intravenous fluid administration or inotropic medication to stabilize or reverse it
3. Tachycardia that requires intravenous fluid administration or inotropic medication to stabilize or reverse it
4. Tachypnea progressing to slow respirations and then apnea
5. Decreased or absent urine output
6. Pale, cool, clammy skin (except in warm-stage septic shock, when skin is warm and flushed)

◙ INTERVENTIONS USED TO TREAT SHOCK

Noninvasive Interventions

1. Control of external hemorrhage via pressure
   a. Description: Application of external pressure over the bleeding site will stop or decrease bleeding.
   b. Use: To control external hemorrhage.
   c. Positive results: Bleeding stops, and vital signs stabilize.
   d. Negative results: Bleeding continues, and vital signs reflect hypovolemic shock.
   e. Nursing cautions
      (1) Apply tourniquets only in dire circumstances; a loss of circulation occurs distal to the tourniquet.
      (2) If you cannot control bleeding with pressure, surgical intervention is necessary. Prepare to send the person to surgery.
2. Use of military antishock trousers or pneumatic antishock garment (see Chapter 37).
3. Use of modified Trendelenburg position (Fig. 12–5)
   a. Description: With the person in a supine position, elevate the feet and legs markedly and elevate the head and shoulders slightly.
   b. Use: To assist venous return to the heart from the legs and to increase blood pressure.
   c. Positive results: Blood pressure increases.
   d. Negative results: Hypotension continues.
   e. Nursing cautions
      (1) The old Trendelenburg position is no longer used

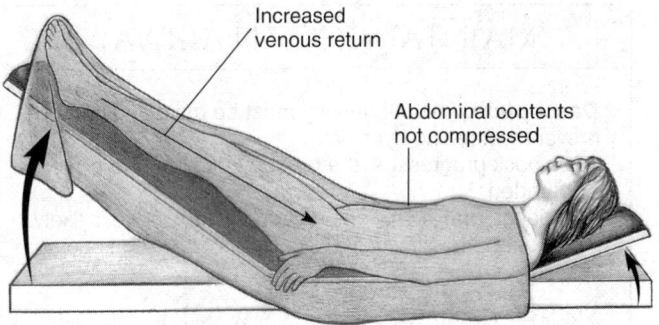

Figure 12–5. Modified shock position.

because shifts in the abdominal organs can decrease lung expansion.
      (2) Assess for spinal cord injury before positioning the person.
4. Use of cardiac monitoring (see Chapter 23)
   a. Description: Continuous monitoring of cardiac rhythm and rate via electrodes and electronic monitor.
   b. Use: To determine cardiac arrhythmias, which may complicate shock and may trigger life-threatening ventricular arrhythmias.
   c. Positive results: Arrhythmias occur.
   d. Negative results: No arrhythmias occur.
   e. Nursing cautions
      (1) Replace electrodes every 24 hours.
      (2) Document arrhythmias by placing a strip of the rhythm measurement in the chart with the identification.
5. Serial electronic blood pressure monitoring (see p. 370 and Chapter 23)
6. Maintain airway and breathing (Fig. 12–6)
7. Frequent physical assessments
   a. Description: Because shock is a progressive syndrome, the person's assessment findings will change over time. Frequent reassessments are mandatory. Intervals between reassessments may be as short as 10 to 15 minutes during rapid progression and as long as 2 to 4 hours during slow progression.
   b. Use: To discover changes in assessment findings, as shock progresses.
   c. Positive results: Assessment findings do not change.
   d. Negative results: The changes noted indicate worsening shock.
   e. Nursing cautions: In early shock, changes in assessment findings are subtle. Be alert for small differences in findings and report them.

Invasive Interventions

1. Exploratory surgery (see p. 372 and Chapter 13)
2. Continuous hemodynamic monitoring (see p. 371 and Chapter 23)
3. Continuous monitoring of mean arterial pressure (see p. 372 and Chapter 23)
4. Administration of intravenous fluids, blood products, and medications
   a. Description: Intravenous fluids, blood products, and

MAINTAINING AN AIRWAY

Description: An open airway must be maintained to prevent worsening hypoxia.
- As shock progresses, the person becomes more obtunded.
- Partial or total airway obstruction by the tongue is likely. Use of an oral airway is indicated if obstruction occurs.

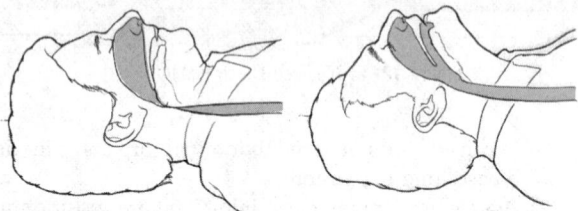

Use: To prevent hypoxia and hypoventilation.
Results:
  Positive: Open airway.
  Negative: Obstructed or partially obstructed airway.
Alert: A drop in oxygen saturation as measured by pulse oximetry may indicate impending obstruction.
Until the cervical spine has been x-rayed and cleared for fractures, use only the jaw thrust maneuver for opening the airway in trauma victims. Do not use the head tilt–chin lift maneuver.

Jaw thrust   **Head tilt and chin lift**

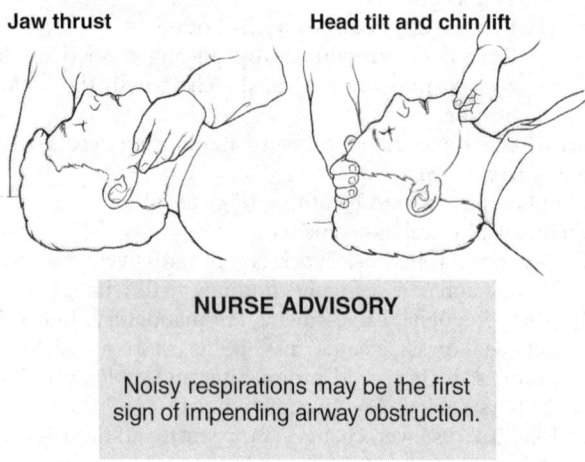

NURSE ADVISORY

Noisy respirations may be the first sign of impending airway obstruction.

Figure 12–6. The jaw thrust maneuver for opening the airway.

medications are helpful in treating shock. These include the following:
  (1) Crystalloids
  (2) Colloids
  (3) Inotropic agents
  (4) Vasopressors
  (5) Vasodilators
  (6) Diuretics
  (7) Antibiotics
  (8) Antihistamines
  (9) Steroids
  (10) Bronchodilators
  b. Use: To arrest and reverse the process of shock.
  c. Positive results: Shock improves.

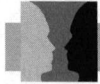
CLINICAL CONTROVERSIES

Fluid Replacement with Colloids

Pros	Cons
Have oncotic properties that decrease fluid movement out of the vasculature, so the chance of producing pulmonary edema and peripheral edema is decreased.	More expensive and less cost-effective. Some may cause allergic reactions. Some may cause coagulopathies.
Are more effective in restoring intravascular volume on a ml per ml basis.	When they leave the vasculature, their oncotic properties pull more fluid into the tissues with them.
Remain in the intravascular compartment longer than crystalloids.	

  d. Negative results: Shock worsens.
  e. Nursing cautions
    (1) Fluid overload is possible.
    (2) Titrate therapeutic drips to stabilize blood pressure and pulse.
5. Oxygen administration
  a. Description: Oxygen is delivered by nasal cannula or face mask. Some people must be ventilated mechanically (see Chapter 22).
  b. Use: To increase delivery of oxygen to tissues and cells and to prevent acidosis from hypoxia.
  c. Positive results: Arterial blood gas values are normal.
  d. Negative results: Arterial blood gas values reflect impaired delivery of oxygen or acidosis.
  e. Nursing cautions
    (1) People in shock may not be able to tolerate an oxygen mask. Use a nasal cannula, if necessary.
    (2) Do not deliver more than 2 liters of oxygen per minute if the person has a history of chronic pulmonary disease.
    (3) Monitor serial arterial blood gas values to assess the patient's response to oxygen therapy.
6. Continuous monitoring of urinary output via indwelling catheter (see p. 371 and Chapter 26).
7. Ventricular assist devices (see Chapter 23)
  a. Description: Centrifugally, pneumatically, or electromagnetically driven devices that provide right, left, or biventricular support.
  b. Use: To augment ventricular output.
  c. Positive results: Ventricular output increases without cardiac workload increasing.
  d. Negative results: Ventricular output does not increase.
  e. Nursing cautions
    (1) Devices may be external or internal.
    (2) Devices may cause thrombosis.
    (3) Devices may increase infection risk.
8. Enteral or parenteral nutritional support (see Chapter 10)
  a. Description
    (1) The person in a state of shock needs a tremendous number of extra calories.
    (2) Unless shock is reversed quickly, the person must be fed enterally through a nasogastric or intestinal tube or parenterally through a central vein.

Table 12–1. Drugs Used in the Treatment of Shock

Drug Classification	Use in Shock
Crystalloids	Used for intravenous fluid replacement (at a ratio of 3 or 4 ml for each 1 ml of blood loss) in the early phases of shock. Ringer's solution, Ringer's lactate, and normal saline are the most commonly used.
Colloids	Used for fluid replacement (at a 1:1 ratio) for fluid loss. Albumin and plasma substitutes (dextran, hetastarch) are recommended for cardiogenic shock but not for hypovolemic shock. Packed red blood cells, whole blood, autotransfusion, and synthetic blood products may be ordered for hypovolemic shock. (See Clinical Controversies, p. 374)
Inotropic agents	Dopamine, dobutamine, norepinephrine. Improve myocardial contractility, increase cardiac output, reverse hypotension, and increase organ perfusion.
Vasodilators	Nitroglycerin, sodium nitroprusside. Used to dilate the coronary arteries, improving myocardial oxygen supply. Reverse vasoconstriction, improving tissue perfusion.
Diuretics	Used to treat oliguria. Increase urine excretion.
Antibiotics	Used in septic shock because they are bactericidal. May be used prophylactically in other forms of shock. Until the source is identified, the physician should order at least a 2-drug combination. When the source is identified, therapy may be tailored to the cause.
Antihistamines	Epinephrine, diphenhydramine hydrochloride (Benadryl). Used in anaphylactic shock. Reverse bronchoconstriction, hypotension, and vasodilation, by blocking the action of histamine.
Steroids	Methylprednisolone sodium succinate. Use in shock is controversial, because their actions have not been substantiated in research. May decrease fluid shifts out of the vasculature by stabilizing capillary walls.
Sodium bicarbonate	May be used to treat the metabolic acidosis that occurs as shock progresses.
Thrombolytics	Tissue plasminogen activator, streptokinase. May be used in cardiogenic shock following a myocardial infarction. Can restore circulation to the ischemic portion of the left ventricle by dissolving the clot that is obstructing blood flow to the area.
Bronchodilators	Aminophylline, atropine, albuterol, epinephrine. Used in anaphylactic shock to relieve bronchoconstriction.
Vagolytics	Atropine. Used in neurogenic shock to counteract the bradycardic effects of the vagus nerve on the heart.

(3) Enteral feeding is the preferred method, because it may decrease bacterial translocation from the gut and inhibit sepsis.
b. Use: To maintain adequate nutrition.
c. Positive results: No muscle wasting, weight loss, or decrease in serum albumin occurs.
d. Negative results: Muscle wasting, weight loss, or decreased serum albumin develops.
e. Nursing cautions
(1) If enteral feeding is used, check gastric residuals and monitor bowel sounds every 4 hours to assess for absorption.
(2) If parenteral feeding is used, check blood glucose levels every 4 to 6 hours and give regular insulin by sliding scale to treat hyperglycemia.

Pharmacologic Interventions

1. Table 12–1 lists drugs used to treat shock.

Experimental Therapies

1. Table 12–2 lists experimental therapies for septic shock.

■ *APPLYING THE NURSING PROCESS*

NURSING DIAGNOSIS: Fluid volume deficit or risk for fluid volume deficit R/T hemorrhage

1. *Expected outcomes*
a. Fluid balance should return to normal as evidenced by normal results on cardiac output, urine output, and vital signs.
b. Hemorrhage should be controlled as evidenced by normal results on vital signs and hematocrit and hemoglobin tests.

NURSE ADVISORY

Hemorrhage is often a life-threatening event. You must be able to recognize the signs and symptoms of hemorrhagic shock.

Table 12–2. Experimental Therapies for Septic Shock

Naloxone	May stop septic shock by interacting with the endogenous opiate system.
Monoclonal antibodies	May stop septic shock by interacting with endotoxin or tumor necrosis factor.
Nonsteroidal anti-inflammatory drugs	May stop septic shock by inhibiting the formation of prostaglandins.
Allopurinol	May stop septic shock by inhibiting the production of toxic oxygen free radicals.
Human endotoxin anti-serum	May stop septic shock by producing antibodies to endotoxin.
Prostacyclin and prostaglandin E_2 analogues	May stop septic shock by increasing peripheral tissue perfusion through vasodilation.

2. *Nursing interventions:* The physiologic effects of hemorrhage must be treated quickly to control shock.
   a. Control external bleeding with direct external pressure on the injured site.
   b. Monitor for early signs and symptoms of internal bleeding.
      (1) Changes in blood pressure: initially, increased or stable systolic with increased diastolic; blood pressure decreases as shock progresses
      (2) Increased pulse and narrowing pulse pressure
      (3) Subtle changes in sensorium
      (4) Positive test result for occult blood in the gastric aspirate; coffee-grounds–colored or bright red emesis
      (5) Positive test result for occult blood in the stool; melena or bright red stools
      (6) Hematuria
      (7) Widening abdominal girth and increased abdominal firmness
      (8) Hemoptysis
      (9) Swelling around a fracture site
   c. Ask the physician to examine the person.
   d. Place the person in the modified Trendelenburg position (see Fig. 12–5).
   e. Keep the person warm and monitor temperature hourly until stable.
   f. Be prepared to send the person to surgery.
   g. Be prepared to apply military antishock trousers, if ordered.
   h. Insert at least 2 large-bore intravenous lines; a central catheter may need to be inserted rapidly.
   i. Draw blood as ordered for laboratory analysis and for type and crossmatch.
   j. Administer intravenous fluids as ordered, starting with crystalloids and advancing to colloids.
   k. Insert an indwelling catheter as ordered and monitor urinary output hourly to assess perfusion.
   l. Administer oxygen as ordered via face mask or nasal cannula.

NURSING DIAGNOSIS: Impaired gas exchange or risk for impaired gas exchange R/T decreased functional alveoli from atelectasis

1. *Expected outcomes*
   a. Breathing pattern will be effective as evidenced by normal respiratory rate, equal aeration of all lung fields on auscultation, normal arterial blood gas analysis, and normal pulse oximetry readings.
   b. Adequate oxygenation will be provided as evidenced by lack of cyanosis or pallor, normal arterial blood gas analysis, and normal pulse oximetry readings.
   c. Atelectasis will resolve as evidenced by equal aeration of all lung fields on auscultation and normal results on chest film readings, arterial blood gas analysis, and pulse oximetry readings.
2. *Nursing interventions:* Retained respiratory secretions are a primary cause of atelectasis, which can promote the following:

• Decrease delivery of oxygen to the tissues and reduce removal of carbon dioxide from the blood
• Result in hypoxemia
• Complicate the recovery period
• Place the person at risk for adult respiratory distress syndrome

   a. Assess for atelectasis (see Chapter 22)
   b. Monitor arterial blood gas results for decreased arterial oxygen content, elevated carbon dioxide content, and decreased pH.
   c. Assess the respiratory system for atelectasis every 4 hours.
      (1) Note the rate and rhythm of respirations.
      (2) Note the color and quantity of sputum.
      (3) Note the development of crackles, rhonchi, or wheezes.
      (4) Note the development of areas of diminished breath sounds.
   d. Observe the person for the following signs and symptoms of hypoxia:
      • Restlessness
      • Confusion
      • Pallor
      • Cyanosis
      • Anxiety
   e. Prevent atelectasis by instituting measures to help the person expectorate secretions from the respiratory tract.
      (1) Prevent airway obstruction by positioning the head (see Fig. 12–6) and by using an oral airway or a nasal trumpet if the patient is obtunded.
      (2) Begin chest physiotherapy with percussion, vibration, and postural drainage to mobilize retained secretions.
      (3) Turn the person every 2 hours to prevent pooling of secretions.
      (4) Administer oxygen as ordered. If necessary, monitor pulse oximetry and transcutaneous oxygen saturation to ensure tissue delivery.
      (5) Encourage the person to use incentive spirometry and to cough and breathe deeply to increase lung expansion (see Chapter 13).

NURSING DIAGNOSIS: Impaired gas exchange R/T hypoventilation

1. *Expected outcomes*
   a. Breathing pattern will be effective as evidenced by normal respiratory rate and depth, equal aeration of all lung fields on auscultation, normal arterial blood gas analysis, and normal pulse oximetry readings.
   b. Adequate oxygenation will be provided as evidenced by lack of cyanosis or pallor, normal arterial blood gas analysis, and normal pulse oximetry readings.
2. *Nursing interventions*
   a. As the person's level of consciousness decreases, the risk for hypoventilation increases, which could result in hypoxemia, leading to tissue damage and death. You should do the following:
      (1) Monitor level of consciousness every 1 to 4 hours.

(2) Be prepared to insert an oral airway or nasal trumpet if noisy respirations indicate that the person is unable to prevent airway obstruction by the tongue.

(3) Suction the upper airway as needed to remove secretions.

b. Elevate the head of the bed, if possible, to assist ventilation.

c. Turn the person every 2 hours.

d. Encourage coughing and deep breathing or use of incentive spirometry.

NURSING DIAGNOSIS: Decreased cardiac output R/T ineffective cardiac function

1. *Expected outcomes*
   a. Cardiac output will return to normal as evidenced by normal pulmonary artery catheter readings, normal vital signs, normal tissue perfusion, and normal heart sounds on auscultation.
   b. Cardiac function will return to normal as evidenced by normal echocardiogram findings.
2. *Nursing interventions*
   a. To correct a lack of circulating volume, administer intravenous fluids to replace lost volume. Ringer's lactate and normal saline solution are the most commonly used replacement fluids.
   b. Monitor urinary output.
   c. Monitor blood pressure, pulse, and cardiac rhythm continuously.
   d. Treat the underlying cause by controlling bleeding, vomiting, and diarrhea. Replace fluids lost because of extensive burns (see Chapter 36). Administer oxygen as ordered.
   e. To correct impaired ventricular function, titrate inotropic agents (dopamine, dobutamine, norepinephrine) and antiarrhythmics (lidocaine, procainamide, bretylium) as ordered to control blood pressure and arrhythmias.
      (1) Monitor hemodynamic parameters of cardiac output, cardiac index, pulmonary artery pressure, pulmonary capillary wedge pressure, central venous pressure, and arterial blood pressure for increases in preload and afterload.
      (2) Be prepared to insert a ventricular assist device to boost ventricular function.
      (3) Administer oxygen as ordered.

NURSING DIAGNOSIS: Risk for aspiration R/T inability to control secretions from decreased level of consciousness

1. *Expected outcomes*
   a. Level of consciousness will increase as evidenced by patient being awake, alert, oriented, and able to clear secretions effectively.
   b. Airway will be protected from aspiration as evidenced by normal chest film readings.
2. *Nursing interventions:* Aspiration of secretions or emesis

may result in pneumonia and can complicate the person's recovery.

a. Proper positioning can prevent aspiration. Once the cervical spine has been cleared for fracture following trauma, turn the person's head to the side if vomiting occurs. If the cervical spine has not been cleared for fracture following trauma, logroll the person to the side if vomiting occurs.

b. If permitted, elevate the head of the bed to a 30-degree angle to prevent aspiration in the unconscious person.

NURSE ADVISORY

> Elevating the head of the bed to a 30-degree angle may not be an appropriate strategy for a person with early hypovolemic shock before fluid replacement. Inadequate circulating volume may make perfusion of the brain impossible, resulting in brain damage.

c. Position the person on the right or left side to decrease the chances for aspiration.

d. Discontinue tube feedings at the following times to prevent aspiration.
   • During chest percussion
   • During vibration
   • During postural drainage
   • When the person is lying flat

NURSING DIAGNOSIS: Risk for infection R/T interruption of skin integrity from invasive procedures and placement of tubes

1. *Expected outcomes*
   a. Infection will be arrested or prevented as evidenced by no outward signs or symptoms of infection, no fever, and normal white blood cell counts.
   b. Puncture sites will remain free from signs and symptoms of infection.
2. *Nursing interventions:* Nosocomial (hospital-acquired) infections complicate recovery, raise the cost of therapy, lengthen the hospital stay, and increase morbidity and mortality.
   • Invasive tubes provide a route for bacteria to enter the body.
   • Urinary tract infections and pneumonias are common nosocomial infections.
   a. You can take precautions to prevent nosocomial infections.
      (1) Wash your hands frequently to prevent transfer of bacteria between patients.
      (2) Use aseptic technique when inserting invasive tubes or changing dressings.
      (3) Monitor insertion sites of invasive tubes for signs and symptoms of infection.
      (4) Do indwelling catheter care every shift.
      (5) Change intravenous catheters every 3 days.
      (6) Identify persons at greatest risk for nosocomial infections—the very old, the very young, the

immunocompromised—and use the preventive strategies listed previously.
b. Checking the following parameters will help you detect the start of a nosocomial infection.
  (1) Monitor temperature every 4 hours and report elevations.
  (2) Monitor serial white blood cell counts for elevations of greater than 10,000 per mm^3.
  (3) Monitor drainage from tubes and wounds for signs and symptoms of infection (odor, change in drainage appearance, induration around the drainage site, appearance of pus).
  (4) Auscultate breath sounds every 2 to 4 hours, and report abnormalities (absence of breath sounds, crackles, rhonchi, wheezes).
  (5) Assess for change in level of consciousness (restlessness, confusion, anxiety, and decreased awareness; inability to arouse person).

NURSING DIAGNOSIS: Fear or anxiety R/T lack of understanding of therapeutic regimen

1. *Expected outcomes*
  a. Patient will demonstrate an understanding of the treatment plan by discussing it with the health care team and by participating in planning and implementation of care.
  b. Fear and anxiety will decrease as evidenced by normal vital signs, calm demeanor, and patient reports of reduced fear and anxiety.
2. *Nursing interventions*
  a. You can allay fear or anxiety by giving a brief, clear, and accurate explanation of the therapeutic procedures.
  b. Begin by determining the person's concept of what has happened, why it happened, and what should be done.
  c. Calmly explain what will be done and what the person will see, hear, and feel during the procedure.
  d. Encourage the person to ask questions and express concerns. Make sure the person understands your explanation.
  e. Include the person in planning care. Negotiate nursing and medical interventions that satisfy both the person and the nursing and medical team.
  f. Arrange for interpreters to explain what you have said to people who have limited English proficiency (see Chapter 4).

NURSING DIAGNOSIS: Impaired skin integrity or risk for impaired skin integrity R/T decreased mobility and impaired oxygenation of the tissues

1. *Expected outcomes*
  a. Mobility will be increased to normal as evidenced by progressive increases to ambulation without incident.
  b. Skin integrity will be maintained through turning and use of pressure relieving and reducing devices as evi-

denced by healing of disruptions in skin integrity and no evidence of additional skin breakdown.
2. *Nursing interventions*
  a. Increase the person's physical mobility as quickly as possible.
    (1) Begin by turning the person every 2 hours, performing passive exercises, and encouraging active range-of-motion exercises while the person remains on bed rest.
    (2) Advance to dangling, chair rest, and progressive ambulation as the person's condition permits.

TRANSCULTURAL CONSIDERATIONS

Families in some religious and cultural groups (e.g., Hindu, Islamic, and Mennonite) consider it their responsibility to assist in patient care. Have the family present when increasing the person's activity level.

    (3) Consult the physical therapy department for assistive devices to help with ambulation.
  b. If the person must remain immobile or minimally mobile for some time, use pressure-relieving devices to prevent skin breakdown (see Chapter 7).
    (1) Begin with egg crate mattresses.
    (2) Advance to air-inflation mattresses or specialty beds if bed rest is prolonged.
    (3) Consult the enterostomal therapy nurse for other suggestions about pressure-relieving devices.
  c. Turn and reposition the person every 2 hours. Give back care, rubbing lotion over bony prominences.

NURSING DIAGNOSIS: Altered peripheral tissue perfusion R/T edema from stasis of blood in the capillaries and vasoconstriction

1. *Expected outcomes*
  a. Edema will disappear as evidenced by decreased swelling at sites of edema.
  b. Peripheral perfusion will return to normal as evidenced by return of normal skin color, normal vital signs, and normal capillary refill time.
2. *Nursing interventions*
  a. Movement of fluid from the vasculature into the tissues results in edema. Determine the extent of edema by doing the following:
    (1) Monitor daily for a positive fluid balance (greater intake than output) and keep a running total of the excess to determine the extent of fluid retention.
    (2) Monitor daily weights for increases indicating fluid retention. Each liter of retained fluid increases weight by 1 kg.
    (3) Assess the skin every 2 to 4 hours to determine the extent and severity of edema.
  b. When fluids flow back into the vessels from the tissues, signs and symptoms of fluid overload can occur

(see Chapter 9). To identify this problem, do the following:
(1) Assess breath sounds for crackles, rhonchi, or wheezes.
(2) Monitor for shortness of breath.
(3) Assess for an extra heart sound (S3) every 2 to 4 hours.
(4) Watch for elevation in central venous pressure above 6 cm/H$_2$O.
(5) Observe for distended jugular veins.

NURSING DIAGNOSIS: Altered nutrition: less than body requirements R/T decreased (or absent) oral intake of nutrients

---

1. *Expected outcomes*
   a. Oral intake of nutrients will return to normal as evidenced by patient tolerating normal daily dietary intake; maintaining or gaining weight; and experiencing no nausea, vomiting, or diarrhea.
   b. Adequate nutrition will be maintained as evidenced by maintenance of total body weight and no decrease in serum albumin or serum transferrin.
2. *Nursing interventions:* Adequate nutrition may not be a priority in the emergency care of the person in shock. If the crisis is resolved quickly, nutritional deficits are not usually a problem. People in a prolonged state of shock require additional calories to maintain an appropriate nutritional status.
   a. Monitor daily weights to identify weight loss.
   b. Request consultation by a nutritionist for recommendations about diet.
   c. Implement the prescribed nutritional therapy by enteral or parenteral route.
   d. Monitor serum blood glucose if the person is on total parenteral nutrition. Remember that blood glucose values may also be elevated secondary to the sympathetic nervous system stimulation that occurs in shock.
   e. Check for gastric residuals every 4 hours if the patient is on enteral feedings. Notify the physician if the residual is greater than 100 ml.
   f. Monitor serum transferrin, serum albumin, and hematocrit and hemoglobin levels to assess the adequacy of nutritional replacement.

NURSING DIAGNOSIS: Ineffective breathing pattern R/T pain

---

1. *Expected outcomes*
   a. Pain will be adequately controlled by pharmacologic and nonpharmacologic means as evidenced by effective breathing, normal vital signs, and patient reports of pain control.
   b. Breathing pattern will be effective as evidenced by normal respiratory rate and depth, equal aeration of all lung fields on auscultation, normal arterial blood gas analysis, and normal pulse oximetry readings.

2. *Nursing interventions:* Shallow breathing leads to atelectasis, decreased lung function, and possibly pneumonia. The person in pain will be reluctant to perform any procedure that will increase the pain.
   a. Improve the person's depth of breathing by controlling pain with analgesics (see Chapter 11).

■ SUPPORTING THE FAMILY

Communicating with the Family

TRANSCULTURAL CONSIDERATIONS

Maintain a broad definition of "family." It often extends beyond blood relatives or relatives by marriage. For example, in many cultures, the oldest male or female in an extended household, not necessarily the patient's spouse, speaks for the family.

1. Maintain open and honest communication with the family.
2. Determine the family's explanatory model to be sure they understand the nursing and medical management (see Chapter 2).
3. Allot time to answer the family's questions.
4. Encourage the family to talk about concerns.

Providing Resources and Assistance

1. If indicated, consult ordained or nonordained clergy or a social worker to help the family resolve any crisis arising from the patient's condition.
   a. Such consultation is especially important if the precipitating event has been sudden or the person is not expected to survive.
   b. In some cases, you may have to consult practitioners of folk religion instead of, or in addition to, practitioners of orthodox religion (see Chapter 2).
2. Help notify extended family of the situation, making sure the information provided is accurate.
3. Liberalize visiting hours, especially if the person's condition is critical.
4. Ensure that family members are getting adequate nutrition and rest. Encourage family members to rotate shifts once the person's condition stabilizes.
5. Help family members appoint a contact person. Allow that person to call the unit as needed to check on the patient's condition. Other family members can then call the contact person for information. In some cases, you may need to appoint multiple contact persons; for example, a blood relative and the patient's partner in a gay relationship.

Bibliography

Books

Alspach JG. *American Association of Critical Care Nurses: Core Curriculum for Critical Care Nursing.* 4th ed. Philadelphia: WB Saunders, 1991.

Bayley EW, and Turcke SA. *A Comprehensive Curriculum for Trauma Nursing.* Boston: Jones & Bartlett, 1992.

Cardona VD, et al. *Trauma Nursing: From Resuscitation Through Rehabilitation.* Philadelphia: WB Saunders, 1988.

Deglin JH, and Vallerand AH. *Davis's Drug Guide for Nurses.* 3rd ed. Philadelphia: FA Davis, 1993.

Dolan JT. *Critical Care Nursing: Clinical Management Through the Nursing Process.* Philadelphia: FA Davis, 1991.

Dossey BM, Guzetta CE, and Kenner CV. *Critical Care Nursing: Body-Mind-Spirit.* Philadelphia: JB Lippincott, 1992.

Guyton AC. *Textbook of Medical Physiology.* 8th ed. Philadelphia: WB Saunders, 1991.

Holloway NM. *Nursing the Critically Ill Adult.* 4th ed. Redwood City, CA: Addison-Wesley, 1993.

Ignativicius DD, and Bayne MV. *Medical-Surgical Nursing: A Nursing Process Approach.* Philadelphia: WB Saunders, 1991.

Kitt S, and Kaiser J. *Emergency Nursing: A Physiologic and Clinical Perspective.* Philadelphia: WB Saunders, 1990.

McCance KL, and Huether SE. *Pathophysiology: The Biologic Basis for Disease in Adults and Children.* St. Louis: CV Mosby, 1990.

Sheehy SB. *Emergency Nursing: Principles and Practice.* 3rd ed. St. Louis: CV Mosby, 1992.

Thelan LA, Davie JK, and Urden LD. *Textbook of Critical Care Nursing Diagnosis and Management.* St. Louis: CV Mosby, 1990.

Urden LD, Davie JK, and Thelan LA. *Essentials of Critical Care Nursing.* St. Louis: CV Mosby, 1992.

Vasquez M, Lazear SE, and Larson EL. *Critical Care Nursing.* 2nd ed. Philadelphia: WB Saunders, 1992.

Wilson RF. *Critical Care Manual: Applied Physiology and Principles of Therapy.* Philadelphia: FA Davis, 1992.

Wright JE, and Shelton BK. *Desk Reference for Critical Care Nursing.* Boston: Jones & Bartlett, 1993.

Journal Articles

Causes of Shock

Broscious SK. Toxic shock syndrome and its potential complications. *Crit Care Nurse* 11(2):28–35, 1991.

Dandan IS. Trauma in the elderly patient. *Top Emerg Med* 14(3):39–45, 1992.

Hazinski MF, et al. Epidemiology, pathophysiology, and clinical presentation of gram-negative sepsis. *Am J Crit Care* 2(3):224–234, 1993.

Stages of Shock

Cerra FB. Multiple system organ failure. *Dis Mon* 38(12):847–889, 1992.

Weil MH, and Desai V. Measuring the severity of shock. *Emerg Med* 24(4):207–209, 1992.

White KM. Sepsis and the systemic inflammatory response syndrome. Lecture notes from 1993 National Teaching Institute and Critical Care Exposition. Anaheim, CA, May 1993.

The Body's Reaction to Shock

Huggins B. Trauma physiology. *Nurs Clin North Am* 25(1):1–9, 1990.

Leor J, et al. Cardiogenic shock complicating acute myocardial infarction in patients without heart failure on admission: Incidence, risk factors, and outcome. *Am J Med* 94(3):265–272, 1993.

Rice V. Shock, a clinical syndrome: An update. Part 1: An overview of shock. *Crit Care Nurse* 11(4):20–27, 1991.

Summers G. The clinical and hemodynamic presentation of the shock patient. *Crit Care Nurs Clin North Am* 2(2):161–166, 1990.

Interventions Used to Treat Shock

Brown KA, and Sheagren JN. Recognition and emergent treatment of septic shock/multiple systems organ failure syndrome. *Intern Med* 11(2):3–11, 1990.

Clevenger FW. Nutritional support in the patient with systemic inflammatory response syndrome. *Am J Surg* 165(2A):68S–73S, 1993.

Klein DM, and Witek-Janusek L. Advances in immunotherapy of sepsis. *Dimens Crit Care Nurs* 11(2):75–88, 1992.

Klein HG. When is transfusion the best option? *Emerg Med* 24(4):59–66, 1992.

Littleton MT. Trends in agents used for the management of sepsis. *Crit Care Nursing Q* 15(4):33–46, 1993.

Meyers KA, and Hickey MK. Nursing management of hypovolemic shock. *Crit Care Nursing Q* 11(1):57–67, 1988.

Schell KH. Current trends in antimicrobial therapy for the critically ill patient. *Crit Care Nursing Q* 15(4):23–32, 1993.

Schumann LL, and Remington MA. The use of naloxone in treating endotoxic shock. *Crit Care Nurse* 10(2):63–71, 1990.

Sympson GM. CATR: A new generation of autologous blood transfusion. *Crit Care Nurse* 11(4):60–64, 1991.

13

Caring for People Undergoing Surgery

◨ OVERVIEW OF PERIOPERATIVE NURSING

Definitions

1. **Preoperative phase.** The nurse provides care for the surgical patient before surgery, including physiologic and psychosocial assessment, education, and physical and psychosocial preparation.
2. **Intraoperative phase.** The nurse provides care for the surgical patient during surgery, including patient positioning, maintaining a surgically clean environment, and caring for the patient under anesthesia.
3. **Postoperative phase.** The nurse provides care for the surgical patient after surgery, including making postoperative assessments during the immediate, intermediate, and extended stages; providing postoperative medications; giving pain management; providing assessment and management of postoperative complications; and teaching and discharge planning.

Classifications of Surgeries

1. Classifications based on purpose
   a. **Diagnostic surgeries** are those in which the surgeon explores an area of the body to make an accurate diagnosis (e.g., exploratory laparoscopy and arthroscopy).
   b. **Curative surgeries** are those in which a disease is arrested or eradicated (e.g., appendectomy and open reduction internal fixation of the hip).
   c. **Restorative surgeries** improve function or partially or fully restore damaged organs to predamaged condition (e.g., repair of an umbilical hernia or atrial-septal defect).
   d. **Palliative surgeries** alleviate symptoms but do not affect the disease (e.g., tracheostomy and creation of an arteriovenous fistula for hemodialysis).
   e. **Cosmetic surgeries** improve appearance (e.g., breast reconstruction and face lifts).
2. Classifications based on need
   a. **Emergency surgeries** are performed immediately (e.g., an abdominal laparotomy to repair a gunshot wound and control bleeding).

b. **Urgent surgeries** are performed within 48 hours (e.g., removal of kidney stones).
   c. **Required surgeries** are performed within weeks or months (e.g., cataract removal).
   d. **Elective surgeries** are performed when the patient desires the surgery (e.g., lipectomy).

Settings for the Surgical Experience

1. Approximately 30 percent of surgeries require hospital-based nursing care postoperatively for more than 24 hours. Most such patients are admitted on the morning of the surgery.
2. Approximately 60 percent of all surgical procedures are performed on an outpatient basis. Advantages for the patient include decreased cost of treatment, convenience, reduction of stress and emotional disturbance because the patient can convalesce at home in a familiar environment, decreased risk of nosocomial infection (less than 5%), and reduced period of dependency and disability.
3. Freestanding surgical facilities called ambulatory surgery centers admit patients for ambulatory day surgery. These centers may be either hospital affiliated or independently owned and operated.

◨ PREOPERATIVE NURSING ASSESSMENT

Physiologic Assessment

1. Major complaint
2. Conditions that increase the risk of surgery
   a. Cardiac conditions
      • Dysrhythmias
      • Angina
      • Hypertension
      • Myocardial infarction
      • Congestive heart failure
      • Endocarditis
      • Valvular heart disease
      • Congenital abnormalities
   b. Respiratory conditions
      • Pneumonia and other respiratory infections
      • Chronic obstructive pulmonary disease

- Emphysema
- Asthma

c. Neurologic conditions
- Seizures
- Myasthenia gravis
- Alzheimer's disease

d. Renal conditions
- Renal insufficiency
- Urinary tract infections
- Prostatic hypertrophy

e. Endocrine conditions
- Diabetes
- Hypothyroidism
- Hyperthyroidism
- Adrenal insufficiency

f. Gastrointestinal conditions
- Esophogeal varices
- Peptic ulcers
- Ulcerative colitis
- Cirrhosis
- Hiatal hernia

g. Musculoskeletal conditions
- Myasthenia gravis
- Fractures
- Contractures

h. Immunologic conditions include allergies to food, drugs, and environmental factors.

i. Hematologic conditions
- Anemia
- Hemophilia
- von Willebrand's disease
- Sickle cell disease
- History of excessive bleeding, easy bruising, or nosebleeds

3. Patient's present lifestyle
a. Diet
b. Exercise
c. Substance abuse of alcohol, tobacco (smoking increases the risk of laryngospasm during emergence from anesthesia), and prescribed, over-the-counter, or illegal drugs
d. Family and social support

4. Nutritional status (see Chapter 10)
a. Obesity
b. Malnutrition or dietary deficiencies (e.g., of fluid, sodium, iron, potassium, and protein that may be dangerous for the surgical candidate)
c. Conditions that may produce nutritional deficiencies
- Cancer
- Organ failure
- Substance abuse
- Chronic illness

5. Status of body systems
a. Cardiovascular (see Chapter 23)
- Blood pressure
- Heart sounds
- Pulses
- Capillary refill
b. Respiratory (see Chapter 22)
- Breath sounds
- Respiration

- Dyspnea
- Clubbed fingers
- Chronic or productive cough

c. Neurologic (see Chapter 18)
- Level of consciousness
- Orientation to time, person, place
- Pupil response
- Decreased reflexes
- Numbness or weakness of extremities
- Dizziness

d. Renal (see Chapter 26)
- Oliguria
- Dysuria
- Hematuria or other discolorations
- Frequency of urination
- Chemistries and ability to clear substances
- Blood urea nitrogen and creatinine levels

e. Endocrine (see Chapter 29)
- Blood glucose levels
- Enlarged glands

f. Gastrointestinal (see Chapter 27)
- Bowel sounds
- Nausea and vomiting
- Gastrointestinal bleeding
- Indigestion
- Ascites
- Jaundice

g. Musculoskeletal (see Chapter 34)
- Muscle weakness
- Range of motion
- Prostheses (e.g., total knee prosthesis)

h. Immunologic (see Chapter 21): Ask about allergies (i.e., patient reactions, including duration, and patient actions that stop reactions).

i. Hematologic (see Chapter 25): Check laboratory values of computer blood count, prothrombin time, and partial thromboplastin time, if indicated.

Psychosocial Assessment

1. Anxiety level (monitor breathing, pulse rate, and blood pressure)
a. Moderate anxiety is normal.
b. Previous surgical and anesthetic experience affect a person's feelings about the present surgery.

2. Fears associated with surgery
a. Fear of prognosis
b. Fear of change in lifestyle or body image (increased need for dependency)
c. Fear of pain
d. Fear of death (especially not awakening from anesthesia)

3. Other emotional issues
a. The person's overall emotional state
b. The person's history of coping
c. The person's social support system (see Chapter 6)
d. Cultural practices and religious beliefs that may affect the patient's attitudes toward surgery

4. Financial concerns
a. Loss of income
b. Cost of hospitalization

LEARNING/TEACHING GUIDELINES
for Preoperative Teaching of the Surgical Patient

General Guidelines

1. Informing patients about postoperative pain and planned pain management helps to decrease their anxiety:
   a. Explain the sensations that the person may experience.
   b. Tell the person not to hesitate to request pain medication when needed.
   c. Describe planned interventions to control postoperative pain.
      (1) Explain that combining invasive and noninvasive measures achieves the highest level of pain relief.
      (2) Discuss and teach noninvasive pain relief measures, such as relaxation, guided imagery, and distraction techniques. (See Chapter 11.) Instruct patients to use such techniques before pain occurs and as soon as pain is noticed.
      (3) Demonstrate the use of the patient-controlled analgesia pump if its use is anticipated. Emphasize that it is more effective to self-administer a small amount of narcotic at the onset of pain than to wait and administer a large dose of narcotic when the pain reaches its peak.
      (4) Point out that narcotics such as morphine or meperidine will be administered intramuscularly as needed. Explain that requesting a narcotic after surgery will not make the person a drug addict. Narcotic studies have proven that patients are addicted only to pain relief and not to the narcotic. When pain relief is achieved, the person does not desire the narcotic.
      (5) Describe electronic pain control devices that may be used postoperatively, such as a transcutaneous electrical nerve stimulator.
2. Demonstrate deep breathing and coughing techniques and explain their benefits (see Fig. 13–1), which include
   a. Decreasing the risk of the development of pneumonia by removing secretions from the lungs
   b. Decreasing the risk of the development of atelectasis
3. Describe leg and foot exercises and their benefits (Fig. 13–2).
4. Explain any invasive devices that the person may return with from surgery. These devices include nasogastric tubes, wound drains, Foley catheters, epidural catheters, and subclavian or intravenous lines.
   a. Tell the person not to pull on any of the devices, that the devices are temporary and will be removed as soon as possible, and that the person may experience some mild discomfort.
   b. Carefully monitor any temporary invasive devices installed during surgery. The anesthetized person cannot be responsible for their removal.

Diagnostic Tests

1. Endoscopic procedures
   a. Bronchoscopy (see Chapter 22)
   b. Esophagogastroduodenoscopy (see Chapter 27)
   c. Proctoscopy, sigmoidoscopy, and colonoscopy (see Chapter 27)
2. Computed tomography and intravenous pyelography (see Chapters 23, 26, 27)

◼ *CARING FOR PEOPLE BEFORE SURGERY*

Preoperative Teaching

1. Teaching in the preoperative period is vital, whether surgery is to be performed on an inpatient or an outpatient basis (Learning/Teaching Guidelines for Preoperative Teaching of the Surgical Patient).
2. In all preoperative teaching, the nurse should remain alert for and sensitive to transcultural differences that may affect patient learning style, educational needs, and responses.
3. The nurse should advise the person about other general issues related to surgery, including

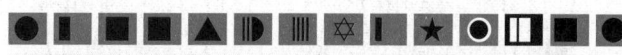

TRANSCULTURAL CONSIDERATIONS

It is important to emphasize that it is acceptable and necessary to express pain. Some cultures maintain a stoic attitude toward pain, which may lead a person to refuse pain medication that may relieve the pain and prevent postoperative complications.

   a. Preoperative tests (see pp. 382 and 387)
   b. Location and size of incision
   c. Awakening in the postanesthesia unit
   d. Physical limitations after surgery
   e. Typical diet after surgery
   f. Areas where family members wait during surgery and where the surgeon will notify them of the results of the surgery

Obtaining Informed Consent

1. The surgeon is responsible for obtaining the person's permission for surgery. The surgeon explains the type of

AREAS OF SURGICAL SKIN PREPARATION

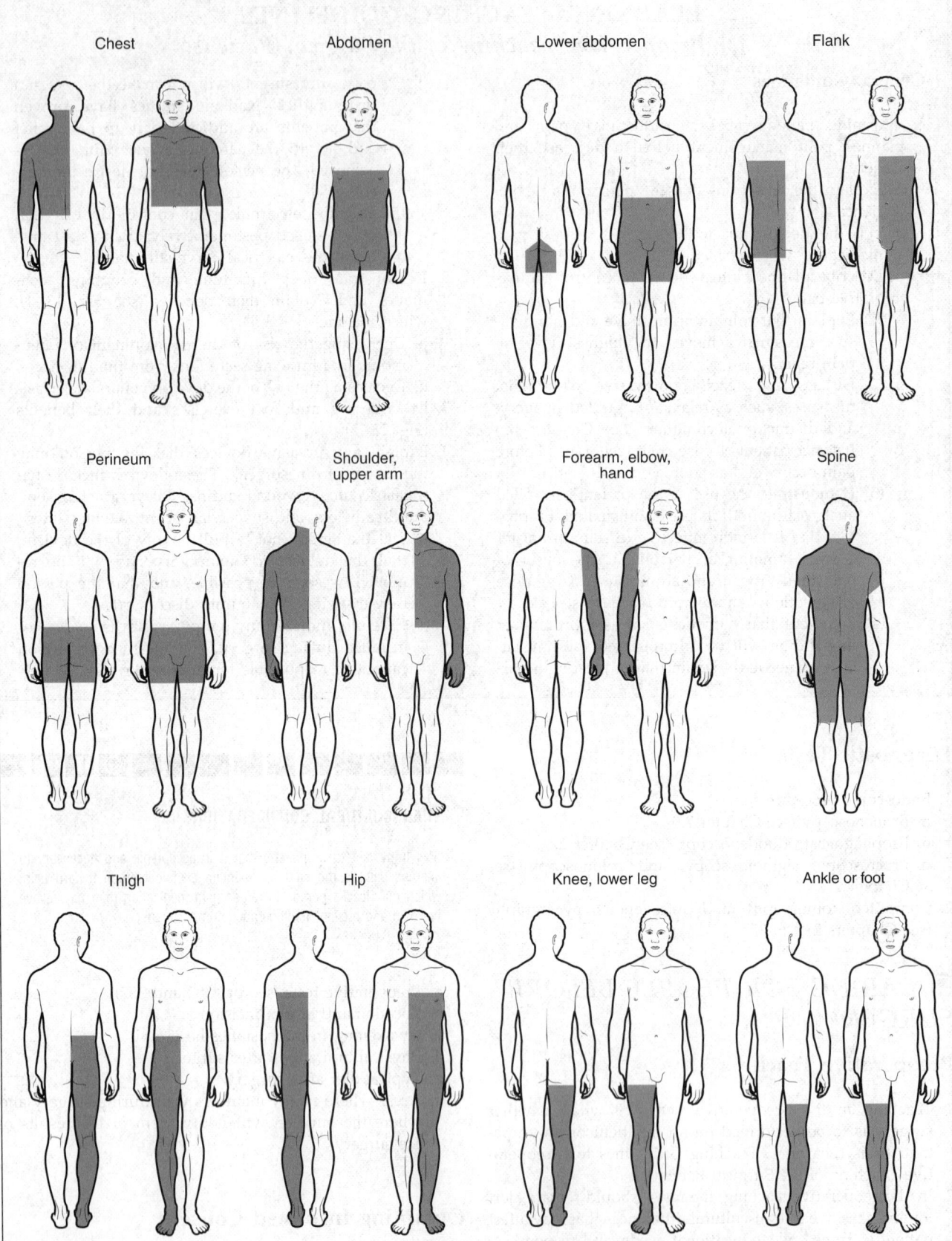

Chest

Abdomen

Lower abdomen

Flank

Perineum

Shoulder, upper arm

Forearm, elbow, hand

Spine

Thigh

Hip

Knee, lower leg

Ankle or foot

Figure 13–1.

surgery to be performed and discusses benefits, risks, and possible complications.

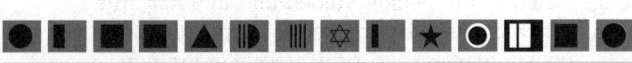

TRANSCULTURAL CONSIDERATIONS

In some cultures, the decision to have surgery is made by the head of the family or a group of elders in the religious community. It is important that they—as well as the patient—understand the surgery and its importance.

2. No sedation can have been administered to the patient before signing.
3. Minors may need a parent or legal guardian's signature.
4. Older people may need a legal guardian's signature.
5. Before you witness the person's signature on the operative permit, make sure the person has understood the surgeon's explanation of the surgery.
6. Document in the nurse's notes that you witnessed the signing of the operative permit after the person acknowledged understanding the procedure.

Physical Preparation

1. Nutritional preparation
   a. Typically, solid foods are withheld for 6 to 8 hours before surgery with general anesthesia (to avoid aspiration of gastric contents) and for 3 hours before surgery with local or regional anesthesia.
   b. All fluids are typically withheld for 4 to 6 hours before general anesthesia is used.
   c. Total parenteral nutrition is administered preoperatively to people who are malnourished, have protein or metabolic deficiencies, or cannot ingest foods.
2. Bowel preparation: If the patient is having intestinal or abdominal surgery, an enema or a laxative or both are administered the night before the surgery.
3. Urinary preparation
   a. If the patient requires a lengthy operation, if urine needs to be monitored hourly or more frequently, or if certain gynecologic procedures are performed, an indwelling Foley catheter may be inserted.
   b. The person should void immediately before surgery. If there is already an indwelling Foley catheter, it should be emptied and the amount of its contents recorded.
4. Respiration preparation. The person should be advised not to smoke for at least 8 to 12 hours before surgery.
5. Skin preparation
   a. The size of the incision and the type of surgery determine the extent of the area to be prepared (Fig. 13–1).
   b. To help reduce transient bacteria in the operative site, the skin is cleansed the night before surgery with a mild antiseptic soap.
   c. Skin is prepared again in the operating room using antimicrobial soap solution and mechanical action, followed by an antimicrobial paint solution.
6. Hair removal
   a. Shaving

CLINICAL CONTROVERSIES

Shaving, once a standard procedure before surgery, has become the center of controversy. According to some recent studies, patients subjected to traditional shaving have the highest rate of infection—higher than those whose hair was clipped, cut with electric razors, or not shaved at all. To minimize the risks of shaving, when necessary, the Centers for Disease Control and Prevention advocates that shaving be done in the operating room immediately before surgery and only after the nurse has assessed the skin to ensure that there are no abrasions, lacerations, or signs of infection in the area to be shaved.

   (1) Hair should be shaved only if it would otherwise interfere with the surgical procedure.

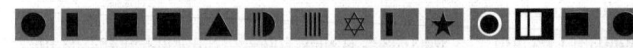

TRANSCULTURAL CONSIDERATIONS

Shaving body hair violates some cultural beliefs and practices. The Sikh religion (East India) forbids cutting or shaving of body hair. In Greece, the concept of manhood is linked to body hair. For Native Americans, body hair may be a sign of health and strength.

   (2) Shaving should be done as soon before the operative time as possible.
   (3) The razor should be sharp.
   (4) A wet shave is preferable.
   (5) Shaving should be done in the direction of hair growth.
   (6) Caution should be used because shaving may cause cuts and epidermal damage.
   b. Electric clipping or use of depilatories
   (1) These methods are preferable to shaving.
   (2) Clippers may cause cuts at skin creases but cause fewer microabrasions.
   (3) Depilatories cause no skin damage but may cause lymphocytic infiltration.
7. Preoperative medication administration
   a. Patients admitted to the nursing unit before surgery are sometimes given "on-call" medications that are administered immediately after the surgery team is ready (Table 13–1).
   b. Tell the person to expect to feel relaxed and drowsy after taking the medications.
   c. After giving the medications, keep the person in bed with the side rails up.
   d. Often, the preoperative medications are administered intravenously in the preanesthesia area because most patients are not admitted to the nursing unit before surgery.

Psychologic Preparation

1. Observe the person's anxiety level and assist in answering any last-minute questions or concerns about the surgery.
2. Allow time and privacy for specific cultural rituals that help prepare the person for surgery.

Table 13–1. Commonly Used Preoperative Medications

Classification and Medication	Desired Effects	Nursing Implications
Sedatives		
Pentobarbital sodium (Nembutal)	Promotes relaxation and sleep	Observe elderly for excitement or confusion.
Narcotics		
Morphine sulfate	Decreases pain; reduces anxiety	Observe for nausea and vomiting.
Tranquilizers		
Diazepam (Valium)	Decreases anxiety and promotes a calm preoperative state	Smoking increases the metabolism of diazepam, so smokers may need a higher dose than nonsmokers.
Anticholinergics		
Atropine sulfate	Reduces secretions and keeps respiratory passages clear and dry	Observe for tachycardia. Smaller doses are indicated for the elderly.
Receptor Antagonists		
Cimetidine (Tagamet)	Decreases the amount of gastric secretions and increases the pH of gastric secretions	Absorption may be decreased by antacids. Observe for confusion in the elderly.
Antiemetics		
Promethazine HCl (Phenergan)	Prevents postoperative nausea and vomiting	Observe for marked sedation and dizziness.

Preoperative Checklist

1. It is your responsibility to review each item on the preoperative checklist (Fig. 13–2) and to make sure that each item is addressed satisfactorily before the person is transported to surgery. The operating room nurse reviews and verifies the information to ensure completeness and accuracy of information.
2. Items on checklist include the following:
   a. Patient identification number
   b. Whether the following consent forms for surgery were signed:
      • For an operative procedure
      • For blood transfusions
      • For disposal of limb
      • For sterilization (including a separate consent form that exempts the institution, physicians, or both for either an ineffective or a nonreversible process)
   c. Whether the history and physical examinations were completed
   d. Whether consultations were done
   e. Whether laboratory results were charted
   f. Blood type and screen or type and crossmatch (if appropriate)
   g. Whether the person voided and at what time
   h. Whether jewelry, makeup, dentures, hairpins, nail polish, glasses, and prostheses were removed

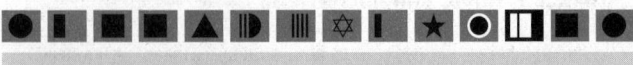

TRANSCULTURAL CONSIDERATIONS

In some cultures, amulets and other jewelry are viewed as religious artifacts and are not to be removed from the body. If they compromise or interfere with the surgical procedure, usually the person will agree to have them placed in contact with another part of the body.

   i. Whether valuables were given to family members or locked in the hospital safe
   j. Electrocardiogram and chest radiograph reports
   k. Whether preoperative medications were given
   l. Vital signs
   m. Whether operating room attire was worn
   n. Last time patient ate or drank

Preanesthesia Care Unit

1. The preanesthesia care unit is a designated area within the surgical suite where persons are brought preoperatively. It is usually located near the main entrance to the suite but away from loud activity.
2. The preoperative holding area was developed to
   a. Humanize surgical patient care
   b. Increase patient comfort and safety
   c. Calm patients outside the operating room
3. Members of the surgical team informally share information with the patient, talk with the patient to alleviate anxiety, and communicate the person's concerns to other surgical team members.
4. The team reviews the patient's chart for completeness by doing the following:
   a. Verifying chart and identification band with the person's verbal response
   b. Reviewing consent forms, history and physical examination information, and allergic reaction information
   c. Reviewing physician's orders and verifying that they were carried out
   d. Determining that all laboratory values and other studies were completed
5. Nurses or other team members initiate intravenous lines.
6. The anesthesia team interviews the patient and instills required anesthesia.

Applying the Nursing Process

NURSING DIAGNOSIS: Knowledge deficit R/T lack of experience with preoperative, surgical, and postoperative routines and procedures

PREOPERATIVE CHECK LIST

PREOPERATIVE ASSESSMENT

ALLERGIES _____ WEIGHT _____

Deaf ☐   Mental status: Alert ☐

Blind ☐   Confused ☐

Jones, Robert   SP   403

#123−45−6789   CATH.

Drs. Albert/Watson   11−11−23

NICKNAME:

PRELIMINARY PREOPERATIVE PREPARATION

LAB WORK	N/A	Initiated	Charted	Sent/Called to OR
CBC		☐	☐	☐
SMA$_{12}$		☐	☐	☐
Urinalysis		☐	☐	☐
Electrolytes	☐	☐	☐	☐
Biocept G	☐	☐	☐	☐
Type and screen	☐	☐	☐	☐
Type and cross	☐	☐	☐	☐
# Units				

DIAGNOSTIC WORK-UP	N/A	Initiated	Charted	Sent/Called to OR
Chest x-ray	☐	☐	☐	☐
ECG	☐	☐	☐	☐
History and physical	☐	☐	☐	☐
Preoperative note		☐	☐	☐
Medical consultation	☐	☐	☐	☐
Consent		☐	☐	☐
Preoperative preparation	☐			

Signature of nurse(s) responsible for completing this segment:

3−11 _____

11−7 _____

7−3 _____

Comments: _____
_____
_____
_____
_____

IMMEDIATE PREOPERATIVE PREPARATION

Check box if present and removed:

Glasses ☐

Nail polish ☐

Contact lenses ☐

Hair pins, beads ☐

Property and valuables ☐

Jewelry ☐

Dentures ☐

Prosthesis ☐

If present check box:

Pacemaker ☐

Hearing aid ☐

Caps ☐

Loose teeth ☐

—Location _____
_____

NPO   Yes ☐   No ☐

Voided   Yes ☐   No ☐

Vital signs:

T _____

P _____

R _____

B/P _____

Preoperative medications: Given ☐   Held ☐   Not ordered ☐

Side rails: In place ☐   Addressograph plate ☐   MAR ☐

Special comments: _____
_____
_____
_____
_____

Checklist reviewed by _____

Doctor please call _____   At phone # _____

To OR at: _____   Received in OR at: _____   Signature: _____

Figure 13−2. Preoperative checklist. (From Seneca C. How we streamlined pre-op paperwork. *RN* 49:3, 1986. © 1986 Medical Economics, Montvale, NJ. Reprinted by permission.)

1. *Expected outcomes:* Following interventions, the person should be able to do the following:
   a. Identify the need for the surgery to be performed.
   b. Express understanding of the events that will occur before, during, and immediately after the surgery and how the body responds at each stage in the process.
   c. Describe ways to facilitate the surgical experience and speed recovery.
2. *Nursing interventions*
   a. Explain the need for surgery and answer any questions about the link between the patient's problem and the surgical procedure.
   b. In combination and consultation with other members of the surgical team, describe the surgical process, including preoperative and postoperative routines, and the likely physiologic responses at each stage.
   c. Teach methods of minimizing postoperative complications, such as coughing, deep breathing, and splinting.

NURSING DIAGNOSIS: Fear R/T to anticipated pain or loss of control postoperatively

1. *Expected outcomes:* Following interventions, the person should be able to do the following:
   a. Express a positive outlook toward the impending surgery.
   b. Demonstrate and use relaxation and other noninvasive techniques to control preoperative anxiety and postoperative pain.
2. *Nursing interventions*
   a. Allow time for the person to talk about concerns and fears related to the surgery.
   b. Teach the patient relaxation techniques to deal with preoperative anxiety and postoperative pain. Emphasize that adequate medicinal pain control will be provided postoperatively.

NURSING DIAGNOSIS: Anticipatory grieving R/T altered body image and loss of control following surgery

1. *Expected outcomes:* Following interventions, the person should be able to do the following:
   a. Describe the rehabilitation process.
   b. Express feelings of personal control regarding rehabilitation.
2. *Nursing interventions*
   a. Describe any temporary or permanent alterations in body appearance or function or lifestyle changes that will result from the surgery.
   b. Explain what the patient can do to speed the recovery process (e.g., coughing, splinting, early ambulation).
   c. Help the patient adapt to permanent changes resulting from surgery (e.g., exploring types of makeup to cover scars or new forms of exercise to accommodate new limitations). If appropriate, arrange for a visit from someone who has undergone the same procedure to provide proof of successful recovery and offer further adaptive suggestions.

CARING FOR PEOPLE DURING SURGERY (INTRAOPERATIVELY)

Promoting Safety

1. Environmental safety
   a. Check the person's identity on transfer to the operating room.
   b. Confirm the site to be operated on.
   c. Support the head at all times.
   d. Avoid hyperextending any joint and dislodging any drains or the infusion needle in the arm.
   e. If a person is prone, relieve pressure on the thorax to facilitate respiration.
   f. Do not obstruct any tubes or monitors.
   g. Be sure you have adequate assistance when moving a patient.
   h. Make sure sponge count is correct. (Approximately 45 percent of all malpractice claims involve foreign objects being left in patients during surgery.)
      (1) When soiled sponges are discarded from the sterile field, the scrub person and circulating nurse should count and bag the sponges in clear plastic bags, which allows for quick, reliable recounting. Throughout the procedure, the scrub person keeps a silent count of all sponges.
      (2) Before the closing of the procedure, the first closing count is made; it is verified by both the scrub nurse and circulating nurse and is reported to the surgeon and recorded.
      (3) The second closing count is made before closure of the subcutaneous layer and is compared with the first count, reported to the surgeon, and recorded.
   i. Count the needles at the same time as the sponges. To ensure their containment, collect the needles on a needle pad or container and then bag and label them with the number of needles contained inside.
   j. Count the instruments
      (1) In the instrument room as the sets are being assembled
      (2) In the operating room (by the scrub person)
      (3) Before the operation and before closure begins (by the circulating nurse)
   k. If there is a conflicting count of sponges, needles, or instruments, the count is repeated. If the count is still inconsistent, the surgeon is notified immediately, and the missing item is sought. If the item is not found, a radiograph is taken and the results noted. If the radiograph is negative, the count is recorded as incorrect and an incident report is filed.
2. Electrosurgery safety
   a. The electrosurgical unit cuts tissue and controls bleeding through the application of heat. A dispersive grounding pad in the electrosurgical unit prevents burns by ensuring proper return of the electrical energy to the unit.

b. Inspect all electrical equipment before and after each use.
c. Power cords should lie flat on the floor or be suspended to prevent obstruction of traffic areas.
d. Avoid the use of extension cords as much as possible.
e. Never operate equipment with wet hands.
f. Return active electrodes to holster when not in use to prevent accidental activation.

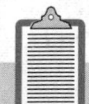

NURSING MANAGEMENT

All persons handling power equipment should be educated about function and proper use of that equipment.

Caring for the Person During Anesthesia

1. Induction and maintenance of general anesthesia
   a. Make sure resuscitative equipment, including the defibrillator, is readily available.
   b. Remain at the person's side to provide protection, assistance, and emotional support.
   c. Monitor oxygen saturation (SaO_2) to give early warning of loss of pulse and to prevent major hypoxia (SaO_2) of less than 90 percent. Pulse oximetry is a noninvasive method for measuring the oxygen saturation of hemoglobin in the blood.
   d. To prevent regurgitation of stomach contents and assist in the visualization of the vocal cords during intubation, apply backward pressure to the cricoid cartilage.
   e. Observe for vomiting, irregular respiratory patterns, or laryngospasm.
   f. Monitor the electrocardiogram.
   g. Monitor the patient's temperature using a skin sensor placed on the patient's forehead, and attempt to keep the patient warm.
      (1) To keep the patient warm, maintain the room temperature at 72 degrees Fahrenheit. (Sometimes the gowned surgical team prefers a cooler room or the procedure requires one.) Keep the patient covered, use warm irrigating fluids and skin preparation solutions, and administer blood through an electron warmer.
      (2) Malignant hyperthermia is a rare but potentially fatal condition triggered primarily by exposure to anesthetic agents (especially succinylcholine) and volatile anesthetic gases (e.g., halothane). If a positive familial history is found during preoperative screening, the anesthesiologist administers alternative anesthetics.
   h. The circulating nurse should do the following:
      (1) Inspect all supplies and instruments for sterility before the procedure begins and observe for maintenance of sterility throughout the procedure.
      (2) Inform team members when there is a break in aseptic technique and assist them in correcting the problem.
      (3) Label, store, and transport specimens.
   i. The scrub person assists the surgeon with the operative procedure by passing the surgical instruments and holding retractors.

2. Emergence from general anesthesia
   a. To prevent aspiration and respiratory obstruction, observe for the following:
      • Retching
      • Vomiting
      • Restlessness
      • Excitation
   b. Help remove drapes, and turn off equipment. Cleanse the patient's skin where solutions have dripped.
   c. Apply dressing using sterile technique.
   d. Assist in the transfer of the patient to the postanesthesia unit, and give a report of the procedure, medications administered, type of dressing, presence of drains, and any instructions by the surgeon regarding postoperative care.

3. Local, regional, or intravenous conscious sedation
   a. The nurse assumes the same responsibilities regarding aseptic technique, maintenance and observation of equipment, and monitoring of patient status as described for the care of the patient receiving general anesthesia.
   b. Psychologic support
      (1) The inability to see but ability to hear during the procedure may increase the person's anxiety.
      (2) Communicate with the person to alleviate anxiety. Provide explanations of the procedure when appropriate.
   c. Each facility may have different policies and procedures regarding the monitoring and administration of intravenous drugs for conscious sedation. In some settings, the nurse may administer only intramuscular medications. In other settings, administration of intravenous medications by the nurse is allowed.

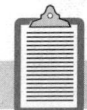

NURSING MANAGEMENT

The nurse who administers intravenous sedation during surgery should have only that responsibility on the case.

   d. Monitor the intravenous site and the general effects of the medications.
   e. Assess the patient's central nervous system for signs of toxicity (e.g., loss of consciousness, drowsiness, disorientation, slurred speech, numbness, convulsions, and coma). Administer thiobarbiturates and succinylcholine to control seizures.
   f. Assess the patient's cardiovascular system for signs of toxicity (e.g., bradycardia, hypotension, and asystole). Administer fluids and vasopressors as needed.
   g. Assess the patient's respiratory system for respiratory arrest. Maintain the airway, and administer oxygen as needed.

Common Surgical Positions

Supine:

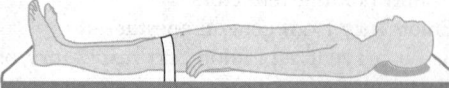

This is the most frequently used position because it is least stressful to the patient, homeostasis is easiest to maintain during it, and it allows access to the face, neck, abdomen, chest, and extremities. Vulnerable pressure points should be padded, such as heels, elbows, and sacrum. The bed strap should be placed 2 inches above the knees to prevent the person from bending the knees during induction and emergence from anesthesia, which could cause an injury. The elbows should not rest on the metal edge of the bed because this may cause pressure to the ulnar nerve. Protect the ear and other bony prominences from pressure. Possible complications include decreases in blood pressure, vital capacities, tidal volume, and potential for venous pooling in the lower extremities.

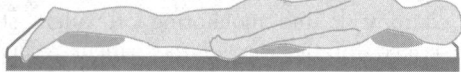

Prone:

This position allows access to the posterior of the neck, back, and extremities. It is frequently used for lumbar laminectomies.

Turn the head to the side or face downward with a foam headrest for protection. Possible complications include difficulty breathing related to body weight against the abdominal wall and decrease in blood pressure if improperly positioned.

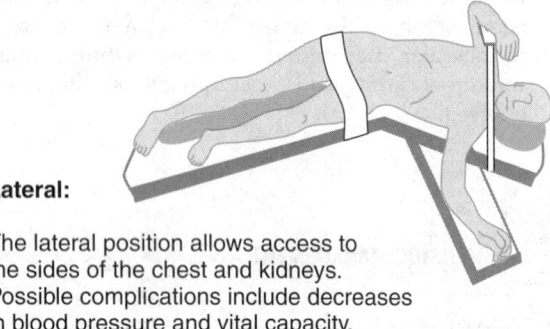

Lateral:

The lateral position allows access to the sides of the chest and kidneys. Possible complications include decreases in blood pressure and vital capacity.

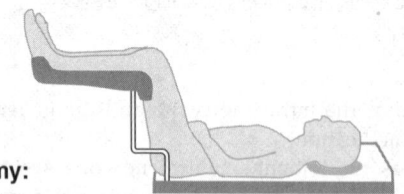

Lithotomy:

This position allows access to perineal and rectal areas. It is used for rectal, gynecologic, and urologic surgeries. Possible complications include decrease in venous return as a result of the pressure by the legs on the abdomen, limited diaphragmatic movements as a result of abdominal pressure against the diaphragm, and nerve damage to the femoral and perineal nerves.

Positions for Specialized Surgeries

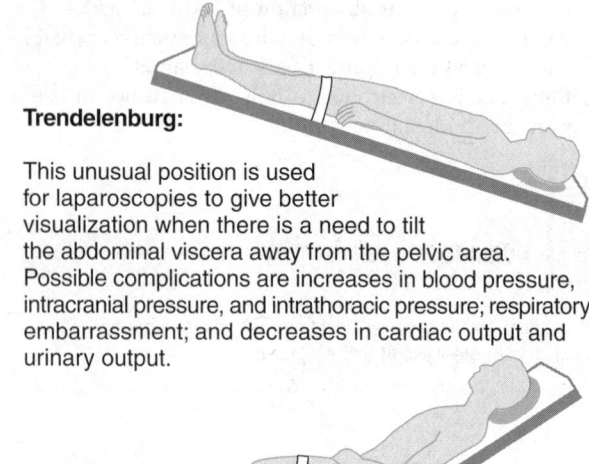

Trendelenburg:

This unusual position is used for laparoscopies to give better visualization when there is a need to tilt the abdominal viscera away from the pelvic area. Possible complications are increases in blood pressure, intracranial pressure, and intrathoracic pressure; respiratory embarrassment; and decreases in cardiac output and urinary output.

Sitting:

Some cervical, ear, and nose surgeries use this position. Pressure areas include the scapula, sacrum, and the ischial tuberosities. Possible complications include decreased blood pressure, venous pooling in lower extremities, and air embolism.

NURSING INTERVENTIONS

1. Confirm the selected position with the surgeon's orders.
2. Make sure adequate assistance is available.
3. When wrist restraints are necessary, the padded cloth clove hitch produces the least trauma. Leather restraints may chafe the skin.
4. To prevent muscle strain due to the flat operating bed, place a small pillow under the small of the back and under the knees.
5. Always place the arm at less than a 90-degree angle to the body with palms up to diminish pressure on the median and ulnar nerves.
6. Support the feet on a padded footboard for long surgical procedures to prevent plantar flexion.
7. Keep the legs uncrossed and parallel to prevent tibial nerve injury and compromised circulation.
8. Protect muscles and joints from strain. When extremities are placed in stirrups or slings, move them simultaneously.
9. Always keep the neck in alignment with the spine and positioned on a foam pillow or towel. Protect the eyes from injury.
10. Place a lifting sheet under the patient for turning. Gently logroll the patient to protect the neck and spine.
11. Use an armboard to support the arms and to protect the IV site.
12. Do not allow any parts of the body to extend over the edge of the operating bed or touch any metal or unpadded surfaces.

Figure 13–3.

Positioning the Person for Surgery

1. The surgeon selects the position for the surgical procedure keeping in mind the following:
   a. Providing adequate visibility for the location of the surgical incision and the operative procedure
   b. Providing access for induction and maintenance of anesthesia
   c. Promoting circulatory and respiratory function
      (1) There should be no constriction around the patient's neck or chest.
      (2) The arms should not be crossed on the chest.
      (3) The ankles or legs should not be crossed, which creates occlusive pressure on blood vessels, nerves, and soft tissue.
      (4) Pressure should not be applied to the peripheral blood vessels.
      (5) Body and restraining straps should not be fastened too tightly.
      (6) At the end of the surgical procedure, the patient's condition should be assessed.
   d. Promoting skeletal alignment
   e. Preventing undue pressure on bony prominences and skin
      (1) Use padding to protect bony prominences from constant pressure by the hard surfaces of the operating room bed.
      (2) Avoid contact with any metal.
      (3) Use bed extensions as necessary (footboard if person is tall, armboard extensions if person is obese).
   f. Preventing unnecessary postoperative discomfort. The anesthetized person lacks protective muscle tone and is susceptible to postoperative discomfort. Strain on the muscles can result in injury or pain, such as a stiff neck from hyperextending the head for a prolonged time.
   g. Providing sterile draping and preserving modesty
      (1) Handle the drapes as little as possible.
      (2) Protect gloved hands by cuffing the ends of sheets.
      (3) Hold the drapes high enough to avoid touching nonsterile areas.
      (4) Once a drape is placed, do not adjust it.
      (5) If a drape is incorrectly placed, discard it.
      (6) Never reach across the bed to drape the opposite side.
2. Figure 13–3 shows 4 common positions for surgery.

Maintaining a Surgically Clean Environment

1. Surgical wound infections may develop as a result of the following:
   a. Microbial contamination, especially from *Staphylococcus aureus*
   b. Condition of the wound at the end of surgery
   c. Susceptibility of the person, which may be affected by factors such as obesity, debilitation, age, complexity and length of surgery, and presence of other diseases
2. Measures to prevent surgical wound infection include the following:
   a. Cleansing the patient's skin before surgery
   b. If appropriate, removing hair from the surgical site
   c. Maintaining a sterile field throughout surgery
3. Figure 13–4 shows common surgical incisions.

◼ CARING FOR PEOPLE AFTER SURGERY

Postanesthesia Assessment

1. The immediate stage, or phase I, is the period 1 to 4 hours after surgery.
   a. During the first few minutes in the postanesthesia care unit, a rapid appraisal on all body systems, with a focus on vital functions is performed. A numeric scoring system assesses patient activity, respiration, circulation, consciousness, and color.
   b. The most important assessment the nurse makes in the immediate stage is that of airway patency and adequate ventilation.
      (1) Prolonged mechanical ventilation during anesthesia may affect postoperative lung function. Extubated persons who are lethargic may not be able to maintain an airway.
      (2) Ascultate lungs, noting rate, depth, and quality of respirations, and observe chest expansion. Rate should be greater than 10 and less than 30.
      (3) Assess breath sounds: stridor, wheezing, or crowing can indicate partial obstruction, bronchospasm, or laryngospasm. Crackles or rhonchi may indicate pulmonary edema.
      (4) Observe chest movement for symmetry and use of accessory muscles.
      (5) Administration of oxygen is standard practice after general anesthesia or heavy sedation.
      (6) To prevent hypoxia, continue pulse oximetry after surgery until an acceptable oxygen saturation level

COMMON SURGICAL INCISIONS

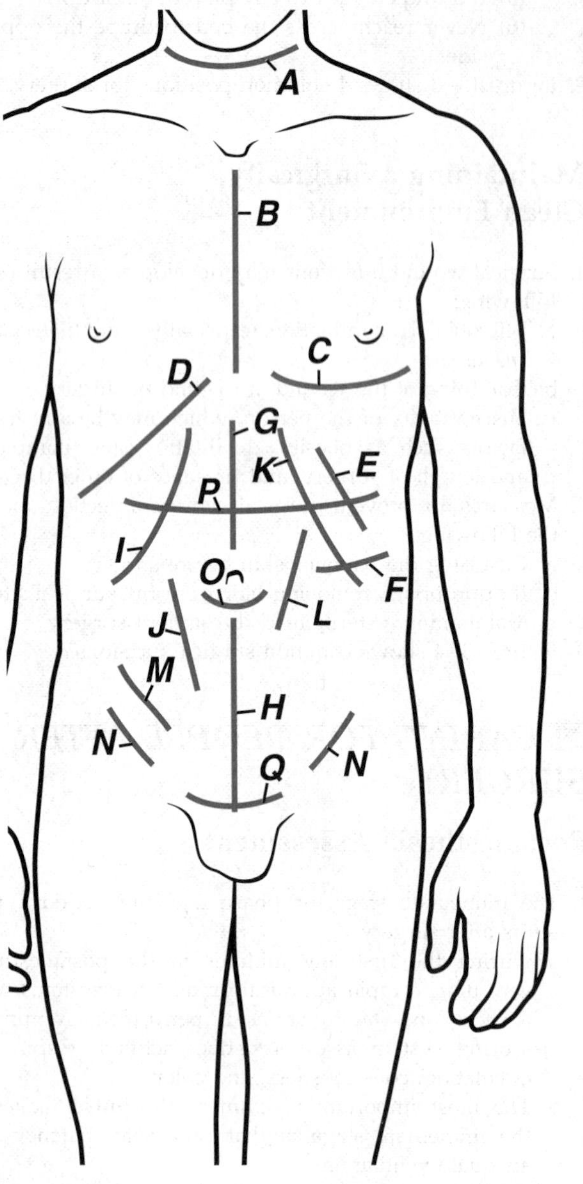

A Collar
B Sternal split
C Lateral
  thoracotomy
D Right subcostal
E Left subcostal
F Horizontal flank
G Upper abdominal
  midline
H Lower abdominal
  midline
I Right upper
  paramedian

J Right lower
  paramedian
K Left upper
  paramedian
L Left lower
  paramedian
M McBurney's
N Inguinal
O Infraumbilical
P Transverse upper
  abdominal
Q Transverse
  suprapubic

Figure 13–4.

(SaO_2 of more than 95 percent) is achieved. Apply blankets and continue oxygen therapy if the person is shivering.

ELDER ADVISORY

Place older persons in a low Fowler's position after surgery to increase the size of the thorax. Administer oxygen until the older patient is fully conscious.

    (7) Observe the person for signs of atelectasis, pneumonia, and pulmonary embolism.
  c. Cardiovascular assessment: Assess vital signs every 15 minutes until baseline readings are maintained.
    (1) Assess pulse for rate, rhythm, and amplitude. Weak, absent, or irregular pulses may reflect hypovolemia, decreased cardiac output, acute myocardial infarction, or cardiac dysrhythmias. A bounding pulse may indicate hypertension, fluid overload, or excitement.
      • Observe for signs of hypertension and hypotension. Monitor cardiac dysrhythmias if the person is on an electrocardiographic monitor.
      • Often persons are hypertensive from pain, agitation, or vasoconstriction secondary to hypothermia.
      • Often persons are hypovolemic secondary to bleeding, insufficiently replaced fluid loss, or third-spacing.
    (2) Assess patient color by observing capillary refill, mucous membranes, and sclera.
    (3) If fulminant hepatic failure is suspected, assess peripheral pulses and edema.
  d. Fluid and electrolytes assessment
    (1) Monitor for signs of hypothermia (e.g., low temperature, extremity cyanosis) that may result from anesthesia, cool operating room temperature, and exposure of skin and internal organs during surgery. If needed, supply warm blankets or warm intravenous solutions.
    (2) Monitor the patient for signs of hypocalcemia, hyperglycemia, and metabolic and respiratory acidosis and alkalosis.
    (3) Continue intravenous therapy until the person can tolerate fluids. When oral fluids are permitted, start with ice chips and water.
  e. Gastrointestinal assessment: Monitor for nausea and vomiting which are common after anesthesia.
    (1) If the person has a history of motion sickness or previous occurrences of nausea and vomiting postoperatively, administer a prophylactic antiemetic.
    (2) Turn the unconscious patient to a side-lying position if vomiting occurs and have suctioning equipment ready.
  f. Renal assessment: Assess bladder for distention.
  g. Musculoskeletal assessment
    (1) Assess the patient for movement of all extremities.
    (2) Assess for pain.

(3) Check redness at pressure points of surgical positioning.
h. Neurologic assessment
(1) Assess level of consciousness by observing how the person responds to verbal commands and touch. Pupil reaction to light and reflexes should be observed.
(2) The patient receiving general anesthesia may be drowsy or unconscious. Never leave the unconscious person unattended. Periodic, frequent attempts to awaken the person should continue until the person awakes. Speak in a soft tone and filter out extraneous noises in the environment.
(3) Review the type of anesthetic and preoperative medications that the person received. Shorter-acting anesthetics used for short procedures yield patients who are more aware.
(4) The most common reasons for a person not to awaken shortly after surgery
• Drug interaction
• Prolonged effect of anesthetics
• Cardiac or respiratory instability
• Preoperative or intraoperative condition
• Fluid and electrolyte imbalances
(5) The nurse should observe the patient for any paralysis and assess respiratory function. The most serious consequence of inadequate reversal of muscle relaxants usually results from intraoperative drug interactions. The nurse should also assess the patient for numbness or tingling sensations.
i. Circulatory assessment
(1) Monitor oxygen (SaO$_2$ should be >90%).
(2) Monitor the electrocardiogram if applicable.
(3) Report vital sign changes, count apical pulse for a full minute, and assess heart sounds.
(4) Observe the person for signs of myocardial infarction, thrombophlebitis, hypotension, hypertension, and shock.
2. The intermediate stage, or phase II, occurs 4 to 24 hours after surgery.
a. For ambulatory or morning admissions without complications, the phase II area is used as the "discharge unit." Persons receiving local or regional anesthesia without complications are admitted to the phase II area directly from the operating room.
b. Generally, the person is ambulatory and able to perform self-care; however, close observation and monitoring of body systems are still required because postoperative changes can occur suddenly.
c. Respiratory assessment
(1) Check the patency of the airway
(2) Verify that lungs are clear on auscultation
d. Cardiovascular assessment
(1) Vital signs are stable.
(2) Circulation is efficient as measured by the presence of peripheral pulses, capillary refill, and absence of edema, numbness, and tingling.
(3) Intravenous lines are infusing.
e. Neurologic assessment
(1) Level of consciousness: The patient is alert and oriented and responsive to commands.

(2) All reflexes are present.
f. Gastrointestinal assessment
(1) There are normal bowel sounds in all 4 quadrants when the abdomen is auscultated and palpated.
(2) Minimal nausea and vomiting occur.
g. Urinary assessment
(1) Urine output is greater than 30 ml per hour.
(2) The patient may have a full bladder as a result of intraoperative fluid administration.
(3) The patient may have bladder distention or pain, especially after spinal or epidural anesthesia, because of the inability to void.
h. Musculoskeletal assessment
(1) There is movement of all extremities; ambulation should be encouraged.
(2) Minimal pain occurs with motion.
i. Metabolic assessment
(1) Monitor for sodium deficit (hyponatremia) caused by vomiting, nasogastric intubation, and diarrhea.
(2) Monitor for potassium deficit (hypokalemia), which is caused by vomiting, diarrhea, nasogastric intubation, and prolonged administration of potassium-free intravenous solutions.
(3) Monitor for acidosis caused by shock, diabetes, hypoventilation, and abdominal distention.
(4) Monitor for alkalosis caused by anxiety, hyperventilation, blood transfusions, pain, and nasogastric intubation.

ELDER ADVISORY

Older people are more susceptible to water intoxication and pulmonary edema because of overhydration resulting from fluid replacement after surgery.

j. Surgical site and drains assessment
(1) There should be minimal bleeding or drainage.
(2) Fluid drains should be patent.
3. The extended stage is the period of at least 1 to 4 days after surgery.
a. Patients with complications from surgery or anesthesia are admitted to a nursing unit. The person at high risk after a surgical procedure because of a preexisting condition may stay several days or longer in the hospital to recover.
b. Throughout the extended stage, assess and observe the patient's body systems as discussed for the intermediate phase, with specialized nursing care being given for complications of 1 or more systems (see pp. 397–398).
c. Observe the patient for signs of infection such as redness, swelling, and tenderness at the surgical site; fever; and leukocytosis.
d. Encourage active range-of-motion exercises every 2 hours (see Chapter 7). Some patients may need passive range-of-motion exercises every 2 hours (Fig. 13–5).
e. Early ambulation, if ordered by the physician, promotes peristalsis and passage of fluids and gas.

f. Before ambulation, instruct the person to sit on the edge of the bed, with feet supported.

g. Ambulation should be increased every day to increase muscle strength.

h. Persons who are unable to walk should be turned every 1 to 2 hours.

i. Antiembolism stockings promote venous return, strengthen muscle tone, and prevent pooling of secretions in lungs.

j. Encourage the person to select foods that are high in protein and vitamin C content to promote wound healing; fresh fruits such as bananas and oranges provide potassium.

k. Encourage the person to perform as many activities of daily living as possible.

Postoperative Interventions

1. Respiratory interventions
   a. Administer humidified oxygen.
   b. If the person is comatose or semiconscious, position on the side and keep an oral airway in place to maintain airway patency.
   c. Remove any secretions by suctioning, if the person is unable to clear the airway by coughing.
   d. Avoid placing the patient in the supine position until the pharyngeal reflexes have returned.
   e. Encourage turning, deep breathing, and coughing to clear inhalation anesthetic agents from the body and prevent pooling of secretions (Fig. 13–6).

2. Circulatory interventions
   a. Maintain intravenous line patency. Titrate fluids to condition, blood pressure, and need for fluid replacement.
   b. If shock develops, elevate the legs. If the person has had spinal anesthesia, do not elevate the legs any higher than placing them on a pillow; otherwise, the diaphragmatic muscles could be impaired.

3. Neurologic intervention: The nurse should observe the patient for deepening of the effects of the anesthesia or the renarcotization as stored narcotic reenters the bloodstream when pain medication is administered.

4. Renal interventions
   a. Observing the color, amount, consistency, and odor of the patient's urine.
   b. Assess catheters for patency.
   c. If there is no catheter, ensure that the person voids within 6 hours after surgery and that the amount is at least 200 ml.
   d. If the person voids within 6 hours, palpate the abdomen and notify the physician if there is distention.
   e. Facilitate voiding by positioning females in the sitting position or males in the standing position, running water, giving the patient water to drink, placing heat on the perineum to promote relaxation, and getting the patient to ambulate.

5. Gastrointestinal interventions
   a. Ensure that the person receives nothing by mouth until the gag reflex and peristalsis return. Then, if ordered, ice chips or sips of water may be given.

LEG EXERCISES

Leg exercises prevent venous stasis of blood and facilitate venous blood return.

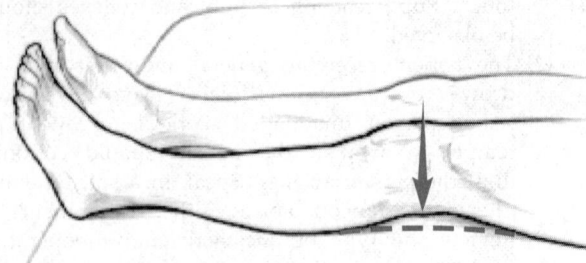

Thigh and Calf Exercises

Instruct the person to press the back of the knee against the bed and then to relax it. This contracts and relaxes the thigh and calf muscles to prevent thrombus formation.

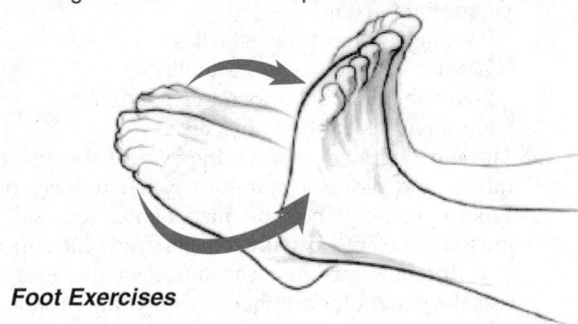

Foot Exercises

Tell the person to rotate each foot in a circle at least 10 times an hour.
If their use is anticipated, explain TED stockings and pneumatic sequential leg wraps.

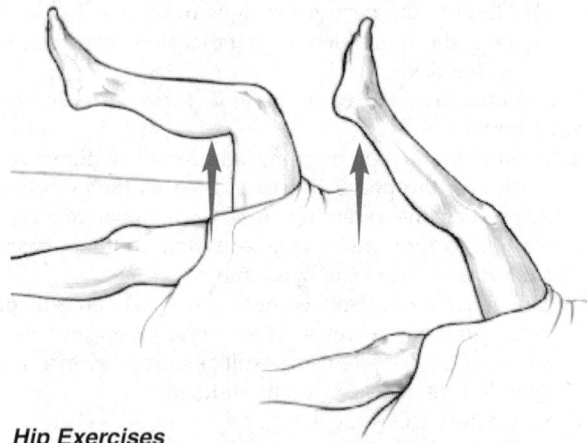

Hip Exercises

Have the person flex the knee and thigh, straighten the leg up in the air, and hold for 5 seconds before lowering. Instruct the patient to perform the exercise 10 times per hour.

Figure 13–5.

COUGHING AND DEEP BREATHING EXERCISES

Explain that the sitting position gives the best lung expansion for this exercise.

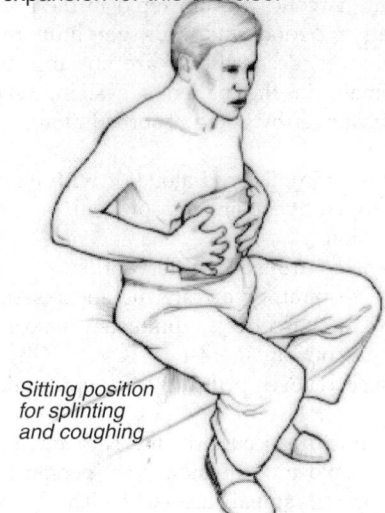

Tell the patient to breathe deeply 3 times, inhaling through the mouth and exhaling through the nose.

The 3rd breath should be held for 3 seconds, then the patient should forcefully cough out 3 times.

Sitting position for splinting and coughing

Have the person perform the exercise every 2 hours after surgery.

Schedule pain medications before exercises.

Explain that a spirometer, a small tool to help maintain alveolar expansion, will be at the bedside to assist in deep breathing.

Show patients having abdominal or thoracic surgery how to support or "splint" the incision.

Alternate sitting position for splinting and coughing

Prone position for splinting and coughing

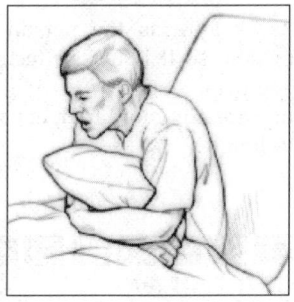
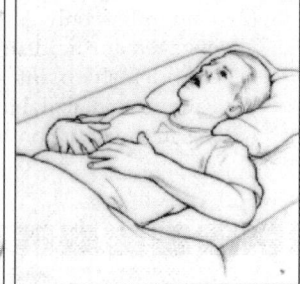

Figure 13–6.

Patients who are nauseated and vomiting should be turned on 1 side, and an antiemetic should be requested.

b. Observe drainage if a nasogastric tube is connected to low suction.

c. Ensure that the person begins on clear liquids and advances to a regular diet as tolerated.

d. Relieve the patient's gas pains by encouraging ambulation, applying heat to the abdomen, positioning the patient, and placing a rectal tube.

e. Administer frequent mouth care to prevent parotitis and promote good oral hygiene.

f. Observe the person for signs of hypovolemia and hypervolemia.

g. Monitor intake and output during every shift.

6. Integumentary interventions
   a. Maintain a dry and intact dressing at the site of the surgical wound. If necessary, reinforce with a sterile dressing and notify physician.
   b. Change dressings as ordered by the physician, noting the amount of bleeding or drainage, odor, and intactness of sutures or staples.
   c. Have obese or debilitated individuals use a binder to prevent rupture of the incision.

Postoperative Medications

1. Antiemetics are given if nausea and vomiting result from the anesthesia or if there has been surgical manipulation of organs.
2. Common antiemetics
   • Hydroxyzine HCl (Vistaril)
   • Droperidol (Inapsine)—used for premedication for surgery, induction, and maintenance in general anesthesia
   • Prochlorperazine (Compazine)
   • Transdermal scopolamine
   • Trimethobenzamide
3. Antibiotics are given to prevent infection of wounds, systemic bacteremia, or pulmonary complications.
4. Common antimicrobials
   • Cephalosporins
   • Penicillins
   • Erythromycin
   • Clindamycin
5. Vitamin C promotes wound healing; multiple vitamins are recommended for older people and persons unable to receive oral nutrition.
6. Cholinergics such as bethanechol chloride aid in the return of peristalsis.
7. Laxatives: Stool softeners such as docusate sodium (Colace) prevent constipation; mineral oil such as Fleet mineral oil softens feces in cases of constipation.
8. Narcotic antagonists (e.g., nalorphine, naloxone, levallorphan) counteract respiratory depression from opiates.
9. Antiarrhythmia drugs include intravenous lidocaine (Xylocaine) or procainamide (Pronestyl) for premature ventricular contractions. Atropine is given for sinus bradycardia.

Postoperative Pain Management

1. Causes of postoperative pain
   a. Cutting, pulling, or manipulation of tissues and organs
   b. Tissue ischemia caused by interference of blood supply to a body part

c. Prolonged surgery requiring the person to be in 1 position for a long period of time, with resultant trauma to the nerve fibers in the skin

d. Stimulation of nerve endings by chemical substances released at the time of surgery

e. Prolonged retraction of muscles

f. Restlessness after anesthesia that causes undue strain on the suture lines

g. Pressure from tissue edema

2. Types of postsurgical pain

a. Incisional pain, described as
   - Sharp
   - Cutting
   - Tearing
   - Stabbing
   - Localized

b. Pain from prolonged stimulation such as tension on sutures, described as a burning pain

c. Somatic pain, usually described as dull and aching

d. Chest pain in patients with preexisting cardiovascular disease, myocardial infarction, or angina

3. Assessment of postoperative pain

a. Pain is whatever the person says it is.

b. Unrelieved pain can prolong convalescence.

c. All pain is not necessarily from the surgical incision.

d. Inquire about the type of pain and location.

e. Ask the person to rate the degree of pain on a scale of 1 to 10, with 10 being the most severe.

f. Ask about the effectiveness of the last pain intervention.

g. Obtain objective data by observing or measuring the following:
   - Facial expressions
   - Body gestures
   - Pulse rate
   - Blood pressure
   - Respirations

4. Invasive interventions (i.e., narcotic analgesics) relieve postoperative pain.

a. The goal is to produce the highest concentration of pain relief consistent with adequate ventilation.

b. The drugs most commonly used for severe postoperative pain are morphine or meperidine.

c. Pain relief through narcotics decreases postoperative complications by increasing compliance with treatment and preventative therapies such as frequent turning, coughing, and deep breathing.

d. Before administering a narcotic, consider the type of anesthesia the person received before and during surgery.

e. During the initial administration of the narcotic, assess the person every 30 minutes for pain relief and respiratory rate. When baseline vital signs have been achieved, assess every 4 hours.

f. Ketorolac (Toradol), a nonsteroidal anti-inflammatory drug, is often given intramuscularly during surgery and greatly decreases the need for postoperative narcotics.

g. The best way to achieve a stable concentration of analgesia—and thereby reduce the total amount of narcotic needed—is to give a continuous infusion of the drug intravenously, especially through use of a patient-controlled analgesic pump (see Chapter 11).

h. Intramuscular administration of narcotics is less desirable because doses are normally too low and too intermittent to sustain pain relief. Most people have trouble absorbing narcotics administered in the immediate postoperative period and thus get little relief from them. Moreover, because they are not absorbed, these drugs remain in the patient's system, where they may pose a danger by being absorbed along with a later dose.

i. Epidural infusions, administered alone or with narcotics, control postoperative pain and prevent narcotic-induced hypotension.

j. Side effects can be controlled by intervention.
   (1) In cases of respiratory arrest, the most serious side effect of narcotics, administer naloxone, which is a narcotic antagonist.
   (2) Naloxone also relieves pruritus from epidural infusions.
   (3) If a dural puncture occurs during catheter insertion for an epidural infusion, the person will likely develop a spinal headache. The person should lie flat for 12 to 24 hours and increase fluid intake.

5. Noninvasive measures to relieve postoperative pain.

a. Effectiveness depends on the person's ability to cooperate and focus. Some anesthetics may leave a postoperative patient unable to perform noninvasive techniques for several hours.

b. Distraction (e.g., rhythmic breathing, singing, conversing or listening to favorite music) can provide relief.
   (1) Distraction aids in decreasing postoperative pain by placing pain on the periphery of awareness.
   (2) Pain relief only lasts as long as the person is engaged in the distraction, so it is most effective for brief, sharp, intense pain.
   (3) Fatigue and irritability are common after engaging in a distraction technique.

◉▐ ▉▣ ▲◖▐ ▦✡⊡▌ ★◉ ❚❙ ▣ ◓

TRANSCULTURAL CONSIDERATIONS

Persons adhering to Eastern religions that emphasize meditation may find relaxation techniques particularly effective in minimizing postoperative pain.

c. Transcutaneous electrical nerve stimulation can be effective (see Chapter 11).

d. Relaxation techniques and guided imagery (see Chapter 11) may reduce or relieve postoperative pain by decreasing anxiety and muscle tension.

e. Basic comfort measures can be extremely helpful in reducing postoperative pain. Examples include the following:
   (1) Proper positioning and frequent repositioning
   (2) Giving back rubs
   (3) Applying frequent oral hygiene
   (4) Encouraging range of motion exercises
   (5) Being available to talk with the person
   (6) Offering fluids frequently
   (7) Providing a quiet and restful environment
   (8) Bathing the patient
   (9) Applying ice therapy
   (10) Providing therapeutic touch

Common Complications in the Immediate Postoperative Stage

1. Aspiration. Regurgitation of gastric contents, food, water, or blood, usually occurs as a result of postanesthesia sedation, producing ineffective reflexes (gag and swallowing).
   a. Assessment: Look for local edema, inflammation, and destruction of the mucosa of the tracheobronchial tree.
   b. Nursing interventions.
      (1) Assess the patient's level of consciousness.
      (2) Position an unconscious person on the right side with the head tilted down.
      (3) Suction the person who is unable to cough.
      (4) If the person has a nasogastric tube, maintain its patency.
      (5) Administer drugs that decrease gastric acidity, if ordered.
2. Airway obstruction by the tongue
   a. Assessment: Check for decreased breath sounds, stridor, snoring, use of accessory muscles for breathing, increased pulse rate, and decreased SaO_2 levels.
   b. Nursing interventions: In a reactive person, verbal and physical stimulation usually correct the problem. In a nonreactive person, hyperextend the head with a chin lift to displace the tongue and open the airway. If this does not correct the problem, insert an airway and position the person on the side. If the problem persists, intubation or tracheotomy is required.
3. Laryngospasm
   a. Assessment: Signs include hypoxia, hypoventilation, absence of breath sounds, crowing sounds with an incomplete spasm, and panic in the conscious person.
   b. Nursing interventions: Remove any irritant or foreign objects. Hyperextend the neck, and supply positive pressure ventilation with oxygen. If ventilation is still inadequate, administer succinylcholine to relax the vocal cords and continue ventilation. Intubation is necessary if the spasm continues.
4. Bronchospasm
   a. Assessment: Look for wheezing, dyspnea, noisy shallow respirations, and tachycardia.
   b. Nursing interventions: Remove the irritant if possible, and administer bronchodilators (such as Bronkosol),

anti-inflammatories (such as intravenous methylprednisolone), and cholinergics (to decrease secretions).
5. Pulmonary edema
   a. Assessment: Examine for shortness of breath; pink, frothy sputum; loud inspiratory and expiratory gurgles; cold, ashen, cyanotic skin; and tachycardia.
   b. Nursing interventions
      (1) Assess hourly for dyspnea, adventitious sounds, alterations in mental status, and cyanosis.
      (2) Supply 100 percent oxygen under positive pressure.
      (3) Administer diuretics, digoxin intravenously, aminophylline intravenously, morphine sulfate intravenously, and vasodilators as ordered.
      (4) Apply rotating tourniquets to extremities if there is no improvement.
6. Shock. Hypovolemia results from hemorrhage or fluid volume deficit.
   a. Assessment: Signs include lethargy, dizziness and weakness, nausea, disorientation, increased pulse rate, decreased blood pressure and urinary output, and slow capillary refill.
   b. Nursing interventions
      (1) Monitor level of consciousness.
      (2) Monitor vital signs for increased pulse or decreased blood pressure.
      (3) Monitor intake and output, measure urine and specific gravity, and weigh the patient daily.
      (4) Assess color, temperature, turgor, and moisture of skin and mucous membranes.
      (5) Monitor SaO_2 and hemoglobin.
      (6) Administer fluids, blood, and colloid solutions as ordered.

Complications in the Intermediate Postoperative Stage

1. Acute respiratory distress syndrome. Acute lung injury results from a response to a pathologic event such as shock, sepsis, disseminated intravascular coagulation, cardiopulmonary bypass, aspiration, or trauma (see Chapter 22).
   a. Assessment: The nurse should check for progressive dyspnea, tachypnea, restriction of thoracic motion, hypotension, cyanosis, decreased breath sounds, audible pulmonary fluid, and decreased SaO_2.
   b. Nursing interventions
      (1) Closely monitor fluid intake and output and daily weight.
      (2) Monitor for increased fluid accumulation in lungs by assessing rales, dyspnea, edema, and jugular vein distention.
      (3) Administer antibiotics as ordered. Supply diuretics to shift and eliminate pulmonary fluid.
      (4) Use mechanical ventilation and apply positive pressure to the lung at the end of exhalation to ensure oxygenation.
2. Urinary retention (especially after spinal and epidural regional anesthesia)

a. Assessment: Look for absence of urine, distended bladder above the symphysis pubis, hypertension, lower abdominal pain, restlessness, and diaphoresis. On percussion, the bladder sounds like a kettle drum.

b. Nursing interventions:
   (1) Monitor for the patient hypertension if the bladder is distended (a hallmark sign of hypertension in postoperative patients).
   (2) Encourage early ambulation.
   (3) Encourage fluid intake, 3000 ml per day.
   (4) Assist the person to void by helping to stand or sit, providing privacy, pouring warm water over the perineum, and allowing the person to hear running water.
   (5) Catheterize the patient, as ordered, after all noninvasive techniques have been attempted.

Complications in the Extended Postoperative Stage

1. Pneumonia and atelectasis. Pneumonia may develop 3 to 5 days postoperatively because of infection, aspiration, or immobility. Atelectasis, the most common postoperative complication, usually occurs 1 to 2 days postoperatively.
   a. Assessment: Factors that increase the risk of pneumonia and atelectasis
      • Chronic obstructive lung disease
      • Age older than 65 years
      • Use of inhalant anesthesia
      • Use of anesthesia longer than 3 hours
      • Decreased chest expansion (as evidenced by shallow respirations or pain on motion)
      • Decreased breath sounds
      • Smoking
      • Sedatives and narcotics
      • Obesity
      • Emergency surgery
      • Upper abdominal or thoracic surgery.
   b. Nursing interventions
      • Percuss the chest.
      • Reposition the patient every hour to prevent aspiration.
      • Provide postural drainage.
      • Encourage early ambulation.
      • Help the patient use the incentive spirometer, cough, and deep breathe.
      • Encourage fluid intake.
      • Suction to clear secretions if the person is unable to cough.

2. Venous thrombosis
   a. Assessment: Venous blood clots may develop without symptoms.
      (1) Phlebothrombosis (thrombus formation without inflammation) occurs mainly in persons who are obese or immobilized, and in postsurgical persons (see Chapter 24).
      (2) If a vein becomes inflamed (thrombophlebitis), the extremity can become swollen, pale, cold, and tender to touch. Increased body temperature is common.

(3) Pulmonary embolism results when a vessel becomes occluded. The nurse should assess the patient for sudden, sharp thoracic or upper abdominal pain, dyspnea, or any sign of shock.

b. Nursing interventions
   (1) Observe legs for swelling, inflammation, cyanosis, pain, tenderness, and venous distention.
   (2) Monitor intake and output.
   (3) Encourage coughing and deep breathing to promote venous return.
   (4) Elevate the leg 30 degrees without allowing any pressure on the popliteal area with pillows or knee gatch of the bed.
   (5) Apply elastic stockings to increase blood flow and prevent venous pooling. Remove stockings twice a day to wash and inspect the legs.
   (6) Apply intermittent pneumatic compression stockings, which may be ordered for persons when on bed rest or when anticoagulant therapy is contraindicated. The stockings are used routinely for patients in high-risk categories.
   (7) If the person is on bed rest, perform passive range-of-motion exercises every 2 hours.
   (8) Encourage early ambulation as ordered by the physician.
   (9) Teach the person not to massage the legs to avoid mobilizing fragments.
   (10) Encourage the person to sit with feet flat on the floor.

NURSE ADVISORY

Postoperative patients with potential or actual venous problems should not be allowed to dangle their feet on the side of the bed.

   (11) Teach the person not to sit in one position for an extended period of time.
   (12) Administer heparin or warfarin as ordered to prevent clotting.

3. Paralytic ileus
   a. Assessment: Assess for nausea and vomiting immediately postoperatively, abdominal distention, and absence of bowel sounds, bowel movement, or flatus.
   b. Nursing interventions
      (1) Monitor intake and output and replace gastric losses, which can be large.
      (2) Give the patient nothing by mouth until bowel sounds return. If such return is prolonged, supply intravenous fluids or total parenteral nutrition for hydration.
      (3) Administer dexpanthenol to increase motility and secretions, if ordered.
      (4) Maintain patency of nasogastric tube.
      (5) Encourage early ambulation.

4. Constipation
   a. Assessment: Check for abdominal distention, absence of bowel movements, anorexia, headache, and nausea.
   b. Nursing interventions

(1) Encourage fluid intake, up to 3000 ml per day, unless contraindicated.

(2) Encourage early and frequent ambulation.

(3) Encourage consumption of fiber and roughage.

(4) Administer stool softeners and mild laxatives if ordered.

(5) Provide privacy and adequate time for bowel elimination.

5. Malnutrition
   a. Assessment
      (1) To assess for return of peristalsis, check for the presence of bowel sounds in all 4 quadrants, the passing of flatus, and belching.
      (2) Assess weight: Loss is possible, as is gain (from fluid retention).
      (3) Other signs of malnutrition include increased blood urea nitrogen and decreased tissue turgor.
   b. Nursing interventions
      (1) Monitor for fluid and electrolyte imbalances.
      (2) If a nasogastric tube is in place, keep tube patent and functioning properly.
      (3) If the person is experiencing nausea and vomiting, give the patient nothing by mouth and administer antiemetics and pain medications as ordered.
      (4) If the person cannot ingest food, provide total parenteral nutrition to supply sufficient calories, fluids, and electrolytes. Intravenous fluids of dextrose, normal saline, or Ringer's lactate do not provide adequate nutritional intake for the postsurgical person.
      (5) If the person can tolerate foods by mouth, provide clear liquids and progress as tolerated by person. Foods should be high in protein and vitamin C.

6. Urinary tract infection
   a. Assessment: Signs include elevated temperature, foul odor to urine, dysuria, frequent urination, and voiding small amounts.
   b. Nursing interventions
      (1) If the person has a Foley catheter, maintain a sterile, closed drainage system.
      (2) Perform periurethral cleansing daily.
      (3) Maintain unobstructed urinary flow.
      (4) Encourage fluid intake.
      (5) Administer antibiotics.

7. Electrolyte complications
   a. Common complications are hyponatremia (especially after transurethral resection of the prostate), hypokalemia, respiratory acidosis, respiratory alkalosis, metabolic acidosis, and metabolic alkalosis.
   b. Assessment
      (1) Signs of hyponatremia are lethargy, anorexia, nausea and vomiting, headache, abdominal cramping, and confusion.
      (2) Signs of hypokalemia are cardiac dysrhythmias, abdominal cramps, increased perioral and digital tingling, and Trousseau's sign (a test for latent tetany).
      (3) Signs of respiratory acidosis are lethargy, weakness, drowsiness, and confusion.
      (4) Signs of respiratory alkalosis are rapid, shallow breathing, light-headedness, dizziness, tingling in the fingers and toes, muscle weakness, positive Trousseau's sign, pH greater than 7.45, and low $Paco_2$
      (5) Signs of metabolic acidosis are disorientation, weakness, nausea, vomiting, diarrhea, abdominal pain, hyperventilation, and asterixis (a hand-flapping tremor).
      (6) Signs of metabolic alkalosis are confusion, stupor, anorexia, nausea, vomiting, hypoventilation, tremors, muscle cramps, and tetany.
   c. Nursing interventions
      (1) Monitor vital signs, noting cardiac rate and rhythm.
      (2) Monitor neurologic status for confusion and level of consciousness.
      (3) Monitor intake and output, noting gastrointestinal losses.
      (4) Monitor the serum sodium and calcium levels.
      (5) Monitor specific gravity.
      (6) Monitor arterial blood gases.
      (7) Monitor the rate of intravenous administration and titrate for volume according to physician's orders.
      (8) Maintain a patent airway.
      (9) Administer oxygen.
      (10) Medicate with analgesics.
      (11) Encourage ambulation.
      (12) Encourage consumption of foods high in protein and fresh fruits.

Postoperative Health Teaching and Discharge Planning

1. All surgical patients need discharge planning. Such planning should begin preoperatively. Most physicians have preprinted instructions that the nurse may modify to the needs of each patient.

a. Be sure to include the patient's family in the teaching.
b. Before beginning teaching, assess the person's readiness to learn, educational level, and desire to change or modify lifestyles. Many older people have no family and may need outside assistance such as that from home health or extended care. Disabled people may also need special assistance.
2. Points of instruction
   a. Care of the incision: If there is a dressing, demonstrate and then have the person demonstrate how to change the dressing before leaving the hospital. Make sure the person is given a 48-hour supply of dressings to take home. Explain how to obtain more supplies.
   b. Complications: Explain the signs and symptoms of possible complications, when to call the physician about a sign or symptom, and how to contact the physician.
   c. Medications: Explain the purpose, dosage, administration, and side effects of each drug. Help patients plan their medication schedules to coincide with their lifestyles.
   d. Diet: Contact the dietitian if a specific diet has been recommended for the person. Reinforce the importance of remaining on the diet. Answer the patient's questions on meal planning.
   e. Activity: Following any major surgery, patients should avoid any heavy lifting for at least 6 weeks. Most patients may return to work in 6 to 8 weeks.

TRANSCULTURAL CONSIDERATIONS

Be sure to assess cultural food practices and beliefs and incorporate them into dietary teaching for postoperative patients.

After any surgery, patients should resume normal activities gradually.
   f. Return appointments: Explain the importance of returning to the physician's office for a checkup, even when the person is feeling well. Make sure disabled persons have transportation.

Applying the Nursing Process

See also page 397.

NURSING DIAGNOSIS: Pain R/T surgical procedure

1. *Expected outcomes*: Following interventions, the person should be able to do the following:
   a. Express satisfaction with pain control.

HOME CARE STRATEGIES

Care of the Postsurgical Patient

Because of the invasiveness of open surgery and early discharge postoperatively, the goal of quality home care assessment and management is to ensure healing without complications.

Visual Assessment

- Observe the incision for any signs of infection, and notify the physician of possible signs.
- Instruct the patient or caregiver, or both, to inspect the incision daily for signs of infection.

Sutures

- Sutures usually are removed per physician's order 7 to 10 days after surgery.
- Tell the patient to cover the incision with plastic when showering. Plastic wrap or a slit clean bread bag taped in windowpane fashion works well.

Staples

- May be removed per physician's order 7 to 14 days after surgery. The area around the staples may become slightly reddened when staples are ready to be removed.
- When showering, the patient should apply antibacterial soap to handle and cleanse the incision well. Rinse thoroughly and pat dry.
- After staples or sutures are removed, Steri-Strips may be applied to give added support. They are especially helpful for incisions on hips, extremities, and large abdomens.

Dressings

- Follow the physician's order regarding dressings. Often incisions are left "open to air" (no dressing) if they are not draining.
- If there is a dressing, instruct the patient or caregiver to change the dressing daily and keep it clean and dry as required.
- Supplies should be assembled and stored in the patient's home in a dry, clean area, away from pets, traffic, and insects. If pets and insects are a problem, find the cleanest place possible and keep dressing packages closed and covered.

Activity

- Instruct the patient to take activity slow and easy. When climbing stairs, take 1 step at a time, resting between steps if needed. Use the hand rail.
- No lifting of 10 pounds or more. No pushing or pulling, especially with abdominal incisions.
- Frequent rest periods are important.

Nutrition

- A well-balanced diet is needed for incisional healing.
- If appetite is poor, the patient may add an oral nutritional supplement.
- Unless on a fluid restriction, the patient should drink 6 to 8 8-ounce glasses of liquid, especially water, per day. This also helps to prevent constipation.

Documentation

Make sure that you document assessment, patient teaching, and patient response in the chart.

b. Demonstrate self-control over pain through use of the patient-controlled analgesic pump or noninvasive pain control techniques.
2. *Nursing interventions*
   a. In cooperation with other team members, ensure that adequate medicinal pain control is available to the patient.
   b. Provide nonmedicinal comfort measures.
   c. Explain the workings of the patient-controlled analgesic pump, if applicable.
   d. Teach noninvasive pain control techniques.

NURSING DIAGNOSIS: Anxiety R/T postoperative treatments and possible alterations in lifestyle

1. *Expected outcomes*: Following interventions, the person should actively participate in the rehabilitation process.
2. *Nursing interventions*
   a. Encourage the patient to express feelings of concern about current loss of control and possible permanent lifestyle changes needed.
   b. Work with the patient and other team members to develop a rehabilitation plan that maximizes patient control and involvement. Explain the need for each step in the rehabilitation process.
   c. Include family members in discussions of the rehabilitation process.
   d. Refer the patient to support groups.

NURSING DIAGNOSIS: Risk for infection R/T surgical wound

1. *Expected outcomes:* Following interventions, the person should be free of infection in the wound area.
2. *Nursing interventions*
   a. Maintain aseptic technique, including frequent hand washing.
   b. Assess the wound area, drains, and dressing frequently for signs of infection.
   c. Monitor for signs and symptoms of infection, and arrange for laboratory studies, as needed.
   d. Administer prophylactic antibiotics, as ordered.

NURSING DIAGNOSIS: Ineffective airway clearance R/T ineffective coughing and deep breathing

1. *Expected outcomes:* Following interventions, the person should be able to use repositioning, coughing, deep breathing, and assistive devices to keep the airway clear.
2. *Nursing interventions*
   a. Monitor for signs of breathing distress.
   b. Assist with repositioning, if necessary.

c. Teach proper coughing and breathing techniques, and have the patient demonstrate these techniques.
   d. Observe for productive coughing.
   e. Encourage fluid consumption.

NURSING DIAGNOSIS: Dysfunctional grieving R/T loss of body part or postsurgical diagnosis

1. *Expected outcomes:* Following interventions, the person should be able to do the following:
   a. Express feelings of loss and grief and share concerns about the future.
   b. Participate actively in the rehabilitation process.
   c. Make decisions for the future.
2. *Nursing interventions*
   a. Encourage person to express feelings of loss and grief.
   b. Meet with the family apart from the patient to discuss their fears and feelings of loss and grief.
   c. Help the person set realistic goals and develop solutions to anticipated lifestyle changes.
   d. Encourage the person to continue with normal activities as long as possible.
   e. Refer to area support groups.
   f. See also the diagnosis for Anxiety and Anticipatory Grieving, and see Chapter 43.

■ CARING FOR PEOPLE UNDERGOING OUTPATIENT SURGERY

Who Has Outpatient (Ambulatory) Surgery?

1. Most surgeries are performed on an outpatient basis.
2. The American College of Surgeons does not have a predetermined list of acceptable ambulatory surgical procedures. The availability of surgeons with a particular expertise and the technology available at the setting play a vital role.
3. Because of its lower costs, ambulatory surgery is preferred by third-party payers and uninsured patients.
4. Factors in patient suitability for ambulatory surgery
   a. Health. The patient's health status is based on the physician's and anesthesiologist's judgment.
   b. Age. Each person is assessed as an individual. Extreme age alone should not be a disqualifier.
   c. Safety. The person should be at low risk to need hospitalization for recovery, and it should be unlikely that complications would develop.

Caring for People Before Outpatient Surgery

1. Most of the preoperative assessment, history and physical examination, and patient teaching discussed in the

preoperative section of this chapter is accomplished before the day of surgery by the office nurse and physician or on a preadmission visit to the hospital the week before surgery.

2. The surgeon explains the surgery, and the person signs the operative permit at the physician's office or hospital and surgical center.

3. Diagnostic and laboratory tests are performed on an outpatient basis before the day of surgery.

4. Patients should wear comfortable casual clothing and leave jewelry and valuables at home.

5. Perioperative nurses must provide postoperative teaching for patients having outpatient surgery.

6. People may learn at home from videotaped instructions, which allow them to learn at their own pace and convenience and reduces hospital costs.

7. The nurse has the person sign for receipt of all preoperative instructions and verifies that the informed consent forms are signed.

NURSE ADVISORY

Videotaped instructions for patients slated to have ambulatory surgery are useful, but they should be accompanied by written instructions.

---

8. Because most patients are discharged shortly after ambulatory surgery, it is important to perform discharge teaching preoperatively.
   a. Discuss common postoperative problems of the surgical procedure.
   b. Discuss common effects of anesthesia, such as muscle aches, headache, mild pain, and nausea and vomiting.

Caring for People During Outpatient Surgery

1. All types of anesthesia (discussed earlier) are administered to outpatient surgical patients.
   a. Selecting the best form of anesthesia to minimize pain, nausea, and vomiting and maximize alertness postoperatively is critical to successful outpatient surgery.
   b. Advantages to regional anesthesia with light sedation in ambulatory surgery include reduced likelihood of vomiting and oversedation and increased residual postoperative analgesia versus general anesthesia. These characteristics also help prevent admission to a hospital nursing unit postoperatively.
   c. When general anesthesia is necessary for outpatient surgery, it most often takes the form of "balanced anesthesia," in which intravenous and inhalation anesthetic agents are combined to produce adequate sedation with minimal aftereffects of nausea, vomiting, and pain.
      (1) Avoid routine preoperative medication if possible. When such medication is necessary, use short-acting agents in small doses (e.g., narcotics such as fentanyl or sedatives such as midazolam). These agents can decrease recovery time becase they de-

crease surgical anesthetic requirements and postoperative pain.
      (2) Administer intravenous anesthetics such as propofol (Diprivan) to maintain general anesthesia. These drugs quickly dissipate, shortening recovery time for awakening, orientation, and ambulation.
      (3) Because it produces a short period of anesthesia, methohexital (Brevital), a barbiturate induction agent, is preferable for simple, quick procedures such as cytoscopy.
      (4) Inhalation agents can provide rapid, safe anesthesia. Nitrous oxide, the most common inhalational agent administered in the ambulatory setting, provides rapid induction of and emergence from anesthesia, but it must be administered in combination with other halogenated agents such as halothane (Fluothane) or desflurane (Suprane).

2. The surgical team observes the same precautions in outpatient surgery as for any operative procedure, including strict adherence to the principles of asepsis.

Discharging People After Outpatient Surgery

1. Criteria for discharge
   a. The patient is alert.
   b. The patient has no respiratory distress.
   c. The patient has voided (sometimes not necessary).
   d. The patient is able to swallow and cough.
   e. The patient is able to ambulate.
   f. The patient has minimal pain.
   g. The patient has minimal nausea and vomiting.
   h. The patient has minimal bleeding from the incisional site.
   i. A responsible adult is available to drive the patient home.
   j. The surgeon has signed a release form.

2. Ambulatory or outpatient surgery discharge instructions
   a. The patient may not drive within 24 hours of general anesthesia or sedation.
   b. The patient may not make any major decisions for 24 hours after surgery.
   c. The patient should call the surgeon, ambulatory center, or emergency department if any postoperative problems occur.
   d. The patient should keep follow-up appointments with the surgeon.

3. A next-day follow-up call by the nurse is essential for assessing and analyzing any potential postoperative problems and allowing communication of any concerns or questions by the patient.

■ *CARING FOR SURGICAL WOUNDS*

Assisting with Surgical Wound Closure

1. Closure, the final step in surgery, is the approximating of wound edges until wound healing is complete. The

more closely the surgeon can approximate the wound edges, the smaller is the chance of scarring.

2. Surgical wounds may be closed with any of a variety of devices, including sutures, staples, skin-closure strips, and zipper-like devices (Fig. 13–7), depending on the procedure, the size and type of the wound, and the surgeon's preference. These closures provide for primary, or first intention, healing (see Chapter 37).

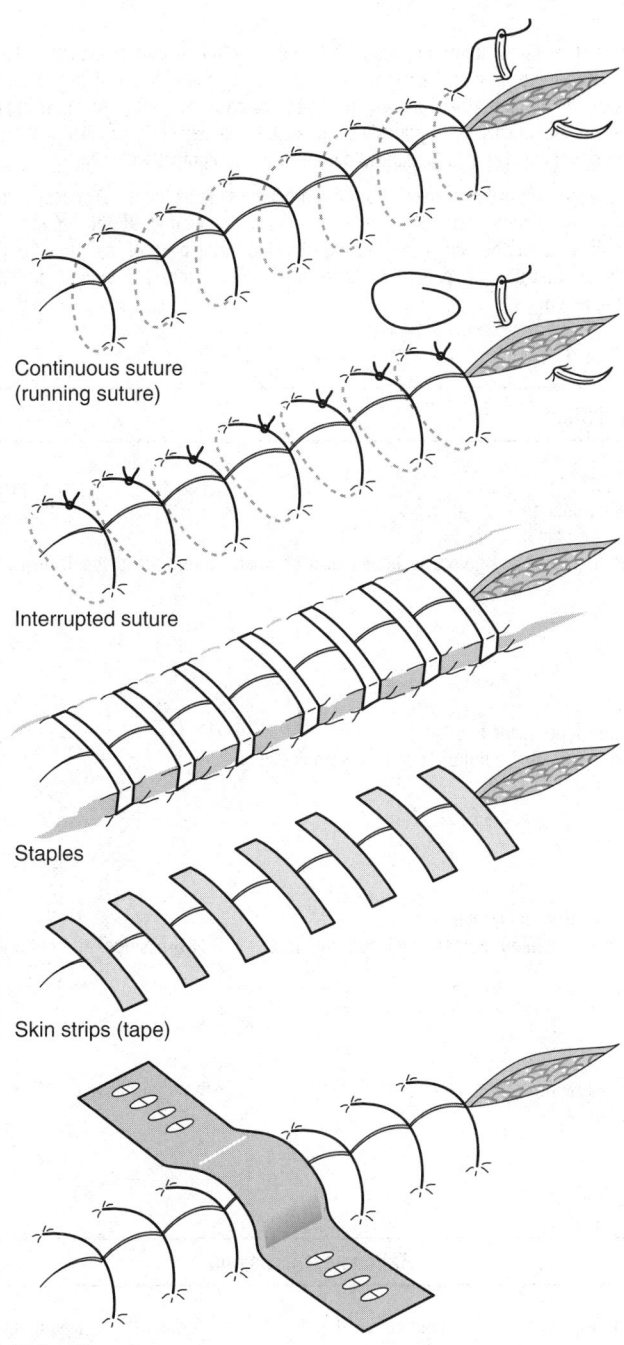

Continuous suture (running suture)

Interrupted suture

Staples

Skin strips (tape)

Retention suture

Figure 13–7. Surgical wound closure devices. (Redrawn from Black JM, and Matassarin-Jacobs E [eds]. *Luckmann and Sorensen's Medical-Surgical Nursing: A Psychophysiologic Approach.* 4th ed. Philadelphia: WB Saunders, 1993, p 427.)

3. After closure, a dressing is applied to the wound. In addition to the traditional functions of absorbing drainage and preventing wound contamination, new dressings speed the healing process.

4. To drain blood, serum, and debris from the wound site that otherwise might delay healing and foster infection, the surgeon may insert a drain. Surgical drains may be free draining, attached to suction, or self-contained drains with suction, depending on the size and type of the wound (see Chapter 27).

Surgical Wound Healing

1. Speed of wound healing depends on the following:
   a. Location of the incision
   b. Type of closure
   c. Patient's overall health and nutritional status
   d. Presence of drains and dressings
2. To promote healing, the nurse should do the following:
   a. Monitor drains and assess drainage amount, color, and consistency.
   b. Observe the wound for
      (1) Approximation of the suture line.
      (2) Edema or bleeding.
      (3) Signs of infection.
   c. Remove drains when the drainage amount becomes insignificant.
   d. Change dressings as needed or as directed (Procedure 13–1).

Complications of Surgical Wounds

1. Complications include infection, wound dehiscence, and wound evisceration.
2. Infection, a serious threat in all wounds, can be averted through proper aseptic technique and monitoring of wounds, drains, and dressings.
   a. Assessment: Look for a fever that spikes in the afternoon and returns to normal by the next morning, tenderness and pain at the wound site, elevated white blood cell count, inflamed and edematous skin, and tight skin sutures.
   b. Nursing interventions
      (1) Monitor drains and ensure that they are patent and functioning properly; keep drains and tubes away from the incision.
      (2) Change dressing as ordered and when it becomes wet.
      (3) Administer antibiotics, as ordered.
   c. High-risk factors for surgical wound infection
      (1) Obesity, which makes approximation of wound edges difficult
      (2) Advanced age, which may be accompanied by lowered defenses against infection
      (3) Presence of debilitating conditions (such as cancer

Procedure 13-1
Changing a Surgical Dressing

Definition/Purposes	To cover wound with a dry gauze sterile dressing. The procedure is done by replacing soiled dressings (usually with physician's permission) for the individual's physical and esthetic comfort. The procedure provides the opportunity to observe wound, assess healing, and remove moist dressing (thus reducing potential for wound contamination). Dressing protects skin around wound, absorbs drainage, and acts as a pressure dressing to minimize bleeding and edema.
Contraindications/Cautions	Avoid communicating any negative personal feelings about the wound. Surgeons often want to change initial postoperative dressings. Nurses usually change subsequent dressings as needed. If dressing is soiled but cannot be changed, reinforce it to protect the wound, monitor drainage, and maintain comfort. Be gentle. Areas around the wound may be hypersensitive to touch, chemicals, and adhesives. If specific sensitivities or allergies are known, avoid precipitating agents. Wound drainage may irritate skin. Minimize drainage contact with skin.
Teaching/Learning Guidelines	Providing information about dressing change importance may promote procedure acceptance. Discuss pain concerns and measures to reduce discomfort. The patient may not want to see the wound. If the wound is observed by the patient or family member, describe signs of healing. Explain principles of asepsis used. Emphasize ways the person can participate. Instruct the patient to keep hands away from the wound during dressing change to prevent wound contamination.

Preliminary Activities

Assessment/Planning	• Verify need for dressing change. • Check chart for orders relative to dressing change. • Note individual preferences on nursing care plan. • Plan activity at the least disruptive time (e.g., not just before or after meals or when visitors are present, or late at night). • Assess type, size, numbers of dressing needed. • Provide privacy. • Create clean, dry work space.
Equipment/Supplies	• Sterile dressing tray • Additional sterile dressings of number and type needed • Solution used to clean wound should be a nonionic solution, such as isotonic saline • Tape, hypoallergenic • Clean gloves—1 pair • Sterile gloves—2 pairs • Generic tape remover, if needed • 1 sterile towel • Waterproof bag to hold used dressing and used equipment • Sterile instrument dressing set, if needed, containing: Forceps, scissors, hemostat, 4 × 4 dressings, and cotton-tipped applicators • Ointment, if prescribed • Gauze ties, if needed
Preparation of the Person	• Explain purposes of dressing change. • Assess with person need for analgesic. Allow time for analgesic to become effective before starting (e.g., 15 to 20 minutes for parenteral, 1 hour for oral).

Procedure

Action	Rationale/Discussion
1. Wash hands carefully.	1. Reduces microorganisms on hands. Reduces potential for wound infection.
2. Screen, position, and drape person properly.	2. Provides privacy. Enhances emotional and physical comfort. Person should be comfortable, with dressing site easily accessible to nurse.
3. Prepare equipment using sterile technique.	3. Prevents infection.
4. Gently fold bedclothes and gown back, exposing dressing.	4. Minimize air currents. Gentleness promotes comfort.

P

Procedure 13–1

(continued)

Action	Rationale/Discussion
5. Loosen tape. Begin at edge away from wound center. Pull skin away from tape, moving in direction toward wound.	5. Prevents wound tension. Pulling skin away (instead of tape away) prevents tearing skin. Pulling in direction away from wound edges would pull apart healing (fibrin network) wound.
6. Remove soiled dressing. Use clean gloves or forceps to remove dressing. Place old dressing inside plastic bag. May use plastic bag that covered sterile dressing set.	6. Dressing is contaminated. Using gloves or forceps prevents organisms from transferring to nurse's hands and being spread. Gentleness and not pulling off adhering (sticking) dressing protects healing and reduces discomfort.
7. If dressing adheres to wound, moisten with sterile saline until dressing lifts off easily.	7. Forceful dressing removal disrupts healing process.
8. Put on sterile gloves.	8. Use sterile gloves to prevent microorganisms from being introduced to the wound surface.
9. Thoroughly assess wound, using your eyes, nose, and gentle palpation.	9. Evaluate for healing progress and complications.
10. If necessary, remove adhesive around wound with generic tape remover. Be gentle.	10. Do not remove adhesive each time unless skin problem is present. Avoid acetone; it may chemically damage the skin or wound.
11. Use sterile isotonic saline (or povidone-iodine or other antiseptic) to clean wound edges and surrounding skin if necessary. Note: antiseptics should be used in the wound bed only in infected wounds and must be ordered by the physician. With each swab, clean downward with a single stroke. Clean from center of wound to periphery. Discard swab after each stroke and use a new swab.	11. Consider wound line cleaner than skin area. Skin pathogens could further infect wound. Intact skin around wound usually provides barrier from infected wound.
12. Apply ointment, if prescribed.	12. Apply ointment to dressing if difficult to apply to wound.
13. Remove gloves and discard into bag with used dressing and swabs.	13. Gloves are contaminated from skin cleansing.
14. Apply sterile dressing after regloving or by using sterile hemostat or forceps. Place small dressing directly over wound. Once dressing is placed, do not reposition it. Cover with larger dressing as necessary. Place additional dressings on dependent parts to collect drainage.	14. Moving dressing after placement moves contaminants from skin to wound. Contains drainage in dressing.
15. Anchor dressing securely with tape or gauze ties.	15. Nonallergenic tape reduces risk of skin breakdown. For dressings needing frequent changing, use Montgomery straps and ties.
16. Replace covers over person and position as needed.	16. Increases comfort.
17. Collect used equipment for removal. Discard disposable equipment into waterproof bag. Wrap nondisposable equipment in sterile towel for return to appropriate area.	17. Soiled dressings and used equipment are contaminated. Prevents spread of pathogens to environment, self, and others.
18. Wash hands thoroughly.	18. Reduces number of microorganisms and contamination of self and others.
19. Gently reposition gown and bedclothes.	19. Movement of air disseminates microorganisms.

Final Activities

Assess individual for comfort and safety. Make sure bed is at desirable height and position and bedside stand with personal effects within reach. Replace side rails if indicated. Return nondisposable instruments and bowl to central service for cleaning and reprocessing; discard towel in laundry. Later, return to room to assess individual and security and comfort of dressing. *Documentation:* drainage character and amount, condition of wound and surrounding tissue, person's responses to dressing change (e.g., emotional response, local pain, generalized discomfort). Note on nursing care plan points of special importance to individual regarding dressing change.

Modified from Bolander VB. *Sorensen and Luckmann's Basic Nursing: A Psychophysiologic Approach.* 3rd ed. Philadelphia: WB Saunders, 1994, pp. 1370–1373.

and malnutrition), chronic diseases (such as diabetes mellitus, ulcerative colitis, and aplastic anemia), or recent therapy with steroids, irradiation, or anticancer drugs, all of which lower resistance to infection

(4) Lengthy, complicated operations, which lower resistance to infection and leave tissues exposed for longer periods of time

(5) Preoperative organ rupture or sepsis, as in the

case of a ruptured appendix or perforated ulcer, which contaminates the wound
3. Wound dehiscence (an opening of the wound edges) and wound evisceration (protrusion of internal organs through an opening in wound edges) are most common among patients who are obese, have abdominal surgery, or have decreased wound healing ability, such as in diabetic patients (Fig. 13–8).
   a. Assessment: Examine for discharge of serosanguineous fluid from a previously dry wound and appearance of loops of bowel or other wound contents. The patient may report a popping sensation after coughing or turning.
   b. Nursing interventions
      (1) Monitor nasogastic tubes for patency.
      (2) Prevent wound infections.
      (3) Prevent vomiting and retching.
      (4) Teach the person to splint the incision when coughing.
      (5) Cover the wound with sterile normal saline.
      (6) If an abdominal wound dehisces, place the person in a low Fowler's position with knees bent to decrease abdominal tension.
      (7) If a wound eviscerates, treat signs of shock and call the surgeon immediately. *Wound evisceration is a medical emergency.*

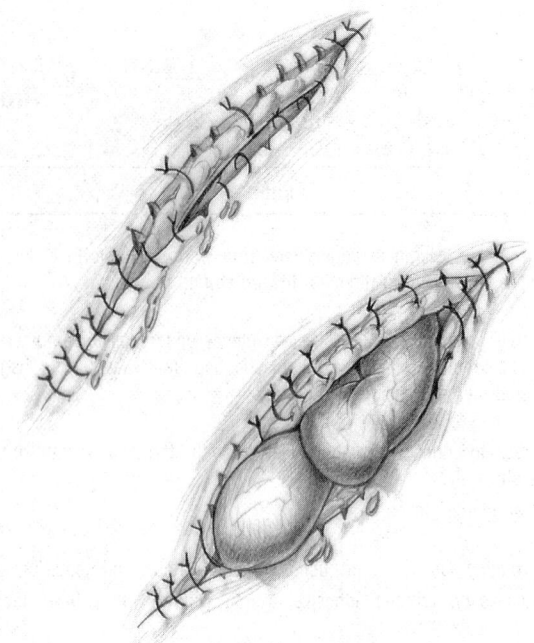

Figure 13–8. Wound dehiscence and evisceration. (Redrawn from Black JM, and Matassarin-Jacobs E [eds]. *Luckmann and Sorensen's Medical-Surgical Nursing: A Psychophysiologic Approach.* 4th ed. Philadelphia: WB Saunders, 1993, p 439.)

Bibliography

Books

Burden N. **Ambulatory Surgical Nursing.** Philadelphia: WB Saunders, 1993.

Burrell L (ed). *Adult Nursing in Hospital and Community Settings.* Norwalk, CT: Appleton & Lange, 1992.

Fairchild S. *Perioperative Nursing: Principles and Practice.* Boston: Jones & Bartlett, 1993.

Flynn J, and Hackel R. *Technological Foundations in Nursing.* Norwalk, CT: Appleton & Lange, 1990.

Frost E. *Post Anesthesia Care Unit: Current Practices.* St. Louis: CV Mosby, 1990.

Groah LK. *Operating Room Nursing: Perioperative Practice.* 2nd ed. Norwalk, CT: Appleton & Lange, 1990.

Kneedler JK, and Dodge GH (eds). *Perioperative Patient Care: The Nursing Perspective.* 3rd ed. Boston: Jones & Bartlett, 1993.

Litwack K. *Post Anesthesia Care Nursing.* St. Louis: CV Mosby, 1994.

Meeker M, and Rothrock J. *Alexander's Care of the Patient in Surgery.* 9th ed. St. Louis: CV Mosby, 1991.

Porth C. *Pathophysiology, Concepts of Altered Health States.* 3rd ed. Philadelphia: JB Lippincott, 1990.

Rothrock J. *Perioperative Nursing Care Planning.* St. Louis: CV Mosby, 1991.

Sabiston D. (ed). *Textbook of Surgery.* 14th ed. Philadelphia: WB Saunders, 1991.

Shekleton M, and Litwack K. *Critical Care Nursing of the Surgical Patient.* Philadelphia: WB Saunders, 1991.

Journal Articles

Caring for People Before Surgery

Chalfin D. Preoperative evaluation and postoperative care of the elderly patient undergoing major surgery. *Clin Geriatr Med* 10(1):51–70, 1994.

Goodwin S. From "my patient" to "our patient." *J Post Anesthesia Nurs* 10(2):65–66, 1995.

Longinow L, and Rzeszewski L. The holding room: A preoperative advantage. *AORN J* 57(4):914–925, 1993.

Yale E. Preoperative teaching strategy: Videotapes for home viewing. *AORN J* 57(4):901–908, 1993.

Caring for People During Surgery

Council on Scientific Affairs. The use of pulse oximetry during conscious sedation. *JAMA* 270(12):1463–1468, 1993.

Rivellini D. Local and regional anesthesia: Nursing implications. *Nurs Clin North Am* 28(3):547–572, 1993.

Caring for People After Surgery

Litwack-Saleh K. The elderly patient in the post anesthesia care unit. *Nurs Clin North Am* 28(3):507–518, 1993.

Mamaril M. Standard of care: Legal implications in the postanesthesia care unit. *J Post Anesth Nurs* 8(1):13–20, 1993.

McCaffery M. Giving narcotics for pain: A problem solver handbook. *Nursing 89* 19:161, 1989.

McGuire L. Administering analgesics: Which drugs are right for your patient? *Nursing 90* 20:34, 1990.

Caring for People Undergoing Outpatient Surgery

Parnass S. Ambulatory surgical patient priorities. *Nurs Clin North Am* 28(3):531–545, 1993.

Pica-Furey W. Ambulatory surgery—Hospital-based vs freestanding. *AORN J* 57(5):1119–1128, 1993.

Renwick P. Time management in a day surgery unit. *Nurs Stand* 7(4):31–34, 1992.

Wiseman S. Patient advocacy: The essence of perioperative nursing in ambulatory surgery. *AORN J* 51:754, 1990.

Agencies and Resources

American Society of Post Anesthesia
  Nurses
11512 Allecingie Parkway
Richmond, VA 23235
(804) 379–5516

Association of Operating Room Nurses
2170 South Parker Road
Suite 300
Denver, CO 80231–5711
(303) 755–6300

Association for Practitioners in Infection
  Control
505 East Hawley Street
Mundelein, IL 60060
(708) 949–6052

Caring for People with Special Developmental Needs and Problems

IV

14
Caring for Families in the Childbearing Cycle

◼ CARING FOR PERSONS SEEKING FAMILY PLANNING HELP

Definitions

1. **Family planning** is usually defined as the purposeful regulation of conception, the voluntary avoidance or delay of pregnancy, or the use of some method or device to avoid pregnancy.
2. Family planning may also refer to preconception planning, wherein the woman or couple gathers information to prepare for pregnancy and parenting.

Transcultural Considerations

1. The value placed on children
   a. The information society middle- and upper-class view of children and childbearing.
      (1) The value of children has increased over the past few years.
      (2) Overall, the birth rate has decreased, and couples have fewer children than in the past.
      (3) The cost of raising a child has increased significantly.
      (4) Each child becomes more important when there are fewer children in a family.
      (5) Many couples are delaying childbearing until later.
      (6) The increased value placed on children has given many people the desire to have a "perfect" child. Parents become very involved in the pregnancy and birth. Many parents expect everything to be perfect if they invest their time and energy. They do not expect problems.
   b. The working-class view of children may vary; however, the following values are commonly held:
      (1) Many families need or want children to fulfill family work roles.
      (2) Having children is seen as an integral aspect of establishing a family.
2. The roles of women and the family
   a. In today's society, women have many options open to them.

   b. A growing number of women are delaying childbearing until they are well into their 30s.
   c. An increasing number of women are entering the work force because they desire to have a career or must work to support their families.
   d. There are a variety of family structures in today's society: single-parent families, childless couples, couples with children, heterosexual and homosexual families, and blended families.
   e. The number of single-parent families is growing.
3. Specific cultural beliefs about family planning
   a. People's views about family planning may be influenced by the following:
      (1) The length of time they have participated in the dominant culture
      (2) Whether they are a 1st-, 2nd-, or 3rd-generation citizen
      (3) The availability of their original cultural support system

Assessment

1. Health history: Ascertain whether the woman has cardiovascular disease, hypertension, or diabetes mellitus; the frequency with which she has urinary tract infections and headaches; whether she has had any sexually transmitted infections; and whether she smokes.
   a. If preconception counseling is the goal, it is important to identify any disease states and provide information regarding maximizing physical and nutritional health status.
   b. If fertility control is the goal, it is important to identify the woman's current health status so that you may provide information on the fertility control methods that are the most appropriate and safest for her.
2. Physical examination: Measure the woman's height, weight, and blood pressure, and examine the thyroid, breasts, uterus, and other reproductive organs.
3. Psychosocial assessment: Explore the woman's or couple's views on childbearing and fertility control.
   a. Is the woman or couple interested in preconception planning or fertility control?
   b. What are the woman's or couple's beliefs and values regarding childbirth?

c. Which member of the couple is responsible for communication?

d. Determine the woman's or couple's beliefs regarding nutrition, the types of food eaten, activity and rest patterns, health-related routines, medications taken, health care providers seen, and specific pregnancy and childbirth practices (e.g., spiritual beliefs, cultural taboos).

e. What are the implications of the woman's or couple's educational level, financial resources, and desire regarding the convenience of the fertility control method used (Table 14-1)?

Contraceptive Options

1. Long-term abstinence: Many teens and young women and men choose abstinence because of philosophic or religious beliefs. These individuals benefit from support from peers and other groups with similar beliefs.

2. Periodic ("rhythm") abstinence, also called the calendar, cervical mucus, or symptothermal method
   a. This method is accepted by all religious groups.
   b. Abstinence from sex is practiced during the time of ovulation in each menstrual cycle. The time of ovulation may be determined by charting the cycle on the calendar, examining the cervical mucus, or using the symptothermal method.
      (1) The characteristics of the cervical mucus are assessed by the woman. Mucus that is abundant, clear, thin, and stringy indicates ovulation. Intercourse is avoided at this time.
      (2) The symptothermal method usually combines examining the cervical mucus method and taking the basal body temperature.
   c. Risks and disadvantages
      (1) Among 100 women using the periodic abstinence method for 1 year, 40 pregnancies are likely to occur.
      (2) Each woman's cycle is variable, and the method depends on some regularity of pattern. If the woman's pattern is variable, the length of time of abstinence may be 14 days or more per cycle.
   d. Implications for postpartum use: Until menses and ovulation are reestablished, the criteria for using the method cannot be met.

3. Barrier methods
   a. Diaphragm
      (1) A round latex device is inserted into the vagina. The diaphragm is placed so that it fits behind the cervix and up under the symphysis pubis.
      (2) Risks and disadvantages
         • The failure rate ranges from 2 to 23 percent.
         • The incidence of side effects is very small, but vaginal irritation from latex rubber or spermicidal cream may occur.
         • Urinary tract infections are twice as common in women who use diaphragms as they are in women who use oral contraceptives.
         • The diaphragm must be inserted before intercourse and left in place for 6 hours. It may be dislodged from the cervix if placed improperly, and pregnancy may result.
         • The diaphragm is best if used in conjunction with a spermicidal jelly or cream.
         • Changes in the size of the vaginal vault with a weight loss of 30 pounds or more require refitting.
      (3) Implications for postpartum use
         • The diaphragm must be refitted after each birth.
         • It may be used while breast-feeding.
   b. Cervical cap
      (1) Before intercourse, a cap is inserted into the vagina and placed over the cervix and may be left in place for up to 36 hours. It must be left in place at least 6 hours past intercourse.
      (2) Risks and disadvantages
         • The failure rate is 18 percent.
         • The cervical cap is more difficult than a diaphragm to insert.
      (3) Implications for postpartum use
         • The cervical cap must be refitted after each birth.
         • The cervical cap may be used while breast-feeding.
   c. Condoms
      (1) There are both male and female condoms.
      (2) The male condom is a latex sheath that is rolled onto the erect penis. The purpose of the male condom is 2-fold: to act as a receptacle for ejaculate during intercourse and to protect both parties from infections.
      (3) The female condom is a larger latex sheath with a large soft ring around the outer edge. The female

Table 14-1. Characteristics of Commonly Used Contraceptive Methods

Method	Unit Cost ($)	Annual Cost (Based on 100 acts of intercourse)	Return of Fertility After Use Is Discontinued	HIV/STD Protection	Use During Lactation
Male condom	$0.50	$50	Immediate	Yes	Yes
Female condom	$2.50	$250	Immediate	Yes	Yes
Diaphragm	$20 plus $50–150 for fitting	$85 if spermicide is used	Immediate	No	Yes
Combined oral contraceptives	$10–20 per cycle	$130–260	Delayed, possibly 2–3 months	No	No
Norplant	$350/kit plus $150–250 for insertion or removal	$130–170 per year if retained for 5 years	Delayed, possibly 2–3 months	No	Yes

LEARNING/TEACHING GUIDELINES
for Self-Care with an Intrauterine Device

General Overview

1. Describe the advantages and disadvantages of using an intrauterine device (IUD) for contraception.
2. Inform the woman that the IUD will be inserted during a menstrual period to ensure that a pregnancy is not currently present. Provide an opportunity for the woman to ask questions and to share concerns regarding the timing of this procedure.

Self-Care Instructions

1. The IUD has a string on the end, which protrudes through the cervix. Immediately after insertion, the care provider clips the string so that it extends just a short distance below the cervix. The woman should check for the presence of the string at the end of each menses by inserting a clean finger into her vagina and feeling for the string. If the string has been cut very short, a pricking type sensation may be felt.
2. If the woman does not feel the string, she should immediately obtain an appointment with her care provider and use an alternative method of contraception until her appointment.

---

condom is inserted into the vagina with the assistance of a plastic device or by hand. The larger outer ring serves to protect the vulva from exposure to any infections that may be present on the male pubic area and to collect the ejaculate during intercourse.

(4) Risks and disadvantages
- The failure rate is 12 percent for the male condom and 18 percent for the female condom.
- The male condom must be placed on the penis after erection, a process some couples find distracting. The condom must be removed carefully after intercourse because the penis is not erect, and if the ejaculate in the condom spills into the vagina, pregnancy may result.
- The female condom must be placed in the vagina just before intercourse, a process some couples may find distracting. It must also be removed carefully after intercourse to avoid spillage of the ejaculate contained within it.
- Some people have difficulty with the manipulating of the penis or vagina that using either the male or the female condom requires.
- Some couples believe that the male condom will come off the penis during intercourse and enter the woman's body.
- Use of the male condom may be discouraged because of the male belief that the condom reduces penile sensation during intercourse and thereby decreases pleasure.

(5) Implications for postpartum use
- No problems have been noted.
- A prescription is not required, and condoms may be used while breast-feeding.

4. Oral contraceptives
   a. Birth control pills contain hormonal substances that suppress ovulation.
   b. Risks and disadvantages
      (1) The failure rate for oral contraceptives is 3 percent.
      (2) Discomforts such as breast tenderness, fatigue, nausea, and breakthrough bleeding may occur for the first 3 cycles.
      (3) More serious risks are blood clots, gallbladder disease, cerebral vascular accident, chlamydial cervicitis, and hepatocellular adenomas.
      (4) Low-dose oral contraceptives may prevent subsequent pregnancy by altering the endometrium rather than suppressing ovulation.
   c. Implications for postpartum use: The minipill needs to be used if lactation is planned.

5. Intrauterine device
   a. An intrauterine device (IUD) is inserted into the uterine cavity by a health care professional and remains in the uterus for a few years.
   b. A string attached to the IUD protrudes through the cervix; the woman can feel for this string on a periodic basis to ascertain that the IUD is still present.
   c. Risks and disadvantages
      (1) The failure rate for IUDs is 3 percent.
      (2) An IUD may increase the risk of infection or may cause increased menstrual flow or cramping.
      (3) An IUD may be expelled from the uterus without the woman's knowing it. The woman needs to be taught to check for the string every month to make sure the IUD is still present (Learning/Teaching Guidelines for Self-Care with an Intrauterine Device).
   d. Implications for postpartum use: The IUD is not recommended for postpartum use.

6. Long-acting steroids
   a. Levonorgestrel implants (Norplant)
      (1) A levonorgestrel implant is a subdermal implant of capsules that contain long-acting, low-dose, reversible progestin.
      (2) Capsules are implanted in the upper inner aspect of the woman's arm under local anesthesia within the first 7 days of the menstrual cycle to ensure she is not pregnant. The implant may remain in place for 5 years.

(3) Risks and disadvantages
  • The failure rate for implants is less than 1 percent.
  • The long-acting drug requires implantation by a skilled health professional.
  • Although the cost of Norplant is approximately half that of a 5-year supply of contraceptive pills, the total cost must usually be paid before insertion.
  • The implant may affect the amount and regularity of menstrual flow for the first 6 to 9 months after insertion.
  • Adolescents may fear the insertion procedure, the visibility of the implant on their arm, and the irregular bleeding. An explanation of the side effects and insertion procedure may reduce fears.
  • Because the implant remains in place for 5 years, the adolescent or woman may not return for ongoing health checks.
  • The implant is contraindicated for persons with hypertension, cardiovascular disease, diabetes, thrombotic disease, acute liver dysfunction, or breast disease.
  • Insertion of Norplant has been court ordered for some women found guilty of child abuse or neglect. Court-ordered insertion of Norplant as a condition of probation, the possibility that insertion may be required to maintain government assistance, and increased use of implants by women of low socioeconomic status and adolescents, raise a variety of ethical dilemmas.
(4) Implications for postpartum use: Current research indicates that Norplant may be inserted within 48 hours after birth with no increased incidence of immediate acute hemorrhage or decrease of hemoglobin at 4 to 6 weeks postpartum. Some women report a significant increase in the incidence of headaches.
  b. Depo-Provera
  (1) Depo-Provera is a progestin-only, long-acting intramuscular injection.
  (2) Effective contraception is maintained for 3 or 4 months.
  (3) Risks and disadvantages
    • The failure rate is less than 1 percent.
    • Depo-Provera requires injections that cannot be reversed for the duration of the medication.
    • Side effects include irregular menstrual bleeding, breast tenderness, weight gain, and depression.
  (4) Implications for postpartum use: Depo-Provera is not recommended for postpartum use.
7. Sterilization: Sterilization is achieved by a vasectomy in the male and a tubal ligation in the female. Both of these surgical methods need to be considered permanent methods of contraception, although some procedures may be used to reverse initial sterilization (see Chapter 31).

Infertility

1. Infertility is the inability of a couple to conceive after 1 year of unprotected intercourse or the inability to carry a pregnancy long enough for the baby to be born and live. Infertility may be primary or secondary.
   a. Primary infertility: The couple has never conceived.
   b. Secondary infertility: The couple has previously conceived but is subsequently unable to conceive within 12 months of unprotected intercourse.
2. Special diagnostic tests: The order in which the tests are completed depends on the woman's history.
   a. A basal body temperature chart helps confirm ovulation, identifies the time of ovulation (immediately after ovulation, a sustained 0.4–0.6 degree Fahrenheit rise in temperature occurs), and provides data to assist in the interpretation of other infertility tests.
   b. Postcoital test
     (1) The postcoital test is completed just before anticipated ovulation.
     (2) The couple refrains from intercourse for 1 to 2 days before the test and then has intercourse without lubricant 2 to 10 hours before an office examination.
     (3) The health care practitioner obtains a sample of vaginal mucus and examines it for the quality of the mucus and the number and quality of sperm.
   c. Semen analysis: Semen analysis is completed on a semen specimen obtained by masturbation or collected in a condom during intercourse. The semen is examined for the following characteristics:
     (1) Volume: 2 to 5 ml
     (2) pH: 7 to 8
     (3) Count: more than 20 million per ml
     (4) Motility: greater than 50 to 60 percent
     (5) Morphology: greater than 50 percent have normal form
     (6) Quality of motion
   d. Endometrial biopsy: Endometrial biopsy is performed late in the menstrual cycle to verify that ovulation has occurred and to determine the adequacy of hormone production after ovulation.
   e. Hysterosalpingogram
     (1) A hysterosalpingogram is obtained by radiograph after menses but before ovulation.
     (2) Dye is placed in the uterus to outline its shape and the patency of the fallopian tubes.
   f. Laser laparoscopy
     (1) Laser laparoscopy is performed early in the menstrual cycle, after menses.
     (2) The laparoscope is inserted into the abdomen through a small incision made near the naval.
     (3) The test permits visibility of the uterus and fallopian tubes and identification of endometriosis, pelvic adhesions or scarring, and tubal disease.
3. Interventions
   a. Artificial insemination
     (1) Semen from the husband or a donor is deposited in the cervix or uterus.
     (2) Artificial insemination allows the sperm to be placed closer to the ovum.
   b. Fertility drugs
     (1) Drugs that may be used to induce ovulation include cyclic estrogen or progesterone, progesterone, clomiphene (Clomid), urofollitropin (Metro-

din), menotropins (Pergonal), and the gonadotropin-releasing hormone pump.

    (2) Luteal-phase support may be treated with human chorionic gonadotropin (Profasi) or progesterone vaginal suppositories.

c. Assisted reproductive technology: Ova are removed from the ovary, and fertilization occurs outside the female's body. The ova may be used immediately or frozen for later use (cryopreservation mechanism). Three types of assisted reproductive technology are currently in use:

    (1) In vitro fertilization, in which the embryo is transferred into the uterus

    (2) Gamete intrafallopian transfer, in which a mature ovum or sperm is transferred into the fallopian tube

    (3) Zygote intrafallopian transfer, in which the zygotes are transferred into the fallopian tube

d. Surrogate mothers

    (1) In some cases, the woman or couple may choose to have another woman become impregnated by donor insemination or oocyte or embryo donation. In this situation, the resulting child has a biologic connection with 1 or both of the requesting parents.

    (2) Surrogacy raises many issues for all parties involved. Extensive screening and counseling are important parts of this process, as is exploration of legal and ethical concerns.

e. Adoption: Some couples seek adoption after a period of unsuccessful infertility treatment.

Unwanted Pregnancies

1. Adoption: Sometimes when an unplanned pregnancy occurs, the teenager or woman chooses to continue the pregnancy but is not able to keep her baby after the birth. Adoption or relinquishment is a choice in this case. Adoption may be open or closed.

a. In open adoption, the mother has the opportunity to maintain contact with the baby and the new parents in a variety of ways.

b. In closed adoption, the mother relinquishes her rights to the child and in many instances does not ever see the child again.

2. Elective termination of pregnancy (induced or therapeutic abortion)

a. Elective termination of pregnancy is legal in the United States through the 2nd trimester.

b. Some teenagers or women who become pregnant do not wish or are unable to continue the pregnancy and may seek an abortion. Most abortions are completed in the 1st trimester (weeks 1–13); fewer are performed in the 2nd trimester.

c. Therapeutic abortion is an emotionally charged procedure for the teen or woman and partner or family, if involved. The decision to abort is rarely made lightly. Abortion is also an emotionally charged issue for health care professionals and for the public at large. As members of society, health care professionals struggle with their own beliefs and values surrounding this issue.

d. Methods

    (1) Before 8 weeks' gestation, aspiration of the uterine contents by vacuum curettage is the current preferred method.

    (2) From 8 to 12 weeks' gestation, curettage and vacuum aspiration or dilation and curettage of the uterus are done.

    (3) In the 2nd trimester (weeks 13–14 through 24), the methods include intra-amniotic prostaglandin injection, intra-amniotic injection of saline and urea, and occasionally a dilation and curettage.

    (4) Mifepristone (RU-486) has been used extensively in France and other European countries for early induced abortion with minimal maternal side effects and is currently being used on an experimental basis in the United States.

Public Health Considerations

1. Preventing teenage pregnancies

a. The number of teenage pregnancies in the United States continues to fluctuate, but in comparison with other industrialized countries, such as England, France, and the Netherlands, it is very high.

b. Teen pregnancy continues to be a complex issue as society tries to find the best approach for prevention.

    (1) Countries with low teen pregnancy rates have some social elements in common, such as offering sex education within the school system and making contraceptive methods available to teens who choose to be sexually active.

    (2) In the United States, some people believe that making sex education and contraceptives readily available would decrease the teen pregnancy rate. Others argue that providing information about sex and making contraceptives available only encourage teen pregnancy, and they would rather devote their energies to promoting abstinence.

2. Promoting the use of contraception

a. Many types of contraceptive devices are currently available. Whether contraceptives are used is influenced by many factors, such as the age and developmental status of the couple, personal beliefs and values, education regarding the various contraceptive methods, and the availability of the methods (including actual availability, access to care, and economic access).

b. The promotion of contraceptive use sometimes brings forward questions regarding philosophical beliefs. You need to be able to acknowledge many belief systems when you are counseling patients. You can do this if you consider the following:

    (1) Your own belief system—It is important that you identify your own beliefs, so that you can prevent them from influencing the information you provide to the teen, woman, or couple.

    (2) The teen's, woman's, or couple's beliefs regarding what methods are acceptable

(3) The availability of and access to information and care

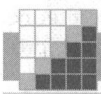

LEGAL AND ETHICAL CONSIDERATIONS

In most all situations, the teen is considered to be in a patient-caregiver situation and can receive information regarding contraceptive methods. If the teen seeks health care, a contraceptive method may be dispensed.

3. Providing public education programs: Information regarding the types and availability of fertility control needs to be available for teens, women, men, and couples who seek to make informed choices in their sexual practices.

NURSE ADVISORY

Professional nurses should note that the 1990 National Academy of Science reported that contraceptive research has essentially come to a standstill in the United States. It takes up to $50 million and 15 years for a new contraceptive to be developed and move through the U.S. Food and Drug Administration approval process, and as of 1990, only 1 pharmaceutical firm was doing research.

◼ OVERVIEW OF THE CHILDBEARING CYCLE

Definitions

1. Pregnancy is 40 weeks in length from the 1st day of the last menstrual period. The 9 calendar months are divided into 3-month segments called the 1st, 2nd, and 3rd **trimesters.** Each trimester is approximately 13 weeks long.
2. Important terms used in maternal-child nursing
   a. Gestation: the number of weeks that have elapsed since the 1st day of the last menstrual period. Note that obstetricians, nurse midwives, and nurse practitioners refer to gestation with this definition. Neonatologists, however, usually refer to gestation by postconception dates. In a woman with a 28-day menstrual cycle this results in a discrepancy of 2 weeks (8 weeks of gestation by menstrual dates is the same as 6 weeks' postconception gestation).
   b. Abortion: a pregnancy that ends before the end of the 20th week of gestation
   c. Term: the expected (normal) length of gestation, which is 38 to 42 weeks
   d. Preterm or premature labor: labor that occurs after the 20th week of gestation and before 37 completed weeks (37 weeks and 7 days) of gestation
   e. Postterm labor: labor that extends past 42 weeks of gestation (or exceeds 294 days past the 1st day of the last menstrual period); may also be referred to as postdate pregnancy.

f. Stillbirth: a fetus that is born dead after 20 weeks of gestation
g. Gravida: a pregnancy, regardless of its duration or outcome
h. Nulligravida: a woman who has never been pregnant
i. Primigravida: a woman who is pregnant for the 1st time
j. Multigravida: a woman who is in her 2nd or subsequent pregnancy
k. Para: a past pregnancy that passed 20 weeks of gestation and resulted in birth, regardless of whether the fetus was born alive or dead and the number of fetuses in that pregnancy. To clarify the term para further, the TPAL labeling system was developed:
   (1) T = term pregnancies
   (2) P = preterm births
   (3) A = abortions
   (4) L = living children born to that woman. For example, a woman pregnant for the 2nd time who has a set of 2-year-old twins at home would be: Gravida-2, Para-1, T-1, P-0, A-0, L-2.
l. Primipara: a woman who has given birth once past 20 weeks of gestation, regardless of whether the fetus or newborn was born alive or dead and regardless of the number of fetuses
m. Multipara: a woman who has had 2 births of fetuses or neonates that developed past the point of viability

Maternal Changes During Pregnancy

Box 14-1 presents the physiologic changes that occur in the mother during each trimester.

1. Reproductive system changes
   a. Uterus
      (1) The prepregnant uterus is small and pear shaped, measures 7.5 × 5 × 2.5 cm, and weighs about 60 gm (2 oz). At the end of pregnancy, the uterus is approximately 28 × 24 × 21 cm and weighs approximately 1000 gm (2.2 lb). The capacity of the uterus increases from 10 ml (2 teaspoons) to 5 liters or more.
      (2) The uterine walls thin as pregnancy progresses. The fetus can be palpated through the uterine wall.
      (3) Braxton Hicks contractions occur intermittently during pregnancy.
   b. Cervix
      (1) The increased estrogen level induces changes in the cervix including softening (Goodell's sign) and hyperemia resulting in a deep bluish color (Chadwick's sign) and softening of the isthmus (Hegar's sign).
      (2) The stimulation of the endocervical glands causes the secretion of mucus, creating a mucus plug and mucorrhea.
   c. Ovaries
      (1) The ovaries cease ovum production because of the high levels of progesterone and estrogen, which causes suppression of follicle-stimulating hormone and luteinizing hormone.

BOX 14–1. Physiologic Changes in Each Trimester

First Trimester
(1–3 months)

- Amenorrhea
- Pregnancy tests may be used from 7–14 days after ovulation
- Breasts begin to enlarge, may feel tender, tingly
- Nausea and vomiting from week 4 through 12
- Urinary frequency develops
- Gestational sac may be seen by ultrasound
- Bluish-purple color of the cervix and vagina (Chadwick's sign)
- Cervix softens (Goodell's sign)
- Softening of lower uterine segment (Hegar's sign)
- Mucus plug forms in the cervix
- Fetal heart rate may be heard by ultrasound at weeks 9–11
- By end of 12th week, weight gain is usually 3 pounds
- Nausea and vomiting usually cease by end of 3rd month

Second Trimester
(4–6 months)

- Quickening occurs by 18–20 weeks
- Fundus at level of umbilicus by 20 weeks
- Fetal heartbeat may be heard by stethoscope
- Blood volume has increased by 30 to 50 percent
- Respiratory rate may increase slightly
- Pulse may rise up to 10 beats per minute
- Expectant woman gains approximately 1 pound per week
- Urinary frequency ceases

Third Trimester
(7–9 months)

- Uterine walls become thinner and fetus can be palpated more easily
- At 31 weeks, fundus is halfway between umbilicus and xiphoid process
- Heartburn becomes more prevalent
- Backache develops due to increasing lordosis
- Expectant women may feel short of breath due to pressure of fundus on diaphragm
- Stretch marks (striae gravidarum) develop
- Linea nigra and chloasma may develop
- Urinary frequency develops
- Braxton Hicks contractions occur more frequently
- Mucus plug is expelled
- Lightening occurs

---

(2) The corpus luteum continues to function until the placenta is fully functioning, at 3 months' gestation.

   d. Vagina

     (1) The increased level of estrogen leads to hypertrophy, increased vascularization, and hyperplasia of the vagina.

     (2) Thickening of mucosa and loosening of connective tissue occur.

2. Cardiovascular system changes

   a. Blood volume begins to increase in the 1st trimester and peaks in the middle of the 3rd trimester at about 30 to 50 percent above prepregnancy volume.

   b. Cardiac output increases by 30 percent during the 1st 2 trimesters. In labor, there is an additional 30 to 40 percent increase in cardiac output from late 3rd-trimester prelabor values during uterine contractions.

   c. Stroke volume increases by about 30 percent.

   d. The heart rate increases by 10 to 15 beats per minute.

   e. Diastolic blood pressure decreases slightly in the 2nd trimester and then rises slowly to the prepregnancy rate at the end of gestation.

   f. The heart is displaced upward and to the left. Heart sounds change: Increased S1, splitting of S1 and S2, an S3 gallop, and a systolic flow murmur are common.

   g. Vasodilation occurs because of an increased amount of progesterone. Vasodilation accommodates the increase in blood volume. Resultant changes in venous pressure lead to the development of hemorrhoids, varicose veins, and dependent edema of the feet.

   h. Hemodynamic changes

     (1) Red blood cell volume increases. Physiologic anemia may occur if the red blood cell increase is less than the increase in plasma volume.

     (2) The fibrin level increases by about 40 percent and fibrinogen increases by 50 percent.

     (3) Leukocytosis (up to $25,000/mm^3$) occurs just before labor.

3. Respiratory system changes

   a. The volume of air breathed in each minute increases by 30 to 40 percent above prepregnant values. Many changes occur to increase the amount of oxygen available.

   b. Dyspnea is experienced by 60 to 70 percent of women.

   c. The diaphragm is elevated by the enlarging uterus.

   d. Edema of the nasal mucosa causes nasal stuffiness.

4. Gastrointestinal changes

   a. Nausea and vomiting in the 1st trimester are associated with human chorionic gonadotropin (hCG) production.

   b. In the 2nd trimester, the increased nutritional needs of the pregnancy are reflected in an increased appetite. The caloric requirement of pregnancy is 200 to 300 kilocalories per day, so the woman needs to add this amount of kilocalories per day to her diet.

   c. Gum tissue may soften and bleed easily.

   d. Gastric emptying time is delayed.

   e. Intestinal motility slows.

   f. Heartburn caused by reflux of gastric secretions

through a relaxed cardiac sphincter is common in the 3rd trimester.
5. Urinary system changes
   a. Dilation of the kidneys and ureters (especially the right ureter) may occur.
   b. The glomerular filtration rate increases by 50 percent, and renal plasma flow increases by 75 percent early in pregnancy.
   c. Excretion of sodium and water is maximized when the woman lies on her side.
6. Integumentary changes
   a. Increased pigmentation is seen in the nipples, areolae, linea nigra, and chloasma. The pigmentation changes are a result of increased levels of progesterone, estrogen, and melanocyte-stimulating hormone.
   b. Vascular changes may include palmar erythema and skin warmth. These changes are the result of increased blood flow secondary to increased estrogen levels.
   c. Striae gravidarum (reddish, wavy stretch marks) may appear on the breasts, abdomen, and thighs. After pregnancy, the color fades to silvery-white.
   d. Vascular spider nevi (small, bright-red, raised areas radiating from a central stem or lesion) may appear on the chest, face, and legs. They disappear after the birth.
7. Skeletal system changes
   a. Postural changes (lordosis and curvature of the thoracic area) occur because of the increasing size of the uterus and changing center of gravity.
   b. Relaxation of the sacroiliac, sacrococcygeal, and pubic joints results in a widened diameter of the pelvis and a waddling gait.
8. Metabolic system changes
   a. The average weight gain is 30 to 35 pounds. The weight is distributed throughout the body as follows: 11 pounds for the fetus, placenta, and amniotic fluid; 2 pounds in the uterus; 4 pounds in increased blood volume; 3 pounds in the breasts; and 5 to 10 pounds in maternal fat stores.
   b. Nutritional changes
      (1) Fats are absorbed more completely.
      (2) Nitrogen retention begins early in pregnancy and continues throughout pregnancy to prepare for lactation.
9. Endocrine system changes
   a. The basal metabolic rate increases by about 25 percent.
   b. Endocrine glands
      (1) The thyroid increases slightly in size.
      (2) The size and secretions of the parathyroid increase throughout pregnancy, paralleling the fetus's need for calcium.
      (3) The anterior pituitary gland produces follicle-stimulating hormone and luteinizing hormone, which make the pregnancy possible. Thyrotropin and adrenotropin alter maternal metabolism so that the pregnancy can be maintained. Oxytocin, which stimulates contractions of the uterus, is produced by the posterior pituitary gland. Prolactin is responsible for initiation of lactation.
10. Hormonal changes
    a. Estrogen and progesterone are secreted first by the corpus luteum and then primarily by the placenta.

Estrogen stimulates growth of tissues, and progesterone promotes smooth muscle relaxation.
    b. The trophoblast secretes hCG early in the pregnancy and promotes the secretion of estrogen and progesterone until the placenta is fully functioning.
    c. Human placental lactogen (hPL), also called **human chorionic somatomammotropin,** is an antagonist of insulin. Its presence results in increased levels of free fatty acids for metabolism, thereby ensuring an adequate energy supply for the fetus.
    d. Relaxin is produced first by the corpus luteum and then by the placenta and decidua. Relaxin promotes relaxation of the uterine muscles and assists in softening the cervix toward the end of the pregnancy, through remodeling of collagen.
11. Changes in the breast
    a. Estrogen and progesterone play a part in stimulating changes in the breast in preparation for lactation after birth.
       (1) Increased estrogen levels stimulate growth of the breast by increasing fat content.
       (2) Progesterone stimulates growth of the lobules and aids in the development of the secretory capacity of alveolar cells. As a result, breast size and nodularity increase. The interaction of estrogen and progesterone works to prohibit milk secretion during pregnancy.
    b. Superficial veins are more prominent, and the areolae darken.
    c. Colostrum is present from about the 12th week of gestation.
    d. Lactation is further stimulated after birth of the baby.
       (1) Prolactin, which is secreted and released from the anterior pituitary gland, stimulates the alveolar epithelium cells to secrete colostrum.
       (2) The suckling of the newborn initiates the letdown reflex, which allows milk to be expressed from the mother's breasts. The sucking action of the newborn stimulates both the production and expression of milk.
12. Changes in sexuality
    a. Physiologic and psychosocial changes during pregnancy may influence the sexuality of both partners.
    b. Box 14–2 presents some possible effects of pregnancy on sexuality.

BOX 14–2. Possible Effects of Pregnancy on Sexuality

During 1st trimester: Nausea, vomiting, and fatigue may lessen the desire for sexual activity

During 2nd trimester: Sexual desire may increase because nausea, vomiting, and fatigue have ceased, and increased vasocongestion of the pelvis, vagina, and vulva may increase sexual pleasure.

During 3rd trimester: Sexual desire may remain increased; however, the increasing size of the uterus may make sexual intercourse more difficult. Intercourse in a side-lying or female dominant position may be more comfortable. With breast stimulation or at the time of orgasm, the woman may feel uterine contractions. The contractions are not a problem for most women.

13. Psychosocial changes (based on research with Western White women): Within Western White culture there is wide variation. Each ethnic or cultural group residing within the United States brings particular values, beliefs, and customs both individually and as a group to the maternal-child setting.
    a. Maternal psychosocial changes
       (1) Ambivalence about the pregnancy and becoming a mother usually develops in the 1st trimester.
       (2) Acceptance of the pregnancy usually occurs early in the 2nd trimester as the pregnancy is validated by ultrasonography, sensation of the baby's movements (quickening), and a change in body size.
       (3) Introversion occurs as the pregnancy progresses. The expectant mother turns inward and focuses on planning and adjusting in preparation for the birth.
       (4) Mood swings are common throughout pregnancy but especially in the 1st trimester.
       (5) Changes in body image occur rapidly during pregnancy.
    b. Maternal developmental changes
       (1) Pregnancy validation: Initial ambivalence occurs as the woman dreams about herself and the pregnancy.
       (2) Fetal embodiment: The expectant mother is introspective and incorporates the fetus into her own body image.
       (3) Fetal distinction: The fetus is conceptualized as a separate entity, and the woman begins to learn child care activities from her own mother, other family members, or friends.
       (4) Role transition: The expectant mother prepares a place for the baby in the home and prepares to separate from the child. She feels ready to take on the role of mother.
    c. Paternal tasks of pregnancy: Within Western White culture there is wide variation. Each ethnic or cultural group residing in the United States brings particular values, beliefs, and customs both individually and as a group to the maternal-child setting.
       (1) Announcement phase: The expectant father experiences ambivalence about becoming a father and explores the expectant-father role.
       (2) Moratorium phase: The expectant father accepts the changes that are occurring in the pregnancy —such as mood swings in his partner and changes in her body size and changes in their relationship patterns—and begins to fantasize about the child.
       (3) Focusing phase: The expectant father assists in the preparations for the child by preparing to be a labor coach, making a place for the child at home, and accepting the approaching father role.

Fetal Growth and Development

1. Gametogenesis
   a. Oogenesis
      (1) Female gametes are produced by a process called oogenesis.
      (2) All the ova (eggs) that the woman will have in her life are present before her birth, in the 6th month of gestation.
      (3) The 1st meiotic division begins in fetal life, stops, and then resumes at the time of puberty. Two cells of unequal size are produced. The larger cell is called the secondary oocyte and the smaller cell the polar body. Each of these cells contains 22 autosomal chromosomes and 1 sex chromosome—an X chromosome—and is referred to as a **haploid cell.**
      (4) The 2nd meiotic division begins at ovulation and continues as the oocyte is propelled into and through the fallopian tube.
      (5) At the time of conception (fertilization) the 2nd meiotic division is completed: 4 haploid cells are the result: 1 ovum and 3 small polar bodies.
   b. Spermatogenesis
      (1) Male gametes are produced by a process called spermatogenesis.
      (2) Spermatogenesis begins at puberty, when the germinal epithelium in the seminiferous tubules of the testes begin producing sperm. The male has the ability to produce gametes on a continuous basis until senescence.
      (3) During the 1st meiotic division, 1 diploid cell (called a primary spermatocyte) divides into 2 haploid cells called **secondary spermatocytes.** During the 2nd meiotic division the 2 haploid cells divide into 4 spermatids, each with 22 autosomal chromosomes and 1 sex chromosome: an X or a Y.
      (4) Spermatids undergo further changes and become sperm, or spermatozoa.
2. Conception and implantation
   a. Fertilization occurs in the ampulla (outer 3rd) of the fallopian tube.
   b. The fertilized cell is called a zygote.
   c. The zygote undergoes rapid mitotic division called cleavage and is now called a blastomere. Cell division continues, and a solid mass of cells called a morula is formed. The morula enters the uterine cavity and floats freely for about 3 days before implantation occurs. At the time of implantation, additional cellular change has occurred, and the morula is developed into a blastocyst. The time from fertilization to implantation is approximately 7 to 9 days.

TRANSCULTURAL CONSIDERATIONS

Conception beliefs vary with different cultural groups. Beliefs may encompass the method of conception, positioning, timing of intercourse, and other practices to ensure conception or a particular desired sex of the infant.

d. Placental development and function: The placenta forms from the trophoblastic cells of the chorionic villi (the embryonic component) and the decidua basalis (the uterine component). It produces hCG, hPL, estrogen, and progesterone.

(1) The placenta develops and begins to have primitive circulation at 3 weeks of embryonic development. It is fully functioning at the beginning of the 3rd month (Fig. 14–1).

(2) The placenta expands until it covers approximately half of the inside of the uterus at the 20th week of gestation.

(3) At term (40th week), the placenta weighs approximately one sixth to one seventh of the weight of the fetus.

(4) The cytotrophoblast thins and becomes the syncytium at the 5th month. The syncytium is in direct contact with maternal blood in the intervillous spaces.

(5) The metabolic functions of the placenta include the production of glycogen, cholesterol, and fatty acids, which are used by the fetus and for hormone production.

STRUCTURE OF THE PLACENTA

The placenta consists of 2 parts: the maternal portion and the fetal portion.

Maternal Portion:
Made up of the *decidua basalis* and its circulation, the maternal portion consists of a rough, red surface that is divided into sections called *cotyledons*.

Fetal Portion:
Consists of the chorionic villi and their circulation. The fetal side has a bluish, shiny appearance because it is covered by the *amnion* (a membrane). The chorionic villi differentiate to 2 layers, the *syncytium* (outer layer) and the *cytotrophoblast* (inner layer).

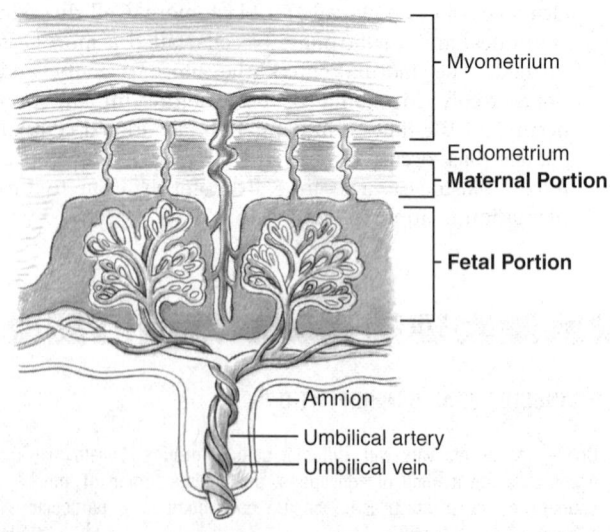

- Myometrium

- Endometrium
Maternal Portion

Fetal Portion

- Amnion
- Umbilical artery
- Umbilical vein

Figure 14–1.

(6) Transport functions are accomplished by 5 mechanisms:

• Simple diffusion (movement of substances from an area of higher concentration to an area of lower concentration) moves substances such as water, oxygen, carbon dioxide, electrolytes, drugs, and anesthetic gases.

• Facilitated transport uses a carrier system to move substances from an area of higher concentration to an area of lower concentration. Glucose, galactose, and some oxygen are transported by this method.

• Active transport moves substances from an area of lower concentration to an area of higher concentration. Substances moved by active transport include amino acids, calcium, iron, iodine, water-soluble vitamins, and glucose.

• Pinocytosis transfers large molecules, such as albumin and gamma globulin.

• Hydrostatic and osmotic pressures provide for the movement of water.

(7) Endocrine functions

• Human chorionic gonadotrophin, an essential hormone, is produced within days of conception. It stimulates the corpus luteum to continue to produce increased amounts of progesterone and estrogen until the placenta is fully functioning, at about 14 weeks.

• The progesterone produced by the placenta exerts a quieting effect on the smooth muscles throughout the uterus and the rest of the body.

• Estrogen stimulates a proliferative function within many tissues, causing enlargement of the breasts and breast glandular tissue and uterus and providing a stimulatory effect on uterine contractions.

• Human placental lactogen (hPL) is similar to human pituitary growth hormone and stimulates changes in the maternal nutritional metabolism so that more protein, glucose, and minerals are available for fetal and tissue growth.

(8) Immunologic aspects of placental development: Progesterone and hCG provide an immunologic masking of the embryo, fetus, placenta, and membranes.

3. Embryonic and fetal development

a. There are 3 stages of development (Fig. 14–2): pre-embryonic (1st 14 days), embryonic (day 15 to the 8th week of gestation), and fetal (the 8th week to the end of pregnancy (called term).

(1) In the pre-embryonic stage, rapid cellular division and differentiation of tissues occur.

(2) In the embryonic stage, differentiation of tissues continues. At 4 weeks, arm and leg buds are visible, the tubular heart is beating, and somites are forming along the midline.

(3) At 8 weeks, the beginning of the fetal stage, the fetus clearly resembles a human. Eyelids begin to fuse, long bones begin to form, movement of large muscles is possible, and all body organs are

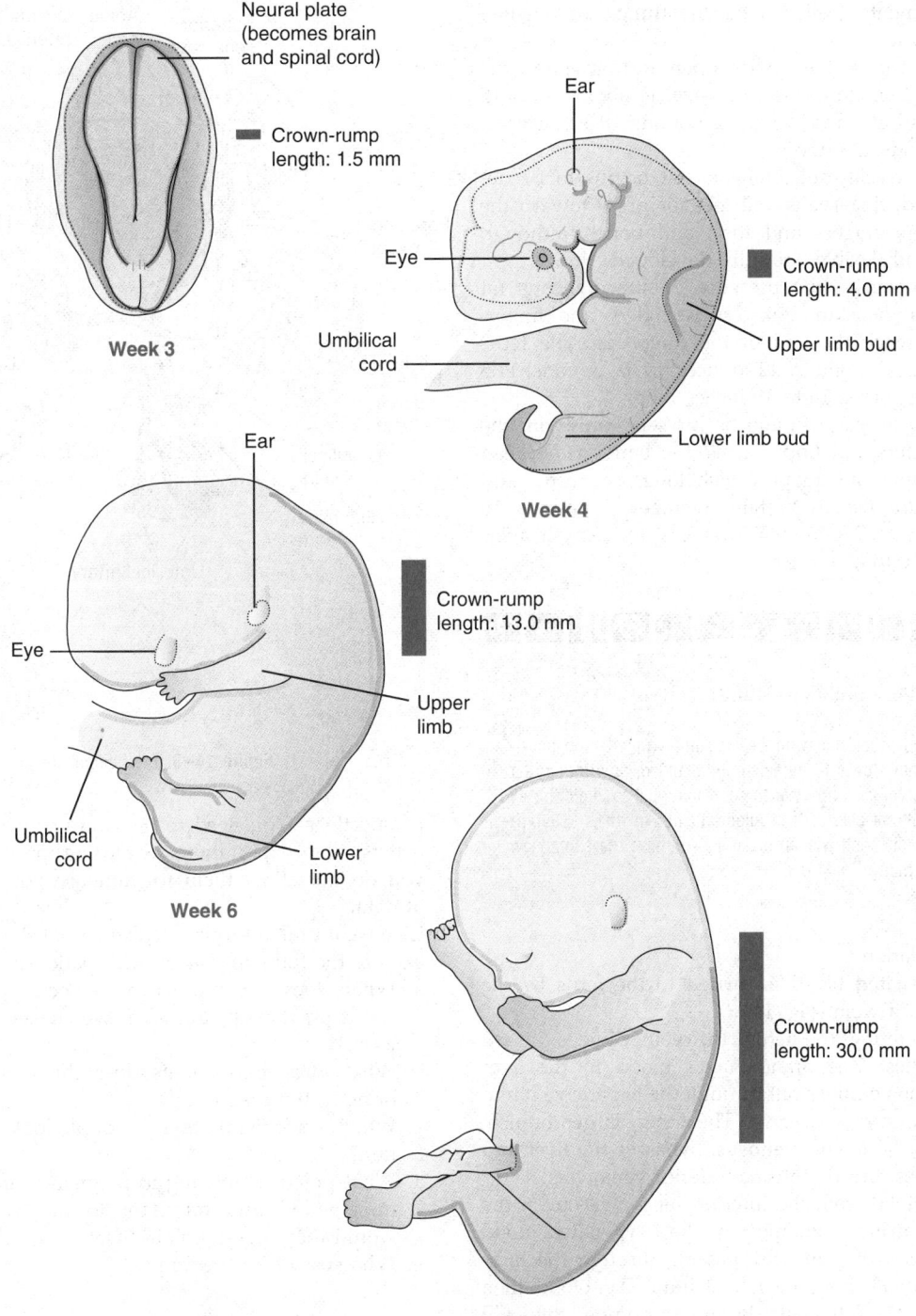

Figure 14—2. Embryonic development from 3 weeks through the 8th week after fertilization. (Modified from Gorrie TM, McKinney ES, and Murray SS. *Maternal Newborn Nursing.* Philadelphia: WB Saunders, 1994, p 102.)

formed. Between 8 and 12 weeks, the fetal heart can be heard with Doppler ultrasonography.

(4) At 12 weeks, the face is well formed, tooth buds appear, the fetus is able to curl its fingers into a fist, and the kidneys begin to produce urine.

(5) At 16 weeks, lanugo develops and active movement is present.

(6) At 20 weeks, the fetus's movements are strong enough that the mother feels them, eyebrows and eyelashes form, the hair on the head is wooly in texture, the fetal heartbeat is auscultated by stethoscope, and the fetus is developing a regular pattern of sleeping and waking cycles.

(7) At 24 weeks, reddish, wrinkled skin covers the body, with little subcutaneous fat present; vernix caseosa covers the body; and fetal respiratory

movements (called fetal breathing movements) begin.

(8) At 28 weeks, the eyelids open and close and the fetus, two thirds its final size, is about 14 to 15 inches long, and weighs 2 pounds 10.5 ounces to 2 pounds 12 ounces.

(9) At 32 weeks, subcutaneous fat begins to be deposited; fingernails and toenails grow toward the ends of fingers and toes; and bones, although soft and flexible, are fully developed.

(10) At 36 weeks, the presence of subcutaneous fat makes the skin look less wrinkled, and fingernails reach the end of the fingertips. The fetus weighs 5 pounds 12 ounces to 6 pounds 11.5 ounces and is 16 to 19 inches long.

(11) At 40 weeks, lanugo is present only on the shoulders and upper arms, the hair on the head is coarse and about 1 inch long, and arms and legs are flexed. Weight averages 6 pounds 10 ounces to 7 pounds 15 ounces and length averages 19 to 21 inches.

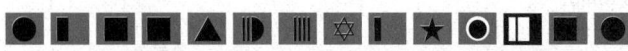

TRANSCULTURAL CONSIDERATIONS

Prenatal practices associated with beliefs about growth and development of the baby, foods to be eaten and avoided, how much rest is needed, how to dress, and what to seek and what to avoid are all based on our cultural beliefs. It is important not to make assumptions that the childbearing woman or family will have the same view of pregnancy as that of the nurse.

b. Fetal circulation
(1) Oxygenated blood is carried to the fetus by the umbilical vein (Fig. 14–3).
(2) On entering the fetus, the vein divides into 2 branches. One branch takes blood to the liver and then empties out through the hepatic vein into the inferior vena cava. The other, larger branch, called the **ductus venosus,** bypasses the liver and empties directly into the inferior vena cava.
(3) The blood from the inferior vena cava enters the right atrium, and most of the oxygenated blood bypasses the lungs by passing through the foramen ovale into the left atrium. The blood then enters the left ventricle and is pumped into the aorta. A small portion of blood does go through to the right ventricle and is circulated to the lungs to provide some nourishment for developing lung tissues. The ductus arteriosus (between the pulmonary artery and the descending aorta) allows most of the blood to bypass the fetal lungs and enter the aorta.

Transcultural Considerations

1. Individuals from different ethic origins approach pregnancy and the growth of a new person with myriad

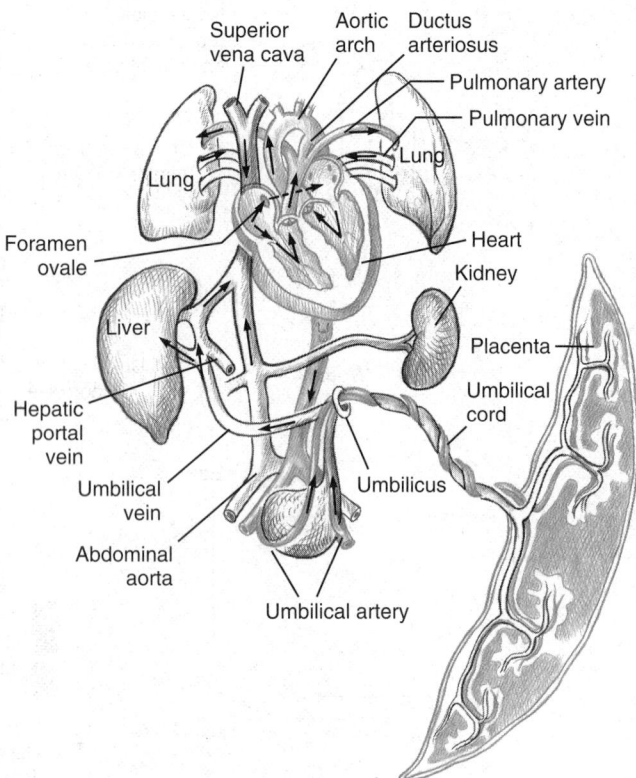

Figure 14–3. Fetal circulation.

perspectives. You need to be aware of your own values, beliefs, and expectations regarding pregnancy, so that you do not allow them to influence your interpretation of data.

2. Glean cultural information from published sources, and explore the following areas with patients:
   a. What does the mother or expectant parents know about pregnancy, and what would she or they like to learn?
   b. What ideas and beliefs does the mother or couple bring to the pregnancy?
   c. Whom does the mother or couple look to for information?
   d. What practices relating to pregnancy and the postpartum period are important to the family and how would they like to obtain them?
   e. Who speaks for the family?

◼ ASSESSING THE WOMAN AND FAMILY DURING PREGNANCY

Signs and Symptoms of Pregnancy

1. Presumptive signs are changes that the woman or examiner can observe, and presumptive symptoms are subjective changes reported by the woman. They are considered presumptive because they are also associated with conditions other than pregnancy.
   a. Presumptive signs
      (1) Amenorrhea (the absence of menstruation) is usu-

ally the 1st presumptive sign. When amenorrhea is caused by pregnancy, it is the result of the maintenance of the corpus luteum through stimulation by hCG and elevated levels of progesterone and estrogen. Amenorrhea is considered presumptive because it is also associated with endocrine conditions (e.g., thyroid or ovarian dysfunction), metabolic conditions (e.g., malnutrition or excessive exercise or weight loss), and systemic disease (e.g., tuberculosis or malignancy).
   (2) Breast engorgement during pregnancy is the result of growth of the secretory ductal system. Breast engorgement may also be caused by premenstrual syndrome and chronic cystic mastitis.
b. Presumptive symptoms
   (1) Nausea and vomiting usually occur in the morning during pregnancy and are associated with the increasing level of hCG. Nausea and vomiting may also be caused by disorders such as anorexia or gastrointestinal disorders.
   (2) Breast tenderness during pregnancy is the result of breast growth. However, breast tenderness may also be caused by premenstrual syndrome and chronic cystic mastitis.
   (3) Urinary frequency during pregnancy is associated with the pressure placed on the bladder by the increasing size of the uterus. Urinary frequency is also associated with such conditions as urinary tract infection and cystocele.
   (4) Quickening (the pregnant woman's perception of fetal movement) is also associated with such conditions as flatus and increased peristalsis.
2. The **probable signs** of pregnancy are objective and may be observed by a health care professional. They are not considered diagnostic, however, because they may also be caused by conditions other than pregnancy. The following are the probable signs of pregnancy:
a. Hegar's sign—softening of the isthmus of the uterus
b. Goodell's sign—softening of the cervix
c. Chadwick's sign—deep red to bluish discoloration of the cervix and the vagina (Chadwick's sign may also be categorized as a presumptive sign)
d. Increased levels of hCG as determined by laboratory tests
e. Increased pigmentation of the skin, such as linea nigra, darkening of the areolae and nipples, and chloasma
f. Abdominal striae
g. Abdominal and uterine enlargement
3. Positive, or diagnostic, signs are objective and are not caused by conditions other than pregnancy. The following are the positive signs of pregnancy:
a. Pregnancy tests
   (1) The diagnosis of pregnancy is based on the presence of hCG. Human chorionic gonadotrophin has alpha and beta subunits, and the most reliable tests are specific to the beta subunit.
   (2) Immunometric tests are specific to the beta subunit of hCG and can reliably detect pregnancy 7 to 10 days after conception (21–24 days past the 1st day of the last menstrual period). A variety of

inexpensive tests are available that use maternal serum or urine and are completed in 1 to 7 minutes. False-negative results are rare.
   (3) Agglutination inhibition slide tests react to hCG but are not specific to the beta subunit. These tests are completed on maternal urine, cost less than immunometric tests, and reliably detect pregnancy 18 to 21 days after conception (32–35 days past the 1st day of the last menstrual period). Agglutination inhibition slide tests are more likely than immunometric tests to have false-negative results.
   (4) Home pregnancy tests are readily available and are frequently used. To enhance their effectiveness, the woman needs to follow test instructions exactly, using the 1st voided urine specimen. The reliability of home pregnancy tests is about 84 percent for positive test results and 64 percent for negative results.
b. Ultrasonography completed with a vaginal probe allows the gestational sac to be seen as early as the 5th or 6th week of gestation. In some instances, such as an ectopic pregnancy, the gestational sac is visible in the fallopian tube and the pregnancy cannot be allowed to continue.
c. The fetal heartbeat can be auscultated by an ultrasound device as early as 10 to 12 weeks and by fetoscope at 17 to 20 weeks.
d. Fetal movements can be felt by a health care professional at about 20 weeks' gestation.

Maternal Health History

1. Previous pregnancies
a. Number of previous pregnancies, abortions (spontaneous and induced), stillbirths or death of a baby in the first 4 weeks after birth, and preterm births (birth before 37 completed weeks of gestation)
b. Number of living children
   (1) Condition of baby at birth, Apgar score, and whether resuscitation efforts were needed
   (2) Weight of baby, neonatal course, type of feeding, and neonatal problems (hypoglycemia, hyperbilirubinemia, isoimmunization, or congenital anomalies)
c. Course of previous pregnancies and births
   (1) Problems associated with pregnancy, such as weight gain, excessive nausea and vomiting, spotting or bleeding, preterm labor, elevated blood pressure, or edema
   (2) Characteristics of labor and birth, such as length of previous labor, type of birth (vaginal birth, forceps- or vacuum extractor–assisted vaginal birth, or cesarean birth), and associated problems and treatment.
   (3) Characteristics of postpartum course, such as normal involution, subinvolution, infection, tissue healing, feeding techniques used and degree of satisfaction or problems with them, and incorporation of new baby into family
2. Gynecologic history

a. Previous infections and surgery
b. Menstrual history (menarche, menstrual pattern, and menstrual problems)
c. Contraceptive history
d. Date of Papanicolaou smear and results
3. History of current pregnancy
a. First day of last menstrual period
b. Types of pregnancy tests the woman has used and the results
c. Recent history of bleeding, cramping, nausea, vomiting, or other problems
4. Medical-surgical history
a. Blood type and Rh factor
b. Childhood diseases (rubella, rubeola, mumps, and chickenpox) and immunizations
c. Medical diseases (diabetes, cardiovascular, pulmonary, kidney, and seizures) and medications used to treat them
d. Previous injuries
e. Previous surgical procedures
f. Previous use of alcohol, recreational drugs, and tobacco
g. Allergies to medications, foods, or other substances
5. Diet history
a. Previous weight pattern
b. Previous problems with maintaining weight or excessive weight gain
c. Dietary customs and practices (vegetarianism or cultural- or religion-associated practices)

Paternal Health History

1. History of any diseases or genetic conditions
2. Blood type and Rh factor
3. Age
4. History of previous or current alcohol, drug, or tobacco use

Determining the Estimated Date of Birth

1. Nägele's rule may be used to calculate the estimated date of birth.
a. Determine the 1st day of the last menstrual period, subtract 3 months, and add 7 days. It is easier to use a number for the month as follows:

$$
\begin{array}{ll}
12/2 & \text{(1st day of the last menstrual} \\
& \text{period was December 2)} \\
-3 & \text{(minus 3 months)} \\
\hline
9/2 & \\
+7 & \text{(plus 7 days)} \\
\hline
9/9 & \text{(estimated date of birth)}
\end{array}
$$

b. Nägele's rule is not helpful if menstrual periods have been very irregular or variant in flow; if conception occurred while the woman was breast-feeding; if conception occurred before reestablishment of menses after cessation of birth control pills; or if the woman has not kept a menstrual calendar or does not define

time spans, such as a menstrual cycle, in the same way as the health care professional.
c. Remember that the calculated estimated date of birth is simply an estimation. Only approximately 5 percent of women give birth on the identified date. A period of 2 weeks before and 2 weeks after the date is considered normal.
2. Ultrasonographic dating
a. Abdominal or endovaginal ultrasonography may be used to see a gestational sac.
b. If the gestational sac is visible in the 7th or 8th week of gestation, the dating of the pregnancy is accurate to plus or minus 5 days.

Physical Examination of the Mother

1. General examination
a. Assess each body system to determine the woman's state of health and identify possible problems. To minimize discomfort, begin the assessment with less invasive areas and then progress to more invasive areas (Table 14–2).

Table 14–2. Antepartum Physical Assessment	
Assessment Area	**Expected Findings**
Vital signs	
Blood pressure	90–140/60–90
Pulse	60–90 beats/min
Respirations	16–22 breaths/min
Temperature	36.2–37.6° C (98–99° F)
Weight	Dependent on body build
Lungs	Breath sounds equal, unlabored respirations, no rales or rhonchi
Breasts	Supple, veins dilated and more prevalent, enlarging size, pigmentation in nipples and aerolae darkening, striae development possible, colostrum possible after 12th wk
Heart	Palpitations possible
Abdomen	Fundal height slightly above symphysis pubis at 10–12 wk, halfway between symphysis pubis and umbilicus at 16 wk, at the level of the umbilicus at 20 wk,; striae gravidarum possible
Fetal status	Fetal heart beat possibly heard by ultrasound at 10–12 wk, fetal movement felt by mother at 18–20 wk, possible for expectant woman to monitor fetal movement from 30 wk, fetal ballotment (fetus rises in amniotic fluid and then returns to original position) during the 4th or 5th month
Pelvis	Skin warm and dry, with no edema present; clear, odorless vaginal discharge; softening of cervix (Goodell's sign); softening of the isthmus of the uterus (Hegar's sign); bluish-purple color with cervix (Chadwick's sign) present at 4–6 wk

b. Blood pressure is usually within the normal limits of 90 to 140 for systolic pressure and 60 to 90 for diastolic pressure. You will increase the accuracy of your assessment if you do the following:
   (1) Give the woman time to rest before you assess blood pressure.
   (2) Maintain the woman in a sitting position with her arm resting on a table at about the level of the heart.
   (3) Make sure you are using the appropriate-sized cuff.
   (4) In determining the diastolic pressure, note both the muffling and the cessation of sound.
c. Assess weight after the woman removes her shoes. Anticipated weight gain is approximately 28 to 35 pounds for the woman at her ideal weight.
d. Breast examination: Assess breasts for nodularity, evidence of previous breast surgery (e.g., removal of cysts or breast reduction or enhancement), and whether nipples are everted or inverted.
e. Abdominal examination (see Table 14–2)
2. External uterine assessment
a. Determine fundal height by measuring the distance in centimeters from the top of the symphysis pubis over the curve of the abdomen to the top of the uterine fundus. The height in centimeters corresponds to the week of gestation; for example, at 22 weeks' gestation the fundal height is 22 cm.
b. Estimate fetal size on the basis of the expected progression of fundal height.
   (1) You can use this method in the 1st two thirds of pregnancy.
   (2) For maximum accuracy, the same examiner should assess the woman's fundal height at each visit, and the woman needs to void just before the examination (Fig. 14–4).
   (3) The ongoing accuracy of measurement is affected by variations in measurements made by different caregivers if more than 1 caregiver sees the woman during prenatal care. In addition, if the woman is very tall, short, or obese, the measurements will differ.
3. Complete a pelvic examination to assess internal and external pelvic tissues and structures, and take measurements that will allow you to determine pelvic adequacy (Fig. 14–5). Some certified nurse midwives and obstetri-

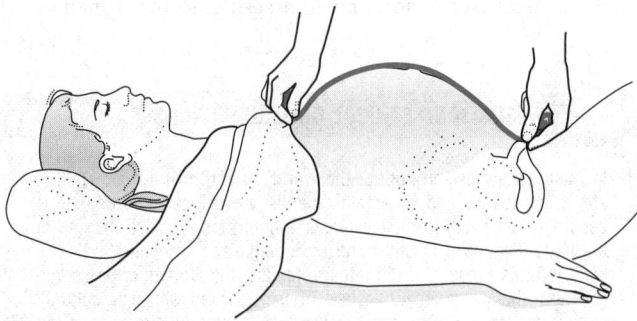

Figure 14–4. Measuring the uterus includes the distance between the upper border of the symphysis pubis and the top of the fundus. (Modified from Gorrie TM, McKinney ES, and Murray SS. *Maternal Newborn Nursing.* Philadelphia: WB Saunders, 1994, p 140.)

PELVIC ADEQUACY

The most critical anteroposterior diameters of the inlet are the **diagonal conjugate, obstetric conjugate,** and **conjugate vera** (true conjugate).

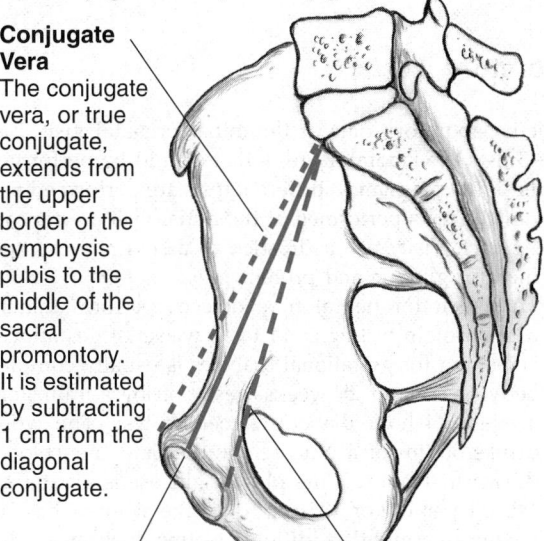

Conjugate Vera
The conjugate vera, or true conjugate, extends from the upper border of the symphysis pubis to the middle of the sacral promontory. It is estimated by subtracting 1 cm from the diagonal conjugate.

Obstetric Conjugate
Extends from the innermost aspect of the upper border of the symphysis pubis to the middle portion of the sacral promontory. It cannot be measured manually but is estimated by subtracting 1.5–2.0 cm from the diagonal conjugate. The obstetric conjugate is the smallest measurement that the fetus must pass through and, therefore, the most important.

Diagonal Conjugate
Estimated manually by measuring from the lower border of the symphysis pubis to the sacral promontory. A normal measurement is 11.5 cm or more.

Estimation of adequacy of the pelvic cavity is made by determining the prominence of the ischial spines and the degree of convergence of the side walls.

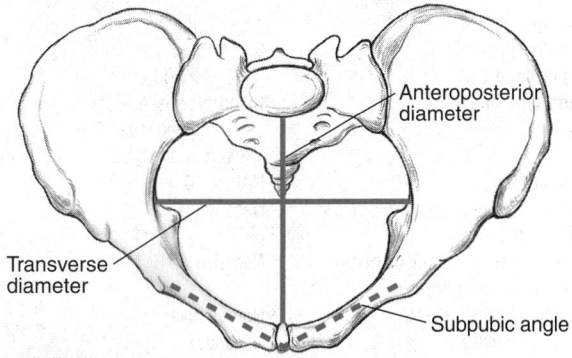

The Pelvic Outlet
The anteroposterior diameter extends from the lower border of the symphysis pubis to the tip of the sacrum and can be measured manually. The normal range is 9.5–11.5 cm. The transverse diameter is measured by placing a closed, gloved fist against the perineum between the ischial tuberosities. The normal measurement is 8–10 cm. The subpubic angle should be 85–90 degrees. It is determined by palpating the bony structure externally.

Figure 14–5.

cians take pelvic measurements on the initial visit to identify the woman who may be at increased risk for cesarean birth. Others wait until later in the pregnancy, when there is greater relaxation of collagen tissues and joints because of the influence of relaxin and progesterone.

Laboratory Tests

1. Obtain laboratory data at the initial prenatal visit. Table 14–3 lists the laboratory tests that should be performed.
2. Later in the pregnancy, different tests are performed and a few of the tests performed at the initial visit are repeated.
   a. At each visit, use a dipstick to assess a urine specimen for glucose and protein.
   b. To screen for neural tube defects, perform maternal α-fetoprotein testing at 14 to 16 weeks of gestation.
   c. Screening for gestational diabetes is usually completed between 24 and 28 weeks' gestation by administering a 50-gm, 1-hour diabetes screening test. The woman drinks 50 gm of a glucose solution and then blood is drawn in 1 hour. If the plasma glucose is greater than 140 ml per dl (or 135 mg/dl if the woman has been fasting overnight), additional testing such as a 3-hour glucose tolerance test is done.
   d. Repeat testing for syphilis (a Venereal Disease Research Laboratory or serologic test for syphilis) at the beginning of the 3rd trimester (about 28 weeks).
   e. If the woman has a history of herpes, continue assessments throughout the pregnancy. If active lesions appear, the lesions and the cervix may be cultured weekly during the last 4 to 8 weeks of pregnancy.

Table 14–3. Laboratory Tests at the Initial Prenatal Visit

Test	Expected Normal Finding
Hemoglobin	12–16 gm/dl
Hematocrit	38–47%
White blood cells	4500–11,000/L
Blood type and Rh	Blood type is A, B or O. Rh is positive or negative. The majority of women are type O, Rh positive
Rubella titer	HAI > 10
Indirect Coombs' test if woman is Rh negative	Negative
Sickle cell preparation or hemoglobin electrophoresis	Negative or HbA only
Syphilis (VDRL or STS)	Nonreactive
Gonorrhea culture	Negative
Urinalysis	Normal color, specific gravity, pH 4.6–8.0. No bacterial growth. Negative for glycosuria and negative for protein
Tuberculin test (PPD) (Do not perform this test for women with previous positive test)	Negative
Papanicolaou smear	Negative

Fetal Assessment

1. Fetal heart rate (FHR) may be assessed as early as 10 to 11 weeks by a hand-held Doppler ultrasonography device. The FHR is usually between 120 and 160 beats per minute. (Note that the fetal heart rate may also be referred to as **fetal heart tones,** but FHR is the more current term.)
2. Presentation of the fetus refers to whether the fetus's head is down in the lower portion of the uterus, a condition called cephalic presentation that occurs in about 97 percent of pregnancies, or whether the buttocks are down in the lower portion of the uterus (called a **breech presentation**). Assess fetal presentation by completing the 4 steps of Leopold's maneuvers (Fig. 14–6).
3. Maternal assessment of fetal movement
   a. Techniques to assess fetal movement are numerous. The Cardiff count-to-ten, daily fetal movement record, and fetal movement diary are a few of the methods.
   b. The woman can start the Cardiff count-to-ten at 28 to 30 weeks of gestation. Instruct the woman to do the following:
      (1) Set aside the same time each day to count fetal movements.
      (2) Count until there are 10 movements and record the time it has taken to achieve this number.
      (3) Note whether the length of time is consistent with the length of time required the previous day or is longer.
      (4) Call the health care provider if the number of movements is decreased or it takes longer to obtain 10 movements.
4. Ultrasonography
   a. Ultrasonography is a useful tool to assess fetal well-being.
      (1) The gestational sac can be seen at 5 to 6 weeks of gestation. The age of the embryo and subsequent calculation of the estimated date of birth if additional ultrasonographic measurements are completed allow an accuracy of plus or minus 1 day.
      (2) Fetal heart rate can be heard by 9 to 10 weeks.
      (3) Fetal breathing movements can be seen by 11 weeks.
      (4) Serial measurements such as crown-rump length and biparietal diameter may be taken to determine fetal growth and validate the estimated date of birth.
      (5) Doppler waveform velocity studies are used to study blood flow changes that occur in maternal and fetal circulation and to assess placental function.

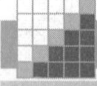

LEGAL AND ETHICAL CONSIDERATIONS

In many countries throughout the world, the birth of a male child is strongly desired, and a female child is viewed as a burden. It is becoming a frequent practice in these countries, to have the sex of the fetus diagnosed in utero and to continue the pregnancy only if a male fetus is present. If the fetus is female, the woman is pressured to abort the pregnancy because of very strong societal, cultural, family, and peer pressure. This practice is carried out to such an extent that the ratio of males to females is beginning to change dramatically in some countries.

ASSESSMENT OF FETAL PRESENTATION: LEOPOLD'S MANEUVERS

1 Stand on the woman's right side while she lies down. Place your hands on the fundus (upper portion) of the uterus to determine if a firm, rounded object (fetal head) or a softer rounded object (fetal buttocks) is present.

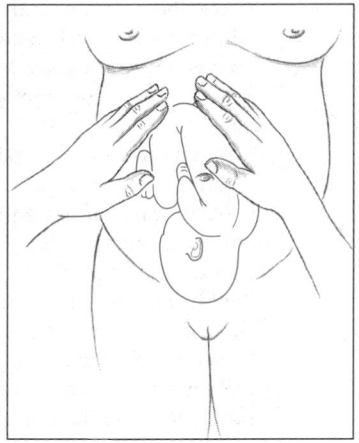

3 Bring your right hand down just above the symphysis pubis and grasp the fetal head to reassess firmness and whether it moves with some gentle pressure.

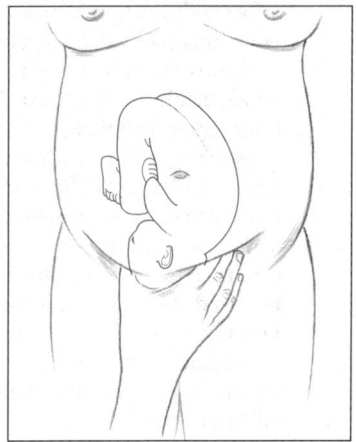

2 Bring your hands down alongside the uterus and attempt to feel a smooth fetal back on one side and smaller parts (elbows, hands, knees, and feet) on the other.

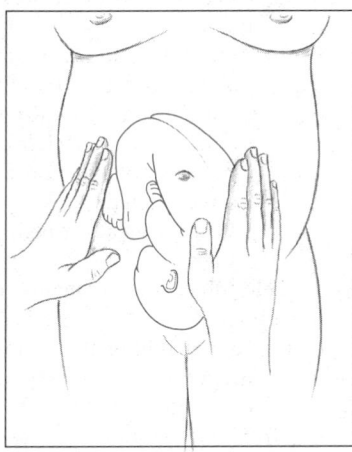

4 Change position so that you are facing the woman's feet. Place both hands at the lower portion of the uterus to assess firmness of the fetal head, whether flexion of the fetal head has occurred, and if the head can be moved with gentle pressure.

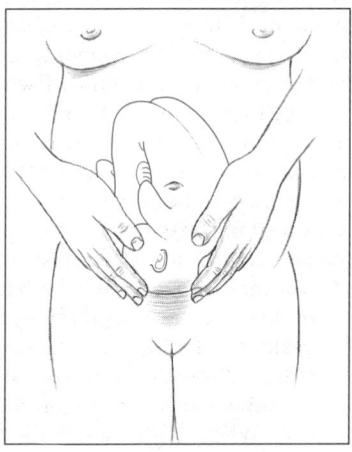

Figure 14–6.

b. Embryoscopy can be performed to observe the embryo for structural problems and to obtain a blood sample for chromosomal and biochemical studies.

5. Amniocentesis
   a. Amniocentesis may be performed between 16 and 18 weeks' gestation for chromosomal and biochemical analysis and between 30 and 36 weeks for assessment of fetal lung maturity.
   b. The procedure entails visualization of the fetus and placenta by ultrasonography, insertion of a needle into the amniotic cavity, and withdrawal of amniotic fluid.
   c. Fetal cells are retrieved from the amniotic fluid and prepared for chromosomal and biochemical analysis. Biochemical studies include enzyme analysis and α-fetoprotein for neural tube defects.
   d. Fetal lung maturity is determined with several tests:
      (1) The lecithin to sphingomyelin ratio: Lecithin and sphingomyelin are phospholipids contained in surfactant. A ratio of greater than 2:1 is associated with fetal lung maturity.
      (2) Phosphatidylglycerol: Phosphatidylglycerol is a phospholipid contained in surfactant. Its presence is associated with fetal lung maturity.
      (3) Creatinine level: Creatinine level is an indirect measure of fetal kidney function and muscle mass. A level of 2 mg per dl is equated with 37 weeks' gestation.

6. Percutaneous umbilical blood sampling
   a. A sample of fetal blood is obtained from the umbilical cord under ultrasonographic guidance.
   b. Tests are then performed for diagnosis of hemophilia, hemoglobinopathies, fetal infections, chromosome abnormalities, nonimmune hydrops, isoimmune hemolytic disorders, and hemoglobin and hematocrit levels.

7. Nonstress test (NST)
   a. The NST is based on observations that fetal movement is accompanied by acceleration of FHR in the normal fetus. Normal movement and acceleration of the FHR suggest that the central and autonomic nervous systems are intact and the fetus is not hypoxic.
   b. The NST is performed on an outpatient basis with an electronic fetal monitor. The monitor records fetal activity in the uterus and the FHR.

c. Results

   (1) A reactive test shows at least 2 accelerations, in a 20-minute period (called a 20-minute window), of at least 15 beats per minute for at least 15 seconds with documented fetal movement. A reactive NST indicates that the fetus is at minimal risk of perinatal death in the next 7 days if there are no intervening problems.

   (2) A nonreactive test shows no accelerations with documented fetal movement. When a test is nonreactive, it is extended for another 30 minutes, and if it is still nonreactive, further testing is indicated. If there is not fetal movement, sound may be used (the fetal acoustical stimulation test or vibratory stimulation test) to awaken the fetus and stimu-late movement, or the woman may be advised to move around, have a snack, and retest in an hour or so.

8. Biophysical profile: The biophysical profile is an assessment of 5 biophysical variables: fetal breathing movement, fetal body movement, fetal tone, FHR reactivity, and amniotic fluid volume. Each variable is assessed and assigned a score of 0, 1, or 2. A score of 10 of 10 or 8 of 10 (as long as amniotic fluid volume received a score of 2) is a normal score. Scores of 6 or lower require further assessment and evaluation.

9. Contraction stress test

a. The contraction stress test assesses the ability of the placenta to oxygenate the fetus and the fetal reserve. In the presence of uterine contractions, the FHR is evaluated for late decelerations, which indicate fetal stress. Uterine contractions are stimulated by infusion of intravenous pitocin or the nipple self-stimulation test. When 3 uterine contractions have occurred in a 10-minute window, the FHR is evaluated for late decelerations.

b. Results

   (1) The absence of late decelerations is a negative test and is the desired result.

   (2) If late decelerations are present with 50 percent or more of the contractions, the test is deemed positive.

   (3) An equivocal (unclear) test is one with late decelerations occurring with fewer than 50 percent of contractions or with late decelerations occurring with contractions that are more frequent than every 2 minutes or last longer than 90 seconds or with a uterine contraction pattern of insufficient quality to allow assessment.

Psychosocial Assessment of the Family

1. Maternal psychosocial status

a. Determine the woman's need for information regarding pregnancy and related self-care, labor and birth, and newborn care. Whether women perceive a need for prenatal care varies according to the number of children they have, their previous postpregnancy outcomes and effectiveness, and their socioeconomic status.

b. Assess the woman's support systems.

   (1) Assess the availability of primary support from the father of the child or other partner.
- Is the relationship supportive and nurturing?
- Are the woman and her partner able to share information and concerns? Is the partner involved and interested in the pregnancy?
- How does the partner get information needs met?
- To whom does the partner turn for information and support?
- What kind of parenting role models does the partner have?
- Does the woman feel safe in her relationship with her partner? Ask the woman about her safety only when she is alone, not in the presence of the partner or any other family members.

   (2) Observe the interactions between the woman and her partner and other support persons. Are they congruent with the woman's verbal report of support?

   (3) Assess the cultural parameters of the family.
- What are the family's expectations regarding childbirth and family life?
- What value do childbearing, mothering, and fathering hold for the family? What role behaviors are expected?
- What are proscribed pregnancy beliefs and routines?

c. Determine the woman's educational and socioeconomic levels.

   (1) Knowledge of the woman's educational and socioeconomic levels may help you plan appropriate educational materials.

   (2) Socioeconomic level can indicate the type of care available.

   (3) Women of lower socioeconomic levels are more likely to have difficulty accessing care and comprehensive follow-through.

   (4) Women of higher socioeconomic levels have more choices regarding the childbearing experience.

2. The father's or other partner's psychosocial status regarding the pregnancy and childbirth is influenced by many factors:

a. Cultural background

b. Educational level

c. Socioeconomic status

d. Desire for information about and involvement in the pregnancy and birth (which may be influenced by cultural views and beliefs)

e. Sense of personal autonomy

f. Presence of a supportive, caring relationship

g. Previous parenting experience

h. Any indicators of current or past abusive relationship or situation

3. Siblings' psychosocial status regarding the pregnancy and the new baby is often determined by their age and developmental status.

a. Because young children's concept of time is not well developed, they need to be told about the pregnancy and the birth of the new baby later in the pregnancy. A young child may be excited or noncommittal regarding the addition of a new baby to the family.

b. A school-aged child may vacillate between excitement, anticipation, resentment, and noncommitment.

c. A child who plans to be present at the birth needs special preparation before the birth.

◼ CARING FOR THE WOMAN AND FAMILY DURING PREGNANCY

Routine Prenatal Care of the Woman

1. Diet
   a. The woman needs an additional 300 kilocalories per day to meet the nutritional demands of pregnancy.
   b. Adding specific foods to her diet will help the woman meet these nutritional demands (Table 14–4).
   c. Elicit cultural and individual food requirements (e.g., vegetarianism) when obtaining the woman's dietary history, and consider these requirements when providing information.
2. Weight control
   a. The recommended weight gain during pregnancy for a woman of normal weight is 25 to 35 pounds (11.5–16.0 kg).
   b. The recommended weight gain for an underweight woman is 28 to 40 pounds (12.5–18.0 kg).
   c. The recommended gain for an overweight woman is 15 to 25 pounds (7.0–11.5 kg).
   d. The typical weight gain pattern is 2 to 5 pounds (1.0–2.3 kg) in the 1st trimester (1–13 weeks), followed by a gain of approximately 1 pound (0.4–0.5 kg) per week for the remainder of the pregnancy.
3. Exercise
   a. Performing physical exercise helps the woman strengthen and maintain muscle tone during pregnancy and birth.
   b. The woman should exercise 3 times a week.
   c. Low-impact exercises such as walking, cycling, swimming, or special low-impact aerobics can usually be maintained as long as the pregnancy proceeds as expected.
   d. It is important that the exercise begin and end with stretching. The exercise period should not exceed 15 minutes, with a maximal pulse rate of 150 beats per minute.
   e. Special exercises may be added to prepare for labor and birth. The pelvic tilt (also called pelvic rock) helps strengthen the lower back and prevent backache during pregnancy (Fig. 14–7). The pelvic tilt may be done in 1 of 3 ways:
      (1) The woman lies on her back on the floor with knees bent and feet flat on the floor. She tightens the abdominal muscles, gently presses the small of her back down to the floor, and then slightly arches her back. This position may be used for the 1st 4 months of pregnancy and then should be avoided because of the risk of supine hypotension (vena caval compression).
      (2) The woman stands with her back against a wall and her knees slightly bent. She gently presses her back to the wall and then arches her back slightly.
      (3) The woman may also do the pelvic tilt on her hands and knees, which allows more curvature of the back. However, encourage the woman to do the exercise in the lying or standing position first, to get the feel of the desired rocking motion. Excessive arching of the back may overstretch rather than strengthen muscles.
4. Rest
   a. Adequate rest is important.
   b. Sleep may be difficult later in the pregnancy because of the enlarged uterus. A side-lying position with extra pillows to support the arms, abdomen, and upper legs increases comfort.
5. Sexual activity
   a. Sexual activity may continue throughout the pregnancy.
   b. Changes in sexual desire and response occur throughout pregnancy. In the 1st trimester, the woman's desire may decrease because of nausea, vomiting, and fatigue. Desire and response may increase in the 2nd trimester because of the increased vascularity of the pelvic organs and vulva. Desire may decrease again in the 3rd trimester because of physical discomfort such as backache.
   c. A back-lying position needs to be avoided, especially after the 4th month. A side-lying position may be used.
   d. Intercourse is contraindicated only if there is rupture of amniotic membranes and preterm labor is present.
6. Lifestyle changes
   a. Most employment may be continued during pregnancy without difficulty. Possible problems include prolonged sitting or standing and exposure to teratogenic or environmental substances that may be harmful.
      (1) If the woman spends most of her time sitting or standing, small changes may need to be made to allow for more frequent position changes or rest breaks.
      (2) If environmental or chemical agents are present, a transfer into another area during pregnancy is advisable.
   b. Travel may be maintained with some modification.
      (1) Long car trips can be handled by arranging frequent rest stops so that the woman can walk for a few minutes. The seatbelt needs to be worn low over the abdomen, across the symphysis pubis. Between rest stops, the woman can do dorsiflexion of the foot to improve blood flow, shift her body weight, and use a small pillow to support the lower back to increase comfort. Maintaining fluid intake is also important.
      (2) Air travel is permitted, but the availability and accessibility of maternal-child care at the destination point need to be considered.

Minor Discomforts of Pregnancy

1. Morning sickness
   a. Nausea and vomiting are associated with increased levels of hCG and changes in carbohydrate metabo-

Table 14–4. Daily Food Plan for Pregnancy and Lactation

Food Group	Nutrients Provided	Food Source	Recommended Daily Amount During Pregnancy	Recommended Daily Amount During Lactation
Dairy products	Protein; riboflavin; vitamins A, D, and others; calcium; phosphorus; zinc; magnesium	Milk—whole, 2%, skim, dry, buttermilk Cheeses—hard, semisoft, cottage Yogurt—plain, low-fat Soybean milk—canned, dry	Four (8 oz) cups (5 for teenagers) used plain or with flavoring, in shakes, soups, puddings, custards, cocoa Calcium in 1 cup milk equivalent to 1 1/2 cups cottage cheese, 1 1/2 oz hard or semisoft cheese, 1 cup yogurt, 1 1/2 cups ice cream (high in fat and sugar)	Four 8 oz cups (5 for teenagers); equivalent amount of cheese, yogurt and so forth
Meat and meat alternatives	Protein; iron; thiamine, niacin, and other vitamins; minerals	Beef, pork, veal, lamb, poultry, animal organ meats, fish, eggs; legumes; nuts, seeds, peanut butter, grains in proper vegetarian combination (vitamin B_{12} supplement needed)	Three servings (1 serving = 2 oz), combination in amounts necessary for same nutrient equivalent (varies greatly)	Two servings
Grain products, whole grain or enriched	B vitamins; iron; whole grain also has zinc, magnesium, and other trace elements; provides fiber	Bread and bread products such as cornbread, muffins, waffles, hotcakes, biscuits, dumplings, cereals, pastas, rice	Six to 11 servings daily: 1 serving = 1 slice bread, 3/4 cup or 1 oz dry cereal, 1/2 cup rice or pasta	Same as for pregnancy
Fruits and fruit juices	Vitamins A and C; minerals; raw fruits for roughage	Citrus fruits and juices, melons, berries, all other fruits and juices	Two to 4 servings (1 serving for vitamin C): 1 serving = 1 medium fruit, 1/2–1 cup fruit, 4 oz orange or grapefruit juice	Same as for pregnancy
Vegetables and vegetable juices	Vitamins A and C; minerals; provides roughage	Leafy green vegetables; deep yellow or orange vegetables such as carrots, sweet potatoes, squash, tomatoes; green vegetables such as peas, green beans, broccoli; other vegetables such as beets, cabbage, potatoes, corn, lima beans	Three to 5 servings (1 serving of dark green or deep yellow vegetable for vitamin A): 1 serving = 1/2–1 cup vegetable, 2 tomatoes, 1 medium potato	Same as for pregnancy
Fats	Vitamins A and D; linoleic acid	Butter, cream cheese, fortified table spreads; cream, whipped cream, whipped toppings; avocado, mayonnaise, oil, nuts	As desired in moderation (high in calories): 1 serving = 1 tbsp butter or enriched margarine	Same as for pregnancy
Sugars and sweets		Sugar, brown sugar, honey, molasses	Occasionally, if desired	Same as for pregnancy
Desserts		Nutritious desserts such as puddings, custards, fruit whips, and crisps; other rich, sweet desserts and pastries	Occasionally, if desired	Same as for pregnancy
Beverages		Coffee, decaffeinated beverages, tea, bouillon, carbonated drinks	As desired, in moderation	Same as for pregnancy
Miscellaneous		Iodized salt, herbs, spices, condiments	As desired	Same as for pregnancy

Note: The pregnant woman should eat regularly, 3 meals a day, with nutritious snacks of fruit, cheese, milk, or other foods between meals if desired. (More frequent but smaller meals are also recommended.) Four to 6 (8 oz) glasses of water and a total of 8 to 10 (8 oz) cups total fluid intake should be consumed daily. Water is an essential nutrient.

From Olds SB, London ML, and Ladewig PA. *Maternal-Newborn Nursing.* 5th ed. Redwood City, CA: Addison-Wesley Publishing, 1996, p 415. Copyright © 1996 by Addison-Wesley Nursing.

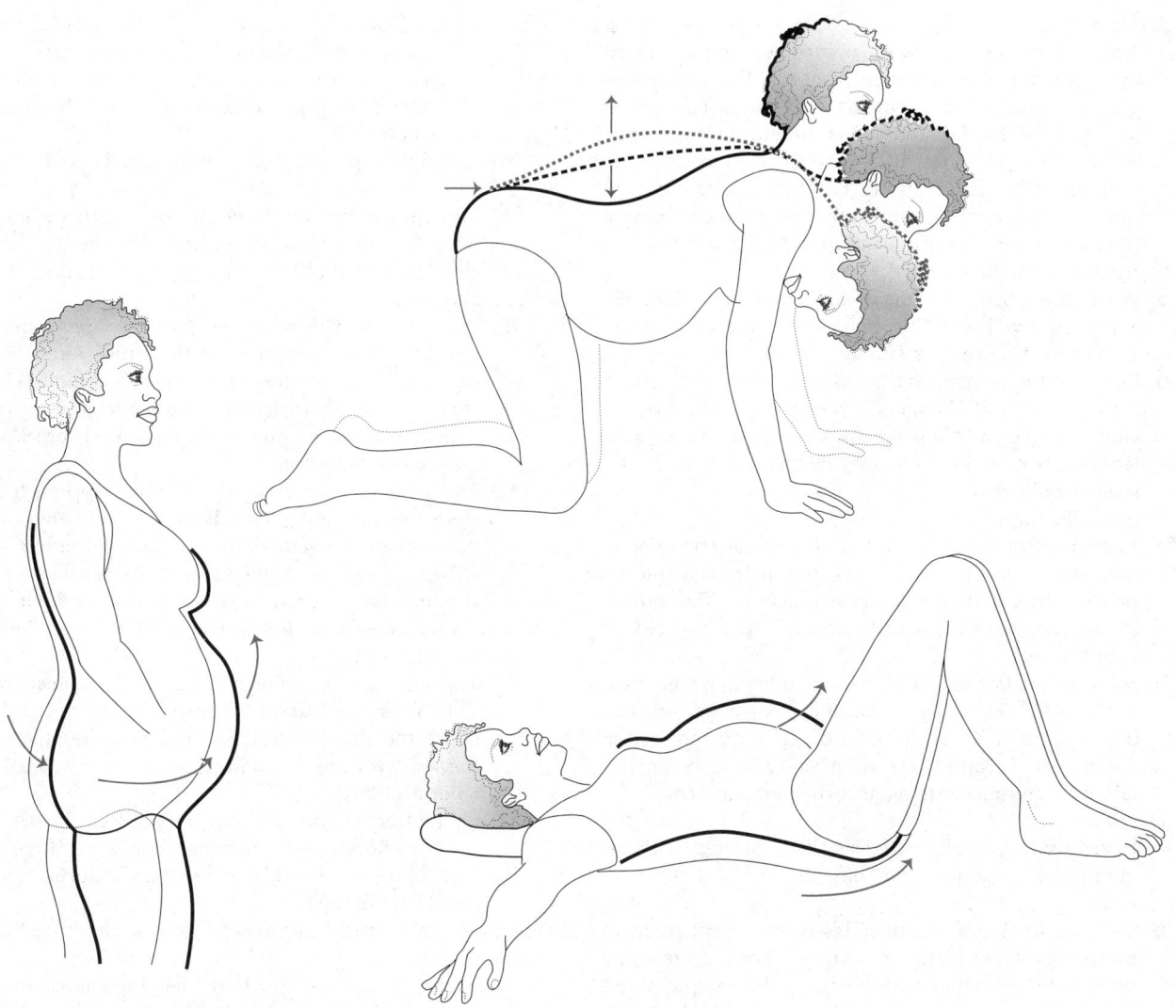

Figure 14–7. Pelvic tilt (or pelvic rock). (Modified from Gorrie TM, McKinney ES, and Murray SS. *Maternal Newborn Nursing*. Philadelphia: WB Saunders, 1994, p 149.)

lism. Morning sickness is most common during the 1st trimester.

b. Nausea most often occurs upon arising, although a few women experience it throughout the day. Most women do not vomit.

c. Self-care measures for morning sickness include eating a dry cracker or toast before getting out of bed, eating small frequent meals, avoiding fatty or spicy foods, rising slowly from a lying or sitting position to avoid orthostatic hypotension, and wearing acupressure wristbands.

2. Tender breasts

a. The breasts are usually tender from early in the pregnancy on, as a result of the increased levels of estrogen and progesterone.

b. Self-care measures for breast tenderness include wearing a well-fitting brassiere, which provides support for the breasts and decreases discomfort, and sleeping with a pillow.

3. Urinary frequency

a. Urinary frequency is present in the 1st trimester and late in the 3rd trimester because of the pressure placed on the bladder by the enlarged uterus.

b. Self-care measures for urinary frequency include emptying the bladder frequently (every 2 hr) and continuing to drink at least 2000 ml of fluids per day.

4. Constipation

a. Constipation may result from the slowing of peristalsis caused by the increased level of progesterone, the displacement of the intestines by the expanding uterus, a lack of activity, and inadequate fluid intake.

b. Self-care measures for constipation include increasing daily fluid intake, including whole grains and roughage in the diet, and exercising regularly.

5. Varicose veins

a. Varicose veins are caused by faulty functioning of the valves or weakening of the walls of the vein.

b. Self-care measures for varicose veins include wearing flat or low-heeled shoes, resting frequently throughout the day with both feet up at hip level, and wearing supportive stockings or hose if prolonged standing is anticipated.

6. Ankle edema
   a. Ankle edema is a common occurrence and is caused by decreased venous return from the feet because of gravity. Ankle edema remains a minor discomfort as long as hypertension and proteinuria are not present.
   b. Self-care measures for ankle edema include elevating the feet at hip level during the day, taking frequent rest periods, wearing supportive hose, and avoiding standing in one position or place for long periods.
7. Shortness of breath
   a. By midgestation, the uterus has risen up out of the abdomen and is exerting pressure on the diaphragm. This change causes pressure on the rib cage.
   b. Reassure the woman that shortness of breath is a normal physiologic change of pregnancy. Self-care includes sitting in an upright position and, if the problem occurs at night, elevating the chest and head with several pillows.
8. Vaginal discharge
   a. Vaginal discharge (called **leukorrhea**) is common in pregnant women, because of the increased mucus production by the endocervical glands. The mucus should be clear or slightly whitish and mucoid in appearance.
   b. Self-care for vaginal discharge includes hygienic measures such as daily cleansing; however, vaginal douching is not recommended. Recommend cotton underwear, because it is absorbent and does not retain heat and moisture against the perineal area.
9. Heartburn
   a. Heartburn, also called pyrosis, is associated with regurgitation of gastric acid contents up into the esophagus.
   b. Self-care for heartburn includes eating small frequent meals, avoiding fatty or spicy foods, remaining upright for 30 minutes after eating, drinking approximately 2000 ml of fluids per day, and taking antacids that contain aluminum hydroxide or a combination of magnesium hydroxide and aluminum hydroxide.

Helping the Family Plan for the Pregnancy and Care of the Newborn

1. The childbearing family has many decisions to make regarding care during pregnancy.
   a. The health care professional may be a certified nurse midwife or obstetrician-gynecologist. The family needs to understand the role of each type of provider.
   b. The place of birth may be a hospital, a free-standing birthing center, or the home.
      (1) Many hospitals now take a more relaxed, family-centered approach to childbirth, which allows the family to participate more in the experience and maintain some control over it.
      (2) Free-standing birth centers are increasing in number and are an option for the low-risk woman. They are usually run by certified nurse midwives and give the woman and family many choices regarding labor and birth.
      (3) Home birth is possible in many parts of the

United States. It is important that the woman have a low-risk status: She must be normotensive; the pregnancy must be a term pregnancy with no bleeding difficulties; membranes must be intact, and so on.
   c. The childbirth preparation method needs to be considered.
      (1) The woman or couple needs to investigate methods of pain relief (in addition to the prepared childbirth method) that are available during labor and birth.
      (2) The woman who takes the psychoprophylaxis, or Lamaze, approach prepares to reduce stress during birth by learning relaxation techniques, increasing her knowledge base concerning pregnancy and birth, and learning paced breathing techniques for labor.
      (3) The woman who takes the Bradley approach focuses on educating herself about pregnancy and birth, learning methods to increase relaxation and reduce stress, and responding to normal body rhythms for breathing techniques during labor.
   d. The family needs to decide whether to have siblings present at the birth.
      (1) The age of the siblings needs to be considered. Very young children (<2 years old) do not understand the process of labor and may become distressed with the discomfort, sights, and sounds of labor and birth.
      (2) If children attend, sibling preparation classes are recommended, and someone should be there for each child so that his or her needs during labor and birth are met.
2. Planning newborn feeding means considering breast and bottle.
   a. Decisions regarding newborn feeding need to be made from a sound, thorough parental knowledge base and consideration of individual values and beliefs.
   b. Explain the advantages and disadvantages of each feeding method to the woman or couple (Table 14–5).

NURSE ADVISORY

It is important that the expectant parents receive accurate, up-to-date information regarding feeding methods. Information needs to be presented in a relaxed manner and the advantages and disadvantages clearly identified.

---

3. Planning for employment means considering child care.
   a. If the expectant woman is employed during the pregnancy, she needs to be informed of the pregnancy needs that must be accommodated by her work setting.
      (1) Prolonged sitting or standing is not advisable. Frequent changes in position are important to promote circulation.
      (2) Fluid intake needs to be considered, and frequent restroom breaks are important.

Table 14–5. *Factors to Consider in Choosing an Infant Feeding Method*

	Breast-feeding	Formula Feeding
Advantages:	Provides antibodies to protect against infections Readily available Easily digestible	Provides adequate calories Easily digestible Baby can be fed by another person
Disadvantages:	Only mother can feed baby (unless milk is expressed) Cost involves increased nutrition for mother	Cost of formula Does not provide antibodies

      (3) The workplace needs to be assessed for environmental hazards.

  b. The woman may be planning to return to the workplace after the birth. If she is planning to breast-feed, she must determine what arrangements need to be made to allow her to do this at work or to store expressed milk safely.

  c. Child care may involve 1 parent remaining at home to provide care. Decisions involve how the care will be shared and perhaps how to choose another person or organization to provide care during a portion of the day.

  d. Assist the expectant parents by helping them focus on some of the critical issues.

      (1) Parental leave may be possible for the 1st few weeks after birth.

      (2) If 1 parent is to remain at home, the couple may want to discuss the aspects of this responsibility and how the other partner can be most supportive.

      (3) Locating a person or daycare facility to provide care will be important.

Public Health Considerations

1. The importance of prenatal visits
  a. Prenatal visits give you opportunities to provide information on self-care, pregnancy changes, and diet and to assess for risk factors and fetal status. At each prenatal visit, specific aspects need to be assessed.
      (1) Maternal assessment
        • Vital signs (blood pressure, pulse, and respirations)
        • Weight
        • Urine sample for glucose and protein
        • Signs of edema, deep tendon reflexes
        • Uterine size
        • The presence of any danger signs
        • The need for additional information
      (2) Fetal assessment
        • Maternal report of quickening at 18 to 20 weeks
        • Fetal heartbeat

        • Fetal movement record (kept by the expectant woman beginning at approximately 30 weeks)

  b. The perceived need for prenatal care varies among women and is influenced by individual or group attitudes, values and beliefs, perceived value or authenticity of the health care system, and access to care.

  c. For every pregnant woman, prenatal care greatly decreases the incidence of maternal, fetal, and neonatal complications. For each dollar spent on prenatal care, at least 3 dollars in treatment of complications after birth are saved.

  d. Even with subsidized care, access to care continues to be a problem for many women. Many health care providers do not accept Medicaid clients or accept very few. Certified nurse midwives are qualified health care providers who are able to provide maternal-child care to low-risk women in a cost-effective manner.

2. The avoidance of substance abuse
  a. Each woman needs to be screened for tobacco use and substance abuse.
  b. If abuse is identified, provide information on its effect on the pregnancy and fetus and refer the woman to appropriate community programs.

3. The incidence of violence for women of childbearing age
  a. One in 3 adolescents and women of childbearing age has been sexually abused in some manner. One in 3 women lives with a partner who abuses her physically, psychologically, or sexually. For 1 in 6 or 7 women, physical violence begins during pregnancy.
  b. It is imperative that each woman be assessed for violence in the home as she enters the health care environment. Nurses have been very successful in establishing the rapport and trust that are needed to obtain accurate information from women regarding the experience of violence.

◼ CONDITIONS THAT COMPLICATE PREGNANCY

Multiple Gestation

1. Definition: Multiple gestation is the presence of more than 1 fetus in the uterus.
2. Incidence and etiology
  a. The incidence of twins is 10 per 1000 births in the United States.
  b. Twins may be dizygotic (2 ova are released from the ovary and fertilized) or monozygotic (1 ovum is released, and after conception the cell divides into 2 separate gestations).
      (1) Dizygotic twins may be of the same sex, or 1 may be female and 1 male. These twins are sometimes referred to as fraternal twins. Each developing fetus has its own amniotic and chorionic membranes and its own placenta. Seventy-five percent of twins are dizygotic.
      (2) Monozygotic twins are always the same sex. The timing of the cell division determines whether

each twin has its own amnion or whether both twins are enclosed in one chorion and amnion and are in direct communication with each other (can touch). Only 25 percent of twins are monozygotic.

3. Clinical manifestations
    a. The uterus grows at an accelerated rate. Frequently, 2 gestational sacs can be seen with ultrasonography at 5 to 6 weeks' gestation. In this case, diagnosis is readily confirmed.
    b. Nausea may be more acute because of increased levels of hCG.
    c. The expectant mother is more likely to have fatigue, backache, varicosities, edema of the ankles, and striae.
    d. The woman is at higher risk for spontaneous abortion, anemia, pregnancy-induced hypertension, placenta previa and abruptio placentae, hydramnios, and cesarean birth.
    e. Monozygotic twins who share 1 chorion but have separate amnions (called monochorionic, diamniotic twins) or who share 1 chorion and 1 amnion (called monochorionic, monoamniotic twins) have an increased risk of mortality.
        (1) When there is only 1 placenta, it is more likely that 1 twin will receive better perfusion than the other. Therefore, a discrepancy in fetal weight may develop. The overperfused twin receives more blood and may be polycythemic. The underperfused twin is lighter and may be anemic.
        (2) Mortality rates for twins vary as follows: Dizygotic twins have a mortality rate of 9 percent; monozygotic twins that are dichorionic and diamniotic have a mortality rate of 9 percent; monochorionic, diamniotic twins have a mortality rate of 25 percent; and monochorionic, monoamniotic twins have a mortality rate greater than 50 percent.
4. Clinical management
    a. Diagnose twins early in the pregnancy to ensure maximum surveillance and support.
    b. Advise the woman about a daily minimum intake of 4000 calories and 135 gm of protein.
    c. Explain that the maternal weight gain pattern is accelerated, with an expected gain of 15 to 20 pounds by

20 weeks' gestation and a total gain of 40 to 60 pounds.
    d. Teach self-care measures for the minor discomforts of pregnancy. All minor discomforts will be exaggerated by the increased size of the uterus.
    e. Provide information on preparation for birth, including preparation for cesarean birth.
    f. Assist the woman or couple in identifying resources and support groups within the community that can provide information that will ease the transition into parenting.

Cardiovascular, Respiratory, and Renal Problems

Table 14–6 explains how various cardiovascular, respiratory, and renal problems can complicate pregnancy and what can be done to counter these complications.

Sexually Transmitted Diseases

Table 14–7 explains how sexually transmitted diseases can complicate pregnancy and interventions for these complications.

Tobacco Use

1. Definition: use of tobacco products during pregnancy
2. Incidence and etiology
    a. Thirty percent of childbearing women smoke cigarettes.
    b. Smoke from cigarettes causes the absorption of nicotine, carbon monoxide, and cyanide. These substances have been linked to vasoconstriction, which decreases the amount of oxygen and nutrition available to the fetus.
3. Clinical manifestations
    a. Smoking presents a serious health hazard to all childbearing women, but during the pregnancy the fetus is also exposed.

Table 14–6. Cardiovascular, Respiratory, and Renal Problems During Pregnancy

Disorder	Implications for Childbearing	Clinical Management
Rheumatic heart disease	The increased blood volume of pregnancy and changes in cardiac output place severe stress on the woman's heart. Congestive heart failure may result.	Monitor pregnancy carefully. Treat congestive heart failure. Plan cesarean birth and avoid stress of labor.
Tuberculosis	If tuberculosis is present in pregnancy, isoniazid may be taken. The expectant woman needs extra rest and limited contact with others until tuberculosis is under control.	Administer isoniazid. If tuberculosis is active, separate mother and baby until the disease is inactive.
Renal disease	Any renal disease precipitates additional stress during pregnancy because of the increased blood and fluid volume. The expectant woman is more likely to develop pregnancy-induced hypertension.	Monitor pregnancy carefully. Monitor kidney status, and watch for development of hypertension.

Table 14–7. Sexually Transmitted Diseases

Disorder	Implications for Childbearing	Clinical Management
Herpes simplex virus type 2 (HSV-2)	Transmission to fetus or neonate may occur with rupture of membranes after 4 hr; passage of the fetus through the birth canal may cause exposure when active lesions are present.	If lesions are active, plan for a cesarean birth. Some physicians treat asymptomatic infants with acyclovir. Herpes culture should be taken before treatment begins.
Chlamydia trachomatis infection	Infection may result in closure of the fallopian tubes, so that pregnancy is not possible. Newborn may have conjunctivitis at birth. Newborn may be born preterm and be at risk for chlamydial pneumonia.	Diagnose and treat chlamydial infection promptly. Provide information about signs and symptoms of infection. Instill erythromycin (Ilotycin) ointment in newborn's eyes within 1 hr of birth.
Gonorrhea *(Neisseria gonorrhoeae)*	Infections at birth may result in ophthalmic neonatorum.	Instill erythromycin (Ilotycin) ointment in newborn's eyes within 1 hr of birth.

b. The woman may have less weight gain than the non-smoking woman, because she may substitute cigarettes for nutritional substances.
c. The fetus may have intrauterine growth retardation or low birth weight.
4. Clinical management
   a. Obtain a history.
   b. Provide information on the effect of tobacco on the woman and the pregnancy.
   c. Provide information on smoking cessation programs.
   d. Review teaching and list of resources.
   e. Provide ongoing support for the woman.

Alcohol Abuse

See Chapter 40 for a discussion of the care of people who abuse alcohol.

1. Definition
   a. Use of alcohol during the prenatal period.
   b. Alcohol abuse during pregnancy carries additional risks.
2. Incidence and socioeconomic impact
   a. The incidence of alcohol use during pregnancy is estimated to be 2 to 70 percent.
   b. In some populations, the high incidence of maternal alcoholism results in an increased number of babies born with fetal alcohol syndrome (FAS). The long-term impact of FAS reaches into all aspects of our society—the educational system, the work environment, and the family structure.
3. Etiology
   a. Alcoholism in women has been associated with early childhood deprivation in the context of the dysfunctional family.
   b. Alcoholism is also associated with the death of a spouse, a child's leaving home, sex role dysfunction, and affective disorders.
4. Clinical manifestations
   a. Poor weight gain
   b. Hypoglycemia
   c. Tremors at rest

d. Nausea
e. Weakness
f. Anxiety
g. Slurred speech
h. Unsteady gait
i. Sweating (palms, forehead, or generalized)
5. Diagnostics
   a. A blood alcohol level of 0.10 (the legal definition of intoxication)
   b. Fetal studies including ultrasonography for growth pattern and signs of congenital problems, the NST, and a fetal biophysical profile.
6. Clinical management
   a. The goals of intervention are identification of the alcohol problem; support and counseling for nutritional needs, self-care, and pregnancy concerns; and referral to community support agencies.
   b. Nonpharmacologic interventions include nutritional counseling and supplementation and education regarding the effects of alcohol on pregnancy.
   c. Pharmacologic intervention entails supplementation with vitamins, ferrous sulfate, and folic acid.
7. Complications
   a. Maternal complications
      (1) Cirrhosis
      (2) Malnutrition
      (3) Withdrawal
      (4) Increased risk of spontaneous abortion
      (5) Megaloblastic anemia as a result of folic acid deficiency
      (6) Increased risk of multiple chemical abuse
      (7) Infectious diseases such as sexually transmitted diseases and parenterally transmitted diseases such as hepatitis.
   b. Fetal complications
      (1) Central nervous system involvement (including mental retardation)
      (2) Facial dysmorphia
      (3) Intrauterine growth retardation
      (4) Failure to thrive
      (5) Stillbirth
      (6) Fetal alcohol syndrome

(7) Microcephaly or microphthalmia
(8) Abnormal development of the central nervous system
(9) Abnormal midline facial features (e.g., a flattened nasal bridge and philtrum, thin upper lip, and short palpebral fissures)
(10) Fetal distress
(11) Low Apgar scores

8. Prognosis
   a. Treatment of alcoholism has varying rates of success.
   b. The child born with FAS usually has additional challenges in life.
9. Applying the nursing process

NURSING DIAGNOSIS: Altered nutrition, less than body requirements, R/T decreased food intake and alcohol consumption

---

   a. *Expected outcomes:* After counseling, the woman should be able to do the following:
      (1) Explain the nutritional needs of pregnancy
      (2) Identify supportive resources within the community
   b. *Nursing interventions*
      (1) Determine current nutritional intake by interviewing the woman, having her keep a 24-hour food diary, or both.
      (2) Provide information on recommended daily nutrition requirements and implications for pregnancy.
      (3) Refer the woman to community resources as needed.
      (4) Monitor weight gain.
      (5) Provide nutritional counseling.
      (6) Assess fetal growth.
      (7) After birth, assess the newborn for signs of withdrawal and FAS.
      (8) Refer for counseling and follow-up.
10. Discharge planning and teaching
    a. Provide information on self-care activities.
    b. Provide information on the effects of alcohol on pregnancy and the developing embryo, fetus, and newborn.
11. Public health considerations
    a. Alcohol is one of the most commonly abused drugs in the world.
    b. The nurse can heighten public awareness regarding alcohol abuse and the availability of community resources for treatment or rehabilitation.

Use of Cocaine

1. Definition: Cocaine can be smoked as crack, taken intranasally, or injected intravenously during pregnancy.
2. Incidence and socioeconomic impact
   a. The incidence of drug use (marijuana, cocaine, or opiates) during pregnancy has been estimated to be 11 to 15 percent.
   b. The incidence of drug use is difficult to determine, because most chemicals are detectable in the blood or urine for only 1 to 5 days after use.
3. Pathophysiology
   a. Cocaine exerts an effect on the nerve terminals, and the reuptake of dopamine and norepinephrine is prevented. This process causes vasoconstriction, tachycardia, and hypertension.
   b. Vasoconstriction in the placenta leads to decreased blood flow to the fetus, may precipitate abruption of the placenta (separation of the placenta before birth of the baby), and stimulates uterine contractions.
4. Clinical manifestations
   a. Irritability
   b. Difficulty sleeping
   c. Anxiety
   d. Gastrointestinal upsets
   e. Headaches
   f. Depression and suicidal tendencies
5. Diagnostics

NURSE ADVISORY

To elicit maternal history related to drug use, use a direct approach. Begin the interview with questions that tend to be neutral and move to more difficult areas.

---

   a. Physical assessment
      (1) Inspect for inflamed nasal alae and intravenous injection sites.
      (2) Look for signs of anemia and malnutrition.
      (3) Note signs of poor dental hygiene, rhinitis, restlessness, dilated or constricted pupils, shortness of breath, and hypertension.
   b. Diagnosis
      (1) Positive urine toxicology screen (detects cocaine ingestion within the past 24 hr)
      (2) Positive toxicology from a meconium test
   c. Diagnostic studies
      (1) Urine or meconium toxicology screening
      (2) Maternal diagnostic studies: complete blood count, Venereal Disease Research Laboratory test, cervical culture for gonorrhea and chlamydia, HIV test, tuberculin skin test, and urinalysis
      (3) Fetal diagnostic studies: serial ultrasonography to determine fetal growth pattern and assess for congenital anomalies, the NST, and a biophysical profile
6. Clinical management
   a. The goals of clinical management are identification of the drug problem and associated complications, support and counseling for nutritional needs, cessation of or decrease in drug use, self-care, pregnancy concerns, and referral to community support agencies.
   b. Nonpharmacologic interventions include counseling and support measures and nutritional supplementation.
   c. Pharmacologic intervention consists of supplementation with vitamins, ferrous sulfate, and folic acid.

7. Complications
   a. The use of cocaine and other chemicals places a woman at increased risk for sexually transmitted infections, parenterally transmitted diseases such as hepatitis and HIV infection, spontaneous abortion, preterm labor (abruptio placentae has occurred moments after nasal or intravenous ingestion of cocaine), seizures, postpartum intracerebral aneurysm, rupture of the ascending aorta, and sudden death.
   b. Fetal complications include congenital anomalies (cardiac, central nervous system, and urinary tract anomalies; nonduodenal intestinal atresia-infarction; and limb reduction defects), perinatal cerebral infarctions, small for gestational age, dysmorphic facial features, and neurobehavioral abnormalities.
   c. Neonatal complications include muscle tone abnormalities as evidenced by overly extended posture and tremulousness, irritability and difficulty being consoled, and abrupt movement from one state to another.
8. Prognosis
   a. The neonate is more likely to have neurobehavioral problems, especially during the 1st year of life.
   b. Drug treatment programs may be effective in providing a method for the woman to cease drug use.
9. Applying the nursing process

NURSING DIAGNOSIS: Risk for injury to the woman and fetus R/T drug use

   a. *Expected outcomes:* After counseling, the woman should be able to do the following:
      (1) Relate the effects of cocaine on pregnancy and discuss the complications for herself, the fetus, and the newborn
      (2) Identify sources of support within the community
   b. *Nursing interventions*
      (1) Provide information on the effects of cocaine on the woman, the fetus, and the newborn.
      (2) Refer the woman to appropriate community agencies.
      (3) Refer the woman to a chemical dependency treatment center.
      (4) Provide counseling regarding nutrition, self-care, preparation for birth, and the effects of cocaine on pregnancy.
      (5) Prevent and treat preterm labor.
      (6) Complete fetal assessment testing to determine fetal condition and allow early recognition of problems.
      (7) Instruct the woman on comfort techniques for the newborn. Tell her to avoid letting the infant reach a frantic cry state. She should allow the newborn to gain control, but if this is delayed, she should swaddle the babe and offer a pacifier. If the irritability does not cease, she should hold the newborn close and rock him or her vertically, offering 1 stimulus at a time.

10. Discharge planning and teaching
    a. Continue to provide support.
    b. Refer the woman to a chemical dependency treatment center.
11. Public health considerations
    a. The use of cocaine has increased among young childbearing women.
    b. The lifelong implications for the child are not clearly understood.

Acquired Immunodeficiency Syndrome

See Chapter 42 for discussion of the care of people with acquired immunodeficiency syndrome (AIDS).

1. Definition
   a. The depressed cell-mediated immunity typical of pregnancy may accelerate the progression of opportunistic diseases during pregnancy.
   b. The HIV-positive woman may therefore be especially vulnerable when pregnant.
2. Diagnostics
   a. Maternal diagnostic studies
      (1) Complete blood count with differential leukocyte count (because anemia, leukopenia, and neutropenia are common)
      (2) Number of T4 cells and T4:T8 ratio (to evaluate immune status)
      (3) Urinalysis (for proteinuria as may be seen with HIV nephropathy)
      (4) Cervical and vaginal smear and cultures (to detect viral infections)
      (5) Chest radiograph (for HIV-related illness); if a chest radiograph is needed, protect the maternal abdomen with a lead apron
      (6) Laboratory abnormalities during HIV infection
         • Decreased T4 count and T4:T8 ratio; leukopenia; lymphopenia; anemia, thrombocytopenia, or both; and elevated serum globulins
         • Possible markers that suggest progression to AIDS. These may be elevated levels of beta$_2$-microglobulin, HIV p24 antigenemia, anemia, low T4 (helper) cell count, high proportion of T8 (suppressor) cells, reduced level of HIV antibody, and elevated level of cytomegalovirus antibody.
   b. Fetal diagnostic studies
      (1) Serial ultrasounds for assessing fetal growth
      (2) An NST and a biophysical profile weekly beginning in the 30th week to assess fetal status
3. Clinical management
   a. Goals of clinical management
      (1) Monitor woman for development of additional infections.
      (2) Monitor pregnancy progress.
      (3) Evaluate for other sexually transmitted diseases.
      (4) Determine T4 cell count at least every trimester. If count is higher than 500, provide regular prenatal care; if count is lower than 500, start therapy with zidovudine (AZT).

(5) Every trimester repeat complete blood count, differential, platelets, and T helper, suppressor, and immunoglobulins.
  b. Nonpharmacologic intervention consists of nutritional counseling to promote most optimal nutrition.
  c. Pharmacologic interventions
    (1) Zidovudine studies are in progress to determine use in pregnancy. Current indications are for use in asymptomatic HIV infection with T4 cell count less than 500 per mm^3, symptomatic HIV infection, or associated infection.
    (2) Sulfamethoxazole-trimethoprim is used to treat *Pneumocystis carinii* pneumonia.
    (3) Pentamidine isethionate may be used after acute treatment of *P. carinii* pneumonia as prophylaxis. The safety of its use during pregnancy is not well known.
    (4) Acyclovir may be used after the birth for maternal human papillomavirus infections.
    (5) Pyrimethamine and sulfadiazine may be used in the 3rd trimester for treatment of toxoplasmosis.
4. Complications
  a. Increased incidence of preterm birth
  b. Intrauterine growth retardation
  c. Premature rupture of membranes (PROM)
  d. Coexistent sexually transmitted diseases
  e. Perinatal transmission to fetus (transplacental) and to newborn through breast milk. Perinatal transmission accounts for 84 percent of pediatric AIDS.
5. Prognosis
  a. If the number of cases continues to increase at the anticipated rate, AIDS will be 1 of the leading 5 causes of death in women of childbearing age.
  b. *P. carinii* pneumonia is the leading cause of maternal mortality in HIV-AIDS–infected women during pregnancy.
6. Applying the nursing process

NURSING DIAGNOSIS: Risk for infection R/T exposure to opportunistic infection and suppression of immune system

  a. *Expected outcomes:* After care the woman should be able to do the following:
    (1) Describe laboratory results necessary to monitor her health status
    (2) State information regarding prevention, treatment, and care of opportunistic infections
  b. *Nursing interventions*
    (1) Assess laboratory results to determine immune system status.
    (2) Provide information regarding prevention, treatment, and care of opportunistic infections.

NURSING DIAGNOSIS: Anticipatory grieving R/T knowledge of disease progression and anticipation of death

  c. *Expected outcomes:* After care the woman should be able to do the following:

    (1) Identify her personal support system
    (2) State the progression of the disease
    (3) Locate supportive resources within the community
  d. *Nursing interventions*
    (1) Establish rapport and provide opportunities for the woman to talk.
    (2) Determine the availability of supportive people in the woman's personal life.
    (3) Refer to community counseling services.
7. Discharge planning and teaching
  a. Provide information on self-care measures, prevention of further infections, and infant care.
  b. Encourage the woman to have protected sexual contact.
  c. Encourage the woman to maintain health care.
8. Public health considerations
  a. The incidence of AIDS is increasing rapidly in women of childbearing age, and perinatal transmission is the major source of infection to children.
  b. HIV-AIDS provides a threat to health care professionals.

Diabetes Mellitus

See Chapter 29 for a detailed discussion of diabetes mellitus.

1. Risk factors
  a. Previous stillbirth
  b. Birth of previous baby weighing over 4000 gm (macrosomia)
  c. History of preeclampsia, recurrent urinary tract infection, chronic hypertension, and hydramnios
2. Pathophysiology
  a. The impact of diabetes on the pregnant woman includes a 25 percent risk of developing preeclampsia, high incidence of infection (monilial vaginitis is common, chorioamnionitis, and postpartum endometritis), and increased risk of cesarean birth.
  b. The impact of diabetes on the fetus includes an increased incidence of congenital anomalies, hypoglycemia, macrosomia, neonatal respiratory distress syndrome, hypocalcemia, and traumatic birth (associated with macrosomia).
  c. The impact of pregnancy on diabetes includes alteration of insulin needs, increased incidence of ketoacidosis, progression of retinopathy, and worsening of nephropathy.
3. Clinical manifestations
  a. Glycosuria is not as reliable a sign in pregnancy.
  b. It may reflect the pregnancy-related lowered renal threshold for glucose.
4. Diagnostics
  a. Maternal assessment
    (1) Clean-catch urinalysis and urine culture each trimester
    (2) Hemoglobin A1c if preexisting diabetes
  b. Fetal assessment
    (1) Fetal activity diary
    (2) Ultrasound test for growth and presence of anomalies

(3) Nonstress test

(4) Fetal biophysical profile

(5) Doppler blood flow studies

(6) Amniotic fluid assessment for fetal lung maturity

5. Clinical management

a. Goals of management

(1) Early recognition of gestational diabetes

(2) Initiation of early treatment

(3) Maintenance of equilibrium between insulin availability and glucose utilization

(4) Education related to disease process, implications of diabetes on pregnancy, and self-care measures

b. Nonpharmacologic interventions

(1) Educate woman regarding prevention of infections, adequate nutrition, testing needed, and administration of insulin if needed.

(2) Emphasize self-care measures that are commonly associated with pregnancy.

c. Pharmacologic intervention

(1) Human insulin may need to be taken. If insulin is required, most women need 2 to 4 injections a day of a mixture of intermediate and regular insulin.

(2) Insulin requirements may fluctuate in early pregnancy and then increase. Insulin requirements may drop precipitously after birth.

6. Complications

a. Maternal complications

(1) Hypertension in 12 to 13 percent of women

(2) A 4-fold increase in pregnancy-induced hypertension (PIH)

(3) Infections (monilial infections are common, and pyelonephritis occurs in 2–12% of women)

(4) Hydramnios in 6 to 25 percent of pregnant women

(5) Intrauterine fetal death rate of 1 to 4 percent

(6) Intrauterine growth retardation in classes D through T of diabetes mellitus

(7) Macrosomic fetus or neonate (especially in classes A–C)

(8) Increased risk of cesarean birth and postpartum hemorrhage

b. Fetal and neonatal complications

(1) A 6 to 12 percent risk of congenital anomalies (3–4 times the risk of general population)

(2) Preterm birth

(3) Hypoglycemia in 20 to 60 percent of neonates

(4) An 8 to 22 percent risk of hypocalcemia

(5) A 15 to 20 percent risk of hyperbilirubinemia

(6) Neonatal respiratory distress syndrome in 3 to 11 percent

(7) An infant of a diabetic mother is more likely to develop diabetes later in life.

7. Prognosis

a. Maternal and fetal or neonatal morbidity depends on the control of the diabetes and the extent of cardiovascular involvement.

b. Maternal mortality is rare unless ischemic heart disease is present.

c. Perinatal mortality is 3.6 to 4.6 percent in women with overt diabetes, a rate 2 to 3 times greater than that in the general population. Congenital anomalies are the most common cause of perinatal death.

8. Applying the nursing process

NURSING DIAGNOSIS: Altered nutrition R/T altered carbohydrate metabolism

a. *Expected outcomes:* As a result of care, the woman should be able to do the following:

(1) Relate the impact of diabetes on nutrition during pregnancy

(2) Select a daily menu that meets her nutritional needs

(3) Identify resources for further assistance when needed

b. *Nursing interventions*

(1) Review the current dietary plan and assess for needed changes related to pregnancy.

(2) Determine the woman's understanding of the impact of pregnancy and diabetes.

(3) Refer for counseling and consultation with nutritionist.

(4) Discuss community resources.

(5) Provide education regarding signs and symptoms, treatment measures, and danger signs.

NURSING DIAGNOSIS: Risk for injury R/T increased fetal glucose levels during gestation

a. *Expected outcomes:* Following care, the newborn should demonstrate the following:

(1) Be within normal weight pattern (average for gestational weight)

(2) Have normal blood sugars after birth

NURSE ADVISORY

To provide comprehensive care of the infant of a diabetic mother, be alert for hypoglycemia, hypocalcemia, hyperbilirubinemia, respiratory distress syndrome, and conditions caused by birth trauma.

b. *Nursing interventions*

(1) Encourage maintenance of recommended dietary intake (30–35 kcal/ideal body weight). If ketoacidosis occurs, caloric intake needs to be increased. Nutritional intake is apportioned as 12 to 20 percent protein, 50 to 60 percent carbohydrate, and 20 to 30 percent fat.

(2) Administer insulin as prescribed.

(3) Monitor blood glucose levels and results of testing such as hemoglobin A1c.

(4) Test urine for ketones if blood sugar is greater than 240 mg per dl or maternal illness is present.

NURSING DIAGNOSIS: Knowledge deficit R/T lack of information regarding expected changes in pregnancy, self-care measures, and danger signs of pregnancy

---

BOX 14–3. Danger Signs During Pregnancy

Advise pregnant woman that any of the following signs and symptoms need to be reported to her care provider immediately.

Vaginal bleeding
Temperature >101° F (38.3° C)
Dizziness, blurring of vision, spots
    before eyes
Edema of hands, face, legs and feet
Epigastric pain
Severe headache

Abdominal pain
Dysuria or oliguria
Absence of fetal movement
Sudden gush of fluid from
    vagina
Persistent vomiting
Convulsions

---

    a. *Expected outcomes:* After prenatal care, the childbearing woman should be able to do the following:
      (1) Maintain a low-risk status during pregnancy
      (2) Attain desired weight gain
      (3) Be knowledgeable regarding self-care measures
    b. *Nursing interventions*
      (1) Determine present level of knowledge.
      (2) Determine educational level and reading ability to obtain and prepare appropriate materials.
      (3) Explore cultural values and beliefs that may affect practices during pregnancy.
      (4) Provide information regarding nutrition.
      (5) Provide information regarding danger signs in pregnancy (Box 14–3).
      (6) Assist the expectant woman (or couple) in obtaining information regarding selecting a caregiver, child birth choices, labor and birth options available in the community, and methods of obtaining comfort or relief.
9. Discharge planning and teaching
    a. Educate the woman regarding the implications of diabetes, treatments, interventions, and self-care measures.
    b. Monitor pregnancy carefully.

◼ COMPLICATIONS CAUSED BY PREGNANCY

Maternal Infections

Table 14–8 lists infections in the mother that may occur during pregnancy.

Pregnancy-Induced Diabetes

1. Definition
    a. Pregnancy-induced diabetes becomes evident during the pregnancy and is called gestational diabetes. The condition may continue after the pregnancy ends.
    b. Insulin may be required during pregnancy.
2. Incidence and etiology
    a. Gestational diabetes occurs in 2 to 3 percent of all pregnant women.
    b. Sixty percent of women who had gestational diabetes develop overt diabetes mellitus within 16 years.
3. Clinical manifestations
    a. The woman may have a history of gestational diabetes in a previous pregnancy, birth of a baby weighing more than 4000 grams, previous stillbirth or baby born with a congenital anomaly, obesity, or a family history of diabetes.
    b. The woman may develop symptoms or may be identified by a screening test.
    c. Glycosuria is not as reliable a sign in pregnancy because it may reflect the pregnancy-related lowered renal threshold for glucose.
4. Clinical management
    a. Screening test for gestational diabetes between 24 and 28 weeks' gestation. Woman ingests 50 gm of glucose. If the plasma glucose level obtained 1 hour after ingestion is higher than 140 mg per dl, further testing is indicated.
    b. Glucose tolerance returns to normal in 98 percent of gestational diabetics after birth.

Hyperemesis Gravidarum

1. Definition: Hyperemesis gravidarum is excessive vomiting during pregnancy and may result in weight loss and fluid and electrolyte problems.
2. Incidence and etiology
    a. The incidence is fairly rare.
    b. The etiology is unclear, but increased estrogen levels, increasing levels of hCG, or both may be contributing factors. Occasionally, psychologic factors may play a part.
3. Clinical manifestations: The expectant woman vomits ex-

Table 14–8. Maternal Infections

Disorder	Implications for Childbearing	Clinical Management
Monilial infection (*Candida albicans*)	Fetus may be infected at birth if infection is active.	Treat pregnant women with clindamycin.
Gardnerella vaginalis	There is an increased risk for premature rupture of membranes and preterm labor.	Treat pregnant women with clindamycin.
Trichomonas vaginalis	If infection is treated with metronidazole and pregnancy is undetected, teratogenic effects may occur.	Treat pregnant women with clindamycin.

cessively, exhibits weight loss, and may develop fluid and electrolyte imbalances.

4. Clinical management
   a. Control of vomiting is an important factor. Some antiemetics may be used.
   b. Fluid loss may need to be replaced with intravenous fluids.
   c. After vomiting is controlled and fluid balance is restored, attention is placed on maintaining adequate nutrition. Frequent, small meals may be tolerated more easily.

Pregnancy-Induced Hypertension

1. Definition
   a. An increase in systolic blood pressure of 30 mm Hg or in diastolic blood pressure of 15 mm Hg over baseline, or both, noted on at least 2 occasions 6 hours or more apart
   b. The presence of proteinuria and edema
   c. One of a number of hypertensive disorders that may occur in pregnancy. The American College of Obstetricians and Gynecologists classifies hypertension as follows:
      (1) Pregnancy-induced hypertension
      (2) Chronic hypertension
      (3) Chronic hypertension with superimposed preeclampsia
      (4) Late or transient hypertension
   d. Also called preeclampsia-eclampsia and classified as mild preeclampsia, severe preeclampsia, or eclampsia
      (1) Mild preeclampsia is characterized by a rise in systolic blood pressure of 30 mm Hg or more or a rise in diastolic pressure of 15 mm Hg or more, or both; generalized edema (feet, lower legs, hands and face); proteinuria 1+ or 2+.
      (2) Severe preeclampsia is characterized by blood pressure of 160/110 or more, proteinuria of 3+ or 4+, oliguria (<400 ml/24 hr or <30 ml/hr), headache, blurred vision, epigastric pain, and hyperreflexia.
      (3) Eclampsia is characterized by grand mal seizure.
2. Incidence
   a. Six to 7 percent of all pregnancies in the United States.
   b. A 15 to 20 percent incidence in Black primigravidas and 30 percent in young primigravidas with a multiple pregnancy.
3. Risk factors
   a. Parity (two thirds of cases occur with primigravidas), family history of PIH
   b. Medical problems such as diabetes mellitus, chronic hypertension, or renal disease
   c. Extremes of age (teenagers or women older than age 35)
   d. Pregnancy problems such as multiple gestation, hydatidiform mole, and hydrops fetalis
4. Etiology
   a. Etology is unknown.

   b. Prevention depends on analysis of risk factors and early detection.
5. Pathophysiology
   a. Increased peripheral vascular resistance (or increased cardiac output)
   b. Rise in blood pressure after 20 weeks
   c. Loss of resistance to angiotensin II and catecholamine
   d. Loss of normal vasodilation of uterine arterioles, resulting in decreased placental perfusion
   e. Decreased renal perfusion
   f. Decreased intravascular volume, leading to increased viscosity of the blood and increased hematocrit
   g. Coagulation abnormalities called HELLP syndrome (*h*emolysis, *e*levated *l*iver enzymes, *l*ow *p*latelet count)
6. Clinical manifestations
   a. Usually develop after the midpoint in pregnancy
   b. Begin with an increase of blood pressure followed by edema and proteinuria
7. Diagnostics
   a. A pregnant woman has PIH when hypertension is present on 2 occasions at least 6 hours apart and edema (exhibited by generalized pitting edema and weight gain) and proteinuria are present. Edema and proteinuria may not be present in the beginning and do not have to be present for clear diagnosis.
   b. Assessment
      (1) History
         • Note the presence of risk factors in prenatal history.
         • Note the pattern and amount of weight gain and blood pressure readings.
      (2) Physical assessment
         • Take blood pressure in sitting position with arm resting on a desk or table. Use appropriate-sized blood pressure cuff, and use phase IV (muffling of sound) as designation of diastolic reading.
         • Inspect for generalized edema, and assess for pitting edema using 0 to 4+ scale (Box 14–4).
         • Use a dipstick for clean-catch urine for protein.
         • Assess deep tendon reflexes (Box 14–5).
         • Assess clonus.
         • Assess for presence of headache, blurred vision, epigastric pain, nausea, and vomiting.
         • Assess the fetus for movement and fetal heart

BOX 14–4. Assessment and Evaluation of Pitting Edema

Uncover the woman's lower leg and press the fingertips of your index and middle finger against the shin and hold pressure for 2 to 3 seconds. Evaluate the depth of the remaining pit as follows:

0	No identification
1+	A slight identation
2+	An indentation approximately 1/4 inch deep
3+	An identation approximately 1/2 inch deep
4+	An identation approximately 1 inch deep

BOX 14–5. Evaluation of Deep Tendon Reflexes and Clonus

1. Expose the woman's lower leg and place 1 hand under the knee to raise it slightly off the bed. Using a percussion hammer, strike the patellar tendon (located just below the patella). The normal response is extension and thrusting of the foot upward.
2. Evaluate the extension in the following way:
    - 0   No response
    - 1+   Diminished
    - 2+   Normal
    - 3+   Increased, brisker than average
    - 4+   Very brisk, hyperactive
3. To detect the presence of clonus, place 1 hand under the woman's knee and bend the knee slightly. Place the other hand on the ball of the foot, and encourage the woman to relax her leg and foot. Sharply dorsiflex the foot. Clonus is present if the foot jerks or taps against your hand. Evaluate as follows:
    - 0   No jerking
    - 1 beat   One jerk or tap
    - 2 beats   Two jerks or taps

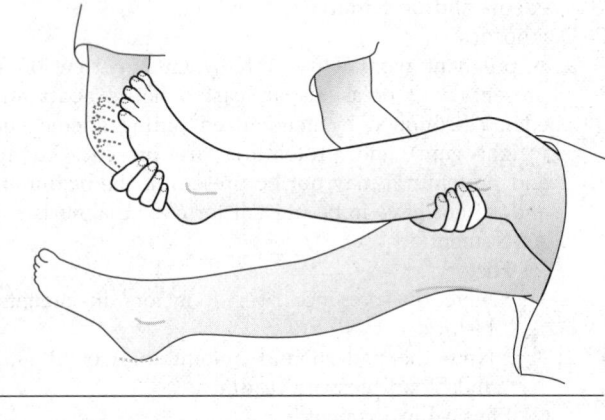

rate. Note the presence of reassuring signs such as average variability, baseline rate between 120 and 160, and the presence of accelerations with fetal movement. Note the presence of nonreassuring signs such as decreased variability, late or variable decelerations, bradycardia or tachycardia, and absence of accelerations with fetal movement.

    (3) Diagnostic studies
- Urinalysis and proteinuria
- Hematologic tests: hemoglobin and hematocrit
- Renal function tests: uric acid, blood urea nitrogen, and creatinine
- Liver function tests: aspartate aminotransferase (AST) and alanine aminotransferase (ALT)
- Coagulation tests: platelets, fibrinogen, prothrombin and partial thromboplastin times, and fibrin degradation products (Table 14–9).

8. Clinical management
  a. Goals of clinical management: Identify women at risk for PIH and provide teaching for self-care, identify presence of PIH, and initiate therapy to treat PIH.
  b. Nonpharmacologic interventions

    (1) Encourage bed rest in a side-lying position to maximize uteroplacental blood flow and renal perfusion, which results in mobilizing body fluids.
    (2) Encourage diet that provides 1 gm protein per kg per day.
    (3) Teach relaxation exercises and stress reduction techniques.
  c. Pharmacologic interventions: Initiate therapy with intravenous magnesium sulfate (Table 14–10).

9. Complications
  a. Maternal complications
    (1) Central nervous system complications
- Eclamptic seizure (from vasogenic cerebral edema)
- Hyperreflexia (from central nervous system irritability)
- Intracerebral hemorrhage (from cerebral edema)
- Blindness (from retinal or cerebral edema or arterial spasm)

    (2) Renal complications include acute tubular necrosis (from underperfusion of the kidneys) and acute cortical necrosis (from destruction of glomeruli).
    (3) The hepatic complication is ischemia, which may result in subcapsular hematoma.
    (4) Cardiac complications may be cardiac failure (resulting from acute increase in afterload).
    (5) The respiratory complication is pulmonary edema (associated with low colloid osmotic pressure and increased capillary permeability).
    (6) Coagulation complications involve consumptive coagulopathy (from endothelial damage).
    (7) HELLP syndrome
- Hemolysis of red blood cells occurs as cells are pressured through vasoconstricted vessels. He-

Table 14–9. Diagnostic Tests for Pregnancy-Induced Hypertension

Tests	Findings in Pregnancy-Induced Hypertension
Hematocrit	Elevated
Renal function tests	
Uric acid	Increased (>5 ml/dl)
Blood urea nitrogen	Increased (>10 mg/dl)
Creatinine	Increased (>1.0 mg/dl)
Liver function tests	
AST	Mild elevation
ALT	Mild elevation
Coagulation studies	
Platelets	Decreased (<150,000)
Fibrogen	Usually normal or slightly elevated
Thrombin time	Prolonged
Prothrombin	Usually normal
Partial thromboplastin time	Usually normal
Fibrin degradation products	Frequently increased

AST, Aspartate aminotransferase; ALT, alanine aminotransferase.

Agent	**Maximum Effect**	**Duration**	**Advantages**	**Disadvantages**

Table 14–10. Pharmacologic Treatment of Severe Preeclampsia

Seizure Prophylaxis

Agent	Maximum Effect	Duration	Advantages	Disadvantages
Magnesium sulfate (MgSO$_4$)	Variable depending on blood level	Variable	Can be titrated based on maternal blood levels	Therapeutic blood level range fairly narrow

Antihypertensive Agents
Direct vasodilators

Agent	Maximum Effect	Duration	Advantages	Disadvantages
Hydralazine	20 min	2–6 hr	Easy to administer. Effect is primarily on resistance vessels so can be used in a hypovolemic woman	Difficult to titrate to woman's blood pressure owing to slower onset and long duration of action. Myocardial oxygen consumption increased due to reflex tachycardia
Nitroprusside	2 min	3–5 min	Rapid onset and short duration of action. Very potent	Intra-arterial monitoring required. Potential for cyanide toxicity with large doses over a long period of time
Nifedipine	15 min	3–5 hr	Hypotension rare. Dilates coronary arteries	Relatively slow onset and long duration. Increases intracranial pressure because the drug increases cerebral blood flow. Causes uterine relaxation. Cannot be used concurrently with magnesium sulfate

Sympatholytic Vasodilator

Agent	Maximum Effect	Duration	Advantages	Disadvantages
Labetalol	10 min	2–8 hr	May be administered easily as a bolus. No reflex tachycardia	Long duration of action. Efficacy is variable

molysis causes a decrease in oxygen-carrying capacity, increased bilirubin level, and an abnormal peripheral blood smear.

- Elevated liver enzymes include an AST of greater than 72 IU per liter.
- Low platelets occur because of the tendency of platelets to aggregate in damaged vascular endothelium. As the platelet count decreases below minimum levels, the risk of maternal hemorrhage increases.

   b. Fetal complications include intrauterine growth retardation (from changes in placental vasculature and decreased placental perfusion), prematurity (from the need to deliver the mother when PIH is severe), and death.

10. Prognosis
   a. Early identification and subsequent aggressive treatment can reduce both maternal and perinatal morbidity and mortality.
   b. Perinatal mortality is increased because of an increased incidence of preterm birth and abruptio placentae.

11. Applying the nursing process

NURSING DIAGNOSIS: Altered tissue perfusion R/T vasoconstriction and decreased intravascular fluid volume

   a. *Expected outcomes:* After intervention, the woman should be able to do the following:
     (1) Maintain blood pressure within acceptable limits

     (2) Maintain a urine output of more than 30 ml per hour
     (3) Be stabilized and have a safe birth
   b. *Nursing interventions*
     (1) Monitor vital signs and signs of worsening condition such as increasing blood pressure, decreasing urine output, increasing hyperreflexia, presence of clonus, decreased respirations, and changing laboratory values indicating development of coagulation problems.
     (2) Initiate and continuously monitor therapy to treat hyperreflexia.
     (3) Initiate and continuously monitor therapy to treat elevation of blood pressure.
     (4) Position the woman on her left side to maximize uteroplacental perfusion.
     (5) Maintain the woman on bed rest.
     (6) Monitor laboratory data.

NURSING DIAGNOSIS: Risk for injury R/T decreased uteroplacental perfusion

   a. *Expected outcomes:* After intervention, the fetus should be able to do the following:
     (1) Maintain reassuring FHR pattern
     (2) Be evaluated to determine whether labor and birth or cesarean birth would be most favorable
   b. *Nursing interventions*
     (1) Monitor FHR on frequent (or continuous) basis as indicated.

(2) Position the woman to maximize uteroplacental blood flow.

(3) Evaluate fetal movement on a frequent basis.

(4) Teach the expectant woman to complete fetal movement record each day.

(5) Perform antepartal testing such as the NST, biophysical profile, Doppler waveform studies, and contraction stress test to determine fetal status.

12. Discharge planning and teaching
    a. Provide information related to risk factors for PIH early in pregnancy.
    b. Teach signs and symptoms of PIH early in pregnancy and provide reinforcement during the pregnancy.
    c. Provide education regarding nutrition and self-care activities.

13. Prognosis
    a. Early identification and subsequent aggressive treatment can reduce both maternal and perinatal morbidity and mortality.
    b. Perinatal mortality is increased because of an increased incidence of preterm birth and abruptio placentae.

14. Public health considerations
    a. Early access to prenatal care is imperative in establishing baselines, assessing for risk factors, and providing opportunities to educate the women regarding self-care measures and signs and symptoms of PIH.
    b. Preparation of qualified physicians, nurse midwives, and professional nurses is critical in providing the critical care this patient and her unborn baby require.

◼ COMPLICATED PREGNANCIES

Hydramnios

1. Definition: presence of more than 2000 ml of amniotic fluid
2. Incidence and etiology
   a. Although the exact cause of hydramnios is unknown, it is associated with congenital anomalies in the fetus.
   b. Hydramnios may be chronic or acute.
      (1) Most cases are chronic, and the increased amount of fluid develops slowly over weeks.
      (2) Acute hydramnios develops over days.
3. Clinical manifestations
   a. There is an accelerated growth rate of the uterus, which places more strain on the back and on returning blood flow from the extremities and pressure on the diaphragm.
   b. The woman may experience backache, edema of the feet, and shortness of breath.
4. Clinical management
   a. Supportive physical and psychologic care is provided.
   b. In case of rapid development of fluid and maternal respiratory distress, fluid may be removed by amniocentesis under ultrasound guidance.
   c. Monitor fetal heart rate carefully when membranes

rupture because of increased risk of prolapsed cord as the fluid escapes from the uterus and out through the cervix and vagina.

Oligohydramnios

1. Definition: less than 500 ml of amniotic fluid between 32 and 36 weeks' gestation.
2. Incidence and etiology
   a. May be associated with leakage of fluid from a tear in the amniotic membrane
   b. May occur in the presence of a congenital anomaly associated with fetal kidneys or urinary tract abnormalities
3. Clinical manifestations
   a. Uterine growth may be delayed.
   b. Ultrasonic measurement of amniotic fluid volume indicates decreased volume.
   c. The fetus is more compressed and unable to move fluid in and out of its lungs, so hypoplastic lungs may develop.
   d. The umbilical cord does not float freely. Cord compression causes a variable deceleration in the FHR and is indicated on an FHR tracing as a variable deceleration.
4. Clinical management
   a. If noted by ultrasound examination during the last trimester, the fetus will be monitored with a minimum of weekly NSTs and biophysical profiles.
   b. If the NST is nonreactive, the biophysical score is diminished because of decreased amniotic fluid volume, and the fetus is at term, labor may be induced. If variable decelerations develop, an amnioinfusion (to replace fluid within the uterus) may be done to increase uterine fluid volume, which floats the umbilical cord and decreases the incidence of cord compression.

Rh Incompatibility and Erythroblastosis Fetalis

1. Definition: Hyperbilirubinemia is an excessive amount of bilirubin in the blood. Erythroblastosis fetalis describes a fetal condition resulting from hemolysis of fetal red blood cells. The fetus is anemic and edematous. Without treatment, the condition may well be fatal.
2. Incidence and etiology
   a. Fetal hyperbilirubinemia is the result of Rh sensitization (Fig. 14–8). This occurs when the expectant woman is Rh negative, the father is Rh positive, and the fetus is also Rh positive.
   b. If an Rh-negative woman has had prior exposure to the Rh-positive factor (previous blood transfusion with Rh-positive blood, previous birth of an Rh-positive baby), she produces immunoglobulin (Ig) G antibody (anti-Rh[D]). At this point, the woman is considered sensitized, and any subsequent exposure to the Rh-positive factor creates an antigen-antibody reaction. The amount of antibody that is produced can be measured (called a titer).

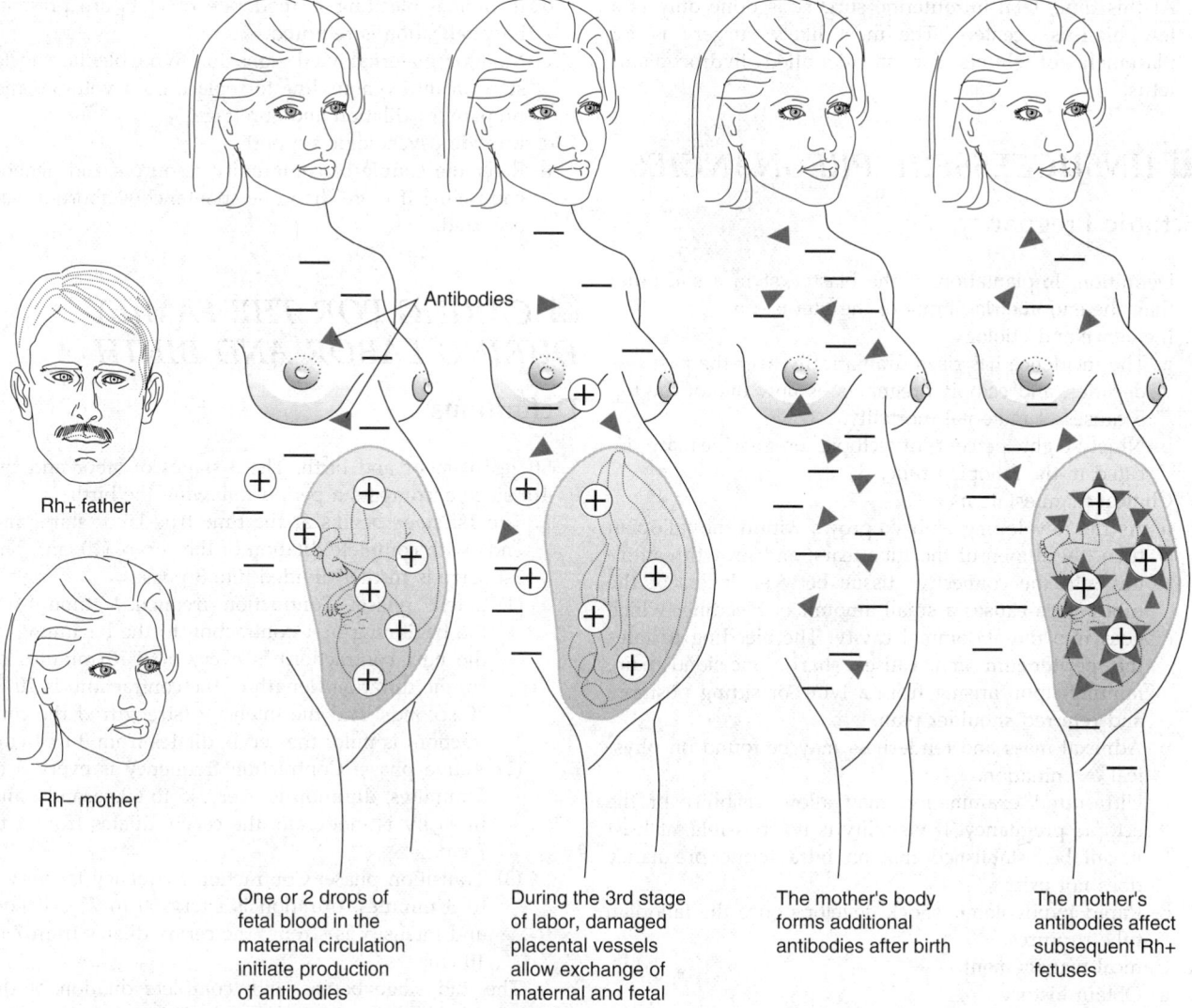

Rh+ father

Rh– mother

Antibodies

One or 2 drops of fetal blood in the maternal circulation initiate production of antibodies

During the 3rd stage of labor, damaged placental vessels allow exchange of maternal and fetal blood

The mother's body forms additional antibodies after birth

The mother's antibodies affect subsequent Rh+ fetuses

Figure 14–8. The process of maternal sensitization to Rh factor. (Modified from Gorrie TM, McKinney ES, and Murray SS. *Maternal Newborn Nursing.* Philadelphia: WB Saunders, 1994, p 695.)

c. During pregnancy, a rising titer or one measured by albumin agglutination techniques that are 16 or more indicates that the fetus may be at risk.

d. In the presence of an Rh-positive fetus, antibodies cross the placenta and cause hemolytic anemia in the fetus by destroying the fetal RBCs. This process results in increased amounts of bilirubin and other by-products of the hemolyzed RBCs. In severe cases, the fetus develops erythroblastosis fetalis.

3. Clinical manifestations: The woman will not be aware of previous exposure or that she has a rising titer.

4. Clinical management

a. Draw a titer during pregnancy for all Rh-negative women. The titer is drawn weekly through the 2nd trimester and then biweekly during the 3rd trimester.

b. If the titer is rising, an amniocentesis is done to obtain amniotic fluid for testing by spectrophotometry. The test result is plotted on a Liley graph for interpretation. The Liley test has 3 zones.

(1) Zone I: The fetus either is not affected or is mildly affected, and no immediate intervention is needed. Another sample of amniotic fluid should be tested in approximately 2 to 3 weeks.

(2) Zone II: The fetus is moderately affected, and more frequent testing should be done.

(3) Zone III: The fetus has severe involvement. If the fetus is at term, birth should occur immediately. If the fetus is preterm, an intrauterine blood transfusion needs to be done.

c. A sample of fetal blood may be obtained directly by percutaneous umbilical blood sampling. This test is done in high-risk centers.

Intrauterine Surgery to Correct Fetal Anomalies

1. Definition: entering the uterus to perform corrective techniques

2. At this time, fetal intrauterine surgery is done only at a few high-risk centers. The most likely surgery is for placement of shunts for an identified hydrocephalic fetus.

▣ UNSUCCESSFUL PREGNANCIES

Ectopic Pregnancy

1. Definition: implantation of the blastocyst in a site other than the endometrial lining of the uterus
2. Incidence and etiology
   a. The incidence has risen dramatically over the past few decades, and ectopic pregnancy is now one of the top 5 causes of maternal mortality.
   b. Ninety-eight percent of ectopic pregnancies are located in the fallopian tube.
3. Clinical manifestations
   a. As the developing embryo grows within the fallopian tube, the lumen of the tube tears, and growth continues into the connective tissue between layers of the tubes. This causes a small amount of bleeding, which goes into the abdominal cavity. The bleeding irritates the peritoneum and causes sharp, one-sided pain, fainting upon arising from a lying or sitting position, and referred shoulder pain.
   b. Adnexal mass and tenderness may be found on physical examination.
   c. Ultrasound examination may allow visibility of the ectopic pregnancy. If visibility is not possible, at least it can be established that an intrauterine pregnancy does not exist.
   d. Rapid hypovolemic shock develops once the fallopian tube ruptures.
4. Clinical management
   a. Obtain history.
   b. Monitor maternal vital signs.
   c. Prepare for surgery.

Spontaneous Abortion

1. Definition
   a. The loss of the embryo or fetus before the 20th week of gestation
   b. Classified as threatened, imminent, complete, incomplete, missed, or habitual
2. Incidence and etiology
   a. The average incidence rate is 43 percent.
   b. The etiology includes many factors, such as chromosomal abnormalities, maternal or fetal infections, teratogenic drugs, placental abnormalities, hormonal imbalance, and faulty implantation.
3. Clinical manifestations: The woman experiences abdominal cramping accompanied by spotting or vaginal bleeding. Once cervical dilation has occurred, the abortion is inevitable.
4. Clinical management
   a. If spotting is small in amount, bed rest is recommended.

b. If vaginal bleeding is moderate or clots are present, hospitalization is required.
c. Monitor maternal vital signs for hypovolemic shock, start an intravenous line to replace fluid volume, and prepare for dilation and curettage.
d. Provide psychologic support.
e. Refer the couple to community resources and genetic counseling if more than one spontaneous abortion has occurred.

▣ CARING FOR THE FAMILY DURING LABOR AND BIRTH

Definitions

1. Stages of labor and birth. The 3 stages of labor and the 4th stage encompass a period following the birth.
   a. The 1st stage begins at the time true labor starts and ends with complete dilation of the cervix (10 cm). The 1st stage is further divided into 3 phases:
      (1) Latent phase: Contraction frequency (time from the beginning of 1 contraction to the beginning of the next contraction) is every 5 to 10 minutes or so; the duration (length of the contraction) is 20 to 30 seconds; and the intensity (strength of the contraction) is mild; the cervix dilates from 0 to 4 cm.
      (2) Active phase: Contraction frequency is every 3 to 5 minutes, duration is every 45 to 60 seconds, and intensity is moderate; the cervix dilates from 4 to 7 cm.
      (3) Transition phase: Contraction frequency is every 2 to 3 minutes, duration is every 60 to 75 seconds, and intensity is strong; the cervix dilates from 7 to 10 cm.
   b. The 2nd stage begins with complete dilation of the cervix and ends with birth of the baby.
   c. The 3rd stage begins with the birth of the baby and ends with the birth of the placenta.
   d. The 4th stage begins with the birth of the placenta and ends 2 to 4 hours after birth.
2. Neonate refers to the baby from the time of birth through the 28th day of life. The terms **newborn** and **neonate** are used interchangeably.
3. Gestation: a pregnancy that ends between the 38th and the end of the 41st week
4. Preterm labor: labor that occurs between 20 weeks and 37 completed weeks
5. Postterm labor: labor that occurs in the 42nd or 43rd week

Assessment

1. Labor and birth practices vary among cultural groups.
   a. Assess wants and desires of the woman in labor.
   b. Determine whether the woman desires any particular activities during labor and birth.
2. The following are critical factors to consider before assessment:

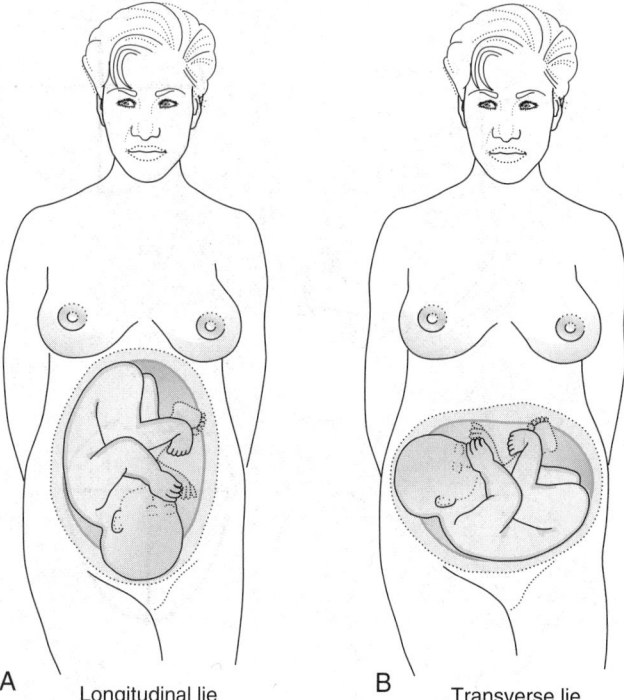

TRANSCULTURAL CONSIDERATIONS

Cultural practices in the labor and birthing area may include the following:

Handling discomfort: may be very stoic and keep a straight face, may cry out, or may breathe with contractions
Use of support person: may want to be alone or may want the support person close by
Touch: may want hand to be held, may want massage, or may want to be left alone
Fluids: may want iced water; others may want lukewarm or warmed fluids

A Longitudinal lie   **B** Transverse lie

Figure 14–9. Fetal lie. *A,* In a longitudinal lie, the long axis of the fetus is parallel to the long axis of the expectant mother. *B,* In a transverse lie, the long axis of the fetus is at right angles to the long axis of the mother. The uterus usually has a wide, short appearance. (Modified from Gorrie TM, McKinney ES, and Murray SS. *Maternal Newborn Nursing.* Philadelphia: WB Saunders, 1994, p 271.)

a. Initiation of labor requires an interplay between progesterone withdrawal and estrogen stimulation, oxytocin stimulation, fetal cortisol, prostaglandins, and uterine distention.
b. Fetal factors include diameters and position of the fetal head, presentation, lie, and position.
 (1) Fetal head diameters are important, as the head is the largest part of the fetus that will pass through the maternal pelvis. When the fetal head is flexed down on the fetal chest, the smallest anteroposterior (suboccipitobregmatic) diameter of the head presents to the maternal pelvis. This diameter averages 9.5 cm in a 7.5-pound baby.
 (2) Fetal presentation refers to the part of the fetal body that 1st enters the maternal pelvis. Presentation is determined by Leopold's maneuvers and by vaginal examination. Normal findings: Cephalic presentation occurs in 97 percent of cases and breech in approximately 3 percent.
 (3) Fetal lie refers to the relationship of the fetal spine to the maternal spine (Fig. 14–9). If the fetal spine lies in the same plane as the mother's, it is called a longitudinal lie. If the fetal spine lies at a right angle to the mother's spine, a transverse lie exists.
 (4) Fetal position refers to the relationship of a particular landmark on the fetal head to the anterior or posterior and the right or left portion of the maternal pelvis. Position: About 75 percent of fetuses are in occipitoanterior position (with left occipitoanterior the most common), and about 25 percent are posterior. Position is assessed by sterile vaginal examination.
c. Maternal pelvis: The 4 major types of pelves are gynecoid, android, anthropoid, and platypelloid (Fig. 14–10). Most women have a gynecoid pelvis, which is more rounded and usually has adequate diameters for birth.
3. Signs of impending labor (also called premonitory signs)
a. Lightening: As the fetus settles down into the maternal pelvis, the uterus moves downward, and the woman can breathe more easily because the uterus does not press on the diaphragm.
b. Braxton Hicks contractions: irregular contractions that do not increase in frequency and do not dilate the cervix.
c. Bloody show: As the cervix changes (becomes more soft and pliable because of changes in collagen fibers) and effacement (thinning out of the cervix) occurs, small capillaries tear and mix with the cervical mucus.
d. Rupture of amniotic membranes: Spontaneous rupture may occur before the beginning of labor.
e. Sudden burst of energy: Some women experience a change in energy level in the day or 2 before labor.
f. Weight loss: Many women lose about 2 to 3 pounds in the week just before the beginning of labor.
4. Signs of active labor
a. Active labor is indicated by regular, rhythmic contractions that increase in frequency, duration, and intensity.
b. Contractions cause the cervix to dilate and efface. Bloody show may be present.
5. Health history: An abbreviated history is obtained at the time of admission to the birthing area.
a. Maternal name and age
b. Gravida, para, and previous pregnancy problems such as long labor, difficult birth, bleeding after birth, or problems that occurred in the newborn
c. Estimated date of birth and whether the dates were confirmed by ultrasound examination
d. Amniotic fluid membrane status: Are the membranes intact or ruptured? If ruptured, what time did it occur and what is the color and amount of the fluid?
e. History of previous illnesses, particularly involving

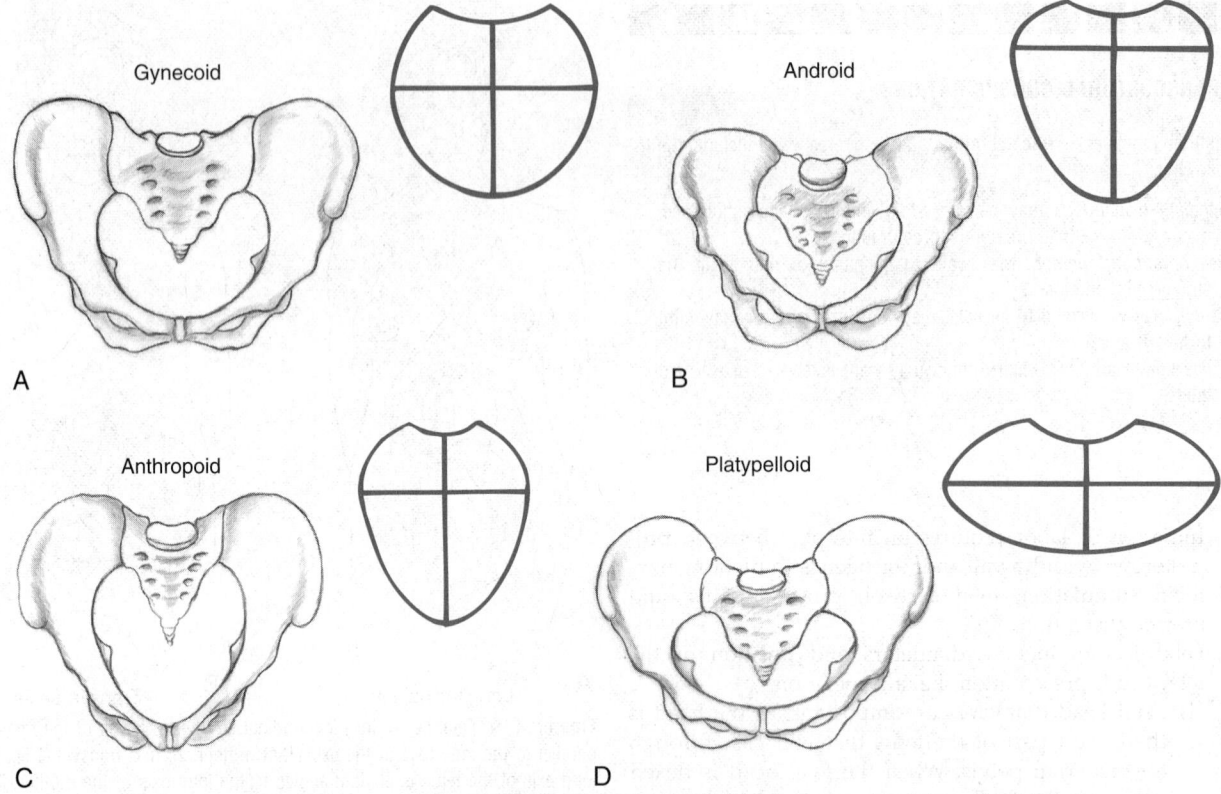

Figure 14–10. Four major pelvic shapes.

the cardiovascular, renal, or pulmonary system or any previous coagulation difficulties

f. Any problems with the present pregnancy such as elevated blood pressure, edema, bleeding, or preterm labor

g. Testing that has been done during the pregnancy such as NST, biophysical profile, or amniocentesis

h. Name of certified nurse midwife or physician and pediatrician or pediatric nurse practitioner

6. Physical examination of the mother
  a. Vital signs
    (1) Blood pressure: 90 to 140/60 to 90, or no more than 15 to 20 mm Hg rise over the baseline blood pressure during early pregnancy.
    (2) Pulse: 60 to 90 beats per minute
    (3) Respiration: 16 to 24 breaths per minute
    (4) Temperature: 36.2 to 37.6 degrees Celsius (98.0–99.6 degrees Fahrenheit).
    (5) Apical pulse: Normal rate and rhythm, including normal pregnancy variation of grade II–IV systolic ejection murmur (secondary to additional blood volume passing through heart valves).
  b. Edema: some edema of the feet normal
  c. Deep tendon reflexes: normal (2+ on most scales)
  d. Clonus: absent
  e. Hydration: skin turgor normal; mucous membranes moist
  f. Fundal height: fundus at xiphoid process at 40 weeks' gestation
  g. Labor status
    (1) Uterine contractions: regular pattern; increasing frequency, duration, and intensity, with normal resting tone between contractions. Labor status is

assessed manually or by electronic fetal monitoring device. Labor can be monitored electronically by external or internal means.

    (2) Dilation of the cervix: progressive dilation from 1 to 10 cm. Nurses need to note that digital examination of the cervix may be inappropriate in Islamic and other cultures. The examination may be completed by a female certified nurse-midwife or physician or nurse only after consultation with the family.
      • Once in active labor, primigravida progresses at average of 1.2 cm per hour, and multigravida progresses at an average of 1.5 cm per hour.
      • Dilation is assessed by sterile vaginal examination.
    (3) Cervical effacement: proceeds from 0 to 100 percent. Effacement is determined by sterile vaginal examination.
  h. Fetal station: progressive fetal descent, proceeds from minus 4 cm down to 0 (ischial spine) then from plus 1, to plus 4, and birth. Fetal station is assessed by vaginal examination (Fig. 14–11)
  i. Amniotic membranes: may rupture before or during labor. Positive findings are indicated by dark blue color on Nitrazine test tape. Amniotic fluid is clear and odorless.

7. Psychosocial assessment
  a. Education
    (1) Recognize that most women have participated in some type of education during the prenatal period.
    (2) Assess information the woman and her support person have and determine their need for further information.

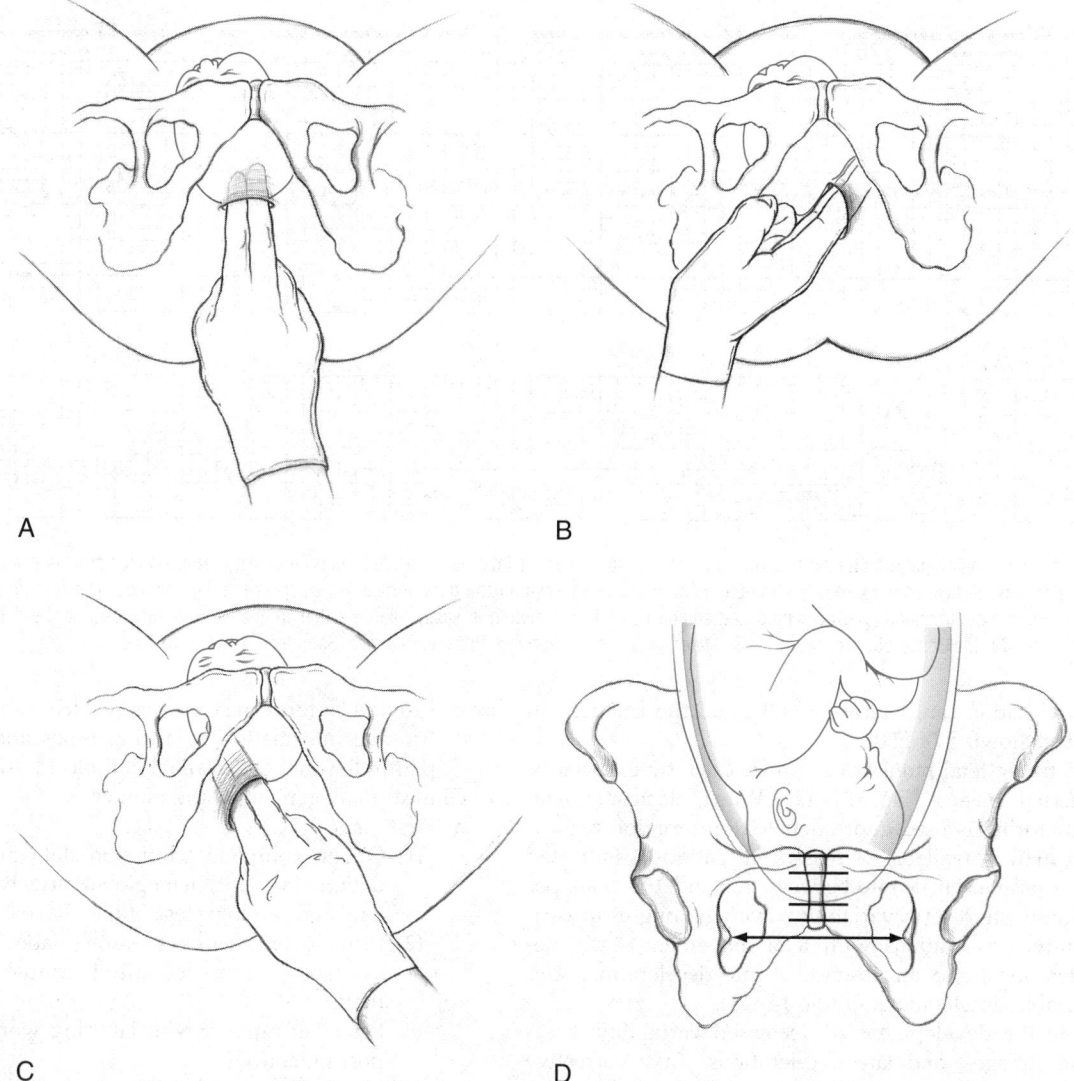

A

B

C

D

Figure 14–11. Fetal station, representing the measurement of fetal descent. The ischial spines are the reference point for estimating station. The level of the ischial spines is a zero station. If the fetal presenting part is above the ischial spines, a negative number describes station. If the fetal presenting part is below the ischial spines, a positive number is assigned to the station.

(3) Determine whether the woman has a birth plan that she has discussed with her physician or certified nurse-midwife during the pregnancy.

b. Support
  (1) The support person may be the father of the baby, a family member, or a friend.
  (2) Assess the relationship and interaction between the laboring woman and the support person. Assess the need for further interaction and support from nursing.

c. Coping with labor
  (1) Assess the woman's anxiety level.
  (2) Assess methods that the laboring woman has to cope with uterine contractions. Does she have a "breathing method" or means to focus during contractions? Is she able to relax between contractions?
  (3) Determine the support system that the woman has available to her.
    • Is the father of the baby or her partner present? Does their relationship seem to be comfortable and supportive?

• What type of prenatal educational experiences does the family have to draw on during the labor and birth process?
• What are the family's desires during labor and birth?

8. Monitoring the fetus
  a. Fetal heart rate can be assessed by auscultation or by electronic fetal monitor.

NURSE ADVISORY

To auscultate the fetal heart rate (FHR), place the Doppler ultrasound device (or fetoscope) on the lower portion of the abdomen in the midline. If the FHR is not heard, move the Doppler to the left, and if the FHR is still not heard move the Doppler again. The FHR will most likely be heard in the woman's left lower portion of her uterus. Once the FHR is heard, palpate the woman's pulse to ensure that you are not listening to her pulse, then count the rate for 1 full minute. It is important to count the rate during the contraction as well as when no contraction is occurring.

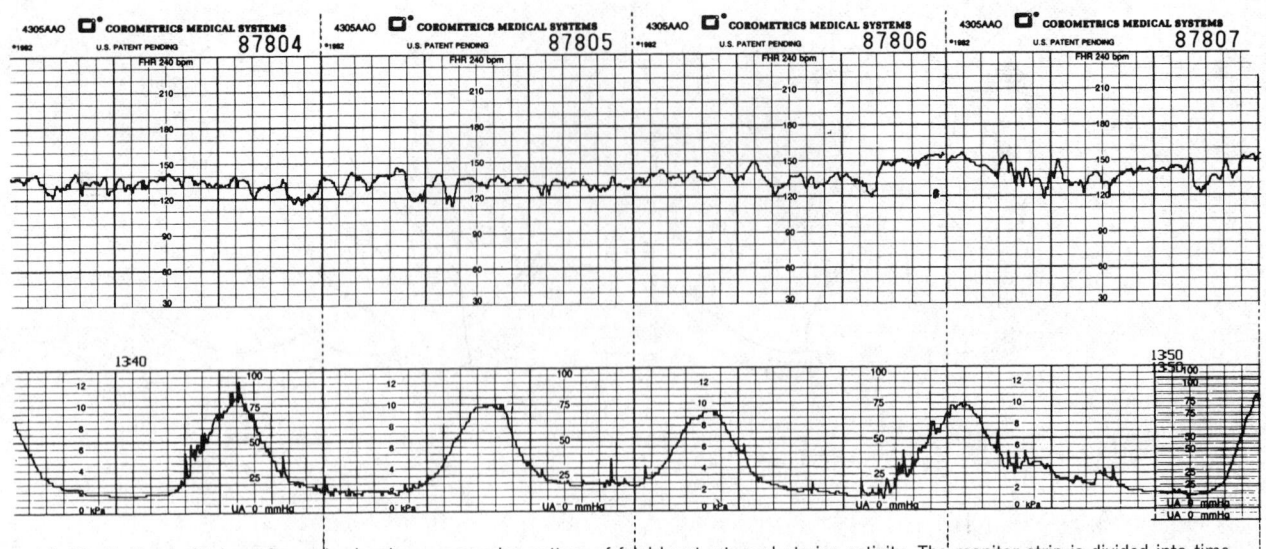

Figure 14–12. Electronic fetal monitor strip showing a reassuring pattern of fetal heart rate and uterine activity. The monitor strip is divided into time segments. The dark vertical lines represent 1 minute. Each small square within the dark vertical lines represents 10 seconds. The bottom portion of the strip depicts uterine contractions. The beginning and ending of each contraction is easily seen, so that frequency and duration may be determined. (Modified from Gorrie TM, McKinney ES, and Murray SS. *Maternal Newborn Nursing.* Philadelphia: WB Saunders, 1994, p 341.)

b. Auscultation can determine FHR, and the listener can detect slowing of FHR.

c. Electronic fetal monitoring can be done by external or internal means (Fig. 14–12). When electronic fetal monitoring is used, more detailed information regarding FHR is available. A reassuring pattern is indicated by a baseline FHR rate between 120 and 160 beats per minute, short-term variability, average long-term variability, accelerations with fetal movement, early decelerations, and an absence of late decelerations and variable decelerations (Table 14–11).

d. Note the development of decreased variability, baseline changes, and late decelerations. Take corrective action immediately if possible.

(1) Position the woman in a side-lying position.

(2) Assess for maternal hypotension.

(3) Provide oxygen and administer intravenous fluids if FHR pattern indicates.

Normal Labor and Birth

1. Pain control

a. Assess current coping ability and tools that the woman has to use during labor.

b. Establish rapport to provide information and support for the laboring woman and her support person.

c. Provide comfort measures as needed and desired.

d. Provide information regarding types and methods of pain relief that are available (Table 14–12).

2. Clinical management of the mother

a. First stage

(1) Obtain complete admission data and laboratory data (hematocrit, hemoglobin, urinalysis, urine protein, and serologic tests if they have not been done).

(2) Provide orientation to room, labor process, and available comfort measure if couple desires information.

(3) Establish rapport with laboring woman and support person.

(4) Monitor maternal, fetal, contraction, and cervical dilation status.

(5) Monitor maternal comfort and need for support and information.

(6) Ascertain whether the woman is open to additional information regarding techniques.

(7) Assess the woman's information base regarding methods to cope with uterine contractions.

(8) Encourage the woman to use comfort-increasing methods that she feels will help her, such as ambulation, changes of position, sitting in the shower, relaxation techniques, distraction, and patterned breathing.

(9) Encourage the laboring woman to make her wishes known.

(10) Stay with the laboring woman to provide support.

(11) Encourage the laboring woman to change position frequently and while lying in bed maintain a side-lying position (to prevent compression of the vena cava, which then leads to a decrease in uteroplacental perfusion).

b. Second stage

(1) Assist the woman with pushing by positioning (on birthing bar, hands and knees, semi-Fowler's

Table 14–11. Characteristics of a Reassuring Fetal Heart Rate

Baseline rate	120–160 beats per min
Variability	
Short term	Present
Long term	Average
Accelerations	Present with fetal movement
Decelerations	Absence of late or variable decelerations

Table 14-12. Selected Analgesic Agents and Regional Anesthetic Blocks

Method	Characteristics	Clinical Management
Butorphanol tartrate (Stadol)	Butorphanol is a mixed agonist-antagonist agent. It is given subcutaneously or by intravenous push during labor for pain relief.	Drug should not be given to the woman who uses drugs, as butorphanol may precipitate acute withdrawal. Monitor the woman's vital signs and response to medication. Monitor fetal heart rate with an external fetal monitor.
Epidural block	Epidural anesthetic block may be given during labor or for cesarean birth. Epidural regional blocks are not associated with a headache because the dura is not punctured (as it is in a spinal block). The most common side effect is maternal hypotension. If severe hypotension occurs, fetal stress and late decelerations may ensue. If an epidural block is given for a cesarean birth, morphine sulfate (Duramorph) or some other type of intrathecal narcotic may be given for pain relief over the next 24 hr.	Monitor maternal and fetal baseline vital signs. Start an intravenous (IV) line and preload with at least 500 ml IV fluid. Monitor maternal vital signs per protocol during and after the epidural. Monitor fetal heart rate continuously with external fetal monitor. Assist the woman with positioning on her side. Assist the woman with pushing in the 2nd stage.
Pudendal block	A pudendal block provides anesthetic effects during the 2nd stage and during repair of an episiotomy. Side effects and complications are rare.	Provide information regarding the block and expected effects.

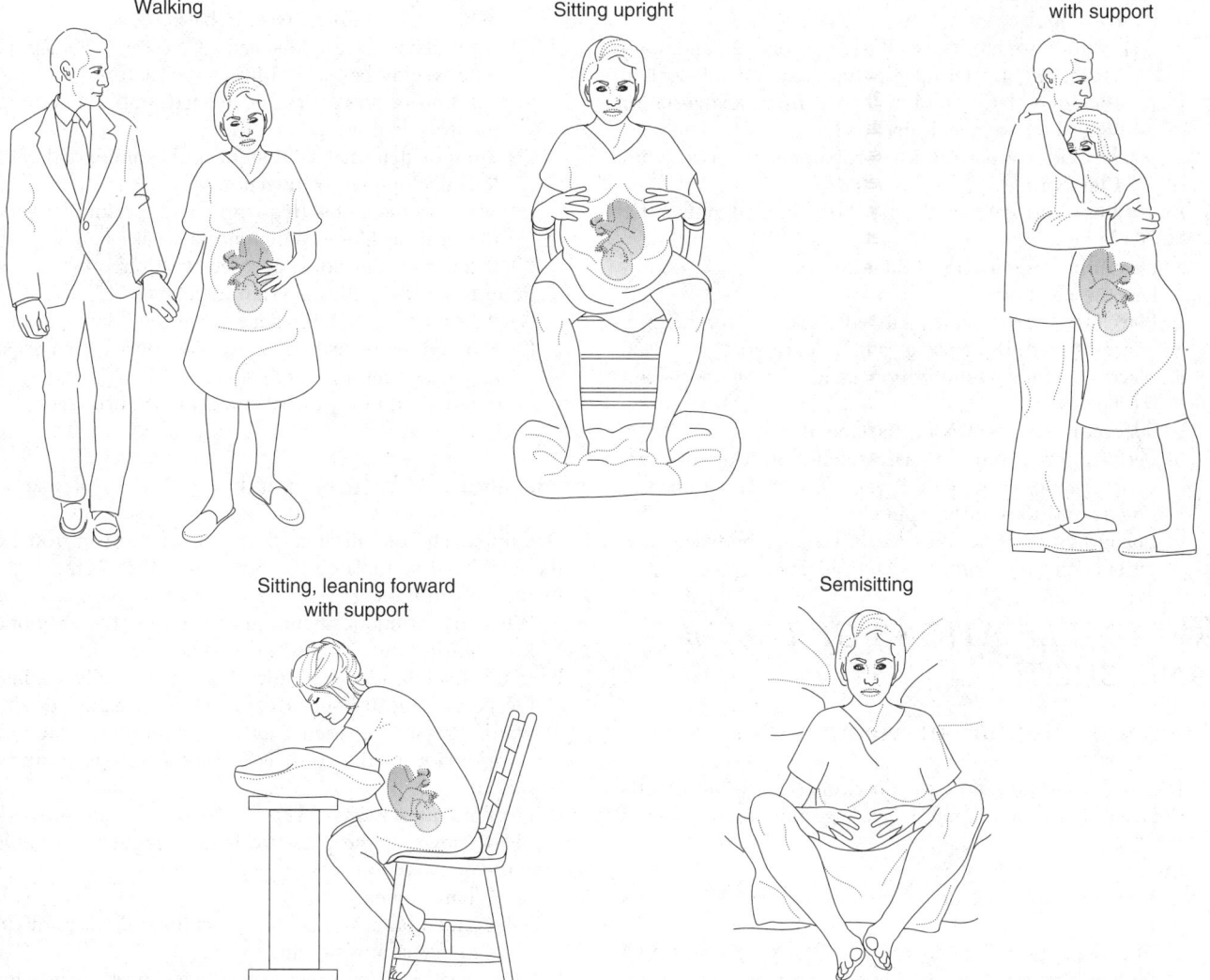

Figure 14-13. Maternal positions for labor. (Modified from Gorrie TM, McKinney ES, and Murray SS. *Maternal Newborn Nursing.* Philadelphia: WB Saunders, 1994, p 311.)

Table 14–13. Apgar Score

Sign	Score 0	Score 1	Score 2
	0	1	2
Heart rate	Absent	Slow—below 100	Above 100
Respiratory effort	Absent	Slow—irregular	Good crying
Muscle tone	Flaccid	Some flexion of extremities	Active motion
Reflex irritability	None	Grimace	Vigorous cry
Color	Pale blue	Body pink, blue	Completely pink

with her knee drawn up to the sides of her abdomen, kneeling) and providing encouragement and support (Fig. 14–13).

    (2) Monitor maternal and fetal status.

    (3) Prepare birthing area.

  c. Third stage

    (1) Continue to provide support to couple.

    (2) Administer oxytocic agent as directed by certified nurse-midwife or physician.

    (3) Examine placenta to determine intactness.

  d. Fourth stage

    (1) Monitor maternal vital signs, position and consistency of uterine fundus, amount of lochia, bladder status, and recovery from analgesia or anesthetic regional block.

    (2) Provide opportunities for parents to bond with newborn.

3. Assessment and care of the newborn immediately after birth

  a. Determine Apgar score (Table 14–13).

  b. Dry the newborn.

  c. Place newborn skin to skin with mother for maintenance of warmth or use a radiant warmer.

  d. Place matching identification bands on newborn and mother.

  e. Suction mouth as needed to remove mucus.

  f. Perform brief physical assessment: position of ears, intact palate, cord with 3 vessels, correct number of fingers and toes, intact spine.

  g. Encourage opportunities for interaction between new parents and newborn.

◼ COMPLICATIONS OF LABOR AND BIRTH

Premature Rupture of Membranes

1. Definition: PROM before the onset of labor. Some experts define PROM before 38 weeks' gestation as preterm PROM.

2. Incidence and etiology

  a. Premature rupture of membranes occurs in 3 to 18.5 percent of births.

  b. The etiology is unknown, but PROM is associated with incompetent cervix, infection, urinary tract infection, hydramnios, and multiple pregnancy.

3. Clinical manifestations: Clear fluid is excreted from the vagina. The fluid tests positive when tested with Nitrazine tape (tape turns a deep blue color), and the ferning test result is positive.

4. Clinical management

  a. Preterm PROM without maternal infection

    (1) Observe for further loss of fluid, and maintain the woman on bed rest.

    (2) Test the amniotic fluid for lung maturity (lecithin to sphingomelin [L/S] ratio and presence of phosphatidylglycerol) on weekly basis.

    (3) Administer betamethasone (Celestone Soluspan) on a weekly basis until lungs are mature.

    (4) Administer tocolytics as needed until fetal lung maturity is present.

    (5) Monitor maternal vital signs and white blood cells for development of infection.

    (6) Monitor the fetus frequently and perform a biophysical profile once or twice a week.

    (7) If infection develops, proceed with birth.

  b. Preterm PROM with maternal infection

    (1) Administer betamethasone (Celestone Soluspan).

    (2) Proceed with birth in 24 to 48 hours if maternal and fetal condition are stable.

  c. Term fetus with or without infection: induce labor.

Prolapsed Umbilical Cord

1. Definition: The umbilical cord falls downward in front of the fetal head or through the cervix into the vagina.

2. Incidence and etiology

  a. When the amniotic membrane ruptures, the amniotic fluid washes out through the cervix.

  b. If the fetal head (or buttocks) are not firmly against the cervix, the umbilical cord can be washed downward. Pressure is then exerted on the cord, causing compression of the cord. Fetal blood flow is compromised.

3. Clinical manifestations: When the cord is compressed, the FHR slows. If the pressure is not relieved, the fetus may die.

4. Clinical management

  a. When membranes rupture, auscultate FHR immediately to detect any slowing.

  b. If an electronic fetal monitor is being used, watch for variable decelerations.

c. Relieve pressure on the cord by placing your gloved index and middle finger in the vagina, against the presenting part and apply gentle pressure. As the pressure on the cord is relieved, the fetal heart rate increases. The examiner's fingers are held in place until an immediate cesarean birth occurs.

Preterm Labor

1. Definition
   a. Uterine contractions and cervical dilation
   b. Labor before 37 completed weeks of pregnancy
2. Incidence and socioeconomic impact
   a. Preterm labor occurs in 8 to 10 percent of all pregnancies. The incidence varies by ethnic grouping with the frequency of delivery at approximately 8 percent for Whites and approximately 15 percent for Blacks.
   b. Preterm labor that proceeds to birth accounts for 50 to 75 percent of perinatal morbidity and mortality.
   c. The major causes of perinatal morbidity are neonatal respiratory distress syndrome and intraventricular hemorrhage. Mental retardation, blindness, and developmental problems are also significant concerns.
   d. There is essentially no increase in maternal morbidity and mortality associated with preterm labor.
   e. Prematurity is one of the major problems in maternal child care today and carries a social cost of more than $1 billion a year.
3. Risk factors
   a. Risk factors can be categorized as economic, cultural-behavioral, biologic-genetic-medical, or reproductive.
      (1) Economic factors include poverty, socioeconomic status, poor access to prenatal care, inadequate access to food, and unemployment.
      (2) Cultural-behavioral factors encompass inadequate health care in general, use of cigarettes, alcohol and drug abuse, being single with minimal support, short interval between pregnancies, physical and psychologic stress, and age younger than 16 or older than 35 years.
      (3) Biologic-genetic-medical risk factors include inadequate nutrition during pregnancy and before pregnancy, short stature, previous preterm birth, and presence of chronic medical illnesses.
      (4) Reproductive factors include presence of a multiple gestation, premature rupture of the membranes, uterine bleeding, PIH, infections, and anemia.
   b. Uterine activity (contractions) is increased by over-distention of the uterus.
4. Etiology
   a. The etiology of preterm labor involves many factors and is not well understood. Of the total incidence: 24 percent is attributed to complications, 10 percent to multiple gestation, 28 percent to elective obstetric intervention, and 38 percent to unknown factors.
   b. Conditions that lead to overdistention are multiple gestation, macrosomia, and hydramnios.
   c. Uterine activity is increased by situations that cause a decrease in uteroplacental blood flow, which leads to decreased placental perfusion. Conditions that cause decreased placental perfusion because of constriction of vessels are PIH, cigarette smoking (more than 10/day), and chronic use of cocaine or similar drugs. Decreased placental perfusion may also be caused by a decrease in blood supply due to compression of vessels, as with supine maternal hypotension and hypovolemia due to hemorrhage or dehydration.
   d. Chorioamnionitis can precipitate preterm labor. The bacterial invasion associated with chorioamnionitis leads to a production of substances such as interleukin-1, tumor necrosis factor, and platelet-activating factor that activate prostaglandin production by the decidua and the amniotic membranes.
5. Pathophysiology
   a. The pathophysiology of preterm labor is unknown.
   b. Mechanisms depend on precipitating factors.
6. Clinical manifestations
   a. Indicators of preterm labor may be subtle and difficult to differentiate from false labor (which does not lead to cervical dilation) and expected discomforts of pregnancy.
   b. Approximately 40 to 60 percent of women report uterine contractions (may be painless or painful), a tightening in the uterus like a "balling up" of 1 area, backache in the lower lumbar and sacral areas, change in vaginal discharge (change of character of discharge or increase in the amount), pelvic pressure, and menstrual-like cramps. Some women report other symptoms such as intestinal cramping, diarrhea, pelvic pain, and urinary frequency.
7. Diagnostics
   a. Preterm labor occurs when the gestation is between 20 and 37 completed weeks, when documented uterine contractions of 4 per 20 minutes or 8 per 60 minutes are present, and when cervical effacement and dilation of at least 2 cm is present (Box 14-6).
   b. Assessment
      (1) History: Note the presence of risk factors. Box 14-7 presents a scoring system of major and minor risk factors. The presence of 1 major factor or 2 minor factors indicates a pregnancy that is high risk for preterm labor.

BOX 14-6. Criteria for Diagnosis of Preterm Labor

Gestation 20-37 completed weeks
and
Documented uterine contractions
(4/20 min, 8/60 min)
and
Ruptured membranes or intact membranes
and
documented cervical change
or
cervical effacement of 80 percent
or
cervical dilation of 2 cm

From Creasy RK, and Resnick R. *Maternal-Fetal Medicine.* 2nd ed. Philadelphia: WB Saunders, 1989, p 448.

BOX 14-7. Major and Minor Risk Factors of the Modified Scoring System for Spontaneous Preterm Labor

Major Factors*	Minor Factors†
Multiple gestation	Febrile illness during pregnancy
Previous preterm delivery	Bleeding after 12 weeks
Previous preterm labor, term delivery	History of pyelonephritis
Abdominal surgery during pregnancy	Cigarette smoking ($>$10/day)
Diethylstilbestrol exposure	One 2nd-trimester abortion
Hydramnios	More than 2 1st-trimester abortions
Uterine anomaly	
History of cone biopsy	
Uterine irritability	
More than 1 2nd-trimester abortion	
Cervical dilation ($>$1 cm) at 32 weeks	
Cervical shortening ($<$1 cm at 32 weeks)	

* Presence of 1 or more indicates high risk.
† Presence of 2 or more indicates high risk.
From Holbrook RH, Laros RK, and Creasy RK. Evaluation of a risk-scoring system for prediction of preterm labor. *Am J Perinatol* 6(1):62–68, 1989.

(2) Physical assessment
- Monitor uterine contractions with an external electronic fetal monitor. Note the frequency and duration of the uterine contractions. Palpate the contractions for intensity.
- Perform a sterile vaginal examination to determine membrane status (ruptured or intact membranes), cervical dilation, effacement, position, and consistency.
- Note the presence of vaginal discharge. Pinkish vaginal discharge (show) may be present with cervical dilation.
- Evaluate fetal status by assessing fetal movement and fetal heart beat characteristics (rate,

variability, presence of accelerations with fetal movement, and presence of decelerations).
c. Diagnostic studies
(1) Perform fetal assessment studies such as the NST and biophysical profile.
(2) Obtain amniotic fluid sample by amniocentesis to determine the L/S ratio and the presence of phosphatidylglycerol and creatinine.
(3) Use ultrasound to obtain fetal measurements to plot serial growth in utero.
(4) Perform laboratory studies to include urinalysis and urine culture and sensitivity, complete blood count with differential, and culture of the cervix.
8. Clinical management
a. Goals of clinical management are to identify women at risk for preterm labor and provide teaching for self-care, identify the presence of preterm labor, initiate therapy to treat preterm labor, and maintain pregnancy to time of fetal lung maturity or term, if possible.
b. Nonpharmacologic intervention
(1) Place the woman in side-lying position to maximize uteroplacental perfusion.
(2) Encourage oral fluids to increase vascular volume.
(3) Encourage the woman to urinate every 2 hours, as a full bladder may increase uterine irritability and contractions.
(4) Teach the woman to monitor fetal activity and complete the fetal kick count (or Cardiff count-to-10).
(5) Teach the woman to self-monitor for signs and symptoms of preterm labor.
c. Pharmacologic intervention
(1) Tocolytic medications commonly used to treat preterm labor include beta-mimetic agents, magnesium sulfate, prostaglandin inhibitors, and calcium channel blockers. Corticosteroids may also be used to accelerate fetal lung maturity.
(2) Table 14–14 outlines major tocolytic agents.
d. Special medical-surgical procedures
(1) Electronic fetal monitoring provides continuous

Table 14–14. Major Tocolytic Agents

Agent	Maternal and Fetal Side Effects	Nursing Considerations
Magnesium sulfate (MgSO$_4$)	*Maternal:* sweating, feeling of warmth, slurred speech, muscular weakness, confusion, respiratory and circulatory collapse *Fetal:* neurologic depression, loss of reflexes and muscular weakness	Carefully monitor respirations, pulse, deep tendon reflexes, and urine output. Assess magnesium blood levels. Assess ability to talk and swallow. Decrease dose for depression of deep tendon reflexes, respirations $<$ 12, urine output $<$30 ml/hr, or blood level above therapeutic range.
Beta-sympathomimetic Ritodrine	*Maternal:* tachycardia, tremors, palpitations, nervousness, shortness of breath, headache, nausea and vomiting, hypokalemia, hyperglycemia, pulmonary edema *Fetal:* tachycardia *Newborn:* hypoglycemia, hypocalcemia	Identify contraindications (hypovolemia, pulmonary hypertension, cardiac disease, diabetes mellitus, chronic renal disease). Maintain continuous electronic fetal monitor and evaluate uterine contractions and fetal heart rate. Assess pulse, respirations, blood pressure, breath sounds. Notify physician if maternal pulse $>$ 120 beats per min, fetal heart rate $>$ 180 beats per min, or both.

data regarding uterine contractions and irritability and characteristics of the FHR.

(2) Use of a tocolytic pump provides a continuous subcutaneous infusion of medication.

(3) Use of at-home uterine-monitoring system detects the presence of uterine contractions.

9. Complications

a. Maternal complications include premature rupture of membranes; infection such as chorioamnionitis; and in some cases the need for prolonged bed rest, hospitalization, or both.

b. Neonatal complications include prematurity, neonatal respiratory distress syndrome, intraventricular hemorrhage, blindness, developmental problems, and mental retardation.

10. Prognosis

a. Early recognition and treatment of preterm labor may reduce the incidence of preterm birth, thereby decreasing the incidence of neonatal complications.

b. Maintenance of the pregnancy to the time of fetal lung maturity significantly reduces the incidence of fetal neonatal respiratory complications.

11. Applying the nursing process

NURSING DIAGNOSIS: Knowledge deficit R/T factors, signs and symptoms of preterm labor, treatment plan, and self-care measures

a. *Expected outcomes:* Following instruction, the woman should be able to do the following:

(1) Demonstrate an understanding of preterm labor by being able to define preterm labor, risk factors, and signs and symptoms and explain the treatment plan

(2) Describe self-care measures

b. *Nursing interventions*

(1) Identify a woman's risk factors.

(2) Determine whether decreasing the risk factors is possible.

(3) Review the woman's knowledge base related to preterm labor.

(4) Provide information related to signs and symptoms of preterm labor and self-care measures.

NURSING DIAGNOSIS: Risk for injury R/T birth prior to fetal lung maturity

a. *Expected outcomes:* Following care, the fetus will remain in the intrauterine environment until lung maturity has occurred.

b. *Nursing interventions*

(1) Date pregnancy by using ultrasonic measurement techniques.

(2) Assist with fetal lung maturity tests such as L/S ratio and phosphatidylglycerol.

(3) Administer betamethasone to enhance fetal lung maturity.

(4) Administer medications to arrest preterm labor.

12. Discharge planning and teaching

a. Provide education regarding risk factors, signs and symptoms, and self-care measures.

b. Provide explanation regarding all treatment modalities and testing procedures.

13. Public health considerations

a. Preterm labor remains a significant obstetric complication in many countries of the world.

b. Efforts to reduce the preterm birth rate need to begin with ensuring access to comprehensive prenatal care for all women.

c. Information regarding pregnancy and preterm labor needs to reach young women before childbearing.

Placenta Previa

1. Definition

a. Placenta previa occurs when the placenta implants in the lower uterine segment.

b. Placenta previa is classified as low lying, marginal (or partial), and complete, depending on the relationship of the placenta to the internal cervical os (Fig. 14–14).

(1) Low lying occurs when the placenta lies low in the lower uterine segment yet does not touch the internal cervical os.

(2) Marginal, or partial, previa occurs when a small edge of the placenta covers the internal cervical os.

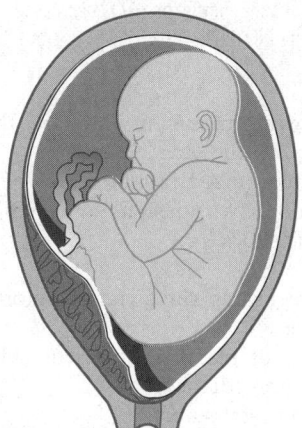 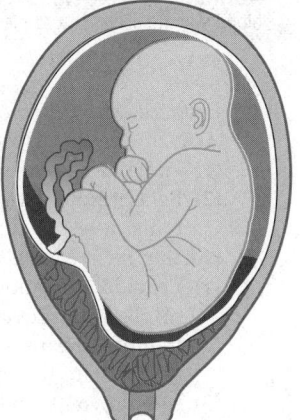 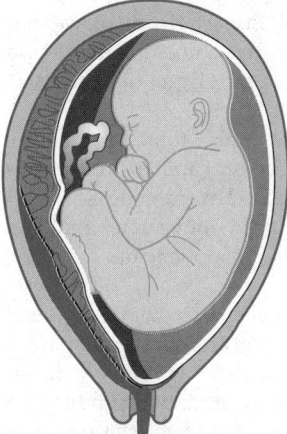 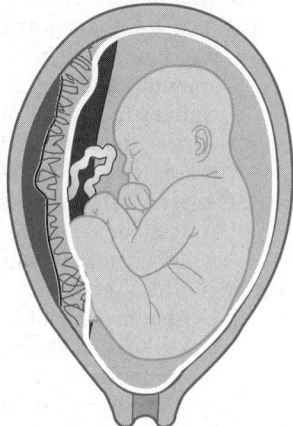

Partial placenta previa   Complete placenta previa   Abruptio placentae marginal   Abruptio placentae concealed

Figure 14–14. Types of placenta previa and abruptio placentae.

(3) Complete placenta previa covers the entire internal cervical os.
2. Incidence and socioeconomic impact
   a. After 24 weeks of gestation, the incidence is 1 in 250 pregnancies.
   b. In nulliparas the incidence is 1 in 1500 and in grand multiparas the incidence is 1 in 20 pregnancies.
3. Risk factors
   a. The presence of some factors seem to increase the risk of placenta previa.
   b. These factors include increased parity, closely spaced pregnancies, previous uterine curettage (unrelated to pregnancy or with a therapeutic abortion), multiple gestation, previous cesarean birth, maternal age older than 35, abnormal fetal presentation (breech, shoulder, and compound), congenital malformations, tumors that distort the uterus, and endometritis.
4. Etiology
   a. A specific etiology is unknown is most cases.
   b. Placenta previa is more frequently found in the conditions listed above.
5. Pathophysiology
   a. Defective or decreased vascularization of the decidua is frequently found.
   b. Mechanisms may depend on precipitating cause.
6. Clinical manifestations
   a. Painless bright red vaginal bleeding after the 28th week of gestation is the classic symptom and is reported by 80 percent of women with placenta previa.
   b. Sixty-five percent of women have their 1st bleed after 30 weeks, and 10 percent of women have their 1st bleed in labor.
   c. The amount of blood loss directly correlates with the type of previa, with the greatest blood loss occurring with complete previa.
7. Diagnostics
   a. Placenta previa may be visible with abdominal ultrasound.
   b. In the 2nd trimester, the incidence of placenta previa is increased, and then there is a conversion to normal placental location by the 3rd trimester in 90 percent of women.
   c. When ultrasound is not available, a gentle speculum vaginal examination may be done by the physician.
   d. Physical assessment
      (1) Assess the amount and characteristics of vaginal bleeding. Weigh pads or chux to determine amount of blood loss. *Note:* 1 gm of weight is equivalent to 1 ml of blood.
      (2) Assess maternal vital signs (blood pressure, pulse, respiration), skin color, capillary refill.
      (3) Assess FHR for reassuring characteristics.
      (4) Assess for presence of fetal movement and any noted changes in amount of movement.
   e. Diagnostic studies
      (1) Disseminated intravascular coagulation panel (complete blood count, prothrombin time, partial thromboplastin time, platelets, fibrinogen, fibrin split products, and fibrin degradation products)
      (2) Kleihauer-Betke stain or Apt test for the presence of fetal blood cells

(3) Nonstress test and biophysical profile to assess fetal status
8. Clinical management
   a. The goals of clinical management are to identify women at risk for placenta previa, provide education related to the signs and symptoms that women should watch for, identify the presence of placenta previa, initiate therapy immediately when a bleed occurs, monitor maternal and fetal status, and, if possible, maintain the pregnancy until fetal lung maturity occurs.
   b. Nonpharmacologic interventions
      (1) Maintain woman in side-lying position to maximize uteroplacental blood flow.
      (2) Maintain adequate nutrition and hydration.
      (3) Monitor fetal status by assessing fetal movement, monitoring FHR, NST, and biophysical profile.
   c. Pharmacologic interventions
      (1) If fetal lungs are not mature (gestational age <36 weeks and/or L/S ratio <2:1 and phosphatidylglycerol not present), administer steroids to accelerate fetal lung maturity.
      (2) Administer tocolytics if the uterus is irritable or preterm labor develops.
      (3) Maintain intravenous infusion of electrolyte solution to keep vein open if bleeding is active.
      (4) Administer oxygen if bleeding is active and hypovolemic shock is present.
      (5) Administer whole type-specific blood for massive active bleeding in the presence of hypovolemic shock.
9. Complications
   a. Maternal blood loss leads to hypovolemia and anemia.
   b. Fetal complications are related to decreased uteroplacental perfusion associated with blood loss and subsequent hypovolemia and hypotension.
10. Prognosis
   a. Perinatal mortality is approximately 10 to 15 percent.
   b. The major cause of perinatal mortality is prematurity.
   c. Maternal mortality is less than 1 percent.
11. Applying the nursing process

NURSING DIAGNOSIS: Altered tissue perfusion R/T decreased blood volume secondary to placental bleeding

   a. *Expected outcomes:* Following treatment and care, the woman should display the following:
      (1) Have any bleeding recognized rapidly
      (2) Be normotensive and have no signs and symptoms of hypovolemic shock
   b. *Nursing interventions*
      (1) Provide education regarding signs and symptoms of placenta previa.
      (2) Identify the presence of placenta previa quickly, and initiate therapy immediately.
      (3) Monitor maternal and fetal status.
      (4) Provide emotional support to woman and her support person.

(5) Review diagnostic studies.

(6) Monitor the amount of blood loss by weighing pads (1 gm = approximately 1 ml).

(7) If acute bleeding episode has ceased, maternal vital signs are within normal range, and fetal lungs are immature, maintain woman on bed rest.

(8) If signs of hypovolemic shock are present, infuse nondextrose crystalloids, monitor urine output, administer oxygen at 8 to 10 liters per minute, monitor maternal vital signs and FHR, and monitor laboratory studies.

NURSING DIAGNOSIS: Anxiety R/T concern for self and fetus

a. *Expected outcomes:* Following care, the woman should be able to do the following:

(1) Verbalize feelings of decreased anxiety and support

(2) Discuss treatment plan and interventions

b. *Nursing Interventions*

(1) Explain all nursing interventions and treatment plan.

(2) Provide support for the woman and her family.

(3) Keep the woman informed regarding fetal status.

12. Discharge planning and teaching

a. Begin teaching when woman is admitted.

b. Refer to community resources as needed.

Abruptio Placentae

1. Definition

a. Separation of the normally implanted placenta occurs after 20 weeks' gestation and before the birth of the baby (Table 14–15; see Fig. 14–14).

b. Marginal separation occurs when an edge of the placenta separates from the decidua. Bleeding occurs and escapes from the vagina.

c. Central (or partial) separation occurs when the center portion of the placenta separates. Resultant bleeding is trapped between the placenta and the uterine wall. Vaginal bleeding does not occur.

d. Complete abruption involves total separation of the placenta from the uterine wall. Massive vaginal bleeding occurs.

e. Other classification terms that may be used include external (marginal or complete) or concealed (central).

2. Incidence and socioeconomic impact

a. Abruptio placentae occurs in 1 percent of pregnancies (1/100).

b. There is a recurrence rate of 5 to 17 percent after the 1st abruption and a 25 percent rate following the 2nd abruption.

3. Risk factors

a. Maternal hypertension

b. High multiparity

c. Poor nutrition, especially folic acid deficiency

d. Smoking more than 10 cigarettes per day

e. Cocaine use

f. Abdominal trauma from a blow or from physical abuse

g. External cephalic version

h. Sudden decompression of the uterus following rupture of membranes

4. Etiology

a. The cause of abruptio placentae is unknown.

b. Rupture of small arterial vessels in the basal layer of the decidua leads to maternal bleeding.

5. Pathophysiology

a. As bleeding occurs, thrombin-rich decidual tissue is infused into the maternal circulation and the coagulation cascade is activated.

b. The result is disseminated intravascular coagulation.

6. Clinical manifestations

a. Marginal abruption placentae is accompanied by vaginal bleeding that is dark in color. Uterine pain and back pain are present in 66 percent of women. Irritability and hypertonicity of the uterus is present in approximately 20 percent of women. Irritability may be exhibited by increased frequency of contractions, increased resting tone between contractions, or both.

b. Fetal demise before admission to the hospital occurs in 25 to 35 percent of women.

7. Diagnostics

a. Physical assessment

(1) Determine the characteristics of vaginal bleeding and the amount of blood loss.

(2) Assess the amount and character of uterine tenderness or pain.

(3) Monitor uterine contractions with an external electronic fetal monitor. Note the frequency and duration of contractions and the resting tone between contractions. Palpate the contractions for intensity. Note the presence of uterine tenderness.

(4) Evaluate fetal status by assessing fetal movement and FHR characteristics (rate, variability,

Table 14–15. Differentiating Placenta Previa and Abruptio Placentae

Characteristic	Placenta Previa	Abruptio Placentae
Onset	Sudden, without warning	Sudden, without warning
Type of bleeding	Bright red	Dark red
Pain	None associated with the previa	May be sharp and intense
Uterine tenderness	None	Present
Fetal heart rate	Usually present	Present or absent

presence of accelerations with fetal movement, and presence of decelerations).

(5) Monitor maternal vital signs and urine output.

b. Diagnostic studies

(1) Ultrasound may be used to see the uterus and placenta.

(2) Laboratory testing usually includes complete blood count, platelets, and disseminated intravascular coagulation screen. An Apt test and Kleihauer-Betke test may be done to identify the source of bleeding (maternal or fetal).

(3) An NST may be done as the contraction pattern and fetal status is monitored.

8. Clinical management

a. Goals are to identify women at risk for abruptio placentae, provide teaching regarding signs and symptoms, identify the presence of abruptio and initiate immediate treatment, and monitor maternal and fetal status.

b. Nonpharmacologic interventions

(1) Position woman in side-lying position to maximize uterine blood flow.

(2) Monitor maternal and fetal status.

(3) Obtain abdominal girth measurements on a regular basis.

(4) Provide support and comfort.

c. Pharmacologic interventions

(1) Maintain intravenous infusion of electrolyte solution to keep vein open if bleeding is active.

(2) Administer oxygen if bleeding is active and hypovolemic shock is present.

(3) Administer whole type-specific blood for massive active bleeding.

9. Complications

a. Complications include anemia, hemorrhage, hypovolemic shock, disseminated intravascular coagulation, Couvelaire uterus, and fetal demise.

b. When disseminated intravascular coagulation occurs, there may be permanent renal damage.

10. Prognosis

a. Maternal mortality is not increased.

b. Perinatal mortality rate is 151 per 1000.

11. Applying the nursing process

> **NURSING DIAGNOSIS:** Altered tissue perfusion R/T hypovolemia secondary to acute blood loss

a. *Expected outcomes:* Following treatment and care, the woman should give evidence of the following:

(1) Normotension

(2) Adequate tissue perfusion

b. *Nursing interventions*

(1) Identify the presence of abruptio placentae, and initiate therapy quickly.

(2) Stabilize the maternal condition.

(3) Monitor maternal and fetal status.

(4) Provide informational and emotional support for the woman and her family.

(5) Start an intravenous line using an 18-gauge needle to enable rapid infusion of solution and administration of whole blood.

(6) Administer whole blood and fluids as directed. Maintain hematocrit at greater than 39 percent and urine output at more than 30 ml per hour.

(7) Monitor laboratory data to determine the maternal response to therapy.

(8) Measure abdominal girth to determine change in size.

(9) Administer oxygen by mask at 8 to 10 liters per minute.

(10) Measure and evaluate blood loss.

(11) Insert an indwelling bladder catheter, and monitor hourly urine output.

(12) Prepare the woman for cesarean birth.

(13) Monitor for signs and symptoms of disseminated intravascular coagulation.

> **NURSING DIAGNOSIS:** Altered tissue perfusion R/T maternal hypovolemia secondary to blood loss

a. *Expected outcomes:* Following treatment and care, the fetus or newborn should display the following characteristics:

(1) Normotension

(2) Normal hematocrit and hemoglobin levels

b. *Nursing interventions*

(1) Maintain the woman in a side-lying position to enhance uteroplacental perfusion.

(2) Monitor FHR continuously by electronic fetal monitor.

(3) Evaluate FHR pattern for reassuring and nonreassuring characteristics.

> **NURSING DIAGNOSIS:** Fear R/T unknown outcome for self and baby

a. *Expected outcomes:* Following treatment and care, the woman should be able to do the following:

(1) Identify supportive people and resources

(2) Verbalize feelings of decreased fear

b. *Nursing interventions*

(1) Provide information regarding interventions and anticipated medical treatment.

(2) Encourage questions and provide an opportunity for the woman to share her feelings.

(3) Provide support to the woman and her family.

12. Discharge planning and teaching

a. Assessment of the need for education is begun on admission.

b. Education regarding management of bleeding episode, subsequent care, postpartum self-care, and infant care is provided as soon as the woman is able to absorb the information.

Induced Labor

1. Definition: initiation of uterine contractions by medical means before the beginning of spontaneous labor to accomplish birth

2. Induction is indicated in the presence of severe preeclampsia, diabetes, prolonged rupture of membranes, chorioamnionitis, postterm gestation, intrauterine fetal death, and previous precipitous labor and birth (labor and birth that occur in 3 hours or less).
3. Induction may also be done for fetal factors such as isoimmunization and intrauterine fetal growth retardation.
4. Clinical management
   a. Obtain a 20-minute electronic fetal monitoring strip to determine whether FHR is reassuring.
   b. Evaluate maternal status.
   c. Begin a primary intravenous line and piggyback in a secondary intravenous line with oxytocin (Pitocin). Regulate oxytocin by infusion pump.
   d. Increase rate of infusion based on American College of Obstetricians and Gynecologists–recommended standards and agency protocol. The goal is to achieve a contraction pattern with a frequency of every 3 minutes, a duration of 60 seconds, and moderate to strong intensity. Once this contraction pattern is reached, the infusion is not advanced any further.
   e. Monitor maternal vital signs, contraction pattern, and characteristics of the electronic fetal monitoring pattern before any increase in flow rate.

Breech Birth

1. Definition: vaginal or cesarean birth of a baby in breech presentation
2. Approximately 3 percent of all fetuses are in breech presentation.
3. Breech presentation is more likely to be associated with congenital anomalies, multiple gestation, low implantation of the placenta, or uterine anomalies.
4. Neonatal morbidity and mortality are increased with vaginal birth of breech presentation because the largest portion of the fetus is the last to pass through the pelvis.
5. Clinical management
   a. External version is attempted at about 38 weeks, to change (convert) the fetus to a cephalic (head down) presentation. Success rate for external versions is about 85 to 87 percent.
   b. If external version is successful, a vaginal birth can be planned.
   c. If external version is unsuccessful, a cesarean birth is usually planned.

Emergency Birth

1. Emergency birth may occur inside or outside of a hospital or birthing setting.
2. Management of emergency birth includes quickly establishing rapport with the laboring woman.
   a. To enhance thinning of the perineal tissues, gently massage the lower border of the vagina as the woman pushes.
   b. As the fetal head crowns, provide gentle pressure on the perineum and ask the woman to pant so the head emerges slowly.

   c. Slide the index finger up along the head to check for nuchal cord (cord around the neck) and remove it, if present.
   d. Encourage the woman to push gently to complete the birth process.
   e. Gently suction the newborn's mouth with a bulb syringe.
   f. Dry the baby and place on the maternal abdomen skin to skin. Cover both the mother and newborn with a warmed blanket.
   g. Determine the Apgar score.
   h. Observe the perineum for any lacerations (tears).
   i. Expect the birth of the placenta within 30 minutes. If it does not occur in this time or if maternal bleeding increases, place the baby at the breast and encourage breast feeding. This releases oxytocin, which stimulates the uterus to contract.
   j. Maintain a record of the birth with the time of birth.

Birth of Multiple Gestation

1. Twins may be born vaginally if the following criteria are met:
   a. The twin that is closest to the cervix is cephalic and is the larger fetus.
   b. Both twins are stable and have reassuring FHRs.
   c. No contraindications for vaginal birth are present.
2. If the above criteria are not met, a cesarean birth is planned.
3. At the time of vaginal birth, special plans need to be made because an emergency cesarean needs to be done quickly if either fetus begins to experience difficulty.
4. The birth of more than 2 fetuses is by cesarean.

Stillbirths

1. Definition: the term used to describe the birth of a baby that has died in utero
2. Ultrasound is used to confirm the death of the fetus. In the examination, no heartbeat is seen and overriding of the cranial sutures is visible.
3. Birth is accomplished by induction.
4. Continuous emotional support is imperative.

■ SURGICAL MANAGEMENT

Amniotomy

1. Definition: a procedure in which the membranes are ruptured artificially by use of a device such as an amnihook. Once the amniotomy is done, amniotic fluid escapes from the vagina.
2. Clinical management
   a. Auscultate or monitor the FHR before and after the amniotomy to detect prolapse of the cord.
   b. Observe the amniotic fluid to determine that it is clear. Meconium may indicate fetal stress.

Median or midline

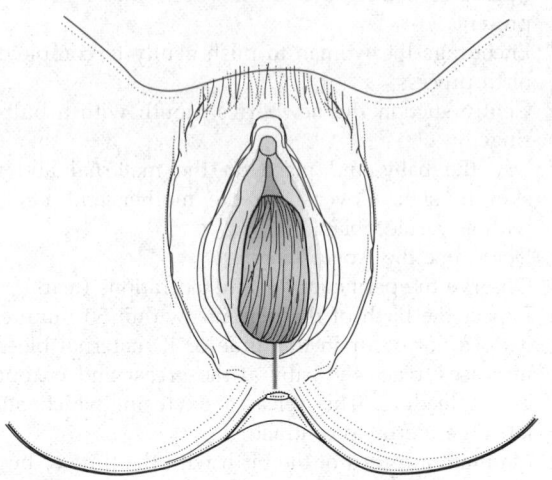

Mediolateral

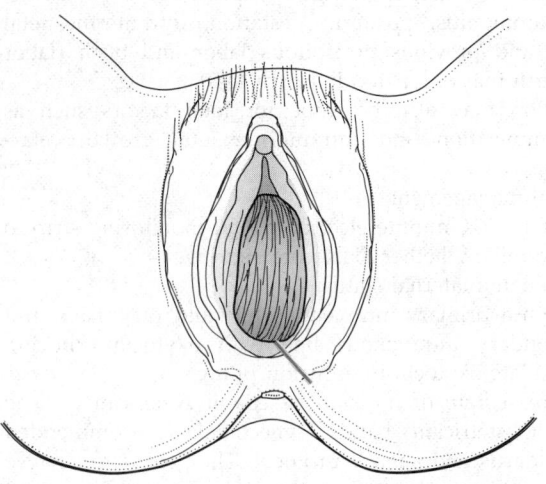

Advantages	*Disadvantages*
Minimal blood loss	An added laceration may ex-
Neat healing with little scarring	tend the median episiotomy
Less postpartum pain than the	into the anal sphincter
mediolateral episiotomy	Limited enlargement of the va-
	ginal opening because peri-
	neal length is limited by the
	anal sphincter

Advantages	*Disadvantages*
More enlargement of the vagi-	More blood loss
nal opening	Increased postpartum pain
Little risk that the episiotomy	More scarring and irregularity
will extend into the anus	in the healed scar
	Prolonged dyspareunia
	(painful intercourse)

Figure 14–15. Types of episiotomies. (Modified from Gorrie TM, McKinney ES, and Murray SS. *Maternal Newborn Nursing.* Philadelphia: WB Saunders, 1994, p 400.)

Episiotomy

1. Definition: a surgical procedure done just before birth to enlarge the vaginal opening. The episiotomy may be midline or mediolateral (Fig. 14–15).
   a. A midline extends from the lower border of the vagina downward toward the anus. The midline is more likely to extend toward the anus during the birth process.
   b. A mediolateral extends from the lower border of the vagina diagonally to the right or left. A mediolateral provides more room (more space for the baby to be born) but is more uncomfortable after birth and heals with more scar tissue.
2. The episiotomy is done after local anesthetic infiltration. The episiotomy is repaired with absorbable suture.

Forceps-Assisted Birth

1. Definition: Forceps are used to assist in the birth of the fetal head. They may be used to shorten the 2nd stage in the presence of maternal or fetal distress or maternal exhaustion. Forceps are classified as outlet, low, or mid.
   a. Outlet forceps: Forceps are applied when the fetal head is on the perineum, the fetal scalp is visible in between contractions, and the sagittal suture is not more than 45 degrees from the midline.
   b. Low forceps: Forceps are applied when the fetal scalp is at +2 station or more.

   c. Midforceps: Forceps are applied to the fetal head when it is engaged but above +2 station.
2. Neonatal risks
   a. Facial edema
   b. Abrasions or bruising of the face

☐ *CESAREAN BIRTH*

Definition

Birth of the fetus through a surgical incision in the maternal abdomen and uterus

Incidence and Socioeconomic Impact

1. Incidence is currently between 20 and 25 percent.
2. Cesarean birth is recommended for conditions such as fetal or maternal distress, placenta previa or abruptio placentae, macrosomic fetus, multiple gestation, and breech presentation.

Clinical Management

1. Provide information regarding the cesarean birth process; need for nothing by mouth status before surgery; methods of anesthesia, with advantages and disadvantages of all; and care following surgery.

2. Provide opportunity for questions.
3. Arrange a tour of the unit to decrease anxiety.
4. Prepare the woman for surgery: abdominal perineal presentation, indwelling bladder catheter, intravenous line, completion of the surgical check list.
5. Monitor maternal and fetal status.

Applying the Nursing Process

NURSING DIAGNOSIS: Ineffective individual coping R/T stress of labor and birth process and lack of coping tools

1. *Expected outcomes:* Following care, the woman will be able to do the following:
   a. Discuss methods that can be used to increase coping skills
   b. State that she feels less stress
2. *Nursing interventions*
   a. Assess current coping ability and tools that the woman has to use during labor.
   b. Establish rapport to provide information and support for the laboring woman and her support person.

NURSING DIAGNOSIS: Pain R/T uterine contractions, birth process, and/or perineal trauma from birth

1. *Expected outcomes:* Following care, the woman should be able to do the following:
   a. Identify pain relief measures
   b. State that her pain level is manageable and that she had a variety of methods to select from
   c. Verbalize support from the nurse during labor and birth
2. *Nursing interventions*
   a. Assess the level of discomfort the woman is experiencing.
   b. Determine the options the woman has for increasing comfort.
   c. Provide support and encouragement to the woman and her support person.
   d. Provide information regarding additional comfort techniques as needed.
      (1) Maintain position of comfort. Encourage the woman to do the following:
      • Ambulate as desired (if membranes are ruptured and presenting part is not well applied to the cervix, the woman may need to remain in bed because of the increased risk of prolapsed cord).
      • Sit up in a rocking chair or other chair that is comfortable.
      • Sit in a whirlpool tub or shower.
      • Stand beside the bed and lean forward over the bed.
      • While in bed, change position every 30 to 60 minutes. The woman can use a side-lying position, a mid to high Fowler's with arms and legs supported with pillows, a hands and knees posi-

tion, or a position with the knees on the bed and the arms up over the back of the bed that has been placed in a high Fowler's.
      • Take care to avoid a supine position as it decreases uteroplacental perfusion.
      (2) Maintain relaxation between contractions.
      • The Mitchell method may be used to enhance relaxation: pull the shoulders down to the floor; place the elbows and arms in a position of comfort, bend the elbows and wiggle them slightly; bend the knees slightly; wiggle them around until a position of comfort is reached; push the heels into the bed and raise the toes toward the ceiling and then release the muscles; let the jaw open and the muscles relax.
      • The woman may use this method during contractions also, but relaxation may be difficult to maintain while she is having the discomfort of uterine contractions. If relaxation can be maintained between contractions, it helps preserve and restore energy.
      (3) During uterine contractions assist the woman to do the following:
      • Use a focal point to help her maintain control.
      • Keep her eyes open, as open eyes help her maintain control.
      • Use a patterned breathing method.
      • Use effleurage (light fingertip stroking over the abdomen in a circular or figure-of-eight pattern).
      • Place a firm support against the lower back if the woman feels severe back discomfort.
      (4) Encourage the woman to urinate at least every 2 hours.
      (5) Encourage the woman to take in some clear fluids, ice chips, or popsicles to maintain hydration.
      (6) Suggest other comfort techniques as needed:
      • Cooling wash cloth on brow or over throat
      • Keeping chux or underpads dry
      • Maintaining a comfortable temperature in the room
      • Encouraging the woman to make sounds if it helps
      • Offering a backrub
      • Holding the woman's hand
      • Offering words of encouragement and support
      • Remaining with the woman or leaving for periods of time as she desires
      (7) Provide support to the coach.
   e. Determine what information the woman has about analgesic agents and regional blocks and her wishes regarding their use.
      (1) Provide additional information as needed.
      (2) Encourage the woman to use these pain relief measures if needed and desired (see Table 14–12).

NURSING DIAGNOSIS: Altered tissue perfusion in the fetus secondary to decreased uteroplacental perfusion

1. *Expected outcomes:* Following care, the fetus should be able to maintain a reassuring FHR pattern.

2. *Nursing interventions*
   a. Encourage the laboring woman to change position frequently and while lying in bed maintain a side-lying position (to prevent compression of the vena cava, which then leads to a decrease in uteroplacental perfusion).
   b. Obtain a fetal-monitoring strip to monitor the FHR.
   c. Monitor maternal vital signs.
   d. Note the development of decreased variability, baseline changes, and late decelerations immediately, and take corrective action if possible.
      (1) Position the woman in a side-lying position.
      (2) Monitor for maternal hypotension.
      (3) Provide oxygen and administer intravenous fluids if the FHR pattern indicates.

Public Health Considerations

1. Although the cesarean birth rate has decreased in the United States over the past few years, the incidence of 20 to 25 percent still remains significantly higher than the 10 to 12 percent incidence of other developed countries such as Great Britain. Continuing emphasis needs to be placed on maintaining low-risk pregnancies and births through promotion of preventive care, prenatal care, and use of certified nurse-midwives.
2. As health care reform continues to evolve, more attention will be placed on the most expeditious and cost-effective method of providing labor and birth services. Freestanding birth centers managed by certified nurse-midwives are being explored as a model that meets the future health care challenges.

■ CARING FOR THE FAMILY IN THE POSTPARTUM PERIOD

Definitions

1. **Postpartum** (also called puerperium) is the 6-week period after birth during which the woman's body returns to essentially the prepregnant physiologic status.
2. **Involution** refers to the progressive descent of the uterus into the pelvic cavity. After birth, descent occurs at about 1 fingerbreadth (approximately 1 cm) per day.

Transcultural Considerations

1. Both the incorporation of the newborn into the family and the designated person with major responsibility for newborn care varies within cultural groups.
2. Preferences for food and fluids differ.
3. Self-care measures such as showering and newborn practices also vary.

Family Assessment

1. Physical examination of the postpartum woman
   a. Vital signs

      (1) Blood pressure: 90 to 140/60 to 90, or consistent with early pregnancy blood pressure
      (2) Pulse: 50 to 90 beats per minute; the slowing of the pulse is normal
      (3) Respirations: 16 to 24 per minute
      (4) Apical pulse: normal rate and rhythm
   b. Lungs: All lobes clear without rales or rhonchi
   c. Breasts: Breasts should be soft and may be filling on day 1 or 2. No redness or nipple cracking should be present.
   d. Abdomen
      (1) Bowels sounds should be normal.
      (2) Diastasis recti (separation of diastasis rectus muscle) may be present. Assess by measuring length and width of separation.
      (3) Assess muscle tone.
   e. Uterine fundus
      (1) Fundal height is located approximately one half of the way between the symphysis pubis and umbilicus immediately after birth. By a few hours after birth, the fundus has risen to the level of the umbilicus, and then it descends 1 fingerbreadth per day.
      (2) The fundus is firm and well contracted.
      (3) The fundus is located in the midline. If the fundus is located toward the woman's right side, assess for bladder distention.
   f. Perineum
      (1) Assess the perineum for bruising and edema.
      (2) Assess the episiotomy for approximation of stitches, edema, and bruising.
      (3) Assess for hemorrhoids.
   g. Lochia
      (1) Lochia rubra is present for the first 2 to 3 days and is followed by lochia serosa.
      (2) A few small clots (the size of a nickel) may be present.
   h. Edema
      (1) Assess the feet, ankles, and lower legs for pitting edema.
      (2) Ask the woman if her rings are tight or if she has noted edema of her hands.
   i. Deep tendon reflex and clonus
      (1) Assess patellar deep tendon reflex, especially if blood pressure is elevated or proteinuria is present.
      (2) Assess for clonus: Normal findings are negative.
   j. Pedal pulse: Pedal pulse should be palpable on both feet.
   k. Urinary output
      (1) Assess urine output until a voiding pattern is established clearly.
      (2) Expect an increase in output in the 1st 12 to 24 hours past birth.
   l. Comfort
      (1) Assess the presence of uterine afterpains, which may be more pronounced in multipara and in breast-feeding mothers.
      (2) Assess the level of discomfort from episiotomy and hemorrhoids.
   m. Fatigue: Assess the patient's level of energy and need for rest.

2. Psychosocial assessment
   a. During the 1st day, the new mother is more interested in her own bodily needs and rest. Assess the need for pain relief, comfort measures, foods and nourishment, quiet time for resting, and information regarding self-care.
   b. During the 2nd day, the new mother moves to more care-taking activities and is more involved in newborn care.
      (1) Assess informational needs regarding newborn care.
      (2) Assess the support structure available for the mother.

Routine Postpartum Care

1. Perineal care
   a. Hygienic measures: Rinse the perineal area after voiding with warm water and pat dry. A peri-bottle or Surgigator may be used.
   b. Comfort measures
      (1) Apply a cool pack (or an ice pack) to the perineum for 20 minutes and then remove the pack for approximately 20 minutes before reapplying. Cool packs are usually used for the 1st 12 hours, and then sitz baths are encouraged. If perineal edema is still present, cool packs may continue to be used.
      (2) Warm sitz baths may be taken 2 or 3 times a day. When at home, a bathtub can be filled with warm water and used as a sitz bath. It is important for the woman to understand that she should not bathe in the water 1st and then sit in it.
      (3) Encourage the woman to sit on a firm chair rather than on a soft cushion.
2. Voiding
   a. After birth, edema of the urethra and urinary meatus is common.
   b. Postpartum diuresis begins in about 12 hours after birth and lasts for approximately a week.

   c. Urinary retention may occur because of edema of the urethra, effects of anesthetic regional blocks, or both.
   d. Each voiding should produce more than 150 ml.

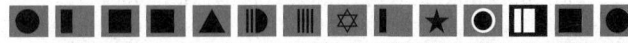

TRANSCULTURAL CONSIDERATIONS

Cultural beliefs and practices in the postpartum period usually center on aspects of newborn care and self-care. The mother may have specific wishes regarding how the baby is handled and what type of interaction people have with her baby. The primary caretaker of the baby may or may not be the mother. The mother may have specific wishes regarding the type of fluids and foods that she wants.

3. Feeding the newborn
   a. Breast-feeding
      (1) Breast-feeding may begin immediately after birth if the mother desires (Procedure 14–1).
      (2) It is currently recommended that the newborn breast-feed on demand and that other fluids or a pacifier not be used. The use of a nipple on a bottle or a pacifier may confuse the newborn in that the sucking action with an artificial nipple is different from that at the mother's breast.
      (3) Most breast-feeding mothers need support and counseling. It is important that the information be presented in a consistent manner.
      (4) The breast-feeding mother may note some discomfort from breast engorgement or nipple soreness for the 1st few days (Box 14–8).
      (5) Problems with nipple soreness, latching on, and engorgement are the most common problems.
   b. Bottle feeding: Many women prefer formula. It is important that the woman who chooses bottle feeding also feels support for her newborn-feeding choice.
4. Fundal checks
   a. Monitor fundal firmness and position every 6 hours.

BOX 14–8. Comfort Measures for Breast Engorgement and Nipple Soreness

The breast-feeding mother may experience discomfort from sore nipples or breast engorgement. Self-care measures that may help are the following:

Nipple Soreness

Position the baby with the ear, shoulder, and hip in straight alignment and with the baby's stomach against the mother's.
Rotate breast-feeding positions.
Break suction with the little finger.
Do not allow the baby to chew on the nipple or to sleep holding the nipple in the mouth.
Nurse frequently.
Apply tea bags soaked in warm water to the nipple.
Begin feeding on the less sore nipple.

Breast Engorgement

Nurse every 1 1/2 to 3 hours around the clock.
Use a supportive, well-fitting bra at all times.
Take a warm shower just before feeding or apply warm compresses.
Alternate breasts during feeding.
Massage breasts before feeding to stimulate let-down.

The uterus is sensitive and needs to be palpated gently. If the fundus is toward the woman's right side, check the bladder for distention.

  b. Teach the woman to assess her own fundus and provide information regarding expected descent.

5. Diet: The postpartum woman needs to continue a nutritious diet to aid restoration of tissues.

6. Rest: Rest is an important aspect of the birth recovery process. The new mother has many demands on her time, both in the birthing facility and at home. It is

Procedure 14–1
Assisting with Breast-Feeding

Definition/Purposes	To help the breast-feeding woman feed the newborn. Breast-feeding provides numerous benefits to the mother and baby. During breast-feeding oxytocin is released, which stimulates uterine contractions and promotes uterine involution. Breast-feeding the newborn provides excellent nutrition and immunologic protection.
Contraindications/Cautions	Major contraindications include the need for ongoing use of medications by the mother that may be passed through the breast milk and be harmful to the newborn; a mother who does not want to breast-feed; and a mother who is positive for the human immunodeficiency virus.
Learning/Teaching Activities	Provide the following information: (a) the variety of positions that may be used to breast-feed; (b) the methods of encouraging the newborn to latch on; (c) the techniques to assess if the newborn is feeding successfully; and (d) the methods of ending the feeding.

Preliminary Activities

Equipment	No special equipment needed
Assessment/Planning	• Assess maternal knowledge and experience base regarding breast-feeding. • Collect breast-feeding handouts and videotapes that may be used for reinforcement of information. • Assess maternal comfort level before breast-feeding and provide analgesic approximately 30 minutes before the feeding if needed.
Preparation of the Mother	• Administer analgesic if needed to relieve pain and discomfort before feeding. • Encourage the mother to wash her hands just before feeding. • Assist the mother to a comfortable position with the newborn. • Have additional pillows on hand, especially if the mother has had a cesarean birth.
Procedure	

Action	Rationale/Discussion
1. Assist mother to a side-lying or sitting position.	1. Maintaining comfort during the feeding will enhance the feeding.
2. In side-lying position, baby may be positioned on a pillow.	2. The baby is raised above bed level.

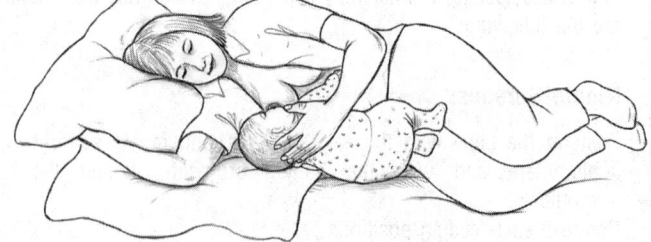

Action	Rationale/Discussion
3. The mother props herself up on her elbow and supports her breast with the opposite hand.	3. Allows the mother to lower her breast to the baby.
4. The baby is pulled close to the mother's breast, and the baby latches on.	4. Baby's position enhances the latching on process.
5. Once the baby is nursing, the mother can lie back.	5. Lying back promotes comfort.
6. To end the nursing, the mother can place her little finger in the side of the baby's mouth to break the suction.	6. To avoid skin damage, the baby should not be pulled off the nipple.

Action	Rationale/Discussion
7. A sitting position may be used.	7. A sitting position is comfortable for most women. The pillow helps support the weight of the newborn.

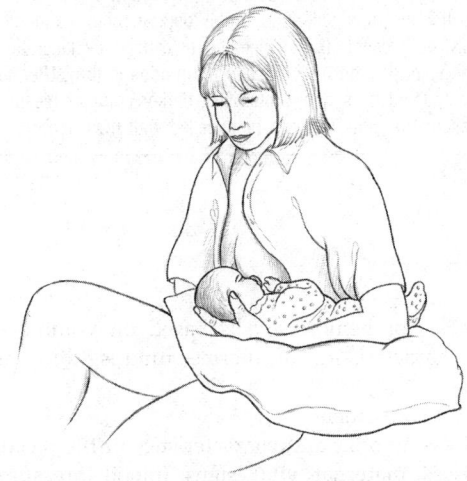

A pillow may be used across the lap to provide support for the baby. The baby's head is cradled in the mother's arm and the baby's body is facing the mother, stomach to stomach.

Final Activities

Assess breast-feeding in view of the mother's comfort level with handling the baby and her physical comfort.

Determine the amount of time the newborn nursed on each breast, and record these figures in the infant record.

Provide support and assistance to the mother as needed.

---

important to provide opportunities for rest in the hospital setting.

7. Postpartum exercises: The woman may begin gentle exercises such as pelvic rock and head lift with bent knees in the 1st few days after birth. It is important not to overdo the exercises.

8. Promoting family bonding
   a. Interaction with newborn
      (1) Attachment behaviors may be indicated by holding the newborn close, eye-to-eye contact, enface position (faces in same plane), talking to the newborn, caretaking activities, looking for similarities and differences in the newborn, selecting a name, and having articles of clothing or other supplies available.
      (2) Attachment behaviors are very individualistic and are influenced by cultural patterns.
      (3) Assess interactional pattern and caretaking activities. Describe observed activities objectively.
   b. Interaction of family members
      (1) Assess the supportive environment around the new mother and the baby.
      (2) Assess her interaction with family members. Is it supportive and helpful? To whom does she look for information? Are referrals to community agencies desired or needed?
      (3) Encourage opportunities for the father, siblings, and family members to interact with the newborn.

9. Resumption of sexual relations
   a. Most women are advised to delay sexual intercourse for about 3 weeks, until the episiotomy has healed and lochia has ceased.
   b. The vagina may have reduced moisture, so a lubricant like K-Y jelly may be needed to increase comfort.

■ POSTPARTUM HEMORRHAGE

Definition

1. Postpartum hemorrhage is the loss of more than 500 ml of blood.
2. Classification

a. Early postpartum hemorrhage occurs within the 1st 24 hours after birth.
b. Late postpartal hemorrhage occurs after the 1st 24 hours.

Incidence and Socioeconomic Impact

1. Postpartum hemorrhage occurs in approximately 4 percent of vaginal births and 6.4 percent of cesarean births.
2. Hemorrhage is a major cause of maternal mortality.

Risk Factors

1. The risk factors associated with vaginal birth include prolonged 3rd stage, preeclampsia, twins, episiotomy, soft-tissue lacerations, and forceps- or vacuum extractor–assisted birth.
2. Risk factors associated with cesarean birth include chorioamnionitis, preeclampsia, prolonged active phase of labor, and general anesthesia.

Etiology

1. In the normal postpartum course, hemorrhage is prevented by constriction of blood vessels in the placental bed and an intact coagulation system.
2. A variety of factors can precipitate postpartum hemorrhage.

Pathophysiology

1. Overdistention of the uterus (twins, macrosomic fetus) and uterine muscle fatigue (long labor, prolonged active phase, or prolonged 3rd stage) may disturb the ability of the blood vessels in the placental bed to contract.
2. Uterine atony (relaxation of the uterus) causes hemorrhage because relaxation of myometrial muscles causes dilation of blood vessels in the placental bed and bleeding occurs. Uterine atony is associated with uterine muscle fatigue and retention of placental fragments or membranes.
3. Soft-tissue damage (lacerations, episiotomy, forceps or vacuum extractor–assisted birth) causes disruption of blood vessels with resultant bleeding. In rare cases, disseminated intravascular coagulation causes a disruption in the body's coagulation system.

Clinical Manifestations

1. More than 500 ml of blood loss
2. Uterine atony: bright red bleeding; boggy, large uterus, clots
3. Vaginal or cervical lacerations, or both: bright red bleeding (unclotted blood) in a steady flow; firm uterus
4. Retained placental fragments: boggy, large uterus (may be firm with massage then become boggy in a short period); bright red bleeding

5. Hypovolemic shock (falling blood pressure, rising pulse rate, cold and clammy skin, air hunger)

NURSE ADVISORY

The major causes of postpartum bleeding are retained placental fragments or retained amniotic membranes, lacerations on the cervix or vagina, and uterine atony. Retained placental fragments prevent the uterus from contracting firmly, so the fundus will feel boggy, the bleeding will tend to be dark in color, and clots will probably be present. If the bleeding is caused by lacerations, the bleeding is bright red in color, and the fundus is firm. Uterine atony is accompanied by a boggy uterus, a darker color of bleeding, and the presence of clots that can be expelled with massage.

Diagnostics

1. Diagnosis of hemorrhage is based on volume of blood lost, characteristics of uterine fundus, and laboratory studies.
2. Physical assessment
   a. Assess amount and characteristics of the bleeding.
   b. Assess maternal vital signs (blood pressure, pulse, respirations) skin color, and capillary refill.
   c. Assess coping state.
3. Diagnostic studies
   a. Complete blood count
   b. Type and cross of blood products for transfusion
   c. Coagulation study workup to determine decreased values of platelets, fibrinogen, prolonged clotting time and prothrombin time, and increase in fibrin split products

Clinical Management

1. Goals of interventions are to identify women at risk, to provide accurate assessments to aid in rapid identification of the problem, and to provide information and support for the woman and her support person or persons.
2. Nonpharmacologic interventions
   a. A boggy (relaxed) uterine fundus is gently massaged.
   b. Ensure that the bladder does not become distended.
   c. Carefully assess maternal stabilization following birth.
3. Pharmacologic interventions
   a. An oxytocic agent (Pitocin or Methergine) may be given following birth to prevent hemorrhage. These medications may also be used when hemorrhage is present.
   b. Oxygen may be administered in the presence of severe hypovolemic shock.
4. Management of early hemorrhage due to retained placenta after the physician or certified nurse-midwife removes the placenta manually:
   a. Massage uterus.
   b. Administer oxytocin (Pitocin) intravenously or intramuscularly.

c. Monitor the uterus for tone.
d. Monitor maternal vital signs.
e. Provide intravenous fluid replacement.

5. Management of early hemorrhage due to vaginal or cervical lacerations after surgical repair of laceration:
   a. Administer oxytocic agent.
   b. Monitor maternal vital signs.
6. Management of late hemorrhage due to retained placental fragments (D & C may be done):
   a. Administer oxytocic agent (Pitocin) as IV infusion per order.
7. Late hemorrhage due to endometritis:
   a. Administer oxytocin orally (usually methylergonovine maleate).
   b. Administer antibiotic if infection is present.
   c. Monitor uterine involution.

Complications

1. Hypovolemic shock
2. Anemia
3. Infection

Prognosis

1. Prognosis is good.
2. Rapid identification and treatment are essential.

Applying the Nursing Process

NURSING DIAGNOSIS: Altered tissue perfusion R/T blood loss

1. *Expected outcomes:* Following care, the woman should display the following characteristics:
   a. Normotension
   b. Informed regarding the bleeding problem
2. *Nursing interventions*
   a. Provide education regarding signs and symptoms, nursing interventions, and treatment measures.
   b. Identify the presence of risk factors.
   c. Monitor maternal status.

Discharge Planning and Teaching

1. Provide information regarding safety measures.
2. Be alert for dizziness on arising.
3. Call for assistance with ambulation for the 1st few hours.
4. Provide information regarding the importance of maintaining a diet high in protein, iron, and vitamin C.
5. Provide information regarding signs and symptoms of infection because hemorrhage increases the risk of infection.

Public Health Considerations

1. Hemorrhage remains a major cause of maternal mortality in the United States.

2. Recognition of risk factors and rapid treatment of hemorrhage is essential.

◼ OTHER POSTPARTUM COMPLICATIONS

Mastitis

1. Definition: Inflammation of the breast. The causative organism is usually *Staphylococcus aureus*. Mastitis usually occurs in breast-feeding women.
2. Clinical manifestations: Reddened, warm painful area on breast, fever, body aches, and flulike symptoms.
3. Clinical management
   a. Increased fluid intake, use of a supportive bra, frequent newborn feedings to empty the breast, analgesics to increase comfort, and application of warm packs.
   b. A 10-day course of antibiotics is recommended.

Puerperal Infection

1. Definition: Most are metritis or endometritis limited to the uterine cavity.
2. Clinical manifestations
   a. Maternal temperature of 100.4 degrees Fahrenheit (38.0 degrees Celsius) or higher, with the temperature occurring on any 2 of the 1st 10 postpartum days
   b. Pain and tenderness over the uterus
   c. Scant or profuse bloody, foul-smelling vaginal discharge
   d. Chills, tachycardia, and subinvolution (classic signs of endometritis)
3. Clinical management: antibiotic therapy

Superficial Thrombophlebitis

1. Definition: presence of a clot in a superficial vein, usually the saphenous; occurs more frequently in the postpartum period than during pregnancy
2. Clinical manifestations: Warmth, redness, tenderness over a portion of the leg, and absence of fever.
3. Clinical management: Application of heat, bed rest, analgesics, and use of elastic hose usually recommended

Subinvolution

1. Definition: A uterus that does not descend at the anticipated rate, with lochia remaining rubra or returning to rubra after a few days
2. Clinical manifestations
   a. Uterus higher than expected in the abdominal cavity
   b. Continued presence of lochia rubra
3. Clinical management
   a. Methylergonovine (Methergine) every 3 to 4 hours for 24 to 48 hours to stimulate uterine contractions

b. Analgesics for the discomfort of increased uterine contractions

Postpartum Depression

1. Definition: depression that occurs in the 1st few days following birth
2. Clinical manifestations: More than 50 percent of women report feelings of weepiness, mild depression, anxiety, difficulty sleeping, headache, and irritability.
3. Clinical management
   a. Provide counseling and support.
   b. Provide opportunities for the mother to talk about her feelings.
   c. Refer to community counseling services if needed.

Infection in Episiotomy

1. Clinical manifestations: Episiotomy exhibits redness, swelling, and tenderness
2. Clinical management
   a. Encourage use of sitz baths 4 times per day.
   b. Antibiotic therapy is warranted.

Postpartum Psychosis

1. Clinical manifestations: restlessness, agitation, hallucinations, insomnia, confusion, irrationality, and delirium
2. Clinical management
   a. Establish rapport.
   b. Refer to professional counseling for treatment.

◼ ASSESSMENT AND CARE OF THE NEWBORN DURING THE FIRST 24 HOURS OF LIFE

Assessment

1. The 1st 4 hours
   a. Axillary temperature is taken and should be between 97.8 and 98.8 degrees Fahrenheit.
   b. A Chemstrip is used to determine blood glucose.
   c. Gestational age is assessed by completing a Ballard gestational assessment.
   d. In many areas, a hematocrit is obtained to assess for hyperviscosity (above 65%).
2. From 4 to 24 hours: Approximately every 6 hours the nurse should complete the following assessments:
   a. Apical pulse (rate and presence of murmurs), respirations (rate, presence of retractions), breath sounds, and bowel sounds
   b. Examine the newborn's head: characteristics of anterior and posterior fontanelles, sagittal suture, presence of caput or cephalhematoma, abrasions, ecchymosis or puncture wounds
   c. Assess eyes and nose for discharge.
   d. Examine the umbilical cord for redness or discharge.
   e. Examine the condition of the skin for dryness, presence of rashes, skin color, and presence of jaundice (determined by blanching skin on tip of nose or over

sternum for a few seconds and then assessing for yellowish tones).
   f. Assess movement of the extremities.
   g. Assess voiding and stool production patterns.

Nursing Care

1. The 1st 24 hours
   a. Complete newborn assessment every 6 hours.
   b. Assist the parents with newborn care.
   c. Apply alcohol to the umbilical cord at least every 6 hours.
   d. Remove the cord clamp when the cord has dried.
   e. Maintain a comforting environment for the newborn.
   f. Reassess the newborn's weight at approximately 12 hours of age.
   g. Complete phenylketonuria and genetic screen testing.
   h. Administer Engerix if ordered by the pediatrician and desired by the parents. (Consent form must be signed.)
   i. Assist parents with newborn feeding.
   j. Be watchful of signs indicating hypoglycemia such as tremulousness and jitteriness of the newborn's hands.
2. Nursing interventions to address a knowledge deficit and teach the woman to describe self-care measures and care for the newborn
   a. Determine the present level of knowledge regarding physiologic changes, self-care needs, and newborn care.
   b. Assess the woman's educational and reading level to assist in preparation of teaching materials best to meet her needs.
   c. Assess the presence of sociocultural factors that will influence the mother's beliefs, values, and practices regarding self-care and newborn care.
   d. Provide information regarding maternal self-care for the following areas:
      (1) Resting frequently during the day to regain strength and energy
      (2) Using comfort measures as needed for afterpains
         • Lie on the stomach with small pillow under abdomen for short intervals.
         • Take prescribed analgesic agent as directed.
         • Drink warm fluids to enhance comfort.
      (3) Using comfort measures for episiotomy discomfort
      (4) Knowing that the uterine fundus should remain firm and descend by 1 fingerbreadth per day
      (5) Explaining about lochia rubra (bright red) remaining for 1st 2 to 3 days, then lochia serosa (pinkish to brownish) from day 3 to day 10, and lochia alba (whitish) for an additional week or so
      (6) Providing information regarding signs that may indicate problems
   e. Provide information regarding newborn care.
      (1) Bathe the newborn 2 to 3 times per week. Do not immerse the newborn in water until the umbilical cord has come off at about 7 to 10 days past birth.
      (2) Feed the newborn on demand but encourage the infant to eat if more than 4 hours has passed.
      (3) Keep a bulb syringe handy to remove nasal secretions or to use in case of choking.
      (4) Take axillary temperature if the baby feels very warm, is lethargic, has diarrhea, vomits, or otherwise does not appear well.

(5) Keep the baby in a car seat while in the car.

(6) Cleanse the perineal area with each diaper change.

(7) Know that the baby should have at least 6 to 8 wet diapers per day.

(8) Apply and wipe alcohol around the umbilical cord 2 to 4 times per day to enhance drying.

3. Nursing interventions to address family coping and potential for growth

a. Discuss feelings regarding the newborn with family members.

b. Discuss anticipated challenges family members think they will encounter.

c. Identify community resources that may be used.

d. Complete the newborn assessments in the mother's room to further acquaint the mother, father, and siblings with the individual characteristics of the baby.

e. Provide opportunities for the mother, father, siblings, and newborn to be together.

f. Encourage rooming in so the family has optimal time to learn caretaking skills and a chance to ask questions.

g. Model caretaking activities.

Public Health Considerations

1. Because early discharge is creating many challenges in the childbearing area, nurses must complete the needed assessments, care, and teaching in a short period.

HOME CARE STRATEGIES

Early Postpartum Discharge

Home health care nurses with obstetric nursing skills make home visits to physically assess mother and infant and continue the teaching begun in the hospital. This assessment and instruction is critical to the health and safety of the mother and infant, especially because hospital stays are so brief.

The physical assessment and management for the mother include the following:

- *Bleeding patterns:* Count pads, and observe for heavy abnormal vaginal bleeding.
- *Postpartum infection:* Take temperature every day for 2 weeks. Report to physician any foul-smelling vaginal discharge, fever, or chills.
- *Breast care:* For the nursing mother, use warm compresses to engorged breasts. Use lanolin cream on cracked or sore nipples. Report flulike symptoms to the physician.
- *Rest:* Rest when the infant and other children nap. Do not lift anything heavier than the baby for the 1st 2 weeks.
- *Nutrition:* Eat from the basic food groups, and drink 6 to 8 glasses of fluid daily.
- *Emotional changes:* Emotional lability is normal. Later feelings of anger, resentment, or hostility toward the baby are abnormal and can be treated.
- *Community resources:* There are various community resources to meet individual needs, such as WIC, Healthy Start, and lactation consultants such as Nursing Mothers and La Leche League.
- *Obstetric follow-up:* Make an appointment for 6 weeks postpartum to discuss returning to work, resumption of sexual activity, and beginning to use birth control.

The physical assessment and management for the infant include the following:

- *Feedings:* Eight to 12 feedings in a 24-hour period is normal if the mother is breast-feeding.
- *Hydration:* One void per day of life is normal. Count stools in a 24-hour period.
- *Sepsis:* Take the infant's temperature at the same time daily for 2 weeks.
- *Jaundice:* Expose the infant to natural light if yellow sclera and sleepiness develop.
- *Pediatric follow-up:* Make an appointment for 2 to 4 weeks to discuss physical assessment, normal growth and development, and establishing baseline data.

BOX 14–9. *Healthy People 2000:* **Maternal and Infant Health**

1. Reduce the infant mortality rate to no more than 7 per 1000 live births. (Baseline: 10.1 per 1000 live births in 1987.)

2. Reduce the fetal death rate (20 or more weeks of gestation) to no more than 5 per 1000 live births plus fetal deaths. (Baseline: 7.6 per 1000 live births plus fetal deaths in 1987.)

3. Reduce the maternal mortality rate to no more than 3.3 per 100,000 live births. (Baseline: 6.6 per 100,000 in 1987.)

4. Reduce the incidence of fetal alcohol syndrome to no more than 0.12 per 1000 live births (Baseline: 0.22 per 1000 live births in 1987.)

5. Reduce low birth weight to an incidence of no more than 5 percent of live births and very low birth weight to no more than 1 percent of live births. (Baseline: 6.9% and 1.2%, respectively, in 1987.)

6. Increase to at least 85 percent the proportion of mothers who achieve the minimum recommended weight gain during their pregnancies. (Baseline: 67% of married women in 1980.)

7. Reduce severe complications of pregnancy to no more than 15 per 100 deliveries. (Baseline: 22 hospitalizations [prior to delivery] per 100 deliveries in 1987.)

8. Reduce the cesarean delivery rate to no more than 15 per 100 deliveries. (Baseline: 24.4 per 100 deliveries in 1987.)

9. Increase to at least 75 percent the proportion of mothers who breast-feed their babies in the early postpartum period and to at least 50 percent the proportion who continue breast-feeding until their babies are 5 to 6 months old. (Baseline: 54% at discharge from birth site and 21% at 5 to 6 months in 1988.)

10. Increase abstinence from tobacco use by pregnant women to at least 90 percent and increase abstinence from alcohol, cocaine, and marijuana by pregnant women by at least 20 percent. (Baseline: 75% of pregnant women abstained from tobacco use in 1985.)

11. Increase to at least 90 percent the proportion of all pregnant women who receive prenatal care in the 1st trimester of pregnancy. (Baseline: 76% of live births in 1987.)

12. Increase to at least 60 percent the proportion of primary care providers who provide age-appropriate preconception care and counseling. (Baseline: data available in 1992.)

13. Increase to at least 90 percent the proportion of women enrolled in prenatal care who are offered screening and counseling on prenatal detection of fetal abnormalities.

14. Increase to at least 90 percent the proportion of pregnant women and infants who receive risk-appropriate care.

15. Increase to at least 95 percent the proportion of newborns screened by state-sponsored programs for genetic disorders and other disabling conditions and to 90 percent the proportion of newborns testing positive for disease who receive appropriate treatment.

From *Healthy People 2000. National Health Promotion and Disease Prevention Objectives.* U.S. Department of Health and Human Services. Public Health Service. DHHS Publication No. (PHS) 91-50213.

---

2. The mother must have an opportunity to recover and regain strength.

3. The new family has a minimal amount of time to become acquainted with the new family member.

4. Box 14–9 lists goals of health care for improved maternal and infant health.

Bibliography

Books and Pamphlets

Arias F. *Practical Guide to High-Risk Pregnancy and Delivery.* 2nd ed. St. Louis: Mosby–Year Book, 1993.

Barber HRK, Fields DH, and Kaufman SA. *Quick Reference to OB-GYN Procedures.* Philadelphia: JB Lippincott, 1990.

Blackburn ST, and Loper DL. *Maternal, Fetal, and Neonatal Physiology: A Clinical Perspective.* Philadelphia: WB Saunders, 1992.

Buckley K, and Kulb NW. *High Risk Maternity Nursing Manual.* Baltimore: Williams & Wilkins, 1990.

Chamberlain G, Dewhurst J, and Harvey D. *Obstetrics.* London: Gower Medial Publishing, 1991.

Chasnoff IS (ed). *Drugs, Alcohol, Pregnancy and Parenting.* Boston: Kluwer Academic Publishers, 1988.

Cunningham FG, et al. *William's Obstetrics.* Norwalk, CT: Appleton & Lange, 1993.

Hatcher R, et al. *Contraceptive Technology 1990–1991.* New York: Irvington Publisher, 1989.

Heppard M, and Garite TJ. *Acute Obstetrics: A Practical Guide.* St. Louis: Mosby–Year Book, 1993.

Hoole J, et al. *Patient Care Guidelines for Nurse Practitioners.* 4th ed. Philadelphia: JB Lippincott, 1995.

Iams JD, and Zuspan FP. *Zuspan and Quilligan's Manual of Obstetrics and Gynecology.* St. Louis: CV Mosby, 1990.

Lader L. *RU486.* Reading, MA: Addison-Wesley Publishing Co, 1991.

Ladrine H. *Bringing Cultural Diversity to Feminist Psychology.* Washington, DC: American Psychological Association, 1995.

Mattson S, and Smith JE (eds). *Core Curriculum for Maternal-Newborn Nursing.* Philadelphia: WB Saunders, 1993.

National Research Council Commission on Behavioral and Social Sciences and Education. *Losing Generations: Adolescents in High-Risk Settings.* Washington, DC: American Psychological Association, 1993.

Olds SB, London ML, and Ladewig PA. *Maternal Newborn Nursing.* Redwood City, CA: Addison-Wesley Publishing Co, 1996.

Reece EA, et al. *Medicine of the Fetus and Mother.* Philadelphia: JB Lippincott, 1992.

Sims LK, et al. *Health Assessment in Nursing.* Redwood City, CA: Addison-Wesley Publishing Co, 1995.

Speroff L, and Darney P. *A Clinical Guide for Contraception.* Baltimore: Williams & Wilkins, 1992.

Stanton AL, and Gallant SJ. *The Psychology of Women's Health.* Washington, DC: American Psychological Association, 1995.

U.S. Department of Health and Human Services, Public Health Service. *Healthy People 2000: National Health Promotion and Disease Prevention Objectives.* Boston: Jones & Bartlett, 1992.

Varney H. *Nurse Midwifery.* Boston: Blackwell Scientific Publications, 1987.

Chapters in Books and Journal Articles

Balcazar H, et al. What predicts breast-feeding intention in Mexican-American and non-Hispanic white women? Evidence from a national survey. *Birth* 22(2):74, 1995.

Bendell A, and Efantis-Potter J. Acquired immune deficiency syndrome in pregnancy. *In* Mandeville LK, and Troiano NH (eds). *High-Risk Intrapartum Nursing.* Philadelphia: JB Lippincott, 1992.

Buckley K. Substance abuse. *In* Buckely K, and Kulb NW (eds). *High Risk Maternity Nursing Manual.* Baltimore: Williams & Wilkins, 1990.

Caufield K. Controlling fertility. *In* Youngkin EQ, and Davis MS (eds). *Women's Health: A Primary Care Clinical Guide.* Norwalk, CT: Appleton & Lange, 1994.

Clarke SC, and Taffel S. Changes in cesarean delivery in the United States, 1988 and 1993. *Birth* 22(2):63, 1995.

Collins JB. Women and the health care system. *In* Youngkin EQ, and Davis MS (eds). *Women's Health: A Primary Care Clinical Guide.* Norwalk, CT: Appleton & Lange, 1994.

Enkin MW, et al. Effective care in pregnancy and childbirth: A synopsis. *Birth* 22(2):101, 1995.

Evans AR, and Benbarka MM. Endocrine disorders. *In* Niswander KR, and Evans AT (eds). *Manual of Obstetrics.* Boston: Little, Brown & Co, 1991.

Gant NF, and Cunningham FG. Management of preeclampsia. *Semin Perinatol* 18(2):94, 1994.

Griffith DR. The effects of perinatal cocaine exposure on infant neurobehavior and early maternal-infant interactions. *In*

Hadlock FP. *Evaluation of Fetal Growth and Size.* Tenth International Symposium on Perinatal Medicine and Obstetrical Ultrasound, Las Vegas, NV, April 9–12, 1990.

Hammill HA, and Murtagh C. AIDS in pregnancy. *In* Knuppel RA, and Drukker JE (eds). *High-Risk Pregnancy.* Philadelphia: WB Saunders, 1993.

Kaye ME, and Chasnoff IF. Substance abuse in pregnancy. *In* Knuppel RA, and Drukker JE (eds). *High-Risk Pregnancy.* Philadelphia: WB Saunders, 1993.

Kulb NW. Disorders of the endocrine system. *In* Buckley K, and Kulb NW (eds). *High-Risk Maternity Nursing Manual.* Baltimore: Williams & Wilkins, 1990.

Lizzi L. Substance abuse in pregnancy. *In* Beck WW (ed). *Obstetrics and Gynecology.* Philadelphia: Harwal Publishing, 1993.

Mandeville LK. Diabetes mellitus in pregnancy. *In* Mandeville LK, and Troiano NH (eds). *High-Risk Intrapartum Nursing.* Philadelphia: JB Lippincott, 1992.

Moore TR. Assessment of amniotic fluid volume in at-risk pregnancies. *Clin Obstet Gynecol* 38(1):78, 1995.

Neal AD, and Bockman VC. Preterm labor and preterm premature rupture of membranes. *In* Mandeville LK, and Troiano NH (eds). *High-Risk Intrapartum Nursing.* Philadelphia: JB Lippincott, 1992.

Niebyl JR. Drugs and related areas in pregnancy. *In* Dilts PV, and Sciarra JJ (eds). *Gynecology and Obstetrics.* Philadelphia: JB Lippincott, 1992.

Paul RH, and Miller DA. Nonstress test. *Clin Obstet Gynecol* 38(1):3, 1995.

Roberts NS. Identification of the high-risk patient. *In* Beck WW (ed). *Obstetrics and Gynecology.* Philadelphia: Harwal Publishing, 1993.

Rotondo L, and Coustan DR. Diabetes mellitus in pregnancy. *In* Knuppel RA, and Drukker JE (eds). *High-Risk Pregnancy.* Philadelphia: WB Saunders, 1993.

Silver HM. Hypertensive disorders. *In* Niswander KR, and Evans AT (eds). *Manual of Obstetrics.* Boston: Little, Brown & Co, 1991.

Silver HM, and Smith LH. The puerperium. *In* Niswander KR, and Evans AT (eds). *Manual of Obstetrics.* Boston: Little, Brown & Co, 1991.

Williams MC. Preterm labor. *In* Niswander KR, and Evans AT (eds). *Manual of Obstetrics.* Boston: Little, Brown & Co, 1992.

15

Caring for Infants, Children, and Adolescents

◼ NORMAL GROWTH AND DEVELOPMENT

Principles of Growth and Development

1. Development is a dynamic, lifelong process of maturation that proceeds in a genetically predictable order.
2. Development proceeds at a specific pace for each child, but the pace varies among children, and every child experiences periods of rapid or decelerated growth.
3. Development is influenced by the person's race, culture, environment, experiences, and intimate relationships. It is an interrelated process, with all dimensions relying on others to form the complex person.
4. Development occurs in a cephalocaudal (head-to-toe) and proximodistal (near to distant) manner and becomes increasingly differentiated.
5. During certain "critical," or "vulnerable," periods, the developing person is more sensitive to the effects of external factors that positively or negatively influence development.

Assessing Areas of Development

1. Physical development is the growth of the body and its structures, including increasing differentiation in both structure and function. Developmental milestones are signposts on which to assess whether the child is developing within the norm (Table 15–1).

◉ ▯ ▰ ▰ ▲ ◨ ▦ ⦀ ✡ ▮ ★ ◉ ▯ ▰ ◉

TRANSCULTURAL CONSIDERATIONS

Children of different cultures grow and develop in slightly different ways, which might not always correspond with Western growth parameters. For example, Asian children in general are smaller than Western children of comparable age, and the gross motor developmental sequence differs (Western children develop psychomotor skills at a slower pace until age 2 years). Teeth erupt earlier in Black children. Cephalocaudal and proximodistal maturation, however, is consistent in children of all cultures.

2. Cognitive development is the development of complex thinking and reasoning skills. Language is the verbal expression of cognitive development. Jean Piaget's theory proposed that as they mature, children develop cognitive intelligence, abstract reasoning, and ability to learn about the environment through a logical, orderly, and sequential process.
   a. After initiating an activity or manipulating an object in the environment, the child creates a mental image, or **scheme,** of the properties of the action or object.
   b. Through the process of **assimilation,** the child incorporates new experiences or properties into already existing schemes, thus learning about new things.
   c. When a new experience does not relate to an existing scheme, the child uses **accommodation** to modify what is known or constructs a new scheme to fit the new experience.
3. Personal and social development
   a. Erik Erikson's theory of psychosocial development explains that personality develops in 8 stages (5 of which apply to children and adolescents). Each stage represents a conflict between the developing person and environmental expectations. Stages and tasks might vary cross-culturally. Positive resolution of the conflict is followed by a new "crisis" with new problems to be mastered. Negative resolution of the conflict may delay development and result in difficulty coping with problems later in life.
   b. Sigmund Freud's theory of personality development explains that the developing personality is an evolving conflict between unconscious, basic impulses (id) and the modifying influences of conscious reality (ego) and conscience (superego). Personality develops in 5 stages associated with different pleasure-seeking behaviors by children at various developmental levels. Personality defects result from inadequate resolution of a particular stage. Freud's theory is used with caution and only in the context of a total approach to child development.
   c. Lawrence Kohlberg's theory of moral development explains that acquiring moral reasoning, or the ability to distinguish right from wrong, is closely related to developing cognitive skills and a sense of justice. Moral development occurs at 3 levels, each containing 2 stages. The process is not so much age related as sequential. Kohlberg's theory is still controversial.

Table 15–1. Theories of Child Development

Developmental Level	Cognitive (Piaget)	Psychosocial		Moral (Kohlberg)
		Erikson	Freud	
Infant (Birth to 1 year)	**Sensorimotor stage:** initial reflex actions become more repetitive and intentional as the infant learns to elicit a response from self or objects in the environment; beginning "object permanence," the ability to understand that an object or person exists even if not seen	**Trust vs. mistrust:** learns to trust the environment through having basic needs met in an adequate and consistent manner	**Oral stage:** increases understanding of the environment through activities associated with the mouth (e.g., sucking, mouthing, chewing)	
Toddler (1 to 3 years)	**Sensorimotor stage (until age 2 years):** learns cause and effect relationships and begins to actively use memory to solve problems; beginning of imitation, speech, and use of symbols; increasing understanding of space and time; advanced concept of object permanence **Preoperational stage (Preconceptual, 2–4 years):** increasing use of symbols in the form of language and imaginative play; egocentric, unable to view situations from another's perspective	**Autonomy vs. shame and doubt:** begins to develop independence and control of physical skills and mental processes with the positive encouragement and support of caregivers	**Anal stage:** develops control over the environment as sphincter control develops	**Preconventional:** determines right and wrong by making decisions according to rules imposed by others or by gratifying impulses; behavior is guided by the expectation of reward or punishment
Preschool (3–6 years)	**Preoperational stage (Intuitive, 4–7 years):** improves language development, which allows the child to gather information through questioning; less egocentric; unable yet to fully understand the changing or reversible properties of objects	**Initiative vs. guilt:** initiates goal-directed exploration and manipulation of the self and the environment, with increasing self-confidence and sense of responsibility for actions	**Phallic stage:** gender identity emerges as a result of unconscious conflict and subsequent identification with the parent of the same sex	
School age (6–12 years)	**Concrete operational stage (7–11 years):** refines logical thought processes by dealing with objects and actions that can be seen and manipulated; develops ability to sort, classify, and order objects, and solve problems systematically and concurrently; understands that certain properties of objects remain the same even though their action or appearance changes (conservation); views a situation from another's perspective	**Industry vs. inferiority:** develops the ability to achieve and the necessary skills to complete activities and projects successfully, with positive feedback from peers and family	**Latency:** resolves previous conflicts and develops greater interest in others	**Conventional:** bases moral behavior on values and expectations of others (e.g., family, peers, teachers) and on respect for authority and established rules
Adolescence	**Formal operational stage (11 years and older):** develops abstract reasoning, hypothetical thinking, deduction, and synthesis of information	**Identity vs. identity diffusion:** develops a positive sense of self, allegiance to a set of values, and mastery of social skills by experimenting with different roles	**Genital stage:** constructs appropriate relationships with members of the opposite sex	**Postconventional (autonomous):** makes moral, rational decisions based on an understanding of law and social order beyond the immediate environment, and considers right and wrong within the context of what is best for the individual as well as society as a whole

4. Temperament results from a combination of genetic and environmental influences and determines how the child responds to people and events
   a. There are 3 major categories of temperament:

(1) Easy child—flexible, adapts readily to new situations, requires little adjustment from parents, cheerful, and friendly
(2) Difficult child—fussy, active, inflexible with rou-

tine, intense and can be negative, exhibits frustration through temper tantrums
(3) Slow-to-warm-up child—sensitive, shy, and aloof with others until comfortable, adjusts slowly to new situations and routines.
b. Temperament positively or negatively affects personality development, and infants who are perceived as "difficult" can be at risk for behavior problems as they develop.
c. More important than the basic temperamental style of the child is the way the family responds. Adapting to the infant's style early minimizes risks as the child matures.

Transcultural Considerations

1. Childrearing practices: Children learn about unique cultural customs, values, and practices through the childrearing approach of parents and extended family members. Major cultures differ in their approach to childrearing according to the following:
   a. Value of the child to the family—the child may or may not be viewed as a welcome addition and sometimes the child's value is related to the child's gender.
   b. Parent involvement—one or the other parent may take on more responsibility for socialization of children, or childrearing may be the primary responsibility of extended family members.
   c. Parental expectations—cultures differ in behavioral expectations of children, as well as in approaches and expectations for reaching developmental milestones, especially in areas of feeding, elimination, sleep, and achievement of adult status in the society.
   d. Child's position in the family—different cultures place different values on children depending on whether the child is the oldest or youngest sibling and the child's relationship with members of other generations.
   e. Types of discipline used—measures include such areas as emphasis on self-control, acceptance of autonomy, amount of openly demonstrated affection, and cooperative decision making.
   f. Religious influences—affect childrearing in areas of dietary practices, religious rituals, accessing health care, and use of religious healers.
2. Cultural comparisons
   a. Native Americans—childrearing practices differ among tribes.
      (1) A major goal is to transmit and preserve Native American history and culture.
      (2) Children are cared for through the cooperative efforts of an extended family and maintain a status equal to other generations. Approach to discipline may be permissive and not understood by health care professionals.
      (3) Native Americans teach their children the interrelationship between humans and nature.
      (4) Religious ceremonies are an integral part of childrearing, promoting health, and treating illness.
   b. Hispanics—people of Mexican, Cuban, Central American, Puerto Rican, and Latin American ethnic backgrounds are included.

(1) Children are highly valued, and extended family members participate in the care of the child. Family members are demonstrative and affectionate toward one another.
(2) Traditionally, men are the authority figures, but women are responsible for child and health care. Discipline is permissive.
(3) Girls are protected until marriage. Boys are encouraged to be assertive and are given more freedom but remain dependent on the family for support and assistance into early adulthood.
(4) A prolonged lying-in period after birth is common. Mothers often bottle feed their babies in the hospital and wait until "milk comes in" before initiating breast-feeding.
   c. Blacks
      (1) Children are welcomed and are encouraged to actively participate in family decision making.
      (2) Good behavior is expected. Crying may be viewed as "being bad."
      (3) Child care is shared by family members. Mothers usually dominate and have a special relationship with their sons. Older people are held in high esteem.
      (4) Adult role-modeling occurs early, and children appear more mature than contemporaries from other cultures. Peer socialization is almost as important as family socialization, especially among inner-city youth.
   d. Asians—people of Chinese, Japanese, Vietnamese, Laotian, Cambodian, and other such ethnic backgrounds are included.
      (1) Respect and love for elders, particularly parents, is of primary importance. Children are often reared in multigenerational families.
      (2) Men are the authority figures, and sons often live with parents into adulthood. The mother-child bond is especially strong.
      (3) The emphasis in childrearing is on respect, discipline, and self-control. Asian children are often toilet-trained very early.
   e. Whites—Childrearing methods usually depend on social stratum, composition of the family, and proximity of extended family members.
3. Cultural attitudes in illnesss prevention
   a. Cultural modalities that influence approaches to illness prevention include the following:
      (1) Traditional and nontraditional medicine
      (2) Prayer
      (3) Diet
      (4) Wearing of amulets or other religious symbols
      (5) Healing properties of foods and herbs
      (6) Rituals
   b. Most Native Americans believe illness is caused by disharmony between the individual and nature (Navajo) or between positive and negative energy forces (Hopi, Cherokee).
      (1) The medicine man addresses both the body and the spirit to heal and restore harmony.
      (2) Other approaches to healing include use of religious rites, amulets, masks, and sand painting.
   c. Hispanics may see health as good luck and consider

illness to be a punishment for having done something wrong.

(1) Consultation with a *curandero* (healer) may be requested. The *curandero* may prescribe a variety of remedies including herbs and teas, which are directed toward restoring the body's balance.

(2) Prayer, pilgrimages, the wearing of medals and religious symbols, and the burning of candles are used. Placing a coin and cloth binder in the umbilical area protects infants against protrusion of the umbilicus.

(3) Hispanics are present time–oriented and may not believe in immunization or respond to anticipatory guidance or adhere to biomedical regimens to prevent future illness. The nurse should provide reminders for appointments and give parents written directions for care.

d. Blacks may believe illness is caused by disharmony with nature or separation of the body and the spirit.

(1) Voodoo, prayer, wearing of amulets or certain jewelry, and use of teas, poultices, and herbs are believed to both prevent and heal disease.

(2) Wearing garlic is believed to get rid of evil spirits.

e. In Asian cultures, health is a balance in the body between the yin and the yang.

(1) Traditional approaches used to restore balance include acupuncture, which balances excess yang, and moxibustion, which balances excess yin. Immunization has been used traditionally for disease prevention. Herbal treatments, diet, and rituals prevent illness.

(2) Overdressing protects the body from exposure or loss of heat, and infants are often brought to the physician's office in many layers of clothing, regardless of weather and temperature.

f. Many Whites believe that health is related to taking care of one's body throughout life and practicing a "healthy lifestyle."

(1) Anticipatory guidance is usually successful because this is a future-oriented cultural group.

(2) Prayer, wearing of religious symbols, good diet, exercise, and herbs are also used to prevent or cure illness. There is widespread use of over-the-counter medications.

Age-Appropriate Assessment

1. Communicating with children: cultural considerations. Children's immaturity and more limited verbal skills can interfere with their ability to communicate. They are often less able to express emotions and feelings precisely when describing signs and symptoms.

a. Children are often unsure of how to behave when interacting with health care professionals who are different culturally. This confusion can create mistrust or suspicion in either the child or the professional. Adaptation of the usual methods of communicating is necessary to provide optimal care to children. Culture-specific communication patterns can be a barrier to achieving successful relationships with people who

are culturally different, particularly in the following areas:

(1) Nonverbal communication—use of touch, eye contact, variations in time orientation, nonverbal expression of emotion

(2) Verbal communication—predominant language not English or extensive use of cultural terminology not understood by others

b. Native Americans—children learn respect for others and demonstrate it through liberal use of nonverbal communication. Long pauses in conversation indicate respect, through careful contemplation of what another is saying. Eye contact may be avoided.

c. Hispanics—the spoken language is usually Spanish. Verbal communication sometimes includes emotional, demanding behavior.

d. Blacks—Black children often communicate with one another in language that would be racist if spoken by non-Blacks. Black children can feel alienated by the dominant cultural system. These feelings are often rooted in the experience of racial prejudice.

e. Asians—many Asian Americans communicate with their children in their native language. Children and adults exhibit limited eye contact with health care professionals out of respect for the professional.

f. Whites—most Whites speak English, which is the primary language spoken by health care professionals in the United States. Various subgroups (e.g., adolescents, people affiliated with certain religious groups) may use alternative ways of communicating (e.g., jargon).

2. Communicating with children: developmental considerations

a. Infants

(1) Approach infants slowly and touch them gently. Be careful touching infants whose parents might have "evil eye" beliefs.

(2) Talk in a low voice at a distance of approximately 10 to 12 inches from the infant's face. Smiling and nodding can elicit a smile or laugh from the infant. Responding in kind to the infant's initial verbal cues encourages additional verbal exchange.

(3) Infants approximately 8 to 9 months old might regard a stranger with concern. Approach these infants in a manner that allows the child to see the parent as well.

b. Toddlers

(1) Get as close to the child's eye level as possible when initiating conversation.

(2) Allow the child to be in physical contact with the parent as much as possible. Do not talk "baby talk" to the child.

c. Preschoolers

(1) Preschoolers often rely on familiar transition objects to help them cope with a strange setting. Allow them to include these objects in the conversation, if desired.

(2) Do not hesitate to get involved with a young child's fantasy play during a well visit or in the hospital setting. Children use fantasy to help them cope with the unfamiliar.

(3) Allow children to examine pieces of equipment and practice using them.

(4) Use words that are familiar to describe sensations (e.g., ouch, owie, tickle, cough, tight). Explain what will happen in words they understand (e.g., "This machine is going to give your arm a hug.").

d. School-age children

(1) Encourage the child to express feelings and emotions if appropriate. The child can use verbal and nonverbal methods (e.g., crying, drawing, singing, storytelling, games, doll play).

(2) Allow the child to ask questions, and answer all questions as honestly as possible.

(3) Prepare children for procedures as close to the time as possible, using words they understand. Tell them what they will experience, for how long, and what they can do to help (e.g., count to 5, take deep breaths, sing a song).

(4) Always verify that the child has understood what you have said or are about to do.

(5) Praise them for cooperation afterward.

e. Adolescents

(1) Encourage adolescents to express their concerns.

(2) Assure confidentiality when appropriate, but do not promise confidentiality for all circumstances. Explain that if the health or welfare of the adolescent is in severe jeopardy, disclosure might be necessary.

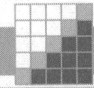

LEGAL AND ETHICAL CONSIDERATIONS

The nurse or physician must obtain informed consent before any procedure or treatment that is potentially harmful to the child. These include immunizations and participation in research. A parent, an adolescent older than 18 years, or an emancipated minor (a minor child who is no longer dependent upon parents for either emotional or financial support) may give consent. Children able to understand the procedure and its implications should be included in the decision making. In certain cultures, the primary caregiver is not the child's legal guardian and cannot give consent. To give culturally sensitive care, include all the child's significant caregivers in the decision-making process.

3. Obtaining a health history—general principles

a. Starting the interview

(1) Begin to establish a trusting relationship by introducing yourself to the parent or caregiver and child. Call the child and caregiver by name throughout the interview.

(2) Verify the caregiver's relationship to the child, and record appropriate information—address, telephone number, birth date, insurance information.

b. Tell the child and parent that you need to ask some questions to find out more about them. Encourage the child to answer whenever possible. Information can be verified by the parent either nonverbally or verbally.

c. Phrase questions using terms appropriate for the child's age and in a manner designed to obtain the

most information, such as, "Can you tell me about any problems you have when you see things?" rather than, "Is your vision good?" If the child or parent has difficulty understanding what is needed, try rephrasing the question using different terms.

d. Allow adolescents to be seen without a parent present if they choose, but tell them you will be talking to the parent as well, to determine any parental concerns.

e. Ask relevant questions about each area of functioning, and elicit concerns, if any. Ask for clarification if needed. Obtain specific information about the following at each well visit:

(1) Activity—level, participation in sports or extracurricular activities, hobbies

(2) Nutrition—method of feeding, amount and types of food and fluids eaten on a regular basis, pattern of eating, vitamins, fluoride (for children up to age 12 years whose water is not fluoridated)

(3) Elimination—bowel and urinary elimination pattern, toilet training, problems with elimination (constipation, diarrhea, enuresis)

(4) Sleep—number of hours, quality of sleep (sound, restless), sleep problems (walking, nightmares, night terrors)

(5) Dentition—tooth eruption, brushing, frequency of dental visits

(6) Senses—same as for adult

(7) Development—physical, fine and gross motor, cognitive, sexual

(8) Social and emotional development—temperament, relationships with parents and peers, adjustment to school

(9) Safety—according to age group (e.g., use of car seats, bicycle helmets, childproofing)

(10) General state of health—exposure to disease such as communicable diseases of childhood (e.g., chickenpox, pertussis), strep-related disease, and sexually transmitted diseases and exposure to health risk factors (e.g., smoking in the home, substance use)

(11) Illness or concerns since last visit (review of systems elicits this information)

f. If this is the first visit for this child, inquire about the following:

(1) Health history

• Pregnancy or prenatal problems

• Birth and neonatal history (including apgar scores, weights, length, color, treatment for any problems such as jaundice, phenylkentonuria screening done)

• Chronic or recurrent acute medical problems and treatments used, surgeries

• Serious accidents or injuries

• Allergies

• Immunization status, screening procedures

• Current medications

• Childhood illnesses

(2) Family history, including number and composition of family members, cultural orientation, relationships, problems

g. Observe interaction between child and parent during

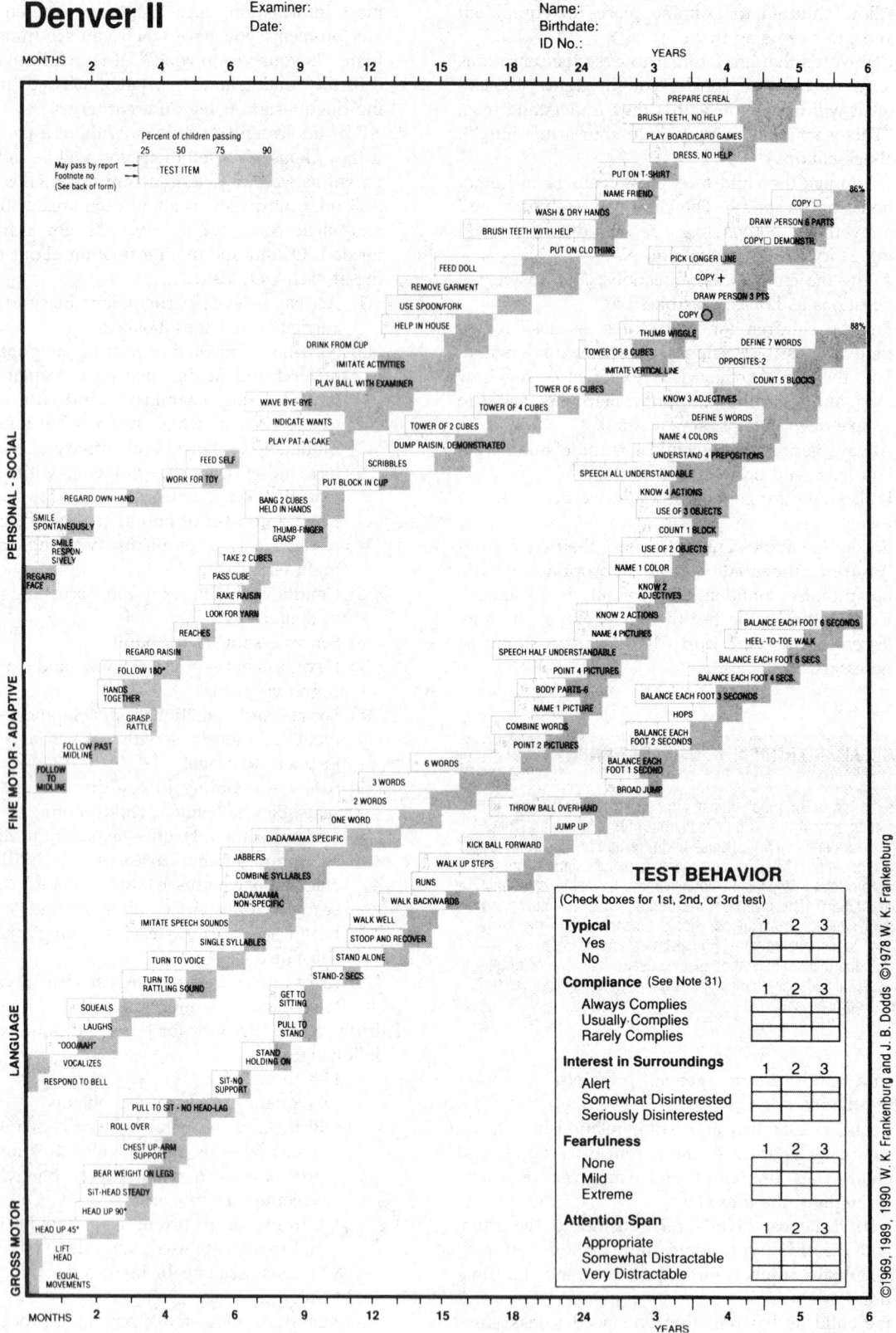

Figure 15–1. Denver Developmental Screening Test (Denver II). (Used with permission from Denver Developmental Materials, Inc., Denver, CO, 1990.)

the interview to gain clues to family dynamics and parenting skills.

h. If the visit is in response to a specific complaint, determine the nature of the complaint, its history and duration, and any remedies that have been tried (see Chapter 4).

4. Physical examination

a. Equipment used for physical examination of infants,

DIRECTIONS FOR ADMINISTRATION

1. Try to get child to smile by smiling, talking or waving. Do not touch him/her.
2. Child must stare at hand several seconds.
3. Parent may help guide toothbrush and put toothpaste on brush.
4. Child does not have to be able to tie shoes or button/zip in the back.
5. Move yarn slowly in an arc from one side to the other, about 8" above child's face.
6. Pass if child grasps rattle when it is touched to the backs or tips of fingers.
7. Pass if child tries to see where yarn went. Yarn should be dropped quickly from sight from tester's hand without arm movement.
8. Child must transfer cube from hand to hand without help of body, mouth, or table.
9. Pass if child picks up raisin with any part of thumb and finger.
10. Line can vary only 30 degrees or less from tester's line. /
11. Make a fist with thumb pointing upward and wiggle only the thumb. Pass if child imitates and does not move any fingers other than the thumb.

      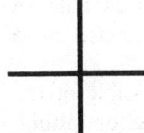   

| 12. Pass any enclosed form. Fail continuous round motions. | 13. Which line is longer? (Not bigger.) Turn paper upside down and repeat. (pass 3 of 3 or 5 of 6) | 14. Pass any lines crossing near midpoint. | 15. Have child copy first. If failed, demonstrate. |

When giving items 12, 14, and 15, do not name the forms. Do not demonstrate 12 and 14.

16. When scoring, each pair (2 arms, 2 legs, etc.) counts as one part.
17. Place one cube in cup and shake gently near child's ear, but out of sight. Repeat for other ear.
18. Point to picture and have child name it. (No credit is given for sounds only.)
    If less than 4 pictures are named correctly, have child point to picture as each is named by tester.

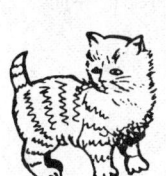 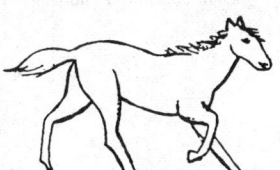 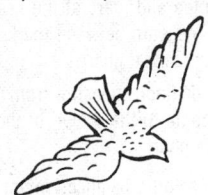 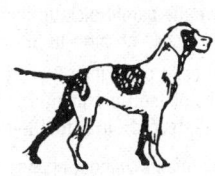 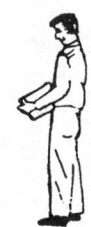

19. Using doll, tell child: Show me the nose, eyes, ears, mouth, hands, feet, tummy, hair. Pass 6 of 8.
20. Using pictures, ask child: Which one flies?... says meow?... talks?... barks?... gallops? Pass 2 of 5, 4 of 5.
21. Ask child: What do you do when you are cold?... tired?... hungry? Pass 2 of 3, 3 of 3.
22. Ask child: What do you do with a cup? What is a chair used for? What is a pencil used for?
    Action words must be included in answers.
23. Pass if child correctly places <u>and</u> says how many blocks are on paper. (1, 5).
24. Tell child: Put block **on** table; **under** table; **in front of** me, **behind** me. Pass 4 of 4.
    (Do not help child by pointing, moving head or eyes.)
25. Ask child: What is a ball?... lake?... desk?... house?... banana?... curtain?... fence?... ceiling? Pass if defined in terms of use, shape, what it is made of, or general category (such as banana is fruit, not just yellow). Pass 5 of 8, 7 of 8.
26. Ask child: If a horse is big, a mouse is __? If fire is hot, ice is __? If the sun shines during the day, the moon shines during the __? Pass 2 of 3.
27. Child may use wall or rail only, not person. May not crawl.
28. Child must throw ball overhand 3 feet to within arm's reach of tester.
29. Child must perform standing broad jump over width of test sheet (8 1/2 inches).
30. Tell child to walk forward, ⟳⟳⟳→ heel within 1 inch of toe. Tester may demonstrate.
    Child must walk 4 consecutive steps.
31. In the second year, half of normal children are non-compliant.

OBSERVATIONS:

Figure 15-1. *Continued*

children, and adolescents is similar to that for adults, with some modifications:
(1) Blood pressure cuffs are available in several different sizes. Select the most appropriate for the child's age and body size (width to cover 50–75% of the body part on which the cuff is positioned, length enough to encircle the part with little overlap).
(2) Choose otoscope specula according to the size of the child and width of the ear canal. The size

giving the widest view with least discomfort is preferable.

   (3) Make the equipment more interesting for children whenever possible (e.g., by attaching a small stuffed animal to the stethoscope, using flavored tongue depressors, incorporating toys and play into the examination). Allowing children to touch the equipment can decrease the child's anxiety during examinations.

b. General procedures

   (1) Proceed from the least to the most threatening or painful part of the examination. For example, elicit the infant's startle reflex, examine the young child's ears and throat, and inspect and palpate the older child's genitals toward the end of the examination. Otherwise, proceed generally in a head-to-toe manner.

   (2) Perform as much as possible of the examination with the parent holding or sitting close to the child. This reduces any fear and subsequent crying.

   (3) Allow the parent to undress an infant or a young child. Encourage preschoolers and older children to undress themselves. Diaper or underpants may be left on. Provide privacy and a gown for older children and adolescents.

   (4) Use inspection, auscultation, palpation, and percussion.

      • Auscultate a young child while the child is quiet. You might want to do this first, before proceeding with the examination.

      • To prevent a "tickle" response to palpation, make sure your hands are warm and distract the child during the procedure (e.g., tell a story, have the child pretend to blow bubbles slowly, sing, concentrate on breathing slowly).

c. Table 5–1 presents the format for head-to-toe physical examination of adults. Table 15–2 presents specific

Text continued on page 481

Table 15–2. Physical Examination: Adaptations for Infants and Children

Assessment Area	Technique	What to Observe
Length/height	Lie infant or child younger than 3 yr old flat and supine on table paper; mark at the crown of the head; with parent holding the head, fully extend one leg and mark at the heel; have the parent pick up the child; measure between marks and record on birth to 36-month percentile chart. Stand child older than 3 yr on scale or floor; measure from base of foot to a point at a right angle to the crown of the head; record on 2- to 18-yr growth chart.	Length increases approximately 1 inch per month for the first 6 months, 50% by the first yr, 2 to 3 inches per yr in older children until the adolescent growth spurt begins.
Weight	Weigh infants without clothes or diaper on a balanced infant scale. Babies may sit unsupported if they are able. Make sure there is no danger of infant rolling, squirming, or falling off of the scale. Weigh older child on balanced standing scale wearing underpants only, or gown. If the child is uncooperative, weigh the parent and child together; weigh the parent alone, then subtract the parent's weight from the combined weight to get the child's weight.	Newborn weight loss of 5–10% is usually regained by age 2 wk; birth weight doubles by 5–6 months, triples by 1 yr. Average weight gain for older children is 5–7 lb/yr.
Head circumference	Measure at the widest point on the head using a paper tape for maximum circumference. Uncooperative children may be held by their parents; otherwise, lay them flat. Record the measurement on the percentile chart.	Excessively small or large head; head growing at faster than normal rate (exceeding percentile curve over a short period of time) might indicate hydrocephalus.

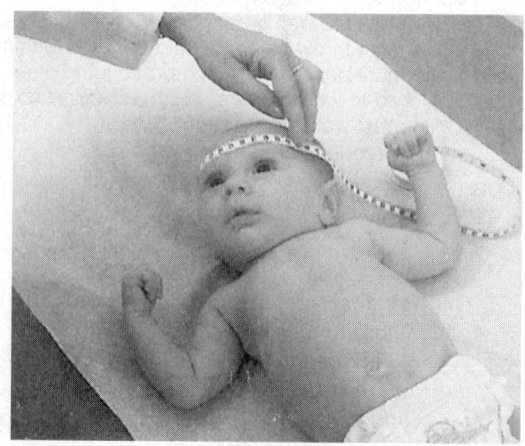

Table 15–2. Physical Examination: Adaptations for Infants and Children (Continued)

Assessment Area	Technique	What to Observe
Temperature	Rectal temperature is most accurate for infants and young children; also use in unconscious or uncooperative children, children with a seizure disorder, or children with a problem affecting the oral cavity. Lay the child prone, or supine holding the legs flexed; insert lubricated rectal bulb no more than 0.5–1 inch; keep in place for 4–5 min, or until temperature registers on digital thermometer; record temperature and route. Oral temperature is acceptable for children older than 5 yr. Insert thermometer under the child's tongue and keep in place for approximately 7 min or until registered on digital thermometer. For axillary temperatures, sit the child on lap and insert thermometer bulb into axillary area; keep arm close to side for approximately 5–6 min or until temperature is registered on digital thermometer. For tympanic temperature, insert the probe gently into the child's outer ear canal; if the child is younger than 3 yr, pull the ear down and back; results are usually available within a minute. Recent research questions the accuracy of tympanic thermometer readings in infants and children younger than 3 yr; it is not as useful for ill children.	Advise parent to call physician immediately for any of the following: Fever associated with difficulty breathing or drooling Fever associated with a stiff neck, lethargy, bulging fontanelle, or irritability Temperature greater than 40.5 degrees Celsius (105 degrees Fahrenheit) Seizure associated with fever Fever accompanied by excessive drooling and difficulty swallowing Fever associated with difficulty breathing. Notify physician if the child has a temperature greater than 38.4 degrees Celsius (101 degrees Fahrenheit) for longer than 72 hr, or if the child has a fever for longer than 24 hr with no other signs of illness. Temperature equal to or greater than 37.8 degrees Celsius (100 degrees Fahrenheit) in child younger than 6 wk old requires immediate evaluation.
Pulse	Apical pulse measured for 1 minute for infants and children younger than age 2 yr; radial pulse for older children.	Average resting pulse rate*: Newborn 133 Infant 140 1–5 yr 113 6–10 yr 95 older than 10 yr 88
Respirations	Watch for irregularities in rate, rhythm, or depth; count for 1 min in infants or if irregular	Average respiratory rate*: Newborn 35 Infant 31 1–5 yr 25 6–10 yr 20 Older than 10 yr
Blood Pressure	Measure with cuff of appropriate size. Blood pressure can be taken in either upper or lower extremities in infants and young children.	Mean blood pressure value*: Newborn 65/41 (Dinamap monitor) Infant 95/58 (Dinamap monitor) 2–5 yr 101/57 (Dinamap monitor) 6–10 yr 105/56 10–13 yr 110/61
Skin	Inspection Palpation	Color: jaundice below the waist in a newborn may need referral for elevated bilirubin count; cyanosis (noticeably best in palms, soles, sclera, lips, nail beds); pallor; flushing; café-au-lait spots (suspect neurofibromatosis). Lesions: Note nevi, vascular lesions (strawberry marks, storkbite mark, port-wine stain). Other lesions (observe and record all as for adult). Accessory structures: hair tuft at base of spine is questionable for spina bifida occulta. Turgor: decreased turgor is assessed by gently pinching the skin on the abdomen and observing for briskness of return; tenting indicates fluid deficit.
Head and neck	Inspection Palpation	Note scaly skin (cradle cap) over anterior fontanel; bald spot in back of head (might indicate infant is left on back most of the time). Palpate fontanels of infants: posterior fontanel closes by 3 months, anterior between 9 and 18 months; observe for any depression or bulging of fontanel.

Table continued on following page

Table 15–2. Physical Examination: Adaptations for Infants and Children (Continued)

Assessment Area	Technique	What to Observe
		Palpate lymph nodes; can be enlarged from severe seborrhea of the head, tick bites, pediculosis; inflamed or painful nodes indicate ongoing infection.
Eyes	Inspection	Note eye placement (too close together or too far apart), presence of epicanthal folds (frequently seen in children of Asian descent), palpebral slant (upward slant seen in children of Asian descent; along with epicanthal folds in White children could indicate Down syndrome).
		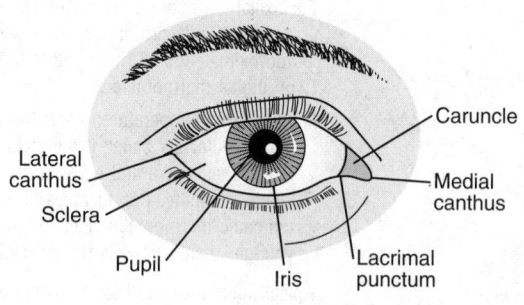
		Note altered eye structures. Deviations (esotropia, exotropia, esophoria, exophoria, nystagmus); signs of disease (conjunctivitis, sty, corneal ulceration); discharge from one eye in the infant suggests blocked lacrimal duct; sudden, persistent, tearing in one eye or appearance of a "film" over the cornea suggests congenital glaucoma.
		Ophthalmoscopic examination, cover test, corneal light reflex.
Ears	Infants can be examined lying on the examination table with head turned and held in position by parent.	Note symmetry and level of ears (low-placed ears can indicate renal disease or other abnormalities); note excessive cerumen.
	Young children are best examined with the child sitting on the parent's lap, head held close to the chest, and turned to the side being examined.	Note color, light reflex, and movement of tympanic membrane; bright red, bulging membrane indicates acute otitis media; gray, retracted membrane suggests fluid in middle ear.
	In examining children younger than 3 yr, pull pinna down and back to straighten canal. In children older than 3 yr, pull pinna up and back.	Perform tympanography if fluid is suspected.
		Observe for presence of any foreign body; children frequently put small objects or toys in their ears.
	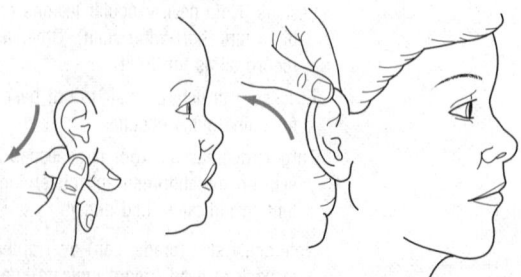	
Nose	Using an otoscope light or small penlight, shine the light at	Nasal mucosa (allergy can cause boggy mucosa); young in-

Table 15–2. *Physical Examination: Adaptations for Infants and Children* (Continued)

Assessment Area	Technique	What to Observe
	the entrance to each nares; ask the child to remain still, or support the child by gently holding the chin.	fants are nose breathers, any blockage of the nasal passageways can interfere with respirations; abnormal, foul-smelling nasal discharge suggests foreign body.
Mouth and pharynx	Avoid using a tongue depressor if possible; examine throat while infant or young child is crying; older children usually can open their mouths wide enough for adequate inspection.	Examine and note the number and condition of teeth. By 13–14 years, the secondary 2nd molars (upper and lower) will have erupted. From 16–20 years, the 3rd molars erupt to complete the set of 32 secondary, or permanent, teeth. Some adults never obtain 3rd molars. ■ Newly erupted (secondary) teeth ▨ Primary teeth ☐ Previously erupted (secondary) teeth Note the size and condition of tonsils and any abnormality of oral mucosa (lesions, ulcerations, white patches that may indicate thrush).
Chest—thorax	Inspection Percussion Palpation	Note the presence of supernumerary nipples in infants; nipple discharge in neonates of both sexes is seen frequently. Asymmetry suggests underlying structural or functional deformity; a one-sided "lump" under the nipple of a 10–14-yr-old prepubertal girl is usually due to breast budding. Perform breast examination on postpubertal adolescents.
Chest—lungs	When auscultating young children, be creative in encouraging them to take deep breaths (e.g., "Pretend you're blowing a very big bubble.").	Abdominal respiratory movements are normal in children younger than 6 yr.
Heart	Use both bell and diaphragm of the stethoscope when auscultating the heart.	Murmurs are graded I–VI, with grade I being faint and obscure when the child is active, and grade VI often being loud enough to be heard without a stethoscope and accompanied by a thrill. Innocent (functional) murmurs differ from organic (pathologic) murmurs in that they occur during systole, are less than grade III in intensity, are low-pitched or musical sounding, are of short duration with no radiation, often disappear as the child grows, and there are no other signs of underlying pathologic condition.
Abdomen	When palpating children's abdomens, encourage them to breathe deeply to avoid eliciting a "tickle" response.	Children younger than 4 yr have prominent, "potbelly" shaped abdomens, which flatten as they get older. Note the condition of the umbilical area in newborns: The cord falls off at approximately 2 weeks of age. The area should be clean and dry, with no drainage.

Table continued on the following page

Table 15–2. Physical Examination: Adaptations for Infants and Children (Continued)

Assessment Area	Technique	What to Observe
		Umbilical hernias are common in infants and usually resolve by age 1 yr.
		Note absent or diminished bowel sounds. Visible peristalsis, particularly in the epigastric area and associated with an "olive" enlargement, could suggest pyloric stenosis.
		Enlargement of the liver or spleen requires referral. A palpable kidney in an older infant requires referral for evaluation of hydronephrosis or other underlying renal abnormality.
Upper extremities	Inspection	Note any discrepancy in muscle strength and tone between right and left sides, joint limitation, and enlargement of joints.
		Document the presence of simian crease on the palm (normally present in low percentage of children, but seen frequently in children with Down syndrome).
Lower extremities	Inspection	Note any discrepancy in muscle strength and tone between right and left sides, joint limitation, and enlargement of joints.
		Observe for leg length discrepancy, toeing in or out, genu varum (bowleg), genu valgum (knock knees).
		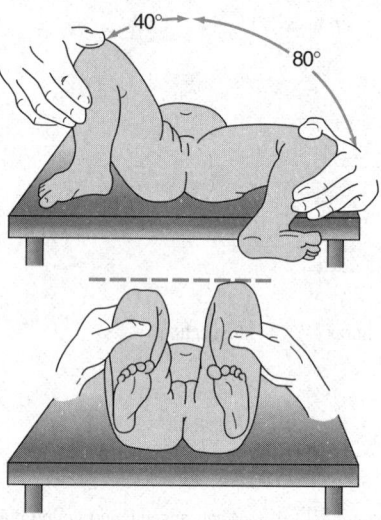
		Presence of the following on hip range-of-motion suggests congenital hip dysplasia: hip click, hip instability, uneven length hip to knee with hips and knees flexed, uneven skin folds on thighs.
		Foot deformities—metatarsus adductus, club foot

Spine	Inspection
	    Standing
	    Bending (have child bend from the waist and touch toes)
		Observe for symmetry of shoulders, scapulas, and hips, especially in adolescents; asymmetry can indicate functional or structural scoliosis.

		Note any abnormal posture or curves from rear and side view (scoliosis, kyphosis).
		From the rear, note any unevenness in the thoracic area, or rotation of ribs or vertebrae that would suggest a scoliosis.
General neurologic		Reflexes and motor function vary according to age group and achievement of developmental milestones (e.g., walking, hopping, jumping, walking backward).
		Particularly observe for altered gait and balance in the walking child, strong hand preference in infants and toddlers, clum-

Table 15–2. Physical Examination: Adaptations for Infants and Children (Continued)

Assessment Area	Technique	What to Observe
		siness, distractibility, hyperactivity, perceptual problems, problems in school.
Male genitalia	Inspection: maintain the child's privacy as much as possible. Palpation: wear gloves if contact with body substances is likely.	Note any abnormal urethral opening, penile curvature, scrotal enlargement, inguinal hernia in infants. Do not force retraction of the foreskin.
		Palpate for undescended testicle. Refer if testicle is not descended by age 1 yr.
		Observe for abnormal drainage, irritation, or inflammation. Yellow "burn-like" area on healing circumcision is normal for several days after the procedure.
		Perform testicular examination in adolescent boys.
Female genitalia		Observe for labial fusion, ambiguous genitalia, feces or urine in vagina, suggesting a fistula.
		Note any abnormal drainage, irritation or inflammation, lesions that might suggest sexual abuse.
		Perform pelvic examination on sexually active adolescents.

* All values from Greene M. *Johns Hopkins' Hospital: The Harriet Lane Handbook.* St. Louis: Mosby–Year Book, 1991.
First figure from Jarvis C. *Physical Examination and Health Assessment.* 2nd ed. Philadelphia: WB Saunders, 1996, p 184; next 3 figures redrawn from Betz CL, Hunsberger M, and Wright S. *Family-Centered Nursing Care of Children.* 2nd ed. Philadelphia: WB Saunders, 1994, pp 478, 483, 347; last figure redrawn from Tachdjian M. *Pediatric Orthopedics.* Philadelphia: WB Saunders, 1972, p 1837.

adaptations for the head-to-toe physical examination of children.
5. Development assessment
  a. Parents are often unnecessarily concerned about their child's development because they compare their child with others the same age or because others tell them the child should be doing certain things at certain ages. Reassurance that some children develop more slowly or quickly than others often allays their concerns.
  b. The Denver Development Screening Test (Denver-II) (Fig. 15–1), a revision of the original DDST, is used along with other screening tests and clinical judgment to assess growth and development and risk for developmental delays.
  c. The Denver II accounts for socioeconomic and environmental differences, but these differences can still affect the child's ability to achieve some of the developmental criteria on some of the standardized measures such as the Denver II. Cautious interpretation of the child's achievement prevents unnecessarily labeling a child from a different culture or socioeconomic background as developmentally delayed, an area of particular concern to Native Americans, Asian Americans, Haitians, and other ethnic groups.
  d. Test administration
    (1) Find a quiet place suitable for testing and comfortable for the child and parent.
    (2) Explain to the parent that this is not an intelligence test, but a method of assessing how the child is developing. Encourage the older child to participate by presenting the tasks as a game and

beginning with a few tasks that the child can easily master.
    (3) After recording pertinent data about the child, calculate the child's chronologic age (adjust for more than 2 weeks' prematurity in children younger than 2 years old and test the child at the adjusted age). Draw a line from top to bottom of the form at the appropriate age.
    (4) Test 3 items in each sector immediately to the left of the age line, all items intersecting the age line, and items to the right of the age line, until the child has 3 failures. Score each item pass, fail, refuse, or no opportunity. Those items marked with an "R" in the left corner are by parent report but should be validated by observation if possible. The child has 3 chances to pass each item.
    (5) For more manageable screening in a limited time frame, identify areas of concern by administering only the 3 items in each sector to the left of the age line. Follow up by administering the complete test if the child fails any of these items.
    (6) At the completion of the test, ask the parent whether the child's behavior is typical and retest at another time if it is not (usually within 2 weeks).
  e. Test interpretation
    (1) Refusal or failure to pass items passed by 75 to 90 percent of the children in the child's age group is cause for concern.
    (2) Refusal or failure to pass items totally to the

left of the age line suggests delays in development.

(3) A child who tests within the norms at an early age may fall behind as achievement of new skills is expected. Testing the child over time, along with index of suspicion from clinical observation and parent report, is a more comprehensive method of developmental assessment than a single screening. Because accurate testing results depend on meticulous administration, use of the Denver II training manual is imperative. The manual and test materials can be obtained through DDM, Inc., P.O. Box 6919, Denver, CO 80206–0919, telephone (800) 419–4729.

f. The Revised Prescreening Developmental Questionnaire (R-PDQ) (Fig. 15–2) is used to screen children quickly for developmental delays. When given with the 12 test items on the Denver II immediately to the left of the child's age line, the test can quickly and accurately identify children of concern.

(1) The test is accompanied by age-appropriate developmental activity suggestions for parents and children to do together.

(2) Four questionnaire forms, divided into ages, contain questions that correspond to the test items on the Denver II. After determining the child's age, give the parent the appropriate form and ask the parent to answer the questions until 3 "no" responses are given.

(3) Review the responses with the parent. "No" answers to those items that 90 percent of the children in the child's age group have passed indicates a delay in that area. For 1 delay, give the activity sheet to the parent and rescreen the child in a month. Screen with the full Denver II if the child has more than 1 delay.

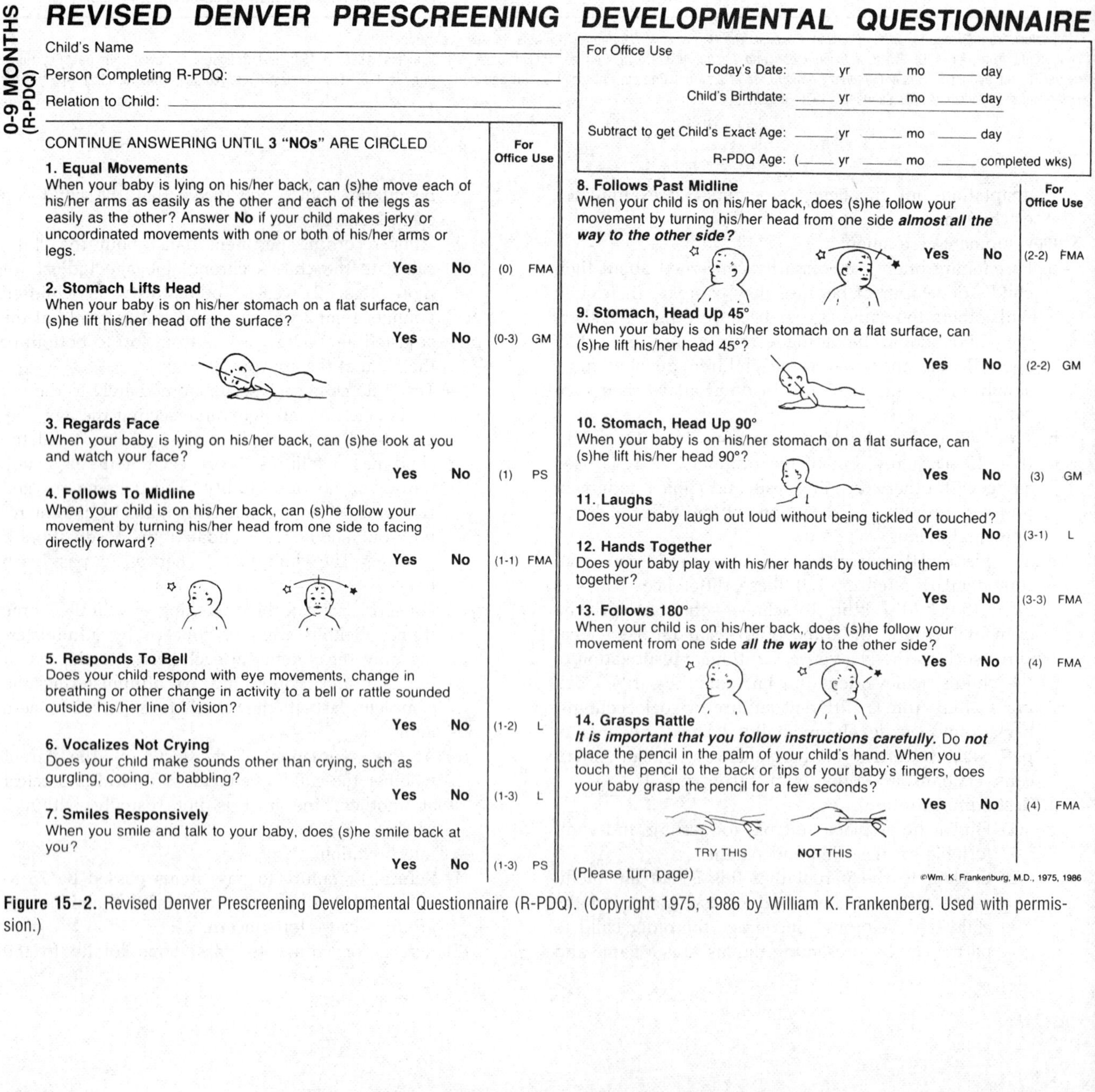

REVISED DENVER PRESCREENING DEVELOPMENTAL QUESTIONNAIRE

0-9 MONTHS (R-PDQ)

Child's Name _____

Person Completing R-PDQ: _____

Relation to Child: _____

For Office Use

Today's Date: _____ yr _____ mo _____ day

Child's Birthdate: _____ yr _____ mo _____ day

Subtract to get Child's Exact Age: _____ yr _____ mo _____ day

R-PDQ Age: (_____ yr _____ mo _____ completed wks)

CONTINUE ANSWERING UNTIL 3 "NOs" ARE CIRCLED   For Office Use

1. Equal Movements
When your baby is lying on his/her back, can (s)he move each of his/her arms as easily as the other and each of the legs as easily as the other? Answer **No** if your child makes jerky or uncoordinated movements with one or both of his/her arms or legs.
Yes   No   (0)   FMA

2. Stomach Lifts Head
When your baby is on his/her stomach on a flat surface, can (s)he lift his/her head off the surface?
Yes   No   (0-3)   GM

3. Regards Face
When your baby is lying on his/her back, can (s)he look at you and watch your face?
Yes   No   (1)   PS

4. Follows To Midline
When your child is on his/her back, can (s)he follow your movement by turning his/her head from one side to facing directly forward?
Yes   No   (1-1)   FMA

5. Responds To Bell
Does your child respond with eye movements, change in breathing or other change in activity to a bell or rattle sounded outside his/her line of vision?
Yes   No   (1-2)   L

6. Vocalizes Not Crying
Does your child make sounds other than crying, such as gurgling, cooing, or babbling?
Yes   No   (1-3)   L

7. Smiles Responsively
When you smile and talk to your baby, does (s)he smile back at you?
Yes   No   (1-3)   PS

8. Follows Past Midline
When your child is on his/her back, does (s)he follow your movement by turning his/her head from one side *almost all the way to the other side?*
Yes   No   (2-2)   FMA

9. Stomach, Head Up 45°
When your baby is on his/her stomach on a flat surface, can (s)he lift his/her head 45°?
Yes   No   (2-2)   GM

10. Stomach, Head Up 90°
When your baby is on his/her stomach on a flat surface, can (s)he lift his/her head 90°?
Yes   No   (3)   GM

11. Laughs
Does your baby laugh out loud without being tickled or touched?
Yes   No   (3-1)   L

12. Hands Together
Does your baby play with his/her hands by touching them together?
Yes   No   (3-3)   FMA

13. Follows 180°
When your child is on his/her back, does (s)he follow your movement from one side *all the way* to the other side?
Yes   No   (4)   FMA

14. Grasps Rattle
It is important that you follow instructions carefully. Do **not** place the pencil in the palm of your child's hand. When you touch the pencil to the back or tips of your baby's fingers, does your baby grasp the pencil for a few seconds?
Yes   No   (4)   FMA

TRY THIS   NOT THIS

(Please turn page)

©Wm. K. Frankenburg, M.D., 1975, 1986

Figure 15–2. Revised Denver Prescreening Developmental Questionnaire (R-PDQ). (Copyright 1975, 1986 by William K. Frankenberg. Used with permission.)

0-9 MONTHS (R-PDQ)

CONTINUE ANSWERING UNTIL **3 "NOs"** ARE CIRCLED

Side #2

For Office Use

15. Sits, Head Steady
When sitting, can your child hold his/her head upright and steady? Answer **No** if his/her head falls to either side or upon his/her chest.

Yes No   (4) GM

16. Stomach Chest Up-Arm Support
When your baby is on his/her stomach on a flat surface, can (s)he lift his/her chest using his/her arms for support?

Yes No   (4-1) GM

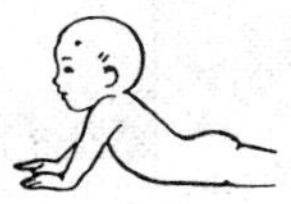

17. Squeals
Does your baby make happy high-pitched squealing sounds which are not crying?

Yes No   (4-2) L

18. Rolls Over
Has your baby rolled over at least 2 times, from stomach to back, or back to stomach?

Yes No   (4-3) GM

19. Regards Raisin
Can your child focus his/her eyes on small objects the size of a pea, a raisin, or a penny?

Yes No   (5) FMA

20. Reaches For Object
Can your child pick up a toy if it is placed within his/her reach?

Yes No   (5) FMA

21. Smiles Spontaneously
Does your child smile at crib toys, pictures, or pets when (s)he is playing by himself/herself?

Yes No   (5) PS

22. Pull To Sit, No Headlag
With your baby on his/her back, gently pull him/her up to a sitting position by his/her wrists. Does your baby hold his/her neck stiffly like the baby in the picture below left? Answer **No** if his/her head falls back like the baby in the picture below right.

Yes No   (6-1) GM

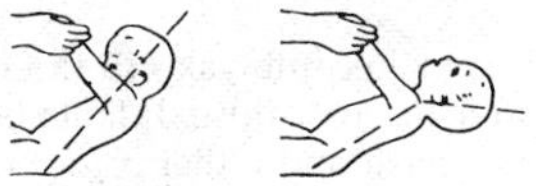

Yes   No

Catalog #1000A

23. Sits, Looks For Yarn
Please follow directions carefully. Get your baby's attention with a scarf, handkerchief, or a tissue and then drop it *out of sight.* Did your baby try to find it? For example, did (s)he look for it under the table or continue to watch where it disappeared?

Yes No   (7-2) FMA

24. Passes Cube Hand To Hand
Can your baby pass something, such as a small block or a small cookie, from one hand to the other? Long objects like a spoon or rattle do not count.

Yes No   (7-2) FMA

25. Sits, Takes 2 Cubes
Can your baby pick up 2 things, such as toys or cookies, and hold one in each hand at the same time?

Yes No   (7-2) FMA

26. Bears Some Weight On Legs
When you hold your baby under his/her arms, can (s)he bear some weight on his/her legs? Answer **Yes** only if (s)he tries to stand on his/her feet and supports some of his/her own weight.

Yes No   (7-3) GM

27. Rakes Raisin, Attains
Can your baby pick up small objects, such as raisins or pieces of food with his/her hand using a raking or grabbing motion?

Yes No   (7-3) FMA

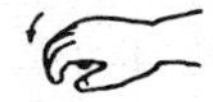

28. Sits Without Support
Without being propped by pillows, a chair, or wall, can your child sit by himself/herself for 60 seconds?

Yes No   (7-3) GM

29. Feed Self Crackers
Can your baby feed himself/herself a cracker or cookie? Answer **No** if (s)he has never been given one.

Yes No   (8) PS

30. Turns To Voice
When your child is playing and you come up *quietly* behind him/her, does (s)he sometimes turn his/her head as though (s)he heard you? *Loud sounds do not count.*

Yes No   (8-1) L

©Wm. K. Frankenburg, M.D., 1975, 1986

Figure 15–2. *Continued*

■ HEALTH PROMOTION FOR INFANTS, CHILDREN, AND ADOLESCENTS

Immunizations

1. Immunizations are scheduled according to the schedule recommended by the Centers for Disease Control and Prevention (Fig. 15–3).
2. Table 15–3 describes the childhood vaccines.

Health Promotion for the 0- to 1-Month-Old Infant

1. Preventive care and health maintenance (Table 15–4)
   a. Scheduling the follow-up—because infants are frequently discharged from the hospital less than 48 hours after birth, early follow-up is necessary to rule

NURSE ADVISORY

Since passage of the National Childhood Vaccine Injury Act and the Vaccine Compensation Amendments, parents must be given written information about vaccines before each immunization. Information must include the benefits of the vaccine, its usual schedule, potential adverse effects, and usual contraindications for using the vaccine. Having read the information and been given the opportunity to ask questions, the parent or guardian must sign permission for each immunization in the child's permanent record. Health providers are required to report any significant adverse effects.

out any problems. Schedule the infant's first visit at 1 to 2 weeks, particularly under the following circumstances:

(1) First babies, particularly if breast-fed
(2) Problem babies—those with jaundice or other neonatal problems, congenital anomalies, and

Text continued on page 494

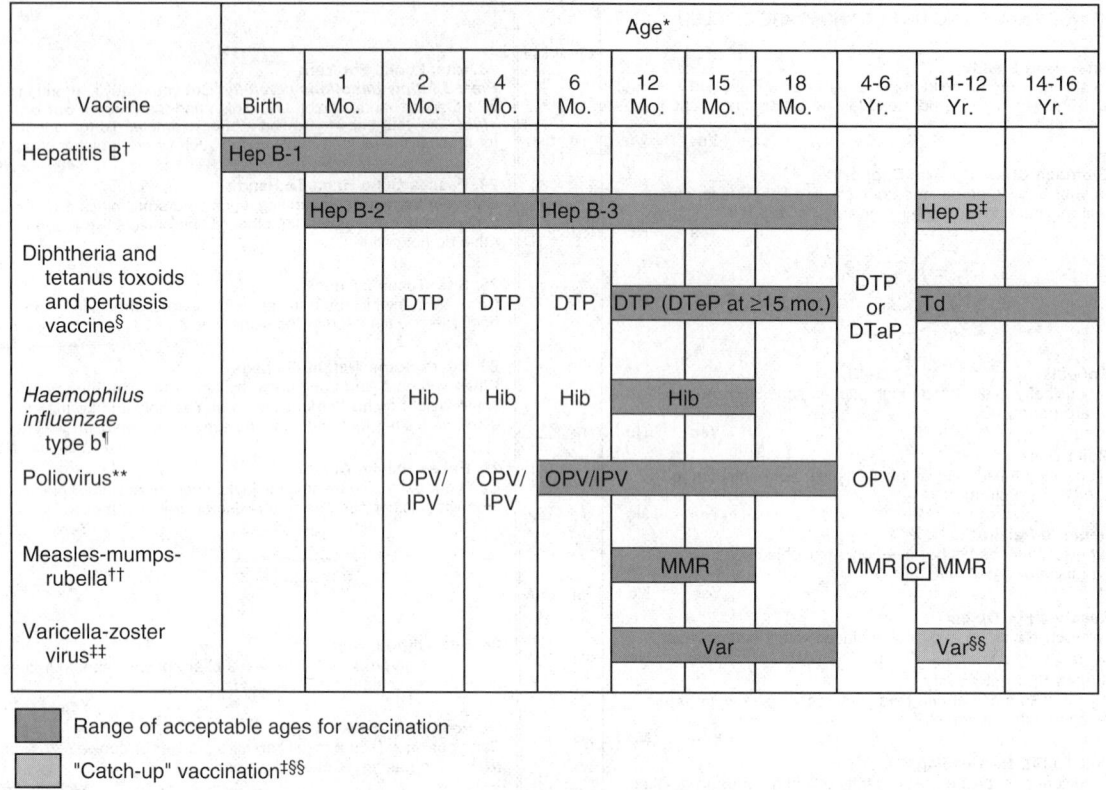

Vaccine	Age*										
	Birth	1 Mo.	2 Mo.	4 Mo.	6 Mo.	12 Mo.	15 Mo.	18 Mo.	4-6 Yr.	11-12 Yr.	14-16 Yr.
Hepatitis B†	Hep B-1										
		Hep B-2			Hep B-3					Hep B‡	
Diphtheria and tetanus toxoids and pertussis vaccine§			DTP	DTP	DTP	DTP (DTeP at ≥15 mo.)			DTP or DTaP	Td	
Haemophilus influenzae type b¶			Hib	Hib	Hib	Hib					
Poliovirus**			OPV/ IPV	OPV/ IPV	OPV/IPV				OPV		
Measles-mumps-rubella††						MMR			MMR or	MMR	
Varicella-zoster virus‡‡						Var				Var§§	

Range of acceptable ages for vaccination

"Catch-up" vaccination‡§§

Figure 15–3. Recommended childhood vaccination schedules—United States—January to June 1996.

* Vaccines are listed under the routinely recommended ages.

† Infants born to hepatitis B surface antigen (HBsAg)-negative mothers should receive 2.5μg of Recombivax HB (Merck & Co.) or 10 μg of Engerix-B (SmithKline Beecham). The 2nd dose should be administered ≥ 1 month after the first dose. Infants born to HBsAg-positive mothers should receive 0.5 ml hepatitis B immune globulin (HBIG) within 12 hours of birth and either 5 μg of Recombivax HB or 10 μg of Engerix-B at a separate site. The 2nd dose is recommended at age 1–2 months and the 3rd dose at age 6 months. Infants born to mothers whose HBsAg status is unknown should receive either 5 μg of Recombivax HB or 10 μg of Engerix-B within 12 hours of birth. The 2nd dose of vaccine is recommended at age 1 month and the 3rd dose at age 6 months.

‡ Adolescents who have not received 3 doses of hepatitis B vaccine should initiate or complete the series at age 11–12 years. The 2nd dose should be administered at least 1 month after the 1st dose, and the 3rd dose should be administered at least 4 months after the 1st dose and at least 2 months after the 2nd dose.

§ The 4th dose of diphtheria and tetanus toxoids and pertussis vaccine (DTP) may be administered at age 12 months, if at least 6 months have elapsed since the 3rd dose of DTP. Diphtheria and tetanus toxoids and acellular pertussis vaccine (DTaP) is licensed for the 4th and/or 5th vaccine dose(s) for children aged ≥ 15 months and may be preferred for these doses in this age group. Tetanus and diphtheria toxoids, absorbed, for adult use (Td) is recommended at age 11–12 years if at least 5 years have elapsed since the last dose of DTP, DTaP, or diphtheria and tetanus toxoids, absorbed, for pediatric use (DT).

¶ Three *Haemophilus influenzae* type b (Hib) conjugate vaccines are licensed for infant use. If PedvaxHIB (Merck & Co.) *Haemophilus* b conjugate vaccine (Meningococcal Protein Conjugate) (PRP-OMP) is administered at ages 2 and 4 months, a dose at 6 months is not required. After completing the primary series, any Hib conjugate vaccine may be used as a booster.

** Oral poliovirus vaccine (OPV) is recommended for routine infant vaccination. Inactivated poliovirus vaccine (IPV) is recommended for persons—or household contacts of persons—with a congenital or acquired immune deficiency disease or an altered immune status resulting from disease or immunosuppressive therapy, and is an acceptable alternative for other persons. The primary 3-dose series for IPV should be given with a minimum interval of 4 weeks between the 1st and 2nd doses and 6 months between the 2nd and 3rd doses.

†† The 2nd doses of measles-mumps-rubella vaccine (MMR) is routinely recommended at age 4–6 years or at age 11–12 years but may be administered at any visit provided at least 1 month has elapsed since receipt of the 1st dose.

‡‡ Varicella zoster virus vaccine (Var) can be administered to susceptible children any time after age 12 months.

§§ Unvaccinated children who lack a reliable history of chickenpox should be vaccinated at age 11–12 years.

Use of trade names and commercial sources is for identification only and does not imply endorsement by the Public Health Service or the U.S. Department of Health and Human Services.

Source: Advisory Committee on Immunization Practices, American Academy of Pediatrics, and American Academy of Family Physicians.

(From Centers for Disease Control and Prevention. *MMWR* 44 [51–52]:992–993, 1996.)

Table 15–3. Childhood Immunizations

DTP: Diphtheria, Tetanus, Pertussis (Intramuscular)

Rationale	Given to protect the child from diphtheria, tetanus, and pertussis (whooping cough); incidence of whooping cough in children is increasing due to underimmunized population.
Side effects	Fever, redness and pain at site, fussiness or drowsiness, lump at site, rarely convulsions (usually febrile).
Contraindications and nursing implications	Take accurate history of neurologic and allergic illness and previous reactions to vaccines; provide information about vaccine effects and answer questions.
	Postpone all vaccines if child has a febrile illness more severe than the common cold, previous allergic reaction or shock, previous convulsion associated with the vaccine, history of progressive or uncontrolled convulsions, high temperature (more than 104 degrees Fahrenheit) after previous DTP vaccination, or episode of persistent inconsolable crying or screaming lasting for more than 3 hr within 48 hr of immunization; use with caution in child with history of febrile seizures; advise prophylactic administration of acetaminophen.

OPV: Oral Polio Vaccine; IPV: Inactivated Polio Vaccine

Rationale	Protects against active polio disease.
Side effects	None known; rarely, paralysis has occurred (1:1.5 million doses) and government recommendations for OPV vs IPV for initial series are being re-evaluated; soreness or redness at injection site of IPV.
Contraindications and nursing implications	Take history of immune depression in child or household contacts. Give IPV to children who are artificially or naturally immune depressed, or who are living with someone who is immune depressed. No OPV is given for hospitalized children. No IPV is given if the child has an allergy to streptomycin or neomycin.

HIB: *Haemophilus influenzae* Type b (Intramuscular)

Rationale	Protects against *Haemophilus influenzae* infection, the leading cause of epiglottitis and meningitis in young children.
Side effects	Mild, if any; low-grade fever, mild tenderness at the site.
Contraindications and nursing implications	None known; vaccine does come mixed with DTP.

Hepatitis B Virus Vaccine (Intramuscular Dose Dependent on Hepatitis Status of Mother)

Rationale	Protects against perinatally acquired hepatitis B, as well as against sexually transmitted hepatitis B during teen years. Children infected with hepatitis B can become hepatitis B virus carriers and experience liver disease during adulthood. Because of increased incidence of hepatitis B in the United States, the American Academy of Pediatrics recommends universal hepatitis B immunization in infancy.
Side effects	Usually minimal, slight soreness at site.
Contraindications and nursing implications	None known (anaphylactic reaction to yeast in older children); use needle of appropriate length to achieve seroconversion.

MMR: Measles, Mumps, Rubella (Subcutaneous Injection)

Rationale	Prevents acquired measles, mumps, or rubella; decreases incidence of fetal malformations from rubella acquired during pregnancy.
Side effects	Low-grade fever, rash, joint aches or inflammation approximately 7–10 days after immunization; rarely shock, allergic reaction, encephalitis.
Contraindications and nursing implications	Previous anaphylactic reaction to eggs or neomycin, conditions causing immune depression (cancer treatment, steroids); children with human immunodeficiency virus should receive MMR; verify that older children are not pregnant or about to become pregnant.

Varicella Vaccine

Not yet given routinely, but is expected to be (probably at age 12 months). Vaccine is unstable; needs to be stored frozen. One dose for children 12 months to 12 yr, 2 doses for children older than 12 yr.

Table 15–4. Health Promotion During Childhood

	Physical Parameters	Developmental Milestones	Preventive Care and Health Maintenance
Newborn to 1 month	Newborn: Average length 19–21 inches, weight 7 1/2 lb, head circumference 13–14 inches; loses 10% body weight in first 3–4 days, regain within 10–14 days (according to race and culture) Two wk to 1 month: Average weight gain nearly 1 ounce/day for the first several months; average length gain 1 inch/month; average head circumference 14 1/4 inches at 1 month	**Personal/Social** Early bonding sets tone for later parent–child relationship—frequent face-to-face contact, gradual touching progressing from fingertip to full arm embrace, reciprocal interaction between parent and infant Newborn—looks at parent's face, begins to fixate and track, has color vision, visual acuity 20/800 Two wk to 1 month—looks at parent's face, begins to smile responsively **Fine Motor** Newborn—reflexes helping to determine normal neurologic function: rooting and sucking, grasping on finger placed in palm, startle to loud noise, moro (extension of arms, head, hands, and fingers, followed by flexion) in response to sudden movement, tonic neck (head turned to 1 side, extension of extremities on that side, flexion of extremities on opposite side) Two wk to 1 month—follows to midline, prefers faces, brightly colored objects, objects with patterns, hands fisted **Language/Cognitive** Newborn—prefers human female voice, hears well, begins to respond to sound of a bell Two wk to 1 month—responds to bell, begins to vocalize soft sounds **Gross Motor** Newborn—has symmetric movements of extremities while lying supine, lifts head while lying prone Two wk to 1 month—lifts head and chin off flat surface	**Immunizations** Hepatitis B vaccine to infants shortly after birth and repeat at age 1 month; infants of hepatitis B positive women also receive one dose of hepatitis B immune globulin as newborns **Health Screening** Screen for phenylketonuria and other metabolic diseases before hospital discharge (capillary sample through heel puncture); may have to repeat if child is discharged before 24 hr old Physical examination (PE) screens for congenital defects and conditions (Table 15–5)
2 months	Average weight 11 lb, average length 22 3/4 inches, average head circumference 15 1/4 inches	**Personal/Social** Watches another's face, smiles in response to facial and voice contact with others; begins to smile spontaneously with no stimulation from another needed **Fine Motor** Follows object to midline; begins to follow past midline toward other side; tonic neck, rooting, stepping reflexes disappear **Language/Cognitive** Vocalizes with soft cooing sounds or short vowel sounds; begins "ooo" and "ah" sounds; beginning voluntary repetitive actions **Gross Motor** Lifts head so face is at 45-degree angle from flat surface	**Immunizations** Diphtheria, tetanus, pertussis (DTP) 1—whole cell pertussis vaccine used in infants; children older than 18 months can receive intramuscular acellular pertussis (DTaP), which has fewer side effects Oral poliovaccine (OPV) or inactivated poliovaccine (IPV) 1 HIB 1—given to prevent *Haemophilus influenzae* infections, the major cause of epiglottitis or meningitis in infants **Health Screening** PE, no additional screening required

Table 15–4. *Health Promotion During Childhood* (Continued)

	Physical Parameters	Developmental Milestones	Preventive Care and Health Maintenance
4 months	Average weight 14 lb, average length 25 inches, average head circumference 16 1/4 inches	**Personal/Social** Smiles spontaneously, stares at own hand, enjoys moving faces **Fine Motor** Grasps a rattle, follows object 180 degrees, binocular vision established, brings hands to middle of body while supine, can hold own bottle **Language/Cognitive** Laughs and squeals out loud, initiates conversation by cooing, turns head to locate sounds **Gross Motor** Lifts head and chest 90 degrees when prone, supports weight on feet when held standing, head steady when sitting with no head lag; might begin to roll prone to supine	**Immunizations** DTP 2, OPV (IPV) 2, HIB 2 **Health Screening** PE, no additional screening required
6 months	Average weight 16 3/4 lb (birth weight usually doubles by 6 months), average length 26 1/2 inches, average head circumference 17 inches	**Personal/Social** Reaches out for toy, interacts readily and noisily with parents and others, beginning caution with strangers **Fine Motor** Rakes objects with the whole hand (grasp reflex has disappeared), puts hands and objects in mouth, looks at raisin placed on contrasting surface **Language/Cognitive** Turns to rattle sound made out of vision on each side, turns to whisper sound on each side, begins to imitate sounds (raspberries, clucking, kissing) and babbles; beginning object permanence, intentional activity, awareness of time sequence **Gross Motor** Rolls over both directions, no head lag, lifts head and chest completely, "swims" or "airplanes" when prone, might get onto hands and knees, might begin to sit unsupported in tripod fashion, bears full weight on legs	**Immunizations** DTP 3, OPV or IPV 3, HIB 3 **Health Screening** PE with lead screening risk assessment
9 months	Average weight 19 1/2 lb, average length 28 inches, average head circumference 17 3/4 inches	**Personal/Social** Stranger wariness, feeds self finger foods **Fine Motor** Transfers objects from one hand to the other, picks up raisin or Cheerio with whole hand or beginning pincer grasp, picks up and holds small block in each hand; actively searches for objects that have fallen out of line of vision (object permanence); beginning depth perception	**Immunizations** Hepatitis B 3 **Health Screening** PE with lead screening risk assessment if not done at 6 months Purified protein derivative if at risk for tuberculosis (recent recommendations advise baseline screening only if at risk)

Table continued on following page

Table 15–4. Health Promotion During Childhood (Continued)

	Physical Parameters	Developmental Milestones	Preventive Care and Health Maintenance
		Language/Cognitive Says single syllables with consonant sounds ("ba," "da," "ma"), beginning to put syllables together ("dada," "baba," "mama"), uses several vowel sounds; beginning to attach meaning to words, understands some symbolic language such as gestures (bye-bye, blowing a kiss) **Gross Motor** Sits without support, begins to get to a sitting position from prone, begins to creep and crawl, pulls self up to stand and stands holding on to furniture; might begin to walk holding on to furniture	
12 months	Average weight 21 3/4 lb, usually triple birth weight, average length 29 3/4 inches, or 50% over birth length, average head circumference 18 1/4 inches	**Personal/Social** Plays pat-a-cake (or claps hands with another), indicates wants without crying, rolls or throws a ball with another person, explores	**Immunizations** Hepatitis B 3, if not given at 9 months, measles mumps rubella (MMR) can be given at this time, varicella vaccine can be given
		Fine Motor Visual acuity 20/40 to 20/60, picks up small objects with developed pincer grasp, can bang two objects together, uses simple toys appropriately	**Health Screening** PE with hemoglobin or hematocrit and lead
		Language/Cognitive Names the appropriate parent, begins to say single words, understands simple requests **Gross Motor** Stands without support for longer periods, begins to climb stairs, walks holding on to a hand, might take first steps unsupported	
15 to 18 months	Steady growth in height and weight, head circumference levels off, anterior fontanel usually closed by 18 months	**Personal/Social** Developing autonomy, negativism, ritualism, increasing tolerance of separation from parents, begins to imitate, feeds self with increasing skill (still rotates spoon), holds a cup, undresses, temper tantrums, has transitional objects, begins to understand gender differences (may begin to masturbate)	**Immunizations** 15 months—MMR 1 (if not given at 12 months), HIB 4 18 months—DTP 4 **Health Screening** Routine PE
		Fine Motor Turns book pages, builds tower with increasing number of blocks, imitates vertical and circular strokes; vision 20/50 at 18 months	
		Language/Cognitive Broadening receptive language, begins to understand and say "no," says single words, may begin to put 2 words together, can point to several body parts and familiar objects; beginning memory, spatial and temporal relationships, increased object permanence; basic moral understanding (reward and punishment)	

Table 15–4. Health Promotion During Childhood (Continued)

	Physical Parameters	Developmental Milestones	Preventive Care and Health Maintenance
		Gross Motor Walks with increasing confidence, begins to run; climbs stairs first by creeping, then walking with hand held; jumps in place, begins to throw ball overhand without falling	
2 yr	Average weight 27 lb (gains approximately 5 lb/yr), average length 34 1/2 inches (approximately half adult height) gains height by approximately 4 inches/yr, head circumference 19 1/2 inches, fontanels closed	**Personal/Social** Imitates household activities and begins to do helpful tasks, uses table utensils without much spilling, drinks from a lidless cup, removes a difficult article of clothing, begins developing sexual identity	**Immunizations** None **Health Screening** PE with hemoglobin or hematocrit and lead screen, baseline cholesterol (if at risk)
		Fine Motor Puts blocks into a cup after demonstration, scribbles spontaneously, dumps a raisin out of a bottle on command after demonstration, builds tower of 4 blocks	
		Language/Cognition Approximately 300 word vocabulary, two-word sentences, points to 6 body parts and pictures of several familiar objects (bird, man, dog, horse, etc); understands cause and effect, object permanence, sense of time, egocentrism	
		Gross Motor Stoops and recovers well, walks frontwards and backwards, climbs stairs holding the railing, runs, jumps, kicks a ball	
3 yr	Weight increases at 4–5 lb/yr, height increases approximately 3 inches/yr	**Personal/Social** Puts on articles of clothing, brushes teeth with help, washes and dries hands using soap and water; notices sexual differences and identifies with children of own sex; knows own name and names one or more friends; increasing independence, may start preschool	**Immunizations** None **Health Screening** PE with hemoglobin or hematocrit
		Fine Motor Vision approaches 20/20; builds a tower of at least 8 blocks; begins purposeful drawing, can imitate a vertical stroke	
		Language/Cognition Increasing vocabulary with intelligible speech, although stuttering is common (thinks faster than can talk); names 4 familiar objects and begins to describe qualities or actions of objects; knows meaning of common adjectives (sleepy, hungry, hot); begins color identification; uses language as symbol; still egocentric; increased concept of time, space, causality	
		Gross Motor Jumps with both feet up and down and over a short distance; throws a ball overhand; balances on each foot for at least 2 sec; begins to ride a tricycle	

Table continued on following page

Table 15–4. Health Promotion During Childhood (Continued)

	Physical Parameters	Developmental Milestones	Preventive Care and Health Maintenance
4 and 5 yr	Weight increases at 4–5 lb/yr, height increases approximately 3 inches/yr	**Personal/Social** Develops a sense of initiative, learns new skills and games, begins problem-solving; develops a positive self-concept; develops a conscience, begins to learn right from wrong and good from bad (based on reward and punishment); learns to understand rules; identifies with parent of same sex, often closely imitating characteristics; independence in self-care; sociable and outgoing (might be aggressive) **Fine Motor** Proficient holding a crayon or pencil, draws purposefully; copies circle, cross, and square, diamond and triangle; draws a person with several body parts; drawings resemble familiar objects or people; may begin to write name or numbers; can tie shoelaces **Language/Cognitive** Begins to understand concepts of size and time (related to familiar events such as meals and bedtime); understands 2 opposites (hot, cold; big, little); can follow several directions consecutively; 4-word sentences using prepositions (e.g., on under, behind); defines 5 words, counts to 5, names 4 colors; begins to see other viewpoints; magical thinking **Gross Motor** Hops on 1 or alternate feet, walks heel to toe (front and back), balances on each foot for longer time; begins to ride bike with training wheels, throws and catches a ball, walks downstairs using alternate feet	**Immunizations** Four-yr-old: DTP 5, OPV (IPV) 4 Five-yr-old: MMR 2 **Health Screening** Four-yr-old: hemoglobin or hematocrit and lead screen, vision, audiometry Five-yr-old: might do baseline tuberculosis screening if not done earlier, vision, hearing
6 to 11 yr	Average weight gain 5 lb/yr with decrease in fat percentage and gain in muscle; average increase in height is 2 1/2 inches/yr until adolescent growth spurt begins; in general, girls are taller than boys of the same age during later years of late childhood	**Personal/Social** Child develops a positive self-esteem through skill acquisition and task completion, doing well in activities and school is important, recognition of accomplishments by others is crucial; peer group is primary socializing force, competition and cooperation with peers assists with developing sense of accomplishment **Fine Motor** Writing and drawing is complex and sophisticated using perspective and depth; performs most self-care tasks—tying shoes, using eating utensils properly, fastening clothes in back; interested in crafts that require fine motor skill—knitting, sewing, building models	**Immunizations** MMR 2 given at entrance to 7th grade, if not given earlier; hepatitis B series if not already immunized **Health Screening** Hemoglobin or hematocrit every 2 yr; vision and hearing screening usually done yearly at school; baseline cholesterol (if not done earlier); scoliosis screening (see Table 15–2); physical examinations every 2 yr unless needed yearly for sports or camp

Table 15–4. Health Promotion During Childhood (Continued)

Physical Parameters	Developmental Milestones	Preventive Care and Health Maintenance

Language/Cognitive

Vocabulary expands, understands different properties of language (e.g., play on words, mnemonics); views issues from other perspectives, accepts rules (but considers them to be imposed by others, rather than self-imposed), uses rules to define cooperative relationships with others; judgments based on what is seen, not yet based on reason; adapts to changing physical properties of objects—volume remains constant even though container shape changes (identity), number operations go in 2 directions (reversibility), developing increased comprehension of time, speed, spacial dimension (reciprocity); improved long-term memory, organizes concepts and relates to past experiences, uses various memory strategies to manage school work; groups, classifies, and relates objects according to several different characteristics (collecting, trading items such as stamps or sports cards is popular)

Gross Motor

Improved muscle mass and hand–eye coordination enable the child to participate in a variety of team and individual sports

Adolescence

Growth spurt weight gain is 50% of adult weight; increase in body fat in girls and muscle mass in boys accounts for large proportion of gain; growth spurt correlates with sexual maturation and occurs approximately 2 yr earlier in girls; average height gain is 20–25% adult height over 2- to 3-yr period; peak height velocity in girls is 6–12 months before menarche

Sexual characteristics: hypothalamic stimulation of the anterior pituitary and gonadotropin stimulation of the gonads to produce estrogen and testosterone initiates puberty

Girls—beginning of growth spurt followed by breast budding and development; pubic and axillary hair appears several months later; menstruation begins approximately 2 yr after first sign of puberty; very little increase in height thereafter

Boys—testicular enlargement, change in color and texture of scrotal skin, and appearance of pubic hair precede growth spurt by several months; penis enlarges and elongates, first ejaculation; gain in height until late adolescence

Personal/Social

Emotional and social turmoil associated with rapid changes in development and altered body image; more interested in establishing relationship with member of the opposite sex (some relationships lead to intimacy too soon); assumes various roles in attempt to integrate social skills with new aspirations; clarifies values and career directions; achieves more stable emotional control

Cognitive/Moral

Becomes future oriented and achieves ability to view the world in broad perspective; hypothesizes several alternatives to problems; thinks and reasons abstractly; develops moral reasoning

Motor

Early awkwardness associated with rapid skeletal growth matures into coordinated motor control

Immunizations

Tetanus/diphtheria (Td) at approximately 15 yr (repeat every 10 yr thereafter)

Health Screening

Hemoglobin or hematocrit every 2 yr; breast or testicular examination (teach self-examination); routine PE every 2 yr, yearly if in sports or camp; pelvic examination if girls are sexually active

whose weight is low or whose parents are concerned about weight gain

(3) Babies with exceptionally nervous or anxious parents whose questions cannot be answered by phone

HOME CARE STRATEGIES

Electronic Monitoring

Many medically fragile children and premature infants are being discharged from the hospital with the need for electronic monitoring devices. It is therefore necessary for all caregivers involved with these children to become skilled and comfortable with equipment such as cardiorespiratory monitors, pulse oximeters, and Dinamaps.

Caregivers should receive basic instruction in the hospital before the child is discharged. A home care nurse can reinforce the instruction and help the family set up the equipment for ease of use and safety. Further instruction in the home should include application of the sensors to the patient, care of the equipment, alarms, troubleshooting, and how to record patient data.

Key issues to keep in mind are the following:

- Many older homes cannot accommodate a 3-prong plug. Carry a 3-prong adapter with you.
- Notify the electric company that there is a patient at home on an electric monitor. They will prioritize service to that address should there be an electrical outage.
- Keep monitors close to the child to eliminate the risk of tripping over wires. The monitors should be on a stable, flat surface at or below the level of the child to prevent injuries from falling equipment.
- Ensure that there are no animals or young children who may chew or bite wires or cords.
- Do not use lotions or oils on the child's skin where the monitor may come into contact.
- Instruct in cardiopulmonary resuscitation and have the caregiver give a return demonstration to ensure the caregiver's ability and understanding.
- Tape the lead wires of the apnea monitor securely in the front of the diaper to prevent accidental pulling.
- Call the supply company immediately if the apnea monitor memory is full. False readings may occur with a full memory.

b. Screen for congenital anomalies (Table 15–5).

2. Anticipatory guidance and teaching parents

a. Nutrition: The decision to breast-feed or bottle feed an infant should be made during pregnancy. Each method has advantages. Breast-feeding enhances bonding, confers immunities, requires no special equipment, is more easily digested, and is more economical. With formula feeding, a father or other family member can more readily participate, allowing the mother to obtain more rest. The mother can return to work, if necessary.

(1) Breast-feeding: Breast-fed infants eat on demand, approximately every 2 to 3 hours for the first several months. Breast-feeding can occur more often if the infant is jaundiced. Methods of breast-feeding are as follows:

- While cradling the infant, hold the infant close and stimulate the rooting reflex to prompt the infant to face the breast. Cup the breast behind the areola, making a "C" with the thumb and forefinger and insert gently into the infant's mouth.

- Let the infant nurse for at least 10 minutes on the first side.
- Break suction by gently inserting a finger between the areola and infant's lips and allow the baby to nurse until satisfied on the second side.
- Alternate the starting side with each feeding
- Burp the infant between sides and at the end of the feeding. Excess breast milk can be pumped and stored in the freezer for later use.

(2) Bottle feeding: Bottle-fed infants require 2 to 3 ounces of iron-fortified formula every 3 to 4 hours. Research linking even mild iron-deficiency anemia with later cognitive difficulties prompted the American Academy of Pediatrics to recommend iron-fortified formula for all bottle-fed infants. Methods of bottle feeding are as follows:

- Use clean equipment and wash hands before preparing formula. Prepare formula immediately before feeding and discard any excess afterward. Do not warm formula in the microwave because the liquid can quickly get hot enough to burn.
- Cradle the infant and stimulate the rooting reflex by touching the nipple to the cheek; insert the nipple into the infant's mouth.
- Feed the infant slowly and burp the infant after every ounce, more often if the baby is "gassy." It is normal for the infant to regurgitate up to an ounce of formula each feeding.

(3) Place infants on their right side after feeding to enhance stomach emptying.

b. Elimination

(1) Urination is adequate if the infant wets at least 6 to 8 diapers per day.

(2) Bowel elimination varies depending on whether the infant is breast-fed or bottle-fed. Breast-fed infants' stools are gold-colored and loose or seedy; bowel movements can occur as often as every feeding, or once every several days. Bottle-fed infants' stools are darker and more varied in consistency.

c. Dentition: breast-feeding mothers need to continue to take prenatal vitamins to ensure adequate source of calcium.

d. Sleep

(1) Newborns and young infants sleep most of the day (16 hours or more) and wake intermittently. Periods awake lengthen as the infant grows.

(2) Take advantage of times awake to play with the infant but be alert to cues that signal that the infant is ready to stop (the infant appears disinterested, turns head away, fusses).

(3) Position the healthy infant on the side or back for sleep. Because research suggests that prone sleep position may be associated with increased incidence of sudden infant death syndrome, the American Academy of Pediatrics recommends avoiding this sleeping position for infants who are unable to roll over.

e. Hygiene

(1) Bathing—sponge bathe the newborn until the cord falls off. Bathe when appropriate using mild

Table 15–5. Conditions Seen in Early Infancy

Condition	Description	Nursing Implications
Hydrocephalus	Enlargement of the brain ventricles resulting from obstruction to the normal circulation of cerebrospinal fluid. Infant's head grows at a rate exceeding the normal head circumference growth curve.	If not treated, results in various degrees of neurologic compromise and mental retardation. Placement of a shunting mechanism reestablishes normal cerebrospinal fluid flow. Most children live normal lives but may need periodic shunt revisions. Often associated with spina bifida.
Spina bifida/ myelomeningocele	Incomplete fusion of the spinal column during fetal development resulting in varying degrees of defect of the spinal cord and cerebrospinal fluid circulation. Depending on location of the lesion, multiple motor and sensory dysfunctions occur, including motor and sensory impairment to lower extremities, absence of bowel and bladder control, and skeletal deformities.	Surgical repair of the defect is required, followed by multidisciplinary follow-up during childhood. Most children do well with support and are able to accomplish many age-appropriate tasks within the limits of their disability. Provide strong emotional support for the family and child.
Developmental dysplasia of the hip	Hip instability or dislocation resulting from inadequate development of the femoral head and acetabulum.	When recognized early, can be treated with hip abduction devices (double diapering, harness, splint). Children with more severe deformity or those not recognized early enough may require traction and immobilization in a spica cast. Keep the cast clean and provide for age-appropriate activities while the child is immobilized, and teach the parents to do the same.
Club foot	Rigid, positional deformity of the foot and ankle that occurs in various degrees. Varus and valgus deformities may be unilateral or bilateral.	Metatarsus adductus, toeing in without rigidity, can be improved with early stretching exercises. True club foot requires serial casting or surgical repair, depending on the severity of the involvement.
Cleft lip and palate	Defects in closure of the lip or soft or hard palate with abnormal opening of various degrees. Cleft lip or palate can occur alone, but most frequently occurs together. They can be unilateral or bilateral.	Depending on severity, they interfere with appearance, feeding, dentition, and speech, and can cause increased episodes of otitis media with resulting hearing deficit. Cleft lip is repaired as soon as possible after birth and the infant has demonstrated stable health status. Cleft palate is closed optimally before the child begins to talk. The repair may be done in stages and may require various adaptive devices for feeding. Later, speech therapy can improve articulation. Provide assistance to the child and family to help them adjust to any cosmetic consequences.
Pyloric stenosis	Caused by hypertrophy of the pyloric sphincter muscle, resulting in obstruction of the upper gastrointestinal tract. More frequently seen in infant boys. Often can be palpated as an olive-sized mass in the epigastric area.	Projectile vomiting, which begins in the 2nd or 3rd week of life, followed by voracious hunger can cause fluid and electrolyte imbalances with weight loss. Surgical repair is necessary.
Anorectal malformations	Failure to develop complete patency of the rectum or anus. Depending on the location of the anomaly, can vary from anal stricture to imperforate anus. Interferes with the passage of stool and with future development of sphincter control.	Dilation of anal stenosis is effective. Surgical repair of imperforate anus may require a temporary colostomy and, if bowel control is not achieved, a permanent colostomy.
Umbilical hernia	Caused by incomplete closure of the umbilical ring. Hernias protrude with crying or exertion. Affects Blacks more frequently.	They usually close spontaneously but require surgery if not closed by school age.
Esophageal atresia/tracheoesophageal fistula	Defect in development of the embryonic foregut that results in anomalies of the esophagus and trachea of several different configurations. Defects range from complete atresia of the esophagus alone to atresia combined with an abnormal connection to the trachea. Type C defect is most common and includes blind esophageal pouch, fistula from the distal esophagus leading from the stomach into the lower trachea. Pneumonitis results from reflux of stomach acid into the respiratory system. Surgical correction connects the two parts of the esophagus and closes the fistula; a gastrostomy may be required until surgical correction is complete.	Meticulous assessment may reveal difficulty with initial breastfeeding, or the infant may find it difficult to handle its secretions (choking, coughing) and may become cyanotic. Nursing care after surgery involves management of gastrostomy and esophagostomy, monitoring for respiratory distress, preventing infection, and maintaining fluid and electrolyte balance. The infant is usually cared for in a special care nursery. Holding the infant for gastrostomy feedings to provide comfort associated with a full stomach is important.
Gastroesophageal reflux	Reflux of stomach contents into the esophagus is related to an inefficient lower esophageal sphincter. Regurgitation is the initial symptom. Complications include failure to thrive, aspiration pneumonia, and esophagitis if the regurgitation is severe.	The goal of treatment is to prevent complications until the cardiac sphincter matures. Carefully monitor hydration status and weight gain. Teach the parent to feed the child in an upright position, burp frequently, and feed slowly. Elevating the head of the crib is controversial, as are thickened feed-

Table continued on following page

Table 15–5. Conditions Seen in Early Infancy (Continued)

Condition	Description	Nursing Implications
		ings. Pharmacologic intervention can include medications that decrease gastric acidity (cimetedine, ranitidine). Surgical treatment is reserved for severely affected infants.
Hypospadias	Urethral meatus abnormally positioned on the penis. Various degrees of penile deformity.	Surgery is required and may consist of several stages, including reconstruction of the penis. The goal of repair is to improve urinary stream and the appearance and function of the penis. Genital surgery is particularly distressing to young children and their parents. Provide as much emotional support as possible. Answer all questions honestly.
Inguinal hernia	Herniation of the peritoneum into the inguinal canal, often reaching the scrotum. Frequently is associated with hydrocele (presence of fluid in the scrotal area).	Surgery is the treatment of choice.
Undescended testicles	Failure of testes to descend into the scrotum. May be unilateral or bilateral. Needs to be differentiated from the cremasteric reflex (the upward movement of the testes and scrotum in response to tactile stimulation to the upper, inner thigh).	Surgical repair is necessary to prevent testicular dysfunction or injury and tumor development. Children are at risk for later testicular cancer and possible fertility dysfunction. Encourage the child and parents to express concerns, and provide support.
Fetal alcohol syndrome	Caused by regular prenatal ingestion of alcohol. Major effects on the infant's neurologic system include mental retardation, altered muscle tone and coordination, delayed development, irritability and hyperactivity. Other manifestations include growth lag, identifiable dysmorphic characteristics (microcephaly, short palpebral fissure, thin upper lip with underdeveloped philtrum). Severely affected infants may seize. Symptoms are irreversible. Depending on severity, the child will experience cognitive difficulties.	Provide appropriate counseling for the mother. Refer for alcohol treatment. Allow for expression of guilt. Assist with public education regarding dangers of prenatal alcohol consumption.
Addicted infants	Habitual drug use during pregnancy causes addiction in newborns. Symptoms are related to drug withdrawal and occur within 24 hr after birth. Symptoms include hyperirritability and hyperactivity, inconsolability, restlessness, poor feeding, gastrointestinal distress, diaphoresis, and tremors or convulsions. Infants exposed to cocaine or "crack" demonstrate decreased length and weight.	Modify the environment to decrease stimuli, use quiet comfort measures, administer anticonvulsants if required, and provide nutritional support. Encourage the mother to express feelings of guilt or anxiety. Refer to social services for counseling and follow-up in community.
Down syndrome	Defect of chromosome 21 (trisomy). Impairment of intelligence and presence of associated dysfunctions. Characteristics are decreased muscle tone with short stature and short, broad neck; distinctive facial features—flat nasal bridge, protruding tongue, presence of epicanthal folds and upward palpebral slant; associated congenital heart defects.	Intellectual potential varies and special education is required. Some children eventually achieve some independence. Health problems include feeding difficulties, increased susceptibility to upper respiratory infections, constipation, atlantoaxial instability (assessed by radiography; if present, precludes participation in any sport activity that exerts stress on the head or neck). Promote maternal–infant attachment, encourage parental expression of feelings and concerns, refer family to support group and for genetic counseling, encourage participation in Special Olympics program and any other activity that develops confidence and positive self-esteem.
Congenital cardiac defects	Any of a number of developmental defects that alter pressure within the cardiac chambers and great vessels, and impact circulation between the right and left sides of the heart (see Table 15–14). Two major consequences include 1. Congestive heart failure—right-sided, left-sided, or both. Demands for increased cardiac output trigger compensatory mechanisms, which eventually fail if the underlying problem is not treated. Symptoms may be subtle at first and include tachycardia, poor peripheral perfusion, diaphoresis, fatigue, feeding difficulties (in infants), signs of progressively worsening respiratory distress, cardiomegaly, cough, orthopnea, pulmonary edema, delayed development, hepatomegaly, and edema.	The goal of cardiac surgery is to correct underlying defects and restore normal pressure and circulatory pattern. Treatment of congestive heart failure includes administration of medications to improve cardiac function (digoxin, captopril) and to increase diuresis (furosemide, spironolactone), fluid restriction if the condition is acute, and decrease of metabolic needs. Major nursing functions include monitoring for signs of congestive heart failure, teaching parents proper medication administration, and helping parents organize the child's activities of daily living to minimize metabolic demands (slow feedings with plenty of rest, adequate warmth, minimization of crying or anxiety). Nursing implications for the hypoxemic child revolve around maintaining adequate hydration, prevent-

Table 15–5. Conditions Seen in Early Infancy (Continued)

Condition	Description	Nursing Implications
	2. Hypoxemia—results from shunting of desaturated blood from the right to left side of the heart and into peripheral circulation. Signs include decreased PaO_2 and arterial oxygen saturation and cyanosis; long-term consequences are polycythemia and clubbing of fingertips and toes.	ing respiratory infection and dealing with body image concerns. Teach parents management of hypercyanotic ("tet") spells (knee-chest or squatting position, notify the physician if such spells are prolonged). Nursing management after cardiac surgery is complex and usually managed initially in the intensive care unit. Reassuring the parent and child both preoperatively and postoperatively is a major nursing function.
Aganglionic megacolon (Hirschprung's disease)	Decreased innervation to the lower colon is caused by an absence of ganglia in the affected bowel segment. Peristalsis is absent. Clinical manifestations include constipation, intestinal obstruction, abdominal distention with palpable mass. Enterocolitis is a complication. The infant may fail to pass meconium. Diagnosis is by rectal biopsy. Treatment is usually surgical resection of the affected segment. A temporary colostomy might be necessary.	Preoperatively, restoring fluid balance is essential. Enemas may be required to clean and sterilize the bowel. Postoperative care is similar to that for any child undergoing surgery. Teach parents colostomy and meticulous skin care.

soap and water or water only. Bathe the infant with dry skin less often. Shampoo gently, keeping soap away from the infant's eyes. Wipe any eye discharge from inner to outer canthus with a cotton ball wet with warm water. Leave the cord area open to dry; apply alcohol with a cotton swab or an alcohol wipe if necessary to promote drying.

(2) Diaper area—Clean the diaper area with each diaper change using water or non–alcohol-based baby wipes. Be sure to wipe girls from front to back; do not retract foreskins of uncircumcised boys. Dry thoroughly before reapplying the diaper. Apply petroleum jelly or other occlusive ointment to irritated areas to prevent skin breakdown. Wash diapers in mild soap and water, with a second rinse if necessary.

f. Safety

(1) Do not smoke around the infant, and preferably eliminate all environmental smoke from the house. Children exposed to environmental smoke have a high incidence of upper respiratory infections and otitis media, and they can develop smoke-related health problems later in life.

(2) Avoiding falls, motor vehicle accidents, and equipment hazards are major safety issues for this age group:
- Never leave an infant unattended in a high place or unstrapped in an infant seat
- Always keep one hand on the infant
- Carry the infant when getting something out of reach
- Use an approved, rear-facing, car safety seat properly secured with the seatbelt
- Make sure all used baby furniture is free of lead-based paint. Cribs should have slats no farther apart than 2⅜ inches, a tight-fitting mattress, and bumper pads.

g. Play: Talk or sing to and smile at the infant frequently; coo in response to the infant's coos; cuddle

and rock after feeding. Using an infant carrier provides a change of scene.

3. Health issues and concerns

a. Lactation: The common concern is that the mother is not producing enough milk, particularly during the 1st 2 weeks of nursing.

(1) Obtain information about the following:
- Frequency of feedings and number of diapers wet daily
- Whether milk has come in (feeling of fullness and tingling in breasts, let-down) and whether breasts are soft after feeding
- Whether the infant is latching properly and the mother can observe sucking and swallowing (infant's ear moves with sucking)
- Whether the mother is relaxed during feeding and drinking enough liquids

(2) The approach to problems of lactation depends on the cause of the problem, but reassurance and encouragement to continue are essential.
- If the infant is not gaining weight properly and decreased milk supply is a legitimate concern, recommend that the mother increase fluid intake and increase the number of feedings (or pump residual milk after feedings). A temporary formula supplement may be necessary if the infant's weight is too low. The father or other family members should be encouraged to feed the formula if required.
- If the infant has problems latching or other mechanical problems such as poor suck, refer to a lactation specialist.
- In general, pacifiers and formula supplements should be avoided in babies who are gaining weight appropriately until lactation is firmly established.

b. Crying: The concern is that the infant cries "all the time" or cries for hours at night.

(1) Obtain the following information:

- Approximate number of hours of crying time, the time of day it most frequently occurs, and whether this is a new behavior for the infant
- Quality of the cry (e.g., high-pitched, angry, irritable, irritating, periodic fussiness)
- Whether it is associated with other symptoms such as gassiness, bowel movements, fever, illness
- General temperament of the infant

(2) The approach to crying problems is as follows:
- Reassure parents that crying is the infant's way of communicating hunger, discomfort, and anger; that most young infants cry up to 2 hours a day for various reasons; that crying is the infant's way of getting needs met; and that infants younger than 2 months old have not yet learned self-consoling activities.
- Parents should respond promptly to the cry and feed the infant only if appropriate; otherwise they should check the infant for a soiled diaper, burp and rock the infant, and put the infant back down when it is settled. If the infant demonstrates the need for additional sucking, a pacifier (not recommended for breast-fed babies) may be tried.
- Infants may be taken for a ride in the car or for a walk using an infant carrier. Playing soft music or a recording of soft mechanical noise (vacuum cleaner, car engine, clothes dryer) may be helpful.
- Refer for evaluation any infant who cries for more than 3 hours a day more than several days a week or if crying is associated with any signs of illness.

c. Colic: The concern is that the infant is "colicky" (gassy, cries all the time, appears to be in pain, draws legs up as if in pain).
(1) Obtain information about the following:
- Pattern and description of crying
- Pattern of feeding
- Relationship of crying to feeding
- Diet of nursing mothers
- Successful or unsuccessful measures used to relieve the problem

(2) The approach to colic is to do the following:
- Advise parents that colic is a set of symptoms with no firmly established cause. Sometimes, infants experience pain associated with milk intolerance. Initially, suggest the following: elimination of milk and milk products from the breast-feeding mother's diet; change formula to a non–milk-based formula (e.g., soy, predigested).
- Try massaging the abdomen or placing the infant prone on the parent's lap with the abdomen resting on a covered heat source (hot water bottle, heating pad) during episodes.
- Try methods for calming a crying infant.
- Provide extra reassurance and support. Advise one caregiver to take a turn caring for the infant, if possible, while the other rests. Reassure the

caregivers that infants usually outgrow the problem by age 3 months.

d. Altered bowel elimination: The concern is that there is a lack of a bowel movement for several days, or diarrhea.
(1) Obtain the following information:
- Time of last bowel movement
- Usual pattern and consistency and whether this represents a change
- Consistency of recent bowel movements
- Whether the infant shows other signs of illness

(2) The approach to altered bowel elimination is to:
- Reassure caregivers that bowel movements vary among infants and that consistency changes as the infant matures. The consistency of the stool is more important than the pattern; some infants have a bowel movement after each feeding and others go several days without one. Often, infants appear to be straining, but the stools are normal. Infant stools usually are loose and should not be confused with diarrhea. As long as the stool is not hard and "pellet-like" and the child is not exhibiting any signs of illness, the parent need not worry.
- Give the following suggestions if stools are hard: give additional fluid, add a small amount of corn syrup to the formula, obtain a rectal temperature to stimulate a bowel movement.

e. Newborn jaundice: The concern is that jaundice in a newborn has a variety of contributing factors that cause hyperbilirubinemia (>12.9 mg/dl), the appearance of yellow-colored skin, and yellowing of the sclera. Severe cases of jaundice can cause kernicterus and neurotoxicity.
(1) Most newborn jaundice is not caused by underlying hemolytic disease (Rh incompatibility, ABO incompatibility), in part because of the administration of Rho immune globulin to unsensitized Rh-negative mothers after each delivery or fetal loss. Jaundice caused by hemolytic disease usually appears before the infant is 24 hours old.
(2) Physiologic jaundice has no known underlying pathologic cause, appears after the first 24 hours, and lasts approximately 5 to 7 days. Bilirubin levels can be markedly elevated (up to 20 mg/dl).
(3) Other causes of jaundice are breast-feeding jaundice (associated with decreased milk intake while breast feeding is being established) and breast milk jaundice (in which jaundice usually does not appear until the infant is 4 to 5 days old).
(4) The approach to newborn jaundice is to reassure parents of mildly jaundiced children that jaundice resolves without intervention; encourage frequent feedings and expose the infant to indirect sunlight (caution against direct sunlight because of the danger of sun burn). Caregivers should contact the physician if jaundice becomes worse or does not begin to resolve after several days.
- Children with severe jaundice and elevated bilirubin levels may need phototherapy treatment (levels usually > 18 mg/dl although protocols

differ). Phototherapy decreases bilirubin levels, but, because the infant is usually hospitalized for the treatment (some infants are candidates for supervised home phototherapy), the treatment can interfere with bonding and breast-feeding (intermittent phototherapy allows for breast-feeding of an infant who has been removed from the lights).

- Warn parents that the child will have an eye shield and will be undressed (the diaper area may be covered with a small diaper for frequent stools).
- Ensure adequate hydration of the infant, keep the infant's skin clean and dry, provide verbal and tactile stimulation, and reassure the parents.

Health Promotion for the 2-Month-Old Infant

1. For preventive care and health maintenance, see Table 15–4.
2. Anticipatory guidance and teaching parents
   a. Nutrition: Breast-feeding should continue on demand, but time between feedings may lengthen somewhat, especially at night. Formula feeding averages 4 ounces given 6 times a day.
   b. Elimination: Bowel movements may decrease in number, but consistency remains the same if breast milk or formula is unchanged. Still wets 6 diapers daily.
   c. Dentition: The breast-feeding mother should continue to take prenatal vitamins and ensure sufficient calcium intake.
   d. Sleep: Grouping of sleep periods occurs, with the infant being awake for longer periods in-between. Many infants obtain a long stretch (5–6 hours) of sleep at night. The infant's crib may be moved to a separate room. Awake times should be used to play with infant.
   e. Hygiene
      (1) Bathe infant several times a week by immersion in a tub of shallow, warm water. Observe for skin dryness, and apply a non–alcohol-based lotion to dry areas (not diaper area).
      (2) Seborrheic dermatitis ("cradle cap") can be treated by applying warm oil to the scalp with a cotton ball, allowing the oil to penetrate the crusts, and shampooing. For more persistent crusting, crusts may be gently loosened with fingernails or a soft comb before shampooing.
   f. Safety: Major safety issues continue to include falls and motor vehicle accidents. Burns become an issue at this age.
      (1) Do not hold an infant while drinking any hot liquid or while smoking. Make sure smoke alarms work.
      (2) Set household water temperature at between 120 and 130 degrees Fahrenheit. Test bath water with the inner aspect of the wrist before immersing the infant.
      (3) If the infant is accidentally burned, immerse the area for several minutes (10–20) in cool water, not ice, then cover loosely with a sterile or clean bandage or cloth. See the physician if the child sustains minor burns (redness only) over a large part of the body or burns that blister, particularly burns on the head, face, hands, feet, and genital area.
   g. Play
      (1) Continue imitating the infant's vocalizations and smile frequently at the baby; change the infant's environment for exposure to a variety of sights and sounds, both indoors and outside; and sing to the infant.
      (2) Make the surrounding environment as interesting as possible, using brightly colored wall hangings, crib accessories, and mobiles; encourage tracking and following; and provide appropriately sized toys of different colors and textures.
      (3) To encourage motor development, place the infant in a sitting position to promote head control and place the infant prone for short, supervised periods to facilitate head lifting.
3. Health issues and concerns: Diaper dermatitis—diaper rash is caused by chemical irritants coming in contact with sensitive skin and made worse by a constantly moist environment.
   a. The concern is that the infant has a reddened diaper area. Obtain the following information:
      (1) Appearance of the rash, including the area affected (folds only, perianal area, spread to lower abdomen), amount of redness and irritation, presence of blisters or associated scattered lesions, whether the skin is oozing or dry
      (2) Type of diapers and diaper covers used
      (3) Whether the child is being given antibiotics (certain antibiotics can contribute to development of a *Candida albicans* infection) and what the parent has used to treat the problem
   b. Approach to diaper dermatitis
      (1) Prevent diaper rash by changing diapers as soon as they are wet, drying the infant thoroughly after cleaning the perineal area, allowing the area to be exposed to air several minutes daily. If diarrhea is a problem, use occlusive ointment (zinc oxide, petroleum jelly, A&D) on noninflamed skin only. Wash off gently and reapply with each diaper change.
      (2) Temporarily change the type of diapers used switching from cloth to disposable, removing the plastic liner from the disposable, or using extra-absorbent diapers, to increase air circulation to the area and decrease skin contact with urine and stool. Avoid plastic pants or other occlusive diaper covers.
      (3) Notify the physician if the diaper rash is severe or not improving. Infants with *C. albicans* infection need to be treated with nystatin ointment or cream to the diaper area and possibly nystatin liquid for oral candidiasis (thrush).

Health Promotion for the 4-Month-Old Infant

1. For preventive care and health maintenance, see Table 15–4.

2. Anticipatory guidance and teaching parents
    a. Nutrition: Maintain breast-feeding schedule. If the mother has returned to work, she may continue breast-feeding on a comfortable schedule, using pumped breast milk in a bottle or formula supplement while she is away. Infants on formula take up to 5 to 6 ounces 5 to 6 times a day.
    b. Elimination: Elimination continues as for a 2 month old.
    c. Dentition: The infant may begin drooling in preparation for tooth eruption.
    d. Sleep: Most infants sleep through the night and are awake more during the day. Total sleep is 15 to 16 hours.
    e. Hygiene: Continue a daily routine of cleanliness.
    f. Safety: Choking becomes a concern as the infant becomes more active.
        (1) Keep all small objects and pieces of food out of the infant's reach.
        (2) Avoid using "teething biscuits," which get smaller as the baby gums.
        (3) Teach older siblings not to give the infant anything small.
        (4) Know how to manage a choking child (see p. 547).
    g. Play
        (1) Continue to talk frequently to the infant; respond verbally, smile, and laugh as the infant does; talk to the infant from various locations so the infant will turn to locate the voice; and sing to the infant frequently.
        (2) Expose the infant to a variety of environments and environmental sounds, and encourage the baby to splash while being bathed.
        (3) Provide rattles, brightly colored plastic rings, or other small, safe toys for the infant to grasp.
        (4) Encourage the infant to sit to increase head control and play standing games, encouraging the infant to bounce while bearing weight on the feet.
3. Health issues and concerns: child care
    a. The concern is that many mothers return to work by the time the infant is 4 months old. Finding appropriate child care is most important. Obtain information about the following:
        (1) How many hours of child care will be necessary
        (2) Parents' financial resources
        (3) Type of child care in which the parent is interested—daycare center, home-based daycare, care of child in own home, cooperative daycare
    b. The approach is to look for the following when considering daycare arrangements:
        (1) Cleanliness of the facility and whether personnel practice and encourage cleanliness; policy for when children become ill
        (2) Number of children cared for and child to staff ratio
        (3) Whether the environment is age-appropriate and appealing, child-proof and safe, and whether equipment is suited to the child's age level
        (4) Whether the provider is willing to maintain the infant's usual schedule, including periods of play and creative learning experiences

    (5) Whether the food provided is appropriate for the child's age and is nutritiously sound
    (6) Whether the provider relates well with infants and children and uses disciplinary measures that agree with the parent's philosophy
    (7) Whether the facility is licensed

Health Promotion for the 6-Month-Old Infant

1. For preventive care and health maintenance, see Table 15–4. Lead poisoning:
    a. Exposure to environmental lead is a problem for infants who have become mobile and who are beginning to put everything in their mouths (Box 15–1).
    b. Homes built before 1960, particularly those with peeling paint or undergoing renovation, pose the greatest danger, although other sources of lead in the environment are also problematic (lead paint on old infant furniture, lead in the drinking water, lead from exhaust fumes, use of lead by family members).

BOX 15–1. Lead Risk Assessment and Management

Assessment

At the 6-month physical examination, assess for environmental exposure to lead. Ask the parent or caregiver (if the child is in daycare on a daily basis, this information should be obtained from the daycare provider as well) whether the child
- Lives in a house built before 1978 with lead pipes or solder or a house built before 1960 that is undergoing renovations. Ask whether the child's house is located near an industry that releases lead into the environment.
- Regularly comes in contact with a household member who works with lead or lead solder (construction and renovation workers, plumbers, stained glass workers).
- Sleeps in or uses old infant furniture or toys.
- Has relatives who have had lead poisoning.
  Test the capillary lead level of any infant who meets any of the above criteria. Further action depends on testing results:
- Lead level less than 10 μg/dl, retest the child at risk every 6 months until 2 tests are less than 10 μg/dl or 3 are less than 15 μg/dl.
- Lead level of 10 to 14 μg/dl, verify with venous lead, retest every 3 to 4 months until venous lead results are as above.
- Lead level of 15 μg/dl or greater, verify with venous lead, retest every 3 to 4 months. Provide educational materials about environmental assessment.
- Venous lead level of 20 μg/dl, refer to a public health agency for environmental testing, modification, and management.

Management

Environmental modification includes identifying sources of lead and keeping child away, covering any peeling surfaces with contact paper, flushing water for several minutes before using for drinking, damp mopping frequently with phosphate-containing detergent, and washing infant's hands, face, and toys frequently.
  Nutritional modification includes providing a diet high in vitamin C, iron, calcium, and zinc and testing hematocrit or hemoglobin if the infant is off formula.
  Chelation is considered for children with a venous lead level of more than 25 μg/dl.

c. Even low levels of lead in the blood can cause later cognitive difficulties. Lead risks are assessed beginning at the 6-month checkup (see Chapter 38).
2. Anticipatory guidance and teaching parents
   a. Nutrition
      (1) Breast-feed 5 or more times a day; bottle-feed 24 to 40 ounces of formula daily.
      (2) Introduce solid foods one at a time (Table 15–6). Give the same food for 4 days before introducing the next, and observe the infant for any adverse reactions. Avoid citrus fruits and juices and egg whites. Do not use commercially prepared mixed

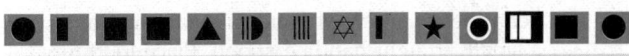

TRANSCULTURAL CONSIDERATIONS

The incidence of lead poisoning is higher in Blacks, Hispanics, and immigrants because they usually live in older housing, particularly in the inner city.

dinners because the protein content is low and it would be difficult to determine the cause of an allergic response or sensitivity.

Table 15–6. Infant-Feeding Guide

Foods	0–4 months	4–6 months	6–8 months	8–10 months	10–12 months
Breast milk	Short, frequent feedings, 8 or more per day	Short, frequent feedings, 5 or more per day	On demand, 5 or more feedings	On demand	On demand
Iron-Fortified Formula	16–32 ounces 5–10 feedings per day	24–40 ounces 4–7 feedings per day	24–32 ounces 3–4 feedings per day	16–32 ounces 3–4 feedings per day Can wean from the bottle	16–24 ounces 3–4 feedings per day Whole milk can be offered after 12 months
Cereals and Bread	None	Boxed rice, oatmeal, or barley (spoon fed) Mix 2–3 teaspoons with formula, water, or breast milk	Most varieties of boxed infant cereal Avoid cereals that are premixed with formula or fruit 1–4 tablespoons, twice a day	Infant cereals, Cream of Wheat, or other plain hot cereals Toast, bagel, or crackers good for teething	Hot or cold unsweetened cereals Bread Rice Noodles or spaghetti
Fruit Juices	None	Infant juice Adult apple juice, vitamin C fortified (Avoid orange and tomato juice) 2–4 ounces per day	Infant juice Adult apple juice, vitamin C fortified Offer juice from a cup 4 ounces per day	All 100% juices	All 100% juices from a cup
Vegetables	None	None	Strained or mashed vegetables Dark yellow or orange (avoid corn) Dark green ½–1 jar or ½ cup per day	Cooked and mashed, fresh or frozen vegetables	Cooked vegetable pieces May have some raw vegetables if the child can chew them well
Fruits	None	None	Fresh or cooked fruits Mashed bananas Applesauce Strained fruits 1 jar or ½ cup per day	Peeled, soft fruit wedges Bananas Peaches Pears Oranges Apples	All fresh fruits, peeled and seeded Canned fruits, packed in water or natural juice
Protein Foods	None	None	Plain yogurt Can be mixed with soft, fresh fruit or applesauce	Lean meat, chicken, and fish (strained, chopped, or small tender pieces) Egg yolk Yogurt Mild cheese Cooked dried beans	Small tender pieces of meat, fish, or chicken Whole egg Cheese Yogurt Cooked dried beans

From the Massachusetts WIC Program, Nutrition Education Task Force, WIC Form #47, Revised 11/85.

(3) Feed the infant slowly and in small amounts with a small, straight-handled spoon. Place food toward the back of the tongue to minimize any remaining tongue-thrust. Hold the infant in the arms or place in an infant seat when feeding.

(4) Begin using a cup, especially for juices.

b. Elimination: Stools become darker and more formed as solid foods are introduced to the diet.

c. Dentition

(1) Tooth eruption is usually preceded by drooling, increased finger-sucking, redness and swelling of the gum, fussiness, and occasionally a low-grade fever (less than 38.4 degrees Celsius, or 101 degrees Fahrenheit).

(2) Tooth eruption usually begins with lower central incisors. Teeth can come in 1 or more at a time.

(3) Begin fluoride supplements, brush erupted teeth with a soft toothbrush without toothpaste. Do not put the infant to bed with a bottle, which can contribute to dental caries.

d. Sleep: The infant sleeps 12 to 16 hours a day, that is, all night, with 2 to 3 naps.

e. Hygiene: Continue the daily routine. Because of increased motor activity, support infants firmly while bathing them.

f. Safety: As the infant becomes more active and begins to explore, falls, motor vehicle safety, burns, and choking assume additional importance. Access to poisonous plants and substances also becomes a concern.

(1) Childproof the home, especially the kitchen and bathroom.

• Remove all dangerous objects, medicines, plants, chemicals, cleansers, toys, utensils, breakable items, and desk accessories (e.g., paper clips, pencils, staples), and place them out of the child's reach. When children learn to crawl and climb, they can reach formerly inaccessible items.

• Use mechanical aids (e.g., gates at the base and top of the stairs and around wood stoves, cabinet and drawer safety latches, doorknob covers, plug fillers).

(2) Keep syrup of ipecac in the home (1 bottle for each child younger than age 5 years). Keep the poison control number on the phone, and call about any questionable ingestion. Follow directions given. Use syrup of ipecac only as directed by the poison control center or the health practitioner.

g. Play

(1) Continue to expose the infant to a variety of sounds, especially different vocal sounds, animal noises, and music; begin playing social games like pat-a-cake, peek-a-boo, bouncing and rocking games, and tickling; provide bath toys, a variety of rattles, a mirror in the crib, soft stuffed animals, or a large ball.

(2) Allow the infant to hold a spoon or cracker while being fed. Encourage the infant to pick up toys and put small blocks in a container.

(3) Encourage the infant to sit unsupported; place in an infant swing or walker when head control is developed. Encourage the infant to rock on hands and knees by placing favorite toy slightly out of reach.

3. Health issues and concerns

a. Teething: the concern is that the infant is often uncomfortable when teething.

(1) Obtain information about the following:

• Any signs of illness—temperature higher than 101 degrees Fahrenheit, pulling at ears, upper respiratory symptoms

• Increase in sucking, mouthing, drooling behaviors

(2) The approach to teething

• Teach parents to observe the infant for any signs of illness and consult the physician if these appear

• Use acetaminophen only if the infant is exceptionally uncomfortable. Give the child a cold, hard, teething ring to gum. Avoid teething biscuits because they can become a choking hazard; if used, observe the infant and remove the biscuit when it becomes too small.

b. Night crying: The concern is that at approximately 6 months old, some infants experience temporary difficulties with sleep. Problems may be related to dreams, temporary illness, the reluctance to separate from the parent at the end of the day, inability to self-console, receiving pleasurable reinforcement from parents when awakening (playing, rocking, or being brought to the parent's bed).

(1) Obtain the following information:

• How often the child wakes and what the parent usually does

• The usual method of settling the infant for the night

• Presence of any signs of illness

(2) The approach to night crying

• Provide a bedtime ritual of rocking, singing, and storytelling, but place the infant in the crib while the infant is still drowsy. Do not allow the infant to fall completely asleep before being put in the crib, either at night or for naps.

• Place a favorite toy or blanket in the crib with the baby

• If infant cries, check every 5 to 15 minutes, without turning on lights, picking the infant up, or taking the infant to another room. Touch gently and talk soothingly for a short time (less than 1 minute).

• If crying persists, rock the infant until asleep, but gradually phase out rocking time.

Health Promotion for the 9-Month-Old Infant

1. For preventive care and health maintenance, see Table 15–4. Tuberculosis screening. Recent recommendations about routine tuberculosis screening in children have changed.

a. Children who live in low-risk areas need not be screened for tuberculosis on an annual basis. One baseline screening with a Mantoux test can be considered sometime before the child enters school.

b. Children who are low risk but who live in a high-risk area can be screened periodically, depending on the local incidence of tuberculosis.

c. Children at high risk should be tested annually with a Mantoux test. High-risk children include those who are in contact with infected adults (or parents who come from areas of the world where tuberculosis is prevalent), those with questionable results on chest radiographs, children infected with human immunodeficiency virus (or those frequently exposed to HIV-infected or at-risk adults) or with other risk illnesses (lymphoma, diabetes mellitus, renal failure), and children who are in jail.

2. Anticipatory guidance and teaching parents
   a. Nutrition: Breast-feeding continues on schedule, with formula being reduced to 16 to 32 ounces per day, continue iron-fortified infant cereal; begin to introduce soft mashed table foods.
   b. Elimination: Urinary and bowel elimination pattern remains consistent.
   c. Dentition: Four teeth are expected to have erupted; recommendations as previously described should be continued.
   d. Sleep: Night waking diminishes if managed appropriately. Review management if night waking remains a problem.
   e. Hygiene
      (1) Pay particular attention to diaper area as the infant's bladder capacity increases and urine becomes more concentrated.
      (2) As the infant begins to use more finger foods, wash the infant's hands and face frequently.
   f. Safety: As infants increase in mobility, falls and drowning become concerns.
      (1) Use nonskid rug liners, socks with nonskid patches, and nonskid strips in the bathtub.
      (2) Keep electrical cords short and wastebaskets covered or out of reach; pad sharp edges and corners of furniture.
      (3) Never leave infant unattended near water or in the bath. Make sure gates surrounding pools are locked. Watch carefully at the beach.
      (4) Do not use electrical appliances (e.g., radios, hair dryers) near water.
   g. Play
      (1) Increase social games; provide the infant with cloth or hard cardboard books and "read" with the infant regularly; continue to hug, rock, and cuddle.
      (2) Promote crawling and walking along furniture by placing a toy out of reach and encouraging the infant to get it or rolling a ball out of reach.
      (3) Allow the infant to use pots and pans and wooden spoons to create new sounds; play "hide-and-seek" games with toys.

3. Health issues and concerns: weaning
   a. The initiation of weaning the infant from breast or bottle to cup depends on parent preference, although infants this age usually are ready to do so. Obtain the following information:
      (1) Desire of the parent to begin weaning. Emphasize to nursing mothers that they may continue to breast-feed if it continues to be mutually enjoyable and beneficial, but they can decrease the number of feedings if desired.
      (2) Signs that the infant is ready to be weaned— eating a well-rounded diet of solid food, eating well from a spoon, drinking from a cup held by parents, beginning to bring cup to mouth
   b. The approach to weaning
      (1) Advise parents to decrease bottle or breast-feeding by 1 feeding at a time while increasing the amount of formula or pumped breast milk given by cup.
      (2) Continue to give iron-fortified formula until the infant is 1 year old.

Health Promotion for the 1- to 3-Year-Old Child

1. Preventive care and health maintenance: iron-deficiency anemia
   a. Hematocrit or hemoglobin should be checked; if not done at 9 months, then it should be checked yearly until age 4 years.
      (1) Iron-deficiency anemia is one of the most common nutritional disorders of childhood.
      (2) Children who are mildly anemic can experience symptoms of subtle behavior changes. For this reason, the American Academy of Pediatrics Committee on Nutrition recommends postponing the replacement of formula or breast-feeding with whole milk until the child is 1 year old and supplementing iron for children who are mildly anemic.
   b. If hemoglobin is less than 11 gm per dl (hematocrit <33%), obtain a complete blood count and reticulocyte count to determine whether the child is iron deficient or has anemia from other causes. Treatment is with supplemental iron (ferrous sulfate) if the child is iron deficient and an increase in dietary iron (dark, leafy vegetables, red meat, egg yolk, raisins, prunes) and vitamin C. Retest the child in 1 month. If hemoglobin is 11 to 11.5 gm per dl (hematocrit 33–35%), recommend vitamins with iron and fluoride and an increase in dietary iron.

℞ DRUG ADVISORY

Some iron preparations can damage children's teeth if precautions are not taken to prevent it. Mix iron preparations with water or fruit juice (preferably juice high in vitamin C) and give to children through a straw (or "sippy cup" for children not able to use a straw). Rinse mouth or brush teeth after the child takes the medication.

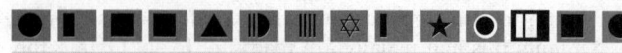

2. Anticipatory guidance and teaching parents
   a. Nutrition
      (1) The child may be given whole milk at age 1 year. Offer a variety of table foods. The first can be whole egg and citrus juices. Do not start the child on low-fat milk until age 2 years. Provide 2 to 3 cups of milk per day, 1 serving of protein, and 4 small servings each of fruits, vegetables, and breads.
      (2) Picky eating and "food jags" begin during this period. Advise parents that these eating habits are normal and that the child will obtain sufficient nutrients if a variety of foods is offered. Make meal time enjoyable by giving children their own dinnerware and utensils.
      (3) Modify diet for children older than 2 years with elevated cholesterol. No more than 10 percent of total calories should be from saturated fat, with 30 percent of total calories from fat. These children should receive less than 300 mg of cholesterol per day. Change to 1% low-fat milk or skim milk; use egg substitutes; choose low-fat meats and cheeses; increase fruits, vegetables, and carbohydrates; decrease added fat; avoid high-calorie, high-fat desserts.
   b. Elimination: Bowel movements decrease in number and become more regular. Increased bladder capacity allows the child to remain dry for several hours. Many children are completely toilet trained by age 3 years.
   c. Dentition: Continue to brush teeth with a soft toothbrush and water or a small amount of fluoride toothpaste. Discourage the child from swallowing the toothpaste. The first dental visit is sometime during this period. Change fluoride supplement to 0.5 mg at age 2 and to 1 mg at age 3 years.
   d. Sleep: Total sleep ranges from 12 to 14 hours a day. The child usually takes 1 nap of several hours in the afternoon and may give up the nap by age 3 years.
   e. Hygiene
      (1) Girls become prone to irritation of the vaginal area from the moist environment. Teach girls to wipe from front to back when toilet training. Adding one-fourth cup of vinegar to the bath water can relieve symptoms of irritation. Girls should wear cotton underwear.
      (2) Foreskin begins to retract in boys at approximately age 2 years. The foreskin should be retracted gently to clean but never forced.
   f. Safety
      (1) Toy safety: Choking causes most toy-related deaths in young children. Common items include marbles, balloon pieces, small balls, and small parts of larger toys. Other injuries caused by toys include falls from moving toys, strangulation from cords that are too long, and trauma from falling toy chest lids. Examine toys and playground equipment on a regular basis for safety. Keep all small parts away from young children.
      (2) Watch the exploring child carefully. The child begins to understand "no" but often does not respond quickly when in danger. Watch the child closely while outside so the child does not dash into the street. Hold the child's hand when walking. Check playground equipment for safety.
      (3) Observe closely while eating that the child does not choke on small pieces of food. Caution the child to sit down while eating.
      (4) Turn pot handles away from edge of the stove.
      (5) When the child weighs 20 pounds, change to a front-facing toddler car safety seat.
   g. Play
      (1) Toddlers like parallel play and find it difficult to share.
      (2) Play begins to become imitative and imaginative.
      (3) Safe toys that appeal to children this age include push–pull toys (with string no longer than 12 inches for safety), various-size balls, colorful picture books, soft stuffed animals or dolls (one may become a transitional object that is taken everywhere), stacking toys, sandbox with pails and shovels, easy wooden puzzles with large pieces, trucks, riding toys, art supplies (large nontoxic crayons, finger paints, paper, clay), child's tape recorder or radio.
3. Health issues and concerns
   a. Temper tantrums (see Learning/Teaching Guidelines for Parents Disciplining Young Children)
      (1) The concern is that rapid cognitive development with still limited ability for verbal expression contributes to frustration and its expression as temper tantrums. Parental attempts at limit setting often conflict with the child's desire for autonomy. Some severe tantrums include breath holding and head banging.
      (2) The approach to temper tantrums is to
         • Set realistic but firm limits to the child's boundaries and behavior. Safety is the first concern, consistency is the most important component.
         • Tell the child and demonstrate what is acceptable behavior. Enforce a few, simple rules that are clear and easy for the child to follow.
         • Use distraction to minimize misbehavior, or physically remove the child from an unsafe situation. Ignore minor behavior problems such as whining and sulking.

LEARNING/TEACHING GUIDELINES
for Parents Disciplining Young Children

General Overview

1. Avoiding conflict can prevent discipline problems before they get out of hand.
2. Use simple rewards—praise, encouragement, being a good role model, hugs and kisses, and positive attention for cooperation. Rewards should be
   a. Appropriate for the child's age and effective for what you want the child to do.
   b. Immediate, particularly for young children who don't have a concept of time.
   c. Consistent.
   d. Gradually phased out.
3. Set a short amount of time aside every day to give attention to the child, regardless of how good or bad a day it was. Let children know you want to be with them during this time. You may do an activity together or just sit and cuddle.
4. Do not always use "time-out" as a disciplinary tactic because children habituate. Vary it with other tactics such as offering choices, using point (sticker, star) system for positive behavior, prescribing a chore for uncooperative behavior, and imposing logical consequences for older children.
5. After an incident, talk with the child to determine how to prevent the behavior from happening again. Show understanding of the child's point of view, and explain your point of view to the child.

Teaching Specifics About "Time-Out"

1. Review the procedure with the child. Select a place in the home for time-out, usually a chair in a hallway or corner. The location must be away from any distraction or anything of interest.
2. Use a timer. Show it to the child and explain that the time-out lasts until the bell rings (or timer buzzes). Time-out should not exceed 5 minutes and should be much shorter for younger children (30 sec, 1 min, 2 min). The time may be increased in increments if the child refuses to remain quiet.
3. Procedure
   a. Determine behaviors for which you will use time-out. When a behavior is observed, give the child directions, using as few words as possible, to stop the behavior immediately. The child should be able to clearly understand the direction.
   b. If the child stops, acknowledge the behavior with praise. If the behavior continues, warn the child by describing what the child is doing wrong and saying, "If you do it again, you'll have to go to time-out."
   c. If the behavior continues and the child does not go voluntarily, take the child to the time-out location. Do not respond to the child during time-out (make sure you monitor the child, however). If the child refuses to stay in the chair, gently restrain with a hand on the thigh.
   d. When time-out is over, distract the child and say something positive as soon as the child displays some positive behavior.

- Give the child a short "time-out" period in a set location if the misbehavior continues. As the child matures, use logical consequences as discipline.
- During a tantrum, make sure the child is safe; then ignore the behavior until it stops. Comfort the child afterward. As the child becomes more verbal, talk about what might have caused the frustration.

b. Toilet training
   (1) The concern is that many parents believe that children should be toilet trained by age 2 years. Some are pressured by their own parents, who insist that toilet training should be completed early.
   (2) The approach to toilet training is to explain to parents that achieving bowel and bladder control is a combination of neurologic maturation and the child's desire. Bowel control usually is achieved first because it is easier to predict when the child will have a bowel movement. Nighttime dryness usually is not achieved until the child is close to 4 years old. Boys often are later at achieving control than girls. Obtain information about the following:
   - Whether the child understands toileting words and can indicate being wet or soiled
   - Whether the child demonstrates behavior that indicates the need for toileting—grunts, points to genital area, pulls down pants, removes diaper, is unable to stand or sit still
   - Whether the child appears to understand the function of the potty chair or toilet
   - Whether the child has regular bowel movements and can stay dry for several hours
   - Whether the child has developed enough sphincter control to wait the time required to get to the bathroom
   (3) Advise parents to be relaxed and progress at the child's pace. Regression is not uncommon, and often children who seem to be doing well return to use of diapers temporarily. The child should understand that this is acceptable until the child is ready to try again.

(4) Put the child in easily removable clothing, but avoid putting the child in training pants or pull-ups until the child begins to demonstrate success.

(5) Have a "potty" chair or modified toilet seat available for the child to sit on as desired. Try to coordinate time on the potty with signals that the child needs to use it. Limit the time that the child stays on the potty initially to no more than 5 minutes.

(6) Praise the child for trying and for success. Demonstrate handwashing after each attempt.

Health Promotion for the 3- to 5-Year-Old Child

1. For preventive care and health maintenance, see Table 15–4.
    a. Hearing screening (audiometry) should begin at age 4 years and be repeated at age 5 years. Most school districts screen for hearing deficits yearly. The child should hear all frequencies (500, 1000, 2000, 4000) at 25 decibels. Occasionally, fluid in the middle ear interferes with the test results, so testing should be repeated at a later date.
        (1) Ask parents whether the child has demonstrated any kind of hearing deficit (needing things turned up loud, asking people to repeat what has been said, indistinct speech).
        (2) Choose a quiet location to administer the test.
        (3) Explain to the child what will be done (e.g., putting ear phones on the child or looking into the child's ear using a hand-held audiometer).
        (4) Describe what the child should do—listen closely for the soft noise, raise a hand when the noise is heard and put it right back down again, keep listening and raising the hand until all the sounds are finished.

NURSE ADVISORY

Children younger than age 5 years sometimes have difficulty understanding the concept of hand raising and lowering. An alternative method is to ask the child to say "hi" to the caregiver each time the noise is heard.

    b. Vision screening begins at age 4 years and is repeated at age 5 years. Vision testing is done in most school systems yearly. Refer to an eye specialist if the child is not able to see at the 20/40 level or if there is a discrepancy of two or more lines between the eyes (e.g., 20/20 left and 20/40 right).
        (1) Ask parents whether the child has demonstrated any signs of decreased vision (squinting, headaches, needing to be close to the television, clumsiness).
        (2) Screen in a well-lighted room with the child standing with heels 20 feet from the eye chart.

The chart should be at a height appropriate for the child's height.
        (3) Choose a chart appropriate for the child's age (Fig. 15–4).
        (4) Show the "E" or pictures to the child before beginning testing and be sure the child can identify the pictures or directions of the "E."
        (5) Have the child cover 1 eye with a small paper cup or commercial disposable occluder. The parent can help. Encourage the child not to peek.
        (6) Point to 1 or 2 pictures on the 20/100 line to verify that the child understands the procedure and can identify the pictures. Then, beginning with the 20/40 line, point to the pictures 1 at a time from left to right.
        (7) If the child identifies more than half the items, continue with lower lines, beginning each at the opposite side and moving in the opposite direction from the line before.
        (8) If the child fails to identify more than half the items, repeat the line in the other direction. If the child continues to fail, move to the next higher line.
        (9) Repeat with the opposite eye.
2. Anticipatory guidance and teaching parents
    a. Nutrition
        (1) Children should eat three to four servings of milk and milk products, two servings of meat, and four servings each of fruits, vegetables, breads.
        (2) Provide nutritious snacks, because the child is often in a hurry to eat at mealtime.
        (3) Begin to emphasize table manners.
    b. Elimination: Bowel movements have decreased to one to two per day; average urinary output is 1000 ml per day. Most children have achieved nighttime control.
    c. Dentition: Continue regular brushing and fluoride, and begin to schedule dental examinations every 6 months.
    d. Sleep: Requirements average 12 to 14 hours a day. The child usually gives up the daytime nap by age 5 years. The child may exhibit night terrors, nightmares, sleepwalking, or talking during sleep.
    e. Hygiene: Begin to teach the child activities that promote good health; such as washing hands and face frequently, especially after toileting and before meals, proper disposal of soiled tissues, and covering the mouth when coughing.
    f. Safety: As the child becomes more independent outside, safety concerns assume greater importance.
        (1) Bicycle safety—bicycle accidents are the most significant cause of head injury in children.
            • Insist that the child wear a bicycle helmet from the time the child first uses a bicycle outside.
            • Teach children to ride on the sidewalk or close to the right-hand side of the road.
            • Be sure the bicycle is the correct size for the child and that the seat level is appropriate (the child should be able to touch the tips of both feet to the ground while sitting on the seat).
        (2) Poisoning: Children occasionally ingest leaves or berries found on various trees or plants. Discour-

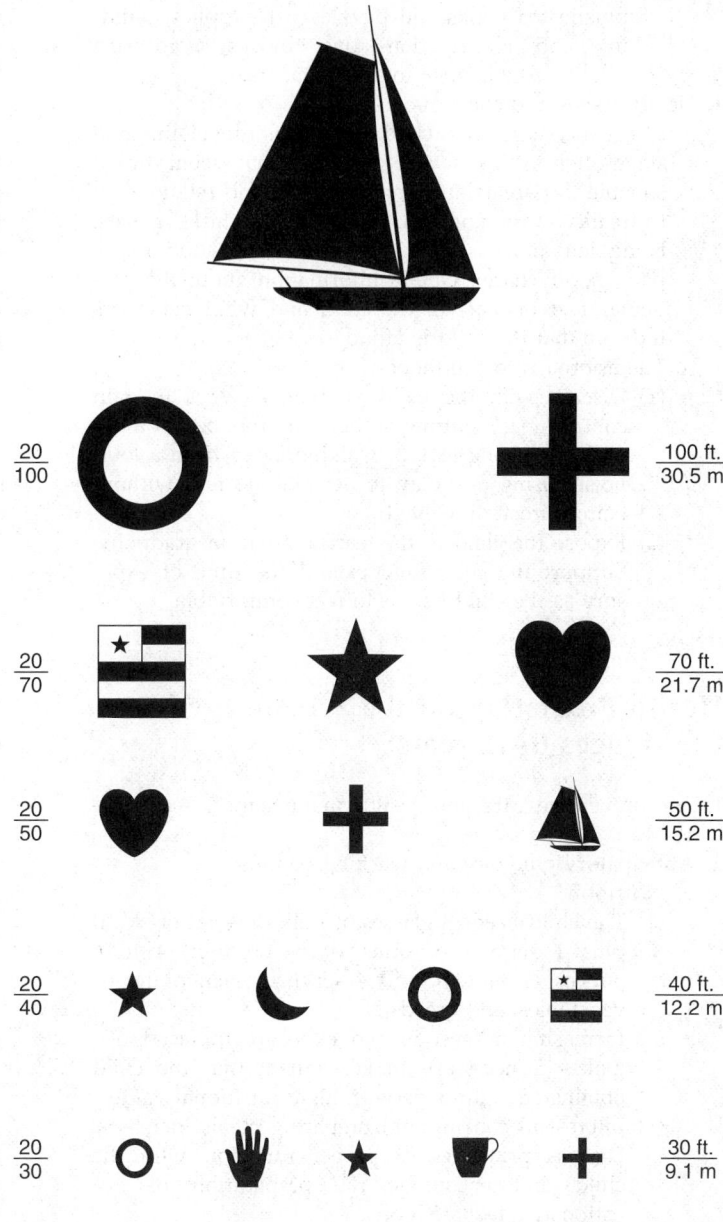

20/100		100 ft. / 30.5 m
20/70		70 ft. / 21.7 m
20/50		50 ft. / 15.2 m
20/40		40 ft. / 12.2 m
20/30		30 ft. / 9.1 m
20/20		20 ft. / 6.1 m

Figure 15–4. Kindergarten vision screening chart. (From ABCO Dealers, La Vergne, TN.)

age children from eating anything found outside without first consulting parents.

(3) Pedestrian safety
  • Begin to teach children to stop and look both ways before crossing the street. Practice this frequently as you walk with the child.
  • Tell the child not to play in the street or to chase another child or ball into the street.

(4) Automobile safety: The child may outgrow a child safety seat (usually at 40 pounds or 40 inches). Keep the child restrained properly in the car using the car safety restrain system. You can use an approved booster seat until the middle of the child's head extends above the back seat of the car.

g. Play
  (1) Imaginative and pretend play peaks at this time. The child often projects misbehavior onto an inanimate object such as a doll or imaginary friend. Encourage the child to be curious and creative. Participate in imaginary play.
  (2) Teach songs and nursery rhymes and read to the child frequently.
  (3) Beginning to comprehend rules makes simple games and sports attractive to the child. Play with the child and begin to teach skills.
  (4) Toys appropriate for children this age include safe playground equipment, plastic sports equipment, riding toys, dolls and doll equipment, toy household and garden tools, dress-up clothes, more so-

phisticated books and puzzles, art supplies, building and construction toys (blocks, cardboard bricks, large Legos), toy instruments.
3. Health issues and concerns: fears
   a. The concern is that children at this developmental stage often exhibit new fears, which may seem unreasonable to parents and appear to have no relationship to reality. Common fears are of the dark, ghosts, being left alone, scary or large animals, loud noise, pain, bodily harm. Obtain information about the particular fear or fears of the child and what behaviors indicate that the child is afraid.
   b. The approach to childhood fears
      (1) Discuss with the child alternative ways to gain control (e.g., putting a light in the bedroom at night, covering ears or walking away from a loud noise, using doll-play to act out the fear without being directly involved).
      (2) Expose the child to the fearful situation gradually. Support the child, and extend the time of exposure as the child begins to feel comfortable.

Health Promotion for the School-Aged Child (ages 6–11 years)

1. For preventive care and health maintenance, see Table 15–4.
2. Anticipatory guidance and teaching parents
   a. Nutrition
      (1) The child needs 3 glasses of milk (low fat or skim) plus 1 serving of other dairy product, 4 to 6 ounces of protein, and 4 servings each of fruits, vegetables, and breads.
      (2) Increasing interest in and exposure to fast foods makes it necessary to be vigilant that the child obtains enough foods with high nutritional value.
      (3) Interest in cooking and preparing meals increases. Discuss principles of proper nutrition with the child and encourage the preparation of nutritiously adequate foods.
   b. Elimination
      (1) Bowel movements are regular according to the child's pattern. Constipated children should increase water intake and intake of fresh fruits and vegetables.
      (2) Occasional night bedwetting is still within the norm. Children with nocturnal enuresis can be helped by a variety of measures:
         • Decreasing fluid intake after supper.
         • Using an enuresis alarm, which awakens the child when urination begins.
         • Prescribing medication: If other measures are unsuccessful and the child experiences decreased self-esteem associated with the problem, the physician can prescribe DDAVP (Desmopressin), an inhaled antidiuretic that decreases urinary output.
   c. Dentition: Regular dental care every 6 months may include application of sealants to protect emerged molars. Continue fluoride supplements until the child is 14.
   d. Sleep: Most children adjust to a sleep pattern that is appropriate for them, with some requiring more sleep than others. Usually, school-aged children are in bed by 9 P.M. and are up by 7 A.M., but this varies, depending on the amount of homework required and the time that the school day (or before school care) starts. Allowing a quiet time before sleep for reading or listening to quiet music helps settle children.
   e. Hygiene
      (1) Resistance to baths and showers is frequently seen early in this stage. Many children are reluctant to take the time away from more interesting activities. It is not unusual to see a child in the same clothes every day, and persuading children to keep their rooms picked up is often unsuccessful.
      (2) Early reluctance to keep clean generally is followed by a period of overcleanliness. The child spends an inordinate amount of time in the bathroom showering and grooming, frustrating other family members. Parents should begin to prepare girls for menstruation by approximately 9 to 10 years old.
   f. Safety
      (1) Review bicycle safety, including the use of helmets, riding on the right side of the road, obeying traffic signals, using hand signals when turning, wearing light clothing, and using reflectors if riding at night.
      (2) Sports injuries are one of the most common sources of injury in children at this developmental level. Of the team sports, gymnastics, cheerleading, football, and basketball cause the most injury to children. Roller skating and skateboarding are the most dangerous of the individual sports, followed closely by bicycling. In addition to encouraging participation in nonorganized athletics, advise parents to examine closely any team sport in which their child is involved. They should look for the following:
         • Coaches with positive attitudes who emphasize skill development and teamwork, rather than winning at all costs
         • Proper division of children by size and maturation level rather than age
         • Correct use of protective and athletic equipment
         • Adherence to safety rules for the particular sport
         • Well-maintained facilities and equipment
         • A required preseason physical examination
         • Proper training of coaches in injury prevention and first aid
   g. Play: In addition to sports, children at this developmental stage enjoy collecting things, playing complicated board and card games, crafts, electronic games, and science-related games.
   h. Self-care: School-aged children can assume responsibility for self-care—bathing, dressing appropriately, keeping fit, not getting overtired, eating nutritious foods, following rules of safety, wearing appropriate protective equipment when participating in sports.

Positive reinforcement for appropriate choices increases the child's confidence and encourages the child to continue the behaviors.

3. Health issues and concerns: Antisocial behaviors
   a. The concern is that antisocial behaviors such as lying, cheating, and stealing (including shoplifting) are not uncommon during this developmental stage but cause parents grave concern. If the problem is minor, discussion with the child may be all that is needed. Obtain the following information:
      (1) Whether the child lies only to get out of a potentially embarrassing situation or to test limits, or whether the lying is becoming a pervasive part of the child's life
      (2) Whether the child is able to differentiate reality from fantasy
      (3) Whether the child is receiving conflicting messages from parents such as "do as I say, not as I do"
   b. The approach to antisocial behavior
      (1) Explore with the child the motivation for the behavior and discuss acceptable ways of avoiding the behavior in the future.
      (2) Never correct the child in front of others. Handle the situation privately and in a nonthreatening manner.
      (3) Insist that the child accept responsibility for the action and make restitution if needed.
      (4) Use logical consequences as discipline. Punishment should be directly related to the offense and should be no more severe.
      (5) Restrict privileges until the child is able to regain trust.
      (6) Refer children with repetitive or severe problems to a mental health counselor.

Health Promotion for the Adolescent

1. For preventive care and health maintenance, see Table 15–4.
2. Anticipatory guidance and teaching adolescents
   a. Nutrition
      (1) Average daily calorie requirements for adolescents range between 2100 and 2800 calories. Active adolescents require additional calories, with very active boys and girls requiring as many as 3000 to 3900 calories daily.
      (2) Emphasize sufficient calcium intake, especially for adolescent girls (to prevent osteoporosis later in life), and increased iron and vitamin intake.
      (3) Adolescents should eat at least 4 servings of milk or dairy products, 9 ounces of protein, and 4 or more servings each of fruits, vegetables, and breads. Foods high in empty calories should be avoided.
      (4) Encourage the adolescent to eat breakfast, even if it is a quick breakfast of an instant drink mixed with milk.
      (5) Many adolescents decide to reduce or eliminate meat from their diets. Adolescents who decide to maintain a vegetarian food program need appropriate nutritional assistance to ensure adequate intake of protein, iron, and other needed nutrients (see Chapter 10).
   b. Elimination: An adult pattern of elimination occurs in adolescents.
   c. Dentition: Encourage adolescents to brush regularly with fluoride toothpaste, to floss daily, and to be seen by a dentist every 6 months. Orthodontic work is often required to correct malocclusion.
   d. Sleep: Patterns vary according to individual need. Adolescents love to sleep late in the morning; they should be encouraged to be responsible for waking themselves in time to get to school.
   e. Hygiene
      (1) Adolescents take responsibility for self-care, cleanliness, and grooming. Emphasize the use of a deodorant and dandruff shampoo if necessary.
      (2) Skin: Adolescent skin is prone to acne caused by overactive sebaceous glands.
         • Advise the use of a mild skin cleanser at least twice a day followed by the application of a mild astringent and the avoidance of vigorous scrubbing of the face.
         • Treat more severe cases with benzoyl peroxide of various strengths, topical tretinoin (retinoic acid), or a topical erythromycin gel (both require a prescription).
         • Discourage squeezing of pustules or comedones.
         • Refer the adolescent to a physician if simple measures are unsuccessful. Systemic therapy with tetracycline or isotretinoin 13-*cis*-retinoic acid (Accutane) may be needed, especially if acne is severe and scarring is likely. Because of the risk for fetal deformities, if Accutane is prescribed for teenaged girls, a pregnancy test must be done before initiating the medication, and stringent precautions are necessary to avoid pregnancy during the treatment and up to 1 month after treatment ceases.
      (3) Menstruation
         • Prepare girls early (usually by 9–10 years) for their first menstruation. Discuss the process in familiar, understandable terms. Demonstrate the use of pads and show where they are kept.
         • Discuss the subtle signs that signal a period is due—breast tenderness, weight gain, increased acne, mild cramping, and feeling "down."
         • Teach the proper use and disposal of sanitary supplies.
         • Older adolescents (older than 15 years) may use tampons, but need instruction for insertion and care, especially the need to wash their hands thoroughly before and after inserting the tampon, change the tampon at least every 4 to 6 hours, depending on the heaviness of flow, and use a pad at night and on days of light flow.
   f. Safety
      (1) Review sports injury risks
      (2) Automobile safety becomes an important issue as adolescents learn to drive.

- Encourage teenagers to always wear safety restraints and to insist that others in the car do so as well.
- Explain the importance of traffic rules, especially those pertaining to speed and stopping at lights.
- Negotiate reasonable curfew times.

(3) Increasingly, school has become an unsafe place for adolescents. Some students bring weapons to school, either for self-defense or the desire to appear powerful.

- Teach adolescents appropriate ways of dealing with anger and threats.
- Enlist the help of school officials to provide crisis management and peer leadership and support.

g. Play: Adolescents participate in sophisticated intellectual games, as well as a wide variety of individual and team sports.

3. Health issues and concerns: Risk behaviors
   a. The concern is that some adolescents engage in a variety of risk behaviors—smoking, sexual intimacy, substance use and abuse. Obtain the following information:
      (1) Recent negative changes in mood; decreased participation in regular activities, activities with friends, or school work; evidence of decreased self-esteem.
      (2) Use of cigarettes, alcohol, drugs
      (3) Overt symptoms of drug or alcohol use (intoxication, experiencing a "high," hallucinations, depression)
      (4) Sexual activity and use of protective measures against sexually transmitted disease and pregnancy (see Chapter 14)
      (5) Deteriorating relationships with parents
   b. The approach to risk behaviors is to prevent them. The health care provider should do the following:
      (1) Discuss these issues at every well checkup.
      (2) Clarify reasons it is important to avoid risk behaviors.
      (3) Encourage development of a comprehensive health education program in the schools that deals with these issues and empowers adolescents to avoid risk behaviors.
      (4) Provide appropriate treatment for sexually transmitted diseases and substance abuse (see Chapters 29, 30, and 40).

■ *CARING FOR THE SICK OR HOSPITALIZED CHILD*

Transcultural Considerations

1. Ethnic background may influence susceptibility to diseases in a number of ways. Several disorders are associated with specific groups and related to identified risk factors:
   a. Environmental adaptation: for example, sickle cell disease in Blacks (hematologic adaptation to malaria)

b. Intermarriage: for example, congenital heart defects in the Amish, hemophilia in western Europeans
c. Ethnicity: for example, Tay-Sachs disease in Ashkenazic Jews
d. Race: for example, cystic fibrosis in Whites
e. Poverty: for example, fetal alcohol syndrome

2. Some serious health problems are associated with specific cultural groups.
   a. Native Americans
      (1) High infant mortality is related to illnesses, such as diarrhea, associated with poverty and decreased access to health care.
      (2) Socioeconomic conditions contribute to the high rates of fetal alcohol syndrome, child abuse, malnutrition, and anemia.
   b. Blacks
      (1) An extremely high neonatal death rate is possibly a result of inadequate prenatal care and poor socioeconomic conditions.
      (2) High incidence of sickle cell trait, hypertension, and anemia may have multiple causes.

3. Major ethnomedical beliefs about the causes of illness in infancy and childhood vary across cultures. Differences include imbalance in the body, disharmony with nature, soul loss, evil spirits, punishment for wrongdoing, hexes and curses, and germs.
   a. Native Americans
      (1) Violating tribal restrictions or disturbing nature generates punishment in the form of illness. Some tribes (e.g., Hopi) believe evil spirits cause disease.
      (2) Nursing implications
         - Accept conversational pauses by a child or family members as a sign of respect.
         - Allow extended family members to participate in the child's care. They may desire to consult with their healer, but the nurse should confirm that the treatment is not harmful to the child.
   b. Hispanic
      (1) Illness may be thought of as being caused by an imbalance between substances symbolically classified as hot and cold or wet and dry.
      (2) *Mal ojo,* or "evil eye," is usually caused by the envy of others. *Mal ojo* occurs in infants who are admired or complimented by others, without the counterbalance of touch (see Chapter 2). *Caida de la mollera* (sunken or fallen fontanel) can be caused by a touch to the infant's head or improper action of the midwife immediately after birth (see Chapter 2). "Soul loss," separation of the spirit from the body, results from fright (see Chapter 2).
      (3) Curative remedies are directed toward restoring balance.
      (4) Nursing implications
         - Use touch when admiring infants, but avoid touching the head.
         - *Do not use the child to translate for the parents.* Because of their inexperience and immaturity, children may provide incomplete or inaccurate information. Children should not be involved in adult decision making.
   c. Blacks

(1) Illness may be thought to result from possession by evil spirits, punishment from God, voodoo, or curses (see Chapter 2).

(2) Illness in children can be viewed as punishment from God for misdeeds by parents or others.

(3) Illness may be thought to be caused by disharmony with nature or separation of the body and the spirit.

(4) Nursing implications
- Because Blacks may perceive illness as being caused by forces outside their control, they may be less amenable to anticipatory guidance and more likely to seek treatment only when children are ill.
- Follow-up by community agencies helps ensure proper care.

d. Asians

(1) Illness may be thought to be caused by an imbalance in the body between the yin and the yang, and treatments often include a balance of hot and cold (see Chapter 2).

(2) Illness may be thought to be caused by improper exposure of the body to the elements.

(3) Use of "coining," "burning," "cupping," and "pinching" as treatments for pain can arouse suspicion of child abuse (Box 15–2).

(4) Nursing implications
- Undress infants slowly, one body part at a time, keeping the infant covered as much as possible.
- Avoid touching the heads of infants and children because some Asian cultures believe the head is the seat of the soul.

e. Whites

(1) Illness may be believed to be caused by germs, abuse of the body, and exposure to harmful agents.

(2) Some Whites believe illness is caused by violating religious prohibitions or regulations.

BOX 15–2. Culturally Determined Healing Methods

Healing methods practiced by certain cultures can be confused with child abuse if the nurse has never before encountered them. Common healing techniques include

Coining: Coins are rubbed on affected areas of the body. Used to treat pain or respiratory symptoms, coining leaves long bruises along the path of the rubbed coin.

Burning: A hot, burning tip of a piece of straw or grass is applied. Used to treat pain, burning leaves areas of burned skin approximately one quarter inch in diameter over affected body parts.

Cupping: A hot, round suction device is applied to draw out pain. Cupping is seen as approximately 2-inch diameter circular burn areas, usually on the chest or back.

Pinching: Pinch marks and small bruises are seen on any area of the body and may be in a specific pattern. Pinching is used to treat a variety of ailments.

Although these are considered acceptable practices in certain cultures, they are harmful to children and can be considered a form of abuse without intent. Advising the caregivers and any involved cultural practitioner of the physical, social, and legal problems inherent in these practices is essential for the protection of the child. Referral to a social service agency may be required.

---

(3) Depending on their level of development, children may view illness as being caused by external forces.

Responses to Hospitalization

1. Children react to hospitalization according to their developmental level (particularly cognitive), presence of supports, and consistency of care.

2. Depending on past exposure to hospitalization or to hospitalized relatives, the hospital may be viewed as a place one goes to die. Parental reaction in this instance might determine the reaction of the child. Often, it is difficult to discriminate causes of behavior, particularly in preverbal children, because the reactions are similar regardless of cause.

3. Being isolated from others in the hospital is an exceptionally frightening experience for a child. Often, gowns and masks are required, leading children to fantasize any number of negative possibilities about what is wrong with them and what is going to happen.

4. Infant responses
   a. Separation from parents
      (1) Protest: The infant screams, cries, actively searches for, or clings to the parent.
      (2) Despair: The infant appears withdrawn, sad, and disinterested and refuses to play.
      (3) Detachment: The infant appears content, plays quietly, no longer searches for parent, and ignores the parent when the parent is present.
   b. Fear: Often communicated to the infant by a fearful parent, fear causes the infant to react by crying, being irritable, refusing to eat, and not sleeping.
   c. Pain: Responses include facial grimacing, avoidance of painful stimulus, increased pulse, and batting at or poking the source of pain.
   d. Loss of control: Loss of control in the infant engenders anxiety and symptoms similar to those caused by separation anxiety.

5. Early childhood (toddler and preschooler) responses
   a. Separation anxiety
      (1) Reactions are similar to those in infants, but are possibly less intense because of object permanence. Tantrums, regression, and anger are not uncommon. The child may repeatedly ask why parents are not present but is somewhat reassured when told they will return.
      (2) Reactions are mitigated by previous separations from parents and by the ability to visualize parents when they are not there.
   b. Fear
      (1) The child may fear machines, strange people, the dark, and loud noises, and may have concerns about body integrity. Young children may demonstrate a negative reaction to any intrusive procedure or procedure that causes bleeding.
      (2) In addition to verbal expressions of fear, children may appear frightened and try actively to avoid the source of the fear. They may also cling to a parent or caregiver.

c. Pain
   (1) Children exhibit increased activity, whimpering, restlessness, crying, and active resistance (screaming, refusing to move, clenching teeth, hitting) in response to pain or the threat of pain.
   (2) Most young children are able verbally to express pain and can respond to pain assessment tools (e.g., pain faces, pain analog scales, color tools, poker chips), but, because they are not cognitively ready to serialize, the pain rating may not be entirely accurate.

d. Loss of control
   (1) Children may be upset by loss of autonomy and disruption of their usual routine.
   (2) Children may react with temper tantrums, resistance, regressive behavior (toileting accidents, thumb sucking, requesting a bottle), or negativism.

6. School-aged child responses
   a. Separation anxiety
      (1) The child often reacts with inappropriate behavior.
      (2) The child is less affected by separation from parents because relationships with peers have assumed increased importance. The child has developed a concept of events or time and can relate parental return to those events (e.g., after a television program, before dinner).
   b. Fear
      (1) Fears center on death or permanent disability, especially disfigurement, mutilation, and procedures affecting the genital area. The child may become frightened at seeing equipment.
      (2) The child is old enough to begin to understand illness causation but may confuse reality with perception of how illness occurred. The child may express guilt about not having done the right things to avoid getting sick.
   c. Pain
      (1) The school-aged child reacts like a younger child, although instead of actively resisting before pain starts, the child is likely verbally to express or demonstrate fear of pain (e.g., "How much will it hurt?" "Tell me what you're going to do." "Where is the needle?") and tries to postpone the inevitable ("I'm not ready yet," and "Can we do this another time instead?").
      (2) The child may want to watch what is being done.
   d. Loss of control
      (1) The child demonstrates helplessness and anger with the loss of independence in self-care and limits to usual activity.
      (2) The child may react with boredom, disinterest, frustration, anger at caregivers, refusal to cooperate with treatments, or depression.

7. Adolescent responses
   a. Separation anxiety: adolescents may be more concerned about separation from peers than parents, but they often like parents to be present during painful treatments or procedures.
   b. Fear
      (1) Adolescents may be most concerned about how illness limits usual activities and whether it will result in significant differences from peers. The

adolescent may be less concerned with the severity of an illness than its effect on appearance or function.
      (2) The adolescent may seek information about consequences of illness and about procedures or treatments required. Adolescents may refuse to cooperate with the treatment regimen if it is difficult to incorporate into their usual lifestyle.
   c. Pain
      (1) The adolescent is less likely to demonstrate anticipatory fear but exhibits muscle tightening along with slightly elevated pulse and blood pressure.
      (2) The adolescent is able to describe the degree of pain and what is needed to alleviate it.
   d. Loss of control
      (1) The adolescent may resist dependence, insist on independence, and actively seek information about what is to happen. Adolescents expect to be treated in an accepting manner.
      (2) The adolescent may attempt to exert control through negative behavior—playing loud music in inappropriate places or at inappropriate times or refusing to follow hospital regulations.
      (3) Adolescents often feel isolated and unable to obtain necessary support.

8. Family member responses
   a. Families experience anxiety about separation, extent of illness, length of course, and prognosis.
   b. Family members feel fear of an unfamiliar environment, the child's pain and discomfort, unfamiliar procedures and treatments, not obtaining accurate and complete information, what is happening at home, and financial difficulties.
   c. Families feel guilt about circumstances of the child's illness or injury and for not paying adequate attention to other family members.
   d. Families experience loss of control when they turn over a child's care to others, they are not able to plan activities except around the ill child's needs, they do not have time together, there is job interruption, and they are waiting for information.
   e. The reaction of family members depends on the effectiveness of usual coping strategies, sociocultural environment, availability of support, seriousness of the illness and its prognosis, willingness of the hospital staff to be honest and communicative, and any prior experiences with illness or hospitalization.

Administering Interventions in the Hospital

1. Communicating with the hospitalized child is similar to communicating with a child who is well (see pp. 474–475). Use of touch (hug, cuddle, rock) should be more liberal, particularly if parents are not present. Explain the treatments or procedures using developmentally appropriate and nonthreatening terminology.
   a. Avoid words such as cut, dye, fix, test, and repair, and complicated medical terminology.
   b. Try to describe what the child will experience, and

relate it to experiences already in the child's repertoire (e.g., "This will feel cold, like ice cream.")

c. Time the explanations about procedures or surgery according to the child's developmental level.

(1) Infant
  - Talk to parents before the procedure and allow for questions.
  - Talk to infants soothingly throughout the procedure, using pain descriptors (ouch, owie, boo-boo) immediately before pain is felt. Comfort the infant afterward.

(2) Early childhood (toddler and preschooler)
  - Talk to parents before the procedure; time explanations to the child as close to the procedure as possible, using simple, descriptive statements and pointing to the part of the body that is affected.
  - If possible, permit the child to handle equipment and to use it on a doll or stuffed animal. Allow the child to keep a security object close by during the procedure.
  - Distract the child with a story, song, or fantasy play. Comfort the child afterward.

(3) School-aged child
  - Describe to the child and parents what will happen before the procedure, showing them the equipment to be used and answering any questions they might have.
  - Explain what the child can do to help make the procedure easier.
  - Provide a measure of control needed by children of this age. Praise the child afterward for cooperation.

(4) Adolescent
  - Explain the procedure in as much detail as the adolescent wishes, focusing on why the procedure is necessary, what will be experienced, how long it will take, and what can be expected afterward.
  - Encourage questions and verify understanding, provide comfort afterward, and encourage verbalization of feelings.

2. Restraints should be used judiciously in the hospital setting because they restrict movement and independence, cause frustration, and may generate more harm than good.

a. Use creative approaches, such as movement play or distraction, to enlist the cooperation of an active child to maintain bed rest or position in bed. Use a crib with a net or plastic bubble to prevent infants from climbing out. A jacket-type restraint can be used for older children, but it can be dangerous if the child is very active in bed.

b. Use restraints only as a final option, after first attempting to enlist the child's cooperation with an imposed restriction. Physically restraining a child for any length of time exacerbates feelings of helplessness and loss of control.

c. Restraints can be used under the following circumstances:

(1) To maintain the position of a precarious intravenous access

(2) To keep the child from removing tubes or dressings or to prevent self-injury (e.g., disturbing an operative site or scratching excoriated skin)

(3) To prevent falls or free access to dangerous items in the environment

d. Types of restraints used with children

(1) A mummy restraint is used to restrain an infant or small child during short procedures to the head or upper body.

(2) Modified mummy restraint (Fig. 15-5) is used to

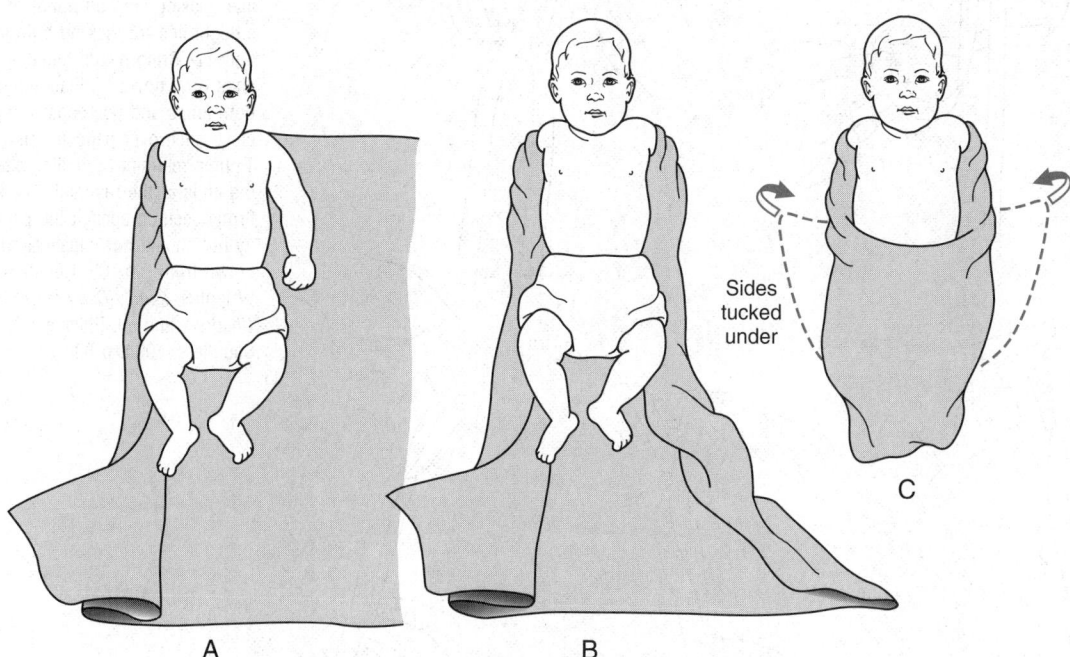

Figure 15-5. Modified mummy restraint. *A,* One side of the blanket is tucked snugly around the arm so that the child is lying on the edge of the blanket. *B,* The other arm is similarly restrained. *C,* The lower edge of the blanket is brought up and tucked under the child. (Redrawn from Betz CL, Hunsberger M, and Wright S. *Family-Centered Nursing Care of Children,* 2nd ed. Philadelphia: WB Saunders, 1994, p 828.)

examine the upper chest with arms secured. The child is placed on a blanket as for the mummy restraint. The first corner is brought over the nearest arm and under the body, and the same is done with the other corner. The lower half of the child is covered with the bottom corner.

(3) A clove-hitch restraint (Fig. 15–6) is used to restrain an arm or leg. Flexible gauze or stockinet is used in a width appropriate to the child's size and of sufficient length to secure to a crib or bed frame.

(4) An elbow restraint (Fig. 15–7) is used to prevent children from reaching up to their face or head. Commercial elbow restraints are available or they can be made out of cardboard tubing of appropriate diameter.

e. Check restraints closely every 1 to 2 hours and release at least every 2 hours. Evaluate the circulatory status and correct the application of the restraint. Be sure to remove restraints when observing the child or when the parent is with the child to give the child the opportunity to play or move about.

f. Positioning the child carefully for certain procedures and treatments protects the child from undue injury and provides a sense of security (see Procedure 15–1).

NURSE ADVISORY

Gloves are to be worn to assist with all procedures involving blood or body fluid exposure.

3. Specimen collection in children is similar to that in adults, with the following modifications:

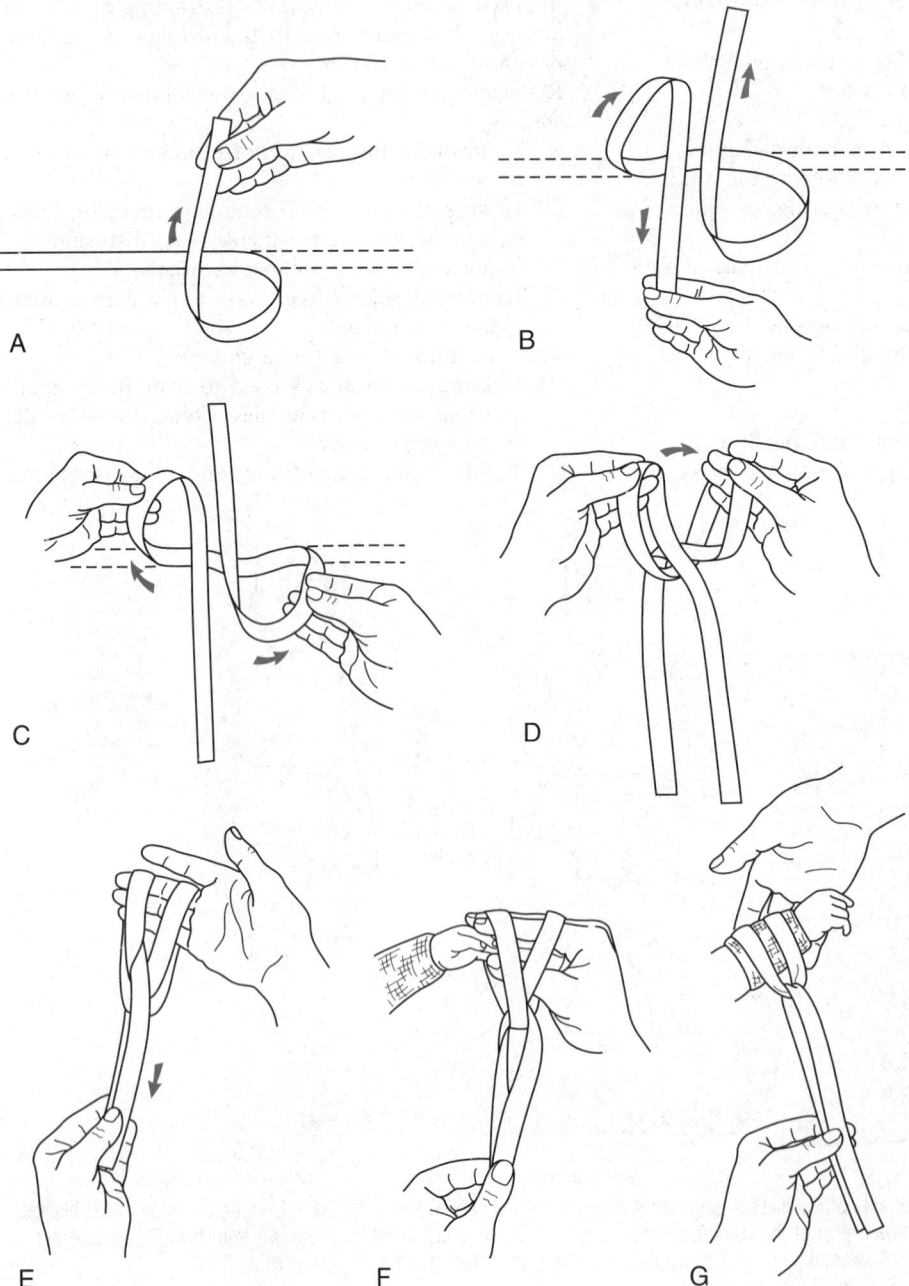

Figure 15–6. Clove hitch restraint. *A,* Lay or hold restraint in a straight line. Make a loop by bringing 1 end across straight line. *B,* Bring other end across straight line, making loop on opposite side of straight line. *C,* Pick up both loops at once. *D,* Bring hands together and let ends drop down. *E,* Place fingers through both loops and pull ends firmly. *F,* Slip clove hitch over padded wrist or ankle. *G,* Tighten restraint by pulling alternately on the ends of the restraint. The knot is firmly secured against the padded extremity but should not impair circulation. (Redrawn from Betz CL, Hunsberger M, and Wright S. *Family-Centered Nursing Care of Children,* 2nd ed. Philadelphia: WB Saunders, 1994, p 830.)

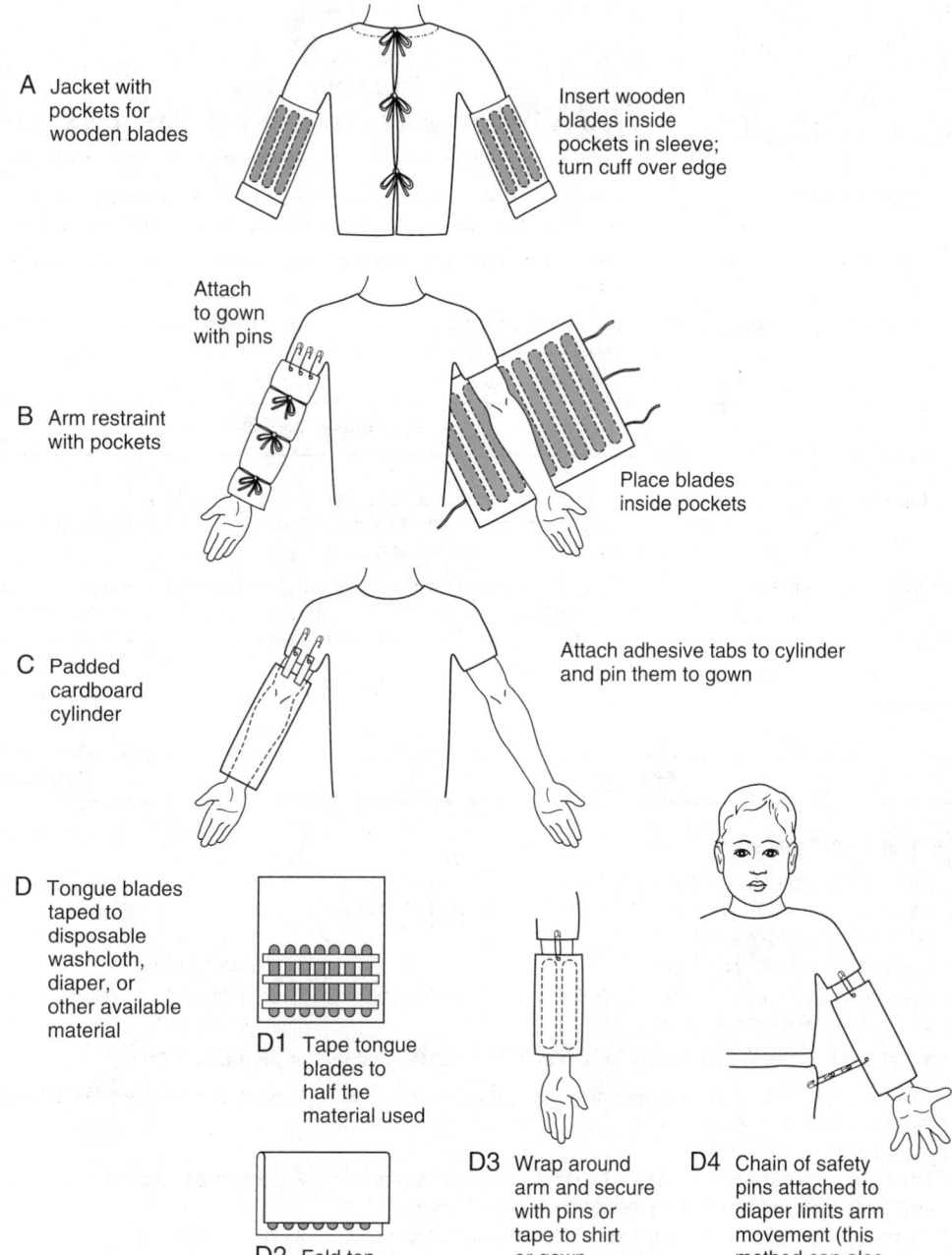

Figure 15–7. Elbow restraints. (Redrawn from Betz CL, Hunsberger M, and Wright S. *Family-Centered Nursing Care of Children*, 2nd ed. Philadelphia: WB Saunders, 1994, p 829.)

A Jacket with pockets for wooden blades

Insert wooden blades inside pockets in sleeve; turn cuff over edge

Attach to gown with pins

B Arm restraint with pockets

Place blades inside pockets

C Padded cardboard cylinder

Attach adhesive tabs to cylinder and pin them to gown

D Tongue blades taped to disposable washcloth, diaper, or other available material

D1 Tape tongue blades to half the material used

D2 Fold top over

D3 Wrap around arm and secure with pins or tape to shirt or gown

D4 Chain of safety pins attached to diaper limits arm movement (this method can also be used for A, B, and C)

a. Urine collection in untrained children
 (1) Aspirate urine directly from a wet diaper or from gauze placed in the diaper, using a 3-ml syringe with no needle. Enough urine can be obtained for routine urinalysis or specific gravity tests.
 (2) Apply a urine collector device (Procedure 15–2).
 (3) For clean-catch urine for culture in the untrained child, do the following:
  • Wash the perineal area as for an adult or older child and apply a sterile urine collector.
  • After removing the bag, peel back the plastic tab and let urine flow into a sterile cup. Refrigerate the specimen if transport to the laboratory will be longer than 30 minutes. If the collecting bag has no tab, insert a sterile needle into the bag to create an opening.

b. Urine collection in toilet-trained children

NURSE ADVISORY

It is not necessary to apply a urine-collecting device to monitor urinary output. Weigh a dry diaper, then weigh the child's wet diaper and compute the difference. The weight difference in grams is equal to the amount of urine (in ml) voided. (Or, the weight difference in ounces converted to ml is the amount voided.)

Procedure 15–1
Positioning for Venipuncture and Other Tests

Definition/Purpose	To position a child safely for a painful procedure so that the child is protected from harm, the procedure can be done more easily and quickly, and the child is not emotionally traumatized.
Contraindications/Cautions	If the child is very large or strong or uncooperative, more than 1 person may be needed to position the child properly.
Learning/Teaching Activities	Tell children who are old enough to understand what is going to be done. Enlist their cooperation if possible. Explain why the procedure is necessary.

Preliminary Activities

Equipment	• Only the equipment needed for the specific procedure • Colorful adhesive bandages that the child can hold during a venipuncture often help the child cooperate. Allow the child to choose the design.
Assessment/Planning	• Enlist the assistance of the child's caregiver if possible to distract the child during the procedure. • Plan an interesting activity for the child to immediately follow the procedure. • Tell the child and caregiver what they can do to help and approximately how long it will be necessary to stay in the same position.

Procedure

Action	Rationale/Discussion
Peripheral Venipuncture	
1. With child lying supine, place arm over the upper part of the unaffected arm and under child's neck in a "hug" position, grasping the upper portion of the unaffected arm.	1. Helps stabilize the child; helps the child feel secure.
2. Hold child's hand with your opposite hand.	2. Stabilizes the site.
3. Warn the child when the needle is to be inserted and ask the child to take a deep breath (sing, say "ow")	3. Gives the child advanced warning to be still; distracts the child during the painful part.
Femoral Venipuncture, Suprapubic Urine Aspiration, or Procedures on the Genital Area	
1. With child lying supine, stand at the child's head. Reach down across the child's arms and secure legs into "frog" position. The child will be looking at you "upside down."	1. Gives young children the feeling of security; stabilizes the site.
2. Make sure the child's genital area is covered appropriately, unless this area needs to be exposed for the procedure (e.g., circumcision).	2. Protects the child's privacy.
3. To stabilize the child's position further, release the unaffected leg and place both hands on the affected leg.	3. Stabilizes the site.
Lumbar Puncture	
1. Infant or child—place the child in a side-lying position with spine close to edge of table or bed.	1. Allows for proper visibility of the lumbar spinal spaces.
2. Wrap 1 arm over the child's neck and the other over the back of the child's knees. Bring both arms close, bending the child so that the spinal area is curved.	2. Stabilizes the child in position and prevents straightening of the spine.
3. Talk soothingly to the child and explain in advance what is to happen.	3. Reassures the child; this position can be frightening for the child because the face is hidden and the child might feel that it is difficult to breathe.
4. Alternate position for the infant—sit infant with buttocks close to table edge, head toward you. This position automatically curves the spinal area. Hold the infant in sitting position by placing hands on sides of thighs and thumbs on back.	4. Small infants are more easily held this way.
Bone Marrow Aspiration	
1. Place the child prone with small pillow under hips to elevate the iliac crest.	1. Bone marrow is taken from the posterior iliac crest area, not the sternum, in most children.

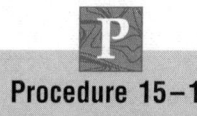

Procedure 15–1

(continued)

Action	Rationale/Discussion
2. Immobilize the child by placing arms over midback and upper thighs. Enlist another person's assistance if possible.	2. Immobilization is more successful when there are 2 people—1 to restrain the upper and 1 the lower parts of the child.
3. Describe each step and explain how it will feel (e.g., iodine feels cold and wet, "pop" and sharp ouch as needle enters the marrow).	3. Prepares the child for what is to come and enhances control.

Final Activities

- Comfort the child and apply the selected Band-aid.
- Involve the child in an enjoyable activity, even if the child needs to remain flat after the procedure.
- Label the specimens properly and send them to the appropriate location for testing.

(1) Recently trained or young children can use a "potty chair" for providing a urine sample. Use words with which the child is familiar to describe what the child should do (e.g., "tinkle," "pee").

(2) A commercially made fitted plastic container that is placed in the toilet under the seat is often more acceptable than a bedpan for collecting urine for the older child.

c. Stool collection for an older child is conducted as it is for an adult. In the untrained child, a small sample of stool is scraped from the diaper with a sterile tongue depressor. The sample is placed in a sterile container for culture, determination of parasitic organisms, or test for occult blood.

4. Measure vital signs in the hospitalized child using the same principles as for a well child (see Table 15–2).

5. Fever control

a. Recent evidence suggests that low to moderate fever enhances the function of the immune system during disease.

b. Treat fever only if it is more than 39 degrees Celsius (102 degrees Fahrenheit), if there is a history of febrile convulsion, or if the fever causes the child discomfort, such as chills, flushing, headache, shivering, or inability to sleep.

c. Administer acetaminophen or ibuprofen in appropriate dosage.

d. Encourage oral fluid intake, particularly cool liquids.

e. Lighten the weight of clothing and apply cool compresses to the forehead at least 30 minutes after administering antipyretics, if the child remains particularly uncomfortable.

f. Do not sponge the child unless the temperature is more than 40 degrees Celsius (104 degrees Fahrenheit) thirty minutes after receiving antipyretic medication. Sponging is done with lukewarm water, one area at a time.

g. Avoid giving aspirin or aspirin-containing medications to children with a febrile illness because of its association with Reye syndrome.

6. Nutrition and feeding

a. Oral feedings

(1) Infant feeding

- Facilitate continuation of breast-feeding in the hospital if at all possible. If the mother is unable to be present, she should be encouraged to pump breast milk, which can be frozen and bottle fed to the infant.
- Follow a bottle-fed infant's usual feeding schedule using the same formula as is used at home.
- Use bottle-feeding technique for the 2-week old infant (see p. 494).
- Obtain information about what solids the infant tolerates and continue feedings with these. Do not introduce new foods to the hospitalized infant, unless the infant is hospitalized for an extended period.

(2) Feeding young children

- Make mealtimes as pleasant as possible for young hospitalized children. Using decorated tableware and allowing them to sit at small tables and chairs with other children normalizes mealtimes.
- Assist bed-ridden children to access the tray.
- Serve small portions and encourage parents to bring favorite foods from home if they are permitted in the child's diet.
- Cut all food into size-appropriate pieces for the child's age and open containers.

b. Gavage and gastrostomy feedings

Procedure 15–2
Applying a Urine-Collecting Device

Definition/Purpose	To obtain a urine sample from an untrained child. To collect urine for 24 hours. To monitor urinary output in the untrained child.
Contraindications/Cautions	Careful monitoring of the device is essential because the bag loosens from the skin easily when the area is moist. For a single urine collection, remove the bag immediately; otherwise, the bag will leak, and the specimen will be lost. Repeated application and removal of a bag can cause skin irritation. To protect the skin from repeated irritation, apply a skin protector such as tincture of benzoin with a cotton applicator before placing the bag.
Learning/Teaching Activities	If the parent or caregiver is with the child, emphasize the importance of quickly reporting any voiding.

Preliminary Activities

Equipment	• Plastic collection bag with adhesive backing. Use sterile pouch for clean-catch urine. Use pouch with tubing for 24-hour collection. • Face cloth, mild soap, water, towel • Tincture of benzoin for 24-hour collection • Disposable diaper • Sterile urine-collecting cup for clean-catch specimen
Assessment/Planning	• Plan to observe child closely if parent or caregiver is not present. • Know and explain to the caregiver why the specimen is necessary.

Procedure

Actions	Rationale/Discussion
1. Lay infant or child supine.	1. Allows for visibility of the site.
2. Wash own hands, then child's perineal area with mild soap and water. Rinse and dry thoroughly.	2. Collecting device will not adhere to a moist surface or a surface that has been powdered or had ointment applied.
3. When area is dry, place bag opening over the urinary meatus. Peel backing off the lower part of the pouch and apply bottom tabs to the child's perineal area. Pull perineal skin in girls slightly taut while sealing the remainder of the bag. If 24-hour collection is desired, apply tincture of benzoin to the perineal area before applying the pouch and allow to dry until tacky. For boys, insert the penis into the pouch opening before sealing (penis and scrotum of very small infants).	3. It is essential to obtain a tight seal to avoid losing the specimen. Tightening the perineal skin while applying the bag reduces traction on the bag after sealing.
4. Poke a small opening in the front of the disposable diaper. Insert the bottom part of the collecting device through the opening. Cuddle the child upright or place in an infant seat.	4. Allows for accurate monitoring of voiding. Timing removal of the pouch as quickly as possible after voiding prevents loss of the specimen or contamination of the bag. Placing in a semiupright position facilitates downward flow of urine into the bag.
5. Remove the pouch and pour urine into appropriate specimen container. Label the container.	5. Proper collection and labeling of specimen is essential for accurate results.

Final Activities

• Replace the child's diaper with a clean one.
• Send labeled specimen to the appropriate location.
• Refrigerate any urine for culture and sensitivity if transport to the laboratory will be longer than 30 minutes.

(1) Children not able to take oral nourishment may require tube feedings.
   • Either insert a gavage tube intermittently or leave it in place, depending on the child's age and comfort level and whether feeding is intermittent or continuous (see Chapters 10 and 27). When inserting a gavage tube, mummy-wrap infants and young children before insertion.

- The type of gastrostomy tube chosen by the surgeon should reflect the child's developmental level and level of activity.
- Use a pump to control the amount and speed of gastrostomy feedings.
  (2) Infants who are being tube fed should be given a pacifier during the feeding to meet sucking needs usually gained through oral feedings.
  (3) Cuddle the infant or young child during the feeding to simulate normal feeding position. The infant should be burped when feeding is complete and placed on the right side to enhance gastric emptying.
7. Fluid and electrolyte balance
  a. Encouraging or restricting oral fluid intake can be a problem in children because their cognitive level often limits comprehension of the reasons for fluid management. Always explain to the child and family the rationale for the approach, and enlist cooperation wherever possible.
    (1) Encouraging fluid intake
    - Choose fluids that the child likes and administer according to the child's usual method (bottle, cup, straw). Administering fluids in solid (gelatin) or frozen form provides a change and makes it more interesting for the child.
    - Give fluids in small, frequent amounts (1–2 oz/hour), rather than in a large amount all at once to increase compliance and decrease the risk of vomiting in an ill child.
    - Arrange a time schedule with the older child for taking fluids (e.g., at each television commercial or before and after certain activities).
    (2) Limiting oral fluids often is more difficult than encouraging them because meticulous cooperation from child and family members is required.
    - Place only the allowed amount of fluid in a bottle or cup to prevent inadvertent intake.
    - Keep all other fluid out of the child's reach and place a sign on the child's bed indicating that fluid restriction is necessary.
    - Include the older child in the planning for fluid intake. Allow the child to choose the type of fluid desired (within dietary restrictions) and the schedule. Provide the fluid promptly at the agreed-on time, and give the child positive reinforcement for following the established schedule.
    - Administer meticulous mouth care to keep mucous membranes moist.
  b. Administering intravenous fluids
    (1) Choose the site that allows the most mobility. The dorsum of the hand or foot is the preferred site for infants. Scalp veins can be used if other areas are inaccessible. The forearm of the nondominant arm is best for older children.
    (2) Select an appropriate-sized needle or catheter. Number 23 or 25 gauge needles are often used for infant intravenous access. Over-the-needle catheters (22 or 24 gauge) provide a more stable intravenous access for older children. Surgical

cutdowns may be necessary for infants with precarious veins.
    (3) Attach solution as ordered. The usual solutions used for children combine dextrose (5–10%) and saline (0.45 or 0.225).
    - Use a pediatric burette that delivers fluid at 60 drops per ml. The number of drops per minute equals the number of ml per hour.
    - Tubing should be clamped between solution container and burette to prevent inadvertent overadministration of fluid. Keep the flow rate clamp out of the child's reach.
    - Use an infusion pump when administering small amounts of fluid hourly. Continue to monitor the infusion as usual.
    (4) Prepare the child and family adequately for intravenous line insertion. Explain that the site will be uncomfortable for only a little while and that the important thing that the child can do to help is to remain still. Use previously discussed distraction techniques during insertion and removal.
    (5) Secure the needle or catheter adequately, using clear plastic tape (Op-Site or Tegaderm) for better visualization of the site. If a board is required for protection of the site, pad it before use. Restrain the child only as a last resort, and release restraints frequently to cuddle the child and allow for mobility.
    (6) Maintain and monitor the intravenous line as you would for an adult, and observe for complications.
  c. Administering total parenteral nutrition (TPN)
    (1) Parenteral nutrition solutions, which contain carbohydrates, amino acids, fats, electrolytes, and other nutrients, support the child's nutritional status under conditions in which absorption through the gastrointestinal tract is limited or when the child's metabolic needs are greatly increased.
    (2) Because parenteral nutrition solutions are highly concentrated and the young child's fluid and metabolic status is more precarious than an adult's, careful monitoring is necessary. Observe for signs of hypoglycemia, hyperglycemia, and electrolyte imbalance.
    (3) Access
    - Peripheral veins are less tolerant of the increased osmolarity of the TPN solution than are the large central veins. If the peripheral vein is used, solution osmolarity should be decreased.
    - Usual placement of a central venous catheter in children is through cutdown into the subclavian or jugular vein and advancement to the junction of the superior vena cava and right atrium.
    - Infusion ports are often used in older children, although the repeated puncturing of the skin to gain access to the port can be uncomfortable. Use of Emla cream 1 hour before access reduces discomfort.
    - Peripherally inserted central catheters (PICC) are being used more frequently in children. Ad-

vantages include surgical placement not necessary, low incidence of complications, and fewer activity restrictions (some children are able to play sports).

(4) Infusion
- Infuse solution intermittently or continuously according to physician direction. Use an infusion pump.
- Monitor the child's tolerance to the concentrations of glucose, fat, and protein while concentrations are being gradually increased.

(5) Maintain the central venous access site according to institution policy for preventing infection and observe for complications as you would for adults (see Chapter 8).

(6) Planning for discharge
- If treatment is to be continued after discharge, teach the caregiver all aspects of care and signs of sepsis. Describe whom to contact and what action to take for mechanical complications (e.g., occlusion, dislodging of the catheter).
- Advise the child to participate in normal, developmentally appropriate activities, but to avoid swimming and contact sports.

8. Administering oxygen
a. Assessment of oxygen status in the child is similar to that in the adult (see Chapter 22). The least invasive method for assessing adequate gas exchange in the child is through pulse oximetry.

(1) Pulse oximetry directly monitors oxygen saturation of the blood using a light probe that measures absorption of light by oxyhemoglobin. The probe is attached to a finger, a toe, or an earlobe and provides continuous or intermittent monitoring of oxygen saturation. The child must remain relatively still while being monitored because the probe measures pulsating light waves (arterial pulses) and extraneous motion confuses the equipment.
- Do not use the same extremity for periodic blood pressure measurements because the constriction of the cuff interferes with peripheral perfusion.
- Use pulse oximetry with caution in premature infants and not at all in children with severe anemia or carbon monoxide poisoning because there may be false or misleading readings.

(2) Another noninvasive monitoring device is the transcutaneous oxygen monitor, which measures oxygen pressure in superficial capillaries. The probe is applied to the skin (usually thorax or abdominal) and set to an ordered temperature. The heat dilates the capillaries, diffusing oxygen molecules across the probe membrane to be measured.
- For continuous measurement, change the probe site every 2 to 4 hours to prevent burning.
- Recalibrate the temperature after each change.

b. Choose the oxygen delivery method according to the condition and developmental level of the child.

(1) Isolette is used for infants who need varying amounts of oxygen and temperature control; it can deliver lower oxygen-flow rates than the Oxy-Hood, but with limited access for care.
- Organize care so that port holes are opened only briefly to avoid loss of oxygen.
- Carefully monitor the ambient temperature.
- Monitor the oxygen concentration frequently.
- While administering care, provide as much tactile stimulation as possible to the infant.

(2) The Oxy-Hood, a clear, plastic hood that covers the infant's head from the neck up, is used for infants. The Oxy-Hood delivers oxygen and mist at least 4 to 5 liters per minute. It restricts access to the infant's head but allows for continuing procedures and treatments not involving the head.
- Frequently monitor oxygen concentration.
- Keep condensation from collecting in the administration tubing.

(3) The nasal cannula (Fig. 15–8) administers oxygen at a flow of 1 to 4 liters per minute (22–40%) for infants and children of all ages. The nasal cannula allows for unrestricted movement during continuous oxygen administration.
- Monitor oxygenation because oxygen concentration cannot be accurately determined.
- Provide frequent mouth care and care of the nares.
- Encourage children to leave the cannula in place.
- To protect the child's skin during continuous administration, patches of stoma adhesive should be applied to the sides of the face and the cannula should be taped to the stoma adhesive.

(4) A mist tent is used primarily for infants and children with croup and delivers cool mist but administers oxygen simultaneously, if required. Mist tents can be frightening to young children

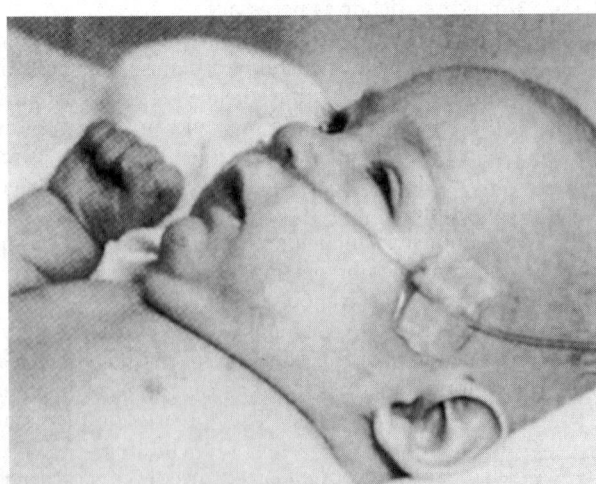

Figure 15–8. Nasal cannula for continuous low-flow oxygen therapy. The cannula is positioned on the philtrum without entering the nares. (From Koops BL, et al. Outpatient management and follow-up of bronchopulmonary dysplasia. *Clin Perinatol* 11(1):101–122, 1984.)

because they create a mechanical barrier between them and others.

- Measure oxygen concentration frequently. Oxygen should flow at a rate of at least 6 liters per minute. Keep unmelted ice in the cooling compartment.
- Tuck the sides of the tent under the mattress tightly; secure the bottom over the older child's legs with a sheet folded over the plastic canopy. *Be sure to raise the side rails of the bed or crib after tucking in the tent.*
- Allow the child to have nonstatic toys in the tent. Encourage parent to be present as much as possible and to reach under the side of the tent to touch and comfort the child.
- Change the child's clothes and bedding frequently because excess moisture can cause chilling.
- Help young children respond better to being in the tent by treating the experience as a game or an exciting pretend adventure. (The tent could be a camp site, pirate ship, space capsule, or whatever the child imagines.)

  (5) An oxygen mask may be used for children but is the most threatening method for delivering oxygen because children feel suffocated. The mask effectively delivers medium to high concentrations of oxygen when temporary, short-term delivery is required.

c. Observe all the usual precautions associated with oxygen therapy. Monitor for complications.

9. For the child in a cast principles of care are similar to those for an adult. Check for comfort, adequate circulation distal to the cast, and signs of complications. The following adaptations are appropriate:

a. Ensuring safety

  (1) Keep all small toys and objects out of the child's reach. The temptation to insert things under the cast is strong if the child is itchy. Using an ice pack over the site of pruritus helps.

  (2) Keep bed rails up because even older children can lose balance while in a cast if they are not accustomed to the additional weight.

  (3) Cover the cast while the child eats to prevent food from lodging under the edges.

b. Meeting developmental needs

  (1) Encourage the child to use unaffected extremities by providing developmentally appropriate toys that require movement (e.g., infant mobiles, bean bag, Nerf ball)

  (2) Once the cast is fully dry, encourage self-care activities.

  (3) Adapt clothing to accommodate the cast. If the child wishes, allow the child or the child's friends to decorate the cast after it is completely dry.

  (4) Explain to the child the sensations experienced with cast removal (e.g., noise of the cutter, heat, vibration), and reassure the child that the cast cutter will not cut the skin. Prepare the child and family for the appearance of the affected limb after removal of the cast.

c. Caring for the child in a hip spica cast

  (1) Before discharge, teach parents how to modify the environment and adapt activities to meet the child's needs, and assist them to obtain any needed equipment for home care.

  (2) Cleanliness

- Protect the cast opening from soiling by inserting sheets of plastic under the cast edges and taping them to the outside of the cast. Change the plastic as needed. Insert sanitary pads or peripads under the plastic and cover the area with a disposable diaper. Some physicians line spica casts with a waterproof liner such as Gore-Tex to prevent moisture from causing skin breakdown.
- Keep an extra-absorbent diaper on an untrained child, and change it immediately if soiled. If the cast is too large for the diaper, keep the diaper in place with a diaper cover with Velcro closures.
- Assist the older child with elimination, to ensure the cast is protected properly.

  (3) Safety

- Turn the child every 2 hours. Do not use the crossbar for turning. Move the child close to you, tell the child when you are going to make the turn ("When I count to three"), lift the cast, and turn away from you.
- Restrain the active, noncompliant child with a wide folded draw sheet secured over the cast. Observe frequently to be sure that the child does not slip down under the restraint.
- Advise the parent to modify the child's car seat to accommodate the cast.

  (4) Feeding

- Support the infant in an elevated position, either in a modified infant seat or high chair or in your lap with a pillow under the cast.
- Allow older children to eat in the prone position if they prefer.

  (5) Development

- Change the child's immediate environment frequently. Carry the infant or child into another room, or move the older child's bed. Some older children prefer to propel themselves into new locations using a low, flat, scooter board.
- Provide developmentally appropriate toys and activities, particularly those that promote muscle motion of the upper extremities.

10. For the child in traction, the principles of management are similar to those for managing a child in a cast but with the following additions:

a. Monitor the child for circulatory compromise, complications of immobility, and signs of infection at pin sites. (Protocol for caring for pin sites varies with the institution.)

b. Safety

  (1) Positioning: because a child weighs much less than an adult, countertraction becomes a problem (children slide easily toward the end of the bed). Reposition the younger child frequently,

and remind the older child to use the overhead trapeze to pull back in the bed. Marking the side-rail with tape indicates the correct position in the bed.

(2) Put the active child in a jacket restraint to maintain position or prevent the child from reaching too far.

(3) If ordered, rewrap elastic bandages on skin traction with a 2nd person holding the traction tapes to prevent slippage.

(4) Check the traction apparatus frequently for proper weight, alignment of ropes on the pulleys, and that weights are off the floor.

c. Types of traction
(1) Skin traction is applied to the skin of the extremity using adhesive traction tapes kept in place with elastic bandage wraps.
  • Bryant traction is used mainly for children younger than 2 years old and is used with caution because of the danger of circulatory compromise. Hips are flexed at a 90-degree angle with both legs straight up.
  • Bucks extension is used in older children, usually for short-term immobilization. Legs are extended straight out.
  • Russell traction is positioned with the leg extended and a sling under the affected knee to elevate the leg.
(2) Skeletal traction is exerted on the affected limb by being attached to pins or wires, which have been secured to bone.
  • A 90-90 traction is used mainly for immobilizing a fractured femur. The hip and knee are flexed at a 90-degree angle, and the lower leg is supported by a sling or is casted.
  • Balance suspension is similar to adult traction.

11. Preparing the child for surgery
a. As much as is possible, surgical intervention for children is provided in an ambulatory surgical setting, where the child's preoperative examination is performed by the pediatrician, the child is admitted directly to the day surgery unit, and the child is discharged to home when stable.
b. Nurse's role in preoperative preparation
(1) Describe what will happen in advance of the surgical procedure and allow time for questions, role-playing, or doll play. Show pictures or diagrams whenever possible and use terminology appropriate for the child's cognitive, not necessarily the chronologic, level (see Learning/Teaching Guidelines for Children Undergoing Surgery).
(2) Provide a visit to the operating room area and recovery room to familiarize the child with the facilities. Many hospitals conduct group tours for children having elective surgical procedures.
(3) Orient the child to the surgical waiting room and recovery room if surgery is planned and demonstrate use of equipment, including masks. Explain what the child will feel like after surgery and where the child will go.

12. Caring for the child after surgery

a. Care of the child after surgery is similar in principle to care of the postoperative adult (see Chapter 13).
b. Modifications for children include the following:
(1) Controlling pain: patient-controlled anesthesia or postsurgical epidural analgesia must be calibrated carefully to meet the needs of the specific child. Oxygen saturations should be conducted, along with hourly respirations for the time that the child is receiving the medications.
(2) Preventing respiratory complications: Some children are reluctant to use incentive spirometers or are cognitively unable to understand their use. Other creative ways of promoting adequate inhalations include blowing bubbles, blowing a ping-pong ball through a straw, or blowing a party favor.
(3) Therapeutic play: Encouraging therapeutic play releases emotions through drawing, writing, and puppet play. Remind the child of activities practiced during preoperative teaching.

Administering Medications to Children

1. Immature body systems in infants and children younger than 2 years old affect the absorption, use, and excretion of drugs. Calibrate dosages and timing of medication administration carefully to avoid complications.
2. Absorption
a. Gastrointestinal tract immaturity delays absorption of orally administered medication for the following reasons:
(1) Drugs take longer to transit the upper gastrointestinal tract and reach the small intestine where most absorption occurs.
(2) Decreased acidity of the gastric contents causes delayed absorption of medications that require an acid environment for optimal absorption.
b. Absorption of parenteral medications depends on adequate perfusion to the muscle or subcutaneous tissue. In young infants with decreased muscle and subcutaneous tissue, absorption can be delayed.
c. Body fluid distribution
(1) Distribution of body fluids affects absorption because the percentage of total body fluid in a neonate or young infant is higher than in an older child or adult.
(2) Dosages based on weight are more dilute in children younger than 2 years old because they have a larger percentage of body fluid in relation to weight.
3. Biotransformation
a. Increased metabolic rate (and subsequently increased drug metabolism) in young children eliminates the medication from the body more rapidly than in the older child or adult. Therefore higher dosages are needed for the same effect.
b. Differences between children and adults in concentration and type of plasma proteins necessary for binding certain drugs results in inconsistent distribution of the drug in the body.

LEARNING/TEACHING GUIDELINES
for Children Undergoing Surgery

General Overview

1. Review with the child and family what they understand about the surgery, its necessity, goals, and expected outcomes.
2. Reassure the child that surgery is not a punishment but something that is needed to help the part of the body work better. Help the child identify the benefits of having the surgery done.
3. Allow the child and parent to express fears and concerns.
4. Review with parents measures that they can use to help the child afterward, such as comforting touch, gentle verbal communication (singing, telling stories).
5. Make sure consent form has been signed and is in order. Contact the physician if there is a problem with consent.

Teaching Specifics About Surgery

1. Explain whether any preoperative scrubs or cleansing procedures are necessary. Describe how many procedures to expect and how they will feel. If shaving the head is necessary, reassure the child that the hair will grow back and discuss creative ways to cover the head after surgery.
2. Tell the child and parent that the child will not be able to eat or drink after a certain time—usually no food after midnight the night before; breast milk or formula and clear fluid intake depends on the age of the child and the preference of the anesthesiologist. General guidelines are
   a. Infants and children up to 3 years may drink fluids up to 2 to 4 hours before surgery.
   b. Children from 3 to 6 years may drink fluid up to 4 to 6 hours before surgery.
   c. Children older than 7 years may drink fluid up to 6 to 8 hours before surgery.
3. Describe the ride to surgery—kind of transportation, how long it will take, whether it will include an elevator ride.
4. Describe the preanesthesia room—what staff and equipment will look like. Explain that the people will be giving the child special medicine to help the child sleep until the surgery is over. Reassure the child that nothing will be felt during the surgery.
5. Explain that the child will wake up after the surgery is done but will not wake up in the hospital room. If possible, show the child the recovery room and introduce the child to the recovery room staff.
6. Tell the child when the parent will leave, where the parent can wait, and when the child can expect to see the parent again.
7. Demonstrate specifics of dressings, treatment devices, tubes, and how the child will look, using any accessory equipment needed—dolls, diagrams, intravenous lines, anesthesia mask, and any other appropriate medical equipment. Practice what the child will be required to do after returning to the hospital room—turning and deep breathing, splinting, keeping the intravenous site still.
8. Discuss what the child can do if in pain.
9. Describe any planned preoperative medication and its effect on the child (sleepiness, dizziness, dry mouth). Save description of any injections until last. Many children become anxious after learning to expect an injection and will not hear the rest of the preoperative teaching.

Adapted from What Children Need to Know About Surgery. *In* Mott S, Rowen James S., and Sperhac A (eds). *Nursing Care of Children and Families.* Menlo Park, CA: Addison-Wesley, 1990.

---

4. Excretion
   a. Immature kidneys are unable to concentrate urine adequately, causing more drug to be eliminated through the dilute urine.
   b. The dehydrated child loses a larger proportion of body fluid because a greater percentage of body fluid is located in the extracellular compartment. Fluid loss combined with decreased fluid intake in an ill child inhibits urinary excretion and enhances retention of a drug.
5. Calculating dosages
   a. Most medications commonly prescribed for children are available in appropriate pediatric concentrations. Dosages usually are computed by multiplying the weight of the drug (usually in milligrams) by the weight of the child (in kilograms).
   b. When attempting to estimate a child's dosage from the known adult dose of the same drug, the following formula is used: body surface area of the child (Fig. 15–9) divided by the body surface area of an adult (average 1.7 m^2) times the usual adult dose.
6. Oral medications
   a. Always administer oral medications with the child sitting in an upright or semiupright position, with the head elevated to prevent aspiration if the child cries or resists.
   b. Never pinch the child's nostrils when administering the medication.
   c. Infants
      (1) Administer pleasant-tasting liquid medication to infants by placing the medication directly into a nipple and allowing the infant to suck. Do not place medication in the bottle.
      (2) Draw the required dose of an unpleasant-tasting medication into a small syringe and place the syringe into the side and toward the back of the

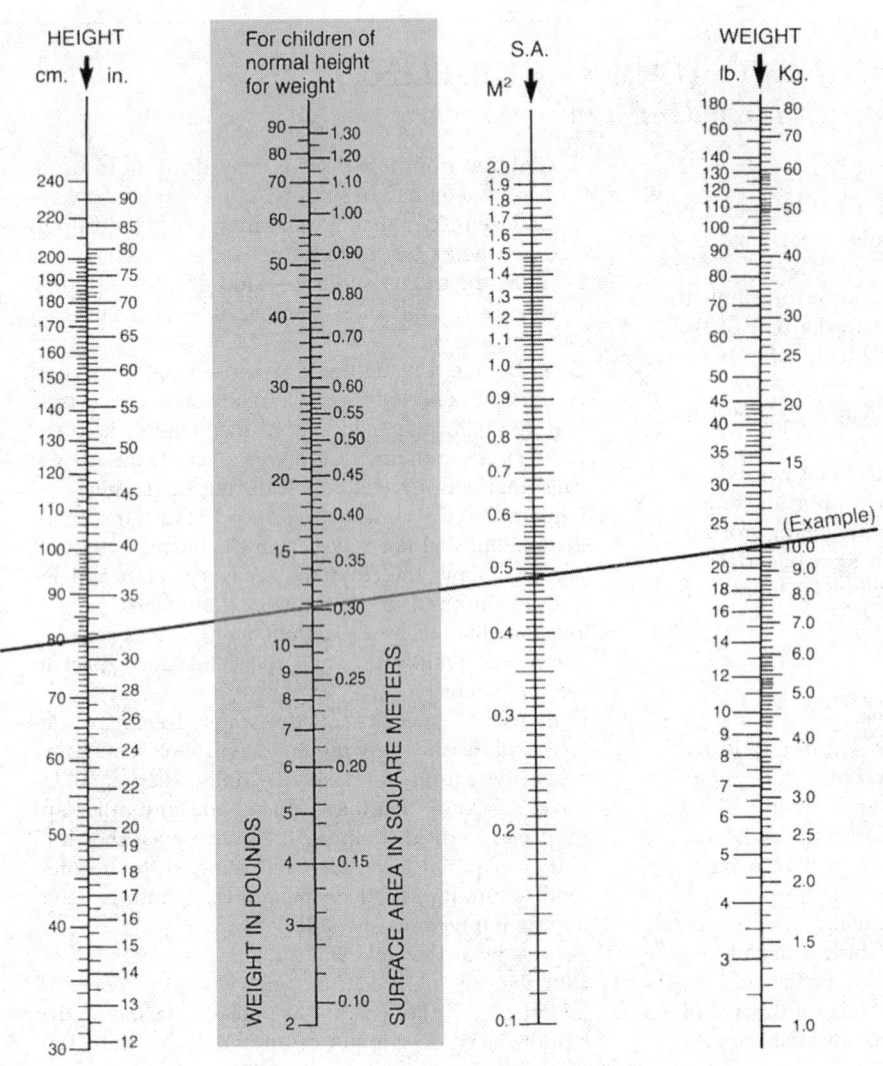

Figure 15–9. Nomogram for estimating body surface area (expressed in m²). Draw a straight line that intersects the child's weight and height Note where the line crosses the surface area. (Redrawn from Bennett JC, and Plum F [eds]. *Cecil Textbook of Medicine.* 20th ed. Philadelphia WB Saunders, 1996. Originally modified from data of E Boyd by CD West.)

infant's mouth. Administer the medication slowly, allowing the infant to swallow according to the pace of administration.

   d. Toddlers and preschoolers

     (1) Place the small child sideways on the lap. The child's closest arm should be placed under the adult's arm and behind the adult's back. Cradle the child's head and hold the child's hand with your hand. Administer medication slowly with a spoon, plastic medication measuring spoon, or small plastic cup.

     (2) Mix liquid medications with a small amount of fluid (less than an ounce) to disguise the taste if necessary. Crush tablets and mix with approximately 1 teaspoon of pureed fruit.

   e. In older children or adolescents, explain the necessity for the medication and what it tastes like if it is a liquid. Children learn to swallow tablets or capsules at varying ages. Chewable tablets are available for some medications.

7. Injections

   a. Choose a needle length and lumen appropriate for the child's size, route of administration, and viscosity of the medication. Generally, a 5/8-inch needle is used to administer subcutaneous injections and intramuscular injections to small infants. One-inch needles (usually 22 or 23 guage) are appropriate for most intramuscular injections in children.

   b. Use a syringe of appropriate size for small doses (1 ml tuberculin, 3 ml).

   c. Select the site—lateral thigh (vastus lateralis muscle) or deltoid for intramuscular injections, upper arm for subcutaneous injections. Avoid the dorsogluteal muscle in children younger than age 5 years.

   d. Gently restrain the young or uncooperative older child.

     (1) For injection in the deltoid, the nurse should sit the child sideways on the parent's or other staff member's lap and instruct the person to hold the child as if oral medication were being administered.

     (2) For injection in the thigh, the nurse should lean over the child and place 1 arm at the level of the child's knees to restrict movement of both legs and the other arm at waist level to restrict arm access to the site. It is helpful to have another

person restrain the child's upper body if the child is particularly resistant.

e. Explain what you are going to do, but follow-up quickly with the injection because many children begin avoidance tactics.

(1) Enlist the help of the older child to remain still. Suggest that the child count slowly or breathe deeply.

(2) Placing an adhesive bandage over the puncture site is important, particularly for toddlers and preschoolers. Use a decorated bandage if possible.

8. Intravenous medications

a. Intravenous medications are less traumatic for the child when round-the-clock parenteral medication is required.

b. Medications may be added to the intravenous bottle or bag, given separately in a burette (usually infused over 1 hour) or injected directly into the intravenous line through a port. Principles for administering intravenous medications to children are similar to those for adults.

c. Because the volume of fluid that dilutes the medication must be added to the total daily intake, children on fluid restriction need special consideration. One of the following methods may be used:

(1) Low-volume intravenous tubing

(2) Retrograde injection: The medication is mixed with the appropriate amount of diluent in a syringe, the intravenous tubing is clamped close to the child, the medication is injected through the port in the direction of the burette, the tubing is unclamped, and the medication is allowed to infuse.

(3) Retrograde administration set: The technique is similar to that for retrograde injection. The volume of medication is usually larger but displaces an equivalent amount of intravenous fluid through use of low-volume tubing and stopcocks. Medication usually takes 30 minutes to infuse.

(4) Syringe pump: A syringe containing the medication is fitted into a pump, which is connected to the intravenous tubing through a Y-connector, and administers the medication slowly over the required period.

d. A heparin lock is used for intermittent intravenous medication administration when additional intravenous fluids are not needed (see Chapter 9).

9. Instillations

a. For children, use a similar technique to that for adults when instilling medication into the eyes or nose.

b. Drop medication into the inner corner of the eye in infants or small children whose eyes are tightly closed.

c. For ear instillations:

(1) Pull the auricle down and back for infants and children younger than 3 years of age.

(2) Pull the auricle up and back for older children.

10. Medication by inhalation

a. Nebulizer

(1) Place the ordered medication in the nebulizer reservoir with saline, then close the reservoir and attach the mouthpiece or mask.

(2) Connect the tubing to the reservoir and start the machine.

(3) Deliver the mist as close to the child's face as possible (infants and young children sometimes resist, so administering the mist through a blow-by mask next to the child might allow for greater inhalation). The older child can place the mouthpiece directly into the mouth. Encourage the child to breathe normally. Children may respond more positively to the treatment while sitting on a parent's lap.

(4) Continue the treatment until all the liquid has aerosolized from the reservoir. Occasionally tapping the sides of the reservoir moves condensation.

b. Metered-dose inhaler and breath-activated device

(1) Shake the inhaler before administration, and attach the inhaler to a spacer device (facilitates more complete administration of the medication). The child should stand or sit upright.

(2) Tell the child to exhale completely (blow out hard), insert the spacer into the mouth, and activate the inhaler by pressing down the pump while inhaling slowly (take a slow, deep breath).

(3) Encourage children to hold their breath for 10 seconds after inhalation.

Applying the Nursing Process

NURSING DIAGNOSIS: Anxiety R/T separation from parents

1. *Expected outcomes*

a. The child should demonstrate decreased anxiety (show increased smiling, more relaxed demeanor, less active protest).

b. The child-parent relationship should continue uninterrupted as much as is possible.

c. The child should maintain a sense of trust.

2. *Nursing interventions*

a. Encourage parents to participate fully in the child's treatment to minimize separation anxiety.

b. Orient the parent and child thoroughly to the hospital setting, including physical facilities, hospital routine, and ways to obtain needed information.

c. Facilitate parental presence by providing appropriate accommodations close to the child, such as a comfortable chair, portable cot, close access to nutritious snacks, and bathing facilities.

d. Include parents in care planning, and plan care to allow for minimal sleep disruption.

e. Assist parents to make arrangements for care of other family members at home and to take breaks as needed.

f. Reassure the child that the parent will return if the parent needs to return home temporarily. Relate the parent's return with an event with which the child is familiar (e.g., time, mealtime, television program, hospital schedule).

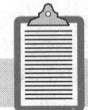

NURSING MANAGEMENT

Assign a primary nurse to any child whose parents are not able to stay and participate in care. Ensure that the initial admission assessment includes all information about the child's usual routine including food preferences, usual mealtimes and utensils used, nap and bedtime schedule, strategies used to comfort or settle the child, words used to describe elimination or body parts, description of any security or transition object or imaginary friend, and names of siblings and best friends. Allow the child to keep security objects and pictures of family members or friends accessible (label all the child's possessions).

NURSING DIAGNOSIS: Anxiety R/T isolation

1. *Expected outcomes*
   a. The child should exhibit decreased anxiety.
   b. The child should demonstrate trust as evidenced by increased ability to wait longer periods for interaction with the nursing staff.
   c. The parent should describe and demonstrate proper precaution technique.
2. *Nursing interventions*
   a. Allow for maximum periods of social interaction with the child. Interventions should be directed toward reducing anxiety.
   b. Explain and demonstrate the required precaution technique to the parent or authorized visitor; verify the skill through return demonstration.
   c. If possible, allow the child to observe what is going on outside the room through a window. Encourage others to smile at or wave to the child frequently. Allow the child to see your face before you put on the mask.
   d. Provide disposable age-appropriate toys or toys that can be properly disinfected.

NURSING DIAGNOSIS: Fear (of bodily harm, pain, death) R/T the unfamiliar environment and potentially threatening events

1. *Expected outcomes*
   a. The child should be able to verbally express the cause of the fear.
   b. The child should be able to engage in play for an appropriate length of time.
   c. The child should be able to sleep restfully.
2. *Nursing interventions*
   a. Provide reassurance to calm the child's fears; use touch (hugging, cuddling, soothing) as an approach.
   b. Use play in the hospital as a primary therapeutic tool

for the child to release feelings of anger or aggression acceptably, to reduce fear, to gain some control over the environment, to act out emotions, to release energy, and to understand the unfamiliar. The following types of play are helpful:
   (1) Role play—acting out situations or emotions
   (2) Doll play—learning about body parts or procedures, releasing aggression, coping with painful or intrusive procedures
   (3) Art—releasing emotions through color, drawing, shaping clay
   (4) Movement play—using a variety of wheeled vehicles (chairs, strollers, gurneys, low trolleys) to move to a new environment such as a playroom; using throwing toys (e.g., bean bags, Nerf balls, Velcro darts) to release aggression or to maintain muscle tone
   (5) Medical play—using real and toy medical equipment to deal with procedures or treatments
   (6) Storytelling—dealing with reality through fantasy
   c. Provide play for all hospitalized children, regardless of whether an official playroom is available. Play equipment suitable for the hospital setting includes the following:
   (1) Infant toys—brightly colored blocks, stacking toys, busy boxes, fabric books, shape sorters, balls, and soft washable stuffed animals
   (2) Art and writing supplies—pencils, paper, glue, crayons, paints, finger paints, fabric scraps, and markers
   (3) Construction toys—large Legos, building blocks, and models
   (4) Social activities—board games, cards, dolls and doll houses, trucks, puppets, Nerf balls, and toy medical equipment
   (5) Quiet activities—books, puzzles, tapes, and craft projects
   (6) Water and sand

NURSING DIAGNOSIS: Powerlessness R/T loss of control

1. *Expected outcomes*
   a. The child should demonstrate continued use of normal routines.
   b. The child should adapt to modification of routine if necessary.
   c. The child should continue to make choices and demonstrate acceptable, controlled behavior.
2. *Nursing interventions*
   a. Preserve the child's usual rituals and routine to enhance feelings of control in an unfamiliar environment.
   b. Take additional measures to decrease the child's feelings of powerlessness:
   (1) Encourage self-care, and include the child in care planning.
   (2) Allow the child to make choices about care within acceptable limits (e.g., deciding a preferred position for receiving an injection, not whether or when the injection is to be given).

(3) Provide adequate explanations and encourage a positive attitude.

(4) Use restraints or physically restrictive devices minimally.

● ▮ ▪ ◼ ▲ ▷ ▦ ⠿ ✡ ▮ ★ ◉ ◫ ◼ ●

TRANSCULTURAL CONSIDERATIONS

Adolescents' approaches to achieving identity sometimes take them out of the "mainstream." Adolescence itself can be a subculture. Allow adolescents as much freedom as possible within the confines of their health problem and hospital regulations. Whenever possible, permit teenagers to wear their own clothes, jewelry, and hairstyles. Listening to music and visiting with friends help adolescents adjust to hospitalization.

NURSING DIAGNOSIS: Pain R/T invasive procedures

1. *Expected outcomes*
   a. The child should be able to describe lessening of pain.
   b. The child should appear more relaxed and calm, able to participate in activities.
   c. The child should point to a face with a low number on the faces scale.
2. *Nursing interventions*
   a. Manage pain (see Chapter 11).
   b. Use the following adaptations to manage pain in children:
      (1) Pharmacologic pain management (Table 15–7)
      • Do not hesitate to medicate children properly for pain. Children experience pain as keenly as adults, and the risk of addiction or respiratory

Table 15–7. Pain Medications for Children

Medication	Administration	Action	Side Effects	Nursing Considerations
Nonsteroidal, nonnarcotics				
Acetaminophen (Tylenol, Panadol)	Oral, rectal	Inhibits transmission of pain impulses Give for mild or moderate pain Not anti-inflammatory	Rare	Use child-resistant caps, overdosage of acetaminophen can cause liver toxicity
Ibuprofen (Advil, Pediaprofen, Motrin)	Oral	Anti-inflammatory, used also to treat fever	Gastric distress, and, rarely, ulceration possible	Do not give ibuprofen to persons with a previous allergic reaction to aspirin
Naproxen (Naprosyn)	Oral	Not for use in children younger than 2 years	Gastrointestinal irritation similar to that associated with ibuprofen	Do not give naproxen to persons with a previous allergic reaction to aspirin
Keterolac tromethamine	Parenteral, oral	Relieves pain by inhibiting prostaglandin synthesis	Drowsiness, sedation, sweating, nausea, gastrointestinal pain, decreased platelet adhesion	Used for short-term pain management (especially after surgery). Can prolong bleeding time. Watch for signs of gastrointestinal bleeding
Narcotic				
Morphine sulphate	Parenteral, multiply established parenteral dose by three to convert to oral dose	Alters pain perception	Mood changes, sedation, dizziness, nausea, vomiting, altered pulse rate, depressed respirations, urinary retention, constipation, agitation, hallucinations	Controlled substance, monitor for effects, especially decreased respirations; institute safety precautions for ambulation; put bed rails up; titrate dose according to effect
Meperidine (Demerol)	Parenteral	Alters pain perception	Sedation, hypotension, nausea, vomiting, constipation, urinary retention	Similar to morphine; use for a short time or for preoperative medication only
Methadone	Oral, parenteral	Alters pain perception	Sedation, euphoria, respiratory depression, visual disturbances, urinary retention	Similar to morphine; often prescribed in sliding scale doses for mild, moderate, and severe pain
Codeine	Oral	Alters pain perception	Sedation, dizziness, dry mouth, respiratory depression, nausea, vomiting, constipation, pruritus, flushing	Often used in combination with appropriate doses of acetaminophen; give with milk or meals

depression from narcotic pain medication is negligible.

- Choose the least intrusive method for administering pain medication that will produce the desired effect (oral, sublingual, dermal, intravenous). Titrate dose to achieve maximum pain relief with minimal sedation.
- Closely monitor vital signs and evaluate level of pain relief.

(2) Nonpharmacologic pain management is similar to that used for adults but is adapted to the child's developmental level. Enlist parent's help and reduce causes of anxiety. Use any of the following alone or together:

- Imagery—use super heroes or fantasy figures to help the young child fight pain. Encourage older children or adolescents to imagine and describe being in a relaxing place and the sensations that they might experience there (e.g., being on the ocean, camping, and looking at the stars).
- Tactile stimulation—stroking, cuddling, rocking, soothing, and rubbing
- Distraction—singing, reading stories, telling jokes, listening to a tape, playing pretend games, and solving verbal puzzles
- Relaxation techniques—rocking, making muscle groups go limp (like cooked spaghetti), rhythmic deep breathing, or slow blowing (pretend to make bubbles, blow up balloons, or blow out birthday candles).

NURSING DIAGNOSIS: Altered family processes R/T disruption of usual family environment and emotional stressors

1. *Expected outcomes*
   a. Family members should be able to demonstrate reduced stress and anxiety.
   b. The family unit should be maintained as a unit as much as possible.
   c. Parents should be able to describe a balance between caring for their hospitalized child and children at home.
   d. Parents should appear more rested and able to cope.
2. *Nursing interventions*
   a. Help parents work out a schedule that addresses their needs as well as the needs of the hospitalized child and any children at home.
   b. Provide appropriate facilities for at least 1 parent to stay with the ill child (sleeping, eating, interaction with others). Encourage siblings to visit or communicate by phone.
   c. Provide uninterrupted time to answer questions, address concerns, and listen to fears and anxieties.
   d. Reassure parents that someone will be with the child as much as possible, if they wish to have some time away.
   e. Explain what is to happen to the child before anything is done, and ask for parent input about the child's coping skills.
   f. Refer to social services to address financial, transportation, and home care problems.

◼ CARING FOR CHILDREN WITH COMMON MEDICAL-SURGICAL DISORDERS

Fluid and Electrolyte and Acid-Base Imbalances

1. Dehydration (see Chapter 9): Management of fluids requires special considerations for children.
   a. Etiology: The primary cause of dehydration in young children is gastroenteritis (see Chapter 27), which can be caused by such organisms as *Shigella*, *Salmonella*, *Staphylococcus aureus*, *Campylobacter*, and *Yersinia*. The most common cause in the United States is rotavirus.
      (1) Some children experience diarrhea without vomiting or other signs of illness for several weeks. The cause is unknown, and, as long as they are retaining fluids, there is little concern about dehydration.
      (2) Members of some ethnic and racial groups give laxatives or purgatives to prevent illness. Related questions should be included in the assessment.
   b. Pathophysiology
      (1) Fluid loss in the child younger than 2 years old can quickly lead to dehydration because of the following factors:
         - A greater proportion of the young child's body fluid is in the extracellular space
         - Other factors such as increased metabolic rate, higher respiratory rate, greater body surface area in relation to weight, and inefficiency of immature kidneys to handle large shifts in fluid volume
         - Decreased plasma volume, causing circulatory collapse in severe cases, with severe fluid and sodium loss from the extracellular compartment
      (2) Dehydration can be hypotonic, hypertonic, or isotonic depending on the relationship of fluid to sodium depletion. Isotonic dehydration (proportional increase or decrease of sodium and water) is the major cause of dehydration in children.
   c. Clinical manifestations: Table 15–8 lists the clinical manifestations of isotonic dehydration in children.
   d. Clinical management
      (1) Oral rehydration therapy is the treatment of choice for children with mild to moderate dehydration. The child takes a rehydrating electrolyte solution (e.g., Rehydralyte, Ricelyte) orally over a 4- to 6-hour period. A small amount is administered frequently to achieve the desired hourly amount and total replacement. A frozen form is available that appeals more to some children.
      (2) Intravenous replacement is instituted for children unable to tolerate enough oral fluids to rehydrate or for those who continue to lose fluid faster than replacement is achieved.
      (3) Prevent skin excoriation from diarrheal stools, especially in the untrained child.
         - Use an occlusive ointment in the diaper area to protect the skin.

Table 15–8. Clinical Manifestations of Isotonic Dehydration in Children

	Fluid Volume Loss	Skin	Urine	Other Signs
Mild dehydration	<50 ml/kg body weight over 24–48 hr	Dry, pale, cool lips and slightly dry, mucous membranes, slightly decreased turgor	Output slightly diminished, increased specific gravity and concentration	Increasing pulse, thirst
Moderate dehydration	50–90 ml/kg	Decreased turgor, grayish color, very dry mucous membranes, cool to touch	Oliguria, concentrated urine, increased specific gravity	Pulse increases, blood pressure decreases, lethargy, absence of tears, eyes sunken, depressed anterior fontanel in child younger than 18 months
Severe dehydration	≥100 ml/kg	Very poor turgor with tenting; cool, mottled, parched mucous membranes; poor peripheral circulation with delayed capillary filling	Anuria	Azotemia, markedly sunken eyes, decreased blood pressure, rapid and thready pulse

• Keep the skin clean and dry (allow to be exposed to air as much as possible).

e. Public health considerations: Keep child with active diarrhea out of daycare until the organism has been identified and the diarrhea has been treated (if treatment is appropriate).

2. Metabolic alkalosis (see Chapter 9): Management of acid-base imbalances involves special considerations for children.

a. Etiology: The primary cause of metabolic alkalosis in children is vomiting caused by pyloric stenosis (hypertrophy of the pylorus), a condition seen in infancy (usually boys). Symptoms include projectile vomiting beginning in the 2nd or 3rd week of life, voracious hunger following vomiting episode, and an "olive" mass in the epigastric area.

b. Clinical management

(1) Surgery and correction of underlying fluid-electrolyte and acid-base imbalances is the treatment of choice.

(2) Home management of vomiting in the older child involves the following:

• Giving the child nothing by mouth for several hours or until vomiting stops

• Giving an electrolyte solution such as Pedialyte in frequent small quantities (1 ounce per hour).

• Gradually advancing the diet as the child retains fluids and having the child avoid milk products if possible because there is a temporary lactose intolerance after diarrhea.

• Calling the physician if the child begins to look dry, complains of thirst, or has decreased urinary output.

Communicable Diseases of Childhood

1. Most communicable diseases of childhood have been eradicated, or their incidence has been reduced drastically as a result of immunization.

2. There have been some recent outbreaks of pertussis in unimmunized young school-age children and of measles in the college-aged population. Administration of a booster measles, mumps, rubella immunization reduces the measles risk.

3. Several relatively benign communicable diseases affect children periodically (Table 15–9).

Childhood Leukemia

1. Definition: One of the most common cancers of childhood, leukemia affects the blood-forming tissues, resulting in abnormal proliferation of immature white blood cells. Leukemia is classified according to the cell line affected. There are several different forms of leukemia, but the 2 seen most often in children are the following:

a. Acute lymphoid leukemia (ALL), which affects the cells in the lymphatic system, the pre-B-cell being the most common cell line affected

b. Acute myelogenous leukemia (AML), which is less common and affects the myeloblasts.

2. Incidence and etiology

a. Incidence: Leukemia affects 4.2 of 100,000 White children younger than age 15 years and 2.4 of 100,000 Black children.

b. The etiology is unknown, although children with trisomy 21 have a much greater chance than other children of acquiring the disease, leading to the belief that there is a genetic component.

3. Clinical manifestations are related to the increased number of immature cells competing with normal cells for sustenance and include the following:

a. Anemia from decreased number of red blood cells

b. Infection from decreased number of white blood cells and ineffectiveness of blast cells to fight infection

c. Bleeding due to decreased number of platelets

d. Infiltration of leukemic cells into the spleen and lymph glands, liver, and central nervous system, generating symptoms related to decreased function of these organs

4. Clinical management

Table 15–9. Most Common Communicable Diseases of Childhood

Disease	Clinical Manifestations	Incubation/ Communicability	Nursing Implications
Varicella (Chickenpox)	Lesions appear after a prodrome of malaise, headache, fever, and stomachache. Lesions first appear on the upper chest or back and spread outward to extremities. They begin as discrete macules and progress to vesicles, which break and scab. The appearance of the lesion is often described as a "dewdrop," with a surrounding erythematous area.	Incubation: 14–21 days Communicable: 24 hr before appearance of lesions until all lesions are scabbed	Pruritus is the most annoying manifestation. Risk of secondary infection increases if the child scratches frequently. Treatment is supportive, with antihistamines given for pruritus. Occasionally, acyclovir is prescribed to lighten the case for exposed high-risk children. Do not administer aspirin for fever management because of its relationship with Reye's syndrome.
Erythema subitum (Roseola)	High temperature (sometimes greater than 104 degrees Fahrenheit) is the initial manifestation. There usually are no other signs of illness. Rash appears when the fever subsides (usually after 3–4 days). Rash is pink, maculopapular, and non-pruritic, appearing on the chest and back and spreading outward to the extremities.	Incubation and communicability: unknown, but incidence is high in children in late infancy and early childhood	Treatment is supportive and directed toward fever management and prevention of febrile seizures.
Streptococcal pharyngitis (Scarlet fever)	Caused by group A β-hemolytic streptococcus. Sore throat, headache, moderate fever, swollen glands, fatigue, anorexia, inflamed pharynx with strawberry-colored tongue. Rash is classic in that it is a diffuse erythematous rash that feels like fine sandpaper. The face appears flushed, and the rash spreads to the trunk and extremities. Desquamation of palms and soles often occurs as the disease resolves.	Incubation: average 3–4 days after exposure Communicable: until 24 hr after initiation of treatment; if untreated, there is risk of development of acute rheumatic fever or poststreptococcal glomerulonephritis	Treatment begins after identification of the organism by rapid strep antigen test or throat culture. Ten days of penicillin (or erythromycin in allergic children) is the treatment of choice. Culture other symptomatic family members. Discourage sharing of eating utensils and bathroom cups. Ensure compliance with therapy. Provide symptomatic relief of sore throat.
Rubeola (Measles)	High fever, cough, conjunctivitis, coryza, light sensitivity, Koplik's spots (prodrome). Dull, red, confluent rash, beginning on the face and spreading to the trunk and extremities after 3–4 days of illness. The child appears very ill.	Incubation: 10–20 days Communicable: from 4 days before to 5 days after the rash appears	Treatment is symptomatic, directed toward fever control and darkening the room. Prevent exposure to others. Complications can be severe and include otitis, pneumonia, and encephalitis.
Rubella (German measles)	Low-grade fever, malaise, headache, cervical lymphadenopathy. Pink, discrete maculopapular rash begins on the face and spreads downward.	Incubation: 14–21 days Communicable: 1 wk before to 5 days after the rash begins	Illness is usually mild. Major danger is to fetuses of exposed pregnant women.
Erythema infectiosum (fifth disease)	Caused by the human parvovirus B19. Rash is preceded by a prodrome of fever, malaise, sore throat, headache. Erythema, or a "slapped-cheek" appearance, is noticed on the face. A characteristic "lacy" rash appears over the next several days and progresses from proximal to distal surfaces of the extremities. The rash gets bright pink when exposed to heat.	Incubation: less than 1 month Communicable: before the appearance of the rash; appearance, disappearance, and reappearance of the rash over approximately 1 month is not unusual, but the child is not considered to be communicable at that time	The disease is benign and self-limiting. It can endanger the fetus of pregnant women who contract the disease during pregnancy. It also can precipitate an aplastic crisis in children with sickle cell disease. Advise pregnant women to avoid situations in which exposure is likely (e.g., entering a school where documented cases have occurred).
Mumps	Fever, pain in front of ear, headache, malaise. Painful enlargement of parotid gland, either unilateral or bilateral.	Incubation: 14–21 days Communicable: immediately before and after swelling starts	Treatment is symptomatic pain relief, increased fluids, and bland foods. Can cause sensorineural deafness and orchitis.
Pertussis (whooping cough)	Upper respiratory tract symptoms followed in several weeks by dry, hacking cough. Coughing spasms become severe with difficult inspiration (whoop), cyanosis, expectoration of mucous plug, and vomiting.	Incubation: 5–21 days Communicable: before onset of spasms	Infants and young children require hospitalization with oxygen. Erythromycin and supportive care is given for older children. Provide humidification and encourage fluid intake.

a. Treatment is based on initial staging of the disease and prognostic factors and includes remission induction with appropriate chemotherapeutic agents (usually corticosteroids, vincristine, L-asparaginase); central nervous system prophylactic therapy with intrathecal methotrexate, cytarabine, and hydrocortisone; and remission preservation.

b. Bone marrow transplants have been successful with some children.

c. The prognosis for properly treated cases of leukemia is excellent.

d. Nursing care is directed toward teaching the child and parent about the disease and its effects, managing the effects of chemotherapy, and providing emotional support to the child and family.

Wilms' Tumor (Nephroblastoma)

1. Definition: An embryonic tumor affecting the kidney that originates from renoblast cells. Some Wilms' tumors are associated with aniridia (congenital absence of the iris) and genitourinary anomalies.

2. Incidence and etiology: Wilms' tumor affects children at an average age of 3 years. There is a genetic component, with siblings and identical twins of affected children having a higher incidence than the general population.

3. Clinical manifestations: The initial manifestation is a large, nontender abdominal mass. Signs and symptoms are related to pressure on the renal system from the mass and might include microscopic hematuria, hypertension, anemia, and anorexia. Metastasis, if it occurs, is usually to the lungs.

4. Clinical management

a. Surgical removal of the affected kidney, followed by chemotherapy, radiation, or both, depending on the staging of the tumor, is the usual treatment. Prognosis with proper intervention is excellent (90% cure rate).

b. Provide teaching and emotional support to the family and child. Avoid palpation of the child's abdomen preoperatively to prevent rupture of the tumor and seeding of the tumor cells elsewhere. Avoidance of contact sports and other activities that might jeopardize the remaining kidney as the child grows is recommended. Teach methods for preventing urinary tract infections.

Neuroblastoma

1. Definition: Neuroblastoma is an embryonal neural crest cell tumor affecting the adrenal medulla and sympathetic ganglia.

2. Incidence and etiology: Neuroblastoma affects mostly children younger than age 2 years, with boys being affected more often than girls. Many children have metastases at diagnosis, most commonly to the liver. Affected children appear ill, and the prognosis for children with stages III and IV is poor. Spontaneous regression in children with stage IV-S is possible.

3. Clinical manifestations (depending on the tissue affected)

a. An abdominal mass that crosses the midline if the adrenal medulla is affected

b. Dual eye color (ophthalmic sympathetic nerves), airway obstruction, and difficulty breathing (mediastinal)

4. Clinical management

a. Treatment depends on staging and includes surgery preceded or followed by radiation and chemotherapy.

b. Nursing care is directed toward caring for the child with cancer and providing emotional support to the family as they come to terms with the diagnosis and possible prognosis.

Seizure Disorders (Epilepsy)

1. Definition: Episodes of abnormal motor or sensory activity caused by abnormal electrical discharges in the brain (see Chapter 18)

2. Incidence and etiology: Most seizures in older children are idiopathic. Certain conditions precipitate seizures in the susceptible child by lowering the seizure threshold. These include fatigue, stress, illness, hypoglycemia, hormone changes, and intermittently flashing lights. Others include the following:

a. Neurologic injury, infection, exposure to toxins (e.g., lead)

b. Birth hypoxia

c. Congenital malformations

d. Fever: Seen predominantly in children younger than age 5 years. Seizure is associated with moderate or high fever. Even repeated episodes usually do not cause permanent neurologic damage.

3. Clinical manifestations (see Chapter 18 for seizure classification): Cognitive or motor delays and behavior problems suggest the need for developmental testing. Contributing factors include the following:

a. Prenatal factors

b. Birth trauma

c. Exposure to toxins

d. Injury or illness

e. Family history of neurologic disease

4. Clinical management

a. The goal of management is maximal control with minimal pharmacologic intervention (Box 15–3).

b. A single anticonvulsant should be used at first, gradually increasing the dose daily until seizure activity ceases or until the child begins to experience adverse effects. Serum levels of the drug should be monitored and a 2nd anticonvulsant added only if necessary. Drugs of choice include those listed in Table 15–10.

BOX 15–3. Home Management for Seizure Disorders

A common nursing diagnosis for a child with a seizure disorder is knowledge deficit about home management of the child with seizures related to initial experience. Expected outcomes include the following:

• The parent, child, or both should describe principles of effective seizure management and compliance with medication administration.

• The child should remain free of injury.

• The child should demonstrate normal growth and development and positive self-image.

Table 15–10. Medications Used to Treat Seizures in Children

Medication	Action	Comments	Side Effects	Nursing Considerations
Phenobarbital	Raises seizure threshold by increasing the threshold for electrical stimulation of the cortex	Status epilepticus, febrile seizures, tonic–clonic, simple partial motor seizures	Drowsiness, hyperactivity in young children, behavior alterations, altered cognitive and motor performance, rare allergic rash, or blood dyscrasia	Monitor child for adverse reactions; encourage routine medication compliance to maintain steady serum level; has additive effect with other central nervous system depressants; toleration develops with continued use
Primidone (Mysoline)	Same as phenobarbital	Same as phenobarbital	Same as phenobarbital	Potentiates action of phenobarbital; dose should be increased slowly; complete blood count and liver function tests obtained every 6 months
Phenytoin (Dilantin)	Limitation of seizure propagation by alteration of sodium ion transport across neurons in the motor cortex	Tonic–clonic, complex partial seizures	Ataxia, slurred speech, decreased coordination, nystagmus, gastrointestinal discomfort, rashes, rarely Stevens-Johnson syndrome or blood dyscrasias, connective tissue alterations including gingival hyperplasia, lymphadenopathy	Action may be altered by other drugs including phenobarbital and valproic acid; can interfere with effect of vitamin D and contraceptives; meticulous oral hygiene required; obtain routine serum levels; physician is consulted for any sign of adverse effects
Diazepam (Valium) Clonazepam (Klonopin)	Sedative effect in limbic system, thalamus, and hypothalamus, fast acting when administered parenterally	Status epilepticus (diazepam), mixed seizure disorder (clonazepam)	Drowsiness, ataxia, confusion, hypotension, gastrointestinal irritation, urinary retention, rare skin rashes, abnormal liver function and blood dyscrasias when administered long term	Intravenous solution administered slowly—no faster than 1 ml/min; monitor for local irritation and phlebitis; use caution when using with other anticonvulsants; obtain frequent complete blood count and liver function tests
Carbamazepine (Tegretol)	Anticonvulsant, exact mechanism unknown	Simple partial, complex partial, secondarily generalized tonic–clonic seizures	Bone marrow depression possible, transient neutropenia frequently seen, allergic rashes, dizziness, drowsiness, nausea, vomiting	Conduct complete blood studies before initiating drug, then weekly during first 3 months and monthly thereafter; warn patient about signs of bone marrow depression; protect from infection
Valproic acid (Depakene) Divalproex sodium (Depakote)	Exact mechanism unknown	Absence, myoclonic, atonic, tonic–clonic, and mixed seizures	Alopecia, increased appetite with weight gain, rare hepatic toxicity and abnormal coagulation	Can potentiate effect of phenobarbital and alter serum levels of other seizure medications; perform liver function and coagulation studies before initiating drug and frequently thereafter
Ethosuximide (Zarontin)	Depresses motor cortex and suppresses electric activity associated with lapses of consciousness	Absence seizures	Gastrointestinal irritation, headaches, hiccups, drowsiness, rare allergic skin rashes and blood dyscrasias	Obtain complete blood count and liver function tests frequently, may increase tonic–clonic seizures

From Matassarin-Jacobs E. *Saunders Review for NCLEX-RN.* Philadelphia: WB Saunders, 1993.

c. Teach parents proper administration of anticonvulsants.
d. Emphasize the necessity to comply with the pharmacologic routine.
e. Teach the side effects of the medication that the child is taking, including gum hyperplasia, and the need for appropriate mouth care.
f. If precipitators are identified, the nurse should encourage their avoidance.

g. Teach parents how to manage a generalized seizure if it occurs.

h. The young child with frequent seizures that cause falls should be advised to wear a protective helmet.

i. The parents need to inform the child's teachers about the child's condition and review emergency management with the teacher.

j. Advise parents to encourage the child to participate in activities that are appropriate for age. Heights and swimming or bicycling alone should be avoided. Most other sports are permitted as long as there is minimal risk for injury if the child has a seizure while participating.

k. Reassure parents that the child can live a nearly normal life with generally few restrictions and that their expectations should be similar as for any child.

l. The family may be referred to an epilepsy support group if desired.

Meningitis

1. Definition: Meningitis is inflammation of the meninges that surround the brain and spinal cord (see Chapter 18).
2. Incidence and etiology
   a. *Haemophilus influenzae* is the most frequent cause of bacterial meningitis in young infants and children, but its incidence has decreased since routine immunization was initiated for infants.
   b. In viral meningitis, an array of viruses produce inflammation. The condition is frequently referred to as aseptic meningitis.
3. Clinical manifestations
   a. In infants, irritability, fever, bulging fontanel, poor feeding, vomiting, and altered consciousness. Infants often resist being held or moved.
   b. In children, fever, severe headache, vomiting, altered consciousness, nuchal rigidity, positive Kernig's and Brudzinski's signs
   c. Petechial rash and shock symptoms with meningococcal meningitis
   d. Complications include permanent damage to cerebrospinal fluid circulation, residual neurologic deficits, developmental delay, deafness, seizures, and death
4. Clinical management
   a. The nurse should document any history of infection or exposure to infection (e.g., otitis media, upper respiratory infection, or tonsillitis) or recent trauma, and ask about the child's immunization status. See Procedure 15–1 for a description of assisting with a lumbar puncture for infants and children.
   b. Parenteral antibiotic therapy should be begun using antibiotics effective against usual causative organisms (ampicillin and cefotaxime for infants younger than age 3 months and cefotaxime or ceftriaxone for infants and children older than 3 months. Therapy should be tailored to the specific organism when culture and sensitivity results return. Antibiotics are usually not used for a child with aseptic meningitis.
   c. Initiate intravenous dexamethasone as ordered before starting antibiotics.

d. Isolate the child for 24 hours after initiation of antibiotics.

e. Other interventions should be directed toward restoring or maintaining fluid and electrolyte balance, reducing fever, preventing or treating seizures, reducing elevated intracranial pressure, and preventing circulatory collapse.

f. Initiate rifampin prophylaxis of household and daycare contacts if there are children younger than 4 years old in those settings who are likely to be exposed and *H. influenzae* is the causative organism. (Use rifampin with extreme caution in pregnant women.) Prophylaxis is required for all contacts of a child with meningococcal meningitis.

Cerebral Palsy

1. Definition: Cerebral palsy (CP) is any of a number of disorders involving impaired neuromuscular coordination and control, language and communication deficits, and perceptual problems. Children with CP may be of normal intelligence or may have learning problems.
2. Incidence and etiology
   a. Cerebral palsy is caused by any of multiple prenatal, perinatal, and acquired problems, with the major contributing factors being prenatal (e.g., exposure to teratogens, genetic abnormalities, intrauterine infections, and placental insufficiency).
   b. Prematurity results in a high incidence of CP.
3. Clinical manifestations
   a. A child with the most common type of CP exhibits spastic hypertonicity of muscle groups and poor posture, balance, and muscle coordination.
   b. Additional manifestations
      (1) Gross and fine motor delays interfering with achievement of developmental milestones
      (2) Infantile reflexes lasting beyond their normally expected disappearance
   c. Associated complications include language delays that may lead to a misdiagnosis of mental retardation, sensory deficits, feeding difficulties, orthopedic and dental problems, and seizures.
4. Clinical management
   a. To prevent orthopedic deformities, health care providers may do the following:
      (1) Provide assistive devices such as braces, walkers, or wheelchairs to promote mobility and independence
      (2) Surgically correct joint deformities and severe contractures
   b. Prevent seizures by prescribing seizure medications.
   c. Enhance communication with picture boards and computers with voice synthesizers.
   d. Refer for the following multimodal services within the community:
      (1) Physical and occupational therapy to promote activities of daily living
      (2) Speech therapy
      (3) Education and recreational activities appropriate for age and developmental level
      (4) Support groups for children and families

Reye's Syndrome

1. Definition: Reye's syndrome is acute encephalopathy with cerebral edema that occurs in tandem with fatty degeneration of the liver and derangement of ammonia metabolism.
2. Incidence and etiology
   a. The cause of Reye's syndrome is unknown, but its appearance in children follows a relatively benign viral infection such as varicella.
   b. Susceptibility to Reye's syndrome appears increased if the child takes aspirin or aspirin-containing products to treat the viral illness. Case incidence has decreased markedly since aspirin warnings were issued in the mid-1980s.
3. Clinical manifestations
   a. Abrupt, progressively more severe vomiting follows what appears to be recovery from a viral illness.
   b. Deteriorating neurologic status concomitant with increasing encephalopathy and cerebral edema and elevated serum ammonia leads to confusion, agitation, and eventual coma.
   c. The condition is self-limiting, but many recovered children manifest neurologic deficits.
4. Clinical management: the child's care is managed in an intensive care unit and is similar to that for anyone with cerebral edema and neurologic and metabolic compromise.

Otitis Media

1. Definition: Otitis media is inflammation or infection of the middle ear with resulting decreased mobility of the tympanic membrane from effusion. Otitis media can be acute or chronic.
2. Incidence and etiology
   a. Usually caused by *Streptococcus pneumoniae,* or *H. influenzae,* otitis media can occur after an upper respiratory infection.
   b. The highest incidence is in children younger than age 5 years. The condition is the most common cause of physician visits during the 1st year of life.
   c. The short, straight eustachian tube in young children (younger than age 3 years) facilitates movement of organisms from the nasopharynx to the middle ear.
   d. The underdeveloped immune system is less able to fight organisms, and flat positioning of young infants allows for pooling of secretions in the nasopharyngeal area.

TRANSCULTURAL CONSIDERATIONS

Native American children have a high incidence of otitis media and require adequate health care to prevent hearing deficits.

3. Clinical manifestations
   a. Moderate fever, irritability, interrupted sleep, decreased appetite, and pain (signified by rubbing or batting at ear by nonverbal children) are initial symptoms. Drainage from the affected ear suggests perforation of the tympanic membrane.
   b. Establish whether the child has had previous upper respiratory infections. Otoscopic examination reveals the following:
      (1) Red, bulging eardrum with absent landmarks and decreased motion of tympanic membrane (acute suppurative otitis media)
      (2) Gray, retracted eardrum with visible fluid, decreased hearing, "popping" sound in ears (otitis media with effusion)
   c. Tympanogram appears flat, revealing absent tympanic membrane mobility. The child may fail audiometric testing.
   d. Recurrent otitis media can cause hearing loss and result in delay in speech development.
4. Clinical management (Table 15-11)
   a. Identification of antibiotic-resistant organisms has prompted a more judicious treatment of episodes of acute otitis media. The condition is self-limiting but should be treated if the child is febrile and uncomfortable. If the child is not in acute discomfort, it may be prudent to wait a few days before initiating treatment.
   b. For acute otitis media, treatment is a 10-day course of antimicrobial therapy.
      (1) Amoxicillin or amoxicillin clavulanate (Augmentin) is the 1st-line drug of choice.
      (2) Cefaclor (Ceclor) can be used for children who are allergic to penicillin.
      (3) Sulfamethoxazole-trimethoprim (Bactrim, Septra) is also prescribed.
   c. For otitis media with effusion, there is usually no treatment unless the condition is prolonged enough to consider tympanostomy tubes.
   d. For recurrent infection, daily prophylactic low-dose sulfisoxazole (Gantrisin) or amoxicillin begins with

Table 15-11. Management of Otitis Media

Nursing Diagnosis	Expected Outcome
Pain related to inflammation	The child should be free from pain, as evidenced by increased ability to rest and play and by decreased episodes of crying. The child should exhibit temperature within normal limits.
Impaired home maintenance management related to incomplete understanding of the treatment regimen	The child should comply with prescribed medication to prevent complications.
Altered growth and development (hearing, speech, language, cognition) related to decreased hearing from repeated incidence of otitis media	The child should demonstrate normal achievement of developmental milestones for language.

the 1st symptoms of an upper respiratory infection and continues until symptoms resolve.

e. Surgical insertion of pressure-equalizing tubes is considered when prophylaxis fails.

f. Nursing interventions

(1) Administer acetaminophen for pain relief every 4 hours as needed.

(2) Have the child with pharyngitis gargle with warm normal saline for comfort.

(3) Have the child with otitis media lie on the affected side and apply external heat if it makes the child more comfortable.

(4) Emphasize to the parent and child that all the medication must be taken. The physician should be notified if there is a problem with the medication or if the child misses a substantial number of doses.

(5) Explain that even though the child feels better, it takes the full course of antibiotics to completely eliminate the organism.

(6) Advise the parent to notify the physician if the child does not improve within 72 hours or if the child has a recurrence after the course of medication is completed.

(7) Encourage the breast-feeding mother to continue nursing the child exclusively for at least 4 months because breast milk confers a protective effect.

(8) Monitor the child's speech and language development at every well visit and refer the child to a specialist if required.

(9) Encourage the parent to keep follow-up appointments after each ear infection to be certain the infection has resolved.

(10) Speak slowly and clearly to the child with diminished hearing.

g. Discharge planning and teaching

(1) Parents should refrain from smoking near the child or in the home. Exposure to environmental smoke increases the incidence of otitis media.

(2) Avoid other children with upper respiratory infections.

(3) Infants should not be fed in a propped position.

(4) Routine hearing screening begins at age 4 years or earlier if a problem is suspected.

Impaired Hearing or Vision

1. The nursing care of the hearing-impaired child is similar to that of the adult (see Chapter 20), but with the following modifications:

a. The nurse should ascertain the child's usual method of communication—signing, lip reading, communication board, or computer—and be sure this is communicated to other staff members.

b. The child's method of communication should be continued when the child is hospitalized.

c. Play may be used to communicate if other methods fail (e.g., using picture books, charts with clock faces, and pictures of hospital routines, procedures, and equipment).

2. Eye trauma and patching after ophthalmologic surgery are the most frequent causes of vision impairment seen in hospitalized children. Because trauma in 1 eye can place stress on the other, both eyes are usually patched. The nursing care of the visually impaired child is similar to that for an adult with the following modifications:

a. Provide a quiet environment so the child is not overwhelmed with hospital sounds. Help the child identify hospital sounds to reduce the stress of the unknown.

b. Describe in detail the surrounding environment to help the child visualize internally; this is especially important when the child is trying to eat.

c. Relate time orientation to familiar events such as television shows.

d. Use audial forms of play such as music and tapes, reading stories, and singing.

e. Promote a sense of control by providing emotional support and encouraging independence in activities of daily living as much as possible.

f. Carefully orient the blind child to the hospital setting in a manner that establishes points of reference and allows the child to cope with the new environment.

Acquired Immunodeficiency Syndrome

1. Definition: Acquired immunodeficiency syndrome (AIDS) is a chronic condition caused by the human immunodeficiency virus (HIV).

2. Incidence and etiology: The primary cause of HIV infection in children is transmission from infected mothers to infants. Considered a chronic disease of childhood AIDS is becoming a major cause of death in children aged 1 to 4 years old.

a. Eighty percent of cases of HIV in children are contracted during perinatal transmission, but the risk of transmission of HIV from mother to child is low (13–40%) and is becoming lower with zidovudine (AZT) treatment of pregnant women with HIV.

b. Diagnosis of HIV infection cannot be made definitively in early infancy because screening tests react to passively transmitted antibody. Most infants serorevert before 24 months of age.

c. There is some evidence that HIV is transmitted through breast milk. Therefore, it is advisable that HIV-infected mothers not breast-feed their infants.

d. Other causes of AIDS in children include blood transfusions (15%) and sexual transmission (1%, and increasing among the teen population).

3. Clinical manifestations

a. One of the first signs of HIV infection in infants is developmental delay and decelerating growth velocity. Encephalopathy can cause regression and loss of previously achieved milestones.

b. Repeated episodes of otitis media, persistent *Candida* infection (oral thrush), or frequent upper respiratory infection should alert the nurse that HIV infection is a possibility, particularly if the child's mother or father is HIV positive or at risk for being HIV positive.

c. Other signs of HIV infection in children include lymphadenopathy, enlargement of the liver and spleen, chronic interstitial pneumonitis, *Pneumocystis carinii* pneumonia, fever, and chronic diarrhea.

d. Antibody tests such as enzyme-linked immunosorbent assay or Western blot are not diagnostic in children younger than 24 months old. To establish a diagnosis, the following must be present:

  (1) In infants younger than 15 months old, HIV antibody accompanied by evidence of immune deficiencies not proved to be caused by any other underlying disorder, and symptoms of HIV infection; clinical manifestations of HIV that meet the Centers for Disease Control and Prevention's definition of AIDS; or positive detection of the virus in blood or tissues.

  (2) In children older than 15 months, detection of the virus in blood or tissues, presence of HIV antibody, or symptoms of AIDS as described by the Centers for Disease Control and Prevention.

e. Decreased CD4 T-cell count and helper to suppressor ratio are diagnostic findings.

4. Clinical management (Table 15–12)

a. To prevent *P. carinii* infection, sulfamethoxazole-trimethoprim (Bactrim) is given orally to children between 1 month and 5 years old or aerosolized pentamidine by nebulizer is given to children older than age 5 years.

b. Zidovudine is given to children with CD4 count alterations as follows:

  (1) Infants less than 1750 per mm^3

  (2) Ages 1 to 2 years, less than 1000

  (3) Ages 2 to 6 years, less than 750

  (4) Ages older than 6 years, less than 500

DRUG ADVISORY

Because antiretroviral agents are absorbed better in a less acidic environment than the acid concentration of gastric contents, most come in buffered form. To increase absorption, give these medications to patients with an empty stomach. Specific recommendations for zidovudine include giving the medication with the child in an upright position and, to avoid esophageal ulceration, giving it with at least 120 ml of water. Crush didanosine tablets to disperse the buffer more accurately, or give unbuffered preparation with Mylanta.

Table 15–12. Management of Acquired Immunodeficiency Syndrome

Nursing Diagnosis	Expected Outcome
Altered growth and development related to disease process and chronic nature of the child's condition	The child should exhibit attainment of developmental milestones.
Altered family processes related to potential death of parent and disease chronicity	The child-parent unit should remain intact for as long as possible. The family should demonstrate positive coping strategies.

c. Supportive nutritional and well-child care is given. Inactive poliovaccine (IPV) instead of oral poliovaccine (OPV) is given. The measles, mumps, rubella vaccine is administered, as are the influenza vaccine, pneumococcal vaccine, and postexposure varicella prophylaxis.

d. Nursing interventions

  (1) Encourage routine well-child care and immunizations and other illness prevention strategies.

  (2) Work with the parent to provide a high-calorie, high-protein diet according to the child's developmental level. Soft or liquid foods are more comfortable for the child with oral candidiasis.

  (3) Refer the family to specialists for any motor, speech, or language delay.

  (4) Demonstrate and encourage positive parenting behaviors—cuddling, rocking, setting limits, allowing autonomy.

  (5) Advise the parent that, when well, the older child may attend school or the younger child may attend daycare.

  (6) Assist the family in the care of the child with a chronic condition.

  (7) Facilitate emotional adjustment and planning for future child care.

  (8) Encourage the parent to seek prompt attention when the child is ill. Give appropriate information about medications and their side effects.

  (9) Refer the family to appropriate resources in the community to meet identified social and emotional needs.

e. Public health considerations: The nurse should become actively involved with disseminating accurate information and preventive guidelines to children and adolescents according to cognitive and developmental level.

Croup (Laryngotracheobronchitis)

1. Definition: Laryngotracheobronchitis is inflammation of the upper airways (larynx, trachea, bronchi).

2. Incidence and etiology

a. Croup has viral origins (rhinovirus, parainfluenza, respiratory syncytial virus).

b. Croup affects children younger than 5 years old and is most commonly seen in early childhood.

3. Clinical manifestations

a. Inflammatory changes in the mucosa of the upper airways cause narrowing and partial airway obstruction and hoarseness initially. These symptoms are followed by a harsh cough and mild inspiratory stridor that is worse at night.

b. Symptoms appear over the course of several days. Fever may or may not be present.

c. Increasing obstruction can cause increased respiratory effort leading to respiratory distress. The child should be observed for

  (1) Stridor, dyspnea, pallor

  (2) Restlessness, tachycardia

  (3) Elevated respirations, retractions, cyanosis

d. A rare complication is complete airway obstruction.
4. Clinical management
   a. Obtain information about course of disease and any treatment method used. Differentiate croup from epiglottitis, which requires emergency treatment. Signs of epiglottitis include the following:
      (1) Rapid onset, over a few hours' time
      (2) Sore throat with excessive drooling and inability to swallow secretions; the child insists on sitting upright
      (3) Moderate to high temperature (more than 38.5 degrees Celsius, 101.5 degrees Fahrenheit) with muffled voice, stridor, and signs of increasing respiratory distress
   b. Observe the child's respiratory status, oxygenation, color, and sound of the associated cough.
   c. For home intervention, humidify the child's environment with a cool mist vaporizer; bring the child outdoors or into a steamy bathroom. Give cool liquids and monitor for signs of respiratory distress.
   d. For hospital intervention
      (1) Administer racemic epinephrine (Table 15–13) if respiratory distress is likely, then admit the child and observe for rebound effect of the medication.
      (2) Place the child in a mist tent with low-dose oxygen if the child is hypoxic.
      (3) Encourage taking clear oral fluids if the child is not in distress. The child may require parenteral fluid therapy.
      (4) Consider steroid treatment.
      (5) Intubate for complete airway obstruction.

Bronchiolitis (Respiratory Syncytial Virus Infection)

1. Definition: Bronchiolitis is inflammation of the lower respiratory tract that causes increased mucus production and inflammation and obstruction of the bronchioles.
2. Incidence and etiology
   a. Respiratory syncytial virus is the causative organism.

Table 15–13. Medications Used for Treating Respiratory Disorders in Children

Medication	Action	Comments	Side Effects	Nursing Considerations
β_2-adrenergic agonists Albuterol (Ventolin, Proventil) Metaproterenol (Alupent)	Relaxes smooth muscles of the airways	Relieves acute bronchospasm	Tremors, nervousness, dizziness, tachycardia, elevated blood pressure, nausea, headache, rebound bronchospasm	Excitement and nervousness is more common in children ages 2–6 yr; effects last up to 6 hr and medication should not be used more frequently than recommended by physician; use of inhaled medication is effective for preventing bronchospasm (especially exercise-induced bronchospasm); teach child use of inhaler; spacer device should be used for young children.
Racemic epinephrine	Bronchodilator, vasoconstrictor	Use for severe croup	Causes increase in cardiac rate and force of contraction, dizziness, palpitations	Monitor vital signs carefully; be alert for rebound effect; child should be admitted to hospital for observation after receiving racemic epinephrine
Methylxanthine Theophylline Aminophylline	Relaxes smooth muscle of bronchial airways resulting in bronchodilation	Use for respiratory conditions involving reversible bronchospasm	Gastrointestinal irritation including nausea, vomiting, epigastric pain, headaches, irritability, tachycardia, dysrhythmias	Give to patients with an empty stomach for maximum absorption but give with full glass of water; monitor vital signs; cardiac monitor required during intravenous administration, theophylline level should be checked regularly and should be less than 20 μg/ml to prevent toxicity; sustained release preparations used for prevention of acute episodes of bronchospasm.
Cromolyn sodium (Intal)	Action not clearly understood; inhibits mediators of allergic/inflammatory response	Use prophylactically to prevent asthma and exercise-induced bronchospasm	Throat dryness or irritation, cough, wheeze, nausea, potential for anaphylaxis	Given by nebulizer or inhaler; must be administered regularly as directed and usually in conjunction with other pharmacologic agents (e.g., bronchodilators).

From Matassarin-Jacobs E. *Saunders Review for NCLEX-RN*. Philadelphia: WB Saunders, 1993.

b. Rapid spread occurs in the pediatric population by droplet dispersion. The organism survives for hours on environmental objects.

c. The peak incidence is during the winter months. Bronchiolitis is particularly severe when it affects infants younger than 6 months old.

3. Clinical manifestations

a. Preceding mild upper respiratory tract infection or otitis media with low fever

b. Signs of progressively increasing respiratory distress with hypoxemia

c. Cough and presence of adventitious respiratory sounds (crackles, wheezes)

d. Hypoxia manifested by decreasing oxygen saturation. Chest radiograph may reveal hyperinflation of the lung and signs of interstitial pneumonitis. Nasopharyngeal culture and smear for respiratory syncytial virus are positive.

e. Complications include apnea, secondary bacterial pneumonia, and potential for future reactive airway disease

4. Clinical management

a. Hospitalization is required for infants with serious disease (as determined by oxygen saturation). Meticulous hand washing and gowns should be used to prevent nosocomial infections.

b. Low concentrations of oxygen are administered for hypoxemia.

c. Use of aerosolized bronchodilators is controversial because of their questionable effectiveness.

d. Recent aerosol trials of the antiviral agent ribavirin (Virazole) have demonstrated some promise in treating severe infection requiring mechanical ventilation. (Pregnant women must not become exposed to ribavirin.)

Asthma

1. Definition: The care of a child or adolescent with asthma is similar to the care of the asthmatic adult (see Chapter 21).

2. Incidence and etiology: The nurse should ask about the following:

a. How the problem has interfered with the child's usual activities, sleep, school, and sports participation.

b. What factors seem to trigger the attacks.

c. Whether the child experiences seasonal inhalant allergies and whether there is a history of allergy in other family members.

d. Whether the child or anyone in the home smokes.

3. Clinical manifestations: Clinical manifestations are similar to those seen in adults. Obtain a baseline peak flow reading when the child is healthy, in a standing position, and using maximal respiratory effort. It may be necessary to use creative approaches when teaching a young child how to use a peak flow meter.

4. Clinical management

a. Inhaled beta agonist (see Table 15–13) is used for acute episodes or before activity to prevent exercise-induced bronchospasm. The child should not use an inhaler more than 4 times a day. The child should use a spacer device to better inhale the entire medication dose.

b. Use an oral beta agonist for children too young to use an inhaler properly.

c. For moderate asthma

(1) Advise child to measure peak flow rate twice a day, once in the morning and once in the evening.

(2) Use an inhaled (or nebulized) beta agonist 4 times a day as needed for symptoms and inhaled cromolyn sodium (see Table 15–13) up to 4 times per day for prevention of episodes. A sustained-release theophylline may be given orally for children who do not respond to 1st-line treatment.

d. For severe asthma

(1) Peak flow measurement is obtained twice daily.

(2) Beta agonist is inhaled 4 times daily.

(3) Cromolyn sodium is inhaled 4 times daily.

(4) Two to 4 puffs of steroid such as beclomethasone (Beclovent, Vancenase) is given 4 times per day. Growth velocity should be measured if steroid is given to young children.

(5) Influenza vaccine should be administered if the child has had at least 1 hospital admission for exacerbated asthma.

e. In cases of exacerbation

(1) Give oxygen if O_2 saturation is less than 95 percent.

(2) Administer nebulized albuterol every 20 minutes for 1 hour, or give continuous nebulized albuterol to children who would require intermittent doses every 15 minutes or for whom respiratory failure appears impending.

(3) If symptoms persist after the 1st nebulizer treatment, 1 dose of an oral prednisone should be given.

(4) If symptoms improve, the child should be sent home and kept on a daily routine of bronchodilators, but with a 3- to 5-day course of oral prednisone substituted for inhaled steroid. There is no need to taper the steroid if the child takes it for less than 1 week.

(5) The child should be admitted to the hospital if oxygen saturation is less than 90 percent.

f. During hospitalization, the following should be administered:

(1) Nebulized beta agonist every 1 to 2 hours

(2) Oral or intravenous methylprednisolone

(3) Intravenous aminophylline is sometimes indicated (with vital signs monitored every 1 hour and a cardiac monitor attached)

(4) Oxygen if needed

(5) Fluid replacement

g. More aggressive therapy should be considered for the patient after discharge.

h. Place the child in cool mist, if warranted.

i. Organize care so the child is disturbed as little as possible. Crying infants may be cuddled. Older children should be taught slow breathing and relaxation techniques. Stress reduction exercises are particularly effective for the child with asthma and are the coping strategies used most frequently by asthmatic children.

j. The nurse can help alleviate anxiety with a gentle, soothing approach to reduce oxygen demands. Encourage rest and quiet activity during acute episodes by playing quietly with the child—telling stories, playing quiet games, listening to tapes.

k. Encourage the child to participate in usual activities when well. Participating in activities as usual, including athletics, helps the child maintain self-esteem.

l. An inhaler may be considered for children with exercise-induced bronchospasm, and the child and family should be taught correct methods of its use. The nurse should observe for side effects.

m. Encourage older children to set goals and reevaluate them frequently. This measure helps prevent noncompliance.

n. Encourage other family members to treat the child normally. Parents should avoid overprotecting the asthmatic child.

o. Teach parents how to allergy-proof the home.

Cystic Fibrosis

1. Definition: Cystic fibrosis is an inherited condition marked by abnormal exocrine gland function and resulting multisystem involvement (mainly respiratory and gastrointestinal systems) in response to thickened mucous secretions and obstruction.
2. Incidence and etiology
   a. Cystic fibrosis has an autosomal recessive inheritance pattern, with a moderate percentage of the general population carrying the gene. The gene locus, on the long arm of chromosome 7, allows for identification of asymptomatic carriers.
   b. Cystic fibrosis predominantly affects Whites.
   c. Cystic fibrosis is a chronic condition of childhood, with an improving prognosis with appropriate treatment. Children live to midadulthood.
3. Clinical manifestations
   a. Respiratory symptoms
      (1) Increased viscosity of bronchial mucus leading to bronchial obstruction with hypoxia, respiratory infection, and chronic obstructive pulmonary disease
      (2) Wheezing, dry cough, increasing respiratory distress, impaired gas exchange, barrel-shaped chest, bronchitis, and pneumonia
   b. Gastrointestinal symptoms
      (1) Meconium ileus in the neonate causing signs of intestinal obstruction
      (2) Mucoid obstruction of the pancreas inhibiting the secretion of pancreatic enzymes needed for digestion
      (3) Bulky, malodorous, "frothy" stools (because of elevated fat content)
      (4) Rectal prolapse is a complication.
   c. Integumentary symptoms
      (1) Sweat containing abnormally high concentrations

of sodium and chloride, making the child taste salty when kissed; the sweat chloride test (pilocarpine iontophoresis) is diagnostic for the condition
      (2) In infants and small children, risk for sodium imbalances
4. Clinical management
   a. Combined therapies to prevent and treat pulmonary and gastrointestinal dysfunction
      (1) Twice daily and as needed chest physiotherapy preceded by administration of aerosolized bronchodilator
      (2) Aerosolized recombinant human deoxyribonuclease, an investigational medication used to thin mucus and promote airway clearance
      (3) Aggressive oral or intravenous antibiotic treatment for respiratory infections
      (4) Replacement of pancreatic enzymes through a high-protein, high-calorie diet and use of multivitamins
   b. Psychosocial support: The nurse should do the following:
      (1) Provide emotional support to the child and family and advice (social and financial) for managing the child with a chronic condition.
      (2) Encourage the child to participate in activities appropriate for age and developmental level; explain that exercise helps mobilize secretions and improves pulmonary health.
      (3) Teach families ways to make the daily therapy interesting and fun for the young child; use play in the approach.
      (4) Teach principles of management to the parents and the child. Refer parents for genetic counseling; put the family in contact with the Cystic Fibrosis Foundation.

Cardiac Defects

See Table 15–14.

Sickle Cell Disease

1. Definition: Congenital hemoglobinopathy. Management of the child with sickle cell disease is similar to that in the adult (see Chapter 25).
2. Incidence and etiology: Seen most frequently in children of African or Mediterranean ethnic groups. The spleen becomes fibrous and nonfunctioning against infection by the time the child is 5 years old.
3. Clinical manifestations: infection can precipitate life-threatening crises.
   a. Vaso-occlusive disease is most commonly seen. It is the abrupt onset of abdominal and joint pain, respiratory distress, or neurologic sequelae resembling stroke. Swelling over the bones of the hands and feet, hand-foot syndrome, is seen frequently in infants and toddlers.
   b. Sequestration affects infants and children younger than 5 years old. Abrupt pooling of large amounts of

Table 15-14. Frequently Seen Congenital Cardiac Defects in Infants

DEFECT	DESCRIPTION	CHARACTERISTIC MURMUR	SURGICAL TREATMENT
Patent ductus arteriosus (PDA)	The ductus arteriosus, present in fetal circulation, fails to close spontaneously after birth, causing circulatory flow from the aorta through the ductus to the pulmonary artery	Machine-like sound, which increases in intensity when infant is lying supine	Administration of indomethacin successfully closes the ductus in some children; otherwise, surgical ligation is necessary
Atrial septal defect (ASD)	Abnormal opening in the atrial septum allows for circulatory flow from the left to the right atrium, increasing the vascular load on the right side of the heart	Systolic ejection murmur at the left upper sternal border	Surgical placement of a Dacron patch, usually before the child reaches school age; cardiopulmonary bypass is necessary
Ventricular septal defect (VSD)	An abnormal opening between the right and left ventricle, which allows blood to shunt from the left to right side and to the pulmonary circulation and increases the vascular load	Pansystolic murmur loudly heard at the left sternal border	Small defects often close spontaneously or are repaired by purse-string suture; recently, repairs have been attempted during cardiac catheterization for children at surgical risk; surgery requires cardiopulmonary bypass and involves closing the defect with a Dacron patch
Coarctation of the aorta	Narrowing of the aorta near the origin of the subclavian artery causes increased pressure proximal to the defect (circulation to head and upper extremities) and decreased pressure distal to the defect (circulation to the lower extremities). Blood pressure between upper and lower extremities is markedly different	None	Excision of the obstruction; if done during infancy, there is the risk of recurrence
Pulmonic stenosis	Stenosis of the opening to the pulmonary artery obstructs blood flow into the pulmonary circulation and causes increased pressure in the right ventricle with right ventricular hypertrophy	Systolic ejection murmur	No treatment if mild; balloon angioplasty during cardiac catheterization is used to dilate the pulmonic valve; surgical intervention widens the pulmonic valve
Tetralogy of Fallot	Combination of 4 separate cardiac defects: ventricular septal defect, pulmonic stenosis, overriding aorta, and right ventricular hypertrophy. Causes altered pressure gradients and either left-to-right or right-to-left shunting, depending on the severity of the pulmonic stenosis and the size of the VSD. Shunting of desaturated blood into both the left ventricle and aorta causes cyanosis and hypoxemia	Radiating ejection click systolic murmur heard best in the 2nd and 3rd interspaces left of the sternum	Goal is complete surgical correction of all underlying defects; in infants who are at surgical risk, a Blalock-Taussig procedure increases pulmonary blood flow until repair is indicated

blood in the spleen causes circulatory collapse and signs of hypovolemic shock.

c. Aplastic anemia is due to decreased marrow production of red blood cells in response to infection (particularly parvovirus, the virus that causes fifth disease) combined with the short circulating life of fragile sickle cells, causing overwhelming anemia.

4. Clinical management
   a. Most states screen newborns routinely for hemoglobinopathies.
   b. Supportive care includes ensuring adequate oxygenation and fluid intake; routine well-child care with vaccine protection against influenza, pneumococcal pneumonia, meningococcal infection, and varicella; and avoidance of crisis precipitators.
      (1) To promote adequate oxygenation to prevent sickling, the child should avoid high altitudes, prolonged stress, strenuous exercise, and unnecessary surgery.
      (2) To conserve energy and decrease metabolic demand during crisis, the child should maintain bed rest with passive exercises. Quiet activities may be conducted with the child as condition improves. Activity as tolerated should be encouraged when the child is well. The child should participate in regular activities but avoid strenuous sports.
      (3) Intake of fluids that the child likes should be increased. To promote hydration at home, parents should do the following:
         • Compute the child's basic fluid requirements, then an amount equal to 1.5 times the basic requirement. This is the daily goal for fluid intake.
         • Identify with the child alternative sources for fluid other than liquid (e.g., frozen desserts, soups, yogurt, gelatins).
         • Make a contract with the child about timing and amount of fluids taken.
         • Remind the child to urinate before bedtime to reduce nocturnal enuresis.
         • Provide a nutritious diet for the child that is high in iron and essential nutrients for growth.
   c. The nurse should teach parents and children about infection prevention methods—avoiding crowds and ill persons, meticulous hand washing, obtaining routine well care and special immunizations against disease, compliance with any antibiotic regimen.
   d. Encourage parents to facilitate normal growth and development, while avoiding precipitating factors.
   e. Refer the child and family for counseling, if appropriate, and encourage parents to seek genetic evaluation.

β-Thalassemia

1. Definition: Inherited hemoglobinopathy produces anemia of varying degrees depending on genetic expression.
2. Incidence and etiology
   a. β-Thalassemia has an autosomal recessive inheritance pattern.
   b. People of Mediterranean descent are usually affected.
3. Clinical manifestations

a. Anemia is of varying degrees, with fatigue, hypoxia, decreased exercise tolerance, splenomegaly, and bone pain; bone marrow hypertrophy causes skeletal malformations.

b. There is a deposition of excess iron from red-cell hemolysis in body tissues (hemosiderosis); skin may have a bronze color.

c. Laboratory tests reveal immature red blood cells, target cells, and decreased hemoglobin and hematocrit. Diagnosis is by hemoglobin electrophoresis, which delineates the type of hemoglobin present in the blood.

4. Clinical management
   a. Management is similar to that for anemia.
   b. Transfusions usually are required for severe forms of the disease but cause greatly increased iron from hemolysis of the transfused cells. Deferoxamine, an iron-chelating agent, can be given to enable excretion of excess iron. Splenectomy may be necessary.
   c. Nursing care is supportive and directed toward ensuring rest, promoting normal growth and development, and care of the family and child with a chronic illness. Family members should be referred for genetic counseling.

Urinary Tract Infection

1. Definition: Microbial invasion of the urinary system causes urinary tract infection (see Chapter 26).
2. Incidence and etiology
   a. Incidence in children is much higher in girls because the urethra is shorter, lessening the transit distance for organisms. Urinary tract infections are more common in uncircumcised boys younger than 1 year of age than in circumcised boys.
   b. Other factors predisposing children to urinary tract infection include the following:
      (1) Willingness of children to ignore the urge to urinate, resulting in urinary stasis, and other conditions resulting in urinary stasis (e.g., neurogenic bladder)
      (2) Presence of congenital mechanical problems of the urinary tract—vesicoureteral reflux, hydronephrosis, urethral stricture, or posterior urethral valves
      (3) Wearing of tight diapers or clothing, or use of bubble bath, conditions causing inflammation of the external area (e.g., vaginitis, pinworm infestation)
      (4) Sexual abuse (suspicious in cases of repeated urinary tract infection)
3. Clinical manifestations
   a. Clinical manifestations in infants and preverbal children are often nonspecific—poor feeding, abdominal discomfort, fever, fussiness, delayed growth, foul-smelling urine, incontinence in a previously trained child.
   b. Urinary tract infection is suspected when an infant demonstrates signs of sepsis without any other demonstrable focus for illness.
   c. It is not unusual for an adolescent girl to experience a urinary tract infection after 1st intercourse.

Table 15–15. Management of Urinary Tract Infection

Nursing Diagnosis	Expected Outcome
Knowledge deficit about prevention of urinary tract infection related to initial experience with the condition	The child and family should be able to describe and demonstrate preventive measures.
Fear of intrusive procedure related to development and cognitive level	The child and family should be able to describe intrusive procedures and cooperate with the procedure as much as possible.

d. Signs of upper urinary tract infection (pyelonephritis) include high fever, chills, flank and abdominal pain, and leukocytosis. The child appears acutely ill.

4. Clinical management (Table 15–15)
   a. A 10-day course of antibiotic therapy is given according to organism sensitivity.
   b. Follow-up culture is obtained 2 to 3 days after completion of the antibiotic regimen.
   c. A complete renal workup (ultrasound, vesicoureterogram, intravenous pyelogram) is ordered for all boys and girls under age 5 after the initial urinary tract infection and for young girls after a 2nd documented case. School-aged and adolescent girls do not generally need a renal workup unless an anatomic problem is suspected.
   d. Nursing interventions
      (1) Explain any proposed procedures thoroughly to the child using visual aids whenever possible.
      (2) Reassure the child that the procedure does not harm the body but is necessary to determine whether anything is not working correctly.
      (3) Encourage the child to breathe deeply and slowly or to sing a song during catheterization. This promotes relaxation of the sphincter.
      (4) Advise parents to avoid using bubble bath or irritating diaper wipes.
      (5) Teach young girls to wipe from front to back after urinating and to keep the area dry. Wearing of cotton underwear allows for adequate air circulation to the area.
      (6) Encourage fluid intake.
      (7) Advise sexually active adolescent girls to urinate after engaging in sexual intercourse.

Nephrotic Syndrome

1. Definition: Nephrotic syndrome is a condition that alters the permeability of the glomerular basement membrane, allowing passage of albumin and other plasma proteins into the glomerulus for urinary excretion.
   a. The protein shift out of the capillaries creates an imbalance between colloidal osmotic pressure and hydrostatic pressure.
   b. Fluid leaks into the interstitial spaces causes edema and hypovolemia. The hypovolemia stimulates the renin–angiotensin mechanism and stimulates the production of antidiuretic hormone, both of which cause reabsorption of sodium and water.
2. Incidence and etiology
   a. The condition affects children primarily younger than 8 years old (but not infants).
   b. The cause is unknown and the course is self-limiting, but some children relapse.
3. Clinical manifestations
   a. Insidious development of edema (periorbital in the morning, ascites), which progresses to generalized swelling
   b. Poor appetite, pale skin
   c. Decreased urine output with dark "frothy" urine and elevated urine protein
   d. True weight loss masked by edema weight
   e. Fatigue
   f. Normal blood pressure
   g. Increased susceptibility to infection from loss of plasma proteins
4. Clinical management
   a. Administration of corticosteroids
   b. Supportive care during acute manifestations includes adequate rest, nutritious diet high in protein, temporary salt restriction, necessary infection prevention, and treatment
   c. Meticulous skin care of edematous areas, particularly the genital area
   d. Reassurance for the child and family

Diabetes

1. Definition: Type 1 insulin-dependent diabetes mellitus is a clinical syndrome characterized by insulin deficiency and is detailed in Chapter 29.
2. Incidence and etiology
   a. Children with insulin-dependent diabetes mellitus often experience their 1st serious episode of hyperglycemia after a mild infection.
   b. In some adolescents with a family history of non–insulin-dependent diabetes, maturity-onset diabetes of youth, a non–insulin-dependent form of diabetes, develops.
3. Clinical manifestations: Because signs of type 1 diabetes are vague in children, the nurse should note the following at every well-child visit:
   a. Any excessive urination (polyuria), particularly if it wakes the child at night or the previously trained child begins to wet the bed
   b. Complaints of persistent thirst (polydipsia)
   c. Gradual weight loss despite increased appetite (polyphagia)
   d. History of *Candida* infections
   e. Family history of insulin-dependent diabetes mellitus
   f. Test urine for glucose and protein at each well visit
4. Intervention (Box 15–4)
   a. Monitor growth velocity.
   b. Check for signs of dehydration.
   c. Insulin requirements vary according to the level of activity at a given time period, during growth spurts,

---

BOX 15–4. Management of Type 1 Diabetes

A common nursing diagnosis for a child with type 1 diabetes is impaired home maintenance management related to disparity of disease restrictions with desired lifestyle.

Expected outcomes include an adolescent who, after teaching, should be able to describe management of the disease and explain how disease management can be adapted to personal lifestyle.

---

at puberty, and when the child is ill or having surgery.

d. Provide a diet of sufficient nutrients for age and growth requirements. Include snacks that are planned around peak action of insulin and before exercise.

e. Encourage regular exercise. Children may participate in school sports.

f. Be particularly supportive to adolescents with diabetes because the desire to conform to peers is important at this developmental level.

g. Encourage the adolescent to express feelings about the disease and its management.

h. If noncompliance becomes a problem, develop a new plan that incorporates the treatments better into the adolescent's lifestyle (e.g., including fast foods in the diet).

i. Be realistic with the adolescent when explaining the importance of lifelong control, pointing out that control does not have to be at odds with lifestyle choices.

j. Encourage the adolescent to take charge of management with some support, and provide frequent positive reinforcement.

k. Assist the family to find support resources in the community and financial help for equipment if needed.

Idiopathic Scoliosis

1. Definition: Idiopathic scoliosis is a lateral curvature of the spine with associated muscle weakness on the convex side of the curve and rotation of the rib cage. The curvature usually becomes apparent during the adolescent growth spurt.
2. Incidence and etiology
   a. The incidence is higher in girls than in boys.
   b. The cause is unknown, although it may be the result of multifactorial or autosomal dominant inheritance pattern.
3. Clinical manifestations include varying degrees of curvatures. Severe curves can cause respiratory compromise.
4. Clinical management
   a. Screening for scoliosis is discussed in Table 15–2.
   b. Treatment for moderate curves includes bracing and exercises. Plastic shell braces are better tolerated than the Milwaukee brace because they can be hidden by loose clothing.
   c. Surgical correction of severe curves includes spinal fusion with placement of rods, wires, or both. Anterior or posterior approach to surgery is used. The

anterior approach requires chest tube placement for several days after surgery.

d. Postoperative nursing care includes logrolling carefully to change the child's position in bed until the child is fitted for a brace; monitoring and treating pain (patient-controlled analgesia is usually used); monitoring circulation, sensation, and motion; and other routine postoperative measures.

e. Emotional support is needed for the adolescent who needs to wear a brace preoperatively or postoperatively. Encourage positive self-esteem.

Legg-Calvé-Perthes Disease

1. Definition: Acquired necrosis of the femoral head causes discrepancy between the femur and the acetabulum. The condition appears in stages over a course of months to years. Stages are avascular, revascularization, reparative, and reformation of the femur head.
2. Incidence and etiology
   a. The disease is seen more frequently in White boys between the ages of 4 and 8 years.
   b. Most cases are unilateral.
3. Clinical manifestations: There is insidious onset of an intermittent limp, stiffness, pain (may radiate down to the knee), and limited range of motion.
4. Clinical management
   a. The goal of management is to contain the femoral head in the acetabulum for proper shaping during regeneration.
   b. The initial period of rest (sometimes with traction) is followed by application of an abduction brace or cast. Ambulation braces are available to allow limited participation in usual activities.
   c. Surgical correction can shorten treatment time.

Osteomyelitis

1. Definition: Osteomyelitis is an inflammation of the bone (see Chapter 34).
2. Incidence and etiology
   a. Osteomyelitis is more common in boys than girls.
   b. It is caused by any one of a number of pathogenic bacteria.
3. Clinical manifestations
   a. Initial symptoms include pain, fever, and malaise.
   b. Later symptoms include swelling, redness, warmth over the bone, irritability, and weakness.
4. Clinical management
   a. Adaptations in nursing care for children with osteomyelitis are directed toward planning with the parent how to meet the child's activity needs as the child's condition improves and providing a high-calorie nutritious diet with sufficient calcium and vitamin D for bone healing and growth.
   b. Children should continue their schooling.
   c. Teach parents how to properly care for the intravenous line and the method for administering intravenous medication at home.

Juvenile Rheumatoid Arthritis

1. Definition: Juvenile rheumatoid arthritis is an inflammatory disease of 1 or more joints, with associated iridocyclitis in some children. The cause may be infectious or an autoimmune process. There are 3 major classifications:
   a. Systemic
   b. Pauciarticular—4 or fewer joints affected
   c. Polyarticular—more than 4 joints affected
2. Incidence and etiology: Occurs mainly in the prepubertal child.
3. Clinical manifestations
   a. Swelling, stiffness, and decreased motion in affected joints, with morning stiffness "gelling" of the joint that improves during the day or after activity.
   b. Fatigue, leukocytosis, positive rheumatoid factor and antinuclear antibodies (depending on the type of arthritis), and elevated erythrocyte sedimentation rate.
4. Clinical management
   a. Management goals include reducing inflammation, reducing pain, and conserving energy while encouraging usual activities.
   b. Nonsteroidal anti-inflammatory drugs help control pain and reduce joint inflammation.
   c. Apply heat modalities (e.g., whirlpool, paraffin, and hot packs) during passive exercise; devices for activities of daily living may need modification.
   d. Teach patients infection prevention and stress reduction measures; provide counseling and support; recommend yearly eye slit-lamp examinations.

Duchenne's Muscular Dystrophy

1. Definition: Duchenne's muscular dystrophy is a childhood-onset condition in which muscle fibers deteriorate, causing deformity and decreased muscle function and strength.
2. Incidence and etiology
   a. An X-linked recessive inheritance pattern causes nearly exclusive incidence in boys.
   b. Average age of onset is 4 years, with progressive deterioration through the teen years; death is usually caused by respiratory or cardiac failure.
3. Clinical manifestations
   a. Muscle weakness that appears subtly and manifests itself through various gross motor delays as the child matures; progresses to muscle atrophy and complete motor disability
   b. Fatty infiltration of calf muscles (pseudohypertrophy)
   c. Mild mental retardation in some affected children
   d. Complications of deformities, scoliosis, contractures, infections, obesity, and late cardiac complications
   e. Elevated creatine phosphokinase and serum glutamic oxaloacetic transaminase; positive biopsy for fatty infiltration of muscle tissue
4. Clinical management: The goals of intervention and plan are similar to those for the child with cerebral palsy.
   a. Goals are to preserve function and prevent deformity.
   b. Encourage mobility without assistance for as long as possible.

   c. Facilitate independence and performance of activities of daily living.
   d. Refer the family for genetic counseling; carrier identification and prenatal diagnoses.
   e. Provide essential services and emotional support.

Dermatitis

1. Definition
   a. Atopic dermatitis (eczema) is inflammation of the skin caused by hypersensitivity to allergens and exacerbated by certain factors in the child's environment (e.g., stress, foods).
   b. Contact dermatitis is skin inflammation caused by contact with an irritant such as plants (e.g., poison ivy, oak, sumac), soaps or detergents, rough clothing, and certain cosmetics such as eye makeup or deodorant.
2. Incidence and etiology: There is usually a genetic predisposition to allergy.
3. Clinical manifestations
   a. In atopic dermatitis, IgE-mediated allergic response causes histamine release into the dermis. The process results in inflammation, edema, skin lesions, and severe pruritus.
   b. In contact dermatitis, allergen (antigen) invasion of the skin causes a T-cell mediated response with delayed inflammatory reaction (2 to 3 days) upon subsequent exposure to the allergen causing localized erythema, severe pruritus, papules, oozing, and crusting of lesions.
   c. Complication: impetigo
      (1) Impetigo is an infection of the skin that is caused by organisms entering through irritated or inflamed tissue.
      (2) Usual causative organisms are *Staphylococcus aureus*, or group A β-hemolytic Streptococcus.
      (3) Highly contagious lesions, which ooze and form a honey-colored crust and can spread quickly to any part of the body.
4. Clinical management
   a. Keep skin moist and lubricated. Reduce pruritus with administration of antihistamines, topical hydrocortisone preparations for nonoozing lesions, and avoidance of precipitating factors.
   b. Teach parents to keep the child's skin lubricated.
      (1) Children should not be bathed every day (except to clean the diaper area in infants).
      (2) Apply bath oil or occlusive moisturizer to wet skin after bathing (seals in moisture). Moisturizer should be used between baths.
      (3) Apply cool compresses to pruritic areas. May use a colloidal oatmeal preparation in the bath water.
      (4) Keep the child's hands clean, and fingernails cut regularly. The child should be encouraged not to scratch or touch infected lesions. The child's hands may be covered with cotton gloves or the infant's hands with soft cotton socks if scratching is a problem.
   c. Secondary infections are treated with topical anti-

infective (mupirocin) or systemic antibiotics depending on severity.

d. Address any body image concerns.

Infestations

1. Definition
   a. Pediculosis is a parasitic invasion by *Pediculus humanus capitis*, or the head louse, usually found in hair on the head.
   b. Scabies is infestation of the body by the *Sarcoptes scabiei*, or itch mite.
2. Incidence and etiology: Lice and mites are transmitted from human to human or from contaminated objects (hair accessories, clothing) to humans.
3. Clinical manifestations
   a. Intense itching at the site of infestation, often keeping the child awake at night
   b. Visible lice or nits (eggs) on the hair shaft (nits closer than one-fourth inch from the scalp indicate active infestation).
   c. Small scabs or tracts on the body with scabies infestation (often seen between fingers and toes)
   d. Associated dermatitis
4. Clinical management
   a. Pediculosis: Treat the child and family members with permethrin shampoo or cream rinse (Nix) and comb out the remaining nits.
   b. Scabies: Treat the child and close contacts with permethrin cream (Elimite).
   c. To prevent the spread of pediculosis and scabies, wash all hats, bedding, hair accessories, jackets, and other articles of clothing in hot water and dry in an electric or gas dryer. Items prone to shrinking can be run dry through a hot dryer cycle for 20 minutes or placed in an airtight plastic bag for 2 weeks.

◘ PEDIATRIC EMERGENCIES

Emergency Equipment

1. Many emergency departments and ambulatory care settings do not have the equipment needed to treat children.
2. Box 15-5 lists basic equipment required to meet the emergency needs of children.

Head Trauma

1. Definition
   a. A skull fracture is usually either linear or depressed.
   b. Concussion is trauma to the head that causes temporary loss of consciousness and usually various degrees of amnesia. Young children are susceptible to post-concussion syndrome—irritability, vomiting, lethargy, without loss of consciousness—within the first 24 to 72 hours after injury.

BOX 15-5. Pediatric Emergency Equipment

Ventilation and Oxygen Equipment

Multisize small airways (infant, small child, small adult)
Oxygen equipment with infant and child-sized masks
Small suction catheters
Laryngoscope blades and handle
Infant and child-sized endotracheal tubes
Nebulizer machine with appropriate administration tubing and reservoir
Pulse oximeter
Peak flow meter

Intravenous Equipment

Small arm boards
Pediatric burettes with tubing
500-ml bags or bottles of various types of intravenous fluid (normal saline, dextrose in half or quarter strength saline, lactated Ringer's solution)
Syringes—tuberculin, 3cc, 5cc, 10cc
Butterfly needles—21, 23, 25 gauge
Straight needles—20, 21, 23 gauge and 5/8, 1 inch long
Small tourniquets or rubber bands to be used as tourniquets
Blood pressure cuffs—infant, child, small adult

Miscellaneous Equipment

Bandages and Band-aids (preferably decorated for young children)
Needle-nosed forceps for removing foreign bodies from the nose
Lumbar puncture tray with small spinal needle
Straight catheters or feeding tubes—8, 10, 12 French

Medications

Epinephrine 1:1000
Albuterol for nebulizer
Saline for nebulizer
Lidocaine
Racemic epinephrine
Aminophylline
Narcan
Digoxin
Sodium bicarbonate
Phenytoin (Dilantin)
Diphenhydramine (Benadryl)
Diazepam (Valium)
Intravenous-methylprednisolone (Solu-Medrol)
Syrup of ipecac
Activated charcoal

---

c. Contusion is bruising or tearing of the brain tissue at the site of impact (coup) or at a site opposite from the impact (contracoup).
d. Hematomas
   (1) Subdural hematoma, which occurs when blood from vessel rupture subsequent to a head injury collects between the dura and the brain. It usually develops slowly over a period of several days and is seen commonly in children ages 2 to 6 months.
   (2) Epidural hematoma occurs when there is bleeding between the dura and the skull. Symptoms appear rapidly after the initial injury. It is not usually seen in children younger than age 4 years.
2. Incidence and etiology
   a. Head injury is 1 of the most frequent causes of childhood morbidity and mortality.

b. Automobile accidents cause the greatest number of head injuries in children, and these are often associated with multiple other types of trauma (e.g., severe abrasions, fractures). Other causes include falls, bicycle accidents, skateboard injuries, and purposefully inflicted head trauma.

c. Open fontanels in children younger than 2 years old assist the brain to absorb mechanical stress better than a rigid cranium. The child's head, however, is larger in proportion to the body than an adult's, and this proportion predisposes the child to injury caused by internal movement of the brain against the skull in response to head trauma.

3. Clinical manifestations: cerebral edema complicates most head injuries.

4. Clinical management: Management of the child is similar to that for the adult (see Chapter 18). Special considerations for children concern effect on future growth and development and prevention of future injury. Children with severe increased intracranial pressure are usually transferred to the intensive care unit, until the condition is stabilized. Children with severe head injury can experience later developmental delays. The patient and family may be referred for early intervention if warranted.

a. Decrease environmental stimuli and keep the child in a dark, quiet room; plan nursing care for minimal disturbance. Talk soothingly to the child to alleviate anxiety, which can exacerbate increased intracranial pressure.

b. The child may experience post-traumatic syndrome up to a year after the injury. Reassure parents that these manifestations usually are self-limiting, but that additional evaluation is required if they last longer than a month. Monitor for the following:
   (1) Poor concentration and problems in school
   (2) Occasional dizziness
   (3) Behavioral alterations, including sleep disturbances
   (4) Seizures (children at risk require anticonvulsants)

c. The circumstances of the injury should be determined, including how it occurred, whether the child lost consciousness, when symptoms began to appear, precautions usually taken to prevent this type of injury (e.g., helmet, other protection measures).

d. Record deviations from the child's normal behavior.

e. Note any complaints of headache, dizziness, nausea, double vision, vomiting, weakness, seizures, confusion, lethargy, and postinjury amnesia.

f. Obtain vital signs at least every 30 minutes, and document any signs of increased intracranial pressure—increasing blood pressure, decreasing pulse and respirations, pupil changes, confused behavior.

g. Perform neurologic assessment, including cranial nerve function, and physical examination to assess the child for associated injuries. Observe the child for clear drainage or bleeding from the ear or nose, which might indicate a skull fracture.

h. Rate the child on the pediatric coma scale for altered consciousness (see Chapter 18).

i. Reinforce safety principles and prevention of injury.

Obstructed Airway

1. Definition: Obstructed airway in children leads to respiratory arrest.

2. Incidence and etiology
   a. The incidence of mechanical airway obstruction is higher in children than adults because young children tend to put things in their mouths and their airways are smaller in diameter. Small parts of toys, balloon pieces, and pieces of food are implicated most frequently.
   b. Infection
      (1) If not recognized and treated quickly, epiglottitis (inflammation of the epiglottis), an infection usually caused by *H. influenzae*, causes airway obstruction. Incidents of epiglottitis have decreased since the advent of the HIB vaccine.
      (2) Severe croup can also cause airway obstruction, but, because the symptoms of croup develop more gradually than those of epiglottitis, intervention usually prevents obstruction before it occurs.
   c. Other causes of airway obstruction include major burns and injury.

3. Clinical manifestations include increased respiratory effort, cyanosis, and cessation of breathing (see pp. 536–537).

4. Clinical management: Endotrachial tube insertion and intravenous steroids may be necessary to prevent airway obstruction in the child with epiglottitis or croup. Removal of obstruction and cardiopulmonary resuscitation are essential for the child with a complete mechanical airway obstruction.

Cardiopulmonary Arrest

See Table 15–16.

Poisoning

1. Definition: Poisoning occurs upon ingestion, inhalation, or contact with a toxic substance or a substance in toxic amounts.

2. Incidence and etiology
   a. Poisonings are a frequent cause of injury in young children.
   b. Use of childproof medicine caps and safety precautions in the home has reduced the incidence, but poisonings tend to occur when parents are temporarily distracted from watching the child. A large number of poisonings occur in grandparents' homes, so parents need to be particularly alert when visiting relatives.

3. Clinical manifestations: Depending on the type of poison, signs can include irritation around the mouth, presence of pills in the mouth, dizziness, lethargy, cyanosis, and burns.

4. Clinical management (see p. 549)
   a. The nurse should obtain the following information from the parent:
      (1) Child's condition—airway, breathing, circulation, level of consciousness, other symptoms

Table 15–16. Cardiopulmonary Resuscitation for Infants and Children

Assessment Data	Management for Infant	Management for Child
Section 1 Child appears cyanotic, not breathing	1. Pinch sole of the foot or flick just beneath sternum to stimulate spontaneous breathing. 2. Call out loud for help. 3. Place infant supine on a hard surface and open the airway by gently tilting the infant's head back at the forehead and lifting the chin (head-tilt/chin-lift).	1. Shake the child, or ask if help is needed. 2. Call out loud for help. 3. Place the child supine on hard surface and tilt the child's head back while lifting the child's chin. 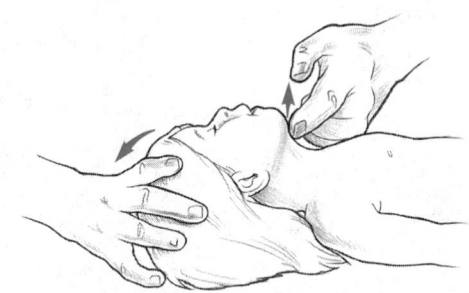
	4. Check for breathing by placing your ear close to the infant's mouth for 3–5 sec; listen and feel for breathing, watch for rise and fall of chest. 5. If there are no respirations, place your mouth over the infant's mouth and nose forming a seal. 6. Give two rescue breaths—slow breaths, each allowing for exhalation in between. If there is no response, reposition and attempt to ventilate again.	4. Same as for infant. 5. If there are no respirations, place your mouth over the child's mouth, forming a seal. Pinch the child's nostrils with the hand that was supporting the forehead. 6. Same as for infant.
Section 2 Obstruction is suspected (child is choking, cannot vocalize, points to throat)	1. Turn infant prone on your lap with head lowered. Administer 5 back blows with the palm of your hand between the scapulas. 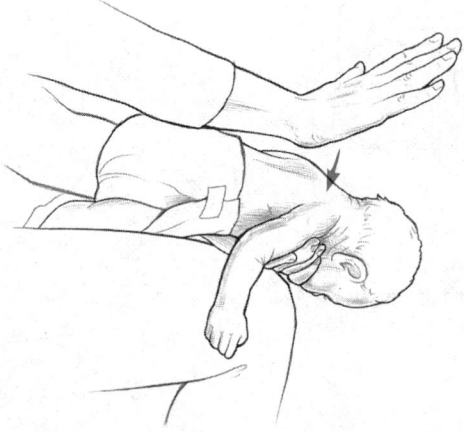	1. Confirm that the child is choking by asking whether help is needed. If the child is coughing or attempting to clear the obstruction, wait.
	2. If object is not dislodged with back blows, turn infant supine, while supporting the infant's head, and administer 5 chest thrusts (compressions) with first two fingers. 3. Alternate back blows with compressions until the object is dislodged. 4. If the infant becomes unconscious, position as for cardiopulmonary resuscitation using jaw lift. Attempt to remove object if visualized. Give rescue breaths and continue with previous steps. Repeat until the object is dislodged or help arrives.	2. Administer the Heimlich maneuver (5 distinct upward subdiaphragmatic abdominal thrusts) if the child is unsuccessful. 3. Persist until the object is dislodged. 4. Same as for infant.

Table continued on following page

Table 15–16. Cardiopulmonary Resuscitation for Infants and Children (Continued)

Assessment Data	Management for Infant	Management for Child
Section 3		
Cyanosis, no pulse	1. See Section 1. 2. Check for pulse (see below). If pulse is present, continue breathing at 1 breath every 3 seconds (20/min). 3. Palpate brachial pulse while keeping the infant's head tilted.	1. See Section 1. 2. For children younger than 8 years, same as for infant; for children older than 8 years, 1 breath every 5 seconds (12/min). 3. Palpate carotid pulse.

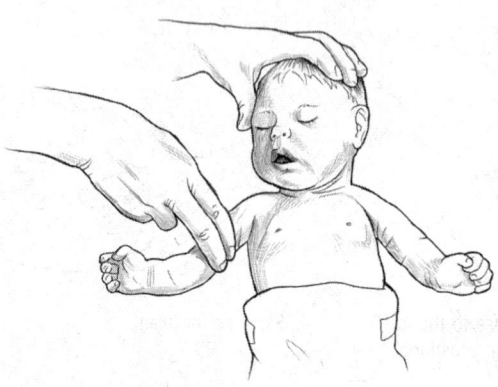

	Management for Infant	Management for Child

	4. Locate site for chest compression:
	  a. Draw an imaginary line connecting nipples.
	  b. Place index finger below the line at sternum, and place the second and third fingers next to it.
		4. Locate site for chest compression:
		  a. Place middle finger on lower rib and follow rib line to sternal notch. Place index finger directly next to and above the notch.
		  b. Place heel of hand on sternum above index finger (two hands for children older than 8 years).

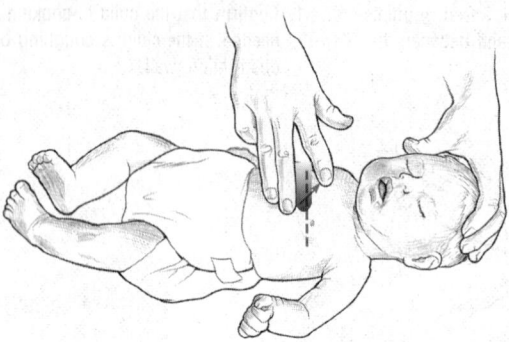
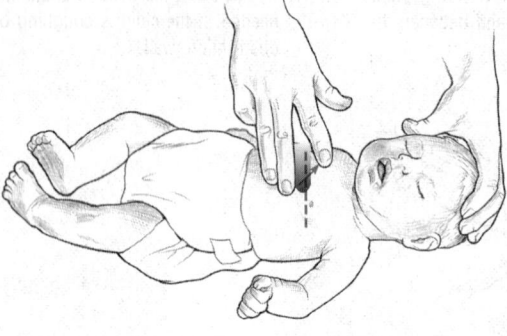

	Management for Infant	Management for Child

	c. Compress 1/2–1 inch at location of 2nd and 3rd fingers at a rate of 100/min.
	
	5. Cardiopulmonary resuscitation cycle
	  a. One rescuer—1 breath per 5 compressions for 20 cycles, check brachial pulse. Reassess every few minutes.
	  b. Two rescuers—same as a.
		c. Compress 1–1 1/2 inches at a rate of 100/min (1 1/2–2 inches at 80–100/min for children older than 8 years).
		5. Cardiopulmonary resuscitation
		  a. One rescuer—1 breath per 5 compressions for 20 cycles, check carotid pulse (children younger than 8 years); 2 breaths per 15 compressions for 4 cycles (children older than 8 years). Reassess every few minutes.
		  b. Two rescuers—1 breath per 5 compressions.

(2) Type of substance involved and amount if known

(3) Route of exposure—oral ingestion, topical contact with skin or eyes, inhaled

(4) Time lapsed since exposure and any first aid administered

(5) Child's age and approximate weight

b. Observations

(1) Obtain vital signs and note level of consciousness.

(2) Record any signs of chemical burning on the lips.

(3) Examine any vomitus for presence of pills.

c. Goals are to

(1) Prevent further absorption of the poison

(2) Prevent secondary complications

(3) Prevent future incidents

d. Emergency management or oral ingestion depends on the type of poison involved. The Poison Control Center or health care provider should be contacted and their instructions followed.

(1) It may be necessary to administer cardiopulmonary resuscitation.

(2) Promote gastric emptying by the following:

- Giving syrup of ipecac followed by 6 to 8 ounces of water to induce vomiting. The water should be given 1st if it appears that the child will refuse the water after the ipecac. Do not induce vomiting for ingestion of petroleum distillates or caustic chemicals, or if the child is unconscious.

- Perform gastric lavage with normal saline if the poisons are rapidly absorbed, if the child is unconscious, or if the child has not vomited for 1 hour after ipecac administration.

(3) Prevent further absorption by administering activated charcoal (1 to 2 gm per kg) orally or through the gavage tube when the stomach is empty. The charcoal may be diluted with water or a cathartic such as sorbitol or magnesium sulfate.

(4) Supportive care is given according to the poison ingested and the child's condition.

e. Emergency management of cutaneous or ocular exposure is performed as follows:

(1) Remove all clothing contaminated with the chemical.

(2) Dilute the poison by flushing with copious amounts of water for a minimum of 15 to 20 minutes.

(3) Burns should be evaluated and treated, eyes should be patched, and the child referred to an ophthalmologist.

f. Teach parents poison prevention and first aid for poisonings.

Drug Overdose and Adolescent Suicide

1. Definition: Adolescents ingest a toxic level of a pharmaceutical.

2. Incidence and etiology

a. Adolescent suicide is becoming one of the leading causes of death in children 15 to 19 years old.

b. Deliberate drug overdose is sometimes used as a method for attempted suicide in adolescents. Often,

adolescents use this method as a "cry for help," hoping that someone will discover that they have taken the drug and get them to emergency assistance.

3. Clinical manifestations vary depending on the substance used. Signs of an impending suicide attempt in an adolescent are similar to those in an adult (see Chapter 41).

4. Clinical management: Treatment is as described for emergency management of the poisoned child (see Chapter 40).

Emergency Management of the Burned Child

1. Definition: Initial burn assessment and management for children is similar to that for adults (see Chapter 36).

2. Incidence and etiology: Special considerations for children with burns are related to fluid balance and body size.

3. Clinical manifestations: Estimating the extent of burns in children differs from that in adults because the child's head is much larger in proportion to the body (see Chapter 36).

a. Minor burns

- Partial-thickness burns that affect less than 10 percent of the body surface are minor.

- Usually, there is no need to admit the child unless the child is younger than 2 years.

b. Moderate burns

- Partial-thickness burns that affect 10 to 20 percent of the body are moderate.

- Moderate burns can be treated and managed at a local hospital with experience in burn care. Children younger than age 4 years or children with burns of the hands, feet, face, or genital area may be transferred to a burn center.

c. Major burns

- Partial-thickness burns that affect more than 20 percent of the body surface are major.

- All full-thickness burns are major burns.

- Burns associated with respiratory tract injury or other internal injuries or illness, and electrical burns are major burns.

- Children with major burns should be admitted to a burn center.

4. Clinical management

a. Maintain life support systems if required. An artificial airway is considered when the burned area involves the face or neck or when there has been significant heat or smoke inhalation.

b. Because the young child's fluid balance is precarious, initiate fluid resuscitation immediately to prevent circulatory collapse.

(1) The goal of fluid replacement is to maintain a urine output of at least 1 to 2 ml per kg per hr.

(2) Intravenous fluid replacement is used for all children with moderate to severe burns. Lactated Ringer's solution is used most frequently.

(3) The resuscitation amount is calculated according to a variety of formulas, but half of the calculated

amount is given within the first 8 hours of the injury, with the remaining half given over the next 16 hours.

   (4) Use of colloids is controversial.

c. For pain management, begin intravenous narcotic administration when the condition is stable.

d. Wound management begins after the child's condition is stable. Excision of eschar, hydrotherapy, and débridement may be necessary.

   (1) Keep the child covered and warm with sterile sheets or dressings until after resuscitation.

   (2) Apply prescribed antimicrobial to burned areas using aseptic technique and sterile dressings.

e. For nutritional management, provide a high-protein, high-calorie diet when the child can take oral feedings (usually after the danger of paralytic ileus has passed). Burns greatly increase the metabolic rate.

f. Subsequent management of the child with a major burn is handled by a burn treatment center. Wound management is particularly complicated. Specialized, expert nursing care is required to prevent physical and severe emotional sequelae.

Sports Injuries

1. Definition: Sports injury results from mechanical stress to muscle ligaments, tendons, or bone.
2. Incidence and etiology: Sports injuries are one of the most common causes of musculoskeletal injury in children (see p. 508).
3. Clinical manifestations
   a. Fractures—obvious deformity, pain, numbness and tingling distal to the injury, limited movement, decreased circulation distal to the injury, and occasional edema. Children are more susceptible to greenstick fractures, which are a bending, rather than break, of bone.
   b. Strain—usually minor injury to the muscle or tendon. It is most often associated with overuse syndromes, and there is slight pain at the site.
   c. Sprain—ligament tear that is often severe. Sprain causes pain and edema at the site, limited movement, and bruising.
   d. Complications—postfracture fat embolism, epiphyseal plate injury that can halt bone growth, and increased potential for reinjury at the site.
4. Clinical management
   a. Obtain information about the pain (intermittent or constant), how the injury occurred, whether there is numbness or tingling, and any treatment measures taken. Definitive diagnosis of a fracture is by radiography of the injured area.
   b. Test for capillary refill distal to the site. Observe for edema, movement limitation, and deformity.
   c. Treatment
      (1) Immobilization by traction, casting, or splinting, depending on the type and extent of the injury
      (2) Open reduction and internal fixation for severe fractures
      (3) RICE (*r*est, *i*ce, *c*ompression, and *e*levation) early

treatment for strains and sprains. Apply ice for 20 minutes an hour for the 1st several hours. Weight-bearing should be limited.

d. The primary goals of nursing care are to prevent further injury and to prevent the hazards of immobility. The child may be immobilized by traction or cast (see pp. 521–522).

Sudden Infant Death Syndrome

1. Definition: Sudden infant death syndrome is the sudden, unanticipated death of an otherwise healthy infant. Autopsy findings provide no explanation for the cause of death, which usually occurs while the infant is sleeping.
2. Incidence and etiology: The cause remains unknown, although extensive research has identified some risk factors:
   a. Peak incidence at 2 to 4 months of age
   b. Male gender
   c. Low birth weight. Preterm infants more susceptible, particularly if Apgar scores are low
   d. Sibling who died of sudden infant death syndrome
   e. Infant in prone sleeping position
   f. Apnea of infancy—apneic spells lasting 20 seconds or longer with color change, suddenly decreased muscle tone, and choking in an infant of normal gestational age (more than 37 weeks)
3. Clinical manifestations
   a. The infant is often brought to the emergency department by ambulance even though already dead.
   b. Autopsy is required to definitively establish the cause of death.
4. Clinical management
   a. Elicit a careful, factual history of the events surrounding the finding of the infant and any resuscitative measures tried.
   b. Protect the parents' privacy and facilitate the grief process.
   c. Assign a primary nurse to remain with the parents and provide a quiet, private area if possible. Expedite the routine information-gathering process. Clarify information given to the parents by the physician about the autopsy and investigation of the death circumstances.
   d. Encourage the parents to ask questions, express feelings, and cry.
   e. The nurse should request appropriate clergy, if parents desire, and offer to contact a funeral home to facilitate arrangements.
   f. The nurse should clean and dress the infant for the parents to say good-bye. Parents should be allowed to hold and cuddle the infant.
   g. Give information about sudden infant death syndrome to the parents and refer them to a local chapter of a support group. Encourage parents to talk to siblings and other family members about sudden infant death syndrome.
   h. Provide other interventions as appropriate for the family of any child who has died.

◼ *PUBLIC HEALTH CONSIDERATIONS*

Health Education in the Public Schools

1. Teaching school-age children about self-care begins at home with parent role modeling and continues through the health education program at school. Parental input into the health education program ensures that the children in a given community receive the information they need.
2. Components of a comprehensive health program focus on the following:
   a. Repetition and reinforcement of information at various age levels and levels of comprehension.
   b. Respect for self and others
   c. Understanding lifestyle factors that contribute to disease.
   d. Principles of preventive health—hygiene, nutrition, exercise, sleep, safety, lifestyle choices, maturation and puberty, and avoidance of risks
   e. Anticipation and discussion of health problems—smoking, substance use, sexuality, and violence
   f. Values clarification, using peers for discussion and support. Refraining from sexual harassment should be emphasized throughout the curriculum.

Identifying and Managing Child Abuse

1. Definition
   a. Child neglect—situation in which multiple family stressors interfere with the proper management of the child's daily needs, including hygiene, warmth, nutrition, rest, and emotional and health care needs.
   b. Child abuse—purposeful physical, sexual, or emotional injury to a child, which results from severe family dysfunction. Child abuse and neglect are illegal in the United States and other countries, and reporting of suspected child abuse is mandatory.
2. Incidence and etiology
   a. Many abusers have been victims of abuse as children and perpetuate the behavior unless stopped by appropriate intervention.
   b. With inappropriate parent-child fit, parental expectations are too high for the child. The child not living up to parental expectations contributes to decreased parental self-esteem.
   c. Decreased knowledge and understanding of parenting skills are often due to becoming a parent at too young an age or lack of effective role models.
   d. With complicated pregnancy or delivery, the infant may be perceived as "difficult." Premature infants are particularly at risk.
   e. Socioeconomic factors include financial stress, emotional illness, separation or divorce, and insufficient social supports. Some families use physical punishment as discipline. Assessment should attempt to discriminate between discipline and abuse.
3. Clinical manifestations
   a. Physical

   (1) Unexplained bruises, lacerations, or unusual marks, particularly on areas of the body that are usually hidden from view
   (2) Fractures (often evidence of old fractures by radiograph)
   (3) Burns, usually regularly marginated
   (4) Head and neck trauma, frequently caused by shaking an infant or young child
   (5) Signs of internal injury and bleeding
   (6) A story about how the injury occurred that is inconsistent with the type of injury sustained or the child's developmental level
   (7) Role reversal in which the child acts protective toward the abusing parent
   (8) Child acting afraid of adults
   b. Emotional
   (1) Failure to thrive, so that the child appears malnourished and listless, and exhibits growth and developmental delay
   (2) Overt signs of low self-esteem
   (3) Overly afraid to make mistakes
   (4) Aggressive behavior or compliant and withdrawn, depending on the child's temperament
   (5) Sleep disturbances, phobias, enuresis, thumb sucking
   (6) Running away, especially the older child who may abuse substances
   c. Sexual
   (1) Abrupt change in behavior, nightmares, sexual "acting out," excessive interest in genital area of self and others, knowledge of adult sexual behavior that is inconsistent with age and developmental level
   (2) Physical signs of sexual abuse, including vaginal discharge, bleeding, rectal bleeding, dysuria, sexually transmitted disease, and signs of trauma in the genital area. Even the young child can give an explicit description of what has happened using terminology appropriate for age and developmental level.
4. Clinical management
   a. The goals for intervention include the following:
   (1) Protecting the child and preventing additional injury
   (2) Assisting the child to obtain or regain emotional stability
   (3) Assisting the family to change abusive behaviors and learn positive parenting skills.
   (4) Preventing abusive behavior in high-risk families
   b. Primary prevention
   (1) Encouraging pregnant women and adolescents to attend prenatal and parenting classes
   (2) Identifying infants at risk through accurate assessment and observation before the infant is discharged from the hospital after birth
   (3) Referring high-risk families to community resources—visiting nurse, adolescent parenting programs, and social services
   c. Secondary prevention
   (1) Assisting with identifying abused or neglected children in the health care setting

(2) Initiating investigation by the department of social services by filing an oral 51A report for all children suspected of being abused or neglected. Many states impose penalties for failure to report. The oral report is followed up with a written report.

(3) Notifying the police if the child appears to be in imminent danger of physical injury

(4) Teaching family members appropriate child care, expected developmental behaviors, management of finances, and problem-solving techniques

(5) Providing extra reassurance and support to the child who has been removed temporarily from the home

(6) Referring family members for counseling and emotional support

Bibliography

Books

American Academy of Pediatrics. *1994 Red Book.* 23rd ed. Elk Grove Village, IL: Author, 1994.

American Academy of Pediatrics. TIPP, the injury prevention program. Elk Grove Village, IL: Author, 1989.

Andrews M, and Boyle JS (eds). *Transcultural Concepts in Nursing Care.* 2nd ed. Philadelphia: JB Lippincott, 1995.

Betz CL, Hunsberger M, and Wright S. *Family-Centered Nursing Care of Children.* 2nd ed. Philadelphia: WB Saunders, 1994.

Frankenburg, WK, et al. *Denver II Screening Manual 1989 Experimental Edition.* Denver CO: Denver Developmental Materials, 1990.

Galanti G. *Caring for Patients from Different Cultures.* Philadelphia: University of Pennsylvania Press, 1991.

Greene M (ed). *Johns Hopkins Hospital: The Harriet Lane Handbook.* 12th ed. St. Louis: Mosby–Year Book, 1991.

Kelly, K. *Transcultural Nursing: Health Care Providers and Ethnically Diverse Clients.* University of Massachusetts Dissertation, 1991, UMI #PUZ9132873.

Lewis K, and Thompson H. *Manual of School Health.* Menlo Park, CA: Addison-Wesley, 1986.

Mott S, James S, and Sperhac A. *Nursing Care of Children and Families.* 2nd ed. Redwood City, CA: Benjamin Cummings, 1990.

National Asthma Education Program. *Executive Summary: Guidelines for the Diagnosis and Management of Asthma.* Washington, DC: US Department of Health and Human Services, Publication 91-3042A, 1991.

National Cholesterol Education Program. *Report of the Expert Panel on Blood Cholesterol Levels in Children and Adolescents.* Washington, DC: US Department of Health and Human Services: NIH Publication 91-2732, September 1991.

North Carolina Nurses' Association. *Advances in Asthma Nursing Care.* New York: SPC Communications, 1992.

Park MK. *The Pediatric Cardiology Handbook.* St. Louis: Mosby–Year Book, 1991.

Reece R. *Manual of Emergency Pediatrics.* 4th ed. Philadelphia: WB Saunders, 1992.

Spector R. *Cultural Diversity in Health and Illness.* 3rd ed. Norwalk, CT: Appleton-Century-Crofts, 1991.

Wong D. *Whaley & Wong's Nursing Care of Infants and Children.* 5th ed. St. Louis: Mosby–Year Book, 1995.

Chapters in Books and Journal Articles

Altieri M, Bellet J, and Scott H. Preparedness for pediatric emergencies encountered in the practitioner's office. *Pediatrics* 85(5):710–714, 1990.

American Academy of Pediatrics Committee on Child Abuse and Neglect. Guidelines for the evaluation of sexual abuse of children. *Pediatrics* 87:59, 1991.

American Academy of Pediatrics Committee on Nutrition. Statement on cholesterol. *Pediatrics* 90(3):469–472, 1992.

American Academy of Pediatrics Committee on Nutrition. The use of whole cow's milk in infancy. *Pediatrics* 89(6):1105–1108, 1992.

American Academy of Pediatrics Task Force on Infant Positioning. Positioning and SIDS. *Pediatrics* 89(6):1120–1126, 1992

American Academy of Pediatrics. Universal hepatitis B immunization. *AAP News* February:13–15, 1992.

Aylward EH, et al. Cognitive and motor development in infants at risk for human immunodeficiency virus. *Am J Dis Child* 146(2):218–222, 1992.

Barnes LP. Managing pain in children: Seek first to understand. *MCN* 20(3):163, 1995.

Barnett E. After the UTI: The pediatrician and the radiologist. Presented at Recent Advances in Diagnosis and Management of Infectious Diseases in Children, March 28, 1992, Boston.

Barnett ED, et al. Otitis media in children born to human immunodeficiency virus–infected mothers. *Pediatr Infect Dis J* 11(5):360–364, 1992.

Bechler-Karsd A. Assessment and management of status asthmaticus. *Pediatr Nurs* 21(4):217–223, 1995.

Belamarich P, and Deckelbaum R. Hypercholesterolemia in children: When to treat. *Physician Assist* 16(2):165–170, 181, 183–184, 1992.

Blum NJ, et al. Disciplining young children: The role of verbal instructions and reasoning. *Pediatrics* 96(2):336–341, 1995.

Bushy A. Cultural considerations for primary health care: Where do self-care and folk medicine fit? *Holistic Nurs Pract* 6(3):10–18, 1992.

Carasso S. Lead law fails to assure proper screening. *AAP News* 8(11):1, 11, 14, 1992.

Carlin S, et al. Host factors and early therapeutic response in acute otitis media. *J Pediatr* 118(2):178–183, 1991.

Casimir G, et al. Atopic dermatitis: Role of food and house dust mite allergens. *Pediatrics* 1993;92(2):252–256, 1993.

Centers for Disease Control. Classification system for human immunodeficiency virus (HIV) infection in children under 13 years of age. *MMWR* 36(15):225–240, 1987.

Chilmonczyk B, et al. Association between exposure to environmental tobacco smoke and exacerbations of asthma in children. *N Engl J Med* 328:1665–1669, 1993.

Chu SY, et al. Impact of the human immunodeficiency virus epidemic on mortality in children, United States. *Pediatrics* 87(6):806–810, 1991.

Clark G. AMA issues annual teen visit guidelines. *AAP News* 9(2):5, 22, 1993.

Clark P and Byrne M. Clinical issues in long-term pediatric HIV disease. *MCN* 18:164–167, 1993.

Cloutier M. Quick: What's first-line therapy for acute asthma? *Contemp Pediatr* 10(3):76–97, 1993.

Committee on Nutrition. Iron-fortified infant formulas. *Pediatrics* 84(6):1114, 1989.

Connor E. Advances in early diagnosis of perinatal HIV infection. *JAMA* 266(12):3474–3475, 1991.

Corbett JV. EMLA cream for local anesthesia. *MCN* 20(3):178, 1995.

Crouch E., and Crouch E. Pediatric vision screening: Why? When? What? How? *Contemp Pediatr* 8:9–30, 1991.

Cruz MN, Stewart G, and Rosenberg N. Use of dexamethasone in the outpatient management of acute laryngotracheitis. *Pediatrics* 96(2):220–222, 1995.

Cunningham A. Antibiotics for otitis media: Restraint, not routine. *Contemp Pediatr* 11(3):17–30, 1994.

Dagan R, et al. Once daily cefixime compared with twice daily trimethoprim/sulfamethoxazole for treatment of urinary tract infection in infants and children. *Pediatr Infect Dis J* 11:198–203, 1992.

Davis K. The accuracy of tympanic temperature measurement in children. *Pediatr Nurs* 19(3):267–271, 1993.

DeRienzo-DeVivio S. Childhood lead poisoning: Shifting to primary prevention. *Pediatr Nurs* 18(6):565–567, 1992.

DeSantis L, and Thomas J. Childhood independence: Views of Cuban and Haitian immigrant mothers. *J Pediatr Nurs* 9(4):258–267, 1994.

Dixon M, Keeling A, and Karrel S. What pediatric hospital nurses know about immunization. *MCN* 19(2):74–78, 1994.

Dixon S, Bresnahan K, and Zuckerman B. Cocaine babies: Meeting the challenge of management. *Contemp Pediatr* 7(6):70–92, 1990.

Drass J. What you need to know about insulin injections. *Am J Nurs* 92(11):40–43, 1992.

Dreifuss F. Classification of epileptic seizures and the epilepsies. *Pediatr Clin North Am* 36(2):265–279, 1989.

Duhaime A, et al. Head injury in very young children: Mechanisms, injury types, and ophthalmologic findings in 100 hospitalized patients younger than 2 years of age. *Pediatrics* 90(2):179–185, 1992.

Duncan B, et al. Exclusive breast-feeding for at least 4 months protects against otitis media. *Pediatrics* 91(5):867–871, 1993.

Ferrante S, and Painter E. Continuous nebulization: A treatment modality for pediatric asthma. *Pediatr Nurs* 21(4):327–331, 1995.

Forster J. Rheumatic fever: Keeping up with the Jones criteria. *Contemp Pediatr* 10(3):51–60, 1993.

Frankenburg WK. Partners in health care programs. *Pediatrics* 93(4):589–593, 1994.

Frankenburg WK. Preventing developmental delays: Is developmental screening sufficient? *Pediatrics* 93(4):586–589, 1994.

Gellis S. (ed). Newer schedule of immunizations for infants under the age of two years recommended by the advisory committee on immunization (ACIP). *Pediatr Notes* 17(48):1, 1993.

Gerber M, and Markowitz M. Streptococcal pharyngitis: Clearing up the controversies. *Contemp Pediatr* 9(10):118–131, 1992.

Gerchufsky M. Diarrhea. *Adv Nurse Practitioners* 3(10):12–16, 1995.

Germain C. Cultural care: A bridge between sickness, illness, and disease. *Holistic Nurs Pract* 6(3):7, 1992.

Hagman LL, and Ryan E. The cardiovascular health profile: Implications for health promotion and disease prevention. *Pediatr Nurs* 20(5):509–515, 1994.

Hall C. Respiratory syncytial virus: What we know now. *Contemp Pediatr* 10(11):92–110, 1993.

Hanna D. The effect of nursing interventions on breastfeeding practices. Presented at conference titled: Toward Research-Based Clinical Practice: 1993 Update. Nashua, NH, May 12, 1993.

Hein K. Risky business: Adolescents and human immunodeficiency virus. *Pediatrics* 88(5):1052–1054, 1991.

Hester N, et al. Excerpts from guidelines for the management of pain in infants, children, and adolescents undergoing operative and medical procedures. *MCN* 17:146–152, 1992.

Hoberman A, et al. Prevalence of urinary tract infection (UTI) in febrile infants. *Pediatr Res* 29 (April):119A, 1991.

Howard B. A guide to how babies—and parents—develop. *Contemp Pediatr* 7(4):12–40, 1990.

Howard B. Parents and child from 3 months to 1 year. *Contemp Pediatr* 7(5):81–98, 1990.

Howard B. Learning independence in the preschool years. *Contemp Pediatr* 7(7):11–26, 1990.

Howard B. Making the grade from 6 to 12. *Contemp Pediatr* 7(8):13–37, 1990.

Hutto C, et al. A hospital-based prospective study of perinatal infection with human immunodeficiency virus type 1. *J Pediatr* 118(3):347–353, 1991.

Intravenous therapy. *Pediatr Nurs* 20(4):341–355, 1994.

Ipp M, and Jaffe D. Physicians' attitudes toward the diagnosis and management of fever in children 3 months. *Clin Pediatr* 32:66–70, 1993.

Jacobsen G. The meaning of stressful life experiences in nine to eleven-year-old children: A phenomenological study. *Nurs Res* 43(2):95–99, 1994.

Johnson C, et al. The role of bacterial adesins in the outcome of childhood urinary tract infections. *Am J Dis Child* 147(10):1090–1093, 1993.

Kachoyeanos M., and Friedhoff M. Cognitive and behavioral strategies to reduce children's pain. *MCN* 18:14–19, 1993.

Kallen R. The management of diarrheal dehydration in infants using parenteral fluids. *Pediatr Clin North Am* 37(2):265–286, 1990.

Kennedy W, Hoyt M, and McCracken G. The role of corticosteroid therapy in children with pneumococcal meningitis. *Am J Dis Child* 145(12):1374–1378, 1991.

Kleiber C, et al. Heparin vs saline for peripheral IV locks in children. *Pediatr Nurs* 19(4):405–407, 1993.

Kline MW, and Shearer WT. A national survey on the care of infants and children with human immunodeficiency virus infection. *J Pediatr* 118(5):817–821, 1991.

Krowchuk D, Tunnessen W, and Hurwitz S. Pediatric dermatology update. *Pediatrics* 90(2):259–264, 1992.

Krugman R. Child abuse and neglect: Critical first steps in response to a national emergency. *Am J Dis Child* 145(5):513–515, 1991.

Kunnel M, et al. Comparisons of rectal, femoral, axillary, and skin-to-mattress temperatures in stable neonates. *Nurs Res* 37(3):162–189, 1989.

Lauer R. Should children, parents, and pediatricians worry about cholesterol? *Pediatrics* 89(3):509–510, 1992.

Lindberg CE. Perinatal transmission of HIV: How to counsel women. *MCN* 20(4):207–211, 1995.

Lovejoy F. Childhood poisonings: What role for ipecac? *Contemp Pediatr* 9(12):99–108, 1992.

Lozoff B, Jiminez E, and Wolf A. Long-term developmental outcome of infants with iron deficiency. *N Eng J Med* 325:687–694, 1991.

Mack R. Toxic plants—winners of our discontent. *Contemp Pediatr* 9(3):133–141, 1992.

Managing pain in infants and children: Meeting the mandate. *MCN* 20(3):141–152, 1995.

Mansson M, Fredrikzon B, and Rosberg, B. Comparison of preparation and narcotic–sedative premedication in children undergoing surgery. *Pediatr Nurs* 18(4):337–342, 1992.

Marciaux M, and Sand E. Promotion of child health. In Doxiadis S. (ed). *Ethical Dilemmas in Health Promotion*. Chichester: John Wiley & Sons, 1987.

Marks M. Early detection and initial management of bacterial meningitis. Lecture for *Practical Reviews in Pediatrics*, May, 1991.

McCarron K. Fever—the cardinal vital sign. *Crit Care Q* 9(1):15–18, 1986.

McMullen A, et al. Heparinized saline or normal saline as a flush solution in intermittent IV lines in infants and children. *MCN* 18(2):78–85, 1993.

Melnyk BM. Coping with unplanned childhood hospitalization: Effects of informational interventions on mothers and children. *Nurs Res* 43(1):50–55, 1995.

Meyers A. Iron deficiency: Diagnosis, treatment, and consequences. Presented through Boston University School of Medicine: Continuing Medical Education, Boston, October 1993.

Millchap J, and Colliver J. Management of febrile seizures: Survey of current practice and phenobarbital usage. *Pediatr Neurol* 7:243–248, 1991.

Neifert M. Screening forms: Aid to breastfeeding. *Pediatr Management* July 1992, pp 24–27.

Nowak A. What pediatricians can do to promote oral health. *Contemp Pediatr* 10(4):90–106, 1993.

Orcutt TA, and Godwin CR. Aerosolized pentamidine: A well-tolerated mode of prophylaxis against *Pneumocystis carinii* pneumonia in older children with human immunodeficiency virus infection. *Pediatr Infect Dis J* 11(4):290–294, 1992.

Oski F, et al. UTI controversies: Circumcision, reflux, and more. *Contemp Pediatr* 9(3):75–101, 1992.

Ostrum G. Sports-related injuries in youths: Prevention is the key—and nurses can help. *Pediatric Nurs* 19(4):333–338, 1993.

Paradise JL. Managing otitis media: A time for change. *Pediatrics* 96(4):712–714, 1995.

Patterson R, et al. Head injury in the conscious child. *Am J Nurs* 92(8):22–27, 1992.

Pelton S. Pediatric HIV infection. *Clinical Care Manual for HIV Infection*. Presented at Infectious Disease Conference sponsored by Boston University School of Medicine, March 28, 1992.

Penticuff J. Ethics in pediatric nursing: Advocacy and the child's "determining self." *Issues Comp Pediatr Nurs* 13:221–229, 1990.

Phillips C. Vaccine update, 1993. *Contemp Pediatr* 10(2):75–95, 1993.

Pike D. Crisis in emergency care. *Pediatr Management* July 1992, pp 12–23.

Plaut T. The peak flow diary: A powerful tool for asthma management. *Contemp Pediatr* 10(5):61–63, 1993.

Pontious SL, et al. Accuracy and reliability of temperature measurement in the emergency department by instrument and site in children *Pediatr Nurs* 20(1): 58–62, 1995.

Porter C, and Villarrual A. Socialization and caring for hospitalized African- and Mexican-American children. *Issues Comp Pediatr Nurs* 14(1):1–15, 1991.

Quinn T, et al. Early diagnosis of perinatal HIV infection by detection of viral-specific IgA antibodies. *JAMA* 266(12):3439–3442, 1991.

Resar L, and Oski F. Cold water exposure and vaso-occlusive crises in sickle cell anemia. *J Pediatr* 118(3):407–409, 1991.

Reynolds E. Controversies in caring for the child with a head injury. *MCN* 17:246–251, 1992.

Reynolds E, and Hoberman A. Diagnosis and management of pyelonephritis in infants. *MCN* 20(2):78–84, 1995.

Rhodes AM. Is mandatory HIV screening for newborns justifiable? *MCN* 20(4):231, 1995.

Ricci L. Photographing the physically abused child. *Am J Dis Child* 145(3):275–281, 1992.

Riesel SK, et al. Effects of communication training on parents and young adolescents. *Nurs Res* 42(1):10–16, 1993.

Risser WL, et al. Medical conditions affecting sports participation. *Pediatrics* 94(5): 757–760, 1994.

Robertson J. Pediatric pain assessment: Validation of a multidimensional tool. *Pediatr Nurs* 19(3):209–213, 1993.

Ross T, and Dickson E. Vertical transmission of HIV and HBV. *MCN* 17(4):192–195, 1992.

Rutstein R. Predicting risk of *Pneumocystis carinii* pneumonia in human immunodeficiency virus–infected children. *Am J Dis Child* 145(8):922–924, 1991.

Ryan-Wanger N, and Walsh M. Childrens' perspectives on coping with asthma. *Pediatr Nurs* 21(4):224–227, 1995.

Sansivero GE. Why pick a PICC? *Nursing 95* 25(7):35–41, 1995.

Savedra MC, et al. Assessment of postoperative pain in children and adolescents using the adolescent pediatric pain tool. *Nurs Res* 42(1):5–9, 1993.

Schechter N, et al. Individual differences in children's response to pain: Role of temperament and parental characteristics. *Pediatrics* 87(2):171–177, 1991.

Schmitt B. Discipline: Rules and consequences. *Contemp Pediatr* 8(6):65–69, 1991.

Schmitt B. Toilet training without tears. *Contemp Pediatr* 9(8):47–49, 1992.

Schmitt B. How to help the trained night crier. *Contemp Pediatr* 9(12):45–49, 1992.

Schmitt B. When your child has a fever. *Contemp Pediatr* 10(6):79–81, 1993.

Schonfeld DJ, and Needham D. Lead: A practical perspective. *Contemp Pediatr* 11(5):64–96.

Schuman A. The truth about teething. *Contemp Pediatr* 9(10):75–80, 1992.

Seideman RV, Kleine PF. A theory of transformed parenting: Parenting a child with developmental delay/mental retardation. *Nurs Res* 44(1):38–44, 1995.

Selekman J. The guidelines for immunization have changed again. *Pediatr Nurs* 20(4):376–378, 1994.

Selekman J, and Snyder B. Nursing perceptions of using physical restraints on hospitalized children. *Pediatr Nurs* 21(5):460–464, 1995.

Shaw K, Bell L, and Sherman N. Outpatient assessment of infants with bronchiolitis. *Am J Dis Child* 145(2):151–155, 1991.

Shoberg D, Ackerman V, and Orr D. Office management of asthma in adolescents. *Adolesc Health Update* 5(4):1–8, 1993.

Spector R, and Sperhac A. Social and cultural influences on the child. *In* Mott S, James S, and Sperhac A (eds). *Nursing Care of Children and Families*. 2nd ed. Redwood City, CA: Benjamin Cummings, 1990.

Standards for pediatric immunization practice. *MCN* 19(2):79–81, 1994.

Stein PR. Indices of pain intensity: Construct validity among preschoolers. *Pediatr Nurs* 21(2):119–123, 1995.

Suri S. Simplifying urine collection from infants and children without losing accuracy. *MCN* 13:438–441, 1988.

Swanson M, and Thompson P. Managing asthma triggers in school. *Pediatr Nurs* 20(2):181–184, 1995.

Teele D. Strategies to control recurrent acute otitis media in infants and children. *Pediatr Ann* 20(11):610–616, 1991.

Thomas S, et al. Long-bone fractures in young children: Distinguishing accidental injuries from child abuse. *Pediatrics* 88(9):471–476.

Tinkelman D. Aerosol beclomethasone dipropionate compared with theophylline as primary treatment of chronic, mild to moderately severe asthma in children. *Pediatrics* 92(1):64–76, 1993.

Trowbridge G, et al. HIV: Recognizing and managing the infant at risk. *Contemp Pediatr* 8(10):118–134, 1991.

Vesley C. Pediatric patient-controlled analgesia: Enhancing the self-care construct. *Pediatr Nurs* 21(2):125–128, 1995.

Vessey J. Improving the primary care pediatric nurses provide to children and their families. *Pediatr Nurs* 20(1):64–67, 1994.

Vessey J. Developmental approaches to examining young children. *Pediatr Nurs* 21(1):53–55, 1995.

Wang W, et al. High risk of recurrent stroke after discontinuance of five to twelve years of transfusion therapy in patients with sickle cell disease. *J Pediatr* 118(3):377–382, 1991.

Wells N, et al. Does tympanic temperature measure up. *MCN* 20(2):95–100, 1995.

Williams J. New genetic discoveries increase counseling opportunities. *MCN* 18:218–222, 1993.

Wilson P, and Testani-Dufour L. Bicycle safety programs: Targeting injury prevention through education. *Pediatr Nurs* 19(4):343–346, 1993.

Wiswell T, and Hachey W. Urinary tract infections and the uncircumcised state: An update. *Clin Pediatr* 32:130–134, 1992.

Wood G. Antiretroviral therapy in infants and children with HIV. *Pediatr Nurs* 21(2):291–296, 1995.

Yager J, et al. Coma scales in pediatric practice. *Am J Dis Child* 144(10):1088–1091, 1990.

Yarcheski A, Scoloveno MA, and Mahon N. Social support and well-being in adolescents: The mediating role of hopefulness. *Nurs Res* 43(5):288–292, 1994.

Yoos L. Children's illness concepts: Old and new paradigms. *Pediatr Nurs* 20(2): 134–140, 1994.

16
Caring for Older People

▣ CHARACTERISTICS OF AGING

Common Characteristics

1. All organisms progressively lose adaptability with the passage of time. This change is the aging process. The loss of adaptability leads the organism to increased vulnerability to internal and external environmental challenges.
2. The aging process is not uniform among individuals because of differences in external and internal factors to which individuals are exposed and because of genetic variation.
3. Although rates of aging vary, all individuals age. **Aging** refers to the biopsychosocial process of change occurring between birth and death.
4. **Senescence** describes the latter part of life. Therefore, although all individuals experience aging, not all encounter senescence.
5. Aging is detrimental to health, system function, and well-being and ultimately results in death.
   a. Intrinsic processes include genetic makeup, individual composition and character, rate and characteristics of aging, and individualized response to the aging process.
   b. Extrinsic elements, such as environment and lifestyle, affect the rate and characteristics of aging. Consistent exposure to secondary cigarette smoke, for example, will create aging changes in the lungs.

Demographics of the Older Population

1. The proportion of older people (those older than 65) is increasing steadily. One out of every 10 Americans is older than 65 years, compared with 1 out of every 50 Americans in 1790. The average life span of Americans (72 years for men and 78 years for women) has increased 300% since 1776 because of disease prevention and management.
   a. Vaccinations affect the spread of communicable diseases such as rubeola, mumps, and pertussis.
   b. Antibiotics control the impact of infectious diseases such as pneumonia and streptococcus B.
   c. Infection control techniques and public health surveillance limit the extensiveness of epidemic outbreaks such as hepatitis A.
2. Persons who live in developed countries have longer average life spans than those in underdeveloped countries.
   a. The average life span is longest for the Japanese, with an average of 79 years.
   b. Individuals in Italy, Switzerland, and Spain have an average life span of 78 years.
3. Women in developed countries have longer average life spans than men, with an average of 7 years longer in Europe and North America.
4. Older people consume 25 percent of all prescription drugs. Cardiovascular drugs are most commonly used, with 26 to 34 percent of older people requiring some type of cardiac medication. Sedative-hypnotics and psychotropics are 2nd in frequency among the prescription medications used by older people.
5. Older people comprise 40 percent of all acute hospital days and expend 30 percent of personal health care dollars and 50 percent of the U.S. health care payments.

Concerns of Older People

1. Poor people may have inadequate income, especially if they are not part of the workforce. Retirement is associated with decline in income and depletion of savings. The degree of dependence on governmental and social systems is correlated to the extent to which older individuals become impoverished.
2. Many older persons are isolated, living alone, and struggling to maintain independence. Because of average female life expectancies that exceed male expectancies, widowhood more often affects women than men. Older women, on the average, have not been economic heads of households, although this situation may change as the baby boomer generation (born 1946–1961) ages. Widowhood often precedes a forced change in living situation.
3. Although many older persons are fully functional, independent, and able to manage financially, functional limitations from chronic illness and disability are frequently associated with aging. Among those 60 to 69 years of

---

ELDER ADVISORY

Avoiding high-risk behaviors can decrease the risk of disease and chronic illness. Behaviors to avoid include the following:
• Smoking
• Falls
• Alcohol use
• Sedentary lifestyle

age, 35 percent have at least 1 chronic condition (e.g., arthritis, hypertension). Approximately 70 percent of those 80 years of age and older have 2 or more chronic conditions.

4. External factors, such as access to social support systems, are known to influence the aging process through behavioral, familial, environmental, and biologic factors that affect how people eat, live, and exercise. Knowledge of and respect for such factors may not extend life but should lead to increased quality of life for older people.

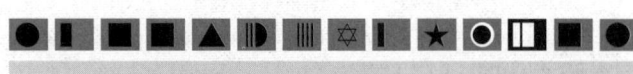

TRANSCULTURAL CONSIDERATIONS

The older population is diverse and heterogeneous. The older person has spent a lifetime developing and therefore, must be considered a unique individual. Nurses must be cautious about imposing their own attitudes toward aging on older people.

◨ STRUCTURE AND FUNCTION OF AGING

Musculoskeletal System

1. Functional changes related to aging occur in all body systems. Some of these changes are listed in Box 16–1. Alterations related to specific structures are summarized in Table 16–1.
2. Posture and stature changes cause a decrease in height of as much as 0.6 cm per decade.
   a. Bone mass changes as bone resorption exceeds bone formation.
      (1) Bone metabolism is primarily responsible for homeostasis of calcium within the body. Aging brings a reduction in calcium absorbed through the gastrointestinal tract. As gastrointestinal absorption of calcium decreases, resorption of calcium from the bones increases.

BOX 16–1. Changes in Musculoskeletal Function with Aging

1. Decreased mobility, range of motion, flexibility, stability, and resilience
2. Decreased relaxation of antagonist muscles
3. Decreased facial expression
4. Increased stiffness
5. Increased latency and relaxation periods
6. Increased liability to degenerative changes
   a. Generalized flexion
   b. Loss of height
   c. Kyphosis of dorsal spine
   d. Slight flexion of head and neck
   e. Bending of upper limbs at elbows and wrists
   f. Slight flexion of hips and knees
   g. Ataxia
   h. Change of gait with shortened step and wider base
   i. Possible arthritic changes

Table 16–1. Musculoskeletal Changes with Aging

Structure	Alteration
Musculature	Decreased number of muscle cells (i.e., motor units) and capillaries Decreased functioning of enzyme systems Decreased amount of elastic tissue Decreased muscle mass, size, and strength Decreased control of antigravity muscles Decreased speed of muscle contraction Increases in collagen Shrinking and sclerosis of muscles
Cartilage	Decreased elasticity Thinning and opacity (yellowish color) Defects over weight-bearing areas, with some calcification
Synovium	Decreased vascularity Increased thickening of synovial fluid
Tendons	Decreased capillary blood supply Increased vulnerability to injury Increased possibility of bone formation in proximal ends of bone Ankylosis of ligaments and joints Shrinkage and sclerosis
Spinal cord	Decreased number of dorsal column fibers Shrinkage of fibroelastic disks between vertebrae Degenerative changes in vertebral column, intervertebral disks, and extrapyramidal nervous system Osteoporosis

---

(2) Osteoporosis is associated with a progressive decline in bone density for both men and women after maturity. Losses in bone density severe enough to cause fracture after minimal trauma account for more than 1 million fractures annually in the United States. By age 65, one third of women have vertebral fractures, and by age 81, one third of women and one sixth of men have suffered hip fractures. Programs of estrogen and calcium supplements and exercise are under investigation for prevention of osteoporosis in women. Such programs are recommended for middle-aged women to improve stress on bones and increased bone formation.

b. Muscle mass decreases and muscles atrophy as the number of muscle fibers declines and organs atrophy.

c. Joint capsule components deteriorate, resulting in inflammation, stiffness, pain, and distortion in joints.

d. Joint diseases include degenerative joint disease, rheumatoid arthritis, osteoarthritis, and gout.

e. Movement slows.

Cardiopulmonary System

1. Energy and endurance diminish.
   a. Lowered tolerance to exercise causes decreased aero-

bic capacity, decreased muscle strength, decreased ventilation, and decreased tolerance to oxygen debt.
   b. Decreased capacity to perform exercise means conditioning takes longer, but performance increases with time. Benefits of exercise are listed in Box 16–2.
2. Respiratory changes with aging include decreased stretch and compliance of chest wall, decreased rib mobility and lung tone, increased anteroposterior diameter, stiffer chest wall, calcification of costal cartilage, and degenerative changes of vertebrae, including kyphosis (curvature of the spine) and upper dorsal scoliosis. Changes in muscles and airways are summarized in Table 16–2. Functional changes are listed in Box 16–3.
3. Cardiovascular changes are summarized in Table 16–3.

Hematologic System

1. In the absence of disease, hemoglobin levels remain within normal ranges but average toward the low end of normal.

2. In the absence of disease, hematocrit levels remain within normal ranges but average toward the low end of normal.
3. Lymphocyte counts may be lower in older people, even in nondisease states.

Integumentary System

1. Changes occur in all layers of the skin and in skin glands, hair, and nails. Specific alterations include the following:
   a. Decreased turgor
   b. Wrinkling
   c. Alterations of facial features
   d. Dry, itchy, cracked skin
   e. Inadequate sweating
   f. Hypopigmentation (gray hair)
   g. Hyperpigmentation (senile lentigo), also called liver spots
   h. Seborrheic and keratosis formations (yellow-waxy)
   i. Senile purpura, leading to tendency for easy bruising
   j. Actinic (senile) keratosis
2. Integumentary changes related to aging are summarized in Table 16–4.

Neurologic System

1. Neurologic changes with aging are summarized in Table 16–5.
2. Changes in neurologic function include changes in proprioception and thermoregulation.
   a. Aging can lead to loss of balance, dizziness, and syncope (along with changes in the vestibular system).
   b. Increased susceptibility to hypothermia is due to decreased sensory input, decreased or absence of shivering, and defective vasoconstriction. When hypothermia occurs in conjunction with bronchopneumonia, myocardial infarction, hemorrhage, gangrene, pancreatitis, or visceral necrosis, the mortality rate is 5 times greater for older people than for the 25 year old.
   c. Increased susceptibility to hyperthermia is due to decreased sweat gland activity, decreased efficiency of hypothalmus, and decreased adaptability to heat in

Table 16–2. Respiratory Changes with Aging

Structure	Alteration
Respiratory muscles	Decreased strength and function
	Decreased efficiency and increased rigidity of thoracic muscles
	Degeneration of myofibrils
	Infiltration of muscles with fatty tissue
Airways	Decreased number of alveoli and interseptal membranes, with some pulmonary capillary destruction
	Decreased diffusion capacity of the lungs
	Decreased total pulmonary surface area
	Decreased size of terminal airways
	Decreased bronchial movement and air flow
	Increased size of alveoli
	Increased airway resistance
	Increased dead space
	Dilation of bronchioles and ducts
	Changes in airway elastin: increase in fibrous connective tissue, increase in number of lymphoid elements, change to collagen tissue (up to 50%)

Table 16–3. Cardiovascular Changes with Aging

Structure or Function	Alteration
Valves	Increased rigidity and thickening (especially aortic and mitral valves) Sclerosis and fibrosis
Vessels	Decreased efficiency of blood return Decreased stroke volume and cardiac output (30% by age 65, 50% by age 80) Decreased elasticity in vessel walls Decreased coronary circulation (30% by age 60) Increased blood circulation time (15 sec in the adult, compared with 27 sec in the 70 year old) Increased peripheral resistance (1% per year after age 60) Increased distensibility (especially aorta and large arteries), with prominent appearance of arteries in head, neck, and extremities and with elongation of the aorta
Muscle	Decreased compliance of the heart (i.e., stiffness) Decreased production of enzymes needed to maintain contraction Increased collagen-elastin ratio
Heart rate	Decreased resting rate (60–84 beats per min) Decreased ability to increase heart rate Diminished effect of catecholamine that increases heart rate Increased time to return to normal after an increase in rate Poor tolerance of a rate of 190 beats per min
Blood pressure	Increase in (140/90–160/100) Increased arterial and systolic pressure with diastolic pressure maintained Increased pulse pressure Increased susceptibility to postural hypotension due to decreased efficiency of venous return
Heart sounds	Decreased intensity Alteration of sounds (possible S4) Onset of cardiac murmurs: systolic murmurs (clinically significant), diastolic murmurs (pathologically significant), dislocation of apical impulse
Electrocardiogram	Increased sensitivity to carotid sinus stimuli leading to dysrhythmias No change in resting electrocardiogram ST depression occurring with activity Depressed P waves and longer QRS segments

general. The result is increased susceptibility to heat stroke.

3. Changes in sleep patterns include increased sensitivity to noises, fatigue, malaise, aches and pains, worry instead of sleeping, and leg cramps. Increased sleeping may be due to boredom, sedation, uremia, or cardiac or renal failure.

a. Sleep apnea is a pause of breathing for more than 10 seconds and more than 5 awakenings per hour. Incidence increases with age, especially with hypertension, smoking, obesity, and cardiac pathology. Affected individuals may awaken 20 to 80 times per hour or 400 to 500 times per night. Males are affected more than females; 50 to 80 percent of older people are affected.

(1) Types of sleep apnea are central (quiet diaphragm), obstructive (active diaphragm with collapsed airway), and mixed (starts as central and evolves to obstructive).

(2) Sleep apnea leads to increased susceptibility to sudden death in people who are given sleeping medication. Older cardiovascular patients have a 50 percent higher mortality rate and die with greatest frequency.

b. Compensatory processes in cases of apnea lead to increased norepinephrine, which leads to high blood pressure, increased oxygen to the tissues, polycythemia, cardiomegaly, and increased risk of cerebrovascular disease (stroke).

Endocrine System

1. With aging, target organs experience a decrease in blood supply, hypothalamic sensitivity, number of receptor cells, tissue response to hormones, and activity of enzyme systems.
2. Decreased secretion of aldosterone contributes to decreased sodium reabsorption.
3. Hormonal changes cause decreased secretion of estrogen, follicle-stimulating hormone, and luteinizing hormone; decreased secretion of progesterone and testosterone;

Table 16–4. Integumentary Changes with Aging

Structure or Function	Alteration
Subcutaneous tissue	Decreased padding and insulation Loss of subcutaneous fat Loss of elasticity
Sebaceous glands	Decreased water content of the skin Gradual atrophy
Vascular supply	Reduction in blood flow to the skin Fragility of capillaries, with decrease in subcutaneous tissue supporting skin capillaries
Pigment cells	Decreased number of functioning pigment cells Hypertrophy of some pigment cells
Epithelium	Thinning epithelium causing increased visibility of blood vessels and localized thickening of the epidermis
Hair	Thinning, balding, or both Atrophy of hair roots Slight growth of hair on upper lip and chin in postmenopausal women (because of decreased estrogen)

Table 16–5. Neurologic Changes with Aging

Structure or Function	Alteration
Brain	Decreased weight (11–40%), water content (5%), and blood flow (20%) Increased size of ventricles Thinning of cortex
Spinal cord	Decreased number of fibers and anterior horn cells (causing muscle weakness) Decreased blood supply Decreased reaction time Increased synaptic delay
Nerves	Decrease in number (1000 per day after age 40) Decrease in myelin (to 50%) Decrease in neurotransmitters and nerve conduction Increased length of dendrites and number of synapses
Reflexes	Decreased reflexes with increased nerve conduction rate Slower (depressed) reflexes, especially deep reflexes General flexion and rigidity
Sleep patterns	Decreased total sleep with earlier risings Decreased stage IV sleep and decreased rapid eye movement Irregular sleep stages, with more and longer awakenings during sleep and greater need for naps Increased number of nightmares, particularly for women Increased nocturnal micturition, particularly for men

and decreased production of renin, angiotensin, and erythropoietin.
4. Decreased secretion of antidiuretic hormone contributes to decreased water reabsorption.
5. Secretion of growth hormone decreases.
6. Decreased secretion of thyroxine contributes to decreased metabolic rate.
7. Decreased secretion of thymosin contributes to decreased immune system response.
8. Decreased secretion of adrenocorticotropic hormone and cortisol leads to decreased efficiency of the stress response.
9. Endocrine changes cause widespread effects on the entire body, with specific changes related to each hormone function.
   a. Increase in mean 2-hour blood sugar level with advancing age
   b. Carbohydrate intolerance
   c. Resistance to insulin on peripheral tissues
   d. Risk of age-related stroke, higher for those at the 80th percentile of serum glucose than for those at the 20th percentile

Gastrointestinal System

1. Physiologic changes in the gastrointestinal system are summarized in Table 16–6. Metabolic changes are listed in Box 16–4.

Table 16–6. Gastrointestinal Changes with Aging

Structure	Alteration
Mouth	Decreased saliva production Increased dryness Pyorrhea and dental caries
Esophagus	Presbyesophagus Achalasia
Diaphragm	Increased weakening of muscles surrounding the hiatus Reflux gastric contents into lower regions of the esophagus
Stomach	Decreased mobility, peristalsis, and gastrointestinal secretions Diminished hunger contractions Delayed emptying time

2. Changes in gastrointestinal function include the following:
   a. Decreased appetite
   b. Decreased thirst
   c. Decreased intake
   d. Decreased need for calories
   e. Increased incidence of gastrointestinal carcinomas
   f. Increased susceptibility to irritation of mucosa or trauma
   g. Increased tendency toward constipation
   h. Difficulty swallowing
   i. Inability to chew food properly
   j. Digestive disturbances
   k. Diarrhea
   l. Lean body weight and basal metabolic rate that can be maintained with exercise
   m. A hiatal hernia rate of 70 percent in 70-year-old people

---

BOX 16–4. Metabolic Changes Related to Gastrointestinal Function in Older People

1. Decreased production of hydrochloric acid
2. Decreased protein metabolism
3. Decreased number of parietal cells
4. Decreased amount of intrinsic factor
5. Decreased absorption of nutrients in general
6. Decreased number of cells on absorbing surfaces of intestines
7. Decreased efficiency of liver functions
8. Decreased liver weight and hepatic blood flow
9. Decreased regenerative capacity
10. Decreased basal metabolism
11. Decreased lean body weight
12. Decreased activity and growth
13. Decreased need for calories
14. Increased pH
15. Increased tendency toward diverticulitis and polyps
16. Increased amount of adipose tissue
17. Increased need for quality nutrients and protein
18. Malabsorption of calcium and iron
19. Degeneration of stomach mucosa
20. Loss of chief cells, resulting in malabsorption of vitamin B_{12}, which decreases the ability to bind iron
21. Slower intestinal peristalsis

Renal System

1. Physiologic changes in the kidney include decreased kidney size and function; decreased efficiency of kidney to concentrate urine, especially at night; decreased blood supply to the kidneys, with deterioration of glomerular arterioles; decreased number of nephrons; and increased deterioration of remaining neurons.
2. Physiologic changes in the bladder include decreased neuromuscular stimulation, decreased emptying, decreased capacity, and increased ease of backflow of urine.
3. Metabolic changes in the renal system include decreased glomerular filtration rate, decreased maximum transport of glucose, decreased secretion of hydrogen ions, and increased plasma urea and uric acid.
4. Changes in renal function include increased residual urine and increased incidence of obstruction, infection, and incontinence. With decreased fluid intake, these conditions may lead to electrolyte and acid-base imbalance, urinary frequency, and nocturia.
5. Fluid and electrolyte changes include decreased fluid intake, decreased potassium, decreased functioning of buffer systems, increased tendency toward dehydration, and increased acidosis.

Special Senses

1. Physiologic changes in vision are summarized in Table 16–7. Changes in visual function include decreased visual acuity; decreased peripheral vision; decreased color vision; decreased visual contrast; increased sensitivity to glare; increased adjustment time to changes in light, especially from light to dark; presbyopia (farsightedness); and cataract formation.

Table 16–7. Changes in Vision with Aging

Structure	Alteration
Pupil	Decreased size and speed of adjusting to changes in light, with decreased amount of light through the pupil
	Smaller pupil, with more sluggish changes
	Decreased number of dilation fibers
	Decreased ciliary muscle efficiency
	Decreased accommodation, especially from light to dark
	Decreased convergence and upper gaze
Lens	Decreased refraction
	Decreased accommodation to near and distant vision
	Decreased flexibility in changing shape
	Decreased color vision but with better vision for warm colors such as red and orange
	Decreased amount of light through the lens
	Increased weight, density (opacity), and thickness, along with yellowing of the lens
Cornea	Change in curvature
Retina	Decreased amount of light
	Deterioration in receptors

Table 16–8. Changes in Hearing with Aging

Structure	Alteration
Cochlea	Deterioration of supporting cells and vascular supply
	Progressive atrophy and increased stiffness
	Decreased perception of high-frequency sounds (consonants show greatest loss); middle-frequency loss (most speech sounds) follows high-frequency loss; low-frequency losses (vowels) follow middle-frequency losses
Hair cells	Increased deterioration of hair cells
Sensory neurons	Decreased number of functioning neurons

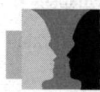 **CLINICAL CONTROVERSIES**

As visual acuity and reflexes diminish, many people are unable to drive safely. Some state laws require recertification of older drivers. Nurses may need to help patients develop alternative methods of transportation when driving is no longer possible.

2. Physiologic changes in hearing are summarized in Table 16–8. Functional changes in hearing include decreased understanding, decreased integration, decreased ability to sort out distractions, increased fatigue, increased central reaction time, and decreased ability to hear high-pitched sounds.
3. Physiologic changes in taste involve changes in the tongue, including reduction in the number of functioning taste buds, tongue furring, and decreased amount of saliva. Changes in sensory neurons involve decreased neuronal input to the brain. Changes in taste function include decreased discernment between unlike tastes, decreased appetite, possible relationship between decreased taste acuity and decreased zinc, increased inability to discern taste of food (sweet and salt flavors tend to be lost before bitter and sour).
4. Changes in smell include decreased smell acuity over age 65 to 80 and decreased number of olfactory neurons after age 20 (1%/year). Changes in the ability to smell involve interference with the ability to taste food, decreased appetite, decreased enjoyment of food, and increased use of spices.
5. Changes in touch involve pain, pressure, and vibration.
   a. Vestibular system changes occur in sensory neurons, with a decrease in efficiency and number of receptors and afferent neurons. The result is a decreased response to changes in the position of the head.
   b. Somatosensory changes in sensory neurons include decreased afferent input and sensitivity, increased deterioration, and decreased function of receptors.
   c. Vascular changes involve decreased blood supply to the spinal cord. Resulting functional changes are listed in Box 16–5.

BOX 16–5. Changes in Touch with Aging

1. Decreased deep sensation (especially visceral)
2. Decreased position sense
3. Decreased vibratory sense
4. Decreased temperature regulation
5. Decreased pain awareness
6. Increased aches and pains, especially in hands and feet
7. Increased pain relief by placebos and pain medications
8. Change in nature, location, and patterns of referred pain

Reproductive System

1. Male
   a. Changes in the testes include decreased testosterone production (possibly), decreased size and firmness of testes, and thickened seminiferous tubules.
   b. Changes in the prostate include symmetric enlargement and rubbery texture. An enlarged prostate may lead to urinary frequency, dribbling, nocturia, and urinary retention with overflow.
   c. Functional changes in the male reproductive system include decreased frequency of intercourse, decreased intensity of sensation, decreased speed of erection, increased dysuria, decreased force of ejaculation, and decreased sperm count.
2. Female
   a. Vaginal changes include decreased muscle and tone; decreased lubrication; thinning and shortening of the vaginal wall; dry, pale, pink color; and secretions that are more alkaline.
   b. Other changes in female reproductive structures include decreased size of labia and clitoris, decreased quantity of pubic hair, shrunken and retracted cervix, atrophied ovaries, and a uterus that becomes smaller and less firm.
   c. Changes in female reproductive function include increased susceptibility to cystocele, increasing atrophic vaginitis, possible painful contractions with intercourse, decreased secretions of hormones (estrogen, progesterone, follicle-stimulating hormone, and luteinizing hormone), and cessation of menses after menopause.

◼ PSYCHOSOCIAL ASPECTS OF AGING

Social Changes

1. The activity theory focuses on the connection among roles, social interactions, and changes with aging.
   a. A person's self-concept is linked to that person's roles in life.
   b. Roles change with age.
   c. Roles that emphasize activity promote healthy responses to aging.
2. Life-course theories are developmental theories of aging.

One is the adjustment theory, which defines aging as a series of adjustments.
   a. To retirement
   b. To grandparenthood
   c. To changes in income
   d. To changes in social life and marital status
   e. To potential deterioration of health and well-being
3. The continuity theory holds that as people age, they try to maintain continuity. People seek familiar strategies to maintain internal and external stability. Continuity during aging is the result of a gentle, gradual change in lifestyle over time.
4. One of the most accepted psychosocial theories of aging is the disengagement theory, which holds that aging individuals lose the quantity and quality of relationships as they age. As a result of the loss of relationships, aging people appear slowly and gradually to withdraw from life.
5. The modernization theory maintains that as civilization occurs, societal attitudes toward older people alter.
   a. In developing countries, the aged are treated with respect.
      (1) Most care is provided by the family in family homes.
      (2) Financial assistance is provided by family members.
      (3) The older person is viewed as powerful and wise, with opinions, views, and decisions to which younger family members adhere.
   b. As countries develop, positive attitudes toward older people change.
      (1) The use of long-term care in institutionalized settings for older people is more accepted in developed countries than in undeveloped countries.
      (2) Older individuals are more likely to become impoverished because of retirement and inadequate fixed income.
      (3) Old age is wrongfully associated with senility and dementia, with the older individual the subject of jokes regarding mental status, frail health, and incontinence.
6. The exchange theory deals with social interactions and withdrawal. Positive and rewarding social interactions or exchanges are believed to be maintained by older people. Exchanges that are not rewarding or beneficial are not cultivated, so that involvement may subside, giving the appearance of withdrawal.
7. The subculture theory looks at the older adult as a member of a social minority group.
   a. Older adults have developed a culture highlighted by such groups as the American Association of Retired Persons (AARP) and the Gray Panthers.
   b. The culture of older adults is in part a response to discrimination against age, common interests and beliefs, and exclusion from other groups.
8. The social competency, or breakdown, theory deals with the self-concepts of older people. Older adults can lose self-confidence for the following reasons:
   a. As health crises occur they feel vulnerable because of a threat to independence.
   b. As they become frail, they lose skills or competencies developed earlier in life.

c. As they take on roles of forced dependence due to economic, health care, or social losses, they lose their independence.

Cognition and Memory

1. Changes in mental functioning
   a. Decreased adaptation, coping with new situations, range of interests, comprehension, perception, and understanding
   b. Increased repetitive thoughts and vulnerability to stress
2. Changes in memory
   a. Decreased number of neurons; blood supply to brain; short-term memory, which is associated with decreased judgment; comprehension; orientation; and insight
   b. Increased central reaction time, with increased time needed to recognize and respond to stimuli
   c. Gradual memory loss during the 6th decade of life with greater memory decline after the mid-7th decade
3. There is lack of consensus about the impact of aging on intelligence but general agreement that learning can improve regardless of age.

Learning and Intelligence

1. Learning may be affected by the aging processes.
   a. Registration of information or reception of new stimuli may be affected through age-associated changes.
      (1) Environmental factors, such as lack of comfort in a situation or distractions, may influence the ability of older people to register new information.
      (2) Sensoriperceptual limitations, such as vision and hearing deficits, may interfere with the older person's capacity to register new information.
      (3) Pacing time may be lengthened with aging, resulting in delayed registration of new information

NURSE ADVISORY

> Learning may be affected by the aging process. Registering new information may be affected by the following:
> • Environmental factors, including a lack of comfort
> • Sensoriperceptual limitations, including vision and hearing deficits
> • Functional and endurance limitations, including the need for pacing and sequencing in the delivery and incorporation of new information

   b. Storage of information includes short- and long-term memory and may be altered through aging processes that slow the peripheral and central nervous systems. Retrieval of information is slowed through aging processes that influence the peripheral and central nervous systems and may result in hesitancy in answering questions or repeating information.

2. Change in intelligence during aging is an area of controversy.

CLINICAL CONTROVERSIES

Some testing reflects declines in intelligence; other studies demonstrate no changes with age.
• Testing with the Wechsler Adult Intelligence Scale (WAIS) reveals declines in intelligence scoring with aging.
• Testing of everyday function does not demonstrate age-related differences in intelligence.

Personality

1. Increased introversion means a focus on the inner rather than the outer world.
2. Acceptance of the environment and circumstances causes older people to make fewer efforts to change their situations.
3. Heightened cautiousness comes with anticipation of change.
4. Self-concept is believed not to be influenced by aging, but life events that occur with age inspire changes in self-concept.

Sociocultural Factors

1. Because older people are the fastest-growing population in the world, they demand special interest groups and changes in attitudes toward participation of older people in work and leisure activities.
2. Role changes occur because of aging. Marital role changes may occur after the death of a spouse, although 50 percent of those older than 65 years are married. Parental role changes continue for 80 percent of older adults. Work role changes occur with aging, with older people retiring from full-time employment, but many older people assume a part-time position to meet economic demands.
   a. First-order role changes (in roles that are central to the individual's well-being) include roles within the marriage and family. Within the marriage, older people experience interdependence. Within the family, they may become dependent.
      (1) With 1 or both spouses home with leisure time, retirement can lead to increased interdependence.
      (2) Relocation may move older people from large homes used for rearing families to smaller, more accessible, homes or to congregate housing.
      (3) Health alterations, with 1 or both spouses coping with chronic illness or physical disability, may leave the other spouse to work as caregiver.
      (4) Within the family, the role of the older parent may change from caregiver to care recipient if care must be accepted from a son or daughter, who in turn may feel obligated to provide care for the aging parent. In these situations, caring for the caregiver takes on significance.

b. Second-order role changes (in roles that are secondary in importance to the older person)
  (1) Leisure activities may change because of increased time available for recreational and avocational endeavors. Leisure may serve as a substitute for employment. Energy, endurance, and functional ability levels will affect leisure activities.
  (2) Friendships may be altered because the older person's friends and associates have also aged.
c. Third-order role changes (in roles that are peripheral to the individual)
  (1) Political affiliations may become stronger in older adults, with more leisure time available. Political activity, including voting, is encouraged through associations for the elderly, such as the AARP.
  (2) Volunteer activities are significant to many retired, older persons. Approximately 14 percent of those aged 65 years and older contribute 40 or more hours a month in volunteer roles.
3. Age staging varies within and between cultures. The United States has no clear definitions for middle age, old age, or very old age. Transcultural attitudes affect the degree to which support systems exist for older adults. For example, in Anglo-American culture, family members may be available and reside close to the older adult with health care needs but may not perceive a responsibility or accountability for providing care. Because people have the ability to modify and transform culture, distinctive cultural differences exist between populations of older people in developing communities and those in developed societies (Table 16–9).
  a. In developing countries, old age is equated with recognition as a community elder and with grandparenthood. Priorities for health care in developing countries include maternal and child care and prevention of disease, with minor focus on the care of older people. Care of older people is provided by family members, friends, and volunteers. The number of nursing homes, long-term care facilities, or outside agencies for the care of older people may be limited.
  b. Because of the emphasis on youth in most developed countries, old age is associated with decline in status in the community. These communities demonstrate a higher degree of acceptance of nursing home placement, with less onus on family responsibilities than in developing countries. Yet in spite of the acceptance of nursing homes, most primary caregivers for older individuals are family members, principally spouses, daughters, and daughters-in-law. Arrangements for the care of older people are provided through social services and institutions, which often rely on professionals with training in gerontology.

Coping With Loss

1. Aging is associated with multiple losses.
  a. Family members and friends, often including the spouse, may have died.
  b. Employment may be viewed as a loss secondary to

Table 16–9. Transcultural Attitudes Toward Aging	
Cultural Group	**Characteristics**
White	May view older people with diminishing respect, so that older people may be assumed to have impaired cognitive and functional capacity. Care needs considered a societal responsibility rather than a family priority. Nursing homes, residential centers, and long-term care facilities for the end of life often deemed commonplace, although less than 10% of older adults are in these facilities.
Black	Older adults viewed with respect. Care needs usually met within the home, by family members, church members, friends, and volunteers.
Hispanic	Older adults seen as respected elders. Care needs met at home by extended family members, friends, and volunteers.
Native American	Older adults treated with respect, although some perceive themselves as intolerable burdens on the community. Therefore, older people may withdraw and look for a swift passing. Care needs provided by the family, as allowed by the older person.
Asian	Older people treated with honor and respect, with younger family members trying to follow their guidance and advice. Care given by other family members.

retirement, which may be perceived as a threat to identity and self-esteem.
  c. Lifestyle may be perceived as a loss because of a fixed income through pension funds and social security.
  d. Health care and physical well-being may be lost after chronic illness or disability.
  e. Community involvement may be threatened due to loss of accessible transportation, causing loss of the ability to choose to participate in community events independently, as the older person must rely on others (usually family members) for transportation.

Elder Abuse and Neglect

1. Elder abuse includes physical, psychologic, financial, and social abuse or violation of an individual's rights (Fig. 16–1).
  a. **Abuse** is the willful inflicting of pain, injury, or debilitating mental anguish. It includes unreasonable confinement or willful deprivation of services, including medical care. Failing to prevent injury is a form of abuse, as is verbal assault or the demand to perform demeaning tasks. Theft or mismanagement of an older person's money or belongings, which often includes denial of rights, also constitutes abuse.

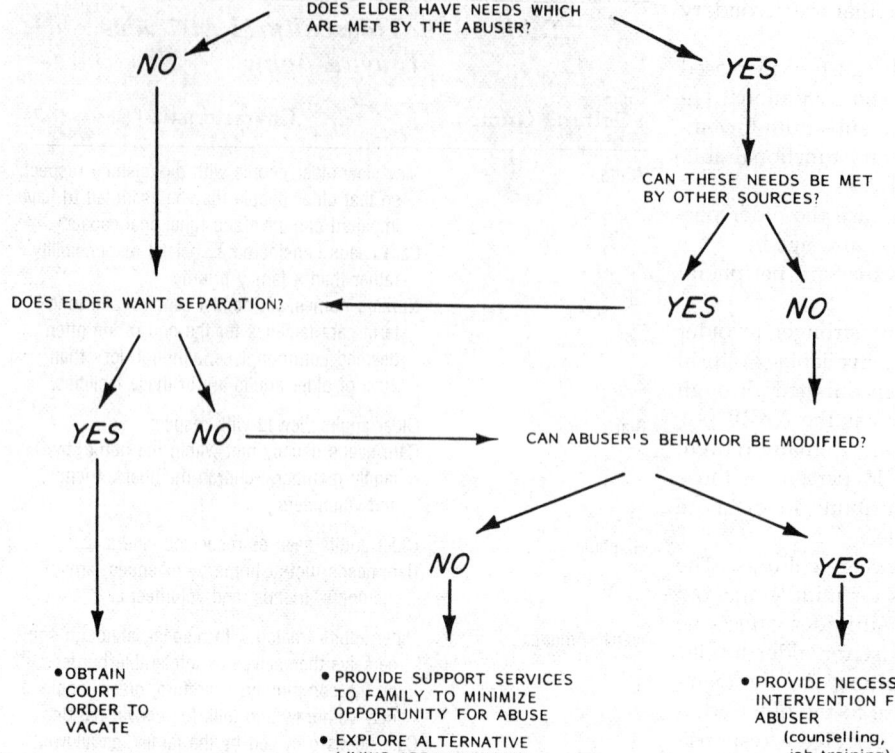

DOES ELDER HAVE NEEDS WHICH ARE MET BY THE ABUSER?

NO   YES

CAN THESE NEEDS BE MET BY OTHER SOURCES?

DOES ELDER WANT SEPARATION?   YES   NO

YES   NO   CAN ABUSER'S BEHAVIOR BE MODIFIED?

NO   YES

- OBTAIN COURT ORDER TO VACATE

- PROVIDE SUPPORT SERVICES TO FAMILY TO MINIMIZE OPPORTUNITY FOR ABUSE
- EXPLORE ALTERNATIVE LIVING ARRANGEMENTS

- PROVIDE NECESSARY INTERVENTION FOR ABUSER (counselling, job training)

Figure 16–1. A guide to decision making in cases of chronic elder abuse or neglect. (From O'Malley TA, Everitt DF, O'Malley H, and Campion E. Identifying and preventing family-mediated abuse and neglect of elderly. *Ann Intern Med* 93[6]:998–1004, 1983.)

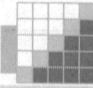

LEGAL AND ETHICAL CONSIDERATIONS

Elderly people, especially those who are isolated, may be vulnerable to abuse by salespeople. Telemarketers and agents for investment companies are sometimes able to charge older people exorbitant fees or convince them to relinquish their savings. Nurses should be aware of state laws that protect consumers and should not hesitate to contact the office of a state attorney general when suspecting this form of abuse.

b. **Neglect** is a lack of services necessary for physical and mental health. Neglect may be active or passive; the difference depends on the caregiver's capacity. Passive neglect means that the caregiver is unable to perform such activities as bathing, dressing, or changing an incontinent older person. Active neglect implies caregiver intent.
c. **Self-neglect** means that the elder person chooses to avoid medical care or other essential services. Older people, unlike children, have the right to refuse care unless they are declared legally incompetent.
d. **Exploitation** is the illegal or improper use of an older adult's resources.
2. Estimates suggest that 2.5 million older adults face abuse or neglect each year. Abuse may occur in any health care setting, including hospitals, and often occurs at home, where older people are under the care of family members.
a. Most at risk are isolated older women on whom the abuser is financially dependent.

b. Other risk factors are advanced age, history of conflict between the older adult and the abuser, alcohol abuse, and caregiver stress. Those at risk for neglect are those most dependent, usually because of confusion, immobility, or need for personal hygiene.
3. All states have enacted mandatory reporting laws, and all have protective service programs for older people. Unfortunately, the indicators of abuse are so similar to the signs and symptoms of many illnesses that cases may go unreported and reported cases may be unsubstantiated. There are, however, some common indicators, as shown in Box 16–6.
a. Nurses in hospitals and nursing homes need to be alert for signs of abuse and neglect and for the family dysfunction that leaves older people vulnerable.

BOX 16–6. Common Indicators of Elder Abuse and Neglect

Abrasions	Injuries inconsistent with history
Lacerations	History of falls
Bruises	Untreated medical problems
Burns	Inappropriate clothing
Sprains	Poor hygiene
Fractures	Excessive drowsiness
Dislocations	Over/undermedication
Pressure sores	Malnutrition/dehydration

From Matteson MA, McConnell ES, and Linton AD. Gerontological Nursing: Concepts and Practice. 2nd ed. Philadelphia: WB Saunders, 1996, p 630.

b. Promoting family functioning and self-care are the best prevention strategies.

c. Nursing has an important role in advocating for the older person. Necessary services are too often in jeopardy, and community leaders may need to learn about the scope of the problem.

4. Factors that contribute to abuse and neglect of older people include long-standing family violence, caregiver stress and impairment, and the older person's increasing dependence.

5. Treatment for abused and neglected older adults includes 5 components: identification, access and assessment, intervention, follow-up, and prevention. Access is often a problem if an older person is at home. The nurse may need to persuade the person and the family that help is needed. A nonjudgmental style and careful negotiation are key skills in gaining access to older people who might be in need of treatment or preventive services.

Questions for planning interventions include the following:

1. Is the person in immediate danger of bodily harm?
2. Is the person competent to make decisions regarding care?
3. What is the degree of impairment?
4. What services might help meet unmet needs?
5. Which family members are involved and to what extent?
6. Are the patient and family willing to accept intervention?

---

a. Interventions available for protection from abuse are, unfortunately, limited. Many older people prefer the abusive situation to institutional care, which is often the only option.

b. Community-based programs that raise awareness of abuse and neglect of older people, together with improved education for health care providers, are the most likely long-term solutions to these problems.

◼ *ASSESSING OLDER PEOPLE*

Special Considerations in Assessment

1. Older people as a group are diverse and heterogenous. The older person has spent a lifetime evolving as a person and therefore must be considered a unique individual. Health care professionals must be cautious of their own attitudes toward older people. Nurses need to find interventions that maintain and enhance self-care ability and independence.

2. Although not all older people are disabled, there is a high incidence and risk of disability with aging.

3. Nurses must seek to make the older person a partner in care, and recognize that habits and behaviors expressed were developed by the older person over a period of decades. In identifying interventions, the nurse should work with the older person to ensure that options selected fit within the older person's lifestyle.

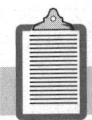

NURSING MANAGEMENT

Nurse managers need to assess the attitudes of nurses and assistants toward older people. Nurses, must focus on interventions to maintain and enhance self-care and independence. It is critical that nurses make older people partners in care and recognize that habits and behaviors expressed by older people have been developed over decades. In identifying interventions, the nurse should work to ensure that options selected fit the older person's lifestyle.

Functional Assessment

1. Because of the frequency of functional impairment in older adults, a systematic functional assessment determines the degree of impact physical disability or chronic illness may have on independence and self-care skills.

2. A variety of functional assessment instruments are available (Table 16–10). Key factors in the selection of instruments are the following:

   a. The tool should be valid and reliable, so that nurses administering the tool will obtain the same result when using the tool on an older individual.

   b. Tools that are short and easy to administer are best for older people because older individuals may have difficulty concentrating during lengthy assessments.

   c. The tool should produce results that can demonstrate improvement or loss of function over time. Summative scales provide a single score that can be used to show improvement or deterioration of function.

3. Assessment of older people should be tailored to their specific needs.

   a. Focus on carefully selected tests of vision, hearing, arm and leg function, urinary continence, mental status, instrumental and basic activities of daily living, environmental hazards, and social support systems.

   b. Use brief questions and easily observed tasks.

   c. Provide for systematic attention to the older person's functional status in addition to a review of systems.

Screening

1. Vision

   a. The presence or absence of cataracts should be assessed.

   b. The capacity for accommodation should be monitored because the capacity can diminish with age.

2. Hearing

   a. Any hearing deficits should be monitored.

   b. Hearing loss without compensation should be identified to prevent false assumptions regarding cognitive status.

   c. Hearing losses can lead to social problems, including isolation, depression, and confusion.

3. Upper extremities

Table 16–10. Instruments for Functional Assessment

Instrument	Date Developed	Activity Measured	Scoring
Activity of Daily Living Instruments			
Katz Index of ADL	1963	Six types of function: bathing, dressing, toileting, transfers, continence, feeding	A total score is obtained.
PULSES profile	1957	Six aspects of function: *p*hysical condition, *u*pper extremities, *l*ower extremities, *s*ensory components, *e*xcretory functions, *s*ocial support factors	A score of 1 (complete dependence) up to 6 (complete independence) is given for each aspect of function. The scores can be tallied to measure progress over time.
Barthel Index	mid-1960s	Function in self-care and mobility. Aspects are coded as follows: (1) can do by myself, (2) can do with the help of someone else, (3) cannot do at all.	A total score is obtained (100 = best score; 0 = worst score) to measure progress over time.
Specific Activity Instruments			
Mini mental state exam	1975	Orientation, short-term memory, attention, registration, and language	A total score (high score indicates cognitive well-being) is obtained to monitor change over time.
Beck Depression Inventory	1961	Conditions of depression	A total score is obtained (low score indicates absence of depression).
GARS Social Resource Scale	1978	Social resources of older adults	Scoring is completed on a 6-point scale (low score indicates excellent social resources).
Global and Comprehensive Instruments			
Functional Independence Measure (FIM)	1986	Provides outcome data reported to a national data bank (Uniform Data System). The tool incorporates 18 components of function, each of which is scored on a scale of 1 to 7 (1 = total dependence; 7 = complete independence).	A total score is obtained and used for monitoring.

a. Proximal functions that should be assessed include raising the arms to comb hair, brushing teeth, and putting on a coat.

b. Distal functions include manual dexterity, writing, and eating with utensils.

4. Lower extremities

a. The tendency to fall should be assessed because this tendency indicates lower extremity strength and balance. Assess trips, falls, and slips. Note any pattern in falls, rate, and circumstances.

b. The older person should demonstrate standing, getting up from a sitting position, and walking 10 feet.

5. Urinary function

a. Urinary continence should be assessed, including frequency and amount.

b. Urinary incontinence occurs in 30 percent or more of the older population and is linked with social isolation.

6. Nutritional status (Table 16–11)

a. The nutritional status of the older person should include hydration and weight.

b. Poor nutritional status may present as acute medical illness, depression, or fatigue and weakness.

c. An older person's ability to maintain nutritional status must be screened, including the ability to self-feed and to shop and cook.

NURSE ADVISORY

Consistently assess nutritional status. Older people are at risk for longer and more expensive hospital stays and at great risk of health complications due to poor nutrition.

7. Psychosocial and environmental concerns

a. Mental status should be assessed through a standardized tool such as the Mini Mental State Examination. Older persons frequently compensate for mental status changes, so the focus of assessment should be on calculational ability and short-term memory.

b. Ask whether or not the older person feels sad or depressed. If the answer is affirmative, use an additional tool such as the Beck Depression Inventory.

c. Assess the home environment, with particular focus on stairs and accessible bathrooms.

d. Review social supports, including identification of actual and potential caregivers, and note anyone for whom the older person is providing care.

Table 16–11. Nutritional Issues for Older People

Nutritional Deficit	Signs and Symptoms	Causes
Anemia	Tachycardia Mucosal pallor Congestive heart failure Cardiac murmurs Headaches Angina	Gastrointestinal tract disorders with inadequate vitamin B_{12} absorption Nutrient deficiency
Undernutrition	Symptoms possibly vague and diffuse Must evaluate several clinical and biochemical markers to identify undernutrition	Low food intake Changes with aging, including lowered hydrochloric acid production Decreases in enzymes and bile salts impairing digestion and absorption
Dehydration	Daily urine output <500 ml Urine with high specific gravity Dry skin Low blood pressure Furrowed tongue Altered mental status	Primary risk factor is inability to self-feed
Anorexia	Weight loss Symptoms of undernutrition	Poor dentition Inadequate desire for food Medications Chronic illness Impaired olfaction and gustation Inactivity
Diarrhea	Frequent loose stools resulting in dehydration and electrolyte imbalance	Lactose intolerance (especially of concern with enteral feedings) Laxative overuse Antibiotics Infections
Constipation	Three or more days without defecation	Laxative overuse Inadequate fluid and fiber intake Decreased bowel tone Inactivity Medications (sedatives and antacids)

From Duchene P, LeSage P. Hydration and nutrition. *In* Corr D, and Corr C (eds). *Nursing Care in an Aging Society.* New York: Springer, 1990. © 1990 Springer Publishing Company, Inc., New York 10012. Used by permission.

◻ MEDICAL-SURGICAL PROBLEMS OF OLDER PEOPLE

Mouth Problems

1. Loss of teeth secondary to periodontal disease is common in older people
   a. Periodontal tissues progressively atrophy with age and infection.
   b. Periodontal disease is caused by failure to remove plaque on the teeth and gums.
2. Osteoporosis occurring with age affects the alveolar bone, resulting in a flattening of the alveolar ridge and causing the bottom lip to draw inward.
3. Diseases of the tongue may increase in frequency with age.
   a. Depapillation, a decrease in papillae around the sides of the tongue
   b. Fissures, such as those seen with anemia

4. Neoplasm of the oral cavity occurs with increasing frequency in those older than 60. Risk factors:
   a. Age 45 years or older
   b. Tobacco use (smoking and chewing)
   c. Regular alcohol consumption
5. Xerostomia, or dry mouth resulting from regressive salivary gland changes, is a frequent problem for older persons.
   a. Dryness of the mouth causes increased plaque formation and a thickening of the saliva.
   b. Dryness may create discomfort, such as consistent burning sensations and unpleasant tastes.

Skin Problems

1. Pruritus is a common problem for older persons and may or may not be linked with underlying pathologic processes.

a. In mild cases, pruritus may constitute an annoyance.
b. In extreme cases, pruritus may be linked with sleep loss and irritability.
c. Causes of pruritus:
 (1) Renal disease
 (2) Biliary disease and obstruction
 (3) Hodgkin's disease
 (4) Anemia
 (5) Hyperthyroidism
 (6) Diabetes
 (7) Malignancy
 (8) Psychosis
2. Dry skin, or xerosis, is so common among the elderly that it is considered universal. The underlying cause of xerosis is uncertain. Xerosis is associated with pruritus and secondary inflammations.
3. Skin cancers occur frequently among older people (see Chapter 17).
 a. Basal cell carcinomas are most frequently the cause of malignant skin lesions. These cancers usually occur in sun-exposed body areas (e.g., face, neck and hands) and grow slowly, sometimes over years.
 b. Squamous cell carcinomas occur more often in fair-skinned, older people. These cancers usually occur in sun-exposed body areas and initially appear as red scaly patches. Ulcerated areas develop as the lesion becomes advanced.
 c. Malignant melanoma occurs most often in persons between 50 and 80 years. Successful treatment depends on early diagnosis. These cancers appear as lesions greater than 7 mm, with varied color.
4. Bullous pemphigoid, a common nonmalignant but distressing skin disorder, is characterized by highly pruritic blisters on reddened or normal skin. This idiopathic condition is immunoglobulin mediated. Therapy includes steroid creams and immunosuppressants (e.g., cyclophosphamide or azathioprine)

Foot Problems

1. Common skin problems involving the foot in older persons include the following:
 a. Dry, scaly, thinning skin that may precipitate peeling, cracking, and fissures of the skin, resulting in infection and inflammation
 b. Stasis dermatitis
 c. Ichthyosis or scaling
2. Treatment for skin problems of the feet
 a. Careful assessment for skin breaks and initial signs of infection and inflammation
 b. Maintenance of foot hydration through application of emollient creams and lotions
 c. Appropriate and well-fitting footwear
3. Common nail problems of the foot
 a. Onychauxis, or hypertrophy of the nails, resulting in nail bed ulcerations and inadequate fit of footwear
 b. Onychogryphosis or "ram's horn" toenails
 c. Onychomycosis
4. Treatment of toenail problems should be done by professional nurses, podiatrists, or physicians to prevent infec-

tion and inflammation and should include careful débridement with appropriate instruments and the use of local anesthesia. Augment treatment through gentle soaks in lukewarm Betadine or Domeboro.

NURSE ADVISORY

To prevent infection and inflammation, toenail problems should be cared for by professional nurses, podiatrists, or physicians. Augment care of the toenails through gentle soaks in lukewarm povidone-iodine (Betadine) or aluminum acetate solution (Domeboro).

---

5. Musculoskeletal problems of the foot are summarized in Table 16–12.
6. Gout (see Chapter 21) typically affects the 1st metatarsophalangeal joint. Exacerbations of gout are linked with trauma and pain.
 a. Systemic treatment includes administration of anti-inflammatory agents, xanthine oxidase inhibitors, or uricosuric drugs.
 b. Nonsystemic treatment involves limitation of joint movement and includes the use of firm-soled shoes and arch supports.
7. Arthritis
 a. Osteoarthritis often affects the 1st metatarsophalangeal joint. Treatment involves limiting joint motion through the use of firm-soled shoes and arch supports. Surgical fusion of the joint may be considered if other methods fail to control pain and promote function.
 b. Rheumatoid arthritis usually affects the forefoot and is associated with joint pain and limitation of function. Treatment includes corticosteroid therapy and wearing adequate, well-fitting footwear.

Mobility Problems

1. Mobility issues for older persons may occur secondary to multiple types of problems and diseases. Limitation in mobility is high among older individuals and varies from slight stiffness to extensive impairment secondary to chronic illness and disability (see Chapter 7).
2. Ambulation may be impaired because of illness or disability.
3. Cardiopulmonary disease may cause energy and endurance limitations of mobility.
 a. Treatment involves correction of the underlying pathologic condition.
 b. Preventing further functional loss and promoting functional potential involves pacing and appropriate use of energy.
 (1) Activities lasting longer than 20 minutes are divided into 20-minute segments.
 (2) Rest breaks of 5 minutes follow 20 minutes of activity.
 (3) Activities requiring high levels of energy are performed midmorning.

Table 16–12. Musculoskeletal Problems of the Foot

Condition	Indications	Treatment
Calluses (plantar keratoses), which affect up to 50% of persons older than 65	Develop under the metatarsal heads and are usually most pronounced under the head of the second and third metatarsal	Largely palliative treatment includes the following: • Appropriate footwear with soft insoles (at least one-eighth inch) • Application of salicylic acid (over-the-counter preparations) • Gentle débridement by a podiatrist or physician
Corns (clavi), which affect around 50% of those older than 65	Caused by the development of hyperkeratotic tissue: • May occur on or between toes • Associated with pressure from poorly fitting footwear • Failure to correct the corn, a risk for sinus tract formation and infection	Treatment of corns includes the following: • Gentle débridement of the hyperkeratotic tissue • Padding of the area • Use of softer, wider shoes • Surgery if the individual's circulatory status is adequate to prevent development of postsurgical complications of infection, inflammation, and gangrene
Heel spurs (plantar fasciitis), which affect the posterior or inferior aspects of the heel and may cause intense pain	Associated with atrophy of the heel pad or in conjunction with systemic diseases (e.g., Paget's disease or rheumatoid arthritis)	Treatment varies with location of the heel spur and includes the following: • Steroid injections for inferior heel spurs • Oral medications such as anti-inflammatories for posterior spurs
Neuroma	Usually presents between the 3rd and 4th or 2nd and 3rd toes and causes severe pain	Nonsurgical treatment includes • Use of wide or open-toed shoes • Use of arch supports Surgical treatment may be considered for individuals without circulatory impairment.
Bunions (hallux valgus), common in people older than 50, occurring 4 times as often in women as in men	Develop because of atrophy of muscles and tissues. Subluxation of the 2nd joint may occur, causing the hammertoe effect. The deformity is not always painful but is visually distressing and can make it difficult to find appropriate footwear.	Treatment includes • Nonsurgical treatment involves finding adequate footwear with sufficient width and depth to accommodate the deformity • Surgical treatment considered if the deformity is painful or if it is difficult to find adequate shoes

(4) Rest periods of at least 30 minutes are maintained in the afternoon, and include true rest, reclining, or napping.

NURSE ADVISORY

> Never do for the older person what that person can do without assistance. Educate caregivers and family members to hold the same philosophy.

4. Musculoskeletal disease requires careful assessment and correction of the underlying cause of disease. Mobility should be maintained through exercise and guided activities.
5. Neurologic disease requires careful assessment and correction of the underlying cause of disease. Mobility should be maintained through exercise and guided activities. Supervision of activities may be necessary if proprioception (position of the body in space) is limited or if the ability to remember instructions is impaired.

NURSING DIAGNOSIS: Impaired physical mobility R/T cerebrovascular accident

1. *Expected outcomes:* Following intervention, the person should be able to do the following:
   a. Achieve an optimal level of physical mobility
   b. Use adaptive devices, as appropriate, to facilitate physical mobility
   c. Attend to safety issues to prevent injury
2. *Nursing interventions*
   a. Monitor limitations to physical mobility with a particular focus on ambulation, gait, balance, coordination, and ability to climb steps and inclines.
   b. Assist the person with a progressive program of physical activity.
   c. Teach the person safety measures:
      (1) Sit and dangle for a minute before standing to prevent falls due to orthostatic hypotension.
      (2) Maintain a clear pathway to the bathroom to prevent falls during the night.
      (3) Use a night-light to prevent falls in the night due to visual problems, which may compound balance and gait deficits.
   d. Teach the person appropriate use of adaptive devices, including repair and maintenance of the devices.

NURSING DIAGNOSIS: Self-care deficit R/T deconditioning

1. *Expected outcomes:* Following intervention and counseling, the person should be able to do the following:
   a. Participate in all aspects of self-care to the extent possible given functional limitations.
   b. Use adaptive and assistive devices, as appropriate, to enhance self-care abilities.
2. *Nursing interventions*
   a. Monitor functional limitations with respect to all self-care abilities:
      (1) Feeding
      (2) Bathing
      (3) Grooming
      (4) Dressing (upper and lower extremities)
      (5) Toileting
      (6) Hygiene
   b. Identify methods modifying self-care activities through adaptive and assistive devices to enhance self-care skills (Table 16–13).
   c. Work with the older person to determine acceptable ways of modifying activities and of incorporating adaptive and assistive devices into self-care routines.
   d. Coach the person through practice sessions with the adaptive and assistive devices.
   e. Never do for the person what that person can do alone. Educate caregivers to hold the same philosophy.

Urinary Problems

1. Neurogenic urinary problems result when illness or injury affects the neurologic innervation of the bladder (see Chapter 26).

   a. Reflex bladder occurs secondary to a spinal cord injury above the T10 level.
      (1) The pattern is a sudden, gushing type of incontinence without warning or awareness.
      (2) The treatment is triggering urine release or managing incontinence with an external urinary collection device.
   b. Uninhibited or functional bladder occurs with an injury to the frontal lobe of the brain.
      (1) The pattern is a sudden need to void. Incontinence may occur, as the individual has little "warning" of the need to void and may be unable to find a restroom or assistance or remove clothing in time to prevent incontinence.
      (2) The treatment is managed by voiding on a consistent schedule, (e.g., every 2 hours, and before and after activity).
   c. Flaccid bladder (retention pattern) occurs with spinal cord injuries below the level of T10.
      (1) The pattern is overflow dribbling and urinary retention.
      (2) The treatment is through intermittent catheterization, usually self-catheterization.
2. Structural bladder problems result from an abnormality in the bladder or the urethral outlet (see Chapter 26).
   a. Detrusor instability may occur because of infection, urinary calculi, or cancer.
      (1) The voiding pattern is incontinence with either complete or partial bladder emptying.
      (2) The treatment is correction of the underlying problem and establishment of a scheduled toileting routine.

Table 16–13. Aids for Promotion of Functional Independence

Functional Deficit	Aids Available	Purchasing Information
Low vision	Single-vision lenses Bifocal glasses and magnifiers Clip-on magnifiers Stand magnifiers Telescopic lenses Prism spectacles	American Foundation for the Blind, Consumer Products Department, 15 West 16th Street, New York, NY 10011, (212) 620–2000
Hearing impairment	Telephone amplifiers Doorbell signalers Fire/smoke alarms Bed vibrators Hearing aids Personal sound-enhancement systems	American Speech-Language-Hearing Association, 10801 Rockville Pike, Department AP, Rockville, MD 20852
Upper extremity mobility deficits	Long-handled reacher Cloth loops on doors Built-up handles on pans and utensils Velcro closures on shoes Apron with pockets for carrying supplies to prevent multiple trips	Fred Sammons, Inc., Box 32, Brookfield, IL 60513 Shalik's Rehab Aids, Box 826, Miami, FL 33143
Lower extremity mobility deficits	Suction mat on stool Raised toilet seat Grab bars around toilet Tub transfer bench	Fred Sammons, Inc., Box 32, Brookfield, IL 60513

b. Outlet incompetence occurs primarily in women and is commonly referred to as "stress incontinence."
   (1) The pattern is sudden incontinence during activity, laughing, or coughing. Usually, the amount of urine is small, and incontinence occurs only when standing or sitting.
   (2) The treatment is usually palliative and involves management of the incontinence through the use of incontinence pads.
c. Outlet obstruction primarily affects men and is secondary to prostate enlargement.
   (1) The pattern is urinary frequency with overflow incontinence and urinary retention.
   (2) The treatment is typically through removal of the obstruction.
3. Mixed bladder problems occur with a combination of a neurologic and a structural deficit (see Chapter 26). The treatment is based on the pattern of incontinence presented.
   a. Incontinence without sufficient warning is managed through the scheduling of voiding times and the use of incontinence products such as pads, briefs, and external collection devices.
   b. Overflow incontinence with urinary retention is managed through the use of external collection devices and intermittent catheterization.

NURSING DIAGNOSIS: Altered urinary elimination R/T functional incontinence (typically a neurogenic type of urinary incontinence, sometimes characterized as "uninhibited")

1. *Expected outcomes:* Following intervention, the person should be able to do the following:
   a. Establish a regular toileting schedule with an absence of breakthrough incontinence.
   b. Become knowledgeable about bladder function, the bladder program, hygiene, and fluid requirements.
2. *Nursing interventions*
   a. Monitor urinary elimination patterns, including intake and output.
   b. Identify contributing factors:
      (1) Distance between chair or bed and bathroom
      (2) Difficulty removing clothing
      (3) Accessibility of assistance with ambulation (caregivers, nurses)
   c. Establish a toileting schedule:
      (1) Every 2 hours
      (2) Before and after activity
      (3) Before and after meals
      (4) Before and after sleep or rest periods
   d. Ensure adequate fluid intake.
   e. Initiate education programs involving the older person and caregivers.

NURSING DIAGNOSIS: Altered urinary elimination R/T reflex incontinence (usually a neurogenic type of urinary incontinence, characterized as a "reflex" pattern)

1. *Expected outcomes:* Following instruction, the person should be able to do the following:
   a. Establish a regular toileting schedule with an absence of breakthrough incontinence.
   b. Become knowledgeable about bladder function, the bladder program, hygiene, and fluid requirements.
2. *Nursing interventions*
   a. Monitor urinary elimination patterns, including intake and output.
   b. Establish a voiding schedule (e.g., every 2–4 hr).
   c. Use triggering mechanisms such as positioning or tapping.
   d. After the person attempts to void, use intermittent catheterization to determine efficacy of the voiding attempt (in many cases, an intermittent self-catheterization program is the urinary management method of choice for this pattern of incontinence).
   e. Ensure adequate fluid intake.
   f. Initiate education programs involving the older person and caregivers.

NURSING DIAGNOSIS: Altered urinary elimination R/T stress incontinence (often a structural bladder problem)

1. *Expected outcomes:* The person should be able to do the following:
   a. Establish a regular toileting schedule with an absence of breakthrough incontinence.
   b. Become knowledgeable about bladder function, the bladder program, hygiene, and fluid requirements.
2. *Nursing interventions*
   a. Monitor urinary elimination patterns, including intake and output.
   b. Identify contributing factors such as coughing, sneezing, laughing, or bladder infection.
   c. Instruct the person about pelvic floor exercises.
   d. Instruct the person about the use of incontinence aids, such as pads and briefs.
   e. Ensure adequate fluid intake.
   f. Initiate education programs involving the older person and caregivers.

NURSING DIAGNOSIS: Altered urinary elimination R/T urinary retention (may be a neurogenic type of urinary impairment, sometimes called a "flaccid" pattern, or a structural problem)

1. *Expected outcomes:* Following instruction, the person should be able to do the following:
   a. Establish a regular toileting schedule with an absence of breakthrough incontinence.
   b. Become knowledgeable about bladder function, the bladder program, hygiene, and fluid requirements.
2. *Nursing interventions*
   a. Monitor urinary elimination patterns, including intake and output.
   b. Instruct the person in the use of the Valsalva maneuver (not recommended for older people with cardiac problems) and Credé's technique. After the person at-

tempts to void, use intermittent catheterization to determine the efficacy of the voiding attempt (in many cases, an intermittent self-catheterization program is the urinary management method of choice for this pattern of incontinence).

   c. Ensure adequate fluid intake.

   d. Initiate education programs involving the older person and caregivers.

Bowel Problems

1. Constipation is the most frequent complaint of older people regarding bowel function.
   a. Assessment of constipation must differentiate between real and perceived constipation. Actual constipation is defined as 3 or more days without defecation. The older person may perceive constipation to be present because of hard stools, straining with defecation, and feelings of incomplete defecation. Assessment of usual bowel habits is essential for effective correction and treatment. Assessment should include the following:
      (1) Frequency of defecation
      (2) Use of laxatives and enemas
      (3) Dietary habits, including consumption of fiber and fluid intake
      (4) Usual time of defecation: Note that when an older person is hospitalized or in a long-term care facility, defecation is sometimes impaired because of immobility and the need to time defecation at the nurse's convenience. Nurses should not try to "reprogram" bowel patterns that have been established over decades. For example, an 80-year-old person who has always gotten up, had a cup of coffee, and gone to the bathroom will do better if nurses try to reestablish the pattern that this person has followed for the past 8 decades.
   b. Causes of constipation
      (1) Medications that slow bowel motility
      (2) Obstruction of the bowel
      (3) Thyroid disease, or hypothyroidism
      (4) Inadequate fiber in the diet
      (5) Inaccessible or unavailable restrooms
   c. Correction of constipation
      (1) Reestablish typical bowel habits to the extent possible.
      (2) Add fiber to the diet.
      (3) Increase fluid intake, giving consideration to cardiac status.
      (4) Use suppositories sparingly, and limit suppository type to glycerin or Dulcolax.
      (5) Avoid long-term use of mineral oil because of problems in absorption of fat-soluble vitamins and potential for aspiration.
      (6) Limit enemas to prevent increased hypotonia of the rectum. The most appropriate type of enema is a small cleansing enema, such as the Fleet or Theravac enemas.
2. Diarrhea is considered frequent defecation of loose or liquid stools.
   a. Acute diarrhea may be unexplained and may be triggered by the same causative factors as those for younger adults.
      (1) Antibiotic-associated diarrhea, such as that caused by *Clostridium difficile,* is a problem for older people, particularly in hospital environments.
      (2) Fecal impaction may cause overflow diarrhea, with stool oozing around the impaction.
      (3) Infections may cause diarrhea.
   b. Chronic diarrhea (lasting >14 days) may be due to inflammation, malabsorption, or medications.
   c. Treatment of diarrhea
      (1) Correction of the underlying pathologic condition (if determined)
      (2) Correction of the fluid deficit and prevention of dehydration
      (3) Monitoring of fluid balance and electrolyte levels
3. Fecal incontinence, like urinary incontinence, may be due to multiple factors, such as diminished sphincter control, rectal distention, and cognitive impairment. Management of fecal incontinence is best accomplished by scheduling and consistent toileting.
   a. Assess and identify premorbid bowel patterns.
   b. Increase dietary bulk and fiber.
   c. Trigger defecation reflex:
      (1) Identify the usual time of defecation. A postprandial time is preferred.
      (2) Employ digital anal stimulation by inserting a gloved, lubricated finger 1 to 2 inches into the rectum. Suppositories (glycerin or Dulcolax) may be used.
      (3) Assist the person to a toilet (no bedpans). Provide privacy if possible, given safety needs and cognitive status.
   d. Time the bowel program to promote effective, regular emptying of the bowel.

NURSING DIAGNOSIS: Constipation R/T inadequate fiber intake

---

1. *Expected outcomes:* Following instruction, the person should be able to do the following:
   a. Determine contributing causes to constipation.
   b. Maintain regular defecation, every 3 days or less.
   c. Report minimal discomfort with defecation.
   d. Articulate the cornerstones of a healthy diet: adequate fluids, high fiber, low fat, and exercise.
2. *Nursing interventions*
   a. Identify bowel habits.
   b. Identify possible causes of constipation.
      (1) Evaluate self-prescribed bowel programs such as use of laxatives or of enemas.
      (2) Evaluate activity levels.
   c. Consider diet habits.
   d. Promote comfort during defecation.
      (1) Provide anal lubricant.
      (2) Add stool softeners to the medication regimen.
      (3) Avoid mineral oil. Ingestion of mineral oil may interfere with absorption of fat-soluble vitamins A, D, E, and K. Also, mineral oil may be aspirated, resulting in pneumonia.

1. *Expected outcomes:* Following intervention and instruction, the person should be able to do the following:
   a. Return to a usual defecation pattern.
   b. Not experience skin impairment around the anal area.
   c. Maintain a stable fluid and electrolyte balance.
2. *Nursing interventions*
   a. Identify defecation patterns.
   b. Identify causative factors and provide antidiarrheal agents.
   c. Monitor fluid and electrolyte balance, and correct as necessary.
   d. Monitor anal skin area for possible impairment of the skin integrity.

NURSING DIAGNOSIS: Bowel incontinence RT decreased cognition

1. *Expected outcomes:* Following instruction and intervention, the person should be able to do the following:
   a. Have a formed, soft stool every 1 to 3 days.
   b. Be continent of stool between bowel programs.
   c. Have intact skin surrounding the anal area.
   d. Experience dignity and privacy at all times throughout the bowel program and during any episodes of incontinence.
2. *Nursing interventions*
   a. Monitor usual bowel habits:
      (1) Frequency of stools
      (2) Any medication or dietary aids taken to trigger the defecation urge
      (3) Time of day in which the individual has usually defecated
   b. Ensure that the lower bowel is empty of formed stool.
   c. Provide a diet high in fiber and adequate in fluids.
   d. Establish a scheduled bowel program, which imitates the usual bowel program closely.
   e. Adopt a philosophy of "scheduled incontinence":
      (1) Plan for fecal incontinence every other day or daily.
      (2) Time the bowel program for shortly after a meal.
      (3) Provide a warm beverage such as coffee, tea, or water with the meal.
      (4) Provide a stimulant such as a glycerin suppository or digital stimulation.
      (5) Assist the individual in sitting on a commode or toilet. Provide privacy, but do not leave the individual unattended.
      (6) After defecation, inspect the condition of the skin surrounding the anus and determine the consistency, quantity, and form of the stool.
      (7) Evaluate the efficacy of the program, and modify as necessary.
      (8) Teach caregivers how to complete the program.

Vision Problems

1. Presbyopia, or the inability to obtain a clear visual focus at less than an arm's lngth, is a common problem in those older than 40 years of age. Presbyopia is attributed to continual growth of lens fibers and results in thickening of the lens. Correction of the deficiency is usually possible by using reading glasses or by switching to bifocal lenses (see Chapter 19).
2. Visual loss
   a. Sudden visual loss may be due to a variety of causes, including occipital lobe or central retinal artery infarcts, subretinal or vitreous hemorrhage, retinal detachment, and ischemic optic neuropathy. Sudden visual loss must be evaluated immediately on an emergency basis by an ophthalmologist.
   b. Gradual visual loss is commonly due to cataracts (see Chapter 19).
3. Glaucoma is caused by increased intraocular pressure. Loss of peripheral vision is gradual and progressive. If disease progresses, intraocular pressure may increase abruptly, resulting in pain. Two percent of adults older than 40 years are affected.
4. Cataracts are lens opacities that begin to form after age 30 years.
   a. The rate of cataract formation varies among individuals. The rate is faster in diabetics and is influenced by exposure to chemicals and environmental toxins.
   b. The treatment of choice is surgical removal of the cataract (see Chapter 19).
5. Age-related macular degeneration is caused by decreased blood supply to the macula, located in the retina, and by accumulation of waste products and tissue atrophy. The macula contains the fovea, the central focusing point for the optic system.
   a. Because the visual loss is central, reading and recognition of objects are impaired. Side vision and mobility remain functional.
   b. Laser therapy may diminish visual loss by sealing off damaged vessels and preventing bleeding, fluid leakage, scar tissue formation, and nerve tissue destruction.

Hearing Problems

1. Vertigo occurs frequently among older people because of inner ear problems. The condition may limit function and ability to perform activities of daily living (see Chapter 20).
2. Presbycusis is hearing loss that commonly affects older people, as many as one fourth of those older than 65. Medical diagnosis of presbycusis is made by ruling out other possible causes. Hearing aids may be of assistance. Selection should include consideration of cognitive status, manual dexterity, compliance, and social activity (see Chapter 20).

NURSING DIAGNOSIS: Sensory/perceptual alteration R/T cerebrovascular accident.

1. *Expected outcomes:* Following instruction, the person should be able to do the following:
   a. Be oriented to person, place, and time.

b. Identify methods of reducing distractions and verbalize the rationale for the treatment approaches used.
2. *Nursing interventions*
   a. Provide reorientation cues throughout the environment, including calendars, clocks, and family photographs.
   b. Encourage participation in self-care activities.
   c. Monitor comprehension levels and provide either written or verbal instructions, depending on which is best comprehended by the older individual.

Cardiovascular Problems

1. Hypertension: Normal changes with aging affect blood pressure, with pulse pressure increasing (widening interval between the systolic and diastolic pressures).
   a. Diagnosis of hypertension is made after 2 or more readings at an elevated level (diastolic 90 or higher and systolic 160 or higher).
      (1) The arm must be at heart level.
      (2) The cuff must be two thirds larger than the size of the arm.
      (3) Readings should not be site dependent to distinguish true hypertension from "white coat" hypertension associated with elevated readings due to anxiety during physician office visits.
   b. Treatment for hypertension is usually indicated when diastolic readings in older adults are greater than 90 to 95 mm Hg.
   c. There is a close association between elevated systolic pressure (160 mm Hg or higher) and cardiovascular disease. Elevated diastolic and systolic hypertension has a compound effect resulting in a significantly higher risk of cardiovascular disease.
   d. Reversible causes of hypertension include hyperthyroidism, which is treatable in older people, and renal artery stenosis due to atherosclerosis, which is treatable through angioplasty.
   e. Irreversible causes include renal impairment, left ventricular hypertrophy, and ischemic heart disease.
   f. Treatment of hypertension in older people
      (1) Nonpharmacologic methods
         • Dietary changes: reduction of salt and alcohol intake and adoption of a low-fat diet
         • Exercise program
         • Weight reduction
      (2) Pharmacologic methods are summarized in Table 16–14.
2. Orthostatic hypotension is defined as a drop of at least 20 mm Hg (systolic blood pressure) or of 10 mm Hg (diastolic blood pressure) on rising from a reclining position. Orthostatic hypotension is measured accurately after 20 minutes of reclining. Blood pressure is checked at 2 minutes and at 5 minutes after standing. Incidence of orthostatic hypotension among older individuals is not clearly documented, but estimates are about 10.7 percent of the population.
   a. Causes of orthostatic hypotension in older people
      (1) Cerebrovascular disease
      (2) Immobility

Table 16–14. Pharmacologic Treatment of Hypertension

Drug	Benefits	Side Effects
Thiazide-like drugs	Low cost Do not contribute to osteoporosis Vasodilation	Hypokalemia Hyperuricemia Impaired glucose tolerance Impotence (occasional)
Beta-adrenergic blockers	Low cost (in generic form) Antianginal action	Fatigue Impotence (occasional)
Calcium antagonists	Vasodilation Antianginal action	Constipation
Converting enzyme inhibitors	Vasodilation	Hyperkalemia Dry cough

   (3) Environmental factors (warm room, warm bed, warm bath or shower)
   (4) Defecation syndrome
   (5) Antihypertensive agents
      • Calcium channel-blocking agents
      • Angiotensin-converting enzyme inhibitors
      • Diuretics
   (6) Antiparkinsonian agents
      • Levodopa
      • Bromocriptine
   b. Correction of orthostatic hypotension
      (1) External support devices such as elastic stockings and abdominal binders
      (2) Gradual changes in position, such as dangling at the side of the bed before standing
      (3) Medications: vasoconstrictors, prostaglandin inhibitors, and beta agonists and β-blockers
      (4) Atrial pacemaker
      (5) Education of the older person on the causes and correction of orthostatic hypotension
3. Coronary artery disease
   a. Coronary artery disease is prevalent among older people.
      (1) Incidence is 50 to 60 percent in men older than 60 years of age.
      (2) Over the past 20 years, the incidence of coronary artery disease has increased in those older than 60 years.
      (3) Coronary artery disease is the most common cause of death in those older than 60 years.
   b. Symptoms of coronary artery disease
      (1) Of persons with coronary artery disease, only 10 to 50 percent are symptomatic.
      (2) Common symptoms
         • Confusion (acute)
         • Dyspnea (acute)
         • Indigestion
         • Heart failure
         • Substernal chest pain
      (3) Infrequent (but misleading) symptoms
         • Pulmonary embolus
         • Heart palpitations

- Deep venous thrombosis
- Syncope
- Stroke
- Vertigo
- Renal failure
  c. Treatment of coronary artery disease
  (1) Dietary changes
  - Reduction of salt intake
  - Reduction of alcohol intake
  - Low-fat diet
  (2) Exercise program
  (3) Weight reduction
  (4) Regular diagnostic testing
  - Stress testing
  - Holter test monitoring
4. Congestive heart failure
  a. Incidence of congestive heart failure increases with age
  b. Causes of congestive heart failure
  (1) Coronary artery disease
  (2) Chronic hypertension
  (3) Valvular disease
  c. Treatment
  (1) Dietary changes
  - Reduction of salt intake
  - Reduction of alcohol intake
  - Low-fat diet
  (2) Exercise program
  (3) Weight reduction
  (4) Regular diagnostic testing
  - Stress testing
  - Holter test monitoring

NURSING DIAGNOSIS: Fluid volume deficit R/T dehydration

1. *Expected outcomes:* Following intervention, the person should be able to do the following:
   a. Demonstrate a balance between fluid intake and output
   b. Have urine specific gravity within normal limits (1.005 to 1.010)
   c. Have normal skin turgor
   d. Develop normally moist mucous membranes
   e. Achieve electrolyte levels within normal ranges
2. *Nursing interventions*
   a. Monitor intake and output
   b. Assess vital signs
   c. Assess electrolyte levels
   d. Monitor weight
   e. Provide adequate fluids

NURSING DIAGNOSIS: Activity intolerance R/T decreased endurance and energy levels secondary to cardiopulmonary disease

1. *Expected outcomes:* Following instruction, the person should be able to do the following:
   a. Express the need to increase activity
   b. Comprehend the need for gradual and progressive increase in activity
   c. Conserve energy with progression of activity
2. *Nursing interventions*
   a. Work with the older person to identify possible activities.
   (1) Discuss factors that effect energy and endurance levels.
   (2) Break up activities into 20-minute or less segments, with time for rest.
   (3) Identify ways to increase activity over a gradual time period.
   b. Monitor the person's response to activity increases.
   (1) Monitor blood pressure
   (2) Monitor fatigue level
   (3) Measure pulse and respiratory rate

Respiratory Problems

1. Pneumonia
   a. Pneumonia is the 5th most common cause of death in older people and the most common infectious cause of death. About 4.4 million hospital days annually are for treatment of pneumonia.
   b. Causes of pneumonia in older people
   (1) Aspiration of pathogens
   (2) Effects of aging: weakened antibacterial defenses, adherence of bacteria to the respiratory tract, impaired mucociliary transport
   (3) Weak cough
   (4) Medications (morphine, sedatives, atropine, corticosteroids)
   (5) Malnutrition
   (6) Comorbidity
   c. Symptoms of pneumonia in older people may be masked by other illnesses. These include confusion, fever (although an estimated 20% of older people are afebrile with pneumonia), cough, and rapid respiratory rate and pulse.
   d. Treatment of pneumonia in older persons should be comprehensive and should include antibiotic therapy, nutritional support, respiratory therapy, and progressive activity, which should be increased to prevent deconditioning due to inactivity.
2. Chronic obstructive lung disease
   a. Older people experience chronic obstructive lung disease more frequently, with 3.3 million of those older than 65 years affected. Chronic obstructive lung disease includes emphysema, chronic bronchitis, and asthma.
   b. Treatment of chronic obstructive lung disease
   (1) Oxygen to correct hypoxemia
   (2) Smoking cessation
   (3) Pacing activities
   (4) Efficiently using energy and endurance levels by breaking up activities into segments of 20 minutes or less
   (5) Nutrition: small, frequent meals to minimize energy used for activity and digestion and a balanced diet to prevent malnutrition

(6) Pharmacologic management
• Theophylline, which causes bronchodilation. Decreased clearance of theophylline (resulting in high blood levels) may occur with old age, hepatic disease, congestive heart failure, acute viral infections, cimetidine use, or erythromycin use. Increased clearance of theophylline (resulting in low blood levels) may occur with phenytoin, phenobarbital, or isoniazid use.
• Beta₂-agonists (inhalers)
• Anticholinergic drugs
• Steroids
• Antibiotics (time limited for specific infections)

NURSING DIAGNOSIS: Ineffective breathing pattern R/T chronic obstructive lung disease

1. *Expected outcomes:* Following instruction and intervention, the person should be able to do the following:
   a. Verbalize the importance of regular pulmonary exercise
   b. Maintain optimum pulmonary function
2. *Nursing interventions*
   a. Monitor respiratory function at rest, during activity, and after activity.
   b. Assist with progressive increase in activity and ambulation.
   c. Pace activity, breaking activities lasting longer than 20 minutes into 20-minute segments with rest periods of 5 minutes or more.
   d. Work with the person in planning activities.
   e. Teach the person methods of improving pulmonary function through controlled breathing and deep breathing

Cancer

1. An estimated 55 percent of cancers occur in people older than age 65. The incidence is higher for women than for men aged 20 to 60. After age 60, the incidence dramatically increases in men more than in women. At age 70, men experience a rate of cancer double the rate in women.
2. Causes of cancer in older people are not always well understood, but some known causative factors include the following:
   a. Smoking and tobacco use
   b. Diets high in fat
   c. Moderate to excessive use of alcohol
   d. Excessive sun exposure
3. Screening for early detection of cancer
   a. Breast (women)
   (1) Self-examination (monthly) at age 20 and older
   (2) Physical examination (annually) over age 40
   (3) Mammography (annually) over age 50
   b. Colon (men and women)
   (1) Sigmoidoscopy (every 3 years) over age 50
   (2) Stool guaiac (annually) over age 50

(3) Digital rectal examination (annually) over age 50
   c. Uterine and ovarian (women)
   (1) Cervical smear (annually) over age 18
   (2) Pelvic examination (annually) over age 18
   (3) Endometrial tissue biopsy (1 time only) at menopause.
4. Treatment of cancer in older people varies with the type of cancer and with comorbidity.
   a. Treatment programs must be tailored to the pharmacokinetic differences in older people.
   b. The principle of treatment in many cases is to start with a low dosage and to increase the dosage slowly.
   c. Side effects of treatments, in addition to potential interaction between premorbid medication regimens and oncology treatment programs, must be monitored.

Endocrine Problems

1. Thyroid disease (see Chapter 29)
   a. Although older people are susceptible to a variety of thyroid diseases, hyperthyroidism and hypothyroidism are most common.
   (1) About one fifth of cases of hyperthyroidism occur in people older than 60.
   (2) Hypothyroidism affects primarily older women.
   • Seventy percent of cases of hypothyroidism occur in people older than 50.
   • Eighty percent of cases of hypothyroidism affect women.
   b. Signs and symptoms of thyroid disease
   (1) Hyperthyroidism
   • Weight loss
   • Heat intolerance
   • Excessive appetite
   • Shortness of breath
   • Palpitations
   • Fine hand tremors
   (2) Hypothyroidism
   • Lethargy
   • Cold intolerance
   • Constipation
   • Psychomotor retardation
   c. Treatment of thyroid disease varies with the underlying cause.
   (1) Treatment in older people may be complicated by coronary artery disease.
   (2) Drug therapy (if indicated) must be tapered to match the blood level with the therapeutic level of effect.
2. Diabetes (see Chapter 29)
   a. The incidence of diabetes increases with age and is estimated to be as high as 40 percent in people older than 65 years. Many people with diabetes who are older than 65 remain undiagnosed.
   b. Signs and symptoms of diabetes mellitus do not differ substantially between older adults and younger people.
   c. Treatment must be balanced and should include the following:
   (1) Patient teaching

(2) Diet counseling (no refined sugars, use of the exchange program, and no fats, with a specific caloric level established every day)

(3) Exercise program

(4) Medication instruction

Pain

1. The incidence of pain is higher in older individuals (see Chapter 11).
   a. People older than 60 report pain twice as frequently as those younger than 60.
   b. Approximately 70 percent of older people who are hospitalized or in long-term care facilities report pain.
   c. Around 80 percent of older people experience pain due to arthritis.
2. Because of the frequency of pain experienced by older people, many health care professionals believe pain to be a normal and an unpreventable aspect of aging.
   a. Such attitudes are incorrect and cause undertreatment of pain.
   b. Education of nurses and health care professionals is essential to prevent failure to treat pain in older adults.
   c. Failure to alleviate or moderate pain in older people leads to functional limitations affecting their ability to perform self-care independently.
3. Standard measures of pain, including verbal descriptor scales and visual analogue scales, have not been established psychometrically for older adults.
   a. The lack of psychometrically sound pain measurement instruments may result in undertreatment or overtreatment of older people's pain.
   b. It is critical, given the incidence of pain in older adults, that nurses use a variety of cues to assess pain.
      (1) Visual cues include agitation, restlessness, moaning, distress, and crying.
      (2) Verbal cues include reports of pain.
   c. Nurses must frequently monitor the older person for pain, and offer some form of alleviation.
4. Nonpharmacologic management of pain
   a. Older people are responsive to common methods of nonpharmacologic pain relief, including the following:
      (1) Relaxation
      (2) Biofeedback
      (3) Distraction
      (4) Massage
   b. Teaching older people self-management of nonpharmacologic pain relief can promote alleviation of pain.
5. Pharamacologic management of pain
   a. Because of pharmacodynamic changes, older people usually require lower doses of analgesics to relieve pain.
   b. Nonsteroidal anti-inflammatory drugs
      (1) Usually the first line of treatment for pain in older people.
      (2) The side effects to which older people are particularly susceptible include renal toxicity, gastric distress, and drug reactions, including headaches, cognitive impairment, and constipation.

   c. Opioid analgesic drugs
      (1) Effective for management and relief of acute pain in older people.
      (2) Smaller dosages are effective in older people and for longer periods.
      (3) Side effects of opioid administration are more pronounced in older people. These effects include respiratory depression, sedation, and urinary retention (of particular concern in older males at risk for prostatic hypertrophy).

NURSING DIAGNOSIS: Pain R/T arthritic joint changes

---

1. *Expected outcomes:* Following intervention, the person should be able to do the following:
   a. Report relief from pain
   b. Report the efficacy of pain relief measures
2. *Nursing interventions*
   a. Identify the pattern of pain.
   b. Implement nonpharmacologic methods of pain relief: relaxation, imagery, distraction, biofeedback.
   c. Implement pharmacologic methods of pain relief.
   d. Monitor efficacy of pain relief measures.

NURSING DIAGNOSIS: Chronic pain R/T osteoarthritis

---

1. *Expected outcomes:* Following intervention, the person should be able to do the following:
   a. Report lower levels of pain
   b. Report less interference from pain
   c. Identify nonpharmacologic methods of pain relief, in addition to appropriate use of pharmacologic methods
2. *Nursing interventions*
   a. Identify the pattern of pain.
      (1) What provokes the pain?
      (2) What is the quality of the pain at the lowest levels experienced, the highest levels experienced, and the usual levels experienced?
      (3) What does the individual use for relief of the pain (including pharmacologic and nonpharmacologic methods of pain relief)?
   b. Monitor activities of daily living and the impact of pain on such activities.
   c. Implement nonpharmacologic methods of pain relief: relaxation, imagery, distraction, biofeedback.
   d. Implement pharmacologic methods of pain relief.
   e. Determine the efficacy of pain relief measures.

▣ *PSYCHIATRIC AND COGNITIVE PROBLEMS IN OLDER PEOPLE*

Depression

1. Depression is a functional disorder of mood that is not linked with aging. Depression may be precipitated by losses related to aging (see Chapter 42).

2. Symptoms of depression
   a. Difficulty concentrating
   b. Feelings of inadequacy, sadness, and pessimism
   c. Difficulty sleeping or excessive sleepiness
   d. Weight gain or loss
   e. Loss of interest in activities
   f. Thoughts of death or suicide
   g. Decreased endurance and energy
3. Treatment includes counseling and medications, usually antidepressants, including imipramine, amitriptyline, fluoxetine, and nortriptyline.

Dementia

1. The incidence of dementia rises with age. Of those age 65 to 74 years, 3 percent experience dementia. Of those age 75 to 84 years, 19 percent experience dementia. Of those age 85 or older, up to 50 percent may experience dementia.
2. The most common type of dementia (39–70% of cases) is Alzheimer's disease (see Chapter 18).
   a. Symptoms of dementia with Alzheimer's disease
      (1) Language disturbance
      (2) Memory loss, especially short-term memory impairment
      (3) Abstract reasoning impairment
      (4) Insidious progression of dementia resulting in complete loss of functional independence, self-care ability, and language comprehension and expression
   b. Treatment of Alzheimer's dementia is oriented around symptom management, promotion of independence, and caregiver support.
      (1) Nonpharmacologic interventions include providing reassurance, redirection, and reorientation. Pharmacologic management involves use of neuroleptics (haloperidol, thioridazine, and thiothixene), while monitoring extrapyramidal side effects (rigidity, tremors, bradykinesia, and restlessness).
      (2) To promote functional independence, guard against learned helplessness by encouraging independence and self-care as long as possible. Provide a structured, predictable daily routine. Communicate with eye contact and direct statements, avoiding complex instructions or questions.
      (3) Caregiver support means identifying the "hidden patient." Respite care is essential to ensure that the caregiver maintains a healthy perspective. Caregiver support groups are available in many areas, and caregivers should be put in connection with other caregivers.
   c. Education of health care providers regarding care of people with Alzheimer's dementia and support of their families is imperative. Care should include the following:
      (1) A team approach for behavior and symptom management
      (2) Maintenance of human dignity
      (3) Identification of planning and therapeutic goals
      (4) Ongoing staff education and support

3. Other diseases, including cerebrovascular disease, may cause dementia.
   a. Symptoms of vascular dementia are similar to those of Alzheimer's disease, except that the onset of deficits are sudden and occur step by step with each infarct.
   b. Treatment of vascular dementia is similar to that for dementia for Alzheimer's disease.

NURSING DIAGNOSIS: Altered thought process R/T multi-infarct dementia

1. *Expected outcomes:* Following intervention, the person should be able to do the following:
   a. Remain oriented to person, place, and time
   b. Not display aggressive or agitated behaviors
   c. Not be harmed and not harm others because of behaviors such as wandering or agitation
2. *Nursing interventions*
   a. Monitor the person to identify degree of orientation to person, place, and time.
   b. Reorient as needed, and provide reorientation cues, such as calendars and clocks.
   c. Approach the person calmly and reassuringly.
   d. For wandering behavior, avoid the use of restraint vests and jackets. Rather use environmental restraints such as closed doors. Rather than restraints in bed, consider the use of a floor bed (mattress on the floor) to eliminate the possibility of falls out of bed.
   e. For agitated or aggressive behavior, approach the person calmly and reassuringly. Identify events that trigger such behaviors, and eliminate, prevent, or prepare for such events. Provide a consistent, predictable routine, and avoid sudden changes.

▣ HEALTH TEACHING AND PREVENTIVE CARE

Nursing Implications for Prevention

1. Older people probably have a greater impact on health care resources and nursing than any other group. People older than 65 years receive the major proportion of health care resources and have unique health care needs and concerns (see Learning/Teaching Guidelines for Older People).
2. The distinctive culture of older Americans has implications for patient education and health care promotion.
   a. The older American must be a "partner in care" for development and implementation of a successful plan of care.
      (1) The nurse works with the older person in identifying health care goals.
      (2) The nurse assesses lifestyle patterns to determine health care maintenance methods most likely to meet with compliance and success.
   b. Older Americans are proud of their self-reliance and perseverance, so that maintaining independence becomes a key motivator.

LEARNING/TEACHING GUIDELINES
for Older People

General Overview

1. Visual aids need to accommodate changes in visual acuity experienced in older people, who need precise discrimination.
2. When presenting information one to one with an older person, stand sufficiently close to promote clarity and strength for sensory stimuli.
3. Maximize auditory input through adjusting the word-per-minute rate of speech to the level best understood by the older person.
4. Work with the older person to identify preferred methods for presenting information (e.g., auditory, visual, tactile, or a combination).
5. Allow the older person to control the presentation pace by selecting the teaching strategies and materials.
6. Ask the older person for feedback throughout the teaching session. Pay special attention to the pace of speech, the intelligibility, and the significance of content.
7. Consult the older person about the appropriate place and time for teaching sessions.
8. Present the person with opportunities for feedback and recall of information presented.
9. Correlate new learning with past and current experiences.
10. Identify opportunities for integration of new behaviors with established behaviors.
11. Establish mutually agreed-on goals with the older person.
12. Identify positive reinforcers for learning and incorporation of new behaviors.
13. Present opportunities for the older person to express feelings and concerns about the information presented.
14. Optimize use of humor throughout the teaching session.

(1) When developing patient education programs, remember that independence is a powerful motivator. Patient education programs that enable the person to complete tasks independently, with minimal risk of error, are likely to promote compliance.

(2) Nurses must remember that the older person's most precious possessions are often dignity and self-respect, which are enhanced by independence.

Immunizations

1. Immunizations against influenza and pneumococcal pneumonia are advised for older people because decreased resistance to disease leads to greater mortality and morbidity. Patients at high risk of developing infections are usually those with chronic conditions and those residing in long-term care facilities.
2. Long-term care facilities and other health care institutions should promote vaccination programs for older people. Community-based programs should be accessible to those living at home as well as to those in nursing homes and hospitals.

Use of Restraints

1. Physical restraints, used to prevent injury, are rarely justified in current nursing practice. Alternatives are usually available.
   a. For the patient at risk for falling out of bed, for example, padding made of foam or pillow cases stuffed with beans or peanuts might be used for positioning. The patient will then slide against a soft, resistant object.
   b. For the patient at risk for removing intravenous lines, a foam football can be placed in the hand, which is then covered with a stockinette. The patient can then retain a degree of mobility.
2. The 2 most common reasons for the use of conventional restraints are legal liability and poor staffing. In these instances, restraints should be accompanied by frequent nursing observation, documentation, and repositioning.

Oral Care

1. Prevention and effective treatment of dental caries is necessary for prevention of tooth loss and tooth disease.
2. Careful tongue cleaning should be included in regular brushing and oral hygiene.
3. Attention to nutritional concerns and prevention of anemia is essential for healthy oral tissues.
4. Replacement of lost teeth should be accomplished through denture prosthodontics.

Smoking

1. Risk of disease can be reduced by eliminating health risks such as smoking.
2. Because older people may have smoked for several decades, many do not plan to stop smoking. In these cases, advise the older person that the best option is to stop smoking. If the person is not willing to stop smoking, recommend smoking low-tar cigarettes, smoking only

part of the cigarette, and reducing the number and frequency of cigarettes smoked.

Sleep

1. As people age, sleep patterns change. Older people require less stage-4 REM rest, less overall rest, and less length of sleep time. Some older people have difficulty sleeping.
2. Use alternatives to sedatives. Warm milk, for example, contains tryptophan, which promotes sleep. Excretion problems with medications include residual "dopey" effects and cloudy mentation. Older people may be incapacitated for days, may doze all day, or may be unable to sleep at night. Inability to sleep may then lead to another dose of sleep medication.
3. Exercise and relaxation techniques are possible alternatives to sleep medication.

NURSING DIAGNOSIS: Sleep pattern disturbance R/T hospitalization

1. *Expected outcomes:* Following intervention, the person should be able to do the following:
   a. Obtain adequate sleep and rest
   b. Describe elements that disrupt or induce sleep
2. *Nursing interventions*
   a. Plan for rest and sleep time.
   b. Reduce distractions and noise as much as possible.
   c. Provide a night light, as older people usually have difficulty accommodating to changes between dark and light.
   d. Provide for toileting needs before sleeping.
   e. Offer a glass of warm or cold milk and a light snack to facilitate sleep.

Scheduling Physical Examinations

1. Physical examinations should be conducted annually after the age of 40 years and should include the following:
   a. Mammography for women
   b. Digital rectal examination
   c. Guaiac stool test
   d. Flu shot
2. At least annually, health counseling should be conducted and should include the following:
   a. Assessment of risk behaviors
      (1) Smoking
      (2) Falls
      (3) Alcohol use
      (4) Sedentary lifestyle
   b. Assessment of over-the-counter and prescription medications
   c. Assessment of dietary habits
   d. Assessment of any perceived health problems or issues as identified by the older person

Preventing Accidents

1. An older person at risk for falls is one with one or more of the following traits:
   a. A past history of falls
   b. A gait disturbance, especially a shuffling gait
   c. Orthostatic hypotension
   d. A loss of lower extremity strength
   e. A number of disabilities
2. To prevent falls:
   a. Eliminate environmental hazards and provide a clear path through the home and rooms.
   b. Maintain the person's mobility through exercise and use of assistive devices.

 HOME CARE STRATEGIES

Modifying the Home Environment to Prevent Falls

Falls in the home are very serious. In order to reduce the risk of falls, home health care providers must be sensitive to older people's reluctance to make changes in their lifestyle and environment. It may take time to establish rapport, which may be necessary before older patients are willing to change their lifestyle and environment, especially because neither may have changed for many years.
   Consequences of falls include the following:
   • Increased fear of falling again, causing depression, confinement, and overall decreased quality of life
   • Debilitating injury, causing limited mobility and decreased independence
   • Death due to the fall itself or complications following the fall
   Identifying and eliminating some or all of the major risk factors associated with falls can greatly reduce the risks of falls in the home and thus prevent serious consequences.
   • Muscle weakness, primarily hip abductors, knee flexors and extensors, ankle dorsiflexors
   • Decreased or poor balance
   • Gait abnormalities
   • Slow response time

• Use and number of medications
• Pathologic conditions such as postural hypotension, stroke, arthritis, Parkinson's disease, and cancer
• Environmental hazards and recommendations
   1. Remove throw rugs, electric cords, and door thresholds.
   2. Clear pathways of furniture and other objects.
   3. Remove and avoid the use of low chairs. Use solid chairs with arm rests.
   4. Provide adequate lighting with accessible light switches. Use a night light.
   5. Adapt bathrooms and kitchens for safety. Consults with an occupational therapist or physical therapist and referral to local resources for equipment may be needed.
   6. Suggest using a cordless phone and obtaining a walker basket to carry it, if necessary.
   7. Consult a physical therapist to instruct in safe techniques to ascend and descend stairs.
   8. Check clothing to avoid floppy shoes, long robes, or other garments that are hazardous.
   9. An occupational therapist consult may be necessary to instruct in safe techniques for performing activities of daily living, such as dressing, toileting, bathing, and meal preparation.

c. Evaluate appropriateness of footwear to ensure that footwear is comfortable, nonskid, and sturdy.
d. Advise the person to change positions slowly, particularly when rising from a prone position after sleeping.

Using Medications Cautiously

1. Because many people take a number of drugs (Table 16–15), it is important for them to know exactly which pills to take each day, including vitamins and over-the-counter and prescription medications (Fig. 16–2).
2. Pharmacokinetics describes absorption, distribution, metabolism, and excretion of drug in the body (Table 16–16). Older people have a normal increase in fat, so that more of a drug can be absorbed and stored in fat for ultimate release.

a. Benzodiazepines (e.g., Valium) bind to fat. This active metabolite may be bound in fat for more than 30 days, causing additive effects when released. The drug, however, is commonly prescribed because it is

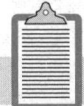

NURSING MANAGEMENT

The nurse manager must be aware of the impact of the nurse on drug therapy. For example, the nurse-patient relationship may have a strong placebo effect and may influence compliance. In addition, if family members have confidence in the nurse, they can facilitate the nurse's ability to provide education by encouraging the older person to listen and heed the nurse's instructions.

Table 16–15. Prevention of Drug Use and Misuse Among Older Individuals

Assessment Area	Precautions
Is drug therapy necessary?	Sleep-inducing medications can be replaced by nonpharmacologic means. Avoid treatment of symptoms without a diagnosis because the additional symptom is sometimes a medication side effect.
Is the dosage appropriate?	Older individuals require lower dosages than younger people. Start low (at a low dosage) and go slow (gradually increasing the dosage). Monitor the person for the desired therapeutic response or toxicity.
What effect will the drug have?	The desired therapeutic response should be identified before treatment.
What undesirable effects may occur?	Identify all possible side effects and monitor for occurrence after any change in the medication regimen.
Is the drug form optimal?	If dysphagia is present, liquid preparations may be best. Slow-release medications may lead to gastric upset. Consider all forms (e.g., liquid, oral, intramuscular, intravenous, suppository).
Is the drug packaging and labeling appropriate?	Make certain that the lids to bottles are removable without causing additional joint stress or making it impossible to comply with the regimen. Labels should be printed large enough, and should be color coded to promote visual recognition of the medication bottle.
Is it possible to guarantee that the medication will be taken appropriately?	The chances of compliance with a medication regimen are increased, if • Three or fewer medications are prescribed • Instructions are in writing • Labels are legible • Old drugs are discarded • The schedule is simple (daily is best)
When should medications be discontinued?	Many drugs are not needed for a lifetime, although medications such as digoxin are commonly prescribed without a time limit. Periodic evaluations of all drugs should be conducted at least semiannually. If in question, a trial period off the drug may be of benefit. Drugs such as steroids, antiparkinsonian agents, and anticonvulsants must be withdrawn carefully and under observation.

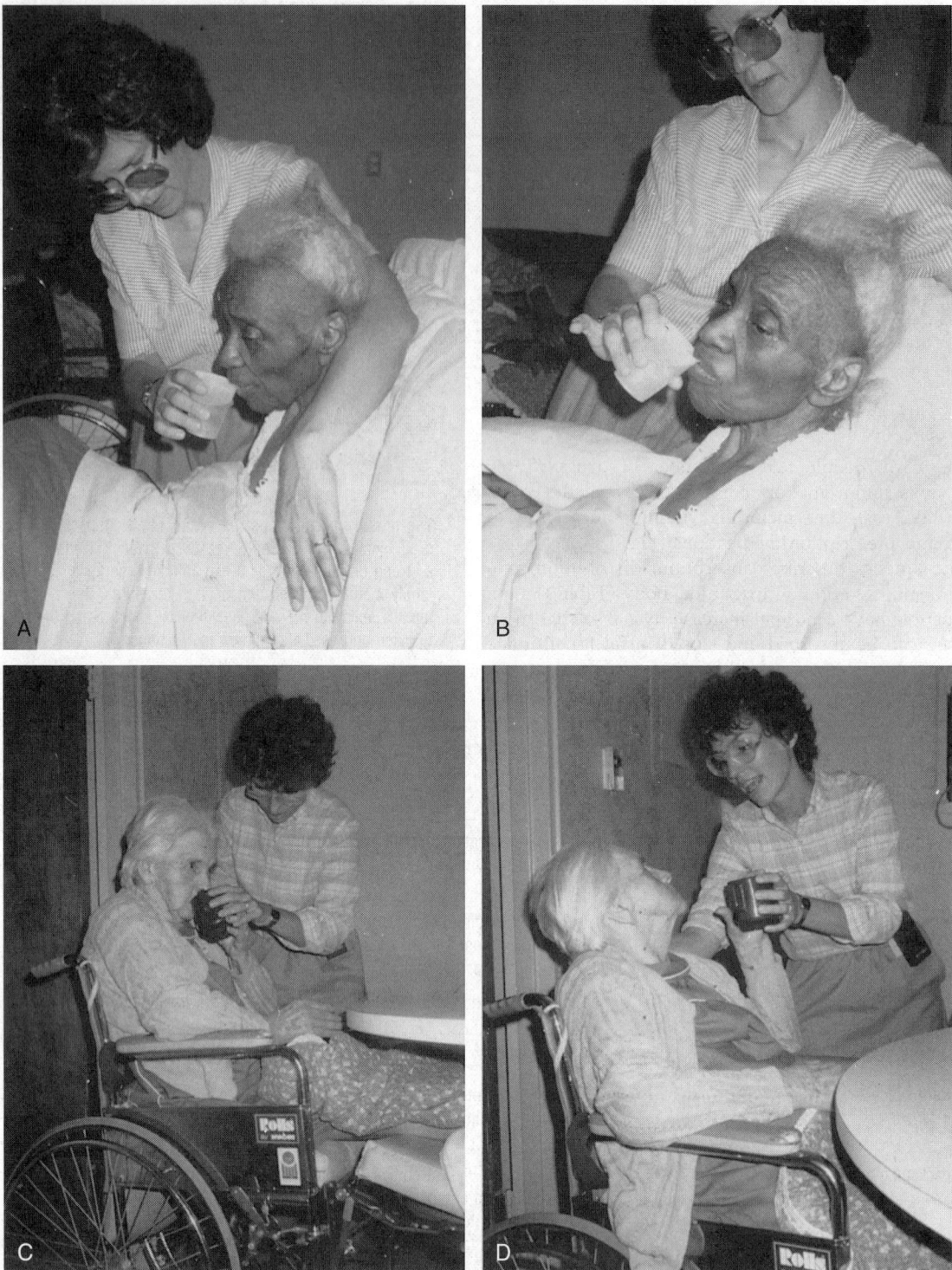

Figure 16–2. *A,* Correct position for medication administration to prevent aspiration in a reclining patient: head forward, neck slightly flexed. *B,* Incorrect position: head back, neck hyperextended. The patient is at high risk for difficulty in swallowing and aspiration. *C,* Correct medication administration position for a seated patient. *D,* Incorrect position. (From Matteson MA, McConnell ES, and Linton AD. *Gerontological Nursing.* 2nd ed. Philadelphia: WB Saunders, 1996.)

cheap and creates a good feeling in the person. Health care providers therefore have difficulty removing the drug from the treatment regimen.

  b. Digoxin is a protein-bound drug and typically a long-term medication; its need decreases with aging. For aging patients, decreasing the dosage may be necessary to prevent digoxin toxicity due to decreased need and decreased excretion.

Table 16–16. Common Adverse Drug Reactions in Older Individuals	
Types of Adverse Reaction	**Possible Causes**
Anxiety	Antacids
Depression	Clonidine Propranolol Methyldopa Digoxin Theophylline
Confusion	Propranolol Antacids Cimetidine (especially in people with renal disease) Antihistamines Theophylline Digoxin (toxicity)
Sedation	Antacids
Tardive dyskinesia	Metoclopramide
Electrolyte imbalance	Diuretics
Gout	Thiazide diuretics
Insomnia	Antacids
Sexual dysfunction	Hydrochlorothiazide Chlorthalidone Propranolol Methyldopa
Hallucinations	Propranolol Digoxin (toxicity)
Headache	Hydralazine
Gastric distress	Reserpine Prednisone Theophylline Laxatives Digoxin (toxicity)
Hypotension	Nitroglycerine Propranolol Furosemide
Parkinson's disease	Reserpine

From Lamy PP. Geriatric drug therapy. *Adv Fam Physician* 34(6):118–124, 1986.

Restricting Alcohol

1. Alcohol may have an increased effect on older people. Ethanol is readily available and water soluble. Ethanol is excreted by being linked to water. In older persons, less water intake plus less water in cells creates a buildup in ethanol effect. In older persons, alcohol has a strong potential for a drug-drug interaction.
2. Alcohol may be used by older people as a self-prescribed sleep aid. Alcoholic drinks may induce sleep initially. Effects of the alcohol wear off shortly after sleep begins. Following initial sleepiness, alcohol may cause recurrent stirrings. Use of alcohol often results in drug tolerance, dependence, and abuse.

Eating a Nutritious Diet

1. Poor nutritional status leads to longer and more expensive hospital stays and greater risk of complications during hospitalization
2. Nutrition screening should include the following:
   a. Body weight
   b. Eating habits
   c. Living environment
   d. Functional status
   e. Height and weight
      (1) The body mass index (BMI) is a ruler to draw a line between height and weight on a scale (see Fig. 10–3).
      (2) In a healthy older adult the BMI is between 24 and 27. A BMI greater than 27 constitutes obesity; a BMI less than 24 means the person is underweight.

Exercising Safely

1. Older people frequently exercise less than younger adults and may lead sedentary lifestyles.
2. Physical and mental health is enhanced through regular exercise.
3. Exercise programs should be prescribed by the person's physician and should consider the person's lifestyle, cardiac status, energy, endurance level, and mobility limitations.
4. Walking programs provide 1 form of exercise that is therapeutic and low risk for most older people.

Controlling Stress

1. Stress management is essential for prevention of disease exacerbation and illness.
2. Stressful events associated with aging include limited financial resources, limited social support systems, inability to get out of the house, loss of friends and family members, and retirement.
3. Stress reduction may be achieved through use of social support systems, relaxation strategies, reframing events, and seeking professional support.

Planning for Illness and Disability

1. Wills should be prepared with legal counsel, and should identify the executor of the estate, address distribution and use of property, and specify plans for burial.
2. Living wills address the withdrawal or withholding of life-sustaining interventions that unnaturally prolong life. A living will identifies the person who will make care decisions if the older person is unable to take action. Living wills are witnessed and signed by 2 people who are unrelated to the older person (see Box 43–2).
   a. Nurses or employees of a facility in which the person is receiving care and beneficiaries of the older person must not serve as witnesses.

b. The older person should discuss the living will with a physician and should review it annually.

c. Copies of the living will should be kept with the medical record, at the physician's office, and in the home of the older person.

3. The older person may delegate power of attorney for aspects of legal business and management of expenses.

a. The power of attorney is not time limited but is invalidated when a person is declared incompetent or unresponsive.

b. Durable power of attorney differs from power of attorney by indicating the older person's intent to delegate power of attorney in the event of an illness or injury affecting the ability to manage personal business.

◪ PLANNING FOR LONG-TERM CARE

Continuum of Care

1. Planning should be completed before the need for self-care assistance.

2. Health promotion planning should include consistency in care providers (i.e., physicians, nurses, and pharmacists) to ensure that all clinicians are aware of the individual's needs and health care issues.

3. Community resources such as home health aides and nurses and social service agencies should be identified and evaluated according to accreditation status, cost of service, scope of service, and referral mechanisms.

Rehabilitation

1. Rehabilitation may be completed in a variety of settings.

a. Inpatient acute rehabilitation units and hospitals

(1) Need for admission may be precipitated by acute illness or injury, including cerebrovascular accident, orthopedic fractures, amputation, or neuromuscular disease.

(2) Admission criteria typically include the need for intensive rehabilitation, up to 3 hours of therapy daily.

(3) Length of stay is usually less than 1 month.

(4) Discharge placement is most often home. A person without a discharge plan may not be admitted.

b. Subacute rehabilitation programs and transitional care units

(1) Need for admission may be precipitated by acute or chronic illness or injury, including cardiovascular disease, pneumonia, or severe cerebrovascular accident.

(2) Admission criteria typically include the need for 1 hour of rehabilitation therapy daily.

(3) Length of stay is usually 1 to 3 months.

(4) Discharge placement may return the person home or to a long-term care facility. A person may be admitted without a firm discharge plan.

2. Determination of appropriate rehabilitation setting should be based on individual preference, cost, accessibility for friends and relatives, and various quality factors such as accreditation status.

a. Quality reports include the incidence of falls (assisted and unassisted), nosocomial pressure ulcers, contracture development, and nosocomial infections, especially methicillin-resistant *Staphylococcus aureus*.

b. Quality issues include the frequency of visits to the community, the percentage of people who are discharged home, and the percentage of people who retain functional progress for 3 months or more after discharge.

Independence and Self-Care

1. Promotion of independence and self-care is critical regardless of setting. Uncorrected self-care limitations will result in increased need for assistance. Independence may be promoted through various strategies.

a. Facilitating self-care through provision of adaptive and assistive equipment

b. Encouraging decision making through building in the perception of control

c. Setting attainable short- and long-term goals with rewards

d. Using contracts to set mutually agreed-on goals

e. Evaluating progress toward goal achievement

Long-Term Care

1. Only 5 percent of those older than 65 reside in long-term care facilities, although up to 30 percent of people may receive some care in a facility.

2. Selection of a long-term care facility should be based on assessment of the following factors:

a. Individual preference

b. Cost

c. Environmental accessibility and design

d. Accessibility for friends and relatives

e. Food quality and variety

f. Quality issues such as the following:

(1) Accreditation and licensure status

(2) Level and amount of nursing care available in the facility, including skill-mix ratio (RNs to NAs), nursing care hours per patient day, and availability of nurse practitioners and clinical nurse specialists

(3) Quality reports on the incidence of falls (assisted and unassisted), nosocomial pressure ulcers, contracture development, and nosocomial infections, especially methicillin-resistant *S. aureus*

(4) Bladder-training protocols, including the incidence of management by indwelling catheters

(5) Access to medical and emergency care

(6) Availability of therapists

(7) Frequency of visits to the community

(8) Percentage of people who are discharged home

Home-Based Care

1. Decentralized care provided to patients at their places of residence is increasingly common for older people. For many of these patients, family members need to be made part of the decision-making and care plans.
   a. Services might include medical care, dental care, nursing, physical therapy, speech therapy, occupational therapy, social work, nutrition, homemaking assistance, transportation, laboratory services, and medical supplies and equipment.
   b. Hospitals often establish their own home care agencies, which can monitor patients and provide continuity of care during hospital stays.
2. Discharge planning is an important link between hospital and home-based care. The process should involve referrals, follow-up, and patient education. Home health agencies and care providers should be identified so that the patient and the home-based caregivers have a resource for answering questions and handling difficulties.
   a. Patients with significant functional disabilities need special attention. The active support of family and friends is often essential to long-term care and rehabilitation. Planning should involve everyone who will participate in the patient's care.
   b. Home health nurses may be direct care providers, managers, and supervisors of paraprofessionals. Coordination of services is a key nursing role, and lack of coordination often means that the patient will do without necessary care.

Bibliography

Books

Burke M, and Walsh M (eds). *Gerontologic Nursing: Care of the Frail Elderly.* Philadelphia: Mosby–Year Book, 1992.

Calkins E, Ford A, and Katz P (eds). *Practice of Geriatrics.* 2nd ed. Philadelphia: WB Saunders, 1992.

Carpenito L. *Nursing Diagnosis: Application to Clinical Practice.* Philadelphia: JB Lippincott, 1993.

Evans J, and Williams T (eds). *Oxford Textbook of Geriatric Medicine.* New York: Oxford University Press, 1992.

Heckheimer E. *Health Promotion of the Elderly in the Community.* Philadelphia: WB Saunders, 1989.

Matteson MA, McConnell ES, and Linton AD. *Gerontological Nursing: Concepts and Practice.* 2nd ed. Philadelphia: WB Saunders, 1996.

Sparks S, and Taylor C. *Nursing Diagnosis Reference Manual: An Indispensable Guide to Better Patient Care.* Springhouse, PA: Springhouse Corporation, 1991.

U.S. Department of Health and Human Services, Public Health Service, Agency for Health Care Policy and Research. *Clinical Practice Guideline: Acute Pain Management: Operative of Medical Procedures and Trauma.* Rockville, MD: Department of Health and Human Services, 1992.

Chapters in Books and Journal Articles

Brown J, Lyon P, and Sellers T. Caring for family caregivers. *In* Volicer L, et al. (eds). *Clinical Management of Alzheimer's Disease.* Rockville, MD: Aspen Publishers, Inc, 1988, pp 29–42.

Duchene P, and Hinderer G. Rehabilitation for clients with disabling or chronic conditions. *In* Ignatavicius DD, and Bayne M (eds). *Medical-Surgical Nursing: A Nursing Process Approach.* Philadelphia: WB Saunders, 1991, pp 490–503.

Duchene P, and LeSage J. Hydration and nutrition. *In* Corr D, and Corr C (eds). *Nursing Care in an Aging Society.* New York: Springer, 1990, pp 92–113.

Folstein M, Folstein S, and McHugh P. Mini-mental state: A practical method for grading the cognitive state of patients for the clinician. *J Psychiatr Res* 12:189–198, 1975.

Lachs M, et al. A simple procedure for general screening for functional disability in elderly patients. *Ann Intern Med* 112(9):699–706, 1990.

Lamy P. Geriatric drug therapy. *Adv Fam Practice* 34(6):118–124, 1986.

McConnell E, and Matteson M. Psychosocial aging changes. *In* Matteson M, and McConnell E (eds). *Gerontological Nursing: Concepts and Practice.* Philadelphia: WB Saunders, 1988, pp 431–479.

Nokes K. Activity exercise pattern. *In* Ferri R (ed). *Care Planning for the Older Adult: Nursing Diagnosis in Long-Term Care.* Philadelphia: WB Saunders, 1994, pp 124–157.

Rheaume Y, et al. Education and training of interdisciplinary team members caring for Alzheimer's patients. *In* Volicer L, et al. (eds). *Clinical Management of Alzheimer's Disease.* Rockville, MD: Aspen Publishers, Inc, 1988, pp 201–224.

Rowe J, and Kahn R. Human aging: Usual and successful. *Science* 237(4811):143–149, 1987.

Saunders D. Pain and impending death. *In* Wall P, and Melzack R (eds). *Textbook of Pain.* New York: Churchill Livingstone, 1994, pp 472–478.

Spreadbury D. Lifestyles: Environmental factors and aging. *In* Christiansen J, and Grzybowski J (eds). *Biology of Aging.* Philadelphia: Mosby, 1993, pp 317–343.

Stone J, Chenitz W. An overview of gerontological nursing. *In* Chenitz W, Stone J, and Salisbury S (eds). *Clinical Gerontological Nursing: A Guide to Advanced Practice.* Philadelphia: WB Saunders, 1991, pp 3–13.

Yen PK. Nutrition—A vital sign. *Geriatr Nurs* 34(1):52–53, 1992.

Agencies and Resources

Alzheimer's Disease and Related
   Disorders Association, Inc.
70 East Lake Street
Chicago, IL 60601
(312) 335–8700
(800) 621–0379

American Association of Retired Persons
1909 K Street, N.W., 5th Floor
Washington, D.C. 20049
(202) 872–4700

American Cancer Society
4 West 35th Street
New York, NY 0001
(212) 736–3030

American Dental Association
211 East Chicago Avenue
Chicago, IL 60611

American Diabetes Association
1660 Duke Street
Alexandria, VA 22314
(800) 232–3472
(703) 549–1500

American Foundation for the Blind
Consumer Products Department
15 West 16th Street
New York, NY 10011

American Heart Association
7320 Greenville Avenue
Dallas, TX 75231
(214) 373–6300

American Lung Association
1740 Broadway
P.O. Box 596
New York, NY 10019
(212) 315–8700

American Speech-Language-Hearing
  Association
Department AP
10801 Rockville Pike
Rockville, MD 20852

Arthritis Foundation
1314 Spring Street
Atlanta, GA 30309

AT&T National Special Needs Center
20001 Route 46
Parsippany, NJ 07054

Fred Sammons, Inc. [Independence aids]
Box 32
Brookfield, IL 60513

General Mills, Inc.
Nutrition Department, Department 45
P.O. Box 1112
Minneapolis, MN 55440

Help for Incontinent People
Department RBC
P.O. Box 544
Union, SC 29379

National Association for the Deaf
814 Thayer Avenue
Silver Spring, MD 20910

National Institute on Aging
Building 31, Room 5C-35
9000 Rockville Pike
Bethesda, MD 20205
(301) 496–1752

Office on Smoking and Health
5600 Fishers Lane
Park Building, Room 1-10
Rockville, MD 20857
(301) 443–1690

Sex Information and Educational Council
Resources Center and Library
32 Washington Place
New York, NY 10011
(212) 673–3850

Shalik's Rehab Aids
Box 826
Miami, FL 33143

Caring for People with Medical-Surgical Disorders

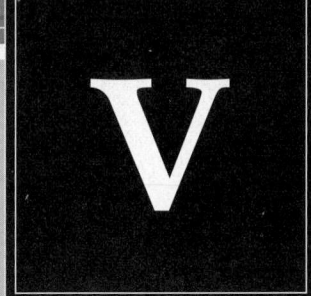

17
Caring for People with Cancer

■ DEFINITIONS

Cancer Terminology

1. **Cancer** is a group of diseases characterized by uncontrolled cellular growth with local tissue invasion and systemic metastasis. Cancer represents more than 100 types of malignant tumors that can occur in individuals of all ages, genders, races, and ethnic and socioeconomic groups. No one is exempt from the potential for developing a cancer.
2. A **benign tumor** is an abnormal growth that does not invade or destroy normal tissue and does not metastasize. Benign tumors are harmful only if they impinge on nerves or compress vital organs.
3. A **malignant tumor** is an abnormal cellular growth that invades the surrounding tissue, usually produces metastases, tends to recur after attempted removal, and causes death unless adequately treated. Malignant tumors, cancer, and neoplasms are synonymous terms.
4. **Metastasis** is the spread of malignant cells from a primary tumor to distant sites through the circulatory or lymphatic system.

Incidence, Mortality, and Survival Rates

1. Descriptive epidemiologic studies provide information to measure the magnitude of the cancer problem (Table 17–1).
2. Incidence, mortality, and survival rates provide data on how many people are ill, have died, or have been cured of cancer. Mortality and survival rates are useful in measuring treatment outcomes. Studies of incidence rates are correlated with various races, ages, and ethnic groups over sufficient time and can give important clues into possible causes of cancer. Incidence, mortality, and survival rates are also important in making decisions about health care policy and the allocation of health care dollars.
   a. On a national level, the cost of cancer is exorbitant when monies spent on cancer research and health care for people with cancer and the loss of productivity of these individuals are combined.
   b. The National Cancer Institute estimates overall costs of cancer to be $104 billion: $35 billion in direct costs, $12 billion in loss of productivity, and $57 billion in mortality cost.
3. Incidence rates

   a. Cancer affects millions of people around the world. It is expected to be the leading cause of death in the United States by the year 2000. It is 2nd only to accidents in the United States as a cause of premature death. In 1996, an estimated 1,359,000 people in the United States were newly diagnosed with cancer. The U.S. cancer incidence rate is 372.5 per 100,000 people. At the present rates, 1 in every 3 Americans will eventually develop cancer.
   b. The cancer incidence rate has been increasing steadily over the past 50 years. The incidence increase is attributed to an aging population and to increases in cigarette smoking.
   c. The most common cancers in 1996 by incidence are prostate (317,100), breast (184,300), lung (177,000), and colon or rectal (133,500). These 4 cancers account for more than 50 percent of the total cancer incidence (Fig. 17–1).
   d. Cancer incidence rates for some specific sites have changed over the past 50 years (Table 17–2).
      (1) The increase in lung cancer is attributed to the significant increase in smoking, especially by women.
      (2) A reduction in stomach cancer has not been explained satisfactorily. Studies correlating the worldwide distribution of the bacterium *Helicobacter pylori* (known to cause stomach ulcers) with the incidence of gastric cancer may provide the answer.
      (3) An increase in breast cancer since 1980 is thought to reflect earlier diagnosis of breast cancer through mammography.
      (4) Increases in lymphoma and brain tumors have not been explained.
      (5) A 10-fold increase of melanoma in Whites is attributed to increased recreational sun exposure.
      (6) Prostate cancer incidence has increased 50 percent between 1980 and 1990. Early diagnosis with prostatic-specific antigen (PSA) testing accounts for this apparent increase.
   e. Data for nationwide incidence rates are obtained from the Surveillance, Epidemiology and End Results (SEER) program, started at the National Cancer Institute in 1973. The SEER program collects incidence data from population-based cancer registries in 9 geographic areas of the United States that represent 9.6 percent of the total population.
4. Mortality rates
   a. In 1996, an estimated 554,000 people died of cancer. The mortality rate is 174 per 100,000 people.

Table 17–1. Terms Used in Reporting Cancer Statistics

Term	Definition
Incidence rate	The number of newly diagnosed cases of all cancers per standard unit of population during a specified period
Mortality rate	The number of cancer deaths per standard unit of population during a specified period
Age (sex, race)-specific rates	Incidence or mortality rates calculated to each variable: age specific, race specific, and so on
Age-adjusted rate	Incidence or mortality rates adjusted to reduce the effect of age distribution in a population. Allows for comparisons of populations not influenced by the age composition of the populations
Observed survival rate	Actual percentage of people with cancer still alive at some specified time after the diagnosis of cancer. Usually reported as a 5-year survival
Relative survival rate	Adjustment of the observed survival rate to remove the effect of causes of death other than cancer

b. Cancer deaths account for 20 percent of deaths in the United States, and cancer is 2nd only to heart disease as a cause of death.

c. The cancer mortality rate has been increasing since 1930 and has been attributed to the increase in cigarette smoking. If lung cancer deaths were excluded, the cancer mortality rate would have decreased 14 percent between 1950 and 1990.

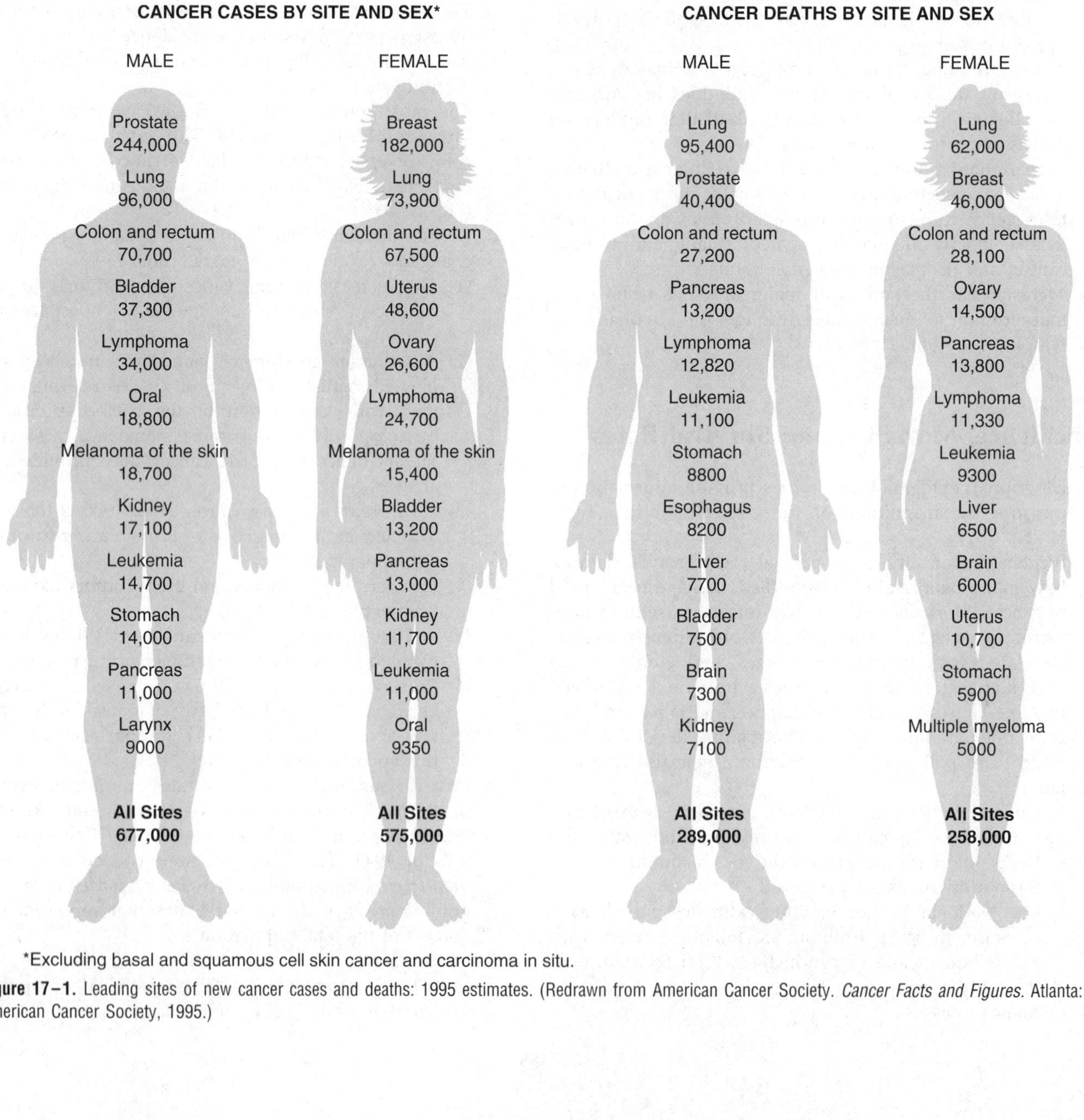

CANCER CASES BY SITE AND SEX*

MALE

Prostate	244,000
Lung	96,000
Colon and rectum	70,700
Bladder	37,300
Lymphoma	34,000
Oral	18,800
Melanoma of the skin	18,700
Kidney	17,100
Leukemia	14,700
Stomach	14,000
Pancreas	11,000
Larynx	9000

All Sites 677,000

FEMALE

Breast	182,000
Lung	73,900
Colon and rectum	67,500
Uterus	48,600
Ovary	26,600
Lymphoma	24,700
Melanoma of the skin	15,400
Bladder	13,200
Pancreas	13,000
Kidney	11,700
Leukemia	11,000
Oral	9350

All Sites 575,000

CANCER DEATHS BY SITE AND SEX

MALE

Lung	95,400
Prostate	40,400
Colon and rectum	27,200
Pancreas	13,200
Lymphoma	12,820
Leukemia	11,100
Stomach	8800
Esophagus	8200
Liver	7700
Bladder	7500
Brain	7300
Kidney	7100

All Sites 289,000

FEMALE

Lung	62,000
Breast	46,000
Colon and rectum	28,100
Ovary	14,500
Pancreas	13,800
Lymphoma	11,330
Leukemia	9300
Liver	6500
Brain	6000
Uterus	10,700
Stomach	5900
Multiple myeloma	5000

All Sites 258,000

*Excluding basal and squamous cell skin cancer and carcinoma in situ.

Figure 17–1. Leading sites of new cancer cases and deaths: 1995 estimates. (Redrawn from American Cancer Society. *Cancer Facts and Figures.* Atlanta: American Cancer Society, 1995.)

d. The 4 cancers causing the greatest number of deaths in 1996 are lung (158,700), colon-rectum (54,900), breast (44,300), and prostate (41,400). The lung cancer rate is almost 3 times greater than that of colon-rectum, the 2nd highest cancer site.

e. Mortality rates between 1973 and 1988 have decreased in children (38%) and for adults under the age of 55. Death rates have increased for people older than 65.

5. Survival rates

a. All people alive who have cancer or who have been treated for cancer are considered to be cancer survivors. Mullan, who coined the term "cancer survivor" described 3 seasons of survival: (1) diagnosis, (2) extended survival, and (3) permanent survival.

b. The observed 5-year survival rate for all cancers is 40 percent (i.e., 40% of people diagnosed with cancer will be alive after 5 years). The relative survival rate

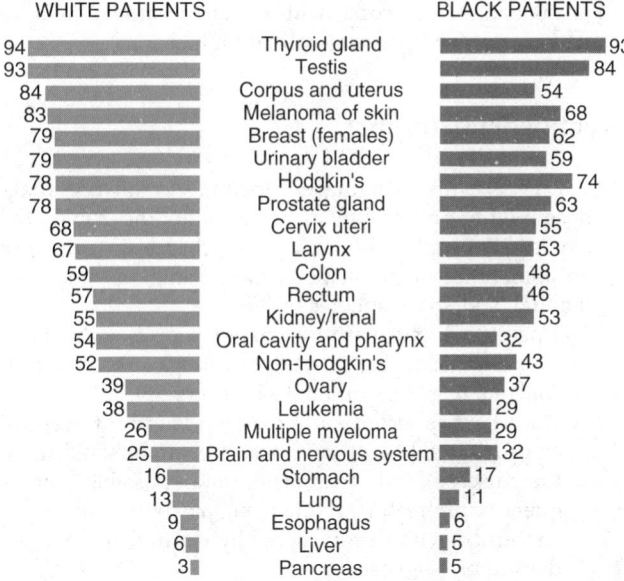

Figure 17–2. Five-year relative survival rates. SEER program, 1983–1988. (Redrawn from American Cancer Society. *Cancer Facts and Figures*. Atlanta: American Cancer Society, 1995.)

is 54 percent (i.e., if death from other causes is removed, 54% of people with cancer will be alive after 5 years).

c. Cancers with the highest survival rates are thyroid, testis, uterine corpus, and melanoma of the skin (Fig. 17–2).

d. Cancers with the poorest survival rates are pancreatic, liver, esophagus, and lung (see Fig. 17–2).

e. Changes in survival rates over time are influenced by improvement in early detection practices and treatment technologies.

> Many people with cancer equate a 5-year survival with cancer cure. Disease recurrence, however, varies with specific type of cancer. For example, testicular cancer rarely recurs after 2 years, whereas breast cancer can recur after 25 years.

■ THE IMPACT OF CANCER

Physical Impact

1. More than 100 types of malignant tumor are represented by the term "cancer." Cancer is an unique experience for each individual.

2. The physical effects can be as minimal as the excision of a small basal cell cancer of the skin, which leaves a minimal scar. At the other extreme, cancer treatment can be mutilating and disfiguring, with devastating changes in physical appearance and function.

3. Cancer treatment can be short or prolonged for years with consequent diminishing of function and quality of life.

Table 17–2. Cancer Sites Ranked by Percentage Change in Mortality and Incidence Rates Between 1973 and 1988

Cancer Site or Type	Percentage Change, 1973–1987	
	Mortality	*Incidence*
Greater than 15% decrease in mortality and incidence		
Hodgkin's disease	−49.5	−15.9
Cervix	−39.6	−36.4
Stomach	−29.4	−20.5
Uterus (endometrium)	−19.8	−26.1
Greater than 15% decrease in mortality but stable or increasing incidence		
Testis	−60.0	39.0
Rectum	−39.9	−3.3
Bladder	−22.7	12.3
Thyroid	−20.6	14.6
Oral cavity and pharynx	−16.2	−1.3
Greater than 15% increase in mortality with increasing incidence		
Lung	34.1	31.5
Melanoma	29.8	83.3
Multiple myeloma	23.6	10.5
Non-Hodgkin's lymphoma	21.7	50.9
Greater than 15% increase in incidence with smaller change in mortality		
Kidney	12.9	27.0
Brain and other nervous system	9.4	23.0
Prostate	7.2	45.9
Breast	2.2	24.2
Fairly stable mortality and incidence		
Esophagus	11.3	12.3
Ovary	−6.4	−6.8
Larynx	−6.0	0.5
Leukemia	−5.6	−10.2
Liver	−4.7	14.5
Pancreas	−2.0	−5.6
Colon	−1.6	10.4
All sites	5.4	14.6

Reprinted with permission from Henderson BE, Ross RK, and Pike MC. Toward the primary prevention of cancer. *Science* 254:1131–1138, 1991. Copyright 1991, American Association for the Advancement of Science.

4. For 50 percent of people with cancer, treatment will be unsuccessful, and survival will be limited.

Psychosocial Impact

1. Cancer is a life-changing experience. For anyone diagnosed with cancer, life is never quite the same. For almost all people with cancer, the diagnosis generates an abundance of problems encompassing the personal, familial, and social spheres of life.
2. The perceived and real problems of people with cancer can be emotional (e.g., negative feelings, uncertainties) or concrete (e.g., loss of job, lack of money).
   a. Uncertainties include an unknown length of survival or prognosis, lack of information or understanding of the disease and treatment, and possible consequences of treatment. Most people with cancer are concerned with death, especially during the first 100 days after diagnosis.
   b. Negative feelings or fear, dread, anxiety, depression, loneliness, shame, guilt, helplessness, hopelessness, powerlessness, anger, and hostility are common for most cancer patients.
   c. Threats to self-esteem depend on the basis of the person's self-esteem. If physical attractiveness is important, then alopecia will be more difficult to accept. Loss of work and the ability to achieve may be more devastating when accomplishments are the basis of self-esteem. Sexuality, or how one perceives oneself as a male or female, is threatened not only by physical problems related to sexual functioning but also by psychologic perceptions of attractiveness.
   d. Loss of control or the ability to manage or influence life's events can be severely limited by cancer. Loss of control can extend from daily living (e.g., inability to do a certain task) to survival.
3. The cancer site affects the type of symptoms the person with cancer experiences. The stage of illness at diagnosis determines the type of treatment and the trajectory of the illness.
4. The goals of treatment dictate the aggressiveness of treatment and the resulting sequelae. Patients undergoing curative regimens may experience body image changes due to radical surgical procedures or long-term effects of radiation therapy.
5. The phase of the cancer experience influences the perception of problems. The emotional issues change as the person goes through diagnosis, treatment, recurrence, or survival.
6. Personality characteristics also define the way the individual perceives problems and their significance and formulates a response. Optimistic people have better coping skills than those who are pessimistic.
7. The person's age and developmental stage influences problem perception. Young people building their careers and futures are more devastated by threatened survival than are older adults. Parents of young children are especially stressed during illness.
8. Cognitive functioning can affect the person's understanding and perspective of the disease and its implications.
9. Previous experiences with family or friends who have had cancer can influence how the individual will respond. Favorable experiences may enhance response, whereas experiences with family members who have had protracted illness with uncontrolled symptoms may have a negative effect.
10. A person's spiritual orientation may give meaning and value to the difficulties experienced.
11. The family structure and relationships as well as those with friends and community members profoundly influence the nature and scope of the person's difficulties. Whether the family is nuclear, extended, or involves significant others may determine the emotional support available to the person with cancer.
    a. The role changes can be significant if the person with cancer is the dominant breadwinner or source of emotional stability. Young adults who once again become dependent on family and friends after achieving independence can be frustrated at a perceived setback. Changes in role occur at least temporarily in almost all families of people with cancer.
    b. The developmental stage of the family influences the problems faced by people with cancer. When a parent with young children has cancer, then responsibility of child care is shifted to the other parent. Elderly people whose children have left home may be without adequate resources.
    c. Relationships and the communication patterns within the family are important. The stresses of illness on a family that may already be dysfunctional can be devastating.
    d. The financial resources of the family alter the magnitude of problems faced by people with cancer. The expenses of medical care added to loss of income may bankrupt a family. Use of savings may deprive the family of planned purchases and financial security. For the individual, the financial impact of cancer can be disastrous. Loss of income, limited health coverage, and the cost of prolonged treatment that may take years can drain all financial resources. If the person does not survive, then the family suffers not only personal loss but also financial depletion.

◼ RISK FACTORS FOR CANCER

Gender

1. For all cancer sites combined, the incidence rate is higher in males (442/100,000) than in females (338/100,000). Males have a higher incidence rate for almost every cancer common to both sexes.
2. The mortality rate is higher in males (228/100,000) than in females (140/100,000).
3. The 5-year survival rate is 46.7 percent for males and 57.0 percent for females.

Age

1. The risk of getting cancer is 10 times higher in people older than 65 than in those younger than 65. Long-term

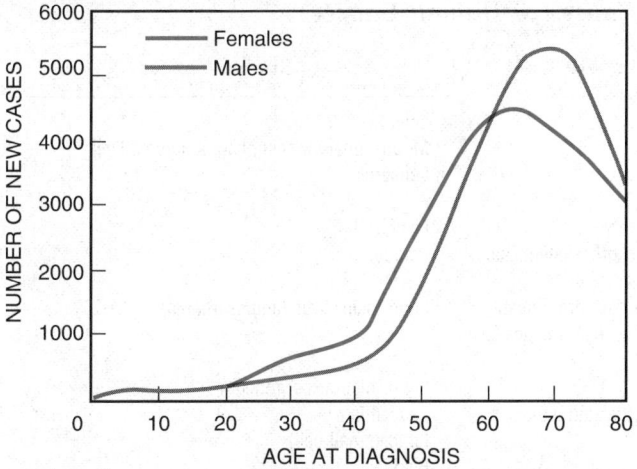

Figure 17–3. Cancer as a disease of the old. (From Kupchella C. *Dimensions of Cancer.* Belmont, CA: Wadsworth Publishing Co, 1987. Data from National Cancer Institute, SEER Program, Bethesda, MD.)

exposure to carcinogens and decreasing immunity with age are believed to explain this increase (Fig. 17–3).
2. The incidence rate is 2013 per 100,000 for those older than 65 and 192 per 100,000 for those younger than 65.
3. More than 50 percent of cancers occur in people older than 67.

Race

1. The incidence of cancer in Black Americans is 8 percent greater than that in White Americans.
2. The percentage of Blacks who survive cancer for more than 5 years (40 percent) is lower than the percentage for Whites (56 percent).

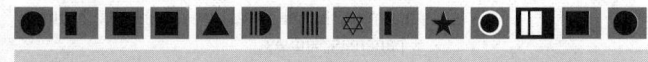

TRANSCULTURAL CONSIDERATIONS

More Blacks (439/100,000) than Whites (406/100,000) develop cancer. More Blacks (228/100,000) than Whites (170/100,000) die of cancer.

Heredity

1. Genetic mutations affecting growth and cell proliferation are the basis for cancer development. Although environmental agents cause genetic mutation in *somatic* cells, mutations in *germ* cell lines can be inherited through dominant or recessive patterns.
2. Cancer families are those in which at least 20 percent of the family members develop cancers at an earlier age than usual and often have multiple cancers. They have an increased incidence of cancer of the colon, breast, ovary, prostate, and uterus. Although cancer families

have been known for some time, the specific genetic defects in these people has only been recently determined.
3. Those individuals born with certain syndromes associated with abnormal chromosomes are at higher risk of developing certain cancers. People with Down syndrome have a 20-fold increase in risk for developing leukemia. Males with Kleinfelter's syndrome have a higher risk of breast cancer. The mechanisms for cancer development in these people are not well understood.
4. In certain people, a normal genetic constitution may make cancer risk higher. For example, fair-skinned people who lack protective pigmented layers are at higher risk of developing skin cancers.

Socioeconomic Status

1. For all cancer sites combined, the cancer incidence is higher in lower educational and income groups, regardless of race.
2. Dietary patterns, tobacco use, and lifestyle behaviors are believed to be influential factors.

Geographic Location

1. New England and the mid-Atlantic states have higher cancer death rates than the western and southwestern states.
2. Utah has the lowest cancer death rate (121/100,000); the District of Columbia has the highest (226/100,000).

Environmental Exposure

1. Air: Both indoor and outdoor air contain a significant number of pollutants. The cancer risk attributed to pollutants has not been defined (Table 17–3).
2. Water: Many potential carcinogens are found in water supplies. Studies have shown some evidence of increased risk of colon, rectum, lung, and urinary bladder cancer from chlorinated water (see Table 17–3). The cancer risk of contaminated ground water has not been determined. Ground waters supply 40 to 50 percent of the U.S. drinking water. Thirty percent of the 8000 sites of industrial waste disposal are above ground water supplies with a permeable soil. Only 40 of the 275 million metric tons of hazardous wastes generated each year are federally regulated.
3. Hazardous wastes: Limited studies have been done to determine the health risks associated with soil and water contamination by hazardous wastes.
   a. Environmental studies relate environmental exposures to cancer risk but are extremely difficult to conduct.
   b. The latency period between environmental exposure and cancer development can be decades long.
   c. Many other variables such as lifestyle, smoking habits, and dietary intake must be excluded.
   d. Few people live in the same location for an extended period of time. Changes occur in any given environ-

Table 17–3. Environmental Causes of Human Cancer

Agent	Type of Exposure	Site of Cancer
Aflatoxin	Contaminated foodstuffs	Liver
Alcoholic beverages	Drinking	Mouth, pharynx, esophagus, larynx, liver
Alkylating agents (melphalan, cyclophosphamide, chlorambucil, semustine)	Medication	Leukemia
Androgen-anabolic steroids	Medication	Liver
Aromatic amines (benzidine, 2-naphthylamine, 4-aminobiphenyl)	Manufacturing of dyes and other chemicals	Bladder
Arsenic (inorganic)	Mining and smelting of certain ores, pesticide manufacturing and use, medication, drinking water	Lung, skin, liver (angiosarcoma)
Asbestos	Manufacturing and use	Lung, pleura, peritoneum
Benzene	Leather, petroleum, and other industries	Leukemia
Bis(chloromethyl)ether	Manufacturing	Lung (small cell)
Chlornaphazine	Medication	Bladder
Chromium compounds	Manufacturing	Lung
Estrogens	Medication	
Synthetic (diethylstilbestrol)		Vagina, cervix (adenocarcinoma)
Conjugated (Premarin)		Endometrium
Steroid contraceptives		Liver, cervix
Immunosuppressants (azathioprine, cyclosporine)	Medication	Non-Hodgkin's lymphoma, skin (squamous carcinoma and melanoma), soft tissue tumors (including Kaposi's sarcoma)
Ionizing radiation	Atomic bomb explosions, treatment and diagnosis, radium dial painting, uranium and metal mining	Most sites
Isopropyl alcohol production	Manufacturing by strong acid process	Nasal sinuses
Leather industry	Manufacturing and repair (boot and shoe)	Nasal sinuses, bladder
Mustard gas	Manufacturing	Lung, larynx, nasal sinuses
Nickel dust	Refining	Lung, nasal sinuses
Parasites	Infection	
Schistosoma haematobium		Bladder (squamous carcinoma)
Clonorchis sinensis		Liver (cholangiocarcinoma)
Pesticides	Application	Non-Hodgkin's lymphoma, lung
Phenacetin-containing analgesics	Medication	Renal pelvis
Polycystic hydrocarbons	Coal carbonization products and some mineral oils	Lung, skin (squamous carcinoma)
Tobacco chews, including betel nut	Snuff dipping and chewing of tobacco, betel, lime	Mouth
Tobacco smoke	Smoking, especially cigarettes	Lung, larynx, mouth, pharynx, esophagus, bladder, pancreas, kidney
Ultraviolet radiation	Sunlight	Skin (including melanoma), lip
Viruses	Infection	
Epstein-Barr virus		Burkitt lymphoma, nasopharyngeal carcinoma
Hepatitis B and C virus		Hepatocellular carcinoma
Human immunodeficiency virus		Kaposi's sarcoma, non-Hodgkin's lymphoma
Human papillomavirus		Cervix, other anogenital tumors
Human T-lymphotropic virus type I		T-cell leukemia and lymphoma
Vinyl chloride	Manufacturing of polyvinyl chloride	Liver (angiosarcoma)
Wood dusts	Furniture manufacturing (hardwood)	Nasal sinuses (adenocarcinoma)

From DeVita JT, Hellman S, and Rosenberg S. *Cancer: Principles and Practice of Oncology.* 4th ed. Philadelphia: JB Lippincott, 1993, p 171.

ment over time as different industries are introduced or as regulations change the kinds of exposures.

e. Good studies are extensive, expensive, and require very long follow-up.

Tobacco

1. Overwhelming evidence supports tobacco use as a cancer-causing agent. Clinical evidence dates back to

---

Scientists at the National Cancer Institute (NCI) and the American Cancer Society attribute the increased incidence in cancer over the past 40 years largely to increases in tobacco smoking and focus their research monies on diagnosis and treatment. Other scientists challenge this assumption, noting that exposure to industrial carcinogens in the air and water has been inadequately studied. Only 1 percent of the total NCI budget is allocated to occupational cancer and cancer prevention.

1761, when John Hill first made the association between snuff use and cancer of the nose. More than 57,000 epidemiologic and animal studies have confirmed the association of lung cancer and cigarette smoking.

2. Tobacco exposure occurs through smoking cigarettes and pipes, use of smokeless tobacco (snuff and chewing tobacco), and exposure to passive smoke.

3. More than 30 percent of cancer deaths are related to tobacco.

4. Smoking: Eighty-five percent of lung cancer is estimated to be caused by cigarette smoking. Smoking is directly related to cancers of the larynx, oral cavity (lip, tongue, salivary glands, mouth and pharynx), and esophagus. There is a synergistic effect between alcohol and tobacco in these cancers. Smoking significantly increases the risk of developing cancer of the bladder and pancreas. Approximately 40 percent of bladder and kidney cancers and 30 percent of the pancreatic cancers are smoking related. Smoking also increases the risk for developing cancers of the liver, anus, penis, and vulva.

    a. International lung cancer mortality rates correlate with cigarette use in the population. Religious groups (e.g., Mormons and Seventh-day Adventists) that prohibit smoking have much lower cancer rates.

    b. A dose-response relationship exists between the number of cigarettes smoked per day, years of smoking, degree of inhalation, and nicotine content of cigarettes and the risk of cancer.

    c. Smokers of 1 or more packs of cigarettes per day have 20 times the risk of nonsmokers.

    d. Nonsmokers exposed to smoke from burning tobacco and exhaled smoke have a modest increase in lung cancer risk.

5. Smokeless tobacco: Chewing tobacco and snuff are known causes of oral cancer and increase the user's risk 4-fold. Studies of snuff users in the rural southern United States and chewing tobacco users in India provide epidemiologic evidence of the cancer-causing potential of chewing tobacco. An alarming number of young American males have taken up chewing tobacco as an alternative to smoking.

Dietary Factors

1. Dietary factors are estimated to cause 35 percent of all cancers. Dietary factors considered most important in cancer causation are fat intake, fiber, and obesity.

2. The evidence supporting dietary factors in cancer risk is not as conclusive as that for tobacco. Epidemiologic and animal studies do not always correlate.

3. Cohort and case studies are limited in dietary studies by the difficulty in obtaining accurate diet histories, especially from early in life. Recall of eating habits 20 to 30 years before the current study is difficult, as is separating other variables within a study group.

4. Fat: International variations in fat consumption per capita correlate directly with increases of incidence in colon-rectal, breast, and prostate cancers. These cancers are prevalent in developed countries and not in underdeveloped countries. Case studies and cohort studies do not always, however, correlate with international studies. A

study of 90,000 nurses, for example, showed no correlation between breast cancer and dietary fat.

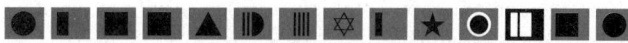

TRANSCULTURAL CONSIDERATIONS

Large differences exist in the worldwide distribution of certain cancers. For example, the incidence of stomach cancer is highest in Japan and lowest in the United States. Over time, people who emigrate to other countries develop the cancer most prevalent in their new country, presumably as a result of dietary and lifestyle changes. The changes in incidence occur too quickly to be attributable to genetic alterations.

5. Obesity: Obesity has been established as a positive risk factor for endometrial cancer and for breast cancer in postmenopausal women.

6. Lack of fiber

    a. The lowest rates of colon cancer are found in Africa and Asia, where high-fiber diets are consumed. The highest rates are found in Western societies, where more refined carbohydrates and less fiber are eaten.

    b. Immigrants from countries of low colon cancer incidence to countries of high colon cancer incidence tend to develop the incidence of the new country as they adopt new dietary patterns.

    c. Seventh-day Adventists, who are lactovegetarians, have significantly lower colon cancer rates.

7. Specific nutrients

    a. Lower consumption of cruciferous vegetables and fresh fruit has been shown to be a predisposing factor to cancer.

    b. Lack of micronutrients (e.g., vitamins C and E, selenium, and calcium) may also be important factors.

    c. No substantital proof is available for coffee as a cause of bladder or pancreatic cancers.

    d. Artificial sweeteners may increase the risk of bladder cancer but only minimally.

Dietary Recommendations to Reduce Cancer Risk

1. Maintain a desirable weight.
2. Eat a varied diet.
3. Include a variety of both vegetables and fruit in the daily diet.
4. Eat more high-fiber foods such as whole-grain cereals, legumes, vegetables, and fruits.
5. Cut down on total fat intake.
6. Limit consumption of alcoholic beverages.
7. Limit consumption of salt-cured, smoked, or nitrite-preserved food.

Medications

1. Hormones: Some daughters of women given synthetic estrogens during pregnancy developed vaginal and uter-

ine cancers during adolescence and early adulthood. Women taking estrogens for menopausal symptoms double their risk for endometrial cancer. Current hormone replacement therapy combines estrogens with progesterone, thereby reducing this risk.
2. Cytotoxic drugs: Certain chemotherapeutic drugs (melphalan, cyclophosphamide, chlorambucil, semustine, busulfan, and others) increase the risk of developing acute nonlymphocytic leukemia in patients treated with these drugs.

Alcohol

1. Alcohol consumption has a synergistic effect with smoking in causing cancers of the oral cavity, pharynx, larynx, and esophagus.
2. Recently, alcohol consumption has been linked with breast and rectal cancer, but a causal relationship has not been definitely established.

Occupation

1. The history of occupational exposure and cancer began in 1775 when Percival Pott, a London surgeon, observed an increased incidence of scrotal cancers among chimney sweeps.
2. Estimates of cancers attributed to occupational exposure range from 4 to 25 percent.
3. Epidemiologic and experimental studies have determined increased site-specific cancer risks with occupational chemicals (see Table 17–3).

Sexual Behaviors

1. Human papillomaviruses have been established as the cause of cervical cancer, establishing it as a sexually transmitted disease.
2. Starting sexual activity before the age of 20 and having multiple sexual partners increase the risk for cervical cancer.

Precancerous Lesions

1. Some pathologic changes have the potential to develop into a cancer.
2. Lobular carcinoma in situ of the breast will become invasive and develop into a frank carcinoma in 35 percent of women.
3. All 3 types of adenomatous polyps of the colon can undergo malignant transformation. Five percent of tubilar adenomas, 22 percent of tubulovillous adenomas, and 40 percent of villous adenomas become malignant.
4. Leukoplakia, a white patch, appearing in the oral cavity is considered precancerous when severe cellular atypia is present. Erythroplakia, red granular patches of mucosa, are more often precancerous lesions of the oral cavity.

■ ETIOLOGY OF CANCER

Radiation

1. Radiation has been recognized as a cause of cancer since the turn of the century, when the 1st associations were made between skin cancer and sunlight. At this same time, scientists were able to produce cancers in animals by radiation exposure.
2. Radiation-induced cancers cause approximately 3 percent of all cancers.
3. Exposure to radiation exists on 3 levels: (1) ionizing or high-frequency radiation associated with medical equipment, occupational exposures (miners), or nuclear warfare; (2) lower-frequency ultraviolet radiation; and (3) very low frequency radiation generated by electrical appliances, electrical transformers, and power lines.
   a. Ionizing radiation
      (1) Many experiences confirming radiation as a carcinogen occurred in the 1930s, before the long-term effects of radiation were recognized. Workers who painted luminous watch dials with radium-containing paints and used their lips to point their paint brushes inadvertently ingested minute amounts of paint. Years later, a significant number of these workers developed bone cancers. Radiologists and dentists using radiographic equipment without protective shielding developed skin cancers and leukemia. People treated with radiation for benign conditions such as ankylosing spondylitis subsequently developed leukemias.
      (2) Survivors of the atomic bomb explosions in Hiroshima and Nagasaki have a higher incidence of leukemias, thyroid, breast, lung, and other cancers.
      (3) Uranium miners have an increased incidence of lung cancer.
   b. Ultraviolet radiation: Skin cancers are more common on exposed skin areas in the Sunbelt region and among "sun worshippers." Fair-skinned people are more susceptible to skin cancers.
   c. Low-frequency radiation: Studies relating exposure to low levels of radiation from electrical transformers, wires, and appliances have been inconclusive to date.

Viruses

1. Until recently it was difficult to confirm viruses as a cause of human cancers. Now, however, it is established that certain forms of human cancers are virally induced.
2. Two classes of viruses can cause cancer in humans: retroviruses and DNA viruses.
3. Human T-cell leukemia virus type 1 (HTLV-1): A retrovirus that produces a rare but virulent leukemia, HTLV-1 is endemic to Japan, parts of Africa, the Caribbean, northern South America, and the southeastern United States. HTLV-1 is the only virus associated with leukemia and appears to be transmitted through sexual activity, breast-feeding, and blood products. Leukemia devel-

ops 20 to 30 years later in 1 percent of infected individuals.

4. Papillomavirus: Of the 60 types of papillomaviruses, several have been found in uterine cancers and have been established as the causative agent. Cigarette smoking, oral contraceptives, and other immune and hormonal factors are involved in producing cervical cancer.

5. Epstein-Barr virus: This virus is strongly associated with Burkitt's lymphoma, a B-cell lymphoma found in African children. Although Epstein-Barr virus is widespread in human populations, it is believed that malaria, which is endemic to Africa, is a cofactor in the production of the lymphoma. The Epstein-Barr virus is found in nasopharyngeal cancer, endemic to areas of southern China, and is thought to be a cofactor in development of those cancers.

6. Hepatitis B virus: Previous infection with hepatitis B is believed to be a cofactor in the development of hepatic cancers. Although rare in the United States, more than 1.2 million cases of liver cancer occur yearly throughout the world.

LEGAL AND ETHICAL CONSIDERATIONS

Because human experimentation is unethical, the cause of cancer must be based on indirect evidence. Three basic sources of information provide evidence for cancer causation: analytic epidemiologic studies that determine associations between agents and their cancer-producing potential; animal experiments; and clinical observations. Whenever evidence from these sources supports the same cause for a specific cancer, the scientific community accepts the cause, even though it has never been confirmed through human experimentation.

Chemical Agents, Drugs, and Hormones

1. Chemicals comprise the largest component of environmental carcinogenic agents. This category includes chemicals found in the air, water, ground, smoke, food, and alcohol, as well as a variety of chemicals used in industrial manufacturing.

2. Estrogen is one of the main hormones associated with cancer. Women using estrogen alone for postmenopausal hormone replacement can develop endometrial and breast cancer.

3. Some chemotherapeutic agents are believed to cause secondary malignancies in previously treated individuals. The alkylating agents in particular are felt to be carcinogenic.

Host Susceptibility

1. Not all people exposed to the same carcinogens develop cancer. Constitutional and genetic factors within an individual promote or hinder cancer development.

2. A person's genetic inheritance may predispose the person to a disease that tends to develop into a cancer (e.g., familial polyposis to colon cancer) or to cancer itself (e.g., cancer families).

3. People whose immune systems are suppressed by drugs (e.g., transplant patients) or by disease (e.g., acquired immunodeficiency syndrome [AIDS]) have a 3-fold increased risk of developing cancers, particularly lymphomas.

4. Metabolism of some carcinogens is genetically determined and may enhance the development of cancers in some individuals.

◼ PATHOPHYSIOLOGY OF CANCER

Carcinogenesis

1. Genetic basis
   a. Normal cell growth, differentiation, and division
      (1) The human body emerges from a single cell in a highly ordered sequence. Germinal cells give rise to specialized stem cells, which become more differentiated with each successive duplication into a variety of specialized cells, organs, and tissues.
      (2) Cell division occurs in a cycle, which is divided into 5 phases (Fig. 17-4).

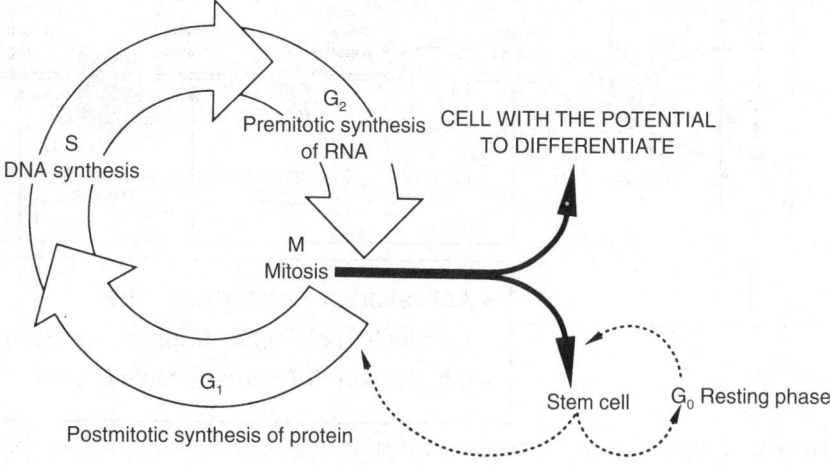

Figure 17-4. Cell cycle. (Redrawn from Maxwell MB, and Maher KE. Chemotherapy-induced myelosuppression. *Semin Oncol Nurs* 8:113-123, 1992.)

(3) Cells in the body are divided into 3 groups based on their proliferation.
- Cells that are constantly renewing are those that must keep up with cell loss (e.g., bone marrow, skin, hair follicles, and mucous membranes). Renewing tissues come from stem cells that operate under various signals that indicate a need for rapid proliferation. Stem cells must renew themselves as well as generate a large family of descendants.
- Cells that renew slowly but proliferate in response to injury (e.g., liver, lung, kidney, endocrine glands, and vascular epithelium)
- Cells that do not divide once they are differentiated (e.g., muscle, brain, bone and cartilage)

(3) The decision for a cell to divide is based on a complex series of signals that come from its environment and from other cells. Signals are transmitted to the cell nucleus, which responds to the signals.

b. Abnormal cell appearance and growth, differing from the normal cell cycle (see Fig. 17–4)
(1) The nucleus of cancer cells is disproportionately larger and shows abnormal mitotic configurations.
(2) Abnormal cells are pleomorphic, with a variety of sizes and shapes.
(3) The cell's surface does not contain normal antigens.

c. Oncogenes
(1) Proto-oncogenes are normal cellular genes found in all species. Proto-oncogenes control normal growth and proliferation of cells.
(2) Oncogenes are mutated proto-oncogenes that produce abnormal growth factors, causing the signals for the cell to proliferate, to remain on, resulting in excessive duplication and abnormal cell growth.
(3) Oncogenes were discovered in retroviruses that were able to transform normal culture cells into cancer cells. Oncogenes are called dominant because the effects occur when only 1 of the 2 inherited proto-oncogenes is damaged.

d. Tumor-suppressor genes are normal cellular genes that suppress the activity of growth-promoting genes. They oppose the activity of proto-oncogenes and are often called antioncogenes. Tumor-suppressor genes are recessive genes (i.e., both copies of the gene must be lost or mutated for the effects to be seen.).

2. Chemical carcinogenesis
a. Tumor formation is a multistep process identified through animal studies over the past 50 years (Fig. 17–5).
b. *Initiation,* the 1st step in chemical carcinogenesis, is an irreversible process in which a permanent change is produced in a cell by a chemical carcinogen. The process is thought to be short and can occur spontaneously. The initiated cell is not a tumor cell and cannot be differentiated from normal cells.
(1) Chemical carcinogens are electrophilic compounds that attach to the electron-rich sites on DNA nucleic acids.
(2) Cells damaged by carcinogens may suffer lethal damage or may be repaired by DNA repair mechanisms. Damaged cells that have not been repaired and undergo replication, however, pass the defect to the daughter cell. This cell is then initiated, and the process is irreversible. In animal models, carcinogenesis is associated with proliferating cells.
c. *Promotion,* the 2nd stage of carcinogenesis, is a process in which the initiated cell undergoes a series of changes under the stimulus of an agent or agents called **promoters.** The process is reversible, at least until the 1st autonomous tumor cell is formed.

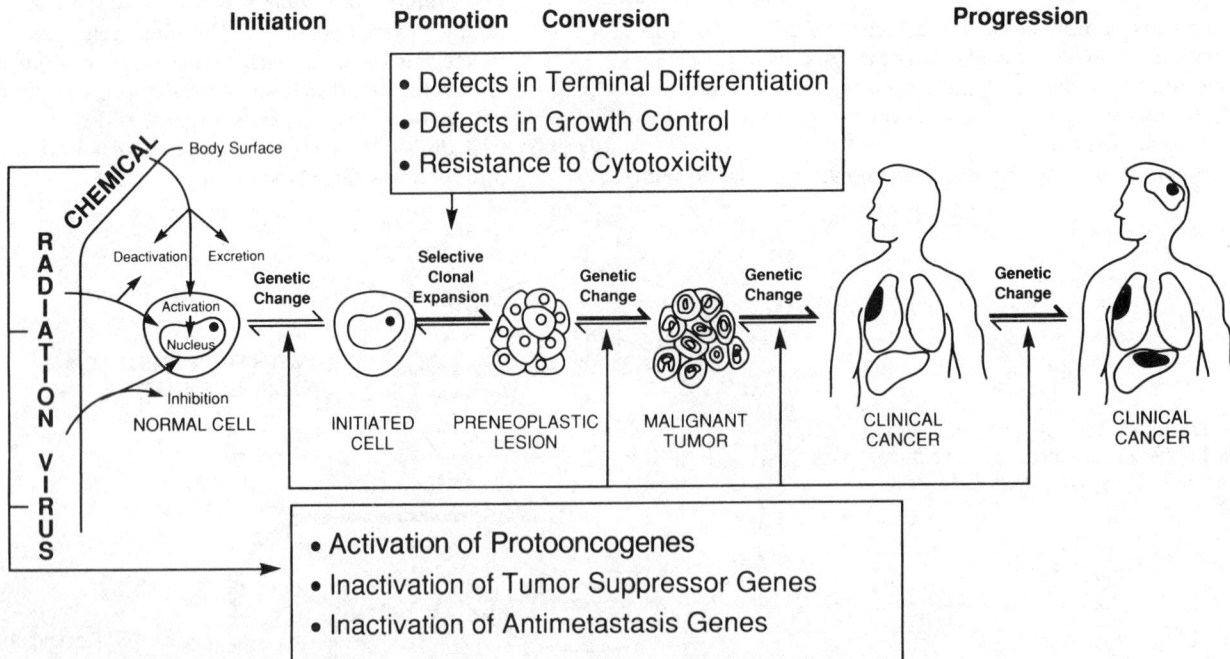

Figure 17–5. Multistep model of carcinogenesis. (From Holleb AI, Fink DJ, Murphy GP [eds]. *American Cancer Society Textbook of Clinical Oncology.* Atlanta: American Cancer Society, 1991.)

---

d. *Tumor progression*, the 3rd stage of cancer development, has been clinically known but only recently studied in animal models. It is an irreversible stage of tumor development in which cellular damage can be detected as the tumor accumulates more malignant characteristics.

3. Radiation carcinogenesis
   a. Carcinogenesis caused by radiation is not as well understood as chemical carcinogenesis. Two modes of damage are believed possible: (1) radiation energy causes direct damage to DNA molecules, or (2) the energy transmitted causes molecules to lose electrons and become electrophilic, thereby acting as a chemical carcinogen.
   b. The stages of promotion and progression in radiation carcinogenesis are not well understood.
4. Viral carcinogenesis
   a. Viruses are believed to cause cancer by direct DNA mutations or by inserting genetic material into the cell, causing a mutation.
   b. The process of viral carcinogenesis is not clear. Apparently DNA viruses need a cofactor in the process (e.g., malarial infection in Burkitt's lymphoma or hepatitis B infection in hepatocellular carcinoma).
5. Role of immunity in carcinogenesis
   a. The role of the immune system in carcinogenesis has not been defined clearly. Some evidence supports the ability of the body to defend against cancer cells. Tumors produce specific antigens as well as tumor-associated antigens.
   b. Many immune cells have cytotoxic capability (e.g., T lymphocytes, natural killer cells, and macrophages). Lymphocyte infiltration is seen at the edge of many tumors. Individuals who are immunosuppressed have a 3-fold increased risk of developing certain cancers, particularly lymphomas and cancers of the skin, lips, vulva, and perineum.

Tumor Biology

1. Tumors are composed of proliferating cells, (i.e., neoplastic cells), stromal cells (i.e., blood vessels and connective tissue), and other cells, such as lymphocytes and macrophages.
2. Tumor growth varies among types of tumors as well as among individual tumors of the same type. Tumor growth is a function of cell growth being greater than cell loss. (Normal cells have a steady state of growth and loss.) Growth depends on 3 factors:
   a. *The growth fraction* or the number of cells that are dividing. As the tumor enlarges, a smaller percentage of cells are in the replicating pool. Most cells in a tumor are not actively proliferating.
   b. *The rate of proliferation.* The cell cycle is similar for many tumors (i.e., 2.0–4.5 hr). Tumor cells do not divide more rapidly than their normal counterparts and often may divide less frequently.
   c. *Tumor cell loss.* Many tumor cells are lost through necrosis and shedding.
3. Tumor-doubling time
   a. The time required for a tumor to double in size may range from 1 month to 1 year.
   b. A tumor measuring 1 cm will have 10^9 or 1 billion cells. This size is reached after approximately 30 doublings. In 10 more doublings, the tumor size will be 10^{12} or 1 kg. This size is 1000 times greater than the 1 cm size (Fig. 17–6).

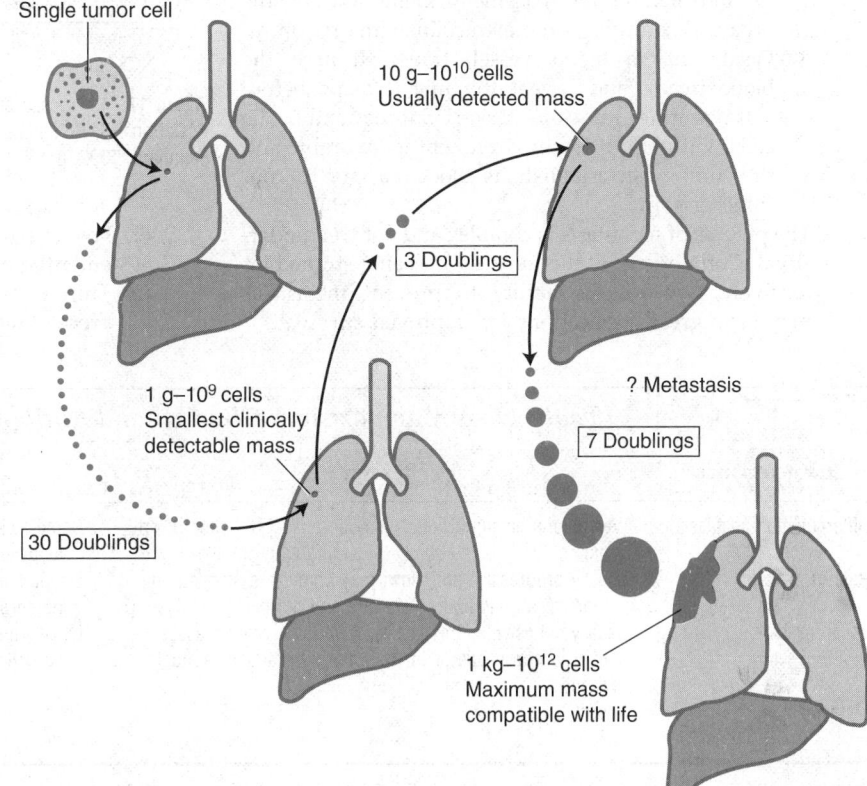

Figure 17–6. Biology of tumor growth. The left panel depicts minimal estimates of tumor cell doublings that precede the formation of a clinically detectable tumor mass. It is evident that by the time a solid tumor is detected, it has already completed a major portion of its life cycle, as measured by cell doublings. The right panel illustrates clonal evolution of tumors and generation of tumor cell heterogeneity. New subclones arise from the descendants of the original transformed cell, and with progressive growth, the tumor mass becomes enriched for those variants that are more adept at evading host defenses and that are likely to be more aggressive. (Adapted from Tannock IF, and Hill RP [eds]. *The Basic Science of Oncology.* 2nd ed. New York: McGraw-Hill, 1992, p 156. Copyright 1992, The McGraw-Hill Companies.)

Single tumor cell

10 g–10^{10} cells Usually detected mass

3 Doublings

1 g–10^9 cells Smallest clinically detectable mass

? Metastasis

7 Doublings

30 Doublings

1 kg–10^{12} cells Maximum mass compatible with life

4. Tumor blood supply
  a. Tumors secrete angiogenic growth factors capable of inducing formation of blood vessels by which the tumor can support itself.
  b. A tumor cannot enlarge more than 1 to 2 mm without developing a blood supply. As tumors enlarge and some cells outdistance their blood supply, necrosis occurs.
5. Tumor heterogeneity
  a. Although a malignant tumor begins with a transformed cell, subsequent mutations produce many subclones, which possess different characteristics (e.g., invasion, metastasis).
  b. Heterogeneity is well established by the time a tumor is clinically detectable (Fig. 17–6).
6. Tumor invasion and metastasis
  a. The capability to invade surrounding tissue and to establish independent tumors in distant sites is the hallmark of malignancy. Most cancers metastasize; a few do not.
  b. Tumors spread by seeding cells within a body cavity (e.g., ovarian cancer with peritoneal metastases), by spreading through lymphatic channels, or by hematogenous mechanisms (i.e., through the bloodstream). Although some tumors follow the natural drainage pathways in spreading, many do not.
    (1) Breast cancers tend to metastasize to the axillary lymph nodes; metastatic colon cancers develop in the liver, the first capillary drainage bed encountered. Many metastases occur in the lung, which is a capillary drainage bed for all body organs. Brain tumors do not metastasize outside the central nervous system.
    (2) Figure 17–7 illustrates the process of hematogenous metastasis. The malignant cell must adhere to and invade the basement membrane of the organ, pass through the extracellular matrix, intravasate into a blood vessel, travel through the bloodstream, and repeat the first 2 steps before extravasating into the tissue. Subsequently, the cells will grow if the environment is favorable and the tumor can establish its blood supply to continue growth.
  c. The process of metastasis is complex and not well understood. Components of this process are being studied intensively, because the ability to prevent metastasis may have great implications for improved survival.

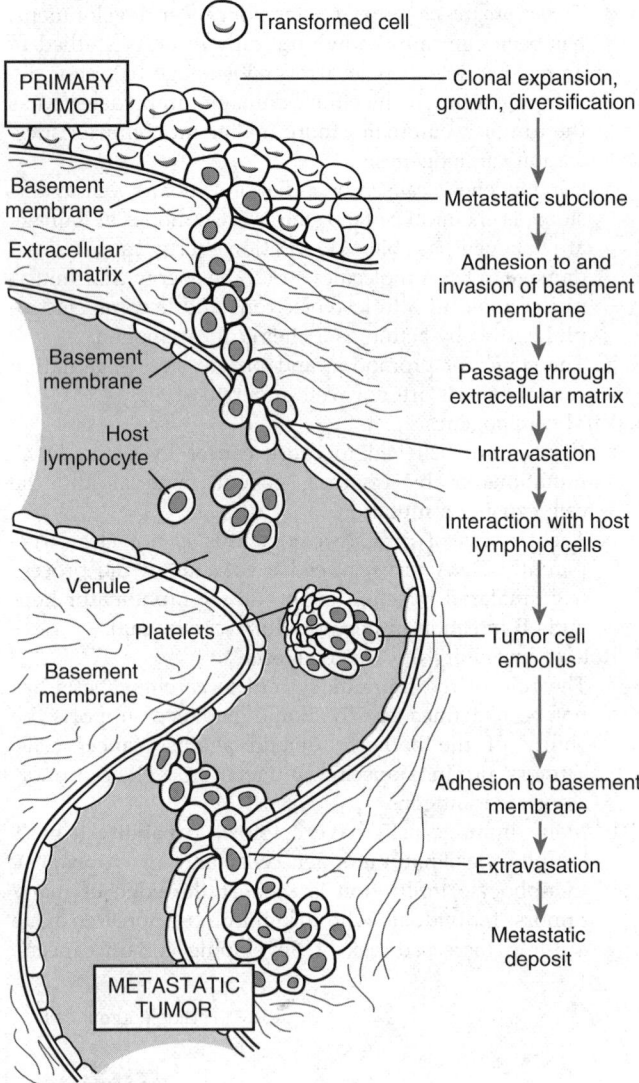

Figure 17–7. Process of hematogenous metastasis. (Redrawn from Kumar V, Cotran RS, Robbins SL. *Basic Pathology.* 5th ed. Philadelphia: WB Saunders, 1992, p 196.)

(1) For every 10,000 cells shed from a tumor that enter the bloodstream, it is believed only 1 survives.
(2) Tumor cells produce a variety of enzymes to break down membranes.

Table 17–4. Comparison of Benign and Malignant Tumors		
Characteristics	**Benign**	**Malignant**
Differentiation-anaplasia	Well-differentiated; structure may be typical of tissue of origin	Some lack of differentiation with anaplasia; structure is often atypical
Rate of growth	Usually progressive and slow; may come to a standstill or regress; mitotic figures are rare and normal	Erratic and may be slow to rapid; mitotic figures may be numerous and abnormal
Local invasion	Usually cohesive and expansile, well-demarcated masses that do not invade or infiltrate the surrounding normal tissues	Locally invasive, infiltrating the surrounding normal tissues; sometimes may seem cohesive and expansile
Metastasis	Absent	Frequently present; the larger and less differentiated the primary, the more likely are metastases

From Kumar V, Cotran RS, and Robbins SL. *Basic Pathology.* 5th ed. Philadelphia: WB Saunders, 1992, p 180.

(3) The nm 23 (nonmetastatic) gene has been identified in some human tumors. In studying breast cancers, individuals with high levels of nm 23 had better survival rates and less metastasis, whereas those with low or absent nm 23 levels had metastasis and poorer survival. How this gene functions remains unknown.

7. Differentiating benign from malignant tumors
   a. Tumors are classified as benign or malignant based on the cell differentiation, rate of growth, local invasion, and metastasis (Table 17–4).
   b. Cell differentiation represents the degree to which the parenchymal tumor cell resembles the normal cell of origin. Benign tumor cells resemble the normal cell of origin. Malignant cells resemble the normal cell and are designated as well differentiated; those that bear little if any resemblance to the normal cell are termed undifferentiated or anaplastic. Intermediate forms of cell differentiation are termed moderately well differentiated or poorly differentiated. The level of differentiation is based on the following criteria:
      (1) Pleomorphism, or variation in cell size and shape
      (2) An abnormal nucleus-to-cytoplasm ratio in which the nuclei are larger than normal cells
      (3) Bizarre-shaped nuclei with a large number of mitoses

Table 17–5. Nomenclature of Tumors

Tissue of Origin	Benign	Malignant
I. Composed of 1 Parenchymal Cell Type		
A. Tumors of mesenchymal origin		SARCOMAS
1. Connective tissue and derivatives	Fibroma	Fibrosarcoma
	Lipoma	Liposarcoma
	Chondroma	Chondrosarcoma
	Osteoma	Osteogenic sarcoma
2. Endothelial and related tissues		
Blood vessels	Hemangioma	Angiosarcoma
Lymph vessels	Lymphangioma	Lymphangiosarcoma
Synovium		Synovium (synoviosarcoma)
Mesothelium		Mesothelioma
Brain coverings	Meningioma	Invasive meningioma
3. Blood cells and related cells		
Hematopoietic cells		Leukemias
Lymphoid tissue		Malignant lymphomas
4. Muscle		
Smooth	Leiomyoma	Leiomyosarcoma
Striated	Rhabdomyoma	Rhabdomyosarcoma
B. Tumors of epithelial origin		CARCINOMAS
1. Stratified squamous	Squamous cell papilloma	Squamous cell or epidermoid carcinoma
2. Basal cells of skin or adnexa		Basal cell carcinoma
3. Epithelial lining		
Glands or ducts	Adenoma	Adenocarcinoma
	Papilloma	Papillary carcinoma
	Cystadenoma	Cystadenocarcinoma
4. Respiratory passages		Bronchogenic carcinoma
		Bronchial "adenoma"
5. Neuroectoderm	Nevus	Melanoma (melanocarcinoma)
6. Renal epithelium	Renal tubular adenoma	Renal cell carcinoma
7. Liver cells	Liver cell adenoma	Hepatocellular carcinoma
8. Urinary tract epithelium (transitional)	Transitional cell papilloma	Transitional cell carcinoma
9. Placental epithelium	Hydatidiform mole	Choriocarcinoma
10. Testicular epithelium (germ cells)		Seminoma
		Embryonal carcinoma
II. More than 1 Neoplastic Cell Type—Mixed Tumors—Usually Derived from 1 Germ Layer		
1. Salivary glands	Pleomorphic adenoma (mixed tumor of salivary origin)	Malignant mixed tumor of salivary gland origin
		Wilms' tumor
2. Renal anlage		
III. More Than 1 Neoplastic Cell Type Derived from More Than 1 Germ Layer—Teratogenous		
1. Totipotential cells in gonads or in embryonic rests	Mature teratoma, dermoid cyst	Immature teratoma, teratocarcinoma

From Kumar V, Cotran RS, and Robbins SL. *Basic Pathology.* 5th ed. Philadelphia: WB Saunders, 1992, p 174.

(4) Lack of architectural patterns of orientation
   c. The rate of growth of benign tumors is generally slow, whereas malignant tumor growth is erratic, from slow to very rapid. Removal of benign tumors is necessary only if they obstruct or impinge on vital structures or nerves or if they are cosmetically unacceptable.
   d. Invasiveness is a major criterion for malignancy. Benign tumors are well-demarcated masses. Malignant tumors invade the surrounding tissue.
   e. Metastasis is one of the hallmarks of malignancy. Benign tumors do not metastasize; malignant tumors do. Generally, undifferentiated or anaplastic tumors and large tumors tend to metastasize.

Tumor Nomenclature

1. **Neoplasm** refers to an abnormal growth of tissue. It is synonymous with the word "tumor" and can refer to either a benign or a malignant tumor.
   a. Most tumors exist in a benign and a malignant form and can arise from any cell type (Table 17–5). Nomenclature is inconsistent. Generally, benign tumors are named by adding the suffix "oma" to the cell type. For example, a fibroma is a benign tumor of fibrous connective tissue. Some of the exceptions are lymphoma, seminoma, melanoma, and mesothelioma, which all refer to malignant tumors. Some tumors are eponyms (e.g., Wilms' tumor and Ewings' sarcomas). The organ or origin is often included (e.g., bile duct carcinoma).
   b. If the cell type is unknown, the designation is poorly differentiated carcinoma or poorly differentiated sarcoma.
2. Carcinomas: Tumors arising from epithelial cells are termed carcinomas. The type of cell is part of the name (e.g., basal cell carcinoma or adenocarcinoma).
3. Sarcomas: Tumors arising from mesenchymal cells have the suffix "sarcoma" added to the cell type (e.g., fibrosarcoma).
4. Leukemias: Leukemias are derived from hematopoietic cells. They are distinguished as acute or chronic and myelogenous or lymphoid (e.g., acute myelogenous leukemia).
5. Lymphomas
   a. Lymphomas arise from lymphoid tissue. The classification of lymphomas undergoes constant revision as new technology allows further differentiation of cell features.
   b. Lymphomas are divided into 2 basic groups: Hodgkins' lymphoma, which is 1 specific disease entity, and non-Hodgkin's lymphoma, which comprises the remaining lymphomas. These may be differentiated as B-cell lymphomas or T-cell lymphomas. Four major groups of lymphomas are currently used:
      (1) Follicular small-cleaved cell lymphoma
      (2) Follicular mixed small-cleaved and large-cell lymphoma
      (3) Diffuse large-cell lymphoma
      (4) Immunoblastic lymphoma

■ ASSESSING PEOPLE FOR CANCER

Key Symptoms and Their Pathophysiologic Bases

1. Cancer symptoms most often are determined by the size and the location of the tumor.
2. Palpable masses located near the body surface are readily detected. Tumors in the breast, extremities, and thyroid are often seen or felt by the patient. Skin cancers are visible as either a new growth or a change in a mole or a wart. Most tumors of the oral cavity can be felt or seen.
3. Bleeding or discharge occurs when tumors have friable surfaces and external egress. Common tumors that can manifest themselves by bleeding are cancers of the lung, colon, uterus, stomach, bladder, and kidneys.
4. Many symptoms related to cancer are produced when a tumor impinges on a structure, partially or totally obstructs a lumen, or interferes with the normal function of the organ.
   a. Brain tumors manifest themselves with specific symptoms caused by pressure on discrete brain areas or by obstruction of the flow of cerebrospinal fluid and production of increased intracranial pressure.
   b. Pancreatic tumors, located near the sphincter of Oddi, causes jaundice by obstructing the common bile duct.
   c. Tumors within the colon cause changes in the caliber of stool or cause constipation and diarrhea, or both.
   d. Inability to swallow food occurs when tumors in the esophagus reach a sufficient size to obstruct the lumen.
   e. Hoarseness can be produced when tumor interferes with the vocal cords or when a thoracic tumor impinges on the recurrent laryngeal nerve and indirectly affects the vocal cord function.
   f. Infection and fever are produced when an overwhelming number of abnormal white blood cells in leukemia reduce the ability of normal cells to provide immunity and resistance.
   g. Pain can be produced when tumor invades nerves or when obstruction is caused. Pain is generally a manifestation of advanced cancer.
5. Fatigue, weight loss, and anorexia are systemic symptoms related to cancer and are seen most often in advanced disease states.
6. Many cancers produce no symptoms and are found inadvertently during routine tests or other procedures.

Cancer's 7 Warning Signals

1. *C*hange in bowel or bladder habits
2. *A* sore that does not heal
3. *U*nusual bleeding or discharge
4. *T*hickening or lump in breast or elsewhere
5. *I*ndigestion or difficulty in swallowing
6. *O*bvious change in a mole or wart
7. *N*agging cough or hoarseness

Table 17–6. Symptom Confusion in Older People		
Symptom or Sign	**Possible Malignancy**	**Aging "Explanation"**
Increase in skin pigment	Melanoma, squamous cell	"Age spots"
Rectal bleeding	Colon/rectum	Hemorrhoids
Constipation	Rectal	"Old age"
Dyspnea	Lung	Getting old, out of shape
Decrease in urinary stream	Prostate	"Dribbling"—benign prostatic hypertrophy
Breast contour change	Breast	"Normal" atrophy, fibrosis
Fatigue	Metastatic or other	Loss of energy due to "aging"
Bone pain	Metastatic or other	Arthritis: "aches and pains of aging"

Reproduced with permission from Hazzard WR, et al. *Principles of Geriatric Medicare and Gerontology.* 2nd ed. New York: McGraw-Hill Information Services, 1992, p 78. Copyright 1992, The McGraw-Hill Companies.

7. The 7 warning signs of cancer publicized by the American Cancer Society alert the public to cancer symptoms. Although many people delay seeking medical attention because of denial, many are unaware of the significance of their symptoms. Older people frequently attribute symptoms to the aging process (Table 17–6).

Health History

1. The standard medical history is used when obtaining information from a symptomatic individual. Attention is given to risk factors that correlate with symptoms and a family history of cancer.
2. Nurses have great opportunities to assess cancer risk and teach early detection to all patients. Early detection of cancer provides optimal treatment and survival. Attention to health habits (e.g., smoking or sunbathing) can provide opportunities to teach cancer prevention. Information and instruction in breast, testicular, and skin self-examination; warning signs of cancer; and recommended screening tests can ultimately save lives.

Physical Examination

1. The standard medical examination provides evaluation for cancer.
2. Attention is given to any palpable masses, hepatomegaly, splenomegaly, lymphadenopathy, and skin lesions.

Special Diagnostic Studies

1. Laboratory Tests
   a. No specific blood test is available to detect cancer. Routine studies (e.g., complete blood count and blood chemistry) provide clues in diagnosis. Anemia can be a result of bleeding from a tumor; leukocytosis or leukopenia may indicate a hematologic malignancy. Elevation of liver enzymes may indicate hepatic involvement.
   b. Tumor markers are antigens, hormones, enzymes, metabolites, oncogenes, and oncogene products secreted by tumors. These substances can be measured in tissue or body fluids. Available tumor markers can be used for screening, diagnosing, and staging and for monitoring response to treatment. No marker is available as a general screening for cancer (Table 17–7). Most markers are used as supportive data in diagnosing cancer or in monitoring the patient's response to treatment. The value of a tumor marker depends on its sensitivity and specificity.
      (1) Sensitivity is the marker's ability to detect cancer in someone who has it. Many markers can be positive in conditions other than cancer, thereby reducing the sensitivity of the test.
      (2) Specificity is the marker's ability to identify people without cancer. If individuals without cancer test positive, the test loses its value.

NURSE ADVISORY

The diagnostic period is one of great anxiety and uncertainty. Anxious patients need simple explanations of procedures and clear directions for test preparation. Informed patients are better able to cope with testing procedures. Delays are very difficult to endure while waiting for a diagnosis. Facilitating efficient test scheduling and result reporting and allowing patients to express their anxieties reduce tension and provide emotional support.

2. Imaging studies: general principles
   a. The patient's presenting symptoms, physical examination results, and presumed location of the tumor direct the choice of imaging studies. Studies can determine size and location of tumors but not their nature.
   b. Imaging studies (radiographs, nuclide scans, ultrasound) are performed to locate a mass for biopsy, to determine extent of disease, to provide a baseline before treatment, or to determine a response to treatment.
   c. All imaging studies use some form of energy (e.g.,

Table 17–7. Selected Tumor Markers

Tumor Marker	Exemplary Malignant Neoplasms	Commonly Associated Nonneoplastic Diseases
Hormones		
Human chorionic gonadotropin (HCG)	Gestational trophoblastic disease, gonadal germ cell tumors (testis)	Pregnancy
Calcitonin	Medullary cancer of the thyroid	
Catecholamines and metabolites	Pheochromocytoma	
Oncofetal Antigens		
Alpha-fetoprotein (AFP)	Hepatocellular carcinoma, gonadal germ cell tumors (especially endodermal sinus tumor)	Cirrhosis, toxic liver injury, hepatitis
Carcinoembryonic antigen (CEA)	Adenocarcinomas of the colon, pancreas, stomach, lung, breast, ovary	Pancreatitis, inflammatory bowel disease, hepatitis, cirrhosis, tobacco abuse
Isoenzymes		
Prostatic acid phosphatase (PAP)	Adenocarcioma of the prostate	Prostatitis; nodular prostatic hyperplasia
Neuron-specific enolase	Small-cell carcinoma of the lung; neuroblastoma	
Specific Proteins		
Prostate specific antigen (PSA)	Adenocarcinoma of the prostate	Nodular prostatic hyperplasia; prostatitis
Immunoglobulin (monoclonal)	Multiple myeloma	Monoclonal gammopathy of unknown significance
CA 125	Epithelial ovarian neoplasms	Menstruation, pregnancy, peritonitis
CA 19-9	Adenocarcinoma of the pancreas or colon	Pancreatitis; ulcerative colitis

From Holleb AI, Fink OJ, and Murphy JP (eds). *American Cancer Society Textbook of Clinical Oncology.* Atlanta: The American Cancer Society, 1991, p 22.

x-ray, sound waves) to create an image on film. Most studies require a contrast medium to enhance images.

   d. All have limited resolution, and masses smaller than a given size will not be detected. For example, most computed tomography (CT) scans cannot detect masses smaller than 1 cm.

   e. Patient preparation

     (1) Studies without contrast usually do not require preparation. Patient preparation for contrast studies is institution specific.

     (2) Optimal preparation of the person with cancer enhances the efficiency of the diagnostic process.

     (3) Sensitivity or allergy to contrast materials should be determined well in advance of the examination so that patients can be premedicated to prevent reactions.

3. Types of imaging studies

   a. Radiograph without contrast

     (1) Chest radiograph

      • This is a 2-dimensional view of a 3-dimensional subject. Two views are taken: an anteroposterior view and a lateral view. Air in the lung provides contrast for the standard chest radiograph.

      • Chest radiographs can reveal tumors of the lung and pleura: pleural and pericardial effusion; peritracheal, hilar, and mediastinal lymph nodes; and rib lesions (Fig. 17–8).

     (2) Skeletal radiographs

      • Skeletal radiographs are usually done to confirm suspicious bone lesions seen on bone scan. The density of the bone provides good contrast, but bone lesions are not usually evident until 30 to 50 percent of the mineral content is lost. There-

fore, a negative result on a bone radiograph does not exclude the presence of a tumor.

      • Skeletal radiographs can demonstrate osteoblastic or osteolytic lesions.

     (3) Mammogram

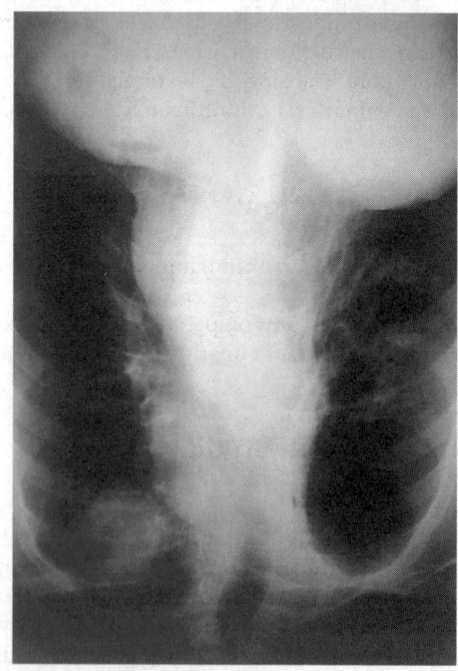

Figure 17–8. Chest radiograph demonstrating a large upper left lobe mass. (Courtesy of Loyola University Medical Center, Maywood, IL.)

- Mammograms are flat films of the breast taken in 2 views: a cranial-caudal view in which the person is sitting and the breast is placed on a block and a lateral view in which the person is standing. The breast is compressed between 2 plastic plates to flatten the tissue to provide better imaging.
- Masses, cysts, distortion of the parenchyma, and calcifications can be seen. Differentiation between benign and malignant calcifications is made of the basis of their distribution, size, and shape. Biopsies can be performed on masses that are suspicious for malignancy if the mass is palpable. Nonpalpable masses can be localized. A localization procedure involves the radiologist's insertion of a dye or a guide wire into the area of calcification. The person is then taken to the operating room where the suspicious lesion is removed. The tissue is radiographed to be certain that the suspected calcification was removed in the biopsy specimen (Fig. 17–9). Ultrasound is often done to differentiate cysts from solid masses seen on mammograms.

b. Radiographs with contrast
  (1) Upper gastrointestinal contrast studies (UGI)
   - A swallowed barium solution provides contrast to outline the esophagus, stomach, and duodenum. Additional serial films can be taken every 30 minutes to demonstrate filling of the small bowel.
   - Upper gastrointestinal studies show abnormalities in the normal anatomic pattern, either by the presence of a mass within the lumen or by extrinsic compression.

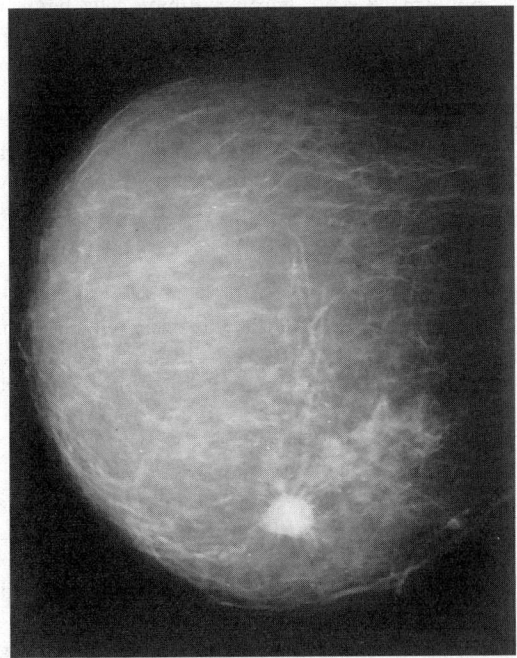

Figure 17–9. Mammogram with a 2-cm stellate mass in the right lateral breast on the cranial caudal view with superimposed benign calcifications. (Courtesy of Loyola University Medical Center, Maywood, IL.)

  (2) Barium enema (BE)
   - Insertion of barium solution through the rectum with spot films taken at intervals as the colon fills. Air can be added during the procedure to improve the contrast.
   - A barium enema can show masses or abnormalities within the colon or lesions causing external compression.
  (3) Intravenous pyelogram (IVP)
   - Intravenous injection of a radiopaque contrast medium outlining the kidneys, ureters, and bladder as the dye passes through them.
   - Intravenous pyelograms can show intrinsic masses and external compression, which compromise the ureters.
  (4) Arteriography
   - Injection of a dye into the arterial system with serial radiographs allowing the visualization of specific arteries.
   - Arteriography is useful to detect hepatic and renal tumors, which often give a typical blush appearance. The procedure is most often used preoperatively in renal or hepatic resections to determine the patient's unique vasculature.
  (5) Lymphangiography
   - Contrast material injected into the lymphatic vessels of the feet. Radiographs are taken 24 hours after injection. The procedure outlines the lymphatic drainage system in the lower extremities and abdomen.
   - Lymphangiography is useful to detect any obstruction, node enlargement, or obliteration of the lymphatic vessels.

NURSE ADVISORY

People experiencing pain should receive enough analgesics to cover them through any diagnostic procedures before they leave the nursing unit.

c. Computed tomography
  (1) These scans combine x-ray tomograms with a computer. As the x-ray beam passes through a tissue, the attenuation (absorption) by each type of tissue is recorded by detectors and read into the computer, which calculates the attenuation coefficient for each tissue and generates the information in the form of an image or digital readout. Intravenous contrast outlines blood vessels, and oral contrast outlines the gastrointestinal tract in a CT scan of the abdomen.
  (2) The CT scans can detect masses greater than 1 cm. The procedure is especially useful for detecting tumors of the liver, pancreas, kidney, pelvis, retroperitoneum, soft tissue, prostate, abdomen, and pelvic lymph nodes.
d. Magnetic resonance imaging (MRI)
  (1) This procedure combines the use of radiofrequency pulses and a powerful magnetic field to

create cross-sectional views of the area. Intravenous paramagnetic contrast agents can be used.

    (2) Magnetic resonance imaging provides optimal imaging of brain, spinal cord, head and neck, and muscle tissue. It has replaced many invasive procedures (e.g., myelogram and pneumoencephalogram) previously used in central nervous system disorders. People with any ferromagnetic implants, pacemakers, pumps, or surgical clips cannot be imaged.

  e. Radionuclide scans (nuclear medicine)

    (1) General concepts

- Nuclear medicine scans are based on the uptake of specific radionuclides by specific organs. The procedure uses a radionuclide (a radioactive isotope) that has been tagged with a chemical compound that has affinity for a specific body tissue. Following injection, the radionuclide is selectively taken up by the tissue and emits radiation from that tissue. A scanner, counter, or gamma camera is passed over the area and converts the radiation emitted into a visual image.

- Radionuclide scans produce images measuring physiologic activity. Radiation exposure from radionuclide scans is minimal. Images created are either positive (hot spots), if the lesion picks up the compound, or negative (cold spots), if the lesion does not pick up the compound.

    (2) Bone scans

- Technetium tagged with phosphorus as a radionuclide is used. Technetium is taken up in greater concentrations in areas of increased bony repair or blood flow. Bone scans are extremely sensitive but not specific. Degenerative, inflammatory, and healing lesions will be demonstrated as well as tumors. Bone uptake is slow. Generally, scanning is done 3 hours after injection of the radionuclide (Fig. 17–10).

- Bone scans are especially useful in staging cancer and demonstrating bony metastasis. Skeletal radiographs are required to confirm the nature of any lesion seen on the bony scan.

    (3) Liver scans

- Technetium 99m sulfur colloid is used as the radionuclide. It is phagocytosed by the Kupffer cell of the reticuloendothelial system and uniformly distributed throughout the liver and spleen. Diseased areas that have no Kupffer's cells show no uptake.

- Liver scans are useful in detecting lesions larger than 2 cm, but they cannot determine the nature of the defects (e.g., tumor, cysts, abscesses, or congenital defects). Computed tomography scanning has largely replaced liver scans in detecting liver metastases.

    (4) Gallium scan

- Gallium Ga 67 citrate is carried in the blood by plasma transferrin and concentrated by cell lysosome. It is taken up by certain tumors.

- Gallium scans are useful in detecting tumors of the lung and breast, lymphoma, and melanoma as well as determining the extent of the disease.

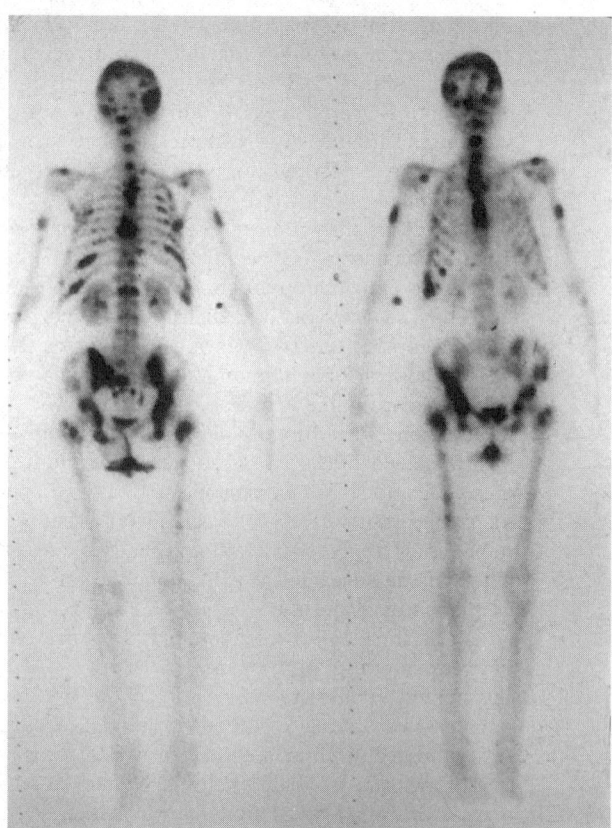

Figure 17–10. Bone scan demonstrating multiple metastases scattered throughout the bony skeleton in a patient with known breast cancer, indicating extensive spread of disease into the bones. (Courtesy of Loyola University Medical Center, Maywood, IL.)

  f. Positron emission tomography (PET)

    (1) These scans measure the function of normal and abnormal tissue. Because tumor cells have higher rates of glycolysis, using a radiopharmaceutical that traces glucose metabolism will identify malignant tissue.

    (2) Positron emission tomography scanning has demonstrated improved detection of a variety of tumors. Radiotracers used in the scan, however, must be produced in a cyclotron and used within a few hours, limiting the facilities available to perform them.

  g. Ultrasound

    (1) High-frequency sound waves (above the limits of hearing) are reflected by different densities of tissue and recorded on an imaging screen. Ultrasound is useful in detecting abdominal, retroperitoneal, and pelvic masses.

    (2) Ultrasound is used endoscopically to determine tumor depth and invasion in gastric, esophageal, and rectal tumors. It is utilized intraoperatively to detect liver metastases before hepatic resections. Transrectal ultrasound is used to guide prostatic needle biopsies.

4. Endoscopy

  a. General principles

    (1) Provides direct visualization of the internal surfaces of a hollow organ or body cavity by inser-

tion of a flexible lighted hollow tube (endoscope). Video cameras reproduce the image on film. Forceps and brushes can be inserted to obtain biopsies.

(2) Endoscopic procedures provide important visual information of the mass and the opportunity to obtain a biopsy during the same procedure.

(3) Local anesthesia and conscious sedation provide sufficient analgesia for all endoscopic procedures except for laparoscopy, thoracoscopy, and mediastinoscopy, which require general anesthesia and inpatient observation.

b. Gastrointestinal tests

(1) Esophagoscopy, gastroscopy, and duodenoscopy allow all parts of the stomach and duodenum to be visualized. Masses can be observed with 95 percent accuracy; the complication rate of perforation is 0.1 percent.

(2) Endoscopic retrograde cholangiopancreatography combines endoscopy and cannulization of the common bile duct and pancreatic duct. After the endoscope is advanced to the duodenum, the ducts are identified and cannulated. A radiocontrast material is inserted. Fluoroscopy provides visibility of the ducts. Serial films are taken of any obstructions or abnormalities. Brushing samples for cytology can be taken during the procedure.

(3) Proctoscopy allows visualization of the colon up to 25 cm, using a flexible or rigid tube.

(4) Colonoscopy provides visualization of the entire colon from rectum to cecum.

(5) Laparoscopy shows the interior of the abdominal cavity through the insertion of a scope through an incision in the abdominal wall. A pneumoperitoneum is created to improve visibility. Peritoneal, hepatic, ovarian, and pelvic masses can be seen.

c. Respiratory tests

(1) Bronchoscopy provides visualization of the larynx and bronchial tree using either a rigid or a flexible bronchoscope. Biopsies can be taken of masses within the bronchi.

(2) Thoracoscopy is accomplished by insertion of an endoscope into the pleural space through a small incision made through the ribs. It allows removal of fluid for cytologic study or biopsy of abnormal lung or pleural tissue.

(3) Mediastinoscopy provides direct visualization of all areas of the superior mediastinum through the insertion of the endoscope into a small incision made over the sternum. Biopsies can be performed on mediastinal lymph nodes to determine whether lung tumors are resectable.

d. Genitourinary tests

(1) Cystoscopy provides visibility of the internal surfaces of the bladder. Biopsy specimens and brushings can be obtained during the procedure.

(2) Colposcopy provides visibility of the cervix and vagina through the magnification of these structures.

5. Cytology and biopsy

a. Cytology

(1) Tumor cell specimens can be obtained from body fluids (ascites, pleural, or pericardial effusions), body secretions (urine or sputum), scrapings or brushings from tissue surfaces (cervix, endometrium, bronchus, or any tumor), or cells obtained by fine-needle aspiration biopsies.

(2) The Papanicolaou test is a cytologic examination of cells scraped from the surface of the uterine cervix. Dysplasia and premalignant changes can be readily identified. The ease of this examination and its widespread use has reduced the death rate from cervical cancer by 70 percent in the past 40 years.

(3) In a fine-needle aspiration biopsy, tumor cells are withdrawn from the tumor mass with a 21-gauge needle and syringe. This procedure is useful for obtaining cells from palpable lesions of the breast and thyroid and, with CT or ultrasound guidance, for obtaining specimens from pancreatic, liver, prostate, and lung tumors.

(4) Cytologic study can establish a diagnosis and avoid a surgical procedure. A negative result on biopsy, however, does not rule out malignancy, as misplaced or inadequate sampling of the tissue may have occurred.

(5) Because the cytology specimen contains cells and not tissue, the invasion or architectural distortion of the cells cannot be determined.

(6) Cytology results are reported as normal, atypical benign, atypical suspicious, probably malignant, malignant, and unsatisfactory.

b. Biopsy

(1) Core needle biopsy uses specially designed needles that have a larger bore than those used in fine-needle biopsy to obtain a tissue sample. The tissue sample is taken from within the body area that will be excised if surgical removal is required. Core biopsies are useful in palpable breast masses, bone marrow sampling, and liver biopsies.

(2) An incisional biopsy takes a sample of tissue with a punch biopsy or scalpel. It can be used during endoscopic procedures or in large soft tissue masses in which the diagnosis must be confirmed before surgical treatment is considered.

(3) An excisional biopsy removes all the tumor mass surgically. It is used for small skin lesions, subcutaneous lesions, and breast tumors. If the surgical specimen margins have no tumor cells, then no further treatment may be necessary.

◼ CANCER DIAGNOSIS, STAGING, GRADING, AND PROGNOSIS

Medical Diagnosis

1. The diagnosis of cancer is made on the microscopic examination of malignant cells from tumor tissue. The source of the tissue sample is determined by the location and size of the tumor, the clinical status of the person with cancer, and the proposed method of treatment.

2. Pathologists have a crucial role in establishing the diagnosis of cancer. They determine the malignant nature of the tumor, the organ and cell subtype from which it arose, and the invasiveness, or extent of the tumor within the sample. Establishing a diagnosis can be difficult. The pathologist may send slides to other experts to obtain a 2nd opinion.

a. Some tumors are so anaplastic that a true source cannot be identified. Approximately 10 percent of people with cancer have an unknown primary tumor.

b. Some tumors may appear histologically malignant but may behave biologically benign and vice versa.

c. Other studies may be done to gain additional information about the tumor.

(1) Histologic staining. Special stains detect the presence of granules, mucin, and other cell products that further define the characteristics of the tumor cell.

(2) Electron microscopy. The high power of the electron microscope can reveal the cell ultrastructure and the presence of specific subcellular structures that will give information concerning the cell origin. Electron microscopy cannot determine whether the cell is malignant.

(3) Immunohistologic staining. Monoclonal antibodies are used to detect the presence of epithelial markers and hormone, estrogen, and progesterone receptors.

(4) Flow cytometry studies. The nuclear DNA content is measured. Diploid refers to normal DNA content, whereas aneuploid refers to nuclear disorganization. The S phase fractionation refers to the number of cells in the S phase, which measures the proliferative capacity of the tumor.

(5) Molecular genetic studies. These detect gene sequences, oncogenes, and tumor suppressor genes.

Staging, Grading, and Prognosis

1. **Staging** determines the extent of the disease. Decisions regarding the curability and appropriate treatment for the person with cancer are based on this evaluation.

a. In addition to the pathologic findings and the clinical evaluation, other tests (e.g., scans and radiographs) are performed to stage the disease. The staging workup chosen is based on the natural history of a particular tumor. Staging for breast cancer may include a bone scan because bone is a common place of metastasis, whereas a surgical laparotomy is often required to determine the extent of Hodgkin's disease.

b. Staging systems have evolved to communicate precise information about tumors as well as to classify and compare groups of patients.

c. The American Joint Committee on Cancer (AJCC) and the International Union contre le Cancer (UICC) have developed similar staging systems based on tumor, regional lymph nodes, and metastasis (TNM). Stages are numeric from I to IV. Stage IV is the most advanced and includes distant metastasis. Each tumor type has its individual staging criteria following the TNM system. The staging criteria for bone cancers is summarized in Table 17–8.

d. Tumors are so varied that no 1 system suffices. The AJCC system is adapted to specific tumor types. Hematologic malignancies, which are disseminated diseases, and brain tumors, which have no lymph node involvement, cannot be staged with the TNM system. Some staging systems used before the development of the TNM system are still used. Among these are Duke's classification for colon cancer, Clark's system for melanomas, and the Ann Arbor system for Hodgkin's disease.

Table 17–8. Staging of Tumors: Bone Cancer

	Abbreviation	Explanation
Primary Tumor (T)	TX	Primary tumor cannot be assessed
	T0	No evidence of primary tumor
	T1	Tumor confined within the cortex
	T2	Tumor invades beyond the cortex
Lymph Node (N)	NX	Regional lymph nodes cannot be assessed
	N0	No regional lymph nodes metastasis
	N1	Regional lymph node metastasis
Distant Metastasis (M)	MX	Presence of distant metastasis cannot be assessed
	M0	No distant metastasis
	M1	Distant metastasis
Histopathologic Grade (G)	GX	Grade cannot be assessed
	G1	Well differentiated
	G2	Moderately differentiated
	G3	Poorly differentiated
	G4	Undifferentiated

Modified from American Joint Committee on Cancer. *Manual for Staging of Cancer.* Philadelphia: JB Lippincott, 1992.

2. Grading
   a. The pathologist determines the aggressiveness of the tumor on the basis of cell differentiation and the number of mitoses.
   b. Grades ranging from I to IV are assigned to the tumor. Grade IV is the most anaplastic and aggressive.
   c. Grading *may* but does not always have prognostic significance.
3. Prognosis: Some people with cancer prefer not to know their prognosis. Oncologists generally wait until the person with cancer indicates a readiness to discuss prognosis before specifying the probability of survival.

Psychosocial Considerations for Cancer Patients

1. Psychosocial assessment must be ongoing and based on observed statements and behavior of individuals. Interviews with open-ended statements promote expression of problems, which is often difficult.
   a. Shock, disbelief, and anxiety are common emotions experienced with the diagnosis of cancer. Anxiety decreases perception. Instructions for the person with cancer must be simple, reinforced, and provided in writing.
   b. Most people are concerned with the fear of death during the first 100 days after diagnosis. Establishing a trusting relationship with the person with cancer and the family members provides emotional support during the very stressful period of diagnosis.
   c. Guilt can be a predominant emotion, if the person believes that lifestyle habits (e.g., smoking) are the cause of the cancer or if the person has delayed seeking treatment.
   d. Abandonment by friends or family can be threatening to the individual. Referral to community agencies that may be helpful is important.

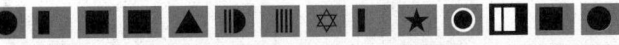

TRANSCULTURAL CONSIDERATIONS

Culture dictates a person's life expectations and influences the response to illness. The American approach of complete disclosure often causes distress when people with cancer are told more than they can integrate without excessive anxiety.

   e. People with cancer and their families need information during the diagnostic period. Often they are seeking 2nd opinions and need guidance in choosing appropriate resources.
2. Coping skills
   a. Coping is a dynamic process that seeks to restore equilibrium and reduce stress. Coping involves conscious actions and differs somewhat from psychologic defense mechanisms, which are unconscious. Coping is often considered a response to a short-term problem, whereas adaptation refers to ongoing adjustments to long-term problems such as chronic disease.
   b. Coping skills are acquired over the person's lifetime and are influenced by personality and life experience. Factors that enable and hinder coping are listed in Box 17–1. Good copers are optimistic, creative, and resourceful; poor copers are pessimistic, rigid, and lack hope.
   c. Some coping strategies can be productive in problem solving, whereas others are counterproductive, closing off options and increasing distress. A comparative analysis of coping strategies is summarized in Table 17–9.
3. Denial is a natural defense mechanism that protects the ego against anxiety. Denial allows a person to ignore or explain away unpleasant or threatening matters. In cancer literature, denial also includes **suppression,** which is a deliberate, conscious decision not to think about the threat, and **repression,** which is unconsciously motivated forgetting.
   a. Denial can only be inferred from the person's observed behavior and statements. Inappropriate optimism or unconcern in the face of a poor prognosis may be evidence of denial.
   b. Extreme denial leads to poor compliance and blocked communication, which adds distress to the family. Partial denial either to parts of the cancer experience or at selective times during the cancer experience is common and can relieve distress for a short time.
4. Family support
   a. Initial role changes in families are required. Whatever the role of the person with cancer in the family, changes must compensate for the loss of that role. If a child has cancer, then many roles are changed to provide support and care during treatment.
   b. Financial concerns may overwhelm the family. Many families do not have adequate insurance to cover a major and long-term illness. Individuals with health maintenance organization coverage may feel frustrated if they are not able to select the "best" cancer specialist.
5. Community support
   a. People with cancer are concerned over loss of friends. Persons who have a severe cancer phobia will indeed desert friends who are diagnosed with cancer.

BOX 17–1. Enabling and Hindering Factors in Coping with Cancer

Enabling Factors	Hindering Factors
Social support systems	Denial
Perception of control	Avoidance
Hardiness	Helplessness
Humor	Powerlessness
Positive appraisal	Hopelessness or despair
Hopefulness	Depression
Positive comparisons	Guilt
Religiosity	Erosion of autonomy
Self-esteem	Isolation or withdrawal
Information seeking	Wishful thinking
Open communication	Anger or hostility
Social skills	Blaming others
Problem-solving ability	Noncompliance

From Dudas S: Alteration in patient coping. *In* Baird SB, McCorkle R, and Grant M. *Cancer Nursing: A Comprehensive Textbook.* Philadelphia: WB Saunders, 1991.

Table 17–9. A Comparison of Coping Strategies

Moos and Schaefer (1984)	Weisman and Worden (1976–1977)	Lipowski (1970)	Penman (1980)
Appraisal-Focused Coping			
Logical analysis	—	Minimization	Rationalizing, reinterpreting (e.g., minimizes; emphasizes self-sufficiency; puts in "perspective")
Cognitive redefinition	Accept, but find something favorable (redefinition).	Denial Rationalization Selective misinterpretation/ interpretation	
Cognitive avoidance	Try to forget; put it out of mind (suppression).		
	Do other things to distract self (displacement).	Avoiding	Avoiding (e.g., withdraws, avoids, seeks distraction)
	Blame someone or something (disown responsibility).	Avoidance Denial	
Problem-Focused Coping			
Seek information or advice	Seek more information about the situation (rational-intellectual).	Vigilant focusing Seek as much information as possible	Tackling and mastering (e.g., seeks information, fights disability, works at problem solving)
	Seek direction from an authority and comply (compliance).		
Take problem-solving action	Take firm action based on present understanding (confrontation).	Tackling Confronting Actively dealing with illness	
Develop alternative rewards	Negotiate feasible alternatives (if *x*, then *y*).		
Emotion-Focused Coping			
Affective regulation	Laugh it off; make light of situation (reversal of affect).		
Resigned acceptance	Withdraw socially into isolation (stimulus reduction).	Capitulating Adapting a passive dependent stance Withdrawal	Capitulating (e.g., accepts stoically; complies passively; expresses futility)
	Submit to and accept the inevitable (fatalism).		
	Blame yourself, sacrifice, or atone (self-pity).		
Emotional discharge	Reduce tension by drinking, overeating, drugs (tension reduction).		Tension-relieving (e.g., expresses and shares feelings; uses humor; blames others)
	Talk with others to relieve distress (shared concern).		
	Do something, anything, however reckless, impractical (act out).		

From Holland JC, and Rowland JH. *Handbook of Psychooncology*. New York: Oxford University Press, 1989, p 52. Copyright © 1989 by JC Holland and JH Rowland. Used by permission of Oxford University Press, Inc.

b. Community resources vary with geographic location. Major metropolitan areas may have wellness communities or other support programs for people with cancer. Persons who live in rural areas, however, may have to be more resourceful. Concerned neighbors may be willing to help the person with cancer.

■ CLINICAL MANAGEMENT FOR CANCER

Goals of Intervention

1. **Cure** is the primary goal for tumors that are localized or have regional lymph node metastasis and for hematologic malignancies that can be treated with curative intent. Few cancers can be cured once they have recurred or are metastatic at the time of diagnosis. **Adjuvant therapy** refers to additional chemotherapy or radiation given after eradication of the tumor to prevent recurrence and therefore improve curability. Adjuvant therapy has proven value in breast and colon cancer.

2. Treatment for noncurable tumors is **palliative** and is directed toward control of tumor growth and relief of symptoms.

Treatment Decisions

1. Tumor-related factors that determine treatment decisions are tumor size, stage of disease, histologic type and grade, natural history of the tumor, and responsiveness of the tumor to various treatment methods.

2. Person-related factors that influence treatment selection

are physical condition, mental status, resources available, and personal preference.
3. Surgery, radiation, and chemotherapy are the primary treatment modalities for cancer. Biotherapy has become the primary treatment for a few specific cancers.
4. Adjuvant treatment includes hormonal therapy, bone marrow transplantation, and some types of biotherapy. These are given in addition to or following primary cancer treatments to effect a cure or to prolong disease-free survival.
5. Most investigational protocols are designed to improve chemotherapy and radiation therapies. Biotherapy, with few exceptions, remains investigational. Gene therapy, photodynamic therapy, and hyperthermia are investigational therapies available in some research centers.

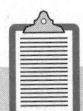

NURSING MANAGEMENT

Health care reform has shifted the care of people with cancer from inpatient to outpatient settings. Short-term and long-term chemotherapy, blood component therapy, invasive procedures, pump maintenance, education, and counseling services are performed in hospital outpatient settings; doctors' offices; 24-hour facilities; and free-standing ambulatory surgery, radiation, and chemotherapy clinics. Eighty to 90 percent of care for people with cancer is delivered in the outpatient setting.

Outpatient nurses are now challenged to provide a higher level of technologic care for people who are sicker, to provide patient support over a 24-hour period, and to provide continuity of care with many caregivers from different health care facilities.

Pharmacologic Interventions: Chemotherapy

1. Chemotherapy is the only systemic primary treatment method that allows curative or palliative treatment of disseminated or localized disease.
   a. Chemotherapy is curative in selected cancers (Table 17–10). Unfortunately, diseases cured by chemotherapy account for only 10 percent of cancers. Lung and colon cancer, 2 of the most common cancers, are minimally responsive to chemotherapy.
   b. Palliative treatment with chemotherapy can reduce tumor bulk and provide relief of symptoms.
   c. Adjuvant chemotherapy describes the administration of chemotherapy for a defined period. Adjuvant chemotherapy follows curative radiation or surgery to eradicate presumed micrometastatic deposits of tumor, which can cause subsequent tumor recurrence.
2. Tumors are believed to grow more rapidly in the early stages of development, before they are clinically evident. Only 1 to 8 percent of cells within a tumor are dividing.
3. Cytotoxic drugs kill only a fixed proportion of tumor cells. Each dose kills a constant fraction of the remain-

Table 17–10. Influence of Chemotherapy on Advanced Cancer

Cure
Gestational trophoblastic tumors
Acute lymphoblastic leukemia
Hodgkin's disease
Non-Hodgkin's lymphoma (children)
Diffuse large cell lymphoma
Burkitt's lymphoma
Testicular tumors

Cure—Adjuvant Chemotherapy
Wilms' tumor
Osteogenic sarcoma
Rhabdomyosarcoma

Complete Remission with Increased Survival
Breast cancer
Small cell carcinoma of the lung
Acute myeloblastic leukemia
Non-Hodgkin's lymphoma, indolent
Prostate cancer
Hairy cell leukemia
Chronic granulocytic leukemia

Response with Some Prolongation of Survival
Multiple myeloma
Ovarian cancer
Endometrial cancer
Neuroblastoma
Colorectal cancer
Liver cancer

Minor Response—No Demonstrable Prolongation of Survival
Non–small cell lung cancer
Head and neck cancer
Stomach cancer
Pancreatic cancer
Cervical cancer
Melanoma
Cancer of the adrenal cortex
Soft tissue sarcomas

Organ Preservation—Neoadjuvant Chemotherapy
Breast cancer
Laryngeal cancer
Bladder cancer
Osteogenic sarcoma
Soft tissue sarcomas
Anus cancer
Esophageal cancer

From Krakoff IH. Systemic treatment of cancer. *CA Cancer J Clin* 46(3):136, 1996.

ing cells. Multiple doses of the drug are therefore required to eradicate tumors (Fig. 17–11).
4. Cytotoxic drugs kill normal as well as tumor cells. The dose of the drug should be large enough to kill tumor cells while inducing only reversible and tolerable side effects from destruction of normal cells.
5. Cytotoxic drugs that interfere with DNA synthesis (S phase) or mitosis (M phase) are cell-cycle or phase specific. Cell-cycle or phase-nonspecific drugs damage DNA directly and are effective during all phases of the cell cycle.

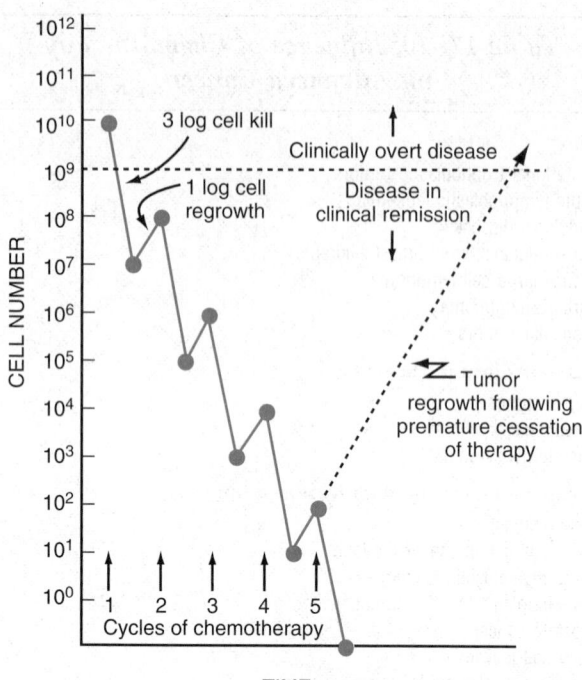

Figure 17–11. Relationship between tumor cell survival and chemotherapy administration. The exponential relationship between chemotherapy drug dosage and tumor cell survival dictates that a constant proportion, not number, of tumor cells is killed with each cycle of treatment. In this example, each cycle of drug administration results in 99.9% (3 log) cell kill, and 1 log of cell regrowth occurs between cycles. The broken line indicates what would occur if the last cycle of therapy was omitted: despite complete clinical remission of disease, ultimately the tumor would recur. (From Murphy GP, Lawrence W Jr, and Lenhard RE Jr. *American Cancer Society Textbook of Clinical Oncology.* Atlanta, GA: American Cancer Society, 1995, p 116.)

6. Because cytotoxic drugs are more effective against proliferating or dividing cells, chemotherapy is more effective when the tumor burden is small and a greater percentage of cells are proliferating.
7. Development of drug resistance is the major cause of chemotherapy failure. Chemosensitive tumors may regress to the point of being clinically undetectable and then regrow while the person is on the same therapy. Many mechanisms of drug resistance are postulated and are under investigation. Cross-resistance to other chemotherapeutic agents occurs even when their mode of action is different. Overcoming drug resistance would improve curability.
8. Cytotoxic drugs are more effective when given in combinations as long as each drug is effective against the tumor as a single agent and the toxicities of the drugs do not overlap.
   a. Combining drugs with different cell cycle activity exposes more cells to damage.
   b. Combination chemotherapy is the standard for most tumors and is given in protocols with specific dosages and administration intervals.
9. The efficacy of chemotherapeutic drugs is measured by tumor shrinkage evident by palpation, imaging techniques, tumor marker measurements, or improvement in performance status. Standard criteria or response are listed in Table 17–11.

10. Only 50 to 60 chemotherapeutic drugs are approved by the U.S. Food and Drug Administration (FDA) as cytotoxic drugs. Although usually classified by similar modes of action, drugs within each group differ in their metabolism, excretion, and administration (Table 17–12).
    a. Alkylating agents are cell-cycle–nonspecific drugs that cause alteration in DNA by forming bonds with electron-rich nucleic acids. These agents cause single- and double-stranded DNA breaks and cross links.
    b. Plant alkaloids are cell-cycle–specific drugs derived from Vinca plants or the May apple plant (VP-16). The *Vinca* alkaloids affect the structure of microtubules during mitosis. The action of VP-16 is not known.
    c. Antitumor antibiotics are cell-cycle–nonspecific drugs derived from the fungus *Streptomyces* or made synthetically. They form free radicals, which induce DNA damage and can interfere in DNA repair.
    d. Antimetabolites are cell-cycle–specific drugs functioning in the S phase of the cell cycle. They compete for or replace metabolites that are essential to DNA formation.
    e. A number of miscellaneous drugs also have varying modes of action.
11. Cytotoxic drugs can be given as single agents or in combination with other drugs or hormones. Most drugs are given at specified intervals to allow for recovery of bone marrow. Depending on the route of administration and institutional policy, chemotherapy can be given by staff nurses, clinical nurse specialists, specifically trained chemotherapy nurses, or physicians.
    a. Routes of administration. Drugs are administered systemically through oral, subcutaneous, intramuscular, or intravenous routes or regionally through topical, intrathecal, intracavitary, or intra-arterial instillations.
    b. The dosage for most cytotoxic drugs is based on body surface area of the person calculated from the height and weight. Accurate measurements are critical to correct dosage.
    c. Intravenous administration is the most common route. Drugs are given intermittently or by continuous infusion with an external or internal implanted pump device.
       (1) Repeated venipunctures that are painful and produce venous injury and sclerosis should be avoided. Chemotherapeutic agents that are vesicants cause severe tissue destruction if extravasation occurs into the surrounding tissue.

Table 17–11. Tumor Response Criteria

Degree of Response	Criterion
Complete response	Complete disappearance of the tumor
Partial response	50% or greater reduction in tumor size
Stable or no response	No change, or less than 50% reduction
Progression	Greater than 50% increase in tumor size

Data from Southwestern Oncology Group (SWOG) criteria.

Table 17–12. Chemotherapeutic Agents

Agent	Trade Name	Abbreviation	Agent	Trade Name	Abbreviation
Alkylating Agents			III. ENZYMES		
I. NITROGEN MUS-TARDS			L-asparaginase	Elspar	L-ASP
Mechlorethamine	Mustargen, nitrogen mustard	HN²	IV. EPIPODOPHYLLOTOXINS		
			Etoposide	Vepesid	VP-16
Cyclophosphamide	Cytoxan, Endoxan	CTX	Teniposide	Vumon	VM-26
			Miscellaneous		
Ifosfamide	Ifex	IFS	I. PLATINUM COORDINATION COMPLEXES		
Phenylalanine mustard	Melphalan, Alkeran	L-PAM	Cis-diamminedichloroplatinum II		
Chlorambucil	Leukeran	CLR	Cisplatin, Platinol	DDP	
II. ETHYLENIMINE DE-RIVATIVES			Carboplatin	Paraplatin	CBP
Triethylenethiophosphoramide	Thiotepa	T-TEPA	II. SUBSTITUTED UREA		
			Hydroxyurea	Hydrea	HXU
III. ALKYL SULFONATES			III. METHYLHYDRAZINE DERIVATIVE		
Busulfan	Myleran	MYL	Procarbazine	Matulane	PROC
IV. NITROSOUREAS			IV. ESTRAMUSTINE PHOSPHATE	Emcyt	Emcyt
Cyclohexyl-chloroethyl nitrosourea	Lomustine, CeeNU	CCNU	V. ACRIDINE DERIVATIVE		
1,3 bis-[2-chloroethyl]-1-nitrosourea	Carmustine, BiCNU	BCNU	Amsacrine	Amsidyl	m-AMSA
Streptozotocin	Zanosar	STZC	**Hormones and Hormone Inhibitors**		
V. TRIAZENES			I. ESTROGENS		
Dimethyl triazeno imidazole carboxamide	Dacarbazine	DTIC	Diethylstilbestrol		DES
			Conjugated estrogens	Premarin	
Antimetabolites			Ethinyl estradiol	Estinyl	
I. FOLIC ACID ANALOGS			II. ANDROGENS		
Methotrexate	Amethopterin	MTX	Testosteraone propionate		TES
II. PYRIMIDINE ANALOGS			Fluoxymesterone	Halotestin, Ora-Testryl, Utandren	
5-fluorouracil	Fluorouracil	5-FU			
Cytosine arabinoside	Cytarabine, Cytosar	ARA-C	III. PROGESTINS		
			17-Hydroxyprogesterone caproate	Delalutin	
III. PURINE ANALOGS			Medroxyprogesterone acetate	Provera	
6-Mercaptopurine	Purinethol	6-MP	Megestrol acetate	Megace	
6-Thioguanine	Thioguanine	6-TG	IV. LEUPROLIDE	Lupron	
Deoxycoformycin	Pentostatin	VM-26	Goserelin acetate	Zoladex	
			V. ADRENOCORTICOSTEROIDS		
Natural or Semisynthetic Products			VI. ANTIESTROGENS		
I. VINCA ALKALOID			Tamoxifen	Nolvadex	
Vinblastine	Velban	VLB	VII. HORMONE SYNTHESIS INHIBITORS		
Vincristine	Oncovin	VCR	Aminoglutethimide	Elipten, Cytadren	
II. ANTIBIOTICS			VIII. ANTIANDROGENS		
Doxorubicin	Adriamycin	ADR	Flutamide	Eulexin	
Mitoxantrone	Novantrone	NOV			
Daunorubicin	Daunomycin	DNR			
Bleomycin	Blenoxane	BLEO			
Dactinomycin	Actinomycin D, Cosmegen				
Mithramycin	Mithracin				
Mitomycin C	Mutarnycin	MITO-C			

From Rubin P, McDonald S, and Qazi R. *Clinical Oncology: A Multidisciplinary Approach for Physicians and Students.* 7th ed. Philadelphia: WB Saunders, 1993.

(2) The use of venous access devices (VAD), developed over the past 15 years, avoids repeated venipuncture and provides stable venous access to minimize drug extravasation. Some factors determining the type of VAD to use are the duration of therapy, complexity of treatment, length of treatment, nature of drugs, person's acceptance, and person's ability to provide maintenance

care (Table 17–13). Long-term VADs can be tunneled to a central vein through the subcutaneous tissue or can be nontunneled central venous lines. Peripherally inserted central catheters are inserted to central veins through antecubital veins. Implantable ports are central catheters with a reservoir implanted in the subcutaneous tissue; these devices require minimal maintenance. Protocols for catheter and site maintenance are institution specific. The most common complications of VADs are catheter occlusion and infection.

(3) Extravasation of vesicant drugs into the surrounding tissue can produce extensive tissue necrosis and damage sufficient to require surgical repair as well as unnecessary pain and disability. Any pain, swelling, erythema, or lack of blood return during infusion may be signs of drug extravasation and must be investigated immediately. Treatment of drug extravasation depends on the drug and the institution. Various protocols are available through the Oncology Nursing Society's *Cancer Chemotherapy Guidelines*.

d. Intrathecal administration. Most systemic chemotherapy drugs do not penetrate the blood-brain barrier and thus make the central nervous system a sanctuary for tumor cells. Drugs can be delivered into the

Table 17–13. Vascular Access Devices

Type	Description	Longevity	Comments
Peripheral Needle Scalp vein Butterfly	• Stainless steel • Single lumen • 27–19-gauge	Minutes to days	• Excellent for short-term access, especially outpatient • Increased risk of infiltration with long-term use
Peripheral Catheter Abbocath Insyte Streamline	• Catheter over needle • Teflon or polyurethane • Streamline is elastomeric hydrogel, which softens and expands one lumen size after insertion • Single and double lumen • 26–14-gauge	Hours to days	• Excellent for multiday infusional therapy • Provides greater patient mobility since less likely to infiltrate • Streamline has been known to remain patent and functioning for 1–2 weeks, due to its softer composition
Nontunneled Central Venous Catheter Subclavian line Arrow	• Polyurethane or silicone catheter • Single, double, and triple lumen	Hours to weeks	• Excellent for emergency need for CVC • Can augment existing VAD for acute care needs • Inserted at bedside by physician • High rate of trauma, infection compared to TCVC and port
Peripherally Inserted Central Catheters (PICCs) C-PICS Per-Q-Cath Groshong PICC	• Silicone elastomer or other polymers • Single and double lumen • 24–16-gauge	Weeks to months	• Excellent for continuous infusion over several weeks or months • Can be inserted at bedside by specially trained nurse • Quick, easy central access without surgical procedure • Requires external site care and routine flushing.
Tunneled Central Venous Catheter Hickman catheter Raaf Cath Groshong catheter	• Silicone catheter with Dacron cuff • Single, double, and triple lumen • 4.2–19.2 Fr; 40–90-cm length • Groshong has slit valve, requiring less flushing	Months to years	• Excellent for long-term, continuous, or intermittent therapy • Preferred for long-term TPN administration • Preferred by many for vesicant infusional therapy • Requires external site care and routine flushing
Implantable Port Port-A-Cath Hickman Port Lifeport	• Titanium, stainless steel, silastic, or plastic portal attached to catheter • Single and double lumen • Access with noncoring needle	Months to years	• Excellent for long-term, intermittent infusional therapy • No site care required, so excellent for patients unable to perform site care • Surgical procedure required for removal
Peripheral Port PAS-Port	• Titanium portal attached to silastic catheter • Single lumen • Access with noncoring needle	Months to years	• Excellent for frequent, intermittent access, particularly for those patients with active lifestyles or body image concerns • No external site care

From Groenwald SL, et al. *Cancer Nursing: Principles and Practice.* 3rd ed. Boston: Jones & Bartlett, 1993. Reprinted with permission.

lateral ventricles through an Omaya reservoir and into the spinal canal through a tap.

    e. Intracavitary administration. Intravesical administration of drugs into the bladder is used in the treatment of superficial bladder cancers. Intraperitoneal infusion is used in the treatment of ovarian and colon cancer. Intrapleural instillation is used in the treatment of pleural malignancies.

    f. Intra-arterial administration. Infusions of drugs into arteries supplying tumors can be accomplished through an external catheter and pump or through an implanted catheter and pump. Intra-arterial drug administration concentrates the drug exposure to the tumor while minimizing systemic side effects. It is most often used in hepatic tumors or metastases.

    g. Topical administration. Cytotoxic drugs can be applied to superficial skin cancers or to cutaneous lesions in T-cell lymphomas.

12. Preparation, handling, and disposal of drugs

    a. Personnel can be exposed to cytotoxic drugs through inhalation of aerosols, absorption through the skin, or ingestion of contaminated materials.

    b. Concern over the exposure of personnel to drugs with carcinogenic potential prompted the establishment of guidelines to minimize drug exposure. Guidelines are available from the Occupational Safety and Health Administration and the Oncology Nursing Society.

13. Because cytotoxic drugs kill or damage normal cells as well as tumor cells, the effects of chemotherapy are seen as acute effects secondary to the effects on self-renewing cell populations and general systemic effects, toxicities occurring in specific organs, and long-term effects of carcinogenesis (Box 17–2). Specific drug and dosage are the most important factors related to toxicity.

14. Acute toxicities to renewing cell populations

    a. Bone marrow suppression

        (1) Hematopoietic stem cells are among the most rapidly proliferating cells in the body, replacing mature leukocytes, platelets, and red blood cells as they are destroyed. When stem cells are destroyed, they are unable to replace lost cells at the normal rate. Blood counts drop. Blood count nadirs occur between the 7th and 14th day after drug administration and recover by the 21st day. Delayed bone marrow suppression caused by some agents begins 4 weeks after drug adminis-

tration. Marrow suppression is greater if active bone marrow sites have been reduced by previous radiation or tumor infiltration.

        (2) Leukocytes survive only 6 hours in the bloodstream. Neutrophils function to localize and neutralize bacteria in the body. When **neutropenia** (a neutrophil count below 1000 cells per mm^3) occurs, the person's response to bacterial infection is severely compromised, and localized infections can progress to septicemia without the usual response of fever or inflammation. Blood counts are monitored at appropriate intervals. The absolute neutrophil count is calculated by multiplying the number of leukocytes by the percentage of neutrophils and bands. Patients are instructed to report promptly any temperatures higher than 100.5 degrees Fahrenheit to the physician or oncology nurse. People with neutropenia *without* fever can be managed as outpatients and are cautioned to avoid crowds and exposure to infected individuals, to maintain good hygiene and hand washing, and to monitor their temperature every 4 hours. Rashes, sore throats, and fevers must be reported. Persons with elevated temperatures or shaking chills are generally advised to contact their physician or return to the hospital immediately or both. Patients with neutropenia and fever constitute a medical emergency and must be treated immediately to avoid sepsis.

NURSE ADVISORY

People receiving chemotherapy must understand that *fever* is the most important symptom to report. Fever with neutropenia is an emergency.

- On hospital admission, a thorough physical examination is performed to determine any sources of infection. Blood cultures and antibiotic therapy are instituted. Because 90 percent of new fevers in people with cancer are bacterial, a combination of a penicillin and an aminoglycoside drug are administered. Colony-stimulating growth factors (see pp. 77–78) may be used to augment leukocyte production.

- Measures to prevent exposure to other sources of infection include reverse isolation; strict hand washing; restriction of fresh fruits and vegetables, plants, and flowers; restriction of visitors; and strict aseptic technique for any invasive procedure.

        (3) Platelets survive 7 to 14 days in the bloodstream. Following drug administration, people are advised to report any symptoms of bleeding gums, tarry stools, dark urine, headache, or shortness of breath, which may indicate **thrombocytopenia**. Platelet counts lower than 50,000 can produce hemorrhage with injury or stimulus. Safety pre-

---

BOX 17–2. Nursing Diagnoses Related to Chemotherapy

- Knowledge deficit R/T the therapeutic plan, efficacy, risks, and benefits, side effects, and symptom management
- Altered nutrition, less than body requirements
- Fatigue
- Altered oral mucous membrane
- Risk for infection R/T neutropenia
- Risk for injury R/T thrombocytopenia
- Altered sexual patterns
- Body image disturbance

cautions to avoid injury are important. Parenteral injections are avoided. People with cancer are instructed not to use aspirin, alcohol, or anticoagulants. Platelet counts lower than 20,000 place the person at risk of spontaneous hemorrhage. Platelet transfusions are usually given.

The risk for bleeding due to thrombocytopenia, secondary to treatment or disease, is related to the following platelet counts:
- Mild risk, 50,000 to 100,000
- Moderately severe risk, 20,000 to 50,000
- Severe risk, under 20,000

---

    (4) Erythrocytes survive 120 days in the bloodstream. Their relatively slow turnover allows time for replacement between chemotherapy cycles. People on chemotherapy, however, usually have hemoglobin levels below normal and consequent anemia. If hemoglobin levels drop below 9 gm per 100 ml of blood, packed cell transfusions may be given, especially if the person has cardiac disease or is symptomatic. People are advised to pace their activities and to take adequate rest periods. Erythropoietin has been used to restore erythrocyte counts.

  b. Mucositis
    (1) Cells of the gastrointestinal lining from the oral cavity to the rectum, which are continuously lost as food and liquids pass through, are replaced from stem cell populations. As chemotherapy destroys stem cells, normal replacement and repair are inadequate.
    (2) Mucositis can occur in any portion of the gastrointestinal tract but is most common in the oral cavity, esophagus, and intestine.

  c. Stomatitis
    (1) Inflammation of the oral cavity ranges from mild discomfort to painful ulcerations. Antimetabolite and antibiotic cytotoxic drugs cause stomatitis more frequently than other drug groups. Drug dosage and duration of treatment affect the degree of stomatitis.
      • Concurrent thrombocytopenia can contribute to mucosal bleeding, and neutropenia may decrease resistance to infection.
      • Decreased saliva and chewing reduce the normal mouth cleansing. Poor oral hygiene, dehydration, poor nutrition, as well as any mechanical, chemical, or thermal irritants intensify stomatitis.
      • Stomatitis becomes a serious problem when it prevents adequate intake of food and liquids, because it leads to dehydration and weight loss.
    (2) Following chemotherapy administration, patients are instructed to maintain good oral hygiene and adequate fluid, and nutritional intake. As stomatitis progresses, additional interventions are used. Institution-specific protocols use the same general principles.

      • Reducing mechanical trauma to the tissue by using soft toothbrushes or gauze. Dentures are cleansed frequently or removed if stomatitis is severe.
      • Maintaining oral hygiene with mouthwashes that are neutral (saline) or oxidizing (hydrogen peroxide/water). The frequency of oral hygiene measure increases with severity of stomatitis.
      • Monitoring for infection with periodic cultures
      • Treating infections with appropriate antimicrobial drugs
      • Reducing pain with topical anesthetics
      • Maintaining lip moisture with lubricants
      • Reducing irritation with diets that are chemical, mechanical, and thermally nonirritating

  d. Enteritis
    (1) Loss of intestinal mucosa can diminish absorption and cause diarrhea.
    (2) Treatment consists of a low-residue diet and antidiarrheal medications to control symptoms. Without complications, enteritis subsides in 7 to 10 days.

  e. Alopecia
    (1) Alopecia can range from scalp hair thinning to total body hair loss. Hair loss occurs most commonly with doxorubicin, cyclophosphamide, and vincristine.
    (2) The proliferating cells at the base of the hair follicle are affected, causing either total destruction or atrophy of the bulb.
    (3) Hair loss begins within 2 to 3 weeks following initiation of chemotherapy. Regrowth begins 4 to 6 weeks after discontinuing treatment.
    (4) Initial regrowth can differ in texture and color, but eventually hair returns to its previous characteristics.
    (5) Hair loss has pronounced negative psychologic effects.
      • Efforts to reduce loss by scalp hypothermia or scalp tourniquets are limited because manufacturers of hypothermia devices were unable to prove efficacy and safety, so the devices have been removed from the market.
      • Reducing the drug concentration to the scalp sets up a potential scalp sanctuary for tumor cells. The possibility of scalp metastasis restricts the use of scalp treatment to noncurative modes of chemotherapy.
      • Instructions that warn the person of sudden hair loss are imperative to prepare the person for the anticipated assault on body image. Wigs for women are reasonably priced and can be improved by styling by a professional hair dresser. The American Cancer Society program Look Good, Feel Better provides consultation with beauticians free of charge.

  f. Gonadal suppression
    (1) Amenorrhea or azoospermia due to cytotoxic effects on reproductive cells can be temporary or permanent.
    (2) People with cancer are advised to use some form

of birth control during chemotherapy as gonadal cell suppression may be incomplete and many agents are teratogenic. Sperm banking can be considered for eligible males. Reproductive function can recur spontaneously, be delayed for many years, or be lost permanently.

15. Acute systemic effects

a. Fatigue: Causes of fatigue are not clear. Weariness, decrease in strength, and weakness are characteristic descriptions of fatigue. Reassurance that fatigue is common during chemotherapy and helping the individual set priorities, redistribute work load, avoid stress, and take frequent rest periods are methods of coping with fatigue.

b. Nausea and vomiting: Nausea is the desire to vomit and is associated with loss of gastric tone and reflux of the duodenal contents into the stomach. Vomiting is the coordinated expulsion of gastric contents.

(1) The emetic center in the medulla oblongata coordinates nausea and vomiting through connections with the respiratory center, vasomotor center, salivatory center, and cranial nerves VIII and X, all of which lie adjacent to it. The emetic center is stimulated by (a) the peripheral, vagal, and sympathetic afferent fibers that come from the gastrointestinal system; (b) the chemoreceptor trigger zone, which detects toxins in the blood believed to be mediated by transmitters such as serotonin, dopamine, histamine, enkephalins, and prostaglandins; and (c) the cerebral cortex.

(2) Nausea and vomiting are described as acute if the condition occurs within 1 to 2 hours after drug administration, delayed if the condition begins more than 24 hours later, anticipatory if it occurs before chemotherapy.

(3) Nausea and vomiting are influenced by the drug and dosage. Cisplatin, dacarbazine, nitrogen mustard, carmustine, lomustine, cyclophosphamide, and streptozocin are the most emetogenic agents. Most cytotoxic drugs produce acute nausea and vomiting, which subsides within 24 hours.

(4) Uncontrolled nausea and vomiting cause 25 to 50 percent of people to delay or refuse further treatment. Inadequate nutritional intake, electrolyte imbalances, and dehydration can occur. Aspiration pneumonia and mucosal tears are possible complications of uncontrolled nausea and vomiting.

(5) Control of nausea and vomiting is achieved by the use of antiemetic drugs (Table 17–14). The phenothiazines, butyrophones, and metoclopramide block dopamine receptors in the chemoreceptor trigger zone. Ondansetron and granisetron are serotonin antagonists. The mechanism of action of the corticosteroids and cannabinoids is not clear. Benzodiazepines are used for their amnestic effect. Antiemetics must be given one-half hour to 24 hours before chemotherapy and should be given on a regular schedule (see Table 17–14).

(6) Other useful measures in reducing nausea and vomiting are reduction of noxious stimuli such as odors, avoidance of spicy and greasy foods, distraction through music or reading, and relaxation.

16. Organ toxicities: Specific cytotoxic drugs produce toxicities in specific organs. Some effects are temporary, whereas others are permanent. They are not always dose related.

a. Cardiac toxicity

(1) Doxorubicin can produce significant cardiomyopathy, causing congestive heart failure. The toxicity is related to the cumulative dose received. Adults are restricted to cumulative doses of 550 mg per m^2; those with previous mediastinal radiation receive only 400 mg per m^2. Myocardial biopsies and measurement of cardiac ejection fractions are performed at intervals to assess cardiac function. The drug is discontinued if myocardial damage is detected or when the cumulative dose is achieved. Daunorubicin produces similar cardiomyopathy. Dexrazoxane, a cardioprotective agent, has been used successfully in clinical trials of women with metastatic breast cancer. Dexrazoxane permitted higher median doses of doxorubicin, with fewer cases of congestive heart failure occurring.

(2) Cardiac toxicities occurring with lesser frequency are cardiac necrosis with high-dose cyclophosphamide, angina with fluorouracil, and congestive heart failure with mitoxantrone.

b. Pulmonary toxicity

(1) Chronic pneumonitis and fibrosis are the most common pulmonary toxicities related to chemotherapy. With some drugs risk factors are cumulative dose, radiation therapy, oxygen therapy, and age. The drugs associated with pulmonary toxicity are bleomycin, mitomycin, busulfan, carmustine, cyclophosphamide, and methotrexate.

(2) Treatment includes discontinuing the drug and managing symptoms. The changes are irreversible. Pulmonary function tests may be obtained before treatment to assess pulmonary function and to determine eligibility for certain drugs.

c. Renal toxicity

(1) Nephrotoxicity occurs most commonly with cisplatin, which can produce acute renal failure with necrosis of the renal tubules. High urine flow during cisplatin therapy achieved by intravenous saline or mannitol provides protection against renal damage. Adequate creatinine clearance function is evaluated before the administration of cisplatin.

(2) The nitrosoureas, streptozocin, methotrexate, and mitomycin can produce renal damage of varying pathologic features.

d. Neurotoxicity

(1) Neural damage can occur to central or peripheral nervous system nerves and to cranial nerves as a direct or indirect effect of cytotoxic drugs. Damage can be reversible or permanent.

Table 17–14. Antiemetic Drugs

Agent	Route of Administration	Side Effect
Phenothiazines		
Prochlorperazine (Compazine)	PO, IM, IV, PR	Extrapyramidal effects, sedation, hypotension
Thiethylperazine (Norzine, Torecan)	PO, IM, IV, PR	
Perphenazine (Triaflon, others)	PO, IM, IV	
Butyrophenones		
Haloperidol (Haldol, others)	PO, IM, IV	Sedation, extrapyramidal effects, hypotension
Droperidol (Inapsine, Innovar, others)	IV	
Corticosteroids		
Dexamethasone (many preparations)	IV, PO	Insomnia, mood change, hyperglycemia
Methylprednisolone (Medrol, others)	IV	
Benzamides		
Metoclopramide (Reglan, others)	IV, IV (continuous), PO	Sedation, extrapyramidal effects, diarrhea, akathisia, bronchospastic reaction
Serotonin Antagonists		
Ondansetron (Zofran)	IV	Headache, hiccups, sedation, diarrhea, dizziness, transient increase in liver transaminases
Granisetron (Kytril)	IV, IV (continuous), PO	
Cannabinoids		
Dronabinol (Marinol)	PO	Sedation, euphoria, hypotension, memory loss, dysphoric reactions, dry mouth, ataxia
Others		
Lorazepam (Ativan, others)	PO, IV	Sedation, hypotension
Diphenhydramine (Benadryl, others)	PO, IV	Sedation, anticholinergic effects
Benztropine (Cogentin, others)	PO, IV	Anticholinergic effects
Combination Therapy (for cisplatin-containing moderate to highly emetic regimens)		
Ondanstron	IV	
Dexamethasone	IV	
Metoclopramide*	IV	
Dexamethasone	IV	
Lorazepam	IV	
Diphenhydramine	IV	

PO, Orally; IV, intravenously; IM, intramuscularly; PR, rectally
* Alternative choice is haloperidol or droperidol.
Modified from Weiss GR (ed). *Clinical Oncology.* Norwalk, CT: Appleton & Lange, 1993.

(2) Vincristine causes peripheral neuropathy with sensory and motor components leading to muscle weakness, foot drop, and atrophy. Damage to nerves of the autonomic nervous system causes ileus, constipation, impotence, and urinary retention. The drug may be withheld until symptoms abate.

(3) Cisplatin can cause peripheral neuropathy and ototoxicity.

(4) Encephalopathies can occur with high-dose methotrexate, cytarabine, and ifosfamide. Cerebellar dysfunction can occur with the use of 5-fluorouracil.

f. Hepatotoxicity: Hepatic damage is uncommon and can range from mild enzyme elevations to cirrhosis. Agents that cause hepatotoxicity are methotrexate (high dose), cytarabine (high dose), and 6-mercaptopurine.

g. Bladder: Cyclophosphamide causes hemorrhagic cystitis, which can range from dysuria to hemorrhage. Good hydration and frequent urination protect the bladder mucosa.

h. Skin: Many cytotoxic agents cause a variety of skin changes. Hyperpigmentation in skin and nail beds, rashes, dermatitis, banding in the nails, erythema, and photosensitivity can be produced by specific agents. Many drugs can produce recall reactions in skin areas that have been irradiated previously.

17. Long-term effects of chemotherapy

a. Development of leukemias can occur as secondary malignancies in 1 to 10 percent of people who have received chemotherapy. Survivors of Hodgkin's disease who have received both chemotherapy and radiation have the highest incidence of secondary malignancies. Alkylating agents, cyclophosphamide, melphalan, carmustine, chlorambucil, and mechlorethamine appear to be the most carcinogenic.

b. Tumors of the bladder, kidney, and ureter have occurred as secondary malignancies.

18. Investigational chemotherapy
    a. Systematic development of chemotherapeutic drugs began in 1954 when the U.S. Congress approved the creation of the Cancer Chemotherapy National Service Center at the National Cancer Institute. Because the side effects of chemotherapy were so distressing and physician case loads were insufficient to study adequate numbers of patients, the study of chemotherapeutic agents became organized into large cooperative study groups that plan, develop, and coordinate large-scale clinical trials.
    b. Animal studies: More than 40,000 chemicals are screened annually for possible antitumor activity. Of these, 10,000 will be laboratory tested with human cell lines. Of these, 10 drugs may be used in human clinical trials.
    c. Clinical trials
       (1) Phase I studies determine the maximum tolerated dose of a drug, its pharmacologic properties (i.e., absorption, metabolism, and excretion and its toxicities). People with disease that has been unresponsive to treatment or advanced disease without beneficial therapy are eligible to receive phase I drugs. These studies are done in selected institutions.
       (2) Phase II studies determine the efficacy of the drug in various tumors as well as toxicity and pharmacologic effects of the drug. Individuals with progressive disease who have completed previous therapies are eligible for phase II studies.
       (3) Phase III studies compare the effectiveness of the drug with that of the standard treatment for specific malignancies. Drugs can be used in combination with other agents. The disease-free survival, overall survival, and quality-of-life measurements are used in this level of study. Large numbers of patients are recruited, generally ones who have had no prior treatment.
       (4) Drugs that have completed clinical trials are submitted for FDA approval.

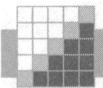

LEGAL AND ETHICAL CONSIDERATIONS

Three basic ethical principles accepted in our cultural tradition guide ethical decision making in health care: autonomy (the right of the individual to choose), beneficence (the obligation of the health care provider to do good and prevent harm), and justice (the notion that each receives a fair share).

Ethical issues related to autonomy are informed consent and truth telling. Choosing one's future presupposes accurate information, comprehension of that information, and absence of coercion or pressure in making a choice. Institutional review boards in health care facilities monitor the informed consent procedures in any research protocol.

Despite safeguards, many ethical issues arise regarding informed consent. How much information must be given to the subject? Does too much information have as great a negative effect as too little? Can the anxious person with cancer really comprehend the volume or the significance of the information? In a choice between consenting to a treatment and death, can the decision be voluntary? There are no clear answers.

NURSING DIAGNOSIS: Risk for injury R/T bleeding due to thrombocytopenia secondary to disease or treatment.

1. *Expected outcomes:* Following intervention, the person with thrombocytopenia should be able to do the following:
    a. Recognize the significance of the risk for bleeding and the relationship among platelets, bone marrow, and bleeding.
    b. Identify observations indicative of bleeding.
    c. Identify monitoring procedures needed during periods of thrombocytopenia.
    d. Identify measures to prevent bleeding.
2. *Nursing interventions*
    a. Monitor appropriate laboratory studies (e.g., platelet count, hemoglobin, and coagulation studies).
    b. Teach the person with cancer about the relationship among platelets, bone marrow and bleeding and about blood tests needed to monitor counts and frequency.
    c. Teach the person to observe signs of bleeding: gross blood, tarry or black stools, red-tinged urine, petechiae, ecchymotic areas, bloody sputum, hematomas.
    d. Teach preventive measures:
       (1) Use soft toothbrush for oral care.
       (2) Avoid activities that predispose to trauma (e.g., contact sports, falling).
       (3) Use an electric razor.
       (4) Avoid enemas and rectal thermometers. Prevent constipation.
       (5) Avoid injections.
       (6) Avoid aspirin or aspirin-containing products.

NURSING DIAGNOSIS: Risk for infection R/T bone marrow depression secondary to chemotherapy

1. *Expected outcomes:* Following interventions, the person with cancer and caregivers will do the following:
    a. Demonstrate knowledge of the signs and symptoms of infection.
    b. Verbalize the person's specific risk for infection.
    c. Describe measures to prevent infection.
    d. State the signs and symptoms to report to the physician and the appropriate timing.
2. *Nursing interventions*
    a. Monitor the person's risk for infection on the basis of tumor type, location, extent, treatment-related factors, and health-related factors.
    b. Teach the person with cancer signs and symptoms of systemic infection (e.g., chills, fever) or localized infection (e.g., redness, swelling, tenderness, pus, foul-smelling discharges).
    c. Instruct the person about signs and symptoms to report to the physician or nurse.
    d. Instruct the person about general measures to prevent infection: frequent hand washing, good nutrition and fluid balance, good body hygiene, avoidance of sick people, aseptic technique for any procedures (e.g., catheter care done at home).
    e. Instruct the person at risk for neutropenia about preventive measures, signs, and symptoms.

BOX 17–3. Nursing Diagnoses Related to Cancer Surgery

- Knowledge deficit R/T the surgical procedure, changes in body function, hospitalization, and symptom management
- Pain R/T the surgical procedure
- Risk for infection
- Altered nutrition R/T the surgical procedure, stress, and hospitalization
- Impaired skin integrity
- Fatigue
- Body image disturbance
- Altered sexual pattern

Surgery

1. Curative surgery: Primary tumors are potentially curable by surgical resection for people with local or regional disease. Forty percent of people with cancer are treated with surgery alone. The goal is adequate removal of the tumor with minimal structural and functional impairment (Box 17–3).
   a. The extent of the excision is based on the type of tumor. Superficial tumors can be treated by a wide local excision. Others that may spread to the regional lymph nodes are removed with an en bloc excision in which the tumor and lymph nodes are removed in continuity.
   b. Techniques are used to prevent dissemination of the tumor into the operative field. Glove changing, instrument cleaning, and wound irrigation with cytotoxic agents are used to prevent cell shedding.
   c. Previous concepts in tumor biology, which presumed cancer to spread in an orderly fashion from tumor to lymph node and then to distant sites, dictated a radical excision as the logical treatment to remove all tumor. Current concepts favor less radical approaches with adjuvant chemotherapy and radiation to eradicate micrometastatic tumors.
   d. Locally recurrent tumors occasionally can be resected to effect a cure, although to a lesser degree. Sarcomas and colon, breast, and skin cancers have been successfully reexcised locally, with resulting cure.
   e. Solitary metastatic lesions in the lungs, brain, or liver can be removed to effect a surgical cure. Decisions to resect metastatic lesions are based on tumor type and natural history, length of the disease-free interval, stability of the lesion, and unresponsiveness of the tumor to chemotherapy and radiation. Metastatic renal cell sarcomas, melanomas, and colon carcinomas have been removed in selected persons, producing cures or prolonged survival times.

ELDER ADVISORY

Older people can tolerate cancer surgery as well as younger people if older patients do not have comorbidity factors such as heart, lung, or kidney disease.

---

2. Palliative surgical procedures are considered if the risk-to-benefit ratio to the person with cancer is positive. Palliative procedures can be done to reduce pain; relieve obstructions in the respiratory, gastrointestinal, or urinary tracts; relieve pressure on the brain or spinal cord; prevent hemorrhage; remove infected or ulcerating tumors; and drain abscesses.
3. Adjuvant surgery: Debulking procedures are performed in large sarcomas or ovarian cancers to reduce the tumor burden and make the tumor more responsive to chemotherapy or radiation.
4. Reconstructive surgery: Following radical curative surgical procedures, people with cancer can have form and function improved with reconstructive surgery. Skin and muscle flaps can be used to cover anatomic defects. Reconstruction in head and neck procedures can be extensive but offer the person with cancer improved cosmesis and quality of life.
5. Prophylactic surgery: People who are at high risk for developing specific cancers may be considered for excision of the target organ.
   a. People with familial polyposis who have a 50 percent risk of developing colon cancer by the age of 40 can undergo subtotal colectomies with little if any alteration in bowel function.
   b. People with long-standing ulcerative colitis also have an increased risk of colon cancer.
   c. Women with high risk factors for breast cancer often elect to have bilateral mastectomies rather than live with the threat of disease.

NURSING DIAGNOSIS: Body image disturbance R/T surgical procedures (head, neck, mastectomy, orchiectomy, pelvic surgery, stomas—colostomy, ileostomy, urinary diversions—limb amputations, disarticulations)

---

1. *Expected outcomes:* Following interventions, the person with cancer should be able to do the following:
   a. Acknowledge the change in image.
   b. Verbalize feelings concerning the change in image.
   c. Identify alternative ways to enhance body image.
   d. Learn self-care activities related to body image change.
2. *Nursing interventions*
   a. Observe for preoccupation with body change, anxiety related to change in lifestyle secondary to body alteration, expression of negative feelings, fear of rejection, and refusal to look at changed body part.
   b. Encourage the person to verbalize feelings regarding body change and lifestyle changes resulting from it.
   c. Encourage the person to look at the affected body part.
   d. Teach self-care activities related to change (e.g., colostomy care, tracheostomy care, crutch walking).
   e. Arrange contacts with persons who have had similar changes, if appropriate (e.g., persons in ostomy clubs).
   f. Inform the person with cancer about resources to improve appearance (e.g., breast prosthesis, wigs, cosmeticians in the American Cancer Society programs "Look Good, Feel Better").

g. Help the person through the grieving process.

h. Whenever possible, discuss changes in body image before they occur.

NURSING DIAGNOSIS: Fatigue R/T cancer treatment

1. *Expected outcomes:* Following interventions the person with fatigue should be able to do the following:
   a. Identify possible causes of fatigue.
   b. Describe methods to maximize energy and limit fatigue.
2. *Nursing interventions*
   a. Monitor nutritional intake, sleep patterns, blood count, and cardiovascular response to activity.
   b. Teach person with cancer the relationship of fatigue to treatment (i.e., chemotherapy, radiation, surgery, or biotherapy).
   c. Explore methods by which the person with cancer can prioritize activities to conserve energy.
   d. Encourage rest periods and naps.
   e. Encourage physical activity consistent with energy reserve.

NURSING DIAGNOSIS: Sexual dysfunction R/T alterations secondary to disease or treatment (surgery, chemotherapy, complications of cancer)

1. *Expected outcomes:* Following interventions, the person with cancer should be able to do the following:
   a. Identify the causes of sexual dysfunction.
   b. Seek the appropriate level of sexual information, counseling, or therapy to meet the need for sexual intimacy.
2. *Nursing interventions*
   a. Establish a therapeutic relationship.
   b. Identify the person's perceived sexual dysfunction through a nursing history.
   c. Consider your own knowledge, value, and comfort in providing appropriate sexual counseling. Interventions can be based on the PLISSIT model (or other available models).
      (1) P—*permission* to introduce the topic of sexual concerns, providing the time to discuss sexual concerns, and being willing to assist the person
      (2) LI—*limited information;* provide information to clarify concerns, dispel myths and misconceptions, and make general suggestions to improve intimacy
      (3) SS—*specific suggestions,* which are provided when general suggestions and limited information are inadequate
      (4) IT—*intensive therapy,* in-depth counseling by a qualified therapist
   d. Provide written materials produced by the American Cancer Society to the person with cancer. These include "Sexuality and Cancer: For the Man Who Has Cancer and His Partner" and "Sexuality and Cancer: For the Woman Who Has Cancer and Her Partner."

Radiation

1. Curative radiation therapy can be used to treat local or regional cancers if the tumor is sensitive to radiation.
   a. Early-stage lymphomas; Hodgkin's disease; carcinoma of the cervix, skin, and eye; and head-neck cancers can often be cured by radiation therapy.
   b. Radiation is chosen for surgically inaccessible tumors and for individuals who are poor candidates for surgery.
2. Adjuvant radiation therapy is used in combination with other treatment methods to improve survival.
   a. Preoperatively, adjuvant radiation can reduce tumor bulk and destroy malignant cells peripheral to the tumor. Postoperatively, tumor cells left in surgical margins can be destroyed.
   b. Radiation in combination with chemotherapy can be used to reduce a large tumor burden, thereby making chemotherapy more effective. It is also effective in destroying tumor in known sanctuaries (i.e., brain and spinal cord) that may not be penetrated by chemotherapy.
   c. Palliative radiation can be used to relieve pain from bony metastases; relieve obstructions of the gastrointestinal, respiratory, and urinary systems; prevent paralysis from spinal cord compression; and relieve neurologic symptoms of seizure, headache, or nerve palsies.
3. Therapeutic radiation uses ionizing forms of radiation.
   a. Electrons, protons, neutrons, alpha particles, negative pi mesons, and high-energy heavy particles are forms of ionizing radiation. Some of these forms of particulate matter are produced in electrical devices, whereas others are emitted from natural radioactive sources.
   b. Electromagnetic x-rays or gamma rays are photons of energy that are the shortest wavelengths of the electromagnetic spectrum. X-rays and gamma rays are the same in physical and biologic function, differing only in their source. X-rays are produced in electrical devices, whereas gamma rays are emitted from radioactive materials such as cobalt.
4. The radiation dosage measures the average energy deposited per unit mass of tissue. The gray (GY) is the standard unit of measurement and represents the energy absorption of 1 joule per kg. One GY equals 100 centigray (cGY). The rad, which was the standard unit before 1985, is equal to 1 cGY. Most therapeutic radiation uses gamma rays or x-rays or electrons. Most particulate radiation generally requires expensive and complicated machinery and is used in investigational studies.
5. Ionizing radiation energy is absorbed as it passes through matter. It interacts with cellular molecules, causing ionization. The electrons acquiring energy from the photons are ejected from their orbits, causing breakage of chemical bonds.
   a. Although not completely understood, ionization is believed either to damage the DNA molecule directly or to react with water in the cell, causing production of free radicals, which diffuse and cause damage to critical structures.
   b. Radiation must produce cell death to be effective. Cells can die immediately if a sufficient dose is given.

Table 17–15. Teletherapy Equipment and Its Use

Equipment	Emission	Beam Characteristics and Radiobiologic Effects	Clinical Application, Advantages, Disadvantages
Kilovoltage			
40–150 kV	X-rays	Superficial, limited range, poor skin tolerance	Skin cancers or other very superficial lesions, if electrons are not available
Orthovoltage			
150–1000 kV	X-rays	Deep penetration, high skin dose, high bone absorption	Limited, owing to poor skin tolerance and potential for bone necrosis
Cesium-137 radioisotope (600 kV)	Gamma rays	Large source size with large penumbra	Long half-life; low energy and output; used in head and neck treatment
Megavoltage or Supervoltage			
Cobalt-60	Gamma rays	Deep penetrating; skin-sparing due to maximum dose build-up beneath the skin; produces penumbra area at edge of beam that receives less dose	Deep-seated tumors; ease of mechanical operation
1.25–2 MeV			Slower dose-rate (longer treatment time) as source decays
Linear Accelerators			
4–20 MeV	Photons	Deeply penetrating; skin-sparing; increased versatility and precision of dose distribution	Deep-seated tumors; large field capability; complex electronics with tendency for "down-time"
6–30 MeV	Electrons (optional)	Electrons give maximum dose on skin and a few centimeters beneath, falling off rapidly thereafter	Skin lesions, chest wall recurrence, superficial nodes
Betatron			
10–30 MeV	Electrons	High-velocity electrons with deep penetration	High dose rate with shorter treatment time; limited field size; bulky equipment; low dose rate photons
18–40 MeV	X-rays	High-energy photons	

From Dow KH, and Hilderley LJ. *Nursing Care in Radiation Oncology.* Philadelphia: WB Saunders, 1992.

Cells that are damaged, however, can die a reproductive death if damage to the DNA renders the cell unable to replicate.

  c. Several factors increase the radiosensitivity of cells:

    (1) Oxygen. The radiation dosage required to kill hypoxic cells is 3 times that of normal cells.

    (2) Cells in the G_2 or M phase of the cell cycle are more radiosensitive.

    (3) Self-renewing cells are the most sensitive to radiation; connective tissue and small blood vessels are intermediate in sensitivity; and nonrenewing cells are most resistant to radiation.

    (4) The radiosensitivity of tumor cells is similar to that of their normal cell of origin.

6. Teletherapy is a radiation technique in which the radiation source is external to the person. The distance allows for more uniform dose distribution. Tables 17–15 and 17–16 list the types of teletherapy equipment available.

Table 17–16. High Linear Energy Transfer (LET) and Heavy Charged Particle Beams

Energy Source	Beam Characteristics and Radiobiologic Effects	Use in Clinical Trials
Fast Neutrons 16–50 MeV deuterons	Fixed field size and beam position; wide penumbra; absorbed dose decreases exponentially with depth; low OER; RBE is higher with small dose increments	Advanced cancers of the head and neck, pelvis, gliomas, and melanoma; esophageal cancer and osteosarcomas
Protons and Helium Ions 600 MeV	Precise dose distribution with ability to deliver very high tumor dose with sparing of adjacent normal tissues; RBE and OER similar to those obtained with gamma and photon sources	Pituitary tumors, chondrosarcoma, cordoma; abdominal and pelvic tumors; soft-tissue sarcomas; head and neck tumors
Negative Pi-Mesons 40–70 MeV	Absorbed dose increases slowly with depth, then rises sharply; lower OER; enhanced RBE	Head and neck tumors, brain, pancreas; skin metastases

OER, Oxygen enhancement ratio; RBE, relative biologic effectiveness.
From Dow KH, and Hilderley LJ. *Nursing Care in Radiation Oncology.* Philadelphia: WB Saunders, 1992.

a. Equipment differs in the type of photon or particle produced, the energy of the photon that determines the depth of tissue that can be penetrated.

b. Older orthovoltage machines produced low-energy x-rays that had poor penetrating ability and deposited the maximum radiation on the skin, causing severe skin damage.

c. Midvoltage machines, the cobalt machine and the linear accelerator, are most commonly used in therapeutic radiation.

  (1) The cobalt machine houses a radioactive cobalt source in the head of the machine. During treatment, the shield is removed and the radiation emitted. Cobalt units have enough penetrating ability to treat brain, head, neck, and bone tumors. The radiation beam can be shaped by means of a collimator (a metal device that bends the radiation beam). The radiation cobalt source decays in approximately 6 years and must be replaced. These units are relatively inexpensive and are commonly used.

  (2) The linear accelerator produces x-rays with electricity and is capable of producing very high energy photons, increasing the ability of the beam to penetrate tissue. The maximum dosage is deposited beneath the skin. X-rays from linear accelerators have sharply demarcated beams; therefore, a more accurate dose can be given (Fig. 17–12).

d. High-voltage machines. Betatrons, cyclotrons, and equipment that produces particulate radiation generally are available only in research facilities.

e. Radiation dosage. The amount of radiation required to eradicate a tumor depends on the cell type of the tumor. Table 17–17 lists typical radiation doses for common tumors. The usual fractionated dosage in curative radiotherapy is 180 to 200 cGy 5 times per week. Individuals with metastatic disease undergoing palliative radiation are usually treated with higher daily dosages in a shorter time interval. The total radiation dose is divided, or fractionated. This basic treatment principle allows for a greater total radiation dose, as opposed to a single dose, to be tolerated and is based on 4 concepts of radiation biology:

  (1) Repair: Cells that have sublethal damage have time to recover, and less tissue damage occurs.

  (2) Reoxygenation: Hypoxic tumor cells that are radioresistant become oxygenated as the tumor shrinks and there is less demand for oxygen.

  (3) Redistribution: Cells that are in the sensitive portions of the cell cycle will be destroyed by the initial radiation treatment. Other cells are then recruited into the replicating pool and will be subjected to radiation at the next dose.

  (4) Repopulation: Normal cells that have repaired sublethal damage are able to duplicate in the intervening time interval.

f. Consultation for treatment. The radiation oncologist

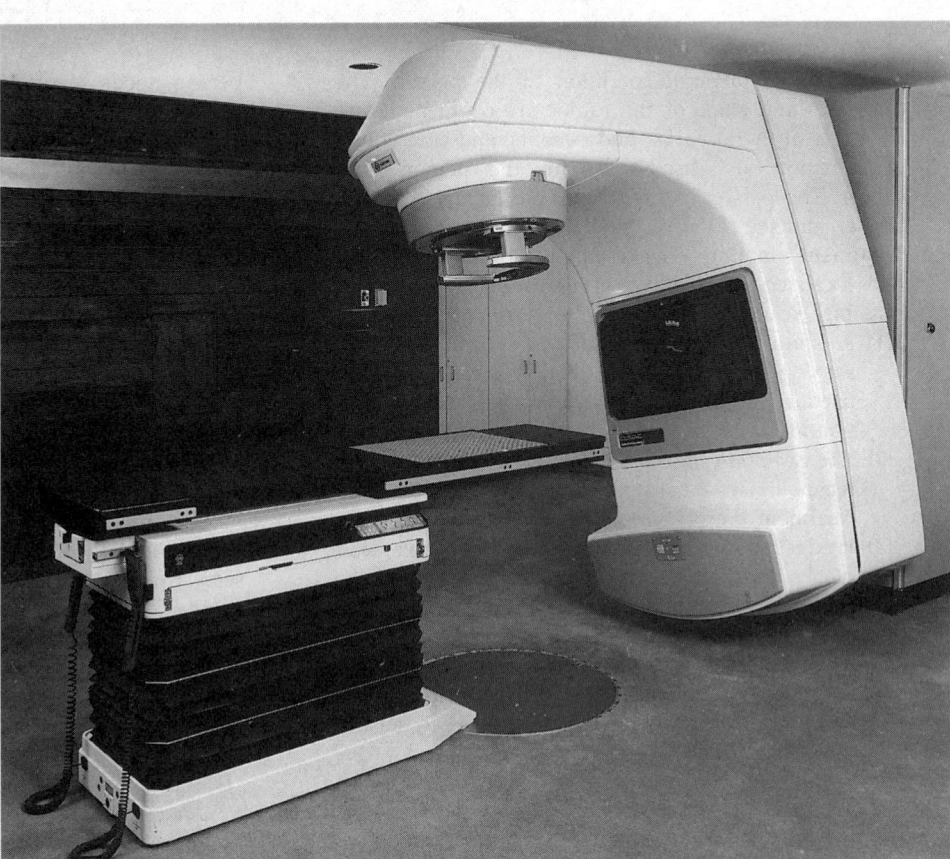

Figure 17–12. A Varian Clinac 2100 C linear accelerator. (Courtesy Varian Oncology Systems.)

Table 17–17. Typical Radiation Doses for Selected Tumors

Tumor	Dose	Remarks
Wilms'	1000–2000 cGy (occasionally up to 3800 cGy)	Used as part of combined modality approach; limited usually to residual disease or patients with unfavorable prognostic signs.
Seminoma	2500–3500 cGy	Primarily applied in stage I or II macroscopic nodal disease or potential microscopic disease below the diaphragm.
Hodgkin's disease	3500–4500 cGy	Used primary modality in most stage I and II and some stage III disease; used for consolidation of some with bulk disease treated with primary chemotherapy.
Non-Hodgkin's lymphoma	3000–5000 cGy	Employed as primary therapy in rare stage I; combined with chemotherapy for cure of certain aggressive histologic types; used as palliation for certain indolent histologic types.
Head and neck	5000–7000 cGy	Used primary treatment for certain stage I and II patients. Combined with surgery in most stage III and IV patients. Offered as palliation in advanced inoperable cases.
Breast	5000–6000 cGy	Combined with lumpectomy for tumors ≤ 4 cm. Used postmastectomy for select patients at high risk for local recurrence.
Esophagus	5000–7000 cGy	Often used alone or with chemotherapy as primary treatment; also as adjunct to surgery pre- or postoperatively.
Cell lung	5000–7000 cGy	Employed as adjunct to surgery with positive nodes or margins, as primary treatment for certain stage I, II, and III patients, as palliation in stage IV.
Small cell lung	5000–6000 cGy (lung) 2400–3000 cGy (brain)	Used as adjunct to chemotherapy in limited disease with chest consolidation and brain prophylaxis; palliative in extensive stage.
Pelvic (cervix, endometrium, bladder, prostate, rectum, anus)	5000–7000 cGy	Whole pelvis often treated to 5000 cGy with boost to macroscopic disease. Often used as adjunct to surgery with positive margins or nodes. Often used externally combined with brachytherapy.
Brain	5000–7000 cGy	Generally combined with surgery and often chemotherapy. Lower doses given for lymphomas and higher doses for gliomas.
Sarcoma	6000–7000 cGy	Used as adjunct to surgery pre- or postoperatively. Sometimes combined with chemotherapy.
Brain and bone metastases	3000–5000 cGy	Accelerated course often appropriate in patients with poor performance status and short longevity.

From Weiss GR (ed). *Clinical Oncology*. Norwalk, CT: Appleton & Lange, 1993.

evaluates the physical condition of the person. The diagnosis and stage of the tumor are confirmed, and the goals of therapy, risk and benefits, and side effects of radiation are discussed with the person with cancer. The person is oriented to the facility, the personnel, and the resources available during treatment.

g. Treatment planning. The treatment volume is defined and localized using physical palpation of tumor (if possible), scans, and x-rays.

(1) A simulator (a diagnostic x-ray unit with the same geometry of the radiation therapy unit) is used to design the radiation ports and tumor volume.

(2) The radiation oncologist, radiation physicist, and technologist determine optimal position and treatment portals.

(3) Wedges to compensate for tissue differences, lead blocks to shield normal tissues adjacent to the tumor, and immobilization casts are created.

(4) Skin markings are done with tattoo or ink to ensure exactly placement of the radiation beam.

(5) A computer simulation is constructed to demonstrate the tumor volume and dosage to ensure precise treatment.

h. Treatment. The person is usually treated with 180 to 200 cGy per day, 5 days a week. Actual radiation time is only a few minutes. Additional time is required if several treatment ports are used and the person needs to be repositioned. The person is seen weekly by the radiation oncologist to monitor progress, make assessment, and treat side effects and reactions. A weekly complete blood count and weight measurement are taken. Dose calculations are frequently checked by the radiation physicist.

NURSE ADVISORY

Reassure people with cancer that although they will be alone during the treatment procedure, they are being monitored on closed-circuit television and are always within someone's view.

i. Posttreatment follow-up. The person with cancer is seen frequently until all acute reactions have subsided. Thereafter, the person is seen every 2 to 3 months during the 1st posttreatment year. If radiation was the primary curative treatment, the person with cancer is seen annually to monitor for late treatment complications.

j. Effects of radiation therapy

(1) Local reactions to radiation occur *only in the irradiated tissue* and are classified as early reactions if they occur during treatment or within several months following treatment and as late or de-

layed effects if they occur any time after 6 months (Box 17–4).

(2) Systemic reactions to radiation (nausea, fatigue, and weakness) occur only during treatment.

(3) The severity of the reaction depends on the total dosage received and the tissue composition. Self-renewing cell systems, skin, bone marrow, and mucosal membranes are most responsive to radiation.

(4) Acute reactions are self-limiting and relate to edema, inflammation, and parenchymal cell death. Acute reactions occur days to weeks after the initiation of therapy and resolve 2 to 4 weeks after the completion of therapy. Some reactions considered acute may occur within a few months of treatment.

(5) Delayed reactions occur in radiated organs secondary to destruction of the endothelial linings of the small blood vessels, which become damaged over time, leading to occlusion, infarction, necrosis, or fibrosis of the affected tissue. Delayed effects are permanent and irreversible. Organs that showed no acute reactions during treatment can have delayed reactions.

k. Acute effects of radiation

(1) Systemic reaction. Fatigue, weakness, and nausea are the most frequently occurring symptoms of systemic reactions to radiation. The cause of these symptoms is unknown. Individuals are advised to pace their activities, avoid exertion, and rest frequently.

(2) Skin reactions: Skin erythema begins 2 to 3 weeks after treatment initiation.

- Reactions can progress from erythema to dry desquamation characterized by dryness, scaling, and itching to moist desquamation (loss of the epidermis), with blistering and weeping of tissue.
- Radiation-induced stimulation of melanocytes causes hyperpigmentation (tanning).
- Hair loss is temporary if the total radiation dose is less than 3000 rads. Hair growth recurs in 6 to 8 weeks, but thickness may be diminished.
- Diminished function in affected sweat and sebaceous glands may produce dryness and anhidrosis.

(3) Interventions for skin reactions

BOX 17–4. Nursing Diagnoses Related to Radiation Therapy

- Knowledge deficit R/T goals of treatment, procedures, risks and benefits, long- and short-term side effects, and symptom management
- Fatigue
- Altered nutrition R/T nausea, vomiting, and stress
- Impaired skin integrity
- Body image disturbance
- Altered sexual patterns

- Skin reactions can be minimized by proper skin care during treatment (Learning/Teaching Guidelines for Skin Care During Radiation Therapy).
- In addition to instruction in routine skin care, people receiving brain radiation must be cautioned to avoid use of electric hair dryers, curlers, and curling rods.

(4) Head and neck radiation reactions: Curative treatment of head and neck tumors requires high doses of radiation. Oral mucositis causes pain, inflammation, and dysphagia. Decreased saliva production causes xerostomia. Saliva becomes thick and acidic, facilitating bacterial growth and tooth decay.

(5) Interventions during radiation

- Symptoms of oral mucositis can be minimized by reducing irritation to the mucosa from any chemical (e.g., alcohol, chewing tobacco, highly seasoned foods, citrus juices, mouthwashes, cough syrups with an alcohol base), mechanical (e.g., hard toothbrushes, partial dentures, foods such as popcorn), or thermal (e.g., hot or cold liquids and foods, cigarette and cigar smoke) stimulus.
- People are advised to eat soft, moist, or pureed foods and to keep their mouths clean by rinsing with tepid solutions (which are institution specific) and using a soft toothbrush.
- Dental consultation for prophylaxis of tooth decay is obtained before radiation therapy and fluoride treatments can be given.
- Mouth dryness can be relieved by frequent gargling with warm water, use of a humidifier during the night, chewing sugarless gum or candy, and eating moist foods with sauces and gravies. Commercial preparations of artificial saliva are available.

(6) Thoracic radiation reactions: Esophagitis with dysphagia can occur if the esophagus is in the radiation port. A dry or sore throat and a dry, persistent cough usually occur. Radiation pneumonitis can occur 1 to 2 months after therapy. The heart is radioresistant, but pericarditis can occur with doses higher than 400 cGY.

(7) Interventions for thoracic radiation reactions

- Dysphagia can be minimized by eating a bland diet with soft, moist foods and avoiding irritants such as alcohol and tobacco smoke. Antacids may be used.
- Dry mouth symptoms are relieved by humidity, adequate fluid intake, sugarless gum, candy, and artificial saliva and frequent rinsing with prescribed solutions.

(8) Abdominal radiation reactions: The radiosensitivity of the epithelium of the small intestine causes diarrhea, bleeding, and cramping as the absorptive capacity of the small intestine is diminished. Gastritis with decreases in the production of gastric secretions can cause anorexia, nausea, and vomiting. Radiation hepatitis can occur when doses higher than 2500 cGY are employed.

LEARNING/TEACHING GUIDELINES
for Skin Care During Radiation Therapy

1. Skin changes during radiation therapy
   a. As radiation passes through the skin, some injury occurs.
   b. Within 2 to 3 weeks, redness, flaking, itching, and tanning can occur.
   c. Skin injury can progress to blistering and weeping, especially in areas where skin overlaps.
   d. Reactions will improve after the radiation is completed.
2. Skin reactions can be minimized by reducing mechanical, chemical, or thermal irritation.
   a. Avoid mechanical irritation with the following precautions:
      (1) Wash the skin gently with lukewarm water.
      (2) Pat the skin dry. Do not rub.
      (3) Protect the skin from friction and rubbing of clothing.
      (4) Wear loose clothing.
      (5) Do not shave skin in the affected area.
   (6) Do not use tape in the affected area.
   b. Avoid thermal irritation with the following precautions:
      (1) Use lukewarm water, no hot or cold water.
      (2) Protect the skin from the sun.
      (3) Do not use hot-water bottles or heating pads on the affected skin.
      (4) Avoid extreme cold or wind.
   c. Avoid chemical irritation with the following precautions:
      (1) Use only mild soap.
      (2) Rinse skin thoroughly.
      (3) Do not use lotions, powders, creams, or perfumes on the affected area unless prescribed by the physician.
3. Do not remove the skin markings.
4. Notify the physician or nurse whenever skin changes cause you discomfort or if any blistering or weeping occurs.

(9) Interventions for abdominal radiation reactions
- Nausea: Eating small, bland, frequent meals high in calories and proteins and avoiding sweet and greasy foods minimizes nausea. Drinking clear liquids (apple and cranberry juice, lemonade, ginger ale, Gatorade, popsicles, and tea) between meals only can usually be tolerated.
- Diarrhea: Fluid intake and calories must be increased to compensate for losses. Eating a low-residue diet of small, frequent meals and avoiding raw fruits and vegetables, gas-producing foods, caffeine, strong herbs and spices, fatty foods, milk, and milk products minimize stimulation of the small intestine. Antidiarrheal medications may be ordered.

(10) Pelvic radiation reactions: Irradiation of the bladder, vagina, and rectum produce irritation and inflammation causing cystitis with frequency, urgency, burning, and hematuria; proctitis with diarrhea, bloody stools, and tenesmus; and vaginitis with dryness and dyspareunia.
- Diarrhea is symptomatically treated, as in abdominal radiation. The rectal area should be cleaned after bowel movements. Sitz baths may be recommended.
- Cystitis can be minimized by increasing intake of fluid, especially cranberry juice, and avoiding substances that irritate the bladder (e.g., caffeine, tobacco products, alcohol, and spices such as pepper and curry). Difficulty in voiding should be reported to the radiotherapist.
- Vaginitis may cause painful intercourse, which may need to be avoided until soreness decreases. Loose cotton underwear, frequent baths, and exposing the perineum to air whenever possible are recommended. Douches, creams, lotions, and sprays should not be used.

l. Late effects of radiation
   (1) The dosage of radiation therapy used to eradicate any tumor is limited by the potential for late effects, which can occur in the normal tissue surrounding the tumor. Effects related to a dosage that is exceeded are seen in Table 17–18. The lens of the eye is the most sensitive, with cataract formation after exposure of 500 cGY.
   (2) Late effects of radiation can be devastating and are generally progressive. Shielding organs during radiation prevents late effects. Comparison of dosages needed to eradicate tumors (see Table 17–17) and doses that produce delayed effects (see Table 17–18) emphasizes the difficulty in designing treatment ports that spare sensitive tissues such as the lungs, kidneys, and liver.
   (3) The most devastating long-term effects of central nervous system radiation are brain necrosis, causing diminished cognition, and transverse myelitis, which results in motor paralysis. Abdominal radiation can cause severe radiation enteritis, necrosis, and fistula formation. Pelvic radiation can cause cystitis and infertility. Osteonecrosis can occur in bones. Pathologic fractures can occur in bones receiving more than 6000 cGY.
   (4) The incidence of secondary malignancies is relatively low following radiation therapy.
7. Brachytherapy is a radiation technique in which radiation sources are placed directly into an organ or tumor.

Table 17–18. Practical Radiation Tolerance of Common Dose-Limiting Organs

Organ	Practical Tolerance	Potential Toxicity
Brain (whole)	6000 cGy	Necrosis, infarction, leukoencephalopathy
Spinal cord (10-cm length)	4500 cGy	Transverse myelitis, necrosis, infarction
Heart (entire organ)	4000 cGy	Pericarditis, myocardiopathy
Heart (25%)	7000 cGy	Pancarditis
Lung (whole)*	2000 cGy	Pneumonitis, fibrosis
Small bowel (400 cm² cross-section)	4500 cGy	Ulcer, perforation, fistula, necrosis
Stomach (100 cm² cross-section)	4500 cGy	Ulcer, perforation, necrosis
Rectum (100 cm² cross-section)	6000 cGy	Stricture, ulcer, necrosis
Liver (whole)	2500 cGy	Acute and chronic hepatitis
Kidney (whole)	2000 cGy	Hypertension, chronic renal failure, proteinuria
Bladder (whole)	6000 cGy	Contracture, ulcer, necrosis
Lens of the eye (whole)	500 cGy	Cataract
Retina (whole)	5500 cGy	Infarction, necrosis
Cornea (whole)	5000 cGy	Ulceration, necrosis
Bone marrow†	250 cGy (whole)	Pancytopenia
	4000 cGy (segmental)	Myelofibrosis

* Smaller segments of the lung may be treated to higher doses without symptomatic pneumonitis. Signficant fibrosis and permanent hypofunction occur for those portions of the lung treated to doses greater than 2000 cGy, but adequate reserve may be available outside the radiation ports.
† If doses to the whole body and therefore to all the marrow exceed 400 cGy, approximately 50% of those so irradiated will die without marrow transplant. For segmental radiation, it is possible that portions of the marrow that exceed 4000 cGy are never repopulated successfully by marrow stem cells owing to myelofibrosis.
From Weiss GR (ed). *Clinical Oncology.* Norwalk, CT: Appleton & Lange, 1993.

Brachytherapy is generally given in addition to teletherapy as a booster dose to increase radiation to the tumor without additional radiation to the surrounding tissue. The principle of inverse square law—the dose to a point is inversely related to the square of the distance between that point and the radiation sources—is the basis for brachytherapy.

a. Radiation sources used in brachytherapy are radioactive isotopes, which are listed in Table 17–19. These sources have low energy and limited tissue penetra-

Table 17–19. Common Radioactive Isotopes Used for Brachytherapy

Isotope	Effective Energy	Half-Life	Application	Source Configuration
Radium (^{256}Ra)	0.83 meV	1622 years	Intracavitary gynecologic Interstitial head and neck Breast and others No longer popular because of radiation safety concerns	Needles, tubes
Cesium (^{137}Cs)	0.6 meV	30 years	Intracavitary gynecologic	Tubes, needles
Iodine (^{125}I)	0.035 meV	60 days	Permanent implant Prostate and others Special high-activity source Temporary brain implants Temporary eye plaque for melanoma	Seeds Plaque
Gold (^{198}Au)	0.42 meV	2.7 days	Prostate and other Permanent implants	Seeds
Iridium (^{192}Ir)	0.38 meV	74 days	Temporary implants Breast, brain, prostate, others	Wire, seeds Ribbon
Cobalt (^{60}Co)	1.25 meV	5.3 years	Ocular melanoma High-activity source in remote afterloading system applied to many tumors	Plaque Tube

From Weiss GR (ed). *Clinical Oncology.* Norwalk, CT: Appleton & Lange, 1993.

tion. Sources can be temporary or permanent, depending on the mode of administration.

b. Intracavitary administration: Application of radiation can be done for any hollow organ, but intracavitary radiation is mainly used for cervical and endometrial cancers. An applicator is placed within the organ in the operating room, and the radiation source is inserted (afterloaded) when the person is returned to the room, thereby limiting radiation exposure to others. Intracavitary radiation is now used to reduce obstructing lung and esophageal tumors that have been radiated previously.

c. Interstitial administration: Wire, needles, or ribbons are placed within the tumor. When placement is deemed satisfactory, radioactive seeds are inserted. This mode is most often used in breast, brain, head, neck, and prostate tumors.

d. Systemic therapy: Thyroid cancer is often treated by systemic therapy based on the affinity of thyroid tissue for iodine. An oral solution of radioactive iodine will be taken up selectively by the thyroid to produce the effect.

e. Procedures to minimize radiation exposure to personnel
(1) The amount of radiation exposure depends on the radiation source. Gamma rays have sufficient penetrating ability to provide a radiation hazard to individuals near the patient. Alpha and beta particles do not penetrate tissue.
(2) The person who conveys radiation risk should be isolated in a clearly marked private room.
(3) Radiation exposure is minimized by reducing the time spent with the person, interposing shielding materials between the person and personnel, and increasing the distance between the person and others. Pregnant personnel and visitors should not be exposed to the person.
(4) Appropriate procedures should be developed with radiation personnel to prevent inadvertent environmental contamination of radioactive materials.

8. Investigational approaches in radiation therapy
a. Use of local or regional hyperthermia immediately following radiation therapy to exploit the ability of hyperthermia to kill oxygen-depleted cells, which are less responsive to radiation.
b. Use of drugs that radiosensitize cells to radiation or radioprotective drugs that protect normal tissues from radiation.
c. Intraoperative radiation given to the tumor bed during surgery to prevent local tumor recurrence has been investigated in cancers of the stomach, pancreas, and retroperitoneal sarcomas.
d. Altered fractionation schedules. Radiation schedules being studied are split-course schedules in which daily radiation is suspended for 2 to 3 weeks after half the dose is given; hyperfractionation, in which treatments are given twice a day; and reduced fractions with fewer doses per week.
e. Development of monoclonal antibodies tagged with radioactive isotopes to carry radiation selectively to tumors.

Adjunctive Therapies

1. Hormonal treatment: Hormone-responsive tumors have been managed empirically for many years by hormone manipulation. The discovery of hormone receptors and the development of receptor assays and synthetic antiestrogens and antiandrogens have improved hormonal treatment. Hormone manipulation is used primarily in the treatment of metastatic breast, prostate, and endometrial cancers and hematologic malignancies.
a. Although hormonal manipulations can cause tumor regressions, the duration of the effect is limited, and eventually the tumor becomes refractory to other manipulations. It is believed that tumors probably contain hormone-dependent and hormone-independent clones and that, as tumor growth progresses and cells become more anaplastic, their dependence on hormones is lost (Box 17–5).
b. Hormonal manipulation can be achieved by adding hormones, suppressing hormones, using antihormones, or surgically removing hormone-producing organs.
(1) Steroid hormones (i.e., estrogens, androgens, progestins, and glucocorticoids) are produced in the adrenal cortex, ovary, and testis. Carried through the blood while bound to plasma proteins, they bind with specific cell receptors that convey them to the cell nucleus, where they affect DNA, RNA, protein synthesis, and cell division. The precise mechanism of hormone action is unknown, but it is thought to affect secretion of tumor growth factors.
(2) Antihormones or synthetic antiestrogens and antiandrogens are hormone antagonists that interfere with the normal hormone-hormone receptor-binding process.
(3) Surgical removal of hormone-producing organs (e.g., testis, ovary, and adrenal glands) also affects hormonal production.
(4) Drugs that suppress hormone production by suppressing gonadotropins can also be used.
c. Breast cancer: Hormonal manipulation in breast cancer is achieved by surgical removal of the ovaries and administration of antiestrogens, estrogens, or androgens. Selection of therapy is based on hormonal receptor status, menopausal state, age of the person with cancer, and extent of disease (see Chapter 33).
(1) Currently, the antiestrogen tamoxifen is most commonly used. Current clinical trials are investigating its use as a chemopreventive agent in women at high risk for breast cancer. Common

---

BOX 17–5. Nursing Diagnoses Related to Hormonal Cancer Therapy

- Knowledge deficit R/T goals of hormonal treatment, risks and benefits, long- and short-term side effects, and symptom management
- Altered sexual patterns
- Body image disturbance

side effects of tamoxifen are hot flashes, nausea and vomiting, vaginitis, and edema. Some evidence suggests that tamoxifen may be a possible cause of endometrial cancer.

(2) Paradoxically, using estrogens often causes tumor regression by an unknown mechanism.

(3) Progestins, megestrol acetate (Megace), and medroxyprogesterone acetate (Provera) also have anti-tumor effects, although the mechanism is unknown. Breast tumors with progesterone receptor–positive receptors respond to progestin administration. Side effects are weight gain, hot flashes, and vaginal bleeding.

(4) Bilateral oophorectomies and hypophysectomies have been used as surgical ablative techniques but are less often used since the development of tamoxifen.

d. Prostate cancer: Prostate cancer depends on androgenic stimulation for its growth. Reducing testosterone levels by surgical removal of the testes or administration of antiandrogens, estrogens, or gonadotropin-releasing hormone agonists can retard tumor growth (see Chapter 30).

e. Endometrial cancer: Progestins are the major hormonal treatment for endometrial cancer, with approximately one third of endometrial cancers responding.

(1) Progestins, medroxyprogesterone acetate (Provera), and megesterol acetate (Megace) are used, but their mechanism of action is unknown.

(2) Side effects of progestins are weight gain, hot flashes, and vaginal bleeding. The increased appetite experienced when using progestins has prompted their prescription for cachectic people.

f. Leukemias and lymphomas: The glucocorticoids, prednisone, and dexamethasone possess antilymphocytic properties that make them useful in treatment of leukemias and lymphomas. They are usually used with other cytotoxic agents.

2. Bone marrow transplantation: Bone marrow transplantation is a supportive therapy used in hematologic malignancies (i.e., leukemia and lymphomas) to restore bone marrow function after eradication of the person's marrow through the use of high-dose chemotherapy and radiation. Long-term remissions and cure can be achieved in some people. In the treatment of solid tumors, bone marrow transplantation allows administration of high-dose chemotherapy to destroy tumor cells of the target organ while preventing the potentially fatal bone marrow destruction associated with high doses. Used most often in the treatment of breast cancer, this treatment remains investigational, although improved survival has been demonstrated for some women with metastatic breast cancer who respond to the chemotherapy (Box 17–6).

a. Sources of bone marrow

(1) Allogeneic: Bone marrow is obtained from a family member or unrelated individual whose marrow is compatible with the person who has cancer. A match is based on human leukocyte antigen (HLA) testing. People receiving allogeneic transplants must be immunosuppressed to prevent rejection.

BOX 17–6. Nursing Diagnoses Related to Bone Marrow Transplantation
- Knowledge deficit R/T the goals of treatment, risks and benefits, treatment procedures, long- and short-term complications, functional capacity after transplant, and symptom management
- Risk for infection
- Risk for injury R/T thrombocytopenia
- Fatigue
- Pain
- Risk for impaired skin integrity
- Altered nutrition
- Altered sexual patterns
- Altered oral mucous membrane
- Risk for altered body temperature

---

(2) Syngeneic: Bone marrow is obtained from an identical twin.

(3) Autologous: Bone marrow is obtained from the person during periods of disease remission. Marrow rejection is avoided with autologous transplantation.
- Bone marrow is harvested from the posterior iliac crest under general anesthesia. Multiple aspirations (150 to 200) are required to obtain sufficient marrow. Following harvest, marrow is screened to remove bone spicules and fat. Autologous marrow can also be treated to remove any residual malignant cells. Erythrocytes are removed from allogeneic marrow if the recipient and donor are ABO incompatible. The marrow is cryopreserved until use.
- Peripheral blood progenitor cells have been harvested from people with hypoplastic marrow. The procedure involves apheresis following marrow stimulation with hematopoietic growth factors.

b. Pretransplantation preparation: Bone marrow transplantation is an aggressive, long, arduous, and stressful treatment that offers a chance of cure or prolonged survival following failure of standard chemotherapy.

(1) Risks of morbidity, mortality, and long-term physical disability are high. The patient and family are given detailed information on the transplantation process, complications, and long-term effects. The ability of the person and family to cope with long-term treatment is evaluated.

(2) Physical evaluation must determine ability to withstand aggressive chemotherapy and includes pulmonary, renal, and cardiac assessment.

c. Transplantation process

(1) Pretreatment: Total-body irradiation and high-dose cyclophosphamide have been the standard conditioning preparation. Conditioning renders the person immunosuppressed and prevents allogeneic transplant rejection. Alternative scheduling of radiation and chemotherapeutic agents (busulfan, cytosine, arabinoside, etoposide, melphalan, and carmustine) is used to minimize the side effects. Radiation is used to destroy malignant cells in the marrow, especially those that may be sanctuaries in the central nervous system.

(2) Transplantation: Bone marrow is transplanted by intravenous infusion 48 to 72 hours after the last chemotherapy dose. The transfused cells find their way to the recipient's marrow.

(3) Engraftment: Transplanted marrow requires 15 to 20 days to become engrafted. Neutrophils may recover in 5 weeks; but thrombocytes may take months. During this time, the person is at high risk for infection and bleeding and must be supported with blood products, fluids, and hyperalimentation. A germ-free environment is established by preventing inhalation of microbes (laminar-flow rooms and isolation), reducing ingestion of bacteria through food preparation (cooked food only), and reducing endogenous microbes (prophylactic antibacterials). Strict aseptic technique is used by all personnel.

(4) Recovery: Allogeneic marrow transplantation requires approximately 35 days of hospitalization. Transplant rejection and acute graft-versus-host disease prolong the recovery period. Autologous transplantation can invoke recovery within 30 days or less. Increasingly, these marrow recipients are managed as outpatients if they reside close to the hospital.

d. Complications: The marrow source, chemotherapy regimen, radiation dosage, and physical condition of the person determine the severity of complications following bone marrow transplantation. Those with allogeneic transplants can develop graft-versus-host disease and graft rejection, whereas those with autologous transplants do not.

(1) Acute complications: Acute complications occur within the first 3 months following transplant. High-dose chemotherapy and radiation can produce all the side effects of those treatments. Toxicities related to renewing cell populations (infection, bleeding, mucositis, diarrhea, and alopecia) and general systemic effects (fatigue, nausea, and vomiting) are intensified by the combination of radiation and high-dose chemotherapy, as are specific organ toxicities. Virtually all patients become infected.

- Graft-versus-host disease occurs in 40 percent of patients with human leukocyte antigen—

compatible donors and in up to 70 percent of those with less compatible donors. The mechanism is thought to be reaction of the donor T cells with recipient tissue antigens. The acute form, which develops during engraftment, manifests as an erythematous maculopapular skin rash over the palms and soles, followed by diarrhea, abdominal pain, and ileus. Liver enzymes are elevated (Fig. 17–13).

- Veno-occlusive disease develops in 10 percent of transplant patients, and 50 percent of those die from it. Occurring in the first 3 weeks after transplant, the syndrome causes ascites, hepatomegaly, and jaundice. No therapy except supportive treatment is available.

- Renal failure occurs in 50 percent of allogeneic transplant patients. Causative factors are mismatched bone marrow, hypovolemia, and reactions to antibiotic therapy and cyclosporine.

- Graft rejection can range from 5 to 60 percent depending on the donor, the age of the patient, and the marrow pretreatment.

(2) Chronic complications: Most chronic complications develop within the 1st year following transplantation. The sequence of complications in allogeneic transplants is seen in Figure 17–13.

- Bacterial, viral, and fungal infections occur during the 1st year following bone marrow transplantation. Cytomegalovirus and *Pneumocystis carinii* pneumonia are not uncommon.

- Chronic graft-versus-host disease occurs in 20 to 40 percent of patients who survive more than 6 months following allogeneic transplant. The chronic form has characteristics of a collagen vascular disorder, affecting joints, esophagus, eyes, lungs, liver, skin, and gut. Most people respond to prednisone treatment.

- Bone marrow transplantation recipients also develop the long-term effects of radiation and chemotherapy, including secondary malignancies.

3. Biotherapy encompasses therapies that augment or manipulate the immune system against cancers (biologic response modifiers), destroy tumors through the use of cytotoxic cytokines, or enhance cell maturation and dif-

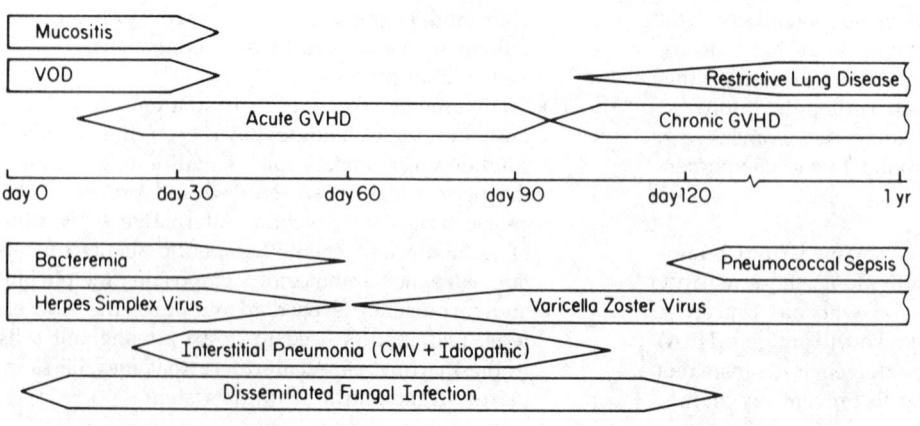

Figure 17–13. Temporal sequence of major complications after allogenic bone marrow transplantation, from day 0 to 1 year after transplantation. (Reprinted from Press OW, Schaller RT, and Thomas ED. *Complications of Organ Transplantation.* New York: Marcel Dekker, 1987, by courtesy of Marcel Dekker, Inc.)

ferentiation by the administration of cytokines. Most biotherapy remains investigational. Despite great promise, the development of biotherapy as the 4th modality of cancer treatment has been slow and frustrating. Only a few biotherapies have been approved by the FDA for specific cancers. Immunotherapy can be active or passive. Cytokine therapy uses specific cytokines that either are cytotoxic or are growth factors involved in cell proliferation and differentiation.

a. Active immunotherapy uses nonspecific agents (e.g., interferons, interleukins) or specific agents (e.g., vaccines) to stimulate a general response.

   (1) Interferon: Interferons are a family of proteins with 3 major groups: alpha, beta, and gamma. Originally discovered by their antiviral activity, interferons also modulate the immune response, enhance the expression of cell surface antigens, and decrease proliferation by lengthening the cell cycle of both normal and tumor cells.

     • Interferon-α is approved by the FDA for use in hairy cell leukemia, Kaposi's sarcoma, and renal cell carcinoma. Other uses in cancer treatment are investigational. Interferon-β and interferon-γ are investigational.

     • Interferon-α is administered subcutaneously, intramuscularly, or intravenously in daily doses ranging from 2 to 9 million units. Individuals are usually taught to self-administer interferon.

     • Toxicities of interferon are an acute flulike syndrome of fever, fatigue, chills, myalgias, and headache; anorexia, weight loss; hypotension, tachycardia, and arrhythmias; and dizziness, lethargy, and depression. The severity and frequency of toxicities are related to the dosage and the age of the person.

   (2) Interleukins: The interleukins (12 are known) are proteins produced by activated lymphocytes or macrophages. They have widespread effects in all phases of T-cell activity. They have no cytotoxic effect.

     • Interleukin-2 is administered intravenously as a bolus or continuous infusion in dosages ranging from 6 to 42 million units per 24 hours. The antitumor activity is dose and schedule dependent.

     • Interleukin-2 has a wide range of toxicities, and most people are treated in intensive care units. The toxicities are reversible after discontinuing the drug. Toxicities include diffuse rash, nausea, vomiting, anorexia, and diarrhea. A capillary leak syndrome of intravascular volume depletion with fluid retention and interstitial edema occurs. Cardiac arrhythmias, myocardial infarction, hallucinations, disorientation, anemia, and thrombocytopenia are other side effects.

   (3) Bacille Calmette-Guérin (BCG): This is a strain of *Mycobacterium bovis*, originally designed as a vaccine against tuberculosis. Its use has been investigated extensively in colon, breast, bladder, and renal cancers and in malignant melanomas, although treatment of bladder cancer is now its sole use.

     • Bacille Calmette-Guérin is administered intravesically in dosages ranging from 10 to 100 million bacilli on a weekly basis for 6 months. People receiving BCG must have a small tumor and be immunocompetent.

     • Systemic side effects include fever, chills, malaise, headache, and weakness. Local side effects are bladder irritability, frequency, urgency, and dysuria.

   (4) Vaccines: Vaccines against cancer have been tested over many years for leukemia; ovarian, lung, and renal cancers; melanomas; and sarcomas. To date, no satisfactory vaccine has been developed.

b. Passive immunotherapy involves transfer of immunologic cells or antibodies that have the ability to mediate antitumor responses.

   (1) Monoclonal antibodies: Unconjugated or "naked" monoclonal antibodies can produce an antitumor effect either by direct cytotoxicity or by activating cytotoxic cells in the immune system.

     • Monoclonal antibodies can be conjugated to drug molecules, toxins, and radionuclides that can deliver cytotoxic products selectively to cancer cells. Clinical studies now are evaluating these methods.

     • Side effects of monoclonal antibody therapy are fever, chills, flushing, urticaria, nausea, and vomiting. Anaphylactic reactions can occur in those with high levels of human antimouse antibodies.

   (2) Cells (i.e., adoptive immunotherapy): Lymphokine-activated cells are produced by exposing peripheral blood mononuclear cells to high concentrations of interleukin-2. These lymphokine-activated cells are capable of lysing tumor cells but do not destroy normal cells.

c. Cytotoxic cytokines. Tumor necrosis factor (TNF) shows dramatic necrosis in established tumors in animals, but this activity has not been demonstrated in human tumors unless TNF is injected directly into the tumor.

   (1) Currently in clinical trials, TNF is used in combination with chemotherapy and biologic response modifiers to eradicate tumors.

   (2) Tumor necrosis factor can be administered intravenously or subcutaneously, although the latter route can produce severe inflammation.

   (3) Side effects are fever, chills, rigors, headache, fatigue, hypotension, and thrombocytopenia.

d. Cytokines (growth factors). Hematopoietic colony-stimulating factors are growth factors essential for the proliferation, differentiation, and maturation of blood cells. Of the many that have been identified and cloned, 3 have FDA approval.

   (1) Erythropoietin is a cytokine produced in the kidneys in response to hypoxemia. Originally used to treat the anemia of end-stage renal disease, erythropoietin is also used to treat the reduced erythrocyte count of myelosuppressed individuals. It is administered 3 times weekly by subcutaneous injection. Side effects are mild hypertension.

(2) Granulocyte-macrophage colony-stimulating factor is produced by T cells stimulating the production of neutrophils, basophils, eosinophils, monocytes, erythrocytes, and megakaryocytes. Its use in clinical trials has shown shortened periods of neutropenia but no effect on thrombocytopenia. Administered intravenously or subcutaneously in varying dosages, it causes such transient side effects as fever, myalgia, bone pain, and nausea.

(3) Granulocyte colony-stimulating factor influences maturation of granulocytes. It has been demonstrated to shorten the period of neutropenia when given to people receiving various cytotoxic drugs. It is approved by the FDA for use in cases of neutropenia associated with chemotherapy. Administered subcutaneously, its mild side effects are bone pain, myalgias, and skin rash.

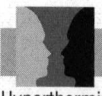 **CLINICAL CONTROVERSIES**

Hyperthermia, the application of heat to tumors, is an investigational therapy based on the greater sensitivity of tumor cells to heat. Investigations, however, have been plagued by technologic difficulties. Photodynamic therapy exploits the selective higher concentration of photosensitizing compounds (porphyrins) by tumor cells. When sensitized cells are exposed to a light source (laser) in the presence of oxygen, a cytotoxic effect occurs. Gene therapy offers new approaches to cancer therapy by repairing cells rather than destroying them. Current investigations are focused on developing safe methods of delivering genes into the cell nucleus.

Cancer Rehabilitation

1. Rehabilitation is a dynamic process directed toward enabling persons to function at their maximum level but within the limitations of the disease or disability. Rehabilitation involves the physical, mental, emotional, social, and economic potential of the person involved.
2. Rehabilitation goals must be determined concurrently with treatment goals. Although rehabilitation may occur after a procedure (e.g., speech therapy after a laryngectomy), it is an ongoing process for most people with cancer.
3. Goals of rehabilitation are preventive measures designed to improve physical functioning and reduce morbidity and disability, restorative measures designed to return the person with cancer to optimal functional status, supportive measures to lessen disability when cancer is persistent, and palliative measures to improve the quality of remaining life when cancer is advanced.
4. Changes that occur from cancer and its treatment can affect all aspects of life: physical, psychologic, social, and economic. Changes can be temporary, permanent, progressive, or static.
   a. Physical changes can include changes in structure and function of particular organs (e.g., colostomy) or general changes in function (e.g., deterioration of muscle strength or fatigue).
   b. Psychologic functioning may be impaired because of cognitive changes related to medications or physical changes. Loss of self-esteem can be related to changes in body image, sexuality, and relationships resulting from changes in appearance or functioning.
   c. Changes can occur in family roles and functioning, work, and friendships.
   d. Economic issues are significant for most people with cancer, if treatment is long-term. Loss of work or other sources of money may intensify the problem.
5. Whereas medical interventions focus mainly on treatment, many nursing interventions are related to rehabilitation and improving the quality of life for people with cancer. Most health care institutions do not have formal rehabilitative services, and nurses can serve as important advocates in meeting rehabilitative needs for people with cancer.

Psychosocial Effects and Intervention

1. The variables that define psychosocial problems are age, developmental stage, personality, cognitive functioning, and spiritual orientation (see p. 592).
2. Psychologic problems during primary treatment can be overwhelming, especially if the duration of treatment is long.
   a. Uncertainties: Survival in cancer is never guaranteed, and the person with cancer knows survival only in retrospect. If initial treatment is successful, then the potential of recurrence may be a constant reminder of vulnerability. Complications from treatment may not be evident for years.
   b. Negative feelings: Maintaining emotional stability is difficult in long-term treatment. People with cancer may feel angry, anxious, discouraged, sad, depressed, and lonely.
   c. Loss of self-esteem: Cancer treatment causes many physical changes in body image (e.g., alopecia from chemotherapy or radiation therapy, changes in secondary sex characteristics from hormone therapy, weight loss, facial edema from steroid therapy, skin changes from radiation). Changes in work function and family and community roles also can cause loss of self-esteem.
   d. Loss of control: Cancer runs the life of people on aggressive, long-term cancer treatment. Work or school schedules, family activities, and daily life can be dictated by treatment schedules. People with cancer struggle to gain some control over their lives while undergoing treatment.
3. Facilitating coping and adaptation
   a. Helping people with cancer cope with uncertainties includes the following:
      (1) Determining the knowledge deficits of the person regarding disease, treatment, symptom management, protocols, routine procedures, and so forth
      (2) Assisting the person with cancer in identifying what information is needed
      (3) Providing appropriate information and resources where information can be obtained
   b. Helping people with cancer cope with negative feelings includes the following:
      (1) Assisting the person in recognizing and expressing feelings

(2) Listening to the person's expression of emotions
(3) Helping the person with cancer identify resources or methods of expression of feelings through support groups; relaxation techniques; humor, art, or recreation; exploring the use of spiritual resources; and conveying an attitude of realistic hope.
c. Helping people with cancer cope with changes in body image includes the following:
(1) Providing anticipatory guidance for body changes that are predictable
(2) Monitoring for statements of self-criticism, ability to look at the changed part, and statements regarding changes
(3) Helping the person to separate physical changes from feelings of self-worth
(4) Promoting an atmosphere of acceptance
(5) Helping the person to identify ways and resources to enhance appearance and minimize defects
(6) Identifying support groups available to people with similar problems (e.g., ostomy, laryngectomy groups)
d. Helping people with cancer cope with loss of control includes the following:
(1) Helping the person identify things that can be controlled
(2) Assisting the person in understanding that physical fatigue and stress reduce decision-making ability
(3) Helping the person to identify long- and short-term goals
(4) Arranging situations in which the person's autonomy is enhanced
(5) Providing resource information for problem resolution

◼ COMPLICATIONS OF CANCER

Cancer Pain

1. The experience or the anticipation of pain is the most feared and dreaded complication of cancer, compromising the quality of life for most people with cancer.
2. Persistent pain occurs in 70 to 90 percent of terminally ill cancer patients. Moderate to severe pain occurs in 40 to 50 percent of patients with early- or intermediate-stage cancer.
3. Cancer pain can be controlled in 90 to 95 percent of cases, but undertreatment of cancer pain is a worldwide phenomenon, with 25 to 80 percent of people with cancer living with uncontrolled pain. Inadequate pain control can result from undertreatment by health care professionals, the person with cancer's fears of addiction, cultural beliefs, or inadequate compliance due to side effects. The magnitude of the problem is evidenced by the worldwide attention paid to pain by the World Health Organization, many state pain initiatives, and professional organizations that address control of pain.
4. Sources of pain
a. Approximately 75 percent of pain is tumor related. Causes of pain are the following:

(1) Tissue damage causing necrosis, ulceration, and infection
(2) Tumor erosion, with infiltration of nerves
(3) Obstruction or infiltration of blood vessels, causing ischemia (arterial) or edema and engorgement (venous)
(4) Obstructions of hollow organs (e.g., bowel obstruction)
(5) Pressure from tumor growth in tight compartments (e.g., pain from stretching of Glisson's capsule in liver metastasis)
b. Cancer therapies account for 20 percent of cancer pain through injuries to nerves or pain-sensitive structures from chemotherapy (peripheral neuropathies), radiation therapy, or surgery (e.g., postmastectomy pain syndrome, postthoracotomy pain syndrome).
c. Pain unrelated to cancer accounts for 5 percent of pain reported by people with cancer. Pressure sores, peptic ulcers, constipation, and osteoarthritis are other causes of pain.
5. Temporal classifications of pain
a. Acute cancer-related pain can be caused by tumor or tumor-related therapies (e.g., postoperative pain). Acute pain is of limited duration, with a defined onset, and is associated with symptoms of sympathetic stimulation (e.g., sweating, tachycardia). The cause of acute pain can usually be determined easily and managed by treatment of the underlying cancer or the use of analgesics, or both.
b. Chronic cancer-related pain persists for more than 3 months. Signs of sympathetic stimulation are absent, but changes in mood, gait, and facial expression are seen. Alterations in appetite, sleep, and concentration and irritability are prominent.
(1) Chronic pain is caused by tumor progression or syndromes related to cancer therapies (e.g., postmastectomy pain syndrome, postherpetic neuralgia).
(2) Pain related to tumor progression increases in severity with tumor infiltration of bone, nerves, and soft tissue adjacent to the tumor. Fear of death and hopelessness are related psychologic factors.
6. Pain assessment
a. Determining the source of pain is accomplished through a detailed medical history with a physical examination and a thorough neurologic examination. Diagnostic tests may be ordered.
b. Determining the nature of the pain is accomplished through a detailed pain history, use of pain assessment tools, and a psychologic evaluation of the person with cancer.
c. Pain assessment should occur regularly and systematically. People's reports of pain should always be believed (see Chapter 11).
7. Pain control requires multimodal treatment with analgesics and other approaches. Removing the cause of pain is limited in treatment-related syndromes. Pain management is difficult and complicated in people with cancer who have had preexisting chronic pain syndromes related to noncancer causes or a history of drug abuse (see Chapter 11).

a. The large numbers of people suffering with cancer pain, along with the known undertreatment of cancer pain, are of sufficient magnitude to consider this a public health problem. To promote better pain management, the Agency for Health Care Policy and Research of the Public Health Service has developed *Clinical Practice Guidelines in the Management of Cancer Pain*, a monograph available free of charge to health professionals and people with cancer.

b. Pain management begins with the analgesic ladder developed by the World Health Organization (Fig. 17–14). As pain increases, stronger opioids are added to the treatment regimen. Additional measures of pain control are added as the pain assessment dictates. Treatment of the cause of the pain by surgery, chemotherapy, or radiation should begin simultaneously whenever possible.

c. Analgesics
   (1) Analgesic ladder. Mild pain is treated with a nonopioid analgesic or nonsteroidal anti-inflammatory drug (NSAID). Adjuvant medications may or may not be added (see Fig. 17–14).
   • An opioid is added if pain persists or if pain is moderate at initial assessment.
   • If pain is severe or persists, the potency or dosage of the opioid should be increased.
   • All medications must be individualized for the person with cancer.
   (2) Routes of administration
   • The simplest and least invasive methods should be used.
   • The oral route is preferred for its convenience and cost effectiveness.
   • If the oral route cannot be used, the least invasive other routes (i.e., transdermal and rectal)

should be considered. If these are ineffective, then intravenous or subcutaneous routes with portable or implanted pumps should be considered.
   • Intraspinal systems (epidural, intrathecal, and intracerebral ventricular routes) should be used only if maximal doses of systemic drugs fail to control pain.
   • Intramuscular administration should be avoided. It is painful and inconvenient, and drug absorption is not reliable.
   (3) Medications should be administered around the clock and not on an as necessary basis. Anticipation and prevention of pain is most effective. Breakthrough pain can occur spontaneously or with a specific activity such as walking or eating. Supplementing the pain prevention regimen with a short-acting analgesic with rapid onset of action controls breakthrough pain.
   (4) Addiction rarely occurs in people with cancer who have chronic cancer pain. Physical dependence and opioid tolerance are expected with long-term treatment and should not be confused with psychologic addiction. Discontinuation of opioids, if necessary, should be done gradually to avoid withdrawal symptoms.
   (5) Side effects
   • Constipation is one of the most common side effects of opioid use. Opioids inhibit peristalsis, requiring use of cathartics if these are not contraindicated. Increased fluid intake, stool softeners, and fiber may be added.
   • Sedation is also a frequent side effect, but tolerance develops. If sedation is persistent, switching to another opioid or administering stimulants (e.g., caffeine) may be helpful.
   • Nausea and vomiting may occur and can be treated with antiemetics.
   • Respiratory depression occurs in long-term opioid users when pain is relieved abruptly and not opposed by the stimulating effects of pain. Respiratory depression can be relieved by the use of naloxone, but this drug must be titrated carefully so as not to reverse the analgesic effect of the opioid with the reversal of respiratory depression.

d. Nonnarcotics. Empiric use of several classes of drugs provides analgesia in specific situations either by direct analgesic effect or by increasing the analgesic effect of the opioids.

e. Noninvasive pain management
   (1) Cutaneous stimulation through massage, acupressure, vibration, and transcutaneous electrical nerve stimulation (TENS) have a role in managing mild pain, often in conjunction with drug therapy.
   (2) Heat and cold applications may be helpful in selected individuals.
   (3) Maintaining mobility and function through recreational, physical, or occupational therapy can prevent pain due to inactivity and immobilization as well as counteract a depressive mood.

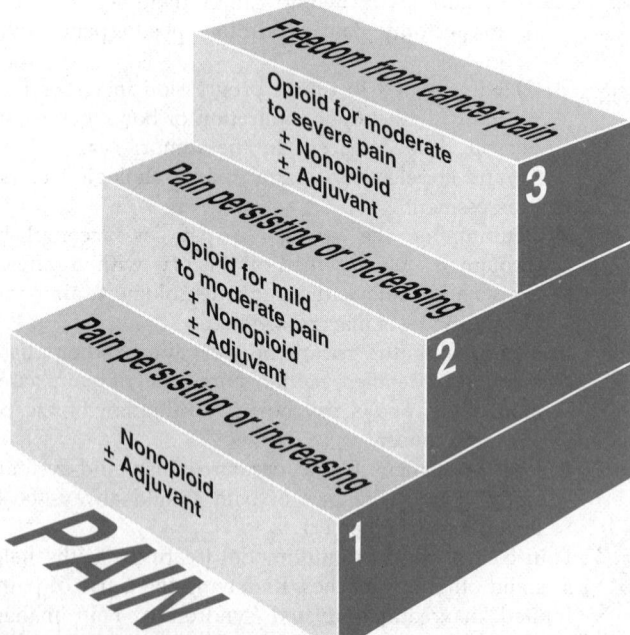

Figure 17–14. The analgesic ladder. (Reproduced by permission of World Health Organization (WHO) from *Cancer Pain Relief*. 2nd ed. Geneva: World Health Organization, 1996.)

f. Invasive pain management: Cancer pain can be treated with anesthetic procedures or with neuroablative and neurostimulatory procedures in selected situations (see Chapter 11).

g. Psychologic pain management: Pain is intensified by many psychologic states such as anxiety and depression. Short-term psychotherapy often can be helpful in providing the person with coping strategies.

Superior Vena Cava Syndrome

1. The superior vena cava is a thin-walled structure with low intravascular pressure. Venous return from the head, chest, and upper extremities can be impeded by extrinsic tumor growth or lymph node enlargement. If the process occurs slowly, collateral circulation develops. If tumor growth has been rapid, an emergency arises. Ninety percent of superior vena cava syndrome cases are caused by malignant tumors, especially lung cancers. Occasionally, this syndrome is the presenting sign of lung cancer.
2. Symptoms of superior vena cava syndrome are chest pain, tachypnea, cough, and hoarseness. Facial swelling and distention of veins over the neck and chest wall are physical signs.
3. Radiation therapy to the obstructing tumor is the usual therapy. Chemotherapy may be used in small-cell lung cancers or lymphomas that are chemoresponsive. Maintaining a high Fowler's position and using oxygen therapy, diuretics, and corticosteroids may be helpful in supportive treatment.

Cardiac Tamponade

1. Impairment of heart filling during diastole can occur when pericardial fluid produced by tumor cells accumulates in the pericardial sac or when the pericardium becomes fibrotic or constricted following radiation therapy. Lung, breast, and esophageal tumors can invade the pericardium directly. If the pericardial fluid accumulates rapidly, circulatory collapse can result.
2. Symptoms of cardiac tamponade are anxiety, chest pain, dyspnea, and cough. Signs of cardiac tamponade relate to rapidity of fluid accumulation. Hypotension, cyanosis, pulsus paradoxus, and pericardial rub are frequent signs.
3. Echocardiography is the most specific and sensitive diagnostic tool. Typical changes are also seen on chest radiograph and electrocardiogram.
4. Treatment of cardiac tamponade depends on its severity. Pericardiocentesis is done as an emergency therapeutic procedure. A pericardial window, pericardiectomy, or sclerosis of the pericardium are other treatment options.

Hemorrhage

1. Bleeding can occur from any tumor surface; occasionally, tumors invade blood vessels and cause profuse bleeding.
2. Gastrointestinal, bladder, pelvic, and head and neck tumors most often cause bleeding problems. Treatment is specific to the site.

Disseminated Intravascular Coagulation

1. Disseminated intravascular coagulation can occur during intensive chemotherapy in leukemia and is thought to be related to the release of tissue thromboplastins, proteases, or interleukins released from blast cells.
2. This condition also occurs as a sequelae of sepsis.

Septic Shock

1. Septic shock causes circulatory collapse, irreversible organ damage, and death unless bacteremia and sepsis are recognized and treated promptly.
2. Myelosuppression from treatment, tumor, poor nutrition, and advanced disease are factors in the development of bacteremia. Sources of infection can be endogenous (e.g., the person's microbacterial flora) or exogenous (e.g., catheters).
3. Early signs of sepsis—fever, shaking, chills, tachycardia, or decreased sensorium—must be recognized in the neutropenic patient. Cultures are drawn, and antibiotic treatment is instituted promptly.

Upper Airway Obstruction

1. Obstruction of the trachea or bronchus can occur at any point. Lung, head and neck, and thyroid tumors and lymphomas most commonly cause airway obstructions.
2. Symptoms depend on the severity of the obstruction.
3. Radiation therapy to the obstructed area with initial high doses can be given. Intraluminal obstruction to the bronchus can be relieved by bronchoscopic laser treatment or photodynamic therapy. Additional chemotherapy is given to responsive tumors (e.g., lymphomas and small cell lung cancers).

Pleural Effusions

1. The quantity of fluid accumulation produced by tumor implants on the visceral and parietal pleura or impairment of fluid drainage by mediastinal tumor varies. Malignant pleural effusions most often result from metastatic breast and lung cancers and lymphomas. They can be asymptomatic or sufficiently large to produce respiratory insufficiency.
2. Dyspnea and unproductive cough are common symptoms.
3. Chest radiographs reveal most pleural effusions.
4. Malignant pleural effusions (usually confirmed by cytologic studies) are treated by thoracentesis. Chest tube drainage and pleural sclerosing may be necessary if fluid reaccumulates.

Hypercalcemia

1. High levels of serum calcium (above 13 mg/dL) can arise when the calcium mobilization from bone exceeds the capacity of the kidneys to excrete it. Bone metastasis is present in 80 percent of patients with hypercalcemia. Some tumors that produce peptides that function as parathormone also produce hypercalcemia without bone metastasis. Tumors of the lung, breast, pancreas, kidney, and ovary, as well as squamous cell head and neck cancers most often produce hypercalcemia.
2. People with hypercalcemia experience fatigue, anorexia, nausea, vomiting, constipation, polyuria, and polydypsia. Untreated hypercalcemia can progress to altered mental status, seizures, coma, and death.
3. Elevated serum ionized calcium levels are diagnostic of hypercalcemia.
4. Treatment depends on the severity of the condition. Hydration with normal saline, plicamycin (mithramycin), calcitonin, corticosteroids, or diphosphonates depends on the person's condition and underlying disease. Long-term control of hypercalcemia is achieved by treatment of the underlying tumor (see Chapter 9).

Hyponatremia

1. The syndrome of inappropriate antidiuretic hormone (SIADH) most often occurs in small-cell lung cancers.
2. Brain metastases or treatment with cyclophosphamide and vincristine can produce this syndrome by disturbing hypothalamic and pituitary function.

Acute Tumor Lysis Syndrome

1. Hyperuricemia, hyperkalemia, hyperphosphatemia, and hypocalcemia occur in acute tumor lysis syndrome. Individuals with highly proliferative tumors, especially leukemia and lymphomas, who are undergoing chemotherapy or radiation that produces a highly volume of destroyed cells can develop this syndrome.
2. Prophylactic treatment with allopurinol to increase uric acid excretion, alkalinization of urine, hydration, and frequent monitoring and correction of electrolyte imbalances can prevent development of acute tumor lysis syndrome and renal dysfunction.

Esophageal Obstruction

1. Obstruction of the lumen of the esophagus most often is caused by primary esophageal cancers, but mediastinal lymphomas and lung cancers can obstruct the lumen by external compression.
2. Increasing dysphagia, weight loss, and aspiration of oral secretions are symptomatic of obstruction.
3. Obstruction is easily identified by esophagogram and esophagoscopy.
4. Treatment depends on the extent of the disease and the size of the obstructing tumor. Surgery, radiation, and chemotherapy may be used. In advanced disease, partial tumor ablation with laser therapy, or stent placement can provide temporary patency.

Bowel Obstruction and Perforation

1. Peritoneal carcinomatosis can produce single or multiple bowel obstructions with an associated risk of perforation. Ovarian, gastrointestinal, and breast cancers are associated with obstructions.
2. Treatment depends on the extent of disease and the condition of the person. Surgical correction is preferred if possible, but may be excluded if extensive abdominal carcinomatosis exists.

Ascites

1. Ascites can be caused by obstruction of the subdiaphragmatic lymphatics or by fluid production of metastatic peritoneal tumors.
2. Hepatic metastases can cause portal hypertension and hypoalbuminemia, resulting in ascites.

Ureteral Obstruction

1. Bilateral ureteral obstruction, which can progress to renal failure, is most often caused by advanced genitourinary tumors (cervical, bladder, or prostate) or by large retroperitoneal tumors.
2. Obstructions can be relieved by percutaneous nephrostomy followed by ureteral stent placement.

Spinal Cord Compression

1. Metastasis to a vertebral body or pedicle with erosion into the anterior or anterolateral epidural space or direct extension by paraspinal tumor can cause spinal cord compression with irreversible damage if untreated. Lung, breast, prostate, and kidney cancers and lymphoma are the most frequent tumors associated with spinal cord compression.
2. Sudden, unusual pain in the back or neck, which can be described as local or radicular pain is the most common symptom. Pain is described as constant and is increased by coughing or straining. Leg weakness, numbness, paresthesias, and loss of bowel and bladder control signal progressive compression.
3. Prompt diagnosis is important to prevent irreversible nerve damage. MRI has replaced myelography as best diagnostic technique.
4. Steroids are given to reduce edema. Radiation therapy is used if the person has not been irradiated previously. Laminectomy and chemotherapy are also therapeutic options for some people.

Severe Depression

1. Clinical depression occurs in approximately 6 percent of the general population. The incidence in cancer patients varies between studies from 4.5 to 50 percent. Persons with pancreatic and head and neck cancers have the highest incidence of depression.
2. The diagnosis of depression in people with cancer is particularly difficult because some of the somatic symptoms of depression are also the symptoms of cancer. The criteria for the diagnosis of major depression are dysphoria (feelings of unhappiness) and anhedonia (lack of pleasure); physical signs such as sleep disorder, appetite change, fatigue, and psychomotor retardation or agitation; and psychologic symptoms such as low self-esteem, guilt, poor concentration, indecisiveness, and suicidal ideation. Any 4 of the physical or psychologic symptoms in combination with dysphoria and anhydonia lasting more than 2 weeks are diagnostic of major depression.
3. The diagnosis of depression is difficult in people with cancer because feelings of sadness are normal responses to losses common with this illness. Many of the medications used in treatment (e.g., steroids) can also cause depression.
4. Diagnosing depression is important in people with cancer because it hinders coping and increases morbidity and overall disability. Likewise, it is a major factor in suicide.
5. People with depressive symptoms should be referred to a psychiatrist for diagnosis and antidepressant therapy when appropriate.

Suicide

1. Although suicide is rare in people with cancer, the relative risk is twice that of the general population.
2. Depression is a major factor in 50 percent of suicides. People with depression are at 25 times greater risk for committing suicide. Advanced illness, poor prognosis, uncontrolled pain, hopelessness, prior suicide attempt, and family history of suicide are other factors.
3. People with risk factors should be assessed for suicide risk and referred for psychiatric consultation. Treating pain, anxiety, and depression and providing social support to help the person cope may prevent suicide and the devastating sequelae on family and friends.

Altered Nutrition and Cancer Cachexia

1. People with cancer vary greatly in the nutritional problems they encounter. Some patients can maintain their food intake and weight throughout their illness, whereas others experience anorexia and weight loss as presenting symptoms.
2. Weight loss and malnutrition can be related to either decreased nutrient intake secondary to cancer treatment or its sequelae or to cancer cachexia.
   a. Decreased nutrient intake related to cancer treatment can be the result of inability to take in food caused by such conditions as nausea, stomatitis, dysphagia, xerostomia, surgical resection of the tongue, pharynx, or stomach or of loss of nutrients through vomiting, diarrhea, fistulas, or surgical procedures that decrease the absorptive surface of the small intestine. Psychologic factors—depression, anxiety, and stress—can also decrease appetite and food intake.
   b. **Cancer cachexia** is a paraneoplastic syndrome characterized by anorexia, early satiety, weakness, weight loss, and muscle wasting.
      (1) Currently, cachexia is believed to be caused by peptides and cytokines that are released from normal cells in response to the tumor. Tumor necrosis factor, interferon-γ, interleukin-1, and interleukin-6 may be involved in cachexia development.
      (2) Diagnosis of cachexia is based on symptoms. Generally, weight loss greater than 10 percent is considered cachexia.
      (3) The severity of cachexia is not correlated to tumor size, type of tumor, or extent of disease. More commonly seen in advanced disease, cachexia also occurs in localized cancers.
      (4) Weight loss in cachexia results from decreased nutrient intake and altered metabolism. Decreased nutrient intake is affected by anorexia and early satiety. Abnormalities in taste and aversion to red meat are common. Increased energy expenditure has been demonstrated in some studies. In normal malnutrition, the body reduces its basal metabolic rate, but in people with cancer, it is elevated. Protein, carbohydrate, and fat metabolism are altered, resulting in increased glucose production, decreases in body fat and protein catabolism, and muscle wasting. (Normal responses to starvation are decreased glucose production and muscle sparing.)
3. Adequate nutrition is vital for maintaining immunocompetence and resisting infection. Assessment of nutritional status is important to determine the need and extent of nutritional support. Although many sophisticated measures are available, simple assessment measures exist.
   a. Malnutrition can be determined if the person exhibits unexplained weight loss of 10 percent or more of body weight, serum transferrin less than 150 mg per dL, and serum albumin less than 3.4 gm per dL. Meeting 2 of the 3 criteria indicates a need for nutritional support.
   b. The subjective global assessment gives a clinical determination of malnutrition (Box 17–7).
4. The goal of nutritional support must be determined before intervention to determine the extent of therapy.
   a. Oral nutrition may suffice for those who are nourished or mildly malnourished but are undergoing

BOX 17–7. Components of the Subjective Global Assessment

History

Weight change over time
Change in dietary intake relative to normal
Presence of gastrointestinal symptoms for over 2 weeks
Change in functional capacity
Concurrent diseases or stress

Physical Examination

Evidence of loss of subcutaneous fat stores
Evidence of muscle wasting
Presence of ascites
Presence of ankle or sacral edema

Diagnostic Categories

Well nourished
Minimally malnourished
Severely malnourished

Abstracted, with permission, from Detsky AS, et al. What is subjective global assessment of nutritional status? *JPEN* 11:8, 1987.

temporary impairment of nutritional intake or increased nutrient losses. Chemotherapy and radiation therapy produce a range of side effects that impair nutrition. Interventions listed in Table 17–20 may assist many people with cancer to maintain adequate intake. Antidepressant therapy can reduce anorexia caused by depression. Symptomatic treatment of stomatitis and mucositis also improves intake. Metoclopramide can be used to improve gastric emptying. Hydrazine, dexamethasone, and megestrol acetate can be used empirically to improve nutritional intake.
  b. Enteral therapy is indicated for those who are unable to maintain adequate oral intake but have a functioning gastrointestinal system. Short-term therapy can be accomplished with a small-bore feeding tube. Long-term management requires a gastrostomy or jejunostomy tube.
  c. Parenteral therapy is indicated for those in whom the gastrointestinal tract cannot provide nutrient intake (e.g., cases of fistulas, obstructions, malabsorption, or severe malnourishment). Peripheral or central venous access can be used to provide parenteral nutrition.

 CLINICAL CONTROVERSIES

The role of total parenteral nutrition (TPN) in therapy for cancer patients is very controversial. No conclusive evidence of improved survival or response to treatment has been determined for TPN use during aggressive chemotherapy and radiation therapy. In the perioperative period and during bone marrow transplantation TPN has been useful for malnourished and high-risk patients. During advanced disease or terminal-stage illness, TPN has not been shown to be effective and may be detrimental. Some evidence shows that nutritional therapy increases tumor growth.

NURSING DIAGNOSIS: Altered nutrition: less than body requirements R/T cachexia (anorexia, early satiety, increased metabolic requirements)

1. *Expected outcomes*: Following interventions, the person with cancer and caregivers will do the following:
   a. Demonstrate knowledge and techniques to maintain adequate nutrition.
   b. Identify the source of the symptom and seek treatment of the cause.
   c. Demonstrate the ability to manage tube feedings, if required.
   d. Verbalize any signs or symptoms that require reporting to the appropriate person in health care.
2. *Nursing interventions*
   a. Evaluate dietary intake or caloric intake.
   b. Measure height, weight, blood chemistries, serum albumin, serum transferrin, and absolute white blood count.
   c. Identify factors related to inadequate intake.
   d. Obtain treatment for causes of inadequate intake, when appropriate.
   e. Teach good oral hygiene.
   f. Teach psychologic techniques (e.g., distraction, imagery, socialization, and relaxation to improve caloric intake).
   g. Teach high-protein, high-calorie diet.
   h. Teach use of antiemetics.
   i. Provide written materials (see Table 17–20 for additional hints).

Paraneoplastic Syndromes

1. **Paraneoplastic syndromes** are symptom complexes that are not produced directly by the tumor or its metastases. Often called remote or systemic effects of malignancy, paraneoplastic syndromes represent a diverse group of symptoms affecting many body systems (Table 17–21).
2. Occurring in 10 to 15 percent of cancer patients, paraneoplastic syndromes can be caused by production of hormones by the tumor affecting the target organ, proteins secreted by the tumor (e.g., colony-stimulating factors), proteins produced by normal cells in response to tumors (e.g., TNF), and antibodies produced in response to the cancer.
3. Paraneoplastic syndromes occur most frequently with lung tumors, although they can occur with any cancer.
4. Paraneoplastic effects can be manifested as endocrine, neuromuscular, cutaneous, hematologic, gastrointestinal, renal, or connective tissue disorders.
5. Although paraneoplastic syndromes have been known clinically for many years, precise causes are now being determined as cellular technology permits identification of tumor genes and proteins.
6. Paraneoplastic syndromes can be the 1st manifestation of a malignancy.
7. Recognition of paraneoplastic syndromes is important. Some can be fatal if not recognized and treated. They can mimic metastatic disease and confuse treatment.
8. Treatment is aimed at tumor control, which also controls the symptoms of the syndrome.

Table 17–20. Suggestions for Improving Nutrition

Symptom	Suggestions
Anorexia	Eat small meals more often Keep snacks for nibbling Rely on foods you love Make food attractive Eat in pleasant surroundings with good company
Taste changes	Use other protein sources (e.g., eggs, chicken, cheese, fish) if taste for red meat is lost Tart foods (e.g., orange juice, pickles, lemonade, vinegar) may enhance flavors Wines, beer, or mayonnaise improves taste of soups and sauces Marinating meat in sweet fruit juices, wines, or Italian dressing improves flavor; use more and stronger seasonings Eat foods that are cold or at room temperature
Early satiety	Eat smaller meals more often Keep nutritional snacks around Chew foods slowly Make sure that liquids you drink have nutritional content Drink liquids 30 to 60 min before meals
Nausea	Eat smaller portions lower in fat content Eat salty foods and avoid overly sweet foods Eat dry foods, especially after getting up in morning Do not eat foods you like when you are nauseated Clear, cool beverages (e.g., clear soups, gelatin, ginger ale, popsicles, ice cubes) are usually retained best Avoid liquids at mealtimes—take 30 to 60 min before eating Loose clothing and fresh air can help Take antinausea medications If the smell of food makes you nauseated, let someone else do the cooking; stay in another room until food is prepared; do not prepare fried foods or those with distinct odors (e.g., coffee); use prepared foods from a freezer that can be prepared at low temperatures If you have pain or a swollen stomach before nausea and vomiting that is relieved by vomiting, call your doctor
Difficulty chewing or swallowing (because of soreness or dryness)	Try a softer diet Use a blender; food tastes better if it is cooked before blended Cut meats into small pieces; add gravy Use butter, gravies, sauces, soft foods (e.g., yogurt, mashed potatoes, custards, cheese); soak foods in coffee, tea, milk Avoid spices, rough coarse foods, hard toast, acidic foods like orange juice and tomatoes Eat lukewarm or cold rather than hot foods; cold foods can be soothing; eat ice cream and popsicles Do not smoke or drink; use a humidifier in your house Rinse your mouth frequently
Diarrhea	Use less fiber; use only cooked vegetables, omitting those with seeds and tough skins (e.g., beans, broccoli, corn, onions, garlic, bread, and nuts) If you have large quantities of diarrhea, you may have lost enough potassium to feel weak; eat foods high in potassium (e.g., bananas, apricot nectar, fish, potatoes, and meat) If you have cramps, stay away from foods that may encourage gas (e.g., carbonated drinks, beer, beans, cabbage, cauliflower, highly spiced foods, sweets, and gum) Avoid fatty foods that are highly spiced Drink liquids between meals Do not skip meals
Constipation	Include fruits, vegetables, whole-grain breads and cereals, dried fruits, and nuts in your diet Add one or more tablespoons of bran to your foods Try high-fiber snack foods, such as sesame sticks or date nut bread Drink 8 to 10 glasses of liquid per day Drink hot lemon water in the morning or prune juice at night

Adapted from National Institutes of Health. *Eating Hints. Recipes and Tips for Better Nutrition During Treatment*. Bethesda, MD: U.S. Department of Health, Education, and Welfare, Publ. No. (NIH) 80-2079, 1980.

Recurrent Cancer

1. Cancer can recur locally at the site of the primary tumor or at a distant site, causing metastasis.
2. Cancer recurrence at the original site of the tumor can be treated; in a small percentage of cases, treatment leads to subsequent cures. Breast cancer can recur locally and be reexcised. Occasionally, radiation therapy is used to treat local recurrence. Recurrent hematologic malignancies can be treated with chemotherapy and subsequent cure.

Table 17–21. Some Neoplastic Syndromes

Clinical Syndromes	Major Forms of Underlying Cancer	Causal Mechanisms
Endocrinopathies		
Cushing's syndrome	Small cell cancer of the lung	ACTH or ACTH-like substance
	Pancreatic carcinoma	
	Neural tumors	
Hyponatremia	Small cell carcinoma of lung	Antidiuretic hormone or atrial natriuretic factor
	Intracranial neoplasms	
Hypercalcemia	Squamous cell carcinoma of lung	PTH-like substance, TGF-α, vitamin D
	Breast carcinoma	
	Renal carcinoma	
Carcinoid syndrome	Bronchial carcinoid	Serotonin, bradykinin, ?histamine
	Pancreatic carcinoma	
	Gastric carcinoma	
Polycythemia	Renal carcinoma	Erythropoietin
	Cerebellar hemangioma	
	Hepatocellular carcinoma	
Nerve and Muscle Syndromes		
Disorders of the central and peripheral nervous systems	Small cell carcinoma of lung	?Immunologic, ?toxic
Myasthenia gravis	Breast carcinoma	
	Thymoma	?Immunologic
Osseous, Articular, and Soft Tissue Changes		
Hypertrophic osteoarthropathy and clubbing of the fingers	Adenocarcinoma of lung	Unknown
Vascular and Hematologic Changes		
Venous thrombosis (Trousseau's phenomenon)	Pancreatic carcinoma	Hypercoagulability
	Lung carcinoma	
	Other cancers	
Nonbacterial thrombotic endocarditis	Advanced cancers	Hypercoagulability

From Kumar V, Cotran RS, and Robbins SL. *Basic Pathology.* 5th ed. Philadelphia: WB Saunders, 1992.

Metastatic Disease

1. Approximately 34 percent of people with cancer have metastatic disease at the time of diagnosis. In addition, 23 percent of persons with local or regional disease will experience a recurrence after initial curative treatment.

2. Most people with cancer die of metastatic disease. The most common sites of metastasis are the lungs, liver, bone, and brain. Lung and liver metastases are common autopsy findings (Table 17–22). Unusual metastatic sites have become more frequent as the length of survival has improved in many cancers.

Table 17–22. Incidence of Metastasis at Diagnosis and Autopsy*

Site of Primary Tumor	Metastatic Site							
	% Bone		% Brain		% Lung		% Liver	
	Diagnosis	Autopsy	Diagnosis	Autopsy	Diagnosis	Autopsy	Diagnosis	Autopsy
Lung	16 (38)†	20–36	18–28 (8–14)†	18–37 (42)†		21–60	17	25–48 (74)†
Breast	20–40	44–73	15	9–20		59–69		56–65
Prostate	20–40	50–70	<1	2	5	15–53	1	5–13
Kidney	6–10	24–50	4	7–8	5–30	50–75	13	27–40
Bladder	5	12–25	<1	<1	5–10	25–30	>5	30–50
Testis (germinal)	<1	20	<1	<10	2–12	70–80	<1	50–80
Colon-rectum	<1	22	4	8	<5	25–40	20–24	60–71
Cervix	<1	8–20	<1	2–3	<5	20–30	<1	20–35
Ovary	<1	9	<1	<1	<5	5–10	<5	10–15
Uterus	<1	5–12	<1	<5	<1	30–40	<1	10–30

* Numbers represent estimates from several sources.
† Represents values for small cell carcinoma.
From Rubin P, McDonald S, and Qazi R (eds). *Clinical Oncology: A Multidisciplinary Approach for Physicians and Students.* 7th ed. Philadelphia: WB Saunders, 1993.

3. Occasionally, metastatic disease can be treated with curative intent. Surgical removal of metastatic lesions in the lung and liver can improve survival. Most metastatic lesions are usually treated if they are symptomatic or potentially disabling.
4. Improving the quality of life and minimizing the side effects of treatment are treatment goals for people with metastatic disease. Cost containment in medical care may limit the use of expensive technologies that neither improve the quality of life significantly nor improve survival.
5. Lung metastasis
   a. Lung metastases are often asymptomatic masses found in the periphery or outer 3rd of the lung parenchyma. Dyspnea may occur with airway obstruction or pleural effusions.
   b. Pulmonary metastases appear as nodular densities on chest radiograph. People with increasing dyspnea without any findings on radiograph may have diffuse lymphangitic metastases throughout the lungs. The standard diagnostic test in defining pulmonary metastases is the CT scan.
   c. Treatment of pulmonary metastases depends on the person's physical condition, the type of tumor, and the extent of disease.
      (1) Surgical resection of a limited number of pulmonary metastases is considered if the primary disease is controlled, no other metastatic lesions are detected, the lesions are resectable, and the person has had a reasonable disease-free survival.
      (2) Chemotherapy may be used in responsive tumors.
      (3) Radiation may be used to reduce obstructing lesions.
6. Liver metastasis
   a. Colon cancer most frequently metastasizes to the liver. Between 15 to 25 percent of patients have liver metastases at the time of diagnosis. An additional 20 to 25 percent will develop metastases after curative resections. Lung, kidney, bladder, and breast cancers also metastasize to the liver.
   b. Although limited hepatic metastases are usually asymptomatic, extensive liver metastasis causes anorexia, nausea, fever, and malaise. Ascites, pain, and jaundice are late signs. Computed tomography scanning provides the best diagnostic technology for the detection of liver metastases.
   c. Surgical resection of liver metastases from colon cancer can be curative in selected patients who have good liver function and a limited number of metastatic lesions. Survival rates of 25 to 40 percent have been reported. Resection of noncolonic tumors does not improve survival. Liver metastases can be treated by systemic chemotherapy or regional hepatic artery infusion with implanted or portable infusion pumps.
7. Bone metastasis
   a. Bone is the 3rd most common site of metastasis, but bone metastases occur in the 3 most common tumors: breast, prostate, and lung. Therefore, the number of people with bone metastases is large. The most common sites are vertebrae, pelvis, femur, and skull. Metastatic lesions can be osteolytic through destruction of bone by osteoclasts or osteoblastic through development of new bone in response to tumor invasion.
   b. Pain is the most common symptom. Described as insidious, aching, and increasing in intensity over time, pain is usually localized to the area of tumor, although extensive bony metastasis can exist without pain. Increasing back pain can represent external compression of the spinal cord or cauda equina by metastatic lesions. Emergency evaluation is needed to prevent irreversible neurologic damage.
   c. Bony metastases are diagnosed by bone scan, which is extremely sensitive to changes in the bone, detecting changes of as little as 5 percent. Specificity, however, is poor. Lesions that are primarily osteolytic will show as cold spots, whereas osteoblastic lesions will appear as hot spots (see Fig. 17–10). Radiographs can detect bone changes after 30 to 50 percent of the bone is destroyed and the lesion is 1.0 to 1.5 cm in diameter. Computed tomography and MRI may be useful in equivocal situations.
   d. Relief of pain and prevention of fractures and disability are treatment goals. Local treatment to bony metastasis with radiation therapy is effective to relieve pain and improve function. Approximately 60 to 90 percent of patients have moderate to severe pain. Chemotherapy and hormonal therapy (in breast and prostate) are used to treat the underlying cancer. Surgical intervention is needed for impending fractures. Internal fixation of the bone with rods and plates and use of bone cement provide stability in weight-bearing bones.
8. Brain metastasis
   a. Brain metastasis occurs in approximately 13 percent of cancer patients. Single metastatic lesions are associated with ovarian cancer, osteogenic sarcoma, breast cancer, and renal cancer, whereas lung cancer, melanomas, and seminomas tend to develop multiple metastatic lesions. Brain metastases generally develop multiple metastatic lesions. Brain metastases generally arise after secondary metastases to the lungs and liver.
   b. The presenting signs and symptoms of brain metastases are headache, focal weakness, mental disturbances, and seizures. Magnetic resonance imaging is the most sensitive diagnostic tool to detect brain metastases, but CT scanning is also excellent.
   c. Maintaining maximum neurologic functioning is the treatment goal in brain metastases. Radiation therapy is the primary mode of treatment. Selected patients with single lesions may benefit from surgical excision. Supportive care with steroids can be helpful. Chemotherapy is limited to the few tumors that respond.

Terminal Cancer

1. Palliative treatment refers to the use of treatment modalities (chemotherapy, surgery, radiation) in incurable cancer to alleviate symptoms caused by persistent tumor growth, new metastatic lesions, and the side effects of

treatment. Palliative care is frequently referred to as the chronic phase of cancer. For people with certain types of cancer, it can extend for many years. Many remain working and productive, functioning in their usual roles.

2. When treatment options have been exhausted and tumor growth is uncontrolled, the terminal phase of cancer begins. Either the tumor is refractory to chemotherapy and radiation, or new metastatic lesions occur in locations that have received maximum radiation dosages. The person might also choose to terminate treatment. The treatment goals then become symptom management.

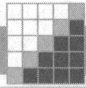

LEGAL AND ETHICAL CONSIDERATIONS

Resuscitation in the metastatic, terminally ill person is a futile procedure, yet both cancer patients and families often request that "everything be done." Likewise, total parenteral nutrition (TPN) in the terminally ill has no proven benefit, may exacerbate symptoms, and may be harmful, yet physicians are frequently pressured to provide TPN. The expense of home TPN ($150,000) per year adds the dimension of justice to the conflict.

   a. Medicare eligibility requirements for hospice care define terminal illness as the last 6 months of life, but many terminally ill people are in this phase for longer periods.

   b. Not all people with metastatic cancer become terminally ill. Some die of complications related to treatment or of other causes (e.g., myocardial infarcts).

3. Physical problems. As the disease advances, physical symptoms increase and require constant evaluation and new treatment strategies.

   a. Pain, anorexia, nausea, vomiting, constipation, and fatigue are common problems resulting either from tumor growth or from side effects of medications. Other physical symptoms vary and relate to organs involved with tumor, dehydration, weakness, immobility, and cachexia.

   b. People who are moribund with imminent death (less than 4 weeks) experience significant anorexia, dysphagia, and weight loss. Respiratory symptoms (e.g., dyspnea and retained secretions) occur near death. Drowsiness, confusion, and changes in consciousness level occur.

   c. The immediate causes of death in people with cancer are infection (47% pneumonia and septicemia), organ failure (25% respiratory, cardiac, hepatic, and renal), infarction (11% heart and lung), carcinomatosis (10% widespread metastatic disease), and hemorrhage (7%).

4. Psychologic issues. Losses predominate the psychologic concerns of the terminally ill. Losses include independence, function, roles, relationships, physical attractiveness, and ability to enjoy simple pleasures (e.g., a walk, a good meal). As people become moribund, cognitive ability is also lost.

   a. Terminally ill people may feel angry, lonely, isolated, anxious, depressed, and fearful. Those who have reconciled their situation may be peaceful and serene.

   b. Many people with cancer can reconcile these losses as they become resigned or accept their fate, but many cannot and maintain unrealistic hope until their death.

   c. The psychologic needs of the family are extremely important. The physical stress of caring for the dying person often leaves family members with little energy to cope with emotions and psychologic issues.

5. Supporting the dying person (see Chapter 43)

   a. Symptom management is the key to quality of life in the terminally ill, and requires constant evaluation and collaboration of the patient, nurse, physician, and family in discerning the true cause of symptoms and appropriate interventions. Good problem solving and persistence are indispensible.

   b. Constant attention to pain control is critical as tumor growth may change the nature and source of pain.

   c. Good control of nausea and vomiting will enable the person to eat. Anorexia and dysphagia limit the ability to maintain adequate nutrition, but some interventions may be helpful (see Table 17–20). In the moribund patient, emphasis on food and hydration is futile. Dying people tolerate dehydration and often are less symptomatic. The beneficial aspects of dehydration are reduced urinary output (less incontinence), reduced gastric secretions (less vomiting), and reduced pulmonary secretions, edema, pleural effusions and ascites.

   d. Maintaining optimal physical functioning is important within the person's limitations. Fatigue is a major limitation to activity, but good pain control and proper timing of activities can be helpful.

   e. Maintaining optimal bowel and bladder function, good skin care, and oral hygiene are ways to promote comfort, as is good, simple physical care (e.g., bathing and massage). These measures can provide distinct comfort for the dying person.

   f. Nurses can help dying people cope by enhancing their autonomy, allowing them to express their feelings and thoughts, providing opportunities and resources for them to talk and reconcile their life, and maintaining their respect and dignity.

   g. The essence of nursing the dying person is care and compassion.

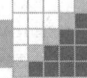

LEGAL AND ETHICAL CONSIDERATIONS

Justice in health care has not been defined by our culture. The rights of the individual to choose often conflict with the equal distribution of health care resources. Are life-saving treatments available to all? If health care is a basic right, who has the responsibility to provide it? People with insurance coverage have access to treatments unavailable to the uninsured.

   Does expending finite health care resources on futile measures demanded by patients and families deny justice to those who might receive life-saving treatments if health care dollars were available?

6. Supporting the family

   a. Families need to be taught the physical care of the dying person. They need constant reassurance that they are providing good care. Information on physical changes occurring during the dying process reduces anxiety of facing unexpected changes.

   b. Families may need guidance and resources for resolution of conflicts or expression of feelings with the dying person. Counseling may be appropriate for some family members.

c. In the final days, families need direction with procedures like death certification and burial.

d. Information and access to 24-hour, on-call nursing coverage also reduce anxiety. Most families are able to manage care of a dying person, no matter how physically exhausting, if they know they can obtain help when they need it.

e. Allowing family members to express feelings and problems as they arise and facilitating problem solving promotes coping for family members.

◼ ISSUES IN LONG-TERM CANCER MANAGEMENT

Discharge Planning and Teaching

1. Discharge planning and teaching provide for the continuity and safe care of the person with cancer. These processes facilitate the transition from hospital to home or to another health care facility.
2. Discharge planning begins when the person is admitted to the hospital. As people are discharged with greater physical needs and technologic interventions, adequate time is needed to arrange for home services and to teach people with cancer and their families specific procedures.
3. The assessment of the discharge needs of the person with cancer is based on physiologic, psychologic, and social factors that define the problems and the resources available (Box 17–8).
4. Discharge planning requires a multidisciplinary effort involving the person with cancer, nurse, physician, and social worker as primary team members and ancillary services whenever they are part of the person's care.
5. During the planning phase of discharge, the person's needs for health maintenance and disease and symptom control are matched with the resources available and the desires of the person with cancer and the family.

BOX 17–8. Discharge Needs in Assessing the Person with Cancer

Physiologic Factors

- The ability of the person to perform activities of daily living
- The complexity of medication regimen, dressing changes, or wound care
- The complexity of symptom management
- The types of equipment needed for monitoring and treatments

Psychologic Factors

- The cognitive ability of the individual
- The coping ability of the individual and family
- Psychologic conditions (e.g., depression, anxiety)

Social Factors

- Presence and support of functional family
- Availability of a home
- Community resources
- Health care resources
- Financial resources

---

a. The physiologic and psychologic needs are determined with appropriate interventions.
b. The availability of equipment, home health agencies, financial coverage, and access to health care facilities for ongoing care is determined.
c. The complexity of needs and the availability of resources determine the place where the person with cancer will receive the next level of care (e.g., home or another health care facility).
d. The teaching plan is formulated to provide instruction to the person with cancer or the family if the person is going home.

 HOME CARE STRATEGIES

Home Chemotherapy

The home care nurse plays a critical role in ensuring positive outcomes for the patient receiving home chemotherapy. It is advisable for all home chemotherapy patients to have a central venous catheter in place, but it is mandatory for patients receiving continuous vesicant infusions. Administration of vesicant chemotherapy through an implanted port is considered one of the higher risk, high-tech home care procedures and requires special vigilance with needle placement.

To ensure proper and secure needle placement, consider the following:

1. Use a bent, noncoring needle (e.g., a Huber) with a short length of extension tubing attached.
2. Stabilize the port septum with your thumb and forefinger while inserting the needle.
3. Insert the needle into the portal septum at a 90-degree angle until you contact the "needle stop" at the bottom of the port reservior. You will feel resistance when you reach this point. With metallic ports, you may hear a faint click when this point is reached.
4. Confirm the correct needle placement by aspirating gently to obtain a blood return.
5. If you are unable to obtain a blood return, try the following:
   - Have the patient change positions, cough, move the arms, and rotate the head.
   - Gently alternate between irrigation and aspiration with a 10-ml saline-filled syringe attached to the Huber needle extension tubing.
   - Reposition or remove the needle and place the new one in a different area of the portal septum.
6. After confirming blood flashback, administer a 10-ml saline fluid bolus through the needle. Observe the pocket around the port for signs of subcutaneous swelling, and ask the patient if he or she notices any burning, stinging, or discomfort with the bolus. If so, hold the chemotherapy and notify the physician. A chest radiograph may be needed to confirm proper catheter tip placement and location of the infusate. (For further troubleshooting interventions, refer to the manufacturer's guidelines for the type of device you are accessing.)
7. Secure the needle and extension tubing well per agency protocol, and use Luer-Lok fittings at all tubing attachment points.

Remember, patients education is *essential* to the success of a home chemotherapy program. Complete verbal and written instructions regarding ambulatory infusion pump function, troubleshooting, handling of chemotherapy waste or leakage, and signs and symptoms to report are a must.

Data from Larkin M (ed). *Intravenous Nursing Standards of Practice.* Belmont, MA: Intravenous Nursing Society, 1990.

6. The nurse's role in implementing the discharge plan is as follows:

a. To collaborate with the physician in determining the person's continuing needs for medical treatment and symptom control

b. To continue ongoing evaluation of the person's self-care potential

c. To provide input to other disciplines concerning the person's capabilities

d. To teach the person and family self-care, treatments, and health maintenance

e. To inform the person and family of appointments, tests, and consultations arranged after discharge. Phone numbers of physicians, nurses, social workers, and agencies involved in the discharge must be given to the person to obtain help or information if needed.

7. With proper planning and teamwork, the discharge of the person with cancer will provide optimal and safe care at the next level.

8. Evaluation of discharge planning from the hospital's perspective will be cost containment for timely and efficient discharge of the person with cancer.

Public Health Considerations

1. Nurses, as individuals, can practice cancer-prevention measures for themselves and their families, serving as role models.

2. Nurses, as professionals, have a great opportunity to educate people at risk for cancer about preventive behaviors and self-examination techniques and to volunteer for their local unit of the American Cancer Society, working in public education programs, especially those related to smoking.

3. Nurses, as citizens, can be proactive in promoting and lobbying for environmental legislation, especially tobacco issues and funding for cancer research and programs.

4. Primary prevention strategies attempt to remove known cancer risks by individual effort or governmental restriction. Because many cancer causes are related to lifestyle, change in individual behavior is an important method of primary prevention. Behaviors that would restrict exposure to carcinogens are

a. Smoking cessation or avoidance of smoke exposure

b. Adherence to dietary recommendations (see p. 595)

c. Reduced exposure to sunlight (i.e., tanning)

d. Restriction of early sexual activity and number of partners

5. Governmental restrictions are important in reducing occupational and environmental exposures. Local smoking restriction laws and food labeling for fat and fiber assist in changing individual behavior.

6. Because behavior changes are difficult and many cancers are not readily detectable at an early stage, efforts have been directed toward intervention in the process of carcinogenesis by administration of chemical compounds or vaccines known to inhibit or reverse cancer. Many of the compounds are micronutrients.

7. Chemoprevention trials are very expensive and must include a large number of subjects. The long latency of cancer makes disease onset impractical to use a study endpoint. Therefore, work is now directed toward measurement of other biologic markers as study endpoints.

8. Chemoprevention trials, being coordinated by the National Cancer Institute (NCI), are done on 3 levels:

a. Prevention of recurrence in people with histories of cancer. For example, administration of betacarotene for those with colon cancer.

b. Prevention of cancer in groups at high risk for specific cancers.

c. Studies in normal risk groups to prevent cancer in all sites. The Women's Health Study will enroll 40,000 nurses in a double-blind study using vitamin E over a 5-year period. Cancer incidence will be compared longitudinally.

9. The effectiveness of a screening program depends on the availability of a test that would be noninvasive or minimally invasive, specific for people with cancer, and sensitive, so that it would be negative in people without cancer. Tests that produce false-positive results add expense and morbidity in searching for a nonexistent cancer. Tests that produce false-negatives miss too many people with cancer and reduce the effectiveness of the screen.

10. No mass screening programs exist. Programs designed or currently in progress address 4 major cancers. The goal is to determine available screening procedures that will be effective.

11. Public education also involves individual screening and self-examination.

a. The NCI and the American Cancer Society (ACS) publish screening guidelines for use by asymptomatic individuals in consultation with private physicians.

b. Screening guidelines are seen in Table 17–23.

c. People with high-risk conditions usually require more frequent monitoring tailored to their individual needs by private physicians.

d. The ACS and the NCI produce educational materials describing self-examination techniques to detect breast, skin, mouth, and testicular cancers. Although the latter is not a common cancer, the ease of examination justifies the educational effort.

e. Unfortunately, few insurance programs provide reimbursement for preventive measures; hence, screening tests are not usually covered.

12. Public education involves 7 warning signs of cancer.

a. Although the warning signs do not always indicate early disease, they at least alert the public to cancer symptoms.

b. People often delay seeking medical attention for 1 to 2 years after symptoms appear. Sometimes this delay is a manifestation of denial, but often people

ELDER ADVISORY

Studies show that older people, especially the poor, less educated, and minorities, have inadequate knowledge of cancer. Cancer is often not perceived as a health concern by people between 60 and 75. Early detection programs must actively address older adults if such programs are to be successful.

Table 17–23. Summary of Recommendations of the American Cancer Society for the Early Detection of Cancer in Asymptomatic People

Test or Procedure	Sex	Age	Frequency
Sigmoidoscopy, preferably, flexible	M and F	50 and over	Every 3–5 yr
Fecal occult blood test	M and F	50 and over	Every yr
Digital rectal examination	M and F	40 and over	Every yr
Prostate examination*	M	50 and over	Every yr
Papanicolaou (Pap) test	F	All women who are or who have been sexually active, or have reached age 18, should have an annual Pap test and pelvic examination. After a woman has had 3 or more consecutive satisfactory normal annual examinations, the Pap test may be performed less frequently at the discretion of her physician.	
Pelvic examination	F	18–40	Every 1–3 yr with Pap test
		Over 40	Every yr
Endometrial tissue sample	F	At menopause, if at high risk†	At menopause and thereafter at the discretion of the physician
Breast self-examination	F	20 and over	Every month
Breast clinical examination	F	20–40	Every 3 yr
		Over 40	Every yr
Mammography ‡	F	40–49	Every 1–2 yr
		50 and over	Every yr
Health counseling and cancer checkup§	M and F	Over 20	Every 3 yr
	M and F	Over 40	Every yr

* Annual digital rectal examination and prostate-specific antigen should be performed on men age 50 and older. If either is abnormal, further evaluation should be considered.
† History of infertility, obesity, failure to ovulate, abnormal uterine bleeding, or unopposed estogen or tamoxifen therapy.
‡ Screening mammography should begin by age 40.
§ To include examination for cancers of the thyroid, testicles, ovaries, lymph nodes, oral region, and skin.
From Mettlin C, et al. Defining and Updating the American Cancer Society guidelines for the related check-up: Prostate and endometrial. *CA Cancer J Clin* 43(1):45, 1993.

are ignorant of the significance of their symptoms. The elderly frequently attribute symptoms of cancer with "growing older" (see Table 17–6).

13. Self-examination of the skin, breast, and testes can promote early detection of specific cancers. (See Chapter 33 for breast self-examination, Chapter 31 for testicular self-examination, and Chapter 35 for skin self-examination.)

14. Nurses can assist the public through education about unproven remedies. The ACS defines unproven methods as "Those diagnostic tests which are promoted for general use in cancer prevention, diagnosis, and treatment and which are, on the basis of careful review by scientists and/or clinicians, not deemed proven nor recommended for current use." Unproven methods are also referred to as questionable, disproven, fraudulent, unorthodox, unconventional, alternative, and complementary.

 a. People with cancer often reveal their use of unproven methods to nurses. While maintaining an open attitude, the nurse can assist the person in evaluating the therapy and its potential harmful side effects (Table 17–24). While respecting the person's right to determine treatment, the nurse should direct the person to accurate sources of information so that the decision is an informed one.

 b. Evaluating the person's rationale for use of unproven methods may reveal inadequacies in the health care system, which can be remedied to provide bet-

ter care, especially more active participation in treatment decisions.

 c. Nurses should report any new unproven methods to the local health authorities and the ACS (see Table 17–24).

 d. Types of unproven methods

Table 17–24. Ten Questions to Ask in Deciding Whether a Treatment Is Questionable

1. Is the treatment based on an unproven theory?
2. Is there a purported need for special nutritional support?
3. Is there a claim for painless, nontoxic treatment?
4. Are claims published only in the mass media and not in reputable, peer-reviewed scientific journals?
5. Are claims for benefit merely compatible with a placebo effect?
6. Are the major proponents recognized experts in cancer treatment?
7. Do proponents claim benefit for use with proven methods of treatment? for prolongation of life? for use as a cancer preventative?
8. Is there a claim that only specially trained physicians can produce results with the drug, or is the preparation secret?
9. Is there an attack on the medical and scientific establishment?
10. Is there a demand by promoters for "freedom of choice" regarding drugs?

From Subcommittee on Unorthodox Therapies, American Society of Clinical Oncology. Ineffective cancer therapy: A guide for the layperson. *J Clin Oncol* 1:154–163, 1983.

(1) Physical methods include biologic materials, chemicals, cells, diets, teas, herbs, and electronic devices.

(2) Psychologic methods includes imagery, visualization, muscle relaxation, meditation, faith healing, and biofeedback. Although some of these methods are believed to reduce stress, some practitioners claim also that they cure cancer.

e. Historically, unproven methods have always been promoted and available. The first recorded case of cancer fraud in the United States occurred in pre-Revolutionary War days. Each decade of the 20th century has had its fad in unproven therapy. The current popular treatments are metabolic treatments, and these support a large industry in Tijuana and other Mexican border clinics. The therapy consists of 3 phases: detoxification, fasting, and bowel cleansing; strengthening the immune system; and treating the cancer with natural and nontoxic chemicals. Coffee enemas, massive doses of vitamins, infusions of Laetrile, and injections of hydrogen peroxide are used.

f. Studies indicate that from 9 to 50 percent of people with cancer use unproven methods of treatment. Five percent abandon standard therapy while using unproven methods. The stereotype of the poor and uneducated person with cancer as a user of unproven methods is inaccurate. Studies demonstrate that White, foreign-born, educated people predominately between 30 and 50 years of age are the most frequent users.

g. People often choose unproven methods because cancer treatment is demanding, exhausting, and the cause of toxic side effects. The lure of a nontoxic, natural treatment attracts many people into unproven methods. Some people have a mistrust of the medical community and find difficulty accepting the treatments offered in standard therapy. Often, physicians are seen as financially motivated. Some physicians themselves recommend unproven methods. Faced with incurable cancer, many people are willing to gamble in an effort to do something. Family pressure for the person with cancer to do everything possible brings some to unproven methods.

h. Most people learn about unproven methods through the media (print, radio, television) or by word of mouth. Inquiries to the official cancer education channels (ACS and NCI) for information are not common. The "sellers" of unproven therapies are optimistic and cheerful. They describe their treatments as "natural." Outside the standard channels of science and medicine, they focus on a conspiracy against them by the scientific community and government. Records are incomplete or nonexistent; they do not require biopsy verification of cancer. Testimonials are frequently used.

i. Standard treatments, in contrast, must meet the following criteria to be accepted as medical treatment:

(1) The therapy is used to treat biopsy-proven cancer.

(2) An adequate number of patients must be treated and compared with a control group.

(3) Effects must be measured and evaluated at appropriate intervals for a sufficient period. Survival outcome should be reported.

(4) Results must be reported in peer-reviewed journals and be available for analysis.

(5) Results should be reproducible by other investigators.

j. Proponents of unproven therapies who believe they have a valid, novel approach to cancer treatment but who are outside the recognized scientific community can receive review and assistance from the NCI in evaluating their method, if their cases are biopsy proven with sufficient documentation. Proponents of therapies who are unwilling to follow the proposed scientific channels should be suspect.

k. Current estimates for spending on unproven methods is $4 billion annually. Additional monies are wasted in government expenditures in investigations to prove the ineffectiveness of some methods. Some unproven methods are physically harmful. Laetrile, for example, can cause death by cyanide poisoning. Biologics used in clinics have been found to be contaminated with hepatitis and other viral and bacterial contaminants.

l. Delay in seeking standard treatment can be harmful if the opportunity for cure has been lost. Many people using psychologic methods for cure feel inadequate when they are unable to control the disease with these methods.

m. The ACS maintains a standing committee on questionable methods of cancer management. Reviews of unproven methods are published regularly in the journal *CA A Cancer Journal for Clinicians*. Information on any specific therapy is available. The NCI, the FDA, and the American Society for Clinical Oncology are additional reviewers of unproven methods.

Challenges of Cancer Survivorship

1. For many years, the problems of those surviving cancer were not recognized. As many more people began to survive longer, they began to organize and advocate to correct the problems they faced.

a. Depending on the treatment, people with cancer can face life-long disfigurement or diminished function. Fatigue and the long-term effects of therapy remain with them. They require long-term follow-up. With sufficient rehabilitation, however, many can return to reasonable functioning.

b. Many face psychologic difficulties because they deal with body image and role changes. Guilt over surviving is experienced or fear of recurrence can plague some individuals.

c. Financial difficulties related to treatment expenditures

BOX 17–9. American Cancer Society
The Cancer Survivors' Bill of Rights

A new population lives among us today—a new minority of 6 million people with a history of cancer. Three million of these Americans have lived with their diagnoses for 5 years or more.

You see these modern survivors in offices and in factories, on bicycles and cruise ships, on tennis courts, beaches, and bowling alleys. You see them in all ages, shapes, sizes, and colors. Usually they are unremarkable in appearance; sometimes they are remarkable for the way they have learned to live with disabilities resulting from cancer or its treatment.

Modern medical advances have returned about half of the nation's cancer patients of all ages (and 59 percent for those under the age of 55) to a normal lifespan. But the larger society has not always kept pace in helping make this lifespan truly "normal": at least, it has felt awkward in dealing with this fledgling group; at most, it has failed fully to accept survivors as functioning members.

The American Cancer Society presents this Survivors' Bill of Rights to call public attention to survivor needs, to enhance cancer care, and to bring greater satisfaction to cancer survivors, as well as to their physicians, employers, families, and friends:

1. Survivors have the right to assurance of lifelong medical care, as needed. The physicians and other professionals involved in their care should continue their constant efforts to be:

• Sensitive to the cancer survivors' lifestyle choices and their need for self-esteem and dignity
• Careful, no matter how long they have survived, to have symptoms taken seriously, and not have aches and pains dismissed, for fear of recurrence is a normal part of survivorship
• Informative and open, providing survivors with as much or as little candid medical information as they wish, and encouraging their informed participation in their own care
• Knowledgeable about counseling resources, and willing to refer survivors and their families as appropriate for emotional support and therapy that will improve the quality of individual lives

2. In their personal lives, survivors, like other Americans, have the right to the pursuit of happiness. This means they have the right:

• To talk with their families and friends about their cancer experience if they wish, but to refuse to discuss it if that is their choice and not to be expected to be more upbeat or less blue than anyone else
• To be free of the stigma of cancer as a "dread disease" in all social relations
• To be free of blame for having gotten the disease and of guilt for having survived it

3. In the workplace, survivors have the right to equal job opportunities. This means they have the right:

• To aspire to jobs worthy of their skills, and for which they are trained and experienced, and thus not to have to accept jobs they would not have considered before the cancer experience
• To be hired, promoted, and accepted on return to work, according to their individual abilities and qualifications, and not according to "cancer" or "disability" stereotypes
• To privacy about their medical histories

4. Since health insurance coverage is an overriding survivorship concern, every effort should be made to ensure all survivors adequate health insurance, whether public or private. This means:

• For employers, that survivors have the right to be included in group health coverage, which is usually less expensive, provides better benefits, and covers the employee regardless of health history
• For physicians, counselors, and other professionals concerned, that they keep themselves and their survivor-clients informed and up-to-date on available group or individual health-policy options, noting, for example, what major expenses like hospital costs and medical tests outside the hospital are covered and what amount must be paid before coverage (deductibles)

From Spingarn ND. *The Cancer Survivors' Bill of Rights*. American Cancer Society, Inc.

may require changes in lifestyle. People with residual difficulties may face job changes or role changes within the family.
2. Obtaining insurance has been difficult, if not impossible, for some people following cancer treatment. The Consolidated Omnibus Budget Reconciliation Act (COBRA) requires employees to provide insurance for 18 months following job loss, and some states provide pooled insurance for people who cannot get conventional coverage. People with cancer who have difficulty in obtaining insurance should do the following:
a. Call their state ACS office or their state department of insurance for information.
b. Obtain the booklet *Facing Forward* from the National Institutes of Health. Detailed information regarding insurance is provided in this booklet.
3. Many people with cancer were terminated from their jobs after the diagnosis of cancer, despite research demonstrating that people with cancer are as productive as other workers. Twenty-five percent of cancer survivors experience some form of employment discrimination. People with cancer are now protected from employment discrimination under the Americans with Disabilities Act. Any person with cancer experiencing job discrimination should contact the ACS, a state department of human rights, or a lawyer (Box 17–9).

Bibliography

Books

American Cancer Society. *Questionable Methods of Cancer Treatment*. Atlanta: Author, 1993.

American Cancer Society. *Cancer facts and figures*. Atlanta: Author, 1995.

American Joint Committee on Cancer. *Manual for Staging of Cancer*. Philadelphia: JB Lippincott, 1992.

Chapman CR, and Foley KM. *Current and Emerging Issues in Cancer Pain*. New York: Raven Press, 1993.

Cooper CL, and Watson M. *Cancer and Stress: Psychological, Biological and Coping Studies*. Chichester: John Wiley & Sons, 1991.

DeVita JT, Hellman S, and Rosenberg S (eds). *Cancer: Principles and Practice of Oncology*. 4th ed. Philadelphia: JB Lippincott, 1993.

Doenges ME, et al. *Application of Nursing Process and Nursing Diagnosis*. Philadelphia: FA Davis, 1995.

Economou SG, et al. *Adjuncts to Cancer Surgery*. Philadelphia: Lea & Febiger, 1991.

Greenwald HP: *Who Survives Cancer*. Berkeley: University of California Press, 1992.

Groenwald SL, et al (eds). *Cancer Nursing—Principles and Practice*. 3rd ed. Boston: Jones & Bartlett Publishers, 1993.

Hazzard WR, et al (eds). *Principles of Geriatric Medicine and Gerontology*. 2nd ed. New York: McGraw-Hill Information Services, 1992.

Holland JC, and Rowland JH. *Handbook of Psychooncology*. New York: Oxford University Press, 1989.

Holleb AI, Fink OJ, and Murphy GP (eds). *American Cancer Society Textbook of Clinical Oncology*. Atlanta: The American Cancer Society, 1991.

Kemp C. *Terminal Illness*. Philadelphia: JB Lippincott, 1995.

Kumar V, Cotran RS, and Robbins SL. *Basic Pathology*. 5th ed. Philadelphia: WB Saunders, 1992.

Kupchella C. *Dimensions of Cancer*. Belmont, CA: Wadsworth Publishing Co, 1987.

Levine C (ed). *Taking Sides: Clashing Views on Controversial Bioethical Issues*. Guilford, CT: The Dushkin Publishing Group, 1995.

McCloskey JC, Bulechek GM. *Nursing Interventions Classification (NIC)*. 2nd ed. St. Louis: Mosby, 1995.

McCorkle R, et al. *Cancer Nursing: A Comprehensive Textbook*. 2nd ed. Philadelphia: WB Saunders, 1996.

McNally JC, et al. *Guidelines for Cancer Nursing Practice*. Orlando: Grune & Stratton, 1985.

Miastkowski C. *Oncology Nursing*. Albany: Delmar Publishers, 1995.

Morris SC. *Cancer Risk Assessment*. New York: Marcel Dekker, 1990.

O'Connor JM, and Ferguson-Smith MA. *Essential Medical Genetics*. 3rd ed. Oxford: Blackwell Scientific Publications, 1991.

Osteen RT (ed). *Cancer Manual*. 8th ed. Boston: American Cancer Society, Massachusetts Division, 1990.

Otto SE. *Oncology Nursing*. 2nd ed. St. Louis: CV Mosby, 1994.

Ries LAG, et al. *Cancer Statistics Review*. Bethesda, MD: National Institutes of Health, National Cancer Institute (NIH Pub. No. 91-2789), 1991.

Roberts R, et al. *A Primer of Molecular Biology*. New York: Elsevier, 1992.

Rubin P, McDonald S, and Qazi R (eds). *Clinical Oncology: A Multidisciplinary Approach for Physicians and Students*. 7th ed. Philadelphia: WB Saunders, 1993.

Stoll BA. *Coping with Cancer Stress*. Dordrecht, Netherlands: Martinus Nijhoff Publishers, 1986.

Tannock IF, and Hill RP (eds). *The Basic Science of Oncology*. New York: McGraw-Hill, 1992.

U.S. Department of Health and Human Services. *Management of Cancer Pain: Clinical Practice Guideline No. 9*. Washington, DC: DHHS, Agency for Health Care and Policy Research, 1994.

Vile, RG (ed). *Introduction to Molecular Genetics of Cancer*. Chichester: John Wiley & Sons, Ltd, 1992.

Weisman AD. *Coping with Cancer*. New York: McGraw-Hill Book Co, 1979.

Weiss GR (ed). *Clinical Onocology*. Norwalk, CT: Appleton & Lange, 1993.

Zenser TV, and Coe RM. *Cancer and Aging*. New York: Springer Publishing Co, 1989.

Chapters in Books and Journal Articles

Epidemiology, Causation, Early Detection, and Prevention

Berger NS. Prostate cancer: Screening and early detection update. *Semin Oncol Nurs* 9(3):180–183, 1993.

Boring CC, Squires TS, and Heath CN. Cancer statistics for African Americans. *CA Cancer J Clin* 42(1):7–17, February 1992.

Early detection of colorectal neoplasia: Obstacles and opportunities. *Mayo Clin Update* 9(2):1–3, 1993.

Epstein S. Evaluation of national cancer program and proposed reforms. *Int J Health Serv* 23(1):15–44, 1993.

Fitzsimmons ML, and Fales L. Colon cancer prevention update. *Semin Oncol Nurs* 9(3):163–168, 1993.

Frank-Stromberg M, and Rohan K. Nursing's involvement in the primary and secondary prevention of cancer. *Cancer Nurs* 15(2):79–108, 1992.

Fraumeni JF, et al. Epidemiology of cancer. *In* Devita JT, Hellman S, and Rosenberg SA (eds). *Cancer: Principles and Practice of Oncology*. 3rd Ed. Philadelphia: JB Lippincott, 1989.

Garfinkel L. Nutrition and cancer: Current status. *CA Cancer J Clin* 41(6):325–327.

Goodwin SC. Gastric cancer and *Heliobacter pylori*: The whispering killer. *Lancet* 342:507–508, 1993.

Henderson BE, Ross RK, and Pike MC.

Toward the primary prevention of cancer. *Science* 254:1131–1138, 1991.

Kelloff GJ, et al. Progress in applied chemoprevention research. *Semin Oncol* 17(4):438–455, 1990.

Kritchevsky D. Diet and cancer. *CA Cancer J Clin* 41:328–333, 1991.

Lippman SM, et al. Recent advances in cancer chemoprevention. *Cancer Cells* 3(2):59–65, 1991.

Mettlin C. Research in cancer prevention and detection. *Curr Issues Cancer Nurs Pract* 1(4):1–9.

Mettlin C. Trends in years of life lost to cancer. *CA Cancer J Clin* 39(1):33–38, 1989.

Mettlin C, et al. Defining and updating the American Cancer Society guidelines for the cancer related checkup: Prostate and endometrial. *CA Cancer J Clin* 43(1):42–46, 1993.

Meyskens FL Jr. Coming of age—The chemoprevention of cancer. *N Engl J Med* 323(12):825–826, 1990.

Potanovich LM. Lung cancer: Prevention and detection update. *Semin Oncol Nurs* 9(3):174–179, 1993.

Smith PE. Breast cancer prevention and detection update. *Semin Oncol Nurs* 9(3):150–154, 1993.

Swanson GM. Cancer prevention in the workplace and natural environment. *Cancer* 62(Suppl):1725–1746, 1988.

Work Study Group on Diet, Nutrition and Cancer. American Cancer Society guidelines on diet, nutrition and cancer. *CA Cancer J Clin* 41(6):334–338, 1991.

Tumor Biology

Fearon ER, and Vogelstein B. A genetic model for colorectal tumorigenesis. *Cell* 61:759–767, 1990.

Knudson AG. Hereditary cancer, oncogenes, and antioncogenes. *Cancer Res* 45:1437–1443, 1985.

Liotta LA. Cancer cell invasion and metastasis. *Sci Am* 266:54–63, 1992.

Pitot HC, and Dragan YP. Stage of tumor progression, progressor agents and human risk. *Proc Soc Exper Biol Med* 202:37–43, 1993.

Weinberg RA. The genetic bases of cancer. *Arch Surg* 125:257–260, 1990.

Weinberg RA. A short guide of oncogenes and tumor-suppressor genes. *J NIH Res* 3:45–48, 1991.

Weinberg RA. Tumor suppressor genes. *Science* 254:1138–1145, 1991.

Yarbro JW. Oncogenes and cancer suppressor genes. *Semin Oncol Nurs* 8(1):30–39, 1992.

zur Hausen H. Viruses in human cancers. *Science* 254:1167–1172, 1991.

Cancer Diagnosis and Treatment

Applebaum FR. The application of hematopoietic colony stimulating factors in cancer management. *Curr Issues Cancer Nurs Pract Updates* 2(2):1–13, 1992.

Cohen MH, et al. Continuous intravenous

narcotic infusions for cancer pain. *Cancer Invest* 11(2):169–173, 1993.

Crouch MA, and Ross JA. Current concepts in autologous bone marrow transplantation. *Semin Oncol Nurs* 10(1):12–15, 1994.

Dachowski LJ, and DeLaney TF. Photodynamic therapy: The NCI experience and its nursing implications. *Oncol Nurs Forum* 19(1):63–67, 1992.

Finkbiner KL, and Ernst TF. Drug therapy management of the febrile neutropenic cancer patient. *Cancer Practice* 1(4):295–304, 1993.

Fletcher DM. Unconventional cancer treatments: Professional, legal and ethical issues. *Oncol Nurs Forum* 19(9):1351–1358, 1992.

Goldenberg DM. New developments in monoclonal antibodies for cancer detection and therapy. *CA Cancer J Clin* 44(12):43–63, 1994.

Haibeck SV. Intraoperative radiation therapy. *Oncol Nurs Forum* 15(2):143–147, 1988.

Hawkins MJ, and Friedman MA. National Cancer Institute's evaluation of unconventional cancer treatments. *J Nat Cancer Inst* 84(22):1699–1702, 1992.

Hooper PJ, and Santas EJ. Peripheral blood stem cell transplantation. *Oncol Nurs Forum* 20(8):1215–1220, 1993.

Jassak PF, Petty J, and Krol MA. Treatment modalities for neoplastic disorders. *In* Black JM, and Matassarin-Jacobs E (eds). *Luckmann and Sorensen's Medical-Surgical Nursing: A Psychophysiologic Approach.* 4th ed. Philadelphia: WB Saunders, 1993.

Jordan LN, and Mantravadi RVP. Nursing care of the patient receiving high dose brachytherapy. *Oncol Nurs Forum* 18(7):1167–1171, 1991.

Kusler DL, and Rambur BA. Treatment for radiation induced xerostomia. *Cancer Nurs* 15(3):191–195, 1992.

Lamkin L. Outpatient oncology settings: A variety of services. *Semin Oncol Nurs* 10(4):227–230, 1994.

Lin EM, Tierney DK, and Stradtmauer B. Autologous bone marrow transplantation—A review of principles and complications. *Cancer Nurs* 16(3):203–213, 1993.

Lucas AB. A critical review of venous access devices: The nursing perspective. *Curr Issues Cancer Nurs Pract* 1(7):1–10.

Maxwell MB, and Maher KE. Chemotherapy induced myelosuppression. *Semin Oncol Nurs* 8(2):113–123, 1992.

McGinnis LS. Alternative therapies, 1990. *Cancer* 67(6, suppl):1788–1792, 1991.

Oettgen HF. Cytokines in clinical cancer therapy. *Curr Opin Immunol* 3:699–705, 1991.

Peters WP. Bone marrow transplantation. *In* Weiss GR (ed). *Clinical Oncology.* Norwalk, CT: Appleton & Langre, 1993.

Ravikumar TS, and Steele GD. Modern immunotherapy of cancer. *In* Cameron JL (ed). *Advances in Surgery.* Vol. 24. St Louis: Mosby–Year Book, 1991.

Rostad ME. Current strategies for managing myelosuppression in patients with cancer. *Oncol Nurs Forum* 18(2, suppl):7–15, 1991.

Savage DE. Principles of radiation oncology. *In* Rosenthal S, Carignan JR, and Smith BD (eds). *Medical Care of the Cancer Patient.* 2nd ed. Philadelphia: WB Saunders, 1992.

Sitton E. Early and late radiation-induced skin alterations. Part I: Mechanisms of skin changes. *Oncol Nurs Forum* 19(5):801–806, 1992.

Sitton E. Early and late radiation-induced skin alterations. Part II: Nursing care of irradiated skin. *Oncol Nurs Forum* 19(6):907–912, 1992.

Storm FK. What happened to hyperthermia and what is its current status in cancer treatment? *J Surg Oncol* 53:141–143, 1993.

Strohl RA. The nursing role in radiation oncology: Symptom management of acute and chronic reactions. *Oncol Nurs Forum* 15(4):429–434, 1988.

Winslow MN, Trammel L, and Campsorrell D. Selection of vascular access devices and nursing care. *Semin Oncol Nurs* 11(3):167–173, 1995.

Wujcik D. An odyssey into biologic therapy. *Oncol Nurs Forum* 20(6):879–886, 1993.

Zalosnik AJ. Unproven (unorthodox) cancer treatments. *Cancer Pract* 2(1):19–24, 1994.

Complications of Cancer

Cohen MF, et al. Continuous intravenous narcotic infusions for cancer pain. *Cancer Invest* 11(2):169–173, 1993.

Melzack R. Tragedy of needless pain. *Sci Am* 262(2):27–33, 1990.

Racolin AA. Metastasis to bone. Incidence, issues, and implications for nursing. *Curr Issues Cancer Nurs Pract Updates* 1(5):1–11, 1992.

Rhymes J. Hospice care in America. *JAMA* 264(3):369–372, 1990.

Sharp JW, and Roncagh T. Home parenteral nutrition in advanced cancer. *Cancer Pract* 1(2):119–123, 1993.

Psychosocial Aspects of Cancer

Cassel EJ. The nature of suffering and the goals of medicine. *N Engl J Med* 306(11):639–645, 1982.

Cella DF. Cancer survival: Psychosocial and public issues. *Cancer Invest* 5(1):59–67, 1987.

Cella DF, and Yellen SB. Cancer support groups. *Cancer Pract* 1(1):56–61, 1993.

Dunphy JE. Annual discourse—On caring for the patient with cancer. *N Engl J Med* 295(6):313–319, 1976.

Ferrell BR, and Rivera LM. Ethical decision making in oncology. *Cancer Pract* 3(2):94–99, 1995.

Glajchen M. Psychosocial consequences of inadequate health insurance for patients with cancer. *Cancer Pract* 2(2):115–120, 1994.

Hoffman B. Employment discrimination: Another hurdle for cancer survivors. *Cancer Invest* 9(5):589–595, 1991.

Jassak PF. Families: An essential element in the care of the patient with cancer. *Oncol Nurs Forum* 19(6):871–876, 1992.

Kristjanson LJ, and Ashcroft T. The family's cancer journey: A literature review. *Cancer Nurs* 17(1):1–17, 1994.

Lane D. Music therapy: A gift beyond measure. *Oncol Nurs Forum* 19(6):863–867, 1992.

Mahon SM. Managing the psychosocial consequences of cancer recurrence: Implications for nurses. *Oncol Nurs Forum* 18(3):577–583, 1991.

Mahon SM, Cella DF, and Donovan MI. Psychosocial adjustment to recurrent cancer. *Oncol Nurs Forum* 17(3, suppl):47–54, 1990.

McMillan SC, Tittle MB, and Hill D. A systematic evaluation of the "I Can Cope" program using a national sample. *Oncol Nurs Forum* 20(3):455–461, 1993.

Padberg RM, and Padberg LF. Strengthening the effectiveness of patient education: Applying principles of adult education. *Oncol Nurs Forum* 17(1):65–69, 1990.

Schneiderman L. Ethical issues and code status in cancer patients. *In* Moosa AR, et al (eds). *Comprehensive Textbook of Oncology.* 2nd ed. Baltimore: Williams & Wilkins, 1991.

Sharp JW, and Toncagli R. Home parenteral nutrition in advanced cancer: Ethical and psychosocial aspects. *Cancer Pract* (1)2:119–123, 1993.

Valente SM, Saunders JM, and Cohen MZ. Evaluating depression among patients with cancer. *Cancer Pract* 2(1):65–71, 1994.

Volker DL. Needs assessment and resource identification. *Oncol Nurs Forum* 18(1):119–122, 1991.

Weisman AD, and Worden JW. The emotional impact of recurrent cancer. *J Psychosoc Oncol* 3(4):5–15, 1985–1986.

Agencies and Resources

Patient Education and Support Service

American Brain Tumor Association
2720 River Road, Suite 146
Des Plaines, IL 60018
(800) 886-2282

American Cancer Society
1599 Clifton Road, NE
Atlanta, GA 30329–4251
(800) ACS–2345
• Reach to Recovery
• International Association of Laryngectomees

• Cansurmount
• I Can Cope
• Look Good, Feel Better
• Man to Man

Candlelighters Childhood Cancer
  Foundation
7910 Woodmount Avenue, Suite 460
Bethesda, ME 20814
(800) 366-2223
(301) 657-8401

Children's Oncology Camps
  of America
c/o Linda Wells, RN
7 Richland Memorial Park, Suite 203
Columbia, SC 29203
(800) 434-3533

Corporate Angel Network
Westchester County Airport
  Building 1
White Plaines, NY 10604
(914) 328-1313

Encore Plus
YWCA of the USA
624 Ninth Street, NW,
  Third Floor
Washington, DC 20001-5394
(202) 628-3636

Leukemia Society of America
600 Third Avenue
New York, NY 10016
(800) 955-4LSA
(212) 573-8484

Make Today Count
c/o Connie Zimmerman
Mid-America Cancer Center
1235 East Cherokee
Springfield, MO 65804-2263
(800) 432-2273

National Brain Tumor Foundation
785 Market Street, Suite 1600
San Francisco, CA 94103
(800) 934-CURE

National Coalition for Cancer Survivorship
1010 Wayne Avenue, Fifth Floor
Silver Spring, MD 20910
(301) 650-8868

National Hospice Organization
1901 North Moore Street, Suite 901
Arlington, VA 22209
(800) 658-8898
(703) 243-5900

National Lymphedema Network
2211 Post Street, Suite 404
San Francisco, CA 94115
(800) 541-3259

United Ostomy Association
36 Executive Park, Suite 120
Irvine, CA 92714
(714) 660-8624
(800) 826-0826

Us Too Prostate Cancer Survivor Support
  Group
Us Too International, Inc.
930 North York Road, Suite 50
Hinsdale, IL 60521-2993
(708) 323-1002
(800) 828-7866

Y-Me National Organization for Breast
  Cancer Information and Support
212 West Van Buren, Fourth Floor
Chicago, IL 60607
(312) 986-8228
(800) 221-2141

Cancer Information Services

American Cancer Society
1599 Clifton Road, NE
Atlanta, GA 30329-4251
(800) ACS-2345

National Cancer Institute
PDQ (Physician Data Query)
ICIC Building
9000 Rockville Pike, Building 31, Room
  10A16
Bethesda, MD 20892
(800) NCI-7890

Cancer Information Service
(800) 4-CANCER

Professional Oncology Nursing Organizations

American Society for Pain Management
  Nurses (ASPMN)
P.O. Box 2162
Tucker, GA 30085

Association of Pediatric Oncology Nurses
  (APON)
5700 Old Orchard Road, First Floor
Skokie, IL 60077
(708) 966-3723

Hospice Nurses Association
5512 Northumberland Street
Pittsburgh, PA 15217-1131
(412) 687-3231

International Society of Nurses in Cancer
  Care
Christopher Bailey, Secretariat
The Royal College of Nursing
20 Cavendish Square
London W1M OAB, England
071-495-6119

Oncology Nursing Society (ONS)
501 Holiday Drive
Pittsburgh, PA 15220-2749
(412) 921-7373

18

Caring for People with Neurologic Disorders

☐ *NERVOUS SYSTEM STRUCTURE AND FUNCTION*

Overview

1. The nervous system is a highly specialized system of cells that controls and integrates the body's many activities.
2. It is divided into 2 major parts: the central nervous system (CNS) and the peripheral nervous system (PNS) (Fig. 18–1).

The Central Nervous System

1. Neuroglia and neurons are the 2 major types of CNS cells (Fig. 18–2).
   a. Neuroglia constitute about 85 percent of the CNS cells.
      (1) They include astrocytes, oligodendroglia, microglia, and ependymal cells.
      (2) They provide support, nourishment, and protection to neurons.
      (3) Primary tumors of the CNS are usually glial tumors.
   b. Neurons transmit nerve impulses. They do not have the capacity to replicate after birth, so they cannot become neoplastic.
      (1) The cell body of the neuron contains the nucleus and cytoplasm, where metabolic activity takes place.
      (2) Dendrites are short processes that extend from the cell body and receive nerve impulses from axons of other neurons.
      (3) Each neuron has a single axon projecting from the cell body and ranging in length from several micrometers to more than 1 meter. The axon carries nerve impulses away from the cell body to other neurons or to end organs (e.g., skeletal muscle and glands).
      (4) A synapse is the structural and functional junction between 2 neurons.
      (5) The presynaptic terminal is the end of an axon where a nerve impulse arrives before being transmitted to another neuron or an end organ.

   (6) The synaptic cleft is the space between the presynaptic terminal and the receptor site on the postsynaptic cell.
   (7) When a nerve impulse reaches the presynaptic terminal, it causes release of a chemical substance (neurotransmitter) from tiny vesicles within the terminal (Fig. 18–3).
   (8) The neurotransmitter then crosses the microscopic space (synaptic cleft) between the 2 cells and attaches to receptor sites of the receiving cell, causing a change in the permeability of the postsynaptic cell to certain ions such as sodium and potassium.
   (9) Some neurotransmitters are excitatory, causing the postsynaptic cell to be more likely to fire an *action potential* (a nerve impulse within a cell).
   (10) Other neurotransmitters are inhibitory, causing the postsynaptic cell to be less likely to fire an action potential.
   (11) The net effect of the synaptic input depends on the number of presynaptic neurons releasing neurotransmitters and their type of influence (excitatory or inhibitory).
   (12) The presynaptic input is summed by the number of presynaptic cells firing (spatial summation) and by the frequency of firing of a single presynaptic cell (temporal summation).
   (13) Neurotransmitters continue to combine with the receptor sites at the postsynaptic cell membrane until they are inactivated by enzymes, taken up by the presynaptic endings, or diffused away from the synaptic region.
   (14) Neurotransmitters can be affected by drugs and toxins, which can modify their function or block their attachment to receptor sites on the postsynaptic membrane.
2. The CNS consists of the spinal cord and the brain.
3. The spinal cord begins at the base of the brain stem and ends between the 1st and 2nd lumbar vertebrae (Fig. 18–4).
   a. Gray matter (gray because it is composed of nerve cell bodies) is centrally located in an H shape and is surrounded by white matter (white because it is composed of myelinated nerve axons).
   b. White matter contains groups of function-specific axons (called tracts) of ascending and descending neurons (Fig. 18–5).

ORGANIZATION OF THE NERVOUS SYSTEM
CENTRAL NERVOUS SYSTEM
- Brain and spinal cord
PERIPHERAL NERVOUS SYSTEM
- Cranial and spinal nerves
SENSORY DIVISION
(afferent)
- Somatic and visceral sensory neurons
MOTOR DIVISION
(efferent)
- Motor neurons
AUTONOMIC NERVOUS SYSTEM
- Involuntary
SOMATIC NERVOUS SYSTEM
- Voluntary, skeletal muscles
SYMPATHETIC DIVISION
"Flight or fight"
-Thoracolumbar
PARASYMPATHETIC DIVISION
"Conserve and restore"
- Craniosacral

Figure 18–1.

STRUCTURE OF THE CNS
Main divisions of the CNS
Cerebrum
Pons
Medulla oblongata
Cerebellum
Cervical
Spinal cord
Thoracic
Lumbar
Sacral
Coccygeal
Neuroglial cells
Support cells of the CNS
Astrocyte
Microglial cell
Oligodendrocyte
Ependymal cell
Neurons
Cell body
Axon hillock
Axon
Neurilemma (myelin sheath of Schwann cell)
Dendrites
Structural classification
Unipolar
Cell body
Axon
Dendrites
Cell body
Dendrites
Axon
Bipolar
Cell body
Dendrites
Axon

Figure 18–2.

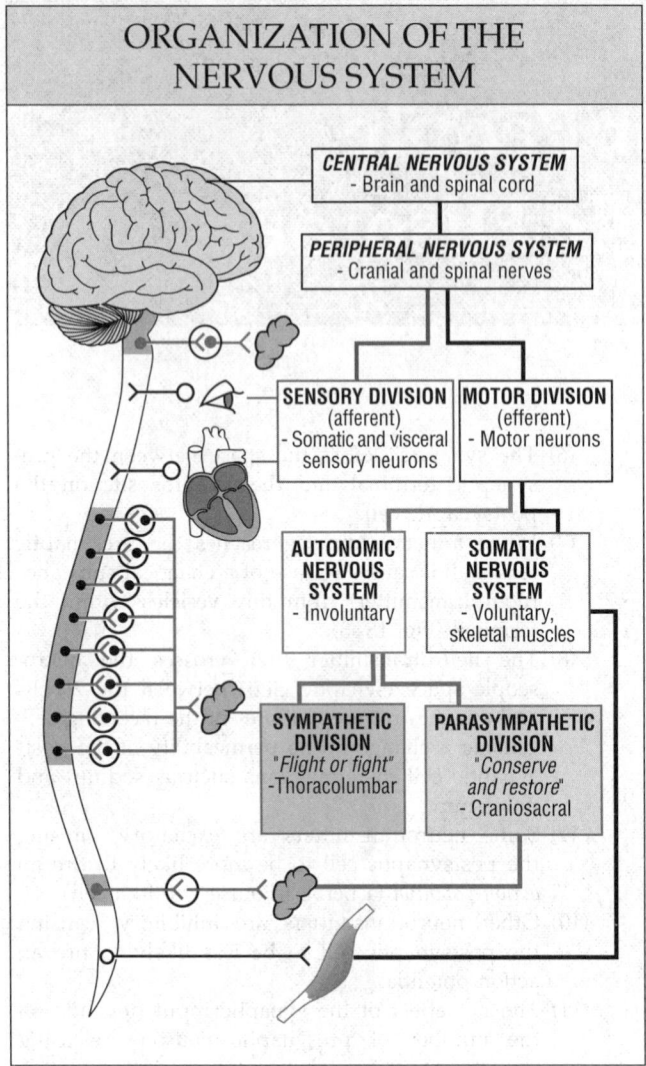

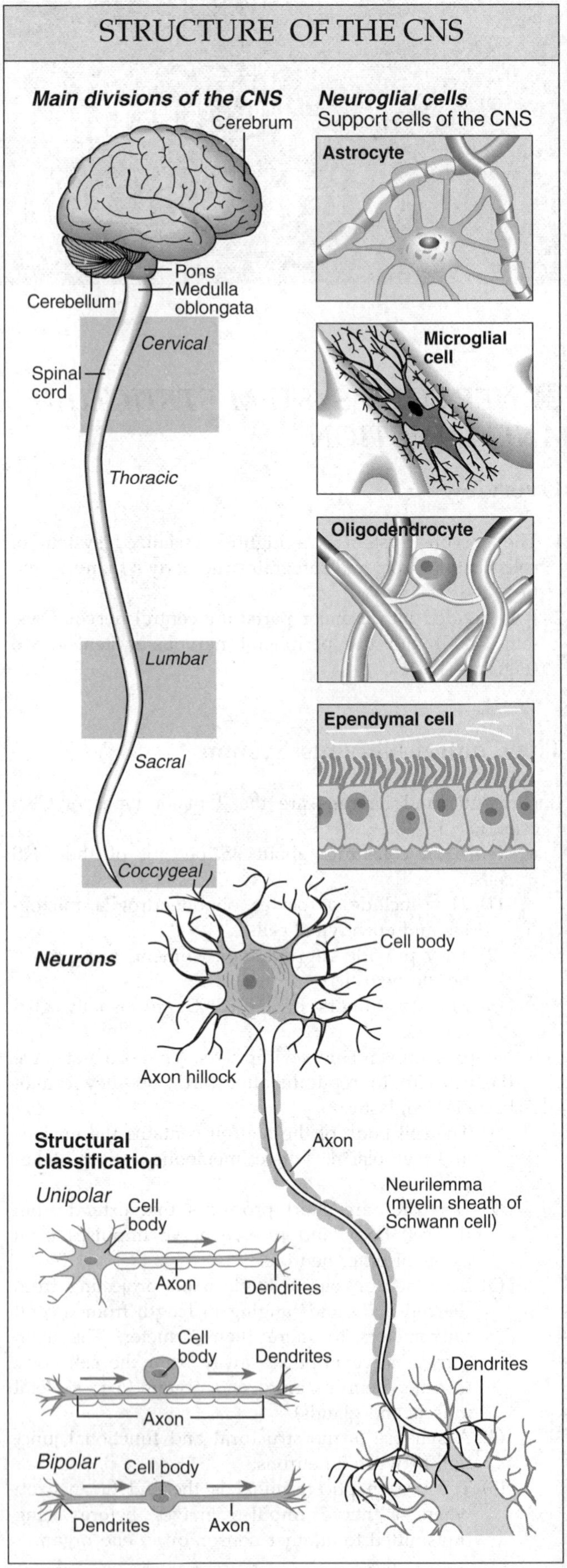

4. The brain is divided into 3 major structures: the brain stem, the cerebellum, and the cerebrum (Fig. 18–6).
   a. The brain stem (made up of the medulla, the pons, and the midbrain) connects the spinal cord to the cerebellum and the cerebrum.
      (1) The brain stem contains the reticular activating system, which regulates arousal, a component of consciousness.
      (2) The cell bodies (nuclei) of cranial nerves (CNs) III through XII are located in the brain stem.
      (3) Vital centers for respiratory, vasomotor, and cardiac function are located in the medulla.
      (4) The brain stem also contains the centers for sneezing, coughing, hiccuping, vomiting, sucking, and swallowing.
   b. The cerebellum is located posterior to the brain stem. (Both structures are located in the posterior fossa.)
      (1) The cerebellum coordinates voluntary movement and maintains trunk stability and equilibrium.
      (2) The cerebellum influences motor activity by connecting to the motor cortex and brain stem nuclei.

STRUCTURE OF A SYNAPSE

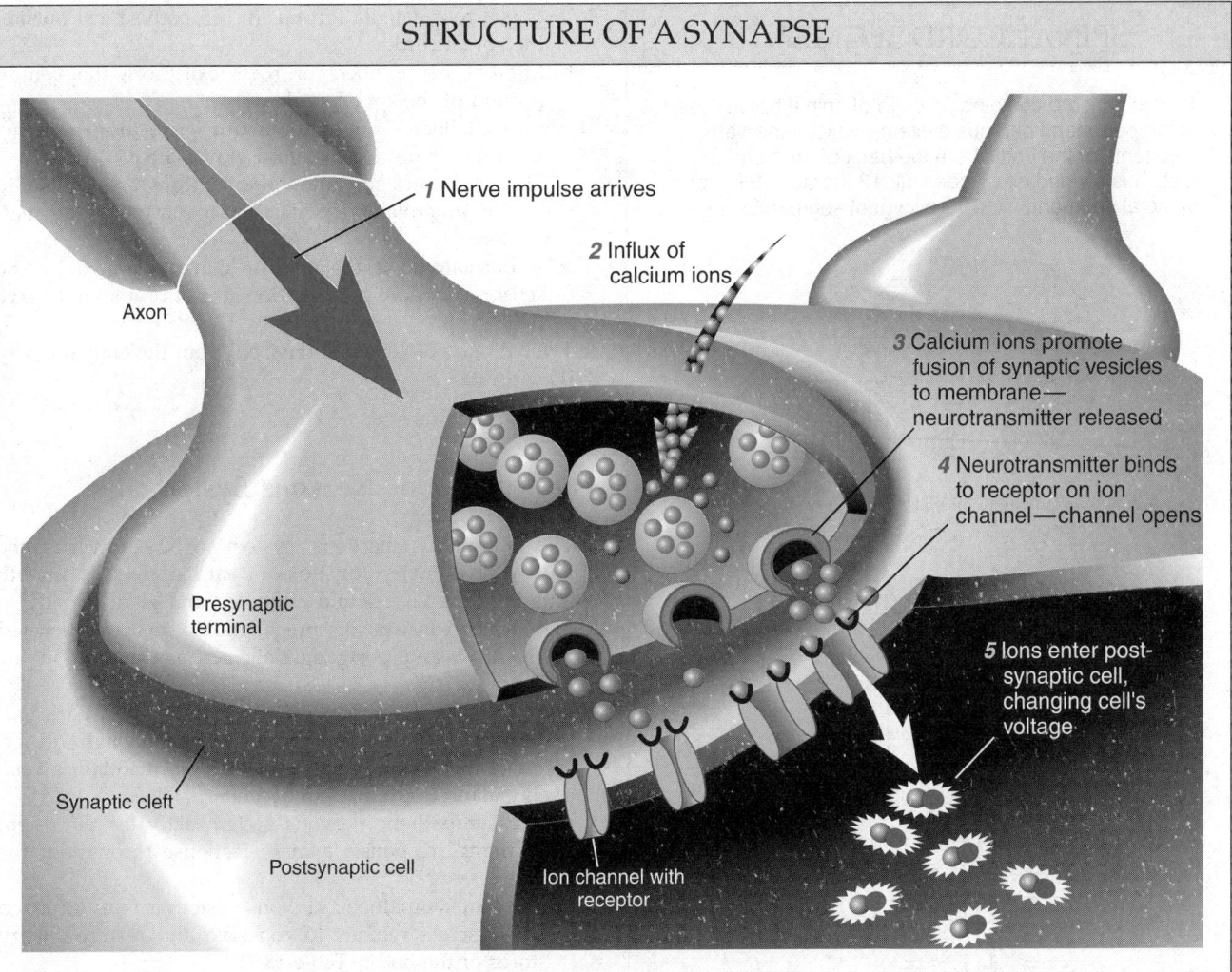

1 Nerve impulse arrives

2 Influx of calcium ions

Axon

3 Calcium ions promote fusion of synaptic vesicles to membrane— neurotransmitter released

4 Neurotransmitter binds to receptor on ion channel—channel opens

Presynaptic terminal

5 Ions enter post- synaptic cell, changing cell's voltage

Synaptic cleft

Postsynaptic cell

Ion channel with receptor

Figure 18–3.

c. The cerebrum is divided into the right and left cerebral hemispheres.
   (1) Each hemisphere has a frontal lobe, a temporal lobe, a parietal lobe, and an occipital lobe.
   (2) The neocortex, the outer layer of the cerebrum, contains neuronal cell bodies (and thus is made up of gray matter).
   (3) Neurons in specific parts of the neocortex are essential for various highly complex and sophisticated aspects of mental functioning, for voluntary movement, and for appreciation and integration of sensory information.
d. The thalamus, which lies directly above the brain stem, is the major relay center for sensory and other afferent (e.g., cerebellar) inputs to the cerebral cortex.
e. The hypothalamus, located just inferior and anterior to the thalamus, regulates the autonomic and neuroendocrine systems.
f. The basal ganglia lie just above the thalamus, although separated somewhat from it by the fluid filled ventricles. They modulate the initiation, exe-

cution, and completion of voluntary movements and automatic movements associated with skeletal muscle activity (e.g., swinging the arms while walking).
g. The limbic system, located near the inner surfaces of the cerebral hemispheres, regulates emotion, aggression, feeding behavior, and sexual response.
5. The ventricles and cerebrospinal fluid (CSF) are illustrated in Figure 18–7.

The Peripheral Nervous System

1. The PNS includes all neuronal structures that lie outside the CNS. Thus, it encompasses the spinal nerves and CNs, their associated ganglia, and peripheral portions of the autonomic nervous system.
2. A pair of spinal nerves exits from each segment of spinal cord to each side of the body.
   a. Afferent nerve fibers or roots enter the dorsal portion of the spinal cord. Their cell bodies are located in the

SPINAL CORD SEGMENTS

The spinal cord contains 31 pairs of spinal nerves (part of the peripheral nervous system), which innervate segments of the body, from the back of the head to the feet. It is divided into 8 cervical, 12 thoracic, 5 lumbar, 5 sacral segments, and 1 coccygeal segment.

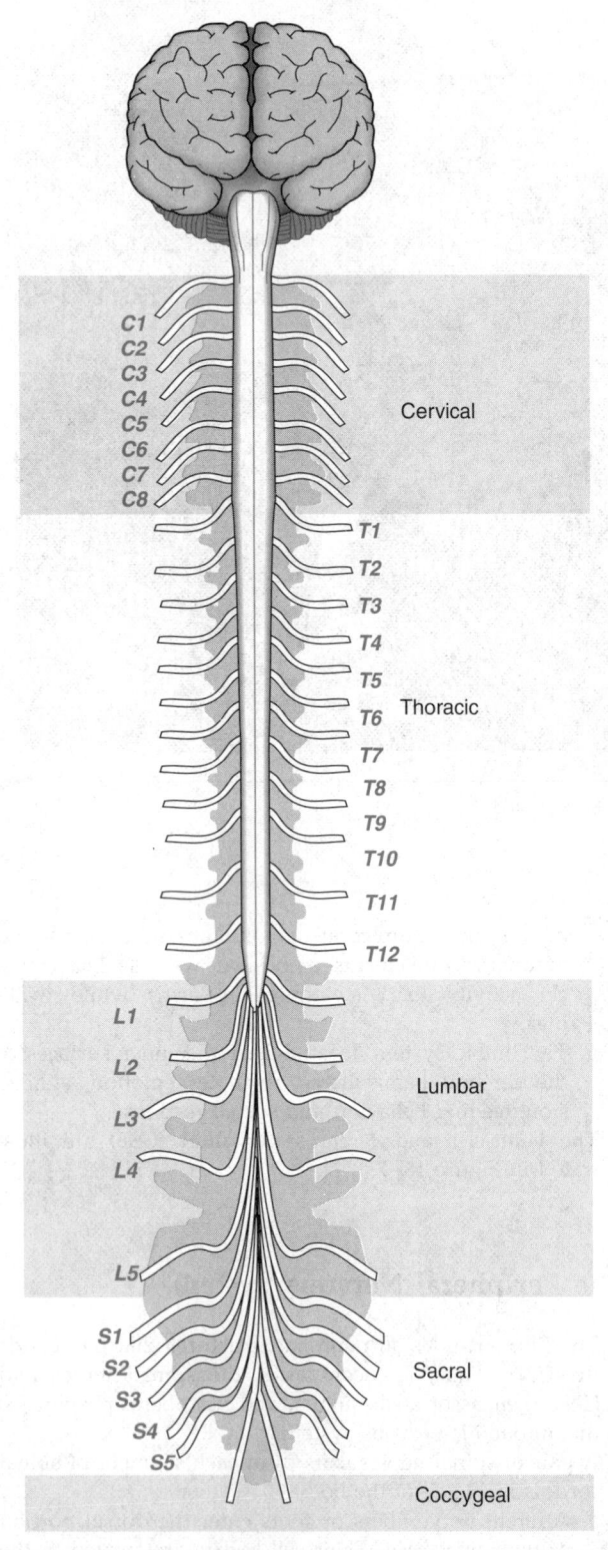

Cervical

Thoracic

Lumbar

Sacral

Coccygeal

Figure 18–4.

dorsal root ganglia (groups of cell bodies) just outside the spinal cord.
   b. Efferent nerve fibers or roots exit from the ventral portion of the spinal cord.
     (1) Cell bodies for motor neurons are located in the anterior horn spinal cord gray matter.
     (2) Cell bodies for autonomic neurons are located in the anterolateral portion of spinal cord gray matter.
   c. A dermatome is the area of skin innervated by the sensory fibers of a single dorsal root of a spinal nerve (Fig. 18–8).
3. Twelve pairs of CNs exit the CNS from the cranial cavity (Fig. 18–9).

The Autonomic Nervous System

1. The autonomic nervous system (ANS) governs the mostly involuntary functions of cardiac muscle, smooth muscle of the viscera and arterioles, and glands.
2. The ANS consists of preganglionic neurons located in the CNS and postganglionic neurons located in the PNS.
3. The ANS has 2 components, sympathetic and parasympathetic, which are anatomically and functionally different. The 2 systems function together to maintain a relatively balanced internal environment.
   a. The sympathetic nervous system activates the "fight or flight" response, a mass response throughout the body.
   b. The parasympathetic nervous system acts in localized and discrete regions to conserve and restore energy stores of the body (Table 18–1).

Cerebral Circulation

1. The blood supply to the brain depends on 2 internal carotid and 2 vertebral arteries (Fig. 18–10).
2. The internal carotid arteries supply the anterior circulation of the brain (anterior and middle cerebral arteries).
   a. The anterior cerebral artery supplies the medial aspect of the frontal lobe.
   b. The middle cerebral artery comes directly off the internal carotid artery.
     (1) It carries 80 percent of the blood going to the cerebral hemispheres.
     (2) It supplies most of the outer surface of the cerebral cortex, including motor and sensory cortex and language centers.
     (3) It has penetrating branches that anastomose with branches of the anterior and posterior cerebral arteries deep within the brain.
3. The two vertebral arteries combine to form the basilar artery and supply the brain stem (these 3 arteries are called the vertebrobasilar system).
4. The posterior cerebral arteries come off the top of the basilar artery and supply the posterior, inferior

SENSORY AND MOTOR PATHWAYS

Ascending tracts carry specific sensory input from special sensory endings (receptors) in the skin, muscles, and joints, viscera, and blood vessels to higher levels of the central nervous system. The spinothalamic tracts carry pain and temperature inputs, and the posterior or dorsal columns carry touch, pressure, vibration, and position sense inputs.

Descending tracts (pyramidal and extrapyramidal) carry impulses that are responsible for muscle movements from higher levels of the central nervous system to skeletal muscle via the spinal cord. These motor tracts terminate on nerve cell bodies called *anterior horn cells*, in the anterior horn of the spinal cord gray matter. These anterior horn cells (and their counterparts in the cranial nerve nuclei of the brain stem) comprise the lower motor neurons, which represent the final common pathway for higher motor centers to influence skeletal muscle. Upper motor neurons, which are located in the brain stem and cerebral cortex, include all supraspinal motor neurons that influence skeletal muscle movement.

SENSORY PATHWAY

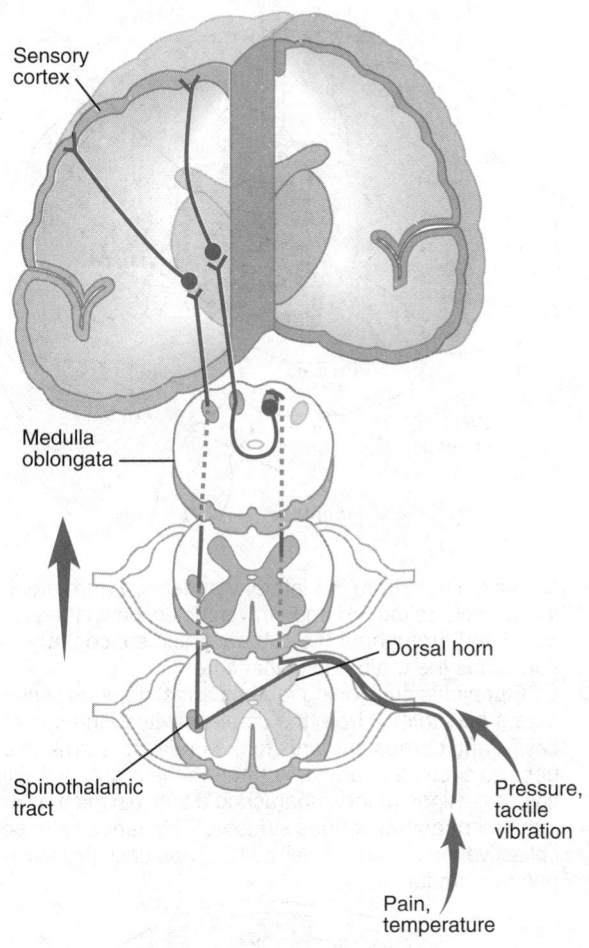

MOTOR PATHWAY

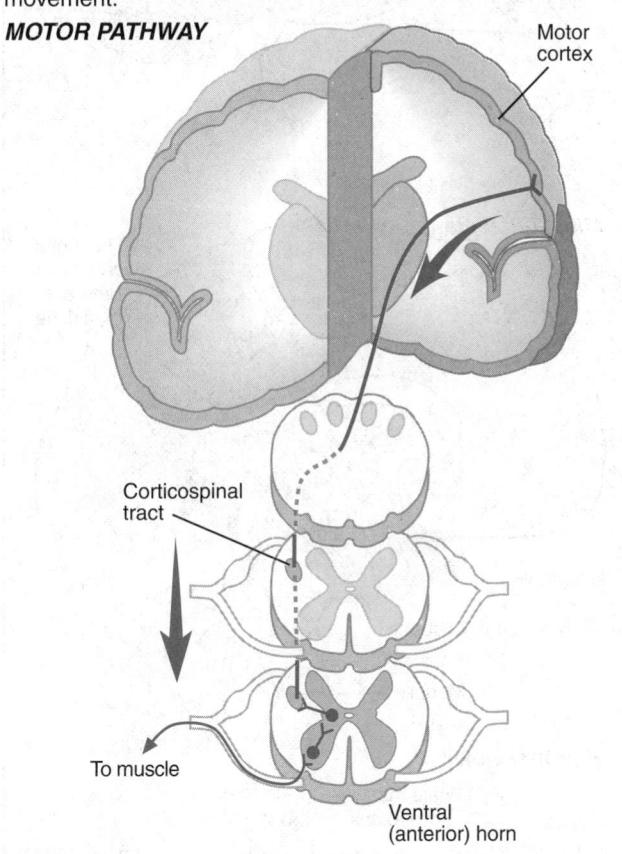

Figure 18–5.

portion of the cerebral hemispheres (occipital cortex, thalamus, mesial temporal lobe). These arteries and the vertebrobasilar system comprise the posterior circulation.
5. The circle of Willis is a ring of vessels at the base of the brain.
   a. It is formed by anastomoses of paired anterior cerebral, internal carotid, posterior cerebral, and communicating arteries.
   b. It provides alternative blood supply to the cerebrum if 1 of the major arteries becomes narrowed or occluded.
6. The blood-brain barrier is a physiologic barrier between blood capillaries and brain tissue. It protects the CNS from changes in its chemical environment.

Protective Structures of the Central Nervous System

1. The CNS is protected by the meninges, skull, and vertebral column (Fig. 18–11).

◼ *ASSESSING PEOPLE WITH NEUROLOGIC DISORDERS*

Key Symptoms and Their Pathophysiologic Bases

1. Nervous system disease can affect consciousness, mentation, movement, sensation, and integrated regulation

BASIC ANATOMY OF THE BRAIN

Lateral view

Motor
Sensory
Parietal
Frontal
Occipital
Temporal

Midsagittal view

Thalamus located just lateral to midline
Cerebrum
Hypothalamus
Brain stem: Midbrain
Pons
Medulla
Cerebellum

Coronal view

White matter—cell axons
Lateral ventricle
Cortex—cell bodies
Thalamus
Hypothalamus
Basal ganglia
3rd ventricle

Figure 18–6.

VENTRICLES OF THE BRAIN AND CEREBROSPINAL FLUID CIRCULATION

The ventricles are 4 fluid-filled cavities within the brain. They connect with one another and with the spinal canal, which descends down the center of the spinal cord.

These chambers and the spinal canal are filled with cerebrospinal fluid (CSF), a total volume of 135 ml.

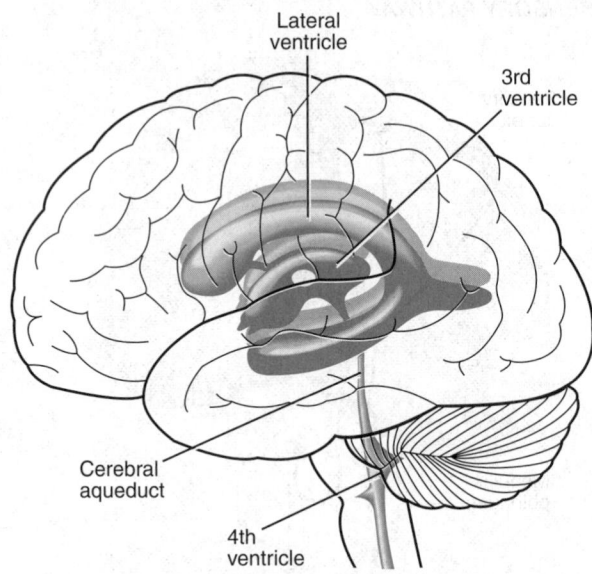

Lateral ventricle
3rd ventricle
Cerebral aqueduct
4th ventricle

CSF circulates from the lateral ventricles, where most of it is formed, to the 3rd and 4th ventricles, down the spinal canal and throughout the subarachnoid space that surrounds the brain and spinal cord.

CSF provides cushioning for the central nervous system, allows fluid to shift from the cranial cavity to the spinal cavity, and carries nutrients to the brain. It returns to the general circulation primarily through the arachnoid villi, tiny projections of the subarachnoid space, which extend into the intradural venous sinuses. The venous sinuses collect venous blood as well as CSF and pass this mixture into the jugular veins.

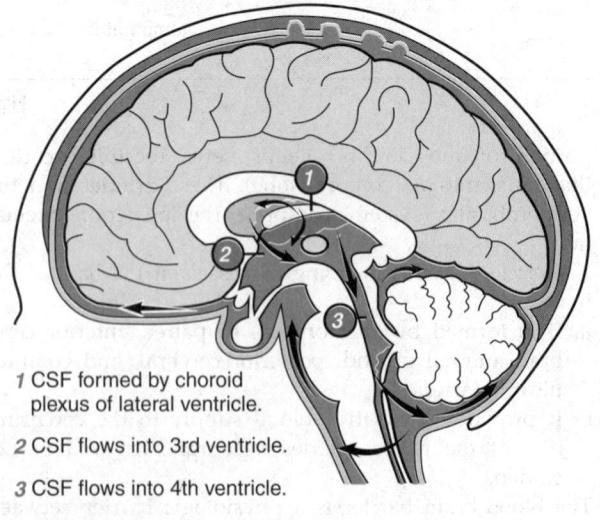

1 CSF formed by choroid plexus of lateral ventricle.

2 CSF flows into 3rd ventricle.

3 CSF flows into 4th ventricle.

Figure 18–7.

DERMATOMES

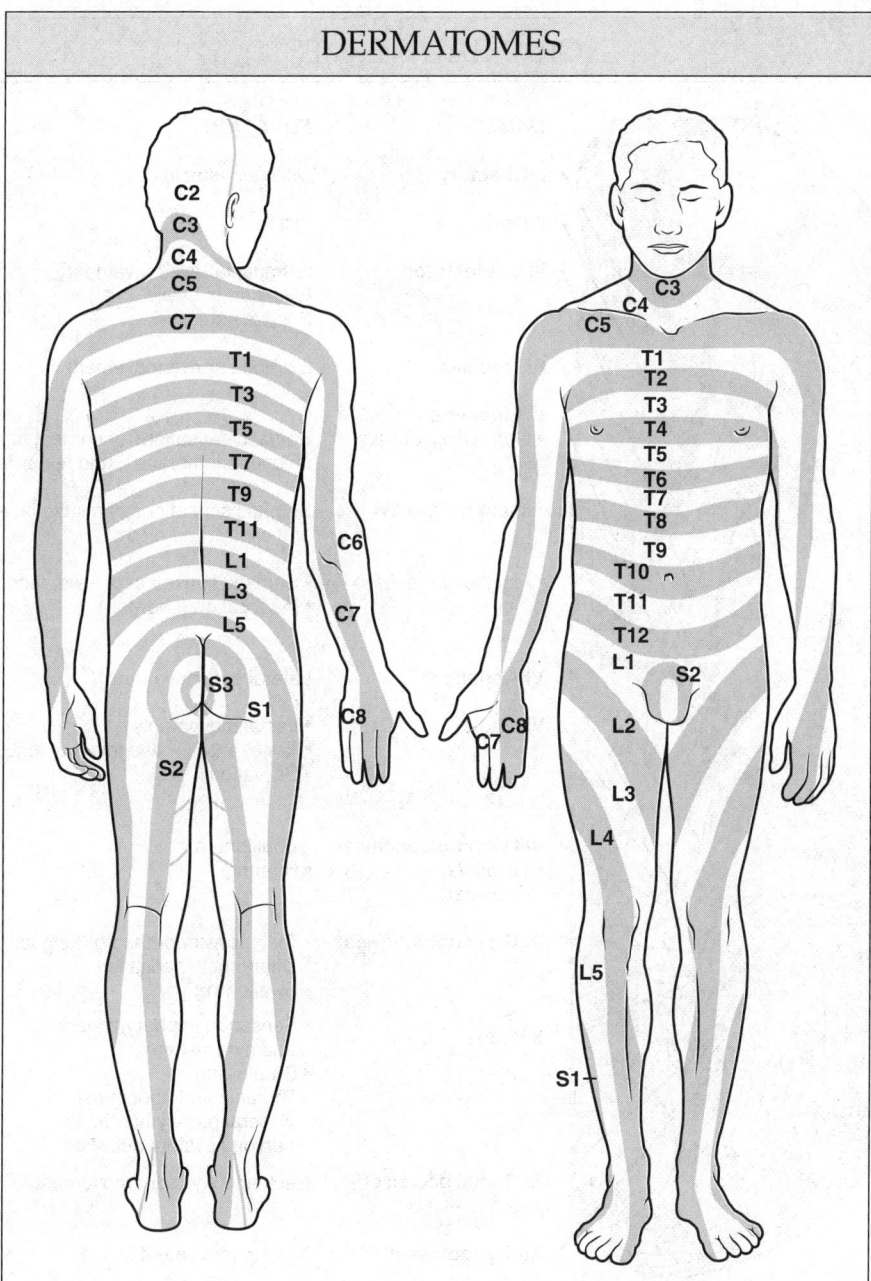

Figure 18–8.

(i.e., breathing, circulation, temperature control, and elimination).

a. Consciousness can be impaired by diseases that affect the brain stem reticular activating system or both cerebral hemispheres, causing, for example, fainting or loss of consciousness.

b. Mentation can be impaired by diseases that affect the cerebral cortex, causing, for example, altered memory, distortions of reality, disorientation, loss of ability to concentrate, or changes in ability to speak or understand language.

c. Movement and coordination can be impaired by diseases that affect any part of the motor pathways (cerebral cortex, descending pyramidal and extrapyramidal tracts, and peripheral nerves) or cerebellum, causing, for example, weakness, loss of coordination, staggering, paralysis, or shuffling gait.

d. Sensation can be impaired by diseases that affect any part of the sensory pathways (peripheral nerves, ascending tracts, thalamus, cerebral cortex), causing, for example, numbness or paresthesias.

e. Breathing can be impaired by disorders that affect the brain and brain stem and spinal nerves affecting accessory muscles of breathing.

f. Circulation can be influenced by local innervation, disorders affecting the ANS regulation, and cortical and brain stem regulatory malfunctions, causing, for example, palpitations, hypotension, or hypertension.

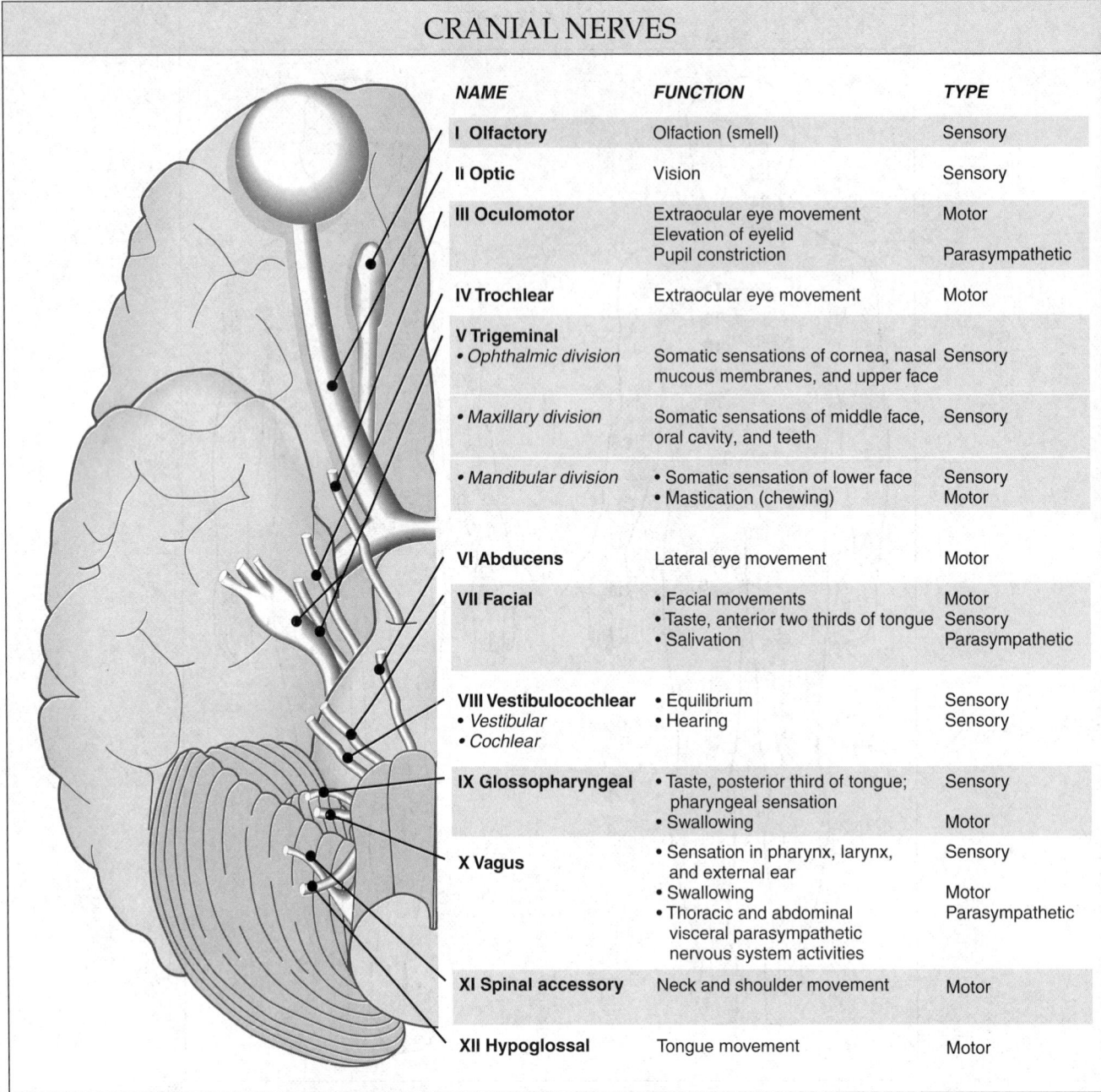

CRANIAL NERVES

NAME	FUNCTION	TYPE
I Olfactory	Olfaction (smell)	Sensory
II Optic	Vision	Sensory
III Oculomotor	Extraocular eye movement Elevation of eyelid Pupil constriction	Motor Parasympathetic
IV Trochlear	Extraocular eye movement	Motor
V Trigeminal • *Ophthalmic division*	Somatic sensations of cornea, nasal mucous membranes, and upper face	Sensory
• *Maxillary division*	Somatic sensations of middle face, oral cavity, and teeth	Sensory
• *Mandibular division*	• Somatic sensation of lower face • Mastication (chewing)	Sensory Motor
VI Abducens	Lateral eye movement	Motor
VII Facial	• Facial movements • Taste, anterior two thirds of tongue • Salivation	Motor Sensory Parasympathetic
VIII Vestibulocochlear • *Vestibular* • *Cochlear*	• Equilibrium • Hearing	Sensory Sensory
IX Glossopharyngeal	• Taste, posterior third of tongue; pharyngeal sensation • Swallowing	Sensory Motor
X Vagus	• Sensation in pharynx, larynx, and external ear • Swallowing • Thoracic and abdominal visceral parasympathetic nervous system activities	Sensory Motor Parasympathetic
XI Spinal accessory	Neck and shoulder movement	Motor
XII Hypoglossal	Tongue movement	Motor

Figure 18–9. (Tabular material from Black JM, and Matassarin-Jacobs E [eds]. *Luckmann and Sorensen's Medical-Surgical Nursing: A Psychophysiologic Approach.* 4th ed. Philadelphia: WB Saunders, 1993, p 630.)

g. Temperature control can be disrupted by impaired hypothalamic function or by denervation of sweat glands (e.g., spinal cord injury).

h. Urinary and bowel elimination (retention or incontinence) can be impaired by disruption of the cortical descending inhibitory pathways (urge incontinence), by spinal cord disease, and by peripheral nerve disease.

i. Eye, ear, nose, and throat function can be impaired by abnormalities in neurologic function, causing, for example, visual loss, diplopia, nystagmus, hearing loss, tinnitus, vertigo, voice change, dysphagia, or changes in taste or smell.

Health History

1. Do the following *before* taking a health history.
   a. Consider the reliability of the patient: Neurologic disease can affect mentation. Obtain the history from a family member or significant other if the patient is unreliable.

Organ	Effect of Sympathetic Stimulation	Effect of Parasympathetic Stimulation
Eye		
Pupil	Dilated	Constricted
Ciliary muscle	Slight relaxation (far vision)	Constricted (near vision)
Glands	Vasoconstriction and slight secretion	Stimulation of copious secretion (containing many enzymes for enzyme-secreting glands)
Nasal		
Lacrimal		
Parotid		
Submandibular		
Gastric		
Pancreatic		
Sweat glands	Copious sweating (cholinergic)	Sweating on palms of hands
Apocrine glands	Thick, odoriferous secretion	None
Heart		
Muscle	Increased rate	Slowed rate
	Increased force of contraction	Decreased force of contraction (especially of atria)
Coronaries	Dilated (β_2); constricted (α)	Dilated
Lungs		
Bronchi	Dilated	Constricted
Blood vessels	Mildly constricted	? Dilated
Gut		
Lumen	Decreased peristalsis and tone	Increased peristalsis and tone
Sphincter	Increased tone (most times)	Relaxed (most times)
Liver	Glucose released	Slight glycogen synthesis
Gallbladder and bile ducts	Relaxed	Contracted
Kidney	Decreased output and renin secretion	None
Bladder		
Detrusor	Relaxed (slight)	Contracted
Trigone	Contracted	Relaxed
Penis	Ejaculation	Erection
Systemic arterioles		
Abdominal viscera	Constricted	None
Muscle	Constricted (adrenergic α)	None
	Dilated (adrenergic β_2)	
	Dilated (cholinergic)	
Skin	Constricted	None
Blood		
Coagulation	Increased	None
Glucose	Increased	None
Lipids	Increased	None
Basal metabolism	Increased up to 100%	None
Adrenal medullary secretion	Increased	None
Mental activity	Increased	None
Piloerector muscles	Contracted	None
Skeletal muscle	Increased glycogenolysis	None
	Increased strength	
Fat cells	lipolysis	None

From Guyton AC. *Textbook of Medical Physiology*. 8th ed. Philadelphia: WB Saunders, 1991, p 672.

b. Avoid suggesting symptoms.

c. Gather information on mode of onset and course of symptoms.

d. Recognize that the history helps to focus the neurologic examination.

2. Obtain the past health history.

a. Ask the person about chronic diseases, trauma, infections, exposure to toxins.

b. Obtain a growth and development history to determine whether neurologic dysfunction was present at an early age.

c. Ask if family members have or have had similar

CIRCULATION OF THE BRAIN

Lateral view of the brain

Middle cerebral a.

Anterior cerebral a.

Posterior cerebral a.

Left internal carotid a.

Vertebral a.

Common carotid a.

Sagittal view of the brain

Anterior cerebral a.

Internal carotid a.

Posterior cerebral a.

Inferior view of the brain

Anterior cerebral a.

Anterior communicating a.

Middle cerebral a. (internal)

Internal carotid a.

Pontine a.

Posterior cerebral a.

Basilar a.

Vertebral a.

Anterior inferior cerebellar a.

Figure 18–10.

PROTECTIVE STRUCTURES OF THE CENTRAL NERVOUS SYSTEM

The meninges are three layers of protective membranes (dura mater, arachnoid, and pia mater) that surround the brain and spinal cord.

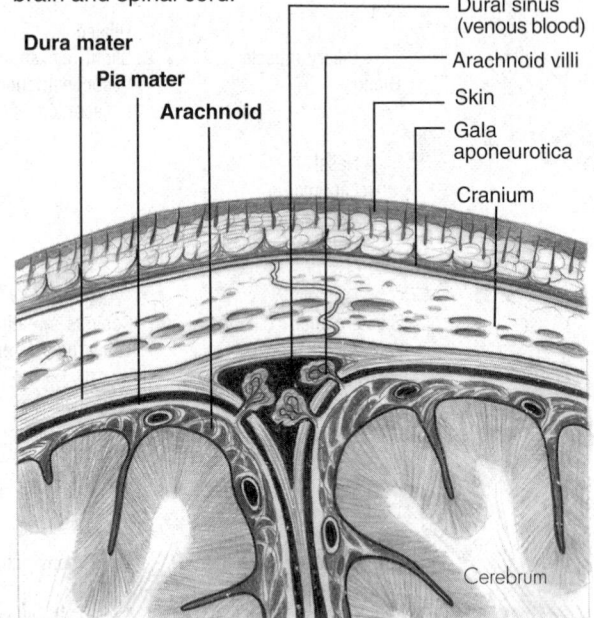

Dura mater

Pia mater

Arachnoid

Dural sinus (venous blood)

Arachnoid villi

Skin

Gala aponeurotica

Cranium

Cerebrum

The bony skull protects the brain from external trauma and is composed of eight cranial bones and 14 facial bones. The vertebral column is made of 33 individual vertebrae: 7 cervical, 12 thoracic, 5 lumbar, 5 sacral (fused into one), and 4 coccygeal (fused into one). It protects the spinal cord, supports the head, and provides for flexibility.

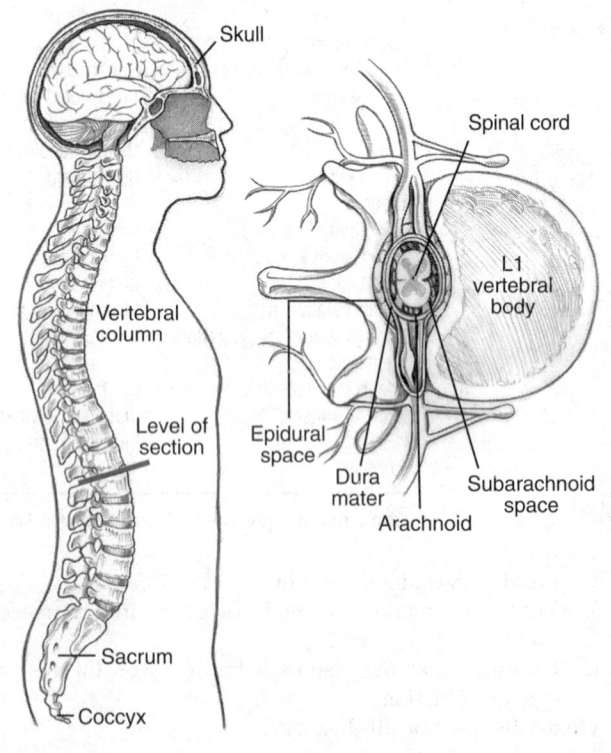

Skull

Spinal cord

Vertebral column

L1 vertebral body

Level of section

Epidural space

Dura mater

Arachnoid

Subarachnoid space

Sacrum

Coccyx

Figure 18–11.

problems to establish a possible hereditary component.

   d. Ask if there have been any changes in daily living routines. All of the following can have neurologic implications.

     (1) Appetite
     (2) Sleep
     (3) Exercise
     (4) Recreation
     (5) Occupation
     (6) Stressors
     (7) Sexual practices

3. Conduct a review of neurologic function related to mentation, movement, sensation, and integrated regulation.

   a. Mentation aspects: Ask the following questions:

     (1) Have you noticed changes in ability to read? Speak? Understand language?
     (2) Is your memory for recent events altered?
     (3) Do you have difficulty concentrating, solving problems, or making good judgments?
     (4) Do you have difficulty managing daily living tasks? Work? Financial affairs?
     (5) Have you ever "blacked out" or lost track of time?

   b. Movement aspects: Ask these questions:

     (1) Have you noticed weakness, tremor, or abnormal movements in one or more limbs?
     (2) Have you fallen? Been off balance?
     (3) Do you have trouble chewing? Swallowing? Pronouncing words clearly?
     (4) Do you have trouble dressing? Doing personal hygiene? Climbing stairs?

   c. Sensation aspects: Ask the following questions:

     (1) Do you have trouble seeing? Hearing? Smelling? Tasting?
     (2) Do you experience abnormal sensations? Burning? Tingling? Aching? Numbness? Where?

   d. Integrated regulation: Ask these questions:

     (1) Do you have trouble with bowel or bladder function? Incontinence? Constipation? Urinary retention? Urgency? Hesitancy?
     (2) Do you have difficulty breathing? Do you snore during sleep? Do you stop breathing during sleep?
     (3) Do you have trouble with sexual response? Inability to sustain erection? Ejaculate? Attain orgasm?
     (4) Do you have disrupted sleep? Excessive daytime sleepiness? Difficulty falling asleep? Awakening early?

   e. Coping aspects: If neurologic dysfunction exists, does person acknowledge problems? Show adaptive capacity? Have good support system?

Neurologic Assessment

1. The type of assessment depends on the clinical situation.

   a. If the person is alert and cooperative and a comprehensive neurologic review is required, perform the complete assessment (see later discussion).

   b. If the person has had recent neurosurgery, for example, lumbar laminectomy, you may want to focus the postoperative assessment on function and sensation of the lower extremities only.

   c. If the person comes into the emergency department after a head injury and is unconscious, focus the assessment on responses to stimuli.

2. The comprehensive assessment includes several major categories.

   a. Mental status

     (1) General appearance and behavior. Is the person well groomed? Well dressed? Unkempt? Agitated, withdrawn, or confused?
     (2) Level of consciousness (see p. 679 and Chapter 6).
     (3) Content of consciousness (see also Chapter 6). Is the person oriented to person, place, time, and situation (e.g., why the person is seeking health care)? Can the person recall newly learned items (e.g., 3 objects after 5 minutes? Recent events? Remote events?)? What is the person's fund of information (general knowledge)? For example, if an American, ask the person to name the most recent presidents of the United States. Can the person perform simple calculations? Complex calculations? Does the person show insight about his or her current situation?
     (4) Mood and affect. Is the person agitated? Angry? Depressed? Euphoric? Are these moods appropriate? Does the person have a flat affect?
     (5) Thought content (see also Chapter 41). Does the person have hallucinations? Delusions? Paranoia? Check for psychiatric history. Check for medications that might cause these symptoms.

   b. Cranial nerve function (see Fig. 18–9)

     (1) Test sense of smell (olfactory nerve [CN I]) if the person complains of lack of smell or altered sense of smell. Ask the patient to close the eyes and sniff from a bottle containing coffee, spice, soap, or another easily recognizable odor. Chronic rhinitis, sinusitis, and heavy smoking can decrease sense of smell and should be included in the health history.
     (2) Test the person's visual field (optic nerve [CN II]). Ask the person to close 1 eye and to look directly at the bridge of your nose. Then, move your finger in from the periphery of each of the 4 visual quadrants until the person tells you he or she can see your finger. Repeat the test for the other eye. The person with intact visual fields should be able to see your finger in the periphery of all 4 quadrants (Fig. 18–12). The nasal side of the visual field is narrower because of the nasal bridge. Lesions of the optic nerve can create monocular vision disturbance. Lesions of the optic chiasm usually create "tunnel vision" or loss of peripheral vision. Lesions of the optic tracts that extend through the temporal, parietal, and occipital lobes may cause a hemianopia (loss of vision in one half of the visual field) or a quadrantanopia (loss of 1 quadrant of the visual field).
     (3) Test visual acuity (optic nerve [CN II]) by asking

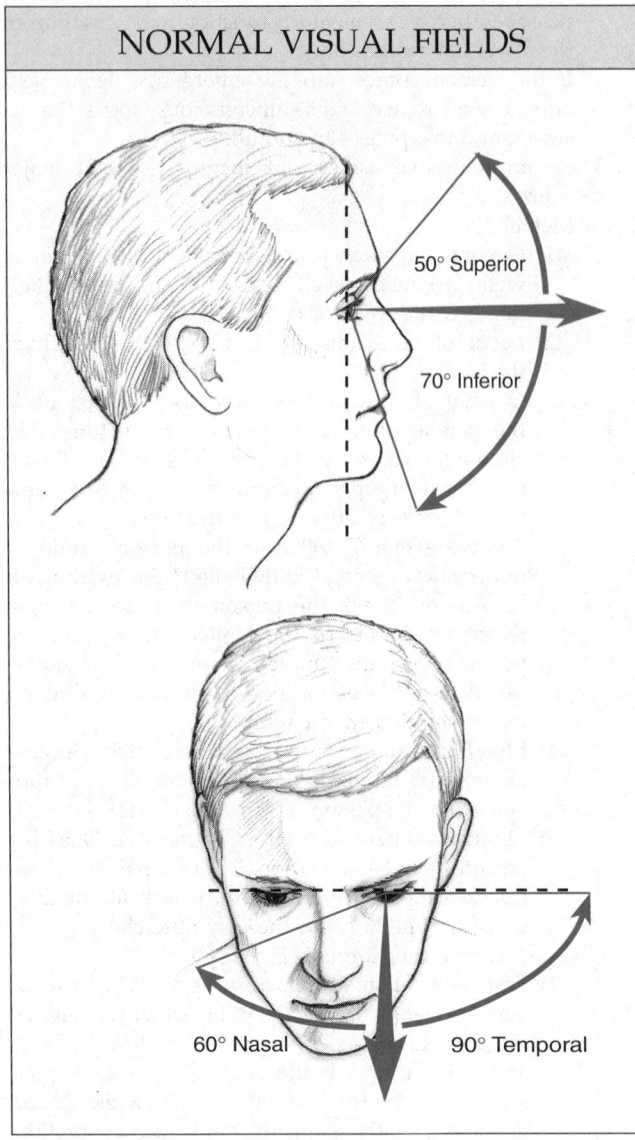

NORMAL VISUAL FIELDS

50° Superior

70° Inferior

60° Nasal   90° Temporal

Figure 18–12.

the person to read newsprint at a comfortable distance (less than arm's length). More formal testing is done with a Snellen chart (see Chapter 19).

NURSE ADVISORY

Allow the person to wear corrective lenses during vision testing.

(4) The oculomotor nerve (CN III) governs 4 of the muscles that move the eyeball. Test it along with the trochlear nerve (CN IV), which controls the superior oblique muscle, and the abducens nerve (CN VI), which controls the lateral rectus muscle of the eyeball.
  • Ask the person to follow your finger as it moves horizontally and vertically—making a

cross—and diagonally—making an X. Failure of the eyes to move symmetrically indicates disconjugate gaze. Jerky movements of the eyes as they track—nystagmus—is usually a sign of vestibulocerebellar dysfunction.
  • Check for pupillary constriction by shining a light into each eye. The pupils normally constrict briskly.
  • Check for convergence (eyes turning inward when focusing on a near object) and for accommodation (pupils constricting when the eyes focus on a near object) by asking the person to focus on your finger as you move it toward the person's nose.
  • Testing for pupillary constriction is an important component of the neurologic assessment of people at risk for herniation syndrome (see Caring for People with Traumatic Brain Injury) because the oculomotor nerve exits at the top of the brain stem, at the tentorial notch, and it can be compressed easily by expanding mass lesions in the cerebral hemispheres.
  • Another function of the oculomotor nerve is to keep the eyelid open. Damage to this nerve can cause ptosis (drooping eyelid).
(5) The trigeminal nerve (CN V) governs sensation of the face, eyes, and oral cavity. It also governs the masseter, temporal, and pterygoid muscles, which open and close the jaw.
  • Test the sensory component of CN V by asking the person to close the eyes and indicate when he or she feels light touch (with a cotton tip applicator) and pinprick in the ophthalmic, mandibular, and maxillary divisions of the nerve on both sides of the face.
  • Test the motor component of CN V by asking the person to clench teeth while you palpate the masseter muscles just above the mandibular angle.
(6) Test facial muscles (facial nerve [CN VII]) by asking the person to raise the eyebrows, close the eyes tightly, purse the lips, draw back the corners of the mouth in an exaggerated smile, and frown. Note any asymmetry in facial movements.
(7) Test taste discrimination of saltiness and sweetness (CN VII) if you suspect a peripheral nerve lesion.
(8) The vestibulocochlear nerve (CN VIII) governs aspects of equilibrium and the special sense of hearing. Usually you will test just the hearing component. Ask the person to discern a ticking watch or the sound of your fingers rubbing together from a few inches away. Formal audiography produces more precise measurements of hearing (see Chapter 20).
(9) Test the glossopharyngeal (CN IX) and the vagus (CN X) nerves together because they both control the pharynx. To test the sensory component of the pharynx (CN IX), check the gag reflex by placing a tongue blade on either side of the soft

palate in the back of the throat. CN X governs the motor part of the gag response and elevation of the soft palate with phonation (tested by asking the person to say *"aaaahhhh"*). Swallowing is a good indicator of the integrity of CNs IX and X.

(10) Test the spinal accessory nerve (CN XI) by asking the person to shrug the shoulders against resistance and to turn the head to either side against resistance.

(11) Test the hypoglossal nerve (CN XII) by asking the person to protrude the tongue, which should be in the midline.

c. Motor function of skeletal muscles

(1) Test muscle strength of all major muscle groups of the upper and lower extremities by asking the person to contract a certain muscle group against your resistance (Fig. 18–13).

(2) Check for pronator drift, a sensitive measure of arm weakness, by asking the person to close the eyes and hold both arms outstretched with palms turned upward. An abnormal response is pronation or downward drifting—or both responses—of the affected arm.

(3) Test muscle tone by passively moving the limbs through range of motion (see Chapter 7). You will feel resistance, rigidity, or spasticity when moving limbs that have increased tone. You will feel limpness or flaccidity when moving limbs that have decreased tone.

(4) Check muscle bulk by comparing the size of one limb with that of the opposite limb. Note any wasting or atrophy.

(5) Check for Babinski's sign, which is an indication of disease somewhere along the voluntary motor pathways (Fig. 18–14).

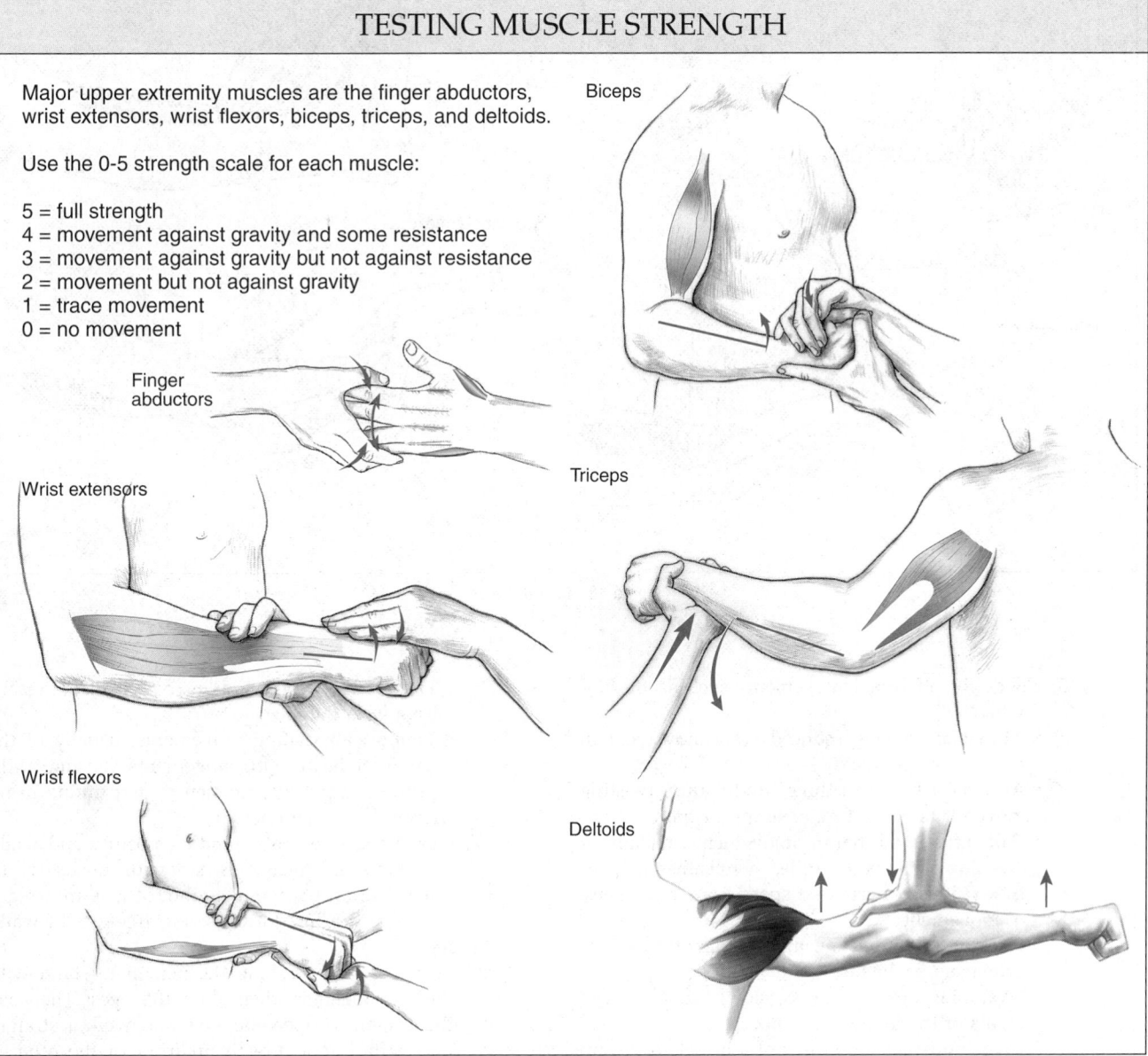

TESTING MUSCLE STRENGTH

Major upper extremity muscles are the finger abductors, wrist extensors, wrist flexors, biceps, triceps, and deltoids.

Use the 0-5 strength scale for each muscle:

5 = full strength
4 = movement against gravity and some resistance
3 = movement against gravity but not against resistance
2 = movement but not against gravity
1 = trace movement
0 = no movement

Finger abductors

Wrist extensors

Wrist flexors

Biceps

Triceps

Deltoids

Figure 18–13.

Illustration continued on following page

TESTING MUSCLE STRENGTH (continued)

Major lower extremity muscles are the hip flexors, quadriceps, hamstrings, foot dorsiflexors, and foot plantar flexors.

"Inversion of foot"

Hip flexors

Quadriceps

Hamstrings

Foot dorsiflexors

Foot plantar flexors

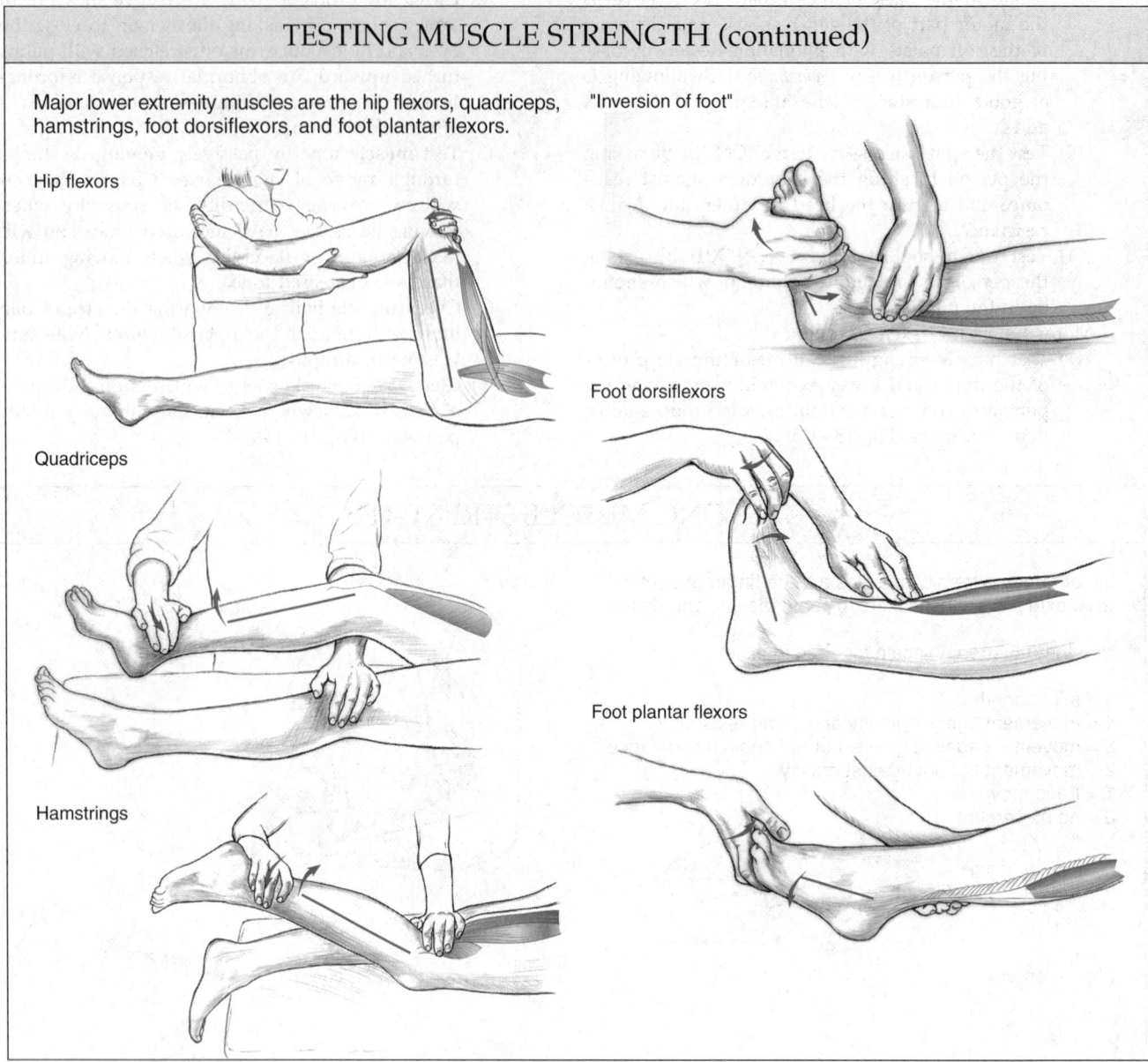

Figure 18–13. *Continued*

(6) Check for abnormal movements such as the following:
- **Akinesia:** severely reduced body movement in the absence of weakness
- **Athetosis:** slow, writhing, undulating, twisting movements of the face or limbs, or both
- **Ballismus:** wild, flailing movements, usually of one side of the body (called hemiballismus)
- **Bradykinesia:** decreased speed and spontaneity of movement
- **Chorea:** jerky, twisting movements of a limb or grimacing of the face
- **Dystonia:** large, distorted, slow, bizarre movements of the limbs and trunk
- **Myoclonus:** a sudden jerk of a muscle or group of muscles

- **Tic:** a stereotyped sudden twitch of a muscle, usually in the face
- **Tremor:** alternating movements, usually of the hands or head, with movements varying in direction, amplitude, frequency, and timing in relation to rest and activity

(7) Observe the person's standing posture and walking. Note if posture is stooped, unsteady, or tilted. Note if pace and rhythm of gait are irregular. Note if arms do not swing freely with walking.

(8) Test balance by asking the person to stand with the feet together, then close the eyes. Then ask the person to open the eyes and walk a straight line with 1 foot directly in front of the other—tandem walking (Fig. 18–15).

TESTING MOTOR PATHWAYS: BABINSKI'S SIGN

Stroke the lateral aspect of the sole of the foot with a semisharp object, e.g., the tip of a key or a splintered tongue blade.

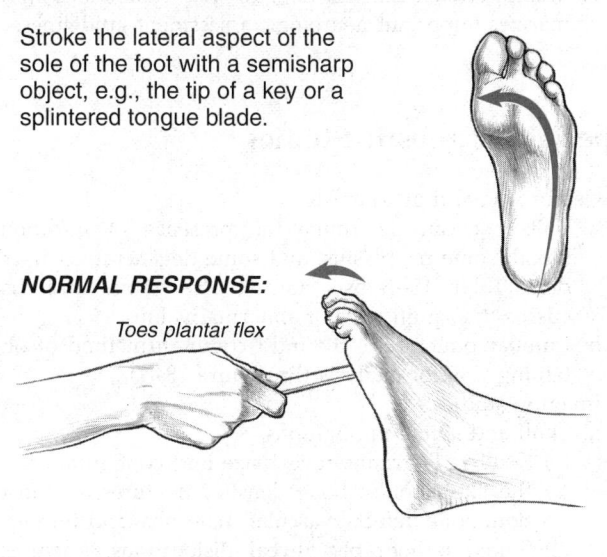

NORMAL RESPONSE:

Toes plantar flex

ABNORMAL RESPONSE:

If the big toe extends, Babinski's sign is present.

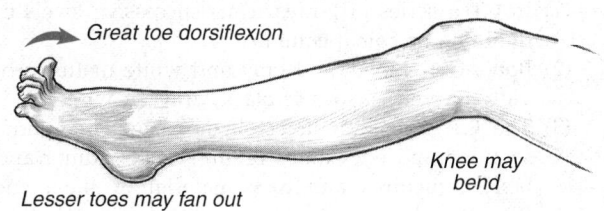

Great toe dorsiflexion

Knee may bend

Lesser toes may fan out

Figure 18–14.

(9) Test coordination of the arms and legs (Fig. 18–16).

d. Sensory function. Assess for possible signs of sensory cortex disorders.

(1) Follow several guidelines.
- Ensure that the person's eyes are closed during testing to avoid visual cues.
- Avoid giving verbal cues, that is, do not ask the person, "Is this sharp?" Rather, ask the person to identify the sensation.
- Apply the sensory stimulus in an irregular pattern so the person does not know what to expect.
- Ask the person to tell you when he or she feels the stimulus.
- Test the hands and feet unless you suspect a specific deficit or the person identifies one.
- If the person has a discrete area of sensory loss, carefully identify the area by presenting the stimulus first in the area of decreased or absent sensation. Then move the stimulus gradually toward the areas of intact sensation until the person positively identifies the stimulus.

(2) Test light touch by gently touching the skin with a cotton wisp or the tips of your fingers.
(3) Test pain by touching the skin with a safety pin. *Do not reuse the pin.*
(4) Test vibration sense by applying a vibrating C-128 tuning fork to the fingernails and bony prominences of the limbs.
(5) Test position sense by having the person close his or her eyes, then moving the person's big toe up or down. Ask the person to tell you which direction the toe moves.
(6) Test cortical integration of sensations by several methods.
- To test **2-point discrimination,** place the 2 points of a calibrated compass on the tips of the person's fingers and toes. The minimum recognizable separation of the 2 points is 4 to 5 mm on the fingertips.
- Test **graphesthesia** by asking the person to identify numbers you trace on the palm of his or her hands when eyes are closed.
- Test **stereognosis** by asking the person to iden-

TESTING BALANCE

Postural Stability:
Patient stands still with eyes closed. Swaying should not be noticeable.

Tandem Walking:
With eyes open, patient walks a straight line, heel to toe. Swaying should not be noticeable.

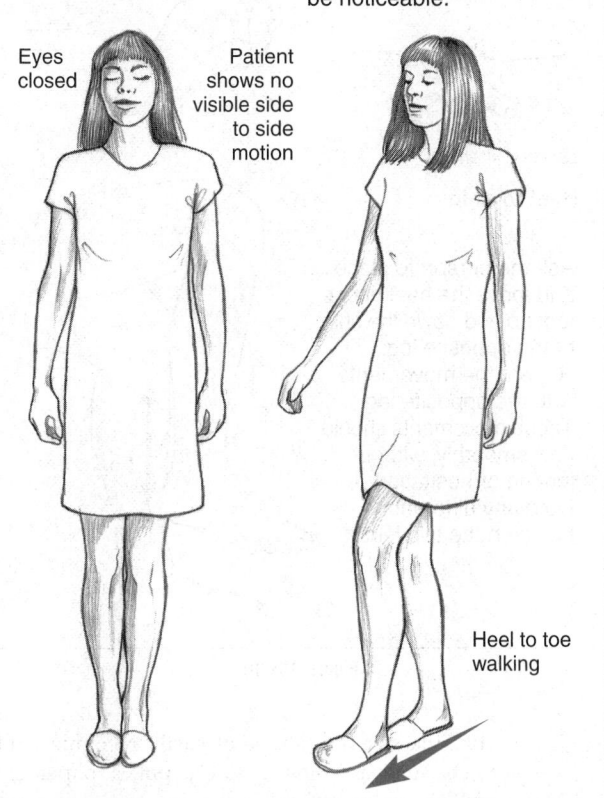

Eyes closed

Patient shows no visible side to side motion

Heel to toe walking

Figure 18–15.

TESTING COORDINATION

Upper extremity:

Finger-to-nose test

Note the speed and accuracy of these movements.
Note tremor or past-pointing.

1. Patient touches examiner's forefinger.
2. Patient touches own nose.
3. Reposition examiner's finger, repeat movements.

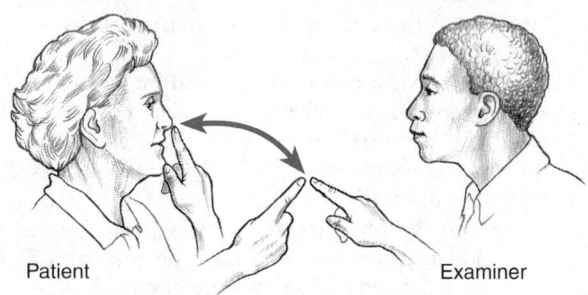

Patient   Examiner

Pronate and supinate one hand rapidly on the palm of the other hand (rapid alternating movements).
Repeat this with the other hand and note any differences between the two hands.

Pronation-supination   **Fine movements**

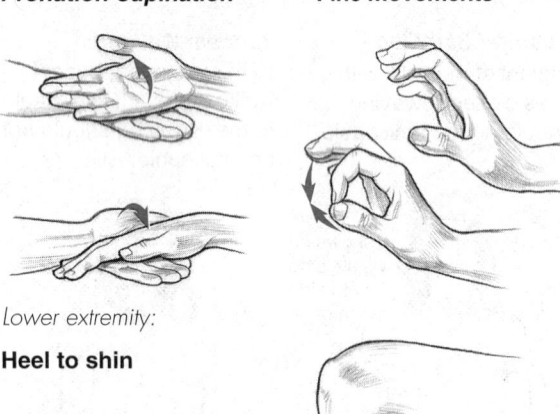

Lower extremity:

Heel to shin

Ask the person to place and move the heel of one foot up and down the shin of the opposite leg. Repeat the movements with the opposite leg. These movements should flow smoothly, without jerking or hesitation. Note any differences between the two legs.

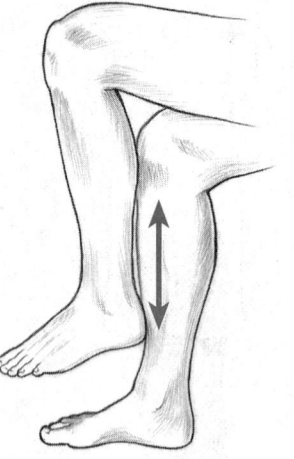

Figure 18–16.

tify the size and shape of easily recognized objects such as coins, a safety pin, a paper clip, which are placed in each hand, with their eyes closed.
· Test **sensory extinction or inattention** by touching both sides of the body simultaneously. An abnormal response is when the person identifies the stimulus on only one side.
e. Muscle stretch reflexes (Fig. 18–17). Table 18–2 summarizes important neurologic assessment guidelines.

Special Diagnostic Studies

1. Cerebrospinal fluid analysis
   a. This test can determine the presence of infection, blood, some neoplasms, and some degenerative disorders. Table 18–3 lists normal CSF values and discusses the significance of abnormal values.
   b. Lumbar puncture is the most common method of obtaining CSF for analysis (Procedure 18–1).
2. Imaging studies
   a. Skull and spinal radiographs
      (1) Skull radiographs reveal size and configuration of the skull bones, bone density, fractures, calcification, bone defects, vascular markings, and tumors.
      (2) Spinal radiographs reveal dislocations, fractures, compressions, curvature, and degeneration of the vertebrae and disks.
   b. Computed tomography (CT) scan
      (1) In CT a series of x-rays scans successive levels of the brain or spinal column.
      (2) Bone, CSF, blood, and gray and white matter provide different shades of black, gray, or white.
      (3) The CT scans can detect hemorrhage, infarction, softened and edematous brain, abscess, tumor and bony structures and disk material of the spine (Fig. 18–18).
   c. Magnetic resonance imaging (MRI) scan
      (1) In MRI magnetic energy with pulses of radio frequency energy causes protons in the body to resonate and change their alignment.
      (2) When the pulse stops, a computer reads the remaining energy field and produces a picture of the nervous system structures.
      (3) The MRI scans can detect brain and spinal cord edema, hemorrhage, infarction, blood vessels, tumor, and bone lesions.
      (4) These scans provide more detailed images of the posterior fossa (brain stem and cerebellum) and more clarity of soft tissue changes (e.g., demyelination) than a CT scan (Fig. 18–19).
      (5) Because MRI requires the person to be very still for up to 1 hour, it cannot be used in uncooperative people or young children without sedation.
      (6) It cannot be used in anyone who has a pacemaker or certain blood vessel clips.
   d. Angiography
      (1) Provides images of blood vessels.
      (2) Identifies aneurysms, vascular malformations, narrowed or occluded vessels, arterial dissections, and vasculitis.
      (3) A catheter is inserted in the femoral artery at the groin and threaded into the carotid or vertebral artery.
      (4) Dye is injected into the catheter.

Text continued on page 671

TESTING MUSCLE STRETCH REFLEXES

Using a reflex hammer, briskly tap the tendon of a stretched muscle.

> Note the response or degree of muscle contraction by using the 0-4 point scale. The normal range is 1 to 3.
>
> **0** = absent response
> **1** = barely perceptible response
> **2** = average response
> **3** = exaggerated or brisk response
> **4** = hyperreflexia with clonus
> (a continued, rapid, rhythmic contraction and relaxation of the muscle after the stimulus is applied)

Brachioradial Tendon:
Test the brachioradial tendon by striking the brachioradial muscles a few centimeters above the wrist while the person's arm is relaxed. The normal response is flexion and supination at the elbow or visible contraction of the brachioradial muscle.

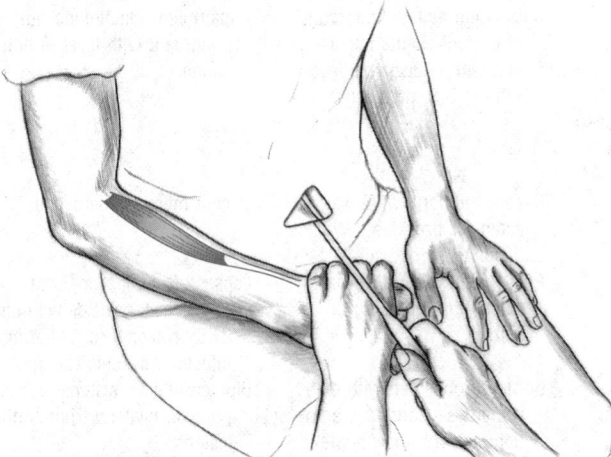

Patellar Tendon:
Test the patellar tendon by striking the tendon just below the knee while the knees are flexed about 90 degrees. The normal response is extension of the leg with contraction of the quadriceps muscle.

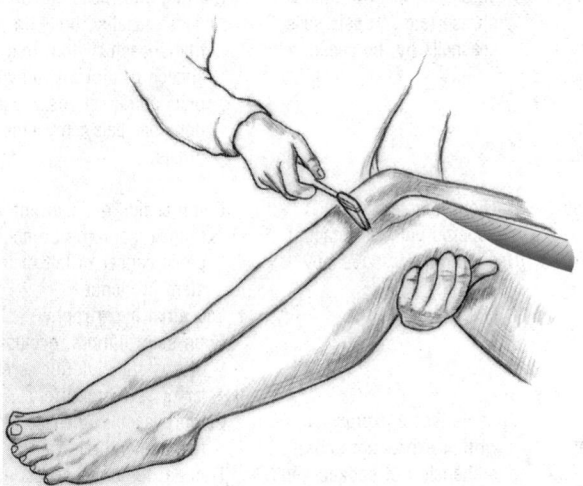

Triceps Tendon:
Test the triceps tendon by striking the person just above the elbow while the arm is partially flexed. The normal response is extension of the arm or visual contraction of the triceps muscle.

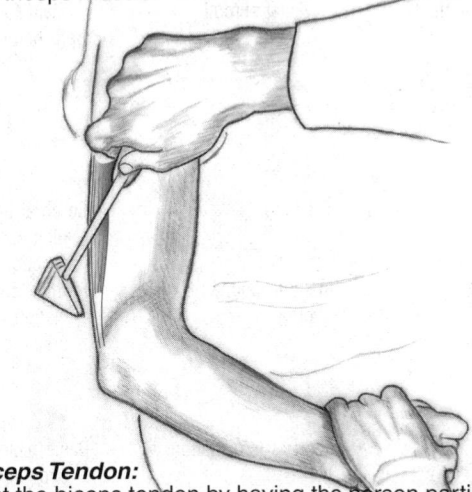

Biceps Tendon:
Test the biceps tendon by having the person partially flex his or her arm, placing your thumb over the biceps tendon in the antecubital space and striking your thumb with the reflex hammer. The normal response is flexion of the arm at the elbow or palpable contraction of the person's tendon under your thumb.

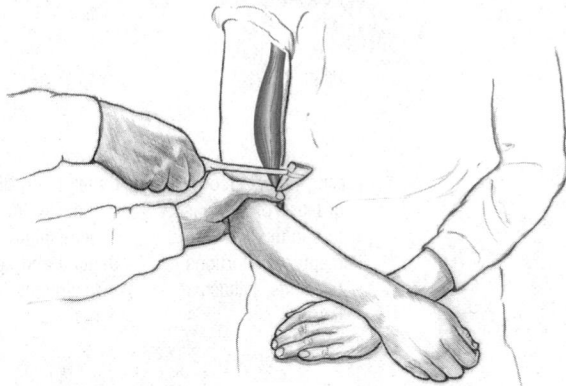

Achilles Tendon:
Test the Achilles tendon by striking the tendon while the knee is flexed and the foot is slightly dorsiflexed. The normal response is plantar flexion at the ankle.

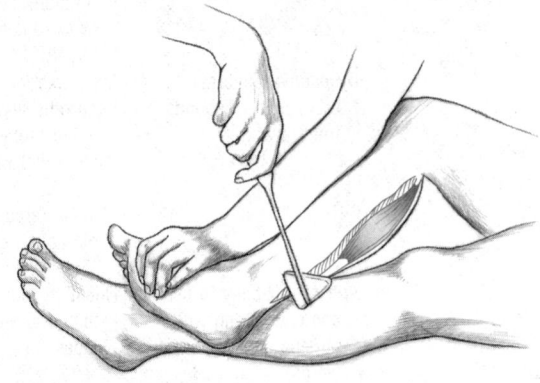

Figure 18-17.

Table 18–2. Neurologic Assessment Guidelines

Functional Category	Specific Category	Areas of Nervous System Involved	Assessment Technique	Examples of Dysfunction
1. Consciousness (awareness of self and environment)	Arousal response to verbal, tactile, and visual stimuli	Reticular activating system (mesencephalon, diencephalon) Both hemispheres	Is client alert? What is attention span? Is there normal response to visual and auditory stimuli? Reaction to loud noises, shaking, deep pressure over eye orbits or sternum? Are vital signs, pupils, and reflexes normal?	Elevation: insomnia, agitation, mania, delirium Depression: somnolence, lethargy, semicoma, coma
2. Mentation	Thinking	Cerebral hemispheres plus specific regional functions	Is client oriented (time, place, person)?	Disorientation
	Insight, judgment, planning	Frontal lobe, with association fibers to other areas of cerebrum	Does client recognize implications of illness? Are goals congruent with abilities? How would client respond to given situation (e.g., house on fire)?	Lack of judgment, inattention to grooming, appearance, and personal habits
	Fund of information	Basic biologic intellect (frontal lobe) integrated into other areas	Calculation ability, knowledge of current events consistent with educational level. Who is U.S. president?	Impairment: functioning not congruent with level of education
	Memory	Temporal lobe and association to most other areas of cortex		
	Recent:		Recent memory: what was eaten for breakfast? What happened 1 day ago?	Recent memory: dementia
	Past:		Past memory: recall of past events during taking of history	Lapses of memory for past events may coincide with past CNS problems (e.g., trauma, infection, psychic trauma)
	Feeling (affect) (congruence of response to stimulus)	General and bifrontal (usually involves both hemispheres)	Compare observed with expected reactions. Are emotions labile? Appropriate?	Blunted affect. Hysteria, schizophrenia, bilateral frontal lobe lesions
	Perceptual distortions (illusions, hallucinations)	General and specific cortical areas in hallucinations	Observations for behavior indicating perceptual problems. Ask client.	Irritative lesions of cortex may → hallucinations. (Occipital cortex → visual, postcentral gyrus → somatic sensation, uncus → smell)
3. Language and speech	*Dysarthria* (defects in articulation, enunciation, and rhythm in speech)	Impairment of muscles of tongue, palate, pharynx, or lips (may be due to ↓ impulses or incoordination) Brain stem, cerebellum, or extraneural causes CN V, VII, IX, X, XII	Have client repeat a difficult phrase (e.g., "Susie sells seashells by the seashore")	Slurring, slowness, indistinctness, nasality, break in normal speech rhythm (e.g., speech of a drunk, amyotrophic lateral sclerosis, pseudobulbar palsy, myasthenia gravis)
	Dysphonia (abnormal production of sounds from larynx)	Many extraneural causes Recurrent laryngeal nerve problems (part of vagus) CN X Medulla (area of nucleus of vagus nerve)	Is client hoarse? Whispered voice is intact Use indirect laryngoscopy findings	Compression of recurrent laryngeal nerve by bronchogenic cancer of left main stem bronchus Left atrial hypertrophy Brain stem tumors, occlusion of posterior inferior cerebellar or vertebral artery
	Aphasia (inability to use and understand written and spoken words)	Fluent (receptive) left temporal and parietal lobes	Observe: vocal expression; written expression; comprehension of spoken and written language and gesture communication	Cerebrovascular disease of middle cerebral artery Trauma, tumor, abscess, etc., in left temporal and parietal lobe areas

Table 18–2. Neurologic Assessment Guidelines (Continued)

Functional Category	Specific Category	Areas of Nervous System Involved	Assessment Technique	Examples of Dysfunction
		Nonfluent (expressive) Broca's area (lateral) inferior portion of frontal lobe of dominant side Global (combined)		
	Agnosia (inability to recognize objects or symbols by means of senses)	Primarily in parietal temporal and occipital areas	Sense organs intact? Can the client recognize objects by sight, touch, hearing, etc?	Cerebrovascular disease
4. Motor function	Expression (facial)	CN VII	Symmetry of smile, frown, raising eyebrows	Central facial weakness (upper motor neuron dysfunction); weakness of lower half of face. Causes: Cerebrovascular accident, corticobulbar tract Peripheral facial weakness (lower motor dysfunction); weakness of entire half of face. Causes: Bell's palsy, brain stem tumor, fracture of temporal bone
	Eating (chewing, swallowing)	CN V, VII, IX, X, XII	Strength of masticator muscles, gag reflexes, ability to swallow	Tetanus, peripheral spasm of muscle. Amyotrophic lateral sclerosis, medullary tumor. Pseudobulbar palsy may be associated with dysarthria
	Eye movements	CN III, IV, VI	Extraocular movement, pupil size, reactivity, pupils equally react to accommodation, diplopia, nystagmus	Cerebral peduncle pressure → CN III dysfunction, cavernous sinus thrombus → CN III, IV, VI, problem Muscular problems (e.g., myasthenia gravis, hyperthyroid), Horner's syndrome (ptosis, constricted pupil), anisocoria
	Moving	Motor precentral gyrus (pyramidal) and cerebellar systems, basal ganglia, CN XI, spinal cord, upper motor neuron (brain → anterior horn cell via corticospinal tract) Lower motor neuron (motor cells of cranial nerves and anterior horn cells → peripheral muscles) Involves brain, midbrain, cerebellum, and spinal cord	Gait, heel-to-toe walking, presence or absence of involuntary movements, coordination, muscle tone, mass, strength, Romberg reflex, ability to shrug shoulders and to rise from chair	*Upper motor neuron* Brain and cord-sparing anterior horn cell Tone ↑ ↑ (spastic) Bulk ↓ due to atrophy of disuse Reflexes ↑ ↑ due to loss of central inhibition No fasciculations Frequent clonus *Lower motor neuron* Segment anterior horn cell peripheral nerve Tone ↓ ↓ (flaccid) Bulk ↓ due to tone loss Reflexes ↓ or absent due to loss of anterior horn cell

Table continued on following page

Table 18–2. Neurologic Assessment Guidelines (Continued)

Functional Category	Specific Category	Areas of Nervous System Involved	Assessment Technique	Examples of Dysfunction
				Fasciculations
				No clonus
				Cerebellar problem → Loss of coordination and balance
5. Sensory function	Seeing	CN II Optic, occipital lobe	Acuity, visual fields, funduscopy	Field test: loss in retina or optic nerve → loss in eye involved, optic chiasm → bitemporal hemianopia. Optic tract → homonymous hemianopia, parietal lobe → quadrant problems (inferior), temporal lobe → superior quadrant problems ↑ ICP → papilledema (raised disk → hemorrhage)
	Smelling	CN I Temporal lobe (uncus)	Ability to detect familiar odors	Usually ↓ smell due to extraneural causes (e.g., upper respiratory infection, allergy, smoking), olfactory groove Meningioma, olfactory hallucinations
	Hearing	CN VIII Cochlear division, temporal lobe	Acuity of hearing, presence or absence of unusual sounds, Weber and Rinne tests	May have conductive (nerve ok) or neural hearing loss. Ménière's syndrome (tinnitus, hearing loss, vertigo, and nystagmus), basilar skull fracture → otorrhea Brain stem vascular dysfunction or tumors → ↓ hearing
	Taste	CN VII, IX	Ability to differentiate sweet, salt, sour, and bitter	Brain stem lesions → ↓ taste Extraneural causes, smoking, poor oral hygiene
	Feeling (sensory)	Peripheral nerves → Dermatomes → Spinal cord → Tracts (leading to) Pain: temperature tactile, anterolateral system, proprioception, stereognosis, dorsal roots thalamus (leading to) somasthetic area (postcentral gyrus) (parietal lobe)	Pain: pinprick Touch: cotton touched to skin Proprioception: check where digit is in space Vibration: place vibrating tuning fork on bony prominence Temperature: test tubes of cold and warm water laid against skin; person identifies whether hot or cold	Polyneuropathy (e.g., diabetes, anemia) Spinal cord lesions → Dermatome alterations Upper pons → thalamus, contralateral loss Thalamus → contralateral loss + paresthesia Thalamus → cortex → cortical sensory loss
6. Bowel and bladder function	Bowel function	Afferent Spinal nerve S3-S5 External sphincter (voluntary control) Internal sphincter Spinal nerve S3-S5 Autonomic nervous system	Check for fecal impaction or incontinence Check muscle tone	Fecal incontinence with lesions of S3, 4, 5 Anal anesthesia—conus medullaris and tabes dorsalis May be extraneural causes

Table 18–2. Neurologic Assessment Guidelines (Continued)

Functional Category	Specific Category	Areas of Nervous System Involved	Assessment Technique	Examples of Dysfunction
	Bladder function	Autonomic nervous system	Feel when bladder is full, complete emptying. Does client have urgency, frequently?	Urinary incontinence
		Afferent		Flaccid bladder
		Spinal nerves T9-L2 and S2-S4		
		Pudendal nerve		
		Efferent		Spastic bladder
		Spinal nerve T11-L2		
		External sphincter (voluntary)		
		Spinal nerve S2-S4		May be extraneural causes

From Black JC, and Barker E. Assessment of clients with neurologic disorders. *In* Black JM, and Matassarin-Jacobs E (eds). *Luckmann and Sorensen's Medical-Surgical Nursing: A Psychophysiologic Approach.* 4th ed. Philadelphia: WB Saunders, 1993, pp 651–655.

(5) Serial radiographs are taken to image the arterial, capillary, and venous phases of blood flow through the cerebral vessels (Fig. 18–20).

(6) Postprocedure nursing care
- Place a sandbag over the groin puncture site to promote hemostasis and prevent hematoma formation.
- Avoid hip flexion for 6 to 12 hours.
- Check pedal pulses at regular intervals. (Remember to check pedal pulses before the procedure, as up to 20% of people have congenitally unpalpable pedal pulses.)

(7) Magnetic resonance angiography (see Chapter 23) is a new noninvasive method of angiography, but it has not yet achieved the sensitivity of invasive angiography.

e. Positron-emission tomography (see Chapter 23)
(1) Positron-emission tomography (PET) is used to assess the metabolic and physiologic function of the brain; to diagnose stroke, brain tumors, and epilepsy; and to monitor the course of Parkinson's disease, Alzheimer's disease, head injury, and some mental disorders.
(2) The patient is injected with doses of strong radio-

Table 18–3. Normal CSF Values and Significance of Abnormal Values

Substance	Normal Value (Conventional Units)	Significance of Abnormal Values
Blood	None; CSF should be clear	Gross blood is seen in CNS hemorrhage. Rarely, there are some blood cells in the 1st tube of CSF collected, because of trauma during the tap. The collection of specimens in sequence should be marked, so that it is possible to determine whether the blood in the 1st tube is more than that in the last tube. If the CSF is grossly bloody, other tests may not be able to be performed.
Cells	0–5 mononuclear	Increased neutrophils may be seen in bacterial infections such as bacterial meningitis. Lymphocytes may be increased in tuberculosis and some viral disorders.
Enzymes (LDH)	10% of serum level	Elevated with inflammations and bacterial meningitis.
Glucose	50–75 mg/dl, should be 20 mg less than serum glucose level	Glucose level is lowered in bacterial infections, because bacteria use sugar. Some types of tumors also lower CSF glucose. Be certain to compare CSF glucose with serum glucose. Ideally, a serum specimen should be drawn 30 min before a lumbar puncture, because it takes glucose about 30 to 60 minutes to diffuse into the CSF.
Protein Albumin	15–45 mg/dl 29.5 mg/dl (80%)	Increased proteins may be seen in degenerative disorders and brain tumors. Lesions that interrupt the blood-brain barrier also increase proteins because there is an increased diffusion from the blood into the brain tissues.
IgG	<14% of total protein	IgG and oligoclonal bands (an abnormal type of protein band seen on immunoelectrophoresis) are often present in multiple sclerosis and neurosyphilis.
Oligoclonal bands	Absent	
Pressure	70–180 mm H_2O	Elevated in bacterial meningitis, cerebral bleeding, and tumors. Decreased in conditions that obstruct CSF flow, such as tumors of the spinal canal.

From Black JC, and Barker E. Assessment of clients with neurologic disorders. *In* Black JM, and Matassarin-Jacobs E (eds). *Luckmann and Sorensen's Medical-Surgical Nursing: A Psychophysiologic Approach.* 4th ed. Philadelphia: WB Saunders, 1993, p 666.

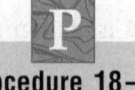

Procedure 18–1
Lumbar Puncture

Definition/Purpose Lumbar puncture involves insertion of a needle into the subarachnoid space of the lumbar spinal column for several purposes: to obtain cerebrospinal fluid for analysis, to measure and relieve cerebrospinal fluid pressure, and to deliver drugs or dye into the spinal column.

Contraindications/Cautions Evidence of increased intracranial pressure and anticoagulation therapy are *relative* contraindications (i.e., in some cases the benefit of the procedure outweighs the risk). Cutaneous or osseous infection at the puncture site is an *absolute* contraindication.

Learning/Teaching Activities The patient should be instructed about the procedure and be reassured that the needle is inserted *below* the level of the spinal cord.

Preliminary Activities

Equipment
- Sterile lumbar puncture set
- Sterile gloves
- Topical anesthetic solution

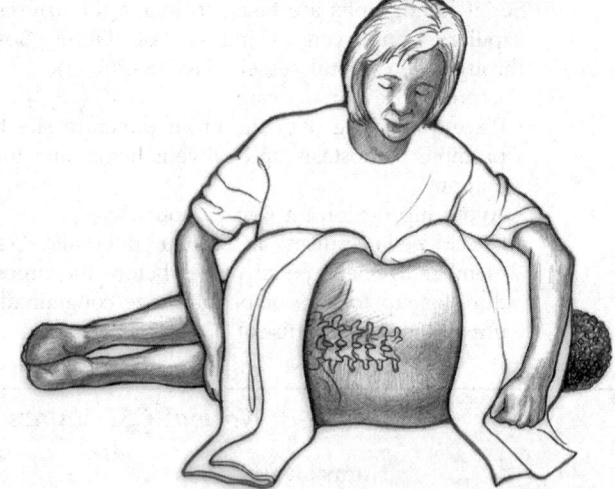

Assessment/Planning
- Know reason for procedure (e.g., diagnostic or therapeutic purpose)
- Explain the procedure to the patient
- Have patient empty bladder immediately before the procedure
- Position patient on side near the edge of the bed with a pillow between the legs, which should be flexed at the hips and knees in a fetal position
- Assist patient in maintaining this position by standing at the bedside (facing the patient's abdomen) and place one hand behind the neck and one hand behind the knees.

Procedure

Actions	Rationale
1. Physician injects local anesthetic into the skin near the third and fourth vertebrae. Once the skin is anesthetized, physician inserts a sterile spinal needle between the third and fourth vertebrae and into the subarachnoid space of the spinal column.	1. Spinal cord terminates between the first and second lumbar vertebrae; therefore, the needle does not come near the spinal cord.
2. Physician attaches a manometer to the spinal needle to record cerebrospinal fluid pressure (the "opening pressure").	2. Normal opening pressure is 60–150 mm H_2O. Higher readings can indicate increased intracranial pressure.
3. Physician removes manometer and collects several tubes of cerebrospinal fluid for laboratory analysis.	3. Cerebrospinal fluid analysis can help diagnose subarachnoid hemorrhage (if blood is found), infection, inflammatory disease, and cancer.
4. At the conclusion of the procedure, physician places a bandage over the puncture site.	

Final Activities

1. Ensure that the patient remains flat in bed for the next 6–24 hours and drinks fluid liberally. Offer oral analgesics for headache, which can occur after lumbar puncture because of cerebrospinal fluid leakage or irritation of the meninges. Lying flat promotes healing of the puncture site and lessens the risk of leakage. Forcing fluids promotes replacement of cerebrospinal fluid if leakage occurs.
2. Record procedure and how patient tolerated it.

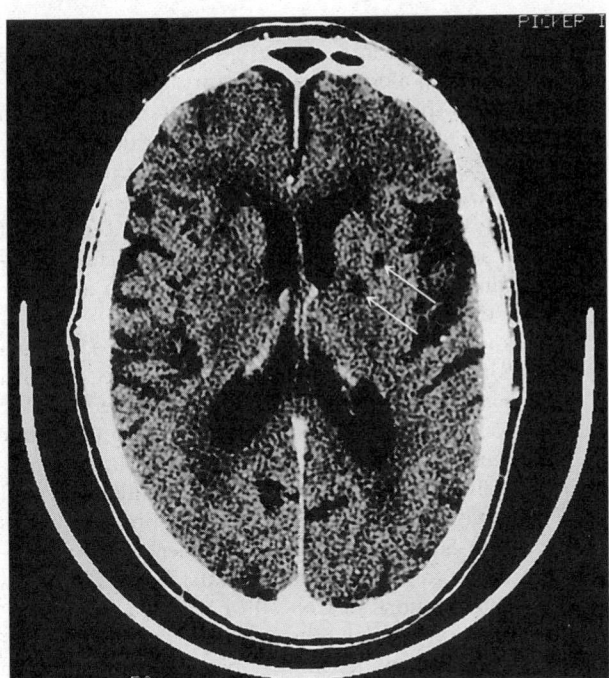

Figure 18–18. Computed tomography scan of the brain. Note two lacunar infarcts in the left basal ganglia.

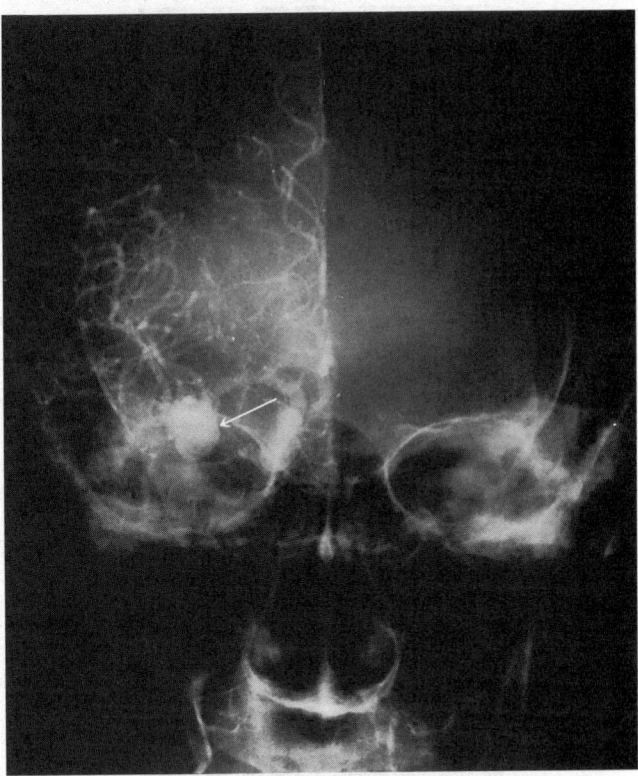

Figure 18–20. Angiogram of right cerebral arteries showing an aneurysm (arrow).

active tracers that release positive electrons. When these positrons contact negatively charged electrons in the body cells, they emit a signal that can be detected by a scanner. These signals are then translated by a computer into patterns that the physician uses to detect cerebral abnormalities.

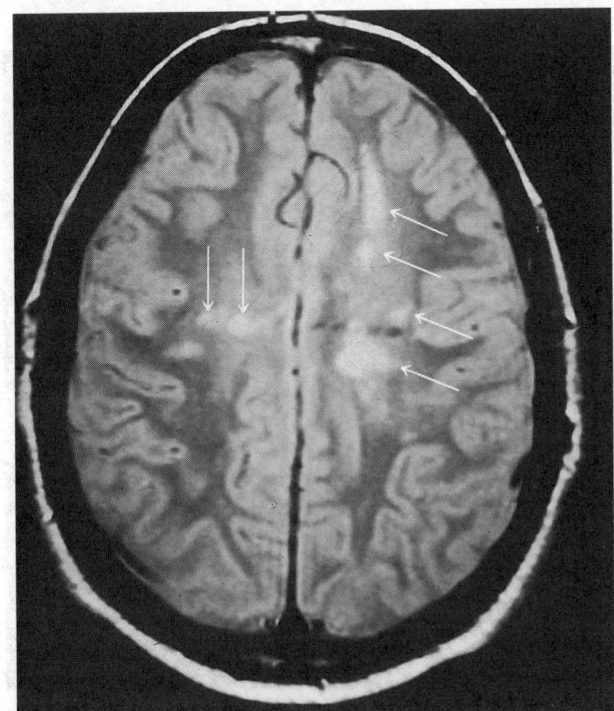

Figure 18–19. Magnetic resonance imaging view of the brain showing plaques of multiple sclerosis (arrows).

f. Myelography
  (1) Provides visualization of the spinal column and subarachnoid space when a spinal lesion is suspected.
  (2) Involves injection of contrast dye via lumbar or cisternal puncture into the subarachnoid space.
  (3) Blockage or narrowing of the dye along the spinal column indicates a lesion such as a tumor or a disk or bony deformity (Fig. 18–21).
  (4) The CT scanning may be done after the dye is injected to provide transverse views of the spinal column (Fig. 18–22).
  (5) Postprocedure nursing care involves keeping the head slightly elevated for 4 to 6 hours to prevent dye from migrating into the cerebrum.
3. Electrographic studies
  a. Electroencephalography
    (1) Records electrical activity of the brain through electrodes placed on the scalp.
    (2) Evaluates the presence of cerebral disease as well as metabolic and systemic disease that affects the brain.
    (3) Continuous electroencephalographic monitoring is used to distinguish seizures from pseudoseizures or to identify a seizure focus in intractable epilepsy.
    (4) Electrodes may be surgically placed directly on the brain surface or deep within the brain for continuous monitoring to identify a seizure focus in intractable epilepsy.
  b. Electromyography and nerve conduction velocity studies

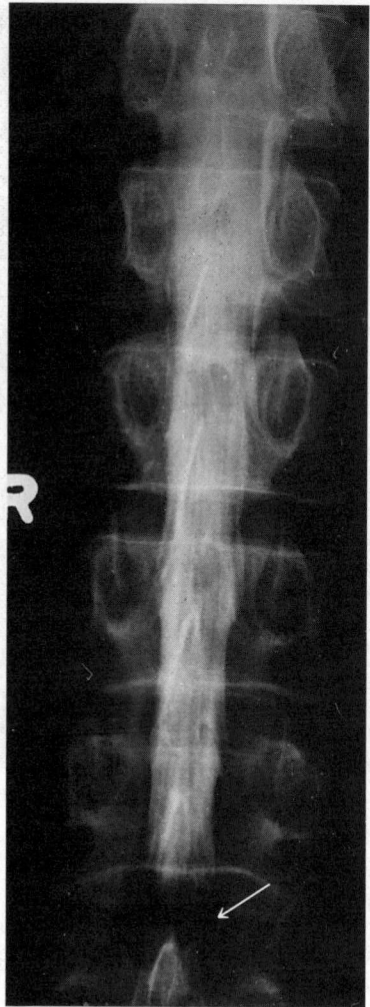

Figure 18-21. Myelogram of the lumbar spine showing blockage of dye at the L4-5 vertebral level (arrow) due to a herniated disk.

(1) For electromyography studies, needles are placed in selected muscles to record electrical activity associated with innervation of skeletal muscle. A normal muscle at rest shows no electrical activity. Typical activity occurs with muscle contraction. Abnormal activity can be seen in disorders of the muscle itself (myopathy) or of muscle innervation (peripheral neuropathy, radiculopathy, or upper motor neuron lesions).

(2) For nerve conduction velocity studies, an accessible nerve is stimulated through the skin by surface electrodes. The resulting action potential is recorded at different sites along the nerve pathway. Because damaged nerves conduct action potentials more slowly, the test provides information about the nature and location of the nerve damage.

(3) Electromyography and nerve conduction velocity studies help diagnose entrapment neuropathies (carpal tunnel syndrome, ulnar entrapment), peripheral neuropathies, radiculopathy, Guillain-Barré syndrome, myasthenia gravis, Eaton-Lambert syndrome, and motor neuron diseases.

c. Evoked potentials

(1) Records electrical activity associated with nerve conduction along specific sensory pathways.

(2) Various peaks in the wave patterns shown in these recordings correspond to conduction of the stimulus through certain points along the sensory pathway.

(3) Increases in the time intervals between the time of the stimulus onset and a given peak (latency) indicate slowed nerve conduction or nerve damage.

(4) Types of evoked potentials

• Visual evoked potentials. Record nerve conduction of a light stimulus (alternating checkerboard patterns on a screen) from the optic nerve to the occipital lobe of the brain. Can diagnose optic neuritis, a common finding in multiple sclerosis.

• Brain stem auditory evoked potentials. Record nerve conduction of a sound stimulus (clicks from headphones) from the inner ear to the auditory cortex in the temporal lobe of the brain. Detect lesions of CN VIII, namely, acoustic neuroma (vestibular schwannoma), and the cerebellopontine angle. Many people with multiple sclerosis have abnormal results on brain stem auditory evoked potentials studies.

• Somatosensory evoked potentials. Record nerve conduction of a painless electrical stimulus on the skin over the median, peroneal, or tibial nerve to the somatosensory cortex in the parietal lobe of the brain. Detect lesions in spinal roots, posterior columns of the spinal cord, and brain stem in such disorders as Guillain-Barré syndrome, multiple sclerosis, and cervical spondylosis.

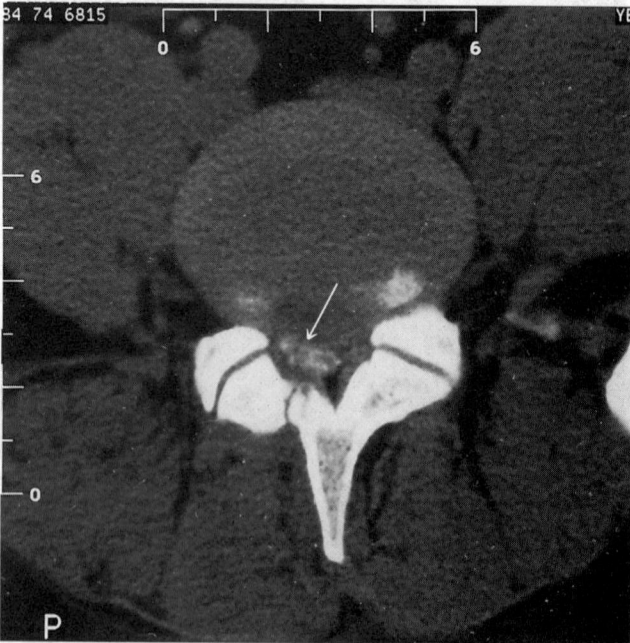

Figure 18-22. Computed tomography scan of the L4-5 disk space after injection of contrast dye (for myelography) showing deviation of the spinal cord (arrow) by a herniated disk (some patient as in Fig. 18-21).

◧ *CARING FOR PEOPLE WITH SPECIAL NEUROLOGIC PROBLEMS*

Increased Intracranial Pressure

1. Definition
   a. Intracranial pressure (ICP) is the pressure created within the cranium (a hard bony container) by its contents. Cranial contents include the following:
      (1) Brain tissue
      (2) Blood
      (3) Cerebrospinal fluid
   b. The ICP is based on CSF measurements.
      (1) The normal range of CSF pressure is 5 to 15 mm Hg or 60 to 200 mm of water.
      (2) Pressure readings above 200 mm of water (approximately 20 mm Hg) are considered abnormally high.
      (3) Like arterial pressure, ICP fluctuates with activity such as performing the Valsalva maneuver; e.g., straining at stool or performing isometric exercises.
2. Etiology
   a. Increased ICP occurs when 1 of 3 intracranial contents (blood, brain, or CSF) increases in volume without a compensatory decrease in the volumes of the others.
   b. Brain injury, like stroke or hemorrhage, can disrupt the normal compensatory mechanisms that keep ICP low.
   c. Increased ICP usually results from the following:
      (1) An expanding lesion, for example, from bleeding due to head injury or a ruptured aneurysm
      (2) Obstructed outflow of CSF due to a growth or tumor
      (3) Cerebral edema due to stroke or lead poisoning, for example
      (4) Intracranial surgery
      (5) Infection or abscess within the brain
3. Pathophysiology
   a. Normal ICP is 60 to 180 mm of water, or 5 to 15 mm Hg as noted above.
   b. Cerebral perfusion pressure (CPP) equals the difference between the mean arterial pressure (MAP) and ICP (CCP = MAP − ICP). The CPP must be at least 50 to 60 mm Hg for adequate neuronal functioning.
   c. Increased volumes of blood (e.g., hemorrhage), CSF, or brain (e.g., edema) cause increased ICP unless there is a corresponding decrease in another of these brain elements, because the brain is enclosed in a rigid skull. Compensatory decreases in these brain elements rarely occur in head injury because the injury occurs so quickly.
   d. Expansion of the brain contents within the rigid skull can also lead to herniation of brain tissue from one compartment to another, resulting in neurologic deficits.
   e. Symptoms arise from the increased ICP exerted on the cerebral blood vessels, pain-sensitive dura mater, and other structures within the brain and in back of the eye (Fig. 18–23).

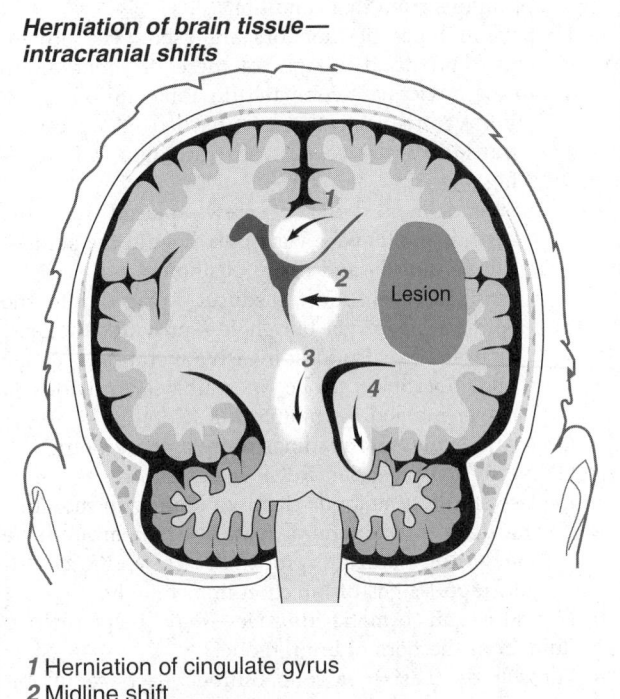

HERNIATION SYNDROMES

Herniation of brain tissue— intracranial shifts

1 Herniation of cingulate gyrus
2 Midline shift
3 Downward displacement of brain stem
4 Herniation of temporal lobe

Figure 18–23.

   f. Cushing's triad—a combination of hypertension, bradycardia, and irregular respiration—is a late manifestation of brain stem ischemia from increased ICP.
4. Clinical manifestations: symptoms are subtle and vary from patient to patient. Symptoms include the following:
   a. Alterations in level of consciousness (see p. 679)
   b. Restlessness, irritability, and confusion
   c. Decrease in the Glasgow Coma Scale score (see Procedure 18–2)
   d. Headache, nausea, and vomiting that may be projectile
   e. Diplopia (double vision) or blurred vision
   f. Changes in pupil size and reaction to light
   g. Papilledema (edema and hyperemia of the optic disk)
   h. Speech, motor, or sensory changes
   i. Changes in pulse rate from bradycardia to tachycardia as ICP rises
   j. Cushing's triad (rising blood pressure, slowness of heartbeat, and irregular respirations)—a late and dangerous sign.
5. Diagnostics
   a. The CT and MRI scans help identify cause of increased ICP.
   b. Continuous ICP monitoring is used both to monitor the level of ICP and to treat increased ICP.
6. Clinical management
   a. Monitor ICP continuously

(1) Continuous ICP monitoring allows for aggressive management of people with actual or potential increased ICP. It can also be used to prevent complications from this condition.

(2) Several types of monitors are used (The advantages and disadvantages of these different monitoring devices are compared in Table 18–4.):
- Intraventricular catheter—attached to a pressure transducer—gives the most accurate ICP reading.
- Subarachnoid bolt or screw—placed into the subarachnoid space via a burr hole in the skull—can be quickly and easily positioned.
- Epidural fiberoptic transducer—placed into the epidural space via burr hole—provides the least accurate but also least invasive method.
- The fiberoptic probe or catheter provides a newer method for monitoring ICP.

(3) Monitor pressure readings at least every hour.

(4) Notify the physician if ICP increases.

(5) Use sterile technique when working with monitoring devices. Maintain a clean dry area around the monitoring catheter, probe, or screw. Watch for and report signs of infection immediately.

b. Mannitol—an osmotic diuretic—may help remove fluid from the normal brain tissue.

c. Furosemide (Lasix)—a loop diuretic—acts to inhibit reabsorption of sodium and chloride at the proximal portion of the ascending loop of Henle. Observe for nausea, vomiting, and fluid and electrolyte imbalances (see Chapter 9).

d. Steroids, although controversial, may help reduce edema—especially edema resulting from brain tumors. Dexamethasone (Decadron) may be ordered.

e. Anticonvulsants such as phenytoin (Dilantin) and phenobarbital help control the seizures that may follow a head injury.

f. Antihypertensive agents may be ordered to control sustained arterial hypertension higher than 160 mm Hg systolic.

g. Large doses of barbiturates are used to sedate the patient with uncontrolled ICP. A comatose state reduces brain metabolism, which in turn reduces cerebral blood flow. The result is reduced ICP.

h. Surgery may be necessary for increased ICP. Procedures include the following:
(1) Surgical placement of a shunt into the lateral ventricle that allows for drainage of CSF.
(2) Reduction surgery, which involves removal of some brain tissue, thereby creating space for expansion of remaining structures within the cranium.

7. Applying the nursing process

NURSING DIAGNOSIS: Altered cerebral tissue perfusion R/T increased intracranial pressure

a. *Expected outcomes:* Following interventions, person should maintain normal ICP.

b. *Nursing interventions*
(1) Monitor ICP and MAP and calculate CPP.
(2) Adjust the head of the bed to optimize CPP. Some individuals' CPP improves with the head of the bed elevated 30 to 45 degrees. Other individuals' CPP improves when the head is lower. Monitor ICP and CPP to determine which position is best.

Table 18–4. Advantages and Disadvantages of Monitoring Devices

Monitoring Device	Advantages	Disadvantages
Intraventricular catheter (IVC)	• Accurate measurement of ICP • Allows drainage or sampling of CSF • Allows instillation of contrast media • Provides reliable evaluation of volume or pressure responses	• Provides additional site for potential infection • Most invasive method for monitoring ICP • Must be balanced and recalibrated frequently • Catheter can become occluded by blood or tissue.
Subarachnoid bolt or screw	• Allows sampling of CSF • Lower infection rates than with the IVC • Quickly and easily placed	• Tendency for dampened waveforms • Less accurate at high ICP • May become occluded by tissue or blood • Must be balanced and recalibrated frequently (i.e., q4h and whenever the client is repositioned)
Subdural, extradural catheter or sensor	• Least invasive • Easily and quickly placed	• Increasing baseline drift over time; therefore, accuracy and reliability are questionable • Does not provide for CSF sampling
Fiberoptic probe or catheter	• Can be placed in subdural or subarachnoid space, in ventricle, or into brain tissue • Easily transported • Requires zeroing only once (during insertion) • Baseline drift to 1 mm Hg/day • No irrigation—less risk of infection • Less waveform artefact • No need to adjust transducer to the client's position	• Does not provide for CSF sampling • Cannot be recalibrated after it is placed • Breakage of the fiberoptic cable

From Gilliam EE. Intracranial hypertension: Advances in intracranial pressure monitoring. *Crit Care Nurs Clin North Am* 2(1):25, 1990.

CLINICAL CONTROVERSIES

Elevating the head to reduce increased intracranial pressure does not always work because compensatory mechanisms may already be at the maximum level. Head elevation may reduce cerebral perfusion pressure in this situation. Establish optimal head positioning for each person individually.

(3) Space nursing care activities to allow rest periods for ICP to return to baseline. Check CPP before initiating activity. Nursing care procedures may safely be performed if CPP is at or above 50 mm Hg.

(4) Ensure optimal suctioning. Hyperoxygenate and hyperinflate lungs before, during, and after suctioning. Limit suctioning to 10 to 15 seconds.

(5) Alleviate conditions that lead to increased intrathoracic pressure (Valsalva maneuver), such as coughing, pain, and straining to defecate.

(6) Maintain alignment of person's head with the trunk. Keep the chin over the sternum. Avoid lateral or forward flexion of the neck. These positions prevent constriction of the jugular veins, thereby promoting drainage of cerebral venous blood. Avoid extreme hip flexion and knee Gatch bed elevation.

(7) Maintain prescribed fluid restriction to avoid increased cerebral volume.

(8) Maintain normothermia.
- Monitor body core temperature.
- Reduce temperature elevations to avoid increased cerebral metabolism. Administer antipyretics as ordered, usually acetaminophen. Employ tepid water baths, ice packs, or cooling blanket as needed. Avoid rapid cooling and prolonged use of a cooling blanket, either of which may cause shivering, which increases cerebral metabolism.

(9) Recognize and treat seizures promptly.
- Maintain a patent airway. Turn person to sidelying position to promote drainage of oral secretions away from airway. Suction secretions.
- Provide supplemental oxygen
- Prevent physical injury

Unconsciousness and Coma

1. Definitions
   a. Unconsciousness is a state of depressed cerebral function that results in an abnormal loss of awareness of the self and surroundings. Although usually a sleeping person can be awakened easily, an unconscious person is difficult or impossible to arouse. Unconsciousness may range from stupor to coma.
   b. Stupor ranges from partial to nearly complete unconsciousness.
   c. Coma is a state of sustained and profound unconsciousness from which the person cannot be aroused. The comatose patient fails to respond to strong external stimuli, such as loud shouting, or to internal stimuli, such as a full bladder.
   d. The vegetative state (according to the Multi-Society Task Force on Persistent Vegetative State [PVS]) is "a clinical condition of complete unawareness of the self and the environment, accompanied by sleep-wake cycles, with either complete or partial preservation of hypothalamic and brain stem autonomic functions." A persistent vegetative state is a "vegetative state present one month after acute traumatic or nontraumatic brain injury or lasting for at least one month in patients with degenerative or metabolic disorders or developmental malformations."

2. Etiology
   a. Head injury
   b. Brain tumor
   c. Brain abscess
   d. Intracerebral hemorrhaging
   e. Drug overdose
   f. Metabolic dysfunction (e.g., diabetic coma, hepatic coma, drug overdosage)

3. Pathophysiology
   a. Coma results from a disturbance or damage to those areas of the brain that are involved in maintaining a conscious state.
   b. Areas of the brain that are primarily affected by coma include parts of the cerebrum, upper parts of the brain stem, and central regions of the brain—in particular the limbic system.
   c. Brain death occurs when there is irreversible damage to cerebrum, cerebellum, and brain stem. Confirmation of brain death occurs when there is evidence that cerebral and brain stem activity has ceased.

4. Clinical manifestations
   a. Manifestations vary depending on the person's level of consciousness. Consciousness may deteriorate from a person's normal alert state in stages that progress from confusion, to disorientation, to lethargy, to obtundation (patient is difficult to arouse), to stupor, to coma.
   b. Level of consciousness varies depending on the underlying etiology of the problem. Patients with structurally induced coma (due to a mass in the brain from a tumor, bleeding, or abscess) experience different manifestations from those with metabolically induced coma (due to diabetic coma, hepatic coma or drug overdose) (Table 18–5).
   c. In addition to the manifestations listed in Table 18–5, comatose patients may also experience the following:
      (1) Changes in respiratory rate and rhythm.
      (2) Increased vulnerability to airway obstruction and aspiration due to missing gag reflex.
      (3) Changes in blood pressure, pulse, and body temperature. Complications such as cardiac arrhythmias and shock may also develop.
      (4) Fluid, electrolyte, and acid-base imbalances.
      (5) Drying of the cornea due to sluggish or absent corneal reflexes and blink response.
      (6) Increased intracranial pressure that may result in Cushing's triad (see p. 675).

5. Diagnostics

Table 18–5. Clinical Manifestations of Metabolically Induced and Structurally Induced Coma

Manifestation	Metabolically Induced Coma	Structurally Induced Coma
History	Behavioral changes	Frontal headache
		Local seizures
Typical problem	Hepatic coma	Tumor or bleeding in one area
	Diabetic ketoacidosis	
Pupillary reaction (CN II)	Preserved	Unequal reaction
Pupillary size	May be midposition and fixed from anticholinergics	May be unequal
	Fixed and dilated from anoxia	Midposition from injury to the midbrain
	Pinpoint from opiates	Pinpoint from injury to the pons
		Large from herniation
Corneal reflex	Present and equal	Unequal, may be absent
Extraocular movement (CN III, IV, VI)	Eyes rove, calorics intact, doll's eyes absent	May have gaze paresis from a trapped CN III
Extremity movement	Moves both sides equally	Weakness or absent movement on one side
Abnormal posturing	Absent	Present (decerebrate, decorticate)
Reflexes	Deep tendon reflexes present and equal	Deep tendon reflexes unequal
	Plantar flexion	Babinski's response
Response to pain	Equal	Unequal

Data from McCance K, and Huether S. *Pathophysiology.* St Louis: CV Mosby, 1990; and Wyngaarden JB, et al. *Cecil Textbook of Medicine.* 19th ed. Philadelphia: WB Saunders, 1992.
From Black JC, and Barker E. Nursing care of patients with loss of protective function. *In* Black JM, and Matassarin-Jacobs E (eds). *Luckmann and Sorensen's Medical-Surgical Nursing: A Psychophysiologic Approach.* 4th ed. Philadelphia: WB Saunders, 1993, p 677.

a. Assess the patient's level of consciousness using the Glasgow Coma Scale—a standardized tool for assessing the level of consciousness. Procedure 18–2 provides a step-by-step method for performing this assessment.

b. Check brain stem reflexes.

(1) Pupillary light reflex. Shine a light into each eye. Observe for presence and briskness of pupillary constriction. Asymmetric or sluggish pupils indicate compression of CN III (oculomotor nerve) at the level of the midbrain. Immediately report changes in size or reaction time of the pupils to physician.

(2) Corneal or lash reflex. Gently stroke the cornea or the eye lash with a wisp of cotton. Sluggish or absent eye closure or blink response implies compression of CN V (trigeminal) or CN VII (facial nerve) at the level of the pons.

(3) Oculocephalic reflex (doll's head maneuver). Briskly turn the head side to side. A normal response is movement of the eyes opposite the direction of head turning. Abnormal response such as passive movement of the eyes in the direction of head turning or lack of conjugate gaze with head turning indicates damage in the brain stem affecting CNs III, VI, and VIII. If no response is obtained, the physician may irrigate the ear with ice water (cold calorics) to test the oculovestibular reflex.

(4) Gag reflex. Absence of a gag reflex indicates damage to CNs IX and X in the region of the medulla. Absence of this reflex and the oculocephalic reflex indicates damage in the lower brain stem where vital respiratory and cardiac functions are regulated and thus is a poor prognosis.

h. Check vital signs.

(1) Check blood pressure and heart rate to ensure adequate perfusion of brain tissue. Bradycardia and hypertension (Cushing's reflex) indicate lower brain stem dysfunction and carry a grave prognosis.

(2) Calculate CPP by subtracting ICP from MAP (see p. 675) to ensure adequate cerebral perfusion.

(3) Assess respiratory pattern. Changes in respiratory pattern are associated with level of brain dysfunction. Cheyne-Stokes respirations occur with hemispheric compression. Other patterns are suggestive of various levels of brain stem dysfunction. Note any change in respiratory pattern, as it can indicate deterioration in neurologic function and may require intervention.

i. Assess motor responses

(1) Compare motor responses of the right and left sides of the body during coma scale assessment.

(2) Note asymmetries in movements.

j. Monitor ICP if indicated (see pp. 675–676)

6. Clinical management

a. Treatment of the underlying cause of the coma; for example, head injury, brain tumor, brain abscess, diabetic coma or hepatic coma.

b. Maintenance of respiration, circulation and arterial blood pressure.

c. Treatment of increased intracranial pressure if it develops (see pp. 675–676).

d. Prevention of the many potential complications produced by a comatose state such as choking, aspiration, pneumonia, malnutrition, fluid and electrolyte

Procedure 18-2
Coma Scale Assessment

Definition/Purpose	To determine level of consciousness and to provide serial assessments for ascertaining deterioration or improvement in the person's neurologic condition.
Contraindications/Cautions	Do not use supraorbital pressure if facial trauma is present or basilar skull fracture is suspected.
Learning/Teaching Activities	Because the patient requiring this type of assessment has decreased consciousness, teaching about the procedure may not be indicated.

Preliminary Activities

Equipment

• Glasgow Coma Scale

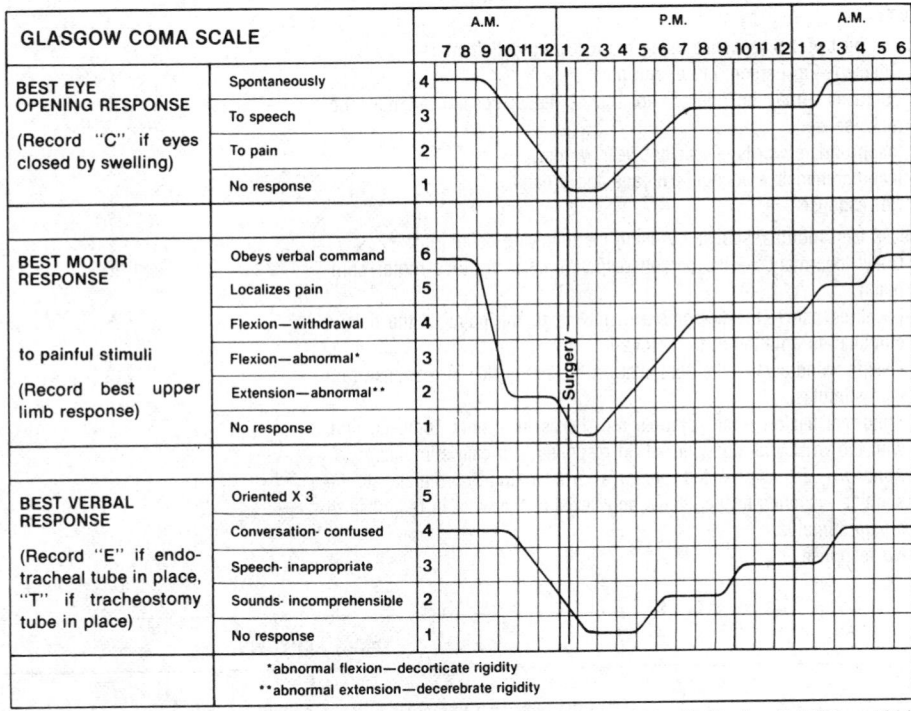

(From Hickey JV: *Neurological and Neurosurgical Nursing.* 2nd ed. Philadelphia: JB Lippincott, 1986, p 121.)

Assessment/Planning

• Know previous coma scale assessments for this patient.
• Note trends in level of consciousness.
• Schedule assessments as determined by patient's condition and physician's orders.

Procedure

Actions	Rationale/Discussion
1. Test the 3 categories of responses, which are listed from the highest level of functioning (which has a higher score) to the lowest level of functioning (which has a lower score). The best total score is 15, and the lowest is 3.	1. Glasgow coma score at the time of admission correlates with outcome (higher score means better outcome).
2. Base subsequent assessment on verbal commands (voice stimulus) 1st, shifting to pain stimuli if there is no response to voice. Use 2 forms of pain stimuli: nailbed pressure and supraorbital pressure. a. Nailbed pressure—place a pen or pencil on the base of the person's	2. Voice is a higher order stimulus than pain and should be used 1st to detect the highest level of brain functioning. Supraorbital pressure presents a pain stimulus more proximal to the brain (i.e., via CN V) and may provoke a response when nailbed pressure may not.

(continued)

Procedure 18–2

(continued)

Actions	Rationale/Discussion

nailbed and squeeze the pen onto the nailbed, using your thumb and forefinger.

b. Supraorbital pressure—if nailbed pressure does not elicit a response after checking all 4 extremities, place your thumb deep in the inner aspect of the person's orbit and press upward toward the top of the head. Do not use supraorbital pressure if facial trauma or basilar skull fracture is present.

3. Assess eye opening by observing 1st if the eyes are already open (eyes open spontaneously). If they are not open, call to the patient by name. If they do not open with this stimulus, apply pain stimuli (see above). Check the box corresponding to the patient's response on the flow sheet.

    3. All responses in the coma scale are arranged from the highest to the lowest level of functioning. Therefore, a higher total score reflects a higher level of functioning.

4. Assess best verbal response using the following definitions:
   a. Oriented—to person, place, and time.
   b. Confused—may be oriented to 1 or 2 items; speaks but does not make sense.
   c. Inappropriate words—usually swear words.
   d. Incomprehensible sounds—moans and groans.
   e. No response

5. Assess best motor response by using the following definitions:
   a. Obeys commands—the person responds correctly to a motor command.
   b. Localizes pain—the person's arm moves to the point of the painful stimulus, in an attempt to remove it.
   c. Flexion withdrawal—the person's arm flexes quickly in response to a pain stimulus.
   d. Abnormal flexion—the person's arm flexes in a slow, tonic fashion, with the wrist and elbow flexed, in response to a pain stimulus.
   e. Abnormal extension—the person's arm internally rotates at the shoulder, extends at the elbow, and flexes at the wrist in response to a pain stimulus.
   f. No response

Final Activities

Call the physician immediately if the patient exhibits a rapidly deteriorating level of consciousness.

imbalances, skin breakdown, corneal drying, contractures, and injury due to seizures or agitation.

7. Applying the nursing process

> **NURSING DIAGNOSIS:** Ineffective airway clearance and impaired gas exchange R/T unconsciousness, and impaired gag and cough reflexes

a. *Expected outcomes:* Following intervention, the person should be able to do the following:
   (1) Maintain an adequate airway.
   (2) Maintain optimal blood oxygen saturation.
   (3) Avoid aspiration.

b. *Nursing interventions*
   (1) Check for signs and symptoms of respiratory distress regularly if person is getting weaker.
   - Dyspnea
   - Pulse less than 70 or greater than 120 beats per minute
   - Rapid, shallow respirations
   - Decreased or asymmetric breath sounds
   - Increased use of accessory breathing
   - Paradoxical respiratory movements
   (2) Check for signs and symptoms of aspiration and pneumonia.
   - Auscultate breath sounds.
   - Observe for increased production of sputum.
   - Monitor body temperature.

(3) Position person alternately in semi-Fowler's position and side-lying position.

(4) Suction secretions as needed.

(5) Encourage coughing and deep breathing if person has sufficient muscle strength.

(6) Anticipate need for intubation and assisted ventilation if respiratory function continues to decline.

NURSING DIAGNOSIS: Ineffective breathing patterns R/T brain stem regulatory dysfunction and immobility

a. *Expected outcomes:* Following intervention, the patient should have the following:

(1) Clear breath sounds

(2) Completely expanded lungs

(3) Effective breathing pattern

(4) Normal blood gases

b. *Nursing interventions*

(1) Assess for the following every 15 to 30 minutes:
  • Altered respiratory rate, rhythm, and quality
  • Rales on auscultation
  • Accumulation of secretions
  • Abnormal blood gases (low PaO_2, high $PaCO_2$, decreased oxygen saturation)

(2) Suction secretions as necessary.

(3) Hyperventilate lungs with 100 percent oxygen before and after suctioning, with physician approval.

(4) Be prepared to assist with intubation, tracheostomy, and mechanical ventilation if necessary (see Chapters 20 and 22).

NURSING DIAGNOSIS: Impaired physical mobility R/T unconsciousness

a. *Expected outcomes:* Following intervention, the patient should experience the following:

(1) Full range of motion

(2) Optimal return of strength and motor control

(3) Maintenance of muscle mass

(4) No evidence of contractures, pressure sores, pneumonia, or deep vein thrombosis

b. *Nursing interventions* (see Chapter 7)

(1) Turn the patient every 2 hours; take care that patient's body is in correct alignment.

(2) Use side-lying positions.

(3) Provide passive range of motion to all extremities at least 4 times daily.

(4) Avoid pressure on bony prominences; massage pressure points every 2 hours.

(5) Support patient's extremities.
  • Support flaccid limbs with splints and pillows.
  • Support spastic limbs opposite their position tendency.
  • Maintain position of function.
  • Prevent flexion contractures of the fingers, wrist drop, and foot drop with appropriate devices such as hand rolls, splints, and casts.

(6) Avoid shearing forces when moving patient in bed.

(7) Keep skin dry and clean.

(8) Request a physical therapy referral.

(9) Promote active range of motion and then mobility with weight-bearing activities once patient regains consciousness.

(10) Prevent pneumonia.
  • Auscultate breath sounds as condition requires.
  • Monitor for change in respiratory pattern, depth, rate.
  • Encourage person to cough, deep breathe, or both at least every 2 hours.
  • Suction as needed.
  • Check placement of feeding tube before administering feeding formula.
  • Check for residual feeding formula in stomach.

(11) Assess for and report signs of thrombophlebitis or deep vein thrombosis; for example, redness, warmth, pain, red streaking on the leg. Apply antiembolus stockings or sequential compression equipment to legs as ordered.

NURSING DIAGNOSIS: Total bathing/ hygiene, feeding, dressing/ grooming, toileting self-care deficit R/T unconsciousness, lack of purposeful movements

a. *Expected outcomes:* Following intervention, the patient should have the following:

(1) Clean body, hair, nose, nails, and teeth

(2) No offensive odors

(3) Adequate intake of nutrients and output of urine and feces

(4) Evidence of fluid and electrolyte balance

(5) On regaining consciousness, ability to perform self-care activities

b. *Nursing interventions* (see Chapter 7)

(1) With a flashlight and tongue depressor, inspect the patient's mouth every day. Observe the lips for crusting and drying.

(2) Provide oral hygiene and lubricate the lips with a water-soluble lubricant at least 3 times a day. Suction excess secretions to prevent the patient from aspirating.

(3) Gently remove encrustations from the nose with an applicator moistened in water or normal saline. Then with an applicator, apply water-soluble lubricant to the nose.

(4) Immediately report bleeding or drainage of a watery substance (CSF) from the nose or ears to the physician.

(5) Do not insert an applicator into the nose or ears of a patient who has had brain surgery or has a head injury.

(6) Bathe the patient daily, clean the nails, and comb the hair. Provide perineal care to unconscious women, especially if they are menstruating.

(7) Skin care, providing nutrients, and toileting are discussed in the nursing diagnoses that follow.

NURSING DIAGNOSIS: Risk for impaired skin integrity R/T immobility, nutritional deficit

a. *Expected outcomes:* Following intervention, the person should be able to maintain skin integrity.
b. *Nursing interventions*
   (1) Monitor skin every few hours; keep skin clean and dry.
   (2) Protect bony prominences from pressure.
   (3) Apply protective padding as needed.
   (4) Teach person to change position at least every 2 hours, or assist person to change position.
   (5) Avoid shearing friction when moving person in bed.

NURSING DIAGNOSIS: Altered nutrition, less than body requirements, R/T unconsciousness

a. *Expected outcomes:* Following intervention, person should maintain normal body weight.
b. *Nursing interventions*
   (1) Monitor daily weight.
   (2) Monitor blood and urine laboratory values for inadequate nutrition and infection.
      • Serum albumin
      • Serum transferrin
      • Thyroxin-binding prealbumin
      • Creatinine height index
      • Total lymphocyte count
   (3) Consult dietitian to calculate caloric requirements.
   (4) Ensure adequate caloric intake.
      • Assess placement of feeding tube regularly.
      • Document actual caloric intake.
      • Assess skin condition.
      • Recognize risk for infection and skin breakdown.

NURSING DIAGNOSIS: Total incontinence R/T brain damage

a. *Expected outcomes:* Following interventions, the following should occur:
   (1) Controlled elimination of urine
   (2) Prevention of bladder overdistention
   (3) Skin and bed linens remain clean and dry
   (4) Maintenance of a patent, clean urinary drainage system
   (5) Once conscious, patient returns to normal voiding pattern
b. *Nursing interventions* (see Chapter 26)
   (1) Assess for urinary retention and an overdistended bladder. Palpate the patient's bladder every 3 hours. Use intermittent bladder catheterization if necessary.
   (2) As a temporary measure, insert an indwelling urethral catheter.
   (3) Assess for urinary infection; monitor the urine for color, odor, and cloudiness.

   (4) Maintain a fluid intake of 2000 ml per day. Carefully monitor intake and output.
   (5) Once the patient regains consciousness, begin a bladder retraining program.

NURSING DIAGNOSIS: Constipation R/T immobility, medications

a. *Expected outcomes:* Following intervention, the person should do the following:
   (1) Defecate every 1 to 3 days
   (2) Have well-formed but soft consistency stool
b. *Nursing interventions*
   (1) Evaluate premorbid elimination pattern.
   (2) Assess abdominal distention or discomfort.
   (3) Check for bowel sounds.
   (4) Check for difficulty passing stool.
   (5) Check consistency of stool.
   (6) Review medications that may contribute to constipation.
   (7) Assess diet and fluid intake.
   (8) Encourage moderate physical exercise on a regular basis once patient is conscious.
   (9) Establish bowel program once patient is conscious.
      • Schedule routine for defecation 30 to 60 minutes after a meal based on the premorbid pattern. Include warm liquids in the meal. Use stool softeners or suppositories as ordered.
      • Encourage fluid intake of 2000 ml per day.
      • Encourage or provide a high fiber diet.
      • Provide privacy for defecation.
      • Use the bathroom or commode instead of a bedpan whenever possible.
      • Allow sufficient time for defecation.
      • Remove feces manually if necessary.

NURSING DIAGNOSIS: Impaired, tissue integrity, R/T drying of the cornea due to absent eye closure or blink response

a. *Expected outcomes:* Following intervention, the patient should be free of corneal abrasion and irritation.
b. *Nursing interventions*
   (1) Moisten cornea by instilling methylcellulose solution.
   (2) Note if corneal reflex is absent, if eyes remain open, or if eyes are irritated. If so, protect eyes with protective eye shields or close eyelids with adhesive strips.

■ CARING FOR PEOPLE WITH TRAUMATIC BRAIN INJURY
(see Chapter 37)

Definition

1. Traumatic brain injury is any injury to the head that results in damage to the brain.

2. Injury can be the result of a blow to the head, acceleration-deceleration, or a projectile, such as a bullet.
3. Types of brain injury
   a. Linear skull fracture appears on plain radiograph of the skull in the form of thin dark lines. It generally does not require treatment unless secondary brain injury occurs.
   b. Depressed skull fracture is the inward depression of the outer table of the skull below the inner table of the skull. Brain damage occurs if bone fragments penetrate the brain.
   c. Basilar skull fracture includes fractures in the skull base that can involve the anterior, middle, or posterior fossa.
   d. Concussion is a transient neuronal dysfunction due to a rapid acceleration-deceleration or a sudden blow to the head.
      (1) Classic concussion is the loss of consciousness, typically for a few minutes.
      (2) Mild concussion results in temporary confusion, disorientation, and sometimes amnesia.
   e. Contusion and laceration (see Chapter 37)
      (1) Contusions involve cortical bruising.
      (2) Lacerations include actual section of blood vessels and brain tissues with subsequent tissue infarction and necrosis.
      (3) Major sites of contusion and laceration are the anterior frontal lobes and the temporal lobes at the temporal tips, owing to the bony ridges on the inner surface of the skull in these areas.
   f. Penetrating injuries cause damage to brain tissue owing to entry of a foreign object (e.g., bullets, knives, and other projectiles) into the brain, which breaks the protective barrier of the skull and meninges.
   g. Closed head injuries do not include penetrating wounds, so there is no break in the integrity of the skull and meninges.
   h. Subdural hematoma results from rupture of the bridging veins in the subarachnoid space caused by trauma.
      (1) Bleeding into the subdural space occurs, forming a hematoma and compressing the brain.
      (2) Three types of subdural hematoma are based on time of injury and onset of symptoms.
         • **Acute:** Symptom onset is within 24 to 48 hours. Rapid deterioration occurs, requiring immediate surgical evaluation.
         • **Subacute:** Onset of symptoms (headache, decreased level of consciousness, focal deficits) is gradual, taking 48 hours to 2 weeks after injury. Surgery is usually indicated.
         • **Chronic:** Symptom onset is gradual (over weeks to months), so etiology is unclear or forgotten. Need for surgical removal depends on size and location of hematoma.
      (3) Elderly people and alcoholics are at high risk for subdural hematoma from falls.
   i. Epidural hematoma occurs when a major epidural blood vessel is ruptured.
      (1) Blood accumulates in the epidural space, compressing the brain underneath it.

      (2) Epidural hematomas are often associated with temporal or parietal skull fractures that rupture the middle meningeal artery.
   j. Intracerebral hematoma, an accumulation of blood within brain tissue, occurs with lacerations in closed head injury or with penetrating injury.

Incidence and Socioeconomic Impact

1. Approximately 5 percent of the United States population sustain a head injury serious enough to result in lost time from normal daily activities.
2. Motor vehicle accidents account for almost 50 percent of all head injuries.
3. Head injury is the leading cause of all trauma-related deaths.
4. Approximately 200,000 people die or are permanently disabled each year from brain trauma.
5. Direct costs for diagnosis, treatment, and rehabilitation and indirect costs to society from lost productivity total more than $5 billion. This figure does not include psychosocial and emotional costs such as pain, suffering, disability, and effects on family and significant others.

Risk Factors

1. Age
   a. Motor vehicle accidents are most common in the 15- to 24-year-old age group.
   b. Falls, another cause of head injury, are most common in older people and in the younger than 15-year-old age group.
2. Gender: Three times as many males as females sustain head injuries.
3. Lifestyle
   a. Alcohol use is the most significant factor in all accidents.
   b. Noncompliance with the use of protective devices such as seatbelts and helmets increases the risk of head injury.

Etiology

1. Motor vehicle accidents
2. Acts of violence (e.g., shootings or direct blows to the head)
3. Falls

Pathophysiology

1. Mechanisms of head injury
   a. Skull deformation
   b. Acceleration-deceleration forces
      (1) Sudden changes in the velocity of head movement cause movement of the brain within the skull.
      (2) This movement can cause injury to brain tissue as the brain bounces against the rigid skull.
      (3) The maximum amount of injury is usually found at the tips of the frontal and temporal poles.
   c. Coup and contrecoup injuries
      (1) A coup injury is one that occurs directly beneath the point of trauma.
      (2) A contrecoup injury occurs at the opposite pole of impact as the brain rebounds and strikes other parts of the skull.
      (3) Both coup and contrecoup injuries result in contusions and lacerations.
   d. Rotational forces
      (1) Rotational forces are created when the head is twisted, flexed laterally, hyperextended, or hyperflexed.
      (2) These forces can occur with acceleration-deceleration mechanisms and severe direct blows to the head.
   e. Several forces occur *within* the brain to cause injury.
      (1) Compression or pushing of tissue together
      (2) Tension or pulling apart of tissue
      (3) Shearing or sliding of portions of tissue over other portions (e.g., gray matter over white matter, fibrous tissue over cerebral tissue)
   f. Diffuse axonal injury
      (1) Diffuse axonal injury is the most severe form of brain injury.
      (2) It leads to severe, widespread damage to the white matter owing to shearing forces within the brain.
      (3) The result is a functional disconnection of the hemispheres from the brain stem's reticular activating system, leading to immediate and prolonged coma.
      (4) Widespread neurologic dysfunction, diffuse white matter degeneration, and global cerebral edema also occur.
      (5) Diffuse axonal injury is termed mild, moderate, or severe based on the degree of damage as evidenced by severity of symptoms and duration of coma.
   g. Disrupted autoregulation
      (1) Autoregulation is a process by which the small arterioles in the brain vasculature adjust their diameter to ensure constant cerebral blood flow throughout a wide range of MAPs, that is, 60 to 160 mm Hg.
      (2) With brain injury, autoregulation is disrupted and cerebral blood flow becomes passively dependent on blood pressure.

Clinical Manifestations

1. Clinical manifestations depend on the degree and location of brain injury and subsequent cerebral edema.

   a. Cerebral edema expands brain volume.
   b. The edema compresses brain tissue in the region, causing neurologic dysfunction governed by that region.
2. Anatomic abnormalities
   a. Scalp lacerations, breaks or depressions in the skull, and bruises on the face may indicate traumatic brain injury.
   b. Blood, or CSF, which is clear, may drip from the nose or ears.
   c. Bruising under the eyes (raccoon eyes) or on the mastoid process (Battle's sign) are signs of basilar skull fracture.
3. Level of consciousness (see p. 675)
   a. Level of consciousness may be mildly impaired in simple concussion.
   b. Coma may be short, as in classic concussion, or prolonged, as in diffuse axonal injury.
4. Cranial nerve dysfunction
   a. Pupils unequal in size; 1 or both pupils may be nonreactive to light.
   b. Absent corneal reflex
   c. Asymmetric face movement
   d. Garbled speech
   e. Impaired cough and gag reflexes
5. Motor dysfunction
   a. Hemiparesis or hemiplegia
   b. Abnormal posturing

Diagnostics

1. Assessment
   a. Obtain details about the circumstances of the injury from witnesses and emergency personnel (see Chapter 37).
   b. Once the person has been evaluated by emergency caregivers and the person is transferred to an intensive care or acute care unit, obtain details about the diagnosis, associated injuries, treatment to date, and special observations and concerns.
   c. Ascertain if family members have been notified.
   d. Perform physical examination to establish baseline neurologic function.
   e. Because most people with head injury serious enough to warrant hospital admission have decreased consciousness, focus the assessment on responses to stimuli and brain stem reflexes.
   f. Check level of consciousness (see p. 675).
   g. Check brain stem reflexes.
      (1) Pupillary light reflex
      (2) Corneal or lash reflex
      (3) Oculocephalic reflex (doll's head maneuver)
      (4) Gag reflex
   h. Check vital signs.
      (1) Check blood pressure and heart rate.
      (2) Calculate cerebral perfusion pressure if ICP is monitored.
      (3) Assess respiratory pattern.
   i. Assess motor responses (see pp. 663, 665).
   j. Monitor ICP if indicated (see pp. 675–676).

2. Medical diagnosis
   a. Diagnosis is based on history, physical examination, and brain imaging, usually CT scan.
   b. Skull radiographs may be used to diagnose skull and facial fractures in the emergency department.
   c. Magnetic resonance imaging is not routinely used because it is not suitable for critically ill people.
      (1) Magnetic resonance imaging takes longer than CT scanning.
      (2) Magnetic resonance imaging cannot accommodate people with ICP monitors or ventilators.

Clinical Management

1. Goals of clinical management
   a. Prevent secondary brain injury.
   b. Provide support.
   c. Correct surgically treatable abnormalities.
2. Nonpharmacologic interventions
   a. Hyperventilation
      (1) Hypocapnia theoretically helps reduce increased ICP by reducing cerebral blood flow.
      (2) Hyperventilation is used to achieve hypocapnia.
      (3) The partial pressure of carbon dioxide is kept at 27 to 33 mm Hg.
      (4) Drawbacks to this therapy are that after head injury, the brain becomes ischemic for a time. Also, inducing hypocapnia and reducing cerebral blood flow when the brain is already ischemic may worsen ischemia (hypoperfusion of the brain). Finally, hyperventilation may be most effective during the hyperemic phase of cerebral blood flow, which peaks approximately 60 hours after injury.

 CLINICAL CONTROVERSIES

Hyperventilation, once advocated as a primary intervention to control increased intracranial pressure, may actually contribute to focal cerebral ischemia.

      (5) Hyperventilation is used only for a few hours, as longer use causes cerebral ischemia.
      (6) Use of hyperventilation is dependent on the person's response to this therapy.
   b. Oxygenation
      (1) People with severe brain injury may need to be intubated and placed on a ventilator to ensure optimal cerebral oxygenation.
      (2) Positive end-expiratory pressure (PEEP) may be needed to prevent collapse of the alveoli at the end of expiration.
      (3) Evaluation of oxygen therapy is achieved by ongoing blood gas analyses and special monitoring devices (e.g., pulse oximetry).
   c. Ventricular drainage
      (1) The neurosurgeon places a ventricular catheter into the lateral ventricle and connects it to a drainage system.
      (2) The drip chamber is set at an established level above the midbrow or other anatomic landmark that approximates the level of the ventricles.
      (3) Cerebrospinal fluid is allowed to drain from the ventricle to decrease brain volume, thus lowering ICP.
   d. Fluid restriction: Restricting fluid intake to half the normal daily volume (i.e., 1500 ml) helps to decrease brain volume, thus lowering ICP.
3. Pharmacologic interventions
   a. Osmotic diuresis with mannitol
      (1) Mannitol creates an osmotic gradient across the blood-brain barrier that draws water from brain tissue into the bloodstream, reducing brain volume and thereby reducing ICP.
      (2) This therapy, like hyperventilation, works only on intact brain tissue. It may not work in severe, diffuse brain injury.
      (3) With prolonged use, mannitol may increase ICP by pulling fluid into edematous brain tissue.
   b. Antiepileptic therapy
      (1) Seizures cause a profound elevation in ICP.
      (2) Phenytoin (Dilantin) is used most often for seizure control because it can be given intravenously and enterally.
   c. Antipyretic therapy
      (1) Fever can aggravate ICP.
      (2) Acetaminophen, aspirin, or a cooling blanket is effective.
   d. High-dose barbiturate therapy
      (1) Administration of general anesthetic doses of pentobarbital puts the person in a coma for prolonged periods, decreasing the metabolic needs of the brain and thus reducing ICP.
      (2) This therapy requires close monitoring in an intensive care setting for several days.
4. Special medical-surgical procedures: Surgical intervention is required for the following injuries (see also Chapter 37):
   a. Depressed skull fracture
      (1) The surgeon removes bone fragments and débrides necrotic tissue.
      (2) A plate may be needed to cover the area of missing bone.
   b. Subdural hematoma
      (1) Blood is evacuated via a burr hole. To create a burr hole, the surgeon makes an opening in the cranium, using a special drill.
      (2) In some cases, the surgeon performs a craniotomy. A craniotomy involves either surgically opening the skull and creating a bone flap or enlarging a burr hole. Craniotomy allows access to the brain and surgical evacuation of the blood.
   c. Epidural hematoma: this condition is surgically treated in the same manner as subdural hematoma.
   d. Large intracerebral hematoma: the hematoma may or may not be evacuated surgically, depending on the extent of the injury.
   e. Missile wounds (e.g., from bullets): treatment depends on the injury and its location. A craniotomy is usually performed, and the wound is débrided.

Complications

1. Cerebral edema, hemorrhage, and increased ICP
   a. Cerebral edema accompanies all serious head injuries.
      (1) Vasogenic edema results from alteration in vascular permeability, allowing fluid to leak from blood vessels into the interstitial space.
      (2) Cytotoxic edema results from tissue hypoxia, allowing fluid into brain cells.
   b. Hemorrhage may occur if head injury forces are severe enough to cause rupture of blood vessels.
   c. These phenomena contribute to development of increased ICP (see p. 675).
2. Infection
   a. Infection is a risk in any penetrating head injury.
   b. Infection may also occur with the use of invasive monitoring devices (e.g., ICP monitor) or surgery.
3. Pulmonary conditions
   a. Pneumonia and atelectasis
      (1) Pneumonia and atelectasis in people with head injuries usually results from immobility and decreased consciousness.
      (2) Aspiration may occur at the time of injury, which predisposes to pneumonia.
   b. Adult respiratory distress syndrome (ARDS)
      (1) In theory, brain injury causes massive sympathetic discharge mediated by the hypothalamus.
      (2) For unknown reasons, diffuse alveolar-capillary membrane damage occurs.
      (3) Interstitial edema develops.
      (4) Alveoli eventually fill with fluid.
      (4) Blood is not oxygenated well, and systemic hypoxemia occurs.
4. Diabetes insipidus
   a. Diabetes insipidus occurs with hypothalamic and posterior pituitary damage, causing decreased secretion of antidiuretic hormone.
   b. Diabetes insipidus is characterized by polyuria with low specific gravity and hypernatremia.
   c. The unconscious person is unable to drink enough water to replace fluid loss and is at risk for serious hypovolemia.
5. Syndrome of inappropriate secretion of antidiuretic hormone (SIADH)
   a. This syndrome is characterized by hyponatremia and hypo-osmolar serum.
   b. It can contribute to cerebral edema.
   c. It can precipitate seizures.
6. Complications of immobility (see Chapter 7)
   a. Decubiti
   b. Contractures
   c. Atelectasis, pneumonia
   d. Deep vein thrombosis
7. Seizures
   a. Early seizures (those occurring within the 1st week after trauma) occur in about 5 percent of people with head injuries.
   b. Recurring seizures from trauma (post-traumatic epilepsy) develop weeks to months to years after trauma and are probably unrelated to early seizures.
   c. The incidence of post-traumatic seizures is higher in people who have suffered a penetrating head injury.
8. Gastrointestinal hemorrhage
   a. Severe trauma can cause an elevation of adrenocorticotropin hormone levels, leading to increased gastric acid secretion, and thus predisposing individuals to gastrointestinal hemorrhage.
   b. Use of steroids to control increased ICP contributes to risk of gastrointestinal hemorrhage.
9. Postconcussion syndrome
   a. Postconcussion syndrome is a common sequela of closed head injury.
   b. It is characterized by headache, dizziness, irritability, fatigability, cognitive difficulties, decreased inhibition, and loss of libido.
   c. It may last several weeks to 1 year after injury.

Prognosis

1. Varies by type of head injury
2. Varies by severity of head injury

Applying the Nursing Process

NURSING DIAGNOSIS: Impaired gas exchange R/T decreased level of consciousness and weakness

1. *Expected outcomes:* Following intervention, person should maintain adequate oxygenation.
2. *Nursing interventions*
   a. Monitor blood gases and pulse oximetry.
   b. Auscultate chest for breath sounds.
   c. Monitor rate, depth, quality, and pattern of respirations.
   d. Suction as necessary.
   e. Position person to facilitate respiratory function.
   f. Turn person at least every 2 hours.
   g. Ensure proper functioning of ventilator.
      (1) Ensure ventilator parameters are set properly.
      (2) Monitor synchrony of person's respirations with ventilator.
      (3) Provide appropriate tracheostomy or endotracheal tube care (see Chapter 20).

NURSING DIAGNOSIS: Altered thought processes R/T head injury, manifested by agitation and aggression in the recovery phase

1. *Expected outcomes:* Following intervention, the person should exhibit appropriate behavior and thought processes.
2. *Nursing interventions*
   a. Identify precipitating factors.
   b. Eliminate or decrease such factors.
   c. Determine and employ interventions that have calming effects, such as music.

d. Redirect the agitated person's attention away from the source of agitation.

e. Consider moving the person to a private room if too much stimulation aggravates the agitation.

f. Use a calming manner when talking to the person.

g. Avoid reprimanding language.

h. Avoid sudden changes and surprises.

i. Increase the person's physical activity to divert energy from agitation.

j. Avoid use of restraints, as they can aggravate agitation by increasing the person's sense of powerlessness and loss of control.

k. During calm periods, discuss with the person aspects of his or her behavior that were inappropriate.

l. Teach the person to recognize loss of control.

m. Teach the person methods of alleviating agitation.
   (1) Walking
   (2) Listening to soft music
   (3) Going to a quiet area

n. Praise all efforts at self-control.

o. Teach family members about managing inappropriate behavior.

NURSING DIAGNOSIS: Impaired physical mobility, R/T hemiparesis, or hemiplegia

1. *Expected outcomes:* Following intervention, the person should be free from the following:
   a. Contractures
   b. Pressure sores
   c. Pneumonia
   d. Deep vein thrombosis
2. *Nursing interventions*
   a. Maintain musculoskeletal alignment.
      (1) Maintain limbs and body in proper alignment and positioning. Support flaccid limbs with splints and pillows. Position spastic limbs opposite their flexion posture.
      (2) Provide active and passive range of motion for all limbs (see Chapter 7).
      (3) Change body position every 2 hours or as needed.
      (4) Promote mobility with weight-bearing activities as soon as possible.
   b. Maintain skin integrity (see Chapter 7).
   c. Prevent pneumonia.
      (1) Auscultate breath sounds as condition requires.
      (2) Monitor for change in respiratory pattern, depth, and rate.
      (3) Encourage person to cough, deep breathe, or both at least every 2 hours.
      (4) Suction as needed.
      (5) Check placement of feeding tube before administering feeding formula.
      (6) Check for residual feeding formula in stomach.

NURSING DIAGNOSIS: Impaired verbal communication R/T damage to language cortex

1. *Expected outcomes:* Following interventions, the person should be able to communicate effectively.
2. *Nursing interventions*
   a. Assess ability to comprehend, speak, read, and write.
   b. For verbal expression deficit with comprehension intact, do the following:
      (1) Ask yes-no questions.
      (2) Anticipate needs.
      (3) Use communication board.
   c. For verbal comprehension deficit with comprehension problems, initiate the following:
      (1) Use pantomime, gestures, or pictures to communicate, and encourage the person to do likewise.
      (2) Speak slowly in short, simple phrases.
   d. Establish a calm, nondistracting environment.
   e. Seek validation of the person's communication.
   f. Allow adequate time for the person to respond.
   g. Collaborate with a speech therapist to establish a communication plan.
   h. Educate family members about communication techniques.

NURSING DIAGNOSIS: Ineffective family coping R/T overwhelming aspects of head injury on family member

1. *Expected outcomes:* Following counseling, family members should do the following:
   a. Report acceptance of head-injured family member.
   b. Report that they are participating in the person's care as appropriate.
   c. Report on the resolution of care issues and financial burdens.
2. *Nursing interventions*
   a. Encourage family members to express feelings and concerns.
   b. Encourage family members to participate in the person's care if they are ready.
   c. Refer family members to a social worker for placement, financial, and counseling concerns.
   d. Refer family members to support groups like those sponsored by the National Head Injury Foundation.

Additional Nursing Diagnosis Commonly Associated with Traumatic Brain Injury

- Altered nutrition, less than body requirements R/T hypermetabolic state of head injury

Discharge Planning and Teaching

1. Educate family about sequelae of head injury.
2. Ensure that prosthetic devices and adaptive aids are available at discharge.
3. Make sure that person, family member, or other caretaker has medications to take home and understands how to administer them.

■ CARING FOR PEOPLE WITH CEREBROVASCULAR DISEASE

Definitions

1. Transient ischemic attack
   a. An episode of transient focal neurologic dysfunction caused by inadequate blood supply to part of the brain.
   b. Lasts less than 24 hours and usually less than 1 hour.
2. Cerebrovascular accident, or stroke
   a. Infarction of a part of the brain due to insufficient blood supply (ischemia) or to rupture of a blood vessel (hemorrhage).
   b. The blood vessel affected determines the area and the extent of brain damage.
   c. Neurologic dysfunction is long-lasting and often permanent.

Incidence and Socioeconomic Impact

1. Prevalence worldwide—500 to 600 per 100,000 persons.
2. Stroke incidence has been declining for the past 30 years, in part because of better control of hypertension, increased diet consciousness, and reduction of smoking in some segments of the population.
3. The incidence of stroke in the United States is 500,000 cases per year, according to the American Heart Association.
4. Of these, 150,000 will die.
5. Of the 2 million people alive who have survived stroke, many require nursing or health care assistance.
6. Estimated direct cost of stroke in the United States in 1993 was $30 billion.

Risk Factors

1. Hypertension (see Chapter 23)
   a. Hypertension is the most important risk factor in stroke.
   b. Cerebral infarction related to atherosclerosis develops 7 times more often in hypertensive people than in normotensive people.
   c. The risk of stroke rises proportionately to blood pressure elevation (both systolic and diastolic).
2. Smoking (see Chapter 40) aggravates atherosclerosis.
   a. Smoking increases the risk of stroke in both men and women.
   b. The relative risk increases directly with the number of cigarettes smoked.
   c. Risk of stroke decreases for people who quit smoking.
3. Hypercholesterolemia (see Chapter 23)
   a. Increased total serum cholesterol levels correlate with increased production of plaques in the arteries.
   b. Reduction of cholesterol and fat intake in the diet can reverse atherosclerosis to some degree.
4. Cardiovascular disease (see Chapter 23)
   a. Cardiovascular disease is the most common cause of death in people with cerebrovascular disease.
   b. Atherosclerosis in the coronary arteries reflects the degree of atherosclerosis in the carotid arteries.
5. Diabetes mellitus (see Chapter 29)
   a. Diabetes promotes atherosclerosis.

b. Diabetes is found in 10 to 30 percent of people with stroke.
6. Race: Incidence of stroke is higher in Blacks than in Whites in the United States.

Etiology

1. Narrowing or occlusion of arteries supplying the brain usually results from atherosclerosis and plaque formation in the artery wall (see Chapter 23).
2. Thrombosis—occlusion of an artery by local disease at the site of occlusion—generally results from atherosclerosis.
3. Embolism
   a. Occlusion of an artery by thrombus, tumor, fat, bacteria, or air bubble that has traveled from its origin and lodged in a narrower vessel.
   b. Common sources of thrombotic emboli are the heart and the carotid arteries.
4. Hemorrhage
   a. Intracerebral bleed
      (1) Caused by rupture of a cerebral vessel that bleeds into brain tissue.
      (2) Is responsible for 10 percent of all strokes.
      (3) Is most often related to hypertension and atherosclerosis, which creates fragile walls of the smaller vessels, making them prone to rupture.
      (4) Is also caused by arteriolar spasm, congenital angiomas, polyarteritis nodosa, toxins, arteriopathies, blood dyscrasias, neoplasms, dural sinus thrombosis resulting in hemorrhage, amphetamine abuse, and alcohol abuse.
      (5) Usually occurs in people between the ages 50 and 70 years.
   b. Aneurysm
      (1) An abnormal localized dilation of the lumen of an artery or a vein.
      (2) Types
         • Congenital (berry, or saccular) aneurysm constitutes more than 90 percent of all aneurysms and is the most common cause of subarachnoid hemorrhage (see p. 693).
         • Atherosclerotic (fusiform or giant)
         • Septic (mycotic)
         • Traumatic
         • Neoplastic (myxoma)
         • Hypertensive microaneurysms
   c. Arteriovenous malformation
      (1) A congenital conglomeration of abnormal arteries, veins, and their connecting channels that causes shunting of blood from the arterial to the venous circulation.
      (2) Varies greatly in size but enlarges slowly over many years.
      (3) Hemorrhage occurs in approximately 50 percent of all arteriovenous malformations, usually in the 3rd decade of life.

Pathophysiology

1. Ischemia of brain tissue leads to temporary dysfunction of some neurons and total destruction of other neurons (infarction).

a. The intracellular sodium-potassium pump fails, allowing the cell membrane to depolarize.
b. Calcium enters the cell, which activates an enzyme that releases free fatty acids and free radicals.
c. Adenosine triphosphate is depleted.
d. Lactic acidosis develops.
e. Electrical activity ceases.
2. Modifiers of ischemia determine whether an arterial occlusion causes ischemia (temporary hypoperfusion) or infarction (permanent cell damage) and, if so, to what extent. Modifiers include the following:
   a. Degree of collateral blood flow to the affected area.
      (1) Collateral blood flow via the circle of Willis or other blood vessels can prevent ischemia if a relatively large vessel is occluded (e.g., internal carotid artery, middle cerebral artery).
      (2) The most distal and the smallest arteries usually do not have a significant collateral circulation, nor do they cause as serious a neurologic deficit as a larger vessel.
   b. Speed of occlusion
      (1) Gradual occlusion (e.g., thrombus formation) of an artery allows time for development of collateral circulation and thus causes a less serious neurologic deficit.
      (2) Rapid occlusion, as with an embolus, does not allow for collateral circulation development. Neurologic dysfunction will be more sudden and often more serious.
      (3) As many as 40 to 50 percent of arteries occluded by thrombus or embolism recanalize spontaneously within 3 to 7 days of occlusion.
   c. Blood pressure
      (1) Low blood pressure after a cerebral insult may not be adequate to maintain collateral circulation.
      (2) High blood pressure, or sharp fluctuations in systolic pressure, may precipitate a hemorrhage through damaged vessel walls.
      (3) In hypertensive people, the upper and lower limits of autoregulation are shifted toward higher pressures. These people have improved tolerance to hypertension and impaired tolerance to hypotension. They develop structural changes in vessel walls, which predispose them to thrombosis and hemorrhage.
   d. Loss of autoregulation in damaged areas of the brain can cause further damage because blood vessels that are still intact are no longer able to adjust their diameter in response to carbon dioxide and oxygen levels in the blood.
   e. Increased blood viscosity (e.g., from dehydration, polycythemia) may cause sludging of blood and adherence of blood particles to atheromatous plaques.
3. Edema
   a. Edema forms in the region of the infarction and contributes to neuronal dysfunction.
   b. The following are two types of edema, both of which can occur with infarction:
      (1) Vasogenic—accumulation of fluid in the interstitial space after breakdown of the blood-brain barrier.
      (2) Cytotoxic—accumulation of fluid within the cell due to failure of cellular metabolism from injury.
   c. Edema can cause compression of brain structures or herniation (displacement of brain tissue into another compartment).
   d. Ischemic brain edema develops within a few minutes of artery occlusion and peaks 3 to 4 days after the event.

Clinical Manifestations

1. The location and extent of infarction determines manifestations.
2. Common manifestations of transient ischemic attack
   a. Weakness or numbness and tingling in 1 limb, or 1 side of the face and 1 limb, or 1 whole side of the body
   b. Blindness in 1 eye, often described as a shade coming down over the eye (also called amaurosis fugax)
3. Manifestations of stroke can include weakness, numbness, speech impairment, visual disturbance, cranial nerve abnormalities, or coordination difficulties.
4. Major stroke syndromes
   a. Ophthalmic artery
      (1) Loss of vision in 1 eye resulting from ischemia or infarction of the retina
      (2) Blindness may be temporary (e.g., amaurosis fugax).
   b. Middle cerebral artery
      (1) Manifestations can result from internal carotid occlusion or middle cerebral artery occlusion.
      (2) Weakness (hemiparesis) or paralysis (hemiplegia) and numbness occur in the contralateral face and arm but may affect the leg somewhat owing to damage of the primary motor and sensory cortex.
      (3) Loss of vision in the contralateral half of the visual field occurs because of damage to the optic radiations.
      (4) Aphasia occurs if the dominant hemisphere is affected.
         • **Receptive aphasia**—the inability to understand language—occurs with damage to Wernicke's area at the frontoparietotemporal junction.
         • **Expressive aphasia**—the inability to express language properly—occurs with damage to Broca's area in the posteroinferior frontal lobe.
         • **Global aphasia** includes both receptive and expressive aphasia and results from widespread hemisphere damage.
      (5) Neglect syndrome (inability to appreciate one's deficits) occurs if the nondominant hemisphere (right side in most people) is affected.
   b. Anterior cerebral artery
      (1) Weakness occurs in the contralateral leg and, to a lesser extent, in the arm.
      (2) Confusion, personality changes, and incontinence may occur owing to loss of frontal lobe function.
      (3) The eyes deviate to the ipsilateral side because of damage to the frontal gaze centers.
   c. Posterior cerebral artery
      (1) Loss of vision in the contralateral field occurs owing to damage to half of the occipital cortex.
      (2) Decreased pain sensation of the contralateral body occurs because of damage to the thalamus.
      (3) Memory of recent events may be impaired owing to damage to the mesial temporal lobe.

(4) Dysphasia, dysnomia, and dyslexia without agraphia may occur if the dominant hemisphere is affected.
(5) Choreoathetosis and hemiplegia may also occur.

d. Penetrating arteries
(1) Strokes of the penetrating arteries are called lacunar infarctions.
(2) They constitute 10 to 30 percent of all strokes.
(3) Signs and symptoms depend on the location of the affected vessel.
(4) Because they involve small arteries, they cause only isolated deficits (e.g., motor or sensory deficits in a contralateral limb).
(5) Hypertension is the most common cause of lacunar infarction. Hyalin materials accumulate in the subintimal layer of the vessel, causing lipohyalinosis (fibrinoid necrosis). The media split, and microaneurysms form. The lumen of the vessel becomes stenotic and then occluded.

e. Brain stem arteries
(1) Basilar artery syndrome. Occlusion of the basilar artery causes infarction of the pons, cerebellum, and midbrain. Signs and symptoms are coma, paralysis of the face and limbs, fixed eyes during head rotation (absent doll's eye response), unreactive or dilated pupils, decerebrate posturing, and some reflex responses.
(2) Posterior inferior cerebellar artery syndrome (Wallenberg's syndrome). Occlusion of this artery causes a wedge-shaped infarction of the lateral medulla. Signs and symptoms are sudden onset of vertigo, nystagmus, dysphagia, ataxia, nausea, and vomiting. There can be loss of pain and temperature sensation on the opposite side of the body.
(3) Occlusion of other branches of the vertebrobasilar system can cause a variety of less common stroke syndromes.

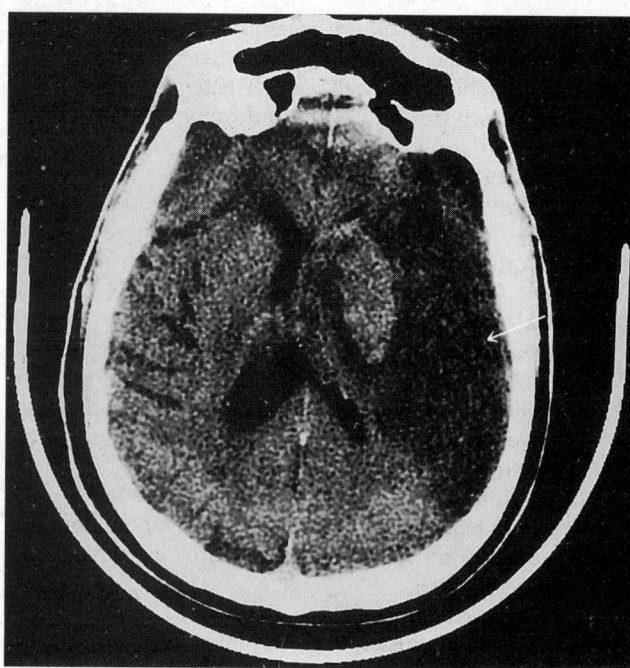

Figure 18–24. Computed tomography scan of brain showing infarction with edema in the left hemisphere (arrow). Note the midline shift and the obliteration of the left ventricle.

Diagnostics

1. History
   a. Assess the nature of the symptoms and their onset and duration.
   b. Assess for risk factors and prior history of stroke or transient ischemic attack.
   c. Check medications.
2. Physical examination
   a. Assess neurologic function.
   b. Check blood pressure.

NURSE ADVISORY

Blood pressure generally should *not* be lowered below 150/90 in normally hypertensive patients who have had a stroke.

3. Diagnostic studies (see Assessing People with Neurologic Disorders)
   a. A CT scan or an MRI view
   (1) May not show ischemic changes until 24 to 48 hours after the event (compare Figs. 18–18 and 18–24).
   (2) Will detect hemorrhage immediately
   b. Carotid duplex
   (1) Involves use of ultrasound with Doppler technology.
   (2) Helps determine presence of plaques and approximate degree of carotid stenosis.
   c. Cerebral angiography is necessary to determine the exact degree of stenosis if endarterectomy is contemplated.
   d. Echocardiography (see Chapter 24) is done if cardiac source of emboli is suspected.

Clinical Management

1. Goals of clinical management
   a. Preserve life
   b. Manage ICP
   c. Maximize neurologic function
   d. Prevent recurrence
2. Nonpharmacologic interventions
   a. Proper positioning can alleviate increased ICP and prevent contractures and aspiration.
   b. Supportive therapy such as physical therapy, occupational therapy, speech therapy, and swallowing therapy can help maximize neurologic function.
3. Pharmacologic interventions
   a. Several drugs are used to prevent thrombotic stroke by reducing blood coagulability.
   (1) Aspirin
      • Prevents platelet aggregation
      • First-line drug for prevention of thrombotic stroke
      • Indicated for prevention of embolic stroke related to chronic atrial fibrillation
   (2) Ticlopidine (Ticlid)
      • Prevents platelet aggregation via a mechanism different from that of aspirin

- Approved in 1992 for use in patients who cannot tolerate aspirin or who have failed aspirin therapy for prevention of thrombotic stroke. Not yet tested in atrial fibrillation.
- Requires complete blood count with differential cell count every 2 weeks for the first 3 months of therapy because of rare but dangerous reactions such as neutropenia and agranulocytosis.

(3) Warfarin (Coumadin)

- Indicated for prevention of thrombotic stroke if aspirin or ticlopidine fails.
- May be used to prevent embolic stroke in atrial fibrillation.
- Check International Normalized Ratio at regular intervals to ensure that it is in the optimal range, because warfarin metabolism can be affected by many drugs. Dosage is aimed at achieving an International Normalized Ratio of 2.0 to 3.5.

NURSE ADVISORY

Thrombolytic therapy for acute cerebrovascular accident must be given within 3 hours of onset of symptoms and after a CT scan has rulled out hemorrhagic stroke.

- The choice of this drug must be weighed against the risk of serious hemorrhage from falls and peptic ulcer disease.
  b. Drugs for acute management of stroke
     (1) Heparin to prevent further extenuation of thrombosis with stroke
     (2) Steroids and osmotic diuretics to reduce increased intracranial pressure
     (3) Antiepileptic drugs if seizures occur
4. Special medical-surgical procedures
   a. Carotid endarterectomy
      (1) Definition: surgical removal of plaque from the carotid artery.
      (2) Carotid endarterectomy is the treatment of choice in symptomatic high-grade (70–99%) carotid stenosis.
      (3) The surgeon makes an incision along the carotid artery and then removes the plaque (or atheroma) from the stenotic carotid artery. In some cases, portions of the carotid artery are removed. Vein grafts or Dacron are used to reconstruct the artery.
      (4) A major risk during surgery is decreased cerebral perfusion due to temporary artery clamping during the procedure. Intervention involves temporarily shunting blood around the surgical site.
      (5) On removal of the plaque, a drain is placed, the incision closed, and a pressure dressing applied to help prevent hematoma formation.
      (6) Complications of carotid endarterectomy include stroke, myocardial infarction, wound hematoma, cranial nerve deficit, and respiratory insufficiency.
      (7) Nursing intervention is the same as for other patients undergoing other types of intercranial surgery (see pp. 737–738).
   b. Aneurysms (see p. 693): Aneurysms require dissection

and surgical clipping, which involves obliteration of the aneurysm with a metal clip.
   c. Arteriovenous malformations are treated with surgical resection, radiation therapy, interventional radiology, or a combination of these.
   d. Large hemorrhages may require surgical removal via burr hole or craniotomy.

Complications

1. Complications related to neurologic outcome depend on the location and extent of infarcted brain.
   a. Brain stem or bilateral hemisphere damage due to edema from a hemispheric stroke can cause coma.
   b. Hemiplegia occurs if the motor cortex or descending motor pathways are affected.
      (1) Hemiplegia may improve to hemiparesis with recovery of brain tissue after the stroke.
      (2) Limbs are usually flaccid initially and later develop spastic or increased tone.
      (3) Contractures can develop if spastic, paralyzed joints are not moved through their range of motion several times daily.
   c. Numbness occurs if sensory cortex or ascending sensory pathways are affected, leading to thermal and traumatic injury due to lack of sensory perception.
   d. Aspiration pneumonia commonly occurs when swallowing and gag reflexes are impaired.
   e. Bowel and bladder urge incontinence occurs if frontal lobes are affected.
2. Increased ICP (see p. 675)
3. Respiratory complications
   a. Atelectasis and pneumonia
      (1) Decreased cough and gag reflexes and decreased mobility contribute to development of atelectasis and pneumonia.
      (2) The presence of a nasogastric tube or an endotracheal tube provides a nidus for nosocomial infection.
   b. Adult respiratory distress syndrome (see Chapter 22)
      (1) Adult respiratory distress syndrome causes ventilation-perfusion abnormalities, obstruction of pulmonary microcirculation, and noncompliant or stiff lungs due to decreased availability of surfactant.
      (2) This syndrome is associated with the aspiration of gastric secretions and pneumonia that can occur with stroke.
   c. Neurogenic pulmonary edema
      (1) This rare condition may occur in stroke associated with brain stem insult or sudden increase in ICP.
      (2) The postulated cause is massive sympathetic outflow, which leads to systemic hypertension and diffuse pulmonary capillary endothelial leak.
   d. Pulmonary embolism may result from immobility and changes in vasomotor tone (see Chapter 22).
4. Seizures
   a. Brain infarction or metabolic derangement in stroke can cause acute seizures.
   b. Damaged areas of the brain become a focus for recurrent seizures or epilepsy in 4 to 10 percent of cases.
5. Deep vein thrombosis (see Chapter 24)

a. Immobility and confinement to bed promotes venous stasis.
b. Deep vein thrombosis may result from such stasis.
6. Hypothalamic syndromes
    a. Syndrome of inappropriate antidiuretic hormone
    b. Diabetes insipidus
    c. Hyperthermia

Prognosis

1. Most recovery occurs within the 1st few weeks after stroke.
2. Minor improvement may occur up to 1 year after stroke.
3. Death may result from the following:
    a. Respiratory compromise (usually from aspiration pneumonia) leading to progressive hypoxia
    b. Depression of the vital centers in the medulla
    c. Brain stem failure resulting from increasing ICP, central herniation, or brain stem hemorrhage
    d. Death is more likely with hemorrhagic stroke and subarachnoid hemorrhage than with occlusive stroke.

Applying the Nursing Process

NURSING DIAGNOSIS: Self-care deficits in bathing and feeding R/T decreased mobility, hemiparesis, or hemiplegia

1. *Expected outcomes:* Following intervention, the person should be able to do the following:
    a. Obtain adequate nourishment
    b. Avoid aspiration
    c. Be as independent as possible in activities of daily living
2. *Nursing interventions*
    a. Bathing and dressing self-care deficit
        (1) Provide adaptive equipment as needed.
        (2) Assist person as needed.
        (3) Encourage independence to extent possible.
        (4) Remind person to attend to body part affected by altered sensation.
    b. Feeding self-care deficit
        (1) Ensure that chewing, swallowing, and gag reflex are intact.
        (2) Provide assistive devices as indicated (e.g., padded utensils, wrist splints, plate guards).
        (3) Assist with meals as needed according to disability.
        (4) Avoid distraction during meals.
        (5) Discourage person from talking while eating.
        (6) Maintain body in bolt upright posture when eating.
        (7) Keep chin flexed while swallowing.
        (8) Ensure safety before allowing person to eat unattended.
        (9) Consult speech therapist as needed.

Additional Nursing Diagnoses Commonly Associated with Cardiovascular Accidents

- Impaired physical mobility R/T paralysis
- Impaired verbal communication R/T aphasia secondary to cardiovascular accident
- Constipation R/T effects of sensorimotor impairment

Discharge Planning and Teaching

1. Educate the person and family members about the disease, the medications, and the warning signs of stroke.
2. Encourage compliance with the treatment for risk factors of stroke (see p. 688).

HOME CARE STRATEGIES

Caring for Stroke Patients

A smooth continuum of care is of special importance with cerebrovascular accident patients to attain optimal adjustment and rehabilitation in the home setting.

Interdisciplinary Coordination

The plan of care and common goals are established and revised with input from all team members—patient; family; physician; nurse; physical, occupational, or speech therapist; nutrition consultant; social worker; and home health aide service. The nurse acts as a case manager or coordinator for the ongoing, accurate exchange of information via joint visits in the home, conferences, telephone calls, and written material.

Direct Nursing Care

- Alter the home environment to allow the patient privacy and the opportunity to observe and be a part of the family.
- Teach safety—clear pathways; suggest adaptive and durable medical equipment; evaluate lighting; keep a phone with large numbers and preprogrammed important, frequently called numbers within reach; suggest a system to call the caregiver; assist in the development of a fire evacuation plan (alert fire department of patient with impaired mobility).
- Teach basic home nursing care
    (1) Personal hygiene
    (2) Turning and positioning schedules
    (3) Transfer techniques
    (4) Bowel and bladder training
    (5) Social stimulation
    (6) Encourage dressing in "street clothes"
    (7) Direct communication to the patient
- Teach special procedures:
    Tube feedings—4 to 5 bolus feedings instead of continual feed on pump.
    Catheter—wear leg bag during the day.
- Provide emotional support and teaching to meet needs and feelings. Major role changes may be involved.

Utilization of Community Resources

- Support groups—"stroke clubs"
- Daycare programs
- Outpatient services—physical therapy, occupational therapy, individual or group speech
- Vocational rehabilitation
- Caregiver support—respite programs, support groups
- State-funded programs for extended services to those who are financially eligible

Public Health Considerations

1. Teach the public to avoid risk factors.
2. Monitor and treat hypertension.

■ CEREBRAL ANEURYSM AND SUBARACHNOID HEMORRHAGE

Definition

1. A cerebral aneurysm is an abnormal dilation of the wall of a cerebral artery.
2. Subarachnoid hemorrhage can result from a ruptured cerebral aneurysm bleeding into the subarachnoid space.
3. Classification by type
   a. Berry or saccular aneurysm
      (1) A saclike dilation of the arterial wall, usually with a neck or stem and a dome, that occurs at the base of the brain at the circle of Willis.
      (2) Likely due to a congenital defect in the anatomic development of the muscle wall.
      (3) Most common type of aneurysm.
   b. Giant or fusiform aneurysm
      (1) A large, irregular dilation of an artery, 3 cm or more in diameter, located on the internal carotid artery or the basilar artery.
      (2) Occurs with widespread atherosclerotic disease.
      (3) Creates a mass effect in the brain, leading to neurologic deficits due to compression of nerve tissue.
      (4) Rarely ruptures
   c. Mycotic aneurysm
      (1) Results when septic emboli that develop from bacterial endocarditis lodge in arterial lumina, causing arteritis.
      (2) Arterial wall weakens and dilates.
      (3) Rare type of aneurysm
   d. Traumatic aneurysm
      (1) Caused by trauma to the arterial wall.
      (2) The weakened wall becomes weaker as pulsating blood expands the aneurysm.
4. Classification by severity
   a. Grade I—minimal bleed
      (1) Asymptomatic
      (2) Alert with minimal headache
      (3) Slight nuchal rigidity (neck stiffness)
      (4) No neurologic deficit
   b. Grade Ia—minimal bleed
      (1) No acute meningeal or brain reaction
      (2) Fixed neurologic deficit
   c. Grade II—mild bleed
      (1) Alert
      (2) Mild to severe headache
      (3) Nuchal rigidity
      (4) Minimal neurologic deficit (e.g., cranial nerve dysfunction)
   d. Grade III—moderate bleed
      (1) Drowsy or confused
      (2) Headache
      (3) Nuchal rigidity
      (4) May have mild neurologic deficits
   e. Grade IV—moderate to severe bleed
      (1) Stupor
      (2) Moderate to severe hemiparesis
      (3) Nuchal rigidity
      (4) Possible early decerebrate posturing
      (5) Vegetative disturbances
   f. Grade V—severe bleed
      (1) Deep coma
      (2) Decerebrate rigidity
      (3) Moribund appearance

Incidence and Socioeconomic Impact

1. Incidence—26,000 new cases every year.
2. Prevalence—an estimated 4 percent of the population have asymptomatic cerebral aneurysms.
3. An estimated 20 percent of people with cerebral aneurysm have more than 1.
4. The highest incidence of subarachnoid hemorrhage from a ruptured cerebral aneurysm occurs between the ages of 35 and 65 years.
5. Ruptured cerebral aneurysm is the cause of subarachnoid hemorrhage in 50 to 75 percent of cases.
6. Eighty-five percent of congenital aneurysms occur in the anterior circulation, which is composed of the distal internal carotid arteries, the middle cerebral arteries, and the anterior cerebral arteries.
7. Fifteen percent of congenital aneurysms occur in the posterior circulation, which is composed of the vertebral arteries, the basilar artery, the posterior cerebral arteries, and the posterior communicating arteries (Fig. 18–25).

Risk Factors and Etiology

1. Hypertension is a risk factor for giant aneurysms.
2. Trauma is a risk factor for traumatic aneurysms.
3. Smoking.
4. Polycystic kidney disease (autosomal dominant disease associated with cerebral aneurysm).
5. The etiology of aneurysm formation is still conjectural.

Pathophysiology

1. Most congenital or berry aneurysms arise from the bifurcation of major proximal cerebral arteries around the circle of Willis.
2. Rupture of a cerebral aneurysm occurs when the following factors overpower the structural integrity of the vessel wall.
   a. Intra-aneurysmal pressure
   b. Aneurysm size
   c. Thinning of the vessel wall
3. Rupture can be precipitated by certain activities.
   a. Sexual intercourse
   b. Sports activities
   c. Valsalva maneuver
   d. Other physical exertion
4. When an aneurysm ruptures, blood leaks into the subarachnoid space, where the major proximal cerebral arteries are located. Further bleeding is stopped by 2 things.
   a. Formation of a fibrin plug at the site of rupture
   b. Local tissue pressure
5. Blood may also leak into the brain tissue (parenchyma) and cause an intracerebral hematoma.

BERRY ANEURYSMS

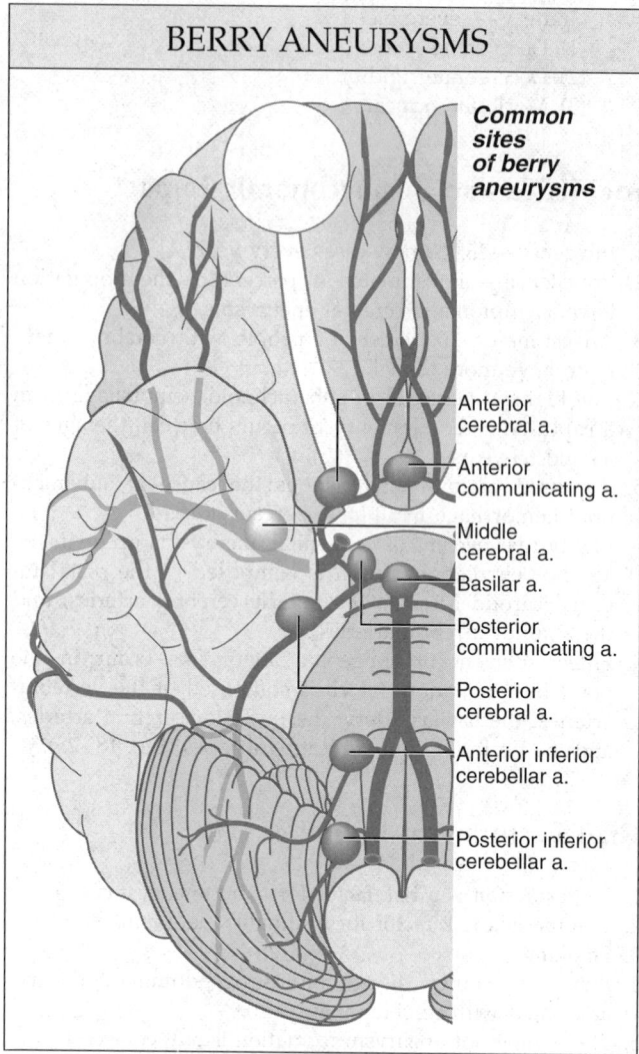

Common sites of berry aneurysms

- Anterior cerebral a.
- Anterior communicating a.
- Middle cerebral a.
- Basilar a.
- Posterior communicating a.
- Posterior cerebral a.
- Anterior inferior cerebellar a.
- Posterior inferior cerebellar a.

Figure 18–25. Common sites of cerebral aneurysm.

6. The following conditions that occur after rupture contribute to neurologic dysfunction.
   a. Increased intracranial pressure due to edema and mechanical distortion of cerebral structures
   b. Altered cerebral metabolism due to exposure of the brain to blood
   c. Vasospasm
      (1) Vasospasm is a pathologic constriction of the cerebral arteries that reduces blood flow to the brain.
      (2) This reduction in blood flow leads to decreased perfusion of brain tissue.
      (3) Vasospasm is a major cause of disability and death from ruptured cerebral aneurysm.
      (4) Vasospasm peaks between day 7 and day 10 after rupture and may persist for weeks.
      (5) The etiology of vasospasm is unclear, although several theories exist, as follows: Substances released from breakdown of red blood cells contribute to vasospasm; immunoreactive and inflammatory processes ensue; vasculopathy develops; and damage to the hypothalamus causes abnormal autonomic nervous system function, which leads to

disrupted cerebral vasoconstriction and vasodilation.
   d. Rebleeding
      (1) Rebleeding from the rupture is a major cause of mortality.
      (2) The risk of rebleeding is highest within the first 24 hours after rupture.
      (3) The next highest risk for rebleeding is during the 2 weeks following rupture.
      (4) Fibrinolysis, or breakdown of the fibrin clot around a ruptured aneurysm, begins a few days after rupture, reaches a peak after the end of the 1st week, and can persist for up to 3 weeks.

Clinical Manifestations

1. Prerupture symptoms occur in 40 to 60 percent of cases and include the following:
   a. Generalized headache with subsequent lethargy
   b. Nuchal rigidity
   c. Diplopia
   d. Vision loss
   e. Eye pain
   f. Ptosis
   g. Seizure
   h. Motor or sensory deficit
   i. Dizziness
   j. Nausea
   k. Vomiting
2. Prerupture symptoms may result from the following:
   a. Expansion of the aneurysm
   b. Minor oozing of blood
   c. Ischemia from vasospasm or vessel occlusion
3. After rupture, symptoms include the following:
   a. Severe, "explosive," headache
   b. Decreased level of consciousness
   c. Cranial nerve deficits if bleeding is minor and restricted to the subarachnoid space
      (1) Optic nerve (CN II): monocular blindness from optic nerve compression and bitemporal visual field deficit from optic chiasm compression
      (2) Oculomotor nerve (CN III): ptosis, diplopia, pupillary dilation, and divergent strabismus (eyes looking outward)
   d. Signs of meningeal irritation due to blood circulating in the CSF of the subarachnoid space
      (1) Nausea
      (2) Vomiting
      (3) Neck and back pain
      (4) Nuchal rigidity
      (5) Photophobia
      (6) Irritability
      (7) Restlessness
   e. Hemiparesis or hemiplegia, if edema compresses motor fibers in the cerebral peduncles at the top of the brain stem
   f. Signs and symptoms of hypothalamic dysfunction. The hypothalamus is adjacent to the subarachnoid space around the circle of Willis, a common site of aneurysm rupture.

(1) Elevated body core temperature
(2) Sweating
(3) Hypertension
(4) Cardiac arrhythmias
(5) Sleep disturbance
(6) Behavior change

Diagnostics

1. History
   a. Obtain history of symptom onset.
   b. Determine if activity precipitated symptoms.
   c. Obtain past medical history for risk factors.
2. Physical examination
   a. Perform neurologic assessment.
   b. Check for signs and symptoms of meningeal irritation.
   c. Perform cardiovascular assessment to detect arrhythmias due to hypothalamic dysfunction.
3. Diagnostic tests
   a. Obtain CT scan to detect hemorrhage.
   b. Obtain cerebral angiogram to determine the following:
      (1) Presence, location, and size of aneurysm for surgical intervention
      (2) Presence of vasospasm
      (3) Presence of other aneurysms
   c. Perform lumbar puncture for CSF analysis to detect the presence of blood *only if*
      (1) The CT scan is negative
      (2) The CT scan is unavailable.

NURSE ADVISORY

Withdrawal of cerebrospinal fluid from the lumbar space may precipitate central herniation or rebleeding from aneurysms.

Clinical Management

1. Goals of clinical management
   a. Prevent further deterioration in function
   b. Prevent complications
   c. Promote recovery of function
2. Nonpharmacologic interventions
   a. Aneurysm precautions
      (1) Complete bed rest
      (2) Quiet environment, free of sudden noises or activities
      (3) Private room
      (4) Limitation of visitors
      (5) Subdued lighting
      (6) No telephone
      (7) Radio or television is permissible.
   b. Controlled hyperventilation
   c. Fluid restriction
   d. Elevation of head of bed
3. Pharmacologic interventions

   a. Antiepileptic drugs to prevent or control seizures
   b. Corticosteroids to reduce cerebral edema and control intracranial pressure
   c. Calcium channel blockers to reduce morbidity, although their role in preventing vasospasm is not proven
   d. Antihypertensives to prevent rebleeding
   e. Analgesics and sedatives to reduce stress, which can cause rebleeding
   f. Antifibrinolytic therapy (e.g., ϵ-aminocaproic acid or AMICAR) to limit lysis of aneurysm clot
      (1) This therapy is controversial.
      (2) It reduces risk of rebleeding by 50 percent.
      (3) It may increase ischemic neurologic deficits.
      (4) It should not be used if surgery will be done within 2 days of the bleed.
      (5) Diarrhea occurs in 24 percent of cases.
   g. Hypervolemic hemodilution
      (1) Goals: Improve cerebral blood flow in the microcirculation and elevate cerebral perfusion pressure.
      (2) Procedure involves adding blood volume expanders (albumin, dextran, fresh frozen plasma) to reduce hematocrit to 30 to 33 percent.
      (3) Theory is that the diluted blood is less viscous and can flow more easily.
      (4) This treatment is controversial.
   h. Sympathomimetic agents to control hypertension
      (1) Maintain systolic blood pressure between 140 and 170 mm Hg.
      (2) Purpose is to promote cerebral perfusion.
      (3) Danger is increased risk of rebleeding.
   i. Stool softeners to avoid straining with defecation
3. Special medical-surgical procedures
   a. Surgery is the treatment of choice in aneurysmal subarachnoid hemorrhage.
   b. Goals of surgery
      (1) Obliterate the aneurysm, usually by clipping the neck of the aneurysm.
      (2) Preserve normal circulation.
      (3) Minimize disruption of brain tissue.
      (4) Remove as much clot as is safely feasible.
   c. Timing of surgery is controversial.
      (1) Advantages of early surgery (within the first 2 days after rupture): prevents rebleeding and prevents ischemic complications due to vasospasm.
      (2) Disadvantage of early surgery is risk of cerebral infarction, because blood pressure must be lowered during surgery to enable safe dissection of the aneurysm.
      (3) Indications for early surgery: the person is admitted to a neurosurgical center soon after rupture; the aneurysm is grade I or II; and little or no blood is seen on CT scan.
      (4) Advantages of delayed surgery (10 to 14 days after rupture): allows time for rebleeding and vasospasm risks to pass and allows time for the person to recover from the rupture.
      (5) Indications for delayed surgery: the aneurysm is grade III or higher (i.e., more severe) and the person's admission to a neurosurgical specialty facility is delayed.

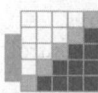
LEGAL AND ETHICAL CONSIDERATIONS

Family members may need to decide about life-sustaining treatments. Ensure that they know their options as surrogate decision makers as well as the institution's policies on end-of-life decision making.

Complications

1. Vasospasm
2. Rebleeding
3. Unresolved cerebral edema
4. Hydrocephalus
   a. Communicating (malabsorptive) hydrocephalus
      (1) Blood in the CSF can block the arachnoid villi, preventing absorption of CSF into the venous sinuses and back into the general venous circulation.
      (2) General signs and symptoms: confusion, gait ataxia, incontinence, and poor balance
      (3) Frontal lobe signs: slowness, mutism, lack of spontaneity and grasping and sucking reflexes
      (4) Onset is slow, taking up to a few weeks after rupture.
   b. Noncommunicating (obstructive) hydrocephalus
      (1) A blood clot in the sylvian aqueduct, which connects the 3rd and 4th ventricles, blocks the flow of CSF.
      (2) Signs and symptoms: loss of pupillary reflexes and downward deviation of the eyes; other brain stem reflexes may remain intact.
      (3) Onset is rapid and can occur within hours or days from the time of rupture.
5. Hyponatremia
   a. May result from loss of salt by an unknown natriuresis (salt-wasting mechanism).
   b. Other causes may be iatrogenic.
      (1) Aggressive antihypertensive therapy may stimulate antidiuretic hormone to save water at the expense of sodium.
      (2) Management of vasospasm may stimulate a substance that causes diuresis and natriuresis.
      (3) Persistent, severe headache, nausea, and vomiting, as well as surgical and anesthetic stress can stimulate excessive antidiuretic hormone secretion.

Prognosis

1. Death rate from aneurysmal subarachnoid hemorrhage approximates 50 percent of cases.
2. One third of patients die before entering the health care system.
3. Permanent neurologic disability occurs in 20 to 50 percent of cases.
4. Risk of rebleeding from a subarachnoid hemorrhage of unknown source is 4 percent in the first 6 months and 0.2 to 0.86 percent per year thereafter.

Applying the Nursing Process

NURSING DIAGNOSIS: Risk for injury R/T altered tissue perfusion from rebleeding or vasospasm

1. *Expected outcomes:* Following intervention, person should be free of secondary brain injury from rebleeding or vasospasm.
2. *Nursing interventions*
   a. Continuously assess neurologic function for changes that indicate deterioration.
   b. Monitor physiologic parameters.
      (1) Central venous pressure (10–12 mm Hg)
      (2) Pulmonary capillary wedge pressure (18–20 mm Hg)
      (3) Arterial oxygenation (>80 mm Hg)
      (4) Hematocrit (30–35%)
      (5) Serum sodium (135–145 mOsm/L)
      (6) Blood pressure (maximal systolic pressure of 160 mm Hg before surgery, 240 mm Hg after surgery)
   c. Enforce procedures to control blood pressure fluctuations.

NURSING DIAGNOSIS: Fluid volume excess R/T hypervolemic hemodilution as manifested by pulmonary congestion, fluid and electrolyte disturbances, and congestive heart failure

1. *Expected outcomes:* Following intervention, person should be free from pulmonary congestion, fluid and electrolyte disturbance, and congestive heart failure.
2. *Nursing interventions*
   a. Assess physical parameters of fluid balance.
      (1) Check breath sounds.
      (2) Note dyspnea, tachypnea.
      (3) Observe for frothy tracheal secretions.
      (4) Check for peripheral edema.
      (5) Monitor and record fluid intake and output (volumes should be equivalent).
      (6) Check for jugular vein distention.
      (7) Check for electrocardiographic changes. Dysrythmias may contribute to heart failure. Tachycardia may be a manifestation of heart failure.
   b. Review laboratory results for the following:
      (1) Hyponatremia
      (2) Hypochloremia
      (3) Decreased serum osmolality
      (4) Decreased hematocrit
   c. Monitor pulse and blood pressure at frequent intervals.
   d. Notify physician of significant changes in status.

NURSING DIAGNOSIS: Pain R/T headache, meningeal irritation, photophobia, fever, nausea

1. *Expected outcomes:* Following intervention, person should be free from pain and discomfort related to meningeal irritation.

2. *Nursing interventions*
   a. Administer antipyretics, analgesics, or antiemetics as ordered.
   b. Maintain a dark, subdued environment.
   c. Plan care to allow rest periods.
   d. Position the patient to promote comfort.

NURSING DIAGNOSIS: Knowledge deficit R/T lack of education about the pathophysiology, diagnosis, and treatment of aneurysms and the need for compliance

1. *Expected outcomes:* Following instruction, the patient and family members should be able to explain the following:
   a. How subarachnoid hemorrhage occurred.
   b. Why presurgical precautions were necessary.
   c. Why surgery was done.
2. *Nursing interventions*
   a. Educate about pathophysiology of aneurysm and need for compliance with presurgical precautions.
   b. Explain diagnostic and treatment procedures.

NURSING DIAGNOSIS: Ineffective individual and family coping R/T seriousness of person's condition

1. *Expected outcomes:* Following counseling, the person and family members should report the following:
   a. Their emotional needs have been addressed.
   b. They know who to call for support.
2. *Nursing interventions*
   a. Encourage the expression of feelings and concerns.
   b. Assess adjustment to hospitalization.
   c. Offer realistic information.
   d. Provide emotional support.
   e. Coordinate support services.

See pages 676–677 for nursing care related to increased intracranial pressure and page 692 for nursing care related to cerebrovascular disorders.

Discharge Planning and Teaching

1. Explain warning signs of complications (e.g., hydrocephalus).
2. Ensure that the person and family members know the following:
   a. Medications, dosages, and their purposes
   b. Proper use of adaptive equipment

◼ CARING FOR PEOPLE WITH SEIZURES OR EPILEPSY

Definitions

1. **Seizure**—a paroxysmal hypersynchronous discharge of neurons in the brain
2. **Epilepsy**—recurring, nonmetabolic seizures

Classifications

1. The international classification of epileptic seizures is based on clinical and electroencephalographic features. Correct classification of a person's seizure is important for determining medication therapy.
2. Partial seizures (focal seizures)—begin locally
   a. Simple partial seizures—conciousness not impaired
      (1) With motor symptoms
      (2) With somatosensory symptoms or special sensory symptoms
      (3) With autonomic symptoms
      (4) With psychic symptoms
   b. Complex partial seizures (temporal lobe seizures or psychomotor seizures)—impair consciousness
      (1) Beginning as simple partial seizures and progressing to impairment of consciousness
         • With no other features
         • With features as in simple partial seizure
         • With automatisms
      (2) With impairment of consciousness at onset
         • With no other features
         • With features as in simple partial seizures
         • With automatisms
3. Generalized seizures (bilaterally symmetric and without local onset)
   a. Absence seizures (petit mal seizures)
      (1) Typical
      (2) Atypical
   b. Myoclonic seizures
   c. Clonic seizures
   d. Tonic seizures
   e. Tonic-clonic seizures (grand mal seizures)
   f. Atonic seizures (drop attacks)
4. Unclassified epileptic seizures (inadequate or incomplete data)
5. Proposed international classification of epilepsies and epileptic syndromes
   a. Localization-related (focal, partial) epilepsies and syndromes
      (1) Idiopathic
         • Benign childhood epilepsy
         • Primary reading epilepsy
      (2) Symptomatic
         • Chronic progressive epilepsia partialis continua of childhood
         • Syndromes characterized by seizures with specific modes of precipitation (e.g., specific sensory stimuli)
      (3) Cryptogenic
         • Cryptogenic epilepsies are presumed to be symptomatic, but etiology is unknown.
         • This category differs from the previous one by the lack of etiologic evidence.
   b. Generalized epilepsies and syndromes
      (1) Idiopathic
         • Benign neonatal convulsions
         • Benign myoclonic epilepsy in infancy
         • Childhood absence epilepsy
         • Juvenile absence epilepsy
         • Juvenile myoclonic epilepsy

- Epilepsy with generalized tonic-clonic seizures on awakening
  (2) Cryptogenic or symptomatic
  - West's syndrome (infantile spasms)
  - Lennox-Gastaut syndrome (combination of atypical absence, tonic, and atonic or myoclonic seizures)
  - Epilepsy with myoclonic-astatic seizures
  - Epilepsy with myoclonic seizures
  (3) Cryptogenic
  - Nonspecific etiology: Early myoclonic encephalopathy or early infantile epileptic encephalopathy with suppression burst.
  - Specific syndromes: Epileptic seizures may complicate many disease states. Includes diseases in which seizures are a presenting or predominant feature.
  c. Epilepsies and syndromes undetermined whether focal or generalized
  (1) With both generalized and focal seizures
  - Neonatal seizures
  - Severe myoclonic epilepsy in infancy
  - Epilepsy with continuous spike waves during slow wave sleep
  - Acquired epileptic aphasia
  (2) Without unequivocal generalized of focal features
  d. Special syndromes
  (1) Febrile convulsions
  (2) Isolated seizures or isolated status epilepticus
  (3) Seizures that occur only when there is an acute metabolic or toxic event due to factors such as alcohol, drugs, eclampsia, or nonketotic hyperglycemia (see discussion of metabolic and nutritional risk factors)

Incidence and Socioeconomic Impact

1. At least 1 seizure: 120 per 100,000 persons
2. Epilepsy: 50 per 100,000 persons
3. Incidence rates may actually be higher because many people do not report seizures owing to the stigma sometimes associated with epilepsy.

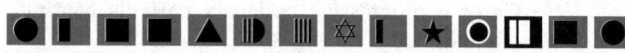

TRANSCULTURAL CONSIDERATIONS

Some cultures believe that seizures are a manifestation of communication by a deity, whereas other cultures believe them to be a sign of evil.

Risk Factors

1. Genetic tendency and chromosomal abnormalities
2. Structural factors
   a. Head injury

b. Cerebrovascular disorders
   (1) Infarction
   (2) Hemorrhage
   (3) Vascular malformations
c. Central nervous system infections
   (1) Encephalitis
   (2) Meningitis
   (3) Brain abscess
   (4) Opportunistic infections from acquired immunodeficiency syndrome (AIDS)
d. Neoplasms
   (1) Primary
   (2) Metastatic
e. Degenerative disorders
   (1) Alzheimer's disease
   (2) Multiple sclerosis
3. Metabolic-nutritional factors
   a. Fluid and electrolyte imbalances
   b. Hypoxia
   c. Acidosis
   d. Toxins and toxic factors
      (1) Heavy metals
      (2) Systemic disorders: uremia and toxemia
      (3) Drug overdose from illicit drugs (e.g., cocaine) or theophylline overdose
      (4) Abrupt drug withdrawal from alcohol, barbiturates, antiepileptic drugs, or diazepam
4. Precipitating factors—increase likelihood of a seizure in a given individual
   a. Physical
      (1) Sensory stimuli: flashing lights, sounds, computer games
      (2) Specific cognitive, affective, or motor activity—precipitants of "reflex epilepsy": reading, laughing, or eating
      (3) Fever or intercurrent illness
      (4) Injury
      (5) Fatigue
      (6) Sleep deprivation
      (7) Inadequate nutrition
      (8) Hyperventilation
      (9) Menses
   b. Psychosocial
      (1) Individual, family, and environmental stressors
      (2) Inadequate support systems

Etiology

1. Unknown in 70 percent of cases
2. Previously mentioned risk factors and other less common etiologies in 30 percent of cases

Pathophysiology

1. Neuronal damage leads to hyperexcitability (so seizures arise from gray matter).
2. Damaged neurons recruit adjacent normal neurons to fire abnormally.
3. Abnormal discharges spread to other parts of the brain.

4. Clinical manifestations occur when a sufficient number of neurons fire abnormally.

Clinical Manifestations

1. Some of those suffering from partial epilepsy report an ability to predict the onset of a seizure based on a special sensation or "aura."
2. Partial seizures
   a. Simple partial seizure
      (1) Motor symptoms usually include jerking of the face or a limb or 1 side of the body.
      (2) Somatosensory symptoms usually include tingling or unusual sensations of a body part. Jerking may "march" along a limb and eventually affect 1 whole side of the body (jacksonian march).
      (3) Special sensory symptoms can include visual, auditory, or olfactory hallucinations.
      (4) Autonomic symptoms are sensations described as a "rush" or "butterflies in the stomach."
      (5) Psychic symptoms can include a feeling of fear or dread or a sense of deja vu.
      (6) Seizure manifestations depend on the location of the abnormally firing neurons or "epileptic focus" in the brain.
   b. Complex partial seizure
      (1) May begin as a simple seizure and progress to impairment of consciousness.
      (2) Includes impairment of consciousness.
      (3) Most commonly involves automatisms—repetitive, stereotyped, semipurposeful movements such as lip-smacking, chewing movements, or picking at clothing.
      (4) Duration ranges from a few seconds to a few minutes.
      (5) Is second to generalized tonic-clonic seizures as the most common seizure type.
3. Generalized
   a. Absence seizure
      (1) Includes a blank stare with little or no movement.
      (2) Produces state of unawareness during the seizure.
      (3) Has sudden onset and sudden termination.
      (4) Usually lasts less than 15 seconds.
      (5) Produces typical 3-per-second spike-and-wave pattern on electroencephalogram.
      (6) Usually occurs only in children.
   b. Atypical absence seizure
      (1) Staring spell usually accompanied by myoclonic jerks and automatisms such as chewing or smacking the lips.
      (2) Produces atypical 2-to-4-per-second spike-and-wave pattern on electroencephalogram.
   c. Generalized tonic-clonic seizure
      (1) Seizure begins with sudden loss of consciousness (unless preceded by a partial seizure that secondarily generalizes).
      (2) Body stiffens (tonic phase) for several seconds; seizure may be accompanied by a cry as air is forced through a constricted airway.
      (3) Extremities produce rhythmic jerking (clonic phase).
      (4) Person may bite the tongue or cheek or be incontinent of urine, or both.
      (5) Entire seizure usually lasts only 1 to 2 minutes.
      (6) Postictal period includes deep sleep for several minutes to several hours.
   d. Myoclonic seizure
      (1) Seizure includes a sudden excessive jerk of the body or extremity, lasting only 1 or 2 seconds.
      (2) Consciousness is preserved.
      (3) Seizures may occur in clusters.
   e. Atonic seizure
      (1) Seizure includes either a myoclonic jerk or, more rarely, a sudden loss of muscle tone, usually causing the person to fall.
      (2) Consciousness is usually preserved.

Diagnostics

1. History
   a. Ask about antecedent events and precipitating factors.
   b. Ask about prior head trauma, family history of seizures, central nervous system infection, growth and development, past medical history.
   c. Determine seizure pattern, duration, and frequency.
2. Physical assessment
   a. Check for asymmetry of limbs, focal weakness, and other neurologic deficits.
      (1) Findings may be evidence of prenatal problems or birth trauma in children.
      (2) Findings may be evidence of brain insult or trauma in adults.
   b. Results of physical assessment are often normal.
   c. Observations during a seizure
      (1) Note date, time of onset, and duration of seizure.
      (2) Note activity of patient at seizure onset.
      (3) Determine if precipitating factors were present.
      (4) Note body parts involved and sequence of motor activity.
      (5) Check for autonomic signs: pupil size and reactivity, respiratory pattern, cyanosis, diaphoresis, incontinence, and salivation.
      (6) Assess level of consciousness through arousability, duration of reduced consciousness, and awareness and memory of the event.
      (7) Check for trauma in the mouth and tongue and in the body.
      (8) Check for postictal paralysis (Todd's paralysis).

NURSE ADVISORY

Be sure to note all aspects of seizure behavior, as the clinical description is the most important aspect of seizure diagnosis.

3. Diagnostic studies
   a. An electroencephalogram is helpful only if epileptic discharges are seen.
      (1) Activation techniques such as hyperventilation,

photostimulation (strobe light), and sleep or sleep deprivation may elicit epileptic discharges.

(2) Use special electrodes. Nasopharyngeal or sphenoidal leads may identify a mesial temporal lobe epileptic focus. Cortical strip electrodes (placed on the surface of the brain) or depth electrodes (placed deep within the brain) may be used for surgical evaluation.

(3) Repeated studies may be necessary to see epileptic discharges.

(4) A normal result on electroencephalogram does not rule out epilepsy.

b. Brain imaging is necessary to rule out neoplasm, infection, vascular abnormalities, and other causes.

c. Laboratory studies identify metabolic and toxic causes.

4. Epilepsy is diagnosed if 2 or more seizures occur without a metabolic or toxic (i.e., reversible) cause.

Clinical Management

1. Goals of clinical management
   a. Seizure control
   b. Minimal drug side effects
   c. Psychosocial adjustment
2. Nonpharmacologic interventions
   a. Avoid precipitating factors.
      (1) Fatigue
      (2) Sleep deprivation
      (3) Stress
      (4) Intercurrent illness
   b. Develop good coping skills.
3. Pharmacologic interventions: antiepileptic drugs
   a. Choice of drug depends on seizure type.
      (1) Partial and generalized tonic-clonic seizures: carbamazepine (Tegretol), phenobarbital, phenytoin (Dilantin), primidone (Mysoline), divalproex semisodium (Depakote)
      (2) Absence and other generalized seizures: clonazepam (Klonopin), ethosuximide (Zarontin), divalproex sodium (Depakote)
      (3) New drugs for partial and generalized tonic-clonic seizures:
         • Felbamate (Felbatol)—approved in 1993 but restricted in 1994 to severe cases owing to high incidence of aplastic anemia and liver toxicity
         • Gabapentin (Neurontin)—approved in 1994
   b. Principles of antiepileptic drug therapy
      (1) Use a single drug first.
      (2) Increase the dose until seizures are controlled or side effects occur.
      (3) Try a 2nd drug if the 1st is unsuccessful.
      (4) Use the therapeutic range of a drug to guide dosing. Therapeutic range is the drug serum level below which *most* people continue to have seizures and above which *most* people experience dose-related side effects.
      (5) Use 2 drugs if a single drug is ineffective.

DRUG ADVISORY

Remember to treat the *patient*, not the serum level of the drug. Some people obtain good seizure control with subtherapeutic drug levels, whereas others require levels above the therapeutic range to achieve seizure control yet experience no adverse side effects.

4. Special medical-surgical procedures
   a. Surgical removal of cerebral cortex may be indicated if the following are applicable:
      (1) The person has disabling, intractable seizures despite having been given therapeutic levels of all major antiepileptic drugs.
      (2) The epileptic focus is clearly identified.
      (3) Removal of the focus will not cause a neurologic deficit (e.g., weakness, aphasia).
   b. Corpus callosotomy (sectioning of the anterior two thirds of the corpus callosum) may be indicated if the person suffers from the following:
      (1) Severe atonic seizures (drop attacks)
      (2) Only mild mental retardation
      (3) Dysfunction related to 1 hemisphere

Complications

1. Status epilepticus
   a. A condition of continuous seizure activity or a series of seizures in which the person does not regain consciousness between seizures.
   b. There are as many forms of status epilepticus as there are seizure types.
   c. More than 50 percent of the cases are due to symptomatic causes (e.g., head trauma, cerebrovascular disease, metabolic disorders, cerebral tumors, infection, drug abuse).
   d. Mortality can reach 20 percent of cases.
   e. Morbidity and mortality are highest with generalized tonic-clonic seizures and young age.
   f. The most common cause of status epilepticus in people with epilepsy is withdrawal of antiepileptic drugs owing to noncompliance.
2. Injuries
   a. Minor injuries such as mouth trauma and sore muscles often accompany a generalized tonic-clonic seizure.
   a. Fractures, bruises, lacerations, or burns may result from falling during a seizure.
   b. Serious burns and mutilation can occur if a seizure occurs while the person is cooking or using dangerous machinery.

Prognosis

1. Approximately 70 percent of people with epilepsy achieve seizure control (5 years without seizures).
2. Mortality is slightly increased, primarily owing to underlying symptomatic causes and accidents related to seizures.

3. Death may occur if a seizure occurs while the person is swimming or even bathing in a tub.
4. A few cases of sudden unexplained death in people with epilepsy have been reported. Death is presumably from a severe seizure that induces cardiac arrhythmia, pulmonary edema, or both.

Applying the Nursing Process

NURSING DIAGNOSIS: Ineffective airway clearance R/T generalized tonic-clonic seizure activity

1. *Expected outcomes:* Following intervention, the person should have a clear airway.
2. *Nursing interventions*
   a. Loosen constricting clothing.
   b. Suction mouth secretions.
   c. Turn person on the side to promote drainage of mouth secretions and allow tongue to fall forward.
   d. *Never* force any objects between the teeth during a seizure of any kind.

NURSE ADVISORY

Do not force anything between the teeth of a person having a seizure, as the risk of injury from this action far outweighs potential injury to the mouth from the seizure itself.

NURSING DIAGNOSIS: Impaired physical mobility R/T postictal effects of seizure activity

1. *Expected outcomes:* Following intervention, person should be able to return safely to baseline motor activity.
2. *Nursing interventions*
   a. Assist with activities of daily living until motor function returns.
   b. Ensure intact motor functioning before allowing person to ambulate.

NURSING DIAGNOSIS: Impaired verbal communication R/T postictal effects of seizure activity

1. *Expected outcomes:* Following intervention, person should be able to communicate effectively.
2. *Nursing interventions*
   a. Reassure person with short, simple statements or gestures.
   b. Stay with person until communication abilities return.

NURSING DIAGNOSIS: Noncompliance with antiepileptic therapy R/T lack of understanding of epilepsy and its treatment

1. *Expected outcomes:* Following intervention, person should be able to take antiepileptic medications as prescribed.
2. *Nursing interventions*
   a. Background
      (1) Noncompliance is the most frequent cause of poor seizure control.
      (2) The following factors contribute to "willful" noncompliance: denial of epilepsy diagnosis; rebellion against the need for long-term, often lifetime, medication, even during seizure-free periods; and medication side effects.
      (3) Other factors contribute to inadvertent noncompliance (i.e., forgetfulness): brain damage that caused the epilepsy; distractions in performing daily living tasks; seizures themselves, if frequent; and complexity of medication regimen.
   b. Interventions for willful noncompliance
      (1) Determine the cause of noncompliance.
      (2) Encourage the person to express his or her feelings about the meaning of epilepsy (see following sections for interventions in cases of fear, denial, and ineffective coping).
      (3) Counsel the person about the need for continuous antiepileptic therapy.
   d. Interventions for inadvertent noncompliance
      (1) Adjust the medication to avoid side effects.
      (2) Simplify the drug regimen.
      (3) Provide written instructions for taking medication.
      (4) Have the person record each dose on a calendar.
      (5) Encourage the use of a pill box or container with compartments for days of the week and, if necessary, times of the day.
      (6) Encourage the person to time medication taking with other daily routines such as meals or daily hygiene or toileting activities.

NURSING DIAGNOSIS: Knowledge deficit R/T the disorder and its consequences

1. *Expected outcomes:* Following instruction, the person should be able to do the following:
   a. Demonstrate an understanding of epilepsy by
      (1) Defining epilepsy
      (2) Describing its potential impact on daily living
      (3) Describing appropriate first aid measures for seizures
      (4) Identifying activity restrictions
   b. Describe the antiepileptic medication regimen.
   c. Explain state law regarding driving.
   d. Identify community resources.
2. *Nursing interventions*
   a. Assess knowledge by asking person to describe what epilepsy means to him or her.
   b. Educate person and significant others about epilepsy.
      (1) Pathophysiology of epilepsy
      (2) Seizure type
      (3) Purpose of medication
      (4) First aid measures for seizures
      (5) Need for follow-up care

LEARNING/TEACHING GUIDELINES
for Self-Management in Epilepsy

General Overview

1. Epilepsy is a chronic disorder that requires long-term—often lifetime—antiepileptic medication and lifestyle changes.
2. People with epilepsy *and their family members* should be educated about how to manage epilepsy effectively through behavioral as well as pharmacologic interventions.
3. The Health Belief Model is a useful framework for organizing a health education approach and motivating people to take an active role in managing their epilepsy.
4. This model holds that people are not likely to take a health action unless they believe the following:
   a. They are susceptible to an illness.
   b. There are adverse consequences of the illness.
   c. There are actions they can take to reduce their susceptibility.
   d. The benefits of these actions outweigh the burdens.

Accepting the Chronic Nature of Epilepsy

1. Explain the anatomy and physiology of normal nerve impulse transmission and abnormal nerve activity in epilepsy.
2. Identify the person's seizure type and the probable cause of the person's seizures, if known.
3. Describe body functions governed by specific brain regions and how the person's seizure behavior is influenced by abnormal nerve activity in these regions.

Accepting Limitations

1. Discuss various categories of limitations: physical injury from a seizure, difficulty finding or maintaining employment, and restriction of driving and some recreational activities.
2. Explain the following to the person and family members:
   a. Persons with *uncontrolled* epilepsy should avoid working with dangerous machinery or in high places; engaging in solitary sports that involve risk, such as swimming or climbing alone; or driving a motor vehicle.
   b. Persons with epilepsy must weigh the risks and benefits of informing their employers about the disorder.
   c. They need to be aware of their state's laws regarding the seizure-free interval required to obtain a driver's license, as laws differ widely from state to state.

Taking Responsibility and Control

1. Explain that seizures beget more seizures, so there is value in controlling seizures early in the disorder.
2. Review with the person and family members the medication regimen and the importance of compliance in controlling seizures.
3. Help the person identify trigger factors and develop ways to avoid them.
4. Train family members in first-aid procedures for seizures. Tell them that calling an ambulance is not appropriate for a routine recurrent seizure that does not include significant trauma.
5. Teach the patient behavioral strategies to cope with epilepsy, such as relaxation, stress management, and participation in self-help groups.

---

   (6) Driving laws
   (7) Activity restrictions
   (8) Community resources

NURSING DIAGNOSIS: Fear R/T risk of injury or death, rejection or prejudice, fetal malformations

1. *Expected outcomes:* Following counseling, person should be able to do the following:
   a. Identify fears related to epilepsy.
   b. Distinguish real grounds for fear from groundless fears.
   c. Describe realistic expectations about epilepsy.
   d. Identify health care and community support services.
2. *Nursing interventions*
   a. Explain activity restrictions based on seizure type and frequency.
   b. Tell the person who has frequent tonic-clonic seizures that he or she should avoid working in high places or around dangerous machinery.
   c. Explain the importance of not swimming or doing any other potentially dangerous recreational activity alone.
   d. Encourage the person to avoid if possible factors that may precipitate a seizure.
   e. Determine the source of the person's fear of rejection (e.g., family, coworkers, employer, schoolmates, general public) and refer to respective counseling source (e.g., family therapist, school counselor, Epilepsy Foundation of America local affiliate for support groups).
   f. Assess fears relating to childbearing and refer to epilepsy specialist for counseling.

NURSING DIAGNOSIS: Ineffective coping, denial R/T stigma, loss of independence, fears of consequences of epilepsy

1. *Expected outcomes:* Following counseling, the person should be able to do the following:
   a. Identify reasons for denial.
   b. Identify manifestations of the denial.
   c. Identify resources to cope with epilepsy.
2. *Nursing interventions*
   a. Determine source of denial.
      (1) Causes include fear of being labeled epileptic, concern about losing independence, and fears listed earlier.
      (2) Denial may manifest as poor compliance, continuation of activities that precipitate seizures, or continuing to drive a motor vehicle in the presence of frequent seizures.
   b. Interventions include counseling and referral to psychologic, social, and community resources.

> **NURSING DIAGNOSIS:** Social isolation R/T fears of rejection, having a seizure in public

1. *Expected outcomes:* Following counseling, person should be able to participate comfortably in social situations.
2. *Nursing interventions*
   a. Help person establish personalized goals.
   b. Encourage person to participate in social activities.
   c. Arrange for role play in a group setting to practice social skills.

> **NURSING DIAGNOSIS:** Altered role performance R/T loss of role as worker, spouse, parent, homemaker, student, athlete

1. *Expected outcomes:* Following counseling, person should be able to maximize role performance within the limitations of epilepsy.
2. *Nursing interventions*
   a. Assess feelings of inadequacy related to loss of job, inability to find work, loss of independence, or inability to participate in previous activities.
   b. Acknowledge person's need to grieve for loss of role.
   c. Offer vocational counseling, family therapy, or referral to local affiliates of the Epilepsy Foundation of America as indicated.

Discharge Planning and Teaching

1. Educate the person about disease, seizure type, medications, avoidance of precipitating factors, and driving laws.
2. See Learning-Teaching Guidelines for Self-Management in Epilepsy

Public Health Considerations

1. Stress need to avoid head injury, stroke, and risky behaviors like climbing, swimming alone, working around dangerous machinery.

2. Educate public about epilepsy to eliminate the social stigma attached to it in some quarters.

■ CARING FOR PEOPLE WITH HEADACHE

Definition

1. A condition of pain in the head.
2. Pain may involve any one or a combination of the following areas (see also Pathophysiology, below):
   a. Pericranial muscles
   b. Neck muscles
   c. Eyes
   d. Jaw
3. The brain itself does not contain pain receptors.
4. Pain may be described as any one or a combination of the following:
   a. Pressure or viselike hold
   b. Throbbing or pounding
   c. Sharp or stabbing
   d. Aching
5. Pain may be episodic or chronic.
6. Pain may be associated with other symptoms.
   a. Nausea, vomiting, or both
   b. Visual disturbance
   c. Hemisensory disturbance
   d. Hemimotor disturbance
   e. Photophobia
   f. Phonophobia
7. Classification—based on International Headache Society Diagnostic Criteria (abbreviated)
   a. Migraine without aura (formerly common migraine)
   b. Migraine with aura (formerly classic migraine)
   c. Episodic tension-type headache (formerly muscle contraction headache)
   d. Chronic tension-type headache (formerly chronic daily headache)
   e. Cluster headache
   f. In addition, headaches may be symptomatic of other disorders (e.g., intracranial tumors).

Incidence and Socioeconomic Impact

1. More than 90 percent of all headaches are benign.
2. Tension-type headache is the most common headache type. One-year prevalence is 63 percent in men and 86 percent in women.
3. Migraine headache is the next most common headache.
   a. Prevalence in women is 11 to 28 percent.
   b. Prevalence in men is 5.3 to 19.0 percent.
   c. Of those experiencing migraines, 85 percent of women and 82 percent of men report some disability from their headache; 47 percent of women and 43 percent of men report moderate to severe disability.
4. Many people have both types of headache.
   a. Sixty-two percent of people with migraine have tension-type headache.

b. Twenty-five percent of people with tension-type headache have migraine.

Risk Factors

1. Family history—present in 60 percent of people with migraine.
2. Precipitating factors in migraine include the following:
   a. Substances containing amines
      (1) Ripened cheeses
      (2) Sausages
      (3) Sauerkraut
      (4) Yeast extracts
      (5) Meat extracts
   b. Chocolate
   c. Red wine
   d. Alcohol other than red wine
   e. Monosodium glutamate
   f. Certain sensory stimuli
      (1) Particular odors
      (2) Bright light
      (3) Wind
      (4) Changes in barometric pressure
      (5) Excessive or inadequate sleep
   f. Emotional stress
   g. Menstrual period

Etiology

1. Etiology of migraine and tension-type headache is unknown.
2. Etiologies of headache not related to migraine or tension-type include the following:
   a. Psychiatric
      (1) Depression
      (2) Anxiety
      (3) Conversion reaction
   b. Vascular
      (1) Acute subarachnoid hemorrhage
      (2) Chronic subdural hematoma
      (3) Temporal arteritis
      (4) Hypertension
   c. Post-traumatic
      (1) Postconcussion syndrome
      (2) Whiplash
   d. Neoplastic
      (1) Brain tumors
      (2) Carcinoid tumors
      (3) Some pancreatic islet tumors
      (4) Pheochromocytoma
   e. Other
      (1) Fever
      (2) Carbon monoxide exposure
      (3) Chronic lung disease with hypercapnia
      (4) Hypothyroidism
      (5) Cushing's disease
      (6) Chronic nitrate exposure
      (7) Birth control pills

Pathophysiology

1. Pain-sensitive intracranial structures
   a. Great venous sinuses
   b. Dural arteries
   c. Proximal 20 percent of the larger arteries forming the circle of Willis.
   d. Pain-sensitive fibers of CNs V, IX, and X and upper cervical nerves.
   e. Parts of the dura mater at the base of the skull.
2. Theories of migraine
   a. Vascular theory
      (1) Superficial temporal arteries have increased pulsatility during experimental migraine.
      (2) Serotonin is the vasoactive agent. Serum serotonin increases during the prodromal phase of migraine and decreases to subnormal levels during the headache phase of migraine.
      (3) Headache is associated with platelet dysfunction (most of the body's serotonin is stored in the platelets).
   b. Neural theory
      (1) Migraine headache is associated with "spreading depression," a neural phenomenon. Studies show a wave of oligemia (diminished cerebral blood flow) beginning in the occipital lobe and spreading forward in the brain at a rate of 2 to 3 mm per minute. Oligemia is accompanied by spreading depression of neuronal activity at the same rate.
      (2) Trigeminal—vascular connection. The trigeminal nerve innervates all of the intracranial and extracranial blood vessels. Research demonstrated that pain fibers connecting the vessels to the brain stem via the trigeminal nerve could pass impulses in both directions. Migraine headache may originate in or be perpetuated by reverberations of impulses in this pathway. In experimental studies, these impulses cause release of substance P and other peptides, resulting in neurogenic inflammation of blood vessel walls.
3. Theories of tension-type headache
   a. Headache is a result of abnormal neuronal sensitivity and pain facilitation.
   b. It is *not* a state of abnormal muscle contraction, because electomyographic activity does not always correlate with tenderness in the pericranial muscles.
   c. Platelet serotonin content in chronic tension-type headache is significantly lower than normal.
   d. People with chronic tension-type headache have low CSF β-endorphin levels.
4. Theories of cluster headache
   a. Extracranial blood vessels dilate.
   b. These vascular changes may be secondary to neuronal discharges in the affected area of pain.
   c. As with migraines, abnormal trigeminal system neuronal activity may contribute to cluster headaches.
   d. Symptoms of cluster headache point to a possible lesion in and around the cavernous portion of the carotid artery.
   e. The periodicity of cluster headache may be due to abnormality in the hypothalamus.

f. Responsiveness of cluster headache to oxygen therapy indicates hypoxemia is a factor in the pathogenesis.
g. Chemoreceptors in the carotid body may be dysfunctional.

Clinical Manifestations

1. Migraine without aura
   a. At least 5 attacks
   b. Duration of 4 to 72 hours
   c. Pain characteristics (at least 2 of 4)
      (1) Unilateral
      (2) Pulsating
      (3) Moderate to severe intensity
      (4) Aggravated by physical activity
   d. At least 1 of the following:
      (1) Nausea or vomiting
      (2) Photophobia or phonophobia
2. Migraine with aura
   a. At least 2 attacks
   b. Aura characteristics
      (1) One or more fully reversible symptoms occur: scotoma or blind spots, jagged lines in visual fields ("fortification spectra"), flashing lights and colors ("scintillating scotomata"), paresthesias, and visual or auditory hallucinations.
      (2) The aura gradually evolves over more than 4 minutes, or 2 or more symptoms occur in succession.
      (3) Duration is shorter than 1 hour, or duration is proportionately increased if there is more than 1 aura symptom.
      (4) Aura is followed by headache within 60 minutes.
3. Episodic tension-type headache
   a. At least 10 previous headache episodes
   b. Duration of 30 minutes to 7 days
   c. Pain characteristics (at least 2 of 4)
      (1) Pressing or tightening quality
      (2) Mild or moderate intensity
      (3) Bilateral location
      (4) No aggravation by physical activity
   d. No nausea or vomiting
   e. No photophobia or phonophobia
4. Chronic tension-type headache
   a. Average headache frequency is greater than 15 days per month for more than 6 months.
   b. Pain characteristics are same as for episodic tension headaches.
   c. May have one of the following:
      (1) Nausea
      (2) Photophobia
      (3) Phonophobia
5. Cluster headache
   a. At least 5 attacks
   b. Duration of 15 to 180 minutes if untreated
   c. Frequency range: 1 every other day to 8 per day
   d. Pain characteristics
      (1) Severe intensity
      (2) Pain is located in 1 or more of the following areas: unilateral orbital, unilateral suborbital, or unilateral temporal.

   e. Headache is associated with at least 1 of the following symptoms:
      (1) Conjunctival injection
      (2) Lacrimation
      (3) Nasal congestion
      (4) Rhinorrhea
      (5) Forehead and facial swelling
      (6) Miosis
      (7) Ptosis
      (8) Eyelid edema

Diagnostics

1. Obtain complete headache history (see Clinical Manifestations, earlier).
2. Obtain complete medical history; be alert to the prospect that chronic headaches may be symptomatic of other disorders.
3. Results of physical assessment are often normal.
   a. Inspect for local infections.
   b. Palpate head and neck for tenderness and muscle tightness.
   c. Check for restricted neck range of motion.
4. If the person has symptoms typical of migraine, tension-type, or cluster headache and results of physical examination are normal, no other diagnostic studies are necessary.
5. If the person has abnormal physical findings or headache pattern changes, cerebral imaging should be done (CT scan or MRI scan).

Clinical Management

1. Goals of clinical management
   a. Provide symptomatic relief of headache. (There is no cure for benign headache.)
2. Check the following baseline laboratory studies before beginning treatment:
   a. Complete blood count
   b. Urinalysis
   c. Sedimentation rate
   d. Blood chemistry profile
3. Nonpharmacologic interventions
   a. Avoid precipitating or trigger factors.
   b. Eliminate unnecessary drugs; seek alternative drugs to those that may contribute to headache.
      (1) Antihypertensives
      (2) Vasodilators
      (3) Contraceptives
      (4) Chronic daily overuse of analgesics or ergotamine
   c. Relaxation training
   d. Biofeedback
   e. Lying quietly in a darkened room
   f. Topical application of ice
   g. Oxygen inhalation, 5 to 8 liters per minute for 10 minutes at onset of headache for cluster headache
4. Pharmacologic interventions (Box 18–1)

BOX 18-1

I. Migraine headache
A. Drugs for acute headache—abortive therapy
1. Ergotamines
2. Isometheptene mucate (Midrin)
3. Nonsteroidal anti-inflammatory agents (NSAIDs), especially naproxen (Naprosyn)
4. Combination drugs (aspirin or acetaminophen with caffeine, butalbital, or both, i.e., Fiorinal, Fioricet)
5. Prochlorperazine (Compazine)
6. Metoclopramide (Reglan)
7. Narcotics
8. Sumatriptan (Imitrex)
9. Intravenous corticosteroids
10. Intravenous dihydroergotamine (DHE 45) with metoclopramide
B. Drugs for prevention of migraine headache—prophylactic therapy
1. Beta blockers—propanolol (Inderal)
2. Calcium channel blockers
a. Verapamil (Calan)
b. NSAIDs
c. Tricyclic antidepressants
d. Cyproheptadine (Periactin)
e. Clonidine (Catapres)
f. Lithium
g. Divalproex sodium (Depakote)
3. Criteria for using prophylactic medication—1 or more of the following features must be present:
a. Two or more migraine headaches per month
b. Headache duration of 2 days or more
c. Headache that disrupts work or daily life

II. Tension-type headache
A. Drugs for abortive therapy
1. Aspirin
2. Acetaminophen (Tylenol)
3. NSAIDs
4. Combination drugs (aspirin or acetaminophen with caffeine, butalbital, or both, i.e., Fiorinal, Fioricet).
5. Anxiolytics
6. Codeine
B. Drugs for prophylactic therapy (same as for migraine prophylactic therapy)
III. Cluster headache
A. Drugs for abortive therapy
1. Ergotamines
2. Intravenous dihydroergotamine (DHE 45)
3. Sumatriptan (Imitrex)
4. Intravenous corticosteroids
B. Drugs for prophylactic therapy
1. Ergotamines
2. Methysergide (Sansert)
3. Corticosteroids
4. Calcium channel blockers
5. Lithium
6. Indomethacin (Indocin)
7. Valproate (Depakene)
C. Importance of prophylactic medication
1. Cluster headache attacks are often too short for abortive therapy to take effect.
2. Abortive medications may delay rather than abort attacks.
3. Abortive treatment of frequent attacks may result in adverse side effects.

 DRUG ADVISORY

Excessive daily use of acetaminophen or aspirin can lead to chronic daily headache and should be avoided.

5. Special medical-surgical procedures
a. There are no special medical procedures for migraine headache or tension-type headache.
b. The following procedures are for cluster headaches:
(1) Blockade of the sphenopalatine ganglion
(2) Injection of methylprednisolone and lidocaine into the occipital nerve
(3) Alcohol injection into the supraorbital and infraorbital nerves
(4) Alcohol injection into the gasserian ganglion
(5) Avulsion of the infraorbital, supraorbital, and supratrochlear nerves
(6) Retrogasserian glycerol injection
(7) Radiofrequency trigeminal gangliorhizolysis
(8) Trigeminal sensory root sections
(9) Section of the greater superficial petrosal nerve
(10) Section of the nervus intermedius
(11) Section or cocainization of the sphenopalatine ganglion

Complications

1. Stroke associated with migraine
a. Stroke usually occurs in posterior circulation.
b. Stroke may also occur in middle cerebral artery circulation.
c. Stroke is rare among people with migraine.
d. Functional impairment is usually mild.
2. There are no common complications of tension and cluster headaches.

Prognosis

1. More than 90 percent of headache sufferers have benign headache.
2. Life expectancy is not altered by benign headache.

Applying the Nursing Process

NURSING DIAGNOSIS: Chronic pain R/T intractable headache

1. *Expected outcomes:* Following intervention, the person should report the following:
a. Successful avoidance of headache triggers
b. Reduced discomfort from chronic headache pain
2. *Nursing interventions*
a. Assist person to identify and avoid possible headache triggers or precipitating factors, includng overuse of headache medication.
b. Collaborate with pain management specialists to develop effective treatment methods and establish a management plan.

NURSING DIAGNOSIS: Ineffective individual coping R/T chronic pain behavior

1. *Expected outcomes:* Following intervention, the person should report the following:
   a. Use of alternative coping strategies
   b. Headache is not a dominating issue in daily living
2. *Nursing interventions*
   (1) Review with the person his or her daily routine and response to headache.
   (2) Support use of alternative ways to cope with headache, which include but are not limited to the following: relaxation and biofeedback exercises, stress management practices, hot or cold packs, massage, meditation, yoga, hypnosis, and acupuncture.
   (3) Educate the person and family members about pain and its management.
   (4) Provide positive reinforcement for health-promoting behaviors and appropriate use of caregivers and support systems.

NURSING DIAGNOSIS: Anxiety R/T lack of knowledge about headache etiology

1. *Expected outcomes:* Following intervention, the person should report feelings of assurance that the etiology of the headache is not life threatening.
2. *Nursing interventions*
   a. Encourage the person to express concerns and fears about the headaches.
   b. Review with the person the medical evaluation of the headaches.
   c. Offer reassurance that headache is not an indication of serious illness, such as brain tumor, if appropriate.
   d. Remind the person that at least 90 percent of headaches are benign.

Health Teaching

1. Ensure that the person and family members know the type of headache and the treatment strategies.
2. Promote avoidance of precipitating or trigger factors.

■ CARING FOR PEOPLE WITH CENTRAL NERVOUS SYSTEM INFECTIONS

Bacterial Meningitis

1. Definition: Bacterial meningitis is an infection of the pia and arachnoid meninges due to an alteration in the person's immune defense system.
2. Incidence and socioeconomic impact
   a. Approximately 20,000 to 25,000 cases are reported each year.
   b. Seventy percent of cases occur in children younger than 5 years old.
   c. Mortality ranges from 5 to 30 percent of treated cases.
   d. Permanent neurologic deficits occur in 20 to 50 percent of cases.
3. Risk factors
   a. Immunocompromised state (e.g., human immunodeficiency virus [HIV] infection or AIDS)
   b. Antecedent viral infection
   c. Age younger than 5 years
   d. Head trauma
   e. Systemic infection or illness
   f. Neurosurgical procedures
   g. Anatomic defects in the skull
4. Etiology
   a. Bacterial infection
   b. Organisms most commonly seen include the following:
      (1) *Haemophilus influenzae*
      (2) *Streptococcus pneumoniae*
      (3) *Neisseria meningitidis*
5. Pathophysiology
   a. The bacteria listed previously exist in the nasopharynx of many people.
   b. The bacteria become pathogenic when the host's resistance is impaired.
   c. Bacteria travel by blood to the brain and infect the meninges and the CSF.
   d. Inflammation of the meninges creates a purulent exudate in the subarachnoid space.
   e. This inflammation produces cytokines that are toxic to CNS tissue.
   f. This series of events leads to the following:
      (1) Edema
      (2) Increased intracranial pressure
      (3) Breakdown of the blood-brain barrier
      (4) Cerebral vascular injury
      (5) Subdural effusion and empyema
      (6) Septic shock
6. Clinical manifestations
   a. Fever and headache—first symptoms
   b. Meningeal irritation
      (1) Stiff neck—resistance of movement of the neck
      (2) Photophobia
      (3) Brudzinski's sign—flexion of thighs and legs with passive flexion of the neck
      (4) Kernig's sign—inability to extend the knee to more than 135 degrees while the hip is flexed
   c. Malaise
   d. Clouding of consciousness
   e. Seizures
7. Diagnostics
   a. Obtain history of symptoms.
   b. Review past medical history for risk factors.
   c. Perform physical examination.
      (1) Check body core temperature.
      (2) Check for meningeal irritation.
   d. Review diagnostic tests.
      (1) Lumbar puncture for CSF analysis. Analysis of the CSF is the only way to diagnose and treat bacterial meningitis. Anticipate the need to treat

brain herniation after lumbar puncture, a common aftereffect.

(2) Cerebrospinal fluid in bacterial meningitis:
- Elevated opening pressure—greater than 180 cm H_2O
- Pleocytosis (increased number of blood cells) ranging from 1000 to 10,000 cells per mm^3 with a predominance of polymorphonuclear cells
- Elevated CSF protein, greater than 100 mg per ml
- Decreased CSF glucose, below 60 percent of simultaneously recorded serum glucose
- Positive Gram stain result in 80 percent of cases
- Bacterial organism growth in CSF cultures

(3) Brain imaging (CT scan or MRI scan) may be performed if signs of brain herniation are present.

8. Clinical management
   a. Bacterial meningitis is a medical emergency requiring *immediate* treatment.
   b. Goals of clinical management
      (1) Eradicate the infection.
      (2) Prevent complications if possible.
      (3) Treat complications quickly.
      (4) Promote recovery.
   c. Pharmacologic interventions
      (1) Antibiotics. The choice of antibiotic depends on the organism. Commonly used antibiotics include penicillin G, ampicillin, ceftriaxone, and cefotaxime. Antibiotics are usually given intravenously over several days.
      (2) Antiepileptic drugs for seizures
      (3) Dexamethasone to treat cerebral edema
      (4) Analgesics for headache

9. Complications
   a. Brain herniation due to increased ICP and cerebral edema
   b. Stroke due to cerebrovascular injury
   c. Seizures due to brain irritation
   d. Hydrocephalus due to clogging of CSF channels by exudates
   e. Cognitive deficits
   f. Behavioral disturbances
   g. Hearing loss
   h. Visual disturbance

10. Prognosis depends on several factors:
    a. Causative organism
    b. Age—neonates and elderly have poor prognosis
    c. Presence of underlying disease
    d. Promptness of treatment

11. Applying the nursing process

NURSING DIAGNOSIS: Hyperthermia R/T infection and abnormal temperature regulation by hypothalamus from increased ICP

---

a. *Expected outcomes:* Following intervention, the person should maintain a body core temperature between 37 and 38 degrees Celsius (98 and 100 degrees Fahrenheit).

b. *Nursing interventions*
   (1) Check body temperature every 2 to 4 hours.
   (2) Keep environmental temperature at 21 degrees Celsius (70 degrees Fahrenheit).
   (3) Employ skin cooling measures.
   - Use light clothing and bedcovers.
   - Give tepid sponge bath.
   - Use hypothermia blanket.
   - Cool the skin gradually.

Other Nursing Diagnoses Commonly Associated with Central Nervous System Infections

- Altered cerebral tissue perfusion R/T infectious process and increased ICP
- Risk for injury to brain R/T increased ICP and cerebral edema
- Impaired physical mobility R/T sedation from infection
- Altered nutrition, less than body requirements, R/T hypermetabolic state of infection

Brain Abscess

1. Definition
   a. A brain abscess is a collection of either encapsulated pus or free pus within brain tissue.
   b. The primary focus of infection is usually outside the brain.

2. Risk factors
   a. Infections of structures near the brain
      (1) Paranasal sinuses
      (2) Middle ear
      (3) Mastoid
   b. Infections in distant sites
      (1) Oral cavity
      (2) Skin
      (3) Lungs
      (4) Bone
      (5) Heart valves
   c. Head trauma
      (1) Penetrating wounds
      (2) Basilar skull fracture
   d. Immune system compromise

3. Etiology
   a. The abscess is caused by the organism at the original site of infection.
   b. Common bacterial organisms include the following:
      (1) *Streptococcus* (60–70% of cases)
      (2) *Staphylococcus aureus* (10–15% of cases)
      (3) *Enterobacter*
      (4) *Haemophilus*
      (5) *Proteus*
      (6) *Escherichia coli*
      (7) *Pseudomonas*
   c. Anaerobic bacteria are the usual cause of otic, dental, and metastatic brain abscesses.

d. Yeast and fungi are responsible for 9 to 17 percent of cases.
4. Pathophysiology
   a. Microorganisms seed necrotic areas of the brain parenchyma by several mechanisms:
      (1) Direct extension of local infection
      (2) Direct brain trauma
      (3) Blood flow from a distant site of infection
   b. The abscess undergoes several stages of evolution.
      (1) Early cerebritis stage (days 1–3): central necrosis, local inflammation, and edema
      (2) Late cerebritis stage (days 4–9): development of pus and enlargement of the necrotic center, which is surrounded by macrophages and inflammatory cells
      (3) Early encapsulation stage (days 10–13): formation of a collagen capsule around the abscess prevents spread of the infection
      (4) Late capsule stage (day 14 onward): the establishment of 5 distinct zones of tissue:
         • Necrotic center
         • Peripheral zone of inflammatory cells and fibroblasts
         • Abscess capsule
         • Zone of neovascularity and cerebritis
         • Surrounding area of edema and reactive gliosis
5. Clinical manifestations
   a. Symptoms depend on the size and location of the abscess, which acts like a mass lesion.
   b. Headache is common in 70 percent of cases.
   c. Nausea and vomiting occur in 25 to 50 percent of cases.
   d. Focal neurologic symptoms occur in 60 percent of cases and include the following:
      (1) Hemiparesis
      (2) Dysphasia
      (3) Visual field deficits
      (4) Ataxia
      (5) Nystagmus
   e. Seizures occur in 30 to 50 percent of cases.
   f. Fever and chills occur in approximately 50 percent of cases.
6. Diagnostics
   a. Obtain history of symptoms.
   b. Review past medical history for risk factors.
   c. Perform physical examination.
      (1) Check for possible sites of infection.
      (2) Check body core temperature.
      (3) Check for neurologic deficits.
   d. Review diagnostic tests.
      (1) Peripheral white blood cell count is usually less than 15,000 cells per mm³.
      (2) Erythrocyte sedimentation rate is elevated.
      (3) Cerebrospinal fluid analysis: mildly elevated protein, normal glucose, and usually negative cultures.
      (4) Brain imaging (CT scan or MRI scan): brain imaging shows a ring-enhancing lesion when contrast dye is used. The ring enhancement will not appear if the abscess is still in its early stages (Fig. 18–26).

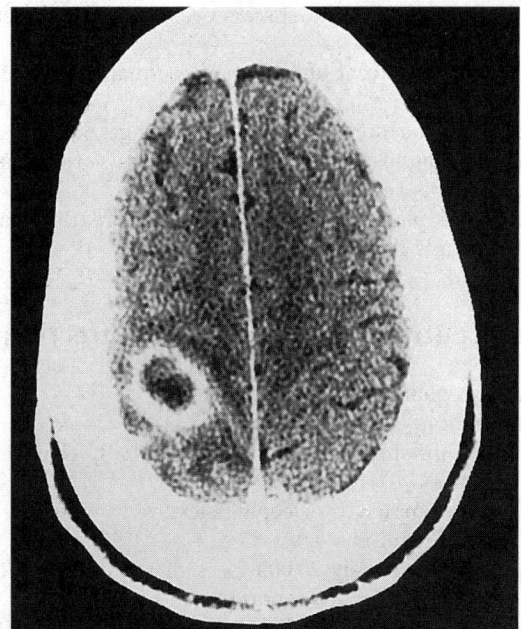

Figure 18–26. Computed tomography scan of a brain abscess.

      (5) Radionuclide imaging can help distinguish brain abscess from other intracranial space-occupying lesions.
      (6) Brain biopsy via needle aspiration through a burr hole may be necessary to obtain a diagnosis.
8. Clinical management
   a. Goals of clinical management
      (1) Eradicate the abscess or abscesses.
      (2) Treat any complications.
      (3) Promote recovery.
   b. Pharmacologic interventions
      (1) Antibiotics. Ideally, antibiotics are chosen on the basis of culture and sensitivity testing, but they may be chosen on the basis of presumed pathogenesis, if culture results are pending or impossible to obtain. Antibiotics are given for 6 weeks.
      (2) Corticosteroids. Corticosteroids may be used to decrease cerebral edema in cases of impending herniation, but because they can decrease the host response to infection, they are not used routinely.
   c. Special medical-surgical procedures
      (1) Serial brain imaging studies are performed to monitor resolution of the abscess.
      (2) Larger abscess may require surgical removal.
8. Complications
   a. Increased ICP from edema
   b. Seizures
9. Prognosis
   a. Early recognition, diagnosis, and treatment have greatly reduced mortality from brain abscess in the last 2 decades.
   b. The condition of the person on presentation is the most significant predictor of response to therapy. Those with stupor or coma have high mortality.
   c. Death is usually from herniation due to mass effect of the abscess or from rupture into the ventricular system.

d. Recurrence of brain abscess occurs in 5 to 10 percent of cases.

e. Up to 50 percent of cases have permanent neurologic deficits.

10. Applying the nursing process. See page 692 for other nursing diagnoses and interventions for various neurologic deficits seen in brain abscess.

11. Discharge planning and teaching: Ensure that patient understands drug regimen.

Other Central Nervous System Infections

1. Viral encephalitis
   a. Definition
      (1) An inflammation of the brain, usually caused by a virus
      (2) Also known as "sleeping sickness"
   b. Incidence and etiology
      (1) Approximately 20,000 cases of acute viral encephalitis a year are reported by the Centers for Disease Control and Prevention. Viral encephalitis is primarily caused by the herpes simplex virus and arboviruses.
      (2) The herpes simplex virus type 1 (which also causes cold sores) is passed from person to person. The resulting condition, herpes simplex encephalitis, is distributed throughout the United States.
      (3) Arboviruses are transmitted to humans via mosquito and tick bites, causing arboviral encephalitis. The mosquito or tick becomes infected when it ingests infected blood from a viremic host—either a horse or bird. The resulting disorders include St. Louis encephalitis (primarily distributed along the Mississippi River), eastern equine encephalitis (observed primarily in the eastern states), and western equine encephalitis (distributed mainly west of the Mississippi River).
   c. Clinical manifestations
      (1) Herpes simplex virus encephalitis
         • Headache
         • Vomiting
         • Fever
         • Seizures sometimes develop
         • Confusion, stupor, and coma if acute condition is not treated aggressively
         • More than 50 percent of these patients may die or develop permanent CNS disabilities.
      (2) Arboviral encephalitis
         • Gradual onset of symptoms
         • Headache
         • Nausea and vomiting
         • Fever
         • Seizures, stupor, and coma within days
         • Photophobia, hemiparesis, and asymmetric reflexes in some cases
         • Two thirds of patients die or suffer from permanent disabling CNS abnormalities.
   d. Interventions
      (1) Administer a 14-day course of intravenous acyclovir (an antiviral agent) for herpes simplex as ordered. The earlier in the illness the patient receives this medication, the better the prognosis.
      (2) Administer corticosteroids for brief periods as ordered to control brain swelling.
      (3) Protect the patient from injury to self due to seizures.
      (4) Protect the patient from the complications of immobility if stupor or coma develops (see Chapter 7).

2. Central nervous system fungal infections
   a. Definition: fungal infections of the CNS that may result in meningitis, meningoencephalitis, intracranial thrombophlebitis, or brain abscess
   b. Incidence and etiology
      (1) Central nervous system fungal infections are rare.
      (2) Fungal infections may arise as complications of leukemia, organ transplants, diabetes, collagen disease, or vascular disease. These disorders suppress the immune response, lowering the person's resistance to infection.
   c. Clinical manifestations
      (1) Fever
      (2) Increased pulse and respirations
      (3) Weakness, confusion, headache
      (4) Other manifestations of bacterial infections (see Chapter 8)
   d. Interventions
      (1) Administer intravenous amphotericin B combined with flucytosine for 4 to 6 weeks as ordered.
      (2) With treatment, the prognosis is excellent unless the patient has advanced leukemia, diabetes, or other potentially fatal disorders.

◼ CARING FOR PEOPLE WITH INTRACRANIAL TUMORS

Definition

1. Intracranial tumors are primary and metastatic neoplasms that affect the brain.
2. Primary tumors develop from cells within the brain.
   a. Tumors are named after their cell of origin (e.g., astrocytoma is a tumor of astrocytes).
   b. The most common types of primary tumor are composed of glial cells, because these cells are capable of mitosis (cell reproduction).
      (1) Glial cell tumors are graded according to degree of cell differentiation.
      (2) Astrocytoma: Cells in grades 1 and 2 are well differentiated. Cells in grades 3 and 4 (also called glioblastoma multiforme) are less well differentiated.
      (3) Oligodendroglioma
      (4) Ependymona
   c. Meningioma
      (1) Tumor that affects the meninges.
      (2) Because it is usually encapsulated (does not invade brain tissue) and easily excised, it is benign.

Table 18-6. Incidence of Intracranial Tumors by Type	
Type	**Percent of Intracranial Tumors**
Gliomas	45
Astrocytoma	
Grades I and II	10
Grades III and IV (glioblastoma multiforme)	20
Oligodendroglioma	5
Ependymoma	6
Medulloblastoma	4
Meningioma	15
Pituitary tumors	7
Vestibular schwannoma (acoustic neuroma)	7
Metastic tumors	10
Craniopharyngioma, dermoid, epidermoid, teratoma tumors	4
Other tumors (sarcoma, angioma, pinealoma, chordoma, granuloma, lymphoma)	12

d. Neurons rarely cause tumors because they generally do not have the ability to reproduce.
e. Some intracranial tumors arise from other brain tissues.
  (1) Colloid cyst
  (2) Craniopharyngioma
  (3) Dermoid cyst
  (4) Medulloblastoma
  (5) Pinealoma
  (6) Pituitary adenoma
  (7) Teratoma
  (8) Vestibular schwannoma
  (9) Cholesteatoma
3. Metastatic tumors arise from neoplasms outside the brain.
  a. Lung and breast neoplasms are the most common origins of metastatic tumors in the brain.
  b. Other brain metastases arise from melanoma and colon, rectal, and kidney cancers.

Incidence

1. In the United States, 10,000 per year
2. See Table 18-6 for incidence by tumor type.

Risk Factors and Etiology

1. There are no known risk factors or etiology for primary intracranial tumors.
2. Most metastatic tumors arise from the spread of neoplasms of the lung and breast.

Pathophysiology

1. Tumor infiltrates or compresses brain tissue (or does both).
2. Compressed brain tissue causes neurologic deficits, headache, and seizures.
3. Surrounding edema leads to increased ICP (see p. 686).

Clinical Manifestations

1. Manifestations depend on location of the tumor and effects of edema
2. Neurologic deficits can include the following:
  a. Weakness
  b. Sensory changes
  c. Visual field deficits
  d. Language disturbance
  e. Gait disturbance
  f. Cognitive impairment
  g. Personality change
3. Headache occurs with increased ICP or pressure of the tumor on pain-sensitive structures in the brain.
4. Seizures may be the first manifestation of a brain tumor.

Diagnostics

1. History
  a. Ask about nature and onset of symptoms.
  b. Check for history of cancer.
2. Physical assessment
  a. Check for the neurologic deficits listed earlier.
  b. Perform neurologic physical assessment
3. Diagnostic studies
  a. Brain imaging, MRI scan, or CT scan (Fig. 18-27)

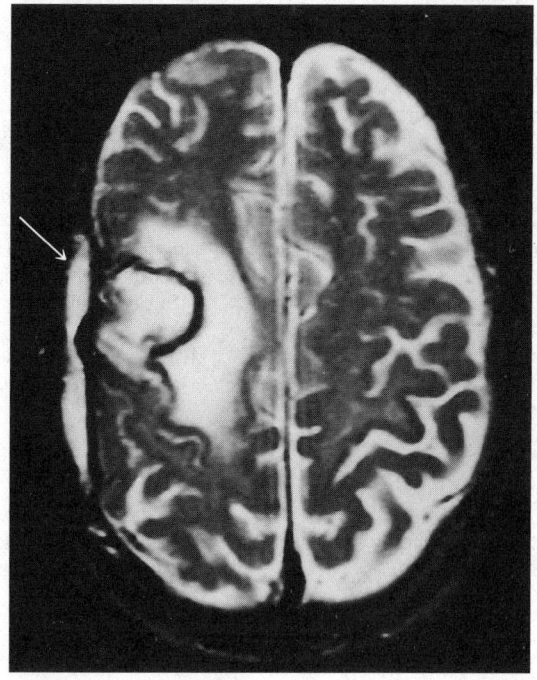

Figure 18-27. Magnetic resonance imaging view of a glioblastoma in the right frontal lobe (arrow) with surrounding edema.

b. Electroencephalogram to check for seizure activity
c. Chest radiograph to check for lung tumor
d. Neuroendocrine tests for pituitary tumors
e. Cerebral angiography to check vascularity of tumor
f. Cerebrospinal fluid analysis for cytology
g. Brain biopsy for histologic confirmation of tumor cell type

Clinical Management

1. Goals of clinical management
   a. Prolong life
   b. Maintain quality of life
2. Nonpharmacologic interventions: radiation therapy (see also Chapter 17)
   a. Conventional therapy is 5000 to 6000 rads (6000 centigray units) of external radiation over 5 to 6 weeks.
   b. Brachytherapy involves radioactive seeds placed in the tumor bed.
      (1) Therapy is administered 5 days per week for a total of 1200 rads.
      (2) Seeds are replaced every few days.
   c. Neurologic side effects
      (1) Acute encephalopathy. Etiology is likely related to associated edema. Symptoms are dose related and can be prevented by pretreatment with high doses of steroids and avoidance of high initial radiation doses.
      (2) Delayed cerebral radiation necrosis occurs several months after radiation therapy. Symptoms include headache, personality change, focal neurologic deficits, and seizures. Treatment includes steroid administration and surgical resection of necrotic brain, although neither is very successful.
3. Pharmacologic interventions
   a. Chemotherapy (see also Chapter 17)

(1) Chemotherapy may be given as primary therapy.
(2) Chemotherapy may be adjunctive to surgery and radiation.
(3) Selection of drugs is based on specificity for certain cell types.
(4) Drugs may be administered intra-arterially, intrathecally, or intraventricularly.
(5) Common drugs (Table 18–7)
   b. Medications
      (1) Antiepileptic drugs are used to control seizures.
      (2) Dexamethasone (Decadron) reduces brain swelling from the tumor and from radiation therapy.
4. Special medical-surgical procedures
   a. Brain biopsy to determine type of tumor
   b. Craniotomy for surgical excision or debulking of the tumor
      (1) Surgery generally precedes other therapies (i.e., radiation, chemotherapy).
      (2) Well-encapsulated tumors in accessible locations (e.g., meningioma) can be removed completely.
      (3) Tumors infiltrating adjacent brain tissue (e.g., glioblastoma) can only be partially removed (debulked) and consequently need further treatment with radiation or chemotherapy.

Complications

1. Permanent neurologic deficits
2. Recurring seizures

Prognosis

1. Prognosis depends on tumor type
   a. Astrocytoma (grades 1 and 2): 6 to 15 years; varies widely due to size and location of tumor

Table 18–7. Chemotherapeutic Agents in the Treatment of Intracranial Tumors

Agents and Usage	Mechanism of Action	Side Effects
Nitrosoureas (BCNU is most common)	Nitrosoureas are cell-cycle specific with alkylating properties. They are lipid soluble and cross the blood-brain barrier.	Nitrosoureas are not neurotoxic in routine doses, but BCNU combined with total brain irradiation can increase neurotoxicity (radionecrosis and cerebral atrophy).
Methotrexate (Used for CNS lymphoma)	Methotrexate is cell-cycle specific. It depletes intracellular folate but has little effect on nondividing cells.	Neurologic side effects of intrathecal administration include the following: • Arachnoiditis (self-limiting) • Myelopathy • Encephalopathy neurologic side effects are R/T concentration of methotrexate and duration of methotrexate exposure to CNS tissue.
Cisplatin (Used in some primary tumors)	Cisplatin binds directly to DNA. It has synergistic action with other antineoplastic drugs and with radiation therapy.	Neurologic side effects are R/T cumulative dose of cisplatin and include the following: • Hearing loss due to cochlear damage. • Primarily sensory peripheral neuropathy, causing paresthesias and decreased sensation in stocking-glove distribution, and severe gait ataxia in severe forms.

BCNU, Carmustine; CNS, central nervous system.

b. Astrocytoma (grades 3 and 4 or glioblastoma multiforme): 6 months to 2 years
c. Oligodendroglioma: 5 or more years
d. Metastatic tumor: poor owing to metastatic nature of cells
e. Pituitary tumor: good with complete removal
f. Vestibular schwannoma: 30 percent mortality after 3 to 4 years with incomplete removal
g. Meningioma: normal life expectancy with total removal; many years with partial removal
2. Death generally results from the following:
   a. Increased ICP
   b. Direct invasion of vital brain stem structures by the tumor

Applying the Nursing Process

NURSING DIAGNOSIS: Altered cerebral tissue perfusion R/T increased ICP after craniotomy

1. *Expected outcomes:* Following intervention, person should be free of signs of increased ICP.
2. *Nursing interventions*
   a. Continually assess person's neurologic status.
   b. Monitor ICP and cerebral perfusion pressure when feasible.
   c. Ensure proper positioning of head.
      (1) Head is usually elevated 30 degrees after supratentorial surgery.
      (2) Head is usually kept flat after posterior fossa surgery.
   d. Administer drugs as indicated.

NURSING DIAGNOSIS: Ineffective breathing pattern R/T decreased level of consciousness, immobility, positioning, and impaired coughing

1. *Expected outcomes:* Following intervention, person should maintain normal respiratory patterns.
2. *Nursing interventions*
   a. Assess respiratory parameters.
   b. Draw and evaluate arterial blood gases as indicated.
   c. Encourage gentle coughing and turning.
   d. Suction mouth and throat briefly if needed. Hyperventilate and hyperoxygenate before and after each session to prevent increased ICP.

NURSING DIAGNOSIS: Self-care deficit R/T decreased level of consciousness or neurologic deficits

1. *Expected outcomes:* Following intervention, the person should maintain the following:
   a. Adequate nutrition
   b. Skin integrity
   c. Good hygiene
2. *Nursing interventions*
   a. Provide for total self-care requirements.

(1) Turn every 2 hours to prevent skin breakdown.
(2) Provide adequate nutrition and hydration (e.g., intravenous fluids, enteral feedings, oral feedings).
(3) Ensure adequate elimination from bowel and bladder. Monitor intake and output, maintain indwelling catheter patency and sterility, and establish a bowel program.
   b. Maintain range of motion of all joints.

NURSING DIAGNOSIS: Anxiety R/T neurologic deficits and prospect of terminal illness

1. *Expected outcomes:* Following counseling, person and family members will report the following:
   a. Their questions and concerns have been addressed.
   b. They have had an opportunity to make an advance directive (living will).
2. *Nursing interventions*
   a. Encourage person and family members to express their feelings and concerns.
      (1) Discuss end-of-life decisions.
      (2) Support making an advance directive, designating a surrogate decision maker, or both.
      (3) Offer reassurance that comfort care (adequate pain control, physical and psychologic comfort) will always be provided.
   b. Provide information about support groups.
   c. Arrange for hospice if indicated.

NURSE ADVISORY

When a patient with an intracranial tumor becomes terminally ill, counsel the patient and family members about hospice and comfort care.

Discharge Planning and Teaching

1. Educate person and family members about the following:
   a. Medical diagnosis
   b. Treatment strategy and side effects of treatment
   c. Signs and symptoms of deterioration
   d. Brain tumor support groups
   e. Hospice
2. Ensure that the person and family members have home adaptive devices and proper training in their use.

◼ CARING FOR PEOPLE WITH ALZHEIMER'S DISEASE

Definition

1. Alzheimer's disease is an irreversible form of senile dementia from nerve cell deterioration.
2. Victims experience cognitive deterioration and progressive loss of ability to carry out the functions of daily living.

Incidence and Socioeconomic Impact

1. Between 1.5 and 2 million people in the United States have Alzheimer's disease.
2. It is very rare in those younger than 60 years of age.
3. Incidence is 10 to 15 percent in people older than 65 years and rises with advancing age (47 percent in people older than 85 years).
4. Approximately 720,000 of the 1.6 million nursing home residents in the United States have dementia (primarily Alzheimer's disease).
5. Men and women are affected equally.
6. The disease poses a tremendous economic, psychologic, and social burden on family members who care for the affected person at home.

Risk Factors

1. Advancing age
2. Head trauma
3. Lack of education
4. Family history: Defects in chromosomes 1, 14, 19, and 21 have been found in families with high rates of Alzheimer's disease.

Etiology

1. Etiology is idiopathic in most cases.
2. Genetic abnormality is the cause in approximately 10 percent of cases.

Pathophysiology

1. Neurons in neocortex and hippocampus develop excessive numbers of senile plaques (abnormal proteins) and neurofibrillary tangles.
   a. A neuritic plaque is a cluster of degenerative nerve terminals that contain amyloid protein.
   b. Neurofibrillary tangles are abnormal neurons within which the cytoplasm is filled with bundles of abnormal protein.
   c. Elderly people without dementia have some plaques and tangles in their brains.
   d. People with Alzheimer's disease have a much higher number of plaques and tangles.
2. Gross atrophy of brain occurs as neurons degenerate and die.
3. Loss of neurons occurs primarily in the neocortex and hippocampus, which are essential structures for normal cognition.
4. Neuronal loss also occurs in the nucleus basalis of Meynert.
   a. These neurons provide the principal cholinergic innervation of the hippocampus and neocortex.
   b. Loss of cholinergic innervation is only 1 of many biochemical changes that occur in Alzheimer's disease.

Clinical Manifestations

1. Progressive impairment of memory and other cognitive skills.
2. Three stages of illness
   a. Stage I (duration of disease 1–3 yr)
      (1) Mild memory impairment
      (2) Some naming errors
      (3) Indifference, occasional irritability
   b. Stage II (duration of disease 2–10 yr)
      (1) Moderate memory impairment
      (2) Spatial disorientation
      (3) Fluent aphasia
      (4) Ideomotor apraxia (difficulty dressing and difficulty using utensils of daily living, such as combs, toothbrushes, or electrical appliances)
      (5) Indifference or irritability
      (6) Delusions in some
      (7) Restlessness, pacing – Agitation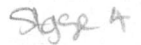
   c. Stage III (duration of disease 8–12 yr)
      (1) Severely impaired cognitive function
      (2) Limb rigidity, flexion posture
      (3) Urinary and fecal incontinence

      Stage 4.

Diagnostics

1. History: Look for a history of gradual memory impairment.
2. Physical examination: Usually normal in initial stages
3. Symptoms should include 2 or more cognitive deficits, of which impaired memory is usually the 1st to appear.
4. Medical diagnosis
   a. Physician arrives at diagnosis by excluding other causes of dementia, which include the following:
      (1) Multiple cerebral infarction
      (2) Central nervous system infection, such as encephalitis, slow virus disease, or HIV infection
      (3) Toxic and metabolic encephalopathies, such as systemic illness, endocrinopathy, deficiency states, drug intoxication, or heavy metal exposure
      (4) Chronic alcoholism
      (5) Neurodegenerative diseases, such as Parkinson's disease, multiple sclerosis, progressive supranuclear palsy, or spinocerebellar degeneration
      (6) Miscellaneous dementia syndromes, such as postanoxic, post-traumatic, neoplastic, depression, or normal pressure hydrocephalus
   b. A CT scan or MRI view can detect brain atrophy.
   c. Neuropsychologic testing can assess the degree and nature of cognitive deficits.
   d. Diagnosis can only be confirmed by postmortem examination of brain tissue.

Clinical Management

1. Goals of clinical management
   a. Help person and family members manage memory deficits and behavioral changes.

LEARNING/TEACHING GUIDELINES
for Teaching Family Members to Care for Patients with Alzheimer's Disease

General Overview

1. Although most late-stage Alzheimer's patients require the care of a nursing home or hospital, patients in earlier stages of the disease generally benefit from a noninstitutional setting.
2. However, those who will care for the patient need practical guidelines to ensure the patient's safety.
3. At the same time, both nursing staff and home care providers should try to identify and reinforce retained skills and to provide here-and-now pleasures for the patient, rather than focusing only on problem behaviors or potentialities.

Coping with Specific Behaviors

1. Wandering
   a. Provide supervision.
   b. Close and secure doors.
   c. Use identification bracelets.
   d. Use electronic surveillance.
2. Feeling lost, searching for something, desire to "go home"
   a. Furnish environment with familiar possessions and family mementos.
   b. Acknowledge the person's feelings.
   c. Reassure the person.
   d. Try distraction.
3. Need to exercise
   a. Provide a secure area for walking.
   b. Make the walking area interesting.
   c. Provide an escort.
   d. Offer active tasks such as sweeping, dusting, errands.
4. Agitation
   a. Intervene early.
   b. Determine the physical and psychosocial precipitants of agitation.
   c. Reassure the person.
   d. Approach the person slowly and calmly, from the front, then speak, gesture, and move slowly.
   e. Remove the person to a less stressful setting.
   f. Remove items that could be hazardous if the person becomes agitated.
   g. Distract the person with questions about the problem and gradually turn attention to something else.
   h. Use touch judiciously and gently.
5. Overreaction to minor stress ("catastrophic reaction")
   a. Recognize early warning signs.
      (1) Flushing
      (2) Restlessness
      (3) Refusal
      (4) Anger
   b. Recognize that behavior is not willful.
   c. Remove precipitating factor.
   d. Avoid arguing or restraining.
   e. Be calm and reassuring.

---

   b. Provide support and resources as needed.
2. Nonpharmacologic interventions
   a. Behavior management

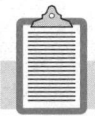

NURSING MANAGEMENT

Remind staff and family members that the agitated behavior of patients with Alzheimer's disease is not willful. Instruct personnel to avoid injury to the patient and to themselves when interacting with the agitated patient.

   b. Caregiver support
      (1) Spouses usually provide care of the demented adult.
      (2) If the spouse is unable to provide care, responsibility for care usually goes to daughters and daughters-in-law.
      (3) Female family members are more likely than male family members to give up or reduce paid employment to provide care.
      (4) The burden of providing care is very stressful, both physically and emotionally.
      (5) Perceived social support strongly influences caregiver well-being.
      (6) For caregiver support, provide verbal and written information about the disease, the diagnostic test results (including neuropsychologic testing), the legal and financial resources, and the social support resources such as Alzheimer's support groups. Establish regular meetings with clinicians and family members to discuss the demands of caregiving and strategies to reduce stress (see Learning/Teaching Guidelines for Teaching Family Members to Care for Patients with Alzheimer's Disease).
3. Pharmacologic interventions
   a. Guidelines for pharmacotherapy in dementia
      (1) Keep use of medications to a minimum.
      (2) Seek nonpharmacologic alternatives.
      (3) Take a careful medication history, including over-the-counter drugs.
      (4) Carefully monitor response to therapy.
      (5) Begin with dosages at one third to one half of normal adult doses.

(6) Increase dosages in small increments.

(7) Avoid multiple drug regimens whenever possible.

(8) Be aware of potential additive drug toxicity.

(9) Monitor side effects regularly.

b. Memory-enhancing drugs

(1) Studies of the effects of acetylcholine precursors (choline and lecithin) and nonspecific anticholinesterase inhibitors (e.g., physostigmine) have shown poor results.

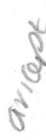

(2) Tacrine (Cognex), approved in 1993, may delay deterioration in cognition. Tacrine works by specifically inhibiting the action of acetylcholinesterase in the brain, which allows more acetylcholine to be available for nerve impulse transmission. Most frequent side effects are elevation of liver enzyme serum glutamic-pyruvic transaminase and nausea and vomiting. Tacrine also can cause cholinergic side effects such as bradycardia, peptic ulcer disease, and diarrhea and can prolong the effects of succinylcholine used in anesthesia.

DRUG ADVISORY

Initiation of tacrine requires biweekly liver function tests for 18 weeks and for 6 weeks after each dose increase.

c. Drugs to manage hallucinations, delusions, combativeness, aggression, and agitation

(1) The neuroleptic drugs haloperidol and thioridazine are used most commonly.

(2) Side effects of neuroleptics include sedation, orthostatic hypotension, anticholinergic side effects, and tardive dyskinesia.

(3) Nonneuroleptic drugs include benzodiazepines, propranolol, trazodone, fluoxetine, buspirone, and carbamazepine.

(4) Dosages should be small initially and increased slowly if needed.

(5) Persons taking these drugs should be weaned off them occasionally to determine whether they are still needed.

(6) Concerns about the misuse of these drugs in nursing home patients led to strict guidelines for their use in the Nursing Home Reform Provisions of the Omnibus Budget Reconciliation Act of 1987.

ELDER ADVISORY

Older people usually require lower doses of medication owing to age-related changes in their ability to absorb, metabolize, and eliminate drugs (see Chapter 16).

d. Drugs to manage depression

(1) Tricyclic antidepressants: nortriptyline (Pamelor), desipramine (Norpramin), and doxepin (Sinequan)

(2) Serotonin reuptake inhibitors: fluoxetine (Prozac), sertraline (Zoloft), and paroxetine (Paxil)

(3) Trazodone (Desyrel)

(4) Monoamine oxidase inhibitors

(5) Lithium

e. Drugs to manage insomnia

(1) Thioridazine (Mellaril)

(2) Temazepam (Restoril)

(3) Lorazepam (Ativan)

(4) Zolpidem (Ambien)

(5) Sedating antidepressants

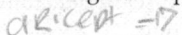

Complications

1. General physical debilitation in later stages
2. Injuries stemming from poor judgment

Prognosis

1. Steady decline in mental and physical function may occur over several years.
2. The person usually needs nursing home placement in the final stage of illness.

Applying the Nursing Process

NURSING DIAGNOSIS: Altered thought processes R/T neuronal degeneration

1. *Expected outcomes:* Following intervention, the person should demonstrate optimal thought processes for the disease stage.
2. *Nursing interventions*

a. Reorient person regularly.

b. Place a calendar and a clock in visible places.

c. Allow person to reminisce.

d. Repeat information as needed.

e. Simplify tasks.

f. Make environment easier to understand.

g. Give positive reinforcement for desired behaviors.

h. Allow plenty of time to complete a task.

i. Maintain familiar routines.

NURSING DIAGNOSIS: Risk for injury R/T impaired judgment and forgetfulness

1. *Expected outcomes:* Following intervention, the person should be free from injury.
2. *Nursing interventions*

a. Develop a monitoring system for the person's whereabouts.

b. Place an identification bracelet on the person.

c. Keep dangerous objects out of reach.

d. Educate family members regarding measures to make the home environment safe.

(1) Remove throw rugs, toxic substances, and dangerous electrical appliances.

(2) Reduce hot water heater temperature.

(3) Maintain adequate lighting.
(4) Secure doors and windows.

NURSING DIAGNOSIS: Impaired verbal communication R/T neuronal degeneration

1. *Expected outcomes:* Following intervention, the person should be able to communicate as much as possible, given the disease stage.
2. *Nursing interventions*
   a. Adapt to the communication level of the person.
   b. Speak slowly and clearly.
   c. Use simple words and short sentences.
   d. Use firm volume with low pitch.
   e. Use a calm, reassuring voice.
   f. Use pantomime gestures if the person is unable to understand spoken words.

NURSING DIAGNOSIS: Self-care deficit R/T neuronal degeneration

1. *Expected outcomes:* Following intervention, the person should be able to provide as much self-care as possible.
2. *Nursing interventions*
   a. Encourage the person to do as much as possible.
   b. Carefully balance helping the person with maintaining his or her autonomy.
   c. Allow plenty of time to complete a task.
   d. Use constant encouragement, urging and reminding in a step-by-step approach.

NURSING DIAGNOSIS: Ineffecive family coping R/T frustration and stress of caregiving

1. *Expected outcomes:* Following counseling family members should report increasing ability to cope.
2. *Nursing interventions*
   a. Encourage family members to express feelings about caregiving.
   b. Provide information about support services.

Discharge Planning and Teaching

1. Provide support for caregivers.
2. Provide community resources (e.g., adult daycare, local support groups).

■ CARING FOR PEOPLE WITH MULTIPLE SCLEROSIS

Definition and Incidence

1. Multiple sclerosis (MS) is a progressive degenerative disease that affects the myelin sheath of neurons in the CNS.
2. Incidence
   a. Prevalence in the United States has a wide range.

(1) 8.8 per 100,000 to 10.5 per 100,000 in Hawaii
(2) 69 per 100,000 in the Seattle-Tacoma area of Washington state
(3) 173 per 100,000 in Rochester, Minnesota
(4) Approximately 250,000 to 300,000 cases in United States as a whole
   b. Accurate data are difficult to obtain.
   (1) Time interval from clinical onset to diagnosis is months to years.
   (2) Medical expertise varies.
   c. Multiple sclerosis is generally more prevalent in temperate than in tropical climates within a geographic region.
   d. Variations from this pattern may be related to genetic and environmental factors.
   e. The onset of MS occurs most often between ages 20 and 40 years.

Risk Factors and Etiology

1. The epidemiology of MS cannot be explained by any single known environmental or genetic factor in isolation.
2. The etiology is unknown, although theories relate to immunogenetic viral disease.
3. Genetics
   a. In 15 percent of cases, MS is familial.
   b. The presence of certain genetic markers increases the risk of developing MS.
4. Viral infection acquired in childhood may contribute to the onset of MS in adulthood, but no specific virus has been identified yet.
5. Faulty immune response
   a. Altered humoral and cell-mediated immunity to viral agents may cause the onset of symptoms and exacerbations.
   b. An autoimmune reaction leads to the destruction of myelin.
6. Precipitating factors of an MS exacerbation
   a. Infection
   b. Stress (possibly)
   c. Pregnancy (postpartum period)
   d. Fatigue
   e. Heat
   f. Heavy metal exposure

Pathophysiology

1. Plaques form along the myelin sheath of nerves within the CNS, causing primary demyelination with preservation of axons.
2. Inflammation, edema, and death of oligodendrocytes (myelin-producing cells) occur.
3. Remission of symptoms is associated with reformation of myelin along nerves.
4. Progressive decline in nervous system function is associated with scarring and destruction of the axons.
5. Two major courses of MS
   a. Relapsing and remitting
   b. Chronic and progressive

Clinical Manifestations

1. Weakness: Most commonly weakness of both lower limbs, although weakness in one lower limb or weakness in one side of the body are also common.
2. Sensory changes
   a. Tingling sensations in one or more limbs
   b. Decreased sensitivity to sensory stimuli on the affected limb
2. Vision deficit
   a. Optic neuritis (inflammation and demyelination of the optic nerve) causing the following:
      (1) Blurred vision
      (2) Decreased visual acuity
      (3) Altered color vision
   b. Internuclear ophthalmoplegia (paresis of intraocular muscles), causing diplopia with lateral gaze
3. Dyscoordination and tremor in face and extremities
4. Bowel and bladder dysfunction
   a. Neurogenic bladder
      (1) Early complaints include hesitancy, urgency, frequency, loss of sensation, incontinence, retention
      (2) End-stage bladder function is usually hyperreflexic with sphincter dyssynergia.
   b. Bowel incontinence
5. Pain
   a. Lhermitte's sign—electric shock feeling passing down the back and legs, precipitated by neck flexion
   b. Dysesthesias—painful sensations on the skin that may be precipitated by mild sensory stimulation
   c. Tic douloureux—paroxysmal, excruciating pain along one or more divisions of the trigeminal nerve (see p. 729)
6. Seizures (in about 20% of people with MS)

Diagnostics

1. History
   a. Obtain detailed history of symptoms.
   b. Obtain past medical history.
   c. Inquire about family history of MS.
2. Physical examination should include detailed neurologic assessment.
3. Diagnostic studies
   a. Brain or spine MRI, or both, to check for MS plaques (see Fig. 18–21)—the most sensitive and specific test for MS
   b. Spinal fluid analysis to check for oligoclonal banding
   c. Brain stem–evoked potentials to check for increased latencies of nerve conduction in optic nerve or auditory pathways
4. Medical diagnosis also requires at least 2 episodes of CNS dysfunction separated by time and location in the CNS.

Clinical Management

1. Goals of clinical management
   a. Manage symptoms.
   b. Prevent complications.
   c. Optimize function.
2. Nonpharmacologic interventions
   a. Physical therapy provides help for ambulation needs and transferring from sitting to standing.
   b. Occupational therapy provides help with personal hygiene, dressing, and feeding.
   c. Speech therapy provides help with dysarthria and impaired swallowing.
3. Pharmacologic interventions
   a. Antispasticity drugs
      (1) Baclofen (Lioresal) inhibits presynaptic and postsynaptic spinal reflexes. It may be ineffective in spasticity of supraspinal origin and may aggravate weakness.
      (2) Dantrolene (Dantrium) inhibits skeletal muscle contraction directly by blocking release of calcium from the sarcoplasmic reticulum. Dantrolene may cause weakness and may lead to hepatic toxicity in women and people older than 35.
      (3) Diazepam (Valium) modulates spasticity through spinal mechanisms. It causes side effects that can worsen the preexisting problems such as fatigue, cognitive impairment, and depression.
   b. Amantadine (Symmetrel) may be used to decrease fatigue.
   c. Pain medications
      (1) Carbamazepine (Tegretol) is useful for tic douloureux, as well as for painful dysesthesias. Carbamazepine blocks entry of sodium into nerve cells, decreasing their firing.
      (2) Tricyclic antidepressants such as amitriptyline (Elavil) have an analgesic effect independent of their antidepressant effect.
   d. Drugs to treat neurogenic bladder
      (1) Propantheline (Pro-Banthīne) is used for detrusor spasms.
      (2) Oxybutynin (Ditropan) has anticholinergic effects as well as smooth muscle relaxant effects on the detrusor muscle.
      (3) Bethanechol (Urecholine) has cholinergic effects to relieve urinary retention.
   e. Drugs to treat exacerbations
      (1) Corticosteroids such as prednisone, methylprednisolone, and adrenocorticotropic hormone have both anti-inflammatory and immunosuppressive properties. Studies of their efficacy in treating acute relapses have not shown great benefit. This therapy is usually offered, despite its marginal efficacy, to give the person a sense that the provider is offering a treatment. Corticosteroids theoretically bring about a faster recovery from a relapse but do not alter the ultimate outcome of the relapse.
      (2) Interferon-β (Betaseron) is a genetically engineered complex protein with both antiviral and immunoregulatory properties. Studies show that it may lessen the number of MS exacerbations. Currently approved for use in people with relapsing and remitting MS who are ambulatory, it is under study in people with chronic and progressive MS.

The drug is self-administered by subcutaneous injection every other day.

Complications

1. Spasticity can cause the following:
   a. Reduced energy
   b. Inhibition of motor control
   c. Interference with self-care
   d. Alteration of sexual activity
   e. Disruption of vocational responsibilities
   f. Inability to pursue recreational activities
   g. Contractures
2. Pressure ulcers
3. Respiratory compromise due to weakness
4. Infection: Lung and bladder are the most common sites.

Prognosis

1. There is no cure for MS.
2. The prognosis depends on the nature of MS.
   a. The exacerbating and remitting type may have a mild course.
   b. The chronic and progressive type will show steady decline and ultimate death due to infections, respiratory complications, or severe debilitation.

Applying the Nursing Process

NURSING DIAGNOSIS: Feeding self-care deficit R/T impaired physical mobility

1. *Expected outcomes:* Following intervention, the person should be able to self-feed effectively to the extent possible.
2. *Nursing interventions*
   a. Provide adaptive aids and assistive devices as needed.
   b. Assist with meals as needed.
   c. For impaired swallowing, do the following:
      (1) Position person bolt upright (head of bed at 90 degrees).
      (2) Keep chin flexed while swallowing.
      (3) Keep bites of food small.
      (4) Do not talk while eating.
      (5) Ensure food forms a good bolus.
      (6) Avoid thin liquids.

NURSING DIAGNOSIS: Bathing and dressing self-care deficit R/T physical immobility

1. *Expected outcomes:* Following intervention, the person should be able to provide self-care regarding bathing and dressing to the extent possible.
2. *Nursing interventions*
   a. Provide privacy and warmth for bathing, grooming, and dressing. (Avoid hot bath water as this may worsen weakness.)
   b. Provide adaptive equipment as needed.
      (1) Consult occupational therapy.
      (2) Teach family members as needed.
   c. Encourage independence.
   d. Assist as needed.

NURSING DIAGNOSIS: Impaired physical mobility R/T weakness and increased muscle tone (spasticity)

1. *Expected outcomes:* Following intervention, the person should be
   a. Free from pain
   b. Free from contractures
   c. Able to use adaptive strategies and devices effectively
2. *Nursing interventions*
   a. Position limbs opposite flexion posture.
   b. Maintain head in midline position.
   c. Utilize spasticity to promote leg strength for transferring from sitting to standing.
   d. Encourage proper use of adaptive strategies and devices.
   e. Prevent complications that increase spasticity.
      (1) Urinary tract infection
      (2) Pressure ulcers
      (3) Constipation
      (4) Deep venous thrombosis

NURSING DIAGNOSIS: Activity intolerance R/T fatigue

1. *Expected outcomes:* Following intervention, the person should be able to do the following:
   a. Schedule activities realistically
   b. Achieve optimal strength and endurance
2. *Nursing interventions*
   a. Teach person to space activities over time to avoid fatigue.
   b. Explain the need to keep environment at moderate temperature.
   c. Describe techniques to avoid infection.

NURSING DIAGNOSIS: Altered urinary elimination R/T neurogenic bladder

1. *Expected outcomes:* Following intervention, the person should be able to do the following:
   a. Manage incontinence with effective procedures
   b. Prevent overdistention of the bladder
   c. Establish a voiding schedule
   d. Express satisfaction with urinary elimination status
2. *Nursing interventions*
   a. Encourage fluid intake of 2000 ml per day.
   b. Establish regular voiding schedule.

c. If ureteral and bladder pressures are below normal, select trigger mechanisms to assist voiding.
   (1) Suprapubic tapping
   (2) Tugging on pubic hair
   (3) Stroking inner thigh
d. Utilize intermittent catheterization if voiding attempts fail.
   (1) Catheterize every 6 hours.
   (2) Catheterize every 4 hours if urine volumes exceed 500 ml.
e. Insert indwelling catheter if necessary.

NURSING DIAGNOSIS: Visual or perceptual alterations R/T optic neuritis

1. *Expected outcomes:* Following intervention, the person should be able to do the following:
   a. Be free of injury
   b. Utilize adaptive strategies
   c. Make necessary lifestyle changes
2. *Nursing interventions*
   a. Assess environment for hazards.
   b. Remove potentially harmful objects.
   c. Promote measures and use of assistive devices to strengthen person's visual ability.
   d. Structure environment and daily routine to maximize self-care ability.
   e. Provide adequate lighting.
   f. Assist person and family members to identify lifestyle changes and develop adaptive strategies.
   g. Consult rehabilitation and community resources.

NURSING DIAGNOSIS: Self-esteem disturbance R/T altered body image

1. *Expected outcomes:* Following intervention, the person should report improved self-esteem.
2. *Nursing interventions*
   a. Assist person to adjust to physical limitations.
   b. Refer to local support groups.
   c. Encourage participation in recreational activities for disabled people.

Additional Nursing Diagnosis

• Constipation R/T immobility and demyelination

Discharge Planning and Teaching

1. Discuss unpredictable course of the disease.
2. Educate about precipitating factors.
3. Ensure that adaptive aids are available at discharge and that person and family members can manage at home.

■ CARING FOR PEOPLE WITH PARKINSON'S DISEASE

Definition and Incidence

1. Parkinson's disease is an idiopathic syndrome involving disability from tremor, rigidity, and bradykinesia.
2. Incidence and prevalence in the United States
   a. Incidence—20 per 100,000
   b. Prevalence—150 per 100,000
   c. More men are affected than women in a ratio of 3:2.

Risk Factors and Etiology

1. Parkinson's disease appears to be genetic in a small portion of cases.
2. The etiology is unknown for the idiopathic form.
3. Symptomatic causes of parkinsonism
   a. Encephalitis epidemic of 1919
   b. Atherosclerosis causing ischemia of basal ganglia
   c. Phenothiazine drugs
   d. Toxins (carbon monoxide, mercury, manganese)
   e. Trauma to midbrain

Pathophysiology

1. Dopamine-producing neurons in substantia nigra of midbrain degenerate.
2. Because neurons in the substantia nigra provide input to the basal ganglia, loss of this input in turn leads to a depletion of dopamine in the basal ganglia and a relative excess of acetylcholine.
3. Deterioration of the basal ganglia leads to declining ability to do the following:
   a. Initiate movement
   b. Control posture
   c. Maintain muscle tone
   d. Engage in automatic movements (e.g., swinging of arms while walking, eye blinking)
5. Symptoms do not appear until 70 to 80 percent of substantia nigra neurons are lost.

Clinical Manifestations

See Figure 18–28 for a summary of clinical manifestations.

Diagnostics

1. History
   a. Determine pattern of symptom onset.
   b. Assess family history.
   c. Check past medical history, including exposure to toxins and medication history.
2. No diagnostic studies are used for Parkinson's disease. Medical diagnosis is based solely on clinical signs and symptoms.

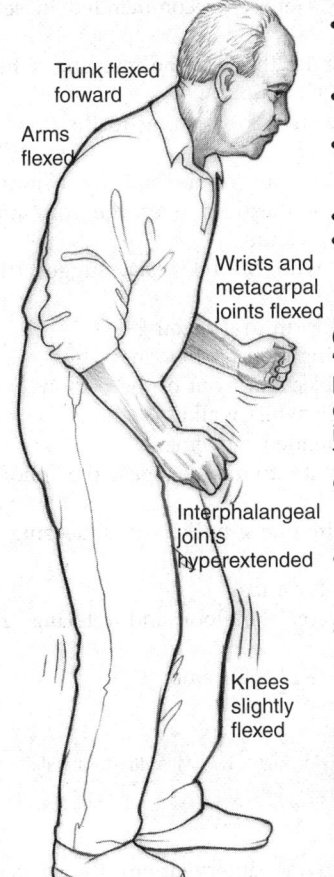

CLINICAL MANIFESTATIONS OF PARKINSON'S DISEASE

Dementia similar to Alzheimer's disease occurs in 15-20% of cases.

Trunk flexed forward

Arms flexed

Wrists and metacarpal joints flexed

Interphalangeal joints hyperextended

Knees slightly flexed

Bradykinesia:
- Slowness of movement
- Masklike face, devoid of expression.
- Drooling may occur due to lack of automatic swallowing.
- Soft voice, with low volume.
- Slow and shuffling gait, with small steps (festination).
- Stooped posture.
- Handwriting becomes small (micrographia).

Tremor:
Coarse, 3-4 per second "pill-rolling" tremor in the hands and arms at rest, disappears with intentional movements. Tremor may affect only one arm, initially.

Rigidity:
- Increased muscle tone (resistance to passive motion).
- Limb has a "cogwheel" or ratchet-like response to passive movement.

Autonomic dysfunction:
- Excessive perspiration
- Seborrhea
- Constipation
- Urinary hesitancy or retention
- Heat intolerance

Figure 18–28.

3. Medical diagnosis can be confirmed by response to medication.

Clinical Management

1. Goals of clinical management
   a. Manage symptoms
   b. Prevent complications
   c. Optimize function
2. Pharmacologic interventions
   a. Selegiline (Eldepryl)
      (1) Used as preventive therapy and as adjunctive therapy
      (2) May slow progression of the disease by reducing oxidative stress caused by dopamine degradation and increasing free radical elimination

(3) Selegiline potentiates levodopa effects in several ways:
   - Irreversibly inhibits monoamine oxidase B, which is the primary metabolizer of dopamine
   - Increases dopamine content in the CNS
   - Inhibits uptake of dopamine and noradrenaline into presynaptic nerve terminals
   - Increases turnover of dopamine
   b. Levodopa or carbidopa (Sinemet)
      (1) Levodopa is the first choice for treatment of Parkinson's disease.
      (2) Mechanism of action: Levodopa is a synthetic metabolic precursor of dopamine, which it provides to the brain.
      (3) It is combined with carbidopa, which prevents peripheral metabolism of levodopa.
      (4) It is indicated for treatment of rigidity and bradykinesia but is less effective for tremor.
      (5) Benefit declines with prolonged use, so drug is usually withheld until symptoms become disabling.

 DRUG ADVISORY

Absorption of levodopa is decreased by protein in the diet. To obtain maximal absorption, protein intake should be limited to the evening meal.

      (6) Side effects are dyskinesias, hallucinations and nightmares, orthostatic hypotension, and nausea and vomiting.
   c. Synthetic dopamine agonists
      (1) Bromocriptine (Parlodel)
      (2) Pergolide (Permax)
   d. Anticholinergics such as trihexyphenidyl (Artane), benztropine bitartrate (Cogentin), and procyclidine (Kemadrin)
      (1) Act by correcting the balance between dopamine and acetylcholine.
      (2) Help control tremor but are less useful for rigidity or bradykinesia.
   e. Amantadine (Symmetrel): an antiviral drug that resembles anticholinergic drugs. Its mechanism of action is unknown.
3. Special surgical procedures
   a. Thalamotomy
      (1) Thalamotomy may be indicated for rigidity and intractable tremor. It is more successful in younger patients.
      (2) This stereotactic surgical technique localizes and destroys specific groups of cells within the thalamus. Stereotactic surgery precisely localizes cells and tissues by using 3-dimensional coordinates that are identified by means of imagery (e.g., CT scan or MRI).
      (3) The ventrolateral nucleus of the thalamus is destroyed by freezing, electrical coagulation, radioactivity, or ultrasound.
   b. Globus pallidus pallidotomy

(1) This experimental stereotactic procedure may be performed for intractable tremor.

(2) The rationale for globus pallidus pallidotomy is that Parkinson's disease (and the accompanying rigidity and tremor) may be caused by overactivity of the globus pallidus. Thus, surgically reducing PSi activity should reduce tremor and improve the patient's motor function.

(3) In 1 study, 14 patients with Parkinson's disease were studied following globus pallidus pallidotomy. Six months following surgery, these patients demonstrated improved motor performance, improved gait, and reduced akinesia (loss of power of voluntary movement). Also, the patients no longer experienced levodopa-induced dyskinesias.

c. Fetal neural tissue transplant to basal ganglia (experimental)

Complications

1. Fluctuations in mobility
   a. Wearing-off effects—predictable episodes of bradykinesia that occur at the end of the drug-dosing interval.
   b. On-off symptoms—unpredictable symptoms that involve rapid fluctuation between dyskinesia ("on" symptoms) and rigidity or bradykinesia ("off" symptoms)
      (1) Transition between these 2 states may be within 1 to 2 minutes.
      (2) Initially, "off" symptoms occur at the end of a dosing interval. Later, the transition may happen at any time and be unrelated to the ingestion of medication.
   c. Psychiatric effects such as confusion, visual hallucinations, and paranoia often occur in combination with dementia related to the disease but may also be side effects of medication.
   d. Sleep disturbance has several features.
      (1) Increased muscle activity during sleep.
      (2) Altered circadian rhythms affecting sleep.
      (3) Disorganization of breathing in sleep, including obstructive and central sleep apnea.
      (4) Rapid eye movement and non–rapid eye movement variations of the nigrostriatal dopamine receptor sensitivity during sleep.

Prognosis

1. There is no cure for Parkinson's disease.
2. Parkinson's disease is slowly progressive.
3. The course varies, but decline usually occurs over several years.

Applying the Nursing Process

NURSING DIAGNOSIS: Impaired physical mobility R/T rigidity, bradykinesia, tremor

1. *Expected outcomes:* Following intervention, the person should exhibit improved physical mobility to the extent possible.
2. *Nursing interventions*
   a. To help the person avoid rigidity and development of contractures, do the following:
      (1) Encourage regular exercise and stretching.
      (2) Teach the person exercises recommended in self-help booklets.
      (3) Suggest exercising 1st thing in the morning, when energy level is high.
      (4) Suggest exercising in bed if getting to the floor is difficult.
      (5) Recommend getting out of a chair by bending over slowly so the head is over the toes and avoiding soft, deep chairs.
   b. To help the person with bradykinesia, suggest the following:
      (1) Rocking back and forth to get going
      (2) Thinking of stepping over an imaginary line
      (3) Throwing small objects in front of the person
      (4) Counting to oneself while walking
      (5) Visualizing the intended movement
   c. To help the person with tremor, suggest the following:
      (1) Holding change in one's pocket or squeezing a small rubber ball
      (2) Using both hands for a task
      (3) Lying face down on the floor and relaxing the entire body
      (4) Sleeping on the side of the tremor

NURSING DIAGNOSIS: Risk for injury R/T falls due to shuffling steps and bradykinesia

1. *Expected outcomes:* Following intervention, the person should be free from injury.
2. *Nursing interventions:* Offer the following suggestions:
   a. Wear good, sturdy shoes.
   b. Use a cane or a walker.
   c. Concentrate on standing upright.
   d. Consciously pick up the feet to take steps.
   e. Remove all throw rugs, electrical cords, and other clutter from the floor.
   f. Ensure adequate lighting.
   g. Arrange essential items within easy reach.
   h. Use a bath chair and a hand-held shower nozzle.
   i. Install grab bars in the bathroom.
   j. Install a raised toilet seat.

NURSING DIAGNOSIS: Impaired verbal communication R/T incoordination and reduced movement of muscles that control respiration, phonation, and prosody (rhythm and intonation)

1. *Expected outcomes:* Following intervention, the person should be able to communicate effectively.
2. *Nursing interventions:* Make the following suggestions:
   a. Pause between every few words.

b. Exaggerate pronunciation of words.
c. Finish saying the final consonant of a word before starting to say the next word.
d. Express ideas in short, concise phrases.
e. Plan what to say.
f. Face the listener.

NURSING DIAGNOSIS: Impaired swallowing R/T reduced movement of throat muscles

1. *Expected outcomes:* Following intervention, the person should be able to do the following:
   a. Maintain adequate oral intake
   b. Avoid aspiration
2. *Nursing interventions*
   a. Teach the person to do the following:
      (1) Think through the steps of swallowing:
         • Keep lips closed.
         • Keep teeth together.
         • Put food on the tongue.
         • Lift the tongue up and back.
         • Swallow.
      (2) Eat slowly with small bites.
      (3) Chew hard and move food around with the tongue.
      (4) Finish 1 bite before taking another.
   d. Suggest that the person do the following for problems with saliva buildup:
      (1) Make a conscious effort to swallow saliva often.
      (2) Keep the head in an upright position so that saliva will collect in the back of the throat and stimulate automatic swallowing.
      (3) Swallow excess saliva before attempting to speak.

Discharge Planning and Teaching

1. Instruct the person and family members about medications and dosing and side effects.
2. Teach adaptive strategies to enhance mobility, communication, and swallowing.
3. Ensure that adaptive aids are available at discharge.

■ CARING FOR PEOPLE WITH MYASTHENIA GRAVIS

Definition

1. Myasthenia gravis is an autoimmune disease.
2. It involves increasing weakness and fatigue with sustained muscle contraction and improves with rest.

Incidence in the United States

1. Incidence—0.4 per 100,000 persons
2. Prevalence—0.5 to 5.0 per 100,000 persons

3. Two peaks of onset
   a. Ages 20 to 30 years: more common in women than in men.
   b. Older than age 50 years: more common in men than in women.

Risk Factors and Etiology

1. No known risk factors
2. Factors that precipitate exacerbations
   a. Emotional stress
   b. Physical stress
   c. Concurrent illness
   d. Hormonal changes
      (1) Disturbance in thyroid function
      (2) Menstrual cycle
      (3) Pregnancy
   e. Drugs
      (1) Alcohol
      (2) Mycin antibiotics (e.g., streptomycin)
      (3) Procainamide
      (4) Quinidine
      (5) Morphine
      (6) Phenothiazines
      (7) Barbiturates
      (8) Tranquilizers
3. Etiology is probably an autoimmune disorder.

Pathophysiology

1. Thymic lymphocytes produce acetylcholine-receptor antibodies that attack the postsynaptic muscle membrane.
2. Loss of acetylcholine receptors on the postsynaptic muscle fiber occurs at the neuromuscular junction.
3. Fewer receptors are available to combine with acetylcholine to trigger a muscle action potential.
4. Eighty percent of people with myasthenia gravis have microscopic abnormality of the thymus gland; 10 percent have thymoma.

Clinical Manifestations

1. Increasing weakness with sustained muscle contraction
2. Ptosis of 1 or both eyes with sustained gaze due to weakness of the levator muscles of the upper eyelid
3. Diplopia due to weakness of the extraocular muscles
4. Dysphagia and nasal speech due to weakness of the muscles of chewing and swallowing
5. Facial muscle weakness, resulting in the following:
   a. Expressionless face
   b. Droopy eyelids
   c. Smoothed facial features
   d. Tendency for the mouth to hang open
6. Limb weakness
7. Fatigue

Diagnostics

1. History of onset of signs and symptoms
2. Physical examination revealing clinical manifestations
3. Diagnostic tests
   a. Edrophonium (Tensilon) test
      (1) Edrophonium (short-acting anticholinesterase drug) is given intravenously.
      (2) A small amount is given initially.
      (3) The remainder of the dose is given only if there is no untoward reaction such as increased weakness, change in cardiac rate or rhythm, nausea, or abdominal cramps.

DRUG ADVISORY

Be sure to have atropine sulfate available for intravenous injection to counteract severe cholinergic reactions to edrophonium chloride.

      (4) A positive response is transitory improvement in muscle strength.
   b. Acetylcholine receptor antibodies
      (1) Titer of acetylcholine receptor antibodies in blood is elevated in 80 percent of people with generalized myasthenia.
      (2) There is no correlation between acetylcholine receptor antibodies titer and clinical severity.
   c. Electromyography
      (1) Record electrical activity from an affected muscle after repetitive electrical stimulation.
      (2) In those with myasthenia gravis, the resulting muscle action potential shows a decrementing response.
   d. Chest CT (to rule out thymoma)

Clinical Management

1. Goals of clinical management
   a. Manage symptoms.
   b. Prevent complications.
   c. Optimize function.
2. Pharmacologic interventions
   a. Anticholinesterase drugs (e.g., pyridostigmine [Mestinon] and neostigmine [Prostigmin]) act by blocking acetylcholinesterase, an enzyme that breaks down acetylcholine at the neuromuscular junction.
      (1) Dosages are highly individualized, based on physiologic response to medication.
      (2) The goal is to achieve maximum muscle strength and endurance with minimal cholinergic side effects.
   b. Corticosteroids (e.g., prednisone) reduce levels of serum acetylcholine receptor antibodies.
      (1) Clinical improvement can occur even when no significant reduction in antibodies occurs.
      (2) Dosage may be decreased after improvement is achieved.
      (3) Antacids may be required to avoid peptic ulcer disease, a possible side effect of prednisone therapy.
   c. Cytotoxic agents include azathioprine (Imuran), cyclophosphamide (Cytoxan), and methotrexate.
      (1) Usually initiated when symptoms are unresponsive to steroids or thymectomy.
      (2) May reduce need for large doses of steroids.
3. Special medical-surgical procedures
   a. Thymectomy
      (1) The thymus gland is located in the superior mediastinum.
      (2) Although it is important during fetal development for development of the immune system, it is usually atrophied and nonfunctioning in the adult.
      (3) Removal of the thymus gland may reduce acetylcholine receptor antibody formation in people with myasthenia gravis.
      (4) Thymectomy is indicated in the following cases: people with thymoma, selected people without thymoma, and selected people with disabling ocular myasthenia gravis.
   b. Plasmapheresis: Discarding plasma separated from a person's blood; adding albumin, normal saline, and electrolytes to the packed red blood cells; and returning the blood to the person.
      (1) The purpose is to remove plasma proteins containing acetylcholine receptor antibodies.
      (2) It is used for people with pending respiratory failure.
      (3) Three to 5 treatments are usually required.

Complications

1. Myasthenic crisis
   a. Sudden worsening of the disease
   b. Occurs in people with moderate or severe bulbar or generalized myasthenia gravis.
   c. Involves severe muscle weakness, which can lead to respiratory paralysis.
   d. Requires immediate endotracheal intubation and respiratory support if injection of anticholinesterase drug is not helpful.
2. Cholinergic crisis
   a. Results from toxic effects of anticholinesterase drugs.
   b. Muscarinic effects include the following:
      (1) Abdominal cramps
      (2) Diarrhea
      (3) Excessive pulmonary secretions
   c. Nicotinic effects include the following:
      (1) Weakness or paralysis of voluntary muscles
      (2) Bronchiolar muscle spasm
      (3) Excessive pulmonary secretions
3. Respiratory distress
   a. Respiratory distress may occur in either myasthenic or cholinergic crisis.
   b. Treatment is the same for both.
      (1) Support with intubation and assisted ventilation until crisis has passed.
      (2) Withhold anticholinesterase drugs in cholinergic crises.

Prognosis

1. There is no cure for myasthenia gravis.
2. Prognosis is good in mild forms but poor in severe forms, with death occurring due to severe weakness and debilitation.
   a. Type 1—ocular myasthenia
      (1) No mortality
      (2) High rate of spontaneous remissions
   b. Type 2A—mild myasthenia
      (1) Low mortality
      (2) Remissions possible
   c. Type 2B—severe myasthenia
      (1) Restricts functional activity
      (2) Low mortality
      (3) Remissions possible
   d. Type 3—fulminating, acute, severe myasthenia
      (1) Rapid deterioration within 6 months
      (2) High mortality due to respiratory muscle weakness and general debilitation
      (3) Thymomas most frequent in this group
   e. Type 4—chronic, late, severe myasthenia
      (1) Severe symptoms develop within 2 years of onset.
      (2) High mortality is due to respiratory muscle weakness and general debilitation.

Applying the Nursing Process

NURSING DIAGNOSIS: Activity intolerance R/T fatigue with sustained muscle activity

1. *Expected outcomes:* Following intervention, the person should report achievement of optimal strength and endurance.
2. *Nursing interventions.* Teach the person to do the following:
   a. Plan rest periods.
   b. Do most essential motor activities early in the day.
   c. Rearrange home environment to help prevent unnecessary energy expenditure.

NURSING DIAGNOSIS: Impaired verbal communication R/T muscle weakness

1. *Expected outcomes:* Following intervention, the person should be able to communicate effectively.
2. *Nursing interventions.* Teach the person to do the following:
   a. Speak in short phrases to conserve energy.
   b. Use hand to support jaw while speaking.
   c. Exaggerate pronunciation of words.

Additional Nursing Diagnoses Commonly Associated with Myasthenia Gravis

• Impaired swallowing R/T facial and throat muscle weakness

• Ineffective airway clearance and impaired gas exchange R/T intercostal muscle weakness and impaired gag and cough reflexes

Discharge Planning and Teaching

1. Educate the person and family members about medications, side effects, and complications.
2. Refer to support services.

■ CARING FOR PEOPLE WITH AMYOTROPHIC LATERAL SCLEROSIS

Definition and Incidence

1. Amyotrophic lateral sclerosis leads to progressive weakness of skeletal muscles.
2. Also called Lou Gehrig's disease, it is the most common of the motor neuron diseases.
3. Incidence in the United States
   a. Incidence—0.4 to 1.8 per 100,000 persons
   b. Prevalence—4 to 6 per 100,000 persons

Risk Factors

1. Approximately 5 to 10 percent of cases are inherited as an autosomal dominant trait.
2. No risk factors are known for the idiopathic type.
3. A higher incidence is found in people with the following:
   a. Hyperparathyroid disorder (see Chapter 29)
   b. Hypothyroid disorder (see Chapter 29)
   c. Immune disorder (see Chapter 21)

Etiology

1. Unknown in idiopathic cases. Theories include the following:
   a. Premature aging of motor neurons accelerated by exogenous factors.
   b. Elevated levels of metals or electrolytes
      (1) Lead
      (2) Aluminum
      (3) Calcium
      (4) Manganese
   c. Viral and immune responses
      (1) Increased cell-mediated immunity to poliovirus antigen
      (2) Presence of circulating immune complexes
   d. Elevated norepinephrine levels
2. Genetic defect in autosomal dominant cases
   a. Defect is on chromosome 21.
   b. Defect is in the gene which encodes cytosolic superoxide dismutase.

c. Superoxide dismutase is responsible for deactivating toxic substances called free radicals in cells.

d. The discovery of this genetic defect may provide ideas for innovative therapies for both familial and idiopathic amyotrophic lateral sclerosis.

Pathophysiology

1. Degeneration and loss of motor neurons occurs in the following:
   a. Cerebral cortex motor neurons
   b. Corticospinal and corticobulbar pathways
   c. Anterior horn cells of the spinal cord
2. Central nervous system process
   a. Neurons replaced by fibrous astrocytes, resulting in gliosis.
   b. Remaining cells shrink and fill with intracytoplasmic lipofuscin.
3. Peripheral nervous system process
   a. Reduction of large myelinated fibers of ventral roots
   b. Acute axonal degeneration
   c. Distal axon atrophy
   d. Loss of or decreased size of endplate terminals
   e. Decrease in choline acetyltransferase and acetylcholinesterase
   f. Depletion of the following receptors in the spinal cord:
      (1) Muscarinic
      (2) Cholinergic
      (3) Glycinergic

Clinical Manifestations

1. Both upper motor neuron and lower motor neuron manifestations
2. Muscle weakness
3. Muscle atrophy
4. Cramps
5. Spasticity
6. Fasciculations
7. Hyperreflexia
8. Bulbar symptoms
   a. Dysarthria
   b. Dysphagia
9. Respiratory compromise due to intercostal muscle weakness
10. Functions that are spared include the following:
    a. Cognition
    b. Sensation
    c. Bowel and bladder function
    d. Autonomic function
    e. Extraocular movements
11. Onset has two major forms.
    a. Weakness in 1 or more limbs
    b. Bulbar symptoms

Diagnostics

1. History
   a. Determine nature and course of symptom onset.

b. Obtain family history.
2. Physical examination
   a. Check motor strength.
   b. Check speech and swallowing functions.
   c. Observe for fasciculations.
   d. Observe for atrophy.
3. Diagnostic tests
   a. Electromyography, the definitive study, produces findings such as the following:
      (1) Chronic motor unit potential changes in multiple nerve roots
      (2) Fibrillations
      (3) Fasciculations
      (4) Normal nerve conduction (sensory) responses
   b. Muscle biopsy shows atrophic fibers interspersed with normal fibers.

Clinical Management

1. Goals of clinical management
   a. Alleviate symptoms
   b. Provide supportive care
2. Nonpharmacologic interventions
   a. Physical therapy to maintain range of motion
   b. Adaptive aids to maximize function
      (1) Leg and hand braces
      (2) Special eating utensils
      (3) Dressing aids
      (4) Communication devices
      (5) Suction device
      (6) Feeding tube
      (7) Ventilator
3. Pharmacologic interventions
   a. Antispasmodic drugs
      (1) Diazepam (Valium)
      (2) Baclofen (Lioresal)
      (3) Dantrolene (Dantrium)
   b. Anticholinergic drugs for sialorrhea
   c. Quinine for cramps
4. Special medical-surgical procedures
   a. Tracheotomy for assisted ventilation, if requested (see Chapter 20)
   b. Percutaneous endoscopic gastrostomy for tube feedings

Complications

1. Hazards of immobility
2. Respiratory compromise resulting in aspiration or pneumonia or both

Prognosis

1. There is no cure for amyotrophic lateral sclerosis.
2. Death usually occurs within 2 to 5 years from respiratory complications.
3. Older age at onset is associated with shorter duration of the disease.
4. Early bulbar symptoms are associated with earlier death.

Applying the Nursing Process

NURSING DIAGNOSIS: Impaired physical mobility R/T either upper motor neuron or lower motor neuron features

1. *Expected outcomes:* Following intervention, the person should be free from the following:
   a. Contractures
   b. Pressure ulcers
   c. Pneumonia
   d. Deep venous thrombosis
2. *Nursing interventions*
   a. Position limbs according to type of weakness.
   b. Provide rest periods between activities.
   c. Refer to occupational therapy and physical therapy for adaptive devices.
   d. Add hand rails and other adjustments in the home for better mobility.
   e. Teach safety precautions.

NURSING DIAGNOSIS: Impaired verbal communication R/T progressive weakness of face and throat muscles

1. *Expected outcomes:* Following intervention, the person should be able to communicate effectively.
2. *Nursing interventions*
   a. Assist person and family members to develop meaningful ways to communicate if voice volume becomes too low.
   b. Suggest use of hand or eye signals or communication devices (consult speech therapist).
   c. See also page 725.

NURSING DIAGNOSIS: Impaired swallowing R/T progressive face and throat muscle weakness

1. *Expected outcomes:* Following intervention, the person should be able to do the following:
   a. Maintain adequate nutrition.
   b. Avoid aspiration.
2. *Nursing interventions*
   a. Encourage frequent, small, high-nutrient feedings.
   b. Allow adequate time to eat.
   c. Put small portions on back of tongue. Use a large syringe with short tubing to place liquid at back of tongue if needed.
   d. Keep suction device nearby.
   e. Anticipate need for Heimlich maneuver if the person chokes and suction is not helpful.
   f. Stabilize head in an upright position with a soft cervical collar.
   g. Provide straws or cup with spout for liquids.
   h. Place papase tablets under the tongue 10 minutes before a meal to thin saliva.
   i. Weigh person weekly.
   j. Anticipate need for nasogastric tube or gastrostomy feedings.
   k. See also page 725.

NURSING DIAGNOSIS: Anticipatory grieving R/T loss of motor function and ultimate death

1. *Expected outcomes:* Following counseling, the person and family members should be able to do the following:
   a. Verbalize expected losses.
   b. Name available support services.
2. *Nursing interventions*
   a. Encourage the person and family members to express losses they are expecting.
   b. Meet with the person and family members separately to allow free expression of concerns.
   c. Encourage family members to take time away from caregiving for themselves.
   d. Encourage the person to continue in a job or other activities for as long as possible.
   e. Refer to support groups in the area.

Additional Nursing Diagnosis Commonly Associated with Amyotrophic Lateral Sclerosis

- Ineffective airway clearance and impaired gas exchange R/T progressive weakness of face, throat, and chest muscles

Discharge Planning and Teaching

1. Discuss hospice care.
2. Encourage the person to develop an advance care directive regarding ventilator support, artificial feeding, and other therapies.

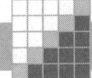 **LEGAL AND ETHICAL CONSIDERATIONS**

Discuss the patient's wishes regarding intubation and use of a ventilator *before* respiratory compromise occurs.

3. Teach use of home adaptive aids (e.g., suction device, dressing aids).
4. Ensure adaptive aids are available at discharge.
5. Refer the person and family members to support groups.

◼ CARING FOR PEOPLE WITH GUILLAIN-BARRÉ SYNDROME

Definition and Incidence

1. Named for the 2 physicians who wrote several papers about it in the early 1900s, Guillain-Barré syndrome is an

illness of generalized weakness and distal paresthesias progressing over several days.
2. Incidence is 0.72 to 2.0 per 100,000 persons.

Risk Factors and Etiology

1. A history of viral infection a few weeks before the onset of symptoms occurs in two thirds of cases.
2. Viral agents include the following:
   a. Epstein-Barr with hepatitis or mononucleosis
   b. *Campylobacter jejuni* enteritis
   c. Cytomegalovirus
   d. Human immunodeficiency virus
   e. *Salmonella typhosa*
   f. *Mycoplasma pneumoniae*
3. Other risk factors (in a small number of cases)
   a. Vaccinations
   b. General surgery
   c. Epidural anesthesia
   d. Drugs
      (1) Thrombolytic agents
      (2) Heroin
      (3) Immunosuppressive agents
   e. Concurrent disease
      (1) Lupus erythematosus
      (2) Hodgkin's disease
      (3) Sarcoidosis
      (4) Infection with HIV
   f. Pregnancy
4. Etiology is unknown, but may be an abnormal immunologic response to a prior infection or other immunologic stimulus.

Pathophysiology

1. Lymphocytic T cells initiate an inflammatory response to prior infection or other immunologic stimulus.
2. Lymphocytes and macrophages surround vessels within the nerve and cause demyelination. Nerve roots are affected most.
3. Circulating antineural antibodies are directed at a number of antigens.
4. Widespread axonal degeneration may occur without demyelination in some cases.
5. The Guillain-Barré syndrome may be the consequence of a variety of different pathologic processes that produce a similar clinical pattern of disease.

Clinical Manifestations

1. Onset involves paresthesias in toes or fingertips.
2. A few days later leg weakness occurs.
3. Weakness progresses to arms and face.
4. Paresthesias extend proximally.
5. Pain may occur in the back, flank, or thighs.
6. Deep tendon reflexes are diminished or absent.
7. In severe cases weakness may affect the following:
   a. Respiration

   b. Eye movements
   c. Swallowing
   d. Autonomic function
      (1) Orthostatic hypotension
      (2) Hypertension
      (3) Pupillary disturbances
      (4) Sweating dysfunction
      (5) Cardiac dysrhythmias
      (6) Paralytic ileus
      (7) Urinary retention

Diagnostics

1. History
   a. Obtain history of prior infection.
   b. Determine pattern of symptom onset.
2. Physical examination: Regularly evaluate neurologic function and vital signs (every 2–4 hr).
   a. To determine if muscle weakness is ascending, evaluate strength in all 4 limbs and in face (including cough, gag, and swallowing).
   b. Assess respiratory function.
      (1) Check vital signs.

NURSE ADVISORY

When Guillian-Barré syndrome is suspected, assess respiratory function regularly and inform the physician *immediately* if respirations become compromised.

      (2) Check breath sounds. Obtain pulmonary function test results (maximal inspiratory force and expiratory vital capacity).
3. Diagnostic studies
   a. Evaluate CSF for the following:
      (1) Elevated protein
      (2) Absence of white blood cells
   b. Review electromyogram for the following:
      (1) Conduction block (muscle action potentials are reduced after stimulation of the distal as opposed to the proximal nerve)
      (2) Temporal dispersion of compound action potentials
      (3) Slowed nerve conduction velocities

Clinical Management

1. Goals of clinical management
   a. Provide supportive care during acute phase.
   b. Prevent complications.
2. Nonpharmacologic interventions
   a. Physical therapy to maintain range of motion
   b. Adaptive aids to maximize function
      (1) Leg and hand braces
      (2) Special eating utensils
      (3) Dressing aids
      (4) Communication devices

(5) Suction device
(6) Feeding tube
(7) Ventilator
3. Pharmacologic interventions
   a. Steroids are no longer considered useful.
   b. Pooled gamma globulin (IgG)
      (1) Administer intravenously.
      (2) Give daily for the first 2 weeks of the disease.
      (3) This therapy may be as beneficial as plasmapheresis and is easier to administer (see later discussion).
4. Special medical-surgical procedures
   a. Plasmapheresis (see p. 724)
      (1) A total of 200 to 250 ml of plasma per kg is removed in 4 to 6 treatments.
      (2) Treatments occur every other day for a total of 10 to 15 days.
      (3) The purpose is to remove antibodies responsible for the syndrome.

Complications

1. Irreversible demyelination leading to permanent neurologic deficit
2. Complications of immobility
3. Respiratory compromise, resulting in pneumonia, aspiration, or both

Prognosis

1. The prognosis varies widely, depending considerably on the availability of skilled nursing care.
2. Eighty-five to 90 percent of patients recover completely.
3. Certain factors are related to poor prognosis.
   a. Very low distal motor amplitude on electromyogram results
   b. Older age
   c. Ventilatory failure requiring mechanical ventilation
   d. Rapidly progressive disease over 1 week or less.

Applying the Nursing Process

NURSING DIAGNOSIS: Impaired physical mobility R/T progressive weakness and paralysis

1. *Expected outcomes:* Following intervention, the person should remain free from complications of immobility.
2. *Nursing interventions*
   a. Assess motor function frequently.
      (1) Test limb strength.
      (2) Evaluate cranial nerve function (see pp. 661–663)
   b. Monitor blood pressure and pulse frequently.
   c. Observe for urinary retention.
   d. Assess respiratory function diligently (see Chapter 22).

NURSING DIAGNOSIS: Fear R/T loss of function and uncertainty about disease outcome

1. *Expected outcomes:* Following counseling, the person should do the following:
   a. Express concerns about the illness.
   b. Demonstrate an understanding of the disease progression and treatments.
2. *Nursing interventions*
   a. Encourage the person to express concerns.
   b. Keep the person informed of health status and treatment plan.
   c. Have a person who has had Guillain-Barré syndrome talk to the person.
   d. Provide realistic encouragement.
   e. Provide diversional activities.

Additional Nursing Diagnoses Commonly Associated with Guillain-Barré Syndrome

- Self-care deficit R/T progressive weakness and paralysis
- Impaired swallowing R/T face and throat muscle weakness (see p. 727)
- Ineffective airway clearance and impaired gas exchange R/T progressive muscle weakness (see p. 725)

Discharge Planning and Teaching

1. Educate person and family members about the disease.
2. Refer them to the Guillain-Barré Foundation for literature and support.
3. Consult a social worker if financial or vocational aspects are a concern.

■ CARING FOR PEOPLE WITH CRANIAL NERVE DISORDERS

Trigeminal Neuralgia (Tic Douloureux)

1. Definition: A syndrome of chronic, intermittent pain, involving one or more divisions of the trigeminal nerve (CN V).
2. Incidence in the United States
   a. Prevalence—1 per 25,000 persons
   b. Incidence—4.3 per 100,000 persons
   c. Peak incidence is between ages 50 and 70 years for the idiopathic form, and between ages 30 and 35 for the symptomatic form.
   d. Women are more often affected than men by a ratio of 3:2.
3. Risk factors
   a. Family history—trigeminal neuralgia is familial in 0.6 to 5.3 percent of cases.
   b. Multiple sclerosis

(1) One percent of people with MS develop trigeminal neuralgia.

(2) People with MS are more likely to have bilateral pain than people without MS.

c. See also etiologic factors listed below.

4. Etiology

  a. Intrinsic lesions of the trigeminal nerve

    (1) Demyelination, as seen in MS

    (2) Proliferated, hypertrophic, or tortuous masses of myelin.

    (3) Herpesvirus infection

  b. Extrinsic lesions impinging on the trigeminal nerve

    (1) Tumors (e.g., meningioma of middle or posterior fossa, vestibular schwannoma [acoustic neuroma], and peripheral nerve tumors involving the trigeminal nerve, including epidermoid tumors, meningioma, and neurofibroma)

    (2) Vascular irregularities, such as arteriovenous malformation, aneurysm, ectatic vertebrobasilar system, or the presence of normal arteries adjacent to the trigeminal nerve (e.g., superior cerebellar artery, posterior inferior cerebellar artery, or anterior inferior cerebellar artery)

    (3) Dental causes, such as diffuse pulpal calcification, dental abscesses, or bone resorption leading to irritation of the trigeminal nerve in the maxilla or mandible

5. Pathophysiology

  a. The current theory is that trigeminal neuralgia is due to chronic irritation of the trigeminal nerve.

  b. Uninhibited ectopic action potentials of the nerve produce paroxysms of pain.

6. Clinical manifestations

  a. Abrupt onset of extreme pain in 1 or more divisions of the trigeminal nerve.

  b. Pain is usually unilateral.

  c. Pain usually involves the mandibular or maxillary division of the nerve (in the lips, gums, cheek, side of nose).

  d. Pain is described as sharp, stabbing, knifelike, or burning.

  e. Pain is accompanied by twitching, grimacing, and frequent blinking and tearing of the eye.

  f. Duration of pain is usually less than 30 seconds but can occur in clusters, with seconds or minutes between attacks.

  g. Pain may be triggered by mild tactile stimulation of the face, including the following:

    (1) Shaving

    (2) Talking

    (3) Chewing

    (4) Biting

    (5) Brushing of teeth

    (6) Exposure to wind

  h. Recurrences of pain are unpredictable. Remission periods may last years but tend to decrease in length with increasing age.

7. Diagnostics

  a. History

    (1) Diagnosis is based on clinical history.

    (2) Note the following aspects of the pain: nature, distribution, severity, and pattern of onset.

b. Results of physical examination are usually normal.

c. Diagnostic studies are rarely useful.

8. Clinical management

  a. Goals of clinical management

    (1) Provide symptomatic relief.

    (2) Prevent future recurrence.

  b. Nonpharmacologic interventions

    (1) Use prophylactic measures, such as wearing a cloth over the face when going outside.

NURSE ADVISORY

Although patients with tic douloureux should be taught to avoid trigger factors when possible, be careful to steer patients away from avoidance techniques that create new health problems (e.g., refusal to talk and socialize, failure to eat, poor dental hygiene).

---

    (2) Biofeedback

  c. Pharmacologic interventions

    (1) Goal is to provide pain relief within 24 to 28 hours of starting medication.

    (2) Drugs include carbamazepine (Tegretol), phenytoin (Dilantin), and baclofen (Lioresal).

    (3) These drugs may lose their effectiveness over time.

  d. Special medical-surgical procedures

    (1) Local nerve block: Nerve is injected with local anesthetic or glycol. Relief may last only a few months.

    (2) Percutaneous radiofrequency rhizotomy: surgical placement of a needle into the trigeminal rootlets adjacent to the pons. Radiofrequency electrical current is supplied through the needle and destroys the nerve. The result is total anesthesia of the unilateral face.

    (3) Microvascular decompression of the trigeminal nerve. Surgeon dissects blood vessels away from the nerve and places a sterile pad between the blood vessel and the nerve. The theory is that certain blood vessels compress the trigeminal nerve, causing pain.

      • Advantage: Relieves pain without residual sensory loss

      • Disadvantage: Requires a posterior fossa or suboccipital craniectomy and thus carries some risk

9. Complications result from a fear of triggering attacks through various activities of daily living.

  a. Social withdrawal caused by the following:

    (1) Fear of speaking

    (2) Fear of moving the face, resulting in stony countenance

  b. Fear of opening the mouth and chewing, resulting in malnutrition

  c. Dental problems resulting from the following:

    (1) Fear of brushing or flossing teeth

    (2) Fear of having face or mouth touched by dentist

10. Prognosis

  a. Without treatment, permanent remission is rare.

b. Surgery provides permanent relief of pain in some but not all cases.
11. Applying the nursing process

NURSING DIAGNOSIS: Chronic pain R/T trigeminal neuralgia

a. *Expected outcomes:* Following intervention, the person should be pain free.
b. *Nursing interventions*
   (1) Support use of prophylactic medication.
   (2) Teach methods of avoiding pain triggers.
      • Use a water jet device instead of a toothbrush.
      • Use temperate water to wash the face.
      • Eat lukewarm, nutritious foods that are soft and easy to chew.
      • For males, grow a beard to avoid shaving-induced pain.
      • Write needs on paper to avoid speaking-induced pain.

NURSING DIAGNOSIS: Social isolation R/T anxiety over pain attacks and desire to avoid pain triggers

a. *Expected outcomes:* Following intervention, the person should utilize positive coping strategies.
b. *Nursing interventions*
   (1) Encourage the person and family members to express feelings about the pain.
   (2) Educate the person about the value of compliance with prophylactic medication.
   (3) Review pain avoidance procedures.
   (4) Refer to social workers or counselors as needed.
   (5) Mention surgery as a therapeutic option if medications fail.
10. Discharge planning and teaching
   a. Support use of prophylactic medication.
      (1) Ensure the person knows the appropriate medication, dose, and schedule.
      (2) Emphasize the importance of compliance to maintain therapeutic serum drug levels.
   b. Provide resources for psychosocial issues.

Bell's Palsy

1. Definition: An idiopathic lesion of the peripheral facial nerve (CN VII) that causes temporary paralysis of 1 side of the face.
2. Incidence in the United States
   a. Twenty per 100,000 persons
   b. Males and females are affected equally.
   c. Paralysis occurs bilaterally in 0.3 percent of cases.
   d. Bell's palsy is recurrent in 7 to 9 percent of cases.
3. Risk factors
   a. Family history—Bell's palsy is familial in 1 to 2 percent of cases.
   b. Pregnancy
   c. Diabetes mellitus
4. Etiology

a. Etiology is unknown, although several factors have been implicated.
   (1) Infection
   (2) Ischemia
   (3) Genetic factors
   (4) Trauma
   (5) Inflammatory reaction
5. Pathophysiology (Fig. 18–29)
6. Clinical manifestations (see Fig. 18–29)
7. Diagnostics
   a. History
      (1) Obtain history of symptom onset.
      (2) Review past medical history, as symptoms may be an indication or result of one of the following:
         • Trauma to face or skull
         • Neurologic conditions, including MS, Guillain-Barré syndrome, and myasthenia gravis
         • Infection, including otitis media, external otitis, and herpes zoster infection of the facial nerve (Ramsay Hunt syndrome)
         • Diabetes mellitus
         • Neoplasms, including cholesteatoma, leukemia, and meningioma
         • Cerebrovascular accident (Note that the facial weakness in stroke involves only the lower half of the face.)
   b. Physical examination. Check for the following:
      (1) Asymmetry of facial features, both at rest and with movement.
      (2) Corneal reflex: The affected eye will not close with corneal stimulation.
      (3) Decreased taste sensation on the anterior two thirds of the tongue on the affected side.
      (4) Hearing impairment: If the lesion is at the level of the internal auditory meatus, CN VIII may be affected.
   c. Although diagnostic studies are not usually necessary, electromyography can provide prognostic information.
8. Clinical management
   a. Goals of clinical management
      (1) Prevent complications.
      (2) Enhance nerve regeneration.
   b. Nonpharmacologic interventions
      (1) Methylcellulose eye drops several times a day prevent corneal damage from incomplete eye blink.
      (2) Patching the eye closed during the night prevents corneal damage from inadequate eyelid closure during sleep.
      (3) Massage of facial muscles promotes circulation and maintains muscle tone.
      (4) Warm, moist heat relieves pain.
      (5) Facial physical therapy exercises speed nerve regeneration if performed 3 times daily for 5 minutes. Some examples are grimacing, wrinkling the brow, forcing the eyes closed, whistling, and puffing the cheeks and blowing air out.
   c. Pharmacologic interventions
      (1) Corticosteroids (e.g., prednisone) decrease pain associated with Bell's palsy and may enhance recovery.

BELL'S PALSY

Pathophysiology:

A lesion of the facial nerve occurs in the facial canal between the internal acoustic meatus and the stylomastoid foramen. Interruption of nerve function can result from (1) edema compressing the nerve and/or (2) ischemia or inflammation causing physiologic disruption.

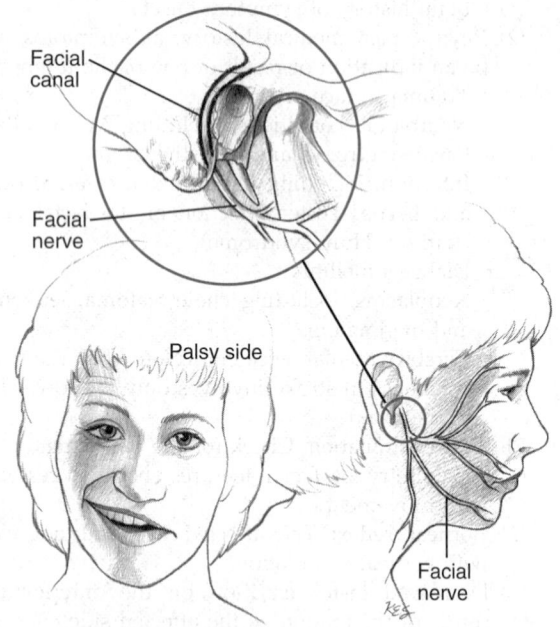

When patient tries to smile, only the unaffected side is mobile.

Clinical manifestations:

Clinical manifestations depend on the location of the lesion on the nerve. The onset of symptoms may be sudden or may occur over a few hours. Recovery of function occurs over several weeks to several months.

The affected side of the face is flaccid:
• Mouth droops.
• Nasolabial fold is flattened.
• Palpebral fissure (distance between upper and lower eyelids) is widened.
• Movements of the face cause characteristic features: eyelids cannot close completely, so the eyeball rolls upward with attempted eyelid closure (Bell's phenomenon).
• Facial expression is asymmetric.
• Saliva may drool from the affected side of the mouth.
• Pain and hyperacusis may occur in the affected ear.
• Excessive tearing may occur in the affected eye.
• Decreased taste may occur on the anterior two thirds of the tongue on the affected side.
• Facial weakness may slowly progress over several days but will reach maximal intensity within 3 weeks.

Figure 18–29.

(2) Analgesics for pain
   d. Special medical-surgical procedures
     (1) Surgical decompression of the nerve
     (2) Electromyographic stimulation
     (3) Both procedures are controversial.
9. Complications
   a. Abnormal regeneration of the nerve is the usual cause of complications.
   b. If autonomic fibers reconnect to the lacrimal ducts instead of the salivary glands, the person will develop excessive tearing while eating ("crocodile tears").
   c. If motor fibers reinnervate inappropriate muscles, abnormal facial movements will occur.
   d. If motor fibers have incomplete reinnervation, spasms, atrophy, and contractures may occur.
   e. If the eyelid muscles do not regain full function, the person may develop keratitis and blindness.
10. Prognosis
   a. Total recovery of function occurs in approximately 85 percent of cases.
   b. Factors indicating good recovery
     (1) Partial facial paralysis
     (2) Recovery of taste within the 1st week of symptom onset
     (3) Lack of nerve degeneration on electromyography done 2 weeks after onset of symptoms
   c. Factors indicating poor recovery
     (1) Total facial paralysis
     (2) Presence of nerve degeneration on electromyography done 2 weeks after onset of symptoms
     (3) Hypertension
     (4) Lack of ear pain
     (5) Age older than 60 years
     (6) Diabetes mellitus
11. Applying the nursing process

NURSING DIAGNOSIS: Pain R/T inflammation of CN VII

   a. *Expected outcomes:* Following intervention, the person should be pain free.
   b. *Nursing interventions*
     (1) Provide warm, moist packs to increase circulation and alleviate pain.
     (2) Encourage reasonable use of analgesics.
     (3) Educate the person about corticosteroid therapy.

NURSING DIAGNOSIS: Altered nutrition, less than body requirements, R/T decreased oral intake due to facial weakness

   a. *Expected outcomes:* Following intervention, the person should maintain adequate nutritional status.
   b. *Nursing interventions*
     (1) Educate the person about how to chew on the side opposite the affected one.
     (2) Encourage good oral hygiene to remove residual food.

(3) Suggest foods that do not require much mouth manipulation.

NURSING DIAGNOSIS: Risk for injury (corneal damage) R/T inability to blink effectively

---

a. *Expected outcomes:* Following intervention, the person should maintain corneal integrity.
b. *Nursing interventions*
   (1) Provide methylcellulose eye drops to the affected eye at least 3 times daily.
   (2) Provide an eye patch to keep the affected eye closed during sleep.

NURSING DIAGNOSIS: Body image disturbance R/T change in facial appearance due to muscle weakness

---

a. *Expected outcomes:* Following intervention, the person should report a positive self-image.
b. *Nursing interventions*
   (1) Reassure the person that facial movement will return in most cases.
   (2) Suggest wearing sunglasses when around others.
   (3) Refer to counseling if facial paralysis is permanent.
12. Discharge planning and teaching
   a. Educate person and family members about the natural course of the disease.
   b. Ensure that the person knows how to prevent complications.
   c. Educate the person about medications—type, dosage, and purpose.

▣ CARING FOR PEOPLE WITH TUMORS OF THE SPINAL CORD AND THE SPINAL COLUMN

Definitions

1. Extramedullary tumors
   a. These tumors arise outside the spinal cord—in the meninges, nerve roots, vertebrae, or soft tissue.
   b. They include extradural and intradural tumors.
      (1) Extradural tumors are located outside the dura in the epidural space, bones of the spinal column, or soft tissue. They include sarcoma, metastases, and lipoma.
      (2) Intradural tumors are located within or beneath the dura mater of the meninges. They include meningioma, neurilemoma, neurofibroma, and lipoma.
2. Intramedullary tumors
   a. Located within the spinal cord itself
   b. Include ependymoma, astrocytoma, and hemangioblastoma
3. Dumbbell tumors are dumbbell shaped and are located

in both the intradural and extradural space of the nerve roots.
4. Classification
   a. Primary tumors arise from epidural vessels, meninges, or glial cells of the spinal cord.
   b. Secondary tumors arise from bones of the spinal columns or metastases of lung, breast, kidney, or gastrointestinal cancers.

Incidence and Socioeconomic Impact

1. Most spinal cord tumors occur in adults.
2. Children have a higher incidence of sarcoma and glioma.
3. Percentage of spinal tumors by location
   a. Thoracic region—50 percent
   b. Lumbar region—25 percent
   c. Cervical region—20 percent
   d. Cauda equina—5 percent
4. Percentage of spinal tumors by classification
   a. Primary tumors—60 to 70 percent
   b. Secondary tumors—20 to 30 percent

Risk Factors and Etiology

1. Metastatic cancer is a risk factor.
2. Etiology of primary spinal cord tumors is unknown. Many secondary spinal cord tumors are caused by bony metastasis from lung, breast, kidney, or gastrointestinal cancers.

Pathophysiology

1. Spinal tumors cause compression, irritation, and traction of spinal nerve roots and the spinal cord.
2. Intramedullary tumors invade the spinal cord and cause destruction of the spinal cord itself.
3. Spinal tumors can obstruct blood supply and interfere with CSF circulation.
5. Slow-growing tumors (usually primary tumors) allow the spinal cord to adjust, causing minimal neurologic symptoms, until the mass becomes so large it compresses the cord against the bony confines of the vertebral column.
6. Fast-growing tumors (usually metastatic tumors) do not allow the spinal cord to adjust and cause rapid deterioration in neurologic function over days to weeks.

Clinical Manifestations

1. Symptoms depend on the vertical and horizontal location of the tumor.
2. Symptoms of extramedullary tumors are due to compression of the spinal cord or its roots (radiculopathic symptoms) and include the following:
   a. Radicular pain (pain that runs through a sensory nerve root)
   b. Paresthesias

c. Muscle weakness and wasting in the distribution of nerve roots.

d. Hyperactive muscle stretch reflexes

e. Brown-Séquard's syndrome
   (1) Contralateral loss of pain sensation, temperature, and strength
   (2) Ipsilateral loss of fine touch proprioception and vibration sense

3. Symptoms of intramedullary tumors are due to destruction of the spinal cord parenchyma (i.e., myelopathic symptoms) and may include the following:
   a. Burning, poorly localized pain
   b. Spotty sensory change
   c. Lower motor neuron weakness early in the course, with muscle wasting and fasciculations
   d. Upper motor neuron weakness later in the course, with hyperactive muscle stretch reflexes

4. Symptoms of tumors in the conus medullaris
   a. Pain, if present, is bilateral and symmetric.
   b. Sensory deficit has a saddle distribution, with dissociated features (loss of pain and temperature with preservation of touch and proprioception).
   c. Weakness is mild and symmetric.
   d. Muscle stretch reflexes of the ankle are absent.
   e. Bowel and bladder dysfunction is present early in the course and is marked.

5. Symptoms of tumors in the cauda equina
   a. Pain is severe, radicular, and in the distribution of sacral nerves.
   b. Sensory deficit has saddle distribution but may be unilateral or asymmetric.
   c. All sensory modalities are affected.
   d. Weakness is marked and asymmetric.
   e. Muscle stretch reflexes in the knee and ankle may be absent.
   f. Bowel and bladder dysfunction occurs late in the course and is less marked.

Diagnostics

1. History
   a. Check nature of progressive motor and sensory deficits.
   b. Inquire about bowel, bladder, and sexual function.
   c. Check for history of lung, breast, kidney, or other cancer.

2. Physical examination. Check the following:
   a. All sensory modalities in area of sensory deficit
      (1) Determine spinal level of sensory modalities.
      (2) Note location of a narrow band of hyperesthesia above the region of sensory deficit, as this often marks the level of the lesion.
      (3) Note dissociation of sensation (pain and temperature loss on 1 side with touch and proprioceptive loss on the other side).
   b. Motor function, including the following:
      (1) Strength of all muscle groups affected
      (2) Coordination of limb movements
      (3) Muscle tone
   c. Muscle stretch reflexes

d. Superficial reflexes

e. Anal sphincter tone

3. Diagnostic studies
   a. Plain radiographs of the spinal column (Fig. 18–30) can show the following:
      (1) Narrowing of the spinal canal
      (2) Bony changes
      (3) Distortion of paraspinal tissues
   b. A CT scan or an MRI scan
   c. Myelography
   d. A lumbar puncture
      (1) The lumbar puncture should be done cautiously if elevated intraspinal pressure is suspected.
      (2) Cerebrospinal fluid analysis can show elevated protein, xanthochromia, and tumor cells
   e. Electromyogram
      (1) An electromyogram is used to rule out other diseases (e.g., MS and amyotrophic lateral sclerosis).

Clinical Management

1. Goals of clinical management
   a. Control of symptoms
   b. Surgical removal of tumor, if possible

2. Pharmacologic interventions
   a. Dexamethasone to control edema of the spinal cord
   b. Antispasmodics to control spasticity
   c. Anticholinergics to control reflex incontinence
   d. Chemotherapy for some metastatic tumors

3. Special medical-surgical procedures
   a. Surgery (see Chapter 34)

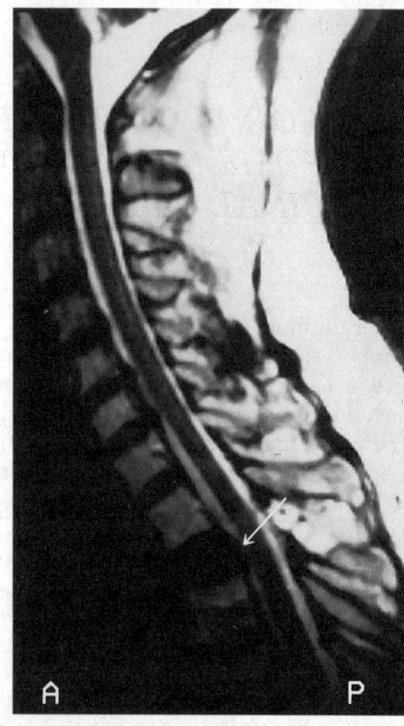

Figure 18–30. Magnetic resonance imaging view of an extradural spinal tumor at the T1 vertebral level (arrow).

(1) Decompressive laminectomy may be done in order to remove intradural tumors and relieve pressure in metastatic tumors or lymphomas.

(2) Surgical removal of some intramedullary tumors is possible.

b. Radiation therapy is employed to shrink the tumor in the following circumstances:

(1) When complete tumor removal is not possible

(2) For most metastatic tumors

Complications

1. Complications depend on the segmental location of the tumor and the type of tumor.
2. Cervical tumors above C4
   a. Can cause respiratory compromise owing to involvement of the phrenic nerve, which innervates the diaphragm.
   b. Can cause quadriparesis, leading to the hazard of immobility.
3. Metastatic tumors
   a. Can cause rapid deterioration in neurologic function.
   b. Surgery may be required to decompress the tumor.

Prognosis

1. Prognosis depends on tumor type.
2. Metastatic tumors imply terminal illness.
3. Benign or slow-growing tumors may cause permanent dysfunction but not death.

Applying the Nursing Process

NURSING DIAGNOSIS: Risk for injury R/T sensory deficit

1. *Expected outcomes:* Following intervention, the person should be free from injury.
2. *Nursing interventions*
   a. Advise the person to check the skin for breakdown or injury of affected body part on a daily basis.
   b. Advise the person to check the position of affected limbs.
   c. Warn the person to check the temperature of objects before allowing them to touch the affected parts of the body.

NURSE ADVISORY

Be sure to avoid pressure and other irritants on the patient's skin below the spinal sensory level.

NURSING DIAGNOSIS: Risk for impaired skin integrity R/T sensory deficits

1. *Expected outcomes:* Following intervention, the person should be able to maintain skin integrity.
2. *Nursing interventions*
   a. Monitor skin every few hours.
   b. Protect bony prominences from pressure.
   c. Apply protective padding as needed.
   d. Teach person to change position at least every 2 hours, or assist person to change position.
   e. Avoid shearing friction when moving person in bed.

NURSING DIAGNOSIS: Altered urinary elimination R/T reflex incontinence due to lesions above the sacral segments

1. *Expected outcomes:* Following intervention, the person should be able to do the following:
   a. Manage incontinence with effective procedures.
   b. Prevent overdistention of the bladder.
   c. Establish a voiding schedule.
   d. Express satisfaction with urinary elimination status.
2. *Nursing interventions*
   a. Initiate intermittent catheterization schedule based on diagnostic tests of bladder function.
   b. Utilize trigger mechanisms to initiate voiding, if necessary (see pp. 719–720).
   c. Maintain fluid intake of 2000 ml per day.
   d. Monitor intake and output.
   e. Control spontaneous urination by using anticholinergic drugs or adjusting intermittent catheterization schedule.
   f. Use external urinary drainage device if continence cannot be maintained.

NURSING DIAGNOSIS: Bowel incontinence R/T damage to sacral nerves that control anal sphincter

1. *Expected outcomes:* Following intervention, the person should be able to do the following:
   a. Maintain skin integrity.
   b. Have regular, planned bowel movements.
2. *Nursing interventions*
   a. Provide adequate padding.
   b. Adjust diet to facilitate normal bowel pattern.
   c. Initiate bowel program.

NURSING DIAGNOSIS: Pain R/T compression of spinal cord and roots by spinal tumor or bony metastases

1. *Expected outcomes:* Following intervention, the person should be able to do the following:
   a. Report satisfactory pain control.
   b. Exhibit a relaxed posture.
2. *Nursing interventions*
   a. Assess location and character of pain.
   b. Administer pain medication to ensure constant analgesic blood levels.
   c. Provide comfort measures.
      (1) Maintain proper body alignment.

(2) Reposition limbs as necessary for comfort.

(3) Provide diversional activities.

(4) Encourage use of noninvasive pain relief measures, such as relaxation, cutaneous stimulation, massage, and hot or cold packs.

(5) Alleviate anxiety.

NURSING DIAGNOSIS: Anticipatory grieving R/T loss of body function and uncertainty about the future

---

1. *Expected outcomes:* Following intervention, the person should do the following:
   a. Express grief.
   b. Share concerns.
   c. Participate in decisions for the future.
2. *Nursing interventions*
   a. Encourage the person to express feelings and concerns.
   b. Correct misinformation and clarify information as needed.
   c. Help the person set realistic goals.
   d. Help the person find ways to cope with grief.
      (1) Diversional activities
      (2) Relaxation
      (3) Meditation
      (4) Yoga
      (5) Spiritual counseling

Additional Nursing Diagnoses Commonly Associated with Tumors of the Spinal Cord and Spinal Column

- Impaired physical mobility R/T weakness or paralysis
- Altered urinary elimination R/T neurogenic bladder due to lesions of the sacral segments
- Constipation R/T immobility from spinal cord damage
- Bowel incontinence R/T damage to sacral nerves that control anal sphincter

Discharge Planning and Teaching

1. Teach use of home adaptive aids.
2. Ensure adaptive aids are available at discharge.
3. Refer the person and family members to support groups.
4. If the person has terminal cancer, discuss the following:
   a. Hospice care
   b. Formulating an advance care directive regarding end-of-life therapies

◼ CARING FOR PEOPLE WITH OTHER NEUROLOGIC DISORDERS

Spinal Cord Injuries

1. Injuries to the spine and spinal cord usually result from severe trauma (falls, diving accidents, automobile acci-

dents). Damage to the spinal cord can produce loss of sensation, muscle weakness, or paralysis.

2. The emergency care of patients with spinal cord injury is discussed in Chapter 37. Long-term care is considered in Chapter 7. Relevant nursing diagnoses are also addressed on pages 735–736.

Huntington's Disease

1. Definition: Huntington's disease (also called Huntington's chorea) is a genetic disorder that is characterized by degeneration of the basal ganglia (see p. 653). The distinguishing characteristic of this disorder is **chorea**—jerky, rapid, involuntary movements.
2. Incidence and etiology
   a. Huntington's disease is rare, developing in approximately 5 per 100,000 individuals in the United States.
   b. The disease is distinguished by an autosomal dominant pattern of inheritance. Thus, the children of patients with this disease have a 50 percent chance of inheriting the disease. The 50 percent of offspring who do not inherit the gene will *not* pass the disease on to their children.
   c. The aberrant gene is found on the short arm of chromosome 4.

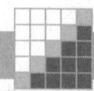 **LEGAL AND ETHICAL CONSIDERATIONS**

Genetic testing for the gene responsible for Huntington's disease has been available since the fall of 1993. Although genetic testing on the basis of linkage analysis was available earlier, the new gene test is highly accurate. However, whereas the new test can predict *who* will develop Huntington's disease, it cannot predict *when* the person will develop symptoms or the severity of the symptoms.

Because the symptoms of Huntington's disease can be devastating, some people at risk would rather not be tested. The decision to decline testing can seriously affect family dynamics and can raise legal and ethical issues should the person have children and then develop the disease.

---

3. Clinical manifestations
   a. The onset of the disease usually occurs in individuals between 35 and 50 years—often after the person (who was unaware of the disease) has had children.
   b. The chorea may be subtle at first and later affect the face, arms, and trunk. The person may twitch, grimace, and appear restless, fidgety, and clumsy. To mask the chorea, patients may constantly scratch their heads and cross and uncross their legs.
   c. Chorea may diminish or disappear when the patient sleeps.
   d. Emotional problems often precede or accompany the chorea. The person may become irritable, suspicious, and moody. Memory loss and inability to make decisions are common. Eventually, the patient may become severely depressed or psychotic.
   e. Dysphagia sometimes develops during the midstage or late stage of the disease, resulting in difficulty in eating and weight loss.

4. Interventions
   a. No treatment to date will cure or halt the course of Huntington's disease.
   b. Haloperidol (Haldol) and diazepam (Valium) may help control the chorea, lessen anxiety, and manage behavioral problems.
   c. Antidepressants may be prescribed to treat depression.
   d. Dietary modifications often lessen the dysphagia and help stabilize the patient's weight.
      (1) Provide the patient with high-calorie foods served in small, frequent feedings.
      (2) Serve foods that are soft and easy to swallow such as custards, scrambled eggs, mashed potatoes, and chopped meat in gravy.
      (3) Have the patient sit up straight when eating. Instruct the person to point the chin down toward the chest when swallowing.
   e. A feeding tube may be necessary for the patient who continues to have difficulty swallowing and who is losing weight.
   f. As the patient's movements are erratic, protect the person from injury (e.g., pad bedrails and wheelchairs, provide the patient with a walker).

◼ CARING FOR PEOPLE UNDERGOING CRANIOTOMY

Definition

1. A craniotomy is an operation on the cranium that allows access to the brain and other intracranial structures.
2. A craniotomy involves either opening the skull surgically and creating a bone flap or enlarging a burr hole (see earlier discussion and Chapter 37).

Purposes

1. Perform a biopsy
2. Remove a tumor
3. Aspirate and drain an abscess or a blood clot
4. Lower increased ICP
5. Stop hemorrhage

Preoperative Nursing Management
(see Chapter 13)

1. Provide the patient and family with information concerning the following:
   a. The rationale for preoperative procedures such as cutting the hair or shaving the head, a procedure that is usually performed in the operating room.
   b. The surgical procedure itself.
   c. The purpose of the recovery room and intensive care unit.
   d. The interventions that will be used to control pain following surgery.

2. Assess the patient for level of consciousness, orientation to time and person, pupil response, numbness or weakness of the extremities, dizziness, sensory abnormalities, edema, indications of dehydration, and visual or auditory alterations. Check vital signs and weigh the patient.
3. Assess for signs of increased ICP, and report your findings immediately to the surgeon.
4. Wash the patient's hair, and neatly braid long hair.
5. Provide emotional support; strive to allay the patient's and family members' anxiety. It may help to have a member of the clergy visit the patient.
6. Withhold solid foods usually 6 to 8 hours before surgery and fluids 4 to 6 hours before surgery.
7. Carefully review your facility's preoperative checklist. On the day of surgery, check off each item before transporting the patient to the operating room. General preoperative care is discussed in Chapter 13.
8. Give preoperative medications as ordered.

Postoperative Care (see Chapter 13 for basic care)

1. Assess the patient immediately following cranial surgery as follows:
   a. Assess vital signs every 15 to 30 minutes for the 1st 8 to 12 hours, then every hour for the next 12 hours, or until stable, and then every 2 hours.
   b. Assess for signs of increased ICP (see p. 675). Notify the neurosurgeon immediately if ICP increases.
   c. Assess neurologic status over the 1st 72 hours following surgery. Also document the patient's intake and output. Monitor fluid and electrolyte levels for signs of sodium imbalance or hypovolemia (see Chapter 9).
   d. Assess the head dressing and notify the neurosurgeon if bleeding, drainage, or loss of spinal fluid is evident. Also note if a drain or catheter is in place. Observe for signs of wound infection, such as abnormal amounts of drainage or foul odor.
   e. Watch for and immediately report to the neurosurgeon any localized or generalized seizure activity. Protect the patient from harm, and carry out interventions to promptly stop the seizures as ordered.
2. Position the patient properly, depending on the site of the surgery.
   a. Supratentorial surgery (above the brain's tentorium): Elevate the patient's head 30 degrees to promote venous outflow through the jugular veins.
   b. Infratentorial surgery (below the brain's tentorium): keep the patient's head flat to prevent pressure on brain stem contents. Turn the person from side to side every 2 hours. Do *not* leave the person in a back-lying position, as this could result in potentially deadly pressure on brain stem structures.
3. Care for the scalp incision, and change the head dressing as needed. Clean the area of the incision with an antiseptic disinfectant followed by an application of antibiotic ointment. The dressing will likely be removed within 3 to 5 days.
4. Observe for the general complications of surgery (see Chapter 13) and for the complications that may follow neurosurgical procedures. Potential neurologic complica-

tions include paralysis, memory loss, visual or speech impairment, and mental confusion.

Applying the Nursing Process

NURSING DIAGNOSIS: Altered cerebral tissue perfusion R/T increased ICP after craniotomy

1. *Expected outcomes:* Following intervention, the patient should be free of signs of increased ICP.
2. *Nursing interventions*
   a. Continually assess person's neurologic status.
   b. Monitor ICP and cerebral perfusion pressure when feasible.
   c. Ensure proper positioning of head. Remember to elevate the head 30 degrees after supratentorial surgery, and keep the head flat after posterior fossa surgery. Administer drugs as indicated.

NURSING DIAGNOSIS: Pain R/T craniotomy and scalp incision

1. *Expected outcomes:* Following intervention, the patient should express satisfaction with pain control measures and should be able to rest and sleep without being disturbed by pain.
2. *Nursing interventions*
   a. In cooperation with other team members, ensure that adequate medicinal pain control is available to the patient.
   b. Keep the patient's environment calm, dark, and quiet. Avoid sudden noises. Take care not to jar the patient's bed.
   c. Provide nonmedicinal comfort measures (see Chapter 13).

NURSING DIAGNOSIS: Risk for infection R/T surgical incision

1. *Expected outcomes:* Following interventions, the person should be free of infection in the wound area.
2. *Nursing interventions*
   a. Maintain aseptic technique, including frequent hand washing.
   b. Assess wound area, drains, and dressing frequently for signs of infection.
   c. Monitor for signs and symptoms of infection, and arrange for laboratory studies, as needed.
   d. Administer prophylactic antibiotics, as ordered.

NURSING DIAGNOSIS: Anxiety R/T postoperative treatments and possible alterations in lifestyle

1. *Expected outcomes:* Following interventions, the person should actively participate in the rehabilitation process.
2. *Nursing interventions*
   a. Encourage the patient to express feelings of concern about current loss of control and possible permanent lifestyle changes needed.
   b. Work with the patient and other team members to develop a rehabilitation plan that maximizes patient control and involvement. Explain the need for each step in the rehabilitation process.
   c. Include family and significant others in the rehabilitation process.
   d. Refer the patient to support groups.
   e. Help the person set realistic goals and develop solutions to anticipated lifestyle changes.
   f. Encourage person to continue with normal activities as long as possible.

Additional Nursing Diagnoses Associated with Craniotomy

- Ineffective breathing pattern R/T decreased level of consciousness, immobility, positioning, and impaired coughing following craniotomy
- Impaired gas exchange R/T decreased level of consciousness and weakness
- Self-care deficit R/T impaired physical mobility
- Impaired verbal communication R/T aphasia following craniotomy

Discharge Planning and Teaching

1. Discharge planning depends on the patient's presurgical diagnosis and the outcome of the surgical procedure.
2. Some patients recover completely following discharge. Other patients must undergo rehabilitation before returning to a normal active life. Unfortunately, still other patients never achieve full neurologic function, and may require ongoing medical intervention, home nursing care, and family support.

Bibliography

Books

Adams RD, and Victor M. *Principles of Neurology.* 5th ed. New York: McGraw-Hill, 1993.
American Association of Neuroscience Nurses. *Core Curriculum for Neuroscience Nursing.* 3rd ed. Chicago: American Association of Neuroscience Nurses, 1990 and 1993.
Cummings JL, and Benson DF (eds). *Dementia, A Clinical Approach.* 2nd ed. Boston: Butterworth-Heinemann, 1992.
Guyton AC. *Textbook of Medical Physiology.* 8th ed. Philadelphia: WB Saunders, 1991.
Haerer AF. *DeJong's The Neurologic Examination.* 5th ed. Philadelphia: JB Lippincott, 1992.
Hickey JV. *The Clinical Practice of Neurological and Neurosurgical Nursing.* Philadelphia: JB Lippincott, 1992.
Matthews WB, et al. *McAlpine's Multiple Sclerosis.* Edinburgh: Churchill Livingstone, 1991.

Morantz RA, and Walsh JW (eds). *Brain Tumors*. New York: Marcel Dekker, 1993.

Rottenberg DA. *Neurologic Complications of Cancer Treatment*. Boston: Butterworth-Heinemann, 1991.

Toole JF. *Cerebrovascular Disorders*. 5th ed. New York: Raven Press, 1990.

Wyllie E. *The Treatment of Epilepsy: Principles and Practice*. Philadelphia: Lea & Febiger, 1993.

Chapters in Books and Journal Articles

Head Injuries

Dinner DS. Posttraumatic epilepsy. *In* Wyllie E (ed). The *Treatment of Epilepsy: Principles and Practice*. Philadelphia: Lea & Febiger, 1993.

Godbole KB, Berbiglia VA, and Goodard L. A head-injured patient, clinical progress and nursing care priorities. *J Neurosci Nurs* 23(5):290–294, 1991.

Lovasik DA, and Kerr ME. Controversial treatments of the traumatic brain-injured patient. *Am J Nurs* 93(suppl):28–33, 1993.

Multi-Society Task Force on PVS. Medical aspects of the persistent vegetative state [First of two parts]. *N Engl J Med* 330(21):1499–1508, 1994.

Nockels RP, and Pitts LH. Diagnosis and treatment of head injury. *In* Grotta JC (ed). *Management of the Acutely Ill Neurologic Patient*. New York: Churchill Livingstone, 1993.

Pylar PA. Management of the agitated and aggressive head injury patient in an acute hospital setting. *J Neurosci Nurs* 21(6):353–356, 1989.

Walleck C. Patients with head injury and brain dysfunction. *In* Clochesy JM, et al. (eds). *Critical Care Nursing*. Philadelphia: WB Saunders, 1993.

Williams MA, and Hanley DF. Intracranial pressure monitoring and cerebral resuscitation. *In* Grotta JC (ed). *Management of the Acutely Ill Neurologic Patient*. New York: Churchill Livingstone, 1993.

Cerebrovascular Disorders

Black JC, and Barker E. Nursing care of patients with loss of protective function. *In* Black JM, and Matassarin-Jacobs E (eds). *Luckmann and Sorensen's Medical-Surgical Nursing: A Psychophysiologic Approach*. 4th ed. Philadelphia: WB Saunders, 1993.

Bladin CF, and Willmore J. Seizures after stroke. *Stroke Clinical Updates* 5(2):5–8, 1994.

European Carotid Surgery Trialists' Collaborative Group. MRC European carotid surgery trial: Interim results for symptomatic patients with severe (70–99%) or with mild (0–29%) carotid stenosis. *Lancet* 337(8752):1235–1243, 1991.

Fihn SD, et al. Risk factors for complications of chronic anticoagulation. *Ann Intern Med* 118(7):551–520, 1993.

Gilliam EE. Intracranial hypertension: Advances in intracranial pressure monitoring. *Crit Care Nurs Clin North Am* 2(1):25, 1990.

Goldstein M. Stroke prevention and health care issues: An American perspective. *Cerebrovasc Dis* 3(suppl 1):29–33, 1993.

Kelly-Hays .M. A preventive approach to stroke. *Nurs Clin North Am* 26(4):931–942, 1991.

Leahy NM. Complications in the acute stages of stroke. *Nurs Clin North Am* 26(4):971–983, 1991.

Marshall RS, and Mohr JP. Current management of ischaemic stroke. *J Neurol Neurosurg Psychiatry* 56:6–16, 1993.

Matchar DB, and Duncan PW. Cost of stroke. *Stroke Clinical Updates* 5(3):9–12, 1994.

Mayberg MR, et al. Carotid endarterectomy and prevention of cerebral ischemia in symptomatic carotid stenosis. *JAMA* 266(23):3289–3294, 1991.

North American Symptomatic Carotid Endarterectomy Trial Collaborators. Beneficial effect of carotid endarterectomy in symptomatic patients with high-grade carotid stenosis. *N Engl J Med* 325(7):446–452, 1991.

Phillips SJ, and Whisnant JP. Hypertension and the brain. *Arch Intern Med* 152:938–945, 1992.

Rothrock JF, and Hart RG. Antithrombotic therapy in cerebrovascular disease. *Ann Intern Med* 115(11):885–895, 1991.

Schnell SS. Nursing care of clients with cerebral disorders. *In* Black JM, and Matassarin-Jacobs E (eds). *Luckmann and Sorensen's Medical-Surgical Nursing: A Psychophysiologic Approach*. 4th ed. Philadelphia: WB Saunders, 1993.

Shafer PO. Cerebrovascular disorders. *In* Patrick ML, et al. (eds). *Medical-Surgical Nursing: Pathophysiological Concepts*. Philadelphia: JB Lippincott, 1991.

Ticlopidine for prevention of stroke. *Med Lett* 43(874):65–66, 1992.

Cerebral Aneurysms and Subarachnoid Hemorrhages

Cook HA. Aneurysmal subarachnoid hemorrhage: Neurosurgical frontiers and nursing challenges. *AACN Clin Issues* 2(4):666–674, 1991.

Day AL, and Salcman M. Subarachnoid hemorrhage. *Am Fam Physician* 40(1):95–105, 1989.

Kassel NF, Shaffrey ME, Shaffrey CI. Cerebral vasospasm following aneurysmal subarachnoid hemorrhage. *In* Appuzzo MLJ (ed). *Brain Surgery*. New York: Churchill Livingstone, 1993.

Kopitnik TA, and Samson DS. Management of subarachnoid hemorrhage. *J Neurol Neurosurg Psychiatry* 56:947–959, 1993.

Manifold SL. Aneurysmal SAH: Cerebral vasospasm and early repair. *Crit Care Nurse* 10(8):62–69, 1990.

Segatore M. Hyponatremia after subarachnoid hemorrhage. *J Neurosci Nurs* 25(2):92–99, 1993.

Seizures and Epilepsy

Lannon S. Epilepsy in the elderly. *J Neurosci Nurs* 25:273–281, 1993.

Legion V. Health education for self-management by people with epilepsy. *J Neurosci Nurs* 23(5):300–305, 1991.

Ozuna J. Intermittent loss of arousal. *In* Mitchell PH, et al. (eds). *AANN's Neuroscience Nursing*. Norwalk, CT: Appleton & Lange, 1988. (revision in press)

Headaches

Broderick JP, and Swanson JW. Migraine-related strokes. *Arch Neurol* 44:868–871, 1987.

Diamond S. Strategies for migraine management. *Cleve Clin J Med* 58(3):257–261, 1991.

Edmeads J. What is migraine? Controversy and stalemate in migraine pathophysiology. *J Neurol* 238:S2–S5, 1991.

Gallagher RM. Headache diagnosis and treatment. *J Am Acad Nurs Pract* 3(1):5–10, 1991.

Gilman S. Advances in neurology. *N Engl J Med* 326(24):1608–1616, 1992.

Mather PJ, et al. The treatment of cluster headache with repetitive intravenous dihydroergotamine. *Headache* 31(8):525–532, 1991.

Mathew NT. Cluster headache. *Neurology* 42(suppl 2):22–31, 1992.

Olesen J. A review of current drugs for migraine. *J Neurol* 238:S23–S27, 1991.

Schulman EA, and Silberstein SD. Symptomatic and prophylactic treatment of migraine and tension-type headache. *Neurology* 42(suppl 2):16–19, 1992.

Silberstein SD. Advances in understanding the pathophysiology of headache. *Neurology* 42(suppl 2):6–10, 1992.

Silberstein SD. Tension-type and chronic daily headache. *Neurology* 43:1644–1649, 1993.

Stewart WF, et al. Prevalence of migraine headache in the United States. *JAMA* 267(1):64–69, 1992.

Whitney CM. New headache classification: Implications for neuroscience nurses. *J Neurosci Nurs* 22(6):385–388, 1990.

Central Nervous System Infections

Ballard NR. Infectious and degenerative neurological disorders. *In* Patrick ML, et al. (eds). *Medical-Surgical Nursing: Pathophysiological Concepts*. Philadelphia: JB Lippincott, 1991.

Berger J, and Levy RM. Infections of the nervous system. *In* Grotta JC (ed). *Management of the Acutely Ill Neurological Patient*. New York: Churchill Livingstone, 1993.

Twomey CR. Brain abscess: An update. *J Neurosci Nurs* 24(1):34–39, 1992.

Intracranial Tumors

Schnell SS. Nursing care of clients with cerebral disorders. *In* Black JM, and Matassarin-Jacobs E (eds). *Luckmann and Sorensen's Medical-Surgical Nursing: A Psychophysiologic Approach*. 4th ed. Philadelphia: WB Saunders, 1993.

Vos H. Central nervous system tumors. *In* Patrick M, et al. (eds). *Medical-Surgical Nursing: Pathophysiological Concepts*. Philadelphia: JB Lippincott, 1991.

Walleck C. Intracranial problems. *In* Lewis SM, and Collier IC (eds). *Medical-Surgi-*

cal Nursing: Assessment and Management of Clinical Problems. St. Louis: Mosby–Year Book, 1992.

Alzheimer's Disease

Davis KL (ed). Neuroscience and socioeconomic challenge of Alzheimer's disease. *Neurology* 43(suppl 4), 1993.

Evans DA, et al. Prevalence of Alzheimer's disease in a community population of older persons. *JAMA* 262(18):2551–2556, 1989.

Karzman R, and Jackson JE. Alzheimer's disease: Basic and clinical advances. *J Am Geriatr Soc* 39(5):516–525, 1991.

Mace NL, Whitehouse PJ, and Smyth KA. Management of patients with dementia. *In* Whitehouse PJ (ed). *Dementia*. Philadelphia: FA Davis, 1993.

Ozuna J. Nursing care of clients with degenerative neurologic disorders. *In* Black JM, and Matassarin-Jacobs E (eds). *Luckmann and Sorensen's Medical-Surgical Nursing: A Psychophysiologic Approach*. 4th ed. Philadelphia: WB Saunders, 1993.

Teri L, and Logsdon R. Assessment and management of behavioral disturbances in Alzheimer's disease. *Compr Ther* 16(5):36–42, 1990.

Multiple Sclerosis

Anderson DW, et al. Revised estimate of the prevalence of multiple sclerosis in the United States. *Ann Neurol* 31(3):333–336, 1992.

de Roin S, and Winters S. Amantadine hydrochloride: Current and new uses. *J Neurosci Nurs* 22(5):322–325, 1990.

Erickson RP, Lie MR, and Wineinger MA. Rehabilitation in multiple sclerosis. *Mayo Clin Proc* 64:818–828, 1989.

Goodin DS. The use of immunosuppressive agents in the treatment of multiple sclerosis. *Neurology* 41:980–985, 1991.

The INFB Multiple Sclerosis Study Group. Interferon beta 1-b is effective in relapsing-remitting multiple sclerosis. *Neurology* 43:655–661, 1993.

Ozuna J. Nursing care of clients with degenerative neurologic disorders. *In* Black JM, and Matassarin-Jacobs E (eds). *Luckmann and Sorensen's Medical-Surgical Nursing: A Psychophysiologic Approach*. 4th ed. Philadelphia: WB Saunders, 1993.

Sadovnick AD, and Ebers GC. Epidemiology of multiple sclerosis: A critical overview. *Can J Neurol Sci* 20(1):17–28, 1993.

Parkinson's Disease

American Parkinson Disease Association. Speech problems and swallowing problems in Parkinson's disease. New York: American Parkinson Disease Association, Inc., 1989.

Askenasy JJM. Sleep in Parkinson's disease. *Acta Neurol Scand* 87:167–170, 1993.

Calne DB. Treatment of Parkinson's disease. *N Engl J Med* 329(14):1021–1027, 1993.

Goetz CG, et al. Neurosurgical horizons in Parkinson's disease. *Neurology* 43:1–7, 1993.

Heinonen EH, Lammintausta R. A review of the pharmacology of selegiline. *Acta Neurol Scand* 84(suppl 136):44–59, 1991.

Lazano MA, et al. Effect of GPi pallidotomy on motor function in Parkinson's disease. *Lancet* 346:1383–1387, 1995.

Ozuna J. Nursing care of clients with degenerative neurologic disorders. *In* Black JM, and Matassarin-Jacobs E (eds). *Luckmann and Sorensen's Medical-Surgical Nursing: A Psychophysiologic Approach*. 4th ed. Philadelphia: WB Saunders, 1993.

The Parkinson Study Group. Effects of tocopherol and deprenyl on the progression of disability in early Parkinson's disease. *New Engl J Med* 328:176–183, 1993.

Propath (The Route to better management of Parkinson's disease). Tips for daily living. East Hanover, NJ: Sandoz Pharmaceuticals, 1992.

Myasthenia Gravis

Lanska DJ. Indications for thymectomy in myasthenia gravis. *Neurology* 40:1828–1829, 1990.

Ozuna J. Nursing care of clients with degenerative neurologic disorders. *In* Black JM, and Matassarin-Jacobs E (eds). *Luckmann and Sorensen's Medical-Surgical Nursing: A Psychophysiologic Approach*. 4th ed. Philadelphia: WB Saunders, 1993.

Perlo VP. Treatment of the critically ill patient with myasthenia. *In* Ropper A (ed). *Neurological and Neurosurgical Intensive Care*. 3rd ed. New York: Raven Press, 1993.

Amyotrophic Lateral Sclerosis

Ringel SP. The natural history of amyotrophic lateral sclerosis. *Neurology* 43:1316–1322, 1993.

Rosen DR, et al. Mutations in Cu/Zn superoxide dismutase gene are associated with familial amyotrophic lateral sclerosis. *Nature* 362:59–62, 1993.

Stone N. Amyotrophic lateral sclerosis: A challenge for constant adaptation. *J Neurosci Nurs* 19(3):166–173, 1987.

Guillain-Barré Syndrome

Murray DP. Impaired mobility: Guillain-Barré syndrome. *J Neurosci Nurs* 25(2):100–104, 1993.

Ropper AH. The Guillain-Barré syndrome. *N Engl J Med* 17(326):1130–1136, 1992.

Thomas PK. The Guillain-Barré syndrome: No longer a simple concept. *J Neurol* 239:361–362, 1992.

Cranial Nerve Disorders

Dalessio DJ. Diagnosis and treatment of cranial neuralgias. *Med Clin North Am* 75(3):605–615, 1991.

Morgenlander JC, and Massey, EW. Bell's palsy. *Postgrad Med* 88(5):157–164, 1990.

Wollenberg SP. Primary care diagnosis and management of Bell's palsy. *Nurs Pract* 14(12):14–17, 1989.

Tumors of the Spinal Cord and Column

Raney DJ. Malignant spinal cord tumors: A review and case presentation. *J Neurosci Nurs* 23(1):45–49, 1991.

Huntington's Disease

Ozuna J. Nursing care of clients with degenerative neurologic disorders. *In* Black JM, and Matassarin-Jacobs E (eds). *Luckmann and Sorensen's Medical-Surgical Nursing: A Psychophysiologic Approach*. 4th ed. Philadelphia: WB Saunders, 1993.

Read AP. Huntington's disease: Testing the test. *Nat Genet* 4:329–330, 1993.

Agencies and Resources

American Brain Tumor Association
3725 North Tallman Avenue
Chicago, IL 60618
(312) 286–5571

American Cancer Society
261 Madison Avenue
New York, NY 10016
(212) 599–3600

The American Parkinson's Disease Association
1256 Hylan Boulevard
Staten Island, NY 10305
(800) 223–2732

Epilepsy Foundation of America
4351 Garden City Drive
Landover, MD 20785–2267
(301) 459–3700

Guillain-Barré Syndrome Foundation International
P.O. Box 262
Wynnewood, PA 19096
(215) 667–0131

Myasthenia Gravis Foundation
53 West Jackson Boulevard, Suite 660
Chicago, IL 60604
(800) 541–5454 or (312) 427–6252

National Alzheimer's Association
919 Michigan Avenue, Suite 1000
Chicago, IL 60661
(800) 272–3900

National Brain Tumor Foundation
323 Geary Street, Suite 510
San Francisco, CA 94102
(415) 296–9303 or 296–0404

National Head Injury Foundation
333 Turnpike Road
Southborough, MA 01772
(800) 444–6443

National Multiple Sclerosis Society
733 Third Avenue
New York, NY 10017
(212) 986–3240

National Parkinson's Foundation, Inc.
1501 N.W. 9th Avenue—Bob Hope Road
Miami, FL 33136
(800) 327–4545

National Stroke Association
8480 East Orchard Road, #1000
Englewood, CO 80111
(800) 787–6537

The Parkinson's Disease Foundation
710 West 168th Street
New York, NY 10032
(800) 457–6676

Parkinson's Support Group of America
13376 Cherry Hill Road, Apartment 204
Beltsville, MD

United Parkinson's Foundation
833 West Washington Boulevard
Chicago, IL 60607
(312) 733–1893

19

Caring for People with Visual Disorders

STRUCTURE AND FUNCTION OF THE VISUAL SYSTEM

Structure

The visual system consists of the ocular adnexa, the external eye, and the internal eye (Fig. 19–1).

Function

1. The function of the visual system is to connect the human body to the environment and other people (Fig. 19–2). It functions interdependently with the other body senses and the nervous system.
2. The ocular adnexa (accessory structures) support and protect the eyes.
   a. The 4 rectus muscles move the eye up and down and from side to side. The 2 oblique muscles work with the rectus muscles to allow the eyeball to rotate in circular movements and to move at angles.
   b. The eyelids protect the eyes by blinking, which also spreads the tear film on the surface of the eyeball.
   c. The lacrimal gland continually produces tears that are drained away by the nasolacrimal duct. The function of tears is to produce a smooth optical surface, protect the cornea and conjunctival surfaces, inhibit the growth of microorganisms, and provide the cornea with nutrition.
3. The function of the external eye structures is to protect the eye and provide optical clarity.
   a. The elasticity of the conjunctiva allows the eye to move in all directions. Its continuity prevents the eye from coming out of the socket.
   b. The convex shape of the cornea refracts (bends) light rays onto the retina. Because it is highly innervated, the cornea protects the eye through its extreme sensitivity.
   c. The sclera's fibrous tissue provides protection for the delicate inner structures of the eye.
4. The function of the internal eye is to convert light rays and images into neural messages to the brain.
   a. The uveal tract is the vascular layer of the eye that provides nourishment to the eye structures.

   (1) The iris constricts and dilates to control the amount of light that enters the eye through the pupil.
   (2) The ciliary body processes produce the aqueous humor.
   (3) The choroid provides nourishment to the retina.
   b. The function of the angle structures is to filter out the aqueous humor and channel that fluid into the bloodstream.
   c. The aqueous humor maintains the intraocular pressure.
   d. The elasticity of the crystalline lens allows it to bring into focus both near and distant objects (accommodation).
   e. The viscosity of the vitreous humor maintains the shape and transparency of the eye.
   f. The retina is responsible for the transmission of light rays into neural impulses. The rods provide for peripheral vision and vision in dim light. The cones provide fine detail and color vision.
   g. The optic nerve fibers synapse in the lateral geniculate body, one of the two elevations of the lateral posterior thalamus.
   (1) They synapse on neurons whose axons terminate in the primary visual cortex of the occipital lobe of the brain.
   (2) Because the ganglion cells of the retina and their axons are part of the central nervous system, the tissue does not regenerate if damaged or severed.

ASSESSING PEOPLE WITH VISUAL DISORDERS

Key Symptoms and Their Pathophysiologic Bases

1. Common symptoms in ocular disorders
   a. *Abnormalities of vision:* May be due to an abnormality in the eye or along the visual pathway. Symptoms include the following:
   (1) Increased glare

THE EYE: External Structures

External Eye Structures

The external eye includes the conjunctiva, cornea, and sclera.

The **sclera**, the white, fibrous outer layer of the eyeball, is approximately 1 mm thick and is continuous with the cornea where it becomes clear.

The **conjunctiva** is composed of a thin, transparent vascular layer of mucous membrane that lines the eyelids and covers the eyeball. The palpebral conjunctiva that lines the eyelids is continuous with the bulbar conjunctiva that covers the eyeball.

The **cornea**, the transparent window of the eye, is avascular, convex shaped, and approximately 0.5 mm thick and approximately 11.5 mm in diameter.

The **eyelids** (palpebrae) are elastic folds of skin composed of areolae, muscle, and fibrous tissue.

Ocular Adnexa,
the external structures surrounding the eye, include the ocular muscles, pads of fat, bony orbit, eyelids, eyebrows, eyelashes, and lacrimal system.

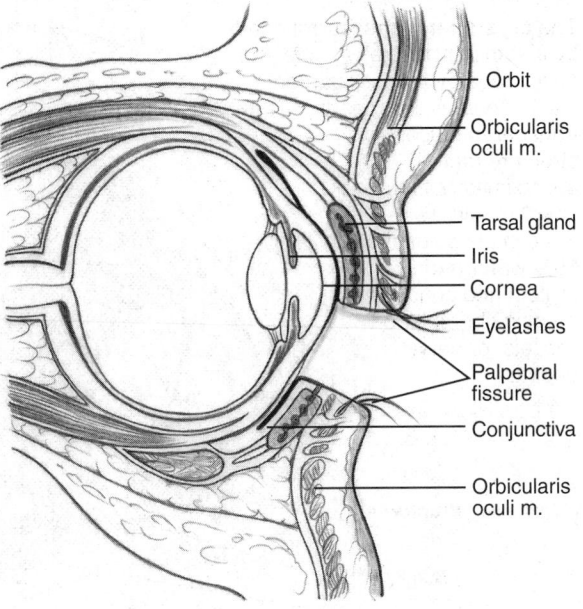

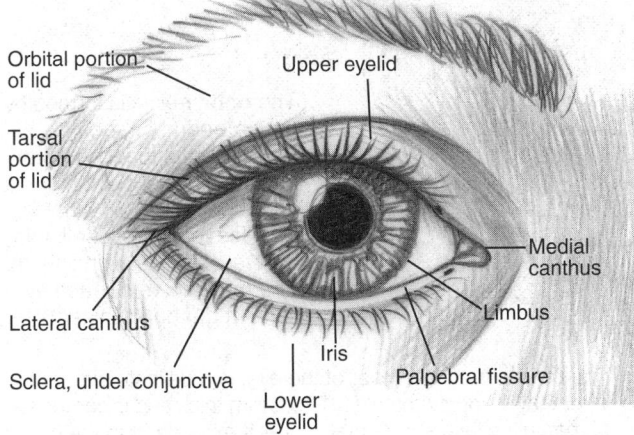

Lacrimal System

The lacrimal apparatus includes the lacrimal gland, accessory glands, the canaliculi, the lacrimal sac, and the nasolacrimal duct.

The tear film is composed of protein, mucin, potassium, sodium, chloride, glucose, and urea. The average pH of the tear film is 7.35.

Ocular Muscles

There are 6 ocular muscles, 4 rectus muscles (medial, lateral, superior, and inferior), and 2 oblique muscles (superior and inferior). The bony orbit has a volume of approximately 30 ml.

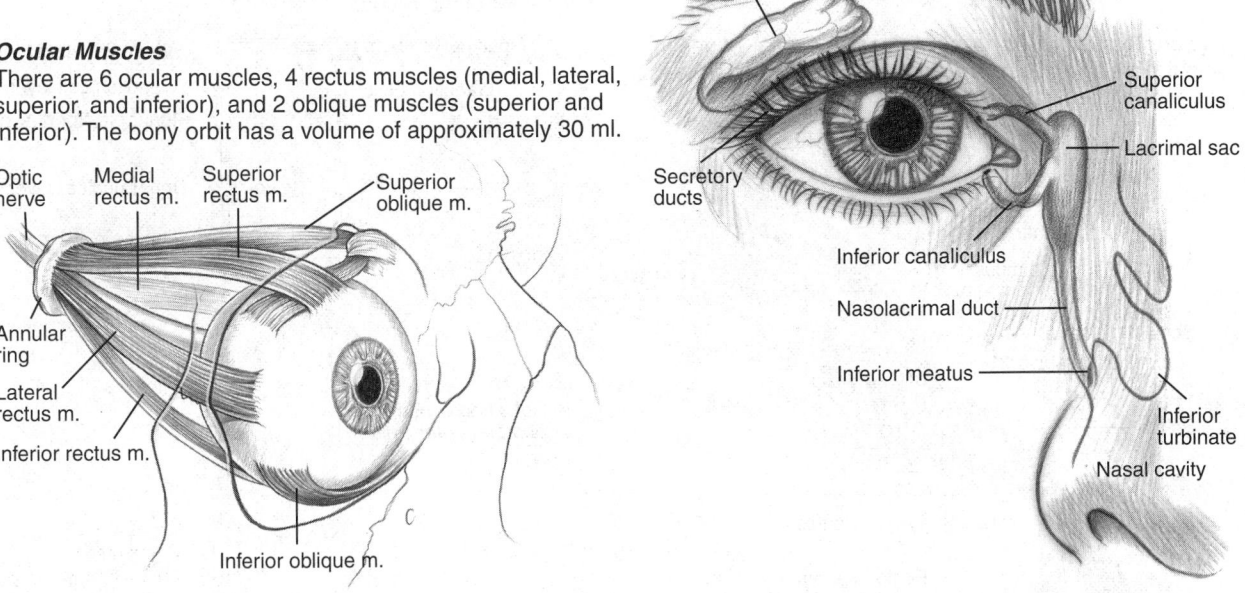

Figure 19–1. Ocular adnexa, lacrimal system, external eye structures, internal eye structures, cross-section of anterior chamber structures, and layers of the retina.

Illustration continued on following page

THE EYE: Internal Structures

Internal Eye Structures

The internal eye is composed of the uveal tract, angle structures, aqueous humor, crystalline lens, vitreous humor, retina, and optic nerve.

The **crystalline lens**, surrounded by a semipermeable capsule and suspended by fibrous ligaments called *zonules*, is a nearly transparent, biconvex structure that is approximately 4 mm thick and 9 mm in diameter. It is composed of about 65% water and 35% protein and contains no pain fibers, blood vessels, or nerve endings.

The **uveal tract**, the middle layer of the eye, includes the iris, the ciliary body, and the choroid. The **iris** is a pigmented tissue composed of sphincter and dilator muscles. Its color is determined by the presence or absence of stromal melanocytes. The **ciliary body**, composed largely of capillaries, is a triangular body that is continuous with the root of the iris, forming a circle behind it. The **choroid**, joined to the ciliary body and firmly attached to the optic nerve, is composed of three layers of blood vessels.

The **angle structures**, located where the outer edges of both the iris and the cornea meet to form an angle, are the trabecular meshwork and Schlemm's canal.

The **aqueous humor** has a composition similar to that of plasma and is a clear, watery liquid that fills the anterior and posterior chambers.

The **vitreous humor** is a clear, gelatinous fluid composed of 99% water and 1% collagen and hyaluronic acid. It fills the space between the lens and the retina, making up nearly two thirds of the volume and weight of the eye.

The **optic nerve** is formed by the gathering of about 1 million axons that come from the ganglion cells of the retina and is about 25–30 mm long. As it leaves the eyeball, it is covered with a myelin sheath. The optic nerve of each eye joins at the optic chiasm.

The **retina,** the inner layer of the eye, is a delicate pigmented layer that is approximately 0.1–0.2 mm thick and is composed of many fine layers of neural tissue. It extends from the ciliary body and gathers at the optic nerve. Located in the retina are the photoreceptor cells, approximately 125 million rods and 6 million cones. The rods are distributed throughout the periphery of the retina and the cones are concentrated in an area about 5 mm in diameter known as the *macula*, near the center of the retina.

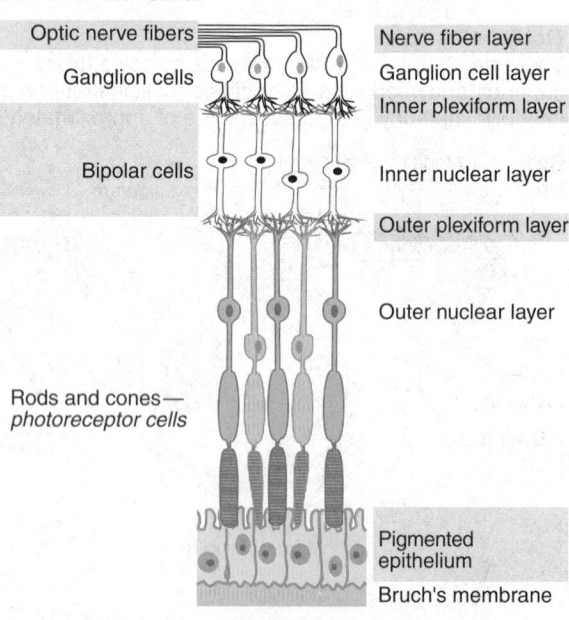

Uveal tract structures:
Iris
Ciliary body
Choroid

Posterior chamber · Optic nerve · Macula · Retina · Cornea · Lens · Zonules · Sclera

Optic nerve fibers — Nerve fiber layer
Ganglion cells — Ganglion cell layer
Inner plexiform layer
Bipolar cells — Inner nuclear layer
Outer plexiform layer
Outer nuclear layer
Rods and cones— *photoreceptor cells*
Pigmented epithelium
Bruch's membrane

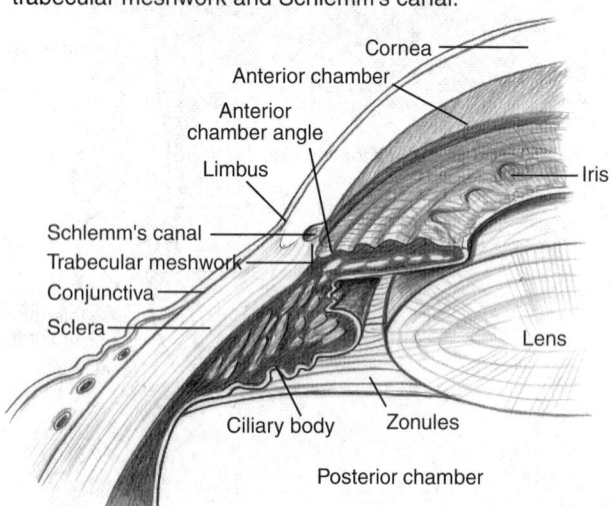

Cornea · Anterior chamber · Anterior chamber angle · Limbus · Schlemm's canal · Trabecular meshwork · Conjunctiva · Sclera · Iris · Lens · Ciliary body · Zonules · Posterior chamber

Figure 19–1. *Continued*

VISUAL PATHWAY

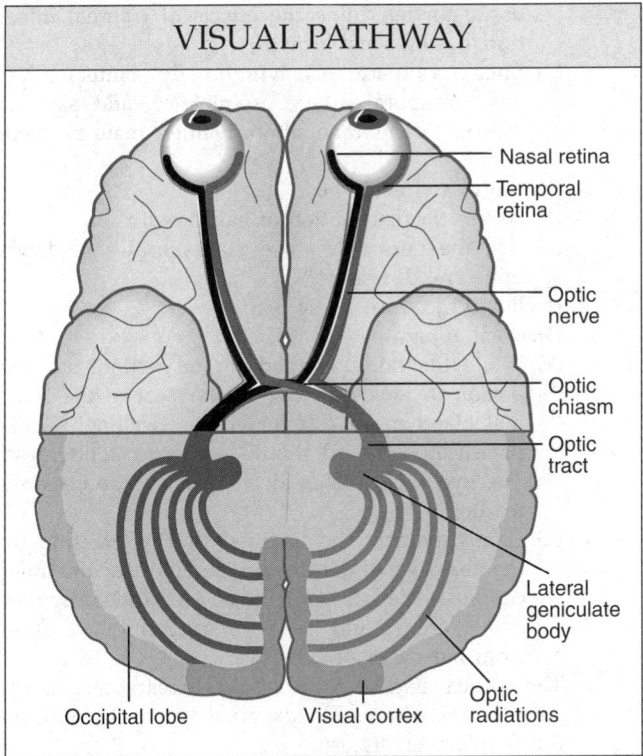

Nasal retina

Temporal retina

Optic nerve

Optic chiasm

Optic tract

Lateral geniculate body

Occipital lobe

Visual cortex

Optic radiations

Figure 19–2.

(2) Flashing lights or halos around lights
(3) Floating spots
(4) Diplopia (double vision)
(5) Blurred vision
(6) Visual field deficits

b. *Abnormalities of appearance*

(1) "Red eye" is the most common abnormal appearance of the eye. It is due to dilated and congested conjunctival vessels. Causes for a reddened eye may be minor or serious and include the following:
   • Minor irritation
   • Subconjunctival hemorrhage
   • Inflammatory disorders
   • Infection
   • Allergy
   • Trauma

(2) Other external changes in appearance include growths, lesions, edema, or abnormal position.

c. *Abnormalities of sensation:* Sometimes these are not well defined. Individuals more often complain of eye strain, pulling sensations, pressure, fullness, or generalized headache. The following are other characteristics of eye discomfort:

(1) The pain or discomfort may be ocular, periocular, or retrobulbar (behind the eye).

(2) *Foreign body sensation* may range from mild grittiness to sharp superficial pain. It is relieved by the application of topical anesthetic.

(3) Deeper internal aching may indicate glaucoma, inflammation, muscle spasm, or infection.

(4) *Photophobia* (sensitivity to light) may indicate cor-

neal involvement but is also found in migraine and viral infection.

(5) *Itching* is usually a sign of an allergy attack.

(6) *Dryness and burning* can occur with dry eyes or corneal irritation.

(7) *Increased tearing* may be due to irritation, allergy, an abnormality of the lacrimal system, or infection.

2. To determine the significance of these symptoms, ask the person the following questions (see also Table 4–2):

a. How long have you experienced the symptom, and how much does it bother you?

b. Have you noticed other symptoms, for example, headache?

c. Does the symptom seem related to any activity or particular incident?

(1) Sports and recreational activities
(2) Work or outdoor activity
(3) Use of new products for cleaning or hygiene, for example, floor or window cleaning sprays, hair gel, or mousse.
(4) Time of day

d. Is there anything that relieves the symptom?

TRANSCULTURAL CONSIDERATIONS

The eyes have a mystical quality unparalleled by any other part of the human body. Throughout history, many cultures have assigned unique powers to the eyes. The concept of the "evil eye"—the ability to cause harm with a glance or by blinking—is regarded with varying degrees of respect in European, Mediterranean, Arabic, Latin American, African, Polynesian, and other cultures.

Other cultural values that relate to eyes may include an inhibition about receiving donor tissue for a corneal transplant or a belief in accepting fate when a particular body part wears out.

Iridology, the practice of diagnosing health problems by the appearance of the iris, has no scientific basis and is not associated with eye disorders. Belief in iridology, however, is related to the mystical powers attributed to the eye.

Health History

1. Chief complaint

a. Ask the person to describe the visual symptom according to duration, frequency, onset, location, and severity.

b. Ask about associated symptoms such as headache or facial pain, which may be related to the ocular symptom.

2. Ocular history: Ask about previous ocular injuries, surgeries, and medications, including the use of eye drops, eye ointments, time-release ocular inserts, and oral agents.

3. Medical history

a. Vascular disorders such as diabetes and hypertension commonly have ocular manifestations.

b. Other systemic diseases with ocular manifestations include rheumatoid arthritis, lupus erythematosus, leukemia, sickle cell disease, thyroid disorders, vitamin deficiency, tuberculosis, leprosy, syphilis, herpes infections, fungal infections, acquired immunodeficiency syndrome, Sjögren's syndrome, Marfan syndrome, multiple sclerosis, and myasthenia gravis.

c. Systemic medications may be responsible for ocular complications.

(1) People taking amiodarone for a cardiac dysrhythmia may develop tiny deposits in the corneal epithelium.

(2) Chloroquine, an antimalarial drug used in the treatment of collagen disorders, causes both corneal and retinal changes.

(3) Long-term corticosteroid therapy can cause chronic open-angle glaucoma, cataracts, and exacerbation of herpes infections.

(4) The use of phenobarbital and phenytoin may produce nystagmus and weakness of convergence (the ability of the eyes to fixate on the same point) and accommodation (the ability of the eyes to adjust between near and far points).

(5) Sedatives, when taken regularly, can decrease tear production, which results in ocular irritation from dry eyes.

(6) Anticholinergics such as atropine and scopolamine dilate the pupils and may induce an attack of acute angle-closure glaucoma in persons with anatomically narrow anterior chamber angles. They also cause blurred vision in presbyopic individuals who are no longer able to adjust vision between near and far objects.

NURSE ADVISORY

Atropine and scopolamine are often prescribed preoperatively for general surgery. These may precipitate an acute attack of angle-closure glaucoma by dilating the pupils.

---

(7) Over-the-counter medications such as antihistamines and decongestants may cause drying of the eyes.

d. Family history is pertinent for ocular disorders such as strabismus, amblyopia, glaucoma, cataracts, retinal detachment, and macular degeneration.

Physical Examination

1. Inspection

a. Symmetry of the eyes and face

(1) Note size and placement of both eyes in relation to each other. Malposition of the globe may indicate orbital disease.

(2) Palpate the bony orbital rim and periocular soft tissue to determine the effects of trauma, infection, or abnormal growth.

(3) Enlarged preauricular lymph nodes, sinus tenderness, temporal artery prominence, and skin or mucous membrane abnormalities may be relevant.

b. Eyebrows and eyelashes

(1) Assess for distribution of hair growth.

(2) Ask the person to raise the eyebrows to determine any difference.

c. Eyelids (Procedure 19–1)

d. Lacrimal apparatus

(1) While the lid is everted for inspection, ask the person to look down so that a part of the lacrimal gland may be observed for swelling. Gentle pressure on the lid should not reveal tenderness. The eye surface should be moist without excess tearing.

(2) Gently palpate the lacrimal sac by pressing on the area over the lower orbital rim near the inner canthus. The area should be free of tenderness, and there should be no regurgitation of fluid from the sac or puncta.

e. The cornea. Each cornea should appear transparent, smooth, and shiny. Cloudy areas or specks may indicate injury or disease.

ELDER ADVISORY

Several eye changes are associated with aging. The eyes of the older person may appear to be sunken because of the loss of subcutaneous fat and the decreased elasticity of the skin. Older individuals are less able to maintain an upward gaze and have more difficulty converging the eyes. Arcus senilis, an opaque ring formed at the edge of the iris, is the result of fatty deposits. The cornea may be less clear, and the pupil size may be diminished. Xanthelasma—yellowish, wrinkled patches on the lids, usually near the inner angle of the eye—represents lipid deposits that normally occur in older people.

---

f. The pupils

(1) Both pupils should appear round and equal in size (see Fig. 19–13).

(2) Abnormal pupil size may indicate neurologic disease, acute intraocular inflammation, surgical alteration, or the effects of systemic or ocular medications.

(3) Normal pupil size is 2 to 6 mm. Pupils smaller than 2 mm are considered constricted. Pupils larger than 6 mm are considered dilated. Some variations in size are benign.

(4) Pupils are assessed for response to light. Pupil reaction may be described as brisk, sluggish, or nonreactive (fixed) (Procedure 19–2).

(5) Assess the pupils for accommodation (Procedure 19–3).

(6) The notation PERRLA stands for *p*upils *e*qual, *r*ound, *r*eact to *l*ight, and *a*ccommodation. Note

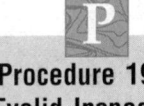

Procedure 19–1
Eyelid Inspection

Definition/Purpose	To examine the palpebral conjunctiva
Contraindications/Cautions	Use a gentle touch and an unhurried approach.
Learning/Teaching Activities	Provide the following information: (a) describe the procedure; (b) explain that it will not cause pain.
Equipment	Cotton applicator stick
Procedure	

Actions	Rationale/Discussion
1. Have the person sit opposite you in good lighting.	1. Maximize comfort and ability to observe.
2. Gently pull down on the lower lid. Observe color, texture, vascularity, secretions, and presence of any foreign body.	2. Extreme paleness or bright red color is abnormal.
3. Place the cotton-tipped applicator on the outside of the upper lid. Gently press down on the applicator stick, and as the upper lid curls up, use gentle pressure with your other hand to push the lid up so that it turns inside out.	
4. To return the eyelid to the normal position, ask the person to look up while you gently pull the eyelashes forward.	

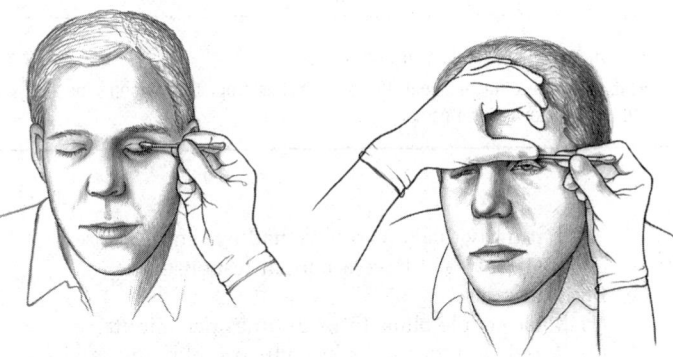

Procedure 19–2
Testing Pupillary Response

Definition/Purpose	To evaluate the response of each pupil to light as well as their response together
Learning/Teaching Activities	Provide the following information: (a) describe the procedure; (b) instruct the person that there is no discomfort involved.

Preliminary Activities

Equipment	Flashlight or penlight
Procedure	

Actions	Rationale/Discussion
1. Dim the lights in the room.	1. Enhances ability to observe pupil response.
2. Have the person sit facing you.	
3. Ask the person to look straight ahead while you quickly bring the beam of light from the side and direct it at the right eye. Watch the speed and amount of the *direct response.*	3. Approximately 25% of all individuals will have unequal pupil size (due to previous eye surgery, trauma, or medications).
4. At the same time, watch the *consensual response* of the left eye to the light in the right eye.	
5. Repeat the procedure in the left eye.	

Procedure 19–3
Testing Pupil Accommodation

Definition/Purpose To evaluate the ability to adjust the focal power of the eye from near to far

Learning/Teaching Activities Provide the following instruction: (a) describe the procedure; (b) instruct the person that there is no discomfort associated with this test.

Preliminary Activities

Equipment None

Procedure

Actions	Rationale/Discussion
1. Have the person sit directly in front of you.	1. As the person's eyes converge while watching your finger, the pupils should constrict equally. The pupil normally constricts when looking at a near object and dilates when looking at an object far away.
2. Hold your index finger about 12 to 18 inches from the person's nose and move it toward the person.	

that individuals who have had eye surgery previously may not have a normal response.
 g. Blink response
  (1) Most people blink 15 to 20 times per minute.
  (2) Rapid, infrequent, or asymmetric blinking is abnormal.
2. Corneal reflex. The corneal reflex is performed to assess

the function of the 5th (trigeminal) cranial nerve (Procedure 19–4).
3. Ocular motility
 a. The objective of ocular motility testing is to evaluate the alignment of the eyes and their movements independently and together.
 b. Impairment of eye movements can be due to a de-

Procedure 19–4
Testing Corneal Reflex

Definition/Purpose To assess the function of the fifth (trigeminal) cranial nerve

Learning/Teaching Activities Provide the following information: (a) describe the procedure; (b) instruct the person that the test will cause discomfort.

Preliminary Activities

Equipment Sterile cotton ball wisp

Preparation of the Person 1. Be sure the individual is not wearing contact lenses.

Procedure

Actions	Rationale/Discussion
1. Have the person sit and look straight ahead with the eyes open.	1. Maintain a comfortable position.
2. Bring the cotton wisp from behind the person's field of vision and very lightly touch it to the cornea.	2. The person should blink and tear, indicating that the nerve function is intact.
3. Use a separate wisp to test the other eye.	3. To prevent cross-contamination.

Procedure 19–5
Testing Corneal Reflection (Hirschberg Test)

Definition/Purpose	To determine the presence or absence of strabismus
Learning/Teaching Activities	Provide the following information: (a) describe the procedure and (b) instruct the person that the test will not cause discomfort.

Preliminary Activities

Equipment	Penlight or flashlight
Procedure	

Actions	Rationale/Discussion
1. Ask the person to look straight ahead.	
2. Stand in front of the person and shine the light directly into both eyes from a distance of about 13 inches.	2. If there is no deviation, the pinpoint of light reflection should appear symmetrically in both eyes.

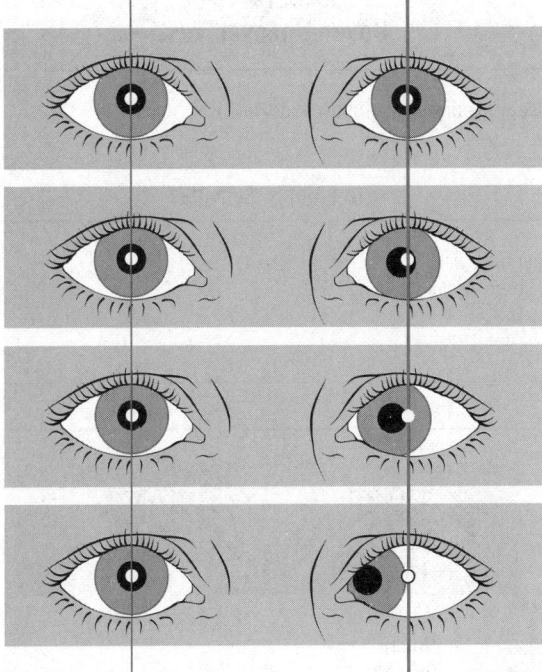

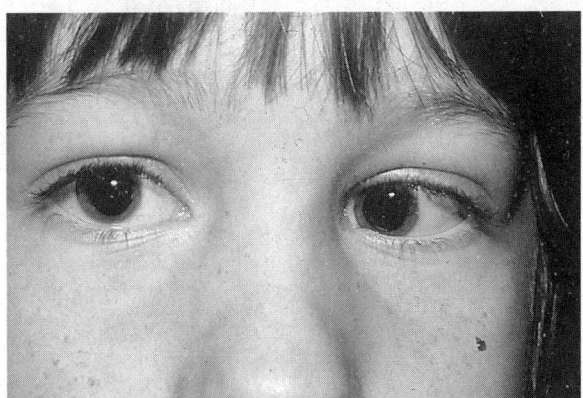

Strabismus in a young child. (Courtesy of the Department of Ophthalmology, W.K. Kellogg Eye Center, University of Michigan, Ann Arbor, MI.)

viation in ocular alignment (strabismus), to neurologic problems (cranial nerve palsy), to primary extraocular muscular weakness (myasthenia gravis), or to muscle entrapment in an orbital floor fracture after trauma.

  c. Ocular motility is evaluated using 3 methods of testing.

    (1) The corneal reflection (Hirschberg's test) determines the presence or absence of strabismus (Procedure 19–5).

    (2) The cover-uncover test is used to determine ocular muscle deviation. Normally, both eyes maintain a parallel position in binocular position (Procedure 19–6).

    (3) The 3rd test for ocular motility is the evaluation of the 6 cardinal positions of gaze (Procedure 19–7). A muscle deviation will prevent an eye from turning to a particular position.

4. Visual acuity

  a. This test assesses macular function using the Snellen chart at a distance of 20 feet or 6 meters (Procedure 19–8). Often a projected chart with letter sizes adjusted for a distance shorter than 20 feet is used. Charts with symbols and objects may be used when individuals are unable to read or to speak English.

  b. Findings are noted at a distance of 20 feet. A finding of 20/30 indicates that the person must be at a distance of 20 feet to see what the average person can see at 30 feet.

Procedure 19–6
Cover-Uncover Test

Definition/Purpose   To assess the presence of muscle deviation

---

Preliminary Activities

Equipment
- Target on a wall
- Eye cover (occluder)

Procedure

Actions	Rationale/Discussion
1. Direct the person to look at a target at eye level with both eyes.	
2. Cover one eye and observe the other.	2. If the other eye moves to focus on the target, it was not previously fixating on the target.
3. Remove the cover and observe the covered eye.	3. The covered eye should have remained in its former position. If the covered eye has a muscle deviation, the eye will drift out of position while covered.

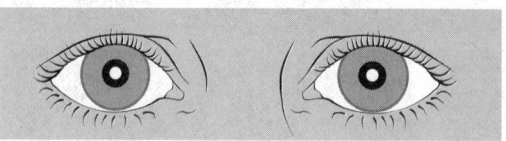

Watch this side

If this eye moves after the other is covered, this eye has a deviation.

Watch this side

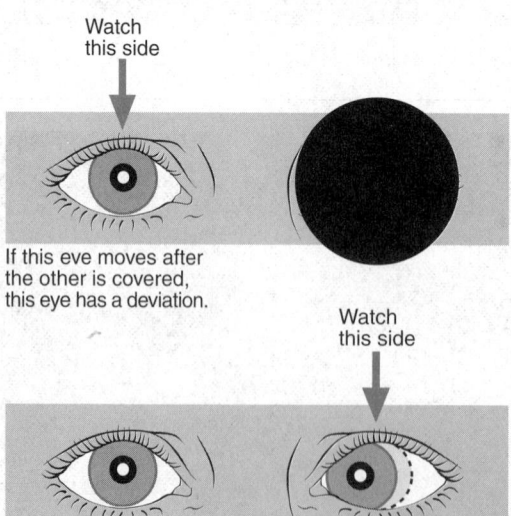

Eye moves while covered

Procedure 19–7
Testing the 6 Cardinal Positions of Gaze

Definition/Purpose   To assess the presence or absence of ocular muscle deviation

Learning/Teaching Activities   Provide the following information: (a) describe the procedure and (b) instruct the person that there is no discomfort with this test.

Procedure

Actions	Rationale/Discussion
1. Using your hand or an object as a guide, ask the person to look with both eyes: • left • right • up and right • up and left • down and right • down and left	1. Both eyes should move together in each direction as far as possible.

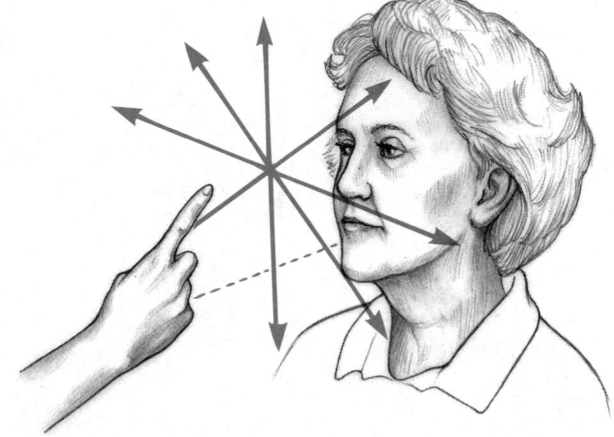

c. Visual acuity should be evaluated both with and without the use of corrective lenses.

d. Pinhole vision testing further evaluates visual acuity. The pinhole occluder placed before the eye eliminates peripheral rays of light, improves contrast, and generally improves vision almost within normal limits (even if the person has a refractive error). The pinhole disk differentiates between visual loss due to refractive error and poor vision due to eye disease.

e. When the person is unable to read the largest letter on the chart, visual acuity is evaluated by holding up fingers at a distance of 2 to 3 feet. The visual acuity is recorded as counting fingers (CF).

f. If the person is unable to count fingers, the visual acuity is documented as hand motion (HM), light perception (LP), or no light perception (NLP).

g. In the United States, the most widely used definition of blindness is that used by the Internal Revenue Service for tax purposes: *central visual acuity 20/200 or less in the better eye with best correction, or widest diameter of visual field no greater than 20 degrees.*

5. Near vision

a. Gross assessment of near visual acuity is evaluated by holding a *Jaeger near card* or a similar card at a distance of 14 inches and asking the person to read the smallest line possible. If the individual is able to read the largest line only by holding the card nearer than 14 inches, the distance at which the person is able to read the largest letters should be noted.

b. Visual acuity is tested with each eye individually and then with both together.

NURSE ADVISORY

Testing vision with the Jaeger near card is often prescribed at frequent intervals (every hour) following plastic and reconstructive surgery of the eyelids, orbital decompression, or optic nerve sheath decompression. These procedures can cause postoperative bleeding or edema that could result in pressure on the optic nerve and permanent vision loss. Notify the physician of a decrease in near vision of 1 line or more. If the individual cannot read, use a card with symbols or pictures.

6. Visual fields

a. Two methods may be used to determine the field of vision or peripheral vision.

(1) The confrontation method requires no special instruments (Procedure 19–9). The examiner must have normal peripheral vision.

(2) The 2nd method of evaluating the visual field involves the use of an automated or a computerized perimeter such as the Goldmann, Humphrey, or Octopus (Fig. 19–3). The person sits with the head on a chin rest facing a large half sphere. Test lights appear in scattered areas. The

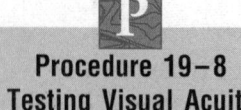

Procedure 19–8
Testing Visual Acuity

Definition/Purpose	To determine clarity of vision, the ability to see and distinguish fine details (macular function), or both
Learning/Teaching Activities	Provide the following information: (a) describe the test; (b) instruct the person that there is no discomfort associated with the test.

Preliminary Activities

Equipment	• Snellen chart • Eye cover (occluder)

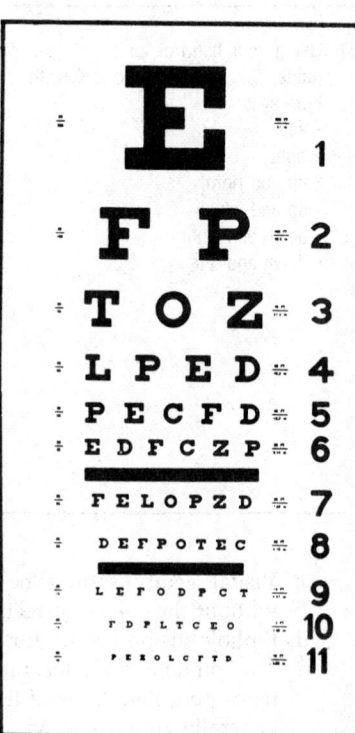

Procedure

Actions	Rationale/Discussion	
1. Ask the person to cover the left eye with the occluder.	1. Using an occluder or a piece of heavy paper instead of the hand prevents the use of the other eye.	DOCUMENTATION OF VISUAL ACUITY
2. With the chart at a distance of 20 feet or the equivalent in chart size, ask the person to read the smallest line possible.	2. If the individual misses letters on the line, record the number of misses (e.g. 20/20 − 2).	V ──── 20/30 $\overline{c}$ ──── 20/40
3. Repeat the test with the opposite eye occluded.		Visual acuity is documented in the medical record. The top reading is always the right eye, and the bottom reading is always the left eye. The abbreviation $\overline{c}$ or $\overline{s}$ under the V indicates whether the reading is with or without correction by glasses or contact lenses.
4. Repeat the test with the person using both eyes.		

person responds verbally or with a hand-held device. This method is able to measure both subtle and gross defects in the field of vision.

    b. Visual field defects occur in glaucoma, retinal de-

tachment, retinitis pigmentosa, and central nervous system disorders such as a brain lesion, syphilis, or stroke.

7. Direct ophthalmoscopy (Fig. 19–4)

Procedure 19-9
Confrontation Testing of Visual Fields

Definition/Purpose	To assess the field of vision or peripheral vision
Learning/Teaching Activities	Provide the following information: (a) describe the procedure; (b) instruct the person that there is no discomfort associated with this test.
Equipment	None
Assessment/Planning	This informal method of testing visual fields assumes that the examiner has a normal field of vision.
Procedure	

Actions	Rationale/Discussion
1. Face the person at a distance of 3 feet.	1. The visual field test is considered normal if the person can see the target at • 90 degrees temporally • 50 degrees nasally • 50 degrees upward • 65 degrees downward
2. Ask the person to cover the left eye and look with the right eye at the left eye of the examiner.	
3. Cover your own right eye.	
4. Using a pencil or a finger as a target, place the target midway between the examiner and the person, beyond the field of vision of both.	
5. Slowly move the target into the line of vision and note when the person can see it.	
6. Repeat at 8 or 10 meridians spaced over 360 degrees.	
7. Repeat the test on the other eye.	

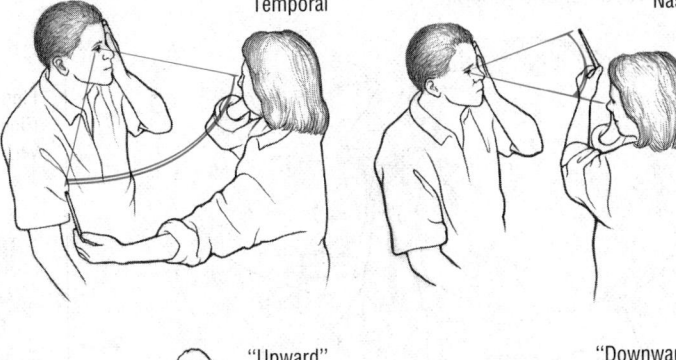

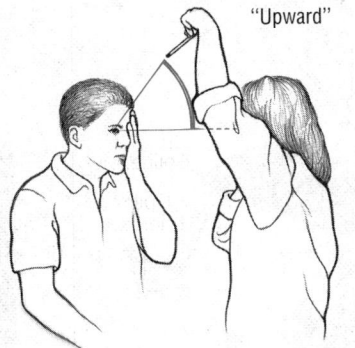
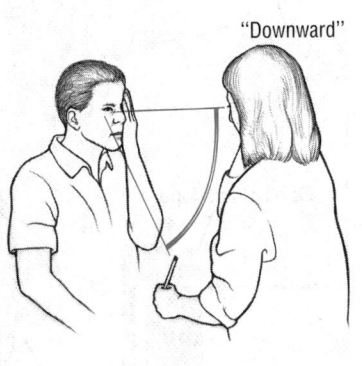

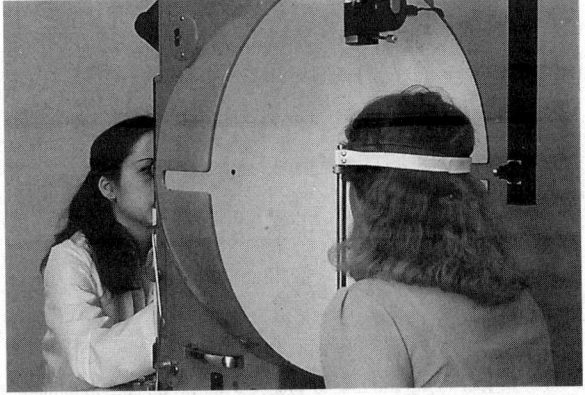

Figure 19-3. Visual field testing using the Goldmann automated perimeter. (Courtesy of Ophthalmic Photography at the W.K. Kellogg Eye Center, University of Michigan, Ann Arbor, MI.)

8. Indirect ophthalmoscopy
   a. This procedure provides a stereoscopic view of the fundus and includes a wider field than that of the direct ophthalmoscope (Fig. 19-5).
   b. The eye must be fully dilated for the examination.
   c. The examiner holds a convex lens in front of the person's eye. Through a viewing device with a light source attached to a headband, the examiner sees a reversed image of the fundus.
9. Tonometry
   a. Normal intraocular pressure is 10 to 22 mm Hg over water.
   b. Intraocular pressure is measured with a variety of instruments.
      (1) Schiotz. A hand-held portable instrument that measures the amount of corneal indentation produced by a preset weight (Fig. 19-6). Resistance

DIRECT OPHTHALMOSCOPY

The hand-held direct ophthalmoscope provides a magnified (15x) image of the fundus, the posterior portion of the eye. A darkened room or the use of dilating drops enhances the visibility of the organs. Note that the view of the fundus may be compromised by a cloudy cornea or a cataract.

1 Holding the ophthalmoscope at arm's length from the person, shine the light directly into the eye. When the ophthalmoscope focuses on the plane of the pupil, the pupil appears to be a bright reddish-orange color. This **red reflex** is the reflection of the fundus color through the clear ocular media (vitreous humor, lens, aqueous humor, and cornea).

2 The ophthalmoscope should be held 1-2 inches from the person's eye to examine the optic disk, retinal vessels, and macula.

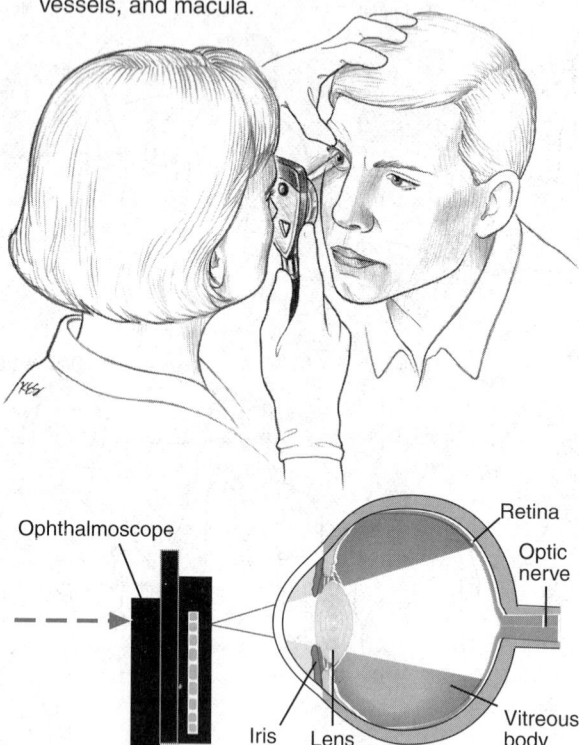

The optic disk should appear round and creamy white with well-defined margins. The average width is 1.5 mm. Retinal veins appear slightly darker than retinal arteries. The macula is a small avascular area that appears to be slightly deeper red than the surrounding fundus. The bright oval reflection in the middle of the macula is the fovea centralis, responsible for fine, detailed vision.

Figure 19-4. Ocular examination using the direct ophthalmoscope.

from a high intraocular pressure will allow less indentation than a low pressure. The cornea must be anesthetized with a topical anesthetic drop. A conversion chart is used to convert the scale reading into millimeters of mercury.

(2) Air puff noncontact tonometer. Measures the indentation of the cornea caused by a puff of air.

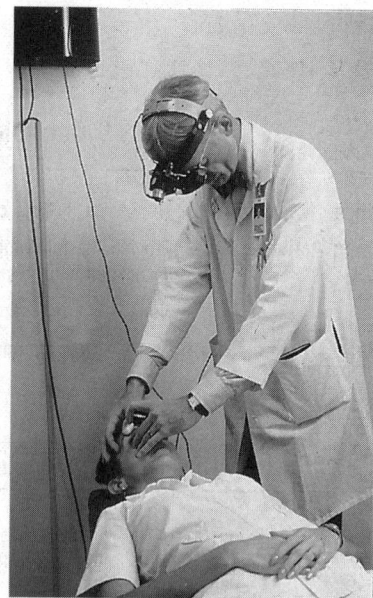

Figure 19-5. Ocular examination using the indirect ophthalmoscope. (Courtesy of Ophthalmic Photography at the W.K. Kellogg Eye Center, University of Michigan, Ann Arbor, MI.)

NURSE ADVISORY

The cornea remains anesthetized for 15 to 20 minutes after the instillation of a topical anesthetic. Advise the person not to rub the eye or scratch the eyelid during this time.

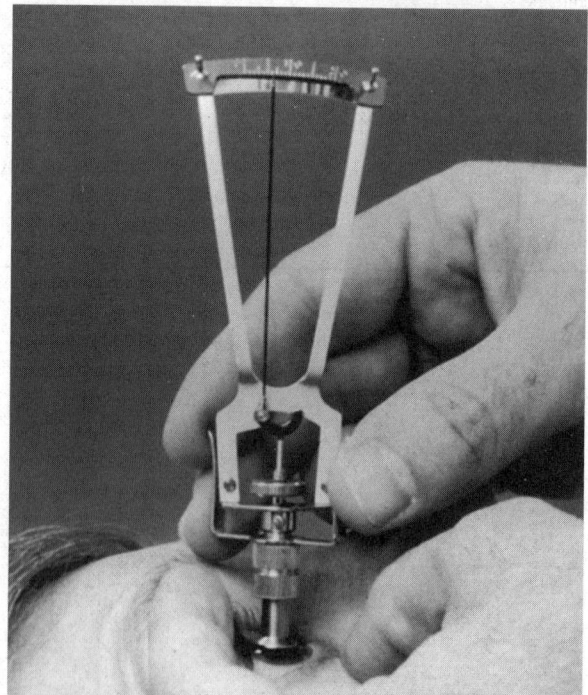

Figure 19-6. Measuring intraocular pressure with a Schiotz tonometer. (From Black JM, and Matassarin-Jacobs E. [eds]. *Luckmann and Sorensen's Medical-Surgical Nursing: A Psychophysiologic Approach.* 4th ed. Philadelphia: WB Saunders, 1993, p 842.)

No anesthetic agent is needed. Results are indicated on a digital screen.

(3) Pneumotonometer. Measures intraocular pressure through the tip of an instrument momentarily touched to the cornea. Topical anesthesia is necessary. Results are indicated on a digital screen.

(4) Applanation tonometer. Measures the amount of force needed to flatten the cornea by a standard amount of pressure (Fig. 19–7). Topical anesthesia is necessary. The measurement on the drum of the instrument is multiplied by 10 to obtain results in millimeters of mercury.

10. Biomicroscope or slit-lamp examination

 a. Provides a magnified view of the external ocular structures, the cornea, the anterior chamber, the iris, and the angle structures to the depth of the anterior vitreous with the use of an adjustable slit beam of light (Fig. 19–8).

 b. Under the highest magnification, the presence of red blood cells, white blood cells, and protein may be visualized. Cells and flare are noted as 0 to 4 +.

 c. The person sits with the head on a chin bar and head strap for stability.

 d. The examiner looks at each eye through the microscope and controls the light beam and magnification.

 e. Fluorescein dye, applied from a paper strip, is used to detect corneal defects. A cobalt (blue) light enhances the staining effects so that irregularities may be visualized.

 f. Hruby lens: A 55-diopter lens held in front of the

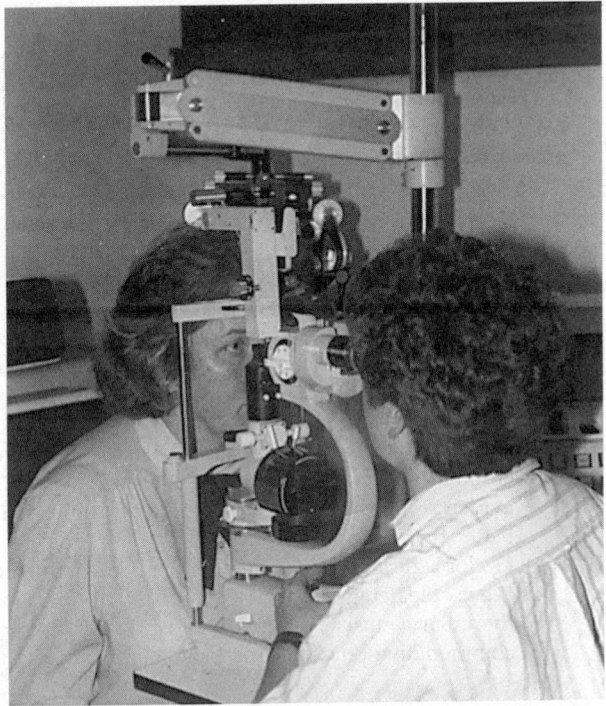

Figure 19–8. Ocular examination at the slit-lamp biomicroscope. (From Ignatavicius DD, Workman ML, and Mishler MA [eds]. *Medical-Surgical Nursing: A Nursing Process Approach.* 2nd ed, Vol 2. Philadelphia: WB Saunders, 1995, p 1306.)

person's eye permits examination of the vitreous body and the fundus with a round beam of light.

 g. Fundus contact lens: The eye is anesthetized, and the lens is coated with a drop or 2 of methylcellulose. By eliminating air between the lens and the eye, the fundus can be visualized with less irregularity.

 h. Pachymeter—an attachment to the slit lamp that measures the thickness of the cornea and the depth of the anterior chamber.

 i. Goniolens—a mirrored lens that allows the examiner to view the angle structures, the ciliary body, and the peripheral retina.

11. Refraction

 a. As it passes through the cornea and lens of the eye, light is bent or refracted. Refraction results in the focusing of images on the retina of the eye, permitting vision.

 b. Refraction is also a method used to characterize and quantify optical errors of the eye and their correction with glasses or contact lenses. Refraction distinguishes between blurred vision caused by refractive error (due to myopia, hyperopia, or astigmatism) and abnormalities or disorders of the visual system.

 c. Refractometry measures refractive error alone. Refraction determines which lens or lenses (if any) should be used to correct refractive error.

 d. Physical optics affecting vision and correction of visual refractive errors include the following:

 (1) Wavelength of light

 (2) Frequency of light waves

 (3) Velocity of light waves

 (4) Refraction index

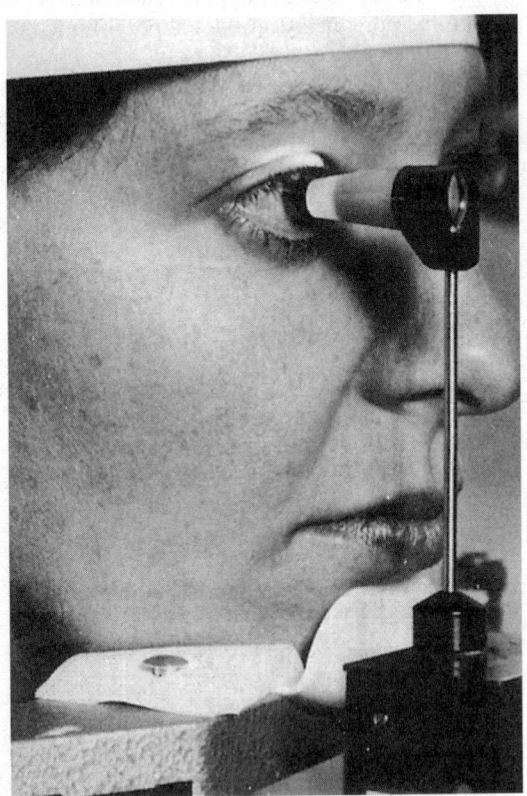

Figure 19–7. Measuring intraocular pressure with an applanation tonometer. (From Vaughan D, Asbury T, and Riordan-Eva P. *General Ophthalmology.* 13th ed. Norwalk, CT: Appleton & Lange, 1992.)

(5) Electromagnetic radiation energy
(6) Loss of light by reflection or absorption
(7) Color of light
(8) Reflection
(9) Refraction of light
e. Refraction techniques
  (1) Retinoscopy—a hand-held instrument that focuses a beam of light onto the retina. The examiner adjusts the plus or minus lens power until reflex created by the light does not move (indicates neutralization of refractive error).
  (2) Subjective refraction. Begins with information obtained with retinoscopy. Requires person to indicate whether added lenses make vision better or worse.
  (3) Automated refraction. Computerized equipment eliminates examiner involvement and bias. No evidence indicates that the automated refractor is better than retinoscopy and subjective refraction.
  (4) Cycloplegic refraction. The eyes are dilated with a cycloplegic agent, which temporarily paralyzes the ciliary muscle. Cycloplegia rules out the accommodative power of the lens fibers.

Special Diagnostic Tests

1. Special studies used to diagnose loss of vision include a variety of tests that may be performed in an office or a clinic, radiographic techniques requiring complex equipment, and diagnostic photography.
2. Nursing responsibilities
   a. Provide the individual with accurate and understandable information about the prescribed test (purpose and procedure).
   b. Schedule the test.
   c. Inform the individual of any necessary preparations (adjustment in diet or medications or need for transportation).
   d. Promote maximum emotional and physical comfort for the individual.
3. Office or clinic tests
   a. Contrast sensitivity
     (1) Tests the ability of the eye to discern subtle degrees of contrast.
     (2) The inability to detect subtle degrees of contrast may be caused by retinal disease, optic nerve disease, or clouding of the optic media (corneal disorders and cataract).
     (3) Contrast sensitivity may become decreased before visual acuity, as indicated by the Snellen test, is affected.
     (4) The individual is evaluated by reading a chart of circles with thick to thin lines that gradually fade into the background.
     (5) Because light affects contrast, the light in the room must be standardized and measured with a light meter.
   b. Glare testing or brightness acuity testing
     (1) Tests the ability to see in the presence of bright light.

(2) Cloudiness of the cornea and cataract disperse rays of light rather than focus them.
(3) The individual is evaluated by reading the Snellen chart through a device that simulates bright light.
c. Amsler grid
  (1) A hand-held chart of vertical and horizontal graph lines (Fig. 19–9).
  (2) Used to test central 20 degrees of visual field.
  (3) A blank spot or missing area of the chart when viewed (scotoma) may indicate age-related macular degeneration or optic nerve disease.
  (4) Wavy distortion of the lines (metamorphopsia) can indicate macular edema or submacular fluid.
  (5) The grid chart can be sent home with the individual to evaluate changes in vision over time.
d. Exophthalmometry
  (1) Measures the distance between the bony orbital rim and the tip of the cornea.
  (2) The examiner uses a hand-held device with a scale and mirrors to measure the distance in millimeters.
  (3) The normal distance ranges from 12 to 20 mm.
  (4) This measurement evaluates the forward protrusion of the eye (exophthalmos) in orbital hemorrhage, neoplasm, inflammation, or edema.
e. Ophthalmodynamometry
  (1) Measures pressure in the ophthalmic artery and the internal carotid artery.
  (2) Both eyes must be dilated and anesthetized.
  (3) The individual is seated while 1 examiner presses the tip of the ophthalmodynamometer on the bulbar conjunctiva at the temporal horizontal meridian of the eyeball. The other examiner visualizes the retinal vessels. The examiner holding the ophthalmodynamometer gradually increases the pressure until the other examiner observes a pulsation in the central retinal artery. Pressure on

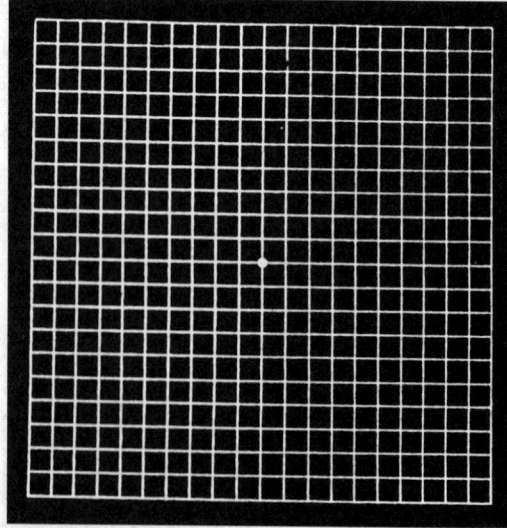

Figure 19–9. Amsler grid. (From Vaughan D, Asbury T, and Riordan-Eva P. *General Ophthalmology.* 13th ed. Norwalk, CT: Appleton & Lange, 1992.)

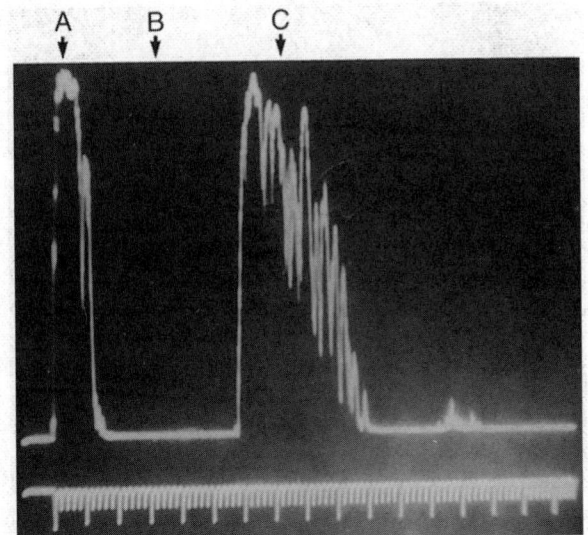

Figure 19–10. Normal A-scan ultrasonography reading. A, Cornea and lens; B, vitreous; C, retina and choroid. (From Black JM, and Matassarin-Jacobs E [eds]. *Luckmann and Sorensen's Medical-Surgical Nursing: A Psychophysiologic Approach.* 4th ed. Philadelphia: WB Saunders, 1993, p 843.)

the conjunctiva is gradually continued until the pulsing of the artery ceases. The 1st reading is the diastolic pressure, and the 2nd is the systolic pressure.
  (4) The readings are recorded in grams.
  (5) A pressure difference of 20 percent or more in the diastolic pressure between the 2 eyes is considered significant.
  (6) Carotid insufficiency may be indicated on the side with the lower pressure.
  (7) Useful in the neurologic evaluation of individuals who complain of "blackout" vision (amaurosis fugax) in 1 eye, spells of weakness on 1 side of the body, or other symptoms of transient ischemic attacks.
  (8) The test is often performed along with angiography and ultrasonography of the carotid arteries.
 f. Ultrasonography
  (1) Evaluates structures of the eye and orbit.
  (2) The eye must be anesthetized.
  (3) A probe containing both the transmitter and the receiver of the sound waves is placed directly on the eye. Various structures in the path of the sound waves reflect separate echoes back toward the probe.
  (4) Findings are visible on an oscilloscope and are captured with a photograph.
  (5) There are 2 methods of clinical ultrasonography: A scan (Fig. 19–10) and B scan. *A scan:* Each returning echo is displayed as a spike on the graph; used most often to measure the distance from the cornea to the retina (axial length). *B scan:* The probe is swept across the eye to give a spatial or 2-dimensional picture; used most often to provide clues to tumor character and location.
 g. Electroretinography

  (1) Measures the electrical response of the retina caused by a diffuse flash of light.
  (2) Reveals disease affecting either the rods or the cones, or both.
  (3) Electrodes are incorporated into a contact lens, which is placed on the anesthetized eye.
  (4) The eyes must be held still during the examination.
  (5) Loss of electrical activity occurs in retained iron, foreign body in the eye, retinitis pigmentosa, vitamin A deficiency, night blindness, and color blindness.
 h. Visual evoked response
  (1) Measures electrical response of the retina resulting from a visual stimulus.
  (2) Scalp electrodes are placed over the occipital cortex.
  (3) The entire visual pathway between the retina and the cortex must be intact to produce a normal reading.
  (4) Objectively evaluates infants and unresponsive individuals.
  (5) An abnormal visual evoked response may indicate poor central visual acuity.
4. Radiographic tests—Computed tomography scans and radiographs are useful in the evaluation of neoplasm, inflammatory masses, fractures, extraocular muscle enlargement associated with Graves' disease, and detection of a foreign body.
5. Magnetic resonance imaging (Fig. 19–11)
 a. Multidimensional views of the eye and orbit are possible.
 b. The individual is not exposed to ionizing radiation.
 c. Used to image edema, trauma, areas of demyelination, and vascular lesions.
 d. Should not be used in the presence of a ferromagnetic foreign body such as a BB.
6. Diagnostic photography

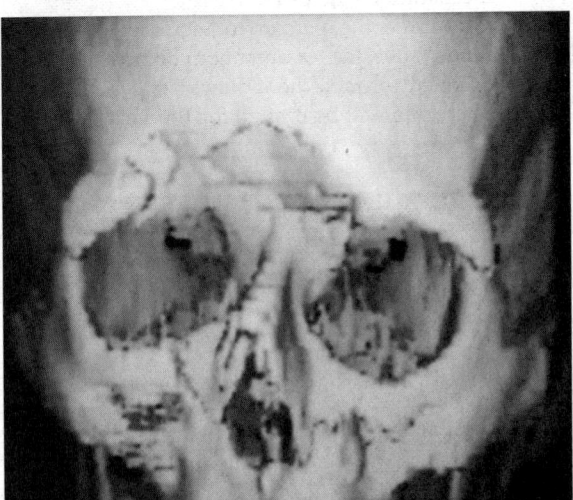

Figure 19–11. Magnetic resonance imaging view. (From Black JM, and Matassarin-Jacobs E [eds]. *Luckmann and Sorensen's Medical-Surgical Nursing: A Psychophysiologic Approach.* 4th ed. Philadelphia: WB Saunders, 1993, p 843.)

a. Fundus photography (see Color Fig. 19–1)
   (1) A camera capable of focusing on the fundus takes a color slide for detailed observation of changes over time.
   (2) The eye must be dilated.
   (3) Most often used to evaluate optic nerve and glaucomatous changes.
b. Specular micrography (Fig. 19–12).
   (1) Evaluates the endothelial surface of the cornea.
   (2) A camera is mounted on a microscope, which focuses on the endothelial layer and magnifies it.
   (3) Because endothelial cells are not regenerated, assessment of the density may indicate ability to heal after cataract or transplant surgery.
c. Fluorescein angiography (Fig. 19–13)
   (1) A rapid sequence of fundus photographs, which document the perfusion of the retinal and choroidal vessels with radiopaque dye.
   (2) Used for documenting changes in diabetic retinopathy.
   (3) The eyes must be dilated.
   (4) The procedure is considered invasive because the fluorescein dye is injected into a vein in the arm.
   (5) Individuals who are allergic to other dyes used in intravenous pyelogram or cholangiogram should be observed carefully or given prophylactic diphenhydramine.

NURSE ADVISORY

Emergency life support equipment should be close at hand to manage occasional vasovagal and possible anaphylactic reactions.

   (6) The person may experience a warm sensation when the dye is injected.
   (7) The person will also experience rapid bright flashes of light from the camera and hear the mechanics of the camera.
   (8) Encourage the person to increase the intake of fluids after the examination because the dye is excreted through the kidneys.
   (9) The urine will be orange for the next 24 hours.

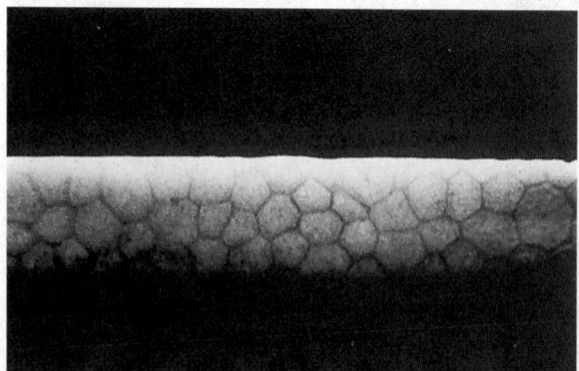

Figure 19–12. Specular micrography. (Courtesy of Ophthalmic Photography at the W.K. Kellogg Eye Center, University of Michigan, Ann Arbor, MI.)

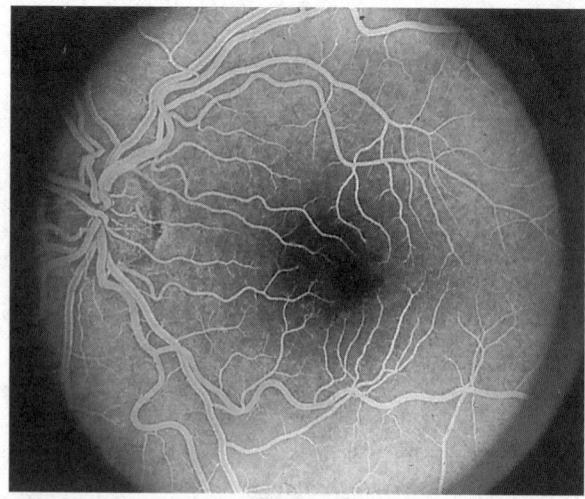

Figure 19–13. Normal fluorescein angiography. (Courtesy of Ophthalmic Photography at the W.K. Kellogg Eye Center, University of Michigan, Ann Arbor, MI.)

   (10) Some people may notice a yellow tinge to the skin and sclera.

◼ REFRACTIVE DISORDERS

Definition

1. Refractive disorders are abnormalities of refraction that occur in the eye (Fig. 19–14).
2. The 3 major types of refractive disorders are as follows:
   a. Myopia, or nearsightedness
   b. Hyperopia, or farsightedness
   c. Astigmatism

Etiology

1. Myopia is usually caused by an eyeball that is longer than normal. This trait may be genetically transmitted.
2. Temporary myopia may result from the administration of some medications (e.g., sulfonamides, acetazolamide, salicylates, and steroids), and it may accompany influenza, typhoid fever, severe dehydration, and large intake of antacids.
3. Hyperopia is caused by an eyeball that is shorter than normal or from a cornea that is less curved than normal.
4. Astigmatism arises when the curvature of the cornea is not perfectly spheric. As a result, the cornea cannot bend the rays of light equally in all directions, and images are not properly focused.

Clinical Manifestations

1. Myopia—the person has poor distance vision.
2. Hyperopia—the person has difficulty doing close work or reading and may suffer from eyestrain, headaches, or both as a result.

REFRACTIVE DISORDERS AND CORRECTION

EMMETROPIA
No optical correction is needed because the eye is naturally in optimal focus.

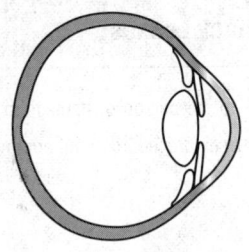

AMETROPIA
Corrective lenses are necessary to bring the eye to a state of optimal focus.
Some forms of ametropia are:

Myopia, nearsightedness, occurs when the focused image is formed in front of the plane of the retina.

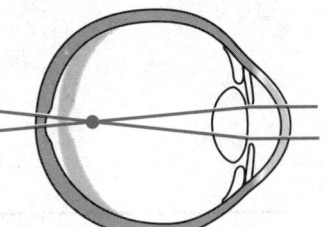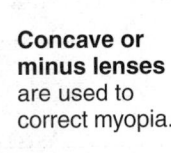

Hyperopia, also called farsightedness, occurs when the focused image is formed behind the plane of the retina.

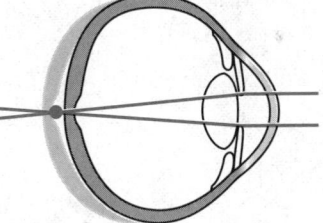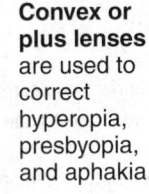

Astigmatism prevents light rays from focusing on the retina owing to the irregular shape of the cornea or lens.

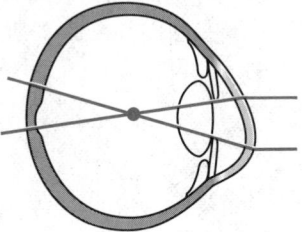

Prism lenses are used to correct extraocular muscle imbalance.
Aphakia is the absence of the lens after removal for cataract.
Anisometropia means that a different refractive error exists in each eye.
Presbyopia is the inability of the lens fibers to accommodate from far to near vision owing to the aging process.

TYPES OF CORRECTIVE LENSES

Lens power is measured in diopters (the reciprocal to the focal length of the lens in meters).

Concave or minus lenses are used to correct myopia.

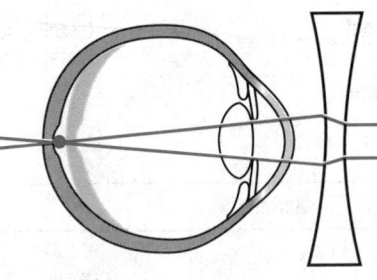

Convex or plus lenses are used to correct hyperopia, presbyopia, and aphakia.

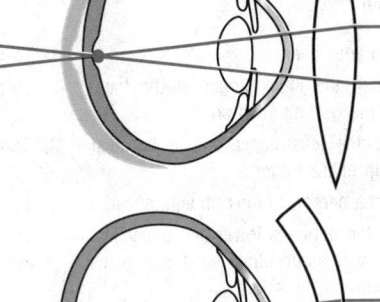

Toric lenses are used to correct astigmatism.

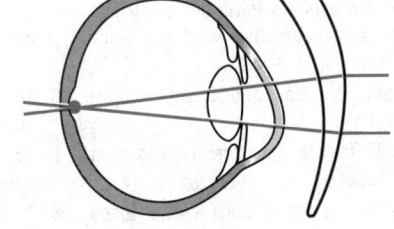

Figure 19–14.

3. Astigmatism—the person has poor distance vision and has difficulty seeing close objects.

Intervention

1. Corrective lenses (see Fig. 19–14)
   a. Myopia—concave or minus lenses
   b. Hyperopia—convex or plus lenses
   c. Astigmatism—toric lenses
   d. Procedure 19–10 provides instructions for inserting and removing contact lenses
2. Medical-surgical procedures
   a. Radial keratotomy

(1) This elective surgical intervention is used to correct some cases of myopia and to reduce or eliminate the need for myopic refractive correction.
(2) In one procedure, the surgeon makes 8 partial-thickness incisions into the cornea with a diamond blade to flatten the curvature of the cornea.
(3) Surgical risks include unsatisfactory correction, corneal glare, and postoperative infection.
(4) Radial keratotomy was once controversial, but owing to its success in correcting myopia, is now accepted widely.
   b. Excimer laser surgery
(1) The excimer laser has recently been approved by

Procedure 19–10
Inserting and Removing Contact Lenses

Definition/Purpose	To insert or remove contact lenses without injury to the person or damage to the lenses
Contraindications/Cautions	Do not insert contact lenses after eye surgery or laser procedures until approved by the ophthalmologist.
Learning/Teaching Activities	Describe the procedure to the person.

Preliminary Activities

Equipment	• Cleaning solution • Storage case
Procedure	

Actions	Rationale/Discussion

HARD CONTACT LENSES

Insertion

1. Wash your hands.
2. Moisten the index finger of the hand with the wetting solution.
3. Place the lens concave side up near the tip of the finger.
4. Ask the person to look straight ahead.
5. Hold the person's lower and upper lids open with your other hand and place the lens on the sclera.
6. Steady the lens and slowly remove your finger.
7. Gently release the lower lid and then the upper lid.
8. Ask the person to blink several times to be sure that the lens is on the cornea.

1. To remove surface microorganisms
2. To provide a surface for the lens
3. Correct position for insertion
4. To position the eye to receive the lens
5. To bring the lens in contact with the eye
6. To leave the lens in the correct position
7. To prevent the lens from being dislodged
8. To prevent accidental loss of the lens

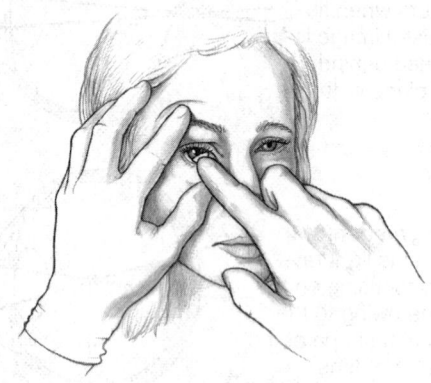

Removal

1. Wash your hands.
2. Fill the lens case with storage solution.
3. Place a towel on the person's chest.
4. Ask the person to look straight ahead and open eyes wide.
5. Place one forefinger on the lower lid and the other on the upper lid.
6. Gently press toward the edges of the contact lens.
7. Ask the person to blink.
8. Place the lens in the correct side of the case.

1. To remove surface microorganisms
2. To keep the lenses moist
3. To prevent loss of a lens
5. To force the lens away from the cornea and onto your hand
7. The lens should dislodge
8. To ensure that the lenses are correctly identified

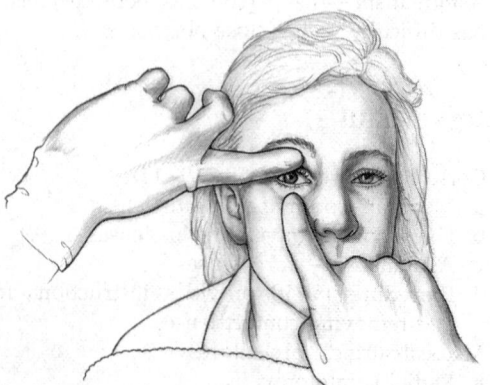

P

Procedure 19–10

(continued)

Actions	Rationale/Discussion

SOFT CONTACT LENSES

Insertion

1. Wash your hands.
2. Moisten the index finger of your hand with the wetting solution.
3. Place the lens concave side up near the tip of the finger.
4. Ask the person to look straight ahead.
5. Hold the person's lower and upper lids open with your other hand and place the lens on the sclera.
6. Steady the lens and slowly remove your finger.
7. Gently release the lower lid and then the upper lid.
8. Ask the person to blink several times to be sure that the lens is on the cornea.

1. To remove surface microorganisms
2. To provide a surface for the lens
3. Correct position for insertion
4. To position the eye to receive the lens
5. To bring the lens in contact with the eye
6. To leave the lens in the correct position
7. To prevent the lens from being dislodged
8. To prevent accidental loss of the lens

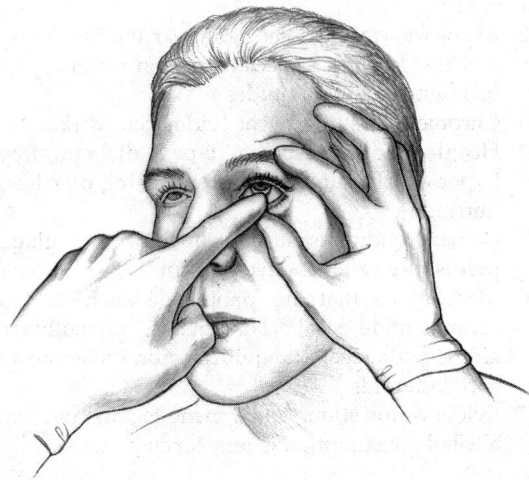

Removal

1. Wash your hands.
2. Fill the lens case with storage solution.
3. Place a towel on the chest of the person.
4. Instruct the person to look up.
5. Pull the person's lower lid down and hold the upper lid open with one hand.
6. Gently touch the sclera with the other forefinger and pull down.
7. Capture the lens between the thumb and forefinger.
8. Place the lens in the correct side of the case.

1. To remove surface microorganisms
2. To keep the lenses moist between wearings
3. To prevent loss of a lens
4. To position the eye to facilitate removal
5. To maximize exposure of the lens
6. Touching the sclera is less sensitive than touching the cornea
7. To secure the lens
8. To ensure that the lenses are correctly identified

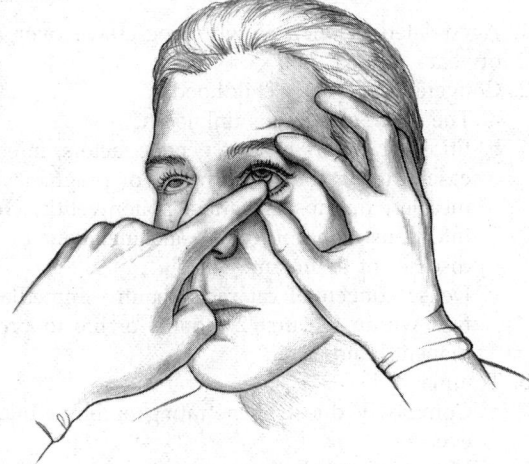

the U.S. Food and Drug Administration for the correction of myopia.

(2) The excimer laser can shave precise cell layers from the corneal surface. This process reshapes the cornea, which improves vision without involving the highly sensitive deeper corneal cells.

■ *CATARACT*

Definition

An opacity of the crystalline lens resulting in visual disturbance (see Color Fig. 19–2).

Incidence and Socioeconomic Impact

1. The most prevalent visually disabling eye disease in the world.
2. Ninety-five percent of persons older than 65 years of age have some degree of lens opacity.
3. More than 1.35 million cataract extractions are performed in the United States each year.

Risk Factors

1. Age
2. Exposure to ultraviolet light over the life span
   a. Outside work, especially out on water
   b. Living at high altitudes
3. Chronic exposure to heat (industrial workers)
4. Health conditions such as type II diabetes, hypertension, hypocalcemia, uremia, life-threatening diarrhea, and malnutrition
5. Ocular conditions such as myopia and glaucoma may predispose cataract development
6. Medications that are phototoxic such as tetracyclines, sulfanilamides, salicylanilamides, phenothiazines, thiazides, psoralens, tranquilizers, oral contraceptives, and corticosteroids
7. Evidence for ethnic and genetic factors and smoking and alcohol consumption is less conclusive.

Etiology

1. Age-related (senile): Slowly progressive over a number of years.
2. Congenital and early childhood
   a. The cause of many is unknown.
   b. Etiologic factors include genetic factors, infectious diseases during the 1st trimester of pregnancy (German measles, mumps, hepatitis, poliomyelitis, chickenpox, infectious mononucleosis), and metabolic or infectious diseases of the infant.
   c. Dense congenital cataracts require immediate extraction within the first 2 months of life to prevent permanent blindness.
3. Trauma
   a. Commonly due to penetrating or blunt injury to the eye.
   b. May also result from overexposure to heat (glassblowers' cataract), x-rays, and radioactive materials or from ingestion of toxic chemicals.

Pathophysiology

1. Because it is encapsulated, the lens is unable to shed dead cells. Over the life span, the lens becomes more dense.
2. Changes in the molecular structure of the cells causes whitish opacities to appear.

3. Ultraviolet radiation causes an increase in the development of fluorescent substances.
4. Along with the increasing density and opacity of the lens, the ability of the lens to absorb ultraviolet light actually protects the retina from light damage. When the lens absorbs ultraviolet light, there is a fluorescent reaction, which results in the yellowing of the lens.

Clinical Manifestations

1. Subjective
   a. Increased glare in bright light
   b. Blurred or distorted images
   c. Altered color perception (the yellowing of the lens acts as a light filter)
   d. Difficulty with night driving
   e. Behavioral changes in children
2. Objective
   a. Reduced visual acuity
   b. Visible opacity of the lens in ophthalmoscopic examination
   c. Leukokoria or "white pupil" is seen only in advanced stages of cataract.

Diagnostics

1. History
   a. Determine the presence of risk factors in the individual's lifestyle.
   b. Assess the individual's cultural and personal beliefs about cataracts and vision loss.
2. Physical assessment
   a. Visual acuity
   b. Penlight examination of pupil and lens
   c. Direct ophthalmoscopy
   d. Slit-lamp biomicroscopy
   e. Refraction and retinoscopy
   f. Glare testing
   g. Contrast sensitivity
3. Medical diagnosis
   a. The decision to perform cataract surgery is made after assessing the following:
      (1) The effect of the cataract on the individual's vision
      (2) The individual's visual needs
      (3) Consideration of risks and benefits associated with surgery
   b. Surgical removal of a cataract is not necessary solely because a cataract is present.

Clinical Management

1. The goal is to restore visual acuity.
2. Pharmacologic intervention: Mydriatic agents may improve vision temporarily in the early stages of cataract development. Pupil dilation can increase vision when the cataract is a small central opacity.

3. Special medical-surgical procedures: Surgical intervention to remove the cataract may be performed using 1 of 3 techniques (Fig. 19–15).
   a. Phacoemulsification and aspiration
      (1) Length of scleral incision is based on whether an intraocular lens implant (IOL) is to be inserted and if so, what type. The IOLs are supplied by a variety of manufacturers in various shapes and designs. Most IOLs require an incision of 7.0 to 7.5 mm. Foldable-style IOLs require an incision of 3.0 to 3.5 mm. The complication rate is much lower for posterior IOLs than for anterior IOLs.

      (2) A titanium needle vibrating at ultrasonic frequencies disrupts the lens nucleus.
      (3) The anterior capsule and lens particles are removed from the eye by irrigation and aspiration through a sleeve around the needle.
      (4) The posterior capsule is left intact to support an IOL.
      (5) The incision may be closed with 1 to 3 sutures or none at all.
   b. Extracapsular cataract extraction
      (1) Instruments are used to remove the anterior capsule and the lens manually.
      (2) The posterior capsule is left intact to support an IOL.
      (3) The incision is usually closed with 1 to 3 sutures.
   c. Intracapsular cataract extraction
      (1) Supporting zonules are dissolved with the enzyme α-chymotrypsin.
      (2) Instruments are used to remove the entire lens and capsule manually.
      (3) Intracapsular cataract extraction is infrequently used because posterior chamber IOLs cannot be supported.

Complications

1. Without surgical intervention, blindness and glaucoma often occur.
2. Postoperative complications include the following:
   a. Posterior capsule opacification
      (1) Frequency of occurrence is higher than 50 percent.
      (2) Forms as the result of remnant or regenerated lens cells. Obstructs vision in the same way as a cataract.
      (3) Often referred to as "after cataract" or "secondary membrane."
      (4) Capsulotomy must be performed to provide a clear visual pathway. Opacity may be effectively excised by neodymium:yttrium-aluminum-garnet (Nd:YAG) laser in an office procedure. May also be removed with a surgical procedure.
3. Other complications that may arise after cataract extraction include the following:
   a. Cystoid macular edema
   b. Pseudophakic bullous keratopathy
   c. Secondary glaucoma
   d. Retinal detachment
   e. Postoperative astigmatism
   f. Postoperative infection
   g. Strabismus

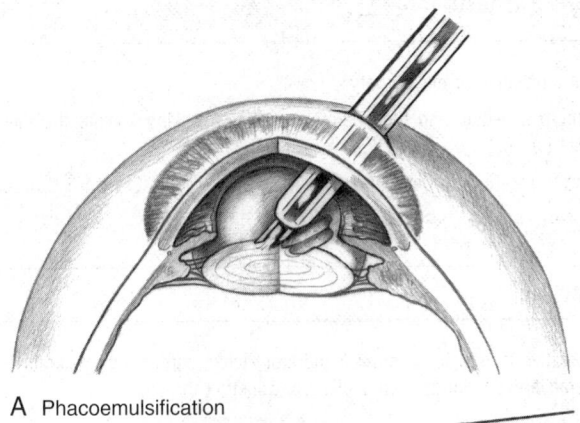

A Phacoemulsification

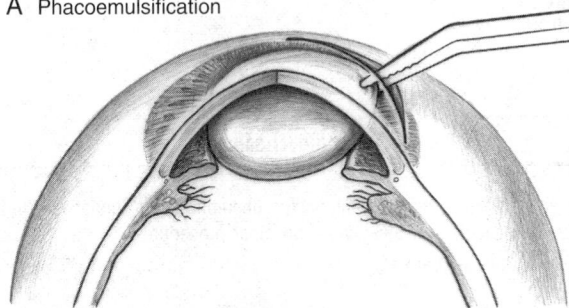

B Intracapsular cataract extraction

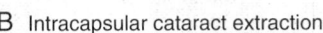

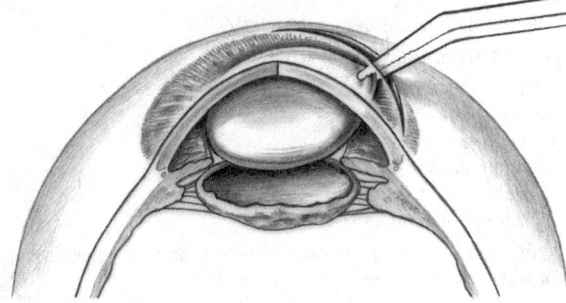

C Extracapsular cataract extraction

Figure 19–15. Surgical techniques for cataract extraction. In phacoemulsification, the lens is aspirated through a series of "scoops."

Prognosis

1. Cataract surgery is a highly successful procedure. Individuals can expect an increase in well-being and quality of life 90 to 95 percent of the time when there are no other complicating eye disorders.

2. Positive outcomes after cataract surgery include the following:
   a. Increased ability to read or do close work
   b. Increased ability to perform activities of daily living
   c. Increased mobility and ability to avoid injury
   d. Increased independence and sense of well-being
   e. Reduced glare disability
   f. Improved depth perception

Applying the Nursing Process

> **NURSING DIAGNOSIS:** Knowledge deficit R/T causes of cataracts and risks and benefits regarding cataract surgery

1. *Expected outcomes:* Following instruction, the individual should be able to do the following:
   a. Describe the causative factors and slow progression of cataract development.
   b. Determine whether the inconvenience and level of disability is greater than the risk associated with surgical intervention.
2. *Nursing interventions* (Procedures 19–11 and 19–12)
   a. Assess the person's current level of knowledge about cataracts and surgery (see Chapter 13).
   b. Discuss visual impairment and limitations in activities of daily living (e.g., working, reading, watching television, driving, cooking, cleaning)
   c. Discuss risks of surgery and anesthesia as well as benefits of surgery.

Procedure 19–11
General Preoperative Care for
Persons Having Eye Surgery

Definition/Purpose	To appropriately and adequately prepare an individual for eye surgery
Contraindications/Cautions	Confirm with the person, the operating room schedule and the operative permit. Checking against the medical record, confirm which eye is the correct eye for surgery.
Learning/Teaching Activities	Ask the person to tell you about the surgical procedure to determine the level of knowledge. Explain and describe any additional information.

Preliminary Activities

Assessment/Planning	• Review the medical record for any preoperative tests or procedures (laboratory tests, photography, examination). • Review the physician's orders for preoperative eye medications (to dilate or constrict the pupil).
Preparation of the Person **Procedure**	The person should be relaxed and comfortable.

Actions	Rationale/Discussion
1. Ask the person to remove all underwear and change into a hospital gown.	1. If an emergency occurs while in the operating room, underwear prohibits the placement of EKG leads and other procedures.
2. Describe the events as they will take place in the operating room, including what will be seen and heard.	2. To allay fear and anxiety.
3. Describe the type of anesthesia and what the person will feel.	3. To avoid surprise or discomfort.
4. Document complete vital signs.	4. Baseline documentation.
5. Instill any eye medications and any other preoperative medication.	5. To prepare the eye and person for surgery.
6. Be sure the person voids when put on call for the operating room.	6. To avoid the need to void during surgery.
7. Review the routine operating room checklist: • ID band on • Dentures removed • Jewelry removed • Hearing aid removed • Note pacemaker or prosthesis	7. To ensure preoperative preparation: • Correct person • Safety precaution • Safety precaution • Avoid damage from preparation solution • To alert operating room staff
8. Review postoperative plan of care, including the following: • Pain and nausea control • Diet • Activity • Eye care	8. To provide a baseline of knowledge so that the information is not new immediately after surgery.
9. Ask the person if there are any anticipated problems with care at home.	9. To allow as much time as possible for problem solving.

Procedure 19–12
General Postoperative Care of the
Person Having Eye Surgery

Definition/Purpose — To provide appropriate and adequate postoperative care after eye surgery

Contraindications/Cautions — Although the operative site is small and the effects of the surgery may seem localized, the nurse should anticipate and observe for both ocular and systemic problems.

Learning/Teaching Activities — Review the postoperative plan of care as described before surgery as well as any alterations.

Procedure

Actions	Rationale/Discussion
1. Take vital signs immediately on return.	1. To determine status.
2. Assess comfort level.	2. Medicate if necessary.
3. Review the physician's orders for postoperative care.	3. To provide appropriate care as ordered.
4. Evaluate the eye dressing for drainage.	4. Note on chart and report any unusual amounts.
5. Assist the person to the bathroom.	5. Person may be unsteady.
6. Obtain a snack or meal for the person.	6. Ensure adequate intake.
7. Discontinue intravenous line if able to tolerate fluids or food.	7. Wait until you are sure the person is stable before discontinuing the line.
8. Review postoperative plan of care in detail with person and with family member.	8. Allow for questions.

d. Describe preparation, surgical procedure, and postoperative course.
e. Allow the individual time to absorb this information and make a decision.

NURSING DIAGNOSIS: Risk for infection R/T surgical incision and self-care after surgery

1. *Expected outcomes:* Following instruction, the person should be able to do the following:
   a. Properly self-administer eye medications.
   b. Cleanse the area around the eye.
2. *Nursing interventions*
   a. Explain the action and importance of eye medications.
   b. Demonstrate eye drop instillation technique and instillation of ophthalmic ointment (Procedures 19–13 and 19–14).

Procedure 19–13
Instillation of Eye Drops

Definition/Purpose — To instill topical medication into the eye

Contraindications/Cautions — Do not touch the tip of the bottle to any part of the eye.
O.D. (Oculus dexter) = right eye
O.S. (Oculus sinister) = left eye
O.U. (Oculus uterque) = both eyes

Learning/Teaching Activities — Provide the following information: (a) describe the procedure; (b) explain that the drop may feel cool to the eye.

Preliminary Activities

Assessment/Planning
• Check the name of the person.
• Check the name of the medication against the physician's order.
• Check the dose of the medication.
• Check the correct eye.
• Check the expiration date of the medication.

Preparation of the Person — The person should be lying or sitting.

Procedure

Procedure continued on following page

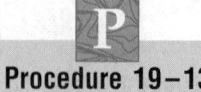

Procedure 19–13

(continued)

Actions	Rationale/Discussion
1. Wash your hands.	1. To remove surface microorganisms
2. Use gloves if secretions are present.	2. Universal precautions
3. Ask the person to tilt the head backward, open the eyes, and look up.	3. To position the head properly
4. Gently pull the lower lid downward against the cheekbone.	4. To create a pocket into which the eye drop will be placed
5. Instill the eye drop.	
6. Instruct the person to close the eyes.	6. To distribute the medication
7. If necessary to inhibit systemic absorption of the medication, press the inner canthus firmly with the forefinger for 5 minutes.	7. To block the upper and lower canaliculi. Excess medication spills out of the eye instead of running down into the nose where it is absorbed by the nasal mucosa.

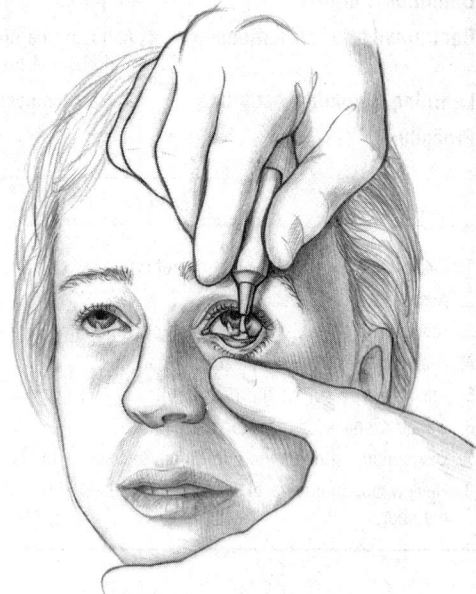

NURSE ADVISORY

When multiple eye drops are prescribed to be given simultaneously, *5 minutes* should be allotted between drops to allow for adequate ocular absorption, for tearing to diminish, and for prevention of washout of the first medication by the second.

c. Ask patient or family member to return the demonstration.
d. Explain cross-contamination and the importance of the tissue integrity of a wound.

NURSING DIAGNOSIS: Risk for injury R/T sensory deficit while operative eye is patched

Procedure 19–14
Instillation of Ophthalmic Ointment

Definition/Purpose	To instill ointment into the eye
Contraindications/Cautions	Do not touch the tip of the tube to the eyelid.
Learning/Teaching Activities	Provide the following information: (a) describe the procedure; (b) explain that the medication may feel cool to the eye.

Preliminary Activities

Assessment/Planning	• Check the name of the person. • Check the name of the medication against the physician's order. • Check the dose of the medication. • Check the correct eye. • Check the expiration date of the medication.
Preparation of the Person	• The person should be lying or sitting.
Procedure	

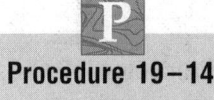

Procedure 19–14
(continued)

Actions	Rationale/Discussion
1. Wash your hands.	1. To remove surface microorganisms
2. Use gloves if secretions are present.	2. Universal precautions
3. Ask the person to tilt the head backward, open the eyes, and look up.	3. To position the head properly
4. Gently pull the lower lid downward against the cheekbone.	4. To create a pocket into which the ointment will be placed
5. Squeeze a one-quarter inch ribbon of the ointment into the pocket.	
6. Instruct the person to close the eyes.	6. To distribute the medication
7. Explain that vision may be blurred for a while.	7. To prevent anxiety and injury

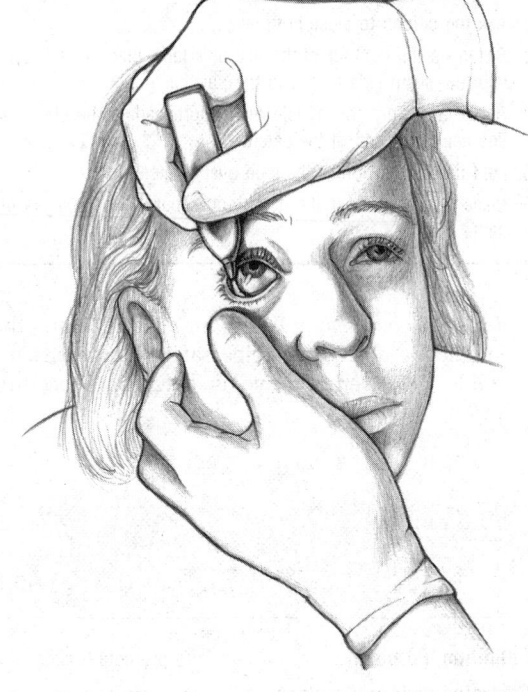

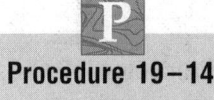

Procedure 19–15
Applying an Eye Patch and Shield

Definition/Purpose	To protect the eye from light and dust, to prevent blinking that promotes healing, and to absorb excess tears.
Contraindications/Cautions	Be sure that the eye is completely closed under the patch and cannot open. Patching the eye is usually contraindicated in the presence of infection. An eye patch worn for several days may cause temporary ptosis (drooping eyelid) due to pressure on the levator tendon.
Learning/Teaching Activities	Provide the following information: (a) describe the procedure; (b) explain the reason for the eye patch.

Preliminary Activities

Equipment	• Two eye patches • Nonallergenic ½-inch tape • Metal or plastic shield
Assessment/Planning	• Note the facial contour of the person and how deep set the eyes are. • Note the integrity and tone of the skin around the eye.
Preparation of the Person	• Person may be seated or lying down.

Procedure continued on following page

Procedure 19–15

(continued)

Actions	Rationale/Discussion
1. Wash your hands.	1. Reduce surface microorganisms.
2. Ask the person to close both eyes.	2. A corneal abrasion may result from an open eye under a patch.
3. Based on the contour of the person's face, place 1 or 2 eye patches flat with the seam side turned to the outside.	3. To promote safety and comfort.
4. Apply tape from the middle of the forehead to the cheek in a diagonal line near each end of the patch.	4. To secure the patch.
5. Fold the top portion of the tape over on itself.	5. To facilitate removal of the tape.
6. Place the shield over the patch and secure with 2 pieces of tape in the same manner.	6. To maximize protection of the eye.

1. *Expected outcomes:* Following instruction, the person should be able to describe safety alterations in behavior while the operative eye is patched (Procedures 19–15 through 19–17).

2. *Nursing interventions*
   a. Instruct the person to sleep on the unoperative side to prevent pressure on the incision.
   b. Explain reduced depth perception when 1 eye is cov-

Procedure 19–16
Applying a Pressure Patch

Definition/Purpose	To promote healing of the epithelium by prohibiting blinking
Contraindications/Cautions	Be sure that the eye is completely closed under the patch and cannot open. Patching the eye is usually contraindicated in the presence of infection. An eye patch worn for several days may cause temporary ptosis (drooping eyelid) due to pressure on the levator tendon.
Learning/Teaching Activities	Provide the following information: (a) describe the procedure; (b) explain the reason for the eye patch.

Preliminary Activities

Equipment	• Two eye patches • Nonallergenic ½-inch tape
Assessment/Planning	• Note the facial contour of the person and how deep set the eyes are. • Note the integrity and tone of the skin around the eye.
Preparation of the Person	• Person may be seated or lying down.
Procedure	

Actions	Rationale/Discussion
1. Wash your hands.	1. Reduce surface microorganisms.
2. Ask the person to close both eyes.	2. A corneal abrasion may result from an open eye under a patch.
3. Based on the contour of the person's face, fold 1 eye patch in half (short ends together) with the seam side turned inside and place over the eye. Place the 2nd patch flat over the folded patch.	3. To promote safety and comfort.
4. Pull the tape snugly so that the cheek is pulled upward.	4. If the pressure patch is appropriately applied, the corner of the mouth on that side should be higher.
5. Apply tape from the middle of the forehead to the cheek in a diagonal line. Cover the patch with overlapping pieces of tape.	5. To secure the patch.
6. Fold the top portion of the tape over on itself.	6. To facilitate removal of the tape.

P
Procedure 19–17
Applying Ocular Compresses

Definition/Purpose   To promote healing, prevent swelling, and provide comfort

Contraindications/Cautions   Always obtain a physician's order for warm or iced compresses for postoperative application.

Learning/Teaching Activities   Explain the procedure to the person.

Procedure

Actions	Rationale/Discussion
1. Wash your hands.	1. Reduce surface microorganisms.
2. For warm compresses, use a washcloth folded in fourths or 2 packages of 4 × 4 pads. Use very warm but not *hot* tap water.	2. Test the warmth on your wrist and ask the person to verify comfort level.
3. For cold compresses, use a washcloth and cold tap water, or fill 2 gloves with a small amount of chipped ice.	3. Large amounts of ice may apply too much pressure.
4. Position the compress over the closed eye.	4. To protect the cornea.
5. Secure with a plastic incontinence pad folded lengthwise and tucked behind the head.	5. To maintain warm or cold temperature as long as possible.
6. Repeat the process when the warmth or cold is no longer effective.	

ered. The individual should exercise caution in reaching for objects or other people, driving, crossing streets, and using appliances.

c. Explain the importance of not touching or rubbing the eye with the hands and of wearing a metal shield or glasses at all times.

Discharge Planning and Teaching

1. After outpatient surgery, individuals need to know the course of postoperative care, what will be experienced, and the expected outcomes (Learning/Teaching Guidelines for Self-Care After Cataract Surgery).

Public Health Considerations: Primary Prevention

1. There is no known medical cure for cataract.
2. Because it is known that the effects of ultraviolet exposure are cumulative over the life span, wearing protective eyewear and a hat or a sunshield may prevent or retard the development of cataracts.
3. Protective eyewear should be encouraged in children.

■ *GLAUCOMA*

Definition

1. Glaucoma is a group of ocular disorders characterized by the following:
   a. Increased intraocular pressure

b. Cupping and atrophy of the optic nerve head (see Color Fig. 19–3)
c. Visual field changes

Incidence and Socioeconomic Impact

1. Glaucoma is the 2nd leading cause of blindness in the United States.
2. Approximately 1 in 50 Americans older than 35 develop glaucoma.
3. Approximately 1 million Americans have glaucoma and are unaware of it.
4. The prevalence of glaucoma in Blacks between the ages of 45 and 65 is at least 5 times that of Whites of the same age range.

Risk Factors

1. Age
2. Heredity
3. Myopia
4. Diabetes mellitus
5. Ocular trauma
6. Ocular surgery
7. Topical and periocular corticosteroids

Etiology

1. Glaucoma is classified as *primary* or *secondary* to another ocular disorder.
2. It is also classified by the anatomic size of the anterior

LEARNING/TEACHING GUIDELINES
for Self-Care After Cataract Surgery

General Overview

1. Using an eye model or a cross-section picture of the eye, point out the lens, describe cataract development, and demonstrate how the lens was removed and replaced by an artificial intraocular lens.
2. Describe the healing process and the expected visual rehabilitation time frame.
3. Discuss the administration of eye drops, including the name of the medication and the rationale for use. Describe the dosage, frequency, and storage of the medication.
4. Demonstrate the instillation of the eye drops, and request a return demonstration by the person and a family member.
5. Describe how to care for the eye dressing at home and the signs and symptoms that indicate the person should notify the physician.
6. Discuss any limitation in activities.
7. Review the date and time of the next visit to the physician as well as expected future visits.

Medications

1. A combination steroid and antibiotic eye drop is usually prescribed 4 times a day in the operative eye for 1 week tapering off after 4 to 8 weeks. The medication is prescribed to reduce inflammation and prevent postoperative infection.

Healing and Visual Rehabilitation

1. Wound healing takes 6 weeks to 3 months.
2. If an intraocular lens has not been implanted, temporary cataract glasses (+10 diopters) may be used if the vision in the other eye is poor or that eye has also undergone cataract extraction without the implantation of an intraocular lens.
   a. Adjustment to these glasses involves teaching the person that the following will be evident:
      (1) A dramatic reduction in the field of vision
      (2) A 30 to 35 percent deficit in the depth perception
      (3) A circular central blind zone, which makes objects appear to jump suddenly into view.
3. Vision may be blurred or markedly improved (if an

intraocular lens is used) on the 1st day and gradually improves over the next month.
4. After 6 weeks to 3 months, glasses or contact lenses may be prescribed for correction.

Eye Dressing and Care

1. The eye is usually patched with a metal or plastic shield taped over the dressing until the next morning.
2. After the dressing is removed, either the glasses or the shield alone should be worn at all times for approximately 6 weeks to protect the eye during the healing process. Remind the individual to put on the shield at bedtime.
3. Removal of the sutures depends on the practice of the ophthalmologist and the manner in which the eye heals. Postoperative astigmatism may be improved by removing 1 or more sutures.
4. Instruct the person that any redness around the eye should gradually resolve. An increase in redness or swelling around the eye should be reported to the physician.
5. Increased tearing is normal after cataract surgery, and a small amount of dried matter may appear on the lashes in the morning or after naps. Instruct the person to use a warm washcloth to remove the matter. If purulent drainage is noted, the person should call the physician.
6. Postoperative discomfort should be relieved by acetaminophen. Unrelieved pain should be reported to the physician (may indicate an increase in intraocular pressure).
7. A sudden or noticeable decrease in vision should also be reported to the physician.

Activity

1. Some ophthalmologists advise lifting and straining restrictions, but most advise individuals to return to normal activities (excluding contact sports).

Postoperative Visits

1. Return visits are usually on the day after surgery, at 1 week, at 2 to 3 weeks, and at 2 months.

---

chamber angle: *open* (or wide) or *angle closure* (or narrow, closed) (Fig. 19–16).

Pathophysiology (see Fig. 19–16)

Clinical Manifestations

1. Primary open-angle glaucoma
   a. A silent, insidious process without discomfort or pain

b. Gradual loss of peripheral vision followed by loss of central vision in the end stage
2. Angle-closure glaucoma: may be intermittent but usually appears with the following:
   a. An acute attack of pain and blurred vision
   b. Blurred vision and rainbow halos around lights
   c. Nausea and vomiting, sometimes accompanied by abdominal pain
   d. Redness of the sclera and conjunctiva
   e. Increased intraocular pressure

PATHOPHYSIOLOGY OF GLAUCOMA

NORMAL FLOW OF AQUEOUS HUMOR

1. Aqueous humor is produced by the ciliary body and flows into the posterior chamber behind the iris.

2. It exits the eye by flowing between the iris and the lens around the pupil edge and into the anterior chamber.

3. The trabecular meshwork filters the aqueous humor into Schlemm's canal, where the fluid is picked up by the episcleral vessels and is mixed with blood.

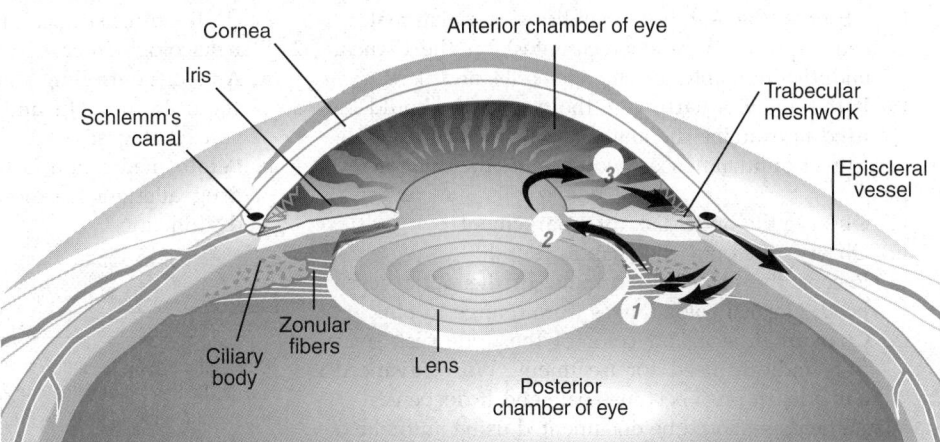

Intraocular Pressure

Intraocular pressure (IOP) is determined by the rate of aqueous humor production by the ciliary body, the resistance to aqueous outflow through the trabecular meshwork, and the level of episcleral venous pressure. It varies with diurnal cycles (the highest pressure is usually upon awakening) and with position of the body (increased when lying down). In the majority of cases, increased IOP is due to an abnormality that prevents outflow rather than an increased rate of production of aqueous. When aqueous humor production exceeds the ability of the trabecular meshwork to filter it out, the IOP inhibits the blood supply to the optic nerve and the retina, causing them to become ischemic and gradually lose function.

GLAUCOMA

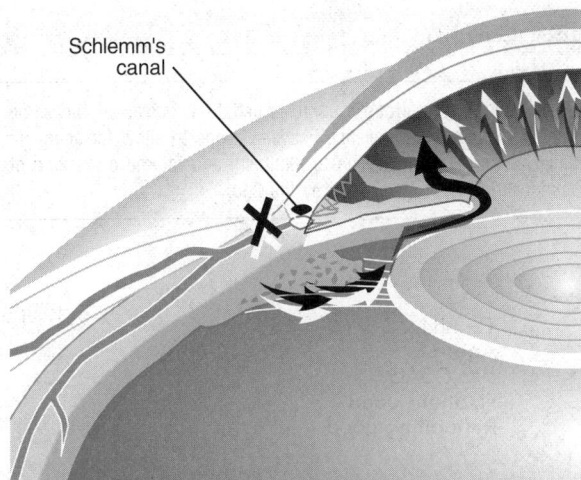

Primary open-angle glaucoma is caused by degenerative changes in the trabecular meshwork that inhibit the outflow of aqueous humor.

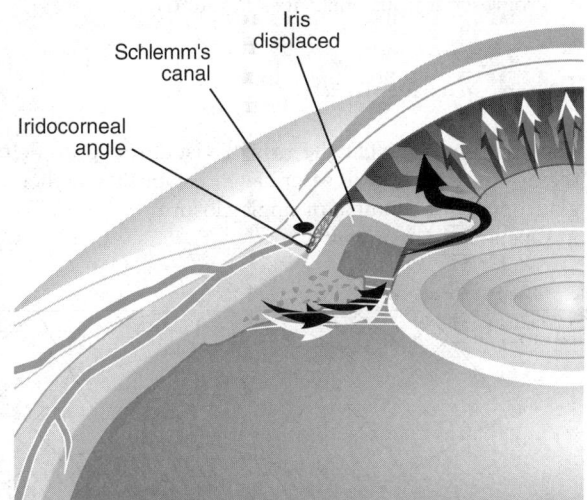

Angle-closure glaucoma occurs in eyes with preexisting anatomic narrowing of the anterior chamber angle and is caused by the forward shift of the iris, which blocks the outflow of aqueous humor from the posterior chamber.

Figure 19–16.

Diagnostics

1. History
   a. Ask the person about ocular symptoms related to glaucoma (pain, redness, halo vision, blurred vision). Also ask about trauma, previous ocular surgery, and ocular disease.
   b. Obtain pertinent information from the general medical history regarding diabetes, hypertension, medications, allergies, and family history of glaucoma and retinal detachment.
2. Physical examination
   a. Tonometry
      (1) Measurement may be taken by any method; how-

ever, because slit-lamp examination is also necessary, the applanation method may be used (see Fig. 19–7).
   b. Slit-lamp examination
      (1) Assess the structures and depth of the anterior chamber.
      (2) Observe the anterior chamber for inflammatory cell deposits (keratic precipitates) on the corneal endothelium, anterior chamber cells, and flare.
      (3) If the angle is narrowed, the goniolens should be used to examine the angle structures further.
   c. Use direct ophthalmoscopy to examine the optic nerve head
      (1) Observe the optic disk for enlargement.
      (2) Observe the optic disk cup for depth.
      (3) Record the color and contour of the optic nerve head. Normal color ranges from orange to pink.
      (4) Changes in size and color of the optic disk over time indicate need for treatment. With advanced damage, the cup becomes pale and it deepens.
   d. Visual fields—should be documented using automated equipment as opposed to the confrontation method (see visual field examination methods, Fig. 19–17).
3. Medical diagnosis
   a. Intraocular pressure is greater than 22 mm Hg.
   b. Anterior chamber depth less than 3 times the corneal thickness is suggestive of narrow-angle glaucoma.
   c. Enlargement, increased cupping, and pallor of the optic disk are noted.
   d. Progressive visual field loss is found.

Clinical Management

1. The goal is to prevent the loss of visual function. Before therapy is begun, it is essential to establish whether the glaucoma is open-angle or angle-closure.
   a. Open-angle treatment

(1) Lower intraocular pressure with medication that facilitates outflow or decreases production of aqueous humor.
      (2) Surgery is required only when medical therapy fails.
   b. Angle-closure treatment
      (1) Requires surgical intervention.
2. Pharmacologic interventions
   a. Aim of controlling intraocular pressure is a range of 16 to 18 mm Hg and lower (11–13 mm Hg) in advanced stages.
   b. Before medication is begun, ask the individual about drug allergies, cardiopulmonary problems, and renal dysfunction.

   c. Initial therapy begins with 1 type of medication at the lowest drug concentration appropriate.
      (1) Higher doses are prescribed as necessary.
      (2) When a 2nd drug is initiated, the 1st is usually discontinued to ascertain whether 1 or both medications are needed to control intraocular pressure.

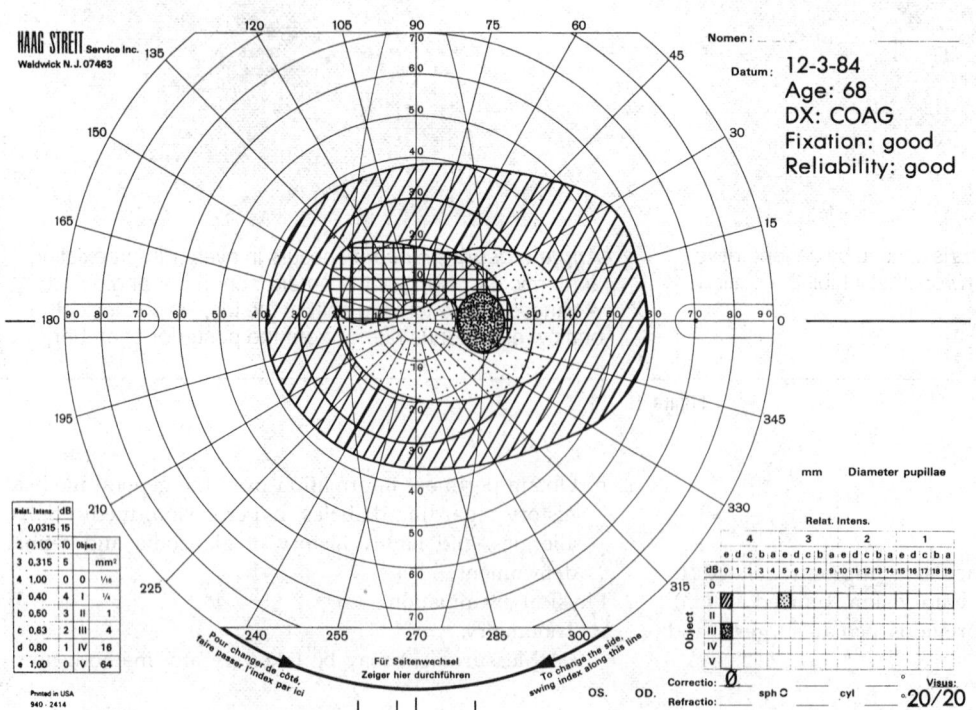

Figure 19–17. Visual field documentation using the Goldmann perimeter. (Courtesy of Humphrey Instruments.)

Table 19–1. Antiglaucoma Medications

Medication	Actions	Comments	Contraindications	Side Effects	Nursing Considerations
Cholinergics					
Pilocarpine	Decreases formation and increases outflow of aqueous humor	Pupillary variation may cause a change in visual field (i.e., decreased peripheral vision).	Acute iritis anterior segment inflammation, or corneal abrasion	Transient brow pain and myopia when initiated. Systemic: sweating, nausea, vomiting, diarrhea, pulmonary edema, salivation, lacrimation, and bronchospasm	Warn the individual about blurred vision.
Carbachol	Widens trabecular meshwork facilitating outflow of aqueous humor	See pilocarpine. Use punctal occlusion to reduce systemic effects.	Same as pilocarpine. Use with caution in persons with Parkinson's, heart failure, or urinary tract obstruction.	See pilocarpine.	Persons who experience side effects may have poor compliance.
Anticholinergics					
Ecothiophate iodide (Phospholine Iodide)	Contracts ciliary muscle, which facilitates outflow of aqueous humor.	Angle-closure glaucoma, uveitis. Causes respiratory paralysis when used with succinylcholine in general anesthesia.	Aggravation of bronchial asthma, diarrhea, vomiting, hypertension, bradycardia, sweating, salivation, and lacrimation.	Same as for carbachol. Drug must be discontinued for 10 days before the administration of general anesthesia.	
Physostigmine	Opens trabecular meshwork by tightening ciliary muscles.	Same as for ecothiophate iodide	Less intense, but same as for ecothiophate iodide	Same as for carbachol	
Adrenergic Agonists					
Epinephrine	Not fully known; stimulates outflow of aqueous	Use with caution in persons with diabetes, cardiovascular disease, hyperthyroidism, or cerebrovascular disease.	Ocular: stinging, redness, eye ache, headache, mydriasis, cystoid macular edema	Warn the person about the possible side effects. Assess compliance.	
Dipivefrin	Inhibits aqueous production and facilitates outflow	Same as for epinephrine	Ocular: stinging, mydriasis, allergic conjunctivitis. Systemic: same as for epinephrine but less intense		
Beta-Adrenergic Antagonists (Sympathomimetics)					
Timolol	Reduces aqueous humor formation and may increase aqueous outflow	Nonspecific β-blocker affecting β receptors in eye, heart, and lungs	Asthma, heart failure, severe cardiac disease, chronic obstructive pulmonary disease	Headache, depression, fatigue, bradycardia, anorexia, syncope, exacerbation of asthma and congestive heart failure; may mask symptoms of hyperglycemia; corneal anesthesia	Evaluate pulse and blood pressure before starting. Monitor side effects closely.
Betaxolol	Reduces aqueous humor formation	Specific β-blocker; does not affect β receptors in lungs	Same as for timolol	Same as for timolol except no corneal anesthesia	Same as for timolol
Levobunolol	Reduces aqueous humor	Nonspecific β-blocker	Same as for timolol	Same as for timolol except no corneal anesthesia	Same as for timolol

Table continued on following page

Table 19–1. Antiglaucoma Medications (Continued)

Medication	Actions	Comments	Contraindications	Side Effects	Nursing Considerations
Carbonic Anhydrase Inhibitors					
Acetazolamide	Decreases aqueous production by inhibiting carbonic anhydrase in the ciliary body		Persons who are allergic to sulfonamides or who have Addison's disease and/or adrenal insufficiency	Tingling paresthesias, anorexia, nausea, vomiting, diuresis, renal colic, stone formation, malaise, depression, confusion, decreased libido	Assess appetite and mental changes, particularly in the older person. Monitor potassium level and instruct person about high potassium foods. Risk for injury with night diuresis.
Methozolamide	Same as for acetazolamide		Same as for acetazolamide	Same as for acetazolamide	Same as for acetazolamide
Hyperosmotic Agents					
Glycerin (oral)	Movement of water from intraocular structures to circulation via plasma osmolarity	More palatable if mixed with chipped ice and flavored with lemon or other tart juice	Severe congestive heart failure, impaired renal function, pulmonary edema, anuria	Increased cardiovascular workload, headache, confusion, nausea, urinary retention, rhinitis, blurred vision, tachycardia	Keep emesis basin near; monitor output
Mannitol (intravenous)	Same as for oral glycerin	Check solution for precipitates before giving. If precipitates are present, warm bottle to dissolve.	Same as for oral glycerin	Same as for oral glycerin	Monitor vital signs during administration. Give through intravenous micron filter.

3. Special medical-surgical procedures
   a. Laser procedures
      (1) Argon and krypton lasers use the heating and disrupting effect of laser energy to create tissue burns or openings that allow for the outflow of aqueous humor.
      (2) The laser produces a sudden tissue expansion with tearing and disruption of tissue by delivering high-powered near-infrared irradiances in small focused spots.
      (3) Laser trabeculoplasty. After topical anesthesia and pupil constriction, a goniolens is placed over the individual's eye. The laser beam is focused on the trabecular meshwork, and an opening is created. The procedure may be performed in 2 stages several weeks apart.
         Follow-up after treatment is important because tissue damage and edema may cause a rise in intraocular pressure. The person should be evaluated during the 1st hour after the procedure, at 24 hours, 1 week, 2 weeks, and 1 month. Antiglaucoma medication is continued along with topical steroid 3 or 4 times a day and is tapered off over 2 weeks. A positive outcome of reduced intraocular pressure may last weeks, months, or years, but treatment usually needs to be repeated.
      (4) Laser iridectomy. The pupil is constricted with pi-

locarpine. After topical anesthetic, the laser beam is aimed at the iris in an area usually covered by the upper lid and fired until a hole is created.
   Follow-up treatment is the same as for laser trabeculoplasty.
   b. Filtering procedures. Surgical procedures that create a bypass in the natural outflow pathways to allow drainage of aqueous from the eye.
      (1) Trephine: A piece of corneoscleral limbus (the area where the cornea and sclera meet) is removed with a trephine instrument.
      (2) Sclerectomy: A partial-thickness incision is made in the sclera at the limbus, and 1 or more openings are made with a punch. The top flap of sclera is closed over the punched holes.
      (3) Thermal sclerostomy: Cautery is applied to the sclera under a corneoscleral flap, which creates an opening.
      (4) Trabeculectomy: A partial-thickness incision is made in the sclera at the limbus, and further section of sclera is removed. The top flap is closed over the opening, creating a "filtering bleb." In some individuals, this filtering bleb heals and closes off the opening. To prevent healing of the opening, 5-fluorouracil or mitomycin is injected, which causes the tissues to scar open.
      (5) Filtering tubes and implants: A tiny plastic device

is sutured to the sclera, and a tube is fed through a sclerectomy into the anterior chamber to drain aqueous out to the conjunctival sac. Some devices have valves for adjusting the flow.

  c. Ciliodestructive procedures: Cyclocryotherapy, the application of a freezing probe to the sclera over the ciliary body that destroys some of the ciliary processes, results in the reduction of the amount of aqueous humor produced.

  d. Cyclodialysis. Through a small incision in the sclera, a spatula-type instrument is passed into the anterior chamber, creating an opening in the angle.

Complications

1. Without pharmacologic or surgical intervention, the following may occur:
  a. Irreparable damage to the optic nerve and retina eventually results in blindness.
  b. Even after blindness occurs, the individual may continue to experience pain, eventually requiring the eye to be removed.

NURSE ADVISORY

In general, people who are blind wish to be as independent as sighted people. It is important to offer assistance to a blind person and to help in a way that preserves dignity and independence. When walking with a blind person, offer your elbow and allow the blind person to grasp it lightly. The blind person will prefer to walk a step behind you, adjusting gait and movement by the changes in your step. Alert the person to upcoming steps or turns in advance. You can assist a blind person with meals by describing the location of different food items on the plate by the hours of the clock (e.g., peas at 3 o'clock and meat at 7 o'clock). Remember to announce yourself as you walk in the room and always speak *before* touching someone. Be sure the call light and other important items are within reach, and describe to the person where they are.

---

2. Postoperative complications include the following:
  a. Development of peripheral anterior senechiae (adhesions of the iris to the cornea)
  b. Corneal damage
  c. Hemorrhage
  d. Iritis
  e. Hypotony (flat anterior chamber)
  f. Cataract formation
  g. Pain
  h. Cystoid macular edema
  i. Atrophy of the eyeball (phthisis bulbi)
  j. Closure of the opening

Prognosis

1. There is no cure for glaucoma.
2. Early detection and treatment maximize the preservation of vision.

Applying the Nursing Process

NURSING DIAGNOSIS: Impaired adjustment to therapeutic regimen R/T individual's lack of acceptance or denial regarding diagnosis

1. *Expected outcomes:* Following instruction, the person should be able to do the following:
  a. Describe the cause of glaucoma and the risks of ineffective treatment.
  b. Relate the importance of treatment when there are no noticeable symptoms.
2. *Nursing interventions*
  a. Explain the causative factors underlying glaucoma as well as the implications of inadequate treatment.
  b. Ask the person to identify events of the day that will help them remember to instill eye drops.
  c. Discuss with the individual and family members the importance of establishing a routine for the administration of medications and of keeping follow-up appointments.

NURSING DIAGNOSIS: Anticipatory grieving R/T progressive vision loss

1. *Expected outcomes:* Following instruction, the person should be able to do the following:
  a. Discuss fears and concerns related to vision loss.
  b. Identify strengths and successful coping skills used in the past.
2. *Nursing interventions*
  a. Provide an open and accepting environment for the individual to discuss concerns.
  b. Explain the grieving process to the person and family members.
  c. Facilitate acknowledgment of fears.
  d. Assist the person to identify strengths and successful uses of coping skills in the past.
  e. Document anxiety manifestations and progress toward expected outcomes.

Discharge Planning and Teaching

1. After laser or surgical procedure for glaucoma control, the person needs to know the course of treatment, what will be experienced, and the expected outcomes (Learning/Teaching Guidelines for Self-Care After Glaucoma Surgery).

Public Health Considerations: Primary Prevention

1. An estimated 2 million Americans have glaucoma, and almost 80,000 Americans are blind from it.
2. Glaucoma testing and public education are imperative to prevent needless loss of vision.

LEARNING/TEACHING GUIDELINES
for Self-Care After Glaucoma Surgery

General Overview

1. Using an eye model or a cross-section picture of the eye, describe the type of glaucoma and how it affects the structures of the eye. Describe the surgical procedure.
2. Describe the healing process and the expected visual rehabilitation time frame.
3. Discuss the administration of eye drops, including the name of the medication and the rationale for use. Describe the dosage, frequency, and storage of the medication.
4. Demonstrate the instillation of the eye drops, and request a return demonstration by the person and a family member.
5. Describe how to care for the eye dressing at home and the signs and symptoms that indicate the person should notify the physician.
6. Discuss any limitation in activities.
7. Review the date and time of the next visit to the physician as well as expected future visits.

Medications

1. Topical steroids are usually prescribed as often as every hour while the patient is awake to reduce inflammation and to keep the filtering bleb from healing closed.

Healing and Visual Rehabilitation

1. Wound healing takes 6 weeks.
2. Initially, vision is decreased due to inflammation; however, it should return to preoperative acuity.

Eye Dressing and Care

1. Laser procedures do not require patching, but a patch and shield are usually applied immediately after a surgical procedure.
2. After the dressing is removed the next morning, either the glasses or the shield alone should be worn at all times for approximately 6 weeks to protect the eye during the healing process. Remind the individual to put on the shield at bedtime.
3. Sutures may be absorbable or a combination of absorbable and nonabsorbable. No sutures are removed.
4. Instruct the person that any redness around the eye should gradually resolve. An increase in redness or swelling around the eye should be reported to the physician.
5. Increased tearing is normal after glaucoma surgery, and a small amount of dried matter may appear on the lashes in the morning or after naps. Instruct the person to use a warm washcloth to remove the matter. If purulent drainage is noted, the person should call the physician.
6. Postoperative discomfort should be relieved by acetaminophen. Unrelieved pain should be reported to the physician (may indicate an increase in intraocular pressure).
7. A sudden or noticeable decrease in vision should also be reported to the physician.

Activity

1. Usually none.

Postoperative Visits

1. Return visits are usually on the day after surgery, at 1 week, at 2 weeks, and at 1 month. Frequency of visits depends on posttreatment stability of intraocular pressure and wound healing.

◼ RETINAL DETACHMENT

Definition

A separation of the neurosensory retina from the pigment epithelium and choroid

Incidence

The incidence increases during the 4th decade of life and peaks during the 5th and 6th decades.

Risk Factors

1. Age
2. Cataract extraction
3. Severe myopia
4. Trauma

Etiology

1. Degenerative changes that occur with aging are the most frequent cause of retinal detachment.

2. Blunt trauma to the head or eye can cause the retina to tear or break.
3. Ocular conditions such as severe myopia, papilledema, choroidal tumor, previous ocular surgery, and many retinal disorders predispose the eye to retinal detachment, even in young individuals.
4. Rhegmatogenous retinal detachment
   a. A spontaneous hole or tear in the retina allows vitreous fluid to collect underneath it (see Color Fig. 19–4).
   b. It occurs in individuals older than 45 and more commonly in males.
5. Hemorrhagic retinal detachment—leakage from the choroid or retinal vessels collects under the retina.
6. Traction retinal detachment—degenerative changes cause fibrous bands to develop in the vitreous, pulling the retina away from the blood supply.
7. Retinal breaks are described as giant when the tear extends 90 degrees or more along the circumference of the globe.

Pathophysiology

1. The most complex of the ocular tissues, the retina is only 0.23 to 0.10 mm thick.
   a. Processing of retinal information proceeds from the photoreceptor layer through the ganglion cell axon to the optic nerve and brain.
   b. The retina receives its blood supply from the following:
      (1) The choriocapillaris on the surface of the retina, which supplies the top third of the retina.
      (2) The central retinal artery, which supplies the lower two thirds of the retina.
   c. With aging, degenerative changes in the vitreous humor apply traction to the retina, tearing it away from its blood supply.
   d. Fluid collects in the space beneath the detachment.
2. Retinal detachments can also occur in systemic conditions such as diabetes, severe hypertension, toxemia of pregnancy, and chronic glomerulonephritis.

Clinical Manifestations

1. People experience photopsia (flashing lights), vitreous floaters (black spots, cobwebs, or lace curtain effect), or both (Fig. 19–18).
2. No pain is associated with a retinal tear.

Diagnostics

1. History
   a. Because retinal detachment usually results in an emergency examination, the nurse should carefully assess the person's level of anxiety.
   b. Ask the individual to describe the character and onset of visual symptoms.
   c. Assess the person's cultural and personal beliefs related to vision loss.

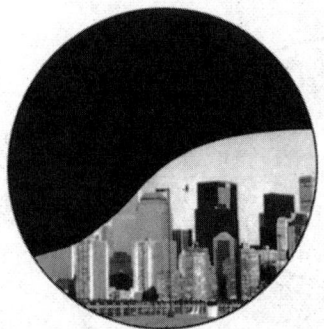

Detached Retina

Figure 19–18. Visual defect seen with a retinal detachment. The detachment is interior and nasal, opposite the visual field defect, which is superior and temporal. (Courtesy of National Industries for the Blind, Wayne, NJ.)

2. Physical examination
   a. Both eyes must be dilated and examined even if only 1 eye has symptoms.
   b. Direct and indirect ophthalmoscopy may be used to visualize the complete fundus.
   c. Slit-lamp examination with the Hruby lens may also be used.
3. Medical diagnosis
   a. Ophthalmoscopy shows that the retina has lost its pink color and appears gray.
   b. If the collection of subretinal fluid is large enough, a ballooning or pouching effect and subsequent folds in the membrane may be visualized.
   c. Tears frequently appear in a horseshoe shape.

Clinical Management

1. The goal is to repair the retinal break to maintain visual reception.
2. Special medical-surgical procedures
   a. Scleral buckling procedure
      (1) Reattachment of the retina is accomplished by aspirating the subretinal fluid and indenting the sclera with an explant of silicone sponge or band (Fig. 19–19). By pushing in the sclera, the retina and choroid can heal together, and the blood supply is restored.
      (2) During the scleral buckling procedure, diathermy (application of heat), cryopexy (application of cold), or the argon laser may be used to create further adhesion of the retina.
   b. Pneumatic retinopexy involves an intraocular injection of air, an expandable gas such as sulfur hexafluoride (SF6), or a combination of both to tamponade the break while healing takes place. The tamponade effect is maximized by positioning the individual postoperatively so that gravity causes the air-gas bubble to rise and press on the affected area.
   c. Vitrectomy
      (1) At the pars plana (space between the retina and ciliary body), 2 1- to 4-mm incisions are made on

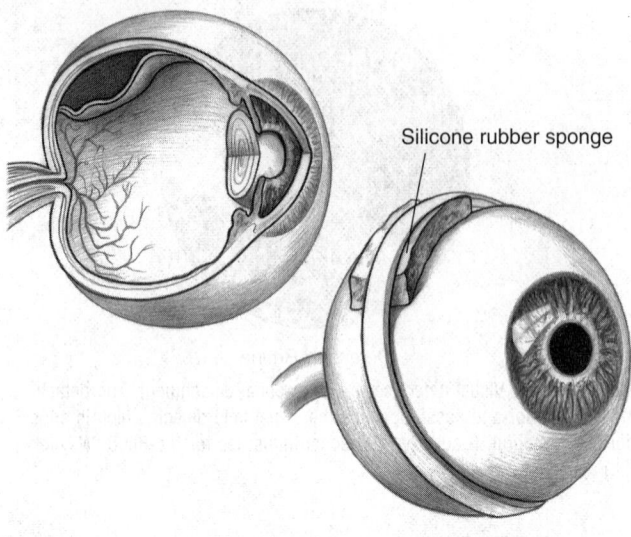

Figure 19–19. Scleral buckling procedure using an encircling band.

each side of the cornea and secured with a scleral plug to allow insertion of surgical instruments.

(2) One incision is used for a fiberoptic light source, and the other is used to introduce instruments to aspirate vitreous, manipulate tissue, or apply diathermy or laser treatment (Fig. 19–20).

(3) A vitrectomy is done most commonly to accomplish the following:
  • Remove vitreous opacified by blood
  • Treat vitreous traction on the retina

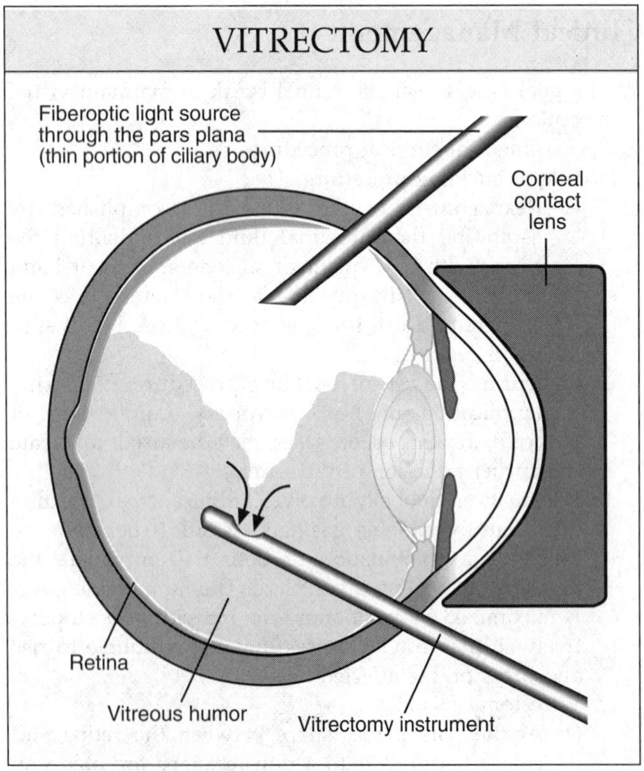

VITRECTOMY

Fiberoptic light source through the pars plana (thin portion of ciliary body)

Corneal contact lens

Retina

Vitreous humor

Vitrectomy instrument

Figure 19–20.

  • Remove membranes that deform or detach the retina
  • Remove vitreous in infections (endophthalmitis) to reduce the population of organisms and instill antibiotics

Complications

1. Untreated, retinal detachment leads to ischemic death of the affected tissues.
2. Resulting blind spots in the retina correspond inversely to the area affected (i.e., a right upper quadrant tear will appear as a lower left visual defect).
3. Peripheral tears result in less debilitating loss than tears near or involving the macula where the cone receptors for central and fine vision are located.
4. Postoperative complications
   a. When an air-gas bubble is used, the expansion may cause a rise in intraocular pressure in the first 12 to 24 hours after surgery. Diuretics such as acetazolamide are often prescribed prophylactically to prevent a rise in intraocular pressure that could endanger the optic nerve. On rare occasions, the person may have to return for a surgical procedure to aspirate some of the air-gas.
   b. Failure of reattachment
   c. Infection

Prognosis

1. Return of vision is directly related to the length of time between the retinal detachment and the surgical repair.
2. Reattachment rates are reported to be 90%, but the amount of vision gained depends on the area of detachment and the ability to heal.

Applying the Nursing Process

NURSING DIAGNOSIS: Knowledge deficit R/T cause, complications, and postoperative program for retinal surgery

1. *Expected outcomes:* Following instruction, the person should be able to do the following:
   a. Describe the causes of retinal detachment.
   b. Verbalize any feelings of guilt or remorse if there was a delay in treatment.
2. *Nursing interventions*
   a. Allow time for questions and verbalization of feelings about the impact on lifestyle.
   b. Assess the current level of knowledge.
   c. Assess the readiness to learn.
   d. Explain the causes of retinal detachment and review preoperative and postoperative expectations.

NURSING DIAGNOSIS: Sensory-perceptual alterations R/T vision loss due to retinal detachment

1. *Expected outcomes:* Following instruction, the person

LEARNING/TEACHING GUIDELINES
for Self-Care After Scleral Buckle Surgery

General Overview

1. Using an eye model or a cross-section picture of the eye, describe the location of the retinal detachment. Describe the surgical procedure.
2. Describe the healing process and the expected visual rehabilitation time frame.
3. Discuss the administration of eye drops including the name of the medication and the rationale for use. Describe the dosage, frequency, and storage of the medication.
4. Demonstrate the instillation of the eye drops, and request a return demonstration by the person and a family member.
5. Describe how to care for the eye dressing at home and the signs and symptoms that indicate the person should notify the physician.
6. Discuss any limitation in activities.
7. Review the date and time of the next visit to the physician as well as expected future visits.

Medications

1. Atropine is usually prescribed for dilating the eye and for cycloplegia.
   a. Dilation is necessary for each return visit and examination. Photophobia is reduced with dark glasses.
   b. Cycloplegia (paralysis of the ciliary muscle) prevents spasm and promotes comfort.
2. Antibiotic eye drops are usually prescribed to prevent infection.
3. Corticosteroid drops are usually prescribed to reduce inflammation.

Healing and Visual Rehabilitation

1. Wound healing takes 6 weeks to 3 months.
2. Initially, vision is decreased owing to inflammation and edema.
3. Vision should gradually improve over the following 2 weeks. Best vision may take as long as 6 months.

Eye Dressing and Care

1. Immediately after surgery the eye will be very red, sometimes ecchymotic, and swollen owing to manipulation during surgery.
2. After the dressing is removed the next morning, either the glasses or the shield alone should be worn at all times for approximately 6 weeks to protect the eye during the healing process. Remind the individual to put on the shield at bedtime.
3. Warm compresses may be applied 4 to 6 times a day to promote healing and provide comfort.
4. Sutures and explant materials (sponge or band) are not removed. Healing around the explant materials takes place in 10 to 14 days.
5. Redness of the conjunctiva may take up to 3 months to clear.
6. Postoperative discomfort should be relieved by acetaminophen. Initially, acetaminophen with codeine may be prescribed. Unrelieved pain should be reported to the physician.
7. A sudden or noticeable decrease in vision should also be reported to the physician.

Activity

1. Heavy lifting (greater than 25 pounds) is usually restricted.

Postoperative Visits

1. Return visits are usually every 2 weeks until the condition is stable.

---

should be able to maintain a safe low-vision environment.
2. *Nursing interventions*
   a. Provide a safe clinical environment, and make modifications to maximize the person's visual ability.
   b. Assess the home environment and explore options for adaptations with the person and family members.

Discharge Planning and Teaching

1. Before discharge, people need to learn about self-care after retinal detachment surgery, including medications, activity restrictions, and signs and symptoms of infection and redetachment (Learning/Teaching Guidelines for Self-Care After Scleral Buckle Surgery and Learning/Teaching Guidelines for Self-Care After Vitrectomy Surgery).

Public Health Considerations: Primary Prevention

1. Home care evaluations are an important consideration when the individual lives alone or with a dependent partner.

CHOROIDAL MELANOMA
Definition

Choroidal melanoma is a malignant tumor of the uveal tract.

HOME CARE STRATEGIES

Modifying the Home Environment for People with Visual Disorders

Many home health care patients are older adults among whom visual disturbances such as glaucoma, cataracts, retinopathy, and macular degeneration are common. Although the home environment is one in which the patient with a visual disorder feels most comfortable, safe, and secure, it is one in which she or he may be at risk for falls and other injuries. Modification of the home environment may enable the patient to be safe and more independent.

Environmental modification must be preceded by a thorough assessment, including the patient's willingness to allow changes to the home. The potential long-term benefits must be weighed against the discomfort and insecurity of disrupting familiar surroundings.

Assess the following areas and suggest modifications as needed:

Lighting
- Examine lighting pattern and daily activities.
- Suggest low-level indirect lighting throughout the home.
- Supplement with direct lighting in work and high-traffic areas.
- Reduce glare from windows with sheer curtains or blinds.
- Use night-lights in halls, bedrooms, and bathroom.

Floors
- Assess condition and coverings.
- Suggest intact light-colored nonglare floor coverings and finishes with contrasting baseboards and stair edge markings.
- Keep floors and stairs clear of throw rugs and other objects.

Kitchen and Laundry
- Inspect appliances and work areas.
- Mark common settings on appliance dials with red tape or nail polish.
- Install direct lighting over work areas, appliances, and sinks.
- Use utensils whose colors contrast with those of tabletops and work surfaces.

Bathroom
- Inspect tub, lighting, and floor.
- Suggest marking faucets and appliances as above.
- Use a night-light.
- Install direct lighting over sink *and* tub.
- Use tub or bath mats whose colors contrast with those of the floor.

Bedroom and Livingroom
- Assess lighting, furniture position, and color.
- Suggest indirect lighting in addition to lamps.
- Position furniture to maintain clear walkways.
- Use furniture coverings that contrast with the floor's color.

Incidence and Socioeconomic Impact

1. Occurs in 0.04 percent of the total population in the United States.
2. Occurs most frequently in White adults after the 5th decade of life.
3. Is rarely bilateral.

Risk Factors

1. Genetic predisposition
2. Presence of ocular melanocytic conditions such as melanosis oculi and oculodermal melanocytosis

3. Light iris color
4. Exposure to ultraviolet light

Etiology

1. Unknown. Posterior uveal melanomas are commonly classified by size.
   a. Small: 5 to 10 mm in diameter and up to 3 mm in thickness
   b. Medium: 10 to 15 mm in diameter and 3 to 5 mm in thickness
   c. Large: 15 to 20 mm in diameter and 5 to 10 mm in thickness
   d. Extra large: greater than 20 mm in diameter and greater than 10 mm in thickness

Pathophysiology

Choroidal malignant melanomas originate in the vascular layer, the choroid, and often erupt in a mushroom shape into the vitreous space.

Clinical Manifestations

1. No pain or discomfort is associated with the growth of the tumor.
2. Vision may be impaired depending on the location of the tumor.

Diagnostics

1. History
   a. Ask the individual to describe vision changes.
   b. Because there is no pain with tumor development, choroidal melanomas are often discovered during routine eye examinations.
   c. Assess the person's cultural and personal beliefs about cancer and vision loss.
2. Physical examination
   a. Tumors are often visible with the direct ophthalmoscope.
   b. Transillumination: In a darkened room, a light source is placed in the conjunctival fornix opposite the lesion. The location and approximate dimensions of the tumor can be visualized by the shadow of the tumor.
3. Medical diagnosis
   a. Fluorescein angiography shows fluorescence of the vessels affected by the tumor and essentially outlines the mass of growth.
   b. Ultrasound demarcates the size and shape of the tumor.

Clinical Management

1. The goal is to stop growth of the tumor and to prevent metastasis.
2. Pharmacologic interventions

a. If the tumor is small and does not threaten central vision, chemotherapy may be prescribed.

b. Antineoplastic agents such as vincristine, doxorubicin hydrochloride (Adriamycin), cytarabine (ara-C), etoposide (VP-16), and dacarbazine (DTIC) are used in the management of ocular tumors; however, there is no conclusive evidence that they are effective.

3. Special medical-surgical procedures
   a. Enucleation
      (1) Usually the treatment of choice for large choroidal melanoma tumors.
      (2) The entire eyeball is removed. The ocular muscles are separated from the globe. The optic nerve and vessels are severed. An implant of silicone, wire mesh, or hydroxyapatite material replaces the eyeball in the orbit. The ocular muscles are reattached to the implant so that the prosthesis will move in concert with the other eye. The conjunctiva is closed over the implant, and a silicone or plastic conformer is placed in the socket until healing occurs (see Color Fig. 19–5).
   b. Exenteration
      (1) Removal of the entire eyeball along with surrounding tissues in the orbit or lids.
      (2) The treatment of choice when there is invasive tumor growth to the lids or paranasal sinuses.
   c. Other interventions
      (1) Photocoagulation: Xenon, argon, and krypton lasers may be used to destroy certain small intraocular tumors.
      (2) Cryotherapy may be used to treat selected small tumors.
      (3) Radiation therapy may be the treatment of choice for certain tumors; however, there are dangers of radiation cataract and retinopathy.
      (4) Radioactive plaque: Radioactive isotope seeds are placed in a dime-sized saucer that is applied to the sclera directly over the tumor. Iodine-125 is most commonly used; however, other isotopes such as cobalt-60, ruthenium-106, and iridium-192 are also used. A lead shield is placed over the eye, and the individual is placed under radiation precautions until the plaque is removed, usually 4 to 5 days later. The length of time that the plaque stays in place is relative to the strength of the radiation source.
      (5) Charged particle radiation. Several days before the 1st treatment, tantalum clips are sutured to the sclera to mark the margins of the tumor. The charged particle beam delivers a more homogeneous dose of radiation energy than does radioactive plaque therapy, and there is less lateral spread of the beam.

Complications

1. Retinal detachment is commonly associated with tumor growth.
2. Spontaneous hemorrhage into the subretinal space or vitreous.

Prognosis

The interval between enucleation and the onset of metastatic disease is often as early as 2 to 4 years in people who develop clinical metastatic disease from choroidal melanoma. The median is 7 years.

Applying the Nursing Process

NURSING DIAGNOSIS: Body image disturbance R/T loss of eye and change in appearance

1. *Expected outcomes:* Following instruction, the person should be able to do the following:
   a. Verbalize feelings about losing an eye.
   b. Describe prosthetic devices and care.
2. *Nursing interventions*
   a. Describe what the individual will see after the dressing is removed for the 1st time. Make sure both the individual and the family member are seated when seeing the surgical site for the 1st time.
   b. Assess the person's current feelings about how the prosthesis will look and how others will think it looks after surgery.
   c. Identify the chief concerns of the individual (e.g., acceptance by family members, fear of frightening other people, ability to take care of the prosthesis and socket), and plan coping strategies.
   d. Describe the process of fitting a prosthesis and its care (Procedure 19–18).

NURSING DIAGNOSIS: Sensory-perceptual alteration R/T singular vision

1. *Expected outcomes:* Following instruction, the person should be able to make adaptations in behavior to compensate for loss of depth perception.
2. *Nursing interventions:* Teach the individual to identify safety factors and apply adaptive methods.
   a. Double-check traffic from the blind side before crossing a street.
   b. When reaching out to shake hands or pick up an object, watch the hand until contact is made.
   c. Use mirrors for driving.
   d. Use handrails on stairs.

Discharge Planning and Teaching

Individuals need to be prepared for hospitalization for scleral plaque therapy or enucleation. Some enucleation procedures are performed on an outpatient basis (Learning/Teaching Guidelines for Self-Care After Enucleation).

Public Health Considerations: Primary Prevention

1. The presence of choroidal melanoma is often detected during a routine eye examination because there are no symptoms when the tumor is small.

LEARNING/TEACHING GUIDELINES
for Self-Care After Enucleation

General Overview

1. Some people do not wish to discuss the details of the surgery and others want to know details. Ask the person before you begin to discuss the surgical procedure and describe the type of implant used.
2. Describe the healing process and the expected time frame.
3. Discuss the administration of medication into the socket, including the name of the medication and the rationale for use. Describe the dosage, frequency, and storage of the medication.
4. Demonstrate the instillation of the medication, and request a return demonstration by the person and a family member.
5. Describe how to care for the dressing at home and the signs and symptoms that indicate the person should notify the physician.
6. Discuss any limitation in activities.
7. Review the date and time of the next visit to the physician as well as expected future visits.

Medications

1. Antibiotic ointment is usually prescribed to be instilled in the socket twice a day for 1 to 2 weeks.

Healing and Rehabilitation

1. Wound healing takes over 6 to 8 weeks.
2. Drainage will be serosanguinous to yellow serous with some mucus.
3. A conformer is worn to maintain the space for the eventual prosthesis. If the conformer falls out, it should be washed with soap and water and reinserted. If the conformer is left out for more than 24 hours, healing may decrease the available space.

Eye Dressing and Care

1. A pressure dressing is usually applied in the operating room and should be left on for 1 to 2 days. When the dressing is removed, a patch may be worn for cosmesis. The dressing removal may be a very difficult and emotional experience. Be sure the person and family member are seated and be prepared to discuss the situation after the dressing change.
2. For evisceration or extenteration, packing may be advanced 3 inches per day, clipped, and covered with a patch until all is removed.
3. Postoperative discomfort should be relieved by acetaminophen. Initially acetaminophen with codeine may be prescribed. Nonsteroidal anti-inflammatory drugs and aspirin should be avoided before and after surgery. Unrelieved pain should be reported to the physician.

Activity

1. Athletic and vigorous activity may be modified for 2 weeks.

Postoperative Visits

1. Return visits are usually every 2 weeks until the condition is stable.

Procedure 19–18
Insertion and Removal of an Ocular Prosthesis

Definition/Purpose	To insert and remove an ocular prosthesis correctly
Contraindications/Cautions	Never clean prosthetics with anything except a mild soap and water. Alcohol and other cleaning solutions will permanently damage the plastic material. Never put one in a sterilizer. Prosthetic devices may need to be revised after orbital reconstructive surgery.
Learning/Teaching Activities	Explain the procedure to the person.

Preliminary Activities

Equipment
- Towel
- Prosthesis

Procedure

Procedure 19–18
(continued)

Actions	Rationale/Discussion

Insertion

1. Wash your hands.
2. Place the towel on the work surface.
3. Remove the prosthesis from the container and rinse with tepid water. The notched edge of the prosthesis is placed closest to the person's nose.
4. Lift the person's upper lid with one hand and slide the prosthesis up under the lid.
5. Release the upper lid and pull down on the lower lid until the bottom edge of the prosthesis slips behind it.
6. Gently position both lids into place. Ask the person to blink.

1. To remove surface microorganisms
2. To provide a clean work surface
3. To facilitate insertion

4. To maximize the area of insertion

5. To position the prosthesis

6. To ensure proper position

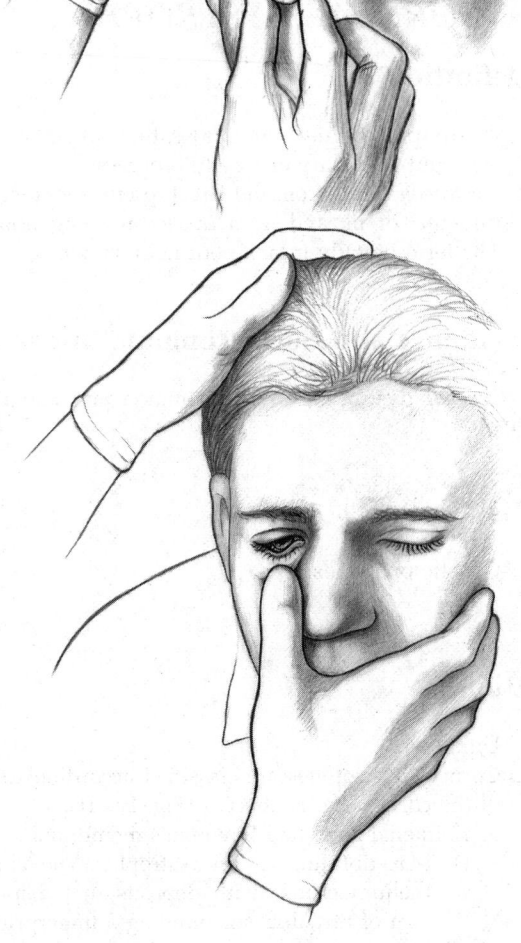

Removal

1. Wash your hands.
2. Have the person sit in front of you or lie down.
3. Pull the lower lid down and to the side.
4. Gently press against the prosthesis and allow it to fall into your other hand.
5. Place the prosthesis in a labeled container.

1. To remove surface microorganisms
2. To facilitate removal
3. To increase the surface area
4. To facilitate removal
5. To prevent loss

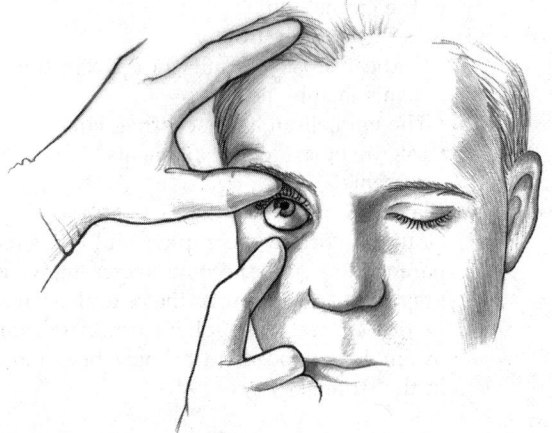

2. The choroid can become a metastatic site when a primary source of malignancy is present in another part of the body. Routine eye examinations by an ophthalmologist should be a part of the follow-up.
3. Clinical centers all over North America have been cooperating for more than 10 years in the Collaborative Ocular Melanoma Study. In this project, individuals with medium-sized melanomas who choose to participate are randomized to either enucleation or iodine-125 plaque irradiation. Before this study, there were no conclusive data that supported either treatment as being more successful in prolonging life.

■ *CORNEAL DYSTROPHIES*

Definition

1. A group of corneal conditions that are inherited, bilateral, and stationary or slowly progressive.
2. *Dystrophy* stems from the Greek prefix *dys,* meaning bad, difficult, or ill, and from *trophe,* meaning nourishment. The term literally means poor nourishment.

Incidence and Socioeconomic Impact

Corneal dystrophies are uncommon and usually hereditary.

Risk Factors

1. Genetic predisposition
2. Age

Etiology

1. Unknown.
2. Corneal dystrophies are classified according to the layer of the cornea that is affected (Fig. 19–21).
   a. Epithelial layer and Bowman's membrane
      (1) Map-dot fingerprint dystrophy: The corneal epithelium erodes with deposits that display a pattern of tiny dots surrounding a fingerprint.
      (2) Meesman's dystrophy: Microcystic areas develop in the epithelium.
      (3) Reis-Bücklers dystrophy
         • Corneal erosion results in opacification of Bowman's membrane.
         • The epithelium becomes irregular.
         • Microscopic "curly filaments" are sometimes present.
   b. Stromal layer
      (1) Granular corneal dystrophy: Multiple small transparent dots that become increasingly white or gray with age appear in the central stroma.
      (2) Lattice corneal dystrophy: Corneal erosions result in amyloid deposits in a linear branching pattern in the stroma.

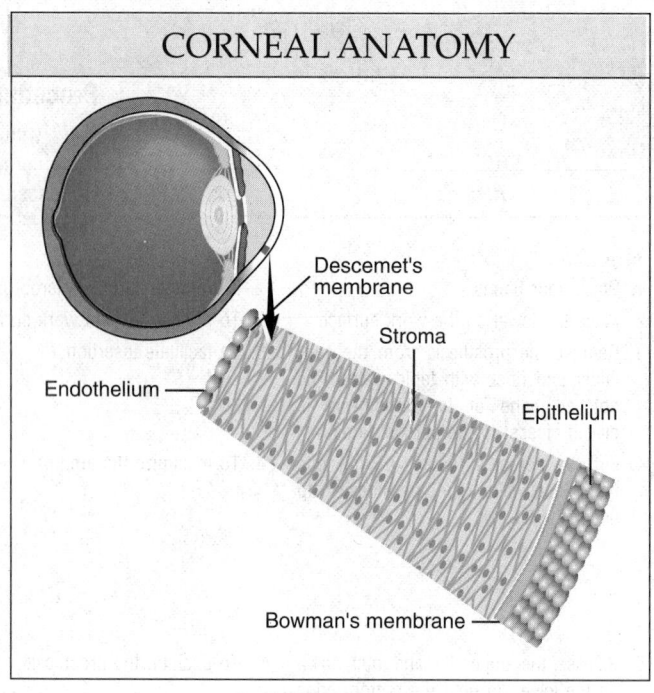

CORNEAL ANATOMY

Descemet's membrane
Stroma
Endothelium
Epithelium
Bowman's membrane

Figure 19–21.

Macular corneal dystrophy
   • Diffuse corneal clouding starts centrally and progresses to affect the whole thickness of the cornea.
   • Dense macules appear at the surface of the cornea and are often elevated.
   c. Endothelial layer and Descemet's membrane
      (1) Fuch's corneal dystrophy: Central wartlike deposits form on Descemet's membrane, along with thickening of the membrane and defects in the endothelium (see Color Fig. 19–6).
      (2) Posterior polymorphous dystrophy: Polymorphous vesicles, lines, and plaques occur in the endothelium and Descemet's membrane.
   d. Ectatic dystrophies—keratoconus
      (1) Thinning of the central cornea results in a cone-shaped cornea (Fig. 19–22).
      (2) Keratoconus is the second leading cause of corneal transplantation.

Pathophysiology

1. The integrity of the cornea is compromised by microscopic erosions, which result in corneal edema.
2. Corneal deposits further irritate tissues.

Clinical Manifestations

1. Corneal vesicles and erosions are painful.
2. Corneal edema causes blurred vision, and the corneal deposits also interfere with vision.
3. Distortion of the cornea results in astigmatic vision.

KERATOCONUS

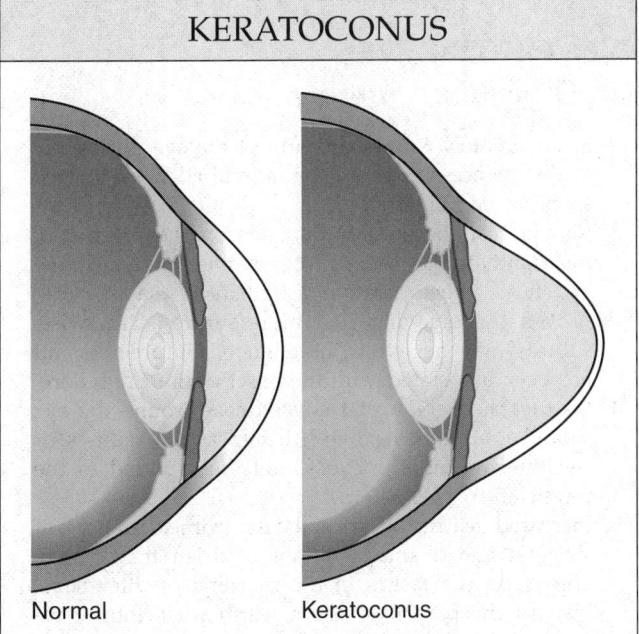

Normal   Keratoconus

Figure 19–22.

Diagnostics

1. History
   a. Ask questions about other family members with similar eye problems.
   b. Ascertain age of onset, frequency, and duration of symptoms.
   c. Assess the individual's cultural and personal beliefs regarding vision loss and transplantation.
2. Physical examination
   a. Visual acuity
   b. Slit-lamp examination—observe the anterior chamber and corneal layers.
3. Medical diagnosis—by identifying characteristics of the particular dystrophy in slit-lamp examination.

Clinical Management

1. The goal is to provide comfort and maximize visual acuity.
2. Pharmacologic intervention—lubricating eye drops and ointments.
3. Special medical-surgical procedures

NURSE ADVISORY

Lubricating eye ointments should be used only at night because they cause blurred vision. Lubricating eye drops should be used during the day.

   a. Scraping the epithelium removes deposits and vesicles in this layer, which regenerates over 24 to 72 hours.
   b. Corneal transplantation (penetrating keratoplasty) (Fig. 19–23).

   c. Lamellar keratoplasty
      (1) Partial-thickness corneal transplant
      (2) More successful with superficial corneal scarring or disease
   d. Complications—graft rejection (see Color Fig. 19–7).
      (1) Occurs in less than 10 percent of grafts.
      (2) The cornea is less disposed to transplant rejection

CORNEAL TRANSPLANTATION

Corneal transplantation (penetrating keratoplasty, or PKP) involves the surgical removal of the diseased or scarred cornea and the replacement with a human donor cornea. The steps are as follows:

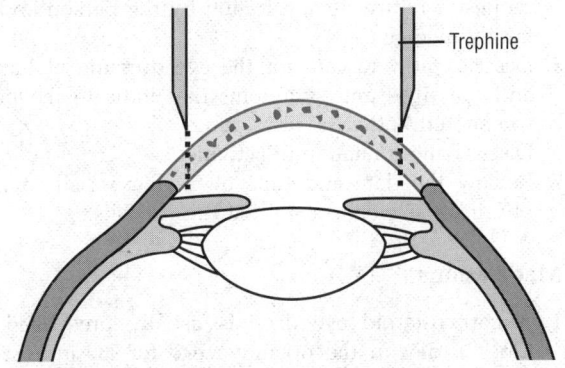

1 The center 7–8 mm of full-thickness diseased cornea is removed by using a trephine.

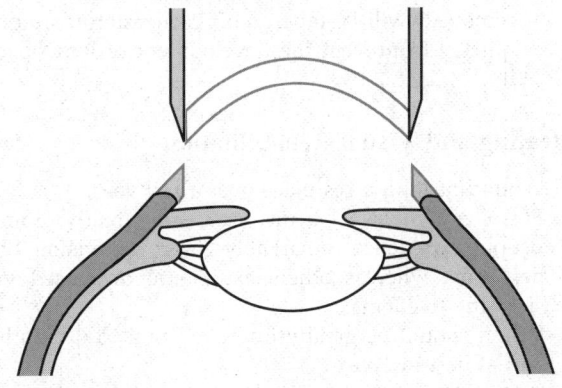

2 The donor cornea is cut at least 0.5 mm wider so that the edges overlap slightly.

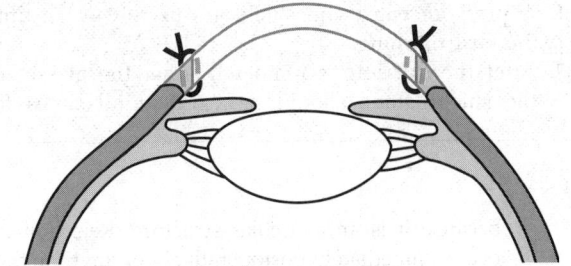

3 The donor cornea is sutured into place with two sets of interlaced running sutures or interrupted sutures.

Figure 19–23.

LEARNING/TEACHING GUIDELINES
for Self-Care After Corneal Transplant Surgery

General Overview

1. Using an eye model or a cross-section picture of the eye, point out the cornea and describe the surgical procedure.
2. Describe the healing process and the expected visual rehabilitation time frame.
3. Discuss the administration of eye drops, including the name of the medication and the rationale for use. Describe the dosage, frequency, and storage of the medication.
4. Demonstrate the instillation of the eye drops, and request a return demonstration by the person and a family member.
5. Describe how to care for the eye dressing at home and the signs and symptoms that indicate the person should notify the physician.
6. Discuss any limitation in activities.
7. Review the date and time of the next visit to the physician as well as expected future visits.

Medications

1. A corticosteroid eye drop is usually prescribed 4 times a day in the operative eye for an indefinite period of time. The medication is prescribed to reduce inflammation and prevent graft rejection.
   a. Phakic individuals (ones whose lens has not been removed) will be tapered off corticosteroids more quickly to prevent the development of lens opacity.

Healing and Visual Rehabilitation

1. Wound healing takes place over a full year.
2. Postoperative visual acuity can vary greatly. Some people experience remarkably improved vision the next day, whereas others experience decreased vision due to edema.
3. Vision should be greatly improved in 4 to 6 months and at best in 1 year.

Eye Dressing and Care

1. A pressure patch and shield are usually worn until the next morning.
2. After the dressing is removed, either the glasses or the shield alone should be worn at all times for approximately 6 weeks to protect the eye during the healing process. Remind the individual to put on the shield at bedtime.
3. Removal of the sutures depends on the practice of the ophthalmologist and the manner in which the eye heals. Postoperative astigmatism may be improved by removing 1 or more sutures. Otherwise, sutures may be left in indefinitely. Suture removal has been associated with the onset of graft rejection.
4. Instruct the person that any redness around the eye should gradually resolve. An increase in redness or swelling around the eye should be reported to the physician.
5. Increased tearing is normal after corneal transplant surgery, and a small amount of dried matter may appear on the lashes in the morning or after naps. Instruct the person to use a warm washcloth to remove the matter. If purulent drainage is noted, the person should call the physician.
6. Postoperative discomfort should be relieved by acetaminophen. Unrelieved pain should be reported to the physician (may be due to increased intraocular pressure).
7. A sudden or noticeable decrease in vision should also be reported to the physician. The person should check vision in the operative eye every day by looking with the operative eye at an object that is always in the same spot and in the same lighting.
8. Teach the individual to remember *RSVP* for signs of graft rejection:

   R = redness

   S = swelling

   V = vision loss

   P = pain

Activity

1. Avoid bumping the eye and contact sports for 1 year.

Postoperative Visits

1. Return visits are usually on the day after surgery, at 1 week, at 2 to 3 weeks, and then every 3 months.

because it is an avascular structure. Rejection may occur immediately postoperatively or anytime thereafter. It can often be resolved with an intense regimen of corticosteroid eye drops (given every 15 or 30 minutes around the clock until the reaction begins to regress).

Complications

1. Corneal scarring
2. Corneal perforation
3. Secondary inflammation or infection

Prognosis

1. There is no cure for corneal dystrophies, although progression in some individuals is very slow.
2. Corneal transplant surgery is successful in more than 90 percent of cases.

Applying the Nursing Process

NURSING DIAGNOSIS: Pain R/T corneal erosions

1. *Expected outcomes:* Following instruction, the person should be able to decrease discomfort.
2. *Nursing interventions*
   a. Instruct the person to use lubricating drops or ointment to decrease friction during blinking.
   b. A pressure patch may be necessary to promote healing of the epithelium.
   c. Encourage the use of acetaminophen or ibuprofen at regular intervals.

Discharge Planning and Teaching

Before discharge, people should learn the signs and symptoms of postoperative infection and graft rejection (Learning/Teaching Guidelines for Self-Care After Corneal Transplant Surgery).

Public Health Considerations: Primary Prevention

1. Availability of corneal tissue for transplant operations has been greatly increased by improved corneal preservation techniques and coordination of donor tissue by the state eye banking systems.
2. Required request regulations have also contributed to availability of tissue.
3. If donated eyes are unsuitable for transplantation (e.g., age, presence of infection), they are used in ophthalmic research.

◼ *DIABETIC RETINOPATHY*

Definition

Progressive microangiopathy characterized by small vessel damage and occlusion.

Incidence and Socioeconomic Impact

1. The leading cause of new cases of blindness in the United States.
2. In type I disease in diabetics who have had diabetes for at least 15 years, the prevalence of proliferative diabetic retinopathy is 50 percent.

Risk Factors

1. Duration of diabetes
2. The relationship of metabolic control of diabetes to diabetic retinopathy is not clear.
3. Hypertension
4. Elevated lipid levels
5. Renal disease

Etiology

1. Although not definitely proven, an accepted cause for diabetic retinopathy is thought to be widespread capillary closure (Fig. 19–24).

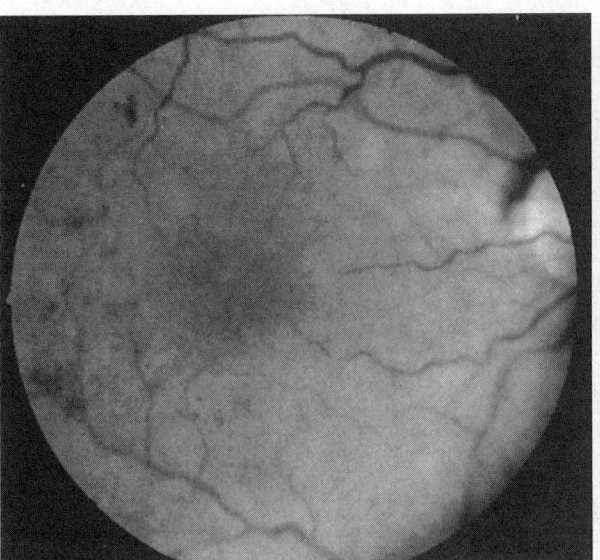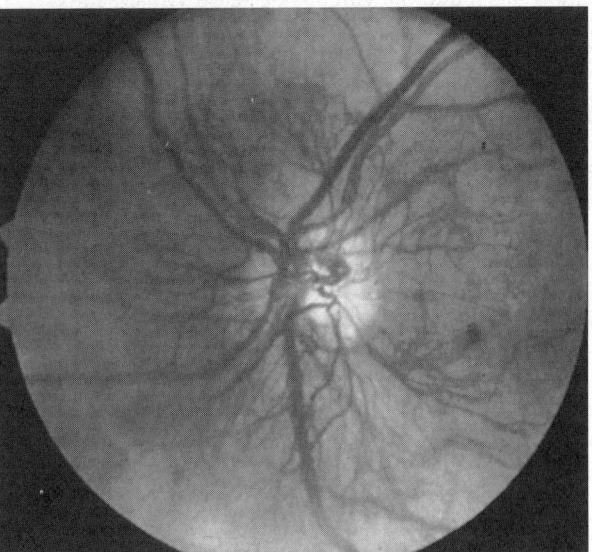

Figure 19–24. Diabetic retinopathy. (From Smith SC. Diabetic retinopathy. *Nurs Clin North Am* 27[3]:745–759, 1992.)

2. Background retinopathy (nonproliferative), which is characterized by the following:
   a. Microaneurysms
   b. Hemorrhages
   c. Soft exudates (cotton-wool spots)
   d. Hard exudates
3. Preproliferative diabetic retinopathy
   a. Characterized by the presence of intraretinal microvascular abnormalities such as shunt vessels, multiple cotton-wool spots, and venous bleeding.
   b. Severe macular edema is present.
   c. Ten to 40 percent of individuals who reach this stage develop proliferative diabetic retinopathy within 1 year.
4. Proliferative diabetic retinopathy
   a. Occurs in 5 percent of individuals with diabetic retinopathy.
   b. Vascular abnormalities appear on the surface of the retina.
   c. Visual loss may be severe.
   d. New blood vessels growing on the surface of the retina and the optic nerve are often attached to the surface of the vitreous body. Vitreous contraction causes hemorrhage.

Pathophysiology

1. Capillary closure results in retinal ischemia, which in turn stimulates the growth of new retinal vessels in an attempt to provide a blood supply to poorly perfused tissue.
2. The greatest amount of pathology is usually temporal to the macula.

Clinical Manifestations

1. Metamorphopsia (distorted lines and shapes) due to macular edema
2. Hemorrhages into the vitreous decrease visual acuity.
3. Color vision testing. In preproliferative diabetic retinopathy, a characteristic blue-yellow color vision develops as a result of electrophysiologic dysfunctions.
4. Contrast sensitivity may be reduced.
5. Visual field testing may demonstrate scotomas.
6. Abnormalities of dark adaptation

Diagnostics

1. History
   a. Ask the person questions about the onset and duration of diabetes.
   b. Note the amount of control and stability of blood glucose levels the person appears to maintain.
   c. Assess the individual's cultural and personal beliefs about vision loss.
2. Physical examination
   a. Direct and indirect ophthalmoscopy reveals the status of retinal vessels.

b. Fundus photographs and fluorescein angiography document changes over time.
3. Medical diagnosis: Diagnosis and staging are determined by the severity of symptoms and manifestations.

Clinical Management

1. The goal is to arrest the progression of the disease and maintain as much visual function as possible.
2. Pharmacologic intervention: Regulate insulin doses to maintain balanced blood glucose levels.
3. Special medical-surgical procedures
   a. Argon laser photocoagulation
      (1) Panretinal photocoagulation can reduce significantly the chance of massive vitreous hemorrhage and retinal detachment by burning and destroying the new and aberrant vessel growth (Fig. 19–25).
      (2) The xenon or argon laser may be used to place between 500 and 2000 microscopic burns around the peripheral retina.
      (3) Every laser burn that is placed to stop retinal vessel growth also destroys the retinal receptors in that area. Extreme caution should be used when placing burns near the macula.
   b. Vitrectomy
      (1) In cases of severe hemorrhage, removal of a portion of the vitreous to clear the debris may be necessary to improve vision.
      (2) Vitrectomy is also performed to loosen and remove fibrous bands and membranes that cause traction detachments or interfere with vision.

Complications

1. With delayed or without surgical intervention:
   a. Retinal detachment
   b. Vitreous hemorrhage
   c. Blindness
   d. Pregnancy can accelerate the progression of retinopathy.

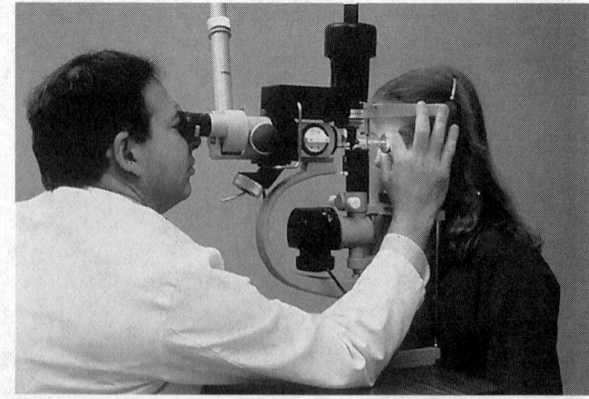

Figure 19–25. Argon laser treatment. (Courtesy of Ophthalmic Photography at the W.K. Kellogg Eye Center, University of Michigan, Ann Arbor, MI.)

LEARNING/TEACHING GUIDELINES
for Self-Care After Vitrectomy Surgery

General Overview

1. Using an eye model or a cross-section picture of the eye, describe the surgical procedure.
2. Describe the healing process and the expected visual rehabilitation time frame.
3. Discuss the administration of eye drops, including the name of the medication and the rationale for use. Describe the dosage, frequency, and storage of the medication.
4. Demonstrate the instillation of the eye drops, and request a return demonstration by the person and a family member.
5. Describe how to care for the eye dressing at home and the signs and symptoms that indicate the person should notify the physician.
6. Discuss any limitation in activities.
7. Review the date and time of the next visit to the physician as well as expected future visits.

Medications

1. Atropine is usually prescribed for dilating the eye and for cycloplegia (paralysis of the ciliary muscle).
   a. Dilation is necessary for visualization of the fundus at each return visit.
   b. Cycloplegia prevents spasm and promotes comfort.
2. Antibiotic eye drops are usually prescribed to prevent infection.
3. A corticosteroid drop may be prescribed 2 to 4 times a day to reduce inflammation.

Healing and Visual Rehabilitation

1. Wound healing takes place over 3 to 6 months.
2. Initially, vision is decreased owing to inflammation and edema.
3. Vision improves slowly. Best vision may take as long as 6 months.

4. If an air or air-gas bubble has been injected, the following will take place:
   a. Air will absorb in 1 week.
   b. SF6 gas absorbs in 1 to 3 weeks.
   c. C3F6 gas absorbs in 3 weeks to 3 months.

Eye Dressing and Care

1. Immediately after surgery the eye will be very red, sometimes ecchymotic, and swollen due to manipulation during surgery.
2. The next morning, after the dressing is removed, either the glasses or the shield alone should be worn at all times for approximately 6 weeks to protect the eye during the healing process. Remind the individual to put on the shield at bedtime.
3. Warm compresses may be applied 4 to 6 times a day to promote healing and provide comfort.
4. Redness of the conjunctiva may take up to 3 months to clear.
5. Postoperative discomfort should be relieved by acetaminophen. Initially, acetaminophen with codeine may be prescribed. Unrelieved pain should be reported to the physician (may indicate increase in intraocular pressure).
6. A sudden or noticeable decrease in vision, the appearance of black spots, or a curtain over the field of vision should also be reported to the physician.

Activity

1. Heavy lifting (greater than 25 pounds) is usually restricted.
2. Vigorous head movements should be avoided.
3. Individuals with an air-gas bubble should avoid high altitudes until the bubble is absorbed.

Postoperative Visits

1. Return visits are usually every 2 weeks until the condition is stable.

2. Postoperative complications
   a. No improvement
   b. Further hemorrhage and retinal detachment

Prognosis

Vitrectomy surgery should be undertaken with careful consideration of potential risks and benefits for the individual.

Application of the Nursing Process

NURSING DIAGNOSIS: Ineffective management of therapeutic regimen R/T nonacceptance of health status change

1. *Expected outcomes:* Following instruction, the person should be able to describe the importance of effective diabetic management.
2. *Nursing interventions*
   a. Review the relationship between diet, exercise, and insulin levels.
   b. Assess home environment and usual activities of daily living.
   c. Encourage the individual to make choices that affect long-term healthy practices.

NURSING DIAGNOSIS: Sensory-perceptual disturbances R/T decreased vision

1. *Expected outcomes:* Following instruction, the person should be able to describe adaptive techniques for handling difficulties experienced in performing activities of daily living.
2. *Nursing interventions*
   a. Assess home environment for lighting and safety hazards.
   b. Suggest use of hand-held magnifier, telescope, large-print publications, and glasses with filters to decrease glare and color distortion.
   c. Refer the individual to a low vision specialist or clinic.

Discharge Planning and Teaching

Before discharge, the person who has had a laser treatment or a vitrectomy needs to know what to expect and how to maximize vision (Learning/Teaching Guidelines for Self-Care After Vitrectomy Surgery).

Public Health Considerations: Primary Prevention

1. Education on the management of diabetes plays a significant role in determining how diabetic persons learn to take care of themselves.
2. In the United States, a diabetic person has more than a 20-fold chance of becoming blind than a nondiabetic person.

■ OCULAR INFLAMMATIONS

Definition

1. Ocular inflammations are marked by tissue irritation and edema; inflammatory disorders can arise in various eye structures.
2. Ocular inflammations include chalazion, blepharitis, and uveitis.
   a. Chalazion is an idiopathic, sterile, chronic, granulomatous inflammation of a meibomian gland. It often points toward the conjunctival surface (see Color Fig. 19–8).
   b. Blepharitis is a chronic bilateral inflammation of the lid margins.
   c. Uveitis is an inflammation of the uveal tract.
      (1) Anterior uveitis (iritis): usually unilateral
      (2) Posterior uveitis: retina may be affected
      (3) Nongranulomatous uveitis: occurs mainly in the anterior portion of the uveal tract (iris and ciliary body). In severe cases, a fibrin clot or hypopyon may form in the anterior chamber.
      (4) Granulomatous: affects all areas of the uvea including the posterior portion (retina). Inflammatory deposits collect on the surface of the cornea. Nodular collections of cells and lymphocytes are present in affected areas.

Incidence and Socioeconomic Impact

Ocular inflammations are common.

Risk Factors

1. Chalazion and blepharitis—none
2. Uveitis
   a. Rheumatoid arthritis and gout
   b. Inflammatory bowel disease
   c. Immunosuppression
   d. Psoriasis
   e. Secondary to ocular surgery or disease

Etiology

Unknown

Pathophysiology

1. Chalazion: obstruction of the meibomian gland
2. Blepharitis: may be associated with scalp seborrhea or *Staphylococcus* infections
3. Uveitis: The proximity of the affected tissues—the iris, ciliary body, and choroid—provides a mechanism for the inflammation to spread from one structure to another.

Clinical Manifestations

1. Chalazion—acute swelling, redness, and pain
2. Blepharitis—irritation, burning, and itching of the lid margins
3. Uveitis
   a. Nongranulomatous
      (1) Acute onset of redness, photophobia, blurred vision, and pain.
      (2) Presence of keratic precipitates, fine white deposits, on the posterior surface of the cornea.
   b. Granulomatous—more insidious onset of pain, redness, photophobia, and blurred vision

Diagnostics

1. History
   a. Ask the person what treatments have been used at home.
   b. Assess the person's cultural and personal beliefs about eye inflammations and vision loss.
2. Physical examination
   a. Penlight examination
   b. Slit-lamp examination
3. Medical diagnosis
   a. Chalazion—size, shape, and location of swelling
   b. Blepharitis

(1) Presence of scales or granulations clinging to lashes

(2) Redness of lid margins

c. Uveitis—presence of inflammatory cells in the anterior chamber accompanying clinical manifestations

Clinical Management

1. The goal is to resolve the inflammatory process.
2. Pharmacologic interventions
   a. Antibiotic (usually sulfonamide) eye drops to arrest and prevent further infection.
   b. Corticosteroid eye drops to reduce inflammation.
   c. Pupil dilation and cycloplegia are necessary in uveitis to keep the iris from forming synechiae and to relieve ciliary spasm.
3. Special medical-surgical procedures: Chalazion may be resolved with frequent warm compresses, or incision and curettage may be necessary.

Complications

1. Chalazion
   a. Spread of local infection
   b. Development of chronic cysts
2. Blepharitis—spread of infection
3. Uveitis
   a. Posterior synechiae (adherence of the iris to the cornea), which may block the flow of aqueous and result in glaucoma
   b. Retinal detachment
   c. Cystoid macular edema

Prognosis

1. Chalazion and blepharitis usually resolve but may recur.
2. Uveitis is often a chronic condition.

Applying the Nursing Process

NURSING DIAGNOSIS: Ineffective management R/T chronic recurrence of condition

1. *Expected outcomes:* Following instruction, the person should be able to describe the importance of effective treatment.
2. *Nursing interventions*
   a. Describe the inflammatory process, and explain that response to treatment is often slow.
   b. Explain that the condition may occur again even after it appears to be resolved.
   c. Discuss the importance of the medications and follow-up appointments.

Discharge Planning and Teaching

1. It is rarely necessary to hospitalize a person with an ocular inflammatory disease.
2. It is important that the person and a family member understand the chronic aspects of the condition and the need for follow-up.

Public Health Considerations: Primary Prevention

1. Unless it is due to an ocular infection, an inflammatory condition is not contagious.
2. Many people who develop uveitis have a history of other inflammatory conditions.

◼ OCULAR INFECTIONS

Definition

1. Invasion of ocular tissues and structures by a variety of microorganisms, resulting in tissue damage and loss of vision
2. Ocular infections include hordeolum, conjunctivitis, keratitis, and dacryocystitis.
   a. Hordeolum (sty) is an acute focal infection of the meibomian glands at the eyelid margin.
   b. Conjunctivitis is an inflammation of the conjunctiva caused by microorganism activity, characterized by vascular dilation, cellular infiltration, and exudation.
   c. Keratitis is an inflammation and infection of the cornea, sometimes resulting in corneal ulcer. Corneal ulcer is a break or open sore in the outer layer of the cornea (see Chapters 36 and 37).
   d. Dacryocystitis is an inflammation and infection of the lacrimal sac.

Incidence and Socioeconomic Impact

1. Mild eye infections such as sty are common and respond well to treatment.
2. Severe eye infections are less common and may result in blindness.

Risk Factors

1. Trauma
2. Surgical procedure
3. Overwear of contact lenses
4. Dry eyes

Etiology

Exposure and susceptibility to microorganisms.

Pathophysiology

Structures of the eye and orbit may be infected with organisms that affect open wounds in any other part of the body. Organisms include bacteria, viruses, fungi, and amoebae.

Clinical Manifestations

1. Redness and swelling around the infected area
2. Sloughing of tissue, particularly in the cornea
3. Presence of purulent drainage—hypopyon (pus in the anterior chamber) (see Color Fig. 19–9)

Diagnostics

1. History
   a. Ask the person what treatments have been used at home.
   b. Assess the person's cultural and personal beliefs about eye infections and vision loss.
2. Physical examination
   a. Examination of lid margins and external eye by penlight, ophthalmoscopy, and slit lamp.
   b. Examination under microscope of tissue smear and staining is performed to obtain preliminary identification of organism.
   c. Culture of drainage or tissues is analyzed.
3. Medical diagnosis
   a. Gram-staining reveals gram-positive or negative bacteria.
   b. Culture report identifies organism
   c. Hypopyon (a layer of white blood cells in the anterior chamber) may be diagnostic of corneal ulceration.

Clinical Management

1. The goal is to arrest or destroy the growth of bacteria and to prevent damage to ocular structures.
2. Pharmacologic interventions
   a. For small infections such as sty, instillation of sulfonamide eye drops is usually prescribed.
   b. For severe infections that affect the cornea, antibiotics and antiviral or antifungal eye drops may be prescribed as frequently as every 15 minutes around the clock.
   c. Often 2 antibiotics may be prescribed to be given alternatively, or together, 5 minutes apart.

ELDER ADVISORY

The thin, delicate facial skin of older adults may become irritated by the constant tearing and application of frequent eye drops. To prevent skin breakdown, coat the skin under the eyelid with a light application of petroleum jelly. Provide for a margin at the lid so that the petroleum jelly does not get into the eye.

d. As the cornea begins to heal, the frequency of eye drops may be reduced to every 30 minutes, then every hour, and so forth.
e. Fortified antibiotics may be prescribed. Fortified (strengthened in dosage) medication is not usually available commercially and must be prepared by a pharmacist. Expiration dates vary but are usually within days or 1 week.
f. Bacteriostatic antibiotics inhibit bacterial growth.

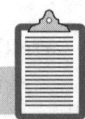

NURSING MANAGEMENT

Managing the workload assignment can be a challenge when 1 or more persons require the administration of frequent eye drops. Sharing the responsibility of administering the eye drops prevents 1 nurse from being occupied nearly totally with eye drop instillation.

1. Post a small sign at the door or at the bedside that shows a clock and the times that alternating drops are to be given.

gentamycin

12

tobramycin   9   3   tobramycin

6

gentamycin

2. Assign 1 nurse to administer the drop on the hour and half hour and a 2nd nurse to administer the drop on the quarter hours.
3. If there is more than 1 person receiving frequent eye drops, consider assigning 4 nurses, 1 to each quarter hour.

g. Bactericidal antibiotics destroy bacteria.
3. Special medical-surgical procedures
   a. If a sty does not respond to warm compresses and antibiotic eye drops, incision and drainage may be necessary.
   b. Anterior or posterior vitrectomy may be performed to obtain a specimen for culture and sensitivity studies.
   c. Conjunctival flap may be performed to maintain corneal integrity if the cornea becomes very thin.
   d. Dacryocystorhinostomy (probing the lacrimal canal) may be necessary if the canal becomes constricted or obstructed after an infection.
   e. Corneal transplant is contraindicated while infection is present.

Complications

1. Endophthalmitis (infection of the entire eyeball)
2. Cellulitis of the orbit and face
3. Encephalitis
4. Septicemia

Prognosis

Directly related to the severity of the infection, the person's immune system's ability to heal, and the availability of effective medication.

Applying the Nursing Process

NURSING DIAGNOSIS: Sleep pattern disturbance R/T instillation of frequent eye drops

1. *Expected outcomes:* Following instruction, the person should be able to identify strengths and coping mechanisms in experiencing fatigue, irritability, anger, increased sensitivity to pain, depression, and sometimes confusion.
2. *Nursing interventions*
   a. Assess normal sleep pattern at home (usual bedtime, number of times up during the night, usual waking time, use of sleep aids, naps during the day).
   b. Ask the person to describe usual bedtime routine.
   c. Establish times for bedtime and nap or rest periods during the day.
   d. During rest times, draw blinds and make room comfortable. Remind the person that the only interruption will be the nurse administering eye drops. If the individual prefers, the nurse administers the eye drops with as little stimulation as possible, that is, with no conversation.
   e. Offer sedative at bedtime and analgesics regularly.
   f. Encourage exercise schedule and other diversional activities during waking times.
   g. Show the individual how to use relaxation techniques such as deep breathing or imagery.

Discharge Planning and Teaching

1. Hand washing before and after touching the eyes is imperative.
2. Instruct persons with an eye infection of any kind to use a separate tissue or washcloth for each eye to prevent cross-contamination.
3. If an individual is going to be sent home on a schedule of frequent eye drops, it will be necessary to mobilize 1 or more friends or family to assist the person with the administration.
4. If the person lives in a small town or community, check the availability of any fortified medication.
5. After a dacryocystorhinostomy, a small pressure dressing is placed over the suture line and is removed after 2 days. The wound should be kept dry. The skin heals in 4 days.

Public Health Considerations: Primary Prevention

1. All eye infections are spread by direct contact and are preventable by hand washing.
2. With universal precautions, isolation of persons with eye infections is no longer necessary.
3. Appropriate cleaning, handling, and wearing of contact lenses (soft or hard) are essential in preventing needless eye infections (See Procedure 19–11).

◼ *OTHER OCULAR CONDITIONS*

Strabismus (see Chapter 15)

Bibliography

Books

Berson F. *Basic Ophthalmology for Medical Students and Primary Care Residents.* San Francisco: American Academy of Ophthalmology, 1993.

Chawla HB. *Ophthalmology.* 2nd ed. Edinburgh: Churchill Livingstone, 1993.

Hoffman J. *Pocket Glossary of Ophthalmologic Terminology.* Thorofare, NJ: Slack, Inc, 1989.

Pavan-Langston D. *Manual of Ocular Diagnosis and Therapy.* 3rd ed. Boston: Little, Brown & Co, 1991.

Pavan-Langston D, and Dunkel E. *Handbook of Ocular Drug Therapy and Ocular Side Effects of Systemic Drugs.* Boston: Little, Brown & Co, 1991.

Phillips EI, et al. *Ophthalmology.* London: Bailliere Tindall, 1994.

Stein H, Slatt B, and Stein R. *The Ophthalmic Assistant.* St. Louis: CV Mosby, 1988.

Vaughan D, Asbury T, and Riordan-Eva P. *General Ophthalmology.* 13th ed. Norwalk, CT: Appleton & Lange, 1992.

Chapters in Books

Buxton J, and Buxton D. Corneal surgery. *In* Collins J (ed). *Ophthalmic Desk Reference,* New York: Raven Press, Ltd, 1991.

Schremp P. Interventions for clients with eye and visual disorders. *In* Ignatavicius, DD, Workman ML, and Mishler MA. *Medical-Surgical Nursing: A Nursing Process Approach.* 2nd ed. Philadelphia: WB Saunders, pp 1297–1349.

Vader L. Nursing care of clients with eye disorders. *In* Black JM, and Matassarin-Jacobs E (eds). *Luckmann and Sorensen's Medical-Surgical Nursing: A Psychophysiologic Approach.* 4th ed. Philadelphia: WB Saunders, 1993.

Journal Articles

Bigar F, and Herbort C. Corneal transplantation. *Curr Opin Ophthalmol* 3:473–481, 1992.

Bigerly J, and Nozik R. Management of uveitis. *Curr Opin Ophthalmol* 3:527–533, 1992.

Cleary M. Helping the person who is visually impaired: Concerns, questions, remedies, & resources. *J Ophthalmic Nurs Technol* 14(5):205–211, 1995.

Edwards M, and Schachat A. Impact of enucleation for choroidal melanoma on the performance of vision-dependent activities. *Arch Ophthalmol* 109:519–21, 1991.

Fishbaugh J. Nursing care of the patient with corneal graft rejection. *Insight* 20(4):34–37, 1995.

Gardner T. Complications of retinal laser therapy and their prevention. *Semin Ophthalmol* 6(1):19–26, 1991.

Glynn-Milley C, and MacKay J. Home care for the postoperative patient. *Insight* 20(4):21–25, 1995.

Harding J. Cataract epidemiology. *Curr Opin Ophthalmol* 1:10–15, 1990.

Huber-Spitzy V, and Grabner G. Degenerative conditions, keratoconus, contact lenses, and dry eyes. *Curr Opin Ophthalmol* 2:402–408, 1991.

Lim A, Chew P, and Jin C. Surgical methods. *Curr Opin Ophthalmol* 1:16–19, 1990.

Masket S. Complications of cataract and intraocular lens surgery. *Curr Opin Ophthalmol* 3:52–59, 1992.

Meissner JE. Caring for patients with glaucoma. *Nursing* 25(1):56–57, 1995.

Pallan L, Eller A, and Friberg T. Pneumatic retinopexy: An overview. *Semin Ophthalmol* 6(1):27–35, 1991.

Rapuano C, and Laibson P. Corneal dystrophies. *Curr Opin Ophthalmol* 3:438–444, 1992.

Sandler RL. Clinical snapshot: Glaucoma. *Am J Nurs* 95:(3):34–35, 1995.

Sawusch M, and McDonnell P. Posterior capsule opacification. *Curr Opin Ophthalmol* 1:28–33, 1990.

Sivalingam E. Glaucoma: An overview. *J Opththalmic Nurs Technol* 15(1):15–18, 1995.

Slakter J. Recent developments in ophthalmic lasers. *Curr Opin Ophthalmol* 3:83–93, 1992.

Smith S. Complications of surgery. *Curr Opin Ophthalmol* 1:34–41, 1990.

Solomon K, and Kostick A. Capsular opacification after cataract surgery. *Curr Opin Ophthalmol* 3:46–51, 1992.

Vader L. Invisible light. *Insight* 17(2):12–14, 1992.

Vader L. Vision and vision loss. *Nurs Clin North Am* 27(3):705–714, 1992.

van Bijsterveld O, and van Hemel O. Bacterial conjunctivitis. *Curr Opin Ophthalmol* 1:323–332, 1990.

Other Publications

American Academy of Ophthalmology. Basic and Clinical Science Course Section 4: Ophthalmic Pathology and Intraocular Tumors, San Francisco, CA: Author, 1992–1993.

American Academy of Ophthalmology. Basic and Clinical Science Course Section 7: Orbit, Eyelids, and Lacrimal System, San Francisco, CA: Author, 1993–1994.

American Academy of Ophthalmology. Basic and Clinical Science Course Section 8: Glaucoma, Lens, and Anterior Segment Trauma, San Francisco, CA: Author, 1989–1990.

American Academy of Ophthalmology. Basic and Clinical Science Course Section 8: Pediatric Ophthalmology and Strabismus, San Francisco, CA: Author, 1994–1995.

Ginsburg L, and Aiello L. Diabetic retinopathy: Classification, progression, and management. *Focal Points*. San Francisco, CA: America Academy of Ophthalmology, September 1993.

U.S. Department of Health and Human Services. *Cataract in Adults: Management of Functional Impairment*. Public Health Service, Agency for Health Care Policy and Research, Clinical Practice Guideline Number 4. Bethesda, MD, 1993.

Agencies

American Foundation for the Blind
15 West 16th Street
New York, NY 10011
(800) 232–5463

Association for Education and
  Rehabilitation of the Blind and Visually
  Impaired
206 North Washington Street, Suite 320
Alexandria, VA 22314
(703) 548–1884

Lions Clubs International
330 22nd Street
Oakbrook, IL 60521
(708) 571–5466

National Eye Institute
National Institutes of Health
Building 31, Room 6A32
Bethesda, MD 20892
(301) 496–5248

National Society to Prevent Blindness
500 East Remington Road
Schaumberg, IL 60173
(800) 331–2020

Talking Books: National Library Service
  for the Blind and Visually Impaired
Library of Congress
Washington, DC 20540
(800) 424–9100

20
Caring for People with Ear, Nose, Throat, Head, and Neck Disorders

◻ *EAR, NOSE, AND THROAT STRUCTURE AND FUNCTION*

The Cranium

1. Eight bones from the **cranium:** the frontal bone, 2 parietal bones, the occipital bone, 2 temporal bones, the sphenoid bone, and the ethmoid bone (Fig. 20–1). Some cranial bones contain sinuses that, along with the mastoid air cells, reduce the weight of the skull.
2. The facial skull has several cavities and forms the basic shape of the face. It provides the surface attachment for muscles controlling the jaw and facial expression.
   a. Thirteen immovable bones form the **facial skeleton:** 2 maxillae bones, 2 palatine bones, 2 zygomatic bones, 2 lacrimal bones, 2 nasal bones, 2 inferior nasal conchae bones, and the vomer bone.
   b. The mandible is the only movable bone in the facial skeleton and is attached to the cranium by ligaments.
   c. Facial muscles are innervated by cranial nerves (CNs) V (the trigeminal nerve) and VII (the facial nerve). (See Chapter 18.)
3. The cranium encloses and protects the brain. It is also the surface to which the muscles that control the jaw and head movements are attached.
4. The **neck** is formed by 7 cervical vertebrae, ligaments, the sternocleidomastoid muscle, and the trapezius muscles (Fig. 20–2).
   a. Mobility is greatest at the level of C4–5 or C5–6.
   b. The relationships of these muscles, bones, and joints are used as landmarks.
      (1) The posterior triangle of the neck is formed by the trapezius and sternocleidomastoid muscles and the clavicles. It contains the posterior cervical lymph nodes.
      (2) The anterior triangle of the neck is formed by the medial borders of the sternocleidomastoid muscles and the mandible. It houses the carotid artery, internal and external jugular veins, and anterior cervical lymph nodes.

The Temporal Bones and Ears

1. The temporal bones
   a. The 2 **temporal bones** house the ears.

b. Each temporal bone is divided into 4 parts: the squamous, the petrous, the tympanic, and the mastoid.
   (1) The squamous part is superior to the external auditory canal (EAC).
   (2) The petrous part is anterior to the EAC and houses the middle and inner ears.
   (3) The tympanic part is inferior to the EAC.
   (4) The mastoid part is posterior to the EAC. It consists of the mastoid process, the mastoid antrum, and the mastoid air cells and communicates with the middle ear.
   c. Each temporal bone articulates with the sphenoid, parietal, and occipital bones.
   d. Each temporal bone protects the EAC and internal auditory canal, the mastoid air cells, the blood vessels, the facial and auditory nerves, the labyrinth, and the cochlea.
   e. Interconnected air-filled cavities in the mastoid help the middle ears adjust to changes in pressure. This system of cavities and air cells also lightens the skull, which is necessary for human posture.
2. The ears
   a. The **external ear** is divided into 3 parts: the pinna or auricle; the EAC, or ear canal; and the tympanic membrane, or eardrum (Fig. 20–3).
      (1) The **pinna** is the visible part of the ear. It is attached to the side of the head by skin and, except for fat and subcutaneous skin in the lobule, is composed of cartilage. The major parts of the pinna are the helix, the concha, the tragus, and the lobule. The pinna collects sound vibrations and directs them to the ear canal.
      (2) The **EAC** is an S-shaped canal, approximately 2.5 cm or 1 inch in length, that extends from the concha to the tympanic membrane. The outer one third of the EAC has a skeleton of cartilage, and the inner two thirds have a skeleton of bone. The skin of the EAC contains sebaceous glands, ceruminous glands, and hair follicles. Ceruminous glands produce cerumen or wax. Wax and fine hairs cleanse the ear of foreign materials, which protects the tympanic membrane.
      (3) The **tympanic membrane** covers the end of the EAC and separates the EAC from the middle ear. It consists of 3 layers of tissue: an outer layer of skin that is continuous with the EAC, a fibrous

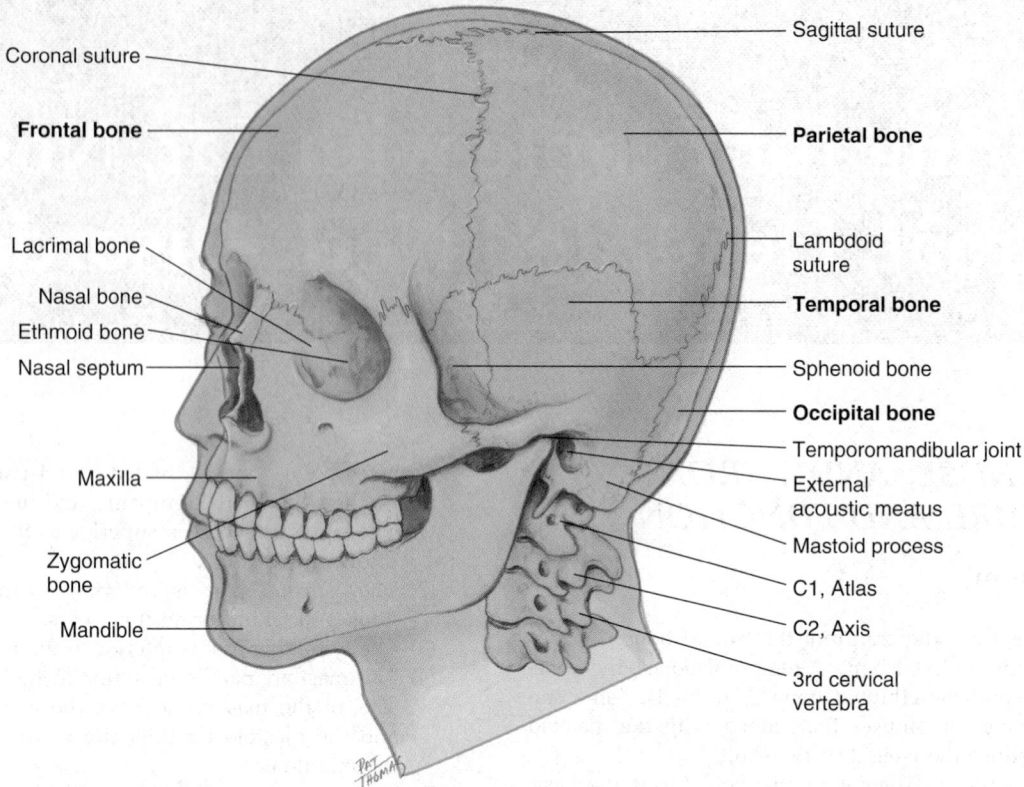

Figure 20–1. Bones of the skull. (From Jarvis C. *Physical Examination and Health Assessment*. 2nd ed. Philadelphia: WB Saunders, 1996, p 268.)

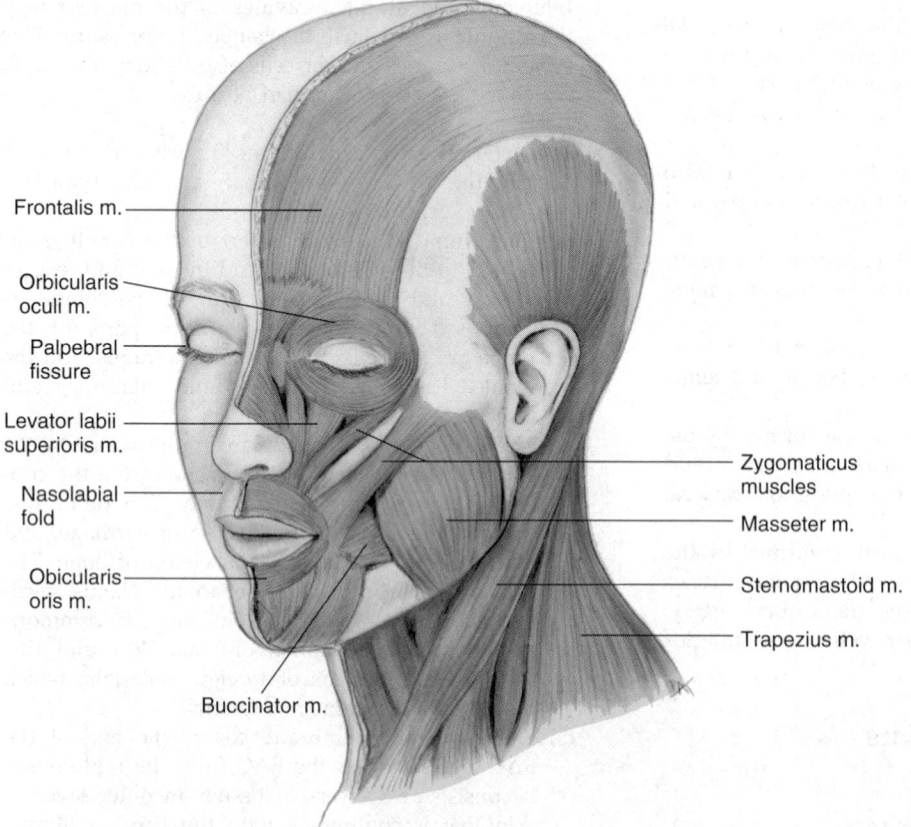

Figure 20–2. Anterior and posterior triangles of the neck and face. (From Jarvis C. *Physical Examination and Health Assessment*. 2nd ed. Philadelphia: WB Saunders, 1996, p 269.)

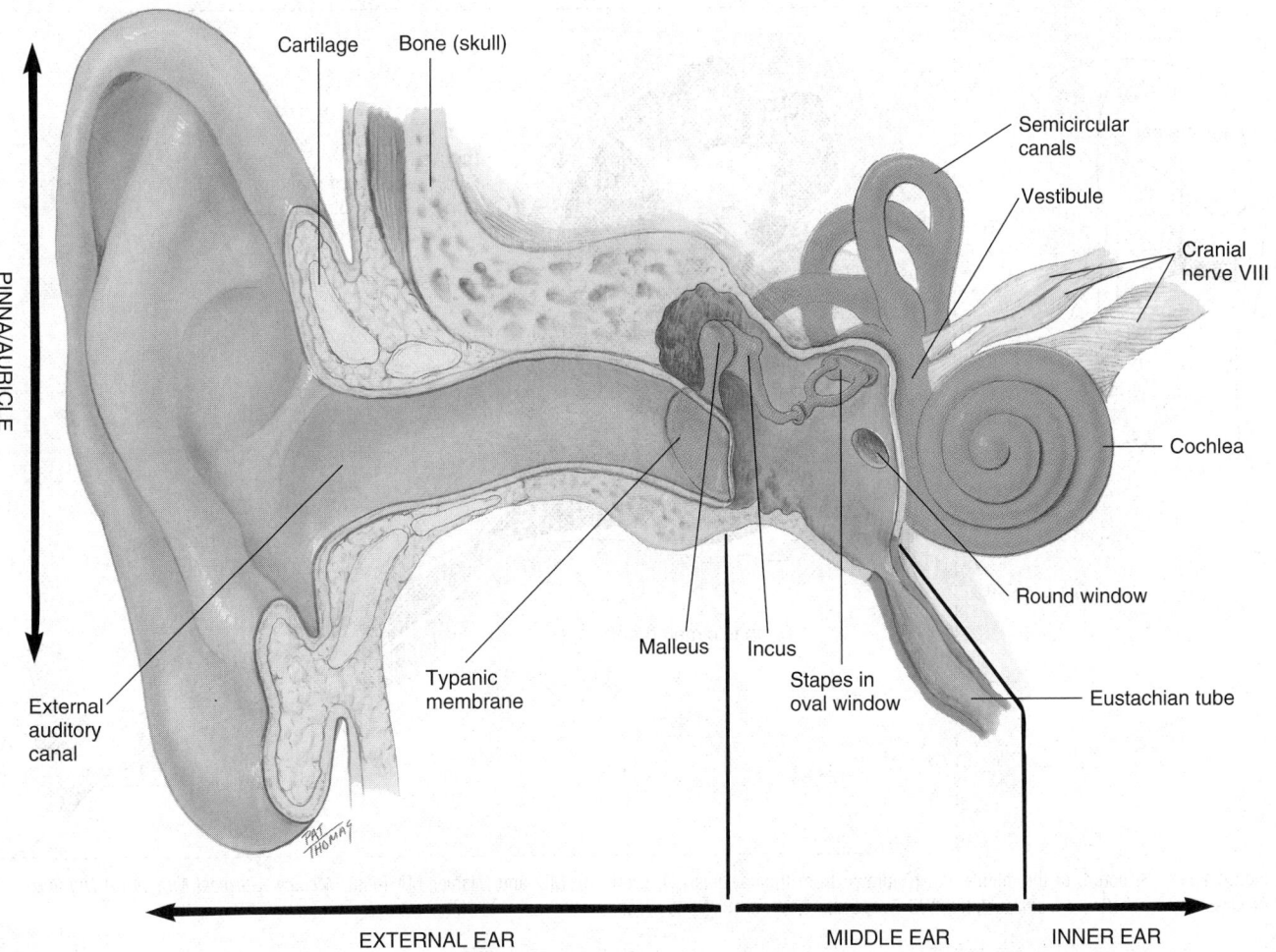

Figure 20-3. Anatomy of the ear. (From Jarvis C. *Physical Examination and Health Assessment.* 2nd ed. Philadelphia: WB Saunders, 1996, p 353.)

supporting layer, and an inner layer of mucosa that is continuous with the middle ear. The distinguishing landmarks of the tympanic membrane are the annulus, the fibrous border that attaches the tympanic membrane to the temporal bone, the short and long processes of the malleus, the umbo of the malleus, the pars flaccida, and the pars tensa. The functions of the tympanic membrane are to protect the middle ear and conduct sound vibrations from the EAC to the ossicles.

b. The **middle ear** contains the ossicles, the oval and round windows, and the eustachian tube. It is located above the jugular fossa, behind the carotid canal, and in front of the mastoid air cells (Fig. 20–4).

(1) The **ossicles** of the middle ear are the malleus, or hammer; the incus, or anvil; and the stapes, or stirrup. The ossicles are held in place by joints, muscles, and ligaments that also protect the inner ear from loud sounds. The ossicles transmit sound vibrations from the external ear, through the middle ear, to the inner ear.

(2) Two windows, named for their shapes, are located in the middle ear. The **oval window,** which is filled by the footplate of the stapes, allows sound vibrations to enter the inner ear. The **round win-**

dow is the exit through which sound vibrations leave the inner ear.

(3) The **eustachian tube** is a narrow channel, 3.5 cm long and 1 mm wide at its narrow end, that connects the middle ear to the nasopharynx. The eustachian tube is composed of fibrous tissue, cartilage, and bone and is lined with mucous membrane. The walls of the eustachian tube touch each other lightly but are forcibly opened during yawning, swallowing, sneezing, and the Valsalva maneuver. The eustachian tube allows air to pass from the nasopharynx to the middle ear and equalizes pressure on both sides of the tympanic membrane.

c. The **inner ear,** or labyrinth, contains the sense organs, or end organs, for hearing and balance and cranial nerves VII and VIII. The **bony labyrinth** surrounds and protects the delicate membranous labyrinth and is composed of the cochlea and the semicircular canals (Fig. 20–5).

(1) The cochlea is a snail-shaped bony tube about 3.5 cm in length that spirals for 2.5 turns. It is divided into the scala vestibuli (the upper compartment), the scala tympani (the lower compartment), and the cochlear duct. Semicircular canals are at right

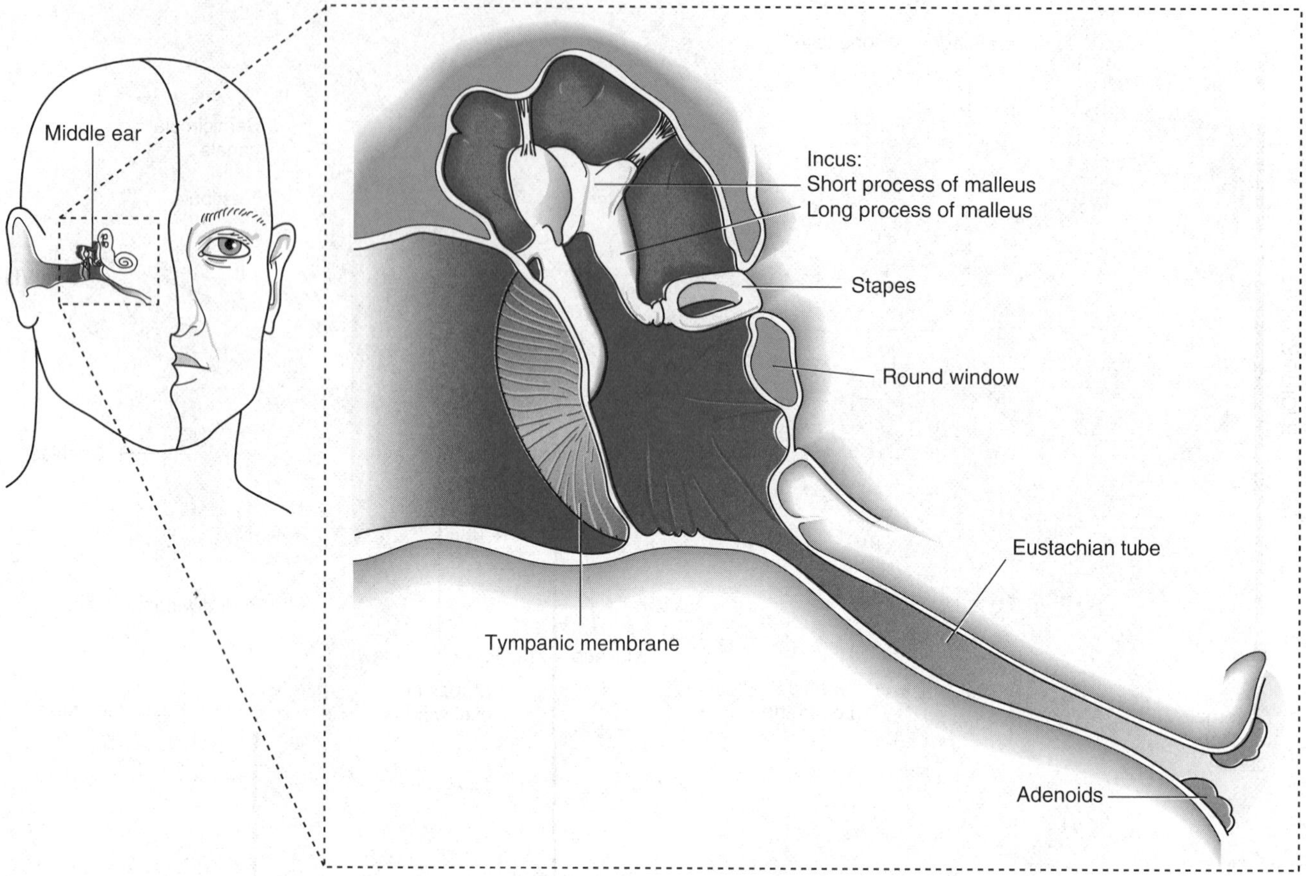

Incus:
Short process of malleus
Long process of malleus

Stapes

Round window

Eustachian tube

Adenoids

Tympanic membrane

Middle ear

Figure 20–4. Structure of the middle ear. (Redrawn from Ignatavicius DD, Workman ML, and Mishler MA [eds]. *Medical-Surgical Nursing: A Nursing Process Approach.* 2nd ed. Philadelphia: WB Saunders, 1996, p 1354.)

angles to each other. They are called the superior, posterior, and lateral (or horizontal) canals.

(2) The **membranous labyrinth** lies within the bony labyrinth but does not completely fill it. It is bathed in perilymph, much like cerebrospinal fluid, and contains endolymph. The membranous labyrinth has several parts, including the utricle,

saccule, membranous semicircular canals, the cochlear duct, and the organ of Corti. The utricle and saccule are vestibular receptors that initiate reflexes to adjust the head's position in response to the pull of gravity and movement. The membranous semicircular canals are arranged to sense rotational movements.

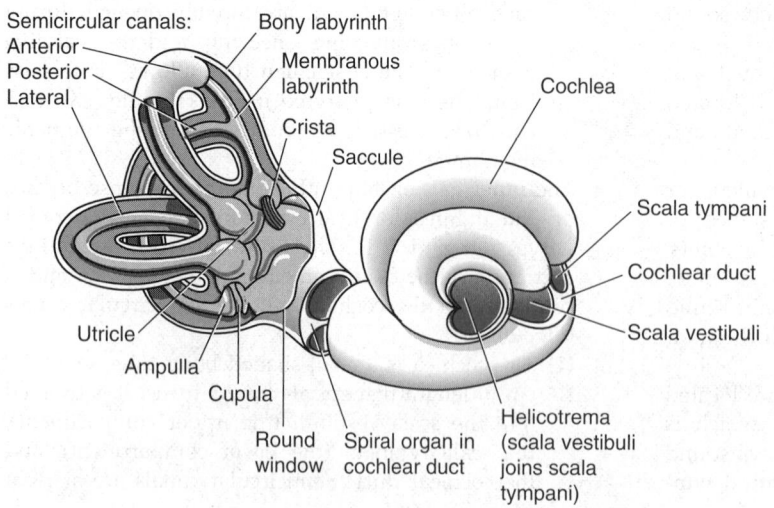

Semicircular canals:
Anterior
Posterior
Lateral

Bony labyrinth

Membranous labyrinth

Crista

Saccule

Cochlea

Scala tympani

Cochlear duct

Scala vestibuli

Utricle

Ampulla

Cupula

Round window

Spiral organ in cochlear duct

Helicotrema (scala vestibuli joins scala tympani)

Figure 20–5. Structure of the inner ear. (Redrawn from Black JM, and Matassarin-Jacobs E [eds]. *Luckmann and Sorensen's Medical-Surgical Nursing: A Psychophysiologic Approach.* 4th ed. Philadelphia: WB Saunders, 1993, p 869.)

(3) The cochlear duct is located between the scala vestibuli and the scala tympani. It contains the organ of Corti.

(4) The functions of the inner ear are hearing and balance.

  • Sound vibrations pass from the stapes footplate through the oval window and move the perilymph. Vibrations of the perilymph are transmitted through the vestibular membrane to the endolymph that fills the cochlear duct. The organ of Corti lies on the basilar membrane. It transforms mechanical sound in neural activity and separates sound into different frequencies. Electrochemical impulses travel from the organ of Corti to the temporal cortex via the acoustic nerve. The impulses are decoded from sound to speech in the cerebral cortex.

  • The utricle, the saccule, and the 3 semicircular canals are the sense organs responsible for body and head position. The semicircular canals sense rotational movement. The utricle and saccule are involved with linear movement.

The Nose

1. The **external nose** consists of a bony section (upper one third) and a cartilaginous section (lower two thirds) covered by skin. The nose is surrounded by the maxilla bones laterally and inferiorly and the frontal bone superiorly. The **nasion** is the point where the nose joins the forehead, the bridge of the nose is called the **dorsum**, and the **base** is where the nose joins the upper lip. The **nares** are separated by the **columella** and allow air to pass into the nasopharynx.

2. The **nasal cavity** (internal nose) lies over the oral cavity (Fig. 20–6). The irregularly shaped nasal cavity is separated in the midline by a **septum**. The lateral walls of the nose are formed by the inferior, middle, and superior turbinates. The muscles of the nose are innervated by cranial nerves I, V, and VII.

3. **Nasal mucosa** lines the nasal cavity with 2 different epithelium. The nares open into the vestibule, which is lined with stratified squamous epithelium, vibrissae (coarse hairs), sebaceous glands, and sweat glands. The nasal cavity is lined with pseudostratified ciliated epithelium containing goblet cells that secrete mucus. The olfactory nerves are located near the roof of the nasal cavity. The posterior nares are funnel-shaped openings that permit air to pass from the nasal cavity into the nasopharynx.

4. The major functions of the nose are to warm, filter, and moisten inhaled air; provide the sense of smell; and serve as the primary passageway for air to the lungs.

The Paranasal Sinuses

1. The 4 pairs of **paranasal sinuses** are frontal, maxillary, ethmoid, and sphenoid (Fig. 20–7).
   a. **Frontal sinuses** are located above the orbit of each eye.
   b. **Maxillary sinuses** (the largest sinuses) lie along the lateral wall of the nasal cavity.
   c. **Ethmoid sinuses** lie near the superior portion of the nasal cavity.
   d. **Sphenoid sinuses** lie deep in the skull, behind the ethmoid sinuses.

2. The paranasal sinuses are sterile air-containing spaces that open and drain into the nasal cavity through the ostia of the middle meatus.

3. The paranasal sinuses lighten the weight of the skull and give timbre and resonance to the voice.

The Pharynx

1. The **pharynx** is a muscular, tube-shaped structure approximately 12.5 cm in length that extends from the base of the skull to the larynx.

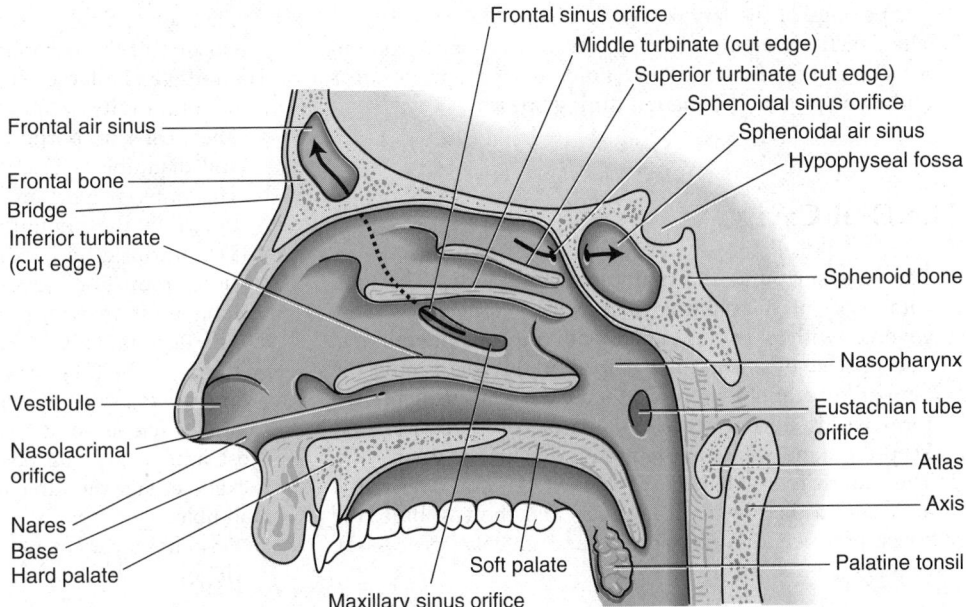

Figure 20–6. Structure of the nose and nasopharynx. (Redrawn from Black JM, and Matassarin-Jacobs E [eds]. *Luckmann and Sorensen's Medical-Surgical Nursing: A Psychophysiologic Approach.* 4th ed. Philadelphia: WB Saunders, 1993, p 901.)

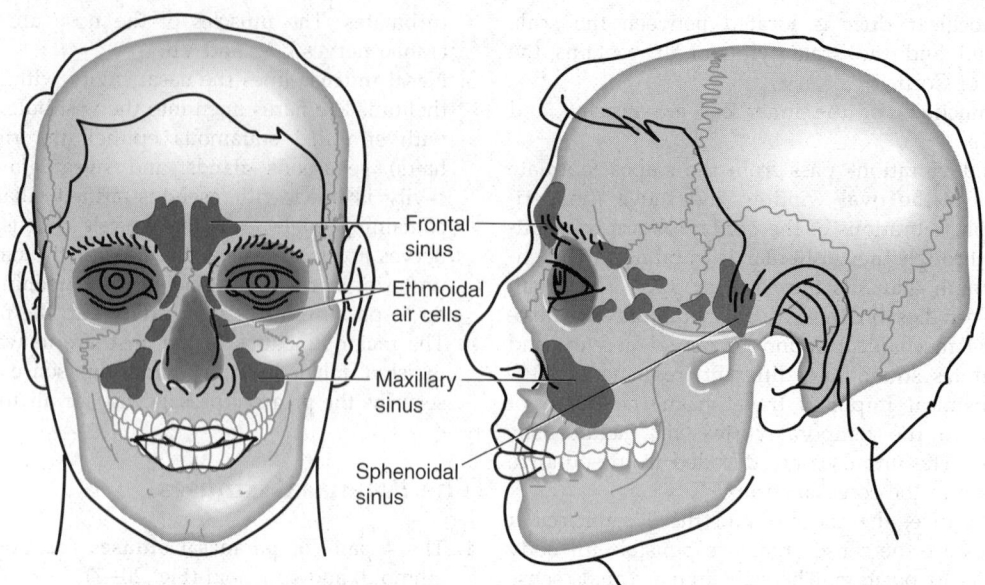

Figure 20-7. Facial sinuses. (Redrawn from Black JM, and Matassarin-Jacobs E [eds]. *Luckmann and Sorensen's Medical-Surgical Nursing: A Psycho-physiologic Approach.* 4th ed. Philadelphia: WB Saunders, 1993, p 901.)

2. The parts of the pharynx are the nasopharynx, the oropharynx, and the laryngopharynx (see Fig. 22–3).
   a. The **nasopharynx,** the superior portion, lies behind the nasal cavities and extends from the posterior nares to the level of the uvula.
      (1) The eustachian tube opens into the nasopharynx.
      (2) Pharyngeal tonsils or adenoids are found on the posterior surface.
   b. The **oropharynx** is located behind the oral cavity and extends from the uvula to the epiglottis.
      (1) The palatine (removed by tonsillectomy) and lingual tonsils are found in the oropharynx.
      (2) The pharyngeal, palatine, and lingual tonsils form Waldeyer's ring, lymphoid tissue that serves as the body's first line of immunologic defense.
   c. The **laryngopharynx** extends from the epiglottis to the openings of the larynx and esophagus.
3. The functions of the pharynx are to serve as a conduit for channeling air, food, and fluids to appropriate areas and to help vowel formation during speech.

The Oral Cavity

1. The **lips** surround the oral cavity anteriorly. They are composed of a sphincter-like muscle (orbicularis oris) covered with skin and lined with mucous membrane. The lips have sensors that help the body determine the temperature and texture of foods. The lips function to form words during speech, aid in facial expression, and keep food and saliva in the mouth during chewing.
2. The **mouth** is divided into 2 cavities: the oral cavity (the area within the alveolar processes) and the vestibule (the space between the lips, cheeks, and alveolar processes). (see Fig. 27–2).

3. The **buccal mucosa** (the cheeks) forms the lateral walls of the oral cavity and is composed of buccinator muscles, fat, areolar tissue, nerves, blood vessels, and buccal glands (mucous glands).
   a. The buccal mucosa plays an important role in chewing by manipulating food in the oral cavity. It also functions to form words during speech and aid in facial expression.
4. The **hard and soft palates** form the roof of the mouth.
   a. The hard palate (bone) is anterior to and attached to the soft palate (muscle), forming a partition between the oral cavity and the nasopharynx.
   b. The **fauces** is the opening in the arch of the soft palate that leads from the mouth to the oropharynx.
   c. The **uvula** is the projection on the posterior border of the soft palate.
   d. The soft palate moves upward during swallowing, closing off the nasopharynx to food and fluid.
5. The **tongue** is a large, muscular organ that occupies most of the oral cavity.
   a. The posterior portion is attached to the hyoid bone and mandible.
   b. The anterior portion is attached to the floor of the mouth by the frenulum.
   c. The intrinsic and extrinsic muscles assist in protrusion, retraction, depression, and elevation of the tongue for chewing, swallowing, and speech.
   d. The taste buds are located mainly on the anterior two thirds of the tongue. The 4 primary sensations of taste are sweet, salty, sour, and bitter. The sense of smell affects the sense of taste.
6. Most adults have 32 permanent **teeth,** which are set in sockets along the alveolar ridges of the maxilla and mandible.
   a. Periodontal ligaments secure the teeth in the alveolar ridges.

b. The gums, or gingivae, cover the alveolar ridges.

c. The teeth cut and mix food, increasing the surface area exposed to digestive enzymes and making the food easier to swallow.

7. The **salivary glands** secrete approximately 1 liter of saliva per day.

a. Saliva moistens food particles, binding them together; acts as a solvent for food chemicals to provide taste; and begins the digestion of carbohydrates.

b. The 3 major pairs of salivary glands are the parotid glands, the submandibular glands, and the sublingual glands.

(1) The parotid glands are the largest and are located anterior to the ears. The parotid ducts are known as **Stensen's ducts.**

(2) The submandibular, or submaxillary, glands are smaller than the parotid glands and are located on the floor of the mouth on the mandible's inner surface. The submandibular ducts are known as **Wharton's ducts.**

(3) The sublingual glands are the smallest of the paired salivary glands and are located under the tongue.

The Larynx

1. The **larynx,** or voice box, is a tubular structure located between the trachea and the pharynx.

a. The larynx has 2 folds that divide it into 3 compartments: the vestibule, the false vocal cords, and the true vocal cords.

b. The larynx is composed of 9 cartilages. Three of these cartilages are paired structures: the arytenoid, the corniculate, and the cuneiform cartilages. Three of these cartilages are unpaired structures: the thyroid, the epiglottis, and the cricoid cartilages. The cricoid cartilage is the only complete ring of cartilage in the larynx.

c. The muscles of the larynx are divided into extrinsic and intrinsic muscles. The extrinsic muscles connect the larynx to adjacent structures of the neck and move the larynx as a whole. The intrinsic muscles connect the cartilages, alter the shape of the laryngeal cavity, and are innervated by the recurrent laryngeal nerve. This innervation is important during endotracheal intubation and during and after thyroid surgery.

2. The larynx functions as a passageway for air between the pharynx and trachea (Fig. 20–8).

a. The larynx warms and filters the air, prevents aspiration, and assists in coughing.

b. The larynx is the organ of voice production as a result of vocal cord vibration.

The Trachea

1. The **trachea,** or windpipe, is a flexible, cylindrical tube, about 2.5 cm in diameter and 11 cm long, that extends

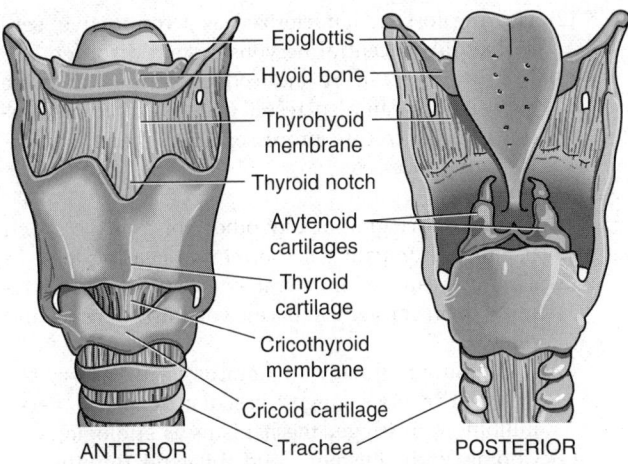

Figure 20–8. Structure of the larynx. (Redrawn from Ignatavicius DD, Workman ML, and Mishler MA [eds]. *Medical-Surgical Nursing: A Nursing Process Approach.* 2nd ed. Philadelphia: WB Saunders, 1996, p 611.)

from the cricoid cartilage of the larynx to the mainstem bronchi.

2. The trachea is composed of C-shaped rings of hyaline cartilage that reinforce, maintain, and protect the airway.

3. The trachea is lined with a ciliated mucous membrane that warms the air and filters and moves entrapped particles upward to the larynx.

4. The trachea functions as a passageway for air to enter the lungs.

The Thyroid and Parathyroid Glands

1. The thyroid gland, the largest of the endocrine glands, lies in the anterior part of the neck.

2. The parathyroid glands are in the posterior part of the thyroid gland. See Chapter 29 for discussions of the thyroid and parathyroid glands.

◼ ASSESSING PEOPLE WITH EAR, NOSE, AND THROAT DISORDERS

The Ear

1. Key symptoms and their pathophysiologic bases. The most common ear symptoms include pain, hearing loss, tinnitus, ear drainage, and vertigo.

a. Pain or otalgia

(1) The most common symptom, pain can be caused by trauma, acute or chronic infection processes, or frostbite.

(2) Pain can be referred from surrounding areas such as the temporomandibular joint or the eustachian tube.

b. Hearing loss

(1) Hearing loss can be congenital or acquired, sudden or gradual, partial or total, and unilateral or bilateral.

(2) Hearing loss is characterized as a conductive, sensorineural, or central nervous system disorder.

(3) Hearing loss can be induced by trauma or noise exposure. It can also result from ototoxic medications, degenerative processes (e.g., aging), or infectious processes.

c. Tinnitus

(1) Tinnitus is ringing or any other noise in the ear. It usually accompanies sensorineural hearing loss.

(2) Tinnitus can be unilateral or bilateral and intermittent or constant and can vary in intensity and pitch.

(3) The pathophysiology of tinnitus is unknown, but different theories suggest vascular disorders, nerve inhibition, or trigger mechanisms as etiologies.

(4) Coping with constant, loud, bilateral tinnitus has tremendous psychosocial implications.

d. Otorrhea (ear drainage)

(1) Otorrhea is usually related to an infectious process or perforation of the tympanic membrane.

(2) The drainage can be clear (serum), sanguinous (blood), serosanguineous (mixed serum and blood), or purulent (pus).

(3) Drainage can be unilateral or bilateral, acute or chronic, and with or without an odor.

(4) Frequently, ear drainage is accompanied by erythema, edema, or lesions of the pinna.

e. Vertigo

(1) A common symptom, vertigo is the sensation of rotating, spinning, or turning or the hallucination of movement.

(2) Vertigo can be intermittent or constant, can come in attacks, and can be position related or spontaneous. It can last a few seconds or several days.

(3) Vertigo can be accompanied by nausea, vomiting, or diarrhea.

(4) Vertigo can cause a decrease in daily activity, uncertainty, anxiety, decreased quality of life, and handicapping effects.

(5) Vertigo associated with the labyrinth is caused by a peripheral ear disorder such as a viral or bacterial infection, decreased circulation, or certain toxic metabolic conditions.

2. Health history: Evaluation of a patient with an ear disorder begins with the patient's history, which can be the most important assessment tool. For discussion of transcultural assessment issues, see Chapter 2. Holistic health assessment is discussed in Chapters 4 through 6. Table 20–1 presents a questionnaire on hearing, tinnitus, drainage, and pain assessment. Figure 20–9 presents a questionnaire on vertigo, balance, and tinnitus.

3. Physical examination: See Chapter 5 for a discussion of the physical examination of the ear.

Table 20–1. Sample Hearing Questionnaire

HEARING QUESTIONNAIRE

1. Do you have any problems with your hearing? _____
2. How long have you had a hearing loss in the   right ear? _____ Years
                                                         left ear? _____ Years
3. Which is your worse ear? (circle)   R   L
4. Have you had extensive ear drainage since childhood? _____
5. Who in your family was hard of hearing before age 50?   Mother   Father   Brother   Sister
6. Did any of your blood relatives ever have ear surgery? If yes, who were the patient and the doctor? _____
7. Are you wearing hearing aids now?
   How old is the right aid?   _____ Years
   How old is the left aid?   _____ Years
8. Have you worked amid loud noise?   _____
   If so, please indicate the number of years.   _____ Years
9. Are you still working amid loud noise? _____
10. Were you in the military, and did you serve around loud noise there? _____
    How many rounds have you fired outside the service? _____
11. Do you have head noise or ringing? _____
12. Is dizziness or unsteadiness a major problem? _____
13. Have you had previous ear surgery? _____
14. If you have had previous ear surgery, please indicate which ear was operated on, the type of surgery, and the physician who performed the surgery.
    Right Ear   19_____   _____   _____
                     19_____   _____   _____
    Left Ear   19_____   _____   _____
                     19_____   _____   _____
15. If you are allergic to any medications, please list them here:
    _____
    _____
    _____

From Sigler BA, and Schuring LT. *Ear, Nose, and Throat Disorders.* St. Louis: Mosby–Year Book, 1993, p 275.

A. Please answer these questions regarding dizziness. "Dizziness" is a broad term used to define many sensations.

1. When did the dizziness first occur?_____
2. Did the dizziness start suddenly or gradually?_____
3. Describe your **first attack** of dizziness._____

4. Is the dizziness constant or does it come in "attacks"?_____
5. Overall, has the dizziness gotten better or worse since starting?_____
6. Describe the sensation that you are having without using the word "dizzy."_____

7. Do any other symptoms occur simultaneously with the dizziness? (for example: nausea, vomiting, ear pressure) Please explain:

8. When was your last attack?_____
9. Describe your **last attack** of dizziness._____

10. How often do the attacks occur?_____
11. How long do the attacks last?_____
12. List anything that will stop or make an attack of dizziness better._____

13. List anything that will bring on an attack or make the dizziness worse._____

14. Are you completely free of dizziness between attacks?_____
15. Does the dizziness occur only in certain positions?_____ If "yes," what positions?

16. Does the dizziness occur only while standing or walking?____
17. Does the dizziness affect your balance or make you walk abnormally?_____
18. Do you support yourself while standing or walking?_____
19. Have you ever fallen because of the dizziness?_____
20. Have you ever injured your head or neck?_____
21. Does stress have any relationship to the dizziness?_____
22. Do you faint, blackout, or experience seizures with the dizziness?_____
23. Are you prone to motion sickness?_____

B. Please answer these questions regarding hearing.
Check "Yes" or "No," and circle which ear when necessary.

Yes No
- [ ] [ ] 1. Do you have any **difficulty hearing**? Right Left Both
  2. How long have you noticed the hearing loss?
  Right ear_____
  Left ear_____
- [ ] [ ] 3. Do you have any difficulty understanding what you hear?
  Right   Left   Both ears
  4. How long have you had **difficulty understanding**?
  Right ear_____
  Left ear_____
- [ ] [ ] 5. Do you have any **noises** in your ears? Right Left Both
- [ ] [ ] 6. Is the noise constantly with you?
- [ ] [ ] 7. Does the noise occur only with the dizziness?
- [ ] [ ] 8. Have you worked in a noisy environment or been exposed to loud noise?

C. Please answer these questions pertaining to your ears.
Check "Yes" or "No," and circle which ear when necessary.

Yes No
- [ ] [ ] 1. Do your ears have pain and/or drainage? Right Left Both
- [ ] [ ] 2. Have you had any surgery on your ears? Right Left Both
  3. List the date of surgery, the reason for surgery, and the operated ear.

D. Please check box for either "Yes" or "No," and circle if "Constant" or "In Episodes."

Yes No
- [ ] [ ] 1. Blurred vision   Constant   In Episodes
- [ ] [ ] 2. Double vision   Constant   In Episodes
- [ ] [ ] 3. Numbness in the hands or feet   Constant   In Episodes
- [ ] [ ] 4. Weakness in the arms or legs   Constant   In Episodes
- [ ] [ ] 5. Numbness or tingling of the mouth or face   Constant   In Episodes
- [ ] [ ] 6. Lack of coordination or confusion Constant   In Episodes
- [ ] [ ] 7. Difficulty with speech   Constant   In Episodes
- [ ] [ ] 8. Difficulty swallowing   Constant   In Episodes
- [ ] [ ] 9. Do you get dizzy after heavy lifting, straining, exertion, or overwork?
- [ ] [ ] 10. Did you get new glasses recently?
- [ ] [ ] 11. Do you get dizzy when you have not eaten for a long time?
- [ ] [ ] 12. For females: Is your dizziness connected with your menstrual cycle?

Figure 20–9. Balance questionnaire. (Courtesy of Linda Schuring, Balance Disorder Clinic, Warren Otologic Group, Warren, OH.)

Illustration continued on following page

The Nose and Sinuses

1. Key symptoms and their pathophysiologic bases
   a. Nasal stuffiness or obstruction

(1) A feeling of a decreased ability or inability to breathe through the nose can be caused by swollen mucous membranes or nasal polyps. Polyps are benign (possibly precancerous), nontender

E. List all medications with the dosages that you are currently taking.

F. List your past medical and surgical history (operations, chronic illnesses, injuries, etc.):

G. In your family (parents, siblings), are there any diseases of the ear or central nervous system (brain tumors, multiple sclerosis, etc)? _____

☐ Yes   ☐ No

If "yes" please explain:

H. Personal History:

Yes No
☐   ☐   1. Married?
☐   ☐   2. Children?
☐   ☐   3. Employed?
☐   ☐   4. Are you physically active (exercise, sports, etc.)?
☐   ☐   5. Habits:
☐   ☐   a. Do you use tobacco in any form?
             How much? _____
☐   ☐   b. Do you use alcohol?
             How much? _____
☐   ☐   c. Do you use caffeine?
             How much? _____
☐   ☐   d. Do you eat a well-balanced diet?
☐   ☐   6. Has the dizziness affected your quality of life?
☐   ☐   7. Do you have a high stress level or tend to worry a great deal?
☐   ☐   8. Have you ever seen a psychiatrist or psychologist for any reason?

Figure 20–9. *Continued*

growths that look soft, pale, and gray. They form gradually as a result of recurrent localized swelling of the sinus or nasal mucosa.

(2) Other symptoms such as shortness of breath, breathing through the mouth, sneezing, and wa-tery eyes may accompany nasal stuffiness or obstruction.

b. Rhinorrhea (nasal discharge)
   (1) Rhinorrhea is the free discharge of a thin nasal mucus.
   (2) Inflammation or infection of the mucous membranes is called **rhinitis.** Rhinitis usually produces a thicker, more purulent discharge than does rhinorrhea.

c. Epistaxis (nosebleeds)
   (1) Epistaxis is usually due to rupture of small vessels overlying the anterior part of the cartilaginous nasal septum.
   (2) Epistaxis is more common in men than in women, and it can increase during winter months if insufficient humidity dries the mucous membranes.
   (3) Epistaxis can be caused by trauma, a foreign body, vigorous nose blowing and nose picking, or disease processes of the nose and sinuses.
   (4) Epistaxis is usually mild and easily controlled, but it can be a symptom of coagulation disorders, hypertension, hemophilia, chronic allergies, or chronic infection.

d. Pain
   (1) Pain can vary from low grade to intense and can radiate to the face, forehead, and ears.
   (2) Negative sinus pressure, exudate, or edema of the nasal tissue can produce pain.
   (3) Pain can be caused by trauma, infection, or a foreign body.

e. Altered sense of smell
   (1) Hyposmia (a decrease in smell sensitivity) or anosmia (the absence of smell sensitivity) can be a symptom of nasal stuffiness or obstruction.
   (2) The senses of smell and taste are closely related.
   (3) Many conditions alter a person's sense of smell, including polyps, nasal obstruction, infection, normal aging, allergies, and head injuries.

2. Health history
   a. A past medical history of frequent colds, sinus infections, nasal stuffiness, allergies, or trauma is solicited.
   b. Current problems with epistaxis, sinus infections, allergies, postnasal drip, sneezing, nasal discharge, pain, obstruction, or decreased sense of smell are noted.
   c. Episodes of epistaxis are explored for etiology (e.g., hypertension), frequency, and previous treatment.
   d. Concurrent medical conditions (e.g., pregnancy) and medication use (e.g., nasal sprays, antihypertensive agents, birth control pills, or antidepressants) that can cause nasal obstruction are evaluated.

3. Physical examination: See Chapter 5 for discussion of the physical examination of the nose and sinuses.

The Throat, Head, and Neck

1. Key symptoms and their pathophysiologic bases
   a. Throat pain

(1) Throat pain can be produced by viral or bacterial infections, inflammation of mucous membranes, cysts or tumors, or injury.

(2) Throat pain varies in intensity, frequency, duration, and other characteristics and can radiate to surrounding structures, such as the ears. It can be related to edema, pressure, or inflammatory or infectious processes.

(3) Other symptoms, such as cervical lymphadenopathy, fever and chills, thick secretions, and headache, can accompany throat pain.

b. Change in voice quality

(1) A change in voice quality can be caused by infection, inflammation, or a benign or malignant tumor.

(2) Chronic hoarseness (i.e., hoarseness that lasts longer than 2 weeks) should be evaluated. Hoarseness can be caused by inflammation of the vocal cords, abnormal movements of the vocal cords, vocal cord abuse (e.g., excessive screaming) or a benign or malignant tumor of the vocal cords.

(3) An abnormal voice can also be the result of vocal abuse.

(4) Associated symptoms are a tickling in the throat, a sensation of having a foreign body in the throat, huskiness, and painful or difficult phonation.

(5) The onset, frequency, duration, and characteristics of the change in voice quality should be assessed.

c. Coughing

(1) Coughing is the explosive expulsion of air from the lungs to propel foreign matter and excess mucus up through the airways and to protect the lungs from aspiration.

(2) Coughing can be acute, chronic, or paroxysmal (i.e., intermittent or uncertain).

(3) The cough can be productive or nonproductive, dry or moist, barking, hoarse, or hacking.

(4) Persistent coughing can be caused by infection, excessive vocalization, allergies, the weather, anxiety, environmental irritants, or body position.

(5) The onset, duration, and amount of coughing should be assessed.

d. Hemoptysis

(1) Hemoptysis is the coughing up of blood or blood-tinged sputum. The source of bleeding can be anywhere in the upper or lower airways or in the lung parenchyma.

(2) Obtain a description of the onset and duration of the hemoptysis and the amount and color of the blood or blood-tinged sputum.

(3) Differentiate between hemoptysis and hematemesis if possible.

(4) The patient's perception of hemoptysis as an indicator of serious illness produces fear and anxiety.

e. Dyspnea

(1) Dyspnea is breathlessness inappropriate to the level of exertion or labored or difficult breathing.

(2) Dyspnea has both physiologic and cognitive components.

(3) Dyspnea associated with throat disorders results from pathologic changes that increase airway resistance, decrease ventilation, or reduce the amount of oxygen in the blood.

(4) Dyspnea can be acute or chronic; episodic or paroxysmal; or related to associated factors, such as the time of day, the weather, environmental irritants, anxiety, or body position (e.g., orthopnea).

(5) Assess the onset, frequency, and duration of the dyspnea and the phase of the respiratory cycle when it occurs.

f. Dysphagia

(1) Dysphagia, or difficulty swallowing, can range from mild discomfort to severe inability to control the muscles needed for chewing and swallowing.

(2) Dysphagia can compromise the patient's nutritional status.

(3) The causes of dysphagia include neuromuscular (incoordination of swallowing) or muscular weakness; esophageal disorders; or a tumor of the oral cavity, pharynx, larynx, or esophagus.

(4) Swallowing is often restricted in throat disorders because of pain or obstruction.

(5) Assess the characteristics of the dysphagia, such as the onset and frequency (whether it occurs each time the patient swallows or intermittently); whether it occurs with solids, liquids, or both; and associated symptoms (e.g., pain).

g. Lumps, enlarged lymph nodes, or swelling in the neck

(1) A lump, enlarged lymph node, or swelling in the neck may be the first sign of head and neck cancer or infection.

(2) Note the location, size, and other characteristics (e.g., tenderness).

(3) Regional lymph node metastasis from a head and neck tumor can be palpable in the neck. Examine the rest of the head and neck area to locate the primary site.

2. Health history

a. The patient has a past medical history of tonsillitis, strep throat infections, and aspiration during swallowing.

b. The patient is currently experiencing alterations in taste, difficulty moving the tongue or chewing, swelling or sores in the mouth, bleeding gums, increased or decreased saliva, changes in articulation, throat pain, coughing, expectoration of blood, difficulty breathing or swallowing, hoarseness, decreased range of motion in the neck, and discomfort or lumps in the neck.

c. Assess the patient's history, such as the use of tobacco, alcohol, or drugs (method, amount, and number of years); dental hygiene; dietary, sleeping, and sexual activity; the date of the patient's last dental examination; and whether the patient was exposed to noxious fumes or chemicals.

d. Assess the family history for cancer, especially head and neck cancers, or other ear, nose, and throat disorders.

e. Evaluate the patient's general medical condition and use of medications.

3. Physical examination: See Chapter 5 for a discussion of the physical examination of the mouth and throat.

Special Diagnostic Studies

1. Audiometry
   a. Audiometry is a hearing test performed by an audiologist with an audiometer to assess the middle and inner ears for hearing.
      (1) The patient wears earphones in a soundproof booth and signals when a tone is heard.
      (2) The responses are plotted on a graph called an **audiogram.**
      (3) Air conduction is achieved by presenting the tones through the earphones.
      (4) Bone conduction is achieved by presenting the tones through an oscillator placed on the mastoid bone.
      (5) Speech testing is achieved by presenting words through the earphones.
   b. Indications for audiometry include all types of hearing impairments, chronic ear infections, trauma, eustachian tube problems, otosclerosis, tinnitus, and retrocochlear disorders. There are no contraindications.
   c. Patient teaching includes explanations of the purpose of the test, the testing procedure, and the results (when appropriate).
2. Impedance audiometry
   a. Impedance audiometry assesses the middle ear pressure and acoustic reflex.
   b. Tympanometry measures the mobility (compliance) and impedance (resistance) of the tympanic membrane and ossicles of the middle ear. It is performed by placing a probe in the external ear canal, which forms a seal. Positive or negative air pressure introduced through the probe plots a distinctive tracing called a **tympanogram.** This test is useful for differentiating problems in the middle ear.
   c. Acoustic reflex is the contraction of the stapedius muscle in response to an intense sound. Stimulation of one ear causes a reaction in both ears. Certain pathologic conditions in the cochlea produce a reduced or absent acoustic reflex.
   d. Indications for tympanometry include all types of hearing impairments, chronic ear infections, trauma, eustachian tube problems, otosclerosis, tinnitus, and retrocochlear disorders.
   e. Patient teaching includes explanations of the purpose of the test, the testing procedure, and the results (when appropriate).
3. Electrocochleography
   a. Electrocochleography is the electrophysiologic measurement and graphic recording of the electric potentials of CN VIII.
      (1) An electrode is placed on the ear canal, tympanic membrane, or promontory of the middle ear, and other electrodes are placed on the head, mastoid process, or ear lobe.
      (2) Electrocochleography indicates whether a hearing loss originates at the level of the cochlea or cranial nerve VIII.
      (3) The indication for electrocochleography is a hearing loss. There are no contraindications.
   b. Patient teaching includes explanations of the purpose

and procedure of the test. Explain that paste is used to apply the electrodes and will be washed off the patient; that the patient may fall asleep during the test; and that pain is minimal, because a very tiny electrode is used.

4. Electronystagmography
   a. Electronystagmography (ENG) is the measurement and graphic recording of the electrical potentials of involuntary eye movement (nystagmus).
   b. It is used to assess the oculomotor and vestibular systems and their interaction.
   c. Electrodes are placed on the skin lateral to each eye, on the bridge of the nose, and above and below 1 eye.
   d. The testing battery is designed to test the function and status of each labyrinth.
   e. Electronystagmography can also detect disorders of the central nervous system.
   f. Indications for ENG are unilateral or bilateral sensorineural hearing loss; conductive hearing loss; or tinnitus with vertigo, imbalance, or abnormal gait. There are no contraindications.
   g. Determine any history of street drugs or alcohol use, which can alter the results of ENG. Also, certain prescribed medications, such as vestibular sedatives, tranquilizers, and pain medications, may affect nystagmus and should be discontinued 24 hours before the test. Patients prone to nausea or vomiting should not eat heavy meals before the test.
   h. Patient teaching includes explanations of the purpose and procedure of ENG. The test requires at least 1 hour and is painless. However, vertigo can occur during the caloric irrigations, which can cause nausea and vomiting.
5. Rotary chair, or rotational test
   a. The rotary chair, or rotational test, is also used to assess the oculomotor and vestibular systems and their interaction.
   b. The patient is seated in a chair that can be rotated at a constant velocity, accelerated smoothly, or brought abruptly to rest. The physical forces applied by the chair on the labyrinth can be measured precisely.
   c. Rotational testing is useful for documenting recovery from a unilateral labyrinthine loss.
   d. Indications are the same as for an ENG. There are no contraindications.
   e. Nursing care is the same as for an ENG.
   f. Patient teaching includes explanations of the purpose and procedure of the test. Explain that the test is painless but can cause vertigo and resultant nausea and vomiting and that the chair is not rotated at high speed.
6. Platform posturography
   a. Platform posturography is a series of tests performed to detect the cause(s) of balance problems.
   b. The patient is placed in a safety harness while standing on sensor plates surrounded by a visual field.
   c. Six different tests are performed to differentiate balance problems caused by the eyes (visual), the ears (vestibular), and proprioceptors (muscles and joints).
   d. The safety harness prevents the patient from falling

when the sensor plates are moved, the visual field is swayed, or the eyes are opened or closed.

    e. Indications are the same as for an ENG. There are no contraindications.

    f. Nursing care is the same as for an ENG.

    g. Patient teaching includes explanations of the purpose and procedure of the test. Explain that the test is painless but can cause vertigo and resultant nausea and vomiting.

7. Auditory brain stem response

    a. Auditory brain stem response evaluates dysfunction of the auditory nervous system at the level of cranial nerve VIII, pons, or midbrain.

    b. Electrodes are placed on the vertex, mastoid process, or earlobes while the patient is seated in a comfortable chair.

    c. Auditory evoked potentials measure electrical activity along the central auditory pathways of the brain stem in response to clicking sounds.

    d. An abnormal test result can suggest a lesion of the acoustic nerve or brain stem.

    e. Indications for auditory brain stem response are unilateral hearing loss, unilateral tinnitus, intracranial tumor, acoustic tumor, or head injury. There are no contraindications.

    f. Patient teaching includes explanations of the purpose and procedure of the test. Explain that the test is painless; that although clicking sounds will be heard, the patient may fall asleep; and that the patient will need to wash the electrode paste from his or her hair.

8. Sialography

    a. Sialography is a radiographic evaluation of the salivary glands and ducts using a radiopaque dye.

    b. Indications for sialography are parotid or submandibular swelling related to narrowing blockage of Stensen's or Wharton's ducts. Contraindications are complete stenosis of either duct, allergy to radiopaque dye, or pregnancy.

    c. Nursing care includes observation for erythema, edema, or drainage at the punctum of the duct and signs of reaction to the dye (rash, hives, itchiness, or breathing difficulties).

    d. Patient teaching includes explanations of the purpose and procedure of the test. Explain that a local anesthetic will be injected and the patient will feel slight pain or discomfort near the duct. Instruct the patient to rinse his or her mouth with half-strength hydrogen peroxide and water after meals and at bedtime and to apply external heat to the gland to reduce discomfort.

9. Nuclear medicine scanning

    a. Nuclear medicine scanning is performed to evaluate the uptake of an isotope by body tissue.

    b. A radioactive isotope specific to the area for scanning is ingested or injected.

    c. The indication for thyroid scanning is to detect enlargement or masses of the thyroid, and the indication for bone scanning is to evaluate for bony metastasis. Pregnancy is a contraindication for scanning.

    d. Nursing care includes assessment of the injection site for erythema, edema, or drainage. Encourage ingestion of plenty of fluids to ensure excretion of the isotope through the kidneys.

    e. Patient teaching includes explanations of the purpose and procedure of the test. The patient is given instructions for the completion of the scan at a specific time. Emphasize that the amount of radiation is minimal and poses no danger to other people.

10. Esophagography, or barium swallow

    a. Esophagography, or barium swallow, evaluates the patient's ability to swallow and reveals any abnormalities of the pharynx or esophagus.

    b. The patient swallows a radiopaque drink or food coated with barium and undergoes a videofluoroscopy while in sitting and lying positions.

    c. Indications for an esophagography are dysphagia and gastroesophageal reflux and to rule out a tumor of the upper aerodigestive tract. Pregnancy is a contraindication.

    d. Patient teaching includes explanations of the purpose and procedure of the test. Explain that no eating or drinking is allowed for 4 hours prior to the test and that chalky liquid will be ingested in sips during the radiographic examination. Encourage plenty of fluids and a laxative to prevent a barium impaction.

11. Angiography

    a. Angiography is the radiographic examination of selected vessels after the injection of a radiopaque dye.

    b. Local anesthesia is injected into the groin, and a catheter is inserted into the femoral artery and threaded up to the carotid artery.

    c. Iodinated dye is injected periodically into the catheter, and radiographs are taken.

    d. Balloon occlusion testing can be performed after angiography to determine the patient's ability to tolerate ligation of the carotid artery.

    e. Embolization of blood vessels feeding a tumor may be performed following angiography.

    f. Indications for angiography are to identify vascular tumors in the head and neck, to show a tumor's proximity to the carotid artery, to identify a tumor's vascular supply, and to embolize an area of bleeding or a vascular tumor. Contraindications are an allergy to the dye, anticoagulant therapy, and a recent embolic or thromboembolic event.

    g. Complications include bleeding, hematoma, and possible allergic reaction to the dye.

    h. Nursing care includes a thorough assessment for allergies to dyes, use of anticoagulants such as aspirin and nonsteroidal anti-inflammatory drugs, impaired renal function, and a history of an embolic or thromboembolic event. Monitor vital signs before, during, and after the procedure. Ensure that the patient keeps the affected leg straight and remains on bed rest for 6 to 8 hours. Assess the catheter insertion site for erythema, edema, or bleeding and place a pressure dressing over the puncture site. Encourage fluids to promote excretion of the dye.

    i. Patient teaching includes explanations of the purpose

and procedure of the test. No eating or drinking for 8 hours before the test. Inform the patient that vital signs are taken frequently, and sensations such as a warm feeling, flushing or pressure are normal and response to questions or commands may be necessary during the procedure.

12. Other imaging studies
    a. Other imaging studies are often necessary for ear, nose, and throat disorders, such as plain-film radiographs, computed tomography, or magnetic resonance imaging, with or without the use of a contrast medium.
    b. Indications for these studies are to establish a baseline condition, to detect changes in a baseline condition, to monitor response to therapy, to detect metallic foreign bodies, to determine the need for more extensive surgery, to diagnose and evaluate tumors of the head and neck, to detect abscesses, to evaluate sinus disease, and to determine upper and lower airway obstruction.
    c. Pregnancy is a contraindication for plain-film radiographs. Pregnancy, allergy to the contrast medium, claustrophobia, weight more than 300 pounds, and implanted metal devices are contraindications for computed tomography and magnetic resonance imaging.

◼ EAR DISORDERS

Permanent Sensorineural Hearing Loss or Impairment

1. Definition
   a. Sensorineural hearing loss is caused by a disorder that affects the inner ear, neural structures, or nerve pathways leading to the brain stem.
   b. Sensorineural hearing loss can be partial or complete and unilateral or bilateral and can range from loss of low tones to loss of high tones.
2. Incidence and socioeconomic impact: Impaired hearing is the most common disability in the United States and the 3rd most prevalent condition among people 65 years of age or older. More than 28 million people in the United States have a hearing impairment, and 90 percent of these people have a permanent sensorineural hearing loss.
3. Risk factors
   a. Genetics
   b. Exposure to noise
   c. Ototoxic drugs (Box 20–1)
   d. Professions that carry a high risk for head trauma
4. Etiology
   a. Heredity
   b. Infectious diseases (measles, mumps, labyrinthitis, or meningitis)
   c. Arteriosclerosis
   d. Ototoxic drugs
   e. Autoimmune reactions
   f. Neuromas of CN VIII

BOX 20–1. Ototoxic Drugs

Aminoglycoside Antibiotics

Amikacin
Gentamicin
Kanamycin
Neomycin
Netilmicin
Streptomycin
Tobramycin

Other Antibiotics

Capreomycin
Erythromycin
Minocycline
Polymyxin B
Polymyxin E
Vancomycin
Viomycin

Chemotherapeutic Drugs

Cisplatin
Nitrogen mustard

Diuretics

Acetazolamide
Ethacrynic acid
Furosemide

Other Drugs

Bleomycin
Quinidine
Quinine drugs
Salicylates

From Schuring L. Assessment of the ear. *In* Phipps W, et al. (eds). *Medical-Surgical Nursing Concepts and Clinical Practice.* 4th ed. St. Louis: Mosby–Year Book, 1995, pp 2113–2126.

---

g. Meniere's disease
h. Otospongiosis
i. Traumatic injury to the head or inner ear
j. Presbycusis, a degenerative process of aging
k. Senile degeneration of the hair cells in the organ of Corti (Table 20–2)

5. Pathophysiology: The pathophysiology of sensorineural hearing loss is damage to the hair cells of the cochlea, the cochlear nerve (CN VIII) or the nerve pathways.
6. Clinical manifestations
   a. Normal tympanic membrane
   b. Sensorineural hearing loss on audiogram that can be progressive, sudden, or fluctuating; unilateral or bilateral; and mild to severe
   c. Decreased discrimination (understanding of words) on audiogram

---

Table 20–2. Otologic Diseases of Aging

Change in Anatomy	Change in Physiology
Decreased vascularity of cochlea	Equal loss of hearing at all frequencies
Loss of cortical auditory neurons	Diminished hearing and speech comprehension
Degeneration of basilar conductive membrane of cochlea	Inability to hear at all frequencies but greater inability at higher frequencies (cochlear conductive loss)
Degeneration of cochlear hair cells	Inability to hear high-frequency sounds (sensorineural loss)
Loss of auditory neurons in spiral ganglia of organ of Corti	Inability to hear high-frequency sounds (sensorineural loss)

Adapted from Sigler BA, and Schuring LT. *Ear, Nose, and Throat Disorders.* St. Louis: Mosby–Year Book, 1993, p 69.

d. Tinnitus (perception of a sound in the absence of an acoustic stimulus)

e. Normal tympanogram

7. Diagnostics

a. History of decreased hearing

b. Pneumatic otoscopy or microscopic examination

c. Rinne and Weber tuning fork tests

d. Audiometry and tympanometry to assess middle and inner ear function

e. Auditory brain stem response test to determine the site of the lesion and the extent to which the auditory nervous system is involved

f. Imaging studies to identify retrocochlear pathology

8. Clinical management

a. The goal of clinical management is aural rehabilitation.

b. Nonpharmacologic interventions

(1) Auditory training (enhances listening skills)

(2) Speech reading (lip reading)

(3) Speech training (conserves, develops, or prevents deterioration of speech skills)

(4) Hearing aids

c. Pharmacologic interventions

(1) Nicotinic acid (niacin), 50 to 300 mg, to dilate blood vessels that supply the inner ear

(2) Sodium fluoride for cochlear otospongiosis

(3) Steroids for autoimmune reactions

d. Special medical-surgical procedures: Cochlear implants can be used for the profoundly deaf patient without any aidable hearing bilaterally.

9. Complications

a. Complete loss of hearing

b. Complete loss of balance

c. Loss of cerebrospinal fluid (CSF)

d. Meningitis

e. Septicemia

f. Dehydration

g. Vertigo

h. Falling

i. Abnormal gait

j. Central nervous system abscess

10. Prognosis: With adequate aural rehabilitation, the prognosis for permanent sensorineural hearing loss or impairment is good.

11. Applying the nursing process

NURSING DIAGNOSIS: Altered auditory sensory perception R/T sensorineural hearing loss

a. *Expected outcomes:* The patient's hearing loss should stabilize.

b. *Nursing interventions*

(1) Obtain the patient's otologic history. Include questions about tinnitus, eliciting information on its subjective loudness, on whether it is steady or fluctuating and continuous or intermittent, on its pitch or frequency; and on whether it affects one or both ears.

(2) Assess the patient's hearing acuity level; assess

the audiogram or tympanogram for the extent of hearing impairment.

(3) Assess the family history of ear disease and ask the patient whether he or she has been exposed to loud noises.

(4) Perform a review of systems, paying special attention to the central nervous system and cardiovascular system.

(5) Assess the patient's dietary habits, alcohol ingestion, use of safety equipment such as ear muffs or plugs, and current prescribed medications.

(6) Assess the patient's auditory acuity level.

(7) Face the person and speak distinctly, without shouting.

NURSING DIAGNOSIS: Anxiety R/T the threat of change or change in interaction patterns

a. *Expected outcomes:* The patient should be less anxious.

b. *Nursing interventions*

(1) Assess the level of anxiety (mild, moderate, severe, or panic).

(2) Assess the patient's perception of needs and expectations.

(3) Help the patient recall coping skills used successfully in the past.

(4) Provide information about tinnitus and its treatment.

(5) Administer antidepressants as ordered.

(6) Suggest psychologic evaluation if appropriate.

(7) Encourage the patient to express feelings and concerns.

NURSING DIAGNOSIS: Impaired verbal communication R/T decreased hearing

a. *Expected outcomes:* The patient should be able to communicate adequately.

b. *Nursing interventions*

(1) Assess the degree of hearing impairment.

(2) Use an adequate alternative method of communication (e.g., raising your voice or writing).

(3) Check the patient's hearing aid for power level, battery, and other problems (Box 20–2).

(4) Get the patient's attention by raising your arm or hand.

(5) Shine a light on your face; face the patient and talk directly to him or her; speak clearly but do not overaccentuate words.

(6) Speak in a normal tone of voice without shouting.

(7) If the patient does not seem to understand what you say, express it differently.

(8) Move closer to the patient and toward his or her better ear.

(9) Write out proper names or any statement the patient may not have understood.

BOX 20–2. Hearing Aids

Care of a Hearing Aid

1. Turn the hearing aid off when not in use.
2. Open the battery compartment at night to avoid accidental drainage of the battery.
3. Keep an extra battery available at all times.
4. Wash the earmold frequently with mild soap and warm water, using a pipe cleaner to cleanse the cannula.
5. Dry the earmold completely before reconnecting it to the receiver.
6. Do not wear the hearing aid during an ear infection.

What To Do If Hearing Aid Fails To Work

1. Check the on-off switch.
2. Inspect the earmold for cleanliness.
3. Examine the battery for correct insertion.
4. Examine the cord plug for correct insertion.
5. Examine the cord for breaks.
6. Replace the battery, cord, or both, if necessary. (Batteries last from 2 to 14 days.)
7. Check the position of the earmold in the ear. If the hearing aid "whistles," the earmold is probably not inserted properly into the ear canal, or the person needs to have a new earmold made.

Adapted from Schuring L. Nursing care of clients with ear disorders. *In* Black JM, and Matassarin-Jacobs E (eds). *Luckmann and Sorensen's Medical-Surgical Nursing: A Psychophysiologic Approach.* 4th ed. Philadelphia: WB Saunders, 1993.

(10) Do not smile, chew gum, or cover your mouth when talking.
(11) Do not show annoyance by careless facial expression.
(12) Encourage the patient to use a hearing aid if one is available; allow the patient to adjust it before speaking.
(13) Do not use the intercommunication system.
(14) Do not avoid conversation with a patient whose hearing is impaired.

NURSING DIAGNOSIS: Diversional activity deficit R/T environmental lack of such activity and decreased hearing

a. *Expected outcomes:* The patient should participate in his or her usual recreational and leisure activities.
b. *Nursing interventions*
(1) Encourage the patient to participate in group social events.
(2) Encourage the patient to talk about his or her anger at having this disability.
(3) Inform the patient of treatment options to increase or maximize hearing and increase effective communication with others.
12. Discharge planning and teaching
a. Explain the cause of the hearing loss and the medical or surgical treatment options.
b. Explain how the hearing loss is related to tinnitus.
c. Explain the signs and symptoms related to the cause of the patient's tinnitus.
d. Teach the patient how to use and maintain a hearing aid, if one is required.

e. Make appropriate referrals for aural rehabilitation, hearing aids, or appointments with an otologist.
f. Encourage the patient to ask questions about anything he or she does not understand.
g. Explain the reason for retrocochlear testing and imaging studies for unilateral tinnitus and hearing loss.
h. Refer the patient for psychologic evaluation if appropriate.

Blocked Ear Canal

1. Definition: A blocked ear canal is an ear canal obstructed by cerumen (earwax) or a foreign object.
2. Incidence and socioeconomic impact: A blocked ear canal is the most common finding of the external ear.
3. Risk factors
a. Frequent use of cotton-tipped applicators to clean the ear, which forces the wax into the ear
b. The presence of an open cavity after mastoid surgery, which predisposes to cerumen and debris accumulation
4. Etiology
a. Cerumen can become impacted as a result of improper cleaning or overproduction. Excess cerumen is a frequent finding in the older population.
b. A wide array of foreign objects fit into the ear canal, such as insects; inorganic material such as cotton tips, small toys, and beads; and vegetable matter such as beans and peas.
5. Pathophysiology
a. Normal wax produced by the ceruminous glands of the cartilaginous canal varies considerably in consistency, amount, and color, but some ear canals tend to self-cleanse less well than others.
b. Foreign bodies are more common in the pediatric population than in the adult population.
c. In adults, pieces of cotton and insects are the most frequent obstructions of the ear canal.
6. Clinical manifestations
a. Hearing loss
b. Aural pressure or fullness
c. Aural discomfort or pain
7. Diagnostics
a. Otoscopic or microscopic examination of the external ear canal
b. Audiometric evaluation of hearing
8. Clinical management
a. The goal of clinical management is removal of the blockage of the ear canal to restore the patency of the external ear.
b. Nonpharmacologic interventions
(1) Wax impaction can be removed by curettage (occasionally requiring the use of a microscope) or irrigation (Box 20–3).
(2) Foreign bodies can be extracted by irrigation, suction, or forceps, sometimes requiring the use of a microscope.
(3) Do not irrigate vegetable foreign bodies with water because the vegetable will swell. Alternative forms of removal should be used.

BOX 20-3. Ear Irrigation

Irrigate the ear to cleanse the external auditory canal or to remove impacted wax, debris, or foreign bodies. Do not give irrigations to patients who have a history of a perforated eardrum or are suspected of having a perforated eardrum.

Warm the irrigating solution (usually water) to body temperature and place it in the irrigating syringe. Protect the patient's clothes with a plastic drape. Place a kidney-shaped basin below the ear to catch the irrigating solution. Have the patient sit with the ear to be irrigated toward you and the head tilted toward the opposite ear. With adult patients, pull the external ear upward and backward. Direct the tip of the syringe along the upper wall of the ear canal.

When charting the ear irrigation, include the nature of the returned solution regarding the amount, texture, and color of cerumen or type of debris. Instruct the patient to report pain, vertigo, or nausea during the procedure.

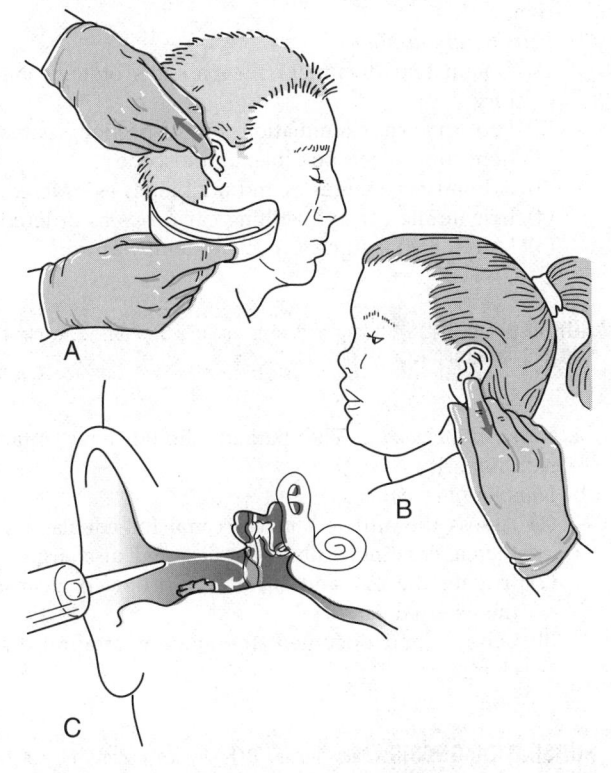

From Black JM, and Matassarin-Jacobs E (eds). *Luckmann and Sorensen's Medical-Surgical Nursing: A Psychophysiological Approach.* 4th ed. Philadelphia: WB Saunders, 1993, p 880. Illustration redrawn from Lammon CB, et al. *Clinical Nursing Skills.* Philadelphia: WB Saunders, 1995, p 314.

    (4) To remove an insect, instill ether, chloroform, or alcohol first to kill the insect.
    (5) Irrigation should not be used for a blocked ear canal if the eardrum is perforated.
  c. Special medical-surgical procedures: Occasionally, because of the patient's age or lack of cooperation or the difficulty of the procedure, general anesthesia may be required for removal of a foreign object.
9. Complications
  a. Hearing loss
  b. Infection
  c. Ossicular trauma
10. The prognosis is excellent with skillful removal of cerumen or the foreign body.

11. Applying the nursing process

NURSING DIAGNOSIS: Altered auditory sensory perception R/T occlusion of the ear canal by cerumen or a foreign body

  a. *Expected outcomes*
    (1) The patient should have a patent ear canal.
    (2) Hearing should be restored to the preblockage level following occlusion removal.
  b. *Nursing interventions*
    (1) Assess for recent changes in hearing acuity.
    (2) Assess audiograms and tympanograms for hearing impairment.
    (3) Speak distinctly without shouting.

NURSING DIAGNOSIS: Impaired skin integrity R/T pressure necrosis

  a. *Expected outcomes:* The patient should have intact skin integrity.
  b. *Nursing interventions*
    (1) Discourage unskilled patients from removing impacted wax or a foreign body themselves.
    (2) Teach the patient how to instill ear drops and irrigate the ear canal.

External Otitis

1. Definition
  a. External otitis is an inflammatory disease of the auricle or external ear canal.
  b. It may be acute or chronic, mild to severe (malignant external otitis) and localized (furuncles, abscesses, and boils) or diffuse.
2. Incidence: External otitis is a very common condition for all ages, especially in the summer (swimmer's ear).
3. Risk factors
  a. Long-term use of earphones, earplugs, earmuffs, or hearing aids, which trap moisture and create a medium for infection
  b. Swimming in contaminated water
  c. Cleaning or scratching the external ear with a foreign object
  d. Chronic use of irritants such as hair spray or hair dye or excessive dirt exposure
4. Etiology
  a. Infection, or dermatosis, or a combination of the two can cause external otitis.
  b. Infection caused by bacteria is usually attributable to *Proteus, Pseudomonas, Staphylococcus,* or *Streptococcus* organisms.
  c. Infection caused by fungus is usually attributable to *Aspergillus* or *Candida* organisms.
  d. Contact or seborrheic dermatitis can cause external otitis from various animals, vegetable or chemical substances, mechanical irritation, or heat or cold irritation.

5. Pathophysiology
   a. Acute external otitis is most commonly caused by the appearance of a *Pseudomonas* organism in the external ear canal after a minor irritation that causes a loss of skin integrity.
   b. Chronic external otitis is related to the frequency of the disorder, and the skin is red and thickened.
   c. **Malignant external otitis** is a rare, lethal type of external otitis. It is a fulminant, bone-destroying infection that must be treated with parenteral antibiotics.
   d. **Furunculosis** is infection of the glands and hair follicles in the area, which can form boils or furuncles.
6. Clinical manifestations
   a. Pain
   b. Tenderness of the pinna or tragus
   c. Decreased hearing
   d. Pruritus
   e. Otorrhea (ear drainage)
   f. Elevated temperature
   g. Lymphadenopathy
7. Diagnostics
   a. Pain when the pinna is greatly pulled or the tragus gently pushed
   b. Inflammation and swelling of the ear canal and excoriation of the skin
   c. Clear drainage (early in the process) or drainage discolored by pus
   d. Sometimes culture of the discharge for identification of the organism
   e. Otoscopic examination may not be possible because of pain, and swelling can prevent visualization of the tympanic membrane.
8. Clinical management
   a. The goals of clinical management are to reduce swelling, relieve pain, regain skin integrity, and control the infection or dermatosis.
   b. Nonpharmacologic interventions: Ear irrigations are performed, usually with boric acid and alcohol to cleanse the external ear canal.
   c. Pharmacologic management
      (1) Local antibiotic or antifungal medications, such as neomycin or polymyxin ear drops, are prescribed.
      (2) Systemic antibiotics are prescribed for severe infections and are determined by the cultured organism.
      (3) A narcotic analgesic such as codeine is prescribed for severe pain.
      (4) Aspirin or acetaminophen is prescribed for minor pain.
   d. Special medical-surgical procedures
      (1) A wick is inserted into the ear canal if the swelling is severe enough to occlude the meatus. The wick transfers the topical medication of hydrocortisone and antibiotics medially.
9. Complications
   a. Abscess
   b. Cellulitis
   c. Discoloration
   d. Hearing loss
   e. Infection of the middle ear
   f. Ischemia or necrosis of the pinna
   g. Lymphadenopathy
   h. Osteitis
   i. Septicemia
   j. Stenosis
10. With early intervention and adequate treatment, the prognosis for external otitis is excellent.
11. Applying the nursing process

NURSING DIAGNOSIS: Risk for Infection R/T impaired skin integrity

   a. *Expected outcomes:* The patient should have no infection.
   b. *Nursing interventions*
      (1) Obtain and document the patient's otologic history.
      (2) Performance examination by inspection; palpations and, when possible, an otoscope.
      (3) Administer analgesics and antibiotics as ordered.
      (4) Irrigate the ear by instilling ear drops as ordered.
      (5) Monitor vital signs, especially temperature.

NURSING DIAGNOSIS: Impaired skin integrity R/T pressure on skin that is causing excoriation

   a. *Expected outcomes:* The patient should have intact skin integrity.
   b. *Nursing interventions*
      (1) Assess the auricle and ear canal for edema, erythema, crusting, scabs, pustules, and discharge.
      (2) Irrigate the ear and instill ear drops to cleanse the external ear.
      (3) Observe and document the amount of aural discharge.

NURSING DIAGNOSIS: Pain (acute) R/T physical factors of ear infection

   a. *Expected outcomes:* The patient should have no pain.
   b. *Nursing interventions*
      (1) Assess the location, intensity, and frequency of otalgia (ear pain) and the need for analgesics.
      (2) Administer analgesics as ordered. Evaluate and document the patient's response.

NURSING DIAGNOSIS: Altered auditory sensory perception R/T blockage of the ear canal as a result of edema, debris, or drainage

   a. *Expected outcomes:* The patient's hearing loss should resolve or stabilize.
   b. *Nursing interventions*
      (1) Assess for a recent change in hearing acuity.
      (2) Speak distinctly without shouting.

12. Discharge planning and teaching
    a. Teach the patient how to avoid getting water in the ears by using earplugs or cotton smeared with petroleum jelly.
    b. Teach the patient how to prevent future external ear infections or swimmer's ear.
    c. Teach the patient how to administer drops, ointment, or ear wash.
    d. Explain the purpose of wicks when the external auditory canal is occluded.
    e. Reassure the patient that hearing loss from an external ear infection is temporary.
    f. If the patient's hearing is decreased, teach him or her alternative communication methods.
    g. Inform the patient of the side effects of any prescribed medications.
13. Public health considerations
    a. Teach the need for thorough drying of the external ear after water gets into the ear canal.
    b. Teach the need to use ear drops (e.g., alcohol or acetic acid) after swimming or bathing to reduce moisture and thus limit growth of organisms and to maintain normal acidity.

Perichondritis

1. Definition: Perichondritis is an inflammation of the auricular cartilage.
2. Incidence and etiology: Perichondritis, a rare finding, can be caused by trauma (e.g., boxing), insect bites, ear piercing, or skin infections, all of which allow bacteria to enter.
3. Pathophysiology
    a. The causative organism is usually a gram-negative rod, frequently a *Pseudomonas* species.
    b. Bacteria causes pus to form between the perichondrium and cartilage.
    c. Perichondritis diminishes the blood supply, resulting in breakdown and necrosis of the cartilage and loss of the auricle's distinctive shape.
4. Clinical manifestations
    a. Erythema of the pinna (except the lobule)
    b. Drainage
    c. Edema of the pinna
    d. Elevated temperature
    e. Skin necrosis or abscess
    f. Pain or tenderness
    g. Lymphadenopathy
5. Diagnostics
    a. Enlarged pinna with a shiny appearance as a result of edema and inflammation
    b. Culture of the discharge for identification of the organism
    c. Possibly imaging studies to rule out tumors or osteitis
6. Clinical management
    a. The goal of clinical management is prompt and aggressive treatment of the infection.
    b. Nonpharmacologic intervention consists of local heat application for pain relief.
    c. Pharmacologic interventions

(1) Systemic parenteral antibiotic therapy, depending on the cultured organism
(2) Local irrigation with antibiotic solutions such as neomycin, polymyxin B, bacitracin, or a combination of antipyretic agents
(3) Analgesics such as aspirin, acetaminophen, or codeine
    d. Special medical-surgical procedures
(1) Incision and drainage of purulent material
(2) Removal of necrotic cartilage
(3) Insertion of a small polyethylene tube for irrigations
7. Complications
    a. Abscess
    b. Cellulitis
    c. Discoloration of the pinna
    d. Disfigurement of the pinna
    e. Ischemia or necrosis of the pinna
    f. Keloid formation
    g. Lymphadenopathy
    h. Osteitis
    i. Septicemia
8. If there is early and aggressive intervention for this rare disorder, the prognosis is fairly good. Otherwise, the disease course is lengthy and very destructive.
9. Applying the nursing process

NURSING DIAGNOSIS: Risk for infection R/T broken skin

    a. *Expected outcomes:* The patient should have no infection.
    b. *Nursing interventions*
(1) Obtain and document the patient's otologic history.
(2) Perform an ear examination by inspection and palpation and, when possible, an otoscope.
(3) Administer analgesics and antibiotics as ordered.
(4) Instill ear drops as ordered.
(5) Monitor vital signs, especially temperature.

NURSING DIAGNOSIS: Impaired skin integrity R/T pressure on skin that is causing excoriation

    a. *Expected outcomes:* The patient should have intact skin integrity.
    b. *Nursing interventions*
(1) Assess the auricle and ear canal for edema, erythema, crusting, scabs, pustules, and discharge.
(2) Instill ear drops to cleanse the external ear.
(3) Observe and document the amount of aural discharge.

NURSING DIAGNOSIS: Pain (acute) R/T physical factors of ear infection

    a. *Expected outcomes:* The patient should have no pain.
    b. *Nursing interventions*

(1) Assess the location, intensity, and frequency of the otalgia and the need for analgesics.

(2) Administer analgesics as ordered. Evaluate and document the response.

10. Discharge planning and teaching

a. Teach the patient how to administer oral and topical antibiotics and anti-inflammatory drugs (i.e., type, amount, frequency, and side effects).

b. Teach the patient the signs and symptoms of abscess and tissue necrosis.

c. Teach the patient how to monitor oral temperature and how to take antipyretic drugs (i.e., type, amount, frequency, and side effects).

d. Inform the patient and family that minor surgery such as incision and drainage or débridement may have to be done if the infection cannot be controlled medically.

Otitis Media

1. Definition

a. Otitis media is an inflammation of the middle ear that most often occurs in infants and young children but can occur at any age.

b. Serous otitis media is the accumulation of serous fluid in the middle ear space.

c. Secretory otitis media is the accumulation of amber, mucoid, or grayish fluid in the middle ear, probably in response to an allergen.

d. Suppurative otitis media is an infection of the middle ear caused by pus-producing bacteria that are trapped in the middle ear.

2. Incidence and socioeconomic impact

a. According to the National Center for Health Statistics, otitis media is the most common diagnosis to children under age 15 at physician office visits.

b. The conductive hearing loss that can occur with otitis media has been associated with delayed language development.

3. Risk factors

a. The inflammation usually results from an infection in the nasopharynx that enters the middle ear via the eustachian tube and involves the lining of the middle ear. Infants and children have shorter, straighter eustachian tubes than adults do, which is a contributing factor.

b. Also, adenoidal tissue can obstruct the opening of the eustachian tube and contribute to the secondary development of otitis media.

c. Any factor that causes eustachian tube dysfunction causes a middle ear vacuum (negative pressure) and eventually middle ear effusion.

4. Etiology and pathophysiology

a. Exudate and edema form in the lining of the eustachian tube and middle ear, resulting in decreased aeration, retraction of the tympanic membrane, and serous exudation in the middle ear. The exudate can become purulent and cause bulging of the tympanic membrane as pus forms. The tympanic membrane can rupture.

b. The usual pathogens are gram-positive cocci, such as *Streptococcus* species and *Haemophilus influenzae*. In an adult, chronic unilateral fluid can indicate carcinoma of the nasopharynx.

5. Clinical manifestations

a. History of an upper respiratory infection

b. Pain

c. Elevated temperature

d. Hearing loss (conductive)

e. Aural fullness or pressure

f. Lack of response to conversation

g. Purulent drainage

h. Change in behavior or irritability

6. Diagnostics

a. Otoscopic or microscopic examination

b. Tympanic membrane abnormality such as retraction, serous bubbles, bulging, or perforation with drainage

c. Culture of purulent drainage to identify causative organisms

d. Audiometry and tympanometry to assess middle ear function

7. Clinical management

a. The goals of clinical management are to restore eustachian tube and middle ear function, eliminate inflammation and infection, and control any allergies.

b. Nonpharmacologic intervention consists of the Valsalva maneuver to open the eustachian tube and force air into the middle ear to equalize pressure. Children can blow up balloons several times per day to accomplish this task.

c. Pharmacologic interventions

(1) Decongestants and antihistamines (though their use is somewhat controversial), such as chlorpheniramine and pseudoephedrine hydrochloride (Sudafed).

(2) Analgesics and antipyretics such as acetaminophen or aspirin.

(3) Antibiotics such as amoxicillin, preparations of trimethoprim and sulfamethoxazole (Septra and Bactrim), penicillin, or ampicillin.

d. Special medical-surgical procedures: Surgery for otitis media is a myringotomy and placement of a transtympanic tube for ventilation. This procedure is minor, and the tubes usually fall out as the tympanic membrane grows in 6 to 9 months. Hearing returns to normal for the patient.

8. Complications

a. Hearing loss with repeated, untreated infections

b. Chronic otitis media

c. Perforation

d. Otorrhea

e. Poor speech development

f. Cholesteatoma (a skin-lined sac)

9. With prompt treatment, the prognosis is very good.

10. Applying the nursing process

NURSING DIAGNOSIS: Risk for infection R/T eustachian tube dysfunction

a. *Expected outcomes:* The patient should have no infection.

b. *Nursing interventions*

(1) Obtain and document the patient's otologic history (such as recent upper respiratory infection, exposure to water, ear trauma, allergy, or ear infections). Pertinent symptoms include otalgia, otorrhea, pruritus, hearing loss, and aural fullness.

(2) Perform and document an otoscopic examination. Check for drainage or debris in the ear canal, note the color and the appearance of the tympanic membrane, and check for fluid in the middle ear.

(3) Administer antibiotic and antipyretic preparations as ordered.

(4) Teach the patient how to instill ear drops or irrigate the ear if ordered; instruct the patient on the administration of medications and their side effects.

(5) Monitor and document the patient's response to drugs.

(6) Instruct the patient about restrictions on water in the ear

---

NURSE ADVISORY

> Instruct the patient that water can cause infection of the ear after transtympanic tube placement. External earplugs can be worn to prevent water from entering the middle ear through the tube. Disposable plugs or custom-made plugs should be worn while bathing or swimming. Advise the patient to also wear a swimmer's cap to ensure retention of the plugs. If plugs are not available, tell the patient to place a piece of cotton in the ear and follow this with a 2nd piece of cotton that has been saturated with petroleum jelly. This method is adequate for bathing but not for swimming.

NURSING DIAGNOSIS: Altered auditory sensory perception R/T fluid in the middle ear

a. *Expected outcomes:* The patient's hearing loss should resolve or stabilize.

b. *Nursing interventions*

(1) Assess and document a recent change in hearing acuity; assess the audiogram or tympanogram for hearing impairment.

(2) Speak distinctly without shouting.

NURSING DIAGNOSIS: Pain R/T infection

a. *Expected outcomes:* The patient should have no ear pain or discomfort.

b. *Nursing interventions*

(1) Assess and document the location, intensity, and frequency of the pain.

(2) Observe the ear canal for inflammation and swelling and the tympanic membrane for redness, bulging, or bubbles.

(3) Administer analgesics as ordered and instruct the patient on the administration and side effects of medications.

(4) Monitor and document the patient's response to analgesics.

11. Discharge planning and teaching

a. Teach the patient the causes, signs, and symptoms of serous otitis media.

b. Stress to the patient that he or she should see a physician about any significant earache and teach the patient how to carry out medical treatment of serous otitis media (antihistamines, decongestants, the Valsalva maneuver, or a combination of these).

c. Inform the patient that minor surgery may be necessary to remove fluid from or to ventilate the middle ear.

d. Reassure the patient that hearing loss caused by serous otitis media is temporary.

Chronic Otitis Media and Chronic Mastoiditis

1. Definition

a. Chronic otitis media results from repeated attacks of acute otitis media. Chronic secondary changes can occur in the middle ear, such as thickening and scarring of the mucosa, perforation of the tympanic membrane, and gradual destruction of the ossicles.

b. Chronic mastoiditis can also result as an extension of repeated middle ear infections.

2. Risk factors

a. Lack of or inadequate treatment of otitis media

b. An infecting organism that is resistant to antibiotics

c. A particularly virulent strain of organism

3. Etiology: Long-term changes are caused by repeated infections in the middle ear and mastoid cavity resulting from eustachian tube dysfunction and bacterial superinfection.

4. Pathophysiology

a. Common causative organisms can be gram-positive cocci, such as *Streptococcus* species or *H. influenzae*, or a gram-negative organism, such as *Pseudomonas*.

b. Chronic infection with perforation can lead to the formation of a cholesteatoma.

c. As the skin from the ear canal grows, debris and desquamation slowly collect inside the middle ear. As the cholesteatoma enlarges, expansion into the mastoid spaces can cause bony necrosis.

d. In the absence of treatment, serious complications can occur, because of the proximity of surrounding structures.

e. Repeated ear infections can also result in tympanosclerosis, a deposit of collagen and calcium in the tympanic membrane or middle ear space.

5. Clinical manifestations

a. History of repeated ear infections

b. Painless otorrhea with or without an odor

c. Perforation of the tympanic membrane with or without ossicular damage, tympanosclerosis, cholesteatoma, or mastoid problems

d. Conductive hearing loss (the loss is greater if the ossicles are involved)

e. Aural fullness or pressure

f. Abnormal tympanogram showing a large volume of perforation

g. Vertigo (with inner ear erosion)

6. Diagnostics
   a. Otoscopic or microscopic examination
   b. Culture or sensitivity of exudate to identify organism
   c. Biopsy to identify any tissue changes (i.e., malignancy)
   d. Audiometry and tympanometry to assess middle ear function
   e. Imaging studies to diagnose the extent of disease or any complications

7. Clinical management
   a. The goals of clinical management are to stop the repeated infections and restore the integrity and function of the tympanic membrane, middle ear cavity, and mastoid cavity.
   b. Nonpharmacologic interventions: none
   c. Pharmacologic interventions
      (1) Chronic ear drainage may not respond as well to systemic antibiotic therapy as acute otitis media does.
      (2) Local treatment is generally used, such as an antiseptic ear wash with antibiotic or anti-inflammatory ear drops (i.e., a boric acid and alcohol ear wash followed by Cortisporin ear drops).
   d. Special medical-surgical procedures
      (1) The most common surgical procedure performed for chronic otitis media is a tympanoplasty with or without an ossiculoplasty. A tympanoplasty is the repair of the tympanic membrane to correct a perforation, retraction pocket, or tympanosclerosis. In addition, polyps, granulomas, and infection are removed.
      (2) An **ossiculoplasty** is the repair or replacement of the ossicles (malleus and incus stapes) for the purpose of restoring middle ear continuity.
      (3) A tympanomastoidectomy is the cleaning and preserving of the mastoid cavity and repair or replacement of the tympanic membrane and ossicles.
      (4) Rarely, a radical or a modified radical mastoidectomy is performed.
      (5) The basic objectives of surgery for chronic otitis media with or without chronic mastoiditis are to clean and remove the causes and results of infection, to prevent recurrent infections, to close a perforation; to provide adequate aeration of the middle ear; and to improve hearing.

8. Complications
   a. Central nervous system abscess
   b. Complete loss of balance
   c. Loss of CSF
   d. Facial nerve paralysis
   e. Complete hearing loss
   f. Infection of surrounding structures
   g. Leukocytosis
   h. Lymphadenopathy
   i. Meningitis
   j. Metastasis of bacteria
   k. Septicemia
   l. Sigmoid sinus thrombosis
   m. Subperiosteal abscess
   n. Vertigo

9. Applying the nursing process

NURSING DIAGNOSIS: Risk for infection R/T by tissue destruction and chronic disease

a. *Expected outcomes:* The patient should have no infection.
b. *Nursing interventions*
   (1) Obtain the patient's otologic history, such as previous ear infections, exposure to water, allergies, and use of earphones or hearing aids. Pertinent symptoms include otorrhea, otalgia, pruritus, hearing loss, and vertigo.
   (2) Perform an otoscopic examination. Check for drainage or debris in the ear canal, note the color and appearance of the tympanic membrane, and whether it is perforated; check for tympanosclerosis and cholesteatoma.
   (3) Administer antibiotic and anti-inflammatory preparations as ordered.
   (4) Teach the patient how to instill ointment, drops, and ear wash if ordered.
   (5) Monitor the patient's responses to all medications.
   (6) Instruct the patient about water restrictions.

NURSING DIAGNOSIS: Pain (chronic) R/T physical factors

a. *Expected outcomes:* The patient should have no pain.
b. *Nursing interventions*
   (1) Assess the location, intensity, and frequency of the pain.
   (2) Use an otoscope to check the tympanic membrane for redness, perforation, or drainage.
   (3) Administer analgesics as ordered.
   (4) Instruct the patient in the administration of analgesics and their common side effects.
   (5) Monitor the patient's response to analgesics.

NURSING DIAGNOSIS: Altered auditory sensory perception R/T to partial or total perforation of the tympanic membrane or destruction of the middle ear ossicles

a. *Expected outcomes:* The patient's hearing loss should resolve or stabilize.
b. *Nursing interventions*
   (1) Assess changes in hearing acuity; assess the audiogram or tympanogram for hearing impairment.
   (2) Face the patient and speak distinctly, without shouting.

NURSING DIAGNOSIS: Impaired verbal communication R/T hearing deficit

a. *Expected outcomes:* The patient should be able to communicate adequately.
b. *Nursing interventions*
(1) Assess the degree of hearing impairment.
(2) Use an adequate alternative method of communication (e.g., raise your voice or write notes).
(3) Speak distinctly, without shouting.

NURSING DIAGNOSIS: Risk for trauma R/T vertigo

a. *Expected outcomes:* The patient should not experience vertigo.
b. *Nursing interventions*
(1) Assess for vertigo by observing for nystagmus, an abnormal gait, a positive Romberg's sign, and an inability to perform the tandem Romberg test (walking heel-to-toe).
(2) Help the patient with ambulation when indicated.
10. Discharge planning and teaching
a. Instruct the patient to avoid getting water in the ears by using earplugs or cotton with petroleum jelly on it.
b. Teach the patient how to use ear drops or ear wash.
c. Teach the patient the causes, signs, symptoms, and treatment of chronic otitis media.
d. Inform the patient that surgery may be needed to remove the infection and restore some degree of hearing.

Otosclerosis

1. Definition
a. Otosclerosis is "hardening of the ear," a disorder of the bone in the otic capsule in which normal bone is replaced by abnormal "spongy bone," causing fixation of the stapes bone.
b. Otosclerosis can be bilateral (75% of cases) or unilateral (25% of cases).
2. Incidence and socioeconomic impact: Otosclerosis is twice as common in women than in men and often progresses during pregnancy. Approximately 5 percent of all people with hearing problems have otosclerosis.
3. Etiology
a. Although the etiology is unknown, about half the patients with otosclerosis have a family history of the disorder. It is usually 1st noticed as a young adult.
b. This disorder is also associated with van der Hoeve's syndrome (blue sclerae, osteogenesis imperfecta [fragile bones], and stapedial fixation).
4. Pathophysiology
a. The pathophysiology that causes otosclerosis is still unclear.

b. During the process, normal bone in the otic capsule is gradually replaced by otosclerotic bone that is highly vascular and described as spongy.
c. One theory suggests that this destruction of normal bone releases enzymes that cause vestibular and cochlear functional impairment. Calcification of the involved area is the body's natural healing reaction.
d. This calcification causes fixation of the stapes bone and immobilization of the footplate in the oval window.
5. Clinical manifestations
a. Conductive hearing loss
b. Normal-appearing tympanic membrane (sometimes a pink blush color is noted through the tympanic membrane; this is called Schwartz's sign)
c. Normal tympanogram
d. Absent acoustic reflex
e. Tinnitus
f. Quiet, well-modulated voice
6. Diagnostics
a. Pneumatic otoscopy or microscopic examination
b. Rinne and Weber tuning fork tests
c. Audiometry and tympanometry to assess middle ear function
d. History of gradual onset of hearing loss
7. Clinical management
a. The goals of clinical management are to prevent additional hearing loss and restore hearing medically and surgically.
b. Nonpharmacologic interventions: A hearing aid can be fitted for the ear to amplify the sound.
c. Pharmacologic interventions: No known medical treatment exists for otosclerosis, but sodium fluoride given daily for 1 to 2 years seems to stabilize the hearing loss.
d. Special medical-surgical procedures
(1) Stapes replacement surgery is the treatment of choice for otosclerosis.
(2) Stapedectomy (removal of the stapes and replacement with a prosthesis) and stapedotomy (opening of the stapes footplate and placement of a prosthesis) are usually performed under local anesthesia, transcanal, and aided by the use of a microscope.
8. Complications
a. Progressive hearing loss
b. Cochlear otospongiosis (a soft form of otosclerosis of the inner ear)
c. Tinnitus
d. Vertigo
9. Prognosis: With a stapedectomy, the prognosis for improved hearing is excellent.
10. Applying the nursing process

NURSING DIAGNOSIS: Altered auditory sensory perception R/T gradual fixation of the stapes footplate in the oval window

a. *Expected outcomes:* The patient should understand that otosclerosis causes progressive loss of hearing.

b. *Nursing interventions*
   (1) Assess the patient's hearing acuity level; assess the audiogram and tympanogram for hearing impairment.
   (2) Assess the tympanic reflex.
   (3) Speak distinctly, without shouting.

NURSING DIAGNOSIS: Impaired verbal communication R/T hearing deficit

a. *Expected outcomes:* The patient should be able to communicate adequately.
b. *Nursing interventions*
   (1) Assess the degree of hearing impairment.
   (2) Use an adequate alternate method of communication (e.g., raise your voice or write notes).
   (3) Speak distinctly, without shouting.

NURSING DIAGNOSIS: Risk for trauma R/T balance difficulties

a. *Expected outcomes:* The patient should understand that he or she is experiencing intermittent vertigo because of the disease.
b. *Nursing interventions*
   (1) Assess for vertigo by observing for nystagmus, an abnormal gait, a positive Romberg's sign, and an inability to perform a tandem Romberg test.
   (2) Help the patient with ambulation when indicated.
11. Discharge planning and teaching
   a. Teach the patient with signs, symptoms, and causes of otosclerosis.
   b. Inform the patient that hearing loss can be helped by surgery, either a stapedectomy or a stapedotomy, or by a hearing aid.
   c. Explain the surgical procedure.
   d. Teach the patient the dosages, administration, and side effects of any medications prescribed.

Meniere's Disease

1. Definition: Meniere's disease is a syndrome characterized by a triad of symptoms: attacks of incapacitating vertigo, sensorineural hearing loss, and tinnitus.
2. Incidence and socioeconomic impact
   a. Meniere's disease affects approximately 545,000 or more people in the United States.
   b. Meniere's disease usually occurs in adulthood and can be unilateral or bilateral.
   c. Although this disease is never fatal, it can have devastating effects during the attacks, which can last for several hours. Initially, the patient is asymptomatic between attacks. However, as the disease progresses, hearing loss and tinnitus can become residual problems.

3. Risk factors
   a. Developmental disorder
   b. Circulatory disorder
   c. Metabolic disorder
   d. Toxicity
   e. Allergies
   f. Emotional factors that can influence the intensity or precipitate the attacks
4. Etiology: The etiology for Meniere's disease of the inner ear is unknown, but it has been likened to that of glaucoma.
5. Pathophysiology
   a. Overproduction and malabsorption of endolymph occur, both of which lead to an excess accumulation of this inner ear fluid.
   b. The increased pressure caused by this fluid collection results in distention and rupture of the membranous labyrinth.
   c. As the disease progresses, morphologic changes occur in sensory and neural structures, which cause permanent losses in auditory and vestibular function.
6. Clinical manifestations
   a. Prodromal symptoms, aural pressure, or tinnitus
   b. Incapacitating attacks of vertigo
   c. Fluctuating sensorineural hearing loss initially in the low frequencies
   d. Tinnitus, initially fluctuating
   e. Autonomic symptoms of nausea, vomiting, diarrhea, increased pulse rate, and diaphoresis
   f. Exhaustion with many hours of sleep after the attack
   g. Absence of symptoms between attacks initially
   h. Abnormal gait (veering in either direction) and change in the ability to estimate spatial relationships between the body and environment
7. Diagnostics
   a. Otoscopic or microscopic examination of the ear
   b. Rinne and Weber tests
   c. Audiometry and tympanometry with acoustic reflex and reflex decay
   d. Electronystagmography
   e. Auditory brain stem response (if abnormal, imaging studies are indicated to rule out retrocochlear pathology)
8. Clinical management
   a. Although no cure is available, the goals of clinical management of Meniere's disease are to control vertigo, preserve hearing, and stabilize tinnitus. However, treatment varies widely among physicians.
   b. Nonpharmacologic interventions
      (1) Labyrinthine compensatory exercises
      (2) Low-sodium diet
      (3) Avoidance of caffeine, nicotine, and alcohol
      (4) Maintenance of a diary of symptoms
      (5) Biofeedback, self-hypnosis, and relaxation techniques for secondary psychologic symptoms
   c. Pharmacologic interventions (Table 20–3)
      (1) Vestibular suppressants
      (2) Diuretics

Table 20–3. Pharmacologic Interventions for Meniere's Disease

Drug (Adult Dose)	Nursing Considerations
Cyclizine (Marezine) 50 mg q 4–6 hr	Drowsiness and dry mouth are common.
Diazepam (Valium) 2–5 mg q 4–6 hr	May be addictive.
Dimenhydrinate (Dramamine) 50 mg q 4–6 hr	Drowsiness is common with continued use.
Haloperidol (Haldol) 0.5 mg PO qid	Drowsiness and dry mouth are common.
Meclizine (Antivert, Bonine) 25 mg tid–qid PRN	Dose is titrated to just below side effect level. Compensation of balance system may not occur with continued use.
Prochlorperazine (Compazine) 25 mg PO or suppositories q 4–6 hr	Has strong antiemetic properties.
Promethazine (Phenergan) 12.5–50 mg q 4–6 hr oral or suppositories	Drowsiness is common; has strong antiemetic properties.
Scopolamine (Transderm Scop) 0.5-mg patch q 3 days	Diminished short-term memory and dry mouth are common; hallucinations have been reported.
Trimethobenzamide (Tigan) 250 mg tid–qid	Is more effective for moderate to severe nausea.

Adapted from Sigler BA, and Schuring LT. *Ear, Nose, and Throat Disorders*. St. Louis: Mosby–Year Book, 1993, p 83.

(3) Vasodilators
(4) Cholinergics
(5) Antiemetics
d. Special medical-surgical procedures
(1) Medical interventions include ototoxic ablation therapy, which is the transtympanic injection of antibiotics that are toxic to the inner ear.
(2) Surgical interventions include conservative procedures, such as endolymphatic sac decompression or endolymphatic shunt, or destructive procedures, such as labyrinthectomy or vestibular nerve section for uncontrollable unilateral Meniere's disease.
9. Prognosis: Most cases (95%) can be controlled (though not cured) either medically or surgically.
10. Complications
a. Partial to total loss of hearing on affected side(s)
b. Constant tinnitus on affected side(s)
c. Permanent balance disability
d. Trauma from falling
e. Dehydration
f. Decreased quality of life
g. Fears, phobias, and panic attacks
11. Applying the nursing process

NURSING DIAGNOSIS: Risk for fluid volume deficit R/T increased fluid output, altered intake, and medications

a. *Expected outcomes:* The patient should maintain a normal fluid-electrolyte balance.
b. *Nursing interventions*
(1) Assess or have the patient assess intake and output (including emesis, liquid stools, urine, and diaphoresis).
(2) Assess indicators of dehydration, including blood pressure (orthostasis) pulse, skin turgor, and mucous membranes.
(3) Encourage oral fluids as tolerated; discourage beverages that contain caffeine.
(4) Administer or teach the administration of antiemetics and antidiarrheal medication as ordered and needed.

NURSING DIAGNOSIS: Risk for injury R/T altered mobility because of gait disturbance and vertigo

a. *Expected outcomes:* The patient should remain free of any injuries associated with imbalance or falls.
b. *Nursing interventions*
(1) Assess for vertigo (history, onset, description of attacks, duration, and any associated symptoms) (see Fig. 20–9).
(2) Assess the extent of disability in relation to activities of daily living.
(3) Teach or reinforce vestibular or balance therapy as prescribed.
(4) Administer or teach the administration of antivertiginous medications or vestibular sedation medication. Instruct the patient on these drugs' side effects.

NURSING DIAGNOSIS: Powerlessness R/T the illness regimen and helplessness in certain situations because of vertigo

a. *Expected outcomes:* The patient should feel an increased sense of control over his or her life and activities.
b. *Nursing interventions*
(1) Assess the patient's needs, values, attitude, and readiness to initiate activities.
(2) Give the patient opportunities to express his or her feelings about having the illness.
(3) Help the patient identify coping behaviors used successfully in the past.

NURSING DIAGNOSIS: Altered auditory sensory perception R/T altered state of the ear

a. *Expected outcomes:* The patient's hearing loss should stabilize.
b. *Nursing interventions*
(1) Assess hearing acuity and audiogram results.

(2) Speak distinctly, without shouting.

(3) Assess for tinnitus.

(4) Assess the history of hearing loss.

NURSING DIAGNOSIS: Risk for trauma R/T difficulties with balance

a. *Expected outcomes:* The patient should reduce the risk of trauma by adapting the home environment and by using rehabilitative devices if necessary.

b. *Nursing interventions*

(1) Assess for vertigo by taking a history and observing for nystagmus, a positive Romberg's sign, and an inability to perform a tandem Romberg test.

(2) Help the patient with ambulation when indicated.

(3) Assess for visual acuity and proprioceptive deficits.

(4) Encourage an increased activity level with or without the use of assistive devices.

(5) Help identify hazards in home environment.

NURSING DIAGNOSIS: Impaired adjustment R/T disability requiring change in lifestyle

a. *Expected outcomes:* The patient should adjust to or modify his or her lifestyle to decrease disability and exert maximum control and independence within the limits imposed by chronic vertigo.

b. *Nursing interventions*

(1) Encourage the patient to identify his or her strengths and roles that can still be fulfilled.

(2) Provide information about chronic vertigo and what to expect.

(3) Assist in selection of self-care practices (e.g., increased aerobic activity and balance exercises).

(4) Include family members in the rehabilitative process.

(5) Encourage the patient to maintain a sense of control by making decisions and assuming more responsibility for care.

NURSING DIAGNOSIS: Anxiety R/T the threat of change or actual change in health status or role functioning

a. *Expected outcomes:* The patient should have less or no anxiety.

b. *Nursing interventions*

(1) Assess the patient's level of anxiety.

(2) Help the patient identify coping skills used successfully in the past.

(3) Provide information about vertigo and its treatment.

(4) Encourage the patient to discuss anxieties and explore concerns about vertigo attacks and decreased hearing.

(5) Teach the patient stress management techniques.

(6) Suggest psychotherapy for the patient who is anxious and depressed.

NURSING DIAGNOSIS: Body image disturbance R/T the biophysical factors of vertigo

a. *Expected outcomes:* The patient should have a positive body image.

b. *Nursing interventions*

(1) Encourage the patient to discuss his or her feelings and concerns about vertigo.

(2) Assess the patient's current perceptions and feelings.

(3) Help the patient identify, label, and express his or her feelings about diagnosis, treatments, and anticipated prognosis.

(4) Promote the acceptance of a positive, realistic body image.

NURSING DIAGNOSIS: Ineffective individual coping R/T vulnerability and unmet expectations stemming from vertigo

a. *Expected outcomes:* The patient should develop the coping skills necessary to decrease his or her vulnerability and unmet needs and will demonstrate effective coping.

b. *Nursing interventions*

(1) Assess the patient's cognitive appraisal of having Meniere's disease and factors that may be contributing to his or her inability to cope.

(2) Provide factual information about treatment and the patient's future health status.

(3) Encourage and help the patient participate in decision making about adjustments in lifestyle.

(4) Encourage the patient to maintain participation in diversional or recreational activities, exercise, and social events.

(5) Help the patient identify his or her strengths and develop coping strategies based on them, on previous successes in dealing with stress, and on situational supports.

(6) Refer the patient to support groups or counseling as indicated.

NURSING DIAGNOSIS: Diversional activity deficit R/T a lack of such activity in the environment

a. *Expected outcomes:* The patient should engage in diversional activities.

b. *Nursing interventions*

(1) Assess the level and type of diversional activity to plan appropriate activities.

(2) Discuss the patient's usual pattern of diversional activities with him or her.

(3) Suggest opportunities to continue meaningful diversional activities.

a. *Expected outcomes:* The patient's fear should decrease as a result of having increased knowledge of vertigo.
b. *Nursing interventions*
   (1) Encourage the patient to talk about his or her feelings, perception of danger, and perception of own coping skills and limitations.
   (2) Replace distorted perceptions and misinformation about vertigo with accurate information.
   (3) Teach therapeutic treatments of vertigo and what to expect.
   (4) Refer the patient to support groups.
   (5) Encourage the use of such comfort measures as music, religious practices, and the company of family and friends.
12. Discharge planning and teaching
    a. Teach the patient and family about the diagnosis and treatment of chronic vertigo.
    b. Discuss the importance of maintaining or resuming activities.
    c. Discuss the importance of a regular exercise schedule that includes aerobic activities.
    d. Discuss the importance of diversional or social activities.
    e. Teach the patient the names, dosages, and side effects of prescribed medications.
    f. Discuss the importance of not allowing anticipation of vertigo to curtail activity when the vertigo is absent.

Other Ear Disorders

1. Benign paroxysmal positional vertigo (BPPV)
   a. Definition: Benign paroxysmal positional vertigo is a benign disorder because it is not life threatening, a paroxysmal disorder because it happens without warning, and a position disorder because it is produced by movement of the head or body.
   b. Etiology
      (1) Four factors predispose to BPPV: advanced age, trauma, inactivity, and ear disease.
      (2) Typically, BPPV is idiopathic or develops secondarily to an inner ear disorder.
      (3) The damage that gives rise to BPPV can be caused by trauma to the head, a whiplash injury, a viral infection, circulatory changes, degeneration of the system related to aging, or an unknown cause.
   c. Clinical manifestations
      (1) In BPPV, a very brief period of incapacitating vertigo occurs during a sudden head movement or change in body position. Most patients experience the imbalance when they are trying to lie down, rise, or turn over in bed.
      (2) Nausea and vomiting may also accompany BPPV.
      (3) The type of movement that produces the symptoms varies according to the position of the vestibular system that has been damaged. Sometimes, rapid movement causes symptoms; for example, a

car passing by or walking up and down a grocery store aisle may produce dizziness or vertigo.
      (4) The symptoms typically are worse in the morning and improve during the day.
   d. Clinical management
      (1) This condition often resolves spontaneously without any need for intervention.
      (2) A common treatment strategy is to wait it out.
      (3) Antivertiginous medicines generally do not prevent the paroxysmal attacks.
      (4) Vestibular habituation exercises are prescribed, and a canalith repositioning procedure may be recommended.
2. Presbyastasis
   a. Definition: Presbyastasis, also known as presbyvertigo, is the balance disorder of aging.
   b. Etiology: Presbyastasis results from the generalized degenerative changes in the labyrinth.
   c. Clinical manifestations
      (1) Constant sensation of imbalance while standing or walking
      (2) Decreased visual acuity and compromised proprioception with vestibular dysfunction
      (3) Falls and subsequent injuries, as a result of having all 3 systems (visual, vestibular, and proprioceptive) involved
   d. Clinical management: Management of the patient with presbyastasis includes physical therapy, the use of canes or walkers, administration of vasodilators, and neurologic referrals. The overall goal of treatment is control, not cure.
3. Vestibular neuronitis
   a. Definition: Vestibular neuronitis is caused by damage to or infection of the vestibular portion of the acoustic nerve.
   b. Incidence and etiology
      (1) Vestibular neuronitis is common.
      (2) It is most often caused by a virus, and many patients have had previous ear, nose, and throat infections. Vascular and demyelinating disorders and toxins are also causes of vestibular neuronitis.
   c. Clinical manifestations
      (1) Vestibular neuronitis is characterized by a sudden onset of severe vertigo without loss of hearing.
      (2) The 1st episode is the worst, with subsequent attacks bringing less and less vertigo.
   d. Clinical management
      (1) Vestibular suppressants are used to treat acute attacks.
      (2) Labyrinthine exercises are prescribed to hasten compensation.
      (3) Recovery can occur without treatment over a period of several weeks to months.
      (4) A less common, chronic form can persist for months to years. This form can be surgically controlled with a vestibular nerve section.
4. Vestibular labyrinthitis
   a. Definition: Vestibular labyrinthitis is an inflammation of the inner ear caused by a bacterial or viral infection.

b. Incidence and etiology
   (1) Viral labyrinthitis is much more common than bacterial labyrinthitis.
   (2) Viral causes include the sequelae of measles, mumps, rubella, encephalitis, upper respiratory infections, and herpetiform disorders of cranial nerves VII and VIII (Ramsay Hunt's syndrome).
   (3) Bacterial causes include otitis media, cholesteatoma that causes erosion of the lateral semicircular canal, and bacterial meningitis.
c. Clinical manifestations
   (1) Sudden onset of severe vertigo
   (2) Varying degrees of sensorineural hearing loss
   (3) Possibly tinnitus
   (4) Acute attacks of vertigo that recur for 5 to 6 weeks.
   (5) Nausea and vomiting
d. Clinical management
   (1) Vestibular suppressants are used to treat acute attacks.
   (2) Labyrinthine exercises are prescribed to hasten compensation.
   (3) Bacterial labyrinthitis is treated with antibiotics.
   (4) Chronic labyrinthitis can be surgically treated by a vestibular nerve section.
5. Tinnitus
   a. Definition
      (1) Tinnitus is a distressing symptom, not a disorder.
      (2) Ringing or any other noises in the ear is called tinnitus.
   b. Etiology
      (1) The pathophysiology of tinnitus is still in the realm of speculation. Some theories involve vascular disorders, nerve inhibition, and trigger mechanisms.
      (2) Tinnitus accompanies most types of sensorineural hearing loss.
   c. Clinical manifestations
      (1) Unilateral or bilateral noise
      (2) Intermittent or constant noise
      (3) Sudden or gradual onset of noise
      (4) Mild to severe intensity of noise
      (5) Possibly unilateral tinnitus as a symptom of retrocochlear pathology
   d. Clinical management: There is no specific therapy for tinnitus, but several treatments can be tried with moderate success.
      (1) Vasodilators
      (2) Steroids
      (3) Hearing aids
      (4) Tinnitus maskers
      (5) Biofeedback
      (6) Electrostimulation
      (7) Self-hypnosis
6. Acoustic neuroma
   a. Definition: Acoustic neuroma is a rare, benign, encapsulated tumor of the acoustic nerve, cranial nerve VIII.
   b. Incidence and etiology
      (1) Acoustic tumors account for only 5 to 10 percent of all intracranial tumors, affect both men and women, and usually occur in the 4th decade of life.
      (2) Neuromas usually arise from the Schwann cells of the vestibular portion of the acoustic nerve; only occasionally do they originate from the cochlear portion.
      (3) Usually only 1 ear is affected, but both ears can be involved in Von Recklinghausen's disease (neurofibromatosis).
   c. Clinical manifestations: The most common symptoms are sensorineural hearing loss, tinnitus, and dizziness. The symptoms are usually gradual in onset, although they can occur suddenly.
   d. Clinical management
      (1) Surgical removal is the treatment of choice for these tumors, because they do not respond well to radiation or chemotherapy. The major objectives are to save the patient's life and remove the tumor while preserving the facial and acoustic nerves.
      (2) One of 4 microsurgical approaches is used, depending on the size and location of the tumor and the patient's hearing: the middle fossa approach; the translabyrinthine approach; the 1-stage, combined translabyrinthine-suboccipital approach; or the suboccipital approach.

Major Ear Surgeries

1. *Myringotomy* with or without placement of transtympanic tubes
   a. Definition: In a myringotomy, an incision is made in the pars tensa of the tympanic membrane, the fluid is suctioned out of the middle ear cavity, and a ventilating tube can be inserted transtympanically.
   b. Indications
      (1) Chronic serous otitis media
      (2) Recurrent serous otitis media
      (3) Eustachian tube dysfunction with middle ear atelectasis
   c. Preoperative care
      (1) Explain the purpose and technique of the procedure.
      (2) Discuss the potential complications.
      (3) Check the operative consent form.
   d. Postoperative care: Discuss water restrictions. The nurse instructs the patient to keep the head dry by not washing the hair or showering for several days postoperatively.
   e. Complications
      (1) Hearing loss
      (2) Injury to the ossicular chain
      (3) Otorrhea
      (4) Tympanosclerosis of the tympanic membrane
      (5) Perforation of the tympanic membrane
      (6) Cholesteatoma
2. *Tympanoplasty*
   a. Definition
      (1) Tympanoplasty is the repair of the tympanic membrane.

(2) Type I: Repair of a perforation of the tympanic membrane only
(3) Type II: Repair of a perforation of the tympanic membrane, and placement of a graft on the long process of the malleus
(4) Type III: Repair of a perforation of the tympanic membrane and placement of a graft on the head of the stapes
(5) Type IV: Repair of a perforation of the tympanic membrane and placement of the graft on the stapes footplate
(6) Type V has been replaced by stapes surgery.
b. Indications
(1) To close a perforation of the tympanic membrane.
(2) To prevent recurrent infections.
(3) To provide adequate aeration of the middle ear.
(4) To improve hearing.
c. Contraindications
(1) Nonfunctioning eustachian tube
(2) Only hearing ear
(3) Necrotizing external otitis
(4) Malignant neoplasm
(5) Several previous tympanoplasty failures
d. Pre- and postoperative care is presented in Box 20–4.
e. Complications
(1) Graft failure
(2) Facial nerve injuries
(3) Taste disturbance
(4) Vertigo
(5) Sensorineural hearing loss
(6) Tinnitus
(7) Dry mouth
(8) Ear infection

3. *Stapes replacement surgery*
a. Definition
(1) Stapes replacement surgery is the replacement of the stapes bone that has become fixed by otosclerosis or tympanosclerosis with a prosthesis to increase hearing.
(2) Stapedectomy is the removal of the stapes superstructure and the stapes footplate and the placement of a graft and prosthesis to increase hearing.
(3) Stapedotomy is the removal of the stapes superstructure, placement of a hole in the stapes footplate, and insertion of a prosthesis in the hole to increase hearing.
b. Indications
(1) Otosclerosis
(2) Tympanosclerosis of stapes footplate
c. Contraindications
(1) Serious medical problems
(2) Small conductive hearing loss
(3) Only hearing ear
(4) Perforation of the tympanic membrane
(5) Infection
d. Pre- and postoperative care is presented in Box 20–4.
e. Complications
(1) Taste disturbance
(2) Dry mouth
(3) Hearing loss
(4) Tinnitus
(5) Facial paralysis
(6) Perforation of the tympanic membrane
(7) Infection
(8) Dislocation of the incus
(9) Perilymphatic fistula or gusher

4. *Mastoid surgeries*
a. Definition

BOX 20–4. Pre- and Postoperative Care for Transcanal Ear Surgeries

Preoperative Care

Explain the surgical procedure.
Explain the rationale for shaving above and behind the ear and the graft site when appropriate.
Review postoperative instructions.
Encourage the patient to express any fears, anxiety, concerns, or questions.
Discuss the risks and complications of surgery.
Advise the patient to wash his or her hair before surgery.
Remove the hearing aid, if any, from the operative ear.
Check the consent form.
Administer preoperative medications.

Postoperative Care

1. Instruct the patient to sneeze or cough with his or her mouth open for 1 week after surgery to prevent dislodgement of grafts or prostheses.
2. Instruct the patient to blow the nose gently one side at a time for 1 week after surgery to prevent dislodgement of grafts or prostheses.
3. Instruct the patient to perform no physical activity for 1 week and then to resume all normal activities.
4. Tell the patient to return to work after 1 week. If work is strenuous, the patient may return to work in 2 to 3 weeks.
5. Inform the patient that a variety of noises such as cracking or popping may be present.
6. Tell the patient that the ear packing decreases hearing in the affected ear and can sound as if the patient is talking in a barrel.
7. Reassure the patient that minor ear discomfort is normal and urge the patient to take the prescribed pain medication. Stress that excessive ear pain should be reported to the ear surgeon.
8. Occasionally, a small amount of bleeding from the ear occurs; reassure the patient that this is normal. Instruct the patient to report excessive ear drainage to the ear surgeon.
9. Remind the patient to change the cotton ball in the ear as ordered.
10. Tell the patient that there is to be no water in the ear for several weeks and the ear should be protected with two pieces of cotton, the outer one saturated with petroleum jelly.
11. Tell the patient that the graft site should be protected for 1 week; usually there are no sutures to be removed.
12. Urge the patient to take antibiotics as prescribed.
13. Remind the patient to wear noise defenders or cotton with petroleum jelly around loud noises.
14. Tell the patient to check with the ear surgeon for instructions for flying.

Postoperative instructions for transcanal surgery vary greatly among ear surgeons. These guidelines are only suggested areas for patient teaching.

Adapted from preoperative care developed from the text from a chapter in Sigler BA, and Schuring LT. *Ear, Nose, and Throat Disorders.* St. Louis: Mosby–Year Book, 1993; postoperative care from same source, p 111.

(1) Mastoid surgeries are performed to eradicate infection of the mastoid, to eliminate cholesteatoma, to restore hearing when possible, and to create access to neural structures in neurologic procedures

(2) Simple mastoidectomy. A simple mastoidectomy is performed to enlarge and clean the mastoid cavity.

(3) Radical mastoidectomy. A radical mastoidectomy is performed to clean and completely exteriorize the mastoid cavity, which sacrifices the middle ear for hearing.

(4) Modified radical mastoidectomy. A modified radical mastoidectomy is performed to clean and partly exteriorize the mastoid cavity, which preserves the middle ear for hearing.

(5) Tympanomastoidectomy. A tympanomastoidectomy is performed to clean but preserve the mastoid cavity, which restores the middle ear for hearing. It combines mastoid surgery with tympanoplasty and ossiculoplasty.

b. Indications
(1) Chronic otitis media
(2) Chronic mastoiditis
(3) Cholesteatoma
(4) Transmastoid labyrinthectomy
(5) Cochlear implantation

c. Contraindications
(1) Only hearing ear
(2) Serious medical problem
(3) Necrotizing external otitis
(4) Infectious systemic disease
(5) Age
(6) Malignant neoplasm

d. Pre- and postoperative care is discussed in Box 20–5
e. Complications

5. *Cochlear implantation*
a. Definition: The internal device, a multichannel electrode, is inserted into the basal turn of the cochlea through a mastoidectomy. The external equipment is applied over the internal device after healing and is held in place by a magnet across the skin. The external device consists of a microphone and a sound processing unit. Extensive cochlear rehabilitation is necessary for a successful outcome.

b. Indications
(1) No useful hearing in either ear
(2) Lack of benefit from a hearing aid
(3) Patient who is emotionally stable and noninstitutionalized
(4) Patient who is able to give informed consent and follow through with rehabilitation
(5) Intact auditory nerve and central auditory pathway

c. Contraindications
(1) Auditory nerve or central auditory pathway that is not intact
(2) Age (few sites in the United States are authorized to perform cochlear implants on children)

d. Pre- and postoperative care is discussed in Box 20–5.
e. Complications
(1) Perforation of the cochlea
(2) Infection or otorrhea
(3) Meningitis

BOX 20–5. Postoperative Care for Transmastoid Ear Surgeries

Preoperative Care

1. Initiate preoperative instruction for the patient and family.
   Explain the surgical procedure and the purpose for shaving above and behind the patient's ear.
   Explain or review the postoperative course.
   Discuss postoperative instructions, such as activity restrictions, head movement, and symptoms. Encourage the patient to express any anxiety, fears, concerns, and questions.
2. Check the operative permission form.
3. Discuss the risks and complications of surgery if appropriate.
4. Withhold food and water for the appropriate length of time before surgery.
5. Wash the patient's hair before surgery.
6. Remove all jewelry, glasses, contact lenses, and hearing aid in the operative ear from the patient.
7. Administer preoperative medications.

Postoperative Care

1. Instruct the patient to sneeze or cough with the mouth open for 1 week after surgery to prevent dislodgement of grafts or prostheses.
2. Instruct the patient to blow the nose gently one side at a time for 1 week after surgery to prevent dislodgement of grafts or prostheses.
3. Instruct the patient to perform no physical activity for 1 week and then to resume all normal activities.
4. Tell the patient to return to work after 1 week. If work is strenuous, the patient may return to work in 2 to 3 weeks.
5. Inform the patient that a variety of noises such as cracking or popping may be present.
6. Tell the patient that the ear packing decreases hearing in the operated ear and can sound as if the patient is talking in a barrel.
7. Reassure the patient that minor ear discomfort is normal and urge the patient to take the prescribed pain medication. Stress that excessive ear pain should be reported to the ear surgeon.
8. Occasionally, a small amount of bleeding from the ear occurs; reassure the patient that this is normal. Instruct the patient to report excessive ear drainage to the ear surgeon.
9. Remind the patient to change the cotton ball in the ear as ordered.
10. Tell the patient that there is to be no water in the ear for several weeks and the ear should be protected with two pieces of cotton, the outer one saturated with petroleum jelly.
11. Tell the patient that the graft site should be protected for 1 week; usually there are no sutures to be removed.
12. Tell the patient to take antibiotics as prescribed.
13. Urge the patient to wear noise defenders or cotton with petroleum jelly around loud noises.
14. Advise the patient to check with the ear surgeon regarding instructions for flying.
15. Inform the patient that temporary facial weakness, taste disturbances, and numbness of the pinna (external ear) can occur, but usually return to normal function.

Postoperative instructions for a transmastoid approach for ear surgeries vary greatly among ear surgeons. These patient teaching guidelines are only suggested areas for education.

Adapted from Sigler BA, and Schuring LT. *Ear, Nose, and Throat Disorders.* St. Louis: Mosby–Year Book, 1993, pp 117–121.

(4) Cerebrospinal fluid leak
(5) Vertigo
(6) Perilymphatic fluid leak
(7) Hemorrhage
(8) Paralysis of facial nerve
(9) Lump behind ear

(10) Failure of device, requiring its removal
(11) Taste disturbance
(12) Tinnitus

☐ *NOSE AND SINUS DISORDERS*

Epistaxis

1. Definition: Epistaxis is bleeding from the nose.
2. Incidence and socioeconomic impact
   a. Epistaxis occurs equally in males and females and affects all age groups.
   b. Children are more likely to have anterior nasal bleeding, and adults are more likely to have posterior nasal bleeding.
3. Risk factors
   a. Chronic nose picking
   b. Overuse of certain medications
   c. Hereditary diseases, such as Rendu-Osler-Weber disease (a hereditary hemorrhagic telangiectasia) or hemophilia
4. Etiology
   a. Trauma
   b. Foreign body
   c. Infection
   d. Inflammation
   e. Blood or coagulation disorder
   f. Tumor
5. Pathophysiology
   a. Anterior nasal bleeding occurs most frequently in Little's area on the anterior nasal septum.
   b. Posterior nasal bleeding usually occurs high on the nasal septum or in Woodruff's plexus under the posterior, inferior turbinate.
   c. Infection of the nose produces inflammation and friable nasal mucosa that bleeds easily.
   d. Blood disorders, such as hemophilia, immunodeficiency, a lymphoproliferative disorder that aggravates or prolongs bleeding or clotting time, or a decreased platelet count, can cause epistaxis.
   e. Chemotherapy, aspirin, and nonsteroidal anti-inflammatory drugs increase the tendency for epistaxis.
   f. Atherosclerosis and hypertension are contributing factors, because blood vessel contraction is altered and blood pressure is elevated.
6. Clinical manifestations
   a. Nasal bleeding
   b. Mouth breathing secondary to nasal obstruction
   c. Hypertension, which alters vessel contraction
   d. Hypotension secondary to blood loss
   e. Increase pulse rate compensatory to blood loss
7. Diagnostics
   a. History of recent trauma, hereditary disease, or nasal surgery
   b. Inspection with the nasal speculum to determine the site of bleeding
   c. Blood evaluation (complete blood count and coagulation studies) to rule out blood dyscrasias
   d. Rhinoscopy to localize the site of bleeding
   e. Naspharyngoscopy to localize the site of bleeding
8. Clinical management

   a. The goal of clinical management is to control the nasal bleeding. The interventions used depend on the source and severity of the bleeding.
   b. Nonpharmacologic interventions
      (1) Pinch anterior nose tightly for a minimum of 10 minutes.
      (2) Apply ice compresses to nose to promote vasoconstriction.
      (3) Assist patient into a sitting position with head slightly forward to prevent swallowing or aspirating blood.
      (4) Insert anterior or posterior nasal packing once bleeding area is identified.
   c. Pharmacologic interventions
      (1) Medications to promote vasoconstriction, allay anxiety, and decrease discomfort
      (2) Topical decongestants to promote vasoconstriction
   d. Special medical-surgical procedures
      (1) Ligation of ethmoid, maxillary, or carotid artery
      (2) Endoscopic cautery to cauterize vessel(s) clinically or electrically
      (3) Laser photocoagulation for Rendu-Osler-Weber syndrome
      (4) Skin graft to nasal septum and lateral walls for Rendu-Osler-Weber syndrome
      (5) Angiogram with embolization in patients unable to have surgery
9. Complications
   a. Otitis media from blocked eustachian tube resulting from nasal edema or packing
   b. Sinusitis related to nasal congestion, blockage of drainage through sinus openings
   c. Rhinitis related to nasal congestion, blockage of drainage through sinus openings
   d. Toxic shock syndrome from the endotoxin of a certain staphylococcal bacteria in the nasal cavity
   e. Hypoventilation as a result of nasal packing
   f. Hypoxia as a result of nasal packing
   g. Cardiac arrest from cardiac arrhythmia
10. Prognosis: good, if adequate treatment is received
11. Applying the nursing process

NURSING DIAGNOSIS: Risk for fluid volume deficit R/T nasal bleeding

   a. *Expected outcomes:* Nasal bleeding should be controlled.
   b. *Nursing interventions*
      (1) Practice universal precautions (wear goggles, gloves, mask, and gown).
      (2) Provide good illumination (headlight or head mirror) and suction equipment.
      (3) Place the patient in a sitting position.
      (4) Administer medications as ordered (e.g., morphine or valium).
      (5) Monitor blood pressure, pulse, and respiratory rate.
      (6) Prepare topical agents (e.g., 4% cocaine hydrochloride, epinephrine 1:1000, or oxymetazoline) for vasoconstriction and anesthesia of the nose.

(7) Prepare the patient for treatment to stop the bleeding.

(8) Assist with the insertion of nasal packing. Plain ribbon gauze coated with antibiotic ointment is inserted tightly into the anterior nasal cavity and remains in place for 48 to 72 hours.

(9) Apply a nasal sling (a 2 × 2 gauze pad folded into thirds with tape placed tightly on either side of the nose).

(10) Inspect the oral cavity for palatal bulging, which may indicate overpacking.

(11) Assist with the insertion of posterior nasal packing (a 14 or 16 Foley catheter and rolled lambs-wool or gauze) (Fig. 20–10 and Box 20–6).

(12) Examine the nasal columella for excoriation and laceration.

(13) Monitor fluid, electrolyte, and hematologic values.

(14) Assess blood pressure, pulse, respirations, and level of consciousness.

(15) Administer intravenous hydration and blood products as ordered.

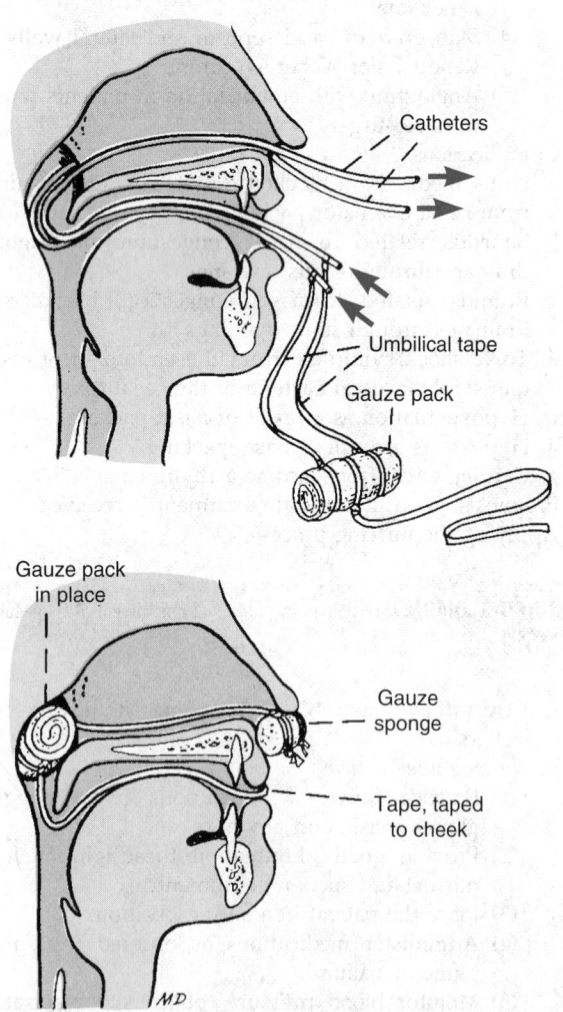

Figure 20–10. Instillation of posterior nose packing. (From Black JM, and Matassarin-Jacobs E [eds]. *Luckmann and Sorensen's Medical-Surgical Nursing: A Psychophysiologic Approach.* 4th ed. Philadelphia: WB Saunders, 1993, p 1013.)

Catheters

Umbilical tape

Gauze pack

Gauze pack in place

Gauze sponge

Tape, taped to cheek

BOX 20–6. Insertion of Posterior Nasal Packing

1. Wear gloves, goggles, a gown, and a mask.
2. Assemble the necessary supplies:
   • Red rubber catheter
   • Nasopharyngeal pack coated with antibiotic ointment
   • Curved Kelly hemostat
   • Anterior nasal packing coated with antibiotic ointment
3. Provide adequate lighting.
4. Insert the catheter through the nose into the nasopharynx.
5. Pull the catheter through the oral cavity with the curved hemo-stat.
6. Tie the strings of the pack to the catheter.
7. Withdraw the catheter through the nose to position the pack in the nasopharynx.
8. Insert the anterior nasal packing in both nares.
9. Untie the strings from the catheter and tie them over the tonsil sponge to secure the packing.

Adapted from Sigler BA, and Schuring LT. *Ear, Nose, and Throat Disorders.* St. Louis: Mosby–Year Book, 1993, p 151.

(16) Elevate the head of the bed.

(17) Apply ice compresses to the nose and face.

(18) Encourage the patient to minimize activity.

NURSING DIAGNOSIS: Risk for aspiration R/T nasal bleeding

a. *Expected outcomes:* The patient should have no aspiration-related complications.

b. *Nursing interventions*

(1) Elevate the head of the bed; maintain the patient in a sitting position.

(2) Encourage the patient to expectorate blood and help the patient with suctioning, should vomiting occur.

NURSING DIAGNOSIS: Risk for infection R/T nasal packing

a. *Expected outcomes:* The patient should exhibit no signs of infection.

b. *Nursing interventions*

(1) Take the patient's axillary, rectal, or otic temperature every 4 hours.

(2) Apply antibiotic ointment to nasal packing before insertion; administer antibiotics, as ordered.

(3) Observe the patient for symptoms of toxic shock syndrome: nausea, vomiting, headache, myalgia, fever, hypotension, and tachycardia. If toxic shock is suspected, obtain a physician's order for blood cultures.

NURSING DIAGNOSIS: Ineffective breathing pattern R/T nasal bleeding and packing

a. *Expected outcomes:* Nasal breathing should be restored.

b. *Nursing interventions*

(1) Monitor respirations and pulse oximetry or arterial blood gases as ordered.

(2) Administer supplemental humidified oxygen (usually at a 40% concentration) as ordered by face mask.

(3) Monitor patients with chronic obstructive pulmonary disease who are receiving supplemental oxygen for possible respiratory depression.

NURSING DIAGNOSIS: Fear R/T possible exsanguination

---

a. *Expected outcomes:* The patient's fears should be reduced.

b. *Nursing interventions*

(1) Allay the patient's anxiety by thoroughly explaining all procedures and providing reassurance.

(2) Investigate the causes of fear and anxieties.

(3) Administer sedatives or antianxiety medications as ordered, while continuing to monitor respiratory status.

12. Discharge planning and teaching

a. Inform the patient of ways to increase humidification, such as using a bedside humidifier, instilling nasal saline sprays, or applying a small amount of ointment to the anterior nasal cavity to lubricate the membranes.

b. Instruct the patient to avoid routine use of nasal decongestant sprays.

c. Instruct the patient to avoid blowing the nose and to sneeze with the mouth open.

d. Encourage the patient to avoid nasal trauma and strenuous activity for 4 to 6 weeks.

e. Provide the patient with information to control other existing medical conditions.

f. Instruct the patient to avoid using aspirin, aspirin-containing products, and nonsteroidal anti-inflammatory drugs.

g. If nasal bleeding occurs, the patient should be instructed to do the following. (The family should also be instructed on this procedure.)

(1) Pinch the nostrils for 10 minutes.

(2) Apply ice compresses to the nose.

(3) Sit upright with the head tilted forward.

(4) Use a nasal decongestant spray to produce vasoconstriction, as ordered.

(5) Seek medical attention if the bleeding does not stop with these measures.

Nasal Deformities

1. Definition

a. A nasal deformity is a condition that causes an alteration in the shape or structure or a malformation of the nose.

b. A deviated nasal septum is a shift of the septum from the midline (Fig. 20–11).

c. A nasal fracture is a break of the nasal bones; it may be associated with fractures of other facial bones.

2. Incidence and socioeconomic impact: Nasal fractures occur more commonly in men than women and are often associated with accidents, sport injuries, and assaults.

3. Risk factors: Participation in contact sports increases the risk of sustaining a nasal deformity.

4. Etiology

a. Nasal septal deviation can be related to congenital disproportion (in which the cartilage is too large for the area), trauma during the birth process, or trauma during the life span.

b. Nasal fractures are always a result of trauma. A "greenstick" nasal fracture can occur in the birth canal during delivery and is easily realigned.

5. Clinical manifestations

a. Obstruction of nasal breathing

b. Mouth breathing

c. Twisting of the nasal septum

d. Excoriation of the nasal mucosa

e. Epistaxis

f. Edema and ecchymosis of the midface

g. Pain and tenderness on palpation

6. Diagnostics

a. Inspection of the nose and face

b. Nasal examination

c. Facial radiographs to diagnose nasal fracture or deviation of nasal septum

d. Skull radiographs to rule out a skull fracture

7. Clinical management

a. The goal of clinical management is to restore nasal breathing.

b. Nonpharmacologic interventions

(1) Elevation of the head of the bed to reduce nasal edema

(2) Application of ice compresses to the nose to stop the bleeding

(3) Increased supplemental humidification

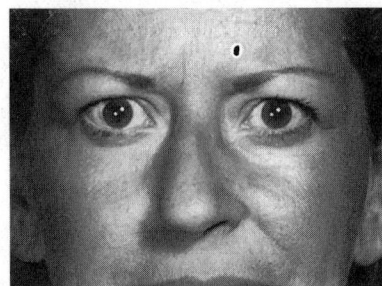
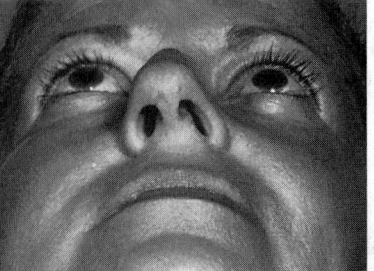

Figure 20–11. Deviated septum. (From McCarthy JG. *Plastic Surgery.* Vol. 3. Philadelphia: WB Saunders, 1990, p 1868.)

c. Pharmacologic interventions
   (1) Systemic decongestant medications to decrease nasal edema
   (2) Topical nasal steroid sprays to reduce nasal edema
   (3) Analgesics to eliminate pain
d. Special medical-surgical procedures
   (1) Reduction of nasal fracture
   (2) Nasal septoplasty to straighten the septum
   (3) Rhinoplasty for cosmetic repair of the nose
8. Complications
   a. Nasal obstruction
   b. Epistaxis
   c. Cosmetic nasal deformity
   d. Sinusitis
9. Applying the nursing process

NURSING DIAGNOSIS: Ineffective breathing pattern R/T nasal obstruction

a. *Expected outcomes:* The patient's nasal breathing should be restored.
b. *Nursing interventions*
   (1) Elevate the head of the bed.
   (2) Administer systemic decongestant medications and nasal sprays as ordered.

NURSING DIAGNOSIS: Risk for fluid volume deficit R/T nasal bleeding

a. *Expected outcomes:* The patient should maintain adequate fluid balance as evidenced by stable vital signs and cessation of hemorrhage.
b. *Nursing interventions*
   (1) Apply ice compresses to the nose after acute injury.
   (2) Pinch the nostrils at the tip for a minimum of 10 minutes if nasal bleeding occurs.
   (3) Increase supplemental humidification.
   (4) Weigh dressings, if necessary, to estimate fluid loss.
   (5) Replace fluid loss as indicated.
10. Discharge planning and teaching
   a. Instruct the patient on ways to decrease nasal edema (e.g., elevating the head of the bed).
   b. Explain techniques to increase humidification, such as using a bedside humidifier, instilling normal saline sprays or using irrigations, or applying ointment to the nose to lubricate the membranes.
   c. Provide information about the side effects of prescribed medications, such as drowsiness from systemic decongestants and rebound swelling from topical decongestants.

Nasal Polyposis

1. Definition: Nasal polyps are swelling of the mucous membranes of the sinus mucosa into the nose and paranasal sinuses (Fig. 20–12).

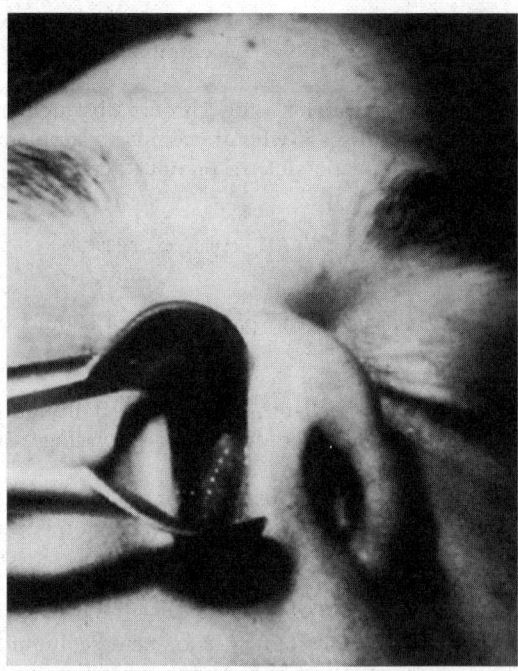

Figure 20–12. Nasal polyp. (From Krause HF. *Otolaryngic Allergy and Immunology.* Philadelphia: WB Saunders, 1989, p 55.)

2. Incidence and socioeconomic impact
   a. The incidence of nasal polyposis is unknown, but it is a common occurrence.
   b. Nasal polyposis occurs twice as often in men as in women.
   c. Nasal polyps are found in all age groups and with ciliary motility disorders, allergies, asthma, chronic rhinitis, chronic sinusitis, and cystic fibrosis.
3. Etiology: The cause of nasal polyps is unknown. They have been suggested to be an inflammatory response as well as the result of chronic viral or bacterial infection.
4. Clinical manifestations
   a. Difficulty breathing through the nose
   b. Mouth breathing
   c. Sensation of having a foreign object in the nose
   d. Grayish growths of tissue visible on nasal examination
   e. Unilateral or bilateral polyps on nasal examination
   f. Decreased or absent sense of smell
   g. Rhinorrhea (watery mucous discharge)
   h. Excessive sneezing
   i. Excessive tearing
5. Diagnostics
   a. Nasal examination
   b. Sinus radiographs showing diffuse mucosal disease or an air-fluid level if sinus is obstructed.
   c. Computed tomographic scan to evaluate the extent of disease.
   d. Immunologic assessment if allergy is considered a causative factor.
6. Clinical management
   a. The goals of clinical management are to remove the polyps and restore nasal breathing.
   b. Nonpharmacologic interventions

(1) Use of a humidifier or nasal saline sprays and increased fluid intake to increase humidity
(2) Elevation of the head of the bed to reduce nasal edema
(3) Avoidance of upper respiratory infections
c. Pharmacologic interventions
(1) Antihistamines to treat allergic symptoms
(2) Antibiotics to treat infections
(3) Corticosteroids to decrease the size of the polyp(s) temporarily. (Because of their side effects, systemic corticosteroids are used only for extremely obstructed airways. Local injection of steroids or local instillation of sprays [Beconase, Vancenese, or Nasacort] is used to reduce the size of the polyps and inflammatory response and to prevent recurrence.)
d. Special medical-surgical procedures
(1) Nasal polypectomy to remove the polyps
(2) Functional endoscopic sinus surgery to remove the polyps
(3) Caldwell-Luc surgery, in which an incision is made in the gingival buccal sulcus to gain entry into the maxillary sinus to remove the polyps
7. Complications
a. Epistaxis
b. Sinusitis
8. Prognosis: Recurrence is probable unless the cause of the nasal polyps is also treated.
9. Applying the nursing process

NURSING DIAGNOSIS: Ineffective breathing pattern R/T nasal obstruction

a. *Expected outcomes:* The patient should be able to breathe through his or her nose with minimal difficulty.
b. *Nursing interventions*
(1) Increase humidification through the use of a humidifier and nasal saline spray and an increase in fluid intake.
(2) Raise the head of the bed.
(3) Instruct the patient to avoid upper respiratory infections.
(4) Instruct the patient in the procedure for administering nasal steroid spray as ordered; explain that the nozzle of the spray must be aimed toward the cheek (sinuses). (Steroid nasal sprays must be used for several days before any change in symptomatology is noticed.)

NURSING DIAGNOSIS: Altered sensory (olfactory) perception R/T nasal obstruction

a. *Expected outcomes:* The patient should be able to distinguish common odors and will use safety measures to compensate for the loss of the sense of smell.
b. *Nursing interventions:* Instruct the patient to make changes in his or her living environment, such as installing smoke detectors, checking the appearance of stored food for signs of spoiling, routinely checking gas lines for leakage, and installing gas detectors.

NURSING DIAGNOSIS: Altered sensory (gustatory) perception R/T weight loss secondary to an altered sense of smell

a. *Expected outcomes:* The patient should maintain his or her body weight.
b. *Nursing interventions*
(1) Consult with a dietitian.
(2) Suggest foods with visual appeal.
(3) Encourage the patient to experiment with various spices and additives to increase the taste of food.

NURSING DIAGNOSIS: Risk for infection R/T nasal obstruction or obstructed sinus ostia

a. *Expected outcomes:* The patient should have no signs of infection.
b. *Nursing interventions*
(1) Instruct the patient to avoid crowds and people known to have an upper respiratory infection.
(2) Instruct the patient in the proper use of antibiotics, including side effects and dosages.
(3) Instruct the patient in the proper use of antihistamines and decongestants, including side effects and dosages.
10. Discharge planning and teaching
a. Teach the patient ways to decrease nasal edema to improve nasal breathing (e.g., elevate the head of the bed).
b. Encourage the patient to use a bedside humidifier and nasal saline sprays and to increase fluid intake.
c. Emphasize the importance of avoiding upper respiratory infections. Encourage the patient to notify the physician if an upper respiratory infection is suspected, so that appropriate therapy may be started.
d. Provide information about all prescribed medications, including their side effects, proper dosages, and administration.
e. Encourage the patient to seek medical attention if polyps recur.

Rhinitis (Common Cold)

1. Definition
a. Rhinitis is an inflammation of the nasal mucous membranes.
b. It can be classified as acute, allergic, vasomotor, or medicamentosa.
(1) Acute rhinitis: the common cold, or coryza
(2) Allergic rhinitis: nasal inflammation caused by allergic response
(3) Vasomotor rhinitis: chronic idiopathic or nonallergic rhinitis
(4) Rhinitis medicamentosa: abuse or overuse of topical agents, such as nasal sprays or cocaine

2. Pathophysiology
   a. Acute rhinitis is most frequently caused by a virus, but it may have a secondary bacterial infection. Acute viral rhinitis is spread by droplet and usually is contagious for 2 to 3 days.
   b. Allergic rhinitis
      (1) Seasonal allergic rhinitis is an acute response to a specific antigen, such as pollen from grass, trees, or flowers. Symptoms are present as long as the specific antigen is present.
      (2) Perennial allergic rhinitis is a chronic disorder in response to antigens constantly present in the environment, such as dust, animal dander, mold, and foods.
   c. The cause of vasomotor rhinitis is unknown, but can be an abnormality of the parasympathetic activity of the nerves. Other contributory factors are tumors, granulomatous disease, septal deviation, nasal polyps, foreign bodies, tuberculosis, sarcoidosis, medications, and pregnancy.
   d. Rhinitis medicamentosa
      (1) Initially, these topical agents cause vasoconstriction and decongestion. However, when used habitually, they have a rebound effect, resulting in mucosal edema.
      (2) The symptoms of rhinitis medicamentosa can be alleviated by discontinuing use of the agents.
3. Clinical manifestations
   a. Nasal obstruction
   b. Rhinorrhea or postnasal drip
   c. Sneezing
   d. Watery, itchy eyes and nose
   e. Altered sense of smell
   f. Headache
   g. General malaise, muscular aches, and chills
   h. "Allergic salute"—the palm of the hand rubbing the nose upward
   i. "Allergic shiner"—dark circles under the eyes and periorbital and eyelid edema
4. Diagnostics
   a. Allergy testing to identify the causative allergen
   b. Culture of nasal drainage to determine the causative organism
   c. Nasal smear to identify eosinophils
   d. Rhinoscopy to visualize edema and drainage
   e. Sinus radiograph or computed tomographic scan to rule out sinusitis
5. Clinical management
   a. The goals of clinical management are to restore the nose to proper functioning, alleviate the symptoms, and identifying the causative agents.
   b. Nonpharmacologic management consists of environmental control to eliminate exposure to allergens.
   c. Pharmacologic management
      (1) Antihistamines to treat allergic symptoms
      (2) Decongestants (oral and topical) to decrease nasal edema
      (3) Anticholinergic medications to control rhinorrhea
      (4) Cromolyn sodium (systemic and topical) to inhibit mast cell degranulation in patients with allergic symptoms

(5) Corticosteroids (systemic and topical) to decrease nasal edema and reduce mucosal inflammation
      (6) Allergic desensitization to treat allergy
   d. Special medical-surgical procedures
      (1) Removal of turbinates to increase breathing space
      (2) Nasal septoplasty to straighten the nasal septum
      (3) Polypectomy to remove polyps
6. Complications
   a. Serous otitis media
   b. Nasal polyps
   c. Sinus infection
   d. Exacerbation of asthma
7. Applying the nursing process

NURSING DIAGNOSIS: Ineffective breathing pattern R/T nasal obstruction

   a. *Expected outcomes:* The patient should have a clear nasal airway.
   b. *Nursing interventions*
      (1) Elevate the head of the bed.
      (2) Increase humidification.
      (3) Instruct the patient on the proper administration, side effects, and dosages of decongestants, antihistamines, and nasal sprays.
      (4) Review environmental control measures with the patient and family to decrease the patient's exposure to allergens.
      (5) Review the medications the patient is currently taking and their side effects to identify drugs that may have caused the rhinitis.
      (6) Identify concomitant medical conditions that may have caused the nasal stuffiness.

NURSING DIAGNOSIS: Altered sensory (olfactory) perception R/T edema of the nasal mucosa

   a. *Expected outcomes:* The patient should be able to distinguish common smells and will use safety measures to compensate for the lack of the sense of smell.
   b. *Nursing interventions:* Instruct the patient to make appropriate changes in his or her living environment (e.g., using smoke detectors), to observe the appearance of stored food for spoilage, and to check gas lines for leaks routinely.
8. Discharge planning and teaching
   a. Give the patient information about prescribed medications, such as routes, dosages, frequencies, actions, and side effects.
   b. Caution the patient against participating in activities that require alertness, such as driving or operating machinery, while taking medications known to cause drowsiness.
   c. Help the patient identify possible causative agents of the rhinitis and help him or her develop strategies for avoiding them.
      • *Pollens:* Instruct the patient to avoid outdoor activities such as lawn work, to keep doors and windows

closed during high pollen seasons, to install electrostatic air filters to filter out pollen, and to schedule vacations so as to avoid peak pollen times.

- *Molds:* Instruct the patient to control dampness in the home to minimize mold growth and to avoid heavy vegetation around the house, which increases humidity in the house.
- *Dust:* Instruct the patient to control household dust, avoid carpeting and down or feather comforters and pillows, and to vacuum the mattress frequently.
- *Animal dander:* Instruct the patient to avoid furred or feathered animals.

d. Review the patient's current medications with him or her to identify those with a side effect of rhinitis (e.g., antihypertensive drugs, birth control pills, and decongestant nasal sprays).

e. Emphasize the importance of avoiding crowds and people known to have an upper respiratory tract infection.

Sinusitis

1. Definition
   a. Sinusitis is an infection of 1 or more of the paranasal sinuses.
   b. Sinusitis can be bacterial, viral, or fungal in origin and acute or chronic in nature.
2. Etiology
   a. Anything that alters the mucociliary transport, including anatomic variations of the nasal cavity that obstruct the ostia, causing retention of secretions, can result in sinusitis.
   b. Swimming and diving can allow a massive influx of contaminated material to enter the sinuses, causing infection.
   c. Dental abscesses or a root canal on a tooth with roots in the maxillary sinus can cause sinusitis.
   d. Prolonged use of nasogastric or nasotracheal tubes and nasal packing can cause increased irritation and edema of the nasal mucosa, resulting in the obstruction of sinus drainage.
3. Pathophysiology
   a. Bacterial sinusitis is associated most commonly with *Streptococcus pneumoniae, H. influenzae,* and *Moraxella catarrhalis.* The latter 2 organisms can produce β-lactamase, causing resistance to penicillin antibiotics.
   b. Viral sinusitis usually follows an upper respiratory infection. The virus infiltrates the normal mucous membrane, causing decreased ciliary transport. The stasis and edema that result can lead to a secondary bacterial infection.
   c. Fungal sinusitis is uncommon and most frequently affects people who are immunocompromised or in a debilitated state. The most common types of fungus that cause sinusitis are aspergillosis, mucormycosis, candidiasis, histoplasmosis, and coccidioidomycosis. Mucormycosis can cause necrosis of the turbinates and death if not treated aggressively.
   d. Acute sinusitis is usually the result of an upper respiratory infection, swimming, allergic rhinitis, or dental

manipulation. All of these disorders cause inflammation and retention of secretions providing a medium for bacteria.

   e. Chronic sinusitis is a persistent infection of the sinuses. Patients with chronic sinusitis can also have allergies and nasal polyps. Repeated acute exacerbations can result in an irreversible loss of the normal ciliated epithelial lining of the sinus cavity.
4. Clinical manifestations
   a. Edema of the face and periorbital area
   b. Facial pain over the affected sinuses
   c. Elevated temperature
   d. Edematous nasal mucosa
   e. Mucopurulent drainage in nose and posterior pharynx
   f. Headache
5. Diagnostics
   a. Sinus radiographs (plain films) or coronal computed tomography revealing opaque sinuses or air-fluid level
   b. Sinus endoscopy showing purulent exudate and edema of the nasal mucosa
   c. Culture and sensitivity to guide the choice of medication
6. Clinical management
   a. The goal of clinical management is to restore the sinuses to normal functioning; to achieve a patent nasal airway; and to rid the sinuses of inflammation, infection, or blockage.
   b. Nonpharmacologic interventions
      (1) Increased humidification to promote nasal drainage
      (2) Raised head of the bed
      (3) Application of warm compresses to improve drainage and promote comfort
   c. Pharmacologic interventions
      (1) Decongestants
      (2) Nasal sprays
      (3) Antibiotic or antifungal agents
   d. Special medical-surgical procedures
      (1) Sinus tap and irrigation for acute sinusitis
      (2) Functional endoscopic sinus surgery
      (3) Caldwell-Luc surgery
      (4) External ethmoidectomy or sphenoethmoidectomy for chronic sinusitis
      (5) Frontal sinusectomy with or without obliteration for chronic sinusitis
7. Complications
   a. Orbital or periorbital cellulitis or abscess
   b. Cavernous sinus thrombosis
   c. Bacteremia or septicemia
   d. Osteomyelitis
   e. Brain abscess
   f. Meningitis
8. Applying the nursing process

NURSING DIAGNOSIS: Ineffective breathing pattern R/T nasal obstruction

a. *Expected outcomes:* The patient should be able to breathe through the nose.

b. *Nursing interventions*
  (1) Increase humidification (to thin the secretions and promote drainage).
  (2) Administer medications as ordered.
  (3) Elevate the head of the bed to decrease edema.

NURSING DIAGNOSIS: Risk for infection R/T sinusitis

a. *Expected outcomes:* The patient should be free of infection.
b. *Nursing interventions*
  (1) Monitor the amount, color, and consistency of the nasal drainage.
  (2) Monitor the patient's temperature.
  (3) Obtain a culture of the drainage or assist with obtaining one.
  (4) Assist with sinus irrigation.
  (5) Observe the patient for orbital complications, such as edema of the eyelids or the area around the eyes, anesthesia or paresthesias, protrusion of the globes, decreased vision, congestion or swelling of the conjunctivae, diplopia, or photophobia.
  (6) Monitor the patient for a decreased pulse rate, which may be caused by oculocardiac reflex.
  (7) Monitor the patient for intracranial complications, such as lethargy or somnolence, a decreased appetite, vomiting, headache, seizures, a change in the level of consciousness, or irritability.
  (8) Administer antibiotics or antifungal agents as ordered.

NURSING DIAGNOSIS: Altered sensory (olfactory) perception R/T nasal edema

a. *Expected outcomes:* The patient should be able to identify common odors and adapt his or her living environment to prevent accidents related to the loss of the sense of smell.
b. *Nursing interventions*
  (1) Instruct the patient to make changes in his or her living environment to compensate for the loss of the sense of smell.

NURSE ADVISORY

Patients with total nasal obstruction experience a loss of the sense of smell. Instruct them to make the following changes in their living environment to compensate for their inability to smell:
- Install smoke detectors and carbon monoxide detectors in the home to monitor for fires and the presence of a carbon monoxide accumulation.
- Examine stored food for evidence of spoilage, such as mold. Label food with the date it is placed in storage.
- Routinely examine gas lines for leaks. Contact the gas company for assistance.
- Install a monitor for detection of gas leaks.

NURSING DIAGNOSIS: Pain (acute) R/T sinus infection

a. *Expected outcomes:* The patient should be free of pain.
b. *Nursing interventions*
  (1) Assess the amount, location, and characteristics of the pain.
  (2) Administer analgesics as ordered and evaluate their effectiveness.
  (3) Encourage the patient to avoid bending, lifting, and stooping.
  (4) Apply warm, moist compresses to the sinus area.
9. Discharge planning and teaching
  a. Give the patient and family information on the anatomy and physiology of the sinuses, the causes of and symptoms of sinusitis, and the proper use and side effects of medications.
  b. Inform the patient that bending and stooping during the acute phase of sinusitis increases pressure and therefore pain.
  c. Encourage the patient to use a systemic decongestant or a decongestant nasal spray (with a physician's order) before flying in a plane to decrease nasal edema and open the eustachian tube and prevent ear discomfort.
  d. Encourage the patient to avoid exposure to cigarette smoke and environmental pollutants when possible.
  e. Encourage the patient to avoid contact with anyone who has an upper respiratory infection.
  f. Encourage the patient to use supplemental humidification procedures, such as keeping a humidifier or vaporizer near the bed, using a nasal saline solution spray, and increasing fluid intake.
  g. Review the dosages, administrations, and side effects of prescribed medications.
  h. Instruct the patient to notify the physician if symptoms of sinusitis or complications of sinusitis occur.

◼ THROAT DISORDERS

Pharyngitis and Tonsillitis

1. Definition
  a. Pharyngitis is acute inflammation of the pharyngeal walls, including the tonsils, palate, and uvula.
  b. Tonsillitis is inflammation of the tonsils.
2. Incidence and socioeconomic impact
  a. Oropharyngeal inflammation is one of the most common reasons adults and children make visits to health care professionals.
  b. Viral pharyngitis makes up 70 percent of cases.
  c. Beta-hemolytic streptococcal pharyngitis forms 15 to 20 percent of cases.
  d. Miscellaneous organisms causing pharyngitis make up 10 to 15 percent of cases.
  e. Beta-hemolytic streptococcal tonsillitis makes up 30 percent of cases.
  f. Pneumococcal organisms, gram-negative organisms, and viruses cause the remainder of cases.

3. Risk factors: Tonsillitis and pharyngitis are communicable by droplet infection or direct contact.
4. Pathophysiology
    a. Beta-hemolytic streptococci, *Neisseria gonorrhoeae, and Corynebacterium diphtheriae* are bacterial organisms that cause pharyngitis.
    b. As mentioned, viral pharyngitis accounts for the majority of acute cases of pharyngitis. Infectious mononucleosis, caused by the Epstein-Barr virus, also produces pharyngitis.
    c. Fungal infections of the pharynx can occur with prolonged use of antibiotics in an immunosuppressed patient, such as a person receiving radiation therapy or chemotherapy, a person infected with the human immunodeficiency virus, or a chronically debilitated person.
5. Clinical manifestations
    a. Throat pain or discomfort
    b. Otalgia
    c. Purulent exudate, redness, and edema of the lymphoid tissue around the palate, tonsils, and uvula
    d. General malaise
    e. Elevated temperature
    f. Cervical lymphadenopathy
    g. Dysphagia or drooling
    h. Bad breath and foul taste
    i. Sensation of having a foreign object in the throat
    j. Gray or white membrane over the pharyngeal and tonsil regions (*C. diphtheriae*)
    k. Vesicles on the pharyngeal walls and tonsils (virus)
    l. Adherent white plaques in the pharynx
6. Diagnostics
    a. Thorough history
    b. Examination of oral cavity
    c. Throat culture to identify the organism
    d. Palpation of the neck
    e. White blood cell count
    f. Heterophil agglutination antibody (Monospot) test
    g. Computed tomographic scan to rule out abscess
7. Clinical management
    a. The goals of clinical management are the absence of infection and the relief of pain.
    b. Nonpharmacologic interventions
        (1) Warm saline throat irrigation
        (2) Increased humidification
        (3) Oral hygiene
    c. Pharmacologic interventions
        (1) Analgesics
        (2) Antibiotics
        (3) Equine antitoxin (diphtheria)
        (4) Antifungal agents (candidiasis)
        (5) Intravenous fluids for dehydration
    d. Special medical-surgical procedures: A tonsillectomy can be performed for recurrent episodes of acute tonsillitis or chronic tonsillitis.
8. Complications
    a. Retropharyngeal abscess
    b. Parapharyngeal abscess
    c. Glomerulonephritis (with β-hemolytic streptococcal infection)
    d. Subacute bacterial endocarditis
9. Applying the nursing process

NURSING DIAGNOSIS: Pain R/T infection

a. *Expected outcomes:* The patient should experience relief from pain.
b. *Nursing interventions*
    (1) Assess the amount, location, and characteristics of the pain.
    (2) Administer analgesics as ordered and evaluate their effectiveness.
    (3) Provide warm saline throat irrigations as ordered.

NURSING DIAGNOSIS: Infection R/T invasion of the oropharynx by a bacteria, virus, or fungus

a. *Expected outcomes:* The patient should show no sign of infection.
b. *Nursing interventions*
    (1) Perform a nursing history, especially questioning exposure to gonorrhea and diphtheria and immunosuppression.
    (2) Assist with or perform a throat culture, as ordered.
    (3) Administer medications as ordered and observe for side effects.
    (4) Monitor vital signs, especially temperature.
    (5) Encourage the patient to rest frequently and avoid strenuous activity.

NURSING DIAGNOSIS: Ineffective breathing pattern R/T oropharyngeal edema

a. *Expected outcomes:* The patient should have no breathing problems.
b. *Nursing interventions*
    (1) Inspect the oropharynx for edema.
    (2) Provide supplemental humidification.
    (3) Assess the rate and depth of respirations.
    (4) Assess breath sounds.
    (5) Observe for signs of respiratory obstruction.

NURSING DIAGNOSIS: Impaired swallowing R/T edema and pain

a. *Expected outcomes:* The patient should maintain weight and hydration.
b. *Nursing interventions*
    (1) Assess the patient's hydration status (evaluate intake and output and skin turgor and dryness).
    (2) Assess the mucous membranes of the oral cavity and lips.
    (3) Assess the patient's ability to swallow.
    (4) Encourage oral fluid intake.
    (5) Administer intravenous fluid as necessary.

10. Discharge planning and teaching
    a. Give the patient information on prescribed medications, including dosages, side effects, and the need to complete the entire course of antibiotics prescribed.
    b. Encourage the patient to seek medical attention if symptoms of pharyngitis or tonsillitis reappear.
    c. Inform the patient that smoking and the use of alcohol can exacerbate symptoms.

Laryngeal Disorders

1. Definition
    a. **Laryngitis** is inflammation of vocal cords caused by upper respiratory infection, vocal cord abuse, smoking, or reflux esophagitis. Edema of the vocal cords, caused by the inflammation, restricts the normal movement.
    b. **Vocal cord paresis or paralysis** is a result of inflammation or injury to the vagus nerve, most commonly the recurrent laryngeal nerve and less often the superior laryngeal nerve. Paresis or paralysis affects the velocity and amplitude of air flow through the cords, resulting in a leak of air through the vocal cords that gives a breathy quality to the voice.
    c. **Spasmodic dysphonia** is a hyperfunctional neuromuscular disorder. The spastic quality of the voice is a result of the inability of the vocal cords to maintain uniform vibration.
    d. **Presbylaryngeus** is the abnormal speech of older people. The aging process causes a loss of muscle tone, resulting in a weakened closure or bowing of the vocal cords.
    e. **Vocal cord lesions** prevent the cords from touching and cause irregular vibrations.
        (1) Vocal cord polyps are edematous mucous membranes attached to the vocal cord. They can be caused by chronic voice abuse, allergies, heavy smoking, or acute infection.
        (2) Vocal cord nodules, also known as "singer's nodules," are benign growths caused by chronic voice abuse.
2. Clinical manifestations
    a. Hoarseness
    b. Aphonia
    c. Breathy quality to voice
    d. Huskiness
    e. Chronic throat clearing
    f. Thick secretions
    g. Chronic cough
    h. Dyspnea
    i. Altered respiratory rate
    j. Restlessness
    k. Aspiration on swallowing
    l. Rhonchi or rales upon auscultation
3. Diagnostics
    a. Indirect laryngoscopy or direct laryngoscopy to observe the vocal cord
    b. Videostroboscopy to observe vocal cord movement during phonation by use of fiberoptic laryngoscopy with a videorecorder to view actual vocal cord motion
    c. Electromyography to determine innervation of vocal cord

    d. Computed tomographic scan to rule out a tumor as the cause of vocal cord paresis or paralysis
4. Clinical management
    a. The goal of clinical management is to restore the voice to an acceptable quality.
    b. Nonpharmacologic interventions
        (1) Increase humidification
        (2) Elevation of the head of the bed
        (3) Ice collar
        (4) Normal saline throat irrigations
    c. Pharmacologic interventions
        (1) Antacids to neutralize gastric acid in gastroesophageal reflux
        (2) Histamine inhibitors to reduce gastric acid in gastroesophageal reflux
        (3) Antibiotics for infection
        (4) Systemic steroids to reduce swelling
        (5) Botulinum toxin injection to paralyze spastic movement
    d. Special medical-surgical procedures
        (1) Direct laryngoscopy with microlaryngoscopy to visualize the vocal cords
        (2) Excision of nodules or polyps with or without the use of a laser to remove lesions
        (3) Injection of Gelfoam or Teflon into the vocal cord to provide bulk to a paralyzed cord
        (4) Thyroplasty, which is the insertion of a stent to move the paralyzed vocal cord into midline position
5. Complications
    a. Aspiration pneumonia
    b. Airway distress
6. Applying the nursing process

> **NURSING DIAGNOSIS:** Impaired verbal communication R/T vocal cord abnormality

a. *Expected outcomes:* The patient should have a normal speaking voice, if possible.
b. *Nursing interventions*
    (1) Investigate factors contributing to the dysphonia, such as vocal cord abuse, smoking, upper respiratory infection, exposure to noxious fumes, or gastroesophageal reflux.
    (2) Consult with a speech therapist who can monitor the range and pitch of the patient's voice and his or her voice abuse patterns and suggest breathing and speech exercises.
    (3) Encourage the patient to rest his or her voice as much as possible and to avoid whispering. Provide the patient with alternative communication methods during this time.
    (4) Increase humidification.
    (5) Promote antireflux activity.
    (6) Have the patient take antacids between meals and at bedtime.
    (7) If the foregoing measures fail, histamine inhibitors may be used.
    (8) Encourage referral to gastroenterologist.
    (9) Provide instruction on the administration, dosages, and side effects of medications (antibiotics, steroids, and mucolytic agents), if indicated.

NURSE ADVISORY

Although gastroesophageal reflux is a disorder of the gastrointestinal tract, symptoms of the disease may cause the patient to visit the ear, nose, and throat specialist. A sore throat, the sensation of having a foreign body in the throat, increased mucus that necessitates continual throat clearing, and hoarseness may be caused by the reflux of gastric acid into the upper esophagus or the airway. The patient may or may not exhibit other symptoms associated with gastroesophageal reflux disorder, such as heartburn, eructation of the gastric contents, and a gastric taste in the mouth. Instruct the patient to take the following noninvasive measures to treat the disorder:
- Elevate the head of the bed on blocks.
- Avoid eating or drinking for 3 to 4 hours before going to bed.
- Avoid caffeine.
- Avoid alcohol, especially before going to bed.
- Do not smoke.
- Do not wear constricting clothing (e.g., tight belts and girdles).
- If overweight, lose weight.

NURSING DIAGNOSIS: Risk for ineffective breathing pattern R/T vocal cord abnormality

a. *Expected outcomes:* The patient should show no signs of airway distress or compromise.
b. *Nursing interventions*
  (1) Assess the patient's respiratory status, including breath sounds, arterial blood gases, pulse oximetry level, and rate and depth of respirations.
  (2) Provide supplemental humidification.
  (3) Elevate the head of the bed.
  (4) Minimize oxygen expenditure by encouraging bed rest and avoidance of strenuous activity.
  (5) Ensure the availability of emergency equipment, such as an endotracheal intubation set and emergency tracheostomy tray.
  (6) Provide comfort measures such as an ice collar, throat irrigations, and cold fluids.
  (7) Instruct the patient to avoid upper respiratory infections to prevent increased edema from inflammation.

NURSING DIAGNOSIS: Risk for aspiration R/T vocal cord paresis or paralysis

a. *Expected outcomes:* The patient should show no signs of aspiration or aspiration-related complications.
b. *Nursing interventions*
  (1) Encourage the patient to eat foods with thick consistency rather than liquids.
  (2) Consult with a swallowing therapist who can evaluate the patient's swallowing problems and determine head and body positions that will minimize aspiration.
  (3) Auscultate the lungs for adequate breath sounds, wheezes, and crackles.
7. Discharge planning and teaching
  a. Instruct the patient to avoid smoking and polluted environments.

b. Review with the patient the possible causes of vocal cord abnormality.
c. Refer the patient to a smoking cessation program, if applicable.
d. Encourage the patient to make follow-up appointments with the physician, speech pathologist, and gastroenterologist, as indicated.
e. Provide supplemental environmental humidity.
f. Instruct the patient on the administration, dosages, and side effects of any prescribed medications.
g. Encourage the patient to avoid upper respiratory infections and strenuous activity, which can increase airway edema, resulting in airway distress.

Foreign Body in the Upper Aerodigestive Tract

1. Definition: A foreign body in the upper aerodigestive tract is the presence in the upper aerodigestive tract of any object that should not be there.
2. Incidence and socioeconomic impact: Both adults and children can accidentally ingest a foreign body. In adults, the foreign body is usually a piece of food that contains small bones that are aspirated or a piece of food that becomes lodged in the esophagus or aspirated into the airway. In children, beans, peanuts, grapes, and toys are the most frequent objects.
3. Risk factors
  a. Swallowing disorders
  b. Alcohol or drug intoxication
  c. Accidental—no known risk
4. Pathophysiology
  a. A foreign body is aspirated into or sticks in the larynx, esophagus, or bronchus.
  b. The object may be aspirated accidentally or before initiation of swallowing, or it may be too large to be swallowed.
5. Clinical manifestations
  a. Recent ingestion of a substance
  b. Coughing
  c. Difficulty breathing
  d. Inability to speak
  e. Coughing up blood or blood-tinged mucus
  f. Inability to swallow
  g. Drooling
  h. Pain and the sensation of pressure in the throat
  i. Edema of the esophagus or airway
6. Diagnostics
  a. Examination of the oral cavity, pharynx, and larynx to visualize the foreign body
  b. Soft tissue radiographs, barium swallow, or computed tomographic scan to visualize the location of the foreign body
7. Clinical management
  a. The overall goal of clinical management is to remove the foreign body without complications.
  b. Nonpharmacologic interventions: The emergency management for complete airway obstruction is the Heimlich maneuver (Figs. 20–13 and 20–14).
  c. Special medical-surgical procedures: Surgical removal of the foreign body is accomplished by endos-

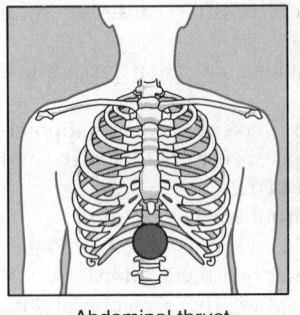

Abdominal thrust

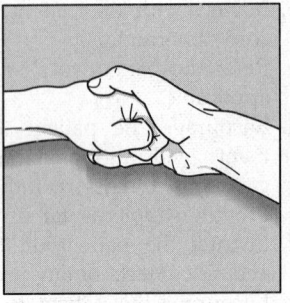

Position of hands from rescuer's view

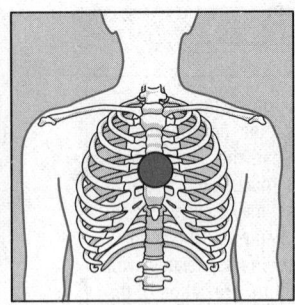

Chest thrust

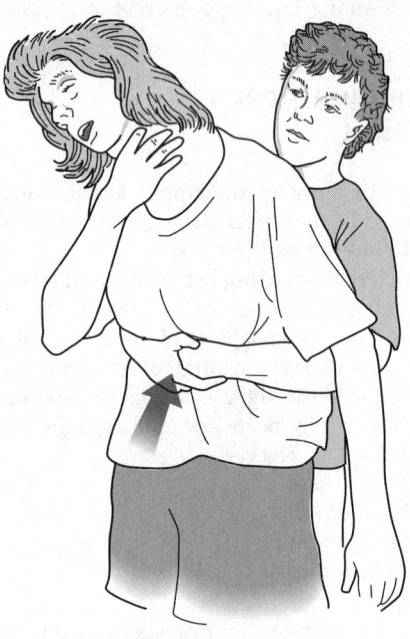

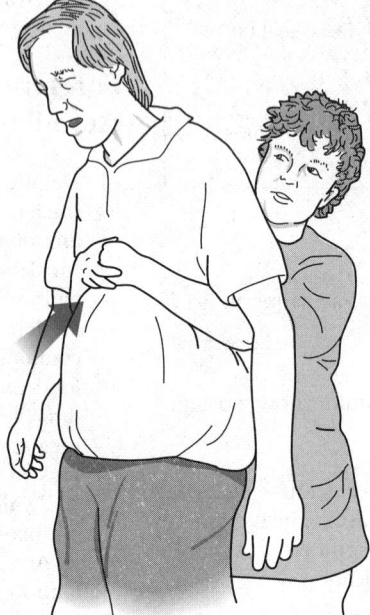

Figure 20-13. Heimlich maneuver for removing a foreign body blocking the upper airway. Vigorously apply upward chest or abdominal thrusts. This creates a force that causes quick changes in air pressure, which produces a rush of air to expel the foreign body. The abdominal thrust is the original Heimlich maneuver. The chest thrust is an adaptation that is useful for obese or pregnant patients. The black dot indicates correct placement of the rescuer's hands. (Redrawn from Black JM, and Matassarin-Jacobs E [eds]. *Luckmann and Sorensen's Medical-Surgical Nursing: A Psychophysiologic Approach.* 4th ed. Philadelphia: WB Saunders, 1993, p 2222.)

copy, which includes direct laryngoscopy, bronchoscopy, or esophagoscopy, depending on the location of the foreign body.

8. Complications
   a. Infection
   b. Airway distress
   c. Death
9. Applying the nursing process

NURSING DIAGNOSIS: Ineffective breathing pattern R/T a foreign body in the airway

   a. *Expected outcomes:* The patient should have a patent airway.
   b. *Nursing interventions*
      (1) Instruct the patient to speak.
      (2) If the patient can speak, instruct him or her to cough deeply. If the patient is unable to dislodge the object, loosen constricting clothes and instruct the patient to lean over the table and cough deeply.
      (3) If the patient is unable to speak or is using the international distress signal, perform the Heimlich maneuver and repeat if necessary.

(4) Prepare the patient for surgical removal of the object, if necessary.
(5) After removal of the foreign body, assess arterial blood gases, respiratory rate and depth, and breath sounds; pulse oximetry should be greater than 90 percent.

NURSING DIAGNOSIS: Impaired swallowing R/T obstruction by food and edema from the trauma of the foreign body

   a. *Expected outcomes:* Patient should swallow normally.
   b. *Nursing interventions*
      (1) Give the patient nothing by mouth if he or she has total obstruction, is unable to swallow, or has difficulty swallowing.
      (2) Force oral fluids if the foreign body has been removed or, if obstruction is minimal, to attempt to dislodge the foreign body.
      (3) Administer analgesics, as ordered, before meals.
      (4) Consult with a dietitian to determine which foods the patient can swallow.
      (5) Place the patient in a high Fowler's position when eating.

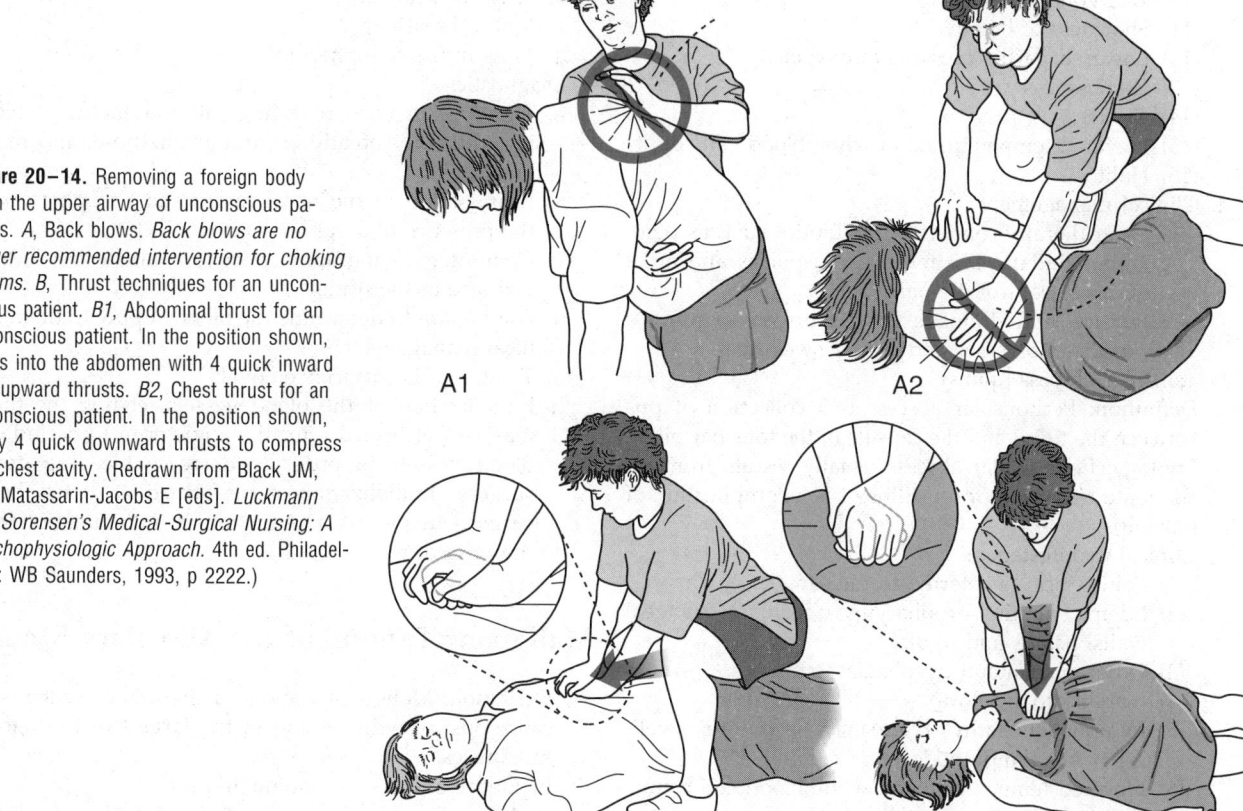

Figure 20–14. Removing a foreign body from the upper airway of unconscious patients. *A,* Back blows. *Back blows are no longer recommended intervention for choking victims. B,* Thrust techniques for an unconscious patient. *B1,* Abdominal thrust for an unconscious patient. In the position shown, press into the abdomen with 4 quick inward and upward thrusts. *B2,* Chest thrust for an unconscious patient. In the position shown, apply 4 quick downward thrusts to compress the chest cavity. (Redrawn from Black JM, and Matassarin-Jacobs E [eds]. *Luckmann and Sorensen's Medical-Surgical Nursing: A Psychophysiologic Approach.* 4th ed. Philadelphia: WB Saunders, 1993, p 2222.)

A1

A2

B1

B2

NURSING DIAGNOSIS: Anxiety R/T breathing difficulty

a. *Expected outcomes:* The patient should be comfortable, without evidence of anxiety.
b. *Nursing interventions*
 (1) Explain all procedures to the patient.
 (2) Offer reassurance.
 (3) Do not leave the patient unattended.
10. Discharge planning and teaching
 a. Provide instruction on the proper use of the Heimlich maneuver.
 b. Encourage the patient to seek medical attention if shortness of breath, difficulty swallowing, or infection occur.
 c. Review nutritional instructions.
 (1) Eat soft, bland foods.
 (2) Increase fluid intake.
 (3) Increase caloric intake.
11. Public health considerations
 a. Complete airway obstruction by a foreign body is an emergency situation that can happen in the home or in any public setting. Teach the international distress signal of placing the hands over the front of the neck to everyone.
 b. Teach the Heimlich maneuver as part of all emergency resuscitation courses. Children and adults

should be required to take a course on emergency resuscitation with biannual review.

Other Disorders of the Nose and Sinuses

1. Ludwig's angina
 a. Definition: Ludwig's angina is an infection or cellulitis of the submental, sublingual, and submandibular spaces.
 b. Incidence and etiology: Trauma, periodontal disease, or periapical abscess occurring around the mandibular teeth can cause the infection to spread into the submental, sublingual, and submandibular spaces. The likelihood of Ludwig's angina increases in persons with untreated dental infection and immunosuppressed persons with dental infection. The causative agents are mixed oral flora, including oral anaerobes.
 c. Clinical manifestations
 (1) Pain, tenderness, and infection in mandibular teeth
 (2) Swelling of the floor of the mouth
 (3) Elevation of the tongue
 (4) Trismus
 (5) Muffled voice
 (6) Dysphagia
 (7) Inability to swallow saliva

(8) Drooling
(9) Dyspnea and stridor
(10) Tachypnea
(11) Shortness of breath
(12) Lowered partial pressure of oxygen
(13) Restlessness
(14) Anxiety
(15) Elevated temperature and white blood cell count
(16) Halitosis
   d. Clinical management
      (1) Drug therapy consists of antibiotics such as penicillin, clindamycin, and cephalosporins and analgesics to control the pain.
      (2) Incision and drainage are performed to remove purulent abscesses and reduce swelling.
2. Peritonsillar abscess (quinsy)
   a. Definition: Peritonsillar abscess is a collection of pus between the tonsil and the capsule of the tonsillar pillar.
   b. Etiology: Peritonsillar abscess usually results from inadequate treatment of tonsillitis; it is a complication of tonsillitis.
   c. Clinical manifestations
      (1) Pain—local or referred to the ear
      (2) Edema of the oropharynx (tonsil, pharyngeal walls, palate, and uvula)
      (3) Odynophagia and dysphagia
      (4) Inability to swallow
      (5) Lymphadenopathy (there may be painful swelling of the lymph nodes)
      (6) Elevated temperature and white blood cell count
      (7) Trismus
   d. Clinical management
      (1) Incision and drainage of the abscess
      (2) Needle aspiration of the abscess
      (3) Intravenous antibiotics
      (4) Tonsillectomy (acute if performed during an episode of peritonsillar abscess and incision and drainage and needle aspiration have not been successful, and elective if performed after infection subsides)

◼ TUMORS OF THE HEAD AND NECK

Juvenile Nasopharyngeal Angiofibroma

1. Definition: Juvenile nasopharyngeal angiofibroma is a benign, slow-growing tumor composed of fibrous stroma and a rich vascular network.
2. Incidence and socioeconomic impact: This tumor primarily affects prepubescent young men.
3. Etiology: unknown
4. Pathophysiology
   a. Juvenile nasopharyngeal angiofibroma arises in the nasopharynx but can expand to fill the nasal cavity, displacing the nasal septum and applying pressure on the bones of the maxillary sinus, sphenoid sinus, infratemporal fossa, and dura of the middle fossa.
   b. The main blood supply to the tumor is the internal maxillary artery.

5. Clinical manifestations
   a. Intermittent nosebleeds
   b. Nasal obstruction
   c. Mouth breathing
   d. Mass in the nasopharynx
6. Diagnostics
   a. Thorough history revealing intermittent nasal bleeding, difficulty breathing through the nose, and mouth breathing
   b. Examination of the nasal cavity and nasopharynx for the presence of a vascular mass
   c. Computed tomographic scan to evaluate the location and size of the tumor
   d. Angiogram to determine the blood supply to the tumor
7. Clinical management
   a. Treatment is surgical removal.
   b. Embolization of the blood vessels feeding the tumor may be performed after the angiogram to occlude the blood vessels in order to decrease bleeding during surgery. Embolization is performed 48 hours before surgery to permit a reduction in inflammation from the procedure.

Malignant Tumors of the Maxillary Sinus

1. Definition: Malignant tumors of the maxillary sinus are cancerous growths arising in the largest of the paranasal sinuses.
2. Incidence and socioeconomic impact
   a. Approximately 2 percent of head and neck tumors originate in the sinus. Eighty percent of sinus tumors are found in the maxillary sinus, and less than 20 percent are found in the ethmoid, sphenoid, and frontal sinuses combined.
   b. There is a higher incidence of sinus tumors in men, and these tumors usually affect older individuals.
3. Etiology
   a. The cause of carcinoma of the paranasal sinuses is not known.
   b. Exposure to carcinogens and metaplasia of the respiratory epithelium caused by chronic infection are possible contributing factors.
4. Pathophysiology
   a. Eighty percent of tumors of the sinus are squamous cell carcinoma.
   b. Twenty percent of sinus tumors are adenocarcinoma, adenoid cystic carcinoma, and mucoepidermoid carcinoma.
5. Clinical manifestations: The clinical manifestations depend on the location of the tumor.
   a. Unilateral nasal obstruction, unilateral nasal bleeding, and drainage if the tumor is on the nasal wall of the sinus
   b. Diplopia, proptosis, and vision changes if the tumor is on the superior wall
   c. Tumor mass palpated on the palate, loosening of maxillary teeth, and ill-fitting dentures if the tumor is on the inferior sinus wall
   d. Edema and asymmetry of the skin of the cheek in anterior wall tumors

e. Paresthesias of the skin of the face in posterior wall tumors invading the infraorbital branch of the trigeminal nerve

f. Trismus, numbness of the face, otitis media, and pain

6. Diagnostics
   a. Thorough history
   b. Examination of the oral cavity, nasal cavity, nasopharynx, ears, and facial skin
   c. Computed tomographic scan to determine the location and extent of the tumor
   d. Magnetic resonance imaging to differentiate the tumor mass from retained secretions

7. Clinical management
   a. The goal of clinical management of tumors of the paranasal sinuses is complete removal of the tumor as evidenced by no recurrence and return of function, that is, no drainage or bleeding and the restoration of nasal breathing.
   b. Pharmacologic interventions
      (1) The use of chemotherapeutic agents in the treatment of sinus tumors may reduce tumor mass, but it has not been proven to cure the disease.
      (2) Radiation therapy is used in combination with surgery to treat tumors of the sinus. Radiation may be used preoperatively to decrease tumor size or postoperatively to treat microscopic disease.
   c. Special medical-surgical procedures
      (1) Surgical excision may consist of a medial maxillectomy (removal of the lateral or nasal wall of the sinus), total maxillectomy (removal of the entire maxillary sinus, including the palate), orbital exenteration (removal of the eye and supporting structures), or craniofacial resection (removal up to the skull base for more extensive tumors).
      (2) A split-thickness skin graft is usually applied to line the cavity after resection. In more extensive resections, a free tissue transfer may be required to replace tissue that has been removed and to improve cosmesis and function.

8. Complications
   a. Bleeding
   b. Leakage of CSF
   c. Infection
   d. Epiphora

9. Prognosis
   a. The prognosis for tumors of the maxillary sinus depends on the stage of disease at diagnosis. The larger the tumor size and the greater the involvement of adjacent structures, the poorer the prognosis.
   b. The TNM system (tumor, lymph node involvement, distant metastasis) for tumor staging is used to stage tumors of the maxillary sinus. In addition, Ohngren's line (a line from the inner canthus of the eye to the angle of the mandible) divides the maxillary sinus into superior and inferior sections. Tumors originating above the line carry a poor prognosis, because of their location and the late development of symptoms.

10. Applying the nursing process

NURSING DIAGNOSIS: Pain (acute) R/T surgical procedure

a. *Expected outcomes:* The patient's pain should be controlled, as evidenced by a verbal expression of a decrease in pain and the absence of nonverbal signs of pain.

b. *Nursing interventions*
   (1) Assess the location, intensity, and characteristics of the pain.
   (2) Identify nonpharmacologic methods useful in controlling pain, such as positioning, relaxation, and imagery.
   (3) Administer analgesics as ordered and evaluate their effectiveness.
   (4) Encourage the patient to use pain relief measures before planned activities.
   (5) See Chapter 11 for details on pain management.

NURSING DIAGNOSIS: Risk for infection R/T surgical incisions, surgical defect, skin graft donor and recipient sites, and possible CSF leak

a. *Expected outcomes:* The patient should be free of infection, as evidenced by normal temperature and white blood cell count, healed incisions, and no evidence of CSF leak.

b. *Nursing interventions*
   (1) Assess incisions, surgical defect, and skin graft donor and recipient sites.
   (2) Observe drainage for color, odor, and consistency.
   (3) Cleanse external incisions with half-strength hydrogen peroxide and water, rinse, and apply antibacterial ointment.
   (4) Provide oral and nasal irrigations as ordered.
   (5) Avoid pressure on the skin graft donor site. Expose it to the air once the outer protective dressing has been removed.
   (6) Allow the patient to soak the donor site in the bathtub once eschar has formed on the site.
   (7) Observe nasal drainage for CSF leak. Test clear drainage with glucose test strips, and send drainage to the laboratory for beta II transferrin.
   (8) Notify the physician if you suspect a CSF leak.
   (9) Monitor the patient's temperature and report an elevation; monitor laboratory testing, especially the white blood cell count and beta II transferrin and report results.
   (10) Administer antibiotics, as ordered.
   (11) Instruct the patient in oral cavity care using half-strength hydrogen peroxide and water.

NURSING DIAGNOSIS: Body image disturbance R/T surgical intervention and changes in appearance

a. *Expected outcomes:* The patient should adjust to changes in body image.

b. *Nursing interventions*
   (1) Assess the patient's body image.
   (2) Describe the physical changes to the patient.
   (3) Evaluate the patient's readiness to observe the surgical defect.
   (4) Encourage the patient to discuss concerns about physical changes.
   (5) Help the patient identify coping strategies used successfully in the past.
   (6) Stay with the patient during the initial viewing of the defect.
   (7) Encourage self-care.
   (8) Teach the patient techniques to minimize the defect.
   (9) Discuss the possible society responses with the patient and family.
   (10) Refer the patient to a support group; if he or she is having difficulty adapting to the changes, make a counseling referral.
11. Discharge planning and teaching
   a. Teach the patient to cleanse suture lines with half-strength hydrogen peroxide and water, rinse, and apply antibacterial ointment.
   b. Instruct the patient in oral and nasal irrigations using a Waterpik or a catheter and syringe. The nose and oral defect may be cleansed with normal saline solution. In addition, the oral cavity defect may be cleaned with half-strength hydrogen peroxide and water to remove crusts and secretions that may produce odor and become infected. The palatal obturator (denture), used to recreate oral-nasal separation following maxillectomy, should be removed after meals to be cleaned and then reinserted (Fig. 20–15). If an obturator has not been used, the defect will require packing.
   c. Instruct the patient to notify the physician of any signs of infection or CSF leak.
   d. Review techniques to camouflage the defect, such as the use of prosthetics, makeup, and dressings.
   e. Provide information on community resources available for support and equipment, such as the American Cancer Society, a home health nursing agency, and a medical supply company.
12. Public health considerations
   a. Because the cause of tumors of the maxillary sinus is not known, it is not possible to caution patients to avoid a specific agent, as may be done with some other cancers.
   b. Encourage the patient to seek medical attention if abnormal symptoms suggestive of a tumor of the maxillary sinus occur. (See "Clinical Manifestations.")

Tumors of the Oral Cavity and Oropharynx

1. Definition
   a. Malignant tumors of the oral cavity are neoplasms arising in the mouth.

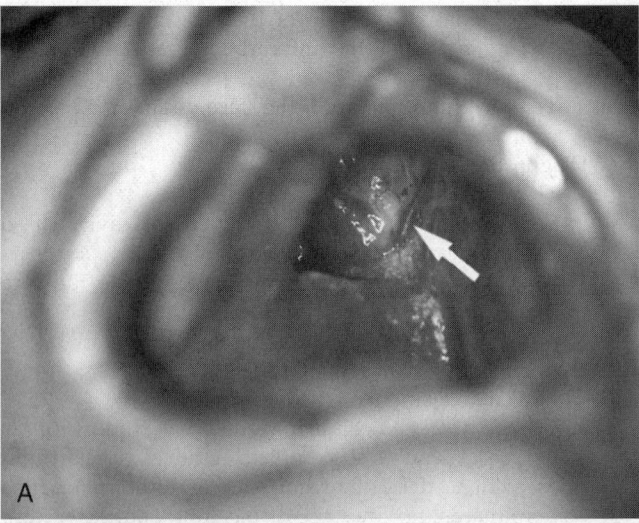

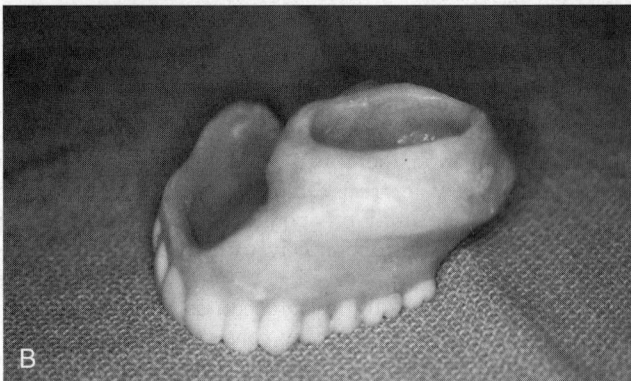

Figure 20–15. *A,* Palatal defect created by maxillectomy. *B,* Obturator, special denture, used to fill defect and restore oral nasal separation.

   b. Malignant tumors of the oropharynx are neoplasms involving the soft palate, the tonsils and tonsillar pillars, the base of the tongue, and the posterior pharyngeal walls.
2. Incidence and socioeconomic impact: Less than 5 percent of all body malignancies occur in the head and neck, with the oral cavity and oropharynx having the highest incidence.
3. Risk factors
   a. Tumors of the oral cavity and oropharynx are related to the use of alcohol and tobacco in any form. Smoking is considered the major etiologic agent of cancer of the head and neck. Alcohol used in combination with tobacco is believed to have a synergistic effect. The use of smokeless tobacco has also been implicated in the development of cancers of the oral cavity.
   b. Other factors that may have a relationship to the development of oral cavity and oropharyngeal cancers include poor oral hygiene; dietary deficiencies, especially deficiencies in riboflavin and iron resulting in Plummer-Vinson syndrome; herpes virus; lichen planus; and inhalation or ingestion of chemicals.
4. Pathophysiology

a. Squamous cell carcinoma is the most common cell type in oral cavity and oropharyngeal tumors.

b. Tobacco causes morphologic changes in the mucosa lining the upper aerodigestive tract. Smokeless tobacco causes these changes to occur in the area where the tobacco is placed.

5. Clinical manifestations
   a. Ulcer or mass in the mouth that does not heal
   b. Changes in speech or swallowing
   c. Ill-fitting dentures or loose teeth
   d. Local pain
   e. Referred pain (otalgia)
   f. Bleeding
   g. Lump in the neck

6. Diagnostics
   a. Thorough history
   b. Examination of the oral cavity, oropharynx, and neck
   c. Chest radiograph to establish a baseline pulmonary status and determine the presence of a lung primary tumor or metastasis
   d. Barium swallow to determine the presence of a second primary tumor of the esophagus and evaluate swallowing function
   e. Computed tomographic scan and magnetic resonance imaging to evaluate the size of the tumor, involvement of adjacent structures, and lymph node metastasis
   f. Endoscopy and biopsy to allow close visualization of the tumor and histologic confirmation of tumor cell type

7. Clinical management
   a. The goal of clinical management is the complete removal of the tumor, as evidenced by no recurrence of the tumor and restoration of function (i.e., speech and swallowing).
   b. Pharmacologic interventions
      (1) Chemotherapy is being used on an experimental basis for tumors of the oral cavity and oropharynx to decrease tumor size and prevent recurrence or distant metastasis. However, it has not been proven to be a definitive treatment for these tumors.
      (2) Radiation therapy may be used as the primary treatment for small tumors of this area, as an adjuvant therapy for large tumors or when there is evidence of regional lymph node metastasis, or as a palliative measure for inoperable or recurrent tumors.
   c. Special medical-surgical procedures
      (1) Tumors of the oral cavity and oropharynx are removed through a transoral (through the mouth) or a transcervical (through the neck) approach, depending on the size of the tumor and the need to remove adjacent structures.
         • If the mandible is involved superficially, a rim of bone may be removed while maintaining the integrity of the mandible. This is a marginal mandibulectomy.
         • If the mandible is invaded by tumor, a segment of the mandible will be removed; this

is a segmental mandibulectomy. Lateral segmental mandibulectomy produces minimal dysfunction; however, anterior segmental mandibulectomy produces severe disability, including an incompetent oral commissure, drooling, speech and swallowing dysfunction, and cosmetic deformity. Immediate reconstruction should be considered for anterior mandible defects. Most oral cavity and oropharyngeal defects can be reconstructed with a primary closure (suturing); a split-thickness skin graft; a regional flap; or, for large defects, a microvascular free tissue transfer.

      (2) Removal of the regional lymph nodes on one or both sides of the neck may be included in the surgical resection if palpable nodes in the neck indicate metastasis or if there is a high incidence of lymph node metastasis from the location of the primary tumor.

8. Complications
   a. Delayed wound healing
   b. Oropharyngeal-cutaneous fistula
   c. Persistent or recurrent tumor
   d. Distant metastasis

9. Prognosis
   a. The prognosis for tumors of the oral cavity and oropharynx depends on the stage of tumor at diagnosis. Early tumors have a good prognosis; however, larger tumors and tumors that have metastasized to the regional lymph nodes or distantly have a poorer prognosis.
   b. Patients who have a cancer of the upper aerodigestive tract have a high incidence of developing multiple tumors in the same area. Long-term follow-up of patients after treatment for a head and neck cancer is essential.

10. Applying the nursing process

NURSING DIAGNOSIS: Ineffective airway clearance R/T postoperative edema and aspiration of secretions.

a. *Expected outcomes:* The patient should maintain a patent airway, as evidenced by clear breath sounds and oxygen saturation within the normal range for the patient.

b. *Nursing interventions*
   (1) Place the patient in a high Fowler's position.
   (2) Monitor respirations and auscultate breath sounds.
   (3) Encourage coughing and deep breathing.
   (4) Suction the oral cavity and oropharynx until the patient is able to swallow secretions.
   (5) Monitor oxygen saturation by arterial blood gases or pulse oximetry.
   (6) Provide supplemental humidification.
   (7) See tracheostomy diagnoses and management.

NURSING DIAGNOSIS: Risk for aspiration R/T the surgical procedure and the presence of a tracheostomy

a. *Expected outcomes:* The patient should not aspirate or develop aspiration-related complications and should maintain nutritional status.
b. *Nursing interventions*
   (1) Give the patient nothing by mouth until he or she is able to swallow secretions and the tracheostomy tube has been removed.
   (2) Administer enteral feedings as ordered.
   (3) Suction the oral cavity.
   (4) Maintain the patient in a high Fowler's position.
   (5) Evaluate the patient for signs of aspiration—coughing, increased mucus, and a change in breath sounds.
   (6) Evaluate tongue movement and strength.
   (7) Assess swallowing reflexes.
   (8) Consult with a swallowing therapist and dietitian.
   (9) Record intake and output and caloric intake.
   (10) Initiate oral feedings. Liquids and foods with a thin consistency are best for anterior oral defects; a thicker (nonpourable pureed) consistency is best for posterior oral defects.
   (11) Advance the diet as tolerated.

NURSING DIAGNOSIS: Risk for altered peripheral tissue perfusion R/T surgical incisions and free tissue transfer used for reconstruction

a. *Expected outcomes:* Surgical incisions and free tissue flaps should heal without complications.
b. *Nursing interventions*
   (1) Assess the oral cavity.
   (2) Assess the viability of the flap (color, warmth, drainage, and blanching time). Notify the physician of any changes.
   (3) Clean the oral cavity 4 times a day as ordered.
   (4) Suction the oral cavity as ordered.
   (5) Avoid putting pressure on the flap or donor site; that is, avoid tracheostomy ties, oxygen ties, and dressings.
   (6) Monitor Doppler signals for microvascular flap viability.

NURSING DIAGNOSIS: Pain (acute) R/T the surgical procedure

a. *Expected outcomes:* The patient's pain should be controlled.
b. *Nursing interventions*
   (1) Assess the location, intensity, and characteristics of the pain.
   (2) Help the patient assume a comfortable position.
   (3) Evaluate nonpharmacologic techniques of pain relief (relaxation, imagery, and positioning).

   (4) Administer analgesics as ordered and evaluate their effectiveness.

NURSING DIAGNOSIS: Impaired verbal communication R/T the surgical procedure and the presence of tracheostomy tube

a. *Expected outcomes:* The patient should be able to communicate effectively.
b. *Nursing interventions*
   (1) Assess the patient's understanding of the changes in his or her oral anatomy that have caused speech changes.
   (2) Consult with a speech therapist who can suggest movement and strengthening exercises for the tongue.
   (3) Encourage the patient to use oral prosthetic devices as ordered. Oral augmentation devices may be used to permit the tongue to touch the palate, to fill in palatal defects, and to create oral-nasal separation.
   (4) See tracheostomy diagnoses and management.

NURSING DIAGNOSIS: Body image disturbance R/T changes created by the surgical procedure

a. *Expected outcomes:* The patient should adapt to the change in body image.
b. *Nursing interventions*
   (1) Identify the patient's concerns.
   (2) Assess the patient's body image.
   (3) Help the patient identify coping mechanisms used successfully in the past.
   (4) Discuss body alterations with both the patient and the patient's family.
   (5) Determine the patient's readiness to participate in self-care activities.
   (6) Remain with the patient during initial self-care activities.
   (7) Discuss possible societal reactions to the altered body image.
   (8) Encourage social interactions during hospitalization.
   (9) Facilitate discussion of sexual concerns between the patient and his or her partner.
   (10) Refer the patient to a support group or organization.

11. Discharge planning and teaching
  a. Teach the patient to perform an oral cavity assessment.
  b. Inform the patient of ways to increase calorie and protein intake.
  c. Reinforce self-care procedures.
  d. Arrange home health services.
  e. Refer the patient to alcohol and smoking cessation programs if appropriate.
  f. See tracheostomy discharge planning and teaching.
12. Public health considerations

a. Tobacco use and alcohol abuse have been shown to be etiologic agents responsible for the development of tumors of the head and neck. Develop smoking cessation programs and make them accessible to the general public. Make referrals to alcohol withdrawal programs and Alcoholics Anonymous when appropriate.

b. The use of smokeless tobacco and cigarette smoking has increased among children. The hazards of smokeless tobacco and cigarette smoking should be presented to local schoolchildren as part of the curriculum. The American Academy of Otolaryngology–Head and Neck Surgery and the Society of Otorhinolaryngology and Head-Neck Nurses have developed programs on the hazards of smokeless tobacco.

Cancer of the Larynx

1. Definition: Cancer of the larynx is a malignant tumor involving any part of the larynx (voice box).
2. Incidence and socioeconomic impact
   a. Cancer of the larynx accounts for about 2 percent of body malignancies and is 2nd only to cancer of the oral cavity and oropharynx in incidence among cancers of the head and neck.
   b. Cancer of the larynx is found more often in men than in women, and the incidence is higher among older age groups.
3. Risk factors
   a. The main etiologic agent of cancer of the larynx is cigarette smoking.
   b. As with cancer of the oral cavity and oropharynx, alcohol appears to be a cocarcinogen and may act to potentiate the effects of tobacco.
4. Pathophysiology
   a. Squamous cell carcinoma is the most common type of tumor of the larynx arising from the squamous epithelium lining the larynx.
   b. The larynx is divided into 3 compartments: The supraglottic larynx is composed of the epiglottis, false vocal cords, ventricle, aryepiglottic folds, and arytenoid cartilages; the glottic larynx is the area of the true vocal cords; and the infraglottic, or subglottic, larynx is the area below the vocal cords.
5. Clinical manifestations
   a. Supraglottic larynx: dysphagia, odynophagia, aspiration on swallowing, foreign body sensation, sore throat, otalgia, and neck mass
   b. Glottic larynx: voice change, hoarseness, unilateral sore throat, and otalgia
   c. Subglottic (infraglottic) larynx: the late symptoms of difficulty breathing, difficulty swallowing, or neck mass when the tumor enlarges
6. Diagnostics
   a. Thorough history
   b. Indirect and direct laryngoscopy with biopsy
   c. Computed tomographic scan to determine the size and location of the tumor, involvement of adjacent

structures, lymph node metastasis, and pulmonary status
   d. Chest radiograph from which to compare future radiographs for improvement, worsening of disease, or no change in disease state and to look for a 2nd primary cancer of the lung
   e. Barium swallow to evaluate the patient's swallowing ability and to look for a 2nd primary cancer of the esophagus
7. Clinical management
   a. The primary goal of clinical management is to cure the disease. The secondary goal is to return the patient to an acceptable quality of life with minimal dysfunction.
   b. Nonpharmacologic interventions
      (1) Initiate smoking cessation measures such as counseling, the use of nicotine gum or patches (as ordered), and support.
      (2) Assess the patient for signs of airway obstruction: stridor, shortness of breath, anxiety, restlessness, and dyspnea with or without exertion.
   c. Pharmacologic interventions
      (1) As with tumors in other areas of the head and neck, chemotherapy is not a 1st-line treatment for cancer of the larynx. Chemotherapy is being used to reduce tumor bulk, as an adjuvant therapy for patients with large tumors, and as a palliative therapy. All modes of chemotherapy are being studied.
      (2) Radiation therapy may be used as the primary treatment for small tumors of the larynx or as a postoperative adjuvant therapy.
   d. Special medical-surgical procedures: Surgery for cancer of the larynx depends on the size and location of the tumor as well as the desires of the patient.
      (1) Supraglottic laryngectomy (horizontal partial laryngectomy) removes the area from the false vocal cords to the epiglottis. Because the epiglottis helps protect the airway when swallowing, the patient must have adequate pulmonary reserves to prevent aspiration-related complications. Speech is nearly normal.
      (2) Vocal cord stripping, with or without the use of the laser, may be used for superficial lesions of the vocal cords (carcinoma in situ, T1). Speech is nearly normal.
      (3) Vertical partial laryngectomy (hemilaryngectomy) removes 1 vocal cord and possibly part of a 2nd vocal cord and is used to treat lesions limited to part of the glottic larynx. Speech has a breathy quality and is low in volume.
      (4) Total laryngectomy is the removal of the larynx and the creation of a permanent tracheostoma. After total laryngectomy there is no connection between the nose, mouth, and lower airway (Fig. 20–16). Normal speech is absent. A primary or secondary tracheoesophageal puncture may be performed to permit air to be shunted from the stoma to the esophagus to produce speech (Fig. 20–17).

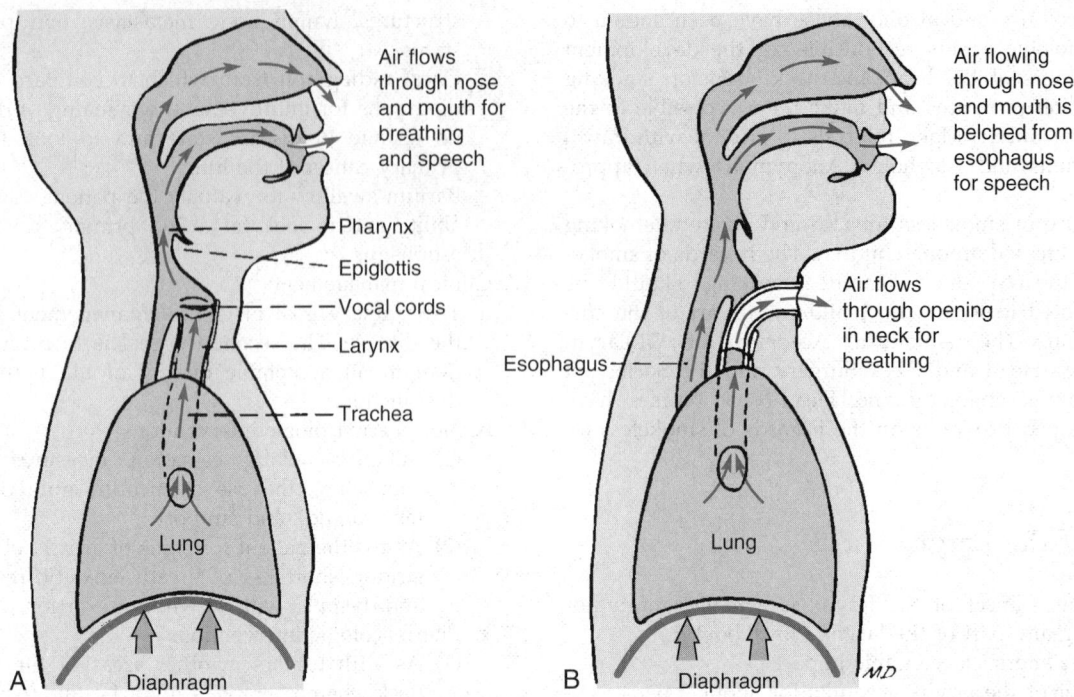

Figure 20–16. *A,* Anatomy of upper airway before total laryngectomy. Air flow is through the nose and mouth. *B,* Anatomy of upper airway after total laryngectomy. Note that there is no longer a connection between the trachea and the upper airway or esophagus.

(5) Removal of regional lymph nodes (neck dissection) may be performed if a palpable neck mass is present. Lymph nodes may be removed prophylactically for supraglottic and infraglottic

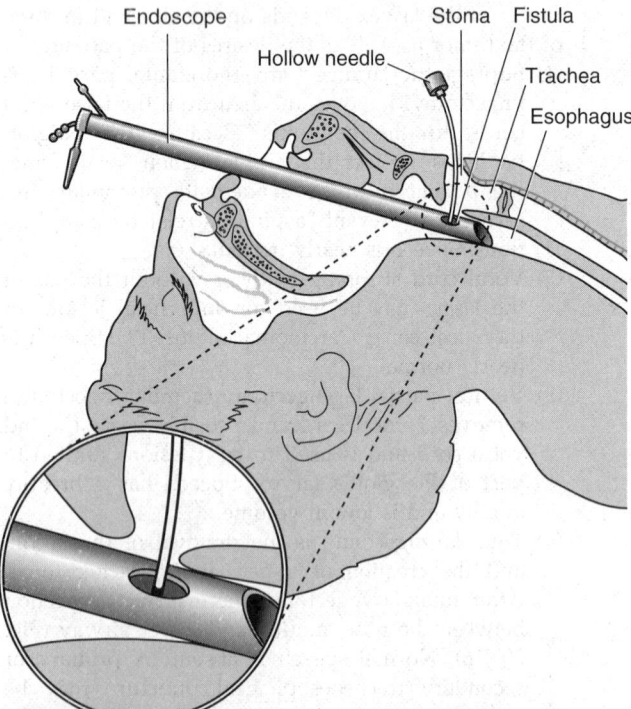

Figure 20–17. Placement of fistula for tracheoesophageal puncture. (Redrawn from Ignatavicius DD, Workman ML, and Mishler MA [eds]. *Medical-Surgical Nursing: A Nursing Process Approach.* 2nd ed. Philadelphia: WB Saunders, 1996, p 657.)

tumors, because the abundant lymphatic drainage channels in these areas increase the possibility of regional metastasis.

8. Complications
   a. Poor wound healing
   b. Bleeding
   c. Pharyngocutaneous fistula
   d. Pharyngeal stricture
9. Prognosis
   a. Small tumors of the larynx have an excellent chance for cure, regardless of the type of treatment used (stripping, laser, radiation, or surgery).
   b. Larger tumors have a poorer prognosis and require more extensive treatment to achieve a cure or to extend the disease-free interval.
   c. Frequent follow-ups are necessary to evaluate for persistent tumor, recurrent tumor, or additional primary tumors.
   d. Patients with cancer of the larynx require multidisciplinary rehabilitative services to restore an acceptable quality of life.
10. Applying the nursing process (Procedure 20–1)

> **NURSING DIAGNOSIS:** Ineffective airway clearance R/T aspiration, increased mucus, ineffective cough, and tracheostomy tube obstruction

   a. *Expected outcomes:* The patient should maintain a patent airway, as evidenced by clear breath sounds, the ability to rid the stoma or tracheostomy tube of mucus, and a clear stoma or tracheostomy tube.
   b. *Nursing interventions*
      (1) Assess the airway and suction the tracheostomy tube as needed.

(2) Assess for a mucus plug by observing for a whistling sound, bloody mucus, dry secretions, and decreased movement of air. Remove the plug if there is one.

(3) Change the permanent tracheostomy tube (total laryngectomy) daily after the cuffed tracheostomy tube has been removed; change the temporary tracheostomy tube per your institution's protocol.

(4) Assess the size of the tracheostoma in the patient who has had a total laryngectomy to determine the need for a tube.

NURSING DIAGNOSIS: Impaired swallowing R/T postoperative edema

a. *Expected outcomes:* The patient should maintain nutritional status by enteral feeding or an oral diet.
b. *Nursing interventions*
(1) Attach the nasogastric tube to low intermittent suction until bowel sounds return or if patient becomes nauseated to remove gastric secretions and prevent vomiting.

Text continued on page 855

Procedure 20–1
Tracheostomy Care

Definition/Purpose	To maintain a patent airway in the patient with a temporary or permanent tracheostomy. Tracheostomy care includes all nursing care performed to ensure a patent airway.
Contraindications/Cautions	1. For most patients with a tracheostomy, this is the only airway. No air is passing through the nose and mouth. 2. Accidental decannulation in the patient with a temporary tracheostomy can be a life-threatening situation. It takes approximately 5 days for a tract to form after the procedure has been performed. Anything that causes removal of the tube before tract formation may precipitate an airway emergency. If traction sutures were placed into the trachea after the surgical procedure, they should be clearly marked and taped to the patient's chest. If the tracheostomy tube is accidentally removed, these sutures are pulled up and away from the stoma in order to reopen it. 3. Before and after the suctioning procedure, the patient should take deep breaths, receive oxygen, or have ventilatory assistance by way of an Ambu bag to replace oxygen removed during the suctioning procedure. Hypoventilation, hypoxia, hypotension, cardiac arrhythmias, and cardiac arrest may occur during the suctioning procedure because of this oxygen removal.
Learning/Teaching Activities	1. Explain the procedure to the patient. 2. Demonstrate coughing and deep-breathing techniques to the patient, if appropriate. 3. Encourage coughing, deep breathing, and ambulation to decrease the need for suctioning. 4. Encourage daily changes of a permanent tracheostomy tube (total laryngectomy). Instruct the patient and family members on the correct technique for changing and reinserting a temporary tracheostomy tube, in case of accidental decannulation.

Preliminary Activities

Equipment	• Stethoscope • Gloves • Goggles for eye protection • Source of negative pressure • Suction catheters (14 or 16 Foley catheter; no larger than half the diameter of the tracheostomy tube) • Two basins for solutions (hydrogen peroxide and sterile water or saline) • Tracheostomy tube brush or pipe cleaners with gauze • Oxygen or Ambu bag • Replacement tracheostomy tube • Gauze sponges (without cotton filling) • Syringe for inflating and deflating tube cuff
Assessment/Planning	• Auscultate the lungs to detect rhonchi, rales, and the need for suctioning. • Observe the patient for evidence of increased secretions from the tracheostomy tube. • Instruct the patient to cough deeply to rid the tracheostomy tube of secretions without suctioning. • Use sterile technique when performing tracheostomy care. You may wish to teach clean technique to the patient when self-care is instituted.
Preparation of Person	• Help the patient assume a semi-Fowler's or high Fowler's position. • Provide a mirror for the patient to observe the procedure during teaching.

(continued)

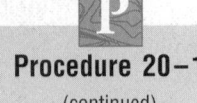

Procedure 20–1

(continued)

Procedure: Suctioning and Inner Cannula Care

Action	Rationale/Discussion
1. Assemble equipment.	1. The tracheostomy care procedure is performed using aseptic technique. All equipment should be assembled before applying gloves.
2. Wash hands; open the suction kit.	2. Good hand washing is mandatory to prevent cross-contamination.

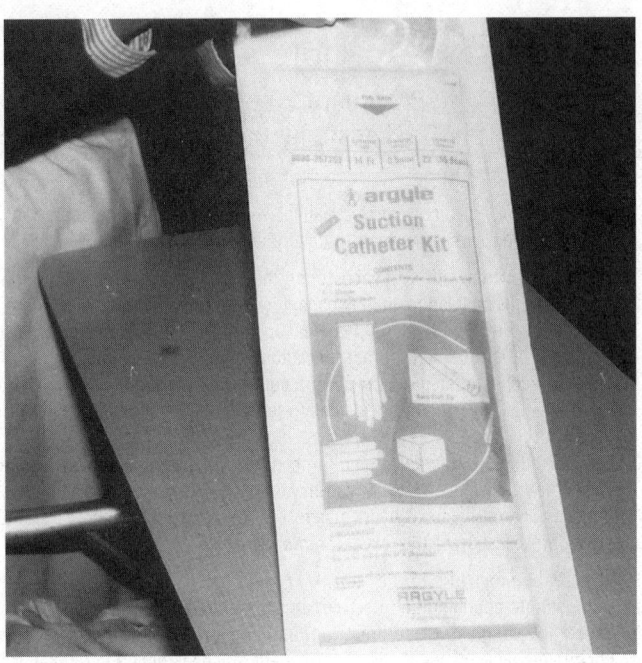

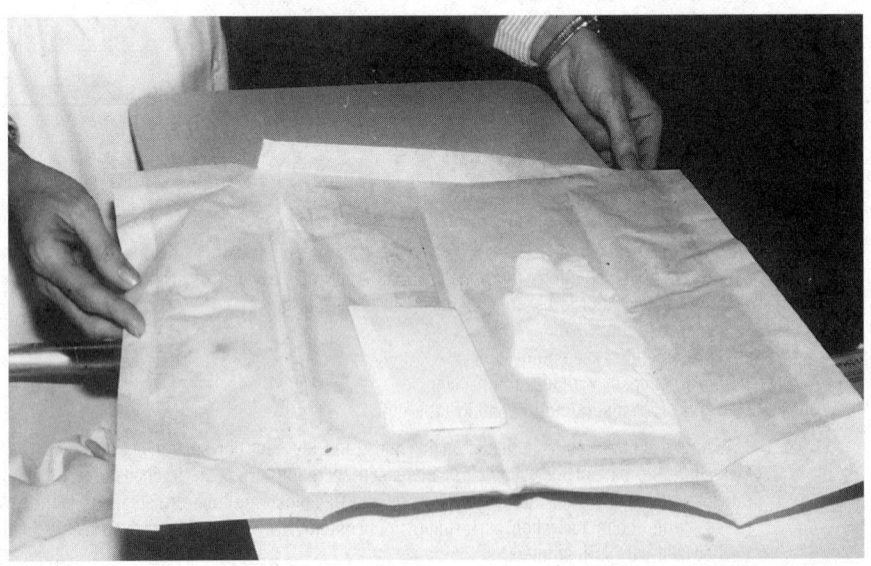

3. Apply gloves and goggles.	3. Prevents cross-contamination and protects you from contact with expectorated secretions.

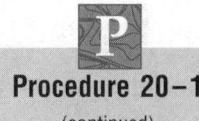

Procedure 20-1

(continued)

Action	Rationale/Discussion
4. Fill one basin with hydrogen peroxide and 1 basin with sterile water or saline.	4. Solutions will be used to clean and rinse the inner cannula of the tube. Sterile water or saline will be used to check the function of the suction and to rinse the catheter during the procedure.

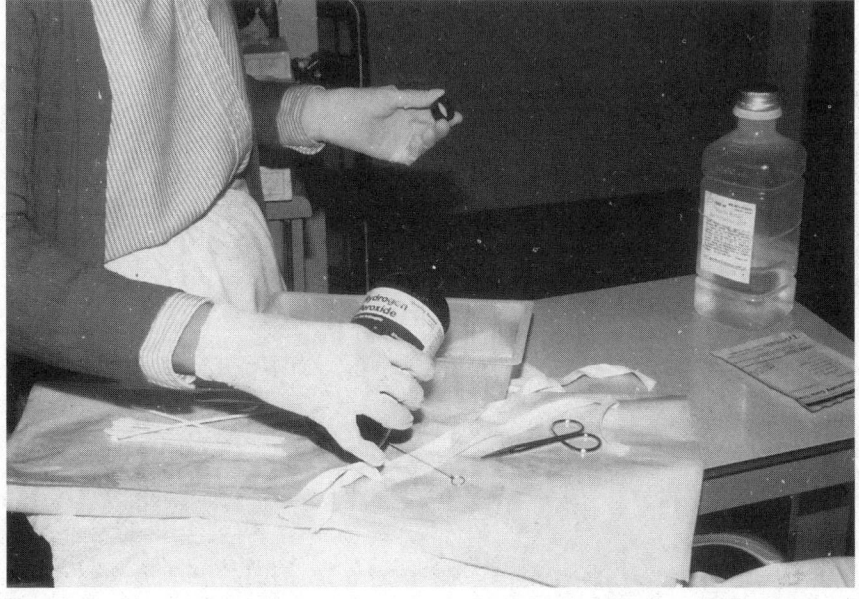

Action	Rationale/Discussion
5. Remove the inner cannula. If it is disposable, discard it. If it is reusable, place it in the basin of hydrogen peroxide to loosen secretions.	5. Removing the inner cannula before suctioning increases the diameter of the outer cannula. *Note:* Suctioning can be performed with the inner cannula in place.
6. Increasing ventilation before suctioning helps to prevent hypoxia.	6. If the patient is unable to take deep breaths, use the Ambu bag or administer oxygen to hyperoxygenate.
7. Lubricate suction catheter tip with sterile saline or water.	7. Permits easier insertion and causes less trauma to the tracheal mucosa.

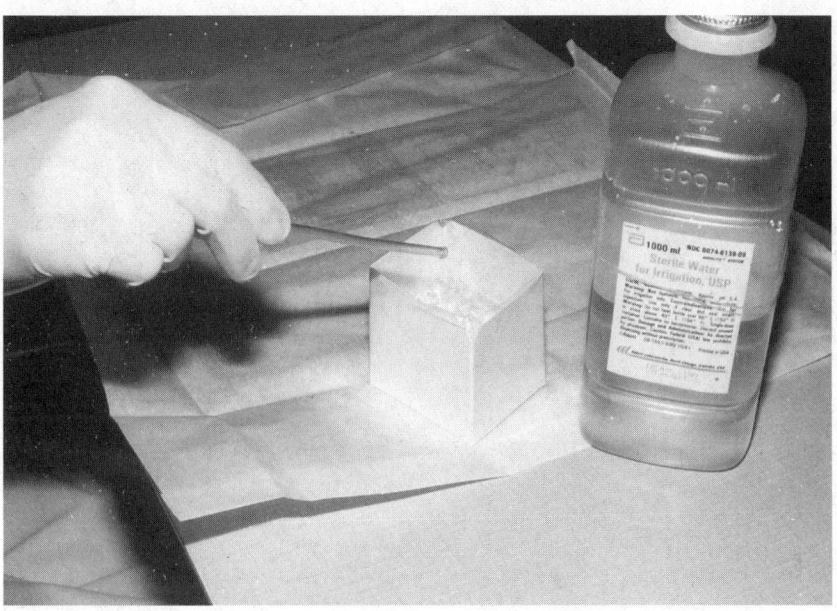

(continued)

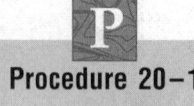

Procedure 20–1

(continued)

Action	Rationale/Discussion
8. Insert the catheter into the tracheostomy tube without applying suction.	8. Minimizes withdrawal of oxygen during suctioning.
9. Apply suction while withdrawing the catheter.	9. Removes secretions.

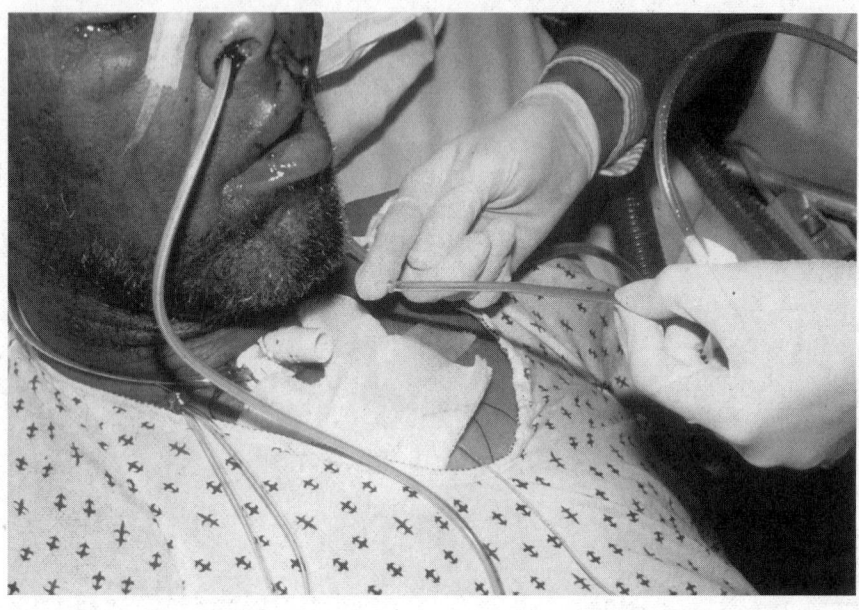

Action	Rationale/Discussion
10. Suction for 5 to 15 seconds.	10. Minimizes removal of oxygen during suctioning.
11. Hyperoxygenate the patient (deep breaths, Ambu bag, and oxygen).	11. Replaces oxygen.
12. Repeat the procedure as necessary.	12. Provides a patent airway without precipitating hypoxia from prolonged suctioning.
13. Clean the inner cannula with a tracheostomy brush and rinse it well. Reinsert it or replace it with a new disposable inner cannula.	13. Prevents residual hydrogen peroxide from irritating the tracheal mucosa.

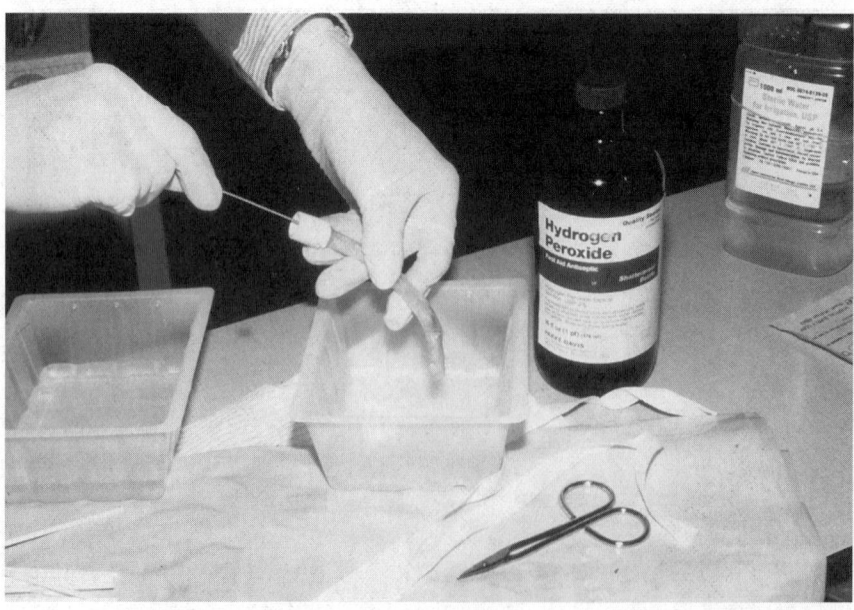

Procedure 20–1

(continued)

Action	Rationale/Discussion

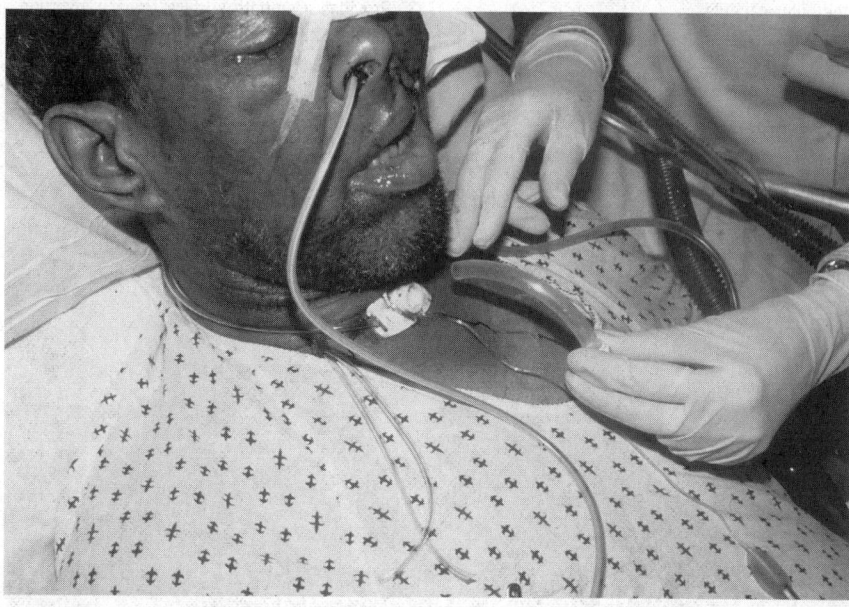

Procedure: Changing the Tracheostomy Tube

Action	Rationale/Discussion
1. Apply gloves and goggles.	1. Prevents cross-contamination and protects you from contamination by secretions.
2. Insert the tracheostomy tube ties into neckplate of the outer cannula. Ties that can be used include shoestrings, intravenous tubing, twill tape, seam binding tape, and Velcro straps.	2. Secures tube upon insertion.

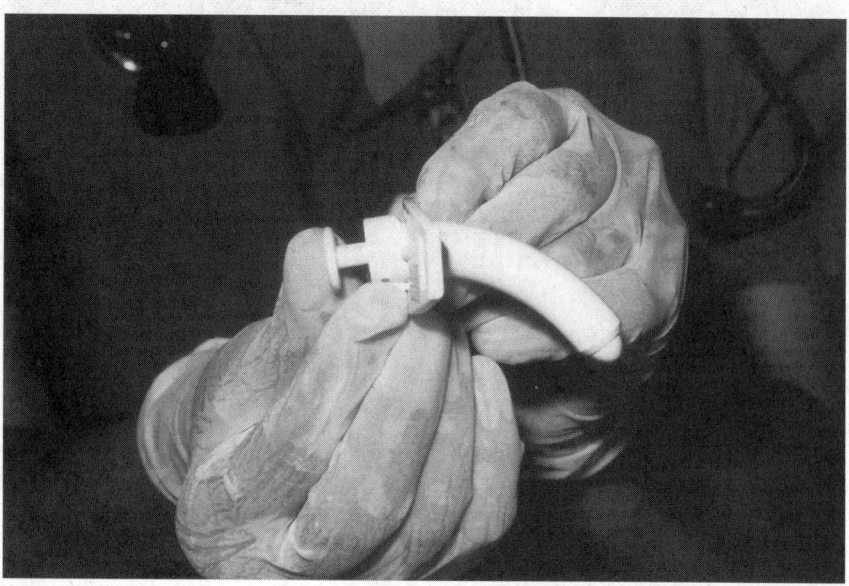

(continued)

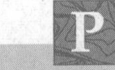

Procedure 20-1

(continued)

Action	Rationale/Discussion
3. Insert the obturator into the outer cannula.	3. Provides a smooth surface to ease insertion and prevents trauma to the tracheal mucosa.

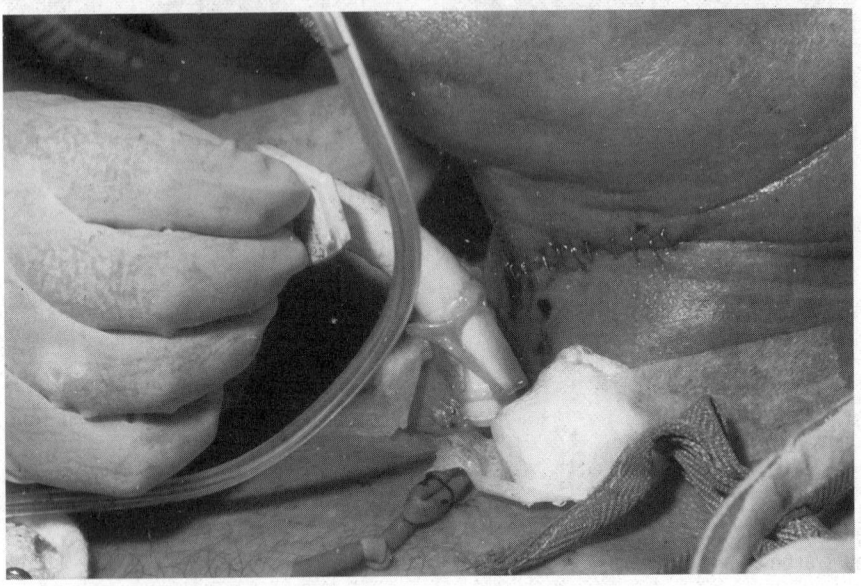

Action	Rationale/Discussion
4. Remove the used tube and remove secretions from the stoma.	4. Prepares the stoma for a new tube and removes crusts and secretions from it.
5. Instruct the patient to take a breath while you insert the tube.	5. The obturator obstructs the opening of the outer cannula.

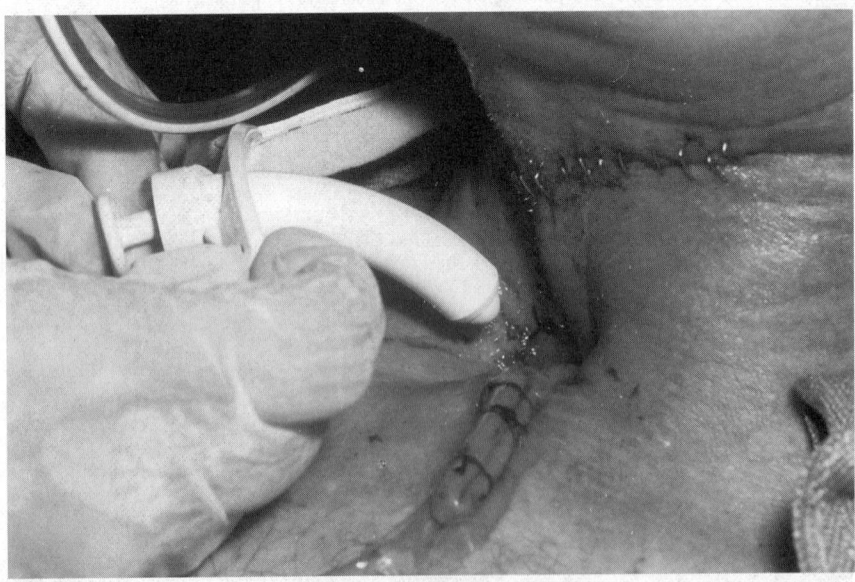

Action	Rationale/Discussion
6. Remove the obturator.	6. Opens airway.

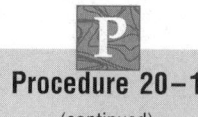

Procedure 20-1

(continued)

Action	Rationale/Discussion

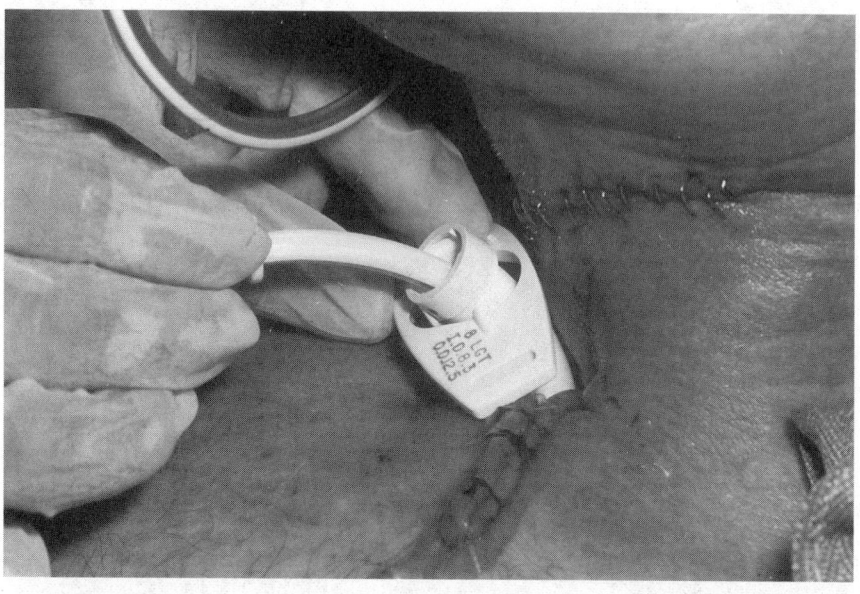

7. Tie the tube in place. Allow 2 fingers to be inserted under ties.

8. Insert the inner cannula, if present.

7. Secures the tube in place without constricting the neck.

8. Prevents accumulation of secretions in the outer cannula.

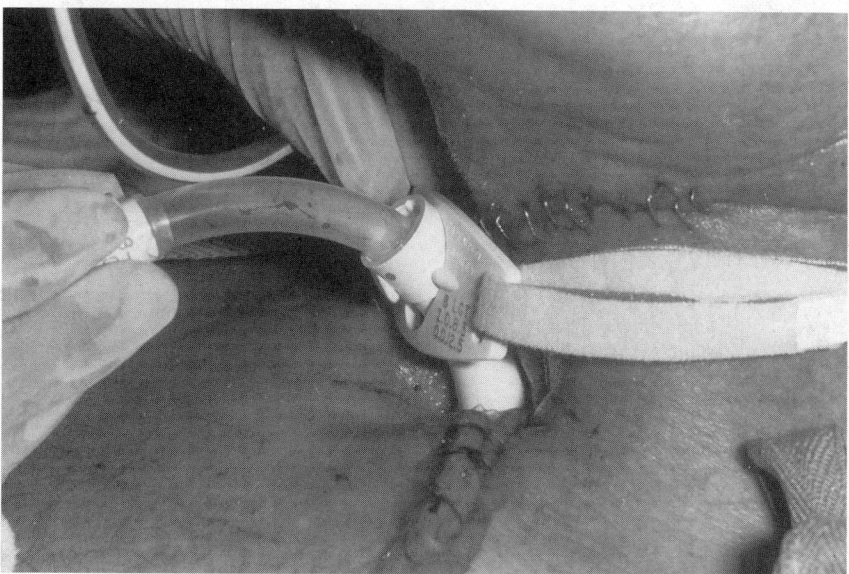

9. Clean or discard the used tube.

9. Some tubes are disposable and are used on only 1 patient. Others such as stainless steel tubes, are used again after thorough cleaning and sterilization.

(continued)

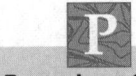

Procedure 20–1

(continued)

Procedure: Changing Tracheostomy Ties

Action	Rationale/Discussion
1. If possible, 2 people should be available to change tracheostomy ties: 1 person to remove and insert the ties, and the other to hold the tube securely in place.	1. Prevents accidental decannulation from coughing or manipulation of tube.
2. Place a slit in one end of the tracheostomy tie; insert the tape from under the neckplate through the opening; pull the other end of the tape through the slit.	2. Secures tube without using knots or any other techniques that will move the tube out of the trachea.
3. Repeat with the other side.	3. Completes the procedure.

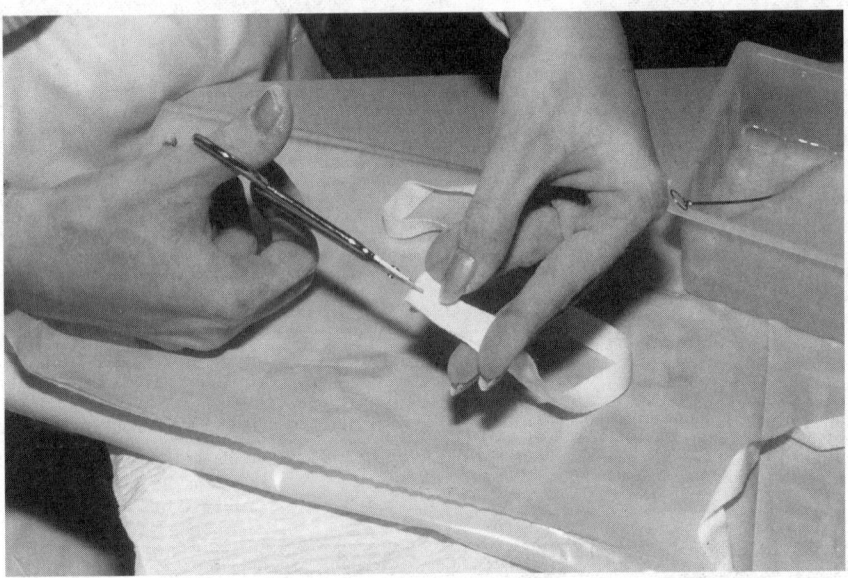

4. Tie tapes on the side of the neck, allowing 2 fingers to be inserted under the tie.	4. Prevents pressure on vertebrae and compression of the neck.

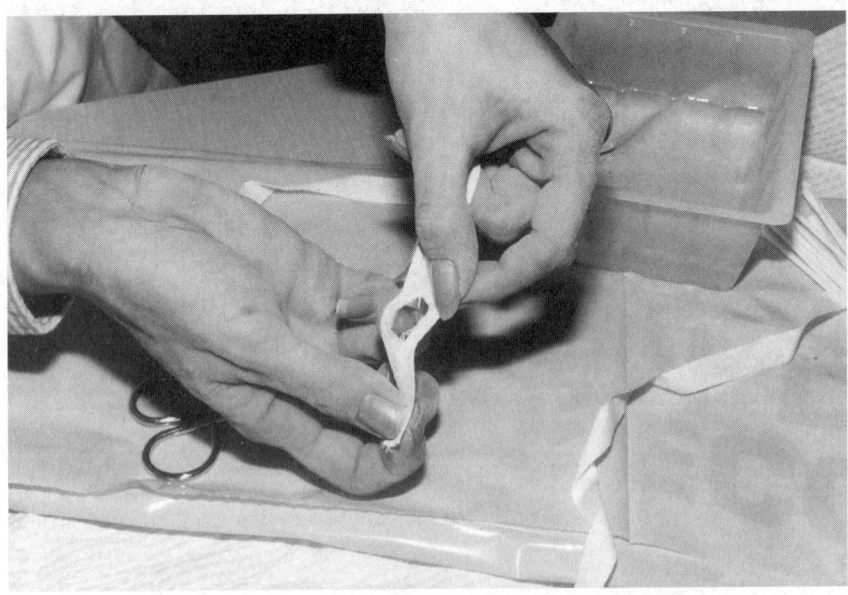

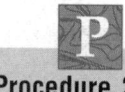

Procedure 20–1
(continued)

Action	Rationale/Discussion
5. If only 1 person is available; insert clean ties before removing soiled ones.	5. Prevents accidental decannulation.

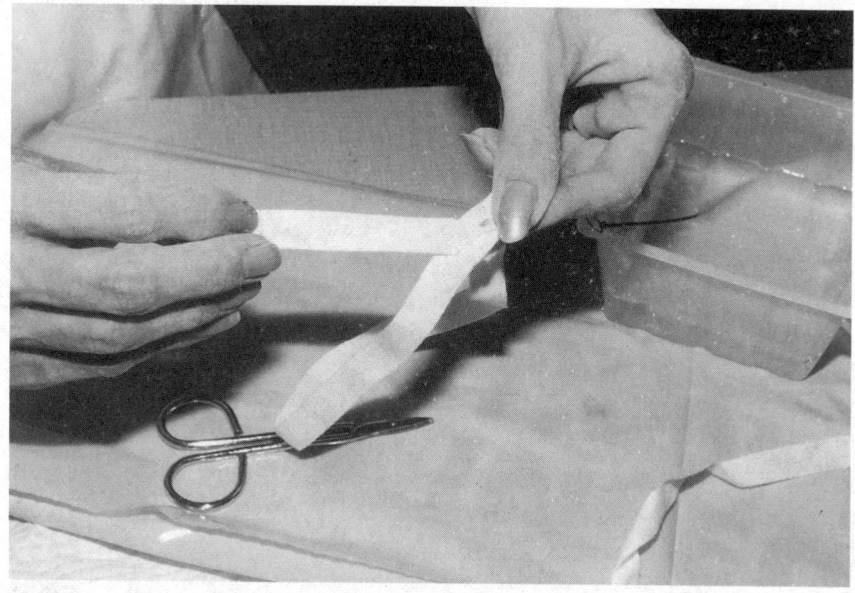

Action	Rationale/Discussion
6. Two people must be available to change Velcro bands, which are inserted using the same technique as described above.	6. Prevents accidental decannulation.

Procedure: Removal of a Mucus Plug

Action	Rationale/Discussion
1. Remove the inner cannula and instruct the patient to cough.	1. A mucus plug is a large amount of mucus or dried mucus that may obstruct the airway. If the mucus plug is larger than the diameter of the cannula, removal of the inner cannula may allow the patient to expel the plug by coughing.
2. Remove the entire tracheostomy tube if the patient has had a *total laryngectomy.*	2. The total laryngectomy patient has a permanent opening (stoma). Removal of the outer cannula may allow the patient to expel the plug by coughing. *This step is not to be performed with the patient who has a temporary tracheostomy.*

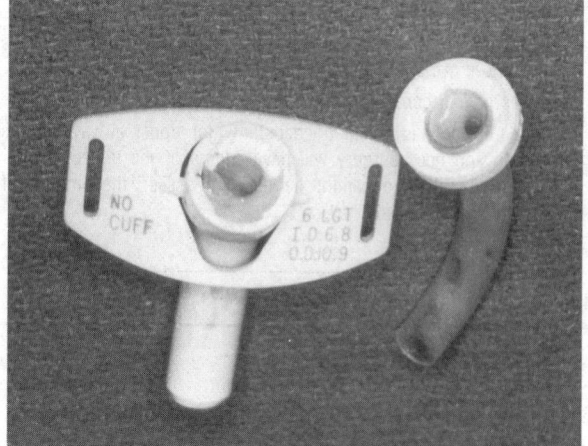

(continued)

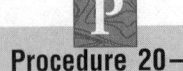

Procedure 20–1

(continued)

Action	Rationale/Discussion
3. Instill 3 to 5 ml of normal saline solution into the tube or stoma. Repeat as needed.	3. Loosens secretions and plug.
4. Suction the stoma.	4. Stimulates movement of the mucus or plug.

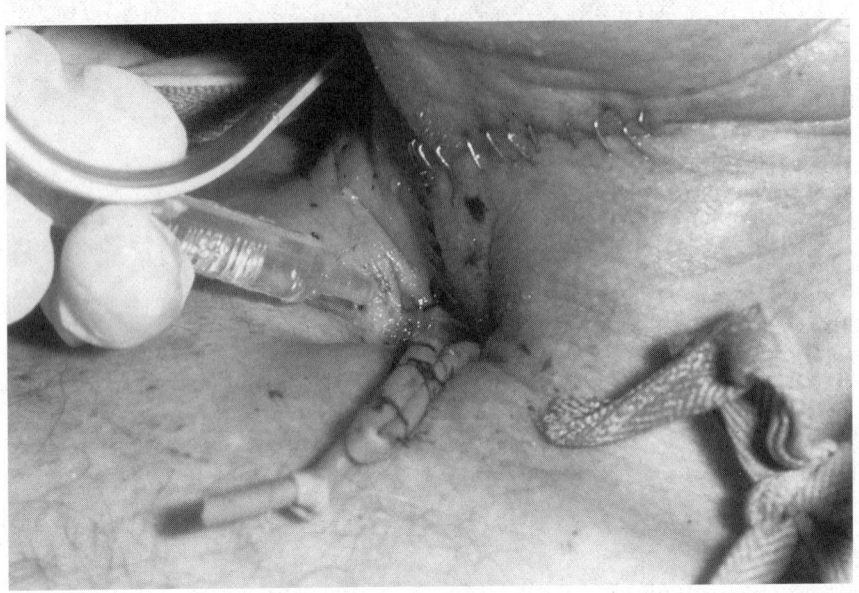

Action	Rationale/Discussion
5. Remove the plug with forceps, if necessary.	5. Removes plug that cannot be removed by previous steps.

Procedure: Deflating and Inflating the Cuff of the Tracheostomy Tube

Action	Rationale/Discussion
1. Suction the tracheostomy tube and mouth.	1. Removes secretions. If you suction the tracheostomy tube before the mouth, use the same catheter unless infection is present. If you suction the mouth before the tracheostomy tube, change the catheter to prevent cross-contamination.
2. Deflate the cuff during exhalation.	2. Prevents aspiration of secretions that accumulate above cuff.
3. Instruct the patient to cough or suction the patient while deflating the cuff.	3. Removes secretions that accumulate above the cuff.
4. Monitor the patient while the cuff is deflated.	4. The patient is at risk of aspiration while the cuff is deflated.
5. Inflate the cuff during inhalation.	5. Increases patient comfort.
6. Insert the amount of air that was removed or has been previously documented. Use a cuff manometer to determine the amount of air needed to inflate the cuff without applying excessive pressure to the tracheal mucosa.	6. The patient who has had a tracheostomy for upper airway obstruction after head and neck surgery will have edema of the upper airway. The minimal-leak technique cannot be used to assess the amount of air needed to inflate the cuff.

Final Activities

- Discard all used equipment.
- Document the procedure and findings.
- Document the patient's tolerance of the procedure.

(2) Administer enteral tube feedings as ordered when bowel sounds return.

(3) Begin oral feedings as ordered. For patients who have had a total laryngectomy or hemilaryngectomy, begin with a full liquid diet and advance as tolerated. For patients who have had a supraglottic laryngectomy, begin with a nonpourable pureed diet; hold liquids until swallowing technique is mastered.

(4) Encourage small, frequent meals and the use of nutritional supplements.

NURSING DIAGNOSIS: Aspiration on swallowing R/T the presence of a tracheostomy tube and removal of the epiglottis

a. *Expected outcomes:* The patient should show no signs of aspiration-related complications; breath signs will be normal, coughing will be effective, and temperature and white blood cell count will be normal.

b. *Nursing interventions*
   (1) If the patient is at risk for aspiration, instruct him or her on the supraglottic swallowing technique:
       • Take a deep breath.
       • Perform a Valsalva maneuver to close the vocal cords.
       • Swallow.
       • Cough to expel food collected on the vocal cords.
       • Swallow.
       • Breathe.
   (2) Consult with a dietitian and swallowing therapist to determine the calorie intake the patient needs and the food consistency best tolerated and for reinforcement of the swallowing technique.

NURSING DIAGNOSIS: Impaired verbal communication R/T surgery on larynx

a. *Expected outcomes:* The patient should be able to communicate effectively.

b. *Nursing interventions*
   (1) See tracheostomy nursing diagnoses and management.
   (2) Review alternative communication devices with the patient and encourage their use (Fig. 20–18).
   (3) Consult with a speech therapist.
   (4) Instruct the patient on the care of the tracheoesophageal puncture (Box 20–7).
   (5) Reinforce instruction provided by the speech therapist.

NURSING DIAGNOSIS: Impaired skin integrity R/T the surgical procedure

a. *Expected outcomes:* The patient's wounds should heal without infection.

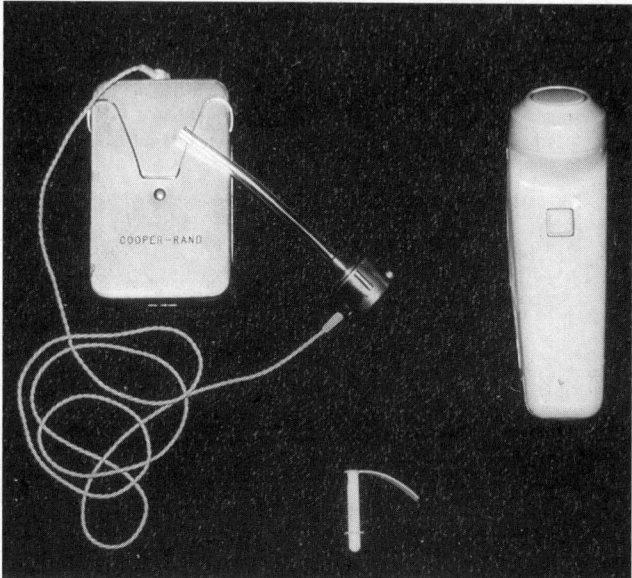

Figure 20–18. Alternate communication devices. *Left,* Cooper Rand intraoral electrolarynx; *right,* Wester electric neck vibrating electrolarynx; *bottom,* tracheoesophageal voice prosthesis.

b. *Nursing interventions*
   (1) Assess the incisions and stoma.
   (2) Monitor the integrity of the incisions, observing their color, drainage, and approximation of wound edges.
   (3) Cleanse incisions with half-strength hydrogen peroxide, rinse with sterile water or saline, and apply antibacterial ointment.
   (4) Evaluate vital signs, especially temperature, and laboratory values, especially the white blood cell count.
   (5) See tracheostomy nursing diagnoses and management.

NURSING DIAGNOSIS: Pain (acute) R/T the surgical procedure

a. *Expected outcomes:* The patient should have minimal pain.

b. *Nursing interventions*
   (1) Assess the pain.
   (2) Help the patient identify nonpharmacologic methods of relieving pain, such as changing position and using relaxation and guided imagery techniques.
   (3) Administer analgesics as ordered and evaluate their effectiveness.

NURSING DIAGNOSIS: Body image disturbance R/T the presence of the stoma

a. *Expected outcomes:* The patient should adapt to the change in body image and perform self-care procedures.

BOX 20–7. Tracheoesophageal Puncture

1. An opening has been made between the tracheostoma and esophagus.
2. Insert a red rubber catheter through the puncture for several days to stent the puncture.

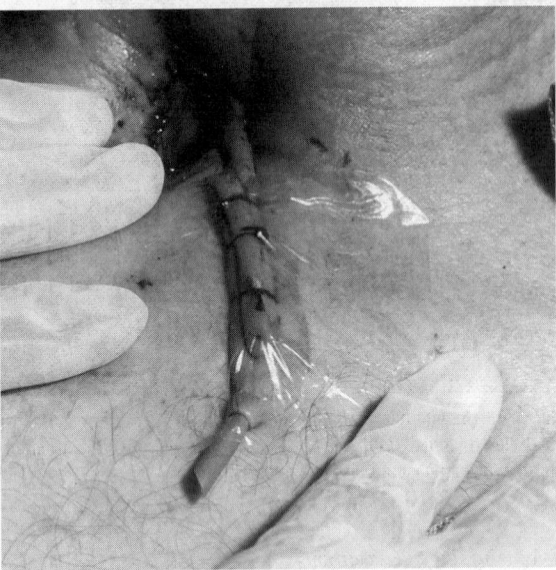

3. Tie a knot in the distal end of the catheter to prevent reflux of stomach contents through the catheter.

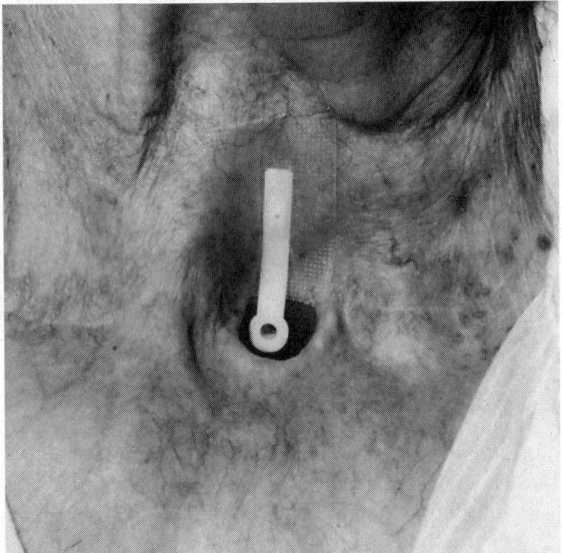

4. To insert the prosthesis:
   - Insert the prosthesis into the puncture site
   - Remove the inserter.
   - Tape the wings of the prosthesis.
5. To use the prosthesis, instruct the patient to cover the stoma with the thumb to shunt air into the esophagus.

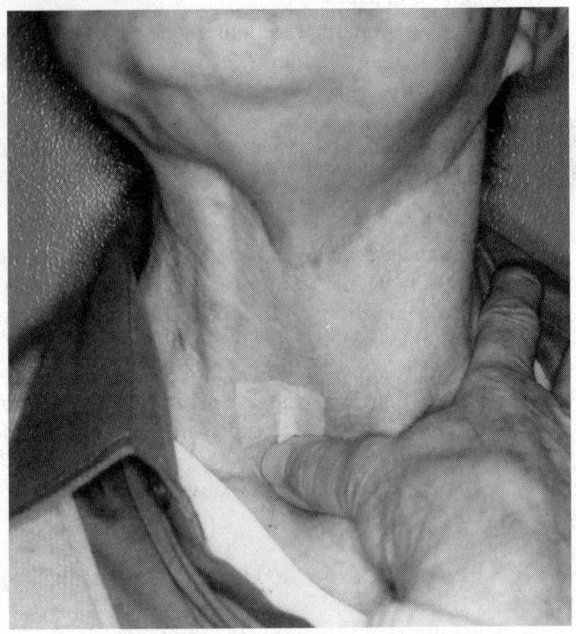

Adapted from Sigler BA, and Schuring LT. *Ear, Nose, and Throat Disorders*. St. Louis: Mosby–Year Book, 1993, p 267.

    b. *Nursing interventions:* See tracheostomy nursing diagnoses and management.
11. Discharge planning and teaching
    a. See tracheostomy discharge planning and teaching.
    b. Give the patient an additional laryngectomy or tracheostomy tube so that he or she can change the tube at home or in the doctor's office.

    c. Reinforce nutritional instructions.
      (1) Use of the supraglottic swallow
      (2) Diet plan and food consistencies
      (3) Use of nutritional supplements
    d. Provide information on obtaining supplies.
    e. Review self-care procedures.
    f. Review tracheoesophageal puncture use and care.

g. Review life activity changes.
   (1) Instruct the patient to avoid getting water in the stoma. The patient may do this by aiming the shower low on the chest, using the sink to wash his or her hair, covering the stoma when shaving to keep lather and hair from entering it, and using a shower shield. Regarding swimming, provide information on the use of a Larkel, a swimming device similar to a snorkel for use by the laryngectomee.
   (2) Inform the patient that no changes in sexual activity are necessary but body hygiene must be maintained.
   (3) Lifting, bowel movements, and childbirth require performing a Valsalva maneuver. After a total laryngectomy, it is not possible to close the vocal cords to perform this maneuver. Changes in these activities may occur.
h. Arrange home health services and equipment.
i. Refer the patient to a support group (e.g., the Lost Chord Club and the American Cancer Society).
j. Support the patient's enrollment in smoking cessation and alcohol withdrawal programs.

12. Public health considerations
   a. There is strong evidence that cancer of the head and neck is related to tobacco and alcohol abuse. Support for alcohol and tobacco cessation programs is mandatory. The nurse is in a key position to provide continuing education and counseling on the hazards of smoking and alcohol abuse and techniques on how to quit and to provide referrals to formal programs.
   b. The patient with a temporary or permanent alteration in breathing or speaking should be encouraged to carry identification informing others that he or she is "neck breathing" or does not have a normal speaking voice in case of an accident or emergency.

Cancer of the Hypopharynx

1. Definition: Tumors of the hypopharynx arise in the pyriform sinus, pharyngeal walls, and posterior cricoid area of the larynx.
2. Incidence and etiology
   a. As with other malignant tumors of the head and neck, squamous cell carcinoma is the most common cell type found in hypopharyngeal tumors.
   b. Excessive tobacco and alcohol use are the etiologic agents related to cancer of the hypopharynx.
3. Clinical manifestations
   a. Dysphagia
   b. Odynophagia
   c. Pain (local and referred)
   d. Hoarseness
   e. Odor secondary to infection
   f. Mass in neck (regional lymph node metastasis)
4. Clinical management
   a. Radiation therapy and chemotherapy are used as adjuvant therapies or palliative treatments for cancer of the hypopharynx, as they are for cancer of the larynx.

b. Surgical removal includes pharyngectomy with or without total laryngectomy.
c. Reconstruction after pharyngectomy may include primary closure or a skin graft for small lesions. If a large resection is necessary, reconstruction may require a pharyngogastric anastomosis (removal of the pharynx and esophagus and mobilization of the stomach to the pharynx to create a new swallowing passage) or a jejunal free flap (in which a portion of the jejunum is used to fill the defect created by the pharyngectomy).
d. Jejunal free flap reconstruction requires a microvascular anastomosis to restore blood supply.
e. Patients who have had a pharyngogastric anastomosis or jejunal free flap require the same care as patients who have had a total laryngectomy as well as care of the free flap.
5. Prognosis: The prognosis for patients with cancer of the hypopharynx is poor.

Congenital Neck Mass

1. Definition: Congenital neck masses are present at birth, are usually remnants of embryologic life, and may not be obvious until later in life.
   a. **Branchial cleft cysts** are remnants of the branchial apparatus (1st, 2nd, or 3rd cleft anomalies determine the location of the cyst in the neck). They are lined with squamous epithelium and may become inflamed after an upper respiratory infection.
   b. **Thyroglossal duct cysts** arise from the duct through which the thyroid gland descends from the base of the tongue to the neck during embryologic life. The duct is lined with squamous epithelium and may become inflamed after an upper respiratory infection.
2. Clinical manifestations
   a. Branchial cleft cyst: a mass in the neck
   b. Thyroglossal duct cyst: a midline neck mass, usually located at the level of the hyoid bone, that moves up and down during swallowing
3. Clinical management
   a. Branchial cleft cyst: Initial treatment is with antibiotics; surgical excision of the cyst and any attached duct is performed once inflammation subsides.
   b. Thyroglossal duct cyst: Initial treatment is with antibiotics; surgical excision of the cyst, duct, and midportion of the hyoid bone is performed once inflammation subsides (the Sistrunk procedure). This cyst has the potential for malignant transformation.

Neoplasms

1. Glomus tumors
   a. Definition: Glomus tumors are usually benign tumors that arise from the chemoreceptor tissue associated with the great vessels. They are also known as **paragangliomas.**
   b. Pathophysiology
      (1) Glomus tumors are usually benign, but they may

be locally aggressive. Malignant changes cannot be determined histologically and are determined by the presence of metastasis.

(2) Some paragangliomas have a familial tendency.

c. Clinical manifestations: Clinical manifestations vary according to the location of the tumor.

(1) Carotid body tumor: a mass in the neck at the area of carotid bifurcation and an audible bruit

(2) Glomus jugulare: a mass in the neck at the jugular bulb and lower cranial nerve deficits—hoarseness, dysphagia, and unilateral tongue atrophy

(3) Glomus vagale: a mass in the neck along the vagus nerve and unilateral vocal cord paralysis

(4) Glomus tympanicum: a bluish mass in the middle ear space, pulsatile tinnitus, conductive hearing loss, and a positive Brown's sign (the bluish mass blanches when pressure is applied to the tympanic membrane with the pneumatic otoscope).

d. Clinical management

(1) Surgical excision of tumor

(2) Possibly radiation therapy for malignant paragangliomas

2. Tumors of the parotid gland

a. Definition: Parotid tumors may be benign or malignant neoplasms of the largest salivary gland.

b. Incidence and socioeconomic impact

(1) The cause of tumors of the parotid gland is unknown.

(2) The majority of parotid gland tumors are benign.

(3) Pleomorphic adenoma (benign mixed tumor) is the most common benign neoplasm; however, it may become malignant.

(4) Mucoepidermoid carcinoma is the most common malignant tumor.

c. Clinical manifestations

(1) Benign tumor: slow-growing, painless mass in the parotid gland

(2) Malignant tumor: slow-growing, painful or painless mass that may involve the facial nerve, causing facial weakness or paralysis

d. Clinical management

(1) Surgical excision is the treatment for both benign and malignant tumors. Superficial lobe parotidectomy removes the outer lobe of the gland, and total parotidectomy removes the entire parotid gland. In any parotid surgery, the facial nerve is at risk of injury that may result in temporary or permanent facial paralysis.

(2) Radiation therapy may be used as adjuvant therapy for malignant tumors.

Cervical Lymph Node Metastasis

1. Definition: Cervical lymph node metastasis is a malignant tumor in the neck, other than lymphoma, that is caused by metastasis to the cervical lymph nodes. The metastasis is usually from a primary tumor in the upper aerodigestive tract, but it can occur from a primary tumor below the clavicles.

2. Risk factors and etiology: The risk factors and etiologic agents are the same as those of the primary tumor.

3. Pathophysiology: Tumor type is the same as the primary tumor.

4. Clinical manifestation: a mass in the neck

5. Diagnostics

a. Thorough history

b. Examination of the oral cavity, oropharynx, nasopharynx, nasal cavity, larynx, pharynx, skin, and neck to look for the primary tumor

c. Endoscopy and biopsy to diagnose the primary tumor

d. Computed tomographic scan and magnetic resonance imaging to diagnose primary tumor, if present, and to evaluate the extent of lymph node involvement

e. Fine-needle aspiration biopsy to identify the histologic tumor type

f. Excisional (open) biopsy if fine-needle aspiration biopsy fails to diagnose the histologic tumor type

6. Clinical management

a. The goal of clinical management is to remove the primary tumor, lymph nodes, drainage channels, and adjacent involved structures.

b. Nonpharmacologic interventions: none

c. Pharmacologic interventions

(1) Radiation therapy and chemotherapy as adjuvant and palliative treatments

(2) Both radiation therapy and chemotherapy to decrease tumor size before surgical interventions

d. Special medical-surgical procedures

(1) The surgery performed to remove lymph node metastasis is called **neck dissection.** A radical neck dissection is an en bloc removal of all the lymph nodes from the clavicle to the mandible, the sternocleidomastoid muscle, the submandibular gland, the internal jugular vein, and the spinal accessory nerve.

(2) A modified neck dissection removes all the structures removed in a radical neck dissection except for the spinal accessory nerve.

(3) A selective neck dissection removes lymph nodes in an area of typical metastasis.

(4) The type of neck dissection performed depends on the staging of the neck mass and the primary tumor's potential for lymph node metastasis.

7. Complications

a. Infection

b. Fistula

c. Wound dehiscence

d. Hematoma or seroma

e. Shoulder dysfunction

f. Recurrent or persistent tumor

g. Airway compromise

8. Prognosis

a. The prognosis after neck dissection depends on the results of the histologic evaluation of the lymph nodes. If no tumor is present in the lymph nodes or if the patient has no evidence of the tumor invading the capsule of the lymph node, the prognosis is that of the primary tumor. If extracapsular invasion is present (the tumor extends to the edges of lymph node or totally replaces lymph node), the prognosis is downgraded.

b. Adjuvant radiation therapy or chemotherapy may improve the prognosis in patients with extracapsular spread of tumor.

9. Applying the nursing process

NURSING DIAGNOSIS: Risk for infection R/T skin incisions from the surgical procedure.

a. *Expected outcomes:* The patient should heal without complications.
b. *Nursing interventions*
   (1) Maintain pressure dressing.
   (2) Assess the surgical incision for color, drainage, temperature, and edema, once the pressure dressing has been removed.
   (3) Maintain the patency of wound catheters, if used (Box 20–8).
   (4) Cleanse the incision with half-strength hydrogen peroxide, rinse with sterile water or saline, and apply antibacterial ointment.
   (5) Avoid hyperextension of the neck.
   (6) Monitor temperature and laboratory values, especially the white blood cell count.
   (7) Place the patient on "Carotid Artery Precautions" if infection or fistula occurs near the carotid artery (Box 20–9).

NURSING DIAGNOSIS: Pain (acute) R/T the surgical procedure

BOX 20–8. Wound Catheter Care

1. Assemble equipment: sterile towel, gloves, angiocatheter or blunt-tipped needle with 10-ml syringe, antimicrobial solution, and hemostats.
2. Apply gloves.
3. Attach the catheter to the source of negative pressure (wall suction or self-containing vacuum container).
4. Maintain suction.
5. Aspirate drainage catheters using aseptic technique, as ordered, with the angiocatheter or the blunt-tipped needle attached to a 10-ml syringe, to remove accumulated secretions.
   • Apply a hemostat (without teeth) to each catheter near the insertion site.
   • Disconnect each catheter from its source of negative pressure.
   • Cleanse the catheter tip with antimicrobial solution.
   • Insert the angiocatheter or blunt-tipped needle into drainage tubing, release the hemostat, and aspirate by pulling back on the syringe.
   • Reapply a hemostat and apply the above-mentioned technique on all drains.
   • Reattach all drains to their negative pressures and remove hemostats.
6. Measure the drainage daily, including the aspirate, and evaluate the consistency.
   • Increased blood drainage may indicate hematoma.
   • Increased serous drainage may indicate seroma.
   • Increased opaque (milky) drainage may indicate a chylous fistula.

BOX 20–9. Carotid Artery Precautions

1. Evaluate the wound for arterial exposure.

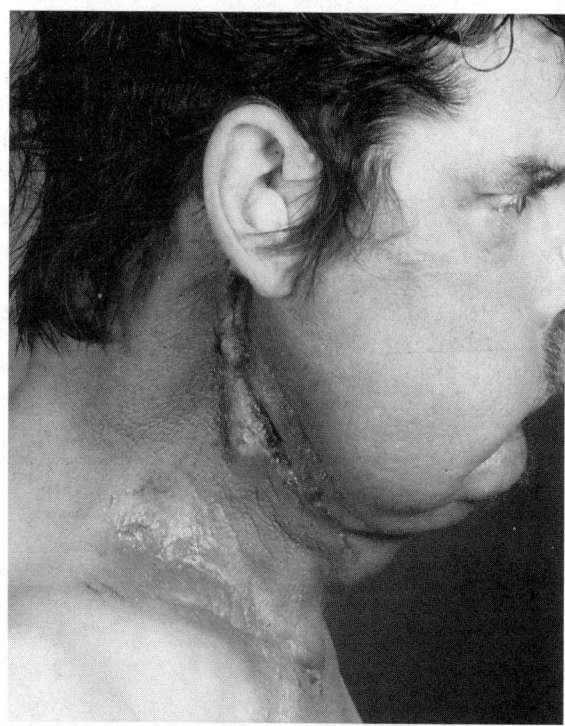

2. Apply a moist sterile dressing to the exposed artery.
3. Notify the physician if any bleeding occurs.
4. Assemble emergency supplies: towels, 4 × 4 gauze sponges, a cuffed tracheostomy tube, hemostats, suction, oxygen, and morphine sulfate injectable.
5. Type and crossmatch the blood.
6. Limit the patient's activity.
7. Instruct the patient to avoid activities that cause an increase in intrathoracic pressure, such as performing the Valsalva maneuver and straining during bowel movements.
8. If bleeding occurs, take the following steps:
   • Apply pressure to the bleeding area.
   • Activate code procedure (unless patient has a "Do Not Resuscitate" order).
   • Maintain the airway.
   • Overinflate the cuff of the tracheostomy tube.
   • Infuse intravenous fluids rapidly.
   • Administer morphine sulfate.
   • Administer blood.
   • Monitor vital signs.
   • Transport the patient to the operating room.
9. Provide psychological support to the patient, family, and health team members present during carotid artery rupture. If a patient is at risk for a carotid artery rupture, all the items listed under nursing interventions should be preordered after discussing with the physician. Once the artery begins to bleed, there is no time to obtain these orders.

---

a. *Expected outcomes:* The patient should be able to verbalize relief of pain or minimal pain in neck and shoulder.
b. *Nursing interventions*
   (1) Evaluate the location, intensity, and characteristics of the pain.
   (2) Elevate the head of the bed and help the patient

assume a comfortable position. Evaluate other nonpharmacologic methods of pain relief (e.g., relaxation and guided imagery).

(3) Administer analgesics as ordered and evaluate their effectiveness.

(4) Support the arm and shoulder on the side on which the surgery was performed with a pillow while the patient is in bed or sitting in a chair; do not allow the arm to be in a dependent position. The patient may use a sling when ambulating, if ordered.

(5) Consult with a physical therapist who can recommend range-of-motion and muscle-strengthening exercises for the arm and shoulder, as ordered. Encourage the patient to continue these exercises after hospital discharge.

(6) Caution the patient about altered sensation in the neck. The patient should avoid using a straight razor or safety razor and a heating pad or hot water bottle, should use heated hair appliances with caution, and should cover the area when outside in cold weather to avoid frostbite.

NURSING DIAGNOSIS: Ineffective airway clearance R/T postoperative edema, hematoma, or seroma formation

a. *Expected outcomes:* The patient should have a clear airway with no evidence of breathing difficulty.

b. *Nursing interventions*
(1) Elevate the head of the bed and avoid flexion of the neck.
(2) Assess respirations: depth, rate, and lung sounds.
(3) Evaluate for signs of airway obstruction: stridor, restlessness, anxiety, and an oxygen saturation level below normal for the patient.
(4) Encourage coughing, deep breathing, and ambulation.
(5) Assess the neck for edema and dressing for tightness.
(6) Monitor wound drainage for an increase in sanguineous, serosanguineous, or serous drainage, which may indicate an accumulation of fluid under the skin flaps.

NURSING DIAGNOSIS: Body image disturbance R/T surgical incisions

a. *Expected outcomes:* The patient should be able to adapt to the changes in his or her appearance and participate in self-care procedures.

b. *Nursing interventions:* See "Tumors of the Oral Cavity and Oropharynx" and "Tracheostomy" for body image disturbance, nursing diagnosis, and management.

10. Discharge planning and teaching
a. Encourage the patient to continue range-of-motion and muscle-strengthening exercises.
b. Instruct the patient to notify the physician if signs of infection, fistula, or bleeding occur.

c. Provide a list of safety measures the patient can take to compensate for altered sensory perception in the neck. Instruct the patient to do the following:
(1) Avoid using heat-producing appliances, such as a heating pad, hair dryer, and heated rollers.
(2) In cold weather, increase protective covering over areas of decreased sensation to prevent frostbite.
(3) Use electric razor.

11. Public health considerations
a. The American Cancer Society's warning signals of cancer include "a mass in the neck or elsewhere." Encourage patients to seek medical attention if they find any of the warning signs of cancer.
b. The fear of being diagnosed with cancer is one reason why people delay medical consultation. Advanced practice nurses, home health nurses, and outpatient nurses are in ideal positions to provide health education about cancer. The knowledge that early diagnosis improves the prognosis may allay some of the fear and anxiety and prompt the patient to see a medical consultant.

Tracheostomy

1. Definition: A tracheotomy is a surgical opening made into the trachea for airway management. A tracheostomy is the surgical creation of a stoma from the trachea to the overlying skin. The terms **tracheotomy** and **tracheostomy** are often used interchangeably. The term **tracheostomy** is used in this chapter.

2. Incidence: unknown

3. Pathophysiology: A tracheostomy is performed for potential or actual airway obstruction, for ventilatory assistance, to protect the airway and provide pulmonary suctioning, to avoid prolonged endotracheal intubation, and to provide an airway for patients with severe obstructive sleep apnea.

4. Clinical manifestations
a. Dyspnea
b. Abnormal arterial blood gas or pulse oximetry readings
c. Stridor with labored respirations
d. Anxiety and restlessness
e. Suprasternal retractions
f. Abnormal voice—a muffled quality of the voice usually indicates an abnormality above the larynx, and hoarseness indicates an abnormality of the glottis (vocal cords) or below
g. Ineffective cough
h. Chronic aspiration

5. Diagnostics
a. Complete history of airway symptoms, including history of trauma, surgery, and possible aspiration of foreign body
b. Indirect and direct laryngoscopy
c. Arterial blood gases
d. Pulse oximetry

6. Clinical management
a. The goal of performing a tracheostomy is to provide a patent airway for the patient with present or potential upper airway distress.

b. Nonpharmacologic interventions
 (1) The patient with potential or present airway compromise should be placed in a high Fowler's position to reduce edema and facilitate chest expansion.
 (2) Increase humidification by administering humidified oxygen by nasal cannula or face mask; administer oxygen directly to the tracheostomy, if it has already been performed.
 (3) Arterial blood gases should be obtained as a baseline, with pulse oximetry used to monitor oxygen levels.
c. Pharmacologic interventions
 (1) Antibiotics may be given to treat infection.
 (2) Steroids may be used to reduce inflammation.
 (3) Medications with a sedating effect or side effect of respiratory depression must be avoided.

NURSE ADVISORY

Anxiety and restlessness are symptoms of airway distress and should be investigated before being treated as a separate diagnosis. Any patient with present or potential airway obstruction should be thoroughly evaluated before receiving narcotic analgesics, antidepressants, or sedatives. These medications may cause respiratory depression. Before administering any medication that may cause respiratory depression, evaluate the patient's respiratory status by monitoring the rate and depth of respirations, auscultating breath sounds, and assessing oxygen saturation by pulse oximetry. If there is any doubt about oxygen status, obtain an order for arterial blood gases.

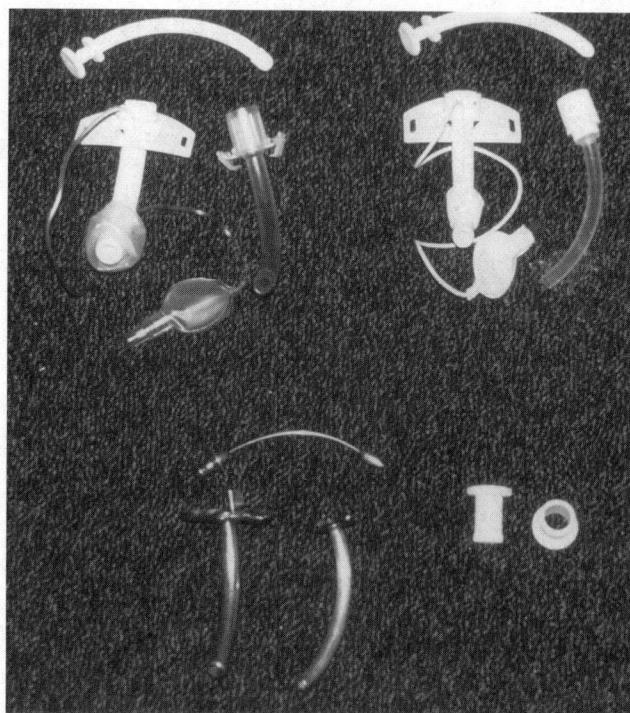

Figure 20–20. *Upper left,* Cuffed tracheostomy tube with disposable inner cannula and obturator; *upper right,* cuffed tracheostomy tube with conventional inner cannula and obturator; *lower left,* Jackson metal uncuffed tube with inner cannula and obturator; *lower right,* tracheostomy button.

d. Procedure: A tracheostomy should be performed in the operating room. The patient is placed in a supine position with the neck hyperextended. The incision is placed between the 2nd and 3rd or 3rd and 4th tracheal rings (Fig. 20–19). Traction sutures—long silk sutures inserted into the trachea above and below the opening—may be inserted for use in opening the stoma in case of accidental decannulation.
e. Types of tracheostomy tubes
 (1) A cuffed tracheostomy tube has an outer cannula, inner cannula, and obturator and a high-volume, low-pressure cuff (Fig. 20–20).
 (2) A cuffless tracheostomy tube has an outer cannula, an open and a plugged inner cannula, and an obturator. These tubes are used for long-term tracheostomy, for evaluating the patient's ability to breathe through the upper airway during the decannulation process, and for the patient no longer at risk for aspiration.
 (3) A laryngectomy tube has an outer cannula, an inner cannula, and an obturator; it is shorter than the standard tracheostomy tube for the patient with a permanent stoma (Fig. 20–21).
 (4) A fenestrated tracheostomy tube differs from the standard tracheostomy tube in that it has an opening along the posterior wall of the outer cannula; when the tube is capped, the patient can breathe through the upper airway and speak. The capped inner cannula cannot be used when the cuff is inflated or for the laryngectomy pa-

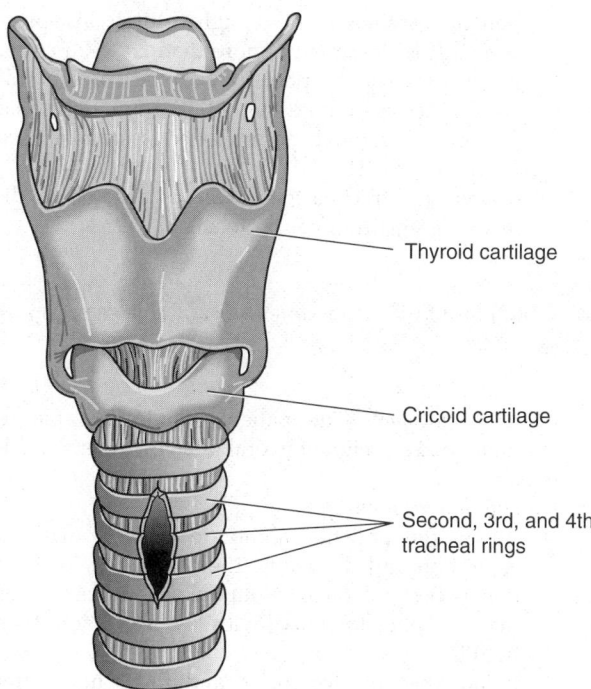

Thyroid cartilage

Cricoid cartilage

Second, 3rd, and 4th tracheal rings

Figure 20–19. Site of insertion for tracheostomy is between the 2nd and 3rd or 3rd and 4th tracheal rings. (Redrawn from Ignatavicius DD, Workman ML, and Mishler MA [eds]. *Medical-Surgical Nursing: A Nursing Process Approach.* 2nd ed. Philadelphia: WB Saunders, 1996, p 658.)

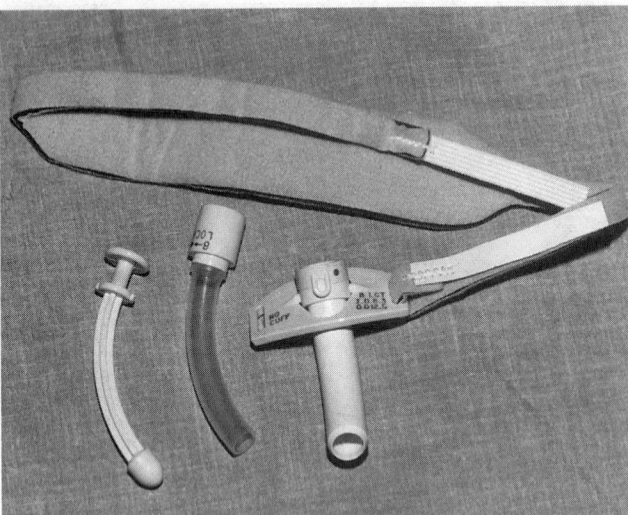

Figure 20–21. Disposable laryngectomy tube; parts left to right include obturator, inner cannula, outer cannula with Velcro ties.

tient, because breathing through the upper airway is impossible (Fig. 20–22).

(5) A tracheostomy with a foam cuff has a tube similar to the standard cuffed tube; however, the cuff is larger and filled with foam, which may apply less pressure to the tracheal mucosa.

(6) The Jackson metal tracheostomy tube has an outer cannula, an inner cannula, and an obturator and comes in standard and short lengths. It can be reused after sterilization (see Fig. 20–20).

(7) The tracheostomy button is a short, straight tube that fits into the stoma but does not enter the trachea; it can be used during the weaning or decannulation process (see Fig. 20–20).

(8) A single cannula tube usually is longer than standard tubes and has an outer cannula and an obturator but no inner cannula. It is used for

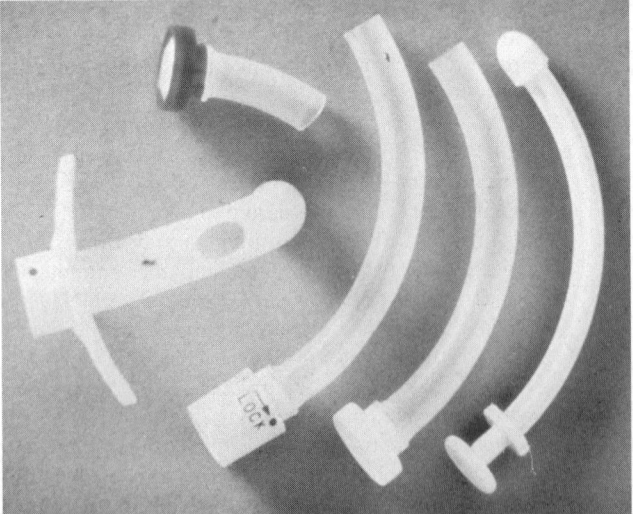

Figure 20–22. Fenestrated uncuffed tracheostomy tube. Note the opening in back of the outer cannula, the short capped inner cannula to allow air to be shunted for speech, the 2 open inner cannulas, and the obturator.

patients with a thick neck, in whom a standard tube would not enter the trachea.

7. Complications
   a. Bleeding
   b. Subcutaneous emphysema
   c. Tracheoesophageal fistula
   d. Pneumothorax
   e. Displaced tracheostomy tube/accidental decannulation.

8. Applying the nursing process

NURSING DIAGNOSIS: Ineffective airway clearance R/T increased mucus, obstruction of the inner cannula of the tracheostomy tube, ineffective cough, and aspiration of secretions

a. *Expected outcomes:* The patient should be able to maintain a patent airway.
b. *Nursing interventions*
   (1) Assess respirations and breath sounds.
   (2) Monitor arterial blood gases or pulse oximetry evaluations.
   (3) Encourage coughing and deep breathing.
   (4) Help the patient assume a high Fowler's position.
   (5) Observe for bleeding, difficulty breathing, an absence of breath sounds, and crepitus in the neck, which are indications of hemorrhage, pneumothorax, and subcutaneous emphysema.
   (6) Provide chest physiotherapy and inhalation treatments as ordered.
   (7) Suction the tracheostomy as needed (see Procedure 20–1).
   (8) If a cuffed tracheostomy tube is used (for assisted or controlled ventilation or to minimize aspiration of secretions), use a high-volume, low-pressure cuff that exerts no more than 20 to 30 cm of water pressure to prevent ischemia of the tracheal mucosa. Deflate the cuff per organizational protocol to remove accumulated secretions (see Procedure 20–1).
   (9) Change the tracheostomy tube as ordered or directed by institutional protocol.

NURSING DIAGNOSIS: Impaired swallowing R/T tracheostomy tube

a. *Expected outcomes:* The patient should be able to maintain body weight by oral diet or enteral feedings.
b. *Nursing interventions*
   (1) Assess the patient's ability to swallow without aspiration and determine the consistency of food that is best tolerated. Nonpourable pureed foods may be better tolerated, with less aspiration, than liquids.
   (2) Inflate the cuff for meals and for 1 hour after meals if the patient is at risk for aspiration.
   (3) Instruct the patient to sit for meals to minimize aspiration.

(4) Consult with a swallowing therapist for a modified barium swallow or body positioning if aspiration occurs.

(5) Monitor the patient's weight and perform a calorie or protein assessment in consultation with a dietitian.

(6) Maintain nothing by mouth status and provide enteral feedings if the patient aspirates with an oral diet.

NURSING DIAGNOSIS: Impaired verbal communication R/T tracheostomy

a. *Expected outcomes:* The patient should be able to communicate effectively.

b. *Nursing interventions*

(1) Assess the patient's understanding of his or her altered anatomy and inability to communicate verbally.

(2) Evaluate the patient's ability to read and write and provide easy-to-use writing materials for communication.

(3) Consult with a speech therapist to determine alternative methods of communication that may be acceptable to the patient, such as paper and pencil, an electrolarynx, a communication board, computer-assisted devices, a speech valve, or a fenestrated tube.

(4) Give the patient using these alternative methods sufficient time to communicate.

(5) Observe for nonverbal communication.

NURSING DIAGNOSIS: Risk for infection R/T the tracheostomy incision

a. *Expected outcomes:* The incision should be free of signs of infection.

b. *Nursing interventions*

(1) Remove the damp dressing, if used, under the neckplate of the tracheostomy tube to avoid excoriation of the skin and infection (Fig. 20–23).

(2) Clean under the neckplate of the tracheostomy tube with half-strength hydrogen peroxide and apply dry dressing.

(3) Assess the stoma and secretions for blood, purulence, and odor.

(4) Monitor vital signs, especially temperature.

(5) Monitor the white blood cell count.

(6) Use sterile technique when providing care and administering supplemental humidification. Instill 3 to 5 ml of normal saline solution into the stoma to stimulate coughing and moisten mucosa (this technique is considered controversial in some institutions). Administer humidified oxygen or air as ordered.

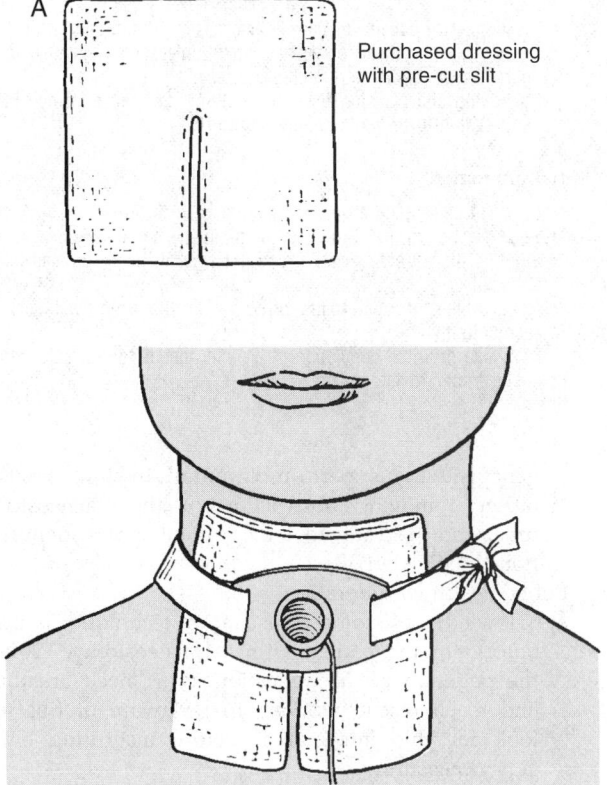

A   Purchased dressing with pre-cut slit

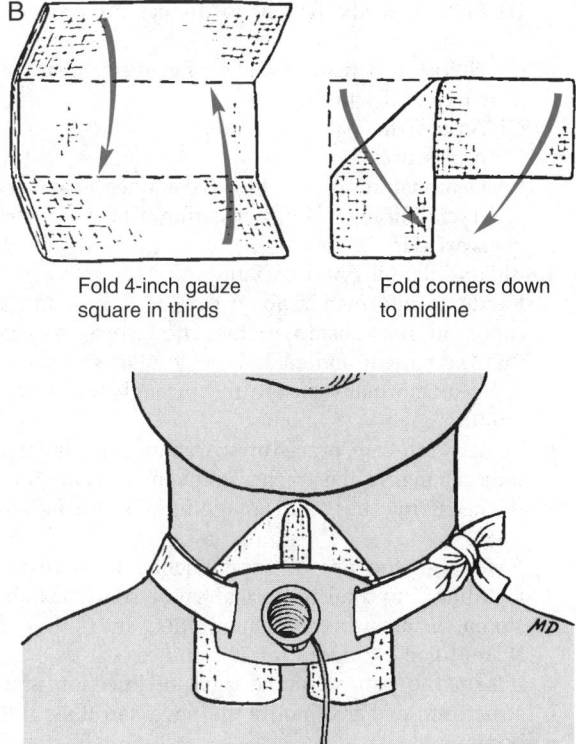

B   Fold 4-inch gauze square in thirds   Fold corners down to midline

Figure 20–23. Tracheostomy dressings. (From Black JM, and Matassarin-Jacobs E [eds]. *Luckmann and Sorensen's Medical-Surgical Nursing: A Psychophysiologic Approach.* 4th ed. Philadelphia: WB Saunders, 1993, p 975.)

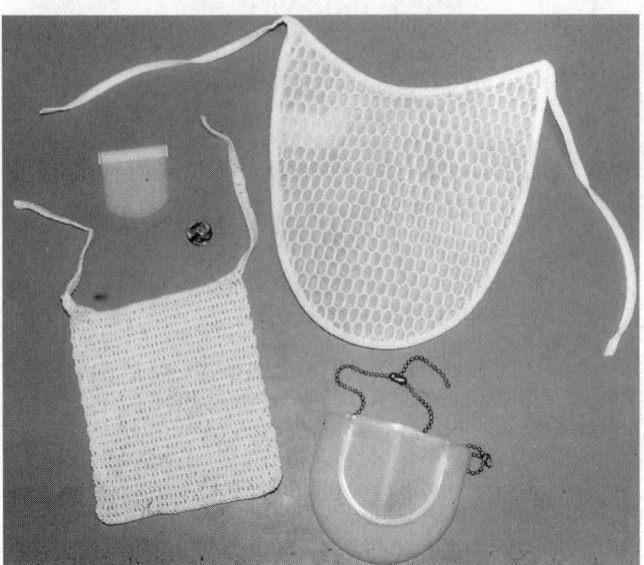

Figure 20–24. Examples of some types of tracheostomy covers.

NURSING DIAGNOSIS: Body image disturbance R/T presence of tracheostomy

    a. *Expected outcomes:* The patient should be able to adapt to the changes in body image and provide self-care.

    b. *Nursing interventions*

       (1) Encourage the patient to discuss his or her concerns.

       (2) Help the patient assess coping mechanisms used successfully in the past.

       (3) Assess the patient's readiness to begin self-care procedures.

       (4) Demonstrate camouflage techniques to cover the tracheostomy, such as wearing a bib, sweater, or scarf (Fig. 20–24).

9. Discharge planning and teaching

    a. Reinforce information about tracheostomy and its location in relationship to the vocal cords to ensure that the patient understands why he or she is unable to speak normally or breathe through the nose and mouth.

    b. Review self-care procedures: cleaning the inner cannula, changing the tracheostomy tube, changing the tracheostomy ties, and plugging the tracheostomy tube.

    c. Encourage the use of supplemental humidification: instilling 3 to 5 ml of normal saline solution into the stoma, using a bedside humidifier, and sitting in a steam-filled bathroom for 20 minutes.

    d. Inform the patient of the signs of infection and instruct him or her to notify the physician if symptoms occur.

    e. Arrange for home equipment and home health nursing before discharge.

    f. Instruct the patient's family on techniques for emer-

HOME CARE STRATEGIES

Tracheostomy Care

There are increasing numbers of home health care patients with tracheostomies who may or may not be ventilator dependent. Long-term care of these patients is being managed in the home. Families may be taught care of the ventilator, tracheostomy care, and signs and symptoms of respiratory distress in the hospital.

The home care nurse should assess the following areas:

Psychosocial

- Assess the coping of patient and family members with care and maintenance of the tracheostomy. Are they comfortable and compliant?
- To alleviate some fears, suggest displaying emergency numbers near all phones.
- A calm, matter-of-fact attitude will ease care.
- If the patient takes time to talk, this relaxes the neck muscles, reduces the respiratory rate, and alleviates caregiver insecurities.
- Suggest plugging the tracheostomy to promote as much patient independence as possible.
- Suggest that the patient continue religious participation, if possible, to promote self-esteem.
- Caregivers may maintain their "sense of self" by maintaining activities during the disruption of the daily lifestyle.

Physical

- Teach assessment of signs and symptoms of infection or distress.
- Observe performance of tracheostomy care.
- Teach clean technique and hand washing.
- Nonsterile gloves are worn, and equipment is reused for up to 72 hours.
- Positioning of patient for care is also assessed and taught.
- Suggest keeping head of bed elevated (unless on ventilator) to improve respirations and decrease stress.
- Suctioning and cleaning the tracheostomy can be performed in this position to promote patient comfort.

Environment

- Assist in developing an escape plan in case of fire.
- Suggest posting "No Smoking" signs in the home.
- Signs to alert fire department and "Oxygen in Use" can also be obtained.
- A humidifier or open pans of water in the room will keep secretions thin.
- Fans also promote circulation of air and patient comfort. Do not direct the fan at the patient.

gency situations: performing mouth-to-stoma resuscitation, removing obstruction of the tracheostomy tube, and ensuring that the patient wears identification (MedicAlert).

10. Public health considerations

    a. Knowledge of stoma resuscitation techniques is mandatory for the patient with a tracheostomy. Provide the patient with identification as a "neck breather" and teach rescue workers to be aware of this and look for this information before instituting emergency measures.

    b. Include stoma resuscitation techniques in basic and advanced courses on cardiopulmonary resuscitation.

Bibliography

Books

Belcher AE. *Cancer Nursing.* St. Louis: Mosby–Year Book, 1992.

Blitzer A, et al. *Surgery of the Paranasal Sinuses.* 2nd ed. Philadelphia: WB Saunders, 1991.

Chips E, Clanin N, and Campbell V. *Neurologic Disorders.* St. Louis: CV Mosby, 1992.

Cummings CW, et al. *Otolaryngology–Head and Neck Surgery.* 2nd ed. St. Louis: CV Mosby, 1993.

Fairbanks DNF. *Antimicrobial Therapy in Otolaryngology–Head and Neck Surgery.* 6th ed. Alexandria, VA: American Academy of Otolaryngology–Head and Neck Surgery, 1991.

Glasscock ME, and Stambaugh GE. *Surgery of the Ear.* 4th ed. Philadelphia: WB Saunders, 1990.

Goldstein JC, Kashima HK, and Kooperman CF. *Geriatric Otolaryngology.* St. Louis: CV Mosby, 1989.

Karb VK, Queener SF, and Freeman JB. *Handbook of Drugs for Nursing Practice.* St. Louis: CV Mosby, 1989.

Kennedy DW. *Sinus Disease: Guide to First-Line Management.* Darien, CT: Health Communications, 1995.

Kim MJ, McFarland GK, and McLane AM. *Pocket Guide to Nursing Diagnosis.* St. Louis: CV Mosby, 1993.

Logemann JA. *Evaluation and Treatment of Swallowing Disorders.* San Diego, CA: College Hill Press, 1983.

McCance K, and Huether SE. *Pathophysiology: The Biologic Basis for Disease in Adults and Children.* St. Louis: CV Mosby, 1990.

Meyerhoff WL, and Rice DH. *Otolaryngology–Head and Neck Surgery.* Philadelphia: WB Saunders, 1992.

Phipps WJ, et al. *Medical-Surgical Nursing: Concepts and Clinical Practice.* 4th ed. St. Louis: CV Mosby, 1991.

Report of the Task Force on the National Strategic Research Plan of the National Institute on Deafness and Other Communication Disorders. Bethesda, MD: National Institutes of Health, 1989.

Seeley RR, Stephens TD, and Tate P. *Anatomy and Physiology.* 2nd ed. St. Louis: CV Mosby, 1992.

Seidel HM, et al. *Mosby's Guide to Physical Examination.* 2nd ed. St. Louis: CV Mosby, 1991.

Sigler BA, and Schuring LT. *Ear, Nose, and Throat Disorders.* St. Louis: CV Mosby, 1993.

Thibodeau GA, and Patton KT. *Anatomy and Physiology.* 2nd ed. St. Louis: CV Mosby, 1993.

Thompson JM, et al. *Mosby's Clinical Nursing.* 3rd ed. St. Louis: Mosby–Year Book, 1993.

Wilson SF, and Thompson JM. *Respiratory Disorders.* St. Louis: Mosby–Year Book, 1990.

Chapters in Books and Journal Articles

Ear

Curtin HD. The use of magnetic resonance imaging in otolaryngology–head and neck surgery. *Adv Otolaryngol Head Neck Surg* 5:71–107, 1991.

Gibbs L. Assessment and management of the allergic patient. *ORL-Head and Neck Nursing* 10(3):10–16, 1992.

Novak MA, Firszt JB, and Meehan K. Cochlear implants in children, part I. *Journal of the Society of Otorhinolaryngology and Head-Neck Nurses* 8(1):22–25, 1990.

Novak MA, Firszt JB, and Meehan K. Cochlear implants in children, part II. *Journal of the Society of Otorhinolaryngology and Head-Neck Nurses* 8(2):12–18, 1990.

Programmed instruction: Patient assessment: examination of the ear. *Am J Nurs* 75:457–476, 1975.

Schuring A, et al. Staging for cholesteatoma in the child, adolescent and adult. *Ann Otol Rhinol Laryngol* 99:256–260, 1990.

Schuring L. Nursing care of clients with ear disorders. *In* Luckmann J, and Sorensen K (eds). *Medical-Surgical Nursing: A Psychophysiological Approach.* Philadelphia: WB Saunders, 1993, pp 865–896.

Schuring LT. Assessment of the ear. *In* Phipps WJ, et al. (eds). *Medical-Surgical Nursing: Concepts and Clinical Practice.* 5th ed. St. Louis: CV Mosby, 1995, pp 2113–2126.

Schuring LT. Clinical standards of practice, *ORL-Head and Neck Nursing* 10(2):5, 1992.

Schuring LT. Management of patients with problems of the ear. *In* Phipps WJ, et al. (eds). *Medical-Surgical Nursing: Concepts and Clinical Practice.* 5th ed. St. Louis: CV Mosby, 1995, pp 2127–2154.

Nose and Throat

Gibbs L. Assessment and management of the allergic patient. *ORL Head Neck Nurs* 10(3):10–16, 1992.

Hereditary Hemorrhagic Telangiectasia Foundation. *Direct Connection* 14(summer), 1995.

Mabry CS, and Mabry RL. Making the diagnosis of allergy. *ORL Head Neck Nurs* 14(1):13–14, 1996.

Mabry RL. A step-by-step approach to the treatment of upper respiratory allergy. *Otolaryngol Head Neck Surg* 107:828–830, 1992.

Mabry RL. Topical pharmacotherapy for allergic rhinitis: new agents. *South Med J* 85:149–154, 1992.

Marsh BR. Foreign bodies in the air and food passages. *Adv Otolaryngol Head Neck Surg* 6:115–147, 1992.

McCall M. It killed George, or managing the peritonsillar abscess patient effectively. *ORL Head Neck Nurs* 11(1):10–13, 1993.

Miller WE. The role of the outpatient nurse in endoscopic sinus surgery. *ORL Head Neck Nurs* 10(3):20–24, 1992.

Slavin RG. Recalcitrant asthma: Could sinusitis be the culprit? *J Respir Dis* 12:182–194, 1991.

Standards of Practice Committee of the Society of Otorhinolaryngology and Head-Neck Nurses. *In Clinical Guidelines for Otorhinolaryngology-Head and Neck Nursing Practice.* New Smyrna Beach, FL: Society of Otorhinolargyngology and Head-Neck Nurses, 1994.

Head and Neck

Bryce JC. Aspiration: causes, consequences, and prevention. *ORL Head Neck Nurs* 13(2):14–23.

Cunningham MF. The management of congenital neck masses. *AM J Otolaryngol* 13:78–93, 1992.

Curtin HD. The use of magnetic resonance imaging in otolaryngology-head and neck surgery. *Adv Otolaryngol Head Neck Surg* 5:71–107, 1991.

Dropkin MJ. Coping with disfigurement and dysfunction after head and neck cancer surgery: A conceptual framework. *Semin Oncol Nurs* 5:213–219, 1989.

Isshiki N. Laryngeal framework surgery. *Adv Otolaryngol Head Neck Surg* 5:37–57, 1991.

Johnson JT. A surgeon looks at cervical lymph nodes. *Radiology* 175:607–610, 1990.

Lockhart JS. Understanding cancer of the larynx. *Focus Geriatr Care Rehabil* 5(6):1–9, 1991.

Lockhart JS, and Bryce JC. Restoring speech with tracheoesophageal puncture. *Nursing '93* 1(1):59–61, 1993.

Lockhart JS, Troff JL, and Artim LS. Total laryngectomy and radical neck dissection. *AORN J* 55:458–479, 1992.

Roberts NK. The selective approach to successful stoma management at home. *ORL Head Neck Nurs* 13(4):12–17, 1995.

Sigler BA. Nursing care of patients with laryngeal carcinoma. *Semin Oncol Nurs* 5:160–165, 1989.

Sigler BA. Nursing care of clients with upper airways disorders. *In* Black JM, and Matassarin-Jacobs E (eds). *Luckmann and Sorensen's Medical-Surgical Nursing: A Psychophysiologic Approach.* 4th ed. Philadelphia: WB Saunders, 1993, pp 993–1019.

Sigler BA, Edwards A, and Wilkerson J. Nursing care of the head and neck cancer patient. *In* Myers EN, and Suen JY (eds). *Cancer of the Head and Neck.* Philadelphia: WB Saunders, 1996, pp 818–839.

Singer MI, and Blom ED. Medical techniques for voice restoration after total laryngectomy. *CA Cancer J Clin* 40:166–173, 1990.

Stam H, Koopmans J, and Mathieson, C. The psychological impact of laryngectomy: A comprehensive assessment. *J Psychosoc Oncol* 9(3):35–57, 1991.

Standards of Practice Committee of the Society of Otorhinolaryngology and Head-Neck Nurses. In *Clinical Guidelines for Otorhinolaryngology-Head and Neck Nursing Practice*. New Smyrna Beach, FL: Society of Otorhinolaryngology and Head-Neck Nurses, 1994.

Strohl RA. The etiology and management of acute and late sequelae of radiation therapy in persons with head and neck cancers. *ORL Head Neck Nurs* 13(4):23–29, 1995.

Wingo PA, Tong T, and Bolden S. Cancer statistics, 1995. *CA Cancer J Clin* 45:8–31, 1995.

Agencies

About Face
(A support and information network for people with facial disfigurement)
99 Crowns Lane, 3rd floor
Toronto, Ontario, Canada M5R 3P4
(416) 944–FACE

Acoustic Neuroma Association
P.O. Box 398
Carlisle, PA 17013
(717) 249–4783

American Academy of Facial Plastic and Reconstructive Surgery
Suite 220
110 Vermont Avenue NW
Washington, DC 20005
(202) 842–4500

American Academy of Otolaryngic Allergy
Suite 745
8455 Colesville Road
Silver Springs, MD 20910
(301) 588–1800

American Academy of Otolaryngology–Head and Neck Surgery
One Prince Street
Alexandria, VA 22314
(703) 836–4444

American Broncho-Esophagological Association
Room 3S35
One Children's Place
St. Louis, MO 63110–1077
(314) 454–2138

American Cancer Society
National Headquarters
1599 Clifton Road NE
Atlanta, GA 30329
(404) 320–3333

American Laryngological Association
Children's Hospital Medical Center
Department of Otolaryngology
300 Longwood Avenue
Boston, MA 02115–5747
(617) 735–6417

American Laryngological, Rhinological, and Otological Society (The Triological Society)
P.O. Box 155
2023 Bethesda Church Road
East Greenville, PA 18041
(215) 679–7180

American Neurotologic Society
Michigan Ear Institute
27555 Middlebelt
Farmington Hills, MI 48334
(313) 476–4622

American Otological Society
Department of Otolaryngology
Loyola University Medical Center
2160 South First Avenue
Maywood, IL 60153
(708) 216–9183

American Rhinologic Society
Long Island College Hospital
340 Henry Street
Brooklyn, NY 11201
(718) 780–1281

American Society for Head and Neck Surgery
John Hopkins University Hospital
Department of Otolaryngology
P.O. Box 41402
Baltimore, MD 21203
(401) 955–5953

American Speech-Language-Hearing Association
Department AP
10801 Rockville Pike
Rockville, MD 20852
(301) 897–5700

American Tinnitus Association
P.O. Box 5
Portland, OR 97207
(503) 248–9985

Association for Research in Otolaryngology
Albert Einstein Medical College
Department of Otolaryngology
Bronx, NY 10461
(718) 430–4082

Council for Better Hearing and Speech Month
3417 Volta Place NW
Washington, DC 20007
(800) 327–9355

Dizziness and Balance Disorders Association of America
1015 NW 22nd Avenue
Portland, OR 97210–5198
(503) 229–7705

International Association of Laryngectomees
c/o American Cancer Society
National Headquarters
1599 Clifton Road NE
Atlanta, GA 30329
(404) 320–3333

National Association of Hearing and Speech Agencies
919 18th Street NW
Washington, DC 20006

National Information Center of Deafness
Gallaudet College
Kendall Green
Washington, DC 20002
(202) 851–5109

National Institute on Deafness and Other Communication Disorders
225 Haverford Avenue #1
Narberth, PA 19072
(610) 664–3135

Oncology Nursing Society
501 Holiday Drive
Pittsburgh, PA 15220–2749
(412) 921–7373

Self Help for Hard of Hearing People
Dept. E
4848 Battery Lane
Bethesda, MD 20814

Society of Otorhinolaryngology and Head-Neck Nurses
116-A Canal Street
New Smyrna Beach, FL 32168
(904) 428–1695

21

Caring for People with Immune and Autoimmune Disorders

■ STRUCTURE AND FUNCTION OF THE IMMUNE SYSTEM

Organs and Tissues of the Immune System

1. The cells, tissues, and organs of the immune system are strategically located throughout the body, ready to react against foreign substances that enter at any site.
2. **Lymphoid tissues** and **organs** are those in which **lymphocytes,** important cells in the specific immune response, are produced, mature, and proliferate (Fig. 21–1).
3. In the primary (central) lymphoid organs—the bone marrow and thymus—stem cell precursors mature into T and B lymphocytes capable of recognizing antigens.
   a. Bone marrow
      (1) Stem cell precursors of both T and B lymphocytes originate from the bone marrow after birth. (The liver performs this function in embryonic and fetal life.)
      (2) Stem cells differentiate into mature B lymphocytes in the spleen and other lymphoid tissues.
      (3) Immature cells destined to become T lymphocytes leave the bone marrow and migrate to the thymus gland.
   b. Thymus gland
      (1) The thymus gland is located in the anterior mediastinum above the level of the heart.
      (2) The thymus is composed of epithelial cells and is divided into 2 lobes, which are surrounded by a capsule. Each lobe is divided into an outer and an inner medulla.
      (3) T-cell precursors leave the bone marrow and migrate into the cortex of the thymus gland. There they differentiate, under the influence of thymic hormones such as thymosin and thymopoietin, into immunocompetent cells capable of recognizing antigens.
      (4) Differentiated T cells leave the cortex and migrate into the medulla from which they exit the thymus gland, enter the general circulation, and are transported to the secondary lymphoid tissues.
      (5) The thymus reaches its maximum size by puberty and then gradually atrophies. This thymic involution has been implicated in the increased frequency of immune disorders in older adults.

4. The secondary lymphoid system—which includes the lymph nodes, spleen, tonsils, appendix, and mucosal lymphatic tissues—has a structure that traps antigens in proximity to the mature T and B lymphocytes residing in these tissues. When lymphocytes encounter antigens, they undergo proliferation and further differentiation. B cells differentiate into antibody-producing plasma cells, and T cells differentiate into a variety of cytotoxic and lymphokine-secreting cells (effector cells).
   a. Lymph nodes
      (1) **Lymph nodes** are round or oval structures, normally less than 1 cm in diameter, located along the lymphatic vessels throughout the body.
      (2) Lymph nodes consist of an outer cortex, a middle paracortex, and an inner medulla. B cells occupy the cortex; T cells occupy the paracortex. The medulla contains both T and B cells.
      (3) Foreign substances (antigens) enter the lymph nodes through the afferent lymphatic vessels. Macrophages that line the lymph node sinuses phagocytose the antigens and present them to T and B lymphocytes in the lymph nodes.
      (4) Those lymphocytes capable of recognizing a particular antigen are stimulated to proliferate and differentiate in germinal centers, causing the lymph nodes to enlarge.
      (5) Lymphocytes (T cells more so than B cells) and antibodies leave the lymph nodes through the efferent lymphatic vessels and circulate in the lymphatic fluid.
      (6) Lymphatic vessels drain into the thoracic duct, which empties into the vena cava. Therefore, lymphocytes and antibodies circulate between the lymphatic fluid and the blood.
   b. Spleen
      (1) The spleen is located in the left upper quadrant of the abdomen behind the stomach.
      (2) The spleen is divided into white pulp and red pulp. White pulp is lymphatic tissue consisting of a central area of T lymphocytes and an outer area of B lymphocytes. Red pulp filters blood and destroys senescent and abnormal red blood cells.
      (3) Antigens that enter the spleen are processed by macrophages, which present them to T and B lymphocytes. The lymphocytes then proliferate and differentiate in germinal centers of the spleen.

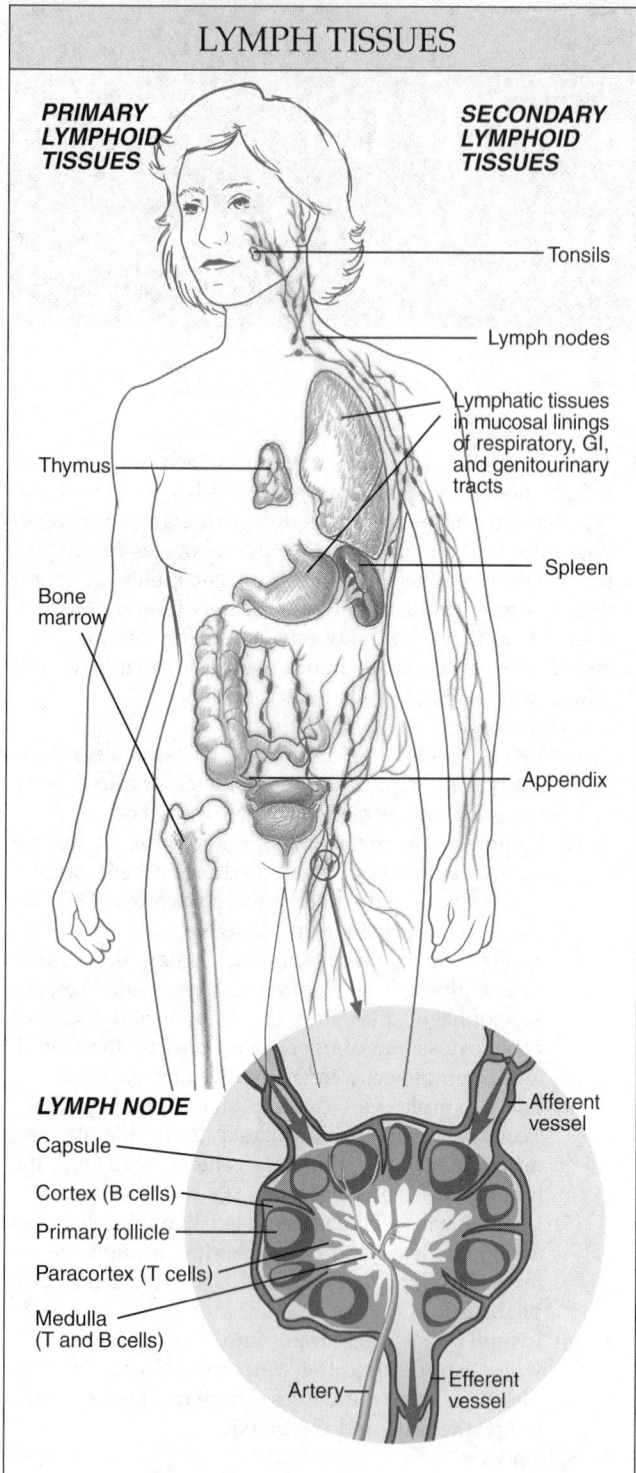

LYMPH TISSUES

PRIMARY LYMPHOID TISSUES

SECONDARY LYMPHOID TISSUES

Tonsils

Lymph nodes

Lymphatic tissues in mucosal linings of respiratory, GI, and genitourinary tracts

Thymus

Spleen

Bone marrow

Appendix

LYMPH NODE

Capsule

Cortex (B cells)

Primary follicle

Paracortex (T cells)

Medulla (T and B cells)

Afferent vessel

Artery

Efferent vessel

Figure 21–1. *Top,* Primary and secondary lymphoid tissues and organs. *Bottom,* Structure of a lymph node.

c. Miscellaneous lymphoid tissues
   (1) Mucosa-associated lymphoid tissues (MALT) are aggregates of T and B lymphocytes and phagocytic cells dispersed throughout the mucosal linings of the respiratory, gastrointestinal, and genitourinary tracts. They are the 1st line of defense against invasion by foreign antigens at points of entry into body cavities.
   (2) Gut-associated lymphoid tissues (GALT) consist of follicles of lymphatic tissue and include the appendix and Peyer's patches in the intestines.
   (3) Follicles of lymphoid tissue are also present in the back of the mouth (lingual and palatine tonsils) and in the pharynx (pharyngeal tonsil).

Nonspecific Body Defenses Against Infection

1. Physical barriers
   a. Physical, or anatomic, barriers are the 1st line of defense against infection.
   b. Physical barriers include intact skin and mucous membranes lining the respiratory, gastrointestinal, and genitourinary tracts.
   c. Conditions that break the integrity of these barriers and increase susceptibility to infection include the following:
      (1) Skin: burns, pressure ulcers, surgical or accidental trauma
      (2) Intestinal tract: intestinal ischemia, prolonged absence of enteral feeding
      (3) Genitourinary tract: bladder catheterization
2. Physiologic barriers: If a foreign substance penetrates the physical barriers, the body often eliminates it by mechanical removal or chemical inactivation before it penetrates into tissues.
   a. Mechanical removal of foreign substances
      (1) Skin sloughing
      (2) Gastrointestinal peristalsis
      (3) Vomiting
      (4) Cough and sneeze reflexes (impaired by general anesthetics and central nervous system depressant drugs)
      (5) Flushing action of tears, saliva, and urine (impaired by urinary stasis)
      (6) Mucocilliary clearance of the airways (impaired by cigarette smoking)
   b. Chemical inactivation of foreign substances
      (1) Lysozyme, an enzyme that hydrolyzes bacterial cell membranes. Lysozyme is present in saliva, nasal and intestinal secretions, tears, and perspiration.
      (2) Acid pH of body secretions: Hydrochloric acid in the stomach results in a pH as low as 1 or 2. This environment is toxic to many ingested microorganisms. This protective mechanism is deficient in individuals who ingest drugs that raise gastric pH (e.g., antacids or cimetidine) and in individuals with achlorhydria. Acid pH of saliva and vaginal secretions also inhibits the proliferation of some microorganisms.
      (3) Cutaneous secretions: Fatty acid secretions by sebaceous glands have antibacterial and antifungal effects. Sweat glands secrete high concentrations of sodium chloride, which inhibits the proliferation of some microorganisms.

(4) Bile: Bile acts like a detergent and decreases surface tension, which weakens the cell membrane of some organisms and makes them more susceptible to hydrolysis by digestive enzymes. Bile provides a protective mechanism against ingested microorganisms.

(5) Normal flora: Normal flora, consisting of microorganisms that colonize the skin, mouth, throat, intestines, and vagina are protective because they control the growth of certain pathogenic microorganisms. The balance of normal flora can be upset during antimicrobial therapy. For example, antibiotic therapy can lead to the overgrowth of fungi or of bacteria resistant to that antibiotic. Normal flora can cause infections if they are transferred from areas they normally colonize to other areas of the body. For example, bacteria that colonize the mouth or throat can cause pneumonia if they are displaced into the lungs during intubation or by aspiration.

3. Cellular barriers: Cells of the immune system consist of leukocytes (white blood cells [WBCs]) distributed throughout the blood, lymph, and tissues of the body. These cells are all derived from stem cells in the bone marrow. Cells are classified into 3 types based on their functions: phagocytic cells, mediator cells, and cells of the specific immune response. The various cell types interact to amplify the immune response and ensure its effectiveness. Regulatory mechanisms keep these cells under control so they do not damage healthy body tissues. In certain disease states, however, these regulatory mechanisms become overwhelmed, and tissue damage results.

a. **Phagocytes:** The function of phagocytic cells is to ingest and destroy foreign substances and cell debris, thereby preventing the spread of infection or toxins and promoting healing. Phagocytic cells accomplish this by producing cytokines, hydrolytic enzymes, and toxic reactive oxygen metabolites (oxygen radicals). Table 21–1 summarizes chemical mediators involved in immune defenses.

(1) **Polymorphonuclear neutrophils (PMNs),** a type of granulocyte, are characterized by a nucleus divided into 3 to 5 lobes. These cells are also called segmented neutrophils. They contain numerous granules in the cytoplasm filled with hydrolytic enzymes that function in phagocytosis. Production of PMNs is stimulated by infection or injury. Only mature PMNs function in phagocytosis. Immature neutrophils are called bands. An increase in the number of circulating bands is called a shift to the left. This shift indicates acute infection. The PMNs leave their site of origin in the bone marrow and circulate in the blood for up to 48 hours. They then migrate into tissues, where they live for a few days and complete their life cycle. Polymorphonuclear neutrophils are very effective phagocytes and an important defense against the spread of infection. They contain receptors for the Fc component of antibodies, and therefore antibody-coated substances are more readily phagocytosed.

They also contain receptors for the activated C3 component of the complement system, and substances coated with complement are also more readily phagocytosed.

(2) **Monocytes and macrophages:** Mononuclear phagocytic cells mature from stem cells in the bone marrow and enter the blood as monocytes, where they circulate for approximately 24 hours. Monocytes then migrate into tissues, where they develop into macrophages and live for several months to years. Macrophages are capable of consuming invading organisms, parasites, and necrotic tissue. Free macrophages circulate through the vascular endothelium and collect at sites of inflammation. Special types of macrophages are located in the liver (Kupffer's cells), connective tissue (histiocytes), kidney (mesangial phagocytes), spleen (dendritic cells), and nervous system (microglial cells). They are also present in peritoneal, pleural, and synovial fluids. Most monocytes are fixed macrophages, or **histiocytes,** which engulf whole microorganisms and debris in the liver, spleen, lungs, lymph nodes, bone marrow, and adrenal and pituitary glands. Macrophages play a central role in the immune response not only because they are effective phagocytes but also because they process and present antigens to T and B lymphocytes, which activates a specific immune response against the antigens. Macrophages contain receptors for the Fc component of antibodies and for complement. Antigens coated with these substances, therefore, are more effectively phagocytosed.

(3) **Eosinophils:** A type of granulocyte, eosinophils contain cytoplasmic granules with enzymes and a basic protein that binds acid dyes such as eosin. Eosinophils are much less effective phagocytes than are the PMNs or macrophages. Eosinophils have 4 main functions:

- Protecting against infections by helminths (parasitic worms) by releasing the toxic contents of their granules into the extracellular space, where they contact and damage the surface of helminths
- Participating in the inflammatory response by secreting proinflammatory chemical mediators (see Table 21–1)
- Controlling inflammatory and allergic reactions by producing histaminases and arylsulfatases, which inactivate some of the chemical mediators that produce the symptoms of inflammation and allergy
- Assisting with the elimination of blood clots through secretion of plasmin, a clot-dissolving enzyme

b. **Mediator cells:** Mediator cells consist of basophils and mast cells, whose primary functions are to synthesize and secrete chemical mediators of inflammation and allergy.

(1) **Basophils:** Circulating in the blood, basophils contain receptors for the Fc component of immuno-

Table 21–1. Chemical Mediators of the Inflammatory and Immune Responses

Mediator	Source	Effects
Histamine	Mast cells Basophils Platelets	Vasodilation, increased vascular permeability, smooth muscle contraction
Serotonin	Platelets Mast cells	Vasodilation, increased vascular permeability
Bradykinin	Plasma kinin system activated by tissue injury	Vasodilation, increased vascular permeability, pain, smooth muscle contraction
Platelet-activating factor (PAF)	Lipid in cell membranes of basophils, neutrophils, macrophages	Platelet aggregation, increased vascular permeability, smooth muscle contraction, neutrophil activation, eosinophil chemotaxis, eicosanoid production
Neutrophil chemotactic factor	Mast cells	Neutrophil chemotaxis
Eosinophil chemotactic factor	Mast cells	Eosinophil chemotaxis
Eicosanoids		
Prostaglandins	Arachidonic acid in cell membranes metabolized by the enzyme cyclooxygenase	Vasodilation or vasoconstriction, increased vascular permeability, pain
Leukotrienes	Arachidonic acid in cell membranes metabolized by the enzyme lipoxygenase	Neutrophil chemotaxis, increased vascular permeability, smooth muscle contraction in bronchioles, increased adhesiveness of endothelial cells
Complement Components		
C3a	Serum complement system	Smooth muscle contraction, degranulation of mast cells
C5a	Serum complement system	Neutrophil and macrophage chemotaxis, neutrophil activation, mast cell degranulation, increased vascular permeability
Reactive Oxygen Metabolites (Oxygen Radicals)		
Superoxide, hydroxyl radical, hydrogen peroxide, singlet oxygen	Neutrophils Macrophages	Structural damage to cell lipids, protein including metabolic enzymes, and DNA
Cytokines		
Interleukin-1 (IL-1)	Macrophages Vascular endothelial cells Lymphocytes Neutrophils Fibroblasts	Fever, drowsiness, eicosanoid production, chemotaxis of neutrophils and macrophages, production of other cytokines, B- and T-cell activation, collagen synthesis, increased endothelial cell adhesiveness
Interleukin-2 (IL-2)	Helper T cells Natural killer (NK) cells	T- and B-cell proliferation
Interleukin-3 (IL-3)	Helper T cells NK cells Mast cells	Proliferation of T cells, mast-cell proliferation and degranulation, growth of bone marrow stem cells
Interleukin-4 (IL-4)	Helper T cells	T- and B-cell proliferation, enhanced phagocytosis by neutrophils and macrophages, decreased production of several other cytokines (anti-inflammatory effect), mast-cell growth factor, decreased adherence of neutrophils to blood vessel wall
Interleukin-5 (IL-5)	Helper T cells	B-cell proliferation and differentiation, maturation of cytotoxic T cells
Interleukin-6 (IL-6)	Helper T cells B cells Macrophages Vascular endothelial cells	B-cell differentiation, T-cell proliferation, fever, production of acute phase reactants, activation of macrophages
Interleukin-7 (IL-7)	Bone marrow	Differentiation of bone marrow stem cells
Interleukin-8 (IL-8)	Macrophages Endothelial cells	Chemotaxis and activation of neutrophils and T cells, decreased neutrophil adherence to blood vessel wall
Interleukin-9 (IL-9)	Helper T cells	T-cell and mast-cell proliferation
Interleukin-10 (IL-10)	Helper T cells B cells	Differentiation of cytotoxic T cells, decreased production of other cytokines
Tumor necrosis factor	Macrophages	Fever, drowsiness, shock (in high concentrations), production of other cytokines, necrosis of tumor cells, B-cell proliferation, increased endothelial adhesiveness, endothelial cell damage, increased vascular permeability
Interferon	Many cell types	Inhibition of viral replication, activation of NK cells
Transforming growth factor beta	Platelets Lymphocytes Macrophages	Tissue repair, decreased oxygen radical production, decreased neutrophil adherence to blood vessel wall, macrophage chemotaxis

globulin E (IgE). When an allergen binds to IgE molecules on the basophil, it cross-links them, increasing the permeability of the basophil-releasing chemicals and causing increased vascular permeability and smooth muscle contraction. Basophils are nonphagocytic cells that secrete heparin, which prevents clot formation. Basophils also secrete **histamine,** which plays a major role in anaphylaxis and other systemic reactions. They also speed removal of lipids from the blood after ingestion of fatty meals.

(2) Mast cells: Rather than circulating in the blood, mast cells are located in most tissues near blood vessels. Mast cells contain receptors for IgE and function in allergic reactions like basophils. Mast cells also function in the inflammatory response.

c. Cells of the specific immune response: Lymphocytes are the cells of the specific immune response. Specific clones of lymphocytes recognize and react to different foreign antigens in an individualized manner. The recognition of antigen occurs through receptors on the lymphocyte cell membrane that have a structure complementary to that of an antigen. Lymphocytes divide into B lymphocytes, or B cells, and T lymphocytes, or T cells, and plasma cells.

(1) **B lymphocytes (B cells):** Originating in the bone marrow and maturing in various secondary lymphoid tissues, B lymphocytes are involved in the humoral immune response, which protects mainly against viral and bacterial infections. When a clone of B lymphocytes is activated by an antigen, usually presented by macrophages, they proliferate and mature into antibody-producing **plasma cells.** They also help form lymphoid follicles of lymph nodes in the spleen and other tissues.

(2) **T lymphocytes (T cells):** T lymphocytes are involved in the cell-mediated immune response, which protects against viral infections, cancer cells, and slow-growing bacteria such as those causing tuberculosis. They also are important in the rejection of transplanted organs. When a specific clone of T lymphocytes is activated by antigen, usually presented by macrophages, the cells proliferate and differentiate into effector and regulator T cells. Effector T cells consist of cytolytic T cells and natural killer (NK) cells, both of which cause the destruction of cells with foreign antigens on their surface. Regulator T cells consist of helper T cells, which amplify the immune response by activating T and B cells, and suppressor T cells, which limit the immune response to prevent tissue injury. T cells contain surface markers or receptors referred to as clusters of differentiation (CD).

- All mature T cells contain CD2, CD3, CD5, and CD7.
- Helper T cells also contain CD4 and are therefore called T4 cells.
- Cytolytic and suppressor T cells also contain CD8 and are therefore called T8 cells.

4. The inflammatory response is an immediate and nonspecific response to tissue injury or infection, that is, the response is the same regardless of the initiating event. Inflammation delivers cells and chemical mediators to a site of injury or infection to wall off the area, destroy toxins, clean the area of cell debris, and repair damaged tissues.

a. Inflammation is triggered by any condition causing tissue injury. The sequence of events is depicted in Figure 21–2. Conditions leading to inflammation include the following:
- Infection: invasion by any pathogenic organism
- Mechanical injury: blunt or penetrating trauma
- Immune reactions: allergic reactions and immune complex formation
- Chemical injury: exposure to strong acids or bases or any corrosive chemical
- Tissue necrosis: cell death due to ischemia, for example
- Thermal injury: burns, frostbite

b. In the vascular phase, an immediate and transient vasoconstriction occurs in response to injury, followed by a more prolonged vasodilation and increased vascular permeability.

(1) Vascular alterations involve the arterioles, capillaries, and venules.

(2) Vasodilation begins within minutes of the initiating event, resulting in an acute increase in blood flow (hyperemia) to the site of injury, making this area warm and red (erythematous).

(3) Early vasodilation is the result of histamine and serotonin released from mast cells (see Table 21–1 for a summary of mediators involved in inflammation).

(4) The increased blood flow delivers cells, oxygen, and metabolic substrates to the area to facilitate immune defenses and healing.

(5) Histamine also causes contraction of vascular endothelial cells, increasing the space between these cells and resulting in increased vascular permeability.

(6) The increased capillary permeability causes fluid to leak out of the vascular compartment into the interstitial space, producing edema. The loss of plasma and subsequent increased viscosity of blood in the area can cause the red blood cells to stack up (rouleaux formation). The edema fluid contains serum proteins that can coagulate and seal off the area.

(7) Late vasodilation, occurring 6 to 12 hours after injury, is the result of a number of chemical mediators, including arachidonic acid metabolites, bradykinin, fibrin degradation products, and cytokines produced by phagocytic cells and lymphocytes.

c. In the cellular phase, the coordinated action of phagocytic cells and lymphocytes begins within 1 hour of the initiating event and lasts up to several days.

(1) The acute cellular phase occurs within the 1st hour of the initiating event and involves the migration of PMNs out of the blood vessels to the site of inflammation.

THE PROCESS OF INFLAMMATION

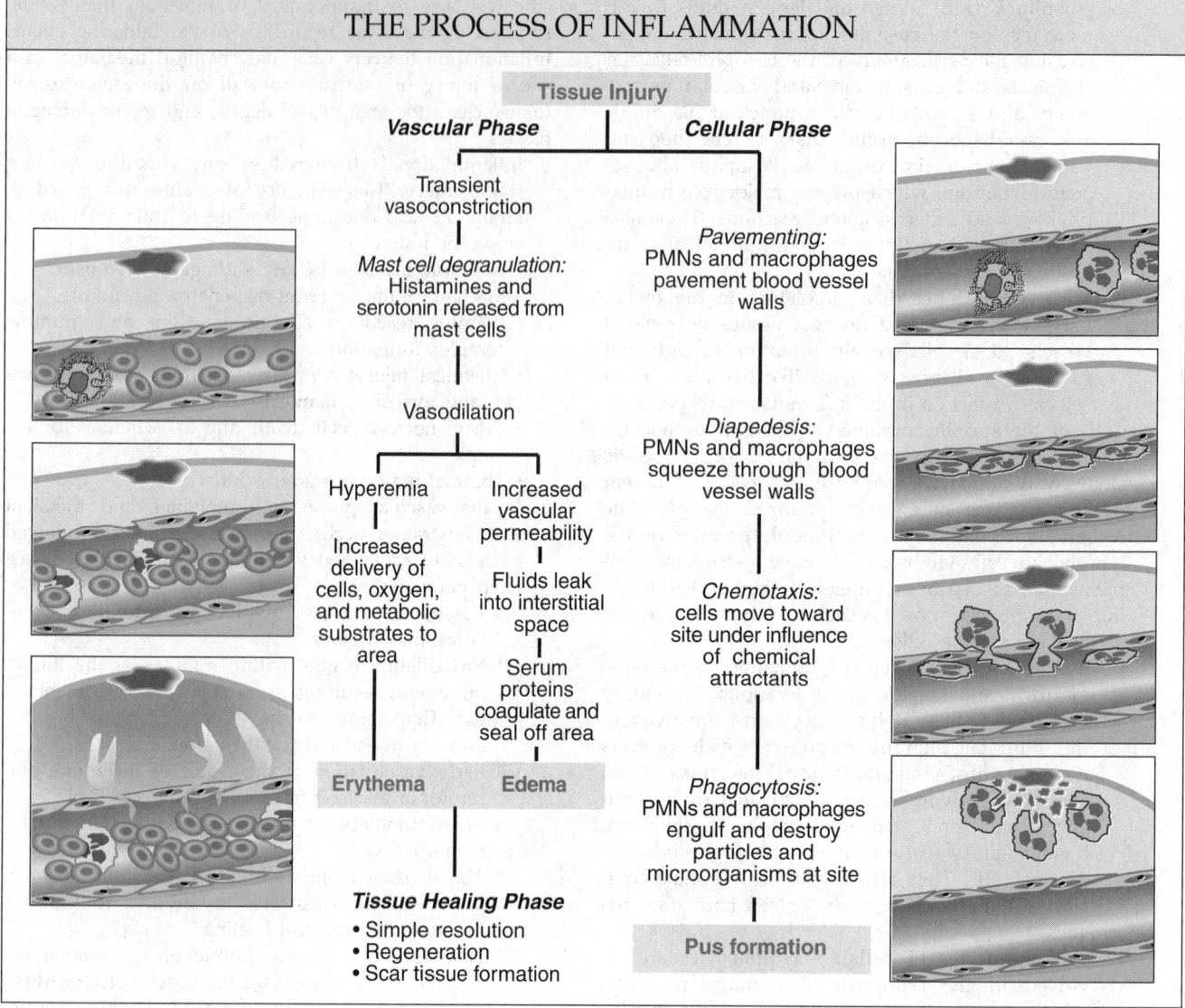

Figure 21–2.

(2) The chronic cellular phase occurs within 6 hours of the initiating event and involves macrophage and lymphocyte infiltration. The lymphocytes initiate a specific immune response.

(3) Mobilization of phagocytic cells in inflammation occurs in the following sequence:
- Pavementing: PMNs and macrophages bind to adhesion receptors on endothelial cells, pavementing a section of the blood vessel.
- Diapedesis: PMNs and macrophages squeeze through the spaces between the adjacent endothelial cells by an ameboid movement. Some red blood cells, platelets, basophils, and eosinophils are passively pushed out into the interstitial space. Hemoglobin released from these red blood cells causes skin discoloration.
- Chemotaxis: Cells move toward the site of inflammation under the influence of chemical attractants such as leukotrienes, complement component C5a, and platelet-activating factor.

- Phagocytosis: Phagocytosis is the process by which cells, such as PMNs and macrophages, engulf and destroy particles and microorganisms. Substances attach to the surface of the phagocytic cell by way of nonspecific receptors or receptors specific for antibody or complement attached to the substance. The phagocytic membrane surrounds the substance and ingests it, forming a phagosome. The phagosome fuses with lysosomes, which are sacks of hydrolytic enzymes. During phagocytosis, the cells undergo a respiratory burst during which they consume increased amounts of oxygen and produce toxic oxygen metabolites (oxygen radicals) that help in the destruction of the substance.

(4) Cell infiltration can localize and inactivate damage caused by the initiating event. If cellular infiltration is not effective, tissue injury can extend to surrounding areas, causing increasing organ dysfunction. If cellular infiltration is not effective in

controlling an infection, microorganisms can invade adjacent tissues and lymphatics, where they encounter additional phagocytic cells and lymphocytes. If the lymphoid system does not adequately control the infection, microorganisms can gain access to the blood and become widely disseminated, causing a systemic infection that can be lethal.

(5) The last phase of the inflammatory response begins approximately 1 day after the initiating event and involves tissue healing.

- Simple resolution occurs when there has been no destruction of tissue, and healing only requires clean-up of the area.
- Regeneration is the replacement of damaged cells with the same type of cells by the process of cell division of the remaining healthy cells. Only tissues with cells capable of mitosis, such as the liver, skin, and epithelium, can heal by regeneration. Regeneration allows for full return of function.
- Scar tissue formation occurs in tissues with cells that are not capable of mitosis, such as the heart and skeletal muscle. Damaged cells are replaced through the proliferation of fibroblasts, which synthesize collagen-forming scar tissue. Scar tissue adds structural integrity but is nonfunctional (e.g., scar tissue in the heart does not contract).

(6) If the cause of inflammation cannot be removed, it can become chronic and last for months or years, with resultant tissue injury and loss of function. Causes of chronic inflammation include continuous presence of microorganisms, persistent presence of antigen-antibody complexes, as in rheumatoid arthritis, and the presence of substances that are not readily phagocytosed, such as silica or asbestos.

(7) Inflammation can occur systemically, producing a condition known as the **systemic inflammatory response syndrome,** which is associated with life-threatening effects resulting from massive tissue injury, systemic vasodilation causing hypotension, and widespread increased vascular permeability causing loss of plasma volume. Conditions that can trigger systemic inflammatory response syndrome include sepsis, multiple trauma, severe burn injury, and pancreatitis.

Immune Response

1. The specific immune response involves individual recognition and reaction to different antigens. Two types of specific immune responses are cell-mediated immunity (CMI), involving T lymphocytes, and humoral immunity (HI), involving B lymphocytes. T and B lymphocytes recognize different antigens through receptors on their cell surface that have a complementary fit to that antigen.
2. The targets of the immune response are antigens. Most often these are protein molecules, but they can also be nucleic acids or polysaccharides. Antigens can be free or attached to a cell surface. In pathologic conditions such as autoimmune disorders, the immune response can also be directed against self-antigens, or human leukocyte antigens (HLAs).
3. The immune response involves cooperation among phagocytic cells, T and B lymphocytes, and a variety of chemical mediators (see Table 21–1).
4. In antigen processing and presentation, foreign antigens enter the body and usually 1st encounter macrophages distributed throughout the blood, lymphoid, and other tissues.
   a. Macrophages ingest and process antigens by combining fragmented antigens with their major histocompatibility (MHC), or self, antigens and transporting the 2 to the cell surface (Fig. 21–3).
   b. Macrophages present the antigen in a form that can be recognized by T and B cells, stimulating their activity. B cells can recognize an antigen without its being associated with an MHC molecule. T cells have receptors for antigen that can recognize antigen only in combination with the MHC antigens of the macrophage. The T cell binds to the macrophage, which secretes interleukin-1 (IL-1). Interleukin-1 stimulates the T cell to secrete IL-2, which drives T cells to proliferate.
5. **Clonal selection** is the process by which a T- or B-cell clone with receptors specific for a particular antigen is activated to proliferate and differentiate. Antigen binds only to those T or B cells with a complementary surface receptor, so that only cells capable of reacting against the antigen are stimulated to proliferate. The result of clonal selection is the production of a large number of lymphocytes capable of reacting to a specific antigen.
6. **Cell-mediated immunity** involves the action of T cells, which are dependent on the thymus for their maturation.
   a. Types of T lymphocytes
      (1) T helper cells, which amplify the immune response of T and B cells
      (2) T suppressor cells, which limit the immune response of T and B cells
      (3) Cytotoxic T cells, which directly attack and rupture cells with foreign antigens on their surface
      (4) Natural killer cells, which are cytotoxic to other cells but do not require prior sensitization to antigen as do the cytotoxic T cells
   b. Cell-mediated immunity is a defense against antigens that enter cells and are not available to attack by antibodies in the extracellular fluid. For example, CMI destroys virus-infected cells and prevents viral replication and infection of other cells. It also recognizes abnormal antigens on cancer cells and destroys the cells. Cell-mediated immunity can cause delayed hypersensitivity reactions.
7. Humoral immunity involves the action of B lymphocytes and the production of antibodies. HI is an important defense against bacteria and other extracellular microorganisms. Each B cell carries 1 type of receptor (actually an antibody molecule) on its surface, and when stimulated by antigen, the B cell proliferates and

ANTIGEN PROCESSING AND PRESENTATION

Activation of T and B lymphocytes

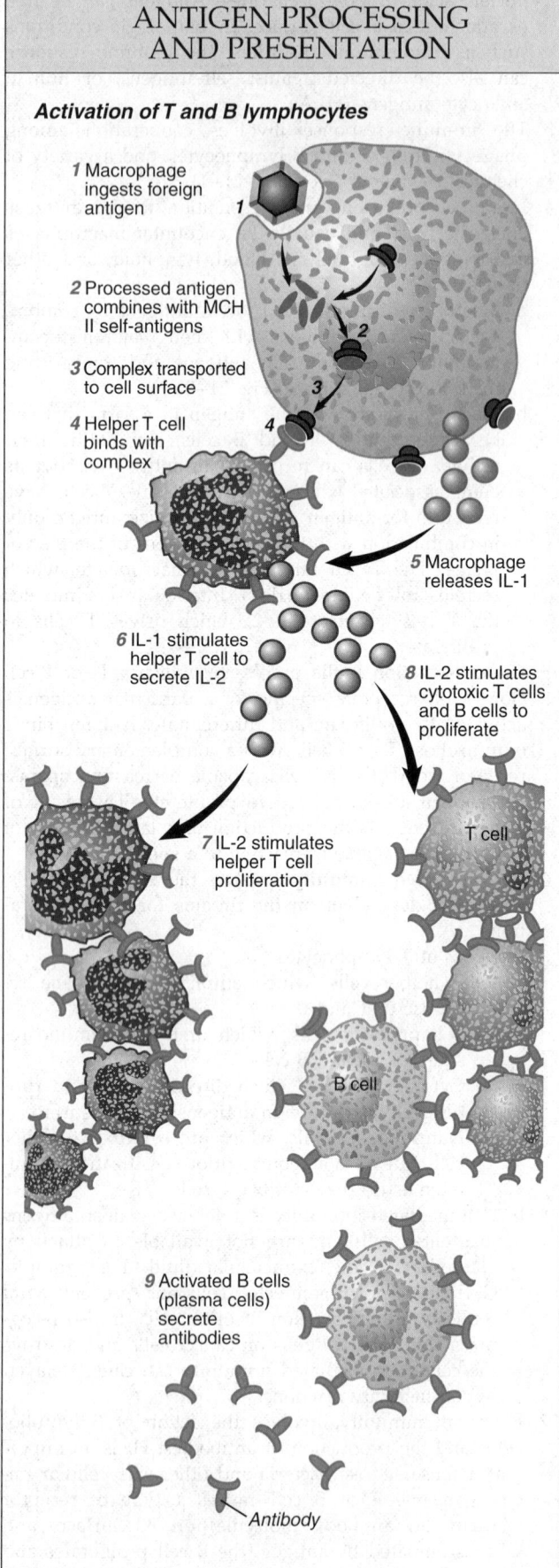

1 Macrophage ingests foreign antigen

2 Processed antigen combines with MCH II self-antigens

3 Complex transported to cell surface

4 Helper T cell binds with complex

5 Macrophage releases IL-1

6 IL-1 stimulates helper T cell to secrete IL-2

8 IL-2 stimulates cytotoxic T cells and B cells to proliferate

7 IL-2 stimulates helper T cell proliferation

T cell

B cell

9 Activated B cells (plasma cells) secrete antibodies

Antibody

Figure 21–3.

differentiates into a plasma cell that produces that same type of antibody. Antibody characteristics are summarized in Figure 21–4. Table 21–2 lists the properties of immunoglobulins.

   a. The **primary immune response** occurs on first exposure to a particular antigen. A lag phase of usually 48 to 72 hours follows exposure to the antigen before antibodies can be detected in the blood. Antibody titers then increase, plateau, and decrease as they are catabolized or consumed in immune complex reactions. IgM is the major antibody of the primary immune response.

   b. The **secondary immune response** occurs upon the 2nd and all subsequent exposures to a particular antigen. The lag phase is much shorter than that in the primary immune response. Antibody titers increase to a higher level and remain elevated longer than in the primary response. IgG is the major antibody of the secondary immune response.

8. After antigenic stimulation, some T and B cells differentiate into memory cells, which are long lived and carry receptors for the antigen that stimulated their produc-

STRUCTURE OF ANTIBODIES

Antibodies (immunoglobulins) consist of 4 chains arranged in the shape of the letter Y. Each antibody unit contains 2 heavy and 2 light chains and has 2 sites where it can bind antigens.

Antibody structure (immunoglobulin molecule)

SS = disulfide bonds

Light chain

Antigen-binding region

Heavy chain

SS

SS

SS

SS

Biologic activity mediation

There are 5 classes of immunoglobulins with different biologic properties. Within each of the 5 classes, there are thousands of different antibody configurations, allowing for interaction with thousands of different antigens.

Antibodies facilitate the destruction of foreign antigens by neutralizing toxins; activating the complement system; opsonizing (coating) antigens and, thus, enhancing phagocytosis; precipitating soluble antigens; and agglutinating cells with foreign antigen on their surfaces.

Figure 21–4.

Table 21–2. Immunoglobulin Levels and Functions

	Isotype				
	IgG	*IgA*	*IgM*	*IgD*	*IgE*
Molecular weight	150,000	160,000 for monomer	900,000	180,000	200,000
Additional protein subunits	–	J and T or S	J	–	–
Approximate concentration in serum (mg/ml)	12	1.8	1	0–0.04	0.00002
Percent of total Ig	80	13	6	0.2	0.002
Distribution	Equal: intravascular and extravascular	Intravascular and secretions	Mostly intravascular	Present on lymphocyte surface	On basophils and mast cells present in saliva, nasal secretions
Half-life (days)	23	5.5	5	2.8	2.0
Placental passage	++	–	–	–	–
Presence in secretion	–	++	–	–	–
Presence in milk	+	+	0 to trace	–	–
Activation of complement	+	–	+++	–	–
Binding to Fe receptors on macrophages and polymorphonuclear cells	++	–	–	–	–
Relative agglutinating capacity	+	++	+++	–	–
Antiviral activity	+++	+++	+	–	–
Antibacterial activity (gram negative)	+++	++ (with lysozyme)	+++ (with complement)	–	–
Antitoxin activity	+++	–	–	–	–
Allergic activity	–	–	–	–	++

J, J chain (peptide chain associated with polymeric immunoglobulins); T, T piece (protein associated with secretory immunoglobulin); S, secretory piece, also known as T piece; +, positive (or reactive); ++, moderately positive (reactive); +++, strongly positive (reactive); –, negative (nonreactive, or not detected).
From Benjamini E, and Leskowitz S. *Immunology: A Short Course.* New York: John Wiley & Sons, 1991. Reprinted by permission of Wiley-Liss, Inc., a subsidiary of John Wlley & Sons, Inc.

tion. On subsequent encounters with that same antigen, T or B memory cells rapidly mount an immune response. Memory cells provide the long-term specific immunity that develops after certain infections and after immunizations.

9. The immune response is regulated by the action of regulatory T cells and a variety of chemical mediators.
   a. Helper T-cell function: Many antigens are T-cell dependent—that is, they require recognition by T as well as B cells to stimulate antibody production. T cells and B cells bind to different sites on an antigen, which links these 2 cells. T cells then secrete a chemical mediator that stimulates the B cells to produce antibodies. Therefore, disorders that directly affect helper T cells (e.g., human immunodeficiency virus [HIV] infection) can indirectly impair B-cell function.
   b. Suppressor T-cell function: Suppressor T cells limit the action of both T and B cells. This process normally prevents the immune response from getting out of control and damaging body tissues. A deficiency in suppressor T cells has been linked to autoimmune diseases.
10. See Figure 21–5 for a review of the complement system.
11. Innate and acquired immunity
   a. **Innate immunity (natural immunity)** is the natural resistance to infection that a person inherits. Components of innate immunity include the physical barriers and nonspecific physiologic and cellular mechanisms. Innate immunity is nonspecific, so that the response to any foreign antigen is similar.
   b. **Acquired immunity (adaptive immunity)** can develop at any time. It protects the body against infection through specific recognition of different foreign antigens and activation of specific populations of T or B cells, or both. Acquired immunity can be active or passive.
   (1) **Active acquired immunity** develops in response to exposure to pathogenic organisms or their products either by natural exposure due to an infection or by artificial exposure during immunizations. Active acquired immunity provides long-term protection due to the production of memory T and B cells capable of recognizing and rapidly activating the immune response against the same foreign antigen on subsequent exposures.
   (2) **Passive acquired immunity** develops after having received antibodies produced in vitro or by another person. This type of immunity does not involve activation of the person's own T or B cells. Passive acquired immunity develops rapidly but is temporary because memory cells are not produced. The immunity lasts only during the life span of the components received, up to a few months at most. Passive immunity includes the following:
   • Transfer of maternal IgG across the placenta to the fetus, which provides an immune defense for the newborn for the 1st few months after birth

THE COMPLEMENT SYSTEM

The complement system is a group of serum proenzymes (inactive enzymes) that interact with one another. The activation of 1 of the proenzymes causes the activation of the next, and so on, resulting in a cascade effect.

Various complement components have different effects:
- Opsonization of antigens
- Chemotaxis of phagocytic cells
- Activation of the inflammatory response
- Lysis of cell membranes

There are 2 pathways of complement activation: classic and alternative.

Classic Pathway
Activated by antigen-antibody complexes, this pathway facilitates the clearance of these complexes. Note that IgG and IgM are the only immunoglobulins that activate this pathway. Enzymes of the classic pathway are designated by the letter C and a number. Fragments of the complement components produced in the cascade reaction are designated with a subscript **a** or **b**, and activated enzymes are designated with a superscript bar. A deficiency in this pathway causes an increased susceptibility to immune complex diseases because this pathway normally facilitates the clearance of immune complexes.

Alternative Pathway
Activated mainly by bacteria with or without the presence of antibody and by complex polysaccharides such as those in bacterial and fungal cell walls, and certain enzymes, this system bypasses some of the early classic pathway components and enters at the point of C3.

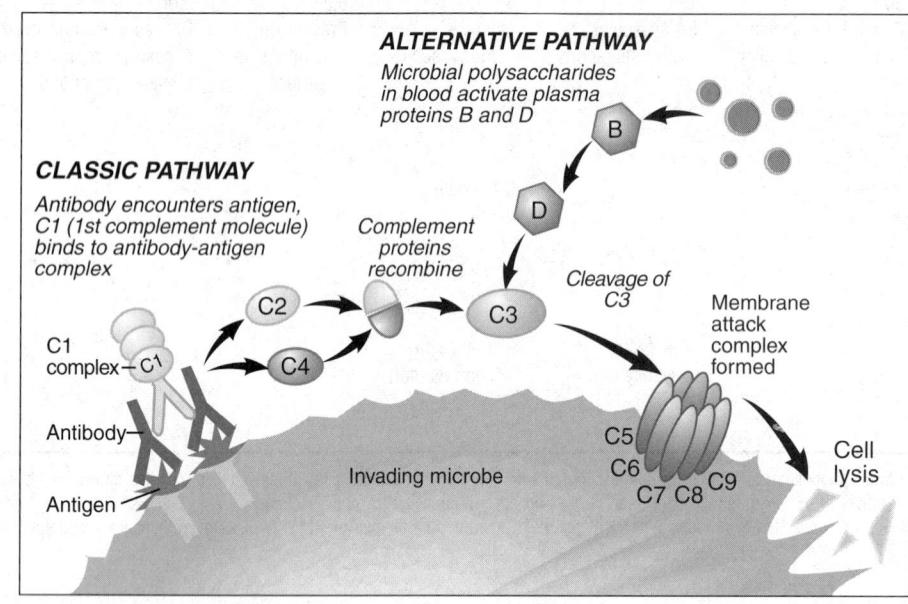

ALTERNATIVE PATHWAY
Microbial polysaccharides in blood activate plasma proteins B and D

CLASSIC PATHWAY
Antibody encounters antigen, C1 (1st complement molecule) binds to antibody-antigen complex

Complement proteins recombine

Cleavage of C3

Membrane attack complex formed

C1 complex — C1
Antibody
Antigen
Invading microbe
C2   C4   C3
C5 C6 C7 C8 C9
Cell lysis

Figure 21–5.

- Maternal IgA transferred to infants in breast milk
- Injection of antibody-enriched serum (antiserum)

Distinguishing Self from Non-self

1. The immune system can distinguish self from non-self, that is, self-antigens from foreign antigens. Self-antigens are proteins on the surface of all nucleated cells. They are called **MHC antigens.** They are also called **human leukocyte antigens** because they were 1st discovered on leukocytes.
   a. The ability to tolerate self **(autotolerance)** is a crucial characteristic of the immune system. Autotolerance allows the body to recognize and attack foreign invaders without attacking its own structures. The **clonal deletion theory** explains this phenomenon. Any immature T or B lymphocytes developing in the thymus or bone marrow, respectively, that are able to react against self are inactivated (become anergic) or are destroyed. Deletion of self-reacting lymphocyte clones occurs because lymphocytes require stimulation of 2 different membrane signal systems when they encounter foreign antigens. In the presence of self-antigens, however, only 1 membrane signal system is stimulated, and the lymphocytes become inactive or die.
   b. Self-reacting immune cells that are not destroyed or inactivated can cause autoimmune diseases.
2. Major histocompatibility antigens
   a. Class I MHC self-antigens are the products of 3 loci on chromosome 6 designated HLA-A, HLA-B, and HLA-C. The many subtypes of these antigens are designated by numbers, such as HLA-A1, HLA-B5.
      (1) Class I antigens are present on almost all nucleated cells and platelets.
      (2) Class I antigens direct cytotoxic T cells to virus-infected cells. T cells recognize MHC antigens when they are in combination with viral antigen on the surface of an infected cell.
   b. Class II MHC antigens are the product of a gene locus designated HLA-D. Class II antigens are present on the surface of antigen-presenting cells (APCs), such as macrophages.
      (1) CD4 (helper) T cells recognize antigen that has been processed by APCs. The foreign antigen on the surface of the APC is presented to T cells in combination with the MHC class II antigens of the APC.

(2) After recognizing foreign antigens, the T cells are stimulated to proliferate under the influence of macrophage mediators such as IL-1.
c. The MHC antigens on cell membranes in transplanted organs trigger an immune response in the recipient that can cause organ rejection. Because of the wide diversity of MHC antigens that can be inherited, usually only identical twins share the exact same pattern of MHC antigens. Tissue typing to assess for similarity of MHC antigens between donor and recipient is important because the greater the difference in these antigens, the more severe the rejection is likely to be.
3. Inheritance of certain MHC antigens is associated with an increased susceptibility to certain diseases. For some diseases this increased risk is greater than for others. Inflammatory, autoimmune, and metabolic enzyme deficiency disorders have been linked to certain MHC antigens (Table 21–3).
a. Several mechanisms have been proposed to explain the association between certain MHC antigens and disease
(1) Genes regulating the expression of certain MHC antigens may also regulate immune responsiveness, leading to an overactive immune response to certain self-antigens or foreign antigens. Tissue injury then occurs.
(2) Certain MHC antigens may have a complementary structure for some viruses that facilitate their attachment and entry into cells.
(3) Microorganisms that have an antigen similar to an MHC antigen may be tolerated by the immune system and avoid attack.
(4) Microorganisms that have an antigen similar to an MHC antigen may activate an immune response that then cross-reacts with cells having the MHC antigen on their surface.
b. Associated diseases do not develop in all individuals with certain MHC antigens because other factors, including gene products and environmental factors, influence disease expression.

Developmental Aspects of the Immune Response

1. Immune function in neonates and infants
a. Humoral immunity: The ability to produce antibodies is immature in the infant at birth and does not reach full capacity until between 6 and 15 years of age. Therefore, neonates and infants have an increased susceptibility to infections, especially those of bacterial origin.
(1) IgG: The neonate's major protective immunoglobulin is maternal IgG transported across the placenta into the fetal circulation in utero (other maternal antibodies do not cross the placenta). Maternal IgG is gradually catabolized and disappears by approximately 9 months of age. The neonate's ability to produce IgG begins shortly after

birth and reaches 60 percent of full capacity by 1 year and full capacity between 6 and 10 years.
(2) IgM: The 1st antibody that the fetus is able to synthesize, beginning at approximately 5 months' gestation, is IgM. Elevated IgM levels in umbilical cord blood indicate an intrauterine infection. IgM production reaches approximately 75 percent of full capacity by the 1st year of life and full capacity by age 2 years.
(3) IgA: The neonate can produce very low amounts of IgA. IgA production is only 20 percent of full capacity by 1 year and reaches full capacity between 6 and 15 years of age.
(4) IgE: Production of IgE reaches full capacity between 6 and 15 years of age.
b. Cell-mediated immunity: The number of T cells and their ability to proliferate in response to antigenic stimulation is comparable to an adult's, but the ability of T cells to destroy antigens is low at birth. The thymus is largest in relation to body size shortly after birth and reaches its greatest weight at puberty.
c. Phagocytic cell function: Phagocytosis by macrophages and neutrophils occurs at adult levels in infants, but chemotaxis by macrophages and neutrophils is decreased.
2. Immune function in older adults
a. Humoral immunity: The number of B cells does not change significantly with aging, but the ability to produce antibodies in response to antigenic stimulation decreases, probably because of decreased activity of helper T cells, which occurs with aging. An increased level of autoantibodies may be associated with the greater incidence of autoimmune disorders with aging.
b. Cell-mediated immunity: The thymus gland atrophies with age, with decreased production of thymic hormones required for T-cell maturation. The decreased ability of T cells to produce IL-2, a T-cell growth factor, is linked to the decreased proliferation of T cells in response to antigenic stimulation. Delayed hypersensitivity reactions (type IV) are diminished. Decreased natural killer cell activity in some older adults is linked to an increased incidence of cancer.
c. Phagocytic cell function: No significant change occurs in healthy, older adults.

Interactions Among Nervous, Endocrine, and Immune Systems: Psychoneuroimmunology

1. A complex bidirectional communication and regulatory network exists between the immune system and the neuroendocrine system. Research demonstrating the link across immune, nervous, and endocrine systems has increased the understanding of disease mechanisms and led to new possibilities for therapy. Many studies have implicated psychologic stressors as causative agents in immunosuppression, resulting in increased susceptibility to diseases such as cancer, autoimmunity, and infection.

Table 21–3. Diseases Showing Positive Human Leukocyte Antigen Associations

	Disease	HLA	Relative Risk*
Rheumatic	Ankylosing spondylitis	B27	69.1
	Reiter's syndrome	B27	37.0
	Acute anterior uveitis	B27	8.2
	Reactive arthritis (*Yersinia, Salmonella,* gonococcus)	B27	18.0
	Psoriatic arthritis, central	B27	10.7
		B38	9.1
	Psoriatic arthritis, peripheral	B27	2.0
		B38	6.5
	Juvenile rheumatoid arthritis	B27	3.9
	Juvenile rheumatoid arthritis, pauciarticular	DR5	3.3
	Rheumatoid arthritis	Dw4/DR4	3.8
	Sjögren's syndrome	Dw3	5.7
	Systemic lupus erythematosus	DR3	2.6
Gastrointestinal	Gluten-sensitive enteropathy	DR3	11.6
	Chronic active hepatitis	DR3	6.8
	Ulcerative colitis	B5	3.8
Hematologic	Idiopathic hemochromatosis	A3	6.7
		B14	26.7
		A3, B14	90.0
	Pernicious anemia	DR5	5.4
Skin	Dermatitis herpetiformis	DR3	17.3
	Psoriasis vulgaris	Cw6	7.5
	Psoriasis vulgaris (Japanese)	Cw6	8.5
	Pemphigus vulgaris (Jews)	DR4	14.6
		A26	4.8
	Behçet's disease	B5	3.8
Endocrine	Insulin-dependent diabetes mellitus (juvenile diabetes mellitus)	DR4	3.6
		DR3	4.8
		DR2	0.2
		BfF1†	15.0
	Graves' disease	B8	2.5
		DR3	3.7
	Graves' disease (Japanese)	B35	4.4
	Addison's disease	Dw3	10.5
	Subacute thyroiditis (de Quervain)	B35	13.7
	Hashimoto's thyroiditis	DR5	3.2
	Congenital adrenal hyperplasia	Bw47	15.4
Neurologic	Myasthenia gravis (without thymoma)	B8	3.3
	Multiple sclerosis	Dw2/DR2	2.7
	Manic–depressive disorder	B16	2.3
	Narcolepsy	DR2	130.0
	Schizophrenia	A28	2.3
Renal	Idiopathic membranous glomerulonephritis	DR3	5.7
	Goodpasture's syndrome (anti-GBM)	DR2	15.9
	Minimal change disease (steroid responsive)	DR7	4.2
	IgA nephropathy (French, Japanese)	DR4	3.1
	Gold/penicillamine nephropathy	DR3	14.0
	Polycystic kidney disease	B5	2.6
Infection	Tuberculoid leprosy (Asians)	B8	6.8
	Paralytic polio	B16	4.3
	Low vs high response to vaccinia virus	Cw3	12.7

* Relative risk $= \dfrac{(\%\text{antigen–positive patients} \times \%\text{antigen–negative controls})}{(\%\text{antigen–negative patients} \times \%\text{antigen–positive controls})}$

† BfF1 is an allele of the complement system that is HLA-linked but is not an antigen.
HLA, Human leukocyte antigens.
From Carpenter CB. The major histocompatibility gene complex. *In* Braunwald E, et al. (eds). *Harrison's Principles of Internal Medicine.* 11th ed. New York: McGraw-Hill Book Co, 1987. Reproduced with permission of the McGraw-Hill Companies.

Thought-induced enhancement of the immune response to control cancer is being investigated. Improved coping mechanisms can increase a person's ability to handle stressors and decrease the risk for certain diseases.

2. Effects of the immune system on the neuroendocrine system
   a. Immune components detect microorganisms and signal the neuroendocrine system to mount a stress response.
   b. Leukocytes affect brain function by secreting chemical mediators. For example, macrophages secrete IL-1, which affects the hypothalamic heat regulatory center, resulting in a fever. Interleukin-1 also increases the secretion of corticotropin-releasing hormone from the hypothalamus.
   c. Antigen activation of the immune system increases firing of neurons in the hypothalamus.
   d. Some immune cells secrete adrenocorticotropic hormone, thyroid-stimulating hormone, and endorphins, which can affect endocrine function.

3. Effects of the neuroendocrine system on the immune system
   a. Lymphoid organs innervated by the sympathetic nervous system include the lymph nodes, thymus, bone marrow, and spleen.
   b. Lymphatic cells in these organs have membrane receptors for the neurotransmitters of the sympathetic nervous system.
   c. The sympathetic nervous system innervates the adrenal gland and stimulates the release of glucocorticoid hormones, which have anti-inflammatory and immune-suppressive properties.

Interaction Between Nonspecific and Specific Immune Defenses

1. The body is constantly exposed to microorganisms both from the external environment and the natural flora. People coexist with microorganisms on the skin, in the gastrointestinal tract, and in body orifices. The immune response normally prevents these organisms from causing serious infection. Components of the immune system cooperate with each other, using cytokines, which act as chemical signals to amplify the immune response in times of infection. (Chapter 8 describes infectious processes.)

2. Immune defenses against bacteria: Bacteria that enter the body usually are checked by phagocytic cells such as macrophages and PMNs.
   a. Antibodies produced by B lymphocytes can neutralize certain bacterial toxins or bind to bacteria and enhance their phagocytosis. Antibodies are especially important in enhancing the phagocytosis of encapsulated bacteria, such as pneumococci, because phagocytic cells do not effectively bind to the polysaccharides in bacterial capsules.
   b. Antibodies bound to bacteria activate the classic complement pathway, resulting in bacterial lysis.

   c. Endotoxin, a lipopolysaccharide component of the cell wall of gram-negative bacteria, directly activates the alternative complement pathway, resulting in bacterial lysis without the need for antibodies.

3. Immune defenses against viruses: Viruses are intracellular pathogens and therefore are not always readily accessible to direct attack by antibodies in the extracellular fluid. Two CMI responses are important in resistance to viral infections.
   a. Cellular cytotoxicity: Large granular lymphocytes, or cytotoxic T cells, recognize viral antigens that become inserted into the cell membrane of virus-infected cells. These infected cells are recognized as non-self and destroyed by the immune cells. In antibody-dependent cell-mediated cytotoxicity, antibodies coat virus-infected cells and enhance their destruction by T cells.
   b. Lymphokine production: In response to viral infections, lymphocytes secrete chemical messengers known as lymphokines. Some lymphokines attract or activate phagocytic cells. Interferon is a lymphokine that protects uninfected cells by stimulating them to produce a substance that inhibits viral replication.

4. Immune defenses against fungi: CMI is a primary defense against fungal infections. In immunocompetent individuals, fungal infections are usually superficial and self-limiting. In individuals with deficient CMI, fungal infections can become systemic and life threatening.

5. Immune defenses against helminths: Helminths (parasitic worms) are multicellular organisms too large to be phagocytosed by white blood cells. Helminthic infections trigger the production of IgE, which causes degranulation of mast cells with release of chemicals, including histamine and eosinophil chemotactic factor. Eosinophils bind to the helminth and discharge their toxic contents onto the organism, damaging its cell membrane.

ASSESSING PEOPLE WITH IMMUNE AND AUTOIMMUNE DISORDERS

Key Symptoms and Their Pathophysiologic Bases

1. Fever: Fever is caused by the release of cytokines from phagocytic cells. These cytokines circulate and reach the temperature control center in the hypothalamus, where they reset body temperature to a higher level.

2. Recurrent infections: The immune response is critical in the defense against invasion by pathogenic organisms. A deficit in components of this system allows these organisms to proliferate uncontrolled.
3. Allergies: Overactivity of the immune system leads to release of chemical mediators, causing the symptoms of allergy.
4. Lymphadenopathy and splenomegaly: Enlargement of the lymph nodes and spleen can be caused by increased proliferation of immune cells in the lymph nodes or spleen, as occurs during an infection.
5. Joint pain: Several autoimmune disorders are associated with inflammation and pain in the joints (e.g., rheumatoid arthritis).

Physical and Psychosocial Health History

1. Determine the chief complaint.
   a. Ask the person the reason for seeking assistance regarding health, and quote the response in the record.
   b. Ask follow-up questions to elicit more information about the chief complaint.
2. Obtain the person's medical history to determine whether a preexisting immune disorder had been diagnosed or if symptoms suggest one.

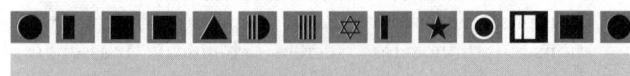

TRANSCULTURAL CONSIDERATIONS

In cultures in which blood plays a central role in health and illness beliefs, patients may understand disease as "bad blood." Be careful, however, to explore the meaning of "bad blood" with the person. Bad blood may mean anything from general vulnerability to infection to a specific sexually transmitted disease.

   a. Ask the person about hypersensitivity disorders such as allergies, asthma, rhinitis, or eczema; when the disorder started; and what the symptoms are.
   b. Ask whether there are recurrent infections, their location, and causative organisms, and whether they developed recently or have been present since childhood.
   c. Ask whether the person has or has had cancer and what type.
   d. Ask whether the person has an autoimmune disease such as rheumatoid arthritis or systemic lupus erythematosus.
   e. Obtain information about immunization history, effectiveness of immunizations, and any adverse reactions.
   f. Ask about treatments that can affect immunity, such as chemotherapy for cancer, radiation therapy, organ transplantation, or splenectomy.
3. Document medications that the person takes, including home remedies and over-the-counter and prescription drugs.
   a. Ask whether the person is taking any immunosuppressant medications, such as corticosteroids, cyclo-

sporine, other drugs to prevent transplant rejection, or cancer chemotherapy.
   b. Ask about the intake of drugs commonly associated with allergic reactions, such as salicylates, penicillins, and cephalosporins.
   c. Ask about alcohol intake because alcohol can cause immunosuppression.
   d. Ask whether the person is using any illegal drugs, such as heroin or cocaine, because intravenous injection of these can increase the risk of infections, including hepatitis and HIV infection.
4. Obtain the family history because some immune disorders are inherited.
   a. Ask whether any family members have a disorder associated with altered immunity, such as recurrent infections, allergies, cancer, or autoimmune disease.
   b. Ask about the outcome of pregnancies and whether there is a family history of early infant deaths, which could be due to severe immune deficiency.

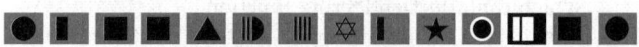

TRANSCULTURAL CONSIDERATIONS

For some ethnic and social groups, especially immigrants from some Third World countries, inquire about the number of pregnancies rather than the number of infants who died. Early infant deaths and stillbirths may not otherwise be counted.

5. Identify the person's occupation, noting possible exposure to allergens or infectious agents in the work environment.
6. Inquire about the person's psychosocial history.
   a. Ask about any major changes in the person's life, such as a birth, death, marriage, divorce, or job change. Also ask about support systems available to help the person cope with stressors. Impaired ability to cope with life's stressors is linked to immune impairment.
   b. Ask about the person's sexual history because homosexuality, bisexuality, or having more than 1 sexual partner increases the risk of acquiring sexually transmitted diseases, including hepatitis and HIV infection.

Physical Examination

1. Examination of the spleen (Fig. 21–6)
2. Examination of the lymph nodes (Fig. 21–7)

Special Diagnostic Studies

1. White blood cell (leukocyte) counts
   a. Total WBC count: The normal total WBC count for an adult ranges from 4500 to 10,000 cells per cubic millimeter of blood (4.5 to 10×10^9/L in system international units). In healthy adults, the WBC count can

SPLENOMEGALY (ENLARGED SPLEEN)

Splenomegaly can develop in immune disorders in which there is increased production or increased destruction of cells in the spleen, for example, in lymphomas, hemolytic anemia, idiopathic thrombocytopenia purpura, and mononucleosis.

Percussion of the Spleen
The spleen is located under the diaphragm posterior to the midaxillary line. Perform percussion to obtain an estimate of the size of the spleen:
1 Percuss along the left lower thorax posterior to the midaxillary line.
2 Percuss over the lowest intercostal space on the left anterior line.
3 Percuss out in several directions from the end of an area of resonance (*lung tissue*) to the area of tympany (*stomach and intestines*).
   Normal-sized spleen: a small area of dullness heard between the 6th and 10th ribs
   Splenomegaly: the normal tympanic sound of the hollow stomach and colon is replaced by dullness, because of the enlarged spleen. Dullness on percussion above the 6th rib or over a large area between the 6th rib and the costal margin also suggests splenomegaly. If dullness is not heard, ask the patient to take a deep breath and percuss this area again. If the spleen is normal in size, the sound elicited usually remains tympanic. However, because deep inspiration pushes the spleen forward, dullness will be heard if the spleen is enlarged.

Palpation of the Spleen
A normal-sized spleen is not palpable because it lies under the rib cage. However, in a few people, the tip of a normal-sized spleen can be palpated, in the presence of a low diaphragm or deep descent of the diaphragm during inspiration, as occurs in disorders of chronic airflow limitation. If you can palpate the spleen, it is usually enlarged 3 times normal size.
1 Stand to the right side of the patient, who should be lying supine.
2 Proceed to palpate gently, because an enlarged spleen is at risk for rupturing.
3 Reach across the patient, placing your left hand under the posterior left lower rib cage and press it forward to lift the spleen anteriorly.
4 Place your right hand under the left costal margin and press in with your fingertips, feeling for the spleen. Feel for a notch along the middle border to differentiate it from an enlarged kidney.
5 Ask the patient to take a deep breath to cause the spleen to descend.
   Normal-sized spleen: will not descend below the 10th intercostal space.
   Splenomegaly: tip of the spleen becomes palpable below the left costal margin during deep inspiration. As splenomegaly progresses, the spleen will descend into the left lower quadrant. A grossly enlarged spleen can extend across the midline.
6 Repeat splenic palpation with the patient lying on the right side with knees and hips flexed. In this position, gravity causes the spleen to descend forward and to the right.

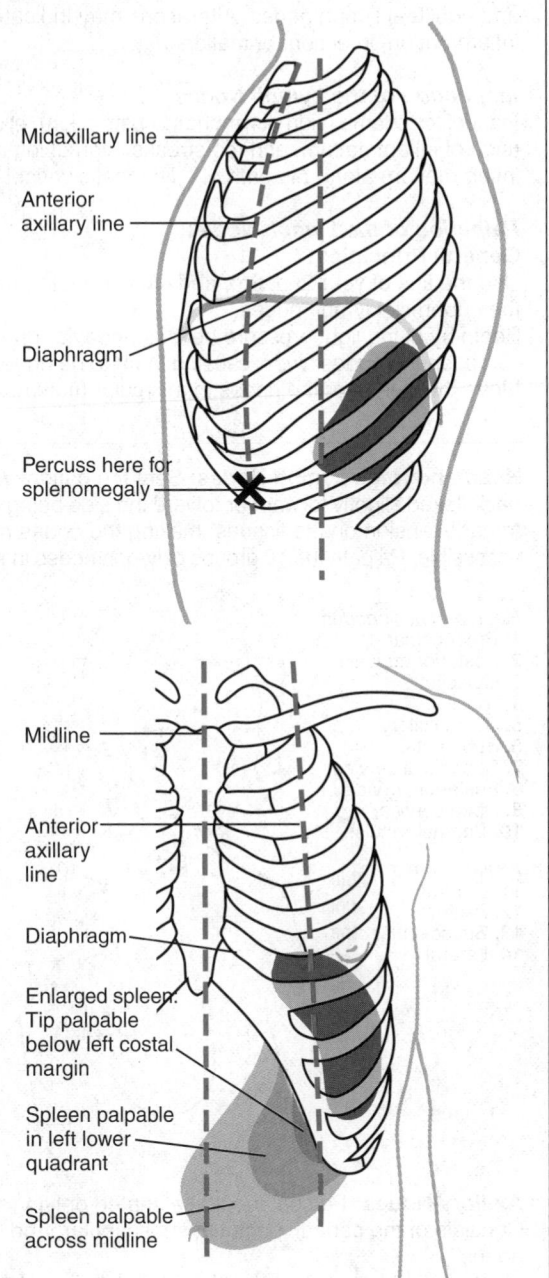

Figure 21–6.

vary from day to day by up to 2000 cells per mm³ as a result of strenuous exercise, stress, or metabolic alterations.
(1) **Leukopenia** is a decrease in the total number of WBCs in the blood.
(2) **Leukocytosis** is an increase in the total number of WBCs in the blood.
b. Differential WBC count: The WBC differential measures the percentage of the 5 different types of WBCs in the blood (Table 21–4). The total WBC count can be normal, increased, or decreased with a change in the percentage of 1 or more cell types. Because the WBC differential provides information about which cell type is altered, it aids in the diagnosis of the underlying disorder.
(1) Assess both the percentage and the absolute number of the different cell types. The percentage of a cell type can increase, but the absolute number of cells can remain normal because of a decrease in the number of another cell type.

Superficial lymph nodes are found in subcutaneous tissues. Examine the head, neck, axillary, epitrochlear, inguinal, and popliteal lymph nodes. Alterations may indicate inflammation, infection, or malignancy.

Inspection of the Lymph Nodes
Inspect for edema (sign of lymphatic obstruction), erythema (sign of inflammation), and red streaks (sign of infection or inflammation) along the path of a lymphatic vessel.

Palpation of the Lymph Nodes
General Principles:
Use the tips of your 2nd, 3rd, and 4th fingers to palpate the superficial lymph nodes.
Begin by using light pressure because heavier pressure can push the nodes away, causing them to be undetected. Move the skin over the nodes in a circular motion.

Compare nodes on each side of the body for
- **Size:** Most lymph nodes are normally too small to palpate. Those that can be palpated in a healthy individual are small (usually less than 1 cm in diameter). If lymph nodes are enlarged (lymphadenopathy), note if this is localized or generalized, that is, involving 3 or more groups.
- **Shape:** should be discrete round or oval structure, not matted together
- **Consistency:** cancerous nodes are harder than normal
- **Mobility:** should be movable, both sideways and up and down, under your fingers and not feel fixed to surrounding tissues
- **Tenderness:** Tenderness on touch or rebound is often an indication of inflammation; cancerous nodes are usually nontender
- **Temperature:** increased warmth often indicates infection or inflammation

---

Head and Neck Lymph Nodes: Seat the patient with the neck flexed slightly forward or toward the side being examined to ease tension on the tissues, making the nodes more accessible. Palpate the 10 groups of lymph nodes in sequence.

Head and neck nodes:
1. Preauricular
2. Posterior auricular
3. Occipital
4. Tonsilar
5. Submaxillary
6. Submental
7. Superficial cervical
8. Posterior cervical
9. Deep cervical
10. Supraclavicular

Axillary nodes
11. Central
12. Pectoral
13. Subscapular
14. Lateral

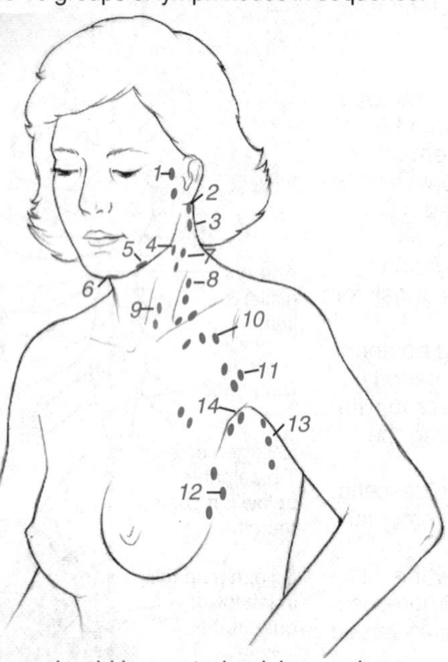

Axillary Nodes: Person should be seated or lying supine. Consists of the central, pectoral, subscapular, and lateral nodes.
Central: Most frequently palpable of the axillary nodes because the other axillary nodes drain into them. Reach deep into the apex of the axilla with your fingers pointing toward the middle of the clavicle and press against the chest wall.
Pectoral (anterior): Palpate inside the anterior axillary fold. Try to feel them between thumb and fingers while gently squeezing the anterior axillary fold.
Subscapular (posterior): Palpate inside the muscle of the posterior axillary fold. Best position to palpate is from behind the patient.
Lateral (brachial): Palpate along the uppermost humerus deep in the axilla, fingers pointing toward the middle of the clavicle, and press against the chest wall.

Epitrochlear Nodes:
Person should be seated or lying supine. Palpate in the medial aspect of the arm 2 to 3 cm above the elbow.

Inguinal and Popliteal Nodes: Place the patient in the supine position with knees slightly flexed.
Inguinal Group:
Horizontal nodes are located in the anterior thigh below the inguinal ligament.
Vertical nodes are located near the upper region of the saphenous vein below the inguinal ligament.
Popliteal Group:
Located behind the knees.

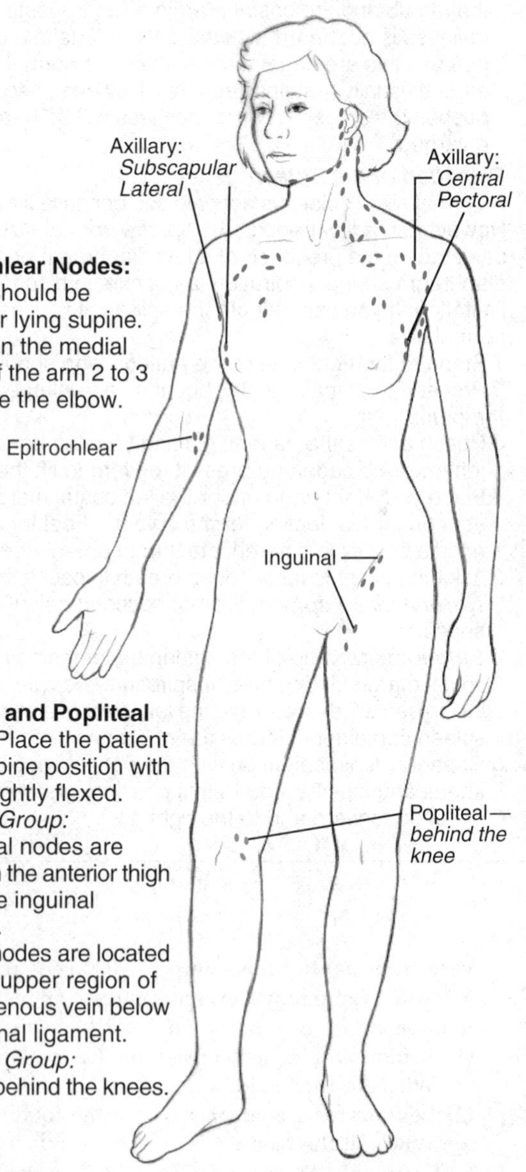

Figure 21–7.

Table 21–4. White Blood Cell Differential

Cell Type	Normal Values*		Factors Causing a Decrease	Factors Causing an Increase
	% of Total Count	Actual Number (cells/mm³)		
Granulocytes				

Neutrophils
  Segmented (mature)
  Banded (immature)
	50–70%	2000–8000	Neutropenia—bone marrow depression, some viral infections, overwhelming infection especially in the immunocompromised or seriously ill, malnutrition, hypersplenism, cancer chemotherapy, some diuretics and antibiotics	Neutrophilia—infections: bacterial, rickettsial, and some viral; severe physical or psychologic stress; corticosteroid therapy; inflammatory conditions; tissue necrosis; renal failure

Eosinophils	1–4%	50–400	Eosinopenia—elevated glucocorticoid levels, severe stress, infectious mononucleosis, indomethacin and procainamide	Eosinophilia—helminthic infections, allergy, adrenocortical insufficiency, splenectomy
Basophils	0.3–2%	25–100	Basopenia—acute allergic reactions, severe stress, chronic corticosteroid therapy, hyperthyroidism	Basophilia—chronic inflammation, recent splenectomy, basophilic leukemia
Monocytes	2–6%	100–600	Monocytopenia—HIV infection, high-dose corticosteroids, hairy cell leukemia	Monocytosis—certain viral, rickettsial, and protozoal infections; recovery stage of acute bacterial infections; tuberculosis; monocytic leukemia; autoimmune collagen disorders
Lymphocytes	20–40%	1000–4000	Lymphopenia—HIV infection and AIDS, bone marrow depression, immunosuppressive drug therapy	Lymphocytosis—viral infection, lymphocytic leukemia, autoimmune disorders, infectious mononucleosis

* Values represent normal ranges for adults.
  HIV, Human immunodeficiency virus; AIDS, acquired immunodeficiency virus.

(2) To obtain the absolute number of cells, the percentage for that cell type is multiplied by the total WBC count. A shift to the left in the WBC differential indicates an increase in the percentage of immature forms of WBCs. An increase in immature WBCs in the blood occurs in acute infections and malignancies of the WBC-forming tissues. A shift to the right in the WBC differential indicates an increase in the percentage of mature forms of WBCs. This shift can occur with an increased number of mature neutrophils needed to clear up tissue damage (e.g., as a result of burns, surgery, electrical or traumatic injuries, ischemia, or malignancy).

2. Studies of immune cell function: In addition to quantifying immune cells, it is important to assess their ability to function in the immune response. A person could have a normal cell number but still have recurrent infections (e.g., because the cells fail to function properly).

   a. Tests of neutrophil function

      (1) Tests of motility: The normal random movement of neutrophils can be assessed by adding a sample of the person's neutrophils to a capillary tube. The tube is observed hourly, and the distance that the neutrophils move from the starting point can be seen with a microscope.

      (2) Tests of chemotaxis: The ability of neutrophils to move toward a chemical attractant is measured and indicates their ability to move toward microorganisms during an infection. Two methods are commonly used to assess neutrophil chemotaxis. In a polarization assay, the neutrophil sample is incubated with a chemotactic factor. A change in shape of the neutrophils, from the spheric shape in a nonstimulated state, indicates a polarized movement toward the chemotactic factor. In Boyden chamber chemotaxis, neutrophils are placed in an upper chamber and are separated from a chemotactic factor in a lower chamber by a filter. Movement of the neutrophils to the lower side of the filter indicates chemotaxis has occurred.

      (3) Tests of phagocytic and killing capacity involve quantifying the number of microorganisms that survive phagocytosis. In assessing phagocytosis of bacteria, neutrophils are exposed to a solution of staphylococci and allowed time to phagocytose them. The unphagocytosed bacteria in the solution are then counted. In assessing phagocytosis of

yeast, neutrophils are exposed to *Candida*, and dead yeast cells are then counted by their inability to exclude a blue dye. In a nitroblue tetrazolium (NBT) test, neutrophils are stimulated to start phagocytosis by the addition of bacterial endotoxin. A yellow dye is added. If neutrophils are undergoing phagocytosis, they will ingest the dye and metabolize it, turning the dye blue. The blue color in the neutrophil is measured spectrophotometrically. At least 80 percent of the neutrophils in the sample should phagocytose the dye.

b. Tests of B lymphocyte function: B-cell function is usually assessed by measuring levels of immunoglobulins, which are the product of mature B cells and the mechanism by which B cells destroy antigens.

(1) A plaque-forming cell test measures the ability of mature B cells to secrete IgG or IgM. These immunoglobulins, in the presence of complement, produce a clear area, a plaque, in a plate of red blood cells because of the lysis of the antigen-sensitized red blood cells.

(2) Immunoglobulin levels: Table 21–2 lists normal immunoglobulin levels. Routine immunoglobulin tests measure levels of IgA, IgG, and IgM by nephelometry, which is based on light scattering caused by particles such as antigen-antibody precipitates or by immunoelectrophoresis. Because little is known about the function of IgD, it is measured only in rare cases (e.g., when an IgD-producing myeloma is suspected). IgE levels are measured in persons suspected of having an atopic (allergic) disorder or an infection caused by helminths because IgE levels are elevated in these 2 conditions. Because IgE levels are lower than those of the other immunoglobulins, they are measured by more sensitive tests such as radioimmunoassay (RIA) or enzyme-linked immunosorbent assay (ELISA).

(3) Detection of autoantibodies: Immunofluorescence is used to measure autoantibodies. If present, autoantibodies become labeled with a fluorescent molecule and can be seen with a microscope that has an ultraviolet light source. A positive result indicates an autoimmune process.

• Indirect immunofluorescence: The person's serum is added to a slice of the type of tissue suspected of being the target of autoantibodies, such as the thyroid, pancreas, or muscle. The tissue slice is then washed to remove any unbound antibodies. Next, the tissue slice is exposed to antihuman immunoglobulins labeled with fluorescein. If the person's serum contains autoantibodies against the tissue tested, the tissue fluoresces and is visible with an ultraviolet microscope.

• Direct immunofluorescence: A biopsy sample is obtained of the person's tissue suspected of being the target of autoantibodies. Antihuman immunoglobulin labeled with a fluorescent molecule is incubated with the biopsy sample. If autoantibodies are present, they bind the fluo-

rescent molecules and can be seen when the tissue is examined with an ultraviolet microscope.

• **Rheumatoid factor** is an IgM molecule that acts against a person's own IgG molecules and is often associated with rheumatoid arthritis. In testing for rheumatoid factor latex beads are coated with IgG and incubated with the person's serum sample. If rheumatoid factor is present in the serum, the latex beads agglutinate.

• Coombs' tests detect antigen-antibody complexes on red blood cells. A **direct Coombs' test** detects antibodies that agglutinate red blood cells. A positive test result occurs in autoimmune hemolytic anemia, drug-induced hemolysis, hemolytic disease of the newborn, and transfusion reactions. An **indirect Coombs' test** detects antibodies that cannot agglutinate red blood cells by themselves because they are present in too low a concentration. The red blood cells agglutinate, however, when an antibody is added. The indirect Coombs' test detects antibodies produced, for example, in response to a previous transfusion or pregnancy.

c. Studies of T lymphocyte function

(1) **Delayed hypersensitivity skin tests** are performed on individuals suspected of having anergy which is cell-mediated (T cell) unresponsiveness. The test involves intradermal injections of a variety of antigens to which most people have been exposed. Antigens used include *Candida*, mumps virus, purified protein derivative from the tubercle bacillus, and streptokinase and streptodornase from streptococci. A normal response is a positive reaction to several of the test antigens, as indicated by erythema and induration at the injection site occurring within 48 hours. If there is no reaction to any of the test antigens, the person likely has deficient T-cell function.

(2) **Antibody-dependent cell-mediated cytotoxicity:** Normal natural killer cells can lyse other cells, including tumor cells and cells infected with intracellular microorganisms coated with antibodies. This action is independent of complement. To assess antibody-dependent cell-mediated cytotoxicity of natural killer cells, the cells are mixed with target cells, usually chicken erythrocytes infected with radioactive-labeled microorganisms. After incubation, the cells are washed to remove the radioactivity from the lysed cells. Then, radioactivity in the remaining intact erythrocytes is counted.

d. T and B lymphocyte transformation tests measure the ability of T and B cells to proliferate in response to a stimulus.

(1) A sample of the person's lymphocytes is incubated with a mitogen, a stimulator of mitosis. Phytohemagglutinin and concanavalin A mainly stimulate T-cell division; pokeweed mitogen mainly stimulates B-cell division.

(2) The proliferation of T or B cells is measured by their uptake of a substance required for DNA synthesis that is tagged with a radioactive label, such

as tritiated thymidine. The radioactivity incorporated into the cells during division is then counted.

e. Complement assays

(1) Complement levels are decreased in genetic complement deficiency disorders and increased in many inflammatory disorders. The most frequently measured complement components and their values are

- C3, 80 to 180 mg per dl
- C4, 15 to 50 mg per dl
- C5, 7 to 17 mg per dl
- C1q, 10 to 21 mg per dl
- factor B, 17 to 27 mg per dl

Complement function tests are based on the ability of the complement system to lyse red blood cells. Results are often reported in CH50 units in which 1 unit equals the amount of patient serum that will lyse 50 percent of the red blood cells added to the assay. **Complement fixation tests** are used mainly in the diagnosis of certain viral, fungal, and rickettsial infections.

- These tests use complement to detect a specific antigen or antibody in a serum sample rather than measuring the person's complement level or activity. The person's complement sample is inactivated before the test.
- A serum sample is added to a solution with either a known antigen or a known amount of complement with antibody present.
- If the serum sample has the corresponding antigen or antibody to the known antibody or antigen used in the test, then antigen-antibody complexes form and bind (fix) complement, so that complement is not available to lyse the red blood cells added in the next step.
- If the antigen or antibody under investigation is not present in the serum sample, complement is not fixed and will be available to bind and lyse the antibody-coated sheep red blood cells added in the next step of the test.

(2) **Complement nephelometry**

- Standard assay antiserum against specific complement components is mixed with the patient's serum sample.
- Antigen (the patient's complement component) and antibody (antiserum against complement) complexes are formed.
- Complement components are quantified by measuring light scattering by the antigen-antibody complexes and comparing this to the amount of light scattering caused by standard solutions of complement.

(3) **Radialimmunodiffusion**

- A serum sample is added to agar gel containing antibody against a specific complement component.
- A ring of antigen-antibody precipitate forms, the size of which is related to the amount of complement present in the sample.

(4) A functional test of the classic complement pathway measures the ability of the patient's complement system to lyse sheep red blood cells coated with antisheep antibodies.

- The patient's serum sample is mixed with the antibody-coated sheep red blood cells, and the mixture is incubated.
- The mixture is centrifuged and the degree of hemolysis is based on changes in light absorbance of the supernatant.

(5) A functional test of the alternative complement pathway uses antibody-coated rabbit red blood cells because they are lysed by the alternative pathway. The remainder of this test is the same as the test of the classic complement pathway.

◼ IMMUNODEFICIENCY DISORDERS

Definition

1. Immunodeficiency disorders are classified according to the component of the immune system affected and whether the condition is primary or secondary. These disorders cause varying degrees of increased susceptibility to infection.
2. Because of interactions among immune system components, a defect in 1 component can indirectly impair the function of other components.

Primary and Secondary Immunodeficiencies

1. Primary immunodeficiency disorders are inherited disorders resulting in developmental failure of 1 or more components of the immune system. Humoral immunity, CMI, the complement system, or phagocytic cells may be affected. Most primary immunodeficiency disorders present as recurrent infections appearing in infancy.
2. Secondary immunodeficiency disorders are characterized by the loss of a previously effective component of the immune response. These disorders can be acquired at any time throughout life. Causes of secondary immunodeficiency include stress, malnutrition, aging, ingestion of immunosuppressive drugs, irradiation, cancer, and overwhelming infections.

Severe Combined Immunodeficiency Disease

1. Severe combined immunodeficiency diseases (SCIDs) are primary immunodeficiency disorders characterized by the absence or severe impairment of T cells (CMI) and B cells (HI). Individuals with SCID are very susceptible to infection with any type of microorganism.
2. Incidence and etiology: The exact incidence of SCID is not known. It is believed that some infants with SCID die in utero or shortly after birth before being diagnosed.

a. The common type of SCID is characterized by impaired CMI and HI and decreased numbers of T and B cells. The basic defect is in the lymphocytic stem cells, but the mechanism responsible for this defect is unknown. Inheritance of this form of SCID can be X-linked or autosomal recessive. The growth of long bones may also be affected, resulting in stunted growth.

b. Severe combined immunodeficiency disease with B lymphocytes is characterized by deficiency of CMI with a decreased number of T cells. B cells are present. These cells, however, may not be able to produce the normal variety of antibodies. The basic defect involves T-cell development and sometimes B-cell development. The mechanism for this disorder is unknown. Inheritance can be X-linked or autosomal recessive.

c. Adenosine deaminase deficiency is characterized by deficiency of CMI and T cells. B cells may or may not be present. If present, B cells have decreased ability to produce antibodies in response to antigens. The basic defect is in the lymphocytic stem cells or in the immature form of T cells and is caused by a deficiency of the enzyme adenosine deaminase. This defect causes accumulation of deoxyadenosine triphosphate in cells, which blocks activity of ribonucleotide reductase, an enzyme necessary for DNA synthesis. Inheritance is autosomal recessive.

d. Purine nucleoside phosphorylase deficiency is characterized by a deficiency of CMI and T cells and deficient antibody production by B cells. The basic defect is impaired maturation of T cells due to a deficiency of the enzyme purine nucleoside phosphorylase. Inheritance is autosomal recessive. The deficiency also causes hypoplastic anemia.

e. Reticular dysgenesis is the most severe form of SCID in which there is a marked deficit of not only T and B lymphocytes but also phagocytic cells. The basic defect is in the hematopoietic stem cell precursor of all WBCs. The mechanism causing this defect is unknown. Inheritance is autosomal recessive.

3. Clinical manifestations

a. Severe combined immunodeficiency disease is associated with deficits in both CMI and HI, resulting in increased susceptibility to infections. The disorder usually becomes apparent within a few months of birth.

b. Some T or B lymphocytes may be present but are not activated by antigens.

c. Two mechanisms are responsible for the immune deficiency of SCID:
   • A defect in stem cell precursors of T and B cells
   • An abnormality or absence of the thymus, which impairs the development of T cells. Because helper T cells are necessary for normal function of B cells, antibody production is also impaired.

d. All forms of SCID, except reticular dysgenesis, have a defect only in stem cell precursors for lymphocytes, so that other WBCs are normal.

e. T and B cells are decreased or absent in both the blood and the lymphoid organs. Serum T cells are therefore absent or severely decreased, and serum B cells are also decreased in most forms of SCID. T or B cells that are present are usually unresponsive to antigens. Lymph node examination reveals small or absent lymph nodes that do not enlarge in response to infection. Lymph node biopsy shows absent or markedly decreased lymphocytes. The thymic shadow is often absent on radiographic examination because of underdevelopment of the thymus.

f. IgG levels may be normal during the 1st few months of life because maternal immunoglobulins cross the placenta and enter the fetal circulation. Because of protection provided by maternal immunoglobulins, the signs and symptoms of infection may not appear until the infant is 3 to 6 months old. In more severe forms of SCID, however, infection may develop in utero or shortly after birth.

g. Typically, the infant with SCID fails to thrive, and recurrent acute and chronic infections such as pneumonia, oral candidiasis, gastroenteritis, otitis media, and sepsis develop. Common childhood infections can be lethal. Many children with SCID die within the 1st year of life of overwhelming infections.

h. Medical diagnosis is usually first based on the presence of recurrent infections during infancy. By sampling amniotic fluid and measuring the enzyme in fetal cells, SCID due to adenosine deaminase deficiency can be diagnosed before birth.

4. Clinical management

a. The goals of clinical management are to prevent infection and restore the immune response.

b. Nonpharmacologic interventions: An infant must be placed in a germ-free environment until curative treatment is attempted. The infant or child with SCID lives in an enclosed unit in which all incoming air is filtered; food, clothes, and toys are sterilized; and contact with others is through a protective shield. The development of the child should be promoted by providing contact and sensory stimulation and encouragement of parent interaction with the child.

c. Pharmacologic interventions: Antimicrobial drugs are used for the treatment of infections. Administration of immunoglobulins is sometimes beneficial.

d. Special medical procedures
   (1) Bone marrow transplantation from a histocompatible sibling may restore immunity. The cell type of donor and recipient must be well matched to prevent graft-versus-host disease (GVHD; see p. 894). In GVHD, the transplanted immune cells react against and reject the cells of the host, which can be fatal. Treatment of donor marrow to remove mature T cells helps to prevent a graft-versus-host reaction.
   (2) For SCID caused by deficiency of adenosine deaminase, clinical trials are studying the effectiveness of insertion of the missing gene for that enzyme into isolated bone marrow cells, which are then reinfused.

NURSE ADVISORY

Do not administer immunizations to infants with severe combined immunodeficiency syndrome because they cannot mount an immune response and serious infection can develop in response to the agent used in the immunization.

(3) Because SCID is a serious genetic disorder, parents should be referred for genetic counseling before initiating another pregnancy. Before successful bone marrow transplantation or gene therapy, parents should be educated about protective isolation and other means of prevention of infection crucial to the child's survival. Long-term survival in a normal environment depends on a successful bone marrow transplant or genetic replacement therapy.

Complement Disorders

1. Definition: Complement disorders consist of a deficiency or dysfunction of 1 or more of the complement components. These disorders may also be the result of a deficiency or dysfunction of a regulatory protein of the complement cascade.
   a. Complement disorders are classified according to the complement component or regulatory protein that is defective or deficient.
   b. Disorders have been identified for each of the components of the classic complement pathway.
   c. Complement components are key factors in the inflammatory and immune responses, and their deficiency or dysfunction results in increased susceptibility to bacterial infections and autoimmune diseases.
      (1) With a disorder of 1 of the components early in the complement cascade, activation of the cascade can only proceed up to the point of the defective component. C3 is especially crucial for defense against bacterial infections because it opsonizes these organisms and recruits phagocytic WBCs. Blockage of the complement cascade at this step also prevents the formation of the C5b–C9 complex, which lyses bacteria. Host resistance is usually not seriously impaired as a result of defects in components C1, C2, or C4 because C3 can also be activated by the alternative pathway. Individuals with defects in the classic complement pathway components have an increased incidence of connective tissue diseases such as systemic lupus erythematosus. The classic pathway interacts directly with immune complexes and functions in their clearance. With increased amounts of immune complexes, which activate the inflammatory response, tissue damage occurs.
      (2) With disorders of late components (C5 through C9) in the complement cascade, some people are asymptomatic. In others, these deficiencies result in recurrent neisserial infections with gonococci or meningococci because bacterial lysis mediated by the late complement components is an important defense against these microorganisms.
2. Incidence and etiology: Primary complement disorders account for less than 1 percent of all primary immunodeficiencies. Complement deficiencies involving components C1 through C4 are the most common.
   a. Primary disorders of the complement system can be inherited as an autosomal dominant or, more frequently, as an autosomal recessive trait.

b. Secondary complement disorders can be acquired as a result of disease processes that cause increased consumption of complement at a rate faster than it can be produced. Such disorders include systemic lupus erythematosus, acute glomerulonephritis, and overwhelming bacterial infections. Secondary complement disorders can also be acquired as a result of protein malnutrition and associated decreased ability to synthesize complement. Such disorders include starvation, severe liver disease, or severe burn injury.
3. Clinical manifestations: Clinical manifestations of complement disorders depend on the component that is defective, on the severity of the defect, and on the acuity or chronicity of the defect. The total serum complement level is decreased if there is a deficiency of 1 of the complement components. Assays of specific complement components identify the deficient component.
   a. Clinical manifestations are primarily related to recurrent infections and connective tissues disorders.
   b. Table 21–5 summarizes specific complement disorders and their associated clinical manifestations.
4. Interventions
   a. Primary complement disorders have no known cure. In the future, genetic replacement therapy may be available. Administration of fresh-frozen plasma replaces complement components, but the effect is only temporary. Bone marrow transplantation is beneficial in some cases. For C1 inhibitor (C1 INH) deficiency, which causes angioedema, partially purified C1 INH can be administered, or anabolic steroids can be used to stimulate production of C1 INH. The importance of preventing infections and the signs and symptoms of infections should be taught to the person or family. Early and aggressive treatment of infections is important.
   b. In secondary complement disorders, management of

Table 21–5. Complement Disorders and Associated Clinical Manifestations

Complement Defect	Clinical Manifestations
C1q, C1r, C1s, C2, or C4	Mild recurrent bacterial infections Increased frequency of immune complex diseases
C3	Recurrent overwhelming bacterial infections, especially with encapsulated bacteria
C5	Recurrent infections, especially of the skin and gastrointestinal tract
C6 through C9 (terminal complement components)	Asymptomatic or increased incidence of neisserial infections
Alternate pathway components	Increased infection rate with encapsulated bacteria
C1 inhibitor (C1 INH)	Hereditary angioedema (edema and dysfunction in the skin, and respiratory and gastrointestinal tracts)
Factor 1 (C3b inactivator)	Recurrent gram-positive and gram-negative infections
Properidin	Recurrent neisserial infections

the underlying disease process restores complement components to normal.

c. The prognosis varies with the severity of the associated infections or immune complex diseases.

Immunoglobulin A Deficiency

1. Definition
   a. IgA is the main immunoglobulin in secretions covering mucosal surfaces in contact with the external environment, including those of the respiratory, gastrointestinal, and genitourinary tracts. Diseases associated with IgA deficiency are manifested primarily in these organ systems. A normal number of IgA type B cells, that is, B cells with IgA on their surfaces, are usually present, but the ability of these cells to transform into plasma cells that synthesize and secrete IgA is decreased.
   b. Selective (isolated) IgA deficiency is present when the serum level of IgA is less than 5 mg per dl. Serum IgA deficiency is also usually associated with an absence or deficiency of secretory IgA. Other immunoglobulins are present in normal or increased amounts.
2. Incidence and etiology: IgA deficiency is one of the most common immunodeficiency disorders in the United States. The incidence varies from 1 in every 600 to 800 individuals. Approximately 40 percent of persons with IgA deficiency have antibodies to IgA, but it is not known whether these antibodies are the cause or the result of the IgA deficiency. Evidence suggests that overactivity of T suppressor cells impairs the maturation of IgA type B cells in some individuals.
   a. Primary selective IgA deficiency has a genetic predisposition and can be inherited by either an autosomal recessive or dominant mechanism. It occurs more frequently in families with histories of other immunodeficiency disorders. IgA deficiency has been linked to the inheritance of human leukocyte antigen patterns A1, A2, B8, and Dw3.
   b. In acquired selective IgA deficiency, the deficiency can be secondary to administration of certain drugs such as penicillamine and phenytoin (Dilantin). IgA levels may return to normal after the drug is discontinued. Selective IgA deficiency can also be secondary to certain viral infections.
3. Clinical manifestations
   a. Some individuals with mild IgA deficiency are asymptomatic, possibly the result of compensatory increases in immunoglobulins of other classes. In more severe forms of IgA deficiency, clinical manifestations are related to recurrent sinopulmonary infections, allergy, autoimmune disease, and cancer. The most common clinical manifestations are related to recurrent sinopulmonary infections of viral or bacterial origin. Allergies, especially those of the respiratory tract, are common. IgA deficiency allows for increased entry of antigens through mucosal surfaces resulting in greater availability of antigens to bind to IgE, triggering an allergic reaction. (See p. 889.)
   b. Serum IgA levels are less than 5 mg per dl. IgA is usually absent in secretions. Serum levels of IgG, IgM, IgD, and IgE are normal or elevated. IgM levels are increased in secretions in some individuals. The number of circulating B cells, including IgA type B cells, is normal. T cells and CMI are normal, but some IgA-deficient individuals have an increased number of suppressor T cells.
   c. Autoimmune disorders, usually rheumatoid arthritis (see p. 898), systemic lupus erythematosus, and pernicious anemia, frequently occur in IgA-deficient individuals. Increased exposure to a variety of antigens, due to IgA deficiency, leads to increased production of other classes of immunoglobulins. Increased immunoglobulin production brings increased risk that some of them will cross-react with self-antigens, producing an autoimmune disease. Autoimmune disease causes elevated levels of autoantibodies characteristic of the disorder (e.g., rheumatoid factor or antinuclear antibodies).
   d. An increased risk of cancer in individuals with IgA deficiency is most likely due to the increased exposure to antigens and associated chronic infections and inflammation, which contribute to malignant transformation of cells. Malignant tumors associated with IgA deficiency most often occur in the respiratory, gastrointestinal, and lymphatic systems.
   e. Gastrointestinal disorders occur with increased frequency in IgA-deficient individuals. Biopsies have detected autoantibodies directed against connective tissue in the intestinal tract. Common gastrointestinal problems are infections, malabsorption syndromes, and ulcerative colitis.
4. Clinical management
   a. Because no replacement or genetic therapy is yet available for IgA deficiency, there is no cure.
   b. The following alternatives are used when an IgA-deficient individual requires a blood transfusion because whole blood contains IgA, which is treated as a foreign substance, possibly triggering an anaphylactic reaction.
      (1) Transfusion with blood from a typed- and cross-matched IgA-deficient donor
      (2) Autotransfusion with blood that the person donated previously
      (3) Use of packed red blood cells washed at least 3 times, although this procedure may not eliminate all IgA

NURSE ADVISORY

Do not administer immunoglobulins to individuals with IgA deficiency. These individuals either have preexisting antibodies against IgA or can produce them when exposed to IgA. In either case, an anaphylactic reaction can develop.

---

   c. The patient should be taught preventive measures against infection (see Chapter 8). The early warning signs of disorders associated with IgA deficiency should be discussed. These include allergies, recurrent infections, cancer, and autoimmune diseases. The person should seek assistance from a health care professional if these develop.

d. Most individuals with moderate to severe IgA deficiency become symptomatic during the 1st decade of life, and early diagnosis of IgA deficiency, prevention of infections, follow-up care, and treatment of complications reduce morbidity. With proper management, many individuals with IgA deficiency live a full life span.

Neutropenia

1. Definition: In neutropenia, the neutrophil count is less than 1800 per mm^3.
2. Incidence and etiology
   a. Decreased neutrophil production
      (1) Cancer chemotherapeutic agents interfere with DNA synthesis in stem cell precursors.
      (2) Cancer cell invasion of bone marrow decreases neutrophil production.
      (3) Phenothiazine tranquilizers inhibit DNA synthesis in stem cell precursors.
      (4) Cimetidine (Tagamet) causes neutropenia in some persons.
   b. Increased neutrophil destruction
      (1) Drug-induced neutropenia: Drug-antibody complex attaches to neutrophils, causing their immune-mediated destruction. This activity is most often caused by penicillin, quinidine, and procainamide.
      (2) Severe alterations in the chemical environment of the blood can cause premature destruction of neutrophils.
   c. Alterations in neutrophil function
      (1) Glucose-6-phosphate dehydrogenase deficiency, an inherited disorder of metabolism, causes decreased production of H_2O_2, which is required for neutrophils to destroy bacteria.
      (2) Myeloperoxidase deficiency, an inherited disorder, causes decreased ability of neutrophils to destroy bacteria and fungi.
      (3) Chédiak-Higashi syndrome, a rare inherited disorder characterized by abnormal cytoplasmic granular inclusions in neutrophils, causes decreased ability to destroy certain microorganisms.

3. Clinical manifestations
   a. The greatest frequency of severe infections occurs when the granulocyte count is less than 100 per mm^3.
   b. With a severe deficiency of neutrophils, the inflammatory response, a classic sign of infection, may be absent.
4. Clinical management
   a. The correction of neutropenia is directed at treatment of the underlying cause. Administration of growth factors, such as granulocyte colony-stimulating factor, stimulates neutrophil production in the bone marrow.
   b. Prevention and early treatment of infections is crucial.

◼ HYPERSENSITIVITY DISORDERS

Allergic Reactions

1. Definition: Increased response to an antigen (either foreign or self) causes tissue damage because it is inappropriate. Hypersensitivity reactions occur after the 1st exposure to an allergen. Allergens are usually high–molecular-weight proteins. Haptens, low–molecular-weight substances that are unable to trigger an allergic response alone, can combine with a larger molecule and then cause an allergic response.
   a. First exposure to an allergen causes primary immune response, which is slow and not severe. This phase is called **sensitization.**
   b. Subsequent exposures cause faster and more severe reactions.
2. Incidence and etiology
   a. Approximately 1 in 4 Americans has serious allergies.
   b. The general cause of hypersensitivity reactions is a decrease in suppressor T-cell activity, an increase in helper T-cell activity, or IgA deficiency, and an increased exposure to antigens. Types of hypersensitivity reactions are summarized in Figure 21–8. Table 21–6 lists chemical mediators in allergic reactions.
3. Clinical manifestations
   a. The medical diagnosis of an allergy often results from the observation or description of the signs and symptoms characteristic of an allergic reaction.

Table 21–6. Chemical Mediators in Allergic Reactions

Clinical Manifestations	Mediators	Actions
Bronchoconstriction, bronchospasm, hypotension, shock, edema, pruritus, nausea, vomiting, diarrhea	Histamines	Increased capillary permeability, bronchial smooth muscle contraction
Bronchospasm	Leukotrienes	Promotes histamine effect on smooth muscle
Bronchospasm, urticaria, erythema, hypotension	Prostaglandins	Bronchial smooth muscle contraction and vasodilation
Angioedema, bronchospasm, pain in area of edema	Kinins	Increased capillary permeability, vasodilation, bronchial smooth muscle contraction
See histamine as a mediator	Activation of the complement system (C3a, C4a, C5a), leading to the ultimate release of histamine	See histamine as a mediator
Hypotension	Vasoactive amines	Vasodilation

HYPERSENSITIVITY (ALLERGIC) REACTIONS

Type I: Anaphylactic (Immediate) Reactions

Type I hypersensitivity reaction can be the most serious form of an allergic reaction. Anaphylaxis is a life-threatening reaction. It is usually triggered by proteins such as animal dander, insect venom, foods, or drugs. Once the allergen enters the body, IgE antibodies are formed to mediate the reaction. IgE immunoglobulins are attracted to mast cells and basophils. Basophils circulate through the bloodstream. Mast cells, found in all body tissues, are most abundant in the nasal area, skin, and lungs.

1 An allergic response begins at the 1st exposure to an antigen/allergen with initial sensitization of B cells to an allergen, which stimulates them to produce IgE.
2 The IgE binds to the Fc receptor on the mast cell or the basophil. Once bound, the IgE molecule is open to bind with the allergen.
3 On the 2nd and all subsequent exposures to the allergen, allergen binding results in cross-linking of IgE molecules and degranulation of mast cells and basophils.
4 Degranulation releases toxic substances, including histamine, and other vasoactive amines.

Clinical Manifestations:
The chemicals released cause increased capillary permeability, leading to edema; vasodilation, leading to hypotension and erythema; and bronchospasm, leading to shortness of breath.

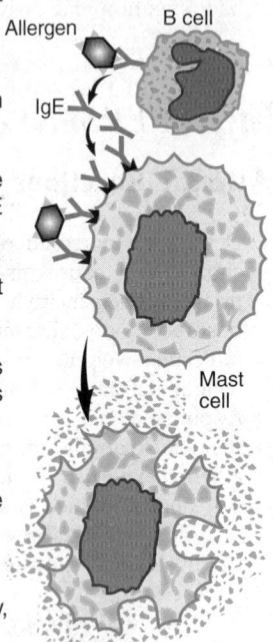

Type II: Cytotoxic Hypersensitivity Reactions

Cytotoxic hypersensitivity reactions occur because antigens on the cell surface react to antibodies in the bloodstream, with resulting cell destruction. A blood transfusion reaction because of ABO or Rh incompatibility is an example.

1 IgG or IgM immunoglobulins are directed against naturally occurring antigens on host cells, most commonly red blood cells.
2 When immunoglobulins affect the cells, the complement system is activated, causing cell lysis, or hemolysis.

Clinical Manifestations:
Due to intravascular hemolysis of red blood cells and include:
• Headache and flank pain
• Nausea and vomiting
• Chest pain
• Tachycardia and hypotension
• Urticaria
• Hematuria

Type III: Immune Complex–Mediated Reactions

Type III reactions cause chronic debilitating diseases such as glomerulonephritis and rheumatoid arthritis. Mediated by IgG and IgM immunoglobulins, this type of reaction results from antigen-antibody complexes deposited in tissues and blood vessels.

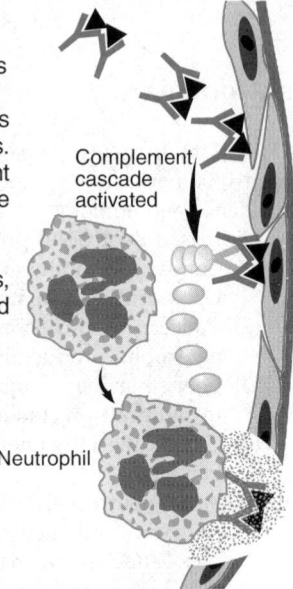

1 Antigen-antibody complexes are deposited in tissues or blood vessels. The complexes are resistant to phagocytosis.
2 They activate the complement system, and phagocytes, like neutrophils, are attracted to the area of deposits.
3 Phagocytes release enzymes, resulting in inflammation and tissue damage.

Clinical Manifestations:
• Urticaria and erythematous rash
• Lymphadenopathy
• Fever
• Angioedema
• Joint pain with objective signs of arthritis
• Headache

Type IV: Delayed Hypersensitivity Reactions

Delayed hypersensitivity reactions include responses to infections by bacteria, fungi, or viruses, contact dermatitis and graft rejections, and tuberculosis skin tests. These reactions develop 12 to 24 hours after exposure to an antigen and are mediated by antigen-sensitized helper T cells after a 2nd exposure to the antigen.

1 Antigens from target cells stimulate production of 2 kinds of T cells, antigen-sensitized cytotoxic Tc cells and delayed hypersensitivity Td cells.
2 Tc cells release lymphotoxins, which destroy cells by directly breaking down the cell membrane, causing lysis of the cell.
3 Lymphokines secreted by Td cells activate macrophages and polymorphonuclear leukocytes, which release enzymes that cause tissue destruction.

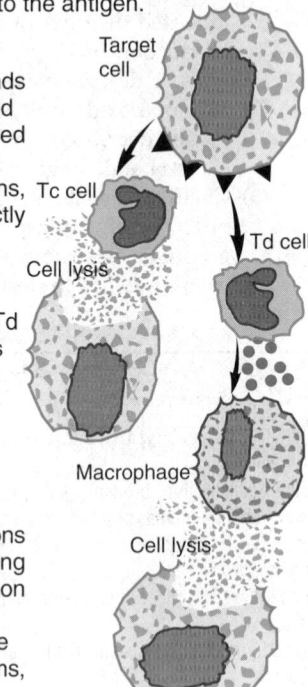

Clinical Manifestations:
• Erythematous vesicular lesions
• Pruritus, burning, and stinging
• Manifestations of graft rejection after transplantation
• General signs are low-grade temperature, flulike symptoms, possible failure of the transplanted organ

Figure 21–8.

In taking a history, ask the person
- To describe the signs and symptoms associated with the suspected allergy, including frequency, duration, and timing
- To list medication history including home remedies and over-the-counter, and prescription medications
- To note where symptoms develop (e.g., at home, work, indoors, or outdoors). Also ask about hobbies because chemicals used in certain crafts can cause allergic reactions.
- To describe any reactions after eating certain foods or after being bitten or stung by an insect.

b. Skin tests are performed to determine a person's sensitivity to specific antigens or allergens placed on or into the skin. If a person is sensitized to that substance and is not immunosuppressed, a visible skin reaction occurs. Three methods of skin testing are the patch test, scratch test, and intradermal test (Table 21–7).
  (1) Reactions to skin testing are common, and minor problems such as discomfort and itching at the test site can be relieved with cool compresses or topical corticosteroids. More serious reactions include ulceration at the test site and, rarely, anaphylactic shock (see pp. 892–893 for interventions related to severe anaphylactic reactions).
  (2) Skin tests should not be performed in areas of skin disorder (e.g., rash, acne, or infection).
  (3) If it is known that the person had an anaphylactic reaction to a particular antigen, that substance should not be used because it is more likely to cause a serious reaction.

c. The use test (also called an elimination test) involves eliminating potential allergenic substances from the person's environment and reintroducing them on a set schedule. After each substance has been reintroduced, the person is monitored for an allergic reaction.

d. Radioallergosorbent test (RAST) detects IgE, helps in identifying causative allergens, and helps in monitoring the effectiveness of therapy.
  (1) A sample of the person's serum is exposed to various allergens attached to different disks. IgE in the serum sample binds to allergens to which the person is sensitive. The radiolabeled antibodies against IgE are added and bind to the IgE attached to allergens on the disks. The radioactivity is measured and is proportional to the amount of IgE present.
  (2) This test requires only a venipuncture to obtain a blood sample and, therefore, generally causes less discomfort than skin tests that elicit a reaction.
  (3) Results are not affected if the person is receiving antihistamine therapy, but the accuracy may be affected if the person had a radioactive scan within the previous week.
  (4) Occasionally, a false-positive or false-negative result occurs.

4. Intervention: See Table 21–8 for the pharmacologic treatment of allergies.

Anaphylaxis and Anaphylactic Shock

1. Definitions: **Anaphylaxis** is a severe, systemic hypersensitivity reaction triggered by exposure to an allergen to which the person is sensitized. **Anaphylactic shock** is the most severe form of anaphylaxis in which a shock stage exists—that is, a generalized state of inadequate perfusion relative to the metabolic demands of tissues.

2. Incidence and etiology
  a. The incidence of anaphylaxis varies depending on the causative agent. Most cases are caused by antibiotics, especially the penicillins and cephalosporins, with 10 to 40 serious reactions occurring per 100,000 injections of penicillin. Insect venom is estimated to cause 1 serious reaction per 10,000 individuals each year.
  b. Anaphylaxis and anaphylactic shock are caused by a severe type I hypersensitivity reaction. The excessive release or activation of chemical mediators including histamines, leukotrienes, prostaglandins, kinins, and complement causes a severe and prolonged allergic reaction (see Table 21–6).
  c. Anaphylactic shock involves maldistribution of vascular volume due to 2 mechanisms:
    (1) The chemical mediators cause massive, systemic vasodilation, resulting in an increased vascular capacity without enough blood to fill it. The end result is hypotension and decreased tissue perfusion.
    (2) Some chemical mediators cause increased capillary permeability, which allows intravascular fluid to leak into tissue spaces, causing hypotension and edema.

3. Clinical manifestations: The onset of clinical manifestations depends on the route of exposure and dose of the allergen. Manifestations can begin within seconds to an hour after exposure. Generally, in more severe reactions, the manifestations appear earlier. Manifestations of anaphylaxis and anaphylactic shock are the result of the actions of chemical mediators (see Table 21–6) that produce vasodilation, increased vascular permeability, and contraction of smooth muscle in the airways and gastrointestinal system. Manifestations are also the result of tissue hypoxia secondary to alterations in gas exchange in the lungs and decreased blood flow.
  a. Generalized manifestations include apprehension, restlessness, flushing, altered level of consciousness, cyanosis, and cool, clammy skin (if shock is present).
  b. Cutaneous manifestations include erythema, hives, edema, and pruritus.
  c. Pulmonary manifestations include wheezing, dyspnea, tachypnea, and tightness in the chest.
  d. Cardiovascular manifestations include tachycardia, dysrhythmias, angina, and hypotension.
  e. Gastrointestinal manifestations include cramps and diarrhea.

Table 21–7. Methods of Skin Testing

Test and Purpose	Method	Interpretation of Results
Patch test: used to identify the allergens producing allergic contact reactions	Choose an area of the skin without hair, such as the forearm, anterior thigh, or scapula. Clean the area with alcohol to remove microorganisms and with acetone to remove dirt and skin oils. Allow the area to dry. Then place the allergen directly on the skin or on a gauze patch; patches saturated with allergens are also available. Cover the patch with tape, using paper tape if the person is sensitive to adhesive tape. Leave in place as directed, usually 48 to 72 hr, and keep the area dry. If more than one patch is used at the same time, place patches at least 5 cm apart so that a reaction from one patch does not interfere with that of another. After removing the patch, wait 20 to 30 min for any irritation from tape removal to subside and evaluate the site.	Results are often observed at multiple time points, such as 48, 72, and 96 hr after application. Possible results are + erythema only, ++ erythema and papules, +++ erythema, papules, and small vesicles, ++++ all of the listed results with bullae and ulceration. False-positive results can occur if a nonallergic skin reaction develops (e.g., from the tape, infection at the site, or contamination from a nearby site). False-negative results can occur if an insufficient amount of antigen was used, the test was read at an incorrect time, or the person was receiving systemic, topical corticosteroids, or antihistamines.
Scratch (tine or prick) test: used to assess a person's response to allergens	Select a site and prepare the skin with the same method used for the patch test. Using a sterile instrument, make a scratch 1 to 4 mm long and approximately 2 mm deep. Immediately apply the solution of allergen. Multiple sites should be at least 5 cm apart. Prepare a control site in the same manner but apply a nonallergenic solution, such as sterile saline, to determine whether a reaction is due to the skin irritation alone.	A positive reaction to the allergen is indicated by erythema or edema appearing within 30 to 40 min. Measure and record the size of the reaction in millimeters.
Intradermal test: used to assess the delayed (type IV) hypersensitivity reaction to recall antigens (i.e., antigens to which the person has been previously exposed and sensitized. Test antigens commonly include those derived from fungi (e.g., *Candida*, blastomyces, or *Histoplasma*), from viruses (e.g., mumps virus), and from bacteria (e.g., *Mycobacterium tuberculosis* or streptococci).	Intradermal tests consist of an injection, with a needle or prolonged lancet, of antigen into the superficial layers of the skin on the forearm or scapula. Clean the area to be tested with the same method used for the patch test. Control tests, consisting of an injection of normal saline or the diluent in which the antigen is dissolved, are usually administered at the same time as the sensitizing agent for comparison. If a needle and syringe are used to administer the antigen, hold the skin taut and insert the needle at a 15-degree angle to the skin and approximately 3 mm below the surface. Inject the solution slowly. A wheal should form as the solution is injected. Do not rub the area after the injection. If a prolonged lancet is used to administer the antigen, the prongs should be firmly and completely pressed into the skin. Circle each injection site and label with the antigen used. Instruct the person not to wash the area.	Read the test in 48 to 72 hr after the injection. The test is positive if a wheal greater than 5 mm in diameter with erythema appears around the site of the allergenic injection. Nothing should appear at the control site. If there is no reaction to any of the test antigens, the person has impaired cell-mediated immunity and is considered anergic.

4. Clinical management
   a. Contact with the allergen should be immediately discontinued if possible. For example, infusion of intravenous drug should be stopped if manifestations of anaphylaxis appear.
   b. A patent airway and adequate oxygenation should be secured by administration of oxygen, bronchodilators, intubation, or performance of a tracheostomy.
   c. Further release of chemical mediators of anaphylaxis can be inhibited and some of their effects counteracted by the administration of epinephrine and antihistamines (Table 21–8).
   d. Hypovolemia should be corrected with fluid therapy. If fluid therapy is not effective in reversing hypotension, vasopressors, such as dopamine, epinephrine, norepinephrine, or isoproterenol, are required.

Table 21–8. Pharmacologic Treatment for Allergies and Anaphylactic Shock

Medication	Action
Methylprednisone	Decreases inflammatory reaction involved in allergy
Epinephrine	Relaxes bronchial smooth muscle and increases cardiac output, counteracting bronchospasm and hypotension
Diphenhydramine	Blocks histamine receptors, thus decreasing bronchospasm and vasodilation
Dopamine	Acts on vascular smooth muscle, causing vasoconstriction and increased tissue perfusion
Aminophylline	Relaxes bronchial smooth muscles, thus increasing airway patency
Norepinephrine	Acts on vascular smooth muscle causing vasoconstriction and increased tissue perfusion
Isotonic IV fluids	Expands vascular volume to increase blood pressure and cardiac filling pressure

e. To prevent protracted or recurrent manifestations of anaphylaxis, corticosteroids and antihistamines should be administered.

f. Assessment should include frequent monitoring of vital signs, mental status, lung sounds, oxygenation (blood gases, oxygen saturation, hemoglobin, skin color), hemodynamic status, and renal status.

g. To prevent future anaphylactic reactions, the person should avoid contact with known allergens, provide a complete history of drug allergies, and wear a Medic Alert tag.

h. To achieve early intervention if a reaction occurs, the person and family members should be taught how to use self-injection kits (e.g., EpiPen or Ana-Kit).

Allergic Rhinitis

1. Definition: Allergic rhinitis is an inflammation of the nasal mucosa, which causes drainage of clear mucus from the nares in response to inhaled allergens. It may be seasonal (e.g., hay fever), occurring at times when pollen and mold are abundant in the environment. It may, however, occur year round in response to animal dander, dust, or air pollution.

2. Incidence and etiology
   a. Rhinitis occurs with some hypersensitivity reactions because mast cells are abundant in the nasal tissue. The degranulation of the mast cells, which causes histamine to be released, causes vasodilation and increased capillary permeability. This process leads to nasal mucosal swelling and a "runny" nose.
   b. Asthma eventually develops in 30 percent of children who have allergic rhinitis.

3. Clinical manifestations include sneezing and nasal congestion, itching of nose and eyes, dark circles under the eyes, and edematous nasal mucosa.

4. Clinical management
   a. Instruct the person on ways to avoid the offending allergen, for example, by eliminating dust-collecting items from the environment, using dust-trapping filters in air conditioner systems and vacuum cleaners, and avoiding wooded areas during pollen seasons.
   b. Teach the person proper administration of prescribed medications such as antihistamines and topical or intranasal corticosteroids.

Urticaria (Hives), Angioedema, and Pruritus

1. Definitions: Urticaria is a skin reaction occurring in the upper dermis and characterized by a wheal (evanescent skin elevation) surrounded by a flare (area of redness due to vasodilation). Urticaria is often associated with pruritis (itching). Angioedema occurs in subcutaneous tissues and is characterized by deeper and larger wheals than in urticaria.

2. Incidence and etiology
   a. Urticaria is more common than angioedema and may occur at some time in as much as 20 percent of the population.
   b. Urticaria and angioedema can occur independently or at the same time.
   c. Urticaria and angioedema are caused by chemical mediators, such as histamine released during an allergic reaction. This process causes inflammation, vasodilation, increased vascular permeability, and transudation of fluid into the tissue spaces.
   d. These reactions can be triggered by drug, food, or chemical allergies. Reactions can be associated with certain diseases such as viral infections and malignancies, or they can be hereditary.

3. Clinical manifestations
   a. Reactions can be mild, involving only wheal and flare reactions in the skin, and be self-limiting.
   b. The person may have the sensation of tightness or burning in the affected area.
   c. Angioedema can occur anywhere, in the skin or in internal organs, but it more commonly develops in the lips, tongue, periorbital area, larynx, and joints.
   d. Angioedema can be life threatening if it causes airway occlusion, which is manifested by hoarseness, stridor, difficulty speaking, and dyspnea.

4. Clinical management
   a. Identify and eliminate, if possible, the agents triggering the reaction.
   b. Administer pharmacologic therapy including antihistamines and corticosteroids.
   c. Apply cold compresses over areas of urticaria to help alleviate swelling and itching.
   d. Administer mild analgesics to relieve pain.

Graft Rejection (Acute or Chronic)

1. Definition: Transplanted tissue is rejected by the recipient's immune system, and a type IV hypersensitivity reaction ensues.

2. Incidence and etiology
   a. Rejection occurs to some degree in most transplantations, except in cases of identical match between donor and recipient which occurs with identical twins.
   b. The rejection is mediated by both CMI and HI responses.

(1) In cell-mediated rejection, cytolytic T lymphocytes directly attack and lyse transplanted cells, or they secrete lymphokines, which recruit macrophages and neutrophils to attack the transplanted tissue. Macrophages also secrete interleukins, which cause T-cell proliferation, resulting in an increased number of T cells attacking the graft.

(2) Helper T lymphocytes activate B lymphocytes to produce antibodies (HI response). These antibodies bind to the histocompatibility antigens on transplanted cells and activate the complement system, which causes cell lysis.

(3) Hyperacute rejection is the result of preformed antibodies present in the recipient before transplantation.

3. Clinical manifestations

NURSE ADVISORY

> When teaching transplant patients to monitor for rejection at home, teach them to monitor temperature, blood pressure, and heart rate daily. For heart and kidney transplant patients, emphasize daily weights to monitor fluid retention. Teach lung transplant patients to check their forced expiratory volume in 1 second and forced vital capacity daily at home with a hand-held spirometer.

Table 21–9. Signs and Symptoms of Specific Organ Rejection

Organ	Signs and Symptoms of Rejection
Heart	Increased central venous pressure as evidenced by jugular venous distention
	Peripheral edema
	Presence of a third heart sound (S_3)
	Hypotension
	Fatigue and general malaise
	Dysrhythmias
Lung	Shortness of breath and dyspnea
	Decrease in lung volumes as measured by pulmonary function testing (FEV_1 and FVC)
	Fatigue and general malaise
	Increased sputum production
	Rhonchi, rales, or wheezing on auscultation
	Fever
Bone marrow	Signs and symptoms of GVHD as described in text
	Maculopapular rash on the skin
	Dry mucous membranes
	Diarrhea, nausea, vomiting
	Jaundice
Kidney	Decreasing urine output progressing to oliguria and anuria
	Tenderness over the site of the graft
	Hypertension
	Electrolyte imbalances
	Fever
Liver	General malaise
	Fever
	Abdominal discomfort
	Ascites

FEV_1, Forced expiratory volume in 1 second; FVC, forced vital capacity; GVHD, graft-versus-host disease.

a. Signs and symptoms depend on the specific organ or tissue being rejected (Table 21–9).

b. General manifestations include fever, fatigue, altered vital signs, and tenderness over the graft site.

4. Clinical management

a. Graft rejection may be prevented or delayed by pharmacologic immunosuppression of the recipient.

b. During an episode of rejection, the dose or variety of immunosuppressant medications is increased.

NURSE ADVISORY

> If organ rejection occurs in transplant patients, in many instances, the corticosteroid dose is increased. There also may be an increase in the doses of other immunosuppressant agents. Often, additional supportive therapy is needed so that the patient can survive the rejection episode. For example, inotropic agents may be needed for heart rejection, supplemental oxygen for lung rejection, and dialysis for kidney rejection.

Graft-Versus-Host Disease

1. Definition: Graft-versus-host disease is a rejection of the recipient's tissues by immune cells in the grafted tissue. It occurs in immunosuppressed recipients whose immune system cannot mount an attack against the transplanted tissue cells. It is most often the result of a bone marrow transplant and can also occur in a severely immunosuppressed person who receives a blood transfusion containing lymphocytes.

2. Incidence and etiology

a. The incidence of GVHD in bone marrow transplant patients is approximately 30%. In severe cases, the mortality rate is as high as 85%.

b. Patients who are at highest risk for development of GVHD are older than 30 years of age, have some degree of histocompatibility antigen mismatch with their donor, and have received marrow from an opposite-sex donor.

c. The recipient's tissues are infiltrated and damaged by the donor's lymphocytes.

d. The acute form of GVHD can occur as early as 1 week after transplantation. Chronic GVHD begins approximately 3 months after transplantation.

e. Medical diagnosis of GVHD is made by biopsy of affected tissue. It is preferable to sample the most accessible organ system, the skin. A sample of gastrointestinal tissue can be obtained by endoscopy.

3. Clinical manifestations

a. Skin GVHD shows an erythematous, maculopapular rash. The rash usually appears on the trunk, ears, palms of the hands, and soles of the feet. The rash may progress to desquamation.

b. Liver GVHD

(1) Hepatomegaly is seen on abdominal examination.

(2) Jaundice occurs as the disease progresses.

(3) Liver function tests are altered. The serum bilirubin, serum transaminases, and alkaline phosphatase increase with GVHD.

c. Gastrointestinal GVHD manifestations include abdominal tenderness, anorexia, nausea, and green, watery diarrhea that may progress to hemorrhagic diarrhea. The gastric mucosa may slough away.

4. Clinical management
   a. Close matching of donor and recipient histocompatibility antigens may prevent GVHD.
   b. Depleting the donor bone marrow sample of T lymphocytes (e.g., by use of monoclonal antibodies against T cells) may prevent GVHD.
   c. Pharmacologic therapy to suppress GVHD may include monoclonal antibodies against T lymphocytes, cyclosporine A, high-dose corticosteroids, azathioprine, and antithymocyte globulin.

Asthma

1. Definition: Asthma is a state of hyperactivity of the lower respiratory tract. It is an obstructive lung disease with episodic and reversible increased resistance to air flow.
2. Incidence and etiology: There is a 12 percent incidence of asthma in children and a 1 percent incidence in the general population. The three types of asthma are extrinsic, intrinsic, and mixed.
   a. **Extrinsic (allergic) asthma**
      (1) Type I (immediate) hypersensitivity reaction is the basis of extrinsic asthma.
      (2) During sensitization to allergens, IgE is produced and binds to mast cells in the bronchial mucosa. On subsequent exposure to allergens, the mast cells degranulate and release chemical mediators that cause bronchospasm, airway inflammation, and excessive mucus secretion, all of which contribute to airway narrowing. Bronchospasm occurs throughout the lungs in large and small airways.
      (3) Perfusion of lung tissue is shunted to areas getting the best air flow to maintain a normal ventilation to perfusion (V/Q) ratio for as long as possible. As an asthma attack progresses, the V/Q ratio becomes abnormal because of decreased ventilation, and the PaO_2 decreases.
      (4) The lungs become overinflated because, as airways constrict and become plugged with mucus, air is trapped in the alveoli. Pressure rising in the lungs and pulmonary arteries can cause a decrease in perfusion of the pulmonary vasculature, impairing gas exchange and subsequently leading to hypoxia of other tissues in the body.
   b. **Intrinsic asthma**
      (1) The trigger for airway narrowing in intrinsic asthma is a nonallergenic irritant, such as respiratory tract infection, exercise, smoke, fumes, and emotional stress.
      (2) The irritants stimulate parasympathetic nerve fibers in the airways, causing bronchoconstriction and activating the inflammatory response.
   c. **Mixed asthma** has characteristics of both extrinsic and intrinsic asthma. Both allergens and nonallergenic triggers can cause an asthma attack.

3. Clinical manifestations
   a. The release of the chemical mediators causes the following clinical manifestations: shortness of breath and tachypnea, a tight feeling in the chest, wheezing, prolonged expiratory phase of respiration, excessive mucus production, use of accessory muscles to breathe (this may include nasal flaring), tachycardia, and anxiety.
   b. The medical diagnosis of asthma is likely to occur with the onset of an asthma attack in childhood. Allergy testing helps determine the cause of some asthma attacks.

TRANSCULTURAL CONSIDERATIONS

Asthma is often not differentiated from other respiratory conditions. Parents sometimes need to learn that children do not outgrow or spontaneously recover from the condition.

   c. Pulmonary function testing in asthmatic patients shows an obstructive pattern—that is, the patients have a decrease in expiratory lung volumes of forced expiratory volume in 1 second (FEV_1), forced vital capacity (FVC), and forced expiratory flow after 25 to 75 percent of vital capacity has been expelled (FEF_{25-75}).
      (1) The FVC is the amount of air forcibly exhaled quickly with maximal effort. This lung volume may be decreased with obstructive lung diseases.
      (2) The FEV_1 is the most accurate pulmonary function test for documenting progression of obstructive lung diseases. The FEV_1 reflects air flow through the large airways during the 1st second of measurement of FVC.
      (3) The FEF_{25-75} reflects the air flow in the middle of the FVC. This measure helps determine the air flow in the smaller airways.
   d. Arterial blood gas analysis may be helpful during an asthma attack.
      (1) Respiratory alkalosis may be seen during the initial stages of an asthma attack. The patient's rapid respiratory rate causes a loss of carbon dioxide (PCO_2) from the system. The oxygen level (PO_2) may also be decreased and lead to hypoxia.
      (2) As the asthma attack progresses, respiratory acidosis develops. As the respiratory muscles become fatigued, carbon dioxide is retained while oxygen levels continue to decrease. These changes coincide with bradypnea, which may lead to complete respiratory failure.
   e. Complications of asthma
      (1) **Status asthmaticus** is an asthma attack that is unresponsive to bronchodilator medications. The normal treatment for asthma does not cause the airways to relax and breathing to return to normal. This condition may result in death. Groups at risk for development of status asthmaticus are individuals between 40 and 60 years of age suffering

from intrinsic asthma without a long history of asthma attacks. Children younger than age 2 years are also at increased risk for the development of status asthmaticus.

(2) Respiratory failure may not be related to status asthmaticus. The respiratory muscles may simply become fatigued during an attack and cause respiratory failure.

(3) Acute respiratory acidosis with high carbon dioxide levels may cause the patient to become unresponsive and unable to maintain the airway spontaneously.

4. Clinical management

a. Interventions that help prevent asthma attacks or limit their severity:

(1) Identifying and avoiding the offending respiratory allergens or irritants

(2) Encouraging use of bronchodilators before exercise, if asthma is triggered by exercise.

(3) Encouraging the person to avoid nonsteroidal anti-inflammatory drugs. Although these agents decrease the production of some chemical mediators, they increase the production of mediators that can trigger bronchospasm in a person with asthma.

NURSE ADVISORY

Warn persons who have histories of asthma to avoid use of aspirin, which is known to precipitate asthma attacks. Aspirin can also cause nasal polyps and rhinitis in these individuals. Warn individuals with asthma about signs and symptoms resulting from complications due to aspirin ingestion.

(4) Teaching the person proper administration of medications such as bronchodilators and corticosteroids

(5) Teaching the person relaxation techniques

(6) Teaching the person the manifestations and appropriate actions to take in the event of mild and serious asthma attacks

b. Interventions during an asthma attack:

(1) Administering bronchodilators, expectorants, and corticosteroids as ordered (Table 21–10)

(2) Administering oxygen as ordered

(3) Placing the person in high Fowler's position to maximize diaphragmatic excursion

(4) Performing nasotracheal suction as needed

(5) Performing postural drainage chest physical therapy as ordered

(6) Assisting with intubation and mechanical ventilation if needed

(7) Monitoring the following:

• Respiratory rate and depth and use of accessory muscles

• Lung sounds for wheezing, crackles, or rhonchi

• Quantity, color, and consistency of sputum

• Changes in level of consciousness

 HOME CARE STRATEGIES

Hypersensitivity Disorders

For patients to function at their optimal ability at home, it is the home care nurse's challenge to help them address complex issues, including chronic pain, weakness, malaise, fatigue, depression, powerlessness, and poor self-esteem. Instruct the patient as follows:

Energy Conservation and Work Simplification

• Before beginning any activity, plan to do it in the easiest, most time-saving way. Start making the bed while still in it.

• Store equipment and supplies within easy reach in the area in which they are most often used. Reorganize the kitchen and bathroom.

• Push or slide objects rather than lifting them. Use a 4-wheeled cart to transport items from room to room.

• Do the most difficult tasks shortly after taking medication.

• Space energy-intensive activities throughout the day.

• Plan rest periods throughout the day. Rest is not necessarily taking a nap—but it is sitting down, putting the feet up, and doing nothing.

Relaxation Techniques

• Meditation or prayer.

• Progressive muscle relaxation. Guide the patient through relaxation of each major body part—tighten, then relax each muscle group. Tape a session for use when you are not there.

• Guided imagery tapes are available for purchase, or assist the patient in creating one. A walk through a pine forest creates a vivid, soothing, pleasurable mental picture.

• Listen to music.

Activities That Support a Positive Self-image

• Help patients identify activities that make them feel good. A warm foot soak in fragrant bubbly water can create a feeling of well-being.

• Encourage patient empowerment. Have patients participate in wellness-related activities and health care decisions.

Home Remedies and Quackery

• Support activities that do not cause harm. Explain and discourage activities that pose health risks.

Symptom Management

• Help patient identify symptom patterns and triggers.

Table 21–10. Pharmacologic Treatment for Asthma

Drug Classification	Medications
Bronchodilators (parenteral)	Epinephrine
	Terbutaline
	Aminophylline
Aerosols	Isoetharine
	Albuterol
	Isoproterenol
Parenteral corticosteroids	Hydrocortisone
	Methylprednisone
Aerosolized corticosteroids	Beclomethasone
Oral corticosteroids	Prednisone

Table 21–11. Blood Transfusion Reactions

Disorder	Incidence and Etiology	Clinical Manifestations	Clinical Management
Allergic (type I) hypersensitivity reactions	Mild allergic reactions are a common result of transfusion. Serious anaphylactic reactions are rare. The allergic reaction is the result of interaction between immunoglobulin E (IgE) produced by the recipient and proteins in the donor's blood, which causes the release of chemical inflammatory mediators. Serious anaphylactic reactions usually occur if an IgA-deficient person (1 in 700 in the United States) who has antibodies against IgA in the donor's plasma. The antibodies are present because of prior sensitization due to foreign IgA exposure through pregnancy or previous transfusion.	Fever is absent. In mild reactions, only urticaria and pruritus are present. In severe reactions, manifestations may include flushing, bronchospasm, laryngeal edema, dyspnea, hypotension, altered level of consciousness, abdominal cramps, diarrhea. These manifestations usually begin shortly after the onset of the transfusion.	Stop the transfusion immediately when the reaction is suspected. Mild reactions, in which only symptoms are urticaria and pruritus, are treated with an antihistamine, such as diphenhydramine (Benadryl). In mild reactions, the transfusion can be continued after the administration of an antihistamine, and the urticaria subsides. Mild reactions can be prevented from recurring through prophylactic administration of diphenhydramine 30 min before transfusion. Serious anaphylactic reactions also require treatment with epinephrine and corticosteroids. Washed red blood cells, which are free of plasma and IgA, should be administered to prevent serious anaphylactic reactions if future transfusions are required.
Acute hemolytic (type II) hypersensitivity reaction	Acute hemolytic reactions are rare, averaging 1 in 7000 transfusions. The mortality rate is 10%. Acute hemolytic reactions are usually caused by an error in blood typing, incorrect labeling of donor blood, or misidentification of the recipient. Acute hemolytic reactions involve transfusion of donor blood that is incompatible with the recipient's blood cell antigens (usually ABO or Rh incompatibility, rarely incompatibility of minor red blood cell antigen system). Antibodies in the recipient's plasma usually recognize an incompatible antigen on donor red blood cells, bind to them, and activate the complement system. This process usually results in hemolysis and the release of inflammatory mediators. Lysed red blood cell–antibody complexes and free hemoglobin cause intravascular occlusion.	Fever and chills (common) Restlessness Hemoglobinemia and hemoglobinuria Chest, back, and abdominal pain Nausea and vomiting Dyspnea Hypotension Renal dysfunction Disseminated intravascular coagulation (DIC) Jaundice Cardiac arrest	Stop the transfusion as soon as the reaction is suspected. Infuse normal saline intravenously. Administer mannitol, Lasix, or other diuretics as ordered to maintain urine output at least 100 ml/hr. Send a sample of the recipient's blood and the donor's blood to the blood bank to recheck the type and crossmatch. Correct complications of hypotension, renal dysfunction, or DIC as needed. Prevent acute hemolytic reactions by proper typing and crossmatching of blood and accurate labeling of blood and patient identification.
Febrile (nonhemolytic transfusion reaction)	Occurs at a rate of 1 in 200 to 500 transfusions. This reaction is usually self-limiting and only reoccurs in 15% of cases. The result of recipient's antibodies causing agglutination or lysis of granulocytes, lymphocytes, or platelets in the donor's blood Occurs in recipients sensitized by prior transfusion or pregnancy Manifestations due to immune-related lysis of white blood cells, causing release of inflammatory mediators	Initial chills and temperature elevation of 1 degree Celsius (1.8 degrees Fahrenheit) or more with flushing, tachycardia, chest discomfort, and neutropenia No evidence of hemolysis Headache and blood pressure instability as later manifestations	Stop the transfusion as soon as the reaction is suspected. Administer antipyretics for fever. To prevent recurrence, administer blood with a microaggregate filter to remove white blood cells or administer washed red blood cells.

- Heart rate and blood pressure (an increasing pulsus paradoxus is a sign of a severe asthma attack)
- Arterial blood gases
  (8) Providing emotional support at the patient's bedside until the acute attack subsides. The patient should not be left alone during an attack.

Blood Transfusion Reactions

1. Blood transfusion reactions occur because of sensitization of the recipient's immune system to a substance in the donor's blood.
2. The 3 types of immune-mediated transfusion reactions are summarized in Table 21–11.

Food and Drug Allergies

1. Definition: Food and drug allergies are usually type I hypersensitivity reactions.
2. Incidence and etiology
   a. A protein in the food or drug usually causes the allergic reaction.
   b. The exact incidence of food allergies is not known, but the estimated range is less than 1%, and up to 7% of the population have some form of food allergy. Foods that commonly cause allergic reactions include the following:
   - Fish and shellfish
   - Milk
   - Eggs
   - Wheat
   - Legumes
   - Mold on fruits or vegetables
   c. The incidence of drug allergies increases with an increasing number of medications. Drugs that commonly cause allergic reactions include the following:
   - Penicillins (most common class of drugs causing allergic reactions)
   - Other antibiotics (cephalosporins, tetracycline, vancomycin, streptomycin, and neomycin)
   - Aspirin
3. Clinical manifestations
   a. The manifestations of a food or drug allergy may occur immediately after exposure to the substance or may be delayed for several hours depending on the amount and route of exposure.
   b. These allergies can cause the following signs and symptoms:
   - Rhinitis
   - Bronchial asthma
   - Urticaria
   - Erythematous skin rashes
   - Nausea, vomiting
   - Diarrhea
   - Anaphylactic shock
4. Clinical management: The interventions for persons with food or drug allergies are similar to those for persons with other type I hypersensitivity reactions.

◼ AUTOIMMUNE DISORDERS

Definition

1. Autoimmune disorders are conditions resulting from the body's production of antibodies directed against its own cells, tissues, or organs (Table 21–12).
2. Autoimmune disorders can affect a single tissue or organ (i.e., are organ specific) or can affect multiple body systems (i.e., are organ nonspecific).
3. The cause of autoimmune disease is unknown, although many theories have been proposed.

Autoimmune Mechanisms

1. Self-antigens can be hidden from birth in body cells and tissues and not be exposed to the body's immune system. If those cells or tissues are disrupted, the self-antigens are released and then recognized by the body as foreign.
2. Partial antigens in the body can combine with a protein and then become complete, causing subsequent production of antibodies.
3. Viral infections can cause immune complex deposits in body tissues and initiate an inflammatory process. Also, foreign antigens from viruses can appear nearly identical to self-antigens, causing subsequent antibody production against that self-antigen.
4. Lymphocytes can produce clones that do not mature and are capable of reacting to self-antigens in the body.
5. Decreased functioning of the suppressor T cells can lead to the inability of the body to tolerate self-antigens.

◼ RHEUMATOID ARTHRITIS

Definition

1. Rheumatoid arthritis is a chronic, systemic, inflammatory disorder.
2. Rheumatoid arthritis primarily involves the connective tissues and synovial membranes of the joints.

Incidence and Socioeconomic Impact

1. Rheumatoid arthritis occurs in women more than men by a ratio of 3:1.
2. Its peak incidence is between ages 25 and 45 years.
3. More than 2 million Americans are affected.
4. The disease occurs in all racial and ethnic groups.

Risk Factors

1. Infectious agents may trigger the disease.
2. Fatigue and emotional stress exacerbate the condition.

Table 21–12. Other Autoimmune Disorders

Disorder	Incidence and Etiology	Clinical Manifestations	Interventions
Sjögren's syndrome, a chronic inflammatory disorder characterized by deficient moisture production of the secretory glands	Primarily affects middle-aged women Etiology unknown	Lacrimal and salivary glands are primarily affected. Disease process leads to decreased gland secretion. Clinical manifestations include dryness of mucous membranes, eyes, nose, and trachea. Parotid gland enlargement is intermittent.	Supportive interventions are based on symptoms. Encourage use of artificial tears, oral fluids for mouth dryness, and avoidance of pharmacologic agents that deplete body fluids.
Scleroderma, a chronic progressive inflammatory disease characterized by swelling and thickening of fibrous tissue	Primarily affects adult females, aged 20–50 yrs Etiology unknown	Connective tissues of the skin and viscera are primarily affected. Clinical manifestations include dry, tough skin, dysphagia, hoarseness, joint stiffness, and pain.	Supportive interventions are based on symptoms. Pharmacologic agents include corticosteroids, immunosuppressives, salicylates, and analgesics. Physical therapy is used to prevent muscle contractures.
Systemic lupus erythematosus, a chronic inflammatory disease affecting multiple body systems	Primarily affects young adult females, aged 20–40 yrs Etiology unknown	There are multisystem effects because autoantibodies produce immune complexes that cluster and produce inflammation and tissue damage. Clinical manifestations vary according to organ involvement and include butterfly facial rash, polyarthritis, glomerulonephritis, vasculitis, and effusions in the pleura, pericardium, and peritoneum.	Interventions are multifaceted and individualized. Advise adequate rest and avoidance of stress and direct sunlight. Complex drug therapy includes corticosteroids, nonsteroidal anti-inflammatory agents, salicylates, cytotoxic agents, and antimalarial drugs. Goals of intervention are preservation of organ function and prevention of organ failure.
Polyarteritis nodosa, an inflammatory vascular disorder of the small- and medium-sized arteries	Primarily affects adults, males more than females Etiology unknown	Tissue ischemia is caused by inflammation and obliteration of small- and medium-sized arteries by circulating immune complexes. Nonspecific symptoms include fever and malaise. Multisystem effects occur in the kidney, heart, lung, gastrointestinal tract, and central nervous system.	Supportive interventions are based on symptoms. Corticosteroids and immunosuppressive drug regimens may be initiated. Physical therapy maintains muscle tone.
Wegener's granulomatosis, a chronic inflammatory disorder characterized by nodular inflammatory lesions of the airways, blood vessels, and glomeruli	Affects both males and females Etiology unknown	Alterations in blood flow are caused by inflammation of the arteries and veins. Symptoms include sinusitis, rhinitis, chest discomfort, pneumonia, and renal failure.	Supportive interventions are based on symptoms. Cytotoxic drugs may be initiated.
Giant cell arteritis, a progressive inflammatory disorder of the large arteries	Primarily effects elderly females Etiology unknown	Necrosis is in the media area of the artery, along with development of multinucleated giant cells. Temporal, retinal, and intracerebral arteries are most frequently affected. Nonspecific symptoms include fever, weight loss, and malaise. Other symptoms depend on the vessel involved. Temporal arteries may be reddened, warm, and painful. Ocular and intracerebral effects include headache and blindness.	Supportive interventions are based on symptoms. Corticosteroids and immunosuppressive drug regimens may be initiated. Physical therapy maintains muscle tone.
Reiter's syndrome, a chronic inflammatory condition	Primarily affects young adult Caucasian males Etiology unknown but disease may result from a myxovirus or mycoplasma infection	Three primary manifestations are arthritis, urethritis, and conjunctivitis. Nonspecific symptoms include fever, weight loss, and malaise.	Antibiotics are used to treat existing infections. Anti-inflammatory agents include corticosteroids. Physical therapy may be used.

Etiology

1. The cause is unknown, but researchers are exploring infectious agents as well as body substances that may activate an autoimmune reaction.
2. Collagen and IgG may stimulate antibody development, forming immune complexes (antigen-antibody complexes) that are deposited within the cartilage.
3. Infection by bacteria, mycoplasma, and viruses may stimulate an immune response in a genetically susceptible person.

Pathophysiology

1. Systemic, inflammatory collagen disease causes pathologic changes within the joint and leads to deformity and disability.
2. Circulating immune complexes in the tissues initiate inflammation.
3. Edema, vascular congestion, fibrin exudate, and cellular infiltrate accumulate in the synovium.
4. Pannus (inflamed projection of granulation tissue) forms at the junction of synovial tissue and articular cartilage, projecting into the joint cavity and causing necrosis (Fig. 21–9).
5. Fibrous ankylosis causes subluxation and distortion of the joint.
6. Bony ankylosis leads to calcification of fibrous tissue, which then changes into osseous tissue.

Clinical Manifestations

1. Onset is insidious or acute.
2. Articular symptoms
   a. Painful, red, swollen, warm, stiff joints
   b. Decreased joint mobility
   c. Involvement of small joints
      (1) At initial presentation, hands, wrists, knees, feet, and ankles are affected (Fig. 21–10).
      (2) As disease progresses, the elbows, shoulders, knees, hips, ankles, and jaw are affected.
   d. Bilateral symmetric deformity and displacement of proximal joints
   e. Morning stiffness, particularly in the hands and feet
   f. Joint tissues that are warm and spongy on palpation
3. Extra-articular symptoms
   • Painless subcutaneous nodules over bony prominences (rheumatoid nodules) affect 25 percent of people with rheumatoid arthritis)
   • Weight loss
   • Anemia
   • Chronic low-grade fever
   • Slight leukocytosis
   • Decreased muscle elasticity and strength
   • Fatigue
   • Anorexia
   • Malaise
   • Neuropathy
   • Lymphadenopathy

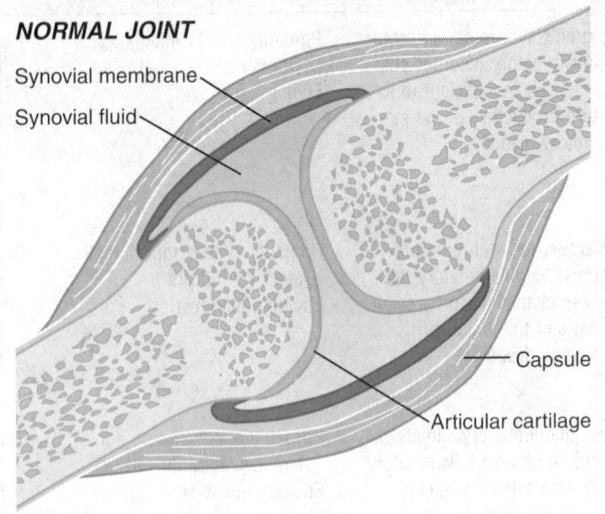

JOINT CHANGES IN RHEUMATOID ARTHRITIS

NORMAL JOINT
Synovial membrane
Synovial fluid
Capsule
Articular cartilage

RHEUMATOID ARTHRITIS

EARLY CHANGES
Inflamed synovium

Loss of cartilage
Pannus
Bone erosion

PROGRESSIVE DISEASE

Figure 21–9.

   • Splenomegaly
   • Vasculitis

Diagnostics

1. Medical diagnosis is made when 5 of the following American College of Rheumatology criteria are met and when these symptoms are present for 6 or more weeks.
   • Morning stiffness that improves during the day
   • Pain or tenderness in at least 1 joint
   • Swelling of 1 joint
   • Swelling of 2nd joint
   • Symmetric joint swelling

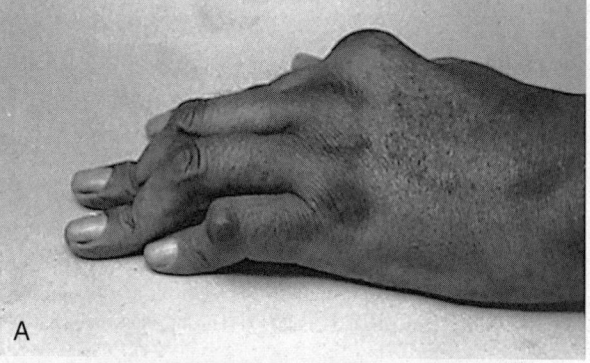
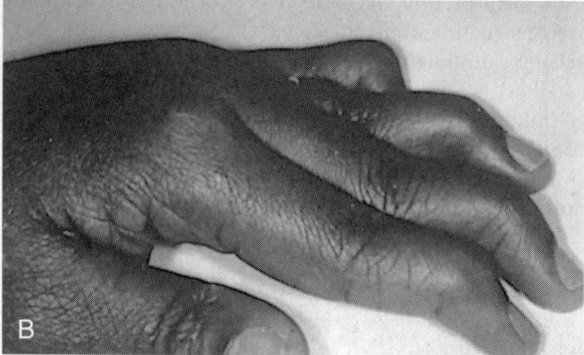
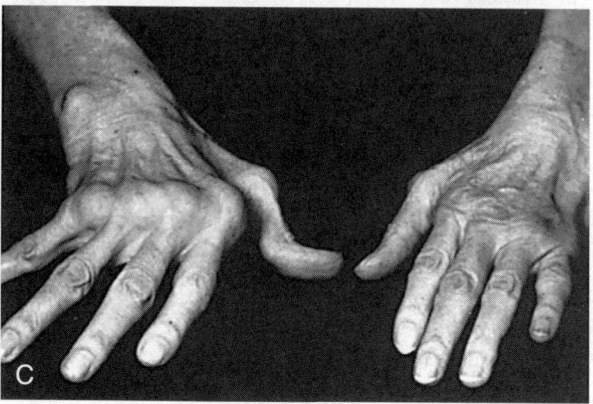

Figure 21–10. Ulnar drift, swan neck, and boutonnière deformities commonly seen in rheumatoid arthritis. (From the Clinical Slide Collection on the Rheumatic Diseases, copyright 1991, 1995. Used by permission of the American College of Rheumatology.)

- Presence of subcutaneous nodules
- Radiographic changes typical of rheumatoid arthritis
- Positive test result for rheumatoid factor
- Poor mucin precipitate in the synovial membrane
- Characteristic histologic changes in the synovial membrane
- Characteristic histologic changes in the subcutaneous nodules

2. Supporting diagnostic tests
   a. A decreased hematocrit, which measures the percentage of red blood cells in the plasma
   b. An increased WBC count, which measures the total number of WBCs in the blood.
   c. The presence of antinuclear antibody, which indicates the presence of antibodies directed against substances found in the nucleus of the cell
   d. A decreased C4 complement component, a measurement of the blood protein involved in the inflammatory response following an antibody–antigen reaction.
   e. An elevated C-reactive protein, a glycoprotein, which appears with inflammatory processes
   f. An elevated erythrocyte sedimentation rate, which is increased in inflammatory processes and measures the speed at which red blood cells settle in anticoagulated blood
   g. A radiograph of the affected joint showing soft tissue swelling and narrowing of joint spaces. In the late stages, radiograph shows erosion of articular surface.

3. The following points should be discussed when interviewing the person with rheumatoid arthritis:
   a. Subjective complaints of pain both at rest and with activity
   b. Inability to perform activities of daily living and work
   c. Complaints of joint stiffness, muscle fatigue, joint swelling
   d. General complaints of fatigue, weight loss, low-grade fever, and morning stiffness

4. During the physical examination, the following should be performed:
   a. Inspection of range of motion for stiff, rigid joints and weak hand grip
   b. Assessment of joint edema and deformity
   c. Observance of gait and stance
   d. Palpation for warmth of joints, swelling, crepitus, and subcutaneous nodules
   e. Assessment of muscle strength, tone, and size

Clinical Management

1. Goals of clinical management are to relieve discomfort, prevent joint destruction, and maintain joint and muscle functioning.

2. Nonpharmacologic interventions
   a. Exercising for joint motion and muscle strengthening
   b. Balancing periods of rest and activity
   c. Using orthopedic splints or braces during acute inflammation to prevent deformity
   d. Using heat or cold therapy
   e. Using paraffin baths, massage, and relaxation techniques
   f. Undergoing orthopedic surgery, including prophylactic procedures (e.g., articular synovectomy, osteotomy,

and arthroscopy or corrective procedures (e.g., joint reconstruction and replacement)
g. Using ambulatory support (e.g., cane, crutches, walker)
h. Applying adaptive devices to assist with activities of daily living
i. Maintaining a well-balanced diet and weight control
3. Pharmacologic interventions
a. Nonsteroidal anti-inflammatory agents (e.g., salicylates and nonsalicylates)

NURSE ADVISORY

Nonsteroidal anti-inflammatory drugs are the treatment of choice for rheumatoid arthritis. Encourage the use of enteric-coated aspirin preparations to decrease gastric symptoms associated with regular aspirin. Measure serum salicylate levels to monitor clinical response and compliance with drug therapy. Assess the person for tinnitus, hearing loss, and platelet inhibition, which can result from high-dose aspirin use. When corticosteroids are part of the therapy, low doses should be used to decrease their multiple side effects, including bone loss.

b. Corticosteroids
c. Remission-inducing agents (e.g., gold salt therapy, penicillamine, and antimalarial agents)
d. Immunosuppressive drugs (e.g., imuran, cyclophosphazide, and methotrexate)
e. Experimental medications (e.g., monoclonal antibodies and interferon)
f. Adjuvant medications
   (1) Calcium supplements
   (2) Drugs to minimize gastric irritation
   (3) Analgesics
4. Special medical-surgical procedures
a. Arthrocentesis (i.e., the withdrawal of fluid from a joint)
b. Plasmapheresis (i.e., the removal of plasma proteins from the blood)
c. Leukapheresis (i.e., the removal of leukocytes from the blood)

Complications

1. Small proteins called cytokines are produced by immune cells. These cytokines are involved in inflammatory and immune reactions. In rheumatoid arthritis, cytokines are believed to stimulate synovial cell production, which leads to cartilage damage in the joint.
2. Destruction of cartilage from inflammatory changes and erosion of bone causes loss of articular joint surfaces, loss of ability to move joints without pain, and resultant muscle atrophy.
3. Inflammation of ligaments and tendons close to the inflamed joints can cause tendinitis and tenosynovitis.
4. Protective immobilization of joints can cause permanent joint deformities, contractures, and partial dislocation of joints (subluxation).

Prognosis

1. Outcomes are variable.
2. Course of the disease varies greatly and is unpredictable, but it tends to be chronically progressive.

Applying the Nursing Process

NURSING DIAGNOSIS: Pain R/T inflammation and joint immobility

1. *Expected outcomes:* Following intervention, the person should be able to do the following:
a. Report elimination or control of discomfort
b. Maintain joint range of motion
c. Maintain baseline activity level
d. Express confidence about knowing enough about the disease and its treatment to manage home care
e. Participate in self-care with the help of equipment as needed
2. *Nursing interventions*
a. Assess pain on a scale of 1 to 10.
b. Assess quality and location of pain.
c. Identify factors that relieve and exacerbate discomfort.
d. Provide nonpharmacologic measures of relief.
e. Provide pain medications as ordered.

NURSING DIAGNOSIS: Impaired physical mobility R/T joint inflammation

1. *Expected outcomes:* Following interventions, the person should be able to do the following:
a. Maintain joint range of motion and muscle strength
b. Maintain baseline physical mobility
c. Move in bed, transfer, and ambulate with minimal assistance
2. *Nursing interventions*
a. Assess joint mobility and joint inflammation.
b. Help the person to change position frequently, alternating sitting, standing, and lying down.
c. Perform range-of-motion exercises according to provided schedule.
d. Maintain proper body alignment with support of joints in extended position.
e. Develop a plan for maintaining physical mobility and balancing rest and activity.

NURSING DIAGNOSIS: Activity intolerance R/T fatigue and anemia

1. *Expected outcomes:* Following interventions, the person should be able to perform activities of daily living without undue fatigue.

2. *Nursing interventions*
   a. Assess relationship of fatigue to activities and symptoms.
   b. Monitor hemoglobin and hematocrit.
   c. Schedule alternating periods of rest and activity.
   d. Investigate sleep patterns and ensure adequate rest.
   e. Encourage adequate dietary intake.

> **NURSING DIAGNOSIS:** Self-care deficit (all activities of daily living) R/T joint pain and deformity

1. *Expected outcomes:* Following intervention, the person should be able to do the following:
   a. Bathe self independently or with minimal assistance
   b. Feed self independently or with minimal assistance
   c. Groom self independently or with minimal assistance
   d. Perform toileting routines independently or with minimal assistance
2. *Nursing interventions*
   a. Monitor joints for pain, swelling, tenderness, and limitation of movement.
   b. Monitor muscle strength and ability to perform daily activities.
   c. Arrange for assistive equipment and adaptive clothing.
   d. Encourage the patient to provide pain control before initiating self-care activities.
   e. Allow the person to determine the self-care routine.
   f. Involve family in learning how to assist the person with self-care deficits.

Discharge Planning and Teaching

1. Assess the person's understanding of the disease process and potential complications of both the disease and the therapy.
2. Provide verbal and written information regarding the disease process and the potential complications of both the disease and the therapy.
3. Explain the purpose, dosage, schedule, and side effects of prescribed medications.

4. Arrange for devices to help the person with daily activities and promote independence.
5. Stress the importance of balancing rest and exercise.
6. Emphasize the need to maintain a well-balanced diet.
7. Provide for physical therapy and application of splints.
8. Advise the person to avoid physical and emotional stress.
9. Stress the importance of follow-up care.
10. Make referrals to community agencies.

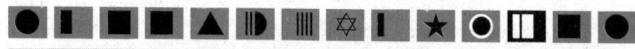

> **TRANSCULTURAL CONSIDERATIONS**
>
> Because of shorter life expectancy in many developing countries from whence immigrants come to the United States, rheumatoid arthritis may not be differentiated from osteoarthritis. Persons aged 25 to 45 years may seem "old" in some parts of the world, and in health teaching, the expected course of illness must be explained.

Public Health Considerations

1. Rheumatoid arthritis is a common, severe health problem in the United States with powerful impact on individuals and their families. An estimated 2,200,000 work days are lost annually, and an estimated $1 billion is spent on unproven and useless remedies.
2. Physical fitness recommendations include 20 minutes of low-intensity aerobic exercise performed 5 times weekly to increase strength of bone and ligaments and nourish cartilage.
3. The person should maintain desirable weight. Increased weight and fat cause increased stress on weight-bearing joints and can cause separation of tendons and ligaments.
4. The person should protect joints by warming up and stretching before physical activity; avoiding injury to muscle, ligament, tendon, and bone; and maintaining proper posture.

Bibliography

Books

Black JM, and Matassarin-Jacobs E (eds). *Luckmann and Sorenson's Medical-Surgical Nursing: A Psychophysiologic Approach.* 4th ed. Philadelphia: WB Saunders, 1993.

Kersten L. *Comprehensive Respiratory Nursing: A Decision-Making Approach.* Philadelphia: WB Saunders, 1989.

McCance K, and Heuther S. *Pathophysiology: The Biologic Basis for Disease in Adults and Children.* St. Louis: CV Mosby, 1994.

Mudget-Grout CL. *Immunologic Disorders.* St. Louis: Mosby–Year Book, 1992.

Phipps WJ, et al. *Medical-Surgical Nursing: Concepts and Clinical Practice.* St. Louis: Mosby–Year Book, 1991.

Roitt IM. *Immunology.* 3rd ed. St. Louis: CV Mosby, 1993.

Sheehan C. *Clinical Immunology: Principles and Laboratory Diagnosis.* Philadelphia: JB Lippincott, 1990.

Smith S. *Tissue and Organ Transplantation: Implications for Professional Nursing Practice.* St. Louis: Mosby–Year Book, 1990.

Thelan LA, Davie JK, and Urden LD. *Textbook of Critical Care Nursing: Diagnosis and Management.* St. Louis: Mosby–Year Book, 1990.

Williams B, Grady K, and Sandiford-Guttenbeil D. *A Manual for Nurses: Organ Transplantation.* New York: Springer, 1991.

Chapters in Books and Journal Articles

Structure and Function of the Immune System

Frey A. The immune system and intravenous administration of immune globulin: Part 1, The immune system. *J Intravenous Nurs* 14(5):315–330, 1991.

Frey A. The immune system: Part 2, Intravenous administration of immune globulin. *J Intravenous Nurs* 14(6):396–405, 1991.

Janeway CA Jr. How the immune system recognizes invaders. *Sci Am* 269(3):73–79, 1993.

Lehman S. Immune function and nutrition: The clinical role of the intravenous nurse. *J Intravenous Nurs* 14(6):406–420, 1991.

Paul WE. Infectious diseases and the immune system. *Sci Am* 269(3):91–97, 1993.

Weissman IL, and Cooper MD. How the immune system develops. *Sci Am* 269(3):64–79, 1993.

Assessing People with Immune and Autoimmune Disorders

Fike DJ. Assays involving complement. *In* Sheehan C (ed). *Clinical Immunology: Principles and Laboratory Diagnosis.* Philadelphia: JB Lippincott, 1990.

Fike DJ. Cellular assays. *In* Sheehan C (ed). *Clinical Immunology: Principles and Laboratory Diagnosis.* Philadelphia: JB Lippincott, 1990.

Immunodeficiency Disorders

Cohen F. The pharmacologic treatment of HIV infection and AIDS in adults. *Nurs Clin North Am* 26(2):315–329, 1991.

Cotran RS, Kumar V, and Robbins SL. Diseases of immunity. *In* Cotran RS, Kumar V, and Robbins SL (eds). *Pathologic Basis of Disease.* 4th ed. Philadelphia: WB Saunders, 1989.

Greenberg P. Immunopathogenesis of HIV infection. *Hosp Pract* 27(2):109–124, 1992.

Greene WC. AIDS and the immune system. *Sci Am* 269(3):99–105, 1993.

Henry SB, and Holzemer WL. Critical care management of the patient with HIV infection who has *Pneumocystis carinii* pneumonia. *Heart Lung* 21(3):243–249, 1992.

Williams AB. The epidemiology, clinical manifestations and health-maintenance needs of women infected with HIV. *Nurse Pract* 17(5):27–34, 1992.

Hypersensitivity Disorders

Barnes PJ. Biochemistry of asthma. *Trends Biochem Sci* Oct:365–369, 1991.

Bochner BS, and Lichtenstein LM. Anaphylaxis. *N Engl J Med* 324(25):1785–1790, 1991.

Crnkovich DJ, and Carlson RW. Anaphylaxis: An organized approach to management and prevention. *J Crit Illness* 8(3):332–345, 1993.

Lichtenstein LM. Allergy and the immune system. *Sci Am* 269(3):117–124, 1993.

Autoimmune Disorders

Crossfield T. Patients with scleroderma. *Nursing* 4(10):19–20, 1990.

Dreisin RB. Wegener's granulomatosis. *Emerg Med* 25(9):61–66, 1993.

Harris ED. Rheumatoid arthritis: Pathophysiology and implications for therapy. *N Engl J Med* 322(18):1277–1289, 1990.

Hooker RS. Clinical characteristics of the seronegative spondyloarthropathies: An increasingly prevalent group of rheumatic diseases that tend to affect young people. *J Am Acad Physician Assist* 5(2):110–120, 1992.

Lash AA. Systemic lupus erythematosus: Diagnosis, treatment modalities, and nursing management. *Medsurg Nurs* 2(5):375–385, 1993.

Shine J. Understanding and treating the symptoms of Sjögren's syndrome. *Arthritis Today* 8(1):10, 1994.

Spiera H. Giant cell arteritis and polymyalgia rheumatica. *Hosp Pract* 25(11):71–82, 1990.

Steinman L. Autoimmune disease. *Sci Am* 269(3):107–114, 1993.

Sullivan JM. Care provided by a nurse managed center: Polyarteritis nodosa. *Dermatol Nurs* 6(1):35–39, 1994.

22

Caring for People with Respiratory Disorders

☐ *RESPIRATORY STRUCTURE AND FUNCTION*

Structures of the Respiratory System

1. Chest wall (Fig. 22–1)
   a. The chest wall resembles a hollow tube composed of bony structures and muscles.
   b. These bony structures and muscles provide a protective, airtight cage around the lungs and heart.
2. Thoracic cavity (Fig. 22–2)
3. Upper airways (Fig. 22–3)
4. Lower airways (Fig. 22–4)

Functions of the Respiratory System

1. Primary function: To provide energy to body cells
   a. To obtain energy, body cells must metabolize glucose, a process that requires a constant supply of oxygen.
   b. Metabolizing glucose also creates waste products (principally carbon dioxide and water) that must be carried away from the cells and out of the body.
2. Two levels of respiration: external (alveolar-capillary level) and internal (tissue-cellular level)
3. The respiratory process (Figs. 22–5 and 22–6)
   a. At rest, pressure (force per unit of area) between the lungs and the atmosphere is equal (is at equilibrium).
   b. On inspiration (inhalation), the diaphragm descends into the abdominal cavity, causing negative pressure in the lungs (pressure lower than that of the atmosphere). This negative pressure draws air (and hence oxygen) from the area of greater pressure (the atmosphere) into the area of lesser pressure (the lungs).
   c. Within the lungs, air passes through the thin-walled terminal bronchioles into the alveoli.
   d. Oxygen from the air diffuses through the respiratory membrane in the alveoli into the surrounding capillaries, which transport it to the left side of the heart. Diffusion is the movement of a substance (in this case, oxygen) from an area of higher concentration to an area of lower concentration.
   e. The heart pumps the oxygenated blood to body tissues and cells, where oxygen and glucose diffuse across the capillary membrane.

f. Within body cells, complex reactions (cellular respiration) involving oxygen and glucose provide energy to the cells.
   g. The cells transfer the waste products from cellular respiration (including carbon dioxide and water) through the capillary membrane to the blood, which returns to the heart and thence to the lungs and alveoli. This process of oxygen moving from the alveoli to the capillaries and carbon dioxide moving from the capillaries to the alveoli is continuous.
   h. Inspiration ends, causing the diaphragm and intercostal muscles to relax and the lungs to recoil.
   i. As the lungs recoil, pressure within the lungs becomes greater than atmospheric pressure, causing air (now containing the cellular waste products carbon dioxide and water) to move from the alveoli in the lungs to the atmosphere. Expiration (exhalation) is a passive process.
4. Maintaining ventilation-perfusion balance (Fig. 22–7)
   a. Ventilation (air flow) is the process during which the air is delivered to the alveoli. The respiratory system maintains ventilation through centers controlling the lungs. Located in the medulla and the pons of the central nervous system, these centers stimulate ventilation in response to elevated levels of carbon dioxide or decreased levels of oxygen.
      (1) The level of carbon dioxide regulates respiration in persons with normal respiratory systems. If the level of carbon dioxide rises, respiration increases to eliminate excess carbon dioxide.
      (2) In contrast, decreased oxygen levels trigger respiration in patients with long-term respiratory dysfunction (e.g., chronic obstructive pulmonary disease [COPD]—see Caring for People with Chronic Obstructive Pulmonary Disease)

NURSE ADVISORY

Patients with chronically elevated carbon dioxide levels should never be given high levels of supplemental oxygen. If the respiratory centers sense elevated oxygen levels, the patient's ventilatory drive may be depressed, leading to respiratory arrest.

b. Perfusion (blood flow) is the blood delivered to the alveoli through the capillary system.

BONY STRUCTURES OF THE CHEST

The 12 ribs, sternum, manubrium, xiphoid process, and spine comprise the bony structures of the chest wall. The ribs are directly attached to the spine, are attached to the sternum by cartilage, and are connected to one another by intercostal muscles. The diaphragm, the largest respiratory muscle, creates the floor of the chest wall.

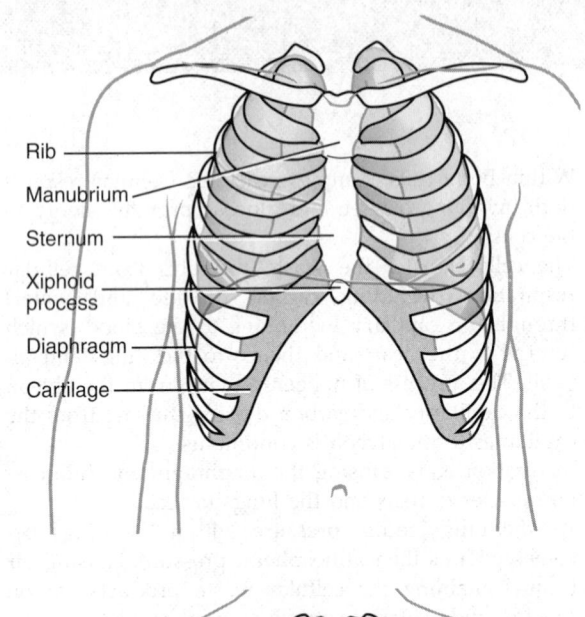

Rib
Manubrium
Sternum
Xiphoid process
Diaphragm
Cartilage

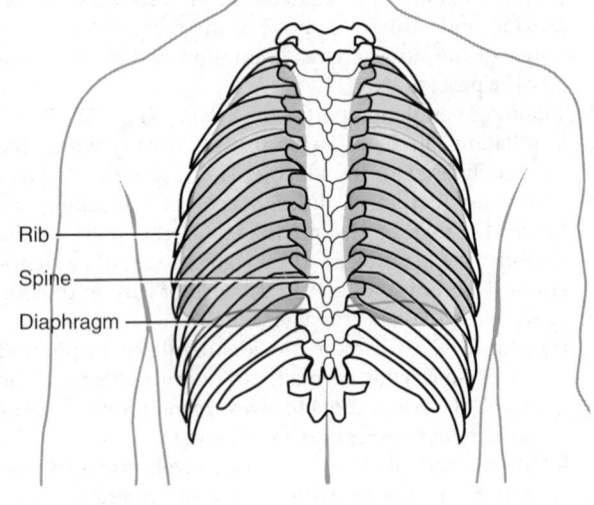

Rib
Spine
Diaphragm

Figure 22–1.

c. Gravity affects perfusion, increasing blood flow to lower lung segments. Ventilation is not affected by gravity, but air flow is greater in upper lung segments because air is less dense than blood.

d. Ventilation and perfusion affect gas exchange by affecting blood flow, air flow, or both.
   (1) Adequate ventilation but inadequate perfusion (as in pulmonary emboli) creates dead-space units that restrict blood flow.
   (2) Adequate perfusion but inadequate ventilation (as in atelectasis) creates shunt units that restrict air flow into the alveoli, which collapse.
   (3) When both perfusion and ventilation are inadequate (as in pulmonary emboli combined with pneumonia or atelectasis), the lung unit is called a silent unit and the alveoli collapse.

5. Regulating acid-base balance
   a. The lungs work to rapidly restore a neutral pH balance in the body.
   b. Changes in carbon dioxide levels in the blood change the pH balance of the body.
      (1) Elevated carbon dioxide levels due to retention of carbon dioxide in the lungs cause respiratory acidosis. The bodies of persons with chronically elevated levels of carbon dioxide retain bicarbonate to maintain a neutral pH.
      (2) Decreased carbon dioxide levels due to hyperventilation cause respiratory alkalosis.

◼ ASSESSING PEOPLE WITH RESPIRATORY DISORDERS

Key Symptoms and Their Pathophysiologic Bases

1. Cough
   a. Coughing is a protective reflex produced in response to tracheobronchial irritations such as foreign bodies, inflammatory agents, and mucus.
   b. It helps to clear secretions from lower bronchial trees and is normal after awakening from a long sleep.
   c. Coughing is the most common symptom of respiratory disease.
   d. It may be described in terms of moisture, frequency, regularity, pitch, and quality.
2. Sputum
   a. The average adult pulmonary system produces approximately 100 ml of mucus per day. Excess mucus is expectorated as sputum.
   b. Note color, consistency, amount, and location of sputum. Sputum characteristics can be suggestive of specific pathologic processes.
   c. Color
      (1) Rust—pneumococcal infection
      (2) Brick red—*Klebsiella* infection
      (3) Salmon colored—staphylococcal infection
      (4) Yellow-green—bacterial infection
      (5) Pink—pulmonary edema
      (6) White—asthma
      (7) Gray—bronchitis
      (8) Brown—aspergillosis
      (9) Anchovy-chocolate—amebic abscess
      (10) Red sputum and saliva—rifampin use
   d. Consistency
      (1) Frothy—pulmonary edema
      (2) Mucoid, sticky—bronchitis
      (3) Thick, purulent, with foul odor—lung abscess or bronchiectasis

THORACIC LANDMARKS AND UNDERLYING LUNG STRUCTURES

The thoracic cavity is contained within the chest wall and is divided into right and left pleural cavities separated by the mediastinum. The mediastinum, located in the center of the chest directly under the sternum, contains the heart, aorta, thymus, esophagus, trachea, bronchi, lymph nodes, and a number of major nerves.

Each pleural cavity contains 1 lung. The right lung consists of 3 lobes, and the left lung consists of 2 lobes and a depression where the heart fits.

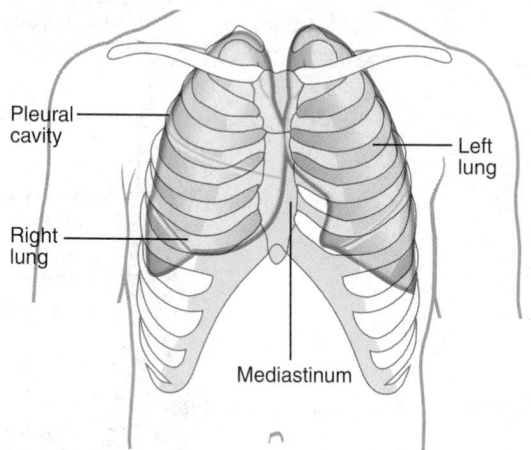

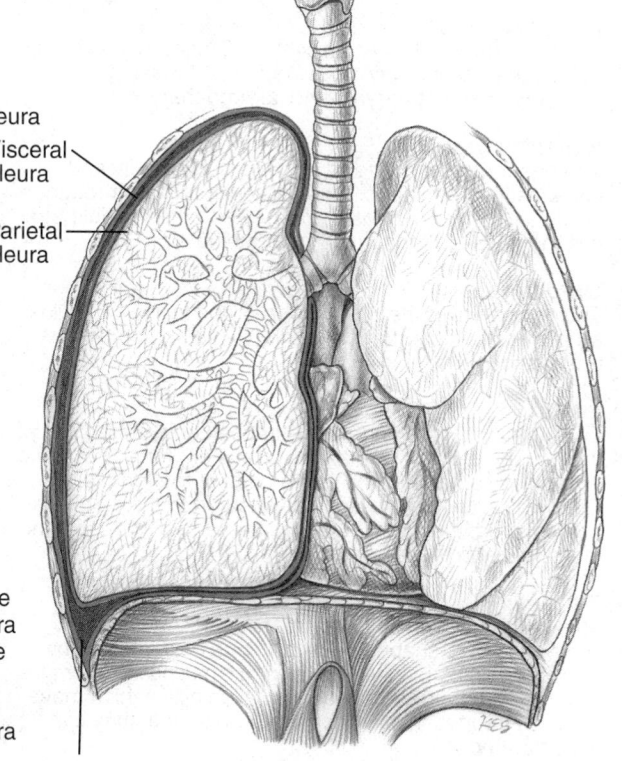

The inside of the pleural cavity and the outside of the lungs are covered by a membrane called the pleura. The 2 layers of pleura are the visceral, which covers the outside of the lungs, and the parietal, which covers the inside of the thoracic cavity and the top of the diaphragm. The area between the pleura contains a lubricating substance, the pleural fluid, which permits the pleura to move over each other without friction. Space between the pleura is negligible, thus the term "potential space."

Figure 22–2.

(4) Tenacious—asthma, COPD
(5) Watery—common cold or allergy
e. Amount
  (1) Profuse—lung abscess
  (2) Increasing amounts over time—chronic bronchitis or bronchiectasis
f. Location
  (1) Clearing throat—sinuses
  (2) Deep, full cough—respiratory tree
3. Hemoptysis: bleeding from anywhere in the respiratory tract, as evidenced by coughing and expectoration of frothy red blood with sputum
a. Common causes of hemoptysis include tuberculosis, bronchiectasis, lung abscesses or malignancies, pneumonia, congestive heart failure, and pulmonary infarction within the respiratory tract.
b. When blood is noted in the sputum, it is necessary to determine if it is from the respiratory tract or the gastrointestinal tract.
4. Chest pain
a. Chest pain in lung disease is usually caused by an inflammation (as in pulmonary infections or infarctions) of the parietal pleura, which is innervated by numerous sensory nerves. (In contrast, the visceral pleura is relatively free of sensory nerves.)
b. Chest pain resulting from an inflamed pleura is characteristically described as a sharp, knifelike pain. It often has an abrupt onset, occurs at the site of the inflammation, and remains localized.
5. Dyspnea: Perceived, labored, or difficult breathing
a. Causes of acute dyspnea
  (1) Inflammation or infection of the respiratory tract
  (2) Obstruction by a foreign object
  (3) Anaphylactic swelling of the respiratory tract
  (4) Trauma to the chest
  (5) Pneumothorax or hemothorax
  (6) Fat embolism
b. Causes of chronic dyspnea
  (1) Congestive heart failure
  (2) COPD
  (3) Pulmonary edema
  (4) Weak respiratory muscles
6. Hoarseness: a rough or raspy quality to the voice
a. Acute hoarseness is usually caused by an inflammatory process such as laryngitis.
b. Chronic hoarseness is usually caused by a benign

UPPER AIRWAY STRUCTURES

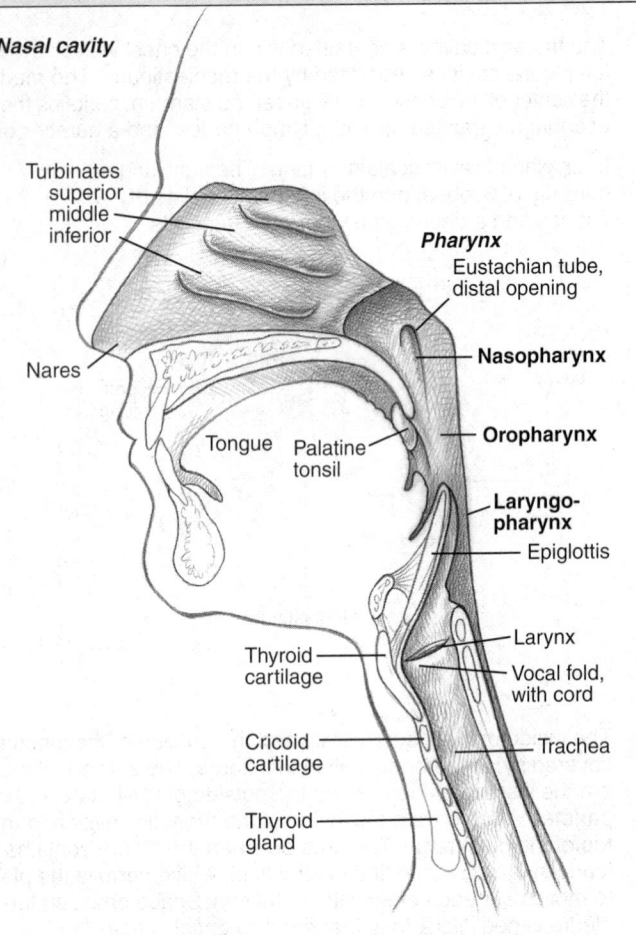

Nasal Cavity:
Two nares are lined by coarse nasal hair and are separated by a septum. Turbinates cover the lateral walls of the nasal cavity.

Pharynx:
The pharynx, which is approximately 5 inches long and lies behind the nasal cavity, is divided into 3 areas: nasopharynx, oropharynx, and laryngopharynx.

Nasopharynx:
The nasopharynx connects with the nasal cavity and contains the opening for the eustachian tubes, through which air from the atmosphere may enter the middle ear. It is the passage for air during breathing.

Oropharynx:
The oropharynx is the passage for air and food and provides an acoustic space during speech. Uvula and soft palate are located here.

Larynx:
The larynx is located above the trachea and at the base of the tongue. It contains the vocal cords or "voice box." The epiglottis is a flap located at the base of the tongue. During swallowing, the larynx is lifted up to the epiglottis and covered; thus food or fluid is prevented from entering the larynx and the trachea.

Trachea:
The trachea, which is approximately 4 inches long, is composed of C-shaped cartilage rings held in place by fibrin elastin membranes. It is lined with mucous membranes covered with hairlike projections called cilia, which move particles trapped in the mucus upward so that they can be expectorated.

Figure 22–3.

tumor such as a polyp, by paralysis of the vocal cords, by a malignant tumor on the true vocal cords, or by a mediastinal lesion.

Health History

1. Chief complaint
   a. Cough
      (1) Onset: sudden or insidious?
      (2) Duration: episodic or constant?
      (3) Characteristics: productive or nonproductive; dry or moist; regular or irregular; barking, hacking, wheezing; brassy, whooping, hoarse?
      (4) Severity
         • Does coughing produce chest pain?
         • Does it disrupt activity?
         • Has it caused nausea, vomiting, or gagging?
         • Is coughing becoming more severe?
      (5) Accompanying symptoms: dyspnea, fever, congestion, chest pain, sore throat, malaise, increased anxiety ("panic attacks")?
      (6) Aggravating factors: activity, weather, position, anxiety, walking, lying down, talking, eating, smoking, time of day?
      (7) Alleviating factors: medication (prescription or nonprescription), vaporizers (warm or cool mist), position change, fresh air, increased fluid intake?
   b. Sputum
      (1) Present or absent?
      (2) Frequency and amount from productive cough?
      (3) Characteristics (see p. 906)
   c. Dyspnea
      (1) Onset: abrupt or gradual?
      (2) Description: shortness of breath, tightness, suffocation, feeling winded or breathless?
      (3) Severity?
      (4) Accompanying symptoms: chest pain or tightness, diaphoresis, dizziness, cough, wheezing, cyanosis, swelling of extremities, anxiety, fatigue?
      (5) Aggravating factors
         • Time of day: increased in the morning or night?
         • Activity tolerance: increased with activity (what kind and how much); worse with eating?

LOWER AIRWAY STRUCTURES

Bronchus:
The bronchus is a large air-conducting passage, which is divided into right and left at the carina, which is located at approximately the level of T5. The right mainstem bronchus is almost vertical from the trachea, slightly larger in diameter and shorter than the left. The left mainstem bronchus makes an abrupt horizontal angle at the carina.

Bronchioles:
Mainstem bronchi continue to divide into lobar and then to segmental bronchioles, which are lined with mucosa and made of smooth muscle rather than the cartilage rings found in the bronchus. Bronchioles end in the terminal bronchioles, which are approximately 1 mm in diameter. Respiratory or acinus units lie at the distal end of the terminal bronchioles.

Acinus Units:
Acinus units, which are composed of respiratory bronchioles and alveolar sacs, are the functional portion of the pulmonary system. Respiratory bronchioles contain occasional alveoli that arise from the bronchiole wall, and alveolar sacs, in turn, may contain many individual alveoli. Alveoli walls are a single cell thick. Alveoli are surrounded by a vast network of capillaries. Alveoli within the alveolar sacs communicate with one another through small openings called pores of Kohn. Gas exchange occurs at this level, and the pores of Kohn allow inspired gas to be distributed evenly throughout the acinus unit.

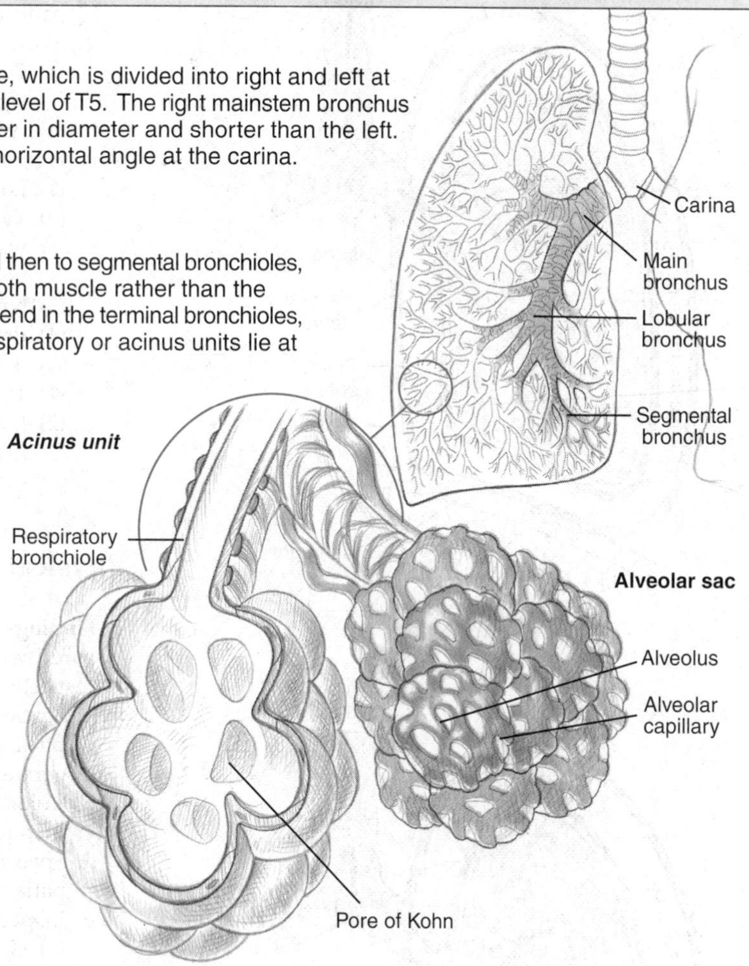

Figure 22–4.

- Body position: increased when lying down; decreased when sitting up or leaning against a wall; number of pillows used when sleeping?
  (6) Alleviating factors: position, medication (prescription or nonprescription), oxygen therapy, increased humidification, resting, coughing?
2. Past medical history
   a. History of pulmonary diseases such as tuberculosis, emphysema, bronchitis, asthma, cystic fibrosis, influenza, pneumonia: How often, how long, and how treated?
   b. Injuries to the face, mouth, nose, neck, throat, or chest?
   c. Immunizations
      (1) What kind?
      (2) Dates received?
      (3) Up to date?
      (4) "Flu shots"? How often?
      (5) Pneumonia vaccination?
   d. Hospitalizations for respiratory surgery or thoracic trauma: blunt trauma, pneumothorax, fractured ribs, use of ventilator or oxygen therapy?
   e. Past chest radiograph or other diagnostic tests: pulmonary function tests, allergy tests, tuberculosis (tine) test?
   f. Medications: prescription (antibiotics, steroids, bronchodilators) and nonprescription (nasal sprays, cough drops)?
   g. Respiratory allergies
      (1) Reactions: tightness in chest, congestion, watery and reddened eyes, rhinitis, wheezing?
      (2) Aggravating factors: food, pollen, smoke, dust, animals, medications, molds?
      (3) Age at which allergies appeared?
      (4) Treatments to prevent or alleviate symptoms?
3. Family history of asthma, cystic fibrosis, pulmonary malignancy, COPD, tuberculosis, allergies
4. Social history
   a. Habits
      (1) Tobacco use: pipes, cigarettes, cigars, smokeless

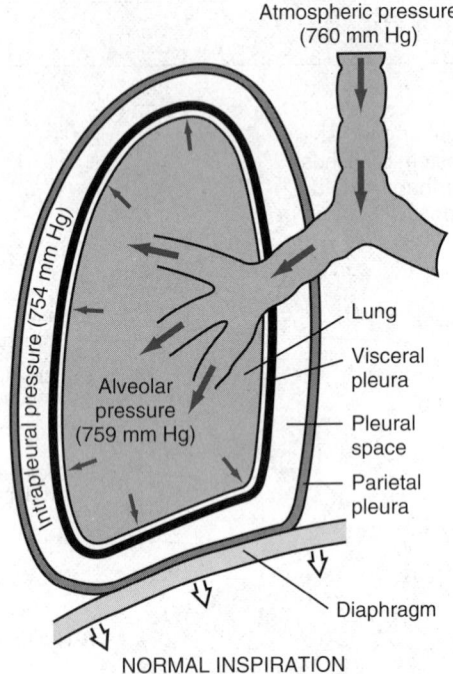

NORMAL INSPIRATION

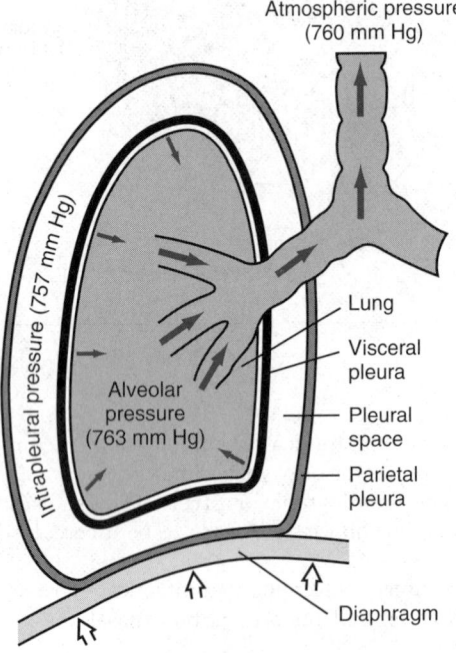

NORMAL EXPIRATION

Figure 22-5. Normal inspiration and expiration. (Redrawn from Black JM, and Matassarin-Jacobs E [eds]. *Luckmann and Sorensen's Medical-Surgical Nursing: A Psychophysiologic Approach.* 4th ed. Philadelphia: WB Saunders, 1993, p 908.)

tobacco? Trying or has tried to quit? Pack-year history (number of years smoked × number of packs per day)?
  (2) Alcohol use: when, how much, how long?
  (3) Recreational drugs: types, share needles, how long?

  b. Exercise: types and duration of regular exercise; activities that cause shortness of breath, coughing, chest pain, wheezing?
  c. Nutrition
    (1) Types of food eaten? How many meals a day? How much eaten at each meal?
    (2) Anorexia? Recent weight loss?
  d. Home environment
    (1) Location?
    (2) Type of house: number of floors, stairs, running water, indoor plumbing, air conditioning, heating, ventilation?
    (3) Number of people living in the house?
    (4) Presence of allergens?
  e. Work environment
    (1) Type of work and how long?
    (2) Exposure to dust, asbestos, silicon, beryllium, animal dander, fertilizers, and chemicals; and grinding, soldering, and welding of metals?

Physical Examination

1. Findings throughout the examination should be compared with those from the opposite side of the chest.
2. Inspection (begin while taking health history)
   a. Signs and symptoms of respiratory difficulty: tachypnea, wheezing, dyspnea, pursed lip breathing, exaggerated use of the accessory muscles, central cyanosis?
   b. Color: pink, dusky, cyanotic?
   c. Inspiratory-expiratory ratio of 1:2?
   d. Speech pattern: How many words or sentences can patient say between breaths?
   e. Inspect head and neck
     (1) Gross abnormalities
     (2) Pursed-lip breathing
     (3) Flared nostrils
     (4) Odor to breath?
     (5) Cough: characteristics?
     (6) Sputum production: color and odor?
     (7) Trachea midline?
   f. Inspect chest wall configuration
     (1) AP-transverse diameter (Fig. 22-8). Normally the transverse diameter is approximately twice the size of the anteroposterior diameter, or a ratio of 5:7 to 1:2.
     (2) Barrel chest: Increased anteroposterior diameter is characteristic of COPD.
     (3) Funnel chest (pectus excavatum): Depressed sternum is characteristic of Marfan syndrome and congenital connective tissue disease.
     (4) Pigeon chest (pectus carinatum): Sternum raised outward is characteristic of atrial and ventricular septal defects, rickets, and Marfan syndrome.
     (5) Kyphoscoliosis: Exaggerated curvature of the spine may result from osteoporosis, rheumatoid arthritis, or poor posture.
   g. Observe breathing pattern (Fig. 22-9)
     (1) Normal respiratory rate is 12 to 22 breaths per minute.

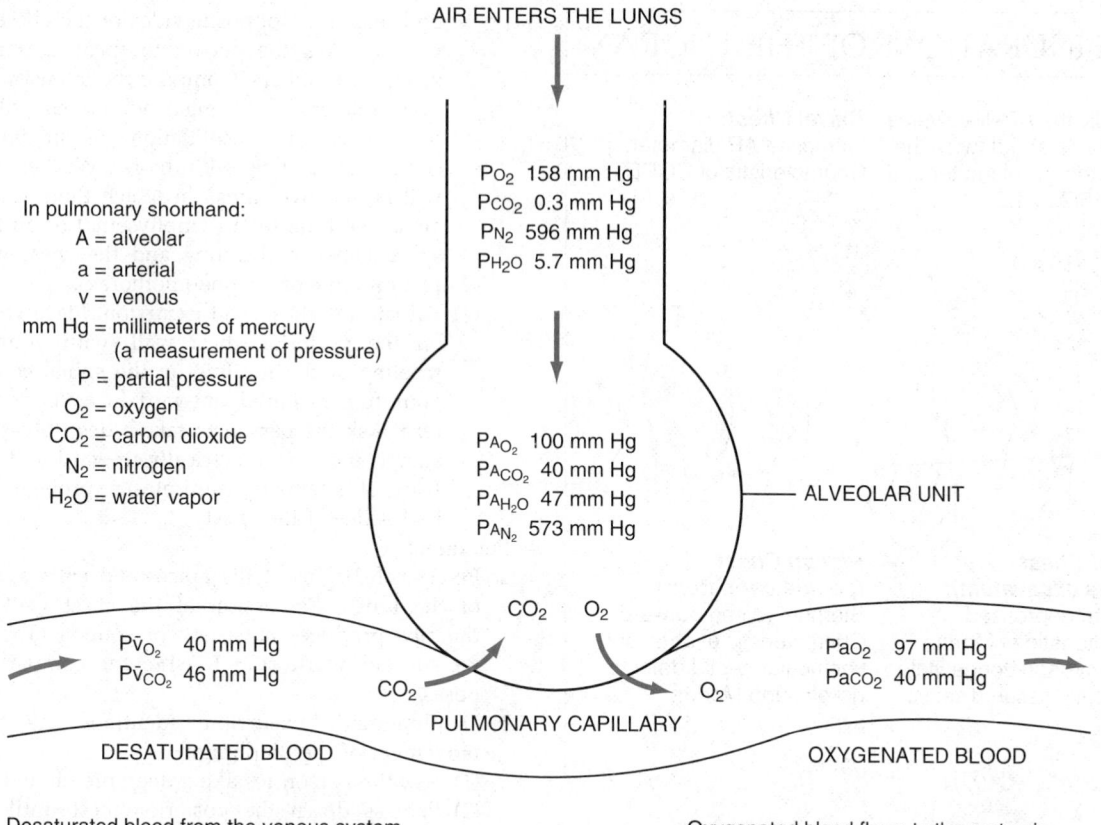

AIR ENTERS THE LUNGS

In pulmonary shorthand:

A = alveolar
a = arterial
v = venous
mm Hg = millimeters of mercury
(a measurement of pressure)
P = partial pressure
O_2 = oxygen
CO_2 = carbon dioxide
N_2 = nitrogen
H_2O = water vapor

P_{O_2} 158 mm Hg
P_{CO_2} 0.3 mm Hg
P_{N_2} 596 mm Hg
P_{H_2O} 5.7 mm Hg

PA_{O_2} 100 mm Hg
PA_{CO_2} 40 mm Hg
PA_{H_2O} 47 mm Hg
PA_{N_2} 573 mm Hg

ALVEOLAR UNIT

CO_2 O_2

$P\bar{v}_{O_2}$ 40 mm Hg
$P\bar{v}_{CO_2}$ 46 mm Hg

CO_2 O_2

Pa_{O_2} 97 mm Hg
Pa_{CO_2} 40 mm Hg

PULMONARY CAPILLARY

DESATURATED BLOOD

OXYGENATED BLOOD

Desaturated blood from the venous system returning to the right ventricle through the pulmonary artery to the lungs bringing carbon dioxide, the waste product of metabolism.

Oxygenated blood flows to the systemic arterial circulation, cells, tissues, and organs of the body.

Figure 22–6. Partial pressures of gases during normal respiration. (Redrawn from Black JM, and Matassarin-Jacobs E [eds]. *Luckmann and Sorensen's Medical-Surgical Nursing: A Psychophysiologic Approach.* 4th ed. Philadelphia: WB Saunders, 1993, p 904.)

(2) Note rate, depth, rhythm, and patterns of respiration and use of accessory muscles.

h. Examine extremities for signs of the following:
(1) Cyanosis
(2) Clubbing (Fig. 22–10): Nail bed angle increases from 160 to 180 degrees, fingers have spoonlike appearance. Clubbing is associated with COPD, cystic fibrosis, lung cancer, bronchiectasis, and congenital heart defects that produce cyanosis.

3. Palpation
a. Trachea
(1) Place thumbs on opposite sides of the trachea, with the trachea at midline.
(2) The trachea should be slightly movable when pushed from side to side and should return to baseline passively.
(3) Abnormalities include masses, crepitus, and deviations.

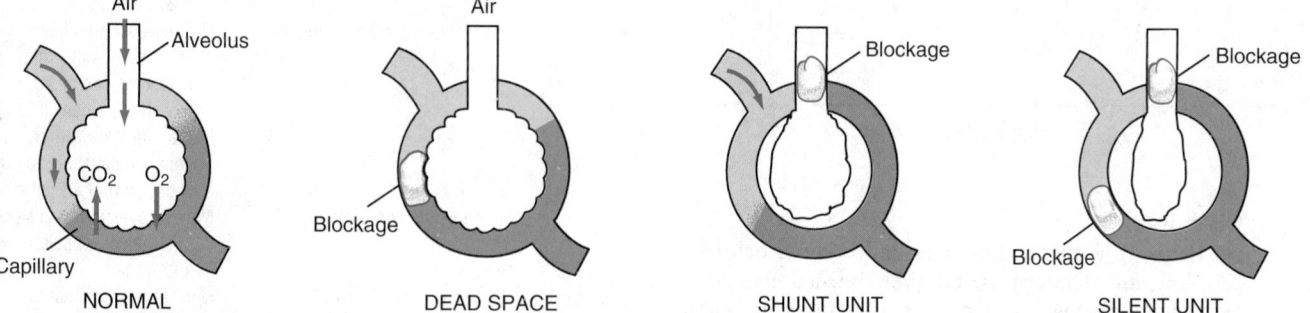

NORMAL   **DEAD SPACE**   **SHUNT UNIT**   **SILENT UNIT**

Figure 22–7. Relationship between ventilation (air flow) and perfusion (blood flow). (Redrawn from Black JM, and Matassarin-Jacobs E [eds]. *Luckmann and Sorensen's Medical-Surgical Nursing: A Psychophysiologic Approach.* 4th ed. Philadelphia: WB Saunders, 1993, p 905.)

CONFIGURATIONS OF THE THORAX

Normally the AP–transverse diameter is about twice the size of the AP diameter or a ratio of 5:7 to 1:2.

Barrel Chest: Increased AP diameter. Characteristic of COPD.

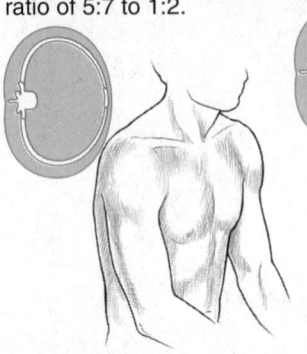
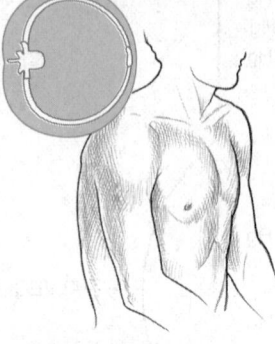

Funnel Chest (pectus excavatum): Sternum depressed. Characteristic of Marfan syndrome and congenital connective tissue disease.

Pigeon Chest (pectus carinatum): Sternum raised outward. Characteristic of atrial and ventricular septal defects, rickets, and Marfan syndrome.

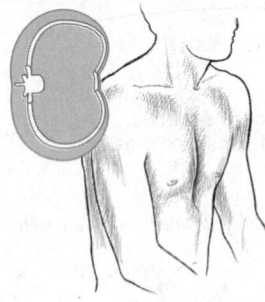
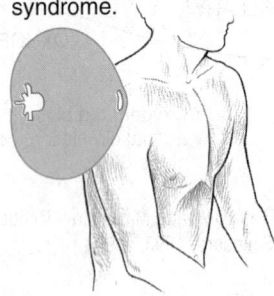

Kyphoscoliosis: Normal curvature of the spine is exaggerated. Causes can include osteoporosis, rheumatoid arthritis, poor posture.

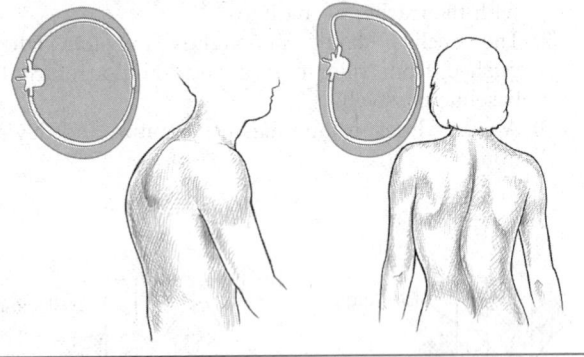

Figure 22–8.

both hands on opposite sides of the chest simultaneously. Ask the person to speak a phrase or a group of numbers. Compare the intensity of vibrations bilaterally. Stronger vibrations will be felt over areas of consolidation (as in pneumonia, compression of tissue, tumors). Weaker vibrations will be felt over areas in which there is increased air in the lung (as in emphysema) or an increased space between the lung and the chest wall (e.g., pleural effusion or pneumothorax).

(4) Palpate for chest wall excursion. Place your hands on the posterior chest wall, with your thumbs meeting at the midline on the spinal column and your fingers flared outward in a "butterfly" pattern. Ask the person to take a deep breath. Hands should move symmetrically upward and outward. Lack of symmetry indicates a problem on 1 or both sides of the chest.

4. Percussion
   a. Percussion begins at the apices and ends at the bases of the lungs. Percussion of the chest wall between the ribs produces a variety of sounds (Table 22–1). Be sure to work side to side for comparison purposes.
   b. Diaphragmatic excursion: identifies the range of movement of the diaphragm
      (1) Ask the person to take a deep breath and hold it.
      (2) Percuss down the posterior chest until the note changes from resonant to dull. Mark this spot.
      (3) Have the person exhale and hold it. Repeat percussion technique.
      (4) Percuss both sides of the chest.

b. Chest wall
   (1) Palpate the thoracic muscles and bony structures.
   (2) Note any tenderness, bulging, retractions, pulsations, crepitus, swelling, or variations in tactile fremitus.
   (3) Tactile fremitus is a vibration perceptible on the chest wall while the patient is speaking. Place

Table 22–1. Sounds Heard at Percussion

Sound Type	Characteristics	Significance
Resonant	Low-pitched, hollow sound	Normal lung tissue
Hyperresonant	Low-pitched, louder than resonant	Normal in children and thin adults. Abnormal in other adults. Indicates excess air in the lung or pleural space (e.g., emphysema or pneumothorax)
Dull	Medium pitched, thudlike	Normal over the liver and heart. Abnormal over other areas of the chest, where it may indicate tumor, consolidation, atelectasis, pleural effusion
Flat	High-pitched, soft	Normal over airless tissue: heavy muscles and bones
Tympanic	High, hollow, drumlike	Normal over stomach. Abnormal on chest, where it may indicate tension pneumothorax

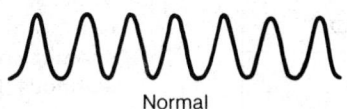
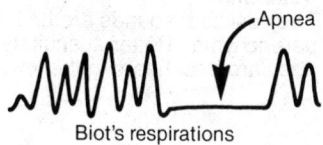
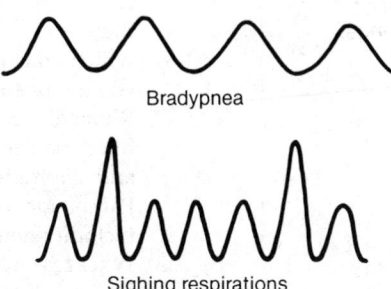
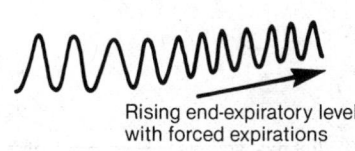

Figure 22–9. Breathing patterns. (Redrawn from Kersten L. *Comprehensive Respiratory Nursing.* Philadelphia: WB Saunders, 1989, p 279.)

(5) Normally, the distance between marks is 3 to 6 cm, with marks higher on the right due to the liver underlying the diaphragm. Emphysema produces little excursion owing to the size of the hyperinflated lungs. A patient with a paralyzed diaphragm will have decreased excursion.

5. Auscultation of the lungs: enables the examiner to assess 3 distinct components—normal breath sounds, adventitious breath sounds, and vocal resonance (transmission of the spoken word through the chest wall)

a. Normal breath sounds are produced by the movement of air within the lungs. There are 3 categories of normal breath sounds: bronchial, bronchovesicular, and vesicular (Fig. 22–11).
   (1) Bronchial: only heard anteriorly over the large airways above the carina; normally louder on expiration
   (2) Bronchovesicular: heard anteriorly and posteriorly over the large airways (e.g., mainstem bronchi); heard equally well on inspiration and expiration

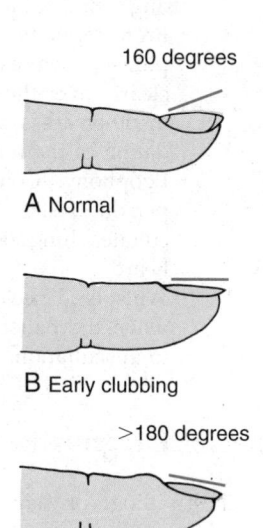
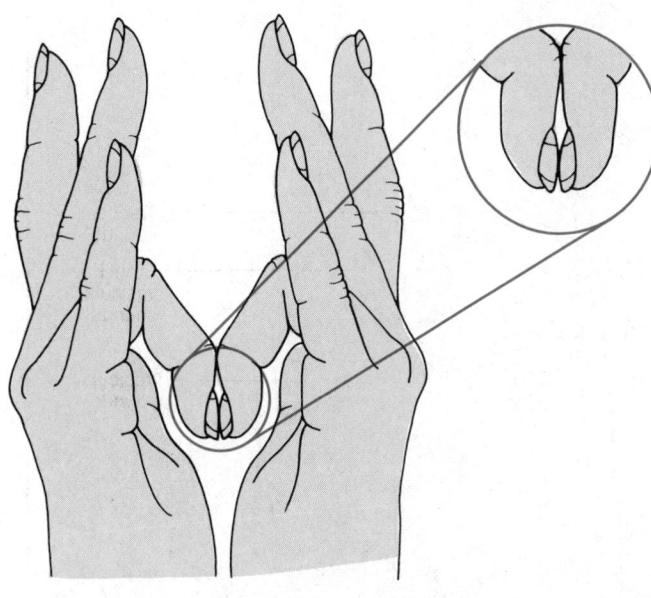

Figure 22–10. Clubbing. (From Black JM, and Matassarin-Jacobs E [eds]. *Luckmann and Sorensen's Medical-Surgical Nursing: A Psychophysiologic Approach.* 4th ed. Philadelphia: WB Saunders, 1993, p 920.)

NORMAL BREATH SOUNDS

Bronchial:
Bronchial breath sounds are only heard anteriorly and are normally louder on expiration. They are heard over the large airways above the carina.

Bronchovesicular:
These breath sounds are heard anteriorly and posteriorly over the large airways, such as the mainstem bronchi, and are heard equally well on inspiration and expiration.

Vesicular:
The vesicular sounds are heard throughout the lung parenchyma. Better auscultated during inspiration, they are best heard in the lower lobes of the lungs.

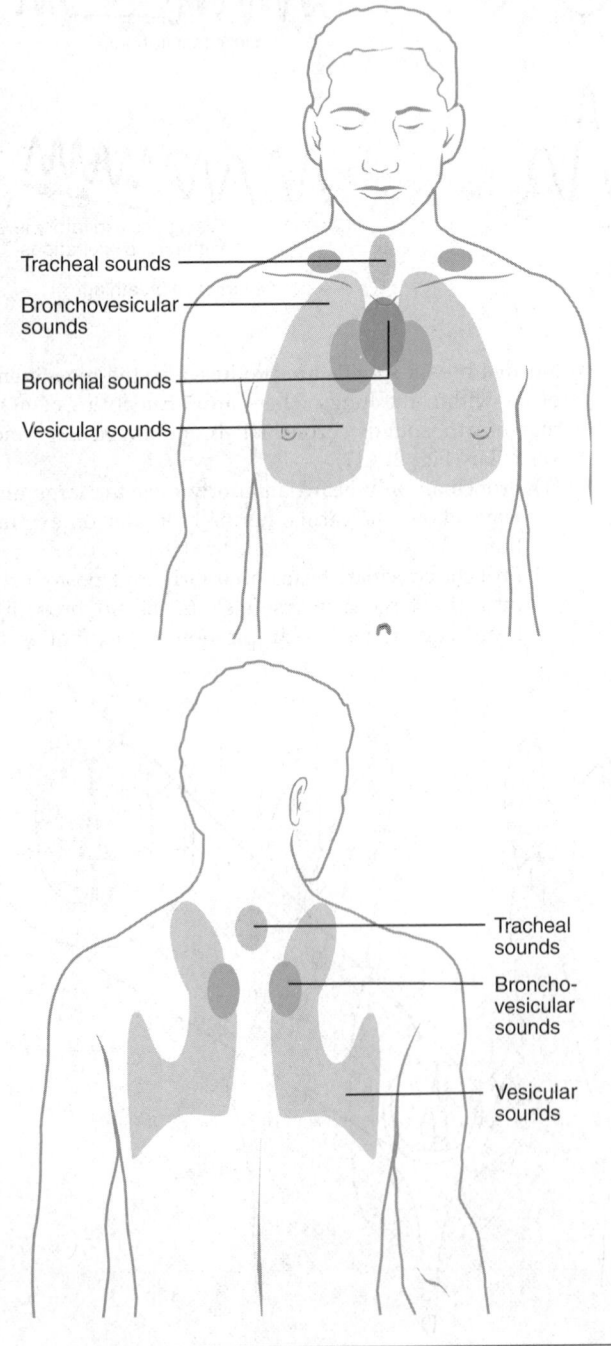

Figure 22–11.

(3) Vesicular: heard through the lung parenchyma but best heard in the lower lobes of the lungs; better auscultated during inspiration
b. Adventitious (abnormal) breath sounds are divided into 4 categories: crackles, rhonchi, wheezes, and pleural friction rubs (Table 22–2).
(1) Crackles, which are heard on inspiration, result from the sudden opening of airways that are filled with fluid. The sound is similar to that produced when hair is rubbed together over the ear. It does not clear with coughing. Atelectatic crackles may be auscultated in people who have shallow respirations. These crackles result from the opening of closed airways and clear with deep breathing; they are nonpathologic. Pathologic disorders in which crackles may be present include pulmonary edema, pneumonia, and pulmonary fibrosis.
(2) Rhonchi occur when air passes through a fluid-filled passageway. They are heard on inspiration and expiration and may be cleared by coughing. Pathologic conditions that may produce rhonchi include pneumonia, bronchitis, and bronchiectasis.
(3) Wheezes result when air passes through a narrowed airway. They have a musical quality that is heard both on inspiration and expiration. Pathologic conditions that produce wheezes include pulmonary edema, foreign bodies, and asthma.
(4) Pleural friction rub is a sound caused by inflamed tissues rubbing together. Heard on inspiration and expiration, the sound has a grating quality to it similar to pieces of leather rubbing together. Pathologic conditions that may cause pleural friction rubs include pleurisy, pleural infarction, pneumonia, and pleural inflammation.
c. Vocal resonance
(1) Normally voice sounds are muffled.
(2) Vocal resonance is louder over the large airways and becomes dampened in the peripheral lung fields.
(3) Consolidation of the lung can be assessed by using 1 of 3 techniques:
• Bronchophony: Assessed when patient speaks a phrase such as "99." Normally, this is heard clearly over the bronchial area. Hearing it clearly in other areas of the lung may indicate consolidation of the lung.
• Egophony: Consolidation is present when the person speaks the letter *A* while the nurse auscultates lung fields, causing the letter *E* to be heard.
• Whispered pectoriloquy: Consolidation is present when the patient whispers a phrase that is clear to auscultation.

Special Diagnostic Tests

1. Chest radiograph (Fig. 22–12)
   a. Uses
      (1) Routinely screen, diagnose, and monitor disorders and abnormalities (e.g., atelectasis, hemotho-

Table 22–2. Adventitious Lung Sounds*

Sound	Description	Mechanism	Clinical Example
Discontinuous Sounds			
Crackles—fine (rales) Inspiration Expiration	Discontinuous, high-pitched, short crackling, popping sounds heard during inspiration that are not cleared by coughing; you can simulate this sound by rolling a strand of hair between your fingers near your ear, or by moistening your thumb and index finger and separating them near your ear	Inhaled air collides with previously deflated airways; airways suddenly pop open, creating crackling sound as gas pressures between the two compartments equalize	*Late inspiratory crackles* occur with restrictive disease: pneumonia, congestive heart failure, and interstitial fibrosis *Early inspiratory crackles* occur with obstructive disease: chronic bronchitis, asthma, and emphysema
Crackles—coarse (coarse rales)	Loud, low-pitched, bubbling and gurgling sounds that start in early inspiration and may be present in expiration; may decrease somewhat by suctioning or coughing but will reappear shortly—sounds like opening a Velcro fastener	Inhaled air collides with secretions in the trachea and large bronchi	Pulmonary edema, pneumonia, pulmonary fibrosis, and the terminally ill who have a depressed cough reflex
Atelectatic crackles (atelectatic rales)	Sound like fine crackles, but do not last and are not pathologic; disappear after the first few breaths; heard in axillae and bases (usually dependent) of lungs	When sections of alveoli are not fully aerated, they deflate and accumulate secretions. Crackles are heard when these sections re-expand with a few deep breaths	In aging adults, bed-ridden persons, or in persons just aroused from sleep
Pleural friction rub	A very superficial sound that is coarse and low pitched; it has a grating quality as if 2 pieces of leather are being rubbed together; sounds just like crackles, but *close* to the ear; sounds louder if you push the stethoscope harder onto the chest wall; sound is inspiratory and expiratory	Caused when pleurae become inflamed and lose their normal lubricating fluid; their opposing roughened pleural surfaces rub together during respiration; heard best in anterolateral wall where greatest lung mobility exists	Pleuritis, accompanied by pain with breathing (rub disappears after a few days if pleural fluid accumulates and separates pleurae)
Continuous Sounds			
Wheeze—high-pitched (sibilant)	High-pitched, musical squeaking sounds that sound polyphonic (multiple notes as in a musical chord); predominate in expiration but may occur in both expiration and inspiration	Air squeezed or compressed through passageways narrowed almost to closure by collapsing, swelling, secretions, or tumors; the passageway walls oscillate in apposition between the closed and barely open positions; the resulting sound is similar to a vibrating reed	Diffuse airway obstruction from acute asthma or chronic emphysema
Wheeze—low-pitched (sonorous rhonchi)	Low-pitched; monophonic (single note), musical snoring, moaning sounds; they are heard throughout the cycle, although they are more prominent on expiration; may clear somewhat by coughing	Airflow obstruction as described by the vibrating reed mechanism above; the pitch of the wheeze cannot be correlated to the size of the passageway that generates it	Bronchitis, single bronchus obstruction from airway tumor
Stridor	High-pitched, monophonic, inspiratory, crowing sound, louder in neck than over chest wall	Originating in larynx or trachea, upper airway obstruction from swollen, inflamed tissues or lodged foreign body	Croup and acute epiglottitis in children, and foreign inhalation; obstructed airway may be life threatening

* Although nothing in clinical practice seems to differ more than the nomenclature of adventitious sounds, most authorities concur on two categories: (1) discontinuous, discrete crackling sounds, and (2) continuous, or musical sounds.

From Jarvis C. *Physical Examination and Health Assessment.* 2nd ed. Philadelphia: WB Saunders, 1996, pp 502–503.

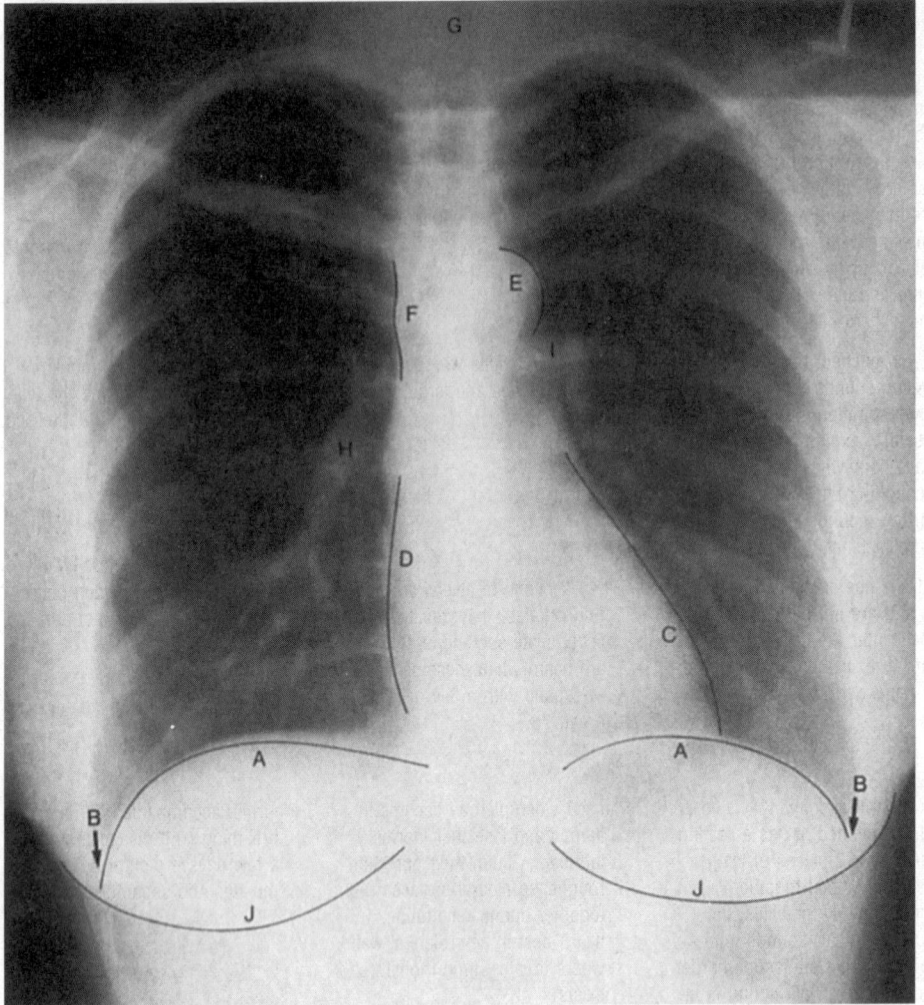

Figure 22–12. Normal chest radiograph taken from a posteroanterior view (PA). The backward L in the upper right corner is placed on the film to indicate the patient's left side of the chest. Some anatomic structures can be seen on the radiographic study. A, Diaphragm; B, costophrenic angle; C, left ventricle; D, right atrium; E, aortic arch; F, superior vena cava; G, trachea; H, right bronchus; I, left bronchus; J, breast shadows. (From Black JM, and Matassarin-Jacobs E [eds]. *Luckmann and Sorensen's Medical-Surgical Nursing: A Psychophysiologic Approach.* 4th ed. Philadelphia: WB Saunders, 1993, p 935.)

rax and pneumothorax, pulmonary edema, pneumonia, pleural effusions, tuberculosis)

 (2) Visualize chest cavity and its contents

 (3) Detect abnormalities not identified by other assessment techniques

 (4) Verify placement of invasive lines and tubes such as central lines, chest tubes, and endotracheal tubes

 b. Procedure: Patient inhales deeply and holds breath.

  (1) Usually obtained while patient is standing or sitting upright facing the film (posteroanterior and posterolateral positions)

  (2) May be taken while patient is in bed, with film placed behind patient (anteroposterior position)

  (3) May locate some abnormalities best by combining posteroanterior or anteroposterior view with lateral views of the chest taken from either the right or the left side of the chest with the patient lying on the side (lateral decubitus view) to distinguish solid from liquid abnormalities: liquids "layer out" or move with gravity; solids remain in their original positions

 c. Normal findings

  (1) Bony structures of the chest (e.g., vertebrae, sternum, ribs, clavicles, scapula)

  (2) Lung fields: appear black

  (3) Hemidiaphragms (located at the bottom of the lung fields): appear as rounded domes on either side of the spinal column, with right hemidiaphragm slightly higher than left

  (4) Junction of the hemidiaphragm and the rib cage (the costophrenic angle): clearly visible

  (5) Heart: appears as a white solid organ that primarily occupies the left side of the chest

  (6) Pulmonary vasculature (hilar region): appears as white lines just above the heart on either side of the spinal column

  (7) Trachea: located midline and bifurcates at the level of the T4 vertebrae

 d. Nursing interventions

  (1) Describe procedure and answer questions.

  (2) Dress patient in hospital gown (no snaps, buttons, buckles).

  (3) Have patient remove all jewelry.

2. Sputum

 a. Examination of sputum is extremely important in patients with pulmonary disease.

 b. Laboratory tests on sputum

  (1) Culture and sensitivity studies identify organisms present and drugs to which the organisms are sensitive. (Gram stains narrow down possible organisms before the culture and sensitivity studies are complete.)

(2) Acid-fast studies (when tuberculosis is suspected): An accurate acid-fast bacilli test requires sputum samples from at least 3 consecutive days.

(3) If a lung malignancy is suspected, a cytologic test is performed.

c. Procedure: To collect sputum, have patient expectorate into a sterile cup or use naso- or endotracheal suction.

d. Nursing interventions

(1) Have client cough up sputum from the lungs. Shallow, throat-clearing coughs will not produce sputum, only saliva.

(2) Collect sputum in the correct container specified for a particular test.

(3) Note color, consistency, amount, and odor of sputum.

(4) Deliver to laboratory immediately.

3. Pulmonary function tests

a. Used to obtain information on lung mechanics and lung volumes

b. Lung mechanics: uses a spirometer to measure flow of air in and out of the lungs and thus evaluate respiratory muscle strength, compliance of the lungs and chest wall, and resistance to airflow

(1) Forced vital capacity (FVC): the greatest volume of air that can be exhaled when the person breathes out forcefully

(2) Forced expiratory volume (FEV_t): greatest amount of air a person can expel in a given time interval (t); FEV_1—the amount of air that a person can forcefully exhale in 1 second

(3) Forced expiratory flow (FEF): rate at which a person can forcibly expel air from the lungs

• $FEF_{200-2000}$: flow rate from 200 to 2000 ml of forcefully expelled air.

• ($FEF_{25-75\%}$): flow rate from 25 to 75 percent when patient performs FVC maneuver

(4) The FVC, FEV, and FEF are stated in terms of predicted volume in view of the patient's age, sex, and height.

(5) Peak expiratory flow rate (PEFR): maximum flow rate when patient performs a FVC maneuver

(6) Maximal voluntary ventilation (MVV): greatest volume of air a patient can voluntarily breathe in 15 seconds

(7) Maximal inspiratory pressure (MIP): peak amount of inspiratory pressure a patient can generate

(8) Maximal expiratory pressure (MEP): peak amount of expiratory pressure a patient can generate

c. Lung volumes and capacities (Fig. 22–13)

(1) Tidal volume (V_T): amount of air inhaled or exhaled during normal respiratory effort (normally 400–700 ml per breath)

(2) Total lung capacity (TLC): amount of air contained in the lungs after maximal inhalation

(3) Vital capacity (VC): maximum amount of air a person can expire after maximal inspiration

(4) Residual volume (RV): amount of air remaining in the lungs after maximal exhalation

(5) Inspiratory capacity (IC): amount of air a person can inhale after normal exhalation

(6) Expiratory reserve volume (ERV): amount of air

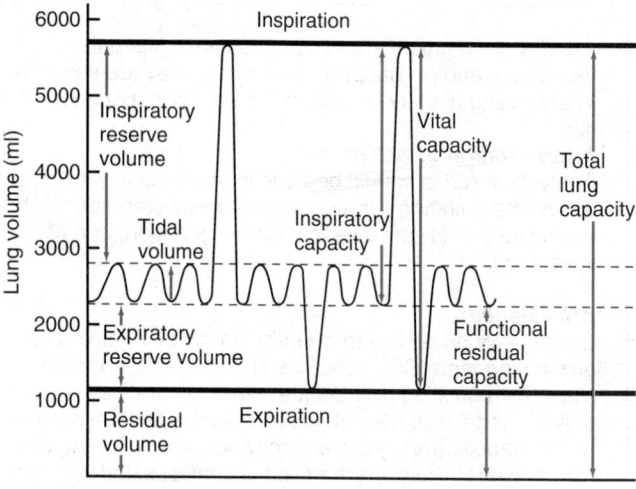

Figure 22–13. Lung volumes and capacities. (From Guyton A. *Human Physiology and Mechanisms of Disease.* 5th ed. Philadelphia: WB Saunders, 1992, p 285.)

a person can forcibly exhale from the end-expiratory phase

(7) Functional residual capacity (FRC): amount of air remaining in the lungs after normal exhalation

(8) Significance: increased lung volumes associated with the "air trapping" and subsequent hyperinflation of the lungs in obstructive lung disease; small total lung volumes associated with constrictions of restrictive disease

4. Ventilation-perfusion scan

a. Uses

(1) Assess lung ventilation and perfusion

(2) Distinguish parenchymal disease (e.g., emphysema, bronchiectasis, bronchitis, tuberculosis) from vascular events (e.g., pulmonary embolism)

b. Procedure: The test is separated into 2 scans, perfusion and ventilation. Matching the 2 scans then helps identify areas of abnormality.

(1) Pulmonary perfusion: Radioactive dye injected into the vascular system causes areas with decreased perfusion to show up on radiographs as areas of decreased radioactivity.

(2) Pulmonary ventilation: Inhalation of a radioactive gas while a scan is performed causes areas that do *not* receive ventilation *not* to be highlighted on radiographs.

5. Pulmonary angiography

a. Uses

(1) Evaluate pulmonary vasculature

(2) Evaluate and diagnose pulmonary embolism, arteriovenous malformations of the lungs, emphysema, carcinomas, and pulmonary hypertension

b. Procedure: Contrast dye is injected through a catheter inserted into the pulmonary artery. A series of radiographs called cineforagraphs are taken simultaneously.

6. Arterial blood gases (Fig. 22–14)

7. Bronchoscopy

Arterial blood gases are used to assess oxygenation, ventilation, and pH balance of the body. They are essential in assessing acutely ill patients with pulmonary disease.

Interpretation of ABGs:
Analysis of ABGs should be done in conjunction with other assessment findings. It requires a step-by-step approach: evaluations of (1) pH balance, (2) oxygenation, and (3) ventilation.

pH Balance:
Lungs respond rapidly to pH imbalances by retaining or eliminating more CO_2, whereas kidneys respond more slowly by regulating bicarbonate levels. Accurate evaluation of ABGs requires systematic assessment of both respiratory and metabolic (renal) system activities. The following are ABG findings in compensated and uncompensated acidosis:

ABG Component	Uncompensated Respiratory Acidosis	Compensated Respiratory Acidosis
pH	7.30 acidotic	7.36 normal
$Paco_2$	50 acidotic	50 acidotic
HCO_3	26 normal	29 alkalotic
Pao_2	90 normal	90 normal

The body usually works to maintain a normal internal environment. If the body becomes either more acidotic or more alkalotic than normal, the buffer systems respond to return the pH to normal. If 1 system becomes acidotic, the other system may become alkalotic to offset the imbalance, resulting in a normal pH. The body does not usually overcompensate.

Oxygenation:
Oxygenation is evaluated by the Pao_2 and the Sao_2. Low levels of both indicate hypoxemia and require administration of supplemental oxygen.

Ventilation:
Ventilation is evaluated by examining $Paco_2$. Increased levels indicate hypoventilation or CO_2 retention, e.g., in COPD's slow and shallow respirations or narcotic overdoses. Decreased levels indicate hyperventilation or increased expiration, or elimination of $Paco_2$ (e.g., in anxiety).

ABG sample is drawn from the radial artery.

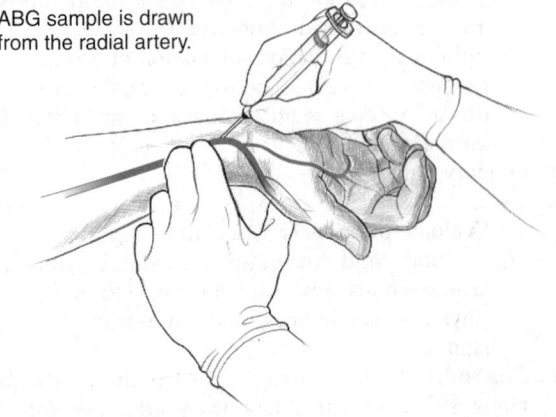

Allen Test:
The Allen test is performed to assess collateral circulation in the hand before obtaining blood from a percutaneous puncture of an artery or from an indwelling arterial catheter.

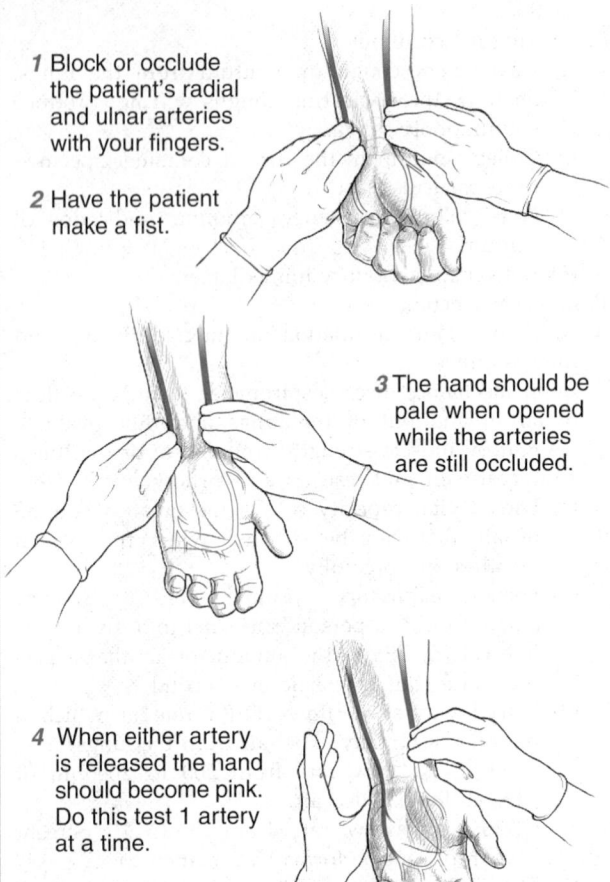

1 Block or occlude the patient's radial and ulnar arteries with your fingers.

2 Have the patient make a fist.

3 The hand should be pale when opened while the arteries are still occluded.

4 When either artery is released the hand should become pink. Do this test 1 artery at a time.

ELDER ADVISORY

Normally, levels of Pao_2 and Sao_2 are lower in older people. The rule of thumb in evaluating ABGs in older adults is to subtract 1 mm Hg from a Pao_2 of 80 for every year that a patient is over age 60 years.

NURSE ADVISORY

Use oxygen cautiously in patients with COPD; they require lower oxygen levels to stimulate breathing.

Figure 22–14.

a. Uses
  (1) Direct visualization of the larger airways
  (2) Diagnostic tool in visualizing bronchial lung tissue, collecting specimens for culture and cytology examination, and evaluating bleeding and tumors
  (3) Therapeutic tool for removing mucus plugs, lesions, and foreign bodies and for correcting atelectasis
b. Procedure: uses a flexible or rigid bronchoscope
  (1) Flexible fiberoptic bronchoscopy: A thin, flexible bronchoscope is passed into the bronchi transnasally, transorally, or through an endotracheal tube. Its small size and flexibility allow visualization of both larger and peripheral airways.
  (2) Rigid bronchoscopy: A hollow metal tube with a light at its end is passed into the bronchi transorally. Currently the tool of choice for use in small children, in retrieving foreign bodies, in treating massive hemorrhages, and in resectioning tumors.
  (3) Tools including forceps and lasers are attached to the end of a bronchoscope in therapeutic use.
  (4) Flexible fiberoptic bronchoscopy may require only local anesthetics or light sedation; rigid bronchoscopy requires full anesthesia.
c. Nursing interventions: preprocedure
  (1) Explain procedure.
  (2) Give patient nothing by mouth for 8 hours before procedure.
  (3) Remove all dentures.
  (4) Administer sedatives, if needed.
  (5) Make sure that a signed consent has been obtained.
d. Nursing interventions: postprocedure
  (1) Assess respiratory status frequently.
  (2) Observe for bleeding.
  (3) Observe for laryngeal swelling.
  (4) Check for gag reflex (no fluids by mouth until the gag reflex is intact).
e. Possible complications and their treatment
  (1) Hypoxemia: Give oxygen.
  (2) Bleeding: Assess amount; notify physician.
  (3) Pneumothorax: Assess breathing; notify physician.
  (4) Bronchial and laryngeal spasm: Administer bronchodilators or humidification.
8. Lung biopsy
  a. Use: obtaining lung tissue samples for microscopic examination
  b. Procedure: may be obtained during bronchoscopy, percutaneously, and by open lung biopsy
    (1) Bronchoscopy: tissue samples from the tracheobronchial tree
    (2) Percutaneous: tissue samples of pleural fluid, mediastinal nodes, and lung lesions taken under local anesthesia in 1 of 2 ways:
      • Transthoracic needle aspiration biopsy: Under a fluoroscope, a long, 18- to 20-gauge needle is inserted percutaneously into a suspected lesion. A syringe is attached to the needle, which is thrust into the mass 2 to 3 times while suction is applied to obtain a specimen. The patient must hold breath 15 to 30 seconds during the procedure.
      • Cutting needle biopsy: A core portion of lung tissue is removed with a Vim-Silverman needle (punch biopsy), a trephine-lung biopsy drill (high-speed drill biopsy), or an Abrams needle (suction excision biopsy). This method carries more risk than needle aspiration but produces a larger tissue sample and can help diagnose problems when other tests fail.
      • Complications: Pneumothorax with either method, hemorrhage in cutting needle biopsies; both require careful postprocedural monitoring
    (3) Open lung biopsy
      • Used only when less invasive methods do not produce adequate tissue samples.
      • Procedure: With the patient under general anesthesia, the surgeon makes a standard thoracotomy incision, inspects the lungs, and removes a tissue sample for biopsy. A chest tube that is connected to water-seal drainage (see pp. 978–979) is inserted and remains in place 1 to 2 days to minimize the risk of pneumothorax. Chest radiographs are generally performed for several days after surgery.
      • Complications: pneumothorax, postoperative respiratory failure, emphysema, chronic bronchopleural fistula; requires careful postsurgery monitoring by the nurse
9. Thoracentesis (Fig. 22–15)
  a. Uses
    (1) Diagnose inflammatory and malignant processes of the lung or pleura
    (2) Remove excess pleural fluid that may be causing respiratory compromise
  b. Procedure: Fluid is removed from the thoracic cavity through a percutaneous puncture made under local anesthesia by a physician. The patient may be sitting or leaning forward (so that pleural fluid accumulates at base of thorax).
  c. Complications: Pneumothorax, hemothorax, subcutaneous emphysema, infection, excessive coughing, or hemoptysis may ensue. If a mediastinal shift occurs owing to the removal of fluid from the thorax, cardiac distress and pulmonary edema may occur.
  d. Nursing interventions
    (1) Describe procedure. Explain need to remain still and not to cough or breathe deeply during the procedure.
    (2) Administer sedatives if needed.
    (3) Assist physician and monitor patient for signs and symptoms of dizziness, changes in skin color, respiratory changes, and heart rate and rhythm changes during the procedure.
    (4) Note color, amount, and consistency of the pleural fluid removed.
    (5) Send pleural fluid for diagnostic evaluation if ordered.
    (6) Immediately following procedure, place patient on the unaffected side.

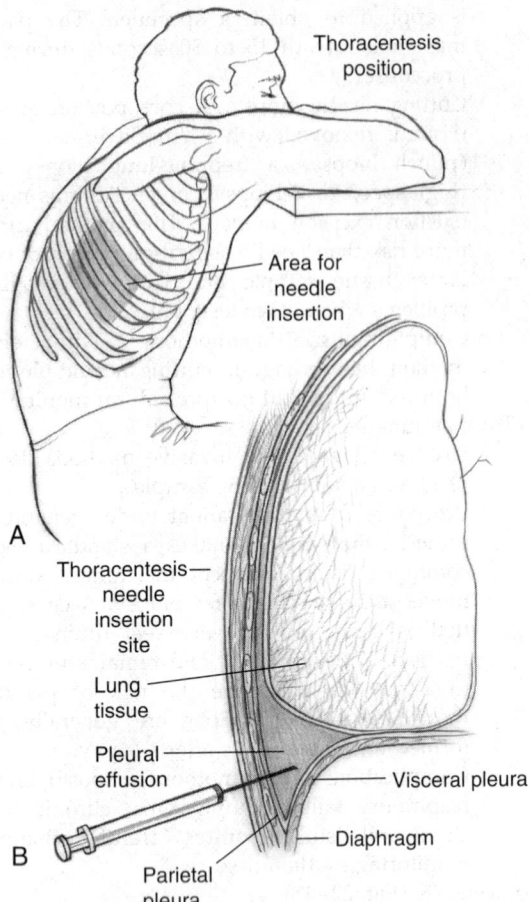

Figure 22–15. Thoracentesis position.

(7) Obtain chest radiograph immediately after the procedure to detect any accidental pneumothorax.

(8) Monitor respiratory status after the procedure.

10. Computed tomography (CT)
   a. Uses
      (1) Provides a 3-dimensional picture of the chest and the structures contained within the thorax
      (2) Helps diagnose peripheral or mediastinal lesions, pulmonary fibrosis, bronchiectasis, and tumors
   b. Procedure
      (1) Patient lies on a table that is then drawn through a tunnel in the scanner.
      (2) A computer divides the thorax into sections (transverse "slices" of chest segments). After taking multiple views of 1 section, the scanner moves to another angle and takes multiple views of another section.
      (3) The computer translates the many radiographs taken as the machine slowly rotates to cover all sides of the patient's body, producing a 3-dimensional picture of the thoracic cavity.
      (4) The procedure takes 10 to 60 minutes, depending on how much of the body is scanned.
   c. Complications: reaction to contrast dye
   d. Nursing interventions
      (1) Explain the procedure, noting the need to lie still, and mention that the table movement and click-

ing sounds heard while the patient is inside the scanner are normal.
      (2) Assess for possible claustrophobic reactions to spending time inside the device.
      (3) Make sure the patient is not wearing jewelry and is wearing only a hospital gown without metal snaps.
      (4) Provide emotional support during the procedure.

11. Pulse oximetry
   a. Uses
      (1) Monitors oxygen saturation, or SaO_2.
      (2) Arterial saturation and pulse oximetry measurements of oxygen closely correlate if the oxygen saturation is greater than 70 percent and the patient does not have peripheral vascular disease.
   b. Procedure (Fig. 22–16)
      (1) A sensor (probe) is placed on the finger, toe, ear, nose, lip, or forehead.

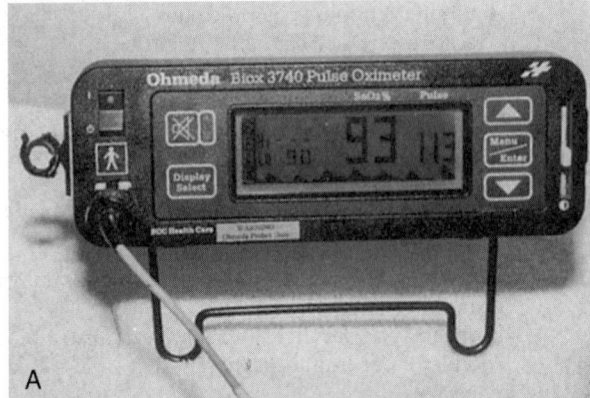
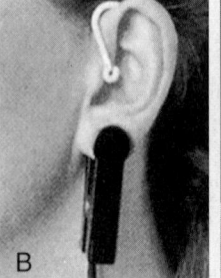
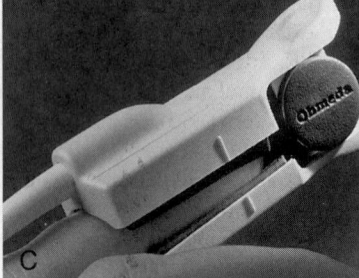

Figure 22–16. Oximetry. Noninvasive monitoring of PaO_2 (oxygen saturation) is done with a pulse oximeter. This unit (*A*) has an ear and a finger sensor. The ear sensor (*B*) is used during measurements of oxygen saturation while exercising. The finger sensor (*C*) is most frequently used for stationary measurements. (Courtesy of Ohmeda, Boulder, CO.)

(2) A beam of red and infrared light passes through the tissue. A photodetector records the amount of each kind of light reflected by oxygen-saturated hemoglobin and displays it on the monitor with each heartbeat.

(3) If levels fall below present minimums, visual or auditory alarms, or both, appear.

c. Limitations of pulse oximetry: Hypothermia, hypotension, and vasoconstriction restrict blood flow; movement of body part with sensor attached skews results.

CARING FOR PEOPLE WITH CHRONIC OBSTRUCTIVE PULMONARY DISEASE

Definition

1. A group of diseases that chronically obstruct bronchial airflow
2. A progressive and irreversible condition characterized by diminished inspiratory and expiratory capacity of the lung
3. Includes chronic bronchitis and emphysema. Bronchial asthma, although often grouped with chronic obstructive pulmonary disorders, differs from them in that asthma is reversible (see Chapter 21).

Incidence and Socioeconomic Impact

1. Approximately 30 million Americans have some form of COPD.
2. Chronic obstructive pulmonary disease is the 5th leading cause of death in the United States. There is no cure for COPD.
3. The death rate for COPD continues to increase. The group with the largest increase in death rate is older men.
4. Most common cause of COPD is smoking, making COPD highly preventable.
5. About 70 to 80 percent of patients who have inherited alpha$_1$-antitrypsin deficiency have COPD.

Risk Factors and Etiology

1. Smoking
2. Middle-aged male
3. Recurrent respiratory infections
4. Air pollutants
5. Industrial irritants
6. Hereditary predisposition characterized by a deficiency in alpha$_1$-antitrypsin levels

Chronic Bronchitis

1. Definition: Inflammation of 1 or more bronchi; frequently involves the trachea as well as the bronchi

2. Pathophysiology
   a. Submucosal glands enlarge, and the number of goblet glands increases, leading these glands to secrete excess mucus.
   b. Consistency of mucus becomes thick and viscous.
   c. Early in the disease process, small airways become inflamed; various degrees of fibrosis may be present.
   d. As the diameter of the airways is reduced, so is airflow from the lungs.
3. Clinical manifestations: May have barrel chest; dyspnea on exertion; on auscultation diminished breath sounds with intermittent wheezes; rhonchi present; consistent, thick, copious sputum production; marked cyanosis; peripheral edema due to cor pulmonale; expiration phase of respiration prolonged; obesity.
4. Diagnostics
   a. Assessment
      (1) History: Check for risk factors (see above), family history of cystic fibrosis, coughing with sputum production, activity intolerance, recurrent respiratory infections, and orthopnea. A diagnosis of chronic bronchitis requires a chronic, productive cough for at least 3 continuous months for 2 consecutive years and sputum production most days for 3 consecutive months in 2 consecutive years.
      (2) Physical examination: Examine for signs of cyanosis, dyspnea, edema, increased jugular vein distention, and obesity. Although percussion note and tactile fremitus are normal, lung sounds include rhonchi and crackles, the expiratory phase of respiration is prolonged, and there is loud S2 in the pulmonic area with a possible S3–S4 gallop.
   b. Medical diagnosis
      (1) Pulmonary function tests: FEF reduced 25–75 percent, FEV reduced, VC decreased, reserve volume increased.
      (2) Chest radiograph reveals increased bronchovesicular markings.
      (3) Arterial blood gases: Elevated $PaCO_2$ with compensation and a decreased PaO_2 as the disease progresses.

Emphysema

1. Definition and classification
   a. Loss of lung elasticity and permanent abnormal enlargement of air spaces distal to the terminal bronchioles
   b. Two types of emphysema: panacinar and centriacinar (Fig. 22–17)
2. Pathophysiology (see Fig. 22–17)
3. Diagnostics
   a. Assessment
      (1) History: Positive family history for alpha$_1$-antitrypsin deficiency, smoking
      (2) Physical examination findings: Increased anteroposterior diameter, position upright or leaning slightly forward (tripod position), dyspnea on exertion, use of accessory muscles of respiration, tachypnea, pursed-lip breathing, normal skin color, decreased diaphragmatic excursion, dimin-

EMPHYSEMA

PATHOPHYSIOLOGY

Emphysema results from a breakdown of elastin by the enzyme elastase. The loss of elastin from the alveolar wall results in diminished elastic recoil of the lungs, which reduces the lung surface area available for gas exchange and which, in turn, causes an altered expiratory flow rate owing to premature closure of the airways.

Elastase is released by 2 of the inflammatory cells within the lung, polymorphonuclear leukocytes and alveolar macrophages. Elastase is usually held in check by the protein alpha$_1$-antitrypsin, but if left unchecked it destroys the alveolar walls. Smoking decreases the efficiency of alpha$_1$-antitrypsin and results in increased levels of elastase.

Types of Emphysema

Panacinar Emphysema:
Panacinar emphysema worsens progressively and is characterized by the enlargement and eventual total destruction of acinar units. Usually, the pattern of lung involvement is diffuse, but it may occur more in the lower lung fields.

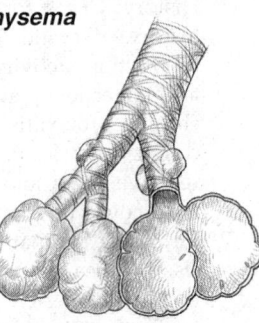

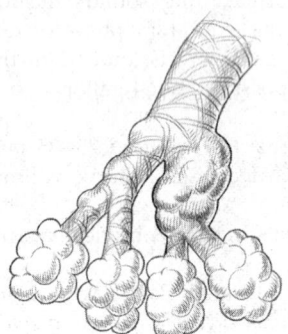

Centriacinar Emphysema:
This type of emphysema is usually seen in smokers. Changes in the acinar unit occur in its proximal portion. The portion of the acinar unit distal to the respiratory bronchioles is usually spared.

CLINICAL MANIFESTATIONS

Good, noncyanotic skin color is maintained because Pao$_2$ remains normal owing to the high minute ventilation. The patient is thin and underweight owing to the increased work of breathing and shortness of breath and has a "barrel chest." The patient is dyspneic, with decreased breath sounds over the entire lung fields. There is a prolonged expiratory phase, and pursed-lip breathing is usually present. There is little or no sputum production unless accompanied by chronic bronchitis or infection.

Figure 22–17.

ished breath sounds throughout, decreased tactile fremitus, decreased chest expansion, prolonged expiratory phase, percussion note hyperresonant, and no adventitious breath sounds.
  b. Medical diagnosis
    (1) Pulmonary function tests

- Increased FRC
- Increased TLC
- Decreased FEV$_1$ (nonreversible with bronchodilators)
- Increased lung compliance
- Decreased diffusion capacity

  c. Arterial blood gases: May be normal or may show slightly decreased Pao$_2$.
  d. Chest radiographic findings: hyperinflated lungs, flattened diaphragm, costophrenic angle greater than 90 degrees

Clinical Management of Chronic Obstructive Pulmonary Disease

1. See pages 958–979 for details on various therapies.
2. Goals of clinical management
  a. Relieve hypoxemia
  b. Decrease carbon dioxide retention
  c. Correct precipitating cause
  d. Facilitate the removal of secretions
  e. Prevent infection
  f. Relieve anxiety
3. Nonpharmacologic interventions
  a. Oxygen therapy
    (1) Treatment of choice for hypercarbia-hypoxia respiratory failure, because maintaining Pao$_2$ above 55 mm Hg decreases dyspnea and pulmonary hypertension, improves activity tolerance, and improves psychologic function.
    (2) If a patient with COPD develops acute respiratory failure, make every effort to avoid intubation and mechanical ventilation, as it is extremely difficult to wean these patients from mechanical ventilation. Indications for mechanical ventilation in this group of clients would include severe hypoxemia, respiratory muscle fatigue, and cardiac compromise.

NURSE ADVISORY

Use oxygen cautiously in patients with chronic obstructive pulmonary disease, because the respiratory drive is regulated by the hypoxic stimulation of the peripheral chemoreceptors. If too much oxygen is present in the blood, these chemoreceptors no longer stimulate breathing, leading to hypoventilation and carbon dioxide retention.

  b. Controlling environmental factors that trigger COPD
    (1) Avoid cigarette smoking.
    (2) Avoid all airborne irritants.
    (3) Monitor air pollution levels, and adjust activities accordingly.
    (4) In cold weather wear a face mask to reduce bronchospasm and dyspnea.
    (5) Avoid exposure to others who have respiratory infections. Avoid large groups of people during "flu season."

c. Maintaining adequate nutrition and fluid balance: Anorexia due to increased dyspnea with eating is common.
   (1) Eat small, frequent meals.
   (2) Supplement diet with vitamins.
   (3) Drink plenty of fluids to liquefy secretions.
   (4) Eat a diet low in carbohydrates, which breaks down into carbon dioxide and thus increases carbon dioxide retention.
d. Ensuring psychologic support: Because dyspnea limits activities, depression is common.
   (1) Encourage patients to be as active as possible.
   (2) Recommend support groups.
4. Pharmacologic interventions (Table 22–3 describes pharmacologic management of respiratory disorders, including COPD.)
   a. Bronchodilators
      (1) Act directly on smooth muscle to relieve bronchospasm
      (2) Divided into 2 groups: β-adrenergic and theophylline preparations
      (3) Common side effects: increased heart rate, palpitations, nausea, anorexia

DRUG ADVISORY

The use of theophylline preparations continues to be controversial. One of the reasons is that the margin between the therapeutic dose and the lethal dose is very narrow. Many factors can influence the metabolism of theophylline. Theophylline is not recommended as a first-line drug for chronic obstructive pulmonary disease. However, it has been beneficial in patients who suffer from nocturnal dyspnea.

   b. Antibiotics
      (1) Used to treat pulmonary infections that may lead to respiratory failure in patients with COPD
      (2) Do not treat viruses (most common cause of pulmonary infections) but help to fight bacterial infections that result from decreased resistance
   c. Adrenal glucocorticoid
      (1) Reduces inflammation that decreases the size of the bronchial lumen
      (2) Decreases responsiveness of cells to allergic stimuli, thus reducing bronchoconstriction
      (3) Aerosolized route provides more benefit by requiring lower dosage of drug
      (4) Acute exacerbation usually treated with intravenous steroids

DRUG ADVISORY

Use adrenal glucocorticoid very cautiously, as it produces a wide range of side effects.

   d. Mucolytics
      (1) Break down the chemical structure of sputum

   (2) Help liquefy secretions
   (3) Benefit patients with abnormal viscid or dry mucous secretions
5. Special medical-surgical procedures: In rare cases, patients who have repeated spontaneous pneumothorax may benefit from bullectomy (removal of large bullae that compress the lung).

Complications

1. Cor pulmonale (right ventricular heart failure secondary to diseased blood vessels in the lungs)
2. Acute respiratory failure
3. Hypoxemia
4. Hypercapnia
5. Polycythemia
6. Dysrhythmias

Prognosis

1. There is no cure for COPD.
2. Lifestyle changes and compliance with the health care regimen can lead to a longer, higher quality of life for those who suffer from COPD.

Applying the Nursing Process

NURSING DIAGNOSIS: Impaired gas exchange R/T decreased ventilation and presence of mucus plugs

1. *Expected outcomes:* Following interventions, the patient should exhibit improved gas exchange, as evidenced by the following:
   a. Arterial blood gases at baseline
   b. Usual skin color (no cyanosis)
   c. Normal mental status
   d. SaO_2 greater than 88 percent
   e. Ability to expectorate sputum effectively
   f. Respiratory rate and heart rate at baseline
2. *Nursing interventions*
   a. Monitor respiratory status: rate, rhythm, and depth and use of respiratory accessory muscles. Report any changes immediately.
   b. Administer oxygen, bronchodilators, or both if indicated.
   c. Monitor ABGs for hypoxemia, hypercapnia, or both.
   d. Auscultate breath sounds every 4 hours.
   e. Monitor SaO_2 via pulse oximeter continually.
   f. Monitor skin color.
   g. Assess for altered level of consciousness due to hypoxia.
   h. Monitor for increased hemoglobin and hematocrit levels.
   i. Assist patient to a comfortable position. A high Fowler's upright position allows full lung expansion and enhances gas exchange.

Table 22–3. *Pharmacologic Management of Respiratory Disorders*

Class	Example	Action	Use	Common Side Effects	Nursing Implications
Antimicrobials					
Penicillins	Penicillin G sodium Procaine penicillin G (Wycillin) Potassium penicillin V (Pen-Vee K) Nafcillin (Unipen) Ampicillin Amoxicillin Carbenicillin Ticarcillin	Bactericidal against a wide variety of gram-positive and some gram-negative organisms Most effective in the treatment of bacterial pneumonia		Allergic reactions (skin rashes, anaphylaxis) Gastrointestinal disturbances (nausea and vomiting, epigastric distress) Central nervous system toxicity (hallucinations, hyperreflexia, seizures when administered in very large doses to patients with neurologic reactions) Hematologic disturbances (thrombocytopenia, agranulocytosis, anemia) Impaired renal function	Check for history of penicillin allergy before administration of drug Observe for allergic manifestations and other side effects Evaluate effects of drug especially when given concurrently with drugs that may increase or decrease its actions; e.g., gentamicin is synergistic to penicillin; probenecid decreases its renal excretion; tetracycline and erythromycin both inhibit bactericidal activity of penicillin Monitor for development of resistant organisms; susceptibility testing should be done before and during the course of therapy
Cephalosporins	Cephalexin (Keflex) Cefamandole (Mandol) Cefazolin (Ancef, Kefzol) Cephalothin (Keflin) Cefoxitin (Mefoxin) Cephapirin (Cefadyl)		Effective against numerous infections but used primarily for *Klebsiella pneumoniae* along with aminoglycoside	Gastrointestinal disturbances Nephrotoxicity (decreased urine output and creatinine clearance, hematuria, proteinuria) Phlebitis with intravenous administration	Assess for allergic reactions to cephalosporins and penicillins; it is controversial whether cephalosporins can be given without causing allergic reactions when there is a known hypersensitivity to penicillin Monitor for toxic side effects Assess effectiveness when administered with bacteriostatic antibiotics, e.g., tetracyclines and erythromycins, which may decrease or destroy their effects
Aminoglycosides	Kanamycin (Kantrex) Neomycin Amikacin sulfate Gentamicin (Garamycin) Tobramycin Streptomycin	Bactericidal against a wide range of gram-positive and gram-negative bacteria and mycobacteria; however, they differ in clinical uses		Ototoxicity Nephrotoxicity Neuromuscular blockade Peripheral neuritis Resistant infection	Assess patient for beginning auditory and vestibular damage, e.g., vertigo, ataxia, roaring in the ears, hearing loss

Table 22-3. *Pharmacologic Management of Respiratory Disorders* (Continued)

Class	Example	Action	Use	Common Side Effects	Nursing Implications
			Streptomycin: used in the treatment of tuberculosis in combination with other tuberculostatic drugs Neomycin: used for reducing intestinal flora and thereby decreasing blood ammonia levels Gentamicin: used to treat bacteremia caused by *Proteus, Pseudomonas, Escherichia coli,* and *Klebsiella* Amikacin and tobramycin: used to treat gentamicin-resistant infection		Monitor renal function, especially when administered to older patients or to those with renal insufficiency Monitor peak and trough levels and drug dosages Assess neuromuscular effects, especially when administered with muscle relaxants and sedatives
Tetracyclines	Chlortetracycline HCl (Aureomycin) Demeclocycline HCl (Declomycin) Doxycycline hyclate (Vibramycin)		Bacteriostatic for many gram-negative and gram-positive organisms, including mycobacteria, rickettsiae, mycoplasma, and agents of psittacosis	Gastrointestinal disturbances Allergic reactions Hepatotoxicity Enamel hypoplasia Permanent staining of teeth when used during tooth development	Avoid use in children, during pregnancy, and when there is impaired hepatic or renal function Do not administer with food, milk, milk products, antacids because they inhibit tetracycline absorption Monitor patient for a developing superinfection Monitor liver function in long-term therapy Instruct patient to avoid direct sunlight because sunburn reaction or erythema is likely to occur
Bronchodilators					
Beta-adrenergics Theophylline	Albuterol (Ventolin) Isoproterenol (Isuprel) Terbutaline (Brethine) Theophylline (Theo-Dur)	Relaxation of constricted airways by stimulating beta-adrenergic receptors Bronchial relaxation by inhibition of the breakdown of cyclic adenosine monophosphate	Symptomatic relief of asthma and bronchial spasms	Gastrointestinal upset Nausea Nervousness, anxiety Urinary frequency Diarrhea Insomnia Tachycardia Palpitations Esophageal reflux Tremors Weakness Hypertension Cardiac Dysrhythmias	Use with caution in patients with hypertension, tachycardia, hypoxemia, glaucoma, hyperthyroidism, benign prostatic hypertrophy, diabetes, congestive heart failure, renal and hepatic disease, pregnancy and lactation Monitor for central nervous system symptoms Give with food or antacids; avoid smoking

Table continued on following page

Table 22–3. Pharmacologic Management of Respiratory Disorders (Continued)					
Class	**Example**	**Action**	**Use**	**Common Side Effects**	**Nursing Implications**
Adrenal glucocorticoids	Prednisone Beclomethasone (Vanceril)	Reduce inflammation and inflammatory response in bronchial walls	Symptomatic relief and preventive care of asthma	With systemic agents —gastrointestinal upset, gastric irritation and ulceration, euphoria, hunger, insomnia, adrenal shutdown	Administer in morning if dosage is 4 times daily; give with food Plan to supplement patients with cortisone agents during periods of stress
Mucolytics	Water Acetylcysteine (Mucomyst)	Thin mucus	Chronic pulmonary conditions that lead to thick, dry sputum	Bronchospasm with Mucomyst	Administer Mucomyst by aerosolized bronchodilator
Antiallergenics	Cromolyn sodium (Intal)	Stabilizes mast cell	Asthma, especially due to exercise or allergen exposure	Headache Rash Cough Worsening of asthma	Require 3 weeks of continuous therapy before they are effective Use in decreased dosages for patients with liver or renal disorders
Antihistamines	Diphenhydramine hydrochloride (Benadryl)	Block action of histamine at H_1-receptor sites, smooth muscles of the blood vessels, bronchioles, and gastrointestinal tract	Relieve symptoms of allergies Adjunct in treatment of anaphylaxis	Sedation Epigastric distress Hypotension Palpitations Tachycardia Thickening of bronchial secretions Vertigo Urinary frequency	Warn about sedation Use carefully in patients with convulsions, hyperthyroidism, cardiovascular and renal disease, hypertension, diabetes Avoid use with alcohol Monitor for dry mucous membranes Give with meals or antacids
	Terfenadine (Seldane)	Specific, selective histamine H_1-receptor antagonist		Dryness of nose, mouth Dysrhythmias when used to toxic levels	Do not use in conjunction with ketoconazole or levamisole (Ergamisole). Use cautiously with erythromycin
Cough preparations Expectorants	Guaifenesin (Robitussin)	Facilitate removal of thick mucus from lungs and act as soothing demulcent by stimulating secretion of a lubricant	Facilitate productive cough	Nausea and vomiting Gastrointestinal irritation Drowsiness Headache Rash	Instruct patient not to use more than 1 week without seeing physician Use high fluid intake and humidity to loosen secretions
Antitussives	Narcotics: any product with codeine Non-narcotics: dextromethorphan	Suppress cough reflex Act centrally on the cough center or peripherally within the tracheobronchial tree to decrease sensitivity to irritant receptors	To treat dry, nonproductive coughs that interfere with sleep or other activities	Dizziness Sedation Sweating Nausea Dry mouth Constipation Urinary retention Palpitations	Caution patient about possible sedation Administer with caution to patients with asthma, COPD, cardiac disease, convulsions, renal or hepatic disease, central nervous system depression, benign prostatic hypertrophy, alcoholism, or hypothyroidism

Table 22–3. *Pharmacologic Management of Respiratory Disorders* (Continued)

Class	Example	Action	Use	Common Side Effects	Nursing Implications
Nasal decongestants	Pseudoephedrine HCL (Sudafed)	Vasoconstriction of respiratory tract mucosa by stimulating α-adrenergic receptors.	Reduces nasal congestion	Restlessness Irritability Headache Insomnia Tachycardia Palpitations	Use with caution in patients with hypertension and coronary artery disease, lactating women, and those who are using monoamine oxidase inhibitors

Modified from Black JM, and Matassarin-Jacobs E (eds). *Luckmann and Sorensen's Medical-Surgical Nursing: A Psychophysiologic Approach.* 4th ed. Philadelphia: WB Saunders, 1993, pp 945–948. Adapted from Matassarin-Jacobs, E. *Saunders Review for NCLEX-RN.* Philadelphia: WB Saunders, 1990.

j. Instruct in coughing techniques.
k. Demonstrate pursed-lip and diaphragmatic breathing.
l. Encourage an intake of 2500 ml of fluid every day.

NURSING DIAGNOSIS: Ineffective airway clearance R/T thick, copious secretions, respiratory muscle weakness, and ineffective coughing

1. *Expected outcomes:* Following interventions, the patient should exhibit improved airway clearance, as evidenced by the following:
   a. Decreased adventitious breath sounds
   b. Effective cough
   c. Ease in handling secretions
   d. Thin secretions
   e. Absence of dyspnea
   f. Normal vital signs
2. *Nursing interventions*
   a. Encourage fluid intake of at least 8 glasses of water per day.
   b. Teach and encourage turning, coughing, and deep breathing.
   c. Perform chest physical therapy and postural drainage.
   d. Provide humidification for the room.
   e. Assess ability to mobilize and expectorate secretions.
   f. Assess lung sounds frequently, especially before and after chest physical therapy and postural drainage or coughing.
   g. Assess respiratory status, rate, rhythm, and depth and use of accessory muscles.
   h. Monitor sputum for changes in color, consistency, amount, and odor.
   i. Administer antibiotics as indicated.
   j. Administer bronchodilators as indicated.

NURSING DIAGNOSIS: Altered nutrition, less than body requirements, R/T decreased appetite and dyspnea

1. *Expected outcomes:* Following interventions, the patient should exhibit improved nutrition, as evidenced by the following:

   a. Albumin level greater than 2.5 gm per dl
   b. Tolerating prescribed diet
   c. Eating three fourths or more of each meal
   d. Weight at calculated ideal body weight
   e. Verbalization of a desire to eat
2. *Nursing interventions*
   a. In consultation with the patient and nutrition team, identify the patient's food preferences and develop a diet that limits glucose, bulk, and fiber. Glucose metabolism results in increased carbon dioxide levels in the body. High bulk and fiber foods create early satiety and may produce intestinal bloating that reduces lung expansion.
   b. Monitor daily weight.
   c. Provide frequent, small meals. Schedule feeding at times of adequate rest.
   d. Assess for nausea and vomiting.
   e. Provide mouth care.
   f. Monitor total protein and albumin levels.
   g. Auscultate bowel sounds.
   h. Provide dietary supplements as needed.

NURSING DIAGNOSIS: Anxiety R/T dyspnea and fear of dying

1. *Expected outcomes:* Following interventions, the patient should demonstrate reduced anxiety as evidenced by the following:
   a. Relaxed appearance
   b. Verbalizing feelings of decreased anxiety
   c. Demonstrating effective use of coping techniques
   d. Demonstrating effective breathing techniques
   e. Normal vital signs
   f. Skin dry
2. *Nursing interventions*
   a. Provide a quiet and calm environment.
   b. Monitor vital signs.
   c. Assess for anxiety. Administer antianxiety medications, if ordered, and evaluate their effectiveness.
   d. Administer sedatives cautiously if indicated.
   e. Position patient for comfort.
   f. Teach breathing techniques to reduce periods of dyspnea.

g. Stay with patient during episodes of acute anxiety. Provide quiet, calm reassurance.
h. Encourage patient to express feelings.
i. Help patient to identify coping mechanisms and support systems.
j. If possible, open doors, windows, and curtains and provide patient with a fan during acute episodes of dyspnea.
k. Explain all procedures.

NURSING DIAGNOSIS: Activity intolerance R/T fatigue, dyspnea

---

1. *Expected outcomes:* Following interventions, the patient should be able to do the following:
   a. Identify realistic goals for activity and properly space activities throughout the day
   b. Improve exercise tolerance
   c. Demonstrate diaphragmatic breathing and coughing techniques
   d. Describe signs and symptoms of activity intolerance
2. *Nursing interventions*
   a. Evaluate degree of activity intolerance.
   b. Encourage the patient to participate as much as possible with activity program. Provide encouragement during periods of activity.
   c. Provide adequate periods of rest.
   d. Instruct the patient about activities that increase oxygen requirements such as walking upstairs, smoking, and rapid changes in temperature.
   e. Help patient space activities throughout the day.
   f. Maintain oxygen therapy during activities if ordered.
   g. Teach breathing techniques that can be utilized during activity (e.g., do work during expiration).
   h. Gradually increase activity as tolerance increases.

NURSING DIAGNOSIS: Risk for infection R/T thick sputum, ineffective coughing, fatigue

---

1. *Expected outcomes:* Following interventions, the patient should be free from infection as evidenced by the following:
   a. No fever
   b. Normal white blood cell count
   c. No change in sputum production, color, or odor
   d. No change in mental status
2. *Nursing interventions*
   a. Monitor vital signs.
   b. Monitor sputum production.
   c. Monitor sputum characteristics for color, amount, consistency, and odor.
   d. Monitor white blood cell count.
   e. Encourage activity as tolerated.
   f. Monitor for signs and symptoms of sepsis.
   g. Send sputum for culture and sensitivity laboratory test if there is a sudden change in its character.
   h. Observe universal precautions.
   i. Encourage increased fluid intake to 2500 ml per day.
   j. Administer influenza inoculation.

Discharge Planning and Teaching

1. Explain the particular disease: its causes, symptoms, and treatment (including medications—dosage, side effects, scheduling).
2. Discuss the possible complications of COPD, their signs, and how to prevent them (e.g., proper hygiene to minimize chances of infection).
3. Instruct the person to avoid things that may induce bronchospasm, such as powders, aerosolized products, and strong odors.
4. Teach breathing and coughing techniques.

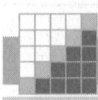

LEGAL AND ETHICAL CONSIDERATIONS

Documenting a patient's wishes regarding life support is extremely important. As chronic obstructive pulmonary disease worsens, so does the patient's overall health. Intubation and mechanical ventilation may be the end result. Patients need to be counseled regarding their rights and responsibilities about advance directives and self-determination (see also Chapter 43).

HOME CARE STRATEGIES

Pulmonary Disease

Although many patients with pulmonary disease are chronically ill, they may achieve a stable status, resulting in a greater level of independence in the home setting. Consider the following:
- Teach the patient and caregiver about nutritional needs and restrictions by actually reviewing the contents of the cupboard with them.
- Instruct the patient regarding energy preservation, particularly during meal time. Talking while eating increases the use of oxygen, resulting in increased shortness of breath.
- Avoid situations that cause energy depletion. Conserving energy enables the patient to maximize the level of independence.
- Intersperse periods of activity and rest in a quiet, comfortable atmosphere. Proceed slowly with activities involving the patient; engage in activities for less than 30 minutes at a time; longer than that tires the patient.
- Develop a successful regimen of bowel treatment for the patient, as constipation results in discomfort and significant anxiety.
- Sleep disturbances and general fatigue may represent side effects of medications or evidence of depression. Explore both possibilities thoroughly.
- Help to prioritize activities so that those that are most important to the patient can be completed without depleting energy. Plan exhausting activities for early morning or the time best suited to the individual patient.
- Encourage patients to use shower rather than taking a tub bath. A shower takes less energy. Using a shower chair conserves energy; using a terry cloth robe just out of the shower reduces energy needed to dry oneself.
- The patient should be encouraged to wear loose-fitting clothing that does not bind or restrict movement and breathing.
- Exercises performed in bed before arising can conserve energy levels.
- Place chairs strategically throughout the house for rest stops during the day. A rolling cart that has shelves can be useful for moving items from 1 room to another with minimal energy consumption.

5. Instruct the patient in diet modification such as lower carbohydrates and higher protein and in the need to take in large quantities of fluids to help liquefy the sputum.
6. Stress the need for ongoing respiratory assessment and yearly consultation with health professionals.
7. Recommend support groups to help patients with COPD and their families deal with the ultimately fatal nature of these disorders and live life as fully as possible.

Public Health Considerations

1. Chronic obstructive pulmonary disease is highly preventable. Emphasis should be on primary prevention: stopping (or not starting) smoking, avoiding environmental pollutants.
2. In addition, patients with COPD can minimize the risks of complications by avoiding large crowds and getting yearly flu shots.

◻ *CARING FOR PEOPLE WITH ACUTE RESPIRATORY FAILURE*

Definition

1. Acute respiratory failure is the sudden inability of the respiratory system to maintain adequate gas exchange due to ventilation failure, oxygenation failure, or a combination of these.
2. Although this is a broad clinical diagnosis, as a general rule a Po_2 less than 50 mm Hg and a rising $Paco_2$ greater than 50 mm Hg with a pH of less than 7.25 define acute respiratory failure.

Risk Factors and Etiology

1. Decreased oxygen transport (decreased cardiac output and decreased hemoglobin content)
2. Chronic pulmonary disorders: COPD, asthma
3. Other acute pulmonary disorders: ARDS, bronchiectasis, pneumothorax, atelectasis, pneumonia, pulmonary embolism
4. Restrictive lung disease
5. Pulmonary contusion
6. Upper airway obstruction
7. Rib fracture
8. Thorax deformities such as kyphoscoliosis
9. Abdominal or thoracic surgery
10. Neurologic disease—stroke, spinal cord injuries above C4, lower motor neuron disease (e.g., amyotrophic lateral sclerosis, myasthenia gravis, multiple sclerosis, polio, and Guillain-Barré)—or dysfunction
11. Aspiration
12. Drugs or toxic agents such as narcotics, barbiturates, anesthetics, and tranquilizers
13. Ascites
14. Obesity

Pathophysiology

1. Three different physiologic mechanisms can cause acute respiratory failure: ventilation failure (hypoventilation), ventilation-perfusion mismatching, and oxygenation problems due to altered diffusion patterns.
2. Ventilation failure: Any change that decreases tidal volume (e.g., overmedication, trauma, ascites, neuromuscular disease) can decrease minute ventilation and produce alveolar hypoventilation. Alveolar hypoventilation results in increased $Paco_2$.
3. Ventilation-perfusion mismatching
   a. Adequate gas exchange depends largely on adequate matching of perfusion and ventilation in the alveoli.
   b. The small amount of dead space normally present within the pulmonary system is compensated for by other lung units.
   c. When diseases such as pulmonary infection, atelectasis, COPD, lung cancer, and pulmonary embolism cause an increase in the number of dead space units, hypoxemia results.
   d. Ventilation-perfusion mismatching in which perfusion is adequate but the lungs receive no ventilation (as in ARDS and pneumonia) produces shunt units and hypoxemia. The degree of hypoxemia is determined by the number of the shunt units.
4. Altered diffusion patterns
   a. Alterations in diffusion patterns occur when the barrier between the alveoli and the capillaries thickens, making it harder for diffusion to occur.
   b. The result is usually hypoxemia because the diffusion of carbon dioxide occurs 20 times faster than that of oxygen.
   c. Diseases that can cause alterations in diffusion patterns include sarcoidosis, interstitial fibrosis, pulmonary fibrosis, and pulmonary edema.
5. In some patients, a combination of ventilation, oxygenation, and ventilation-perfusion problems may lead to acute respiratory failure.

Clinical Manifestations

1. Hypercapnia or hypoxemia
2. Other respiratory manifestations: dyspnea, tachypnea, paradoxical breathing patterns, use of accessory muscles of respiration
3. Cardiovascular manifestations: change in heart rate (bradycardia or tachycardia), change in blood pressure (hypotension or hypertension), dysrhythmias, chest pain, palpitations
4. Integumentary manifestations: pallor; cyanosis; cool, clammy skin
5. Increased jugular vein distention
6. Changes in levels of consciousness
7. Seizures
8. Anxiety, restlessness, or both

9. Decreased urinary output related to sympathetic nervous system stimulation

Diagnostics

1. Assessment
   a. History: dyspnea or increased work of breathing; COPD, restrictive disorders, or neuromuscular defects; family history of pulmonary disease
   b. Physical examination findings (in addition to clinical manifestations noted earlier)
      (1) Increased anteroposterior diameter
      (2) Intercostal retractions
      (3) Spinal or chest wall deformities
      (4) Characteristics of respiration: note rate, rhythm, depth, inspiratory to expiratory (I:E) ratio, lung expansion
      (5) Fremitus: increased with consolidation and decreased with blockage of airways
      (6) Percussion results: dullness with consolidation (e.g., pneumonia), hyperresonance with overinflation (e.g., COPD)
      (7) Pleural friction rub on auscultation
      (8) Pitting edema
   c. Diagnostic studies
      (1) Arterial blood gases: $PaCO_2$ greater than 50 mm Hg, PaO_2 less than 50 mm Hg, or both; acute if pH is less than 7.25; chronic if pH is normal with elevated buffers
      (2) Chest radiograph: depends on disease process
      (3) SaO_2 less than 90 percent
      (4) Intrapulmonary shunt greater than 15 percent

Clinical Management

1. See pages 958–979 for details on therapies.
2. Goals of clinical management
   a. Restore ABG levels, breathing patterns, and lung sounds to baseline
   b. Eliminate cyanosis
   c. Return level of consciousness to baseline
3. Nonpharmacologic interventions
   a. Deep breathing with incentive spirometry to promote adequate ventilation
   b. Chest physiotherapy or postural drainage to loosen and remove retained secretions
   c. Coughing and expectoration of retained secretions
   d. Maintenance of a patent airway
4. Pharmacologic interventions
   a. Bronchodilator therapy to open closed airways
   b. Antibiotics to treat pulmonary infection
5. Special medical-surgical procedures
   a. Nasotracheal suctioning to remove retained secretions if the patient is unable to produce an effective cough
   b. High-flow oxygen delivery systems and mechanical ventilation to relieve hypoxemia and hypercapnia

NURSE ADVISORY

Administration of 100 percent oxygen will not improve hypoxemia resulting from shunt units and may cause deterioration.

   c. Enhancement of oxygen delivery by transfusion of packed red blood cells if hemoglobin is less than 12

Complications

1. Respiratory arrest
2. Cardiac arrest
3. Myocardial infarction
4. Renal failure
5. Cor pulmonale
6. Gastric and intestinal ulcerations
7. Pulmonary hypertension

Prognosis

Depends on the physiologic cause of acute respiratory failure and the speed of treatment

Applying the Nursing Process

NURSING DIAGNOSIS: Ineffective breathing pattern R/T respiratory muscle fatigue, chronic airflow limitations, and chest wall restrictions

1. *Expected outcomes:* Following interventions, the patient should exhibit an improved breathing pattern, as evidenced by the following:
   a. Respiratory rate within normal range of 12 to 20 breaths per minute
   b. Arterial blood gas levels within normal limits for the patient
   c. Breath sounds clear
   d. Symmetric chest excursion
2. *Nursing interventions*
   a. Assess breathing pattern.
   b. Monitor respiratory characteristics and lung sounds.
   c. Obtain ABGs as indicated.
   d. Monitor oxygen saturation, and administer oxygen as needed.
   e. Monitor sputum production, and use endotracheal suction as indicated to remove secretions.
   f. Position for comfort and efficient use of the diaphragm.
   g. Administer bronchodilators as ordered.
   h. Position for comfort and efficient use of respiratory muscles.
   i. Assess for anxiety and implement strategies to reduce anxiety if present.
   j. Teach diaphragmatic breathing.
   k. Teach pursed-lip breathing.

l. Teach positions that ease respiratory effort.

m. Administer theophylline, and maintain blood levels in therapeutic range.

NURSING DIAGNOSIS: Impaired gas exchange R/T diffusion impairments and ventilation-perfusion mismatch due to shunting

1. *Expected outcomes:* Following interventions, the patient should experience improved gas exchange, as evidenced by the following:
   a. Arterial blood gas levels returned to baseline
   b. Absence of cyanosis
   c. Baseline mental status
   d. Airways clear to auscultation
   e. Oxygen saturation greater than 90 percent
   f. Normal vital signs
2. *Nursing interventions*
   a. Monitor respiratory status, noting rate, rhythm, and depth and use of accessory muscles.
   b. Assess lung sounds frequently.
   c. Assess for changes in level of consciousness.
   d. Check for central and peripheral cyanosis by assessing color of lips and nail beds.
   e. Monitor vital signs.
   f. Monitor ABGs, hemoglobin, hematocrit, SaO_2, lactic acid, chest radiographs.
   g. Monitor oxygen saturation, and administer oxygen as appropriate.
   h. Perform nasotracheal or endotracheal suctioning as needed to clear airways.
   i. Administer diuretics if needed for fluid overload.
   j. Assist patient to turn, cough, and deep breathe.
   k. Perform chest physical therapy and postural drainage as indicated.
   l. Provide an environment conducive to rest.

NURSING DIAGNOSIS: Ineffective airway clearance R/T thick sputum, bronchospasm, respiratory muscle fatigue, pulmonary fibrosis, chest wall deformities, and/or pain

1. *Expected outcomes:* Following interventions, the patient should exhibit effective airway clearance, as evidenced by the following:
   a. Clear breath sounds
   b. Thin sputum
   c. Chest radiograph clear
   d. Arterial blood gases returned to baseline
   e. Absence of respiratory distress
2. *Nursing interventions*
   a. Assess lung sounds for rhonchi, crackles, and wheezes.
   b. Administer bronchodilators as indicated.
   c. Monitor chest radiograph.
   d. Monitor for signs or symptoms of infection that may lead to thick, tenacious sputum.
   e. Note color, consistency, amount, and odor of any sputum. Obtain sputum for culture and sensitivity if indicated.

f. Maintain patent airway.

g. Perform chest physical therapy and postural drainage to mobilize and expectorate sputum.

h. Suction if cough is ineffective.

i. Assist patient in turning, coughing and deep breathing.

j. Position for comfort and efficient use of the respiratory muscles.

NURSING DIAGNOSIS: Anxiety R/T dyspnea and fear of dying

See "Nursing Diagnosis: Anxiety" on page 927.

NURSING DIAGNOSIS: Altered nutrition, less than body requirements, R/T dyspnea, decreased appetite from drugs, and generalized weakness

1. *Expected outcomes:* Following interventions, the patient should exhibit such signs of proper nutrition as the following:
   a. Albumin level greater than 2.5 gm per dl
   b. Positive nitrogen balance
   c. Weight within calculated ideal body weight
2. *Nursing interventions*
   a. Assess dietary history.
   b. In consultation with patient and nutrition specialist, identify patient's food likes and dislikes and develop a diet that limits foods high in glucose. (Glucose breaks down into carbon dioxide, which increases levels of carbon dioxide in the body.)
   c. Provide frequent small meals. Schedule feedings around periods of rest.
   d. Monitor albumin and prealbumin levels.
   e. Weigh daily.
   f. Auscultate bowel sounds every shift.

Discharge Planning and Teaching

1. Describe causes of acute respiratory failure, signs and symptoms of infection and respiratory distress, and importance of seeing a health care provider as soon as these symptoms appear.
2. Explain pharmacologic regimen—how to take medications as well as the possible adverse side effects.
3. Discuss the need for the patient to take additional precautions: stop smoking, get flu shots regularly, avoid air pollution as much as possible, maintain proper nutrition, get adequate exercise, avoid becoming exhausted.
4. Help patient identify physiologic needs and status (e.g., dyspnea and exercise intolerance).
5. Discuss patient's resources in meeting those needs caused by acute respiratory failure.
   a. Strong positive support system, ideally including family members who are able and willing to learn to care for the patient
   b. Financial resources
   c. Environmental resources

6. Arrange for specific professional resources (e.g., home care professionals), as needed.

■ CARING FOR PEOPLE WITH ADULT RESPIRATORY DISTRESS SYNDROME

Definition and Incidence

1. Adult respiratory distress syndrome (ARDS) is a sudden progressive pulmonary disorder characterized by reduced perfusion and increased capillary permeability in the lungs.
2. About 150,000 Americans develop ARDS each year.

Risk Factors

1. Can arise from any condition or event that traumatizes the lung tissue directly or indirectly
   a. Pulmonary trauma: lung contusions, fat emboli, pneumonia, aspiration (of smoke, toxins, foreign material, water, vomitus)
   b. Other disorders: sepsis, shock, head trauma, drug overdose, anaphylaxis, pancreatitis, uremia, disseminated intravascular coagulation, eclampsia
   c. Iatrogenic causes: cardiovascular bypass surgery, radiation therapy, massive blood transfusions

Pathophysiology

1. Symptoms may appear within hours of injury to the lungs (as in lung contusion) or not for many days afterward (as in sepsis).
2. Regardless of onset or cause, the body's response sequence in ARDS is the same:
   a. Some form of trauma (see risk factors above) reduces blood flow to the lungs. Platelets aggregate at the site of the injury, releasing histamine, serotonin, and bradykinin.
   b. These substances inflame and damage the alveolar-capillary membrane. This damage increases capillary permeability and allows fluid to move into the interstitial space while proteins and other fluid leak out. Pulmonary edema develops.
   c. Surfactant production falls as fluid builds up in the alveoli and blood flow falls. Without surfactant, alveoli begin to collapse, impairing gas exchange. Lungs become stiff as compliance decreases.
   d. Despite increased respiration rates, sufficient oxygen is unable to pass through the alveolar membrane, while carbon monoxide passes through more easily than normal and is lost on exhalation. As a result, blood levels of both oxygen and carbon dioxide fall.
   e. Left untreated, pulmonary edema worsens, inflammation causes fibrosis (further impairing gas exchange), and hypoxemia and death result.

Clinical Manifestations

1. Tachypnea
2. Dyspnea
3. Hypoxemia
4. Cyanosis
5. Hypocapnia (late sign)

Diagnostics

1. History: Check for recent trauma (see risk factors, above)
2. Physical examination findings (in addition to their clinical manifestations, above)
   a. Findings on both physical examination and diagnostic studies depend on stage of syndrome
   b. Sounds ranging from fine crackles to rhonchi to widespread crackles on auscultation
   c. Tachycardia
   d. Mental sluggishness
   e. Apprehension, restlessness
   f. Impaired motor skills
3. Diagnostic studies
   a. Decreased serum pH and PaO_2 levels
   b. Increased $PaCO_2$ level
   c. Chest radiographs: diffuse, bilateral, rapidly progressing interstitial or alveolar infiltrates

Clinical Management

1. Goals of clinical management
   a. Provide respiratory support
   b. Halt progression of ARDS
   c. Prevent complications
   d. Correct cause of ARDS (see specific disorders for therapies)
2. Nonpharmacologic interventions
   a. Placing patient in semi-Fowler's position to ease respiration
   b. Fluid restrictions to reduce edema
   c. Ample periods of rest
3. Pharmacologic interventions
   a. Sedatives to reduce anxiety and restlessness (especially when mechanical ventilation is in use)
   b. Inotropic agents to improve cardiac output and increase systemic blood pressure
   c. Antibiotics for infection
   d. Diuretics to reduce edema
4. Special medical-surgical procedures
   a. Endotracheal intubation, mechanical ventilation, and oxygen therapy delivered by positive end-expiratory pressure to maintain blood oxygen levels (see pp. 958–979 for details on procedures)
   b. Suctioning, as needed

Complications

1. Hypoxemia
2. Lung fibrosis

Prognosis

1. In 60 to 70 percent of cases ARDS is fatal.
2. About 90 percent of deaths occur within 2 weeks of onset.
3. Patients who do recover generally have little or no permanent lung damage.

Applying the Nursing Process

NURSING DIAGNOSIS: Ineffective breathing pattern R/T decreased compliance of lungs

1. *Expected outcomes:* Following interventions, the patient should exhibit an improved breathing pattern, as evidenced by the following:
   a. Decreased apnea and dyspnea
   b. Decreased $PaCO_2$ level
   c. Decreased anxiety level due to improved breathing pattern
2. *Nursing interventions*
   a. Monitor respiration rate, rhythm, and depth.
   b. Assess skin for change in color, cyanosis, and the like.
   c. Assess for changes in mental state.
   d. Identify alternative pathologic conditions (e.g., pain, weakness, impaired airway clearance).
   e. In conjunction with physician, institute mechanical ventilation, if needed.
   f. Encourage patient to use pursed-lip breathing.
   g. Position patient in semi-Fowler's to ease breathing.
   h. Protect patient from secondary infections.

NURSING DIAGNOSIS: Ineffective airway clearance R/T pulmonary edema

1. *Expected outcomes:* Following interventions, the patient should exhibit improved airway clearance, as evidenced by the following:
   a. Decrease in abnormal breath sounds (e.g., rales, rhonchi, and wheezes)
   b. Skin tones that are normal and not bluish (cyanotic)
   c. Respirations at a more normal rate of 10 to 20 breaths per minute and quiet
2. *Nursing interventions*
   a. Monitor respiration rate, rhythm, and depth.
   b. Maintain patent airway.
   c. Monitor pulmonary artery pressure and pulmonary capillary wedge pressure.
   d. Monitor fluid intake in relation to pulmonary capillary wedge pressure.
   e. Encourage patient to turn, cough, and breathe deeply.
   f. Suction patient as indicated.

NURSING DIAGNOSIS: Impaired gas exchange R/T impaired alveolar-capillary membrane

1. *Expected outcomes:* Following interventions, the patient should exhibit improved airway clearance, as evidenced by the following:
   a. Arterial blood gas levels return to normal (see Appendix C).
   b. Heart rate is 70 to 80 beats per minute and regular.
   c. Pulse oximetry indicates adequate arterial oxygen saturation (greater than 90%).
2. *Nursing interventions*
   a. Monitor arterial blood gases (ABGs), pulmonary artery pressure, pulmonary capillary wedge pressure, and vital signs.
   b. Monitor for signs of cor pulmonale and arrhythmias.
   c. Record input and output.
   d. Administer oxygen, as indicated.
   e. Administer respiratory medications, as indicated.

Discharge Planning and Teaching

1. Provide information on ARDS: its causes, signs and symptoms, interventions (including medications and how and when to take them), and consequences of failure to comply with treatment program.
2. Teach breathing techniques. Stress the need to turn, cough, and breathe deeply on a regular basis.
3. Work with the patient to develop a schedule that provides adequate periods of exercise and rest.

■ CARING FOR PEOPLE WITH ATELECTASIS

Definition and Incidence

1. The collapse or incomplete expansion of alveoli or lung segments, resulting in a state of airlessness of the lung; may be acute or chronic
2. One of the most common respiratory disorders in hospitalized patients—and one of the most preventable complications

Risk Factors

1. Abdominal or thoracic surgery
2. Pain in the abdomen or thoracic region
3. Immobility
4. Narcotic administration

Etiology

1. Hypoventilation due to abdominal or thoracic surgery
2. Other pulmonary disorders: pleural effusion, pneumothorax, hemothorax, emphysema, bronchiectasis
3. Compression of the lung by tumor
4. Mucus plugs
5. Interstitial fibrosis
6. Chest wall deformities

7. Impaired diaphragmatic movement as in obesity, ascites, or both
8. Central nervous system dysfunction
9. Decreased levels of surfactant as a result of oxygen toxicity, smoke inhalation, aspiration

Pathophysiology

1. Atelectasis can be caused by 3 factors: obstruction of the airways, ineffective ventilation, or decreased surfactant production.
2. Obstruction of the airways
   a. When obstruction of the airways occurs, the gas distal to the obstruction is absorbed into the circulation (resorption atelectasis)
   b. Absorption occurs because the oxygen pressure in the capillaries is lower than that of the alveoli. (As noted earlier, oxygen diffuses from an area of higher concentration to an area of lower concentration.)
   c. Because the gas is moving into the capillaries and the alveolar gas is not being replaced by atmospheric gas, the alveoli collapse.
   d. Obstruction of the large lobar and segmental branches of the lung will cause collapse of the lung tissue distal to the obstruction.
   e. Obstructions closer to the periphery of the lung usually do not cause collapse, as the collateral circulation of the alveolar sacs through the pores of Kohn keeps obstructed alveoli from collapsing.
3. Ineffective ventilation
   a. Ineffective ventilation is the main factor in postoperative atelectasis.
   b. Poor inspiratory effort leads to decreased tidal volumes, which in turn decrease lung volume and increase compliance.
   c. Stasis of secretions due to poor inspiratory effort also contribute to postoperative atelectasis.
4. Decreased surfactant levels
   a. Because surfactant is the substance that keeps alveoli open, decreased levels of surfactant result in the collapse of alveoli and thus lung tissue.
   b. Decreased blood flow and poor expansion of the lungs usually lead to decreased surfactant levels.

Clinical Manifestations

1. Tachypnea
2. Nasal flaring
3. Retractions
4. Dyspnea
5. Signs of hypoxemia
6. Decreased chest expansion
7. Cyanosis
8. Fever
9. Tachycardia

Diagnostics

1. Assessment
   a. History: History of any risk factor (see earlier discussion)

   b. Physical examination: In addition to checking for clinical manifestations (listed above), be alert for the following:
      (1) Shift of the trachea to the affected side (result of large atelectasis)
      (2) Decreased chest movement on the affected side
      (3) Decreased fremitus on the affected side
      (4) Lung sounds over the affected area: absent or including crackles with deep inspiration
2. Medical diagnosis
   a. May be based on signs and symptoms present during the physical examination, with chest radiograph to confirm.
   b. Chest radiograph reveals decreased lung markings over the affected area and sometimes elevated hemidiaphragm on the affected side.
   c. Arterial blood gas measurements reveal decreased PaO_2 with normal or decreased $PaCO_2$. Extensive atelectasis may result in respiratory acidosis.

Clinical Management

1. See pages 958–979 for details on therapies.
2. Goals of clinical management
   a. Reinflate collapsed airways
   b. Reduce obstruction
   c. Promote circulation to the lung tissue to prevent decreased surfactant levels
   d. Correct the cause (e.g., remove tumor or drain empyema) of compression atelectasis
3. Nonpharmacologic interventions
   a. Turn, cough, and deep breathe to expand lungs and to stimulate surfactant production.
   b. Perform chest physical therapy and postural drainage to maintain airway patency.
   c. Provide humidification and hydration to prevent thick and tenacious secretions, which may obstruct airways.
   d. Maintain adequate nutrition to prevent muscle atrophy, which may result in weakened inspiratory muscle effort.

NURSE ADVISORY

Postoperatively, patients who have undergone abdominal surgery are at high risk for developing atelectasis. To reduce this risk, provide adequate pain relief to facilitate deeper respirations. In addition, encourage early ambulation and the hourly use of the incentive spirometer.

4. Pharmacologic interventions: bronchodilator therapy to promote the opening of constricted airways
5. Special medical-surgical procedures
   a. Bronchoscopy
      (1) Used to diagnose and treat some causes of atelectasis
      (2) Used to directly visualize and remove mucus plugs and foreign bodies that can lead to resorption atelectasis
   b. Oxygen therapy to treat hypoxemia, if present

c. Endotracheal intubation and mechanical ventilation
   (1) Used in some cases of atelectasis
   (2) Positive end-expiratory pressure and large tidal volumes to fully expand lungs and maintain them in an open position

Complications

1. Pneumonia
2. Hypoxemia
3. Ventilation-perfusion mismatching
4. Respiratory distress
5. Shifting of mediastinum (if area of atelectasis is large)
6. Pneumothorax

Prognosis

1. Can be fatal if untreated
2. Depends on site and degree of blockage and on prompt treatment: removal of airway obstruction, reexpansion of lung, elimination of hypoxia

Applying the Nursing Process

NURSING DIAGNOSIS: Impaired gas exchange R/T obstruction of airways

1. *Expected outcomes:* Following interventions, the patient should demonstrate improved gas exchange, as evidenced by the following:
   a. Normal ABG levels
   b. Patent airways
2. *Nursing interventions*
   a. Monitor ABGs; respiratory rate, rhythm, and depth; and use of accessory muscles.
   b. Assess for changes in mental status.
   c. Have patient turn, cough, and deep breathe.
   d. Encourage ambulation and frequent position changes.
   e. Teach patient to use incentive spirometry.
   f. Perform chest physical therapy and postural drainage.
   g. Administer oxygen if indicated.
   h. Apply continuous positive airway pressure mask or use nasotracheal suctioning if necessary.

NURSING DIAGNOSIS: Ineffective breathing pattern R/T pain, central nervous system dysfunction, and impaired diaphragmatic movement

1. *Expected outcomes:* Following interventions, the patient should exhibit an effective breathing pattern, as evidenced by the following:
   a. Respiratory rate of 12 to 25 breaths per minute
   b. Full, equal breath sounds
   c. Symmetric chest expansion
   d. Absence of use of accessory muscles
2. *Nursing interventions*

a. Assess respiratory rate, rhythm, depth, and use of accessory muscles.
b. Auscultate breath sounds.
c. Note the presence of adventitious breath sounds.
d. Have patient turn, cough, and deep breathe.
e. Encourage deep and slow respiratory patterns.
f. Elevate head of bed to improve diaphragmatic movement.
g. Administer pain medication before pulmonary procedures.

Discharge Planning and Teaching

1. Teach signs and symptoms of atelectasis (e.g., persistent cough, elevated temperature, dyspnea) and when to seek medical treatment.
2. Instruct on techniques of turning, coughing, and deep breathing and use of the incentive spirometer.
3. Encourage daily exercise in moderation.

■ CARING FOR PEOPLE WITH PULMONARY EMBOLISM AND INFARCTION

Definition

1. A pulmonary embolism is an obstruction of a branch of the pulmonary artery by a clot (usually part or all of a thrombus) brought by the blood from another vessel and forced into a smaller lumen, thus obstructing the vessel.
2. A pulmonary embolus is usually a blood clot dislodged from a peripheral vein (most commonly in the deep veins of the leg, pelvis, and right side of the heart).
3. Pulmonary infarction refers to the local necrosis resulting from vascular obstruction.

Incidence and Socioeconomic Impact

1. Pulmonary embolisms and infarctions account for 5 percent of all sudden deaths.
2. True incidence is hard to define owing to difficulties in clinical diagnosis.

Risk Factors

1. Many risk factors are related to impaired mobility: obesity, chronic diseases (e.g., sickle cell anemia, heart disease, cancer, history of pulmonary embolism), fractures of the legs or pelvis, pelvic surgery, old age.
2. Other factors are linked to clot production: use of oral contraceptives, clotting abnormalities, varicose veins, pregnancy, and recent childbirth.
3. Sickle cell anemia results in sickle-shaped cells that tend to occlude the blood vessels.
4. Wearing restrictive clothing, smoking, and abdominal infections are also linked to pulmonary embolisms and infarctions.

Etiology

1. The primary cause of emboli is clots (especially in the thigh and pelvis).
2. Nonthrombotic causes of emboli include air, fat, malignant cells, amniotic fluid, and pericardial vegetations.

Pathophysiology

1. Thrombi formed in blood vessels are dislodged by activities such as standing, turning, coughing, and walking.
2. Once dislodged, an embolus travels through the venous system to the right side of the heart and lodges in the pulmonary arteries, occluding blood flow to the distal pulmonary vasculature.
3. Perfusion to the alveoli distal to the obstruction ceases and dead space increases.
4. Reflex bronchospasm occurs in the affected area, leading to an increase in pulmonary resistance and a decrease in lung compliance.
5. In the affected area, reflex bronchospasms compensate for decreased perfusion, but in adjacent areas they may result in a ventilation-perfusion mismatch, leading to hypoxemia.
6. If the embolism is large enough, it may reduce pulmonary perfusion sufficiently to cause pulmonary hypertension.
7. Pulmonary infarction most often results from occlusion of the mediastinal arteries.

Clinical Manifestations

Clinical manifestations of pulmonary embolism are dyspnea (most common manifestation), tachypnea, tachycardia, persistent cough, hemoptysis, pleuritic pain, apprehension, cyanosis, shock, fever, palpitation, syncope, and diaphoresis.

Diagnostics

1. Assessment
   a. History (in addition to risk factors listed above)
      (1) Have patient describe dyspnea, elaborating on onset, duration, and whether it occurs with activity or rest. Answers will vary, depending on the size of the pulmonary embolism. Dyspnea is usually precipitated by physical activity.
      (2) Have patient describe the chest pain, elaborating on location, duration, severity, radiation, characteristics, and frequency. Chest pain is present if occlusion is greater than 50 to 60 percent owing to pulmonary hypertension. Pleuritic pain that is greater on inspiration and is relieved when the patient is in an upright position may indicate pulmonary infarction.
   b. Physical examination
      (1) Check for clinical manifestations (see previous discussion), bearing in mind that manifestations vary depending on the extent to which the lung is involved, the size of the clot, and the general condition of the patient.
      (2) Auscultation findings: increased intensity of the S2 heart sound in pulmonary hypertension and tricuspid or mitral murmurs.
      (3) Other findings: distended neck veins, nonspecific ST changes, peripheral edema, signs or symptoms of phlebitis, hypotension and cyanosis resulting from right-sided heart failure.
      (4) Pulmonary infarction results in a cough with hemoptysis, pleural effusions, and possibly a pleural friction rub.
   c. Diagnostic studies
      (1) Laboratory findings: Tests of serum enzymes, bilirubin, and ABGs are nonspecific and should not be used in the diagnosis of pulmonary embolus.
      (2) Electrocardiogram: Helps to differentiate between myocardial infarction and pulmonary embolism; usually gives normal results in patients with pulmonary embolism.
      (3) Chest radiographs: Help in determining other causes for patient's condition and interpreting lung scan findings; abnormalities are nonspecific for emboli.
      (4) Lung scan
         • A normal perfusion scan result excludes the diagnosis of pulmonary embolism; an abnormal result is nonspecific and may result from other underlying conditions.
         • If a perfusion defect is localized to a lobe or segment of the lung, chances of a pulmonary embolus causing the defect are greater. If there is a perfusion deficit, then the ventilation scan must be performed.
         • If there are ventilation defects in the same area as perfusion deficits, then the ventilation-perfusion abnormality is usually related to an underlying pulmonary disorder. If there are no ventilation defects in the area of a perfusion defect, suspect a pulmonary embolism.
      (5) Pulmonary angiogram: Used to confirm diagnosis of a pulmonary embolism, this invasive procedure involves catheterization of the right side of the heart. A radiopaque dye is injected into the pulmonary artery while serial radiographs are taken. Occlusions cause interruptions in the flow of dye. Although a relatively safe procedure, possible complications include tachyarrhythmias, myocardial injury, and hypersensitivity reaction to the injected dye.

Clinical Management

1. See pages 958–979 for details of therapies.
2. Goals of clinical management
   a. Alleviating symptoms
   b. Supporting cardiopulmonary function
   c. Preventing the spread of further clots
3. Nonpharmacologic interventions

a. Using sequential compression devices.
b. Wearing antiembolic stockings
c. Performing range of motion exercises while immobile
d. Turning frequently
e. Positioning for comfort
4. Pharmacologic interventions
   a. Heparin and oral anticoagulants
      (1) Intravenous administration of heparin can reduce the size of the embolizing thrombi, slow detachment of emboli from thrombi, and help maintain cardiopulmonary stability.
      (2) Administration proceeds until partial thromboplastin time is 2 to 2.5 times the baseline prothrombin time.
      (3) Several days before discontinuing heparin, oral anticoagulants (warfarin sodium) are usually begun to provide a transition to their exclusive use.
      (4) Patients remain on oral anticoagulants for 3 to 6 months.

DRUG ADVISORY

The patient on oral anticoagulant therapy should be instructed to refrain from eating dark green leafy vegetables, because these contain Vitamin K, which will counteract the anticoagulant.

b. Thrombolytic therapy: indicated for patients with life-threatening pulmonary emboli
   (1) Rapidly dissolve clots and restore hemodynamic stability (most often streptokinase and urokinase).
   (2) After these drugs are discontinued, intravenous heparin therapy should begin.
   (3) Drawbacks to thrombolytics include cost and increased risk of bleeding.
5. Special medical-surgical procedures
   a. Vein ligation to prevent the embolus from traveling to the heart
   b. Insertion of a venacaval umbrella or screen to catch an embolism before it reaches the lungs
   c. Embolectomy to remove an embolus from the pulmonary vasculature

Complications

1. Pulmonary hypertension
2. Pulmonary infarction
3. Shock
4. Pulmonary hemorrhage
5. Cor pulmonale
6. Atelectasis

Prognosis

Untreated pulmonary embolisms have mortality rates of 20 to 35 percent. Treatment reduces this figure to 8 percent.

Applying the Nursing Process

NURSING DIAGNOSIS: Impaired gas exchange R/T reduced cardiac output and reduced blood flow to lung region

1. *Expected outcomes:* Following interventions, the patient should exhibit improved gas exchange, as evidenced by the following:
   a. PaO_2 greater than 80 mm Hg or baseline value
   b. SaO_2 greater than 90 percent
   c. Absence of cyanosis
   d. Absence of mental status disturbances
   e. Normal heart rate and rhythm
   f. Absence of hemoptysis
2. *Nursing interventions*
   a. Assess lung sounds and monitor for sudden changes.
   b. Assess mental status.
   c. Monitor laboratory values (ABGs, SaO_2, hematocrit, hemoglobin).
   d. Monitor respiratory status, noting rate, rhythm, and characteristics.
   e. Monitor vital signs.
   f. Monitor cardiac output.
   g. Limit activity.
   h. Provide a quiet and restful environment.
   i. Administer oxygen as indicated.

NURSING DIAGNOSIS: Altered tissue perfusion R/T embolus in pulmonary vasculature

1. *Expected outcomes:* Following interventions, the patient should exhibit signs of normal tissue perfusion:
   a. Normal respiratory rate
   b. Absence of dyspnea
   c. No complaints of chest pain
   d. Normal heart rate and rhythm
   e. Normal heart sounds
2. *Nursing interventions*
   a. Monitor for bleeding. Check stool and urine specimens for blood.
   b. Monitor electrocardiogram for changes in rate and rhythm.
   c. Auscultate heart sounds frequently.
   d. Administer anticoagulant therapy if indicated.
   e. Administer thrombolytic if indicated.
   f. Monitor prothrombin time and partial thromboplastin time to evaluate effectiveness of anticoagulant therapy.

NURSING DIAGNOSIS: Pain R/T decreased perfusion of pulmonary tissue

1. *Expected outcomes:* Following interventions, the patient should experience decreased pain, as evidenced by the following:
   a. Patient verbalizes a decrease in pain
   b. Normal vital signs

c. Absence of nonverbal expressions of pain
d. Absence of diaphoresis
2. *Nursing interventions*
   a. Assess for pain every 2 hours.
   b. Note any nonverbal expressions of pain.
   c. Administer pain medication as indicated.
   d. Position for comfort.
   e. Note precipitating, aggravating, and alleviating factors of pain.
   f. Utilize nonpharmacologic methods to reduce pain, if appropriate (e.g., distraction, massage).

NURSING DIAGNOSIS: Risk for decreased cardiac output R/T increased pulmonary vascular resistance

1. *Expected outcomes:* Following interventions, the patient should experience a return to normal cardiac output as evidenced by the following:
   a. Stable cardiac output
   b. Stable vital signs
   c. Peripheral pulses present
   d. Skin warm and dry
   e. Absence of jugular venous distention
2. *Nursing interventions*
   a. Monitor vital signs frequently.
   b. Monitor cardiac output and cardiac index, if available.
   c. Monitor intake and output.
   d. Monitor daily weight.
   e. Monitor skin for color and moisture.
   f. Monitor for change in mental status.

Discharge Planning and Teaching

1. Describe the causes, signs, and symptoms of pulmonary embolism or infarction and their complications. Warn patients to seek professional help if they notice any abnormal bleeding or experience an acute onset of chest pain.
2. Teach the patient ways to reduce venous stasis of blood such as leg exercises, wearing antithrombotic stockings, walking, and avoiding sitting in one position for prolonged periods.
3. Emphasize the importance of sound health practices (e.g., quitting smoking, maintaining normal weight).
4. If the patient is a woman, have her consider using non-hormonal forms of birth control.

◾ *CARING FOR PEOPLE WITH BRONCHIECTASIS*

Definition and Incidence

1. A form of obstructive lung disease, this chronic dilation of the bronchus and bronchioles often begins in childhood.
2. It includes a secondary infection usually involving the lower lobes of the lungs.

3. Widespread use of antibiotics for childhood respiratory infections is causing this disease to vanish rapidly.

Risk Factors and Etiology

1. Childhood lower respiratory tract infections that develop as complications of measles, whooping cough, or influenza
2. Bronchial obstructions that result from neoplasms or foreign bodies
3. Cystic fibrosis
4. Bronchitis in the upper lobes associated with tuberculosis
5. Kartagener's syndrome (destroys mucociliary transport)

Pathophysiology

1. Chronic inflammation weakens bronchial walls.
2. Purulent secretions collect in the weakened areas.
3. Stasis of secretions in these areas leads to persistent infections.
4. Chronic infections cause increased irritation to the bronchial walls, creating a cyclic pattern of inflammation.

Clinical Manifestations

1. Chronic, loose, productive cough
2. Large amount of purulent, foul-smelling sputum (as much as 200 ml/day)
3. Coughing (may increase when patient changes positions)
4. Hemoptysis
5. Clubbing of nails
6. Night sweats
7. Fever
8. Late-stage changes: cor pulmonale and dyspnea on exertion

Diagnostics

1. Assessment
   a. History: multiple, recurrent infections in childhood; history of measles, whooping cough, pneumonia
   b. Physical examination findings (in addition to clinical manifestations) are fatigue, weakness, loud, bubbly rhonchi on auscultation.
   c. Diagnostic tests
      (1) Chest radiograph reveals air-fluid levels and thickened bronchi.
      (2) Computed tomography scan delineates the bronchiectasis areas well.
2. Medical diagnosis: Commonly made by physical examination

Clinical Management

Clinical management goals and interventions are the same as those for COPD, with the addition of surgically resecting localized areas of bronchiectasis as a palliative measure.

Complications

Complications depend on the extent of involvement of lung tissue.

Prognosis

The prognosis is the same as that for COPD.

Applying the Nursing Process

Nursing diagnoses, expected outcomes, and nursing interventions are the same as those for COPD.

Discharge Planning and Teaching

Discharge planning and teaching are the same as those for COPD.

Public Health Considerations

1. Monitor children for signs and symptoms of respiratory infections.
2. Treat applicable childhood respiratory infections aggressively with antibiotic therapy.

◼ CARING FOR PEOPLE WITH PLEURISY

Definition

Inflammation of the pleura that may or may not include a pleural effusion.

Etiology

1. Extension of a localized disease such as pneumonia, esophageal rupture, pericarditis, subphrenic abscess, tuberculosis, neoplasm of the pleura, postcardiac injury syndrome, sarcoidosis, pancreatitis, pneumothorax, pulmonary embolism, asbestos pleural effusion, and uremic pleural effusion
2. Complication of a systemic disease such as lupus erythematosus
3. Direct trauma to the chest wall

Clinical Manifestations

1. Chest pain occurs with respirations and may range from mild to severe depending on the extent of the inflammation.

2. Chest pain is worse with coughing, deep breathing, sneezing, laughing, or in some cases talking.
3. Chest pain is described as sharp, shooting, or stabbing in nature.
4. Dyspnea
5. Shallow, rapid breathing
6. Ipsilateral restriction of chest wall motion
7. Pleural friction rub
8. Dull percussion note due to pleural effusion or consolidation
9. Fremitus will be increased or decreased depending on the presence or absence of consolidation.

Clinical Management

1. Goals of clinical management
   a. Treat the underlying cause of the pleural inflammation
   b. Reduce the amount of pleural inflammation
   c. Reduce the pain associated with the plural inflammation
2. Nonpharmacologic interventions
   a. Splint the chest wall with a chest binder or holding a pillow tightly against the chest when coughing or sneezing
   b. Having the patient lie on the affected side
3. Pharmacologic interventions
   a. Analgesics, usually nonsteroidal anti-inflammatory drugs, to reduce chest wall pain. This promotes deeper breaths and reduces the risk of atelectasis
   b. Antibiotics appropriate to treat the causative organism if the inflammation of the pleura is determined to have an infectious origin
   c. Corticosteroids to treat pleural inflammation resulting from lupus erythematosus or postcardiac injury syndrome
4. Special medical-surgical procedures
   a. Chest radiograph to confirm the diagnosis of pneumothorax, esophageal rupture, pancreatitis, pneumonia, or hepatic or splenic abscesses
   b. Pleural fluid analysis is the most helpful tool in determining the cause of the pleural inflammation. A thoracentesis is performed to remove fluid from the pleural space.
      (1) Bloody effusions are indicative of pulmonary embolism, neoplasms involving the pleura, postcardiac injury syndrome, or asbestos-related effusions.
      (2) The presence of pus in the pleural fluid is found with esophageal rupture.
      (3) Elevated pleural amylase suggests pancreatitis or an esophageal rupture.
      (4) Elevated white blood count in the pleural fluid suggests bacterial pneumonia, esophageal rupture, pancreatitis, or a subphrenic abscess.
      (5) Decreased number of white blood cells in the pleural fluid is usually a result of inflammation caused by tuberculosis.
   c. Ventilation-perfusion scan to diagnose pulmonary embolism

d. Pleural biopsy to confirm the presence of tuberculosis
e. Radiographic contrast study of the esophagus to confirm esophageal rupture
f. Abdominal CT scan to verify the presence of a subphrenic abscess
g. Drainage of the pleural space is needed if the pleural inflammation is caused by subphrenic abscess or esophageal rupture.

■ CARING FOR PEOPLE WITH PLEURAL EFFUSION

Definition and Incidence

1. Pleural effusion is the accumulation of fluid in the space between the parietal and visceral pleura.
2. Approximately 1 million cases of pleural effusion occur annually in the United States.

Risk Factors and Etiology

1. Nearly always secondary to other diseases
   a. Cardiovascular conditions: congestive heart failure, pericardial disease
   b. Cirrhosis
   c. Pulmonary emboli
   d. Neoplastic disease
   e. Tuberculosis
   f. Bacterial or fungal infection
   g. Uremia
   h. Pancreatic disease
2. May also arise following radiation therapy or abdominal surgery

Pathophysiology

1. Normally, the space between the lung and the chest wall contains a small amount of fluid that prevents friction. This pleural fluid enters the space from the capillaries lining the parietal pleura. Any excess fluid is absorbed into the visceral pleura capillaries and the surrounding lymphatics.
2. Conditions that alter the secretion or drainage of excess pleural fluid may lead to a pleural effusion.
3. Types of fluids contained in a pleural effusion are transudates, exudates, and pleural empyema.
   a. Transudates: substances that have passed through a membrane or tissue.
      (1) Transudates accumulate when pulmonary venous pressure rises, a condition that favors movement of fluid out of the vessels.
      (2) These fluids tend to accumulate at the base of the lungs owing to the force of gravity.
      (3) Transudates occur principally in conditions involving protein loss and low protein content (e.g., cirrhosis, left ventricular failure, nephrosis).
   b. Exudates: substances that have escaped from blood vessels

      (1) Exudates accumulate secondary to inflammation or malignant growth, processes that increase capillary permeability, decrease lymphatic drainage, or both.
      (2) Exudates have a higher specific gravity and protein content than transudates owing to passing through injured vessel walls; they also contain high levels of lactic dehydrogenase.
      (3) Exudates occur principally when there is an increase in capillary permeability.
   c. Pleural empyema: a purulent, pus-containing pleural effusion
      (1) Pleural empyema is usually a complication of pneumonia, lung abscesses, or perforation of a carcinoma in the pleural cavity.
      (2) If not drained, empyema may form fibrotic adhesions that fix the parietal and visceral pleuras together.

Clinical Manifestations

1. Manifestations depend on the amount of fluid present and the severity of lung compression.
2. Effusions of less than 250 ml are usually asymptomatic.
3. Effusions of more than 250 ml cause greater lung compression and may lead to dyspnea, tachypnea, and shallow respirations.
4. If lung compression is severe enough to impair gas exchange, cyanosis, restlessness, and diaphoresis may be present.
5. Other signs include pleuritic pain, trachea deviated away from effusion, bulging of intercostal spaces (large effusion), and decreased chest movement over the area of effusion.

Diagnostics

1. Assessment
   a. History: Check for risk factors (see above).
   b. Physical examination findings (in addition to clinical manifestations, above)
      (1) Decreased chest expansion over the affected area
      (2) Flat percussion note over the affected area
      (3) Egophony present over the compressed lung
      (4) Diminished vocal and tactile fremitus over the area of effusion
      (5) Diminished breath sounds over the area of effusion
2. Medical diagnosis
   a. The possibility of a pleural effusion should be considered in any patient who has an abnormal result on chest radiograph.
   b. Differential diagnosis requires removal of pleural fluid for analysis (thoracentesis).
      (1) Exudates: pleural fluid protein to serum protein greater than 0.5; pleural fluid lactic dehydrogenase to serum lactic dehydrogenase greater than 0.6; pleural fluid lactic dehydrogenase greater then 200 IU.
      (2) Transudates: pleural fluid protein to serum protein less than or equal to 0.5; pleural fluid lactic

dehydrogenase to serum lactic dehydrogenase less than or equal to 0.6.

(3) Empyema: pleural fluid contains pus, low pH (<7.30).

(4) Pleural fluid may be hemorrhagic (bloody—suspect trauma, carcinoma, pulmonary infarction, pulmonary embolism, tuberculosis), chylous (thick and white colored—suspect lymphatic obstruction), or high in cholesterol (suspect a recurrent infection related to tuberculosis or rheumatoid arthritis).

Clinical Management

1. Goals of clinical management
   a. Improve gas exchange
   b. Remove excess fluid
   c. Prevent fibrotic lesions
   d. Prevent reaccumulation of excess pleural fluid
2. Nonpharmacologic interventions—none
3. Pharmacologic interventions—none
4. Special medical-surgical procedures: draining of excess pleural fluid by thoracentesis (see p. 919) or with chest tubes (see p. 976)

Complications

1. Lung compression leading to impaired gas exchange
2. Mediastinal shift causing decreased cardiac output
3. Pneumonia
4. Pneumothorax

Prognosis

Pleural effusions may recur in some cases, despite aggressive intervention (e.g., in malignancy-induced effusions). Treatment involves obliteration of the pleural space, which may leave the patient with permanent compromised pulmonary function.

Applying the Nursing Process

NURSING DIAGNOSIS: Impaired gas exchange R/T ventilation-perfusion mismatch from atelectasis

1. *Expected outcomes:* Following interventions, the patient should exhibit improved gas exchange, as evidenced by the following:
   a. Alert and fully oriented state
   b. Stable vital signs
   c. Stable ABGs
   d. Absence of cyanosis
2. *Nursing interventions*
   a. Monitor respiratory status, arterial blood gases, hemoglobin, hematocrit, SaO_2, and vital signs.
   b. Assess patient for symmetry of chest movement.
   c. Assess for changes in mental status.

d. Monitor chest tube drainage system, watching for color, consistency, amount, and fluctuation of drainage.
e. Administer diuretics as indicated.
f. Position for comfort and ease of respirations.

NURSING DIAGNOSIS: Impaired breathing pattern R/T thoracic pain and altered respiratory mechanics

1. *Expected outcomes:* Following interventions, the patient should exhibit improved breathing, as evidenced by the following:
   a. Stable vital signs
   b. Unlabored respirations
   c. Full and equal breath sounds.
   d. Symmetric chest expansion.
   e. Minimal or absent atelectatic crackles.
2. *Nursing interventions*
   a. Monitor ventilation and oxygenation by following serial ABGs.
   b. Assess respiratory rate, rhythm, and pattern.
   c. Monitor for respiratory fatigue.
   d. Note use of accessory muscles of respiration.

NURSING DIAGNOSIS: Pain R/T pleuritic irritation

1. *Expected outcomes:* Following interventions, the patient should be free from pain, as evidenced by the following:
   a. Maintenance of a tolerable pain level
   b. Absence of nonverbal signs of pain
2. *Nursing interventions*
   a. Determine how client usually copes with pain.
   b. Note precipitating, aggravating, and alleviating factors of pain.
   c. Administer pain medication as indicated.
   d. Note pain relief with pain medication.
   e. Offer nonpharmacologic pain relief measures.
   f. Assess for nonverbal indications of pain.

Discharge Planning and Teaching

1. Describe the causes, signs and symptoms, and treatment of pulmonary effusion.
2. Prepare the patient for thoracentesis or chest tube insertion, if needed.
3. Explain the importance of positioning for greater breathing comfort and deep breathing and coughing to prevent complications.

◼ *CARING FOR PEOPLE WITH PULMONARY HYPERTENSION AND COR PULMONALE*

Definition

1. Pulmonary hypertension is the elevation of pressure within the pulmonary vasculature.

2. Cor pulmonale is hypertrophy of the right ventricle, leading to heart failure. The primary cause of cor pulmonale is pulmonary hypertension.

Incidence and Etiology

1. Most common cause (75% of cases) of cor pulmonale is COPD, but a significant number of cases of cor pulmonale are caused by multiple pulmonary emboli. Asthma, bronchitis, interstitial lung disease, and pulmonary hypertension are also causes in some cases.
2. Pulmonary hypertension is usually caused by left-sided heart failure or mitral valve stenosis but may also result from COPD, interstitial lung disease, and sleep apnea where hypoxia causes pulmonary vasoconstriction.

Risk Factors

1. Smoking
2. Chronic obstructive pulmonary disease
3. High altitudes

Pathophysiology

1. The pulmonary vasculature is a low-pressure, low-resistance system that allows for a large increase in blood volume without an increase in vascular resistance.
2. When vascular resistance forms in the pulmonary vasculature due to hypoxia or increased volume, pressure within the system increases.
3. As the resistance within the pulmonary vasculature system increases, so does the workload of the right side of the heart, which pumps blood into the system.
4. To compensate for the increased pressure, the right ventricle hypertrophies (becomes larger).
5. When the pressure within the pulmonary system becomes too great for the right ventricle to eject all of its volume, it fails, causing stasis of venous blood in the systemic circulation.

Clinical Manifestations

1. Peripheral edema
2. Cyanosis
3. Changes in mental status
4. Dyspnea
5. Increased jugular venous distention
6. Fatigue
7. Ascites
8. Nocturia
9. Weight gain
10. Anorexia and nausea

Diagnostics

1. History: Check for risk factors (see above).
2. Physical examination findings (in addition to clinical manifestations, above)

a. Wheezing on auscultation
b. Loud S2 in pulmonic area
c. S3–S4 gallop
3. Diagnostic tests
a. Pulmonary artery catheter pressure (20/10 = normal) of 30/15 indicates pulmonary hypertension.
b. Chest radiograph reveals an enlarged right ventricle.
c. Arterial blood gas levels reveal decreased PaO_2 and increased $PaCO_2$.
d. Laboratory studies show increased hematocrit and hemoglobin as a result of chronic hypoxemia.

Clinical Management

1. Goals of clinical management
a. Decrease fluid overload
b. Decrease pulmonary vascular resistance
c. Ease workload of the heart
d. Improve oxygenation
2. Nonpharmacologic interventions
a. Nutritional support to prevent malnutrition
b. Low salt diet to reduce fluid retention
c. Rest periods to conserve energy
3. Pharmacologic interventions
a. Bronchodilators (e.g., theophylline) to improve aeration of lungs and reduce afterload
b. Diuretics to remove excess fluid, thus reducing pulmonary hypertension
c. Oxygenation to reduce bronchial constriction related to hypoxemia
4. Special medical-surgical procedures: echocardiogram to evaluate degree of right ventricle dysfunction

Complications

1. Abdominal pain
2. Hepatomegaly
3. Splenomegaly
4. Malnutrition
5. Pulmonary edema
6. Pulmonary infarction

Prognosis

Heart failure may or may not accompany cor pulmonale.

Applying the Nursing Process

NURSING DIAGNOSIS: Impaired gas exchange R/T pulmonary vascular resistance and fluid overload

1. *Expected outcomes:* Following interventions, the patient should exhibit improved gas exchange as evidenced by the following:
a. Arterial blood gases at baseline levels

b. Absence of cyanosis
c. Respiratory rate of 12 to 20 breaths per minute
d. Absence of dysrhythmias
e. Mental status at baseline
f. Pulmonary artery pressure within normal limits
2. *Nursing interventions*
   a. Monitor ABGs; pulmonary artery pressure; respiratory rate, rhythm, and depth; and use of accessory muscles.
   b. Monitor for dysrhythmias.
   c. Note skin color and moisture.
   d. Monitor for mental status changes.
   e. Administer bronchodilators as indicated.
   f. Administer oxygen as indicated.

NURSING DIAGNOSIS: Fluid volume excess R/T impaired cardiac function

---

1. *Expected outcomes:* Following interventions, the patient should exhibit reduction of fluid volume, as evidenced by the following:
   a. Absence of edema
   b. Weight at baseline or ideal body weight
   c. No crackles noted
   d. Electrolytes within normal limits
2. *Nursing interventions*
   a. Weigh daily.
   b. Monitor edema and ascites.
   c. Monitor for jugular venous distention.
   d. Monitor electrolytes, and replace as indicated.
   e. Monitor intake and output. Restrict fluids if necessary.
   f. Administer diuretics as indicated.
   g. Instruct the patient in the elements of a low sodium diet.

Discharge Planning and Teaching

1. Instruct the patient in the signs and symptoms of right-sided heart failure.
2. Explain the importance and the elements of a low salt diet.
3. Instruct the patient in balancing rest and activity.
4. If the patient has a tendency toward sleep apnea, develop a diet plan to reduce weight.
5. If the patient is going home on oxygen, instruct the patient and family members in proper use of oxygen and oxygen therapies.

Public Health Considerations

Because cigarette smoking is the primary contributor to cor pulmonale and pulmonary hypertension, emphasis should be on primary prevention by urging people to stop (or not start) smoking.

◼ CARING FOR PEOPLE WITH PNEUMOTHORAX, TENSION PNEUMOTHORAX, AND HEMOTHORAX

Definition and Incidence

1. Pneumothorax is the accumulation of air or gas in the pleural cavity, resulting in the collapse of the lung on the affected side. The condition may occur spontaneously or may follow trauma to, or perforation of, the chest wall or lung parenchyma.
2. Hemothorax is the collection of blood in the pleural cavity, which causes the collapse of the lung on the affected side.
3. Tension pneumothorax occurs when air enters the pleural cavity and cannot escape. Pressure builds up in the chest cavity, causing a shift in the mediastinum away from the affected side. *It is considered a medical emergency.*
4. Spontaneous pneumothorax may occur in apparently healthy individuals 20 to 40 years old.

Risk Factors and Etiology

1. Risk factors for tension pneumothorax include chest trauma and mechanical ventilation.
2. Etiology varies, but includes unintentional puncture of the lung (e.g., central line insertion); mechanical ventilation with positive end-expiratory pressure; thoracentesis; bullae on the lung surface, which rupture; chest trauma.

Pathophysiology

1. Normally, between the chest wall and the lung lies an airtight ''potential space'' with a slightly negative pressure.
2. If this normal subatmospheric pressure is lost, the lung, which has a natural tendency to recoil, collapses.
3. Pneumothoraces and tension pneumothoraces
   a. The severity of the lung's collapse and its impact depends on the amount of air that fills the pleural space. Small amounts of air may cause few, if any, symptoms. Large amounts of air may cause cardiopulmonary collapse.
   b. In a pneumothorax, collapse of a lung creates a void on the affected side, causing the mediastinum to shift toward that side.
   c. In a tension pneumothorax, air that enters the pleural cavity cannot exit. This one-way movement of air increases intrapleural pressure on the affected side and causes the mediastinum to shift toward the unaffected side.
4. In a hemothorax, blood enters the pleural cavity. Small hemothoraces (<300 ml) resolve spontaneously as the body gradually reabsorbs the blood. Large hemothoraces (>1500 ml) cause lung collapse, leading to increased tension and hypovolemia.

Clinical Manifestations

1. Clinical manifestations vary with the size of the thorax.
2. Pneumothorax
   a. Acute onset of chest pain, with pain radiating to the shoulders
   b. Dyspnea
   c. Pleuritic pain
   d. Trachea deviated toward the affected side
   e. Tachycardia
   f. Cyanosis
   g. On the affected side: diminished breath sounds, diminished chest expansion, and hyperresonance to percussion
3. Tension pneumothorax
   a. Severe respiratory distress
   b. Apprehension
   c. Agitation
   d. Tachycardia
   e. Hypotension
   f. Cyanosis
   g. Trachea shifted away from the affected side
   h. Increased jugular vein distention
4. Hemothorax
   a. Dullness to percussion on the affected side
   b. Tachycardia
   c. Trachea shifted away from the affected side (in large hemothoraces)
   d. Flat percussion note on the affected side
   e. Absent breath sounds over the affected area
   f. Hypotension
   g. Shock

Diagnostics

1. General: Auscultation of the lung fields reveals unilateral decreased breath sounds.
2. Pneumothorax
   a. History of previous pneumothorax
   b. Physical examination findings (in addition to clinical manifestations, above)
      (1) Asymptomatic if pneumothorax is small
      (2) Chest trauma
      (3) Tachypnea
      (4) Deviation of the trachea toward the unaffected side
      (5) Diminished fremitus over the affected area
      (6) Subcutaneous emphysema
3. Tension pneumothorax
   a. History: see risk factors, above
   b. Physical examination findings (in addition to clinical manifestations, above)
      (1) Dyspnea
      (2) Chest pain radiating to the shoulder
      (3) Tachypnea
      (4) Hyperresonance over the affected area
      (5) Decreased fremitus over the affected area
      (6) Diminished breath sounds over the affected area
4. Hemothorax

   a. History: presence of risk factors, including chest trauma, carcinoma, and central line insertion
   b. Physical examination findings (in addition to clinical manifestations, above)
      (1) Dyspnea
      (2) Chest pain
      (3) Chest trauma
      (4) Tachypnea
      (5) Signs and symptoms of shock
5. Diagnostic tests: Chest radiograph will reveal areas of collapsed lung or fluid accumulation and a shift of the trachea from the midline.

Clinical Management

1. Goals of clinical management
   a. Re-expand lung
   b. Remove blood from the pleural cavity
   c. Restore negative intrapleural pressure
2. Nonpharmacologic interventions—none
3. Pharmacologic interventions—none
4. Special medical-surgical procedures:
   a. Emergent decompression of tension pneumothorax with a large-bore catheter
      (1) A large-bore (14 gauge or larger) catheter is placed in the 2nd intercostal space on the affected side.
      (2) Tube thoracostomy is performed following thoracic decompression with the large-bore catheter.
   b. Chest tubes and drainage systems; see page 978.

Complications

1. Impaired gas exchange
2. Cardiovascular collapse
3. Hypovolemia (hemothorax)
4. Atelectasis
5. Pulmonary embolus
6. Infection

Prognosis

If treated early, full recovery is usually possible without residual deficits.

Applying the Nursing Process

NURSING DIAGNOSIS: Ineffective breathing pattern R/T thoracic pain

1. *Expected outcomes:* Following interventions, the patient should exhibit improved breathing patterns, as evidenced by the following:
   a. Respiratory rate of 12 to 20 breaths per minute
   b. Equal lung sounds bilaterally

c. Symmetric chest expansion

d. No use of accessory muscles

2. *Nursing interventions*

a. Monitor characteristics of respiration.

b. Monitor vital signs frequently.

c. Auscultate lung sounds.

d. Monitor ABGs and SaO_2.

e. Position for comfort and ease of respiration.

f. Medicate for pain, as indicated.

NURSING DIAGNOSIS: Impaired gas exchange R/T collapsed or compressed lung tissue and ventilation-perfusion mismatch

---

1. *Expected outcomes:* Following interventions, the patient should exhibit improved gas exchange, as evidenced by the following:

a. Stable vital signs

b. Arterial blood gas levels at baseline

c. Normal skin color and moisture

d. SaO_2 greater than 90 percent

e. Absence of restlessness, irritability, and confusion

2. *Nursing interventions*

a. Monitor characteristics of respiration.

b. Assess lung sounds.

c. Monitor ABGs.

d. Establish baseline mental status and monitor for changes.

e. Assess skin color and temperature.

f. Administer oxygen as indicated.

g. Maintain proper functioning of chest tube, if present.

h. Encourage patient to turn, cough, and deep breathe.

NURSING DIAGNOSIS: Pain R/T insertion of chest tube

---

1. *Expected outcomes:* Following interventions, the patient should experience decreased pain as evidenced by the following:

a. Absence of nonverbal signs of pain

b. Verbalization of a reduction in pain

c. Vital signs at baseline

2. *Nursing interventions*

a. Administer pain medication as indicated.

b. Assess effectiveness of pain medication.

c. Position for comfort.

d. Assess for anxiety.

e. Administer sedatives as indicated.

f. Provide nonpharmacologic methods of pain relief such as distraction, massage, and relaxation.

Discharge Planning and Teaching

1. Teach signs and symptoms of pneumothorax in case of recurrence.

2. Teach range-of-motion exercises for the affected side (see Chapter 7).

3. Work with the patient to establish a gradual exercise program.

4. Teach the patient breathing techniques to improve lung expansion.

5. Instruct the patient to avoid persons with respiratory tract infections or influenza.

6. Stress the need for the patient to space out activities and avoid any strenuous activity until healing is complete.

7. Emphasize the strong need for patients with these problems to avoid high altitudes, flying in unpressurized aircraft, and scuba diving.

Public Health Considerations

As with most lung diseases, primary prevention focuses on persuading people not to use tobacco products.

◼ CARING FOR PEOPLE WITH PNEUMONIA

Definition and Incidence

1. Pneumonia is an infection and inflammation of the lung parenchyma with consolidation and exudation.

2. Though pneumonia was once a common cause of death that killed 1 out of 4 victims, antibiotic therapy has reduced the morbidity and mortality rates.

3. It remains a severe disease in infants and the elderly, however, and accounts for approximately 10 percent of hospital admissions.

ELDER ADVISORY

Changes in the pulmonary system of older people include diminished gas exchange, reduced ventilation, and a weakened immune system. These changes predispose older people to pneumonia. Older clients usually recover from pneumonia, but most will not be able to attain their previous level of health.

Risk Factors

1. Older age

2. Chronic obstructive pulmonary disease

3. Residence in a nursing home or other crowded living quarters

4. Diabetes

5. Alcohol abuse

6. Malnutrition

7. Neurologic impairments

8. Lung abscess

Etiology

1. **Bacteria,** including *Streptococcus pneumoniae, Staphylococcus aureus, Haemophilus influenzae, Pseudomonas aeruginosa, Klebsiella pneumoniae,* anaerobic bacteria, atypical bacteria such as *Legionella,* and *Mycoplasma pneumoniae*

2. **Viruses,** including influenza and adenovirus
3. **Fungi:** *Candida, Histoplasma, Aspergillus, Coccidioides,* and *Cryptococcus*
4. Protozoa: *Pneumocystis carinii*
5. Aspiration of gastric contents
6. May follow influenza

Pathophysiology

1. In an attempt to combat an infection, inflammatory cells, edema, and fibrin move into the alveolar spaces of the lungs. (Less commonly, bacteria may reach the lungs via the bloodstream.)
2. As defense mechanisms weaken, their effectiveness is lost. The infectious agent then advances to the lower airways and begins to proliferate.

Clinical Manifestations

1. Fever, chills, or both
2. Cough nonproductive to very productive
3. Dyspnea
4. Tachypnea
5. Tachycardia
6. Pleuritic pain
7. Diaphoresis
8. Headache
9. Fatigue

Diagnostics

1. History: Assess for risk factors (above).
2. Physical examination findings (in addition to clinical manifestations, above)
   a. Bronchial breath sounds over the affected area
   b. Whispered pectoriloquy present
   c. Tactile fremitus increased over the affected area
   d. Percussion note dull over the affected area
   e. Unequal lung expansion over the affected area
3. Diagnostic studies
   a. Tests to identify organism responsible: sputum culture and sensitivity, arterial blood gases, blood cultures
   b. Chest radiograph to define location and extent of pneumonia (affected areas appear white or opaque)
   c. Skin test for tuberculosis

Clinical Management

1. See pages 958–979 for details on therapies.
2. Goals of clinical management
   a. Maintain adequate gas exchange
   b. Clear infection
   c. Promote airway clearance
3. Nonpharmacologic interventions
   a. Turn, cough, and deep breathe to remove secretions.
   b. Perform postural drainage and chest physiotherapy.
   c. Ensure proper nutrition to keep immune system functioning properly.

   d. Promote activity such as walking as tolerated.
   e. Isolate immunocompromised patients to prevent continued exposure to infective organism.
4. Pharmacologic interventions (see Chapter 8)
   a. Antibiotic therapy specific to infectious organism.
   b. Employ oxygen therapy to prevent or treat hypoxemia.
5. Special medical-surgical procedures: Bronchoscopy to directly visualize the affected areas, to remove sputum by lavage, and to obtain tissue biopsies.

Complications

1. Respiratory failure
2. Abscess formation
3. Empyema
4. Pleural effusion
5. Bacteremia
6. Septicemia
7. Pulmonary edema
8. Atelectasis
9. Arthritis

Prognosis

Prognosis is good with early aggressive medical intervention.

Applying the Nursing Process

NURSING DIAGNOSIS: Ineffective airway clearance R/T copious sputum production

1. *Expected outcomes:* Following interventions, the patient should exhibit improved airway clearance, as evidenced by the following:
   a. Patent airway
   b. Adequate cough reflex
   c. Clearing secretions
   d. Clear lung sounds
2. *Nursing interventions*
   a. Monitor sputum production, noting color, consistency, amount, and odor.
   b. Provide adequate humidification and hydration to loosen secretions.
   c. Stress the importance of activity and exercise.
   d. Teach the patient to turn, cough, and deep breathe.
   e. Provide chest physical therapy and postural drainage, if indicated.
   f. Administer nasotracheal suction, if indicated.
   g. Administer bronchodilators, if indicated.
   h. Administer antibiotics, if indicated.

NURSING DIAGNOSIS: Ineffective breathing pattern R/T chest pain and hypoxia

1. *Expected outcomes:* Following interventions, the patient should exhibit improved breathing patterns, as evidenced by the following:
   a. Lack of dyspnea
   b. Respiratory rate of 12 to 20 breaths per minute
   c. Lung sounds equal bilaterally
   d. Equal, bilateral chest expansion
2. *Nursing interventions*
   a. Monitor ABGs as indicated.
   b. Monitor respiratory rate, rhythm, and depth and use of accessory muscles.
   c. Position for comfort with head of bed elevated to facilitate efficient use of diaphragm.
   d. Administer pain medication as needed.
   e. Administer oxygen as indicated.

Additional Nursing Diagnosis

- Impaired gas exchange R/T ventilation-perfusion mismatch

Discharge Planning and Teaching

1. Teach turning, coughing, and deep breathing techniques.
2. Instruct the patient to take the full course of any antibiotics prescribed.
3. Help the patient plan rest with gradual increase in activity as tolerated and avoid overworking.
4. Teach the patient to be aware of complications and recurrence of infection—dyspnea, fever, sweating, chest pain.
5. Instruct the patient to drink large amounts of fluids.
6. Explain the importance of good health practices in avoiding pneumonia: hand washing, proper diet, regular activity, avoidance of smoking, avoidance of large crowds during flu season, getting flu shots. High-risk patients should get the pneumococcal vaccine.

Public Health Considerations

Primary prevention focuses on stopping smoking and encouraging good hygiene practices (see Discharge Planning and Teaching, above).

■ CARING FOR PEOPLE WITH INFLUENZA

Definition and Incidence

1. Influenza ("flu") is an acute viral infection of the respiratory tract.
2. Every year, 10,000 to 20,000 people die from influenza. Most deaths occur because pneumonia is contracted or cardiopulmonary disorders resulting from the influenza are exacerbated.
3. Those aged 65 or older make up 80 to 90 percent of influenza deaths.

Risk Factors and Etiology

1. Persons aged 65 or older residing in a nursing home or other long-term care facility, or suffering from chronic disorders of the respiratory or cardiovascular system are at greatest risk.
2. Influenza is called by 1 of 3 airborne infection types: A, B, or C. Types A and B cause the most serious complications.

Pathophysiology

1. An airborne viral infection enters the body through the upper respiratory tract and invades bronchial, nasal, and tracheal mucosal cells, where it incubates for 3 days.
2. The virus causes necrosis and shedding of the serous ciliated cells that line the respiratory tract. As these cells die, they leave holes that expose underlying basal cells.
3. Extracellular fluid escapes through these holes, causing the "runny nose" associated with influenza. Damage to the ciliated epithelium also leaves people vulnerable to secondary infections such as those from pneumonococci, staphylococci, and streptococci.
4. During the recovery phase of the illness, the body produces serous cells more quickly than ciliated cells, resulting in mucus production without the built-in clearance mechanisms. Thus, patients must cough frequently to clear secretions.
5. Symptoms peak in 3 to 5 days and usually end by day 10.

Clinical Manifestations

1. Rapid onset of profound malaise
2. Fever
3. Chills
4. Generalized myalgia
5. Headache
6. Sore throat
7. Nonproductive cough
8. Flushed face
9. Erythema in oral cavity

Diagnostics

1. History: Any recent exposure to someone with influenza?
2. Physical examination findings (in addition to clinical manifestations, above)
   a. Watery eyes
   b. Runny nose
   c. Lung sounds clear
   d. Normal percussion over chest
3. Diagnostic tests
   a. Sputum tests early in the disease
   b. Serology

Clinical Management

1. Goals of clinical management
   a. Prevent complications

b. Treat symptoms
c. Limit infection to upper respiratory tract
2. Nonpharmacologic interventions
   a. Rest: decreases oxygen requirements
   b. Keep warm: maintains respiratory epithelium at core body temperature, which inhibits viral replication
   c. Adequate hydration: keeps respiratory tract lining functioning
3. Pharmacologic interventions
   a. Amantadine (Symmetrel) is available for the treatment of influenza A.
   b. It must be administered for the entire period in which the patient is at risk.
   c. If initiated early in the course of the disease, it will significantly reduce the severity of symptoms.

DRUG ADVISORY

Amantadine (Symmetrel) is primarily a preventive therapy. It does not help to "cure" the flu once it has been contracted. After infection by the influenza A virus has occurred, amantadine only helps to lessen some of the symptoms.

Complications

1. Sinusitis
2. Otitis media
3. Bronchitis
4. Bronchial pneumonia
5. Reye's syndrome

Prognosis

1. Prognosis depends on the condition of the patient before the illness.
2. Usually full recovery is made without treatment.
3. Recovery may be quicker if the illness is treated aggressively early in the course of the disease.

Applying the Nursing Process

NURSING DIAGNOSIS: Risk for fluid volume deficit R/T high fever and malaise

1. *Expected outcomes:* Following interventions, the patient should exhibit the following:
   a. Adequate skin turgor
   b. Weight within normal range
   c. Ability to tolerate fluids
   d. Adequate urine output
   e. Normal mental status
2. *Nursing interventions*
   a. Monitor skin turgor.
   b. Monitor intake and output.
   c. Monitor for mental status changes.

d. Weigh daily.
e. Encourage fluid intake. Administer intravenous fluids, if indicated.

NURSING DIAGNOSIS: Ineffective airway clearance R/T impaired primary defense mechanism

1. *Expected outcomes:* Following interventions, the patient should exhibit effective breathing, as evidenced by the following:
   a. Patent airway
   b. Absence of purulent sputum
   c. Arterial blood gases at baseline
2. *Nursing interventions*
   a. Monitor cough reflex.
   b. Monitor sputum production.
   c. Monitor ABGs as indicated.
   d. Encourage the patient to turn, cough, and deep breathe.
   e. Administer oxygen as indicated.
   f. Suction if necessary.
   g. Promote hydration.
   h. Supply humidification.

NURSING DIAGNOSIS: Hyperthermia R/T increased metabolic rate

1. *Expected outcomes:* Following interventions, the patient's temperature should be within the normal range and the patient should be seizure-free.
2. *Nursing interventions*
   a. Monitor temperature and other vital signs.
   b. Monitor for seizures.
   c. Note skin color and moisture.
   d. Monitor for mental status changes.
   e. Administer fluids as recommended.
   f. Administer antipyretic as indicated.
   g. Give sponge bath or utilize cooling blanket to reduce fever.

Discharge Planning and Teaching

1. Instruct patient to report any persistent, elevated temperature.
2. Instruct the patient in the treatment of symptoms.
3. If ordered, teach the patient side effects of Symmetrel (e.g., insomnia, irritability, lightheadedness).
4. Help the patient establish a daily routine that includes periods of rest until the symptoms decrease.

Public Health Considerations

1. Educate the public about (and administer, as ordered) the influenza vaccine, an inactivated influenza vaccine prepared yearly to reflect strains of influenza A and B that are currently circulating. It is highly purified and minimally reactive.

2. Although available to all, those who should most strongly consider receiving the vaccine include the following:
   a. Adults and children with chronic disorders of the cardiovascular and pulmonary system, chronic metabolic disease, renal dysfunction, anemias, or immunosuppression.
   b. Residents in nursing homes.
   c. Persons older than 65 years.
   d. Children receiving long-term aspirin therapy.
   e. Health care workers and others who provide care for persons at high risk of infection.
   f. Pregnant women after the 1st trimester.

■ CARING FOR PEOPLE WITH TUBERCULOSIS

Definition

1. A chronic inflammatory disease caused by a bacterium, usually *Mycobacterium tuberculosis* (a slow-growing, acid-fast aerobic bacterium)
2. Primarily affects the pulmonary system but can affect other areas as well
3. Characterized by granulomas in the lung tissue

Incidence and Socioeconomic Impact

1. The single largest cause of death in Europe and the United States in 1900, tuberculosis became relatively rare in the developed countries with the advent of antibiotics.
2. In recent years, a multidrug-resistant strain of tuberculosis (MDR-TB) has appeared as a result of improper or noncompliant use of treatment regimens, causing a sharp rise in reported cases. Incidence of MDR-TB has been a particular problem in developing countries.
3. Approximately 20,000 new cases of tuberculosis are reported in the United States each year.

Risk Factors and Etiology

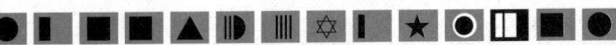

TRANSCULTURAL CONSIDERATIONS

In most developing countries, tuberculosis is a major health care problem. In the United States, rates of tuberculosis infection vary among various ethnic and racial groups. Hispanics, Native Americans, and Blacks have higher rates than do Whites. Blacks and Hispanics, who have experienced the greatest rise in incidence of tuberculosis, also have the highest rates of human immunodeficiency virus infection, which increases the risk of contracting tuberculosis and developing the active disease.

1. Tuberculosis is more common among the homeless, refugees, older people, and prison inmates (either past or present).

2. Alcoholism, intravenous drug use, malnutrition, and infection with the human immunodeficiency virus increase the risks of developing tuberculosis.
3. Children younger than 5 years are at high risk.
4. Living in close contact with a person who has tuberculosis increases the chances of contracting it.
5. Drinking unpasteurized milk increases the risk. (Cows may be infected with bovine tuberculosis.)

Pathophysiology

1. An infected person coughs, sneezes, or laughs, causing droplets containing tuberculosis bacteria to enter the air. A noninfected person who is nearby may inhale these droplets. (Alternatively, bacteria may be ingested in contaminated milk; this problem exists primarily in developing countries.)

NURSE ADVISORY

A positive result on skin testing does not mean that a person has active tuberculosis—only that the individual has had a cell-mediated response to the organism from prior exposure to the bacilli.

---

2. Droplets enter the lungs, where the bacteria form a tubercle (lesion). In most people (85–90%), the body's defense systems are adequate to encapsulate the tubercle, leaving only a scar.
3. In 5 to 15 percent of the population, however, encapsulation fails, and some of the bacteria enter the lymph system, travel to the lymph nodes, and trigger an inflammatory response called granulomatous inflammation.
4. Other bacilli are attacked and surrounded by macrophages and form lesions. These are termed primary lesions, because this is the first (primary) successful infection of a previously noninfected person.
5. In all but about 5 percent of persons, the lesions become dormant but can be reactivated (become a secondary infection) on reexposure to the bacterium in the future, especially persons with suppressed or compromised immune systems.
6. In its active phase (not to be confused with mere infection), tuberculosis causes necrosis and cavitation in the lesions (leading to caseation). Rupture of caseated lesions spreads necrotic tissue, which leads to new lesions, new necrosis, and new cavitation, damaging various parts of the body.
7. Because it is caused by an aerobic bacterium, tuberculosis usually affects the lungs, specifically the upper lobes, in which oxygen content is greatest, but it may affect other organs as well: the brain, intestines, peritoneum, kidney, joints, and liver.

Clinical Manifestations

1. Often asymptomatic in primary infections
2. Fatigue

3. Anemia
4. Weight loss
5. Low-grade fever
6. Chills
7. Night sweats
8. Cough that progresses from dry to wet or bloody (hemoptysis)

Diagnostics

1. History: Check for risk factors (see above).
2. Physical examination findings (in addition to clinical manifestations, above)
   a. Dyspnea
   b. In advanced disease: rhonchi on auscultation, trachea deviation, crackles, and apical dullness
3. Diagnostic tests
   a. Tuberculin skin test: Detects the presence of tuberculin, a protein from the tubercle bacilli
      (1) If the test result is positive, it will be positive in any future tests.
      (2) Mantoux test (standard test for tuberculosis): 0.1 ml or 5 units of tuberculin purified protein derivative (PPD) injected into the intradermal layer of skin; reactive or raised skin greater than 10 mm after 48 to 72 hours is considered a strong indication of tuberculosis.

   b. Chest radiograph: Not definitive on its own, but multinodular infiltrates with calcification in the upper lobes of the lungs suggest tuberculosis.
   c. Cultures (confirm active tuberculosis): from sputum or other sources such as urine, cerebrospinal fluid, or gastric washing

Clinical Management

1. Goals of clinical management
   a. Control symptoms of tuberculosis and degeneration
   b. Prevent transmission of tuberculosis
2. Nonpharmacologic interventions: See Chapter 8 for information on isolating patients with active tuberculosis.
3. Pharmacologic interventions
   a. Treatment of the tuberculosis bacterium is difficult because the bacterium carries a waxy substance on the capsule that makes penetration and destruction very difficult.
   b. Treatment of lesions depends on whether the person has active tuberculosis or has merely been exposed to it.

   c. Patients with active disease are usually treated with combination drug therapy.
      (1) Mutations in the tubercle bacilli inherent in the disease make them resistant to different drugs at different times. For this reason drugs are combined.
      (2) Primary drugs used to treat tuberculosis include isoniazid (INH), ethambutol, rifampin, and streptomycin. Drugs used to treat MDR-TB include capreomycin, ethionamide, cycloserine, and para-aminosalicylic acid.
      (3) Treatment of patients with active tuberculosis usually takes 6 to 9 months. For patients with human immunodeficiency virus infections, it may take longer.
      (4) Effective drug therapy requires very strict adherence to the prescribed regimen.

   d. Treatment for those who have been exposed to active tuberculosis is preventive isoniazid therapy, which lasts 9 to 12 months.
4. Special medical-surgical procedures
   a. Surgery for the resection of a cavity lesion that has persisted even with aggressive therapy
   b. Surgical interventions for severe complications of active tuberculosis (e.g., hemoptysis, pneumothorax, intestinal obstruction)

Complications

1. Respiratory failure
2. Malnutrition
3. Pleurisy with effusion
4. Hemoptysis
5. Tuberculous pneumonia
6. Bronchopleural fistula
7. Empyema
8. Gastrointestinal tuberculosis
9. Atelectasis
10. Pneumothorax
11. Tubercular meningitis

Prognosis

Excellent if treated early and aggressively

Applying the Nursing Process

NURSING DIAGNOSIS: Risk for transmission R/T inadequate body substance isolation

1. *Expected outcomes:* Following interventions, the patient with active tuberculosis should not infect others.
2. *Nursing interventions*
   a. Isolate patient until treatment is well established (7–10 days).
   b. Educate family and close contacts about transmission prevention.
   c. Instruct patient to cover the mouth and nose when coughing, sneezing, or laughing.
   d. Explain the importance of taking medicines as ordered—strictly adhering to the schedule.
   e. Perform purified protein derivative test on all known contacts.

NURSING DIAGNOSIS: Ineffective airway clearance R/T thick or bloody secretions

1. *Expected outcomes:* Following interventions, the patient should exhibit normal breathing patterns, as evidenced by the following:
   a. Patent airway
   b. No cyanosis
2. *Nursing interventions*
   a. Monitor vital signs.
   b. Auscultate lung sounds to evaluate air movement.
   c. Monitor sputum production. Monitor sputum culture and sensitivity tests.
   d. Note color, consistency, amount, and odor of sputum.
   e. Monitor chest radiographs.
   f. Position the patient for comfort and ease of respirations.
   g. Encourage patient to turn, cough, and deep breathe.
   h. Provide humidification and hydration to prevent retention of thick secretions.

NURSING DIAGNOSIS: Impaired gas exchange R/T cavity disease

1. *Expected outcomes:* Following interventions, the patient should exhibit improved gas exchange, as evidenced by:
   a. Arterial blood gases at baseline levels
   b. No cyanosis
   c. No mental status changes
2. *Nursing interventions*
   a. Note respiratory rate, rhythm, depth, and use of accessory muscles.
   b. Note skin color and moisture.
   c. Monitor ABGs.
   d. Monitor for changes in mental status.
   e. Monitor vital signs, especially heart rate and rhythm.
   f. Monitor pulse oximetry.
   g. Administer oxygen, if indicated.

Discharge Planning and Teaching

1. Explain the importance of covering the mouth and nose when coughing or sneezing and of properly disposing of tissues.
2. Describe the treatment regimen (including side effects) and consequences of failing to adhere strictly to it.
3. Describe the complications of tuberculosis and signs of recurrence (e.g., hemoptysis, fatigue, chest pain, shortness of breath).
4. Stress the importance of good nutrition, and instruct in diet as needed.
5. Explain the need to test all close contacts for tuberculosis.

Public Health Considerations

1. Preventing primary infection: Educate the public on the need to avoid high-risk activities such as intravenous drug use and alcohol abuse, on the need to be aware of one's status as a high-risk group member (if applicable), and on how tuberculosis is transmitted. Educate patients with tuberculosis on how *not* to spread the disease.
2. Preventing secondary infections: Educate patients on the need to avoid situations or disorders that compromise the immune system and contact with others who have active tuberculosis.

◼ CARING FOR PEOPLE WITH PNEUMOCONIOSIS

Definition and Incidence

1. Pneumoconiosis describes a group of occupational lung diseases caused by inhaling inorganic dusts and particles.
2. Silicosis results from inhaling silicon particles, which are found primarily in ceramics, paints, building materials, and some kinds of mining.
3. Asbestosis results from inhaling asbestos particles. Though largely banned in the United States now, at one time asbestos was widely used in fireproofing and insulating buildings (see Chapter 38 for a detailed discussion).
4. Coal workers' pneumoconiosis (commonly called "black lung") results from inhaling coal particles. It is more often found among those mining hard coal (anthracite) than those mining soft coal (bituminous).

Risk Factors and Etiology

1. Risk factors: Working in an environment in which fine airborne particles are present
2. Etiology: Effects vary, depending on cause and patient response
   a. Size of dust particles
   b. Chemical nature of particle
   c. Concentration of dust
   d. Length of exposure to dust
   e. Smoking
   f. Presence of underlying pulmonary disorder

Pathophysiology

1. Normally, particles that enter the oropharynx or nasopharynx are trapped in the upper airways in the mucous lining and removed by the mucociliary system.
2. Very small particles bypass this primary defense mechanism and go directly to the alveoli of the lung, which has no defense mechanism for rapid removal of invading material.
3. The particles in the alveoli must be cleared by macrophages, a slow process that gives irritating particles an opportunity to cause damage. Moreover, during the process of phagocytosis (see Chapter 17), the macrophages themselves may be damaged or destroyed by the particles.
4. Silicosis
   a. Silicon particles destroy the macrophages and cause release of substances that produce fibrosis, which leads to stiff, noncompliant lung tissue with nodules or fibrotic lesions.
   b. These lesions are surrounded by damaged lung tissue, resulting in emphysemic changes.
   c. Asymptomatic in mild forms, silicosis can become severe with years of exposure or even short periods of very heavy exposure (as with sandblasting), producing progressive massive fibrosis.
5. Asbestosis
   a. Cellular ingestion of asbestos particles swells the alveolar walls, usually in the lower lungs, by a mechanism not fully understood.
   b. As in silicosis, asbestosis produces fibrosis, but unlike silicosis, the result is nonnodular. Rather, pleural thickening, calcification, and effusion may occur, along with plaque formation. Lung cancers often arise from asbestosis when those exposed to asbestos are also smokers.
   c. Asbestosis symptoms usually appear only after prolonged exposure (10 years or more) to this material.
6. Coal workers' pneumoconiosis
   a. Like silicon, coal dust particles destroy the macrophages of the lungs and overwhelm the pulmonary defense system.
   b. Although not fibrous in themselves (unlike silicon and asbestos), coal dust particles create fibroblasts and lay a thin network of reticulin fibers that trap macrophages and dust particles. These so-called coal macules appear as black dots on the lungs.
   c. As in asbestosis, coal workers' pneumoconiosis is slow to develop, requiring 10 to 12 years of exposure to produce symptoms.

Clinical Manifestations

1. Often asymptomatic
2. Tachypnea
3. Dyspnea that increases gradually over time
4. May or may not have a dry cough
5. May develop cor pulmonale

Diagnostics

1. History: Working in a high-risk environment for exposure to dangerous particles (see earlier discussion)
2. Physical examination findings (in addition to clinical manifestations, above)
   a. Decreased chest expansion
   b. Decreased breath sounds, unequal rhonchi
   c. May have either dullness or hyperresonance to percussion
   d. Increased sputum production
   e. Mental status changes with hypoxemia
3. Diagnostic studies
   a. Chest radiograph of silicosis reveals nodules early in the course of the disease. Late changes include compression of upper lobes (with emphysemic changes) and lower lobes.
   b. Arterial blood gas levels are normal early in the disease. Late changes include hypoxemia and hypercapnia.
   c. Pulmonary function tests reveal decreased static lung compliance, decreased TLC, decreased FVC, and decreased FEV_1.
   d. Biopsy for evaluation of disease

Clinical Management

1. See pages 958–979 for details on therapies.
2. Goals of clinical management
   a. Halt progression of disease
   b. Prevent infection
   c. Improve oxygenation
3. Nonpharmacologic interventions
   a. Chest physical therapy and postural drainage to remove excess sputum and increase gas exchange
   b. Improved nutrition to help fight disease
4. Pharmacologic interventions: Oxygen to improve tissue oxygen levels
5. Special medical-surgical procedures: none

Complications

1. Respiratory failure
2. Fibrosis of lung tissue
3. Emphysema
4. Pulmonary hypertension
5. Cor pulmonale
6. Infections

Prognosis

If caught early, complications can be minimized.

Applying the Nursing Process

NURSING DIAGNOSIS: Impaired gas exchange R/T structural changes in the lung tissue

1. *Expected outcomes:* Following interventions, the patient should exhibit improved gas exchange, as evidenced by the following:
   a. Arterial blood gases at baseline levels
   b. Mental status at baseline level
   c. Absence of cyanosis
   d. SaO$_2$ greater than 90 percent
2. *Nursing interventions*
   a. Obtain ABGs as indicated.
   b. Note respiratory rate, rhythm, and depth and use of accessory muscles.
   c. Auscultate breath sounds.
   d. Monitor vital signs.
   e. Monitor for dysrhythmias.
   f. Monitor pulse oximetry.
   g. Monitor skin color and moisture.
   h. Monitor for mental status changes.
   i. Administer oxygen as indicated.
   j. Position for ease of respirations.
   k. Instruct patient in turning, coughing, and deep breathing.

NURSING DIAGNOSIS: Risk for infection R/T impaired primary defense mechanism

1. *Expected outcomes:* Following intervention, the patient should be free from signs of infection.
2. *Nursing interventions*
   a. Monitor white blood count.
   b. Monitor sputum production, noting changes in amount, color, consistency, and odor.
   c. Monitor vital signs.
   d. Instruct patient to avoid known infectious sources.

NURSING DIAGNOSIS: Knowledge deficit R/T new disease process

1. *Expected outcomes:* Following interventions, the patient should be able to do the following:
   a. Explain the causes, signs, and symptoms of pneumoconiosis and silicosis as well as their management
   b. Minimize further exposure to risk factors
   c. Recognize and act on the need to seek frequent, regular medical care and comply with treatment regimens
2. *Nursing interventions*
   a. Assess level of understanding.
   b. Describe the causes, signs, and symptoms of these diseases.
   c. See "Discharge Planning and Teaching," below.

Discharge Planning and Teaching

1. Explain that masks should be worn at work. Demonstrate proper fitting techniques.
2. Teach the importance of not smoking. Give information on smoking cessation programs if appropriate.
3. Teach signs and symptoms of infection and when to seek medical assistance.

4. Instruct in proper breathing techniques and validate learning by a return demonstration.
5. Describe the complications of pneumoconiosis.

Public Health Considerations

Focus is on prevention through educating workers in high-risk industries on the need for sound nutrition, influenza vaccine, wearing masks and other protective equipment at work, and using caution when handling material covered with dust.

■ CARING FOR PEOPLE WITH LUNG CANCER

Definition and Incidence

1. Lung cancer is a malignant growth in the lung.
2. It affects an estimated 157,000 people in the United States, most aged 50 to 75.
3. Lung cancer is the leading cause of cancer death in men and women in the United States.
4. Lung cancer strikes more Blacks than Whites in the United States; although more men than women contract it, the gap is closing.

NURSE ADVISORY

Short-term exposure to an organism does not usually result in contracting a disease; repeated or prolonged exposure is usually necessary to break down the body's defenses.

5. See "Pathophysiology," below, for details on incidence of specific lung cancers.

Risk Factors and Etiology

1. Cigarette smoking (about 85% of lung cancer can be attributed to cigarette smoking)
2. Exposure to asbestos
3. Air pollution

Pathophysiology

1. Bronchogenic carcinoma, which makes up 90 to 95 percent of lung cancers, is aggressive, locally invasive, and metastatic. These tumors usually originate from the epithelial lining of the major bronchi.
2. Bronchogenic carcinoma can synthesize bioactive products and produce paraneoplastic syndrome. It can form intraluminal masses that invade the bronchial mucosa and the peribronchial connective tissue.
3. Some tumors advance into the pleural space, pleural cavity, and other thoracic organs.
4. Some large tumors have necrosis at the core that can lead to hemorrhage. Hemorrhage may also occur if a tumor extends into a blood vessel.

5. Bronchogenic carcinomas may occur as non–small-cell carcinomas, as small-cell carcinomas, or as a combination of the two.
6. Non–small-cell lung cancers include the following:
   a. Squamous cell carcinomas, which make up 35 percent of all lung cancers, spread centrally to the main bronchi, where they may form obstructions. They then metastasize gradually to areas outside of the chest cavity (albeit later than other types of non–small-cell carcinoma). Approximately 90 percent of such cancers are found in men.
   b. Adenocarcinomas (including bronchoalveolar carcinomas) are slow-growing tumors usually found in the periphery at the site of fibrous scarring from previous damage to the lung. They produce small masses but often spread to the lymph system and metastasize to the brain and other organs.
      (1) Adenocarcinomas are equally common in men and women.
      (2) The correlation between smoking and this type of lung cancer is less than that between smoking and other cancers.
   c. Large-cell carcinomas (including giant and clear cell carcinomas), although most often subpleural and peripheral, can arise in other parts of the lung.
      (1) Slow-growing but rapidly metastatic, over half of all large-cell carcinomas have spread to the central nervous system by the time of diagnosis.
      (2) Large-cell carcinomas generally produce larger masses than adenocarcinomas.
7. Small-cell (oat cell) lung cancers are the most aggressive of all cancers, growing and metastasizing rapidly. They make up about 10 percent of all lung tumors.

Clinical Manifestations

1. May be similar to other forms of lung disease
2. Chronic cough
3. Shortness of breath
4. Wheezing
5. Hemoptysis
6. Dull, intermittent, poorly localized pain
7. Hoarseness and dysphagia (if tumor invades the mediastinum)
8. Pleural effusion that can lead to atelectasis and dyspnea
9. Fever
10. Pleural friction rub
11. Fatigue
12. Weight loss

Diagnostics

1. History: Check for risk factors (see above)
2. Physical examination findings by tumor site (also depend on extent of tumor)
   a. Centrally located tumors: chronic cough; hemoptysis (coughing up blood); shortness of breath; wheezing; sharp, severe localized pain when the tumor invades the pleura

   b. Tumors that invade the mediastinum: hoarseness; dysphagia; stridor; dull, achy, poorly localized pain; decreased draining of blood from the head, neck, and chest due to compression of the superior vena cava
   c. Tumors that invade the pleura: sharp, localized, severe pain; pleural effusion; decreased breath sounds over affected area; dullness to percussion; fever; pleural friction rub
3. Diagnostic tests
   a. Chest radiograph
   b. Sputum cytology
   c. Computed tomography scan
   d. Bronchoscopy for central lesions
   e. Bronchial lavage to obtain cells for cytology
   f. Percutaneous needle biopsy
   g. Open lung biopsy
   h. Thoracentesis
   i. Nuclear scan to check for metastasis to brain, bones, liver
   j. Magnetic resonance imaging
   k. Ultrasound
   l. Carcinoembryonic antigen titer produced by undifferentiated lung tumors: Increased titers suggest extensive disease.
   m. Positron emission tomography (PET) scan.
4. Staging of tumors (Box 22–1 and Chapter 17) is necessary to plan treatment and establish prognosis.

Clinical Management

1. See also Chapter 17.
2. Goals of clinical management
   a. Completely remove the tumor
   b. Restore the patient to a previous state of health or, if not possible, provide palliative treatment to increase the quality of life
3. Nonpharmacologic interventions
   a. Ensure proper nutrition.
   b. Position for comfort and ease of respiration.
   c. Have patient use diaphragmatic breathing for easier respiration.
4. Pharmacologic interventions
   a. Chemotherapy
      (1) Used because of lung cancer's tendency to metastatize
      (2) Treatment of choice in small-cell tumors because of their rapid growth rate
      (3) Usually involves a combination of several chemotherapy drugs
      (4) Frequently used adjunct to radiation therapy or surgery
5. Special medical-surgical procedures
   a. Radiation therapy
      (1) Can be used as the sole treatment, combined with surgery or chemotherapy, or for palliation of symptoms
      (2) Procedure: Exact location of tumor is confirmed with CT scan, and markings are made on the area to be radiated. Precise marking maximizes the ef-

Box 22–1. Classification of Pulmonary Malignancies

Primary Tumor (T)

T_x Tumor proven by presence of malignant cells in bronchopulmonary secretions but not visualized roentgenographically or bronchoscopically, or any tumor that cannot be assessed as in a retreatment staging

T_0 No evidence of primary tumor

T_{is} Carcinoma in situ

T_1 A tumor that is 3 cm or less in greatest dimension, surrounded by lung or visceral pleura and without evidence of invasion proximal to a lobar bronchus at bronchoscopy

T_2 Tumor more than 3 cm in greatest dimension or a tumor of any size that either invades the visceral pleura or has associated atelectasis or obstructive pneumonitis extending to the hilar region; at bronchoscopy, the proximal extent of demonstrable tumor must be within a lobar bronchus or at least 2 cm distal to the carina; any associated atelectasis or obstructive pneumonitis must involve less than an entire lung

T_3 A tumor of any size with direct extension into the chest wall (including superior sulcus tumors), the diaphragm, or the mediastinal pleura or pericardium without involving the heart, great vessels, trachea, esophagus, or vertebral body; or a tumor in the main bronchus within 2 cm of the carina without involving the carina

T_4 A tumor of any size with invasion of the mediastinum or involving the heart, great vessels, trachea, esophagus, vertebral body, or carina in the presence of malignant pleural effusion

Nodes (N)

N_0 No demonstrable metastases to regional lymph nodes

N_1 Metastasis to lymph nodes in the peribronchial or the ipsilateral hilar region or both, including direct extension

N_2 Metastases to ipsilateral mediastinal lymph nodes and subcarinal lymph nodes

N_3 Metastasis to contralateral mediastinal, contralateral hilar, ipsilateral or contralateral scalene, or supraclavicular lymph nodes

Distant Metastasis (M)

M_0 No (known) distant metastasis

M_1 Distant metastasis present, specify site(s)

From Mountain CF. A new international staging system for lung cancer. *Chest* 89:225s–233, 1986.

fectiveness of the radiation while minimizing tissue damage to surrounding structures.

   (3) Doses: Regulated by tissue tolerance and other structures located in the treatment area; administered over 5 to 6 weeks

b. Surgical removal of tumors

   (1) Used to remove small, localized tumors

   (2) Treatment of choice in non–small-cell lung cancers

   (3) Procedures: Wedge resection, segmental resection, lobectomy, and pneumonectomy are common. Choice depends on tumor type, location, and patient condition. The goal is to remove all of the tumor while damaging as little surrounding tissue as possible.

     • *Wedge resection* removes small tumors just under the lung tissue with minimal damage to lung structure.

     • *Segmental resection* removes a segment of lung tissue. This segment includes bronchi and alveoli.

     • *Lobectomy* removes a complete lobe of the lung.

     • *Pneumonectomy* removes an entire lung. Serous fluid accumulates in the space and consolidates, preventing mediastinal shifts.

Complications

1. Airway obstruction
2. Paraneoplastic disorders
3. Atelectasis
4. Pleural effusion
5. Pulmonary abscess
6. Pneumonia

Prognosis

1. Prognosis is generally poor; only 13 percent of patients with lung cancer survive 5 years.
2. Prognosis depends on the spread of tumor before the diagnosis; thus, it is especially poor for large-cell and small-cell carcinomas, which metastasize rapidly.

Applying the Nursing Process

NURSING DIAGNOSIS: Ineffective breathing pattern R/T compression of lung tissue

1. *Expected outcomes:* Following interventions, the patient should exhibit improved breathing patterns, as evidenced by the following:
   a. Respiratory rate 12 to 20 breaths per minute
   b. Breathing without use of accessory muscles
   c. Oxygen saturation greater than 90 percent
   d. No reports or signs of anxiety over breathing
   e. Mental status normal
2. *Nursing interventions*
   a. Monitor respiratory rate, rhythm, and depth and use of accessory muscles.
   b. Monitor oxygen saturation.
   c. Monitor for changes in mental status.
   d. Teach and assist the patient with turning, coughing, and deep breathing.
   e. Encourage use of diaphragmatic breathing.
   f. Position for comfort and ease of respirations.

NURSING DIAGNOSIS: Impaired gas exchange R/T retained secretions and occluded bronchioles

1. *Expected outcomes:* Following interventions, the patient should exhibit improved gas exchange, as evidenced by the following:
   a. Arterial blood gases at baseline levels
   b. Mental status normal
   c. Absence of cyanosis
   d. SaO_2 greater than 90 percent

2. *Nursing interventions*
   a. Assess ABGs as indicated.
   b. Note respiratory rate, rhythm, and depth and use of accessory muscles.
   c. Auscultate lung sounds frequently.
   d. Monitor vital signs.
   e. Monitor SaO_2.
   f. Administer oxygen as indicated.
   g. Suction as indicated.
   h. Position for ease of respirations.
   i. Encourage rest periods throughout the day.

NURSING DIAGNOSIS: Altered nutrition, less than body requirements, R/T dyspnea, fatigue, and side effects of chemotherapy

1. *Expected outcomes:* Following interventions, the patient should exhibit signs of proper nutrition, including the following:
   a. Absence of nausea or vomiting
   b. Serum albumin greater than 2.8 gm per dl
   c. Weight at the calculated ideal body weight
   d. Good appetite
2. *Nursing interventions*
   a. Monitor intake and output.
   b. Monitor laboratory values such as total protein and albumin.
   c. Auscultate breath sounds every shift.
   d. Monitor for nausea and vomiting, and administer antiemetic, as indicated.
   e. Weigh daily.
   f. In conjunction with the dietary team or registered dietitian and the patient, determine the patient's food likes and dislikes and develop a diet plan that meets the patient's needs.
      (1) Involve family members in food choices and preparation, if possible.
      (2) Offer smaller, more frequent meals.
      (3) Coordinate meal times around periods of rest and medication schedule.
      (4) Have meals served at the proper temperature and appropriate seasoning to suit the patient's taste.
      (5) Provide a pleasant environment at meal times.

NURSING DIAGNOSIS: Impaired physical mobility R/T dyspnea and pain

1. *Expected outcomes:* Following interventions, the patient should be able to do the following:
   a. Report that pain is under control
   b. Be free of skin breakdown
   c. Demonstrate increased mobility and strength
2. *Nursing interventions*
   a. Assess for any deterioration from previous activity and mobility level.
   b. Examine skin frequently for signs of breakdown; massage reddened areas to promote circulation.
   c. Encourage ambulation, assisting as necessary.
   d. Turn frequently while in bed.

   e. Provide analgesics, as ordered.
   f. Teach and encourage performance of range-of-motion exercises.
   g. Encourage activities that allow for adequate rest periods.
   h. Consult physical therapist for additional therapy.

Discharge Planning and Teaching

1. Describe the causes, symptoms, and progression of lung cancers.
2. In conjunction with the physician and other team members, answer the patient's questions regarding treatment options and procedures.
3. Stress the importance of quitting smoking.
4. Teach coughing and breathing exercises, and have the patient return the demonstration.
5. Supply information on support groups.

Public Health Considerations

1. Lung cancer is *highly* preventable.
2. Educate the public about the need to avoid smoking and methods of quitting; monitor patients who smoke for early signs of lung cancers.
3. Teach workers in high-risk industries to use precautions (e.g., masks, gloves) when dealing with dangerous materials.

■ CARING FOR PEOPLE WITH LUNG ABSCESSES

Definition and Incidence

1. A lung abscess is a localized collection of pus in the lung followed by the disintegration of tissue.
2. Its incidence is declining due to widespread use of antibiotics.

Risk Factors and Etiology

1. Aspiration
2. Dental infections
3. Pneumonia
4. Tumors
5. Pulmonary embolus
6. Vasculitis
7. Immunocompromised host
8. Debilitating conditions such as congestive heart failure, malnutrition, and alcoholism

Pathophysiology

1. Location of abscess depends on position at time of inhalation. The inhaled substance is affected by gravity and migrates to the lowest portion of the lung.

2. As the material settles in the lung, it is surrounded by fibrin and forms a pocket that fills with pus.
3. When pressure from increasing pus within the abscess becomes too great, the pocket ruptures, spreading the infectious pus throughout the lung region.
4. Sometimes the rupture of a simple abscess results in the healing of the area. Other times it leads to multiple other formations of pus-filled pockets.
5. In early stages, lung abscesses resemble pneumonia. However, if untreated, the resultant pus formation and obstruction may lead to necrosis of the surrounding tissue.

Clinical Manifestations

1. Chills
2. Fever
3. Pleuritic pain
4. Cough
5. Purulent, foul-smelling sputum after rupture of abscess
6. Hemoptysis after rupture of abscess
7. Anorexia

Diagnostics

1. History: Check for risk factors (see above)
2. Physical examination findings (in addition to clinical manifestations, above)
   a. Crackles or decreased or absent breath sounds over affected area
   b. Pleural friction rub
   c. Weight loss
   d. Dullness to percussion
3. Diagnostic studies
   a. Chest radiograph: shows lobar consolidation with intact abscess; reveals fluid levels with ruptured abscess
   b. Sputum culture and sensitivity: to determine specific organism for treatment
   c. Bronchoscopy: allows direct visualization of abscess to determine its severity
   d. Blood tests: to detect anemia

Clinical Management

1. See pages 958–979 for details of therapies.
2. Goals of clinical management
   a. Eliminate signs and symptoms of infection
   b. Halt abnormal sputum production
   c. Relieve respiratory distress
3. Nonpharmacologic interventions
   a. Chest physical therapy and postural drainage to aid in drainage of abscess
   b. Meticulous oral care to avert risk of bacterial overgrowth with antibiotic therapy
   c. Teaching of turning, coughing, and deep breathing exercises
4. Pharmacologic interventions
   a. Antibiotic therapy

(1) Drug of choice is usually penicillin. More specific antibiotics may be ordered after the sputum culture and sensitivity report is done.
(2) Continue until all signs of the abscess are gone according to the chest radiograph. Therapy may take as long as 6 weeks.
5. Special medical-surgical procedures
   a. Bronchoscopy to visualize the abscess, remove foreign matter, and drain the abscess
   b. Surgery (if damage from the abscess is severe): may range from a small portion of the lung to a pneumonectomy

Complications

1. Pleural effusion
2. Pulmonary hemorrhage
3. Empyema

Prognosis

Antibiotic therapy usually controls the infectious process within 6 weeks. In severe cases, however, a portion of the lung or the entire lung may need to be removed surgically to control infection.

Applying the Nursing Process

NURSING DIAGNOSIS: Ineffective airway clearance R/T purulent sputum

1. *Expected outcomes:* Following interventions, the patient should exhibit improved airway clearance, as evidenced by the following:
   a. Absence of cough and sputum production
   b. Breath sounds equal and clear bilaterally
2. *Nursing interventions*
   a. Assess sputum production for color, amount, consistency, and odor.
   b. Auscultate lung sounds frequently.
   c. Maintain a patent airway.
   d. Perform chest physical therapy and postural drainage on the patient.
   e. Perform nasotracheal suctioning as indicated.
   f. Administer antibiotics as ordered.
   g. Provide adequate humidification and hydration to help liquefy sputum.
   h. Instruct the patient in turning, coughing, and deep breathing techniques.

NURSING DIAGNOSIS: Impaired gas exchange R/T stasis of pulmonary secretions

1. *Expected outcomes:* Following interventions, the patient should exhibit improved gas exchange as evidenced by the following:

a. Arterial blood gases within normal limits for the patient
b. Absence of cyanosis
c. Mental status at baseline
d. Respiratory rate 12 to 20 breaths per minute
e. SaO$_2$ greater than 90 percent

2. *Nursing interventions*
a. Monitor vital signs and respiratory rate, rhythm, and depth and use of accessory muscles.
b. Monitor skin color, temperature, and moisture.
c. Monitor for dysrhythmias.
d. Monitor pulse oximetry.
e. Assess for mental status changes such as restlessness, confusion, and irritability.
f. Obtain ABGs as indicated.
g. Administer oxygen if indicated.

Discharge Planning and Teaching

1. Describe the signs and symptoms of infection; explain the importance of taking the full course of antibiotic therapy.
2. Teach turning, coughing, deep breathing, postural drainage, and chest physical therapy techniques.
3. Educate the patient regarding good oral hygiene to prevent superinfections of the mouth.
4. Help patient develop a nutritionally sound, balanced diet.

◼ THERAPIES AND TECHNIQUES FOR IMPROVING OXYGENATION

Chest Physiotherapy and Postural Drainage
(Procedure 22–1)

Procedure 22–1
Chest Physiotherapy and Postural Drainage

Definition/Purpose — Chest physiotherapy (CPT) and postural drainage (PD) are techniques that when combined promote the mobilization of secretions from the lung periphery to the central airways. They also help the respiratory muscles to be more efficient and to re-expand collapsed areas of the lungs.

Contraindications/Cautions — Contraindications for use would include (1) unstable vital signs, (2) increased cyanosis with use, (3) bronchospasm with use, (4) excessive pain during the procedure, (5) possibility of loosened secretions obstructing the airways, and (6) elevated intracranial pressure.

Learning/Teaching Activities — Teach the patient and family members the proper techniques. Inform the patient that it may take a couple of weeks before any benefit will be experienced. Perform CPT 2 hours after a meal to prevent vomiting.

Preliminary Activities

Equipment
- Pillows
- Towels
- Emesis basin
- Tissues
- Oral hygiene utensils and accessories

Assessment/Planning
- Make sure that it has been at least 2 hours since the patient has had any food.
- Assess lung sounds and sputum production.
- If the patient is tube fed, turn off the feeding tube 2 hours before beginning procedure.
- Assess the patient's tolerance.
- Medicate for pain before the treatment if necessary.
- The patient may benefit from bronchodilator therapy before beginning the treatment to open the airways.
- Assess the patient's ability to move from side to side and maintain adequate oxygenation.

Preparation of the Person
- The individual should be stable, relaxed, and positioned with pillows supporting the limbs.
- A towel should be placed over the area to be percussed or vibrated.
- Oxygen saturation should be monitored if the patient has been known to desaturate with therapy.

Procedure

Action	Rationale/Discussion
1. Auscultate lung sounds.	1. Provides baseline data for later assessments.
2. Assess vital signs.	2. Provides baseline data for later assessments.

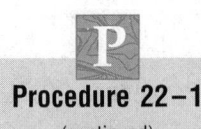

Procedure 22–1

(continued)

Action	Rationale/Discussion
3. Determine the time that the patient last ate or was tube fed.	3. Should be at least 2 hours after the last feeding to help prevent vomiting.
4. Inform the patient of any adverse side effects such as bronchospasm, tachycardia, tachypnea, pain in the chest, and nausea and vomiting.	4. If any of these occur, the therapy should be stopped immediately.
5. Administer medications that may decrease pain perception.	5. Allows the patient to tolerate the procedures for a longer period of time, thus increasing the benefit.

Postural Drainage

1. Remove clothing and replace with a loose-fitting gown.

   1. Allows for ease of movement.

2. Provide the patient with tissues and an emesis basin.

   2. Aids in the collection and disposal of expectorated sputum.

3. Place the patient in the best position for drainage of the targeted lung segment.

   3. Gravity is utilized to drain specific lung segments.

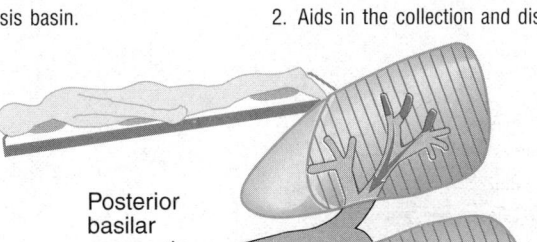

Posterior basilar segments

4. Use a pillow to support limbs and maintain the proper body alignment.

   4. Provides comfort to the joints and maintains the proper position.

5. Maintain each position for at least 5 to 10 minutes or for as long as the patient can tolerate.

   5. Allows for adequate drainage of sputum from each lung segment.

6. Encourage coughing and deep breathing while in each position.

   6. Promotes the mobilization and expectoration of retained secretions.

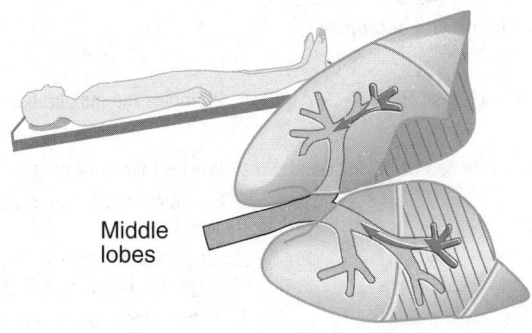

Middle lobes

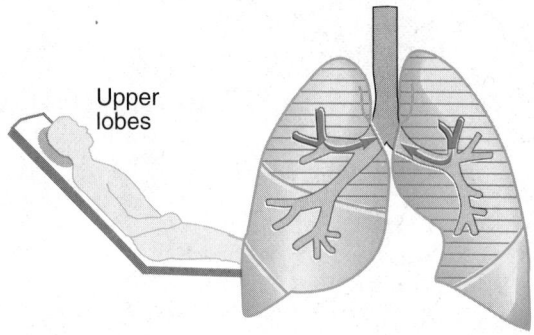

Upper lobes

Chest Physiotherapy

1. While the patient is in the proper postural drainage position, stand on the opposite side of the patient from the side to be percussed.

   1. Provides the best possible alignment of the hand on the chest or back.

2. Have the patient place both hands over the head.

   2. Provides the best possible exposure of the chest while stretching the chest wall and allowing the vibration to be transmitted to the lung tissue.

(continued)

P

Procedure 22–1

(continued)

Action	Rationale/Discussion
3. Place a towel over the area of the chest to be percussed.	3. Protects the chest wall from uncomfortable contact from the hands.
4. Clap the chest wall with a cupped hand, using a rhythmic pattern.	4. Creates a vibration in the chest wall that transmits to the lung tissue and aids in the loosening of secretions.
5. Perform this technique for 2 to 4 minutes over each area.	5. Helps to loosen secretions.

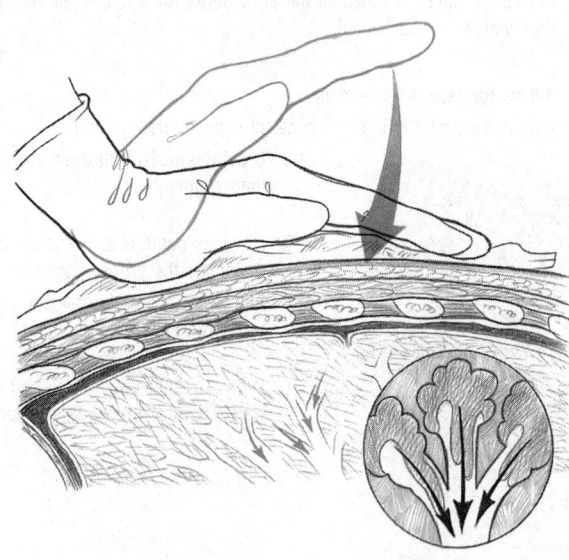

Mobilizing secretions

Action	Rationale/Discussion
6. Encourage coughing and deep breathing after each session.	6. Promotes the mobilization and expectoration of loosened secretions.

Vibration

Action	Rationale/Discussion
1. Place 1 hand flat on the chest and the other on the top of the 1st hand.	1. Provides firm, full contact with the chest wall.
2. Have the patient take in a deep breath.	2. Promotes maximal expansion of the lungs and helps to fully open the airways.
3. Have the patient exhale through pursed lips.	3. Lengthens the time of expiration and creates a "back" pressure in the lungs that helps to facilitate keeping the airways open.
4. During exhalation, vibrate your hands on the selected areas.	4. Helps to facilitate the loosening of secretions.

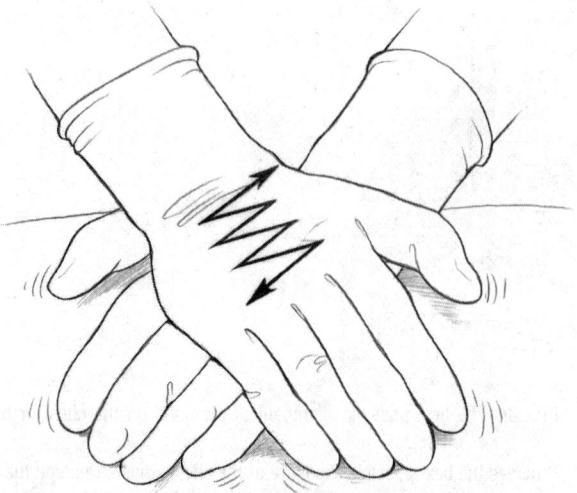

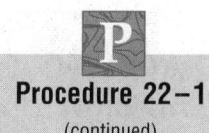

Procedure 22–1

(continued)

Action	Rationale/Discussion
5. Repeat the above procedures to each segment of the lungs.	5. Promotes mobilization and expectoration of sputum from each lung segment.

Final Activities

Reassess vital signs and respiratory status. Return the patient to the most restful position. Perform oral hygiene. Return the bed to the low position if needed. Record the patient's response to therapy.

Exercise and Breathing Retraining

1. Gradually increasing the exercise regimen prevents further deterioration and improves the patient's ability to perform activities of daily living.
2. The use of a treadmill or an exercise bike may be the best form of exercise for this group of patients.
3. The patient should perform the exercise regimen 3 to 4 times a week, with the duration of each exercise session limited by dyspnea, not by time.

Breathing Techniques

1. Diaphragmatic breathing (Learning/Teaching Guidelines for Diaphragmatic Breathing)
2. Pursed-lip breathing (Learning/Teaching Guidelines for Pursed-Lip Breathing)

Incentive Spirometer

1. Definition: a deep-breathing exercise that incorporates visual references to help set goals
2. Used postoperatively to increase the patient's lung expansion through deep breathing
3. Procedure
   a. Help the patient assume a position that is comfortable, usually a semi-Fowler's with the knees slightly bent (Fig. 22–18).
   b. Have the patient place the mouth over the mouthpiece of the incentive spirometer and seal the lips around it.
   c. Instruct the patient to inhale through the spirometer with a strong and steady breath.
   d. At the end of inhalation, the patient should hold inhaled breath briefly to allow for expansion of the lungs.
   e. Have the patient perform this maneuver 10 to 15 times per session, 5 to 6 sessions per day for the 1st 2 to 3 days postoperatively.

Turning, Coughing, and Deep Breathing with Splinting

1. Importance: Turning aids in mobilizing retained secretions. Coughing mobilizes sputum and aids in expectoration. Deep breathing expands the lungs, increases the surface area for gas exchange, and opens closed airways that may be pooling secretions. Splinting provides external pressure to the chest and abdominal wall, which stabilizes these areas, thus decreasing pain when coughing and deep breathing.
2. Indications: primarily used for patients during the imme-

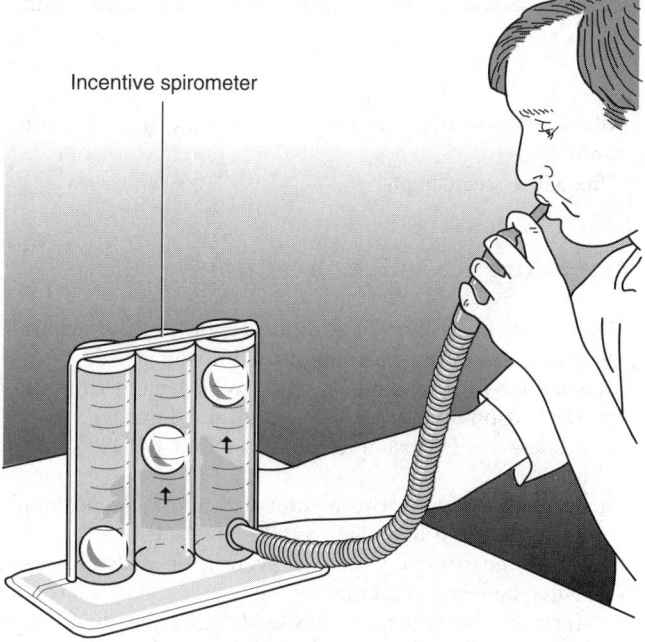

Incentive spirometer

Figure 22–18. Incentive spirometer encourages voluntary deep breathing by providing a visual cue to the patient about the efficiency of deep breathing. (Redrawn from Black JM, and Matassarin-Jacobs E [eds]. *Luckmann and Sorensen's Medical-Surgical Nursing: A Psychophysiologic Approach.* 4th ed. Philadelphia: WB Saunders, 1993, p 957.)

LEARNING/TEACHING GUIDELINES
for Diaphragmatic Breathing

1. Clear the upper and lower airways of excessive sputum or congestion. Many nurses find it necessary to administer aerosol treatments, have the patient turn, cough, and deep breathe, or institute postural drainage to clear airways.
2. Instruct the patient to assume a comfortable position. Optimal positions are those that allow for the relaxation of the abdominal muscles and diaphragm. These positions may include the supine or semi-Fowler's. Ask the patient to bend the knees slightly to further relax the abdominal muscles.
3. Have the patient inhale deeply through the nostrils, keeping the mouth closed.
4. Encourage the patient to concentrate on moving the diaphragm down and the abdominal wall outward. This can be visualized by the patient placing a hand on the abdomen and trying to push it out when inhaling.
5. Instruct the patient to pause at the end of inspiration to allow for maximal expansion of the lungs.
6. Instruct the patient to exhale passively through pursed lips. This should be a natural, quiet, relaxed exhalation procedure.

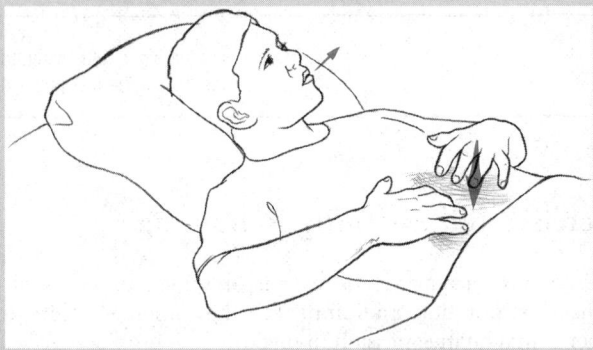

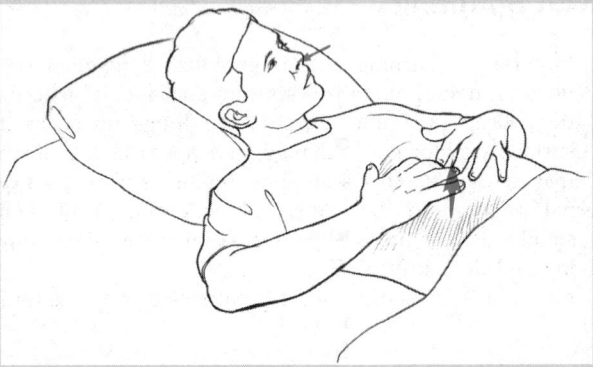

7. Encourage the patient to use the abdominal muscles and diaphragm to help push air out at the end of expiration. The patient should be able to feel the abdominal muscles tighten.
8. Exhalation should take 3 times longer than inhalation.
9. The patient should perform this technique for 15 to 20 minutes, 4 to 5 times a day until this pattern of breathing becomes second nature.

---

diate postoperative period or until they are ready to ambulate
3. Procedure: see Chapter 13

Inspiratory Resistive Breathing

1. Definition: imposition of additional work on the inspiratory muscles during diaphragmatic breathing
2. Indications for use: patients who would benefit from improved inspiratory muscle strength and improved exercise tolerance; for example, patients with COPD
3. Procedure
   a. Instruct the patient to assume a comfortable position, usually sitting in a chair or at the bedside.
   b. Have the patient place a flow resistor with a 1-way valve between closed lips.
   c. Instruct the patient to inhale through the device by using diaphragmatic breathing. As the patient inhales slowly, the 1-way valve closes, forcing the air to be drawn through the resistive opening.
   d. On exhalation, the valve opens to allow for passive exhalation of air against minimal resistance.
   e. When beginning to use the resistive device, set the resistive opening at the lowest level possible.
   f. Instruct the patient to inhale and exhale slowly through the device. Respirations should not exceed 15 breaths per minute.
   g. Encourage the patient to use the device 4 to 5 times daily for 15 minutes per session. As strength and endurance improve, gradually increase the exercise time and inspiratory resistance.

Positioning and Posture

1. Importance: Patients with respiratory dysfunction often breathe more easily with their head and chest elevated. Such positioning allows better expansion of the lungs and more efficient use of the respiratory muscles.
2. Procedure
   a. Instruct the patient to assume a comfortable position from which the shoulders can be rotated upward and backward. This position enables the diaphragm to move freely.
   b. Have the patient sit in a chair or at the side of the bed (orthopneic position).

LEARNING/TEACHING GUIDELINES
for Pursed-Lip Breathing

1. Have the patient assume a comfortable position.
2. Instruct the patient to inhale slowly and deeply through the nostrils. It is helpful to demonstrate the method yourself.
3. Have the patient pause at the end of inspiration to allow for maximal expansion of the lungs.
4. Have the patient exhale slowly through pursed lips. Pursed lips look very much like the lips of someone who is whistling. This technique maintains a slight positive pressure (i.e., higher than the closing pressure) in the airways, which helps keep them open throughout the exhalation phase. This technique ensures that more air will be exhaled, eliminating some of the air trapping associated with chronic obstructive pulmonary disease.
5. Explain that exhalation should be twice as long as inhalation.
6. This technique should be utilized most of the time but especially during episodes of increased dyspnea.

---

c. Support the back and head with pillows. Be careful not to tilt the head forward, which may occlude the airway.
d. Have patients with severe dyspnea sit up and lean forward on an overbed table. Have them rest their arms on the table to increase the effectiveness of the secondary muscles of respiration.

Relaxation

1. Importance: To develop maximal breathing control, the patient must learn to relax.
2. In helping the patient to relax, the caregiver should have an unhurried and calm manner.
3. For maximal relaxation, the patient should do the following:
   a. Wear comfortable, loose-fitting clothes
   b. Assume positions that decrease dyspnea (e.g., sit in a chair with shoulders rotated backward, lean on an overbed table, lean against a wall with the chest slightly forward)
4. Instruct the patient in the following:
   a. Diaphragmatic breathing
   b. Use of relaxation tapes and books
   c. Use of relaxation exercises such as the following:
      (1) Roll head from side to side in a circular motion while utilizing diaphragmatic breathing. Inhale as the head moves from the right to the left; exhale as the head moves back from the left to the right.
      (2) Coordinate diaphragmatic breathing while rotating the shoulders backward and forward. Inhale while the shoulders move backward, and exhale as the shoulders move forward.
      (3) Tighten all muscles from the head to the toes while inhaling, and relax all muscles while exhaling.

Oxygen Therapies

1. Oxygen therapy is used to treat harmful and possible lethal complications related to hypoxemia (inadequate supply of oxygen to the tissues).

Oxygen is a drug and should be used with caution. Oxygen alone will not cure a disease. Diseases that benefit from oxygen therapy include chronic obstructive pulmonary disease, airway obstruction, pulmonary edema, acute respiratory distress, metabolic disorders, cardiac disorders, and shock.

Although oxygen therapy may be helpful for some disorders, too much may be fatal. Never withhold oxygen from a hypoxic patient. Evaluate each patient individually and then administer oxygen at levels that are appropriate for the given situation.

---

2. There are 3 major indications for oxygen therapy: reduced arterial blood oxygen levels (ABGs show blood oxygen levels below 80 mm Hg), increased work of breathing, and need to decrease myocardial workload.
   a. Reduced arterial blood oxygen levels: Supplemental oxygen will correct hypoxemia if the cause is purely hypoventilation or small ventilation-perfusion deficits.
   b. Increased work of breathing
      (1) The body responds to hypoxemia by increasing respiratory rate and depth of respirations, thus placing a greater demand on the respiratory muscles, which in turn use more oxygen.
      (2) Supplemental oxygen may relieve hypoxemia, thus decreasing respiratory effort and restoring a normal breathing pattern.
   c. Need to decrease myocardial workload
      (1) The heart compensates for hypoxemia by increasing cardiac output to deliver more oxygen to the tissues.
      (2) Increased cardiac output increases myocardial oxygen consumption.
      (3) Increased myocardial workload increases stress on the heart, which may ultimately damage the heart's ability to circulate adequate blood volume.
      (4) Improved oxygenation will decrease hypoxemia, decreasing the myocardial workload.
3. Nursing management of oxygen therapy
   a. Nurses who are responsible for oxygen therapy must be knowledgeable about the various kinds of oxygen delivery devices (see below), both to explain them to patients (and family members) and to use them, as indicated.

Box 22−2. Oxygen Delivery Systems

Nasal Cannula

1. Assess patient's respiratory status, mental status, most recent arterial blood gas (ABG) levels, and SaO_2.
2. Connect a humidifying bottle to an oxygen flow meter, and fill with sterile water to the appropriate level (optional).
3. Explain to the patient how it will be placed on the face.
4. Explain why supplemental oxygen is needed.
5. Adjust the oxygen to the prescribed oxygen flow rate.
6. Listen for the oxygen flowing through the cannula.
7. Place the nasal prongs in the nares, drape tubing over the ears, and loosely tighten the tubing below the chin.
8. Position the cannula for comfort. May need to place gauze behind the ears to reduce friction caused by the tubing.

Simple Facemask

1. Assess the patient's respiratory status, mental status, most recent ABG levels, and SaO_2.
2. Attach a humidifying bottle to a flow meter, and fill with sterile water to the appropriate level (optional).
3. Turn the oxygen flow meter to the prescribed oxygen flow rate.
4. Show the mask to the patient, explain how the mask works, and explain why oxygen supplementation is necessary.
5. Listen for the oxygen flowing through the mask.
6. Place the mask over the nose and mouth. Pinch the metal clip on the nose portion of the mask until the mask fits snugly. Adjust the straps to ensure that the mask remains secure.

Simple Facemask with Nebulized Humidity

1. Assess the patient's respiratory status, mental status, ABG levels, and SaO_2.
2. Assess for the production of thick, tenacious sputum.
3. Connect a nebulizer to a flow meter, and attach a heating unit to the nebulizer.
4. Adjust the nebulizer oxygen flow rate to the prescribed oxygen level.

5. Observe for the presence of mist coming from the facemask.
6. Explain the need for oxygen to the patient, and point out that the high humidity helps to loosen and liquefy the sputum.
7. Place the mask over the nose and mouth of the patient, and secure the mask to the face with head straps and a nose clip.
8. Make sure that the fit of the mask is snug and that mist can be seen coming from the holes in the side of the mask.

Nonrebreathing Facemask

1. Assess the patient's respiratory status, mental status, ABG levels, and SaO_2.
2. Connect a humidifier to an oxygen flow meter (optional).
3. Adjust the flow meter to the prescribed flow rate.
4. Make sure that the reservoir bag is completely expanded.
5. Assess to see that air flow is reaching the mask.
6. Explain the need for oxygen therapy to the patient and how the mask works.
7. Place the mask on the patient, making sure that the mask has a snug fit.
8. Observe the reservoir bag immediately after placing the mask on the patient, making sure that the bag does not collapse more than half its full position.

Venti Mask

1. Assess the patient's respiratory status, mental status, ABG levels, and SaO_2.
2. Connect a humidifier to an oxygen flow meter (optional).
3. Select the proper adapter for the FiO_2 that is prescribed.
4. Adjust the flow meter to the rate specified for the prescribed FiO_2.
5. Make sure oxygen flow is coming through the mask.
6. Explain the procedure to the patient.
7. Place the Venti mask securely over the nose and mouth.
8. Observe the patient for the initial reaction to the Venti mask.

---

b. Nursing interventions during oxygen therapy may include the following:
   (1) Educating and providing psychosocial support to the patient and family members regarding oxygen therapy by explaining the process and expected outcomes of the oxygen therapy and demonstrating the equipment
   (2) Correctly administering the prescribed amount of oxygen
   (3) Maintaining a patent airway
   (4) Providing frequent oral and nasal care
   (5) Closely monitoring the patient for the 1st hour after therapy has been initiated (the time when oxygen-induced hypoventilation will most likely occur)
c. Oxygen delivery systems (Box 22−2)
   (1) Low-flow systems: These common, easy-to-use systems include nasal cannulas (Fig. 22−19*A*), simple facemasks (Fig. 22−19*B*), partial nonrebreathers (Fig. 22−19*C*), and face tents. They deliver a wide range of oxygen concentrations. Variables that control the percentage of inspired oxygen are capacity of the anatomic reservoir, type of reservoir system (nose, mask, or reservoir bag), oxygen flow rate (L/min), and ventilation pattern of the patient.

   (2) High-flow systems: These systems include Venti masks (Fig. 22−19*D*) and continuous positive airway pressure masks (Procedure 22−2). These systems provide a constant and accurate delivery of oxygen concentration (FiO_2) at a flow rate and with a reservoir capacity adequate to meet the total inspiratory needs of the patient. They can deliver either high or low concentrations of oxygen. Three advantages over low flow systems are consistent delivery of a precise FiO_2, control of the entire inspiratory atmosphere, and ease of analysis with an oxygen analyzer.

Artificial Airways

1. Definition: Artificial airways are used to provide a patent passageway from the atmosphere to the lungs. They can be inserted through the mouth or nose (endotracheal) or directly through the trachea (tracheostomy). They can be used to administer oxygen and to facilitate removal of secretions (see Chapter 20).
2. Indications
   a. Upper airway obstruction
   b. Respiratory failure

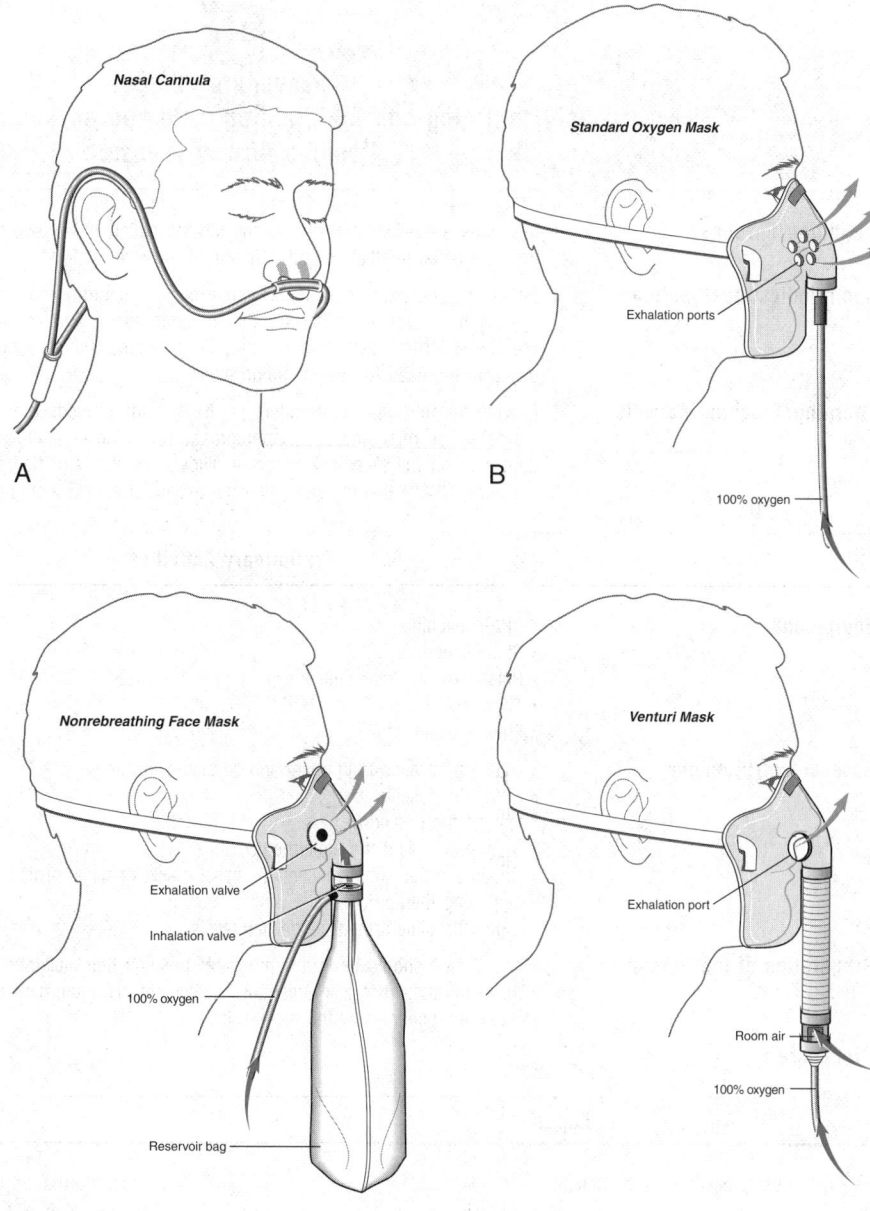

Figure 22–19. Oxygen delivery systems. *A*, Nasal cannula; *B*, simple face mask; *C*, partial nonrebreathing mask; *D*, Venturi mask, a high-flow oxygen system.

c. Chest wall injury or deformity
d. Central nervous system depression
e. Prevention of aspiration
f. Facilitation of tracheal suctioning
g. Facilitation of artificial ventilation
3. Airways: Endotracheal tubes (Fig. 22–20)
   a. Long, slender tubes of polyvinyl chloride are inserted through the oral (orotracheal tube) or nasal (nasotracheal tube) passages and pass through the nasal canal, with the distal tip positioned just above the bifurcation of the mainstem bronchus (carina).
      (1) Endotracheal tubes vary in length depending on the size of the patient (inner lumen of 6.0–10.0 mm in adults)
      (2) All endotracheal tubes have a cuff at the distal end that is inflated after placement to seal the tube in the trachea. Cuffs are regulated at high volume and low pressure to prevent necrosis of the tracheal tissue due to excessive pressure.
   b. Orotracheal tubes
      (1) Usually used for short-term airway management
      (2) Large lumen tubes can be used if necessary.
      (3) Advantages: easier to insert owing to direct visualization of the vocal cords; allow easier removal of thick, tenacious secretions
      (4) Disadvantages: decreased client comfort, increased gag sensation, increased oral secretions, difficult to form words with lips, and decreased integrity of oral cavity owing to pressure of the tube in the mouth

Procedure 22-2
Initiating and Maintaining a Person on Continuous Positive Airway Pressure

Definition/Purpose	Maintains a positive pressure in the airway, which helps to prevent airway collapse during expiration. Utilized to promote better ventilation and diffusion at the alveolar level.
Contraindications/Cautions	Should not be used in patients with excessive sputum production. Patients with chronic obstructive pulmonary disease may experience barotrauma, pneumothorax, and cardiovascular compromise owing to increased airway pressures. Intracranial pressures may be increased. Patients who are claustrophobic may not tolerate the therapy owing to the need for a tight-fitting mask.
Learning/Teaching Activities	Provide the following information: (1) Explain the procedure and the reason for initiating the therapy. (2) Instruct the patient to relax and use diaphragmatic breathing techniques. (3) Explain to the patient the need to maintain a tight seal on the facemask or nasal pillows. (4) Explain the complications related to continuous positive airway pressure (CPAP) therapy and when the patient should discontinue therapy.

Preliminary Activities

Equipment	• CPAP machine • Stethoscope • Pulse oximetry machine • Tissues • Emesis basin
Assessment/Planning	• Obtain a baseline pulmonary and cardiac assessment. • Know the baseline SaO_2. • Explain the procedure. • Show the patient the equipment. • Obtain a proper fitting facemask, nasal mask, or nasal prongs. Make sure that there is a good fit before beginning therapy. • Obtain baseline arterial blood gas levels.
Preparation of the Person	• The person should be in a comfortable position that facilitates an effective breathing pattern. • Allow the patient to ask questions and handle the equipment before use. • Show the patient how the mask will fit.

Procedure

Action	Rationale/Discussion
1. Explain the procedure to the patient.	1. Provides information for the patient and reduces anxiety.
2. Assess the patient's respiratory, cardiovascular, and mental status. Obtain baseline arterial blood gas levels and SaO_2.	2. Provides baseline data for later assessments.
3. Set the prescribed setting on the CPAP generator.	3. Ensures that the CPAP device will be properly adjusted when therapy is initiated. Minimizes the risk of atelectasis and hypoxia.
4. Place the CPAP mask on the patient, making sure that the seals are snug and tight fitting.	4. For the continuous positive pressure to be effective, the mask must be tight fitting to maintain a positive pressure within the airways. The most comfortable delivery devices are the nasal mask and nasal prongs. However, because these devices do not cover the mouth, the patient must keep the mouth closed. The full facemask provides the best seal but is less well tolerated because it covers the mouth and nose. With this device, it is difficult for the patient to eat, drink, or expectorate sputum.
5. Monitor for initial signs of respiratory and cardiac compromise.	5. Because of the change in airway pressure and a tight-fitting mask, the patient may experience a decompensation in the respiratory and cardiac systems.

Final Activities

Stay at the bedside until the patient has adequately adjusted to the CPAP device. Monitor continuous SaO_2 until stable. Reassess vital signs.

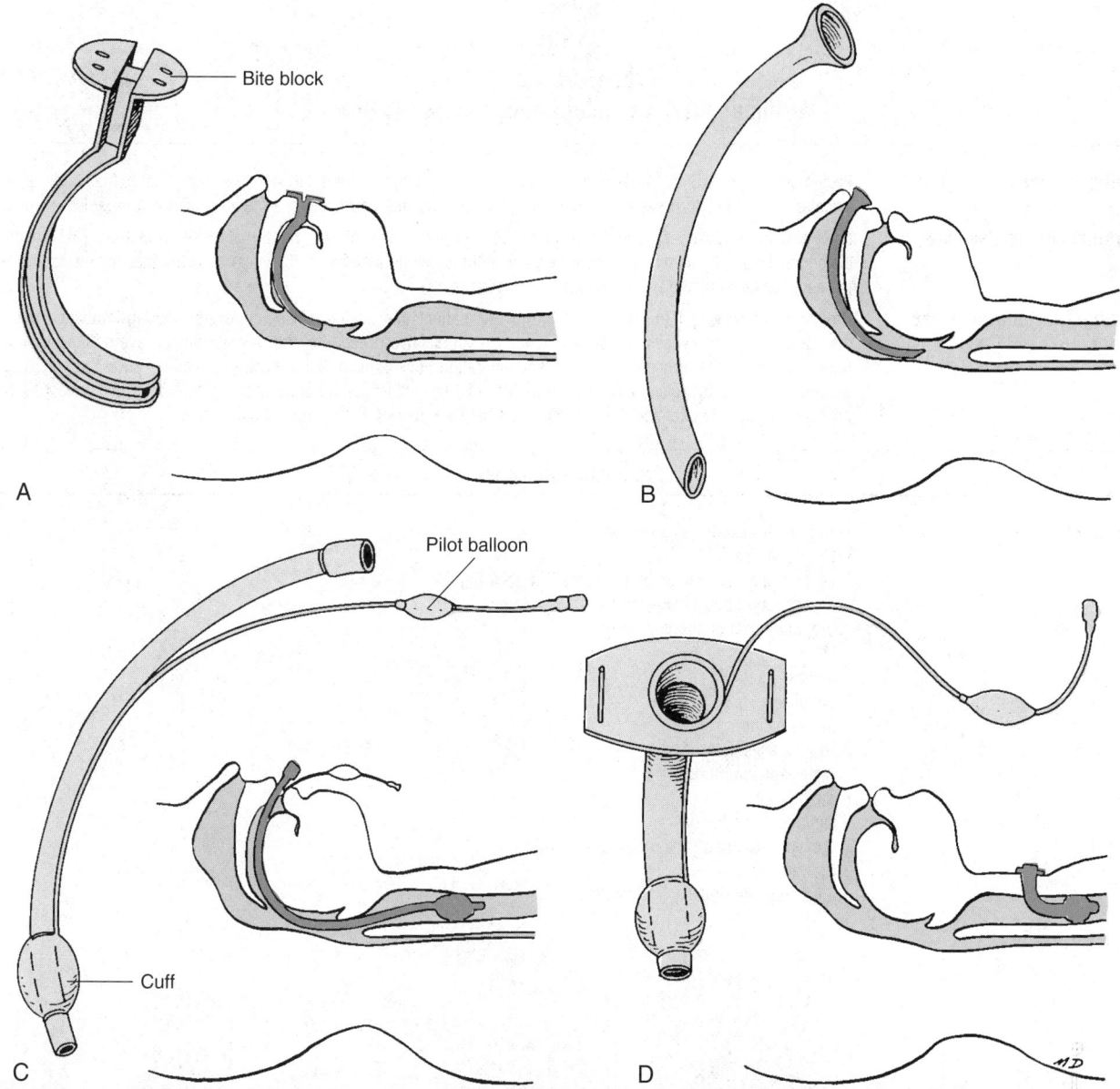

Figure 22–20. Artificial airways. *A*, Oral airway; *B*, nasal airway; *C̄*, endotracheal tube; *D*, tracheostomy tube. Endotracheal tubes have several parts: 15-mm adapter on the proximal end, pilot balloon, radiopaque pilot line, and cuff. All respiratory therapy and anesthesiology equipment is designed to connect with a 15-mm adapter. Consequently, a patient can easily be manually ventilated, mechanically ventilated, or anesthetized via the same endotracheal tube. (From Black JM, and Matassarin-Jacobs E [eds]. *Luckmann and Sorensen's Medical-Surgical Nursing: A Psychophysiologic Approach.* 4th ed. Philadelphia: WB Saunders, 1993, p 963.)

c. Nasotracheal tubes
  (1) Advantages: more comfortable, easier to secure than oral tubes, and lower risk of extubation
  (2) Disadvantages: increased risk of sinusitis, sharp angle at the back of the nasopharynx may kink the tube, smaller lumen tube must be used owing to limited size of nasal cavity, and increased risk for necrosis of the nasal cavity
d. Intubation: insertion of an orotracheal or a nasotracheal tube (Procedure 22–3)
e. Extubation: removal of an oral or a nasal endotracheal tube (see Procedure 22–3); performed when the underlying problem or reason for intubation has been resolved and only after evaluation of the following:
  (1) Lung mechanics (MIP, PEP, VC, spontaneous minute ventilation)
  (2) Level of consciousness
  (3) Hemodynamic stability (heart rate and blood pressure)
  (4) Adequate and effective cough
  (5) Arterial blood gases within the acceptable range for the particular patient
  (6) Absence of infection
  (7) General physical condition

Text continued on page 972

Procedure 22–3
Artificial Airways, Intubation, and Extubation

Definition/Purpose	Placement of an artificial airway to establish and maintain a patent airway; to establish and maintain adequate alveolar ventilation; to prevent the retention of secretions that can provide a medium for microorganism growth
Contraindications/Cautions	Care should be taken to avoid the following: (1) intubation of the right mainstem bronchus; (2) broken or dislodged teeth; (3) cardiac dysrhythmias; (4) hemodynamic instability; (5) vocal cord trauma; (6) bronchospasm; (7) esophageal intubation; (8) hypoxia; (9) aspiration.
Learning/Teaching Activities	Provide the following information: (1) Inform the patient that talking will be impossible during intubation because the vocal cords are bypassed. (2) If intubation is an elective procedure, the patient should have nothing by mouth 6 hours before the procedure to prevent aspiration. (3) Explain the procedure, making sure that the patient understands that the discomfort will be brief. (4) The patient should be assured that after the tube has been properly placed, oxygenation should improve and the sense of well-being should improve.

Preliminary Activities

Equipment	• Endotracheal tube (ET) with stylet • 10-ml syringe • 1-inch adhesive tape or other method of securing ET • Resuscitation bag connected to 100% oxygen • Oropharyngeal suctioning equipment • Mask • Gloves • Goggles • Sterile saline • Topical anesthetic • Water-soluble lubricant • Stethoscope • Laryngoscope handle • Curved and straight laryngoscope blades • Oral airway • Single-use end-tidal CO_2 detector

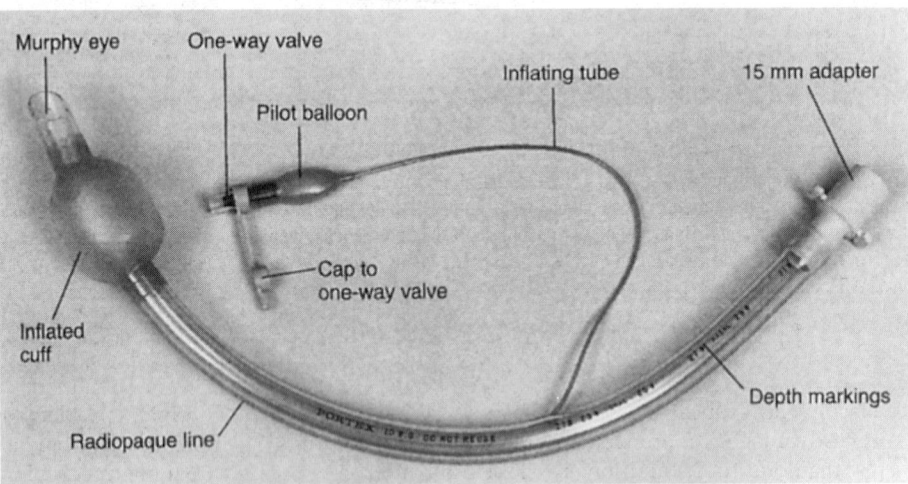

Assessment/Planning	• Obtain baseline arterial blood gas levels. • Obtain baseline vital signs. • Obtain baseline oxygen saturation (SaO_2). • Auscultate the lungs and heart for baseline data. • Obtain the proper size ET. • Ensure that there is functioning suction equipment available. • Have an emergency cart available.
Preparation of Person	• The individual should be sitting upright until just before the insertion of the ET, then placed in a supine position. • Explain the procedure to the patient.

P

Procedure 22-3

(continued)

- Medicate with sedatives if required.
- Remove all dental bridge work and plates.

Procedure

Action	Rationale/Discussion
1. Monitor the patient's respiratory status, mental status, arterial blood gas levels, and Sao₂.	1. Establishes a baseline assessment.
2. Explain the procedure to the patient.	2. Promotes understanding and better compliance during the procedure. Allows the patient to have an opportunity to ask questions and to clarify perceptions.
3. Arrange equipment.	3. Facilitates a rapid and smooth intubation procedure.
4. Obtain the proper style laryngoscope and make sure that the light on the end is functioning properly.	4. Proper functioning laryngoscope is necessary to visualize the vocal cords and epiglottis.
5. Connect the tonsillar suction catheter to a functioning suction source.	5. It may be necessary to clear the oral cavity of secretions to visualize the epiglottis. May help to maintain a patent airway if the patient vomits.
6. If the procedure is elective, it may be helpful to premedicate the client with a sedative.	6. May help the client better tolerate the procedure by reducing anxiety.
7. Select an ET (6.0–10.0 mm), preferably 7.5 mm or greater.	7. All ETs increase the work of breathing, but the larger the tube, the less the resistance to airflow.
8. Inflate and deflate the ET cuff.	8. To check for leaks and to ensure that the cuff is functioning properly.
9. Insert a sterile stylet into the ET.	9. The stylet stiffens the ET, making it easier to insert.
10. Lubricate the end of the ET with sterile water-soluble lubricant.	10. Makes it easier to pass the ET through the epiglottis into the trachea.
11. Position the patient in a supine position with a pillow or towel under the neck.	11. This position helps to align the airway structures, making insertion of the ET easier and less traumatic to the tissue.
12. Put on a mask and gloves.	12. Provides protection from microorganisms during the intubation procedure.
13. Administer 100% oxygen via a resuscitation bag for 2 minutes before intubation.	13. Reduces the risk of hypoxia during the intubation procedure.
14. The individual inserting the ET should place it at least 5 to 6 cm past the vocal cords.	14. Ensures that when the ET cuff is inflated it will not damage the vocal cords.
15. The actual insertion procedure should not take longer than 30 to 60 seconds.	15. The patient is without oxygen during the actual intubation attempt. If this attempt takes longer than 30 to 60 seconds, hypoxia could occur.

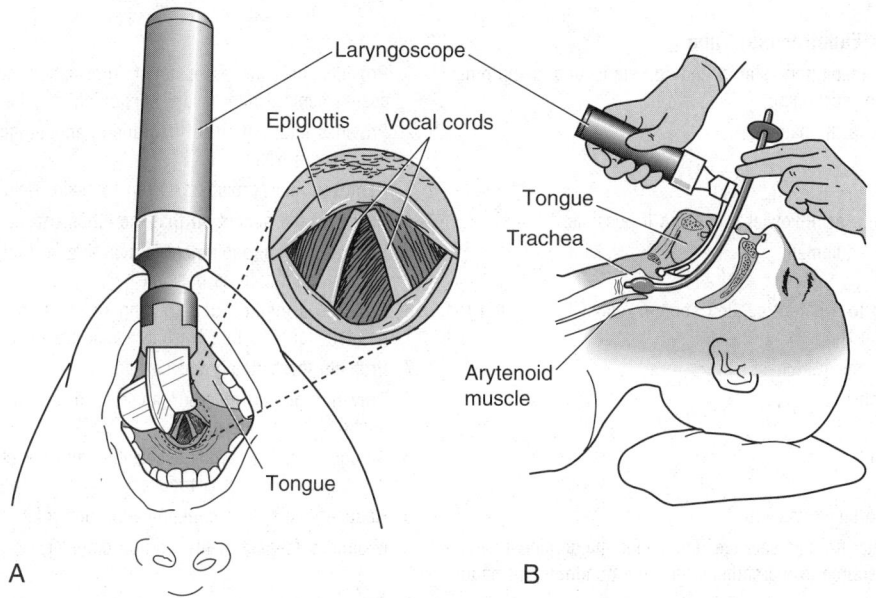

A   B

(continued)

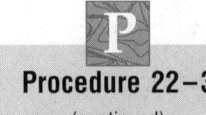

Procedure 22–3

(continued)

Action	Rationale/Discussion
16. After intubation, inflate the cuff of the ET until no air leak is noted during manual resuscitation bag inflations.	16. Prevents aspiration of oral or gastric secretions. Prevents air from leaking out around the ET. Ensures that the ET cuff is tight enough to secure the tube in the trachea but not so tight that it causes necrosis of the tracheal mucosa.
17. While inflating the lungs with the manual resuscitation bag, auscultate the lung fields bilaterally.	17. While inflating the lungs with the manual resuscitation bag, auscultate the lung fields bilaterally.
18. Attach single-use end-tidal CO_2 detector to ET and observe for color change during exhalation.	18. End-tidal CO_2 detectors assist in confirming ET placement in the trachea. There is no color change if the esophagus is intubated.
19. Secure the ET at the proper placement with tape or another method that will prevent its accidental displacement.	19. Prevents the migration of the ET out of the trachea or down into the right mainstem bronchus.
20. After verifying placement with the auscultation of bilateral lung sounds, obtain a chest radiograph.	20. Always done to verify proper placement of the ET. The tip of the ET should be 2 to 4 cm above the carina.
21. After proper placement has been confirmed, mark the ET as it exits the mouth with tape or an indelible marker.	21. Establishes the proper placement of the tube, which can be used as a reference for future caregivers.
22. Record the placement of the ET on the patient's flowsheet.	22. Facilitates the frequent assessment of proper tube placement.

Endotracheal Tube Cuff Inflation (Minimal Leak Technique)

Action	Rationale/Discussion
1. Withdraw all of the residual air from the ET cuff.	1. Ensures that all air is out of the cuff at the beginning of the procedure.
2. Place the diaphragm of the stethoscope over the patient's trachea.	2. Enables the examiner to listen to the air movement in the trachea.
3. Attach a manual resuscitation bag to the ET.	3. Enables the examiner to apply positive pressure air flow through the ET during inspiration.
4. During inspiration, slowly inject air through the 1-way valve on the pilot balloon of the ET with a syringe.	4. Fills the ET cuff with air.
5. Auscultate the neck area above the cuff while providing positive pressure breaths with the manual resuscitation bag. An audible air leak should be noted until the ET cuff is occluding the trachea.	5. Enables the examiner to auscultate any air leaks that are present around the ET cuff. Hearing an air leak ensures that the ET cuff has not been overinflated.
6. Slowly inject air into the ET cuff until the air leak is no longer present during inhalation.	6. The cuff has completely sealed the trachea around the ET when an air leak can no longer be heard.
7. When an air leak is no longer auscultated, remove a small amount of air from the cuff until a small air leak is auscultated over the trachea.	7. Complete occlusion of the trachea by the ET cuff may create too much pressure on the tracheal mucosa, leading to necrosis in that area. A small air leak ensures that the ET cuff is not overinflated.
8. Once the minimal leak is attained, measure the cuff pressure with a manometer.	8. Ensures that the pressure within the ET cuff is no higher than the pressure known to cause tracheal mucosal damage.
9. Routinely measure and document ET cuff pressures.	9. Ensures that the pressures within the ET cuff are maintained at safe levels.

Suctioning Through an Endotracheal Tube

Action	Rationale/Discussion
1. Assess the patient's respiratory status and for signs and symptoms that indicate a need for suctioning.	1. Provides baseline assessment information, which is useful for future assessments. Unnecessary suctioning may be avoided.
2. Explain the procedure to the patient.	2. Provides information to the patient, encourages participation, and helps to reduce anxiety.
3. Wash hands.	3. Removes microorganisms from the skin. Helps to prevent infection.
4. Position the patient in a semi-Fowler's position if possible.	4. Positions the patient so that the lungs can be maximally expanded.
5. Assemble the suction equipment.	5. Ensures that all equipment is available so that the suctioning procedure will be as smooth as possible.
6. Attach suction tubing to a patent suction source. Adjust the suction to no more than 120 mm Hg.	6. Provides a method of removing retained secretions. Suction pressures greater than 120 mm Hg may cause tracheal mucosa damage.
7. Place a towel on the patient's chest.	7. Protects the clothing and bed linen.
8. Put on mask and goggles.	8. Prevents getting microorganisms in the mouth or eyes during the suctioning procedure.
9. Open sterile equipment.	9. All equipment is readily accessible, and the chance of contamination of the respiratory tract is reduced.
10. Glove both hands in a sterile fashion.	10. Reduces the risk of contamination and infection in the respiratory tract.
11. Remove suction catheter from its package, and hold in the dominant hand. Connect the suction source to the catheter with the nondominant hand.	11. Maintains sterility of the suction catheter.
12. With the nondominant hand, remove the oxygen source from the ET.	12. Prevents introduction of microorganisms into the ET.

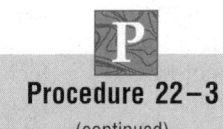

Procedure 22–3

(continued)

Action	Rationale/Discussion
13. With the nondominant hand, connect the manual resuscitation bag to the ET and preoxygenate and hyperventilate with 100% oxygen for 2 minutes before suctioning.	13. Reduces the risk of atelectasis and hypoxia during the suctioning procedure.
14. Using the sterile hand, insert the suction catheter into the ET without applying suction until resistance is met or the patient begins to cough forcibly.	14. Suction is not applied until catheter is fully advanced to reduce the risk of hypoxia. Meeting resistance or coughing usually indicates that the catheter has been advanced to the carina.
15. Withdraw the catheter approximately 2 to 3 cm, and place nondominant hand over the suction port of the catheter to apply suction.	15. Withdrawing the catheter slightly helps to prevent the respiratory tract mucosa from getting caught in the catheter when the suction is applied.
16. While applying suction, remove the catheter from the ET using a rotating motion. The entire suctioning pass should not exceed 10 to 15 seconds.	16. Rotating the catheter on the way out helps to cover all portions of the airway. If the suctioning procedure takes longer than 10 to 15 seconds, hypoxia may occur.
17. Hyperoxygenate and hyperinflate with 100% oxygen for 1 to 2 minutes after each suction pass.	17. Prevents atelectasis and hypoxia from occurring during the suctioning procedure.
18. Repeat as often as needed to clear airway.	18. Airway must be clear for proper ventilation to occur.
19. Reconnect the patient to the oxygen source, and reassess respiratory status.	19. Assesses if suctioning was beneficial and if respiratory status has improved.

Connecting Endotracheal Tube to an Oxygen Source and Endotracheal Tube Cuff Deflation

Action	Rationale/Discussion
1. Explain the procedure to the patient.	1. Provides information to the patient, allows the patient to participate as much as able, and helps to lessen anxiety.
2. Follow the procedure for ET suctioning.	2. The pulmonary tree should be as clear of secretions as possible to prevent complications related to obstructed airways.
3. Connect a tonsillar suction catheter to a suction source, and use to remove oral secretions.	3. Helps to prevent the aspiration of oral secretions when the ET is removed.
4. Advance a sterile suction catheter through the ET to approximately the distal tip of the ET. Deflate the ET cuff while applying suction to the suction catheter.	4. Prevents any secretions that may have collected above the cuff from being aspirated.
5. Suction oropharynx again.	5. Removes any oral secretions that may be aspirated.

Endotracheal Tube Extubation

Action	Rationale/Discussion
1. Explain the procedure to the patient.	1. Provides information to the patient, allows participation as much as able, and lessens anxiety.
2. Follow the procedure for endotracheal suctioning.	2. Removal of retained secretions promotes better ventilation of the respiratory system.
3. Remove tape or other device that was used to hold the ET in place.	3. Allows for the quick removal of the ET after the cuff has been deflated.
4. Follow the procedure for ET cuff deflation.	4. The cuff must be deflated before removal to avoid damage to the vocal cords.
5. Have the patient breathe out forcefully as the ET is removed.	5. Any secretions retained around the ET cuff will be moved up into the oropharynx and removed by expectoration or tonsillar suction.
6. Place the patient on oxygen immediately after extubation of the ET.	6. Prevents the possibility of hypoxia.
7. Assess the patient's respiratory status.	7. Assess for respiratory distress and hypoxia. If these are present, it may indicate the need for reintubation.

Final Activities

After intubation, verify placement of the ET with frequent respiratory assessments. Monitor oxygen saturation and arterial blood gases as indicated. Verify ET placement by checking the mark on the tube where it enters the mouth to make sure that the tube has not advanced or moved out. Monitor the ET cuff pressure frequently to ensure that the proper pressure is being maintained. After extubation, monitor closely for laryngospasms and bronchospasms. Monitor for signs of respiratory distress and hypoxia such as restlessness, tachycardia, irritability, and a decreased SaO_2. The presence of these signs might indicate the need for reintubation.

Illustration redrawn from Black JM, and Matassarin-Jacobs E (eds). *Luckmann and Sorensen's Medical-Surgical Nursing: A Psychophysiologic Approach.* 4th ed. Philadelphia: WB Saunders, 1994, p 964.

f. Complications of endotracheal tubes (Fig. 22–21): Complications include the following: intubation of right mainstem bronchus, cuff rupture, necrosis of trachea, tracheal stenosis, erosion of the innominate artery, accidental extubation, sinusitis, vocal cord edema, vocal cord paralysis, tracheoesophageal fistula, cuff leak, esophageal lacerations, bronchospasms, tube obstruction, aspiration, tube displacement after intubation, and cardiac dysrhythmias.

4. Airways: tracheostomies
  a. Definition: Creation of an opening into the trachea that totally bypasses the upper airway by going through the neck at the level of the 2nd to 3rd cartilage rings; the surgical insertion of an indwelling tube when endotracheal tubes prove inadequate
  b. See Chapter 20 for a detailed discussion of tracheostomy tubes and related patient care.

Suctioning

1. The goal of suctioning is to remove secretions and to stimulate productive coughing without creating complications.
2. Indications
  a. Restlessness
  b. Desaturations

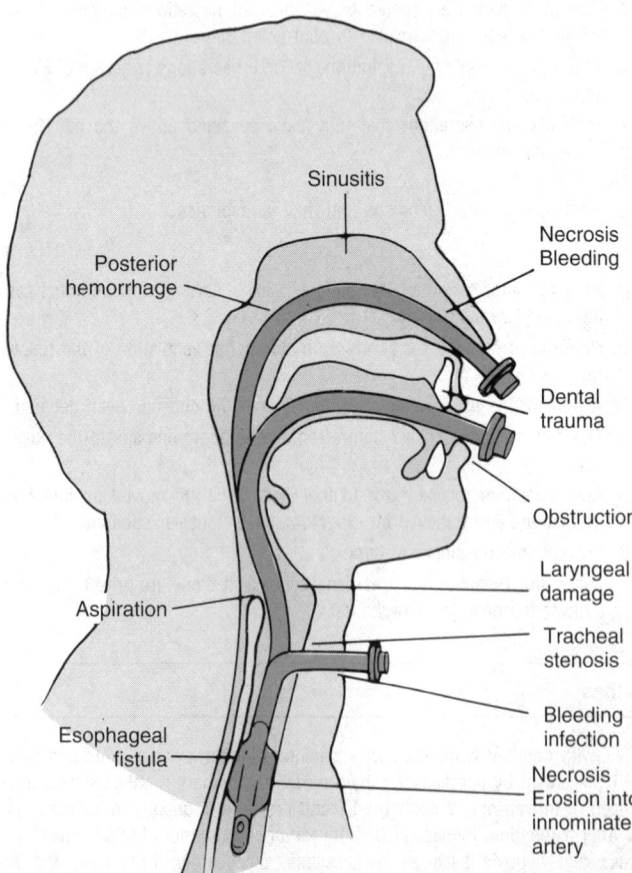

Figure 22–21. Complications of endotracheal intubation and tracheostomy. (From Marino P. *The ICU Book*. Philadelphia: Lea & Febiger, 1991.)

Sinusitis

Necrosis
Bleeding

Posterior
hemorrhage

Dental
trauma

Obstruction

Laryngeal
damage

Aspiration

Tracheal
stenosis

Bleeding
infection

Esophageal
fistula

Necrosis
Erosion into
innominate
artery

c. Labored respirations
d. Elevated blood pressure and heart rate
e. Increased diaphoresis
f. Increased adventitious breath sounds
g. Increased peak inspiratory pressure in patients on mechanical ventilation (see later discussion)

3. Procedure
  a. Removal of sputum by turning, coughing, and deep breathing on the patient's part is the preferred method.
  b. If the patient is unable to clear the sputum, tracheal suctioning through an endotracheal or tracheostomy tube may be necessary (see Procedure 22–3).

4. Complications
  a. Hypoxemia
  b. Dysrhythmias
  c. Bronchospasms
  d. Airway trauma
  e. Infection
  f. Atelectasis or lobar collapse

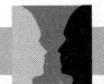

CLINICAL CONTROVERSIES

The routine use of saline to loosen secretions has been a common practice in many institutions. However, some studies have shown that instilling saline may actually *increase* the pooling of secretions and that retained saline may provide a medium in which bacteria can grow. Thus, some institutions are now using saline to loosen secretions only as a latter intervention.

Mechanical Ventilation

1. Definition: use of an artificial airway and a mechanical ventilator to create a flow of gas into and out of the lungs in patients who are unable to ventilate their lungs adequately
2. Goals of mechanical ventilation
  a. Maintain alveolar ventilation
  b. Deliver precise levels of oxygen
  c. Maintain adequate lung expansion
  d. Reduce the work of breathing
3. Indications
  a. Inadequate ventilation
    (1) Inadequate ventilation may result from apnea or hypoventilation.
    (2) Hypoventilation may lead to increased levels of $PaCO_2$ and acidosis.
    (3) Gradually or acutely rising carbon dioxide levels may be an indication for instituting mechanical ventilation, but it is not used as a single criterion.
    (4) The pH is the most important indicator of need for mechanical ventilatory support. Mechanical ventilation is usually needed for patients with respiratory acidosis and a pH of 7.2 or lower, although it may be necessary for some patients with a pH above 7.2.
  b. Hypoxemia: In severe cases that cannot be controlled by noninvasive methods of oxygenation, mechanical ventilation provides high levels of oxygen while reducing the work of breathing.

c. Increased intracranial pressure: Mechanical ventilation may facilitate hyperventilation, leading to hypocapnia and thus an initial lowering of intracranial pressure.

d. Deterioration of clients with neuromuscular disease (e.g., myasthenia gravis, and Guillain-Barré)

e. Flail chest

f. After surgery until anesthesia has worn off

4. Types of mechanical ventilation

a. Volume ventilation: A preset volume of gas is delivered via a tube sealed securely in the trachea. This amount of gas is delivered regardless of the pressure required (i.e., changes in lung compliance do not affect the volume of gas to be delivered).

b. Pressure ventilation: Gas is delivered until a preset pressure is reached. When this preset pressure is reached, it is held for the length of time set on the ventilator or for as long as the patient desires, depending on the mode being utilized (see below). The volume of gas delivered depends on compliance of the lung and pressure level selected.

5. Modes of ventilation

a. Assist-control ventilation

(1) The ventilator has a preset V_T, FiO_2, and rate. This minimum preset number of breaths per minute is delivered regardless of patient effort.

(2) If the patient initiates spontaneous breaths above the preset minimum, the ventilator will sense this effort and will deliver an additional breath to the client at the preset V_T and FiO_2.

(3) Patients cannot vary or control the volume of spontaneously initiated breaths. Every breath will be at the machine-set V_T.

b. Intermittent mandatory ventilation

(1) The ventilator has a preset V_T, FiO_2, and rate. This minimum preset number of breaths per minute is delivered regardless of patient effort.

(2) In intermittent mandatory ventilation, unlike in assist-control ventilation, any spontaneous breaths above the preset minimum will be at any V_T the patient can generate. FiO_2 remains at the preset level.

c. Pressure-controlled inverse ratio ventilation

(1) A preset pressure is selected based on the amount of pressure needed to deliver a predetermined V_T. The gas is delivered under this preset pressure and held in the lungs for a preselected period of time (ratio of inspiration to expiration is 2:1 up to 4:1).

(2) It is believed that holding the gas in the chest longer than normal allows for better distribution to collapsed alveoli.

(3) Normally this mode is used in patients with stiff, noncompliant lungs for whom conventional modes of ventilation have failed.

d. Pressure support ventilation

(1) This mode of ventilation augments spontaneous inspiratory efforts by delivering a set level of positive airway pressure at a preset FiO_2.

(2) When the patient initiates a breath, the ventilator senses the effort and a rapid flow of gas is delivered. This pressure remains constant throughout the inspiratory cycle until the inspiratory flow rate decreases to one fourth the original flow rate.

e. Positive end-expiratory pressure (PEEP)

(1) In PEEP the ventilator provides positive pressure throughout expiration, allowing the alveoli to remain open throughout the entire ventilatory cycle.

(2) Positive end-expiratory pressure can be used in conjunction with assist-control ventilation, intermittent mandatory ventilation, or by itself. It is used especially in patients with oxygenation problems such as atelectasis, pulmonary edema, or ARDS.

(3) Commonly, PEEP is used on ventilated patients at low levels, such as 5 cm H_2O. This level of PEEP is believed to be similar to physiologic PEEP. The use of PEEP may permit reducing FiO_2 to safe levels (below 40%) while maintaining adequate PaO_2 levels.

NURSE ADVISORY

> Positive end-expiratory pressure greater than 10 cm H_2O should rarely be interrupted.

f. Continuous positive airway pressure (CPAP)

(1) CPAP has the same physiologic characteristics as PEEP. CPAP therapy can be used for intubated and nonintubated patients.

(2) When placed on CPAP, the intubated patient breathes spontaneously without the aid of a mechanical rate or V_T delivered by the ventilator.

(3) For intubated patients, this mode of therapy is primarily used during meaning from mechanical ventilation.

(4) For use of CPAP therapy in nonintubated patients see page 966.

6. Complications of mechanical ventilation

a. Decreased cardiac output: The increased intrathoracic pressure produced by positive pressure ventilation decreases venous return to the heart, resulting in a lower cardiac output. This effect is particularly strong with PEEP; monitor heart rate and blood pressure carefully when increasing PEEP settings.

b. Gastric ulcers: Positive pressure ventilation causes the diaphragm to descend into the abdomen during inspiration. Blood flow to the splanchnic area decreases, leading to ischemia of the gastric mucosa.

c. Increased fluid retention: Decreased blood flow to the splanchnic area decreases blood flow to the kidneys. Decreased blood flow to the kidneys signals the posterior pituitary gland to increase secretion of vasopressin or antidiuretic hormone. Antidiuretic hormone increases water retention and stimulates the renin-angiotensin-aldosterone mechanism.

d. Barotrauma: This is the presence of extra alveolar air caused when alveoli are overdistended by positive pressure, increased respiratory rate, and larger V_Ts.

(1) Incidence of barotrauma increases in the elderly and in persons with COPD.

Procedure 22–4
Establishing and Maintaining Mechanical Ventilation
and Managing the Patient Who Is Being Weaned
from Mechanical Ventilation

Definition/Purpose

To provide adequate ventilation to the respiratory system utilizing the method that is best tolerated by the patient. Mechanical ventilation causes air to flow in and out of the lungs by changing the airway pressures. The purpose of mechanical ventilation is to maintain alveolar ventilation, deliver a reliable concentration of oxygen, and reduce the work of breathing.

Contraindications/Cautions

Cautions for mechanical ventilation include (1) monitoring the patient closely for signs of respiratory distress and hypoxia, (2) setting alarms at appropriate levels, (3) monitoring for cardiac complications that may result from hypoxia, and (4) assessing the cardiovascular system for decompensation due to the positive intrathoracic pressure created by the ventilator.

Learning/Teaching Activities

Provide the following information: (1) Explain the operation of the ventilator to the patient. (2) Explain that the patient will not be able to talk while intubated and on the ventilator. Establish a reliable method of communication. (3) Explain the suction procedure and why and when it may be necessary to use it. (4) Explain the alarms and the sound of the ventilator.

Preliminary Activities

Equipment

- Ventilator
- Pulse oximetry
- Gloves
- Mask
- Goggles
- Stethoscope

Assessment/Planning

- Know the baseline vital signs for the client.
- Know the baseline arterial blood gas levels.
- Obtain a baseline pulmonary and cardiac assessment.
- Know the reason for instituting mechanical ventilation in this patient.
- Review any underlying pulmonary or cardiac pathologic condition that may be present before instituting the mechanical ventilation.
- Know what settings are to be used on the ventilator.

Preparation of the Person

- Explain how the ventilator works.
- May require sedation to tolerate the ventilator at first.
- Must be intubated before establishing mechanical ventilation.

Procedure

Action	Rationale/Discussion
1. Explain the need for mechanical ventilation to the patient.	1. Provides information to the patient and helps to reduce anxiety.
2. Put on mask, gloves, and goggles.	2. Protects from microorganisms.
3. Preset the ventilator with the desired settings.	3. Ensures that the patient will receive an adequate oxygen level, tidal volume, and respiratory rate when mechanical ventilation is instituted.
4. Attach pulse oximeter to the patient.	4. Provides an objective assessment of oxygenation.
5. Connect the ventilator tubing to the endotracheal tube or tracheostomy tube.	5. Institutes a positive pressure within the airway, which causes air to move into the lungs.
6. Assess respiratory status, respiratory effort, breath sounds, and equal chest expansion.	6. Regular ongoing assessment is necessary to determine early problems with oxygenation and establish a baseline of therapy.
7. Assess for changes in mental status and increased anxiety.	7. Changes in mental status and increases in anxiety may indicate oxygen desaturation or carbon dioxide retention, or both.
8. Auscultate lungs for the presence of adventitious breath sounds.	8. Adventitious breath sounds indicate the need for suctioning.
9. Suction as needed, hyperoxygenating with 100% oxygen before and after the procedure. Limit suctioning pass to 10 to 15 seconds.	9. Removal of secretions ensures a patent airway. Preprocedure and postprocedure oxygenation and limitation of the suctioning pass to 10 seconds prevent hypoxemia related to suctioning.

P

Procedure 22–4
(continued)

Action	Rationale/Discussion
10. Monitor chest radiograph daily.	10. Ensures proper placement of endotracheal tube, bilateral lung expansion, and presence of fluid or infiltrates.
11. Monitor arterial blood gas levels with each ventilation setting change.	11. Ensures that the proper settings are being utilized on the ventilator. The pH reflects the overall acid-base balance of the body.
12. Reposition the patient frequently.	12. Prevents accumulation and pooling of secretions, which may provide a medium for bacteria or occlude the airways.
13. Monitor peak inspiratory pressure.	13. Increased peak inspiratory pressure may indicate the presence of an airway obstruction. This obstruction may be the result of mucus plugs, kinking of the endotracheal tube, or the patient's biting of the tube.
14. Check position of the endotracheal tube at the lips or nares at least every 2 hours.	14. Correct positioning of the endotracheal tube is necessary to maintain bilateral lung expansion and patent airways.
15. Sedate the patient as needed.	15. Anxiety or pain increases metabolism, which increases oxygen utilization, leading to decreased oxygen available to the rest of the body. Anxiety may cause the patient to fight against the ventilator, making it less efficient.
16. Provide adequate nutrition via a nasogastric tube or hyperalimentation.	16. Nutrition provides the necessary components of metabolism to fight disease processes and regain respiratory muscle strength.
17. Assess and document cardiovascular status.	17. Positive pressure ventilation increases intrathoracic pressure, which decreases venous return and cardiac output, resulting in hypotension. Decreased oxygenation to the myocardium may result in an increase in cardiac dysrhythmias.
18. Monitor for signs and symptoms of infection.	18. Infection increases metabolism, which in turn increases oxygen requirements.
19. Monitor fluid volume balance with intake and output and daily weights.	19. Ongoing assessment helps to determine fluid volume balance. Monitoring hydration is essential to offset the reduction of venous return to the heart.
20. Insert and monitor nasogastric tube.	20. Often utilized in patients with mechanical ventilation due to increased incidence of stress ulcers and increased risk of aspiration. Used for the decompression of the stomach as well.
21. Monitor laboratory values (hemoglobin, hematocrit, arterial blood gases, complete blood count, serum electrolytes, blood urea nitrogen, creatinine).	21. Indication of oxygen status. Indicates the ability of the body to utilize available oxygen. Indicates the presence of infection. Helps to determine kidney function.
22. Monitor for signs and symptoms of pneumothorax.	22. Pressure generated by positive pressure mechanical ventilation may rupture the alveolar walls. Tracheal shifts may occur to the affected side. Chest tube insertion may be necessary in these cases.
23. Monitor heart rhythm closely during suctioning.	23. Hypoxemia related to suctioning may cause cardiac dysrhythmias.
24. Use nonverbal and verbal communication.	24. Intubated patients often experience fear, helplessness, and despair.
25. Inflate endotracheal tube using the minimal leak technique.	25. The endotracheal tube cuff must be adequately inflated to provide a sufficient seal. Underinflation may lead to aspiration of gastric contents. Overinflation may lead to tracheal necrosis.

Managing the Patient's Weaning from Mechanical Ventilation

Action	Rationale/Discussion
1. Assess ventilatory status.	1. Tests that evaluate pulmonary function are important in determining a patient's ability to wean. Strong respiratory muscles must be present for successful weaning to occur.
2. Assess hemodynamics.	2. Alterations in tissue perfusion alter oxygen delivery, which affects the patient's ability to wean.
3. Monitor for signs and symptoms of infection.	3. The inflammatory process of infection utilizes a great deal of energy, which then cannot be used to improve respiratory muscle strength and endurance.
4. Provide adequate nutrition.	4. Protein and amino acids must be available for the muscles to grow and strengthen, which will result in an increase in endurance.
5. Assess oxygenation.	5. Hemoglobin, cardiac output, and PaO_2 must be optimized before weaning can be successful.

(continued)

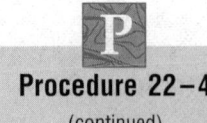

Procedure 22–4

(continued)

Action	Rationale/Discussion
6. Monitor vital signs.	6. The stress of weaning may lead to hypertension or hypotension and tachycardia. These changes may ultimately lead to decreased tissue perfusion.
7. Monitor heart rhythm.	7. Hypoxemia may lead to dysrhythmias.
8. Assess mental status.	8. Increased carbon dioxide retention may lead to lethargy, slurred speech, and headaches.
9. Assess anxiety level.	9. Increased anxiety leads to increased metabolism and increased work of breathing. This may result in an unsuccessful weaning attempt.
10. Monitor response to weaning schedule.	10. Weaning is very individual, and each plan must be customized to meet the needs of each patient.
11. Provide adequate periods of rest.	11. Increased rest promotes an increase in respiratory muscle strength and endurance.
12. Monitor systemic hydration with adequate fluid balance.	12. Adequate hydration prevents mucus plugging and the formation of thick, tenacious sputum. Fluid overload may lead to increased work for the heart, leading to congestive heart failure.
13. Assess psychologic readiness for weaning.	13. A patient with a positive attitude toward the weaning process has better success with weaning. A positive attitude provides a sense of control over one's own environment.
14. Position for comfort.	14. Increased comfort levels decrease anxiety. Increased anxiety leads to an increased demand on respiratory muscles. Sitting in a semi-Fowler's position allows the diaphragm to descend freely, creating efficient use of this muscle.
15. Keep accurate records of weaning plan and patient's response.	15. A reasonable, progressive plan allows for the gradual retraining of the respiratory muscles.

Final Activities

Assess how the patient tolerates the mechanical ventilator, and make changes accordingly. Identify the areas that need to be addressed and that are impediments to weaning, and correct those areas. Obtain arterial blood gas levels and make changes in the ventilator settings if needed.

(2) Signs and symptoms include a shift of the mediastinum, decreased breath sounds, and increased peak inspiratory pressure.

(3) The biggest danger from barotrauma is the development of a tension pneumothorax, which can be treated by placing a chest tube on the affected side.

e. Tracheal mucosal damage: Increased pressure in the endotracheal tube cuff can result in compression of the tracheal mucosa, leading to tissue ischemia and necrosis. Incidence of tracheal mucosal damage has been greatly decreased by the low-pressure cuffs now utilized.

f. Psychologic problems: Difficulty in communication may result from inability to vocalize desires. Increased stress and anxiety may result from dependency on machines to breathe.

7. Nursing care of patients needing mechanical ventilation: establishing, maintaining, and weaning procedures (Procedure 22–4)

Thoracic Surgery

1. Definition: Thoracic surgery is any surgical procedure that requires entry into the chest cavity.
2. Indications
   a. Evidence of intrathoracic damage
   b. Disease process within the chest wall
   c. Chest wall abnormalities
3. Types of surgery
   a. Wedge resection
      (1) Most conservative type of thoracic surgery
      (2) Removes only a small section of lung tissue
      (3) Surgery of choice on small, peripherally located tumors
      (4) Requires chest tubes postoperatively
   b. Segmental resection
      (1) Removes a particular bronchovascular segment of a diseased lung; remaining tissue expands to fill void
      (2) Performed on lesions that are peripherally located and show no signs of metastasis

(3) Requires chest tubes postoperatively
c. Lobectomy
(1) Surgery of choice with tumors that are neatly contained in a single lobe
(2) Procedure similar to segmental resection
(3) Requires chest tubes postoperatively
d. Pneumonectomy
(1) This procedure is used for patients with disease extending beyond 1 lobe of a lung.
(2) Procedure: Removal of entire lung; simple pneumonectomy removes only the lung tissue; radical pneumonectomy removes surrounding lymph nodes, too. To maintain equal bilateral pressure within the thoracic cavity, serous exudate is allowed to fill the void left by removal of lung tissue. This fluid eventually solidifies, preventing a mediastinal shift (Fig. 22–22).
(3) Mortality is substantially higher than with other thoracic surgeries.
(4) Chest tubes are not needed postoperatively.
4. Complications
a. Decreased lung function: decreased VT, VC, and functional residual capacity
b. Ineffective coughing and clearing of secretions
c. Chest wall dysfunction
d. Atelectasis
e. Pain
f. Diaphragm dysfunction
g. Risk for thrombophlebitis, infection, cardiac dysrhythmias
5. Applying the nursing process

> **NURSING DIAGNOSIS:** Ineffective breathing pattern R/T compression of lung tissue

a. *Expected outcomes:* Following intervention, the person should have the following:
(1) Respiratory rate of 12 to 20 breaths per minute
(2) No use of accessory muscles
(3) Oxygen saturation greater than 90 percent
(4) No anxiety
(5) No change in mental status
b. *Nursing interventions*
(1) Monitor respiratory rate, rhythm, and depth and use of accessory muscles.
(2) Monitor for changes in mental status.
(3) Teach and assist the patient with turning, coughing, and deep breathing.

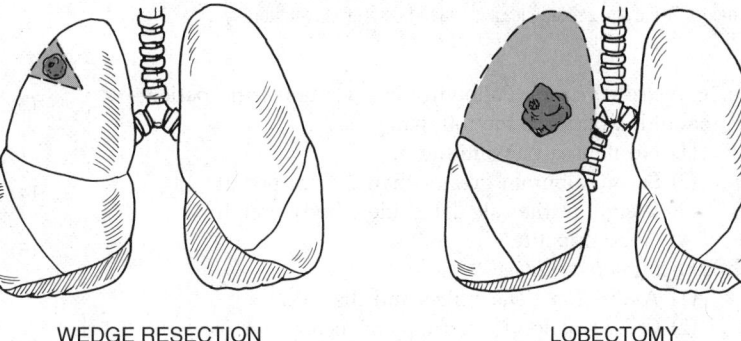

WEDGE RESECTION   LOBECTOMY

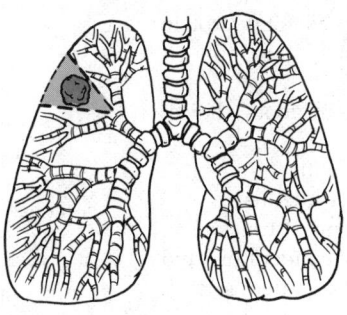

SEGMENTAL RESECTION

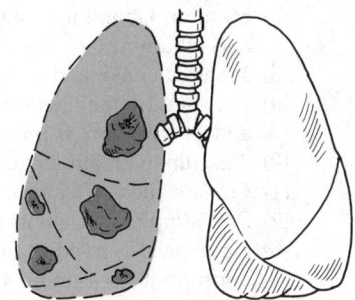

PNEUMONECTOMY

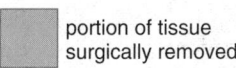

portion of tissue surgically removed

Figure 22–22. Types of surgery to remove pulmonary tumors. (From Black JM, and Matassarin-Jacobs E [eds]. *Luckmann and Sorensen's Medical-Surgical Nursing: A Psychophysiologic Approach.* 4th ed. Philadelphia: WB Saunders, 1993, p 1065.)

(4) Encourage use of diaphragmatic breathing.
(5) Position for comfort and ease of respirations.
(6) Monitor oxygen saturation.

NURSING DIAGNOSIS: Impaired gas exchange R/T retained secretions and occluded bronchioles

a. *Expected outcomes:* Following intervention, the patient should have the following:
   (1) Arterial blood gases at baseline
   (2) No change in mental status
   (3) No cyanosis
   (4) SaO_2 greater than 90 percent
b. *Nursing interventions*
   (1) Assess ABGs as indicated.
   (2) Administer oxygen as indicated.
   (3) Note respiratory rate, rhythm, and depth and use of accessory muscles.
   (4) Auscultate lung sounds frequently.
   (5) Monitor vital signs.
   (6) Monitor SaO_2.
   (7) Position for ease of respirations.
   (8) Suction as indicated.
   (9) Encourage rest periods throughout the day.

NURSING DIAGNOSIS: Altered nutrition less than body requirements R/T dyspnea, fatigue, and side effects of chemotherapy

a. *Expected outcomes:* Following interventions, the patient should experience the following:
   (1) No nausea or vomiting
   (2) Serum albumin greater than 2.8 gm per dl
   (3) Weight at the calculated ideal body weight
   (4) Good appetite
b. *Nursing interventions*
   (1) Assess for dietary likes and dislikes.
   (2) Offer smaller, more frequent meals.
   (3) Monitor for nausea and vomiting.
   (4) Administer antiemetic.
   (5) Coordinate meal times around periods of rest and medication schedule.
   (6) Weigh daily.
   (7) Monitor laboratory values such as total protein and albumin.
   (8) Monitor intake and output.
   (9) Get family members involved in food choices and preparation, if possible.
   (10) Auscultate breath sounds every shift.
   (11) Consult dietary team or registered dietitian.
   (12) Provide pleasant environment at meal times.
   (13) Have meals served at the proper temperature and appropriate seasoning to suit the patient's taste.

NURSING DIAGNOSIS: Impaired physical mobility R/T dyspnea and pain

a. *Expected outcomes:* Following intervention, the patient should have the following:

(1) Controlled pain
(2) No skin breakdown
(3) Increased mobility
(4) Increased strength
b. *Nursing interventions*
   (1) Encourage ambulation; assist as necessary.
   (2) Turn frequently while in bed.
   (3) Note skin or signs of breakdown.
   (4) Massage reddened areas of skin to promote circulation.
   (5) Teach and encourage range-of-motion exercises.
   (6) Encourage activities that allow for adequate rest periods.
   (7) Consult physical therapist for additional therapy.
   (8) Assess for any deterioration from previous activity and mobility level.
6. Chest tubes and drainage systems
   a. Uses
      (1) To reexpand a collapsed lung by restoring negative intrapleural pressure
      (2) To assess drainage from the intrapleural space
      (3) To measure drainage from the intrapleural space
      (4) To reestablish an adequate ventilation-perfusion ratio
   b. Principles of the chest drainage system
      (1) Allows air and fluid to be removed from the intrapleural space.
      (2) Movement of air and fluid is unidirectional. Both move from an area of high pressure (intrapleural space) during expiration to an area of low pressure (drainage system).
      (3) The amount of negative pressure generated by the drainage system depends on the water depth in the water seal system.
      (4) The usual water depth in a water seal system is 2 cm.
      (5) This level creates the slightly negative atmosphere that is present normally in the intrapleural space.
      (6) Too much water (pressure) in the water seal chamber does not allow for pressure that is building up in the intrapleural space to be relieved.
      (7) Maintenance of a water seal chamber prevents the retrograde flow of air or fluid back into the intrapleural space during inspiration.
      (8) Fluctuation of fluid in the chest tube drainage system or in the water seal chamber should be present with each respiration as the pressure in the pleural space changes. Absence of fluctuation can indicate loss of patency in the chest tube or re-expansion of the lung.
   c. Types of drainage systems
      (1) One-bottle system: Water seal and collection of drainage occurs in the same bottle. Used for simple pneumothorax. It incorporates the use of 1 bottle with an air vent. This air vent allows for air that has escaped from the intrapleural space to be expelled into the atmosphere, which prevents a pressure buildup within the system. Because there is only 1 bottle in this system, this container also collects fluid that is drained from the intrapleural space. If fluid drains

into the bottle, the level of the fluid in the system increases. This causes an increase in pressure within the system. The increase in pressure causes resistance to drainage of air and fluid.

(2) Two-bottle system: Water seal and collection of drainage are in separate bottles. The 1st bottle, which is directly attached to a client, serves as the collection container for fluid. The 2nd bottle serves as the water seal container, as in the 1-bottle system. This system is used when drainage from the intrapleural space is expected. The collection container prevents the buildup of pressure within the system that can occur with the 1-bottle

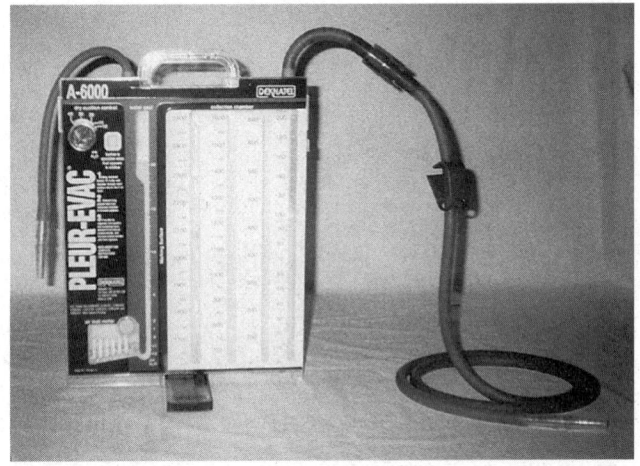

Figure 22–24. Pleur-evac, a 3-bottle chest tube drainage system. (Courtesy of Deknatel, Division of Howmedica, Floral Park, NY.)

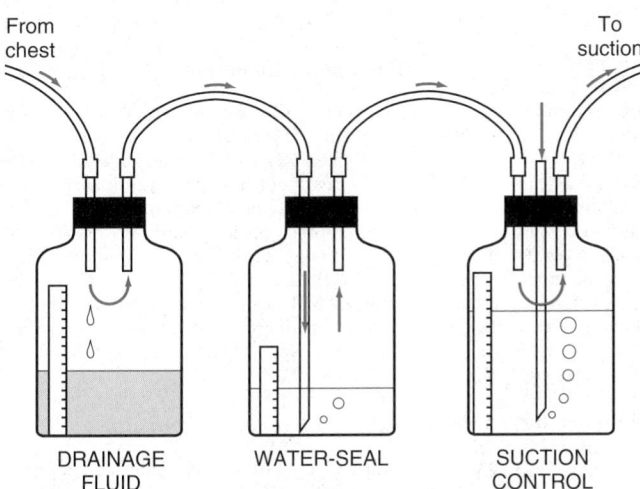

Figure 22–23. Chest tube drainage (3-bottle system). (Redrawn from Black JM, and Matassarin-Jacobs E [eds]. *Luckmann and Sorensen's Medical-Surgical Nursing: A Psychophysiologic Approach.* 4th ed. Philadelphia: WB Saunders, 1993, p 1067.)

system. The exact amount of drainage can be measured from the drainage container.

(3) Three-bottle system: Water seal, collection of drainage, and suction control are in separate bottles (Fig. 22–23). If there is a large amount of drainage or air in the intrapleural space, suction may be required for adequate removal. The amount of suction is determined by the depth of water in the suction container. The collection bottle and water seal bottle function the same as those in the 2-bottle system.

(4) Pleuravac system (Fig. 22–24) Same as the 3-bottle system but incorporated into a single, easily moveable unit. Disposable, so there is no possibility of contacting contaminated drainage. Markings on the side of the collection chambers make it easy to record the amount of drainage.

Bibliography

Books

Carpenito LJ. *Nursing Care Plans and Documentation.* Philadelphia: JB Lippincott, 1991.

Carpenito LJ. *Nursing Diagnosis: Application to Clinical Practice.* 4th ed. Philadelphia: JB Lippincott, 1992.

Dolan JT (ed). *Critical Care Nursing: Clinical Management Through the Nursing Process.* Philadelphia: FA Davis, 1991.

Hartshorn J, Lamborn M, and Noll, ML. *Introduction to Critical Care Nursing.* Philadelphia: WB Saunders, 1993.

Jarvis C. *Physical Examination and Health Assessment.* 2nd ed. Philadelphia: WB Saunders, 1996.

Marino P. *The ICU Book.* Philadelphia: Lea & Febiger, 1991.

McPherson SP, and Spearman CB (eds). *Respiratory Therapy Equipment.* 4th ed. St. Louis: CV Mosby, 1990.

Porth CM. *Pathophysiology: Concepts of Altered Health States.* 4th ed. Philadelphia: JB Lippincott, 1994.

Sexton, DL. *Nursing Care of the Respiratory Patient.* Norwalk, CT: Appleton & Lange, 1990.

Waite LG, and Krummberger JM. *Noncardiac Critical Care Nursing.* Milwaukee, WI: Delmar, 1994.

Weilitz PB. *Pocket Guide to Respiratory Care.* St. Louis: CV Mosby, 1991.

West JB. *Pulmonary Pathophysiology: The Essentials.* Baltimore: Williams & Wilkins, 1987.

Wyngaarden JB, Smith LH Jr, and Bennett JC (eds). *Cecil Textbook of Medicine.* 19th ed. Philadelphia: WB Saunders, 1992.

Chapters in Books and Journal Articles

Diagnostics

American Thoracic Society. Diagnostic standards and classification of tuberculosis. *Am Rev Respir Dis* 142:725–735, 1990.

Carpenter KD. Oxygen transport in the blood. *Crit Care Nurse* 11:20–33, 1991.

Egloft ME. Assessment of clients with respiratory disorders. *In* Black JM, and Matassarin-Jacobs E (eds). *Luckmann and Sorensen's Medical-Surgical Nursing: A Psychophysiologic Approach.* 4th ed. Philadelphia: WB Saunders, 1993.

Kubribayashi L. Pleural effusions. *In* Rakel RE (ed). *Saunders Manual of Medical Practice.* Philadelphia: WB Saunders, 1996.

Nield M. Structure and function of the respiratory system. *In* Black JM, and Matassarin-Jacobs E (eds). *Luckmann and Sorensen's Medical-Surgical Nursing: A Psychophysiologic Approach.* 4th ed. Philadelphia: WB Saunders, 1993.

Rueden KT. Noninvasive assessment of gas exchange in the critically ill patient. *AACN Clin Issues Crit Care Nurs* 1:239–247, 1990.

Sonnesso G. Are you ready to use pulse oximetry? *Nursing 91* 21(8):60–64, 1991.

Interventions

Alderfer S. Common respiratory interventions. *In* Black JM, and Matassarin-Jacobs E (eds). *Luckmann and Sorensen's Medical-Surgical Nursing: A Psychophysiologic Approach.* 4th ed. Philadelphia: WB Saunders, 1993.

Ashworth LJ. Pressure support ventilation. *Crit Care Nurse* 10:20–27, 1990.

Benditt J. Pneumothorax. *In* Rakel RE (ed). *Saunders Manual of Medical Practice.* Philadelphia: WB Saunders, 1996.

Bolgiana CS, et al. Administering oxygen therapy: What you need to know. *Nursing 90* 20(6):47–51, 1990.

Burns SM, Burns JE, and Truwit JD. Comparison of five clinical weaning indices. *Am J Crit Care* 3(5):342–352, 1994.

Caminiti SP, and Young SL. The pulmonary surfactant system. *Hosp Pract* 26(A):87–100, 1991.

Eickhoff RC. Current immunization practices in adults. *Hosp Pract* (10A):114–115, 1990.

Fedorovich C, and Littleton MT. Chest physiotherapy: Evaluating the effectiveness. *Dimens Crit Care Nurs* 9(2):68–74, 1990.

St. John RE, and Eisenberg P. Nutrition and use of metabolic assessment in the ventilator-dependent patient. *AACN Clin Issues Crit Care Nurs* 2:453–462, 1991.

Chronic Obstructive Pulmonary Disease

Dorca J. Acute bronchial infection in chronic obstructive pulmonary disease (review). *Monaldi Arch Chest Dis* 50(5):366–371, 1995.

Owens GR. Advances in the treatment of chronic obstructive pulmonary disease. *Hosp Formulary* 27:1012–1027, 1992.

Schapira RM, and Reinke LF. The outpatient diagnosis and management of chronic obstructive pulmonary disease: Pharmacotherapy, administration of supplemental oxygen, and smoking cessation techniques (review). *J Gen Intern Med* 10(1):40–55, 1995.

Siafakas NM, et al. Optimal assessment and management of chronic obstructive pulmonary disease (COPD). The European Respiratory Society Task Force. *Eur Respir J* 8(8):1398–1420, 1995.

Standards for the diagnosis and care of patients with chronic obstructive pulmonary disease (review). American Thoracic Society. *Am J Respir Crit Care Med* 152(5 Pt 2):S77–121, 1995.

Whatling J. Managing chronic obstructive disease. *Nurs Stand* 10(8):34–37, 1995.

Infectious Respiratory Disorders

Belmonte R, and Crowe HM. Pneumothorax in patients with pulmonary tuberculosis (letter). *Clin Infect Dis* 20(6):1565, 1995.

Cohn DL. Treatment of multidrug-resistant tuberculosis. *J Hosp Infect* 30(Suppl):322–328, 1995.

Douglas RG. Prophylaxis and treatment of influenza. *N Engl J Med* 322:443–450, 1990.

Finegold SM. Aspiration pneumonia. *Rev Infect Dis* 13(Suppl 9):S737–742, 1991.

Jereb JA, et al. Tuberculosis morbidity in the United States: Final data, 1990. *MMWR* 40(No. SS-3):24–26, 1991.

Lambregts-van Weezenbeek CS, and Veen J. Control of drug-resistant tuberculosis. *Tuber Lung Dis* 76(5):455–459, 1995.

Maloney SA, et al. Efficacy of control measures in preventing nosocomial transmission of multidrug-resistant tuberculosis to patients and health care workers. *Ann Intern Med* 122(2):90–95, 1995.

Masden LA. Tuberculosis today. *RN* 53(3):44–50, 1990.

Serkey JM. Multidrug-resistant tuberculosis: A new era in prevention and control. *Dimens Crit Care Nurs* 14(5):236–244, 1995.

Small PA Jr. Influenza: Pathogenesis and host defense. *Hosp Pract* 25(11A):51–62, 1990.

Lung Cancer

Faber LP. Lung cancer. *In* Hollieb AI, Fink DJ, and Murphy GP (eds). *Clinical Oncology.* Atlanta, GA: American Cancer Society, 1991, pp 194–212.

Held JL. Caring for a patient with lung cancer. *Nursing* 25(10):34–43, 1995.

Lin AY, and Ihde DC. Recent developments in the treatment of lung cancer. *JAMA* 267:1661–1664, 1992.

Marrie TJ. Pneumonia and carcinoma of the lung. *J Infect* 29(1):45–52, 1994.

Petty TL. Lung cancer screening (review). *Compr Ther* 21(8):432–437, 1995.

Rostad M. Advances in nursing management of patients with lung cancer. *Nurs Clin North Am* 25(2):393, 1990.

Wolpaw DR. Early detection in lung cancer. Case finding and screening (review). *Med Clin North Am* 80(1):63–82, 1996.

Pneumothorax

Boutin C, et al. Thoracoscopy in the diagnosis and treatment of spontaneous pneumothorax (review). *Clin Chest Med* 16(3):497–503, 1995.

Rutter KM. Tension pneumothorax. *Nursing* 25(4):33, 1995.

Pulmonary Embolism

Goldhaber SZ. Managing pulmonary embolism. *Hosp Pract* 26(9A):37–48, 1991.

Goldhaber SZ, and Morpurgo M. Diagnosis, treatment and prevention of pulmonary embolism: Report of the WHO/International Society and Federation of Cardiology Task Force. *JAMA* 268:1727–1733, 1992.

Stratton MB. Ventilation-perfusion scintigraphy in diagnosis of pulmonary thromboembolism. *AACN Focus Crit Care* 17:287–293, 1990.

Other Pulmonary Disorders

Aldrich J. Pulmonary edema. *Nursing* 24(10):33, 1994.

Crystal R. Alpha$_1$-antitrypsin deficiency: Pathogenesis and treatment. *Hosp Pract* 26(2A):81–94, 1991.

Murray JF. New presentations of bronchiectasis. *Hosp Pract* 26(3A):55–74, 1991.

Rubin LJ. Approach to diagnosis and treatment of pulmonary hypertension. *Chest* 96:659, 1989.

Stauffer JL. Pulmonary diseases. *In* Schroeder SA, et al. (eds). *Current Diagnosis and Treatment.* Norwalk, CT: Appleton & Lange, pp 189–201, 229–230, 232–238, 255–261.

Agencies and Resources

Allergy and Asthma Network/Mothers of Asthmatics (AAN/MA)
3554 Chain Bridge Road,
Suite 200
Fairfax, VA 22030–2709
(800) 878–4403

American Association for Cancer Education (AACE)
Department of Epidemiology, 189
1515 Holcombe Boulevard
Houston, TX 77030
(713) 792–7756 or (713) 792–3020

American Lung Association (ALA)
1740 Broadway
New York, NY 10019–4374
(800) LUNG–USA

Congress of Lung Association Staff (CLAS)
1726 M Street, N.W., Suite 902
Washington, DC 20036–4502
(202) 785–3355

Cystic Fibrosis Foundation (CFF)
6931 Arlington Road, Suite 200
Bethesda, MD 20814
(800) 344–4823

Group Against Smokers' Pollution (GASP)
P.O. Box 632
College Park, MD 20741–0632
(301) 459–4791

National Jewish Center for Immunology and Respiratory Medicine
1400 Jackson Street
Denver, CO 80206
(800) 222–LUNG

23
Caring for People with Cardiovascular Disorders

◻ *CARDIOVASCULAR STRUCTURE AND FUNCTION*

The cardiovascular system consists of the heart, arteries, arterioles, capillaries, veins, and lymphatics (Fig. 23–1).

Heart

1. Structure (Fig. 23–1)
2. Function (see Fig. 23–1)

Coronary Artery System

1. Structure (Fig. 23–2)
2. Function (see Fig. 23–2)

Noncoronary Artery, Venous, Capillary, and Lymphatic Systems (see Chapter 24)

Conduction System of the Heart

1. Structure (Fig. 23–3)
   a. The sinoatrial (SA) node lies near the superior vena cava in the right atrium and is the "pacemaker" of the heart.
   b. The atrioventricular (AV) node lies at the base of the right atrium.
   c. The bundle of His connects the atria to the ventricle.
   d. Purkinje fibers are atypical muscle fibers that form the electric impulse—the conduction system.
2. Function
   a. Electrophysiologic properties
      (1) Excitability is the ability of a nerve to produce an action potential.
      (2) Automaticity is the spontaneous depolarization and the generation of an action potential.
      (3) Conductivity is the electric conduction ability.
      (4) Refractoriness is resistance to stimulation. A stronger stimulus is required to cause a response.
   b. Transmission of a cardiac impulse
      (1) Although the heart has the ability to initiate an impulse in any cell spontaneously, a normal car-

diac impulse begins in specialized pacemaker cells in the SA node.
      (2) The start of an impulse causes cells in the atrial myocardium to depolarize (become excited) spontaneously.
      (3) The impulse then spreads to the AV node (1.0–1.2 m/sec). Impulses travel more slowly through the AV node (0.02–0.05 m/sec), which allows blood to flow from the atria into the ventricles before ventricular contraction.
      (4) Impulses travel very rapidly (2.0–4.0 m/sec) through the bundle branches and into the Purkinje fibers, finally resulting in the systematic contraction and emptying of the ventricles.

Cardiac Cycle

1. A series of electric and mechanical events occur in a single heart beat.
2. The complete series is called a cardiac cycle.

Cardiac Output

1. Cardiac output is the total volume of blood pumped through the heart in 1 minute (normal = 4–8 L/min).
2. Variables affecting cardiac output
   a. Autonomic nervous system (see Chapter 18)
      (1) Vagal nerve stimulation leads to decreased firing rate of the SA node, decreased contractile force of atrial muscle, and decreased impulse speed through the AV node.

Cardiac output = stroke volume × heart rate

---

      (2) Sympathetic nerve stimulation leads to increased heart rate and increased strength of cardiac contractibility.
   b. Heart rate
      (1) The faster the heart rate, the less time the heart has for filling, and cardiac output decreases.
      (2) An increase in heart rate also increases oxygen consumption.

STRUCTURE AND FUNCTION OF THE HEART

Structure of the Heart:
The heart is located in the mediastinum, the space in the thoracic cavity between the lungs and above the diaphragm. It is a cone-shaped, hollow, muscular, contractile organ weighing about 300 gm (11 ounces).

Four vessels provide for blood flow into and out of the heart.

Superior vena cava drains blood from the upper body into the right atrium.

Coronary sinus drains blood from the cardiac veins into the right atrium.

Aorta carries blood from the left ventricle into the systemic circulation.

Inferior vena cava drains blood from the lower body into the right atrium.

Each side of the heart contains 2 chambers: the atrium and the ventricle.
Atrium: The atrium is a thin-walled upper collecting chamber.
Ventricle: The ventricle is a thick-walled lower pumping chamber.
The septum, a muscular wall, separates the chambers on the right side of the heart from those on the left side.

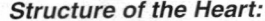

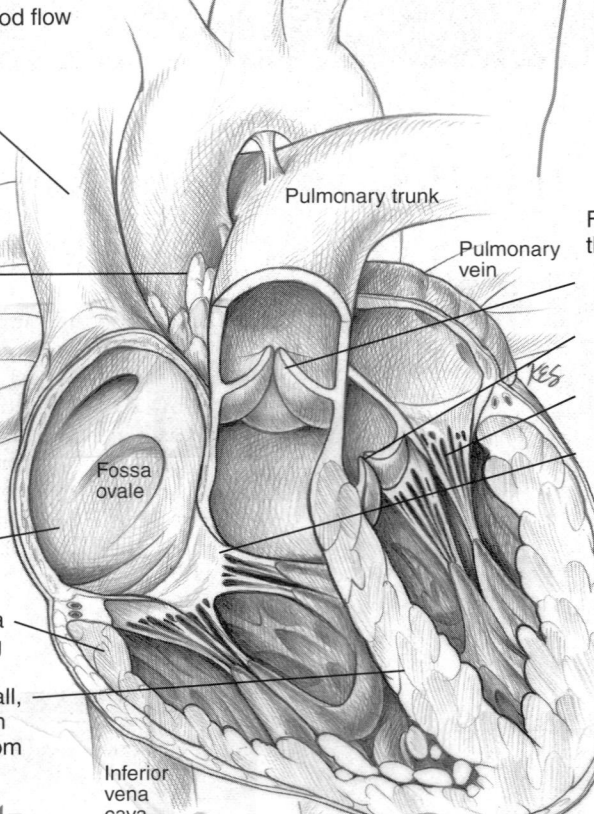

Four valves control blood flow through the heart.

Pulmonary valve: between the right ventricle and the pulmonary artery

Aortic valve: between the left ventricle and the ascending aorta

Mitral valve (bicuspid valve): between the left atrium and ventricle

Tricuspid valve: between the right atrium and ventricle

The heart consists of 3 layers of tissue:
Epicardium: The epicardium is a thin, transparent structure that covers the outer surface of the heart.
Myocardium: The myocardium is the middle layer and the contracting muscle of the heart, consisting of striated muscle fibers interlaced into bundles.
Endocardium: The innermost layer, the endocardium consists of thin endothelial tissue that lines the inner chambers and the heart valves.

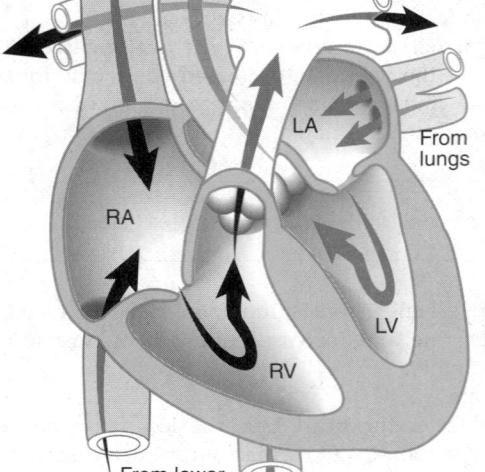

Functions of the Heart:
The pumping action of the heart is the result of muscles in the heart's chambers alternately contracting and relaxing. Contraction of the heart chambers is called systole. Diastole is the relaxation of the heart chambers with resultant dilation and filling.

1 The heart collects deoxygenated blood from the venous system and pumps it to the lungs for reoxygenation. The right atrium receives deoxygenated blood from the body via the superior and inferior vena cava and from the heart muscle via the coronary sinus and pumps it through the tricuspid valve into the right ventricle. The right ventricle, a flat muscular pump, receives deoxygenated blood from the right atrium and pumps it through the pulmonary valve, against low resistance, into the pulmonary artery and into the lungs.

2 The heart pumps oxygenated blood into the systemic circulation, which carries it to the cells. The left atrium receives oxygenated blood from the lungs, via the pulmonary veins, and pumps it through the mitral valve to the left ventricle. The left ventricle, the heart's largest, most muscular chamber, receives oxygenated blood from the lungs via the left atrium and pumps it through the aortic valve against high systemic pressure into the aorta and into the systemic circulation.

Figure 23–1.

STRUCTURE AND FUNCTION OF THE CORONARY ARTERY SYSTEM

Structure of the Coronary Artery System
The coronary artery system, which supplies blood to the myocardium, consists of 2 main coronary arteries: the left coronary artery (LCA) and the right coronary artery (RCA). The LCA divides into 2 branches: the left anterior descending (LAD) branch and the circumflex (CX).

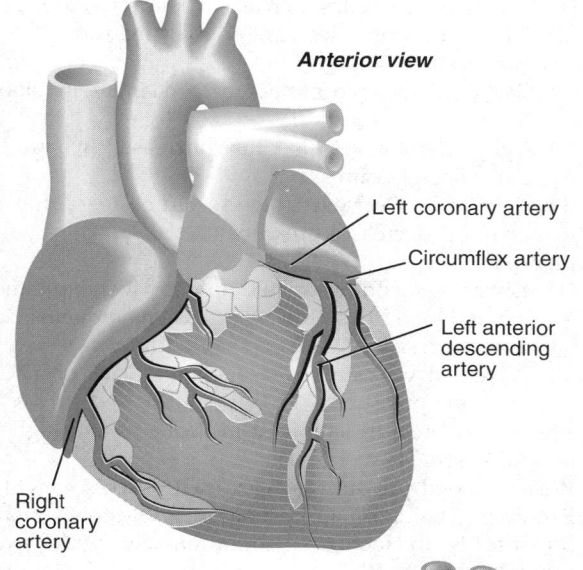

Anterior view

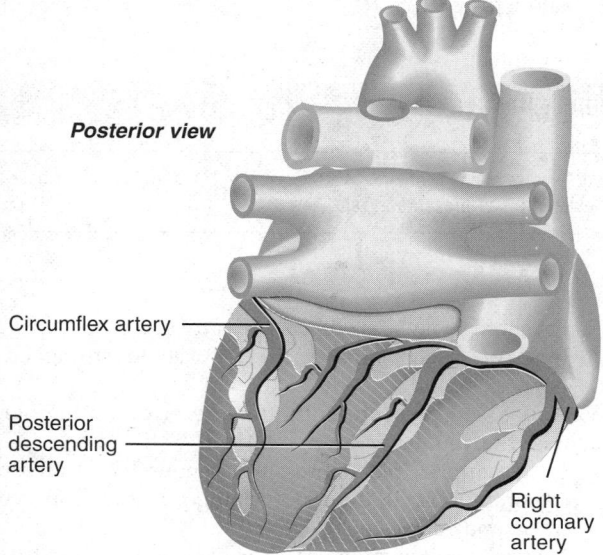

Posterior view

Function of the Coronary Artery System
The LAD branch supplies blood to the left ventricular walls and to the anterior and apical portions of the interventricular septum. The CX supplies blood to the lateral aspects of the left ventricle. It also supplies the sinoatrial (SA) node in 40–50% of people and the atrioventricular (AV) node in 10% of people. The RCA supplies blood to the right ventricle and the inferior wall of the left ventricle. It also supplies the SA node in 50–60% of people and the AV node in 90% of people.

Figure 23–2.

TRANSMISSION OF CARDIAC IMPULSE

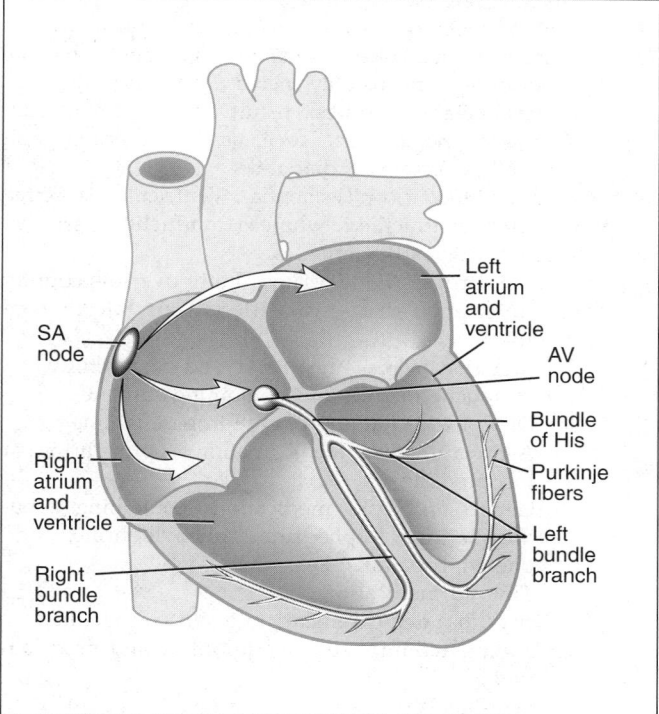

Figure 23–3.

c. Stroke volume: the amount of blood ejected from the left ventricle with each contraction (normal = 70–130 ml/beat). Stroke volume is affected by the following:
   (1) Preload—the volume of blood stretching the left ventricle at the end of diastole. Preload is determined by total circulating blood volume. Preload is increased by an increase in venous return to the heart. Factors affecting preload include exercise and anxiety, both of which increase venoconstriction and reduce peripheral vascular resistance.
   (2) Frank-Starling principle—states that the more the heart fills within reasonable limits during diastole, the greater the force of the contraction during systole and the greater the stroke volume. This mechanism allows the heart to respond to different amounts of incoming blood. The exception to the principle is during heart failure, when increasing blood volume into the ventricle decreases stroke volume.
   (3) Afterload—the force against which the heart has to pump to eject blood from the ventricle. Factors that impede blood flow, such as aortic stenosis, arterial constriction and polycythemia, increase left ventricle afterload. Afterload is increased by pulmonary hypertension and chronic obstructive pulmonary disease.
   (4) Contractility—the intrinsic ability of the heart muscles to contract affects stroke volume.

d. Myocardial oxygen demand: Anything that increases the need for myocardial oxygen, such as exercise and elevated temperature, increases heart rate.

e. Metabolic rate (see Chapter 29)
   (1) Hypermetabolic states: result in abnormally increased metabolism, such as fever and salicylate poisoning, and usually increase cardiac rates
   (2) Hypometabolic states: result in abnormally decreased metabolism, such as hypothermia, and usually decrease cardiac rates

f. Coronary blood flow (ischemia): Ventricular ischemia may affect contractility, whereas conduction tissue ischemia affects cardiac rate.

g. Effect of drugs: Many drugs, both over-the-counter and prescription drugs, can affect heart rate or contractility.
   (1) Drugs that increase heart rate and contractility
       • Headache medications containing caffeine
       • Diet pills containing phenylpropanolamine
       • Asthma medications containing epinephrine or theophylline
       • Cough and cold medications containing pseudoephedrine, ephedrine, phenylephrine, and phenylpropanolamine
       • Thyroid medication
   (2) Drugs that decrease heart rate and contractility
       • Antiarrhythmics such as quinidine and procainamide
       • Beta-blockers
       • Calcium channel blockers such as verapamil and diltiazem
       • Diet pills containing phentermine

h. Oxygen levels: Hypoxia initially increases heart rate, which then decreases as hypoxia continues.

i. Carbon dioxide (CO_2): Elevated levels of carbon dioxide in the blood, as occurs in respiratory failure, increase heart rate.

j. Electrolytes: Imbalances in levels of potassium, sodium, magnesium, and calcium may all influence cardiac functioning (see Chapter 9).

k. Body temperature
   (1) Hypothermia decreases heart rate.
   (2) Hyperthermia increases heart rate.

l. Acid-base balance
   (1) Acidosis increases heart rate and can progress to ventricular fibrillation.
   (2) Alkalosis can lead to ventricular fibrillation.

Blood Pressure

1. Blood pressure measures the force exerted by the blood against the walls of the blood vessels. Arterial blood pressure, the most common measure, is the force exerted by the blood against the arterial walls.
   a. Systolic pressure is the maximum force of the blood exerted against the artery walls when the heart contracts, normally 100 to 140 mm Hg.
   b. Diastolic pressure is the force of the blood exerted against the artery walls when the heart relaxes (fills), normally 60 to 90 mm Hg.

2. Arterial blood pressure can be measured indirectly (by sphygmomanometer) or directly (by arterial catheter). Readings are expressed as systolic/diastolic (e.g., 120/80). Procedure 23–1 describes measuring blood pressure at the brachial pulse site.

3. Circulatory factors that affect arterial pressure
   a. Cardiac output
      (1) Increased output increases arterial pressure.
      (2) Decreased output decreases arterial pressure.
   b. Peripheral vascular resistance
      (1) Narrowed arterioles increase arterial pressure.
      (2) Dilated arterioles decrease arterial pressure.
   c. Arterial elasticity
      (1) Elastic vessels accommodate to changes in blood flow.
      (2) Rigid sclerotic vessels cause increases in systolic and pulse pressures.
   d. Blood volume: Decreased blood volume (e.g., due to hemorrhage) decreases pressure.
   e. Blood viscosity
      (1) Increased blood viscosity, due to overabundance of red blood cells (RBCs) or plasma proteins, increases pressure
      (2) Decreased viscosity, from anemia or lack of RBCs, decreases pressure
   f. Age: Blood pressure is lowest in neonates and highest in adults (see Chapter 5).
   g. Weight: Blood pressure increases with excess weight.
   h. Exercise: The normal response of systolic blood pressure is to increase proportionately with heart rate.

NURSE ADVISORY

Athletes, due to heightened cardiovascular conditioning, often have lowered blood pressure at rest.

   i. Psychologic factors: Blood pressure increases with release of catecholamines in response to strong emotions or stress.

4. Venous blood pressure is the force exerted by the blood against the venous walls.
   a. Unlike arterial blood pressure, venous blood pressure is continuous. It does not change as the heart contracts and relaxes.
   b. Normal venous pressures are highest in the extremities (5–14 cm H_2O in the arm) and lowest closest to the heart (6–8 cm H_2O in the inferior vena cava).
   c. Factors that affect venous pressures
      (1) Blood volume: Decreased blood volume (e.g., due to hemorrhage) decreases venous pressure.
      (2) Tone of the vessel wall: Elastic vessels accommodate changes in blood flow, and rigid sclerotic vessels increase venous pressure.
      (3) Competence of valves: Incompetent valves, that is, those that allow blood to flow backward into the veins, increase venous pressure.

Definition/Purpose	To measure systolic and diastolic blood pressure.
Contraindication/Cautions	• For those who have had a unilateral mastectomy, blood pressure should not be measured on the affected side to avoid the possibility of lymphedema. For those who have had bilateral mastectomies, thigh readings should be taken.
	• For those who have renal dialysis catheters or shunts, blood pressures should not be measured on the extremity with the shunt.
Learning/Teaching Activities	As appropriate, discuss signs and symptoms of hypertension and the need for monitoring.

Preliminary Activities

Equipment	• Stethoscope
	• Mercury or aneroid sphygmomanometer
	• Appropriate-sized cuff—20 cm wider than the limb
Assessment Planning	• Identify normal blood pressure for the person.
	• Understand the reason for measuring blood pressure on this person (e.g., routine vital signs, postoperative care).
	• Be aware of the latest series of vital sign readings for this person and be cognizant of trends.
	• Postpone blood pressure reading for at least 10 minutes for a person who is angry or anxious, or who has just ambulated.
	• Postpone blood pressure reading on a crying infant or child.
	• Schedule frequency for obtaining blood pressure readings as determined by the person's condition and any physician's orders.
Procedure	

Actions	Rationale/Discussion
1. Whether the person is sitting or lying down, place the arm so that it is well supported and positioned at the level of the heart.	1. If the arm is above the level of the heart, a falsely low reading is produced. An arm below heart level produces falsely high readings.
2. Position yourself no more than 3 feet away from the sphygmomanometer, directly in front of the aneroid model, and at eye level with the meniscus of the mercury model. On a portable model, the mercury column should be vertical.	2. A position of more than 3 feet away produces inaccuracies. Looking up at the meniscus gives a falsely high reading. Looking down on the meniscus gives a falsely low reading. Tilting a portable mercury model gives a falsely high reading.
3. If using a mercury manometer, ensure that the level of mercury is at zero before cuff inflation.	3. This ensures proper calibration and an accurate reading.
4. Center the arrow marking on the cuff over the brachial artery, located at the medial side of the antecubital fossa (inner aspect of the elbow).	4. You must apply cuff pressure directly to the artery to occlude blood flow.
5. Expel any air in the cuff and wrap with lower edge 2.5 to 5 cm above the maximal brachial artery pulsation. Avoid contact with clothing. The cuff edge should be high enough to avoid covering the stethoscope.	5. An uneven or too loose cuff gives a falsely high reading because excessive amounts of pressure are needed to occlude the brachial artery. Accidental contact with clothing or tubing produces confusing extraneous noises.
6. Locate the brachial pulse and place the bell of the stethoscope over the artery using light pressure.	6. Heavy pressure may occlude the artery.
7. Palpate the radial artery (on flex or surface of wrist) and inflate the cuff 20 to 30 mm Hg above the point where the pulse disappears. (Systolic pressure is estimated to be the point where radial pulsation is no longer felt.)	7. Counterpressure occludes blood flow. If you do not inflate the cuff high enough, you may miss true systolic pressure. This is especially significant for the person who has an auscultatory gap. In contrast, inflating the cuff too high causes unnecessary pain.
8. Slowly deflate the cuff (by 2 to 3 mm Hg per second) and note the point where initial tapping is heard (systole) and when the tapping disappears (diastole).	8. Rapid cuff deflation may result in a falsely low reading, as initial sounds may be missed.

Final Activities

1. Document systolic and diastolic blood pressure.
2. Consider taking blood pressure in other limbs. Differences between arms and between arms and legs may have important diagnostic implications.

(4) Failure of the right side of the heart increases venous pressures.

■ *ASSESSING PEOPLE WITH CARDIOVASCULAR DISORDERS*

Key Symptoms and Their Pathophysiologic Bases

1. To determine the significance of symptoms, ask the following questions:
   a. Where did the symptom originate? Did it radiate? Where to?
   b. How long have you experienced the symptom? Was it of sudden or gradual onset?
   c. How much does the symptom bother you? Is it mild, moderate, or severe?
   d. Does any particular type of incident, episode, or activity bring on the symptom?
   e. What impact does the symptom have on your lifestyle?
   f. What activities or interventions (e.g., resting, medication) alleviate the symptom? What activities (e.g., exertion, deep breathing) aggravate it?
   g. What do you think is the cause of the symptom (e.g., heart attack, heartburn, indigestion)? See Chapter 2 for a discussion of patient's explanatory model.
2. Major symptoms in cardiovascular disorders include chest pain, dyspnea, and syncope (Table 23–1).

> The symptoms of cardiac disorders are related to 1 or all of these 3 physiologic disturbances: cardiac ischemia, pump insufficiency, and rhythm disturbance.

NURSE ADVISORY

> Absence of chest pain does not rule out a cardiac event.

a. Chest pain
   (1) Common descriptive phrases for chest pain are crushing, strange feeling, indigestion, dull heavy pressure or tightness, burning, constricting, aching, and stabbing or sharp. The classic description for ischemic or myocardial infarction (MI) pain is "an elephant sitting on my chest."
   (2) Pain typically radiates down the ulnar surface of the arm. It may radiate to the jaw, teeth, or neck; the left shoulder, arm, or elbow; both arms; or the back.
   (3) To note duration of pain, observe when chest pain begins and ends. Generally, the pain of an MI lasts longer than 1 hour or until interventions are

instituted. Conversely, anginal pain typically lasts less than 20 to 30 minutes and is relieved by rest.

NURSE ADVISORY

> To determine duration, instruct the person to note the time of onset of chest pain whenever possible.

   (4) To deduce severity of pain, ask the patient to rate the pain on a scale of 1 (least severe) to 10 (most severe). For example, the person may experience 10/10 pain upon admission and then experience 3/10 pain the following day.
   (5) Precipitating or aggravating factors include emotional excitement, temperature extremes, exertion, deep sleep, position changes, deep breathing, straining with defecation, and eating.

TRANSCULTURAL CONSIDERATIONS

> Causes or explanations for radiating pain are often called "malaise" in Hispanic groups, "wind" in Asian groups, and "gas" in Caribbean Black cultures.

   (6) Associated symptoms include anxiety, shortness of breath, nausea, diaphoresis, vertigo, and palpitations.
   (7) Alleviating factors include rest, sublingual nitroglycerin, oxygen, and change in position.

NURSE ADVISORY

> Pain that is not relieved with these interventions strongly suggests a myocardial infarction.

   (8) Chest pain occurs primarily in myocardial ischemia, MI, and pericarditis (see Chapter 37 for a table that compares selected cardiac conditions that are important in the assessment of chest pain).
b. Dyspnea (shortness of breath)
   (1) Dyspnea is labored or difficult breathing. It can stem from cardiac or respiratory problems. It may be a subjective feeling.
   (2) Types of dyspnea include orthopnea (breathing difficulties when lying flat in bed), paroxysmal nocturnal dyspnea (awakening at night with a sense of suffocation), and dyspnea on exertion (difficulty in breathing with minimal exercise).
   (3) Dyspnea associated with cardiac insufficiency may result from anxiety associated with pain, congestive heart failure, or resultant pulmonary edema.

Table 23–1. Cardiovascular Symptoms and Their Pathophysiologic Bases

Symptom	Pathophysiologic Basis
Chest pain	Ischemia to the myocardium
Shortness of breath (dyspnea)	Left ventricular failure causes damming up of blood behind the left ventricle. Increased pressure in pulmonary capillaries leads to fluid extravasation and pulmonary edema. Increased lung fluid leads to stiffer lungs and increased work of breathing.
Shortness of breath while sleeping that awakens the person (paroxysmal nocturnal dyspnea)	In the recumbent position, there is reduced pooling of blood in the lower extremities and abdomen. Venous blood return to the heart increases. Edema in the legs is slowly reabsorbed and increases blood volume. The failing left ventricle cannot pump the extra amount of volume effectively and fluid extravasation occurs in the lungs, leading to dyspnea. During sleep, there is decreased sympathetic stimulation and support to the heart, which depresses pumping ability and the respiratory center.
Dizzy or fainting spells (syncope)	Transient reduction of blood flow to the brain may be caused by several cardiac diseases. Cardiac dysrhythmias may cause a transient drop in cardiac output and decreased blood flow to the brain. Critical reduction of cardiac output due to obstruction of blood flow within the heart may be caused by aortic stenosis or hypertrophic obstructive cardiomyopathy.
Unexplained weakness or fatigue	Depressed cardiac output may cause poor perfusion of skeletal muscles, resulting in weakness or fatigue. Drug therapy such as β-blockers, excessive blood pressure reduction, excess diuresis, or diuretic-induced hypokalemia may also cause fatigue.
Weight loss or weight gain	Right ventricular failure causes damming up of blood behind the right ventricle. Increased systemic venous pressure causes fluid extravasation, leading to dependent edema and weight gain. Hepatic and intestinal edema may also occur, leading to anorexia, nausea, feelings of fullness, and thus weight loss.
Dependent edema	Right ventricular failure causes damming up of blood behind the right ventricle. Increased systemic venous pressure causes fluid extravasation and edema in the mobile person; it starts in the legs and, as it progresses, it ascends upward. In a bedridden person, the edema localizes in the sacral area.
A need to sleep on more than 1 pillow to breathe comfortably (orthopnea)	In the recumbent position, there is reduced pooling of blood in the lower extremities and abdomen and venous blood return to the heart increases. The failing left ventricle cannot pump the extra volume of blood effectively. Increased pressure in the pulmonary capillaries leads to fluid extravasation in the lungs and dyspnea.
Coughing at night	The mechanism leading to orthopnea, pulmonary congestion in the recumbent position, may lead to a nocturnal, nonproductive cough.
Coughing up blood	Severe congestion in pulmonary capillaries may allow red blood cells to leak into alveoli. Frothy, blood-tinged sputum then fills the airways.
Rapid heartbeat or palpitations	Palpitations may be caused by a change in the cardiac rhythm or rate, including tachycardias, premature beats, pauses, and sudden bradycardia.
A need to urinate several times during the night	A person with heart failure may have decreased urine output during the day due to redistribution of cardiac output away from the kidneys during activity. When the person rests at night, cardiac output to the kidneys increases, causing increased urine output at night.
Pain or cramps in the legs while walking that is relieved by rest (intermittent claudication)	Obstruction of arterial vessels in the legs causes decreased blood flow. During exercise, decreased blood flow decreases oxygen delivery to the muscles and slows the removal of metabolic wastes, such as lactic acid, from the muscle. Pain results from an accumulation of metabolic wastes in the muscle tissue.

(4) Dyspnea associated with an MI may indicate congestive heart failure.
 c. Syncope
  (1) Syncope is a transient loss of consciousness.
  (2) Causes of syncope
   • Decreased cardiac output related to heart rate (as in tachycardias, bradycardias, and heart blockages)
   • Decreased cardiac output related to obstruction (as in aortic stenosis, hypertropic cardiomyopathy, atrial myxoma, and pulmonary embolisms)
   • Systemic vascular problems (as in orthostatic hypotension, volume depletion, decreased vascular resistance, and vasovagal response)

Health History

1. Congenital abnormalities
   a. Congenital cardiac anomalies may cause symptoms including: dyspnea, severe fatigue, atrial and ventricular arrhythmias, congestive heart failure, and cyanosis (due to shunting).

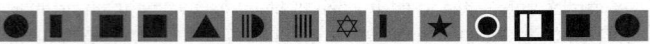

TRANSCULTURAL CONSIDERATIONS

Congenital disorders can be viewed as having supernatural causation—punishment of adults by inflicting illness upon the children. This belief can be found in Black, Appalachian, and Islamic health cultures.

   b. The most common congenital abnormalities seen in the adult are patent ductus arteriosus, atrial septal defect, ventricular septal defect, and pulmonic valvular stenosis.
   c. The patient may not be able to identify a congenital cardiac anomaly by name. Symptoms that may have been present since childhood and may be indicative of disorders include the following:
      (1) Shortness of breath (due to congestive heart failure)
      (2) Severe fatigue (due to hypotension or hypoxia)
      (3) Palpatations (due to arrhythmias)
      (4) Cyanosis (due to shunting)
2. Illnesses and hospitalizations that should be investigated include the following:
   a. Childhood and infectious diseases: Ask specifically about rheumatic fever and severe streptococcal infections, which can result in structural heart diseases, particularly valvular defects (see p. 1055 and Chapter 15).
   b. Diabetes mellitus
   c. Chronic obstructive pulmonary disease
   d. Kidney disease
   e. Anemia
   f. Hypertension
   g. Stroke
   h. Thrombophlebitis
   i. Collagen diseases
   j. Bleeding disorders
   k. Hospitalizations and operative procedures
3. Medical devices
   a. Ask whether the person has a permanent pacemaker.

If so, determine the date it was inserted, the type of pacemaker, and the reason for insertion.
   b. If an intrauterine device is in place, identify the type and date of its insertion.
4. Medications
   a. Ask the patient to list all medications being taken and note the dosage and times of administration.

   b. Ask specifically about cardiac prescription medications that affect the overall performance of the cardiovascular system including antihypertensives, diuretics, vasodilators, and cardiotonic drugs. Persons on digoxin should be carefully evaluated for signs and symptoms of digitalis toxicity.

   c. Ask about noncardiac prescription medications. They can have secondary effects on cardiovascular performance.
      (1) Tricyclic antidepressants and other psychotropic drugs may cause arrhythmias.
      (2) Oral contraceptives may increase the incidence of thrombophlebitis. The overall effect on coronary artery disease is under review, but it is believed that they increase the risk of MI by a minimum of 2-fold.
      (3) Steroids may increase fluid retention.
      (4) Bronchodilators may cause tachycardias and increase myocardial oxygen demand.
   d. Over-the-counter drugs such as aspirin (which may affect bleeding times) and cold remedies (which may include stimulants or sedatives) can affect cardiovascular function.

5. Risk factors
   a. Evaluate the patient for nonmodifiable risk factors.
      (1) Age: As a person ages, cardiovascular disorders increase, with the risk of coronary artery disease increasing significantly after age 45 years in men and age 55 years in women. Coronary artery disease in persons younger than 30 years of age is usually associated with hyperlipidemia, hypertension, and smoking.
      (2) Gender: Males have a higher risk of cardiovascular disease than women until women reach menopause.
      (3) Race: Blacks have a higher risk of death from cardiovascular diseases. Black males are 3 times more likely to die of strokes and twice as likely to die from coronary artery disease than White males.
      (4) Family history. Persons whose parents died of coronary artery disease have a 30 percent increase in risk of disease development before they are 60 years old.
   b. Evaluate the patient for modifiable risk factors.
      (1) Stress level: High stress levels are strongly correlated with cardiovascular symptoms and disorders (see Chapter 6).
      (2) Personality type: "Type A" lifestyles may be more vulnerable to the development of coronary artery disease. They are characterized by extreme competitiveness and aggression—the so-called fast-track lifestyle.
      (3) Level of exercise: Ask the person about the type and amount of exercise routinely engaged in during an average week. Routine aerobic exercise (15–20 min, 3 or 4 times a week) may decrease the likelihood of a coronary event. A sedentary lifestyle is considered a significant risk factor in the development of coronary artery disease.

ELDER ADVISORY

Cardiac improvement occurs at lower levels in older people. Walking for 30 minutes with a target heart rate of 100 beats per minute can have significant benefit.

      (4) Diet
         • Assess the patient for excess or deficit in caloric intake in relationship to the person's sex, height, weight, and age. Alterations in nutritional status such as obesity can increase risk of coronary artery disease.
         • Assess the patient for the approximate intake of foods high in sodium, cholesterol, and saturated fat content because these foods are closely linked to the development of atherosclerosis and hypertensive disease.
         • Examine the person's economic status, attitudes, and cultural beliefs toward food and resistance toward therapeutic alterations in diet.
      (5) Drug use and habits
         • Cigarette smoking significantly increases the risk of coronary artery disease and worsens hypertension. If the person smokes, determine the duration of this habit and the number of cigarettes smoked on a daily basis.
         • Assess the patient's intake of caffeine. Caffeine is a stimulant and can increase heart rate and blood pressure.
         • Excessive alcohol intake can have adverse effects on cardiovascular performance. If the person drinks alcoholic beverages, determine approximate daily and weekly alcohol consumption.
         • Assess the patient for use of illegal or recreational drugs, especially cocaine, which has significant cardiac effects.
      (6) Occupation: The patient's job may have an effect on stress level, sleep and wake patterns, and diet.
6. Psychosocial history (see Chapter 6)

Physical Examination

1. General assessment (see Chapter 5). Note the patient's general appearance. Does the person appear generally comfortable and healthy or in pain and uncomfortable?
2. Evaluate body posture and position.
   a. Does the person lie quietly in bed or is the person restless and moving about continuously, demonstrating signs of pain or hypoxia?
   b. What is the person's posture? Can the person lie flat in bed or tolerate only an upright or erect position reflective of dyspnea or pain?
   c. What is the facial expression? Are there grimaces of pain or obvious signs of respiratory distress?
3. Level of consciousness: Observe the person's general level of consciousness to assess adequacy of cerebral perfusion and oxygenation.
4. Level of anxiety: Monitor anxiety both as a possible symptom of hypoxia and for its effect on the cardiovascular system. Are there obvious signs of anxiety, fear, depression, or anger related to a cardiovascular complaint?
5. Assess the patient's physical characteristics
   a. Are there signs of significant cyanosis or pallor?
   b. Is there clubbing of fingers?
   c. Are there signs of peripheral edema? Is it pitting edema? To assess the edema, press on the skin of a dependent extremity (or the sacral area if the patient is bedridden) for 5 seconds and note the time for any indentation to disappear using the scale in Table 23–2.
   d. Is there jugular venous distention?

Table 23–2. Pitting Edema Rating Scale

0 =	None
+1 =	Minimal: rapidly resolves
+2 =	Moderate: resolves within 15–30 sec
+3 =	Deep: resolves within 1–2 min
+4 =	Very deep: still obvious after 5 min

6. Cardiac assessment
   a. Heart rate and rhythm: Evaluate and document apical rate and rhythm (see Chapter 5).
   b. Pulses
      (1) Evaluate and document pulses in all extremities.
      (2) Compare apical pulse rate with pulses in extremities.
      (3) Evaluate amplitude of pulses as follows:
         • 0 = not palpable
         • +1 = weak / faint
         • +2 = palpable / normal
         • +3 = bounding
      (4) Evaluate the character of the pulse (Fig. 23–4).
         • In pulsus alternans, rate is regular but pulse alternates in size or quality. It is seen in congestive heart failure.
         • In pulsus paradoxus, rate is regular, but the amplitude of the pulse decreases with inspiration and increases with expiration. It is seen in constrictive pericarditis, pericardial effusions, and severe chronic obstructive pulmonary disease.
      • In bigeminal pulse, a normal beat is followed by a premature contraction. The 2nd beat demonstrates decreased amplitude due to the reduced cardiac output of the ectopic beat.
      • In bounding pulse, there is a rapid upstroke and a fast downstroke. It is seen in anxiety, anemia, aortic regurgitation, and hypertension and in the elderly with arteriosclerosis.
      • In weak pulses, there is decreased pressure with a gradual upstroke and a prolonged downstroke. Weak pulse is seen in aortic stenosis and left ventricular failure.

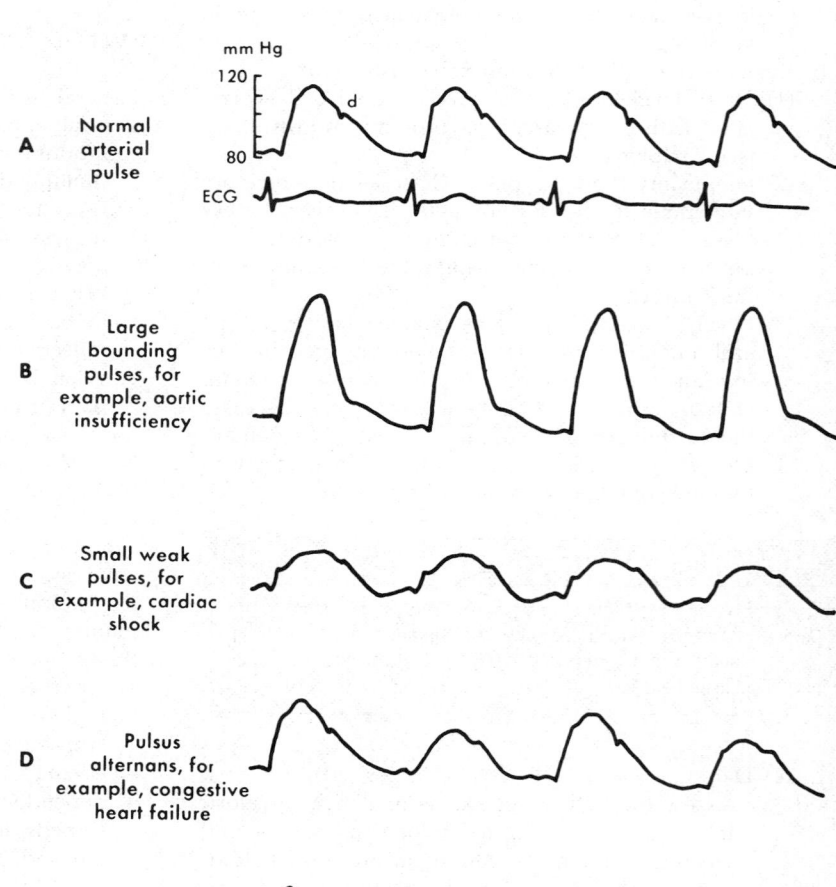

Figure 23–4. Characteristics of pulses. (From Kinney MR, and Packa DR. *Andreoli's Comprehensive Cardiac Care*. 8th ed. St. Louis: CV Mosby, 1996.)

CARDIAC AUSCULTATION SITES

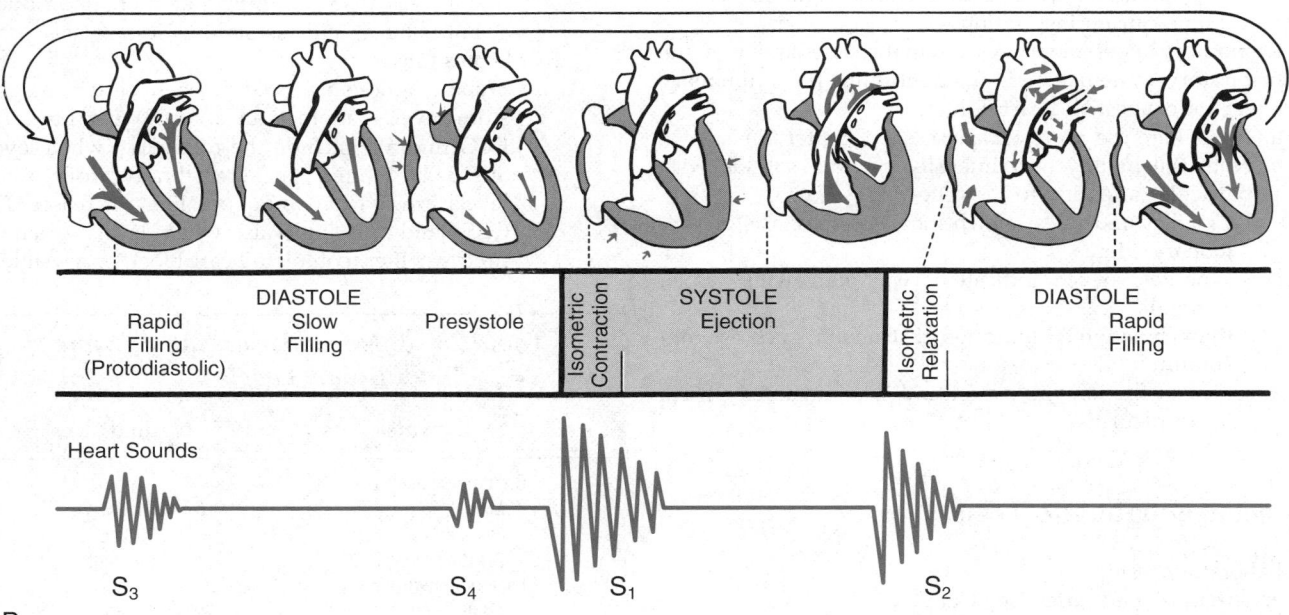

Aortic area

Pulmonic area

Third left interspace

Mitral area

Tricuspid area

A

Figure 23–5*A.*

Table 23–3. Intensity of Murmurs

Grade	Description
I	Difficult to hear, even with a stethoscope; very faint
II	Quiet, heard with a stethoscope
III	Moderately loud, no thrill
IV	Loud, may have a thrill
V	Very loud, can be heard with a stethoscope partially off the chest wall; has a thrill
VI	Can be heard with a stethoscope off the chest wall; has a thrill

c. Cardiac auscultation. At each of 5 locations (Fig. 23–5), evaluate the patient for the following:

(1) First heart sound (S_1): S_1 represents closure of mitral and tricuspid valves at systole.

(2) Second heart sound (S_2): S_2 represents closure of aortic and pulmonic valves at diastole.

(3) Extra systolic heart sounds
- A systolic click indicates mitral prolapse.
- Ejection sounds are characteristic of deformed semilunar valves.

(4) Extra diastolic heart sounds
- A 3rd heart sound (S_3) may occur early in diastole. Although it is normal in adolescents and children, it indicates myocardial failure in adults.
- A 4th heart sound (S_4) may occur late in diastole. It indicates hypertension, coronary artery disease, myocardiopathy, aortic stenosis, and MI.

(5) Systolic and diastolic murmurs: Describe murmurs in terms of their location, pitch, quality, intensity, and timing (Table 23–3).

(6) Extra cardiac sounds, such as pericardial friction rub, which is the sound of inflamed pericardial surfaces rubbing together

DIASTOLE			Isometric Contraction	SYSTOLE	Isometric Relaxation	DIASTOLE
Rapid Filling (Protodiastolic)	Slow Filling	Presystole		Ejection		Rapid Filling

Heart Sounds

S_3 S_4 S_1 S_2

B

Figure 23–5*B.* Heart sounds. (From Jarvis C. *Physical Examination and Health Assessment.* 2nd ed. Philadelphia: WB Saunders, 1996, p 519.)

d. Blood pressure: The most accurate arterial blood pressure reading is one that is taken while the individual is in a restful state, free of all stressful physical and emotional stimuli. The technique for measuring blood pressure at the brachial pulse site is described in Procedure 23–1.

NURSE ADVISORY

Some people are prone to "white coat hypertension," that is, hypertension that results from nervousness at having their blood pressure checked, especially by physicians. Ask "nervous" people to sit or lie quietly and to practice relaxed breathing for at least 15 minutes before blood pressure measurement.

---

(1) "Normal" blood pressure for adults younger than 50 years of age ranges from 100 to 140 mm Hg for systolic pressure, and from 60 to 95 mm Hg for diastolic pressure.
(2) Postural hypotension, a decrease in systolic blood pressure of more than 15 mm Hg and an increase in heart rate of more than 15 percent usually accompanied by dizziness and syncope, indicates volume depletion, inadequate vasoconstrictor mechanisms, and autonomic insufficiency. When changing positions from lying to sitting to standing, care must be taken to provide adequate support in case of symptomatic response such as lightheadedness and syncope.
(3) Pulsus paradoxus is an exaggeration of the normal decrease in blood pressure during inspiration, which reflects an impairment of venous return usually associated with chronic obstructive pulmonary disease, pericardial effusion, severe hypovolemia, pulmonary embolism with acute cor pulmonale, positive pressure ventilation, and cardiac tamponade that reduces left ventricular stroke volume during inspiration.

7. Respiratory assessment: A systematic assessment of the respiratory system assists in identifying the pulmonary effects of congestive heart failure.
   a. Auscultate the posterior chest (see Chapter 22).
   b. Note the quality and intensity of lung sounds with particular attention to the following:
      • Crackles and rales, which indicate atelectasis or pulmonary edema
      • Wheezes, which indicate airway narrowing (as in asthma)
      • Rhonchus, which indicates obstruction, such as from sputum
      • Pleural friction rub, which indicates inflamed pleura (as in pleuritis)

Special Diagnostic Tests

1. Laboratory tests
   a. Arterial blood gases (see Chapter 22)
   b. Cardiac enzymes

(1) Purpose: Cardiac enzymes are organ-specific enzymes that are present in high concentration in myocardial tissue. Myocardial tissue damage causes a release of enzymes from their intracellular storage areas. Drawing enzymes determines whether myocardial damage has occurred. The patterns and timing of elevations for each enzyme indicate the magnitude and timing of the injury.
(2) Procedure: Blood is drawn at prescribed intervals and analyzed for the presence of cardiac enzymes.
(3) Findings and results are listed in Table 23–4.
(4) Nursing interventions: Ensure that blood is drawn at specific time intervals as ordered.

c. Electrolyte assessment: Fluid and electrolytes are discussed in Chapter 9. Effective cardiac functioning requires that electrolyte levels remain within a narrow range. The major electrolytes that affect cardiac functioning are potassium, sodium, magnesium, and calcium.
(1) Potassium
   • Hyperkalemia occurs when plasma concentration is more than 5.0 mEq per liter. Electrocardiogram (ECG) findings include peaked T waves and shortened QT intervals when plasma concentrations reach 6 mEq per liter and widened QRS intervals, and progression to ventricular fibrillation or asystole when concentrations exceed 7 or 8 mEq per liter.
   • Hypokalemia occurs when plasma concentration is less than 2.5 mEq per liter. The ECG findings include a flat broad T wave, enlarged U wave, ST-segment depression, and progression to ventricular fibrillation.
(2) Sodium
   • Hypernatremia occurs when serum sodium level is more than 145 mEq per liter. It produces fluid overload and can precipitate heart failure.
   • Hyponatremia occurs when plasma concentration is less than 136 mEq per liter. It produces volume deficit and resultant tachycardias.
(3) Magnesium
   • Hypermagnesemia occurs when serum magnesium level is more than 2.1 mEq per liter. The ECG findings include the following: when levels are 3 to 5 mEq per liter, bradycardia; when levels are 5 to 10 mEq per liter, increased PR, QRS, and QT intervals; when levels reach 25 mEq per liter, complete heart block or asystole.

Table 23–4. Normal Cardiac Enzyme Blood Levels	
Enzyme	**Normal**
Creatine kinase	
Male	57–374 U/L
Female	35–230 U/L
Creatine kinase-MB	0–3 percent
Lactate dehydrogenase	
Adult	297–537 U/L

- Hypomagnesemia occurs when plasma concentration is less than 1.6 mEq per liter. The ECG findings include paroxysmal supraventricular tachycardia and ventricular irritability, including fibrillation.
(4) Calcium
- Hypercalcemia occurs when plasma concentration is more than 16 mg per 100 ml. The ECG findings include shortened QT interval, sagging ST segment, inverted T waves, and ventricular dysrhythmias.
- Hypocalcemia occurs when plasma concentration is less than 6.1 mg per 100 ml. The ECG findings include prolonged QT interval, increased ST segment, flat or inverted T wave, and various dysrhythmias.
2. Chest radiograph
   a. Purpose: A visual image is made of heart location and size, relative position of major vessels, presence of calcification, and lung fields, which may indicate congestion, pulmonary hypertension, or pleural effusion.
   b. Procedure: Films may be obtained with the patient in a variety of positions, either in the radiology department or at the bedside.
   c. Nursing interventions
      (1) Inform the patient about the procedure.
      (2) Assist the patient with positioning.
      (3) Ask female patients whether they are or might be pregnant.
3. Electrocardiogram
   a. An ECG provides a diagrammatic representation of the cardiac cycle by showing the electric activity of the myocardium (Fig. 23–6).
   b. Obtaining an ECG is done by placing electrodes on the extremities or the chest wall to provide a tracing that shows the transmission of the electric impulse through the conductive tissue of the heart. Recording the electric impulses of the heart from different positions, called leads, allows trained personnel to pinpoint cardiac pathology (Procedure 23–2). When the 6 limb leads and 6 chest leads are combined together, these recordings produce a 12-lead ECG (Fig. 23–7).
   c. Electrocardiogram waveforms
      (1) The P wave is a sinus node impulse and depolarization of the atria. Excitation of the cells results in atrial contraction.

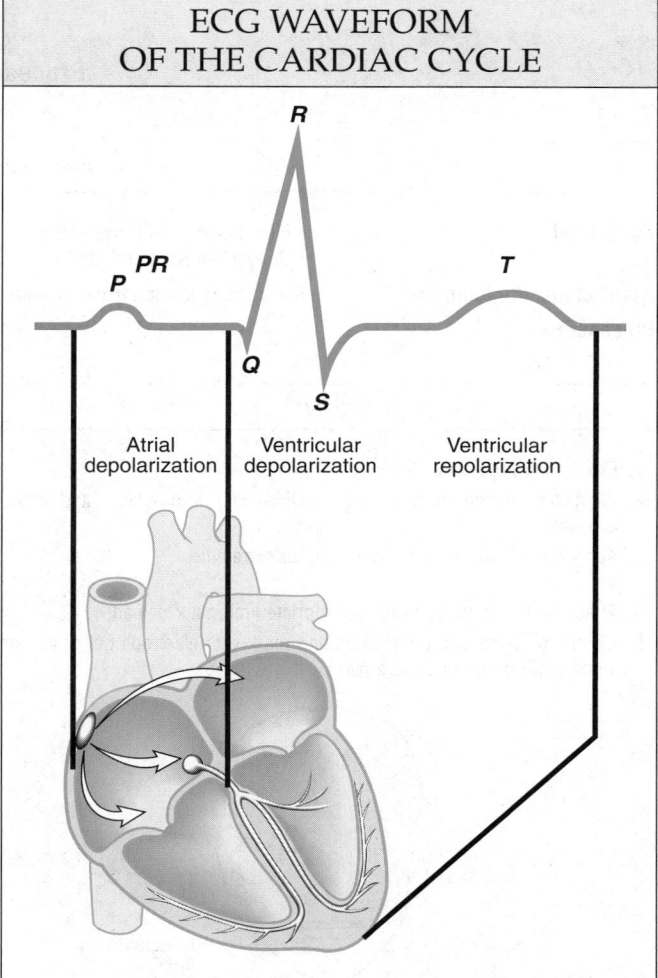

ECG WAVEFORM OF THE CARDIAC CYCLE

Figure 23–6.

(2) The PR interval is the time it takes an impulse to travel to the ventricles (normal duration = 0.12 → 0.20 second).
(3) The QRS complex is depolarization and contraction of ventricles (normal duration = 0.04 → 0.10 second).
(4) The ST segment is the time between the end of

![P]

Procedure 23–2
Taking a 12-Lead Electrocardiogram

Definition/Purpose	To obtain a record of cardiac electric activity. Provides identification of damaged areas of the myocardium, dysrhythmias, intraventricular conduction defects, and other abnormalities.
Contraindication/Cautions	None
Learning/Teaching Activities	Discuss the rationale for the procedure.

(continued)

Procedure 23–2

(continued)

Preliminary Activities

Equipment
- Electrocardiogram machine
- Conductive pads and plates

Assessment Planning Procedure

Know the rationale for the procedure.

Actions	Rationale/Discussion
1. Explain the procedure.	1. Ensures person's cooperation.
2. Place the person in a supine position with arms, legs, and chest exposed.	2. Allows access for lead placement.
3. Apply conductive pads or limb leads to extremities.	3. To minimize artifact—extraneous notations made by muscle twitching—choose a flat, nonbony site distal on the extremity.
4. Attach limb lead wires to the appropriate limb plate or pad.	4. Each wire is labeled and color coded for easy identification.
5. Identify placement of chest leads and mark with electrode gel or ink, or apply a prepared conductive pad.	5. A single-channel ECG machine has 1 chest lead that is moved across the chest as each lead is recorded. A multiple-channel ECG machine has 6 individual chest leads that are placed simultaneously on the chest. If the patient has large, pendulous breasts, the breasts may need to be positioned out of the way before electrode placement.

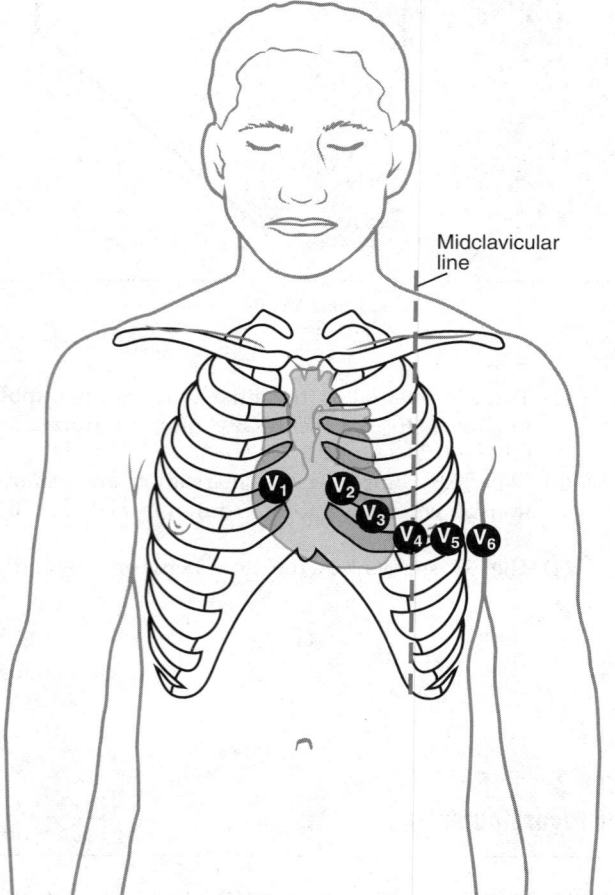

Midclavicular line

6. Drape all wires away from the chest.	6. This minimizes artifact. Otherwise, respirations may cause a wandering baseline.
7. Set paper speed at 25 mm per second and check deflection size by activating the standardization mechanism.	7. Deflection should be set at 10 mm for 1 mV or 10 small squares high on ECG paper.

P

Procedure 23-2

(continued)

Action	Rationale/Discussion
8. Turn on machine.	8. Power source may be battery or electric.

9. Record ECG tracing.
  a. If using a single-channel machine:
    (1) Set lead selector at "Lead I."
    (2) Turn on paper feeder.
    (3) Document lead being recorded by use of approved code or handwritten note on the ECG paper.
    (4) Record approximately 10 seconds of ECG.
    (5) Repeat procedure for each limb and chest lead.
  b. If using a multiple-channel machine:
    (1) Press "auto on" button and the machine automatically records and identifies each lead.
	9. Single-channel and multiple-channel ECG machines operate differently.

10. Turn off ECG machine.	10. Conserves power in battery-operated machines.
11. Remove completed ECG from the machine.	11. ECG recording is part of person's medical record.
12. Disconnect limb leads and chest electrodes.	12. Leads may be left in place briefly if multiple ECG recordings are needed.
13. Wipe skin with tissue or gauze to remove gel.	13. Gel is uncomfortable if left on person's skin.

Final Activities

1. Label ECG recording with name, medical record number, date, and time of recording.
2. Document completion of procedure in the person's record.
3. Document the presence of chest pain or respiratory difficulty during the procedure.
4. Ensure that ECG electrodes and limb straps and wires are cleaned before returning the machine.
5. If doing a 12-lead ECG for episode chest pain or if changes are noted in the rhythm strip, notify the physician at completion of the ECG.

depolarization and the start of repolarization—returning of the cells to a resting state—of the ventricles.

(5) The T wave is the recovery or repolarization phase of the ventricles.

  d. Electrocardiographic analysis

(1) An ECG should be analyzed in a systematic manner.

(2) Calculate heart rate by calculating the atrial rate (count P waves) and calculating the ventricular rate (count QRS complexes).

(3) Determine regularity of rhythm by evaluating the regularity of P waves (measure P to P intervals). Evaluate the regularity of QRS complexes (measure QRS to QRS intervals).

(4) Determine whether there is a P wave before each QRS complex.

(5) Determine whether the P waves and QRS complexes are identical and normal in configuration.

(6) Calculate the PR interval.

(7) Calculate the QRS interval.

(8) Identify the ST segment and T wave.

(9) Label the rhythm as sinus, atrial, junctional, or ventricular (see Types of Dysrhythmias).

  e. Continuous ECG monitoring is ongoing cardiac monitoring of the electric activity of the heart that provides immediate feedback regarding cardiac status.

  f. Exercise stress testing

(1) An ECG is done while the person is walking on a treadmill or riding a stationary bicycle for 30 to 60 minutes to determine how the heart reacts when it is forced to work harder under the stress of exercise. Exercise stress tests can detect and quantify the degree of ischemic heart disease, as well as a person's cardiovascular fitness before the start of an exercise program.

(2) Attach ECG electrodes and cables to monitoring equipment.

(3) Assist the patient onto the treadmill or bicycle and explain the safety features of the equipment.

(4) Monitor the patient for chest pain, leg cramps, shortness of breath, or dizziness while the patient walks or pedals as long and as hard as possible.

(5) Monitor vital signs, physical status, and ECG during the procedure. Particular emphasis should be given to ST elevation, ST depression, and dysrhythmias.

(6) When the person is too tired to continue or when

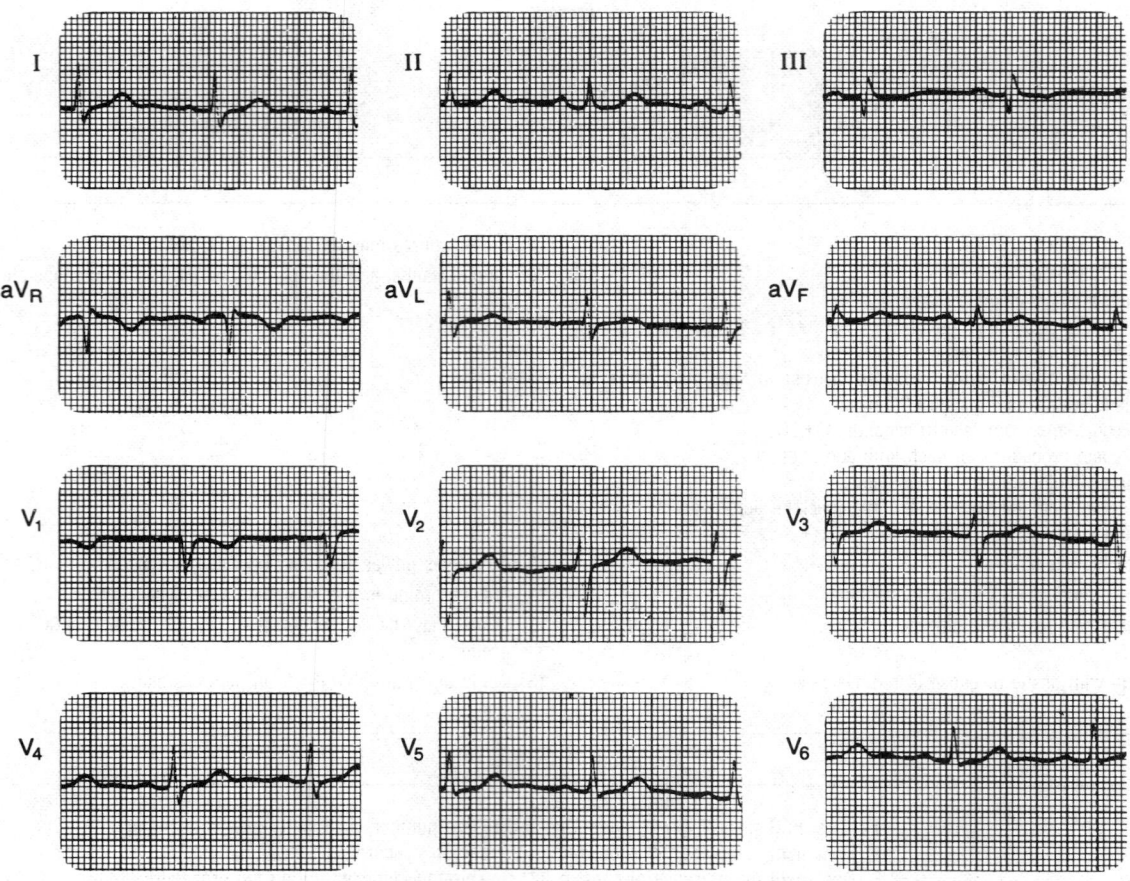

Figure 23–7. 12-lead electrocardiogram. (From Dolan JT. *Critical Care Nursing*. Philadelphia: FA Davis, 1991, p 803.)

significant symptoms or ECG changes occur, help the person to a resting area and continue to monitor the ECG and vital signs until they are stable.

NURSE ADVISORY

Contraindications for exercise stress testing include the following:
- Recent MI. However, a submaximal test may be performed in the first 4 to 6 weeks after the infarction.
- Rapid dysrhythmias
- Heart failure
- Severe aortic stenosis
- Hypertension before the start of the procedure
- Third-degree heart block

---

g. Persantine thallium stress test
   (1) Many patients are unable to walk on a treadmill or ride a stationary bicycle because of orthopedic problems, pulmonary disease, or peripheral vascular disease. The alternative is to perform pharmacologic stress testing using an intravenous coronary vasodilator such as Persantine to detect ischemic heart disease.
   (2) At the point of maximum vasodilation, thallium (a radionuclide used to determine the degree of myocardial perfusion) is injected.

   (3) The nuclear imaging thallium scan allows evaluation of underperfused tissue.
h. A signal-averaged electrocardiography tracing is analyzed using computer filters to critically evaluate the cardiac cycle, particularly the terminal portion of the QRS complex. The risk of sudden cardiac death from sustained ventricular tachycardia can then be determined.
i. Vectorcardiogram is a 3-dimensional ECG produced by placing 7 electrodes on the body. It is used for the following:
   (1) Evaluation of the state of the myocardium
   (2) Detection of exercise-induced ischemia
   (3) Detection and location of an MI
j. Ambulatory electrocardiography (Holter monitoring) is the continuous ECG monitoring of a person going about normal activities.
   (1) Patients wear a miniaturized single- or double-lead system attached to a belt or shoulder strap.
   (2) Patients record their activities, noting the time and any symptoms present.
   (3) Comparing the ECG record with the diary of activities documents rhythmic changes related to specific activities.
   (4) Ambulatory ECGs also help to diagnose dysrhythmias and evaluate the effectiveness of drug therapies.
4. Hemodynamic monitoring

P

Procedure 23-3
Drawing a Blood Sample from an Arterial Line

Definition/Purpose	To draw arterial blood samples for diagnostic testing.
Contraindication/Cautions	Procedure may dampen arterial waveform.
Learning/Teaching Activities	As appropriate, explain rationale for blood tests.

Preliminary Activities

Equipment	• Sterile syringes (one 5 ml for discard; one sized by amount of blood to be drawn) • Sterile stopcock cover • Sterile gauze pads • Blood tubes appropriate to tests ordered
Assessment Planning	• Evaluate arterial waveform. • Evaluate total blood volume requirement for tests ordered.

Procedure

Actions	Rationale/Discussion
1. Turn off monitor alarm.	1. Alarm will sound during procedure unless suspended.
2. Remove stopcock cap from blood drawing port at stopcock closest to insertion site.	2. Minimizes blood loss.
3. Wipe off stopcock with sterile swab.	3. Decreases risk of contamination.
4. Attach 5-ml sterile syringe to port.	4. Needed for removal of heparinized fluid.
5. Turn stopcock OFF to transducer.	5. Opens blood flow to syringe.
6. Allow 5 ml of blood to flow into syringe.	6. Allow blood to flow under the arterial pressure.
7. Turn stopcock OFF to blood drawing port.	7. Prevents blood loss through draw port that would dilute the sample.
8. Remove syringe and discard.	8. This blood includes heparinized flush solution.
9. Attach sterile syringe.	9. Size of syringe depends on amount of blood required.
10. Turn stopcock OFF to transducer.	10. Reopens blood flow to syringe while preventing blood from entering the transducer.
11. Collect blood amount required for testing.	11. This will vary based on test.
12. Turn stopcock OFF to blood drawing port.	12. Prevents blood loss through drawing port.
13. Remove syringe and fill blood tubes.	13. Vacutainer adaptors may be used instead of syringes.
14. Flush line and stopcock.	14. Replaces heparinized solution in line to maintain patency.
15. Clean stopcock with sterile gauze pad.	15. Dried blood can serve as a medium for infection.
16. Attach sterile stopcock cover.	16. Prevents contamination of line.
17. Turn on monitor alarm.	17. Ensures safe monitoring of person's blood pressure.

Final Activities

1. Recalibrate the arterial line.
2. Monitor arterial waveform.
3. Ensure that all connections are tight and stopcocks are in OFF position.

---

a. Arterial pressure measurement
   (1) Direct and continuous blood pressure is measured by placing an indwelling catheter into a major artery, allowing for accurate measurements, early recognition of blood pressure changes related to therapies or disease processes, and ease in obtaining blood samples (Procedure 23-3).

   (2) Complications include hemorrhage, hematoma at the insertion site, infection, false aneurysm, air embolism, and loss or diminished pulse distal to the insertion site.
   (3) Nursing interventions
      • Inform the patient about the procedure.
      • Determine whether circulation in the extremity

has been evaluated and documented before catheter insertion.
- Maintain aseptic technique during insertion of the catheter.
- Instruct the person to limit movement of the affected extremity and to monitor position.
- Change dressing and flush solution as required by policy.
- Ensure that all connections are tight to avoid blood loss or embolism.
- Observe the patient for signs of inflammation or infection.
- Calibrate and zero balance pressure monitoring system; monitor and record the systole, diastolic, and mean pressures by observing the digital readout of the monitor.

NURSE ADVISORY

> Intra-arterial pressure readings are at least 10 mm Hg higher than cuff blood pressure readings.

- Monitor waveform for signs of dampening.
- Keep high and low monitor alarms turned on and at set levels determined by policy.
b. Pulmonary artery pressure measurement (Box 23–1)
  (1) If a patient shows signs of altered ventricular function, a physician may insert a pulmonary artery catheter to allow monitoring of
  - Pulmonary arterial pressure—the result of right ventricular output and the vascular resistance in the pulmonary arterial system (normal peak systolic = 15–30 mm Hg/end diastolic = 3–12 mm Hg)
  - Pulmonary capillary wedge pressure—indirect measure of left atrial functioning (normal = 1–10 mm Hg)
  - Central venous pressure (CVP)—reflection of right ventricular filling pressure (normal = 0–8 mm Hg)
  - Cardiac output—indication of the pumping function of the heart (normal = 4–8 liters per minute)
  (2) Findings
  - Elevated pulmonary artery pressures result from an increase in pulmonary vascular resistance. This occurs in hypervolemia, pulmonary hyper-

tension, pneumothorax, hemothorax, mitral stenosis, left ventricular failure, and chronic obstructive pulmonary disease.
- Decreased pulmonary artery pressures result from a decrease in pulmonary vascular resistance. This occurs in hypovolemia and β_2-adrenergic stimulation.
  (3) Complications may include infection, pulmonary thromboembolism, pulmonary infarction, pulmonary artery rupture, catheter kinking, dysrhythmias, and air embolization.

NURSE ADVISORY

> When the balloon-tipped flow-directed pulmonary artery catheter passes through the ventricle, it may cause ventricular irritability. Although the irritability is usually transient and resolves spontaneously with the passage of the catheter, the nurse should be prepared to defibrillate if necessary.

  (4) Nursing interventions
  - Inform the patient about the procedure.
  - Maintain aseptic technique during insertion and change dressing and tubing according to hospital policy and procedure.
  - Monitor for and report any signs of infection such as pain, redness, drainage, swelling, or warmth.
  - Obtain readings at the level of the phlebostatic axis and report changes as appropriate.
c. Central venous pressure measurement: Monitoring CVP provides a direct reading of right atrial pressure as well as an indirect reading of right ventricular end-diastolic pressure. Central venous pressure measurements are indicated when there are anticipated disturbances in blood volume, venous tone, or right ventricular function (Fig. 23–8 and Procedure 23–4).

BOX 23–1. Indications for Insertion of a Pulmonary Artery Catheter

- Cardiogenic shock
- Complicated myocardial infarction
- Multisystem organ failure
- Sepsis
- Acute respiratory failure
- Severe multiple trauma
- Pulmonary contusion
- Perioperative monitoring of complex surgical patients

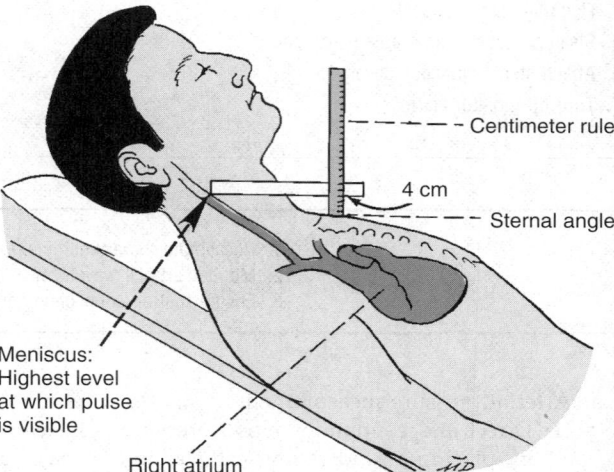

Figure 23–8. Estimating central venous pressure. (From Black JM, and Matassarin-Jacobs E [eds]. *Luckmann and Sorensen's Medical-Surgical Nursing: A Psychophysiologic Approach.* 4th ed. Philadelphia: WB Saunders, 1993, p 1113.)

Procedure 23-4
Taking a Central Venous Pressure Measurement

Definition/Purpose   To assess intravascular fluid status. To administer large volumes of fluids. To administer medications that irritate veins (e.g., potassium chloride, vasopressors, antibiotics, and total parenteral nutrition). When no other site is available, it may be used to draw blood samples.

Contraindication/Cautions   None, although it is important to remember that central venous pressure does not provide an accurate reflection of left ventricular function. Central venous pressure may remain normal until right ventricular dysfunction occurs.

Learning/Teaching Activities   As appropriate, discuss rationale for obtaining central venous pressure readings.

Preliminary Activities

Equipment
- Patent central venous line with connected intravenous setup
- Three-way stopcock
- Manometer

Assessment Planning
- Identify baseline vital signs.
- Know the reason for obtaining central venous pressure readings based on condition and physician orders.

Procedure

Actions	Rationale/Discussion
1. Check the patency of central venous pressure catheter.	1. Kinking of tubing gives a false reading.
2. Evaluate any drugs infusing into the main line.	2. Distribution of flow may affect status.
3. Place patient in a supine position with head of the bed flat. If this position is contraindicated, ensure that all central venous pressure readings are performed with the person in the same position.	3. The level of the person's head and the zero point must remain constant for readings to be reliable.
4. Locate and mark the zero point at the phlebostatic axis level of the right atrium (i.e., 4th intercostal space at the midclavicular line).	4. Measurements are made from this point.

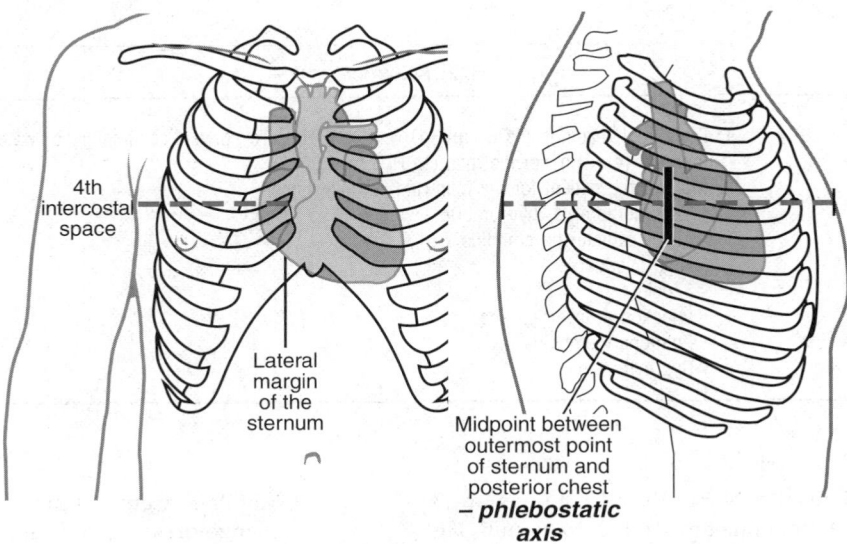

4th intercostal space

Lateral margin of the sternum

Midpoint between outermost point of sternum and posterior chest – *phlebostatic axis*

5. Using sterile technique, attach central venous pressure manometer to the 3-way stopcock so that intravenous fluid goes into the manometer. Close the port to the person. Fill the manometer to approximately 10 mm Hg above the expected reading.	5. Do not fill all the way to the top of the manometer to avoid risk of contamination.
6. To determine central venous pressure measurement, turn the stopcock so that fluid in the manometer runs into the person (the port to the intravenous fluid is closed). The fluid in the manometer decreases until its equilibrium levels with the right atrial pressure.	6. Fluid level fluctuates with the person's respirations because of changes in intrathoracic pressure.

(continued)

Procedure 23–4

(continued)

Actions	Rationale/Discussion
7. Obtain a central venous pressure reading during exhalation.	7. This is the point of lowest intrathoracic pressure.
8. After making the reading, close the port to the manometer, which opens the fluid to the person.	8. Maintains patency of line.
9. Trouble shooting	9. Approach to trouble shooting should be systematic.
a. Question any reading that varies greatly from previous readings.	
b. A high reading may be due to	
(1) Obstruction in the catheter.	(1) If fluid flow through the system is slow and obstruction is suspected, attempt to aspirate approximately 5 ml of blood from the catheter using a small-bore syringe. Discard blood. Then flush the line and measure the central venous pressure.
(2) Zero point too low	(2) Recalibrate.
(3) The person being restless, straining, or coughing	(3) Attempt to calm the patient. Wait until coughing subsides.
(4) The person needing suctioning or hyperventilating	(4) Check radiograph.
(5) Other factors:	(5) Discuss with the physician.
• Catheter is not in proper position.	
• There is volume overload.	
• The patient has chronic obstructive pulmonary disease.	
• The patient has right heart failure.	
• The patient has the cardinal sign of pericardial tamponade.	
• Mechanical ventilation is in progress.	
c. Low reading may be due to:	
(1) Zero point too high	(1) Recalibrate.
(2) Loose or disconnected tubing	(2) Tighten all connections.
(3) Other factors:	(3) Discuss with the physician.
• Volume depletion	
• Hemorrhage	
• Vasodilation	
• Increased contractility of the heart	

Final Activities

1. Document readings (1.36 cm H_2O = 1 mm Hg). To convert centimeters of water (cm H_2O) to millimeters of mercury (mm Hg), divide total cm H_2O by 1.36.
2. Monitor the patient for the following complications:
   • Pneumothorax or hydrothorax
   • Air or catheter tip embolus
   • Fluid overload
   • Sepsis
   • Infection at insertion site
   • Pulmonary embolus
   • Dysrhythmias

---

(1) Findings and results: Normal CVP readings are 3 to 8 cm H_2O (manometer) and 2 to 6 mm Hg (pressure transducer).

(2) Complications include pneumothorax, hemorrhage, hematoma at the insertion site, infection, air embolism, perforation of the right ventricle, and migration of the catheter into the right ventricle, causing ectopy.

(3) Nursing interventions
   • Inform the patient about the procedure and its purpose.

• Maintain aseptic technique during insertion and change dressing and tubing according to hospital policy and protocol.
• Ensure that all connections are tight to avoid blood loss or air embolus.
• Monitor for and report any signs of infection such as pain, redness, drainage, swelling, or warmth.

5. Cardiac catheterization and coronary angiography
   a. Cardiac catheterization is used most often to refer to the combined procedures of cardiac catheterization and coronary angiography (arteriography).

b. Cardiac catheterization uses a radiopaque catheter inserted into the chambers of the heart to evaluate ventricular function and wall motion and to obtain chamber pressures.

c. Coronary angiography involves the injection of contrast media into the coronary vessels to determine blood flow (Procedure 23–5).

6. Electrophysiologic studies
   a. Electrophysiologic studies are similar to cardiac catheterization in the right side of the heart and are used to do the following:
      (1) Evaluate for cardiac etiology of syncope
      (2) Measure conduction intervals
      (3) Localize disturbances in the atrioventricular conduction system
      (4) Localize ectopic foci
      (5) Evaluate antiarrhythmic treatment modalities
   b. Types of electrophysiologic studies
      (1) Bundle of His electrography in which an electrode-tipped catheter is inserted into the heart to record the electric activity of the conduction system.
      (2) Ventricular mapping (programmed electric stimulation) in which up to 6 electrode-tipped catheters are inserted into the heart. The conduction system is stimulated by pacing or drugs to induce and document dysrhythmias. Once the dysrhythmia is identified and localized, the effectiveness of pharmacologic and nonpharmacologic (implantable defibrillator or pacemaker) measures is determined.
   c. Postprocedure care is similar to that provided after cardiac catheterization.

d. Complications include dysrythmias, which may require defibrillation, hemorrhage at the catheter site, thrombolitic or pulmonary emboli, puncture of vessel or myocardium, infection, and pneumothorax.

e. Nursing interventions
   (1) Provide the person with accurate and understandable information about the purpose and procedure. Review the need for complete cooperation during the procedure, particularly regarding coughing to terminate arrythmias.
   (2) Make a complete nursing assessment with particular attention to pulses and allergies.
   (3) Ensure that foods and fluids are restricted for 6 to 12 hours before the procedure.
   (4) Provide psychologic support and monitor for complications during and after procedure.
   (5) Provide instructions regarding immediate postprocedure immobility.
   (6) Provide discharge teaching based on findings and planned interventions.

7. Magnetic resonance imaging (MRI)
   a. A noninvasive technology, MRI is used for evaluation of cardiac anatomy and function.
   b. The MRI uses a strong magnetic field and radio waves to detect differences between healthy and diseased tissues.
   c. Because MRI provides a 3-dimensional image, it can show the heart beating and the blood flowing.
   d. Because this test uses a strong magnet, patients should be evaluated to ensure the following:
      (1) They are wearing comfortable clothes or a hospital

Table 23–5. Other Assessment Techniques

	Echocardiography	Transesophageal Echocardiogram	Phonocardiography
Method	Uses high-frequency sound waves to visualize cardiac structures	A specialized form of echocardiogram that uses a transesophageal probe	Records heart sounds using • A microphone and pulse waves vs time • Microphones placed at the base or apex of the heart • ECG leads or echocardiography
Purpose	Noninvasive assessment for • Dimensions of ventricles • Size and motion of intraventricular septum • Left ventricle wall motion • Valve anatomy and motion • Blood flow characteristics • Evidence of pericardial fluid, tumors, blood clots	To visualize cardiac structures from the perspective of the esophagus and stomach	Examination of the timing of sounds assists in diagnosing and differentiating among heart sounds and murmurs
Complications	None	Vomiting, aspiration, and esophageal bleeding or rupture	None
Nursing Responsibilities*	Instruct persons that they may feel some discomfort from the level of pressure used in holding the transducer against the chest wall.	• Give nothing by mouth at least 4 hours before procedure. • Position the patient to maintain the airway. • Monitor for vomiting, effects of sedation	Instruct persons that they may feel some discomfort from the level of pressure used in holding the transducer against the chest wall.

* In all cases, explain the procedure and determine whether consent is signed.

P

Procedure 23-5
Cardiac Catheterization

Definition/Purpose

Cardiac catheterization provides a precise evaluation of the cause, severity, and prognosis of cardiac disease. It provides physiologic data regarding the following:
- Cardiovascular hemodynamics
- Anatomy of coronary arteries, vessels, and chambers
- Ventricular function and wall thickness
- Cardiac output
- Oxygen saturations within chambers
- Gradients across cardiac valves

Contraindication/Cautions

Serious complications occur in approximately one in every 1000 catheterizations. Major complications resulting from cardiac catheterization include the following:
- Allergic reaction to contrast media
- Occlusion of access artery with loss of peripheral pulse. This may lead to loss of limb.
- Hemorrhage at insertion site
- Stroke
- Myocardial infarction
- Myocardial perforation or rupture
- Ventricular fibrillation
- Death

Learning/Teaching Activities

- Inform the patient about the procedure.
- If possible, allow the patient to tour the catheterization laboratory.
- Provide written materials as available.
- Teach relaxation techniques such as breathing exercises and guided imagery.

Preliminary Activities

Assessment Planning

- Obtain chest radiograph.
- Obtain laboratory tests, including hemoglobin, hematocrit, complete blood count (with differentials), and urinalysis.
- Obtain ECG.
- Provide nothing by mouth for 8 to 12 hours before the procedure.
- Determine that the person's bladder is empty.
- Premedicate the patient as ordered.
- Evaluate the emotional state and level of understanding regarding the procedure.
- Determine whether the patient has any allergies or hypersensitivities to shellfish, iodine, or contrast media.

Procedure

Actions	Rationale/Discussion
1. Wash (may include antimicrobial scrub) and shave the catheter site.	1. Proper site preparation reduces infection risk.
2. Inject the catheter site with local anesthetic.	2. Allows for pain free catheter insertion.
3. A radiopaque catheter is inserted into the heart using direct exposure of a vein and artery (usually the brachial artery and basilic vein) or by the percutaneous Seldinger technique (usually the femoral artery and vein).	3. Site selection is influenced by person's vascular condition.
4. The catheter is advanced while taking blood samples and hemodynamic measurements through the vena cava into the right atrium, right ventricle, pulmonary artery, and distal pulmonary vessel.	4. Serial blood samples are used in the diagnostic process.
5. For left heart catheterization, the right heart catheter may be left in place so that simultaneous waveform readings can be obtained.	5. Simultaneous waveform readings are also used diagnostically.
6. Blood samples may be taken as the catheter is removed to evaluate for the presence of left-to-right shunts.	6. Septal defects may cause a left to right shunt.
7. When catheters are withdrawn, apply 20 minutes of direct pressure then place a pressurized dressing over the puncture sites.	7. Person is at risk for hemorrhage.
8. Continue to provide emotional and psychological support.	8. Cardiac catheterization is an invasive procedure and may be frightening to the person.

P

Procedure 23–5

(continued)

Final Activities

1. Monitor the patient's vital signs every 15 minutes for 2 hours, then every 30 minutes for 1 hour, and then 1 hour for 3 hours or until they are stable.
   - A mild sinus tachycardia (100 to 200 beats per minute) is not unusual due to anxiety, fluid loss, or medications. Evaluate heart rates of more than 120 beats per minute for other causes.
   - Obtain an ECG to identify bradycardia: correlate ECG findings with blood pressure.
   - Paradoxical pulses may indicate pericardial tamponade related to perforation. Assess the patient for paradoxical pulses with each blood pressure reading.
   - Contrast media acts as an osmotic diuretic. Monitor the patient for signs of volume depletion such as orthostatic hypotension and tachycardia.
   - Hypotension (70–80% of baseline) indicates the need to evaluate for hemorrhage.
2. Check the catheterization site for bleeding, hematoma, and swelling, and the circulatory status of the limb every 30 minutes for 3 hours, then every hour for 3 hours.
3. Notify the physician of any of the following:
   - Chest pain
   - Hematoma
   - Decreased or absent pulses
   - Heart rate greater than 120 beats per minute
   - Blood pressure of less than 90 mm Hg
   - Temperature greater than 38 degrees Celsius (100.4 degrees Fahrenheit)
   - Bleeding
4. Medicate the patient as needed.
5. Maintain the patient on bed rest for 2 to 3 hours for the brachial approach and 6 to 8 hours for the femoral approach. Keep the head of the bed at less than a 45-degree angle.
6. Instruct the person not to bend or hyperextend the affected limb for 24 hours with the brachial approach or 2 to 3 hours for the femoral approach.

---

gown without any metal on them (e.g., zippers, snaps).
   (2) They have removed all jewelry, watches, hairpins, clips, barrettes, wigs, and removable dental work before the test.
   (3) They have no metal prostheses, implants, plates, pacemaker, aneurysm clips, or metal fragments anywhere in the body.
e. Because the test requires patients to lie still in a highly enclosed environment for 45 to 60 minutes,
   (1) Ask if they are claustrophobic and arrange sedation if necessary.
   (2) Assure them that very loud buzzing and thumping noises are normal during the test. Ear plugs may be offered.
   (3) Arrange to have a family member present if the patient is too apprehensive.
f. Nursing interventions
   (1) Provide the person with accurate and understandable information about the procedure and its purpose.
   (2) If the patient is female, inquire whether she is or might be pregnant if MRI is contraindicated in pregnancy.
8. Radioisotope evaluation
a. Radioisotope evaluation is a group of tests that pro-

vide qualitative and quantitative evaluation of cardiac functioning and perfusion. Tracking and measuring the intravenously administered radionuclide with a noninvasive cardiac scanner enables areas of fibrosis (caused by an old MI) as well as poor or no perfusion to be identified.
b. Thallium 201 imaging ("cold spot" or "cold spotting")
   (1) Areas of poor uptake of thallium 201 are shown on the computer image as dark or "cold" spots.
   (2) Imaging evaluates myocardial blood flow and determines the status of myocardial cells as in infarction and transient ischemia.
c. Technetium 99m pyrophosphate heart scan ("hot spot" or "hot spotting")
   (1) Normal myocardial tissue does not take up this isotope. Necrotic tissue does and is seen on the scan as a "hot spot."
   (2) Technetium 99m pyrophosphate scanning is used to identify the extent of myocardial damage in the peri-infarct period (until 1 week after infarct), determine the age of infarction, evaluate the patency of bypass grafts, and evaluate the effectiveness of balloon angioplasty.
d. Blood pool scanning (imaging)
   (1) Blood pool scanning, also called radionuclide angiography, involves isotopes that stay in the

Text continued on page 1008

Table 23–6. Dysrhythmias

Type of Dysrhythmia	Characteristics	Etiology	Clinical Manifestations	Complications/ Implications	Intervention
Atrial Origin					
Atrial fibrillation	Atrial rate: Multiple foci → 350 bpm Ventricular rate: 120–200 bpm Rhythm: irregular P waves: replaced by fibrillatory waves PR interval: irregular QRS complex: normal	Increased vagal tone Digoxin effect	None	Rate dependent Congestive heart failure	American Heart Association tachycardia algorithm Cardioversion
Atrial flutter	Atrial rate: 250–350 bpm Ventricular rate: 2:1/3:1 block P waves: replaced by flutter waves PR interval: irregular QRS complex: normal PP interval: none RR interval: varies by degrees of block	Coronary artery disease Rheumatic heart disease	Angina Hypotension Shock	Rate dependent May lead to congestive heart failure within minutes with a 1:1 conduction	American Heart Association tachycardia algorithm Carotid sinus massage
Paroxysmal supraventricular tachycardia	Rate: 150–200 bpm Rhythm: regular P waves: abnormal, may be buried in preceding T wave PR interval: short <0.12 sec QRS complex: usually normal	Not usually indicative of organic heart disease Most common in young adults due to emotional upset or stimulants such as Tobacco Caffeine Alcohol Sympathomimetics	Chest pain Shortness of breath Hypotension Diaphoresis	Dependent on rate and duration Syncope Congestive heart failure	If stable, rest and consider sedation Eliminate cause American Heart Association tachycardia algorithm
Premature atrial contraction	Rate: varies by number of premature atrial contractions Rhythm: irregular P waves: different configurations PR interval: normal, prolonged or blocked QRS complex: may be aberrant	Ischemia of SA node Electrolyte imbalance Atrial infarction	Usually none	Dependent on frequency	Usually none

		Signs and Symptoms	Complications	Treatment
First-degree AV Block	Rate: normal Rhythm: regular P waves: precedes each QRS complex PR interval: > 0.20 QRS complex: normal Conduction: delay at AV node P-P interval: regular R-R interval: regular	Increased vagal tone Digoxin effect Coronary artery disease	None	Can progress to higher levels of block	If digoxin effect, discontinue Monitor for progress
Mobitz Type I Wenckebach	Rate: atrial rate greater than ventricular rate P waves: one or more p waves precede QRS complex PR interval: progressive prolongation until one impulse is blocked QRS complex: normal when present Conduction: progressive delay through AV node PP interval: regular RR interval: shortens until one QRS complex is missed	Coronary artery disease Digitalis toxicity Rheumatic fever Viral infection Myocardial infarction, usually inferior wall	Rate dependent—see Sinus Bradycardia	Rate dependent—see Sinus Bradycardia May progress to third-degree heart block	If asymptomatic, monitor for progression If symptomatic: Correct underlying cause Increase rate to maintain effective cardiac output American Heart Association bradycardia algorithm
Mobitz Type II	Rate: atrial rate greater than ventricular rate P waves: usually 2 or 3 waves precede QRS complex PR interval: constant when QRS is present QRS complex: normal or slightly prolonged Conduction: impulse is blocked below the AV node PP interval: regular RR interval: varies	Anterior wall myocardial infarction Response to digitalis and/or quinidine Ischemia	Rate dependent—see Sinus Bradycardia	Rate dependent—see Sinus Bradycardia	Pacemaker American Heart Association bradycardia algorithm
Third-degree heart block	Rate: usually 60–90 bpm Ventricular rate: usually 30–40 bpm PR interval: atria and ventricle are beating independently QRS complex: normal or widened Conduction: failure of AV node to conduct impulses PP interval: usually regular RR interval: usually regular	Coronary artery disease Fibrosis of conduction system Toxic response to Digitalis Procainamide Verapamil Quinidine Myocardial infarction	Angina Hypotension Syncope	Potentially lethal dysrhythmia Cardiopulmonary arrest Congestive heart failure	Pacemaker American Heart Association bradycardia algorithm

Table continued on following page

Table 23–6. Dysrhythmias (Continued)

Type of Dysrhythmia	Characteristics	Etiology	Clinical Manifestations	Complications/Implications	Intervention
Junctional (Nodal) Origin					
Junctional escape rhythm	Rate: <60 bpm Rhythm: irregular P waves: present PR interval: <0.11 sec or absent QRS complex: normal or aberrant	Digitalis toxicity Ischemia of AV node Complete heart block	Chest pain Shortness of breath Hypotension Decreased level of consciousness Congestive heart failure Premature ventricular contractions Escape rhythms	Myocardial ischemia Congestive heart failure	If toxic, discontinue drug American Heart Association bradycardia algorithm Pacemaker
Premature junctional contraction	Rate: varies by number of premature ventricular contractions Rhythm: irregular P waves: retrograde conduction may cause negative or inverted P waves PR interval: usually less than 0.12 sec QRS complex: may vary	Digitalis toxicity Ischemia of AV node	Usually none	Dependent on frequency	If toxic, discontinue drug
Sinus Origin					
Sinus bradycardia	Rate: <60 bpm Rhythm: regular P waves: precede each QRS complex PR interval: normal QRS complex: normal	Increased parasympathetic tone Digitalis toxicity Increased intracranial pressure Hypothermia Anorexia nervosa Hypoendocrine states: Addison's disease Hypopituitarism Myxedema Physical conditioning Decreased blood flow or damage to the SA node	Chest pain Shortness of breath Hypotension Decreased level of consciousness Congestive heart failure Premature ventricular contractions Escape rhythms	None unless rate results in decreased cardiac output In the setting of an acute MI, can deteriorate into serious dysrythmias such as third-degree heart block	American Heart Association bradycardia algorithm Pacemaker

Dysrhythmia	ECG Characteristics	Causes	Clinical Manifestations	Complications	Treatment
Sinus tachycardia	Rate: 100–160 bpm P waves: precede each QRS PR interval: varies with rate	Exercise Anxiety Fever Pain Hypovolemia Shock Anemia Congestive heart failure Sympathomimetic/parasympatholytic drugs	Chest pain Shortness of breath Diaphoresis Hypotension	Rate dependent Congestive heart failure Syncope	Cardioversion (see Procedure 23–7) American Heart Association tachycardia algorithm
Sinus dysrhythmia	Rate: 60–100 bpm Increases with inspiration Decreases with expiration P waves: precede each QRS PR intervals: normal QRS complex: usually normal Conduction: usually normal	Normal phenomenon	Usually none	None	None
Ventricular Origin					
Premature ventricular contraction	Rate: varies by number of premature ventricular contractions Rhythm: irregular, most premature ventricular contractions are followed by a compensatory pause that allows the atria to reset P waves: normal or retrograde PR interval: varies QRS complex: abnormal, wide	Myocardial ischemia or infarct Digitalis toxicity Electrolyte imbalance	Rate dependent	Can progress to ventricular tachycardia or ventricular fibrillation	In digitalis toxicity, discontinue drug Atropine or pacemaker if due to bradycardia Correct electrolyte imbalance American Heart Association tachycardia algorithm
Ventricular fibrillation	Rate: quivering heart Rhythm: absent P waves: none PR interval: none QRS complex: none	Ischemia Trauma Electrocution Drug toxicity Electrolyte imbalance	Rapid onset of unconsciousness	Cardiopulmonary arrest	Early recognition Early defibrillation Early CPR American Heart Association ventricular fibrillation algorithm
Ventricular tachycardia	Atrial rate: normal Ventricular rate: >100 bpm Rhythm: varies P waves: usually absent QRS complex: wide (>0.12 sec) and bizarre	Myocardial irritability Congestive heart failure Acute MI Arthrosclerotic heart disease Digitalis toxicity Drug reaction Quinidine Procainamide Disopyramide	Varies by rate and duration Chest pain Shortness of breath Hypotension	Can lead to cardiopulmonary arrest	American Heart Association ventricular tachycardia algorithm Cardioversion

bloodstream and are not picked up by the myocardium.
    (2) These studies, including multiple-gated acquisition (MUGA) scan, evaluate left ventricular function and produce an estimate of ejected fraction.
  e. Positron emission tomography
    (1) Metabolic activity of the heart is determined by the uptake of different radioactive positron-emitting substances.
    (2) It is used to assess myocardial perfusion and metabolism, particularly when revascularization procedures such as pulmonary transluminal coronary angioplasty are being considered.

NURSE ADVISORY

Due to the short half-lives of these radioisotopes, there is no need for isolation or special precautions for disposal of urine.

---

9. Other assessment techniques are listed in Table 23–5.

◨ DYSRHYTHMIAS

Overview

1. Definitions
  a. A dysrhythmia (arrhythmia) is a disturbance in the electric cycle of the heart.
  b. Asystole is the absence of all myocardial electric activity.
2. Incidence and socioeconomic impact
  a. Approximately 90 percent of persons who have an acute MI experience dysrhythmias.
  b. Thirty to 60 percent of deaths from coronary artery disease result from ventricular fibrillation.
3. Risk factors
  a. Coronary artery disease
  b. Electrolyte imbalances
  c. Stress
  d. Congenital anomalies
  e. Substance abuse (smoking, alcohol, drugs, caffeine)

Types of Dysrhythmias

1. See Table 23–6 for key data on the most common dysrhythmias (Fig. 23–9).
2. Atrial origin
  a. Atrial fibrillation is the disorganized twitching of the atria at a rate greater than 350 beats per minute. Ventricular response is varied and irregular because only a percentage of atrial impulses are conducted. Rates can achieve 120 to 200 beats per minute. P waves are replaced by fibrillatory (F) waves, which are of varied configurations because they arise from different atrial foci.
  b. Atrial flutter is a single atrial ectopic focus firing at a rate of 250 to 350 beats per minute resulting in a

ventricular response that is slower, usually a multiple of the atrial rate. P waves are replaced by flutter waves that take on a "sawtooth" appearance. Atrioventricular node usually blocks some impulses. The most common block is 2:1. Blocks can be at a fixed rate (e.g., 2:1, 3:1) or at a variable rate.
  c. Paroxysmal supraventricular tachycardia occurs as the following rapid rhythms originating in the atria:
    (1) Paroxysmal atrial tachycardia
    (2) Multifocal atrial tachycardia
    (3) Wolff-Parkinson-White
  d. Premature atrial contraction is an ectopic beat originating from a site in the atria outside of the normal cardiac cycle.
3. Conduction origin: Atrioventricular or sinus exit blocks are categorized into 3 levels:
  a. First-degree atrioventricular block is a slight delay of the electric impulse through the sinoatrial node.
  b. Second-degree atrioventricular block occurs when some, but not all, atrial impulses are conducted through the atrioventricular node.
    (1) Mobitz type I block (Wenckebach's phenomenon) is the most common form of 2nd-degree atrioventricular block in which there is a cyclic prolongation of the P-R interval until a P wave is finally blocked completely.
    (2) Mobitz type II block is a less common but more serious block in which occasional P waves are completely blocked at the atrioventricular node. It is often followed by complete heart block.
  c. Third-degree atrioventricular block is a complete block between the atria and ventricles. The sinoatrial node continues to pace the atria, while an escape focus within the atrioventricular node (idionodal pacemaker) or ventricular muscle (idioventricular pacemaker) controls the ventricular rate.
4. Junctional origin
  a. Junctional (nodal) rhythms
    (1) Junctional escape rhythm occurs when the atrial rate is slow, usually less than 30 beats per minute, and the atrioventricular node assumes responsibility for pacing the heart at a rate of 35 to 60 beats per minute.
    (2) Junctional tachycardia occurs when the atrioventricular node becomes irritable and "overrides" the sinus impulse, becoming the primary pacemaker at a rate of greater than 60 beats per minute.
  b. Premature junctional contraction occurs when an ectopic beat originates from a site in the atrioventricular junction (node) outside of the normal cardiac cycle.
5. Sinus origin
  a. In sinus bradycardia, a heart rhythm is initiated in the sinoatrial node at a rate of less than 60 beats per minute.
  b. In sinus tachycardia, a heart rhythm is initiated in the sinoatrial node at a rate greater than 100 beats per minute.
  c. Sinus arrhythmia is a normal phenomenon in children and older persons, as well as in those with slow heart rates and those with increased vagal tone. It relates to the effect of respiration on the rate of vagus nerve

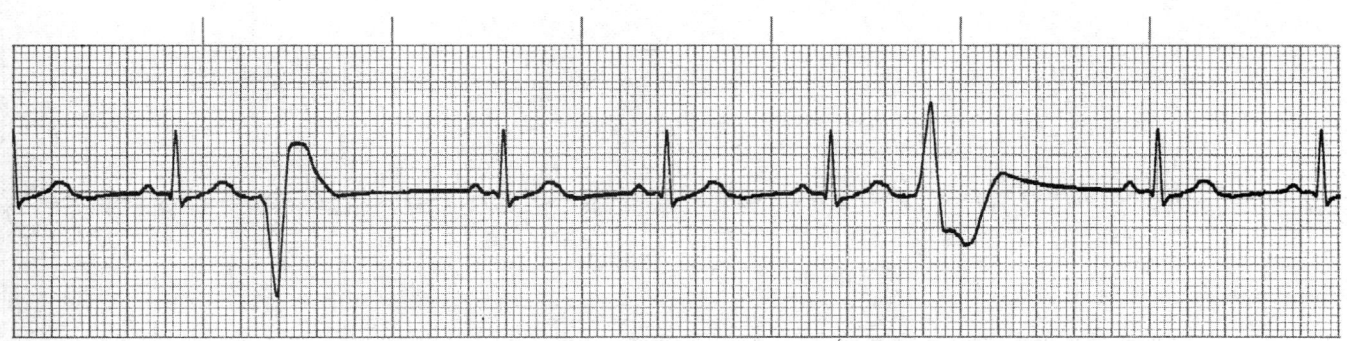

A Premature ventricular contractions—note wide and bizarre QRS complexes

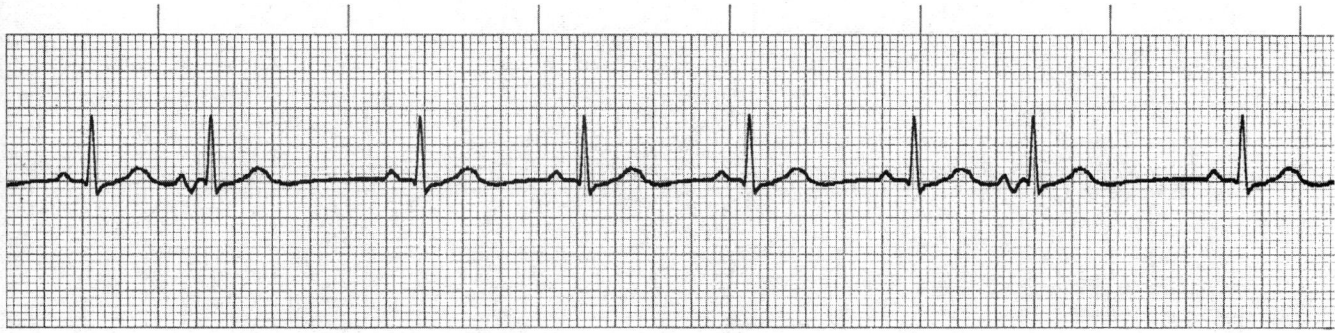

B Premature atrial contractions—note irregular rhythm produced by early complexes

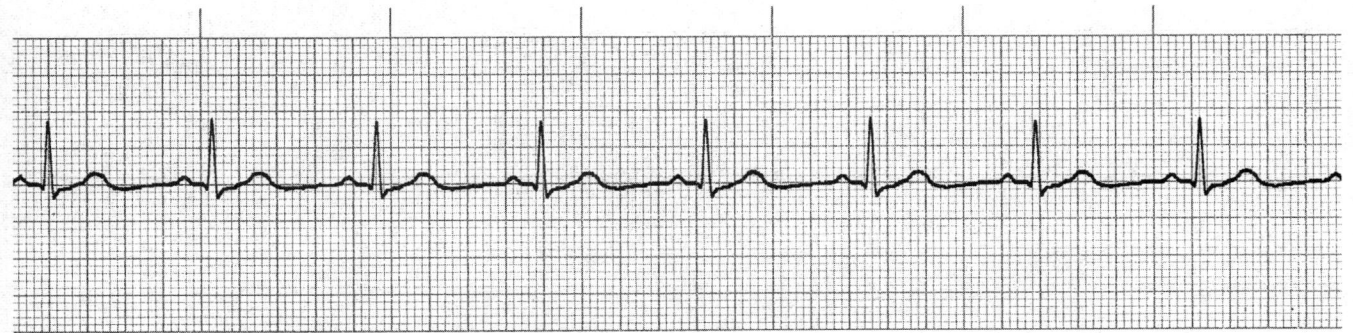

C Normal sinus rhythm

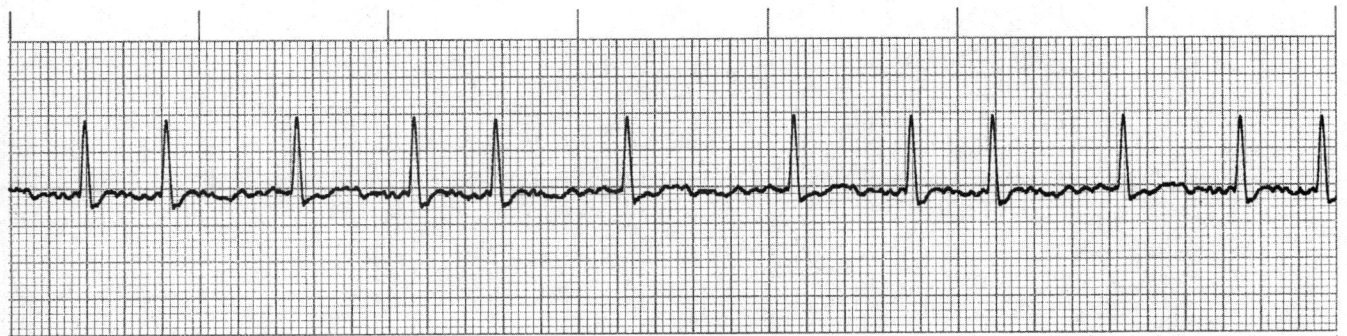

D Atrial fibrillation—note fine fibrillation waves and absent PR interval

Figure 23–9. Dysrhythmias.

Illustration continued on following page

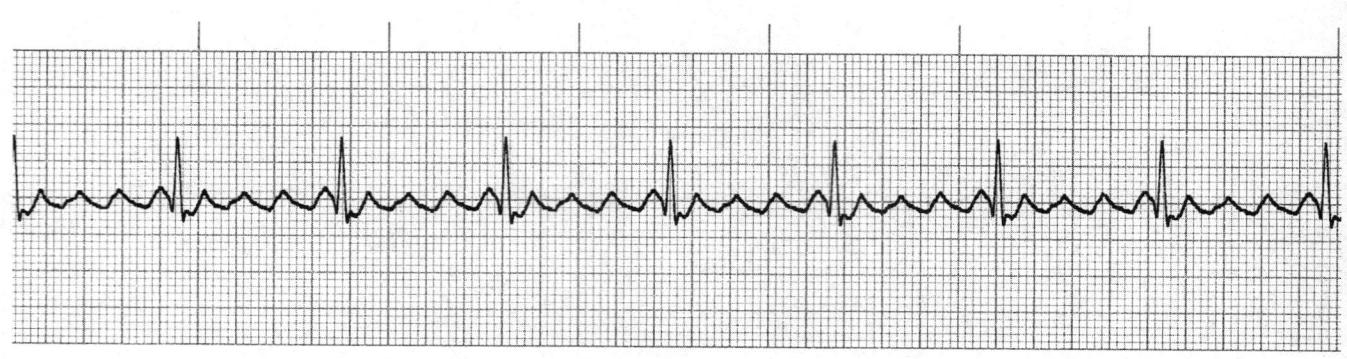

E Atrial flutter—note saw-tooth flutter waves and absent PR interval

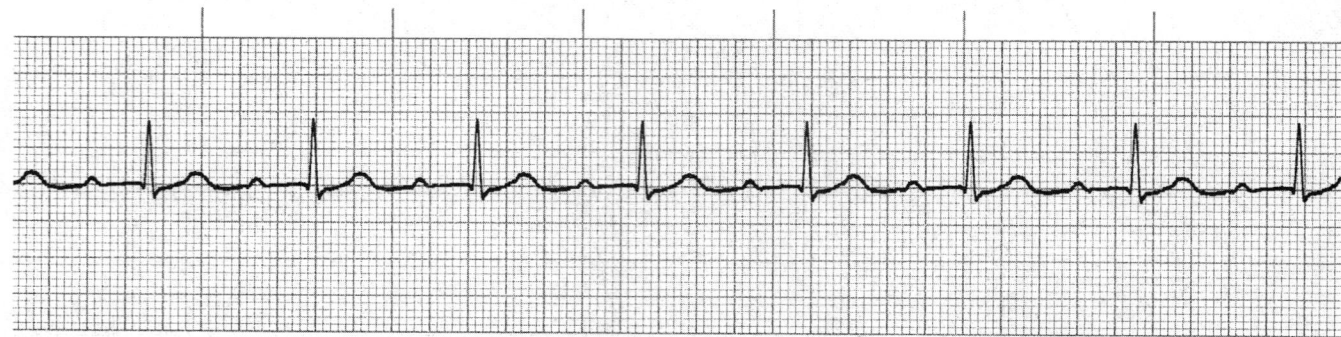

F First-degree atrioventricular heart block—note prolonged PR interval (>20 seconds)

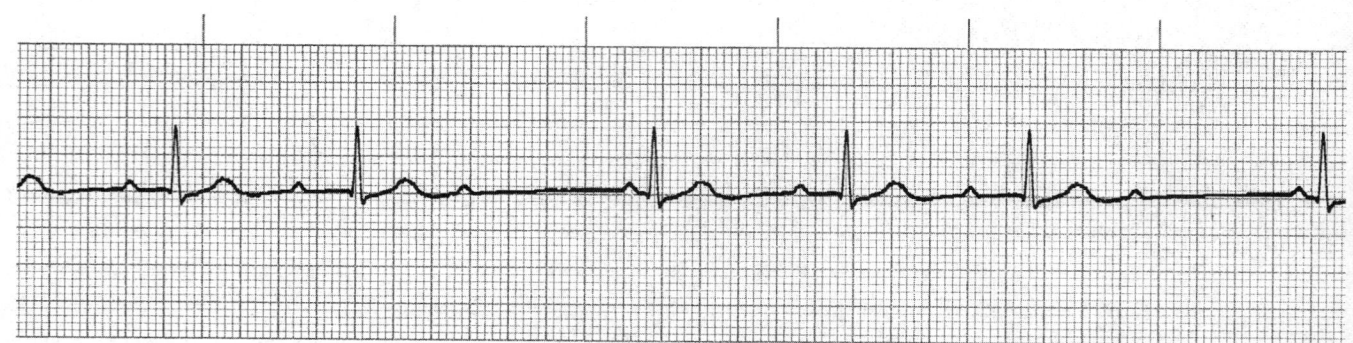

G Second-degree heart block, Mobitz type I (Wenckebach)—note progressively lengthened PR interval before missed complex

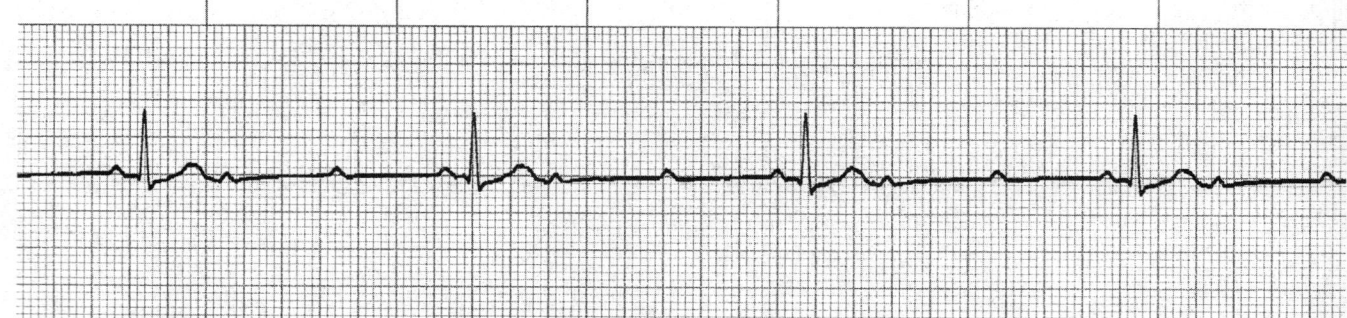

H Second-degree heart block, Mobitz type II—note consistent PR interval and abruptly missed complex

Figure 23–9. *Continued*

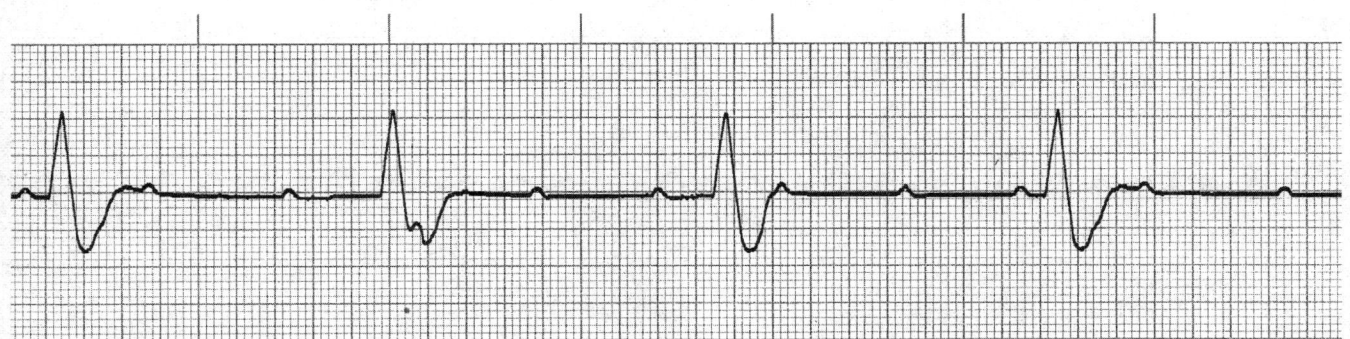

I Third-degree atrioventricular heart block: Complete heart block—note dissociation of P waves and wide QRS complexes

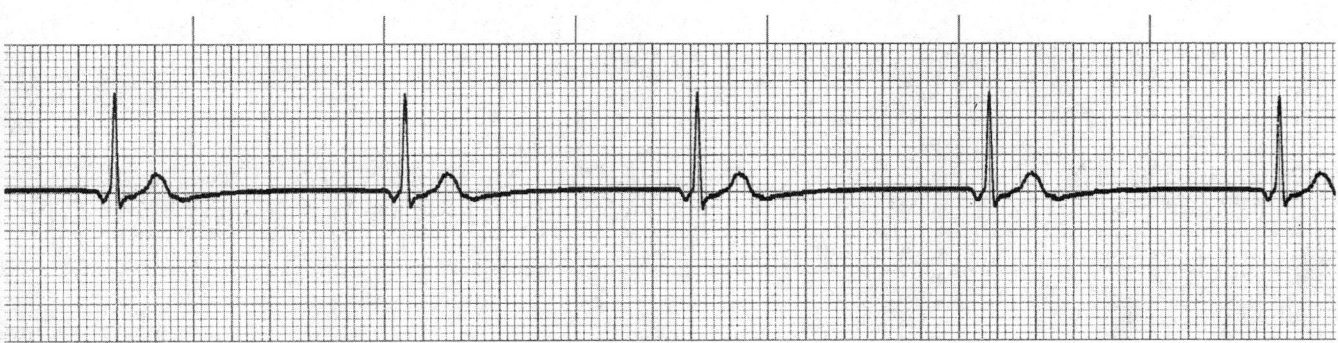

J Junctional (nodal) rhythm—note absent P waves and slow regular rhythm

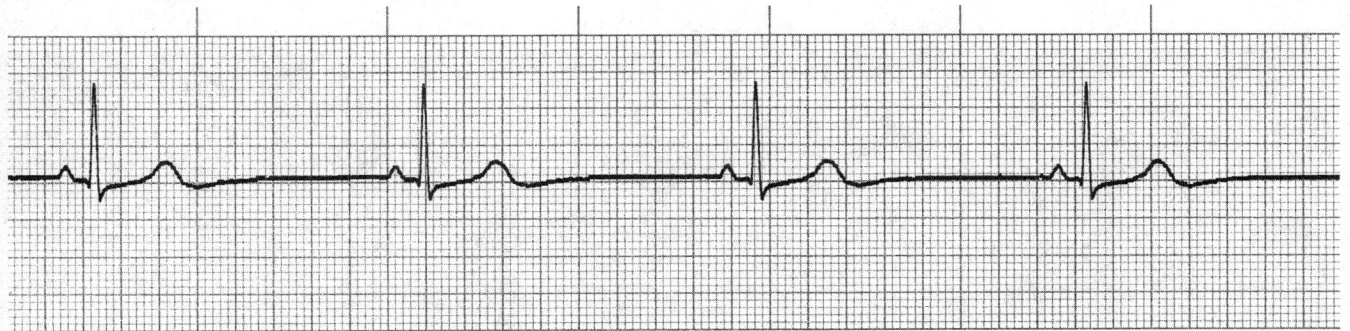

K Sinus bradycardia

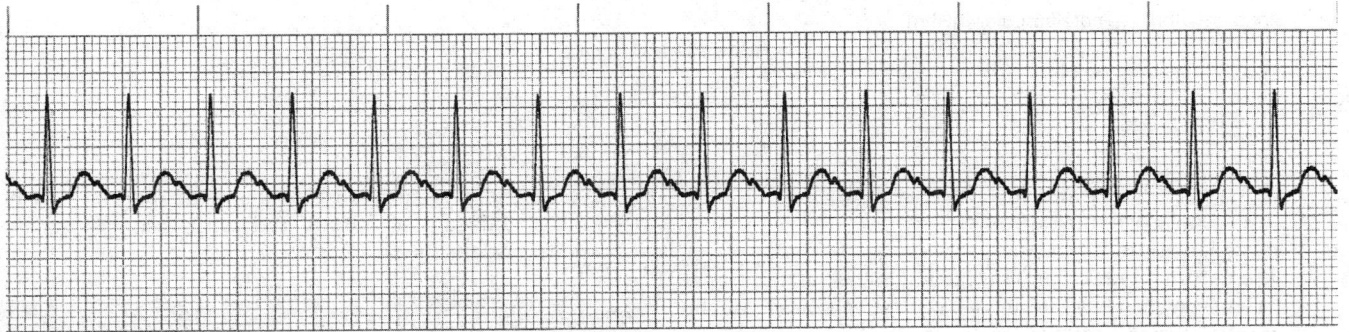

L Sinus tachycardia

Figure 23-9. *Continued*

Illustration continued on following page

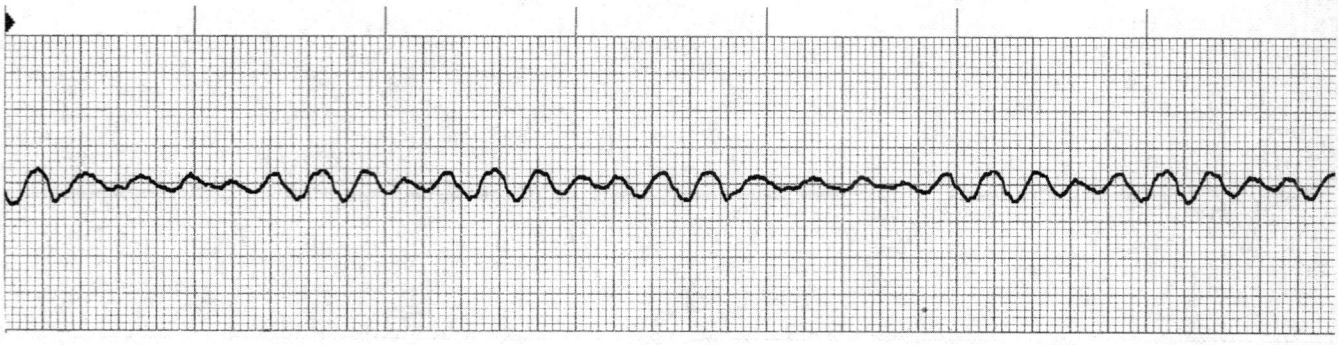

M Ventricular fibrillation—note chaotic electrical discharge

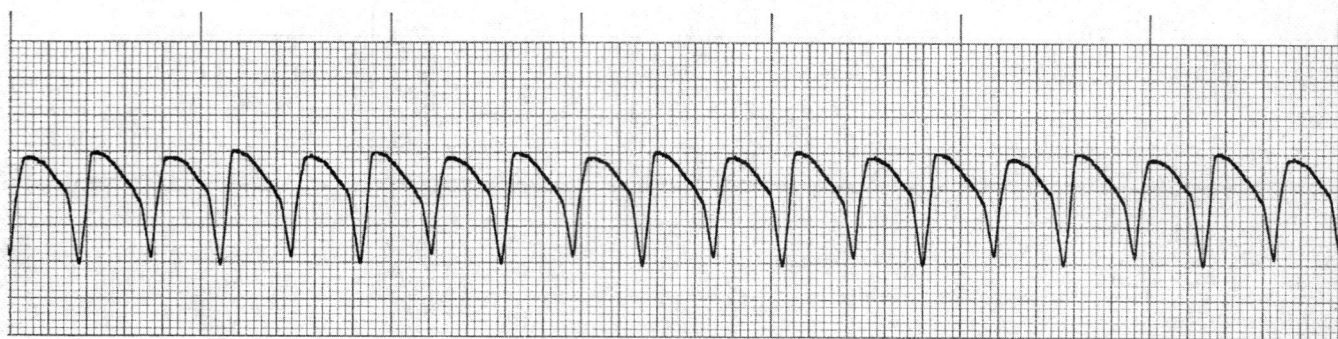

N Ventricular tachycardia—note rapid, wide QRS complexes

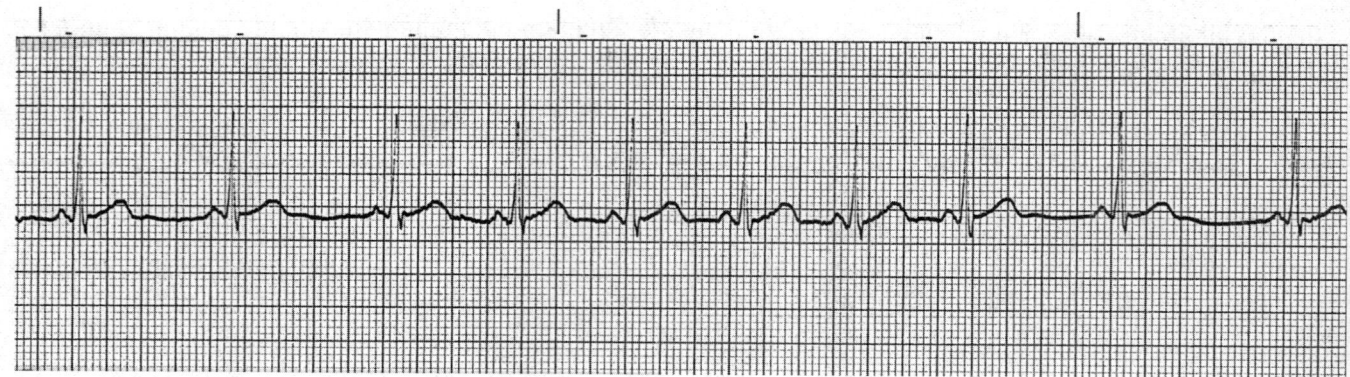

O Sinus arrhythmia—note irregular rhythm

Figure 23–9. *Continued*

discharge. The heart rate increases with inspiration and decreases with expiration.
6. Ventricular origin
   a. Premature ventricular contraction is an ectopic beat originating from a site in the ventricles outside of the normal cardiac cycle.
   b. If a premature ventricular contraction falls on a T wave, it may precipitate ventricular fibrillation. This is called the R-on-T phenomenon.
   c. Ventricular fibrillation occurs as chaotic ventricular

contractions or quivering of the heart muscle with no associated cardiac output and with resultant cardiopulmonary arrest.

NURSE ADVISORY

Early defibrillation is the single most important factor for successful resuscitation.

Table 23–7. Pharmacologic Interventions for Dysrhythmias

Actions	Indications	Adverse Reactions	Special Considerations
Adenosine (IV) Slows conduction in the AV node and inhibits reentry pathways	Narrow-complex paroxysmal supraventricular tachycardia (PSVT) and Wolff-Parkinson-White syndrome	Flushing Chest pain Dyspnea Brief periods of asystole or bradycardia	Avoid if using dipyridamole or theophylline Used to clarify diagnosis in atrial flutter, atrial fibrillation, and ventricular tachycardia by slowing ventricular rate
Amiodarone hydrochloride (IV/PO) Prolongs refractory period and action potential Decreases repolarization period	Ventricular and supraventricular tachycardias Atrial fibrillation and flutter	Dysrhythmias Congestive heart disease Pneumonitis Alveolitis Malaise, fatigue Nausea, vomiting Altered liver status Photosensitivity Corneal microdeposits	Use extreme caution with other antidysrhythmics. May decrease renal and liver clearance Monitor for pulmonary toxicity Can be fatal Advise use of sunscreen
Atropine sulfate (IV) Blocks vagal stimulation Increases heart rate	Bradycardia with hypotension or ventricular ectopy	Increasing heart rate can increase myocardial oxygen demand	Use cautiously in the presence of an acute MI
β-Blockers (such as atenolol, metoprolol, and propranolol) (IV/PO) Blocks β-adrenergic receptor sites Increases refractory period of AV node Decreases automaticity, conduction velocity, myocardial ischemia/excitability, contractility, O_2 consumption, and cardiac output Lowers blood pressure	Wolff-Parkinson-White and digitalis toxic rhythms Ventricular rhythms refractory to other drugs Thyrotoxicosis Hypertension Angina Hypertrophic cardiomyopathy Pheochromocytomas	Hypotension Bradydysrhythmias Asystole Severe bronchoconstriction Cardiac decompensation	Contraindicated in chronic obstructive pulmonary disease, asthma, AV block, congestive heart failure, bradycardia, and cardiogenic shock Use caution with diabetes, renal or liver failure Do not give with calcium channel blockers
Bretylium tosylate (IV) Raises ventricular fibrillation threshold Suppresses ventricular ectopic activity	Ventricular tachycardia or fibrillation resistant to defibrillation and first-line drugs	Initial effect: increased heart rate, blood pressure and premature ventricular contractions Subsequent effect: hypotension, bradycardia, nausea and vomiting	Enhances effect of catecholamines Keep the patient flat Adjust dose in renal failure Contraindicated with digitalis toxicity or fixed cardiac output
Digoxin (PO/IV) Increases contractility and cardiac output Slows AV conduction to reduce ventricular rate	Congestive heart failure Atrial flutter or fibrillation Supraventricular tachycardias	Frequent premature ventricular contractions AV blocks Dysrhythmias Nausea and vomiting Anorexia Diarrhea Mental confusion	Decreased dose with severe respiratory disease, hepatic or renal failure, or hypothyroidism If toxic, monitor cardiac rhythm and correct abnormal electrolytes; may need AV pacing
Diltiazem (IV) Calcium channel blocker	Atrial fibrillation or flutter with rapid ventricular response Narrow-complex PSVT refractory to other medications	Hypotension Congestive heart failure Headache Drowsiness Fatigue Nausea	Not for use in wide-complex tachycardias of unknown origin, or with β-blockers Use caution in older persons because duration of action may be prolonged
Disopyramide (PO) Prolongs action potential Membrane-stabilizing effect	Premature ventricular contractions Ventricular tachycardia not requiring cardioversion Atrial fibrillation or flutter	Hypotension Congestive heart failure Dysrhythmias Heart block	Avoid use in congestive heart failure and heart block Use with caution with urinary tract disease, liver and renal

Table continued on following page

Table 23–7. Pharmacologic Interventions for Dysrhythmias (Continued)

Actions	Indications	Adverse Reactions	Special Considerations
		Blurred vision Dry eyes Constipation	impairment, or narrow-angle glaucoma Manage constipation with diet and laxatives
Epinephrine (IV/ET) Stimulates α- and β-adrenergic receptors Increases heart rate, contractility, automaticity, arterial blood pressure, and blood flow to carotid and coronary arteries	First-line drug for ventricular fibrillation, pulseless ventricular tachycardia, and asystole	Ventricular fibrillation Increased myocardial oxygen consumption	Not to be given in an alkaline solution Avoid intracardiac injection if an intravenous line is available
Flecainide (IV/PO) Depresses phase O without change in action potential Membrane-stabilization effect	Use only in immediately life-threatening ventricular dysrhythmias	New or worsening dysrhythmias Dizziness Headache Visual disturbances Dyspnea	Avoid with heart block Use caution with congestive heart failure, blood dyscrasia, renal and hepatic disease
Lidocaine hydrochloride (IV) Suppresses ventricular dysrhythmias Raises ventricular fibrillation threshold	Frequent, multifocal, paired, or R-on-T premature ventricular contractions Ventricular tachycardia Ventricular fibrillation Acute MI	Confusion/agitation Drowsiness Hearing loss Paresthesias Seizures Heart block	Decrease dose with congestive heart failure, impaired liver function, or age older than 70 years Monitor for toxicity
Magnesium sulfate (IV) Treats hypomagnesemic states Dilates coronary arteries	Torsades de pointes Refractory vs. fibrillation Cardiac arrest or ventricular dysrhythmias due to digitalis toxicity, tricyclic overdose, or hypomagnesemia	Hypotension with rapid administration	Use caution with renal failure
Procainamide hydrochloride (IV) Slows cardiac conduction Decreases cardiac excitability	Ventricular ectopy when lidocaine is ineffective or contraindicated	Hypotension Widening QRS and prolonged QT Heart block Heart failure Agranulocytosis Anorexia Diarrhea Nausea and vomiting	Use with caution with acute MI and renal failure
Quinidine (IV/PO) Depresses phase O and prolongs action potential Membrane-stabilizing effect	Atrial fibrillation and flutter PSVT	Hemolytic anemia Thrombocytopenia Agranulocytosis Vertigo/tinnitus Headache Hypotension Congestive heart failure Ventricular dysrhythmias Nausea and vomiting Diarrhea	Contraindicated with AV conduction defects May increase risk of digitalis toxicity Gastrointestinal symptoms are signs of toxicity Monitor apical pulse and blood pressure
Tocainide (PO) Depresses phase O and shortens action potential Membrane-stabilizing effect	Symptomatic ventricular dysrhythmias	Blood dyscrasias Lightheadedness Tremors New or worsening dysrhythmias Congestive heart failure Pulmonary edema	Considered "oral lidocaine" Contraindicated if lidocaine-sensitive Use with β-blockers; decreases contractility and increases central nervous system toxicity

Table 23–7. Pharmacologic Interventions for Dysrhythmias (Continued)

Actions	Indications	Adverse Reactions	Special Considerations
		Respiratory arrest Nausea and vomiting Epigastric pain	Tremors may indicate approach of maximum dose
Verapamil (IV) Slows AV conduction and refractoriness Inhibits Ca^{2+} flow into cardiac and smooth muscle Decreases SA node discharge Reduces cardiac contractility and myocardial O_2 demand Peripheral arteriolar and coronary artery dilatation	Sinoventricular tachyarrhythmias other than sinus tachycardias Angina due to coronary artery spasm Refractory chronic angina	Hypotension Lightheadedness Headache Dizziness Nausea Sinus bradycardia AV heart block Ventricular fibrillation Asystole Heart failure	Monitor blood pressure, cardiac rhythm, and PR interval Contraindicated with Wolff-Parkinson-White, severe left ventricular failure, and disturbances of the AV node Use with caution with liver and renal insufficiency and in those taking digitalis or β-adrenergic blockers

IV, Intravenous; PO, by mouth.

NURSE ADVISORY

> In some ECG leads, ventricular fibrillation can be mistaken for asystole. Therefore, confirm rhythm as asystole in 2 different ECG leads.

d. Ventricular tachycardia is a consecutive series of 3 or more ventricular premature beats at a rate usually between 150 and 200 beats per minute.
  (1) Torsades de pointes (or polymorphous ventricular tachycardia) is an unusual form of ventricular tachycardia in which the QRS configuration is constantly changing and the QT interval is prolonged (>0.40 sec).
  (2) It is usually associated with an idiosyncratic reaction to quinidine, procainamide, or disopyramide.

Pharmacologic Interventions for Dysrhythmias (Table 23–7)

Pacemakers

1. A pacemaker is a battery-powered device that provides electric stimulation to the myocardium when the intrinsic pacing and conduction system of the heart fail to provide a perfusing rhythm.
2. Pacemakers may be used for the following:
  a. Atrial pacing
  b. Ventricular pacing
  c. Atrioventricular sequential and physiologic pacing by setting the time between atrial and ventricular stimulation
3. Pacemakers can be set to do the following:
  a. Sense the persons' rhythm and pace only if the person's intrinsic rate declines below the set pacemaker rate (synchronous)
  b. Pace at a preset rate, regardless of the person's rhythm (asynchronous). This mode is rarely used because the pacemaker could fire on the T wave and cause ventricular arrhythmias.
  c. Provide an increased rate in bradyarrhythmias
  d. Overdrive and suppress the underlying rhythm in tachyarrhythmias
4. Indications for pacing
  a. Symptomatic bradyarrhythmias
    (1) Severe sinus bradycardia
    (2) Second- and 3rd-degree heart blocks
    (3) Sinus arrest
    (4) Sick sinus syndrome
  b. Symptomatic tachyarrhythmias
    (1) Atrial flutter
    (2) Junctional rhythms
    (3) Ventricular rhythms (not used if very rapid rate)
  c. Asystole
  d. Prophylaxis in persons with high risk for significant bradycardia, such as persons
    (1) With MI with new bifascicular block
    (2) Who have undergone cardiac surgery
  e. Diagnosis or assessment of dysrhythmias during electrophysiologic testing
  f. Other disorders
    (1) Myocardial ischemia
    (2) Myocardial infarction
    (3) Electrolyte imbalances
    (4) Drug toxicity
    (5) Cardiac trauma
5. Types of pacemakers (Fig. 23–10)
  a. Temporary pacemakers
    (1) In endocardial (also called transvenous) pacemakers, a pacing lead wire is inserted through a central vein into the right atrium (for atrial pacing) or right ventricle and positioned in contact with the endocardium. The wire is then connected to a

TYPES OF PACEMAKERS

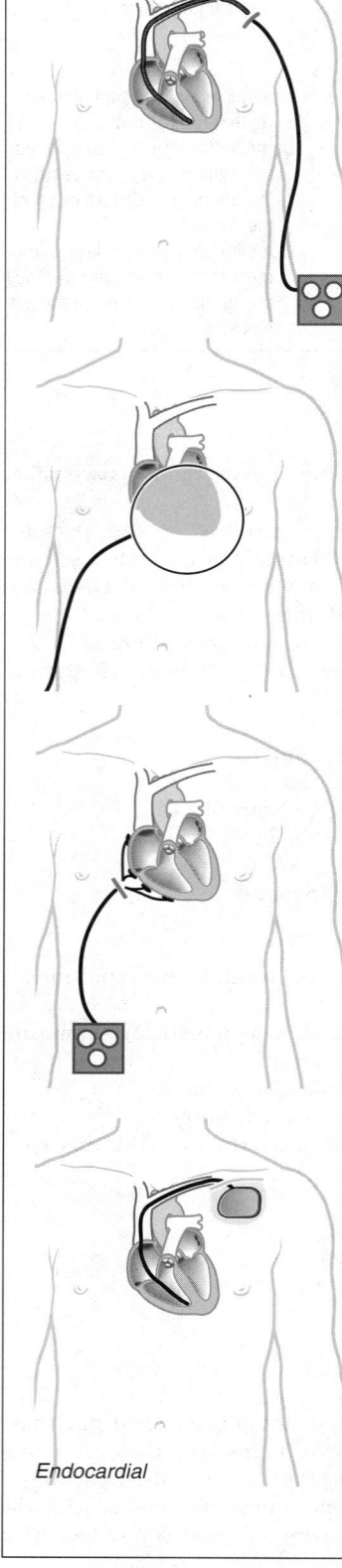

Temporary Pacemakers:

Endocardial Pacemaker
This is the most common method of temporary pacing, also called a transvenous pacemaker. A pacing lead wire is inserted through a central vein into the right atrium, for atrial pacing, or right ventricle and is positioned in contact with the endocardium. The wire is then connected to a pulse generator.

Transcutaneous Pacemaker
Used in emergency situations when pacing wires have not been inserted or when invasive procedures are contraindicated. This is also called an external pacemaker. It delivers energy through the chest wall via surface electrodes.

Epicardial Pacemaker
Epicardial wires are sutured on the epicardium during open heart surgery and brought through the chest wall, where they can be attached to a pulse generator.

Permanent Pacemakers:

Usually the pacing wire is surgically inserted into the right ventricle using the transvenous approach and is positioned in the endocardium. The wire is attached to a small, sealed, battery-powered pulse generator, which is inserted into the chest wall or abdominal cavity. The batteries used in permanent pacemakers last for 4–12 years, depending on the type of pacemaker and the pacemaker function.

Endocardial

Figure 23–10.

pulse generator. This is the most common method of temporary pacing (Procedure 23–6).

    (2) In transcutaneous (also called external) pacemakers, energy is delivered through the chest wall via surface electrodes. It is used in emergency situations when pacing wires have not been inserted or when invasive procedures are contraindicated.

  b. Permanent pacemakers

    (1) The pacing wire is usually surgically inserted into the right ventricle using the transvenous approach and is positioned in the endocardium. The wire is attached to a small sealed battery-powered pulse generator inserted in the chest wall or abdominal cavity.

    (2) The batteries used in permanent pacemakers last for 4 to 12 years depending on the type of pacemaker and pacemaker function.

6. Complications include infection, perforation of myocardium, pneumothorax and hemothorax, dysrhythmias, thrombosis, and embolus.

  a. Failure to capture occurs when the pacing spike is not immediately followed by a QRS complex (or P wave if it is an atrial pacemaker). Failure to capture may be due to battery or pulse generator failure, increased milliamperage requirements, or poor lead wire position.

  b. Failure to sense occurs when a synchronous pacemaker fails to sense and fires without regard for the person's own rhythm. It may be due to sensitivity set too low or failure of the sensing mechanisms in the pulse generator.

  c. Microshock is a low electric current that passes on or through the body unnoticed by the individual. A person with an external transvenous pacemaker has a direct line to the myocardium that could conduct stray electric current from surrounding equipment.

7. Diagnostics

  a. Determine rhythm using ECG lead II.

  b. If rhythm is 100 percent paced, use programmer-analyzer to determine the following:

    (1) Paced rate

    (2) Capture (i.e., each pacemaker spike is followed by a contraction)

    (3) Impulse-to-impulse interval

    (4) Pulse duration

  c. With the physician present, lower the pacer rate to determine and document underlying rhythm.

  d. If there are mixed pacer and intrinsic beats, evaluate the following:

    (1) That each pacemaker is sensing all beats and firing appropriately

    (2) That each pacemaker spike is followed by a contraction

  e. If there are no paced beats, with the physician present, test the pacemaker by increasing rate to slightly faster than the resting heart rate and evaluate for capture.

8. Applying the nursing process

NURSING DIAGNOSIS: Decreased cardiac output R/T pacemaker malfunction

P

Procedure 23–6
Assisting with the Insertion of a Temporary
Transvenous Pacemaker

Definition/Purpose	To deliver electric stimuli to the heart resulting in cardiac depolarization and contraction.
Contraindication/Cautions	Insertion of a catheter may result in a pneumothorax, cardiac tamponade, ventricular irritation, and ectopy.
Learning/Teaching Activities	• Explain the procedure to the patient. Emphasize that sterile drapes will be placed over the insertion site and not to touch this area. • Explain that a local anesthetic will be injected into the insertion site. If the person feels pain during the procedure, the person should inform the nurse.

Preliminary Activities

Equipment	• Percutaneous sheath introducer kit • Sterile towels and drapes • Sterile gloves, gowns, masks, surgical caps • Povidone-iodine • 4 × 4 gauze sponges • Pacing catheter • Temporary pacemaker pulse generator with a new 9-volt battery and patient extension cable • Materials for sterile dressing • Cardiac monitor and defibrillator • 12-lead ECG machine • Alligator clamp (optional)
Assessment Planning	• Know whether the physician prefers to insert the pacing catheter under fluoroscopic guidance, necessitating transport of the person to the procedure room where there is fluoroscopic equipment. • Know whether the physician prefers to insert the pacing catheter under ECG guidance, necessitating an alligator clip and a 12-lead ECG machine. • Know the size of the pacing catheter, the type of pulse generator, and the insertion site to be used. • Examine the pulse generator and extension. Identify the connector terminals for the pacing catheter, rate, MA, and sensitivity dials and be prepared to connect the pacemaker with settings adjusted as directed. • Ensure that the person has a patent intravenous line in case emergency drugs are needed. • Ensure that an emergency cart with emergency drugs, airway equipment, and defibrillator is readily available.

Procedure

Actions	Rationale/Discussion
1. Place the patient in a supine position.	1. This position decreases risk of air embolism.
2. If the jugular or subclavian site is to be used, place a rolled towel between the scapulae.	2. This helps distend the vein and prevent pneumothorax.
3. Connect the cardiac monitor.	3. An ECG should be displayed during insertion.
4. Cleanse the insertion site with povidone-iodine solution.	4. Aseptic technique prevents catheter-related infection.
5. Provide all personnel at bedside with cap and mask.	5. Reduces risk of site contamination.
6. Provide the physician with sterile gown and gloves.	6. Maintains asepsis.
7. Pass equipment to the physician to prepare a sterile field.	7. Sterile field is required for asepsis.

8. Assist the physician as needed as the following are done:
  a. Infiltrate the site with Xylocaine.
  b. Obtain venous access and insert the introducer.
  c. Advance the pacemaker catheter.
    (1) If fluoroscopy is used, assist as needed.
    (2) If ECG guidance used, be prepared to connect one end of the alligator clip to the V lead of the ECG machine and the other end to the negative lead of the pacing catheter.
	8. Ensures person's safety and comfort.
	
	    (2) Lead V displays the intracardiac ECG so that location of the catheter can be determined.

9. Monitor the ECG display throughout insertion.	9. The catheter may irritate the ventricle and cause ectopy.

(continued)

Procedure 23-6
(continued)

Actions	Rationale/Discussion

10. After the catheter is inserted, the physician will ask the person to
   a. Connect the pacing catheter leads to the appropriate connector terminals
   b. Adjust pacemaker settings
	
	b. Settings are adjusted to achieve optimal function.

Final Activities

1. After the catheter is sutured in place, apply a sterile dressing.
2. Place the pulse generator in a secure place (such as hung on an intravenous pole), to prevent any tension on the pacing catheter.
3. Obtain a chest radiograph and a 12-lead ECG.
4. Document the type of pacemaker, insertion site, name of physician, pacemaker settings, and patient's tolerance of the procedure.
5. Monitor the patient for signs of ventricular irritability, cardiac tamponade, and pneumothorax.

a. *Expected outcomes:* Following instruction, the person should be able to do the following:
  (1) Demonstrate an understanding of symptoms of decreased cardiac output
  (2) Know the classification of the pacemaker if it is permanent
b. *Nursing interventions:* Symptoms of pacer failure vary; therefore, teach the patient to be alert for the same symptoms of decreased cardiac output that occurred before the pacer was inserted, such as altered level of consciousness, hypotension, irregular pulse, shortness of breath, chest pain, and dizziness.

NURSING DIAGNOSIS: Anxiety R/T potentially life-threatening dysrhythmia

a. *Expected outcomes:* Following counseling, the person should be able to do the following:
  (1) Verbalize a better understanding of pacemaker therapy
  (2) Demonstrate verbal and nonverbal signs of reduced anxiety
b. *Nursing interventions*
  (1) Assist person to identify fears related to pacemaker.
  (2) Provide written and verbal information about what to expect and how to maintain pacemaker function.
  (3) Monitor anxiety level.

NURSING DIAGNOSIS: Risk for injury R/T microshock (temporary pacemaker)

a. *Expected outcomes:* Following interventions the person should remain free of injury in an electrically safe environment.
b. *Nursing interventions:*
  (1) Assess electric equipment in environment for signs of malfunction and frayed cords.
  (2) Ensure that all equipment in the environment is grounded.
  (3) If pacing leads (e.g., epicardial wires) are not in use and not connected to the pacemaker, place them in a rubber glove or glass phlebotomy tube and secure.
9. Discharge planning and teaching
  a. Before discharge, instruct the patient on the following:
    (1) Reason for pacemaker
    (2) Signs and symptoms of malfunction
    (3) How to check pulse
    (4) Precautions regarding electric equipment
    (5) Activity restrictions
    (6) Follow-up care (see Learning / Teaching Guidelines for Persons with a Permanent Pacemaker)
  b. Review the importance of carrying a MedicAlert card and provide ordering information.
  c. Provide direction on the use of transtelephonic system (if available) to check pacemaker function.
  d. Encourage the person and family to call if they have any questions or concerns.

Other Electronic Interventions for Dysrhythmias

1. Definitive therapy for many dysrhythmias includes application of an electric countershock that causes a mo-

LEARNING/TEACHING GUIDELINES
for People with a Permanent Pacemaker

General Overview

1. Explore the person's feelings about having a pacemaker. Many persons fear depending on a pacemaker for their life or fear dying from pacemaker failure. This may affect their ability to learn.
2. Use written patients education material and pictures provided by the pacemaker manufacturers.
3. Briefly explain the rationale for the pacemaker:
   a. The heart works as a pump to deliver blood with oxygen and nutrients to cells in the entire body.
   b. The natural pacemaker of the heart produces regular electric impulses that stimulate the heart to contract and pump.
   c. Describe the alteration in the natural pacemaker system of the heart and how the artificial pacemaker will help.
4. Describe features of the pacemaker that the person has:
   a. Atrial, ventricular, or both
   b. Rate setting (fixed or demand)
   c. Parts of the pacemaker system (e.g., pulse generator wire, lead on heart)
5. Explain that the person should carry a pacemaker identification card at all times. Wearing a Medic-Alert bracelet or tag is advisable.
6. Instruct the person about pulse checks
   a. Explain that the pulse can serve as a gauge of pacemaker function. Inform the person what the range of pulse rate should be, depending on the type of pacemaker.
   b. Demonstrate how to take a pulse and ask the person to do a return demonstration.
   c. Give the person the following guidelines:
      (1) Take the pulse every day, preferably at the same time, such as 1st thing in the morning.
      (2) Be relaxed or at rest when counting the pulse. It may be necessary to rest for approximately 5 minutes before starting.
      (3) Count for 1 full minute using a clock or watch with a second hand.
      (4) Record the results in a special diary that lists rate, date, and time of day.
      (5) Notify the physician if a problem with the pulse rate persists.
7. Describe the following signs and symptoms that may indicate pacemaker malfunction. If any of these symptoms occur, check the pulse rate and call the physician.
   a. Dizziness or fainting spells
   b. Prolonged weakness or fatigue
   c. Swelling of ankles or legs
   d. Chest pain
   e. Shortness of breath
8. Explain electromagnetic interference
   a. The pacemaker is shielded from interference from most other electric devices
   b. Most electric items can be used without any problem including microwave ovens, radio, television, kitchen appliances such as toasters, electric blankets and heating pads, and hair dryers.
   c. Consult the physician for special situations involving strong electric or magnetic fields, including working with high-current industrial equipment, powerful magnets, arc welders, power transmitters, or radar towers.
   d. If the person experiences any symptoms while near an electric device, move away from the device and count the pulse. The pulse should return to normal when the person moves away.
   e. Tell doctors or dentists about the pacemaker before undergoing medical procedures or tests so that equipment that may cause interference can be avoided.
   f. The pacemaker may set off airport security detectors. Present the pacemaker identification card to airport security and ask for clearance.
9. Instruct the person to follow the physician's guidelines regarding physical activity. Most persons are encouraged to resume previous activity level with the possible exception of contact sports, which may damage the pacemaker.
10. Emphasize the need for continued medical follow-up to make sure that the pacemaker continues to work properly.

mentary depolarization of heart fibers, terminating ectopic activity and allowing the sinus node to reestablish itself as the pacemaker of the heart.

2. Cardioversion is the use of synchronized direct current shock for the elective treatment of atrial rhythm disturbances or ventricular tachycardias. With a synchronized method, the equipment "senses" the patient's intrinsic rhythm and avoids delivering the shock during the vulnerable phase of ventricular excitability following systole. Shocks given during this phase may actually precipitate ventricular fibrillation (Procedure 23–7).

3. Defibrillation is the use of unsynchronized (there is no rhythm to synchronize with) direct current shock to convert ventricular fibrillation into a perfusing rhythm. This shock can be delivered by 2 methods: automated external defibrillation (Procedure 23–8) and conventional defibrillation (Procedure 23–9).

Text continued on page 1024

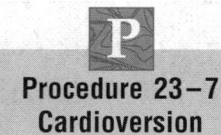

Procedure 23–7
Cardioversion

Definition/Purpose	To convert tachydysrhythmias that are unresponsive to medical therapy to a perfusing sinus rhythm by means of a synchronized electric charge.
Contraindication/Cautions	1. Cardioversion enhances the effects of digitalis and may lead to lethal dysrhythmias. a. Patients on maintenance doses of digitalis should have their digitalis withheld for at least 24 hours before elective cardioversion. b. Emergency cardioversion is usually not indicated for digitalis-toxic dysrhythmias. c. If cardioversion is to be used for digitalis toxicity, ensure that electrolyte imbalances have been corrected and that initial attempts are begun at low energy levels. 2. Obtain serum potassium levels before elective cardioversion. Hypokalemia enhances electric instability and increases the risk of further dysrhythmias. 3. Monitor the patient for respiratory depression or arrest from oversedation. 4. If the patient converts into ventricular fibrillation, turn OFF the synchronizing mode and defibrillate immediately. 5. Monitor the patient for pulmonary or systemic emboli.
Learning/Teaching Activities	As appropriate, review cardiac status and rationale for the procedure.

Preliminary Activities

Equipment	• Cardioverter–defibrillator • Electrocardiogram monitor • Prepared conductive pads • Emergency equipment • Oxygen therapy equipment • Stand-by pacing equipment
Assessment Planning	1. Obtain and evaluate recent serum electrolyte levels and digitalis level, if appropriate. 2. Determine whether digitalis has been given in the last 24 hours. 3. For elective cardioversion, determine whether the person has had anything by mouth for approximately 8 hours. 4. Assess the intravenous line to ensure its patency. (If an intravenous line is not in place, insert one before proceeding.) 5. Assess vital signs, level of orientation, and respiratory status.

Procedure

Actions	Rationale/Discussion
1. Obtain a baseline ECG.	1. Used for comparison after cardioversion.
2. Remove the patient's dentures or dental bridges if appropriate.	2. Evaluate the risk of airway obstruction versus the potential loss of complete seal for bag–valve–mask units if dentures are removed.
3. Administer prescribed sedation such as intravenous diazepam (Valium).	3. If a short-acting anesthetic is needed, an anesthesiologist should be in attendance to monitor airway and respirations.
4. Administer oxygen as ordered before cardioversion.	4. Discontinue oxygen administration at the time of cardioversion, because oxygen is potentially combustible.
5. Prepare equipment	5. Proper equipment preparation facilitates carrying out procedure and ensures patient safety.

a. Plug equipment into an electrical outlet (even if battery operated).
  b. Turn on power.
  c. Connect limb leads.
	c. Ensure that the monitoring lead produces a tall R wave of sufficient amplitude to trigger the synchronizing circuit.

d. Check for artifact. If artifact is present, check electrode placement or the contact and alter as needed to ensure that no artifact is present.	d. Artifact may be interpreted by the cardioverter as an R wave and could allow electric current to be delivered at an incorrect time, which could result in ventricular fibrillation.
e. Activate the synchronizer.	e. If the synchronizer is not activated, electric discharge occurs when the paddle buttons are pressed, regardless of R wave.
f. Check the synchronizing circuit.	f. Most units have a light that flashes on the R wave or may have an auditory tone that beeps with the R wave to demonstrate the cardioverter is *in synchrony* with the cardiac cycle.
6. Select the energy level.	6. Energy levels are determined by clinical presentation, body type, and medications recently taken.
7. Activate the charge button.	

P

Procedure 23–7

(continued)

Actions	Rationale/Discussion
8. Check that the cardioverter is fully charged to the set level.	
9. Make sure the chest is free of any moisture.	9. Moisture may cause arcing and decrease the amount of delivered energy.
10. Apply "hands-off" pads or place paddles firmly on the chest, using 25 pounds of pressure per paddle: a. Standard placement. Place 1 paddle to the right on the sternum below the clavicle. Place the other paddle to the left of the nipple in the midaxillary line. b. In anterior–posterior placement, one paddle is placed at the posterior intrascapular area and the other is placed at the anterior precordial area.	10. Use "hands-off" pads whenever possible.

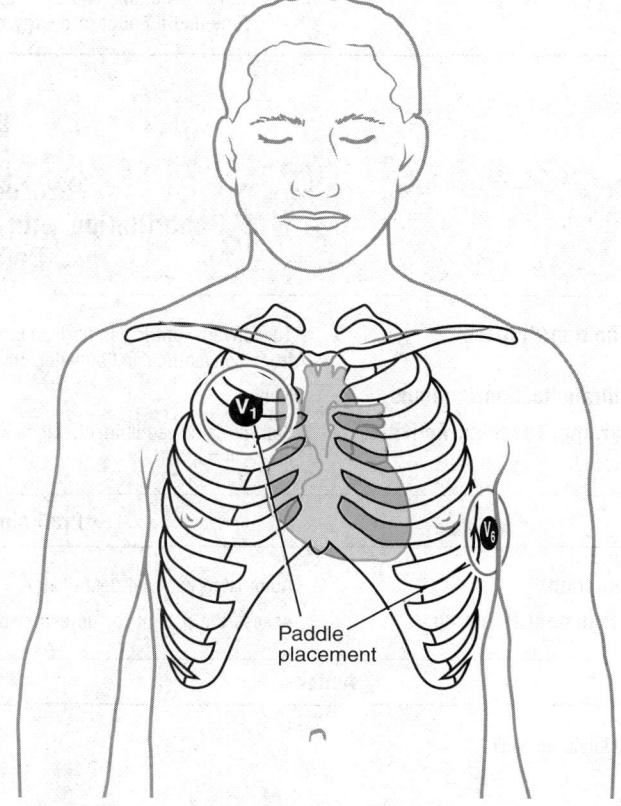

Paddle placement

11. Direct all personnel to stand clear of the bed and release hold on any equipment that is in contact with the person or bed.	11. Confirm that everyone is clear by looking around the bed.
12. Press the discharge buttons and hold until energy is released.	12. Firm contact with the person's chest prevents arcing and ensures charge delivery.
13. Assess the patient's pulse, vital signs, and ECG rhythm.	13. Confirms person's response to procedure.
14. If dysrhythmia persists, check equipment for the following potential causes of failure to cardiovert: • Nonsynchronized mode • Artifact interference • Battery failure (if equipment is not plugged in) • Inadequate pressure on paddles during cardioversion	14. Failure to transmit charge may have multiple causes.
15. If dysrhythmia persists, increase the energy level in increments as prescribed by the physician. The interval between shocks should be at least 3 minutes.	15. Ensure that adequate conductive medium is on the paddles for repeated countershocks.

Final Activities

1. Complete postcardioversion assessment by checking ECG rhythm, vital signs, and airway patency.
2. Obtain a postcardioversion 12-lead ECG.
3. Orient the person to the surroundings and give results of the cardioversion.

(continued)

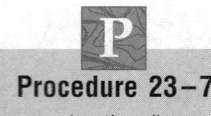

Procedure 23–7

(continued)

Final Activities

4. Monitor the ECG for at least 2 hours after the procedure.
5. Document the person's status before and immediately after the procedure, including the following:
   - Electrocardiogram rhythm
   - Vital signs
   - Level of consciousness
   - Name, dose, and route of sedation administered
   - Time and amount of energy delivered with each shock

Procedure 23–8
Defibrillation with an Automated External Defibrillator

Definition/Purpose To convert ventricular fibrillation into a perfusing rhythm. An automated external defibrillator (AED) differentiates from nonventricular fibrillation rhythms and allows for early defibrillation by first responders.

Contraindication/Cautions None

Learning/Teaching Activities Before using equipment: None. After successful resuscitation: Explain the event and provide emotional and physical support.

Preliminary Activities

Equipment Automated external defibrillator

Assessment Planning Assess the patient for unresponsiveness, breathlessness, and pulselessness.

Actions	Rationale/Discussion
1. Obtain an AED.	1. Immediate attachment and use of the AED is key to successful defibrillation. If an AED is available and only 1 rescuer is available, the American Heart Association recommends obtaining the AED before initiation of cardiopulmonary resuscitation (CPR). If 2 rescuers are available, 1 obtains the AED while the other initiates CPR.
2. Attach AED leads to the patient as indicated on the machine.	2. Ensures effectiveness and person's safety.
3. Turn on the AED.	3. The AED will not discharge unless power is on.
4. Push button to activate the analyzer.	4. Ensures person's and responder's safety.
5. Follow instructions given for the AED, usually to "assess," "stand back," "shock," and "reassess."	5. If there is no ventricular fibrillation, initiate basic life support and advanced cardiac life support therapies as indicated.
6. Evaluate for return of a pulse. If a pulse is present, provide supportive therapy (e.g., oxygen or intravenous medications). If the patient is pulseless, repeat steps 4, 5, and 6 up to 3 times, then perform CPR for 1 minute. Repeat if the patient remains pulseless.	6. Confirm the presence or absence of a pulse after every intervention.
7. Initiate advanced cardiac life support when a qualified responder arrives.	7. Most facilities adhere to American Heart Association protocols.

Final Activities

1. Attach the patient to a cardiac monitor.
2. Evaluate and document the patient's vital signs.
3. Assess the patient for cause of dysrhythmia.
4. Provide ongoing physical and emotional support.
5. Document initial assessment, actions taken, and response to intervention.

Procedure 23-9
Defibrillation

Definition/Purpose	To terminate ventricular fibrillation or pulseless ventricular tachycardia by means of a direct electric discharge. Early defibrillation has been shown to significantly increase the likelihood of successful resuscitation.
Contraindication/Cautions	• Ensure that the person is pulseless and apneic. • Use care in paddle placement to avoid skin burn from defibrillator paddles.
Learning/Teaching Activities	None

Preliminary Activities

Equipment	• Defibrillator • Prepared conductive pads • An ECG machine
Assessment Planning	• Make sure that the person is pulseless. • Remember to not treat the monitor; always assess the person after each intervention.

Procedure

Actions	Rationale/Discussion
1. Evaluate pulselessness and cardiac rhythm.	1. Evaluation of cardiac rhythm should demonstrate ventricular fibrillation or pulseless ventricular tachycardia.
2. Place defibrillator so that paddles can easily reach chest.	2. Facilitates procedure.
3. Turn on machine.	3. Most defibrillators have a synchronization circuit that must be in the OFF or inoperative mode for treatment of ventricular fibrillation.
4. Wipe all moisture off the patient's chest.	4. Water is a good conductive medium and will disperse electric charge.
5. Place "hands-off" or prepackaged defibrillation pads on chest at V_1 and V_6 electrode positions.	5. Allows for most effective charge delivery.
6. Select the correct energy level based on institutional standards.	6. Most institutions adhere to American Heart Association ACLS protocols.
7. Press the charge button (located either on the machine or on the paddles).	7. Allows pads to charge.
8. Watch the charge meter needle until it shows the specified charge.	8. Confirms proper charge level.
9. If not using "hands-off" pads, position the paddles on top of the defibrillator pads using firm, even pressure.	9. Firm pressure facilitates charge delivery and decreases arcing.
10. Direct all personnel to stand clear and release hold on any equipment that is in contact with the person or bed.	10. Confirm that everyone is clear by looking around the bed.
11. If using "hands-on" paddles, apply greater than 20 pounds of pressure on the paddles and simultaneously press the knobs on the paddles to release electric charge. If using "hands-off" pads, push the discharge button.	11. Paddles will discharge and may result in chest wall muscle contraction.
12. Check for return of a palpable pulse.	12. Confirms person's response.
13. Assess postdefibrillation ECG pattern. Continue CPR during any delays.	13. Care should be taken to minimize CPR interruptions.
14. If the rhythm is unchanged, repeat steps 6 through 13 at up to 360 joules.	14. Resistance to charge delivery by the chest wall decreases with each attempt.
15. If a 3rd attempt at defibrillation is unsuccessful, resume CPR and initiate antidysrhythmic therapy.	15. Antidysrhythmic therapy increases the effectiveness of subsequent defibrillation attempts.

Final Activities

1. Document the initial rhythm and clinical condition before intervention.
2. Document defibrillation attempts including energy settings, time, and response.
3. Once a rhythm is established, monitor and record vital signs.
4. Orient the person to surroundings.

4. Automatic implantable cardioverter defibrillators are surgically implanted in patients at a high risk of sudden cardiac death. The device monitors heart rhythm and discharges when rate or rhythm requires it.

Other Nonelectronic Interventions for Dysrhythmias

1. Carotid sinus massage: Occasionally, the ventricular rate is so rapid that flutter waves are obscured. Carotid sinus massage may be used. When massaged, the ventricular response may be slowed and the flutter waves identified.

NURSE ADVISORY

Carotid sinus massage should only be performed by a physician. It may precipitate complete heart block or neurologic impairment if the person has carotid artery disease.

---

2. Radio frequency ablation: In disorders such as the paroxysmal supraventricular tachycardias, radio frequency ablation is used to eliminate aberrant conduction pathways.
   a. While undergoing an electrophysiologic study, a platinum-tipped catheter is used to deliver a low-voltage, high-frequency current that cauterizes the aberrant conduction pathway.
   b. Studies have documented up to a 99 percent success rate in initially eliminating the dysrhythmia; however, in 9 percent of the cases, Wolff-Parkinson-White syndrome can return if the pathway has not been completely ablated.
   c. Complications are those associated with electrophysiologic studies and occur in approximately 1.8 percent of the cases.

Applying the Nursing Process

NURSING DIAGNOSIS: Decreased cardiac output R/T alteration in heart rate or rhythm

1. *Expected outcomes:* Following interventions, the person should exhibit a controlled heart rate and rhythm and an adequate cardiac output as demonstrated by the following:
   a. Stable vital signs with a systolic blood pressure between 90 and 110 mm Hg and respiratory rate between 10 and 20 respirations per minute
   b. Warm, dry skin
   c. The ability to carry out prescribed activities without dyspnea or pain
2. *Nursing interventions*
   a. Perform and document initial and ongoing cardiovascular assessments; monitor the patient for dysrhythmias and signs of heart failure. Frequency of assessments should be determined by condition and should include the following:
      (1) Vital signs
      (2) Breath sounds
      (3) Heart sounds
      (4) Cardiac rhythm
   b. Assess, document, and report any signs of decreased cardiac output including the following:
      (1) Chest pain
      (2) Decrease in systolic blood pressure or a systolic reading of less than 90 mm Hg
      (3) Abnormal heart rhythm or increasing rate
      (4) Presence of murmurs or S_3 on auscultation
      (5) Labored respirations or rate increased to more than 20 respirations per minute
      (6) Presence of rales on auscultation
      (7) Decrease in urinary output to less than 30 ml per hour
      (8) Change in level of consciousness, dizziness, confusion, restlessness, and expression of a sense of doom
      (9) Cool, clammy skin
   c. Administer medications as ordered and monitor and report side effects. Draw blood levels as ordered. Document the effectiveness of pharmacologic and nonpharmacologic interventions in measurable terms.
   d. Monitor laboratory data, especially potassium and magnesium levels.
   e. Be prepared to respond to life-threatening dysrhythmias if they occur.

Discharge Planning and Health Teaching

1. Make an appointment for follow-up care and provide the patient with a written reminder.
2. Make certain that the person understands the importance of taking all medications on time. Ensure that medications are available for discharge. Review the name, purpose, and side effects of each medication with the patient and provide written instructions.
3. Review any dietary or activity limitations with the person and family members. Emphasize the need to stop activity and to rest if symptoms occur.
4. Teach the person and family member how to monitor the heart rate by checking the pulse. Allow time for practice and return demonstrations.
5. Encourage the person to call if there are any questions or concerns. Provide telephone numbers.

■ ARTERIAL HYPERTENSION (HIGH BLOOD PRESSURE)

Definition

1. Arterial hypertension is a persistent elevation of the systolic blood pressure above 140 mm Hg and of the diastolic pressure above 90 mm Hg.
   a. In systolic hypertension, systolic pressure is greater than 140 mm Hg.
   b. In diastolic hypertension, diastolic pressure is greater than 90 mm Hg.

2. A hypertensive crisis includes any clinical condition requiring immediate reduction in blood pressure, such as accelerated hypertension, hypertensive encephalopathy, toxemia of pregnancy, dissecting aortic aneurysm, pheochromocytoma crisis, and intracranial hemorrhage.

Incidence and Socioeconomic Impact

1. Primary hypertension
   a. Primary hypertension affects at least 15 percent of the adult population of the United States and is a leading cause of death and disability among adults.

> **ELDER ADVISORY**
>
> Owing to age-related arterial stiffening, older people are at a significant risk for hypertension. Those older than age 65 years have an approximate 50 percent incidence rate.

   b. Primary hypertension encompasses 90 to 95 percent of all cases of hypertension.
   c. At least 25 percent of the hypertensive population remain undiagnosed.
   d. Hypertension is considered to be the most significant predictor of developing coronary artery disease.
   e. Hypertension is the major risk factor for the coronary, cerebral, renal, and peripheral vascular diseases that account for more than half of all deaths in the United States.
   f. Incidence is greater in Blacks and in males.
2. Secondary hypertension affects 5 to 10 percent of the hypertensive population.

Risk Factors

1. Primary hypertension risk factors
   a. Advancing age
   b. Family history
   c. Black race, males in particular
   d. Obesity
   e. Tobacco use
   f. Stress
2. Secondary hypertension occurs in the following circumstances:
   a. Secondary to a primary disease of the cardiovascular system, renal system, or endocrine system

> **TRANSCULTURAL CONSIDERATIONS**
>
> Because Blacks, especially males, are at high risk of development of hypertension, instruct them to do the following:
> • Frequently monitor their blood pressure or have regular blood pressure checks
> • Keep salt intake low
> • Avoid obesity
> • Promptly seek medical intervention if blood pressure increases

   b. Secondary to pregnancy
   c. Secondary to certain drugs such as estrogen-containing oral contraceptive pills or the monoamine oxidase inhibitors that are used to treat depression.

Etiology

1. Primary hypertension, also known as essential or idiopathic hypertension, is of unknown origin.
2. Secondary hypertension is the result of an identifiable cause.

Pathophysiology

1. Primary hypertension
   a. Large vessel (e.g., aorta, coronary arteries, basilar artery to the brain) damage results in decreased blood flow to the heart and brain, and eventual occlusion or hemorrhage.
   b. Small vessel damage is equally dangerous and results in structural damage in the heart, kidneys, brain, and peripheral vessels, causing progressive impairment of these target organs and tissues.
   c. Systolic hypertension
      (1) In older people, systolic hypertension develops due to loss of elastic tissue and to arteriosclerotic changes that occur in the aorta and other large blood vessels.
      (2) In younger persons, systolic hypertension may reflect an increased cardiac output secondary to overactivity of the sympathetic nervous system.
   d. Diastolic hypertension develops due to decreased arteriolar caliber (as seen with atherosclerosis and vasoconstriction) and increased blood viscosity.
   e. Hypertensive crisis
      (1) Accelerated hypertension constitutes a medical emergency, in which target organ damage (brain, heart, retina of the eye) occurs in a very brief period.
      (2) Death is initially caused by stroke or renal failure, and later is caused by cardiac disease.
2. Secondary hypertension
   a. Pathophysiology depends on the underlying cause.
   b. If the event is time limited, as in pregnancy or drug effects, then permanent damage may be avoided.

Clinical Manifestations

1. Primary hypertension
   a. Usually, no symptoms are present during the early phase of the disease.

> **NURSE ADVISORY**
>
> Hypertension is usually asymptomatic. Therefore, if a hypertensive person's chief complaint is headache, dizziness, chest pain, ringing in the ears, or anxiety, consider differential diagnoses such as angina and tinnitus.

b. Many adults with hypertension remain untreated until complications develop that severely affect the target organs, causing severe symptoms.

2. Secondary hypertension
   a. Manifestations vary based on the primary disorder. (See Chapters 14, 26, and 29.)
   b. Because the diagnosis and treatment of secondary hypertension depends on the organs involved and its causation, the remainder of the discussion on hypertension focuses on primary hypertension.

Diagnostics

1. History
   a. A family history of hypertension, diabetes mellitus, or cardiovascular disease is significant.
   b. Previous documentation of high blood pressure should include age of onset.
   c. Patient history of weight gain and sodium intake should be documented.

2. Physical examination
   a. Measure blood pressure 2 or more times on both arms with the person in a supine (or seated) and in a standing position.
   b. Target organs
      (1) Examine the retina of the eye for hemorrhages, exudates, and papilledema.
      (2) Examine neck for distended veins.
      (3) Examine heart for increased heart rate, dysrhythmias, and enlargement.
      (4) Examine neurologic system for cerebral thrombosis or hemorrhage (see Chapter 18).

3. Diagnostic studies
   a. Complete blood count and urinalysis
   b. Serum potassium and sodium measurement
   c. Fasting blood sugar measurement
   d. Serum cholesterol level
   e. Blood urea nitrogen
   f. Serum creatinine
   g. Electrocardiogram
   h. Chest radiograph

4. Medical diagnosis
   a. Hypertension occurs in the following circumstances:
      (1) When the average of 2 or more diastolic blood pressure readings, on at least 2 subsequent visits, is 90 mm Hg or higher
      (2) When the average measurement of multiple systolic blood pressure over several visits is greater than 140 mm Hg

> Because blood pressure varies widely with emotional and physical activity, a single elevated reading does not indicate hypertension.

b. The Joint National Committee on Detection, Evaluation, and Treatment of High Blood Pressure classifies hypertension by ranges of both systolic and diastolic blood pressure (Table 23-8).

Table 23-8. Classification of Blood Pressure for Adults Aged 18 Years and Older*

Category	Systolic, mm Hg	Diastolic, mm Hg
Normal	<130	<85
High normal	130-139	85-89
Hypertension		
Stage 1 (mild)	140-159	90-99
Stage 2 (moderate)	160-179	100-109
Stage 3 (severe)	180-209	110-119
Stage 4 (very severe)	≥210	≥210

* Not taking hypertensive drugs and not acutely ill.
From The Fifth Report of The Joint National Committee on Detection, Evaluation, and Treatment of High Blood Pressure. *Arch Intern Med* 153:154-183, 1993.

Clinical Management

1. The goal of clinical management is to reduce the person's elevated blood pressure to the extent that cardiovascular risk and target organ damage lessens substantially.

> Adults with systolic pressure of 120 to 140 mm Hg have twice the risk of development of coronary heart disease than do adults with pressures less than 120 mm Hg.

2. Nonpharmacologic interventions. Lifestyle modifications are initial and definitive therapy for hypertension. If blood pressure cannot be successfully decreased after a reasonable trial (1-3 months), pharmacologic treatment is initiated. Nonpharmacologic interventions include the following:
   a. Weight reduction if necessary
   b. Sodium restriction to a level of 70 to 90 mg per day (approximately 2 gm of sodium or 5 gm of salt) (Table 23-9)

ELDER ADVISORY

> Isolated hypertension in older people is usually volume related. Sodium restriction alone may decrease blood pressure.

   c. Moderation in alcohol and caffeine consumption
   d. Gradual initiation of a regular aerobic exercise program (e.g., walking, jogging, and swimming)
   e. Avoidance of smoking

NURSE ADVISORY

> Because of the direct relationship between obesity and hypertension, weight reduction alone may reduce blood pressure in persons with mild uncomplicated primary hypertension.

Table 23-9. High-Sodium Foods to Avoid*

Canned Foods

Canned meats
  Sardines
  Corned beef
  Corned beef hash
  Chopped ham
  Chili
Canned vegetables
  Beets
  Hominy
  Spinach
  Sauerkraut
  Tomato sauce
  Pork and beans
Bottled sauces
  Catsup
  Chili sauce
  Soy sauce
  Steak sauce
Soups
Olives
Pickles
Relishes

Processed Meats and Cheeses

Ham
Bacon
Sausage
Wieners
Salt pork
Chipped beef
Cheese foods
Cheese spreads
Processed cheeses
Luncheon meats

Convenience Foods

Frozen vegetables with sauce
Pot pies
TV dinners
Soup mixes
Bouillon cubes
Rice mixes
Pasta mixes
Gravy mixes
Sauce mixes
Flour mixes
Coating mixes

Cooking Ingredients

Accent
Baking soda
Baking powder
Meat tenderizer
Monosodium glutamate (MSG)
Any seasoning with salt in the name

Snack Foods

Corn chips
Potato chips
Salted nuts
Salted crackers
Salted popcorn
Salted pretzels
Party dips
Frozen pizza
Frozen pizza rolls
Frozen egg rolls

* Many foods contain large amounts of hidden sodium. If a food fits into one of these groups, suspect that it has an elevated sodium content.

f. Alternative medical therapy such as relaxation techniques and biofeedback therapy, or a combination of these treatments to decrease both systolic and diastolic blood pressure
g. Maintenance of ideal body weight
h. Elimination of unnecessary medications such as oral contraceptives that may increase blood pressure
3. Pharmacologic interventions
a. Medications commonly used to treat hypertension include diuretics, sympatholytic agents, vasodilators, angiotensin-converting enzyme inhibitors, and calcium channel blockers (Table 23-10).
b. The stepped-care approach minimizes side effects (Table 23-11).
  (1) A monotherapy (single drug) approach is preferred. The clinician initiates the therapeutic program with a small dosage of an antihypertensive drug, and then increases the dosage of that drug until blood pressure comes under adequate control.
  (2) If the person's blood pressure does not decrease sufficiently, the physician adds another medication (2nd-step therapy) in gradually increasing doses

until achieving the desired blood pressure or the maximum dose is reached.

ELDER ADVISORY

A decrease in the treated blood pressure of older people below 85 diastolic may increase the risk of dangerous irregular heartbeats, especially in older persons who have a thickened heart muscle due to long-time hypertension.

  (3) The overall treatment plan proposed by the Joint National Committee on Detection, Evaluation, and Treatment of High Blood Pressure includes pharmacologic interventions in a stepped-care algorithm to minimize side effects (Fig. 23-11).
4. Special medical-surgical procedures. Systemic intra-arterial pressure monitoring provides continuous detection of arterial blood pressure in seriously ill individuals via an indwelling catheter. It allows for continuous monitoring of people with low cardiac output, fluctuating hemodynamic status, and excessive peripheral vasoconstric-

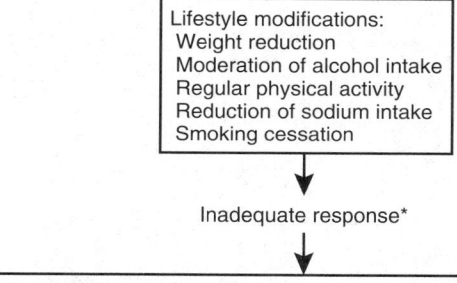

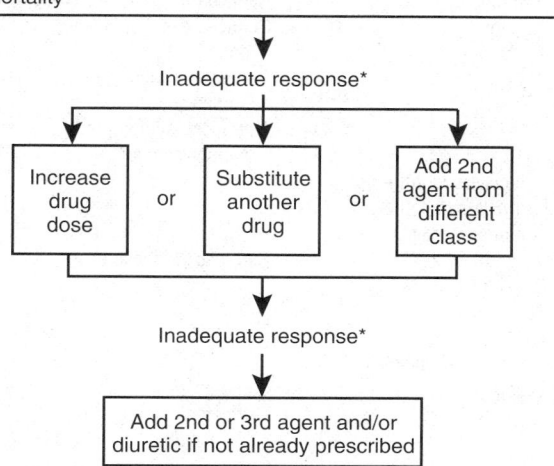

Figure 23-11. High blood pressure treatment algorithm. The asterisk indicates that the patient did not achieve goal blood pressure or is not making considerable progress toward this goal. ACE, Angiotensin-converting enzyme. (From the Fifth Report of the Joint National Committee on Detection, Evaluation, and Treatment of High Blood Pressure (JNC V). *Arch Intern Med* 153:154–183, 1993.)

Table 23–10. Pharmacologic Interventions for Hypertension

Drug	Adverse Reactions	Special Considerations
First-Line Interventions		
Diuretics		
Thiazide and related agents		
Bendroflumethiazide	Aplastic anemia	More effective than loop diuretics, except with elevated creatine
Benzthiazide	Hypokalemia	Increased risk of digitalis and lithium toxicity
Chlorothiazide	Hyponatremia	Enhanced hypotensive effect with antihypertensives, nitrates, alcohol
Chlorthalidone	Hypophosphatemia	May induce gout
Hydrochlorothiazide	Hypercalcemia	Additive hypokalemia with glucocorticoids, mezlocillin, piperacillin, ticarcillin, or amphotericin B
Hydroflumethiazide	Hyperlipidemia	
Indapamide	Dehydration	
Methyclothiazide	Hypotension	
Metolazone	Blood dyscrasias	
Polythiazide		
Quinethazone		
Trichlormethiazide		
Loop diuretics		
Bumetanide	As above, without hypercalcemia	Increased risk of ototoxicity with aminoglycosides and of lithium toxicity
Ethocrynic acid		May need higher doses with congestive heart failure or renal impairment
Furosemide		
Torsemide		
Potassium-sparing diuretics		
Amiloride	Anorexia	Usually used with other diuretics to avoid hypokalemia.
Spironolactone	Headache	Avoid with elevated creatinine.
Triamterene	Hyperkalemia	Increased risk of hyperkalemia with ACE inhibitors or potassium supplements; nephrotoxicity with NSAIDs and Indomethacin; nephrolithiasis with Triamterene.
	Nausea	
	Vomiting	
	Diarrhea	
	Rash	
	Gynecomastia	
Adrenergic Inhibitors		
Beta-blockers		
Atenolol	Bradycardia	May aggravate COPD, CHF, and peripheral arterial insufficiency.
Betaxolol	Heart block	Additive bradycardia with verapamil, digitalis, and reserpine.
Bisoprolol	Hypotension	Additive hypotension with other antihypertensives, alcohol, or nitrates.
Metoprolol	Heart failure	Decreased effect with thyroid medications.
Nadolol	Weakness/fatigue	Abrupt withdrawal may precipitate angina.
Propranolol	Reduced libido	
Timolol	Reduced exercise tolerance	
	Peripheral vascular insufficiency	
	May mask symptoms of hypoglycemia.	
Beta-blockers with intrinsic sympathomimetic activity		
Acebutolol	Same as β-blockers	Same as β-blockers. Used in patients with bradycardia if a β-blocker is required.
Carteolol		
Penbutolol		
Pindolol		
Alpha- and beta-blocker		
Labetalol	Same as β-blockers	Same as β-blockers
	Orthostatic hypotension	Absorption increased with food

Table 23–10. Pharmacologic Interventions for Hypertension (Continued)

Drug	Adverse Reactions	Special Considerations
Alpha₁-receptor blockers		
Doxazosin	Orthostatic hypotension	Hypertension potentiated by other antihypertensives, alcohol, and nitrates
Prazosin	Dizziness or syncope	Use with caution in older patients
Terazosin	Headaches	
	Tachycardia	
	Palpitations	
	Fluid retention	
Angiotensin-Converting Enzyme Inhibitors		
Benazepril	Bronchospasm	Used with coexisting congestive heart failure
Captopril	Hyperkalemia	Use caution with renal failure
Enalapril	Laryngitis	Hyperkalemia with renal impairment or when taking potassium supplements or potassium-sparing diuretics
Fosinopril	Cough	Nonsteroidal anti-inflammatory drugs can decrease effect and increase edema
Lisinopril	Dizziness	
Quinapril	Proteinuria	
Ramipril	Leukopenia	
	Rash	
Calcium Antagonists		
Diltiazem	Bradycardia	Use caution with heart failure
Verapamil	Headache	May increase digoxin levels and cyclosporine or carbamazepine toxicity
	Fatigue	Verapamil may increase theophylline levels
	Dizziness	Can cause bradycardia and heart block, worse if used with β-blockers
	Depression	Contraindicated in 2nd- or 3rd-degree heart block or sick-sinus syndrome.
	Edema	
Dihydropyridines		
Amlodipine	Headache	More potent than diltiazem and verapamil; dizziness, edema, and headache may be worse
Felodipine	Dizziness	
Isradipine	Edema	May increase cyclosporine level
Nicardipine	Tachycardia	May decrease effectiveness with phenytoin/phenobarbital
Nifedipine	Gingival hyperplasia	Toxicity may increase with cimetidine and propranolol
Supplemental Interventions		
Centrally Acting α_2-Agonists		
Clonidine	Dry mouth	Abrupt withdrawal can cause rebound hypertension; avoid in noncompliant patients
Guanabenz	Fatigue	Beta-blockers worsen severity of clonidine withdrawal
Guanfacine	Drowsiness	Monoamine oxidase inhibitors and tricyclic antidepressants decrease effect
Methyldopa	Impotence	Methyldopa can cause liver damage and hemolytic anemia
	Dizziness	
Peripherally Acting Adrenergic Antagonists		
Guanethidine	Dizziness and syncope	Potentiates central nervous system depression with other central nervous system depressants
Guanadrel	Orthostatic hypotension	Decreased effect with tricyclic antidepressants or monoamine oxidase inhibitors
	Drowsiness	Increased dysrhythmias with digitalis, quinidine, procainamide
	Dyspnea	
	Impotence	
	Diarrhea	
	Edema	
Rauwolfia alkaloids		
Rauwolfia root	Lethargy	Contraindicated in depression and peptic ulcer disease
Reserpine	Depression	Even when not taken regularly, reserpine has a prolonged duration of action.
	Nasal congestion	
	Bradycardia	
	Gastrointestinal bleeding	
Direct Vasodilators		
Hydralazine	Headache	Used with severe hypotension
Minoxidil	Increased heart rate	Beta-blockers are used to counteract reflex tachycardia and fluid retention
	Angina	Increased hypotension with monoamine oxidase inhibitors
	Fluid retention	

LEARNING/TEACHING GUIDELINES
for Self-Care in Hypertension

General Overview

1. Describe the disease process and explain that hypertension initially produces few symptoms until target organs (heart, lung, kidneys, and the brain) have suffered serious damage.
2. Discuss dietary modifications including sodium, calorie, saturated fat, and cholesterol restrictions (if indicated).
3. Point out the importance of starting and maintaining a moderate exercise program as recommended by the physician.
4. Describe the proper administration of prescribed antihypertensive drugs, stating the name of each and explaining the rationale for its use. Also describe dosage, frequency, potential side effects, and measures used to minimize side effects.
5. Help the person and family plan ways to reduce stress and tension at home and at work.
6. Demonstrate proper blood pressure measurement technique for home monitoring.
7. Emphasize the importance of lifelong medical follow-up for control of hypertension.

Medication Administration

1. Instruct people who are going to self-administer medications to do the following:
   a. Never adjust the dosage or discontinue a drug without consulting the physician because congestive heart failure or rejection may develop.
   b. Always take the drug on time; never skip doses. Incorporate medication administration into daily routines such as coffee breaks, shaving, and mealtimes to avoid missed doses, or purchase a pill box that is divided into the days of the week.
   c. Always report untoward effects to the physician.
   d. Avoid any over-the-counter medication unless approved by physician.
   e. Do not stop taking medication even when feeling better.

Low-Sodium Diet

1. Point out the following important facts about sodium:
   a. Sodium is found in almost all foods and beverages, including water. It is present in large amounts in baking powder, baking soda, monosodium glutamate, meat tenderizer, and soy sauce, and it is often added to canned, boxed, and some frozen foods. (Frozen fruits and vegetables are usually acceptable.) Sodium is also found in many over-the-counter medications, in particular, in antacids, cough remedies, and laxatives.
   b. Sodium cannot be seen and often is not tasted.
   c. Table salt is sodium chloride (40% sodium). There are 388 mg of sodium in every 1 gm of salt.
   d. Average adult daily intake of salt is 5 to 15 gm.
   e. Therapeutic effects on blood pressure do not take place until salt intake is reduced below 5 gm per day.
2. Tell the person and family members how to avoid foods high in sodium and prepare low-sodium meals:
   a. Read the labels of foods and drugs carefully for "sodium," "Na$^+$," "NaCl," and "MSG," because these are all sources of sodium.
   b. In restaurants, choose foods that are baked, boiled, or roasted without salt gravies or juices. Avoid soups and salad or cheesy dressings.
   c. Do not add salt at the table.
   d. Use no salt or herb salts (celery, onion, and garlic) during food preparation.
   e. Prepare canned vegetables (if eaten) by draining off the canned liquid and heating the food in tap water. Some canned vegetables and tomato products marked "No added salt" or "Low sodium" are available.
   f. Choose low-sodium foods. For example:
      (1) Unprocessed meats, fresh or frozen
      (2) Fresh vegetables
      (3) Vegetables frozen without sauce
      (4) Fruits, fresh, frozen, or canned
      (5) Beans and peas, fresh or dried
      (6) Pasta, fresh or dried
   g. Avoid high-sodium foods (see Table 23–9).
   h. Obtain a low-sodium cookbook (available from the American Heart Association). See also Chapter 10.

Exercise

1. Point out the following physical and psychologic benefits of exercise:
   a. Exercise benefits cardiovascular health and is an aid in lowering blood pressure and heart rate.
   b. By burning calories, exercise helps to reduce or avoid excess body weight and increased percentage of body fat.
   c. Exercise programs may heighten the person's sense of well-being, provide an outlet for emotional tensions, and increase the levels of high-density lipoproteins relative to total blood cholesterol.
2. Give the person the following instructions for starting an exercise program:
   a. Maintain close medical supervision.
   b. Begin the exercise program gradually, increasing its intensity and duration at intervals as tolerated.

LEARNING/TEACHING GUIDELINES
(continued)

c. Be aware that the most suitable exercises for stimulating cardiovascular and respiratory fitness include walking, jogging, swimming, cross-country skiing, and bicycling.
d. Avoid heavy weight lifting and isometric exercises.

Home Blood Pressure Recordings

1. Inform the person about the merits of home blood pressure monitoring.
   a. People who monitor and record their own blood pressure at home tend to be more involved in managing their disease.
   b. Home blood pressure monitoring fosters compliance to intervention, thereby reducing the risk of complications.

c. Monitoring reveals trends in the person's blood pressure and thus may represent the person's condition more accurately than recordings taking in a physician's office.
2. Instruct the person in how to take a home blood pressure recording.
   a. Demonstrate how to do the following:
      (1) Wrap the cuff around the arm
      (2) Position the arm at heart level
      (3) Listen for systolic and diastolic sounds
      (4) Record the pressures
   b. Have the person give a return demonstration.
   c. If economically feasible, suggest the purchase of a blood pressure kit with digital readouts that is used by wrapping the apparatus around the arm, turning it on, and recording the printout.

---

tion, and in whom cuff blood pressure measurements are undetectable.

Complications

1. Complications damage the heart, brain, kidneys, eyes, and peripheral vessels.
2. Major complications
   a. Cardiac disorders, including infarction
   b. Acute pulmonary edema
   c. Hypertensive encephalopathy
   d. Cerebrovascular accident (stroke)
   e. Retinal changes, including hemorrhage
   f. Renal failure

Prognosis

1. Nearly one half of untreated hypertensive people die of heart disease, one third die of stroke, and the remainder die of renal failure.
2. Effective antihypertensive agents have dramatically reduced the mortality rate associated with hypertension.
3. An estimated 40 to 60 percent of people with hypertension fail to comply with prescribed therapy for the following reasons:

a. The disease is initially asymptomatic.
b. Therapeutic regimens demand difficult lifestyle changes such as low-sodium and low-calorie diets.
c. Many antihypertensive agents have annoying side effects and are expensive.

Applying the Nursing Process

NURSING DIAGNOSIS: Knowledge deficit R/T hypertension and self-care, including self-administration of antihypertensive drugs, low-sodium diet preparation, exercise, and home blood pressure measurement

1. *Expected outcomes:* Following instruction, the person should be able to do the following:
   a. Demonstrate an understanding of the hypertensive disease process by being able to define hypertension and explain how uncontrolled hypertension damages the major body systems
   b. Properly self-administer antihypertensive medications
   c. Describe how to shop for and prepare low-sodium meals
   d. Plan a safe exercise program and a realistic schedule for exercising
   e. Demonstrate how to take own blood pressure.
2. Nursing interventions (see Learning/Teaching Guidelines for Self-Care in Hypertension)

NURSING DIAGNOSIS: Ineffective individual coping R/T stress at work and at home

1. *Expected outcomes:* Following counseling, the person should be able to do the following:
   a. Report practicing at least 1 relaxation technique every day
   b. Report a reduction in the number of stress-inducing situations encountered daily

Table 23–11. Stepped-Care Approach to Hypertension

First Step	Second Step
Thiazide diuretic	Beta blocker, angiotensin-converting enzyme (ACE) inhibitor or calcium antagonist
Beta-blocking agent	Thiazide diuretic
ACE inhibitor	Thiazide diuretic
Calcium antagonist	Thiazide diuretic

c. Have a more relaxed facial expression and appear less hurried when speaking

2. *Nursing interventions*
   a. Teach the person how to incorporate relaxation techniques such as medication and yoga into daily routines.
   b. Help the person to identify stressful situations that occur on a regular basis and suggest specific ways to reduce or eliminate factors causing stress.
   c. Ask the person to keep a diary that documents how well each strategy for reducing stress is working.

Discharge Planning and Teaching

1. Make an appointment for the person to have a professional blood pressure checkup after being discharged. Stress the importance of follow-up care.
2. Give the patient a booklet in which to record home blood pressure readings.
3. Make certain that the person has medications to take home and understands how to self-administer them.
4. Give the person a packet of low-sodium meal suggestions and menus.
5. Encourage the person and family to call if they have questions or concerns.

Public Health Considerations

1. Primary prevention
   a. The high incidence of hypertension and the number of undiscovered cases constitute a national public health problem that can only be corrected by a national public health effort.
   b. National efforts involve enlisting governmental support, as well as the support of business and industry, labor organizations, health care institutions, voluntary associations, and local communities.
   c. The National High Blood Pressure Education Program, initiated by the National Heart, Lung, and Blood Association in 1972, is primarily responsible for the successful growth in public awareness and action.
   d. To help identify people at risk for hypertension, organized community screening programs are located in public settings such as shopping malls, schools, and workplaces.
   e. Nurses working in screening programs need to inform people in writing of their blood pressure, its significance, and, if necessary, the importance of follow-up evaluation.

◼ *CORONARY ARTERY DISEASES*

Coronary Artery Disease

1. Definition: Coronary artery disease is a process in which the coronary artery vasculature is partially to totally occluded by an atherosclerotic plaque, resulting in disruption of blood flow to the heart muscle (Fig. 23–12).

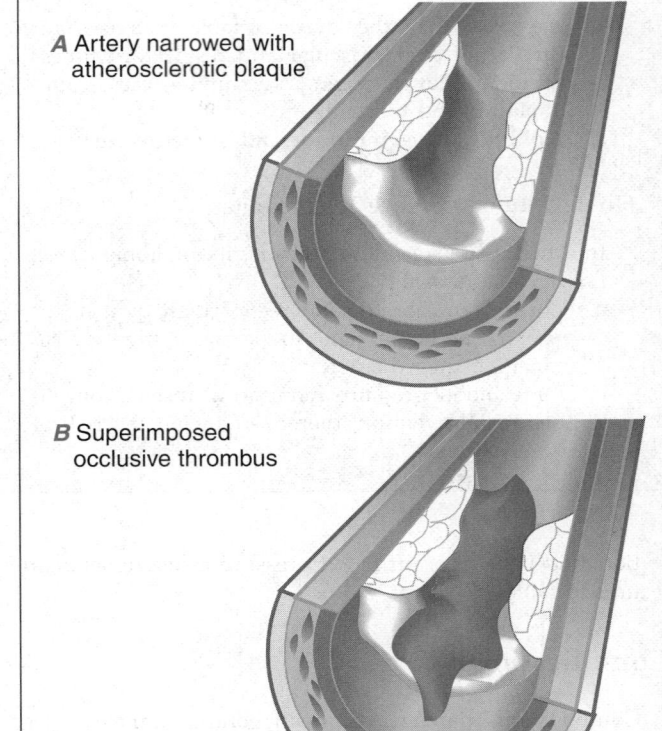

CORONARY ARTERY DISEASE

A Artery narrowed with atherosclerotic plaque

B Superimposed occlusive thrombus

Figure 23–12. Atherosclerosis of coronary arteries.

2. Incidence and socioeconomic impact
   a. Coronary artery disease and its complications are the leading cause of death in the United States, accounting for more than 500,000 deaths annually.
   b. Five million Americans are diagnosed with coronary artery disease each year.
   c. It is estimated that coronary artery disease has a $60 to 100 billion economic impact associated with illness, hospitalization, and lost wages.
3. Risk factors
   a. Modifiable risk factors
      (1) Hyperlipidemia. Elevated cholesterol, especially high low-density lipoprotein and low high-density lipoprotein levels are directly related to the development of coronary artery disease.
      (2) Smoking: Smokers have approximately twice the incidence as nonsmokers. Nonsmokers may be exposed to increased risk by passive exposure to cigarette smoke. Persons who stop smoking markedly decrease their risk. Risk decreases by 50 percent the first year and approaches that of a nonsmoker in 2 to 10 years. Smoking stimulates the sympathetic nervous system, resulting in increased heart rate and blood pressure, and sys-

temic vasoconstriction. Smoking has an adverse effect on cholesterol and triglyceride levels. Smoking may contribute to thrombus development. Smokers have increased platelet aggregation and higher fibrinogen levels.

(3) Hypertension (see p. 1024): Persons with hypertension (blood pressure greater than 160/95) have twice the risk of coronary artery disease. Persons with borderline hypertension (140/159 systolic) have a 50 percent increase in risk.

(4) Diabetes: Atherosclerosis is usually more severe and more extensive in diabetic patients. Coronary artery disease is the leading cause of death in diabetic adults.

◉▐▮▬▲◗▥✡▌★◉▯▬◐

TRANSCULTURAL CONSIDERATIONS

Diabetes is a primary risk factor for coronary artery disease in Hispanics.

(5) Physical inactivity: Evidence indicates that regular and moderate physical activity is beneficial in preventing coronary artery disease. Physical activity has beneficial effects on other risk factors including hyperlipidemia, hypertension, diabetes, obesity, and stress.

(6) Obesity (increase of 20% above ideal body weight). It is often associated with other risk factors of hypertension, diabetes, and hyperlipidemia. Truncal obesity (apple-shaped body) may be more detrimental than peripheral obesity (pear-shaped body) (Fig. 23-13).

(7) Stress and type A personality. Having a type A personality—aggressive, competitive, time focused—or prolonged emotional stress has been shown to predispose a person to coronary artery disease.

> High stress levels and a "type A personality" are strongly correlated with cardiovascular disorders, including hypertension.

b. Nonmodifiable risk factors

(1) Family history: Parental or sibling history of coronary artery disease is strongly associated with increased risk.

(2) Age: Increased age is associated with increased risk and is probably related to duration of exposure to risk factors.

(3) Gender: Men have a greater risk of MI than women, but heart disease is the leading cause of death among women in the United States. Studies have shown the presence of "gender bias" symptoms in women are often interpreted as psychosomatic and women are less likely to be referred for angiogram. Special risk factors in women include the following:

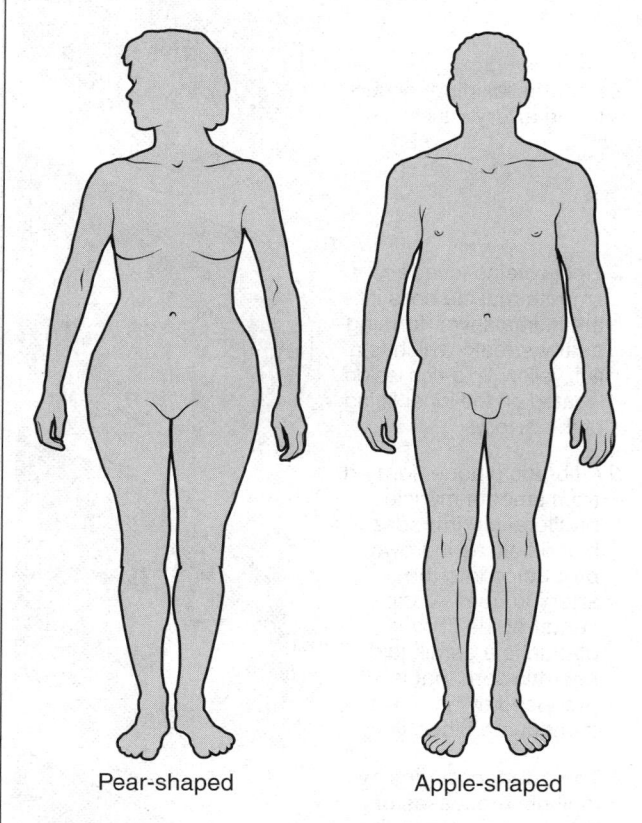

BODY TYPE AND CORONARY ARTERY DISEASE

Pear-shaped   Apple-shaped

Figure 23-13.

- Menopause—heart disease increases after menopause due to decreased estrogen levels.
- Stress—the multiple roles assumed by women (e.g., work and child care) may mean increased risk of heart disease.
- Oral contraceptives affect cholesterol and increase blood pressure and are associated with increased coronary artery disease, especially if a woman smokes.

> Impairment of the coronary circulation by arteriosclerosis is the major cause of heart disease.

4. Etiology

a. Coronary artery disease is caused by atherosclerosis, the most common cause of arterial disease. Over a period of years, the development of atherosclerotic plaques obstruct the arterial lumen (Fig. 23-14).

b. It is not known how atherosclerosis begins.

5. Pathophysiology

a. The pathophysiology of arterial disorders is best understood by considering the circulatory needs of

THE PROCESS OF ATHEROSCLEROSIS

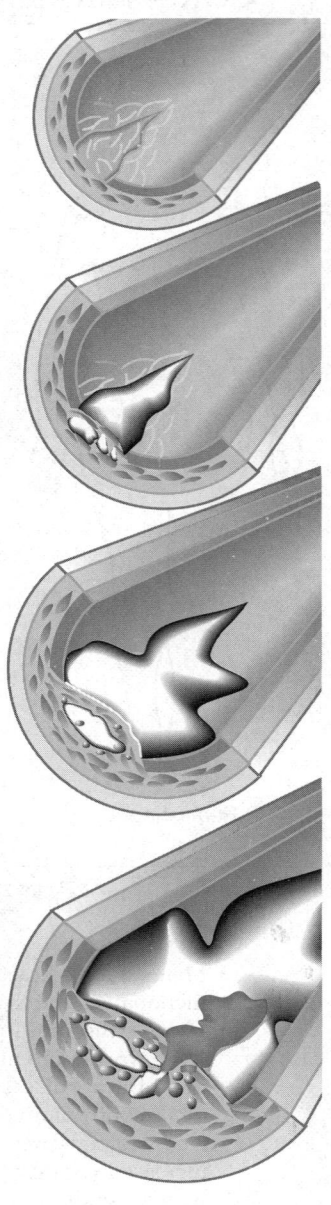

1 Endothelial injury occurs to the artery wall.

2 Lipoproteins invade smooth muscle cells in the intimal layer, forming a fatty streak, which is a flat, yellow, lipid-rich lesion located on the inner lining of the artery.

3 A fibrous plaque, formed from smooth muscle proliferation, impedes blood flow as it grows, protruding into the artery lumen. At the center of the fibrous plaque is a semiliquid necrotic core that is produced by an inadequate blood flow.

4 The artery occludes by multiple processes of hemorrhage, ulceration, calcification, and thrombosis. As the fibrous plaque continues to grow, it can rupture and form a clot or thrombus, which consists of platelet aggregation at the rupture site. If the blockage at the vessel site is great enough, the thrombus may cause total occlusion of the artery.

Figure 23–14.

body tissues. A reduction or occlusion of blood flow occurs in all types of arterial disease.

b. Arteriosclerosis occurs when arteries, either through aging, pathologic processes, or both, lose their elasticity and become hardened.

   (1) Loss of elasticity negatively affects the flow of blood through the vascular channels.

   (2) Changes in the intima of the arteries by the hardening process promote a rough surface inside the artery where plaque forms and platelet aggregation develops.

c. Atherosclerosis is the most common cause of peripheral arterial disease.

d. No one has yet determined the exact cause of atherosclerosis. The reaction-to-injury theory suggests the following sequence of events:

   (1) Endothelial injury occurs to the artery wall.

   (2) Lipoproteins invade smooth muscle cells in the intimal layer, forming a fatty streak. The fatty streak is the earliest lesion of atherosclerosis and may be found in infants and young children. It is a smooth yellow lipid-laden lesion located on the inner lining of the artery.

   (3) The fibrous plaque, the advanced lesion of atherosclerosis, generally appears in early adulthood and progresses with age. It is white, protrudes into the lumen of the artery, and may compromise blood flow if large enough. These lesions are characterized by proliferation of smooth muscle cells covered by fibrous cap of connective tissue covering lipid and cell debris. At the center of the fibrous plaque is a semi-liquid necrotic core that is produced by an inadequate blood flow.

   (4) The artery occludes by multiple processes of hemorrhage, ulceration, calcification, and thrombosis (see Fig. 23–14). As the fibrous plaque continues to grow, it can rupture and form a clot or thrombus, which consists of platelet aggregation at the rupture site. If the blockage at the vessel site is great enough, then the thrombus may cause total occlusion of the artery.

e. Primary sites of atherosclerosis involvement are the large and medium-sized arteries such as the abdominal aorta and iliac arteries.

f. Lesions can be seen throughout the arterial system in segments in varying degrees.

g. The most common sites of atherosclerosis in the lower extremities include aortoiliac, superficial femoral, and tibial arteries (Fig. 23–15).

6. Clinical manifestations

a. Symptoms become evident when the coronary artery lumen is occluded to the point that inadequate blood supply to the muscle occurs, causing ischemia.

b. The most common clinical manifestation of myocardial ischemia is chest pain.

c. Some persons have "silent" ischemia and experience no chest pain.

d. An ECG provides evidence of various degrees of myocardial response to decreased blood flow.

   (1) Ischemia: When blood flow is reduced somewhat but not enough to cause myocardial cell death, the ECG may demonstrate ST segment depression or T wave inversion. When blood flow returns to normal, so does the ST segment.

NURSE ADVISORY

Not all persons having a myocardial infarction experience ECG changes. Approximately 12 percent of persons demonstrate atypical or no changes.

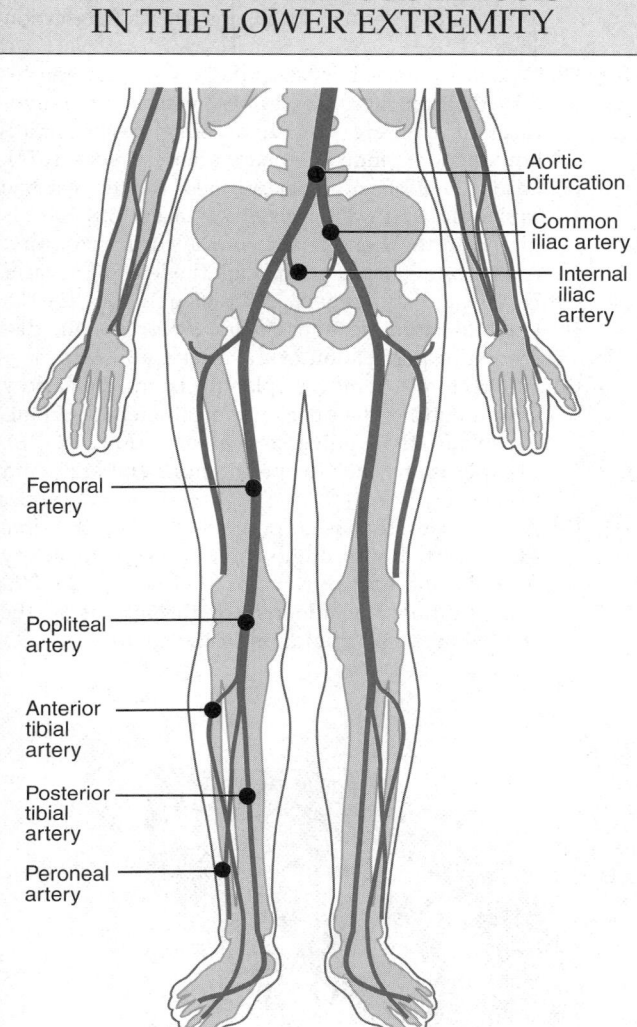

SITES OF ATHEROSCLEROSIS IN THE LOWER EXTREMITY

Aortic bifurcation

Common iliac artery

Internal iliac artery

Femoral artery

Popliteal artery

Anterior tibial artery

Posterior tibial artery

Peroneal artery

Figure 23–15.

(2) Infarction: Within hours after blood flow is occluded, cell injury results in ST segment elevation. This is followed by T wave inversion. Lastly, a Q wave appears, indicating cell necrosis.

7. Diagnostics
   a. History
      (1) Assess the patient for the presence of the primary symptoms of cardiovascular disease: chest pain or discomfort, palpitations, dyspnea, syncope, edema, cough or hemoptysis, and excessive fatigue.
   b. Physical examination. Findings are often normal during asymptomatic periods but vary depending on the specific complication.
   c. Diagnostic studies
      (1) Electrocardiogram
      (2) Exercise tolerance test
      (3) Radionuclide imaging
      (4) Holter or ambulatory ECG monitoring
      (5) Coronary angiography
      (6) Cardiac enzymes test
      (7) Blood lipid levels
      (8) Positron emission tomography
   d. Medical diagnosis
      (1) The presence of atherosclerotic lesions identified during cardiac catheterization is the most definitive source for diagnosis.
      (2) Coronary artery stenosis (narrowing) is usually considered significant if the luminal diameter of the left main artery is reduced at least 50 percent or if any major branch is reduced at least 75 percent.
8. Clinical management
   a. The goal of clinical management is to alter the atherosclerotic progression.
   b. Nonpharmacologic interventions: It is possible to reduce the impact of risk factors by changes in lifestyle (Table 23–12).
   c. Pharmacologic interventions: Drugs can be used to mediate the effects of hypertension and elevated cholesterol levels (Table 23–13).
   d. Special medical-surgical procedures
      (1) Percutaneous transluminal coronary angioplasty is performed in the cardiac catheterization laboratory, where a balloon-tipped catheter is placed

Table 23–12. Nonpharmacologic Interventions to Reduce the Impact of Risk Factors for Coronary Artery Disease

Risk Factor	Nonpharmacologic Intervention
Smoking	Physician emphasis
	Stop smoking programs
	Group support
	Hypnosis
Hypertension	Weight reduction
	Dietary salt restriction
	Exercise
	Stress reduction techniques
	Alcohol restriction
Cholesterol	Diet: <30% total calories from fat
	<200 mg cholesterol/day
	Exercise
Diabetes mellitus	Diet
	Weight control
Stress	Biofeedback
	Medication
	Stress management education
	Exercise
	Behavioral programs
	Counseling
	Relaxation techniques
Physical inactivity	Exercise prescription and instruction
Obesity	Diet counseling and restriction
	Surgery—gastric bypass (controversial)

Table 23–13. Pharmacologic Management Used to Mediate the Effects of Hypertension and Elevated Cholesterol Levels on Coronary Artery Disease

Clinical Management	Rationale
Nitrates	Dilate coronary arteries Decrease preload and afterload
Calcium channel blockers	Dilate coronary arteries and reduce vasospasm
Cholesterol-lowering drugs	Reduce development of atherosclerotic plaques
Elimination of oral contraceptives	Use can cause increased blood pressure and cholesterol levels

in the stenotic area of the coronary artery. To increase blood flow to the myocardium, the balloon is inflated and compresses the plaque against the walls of the artery and dilates the vessel (Fig. 23–16). Potential complications include dysrhythmias, MI, dissection of the coronary artery, acute coronary occlusion due to spasm, restenosis of the artery within the first 6 months, hematoma and vascular problems at the insertion site.

(2) Coronary artery bypass graft is a surgical procedure that improves blood flow to areas of the myocardium that are at risk of ischemia or infarction due to occluded coronary arteries (see p. 1074).

(3) Laser angioplasty is performed in the cardiac catheterization laboratory. A laser catheter is placed in the stenotic area of the coronary artery. As the catheter passes through the lesion, the laser is activated and vaporizes the plaque (Fig. 23–17). Potential complications include reocclusion, dissection or perforation of the artery, and MI.

(4) Atherectomy removes plaque from the artery with a cutting chamber on the catheter or a rotating blade that pulverizes plaque (Fig. 23–18). Complications include perforation, embolus, and restenosis.

(5) A vascular stent is a permanent noncollapsible tube inserted after angioplasty to keep the artery from closing and prevent restenosis (Fig. 23–19). Complications include risk of thrombosis of the stented area and migration of the stent.

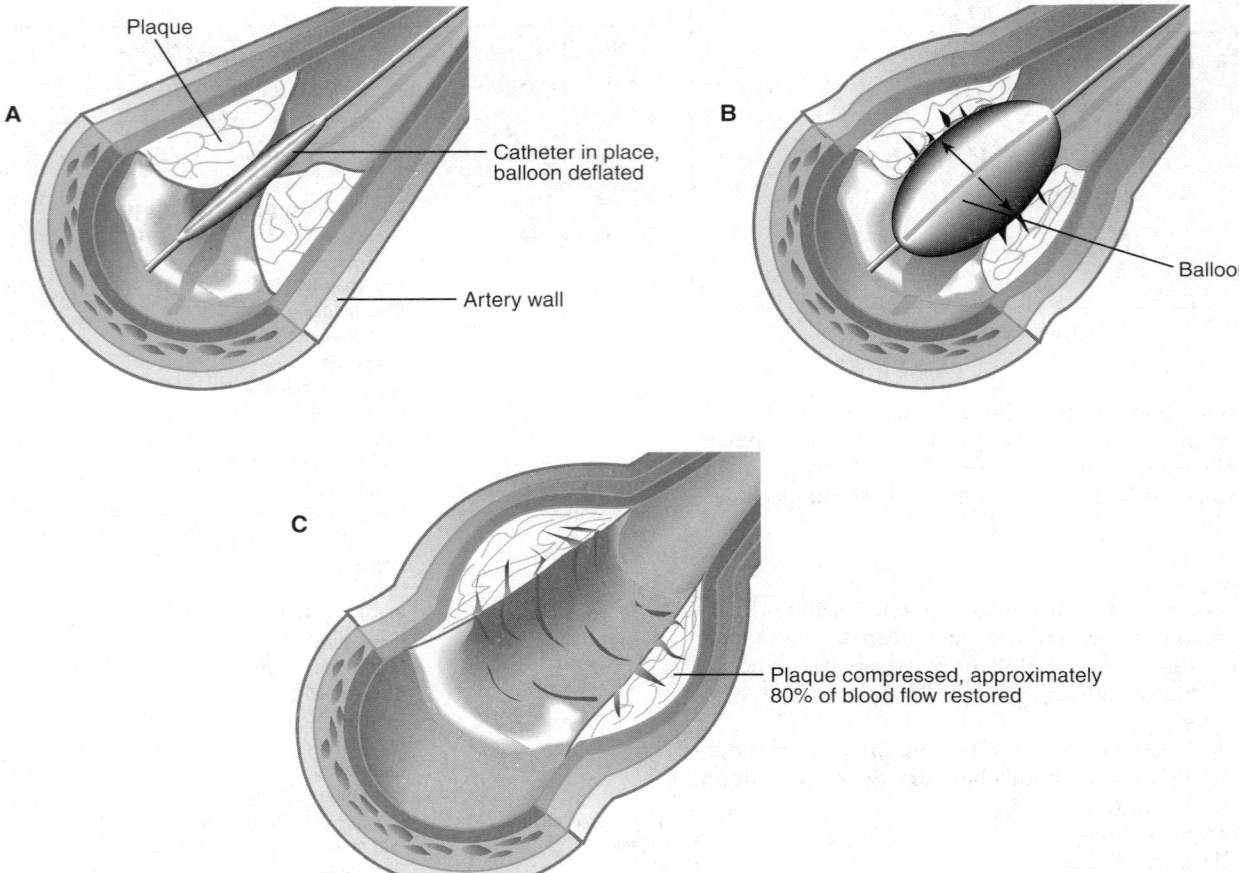

Figure 23–16. Percutaneous transluminal coronary angioplasty.

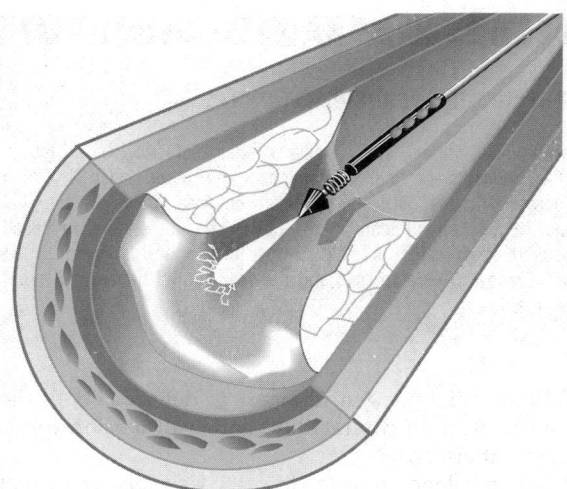

Figure 23-17. Laser angioplasty.

9. Complications from coronary artery disease
   a. Angina
   b. Myocardial infarction
   c. Congestive heart failure
   d. Dysrhythmias
   e. Sudden death
   f. Asymptomatic coronary disease (silent ischemia)
10. Prognosis: The prognosis depends on the complications of the disease.
11. Applying the nursing process

NURSING DIAGNOSIS: Knowledge deficit R/T risk factors for coronary artery disease

a. *Expected outcomes:* Following instruction, the person should be able to demonstrate an understanding of the risk factors associated with coronary artery disease by doing the following:
   (1) Listing the major modifiable risk factors
   (2) Discussing strategies to reduce these risk factors

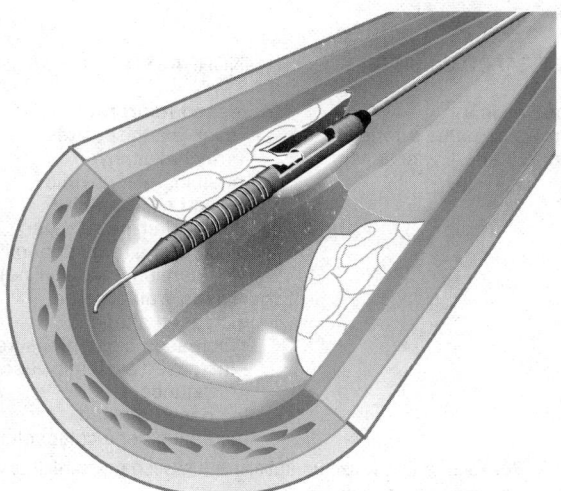

Figure 23-18. Atherectomy.

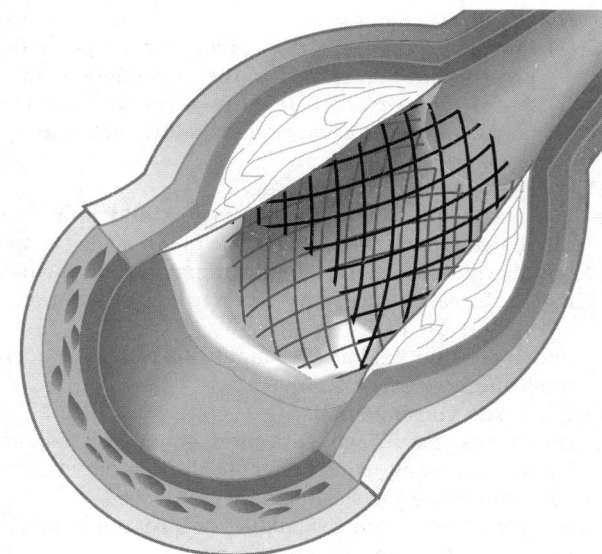

Figure 23-19. Coronary stent.

using exercise, diet, smoking cessation, and stress reduction
b. *Nursing interventions*
   (1) Provide written materials on exercise, diet, smoking cessation, and stress reduction.
   (2) Encourage the person to set reasonable targets for lifestyle changes and measure improvement over time.
   (3) Review the available community resources for exercise and smoking reduction. These may include employee wellness programs at work, American Heart Association programs, and programs based at the YMCA or other community organizations.

NURSING DIAGNOSIS: Noncompliance R/T unwillingness to adhere to the therapeutic plan

a. *Expected outcomes:* Following counseling, the person should be able to do the following:
   (1) Describe their personal barriers to compliance such as the need for business lunches, the cultural impact on cooking habits such as the use of salt or oils, or the use of food as a response to stress or other emotions. Work schedules or family commitments may impact time available for exercise.
   (2) Identify a routine or system that will modify these barriers and provide positive rather than negative reinforcement. Examples include use of support groups, scheduling walks at lunch with coworkers, and involving family members in the risk-modification activities.
   (3) Articulate a daily schedule consistent with a healthy lifestyle including making appropriate dietary choices from sample menus, including time for stress reduction activities and exercise in the plan, and stating that these changes are not temporary but must be maintained for life.

b. *Nursing interventions*
   (1) Encourage the person to identify barriers or express frustration related to the therapeutic plan.
   (2) Assist the person to identify ways to overcome barriers and incorporate therapeutic plan into everyday life.
12. Discharge planning and teaching
  a. Instruct people about the risk factors and how they can be modified, as well as the pharmacologic and nonpharmacologic therapeutic regimens for mediating the effects of coronary artery disease (see Tables 23–12 and 23–13).
  b. Encourage the person and family to call with questions and concerns.
13. Public health considerations
  a. In schools, encourage education about risk factors, enforce smoking bans, offer healthy food choices, and emphasize physical activity.
  b. At work, encourage risk reduction programs including risk factor education and screening.
  c. In the community, participate in education and screening programs.

Angina

1. Definition
  a. Angina pectoris (literally translated, "strangling chest") is chest pain due to transient myocardial ischemia without development of myocardial necrosis.
  b. Classifications include stable angina pectoris (also called exertional angina, angina of effort, or typical angina); variant angina (also called Prinzmetal's angina or vasospastic angina), which results from cyclical coronary artery spasm that is relatively unresponsive to antianginal medications; unstable angina (also called preinfarction angina or acute coronary insufficiency), which refers to the prodromal syndrome of acute MI.
2. Incidence and socioeconomic impact
  a. Approximately 2.5 million people in the United States suffer from some form of angina.
  b. Approximately 3 million new cases of angina are identified each year.
3. Risk factors
  a. Risk factors for stable and unstable angina are the same as those for coronary artery disease (see p. 1032).
  b. Risk factors for variant (Prinzmetal's) angina are unknown.
4. Etiology
  a. Angina is caused by an imbalance between myocardial oxygen supply and demand.
  b. Obstruction of coronary blood flow due to atherosclerosis is the usual cause, but coronary artery spasm and conditions increasing myocardial oxygen consumption may also contribute.
5. Pathophysiology
  a. Myocardial oxygen supply is determined by coronary artery blood flow.

b. Myocardial oxygen demand is determined by heart rate, vigor of contractility, and wall tension (preload and afterload).
c. An imbalance due to decreased supply or increased demand or a combination of both may precipitate anginal episodes (Fig. 23–20).
d. In stable angina, an atherosclerotic plaque partially occludes the coronary artery lumen. This causes a "fixed supply" of oxygen to the myocardium. When oxygen demand increases (e.g., with exercise), supply cannot increase to meet the increased demand.
e. In variant angina, intense coronary artery vasospasm occludes the coronary artery lumen, causing a decreased supply of oxygen to the myocardium.
f. In unstable angina, patients have severe obstructive coronary artery disease. Intermittent platelet aggregation at the plaque site and coronary vasoconstriction are thought to occlude the coronary artery lumen and cause a decreased myocardial oxygen supply.

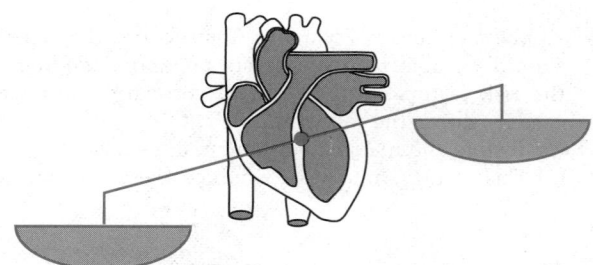

DECREASED O₂ SUPPLY

Atherosclerosis
Narrows coronary arteries
Coronary artery vasospasm

INCREASED O₂ DEMAND

Increased heart rate
Fever, exercise, stress, arrhythmias, hypoxia, anemia, hyperthyroid
Increased contractility
Catecholamine release
Medications (e.g., dopamine, dobutamine, theophylline)
Increased wall tension
Increased afterload
• Increased blood pressure
• Increased systemic vascular resistance
Increased preload
Increased ventricular volume

Figure 23–20. Factors that cause an imbalance between myocardial oxygen supply and demand, resulting in angina.

6. Clinical manifestations
   a. The clinical manifestation of angina is chest discomfort characterized as squeezing substernal pain. Pain may radiate to the shoulders, arms, neck, or back, with a duration of 5 to 15 minutes (see Chapter 37).
   b. Stable angina
      (1) Chest pain occurs with activities that increase oxygen demand such as exertion or emotional excitement.
      (2) The pain is relieved with rest or nitroglycerin.
   c. Variant angina
      (1) Chest pain is not associated with increased myocardial oxygen demand and may occur during rest, usual activity, or sleep.
      (2) Pain is relieved with nitroglycerin.
   d. Unstable angina
      (1) A change in the pattern of angina occurs.
         • Chest pain develops with minimal increase in oxygen demand or at rest.
         • Chest pain develops with increased frequency.
         • Chest pain is more severe and harder to relieve.
      (2) Pain may not be relieved with nitroglycerin.

TRANSCULTURAL CONSIDERATIONS

In Hispanic, Islamic, and Asian ethnic groups, when the heart is seen as the repository of emotion, angina can be perceived as being related to extreme emotion.

7. Diagnostics
   a. The diagnosis is initially made from a characteristic history. If angina is suspected, other diagnostic tests may be done.
   b. History
      (1) Obtain a detailed description of the chest discomfort (see p. 986).
      (2) Note the presence of risk factors for coronary artery disease.
   c. Physical examination
      (1) If the patient is not having pain, the physical assessment may be unremarkable.
      (2) During anginal episodes, patients may appear distressed. Skin may be cool and clammy.
      (3) Signs of ventricular failure such as hypotension, tachycardia, and rales may be noted.
      (4) Blood pressure may be increased and may precipitate or be caused by an angina attack.
      (5) S_4 is often auscultated.
      (6) A transient systolic murmur due to papillary muscle dysfunction is common.
   d. Diagnostic studies
      (1) Electrocardiogram. The ECG results are normal during rest. During an angina episode, the ECG often shows ST segment depression, T wave inversion, or both. Changes resolve when the episode resolves. Variant Prinzmetal's angina is diagnosed by ST segment elevation during the angina episode, which returns to normal after the episode resolves.
      (2) Exercise test
      (3) Radionuclide imaging
      (4) Echocardiography
      (5) Holter monitoring
      (6) Cholesterol level measurement
      (7) Cardiac enzymes test, which are normal in angina and differentiate angina from MI
      (8) Ergonovine test, which induces vasospasm in patients with variant angina and is done in the cardiac catheterization laboratory
      (9) Cardiac catheterization for a definitive diagnosis

8. Clinical management
   a. The goal of intervention is to correct the imbalance between myocardial oxygen supply and demand (Table 23–14).
   b. Nonpharmacologic interventions for unstable angina
      (1) Bed rest
      (2) Emotional rest
      (3) Rule out MI with cardiac enzymes tests and serial ECGs.
      (4) Place on cardiac monitor or telemetry.
      (5) Monitor for chest discomfort.
   c. Pharmacologic interventions for unstable angina
      (1) Intravenous nitroglycerin
      (2) Aspirin
      (3) Intravenous heparin
      (4) Oxygen, 3 liters by nasal cannula
   d. Special medical-surgical procedures
      (1) Percutaneous transluminal coronary angioplasty (see p. 1035)
      (2) Coronary artery bypass graft (see p. 1036)
      (3) Laser angioplasty (see p. 1036)
      (4) Atherectomy (see p. 1036)
      (5) Coronary stents (see p. 1036)

9. Complications
   a. Dysrhythmias
   b. Sudden death
   c. Heart failure
   d. With prolonged ischemia, MI

10. Prognosis
   a. Negative findings during exercise testing are associated with an increased mortality rate.

Table 23–14. Pharmacologic Management of Persons with Angina

Clinical Management	Rationale
Increase Myocardial Oxygen Supply	
Nitrates	Dilate coronary arteries
Calcium channel blockers	Dilate coronary arteries and reduce coronary artery vasospasm
Decrease Myocardial Oxygen Demand	
Nitrates	Decrease preload and afterload
Calcium channel blockers	Decrease afterload, heart rate, contractility

b. Individuals who perform poorly during exercise testing are considered at high risk and should receive aggressive treatment.

11. Applying the nursing process

NURSING DIAGNOSIS: Pain R/T an imbalance between myocardial oxygen supply and demand

---

a. *Expected outcomes:* Following interventions, the person should be able to do the following:
   (1) Verbalize relief of pain
   (2) Demonstrate a decrease in the number and severity of pain episodes
b. *Nursing interventions*
   (1) Instruct the person to inform the nurse if pain occurs. Assess, document, and report any episode of pain, including its location, duration, radiation, severity, associated signs and symptoms, and precipitating factors such as activity, eating, emotional disturbance, and timing of medication dose.
   (2) During episodes of pain, do the following: immediately limit activity and assist the person into a position of comfort, obtain vital signs and a 12-lead ECG, and administer pain medication including oxygen as ordered and monitor its effectiveness.
   (3) Plan nursing care to reduce myocardial oxygen demand. Assist the person with activities as needed. Monitor the person's bowel pattern and provide stool softeners as needed to avoid straining during bowel movement. Provide for frequent rest periods and minimize stimulation and stress.
   (4) Modify care as indicated by factors precipitating pain: monitor visitors, provide small frequent feedings, teach relaxation techniques, and limit the person's activities.

NURSING DIAGNOSIS: Knowledge deficit R/T angina including disease process, precipitating factors, medications, and actions to take when pain occurs

---

a. *Expected outcomes:* Following instruction, the person should be able to do the following:
   (1) Discuss risk factors and the measures necessary to modify weight, cholesterol level, smoking, and stress level
   (2) Describe prescribed medications including name, purpose, dose, and side effects
   (3) Articulate the need to avoid or modify angina-precipitating events such as eating heavy meals, straining during bowel movements, smoking, becoming emotionally upset, overexertion, and experiencing temperature extremes
   (4) Teach the following actions to take if chest pain occurs: stop activity and rest, take nitroglycerin

as ordered, and report to the physician if pain persists after nitroglycerin is taken as ordered
   (5) Explain the need to call the physician for any change in pattern of pain such as if the pain increases in frequency, occurs at rest, or is more difficult to relieve
b. *Nursing interventions*
   (1) Provide information in a calm and culturally relevant manner that is understandable to the person and family.
   (2) Develop a teaching plan that promotes lifestyle changes and reduces risk factors.
   (3) Encourage the person to call a health care provider with any questions or concerns.

12. Discharge planning and health teaching
   a. Make an appointment for follow-up care and provide a written reminder.
   b. Assess the need for assistance at home if the person's activities are limited. Identify available supports and, if necessary, schedule visits from a home care agency.
   c. Provide written materials on the following:
      (1) Take-home medications. Ensure that medications are available and that the person and family members understand how to administer them.
      (2) Activity limitations
      (3) When to call the physician

13. Public health considerations. See coronary artery disease, page 1038.

Hyperlipidemia

1. Definition
   a. Hyperlipidemia is a term used to describe above-normal levels of cholesterol or triglycerides. This condition augments atherosclerotic changes.
   b. Hyperlipidemia may be primary (phenotypic, or Frederickson, classification or genetic classification) or secondary.

2. Incidence and socioeconomic impact
   a. Of MI survivors younger than 60 years old, 5 percent have a family member with hyperlipidemia.
   b. Of MI survivors older than 60 years old, 15 percent have a family member with hyperlipidemia.
   c. Hyperlipidemia increases the risk of coronary artery disease.
   d. Each 1-percent decrease in cholesterol decreases the risk for coronary artery disease by 2 percent.

3. Risk factors
   a. Family history
   b. Risk factors of coronary artery disease that affect low-density lipoproteins and high-density lipoproteins—diet, obesity, smoking, lack of physical activity, use of oral contraceptives, and diabetes.

4. Etiology
   a. Primary causes of hyperlipidemia
      (1) Common (polygenic) hypercholesterolemia
      (2) Familial combined hypercholesterolemia
      (3) Familial hypercholesterolemia
      (4) Remnant (type III) hyperlipidemia

Table 23-15. National Cholesterol Education Program Guidelines

Serum Level	Degree of Risk	Recommendation
Cholesterol		
<200 mg/dl	Low	Recheck cholesterol every 5 years
200–239 mg/dl with congestive heart failure or other high-risk factor	Borderline High	Recommend restriction of dietary saturated fat, cholesterol, and calories if overweight
		Recheck cholesterol annually
		Lipoprotein profile optional
200–239 mg/dl with congestive heart failure or at least 2 other risk factors	High	Obtain lipoprotein profile
		Goals of therapy are based on LDL cholesterol and should begin with diet. If LDL-cholesterol level remains ≥190 mg/dl after 3 to 6 months of diet, consider drug therapy
≥240 mg/dl	High	Same as above
Low-density lipoproteins (LDL) <150 mg/100 ml	Normal	
High-density lipoproteins (HDL) <50 mg/100 ml	Desirable	

(5) Familial hypertriglyceridemia
(6) Chylomicronemia syndrome
b. Secondary causes of hyperlipidemia
   (1) Hypothyroidism
   (2) Diabetes mellitus
   (3) Nephrotic syndrome
   (4) Renal failure
   (5) Liver disease
   (6) Alcohol abuse
   (7) Anorexia nervosa
   (8) Certain antihypertensives such as loop or thiazide diuretics
   (9) Estrogens
   (10) Corticosteroids
5. Pathophysiology
  a. Total cholesterol is a collection of fat particles called lipoproteins (see Chapter 10).
  b. Very low-density lipoproteins, low-density lipoproteins, and high-density lipoproteins make up the total cholesterol level.
  c. Low-density lipoprotein ("bad cholesterol") is the most atherogenic lipoprotein and is associated with an increased risk of coronary artery disease. It is believed that this occurs because elevated levels of low-density lipoprotein infiltrate the intima and cause injury to the endothelial lining of the artery.
  d. High-density lipoprotein ("good cholesterol") lowers the risk of coronary artery disease by facilitating removal of cholesterol from the body.
6. Clinical manifestations
  a. Patients may be asymptomatic.
  b. Patients may exhibit signs of coronary artery disease such as chest pain.
7. Diagnostics
  a. History
   (1) Question the person about family history.
   (2) Review the person's current dietary intake of fats.
   (3) Note the presence of other risk factors for coronary artery disease.

  b. Physical examination
   (1) Xanthoma is a lipid deposit in the skin.
   (2) Corneal arcus is a white band around the cornea.
  c. Diagnostic studies. Table 23-15 lists the range of cholesterol levels and degrees of risk.
8. Clinical management
  a. The goal of clinical management is to lower cholesterol.
  b. Nonpharmacologic interventions
   (1) Diet (see Chapter 9)
   (2) Weight loss, which decreases triglyceride levels
   (3) Exercise, which increases the level of high-density lipoproteins
   (4) Cessation of smoking
  c. Pharmacologic interventions are listed in Table 23-16.

Table 23-16. Pharmacologic Interventions for Hyperlipidemia

Type	Side Effects
Bile acid sequestrants	Constipation
Cholestyramine (Questran, Cholybar)	Bloating
Colestipol (Colestid)	
Nicotinic acid	Gastrointestinal distress
Niacin	Flushing hepatic toxicity pruritus
HMG-CoA reductase inhibitors	Mild gastrointestinal symptoms
Lovastatin (Mevacor)	Increased liver function tests
Simvastatin (Zocor)	
Pravastatin (Pravachol)	
Fibric Acid Derivatives	Increased gallbladder disease
Gemfibrozil (Lopid)	Increased gastrointestinal cancer
Clofibrate (Atromid-S)	Increased liver function tests
Probucol	Diarrhea
Lorelco	
Fish oils	Halitosis
Promega	

9. Complications include atherosclerosis and coronary artery disease.
10. Prognosis
    a. The prognosis varies by type of hyperlipidemia and by compliance with therapeutic regimen.
    b. The risk of coronary artery disease for a person with a cholesterol level of 240 mg per dl is double that of a person with a level of 200 mg per dl.
    c. Persons with a cholesterol level below 175 mg per dl have half the risk of death as someone with a level of 250 mg per dl or greater.
11. Applying the nursing process

NURSING DIAGNOSIS: Knowledge deficit R/T causes and complications of hyperlipidemia

    a. *Expected outcomes:* Following counseling, the person should be able to articulate the following:
        (1) The need for a life-long commitment to modifying risk factors with particular emphasis on diet and exercise. (Even on drug therapy, the person must remain on a low-fat, low-cholesterol diet and continue to exercise.)
        (2) The causes of hyperlipidemia
        (3) The early warning signs of 1 of the major complications of the disease, coronary artery disease, and when to notify the physician for chest pain and other symptoms of an MI
        (4) That exercise and diet will not significantly reduce cholesterol levels for up to 6 months. (If levels are measured during this time frame, the person should not become frustrated with the apparent lack of progress.)
    b. *Nursing interventions*
        (1) Provide written materials on disease, risk factors, diet, exercise, and medications, if prescribed.
        (2) Involve the person and family in developing a plan for lifestyle changes that incorporates their understanding of the disease and the prescribed therapeutic modalities.

NURSING DIAGNOSIS: Noncompliance R/T unwillingness to comply with dietary restrictions

    a. *Expected outcomes:* Following counseling, the person should be able to do the following:
        (1) Establish a target diet and monitor and report adherence
        (2) Articulate situations that present a personal challenge for adhering to the established diet and describe at least 1 healthy alternative choice for dealing with that situation
        (3) Describe how family members and friends can serve as a support system for risk factor modification
    b. *Nursing interventions*

        (1) Provide written materials on a low-fat, low-cholesterol diet.
        (2) Schedule a follow-up appointment with the physician and dietitian, if available.
        (3) Encourage the person and family to call with any questions or concerns.
12. Discharge planning and teaching
    a. Reinforce the concept that hyperlipidemia is a "silent disease" that is present for life and that can be treated.
    b. Provide written information on dietary limitations (see Chapter 9).
    c. Help the person develop a plan to comply with the therapeutic regimen and implement lifestyle changes to optimize health.
13. Public health considerations
    a. The primary prevention goal is to lower the cholesterol levels in the entire population.
    b. The National Cholesterol Education Program has published guidelines to detect, treat and monitor patients (see Table 23–15).
    c. Identify persons at risk for development of coronary artery disease due to hyperlipidemia.

Myocardial Infarction

1. Definition
    a. An MI is death of myocardial tissue due to prolonged myocardial ischemia.
    b. Q-wave infarct (transmural MI) usually involves the full thickness of the myocardial wall (Fig. 23–21) and is usually larger and associated with a higher incidence of complications such as shock or myocardial rupture and with higher in-hospital mortality.
    c. Non–Q-wave infarct (nontransmural or subendocardial MI) is usually subendocardial (see Fig. 23–21) and is associated with fewer complications in the

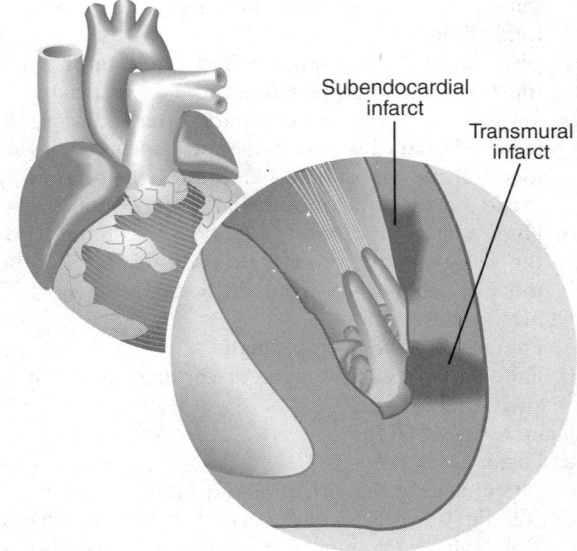

Figure 23–21. Transmural-subendocardial infarction.

acute hospital phase but a higher incidence of rein-farction and recurrent angina.

2. Incidence and socioeconomic impact
   a. Approximately 1.5 million persons have an acute MI annually. Many die before they reach the hospital because they do not seek help quickly enough.
   b. One fourth of all deaths in the United States are due to an acute MI.
   c. Forty-five percent of all acute MIs occur in persons younger than age 65 years.

3. Risk factors
   a. See Coronary Artery Disease for a discussion of risk factors.
   b. Precipitating factors triggering an MI are not clearly understood.
      (1) Half of all persons with an MI have no identified precipitating factors.
      (2) Most (51%) MIs occur at rest. Thirteen percent occur during heavy exertion and 8 percent during sleep.
      (3) Q-wave infarctions often occur in the morning after awakening.
   c. Other precipitating factors
      (1) Emotional stress and upsetting life events such as death of a spouse
      (2) Surgical procedures associated with acute blood loss
      (3) Cocaine use
      (4) Increased myocardial oxygen demand secondary to fever, tachycardia, agitation, hypoglycemia, pulmonary embolus, myocardial trauma, or stroke

℞ DRUG ADVISORY

Thyroxin therapy increases the risk of ischemic heart disease and can precipitate a myocardial infarction in persons with a history of cardiac disease.

4. Etiology
   a. Almost all MIs are caused by atherosclerosis of the coronary arteries, with a superimposed thrombus in the affected area.
   b. The atherosclerotic plaques cause a narrowing of the coronary artery lumen, and the thrombus further narrows or completely obstructs the artery.
   c. Location of infarct
      (1) Most myocardial infarctions occur in the left ventricle. The sites (Fig. 23–22) are
         • Inferior—resulting from occlusion of the right coronary artery
         • Posterior—may occur with right coronary artery occlusion (80–90%) or left circumflex (10–20%)
         • Anterior—occurring with occlusion of the left anterior descending coronary artery
         • Lateral—resulting from occlusion of the left circumflex coronary artery
      (2) Knowing the location of an MI allows the caregiver to anticipate problems and prognosis (Table 23–17).

5. Pathophysiology
   a. The cause of the thrombus is not completely understood. Thrombosis usually results from plaque rupture or endothelial injury, resulting in hemorrhage, platelet aggregation, and release of substances causing vasoconstriction.
   b. Ischemia and resulting necrosis usually proceed from the endocardium to the epicardium in a wave front fashion that is time related (Fig. 23–23).
   c. Irreversible injury occurs in the subendocardium after 20 minutes of cessation of blood flow and in the subepicardium after 3 to 6 hours without blood flow.

6. Clinical manifestations
   a. Chest pain is the most common presenting symptom of an MI (see p. 986).
   b. Characteristic pain is substernal, radiates to the arms, neck, or back, is crushing or squeezing, is severe, is not relieved by rest or nitroglycerin, and lasts longer than 30 minutes.
   c. Associated symptoms may include nausea.
   d. Some persons, most often those with diabetes or hy-

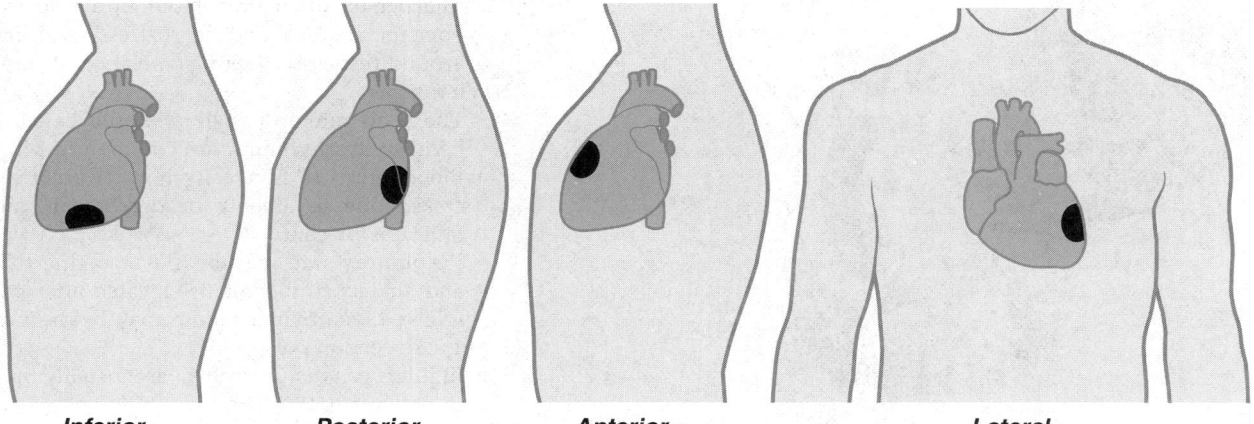

Inferior   *Posterior*   *Anterior*   *Lateral*

Figure 23–22. Location of myocardial infarctions.

Table 23–17. Complications by Type of Infarct

Type of Infarct	Structures Supplied by Coronary Artery	Complications

Anterior
  Left anterior descending
    coronary artery
	Anterior wall of left ventricle
	
	Anterior two thirds of septum
	Bundle of His
	Right bundle branch
	Anterior–superior division of left
	    bundle branch
		Heart failure and shock
		Myocardial rupture
		
		Ventricular septal defect
		Second-degree heart block, type
		    II
		Right bundle branch block
		Left anterior hemiblock
		Bifascicular block

Inferior
  Right coronary artery
	SA node (55%)
	AV node (90%)
	Bundle of His
	Right atrium and right ventricular
	Inferior or diaphragmatic surface
	    of left ventricle
	Posterior 3rd of septum
	Posterior–inferior division of left
	    bundle branch
		Sinus bradycardia
		First-degree AV block
		Second-degree heart block, type I
		Right ventricular infarct
		Papillary muscle rupture
		Left posterior hemiblock

ELDER ADVISORY

Older people with myocardial infarctions are particularly likely to present with atypical symptoms such as heart failure or severe weakness rather than chest pain.

pertension, have no chest pain, or "silent" MI detected only by ECG.

7. Diagnostics
  a. History

(1) A characteristic history is the most valuable finding in initial diagnosis of an MI.
(2) Obtain a detailed description of the chest pain discomfort and associated signs and symptoms (see p. 986).
(3) Ask the person to quantify the pain using a scale of 1 (least severe) to 10 (most severe). This helps establish a baseline for future assessment.
(4) Note the presence of coronary artery disease risk factors.
(5) Note any previous cardiac problems.
(6) Note the patient's perception of the cause of the problem for possible transcultural considerations.
  b. Physical examination
    (1) General appearance
      • The person may appear healthy and complain only of chest pain or be gravely ill with signs of heart failure.
      • The person often breaks out in a cold sweat, appears anxious and in distress, and moves around restlessly, seeking a position of comfort.
    (2) Vital signs
      • The heart rate and rhythm should be assessed because dysrhythmias are common in MI.
      • Blood pressure is usually normal but may increase due to anxiety or decrease if cardiac failure is present.
      • Respiratory rate may be elevated due to pain and anxiety. If it remains elevated after pain is relieved, ventricular failure may be the cause.
    (3) Jugular venous pulse
      • Jugular venous pressures are usually normal in patients with MI.
      • Marked jugular venous distention may occur with a right ventricular infarct.

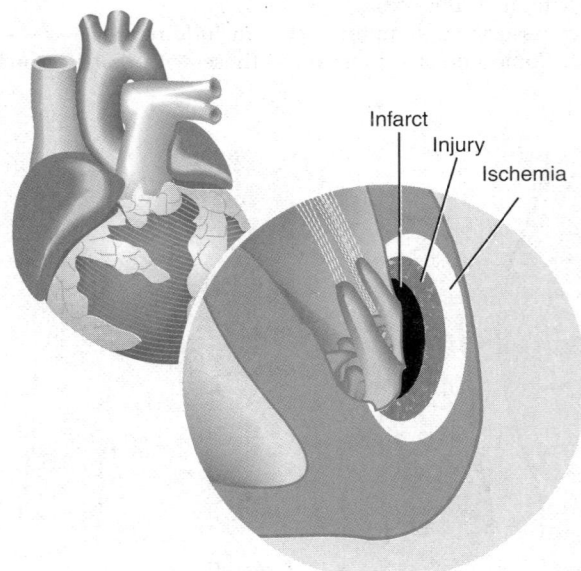

Figure 23–23. Myocardial ischemia and necrosis.

BOX 23-2. Enzymes Used to Detect a Myocardial Infarction

The enzymes most commonly used to detect MI are creatine kinase (CK), lactic dehydrogenase, and aspartate aminotransferase.

Creatine kinase is an enzyme specific to cells of the myocardium, brain, and skeletal muscle.
- Creatine kinase-MM (CK-MM) is the muscle isoenzyme.
- Creatine kinase-MB (CK-MB) is the myocardium isoenzyme.
- Creatine kinase-BB (CK-BB) is an enzyme specific to the brain, lung, stomach, prostate, and smooth muscle of the gastrointestinal tract and bladder.

Lactic dehydrogenase (LD) is an enzyme that catalyzes the reversible conversion of lactate to pyruvate during periods of anaerobic metabolism. The pattern of LD isoenzymes, particularly LD-1 and LD-2, can indicate an acute MI.

Aspartate aminotransferase (AST, GOT, SGOT) is an enzyme found in liver, skeletal muscle, kidney, red blood cells, and the myocardium.

(4) Lungs
- Rales are heard with left ventricular failure.
- The Killip classification (Table 23-18) describes cardiac failure and pulmonary congestion.

(5) Cardiac auscultation
- Heart sounds may be soft.
- A 4th heart sound is almost always present with an MI.
- A 3rd heart sound in MI reflects left ventricular failure.
- A friction rub may be heard in 10 percent of cases, usually on the 2nd or 3rd day after the MI.
- Systolic murmurs may occur due to papillary muscle dysfunction, causing mitral regurgitation. A new prominent holosystolic murmur may occur with papillary muscle rupture or a ventricular septal defect.

c. Diagnostic studies

(1) Cardiac enzymes (see p. 992)
- Irreversibly injured myocardial cells release enzymes into the circulation in a characteristic pattern (Box 23-2).
- The CK-MB isoenzyme is the most sensitive enzyme indicator for myocardial injury because it is present predominantly in cardiac tissue. The CK-MB elevates in MI, myocardial contusion, and cardiac surgery.

Table 23-18. Killip Classification

Class	Description
I	No pulmonary rales
II	Mild to moderate rales
	Possible S$_3$
III	Rales more than halfway up the lung fields
	S$_3$ gallop
IV	Cardiogenic shock

Table 23-19. Enzyme Patterns in Acute Myocardial Infarction

Enzyme	Initial Rise, Hours	Peak Hours	Return to Normal, Days
CK (Creatine kinase)	6-15	24	1-4
CK MB (Isoenzyme of CK)	3-15	12-24	<1-3
LD (Lactic dehydrogenase)	24	48-72	7-14

- Lactate dehydrogenase may increase in noncardiac conditions such as anemia, leukemia, liver disease, and renal disease because it is found in other tissues.
- The CK may elevate in conditions such as with muscle trauma, pulmonary embolus, or cardioversion, or after intramuscular injections.

Because of the enzymes' lack of specificity, the American Heart Association recommends using LD plus CK levels to establish occurrence of MI.

- Non–Q-wave infarcts also produce positive enzyme study results.
- Patterns and timing of the elevation of enzymes are predictable with an MI (Table 23-19 and Fig. 23-24).

(2) Electrocardiogram
- Serial 12-lead ECGs are done to detect and localize an MI (Table 23-20).
- The ECG changes in a Q-wave infarction include ST elevation and Q-wave development.
- The ECG changes in a non–Q-wave infarction are usually persistent ST depression, T wave inversion, or both.
- A right-sided ECG (precordial leads on the right side of the chest) is done to detect a right ventricular infarct.

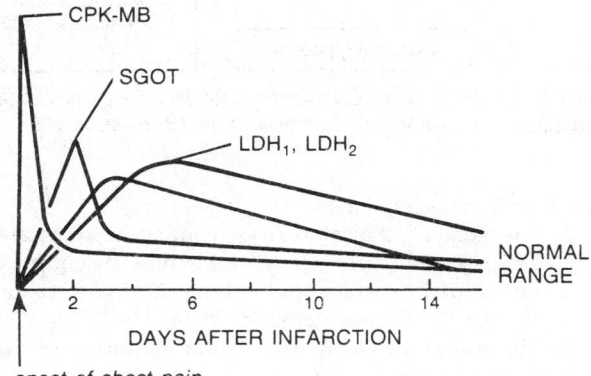

Figure 23-24. Pattern and timing of enzyme elevation with a myocardial infarction. (From Dolan JT. *Critical Care Nursing.* Philadelphia: FA Davis, 1991, p 901.)

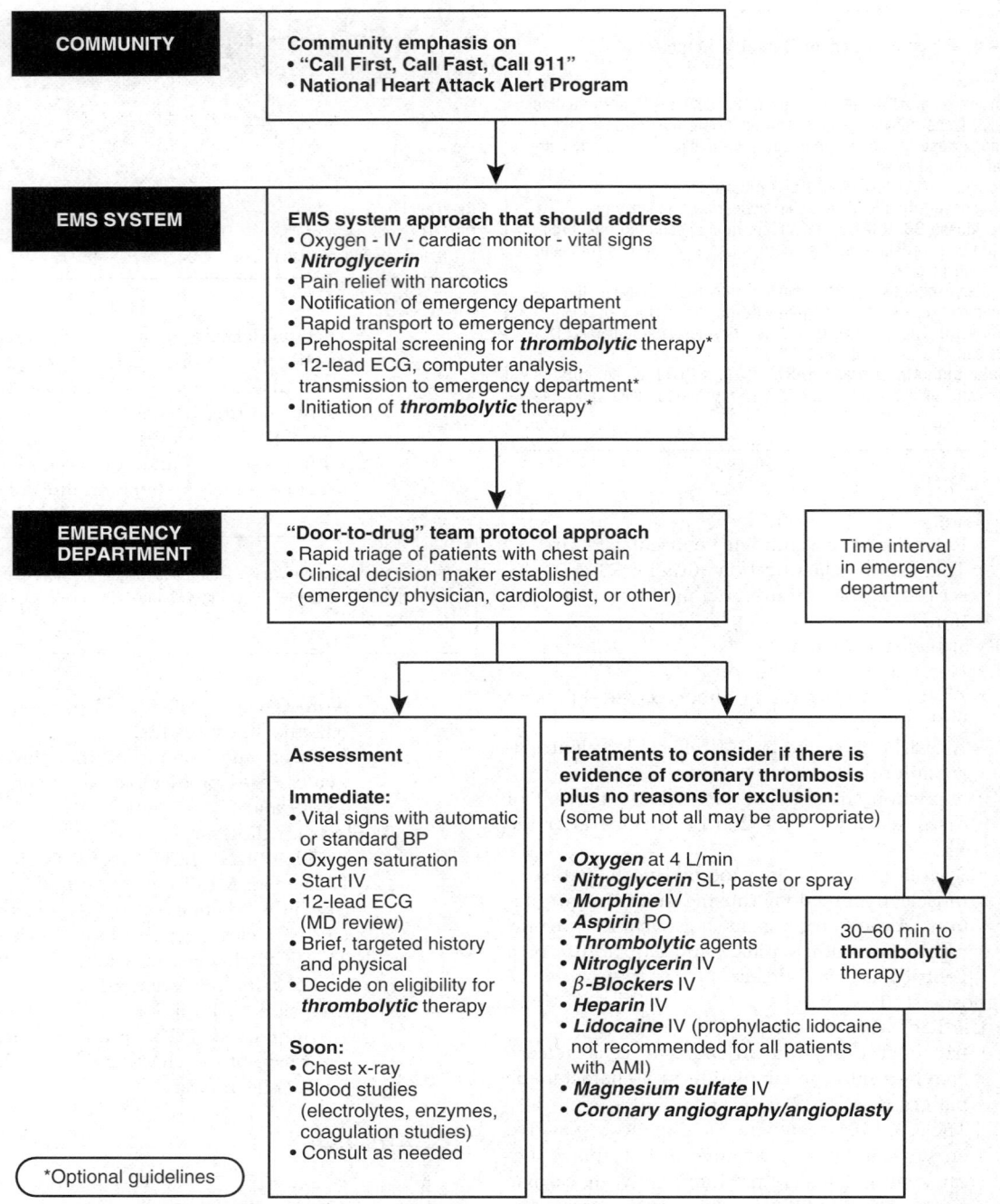

Figure 23–25. Acute myocardial infarction algorithm. Recommendations for early management of patients with chest pain and possible acute myocardial infarction. (From *Guidelines for Cardiopulmonary Resuscitation and Emergency Cardiac Care.* Copyright 1992, American Medical Association.)

8. Clinical management
   a. The goal of clinical management is to eliminate or decrease the size of the infarction by improving myocardial oxygen supply (Table 23–21) or reducing myocardial oxygen demand (Table 23–22).
   b. The American Heart Association algorithm for MI is shown in Fig. 23–25.
   c. Nonpharmacologic interventions
      (1) Cardiopulmonary resuscitation (CPR) (Procedure 23–10)
      (2) Intra-aortic balloon pumping (see p. 1081)
   d. Pharmacologic interventions
      (1) Thrombolytic therapy with agents such as urokinase, streptokinase, and tissue plasminogen activator are used to dissolve clots and allow blood flow to the myocardium.
      (2) Indications include chest pain consistent with MI and greater than or equal to 1 mm ST elevation in 2 contiguous ECG leads.
      (3) It is critical to rapidly recognize and assess persons who may benefit from thrombolytic therapy. Early administration of thrombolytic ther-

Table 23–20. Localizing a Myocardial Infarction: ECG Changes Associated with Location of Infarct

Infarction Site	Leads Affected
Inferior wall	II, III, aVF
Anterior wall	V_3, V_4
Anteroseptal wall	V_1, V_2, V_3, V_4
Anterolateral wall	I, VL, V_3–V_6
Lateral wall	I, aVL, V_5, V_6
Posterior wall*	V_1, V_2
Right ventricle	V_4–R, V_5–R, V_6–R†

* Because no leads are placed on the posterior surface of the heart, V_1–V_2 are assessed for reciprocal charges—ST depression and tall R waves.
† Right-sided ECG.

Table 23–22. Reducing Myocardial Oxygen Demand

Clinical Management	Rationale
Bed rest	Reduces increased oxygen demand secondary to activity
Pain relief	Should decrease sympathetic nervous system response, heart rate, blood pressure, anxiety
Electrocardiographic monitoring	Detects dysrhythmias that may increase oxygen demand
Beta blockers	Decrease heart rate, contractility
Morphine	Relieves pain Decreases preload
Nitrates	Reduce preload, afterload
Calcium channel blockers	Reduce afterload, heart rate contractility
Intra-aortic balloon pump	Reduces afterload

CLINICAL CONTROVERSIES

Traditionally, when prescribing bed rest after an acute myocardial infarction, many physicians have insisted that patients use the bedpan or urinal rather than a bedside commode. At the same time, patients have insisted that they would much prefer to get up and use the commode.

Two studies have challenged the tradition of in-bed toileting. In 1950, Benton and colleagues reported that patients who used the bedpan *expended 50 percent more energy* than patients who used the bedside commode. In 1984, Winslow, Land, and Gaffney published data demonstrating that "no physiologically important differences were found between in-bed and out-of-bed toileting." They concluded that medical patients who can tolerate postural changes *should be allowed to use the commode.*

Data from Benton JG, Brown H, and Risk HA. Energy expended by patients on the bedpan and bedside commode. *JAMA* 144:1443–1447, 1950; Winslow EH, Land LE, and Gaffney FA. Oxygen uptake and cardiovascular response in patients and normal adults during in-bed and out-of-bed toileting. *J Cardiol Rehabil* 4(6):348–354, 1984.

apy reduces morbidity and mortality rates in acute MI. For best results, administer thrombolytic therapy within 6 hours of pain onset. "Time is muscle"; therefore, the earlier the better. By opening the artery, some benefit may occur for up to 24 hours, although there will be permanent myocardial damage due to the already dead myocardial tissue.

    (4) Contraindications for thrombolytic therapy are listed in Table 23–23.

    (5) Complications include bleeding, reocclusion of artery, allergic reaction, and dysrhythmias.

  e. Special medical-surgical procedures

    (1) Hemodynamic monitoring may be initiated with an intra-arterial and pulmonary artery catheter in complicated MIs.

Table 23–21. Increasing Myocardial Oxygen Supply

Clinical Management	Rationale
Oxygen	May improve myocardial oxygenation
Electrocardiographic monitoring	Detect dysrhythmias that may affect cardiac output or coronary perfusion
Thrombolytic therapy	Dissolve thrombus and restore coronary blood flow
Nitrates	Dilate coronary arteries
Aspirin	Prevent platelet aggregation
Heparin, intravenously	Prevent thrombus formation
Calcium channel blockers	Dilate coronary arteries and reduce vasospasm
Percutaneous transluminal coronary angioplasty	Open occluded artery
Intra-aortic balloon pump	Increase coronary artery perfusion pressure
Coronary artery bypass graft	Revascularize myocardium

Table 23–23. Contraindications of Thrombolytic Therapy

Absolute	Relative
Active or recent (< 2 weeks) bleeding	Relatively recent trauma or surgery (> 2 weeks)
History of cerebral hemorrhage	History of nonhemorrhagic cerebrovascular accident with complete recovery
Blood pressure > 200/120 mm Hg	Active peptic ulcer
Suspected aortic dissection or pericarditis	Hemorrhagic retinopathy
Pregnancy	History of severe hypertension with diastolic blood pressure > 100 mm Hg
Recent (< 2 weeks) surgery	Bleeding disorder or use of anticoagulants
Allergy to drug	Previous treatment with streptokinase or streptokinase activator
Prolonged traumatic CPR	
Intracranial neoplasm or recent head trauma	

Procedure 23–10
One-Rescuer Cardiopulmonary Resuscitation

Definition/Purpose	To maintain perfusion of vital organs after cardiac or respiratory arrest until definitive therapy can be initiated.
Contraindication/Cautions	• Ensure that the person is pulseless and apneic before initiating CPR. • To avoid transmission of infectious diseases, use of a face shield or barrier device is strongly recommended.
Learning/Teaching Activities	None

Preliminary Activities

Equipment	Face shield or barrier device.
Assessment Planning	• Assess the patient for unresponsiveness. Ensure breathlessness and pulselessness. • Person is pulseless. • Remember to not treat the monitor; always assess the person after each intervention.

Procedure

Actions	Rationale/Discussion
1. Determine unresponsiveness by gently shaking the person and shouting "Are you OK?".	1. CPR should not be initiated until need is established.
2. Activate the Emergency Medical System.	2. Shortens the Emergency Medical System's response time.
3. Place persons on their back. If neck or back injury is possible, maintain alignment and turn the body and head as a unit.	3. Improper movement may result in spinal cord injury.
4. If the person is unresponsive, open the airway using the head tilt–chin lift method.	4. The tongue is the most common cause of airway obstruction.

5. Evaluate the person's breathing.
  a. If the person is breathing, maintain the airway.
  b. If the person is not breathing, apply a barrier device if available and give two breaths.
    (1) If unable to ventilate the person, reposition the head and attempt to ventilate again.
    (2) If still unable to ventilate the person, attempt to clear the airway using foreign-body airway obstruction maneuvers:
    • Heimlich maneuver with victim standing or sitting
    • Heimlich maneuver with victim lying down
    • Self-administered Heimlich maneuver
    • Chest thrusts with victim lying down
    • Finger sweep
    • With properly trained persons and direct visualization of the foreign body, use of a Kelly clamp or Magill forceps
	5. Improper head position is the most common problem with difficult ventilation.
	
	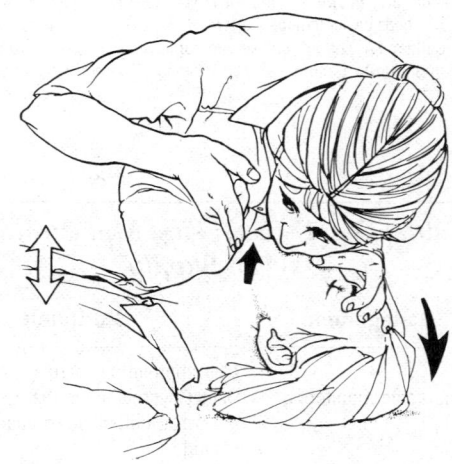

6. Evaluate the person's circulation; check for a pulse.
  a. If the pulse is present and breathing is absent: ventilate with 1 breath every 5 to 6 seconds.
  b. If pulse and breathing are both present, place the person in a recovery position (i.e., roll persons onto their side by moving the head, shoulders, and torso as 1 unit).
  c. If the pulse is absent, initiate CPR.
    (1) Locate proper hand position.
    (2) Provide 15 chest compressions at a rate of 80 to 100 compressions per minute.
	6. The carotid artery is most accessible and reliable.
	
	b. The airway is most likely to remain open in the recovery position.
	
	c. Proper hand position will decrease the risk of rib fracture. The sternum should be compressed 1½ to 2 inches with each compression. Each compression should be released completely to allow for cardiac filling.

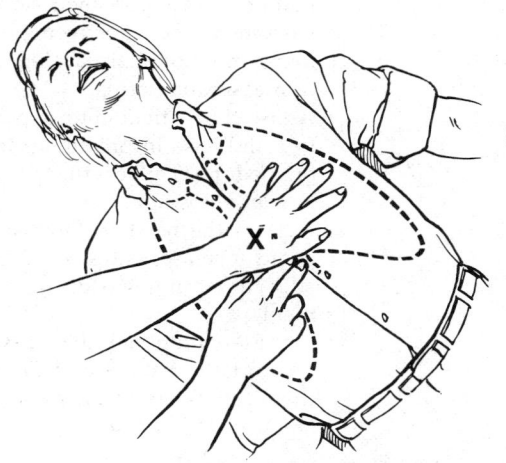

Procedure 23--10
(continued)

Actions	Rationale/Discussion

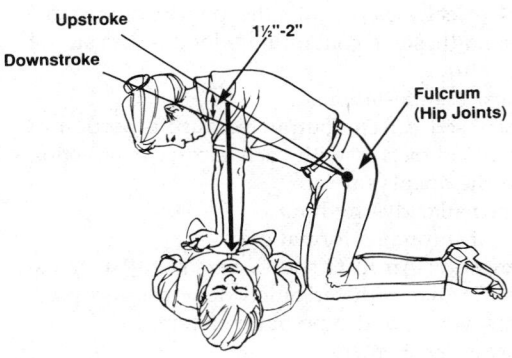

(3) Open the airway and ventilate with 2 breaths lasting 1½ to 2 seconds each.

(4) Replace hands in correct position and provide 15 more compressions at a rate of 80 to 100 per minute.

(5) Repeat for 4 cycles of 15 compressions and 2 ventilations.

7. Reassess

After completion of the 4 cycles of 15 compressions and 2 ventilations, reevaluate the patient for 3 to 5 seconds for return of the carotid pulse.

a. If the pulse is present, check breathing.

(1) If the person is breathing, monitor closely.

(2) If the person is not breathing, provide rescue breathing 10 to 12 times per minute.

b. If the pulse is absent, continue CPR and reassess every few minutes for return of the pulse.

Illustrations redrawn from *Textbook of Basic Life Support for Healthcare Providers*, 1994. Copyright American Heart Association.

(2) Tables 23–21 and 23–22 list other procedures that may be considered to increase supply or decrease demand for myocardial oxygen.

9. Complications: Certain complications are frequently associated with particular types of myocardial infarctions (see Table 23–17): dysrhythmias, ventricular aneurysm, ventricular rupture, ventricular septal ruptures, papillary muscle rupture, left ventricular wall thrombus, pericarditis, right ventricular infarct, cardiogenic shock, and postinfarction angina.

a. Dysrhythmias are seen in 72 to 96 percent of MI patients (see p. 1008).

b. Ventricular aneurysm

(1) Definition: A ventricular aneurysm is a persistent localized weakening of some portion of a ventricular wall (Fig. 23–26).

(2) Types include ventricular aneurysm, chronic left ventricular aneurysm, and false aneurysm.

(3) Incidence and socioeconomic impact: A ventricular aneurysm occurs in approximately 15 percent of persons with MI.

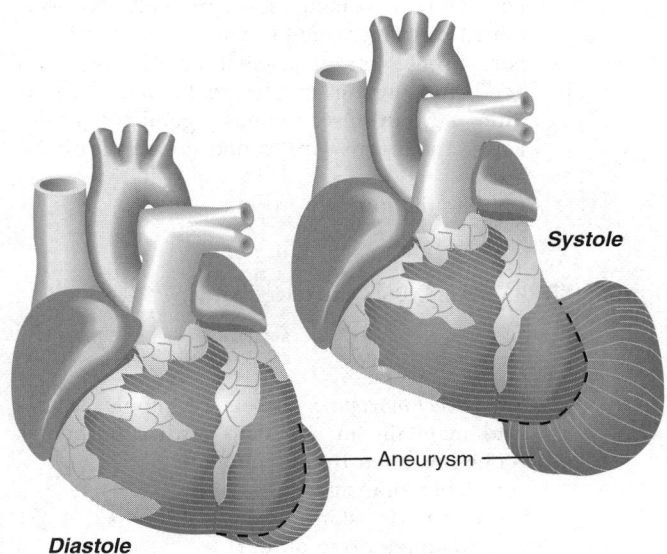

Figure 23–26. Ventricular aneurysm.

(4) Risk factors and etiology: Ventricular and chronic aneurysms usually develop in the 1st 2 weeks after an MI. False aneurysms occur when there is a containment by the pericardium of a ventricular rupture.

(5) Pathophysiology: In ventricular and chronic aneurysms, the necrotic myocardium develops a fibrous scar. Over time, this scar balloons out in response to ventricular pressures. With the decrease in contracting musculature, cardiac output decreases. In false aneurysms, a ventricular rupture leaks blood into the pericardium. Pericardial adhesions contain the blood at the site of the rupture.

(6) Clinical manifestations
  • Decreased cardiac output because a portion of the blood ejected with each cardiac contraction fills the aneurysm
  • Ventricular dysrhythmias
  • Site of thrombus formation

(7) Diagnostics: An ECG shows persistent ST elevations. Cardiac catheterization demonstrates presence, severity, and type of aneurysm.

(8) Clinical management
  • Goals of clinical management should be based on severity to minimize symptoms, avoid embolization, and maintain cardiac output.
  • Nonpharmacologic interventions include sodium restriction for congestive heart failure and restricted activities to avoid exertion.
  • Pharmacologic interventions include, for congestive heart failure, diuretics, digitalis, and oxygen; for potential embolization, anticoagulation.
  • Special medical-surgical procedures include surgical repair of the aneurysm.

(9) Complications include congestive heart failure, dysrhythmias, systemic emboli, ventricular rupture, and sudden cardiac death.

(10) Prognosis
  • For ventricular aneurysms, prognosis is determined by percentage of ventricle involved.
  • For chronic left ventricular aneurysms, with good functioning of the remaining myocardium, surgical resection has a good prognosis.
  • False aneurysms are prone to rupture (see above).

(11) Applying the nursing process

NURSING DIAGNOSIS: Decreased cardiac output R/T ventricular aneurysm

(a) *Expected outcomes:* The person should be able to maintain an adequate cardiac output as demonstrated by the following:
  • Stable vital signs
  • Warm, dry skin
  • Adequate urine output
  • Appropriate mentation
(b) *Nursing interventions*

  • Provide education in understandable terms regarding disease process, therapeutic interventions, and potential for surgical intervention.
  • Document initial cardiovascular assessment including ability to perform activities of daily living.
  • Administer medications as ordered and monitor and report their side effects.
  • Document the effectiveness of pharmacologic and nonpharmacologic interventions in measurable terms.
  • Assist the patient into a position of comfort and ease in breathing. If the patient is on bed rest, place the patient in a high Fowler's position.
  • Explain the need to limit activities and to avoid increased stress on the heart muscle, such as straining during a bowel movement.
  • Provide emotional and psychologic support for the patient and family. Encourage them to talk about their concerns.

NURSING DIAGNOSIS: Fluid volume excess R/T congestive heart failure

(a) *Expected outcomes:* The person should achieve a normal fluid volume as demonstrated by the following:
  • Body weight at person's normal range
  • Clear breath sounds
  • No peripheral edema
  • Absense of S_3 heart sound
(b) *Nursing interventions*
  • Weigh person daily.
  • Monitor intake and output.
  • Auscultate heart and lungs.
  • Assess legs and dependent areas for edema.
  • Administer medications as indicated and monitor and report response.

(12) Discharge planning and teaching
  • Provide written materials on disease process, clinical manifestations, and complications.
  • Make sure the patient is educated regarding medications and can list name, dose, effect, and any complications for each.
  • Provide materials on diet, activity, and fluid restrictions.
  • Provide a written list of symptoms, such as increasing pain and shortness of breath, that indicate the need to contact the physician.

c. Ventricular rupture
  (1) Definition: Ventricular rupture is a breaking apart of the myocardium.
  (2) Incidence and socioeconomic impact
    • Ventricular rupture occurs in 3 to 24 percent of deaths from MI.
    • It is more common in women, elderly persons, and those with hypertension.

- It is more frequent after the 1st rather than subsequent infarctions.
(3) Risk factors and etiology
  - Myocardial infarction
  - Ventricular aneurysms
(4) Pathophysiology: A necrotic section of myocardium breaks down under ventricular pressure.
(5) Clinical manifestations include chest pain, signs of cardiac tamponade, profound hypotension, and cardiopulmonary arrest.
(6) Diagnostics
  - Clinical presentation includes cardiac tamponade and shock.
  - Initial electrocardiogram shows no changes or slight tachycardia. Terminal rhythm shows pulseless electrical activity.
(7) Clinical management
  - Goals of clinical management are early recognition and treatment.
  - There are no nonpharmacologic interventions.
  - There are no pharmacologic interventions.
  - Special medical-surgical procedures include surgical exploration and closure.
(8) Complications include false aneurysm, if contained, and sudden cardiac death.
(9) Prognosis depends on early identification and intervention.
(10) Applying the nursing process

NURSING DIAGNOSIS: Decreased cardiac output R/T cardiac rupture

---

(a) *Expected outcomes:* The person should be able to maintain an adequate cardiac output as demonstrated by the following:
  - Stable vital signs
  - Warm, dry skin
  - Urine output of greater than or equal to 30 ml per hour
  - Appropriate mentation
(b) *Nursing interventions*
  - If the situation allows, provide education in understandable terms regarding disease process, therapeutic interventions, and potential for surgical intervention.
  - Administer medications as ordered and monitor and report their side effects.
  - Document the effectiveness of pharmacologic and nonpharmacologic interventions in measurable terms.
  - Explain the need to limit activities and to avoid increased stress on the heart muscle, such as straining during a bowel movement.
  - Provide emotional and psychologic support for the patient and family. Encourage them to talk about their concerns.
  - Prepare for surgical intervention and initiate basic life support and advanced cardiac life support if needed.

NURSING DIAGNOSIS: Anxiety R/T early symptoms of chest pain, tachycardia, and hypoxia

---

(a) *Expected outcomes:* Following counseling, the patient should be able to do the following:
  - Demonstrate a demeanor consistent with the clinical situation
  - If able, articulate information related to condition, interventions, and preoperative instructions
(b) *Nursing interventions:* Maintain a calm and professional manner while preparing for emergency interventions.
(11) Discharge planning and teaching: If surgical repair is successful, provide routine postcardiac surgery instructions (see p. 1077).
d. Ventricular septal ruptures
  - Ventricular septal ruptures are less common than myocardial rupture.
  - Ventricular septal ruptures occur in multivessel coronary artery disease.
  - Transmural anterior infarcts may cause apical ruptures.
  - Transmural inferior infarcts may cause basal ruptures.
e. Papillary muscle rupture: When a papillary muscle infarcts, it can rupture, causing incomplete closure of the mitral valve and resulting in sudden-onset of congestive heart failure.
f. Left ventricular wall thrombus
  (1) Left ventricular wall thrombus occurs in 20 to 40 percent of anterior MIs.
  (2) The thrombus may break off and embolize.
  (3) Anticoagulation reduces thrombus formation.
g. Pericarditis (see p. 1063)
  (1) Pericarditis is an inflammatory process that can accompany transmural infarcts, usually anterior infarcts.
  (2) Pericardial effusion is commonly associated with pericarditis.
  (3) It usually occurs 2 to 7 days after infarct.
  (4) Dressler's syndrome develops 7 days to 12 weeks after an MI. Symptoms include pericardial pain, pericardial friction rub, pleural effusion, and fever.
h. Right ventricular infarct
  (1) Right ventricular infarct occurs in up to 57 percent of patients with inferior MI.
  (2) The usual presentation includes hypotension and jugular venous distention with clear lungs. It is often asymptomatic.

NURSE ADVISORY

A dextrocardiogram, a right-sided ECG, should be obtained in any person who has had an acute inferior myocardial infarction.

---

  (3) Treatment consists of volume loading to increase cardiac output. Dobutamine may be used to increase contractility.

i. Cardiogenic shock: A full discussion of shock and shock states is included in Chapter 12. Cardiogenic shock occurs in 5 to 15 percent of patients following an MI and is caused by the inability of the heart to pump adequately and maintain tissue perfusion. Severity of the shock is related to the size of the infarct. In-hospital mortality rate ranges from 70 to 100 percent. The 5-year survival rate for those who leave the hospital is approximately 40 percent. This disorder is most commonly related to the following:

  (l) Extensive left ventricular damage
- An acute MI with damage to at least 40 percent of the left ventricular myocardium
- An anterior infarct because the left anterior descending artery supplies the largest myocardial mass

  (2) Mechanical defects
- Ventricular septal rupture
- Ventricular wall rupture
- Ruptured papillary muscle causing severe mitral stenosis

  (3) Scarring from a previous MI or a small MI in the same location as myocardial damage from a previous MI

j. Postinfarction angina
  (1) Postinfarction angina occurs in 18 percent of MIs.
  (2) It is more common in non–Q-wave infarctions and in postthrombolytic and multiple risk factor patients.
  (3) Symptoms include chest pain similar to original MI pain, with or without transient ST-T changes, occurring 24 hours or more after the MI.

NURSE ADVISORY

Chest pain after a myocardial infarction is an important complication, associated with twice the risk of reinfarction and a 2 to 4 times higher mortality rate at 1 year.

---

10. Prognosis
   a. Sixty percent of deaths occur in the 1st hour and are usually due to ventricular fibrillation.
   b. In-hospital deaths are usually due to cardiogenic shock.
   c. In-hospital mortality is lower in a non–Q-wave MI, but the long-term prognosis is similar to a Q-wave MI.
   d. Long-term prognosis is related to degree of left ventricle function and incipient ischemia.
11. Applying the nursing process

NURSING DIAGNOSIS: Pain R/T an imbalance between oxygen supply and demand—myocardial ischemia

a. *Expected outcomes:* Following interventions, the person should be able to verbalize an absence of pain and appear to be comfortable.

b. *Nursing interventions*
   (1) Explain the importance of reporting any pain immediately. Carefully assess and document any complaints of pain, including description of pain, factors that aggravate or relieve pain, vital signs, and any ECG changes.
   (2) To monitor the effectiveness of therapeutic interventions over time, instruct the person on the use of a rating scale to quantify the severity of pain.
   (3) Administer oxygen, morphine, nitroglycerin, and other drugs as ordered and document the response.
   (4) Monitor activity and comfort level. Schedule treatments and assessments to provide for periods of uninterrupted rest.

NURSING DIAGNOSIS: Decreased cardiac output R/T dysrhythmias, decreased myocardial contractility, or ventricular dysfunction such as papillary muscle rupture, ventricular septal defect, or ventricular aneurysm

---

a. *Expected outcomes:* The person should be able to maintain an adequate cardiac output as demonstrated by the following:
   (1) Stable vital signs with a systolic blood pressure between 90 and 110 mm Hg and respiration rate between 10 to 20 respirations per minute
   (2) Warm, dry skin
   (3) Urine output of 30 ml or greater per hour
   (4) Appropriate mentation
   (5) Ability to carry out prescribed activities without dyspnea or pain
b. *Nursing interventions*
   (1) Perform and document initial and ongoing cardiovascular assessments. Monitor the patient for dysrhythmias and signs of heart failure. Frequency of assessments should be determined by condition but should be done no less than every 4 hours and should include vital signs, breath sounds, heart sounds, and cardiac rhythm.
   (2) Assess, document, and report any signs of decreased cardiac output including the following:
   - Decrease in systolic blood pressure or a systolic reading below 90 mm Hg
   - Abnormal heart rhythm or increasing rate; presence of murmurs or S_3 on auscultation
   - Labored respirations or rate increased above 20 respirations per min; presence of rales on auscultation
   - Decrease in urinary output to below 30 ml per hour
   - Change in level of consciousness, confusion, restlessness, and expression of a sense of doom
   - Cool, clammy skin
   (3) Administer medications as ordered and monitor and report their side effects. Document the effectiveness of pharmacologic and nonpharmacologic interventions in measurable terms.

LEARNING/TEACHING GUIDELINES
for People After Myocardial Infarction

General Overview

1. Explore the person's feelings about myocardial infarction (MI). Fear, anxiety, denial, depression, and anger may occur and affect the person's ability to learn.
2. Describe the pathophysiology of an MI and explain the healing process.
3. Explain the importance of risk factor modification, including smoking cessation, maintaining normal weight, exercising as prescribed, reducing stress, and controlling high blood pressure, diabetes, or high cholesterol.
4. Discuss activity guidelines as directed by the physician and the importance of starting slowly.
5. Teach the person about medications, including the name, dose, and reason for taking the drug, how to take the drug, potential side effects, and what to do if side effects occur.
6. Explain what to do if chest pain occurs.
7. Discuss dietary modifications that may include fat, sodium, or calorie restrictions.
8. Provide information about and encourage a cardiac rehabilitation program.

Pathophysiology of Myocardial Infarction

1. Explain that an MI is caused by buildup of atherosclerotic plaques inside the arteries that carry blood to the heart muscle. A blood clot forms in the narrowed artery and blocks blood flow and oxygen supply to the heart muscle, causing a small part of the heart to be damaged.
2. Because part of the heart muscle was damaged, it does not pump as well as usual.
3. As the damaged area heals, a scar forms. Usually it takes 4 to 6 weeks to heal.
4. The physician describes the gradual building up of activity while the heart heals.

Medications

Instruct patients who are going to self-administer medications to do the following:

1. Know the name, dose, and purpose of all medications.
2. Plan the medication schedule, taking into account the reason for the medication and the person's activity, sleep, and work patterns.
3. Take medications exactly as prescribed.
4. Avoid over-the-counter medications without consulting the physician.

Activity Guidelines

1. Follow the physician's instructions regarding progression of activity.
2. Start slowly and pace activities for the first few weeks.
3. Stop activity if extreme fatigue, shortness of breath, dizziness, or chest pain occurs.
4. Explore with the patient the activity required in the work environment and modifications that might be needed.
5. Discuss resuming sexual activity.
   a. Sexual activity can usually be resumed 3 to 4 weeks after an MI.
   b. Explain that the amount of energy exerted during sexual activity corresponds to climbing 2 flights of stairs and that people rarely suffer heart problems during sexual intercourse.
   c. Depression or anxiety after MI may affect libido. Inform the physician if sexual difficulty persists.
   d. Recommendations may include the following:
      (1) Adopting positions that are most comfortable
      (2) Taking nitroglycerin before sexual intercourse
      (3) Resting before sexual intercourse
      (4) Avoiding sexual intercourse after a large meal, when extremely fatigued, when pressured for time, or in extremes of temperature
   e. Advise that sex with an unfamiliar partner may be more stressful.
   f. Inform the physician if symptoms such as fatigue, chest pain, or dyspnea occur after sexual intercourse.

Managing Chest Pain

1. Explain that the person may be especially aware of every ache and worry that it is the heart.
2. Help the person to differentiate chest pain due to myocardial ischemia from other pain.
3. Instruct the person to identify and anticipate things that precipitate pain.
4. Most persons are instructed by the physician to take nitroglycerin for chest discomfort. Relate the following instructions:
   a. Place the nitroglycerin tablet under the tongue and let it dissolve. Do not swallow the tablet or drink liquids while it dissolves.
   b. The tablet should cause a burning sensation. If it does not, the tablet may no longer be effective.
   c. Follow the physician's instructions regarding the number of tablets to take. The usual instruction is 1 tablet every 3 to 5 minutes. If discomfort is not relieved after 3 tablets taken over 15 minutes, then call an ambulance.
5. Review the following usual signs of an MI with the person:
   a. Uncomfortable pressure, squeezing, or pain in the chest that lasts more than a few minutes and is unrelieved by nitroglycerin
   b. Pain radiates to the shoulder, neck, jaw, or arms

(continued)

LEARNING/TEACHING GUIDELINES
(continued)

c. Associated symptoms of dizziness, sweating, nausea, and shortness of breath
6. Denial is a common psychologic response.
7. Prompt help can minimize damage and save lives.

Cardiac Rehabilitation

1. Provide information and resources for cardiac rehabilitation.
   a. A formal cardiac rehabilitation program provides education about heart disease, risk factors, nutrition, and exercise as well as psychologic support.
   b. Cardiac rehabilitation is described in 3 phases:
      (1) Phase I, inpatient
      (2) Phase II, supervised outpatient education program and exercise, usually starting 3 weeks after MI, lasting 12 weeks, and being conducted at a medical facility

   (3) Phase III, long-term continuing exercise program that may or may not be conducted at a medical facility
   c. Emphasize the benefits of exercise, including improved self image, increased cardiac efficiency and strength, and prolonged life and improved quality of life.
2. Relate the following guidelines regarding exercise:
   (1) Wait 2 hours after eating before exercising.
   (2) Do not exercise if ill or having a fever.
   (3) Wear appropriate clothing and shoes.
   (4) Avoid outside exercise in very cold or hot weather.
   (5) Start slowly and progress gradually.
   (6) Inform the physician before continuing the exercise program if chest pain, faintness, extreme fatigue, or shortness of breath occurs.

---

(4) Assist the patient into a position of comfort and ease in breathing. If the patient is on bed rest, place the patient in a semi-Fowler's position.
(5) Explain the need to limit activities and to avoid increased myocardial oxygen demand, such as straining during a bowel movement.

NURSING DIAGNOSIS: Anxiety R/T diagnosis of an MI and fear of death

a. *Expected outcomes:* Following interventions, the person should be able to do the following:
   (1) Express absence of anxiety
   (2) Appear relaxed, be able to rest quietly, and demonstrate appropriate verbal and nonverbal behaviors
b. *Nursing interventions*
   (1) Assess the patient for signs of anxiety such as verbal expression of anxiety, restlessness or sleeplessness, elevated blood pressure or heart rate, and inappropriate verbal or nonverbal communication, including shouting or withdrawing behaviors.
   (2) Provide education in understandable terms regarding disease process and therapeutic interventions.
   (3) Provide nursing care in a calm, caring, and competent manner. Provide a restful environment and administer sedatives as ordered to allow for rest and sleep.

(4) Instruct the patient in relaxation and diversional techniques such as muscle relaxation, listening to music, and visual imaging.
(5) Provide emotional and psychologic support to the patient and family. Encourage them to talk about their concerns. Provide spiritual referral, if desired.
12. Discharge planning and teaching
    a. Before discharge, actively involve the person and family members in the care planning process. At discharge, the person should be able to do the following:
       (1) Explain the disease process and the need for modification of risk factors
       (2) Articulate guidelines for activity
       (3) Properly administer medications
    b. Emphasize the importance of follow-up with the physician. Schedule the next appointment and provide a written reminder.
    c. Review warning signs (e.g., prolonged pain unrelieved by nitroglycerin, change in the character of pain, or pain accompanied by shortness of breath) that require contact with a physician or return to an emergency department.
    d. If appropriate, obtain a referral to a comprehensive cardiac rehabilitation program that includes exercise, dietary instruction, stress management, and lifestyle modification.
    e. If the patient is employed, discuss job duties and be sure the person knows when to return to work and whether modification in duties will be needed (see Learning/Teaching Guidelines for Persons After Myocardial Infarction).

f. Encourage the person or family to call if they have any concerns. Provide telephone numbers to caregivers.
13. Public health considerations. The American Heart Association emphasizes the need for public education.
   a. Recognize the signs of heart attack.
   b. Understand the importance of prompt attention (see p. 1046).
   c. Know how to obtain emergency medical assistance.

■ *VALVULAR DISORDERS*

Definitions

1. Aortic stenosis is a narrowing of the aorta that results in an obstruction to the blood flow from the ventricle during systole.
2. Aortic regurgitation (aortic insufficiency) describes leakage of blood from the aorta back into the left ventricle due to an incompetent aortic valve.
3. Mitral stenosis is a narrowing or thickening of the mitral valve.
4. Mitral regurgitation (mitral insufficiency) describes blood flow back through an incompetent mitral valve into the left atria.
5. Mitral valve prolapse is a bulging, billowing upward and backward of 1 or both of the valve leaflets into the left atrium during ventricular systole.
6. Tricuspid stenosis is a narrowing or thickening of the tricuspid valve.
7. Tricuspid regurgitation (tricuspid insufficiency) describes blood flow back from the right ventricle into the right atria through an incompetent tricuspid valve.
8. Pulmonic stenosis is a narrowing or thickening of the pulmonic valve.
9. Pulmonic regurgitation describes leakage of blood from the pulmonary artery back into the right ventricle.
10. See Table 23–24 for a summary of the differences among the valvular disorders.

Prognosis

1. The prognosis depends on the severity of disease and therapeutic intervention. Symptoms and limitations in activities of daily living are directly related to the severity of the stenosis or regurgitation.
2. Without valve replacement, death often occurs within 5 years after symptoms of congestive heart failure occur.
3. Sudden death can occur in severe cases.

Applying the Nursing Process

NURSING DIAGNOSIS: Decreased cardiac output R/T incompetence of valve

1. *Expected outcomes:* The person should be able to maintain an adequate cardiac output as demonstrated by the following:
   a. Stable vital signs
   b. Warm, dry skin
   c. Urine output greater than or equal to 30 ml per hr
   d. Appropriate mentation
2. *Nursing interventions*
   a. Provide education in understandable terms regarding disease process, therapeutic interventions, and potential for surgical intervention.
   b. Document initial cardiovascular assessment including ability to perform activities of daily living. Monitor the patient for signs of progressing failure.
   c. Administer medications as ordered. Document the effectiveness of both pharmacologic and nonpharmacologic interventions in measurable terms.
   d. Assist the patient into a position of comfort and ease in breathing. If the patient is on bed rest, place the patient in a high Fowler's position.
   e. Explain the need to limit activities and to avoid increased stress on the heart muscle, such as straining during a bowel movement.
   f. Provide emotional and psychologic support to the patient and family. Encourage them to talk about their concerns.

NURSING DIAGNOSIS: Fluid volume excess R/T congestive heart failure

1. *Expected outcomes:* See endocarditis.
2. *Nursing interventions:* See endocarditis.

NURSING DIAGNOSIS: Anxiety R/T disease process

1. *Expected outcomes:* See endocarditis.
2. *Nursing interventions:* See endocarditis.

Discharge Planning and Teaching

1. Explain the disease process, clinical manifestations, and complications.
2. Provide education regarding medication, including name, dose, effect, and potential complications.
3. Explain diet, activity, and fluid restrictions.
4. Provide a written list of symptoms that should be brought to the attention of a physician.

Public Health Considerations

Provide close monitoring and early intervention in persons with rheumatic fever or congenital defects.

Table 23–24. Valvular Disorders

Disorder	Incidence/ Etiology	Clinical Manifestations	Diagnostics	Clinical Management	Complications
Aortic stenosis	*Congenital* Occurs in 1% of the population Occurs in males 3 times more often than in females *Acquired* Rheumatic fever	Angina Syncope Exertional dyspnea Orthopnea Fatigue Symptoms of congestive heart failure (CHF)	*Auscultation* Loud systolic murmur at aortic area Palpable systolic thrill at base of heart *ECG* Left ventricle hypertrophy and/or atrioventricular conduction defects *Chest radiograph* Left ventricular enlargement, pulmonary congestion *Echocardiogram* *Cardiac catheterization*	*For CHF* Diuretics Digitalis Oxygen Sodium restriction *For infective endocarditis* Antibiotics *Special procedures* Valve replacement	CHF Conduction defects With severe stenosis, sudden death
Aortic regurgitation	Occurs more often in males *Congenital* Malposition of papillary muscles Incompetent valve Valvular abnormalities *Acquired* Infective endocarditis Connective tissue disease (Marfan syndrome) Rheumatic fever Syphilis	Angina Syncope Orthopnea Fatigue Exertional dyspnea CHF Diaphoresis Warm, flushed skin	*Auscultation* Blowing diastolic murmur Palpable diastolic thrill at lower left sternal boarder Widened pulse pressure *ECG* Left ventricular hypertrophy *Chest radiograph* Left ventricular hypertrophy Aortic calcification *Echocardiogram* *Cardiac catheterization*	Same as aortic stenosis	CHF
Mitral stenosis	Rheumatic heart disease Bacterial vegetation Atrial myxomas, a tumor of the connective tissue	*Usually occurs when orifice reduced by 50%* Dyspnea Orthopnea Paroxysmal nocturnal dyspnea *In severe cases* Resting tachycardia Increased respirations Narrowed pulse pressure Distended neck veins	*Auscultation* Loud 1st heart sound Opening snap Soft, low-pitched, rumbling, diastolic murmur *ECG* Atrial fibrillation Broad, notched P waves, called "P-mitrale" Tall R waves in lead V_1 *Chest radiograph* Left atrial enlargement *Echocardiogram* *Cardiac catheterization*	Same as aortic stenosis *For atrial fibrillation* Antidysrhythmics Anticoagulants *Special procedures* Commissurotomy, opening of the leaflets Valve replacement *For myxoma* Surgical removal	CHF Atrial dysrhythmias
Mitral regurgitation	Rheumatic fever Mitral valve prolapse, an inherited disorder resulting in a "floppy" valve	*Mild* May be asymptomatic *Moderate* Dyspnea Systemic embolization Jugular venous distention Fatigue Hepatomegaly Peripheral edema *Severe* Acute signs of pulmonary edema	*Auscultation* Pansystolic murmur— best heard at apex, radiates to axilla Split second heart sound *Physical findings* Abnormally large apical impulse *ECG* Atrial fibrillation Left ventricular hypertrophy *Chest radiograph* Left atrial and ventricular enlargement *Echocardiogram* *Cardiac catheterization*	Same as mitral stenosis	Acute onset of CHF Sudden cardiac death

		Table 23–24. Valvular Disorders (Continued)			
Disorder	**Incidence/ Etiology**	**Clinical Manifestations**	**Diagnostics**	**Clinical Management**	**Complications**
Mitral valve prolapse	Most common valve disorder Occurs in 5–10% of adults May be familial May be an isolated abnormality or may occur with endocarditis, myocarditis, trauma, systemic lupus erythematosus, Wolff-Parkinson-White syndrome, muscular dystrophy	May be asymptomatic May experience varying degrees of • Chest pain, unrelated to exertion and unrelieved by rest or nitroglycerin • Dizziness • Syncope • Dyspnea • Palpitations not usually associated with premature beats	*Auscultation* Midsystolic click and/or apical systolic murmur. Click and murmur effected by postural changes that decrease venous return Physical findings "Funnel" chest "Pigeon" chest Scoliosis Kyphosis *ECG* Usually normal, but supraventricular and ventricular abnormalities may occur *Echocardiogram* Shows abnormal valve movement	Most patients with idiopathic mitral valve prolapse do not require medical treatment Reassure patient that condition is usually benign Dyspnea and chest pain may be treated with propranolol Consider antibiotic prophylaxis	Mitral regurgitation
Tricuspid stenosis	Rheumatic heart disease Right atrial myxoma (rarely)	*Symptoms of decreased cardiac output* Fatigue Effort intolerance Hepatomegaly Ascites Peripheral edema	*Auscultation* Rumbling diastolic murmur *Physical findings* Jugular venous distention with clear lung fields *ECG* Prolonged PR Tall peaked P wave *Echocardiogram* *Cardiac catheterization*	Same as aortic stenosis	CHF Liver failure
Tricuspid regurgitation	Right ventricular dilation distorts the valvular ring Infective endocarditis Trauma Carcinoid syndrome from a serotonin-producing tumor	*Mild* Usually asymptomatic *Severe* Ascites Hepatomegaly Pleural effusions Peripheral edema	*Auscultation* Pansystolic murmur best heard at the left sternal border 4th intercostal space *ECG* May show atrial fibrillation *Chest radiograph* *Echocardiogram*	Same as aortic stenosis	CHF Liver failure
Pulmonic stenosis	Usually congenital Rheumatic fever	*Mild* May be asymptomatic *Severe* Dyspnea Fatigue Syncope Ascites Hepatomegaly Peripheral edema	*Auscultation* Systolic thrill best heard at the left sternal boarder Normal S_1 and split S_2 Systolic ejection click *ECG* In severe cases, large R waves in V_1 *Chest radiograph* *Cardiac catheterization*	*For CHF* Digitalis Diuretics Low sodium diet *For infective endocarditis* Antibiotics *Special procedure* Pulmonary valve commissurotomy	CHF Liver failure
Pulmonic regurgitation	Infective endocarditis Dilation of the valvular ring from pulmonary hypertension Mitral stenosis Chronic obstructive pulmonary disease Carcinoid syndrome Congenital malformation	Same as pulmonary stenosis	*Auscultation* Moderately pitched, diastolic murmur best heard at left sternal boarder *Chest radiograph* *Cardiac catheterization*	*For CHF* Digitalis Diuretics Low-sodium diet *For infective endocarditis* Antibiotics *Special procedures* Valve replacement	CHF Liver failure

■ ANATOMIC DISORDERS

As surgical procedures have improved, the number of persons with congenital heart diseases who reach adulthood has increased. Although most lead normal lives, some require close observation or treatment (see Chapter 15).

Atrial Septal Defect

1. Atrial septal defect is an opening between the right and left atria that causes blood to flow from the higher-pressured left atria to the lower-pressured right atria (see Chapter 15).

2. Atrial septal defect allows oxygenated and deoxygenated blood to mix in the right atria.
3. Atrial septal defect may cause second degree atrioventricular block, Mobitz type I, in adults.

Ventricular Septal Defect

1. A ventricular septal defect is an abnormal opening in the wall between the right and left ventricles (see Chapter 15).
2. Ventricular septal defect allows blood to flow from the higher-pressured left ventricle to the lower-pressured right ventricle.

Table 23-25. Comparison of Cardiomyopathies by Type

Dilated	Hypertrophic	Restrictive
Risk Factors/Etiology		
Alcohol		
Viral	Genetically acquired	Myocardial fibrosis
Bacterial		Amyloidosis
Chemotherapy		Neoplastic disorders
Peripartum		
Diagnostics		
Auscultation:		
Apical systolic murmur of mitral regurgitation	Harsh, crescendo–decrescendo systolic murmur	
3rd and 4th heart sounds		
Apical impulse displaced laterally		
ECG:		
Sinus tachycardia	Left ventricular hypertrophy	Signs of pulmonary and systemic congestion
Conduction defects	Atrial–ventricular dysrhythmias	without cardiomegaly
Clinical Management Goals		
Minimize symptoms	Same	Same
Avoid systemic emboli		
Maintain cardiac output		
Nonpharmacologic Interventions		
Sodium restriction for CHF	Same	Same
Restrict activities to avoid exertion		
Oxygen, if needed		
Pharmacologic Interventions		
For inotropic action:	For dysrhythmias:	Same as dilated, *except* avoid vasodilators or
Digitalis	Antidysrhythmics	drugs that reduce venous pressure, because
Sympathomimetics		they may decrease blood pressure and cardiac output
To reduce preload:	To prevent endocarditis:	
Diuretics	Antibiotics	
Nitrates		
To reduce afterload:	To prevent and treat emboli:	
Vasodilators	Anticoagulants	
To prevent and treat emboli:	To reduce hypertrophic response:	
Anticoagulants	Verapamil	
	Propranolol	
Special Medical-Surgical Procedures		
Cardiac transplantation	Myectomy with muscle resection	Resection of endomyocardial tissue
	Transaortic ventriculomyotomy	Repair and replacement of AV valve
Prognosis		
Death usually occurs within 6 months to 5 yr after symptoms appear	High incidence of death due to dysrhythmias	Generally poor

3. The left-to-right shift of blood causes an increase in pulmonary vascular resistance and pulmonary hypertension.
4. In 1 percent of all cases, an MI can lead to an ischemic portion of the ventricular septum and ventricular septal rupture.

Other Congenital Disorders

1. Pulmonic valvular stenosis
   a. Pulmonic valvular stenosis is a narrowing of the pulmonic valve.
   b. This narrowing causes increased right ventricular pressures and hypertrophy.
   c. Depending on the degree of the defect, previous surgical interventions may have been undertaken or may be needed in adulthood.
   d. Drug therapy is determined by the clinical symptoms and degree of ventricular failure.
2. Patent ductus arteriosus
   a. Patent ductus arteriosus is a failure of the ductus arteriosus to close at birth, causing a left-to-right shift of blood through the ductus into the pulmonary artery.
   b. Patent ductus arteriosus increases pulmonary pressures and right ventricular workload, which can lead to heart failure.

Cardiomyopathies

1. Definition
   a. Cardiomyopathies are disorders of the heart muscle categorized by their structural and functional abnormalities.
   b. Dilated cardiomyopathy occurs more frequently in men aged 40 to 60 years and in Blacks.
      (1) All 4 chambers of the heart are dilated owing to an interference with calcium uptake in the mitochondria, reducing contractility.
      (2) A decrease in the left ventricular ejection fraction leads to a decreased stroke volume and an increased left ventricular end diastolic volume.
      (3) Increased left ventricular end diastolic volume increases pulmonary congestion.
      (4) Bilateral ventricular failure ensues.
   c. In hypertrophic cardiomyopathy, left ventricular hypertrophy causes a malalignment of the papillary muscles, a distortion of the mitral valve leaflets, and an obstruction to the left ventricular outflow. Left ventricular end-diastolic pressure (LVEDP) increases, cardiac output decreases, and atrial dilation develops.
   d. In restrictive cardiomyopathy the myocardium is made rigid and noncompliant by eosinophilic inflammatory infiltration.
      (1) Small increases in diastolic volume result in marked increases in pressures.
      (2) Tachycardia occurs in an attempt to compensate.
      (3) Eventually, atrial dilatation and system and pulmonary congestion occurs.
2. Clinical manifestations
   a. Dyspnea
   b. Angina
   c. Palpitations
   d. Dizziness and syncope
3. Table 23–25 lists risk factors and etiology, diagnostics, clinical management, and prognosis.

 DRUG ADVISORY

In hypertrophic cardiomyopathy, avoid any drugs that increase contractility or decrease left ventricular volume because they may increase obstruction. This includes digitalis, diuretics, and nitrates.

4. Complications
   a. Congestive heart failure
   b. Cardiogenic shock
   c. Dysrhythmias, especially ventricular
5. Diagnostic tools
   a. Echocardiography
   b. Angiography
   c. Cardiac catheterization
6. Applying the nursing process. See aortic stenosis.
7. Discharge planning and teaching. See aortic stenosis.

■ *INFLAMMATORY PROCESSES*

Rheumatic Heart Disease

1. Definition: Rheumatic heart disease is residual damage to the heart by 1 or more episodes of rheumatic fever.
2. Incidence and etiology (see Chapter 15)
3. Clinical manifestations
   a. Valvular damage
   b. Compensatory mechanisms for valvular regurgitation and stenosis
   c. Congestive heart failure
   d. Pericarditis
   e. Bacterial endocarditis
   f. Atrial fibrillation
4. Clinical management
   a. Antibiotics for infections and as prophylaxis after dental work and other invasive procedures
   b. Inotropic medications for congestive heart failure
   c. Valve replacement

Endocarditis

1. Definition
   a. Infective endocarditis is an inflammation of the endocardium. It can affect the heart valves, the inner lining of the heart, and the intima of the great vessels.
   b. Libman-Sacks endocarditis is a nonbacterial imflammation that is a complication of systemic lupus erythematosus.

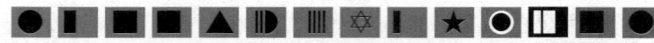

2. Classification
   a. Acute endocarditis occurs with more virulent organisms. It occurs quickly and produces significant heart damage, embolization, and toxemia.
   b. Subacute endocarditis (also known as subacute bacterial endocarditis) occurs with less virulent organisms over a prolonged period of time and is less damaging.
   c. Endocarditis may also be classified by valve type (native versus prosthetic) and or organism, e.g., *Streptococcus viridans* endocarditis, native valve.
3. Incidence and socioeconomic impact
   a. Infective endocarditis occurs in 50 to 60 percent of patients with previous valvular disorders
   b. Libman-Sacks endocarditis occurs in 50 percent of people with systemic lupus erythematosus late in the course of the disease process.
4. Risk factors
   a. For infective endocarditis, the following are risk factors:
      (1) Preexisting valvular damage
      (2) Presence of infective organism
      (3) Drug abuse
   b. For Libman-Sacks endocarditis, systemic lupus erythematosus is a risk factor.
5. Etiology
   a. Organisms that cause subacute and acute infective endocarditis are listed in Table 23–26. In subacute cases, more than 90 pecent are caused by alpha-hemolytic and nonhemolytic streptococci.
   b. In Libman-Sacks endocarditis, vascular injury from systemic lupus erythematosus is a cause.
6. Pathophysiology
   a. Subacute infective endocarditis
      (1) Irregular superficial endocardial valvular lesions called vegetations develop slowly and are easily detached from the valves.
      (2) Infection causes thinning of the valve, leading to valve destruction and regurgitation. Chordae tendineae, papillary muscle, and the conduction system may be involved.
      (3) As the valves heal, calcification and scarring can occur.
   b. Acute infective endocarditis
      (1) Large, soft, rapidly developing vegetations attach to the valves. They have a tendency to break off, causing emboli and leaving ulcerations on the leaflets.
      (2) Chordae tendineae, papillary muscle, and the conduction system may become damaged.
7. Clinical manifestations (related to infection, emboli, and vegetation)
   a. Cardiac murmur
   b. Pericardial friction rub
   c. Fever
   d. Anorexia
   e. Malaise
   f. Clubbing of fingers
   g. Neurologic sequelae of emboli
8. Diagnostics
   a. Auscultatory findings include murmurs in 85 to 95 percent of cases. The type of murmur varies by location and extent of inflammation. Most common are murmurs of regurgitation but they may also reflect stenosis.
   b. Electrocardiogram may demonstrate ST elevations similar to ischemia. Other dysrythmias and conduction disturbances depend on the valve involved.
   c. Laboratory findings include positive blood cultures; normochromic, normocytic anemia; and elevated leukocytes.
   d. Echocardiography reveals vegetation and functioning of valves.
9. Clinical management
   a. Goals of clinical management
      (1) Treat infection
      (2) Maintain cardiac output
      (3) Treat emboli
   b. Nonpharmacologic interventions
      (1) Monitor vital signs frequently and respond to changes
      (2) Provide adequate rest to avoid exertion
      (3) Ensure adequate nutritional intake
   c. Pharmacologic interventions include long-term antibiotic therapy, antipyretics, and anticoagulants.
   d. Special medical-surgical procedures include valve replacement.
10. Complications
    a. Congestive heart failure
    b. Myocardial ischemia and infarction
    c. Pericarditis
    d. Cardiac tamponade
    e. Cerebrovascular accident
    f. Pain in the joints (arthralgia)
    g. Gastrointestinal infarctions
    h. Renal infarctions

Table 23–26. Organisms That Cause Infective Endocarditis

Subacute	Escherichia coli
Streptococcus viridans	*Proteus*
Nonhemolytic streptococcus	*Klebsiella*
Streptococcus faecalis	*Pseudomonas*
	Salmonella
Acute	*Haemophilus*
Staphylococcus aureus	*Serratia*
Diplococcus	*Listeria*
Streptococcus pyogenes	*Bacteroides*
Neisseria gonorrhoeae	*Candida*
Neisseria meningitidis	*Aspergillus*

11. Prognosis varies based on type, organism, when the disease was diagnosed, and when treatment was begun.
12. Applying the nursing process

NURSING DIAGNOSIS: Fluid volume excess R/T congestive heart failure

a. *Expected outcomes:* Following interventions, the patient should be in fluid balance as evidenced by the following:
  (1) Stable vital signs, with no tachycardia
  (2) Clear lung sounds, without rales
  (3) Absence of dyspnea and shortness of breath
  (4) No signs of peripheral edema or cyanosis
b. *Nursing interventions*
  (1) Monitor the patient's vital signs; resting tachycardia can be an early sign of congestive heart failure.
  (2) Monitor the patient's intake and output.
  (3) Weigh the patient daily on the same scale and at the same time of the day.
  (4) Evaluate the patient's heart sounds for new or changed murmurs or additional heart sounds such as an S_3 or S_4 that indicates failure.
  (5) Evaluate the patient's lung sounds for presence of rales.
  (6) Provide for frequent rest periods.

NURSING DIAGNOSIS: Anxiety R/T disease process and long-term hospitalization

a. *Expected outcomes:* Following counseling, the patient should be able to do the following:
  (1) Demonstrate an understanding about the disease process and procedures by defining endocarditis and describing in simple terms the procedures involved in daily care
  (2) Describe a daily routine that allows for rest and diversional activities
  (3) Present a calm and relaxed demeanor and report practicing at least 1 relaxation technique each day
b. *Nursing interventions*
  (1) Explain all procedures in a simple and culturally sensitive manner.
  (2) Involve the person and family in scheduling the daily routine activities. Allow the patient and family to provide as much care and as homelike an environment as possible during a prolonged hospitalization.
  (3) Teach the person how to use relaxation techniques such as meditation, visualization, or guided imagery to cope with stressful situations, to assist them during painful procedures, or to help them to relax or sleep.

NURSING DIAGNOSIS: Infection R/T specific infective organism

a. *Expected outcomes:* Following interventions, the person should be free of infection.
  (1) During diagnosis, serial blood cultures are drawn to demonstrate a sustained rather than transient bacteremia. The person should be able to verbalize an understanding of the need for and frequency of blood cultures.
  (2) Long-term intravenous antimicrobial therapy should be administered in a consistent manner. The person should be able to verbalize an understanding of the need for long-term therapy and express commitment to the process.
  (3) Clinical improvement should be noted. Temperature should be normal. Blood cultures should be negative. The person should describe improvement in condition including improvement in appetite and decrease in fatigue and malaise.
  (4) The person should be without complications from antimicrobial therapy and should be able to verbalize the need to report any symptoms of adverse drug reaction such as rash, itching, diarrhea, or symptoms of anaphylactic shock including shortness of breath; dizziness and hearing loss when taking streptomycin; or renal complications when taking gentamicin.
b. *Nursing interventions*
  (1) Obtain blood cultures as indicated.
  (2) Monitor temperature for elevation.
  (3) Maintain intravenous access for antibiotic drug administration. Monitor for phlebitis or infiltration.
  (4) Administer antimicrobial therapy as indicated.
  (5) Monitor for adverse effects of antimicrobial therapy.
13. Discharge planning and teaching
a. Antibiotic therapy usually requires several weeks of intravenous treatment. This may be provided in the hospital or, in some cases, in an ambulatory or home setting.
b. Teaching should include the following:
  (1) Explanation about the disease and the need for long-term therapy
  (2) Causative factors and the need to avoid problem-prone behaviors such as intravenous drug abuse
  (3) The need for prophylactic antibiotics before dental work and other invasive procedures such as genitourinary and gastrointestinal procedures. Prophylaxis minimizes the risk of microorganisms entering the bloodstream during the procedure and multiplying in the myocardium.
  (4) Symptoms such as fever, tachycardia, dyspnea, and shortness of breath, which may indicate a recurrence and necessitate contacting the physician (see Learning/Teaching Guidelines for Persons at Risk for Infective Endocarditis)
14. Public health considerations. The healthcare provider should do the following:
a. Recognize high-risk populations
b. Provide education on avoiding high-risk behaviors
c. Provide prophylactic antibiotic therapy before dental work or invasive procedures

LEARNING/TEACHING GUIDELINES
for People at Risk for Infective Endocarditis

General Overview

1. Review the heart condition that places the person at risk for infective endocarditis.
2. Point out that infective endocarditis is a serious illness that may require hospitalization or even cardiac surgery.
3. Emphasize the susceptibility to reinfection. Advise the person to tell all physicians and dentists about having the heart condition. Some surgical treatments and dental work such as teeth cleaning can cause an infection if antibiotic prophylaxis is not initiated before treatment.
4. Keep teeth and gums healthy by brushing and rinsing after meals and seeing the dentist regularly. Avoid trauma to the gums by not using toothpicks or other devices that might cause gums to bleed.
5. Always carry the MedicAlert card, which tells about the underlying heart condition.
6. Emphasize the need to take the antibiotic medicine exactly as described on the container or as instructed by the physician.
7. Provide instructions about the need to contact the physician at the 1st sign of fever or other signs and symptoms of endocarditis such as chills, fatigue, weight loss, or anorexia.
8. If the person uses needles or syringes, instruct them not to use someone else's and not to reuse their own. The germs from them can carry an infection through the bloodstream to the heart and damage heart valves.

Myocarditis

1. Definition
   a. Myocarditis is an inflammation of the myocardium.
   b. It may be acute or chronic.
   c. Inflammation may be diffuse or characterized by focal lesions.
2. Incidence and socioeconomic impact
   a. Myocarditis can occur at any age.
   b. Impact varies with cause and severity.
3. Risk factors and etiology
   a. Most commonly idiopathic
   b. Rheumatic fever
   c. Radiation therapy
   d. Drug reaction
   e. Metabolic disorders
   f. Infection
4. Pathophysiology
   a. A myocardial toxin or antibody is produced secondary to the causative agent.
   b. Response can be diffuse or localized.
5. Clinical manifestations depend on the extent of inflammation.
   a. If localized, manifestations depend on location. If inflammation is along conduction pathways, blocks and dysrhythmias may result.
   b. If diffuse, signs and symptoms of heart failure may result, such as fatigue, dyspnea, tachycardia, and chest pain.
6. Diagnostics
   a. A careful history and review of symptoms provide valuable data for diagnosis.
   b. Auscultatory findings
      (1) A murmur that sounds like fluid passing an obstruction
      (2) Pericardial friction rub
      (3) A gallop rhythm (combined S_3 and S_4)
   c. Physical examination findings
      (1) Pulsus alternans
      (2) Fever
      (3) Tachycardia
   d. Radiography shows evidence of cardiomegaly.
7. Clinical management
   a. Goals of clinical management are to do the following:
      (1) Treat the underlying disease
      (2) Reduce the workload of the heart
      (3) Maintain cardiac output
      (4) Prevent emboli
      (5) Monitor for dysrhythmias
   b. Nonpharmacologic interventions
      (1) Limit physical activities to avoid exertion
      (2) Supply oxygen if needed
      (3) Provide continuous monitoring
      (4) Be prepared for emergency resuscitation
   c. Pharmacologic interventions
      (1) Digitalis

℞ DRUG ADVISORY

The person with myocarditis is extremely sensitive to digitalis. Monitor the patient for signs of digitalis toxicity.

      (2) Antiarrhythmics
      (3) Pain medications
      (4) Antibiotics to treat the causative organism
   d. There are no special medical-surgical procedures.
8. Complications
   a. Congestive heart failure
   b. Venous thrombosis
   c. Mural thrombi
   d. Cardiomyopathy
9. Prognosis varies by etiology and extent of involvement.
10. Applying the nursing process

NURSING DIAGNOSIS: Anxiety R/T disease process

a. *Expected outcomes:* Following counseling, the person should be able to do the following:
   (1) Explain the disease process and procedures in a manner that is understandable and relevant
   (2) Describe a preferred mechanism to reduce stress and decrease anxiety, which may include use of relaxation tapes or guided imagery
   (3) Appear comfortable, without signs and symptoms of pain, fatigue, or cardiac failure
b. *Nursing interventions*
   (1) Explain all procedures in simple and easy to understand terms. Ask for frequent feedback from the person and family to ensure that they have understood the information.
   (2) Describe relaxation and diversional techniques and assist the person in using them during times of stress.
   (3) Ensure that the daily schedule includes time for uninterrupted rest several times during the day.

NURSING DIAGNOSIS: Pain R/T inflammation

a. *Expected outcomes:* The person should be able to do the following:
   (1) Demonstrate an understanding of disease process by limiting activities to avoid exertion
   (2) Position self so as to provide physical support and minimize pericardial discomfort
   (3) Take medication on time and as ordered to maintain a therapeutic blood level
b. *Nursing interventions*
   (1) Give medications—analgesics, salicylates, and nonsteroidal anti-inflammatory agents—as ordered to reduce pain, fever, and inflammation.
   (2) Assist the patient into a position of comfort, such as sitting up or leaning forward. If the patient is on bed rest, place the bed in a high Fowler's position and have the person lean forward with arms resting on a pillow placed on the overbed table.
   (3) Allow for frequent periods of rest.
11. Discharge planning and teaching
   a. Base teaching on causative factor and degree of myocardial damage.
   b. Provide specific instructions regarding the medications ordered (which may include antibiotics and digoxin), the symptoms that require referral to a physician, and activities that increase myocardial demand and thus should be avoided. (These may include stair climbing, exercising, and experiencing temperature extremes.)
12. Public health considerations: Educate the public to avoid behaviors that may predispose them to infections.

Pericarditis

1. Definition
   a. Pericarditis is an inflammation of the pericardial lining of the heart, the pericardium.
   b. Classification
      (1) By cause, pericarditis is infectious, nonspecific, drug induced, and autoimmunity and hypersensitivity related.
      (2) By type, pericarditis is acute with effusion, and chronic and constrictive.
2. Incidence and socioeconomic impact: Pericarditis occurs in up to 15 percent of persons with a transmural infarction.
3. Risk factors and etiology: vary by cause (Table 23–27).
4. Pathophysiology
   a. The membranous sac around the heart becomes inflamed from a variety of causes.
   b. Constrictive pericarditis is a chronic inflammatory thickening of the pericardium that constricts the heart, causing compression and keeping the heart from expanding in diastole.

Table 23–27. Etiology of Pericarditis

Infectious	Autoimmune/ Hypersensitivity	Drugs	Nonspecific
Most common with rheumatic fever and pneumonia	Systemic lupus erythematosus	Hydralazine	Trauma
Bacteria	Polyarteritis nodosa	Procainamide	Neoplastic disorders
Staphylococcus	Scleroderma	Anticoagulants	Radiation therapy
Meningococcus	Dressler's syndrome		Myocardial infarction
Streptococcus	Postcardiotomy		Idiopathic
Pneumococcus			Uremia
Gonococcus			Myxedema
Fungus			Anemia
Virus			Aortic dissection
Tuberculosis			
Parisitic			

c. Dressler's syndrome is a combination of pericarditis, pericardial effusion, and pleural effusions, which, for reasons that are unclear, occur several weeks to months after an MI.
5. Clinical manifestations. Pain, which varies in intensity, is located in the anterior chest, precordial. It may be relieved by leaning forward (Table 23–28).
6. Diagnostics
   a. Auscultatory findings include a pericardial friction rub, a scratchy, creaking sound best heard using the diaphragm of the stethoscope during forced expiration. It may help to have the person leaning forward with hands on knees. The rub may occur during atrial systole, S_4; the apex of ventricular contraction; or the diastolic phase of rapid filling, S_3.
   b. Physical examination findings
      (1) Pulsus paradoxus is an exaggeration of normal respiratory variations in blood pressure readings (see Fig. 23–6).
      (2) The person is usually unable to lie flat without pain or dyspnea.
   c. Chest radiograph shows the following:
      (1) An enlarged heart
      (2) Clear lung fields
      (3) Pericardial fluid
   d. Electrocardiogram shows the following:
      (1) Depressed P–R interval
      (2) Elevated ST segment
      (3) A QRS of low voltage or changing amplitude beat to beat (electrical alterations)
      (4) Flat and inverted T wave
   e. Echocardiography indicates the presence and size of pericardial effusion.
   f. Laboratory tests
      (1) Complete blood count with differential reflects an infectious process.
      (2) Sedimentation rate is usually elevated.
7. Clinical management
   a. Goals of clinical management
      (1) Relieve pain
      (2) Avoid or resolve pericardial effusion
      (3) Treat the underlying disease
      (4) Maintain cardiac output
   b. Nonpharmacologic interventions
      (1) Monitor the person for dysrhythmias.

(2) Supply oxygen as necessary.
(3) Limit the person's activity to avoid exertion.
(4) Assist the person into a position of comfort (consider a high Fowler's position or having the person lean forward with arms supported on an overbed table).
   c. Pharmacologic intervention varies depending on etiology. In all cases, consider the following:
      (1) Meperidine or morphine for pain
      (2) Salicylates for pain and to assist in reabsorption of effusion due to rheumatic pericarditis
      (3) Nonsteroidal anti-inflammatories
      (4) Corticosteroids to control symptoms
   d. Special medical-surgical procedures
      (1) Pericardiocentesis (Procedure 23–11) is used to drain any pericardial effusion.
      (2) In a pericardial window, a thoracotomy allows an open drainage of the pericardial effusion. Cultures of the pericardium can be obtained.
      (3) Pericardiectomy, or surgical removal of the pericardium, is used most often when myocardial fibrosis and ventricular atrophy are in their early stages.
      (4) Dialysis is used in cases of uremic pericarditis.
8. Complications
   a. Dysrhythmias
   b. Pericardial effusion—a filling of the pericardial space with fluid with accumulation occurring over time or abruptly and may advance to pericardial tamponade (Fig. 23–27).

NURSE ADVISORY

A rapidly developing pericardial effusion is a true cardiac emergency. The pericardial space can accumulate up to 100 to 150 ml of fluid, leading to cardiac tamponade and decompensation.

9. Applying the nursing process

NURSING DIAGNOSIS: Anxiety R/T pain and lack of knowledge of disease process

   a. *Expected outcomes:* Following counseling, the person should be able to do the following:
      (1) Demonstrate an understanding of the disease process by defining pericarditis as an inflammation of the outer layer of the heart
      (2) Describe the use of 1 relaxation technique such as music therapy or guided imagery that can be used when the patient is anxious, in pain, or during procedures
      (3) Have periods of uninterrupted rest
   b. *Nursing interventions*
      (1) Explain the usual treatment plan and expected course of the disorder.
      (2) Explain all procedures in understandable terms to the person and the family.
      (3) Review use of relaxation methods.

Table 23–28. Comparison of Symptoms in Acute and Chronic Pericarditis

Acute	Chronic (Constrictive)
Fever—low grade	Afebrile
Chills	Fatigue
Restlessness	Orthopnea
Anxiety	Dyspnea
Dysphagia	Cough
Tachypnea	Peripheral edema
Dyspnea	Ascites
	Hepatomegaly

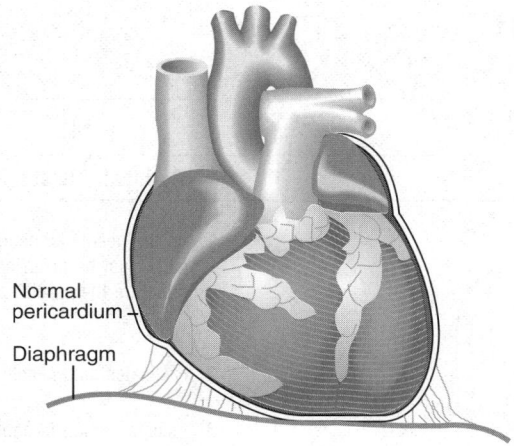

Normal
pericardium

Diaphragm

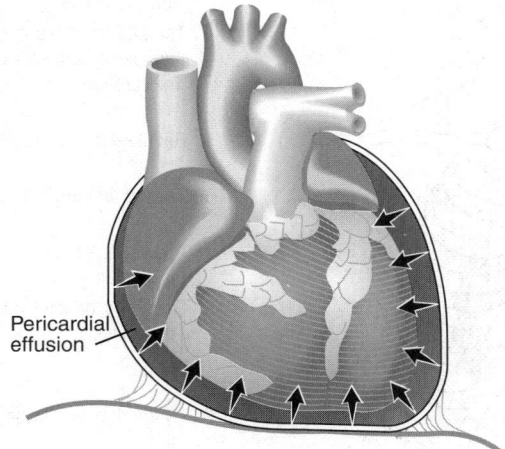

Pericardial
effusion

Figure 23–27. Pericardial effusion.

NURSING DIAGNOSIS: Pain R/T pericardial inflammation

a. *Expected outcomes:* Following interventions, the person should be able to do the following:
   (1) Be comfortable and able to cooperate with the plan of care
   (2) Be able to breathe deeply without splinting
   (3) Be able to sleep without interruption from pain
b. *Nursing interventions*
   (1) Give medications—analgesics, salicylates, and nonsteroidal anti-inflammatory agents—as ordered to reduce pain, fever, and inflammation.
   (2) Assist the patient into a position of comfort, such as sitting up or leaning forward. If the patient is on bed rest, place the bed in a high Fowler's position and have the patient lean forward with arms resting on a pillow placed on the overbed table.
   (3) Allow for frequent periods of rest.

NURSING DIAGNOSIS: Decreased cardiac output R/T pericardial effusion

a. *Expected outcomes:* Following interventions, the person should be able to do the following:
   (1) Be free of the signs and symptoms of pericardial effusion such as pericardial friction rub, tachycardia, and hypotension
   (2) Be able to describe the symptoms of pericardial effusion, including pain made worse by coughing or lying down, and shortness of breath

P

Procedure 23–11
Pericardiocentesis

Definition/Purpose	To relieve pericardial effusion or cardiac tamponade by removing fluid or blood from the pericardial sac, which has accumulated secondary to pericarditis, trauma, acute rheumatic fever, malignant neoplasm or lymphoma.
Contraindication/Cautions	Previous pericardial exploration.

Preliminary Activities

Equipment	• Skin antiseptic • Local anesthetic drug • Small syringe and needle for local anesthesia • Sterile drapes and gloves • Cardiac monitor • Defibrillator • Syringe (20 ml) • Cardiac needle • Small sterile dressing
Assessment Planning	• Know the patient's baseline vital signs. • Know the physiology of cardiac tamponade. • Prepare emergency equipment for resuscitation.

(continued)

Procedure

Actions	Rationale/Discussion

1. Inform the person about the procedure and the importance of remaining immobile.

2. Position the person supine with head elevated 60 degrees.

3. Premedicate the person as indicated.

4. Connect the person to the cardiac monitor.

5. Expose the chest and prepare the site with skin antiseptic.

6. Drape the area with sterile towels.

7. The site is injected with local anesthetic.

8. The cardiac needle is attached to a 20-ml syringe and is advanced by the physician until fluid is obtained.

9. Monitor the person's vital signs and cardiac status during procedure.

10. Evaluate the color and clotting ability of aspirant.

11. Monitor the person for signs of recurrent tamponade.

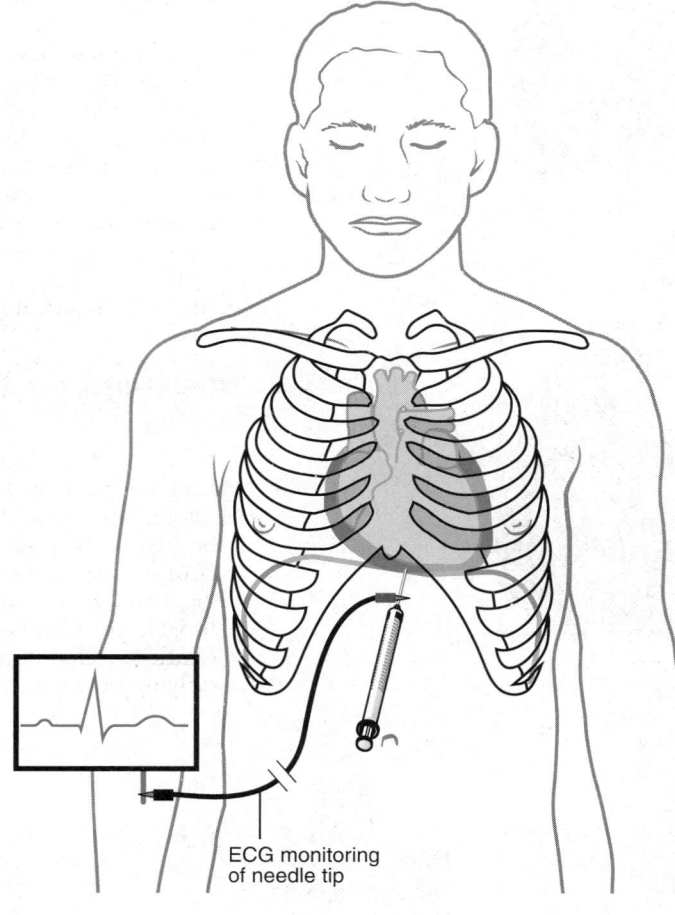

ECG monitoring of needle tip

1. As the needle is inserted, care must be taken not to puncture the cardiac artery.

2. Facilitates safe needle entry.

3. Assists person in cooperating with procedure.

4. The ECG changes occur as the needle connects with the myocardium.

5. Reduces risk of infection.

6. Asepsis is required.

7. Allows for pain-free needle insertion.

8. Fluid may be sent for laboratory analysis.

9. Dysrhythmias can be a complication.

10. Pericardial fluid may be caused by trauma. Pericardial blood does not clot, whereas blood obtained from inadvertent puncture of 1 of the heart chambers does clot.

11. Signs include decreasing blood pressure, narrowing pulse pressure, paradoxical pulse, apprehension, dyspnea, cyanosis, distended neck veins, and muffled heart tones.

Final Activities

1. Continue to monitor cardiac status and vital signs.
2. Assess for other complications such as:
   - Puncture of the heart
   - Dysrhythmias
   - Puncture of the lung, stomach, or liver
   - Laceration of the coronary artery or myocardium
3. Document the following:
   a. Any visible signs of tamponade, as well as cardiac status and vital signs before the procedure.
   b. How the procedure was tolerated.
   c. Any complications during or after the procedure.
   d. The total amount and type of fluid aspirated.
   e. Cardiac status and vital signs during and after the procedure.

(3) Know to call for assistance with any worsening of symptoms that may indicate the beginning of cardiac tamponade

b. *Nursing interventions*

(1) Explain signs and symptoms of worsening pericardial effusions.

(2) Monitor the patient for signs of cardiac tamponade such as hypotension, pulsus paradoxus, and muffled heart sounds.

(3) Monitor the ECG for increasing tachycardia or a decrease in QRS amplitude, which may indicate cardiac tamponade.

(4) If signs of decreasing cardiac output are observed, prepare the patient for rapid infusion of volume expanders such as saline or blood products, pericardiocentesis, or emergency resuscitation.

10. Discharge planning and teaching

a. Provide the person with written materials about medications and their side effects.

b. Review symptoms that require immediate contact of a physician: worsening dyspnea, increasing pain, orthopnea, or signs of hypotension, such as dizziness.

c. Explain the need to avoid upper respiratory infections and the importance of reporting any symptoms of colds, cough, or sore throat.

d. Make an appointment and provide a written reminder for follow-up care. Stress the importance of keeping all appointments.

e. Encourage the person and family to call with any questions or concerns.

Cardiac Tamponade

1. Definition: Cardiac tamponade develops when fluid accumulation in the pericardial cavity restricts ventricular filling. Cardiac tamponade is a true cardiac emergency requiring prompt intervention.

2. Risk factors

a. Presence of an underlying cause

b. Volume of fluid accumulation

c. Condition of pericardium and whether it is thick from disease and nondistensible

d. Rapidity of fluid accumulation. Slow accumulation (as in a chronic condition) allows time for the normal pericardial sac to stretch and accommodate the volume. Up to 1000 ml may accumulate without hemodynamic effects. If fluid accumulates rapidly (as in chest trauma), as little as 100 to 250 ml can cause cardiac tamponade.

3. Etiology

a. Cardiac tamponade may occur with any form of pericarditis, but it is most common in malignancy such as neoplastic pericarditis, idiopathic or viral pericarditis, and uremia.

b. Hemopericardium, accumulation of blood in the pericardial cavity, may occur with trauma to the chest via gunshot wound, stab wounds, or perforation during pacing and cardiac catheterization procedures; postcardiac surgery; rupture of the heart after an MI; aortic dissection; rupture of aortic aneurysm; and anticoagulant therapy.

4. Pathophysiology

a. Fluid accumulation in the pericardium raises pericardial pressure.

b. When pericardial pressure exceeds diastolic filling pressures in the heart, ventricular filling is restricted, stroke volume decreases, and cardiac output decreases.

5. Clinical manifestations

a. Anxiety

b. Jugular venous distention

c. Tachypnea, dyspnea, or orthopnea

d. Tachycardia

e. Sweating

f. Pulseless electric activity, in severe cases

6. Diagnostics

a. History: Note the presence of causes of cardiac tamponade.

b. Physical examination

(1) General appearance: the person may appear anxious, sweating, and dyspneic and may assume a sitting position. Distended neck veins are observed.

(2) Vital signs: Decreased systolic blood pressure and a pulsus paradoxus are present. Pulse rate is increased. Respirations are increased.

(3) Heart sounds may be distant.

(4) Pericardial rub may be present.

c. Diagnostic studies

(1) Chest radiograph

(2) Electrocardiogram

(3) Cardiac catheterization

(4) Echocardiogram, which is the best way to diagnose the cardiac tamponade and should be done before pericardiocentesis, if time permits

7. Clinical management

a. The goal of clinical management is to relieve cardiac compression by removing fluid from the pericardial cavity.

b. Nonpharmacologic interventions include bed rest and high Fowler's position.

c. Pharmacologic interventions include oxygen and volume expansion to raise venous pressure above pericardial pressure.

d. Special medical-surgical procedures include pericardiocentesis (see Procedure 23–11), which removes excess fluid or blood from the pericardial sac.

NURSE ADVISORY

If a person is at risk for cardiac tamponade, equipment for a pericardiocentesis should be kept immediately available at the bedside.

---

8. Complications include cardiogenic shock and circulatory collapse.

9. Prognosis: Immediate prognosis is good with prompt

treatment. Long-term prognosis depends on the underlying cause of the cardiac tamponade.
10. Applying the nursing process

NURSING DIAGNOSIS: Decreased cardiac output R/T restricted ventricular filling

a. *Expected outcomes:* The person should be able to maintain a cardiac output that allows for adequate tissue perfusion as demonstated by the following:
   - Stable vital signs
   - Warm, dry skin
   - Adequate urine output
   - Appropriate mentation
b. *Nursing interventions*
   - Continually assess the patient for early signs and symptoms of cardiac tamponade.
   - If the situation allows, provide education in understandable terms regarding disease process, therapeutic interventions, and potential for surgical intervention.
   - Administer medications and fluids as ordered. Monitor and report side effects and document effectiveness of pharmacologic and nonpharmacologic interventions in measurable terms.
   - Explain the need to limit activities and to avoid increased stress on the heart muscle, such as straining during a bowel movement.
   - Provide emotional and psychological support to the patient and family. Encourage them to talk about their concerns.
   - Prepare for pericardiocentesis or surgical intervention. Initiate basic life support and advanced cardiac life support if needed.

NURSING DIAGNOSIS: Anxiety R/T pain, shortness of breath, or an emergency situation

a. *Expected outcomes:* Following counseling, the person should be able to demonstrate a demeanor consistent with the clinical situation, and if able, articulate information related to the condition, interventions, and preoperative instructions.
b. *Nursing interventions*
   - Maintain a calm and professional manner while preparing for emergency interventions.
   - Prepare the person and family for pericardiocentesis or surgical intervention using understandable terms.
   - If time and condition allow, permit family members to visit.
11. Discharge planning and teaching
   - If time allows, explain all procedures and treatments to the person and family.
   - Additional teaching depends on the underlying cause of cardiac tamponade.

■ CONGESTIVE HEART FAILURE

Definition

1. Congestive heart failure (CHF) describes the syndrome of pulmonary and systemic congestion. The heart fails to pump enough blood to meet the metabolic needs of the body.
2. Classification
   a. Direction of blood flow determines forward versus backward heart failure.
      (1) In forward failure, inadequate output of affected ventricle causes decreased perfusion of vital organs, resulting in symptoms such as mental confusion, muscle weakness, and altered kidney function.
      (2) In backward failure, damming up of blood behind the affected ventricle causes increased pressure in the atrium behind the affected ventricle, increased pressure in the venous and capillary system behind the atria, and movement of fluid from capillary into the interstitium, resulting in symptoms such as pulmonary edema.
      (3) Both backward and forward failure occur in most patients with chronic heart failure.
   b. The right or left side of the heart may be involved.
      (1) Right-sided heart failure and left-sided heart failure are terms used to describe conditions in which the primary problem is on the right or left side of the heart.
      (2) Right-sided heart failure refers to signs and symptoms of increased pressures and congestion in the systemic veins and capillaries.
      (3) Left-sided heart failure refers to signs and symptoms of elevated pressure and congestion in pulmonary veins and capillaries.
      (4) Failure of 1 ventricle often produces changes in the other ventricle, leading to biventricular failure.
   c. Congestive heart failure may be acute or chronic.
      (1) Acute CHF may result in acute decompensation and circulatory collapse (e.g., papillary muscle rupture with acute mitral regurgitation or massive pulmonary embolus).
      (2) Chronic CHF develops over time (e.g., right-sided heart failure from chronic obstructive pulmonary disease).
      (3) A person with chronic heart failure may experience an acute episode.
   d. Low output and high output may be used to classify heart failure.
      (1) Most heart failure is low output, wherein not enough cardiac output is available to meet usual needs. The person shows evidence of impaired circulation and vasoconstriction with cool, pale extremities.
      (2) High-output failure occurs when a condition causes the heart to work harder to meet increased needs (e.g., thyrotoxicosis, sepsis, anemia, and pregnancy). The person appears warm and flushed.
   e. Systolic and diastolic heart failure are terms used to classify heart failure.

(1) Systolic failure is an abnormality in systolic function leading to a problem with contraction and ejection of blood (e.g., dilated cardiomyopathy).

(2) Diastolic failure is an abnormality in diastolic function leading to a problem with the heart relaxing and filling with blood (e.g., hypertrophic cardiomyopathy).

(3) The person may have both a systolic and a diastolic problem (e.g., when a scar from a previous myocardial infarction does not contract—systolic—and is stiff and nondistensible—diastolic).

f. The New York Heart Association Functional Classification is listed in Table 23–29.

Incidence and Socioeconomic Impact

1. Three million people in the United States have heart failure and an additional 400,000 Americans are diagnosed each year.
2. Heart failure occurs in 1 percent of people over age 65 years, 5 percent of those older than age 75 years, and 10 percent of those older than 80 years of age.
3. Heart failure is the most common medical discharge diagnosis for persons older than 65 years of age.

Risk Factors and Etiology

1. Underlying conditions can cause heart failure (Table 23–30).
2. Major etiologies
   a. Coronary artery disease, which causes approximately 60 percent of the cases of heart failure
   b. Myocardial infarction, which increases the risk of heart failure by 4 to 6 times with a history of an MI
   c. Primary cardiomyopathy
   d. Hypertension
   e. Valvular heart disease, particularly aortic
3. Precipitating factors
   a. Noncompliance with therapeutic regimen
   b. Dysrhythmias
      (1) Tachydysrhythmias reduce time for ventricular filling, increase myocardial oxygen demand, and may cause myocardial ischemia.
      (2) Bradydysrhythmias may critically decrease cardiac output.
      (3) Atrial-ventricular dissociation results in loss of atrial kick.

Table 23–29. New York Heart Association Functional Classification of Heart Failure

Class 1	No symptoms with ordinary physical activity.
Class 2	Symptoms with ordinary activity. Slight limitation.
Class 3	Symptoms with less than ordinary activity. Marked limitation of activity.
Class 4	Symptoms with any physical activity or even at rest.

Table 23–30. Underlying Causes of Heart Failure

Intrinsic Myocardial Disease
Coronary artery disease
Cardiomyopathy
Infiltrative disorders (amyloidosis, sarcoidosis)

Excess Volume Load
Aortic regurgitation
Mitral regurgitation
Tricuspid regurgitation
Left to right shunt

Excess Resistance to Ejection
Hypertension
Aortic stenosis
Pulmonic stenosis
Hypertrophic cardiomyopathy

Increased Body Demands
Thyrotoxicosis
Anemia
Pregnancy

Iatrogenic Myocardial Damage
Drugs (e.g., Adriamycin)
Radiation for mediastinal tumors

---

c. Infection
   (1) Infection burdens the heart by increasing metabolic demands.
   (2) Fever causes tachycardia, the discomfort of which increases myocardial oxygen demand.
d. Pulmonary embolism
e. Physical and emotional exertion
f. Cardiac infection
g. Uncontrolled hypertension
h. Myocardial infarction
i. Medications, such as the following:
   (1) Myocardial depressants (e.g., β-blockers, verapamil, and many antiarrhythmic agents)
   (2) Salt-retaining medications (e.g., estrogens, steroids, nonsteroidal anti-inflammatory agents)
   (3) Chemotherapy agents
j. Renal disease, causing decreased sodium and volume excretion
k. Excessive transfusions or intravenous fluids

Pathophysiology

1. In left-sided heart failure, increased left ventricular pressure or volume leads to increased left atrial pressure, which increases pulmonary capillary pressure, resulting in pulmonary edema. Increased pulmonary pressures may cause the right side to fail.
2. In right-sided heart failure, increased right ventricular pressure or volume leads to increased right atrial pressure, which increases sytemic venous pressure, resulting in peripheral edema and hepatic congestion.
3. Decreased cardiac output leads to changes caused by the

renal compensatory and sympathetic nervous systems (Fig. 23–28).

Clinical Manifestations

1. Left ventricular failure manifestations
    a. Dyspnea, which may progress as follows:
        (1) Dyspnea on exertion
        (2) Orthopnea
        (3) Paroxysmal nocturnal dyspnea
        (4) Dyspnea at rest
        (5) Pulmonary edema
    b. Dry, hacking cough, especially when lying down.
    c. Fatigue and weakness
    d. Urinary symptoms, including nocturia, early in the course of failure, and oliguria, late in the course
    e. Cerebral symptoms, including confusion and memory loss

f. Tachycardia
    g. Rales that do not clear with coughing
    h. S_3 and S_4 heart sounds
2. Right ventricular failure manifestations
    a. Peripheral edema without venous insufficiency
    b. Weight gain
    c. Pleural effusions
    d. Anorexia and bloating
    e. Right upper quadrant pain
    f. Neck vein distention
    g. Hepatomegaly
    h. Ascites
    i. Positive hepatojugular reflex

Diagnostics

1. History
    a. Note the presence of symptoms of heart failure.

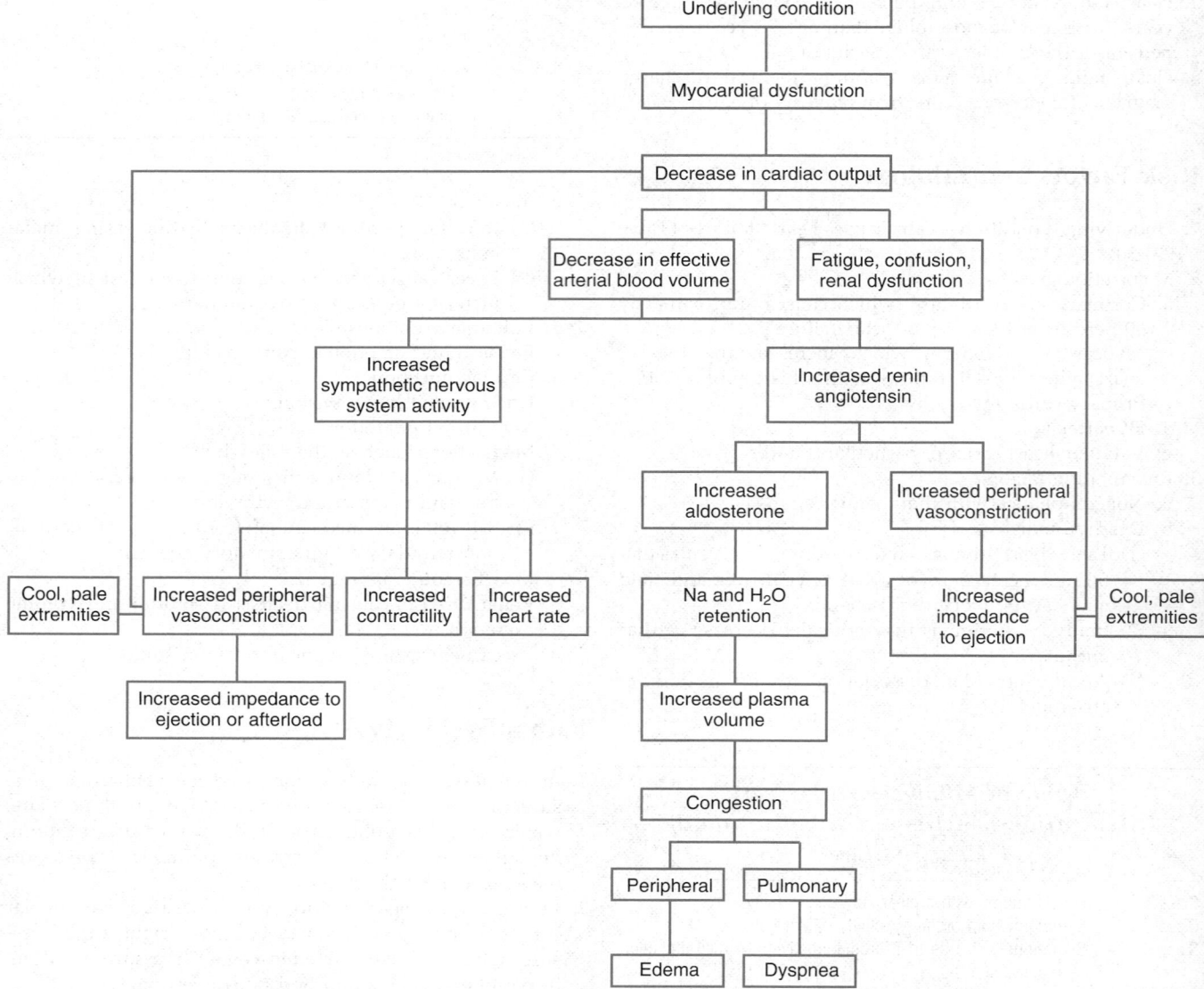

Figure 23–28. Pathophysiology of low-output heart failure.

b. Obtain a detailed description of each symptom. Symptoms such as dyspnea or weakness may occur in response to other diseases.

c. Try to determine the possible underlying cause of heart failure (e.g., history of MI or rheumatic heart disease).

d. Try to determine the precipitating factors in this episode of heart failure.

2. Physical examination

  a. General appearance

    (1) The person may appear breathless at rest, with activity, or be unable to lie flat.

    (2) The person with chronic severe heart failure, especially right sided, may appear thin and undernourished.

    (3) Distended neck veins may be evident in right-sided failure.

  b. Vital signs

    (1) Respirations may be rapid and shallow. Cheyne-Stokes pattern may be observed.

    (2) Pulse

     • Rate and rhythm. Tachycardia may occur as a compensatory mechanism or be a precipitating factor. Irregular or slow rhythms may indicate a precipitating dysrhythmia.

     • Character. Pulsus alternans is a sign of heart failure.

  c. Assess the lungs for rales, cough, pink-tinged sputum, or decreased breath sounds due to pleural effusions or pulmonary edema.

  d. Heart

    (1) Palpate point of maximal impulse, which may be displaced to the left.

    (2) Auscultation may reveal an S_3, a sign of heart failure. An S_4 may occur in people with coronary artery disease. A murmur may indicate a valvular problem.

  e. Assess the abdomen for hepatomegaly and ascites.

  f. Edema

    (1) Assess the patient for the presence of edema in the dependent areas.

    (2) If the person is upright, edema starts in the feet or ankles and moves upward. If the person is in bed, edema accumulates in the sacral, lumbar, and posterior thigh region.

  g. Assess the extremities for color and temperature.

3. Diagnostic studies

  a. Laboratory tests

    (1) Blood chemistry

    (2) Complete blood count

  b. Chest radiograph

  c. Electrocardiogram

  d. Radionuclide studies

  e. Echocardiogram

  f. Right heart catheterization

  g. Ambulatory (Holter) ECG monitoring

Clinical Management

1. Goals of clinical management

  a. Prevent progression of heart failure

  b. Reduce the workload of the heart

  c. Improve pump performance of the heart

  d. Control excessive salt and water balance

  e. Remove the underlying cause of heart failure

  f. Remove precipitating causes

2. Nonpharmacologic interventions are listed in Table 23–31.

3. Pharmacologic interventions are listed in Table 23–32.

Table 23–31. Nonpharmacologic Interventions in Congestive Heart Failure

Goal	Intervention
Prevent progression of failure	Risk factor reduction to slow artherosclerosis
Reduce myocardial workload	Activity modification
	Emotional rest
	Weight reduction
	Intra-aortic balloon pump
Improve pump performance of the heart	Alcohol restriction
Control excess salt and water retention	Dietary salt restriction
	Fluid restriction
	Mechanical removal of fluid with dialysis, paracentesis, or thoracentesis

Table 23–32. Pharmacologic Manipulation of Pump Performance

Decrease Preload
Diuretics
Venous dilators
Morphine
Nitroglycerin

Increase Preload
Fluid administration

Decrease Afterload
Vasodilators
Nitroprusside
Nitroglycerin

Increase Afterload
Vasopressor
Norepinephrine

Increase Contractility
Sympathetic agents
Dobutamine
Dopamine
Phosphodiesterase inhibitors
Amrinone
Digitalis

Decrease Contractility
Calcium channel blockers
Beta blockers

Heart Rate and Rhythm
Correct dysrhythmias with appropriate agent
See specific dysrhythmia algorithms

4. Special medical-surgical procedures
   a. Intra-aortic balloon pump (see p. 1081)
   b. Ventricular assist devices
   c. Hemodynamic monitoring
   d. Cardiac transplantation
   e. Dialysis
   f. Cardiomyoplasty

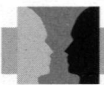

CLINICAL CONTROVERSIES

Researchers at 5 medical centers are studying the use of cardiomyoplasty as an alternative to heart transplants and artificial hearts in treating congestive heart failure.

In cardiomyoplasty, the person's own latissimus dorsi is removed, wrapped around the heart, and stimulated by a pacemaker. The pacemaker trains the muscle to constrict simultaneously with the heart and assist the ventricles, thus increasing cardiac output. The procedure eliminates the risk of tissue rejection and has less mechanical concerns than an artificial heart.

Complications

1. Death. Progression of CHF causes death, or, in up to one half of cases, death is sudden, probably from a dysrhythmia.
2. Acute pulmonary edema
   a. Definition
      (1) Cardiogenic (hydrostatic) pulmonary edema occurs when there is an abnormal accumulation of fluid within the interstitial air spaces of the lungs.
      (2) Pulmonary edema is a physical finding, not a symptom, and gives rise to the most severe form of dyspnea.
   b. Risk factors and etiology
      (1) Mitral stenosis
      (2) Mitral regurgitation
      (3) Left ventricular failure
      (4) Spontaneously, after exercise or during excitement
   c. Pathophysiology: Elevated left atrial and pulmonary capillary pressures lead to severe pulmonary congestion. This interferes with oxygen exchange in the lungs and decreased PO_2.
   d. Clinical manifestations
      (1) Extreme breathlessness, orthopnea, and dyspnea with an increased respiratory rate, which can predispose the patient to hypocapnia. Symptoms include muscle cramps, weakness, dizziness and paresthesia.
      (2) Tachycardia
      (3) Extreme anxiety and or agitation. The patient may complain of a sense of drowning, suffocation, or smothering.
      (4) Cough, with productive pink frothy sputum resulting from intra-alveolar mixture of fluids, red blood cells, and air.
      (5) Rales to apices
      (6) S_3 heart sound
      (7) Profuse sweating
      (8) Cold, clammy, pale, cyanotic skin
      (9) Elevated pulmonary capillary wedge pressure

e. Clinical management
   (1) Goals of clinical management
      • Decrease pulmonary capillary wedge pressure
      • Decrease venous return (preload)
      • Decrease circulatory blood volume
      • Decrease systemic blood pressure (afterload)
      • Increase contractility
   (2) Nonpharmacologic interventions
      • Assist the patient into a position that maximizes comfort and lung expansion, such as a sitting position with legs dangling
      • Surgical intervention may be indicated if pulmonary edema results from mitral stenosis or mitral regurgitation.
   (3) Pharmacologic interventions
      • Oxygen, which improves oxygen delivery to tissues. To improve gas exchange and pulmonary function, intubation and treatment with positive end-expiratory pressure therapy may be necessary.
      • Morphine—the most effective drug in treating pulmonary edema. Morphine provides vasodilation and sedation, which fosters muscle relaxation while decreasing anxiety and myocardial oxygen demand. It may cause respiratory depression or hypotension.
      • Diuretics, usually furosemide, to decrease circulating volume and venous return.
      • Vasodilators, including nitroprusside, nitroglycerin, and nitropaste, to increase cardiac output by decreasing left ventricular pressure. They may cause hypotension and hypoxemia. Nitroprusside may increase myocardial ischemia.
      • Bronchodilators, usually aminophylline, to increase diuresis, cardiac output, and improve PaO_2.
      • Inotropic agents, including digoxin, dopamine, and dobutamine, to increase cardiac output by increasing myocardial contractility and decreasing left ventricular preload. However, these drugs increase myocardial oxygen consumption and should be used with caution in the presence of an MI.

Prognosis

1. In moderate nonprogressive cardiac failure, the annual mortality rate is 10 to 15 percent.
2. In severe progressive heart failure, the annual mortality rate is 50 percent or greater.
3. Prognosis is worse if left ventricular ejection fraction is less than 20 percent, disabling symptoms are present, and exercise tolerance is decreased.

Applying the Nursing Process

NURSING DIAGNOSIS: Decreased cardiac output R/T inability of the heart to pump effectively

LEARNING/TEACHING GUIDELINES
for People with Congestive Heart Failure

General Overview

1. Explore the person's feelings about heart failure. People often feel depressed about lifestyle changes and fear about death, disability, and loss of independence. This may affect the person's readiness to learn.
2. Describe the pathophysiology of heart failure and that, when the heart does not pump effectively, blood flow to the body is reduced, causing symptoms such as weakness (not enough blood to muscles). Also, blood may back up, causing fluid to leak out of the blood vessels and causing symptoms such as breathing difficulty (fluid in lungs) or swollen feet and legs.
3. Discuss things the person can do to reduce risk factors such as avoiding tobacco, maintaining a normal weight, controlling blood pressure, managing stress, and taking medication as ordered.
4. Teach the person about medications including the name, dose, reason for taking the drug, how to take it, potential side effects, and what to do if side effects occur.
5. Discuss dietary modifications including sodium restriction, potassium sources, and calorie, fat, and cholesterol restrictions (if indicated).
6. Discuss activity modifications and pacing of activities, rest periods, and exercise as directed by physician.
7. Instruct the person to report symptoms of fluid retention or heart failure, such as edema or weight gain, to the physician.
8. Provide written materials to reinforce verbal instruction.

Medication Administration

Instruct persons who are going to self-administer medications to do the following:

1. Never skip, change dose, or stop taking medications, even if side effects occur or symptoms increase or go away.
2. Notify the physician if side effects occur, or if medication does not seem to be working.
3. Incorporate medications into daily routine such as mealtimes, bedtime, or breaks to avoid forgetting a dose. A pill box divided into the days of the week may be helpful.
4. Avoid over-the-counter medications without consulting the physician.
5. Contact the physician if unable to take medications due to illness (e.g., nausea and vomiting).
6. Bring all medications whenever visiting the hospital or physician.

Diet

1. Diet modifications may vary depending on each person's disease process.
   a. Most persons are instructed to eat less sodium to help reduce fluid retention (see Table 23–9).
   b. A low-fat or low-cholesterol diet may be prescribed for patients with a high blood cholesterol.
   c. Caffeine may cause irregular heart rhythm in some persons. If directed by the physician to limit caffeine, the person should avoid large amounts of coffee and tea. Caffeine may also be found in cocoa, chocolate, and some carbonated drinks.
   d. The physician may advise limitation of alcohol in some persons.
   e. Persons on diuretics may be advised to eat more foods containing potassium, such as bananas, apricots, tomatoes, citrus fruits, and raisins.
   f. Fluid may be restricted to decrease fluid buildup.
      (1) Spread fluid intake throughout day.
      (2) Measure and record all fluid intake.
      (3) Rinse mouth or suck on hard candy to reduce thirst.
   g. If the person is overweight, calories may be restricted. Most foods with high calories contain fat or sugar.
2. Help the person to identify substitutes or modifications of favorite foods that do not meet dietary guidelines.
3. Encourage small, frequent, nutritious meals and allow adequate time for meals eaten in a pleasant environment. Heart failure may cause loss of appetite, symptoms of anorexia, or a bloated feeling.

Activity

1. Follow the physician's instructions regarding activities.
2. Space periods of activity with rest.
3. Avoid extremely hot or cold temperatures.
4. Try to get enough sleep at night.
5. Increase activity gradually. Stop if difficulty breathing, dizziness, palpitations, or chest pain occurs. Sit down or lie down until symptoms go away. If symptoms do not go away in a few minutes, call the physician.
6. Avoid isometric activities. This increases pressure inside the heart.
7. Identify ways to conserve energy during the daily routine:
   a. Schedule and space activities.
   b. Sit down when possible, for example, to shave or fix hair.

(continued)

LEARNING/TEACHING GUIDELINES
(continued)

c. Allow plenty of time. Avoid rushing.

d. Delegate chores and ask for help.

Symptoms of Heart Failure or Fluid Retention

1. Explain the importance of recording weight every day to detect sudden weight gain due to fluid retention, which indicates the heart is not pumping well.
   a. Weigh self every day, 1st thing in the morning after urinating and before breakfast.
   b. Wear no clothes or the same amount of clothes.
   c. Use the same scale.
   d. Record weight on a special chart or diary.
   e. Contact the doctor if a weight gain of more than 2 pounds occurs in 24 hours.

2. Instruct the person how to check edema by pressing the thumb against the shinbone of the leg. If a dent occurs where the thumb was placed, edema is present. Also, shoes may feel tight, and clothes may feel tight if fluid is accumulating in the abdomen.

---

1. *Expected outcomes:* The person should have improved cardiac output as evidenced by the following:
   a. Stable vital signs, hemodynamic measurements within acceptable limits, and urine output greater than 30 ml per hour
   b. Absence of dyspnea, rales, S_3, and edema
2. *Nursing interventions*
   a. Assess vital signs, breath sounds, heart sounds, hemodynamics, respirations, and peripheral pulses, at least every 4 hours.
   b. Monitor ECG rhythm continuously.
   c. Administer medications to optimize preload and afterload contractility as ordered.
   d. Provide a quiet environment, frequent rest periods, and emotional support.
   e. Provide oxygen therapy as ordered.
   f. Report and document any signs of decreased cardiac output, including dyspnea, confusion, or cough.

NURSING DIAGNOSIS: Fluid volume excess R/T decreased renal blood flow, causing increased levels of aldosterone and antidiuretic hormone

1. *Expected outcomes:* Following interventions, the person should exhibit the following:
   a. Decreased weight (toward normal)
   b. Absence of edema
   c. Clear breath sounds
   d. Absence of S_3 and distended neck veins
2. *Nursing interventions*
   a. Assess, document, and report signs of fluid retention, including sudden weight gain, dyspnea, rales, S_3, edema, distended neck veins, and low serum osmolality.
   b. Regulate fluids. Maintain fluid restriction. Work with the person to plan distribution of fluid throughout the day. Provide hard candy to decrease thirst. Avoid giving unnecessary intravenous fluids. Concentrate intravenous medications as much as possible. Restrict sodium as indicated.
   c. Administer diuretics as indicated and monitor their effectiveness.

d. Monitor the patient's intake and output closely.

e. Weigh the patient daily on same scale in same clothing.

Discharge Planning and Teaching

1. Before being discharged, patients need to learn to avoid foods high in sodium, to eat potassium-rich foods, to recognize symptoms that indicate worsening failure, to take prescribed medications, and how to check their pulse.
2. Evaluate the person's daily activity routine to determine the need for assistance with activities or to provide ideas about modification of activities.
3. Collaborate with appropriate resources to develop a rehabilitation plan. Make an appointment for follow-up care. (See Learning/Teaching Guidelines for Persons with Congestive Heart Failure.)

■ CARDIAC SURGERY

Coronary Artery Bypass Graft

1. The procedure is used to do the following:
   a. Revascularize a section of myocardium
   b. Relieve angina
   c. Preserve myocardial function

 CLINICAL CONTROVERSIES

A study of 1498 persons who underwent coronary artery bypass graft from 1985 to 1989 indicated that, in persons older than 75 years of age, the greatest improvement occurred in those with an ejection fraction of less than 50 percent. Although persons with an ejection fraction of less than 50 percent have been considered to be at highest risk for coronary artery bypass graft, the study questions this assumption in this age group. Overall, mortality rate was 9 percent with a mortality rate of 8 percent for elective cases and 50 percent for emergent cases. Given these results, consideration should be given to increasing the use of elective coronary artery bypass graft for select persons older than age 75 years.

Data from Smith TW, Braunwald E, and Kelly RA. The management of heart failure. *In* Braunwald E (ed). *Heart Disease.* 4th ed. Philadelphia: WB Saunders, 1992.

2. Indications: Controversy exists about who benefits from coronary artery bypass graft; in general, most agree that it is advantageous in people with the following:
   a. Left main coronary artery disease
   b. Severe (>70% obstruction), triple-vessel disease with good distal runoff
3. Cautions and contraindications
   a. Bleeding disorders
   b. Cardiomegaly
   c. Recent MI
   d. Severe congestive heart failure
4. Incidence and socioeconomic impact
   a. Coronary artery bypass graft is the most common type of cardiac surgery with more than 330,000 procedures performed per year.
   b. Six to 18 percent of revascularizations are reoperations for recurrence of progressive coronary artery disease.
5. Procedure: A blood vessel, usually the saphenous vein or internal mammary artery, is harvested and anastomosed to the affected coronary artery, thereby bypassing the obstruction (Fig. 23–29).
6. Complications
   a. Those related to surgical intervention
      (1) Bleeding
      (2) Infection
      (3) Gastric distention
      (4) Respiratory distress
      (5) Transient hyperglycemia
      (6) Postcardiotomy delirium and postoperative sensory disturbances. This usually develops immediately postoperatively and lasts 2 to 3 days. It is directly related to the level of preoperative anxiety and is manifested by changes in behavior, confusion, and, in severe cases, acute psychosis. Postcardiotomy delirium requires frequent explanations, reorientations, and visits from family members.
   b. Those related to use of cardiopulmonary bypass equipment
      (1) Blood dyscrasias
      (2) Pulmonary edema and atelectasis
      (3) Microemboli to the brain
   c. Those related to thoracotomy
      (1) Mediastinitis—a potentially life-threatening complication that involves infection of the mediastinum and that may require drainage, débridement, and antibiotic therapy.
      (2) Hemothorax
      (3) Pneumothorax
      (4) Pericarditis
      (5) Cardiac tamponade
   d. Graft closure
   e. Myocardial infarction
   f. Dysrhythmias
   g. Renal failure
7. Applying the nursing process

NURSING DIAGNOSIS: Knowledge deficit R/T upcoming surgery

---

a. *Expected outcomes:* Following instruction, the person should be able to articulate the following:
   (1) The anticipated preoperative preparation
      • Shave from chin to toes
      • Shower with antimicrobial agent
      • Preoperative studies including complete blood count, electrolytes study, cardiac enzymes test, blood urea nitrogen, creatinine, bleeding studies, arterial blood gases, urinalysis, chest radiograph, ECG, pulmonary function tests, and blood type and crossmatch
   (2) The fact that the intensive care unit environment can be noisy, lights are usually on, and that there may be some limitations on family visits
   (3) The equipment and procedures to be used:
      • An endotracheal tube is in place for 8 to 24 hours, during which time the person is unable to speak, may feel breathless when suctioned, and may have the hands lightly restrained to keep the person from pulling out the tube.
      • A Foley catheter is in place, usually for 24 hours.
      • An arterial line and pulmonary artery catheter are in place, usually for 24 hours.
      • Chest tubes are in place, usually for 2 days.
      • Pacemaker wires may be in place, either attached to a generator or available as a precaution.
      • A nasogastric tube is in place until bowel sounds return.
      • Turning, coughing, and deep breathing are encouraged. It is helpful to hold a pillow as a splint over the chest incision during these exercises.
      • Early ambulation is expected.
      • Pain medication will be available.

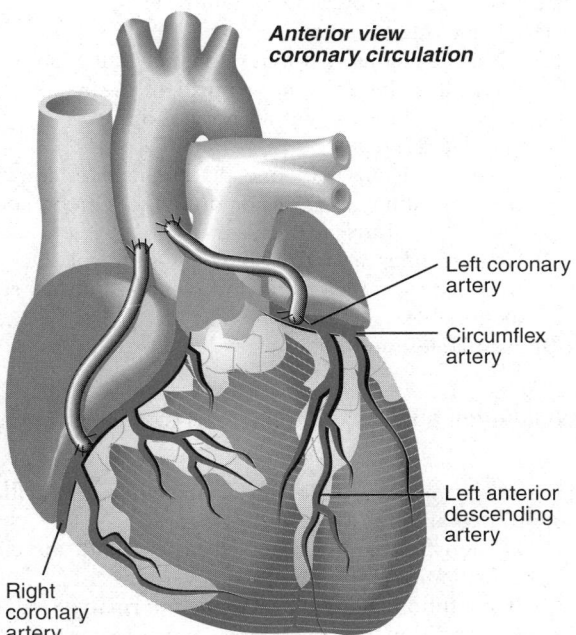

Anterior view coronary circulation

Left coronary artery

Circumflex artery

Left anterior descending artery

Right coronary artery

Figure 23–29. Coronary artery bypass graft.

b. *Nursing interventions*
(1) Provide an explanation of operative procedures and anticipated experiences in a manner that is understandable and culturally relevant to the patient and family.
(2) If possible, provide the patient and family with a tour of the intensive care unit, pointing out equipment and introducing the staff members. If the patient is on bed rest, a video of the intensive care unit may be shown.
(3) Encourage the patient and family to ask questions and express concerns.

NURSING DIAGNOSIS: Decreased cardiac output R/T surgery

a. *Expected outcomes:* The person should be able to maintain a cardiac output that allows for adequate tissue perfusion as demonstrated by the following:
(1) Stable vital signs
(2) Warm, dry skin
(3) Adequate urine output
(4) Appropriate mentation
b. *Nursing interventions*
(1) Monitor hemodynamic parameters by protocol, usually every 5 minutes until temperature returns to normal, then every 15 minutes until the condition is stable.
(2) Complete a full body assessment every hour until the condition is stable.
(3) Monitor the ECG for changes indicative of intraoperative MI or dysrhythmias associated with ventricular irritability.
(4) Monitor hourly the amount and type of chest tube and incisional drainage and record the amounts.
(5) Monitor postoperative laboratory work with particular emphasis on electrolytes, hemoglobin, and hematocrit.
(6) Administer medications and fluids as ordered. Monitor and report side effects and document the effectiveness of pharmacologic and nonpharmacologic interventions in measurable terms.
(7) Notify the physician of changes in status (Box 23–3).
(8) Be prepared for emergency situations such as cardiac tamponade. Initiate basic life support and advanced cardiac life support if necessary.

BOX 23–3. Changes Following Coronary Artery Bypass Graft That Require Notification of Physician

Notify the physician when the following occur:
• Systolic blood pressure: <80 or >180 mm Hg
• Diastolic blood pressure: >100 mm Hg
• Mean arterial pressure: <60 or >100 mm Hg
• Central venous pressure: <5 or >15 mm Hg
• Heart rate: <60 or >100 beats per minute
• Urine output: <30 ml per hour
• Chest tube drainage: >100 ml per hour
• Electrocardiographic changes
• Absence or decrease in pulses

NURSING DIAGNOSIS: Ineffective breathing pattern R/T pain, medication, and intubation

a. *Expected outcomes:* The patient should be able to maintain adequate respiratory function as evidenced by the following:
(1) Normal values on arterial blood gases
(2) Clear lung fields without rales, rhonchi, or diminished breath sounds
(3) Absence of tachypnea or other signs of respiratory distress
b. *Nursing interventions*
(1) Monitor respiratory functions including the following:
• Lung sounds: Unilateral absence of breath sounds suggests atelectasis or malposition of the endotracheal tube.
• Respiratory rate
• Ventilator pressures
• Arterial blood gases
(2) Use suction as necessary. Explain to patients that they may feel a momentary sense of breathlessness during suctioning.
(3) Medicate for pain to prevent tachypnea but not to the point of respiratory depression.
(4) Assist the patient to turn, cough, and deep breathe frequently to avoid atelectasis and to mobilize secretions.
(5) Wean the patient from the ventilator by protocol or by physician order.

NURSING DIAGNOSIS: Risk for infection R/T incisions, multiple line placement sites, and indwelling catheters

a. *Expected outcomes:* The patient should remain infection free as evidenced by the following:
(1) Normal temperature
(2) Clean incisions without signs of infection (e.g., warmth, redness, pain, or purulent drainage)
(3) Laboratory results within normal limits
b. *Nursing interventions*
(1) Assess incisions and line placement sites for redness, swelling, warmth, or drainage. Obtain specimens for culture as necessary.
(2) Change lines and dressings by protocol. Discontinue Foley catheter and intravenous lines as soon as possible.
(3) Administer antibiotics as ordered.

NURSING DIAGNOSIS: Anxiety R/T surgical intervention

a. *Expected outcomes:* Following counseling, the patient should be able to do the following:
(1) Demonstrate a demeanor consistent with the clinical situation
(2) If condition allows, articulate information related to condition, interventions, and preoperative instructions

LEARNING/TEACHING GUIDELINES
for Care of People After Coronary Artery Bypass Graft

General Overview

1. Review the surgical procedure preferred.
2. Evaluate the preoperative functional level and how it relates to the anticipated postoperative functional level.
3. Cardiac rehabilitation has a positive impact on long-term functioning.
4. Review the following teaching outline for information that can be provided to persons who have had a coronary artery bypass graft.
   a. Emotions: After surgery, persons may feel "let down" or depressed. They may feel like crying. These feelings are normal.
   b. Coughing and deep breathing: Fluid can build up in the lungs and cause pneumonia. Coughing and deep breathing help to keep the lungs clear. Because coughing and deep breathing may hurt, it may help to sit the person up and hold a pillow to the chest.
   c. Bathing: The person can shower after 5 days. Staples will still be in, but water will not hurt them. Instruct persons to not use water that is too hot because it may make them feel weak or dizzy. When the chest and legs heal, a tub bath can be taken.
   d. Wound care: The suture line needs to be kept clean and dry.
   e. Warning signs: Instruct persons to call the physician in the following circumstances:
      (1) They have a temperature of more than 101 degrees Fahrenheit for 24 hours.
      (2) The suture line is separating.
      (3) There is drainage or a bad smell from the suture line.
      (4) There is redness or swelling of the suture line.
   f. Support stockings: The physician may order support stockings.
      (1) This helps blood move through the legs and avoid swelling.
      (2) Make sure the person has 2 pairs of stockings.
      (3) Instruct the person to do the following:
         (a) Wear the stockings every day.
         (b) Wash them in warm, soapy water and hang them up to dry. Do not put them in the clothes dryer.
   g. Getting into shape
      (1) The person might feel weak and tired at first. This is from lack of sleep, surgery, medicine, and staying in bed.
      (2) It is important for the person to get out of bed every day. Tell persons to build up slowly, to not overdo it, and to stop if they get too tired.

      (3) If legs swell, instruct the person to sit down and put feet on the chair or stool. If legs remain swollen, call the physician immediately.
      (4) Instruct the person to not cross the legs.
   h. Walking
      (1) Persons should walk daily to increase their strength and improve their sense of well being.
      (2) During extremes in weather or temperature the person should walk in a climate-controlled environment such as a shopping mall or fitness center.
      (3) The person should try to go a little farther during each walk.
   i. Lifting and straining
      (1) The chest bone needs to heal. Tell the patient *not* to do the following:
         (a) Lift anything more than 10 pounds (e.g., grocery bags or suitcases) for the first 2 to 3 months
         (b) Lift children, rather sit down and let them sit in the patient's lap
         (c) Strain (e.g., by opening a jar or pushing a heavy door)
         (d) Strain during a bowel movement (a laxative may be needed)
   j. Sexual activity
      (1) The person might worry whether sexual activity will harm the heart. If the person feels well after climbing 1 flight of stairs, sexual activity should not be a problem.
      (2) To minimize any potential problems during sexual activity, tell the patient to do the following:
         (a) Wait 2 hours after a meal or ingesting alcohol
         (b) Wait until feeling rested
         (c) Keep the room at a mild temperature
         (d) Use a comfortable position
   k. Traveling
      (1) Patients should not drive for 4 to 6 weeks.
      (2) Patients should check with the physician before taking a long trip.
      (3) If traveling, the patient should stop every hour and walk.
   l. Work
      (1) The decision to return to work will be based on physical condition and the work environment.
      (2) If persons lift heavy things or work outside, the physician may want them to stay home longer.
   m. Emphasize that if the person has chest pain, diz-

(continued)

LEARNING/TEACHING GUIDELINES

(continued)

ziness, or trouble breathing, he or she should *stop* the current activity and sit or lie down.

n. Chest pain
   (1) One nitroglycerin pill is put under the tongue.
   (2) After 5 minutes, another one is placed under the tongue if there is still pain.
   (3) If there is still pain after 5 more minutes, another tablet is used.
   (4) If there is still pain, the physician should be called or the patient should go to the hospital.

o. Drinking
   (1) If persons drink alcohol, they should not have more than 2 drinks in 1 day.
   (2) They should not drink alcohol if they are taking pain pills or sleeping pills.

p. After surgery, the person may be given a special low-fat diet.

q. Weight should be recorded every day at the same time. A gain of 3 pounds in 1 day is cause to notify the physician immediately.

r. Medications: Make sure patient knows the following:
   (1) How to take medicine before going home (e.g., what time of day to take medicine and how many pills to take).

(2) To never take more or less medicine than ordered.
(3) To never stop taking medicine without consulting the physician.

s. Lifestyle and risk factors
   (1) Smoking: Smoking increases the chance of death or of having another heart attack. Smoking makes the heart beat faster and work harder and elevates blood pressure.
   (2) High blood pressure: Remind persons that they may feel fine even though their blood pressure is too high. They must take their medicines to control it.
   (3) High cholesterol: Stress the importance of limiting fatty foods.
   (4) Weight: Being overweight is a risk factor for heart attacks, high blood pressure, and diabetes.
   (5) Stress: When upset or angry, the heart beats faster and blood pressure increases. The nurse should provide information on what can be done to control stress.

5. Remind persons to keep all appointments with their physician.

---

b. *Nursing interventions*
   (1) Maintain a calm and professional manner and use understandable terms with the patient and family while preparing the patient for surgery.
   (2) If condition and time allow, permit family members to visit.
8. Discharge planning and teaching: see Learning/Teaching Guidelines for Care of Patients After Coronary Artery Bypass Graft
9. Prognosis
   a. Overall mortality rate is 3 percent.
   b. Preoperative left ventricular function is the most important indicator of survival. It can be determined through radionuclide studies that measure the fraction of blood ejected from the left ventricle with each contraction of the heart compared with the amount of blood in the ventricle at the beginning of diastole (Table 23–33).
   c. Perioperative MIs influence the overall prognosis following surgery. Monitoring creatinine kinase and creatinine kinase-MB enzymes provides evidence of this untoward event.
   d. Improvement in preoperative symptoms occurs as follows:
      (1) Eighty to 90 percent of patients are pain free at 1 year.
      (2) Seventy percent are pain free at 5 years.
      (3) Fifty percent return to work.

Valvular Surgery

1. The purpose of valvular surgery is to repair or replace incompetent valves. Valve repair, if feasible, is preferred to replacement.
2. Indications
   a. In cases of aortic stenosis or regurgitation, valvular replacement is indicated once heart failure, angina, and syncope are anticipated or present.
   b. Mitral stenosis or regurgitation
      (1) Mitral valve replacement is used when there is severe stenosis, regurgitation, or extensive calcification.
      (2) Closed mitral commissurotomy is used rarely, but is considered in persons with good valvular mobility.

Table 23–33. Risk Level for Coronary Artery Bypass Graft by Left Ventricular Function

Ejection Fraction	Risk Level
>55%	Low
30–35%	High
20–25%	Very high

(3) Open mitral commissurotomy is used when there is minimal or no regurgitation and leaflets are pliable without calcification.

(4) Mitral valve reconstruction may also be used when feasible.

3. Cautions: Care must be taken to ensure that the conduction system and circumflex artery are not damaged during valve replacement.

4. Procedure
    a. The damaged valve is surgically removed.
    b. The prosthetic valve is inserted.
        (1) Mechanical valves require lifelong anticoagulation.
        (2) Tissue valves are considered in older people, women in their childbearing years, and confused people who would have problems with compliance or with anticoagulants.

5. Complications
    a. Thromboembolic events
    b. Endocarditis
    c. Systemic infection
    d. Bleeding

6. Nursing interventions
    a. Primary considerations are those associated with cardiac surgery, endocarditis, and anticoagulation.
    b. In addition, reassure the person that hearing the opening "click" of the new prosthetic valve is normal.

7. Prognosis
    a. The overall mortality rate is 3 to 5 percent.

b. Left ventricular function is an important indication of survival.
    c. Most patients show significant clinical improvement and can return to normal activities with few or no limitations.

Cardiac Transplantation

1. The purpose of cardiac transplantation is to replace a heart that is extensively damaged and unable to maintain an adequate perfusion pressure.

2. Indications
    a. Advanced idiopathic cardiomyopathy
    b. Inoperable end-stage coronary artery disease
    c. Congenital heart disease
    d. Endocarditis

3. Cautions and contraindications
    a. Age older than 59 years
    b. Irreversible organ failure
    c. Acute infection
    d. Malignancy
    e. Known noncompliance
    f. Inability to tolerate immunosuppression
    g. Severe pulmonary dysfunction unless combined heart-lung transplant is considered

4. Incidence and socioeconomic impact. The International Society for Heart Transplantation reports that there have

 HOME CARE STRATEGIES

Care of the Cardiac Surgery Patient

Owing to shortened hospital stays for cardiac surgery patients, home health care may be ordered briefly until the patient starts cardiac rehabilitation. You should be aware of the special needs of these patients who have had cardiac surgery.

Assessment

- Hypotension or hypertension may occur as patients become accustomed to β-blockers.
- Heart rate should be regular.
- Low-grade fever may be present. Notify the physician if the temperature elevates past 100.5–101.0 degrees Fahrenheit.
- Breath sounds may be diminished with basilar rales. Patients should use the incentive spirometer or cough and deep breathe.

Incisions

- Legs may be edematous. Mild erythema may be present. Leg incisions may drain up to 3 weeks postoperatively. Report bright red or purulent drainage. Antiembolic stockings are frequently ordered to provide postoperative incisional support and to limit edema.
- Chest incisions should not drain. The sternum should feel firm. If the internal mammary artery is used there may be slight swelling and tingling on the side used. Patients may feel their sternum "shifting" or "popping", particularly if they are lying on their side. Women should wear a bra for incisional support and place a 4 × 4 gauze dressing pad under the bra to prevent irritation of the incision.
- Chest tube sites may appear moist and may drain small amounts of serosanguineous fluid.

- The incisions should be cleansed regularly with antibacterial soap.

Nutrition

- Patients may be anorexic and may experience taste changes. They can expect to lose 5 to 10 pounds secondary to diuresis. Report a 2 to 3 pound weight gain for 2 days, and watch for signs or symptoms of congestive heart failure.
- Patients may experience constipation and should be instructed on how to manage it.

Activity

- Patients will have limited endurance and will experience dyspnea with little activity. Encourage a balance of rest, activity, and a home exercise program.
- Arm exercises will help the back or shoulder pain they may experience.

Psychosocial

- Patients may have difficulty sleeping. Instruct in use of pain medication at bedtime and lying on the back with the head and chest elevated. Depression may occur.

Education

- Review all teaching materials. In addition to postoperative care, include information on cardiac risk factors and lifestyle changes as patients prepare for cardiac rehabilitation.

LEARNING/TEACHING GUIDELINES
for Cardiac Transplantation

General Overview

1. Describe the physiologic and psychologic changes that follow transplantation.
2. Emphasize the need to continue with long-term medication therapy and lifelong medical follow-up.
3. Demonstrate proper administration of medication.
4. Discuss the importance of monitoring for signs of rejection, infection, and side effects of medication.
5. Review the need for sequential endomyocardial biopsies to monitor for rejection.
6. Promote self-care and independence.
7. Encourage daily exercise to promote reconditioning.

Medication Administration

1. Instruct persons who are going to self-administer medications to do the following:
   a. Never adjust dosage without consulting the physician.
   b. Always take the drug on time; never skip doses. Incorporate medication administration into daily routines such as coffee breaks, shaving, and mealtimes to avoid missed doses, or to purchase a pill box that is divided into the days of the week.
   c. Not discontinue a drug without the physician's permission, because congestive heart failure or rejection may develop.
   d. Always report untoward effects to the physician.
   e. Avoid any over-the-counter medication unless approved by the physician.

Exercise

1. Point out the following physical and psychologic benefits of exercise:
   a. Exercise benefits cardiovascular health, and is an aid in lowering blood pressure and heart rate.
   b. By burning calories, exercise helps to reduce or avoid excess body weight and increased percentage of body fat.
   c. Exercise programs may heighten the person's sense of well-being, provide an outlet for emotional tensions, and increase the levels of high-density lipoproteins relative to total blood cholesterol.
2. Give the person the following instructions for starting an exercise program:
   a. Maintain close medical supervision.
   b. Begin the exercise program gradually, increasing its intensity and duration at intervals as tolerated. Encourage participation in a formalized cardiac rehabilitation program.
   c. Be aware that the most suitable exercises for stimulating cardiovascular and respiratory fitness include walking, jogging, swimming, cross-country skiing, and bicycling.
   d. Avoid heavy weight lifting and isometric exercises.

Daily Care

1. Instruct people to assume responsibility for the following:
   a. Daily weight
   b. Daily temperature readings
2. Point out the importance of the following:
   a. Maintaining fluid restriction
   b. Restricting sodium intake
   c. Avoiding people with infections

---

been more than 10,000 cardiac transplantations since 1967.
5. Procedure
   a. Suitability of the recipient is evaluated through the following:
      (1) Laboratory studies

TRANSCULTURAL CONSIDERATIONS

In any surgery involving transplantation of human organs, the recipient's explanatory model should be assessed. Specific assessment should focus on beliefs about taking on the characteristics of the donor (e.g., skin color, cross-gender traits, becoming like the donor person, or taking on the donor's personality, and acquiring responsibilities for the donor's sins or shortcomings).

(2) Physical status
(3) Medical history
(4) Laboratory studies
(5) Comparison of the physical makeup of the donor and recipient, including height, weight, chest size, and age.
(6) Psychologic status
(7) Social supports
(8) Ability to maintain ongoing medical regimen
   b. Usual preparation for cardiac surgery is completed.
   c. Transplantation technique is chosen.
      (1) In heterotopic procedures, the donor heart is anastomosed to the native heart.
      (2) In orthotopic procedures, the native heart is removed and the donor heart implanted.
6. Complications
   a. Initial complications
      (1) Cardiac dysfunction
      (2) Fluid imbalances

(3) Blood dyscrasias
(4) Respiratory distress
(5) Infection
(6) Rejection
b. Long-term complications
(1) Chronic rejection (accelerated graft atherosclerosis)
(2) Psychologic problems
7. Nursing considerations are those associated with the following:
a. Organ rejection (see Chapter 26)
b. Cardiac surgery
c. Compliance with long-term therapy (see Learning/Teaching Guidelines for Cardiac Transplantation)
8. Prognosis
a. Varies based on the suitability of donor and recipient, and operative technique used
b. Since 1967, survival rate has increased due to improvements in techniques, medications, and patient selection.
c. Survival rates
(1) Approximately 91 percent of patients survive at least 30 days.
(2) The 5-year survival rate varies by procedure:
• Orthotopic, 73.9 percent
• Heterotopic, 54.1 percent

Intra-aortic Balloon Pumping

1. An intra-aortic balloon pump is a circulatory assist device used during periods of acute cardiac failure to provide temporary assistance to the heart until the underlying problem is corrected. It consists of a balloon catheter inserted percutaneously or surgically into the femoral artery, threaded up the descending thoracic aorta, and positioned in the aorta distal to the subclavian artery (Fig. 23–30). The catheter is attached externally to a console that synchronizes the inflation and deflation of the balloon with the cardiac cycle.
2. Indications include the need to do the following:
a. Decrease myocardial ischemia
b. Improve cardiac output
c. Decrease myocardial workload
d. Stabilize hemodynamic status
3. An intra-aortic balloon pump improves myocardial oxygen supply and reduces cardiac workload using the principle of counterpulsation. Counterpulsation provides 2 functions.
a. Diastolic augmentation: At the beginning of diastole, the intra-aortic balloon inflates, forcing blood in the aortic arch back into the coronary arteries, thereby improving cardiac oxygenation and perfusion.
b. Diastolic unloading: Just before systole begins, the intra-aortic balloon deflates, decreasing pressure against which the left ventricle must pump in order to open the aortic valve. This decreases myocardial oxygen demand and improves cardiac output.
4. Contraindications
a. Aortic and thoracic aortic aneurysm
b. Aortic regurgitation
c. Peripheral vascular disease
d. Bleeding disorders
5. Complications
a. Dissection of the aorta
b. Thrombocytopenia
c. Infection

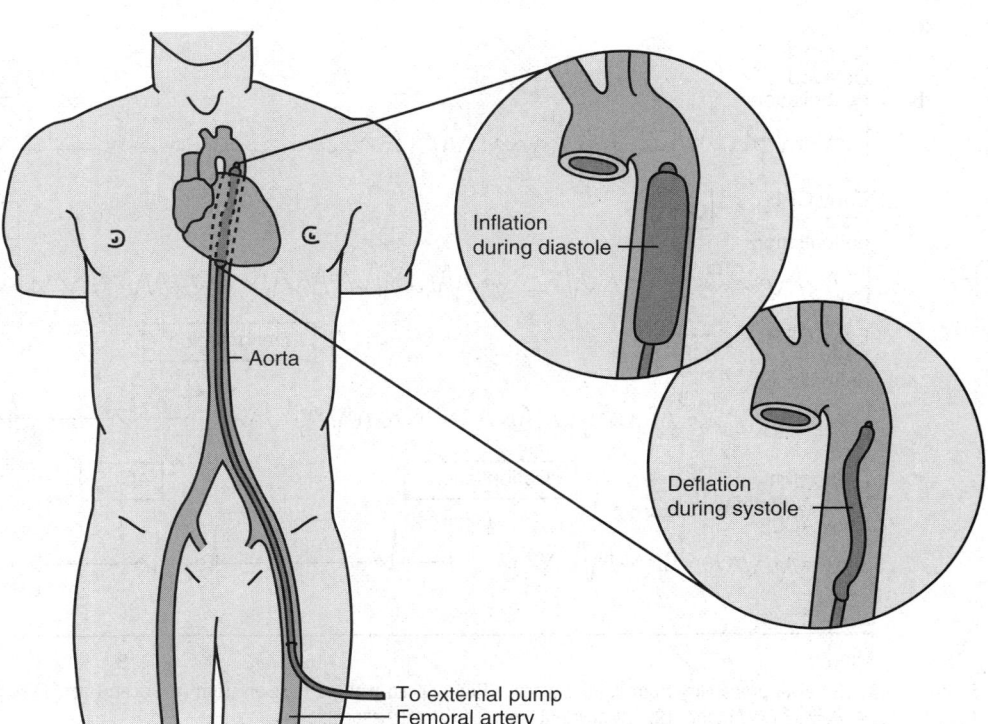

Figure 23–30. Intra-aortic balloon pumping. An intra-aortic balloon catheter is inserted into the femoral artery and advanced into the descending aorta. The polyethylene balloon lies just distal to the left subclavian artery. Immediately after it is inserted, the catheter is connected to the external pump. (Redrawn from Ignatavicius DD, Workman ML, and Mishler MA [eds]. *Medical-Surgical Nursing: A Nursing Process Approach.* 2nd ed. Philadelphia: WB Saunders, 1996, p 1001.)

Inflation during diastole

Deflation during systole

Aorta

To external pump
Femoral artery

d. Ischemia of the extremity distal to the arterial insertion site due to blood flow obstruction by the catheter.

e. Compromise of renal, cerebral, or left arm circulation due to malposition of the catheter occluding the arterial supply.

6. Nursing interventions are those associated with any cardiovascular surgery with particular emphasis on the technical needs of the equipment and the psychologic needs of the patient and family.

   a. Assess cardiovascular status and hemodynamic parameters every 15 to 30 minutes.

   b. Monitor peripheral circulation, particularly in the affected limb, for signs of occlusion such as coolness, mottling, pain, tingling, or decrease in strength of pulse, and report changes immediately.

   c. Anticoagulation is used to prevent clot formation. Monitor for signs of bleeding, particularly at the insertion site.

   d. The patient will be on bed rest, with the affected limb immobilized. Avoid complications of immobility by

     (1) Repositioning the patient frequently

     (2) Log rolling the patient from side to side every 2 hours

     (3) Performing range-of-motion exercises to all extremities except the affected limb

   e. Provide a supportive environment for the patient and family.

     (1) Explain all equipment and procedures in simple terms. The equipment can be noisy. Describe sounds and sensations associated with the normal functioning of the equipment to allay fears.

     (2) Schedule routine care to allow for frequent periods of uninterrupted rest and adequate time for family visits.

(3) Encourage the patient and family to ask questions and express their fears and concerns.

◼ CARDIOPULMONARY RESUSCITATION—ADVANCED CARDIAC LIFE SUPPORT

Maximization of Resuscitation

Maximizing the likelihood of successful resuscitation depends on a series of critical interdependent interventions (Fig. 23–31).

1. Early access
   a. Early warning signs are recognized.
   b. Advanced cardiac life support providers are notified rapidly.
   c. There is rapid dispatch of providers.
   d. Providers arrive quickly.
   e. Providers arrive with all necessary equipment.
   f. Arrested state is verified.
2. Early CPR. Procedure 23–10 describes how to perform 1-rescuer CPR.
3. Early defibrillation
   a. Eighty to 90 percent of persons with sudden, nontraumatic cardiac arrest are found to be in ventricular fibrillation.
   b. Early defibrillation is the one action most likely to improve survival.
   c. Defibrillation is discussed on pp. 1019, 1022–1024.
4. Early advanced cardiac life support
   a. Regardless of the setting (in-hospital or in the community), the goal should be to provide definitive care

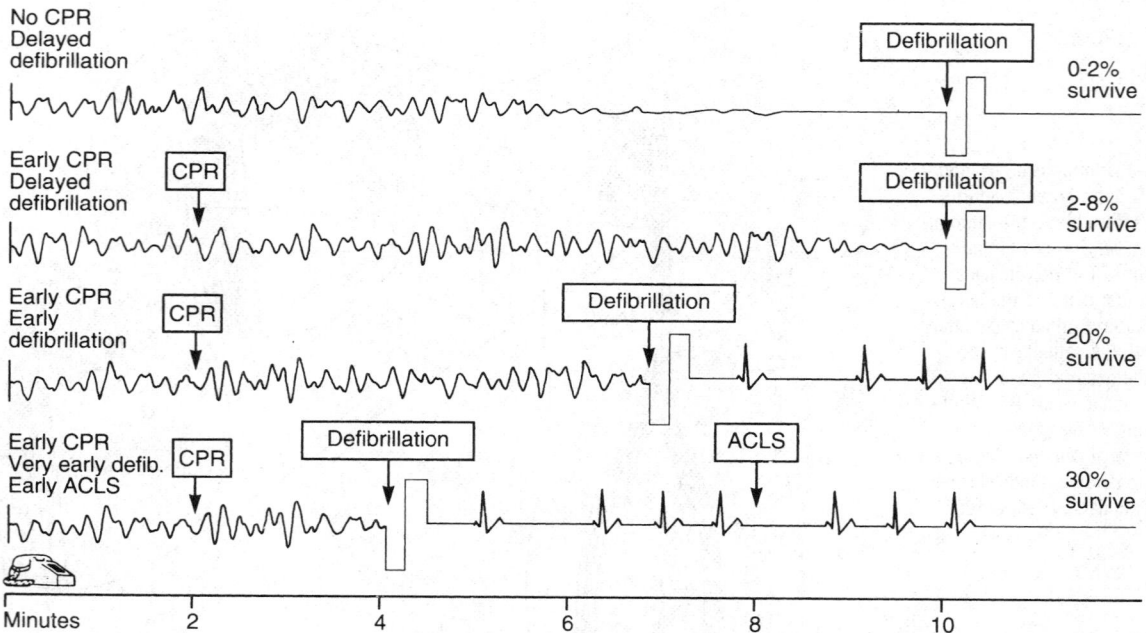

Figure 23–31. Survival probability from cardiac arrest. (Reproduced with permission from American Heart Association. *Textbook of Advanced Cardiac Life Support,* 1994. Dallas, TX: Author, 1994. Copyright American Heart Association.)

(advanced cardiac life support) within 8 to 10 minutes of recognition of arrest.

b. Medications are considered a secondary intervention after CPR, defibrillation, and airway management. Various routes can be used to administer medications. Considerations include the following:
  (1) Central versus peripheral lines
   • Because CPR would be interrupted for a central line insertion, peripheral veins are the 1st choice.
   • When drugs are given peripherally, administer them rapidly and follow with 20 ml of fluid. Elevate extremity in which peripheral intravenous catheter is placed to improve drug circulation. Allow 1 to 2 minutes for the drugs to reach central circulation. If spontaneous circulation does not occur after the initial round of drugs, a central line can be attempted. Defibrillation for ventricular fibrillation or ventricular tachycardia should not be delayed for central line placement.
  (2) Endotracheal drug administration
   • If an endotracheal tube is in place, epinephrine, lidocaine, and atropine can be given via the tube.
   • Medications should be given at 2 to 2.5 times the usual dose.
   • Medication should be diluted in 10 ml of saline or distilled water.
   • To administer, insert a catheter past the tip of the endotracheal tube. Stop chest compression and instill the drug quickly. Give several quick insufflations with the bag-valve-mask unit to hasten absorption. Restart chest compressions.
  (3) Intraosseous administration
   • This route is an alternative route when intravenous access is not available.
   • It is an excellent route in children.
   • The dose is the same as that given intravenously, although higher doses of epinephrine may be considered.
c. Current American Heart Association treatment algorithms are designed to provide guidelines to prevent and treat acute cardiovascular situations.
  (1) Myocardial infarction
  (2) Ventricular fibrillation and pulseless ventricular tachycardia
  (3) Tachycardia
  (4) Electrical cardioversion
  (5) Bradycardia
  (6) Asystole
  (7) Pulseless electrical activity

Organization of Resuscitation

1. Phase I of response is anticipation as follows:
   a. Analyze available data.
   b. Gather team.
   c. Identify team leader.
   d. Delineate responsibilities.
   e. Assemble equipment.
   f. Position team members relative to the victim.
2. Phase II of response is entry.
   a. Obtain vital signs.
   b. Team leader obtains report.
   c. Gather history.
   d. Obtain vital signs again.
3. Phase III of response is resuscitation.
   a. The team leader
    • Focuses on airway, breathing, and circulation (ABC).
    • Maintains calm and quiet.
   b. Team members
    • Monitor vital signs.
    • Report as orders are implemented.
    • Request clarification of orders as needed.
    • Reevaluate as needed.
4. Phase IV of response is maintenance.
   a. Stabilize the condition.
   b. Monitor and support ABC.
5. Phase V of response is family notification. Report with honesty, sensitivity, and promptness. When appropriate, family presence may be allowed during some portion of the resuscitation efforts.
6. Phase VI of response is transfer. If necessary, the patient may be transfered to an appropriate unit.
7. Phase VII of response is critique.
   a. Review performance.
   b. Allow for education.
   c. Provide critical incident stress debriefing.

Postresuscitation Care

1. General principles
   a. Provide cardiorespiratory support to maximize tissue perfusion.
   b. If necessary, transport the patient to an appropriately equipped critical care unit.
   c. Identify the causative factor.
   d. Treat the cause to prevent recurrence.
2. Cerebral resuscitation
   a. When CPR or definitive care is delayed, the cerebral cortex, responding to hypoxia, is irreversibly damaged, resulting in death or severe neurologic damage.
   b. Cerebral resuscitation is an area of ongoing research. Current accepted methodologies to optimize cerebral perfusion pressures include the following:
    (1) Maintaining a normal or slightly elevated mean arterial pressure.
    (2) Reducing intracranial pressure if elevated.

(3) Maintaining normothermia because hyperthermia increases oxygen demand of the brain.

(4) Avoiding seizures by use of phenobarbital, phenytoin, or diazepam because seizures increase oxygen demand.

(5) Elevating the head approximately 30 degrees to increase venous drainage.

(6) Preoxygenating before suctioning to avoid increases in intracranial pressure.

c. Specific postresuscitation actions

(1) Cardiac monitoring including baseline and serial 12-lead ECG.

(2) Supplemental oxygen

(3) Therapeutic interventions
 • For bradycardia, pacemaker
 • For hypoxemia and acidosis, ventilation

(4) Medications as appropriate
 • For hypoglycemia, glucose
 • For dysrhythmias, antidysrhythmics
 • For MI, thrombolytics

• For electrolyte imbalance, infusions as needed
• For hypotension, vasopressors
• Intravenous access, if not already in place
• Laboratory tests (cardiac enzymes, arterial blood gases, electrolytes including magnesium and calcium, glucose, and creatinine)

Public Health Considerations

1. Early CPR has been shown to have a significant positive effect on survival.
2. Widespread training in CPR is recommended.

a. Communities need to recognize the importance of training as many people as possible in CPR and removing any barriers that discourage learning and using CPR.

b. Emphasis in citizen CPR should be placed on recognizing unresponsiveness, calling 911 for help, and initiating CPR.

Bibliography

Books—General

Braunwald E (ed). *Heart Diseases*. 5th ed. Philadelphia: WB Saunders, 1996.

Dossey BM, et al. *Critical Care Nursing: Body—Mind—Spirit*. 3rd ed. Philadelphia: JB Lippincott, 1991.

Dracup K. *Meltzer's Intensive Coronary Care: A Manual For Nurses*. 5th ed. Norwalk, CT: Appleton & Lange, 1995.

Dressler DK (ed). *Cardiovascular Critical Care Nursing*. Albany, NY: Delmar, 1994.

Eagen J, Stewart S, and Vitello-Cicciu J. *Quick Reference for Cardiac Critical Care Nursing*. Gaithersburg, MD: Aspen, 1991.

Guzzetta CE, and Dossey BM. *Cardiovascular Nursing—Holistic Practice*. St. Louis: Mosby–Year Book, 1992.

Hazinski MF, and Cummins RO (eds). *The 1996 Handbook of Emergency Cardiac Care*. St. Louis: Mosby–Year Book and The American Heart Association, 1996.

Hurst JW, et al (eds). *The Heart*. 8th ed. New York: McGraw-Hill, 1994.

Kinney MR, and Packa DR (eds). *Andreoli's Comprehensive Cardiac Care*. 8th ed. Philadelphia: Mosby–Year Book, 1996.

Kinney MR, et al. *AACN's Clinical Reference for Critical Care Nursing*. 3rd ed. St. Louis: Mosby–Year Book, 1993.

National Heart, Lung, and Blood Institute. *Morbidity and Mortality: Chartbook on Cardiovascular, Lung, and Blood Diseases*. Rockville, MD: U.S. Department of Health and Human Services, National Institutes of Health, 1994.

1995 Heart and Stroke Facts. Dallas: American Heart Association, 1995.

Vinsant M, and Spence M. *Commonsense Approach to Coronary Care*. 6th ed. St. Louis: CV Mosby, 1995.

Underhill SL, et al. *Cardiac Nursing*. 3rd ed. Philadelphia: JB Lippincott, 1995.

Cardiovascular Structure and Function

Books

Guyton AC. *Textbook of Medical Physiology*. 9th ed. Philadelphia: WB Saunders, 1996.

Memmler RL, et al. *Structure and Function of the Human Body*. 6th ed. Philadelphia: JB Lippincott, 1996.

Chapters in Books

Kemp D, and Dolan JT. Anatomy and physiology of the cardiovascular system. In Dolan JT (ed). *Critical Care Nursing—Clinical Management Through the Nursing Process*. Philadelphia: FA Davis, 1991.

Cardiovascular Assessment

Books

Erickson B. *Heart Sounds and Murmurs: A Practical Guide*. 2nd ed. St. Louis: Mosby–Year Book, 1992.

Tilkian A, and Conover M. *Understanding Heart Sounds and Murmurs: with an Introduction to Lung Sounds*. 3rd ed. Philadelphia: WB Saunders, 1993.

Chapters in Books and Journal Articles

Anderson FD, and Maloney JP. Taking blood pressure correctly—It's no off-the-cuff matter. *Nursing* 24(11):34–40, 1994.

Dolan JT. Cardiovascular assessment. In Dolan JT (ed). *Critical Care Nursing—Clinical Management Through the Nursing Process*. Philadelphia: FA Davis, 1991.

Fabius DB. Solving the mystery of heart murmurs. *Nursing* 24(7):39–44, 1994.

Fabius DB. Uncovering the secrets of snaps, rubs, and clicks. *Nursing* 24(7): 45–50, 1994.

Green E. Solving the puzzle of chest pain. *Am J Nurs* 92(1):32–37, 1992.

Ishii K. Physical capacity assessment of the cardiovascular patient in the acute setting. *J Cardiovasc Nurs* 9(4):53–63, 1995.

Kirton CA. Assessing normal heart sounds. *Nursing* 26(2):56–57, 1996.

Lohrman JM, and Kinkade SL. Cardiovascular competency standards. In Lohrman JM, and Kinkade SL (eds). *Competency Based Orientation for Critical Care Nursing*. St. Louis: Mosby–Year Book, 1992.

Morton P. *Health Assessment in Nursing*. 2nd ed. Springhouse, PA: Springhouse Corp, 1993.

Raimer F. How to identify electrolyte imbalances on your patient's ECG. *Nursing* 24(6):54–58, 1994.

Registry Committee of the Society for Cardiac Angiography and Interventions: Complications of cardiac catheterization. *Cathet Cardiovasc Diagn* 17:5–21, 1989.

Yancone-Morton L. Perfecting the art of cardiac assessment. *RN* 54(12):28–34, 1991.

Special Diagnostic Procedures

Books

Daily EK, and Schroeder JS. *Techniques in Hemodynamic Monitoring*. 5th ed. St. Louis: CV Mosby, 1994.

Malarkey LM, and McMorrow ME. *Nurse's Manual of Laboratory Tests and Diagnostic Procedures.* Philadelphia: WB Saunders, 1996.

Stillwell SB, and Randall EM. *Pocket Guide to Cardiovascular Care.* 2nd ed. St. Louis: Mosby–Year Book, 1994.

Journal Articles

Dault LH, et al. Helping your patient through cardiac catheterization. *Nursing* 22(2):52–55, 1992.

Dennison RD. Making sense of hemodynamic monitoring. *Am J Nurs* 94(8):24–31, 1994.

Franklin BA. Diagnostic and functional exercise testing: Selection and interpretation. *J Cardiovasc Nurs* 10(1):8–29, 1995.

Hochrein MA, and Sohl L. Heart smart: A guide to cardiac tests. *Am J Nurs* 92(12):22–25, 1992.

Merva J. SAECG: A closer look at the heart. *RN* 56(5):50–54, 1993.

Olbrych D. Interpreting CPK and LDH results. *Nursing* 23(1):48–49, 1993.

Owen A. Tracking the rise and fall of cardiac enzymes. *Nursing* 25(5):35–38, 1995.

Sullivan-Witterschein K, et al. Using transesophageal echocardiography to assess the heart. *Nursing* 22:63–64, 1992.

VanBuskirk MD, and Gradman AH. Monitoring blood pressure in ambulatory patients. *Am J Nurs* 93(6):44–47, 1993.

Electrocardiograms

Books

Catalano JT. *Guide to ECG Analysis.* Philadelphia: JB Lippincott, 1993.

Conover MB. *Understanding Electrocardiography: Arrhythmias and the 12-Lead ECG.* 7th ed. St. Louis: Mosby–Year Book, 1996.

Zimmerman FH. *Clinical Electrocardiography.* New York: McGraw-Hill, 1994.

Chapters in Books and Journal Articles

Ide B. Bedside electrocardiographic assessment. *J Cardiovasc Nurs* 9(4):10–23, 1995.

Interpreting ECG waveform components. *Nursing* 25(6):32c–32f, 1995.

Stein E. *Rapid Analysis of Electrocardiograms: A Self-Study Program.* Philadelphia: Lea & Febiger, 1992.

Toledo L, and Dolan JT. Electrocardiography: An overview. *In* Dolan JT (ed). *Critical Care Nursing—Clinical Management Through the Nursing Process.* Philadelphia: JB Lippincott, 1991.

Dysrhythmias

Books

Kay GN, and Bubien RS. *Clinical Management of Cardiac Dysrhythmias.* Gaithersburg, MD: Aspen, 1992.

Lonsbury PS, and Frye SJ. *Cardiac Rhythm Disorders: A Nursing Process Approach.* 2nd ed. St. Louis: Mosby–Year Book, 1992.

Chapters in Books and Journal Articles

Angelini KM, and Boecklen A. Take it to heart: How to operate an automated external defibrillator. *Nursing* 24(3):50–53, 1994.

Arbour R. Complete heart block: Reacting quickly to prevent asystole. *Nursing* 24(8):33, 1994.

Babien RS, et al. What you need to know about radiofrequency ablation. *Am J Nurs* 93(7):30–37, 1993.

Boltz MA. Nurse's guide to identifying cardiac rhythms. *Nursing* 24(4):54–58, 1994.

Campbell CD, and Newsome JA. Treating a lethal arrhythmia. *Nursing* 22:33, 1992.

Collins MA. When your patient has an implantable cardioverter defibrillator. *Am J Nurs* 94(3):34–38, 1994.

de Buitler M, et al. Reduction in medical care costs associated with radiofrequency catheter ablation of accessory pathways. *Am J Cardiol* 68:1656–1661, 1991.

Elder AN. Sinus bradycardia: Elevating a slow heart rate. *Nursing* 24(11):48–50, 1994.

Elder AN. Sinus tachycardia: Lowering a high heart rate. *Nursing* 24(12):62–64, 1994.

Emergency Cardiac Care Committee and Subcommittees, American Heart Association. Guidelines for cardio-pulmonary resuscitation and emergency cardiac care. *JAMA* 268:2172–2302, 1992.

Hudak C, and Gallo B. *Critical Care Nursing.* 6th ed. Philadelphia: JB Lippincott, 1994, pp 175–186.

Lowen B, et al. Unresolved problems in coronary care. *Am J Cardiol* 20:494–508, 1967.

Mee CL. ActionStat: Bradycardia. *Nursing* 26(4):25, 1996.

O'Neil PA. Tachycardia: Restoring a normal heart rate. *Nursing* 25(6):33, 1995.

Sandler RL. Atrial fibrillation. *Am J Nurs* 94(12):26–27, 1994.

Stahl L. How to manage common arrhythmias in medical patients. *Am J Nurs* 95(3):36–41, 1995.

Starks-Bledsoe DS, and Vespe M. Heading off sudden cardiac death. *Nursing* 22:52–56, 1992.

Toledo L, and Dolan JT. Electrocardiography: An overview. *In* Dolan JT (ed). *Critical Care Nursing—Clinical Management Through the Nursing Process.* Philadelphia: JB Lippincott, 1991.

Arterial Hypertension

Books

American Heart Association. *Blood Pressure.* Dallas: American Heart Association, 1993.

National Institutes of Health. *The Fifth Report Of The Joint National Committee on Detection, Evaluation, and Treatment of High Blood Pressure.* NIH Publication No. 93-1088. Rockville, MD: U.S. Department of Health and Human Services, 1992.

Chapters in Books and Journal Articles

Blanchard EB. Biofeedback treatment of essential hypertension. *Biofeedback Self Regul* 15(3):209–228, 1990.

Cuddy RP. Hypertension: Keeping dangerous blood pressure down. *Nursing* 25(8):35–41, 1995.

Hahn YB, et al. The effect of thermal biofeedback and progressive muscle relaxation training in reducing blood pressure of patients with essential hypertension. *Image* 25(3):204–207, 1993.

The Joint National Committee on Detection, Evaluation, and Treatment of High Blood Pressure. The fifth report of the Joint National Committee on Detection, Evaluation, and Treatment of High Blood Pressure. *Arch Intern Med* 153:154–183, 1993.

Kannel WB, et al. A general cardiovascular risk profile: The Framingham Study. *Ann Intern Med* 85:447, 1976.

Leutwyler K. The price of prevention. *Sci Am* 272(4):124–129, 1995.

Manolino TA, et al. Trends in pharmacologic management of hypertension in the United States. *Arch Intern Med* 155:829–837, 1995.

Naji PM. Nursing management of the patient with coronary artery disease, angina pectoris, or myocardial infarction. *In* Dolan JT (ed). *Critical Care Nursing—Clinical Management Through the Nursing Process.* Philadelphia: FA Davis, 1991.

Nash CA, and Jensen PL. When your surgical patient has hypertension. *Am J Nurs* 94(12):39–44, 1994.

Pheley AM, et al. Evaluation of a nurse-based hypertension management program: Screening, management, and outcomes. *J Cardiovasc Nurs* 9(2):54–61, 1995.

Schwob AC. Elevated blood pressure/hypertension. *In* Loftis P (ed). *Decision Making in Geriatrics.* Toronto: BC Decker, 1992.

Solomon J. Hypertension: New guidelines, new roles. *RN* 23:54–59, 1993.

Van Buskirk MD, and Gradman AH. Monitoring blood pressure in ambulatory patients. *Am J Nurs* 93(6):44–47, 1993.

Wallace PL. Nursing management of the patient with heart failure. *In* Dolan JT (ed). *Critical Care Nursing—Clinical Management Through the Nursing Process.* Philadelphia: FA Davis, 1991.

Coronary Artery Disease

Books

American Heart Association's Educational Task Force of the ACLS Subcommittee.

Advanced Cardiac Life Support Algorithms and Drugs. Dallas: American Heart Association, 1993.

Emergency Department: Rapid Identification and Treatment of Patients with Acute Myocardial Infarction. Bethesda, MD: National Heart, Lung and Blood Institute, 1993.

National Cholesterol Education Program. *Report of the Expert Panel on Detection, Evaluation, and Treatment of High Blood Cholesterol in Adults.* Bethesda, MD: National Heart, Lung and Blood Institute, 1988.

Schlant RC (ed). *The Year Book of Cardiology.* St. Louis: Mosby–Year Book, 1992, pp 1–39.

Wenger NK, and Hellerstein HK, eds. *Rehabilitation and the Coronary Patient.* 3rd ed. New York: Churchill Livingstone, 1992.

Chapters in Books and Journal Articles

Barbiere C. PTCA: Treating the tough cases. *RN* 54(2):38–43, 1991.

Becker RC. Medical therapy for acute myocardial infarction: Where do we go from here? *J Intensive Care Med* 10(2):51–53, 1995.

Benton JG, Brown H, and Risk HA. Energy expended by patients on the bedpan and bedside commode. *JAMA* 144:1443–1447, 1950.

Blankn FSJ, et al. Decreasing "door to thrombolysis" time at one busy acute care hospital. *J Emerg Nurs* 21(3):202–206, 1995.

Callahan LL, and Frohlich GC. Understanding nonsurgical coronary revascularization procedures. *Am J Nurs* 95(5):52h–52k, 1995.

Chaitman BR (for TIMI investigators). Impact of treatment strategy on predischarge exercise test in the thrombolysis in myocardial infarction (TIMI) II trial. *Am J Cardiol* 71:131–138, 1993.

Das B, and Banka V. Coronary artery disease in women: How it is—and isn't—unique. *Postgrad Med* 91(4):197–206, 1992.

Fair JM, and Berra K. Life-style changes and coronary heart disease: The influence on nonpharmacologic intervention. *J Cardiovasc Nurs* 9(2):12–24, 1995.

Fischman DL, et al. A randomized comparison of coronary stent placement and balloon angioplasty in treatment of coronary artery disease. *N Engl J Med* 331:496–501, 1994.

Foley JJ. Drug update: Significant changes in advanced cardiac life support medication guidelines. *J Emerg Nurs* 19(6):516–518, 1993.

Fowler JP. How to respond rapidly when chest pain strikes. *Nursing* 26(4):42–43, 1996.

Froelicher ES, et al. Risk profile screening. *J Cardiovasc Nurs* 10(1):30–50, 1995.

Funk M, et al. Frequency of long-term lower limb ischemia associated with intra-aortic balloon pump use. *Am J Cardiol* 70:1195–1199, 1992.

Gawlinski A, and Jensen G. The complications of cardiovascular aging. *Am J Nurs* 92(11):26–30, 1991.

Grab C. The cutting alternative to PTCA. *RN* 55(7):22–26, 1992.

Grines CL. (for the Primary Angioplasty in Myocardial Infarction Study Group). A comparison of immediate angioplasty with thrombolytic therapy for acute myocardial infarction. *N Engl J Med* 328:673–679, 1993.

Gurbel PA, and Haber HL. The use of anti-thrombolitics in clinical cardiology: Risks vs. benefits. *J Outcomes Manage* 3:11–12, 1996.

Holcomb S. Atherectomy. *Nursing* 23(2):44–47, 1993.

Hunninghake DB, et al. The efficacy of intensive dietary therapy alone or combined with lovastatin in outpatients with hypercholesterolemia. *N Engl J Med* 328:1213–1219, 1993.

Karnes N. Adenosine: A quick fix for PSVT. *Nursing* 25(7):55, 1995.

Lanau C, Lange RA, and Hillis LD. Percutaneous transluminal coronary angioplasty. *N Engl J Med* 330(14):981–993, 1994.

Littrell K, Walker D, and Worthy C. Myocardial infarction and the non-diagnostic ECG: Strategies to meet the challenges. *J Emerg Nurs* 21(4):287–293, 1995.

Loscalzo J. An overview of thrombolytic agents. *Chest* 97(Suppl 4):1179–1239, 1990.

Lothian C. Laser angioplasty. *Nursing* 22(1):62–64, 1992.

Martin J. Nursing actions can limit myocardial damage and save lives: The importance of time to treatment in acute MI. *Saving Lives with Thrombolytic Therapy: A Supplement to AJN.* 94(5):3–8, 1994.

Matrisciano L. Unstable angina: An overview. *Crit Care Nurse* 12(8):30–38, 1992.

O'Neal PV. How to spot early signs of cardiogenic shock. *Am J Nurs* 94(5):36–40, 1994.

Scherck KA. Coping with acute myocardial infarction. *Heart Lung* 21:327–334, 1992.

Stoy D. Pharmacotherapy for hypercholesterolemia: Guidelines and nursing perspective. *J Cardiovasc Nurs* 3(2):34–43, 1991.

Strimike CL. Caring for a patient with an intracoronary stent. *Am J Nurs* 95(1):40–45, 1995.

Sytkowski PA, et al. Changes in risk factors and the decline in mortality from cardiovascular disease: The Framingham Heart Study. *N Engl J Med* 322:1635–1642, 1990.

Titler MG, and Petit DM. Discharge readiness assessment. *J Cardiovasc Nurs* 9(4):64–74, 1995.

White E. Managing hyperlipidemia: New approaches to an old problem. *Nursing* 24(8):66–69, 1994.

Winslow EH, Land LE, and Gaffney FA. Oxygen uptake and cardiovascular response in patients and normal adults during in-bed and out-of-bed toileting. *J Card Rehabil* 4(6):348–354, 1984.

Valvular Disorders

Books

Fink BW. *Congenital Heart Disease: A Deductive Approach to Diagnosis.* 3rd ed. St. Louis: Mosby–Year Book, 1991.

Schlant RC (ed). *The Year Book of Cardiology.* St. Louis: Mosby–Year Book, 1992, pp 55–100.

Journal Articles

Davis JS, and Small BM. Advances in the treatment of aortic stenosis across the lifespan. *Nurs Clin North Am* 30(2):317–332, 1995.

Miner PE. Infective endocarditis: Implications for care of the adult with congenital heart disease. *Nurs Clin North Am* 29(2):269–284, 1994.

Sparachino PSA. Adult congenital heart disease. *Nurs Clin North Am* 29(2):213–219, 1994.

Anatomic Disorders

Chapters in Books and Journal Articles

Gilworth DL. Cardiomyopathy. *In* Mims BC (ed). *Case Studies in Critical Care Nursing.* Baltimore: Williams & Wilkins, 1993.

Handerhan B. Managing patients with cardiomyopathy. *Nursing* 25(1):32c–32e, 1995.

Luquire R, and Houston S. Cardiomyopathy: How to buy time. *RN* 56(5):28–33, 1993.

Inflammatory Process

Journal Articles

Handerhan B. Managing patients with cardiomyopathy. *Nursing* 25(1):32c–32f, 1995.

Congestive Heart Failure

Chapters in Books and Journal Articles

Borcherding L. Congestive heart failure. *In* Mims B (ed). *Case Studies in Critical Care Nursing.* Baltimore: Williams & Wilkins, 1993.

Brown L. Boosting the failing heart with inotropic drugs. *Nursing* 23(4):34–43, 1993.

Dracup K, et al. Rethinking heart failure. *Am J Nurs* 95(7):23–28, 1995.

Fowler JP. From chronic to acute: When CHF turns deadly. *Nursing* 25(12):54–55, 1995.

Letterer R, et al. Learning to live with congestive heart failure. *Nursing* 22(5):34–41, 1992.

Lewandoski DM. Congestive heart failure. *Am J Nurs* 95(5):36–37, 1995.

Robinson K. Reversing pulmonary edema. *Am J Nurs* 93(12):45, 1993.

Sullivan MJ, and Hawthorne MH. Non-pharmacologic interventions in the treatment of heart failure. *J Cardiovasc Nurs* 10(2):47–57, 1996.

Venner GH, and Steelbinder JS. Team management of congestive heart failure across the continuum. *J Cardiovasc Nurs* 10(2):71–84, 1996.

Wallace PL. Nursing management of the patient with heart failure. *In* Dolan JT (ed). *Critical Care Nursing—Clinical Management Through the Nursing Process.* Philadelphia: FA Davis, 1991.

Weeks SM. Caring for patients with heart failure. *Nursing* 26(3):52–53, 1996.

Vacone-Morton LA. Cardiovascular drugs. First-line therapy for CHF. *RN* 58(2):38–43, 1995.

Cardiac Surgery

Chapters in Books and Journal Articles

Allen JK. Physical and psychosocial outcomes after coronary artery bypass graft surgery: Review of the literature. *Heart Lung* 19:49–56, 1990.

Davids D, and Verderber A. Functional outcomes of cardiac surgery for the elderly. *J Cardiovasc Nurs* 9(4):96–101, 1995.

Good M. Relaxation techniques for surgical patients. *Am J Nurs* 95(5):39–42, 1995.

Grumbach J, et al. Regionalization of cardiac surgery in the United States and Canada. *JAMA* 274(16):1282–1288, 1995.

Halfman-Franey M. Coronary artery bypass graft. *In* Mims BC (ed). *Case Studies in Critical Care Nursing.* Baltimore: Williams & Wilkins, 1993.

Hawthorne MH. Gender differences in recovery after coronary artery surgery. *Image* 26(1):75–80, 1994.

Keller SM. Nursing management of the cardiac surgical patient. *In* Dolan JT (ed). *Critical Care Nursing—Clinical Management Through the Nursing Process.* Philadelphia: JB Lippincott, 1991.

Knapp-Spooner C, and Yarcheski A. Sleep patterns and stress in patients having coronary bypass. *Heart Lung* 21:342–349, 1992.

Palarski V, and Washburn S. Overcoming LVD in cardiac rehab. *Am J Nurs* 92(9):52–57, 1992.

Possanza CP. What you should know about coronary artery bypass graft surgery. *Nursing* 26(2):48–50, 1996.

Smith JM, et al. Coronary artery bypass grafting in the elderly: Changing trends and results. *J Cardiovasc Surg* 33:468–471, 1992.

Resuscitation

Books

Basic Life Support Heartsaver Guide. Dallas: American Heart Association, 1993.

Textbook of Advanced Cardiac Life Support. 4th ed. Dallas: American Heart Association, 1994.

Journal Articles

Bailey MM. Emergencies handbook. *Nursing* 26(3):61–64, 1996.

Bedell S, et al. Survival after cardiopulmonary resuscitation in the hospital. *N Engl J Med* 309(10):569–576, 1983.

Dimmitt MA, and Griffiths SE. What's new in prehospital care. *Nursing* 22:58–61, 1992.

Eichhorn DJ, et al. Family presence during resuscitation. It is time to open the door. *Capsules Comments in Crit Care Nurs* 3(1):8–12, 1995.

Emergency Cardiac Care Committee and Subcommittees, American Heart Association. Guidelines for cardiopulmonary resuscitation and emergency cardiac care. *JAMA* 268(16):2171–2302, 1992.

Foley JL. Drug update significant changes in advanced cardiac life support medication guidelines. *J Emerg Nurs* 19:516–518, 1993.

Green E. How codes are really managed. *Nursing* 23:58–61, 1993.

Newman MM. Survival: A matter of timing. *Curr Emerg Cardiac Care* 4(1):1–3, 1993.

Walsh SM. Resuscitation decisions: Showing a family the way. *Nursing* 25(8):51–52, 1995.

Pacemakers

Chapters in Books and Journal Articles

Aufderheide TP. Pacemakers and electrical therapy during advanced cardiac life support. *Resp Care* 40(4):364–376, 1995.

Bush DE, and Finucane TE. Permanent cardiac pacemakers in the elderly. *J Am Geriatr Soc* 42(3):326–334, 1994.

Cross J, and McErlean E. Artificial cardiac pacemakers. *In* Boggs R, and Woolridge-King M. *AACN Procedure Manual for Critical Care.* Philadelphia: WB Saunders, 1993.

Hasemeier CS. Clinical snapshot: Permanent pacemakers. *Am J Nurs* 96(2):30–31, 1996.

McErlean E, and Whitman G. Therapeutic modalities in the treatment of the patient with cardiovascular dysfunction. *In* Dolan J (ed). *Critical Care Nursing—Clinical Management Through the Nursing Process.* Philadelphia: FA Davis, 1991.

Merva J. Temporary pacemakers. *RN* 55(5):28–33, 1992.

Owen A. Keeping pace with temporary pacemakers. *Nursing* 21(4):58–64, 1991.

Pool NP. Initiating temporary transvenous dual-chamber pacing. *Nursing* 24(5):48–50, 1994.

Teplitz L. Transcutaneous pacemakers. *J Cardiovasc Nurs* 5(3):44–57, 1991.

Cardiovascular Drugs

Books

Lehne RA, et al. *Pharmacology for Nursing Care.* 2nd ed. Philadelphia: WB Saunders, 1994.

Nursing 96 Drug Handbook. Springhouse, PA: Springhouse Corp, 1996.

Textbook of Advanced Cardiac Life Support. 4th ed. Dallas: American Heart Association, 1994.

Chapters in Books and Journal Articles

Aragon D, and Martin M. What you should know about thrombolytic therapy for acute MI. *Am J Nurs* 93(9):24–31, 1993.

Braun A. Drugs that dissolve clots. *RN* 54(6):52–57, 1991.

Cronin L. Beat the clock: Saving the heart with thrombolytic drugs. *Nursing* 23(8):34–41, 1993.

Karnes N. Adenosine: A quick fix for PSVT. *Nursing* 25(7):55–56, 1995.

Morse GD, and Meisel SB. Drugs commonly used in the critical care setting. *In* Dolan JT (ed). *Critical Care Nursing—Clinical Management Through the Nursing Process.* Philadelphia: JB Lippincott, 1991.

Redeker NS, and Sadowski AV. Update on cardiovascular drugs and elders. *Am J Nurs* 95(9):34–40, 1995.

Schneeweiss A. Cardiovascular therapy in the elderly. *In* Messerli FH (ed). *Cardiovascular Drug Therapy.* Philadelphia: WB Saunders, 1990, pp 140–180.

Technical Skills

Books

Kinkade SL, and Lorhman J (eds). *Critical Care Nursing Procedures: A Team Approach.* Toronto: BC Decker, 1990.

Technical Skills Manual. Dallas: Parkland Memorial Hospital, 1990.

Textbook of Advanced Cardiac Life Support. 4th ed. Dallas: American Heart Association, 1994.

Chapters in Books and Journal Articles

Daily EK. Hemodynamic monitoring. *In* Dolan JT (ed). *Critical Care Nursing—Clinical Management Through the Nursing Process.* Philadelphia: JB Lippincott, 1991.

Jones A. Assisting with pericardiocentesis. *In* Boggs R, and Woolridge-King M.

AACN Procedure Manual for Critical Care. Philadelphia: WB Saunders, 1993.

Lynn-McHale D, and McGrory J. Intra-aortic balloon pump management. *In* Boggs R, and Woolridge-King M. *AACN Procedure Manual for Critical Care.* Philadelphia: WB Saunders, 1993.

McErlean ES, and Whitman GR. Therapeutic modalities in the treatment of the patient with cardiovascular dysfunction. *In* Dolan JT (ed). *Critical Care Nursing—Clinical Management Through the Nursing Process.* Philadelphia: JB Lippincott, 1991.

Nursing Assessment

Books

Dossey BM, et al. *Holistic Healing: A Handbook for Practice.* 2nd ed. Gaithersburg, MD: Aspen, 1995.

Guzzetta CE, et al. (eds). *Clinical Assessment Tools for Use with Nursing Diagnoses.* St. Louis: CV Mosby, 1989.

Neal MC, et al. *Diseases and Disorders of the Circulatory System: Nursing Diagnosis Care Plans.* Boston: Jones & Bartlett, 1990, pp 58–74.

Wesornick B. *Standards of Nursing Care: A Model for Clinical Practice.* Philadelphia: JB Lippincott, 1993.

Transcultural Considerations

Books

Geissler EM. *Pocket Guide to Cultural Assessment.* St. Louis: Mosby–Year Book, 1994.

Giger JN, and Davidhizer RE (eds). *Transcultural Nursing: Assessment and Intervention.* 2nd ed. St. Louis: Mosby–Year Book, 1995.

Silent Epidemic: The Truth About Women and Heart Disease. Dallas: American Heart Association, 1989.

Spector RE. *Cultural Diversity in Health and Illness.* 4th ed. Norwalk, CT: Appleton & Lange, 1996.

Journal Articles

Ayanian J. Differences in use of procedures between women and men hospitalized for coronary heart disease. *N Engl J Med* 325:221–225, 1991.

Bailey E. Hypertension: An analysis of Detroit African-American health care treatment patterns. *Hum Organ* 50(3):287–296, 1991.

Becker LB, et al. Racial differences in the incidence of cardiac arrest and subsequent survival. *N Engl J Med* 329:600–606, 1993.

Giger JN, Davidhizer R, and Cherry B. Biological variations in the black patient. *NSNA/Imprint.* 38(2):95–105, 1991.

Resources

Agency for Health Care Policy and Research (AHCPR)
(clinical practice guidelines available in versions for both health care providers and consumers)

AHCPR Publications Clearinghouse
P.O. Box 8547
Silver Springs, MD 20907
(800) 358–9295

American Association of Critical Care Nurses
(for nursing standards of care)

American Association of Critical Care Nurses
1 Civic Plaza
Newport Beach, CA 92660
(714) 644–9310

American Dietetic Association
(for information on dietary issues)

American Dietetic Association
430 North Michigan Avenue
Chicago, IL 60611
(312) 280–5000

American Heart Association
(for professional and general public education and research)

American Heart Association
7272 Greenville Avenue
Dallas, TX 75231
(800) 553–6321
(214) 750–5442

American Heart Association
Texas Affiliate, Inc.
P.O. Box 15186
Austin, TX 78761
(to obtain copies of "RISKO, a Heart Hazard Appraisal")

American Lung Association
(for information about smoking cessation programs)

American Lung Association
1740 Broadway
New York, NY 10019
(212) 245–8000

Cardiac Pacemakers, Inc. (subsidiary of Eli Lilly)
(for a generic video describing electrophysiologic testing)

Cardiac Pacemakers, Inc.
4100 Hamline Avenue North
St. Paul, MN 55223
(800) 227–3422

C. R. Bard, Inc.
(for free colorful posters that depict both the normal conduction system and a variety of conduction abnormalities)

C. R. Bard, Inc.
P.O. Box M
Billerica, MA 02821
(800) 322–2273

DuPont Pharmaceuticals
(for free brochures that describe specific dysrhythmias; brochure on atrial fibrillation also available in Spanish)

DuPont Pharmaceuticals
P.O. Box 80026
Wilmington, DE 19880–0026
(302) 992–4240

Knoll Pharmaceuticals
(for a poster of the heart showing normal conduction)

Knoll Pharmaceuticals
30 North Jefferson Road
Whippany, NJ 07981
(201) 887–8300

Krames Communications
(for copies of teaching tools including patient education booklets in both English and Spanish)

Krames Communications
1100 Grundy Lane
San Bruno, CA 94066–3030
(800) 333–3032

Mansfield Scientific
(for free colorful posters that depict both the normal conduction system and a variety of conduction abnormalities)

Mansfield Scientific
135 Forbes Boulevard
Mansfield, MA 02048
(800) 225–2732

National Heart, Lung, and Blood Institute
(for a complimentary copy of "Emergency Department: Rapid Identification and Treatment of Patients With Acute Myocardial Infarction" [NIH Publication No. 93-3278])

NHLBI Information Center
P.O. Box 30105
Bethesda, MD 20824–0105
(301) 251–1222

National High Blood Pressure Education Program
Office of Prevention, Education, and Control
National Institutes of Health
Bethesda, MD 20892
(301) 951–3260

Pritchett & Hull Associates, Inc.
(for copies of patient education books and posters in both English and Spanish on cardiology, exercise, and nutrition; staff educational materials also available)

Pritchett & Hull Associates, Inc.
340 Oakcliff Road
NE STE 110
Atlanta, GA 30340–3079
(800) 752–0510

U.S. Government Printing Office
(clinical practice guidelines available for
   purchase only)

U.S. Government Printing Office
Superintendent of Documents
Washington, DC 20402
(205) 512–1800

Webster Laboratories, Inc.
(for free colorful posters that depict both
   the normal conduction system and a
   variety of conduction abnormalities)

Webster Laboratories, Inc.
5114 Commerce Drive
Baldwin Park, CA 91706
(818) 960–6404

Caring for People with Peripheral Vascular and Lymphatic Disorders

◼ *VASCULAR STRUCTURE AND FUNCTION*

Structure of the Vascular System

The vascular system consists of the arteries, arterioles, capillaries, venules, veins, and valves (Fig. 24–1).

Functions of the Vascular System

1. The vascular system is a conduit for circulating blood to all body tissues.
2. Blood flow is constantly changing. The circulatory needs of tissues determine the percentage of blood flow delivered by the vascular system.
   a. The arteries transport oxygenated blood under high pressure to the tissues. (The only exception is the pulmonary artery, which carries deoxygenated blood from the heart to the lungs.)
   b. Arterioles control the blood flow into the capillaries. An arteriole's muscular structure allows it to close completely or to dilate to several times its size to regulate the amount of blood flow to the capillaries.
   c. Capillaries are a vital part of the circulatory system. They allow exchange of fluid and nutrients between the blood and the interstitial spaces.
   d. Venules receive blood from the capillary bed and move blood into the veins.
   e. Veins transport deoxygenated blood from the tissues back toward the heart and lungs for oxygenation. (The only exception is the pulmonary vein, which carries oxygenated blood from the lungs back to the heart.)
   f. Valves help return blood to the heart against the force of gravity (Fig. 24–2).

Structure of the Lymphatic System

The lymphatic system is composed of lymphatic capillaries, lymphatic vessels, lymphatic fluid, lymph nodes, and lymphoid organs (spleen, thymus, and tonsils) (Fig. 24–3). (Lymphoid organs are discussed in Chapter 21.)

Functions of the Lymphatic System

1. Produces lymphocytes, which are key cells in controlling the immune response
2. Filters out foreign particles from the lymphatic fluid, helping to prevent the spread of infection
3. Absorbs fat from the small intestine
4. Drains the tissue and returns the tissue fluid to the blood

◼ *ASSESSING PEOPLE WITH ARTERIAL DISEASE*

Key Symptoms and Their Pathophysiologic Bases

1. Pain in the extremities after exercise or activity or during rest
   a. Occurrence
   b. Characteristics
   c. Location
   d. Duration
   e. Severity
   f. Precipitating or aggravating factors
   g. Associated symptoms
   h. Alleviating factors
2. Changes in skin appearance and temperature of the extremities
   a. Through *h.*
3. Diminished sensation.
   a. Through *h.*
4. Diminished or absent pulses
   a. Through *h.*
5. History of slow wound healing
   a. Through *h.*
6. Skin breakdown or ulcers
   a. Through *h.*
7. Mild edema
   a. Through *h.*
8. The pathophysiologic basis for all of these symptoms is decreased or absent tissue perfusion due to partial or total obstruction of 1 or more arteries.

STRUCTURE OF THE VASCULAR SYSTEM

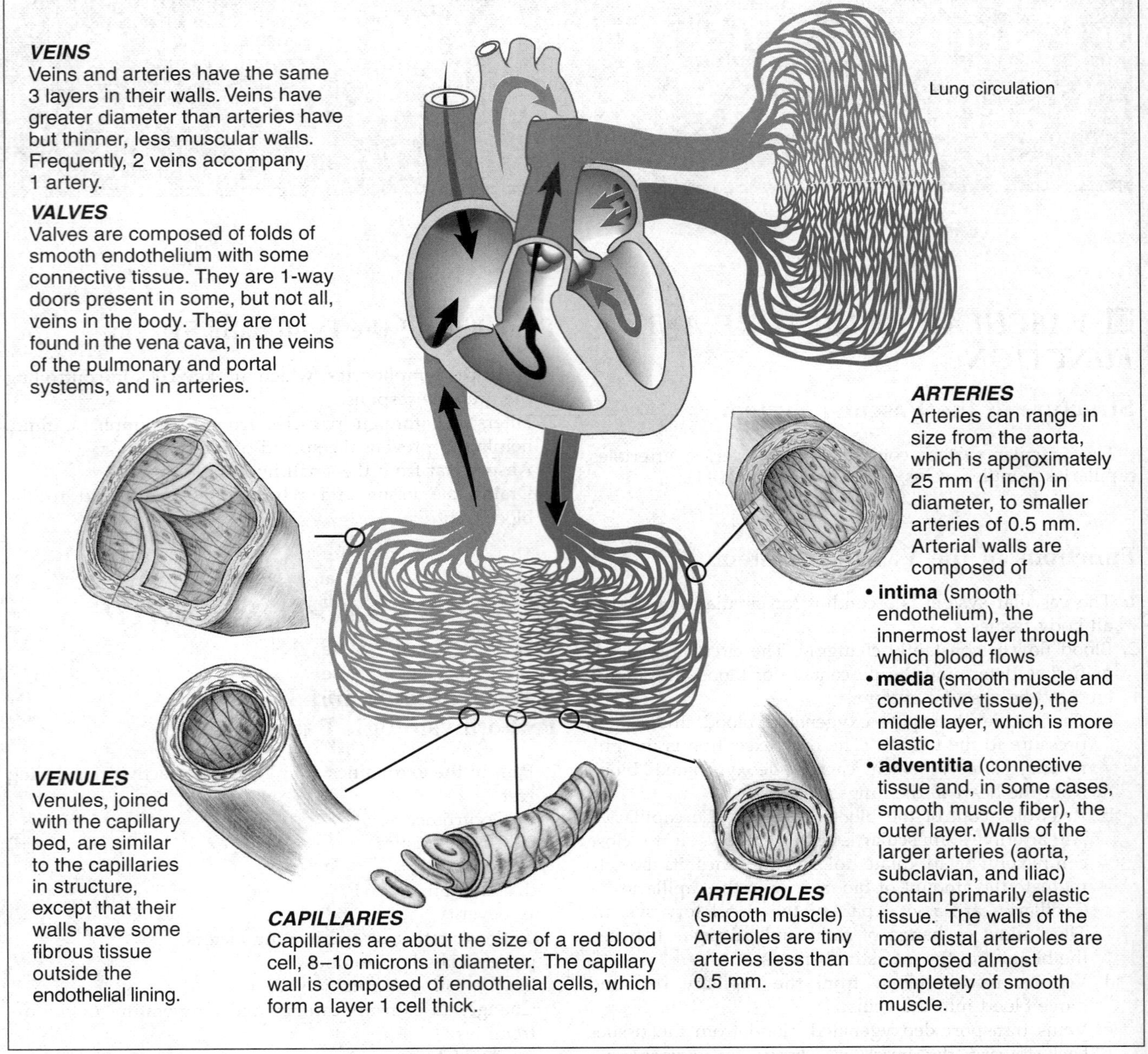

VEINS

Veins and arteries have the same 3 layers in their walls. Veins have greater diameter than arteries have but thinner, less muscular walls. Frequently, 2 veins accompany 1 artery.

VALVES

Valves are composed of folds of smooth endothelium with some connective tissue. They are 1-way doors present in some, but not all, veins in the body. They are not found in the vena cava, in the veins of the pulmonary and portal systems, and in arteries.

Lung circulation

ARTERIES

Arteries can range in size from the aorta, which is approximately 25 mm (1 inch) in diameter, to smaller arteries of 0.5 mm. Arterial walls are composed of

- **intima** (smooth endothelium), the innermost layer through which blood flows
- **media** (smooth muscle and connective tissue), the middle layer, which is more elastic
- **adventitia** (connective tissue and, in some cases, smooth muscle fiber), the outer layer. Walls of the larger arteries (aorta, subclavian, and iliac) contain primarily elastic tissue. The walls of the more distal arterioles are composed almost completely of smooth muscle.

VENULES

Venules, joined with the capillary bed, are similar to the capillaries in structure, except that their walls have some fibrous tissue outside the endothelial lining.

CAPILLARIES

Capillaries are about the size of a red blood cell, 8–10 microns in diameter. The capillary wall is composed of endothelial cells, which form a layer 1 cell thick.

ARTERIOLES

(smooth muscle) Arterioles are tiny arteries less than 0.5 mm.

Figure 24–1. Vascular circulation. Oxygen-rich blood leaves the heart and passes through the aorta to all arteries in the arterial system; an exchange of gases and nutrients takes place within the capillaries. Deoxygenated blood returns through the venous system to the heart to begin the cycle again.

Health History

To determine the significance of the symptoms of arterial disease, ask the following key questions:

1. How far can you walk before you have discomfort?
2. What is the quality of the discomfort? Is it cramping, burning, aching, sharp, dull, stinging, numbness?
3. Rate the intensity of the discomfort on a scale of 0 to 10, with 0 representing little or no pain and 10 representing severe pain.
4. Show me where you are experiencing the discomfort.
5. What activities, if any, cause the discomfort?
6. Does the discomfort subside with rest? How long do you have to rest before the pain disappears?
7. Have you had any problems in the past with slow wound healing? If so, please describe.
8. Do you have any family history of arterial disease?

Physical Examination

1. Inspect skin texture for changes. Skin may be shiny, taut, thin, scaly, lacking hair, or dry.
2. Inspect for lesions or ulcerations.
3. Inspect nail beds for trophic changes such as thickened, missing, or brittle nails.
4. Palpate all peripheral pulses (Table 24–1; Fig. 24–4).
5. Palpate skin to assess for changes in temperature or presence of edema.
6. Assess capillary filling time.
   a. Apply pressure to the nail bed.
   b. Release pressure on the nail bed and observe to see how quickly the original color returns.
      (1) Normal capillaries refill in 1 to 3 seconds.
      (2) Delay of more than 3 seconds is referred to as "sluggish" refill.

Table 24–1. Grading Scale for Peripheral Pulses

Nurse's Finding on Examination	Nurse's Evaluation
Pulse is absent, not palpable	0
Pulse is diminished, barely felt	+1
Pulse is easily palpated	+2
Pulse is full, increased	+3
Pulse is bounding	+4

7. Auscultate over the aorta and over the carotid, subclavian, and femoral arteries for bruits.
   a. A **bruit** is a low-pitched blowing sound best heard with the bell of the stethoscope.
   b. Narrowing of an artery produces turbulent blood flow; therefore, a bruit may indicate arterial disease.

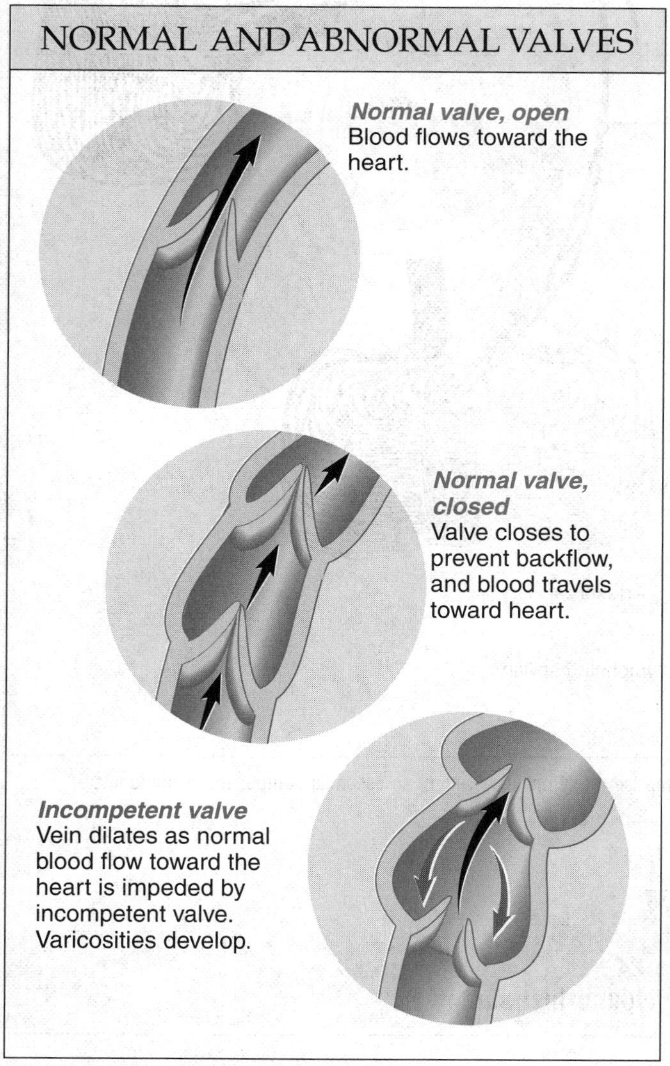

Special Diagnostic Studies

1. Noninvasive testing
   a. Goals of noninvasive testing
      (1) Determine the severity of the disease that is present in the artery.
      (2) Locate the main areas of blockage within the extremity.
      (3) Establish the level of functional impairment created by the disease process.
   b. Specific tests to diagnose arterial disease
      (1) **Doppler ultrasound** sends continuous low-intensity sound waves through tissue. Reflected sound, indicating blood flow through a blood vessel, is detected and amplified as an audible sound and then recorded. In persons with arterial stenoses, the amplitude of sound waves will be diminished; in occlusive disease, sound may be absent (Procedure 24–1).
      (2) **Segmental plethysmography** detects blood-volume changes, then graphs blood flow in the limb. Testing is performed by a nurse or other medical personnel who have received advanced training in vascular technology (Fig. 24–5).
      (3) With **duplex ultrasound,** images of scanned blood vessels appear on a screen as they function.
      (4) The **ankle-brachial index (ABI)** is an assessment tool (Procedure 24–2) that indicates the severity of arterial disease (Table 24–2).

NORMAL AND ABNORMAL VALVES

Normal valve, open
Blood flows toward the heart.

Normal valve, closed
Valve closes to prevent backflow, and blood travels toward heart.

Incompetent valve
Vein dilates as normal blood flow toward the heart is impeded by incompetent valve. Varicosities develop.

Figure 24–2. Normal and abnormal valve function in veins. Competent vein, showing the valve in open and in closed positions. The incompetent valve in the vein is unable to prevent the backward flow of blood.

Table 24–2. The Ankle-Brachial Index (ABI) in Assessment of Arterial Disease

	Normal	Mild Disease	Moderate Disease	Severe Disease
Resting ABI	>0.95	0.8–0.95	0.5–0.79	<0.5

STRUCTURE OF THE LYMPHATIC SYSTEM

Lymph
Lymph is interstitial fluid that is almost identical to tissue fluid. It moves through the lymphatic system
- by the milking action of the skeletal muscles on lymphatic vessels and capillaries as well as intrinsic pressure gradients
- by the closure of valves in the lymphatic system that prevent the reverse flow of lymph
- with the aid of contractions of lymphatic vessel walls moving the lymph along through the system
- with changes in thoracic pressure from breathing, which cause movement of the lymph into the upper thorax

Lymphatic vessels
Lymphatic vessels have similar wall composition to that of veins, except that lymphatic vessel walls are slightly thinner. Also, lymphatic vessels have more valves than veins do. Lymphatic vessels connect with the lymphatic capillaries to empty lymph into the jugulo-subclavian veins.

Lymph nodes
Lymph nodes, oval-shaped bodies containing collections of lymphatic tissue, are found at intervals in the course of lymphatic vessels in the neck, axillae, mediastinum, abdomen, pelvis, and inguinal regions. Physical examination can reveal lymph nodes in the neck, the axillae, and the inguinal area.

Lymphatic capillaries
Lymphatic capillaries are endothelial tubes that form complex networks within the tissues, where they originate and collect tissue fluid. They are distributed unevenly throughout the body, traveling within loose connective tissue between organs, in the subcutaneous and subserous tissues, and in the submucosa of the digestive, respiratory, and urogenital tracts. Lymphatic capillaries are even more porous than venous capillaries.

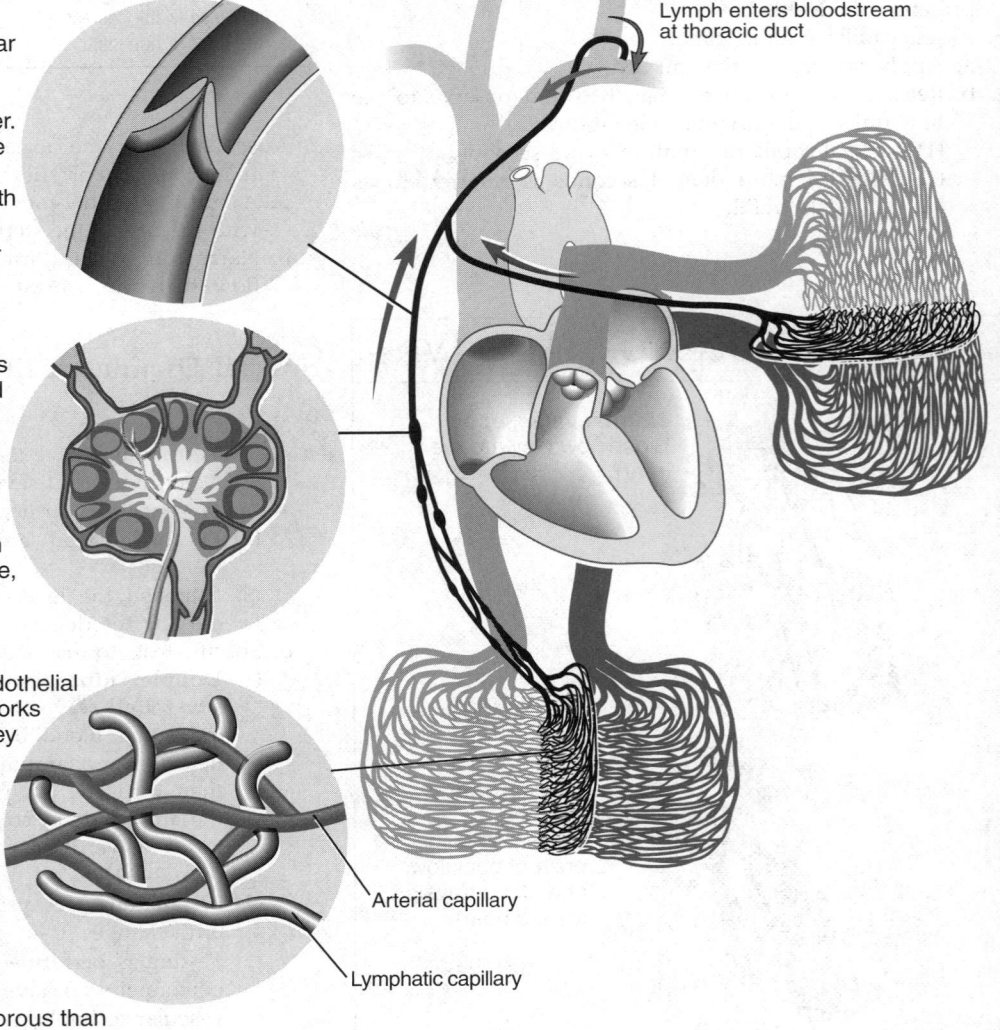

Lymph enters bloodstream at thoracic duct

Arterial capillary

Lymphatic capillary

Figure 24–3. Lymphatic channels include vessels and tissue that comprise the lymphatic system, an essential component of immunity.

P

Procedure 24–1
Using A Doppler Ultrasound Instrument

Definition/Purpose: For assessment of arterial blood flow by audible detection of an arterial pulsation

Learning/Teaching Activities: Provide the following information: (a) describe the procedure; (b) instruct the person that the test will not cause discomfort.

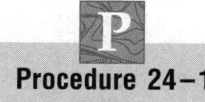

Procedure 24-1
(continued)

Preliminary Activities

Equipment
- Doppler ultrasound instrument
- Acoustic transmission gel

Procedure

Actions	Rationale/Discussion
1. Locate the arterial pulsation by palpation.	1. Usually the dorsalis pedis, posterior tibial, popliteal, or femoral pulses are assessed, or a combination of these.
2. Apply acoustic transmission gel over the arterial pulsation.	2. A beam of ultrasound is sent into tissues through the acoustic transmission gel placed on the skin.
3. Turn the Doppler ultrasound to the "on" position, and place the attached stethoscope earpieces into the ear.	3. Reflected sound from moving blood cells is detected, then amplified as audible sound.
4. Apply the Doppler probe to the area over the arterial pulsation.	4. Arterial blood flow can be distinguished by the pulsatile quality of the blood flow.
5. Listen for audible sounds with pulsatile quality.	5. The presence of audible arterial blood flow is an indicator of arterial patency.

Procedure 24-2
Calculating an Ankle-Brachial Index

Definition/Purpose: To evaluate the patency of the vascular system

Learning/Teaching Activities: Explain the procedure to the patient. Locate the pedal pulses with the Doppler, and mark their sites. *Note:* Use either the dorsalis pedis or the posterior tibialis pulse, whichever is heard loudest with the Doppler. Instruct the person that the test will not cause discomfort.

Preliminary Activities

Equipment
- Blood pressure cuff
- Doppler ultrasound instrument
- Acoustic transmission gel

Procedure

Actions	Rationale
1. Obtain the brachial systolic blood pressure measurement with the Doppler ultrasound and record.	1. The Doppler provides a more accurate blood pressure measurement than the stethoscope.
2. Obtain systolic measurements in both arms, and record the highest reading.	2. Blood pressure can vary in the arms with the presence of underlying vascular disease.
3. Apply an appropriately sized blood pressure cuff over the ankle and the arm.	3. This prevents false readings.
4. Inflate the blood pressure cuff, and place the Doppler probe over the pulse site (dorsalis pedis or posterior tibialis) until the pulse is no longer audible with the Doppler, and then continue to inflate 20 mm Hg higher than this number.	4. In patients with vascular disease, ankle pressures may vary widely. This measurement will be a baseline ankle pressure.

(continued)

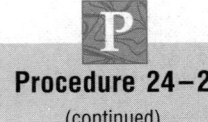

Procedure 24-2

(continued)

Actions	Rationale
5. Deflate the cuff, listening for the arterial pulsation. Record this measurement.	5. This is the systolic blood pressure for the limb segment.
6. To calculate the ankle-brachial index (ABI), divide the ankle systolic pressure by the brachial systolic pressure.	6. $\dfrac{\text{ankle pressure}}{\text{brachial pressure}}$ = A-B ratio
7. Refer to Table 24-3 for using ABI as an assessment of arterial disease.	

(5) Exercise testing helps to further establish the functional impairment caused by the disease process. Instruct the person to walk on a treadmill with a slight (10%) incline at a rate of 1.5 miles per hour. If disease is present, a decrease in the ABI and changes in the amplitude and contour of pulse volume waveforms will occur after exercise.

(6) Leg measurements are used to detect edema in an extremity (Procedure 24-3).

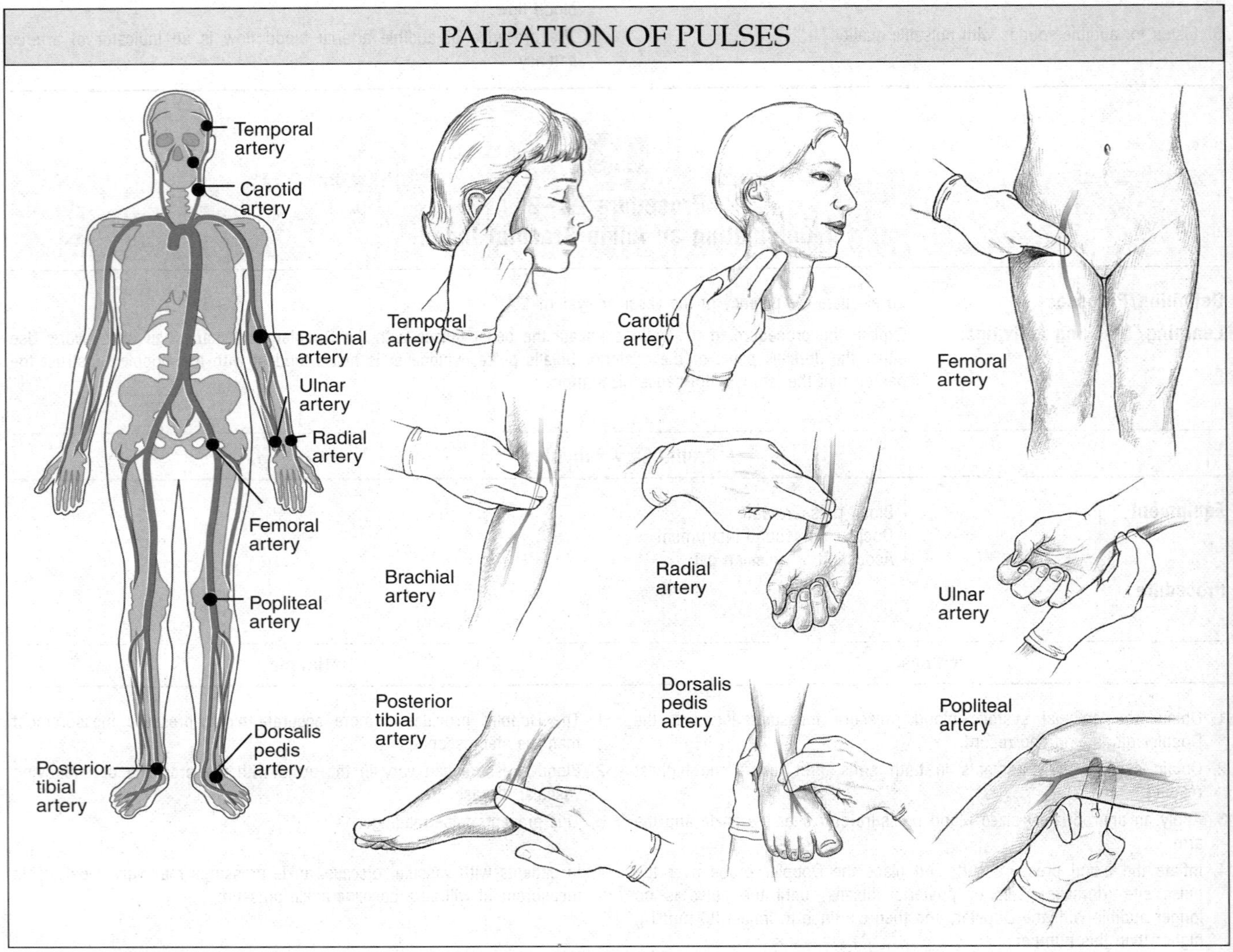

PALPATION OF PULSES

Temporal artery

Carotid artery

Brachial artery

Ulnar artery

Radial artery

Femoral artery

Popliteal artery

Dorsalis pedis artery

Posterior tibial artery

Temporal artery

Carotid artery

Brachial artery

Radial artery

Posterior tibial artery

Femoral artery

Ulnar artery

Dorsalis pedis artery

Popliteal artery

Figure 24-4. Peripheral pulses frequently assessed include dorsalis pedis, posterior tibial, and femoral pulses.

SEGMENTAL PLETHYSMOGRAPHY

In segmental plethysmography, recordings are made by placing blood pressure cuffs on the thigh, calf, and ankle. Waveforms are produced when the volume of blood flowing through the limb increases during systole. Pulse waveforms are evaluated by their amplitude and contour. A dicrotic notch, an indication of the blood vessel's elasticity, should be present.

Its absence, along with a rounding of the systolic peak of the waveform, is a sign of early disease in the blood vessel. A near flattened or flat waveform indicates severe disease with little or no flow through the blood vessel.

Normal waveform

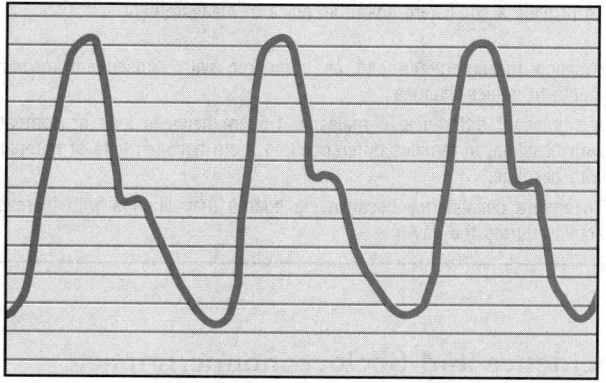

Abnormal waveform

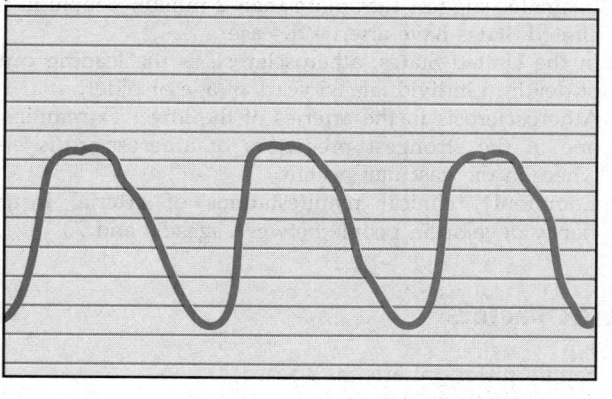

Figure 24–5. Normal pulse waveform and abnormal waveform. The abnormal waveform indicates arterial disease.

2. Invasive testing
   a. An **arteriogram** is a series of x-ray films made when a radiopaque dye is injected into an artery, allowing arterial stenoses or occlusions to be seen.

NURSE ADVISORY

Assessment for any procedure that uses a radiopaque dye should include any history of allergy to contrast medium or shellfish (which contain iodine).

   (1) The test is performed in a special procedures room under sterile conditions.
   (2) Premedication is usually given 30 to 60 minutes before the procedure.
   (3) Local anesthesia is administered in the area of the injection site.
   (4) A catheter is inserted percutaneously into an artery, and radiopaque contrast medium is introduced.
   (5) Serial pictures of the movement of the dye allow visualization of stenoses and arterial occlusions.
   (6) Postprocedure nursing care includes frequent monitoring of vital signs; monitoring of pulses distal to the puncture site; assessing the pressure dressing placed over the arterial puncture site for bleeding or hematoma; and providing pain medication, especially for the relief of site or back discomfrt (common with 4–6 hours of required bed rest after arterial puncture).

NURSE ADVISORY

After arteriography, be alert to changes that indicate bleeding or hematoma formation: change in sensorium, increased restlessness, sensation of wetness at the site of arterial puncture, drop in blood pressure, increased pulse rate, or decrease in peripheral pulse.

   b. In **digital subtraction angiography,** a series of x-ray films allows either the arterial or the venous system to be seen.

Procedure 24–3
Detection of Edema in an Extremity
by Leg Measurements

Definition/Purpose: To determine the presence or absence of swelling in the lower extremities

Learning/Teaching Activities: Provide the following information: (a) describe the procedure; (b) instruct the person that the procedure will not cause discomfort.

(continued)

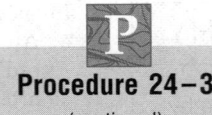

Procedure 24–3
(continued)

Preliminary Activities

Equipment
• Flexible measuring tape in centimeters and inches

Procedure

Actions	Rationale/Discussion
1. Ask the person to lie down.	
2. Mark and measure the widest parts of the ankle, calf, and thigh on each extremity.	2. To provide a consistent anatomic place of measurement.
3. Record baseline measurements with date and time.	3. Baseline measurements can be compared with subsequent measurements to detect changes.
4. Compare measurements of 1 leg with those of the other.	4. A significant difference in males is 1.5 cm between legs or compared with baseline. In females difference is 1.2 cm between legs or compared with baseline.
5. Repeat measurements at the same time of the day.	5. To ensure consistency because leg edema may change with increased activity during the day.

(1) Radiopaque dye is injected into a vein.
(2) A digital computer processor receives x-rays that pass through the body, strike the image intensifier, and are converted to light. These images are then converted into electronic signals sent to the computer.
(3) The digital subtraction technique eliminates all background structures, including bone and gas, leaving only the contrast-containing structures.
(4) Smaller amounts of contrast medium can be used to visualize blood vessels, minimizing the "dye load" needed. In individuals who cannot tolerate a high "dye load" (e.g., those with renal insufficiency), digital subtraction angiography may be a preferred option.

◼ ARTERIAL DISEASE

Definition

1. Arterial disease occurs when there is atherosclerotic narrowing or obstruction of the lumen of the arteries that supply blood to the lower extremities.
2. Stages of arterial disease. The Fontaine classification describes the progression of atherosclerosis of the arteries to the lower extremities.
   a. Stage 1: pathologic changes within the arteries but no symptoms
   b. Stage 2: intermittent claudication
   c. Stage 3: rest pain–indicative of more severe atherosclerotic disease
   d. Stage 4: necrosis and trophic lesions

Incidence and Socioeconomic Impact

1. Estimates suggest that more than 2 million people in the United States have arterial disease.
2. In the United States, atherosclerosis is the leading cause of death in individuals 65 years of age or older.
3. Atherosclerosis in the arteries of the lower extremities is one of the strongest predictors of atherosclerosis elsewhere in the vascular system.
4. Commonly, clinical manifestations of arterial insufficiency develop in people between ages 50 and 70.

Risk Factors

1. Family history of arterial disease
2. Age older than 50 years
3. Hyperlipidemia
4. Smoking or tobacco use in other forms (e.g., chewing tobacco, snuff)
5. Hypertension
6. Diabetes mellitus
7. Sedentary lifestyle
8. Obesity
9. Stress

Etiology

1. Atherosclerosis is the most common cause of arterial disease (see Chapter 23).
2. Arteriosclerosis is another cause, typically seen in the older population.

Pathophysiology

1. The pathophysiology of arterial disorders is best understood by considering the circulatory needs of body tissues. A reduction or occlusion of blood flow occurs in all types of arterial disease.
2. Arteriosclerosis occurs when arteries—through aging, pathologic processes, or both—lose their elasticity and harden.
   a. Loss of elasticity negatively affects the flow of blood through the vascular channels.
   b. The hardening process causes changes in the arterial intima that create a rough surface inside the artery, where plaque formation and platelet aggregation develop.

Clinical Manifestations

1. Intermittent claudication: muscle cramping, burning, or pain that occurs with exercise or activity and is relieved by rest
   a. The discomfort occurs when blood flow is insufficient to meet the needs of the muscles and tissues. Lactic acid and carbon dioxide then accumulate.
   b. Symptoms can be seen in any major muscle group below the site of the atherosclerotic stenosis.
      (1) In aortoiliac disease, claudication is seen in the buttocks, hips, or thighs on the side where the lesion is found.
      (2) In femoral-popliteal disease, calf claudication is noted in the affected extremity.
   c. Intermittent claudication is seen when blood flow with exertion is inadequate to meet the needs of tissues.
2. Rest pain occurs when blood flow is inadequate, even with no activity, to meet the needs of tissues in the extremities.
   a. Rest pain often is described as a sensation of burning or numbness aggravated by leg elevation.
   b. Rest pain can sometimes be relieved by dangling the affected extremity off the side of the bed. Dangling pools blood in the extremity and thereby improves the oxygen supply to the tissues.
3. With severe stenosis or occlusion, trophic changes in the involved limb occur along with skin breakdown, ulcers, and ultimately, gangrene.

Diagnostics

1. Assessment
   a. History
      (1) Family history of vascular disease, hypertension, hyperlipidemia, cardiovascular disease, or diabetes mellitus
      (2) Risk factors
      (3) Any past vascular surgery or trauma
      (4) Presence or history of slow, nonhealing wounds
      (5) Approximate intake of foods high in cholesterol, attitudes toward food, and resistance toward therapeutic alterations in the diet
      (6) Actual weight compared with ideal weight for height and age
      (7) Tobacco history, habits, and attitudes
      (8) Exercise tolerance and preferred form of exercise
      (9) Activity patterns required in work setting
      (10) Preferred leg position for sleep (e.g., legs in a dangling position)
   b. Physical examination (see p. 1093)
2. Medical diagnosis determines the location of the arterial disease, severity of the disease process, degree of ischemia, and adequacy of collateral circulation.

Clinical Management

1. Goal of clinical management: to control the progress of the disease
2. Nonpharmacologic interventions focus on risk factor modification
   a. Cessation of tobacco use
   b. Dietary changes to control hyperlipidemia. Goals are reduction of saturated fat intake and increased use of polyunsaturated varieties, reduction of total fat intake to no more than 30 percent of total calories, and reduction of cholesterol intake to no more than 300 mg per day
   c. Blood pressure control through relaxation techniques, imagery, or biofeedback
   d. Initiation of an individualized exercise program, for example, walking on a level surface for 20 minutes at least 3 times a week. Also, to promote circulation in the lower extremities, teach the person how to perform Buerger-Allen exercises (Learning/Teaching Guidelines for Performing Buerger-Allen exercises).
3. Pharmacologic interventions
   a. Vasodilators
      (1) Vasodilators have not proved particularly successful in treatment of the disease process because peripheral vasodilation normally occurs distal to sites of significant arterial stenosis.
      (2) An example of a vasodilator is papaverine hydrochloride.
   b. Pentoxifylline improves blood flow by decreasing blood viscosity and increasing red blood cell flexibility.
   c. Platelet inhibitors
      (1) These drugs inhibit platelet adhesion to subendothelium and have been reported to decrease progression of atherosclerosis.
      (2) Examples of these medications include aspirin, dipyridamole, and ticlopidine.
      (3) The effectiveness of platelet inhibitors in the treatment of vascular disease continues to be established through research.
   d. Thrombolytic agents
      (1) Thrombolytic agents activate the conversion of plasminogen to plasmin.
      (2) Normally, the body takes days to break down a blood clot. Thrombolytic agents speed the process to reestablish blood flow to affected tissues.

LEARNING/TEACHING GUIDELINES
for Performing Buerger-Allen Exercises

Purpose

1. To teach an individual active exercises that will alternatively fill and empty the blood vessels, promoting circulation.

Caution

1. These exercises are prescribed according to the condition of the person and the extremity.
2. The individual must be able to comprehend and follow commands.
3. Continued and prolonged severe pain in the affected extremity is a contraindication.
4. Other vascular conditions for which these exercises are not indicated include deep vein thrombosis, cellulitis, and ischemic changes of gangrene.

Guidelines for Teaching Buerger-Allen Exercises

1. Ask the person to lie flat, then elevate the legs above the heart for 2 minutes or until blanching of the skin occurs.
2. Allow the legs to be dependent; exercise the feet approximately 3 minutes or until the legs are pink.
3. Instruct the person to lie flat for approximately 5 minutes.
4. Repeat steps 1, 2, and 3 a total of 5 times.
5. Do the entire set 3 times each day.

---

(3) Thrombolytic agents include streptokinase, urokinase, and tissue plasminogen activator (TPA).

e. Anticoagulants

(1) Anticoagulants prevent propagation of a clot but do not enhance clot lysis.

(2) Anticoagulants are also used prophylactically to prevent the development of clots.

(3) Heparin acts by binding to thrombin and inhibiting conversion of fibrinogen to fibrin.

DRUG ADVISORY

Adverse effects of heparin

1. Bleeding—overall risk around 9 percent. The risk is dose related.
2. Osteoporosis—seen with doses greater than 15,000 units per day for 5 to 6 months.
3. Thrombocytopenia—generally transient. Clotting times return to normal within 2 to 4 days after infusion is stopped.
4. Hypercoagulable states—increased risk of reclotting after 3 days of heparin therapy. Hypercoagulability is the therapeutic reason for overlapping heparin and warfarin therapies.

(4) Warfarin inhibits synthesis of vitamin K–dependent factors (II, VII, IX, X) and vitamin K–dependent anticoagulants (protein C and protein S).

DRUG ADVISORY

Adverse effects of warfarin

1. Bleeding—occurs in 4 percent of people when the prothrombin time (PT) is 1.3 times control and in 22 percent of people when the PT is 1.4 to 2.0 times control.
2. Fetal abnormalities—warfarin crosses the placental barrier and may place the fetus at risk for either hemorrhage or teratogenic effects.
3. Purple toe syndrome—occurs infrequently. Purple toes are seen 3 to 8 weeks after initiation of therapy and are felt to be related to cholesterol microembolization.

f. Antihypertensive agents

(1) Limits further vascular injury due to hypertension

4. Special medical-surgical procedures

a. Percutaneous balloon angioplasty (PTBA)

(1) This procedure involves inserting a catheter percutaneously (usually in the femoral artery) and passing it into the stenotic area (see Fig. 23–16).

(2) The physician then inflates the catheter's balloon, compressing the plaque against the wall of the artery.

b. Laser angioplasty

(1) A fiberoptic laser catheter, with or without a balloon tip, is used to open localized, short occlusions of the iliac artery, superficial femoral artery, and above-the-knee popliteal arteries.

(2) The procedure has a relatively high rate of restenosis when compared with that of PTBA. Studies are continuing on its effectiveness.

c. Atherectomy

(1) Atherectomy is a percutaneous procedure in which a special atherectomy catheter with a rotating tip selectively pulverizes atheromatous plaque.

(2) In studies to date, the restenosis rate has been higher with atherectomy than with PTBA.

(3) Although atherectomy is not widely used, the U.S. Food and Drug Administration has approved its limited use in clinical practice.

d. Flexible coil stents

(1) A **stent** is a continuous strand of surgical-grade stainless-steel wire.

(2) The wire is folded back and forth to form a series of loops (like the spring inside a ballpoint pen), then wrapped around a compliant balloon catheter to form a cylinder or tube of interdigitating loops.

(3) In arteries considered prone to restenosis after PTBA, the flexible coil stent can be implanted to prevent arterial closure.

(4) Stents are currently used in coronary, renal, iliac, and femoral arteries.

e. Bypass surgery

(1) The goal of bypass surgery is to restore blood flow by bypassing the occluded artery segments.

(2) Materials used for bypass grafting include autogenous vein (vein from the person's body) and synthetic graft material (Dacron or Teflon).

(3) Bypass procedures are performed under general or regional anesthesia, depending on the patient's age and general medical history and the estimated period required for the procedure. Minimizing cardiovascular stress during surgery is an important goal.

ELDER ADVISORY

Because atherosclerosis in the lower extremities is often a predictor of atherosclerosis elsewhere, older people undergoing vascular bypass procedures should be observed carefully for development of cardiac or cerebrovascular symptoms.

---

(4) Preoperative angiography establishes the exact location of stenosis and allows the surgeon to select the best site for placement of the proximal and distal anastomoses.

(5) Bypass procedures are classified according to the area where the graft is placed: proximal (above the site of stenosis) or distal (below the stenosis).

(6) Commonly performed bypass procedures include aortobifemoral, femoral to femoral, femoral-popliteal, and femoral-tibial (Fig. 24–6).

(7) Amputation: After attempts at limb salvage fail, amputation may be the only way to eliminate rest pain, infection, or extensive gangrene.

Five levels of lower extremity amputation are currently used: foot and ankle, below-knee, knee disarticulation, above-knee, and hip disarticulation.

Complications

1. Arterial disease can significantly reduce the quality of life.
2. Arterial disease can affect any of the arteries of the lower extremities, leading to skin breakdown, ulcer formation, and, ultimately, gangrene requiring amputation.
3. Between 30,000 and 100,000 people in the United States undergo lower extremity amputation annually.

Prognosis

1. Early detection and treatment allow people with arterial disease to live normal lives.
2. For persons who are treated medically with regular follow-up visits that allow early detection and treatment of potential complications, the amputation rate is only about 7 percent.

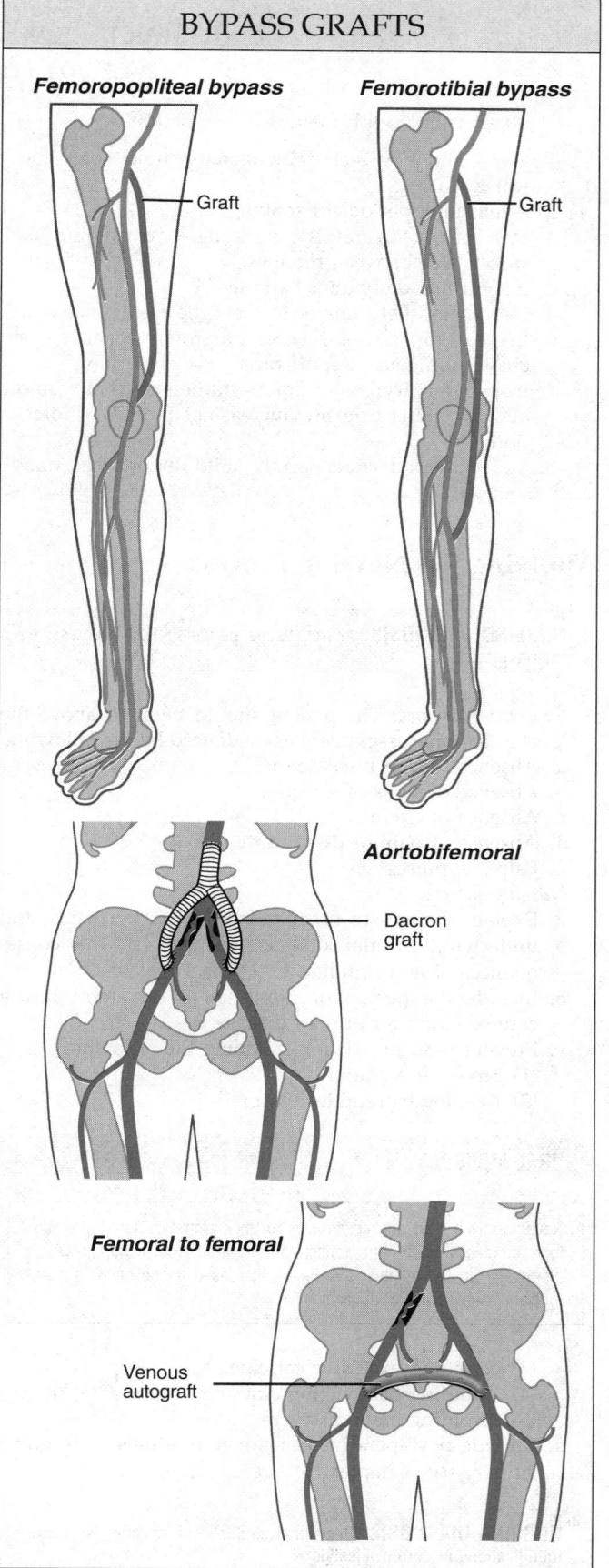

BYPASS GRAFTS

Femoropopliteal bypass

Graft

Femorotibial bypass

Graft

Aortobifemoral

Dacron graft

Femoral to femoral

Venous autograft

Figure 24–6.

LEARNING/TEACHING GUIDELINES
for Foot Care

Instruct people with Buerger's disease to

1. Wash and dry feet daily using a mild soap and warm water.
2. Avoid long periods of soaking.
3. Dry each foot carefully, avoiding hard rubbing. Be sure to dry between the toes.
4. Inspect feet daily after bathing.
5. Use a hand-held mirror to view the feet, if needed.
6. Inspect for blisters, sores, ingrown toenails, or changes in color. Report these to a physician.
7. Inspect for dryness or cracks in the skin that would allow bacteria to grow, increasing the risk of infection.
8. To prevent dryness, apply mild lotion that does

not contain alcohol. Avoid putting lotion of any type between toes or in open sores.
9. Use correct technique for toenail clipping: cut nails straight across; do not dig around corners; file toenails with an emery board to the contour of the toe. Treat cracked or split nails with mineral oil.
10. Pad overlapping toes with cotton.
11. Inspect shoes for proper fit. Shoes that allow ½ to ¾ inch of toe room are recommended. Shoes with hard soles and soft tops are best.
12. Avoid clothing such as girdles, garters, tight socks, or pantyhose, which can restrict circulation.
13. Avoid walking in bare feet.
14. Do not use heating pads.

Applying the Nursing Process

NURSING DIAGNOSIS: Altered tissue perfusion R/T progressive arterial disease

1. *Expected outcomes:* The patient should be at or above the level of baseline assessment as evidenced by the following:
   a. Absence of skin breakdown
   b. Absence of signs of infection
   c. Absence of edema
   d. Absence of pain or discomfort
   e. Palpable pulses
2. *Nursing interventions*
   a. Explain the causes of decreased tissue perfusion and underlying arterial disease, as well as the consequences of noncompliance.
   b. Include the person or family in a long-term health care program for arterial disease.
   c. Prevent vasoconstriction by doing the following:
      (1) Smoking cessation
      (2) Keeping extremities warm

NURSE ADVISORY

Never apply a heat source directly to an extremity. Tissue metabolism increases with heat application. In arterial disease, in which blood flow to the tissues is reduced, increased tissue needs are not met and ischemia may develop.

      (3) Avoiding excessive caffeine
      (4) Avoiding constricting clothing or shoes
      (5) Avoiding emotional stress
   d. Provide postoperative care for individuals undergoing surgery (see Chapter 13).

NURSING DIAGNOSIS: Decisional conflict R/T making risk factor modifications in current lifestyle

1. *Expected outcomes:* The person should be able to do the following:
   a. Acknowledge fear and anxiety regarding ability or desire to make needed changes
   b. Identify and draw on personal, cultural, and religious values to assist in decision making regarding changes
   c. Solve problems, make decisions, and express satisfaction with plans
2. *Nursing interventions*
   a. Assess strengths and weaknesses for coping with needed lifestyle changes; then alter the plan of care, if necessary.
   b. Correct misconceptions by providing information about risk factor modifications.
   c. Provide opportunities to make small decisions in regard to changes. Accept the patient's choices.
   d. Encourage verbalization of fears and anxieties regarding lifestyle modifications.
   e. Encourage the person to ask questions and to keep follow-up appointments with the physician.
   f. Refer to other resources as needed (e.g., smoking cessation programs, weight management programs, vascular rehabilitation programs, clergy, clinical nurse specialist, or psychologist).

Discharge Planning and Teaching

1. Before discharge, people need to learn about arterial disease and its treatment, including risk factor modification principles, exercise, foot care, and medications (Learning/Teaching Guidelines for Foot Care).
2. Make referrals to smoking cessation groups.
3. Enlist dietary consults to aid in meal planning, weight control, and special diets (e.g., diabetic, low-cholesterol, low-sodium, low-fat, or low-caffeine).
4. Make referrals for outpatient exercise programs.

Public Health Considerations

1. Morbidity figures show a high incidence of atherosclerosis in the United States.

HOME CARE STRATEGIES

Peripheral Vascular Disease

Home care provides an opportunity for patients with peripheral vascular disease (PVD) to control their symptoms through informed decision making.

ASSESSMENT

Cardiovascular Status

- Ask to have television, vacuum cleaner, and other noise-making appliances turned off when listening to heart and lung sounds.
- Mark a spot with indelible ink and measure edema. Instruct the home health aide to re-mark the spot when bathing. Show the patient "thumbprints" for baseline.
- Use the scale in the home, if available, to weigh the patient.

Medication

- Evaluate availability and storage.
- A weekly pillbox can serve as a reminder to the patient and a monitoring device to the nurse.
- Have the patient tell you why he or she takes each drug and what is different after taking it.

Diet

- Seek the opinion of the patient and caregiver on how they feel they are doing regarding diet compliance.
- Check cupboards and refrigerator. Ask specific questions about food preferences.

PATIENT TEACHING

When to Call the Physician

- Pain worse than usual.
- Blue extremities that do not improve with elevation.
- Side effects of medication that interfere with compliance. For example, furosemide (Lasix) taken twice a day prevents going out to dinner.
- Weight gain of 3 pounds in 1 day or worsening "thumbprints."

Prevention of Recurrence

- Stress how medication controls the disease and what activities become more feasible.
- Make a written schedule based on the patient's lifestyle.
- Explain the interaction of medication with food or other drugs (e.g., Coumadin and spinach).
- Explain how to manage the side effects of medication. For example, increase roughage and fluids to combat analgesic-induced constipation.

Diet is Usually Low Sodium and Cholesterol

- Discuss the relationship among sodium, cholesterol, and PVD.
- With patient and caregiver, read labels from their own cupboard and refrigerator.
- Help patient make choices and substitutions using favorite foods.
- Limit changes to 1 per week.

Reevaluate with Patient and Caregiver

- Stick with what works and question why something has not worked. Then modify and try again.

2. Many cases of arterial disease go undiscovered because of lack of public knowledge and understanding of the disease.
3. National efforts involve enlisting public and private support to increase public awareness of the disease.
4. To control the disease, health care providers need to direct interventions toward early primary prevention, especially risk factor modification.

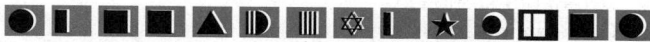

TRANSCULTURAL CONSIDERATIONS

With the lack of overt signs and symptoms in the early stages of arterial disease, members of many ethnic and racial groups seldom believe that any pathology is present without functional impairment. More public education is needed to increase public awareness and emphasize the need for early primary and secondary prevention.

ACUTE ARTERIAL OCCLUSION AND EMBOLISM

Definition

1. **Arterial occlusion** is the complete blockage of an artery by embolism, thrombosis in an already narrowed artery, or trauma.
2. **Thrombosis** is the development of a blood clot.
3. **Embolism** is a piece of a thrombus that has broken off at the point of formation and traveled through a blood vessel to another part of the circulatory system.
4. **Ischemia** is a condition in which blood supply is inadequate to meet the metabolic needs of the tissues.
5. **Gangrene** is the necrosis or death of tissue as a result of deficient or absent blood supply.

Incidence and Socioeconomic Impact

1. Sudden arterial occlusion occurs in approximately 10 percent of cases of arterial disease.
2. The primary risk is limb loss, which can be prevented if circulation to the extremity is restored before the development of irreversible ischemia.
3. Another effect is prolonged length of stay for already hospitalized patients.
4. Emergency medical intervention is required to successfully treat arterial occlusion and prevent limb loss.

Risk Factors

Risk factors are conditions or disease processes that predispose an individual to thrombosis or embolization, such as the following:

1. Atrial fibrillation
2. Acute myocardial infarction

3. Rheumatic mitral stenosis
4. Atherosclerosis
5. Prosthetic cardiac valves
6. Shock
7. Congestive heart failure
8. Abnormal blood coagulation
9. Use of birth control pills
10. Infection
11. Trauma
12. Arterial dissection
13. Collagen diseases (e.g., lupus erythematosus, rheumatoid arthritis)
14. Bacterial endocarditis
15. Aneurysm
16. Advanced metastatic disease
17. Immobility
18. Post parturition

Etiology

1. The primary cause of acute arterial occlusion is arterial embolism.
2. Arterial emboli most often originate in the left side of the heart during an episode of atrial fibrillation.
3. Less frequently, emboli arise from atherosclerotic plaque or an aneurysm within the arterial tree.

Pathophysiology

1. Acute arterial occlusion reduces blood flow to areas within the arterial tree below the level of obstruction.
2. The limb area below the obstruction develops ischemia.
3. The degree of ischemia depends on the size of the occluded artery and the extent of collateral circulation.
4. In general, the larger the occluded artery, the greater the degree of ischemia in the distal limb segment.
5. It is theorized that the embolus releases vasoactive factors (e.g., serotonin) at the site of occlusion and that vasospasm further aggravates the ischemia.
6. Prolonged irreversible ischemia can lead to gangrene in the affected extremity.

Clinical Manifestations

1. Sudden cessation of blood flow to an extremity, which produces severe pain in about three fourths of cases
2. Muscle weakness
3. Loss of pulses below the occlusion
4. Possible paralysis
5. Cyanosis, pallor, and coldness in the affected extremity
6. Paresthesia (numbness or tingling sensations)

Diagnostics

1. Assessment
   a. History
      (1) Note any risk factors.

(2) Ask the patient for a detailed pain description.
   b. Physical examination
      (1) Assess skin for pallor, cyanosis, or coldness of any extremities.
      (2) Palpate all peripheral pulses.
      (3) Check motor and sensory function of the extremities.
2. Medical diagnosis
   a. Diagnosis rests on the clinical manifestations of the disease process.
   b. Commonly, diagnosis is based on the sudden onset of pain and ischemia in an extremity.
   c. Arteriography is used to confirm the diagnosis, establish the location and extent of the blockage, and determine the extent of collateralization.

Clinical Management

1. Goal of clinical management: to restore patency of the occluded artery
2. Nonpharmacologic interventions
   a. Bed rest
   b. Limb placed in a slightly dependent position
   c. Bed cradle
3. Pharmacologic interventions
   a. A thrombolytic agent is administered in persons having no contraindications to thrombolytic therapy. In smaller arteries that are occluded or in persons who are not good surgical candidates, an infusion of either intravenous or intra-arterial thrombolytic agents can be used.

 DRUG ADVISORY

Contraindications to Thrombolytic Therapy

Absolute Contraindications
- Active internal bleeding
- Known coagulation disorder (e.g., hemophilia)
- Recent cerebrovascular accident
- Brain tumor, arteriovenous malformation, or aneurysm
- Recent intracranial or intraspinal surgery
- Recent major trauma
- Recent major surgery

Relative Contraindications
- Severe uncontrolled hypertension
- Recent gastrointestinal bleeding
- Hemorrhagic diabetic retinopathy
- Severe liver or kidney disease
- Pregnancy
- Bacterial endocarditis

---

   b. Streptokinase, produced by hemolytic streptococci, is the oldest of the 3 thrombolytic agents used today.
      (1) Streptokinase is not clot specific; instead it breaks down clots throughout the body.
      (2) After a single use, antibodies are formed to the drug, often rendering it ineffective for future therapy.

LEARNING/TEACHING GUIDELINES
for People on Warfarin

Patients on warfarin should follow these guidelines:

1. Always remember—you are a vital part of the health care team!
2. Warfarin is an anticoagulant, a "blood thinner," that interferes with the blood's ability to clot, thus preventing blood clots from forming in your arteries or veins. Warfarin does not dissolve clots that are already present.
3. Warfarin comes in different-strength tablets that are color coded and inscribed with the dosage: 2 mg (lavender), 2½ mg (green), 5 mg (peach), 7½ mg (yellow), and 10 mg (white).
4. While you are taking warfarin, you must see your physician regularly.
5. The physician determines if your blood clots too slowly or too quickly with laboratory tests, prothrombin time (sometimes abbreviated PT or protime) or INR (international normalized ratio).
6. The laboratory tests PT or INR measure the blood's ability to clot.
7. Each time your blood is tested by the laboratory, your physician's office or clinic will let you know if you are to make any changes in the dosage of warfarin. Your physician will do one of the following: increase, decrease, or keep your dose of warfarin the same.
8. Bleeding is the main side effect that you must watch for. Notify your physician if you notice any of the following symptoms: nosebleeds, bleeding gums, blood in the urine or stool, coughing up blood, sudden appearance of numerous bruises over the body, or any other kind of bleeding without apparent cause.
9. Many medications, both prescription and nonprescription, can interact with warfarin. For example, over-the-counter cold preparations containing aspirin can increase the effect of warfarin, whereas certain sleeping pills can slow its effects.
10. Check with your physician or pharmacist before taking any new medications to be sure they will not interact with warfarin.
11. Tell your physician before stopping or starting any medications, including vitamins.
12. Vitamin K counteracts warfarin's effect on blood clotting.
13. Vitamin K is found in green leafy vegetables and in some vitamins. You do not have to avoid these foods or vitamins. Simply let your physician know if you change your diet pattern or begin taking vitamins so your dosage of warfarin can be regulated accordingly.
14. Alcohol (mixed drinks, beer, and wine) increases the effect of warfarin. Check with your physician for guidelines.
15. Take the dose of warfarin at the same time every day. If you forget a dose, do not double the next dose. Call your physician for instructions.
16. Before undergoing any invasive procedure, notify your dentist, nurse, or physician that you are taking warfarin.
17. Carry identification in your wallet or purse stating that you are on warfarin.
18. Do not stop taking warfarin unless advised to do so by your physician.

Table 24–3. Anticoagulation Agents

	Heparin Sodium	Warfarin
Actions	Inhibits reactions that lead to the formation of fibrin clots.	Inhibits the synthesis of vitamin K–dependent coagulation factors.
Route	Administered IV or subq—is not absorbed orally.	Administered only orally.
Comments	Used for short-term therapy. Does not cross the placental barrier.	Has a lag period of 2–3 days before the effect is noticeable.
Laboratory tests	PTT to measure clotting.	PT or INR to measure clotting.
Laboratory values	Goal is to attain PTT 1.5–2.5 times the normal control value.	Goal is to attain PT 1.3–2.0 times the normal control value or INR of 2.0–3.0.
Adverse effect	Bleeding	Bleeding
Nursing considerations	Correct technique for subq injections: grasp roll of skin gently; inject needle quickly at a right angle; avoid rubbing skin, but press alcohol wipe to site. Rotate sites.	Many different drugs interact with warfarin. Some drugs increase the effect of warfarin (e.g., salicylates) while others decrease its effect (e.g., barbiturates).
Antidote	Protamine sulfate	Vitamin K

IV, Intravenously; subq, subcutaneously; PTT, partial thromboplastin time; PT, prothrombin time; INR, international normalized ratio.

(3) Streptokinase is antigenic in some persons; fever and allergic reactions may occur. Some reactions can be life threatening.

c. Urokinase is not a foreign protein and is produced from human sources.

(1) Urokinase does not cause antibody formation and can be used repeatedly in the same person without inactivation.

(2) Compared with streptokinase, urokinase has a lower incidence of bleeding-related complications.

d. Tissue plasminogen activator is a naturally occurring plasminogen activator secreted by the vascular endothelium of many tissues.

(1) This activator is produced by recombinant DNA techniques and has a short half-life (3–7 min).

(2) Unlike streptokinase and urokinase, TPA is clot specific.

(3) The specific agent, dosage, and duration of therapy are individualized based on clinical presentation and body weight.

(4) Anticoagulant therapy is recommended at the end of thrombolytic therapy. For example, heparin infusion followed by oral anticoagulation with warfarin can prevent recurrent thrombosis (Table 24–3).

NURSE ADVISORY

Bleeding is a common complication of heparin and warfarin use. Protamine sulfate is used to terminate heparin's activity almost immediately. Vitamin K is used to counteract the effects of warfarin by returning the clotting time to normal control values within 4 to 24 hours.

---

4. Special medical-surgical procedures

a. Surgical embolectomy is the preferred treatment when larger arteries are occluded.

b. Balloon embolectomy is performed to remove the thrombus (Fig. 24–7 and page 1107 for postoperative nursing care).

c. The etiology of the acute occlusion, the duration of occlusion, the presence of distal embolization, and the severity of ischemia influence the choice of treatment.

Complications

1. Possible loss of an organ, limb, or life
2. Embolization in another part of the body

Prognosis

1. Early intervention is critical because muscles and nerves develop irreversible damage within 4 to 8 hours after acute arterial occlusion.
2. Several other key factors play a role in the outcome: the age and general health of the patient, the size of the

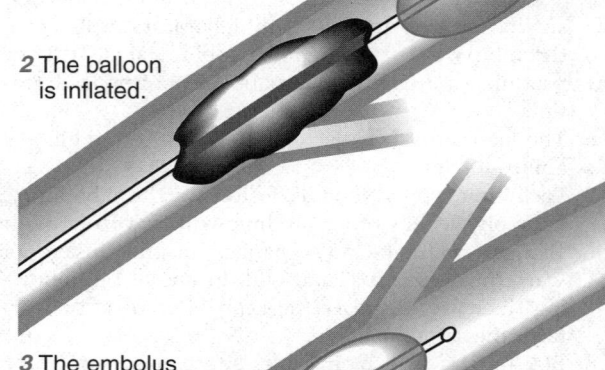

BALLOON EMBOLECTOMY

1 Deflated balloon catheter is passed in the vessel beyond the embolus.

Embolus

Balloon catheter

2 The balloon is inflated.

3 The embolus and its thrombus are removed.

Figure 24–7. A deflated balloon catheter is passed in the vessel past the embolus (1); the balloon is inflated (2); and the embolus and its thrombus are removed (3).

artery involved, the presence of distal embolization, and the extent of collateral circulation.

Applying the Nursing Process

NURSING DIAGNOSIS: Altered tissue perfusion R/T acute arterial occlusion

1. *Expected outcomes:* After intervention, the patient should exhibit the following signs of normal tissue perfusion:

a. Return of audible Doppler signal or palpable pulse
b. Return of normal color, sensation, and motor function
c. Significant decrease in or absence of pain
2. *Nursing interventions*
   a. Provide routine postoperative care for patients undergoing surgical procedures (see Chapter 13).
   b. Assess peripheral pulses every 1 to 2 hours and as needed.
   c. Assess sensory and motor function of the affected extremity every 4 hours and as needed.
   d. Assess the pain level and provide pain relief medications as indicated.
   e. Monitor vital signs every 4 hours and as needed.
   f. Maintain the person on strict bed rest initially; then allow activity as indicated and tolerated.
   g. Administer anticoagulant and thrombolytic agents as ordered.
   h. Monitor prothrombin time, partial thromboplastin time, hemoglobin, hematocrit, international normalized ratio, and platelet counts daily or as ordered, depending on type of anticoagulant therapy.

NURSING DIAGNOSIS: Fear R/T possible limb loss

1. *Expected outcomes:* The person should be able to do the following:
   a. Freely discuss fears, questions, and concerns regarding potential limb loss
   b. Verbalize basic knowledge of arterial occlusion and the treatment plan
   c. Participate in planning care
2. *Nursing interventions*
   a. Acknowledge and encourage discussion of fears of limb loss. Help distinguish between healthy and unhealthy fears.
   b. Actively listen to the individual's concerns.
   c. Provide information and teaching regarding acute arterial occlusion.
   d. Correct any misconceptions about care and treatment.
   e. Include the individual and family members in planning care.
   f. Review the use of antianxiety medications and provide as ordered.

Discharge Planning and Teaching

Before discharge, people need to learn about arterial occlusive disease and its treatment; they need information about activity, wound care, foot care, and medications (Learning/Teaching Guidelines for Foot Care and Learning/Teaching Guidelines for Persons on Warfarin).

Public Health Considerations

1. Educate the public to seek early medical intervention and not delay treatment.
2. Medical personnel should be familiar with the clinical manifestations so that triage occurs quickly (i.e., time is muscle).

3. More research is needed to determine whether and when low-dose anticoagulation is indicated in individuals at high risk for acute arterial embolism.

■ ABDOMINAL AORTIC ANEURYSMS

Definition

1. An **abdominal aortic aneurysm** is an abnormal dilation, resulting from localized weakness and stretching of the arterial wall. The aneurysm can be located anywhere along the abdominal aorta.
2. Classifications (Fig. 24–8)
   a. A **fusiform aneurysm** is a diffuse dilation that in-

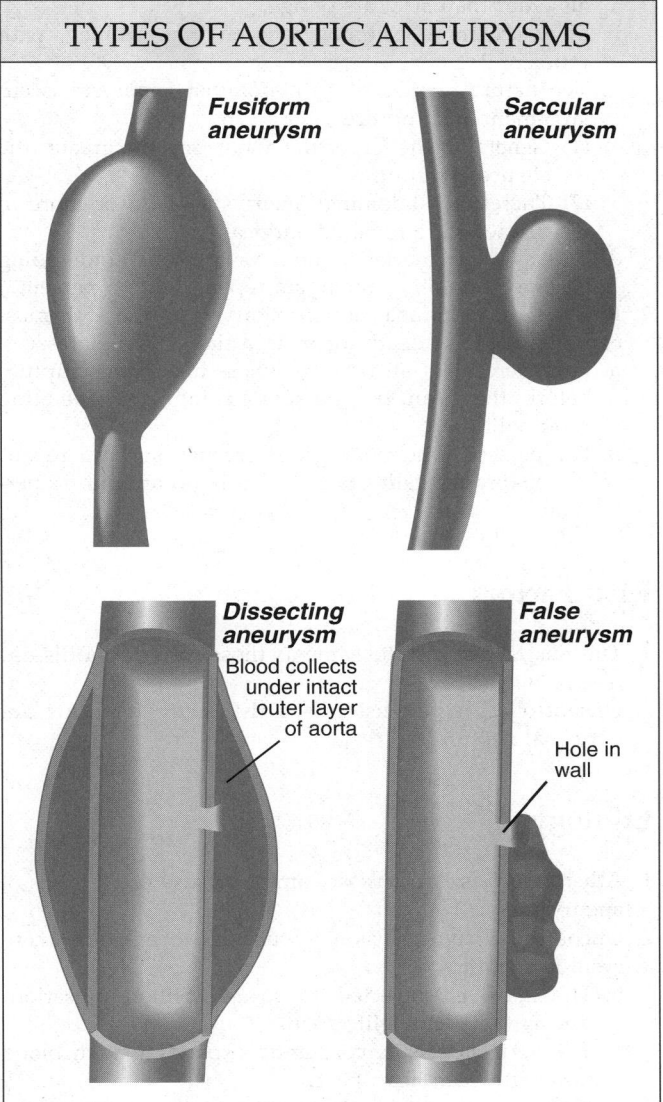

Figure 24–8.

volves the entire circumference of the arterial segment.

b. A **saccular aneurysm** is a distinct, localized outpouching of the artery wall.

c. A **dissecting aneurysm** is created when blood separates the layers of an artery wall, forming a cavity between them.

d. A **false aneurysm (pseudoaneurysm)** occurs when the clot and connective tissue are outside the arterial wall. A false aneurysm is a pulsating hematoma formed after complete rupture of an artery and subsequent formation of a scar sac, composed of connective tissue and old blood clot.

Incidence and Socioeconomic Impact

1. Approximately 36.5 abdominal aortic aneurysms are diagnosed per 100,000 individuals.

   a. Abdominal aneurysms are most common in individuals older than 50 years of age.

   b. They are more common in men than women, with ratios of 2:1.

   c. The natural course of an abdominal aneurysm is enlargement and rupture.

   (1) Generally, the larger the aneurysm, the greater the chance of rupture.

   (2) Therefore, abdominal aneurysms 4 cm or more in diameter are repaired surgically.

   d. The average mortality rate for persons undergoing elective abdominal aneurysm repair is 4 to 5 percent.

2. Rupture of abdominal aortic aneurysm is the 15th most common cause of death for men in the United States.

   a. Fifty percent of all persons whose aneurysms rupture before they can be transported into the operating room will die.

   b. For persons who undergo emergency surgical repair, the 30-day mortality rate is also high, around 54 percent.

Risk Factors

1. The risk factors are the same as those for arterial disease (see p. 1098).

2. Uncontrolled hypertension is a risk factor for acute aneurysmal rupture.

Etiology

1. Atherosclerosis is the most common cause of all types of aneurysms.

2. Uncontrolled hypertension is believed to enhance aneurysm formation.

   a. The aorta is subjected to several billion pulsations during the average life span.

   b. The aorta is elastic, constantly expanding with blood flow with each heart beat.

   c. Hypertension causes destruction of the media of the aorta and decreased intimal adherence.

d. With prolonged and uncontrolled high blood pressure, the wall of the aorta weakens, enhancing aneurysm formation and possibly rupture.

3. Less commonly, abdominal aortic aneurysms are seen with inherited or congenital syndromes, such as Marfan syndrome or Ehlers-Danlos syndrome.

4. Infection can cause aortic aneurysms when septicemia seeds a preexisting arterial lesion.

   a. The process of infection weakens the medial layer of the aorta, leading to the aneurysm formation.

   b. In the late stages of syphilis, arterial inflammation and medial wall necrosis weaken the aortic wall.

5. Blunt or sharp trauma, including operative trauma, can damage the aortic wall.

Pathophysiology

1. Most commonly, atherosclerotic plaque collects on the intimal surface of the aorta.

2. The medial layer of the aorta weakens owing to a number of factors, including wear and tear and impaired nutrition.

3. The destruction of the medial layer of a segment of the aorta containing the elastic fibers is believed to lead to aneurysm formation.

4. The most common sites of aneurysm formation are shown in Figure 24–9.

Clinical Manifestations

1. One third of all abdominal aneurysms are found on routine physical examination as a prominent pulsation at or above the umbilicus.

TRANSCULTURAL CONSIDERATIONS

In Hispanic ethnomedicine an abdominal mass is often diagnosed as an *empacho*, a mass or bolus of ingested food believed to be stuck to the stomach or intestinal wall, producing abdominal pain and swelling, nausea, vomiting, anorexia, and diarrhea. Ethnomedicinal treatment consists of vigorous massage of the abdomen and back until a popping or loud cracking sound is heard, indicating dislodgement of the mass. Massage can be done by a family member or traditional healer.

If an abdominal aortic aneurysm is present, education is essential to correct misperceptions that could result in inappropriate or potentially harmful therapy.

2. Many people have no presenting symptoms.

3. When symptoms are present, abdominal or lower back pain is most commonly reported.

4. Tenderness over the site of the aneurysm may be present.

COMMON SITES OF ANEURYSMS

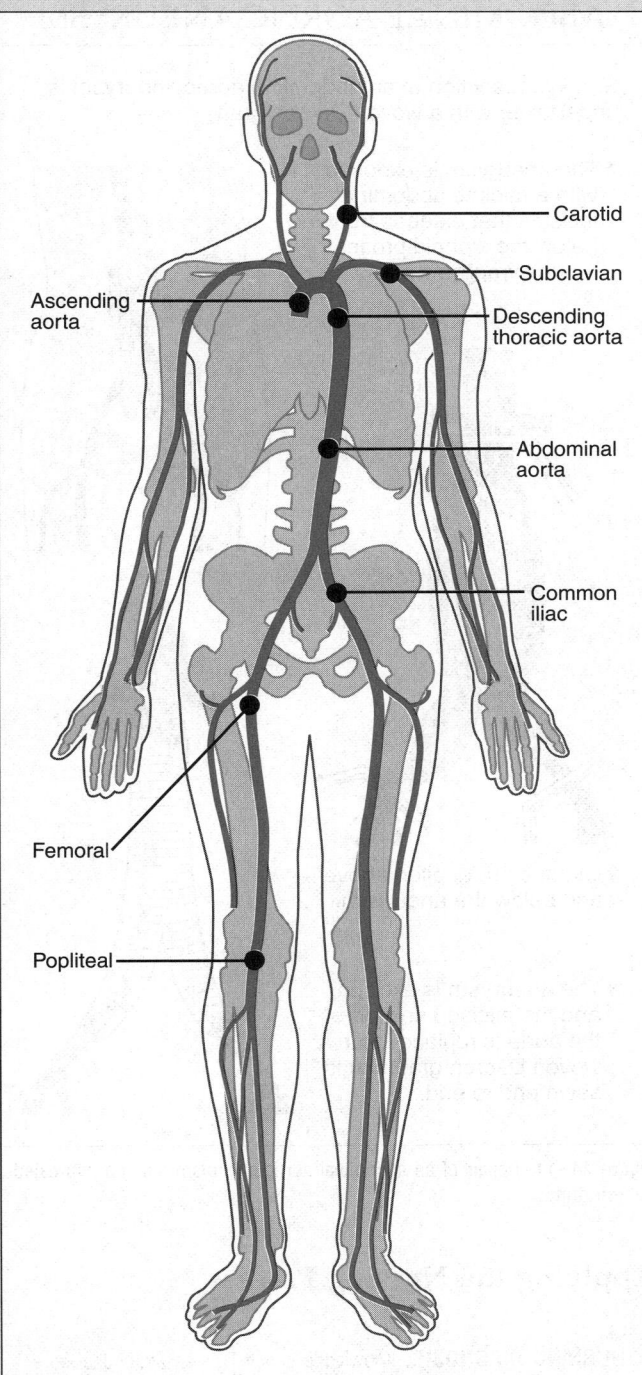

Carotid

Subclavian

Ascending aorta

Descending thoracic aorta

Abdominal aorta

Common iliac

Femoral

Popliteal

Figure 24-9.

5. Tenderness is often seen in the presence of an enlarging aneurysm.
6. Rupture of the aneurysm may be preceded by severe abdominal or back pain, hypotension, and shock.
7. Thrombi may form and then embolize, traveling to other arteries and causing ischemia to develop in the affected limb or limbs.

Diagnostics

1. Assessment
   a. History
      (1) All risk factors for the arterial disease process (see p. 1096)
      (2) Positive family history
      (3) Any back or abdominal pain
      (4) Any sensation of pulsation in the abdominal area
      (5) Any vascular surgical operation or trauma
      (6) Presence or history of slow or nonhealing wounds
   b. Physical examination
      (1) Assess baseline vital signs. Elevated blood pressure places the person at increased risk for rupture due to increased strain on the arterial wall. Sudden development of pain, hypotension, and increased pulse rate could signal aneurysm rupture.
      (2) Inspect the skin for signs of preexisting vascular disease.
      (3) Inspect for skin breakdown.
      (4) Palpate all peripheral pulses.
      (5) Palpate over the umbilicus for a pulsatile abdominal mass (Fig. 24-10).
      (6) Note any tenderness over the aneurysm.
      (7) Auscultate over the aorta and femoral arteries for bruits using the bell of the stethoscope.
2. Medical diagnosis
   a. Often, a palpable mass is felt on routine physical examination.
   b. Several different diagnostic tests may be ordered to confirm the presence and size of the abdominal aneurysm.
      (1) **Abdominal ultrasound** is a noninvasive technique that provides information about the size and location of the aneurysm. Abdominal ultrasound is often used to follow smaller aneurysms and to allow for early detection of enlargement.
      (2) **Computed tomography** is another noninvasive diagnostic tool that allows the clinician to identify the arterial wall of the aorta as well as structures around the aorta.

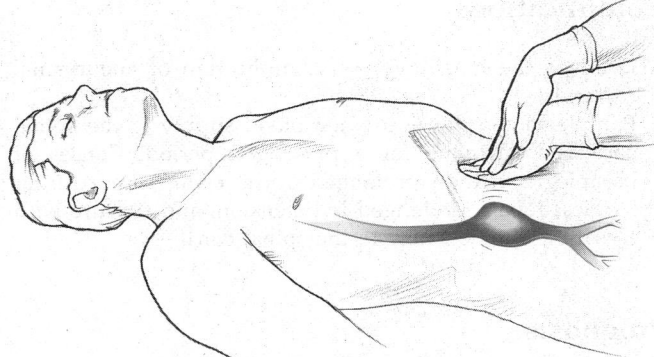

Figure 24-10. Palpation of an abdominal aortic aneurysm. Palpation of an abdominal aortic aneurysm is done by placing the tips of the fingers inward, over the area of the umbilicus. The examiner feels a pulsation against the fingers when an aneurysm is present.

(a) Computed tomography scans are also used to screen and follow aortic aneurysms.

(b) These scans can be used to evaluate postoperative complications, such as graft occlusion, hemorrhage, or abscess formation following repair of the aneurysm.

(3) **Arteriography** is an invasive test used by the vascular surgeon to plan the surgical repair procedure.

Clinical Management

1. Goals of clinical management
   a. Limiting the progression of the disease process by modifying risk factors
   b. Controlling hypertension to prevent further strain on the aneurysm
   c. Recognizing aneurysms early with diagnostic testing
   d. Preventing sudden death from rupture of the abdominal aortic aneurysm by early medical intervention
2. Nonpharmacologic interventions
   a. Modify risk factors (see p. 1099).
   b. Instruct the person to have regular medical checkups, including noninvasive testing, to follow the size of the abdominal aneurysm.
   c. Teach the individual or family members how to take blood pressure and recommended frequency of monitoring.
   d. Educate the individual and family about seeking early medical intervention for any of the following: severe onset of back or abdominal pain, soreness over the umbilicus, sudden development of extremity ischemia, and persistent elevation of blood pressure above baseline measurements.
3. Pharmacologic interventions: Antihypertensive agents to maintain blood pressure within normal limits (see Chapter 23). Keeping blood pressure in the normotensive range decreases strain on the aneurysm.
4. Special medical-surgical procedures (Fig. 24–11 and page 1111 for postoperative nursing care).

Complications

1. Death is the most common complication of aneurysmal rupture.
2. Paraplegia can develop when blood supply to the spinal cord is inadequate for a prolonged period. Causes of paraplegia include prolonged aortic clamp time during surgical repair, prolonged hypotension, and rupture with cessation of blood flow to the spinal cord.

Prognosis

1. With early diagnosis and treatment, the prognosis is good.
2. When the aneurysm ruptures, survival drops dramatically, to below 50 percent.

REPAIR OF ABDOMINAL AORTIC ANEURYSM

Surgical resection of an abdominal aortic aneurysm is undertaken with a woven Dacron graft.

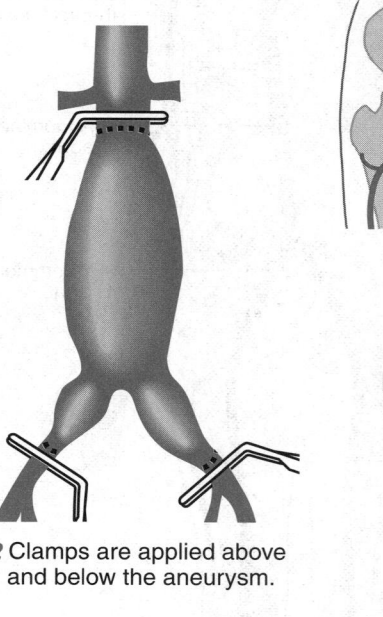

1 The aneurysm is exposed with a midline abdominal incision that extends from below the xiphoid process to the symphysis pubis.

2 Clamps are applied above and below the aneurysm.

3 The aneurysm is excised, and the excised section of the aorta is replaced with a woven Dacron graft that is sewn end to end.

Figure 24–11. Repair of an abdominal aortic aneurysm using a bifurcated Dacron graft.

Applying the Nursing Process

NURSING DIAGNOSIS: Knowledge deficit R/T an abdominal aortic aneurysm and its treatment

1. *Expected outcomes:* After instruction, the person should be able to do the following:
   a. Verbalize understanding of the disease process and treatment
   b. Actively participate in learning and feel free to ask questions
2. *Nursing interventions*
   a. Develop a teaching plan to correct knowledge deficits.

b. Include family in teaching.
c. Provide preoperative and postoperative teaching with written guidelines for persons undergoing surgical resection of the aneurysm (see Chapter 13).
d. Provide information about risk factor modifications.
e. Teach how to measure blood pressure.
f. Instruct about medication regimen: indications, side effects, drug or food interactions, and dosing.
g. Teach the individual when to seek medical intervention.
h. Encourage questions and provide information about additional learning resources.

NURSING DIAGNOSIS: Altered tissue perfusion R/T an abdominal aortic aneurysm and its postoperative treatment

1. *Expected outcomes:* The patient should exhibit signs of normal tissue perfusion, which include the following:
   a. Postsurgical wound healing without evidence of ischemia or infection
   b. Palpable or audible peripheral pulses on Doppler ultrasonography
2. *Nursing interventions*
   a. Monitor vital signs and hemodynamic parameters every hour after the person arrives from the operating room.
   b. Maintain systolic blood pressure below 120 mm Hg to avoid strain on the operative suture lines.
   c. Assess peripheral circulation for presence of pulses, temperature, color, and rate of capillary refill.
   d. Check sensory and motor function of extremities.
   e. Observe for signs of hemorrhage or hypovolemia: hypotension, tachycardia, weak pulses, altered mental status, and decreased hemoglobin and hematocrit.
   f. Monitor electrocardiogram (ECG) for signs of ischemia, myocardial injury, or arrhythmias.
   g. Monitor for organ or limb ischemia that may result from clamping of the aorta during aneurysm resection. Signs include the following:
      (1) Viscera: persistent absence of bowel sounds after 48 to 72 hours; rigidity of abdominal wall
      (2) Spinal cord: decreased reflexes; lost or decreased motor function, sensory function, or both
      (3) Kidneys: decreased or absent urine output, elevated serum blood urea nitrogen (BUN) or creatinine, or increased or fixed urine specific gravity
      (4) Peripheral nervous system: loss of pulses, paresthesias, pallor, pain, or sudden paralysis
   h. Monitor respiratory status during mechanical ventilation and after extubation; then encourage coughing and deep breathing to prevent complications.
   i. Check laboratory tests for abnormalities (e.g., hemoglobin, hematocrit, electrolytes, and arterial blood gases [ABGs]).
   j. Observe for any signs of infection: elevated temperature, sudden elevation in white blood cell count, or change in the appearance of the wound.

NURSING DIAGNOSIS: Anxiety R/T perceived threat of aneurysm rupture and death

1. *Expected outcomes:* The patient should be able to do the following:
   a. Discuss feelings regarding the perceived threat
   b. Identify appropriate problem-solving techniques to deal with anxiety
   c. State that any anxiety is at a level tolerable to the individual
2. *Nursing interventions*
   a. Assess level of anxiety.
   b. Encourage verbalization of fears.
   c. Offer realistic assurances, correcting misperceptions.
   d. Provide antianxiety medications as ordered when appropriate.
   e. Obtain consultations (e.g., psychiatric clinical nurse specialist, psychologist, or clergy).
   f. Allow problem solving by identifying measures used successfully to deal with anxiety in the past.

Discharge Planning and Teaching

1. Provide information about risk factor modification.
2. Discuss the importance of maintaining blood pressure within normal limits with medications, diet, or stress reduction.
3. Review signs and symptoms to report to the physician, including abdominal or back pain.
4. Reinforce the importance of keeping appointments for follow-up monitoring.
5. Inform the person about principles of foot care (see Learning/Teaching Guidelines for Foot Care).
6. Review medications that are to be taken at home.
7. For people who have undergone surgical resection, discuss the following:
   a. Activity restrictions
   b. Wound care procedures
   c. Bathing or showering restrictions
   d. Need to call the physician: fever greater than 101 degrees Fahrenheit, excessive wound drainage, redness at the site, wound separation, or sudden onset of pain

Public Health Considerations

Regular medical visits are the most reliable way to detect abdominal aortic aneurysms. Encouraging adults older than 50 years of age to have an annual physical examination appears to be the key to early diagnosis.

◼ *RAYNAUD'S DISEASE*

Definition

1. In **Raynaud's disease,** episodic vasospasm produces closure of the small arteries in the distal extremities in response to cold, vibration, or emotional stimuli.
2. Referred to as Raynaud's disease when the disorder is primary without underlying cause and as Raynaud's phenomenon (see p. 1115) when secondary to another disease or underlying cause.

Incidence and Socioeconomic Impact

1. Raynaud's disease is seen primarily in women in their teens or early twenties.
2. It is frequently seen in cold climates during the winter months.
3. It is a chronic condition requiring lifestyle and, possibly, job modifications.

Risk Factors

1. Age: more common in persons 11 to 45 years of age
2. Gender: more common in women
3. Evidence of vasospasm in the digits with exposure to cold, stress, or vibration

Etiology

The etiology is unknown.

Pathophysiology

1. An episode manifests with the classic 3-color presentation of Raynaud's disease. Initially, pallor (white color) develops, caused by intense vasoconstriction or spasm in the digital arteries.
2. As the episode progresses, vasoconstriction becomes less severe, with some filling of the capillaries and veins with deoxygenated blood, resulting in peripheral cyanosis (blue color).
3. When the digits rewarm, cyanosis is replaced with an intense rubor (red color) associated with termination of vasospasm and increased blood flow into the dilated capillary bed.

Clinical Manifestations

1. Interruption of circulation to the digits with the classic 3-color presentation of Raynaud's disease
2. Vasospasm and pain in the digits with exposure to cold, vibration, or stress
3. Ulcerations at the fingertips or around the nail bed
4. Changes in the nails
   a. Slow growth
   b. Brittleness or deformity
   c. Poor healing of infections around nail beds
5. Changes in the skin of the affected digit
   a. Hair loss
   b. Tightness or thinning of the skin
   c. Slow healing of injuries or cuts

Diagnostics

1. Assessment
   a. History: Ask the following:
      (1) Describe the location of the symptoms.
      (2) Describe the severity of the symptoms.
      (3) When do the symptoms occur, and how long do they last?
      (4) What are the symptoms like?
      (5) Are there any precipitating factors?
      (6) Is the episode brought on by exposure to cold?
      (7) Is the episode brought on by mechanical activity with exposure to vibration?
      (8) Does emotional stress bring on symptoms?
      (9) Are the symptoms relieved by rewarming the affected digits?
      (10) Give details of your medical history, noting any conditions that are associated with Raynaud's phenomenon.
      (11) Provide information on your medication history.
      (12) Has there been any exposure to chemicals (e.g., polyvinyl chloride)?
   b. Physical examination
      (1) Note any skin changes on the affected digits.
      (2) Note any changes in the nail or nail beds.
      (3) Note any ulcerations at the tips of the digits.
      (4) Palpate for diminished or absent peripheral pulses.
   c. Special diagnostic studies
      (1) Testing performed in the vascular laboratory measures fingertip recovery after digital ice-water exposure (10–15 degrees Celsius). A negative result does not totally exclude Raynaud's disease.
      (2) Arteriography, if performed, usually reveals normal major arteries with spasm of the digital arteries.
2. Medical diagnosis
   a. Diagnosis is based on the history of vasospastic episodes in the digits with exposure to cold, stress, or vibration.
   b. Differentiation between Raynaud's disease and Raynaud's phenomenon is based on exclusion of disorders known to cause Raynaud's phenomenon, which is a secondary condition.

Clinical Management

1. Goal of clinical management: to decrease the number of vasospastic episodes through identification of precipitating factors and lifestyle modification.
2. Nonpharmacologic interventions
   a. If possible, avoid precipitating factors that produce vasospasm.
   b. Prevent injury to the affected digits.
   c. Apply protective measures to minimize exposure to cold or vibration (e.g., wearing protective gloves).
   d. Stop using tobacco.
3. Pharmacologic interventions: The goal of drug therapy is to produce vascular smooth muscle relaxation.
   a. Nifedipine, a calcium antagonist, is the drug of choice.
   b. Smooth muscle contractility is reduced by inhibiting the movement of calcium ions in slow channels.
   c. Side effects include headache, flushing, peripheral edema, and postural hypotension.

Complications

Rarely, in cases with severe progression, complete obstruction of the arteries in the affected digits occurs with gangrene of the tips of the digits.

Prognosis

The prognosis is excellent for persons who adhere to the prescribed medical and nursing regimens.

Applying the Nursing Process

NURSING DIAGNOSIS: Altered tissue perfusion R/T peripheral vasospasm

1. *Expected outcomes:* The patient should exhibit signs of improved tissue perfusion, which include the following:
   a. Decreased frequency of vasospastic episodes
   b. Ability to carry out activities of daily living with minimal discomfort or pain
   c. Absence of fingertip or nail bed ulcerations.
2. *Nursing interventions*
   a. Assess causative factors and develop plan for lifestyle modifications.
   b. Limit digital exposure to cold and vibration.
   c. Wear warm clothing to protect digits in cold weather.
   d. Avoid tobacco use, as tobacco produces cutaneous vasoconstriction.
   e. Use potholders when handling either hot or cold items during food preparation.
   f. Avoid injury to affected digits.

NURSING DIAGNOSIS: Body image disturbance R/T physical changes caused by Raynaud's disease

1. *Expected outcomes:* The patient should be able to do the following:
   a. Verbalize understanding of changes in body image
   b. Freely discuss feelings with health care professionals and family
   c. Demonstrate appropriate problem-solving techniques for coping with body changes
2. *Nursing interventions*
   a. Encourage discussion of feelings about change in body appearance from the disease process.
   b. Correct misperceptions about the disease process.
   c. Assess ethnic and transcultural perceptions.
   d. Discuss fear and anxiety related to changes in body image, noting depression.
   e. Suggest ways to minimize appearance of body changes (e.g., makeup or clothing).
   f. Offer sources of counseling: psychologist, clergy, and support groups.

Discharge Planning and Teaching

1. Smoking cessation
   a. The effects of tobacco on the blood vessels
   b. Basic principles of smoking cessation
   c. Availability of smoking cessation programs in the community
2. Protection of the affected extremities from cold and injury
3. Foot care principles (see Learning/Teaching Guidelines for Foot Care)

Public Health Considerations

Regular physical examinations are important for early recognition and treatment.

■ *OTHER ARTERIAL DISEASES*

Thoracic Aneurysms

1. Definition: A **thoracic aneurysm** is an abnormal dilation along the thoracic aorta caused by localized weakness and stretching of the arterial wall.
2. Incidence and etiology
   a. The thoracic aorta is the most common site of aortic dissection.
   b. Thoracic aneurysms occur more often in men between the ages of 40 and 70.
   c. Thoracic and abdominal aneurysms are diagnosed at a 1:4 ratio.
   d. Atherosclerosis is the most common cause.
   e. Thoracic aneurysms may also be caused by cystic medial degeneration, which involves the proximal aorta and results in degeneration of the elastic tissue in the medial layer of the aorta.
   f. Thoracic aneurysms are commonly seen in Marfan syndrome and in connective tissue disease.
   g. Infection is a possible cause.
      (1) Untreated syphilis was a frequent cause of thoracic aneurysms in the pre-antibiotic era.
      (2) Late-stage syphilis produces arterial inflammation.
      (3) The spirochetes of syphilis attack the thoracic aorta, producing medial necrosis.
      (4) The wall of the thoracic aorta weakens, and an aneurysm forms.
   h. Trauma is a possible cause.
      (1) Falls
      (2) Any injury to the chest
3. Clinical manifestations: Symptoms are related to compression or obstruction of adjacent body structures. The most common presenting symptom is chest pain or pressure.
   a. Hoarseness or coughing is due to stretching of the left recurrent laryngeal nerve.
   b. Dyspnea is caused by tracheal displacement.
   c. Hemoptysis is an ominous sign, indicating erosion into the trachea.

d. Ascending thoracic aneurysms that damage the aortic valve produce aortic insufficiency.

e. Dysphagia results from esophageal compression.

f. Spinal cord compression produces paraplegia or paralysis.

g. Dilated superficial veins on the chest, the neck, or the arms, possibly associated with cyanosis, are evident when large veins of the chest are compressed.

h. Unequal pupil size (anisocoria) occurs with pressure against the cervical chain of lymph nodes in the neck.

i. Shock occurs with rupture.

4. Clinical management

a. Modify existing risk factors for atherosclerosis to reduce the progression of the disease.

b. Control hypertension to decrease stress and tension on the aorta.

c. Promote early diagnosis to permit prompt intervention.

d. Encourage regular follow-up visits with the primary physician to detect enlargement of small thoracic aneurysms that are followed on an outpatient basis.

Aortic Dissection

1. Definition: a circumferential or transverse tear in the intima of the aorta, classified according to the anatomy of the aorta involved. In 1965, DeBakey and associates initially divided aortic dissections into 3 types based on the extent of dissection. Today, a 2-type classification is common.

a. Type A dissections

(1) Include types I and II of DeBakey's classification

(2) Involve the ascending aorta or the ascending and descending aorta

(3) Are the most common and lethal type

b. Type B dissections

(1) Do not involve the ascending aorta

(2) Begin distal to the subclavian artery and extend downward into the descending and abdominal aorta

(3) Are also known as type III of DeBakey's classification

2. Incidence and etiology

a. Approximately 60,000 cases are diagnosed each year in the United States.

b. Incidence is higher in men than women by a ratio of at least 3:1.

c. Most aortic dissections develop in the inner one third to one half of the aortic wall.

d. Marfan syndrome

(1) An inherited connective tissue disorder

(2) Associated increase of elasticity in the wall of the aorta due to deficiency of connective tissue and ineffective cross-linking of collagen

e. Congenital heart disease (e.g., aortic coarctation, bicuspid aortic valve disease)

f. A history of hypertension (present in about 80–90% of persons)

g. Pregnancy: approximately 50 percent of all aortic dissections in women younger than 40 occur during pregnancy.

(1) It is believed that hormonal changes, along with increased blood volume and hypertension, produce disruption in the medial layer of the aorta.

(2) The greatest risk of dissection is in the last trimester of pregnancy.

h. Atherosclerosis

i. Trauma

j. Deceleration injuries from automobile or airplane accidents

(1) Deceleration forces produce injury when the body stops suddenly but the internal organs continue moving forward.

(2) To rupture the aorta, a pressure force of 1000 to 3000 mm Hg is required.

k. Iatrogenic injuries to the aorta can occur during cardiopulmonary bypass procedures, aortography, or intra-aortic balloon pump procedures.

3. Clinical manifestations

a. Sudden onset of pain that is described as severe and tearing. The pain is typically associated with diaphoresis.

b. Location of the pain depends on the site of the dissection.

c. Typically, the pain is localized to either the front or the back of the chest.

d. The pain may migrate along the direction of the dissection.

e. Other physical findings can include any of the following:

(1) Hypertension or hypotension

(2) Absence of peripheral pulses

(3) Aortic regurgitation from damage to the aortic valve

(4) Pulmonary edema

f. Neurologic findings are due to dissection of major arteries.

(1) Carotid artery obstruction produces hemiplegia or hemianesthesia.

(2) Spinal cord ischemia can cause paraplegia.

g. Compression of adjacent structures from the widening dissection can cause any of the following: superior vena cava syndrome, hoarseness, dysphagia, and tracheal displacement.

h. Cardiac tamponade

4. Clinical management

a. Slow or stop progression of the dissection through blood pressure and pain control.

b. Treat the dissection either medically or surgically.

(1) Type A dissections usually are repaired surgically with resection and replacement of the aortic segment with a woven Dacron graft.

(2) Type B dissections often are managed medically.

c. Reduce hypertension to decrease the risk of rupture.

d. Suggest relaxation techniques, imagery, biofeedback, or a combination thereof to decrease stress.

(1) Provide a quiet, calm environment.

(2) Educate the person about the plan of care.

(3) Allow the person to verbalize feelings and fears.

e. Provide analgesics (e.g., morphine sulfate) to decrease pain.

Thromboangiitis Obliterans (Buerger's Disease)

1. Definition: a recurring inflammation of the small and medium-sized arteries and veins of the upper and lower extremities that results in thrombus formation and occlusion of blood vessels
2. Incidence and etiology
   a. This disorder is most often found in men between 20 and 40 years of age.
   b. Incidence is higher in Israel, the Orient, and India than in the United States.
   c. Buerger's disease is not a well-understood disease process, and the diagnosis is often missed or confused with early forms of atherosclerosis.
   d. There is a higher incidence of limb loss in Buerger's disease than in atherosclerosis.
   e. Risk factors
      (1) Family history of the disease
      (2) Cigarette smoking
3. Clinical manifestations
   a. Small and medium-sized arteries and veins are affected in a segmental fashion.
   b. Acute lesions form with proliferation of the intima and thrombosis.
   c. In the later stages, lesions become less cellular and are transformed into a dense scar.
   d. Commonly, lesions of varying stages of progression can be seen in the same vessel.
   e. Pain, the most common symptom, is present in 1 or more digits.
   f. Superficial thrombophlebitis is commonly seen in the affected extremity before arterial symptoms appear.
   g. The pain is accompanied by signs of ischemia (color or temperature changes).
   h. Numbness and tingling of the extremities is a result of ischemic neuropathy.
   i. Occlusion of the distal arteries of the upper and lower extremities is demonstrable on angiography.
   j. Ulcers in the extremities develop spontaneously or as the result of trauma.
   k. Secondary infection of the ulcer site with partial amputation is not unusual.
   l. Edema of the foot is common.
   m. Pulses in the distal limbs—radial, ulnar, dorsalis pedis, and posterior tibial arteries—are diminished or absent.
      (1) Normal pulses are palpable in the proximal arteries.
      (2) The difference between proximal and distal pulsations is another point of contrast with atherosclerosis.
   n. Exercise-related cramping in the feet and legs is relieved with rest.
4. Clinical management
   a. Slow the progression of the disease.
   b. Control pain (see Chapter 11).
   c. Protect the extremity from extremes in temperature and from injury.
   d. Cease tobacco use in any form. Consult national or local agencies for information about smoking cessation programs.
   e. Teach foot care principles (see Learning/Teaching Guidelines for Foot Care).
   f. To promote circulation in the lower extremities, teach the person how to perform Buerger-Allen exercises (see Learning/Teaching Guidelines for Performing Buerger-Allen Exercises).
   g. Provide information about noninvasive pain relief techniques (see Chapter 11).

Raynaud's Phenomenon

1. Definition: a condition characterized by episodes of pallor and cyanosis in the digits brought on by exposure to cold or emotional stress that is always secondary to another disease, such as lupus erythematosus, scleroderma, or atherosclerosis.
2. Incidence and etiology
   a. Raynaud's phenomenon commonly occurs in individuals older than 30 years.
   b. Raynaud's phenomenon can be a manifestation of any of the following conditions:
      (1) Raynaud's disease, the underlying cause in 60 percent of cases (see p. 1111)
      (2) Occlusive arterial diseases
         (a) Arterial embolism or thrombosis
         (b) Buerger's disease
         (c) Arteriosclerosis
      (3) Connective tissue diseases
         (a) Lupus erythematosus
         (b) Scleroderma
         (c) Rheumatoid arthritis
      (4) Repetitive minor vascular injuries
      (5) Neurogenic lesions
         (a) Spinal cord disease
         (b) Thoracic outlet compression
         (c) Carpal tunnel syndrome
      (6) Exposure to certain chemicals or drugs that produce vascular smooth muscle contraction
         • Polyvinyl chloride
         • Beta-adrenergic blocking agents (propranolol)
         • Ergotamine
         • Antimetabolite drugs (cisplatin, vinblastine, or bleomycin)
      (7) Intravascular aggregation or coagulation of blood elements
3. Clinical manifestations
   a. Symptoms are unilateral, usually affecting only 1 or 2 digits
   b. Symptoms of Raynaud's disease (see page 1112), with the distinction between the 2 based on the presence of disorders known to cause Raynaud's phenomenon
4. Clinical management
   a. All of the interventions for Raynaud's disease (see p. 1112)
   b. Careful management of the underlying disease by the primary care provider to avoid exacerbations of Raynaud's phenomenon

c. When secondary to systemic disease (e.g., connective tissue disorder), consultation with a vascular specialist may be indicated

ASSESSING PEOPLE WITH VENOUS DISEASE

Key Symptoms and Their Pathophysiologic Bases

1. Sharp or deep muscle pain that may be relieved by elevation
   a. Occurrence
   b. Characteristics
   c. Location
   d. Duration
   e. Severity
   f. Precipitating or aggravating factors
   g. Associated symptoms
   h. Alleviating factors
2. Aching pain in the leg, particularly with prolonged standing
   a. Through h.
3. Edema
   a. Through h.
4. Diminished pulses
   a. Through h.
5. Changes in skin temperature or appearance
   a. Through h.
6. Skin breakdown, ulcers, or scars indicating healed ulcers
   a. Through h.
7. Prominence of superficial veins
   a. Through h.
8. The pathophysiology of venous disease is related to reduction or occlusion of venous blood return to the heart, usually in one or a combination of the following ways:
   a. Thrombus or thrombophlebitis can obstruct a vein, producing acute pain or throbbing as a result of the inflammatory process.
   b. Reduction of venous blood flow can result from incompetent valves in the veins, producing edema from increased venous and capillary pressure, with fluid seeping out into the surrounding tissues.
   c. Gravitational pressure of standing adds to the strain on veins because hydrostatic pressure increases venous pressure. Lying down lowers hydrostatic pressure and therefore venous pressure.
   d. Venous stasis occurs with immobilization or impairment of the pumping action of the calf muscles. Conditions causing stasis include immobility, obesity, prolonged standing or sitting in one place, and pregnancy.
   e. Conditions that produce hypercoagulability (elevated platelet count, increased clotting factors, increased blood viscosity) can lead to the formation of thrombus that occludes venous circulation. Such conditions include blood dyscrasias, use of birth control pills, malignant neoplasms, and pregnancy.
   f. Injury to the vein or vein wall can lead to decreased

blood flow and can result from a variety of conditions, including surgical and nonsurgical trauma, chemical sclerosing agents, and radiopaque dyes.

Health History

To determine the significance of the symptoms of venous disease, ask the following key questions:

1. Do you have any family history of venous disease?
2. Have you undergone any surgical procedures involving the affected extremity?
3. Have you recently been on prolonged bed rest following surgery, illness, or pregnancy?
4. Do you have any history of leg trauma?
5. Do you use oral contraceptives?
6. Do you have a history of blood clots or superficial phlebitis?
7. Do you sit or stand in one position for prolonged periods?
8. Have you noticed any episodes of limb swelling?
9. Show me where you are experiencing any pain or heaviness in your limbs. Describe your pain.
   a. Occurrence
   b. Characteristics
   c. Location
   d. Duration
   e. Severity
   f. Precipitating or aggravating factors
   g. Associated symptoms
   h. Alleviating factors
10. Rate your pain on a 0 to 10 scale, with 0 representing little or no pain and 10 representing severe pain.
11. Have you noted any changes in skin temperature or appearance?
12. Have you had any skin breakdown or ulcers on your extremities in the past?

Physical Examination

1. Inspect for skin breakdown, noting any scars from healed ulcers.
2. Inspect both extremities for edema and, if present, palpate for pitting edema.
3. Inspect and palpate for varicosities (tortuous or dilated veins), best seen in the standing position, when the gravitational pressure is greatest. Palpate for hard, cordlike segments along the veins that are superficial venous thrombosis.
4. Palpate all peripheral pulses.
5. Palpate the feet and legs to detect any changes in skin temperature.
6. Dorsiflex each foot and note any pain (positive Homans' sign).

Special Diagnostic Studies

1. Noninvasive testing
   a. **Doppler ultrasound** detects obstruction or alteration

of blood flow in the venous system through changes in the frequency of sound waves sent and received by the probe (see Procedure 24–1).

    (1) Venous sounds are low pitched.

    (2) Venous sounds are phasic; they decrease with inspiration and increase with expiration.

b. **Impedance plethysmography** measures changes in venous volume. Decreased flow suggests thrombosis in the extremity.

    (1) Impedance plethysmography measures volume changes specifically in the thigh and calf.

    (2) A thigh cuff is inflated only enough to occlude venous return without affecting arterial inflow.

    (3) The calf cuff measures the increased blood volume, or segmental venous capacitance (SVC).

    (4) Once the plethysmography tracing indicates that maximum calf vein distention has been reached, the thigh cuff is released.

    (5) At this point, the venous volume is measured and is referred to as the maximum venous outflow (MVO).

    (6) Venous obstruction is seen with depressed SVC and MVO.

c. **B-mode ultrasonography** is a relatively new technique that provides a 3-dimensional representation of the deep veins below the iliac crest. This technique allows for visualization of vein size, compressibility, flow patterns, presence of thrombus, and valve competence.

d. A **Trendelenburg test** is used to assess for the presence of varicose veins.

    (1) Have the person lie down.

    (2) Elevate the leg to empty the veins.

    (3) Apply a tourniquet to occlude the superficial veins.

    (4) Instruct the person to stand.

    (5) Release the tourniquet.

    (6) If the veins are incompetent, they immediately become distended because of backflow.

2. Invasive testing: A **venogram** is used to locate and assess the severity of venous obstruction.

a. Local anesthesia may be given over the injection site, and then a catheter is introduced percutaneously.

b. X-ray films are made when a radiopaque dye is injected into a vein that has been previously emptied by gravity.

c. Injection of the contrast medium can be painful because of its irritating effect on the veins.

d. Obstructions or thrombus is seen on the x-ray films.

◼ *DEEP VENOUS THROMBOSIS*

Definitions

1. **Phlebitis** is an inflammation of the walls of a vein.
2. **Venous thrombosis** is the formation of a blood clot that either partially or totally occludes a blood vessel.
3. **Deep vein thrombosis (DVT)** affects the deep, rather than superficial, veins in the lower extremities.

4. In **thrombophlebitis,** a clot forms in a vein as a result of phlebitis or partial obstruction of the vein.

Incidence and Socioeconomic Impact

1. Deep vein thrombosis is a common venous disorder that affects approximately 30 percent of persons older than 40 who have undergone major surgery or have had a myocardial infarction.
2. This disorder costs the health care industry millions of dollars annually by prolonging hospital stays by up to 7 to 10 days.
3. Pulmonary embolus from DVT causes an estimated 50,000 to 200,000 deaths per year in the United States alone.

Risk Factors

1. General surgery (for persons older than 40)
2. Medical conditions requiring prolonged bed rest (e.g., myocardial infarction, stroke)
3. Pregnancy
4. Estrogen use
5. Previous episodes of DVT or venous insufficiency
6. Leg trauma (fractures, casts, joint replacement)
7. Malignancy with altered blood coagulation
8. Obesity

Etiology and Pathophysiology

The exact etiology is unknown, but venous stasis, injury to the venous wall, and a hypercoagulable state have all been implicated.

1. Veins are classified as superficial (greater and lesser saphenous veins) or deep (femoral and popliteal veins). They are joined together by smaller perforator veins (Fig. 24–12).
2. The perforator veins are believed to be important in the pathophysiology of venous stasis.
3. Venous stasis occurs when blood flow to the veins is slowed.
4. Bed rest is known to decrease blood flow in the venous system by at least 50 percent.
5. Hypercoagulability is believed to be produced by any of the following: increased levels of clotting factors, activation of clotting factors (as in cancer), reduced level of clotting inhibitors, and impaired fibrinolysis.
6. The vein wall can be injured either by direct trauma (e.g., during surgery for hip pin placement) or by previous thrombosis.

Clinical Manifestations

1. The first clinical sign may be pulmonary embolism.
2. There may be pain on dorsiflexion (Homans' sign) in the affected extremity.

VEINS OF THE LOWER EXTREMITY

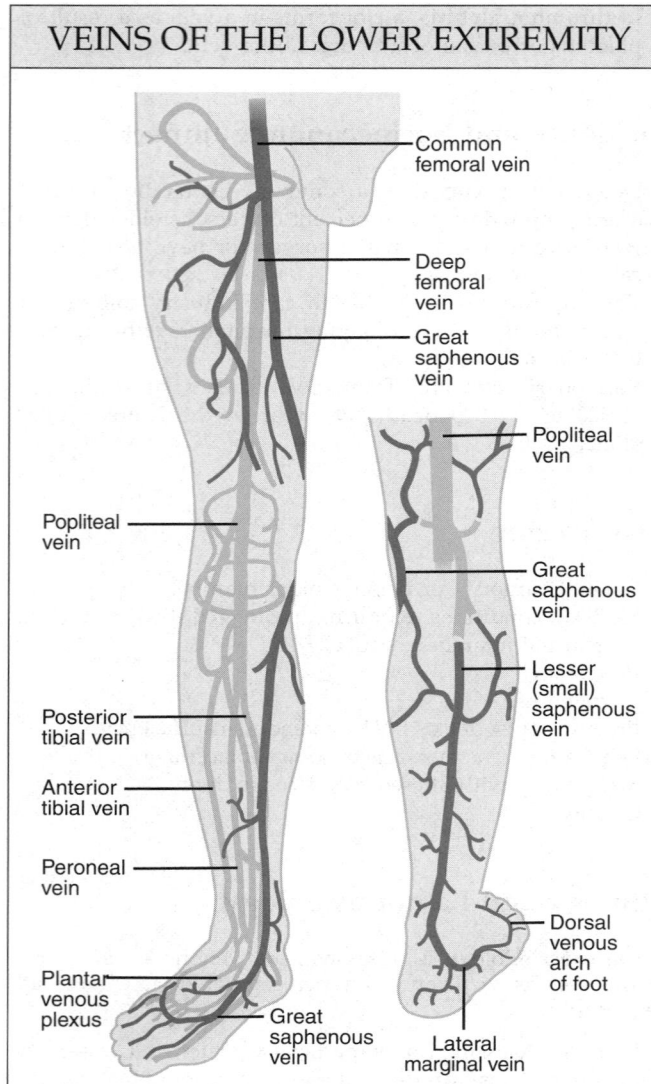

Figure 24–12. The venous system has deep and superficial veins that carry deoxygenated blood back toward the heart.

3. Edema often is seen with venous disorders and can be bilateral or unilateral.
4. Stasis ulcers result from rupture of small skin veins that then necrose to form an ulcer.

Diagnostics

1. Assessment
   a. History: Note any risk factors.
   b. Physical examination
      (1) Clinical findings are highly variable; 50 percent of cases go undetected.
      (2) Assess for a positive Homans' sign.
      (3) Inquire about any sudden onset of pain or swelling in the affected extremity.
2. Medical diagnosis
   a. Both invasive and noninvasive testing may be required.
   b. Deep vein thrombosis is definitively diagnosed by venography.

Clinical Management

1. The goal of clinical management is to prevent the development of thrombosis and decrease the risk of pulmonary embolism.
2. Nonpharmacologic interventions
   a. Minimize edema of the affected extremity.
      (1) Leg elevation (lying flat with the affected extremity elevated above the heart)
      (2) Support stockings to reduce venous stasis and assist in return of venous blood to the heart
      (3) Avoidance of prolonged sitting or standing. Gradual walking on level surfaces.
   b. Sodium restriction to 4 gm per day.
   c. Weight reduction by restricting calories.
   d. Foot care principles (see Learning/Teaching Guidelines for Foot Care).
3. Pharmacologic interventions
   a. Anticoagulation agents are the medications of choice for venous thrombosis (see Table 24–3).
   b. Thrombolytic agents are occasionally used in the treatment of acute thrombosis of the deep veins in the extremities.
   c. Diuretics are used to control lower extremity edema.
   d. Analgesic agents are given for pain.
4. Special medical-surgical procedures
   a. Surgical vein stripping, once a common procedure, is not done as often, primarily because of the high incidence of cardiovascular disease in these patients and the need to preserve vein conduit for possible bypass operations.
   b. Venous thrombectomy involves removal of a clot through an incision in the affected vein.
   c. Inferior vena caval interruption is a technique that prevents embolization.
      (1) In the most common procedure, a filtering device is placed percutaneously within the vena cava for filtration of clots without interruption of blood flow.
      (2) Surgical placement of a Teflon clip on the vena cava is seldom performed.

Complications

1. Pulmonary embolism is a frequent complication of DVT that can lead to death.

NURSE ADVISORY

Observe and report any signs of pulmonary embolism (sudden onset of dyspnea, chest pain, or hemoptysis) in patients with deep vein thrombosis.

2. Deep vein thrombosis can lead to disability if the person's job requires prolonged standing.
3. Inadequate perfusion can produce leg ulcers that are difficult to heal.

Prognosis

1. The prognosis is good for individuals who follow their therapeutic regimen.
2. Hospitalization for DVT generally is 7 to 10 days. Return to work depends on the rate of recovery.
3. Recurrence is rare.

Applying the Nursing Process

NURSING DIAGNOSIS: Impaired skin integrity R/T lower extremity edema

1. *Expected outcomes:* The patient should be able to do the following:
   a. Verbalize understanding concerning the cause and complications of the disorder, medications, diet, activity, and potential complications
   b. Actively participate in planning care
   c. Comply with therapeutic regimen and alter lifestyle as indicated
   d. Avoid skin breakdown or, if skin ulcer is present, show evidence of healing
2. *Nursing interventions*
   a. Discuss ways to cope with swelling in the legs.
   b. Teach the person how to inspect the legs for edema, noting puffiness, stretched skin, pitting, and hardness to touch.
   c. Have the person measure and record leg circumferences to detect asymmetry (see Procedure 24–3).
   d. Teach the person to elevate the legs every few hours for 10 to 20 minutes during the day.
   e. Explain that, to increase venous return, the legs should be higher than the heart.
   f. Inquire about activity patterns both at home and at work. Encourage the person to avoid prolonged standing or sitting.
   g. Recommend a progressive walking program of 10 to 15 minutes a day.
   h. Teach the person and family about elastic stockings (hazards and application technique) if recommended by the physician or nurse practitioner.

Discharge Planning and Teaching

1. Before discharge, people need to learn about DVT and its treatment (see Learning/Teaching Guidelines for Foot Care and Learning/Teaching Guidelines for Persons on Warfarin).
2. A social services consultation may be beneficial if the person's job requires prolonged standing or sitting. Vo- cational counseling may be needed if the person is unable to continue in the same job.

Public Health Considerations

1. High incidence of DVT for individuals older than 40 undergoing major surgery could be decreased with increased public and health care industry education.
2. Nurses and physicians need to screen persons undergoing major surgical procedures to identify those at high risk for DVT.
3. Early mobilization after surgery or long-term illness or injury is important.

■ *VARICOSE VEINS*

Definition

Varicose veins are dilated, tortuous superficial veins that result from incompetent venous valves.

Incidence and Socioeconomic Impact

1. Approximately one fifth of all adults develop varicose veins.
2. Ten to 15 percent of those who develop varicose veins have family members with this disorder.
3. In most people, varicose veins are a relatively benign disorder, producing only an undesirable cosmetic effect.
4. Varicose veins are a risk factor for deep venous thrombosis and chronic venous insufficiency.

Risk Factors

1. Family history
2. Pregnancy
3. Occupations requiring prolonged standing
4. Obesity
5. Old age with loss of tissue elasticity
6. Trauma to the legs

Etiology

1. Congenitally absent or defective venous valves
2. Sustained elevations of venous pressure from any disorder that obstructs a vein
3. Incompetent venous valves (see Fig. 24–2)

Pathophysiology

1. Defective venous valves allow reflux of blood from the more proximal deep veins into the superficial system.
2. As a result, hydrostatic pressure is transmitted from the long column of blood in the inferior vena cava, iliac

vein, and femoral vein to the walls of the saphenous vein.

3. Venous dilation is produced in the saphenous system, resulting in prominent varicose veins.

Clinical Manifestations

1. Many individuals are asymptomatic.
2. Prominent, tortuous veins in the lower extremities produce an undesirable cosmetic effect.
3. Varicose veins lead to edema and leg fatigue, especially after prolonged standing.
4. Aching and heaviness in the legs are usually relieved by elevation or elastic stockings.

Diagnostics

1. Assessment
   a. History
      (1) Risk factors for the disorder
      (2) Description of pain
   b. Physical examination
      (1) Inspect legs for distention of any varicosities by examining the person in a standing position under a good light.
      (2) Assess skin for any discoloration or ulceration.
2. Medical diagnosis
   a. Physical examination is sufficient to make a diagnosis.
   b. Trendelenburg's test identifies defective or incompetent communicating veins.
   c. Noninvasive venous studies or venography establishes the patency of the deep venous system.

Clinical Management

1. Goal of clinical management: to reduce symptoms and limit disease progression
2. Nonpharmacologic interventions
   a. Compression bandages or elastic support stockings.
   b. Avoid tight or constrictive clothing.
   c. Weight reduction in overweight patients.
   d. Regular exercise (e.g., walking 15–20 min 3 times a week).
3. No pharmacologic interventions are available.
4. Special medical-surgical procedures can relieve the condition.
   a. Surgical vein stripping
      (1) **Surgical vein stripping** is a procedure in which small incisions are made at the ankle and groin over the saphenous vein. A nylon wire is then threaded through the lumen of the vein from ankle to groin, and the wire, along with the vein, is pulled from the ankle incision.
      (2) Because of the need for a saphenous vein conduit in coronary artery bypass procedures, this procedure is not recommended frequently.
   b. Sclerotherapy
      (1) In **sclerotherapy,** a small amount of a sclerosant

chemical is injected into the lumen to destroy the venous intima.
      (2) Sclerotherapy is used more commonly for small prominent varicosities that are of cosmetic concern.
      (3) Because of the potential for pulmonary embolism, this procedure is not widely used.

Complications

1. Trauma leading to rupture of a varicose vein
2. Deep vein thrombosis or chronic venous insufficiency
3. Leg edema
4. Skin breakdown and ulceration

Prognosis

1. The prognosis is good for individuals who adhere to the treatment plan.
2. Many individuals will have chronic swelling.

Applying the Nursing Process

NURSING DIAGNOSIS: Knowledge deficit R/T management of varicose veins

1. *Expected outcomes:* Following instruction, the patient should be able to verbalize understanding of varicose vein management.
2. *Nursing interventions*
   a. Assess the individual's knowledge about varicose veins.
   b. Provide the individual and family with information about the care of varicose veins.
   c. Teach the correct application of support stockings:
      (1) Apply in the morning before edema is present.
      (2) Apply while lying down, if possible.
      (3) Apply the stockings or compression bandages from foot to ankle and up the calf.
      (4) Check for proper fit and comfort.
      (5) Remove if fit is improper or cyanosis is observed in the extremities.
   d. Stress the importance of avoiding excessive weight gain.
   e. Emphasize how to avoid obstruction of veins by constrictive clothing. For example, avoid wearing tight garters, socks, stockings, or girdles.
   f. Encourage the individual to elevate the leg whenever possible to prevent or decrease leg edema.
   g. Discourage long periods of standing or sitting in one position. Encourage brief periods of walking (5–10 min) throughout the day.
   h. Instruct the individual to avoid sitting with legs crossed for prolonged periods, as this position promotes venous stasis.

i. Educate the person to seek medical intervention if skin breakdown develops.
j. Provide information about the signs and symptoms of DVT, as well as the importance of early medical intervention.

Discharge Planning and Teaching

1. Provide information about the disorder and its management.
2. Varicose veins usually are not treated on an inpatient basis, so outpatient therapy is designed to promote comfort, decrease edema, and prevent complications.

Public Health Considerations

Regular medical follow-up is important to prevent possible complications.

◼ *VENOUS STASIS ULCERS*

Definition

1. **Venous stasis ulcers** result from postphlebitic valvular incompetence or valve dysfunction secondary to varicose veins.
2. Over time, excessive venous pressure in small skin veins results in erythema, dermatitis, hyperpigmentation, and skin ulceration.

Incidence and Socioeconomic Impact

1. About 75 percent of all leg ulcers are associated with venous disease.
2. Approximately 1 percent of Western populations are affected by venous ulcerations.
3. Venous stasis ulcers are chronic, slow healing, and disfiguring.

Risk Factors

1. Varicose veins
2. Obesity
3. Deep vein thrombosis
4. Congenital incompetence or absence of 1 or more of the deep or perforator veins
5. Venous insufficiency

Etiology

1. Infection
2. Trauma to the extremity
3. Pressure in the affected area
4. A burn in the affected area

Pathophysiology

1. Poor exchange of oxygen and other nutrients in the tissue leads to tissue necrosis.
2. Often, a break in the integrity of the skin leads to skin ulceration and secondary bacterial infection.
3. Once the ulcer stops enlarging, granulation tissue develops.
4. Fibrin exudate in the ulcer stimulates deposition of collagen. White blood cells then remove necrotic tissue and bacteria.
5. The edges of the ulcer form scar tissue, which reduces wound size. Epithelial cells then move in across the ulcer.
6. New endothelial tissue is fragile until it has time to thicken and keratinize as granulation tissue contracts.

Clinical Manifestations

1. Brawny pigmentation in the lower leg
2. A break in the integrity of the skin with the development of an ulcer
3. Commonly seen in the distal 3rd of the leg, above the medial malleolus
4. Cellulitis characterized by diffuse erythema of the entire lower leg

Diagnostics

1. Assessment
   a. History
      (1) Previous treatment of venous ulcers
      (2) History of DVT
      (3) Trauma to the affected extremity
   b. Physical examination
      (1) Inspect the extremities for skin color and presence of varicose veins.
      (2) Inspect the venous stasis ulcer.
      (3) Palpate pulses in the extremities to assess circulation and potential for healing.
      (4) Assess sensory function of the extremities.
2. Medical diagnosis: The diagnosis is based on the physical examination

Clinical Management

1. Goal of clinical management: To promote healing and prevent infection of the venous stasis ulcer
2. Nonpharmacologic interventions
   a. Proper nutrition to promote wound healing
   b. Limb compression therapy to decrease edema in the affected extremity
      (1) Elastic stockings
      (2) Unna boot
      (3) Occlusive or semiocclusive dressings
      (4) Intermittent pneumatic compression
   c. Mechanical débridement of the ulcer to remove necrotic tissue and promote healing

d. Avoidance of activities or clothing that produces venous obstruction
e. Injury prevention
3. Pharmacologic interventions
   a. Antibiotic therapy to treat cellulitis or infections
   b. Topical wound care products (e.g., Silvadene)
4. Special medical-surgical procedures
   a. Surgical débridement of the ulcer
   b. Skin grafting if conservative measures fail

Complications

1. Recurrent episodes of cellulitis
2. Septicemia
3. Limb loss

Prognosis

1. The prognosis is good for individuals who adhere to the prescribed treatment regimen.
2. Venous stasis ulcers can become chronic or recur, requiring periodic medical follow-up.
3. Healing of ulcers is a slow, frustrating process for many individuals.

Applying the Nursing Process

NURSING DIAGNOSIS: Altered tissue perfusion R/T skin breakdown caused by venous disease and secondary infection

1. *Expected outcomes:* The patient should exhibit signs of normal tissue perfusion, which include the following:
   a. Absence of signs of erythema at ulcer site
   b. Absence of fever
   c. Granulation tissue at ulcer site, indicating healing
   d. Decreased swelling
2. *Nursing interventions*
   a. Assess pedal pulses on admission, then daily.
   b. Weigh daily.
   c. Monitor vital signs.
   d. Elevate legs higher than the heart.
   e. Clean skin.
   f. Provide wound care.
   g. Protect wound until healing can begin.
   h. Avoid friction on the skin.
   i. Maintain proper body positioning while in bed.

NURSING DIAGNOSIS: Knowledge deficit R/T care of venous stasis ulcer after discharge.

1. *Expected outcomes:* Following instruction, the patient and family should be able to do the following:
   a. Demonstrate correct dressing technique
   b. List supplies required for wound care
   c. State when to call the physician or nurse practitioner
   d. Ask questions freely

2. *Nursing interventions*
   a. Teach about wound healing.
   b. List needed supplies for wound care.
   c. Demonstrate correct technique for wound care.
   d. Provide step-by-step written instructions.
   e. Review instructions at discharge.
   f. Teach the person to contact the primary care provider when necessary.

NURSING DIAGNOSIS: Anxiety R/T venous stasis ulcer and possible limb loss

1. *Expected outcomes:* The patient should be able to do the following:
   a. Discuss fears of limb loss
   b. Ask questions about care
   c. State that anxiety has lessened
2. *Nursing interventions*
   a. Identify perception of the threat.
   b. Acknowledge fear and anxiety.
   c. Identify coping skills that are effective.
   d. Teach about the course of vascular disease.
   e. Listen attentively.
   f. Encourage questions about care.

Discharge Planning and Teaching

1. Wound care as prescribed by the physician or nurse practitioner
2. Foot care principles (see Learning/Teaching Guidelines for Foot Care)
3. Prevention of leg edema
4. Prevention of injury and trauma
5. Avoidance of constrictive clothing and shoes

Public Health Considerations

Close medical observation is required for individuals with venous stasis ulcers.

■ ASSESSING PEOPLE WITH LYMPHATIC DISORDERS

Key Symptoms and Their Pathophysiologic Bases

1. Edema of the extremity, usually unilateral. Edema is believed to result from blockage of lymph channels.
   a. Occurrence
   b. Characteristics
   c. Location
   d. Duration
   e. Severity
   f. Precipitating or aggravating factors
   g. Associated symptoms
   h. Alleviating factors

2. Inflammation of larger lymphatic vessels; lymph node swelling or tenderness. Inflammation results most often from bacterial or viral infection.
   a. Through *h*.

Health History

To determine the significance of the symptoms of lymphatic disease, ask the person the following key questions:

1. Do you have swelling in your extremities? If so, how long has it been present?
2. Does the swelling go down with elevation of the extremity or overnight?
3. Have you had any bouts of elevated temperature without apparent cause in the last several years?
4. Do you have pain in the affected limb?
   a. Occurrence
   b. Characteristics
   c. Location
   d. Duration
   e. Severity
   f. Precipitating or aggravating factors
   g. Associated symptoms
   h. Alleviating factors
5. Rate your pain on a scale of 0 to 10, with 0 representing little or no pain and 10 representing severe pain.

Physical Examination

1. Inspect for any signs of inflammation (red streaks) extending along the course of lymphatics as they drain.
2. Palpate lymph nodes for enlargement or tenderness.
3. Palpate the lower extremities for edema. Note any pitting edema.

Special Diagnostic Studies

1. A complete blood count (CBC) measures the white blood cell count and aids in diagnosing infection.
2. If infection is present, blood cultures may aid in identifying the specific organism producing the infection and directing appropriate antibiotic therapy.
3. **Lymphangiography,** a radiologic examination, is occasionally indicated to examine lymphatic circulation.
   a. Local anesthesia may be given over the injection site. A catheter is then introduced into a vein percutaneously.
   b. Radiographs are made when a radiopaque dye is injected into a lymphatic vessel of the hand or foot.
      (1) Injection of the contrast medium can be painful because of its irritating effect on the lymphatics.
      (2) Obstructions or thrombus is seen on the radiographs.
4. **Lymphoscintigraphy** is rarely indicated.
   a. The procedure involves the injection of a radioactively labeled technetium-containing colloid.
   b. The test is used to confirm that edema is of lymphatic origin.

c. Technetium 99m is injected into the distal subcutaneous tissue of the affected extremity.
d. The area is scanned 30 to 60 minutes later.
e. Lymphedema is characterized by decreased or absent uptake of the radioactive isotope in the regional lymph nodes.

▣ *LYMPHEDEMA*

Definition

1. **Lymphedema** is often a chronic condition manifested by swelling in an extremity caused by accumulation of lymph (Fig. 24–13).
2. Primary lymphedema (a congenital disorder) is of unknown etiology and believed to be inherited.
3. Secondary lymphedema is caused by lymphatic injury or obstruction from an identifiable cause:
   a. Recurrent episodes of bacterial infection, usually from streptococcus
   b. Radiation trauma following treatment for malignancy or tumor
   c. Trauma or excision of lymphatic pathways during surgical procedures
   d. Parasitic invasion (filariae)

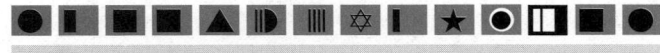

TRANSCULTURAL CONSIDERATIONS

Lymphatic obstruction caused by a parasite, filaria, is seen more frequently in tropical areas.

Incidence and Socioeconomic Impact

1. The exact incidence of lymphatic disorders is not known.
2. Estimates suggest that the incidence of primary lymphedema is 1 per 10,000 persons.
3. Lymphedema is more commonly seen in women older than age 40.

Risk Factors

1. Obstructive tumors or malignancy
2. Injury from surgery or radiation
3. Infections
4. Family history of the disease
5. Travel in tropical areas where filariasis is present

Etiology

1. Primary lymphedema is inherited as an autosomal dominant trait.

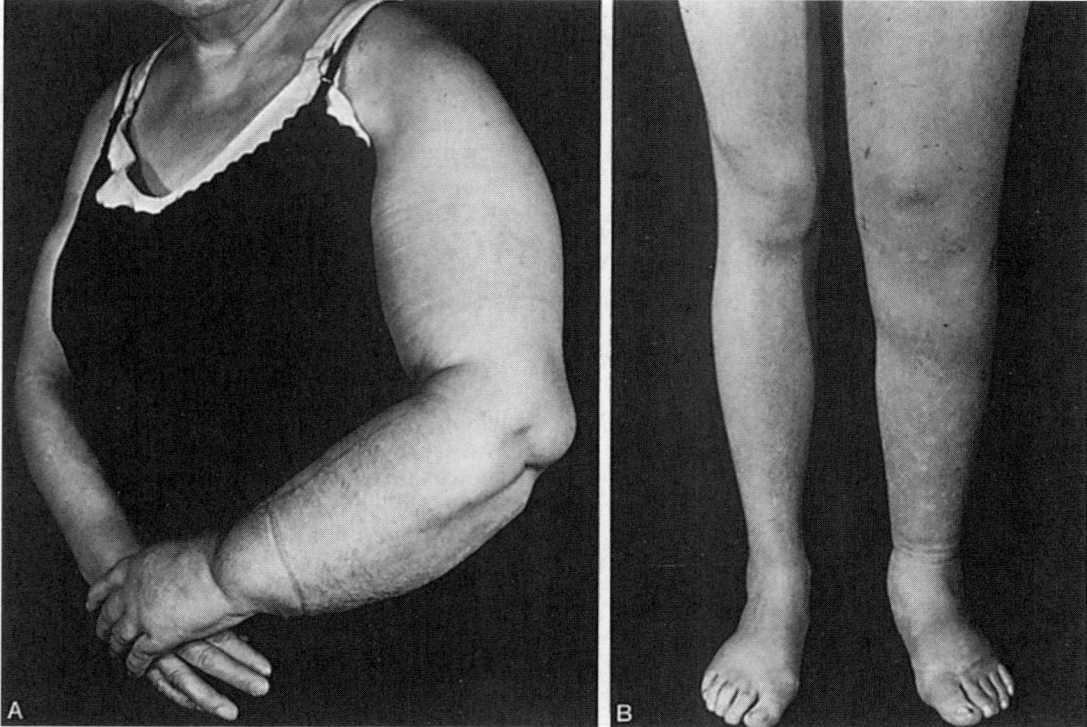

Figure 24–13. Types of lymphedema. *A,* Secondary lymphedema of the arm following mastectomy. *B,* Primary lymphedema. (From Black JM, and Matassarin-Jacobs E [eds]. *Luckmann and Sorensen's Medical-Surgical Nursing: A Psychophysiologic Approach.* 4th ed. Philadelphia: WB Saunders, 1993, p 1311.)

2. Secondary lymphedema is related to some form of damage or obstruction of the lymphatic system.

Pathophysiology

1. An impaired lymphatic transport system allows plasma proteins to accumulate in the interstitial fluid.
2. An increase in colloid osmotic pressure occurs. The body attempts to compensate and reduce the elevated pressure by drawing water into interstitial areas.
3. Lymphatic channels dilate, and lymphatic valves become incompetent.
4. The extra fluid is no longer drained appropriately and accumulates in the tissues.

Clinical Manifestations

1. Permanent swelling of the lower extremities, usually unilateral; if bilateral, the swelling is asymmetric.
2. A chronic, dull, heavy sensation develops in the affected extremity.
3. Edema starts in the foot but gradually progresses up the leg so that the entire leg becomes edematous.
4. In chronic peripheral lymphedema persons often present for treatment because of concern over the appearance of the affected extremity.
5. In the later stages of the disease, the affected limb loses

its normal contour because of swelling. The toes appear square.

Diagnostics

1. Assessment (see p. 1122)
2. Medical diagnosis (see p. 1123)

Clinical Management

1. Goal of intervention: To control the symptoms produced by the lymphatic disorder
2. Nonpharmacologic interventions
   a. Decrease edema and promote lymphatic drainage.
      (1) Pneumatic pumps
      (2) Elastic stockings
   b. Teach meticulous foot care to prevent infection (see Learning/Teaching Guidelines for Foot Care).
   c. Encourage activity (e.g., walking) rather than prolonged standing or sitting.
3. Pharmacologic interventions
   a. Treat infections with appropriate antibiotic therapy as prescribed by the physician or nurse practitioner.
   b. Diuretic therapy usually is avoided in long-term therapy because it can deplete intravascular volume and produce metabolic abnormalities.

Complications

The patient may experience disfiguring changes to the extremities.

Prognosis

Lymphedema is a chronic progressive disease with no cure. Over a prolonged course, it causes disfiguring edema.

Applying the Nursing Process

NURSING DIAGNOSIS: Body image disturbance R/T physical changes produced by chronic peripheral lymphedema

1. *Expected outcomes:* The patient should be able to do the following:
   a. Verbalize understanding of the disease process and the therapeutic regimen
   b. Actively participate in planning care
   c. Demonstrate correct technique for use of lymph-reduction devices
2. *Nursing interventions*
   a. Assess the person's strengths and weaknesses for coping with the alteration in body image.
   b. Encourage the person to ventilate feelings about the disease process and its effect on body image.
   c. Be available for talking and listening.
   d. Help the person identify new methods of coping with the disease process.
   e. Assist the person in developing an exercise program to reduce anxiety and improve lower extremity circulation.
   f. Refer for counseling (e.g., clergy, support group, or psychologist).

Discharge Planning and Teaching

1. Assist the person to problem-solve for ways to maximize extremity elevation and minimize edema at home.
2. Encourage regular follow-up visits with the primary care provider.

Public Health Considerations

1. Because lymphedema can be disfiguring, national support groups could be formed to provide information and counseling to assist persons and their families to cope with the disease.
2. Health information hotlines with toll-free numbers could be established by the health care industry so people could obtain information about lymphatic disorders easily.

■ OTHER LYMPHATIC DISORDERS

Lymphangitis

1. Definition: an acute inflammation of the peripheral lymphatic system
2. Incidence and etiology
   a. The exact incidence is not known, but lymphangitis is uncommon.
   b. Acute infection or inflammation in or around the lymphatic channels.
      (1) Bacteria enter the lymphatic system through a break in the skin (e.g., from an ingrown nail, fungal infections, ulcers, or local trauma).
      (2) The most common causative bacteria are hemolytic streptococci and coagulase-positive *Staphylococcus aureus.*
3. Clinical manifestations
   a. Red streaks that outline the lymphatic system in the affected extremity
   b. Chills, fever, malaise
   c. Enlarged, tender lymph nodes in the region of the affected extremity
4. Clinical management
   a. Wound and blood cultures to identify the causative organism
   b. Administration of antibiotics appropriate for the infective organism
   c. Local care of the extremity
      (1) Analgesics to control pain
      (2) Elevation of the affected extremity
      (3) Warm, wet dressings
   d. Surgical drainage of the infected area

Bibliography

Books

References for all of the vascular disorders: arterial, venous, and lymphatic.
Bates B. *A Guide to Physical Examination and History Taking.* 6th ed. Philadelphia: JB Lippincott, 1995.
Canobbio MM. *Cardiovascular Disorders.* St. Louis: CV Mosby, 1990.
Clement DL. *Vascular Diseases in the Limbs: Mechanisms and Principles of Treatment.* St. Louis: Mosby–Year Book, 1993.

Fahey VA. *Vascular Nursing.* 2nd ed. Philadelphia: WB Saunders, 1994.
Helman CG. *Culture, Health, and Illness.* London: Wright, 1990.
Ignatavicius DD, and Bayne MV (eds). *Medical-Surgical Nursing: A Nursing Process Approach.* Philadelphia: WB Saunders, 1991.
Isselbacher KJ, et al. (eds). *Harrison's Principles of Internal Medicine.* 13th ed. New York: McGraw-Hill, 1994.
Koda-Kimble MA, and Young LY (eds). *Applied Therapeutics: The Clinical Use of*

Drugs. Vancouver, Canada: Applied Therapeutics, Inc, 1992.
Moore WS (ed). *Vascular Surgery: A Comprehensive Review.* Philadelphia: WB Saunders, 1993.
Sherry S. *Fibrinolysis, Thrombosis, and Hemostasis: Concepts, Perspectives, and Clinical Applications.* Philadelphia: Lea & Febiger, 1992.
Wyngaarden JB, Smith LH Jr, and Bennett JC (eds). *Cecil Textbook of Medicine.* 19th ed. Philadelphia: WB Saunders, 1992.

Chapters in Books and Journal Articles

Arterial Disease

Ahn SA. Status of peripheral atherectomy. *Surg Clin North Am* 72(4):869–879, 1992.

Bright LD, and Georgi S. Peripheral vascular disease: Is it arterial or venous. *Am J Nurs* 92(9):34–43, 1992.

Cooke JP, and Ma AO. Medical therapy of peripheral arterial occlusive disease. *Surg Clin North Am* 75(4):569–580, 1995.

Emma LA. Chronic arterial occlusive disease. *J Cardiovasc Nurs* 7(1):14–24, 1992.

Green D, and Miller V. The role of dipyridamole in the therapy of vascular disease. *Geriatrics* 48(1):46–58, 1993.

Henderson LJ, et al. Angioplasty with stent placement in peripheral vascular occlusive disease. *AORN J* 61(4):669–671, 1995.

Kerner M. Noninvasive testing in the evaluation of peripheral vascular disease. *Orthop Nurs* 11(2):50–54, 1992.

Lawrence PF, and Goodman GR. Thrombolytic therapy. *Surg Clin North Am* 72(4):899–917, 1972.

McDermott MM, and McCarthy W. Intermittent claudication: The natural history. *Surg Clin North Am* 75(4):581–592, 1995.

Murray KK. Angiography of the lower extremity in atherosclerotic vascular disease: Current techniques. *Surg Clin North Am* 72(4):767–789, 1972.

Sabiston DC. Disorders of the arterial system. *In* Sabiston DC (ed). *Textbook of Surgery: The Biological Basis of Modern Surgical Practice*. 14th ed. Philadelphia: WB Saunders, 1991, pp 1523–1537.

Wagner MM. Pathophysiology related to peripheral vascular disease. *Nurs Clin North Am* 21(2):195–205, 1986.

Williamson VC. Amputation of the lower extremity: An overview. *Orthop Nurs* 11(2):55–65, 1992.

Aortic Aneurysms

Bright LD, and Georgi S. Peripheral vascular disease: Is it arterial or venous. *Am J Nurs* 92(9):34–43, 1992.

Fellows E. Abdominal aortic aneurysm: Warning flags to watch out for. *Am J Nurs* 95(5):27–32, 1995.

Katz DA, et al. Management of small abdominal aortic aneurysms: Early surgery vs watchful waiting. *JAMA* 268(19):2678–2685, 1992.

Sabiston DC. Abdominal aortic aneurysms. *In* Sabiston DC (ed). *Textbook of Surgery: The Biological Basis of Modern Surgical Practice*. 14th ed. Philadelphia: WB Saunders, 1991.

Sandler RL. Abdominal aortic aneurysm. *Am J Nurs* 95(1):38–39, 1995.

Warbinek E, and Wyness MA. Caring for patients with complications after elective AAA surgery: A case study. *J Vasc Nurs* 12(3):73–79, 1994.

Wolfe WG. Aneurysm of the thoracic aorta. *In* Sabiston DC (ed). *Textbook of Surgery: The Biological Basis of Modern Surgical Practice*. 14th ed. Philadelphia: WB Saunders, 1991.

Wolfe WG. Dissecting aneurysms of the aorta. *In* Sabiston DC (ed). *Textbook of Surgery: The Biological Basis of Modern Surgical Practice*. 14th ed. Philadelphia: WB Saunders, 1991.

Wolfe WG. Traumatic aneurysms of the aorta. *In* Sabiston DC (ed). *Textbook of Surgery: The Biological Basis of Modern Surgical Practice*. 14th ed. Philadelphia: WB Saunders, 1991.

Raynaud's Disease

Davis E. The diagnostic puzzle and management challenge of Raynaud's syndrome. *Nurs Pract* 18(3):21–22, 25, 1993.

Transcultural Considerations

Alford JW. The role of culture in grief. *J Soc Psychol* 135(1):25, 1993.

Crowe CC. Cultural issues. *Aust Fam Physician* 24(8):1464–1466, 1995.

Gelo F. Spirituality: A vital component of health counseling. *J Am Coll Health Counseling* 44(1):38–40, 1995.

Remland MS, et al. Interpersonal distance, body orientation, and touch: Effects of culture, gender, and age. *J Soc Psychol* 135(3):281–329, 1995.

Villarrue AM. Mexican-American cultural meanings, expressions, self-care and dependent-care associated with experiences of pain. *Res Nurs Health* 18(5):427–436, 1995.

Venous Disease

Bright LD, and Georgi S. Peripheral vascular disease: Is it arterial or venous. *Am J Nurs* 92(9):34–43, 1992.

Erickson CA, et al. Healing of venous ulcers in an ambulatory care program: The roles of chronic venous insufficiency and patient compliance. *J Vasc Nurs* 22(5):629–636, 1995.

Harris AH, et al. Managing vascular leg ulcers. Part 1: Assessment. *Am J Nurs* 96(1):38–43, 1996.

Harris AH, et al. Managing vascular leg ulcers. Part 2: Treatment. *Am J Nurs* 96(2):40–46, 1996.

Hobson RW, et al. Diagnosis of acute venous thrombosis. *Surg Clin North Am* 70(1):143–156, 1990.

Kerner M. Noninvasive testing in the evaluation of peripheral vascular disease. *Orthop Nurs* 11(2):50–54, 1992.

Lymphatic Disorders

Browse NL. Primary lymphedema. *In* Ernst CB, and Stanley JC (eds). *Current Therapy in Vascular Surgery*. Toronto: BC Decker, 1987.

Wolfe JH. Diagnosis and classification of lymphedema. *In* Rutherford RB (ed). *Vascular Surgery*. 3rd ed. Philadelphia: WB Saunders, 1989.

Agencies and Resources

American Cancer Society
1599 Clifton Road NE
Atlanta, GA 30329
(800) 227–2345

American Heart Association
7320 Greenville Avenue
Dallas, TX 75231
(214) 750–5300

American Association of Critical Care Nurses (AACN)
1 Civic Plaza, Suite 330
Newport Beach, CA 92660
(714) 644–9310

Society for Peripheral Vascular Nursing (SPVN)
309 Winter Street
Norwood, MA 02062
(617) 762–3630

25
Caring for People with Blood Disorders

▣ HEMATOLOGIC STRUCTURE AND FUNCTIONS

Structure of the Hematologic System

1. The hematologic system consists of blood, bone marrow, and the lymphatic system. Accessory organs of the hematologic system are the liver and spleen (see Chapter 28.)
2. Blood is composed of 3 types of cells: **erythrocytes** (red blood cells, RBCs), **leukocytes** (white blood cells, WBCs), and **thrombocytes** (platelets). These cells are suspended in a solution called **plasma,** which consists of water, serum, and protein substances that help maintain intracellular chemical balances. The normal composition of 1 cubic millimeter (mm^3) of blood is presented in Table 25–1.
3. **Bone marrow** is the soft tissue substance that fills the hollow center of long and flat bones. It is made up of red marrow and yellow fatty marrow. **Hematopoiesis** is the formation of blood in the bone marrow, primarily in the flat bones of the sternum, ribs, vertebrae, and pelvic and shoulder girdles (Fig. 25–1).
4. The **lymphatic system** consists of nodes and channels through which fluids and cells circulate in patterns similar to those in the venous system. **Lymph** is an alkaline fluid that is formed in tissue spaces all over the body. It gathers into the small channels and flows back centrally. Lymph node groups are concentrated in the neck, axilla, epitrochlear, and inguinal areas and are palpable when distended. Lymph nodes also are concentrated in the thoracic, abdominal, and popliteal areas, but they are not usually palpable in these areas.

Functions of the Hematologic System

1. The function of blood is to deliver oxygen and nutrients to and remove wastes from all tissues.
2. Erythrocytes transport hemoglobin, which carries oxygen to tissues, and carry carbon dioxide. In addition, they play a role in the regulation of acid-base balance and in the formation of bile pigments, which are derived from

the decomposition of hemoglobin. The life span of the average RBC is 120 days. Box 25–1 describes anemias, conditions involving a decrease in the number of RBCs.
3. Leukocytes fight infection. They react against foreign tissue or substances within the body and participate in responses to tissue injury. Box 25–2 describes changes in numbers of WBCs. Table 25–2 lists etiologies of leukocytosis. Cells involved in the immune response are described in Chapter 21.
4. Platelets play a major role in blood coagulation, hemostasis, and thrombus formation. They are functional for about 10 days and then die. Platelets aggregate to injured small vessels, sticking to one another and to the edges of the injury. Groups of platelets form a plug that covers the injured area and stops the flow of blood. Approximately two thirds of the body's platelet mass circulates in the bloodstream. The other third is stored in the spleen. Platelets also release clotting factors III and IV and **serotonin,** which promotes vasoconstriction and thus decreases blood flow. Any abnormality in various vascular, platelet, and plasma factors can affect coagulation and cause **coagulopathy,** problems in the process by which the body maintains **hemostasis,** the balance between blood clotting and active bleeding. Mechanisms involved in coagulation include vasoconstriction, platelet plug formation, and blood clotting (Fig. 25–2).
5. Red bone marrow is responsible for producing most blood cells through hematopoiesis. Yellow fatty marrow can convert to hematopoietic tissue if necessary. (See Chapter 34 for further discussion of bone marrow.)

ELDER ADVISORY

By age 65, up to 50 percent of the body's bone marrow has converted to inactive, yellow, fatty marrow. This change may account for the mild anemia seen in many older adults. This marrow can convert to hematopoietic tissue if necessary.

6. The lymphatic system helps preserve the body's internal fluid environment by producing, filtering, and transport-

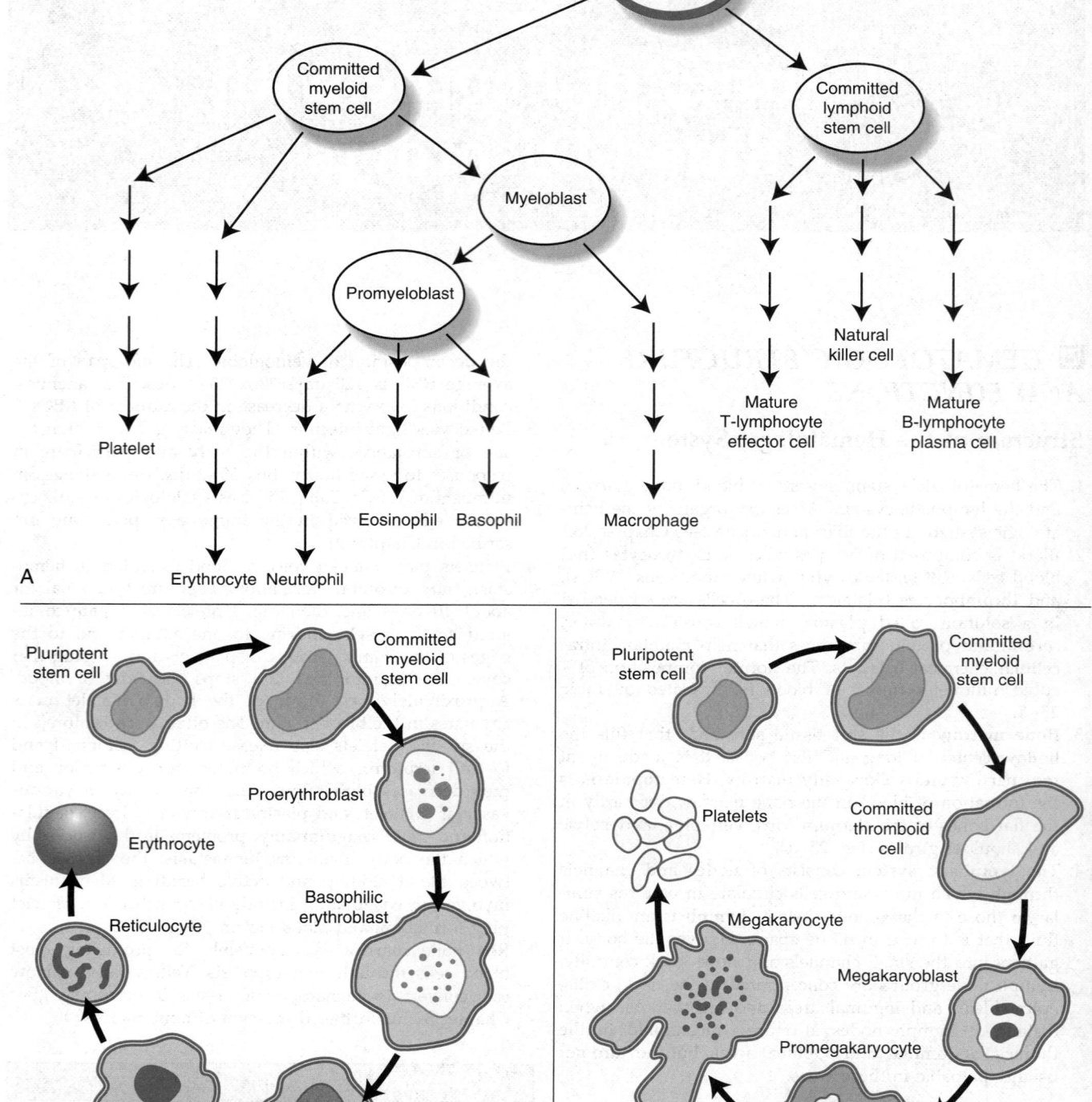

Figure 25–1. *A,* Bone marrow cell differentiation and maturational pathways; *B,* erythrocyte maturational pathway; *C,* platelet maturational pathway. (Copyright 1992 by M. Linda Workman. All rights reserved.)

Table 25–1. Normal Composition of 1 mm³ of Blood

Blood Component

Red blood cells
  Men: 4.5–6.2 million
  Women: 4.2–5.4 million
White blood cells: 4000–10,000
  Granulocytes
    Basophils: 0.5–1%
    Eosinophils: 1–4%
    Juvenile neutrophils: 3–5%
    Mature neutrophils (segmented): 57–65%
  Agranulocytes
    Monocytes: 2–6%
    Lymphocytes: 20–40%
Platelets: 150,000–350,000

BOX 25–2. Changes in the Number of White Blood Cells

Leukocytosis is an increase in the number of leukocytes, or white blood cells (WBCs), to more than 10,000 per mm³ of blood. Generally, this increase is due to infection, but it also can be caused by other conditions. Diseases that cause leukocytosis include infections (not usually viral), leukemias, and other malignancies. Other conditions that cause leukocytosis are extensive surgeries, certain allergies, some toxoids, and hemorrhage.

Leukopenia is an abnormal decrease of leukocytes (WBCs) to less than 5000 per mm³. Conditions that cause leukopenia include agranulocytosis, which can be idiopathic, drug or toxoid induced, or caused by radiation, and immunosuppression. Immunosuppression in certain diseases, such as cancer, occurs as a result of treatments such as chemotherapy or radiation therapy. Immunosuppression can also be intended, as in organ transplant patients. Immunosuppression in acquired immunodeficiency syndrome is the result of viral-induced destruction of many WBC populations.

ing lymph. Through a 1-way network of channels, lymph passively drains excess fats, proteins, fluids, and other substances from body tissue and epithelial spaces. Lymph nodes produce lymphocytes and monocytes and filter matter, especially bacteria, to prevent its access to the bloodstream. Lymph nodes may filter cancer cells, but they may also be the site of origin for some cancers.

7. The liver and spleen service the hematologic system by destroying aged blood cells. The liver synthesizes plasma proteins and some clotting factors. The spleen serves as a warehouse for storing excess blood cells.

◼ ASSESSING PEOPLE WITH HEMATOLOGIC DISORDERS

Key Symptoms and Their Pathophysiologic Bases

1. The hematologic system affects every other body system, making the signs and symptoms of hematologic disorders difficult to identify. An increase in the severity of the blood disorder is reflected by an increase in the severity of symptoms.
2. Low RBC counts result in shortness of breath because of the blood's reduced oxygen-carrying capacity. Weakness,

BOX 25–1. Anemias: Decreases in the Number of Red Blood Cells

Anemia is a frequently occurring clinical condition caused by an abnormality in either the red blood cells (RBCs) or the bone marrow. It may also be a manifestation of an underlying systemic disorder. Anemia involves a decrease in the number of circulating RBCs or a hemoglobin (Hgb) deficiency, with the criteria for diagnosis usually being an Hgb level lower than 12 gm per dl and a hematocrit (Hct) level lower than 36 percent in females and an Hgb level lower than 14 gm per dl and an Hct level lower than 42 percent in males. The clinical manifestations of anemia vary, depending on the etiology, degree of pathology, rapidity of onset, and other underlying medical problems. The more rapid the onset of the anemia, the more severe the symptoms will be. Symptoms are related to tissue hypoxia and include fatigue, headache, dyspnea, tachypnea, weakness, lightheadedness, and angina. Pallor and tachycardia may be indicative of severe anemia. Even severe anemia may be well tolerated if the onset is slow. Anemia may have multiple origins, and treatment needs to be directed toward each.

Hypoproliferative anemia is a decrease in Hct and Hgb levels with an inadequate bone marrow response to the need for RBCs. The marrow fails to increase the number of reticulocytes. Most clinical anemias are due to marrow failures. Many forms of hypoproliferative anemias exist, including aplastic anemias, ineffective hematopoiesis, and hypochromic anemias.

Hemoglobinopathic anemias are inherited disorders of the structure, function, or production of Hgb. The abnormality can be heterozygous or homozygous. These anemias range in clinical severity from asymptomatic conditions to profound multisystem syndromes that result in death. The hemoglobinopathies are the most common inherited disorders of humans. Forms of hemoglobinopathies include sickle cell anemias and thalassemias.

Table 25–2. Etiologies of Leukocytosis

White Blood Cell Type	Cause of Elevation
Basophils	Chronic inflammation Some cancers Hematologic disorders
Eosinophils	Asthma Parasitic infections Allergic reactions Some cancers Skin problems
Neutrophils	Inflammation Acute bacterial infections Stress response Some tumors and cancers
Monocytes	Liver disorders Chronic infections
Lymphocytes	Cancers Some viral infections

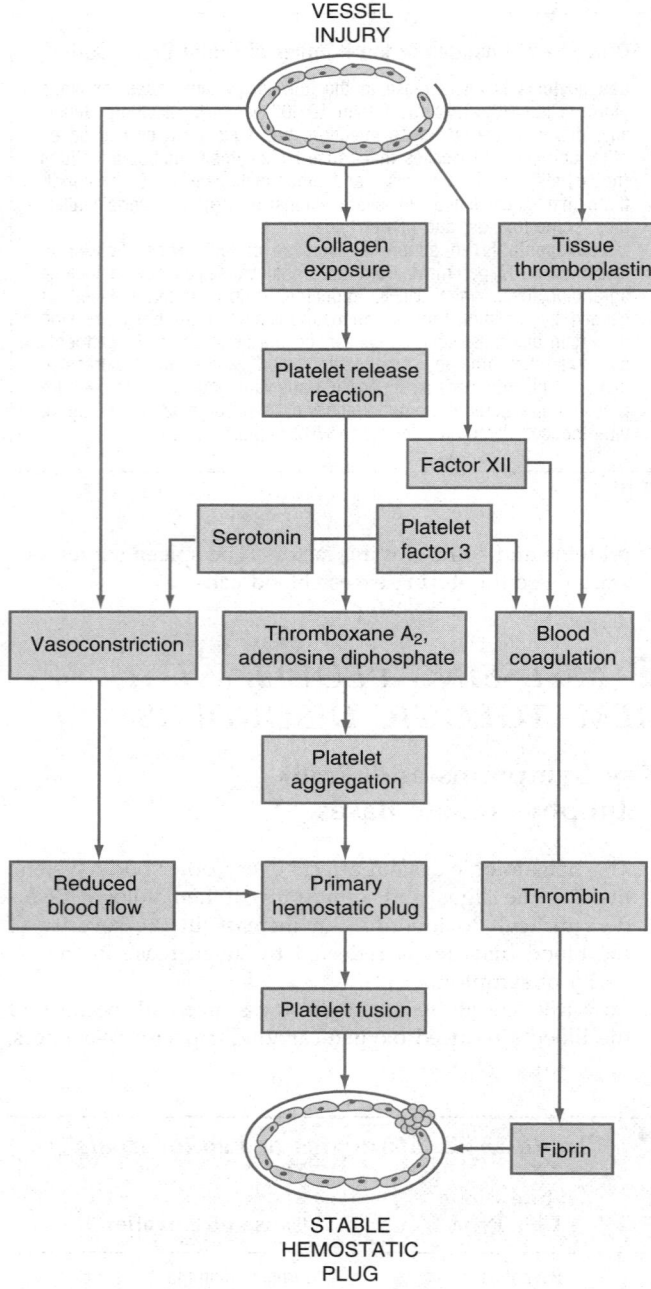

VESSEL
INJURY

Collagen exposure

Tissue thromboplastin

Platelet release reaction

Factor XII

Serotonin

Platelet factor 3

Vasoconstriction

Thromboxane A$_2$, adenosine diphosphate

Blood coagulation

Platelet aggregation

Reduced blood flow

Primary hemostatic plug

Thrombin

Platelet fusion

Fibrin

STABLE HEMOSTATIC PLUG

Figure 25–2. Blood clot formation. A chain reaction of clotting factors produces the formation of a blood clot. Various conditions such as tissue injury, vascular injury, or the presence of a foreign body in the vascular bed can activate the clotting cascade mechanism. (Redrawn from Black JM, and Matassarin-Jacobs E [eds]. *Luckmann and Sorensen's Medical-Surgical Nursing: A Psychophysiologic Approach.* 4th ed. Philadelphia: WB Saunders, 1993, p 1323.)

malaise, and fatigue could indicate a low RBC or WBC count. Abdominal, bone, and joint pain may mean infiltrating proliferating leukocytes, as in leukemias or plasma cell myelomas, or hemolysis.
3. Unusual or prolonged bleeding may indicate a defect in the clotting mechanism.
4. Fever may be caused by infection resulting from a low

WBC count or malfunctioning WBCs. If the infection is of a viral origin, the lymphocyte count will be elevated.
5. Swollen lymph nodes could indicate an elevated lymphocyte count as a result of leukemia or lymphoma or could indicate inflammation as a result of infection.

Health History

1. Careful history taking provides information critical to the diagnosis of the cause of the hematologic disorder. Ask questions in a systematic manner and use your institution's forms to prevent inadvertent omission of information.
2. Include the following in your database:
   a. The time of onset and duration of symptoms and whether symptoms are continuous or intermittent
   b. A history of similar signs and symptoms in a parent or sibling
   c. A history of jaundice or anemia in a parent or sibling
   d. A history of blood loss, bruising, petechiae, or nosebleeds
   e. The patient's typical dietary pattern
   f. The patient's occupational history (some jobs involve exposure to causative agents in hematologic disorders; a list is presented in Table 25–3)
   g. Medication history (some blood disorders are caused by both prescription and nonprescription medications)
   h. Risk factors for hematologic disorders: age, sex, marital status, religion, race and ethnic background, and recent illnesses and treatments
   i. Family history of illnesses for both living and deceased relatives as well as causes of death
   j. Sexual habits: promiscuity, male homosexuality and bisexuality, and partner's sexual habits

Table 25–3. Occupational Causes of Hematologic Disorders	
Chemicals and Compounds	**Affected Occupations**
Insecticides	Exterminators
chlordane	Farmers
DDT	Nursery workers
lindane	Horticulturists
parathion	
arsenic compounds	
pentachlorophenol	
Metal-based dyes in paints	Artists, pottery workers
Resins	Factory workers making artificial limbs
Aromatic hydrocarbons	House painters
benzene	Factory workers in plastics and varnish
toluene	production
carbon tetrachloride	Gasoline station attendants
	Artists

k. Drug abuse history
l. Medical history, including malignancies

Physical Examination

1. Include every body system in your assessment.
2. Table 25–4 lists possible abnormalities associated with hematologic disorders.

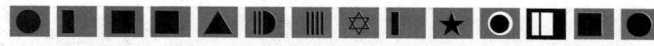

TRANSCULTURAL CONSIDERATIONS

Note that certain religious groups prohibit the transfusion of blood or blood products. For example, Jehovah's Witnesses believe that the body's integrity should be maintained. They believe that no bodily substances should leave the body and no foreign substances should be introduced into it.

Table 25–4. Indicators of Hematologic Disorders

Body System	Signs and Symptoms
Neurologic system	Change in level of consciousness: confusion, inability to concentrate, or drowsiness Mood changes, personality alterations, or worsening dementia Lightheadedness, dizziness, syncope, or vertigo Muscle weakness or facial drooping Paresthesias Inability to sleep Headaches Tinnitus Cold sensitivity
Cardiovascular system	Increased pulse or increased pulse pressure Systolic ejection murmurs Angina Peripheral edema Orthostatic hypotension Bruising or petechiae Intermittent claudication Lymphadenopathy (enlargement and redness) Slow capillary refill
Pulmonary system	Dyspnea Tachypnea Diminished breath sounds
Gastrointestinal system	Abdominal pain or distention Anorexia, nausea, or vomiting Diarrhea or constipation Hematemesis Melena Hepatomegaly and rubs Splenomegaly and rubs Pica (consumption of substances such as ice, starch, and clay) High-pitched, tinkling bowel sounds indicating bowel obstruction
Genitourinary system	Hematuria Impotence Priapism (persistent, usually painful erection of the penis) Bladder dysfunction Abnormal menstrual bleeding Flank pain
Musculoskeletal system	Bone and joint pain Sternal tenderness
Integumentary system	Pallor, jaundice, cyanosis, or plethora (ruddy color): In darker-skinned people, look at the oral mucosa, palms, and soles; inspect the sclerae in all people Bruising or petechiae: Inspect the oral mucosa, sclerae, and conjunctivae; use an ophthalmoscope to examine the retinas Coarse, dry skin: Ask about itching Ulcerations, especially on legs: Ask about wound healing Smooth or ulcerated tongue Gum infections, abscesses, or oral infections such as *Candida* or hairy leukoplakia Nail abnormalities: spoon nails (koilonychia); broad, flat nails (platyonychia); clubbing; or longitudinal striation

Table 25–5. Blood Tests

Test	Purpose	Normal Findings	Collection Procedures
Red blood cell (RBC) count, or erythrocyte count	Measures the total number of RBCs in 1 mm³ of whole blood. Is used to complete erythrocyte indices and help diagnose anemias and polycythemias.	Men: 4.5–6.2 million. Women: 4.2–5.4 million.	Collect blood specimen in purple-top tube.
Reticulocyte count	Measures the percentage of reticulocytes in the total RBC count as a direct indicator of RBC production by the marrow. Is used to evaluate the effectiveness of erythropoiesis and bone marrow function.	Infants from birth to 2 wk: 1.0–2.0% of total RBC count. Adults: 0.5–2.0% of total RBC count.	Collect blood specimen in purple-top tube.
Hemoglobin (Hgb)	Measures the grams of Hgb in 100 ml of blood. Is used to evaluate sufficiency of iron content and oxygen carrying capacity.	Newborns: 17–22 gm/ml. 1-wk-old infants: 10–20 gm/ml. 1-month-old infants: 11–15 gm/ml. Children: 11–13 gm/ml. Men through middle age: 14–18 gm/ml. Men after middle age: 12.4–14.9 gm/ml. Women through middle age: 12–16 gm/ml. Women after middle age: 11.7–13.8 gm/ml.	Collect blood specimen in purple-top tube.

ELDER ADVISORY

The hemoglobin level falls after middle age, with the lowest levels found in the oldest patients. Iron deficiency is the most frequent type of anemia found in older persons. Reduced dietary intake of iron-rich foods may be a contributing factor, but great care should be taken to rule out other causes. Studies indicate that older people absorb iron adequately but do not use oral iron supplements as often as younger people.

Test	Purpose	Normal Findings	Collection Procedures
Hgb electrophoresis	Separates normal Hgb (HbA, HbA2, and low levels of HbF) from certain abnormal Hgb (HbS, high levels of HbF, homozygous HbC, and heterozygous HbC). Is used to measure abnormal Hgb consistent with thalassemia and sickle cell disease.	Neonates: 50% of Hgb is HbF; no other Hgb types are normally found. Adults: more than 99% of Hgb is HbA, 2–3% is HbA2, and less than 1% is HbF.	Collect blood specimen in purple-top tube.
Hematocrit (Hct)	Measures the volume of RBC mass in 100 ml of plasma and is usually expressed as the percentage of red cell mass in blood volume.	Findings vary with the amount of extracellular fluid present: If the person is dehydrated or has polycythemia, the Hct level rises; if the person is excessively hydrated or has anemia, the Hct level falls. Normal ranges: Men: 42–54%. Women: 38–46%. Children: 36–40%.	Collect blood specimen in purple-top tube.
Erythrocyte (RBC) indices Mean corpuscular volume	Reflects the average size of RBCs: Normal-sized cells are called **normocytic;** smaller than normal cells are called **microcytic;** larger than normal cells are called **macrocytic.**	Normal range: 84–99 μm³	Collect blood specimen in purple-top tube.
Mean corpuscular Hgb	Measures the weight of Hgb in an average cell. Is used to help classify anemias.	Normal range: 26–32 pg.	Collect blood specimen in purple-top tube.
Mean corpuscular Hgb concentration (MCHC)	Reflects the concentration of Hgb in each RBC. Is determined through the ratio of Hgb weight to Hct. Is reduced in hypochromic anemias.	Normal range: 30–36 gm/dl.	Collect blood specimen in purple-top tube.
Erythrocyte sedimentation rate (ESR)	Measures the degree of erythrocyte settling during a specified period.	Range: 0–20 mm/hr, depending on the method used.	Collect blood specimen in purple-, black-, or blue-top tube, de-

Table 25–5. Blood Tests (Continued)

Test	Purpose	Normal Findings	Collection Procedures
	Factors that affect ESR include RBC volume, surface area, density, aggregation, and surface charge. Is used to monitor inflammatory or malignant disease and to assist in detection and diagnosis of diseases not yet manifested in other ways.	A nonspecific but very sensitive test, ESR often rises before any other chemical or physical change occurs.	pending on laboratory procedure.
Osmotic fragility	Measures RBC resistance to hemolysis. Is used to confirm morphologic RBC abnormalities and to help in diagnosis of hereditary spherocytosis.	Normal RBCs resist hemolysis until exposed to a saline solution of 0.50% or greater.	Collect blood specimen in green-top tube.
Erythrocyte (RBC) survival	Measures the survival time of RBCs in circulation and identifies any areas of abnormal RBC pooling and destruction. Uses the patient's own RBCs, which are radioactively tagged and injected into him or her. Over 3–4 weeks, blood samples are drawn and the percentage of labeled cells is measured. During this time, the person is scanned with a gamma camera to detect areas of the body that indicate sequestration and destruction of labeled Hgb.	Normal scans may show slight radioactivity in the spleen, liver, and bone marrow during the 3–4 wk of the test. Increased sequestration of RBCs is abnormal. Decreased RBC survival time is consistent with hemolytic diseases.	Collect blood specimen in green-top tube.
Sickle cell (hemoglobin S) test	Indentifies RBCs that severely deform in the presence of low pH, low oxygen tension, high osmolarity, and elevated temperature. Is used to screen for sickle cell disease and sickle cell trait.	Can have erroneous results. Serum electrophoresis should also be performed if sickle cell disease is strongly suspected.	Collect blood specimen in purple-top tube.
Coagulation screening			
Activated partial thromboplastin time	Measures the time required for formation of a fibrin clot in plasma when chemicals are added by evaluating all clotting factors of the intrinsic pathway. Is used to screen for deficiencies of clotting factors in intrinsic pathway and to monitor heparin therapy.	Normal ranges vary across laboratories; a common range is 16–25 sec.	Collect specimen in blue-top tube.
Prothrombin time	Measures the time it takes a fibrin clot to form in plasma when chemicals are added by evaluating extrinsic coagulation factors V, VII, and X; prothrombin; and fibrinogen. It is used to evaluate the effectiveness or activity of a variety of clotting factors.	Normal ranges vary across laboratories; a common range is 9.5–11.5 sec.	Collect blood specimen in blue-top tube.
Platelet count, size, and shape	Is an important screening test for platelet function. Is used to evaluate platelet production, assess the effects of chemotherapy or radiation therapy, and aid in the diagnosis of thrombocytopenic disorders.	Range: 150,000–350,000. A count below 20,000 can cause spontaneous bleeding. A count above 400,00 can cause vascular thrombosis with organ failures.	Collect blood specimen in purple-top tube.
Bleeding time	Gives information on the platelets' ability to perform clotting function and the capillaries' ability to constrict. After written procedures, the test involves timing how long it takes a clot to form after puncture with a lancet.	Normal range is 3–10 min in most laboratories, but values vary, depending on the method used.	
Fibrinogen level	Aids in diagnosis of clotting or bleeding disorders. Restricts clotting system by dissolving fibrin clots after vascular repair.	Range: 195–365 mg/dl.	Collect blood specimen in blue-top tube.

Table continued on the following page

Table 25–5. Blood Tests (Continued)

Test	Purpose	Normal Findings	Collection Procedures
Factor assays	Gives information on the coagulation of specific factors. Is used to study persons with congenital or acquired coagulation defects.	Reference range for most factors: 50–150% of normal activity.	Collect blood specimen in blue-top tube.
Agglutination ABO blood typing	Determines the classification of blood types according to the presence of the major antigens A and B on the surface of the RBC and the presence of anti-A or anti-B antibodies in the serum. Is used to establish blood group and to assess the compatibility between the donor and recipient before transfusion of blood products.		Collect blood specimen in red-top tube.
Rh typing	Establishes the presence or absence of the $Rh_o(D)$ antigen on the surfaces of RBCs. Is used to establish the Rh type and compatibility of the donor before transfusion of blood products and to determine whether the recipient will need injections of Rh immune globulin.		Collect blood specimen in red-top tube.
Crossmatching	Establishes the compatibility of the donor's and recipient's blood after ABO blood type and Rh factor type are established. Detects the presence of antibodies that would destroy the donor's RBCs, causing a transfusion reaction. ABO typing, Rh typing, and crossmatching are all performed together.		Collect blood specimen in red-top tube.
Direct Coombs' test (direct antiglobulin test)	Detects antibodies (immunoglobulins) on the surfaces of RBCs. Agglutination occurs if these antibodies are present. Detects hemolytic disease in newborns. Is used to examine hemolytic transfusion reaction and to aid in the diagnosis of different hemolytic anemias.	A negative result is normal and means that no antibodies or complement appears on the RBCs.	Collect blood specimen in red-top tube.
Indirect Coombs' test (antibody screening, an indirect antiglobulin test)	Detects unknown circulating antibodies in the serum. Agglutination occurs if the serum has any antibodies to the antigens on RBCs of type O blood.	A negative result is normal, indicating that no agglutination has occurred and the serum has no antibodies (except perhaps anti-A or anti-B).	Collect blood specimen in red-top tube.
Leukoagglutination	Identifies any leukoagglutinins (antibodies that react to white blood cells [WBCs]). Is used to determine whether a transfusion reaction is hemolytic or nonhemolytic. May indicate the need for the blood recipient to receive leukocyte-poor transfusions in the future.		Collect blood specimen in red-top tube.
Leukocyte (WBC) count	Determines the number of WBCs in a 1 mm³ of whole blood. Is used to identify infection and inflammation, to determine the need for further testing, and to monitor the response to chemotherapy and radiation therapy.	Range: 4000–10,000/mm³ of blood; the count can differ by as much as 2000 in a single day. Can rise or fall because of disease but must be interpreted with the WBC differential to be of any diagnostic value.	Collect blood specimen in purple-top tube.
WBC differential	Differentiates the WBCs into five major groups of leukocytes—neutrophils, eosinophils, basophils, lymphocytes, and	Normal ranges: neutrophils: 60–70% eosinophils: 1–4%	Collect blood specimen in purple-top tube.

Table 25–5. Blood Tests (Continued)

Test	Purpose	Normal Findings	Collection Procedures
	monocytes—and determines the percentage of each type. Is used to determine the body's ability to fight infection, to diagnose various types of leukemias, to determine and stage the severity of infections, and to detect allergic reactions.	basophils: 0.5–1% lymphocytes: 20–40% monocytes: 3–6% Abnormal percentages are diagnostic and associated with specific diseases.	
Serum unconjugated (indirect) and conjugated (direct) bilirubin	Bilirubin is the main production of Hgb destruction. Unconjugated (prehepatic) bilirubin and conjugated (posthepatic) bilirubin are measured to determine the effectiveness of the hepatobiliary and erythropoietic functions. These tests are used to help diagnose jaundice, hemolytic anemia, and liver function.	Ranges: Unconjugated bilirubin: 0.2–0.8 mg/dl Conjugated bilirubin: 0.0–0.2 mg/dl	Collect blood specimen in red-top or red-marbled (tiger)-top tube.
Urine hemoglobin	**Hemoglobinuria,** or Hgb in the urine, usually occurs when there is large or rapid destruction of RBCs and the reticuloendothelial system cannot metabolize or store the free Hgb. Is used to diagnose transfusion reactions and hemolytic anemias.	Normally, the urine is negative for Hgb.	Collect the random urine specimen in a container with no preservatives.

Special Diagnostic Studies

1. Blood tests: Table 25–1 summarizes the composition of blood. Table 25–5 lists blood tests. Procedure 25–1 explains the technique for drawing blood.
2. Radiologic studies
   a. Computed tomography (CT): The scan can be of the total body or limited to specific areas of interest. The absorption of x-rays by body tissue is analyzed by the computer, with the results displayed on the screen. The amount of absorption depends on tissue density. The views are cross-sectional and 3-dimensional. The person lies on a table that slides through a large ring. The ring houses the source and receptor of the x-ray beam and rotates around the person, making the necessary images. The patient may feel claustrophobic.
      (1) The individual may receive an intravenous (IV) contrast medium. Be sure to ask questions regarding sensitivity to seafood, iodine, and other contrast dyes. Watch for allergic reaction in all patients receiving contrast dyes. If contrast dye is used, the person may have nothing by mouth during the 4 hours before the test.
      (2) A signed informed-consent form is necessary if contrast medium is used.
   b. Gallium scan: A total-body scan is usually done 24 to 48 hours after an IV injection of radioactive gallium citrate. The liver, spleen, bones, and large bowel normally take up gallium, but some neoplasms and inflammatory lesions also absorb it. Gallium scans are used to detect primary and metastatic neoplasms and inflammatory lesions and to evaluate malignant lymphoma after treatment.
      (1) No food or fluid restrictions are required with the test.
      (2) Scanning takes 30 minutes to 1 hour.
      (3) A signed informed-consent form is necessary.
   c. Lymphangiography: A radiographic examination of the lymphatic system follows injection of an oil-based contrast medium into the lymph vessels in the region to be studied. Radiographs are taken immediately after the injection and again 24 hours later. Lymphangiography is used to detect and stage lymphomas, identify metastatic involvement of nodes, and suggest whether surgical treatment is warranted.
      (1) Assess the patient for sensitivity to seafood, iodine, and other contrast dyes. Watch for allergic reactions.
      (2) The test takes about 3 hours.
      (3) There is no need to restrict food or fluid.
      (4) A signed informed-consent form is necessary.
3. Lymph node biopsy
   a. Biopsy of cervical, supraclavicular, axillary, or inguinal nodes is performed. Usually a needle biopsy is performed, as opposed to incision and removal of a node.
   b. Histologic examination of the node helps the physician determine whether the enlarged node is a result of cancer or a noncancerous disorder. It is also used to stage lymph node cancer.
   c. Assess the patient for sensitivity to local anesthetic.
   d. Person can take nothing by mouth for 12 hours if general anesthesia is used for surgical excision of a node. A clear liquid diet is permitted in the morning if local anesthetic is used for excision. No restrictions are necessary if the biopsy is an aspiration biopsy.

Procedure 25–1
Obtaining Blood Samples Through Phlebotomy

Definition/Purpose	Phlebotomy is the removal of blood from a vein. It is performed to obtain serum samples for ordered blood tests.
Contraindications/Cautions	Do not take blood samples from extremities that contain arteriovenous shunts or loops. After mastectomy or axillary node dissection, do not perform phlebotomy on upper extremities from the same side of the body from which the breast was removed. In addition, blood samples should not be drawn from an arm with an intravenous infusion. In certain cases in which there is absolutely no other option, the infusion may be turned off for several minutes, allowing the sample to be taken.
Learning/Teaching Activities	Provide the following information: (a) Describe the procedure, regardless of the person's level of consciousness; (b) explain that the tourniquet may feel tight for several minutes; (c) let the individual know that remaining still is essential during the procedure; and (d) explain the indications for the specific blood test.

Preliminary Activities

Equipment	• Tourniquet • Phlebotomy needle—This may be a Vacutainer needle or a butterfly needle. • Vacutainer • Vacutainer collection tubes—Different tests require different collection tubes. The color of the rubber stopper at the top of the tube reflects the type of preservative and type of tube: A purple-top tube is used for a complete blood count; a blue-top tube is used for prothrombin time, partial thromboplastin time, and a hemostasis profile; a gold- or ghost-top tube is used for chemistries; and a red-top tube is used for most drug levels and blood typing and crossmatching. • Alcohol swabs • Cotton balls or 2 × 2 gauze • Small bandage • Nonsterile gloves
Assessment/Planning	• Review the physician's order for the specific blood test to be obtained. • Coordinate the sequencing of venipuncture with ordered tests to prevent multiple, frequent sticks as much as possible. • Determine the time the sample is to be drawn—for example, after fasting, for morning laboratory work, at random, or in timed sequence (as in peak and trough drug levels). • Assess the upper extremity for an appropriate vein for venipuncture.
Preparation of Person	• The person should be in a stable, relaxed, sitting or lying position. • For a child, have the parent hold the child with his or her arm extended and secured. Do not allow the child to see the needle.

Procedure

Action	Rationale/Discussion
1. Identify the patient.	1. Prevents laboratory draw on the wrong patient.
2. Explain the procedure.	2. Decreases anxiety.
3. Wash your hands.	3. Maintains universal precautions.
4. Prepare the equipment before entering the room. Screw the phlebotomy needle into the top of the plastic Vacutainer.	4. Decreases anxiety.
5. Identify the arm for venipuncture. The arm should be in a dependent position.	5. Allows blood to pool in venous structures.
6. Position yourself next to the arm for venipuncture.	6. Facilitates convenience and allows a good view of the vein.
7. Apply the tourniquet above the elbow.	7. Offers the largest vein for repeated phlebotomy.
8. Palpate for the vein.	8. Determines the site for the initial stick of the needle.
9. Put on gloves.	9. Maintains universal precautions.
10. Cleanse the skin with alcohol.	10. Decreases skin flora.
11. Insert the needle bevel up into the vein approximately one fourth of an inch. There will be no blood return.	11. Reduces trauma to the vein and keeps the needle from clotting with blood and tissue. (The rubberized end of the phlebotomy needle prevents blood return.)

P

Procedure 25–1

(continued)

Action	Rationale/Discussion
12. Push the Vacutainer tube up into the Vacutainer and onto the rubberized end of the needle.	12. Initiates the flow of blood for collection into the tube.
13. Hold the Vacutainer and needle still during application and removal of tubes.	13. Prevents dislodging or further insertion of the needle.
14. When the tube is full, gently remove it from the end of the rubber needle. Rotate the tube if indicated.	14. Stops the flow of blood for collection in that tube and prevents clotting of the sample.
15. If multiple tubes are to be collected, repeat steps 12 and 13.	15. Allows for multiple collections.
16. When collection is complete, remove the tourniquet.	16. Prevents the formation of a hematoma.
17. Quickly remove the needle from the vein while applying pressure to the site with a cotton ball or 2 × 2 gauze.	17. Prevents bleeding from the site.
18. After the site clots, apply a small bandage or leave the site open to air.	18. Prevents infection.
19. Label each tube collected with the person's name, the date and time of the phlebotomy, the test to be performed, and your initials.	19. Properly identifies the sample for the laboratory.
20. Dispose of the needle and Vacutainer into a sharps container. *Do not recap.*	20. Prevents risks of needle exposure and stick.

Final Activities

Remove gloves and discard them, thereby applying universal precautions. Then wash your hands. Check to ensure that the site of the needle stick is free of oozing or hematoma. Ensure patient safety.

---

e. A signed informed-consent form is necessary.
4. Bone marrow aspiration and needle biopsy
   a. Aspiration collects marrow fluid with bone marrow cells in suspension.
   b. Needle biopsy recovers a core of marrow, which contains cells.
   c. Together, these 2 tests provide valuable diagnostic information regarding hematopoiesis and hematologic disorders.
   d. Sites used for these procedures include the posterior superior iliac crest, the spinous process of vertebrae, the tibia (in infants), and the sternum (which involves the most risks and is not often used).
   e. Complications include soreness at the biopsy site, bleeding, and infection.
   f. Monitor the site for bleeding. Monitor pulse, blood pressure, and temperature elevation. Instruct the patient to keep the site dry for 24 hours. Watch for redness, swelling, drainage, and temperature elevation at the site.
   g. A signed informed-consent form is necessary.

◼ *APLASTIC ANEMIAS*

Definition

1. In inherited aplastic anemia, RBCs are no longer being produced by the bone marrow. Most forms of the disorder are accompanied by cessation of leukocyte and thrombocyte production as well. This condition is called **pancytopenia.** Most aplastic anemias are idiopathic rather than inherited.
2. In acquired aplastic anemia, the person was exposed to chemical compounds or drugs that have deleterious effects on the bone marrow, with the result that the marrow no longer produces RBCs. Most acquired aplastic anemias include a reduction in leukocyte and thrombocyte formation as well.

Incidence and Socioeconomic Impact

1. Idiopathic aplastic anemia is generally a disease of the young, with the median incidence at 25 years of age.
2. Acquired aplastic anemia is frequently seen as a result of chemotherapy and radiation therapy treatments for cancer, but it is dose dependent and usually reversible.

Risk Factors

1. Use of drugs that have a high incidence of causing aplasia (see Etiology)
2. Employment in industries that use or produce chemicals, especially benzene, known to be associated with aplastic anemias

Etiology

1. Idiopathic impairment of stem cell development within bone marrow constitutes 80 percent of the aplastic anemias.
2. Drug-induced anemias constitute 10 percent of aplastic anemias. The offending substances include benzenes, kerosenes, paint solvents, butazones, insecticides, gold, anticonvulsants, chlorpromazine, chloramphenicol, cytotoxic cancer drugs, and radiation exposure.
3. Illnesses such as hepatitis C and those caused by Epstein-Barr virus, parvovirus, and cytomegalovirus account for another 10 percent of aplastic anemias.

Pathophysiology

1. An abnormality occurs in the production of stem cells in the bone marrow, but no changes occur in the structure of the marrow. Red blood cell indices show normocytic or macrocytic cells. The abnormality could be due to immunologic suppression of hematopoiesis and damage to stem cells. Marrow biopsy shows mainly fat, with hematopoietic cells constituting only 25 percent, and sometimes as little as 0 to 5 percent, of marrow.
2. These changes are associated with leukopenia and thrombocytopenia.

Clinical Manifestations

1. Manifestations vary with the severity of the disease and underlying disease processes.
2. Signs and symptoms are listed in Box 25–3.

BOX 25–3. Signs and Symptoms of Aplastic Anemia

Fatigue
Malaise
Pallor of the skin and conjunctiva
Headache
Dyspnea
Tachypnea
Palpitation
Tachycardia
Ecchymoses
Petechiae
Bleeding
Fever
Infections
Confusion
Inability to concentrate
Lightheadedness
Dizziness
Paresthesias
Smooth tongue
Sore tongue
Angina
Pica (consumption of such substances as ice, starch, or clay)
Anorexia
Disruption of sleep patterns
Tinnitus
Worsening or new-onset claudication
Increased pulse pressure
Systolic ejection murmur
Mild peripheral edema and progressive weakness

Diagnostics

1. The history and physical examination reveal the signs and symptoms noted in Box 25–1. Pay particular attention to the signs and symptoms of infection and bleeding.
2. A bone marrow biopsy demonstrates the etiology of aplasia. The biopsy demonstrates a fatty, empty marrow.
3. Hematocrit (Hct) and hemoglobin (Hgb) levels, RBC indices, a WBC count with differential, a reticulocyte count, and a platelet count are used to diagnose aplastic anemia. The Hct and Hgb levels and platelet count will be low. The lymphocyte count may be normal or low.

Clinical Management

1. The goals of clinical management are support, remission, and cure.
2. Nonpharmacologic interventions
   a. Drugs associated with onset of the disease should be discontinued.
   b. Transfusions with packed RBCs and platelets to keep Hgb at 7 to 8 gm per dl and the platelet count above 10,000 to 20,000 per μl are recommended. To avoid increased risk of bone marrow graft rejection, transfusions from family members should be avoided if a bone marrow transplant is anticipated. All RBCs should be delivered through leukocyte filters to prevent sensitization against human leukocyte antigens.

TRANSCULTURAL CONSIDERATIONS

Some ethnic and racial groups consider blood to be the carrier of the life force, and thus patients and families in these groups may be hesitant to either donate or receive bone marrow.

---

   c. People known to have been exposed to drugs that cause aplastic anemias require close monitoring.
   d. In patients younger than 20, bone marrow transplantation is 80 percent successful. Graft-versus-host disease increases progressively with age and occurs in 90 percent of adults older than 30. (See Chapter 21.)
   e. In older adults, secondary opportunistic infections and interstitial pneumonitis are significant complications. Therefore, marrow transfusions are not recommended for older patients.
3. Pharmacologic interventions include antithymocyte globulin therapy (immunosuppressive therapy), corticosteroids, androgen therapy, and hematopoietic growth factor.

Complications

1. High output cardiac failure in slowly developing anemias

2. Severe postural hypotension, fall in cardiac output, sweating, restlessness, thirst, and air hunger
3. Retinal hemorrhages
4. Development of pancytopenia and its complications, including hemorrhages, infection, and death

Prognosis

1. The prognosis is determined by the degree of blood count depression. The natural course for severe untreated disease is rapid deterioration and death due to infection and hemorrhage.
2. Bone marrow transplants give an 80 percent survival rate to patients younger than 20. The survival of patients ages 20 to 40 depends largely on general clinical condition and previous transfusions. Immunosuppressive therapy has outcomes similar to those of transplant, except in persons with severe neutropenia.

Applying the Nursing Process

NURSING DIAGNOSIS: Activity intolerance R/T fatigue and shortness of breath due to the blood's decreased oxygen-carrying capacity

1. *Expected outcomes:* After instruction, the person should be able to do the following:
   a. Demonstrate the ability to monitor pulse, respirations, and blood pressure
   b. Verbalize and demonstrate an understanding of how to decrease fatigue
   c. Demonstrate an increased tolerance for performing activities of daily living (ADLs)
2. *Nursing interventions*
   a. Monitor pulse and respirations before and during an ADL.
   b. Stop the ADL if pulse rate becomes tachycardic and respiratory rate rises above normal values. Provide oxygen if necessary.
   c. Monitor blood pressure every 4 hours and when the patient is shifting from sitting to standing or from lying to sitting or standing.
   d. Teach the person to move slowly when changing position, to decrease orthostatic hypotensive episodes.
   e. Between ADLs, allow a 90-minute rest period with vital signs maintained at patient's baseline. (Do not count the period during which vital signs are changed because of activity as part of the rest period.)
   f. Monitor the patient for other signs and symptoms of decreased oxygenation. For example, note dyspnea, dizziness, lightheadedness, headaches, and palpitations.
   g. Teach the person to assess for the same signs and symptoms.
   h. Teach the person the techniques for monitoring pulse, respirations, and blood pressure.

NURSING DIAGNOSIS: Risk for infection R/T decreased capability for immunologic response

1. *Expected outcomes:* After intervention, the patient should be able to do the following:
   a. Prevent infections while in the hospital
   b. Prevent infections after discharge
   c. Verbalize an understanding of preventing infections
2. *Nursing interventions*
   a. Use universal precautions carefully with these patients (see Box 8–3). Teach the patient and all visitors to follow the same universal precautions. Some institutions use reverse isolation.
   b. Monitor the patient for signs and symptoms of infection.
   c. Provide meticulous skin care to maintain the skin's integrity.
   d. Teach and encourage pulmonary toilet, to prevent respiratory infections.

NURSING DIAGNOSIS: Knowledge deficit R/T the etiology and treatment of this life-threatening condition and prevention of its recurrence

1. *Expected outcomes:* After instruction, the person should be able to do the following:
   a. Verbalize understandings of the etiology and treatment of the condition and ways to prevent future exacerbations
   b. Demonstrate compliance with the treatment regimen
2. *Nursing interventions*
   a. Identify the patient's level of knowledge, readiness to learn, and capacity to understand.
   b. Include family members and friends in the teaching when appropriate.
   c. Deliver information verbally, assessing for understanding during the presentations. Keep teaching periods short enough that they do not tax the individual's strength.
   d. Give the person literature to read and to take home. Be sure to follow up and determine whether the person has any questions regarding the information you presented orally or the written literature.
   e. Teach the patient about his or her diet and nutritional needs.

Discharge Planning and Teaching

1. Assess for the need for appointments with a dietitian and with a social worker for help in obtaining needed assistance at home.
2. Encourage the patient to make a follow-up appointment with health care professionals.

Public Health Considerations

1. Teaching people at risk can help reduce exposure to chemical compounds that lead to acquired aplastic anemia.

2. Government regulation of industries will decrease the exposure of employees to potentially dangerous compounds and, consequently, the incidence of acquired aplastic anemia.
3. There are no known primary prevention strategies for idiopathic aplastic anemia.

◼ *HYPOCHROMIC, IRON-DEFICIENCY ANEMIA*

Definition

1. Hypochromic anemia occurs when the body's stores of iron become inadequate for sufficient erythropoiesis. Anemia occurs only after stores of iron have been exhausted. Anemia is therefore a late stage of iron deficiency.
2. Normocytic and normochromic cells appear at the beginning of the disease but become microcytic and hypochromic as the disease progresses. Laboratory values indicate low plasma iron and ferritin levels.

Incidence and Socioeconomic Impact

1. Iron deficiency is the most common cause of anemia in the world. In most developed nations, 3 percent of the men, 20 percent of the women, and more than 50 percent of the pregnant women are deficient in iron according to plasma iron levels.
2. In the United States, 90 percent of the cases of iron-deficiency anemia are found in women.

Risk Factors

1. Chronic blood loss as a result of menstruation is the leading cause of iron-deficiency anemia in women; chronic blood loss caused by gastrointestinal bleeding is the leading cause in men.
2. Iron-poor diets contribute to the incidence. Pregnancy, lactation, infancy, and adolescence place increased demand on the body for iron and can therefore lead to the development of iron-deficiency anemia.

Etiology

1. Loss of blood is usually the underlying cause of the disease. An imbalance between demand and dietary intake also causes iron-deficiency anemia during such times as infancy, adolescence, and pregnancy, when more iron is needed for growth. Iron is routinely lost through the loss of cells that contain iron from the gastrointestinal tract, urinary tract, and the skin. The usual loss is 1 mg per day. Menstruation, childbearing, and lactation are routes of iron loss. An increase in this blood loss can lead to disease.

2. Decreased iron absorption, as is found in patients with celiac disease and postgastrectomy patients, can lead to iron-deficiency anemia.

Pathophysiology

1. Hemoglobin levels fall below normal and continue to fall as the disease progresses. Serum ferritin levels are less than 12 μg per dl (normal is 13–300), serum iron levels are usually low (<60 μg/dl), and total iron-binding capacity is increased (>360 μg/dl). Mean corpuscular volume is usually normal early in the disease and decreases later.
2. Red blood cells are normocytic at the start of the disease and become microcytic and hypochromic as the disease progresses.
3. Bone marrow that shows loss of staining for iron is the definitive test for iron deficiency, but this test is not usually needed for diagnosis.

Clinical Manifestations

1. Manifestations vary with the severity of the disease and underlying disease processes.
2. Signs and symptoms are listed in Box 25–4.

Diagnostics

1. A history of the clinical picture and a physical examination are needed. Careful history taking is important to ensure that the anemia does not have multiple sources.

BOX 25–4. Signs and Symptoms of Iron-Deficiency Anemia

Fatigue
Malaise
Pallor of the skin and conjunctiva
Headache
Dyspnea
Tachypnea
Palpitations
Tachycardia
Confusion
Inability to concentrate
Lightheadedness
Dizziness
Paresthesias
Smooth tongue
Sore tongue
Angina
Pica
Anorexia
Disruption of sleep patterns
Tinnitus
Worsening or new-onset claudication
Increased pulse pressure
Systolic ejection murmur
Mild peripheral edema
Progressive weakness

Laboratory data include Hgb and Hct levels, RBC indices, total iron-binding capacity, ferritin levels, WBC with differential, and bone marrow biopsy and aspiration.
2. Identify the source of bleeding and any evidence of **pica** (consumption of substances such as starch, ice, or clay).
3. Document the patient's response to iron therapy.

Clinical Management

1. Goals of intervention
   a. Identify the cause of iron deficiency.
   b. Increase Hct and Hgb levels to within normal ranges.
   c. Prevent recurrence.
2. Nonpharmacologic interventions
   a. Increase dietary intake of iron. (Dietary intake can supply only normal daily losses of iron. It cannot supply enough iron to restore Hct and Hgb levels to normal.)
   b. Correct the cause of blood loss. For example, if the cause is gastrointestinal or uterine bleeding, surgery may be possible to stop the blood loss.
3. Pharmacologic interventions
   a. Oral therapy is with ferrous sulfate. Ferrous gluconate and ferrous fumarate are alternative oral therapies.
   b. For patients with poor absorption or intolerance of oral iron, parenteral iron therapy can be given with IV or intramuscular (IM) iron dextran. Because the IV and IM routes bring complications such as pain and phlebitis, the oral route is preferred. Parenteral therapy does not usually correct the anemia faster than oral therapy.

Complications

1. High output cardiac failure in slowly developing anemias
2. Severe postural hypotension, fall in cardiac output, sweating, restlessness, thirst, and air hunger

Prognosis

1. Complete recovery is usual if the source of bleeding is found and controlled.
2. The person must follow instructions regarding diet and iron therapy.

Applying the Nursing Process

NURSING DIAGNOSIS: Activity intolerance R/T the blood's decreased oxygen-carrying capacity

NURSING DIAGNOSIS: Fatigue R/T the blood's decreased oxygen-carrying capacity

1. *Expected outcomes:* After instruction, the patient should be able to do the following:

   a. Demonstrate and verbalize an understanding of how to decrease episodes of fatigue
   b. Demonstrate increased tolerance for performing ADLs
   c. Demonstrate the techniques for monitoring pulse, respirations, and blood pressure
   d. Verbalize an understanding of the prescribed medications and how to take them
2. *Nursing interventions*
   a. Monitor pulse and respirations before and during an ADL.
   b. Stop the ADL if the pulse rate becomes tachycardic and respiratory rate increases above normal values. Teach the patient to pace ADLs and take appropriate rest periods. Provide oxygen if necessary.
   c. Monitor blood pressure every 4 hours and when the person shifts from sitting to standing or from lying to sitting or standing.
   d. Teach the person to move slowly when changing position, to decrease orthostatic hypotensive episodes.
   e. Between ADLs, allow a 90-minute rest period with vital signs maintained at patient's baseline. (Do not count the period during which vital signs are changed because of activity as part of the rest period.)
   f. Monitor the patient for other signs and symptoms of decreased oxygenation. For example, note dyspnea, tachypnea, dizziness, lightheadedness, headaches, change in level of consciousness, and palpitations.
   g. Monitor for and report angina.
   h. Teach the patient to observe for signs and symptoms of anemia and to notify you or the physician.
   i. Administer iron supplements as prescribed. If the person complains of nausea, give oral iron with food. Warn the person about the signs and symptoms of toxicity: severe nausea and vomiting, abdominal cramping, diarrhea, and fever.
   j. Do not give oral iron supplements with milk or antacids, which reduce the absorption of iron.
   k. Give oral iron supplements with orange juice, because vitamin C increases the absorption of iron.
   l. Give IM iron supplements using the Z-track method.
   m. Give IV iron supplements slowly to reduce phlebitis.
   n. Increase the amount of fluid intake, as well as fruits and vegetables, to help prevent constipation caused by iron.
   o. Teach the person that iron supplements may cause stools to be dark.
   p. If an elixir is used, prevent staining of teeth by teaching the patient to drink the solution through a straw.

NURSING DIAGNOSIS: Altered nutrition: less than body requirements R/T malaise, fatigue, sore tongue, and resulting anorexia

1. *Expected outcomes:* After instruction, the patient should be able to do the following:
   a. Consume an adequate diet
   b. Stabilize or increase weight
2. *Nursing interventions*

a. Weigh the patient daily, at the same time.
b. Encourage small, frequent meals.
c. Give oral care before and after meals to offer relief from tongue soreness.
d. Encourage family members to bring the patient's favorite foods from home.
e. Avoid highly spiced or acidic foods and extremely hot or cold foods while the tongue is sore.
f. Provide pain medications as needed.

NURSING DIAGNOSIS: Knowledge deficit R/T the etiology and treatment of the disease and prevention of recurrence

1. *Expected outcomes:* After instruction, the person should be able to do the following:
   a. Verbalize an understanding of the etiology and treatment of the disease
   b. Demonstrate compliance with the treatment regimen
2. *Nursing interventions*
   a. Explain the cause, symptoms, and treatment of the disease.
   b. Detail how to prevent recurrence.
   c. Give information in both oral and written forms.
   d. Include family members in the plan of care.
   e. Teach signs and symptoms for which the patient should watch.
   f. Encourage the patient and family to ask questions.

Discharge Planning and Teaching

1. Include the family in the planning and preparation of a diet with adequate iron content, such as a diet of red meat, green vegetables, and dried fruit.
2. Stress the importance of taking iron supplements as prescribed, regardless of increased feelings of well-being, and the importance of keeping follow-up appointments with health care professionals.

Public Health Considerations

1. Primary prevention of iron-deficiency anemia should be taught in health classes as part of grade school education.
2. Groups at risk—women, pregnant women, infants, and adolescents—should have literature available at their primary care physician's office, in schools, and in day-care facilities.

◧ SICKLE CELL DISEASE AND SYNDROMES

Definition

1. All sickle cell disorders are due to the inheritance of a gene for a structurally abnormal portion of the Hgb chain.

2. The beta globin subunit of the adult Hgb chain is structurally abnormal and is called hemoglobin S (HbS). Heterozygous HbS (sickle cell trait) confers immunity to some forms of malaria, and so the incidence of sickle cell trait in equatorial Africa is high (see Etiology).
3. People with homozygous HbS have sickle cell disease of varying severity.

Incidence and Socioeconomic Impact

1. Sickle cell disease affects 1 in 400 Blacks in the United States. This means that the homozygous disease occurs in 1 out of 375 births.
2. Eight to 10 percent of the Black population in the United States has sickle cell trait (and is heterozygous).
3. Sickle cell disorders are found most frequently in Blacks of African descent but have also been found in people of Mediterranean ancestry, in Saudi Arabia, and in India.

Risk Factors

1. Having parents heterozygous for HbS
2. Being Black and of African ancestry

Etiology

1. The heterozygous state for sickle cell syndrome evolved in equatorial Africa.
2. Cell sickling evolved because it confers a biologic advantage against malarial infection.

Pathophysiology

1. The disease results from the concentration and polymerization of HbS molecules inside RBCs. The amount of HbS polymer increases as the amount of oxygen in the RBC decreases. The polymerization process changes the liquid content of the RBC into a viscous gel, which decreases the cell's flexibility. The cell assumes a sickle shape.
2. The process is reversible, but after repeated sickling, the cell becomes permanently sickled.
3. Vaso-occlusion occurs when sickled cells aggregate in small vessels. This process can lead to infarction of any organ.
4. Dehydration can cause a crisis by increasing the blood's viscosity.

Clinical Manifestations

1. Growth and development are delayed.
2. The person is susceptible to infections.
3. Pain crises occur, usually in the back, ribs, and extremities. A person's pain patterns are usually the same from crisis to crisis.
4. Aplastic crisis, a sudden decrease in Hgb level and retic-

ulocyte counts, occurs, usually in association with viral illness.

5. Sequestration crisis, in which blood is sequestered in the spleen, occurs. Signs and symptoms include sudden splenomegaly, hypotension, and shock.
6. Acute chest syndrome—vaso-occlusion of the pulmonary vessels—is demonstrated by chest pain, pulmonary infiltrates, leukocytosis, and hypoxia. Abdominal pain and joint pain are common.
7. When vaso-occlusion occurs in other organs, signs and symptoms are related to that organ.

Diagnostics

1. Follow the assessment guidelines presented earlier in this chapter. Obtain information regarding family history and history of illness.
2. Assess for an event precipitating sickle cell crisis, such as emotional stress, respiratory infection, or gastrointestinal upset, so that the underlying problem can be addressed.
3. Pay particular attention to the pain pattern. If the pattern has changed from what is usually experienced, report this finding to the physician.
4. Measure temperature so that elevations in temperature can be quickly treated.
5. Obtain baseline weight so that intake and output monitoring can be augmented with daily weights.
6. Monitor laboratory values: An Hgb level of 5 to 10 gm per dl, a slightly elevated mean corpuscular volume (due to an increased reticulocyte count of 10–25%), and indirect hyperbilirubinemia are commonly associated with crises.
7. Peripheral blood smear shows classic distorted sickled erythrocytes. The screening test for HbS is positive, and Hgb electrophoresis demonstrates HbS.

Clinical Management

1. Goals of clinical management
   a. Maintain optimal health and prevent sickle crises.
   b. Reduce the clinical manifestations of sickle cell crisis.
2. Nonpharmacologic interventions
   a. Prevent or reverse dehydration with oral or IV fluids. Large volumes (2–3 times normal maintenance) of hypotonic or alkaline solutions are administered intravenously.
   b. Reduce fever with tepid baths.
   c. Apply warmth to painful areas.
   d. Encourage bed rest and help with ADLs to decrease the oxygen demands.
   e. Promote annual ophthalmic examinations and laser therapy as indicated for retinopathy.
   f. Perform transfusion in aplastic crisis; after a cerebrovascular accident; or after severe, frequent pain crises that are refractory to conventional therapy.
3. Pharmacologic interventions
   a. Folic acid is given to children and adults.
   b. Penicillin VK is given to children 3 to 5 years of age to prevent infections.

c. A polyvalent pneumococcal vaccine is given yearly after age 3.
d. Fever is treated promptly with aspirin, acetaminophen, or both.
e. Analgesics, usually narcotics, are given during pain crises.
f. Oxygen therapy is used to correct hypoxia. Do not give oxygen if the patient is not hypoxic, because it may reduce erythropoiesis.
g. Antibiotics are used for acute chest syndrome only if it is associated with bacterial infection.

Complications

1. Osteomyelitis
2. Leg ulcers
3. Priapism
4. Cholelithiasis
5. Renal tubular defects
6. Cardiomyopathy
7. Cerebral ischemia and cerebrovascular accidents
8. Aseptic necrosis of femoral and humeral heads

Prognosis

1. The prognosis for people with sickle cell anemia is variable, but a significant number of infants with the disease die in the first 2 to 3 years of life, as a result of overwhelming sepsis or acute splenic sequestration crisis.
2. Those who survive early childhood have a mean survival to the 4th decade of life, with death resulting from cardiopulmonary complications or renal insufficiency.

Applying the Nursing Process

NURSING DIAGNOSIS: Sickle cell crisis R/T fluid volume deficit

1. *Expected outcomes:* After intervention, the following should occur:
   a. The patient's weight will increase as hydration returns to normal.
   b. Intake and output will balance. (Output will match intake.)
   c. Symptoms of crisis will subside.
2. *Nursing interventions*
   a. Weigh the patient daily, at the same time.
   b. Assess mucous membranes.
   c. Monitor intake and output.
   d. Remember that the individual may need 2 to 3 times normal maintenance fluid and that, because of dehydration, output will not initially match intake.
   e. Encourage oral fluid intake.
   f. Request additional IV fluid replacement if oral intake is not sufficient.
   g. Monitor for abatement of the signs and symptoms of crisis.

NURSING DIAGNOSIS: Pain R/T the disease process, dehydration, and lack of oxygenation

1. *Expected outcomes:* After intervention, the following should occur:
   a. The patient should verbalize a reduction in the level of pain.
   b. The pain should remain at a tolerable level and require less narcotics to do so.
2. *Nursing interventions*
   a. Assess pain by asking the patient to indicate how much pain he or she is experiencing on a pain scale from 0 to 10, with 0 representing no pain and 10 representing the worst pain imaginable.
   b. Take a proactive approach to the pain, offering medication as soon as the physician's orders allow the patient to receive it and obtaining new orders if the ordered medication does not adequately relieve the pain.
   c. Apply warm soaks to painful areas.
   d. Encourage bed rest to minimize oxygen consumption.
   e. Encourage oral fluids to decrease dehydration, which contributes to sluggishness of blood and therefore causes increased pain. Supplement with IV fluids if oral intake is inadequate.
   f. Monitor vital signs, especially temperature, because infection may be a cause of pain.

Discharge Planning and Teaching

1. Teach the patient to avoid exacerbations of the disease process by doing the following:
   a. Avoiding strenuous exercise.
   b. Avoiding cold temperatures and swimming in cold water.
   c. Avoiding medications that cause vasoconstriction.
   d. Avoiding high altitudes or unpressurized airplanes.
2. Promote good general health by teaching the patient to do the following:
   a. Obtain yearly immunizations for prevention of pneumonia.
   b. Eat a well-balanced diet, including foods high in iron.
   c. Drink plenty of fluids.
3. Support the parents of a child with sickle cell disease.
   a. Allow for verbalization of possible feelings of guilt over having "given" the disease to the child.
   b. Monitor the need for information on coping with a chronically ill child.

Public Health Considerations

1. Genetic counseling of identified heterozygotes alerts couples to the possibility of having children with sickle cell disease.
2. Pregnant women who have sickle cell disease or sickle cell trait should be referred to prenatal diagnostic services.

◼ OTHER ANEMIAS

Chronic-Disease Anemia

1. Definition
   a. Chronic-disease anemia is a form of hyproproliferative, hypochromic anemia. It is a mild to moderate anemia associated with chronic disease states.
   b. The RBCs are normocytic and not always hypochromic; the anemia is most often associated with low ferritin levels.
2. Incidence and etiology
   a. Chronic infections, such as tuberculosis and lung abscesses, and chronic inflammatory diseases, such as rheumatoid arthritis, systemic lupus erythematosus, and inflammatory bowel disease, often lead to the development of anemia.
   b. Malignancies are associated with chronic-disease anemia.
   c. Individuals who require hemodialysis can develop chronic-disease anemia.
   d. Because chronic disease is so prevalent, chronic-disease anemia may be 2nd only to iron-deficiency anemia in overall incidence.
3. Clinical manifestations: The anemia is usually mild. The Hct level generally remains between 25 and 40 percent, although in 10 percent of patients the Hct level falls below 20 percent. The signs and symptoms of the chronic disorder usually overshadow the presentation of the anemia. Signs and symptoms vary with the chronic disease process. There is usually no jaundice or serum bilirubin elevation.
4. Clinical management: Treatment is directed at controlling the underlying chronic disease and preventing exacerbating factors, such as nutritional deficiencies and marrow-suppressive drugs, from causing further problems. Erythropoietin is in investigational use in many of these situations. It is currently being used to treat hemodialysis patients who have anemia.

Thalassemias

1. Definition
   a. Thalassemias are hemoglobinopathic hereditary anemias that occur because of mutations that affect Hgb structure. Reduced synthesis of part of the Hgb results in hypochromic and microcytic RBCs.
   b. The most common form is thalassemia trait (a heterozygous form), which is a mild, clinically insignificant anemia that seems to protect individuals from malaria.
   c. The homozygous forms of the thalassemias are more severe. Individuals with these forms of the disease have an average life span of 17 years.
2. Incidence and etiology
   a. In the United States, β-thalassemia affects mainly persons from the Mediterranean area and parts of Africa and Asia. The α-thalassemias affect persons of Asian descent.

b. Approximately 1000 people in the United States are known to have the more severe forms of thalassemia.
3. Clinical manifestations
   a. Clinical manifestations depend on the severity of the disease. Mild cases have clinically insignificant findings. Severe cases can lead to death.
   b. Intermediate forms demonstrate varying degrees of oxygen deprivation; osteoporosis; and organ dysfunction, including cardiac disease.
   c. Severe thalassemia manifests with signs and symptoms of oxygen deprivation, pallor, growth retardation, hepatosplenomegaly, cardiac disease, bone marrow expansion, and bone deformities.
4. Clinical management
   a. Transfusions adequate to sustain life are given.
   b. Splenectomies are performed after the age of 6 years.
   c. Iron chelation therapy is administered.
   d. Nutritional supplementation with vitamin C is given to increase iron secretion. Administration of folic acid and vitamin E is also recommended.
   e. Organ complications are treated individually as they develop.

Hemolytic Anemias

1. Definition
   a. Premature destruction of RBCs occurs either because the RBCs are inherently defective or because noxious factors are present in intravascular compartments.
   b. Forms of hemolytic anemia include hereditary and acquired groups. Intrinsic abnormalities are in RBC membranes and are usually hereditary. Environmental abnormalities that end RBC life are acquired.
   c. Hereditary forms include hereditary spherocytosis (congenital hemolytic jaundice), hereditary elliptocytosis, hereditary pyropoikilocytosis, and South East and Asian ovalocytosis.
   d. Acquired forms include sequestration hemolysis (hypersplenism) and immune hemolysis.
2. Incidence and etiology
   a. Hereditary spherocytosis occurs in all races, but it is especially common in northern Europeans, among whom its incidence is 1 in 5000. Most cases (75%) are autosomal dominant; the rest are a nondominant (most likely autosomal recessive) form.
   b. Sequestration hemolysis anemia (hypersplenism) occurs in conjunction with other hemolytic anemias, chronic leukemias, lipid storage diseases, and rheumatoid arthritis.
   c. Immune hemolysis anemia occurs because antibodies or complement components bind to the erythrocyte membrane, destroying RBCs. This process occurs as a result of autoimmunization, alloimmunization, or exposure to certain drugs.
3. Clinical manifestations
   a. The clinical manifestations of hereditary and acquired hemolytic anemias do not differ from one another.
   b. Jaundice, pallor, and splenomegaly are common and occur in addition to signs and symptoms of other anemias.

4. Clinical management
   a. Treatment for hereditary spherocytosis, if required, includes splenectomy and long-term folic acid administration.
   b. Treatment of acquired hemolytic anemias is directed at controlling the underlying disease process. Splenectomy is rarely used.
   c. Treatment of immune hemolysis anemia for warm-reacting antibodies (IgG) includes curing the underlying disease; administering glucocorticoids and immunosuppressive and cytotoxic drugs; and performing transfusions and, if necessary, a splenectomy.
   d. Treatment of immune hemolysis anemia for cold-reacting antibodies (IgM) includes treating the underlying disease, administering chlorambucil, performing plasmapheresis, and possibly administering blood transfusions.
   e. Treatment of drug-induced immune hemolysis anemia is directed at withholding the offending drug.

Ineffective Hematopoiesis (Megaloblastic) Anemias

1. Definition: Vitamin B_{12}–deficiency anemia (cobalamin deficiency) and folic-acid–deficiency anemia (folate-deficiency anemia)
   a. A deficiency of vitamin B_{12} alters the synthesis of DNA, which results in the production of defective RBCs, WBCs, and platelets (ineffective hematopoiesis). There are many causes of vitamin B_{12} deficiency. When the cause is a gastric defect that prevents the absorption of vitamin B_{12}, the term **pernicious anemia** is applied. This term is often used to refer to all vitamin B_{12}–deficiency anemias but should not be. Pernicious anemia occurs only when a gastric defect prevents vitamin B_{12} absorption.
   b. A deficiency of folic acid prevents normal RBC production. This cause of ineffective hematopoiesis results in folate-deficiency anemia.
2. Incidence and etiology
   a. Vitamin B_{12}–deficiency anemia
      • Ten percent of people older than 70 have vitamin B_{12}–deficiency anemia.
      • Pernicious anemia is the greatest cause of vitamin B_{12}–deficiency anemia in all ages and ethnic groups.
      • One percent of all Americans will develop pernicious anemia. A genetic basis for the condition is suggested by its high incidence in inbred populations and its occurrence in families.
      • Surgical gastrectomy, ileitis or ileal resection, and pancreatic insufficiency cause Vitamin B_{12}–deficiency anemia. It is also seen in patients with diverticula of the small intestine and older persons with atrophic gastritis.
   b. Folate-deficiency anemia
      • Lack of dietary folate can cause folate-deficiency anemia.
      • The incidence of folate-deficiency anemia is not well established, but increases are seen in alcoholism,

malabsorption syndromes, and pregnancy, because of the increased use of folic acid that occurs in these conditions.

- Increased use of pharmacologic agents (e.g., trimethoprim, pyrimethamine, methotrexate, sulfasalazine, oral contraceptives, and anticonvulsants) has increased the incidence of folate-deficiency anemia. Folate deficiency is consequently the most common cause of megaloblastic anemias in the Western Hemisphere.

3. Clinical manifestations
   a. Vitamin B_{12}–deficiency anemia develops slowly, over several years. Symptoms are those related to tissue hypoxia but can also include decreased vibratory and positional sense, ataxia, paresthesias, confusion, and dementia.
   b. Folate-deficiency anemia can develop rapidly, over a period of several months. Symptoms are those related to tissue hypoxia but can include glossitis, jaundice, and splenomegaly.

4. Clinical management
   a. The treatment for vitamin B_{12}–deficiency anemia is to give cyanocobalamin (vitamin B_{12}).
   b. The treatment for folate-deficiency anemia is to administer folic acid every day until the deficiency is corrected. High doses may be administered to patients with malabsorption problems.

Posthemorrhagic Anemia

1. Definition
   a. Posthemorrhagic anemia is anemia caused by the loss of a large amount of blood as a result of trauma or an underlying disease that affects blood vessels or coagulation.
   b. Hemoglobin and Hct levels are lower than the normal ranges because of acute or chronic blood loss.

2. Incidence and etiology
   a. The causes of blood loss are many and varied. Surgery, gastrointestinal hemorrhage, coagulation disorders, fractures, and anticoagulation therapy are some causes of blood loss.
   b. Anemia may result from acute or chronic blood loss.

3. Clinical manifestations
   a. Anemia may not be detected during the 1st phase of acute blood loss, which is 1 to 3 days long. The body has had no opportunity to re-expand blood volume; therefore, Hct and Hgb levels appear to be within normal limits.
   b. Anemia appears during the 2nd phase of acute blood loss, when blood volume is restored and laboratory work reveals low Hct and Hgb levels as well as reticulocytosis.
   c. The presenting symptoms of anemia resulting from acute blood loss depend on the rate and volume of blood loss. Symptoms include tachypnea, dyspnea, vertigo, rapid thready pulse, hypotension, pallor, headache, restlessness, and disorientation.
   d. Anemia resulting from chronic blood loss causes lower than normal Hct and Hgb levels. Laboratory

---

BOX 25–5. Treating Posthemorrhagic Anemia

Hypovolemic Stage—An Emergency Situation

The hypovolemic stage occurs when 30 to 40 percent of the blood volume has been lost. In adults, this is approximately 1500 to 2000 ml of blood. The 1st step is to stop the bleeding. This may not be possible until the patient is taken to surgery. The 2nd step is to replace the blood volume with either crystalloid solutions (e.g., Ringer's lactate) or normal saline with 90 mOsm of sodium bicarbonate added per liter. Another choice is to restore the volume of blood lost with colloid solutions (plasma protein, albumin, dextran, or fresh whole O– blood). The initial infusion of crystalloid solutions will be 2 to 3 times the estimated volume of blood loss.

The administration of 3 liters of crystalloid solutions over a period of 15 to 20 minutes is generally adequate to revive anyone in hemorrhagic shock if the hemorrhage has been stopped. Continued signs of hypovolemia generally mean that the bleeding is still active and surgery is needed to stop it.

Anemic Stage—A Nonemergency Situation

Once the hypovolemic emergency has been corrected and the patient is stabilized, the patient may require rapid correction of the resulting anemia. For example, surgery may not be delayed, and blood transfusions can be started after type matching and cross-matching of blood. If there is no need to correct the situation rapidly, anemia from hemorrhage rarely needs therapy beyond initiating a high-protein diet and oral iron supplements.

---

work will also indicate reticulocytosis until the chronic blood loss has depleted the body's iron stores.
   e. Blood volume remains normal in anemia caused by chronic blood loss.

4. Clinical management
   a. Anemia resulting from chronic blood loss rarely requires more than oral iron supplementation and a high-protein diet. Further measures are summarized in Box 25–5.
   b. Anemia resulting from acute blood loss requires correction of the underlying cause of hemorrhage and the possible administration of transfusion therapy.

◼ HYPERPROLIFERATIVE BLOOD DISORDERS

Definition

1. **Polycythemia** is an elevation of RBC, Hgb, and Hct beyond their normal ranges.
2. An increase in the actual number of RBCs, or absolute erythrocytosis, is caused by an abnormal increase in bone marrow activity. Red blood cell production is apparently autonomous, in that the increased RBC production occurs despite a low or undetectable level of erythropoietin. This condition is called **polycythemia vera.** Polycythemia vera must be differentially diagnosed from other polycythemias.
   a. Polycythemia may be caused by reduction in plasma volume.
   b. If the RBC count is at the upper end of the normal range and plasma volume is at the lower end of the

normal range, the condition is **spurious polycythemia,** also known as **relative erythrocytosis** and **stress erythrocytosis.** The most common cause is dehydration.

   c. Polycythemia may be secondary to other disease processes. Normal bone marrow is stimulated by an increase in erythropoietin or another erythrostimulating substance. Polycythemia may be an appropriate physiologic response to inadequate tissue oxygenation (e.g., in high-altitude polycythemia or in pickwickian syndrome seen in obese male smokers with cardiopulmonary disease). Polycythemia may be due to an inappropriate physiologic response to tissue oxygenation (e.g., in renal, adrenal, or ovarian carcinoma).

Incidence and Socioeconomic Impact

1. Polycythemia vera is a disease of later life, with 60 the median age of diagnosis.
2. Polycythemia vera is slightly more common in males than in females.
3. The frequency of polycythemia vera is somewhat increased in persons of Jewish ancestry.

Risk Factors

1. Genetic predisposition (minimal role in disease transmission)
2. Jewish ancestry

Etiology

1. The etiology is unknown.
2. Recent studies indicate a possible viral connection.

Pathophysiology

1. Increased bone marrow production of erythroid, myeloid, and megakaryocytic cells occurs in the absence of increased erythropoietin.
2. Frequently peripheral granulocytes and platelets are elevated. This elevation is postulated to occur as a result of markedly increased sensitivity to erythropoietin, as opposed to being totally independent of control by erythropoietin.
3. The malignant disorder can be traced to a single stem cell clone.

Clinical Manifestations

1. Most clinical manifestations result from expanded blood volume and increased blood viscosity. Expanded blood volume leads to generalized vascular expansion and venous engorgement, which is demonstrated as a ruddy cyanosis of the skin and mucous membranes and a feeling of fullness in the head and neck. There is an increased occurrence of thrombotic events, specially cerebral events, in response to the increase in viscosity and blood volume.
2. The elevated Hct level leads to decreased cerebral blood flow, which results in headaches, tinnitus, blurred vision, vertigo, and lightheadedness.
3. Epistaxis, spontaneous bruising, and upper gastrointestinal bleeding occur as a result of hypervolemia and platelet dysfunction.
4. As a result of the increased viscosity, hypervolemia, and erythrocytosis, cardiac output and regional blood flow may decrease, leading to tissue hypoxia.
5. Pruritus, sometimes severely disabling, may be related to the increase in histamine release secondary to excessive turnover of granulocytes and basophils.
6. Sweating and weight loss occur and may be due to a hypermetabolic state.
7. Severe pain is experienced in the feet.

Diagnostics

1. Medical diagnosis is based on physical assessment manifestations and findings.
2. Assess for plethora (dusky cyanosis) of hands, feet, face, and mucous membranes and for engorgement of conjunctiva and retinal veins as well as for retinal hemorrhages. Other manifestations include mild hypertension; splenomegaly; and bone pain and tenderness upon palpation, especially of the sternum and ribs.
3. Laboratory findings usually indicate an elevated Hct level of 48 to 60 percent. The platelet count is greater than 400,000 per μl, and WBC count is greater than 12,000 per ml. Leukocyte alkaline phosphatase is greater than 100, serum B_{12} is greater than 900 pg per ml, and uric acid may be elevated. To be consistent with diagnosis of polycythemia vera, the serum erythropoietin level should be zero.
4. Computed tomography demonstrates an enlarged spleen.
5. Assay of bone marrow erythroid colony growth should demonstrate an increase of erythroid colonies independent of added erythropoietin.

Clinical Management

1. Goals of clinical management
  a. Reduce the Hct level to 45 percent
  b. Reduce the incidence of complications
  c. Provide at least 10 years of active life from point of diagnosis
  d. Decrease bone marrow production
2. Nonpharmacologic interventions
  a. Phlebotomies that remove 350 to 500 ml of blood every 2 to 3 days as necessary to reduce the Hct level to 45 percent or lower.
  b. After multiple phlebotomies, the individual may experience a reduction in the number of RBCs produced, because iron stores have been depleted; this reduces the number of phlebotomies needed.
3. Pharmacologic interventions

a. Low-dose aspirin reduces the effectiveness of the increased number of platelets. Monitor for potential problems of hemorrhage.
b. Myelosuppression is induced with radioactive phosphorus or with an alkylating agent such as chlorambucil, busulfan, or hydroxyurea.
c. Interferon or anagrelide has been used when other treatments do not reduce thrombocytosis.
d. H_1 or H_2 blockers (cyproheptadine or cimetidine) are used to reduce pruritus.
e. Allopurinol reduces hyperuricemia.

Complications

1. Thrombotic episodes attributed to increased viscosity or thrombocytosis
2. Hemorrhagic episodes of the upper gastrointestinal system
3. Development of cytopenias, myelofibrosis, and metaplasia after a "spent" phase (a stable period during which a relatively normal blood count is maintained without therapy)
4. Transformation to acute leukemia
5. Gout from excessive hyperuricemia from RBC breakdown

Prognosis

1. Careful control of blood volume and viscosity through phlebotomy supplemented with judicial use of myelosuppressives can ensure most persons a prolonged period of relatively symptom-free survival.
2. Median survival now exceeds 10 years.
3. Symptom-free survival of 15 to 20 years is no longer uncommon.

Applying the Nursing Process

NURSING DIAGNOSIS: Pain R/T headaches, bone pain especially in the ribs and sternum, and foot pain due to blood viscosity and erythrocytosis

1. *Expected outcomes:* After intervention, the person should be able to do the following:
   a. Verbalize a reduction in headaches with reduction in viscosity of the blood
   b. Report a decrease in bone pain in the ribs and sternum
2. *Nursing interventions*
   a. Monitor pain by having the patient complete a pain scale before and after interventions intended to reduce the pain.
   b. Administer IV fluids and encourage oral fluids if possible.
   c. Perform phlebotomies as ordered.
   d. Administer pain medications in a proactive manner.

e. Use nonpharmacologic pain reduction measures, such as relaxation and distraction.
f. Administer myelosuppressive agents as ordered.
g. Prevent prolonged pressure on the ribs by frequently turning the patient with a turn sheet.

NURSING DIAGNOSIS: Altered tissue perfusion (peripheral and cerebral) R/T increased viscosity of blood and increased platelet count

1. *Expected outcomes:* After intervention, the person should be able to do the following:
   a. Experience a return of blood viscosity to normal limits
   b. Suffer no permanent damage from altered tissue perfusion
2. *Nursing Interventions*
   a. Monitor for peripheral thrombosis (e.g., pain and tenderness in the calves, tingling, burning, a decrease in sensation, claudication, cyanosis, pallor, or a change in temperature).
   b. Monitor for cerebral thrombosis (e.g., a change in level of consciousness, mood, restlessness, lightheadedness, vertigo, unilateral extremity weakness, dysphagia, dysphasia, or facial drooping).
   c. Monitor for cardiac thrombosis (note chest pain at rest or with activity).
   d. In the event of thrombosis, return the patient to bed rest or keep him or her on bed rest. Notify the physician and apply oxygen therapy.
   e. Monitor Hct and Hgb levels and intake and output.
   f. Administer myelosuppressive treatments as ordered.
   g. Perform phlebotomies as ordered.

Discharge Planning and Teaching

1. Explain the disease process, noting that lifelong treatment is required.
2. Describe the medications to be taken specifying their names, purposes, and doses; the times they are to be taken; and precautions in taking them.
3. Caution the person not to take multivitamins with iron, because the iron supplement may increase the number of RBCs produced. Clarify the need for the person to consume a balanced diet but to refrain from including iron-rich foods.
4. Stress the importance of keeping a follow-up appointment with health professionals.
5. Explain the necessity of informing health professionals about an increase in symptoms or any new symptom experienced.

Public Health Considerations

1. There is no known way to prevent polycythemias.
2. Inform the public of the importance of contacting a physician if symptoms of polycythemia occur.

■ *LEUKEMIAS*

Definition

1. **Leukemia** is a disease characterized by proliferative growth of leukocytes and their precursors in the tissues. It affects the bone marrow and the lymph tissue, resulting in a decrease in function of normal WBCs.
2. Leukemias are classified by rapidity of onset (acute or chronic) and by the type of cell type that proliferates: myelocytic (granulocytes or monocytes proliferate) or lymphocytic (lymphocytes proliferate).
   a. Acute leukemias are abnormal proliferations of immature WBCs within a short time frame, usually 1 to 5 months. Blast cells are seen with this disease form. Chronic leukemias are excessive accumulations of more mature appearing but still ineffective WBCs. This process occurs over a longer time frame, even 2 to 5 years. Generally, patients have a longer survival with this form of the disease.
   b. Four major leukemia types exist: acute myelocytic leukemia, acute lymphocytic leukemia, chronic myelocytic leukemia, and chronic lymphocytic leukemia. Other names for myelocytic leukemia are **myelogenous, myeloblastic,** and **myeloid leukemia.** Other names for lymphocytic leukemia are **lymphoblastic** and **lymphoid leukemia.** Acute myelocytic and acute lymphocytic cell types are classified further in the French, American, British classification system (Table 25–6).

Incidence and Socioeconomic Impact

1. Leukemia represents about 10 percent of all cancers.
2. Approximately 28,000 new cases occur in the United States each year.

Table 25–6. Classification of Acute Leukemias

Type	Subtype
Acute lymphoblastic leukemia (ALL)	L1: Common childhood leukemia L2: Adult ALL L3: Rare subtype with blasts resembling those in Burkitt's lymphoma
Acute myeloblastic leukemia	Granulocytic 　M1: Myeloblastic leukemia without maturation 　M2: Myeloblastic leukemia with maturation 　M3: Promyelocytic leukemia 　M3: Variant Monocytic 　M4: Myelomonocytic leukemia 　M4E: Myelomonocytic leukemia with eosinophils 　M5: Monocytic leukemia, with subtypes A and B Erythroid 　M6: Erythroleukemia Megakaryocytic 　M7: Megakaryocytic

3. The disease affects many more adults than children, almost an 8:1 ratio. Although children have a better prognosis than adults do, leukemia is the 2nd leading cause of death among children ages 4 to 14.
4. The most common leukemias in adults are acute myelocytic leukemia and chronic lymphocytic leukemia. The most common leukemia in children is acute lymphocytic leukemia.

Risk Factors

1. Leukemia has no known cause, but certain risk factors can predispose a person to development of the disease. People exposed to radiation have an increased incidence of leukemia.
2. Research on predisposing chromosomal abnormalities is in progress. Children with Down syndrome have an increased incidence of acute leukemia.

Etiology

1. Certain chemicals have also been associated with an increase in pancytopenia and leukemia.
2. Some chemotherapeutic agents, including some of the alkylating agents, the antibiotic chloramphenicol, and phenylbutazone, have been associated with an increased risk of leukemias, especially acute myelocytic leukemia.

Pathophysiology

1. As a result of immature or defective cells, a decrease of normal leukocytes, erythrocytes, and platelets occurs.
2. This process produces a pancytopenic condition characterized by anemia, susceptibility to infection, and bleeding tendencies (unexplained petechiae and ecchymoses) (Table 25–7).

Clinical Manifestations

1. Infections commonly recur in the skin, gingiva, perianal tissues, the lungs, and the urinary tract.
2. Abdominal discomfort and bone pain can result from the infiltration of immature or defective cells into bone marrow, liver, spleen, and lymph tissues.

NURSE ADVISORY

Blast crisis is a proliferation of immature myeloblasts in the blood and bone marrow of patients with chronic myeloblastic leukemia (CML). Increased fibrotic marrow, leukopenia, thrombocytopenia, and anemia are some symptoms. Blast crisis is usually fatal within 6 months. Treatments include intensive chemotherapy similar to that used to treat acute leukemias. The choice of drugs depends on the cell line that is proliferating. Bone marrow transplant for blast crisis has had poor results. Providing intensive therapies during CML's chronic stage is an experimental form of prevention of blast crisis.

Table 25–7. Etiology, Pathology, and Prognosis of Leukemias

Acute Myeloblastic Leukemia	Acute Lymphocytic Leukemia	Chronic Myeloblastic Leukemia	Chronic Lymphocytic Leukemia
Makes up 90% of all adult cases Increases in incidence with age Makes up half of all cases Is associated with secondary cancer Can occur after aggressive chemotherapy for Hodgkin's disease, multiple myeloma, ovarian cancer, non-Hodgkin's lymphoma, or breast cancer	Occurs predominantly in children Peaks in incidence between ages 2 and 10 Comprises 10–20% of adult leukemias Most frequently occurs from middle age onward Small predominance in males over females Small predominance in Whites over Blacks	Represents 20% of all leukemias Peak age of onset is between 50 and 60 Small predominance of males over females Rises in frequency after exposure to ionized radiation	Is a disease of adults, usually those older than 50 Is more common in males than in females Is usually diagnosed incidentally during a physical examination Makes up about 20% of all leukemias
Stem cells differentiate into myeloid cells (erythrocytes, granulocytes, and thrombocytes) Myeloblasts (immature precursor cells) proliferate in the bone marrow; lymph nodes and spleen are then invaded	A single defective lymphoid stem cell clones itself Defective cells then proliferate in the lymph nodes, spleen, and thymus Cells infiltrate into the central nervous system early in the disease	Abnormal growth of granulocyte precursors occurs in bone marrow, peripheral blood, and body tissues The least progressive leukemia, with anemia or bleeding abnormalities acute or terminal: blast crisis occurs where myeloblasts proliferate rapidly, causing obstruction of the microvascular circulation in the central nervous system or lungs The only leukemia linked to an abnormal chromosome, the Philadelphia (Ph1) chromosome, which serves as a diagnostic marker. The chromosomal defect could be caused by radiation or carcinogenic agents	Uncontrolled spread of abnormally small lymphocytes occurs in lymph tissue, blood, and bone marrow This life-threatening leukemia may produce few signs and symptoms
Remission occurs in 75% of cases, but relapse eventually occurs in most cases Five-year survival rate is 20–25% without bone marrow transplant and increases to 50% with bone marrow transplant Severe infections from disease or treatment are primary cause of death Death can occur from uncontrolled bleeding	Best prognosis in children: remission occurs within 2 yr of chemotherapy and there is a less than 10% chance of relapse Remission is complete in 90% of children and 65% of adults Longer survival is seen in females and Whites than in males and non-Whites Positive outcome decreases with obesity and central nervous system involvement	Life expectancy is 3–4 yr after chronic phases, 3–6 months once acute (blast or terminal) phase has begun Bone marrow transplant can increase 2-yr survival 40–50% during chronic phase During blast crisis, bone marrow transplant increases 2-yr survival 15–20%	Best prognosis of all types of leukemia: 4–10 yr Life expectancy depends on response to therapy Poor prognosis with anemia, thrombocytopenia, neutropenia, severe lymphocytosis

3. Headaches, nausea, vomiting, dizziness, visual disturbances, seizures, and disorientation are related to meningeal infiltration.
4. Other signs and symptoms include easy bruising, fatigue, fever, hepatomegaly, splenomegaly, weight loss, and sternal tenderness.

Diagnostics

1. Leukemia is initially suspected with clinical complaints and a complete blood count that shows an abnormal WBC count. Leukocyte (WBC) levels may be normal, below normal, or extremely elevated (above 400,000/mm³).

Neutropenia is frequently present. Platelet counts will be below normal. Hemoglobin and Hct levels will also be low. Other tests might include lumbar puncture, chest radiographs, CT and magnetic resonance imaging scans, lymphangiography, and lymph node biopsy. Blood chemistries should be obtained to look for increased uric acid levels and increased lactic dehydrogenase levels.

2. Medical diagnosis is confirmed, classified, and staged by bone marrow aspiration, biopsy, or both. Differentiation among the types of leukemia is essential because of the markedly different treatments and prognoses.
3. The history includes assessment for weight loss and early satiety, fatigue, dizziness, bleeding tendencies, easy bruising, or frequent or recurring infections.

4. Assess for signs and symptoms of anemia, including fatigue, malaise, edema, pallor, headache, tinnitus, dyspnea, palpitations, and tachycardia.
5. Assess for visual changes such as diplopia, blurring, unequal pupils, and retinal changes.
6. Check for renal insufficiency, indicated by decreased urine output and elevated blood urea nitrogen and creatinine. Also check for flank pain.
7. Palpate for abdominal discomfort and enlarged liver and spleen.

Clinical Management

1. Goals of clinical management
   a. In acute leukemias, complete remission must be induced and maintained. Remission is defined as less than 5 percent of blasts in the marrow, with counts restored to normal. This status is usually achieved with chemotherapy. After initial remission, postremission therapy is essential. In cases of complete bone marrow suppression, bone marrow transplantation may be performed.
   b. Treatment for acute leukemias has 2 components:
      • Induction therapy uses cell-cycle–specific antimetabolites and anthracyclines.
      • Postremission therapy (also known as **consolidation, maintenance,** or **intensification therapy**) is necessary, because although patients do achieve remission, they do not remain in remission for long without further chemotherapy.
   c. In chronic leukemias, complete remission often necessitates bone marrow transplant. Chemotherapy will not always prolong life. Management includes restoring leukocyte counts to normal, treating infection and bleeding episodes, and performing symptomatic interventions for other aspects of the disease.
2. Nonpharmacologic interventions
   a. Blood and blood product transfusions are performed to maintain hemostasis and prevent or minimize bleeding episodes.
   b. Some patients with chronic lymphocytic leukemia receive radiation to the lymph nodes. Some patients with acute lymphocytic leukemia receive cranial radiation.
   c. For patients with chronic myelocytic leukemia, bone marrow transplant may offer a chance for cure.
3. Pharmacologic interventions
   a. Rigorous chemotherapy is administered in multiple-dose regimens over several courses. This includes induction and maintenance or consolidation therapy.
   b. Antibiotics are used to treat infections.
   c. Intense antiemetic therapy treats the side effects of chemotherapy and radiation.
   d. Pain management involves narcotics and sedatives. Ativan may also counteract nausea.
   e. In acute lymphocytic leukemia, the goal of treatment is to achieve a cure. Most relapses occur within the first 2 years. Half of relapsed patients can achieve a 2nd remission by repeating the initial induction regimen. Treatment is divided into 3 stages.

   (1) Induction may include vincristine, prednisone, and L-asparaginase with children. These agents alone can induce initial remission of 36 to 67 percent. Therapy may begin with inpatient treatment but later may be switched to outpatient therapy. The addition of daunorubicin can increase remission rates up to 80 percent.
   (2) Central nervous system prophylaxis with intracranial radiation and intrathecal methotrexate is then undertaken. An Ommaya reservoir may be inserted for easy access to the cerebrospinal fluid.
   (3) Maintenance may involve methotrexate and 6-mercaptopurine.
   f. In acute myelocytic leukemia, treatment requires control of the bone marrow and systemic disease. Treatment may involve cytarabine with an anthracycline (e.g., daunorubicin or the newer idarubicin).
   g. In chronic myelocytic leukemia, the only chance for a cure is to eradicate the Ph_1 chromosome with high-dose chemotherapy followed by a bone marrow transplant. In its chronic stage, this leukemia may be treated with hydroxyurea and oral busulfan. In blast crisis, high doses of cytosine arabinoside, anthracyclines, amsacrine, 6-thioguanine, and hydroxyurea are administered. Overall, response rates are low. Newer treatments under investigation include interferon and growth factors such as interleukins, tumor necrosis factor, and colony-stimulating factor.

Rx DRUG ADVISORY

Biologic response modifiers are new drugs such as interleukin-2, colony-stimulating factors, and other growth factors. These relatively new agents are used to treat leukemia and other hematologic malignancies. A condition known as **pulmonary capillary leak syndrome** has begun to manifest more frequently with use of these agents. In this syndrome, fluid shifts and accumulates interstitially in the lungs. Intravascular volume is depleted, leading to decreased organ perfusion, yet volume appears overloaded. With a decreased systemic vascular resistance, hypotension and noncardiac pulmonary edema result. This condition is exacerbated with the use of cytosine arabinoside or cyclophosphamide.

   h. In chronic lymphocytic leukemia, the main decision is when to initiate treatment. Most patients fall into an intermediate phase in which treatment can be delayed for several years. Patients should be observed for 3 to 6 months so that the clinical aggressiveness of the disease can be assessed. Chlorambucil, an alkylating agent, is the most commonly used and best tolerated. Cyclophosphamide is used for patients who do not respond to chlorambucil. Fludarabine is a new drug to treat refractory B-cell chronic lymphocytic leukemia. Also, corticosteroids help to control leukocytosis.
   i. Keep in mind that pharmacologic advances in chemotherapy rapidly continue to produce new agents for treatment, with the results that regimens may quickly become outdated.
4. Special medical-surgical procedures: See Learning/Teaching Guidelines for Psychosocial Aspects of Bone Marrow

LEARNING/TEACHING GUIDELINES
for Psychosocial Aspects of Bone Marrow Transplant

General Overview

1. Bone marrow transplant consists of the harvesting of bone marrow from a carefully matched donor (creating an allogenic graft) or the patient (creating an autologous graft) and transplanting it into someone affected with life-threatening disease. The goal of therapy is to eradicate the disease.
2. These diseases might be leukemia, aplastic anemia, breast cancer, non-Hodgkin's lymphoma, multiple myeloma, or another immune deficiency disorder.
3. Often, the donor is a sibling or twin of the recipient.
4. Because of the threat of death from the underlying disorder, bone marrow transplant is usually a major, sometimes frightening decision for the patient.

Topics for Consideration

1. Take care to explain fully everything that will occur before, during, and after the procedure. Provide printed literature on the procedure or a video of it. Audiovisual material enhances learning. Give the patient and family time to ask questions.
2. Awaiting a donor match, if autologous transplant is not possible, is very anxiety producing. Siblings and relatives may feel guilty if they do not match. Nontwin siblings have a 25 percent chance of matching completely. Unrelated donors have only a 1 in 20,000 chance of matching.
3. Initial human leukocyte antigen testing involves only blood sampling through phlebotomy. Harvesting the marrow involves an outpatient procedure, usually performed under a local anesthetic. Donors should expect some soreness in their hips after the harvest. Prepare the donor or the patient for this discomfort.
4. Preprocedure care of the recipient can be uncomfortable and draining. Many patients experience nausea and discomfort from the total-body irradiation or chemotherapy. Be proactive in pain and nausea management. Many patients are not assertive enough in requesting medicine for their discomfort.
5. In addition, the recipient must be infection free. Waiting until this state is achieved to have the transplant can be anxiety producing and emotionally frustrating. Allow the patient to vent his or her feelings and encourage hope.
6. Once admitted for the transplant, the patient will be in reverse isolation because of his or her extremely immunosuppressed state. Loneliness and feelings of isolationism may ensue during this period.
7. After the transplant, the patient will be hospitalized for 4 to 6 weeks until the marrow is fully engrafted and the pancytopenia subsides. Again, watch for loneliness and feelings of isolation. This period is also anxiety producing because of the ever-present fear of graft rejection. There is also a fear of graft-versus-host disease and development of further infections due to the pancytopenia. (See Chapter 21 for discussion of graft-versus-host disease.)
8. There is also physical discomfort. Side effects from medications may alter body appearance. Some patients develop the Cushingoid side effects (water retention, altered fat distribution, and facial hair) from steroids. In addition, patients usually lose their hair from the intense chemotherapy. Diarrhea is also a problem. Amid the joy of a successful transplant there is much discomfort. Prepare the patient for possible depression and irritability.
9. Involve the patient and family in care. One strategy is to teach the patient to calculate significant blood levels and what they mean. A frequently calculated record of progress is the absolute neutrophil count (ANC), which indicates a percentage differential between "fighter" leukocytes (neutrophils) and "other" leukocytes (immature neutrophils or bands). ANC = (percent of segmented neutrophils + percent of band neutrophils) × WBC.
10. Remember that individuals affected with life-threatening illnesses and their families are under great duress. They may vacillate between disbelief, anger, denial, acceptance, hope, and resilience. When preparing to teach, recognize that learning does not take place during denial. To ensure an adequate milieu for care and intervention, carefully assess the emotional roller coaster that patients and families experience.
11. Because of the high mortality rates and the long-term relationships that caregivers establish with patients undergoing bone marrow transplant and their families, nurses also need support and time to express their feelings.

Transplant and Chapter 17 for information about bone marrow transplant and cancer care.

Complications

1. Main complications are anemias, potentially fatal infections, and bleeding that leads to hemorrhage.

NURSE ADVISORY

Graft-versus-host disease is a life-threatening complication of some allogenic bone marrow transplants. (See Chapter 21.) The donor T cells from the new marrow attack the recipient usually in the skin, intestinal mucosa, liver, and lymph system. Graft-versus-host disease may be acute or chronic and is staged according to its severity.

BOX 25-6. Tumor Lysis Syndrome

Persons with acute lymphocytic leukemia, high-grade lymphoma, or any massive tumor burden with an extremely high white blood cell count are at great risk for tumor lysis syndrome, particularly as chemotherapy is started and afterward. Large number of proliferating cells are lysed open during chemotherapy. As the cell membrane ruptures, intracellular potassium, phosphorus, and nucleotides are released into the bloodstream, resulting in hyperkalemia, hyperphosphatemia, and hyperuricemia. The phosphorus released binds with the calcium, resulting in hypocalcemia. These imbalances precipitate an acute condition with serious complications, such as acute renal failure. Acute renal failure can be avoided if the urine is alkalinized by keeping the urine pH level above 7. Alkaline urine is maintained with intravenous fluid hydration and sodium bicarbonate. Allopurinol may also be used preventably to decrease uric acid levels.

2. Other complications include renal insufficiency, lymphadenopathy, hypermetabolism, veno-occlusive disease, and tumor lysis syndrome (Box 25–6).

Prognosis

1. Untreated, leukemias are fatal. Death can occur within 2 to 3 months.
2. See Table 25–7 for the prognoses of the different leukemias.

Applying the Nursing Process

NURSING DIAGNOSIS: Decreased cardiac output R/T high risk for blood dyscrasias and hemorrhage

1. *Expected outcomes:* After intervention, the patient should maintain a normal cardiac output, as indicated by the following:
   a. Blood counts and values are normal.
   b. Vital parameters are within normal limits.
   c. No bleeding tendencies are noted.
2. *Nursing interventions*
   a. Check vital signs every 4 hours.
   b. Monitor temperature every 4 hours.
   c. Assess for bleeding tendencies.
   d. Maintain IV access.
   e. Administer blood and blood products as ordered. Maintain current type and crossmatch.
   f. Monitor intake and output and daily weights.

NURSING DIAGNOSIS: Pain R/T side effects of chemotherapeutic medications and radiation

1. *Expected outcomes:* After intervention, the person should experience minimal pain during and after administration of chemotherapeutic agents and radiation.
2. *Nursing interventions*
   a. Medicate for pain frequently and proactively.

   b. Monitor diffuse pain by having the patient rate the pain on a scale from 0 to 10.
   c. Premedicate the patient for nausea before chemotherapy and radiation, if necessary.
   d. Minimize patient disturbances. Allow the patient to perform ADLs as able unless platelet counts are too low.
   e. Monitor IV site for extravasation of chemotherapeutic agent.

NURSING DIAGNOSIS: Risk for infection R/T neutropenic condition

1. *Expected outcomes:* After intervention, the person should be able to do the following:
   a. Remain free of infection, as indicated by a WBC count within normal limits, no increase in temperature, and negative blood cultures
   b. Remain free of secondary infections of a fungal or viral nature
2. *Nursing interventions:* Institute neutropenic precautions as necessary, including a neutropenic diet (Box 25–7).

NURSING DIAGNOSIS: Knowledge deficit R/T lack of information about the disease process, complications, medications, and side effects of medications and treatments

1. *Expected outcomes:* After instruction, the patient and family should be able to do the following:
   a. Describe the disease process, progression, treatment, and prognosis
   b. Identify medications used for treatment and their potential side effects
   c. Explain potential complications, the warning signs of complications, and when to call the physician
2. *Nursing interventions*
   a. Provide the patient and family with information about the disease process. Include printed materials.
   b. Ensure that the physician takes the time to explain the disease and its prognosis in detail before you begin the patient education process.
   c. Review the patient's readiness for learning according to the stage of grief and coping present.
   d. Determine the style of learning the patient and family prefer. Also, determine their literacy levels.

BOX 25-7. Neutropenic Precautions

When patients are immunocompromised from disease processes, chemotherapy, or radiation producing low neutrophil counts, it often is necessary to institute neutropenic precautions. This form of isolation requires a private room, if possible, and universal precautions, as usual. Family and caregivers with colds or coughs should not be allowed access to the patient. Visitors should be instructed to check with the nurse before entering the room to receive instructions on universal precautions and handwashing. All persons should complete thorough handwashing with antimicrobial soap. Certain dietary restrictions may also be implemented. A neutropenic diet consists of only thoroughly cooked foods. No raw fruits, vegetables, or salad items are allowed.

e. Fully explain all procedures, including diagnostics and treatments. Ask for verbalization of understanding. Provide literature if possible.

f. Provide information on medications being used. Explain the side effects of medications, treatments, and interventions to prevent untoward effects.

g. Teach the family methods for coping with life-threatening illness. Encourage open communication.

h. Refer the family to support agencies.

NURSING DIAGNOSIS: Ineffective individual and family coping R/T life-threatening illness

NURSING DIAGNOSIS: Anxiety R/T life-threatening illness

1. *Expected outcomes:* After instruction, the patient and family should be able to do the following:
   a. Demonstrate alternative coping techniques to decrease anxiety
   b. Show no signs or symptoms of acute anxiety
2. *Nursing interventions*
   a. Allow the patient to make some decisions regarding the care regimen.
   b. Keep the patient and family informed and educated about the care regimen.
   c. Teach relaxation techniques.
   d. Provide diversional activities as tolerated and warranted.
   e. Monitor patterns of communication between the patient and family members.
   f. Address spirituality and fears of dying when appropriate.
   g. Refer the patient to counseling services and clergy as needed.

NURSING DIAGNOSIS: Impaired skin integrity R/T side effects of medications

1. *Expected outcomes:* After intervention, the patient's skin should remain intact and free of injury.
2. *Nursing interventions*
   a. Monitor the skin frequently for signs of breakdown.
   b. Be careful to avoid causing shear force injuries during transfers to wheelchairs, stretchers, and beds.
   c. Avoid harsh soaps. Use lotions with baths and for maintenance.
   d. Encourage a high-protein diet and dietary items rich in vitamins A and C.
   e. Help the patient cope with the alteration of his or her physical appearance as a result of swelling, petechiae, and bleeding tendencies.
   f. Have the patient use saline and alkaline mouthwashes to gargle every 2 to 4 hours. This type of mouthwash helps inhibit infection. Do not use commercial mouthwashes.
   g. Brush the patient's teeth at least 4 times daily with a soft-bristle toothbrush or tooth sponge.

Discharge Planning and Teaching

1. Teach the signs and symptoms of bleeding tendencies and when the physician should be called.
2. Teach the signs and symptoms of infection and when the physician should be called.
3. Teach about laboratory values, normal values, and their significance.
4. Explain the side effects of chemotherapeutic agents and discharge medications and modalities to cope with these effects.
5. Encourage rest and comfort measures.
6. Provide instruction on eating a high-calorie, high-protein diet. Small, frequent meals may be indicated.
7. Teach the signs and symptoms of disease recurrence (abdominal discomfort and swelling in lymph tissues) and the importance of contacting the physician immediately.
8. Teach the procedure for central line care.
9. Refer the patient to a hospice for end-of-life care when the patient is approaching death.

HOME CARE STRATEGIES

Drawing Blood Work in the Home

Drawing blood work in the home is 1 way that the nurse and the physician can monitor patients with blood disorders. Other indications include monitoring blood levels of certain medications; monitoring protimes for patients on warfarin (Coumadin) therapy; or monitoring blood chemistries such as blood sugars, sodium, and potassium levels.

Some factors to take into consideration when drawing blood in the home:

- Familiarize yourself with the patient's history.
- Inform the patient that you will be drawing blood. Patients that have blood work done on a regular basis probably know what is supposed to be done and may question you. Patients that have blood work done infrequently may ask why you are drawing blood and what you expect to find. Patients will also tell you what is a good site to draw from.
- Organize all supplies. Substitutions may be needed. A blood pressure cuff, a shoestring, or a necktie may be used for a tourniquet. Penlights, flashlights, or sunlight may be used in homes with poor lighting. Patients with poor hygiene may need the site washed with soap and water or you may expect to use several alcohol wipes.
- Agency or laboratory guidelines need to be followed for disposal of needles and storing and transporting blood. Cooling may be needed, especially if the blood will not be taken directly to the laboratory, or if the weather is warm. A small cooler with an ice pack, a waterproof bag with ice, or a fast food drink cup with ice may be used.
- A laboratory that will run the blood work and report the results in a timely manner is essential. Directions need to be clearly stated on the requisition to fax, mail, or telephone laboratory results to the agency and physician. Call the laboratory to obtain results, then call the physician to verify that the results were communicated. Record the results in the patient's record.

Public Health Considerations

1. Teach people to avoid exposure to toxic chemical agents.
2. Teach people the hazard of radiation exposure.

◼ OTHER LEUKEMIAS

Hairy Cell Leukemia

1. Definition: Hairy cell leukemia is a rare, chronic lymphoproliferative disorder characterized by morphologic hairlike projections on cells of the bone marrow.
2. Incidence and etiology
   a. Hairy cell leukemia represents less than 2 percent of all adult leukemias and is usually seen in middle-aged patients.
   b. The etiology is unknown. No association has been made to radiation or other environmental factors.
3. Clinical manifestations
   a. There is excessive infiltration of hairy cells into the bone marrow or spleen. Underproduction or excessive peripheral sequestration of circulating cells shows granulocytopenia, anemia, or thrombocytopenia.
   b. Initial signs and symptoms are weakness, lethargy, or fatigue.
   c. Ninety percent of patients have splenomegaly.
4. Clinical management
   a. Hairy cell leukemia is highly treatable and sometimes curable with interferon-α in low, well-tolerated doses. Deoxycoformycin and cladribine (Leustatin) are also effective.
   b. Splenectomy, the old treatment, is no longer considered effective.

Myelodysplastic Disorders

1. Definition
   a. Myelodysplastic disorders are a group of 5 distinct pathologies: refractory anemia, refractory anemia with ringed sideroblasts, chronic myelomonocytic leukemia, refractory anemia with excess blasts, and refractory anemia with excess blasts in transition.
   b. Severity ranges from mild to leukemic.
2. Incidence and etiology
   a. Myelodysplasia is a disease of the elderly. It is rarely seen in people younger than 30.
   b. The etiology is unclear. Possible links are exposure to benzene, radiation, and chemotherapy (especially alkylating agents).
3. Clinical manifestations
   a. Severe cytopenia or pancytopenia is present.
   b. Infections, especially respiratory or gram-negative septicemias, are seen initially. Bleeding may also be present.
4. Clinical management
   a. Persons with mild anemias may be treated with transfusions.
   b. Allogenic bone marrow transplant is the only curative approach for patients with severe cases; however, patients are generally too old to be considered candidates.
   c. Chemotherapy is only marginally successful. Many patients die during this treatment. Research is being done on the use of growth factors.

◼ AGRANULOCYTOSIS

Definition

1. Agranulocytosis is 1 of several forms of leukocytopenia.
2. It is an acute disease in which the WBC count drops to dangerously low levels and neutropenia is pronounced.

Incidence

The incidence of agranulocytosis is variable and depends on whether the etiology is idiopathic or exposure-related.

Risk Factors

1. Exposure to toxic chemicals
2. Certain psychotropic medications
3. Overexposure to ionized radiation

Etiology

1. Agranulocytosis can be idiopathic.
2. It can also develop as an adverse reaction to exposure to certain drugs (e.g., some psychotropic medications) and toxic chemicals.

Pathophysiology

1. Agranulocytosis is a pathologic state in which the neutrophil count is below 300 per mm^3.
2. It is considered the most severe form of granulocytopenia.
3. The disorder is severe because neutrophils normally make up 55 to 75 percent of all leukocytes and are considered the body's most powerful line of defense against invading microorganisms.

Clinical Manifestations

1. High fever, no fever, or temperature below normal
2. Weakness to the point of prostration
3. Necrotic ulcerations of the mouth, rectum, and vagina
4. Muscle ache and headache
5. Sore throat
6. Tachycardia

Diagnostics

1. Initial complaint of symptoms
2. A complete blood count with differential
3. A thorough history, including questions about exposure to chemical toxoids and medications consumed
4. A thorough assessment of the mouth, gums, and throat

Clinical Management

1. Goals of clinical management
   a. Treatment measures to correct the underlying disorder
   b. Treatment of any developing infections
2. Nonpharmacologic interventions
   a. Possible protective isolation
   b. Possible use of a low-microbial (neutropenic) diet
3. Pharmacologic interventions
   a. Adjustment of therapeutic medications to correct the underlying cause
   b. Antibiotics, antivirals, and antifungals to treat infection

Complications

Development of potentially fatal infections, including bacterial, viral, or fungal infections

Prognosis

1. The disorder can be fatal.
2. Complications may be severe if the disease is not treated early.

Applying the Nursing Process

NURSING DIAGNOSIS: Risk for infection R/T neutropenia

1. *Expected outcomes:* After interventions, the patient should remain free of infection.
2. *Nursing interventions*
   a. Perform careful handwashing.
   b. Maintain isolation of the patient from infectious persons.
   c. Monitor the patient's leukocyte count (see Box 25–7).

NURSING DIAGNOSIS: Risk for impaired skin integrity (stomatitis) R/T pancytopenia

1. *Expected outcomes:* Following interventions, the patient's mouth and mucosa should remain intact.
2. *Nursing interventions*
   a. Débride necrotic lesions.
   b. Have the patient swish and swallow with special non-alcohol mouthwash (e.g., a Peridex, Nystatin, or Mycelex troche) at least every 2 hours.
   c. Avoid acidic foods and drinks.
   d. Administer an ice collar and lozenges for the patient's sore throat.
   e. Encourage a soft, high-protein diet to maintain electrolyte balance and promote healing. Consider a low-microbial diet.

Discharge Planning and Teaching

1. Instruct the patient to avoid exposure to toxic chemicals.
2. Explain the importance of rest and relaxation to ward off fatigue.
3. Teach the signs and symptoms of agranulocytosis to prevent acute complication.

Public Health Considerations

1. Occupational health professionals should educate workers at work sites regarding potential exposure to chemicals.
2. Rural public health professionals should educate farmers and crop dusters who work with toxic chemicals.

◾ *MONONUCLEOSIS*

Definition

1. Mononucleosis is an infectious viral disease in which there is more than the normal number of mononuclear leukocytes in the blood.
2. It is also referred to as the "kissing disease."

Incidence and Socioeconomic Impact

1. Mononucleosis primarily affects children ages 3 to 5 and young persons ages 15 to 25.
2. The disorder occurs as isolated cases or in epidemics.

Risk Factors

1. Exposure to individuals with mononucleosis
2. Exposure to persons incubating the disease

Etiology

1. The disease is believed to be caused by the Epstein-Barr virus.
2. It is thought that the virus is transmitted in the secretions of the mucous membranes of the mouth, gastrointestinal tract, and respiratory tract.

Pathophysiology

1. Mononucleosis primarily affects lymphoid tissue.
2. A large number of immature or abnormal leukocytes congregate in the lymph nodes and spleen.
3. Symptoms are manifested after a 30- to 40-day incubation period.

Clinical Manifestations

1. In the acute phase of mononucleosis, a triad of symptoms is seen in most patients: fever, tender lymph nodes, and sore throat.
2. The spleen enlarges, with pain to the upper left quadrant.
3. Other flulike symptoms are malaise, generalized fatigue and weakness, and anorexia.

Diagnostics

1. Within a week of initial symptoms, a WBC count with differential reveals leukocytosis. The differential count reveals elevations of lymphocytes and monocytes of greater than 50 percent, with 10 to 20 percent atypical lymphocytes.
2. An antibody test for heterophils or Epstein-Barr virus is positive. One third of patients have positive β-hemolytic streptococcus cultures of the throat. Some individuals have elevated liver function studies with liver involvement.
3. Assessment includes palpation of lymph nodes; measurement of vital signs, including temperature; throat inspection; and questions regarding fatigue, weakness, and malaise (Box 25–8).

Clinical Management

1. Goals of clinical management
   a. Management is mostly on an outpatient basis and ensures rest, nutrition, and fluids.
   b. Isolation is not required.
2. Nonpharmacologic interventions
   a. There is no specific regimen.
   b. Bed rest and decreased activities for 2 to 3 weeks are required.
3. Pharmacologic interventions
   a. Antibiotics are not useful, because of the viral nature of the disorder.
   b. Analgesics are given for comfort and fever reduction.
   c. Steroids are prescribed for serious complications of swelling or hemolytic anemia.

Complications

1. Complications are rare.
2. Possible complications include pneumonia, airway obstruction from dysphagia, and splenic rupture.

Prognosis

1. The prognosis is very good if the person experiences no relapse or complications.
2. Adults generally are at greater risk for complications than are children. Complete resolution takes longer for adults than for children.

Applying the Nursing Process

NURSING DIAGNOSIS: Fatigue R/T the disease process

BOX 25–8. Chronic Fatigue Syndrome

A disease defined by the Centers for Disease Control and Prevention (CDC) that continues to elude prompt diagnosis and intervention is chronic fatigue syndrome. This disorder is characterized by myalgias, generalized fatigue, headaches, dizziness, low-grade fever, insomnia, depression, and even confusion. These symptoms seem to be triggered after flulike symptoms.

Often, patients complain to their family or general physician of a flulike illness that persists, mixed with an inescapable fatigue. After a barrage of diagnostic tests, which often come back inconclusive, many physicians write this disorder off as psychologic. Recent attention in the literature has discouraged this practice by providing more specific guidelines for diagnosis (see Fig. 25–4).

This disease has been called many things: **chronic Epstein-Barr virus, acute infective encephalomyelitis, myalgic encephalomyelitis** (in Great Britain), and many other names. The working definition was announced by the CDC in 1988.

At one time, this disorder was believed to originate as part of the Epstein-Barr virus. Research pointed out, however, that most (as many as 85%) of the general population shows a positive titer to Epstein-Barr. Therefore, that diagnostic criterion was not included in the CDC's definition.

Currently, chronic fatigue syndrome can best be described as a collection of fatigue and flulike symptoms somehow influenced by psychoimmunologic risk factors that converge to the final pathway of chronic fatigue. Further research on etiology and treatment is warranted.

Most clinicians agree that the key to diagnosis is a thorough history and physical examination. A detailed psychologic evaluation should be performed, not only for exclusion but also in preparation for long-term support and management of the disease. The longer the duration of chronic fatigue and the greater the number of symptoms, the less the need for extensive diagnostic tests to support the diagnosis. Look for other diagnoses only if the clinical picture is dominated by a single symptom. The two disorders that must be differentiated out are fibromyalgia and depression.

Management should be tailored to the patient's symptomatology. Some beneficial interventions include good dietary and sleep habits and a progressive exercise program (frequent and low intensity) as tolerated. Low-dose antidepressants at bedtime can reduce depression, enhance sleep, and treat myalgias. Some nonsteroidal anti-inflammatories may also help with discomforts. Acyclovir, once used in treatment, is no longer believed to be beneficial. In addition, cognitive-behavioral therapy and support groups to promote a positive outlook and improve overall disability may be valuable.

Most chronic fatigue syndrome patients experience misdiagnosis, being told that their illness is all in their head, and fragmented interventions, with the result that they feel frustrated and humiliated. In general, caregivers and practitioners must show these patients consistent efforts, patience, education, and commitment.

---

1. *Expected outcomes:* After instruction and intervention, the patient should obtain adequate rest so that recuperation may take place.
2. *Nursing interventions*
   a. Encourage bed rest.
   b. Monitor for signs and symptoms of complications.

Discharge Planning and Teaching

1. Resolution of the disease is seen when fatigue diminishes and laboratory values return to normal.
2. Stress the importance of follow-up to ensure resolution and prevent relapse.
3. Instruct the patient to avoid communicable contact with individuals complaining of flulike symptoms.

Public Health Considerations

1. The patient remains infective for 18 months.
2. Explain transmission of the disease.

◼ *HODGKIN'S DISEASE*

Definition

1. Hodgkin's disease is a malignant disorder that usually starts in the lymph nodes. It is defined by the presence of the Reed-Sternberg giant cell. It is not a granulomatous infection or a chronic immunologic disorder.
2. Hodgkin's disease spreads to many body areas—including the mediastinum, bone, liver, spleen, ureters, and bronchi—through the lymph nodes and eventually the blood.

Incidence and Socioeconomic Impact

1. The number of new cases in the United States per year approximates 7000, and approximately 1600 deaths due to Hodgkin's disease occur per year. More males than females have the disease.
2. The average age for an individual with Hodgkin's disease is 32 years. The incidence of this disease has an unusual bimodal pattern. The 1st peak incidence occurs between 15 and 35 years of age; the 2nd occurs after the age of 50 years.

Risk Factors

Young adults who have a sibling with Hodgkin's disease have a 7 times greater risk of developing the disease.

Etiology

1. The etiology of Hodgkin's disease is unknown. There is no confirmation of a bacterial, viral, or fungal cause, although it has been suggested that the disease may be an age-dependent host response to a common infection.
2. There is no evidence for a contagious etiology.

Pathophysiology

1. Controversy over the cell of origin is not resolved.
2. A previously unrecognized early myeloid-monocytoid cell may be the precursor of the Reed-Sternberg cell, which is the diagnostic cell of Hodgkin's disease.

Clinical Manifestations

1. The initial presentation and clinical course are greatly variable, depending on when the patient first presents to health care professionals.

2. Adenopathy, an enlarged painless mass that is often rubbery, firm, and freely moveable, is usually found in the neck. An adenopathy or adenopathies may also be found in the axilla and inguinal areas. Most often, adenopathy is the only finding, although some individuals in the older groups present without any adenopathy.
3. A fever of unknown origin is common. The fever is persistent and is often accompanied by night sweats.
4. Fatigue and weight loss are common manifestations.
5. Pruritus is manifested. Beginning in a mild and localized form, it usually progresses to a generalized, severe form, at which point it often results in excoriation and the inability to sleep.
6. Patchy pulmonary infiltrates are found in about 10 to 20 percent of persons at diagnosis.
7. Bone pain is common.

Diagnostics

1. Medical diagnosis is made by biopsy of involved tissue.
2. The classic presentation is an asymptomatic lymph node, often found during a routine physical examination but sometimes found by the individual. It is common for the node to have been present for several weeks to many months or even years, waxing and waning in size, before presentation.
3. Ask about night sweats and weight loss (the loss of more than 10% of baseline weight is especially critical). Assess for a persistent dry cough, dyspnea, orthopnea, headaches, vertigo, and drowsiness. These may indicate central venous or lymphatic compression. If the symptoms are new, be sure to notify the physician promptly. Additional signs and symptoms may be caused by nodes pressing on adjacent structures or by cancer infiltrating body organs. It is critical to get all information so that staging of the disease and treatment are accurate.
4. Neck or back pain, numbness, tingling or weakness of an extremity, or bowel or bladder dysfunction could indicate cord compression and constitutes a medical emergency. Permanent damage can be prevented if the condition is addressed early.
5. Chest radiographs can disclose lymphadenopathy.
6. Blood tests may include RBC indices and a WBC count with differential as well as blood chemistries.
7. A lymph node biopsy, lymphangiography, a CT scan of the abdomen, a gallium scan, and bone marrow biopsies are commonly performed in the effort to diagnose and stage the disease. Liver biopsies, spleen biopsies, and even exploratory laparotomies are performed to help with staging. Staging of Hodgkin's disease is critical to assess the extent of disease, facilitate the selection of treatment, provide a prognosis, and establish a baseline for reevaluation after treatment.

Clinical Management

1. Goals of intervention
   a. Cure is the goal for all stages, histologic subtypes, and extranodal sites of the disease.

b. The 5-year survival rate has increased to at least 75 percent today.

2. Nonpharmacologic interventions: Radiation therapy is used in tumoricidal doses to treat tumors and adjacent areas and is used prophylactically to treat apparently uninvolved areas for subclinical disease. Radiation therapy is combined with 1 of the chemotherapy regimens for combined-modality treatment of Hodgkin's disease.
3. Pharmacologic interventions
   a. Chemotherapy combinations are used.
   b. Included are MOPP (nitrogen mustard, vincristine, procarbazine, prednisone) and BCVPP (BCNU [carmustine], cyclophosphamide, vinblastine, procarbazine, prednisone). There are other 4- and 5-drug combinations, but they have not been demonstrated to be superior to MOPP or BCVPP.
4. It is essential to administer the full dose at prescribed times. The therapy is given every 4 weeks for a minimum of 6 cycles. An additional 2 cycles are administered after remission has been achieved.
5. Patients who relapse after MOPP can receive ABVD (Adriamycin, bleomycin, vinblastine, dacarbazine), which has a 30 to 60 percent remission rate.

Complications

1. Superior vena caval obstruction or compression of the upper airway by mediastinal disease
2. Pericarditis, pericardial effusions, or both
3. Spinal cord compression
4. Bone marrow suppression from chemotherapy and radiation therapy
5. Sterility, especially in males, from the chemotherapy (sterility can be permanent)
6. Secondary malignancies, such as acute myelocytic leukemia, after cure of lymphoma related to therapy

Prognosis

1. The past 2 decades have seen dramatic improvement in the prognosis for persons with Hodgkin's disease. Cure is a potential for all people diagnosed.
2. A weight loss greater than 10 percent of baseline before diagnosis leads to a poorer prognosis.

Applying the Nursing Process

NURSING DIAGNOSIS: Activity intolerance R/T poor tissue perfusion and neutropenia

1. *Expected outcomes:* After intervention, the person should be able to maximize performance of ADLs without overt fatigue.
2. *Nursing interventions*
   a. Space ADLs out by allowing short intervals between them.

b. Allow for frequent rest periods.
   c. Provide supplemental oxygen as ordered and as necessary.
   d. Provide for independence as much as possible.

NURSING DIAGNOSIS: Impaired swallowing R/T stomatitis from chemotherapy and radiation

1. *Expected outcomes:* After intervention, the person should be able to swallow satisfactorily and obtain adequate nutrition.
2. *Nursing interventions*
   a. Encourage the person to use prescribed mouthwashes and rinses as ordered.
   b. Discourage consumption of acid-based foods and beverages.
   c. Provide soft foods. Avoid extremely crunchy foods.
   d. Do not puree diet (unless absolutely necessary).

Additional nursing diagnoses include the following:
- Impaired skin integrity R/T side effects of radiation therapy
- Anticipatory grieving R/T change in lifestyle and life-threatening illness
- Knowledge deficit (disease, treatment, and prognosis) R/T lack of information
- Altered nutrition (less than body requirements) R/T increased metabolic needs due to cancer
- Risk for infection R/T neutropenia caused by chemotherapeutic agents

Discharge Planning and Teaching

1. Teach the patient about the disease process.
2. If chemotherapy and radiation treatments are to be administered on an outpatient basis, teaching must address the anticipated nausea, fatigue, signs and symptoms of infection, stomatitis, skin care, and alopecia.
3. The patient and family need to be given the name and phone number of at least 1 resource person to call when questions and concerns arise. If indicated, refer the patient to a visiting nurse or home health nurse resource.
4. Counsel the patient regarding the potential of birth defects if conception occurs during courses of chemotherapy and radiation. If indicated, educate couples interested in conceiving at a later date about the availability of sperm banks. (Men who undergo chemotherapy and radiation therapy are at risk for becoming permanently sterile.)

◾ *NON-HODGKIN'S LYMPHOMA*

Definition

1. Non-Hodgkin's lymphoma is a neoplasm of lymphoid tissue that is not Hodgkin's disease. The condition is

characterized by lymphatic proliferation of malignant cells other than Reed-Sternberg cells.
2. There are more than 10 distinct disease entities of non-Hodgkin's lymphoma, including Burkitt's lymphoma, lymphoblastic lymphoma, and adult T-cell leukemia or lymphoma.

Incidence and Socioeconomic Impact

1. Non-Hodgkin's lymphoma is much more common than Hodgkin's disease. It occurs at any age, although it is rare during the 1st year of life. The incidence increases steadily beginning in the 4th decade of life. Each year, 27,000 cases are diagnosed in the United States.
2. Males have a higher incidence than females, and more males than females are young and have aggressive types of lymphoblastic and Burkitt's lymphomas.

Risk Factors

1. A preceding immune dysfunction has been associated with aggressive forms of non-Hodgkin's lymphoma.
2. Some congenital immunodeficiency states are associated with lymphomas.
3. Transplant recipients and patients with acquired immunodeficiency syndrome have an increased risk for the disease, as a result of suppressed immune function.

Etiology

1. The etiology of non-Hodgkin's lymphoma is unclear.
2. The Epstein-Barr virus has been implicated in the pathogenesis of Burkitt's lymphoma. A unique human retrovirus, human T-cell leukemia-lymphoma virus, has been associated with a newly recognized adult T-cell leukemia-lymphoma.
3. Chromosomal translocations are found in most non-Hodgkin's lymphomas.

Pathophysiology

1. Many different classifications have been proposed. Most are based on a cell of origin, a specific chromosomal translocation, or the presence of antibodies.
2. The disease ranges from an aggressive fatal form to an indolent condition.

Clinical Manifestations

1. The clinical manifestations of non-Hodgkin's lymphoma are the same as those of Hodgkin's disease. Symptoms usually present at an advanced state.
2. Large, painless lymph nodes may be associated with enlarged tonsils or adenoids.
3. Back pain (and possibly ascites) result from enlarged retroperitoneal nodes.

Diagnostics

1. The history includes assessment of all systemic symptoms.
2. Analyze predisposing epidemiologic factors.
3. Obtain a tumor tissue sample for examination.
4. Perform diagnostic tests. Blood laboratory work includes a complete blood count with differential, platelets, RBC count and indices, blood chemistries, and a Coombs test if the person is anemic. Other tests include abdominal and pelvic CT and bone scans, chest radiographs to disclose lymphadenopathy, serum immunoglobulins in low-grade stages and antibody for HTLV-I or HTLV-II, and liver and renal function tests.

Clinical Management

1. Goals of intervention
   a. Interventions are based on whether the lymphoma is slowly progressive or rapidly aggressive and fatal without treatment.
   b. Remission is the goal of treatment in all cases.
2. Nonpharmacologic interventions
   a. Regional radiation therapy may be administered.
   b. Whole-body radiation may be administered.
   c. Treatment may be deferred for some low-grade, slowly progressive lymphomas. The physicians will wait until the disease worsens, because there seems to be no advantage to early treatment.
3. Pharmacologic interventions
   a. A single chemotherapeutic agent may be used.
   b. Multiagent chemotherapy may be used. The most successful current program is ProMACE-MOPP (prednisone, methotrexate, Adriamycin, cyclophosphamide, etoposide, mechlorethamine, Oncovin, procarbazine, prednisone) followed by total lymphoid radiation. Investigational drugs may also be tried.
   c. Other multiagent therapies include MACOP-B (methotrexate, Adriamycin, cyclophosphamide, Oncovin, prednisone, bleomycin, co-trimoxazole), CHOP-B (cyclophosphamide, hydroxydaunomycin/Adriamycin, Oncovin, prednisone, bleomycin), and m-BACOD (methotrexate, bleomycin, Adriamycin, cyclophosphamide, Oncovin, dexamethasone).

Complications

1. In up to 50 percent of people with low-grade non-Hodgkin's lymphoma, a shift to a more aggressive form occurs by the 8th year after diagnosis.
2. Tumor doubling can occur in 3 days. The tumor can then obstruct the gastrointestinal tract, ureters, nerve roots, or spinal cord.
3. Renal failure occurs.

Prognosis

1. Most patients with non-Hodgkin's lymphoma respond well to treatment but are less likely than those with

Hodgkin's disease to respond with remissions and cures.
2. At 5 years, 60 percent of all patients are alive and disease free.
3. After 8 years, many patients with low-grade disease become progressively worse whereas those who had higher grade disease at the time of diagnosis remain disease free.

Applying the Nursing Process

See Applying the Nursing Process for Hodgkin's disease.

> Additional nursing diagnoses include the following:
> • Impaired skin integrity R/T side effects of radiation therapy
> • Anticipatory grieving R/T change in lifestyle and life-threatening illness
> • Knowledge deficit (disease, treatment, and prognosis) R/T lack of information
> • Altered nutrition (less than body requirements) R/T increased metabolic needs due to cancer
> • Risk for infection R/T neutropenia caused by chemotherapeutic agents

Discharge Planning and Teaching

1. If the person has a low-grade non-Hodgkin's lymphoma and no treatment is to be given at the time of diagnosis, the person and family members must be taught all the signs and symptoms that might occur. The person must be taught when it is necessary to return to see health care professionals and must understand that return appointments are extremely important for monitoring the progress of the disease and determining when treatment becomes necessary.
2. When the patient is undergoing chemotherapy or radiation therapy, the health teaching is the same as that for Hodgkin's disease.

◨ *HEMOPHILIA*

Definition

1. Hemophilia is a disease in which bleeding time is greatly increased because the blood's coagulability is impaired.
2. Abnormal hemorrhaging can occur if blood fails to clot.

NURSE ADVISORY

> Alterations in coagulopathy originating from platelet disorders can be congenital or acquired. Congenital disorders result from defective platelets produced from the bone marrow. The effects of drugs such as aspirin and carbenicillin and systemic diseases such as uremia can precipitate the acquired form. Replacement of platelets is the only effective treatment.

Incidence and Socioeconomic Impact

1. The disease affects approximately 0.01 percent of the U.S. population, or about 20,000 Americans.
2. Hemophilia A (deficient or absent factor VIII) makes up 80 percent of cases. Hemophilia B (Christmas disease, deficient factor IX) makes up about 15 percent of cases.
3. Up to 30 percent of persons with hemophilia have no notable family history of the disease, suggesting that the condition could be caused by a new gene mutation.

Risk Factors

1. Being male.
2. Having a mother who is a carrier.

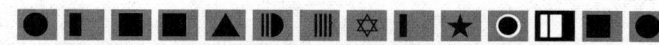

TRANSCULTURAL CONSIDERATIONS

In ethnic and racial groups who rely heavily on a supernatural relationship with religion, the idea that certain blood disorders are hereditary may impart tremendous guilt feelings in the mother. It may be helpful to deal with these feelings by allowing the incorporation of customary rituals to remove the cause.

Etiology

1. Hemophilia is an inherited x-linked recessive disorder. A female carrier has a 50 percent chance of transmitting the defective X chromosome to each son or daughter.
2. The son who inherits the gene will have hemophilia. The daughter who inherits the gene will be a carrier.

Pathophysiology

1. Clotting factor deficiency impairs the hemostatic response, preventing stable clot formation.
2. The severity of the bleeding tendency varies with the degree of clotting factor deficiency as well as with the specific cause and location of each bleeding episode.

Clinical Manifestations

1. Spontaneous bleeding episodes occur throughout life.
2. Musculoskeletal and skin sites that are stressed or receive direct trauma are at risk.
3. Excessive bleeding after circumcision leads to a suspicion of hemophilia.
4. Moderate hemophilia produces prolonged bleeding after dental or surgical procedures and childbirth.
5. Hematomas, either subcutaneous or muscular, can lead to pressure on vital organs and produce damage.

6. A significant number of persons with hemophilia who received blood transfusions before 1984 became infected with the human immunodeficiency virus. This risk has been diminished because of vigorous testing of blood and blood products.

NURSE ADVISORY

Von Willebrand's disease (also known as **pseudohemophilia**) is an inherited or acquired autosomal-dominant coagulation disorder with localized prolonged bleeding times and factor VIII deficiency. Symptoms are mild and generally not diagnosed until some type of injury or surgical procedure precipitates the condition. Treatment consists of local control of bleeding. If that is not effective, cryoprecipitate may be ordered.

Diagnostics

1. Does the patient have a history of prolonged or spontaneous bleeding? Ask about a family history of disease or prolonged bleeding.
2. Look for or ask about easy bruising, epistaxis, and hematomas.
3. During the acute phase, assess for swollen joints, localized and prolonged bleeding, bleeding from the gums, abdominal distention, hematemesis or melena, pallor, weakness, restlessness, increased pulse, and decreased blood pressure.
4. In hemophilia A, factor VIII assay is 0 to 30 percent of normal; activated partial thromboplastin time is prolonged; and platelet count, bleeding time, and prothrombin time are normal.
5. In hemophilia B, factor IX assay is deficient; platelet count, bleeding time, and prothrombin time are baseline; and factor VIII level is normal.
6. The degree of factor deficiency determines the severity of the hemophilia. During bleeding episodes, assessment might include endoscopies for gastrointestinal bleeds, CT scans for intracranial hemorrhage, and arthroscopies for hemarthrosis.

Clinical Management

1. Goals of clinical management
   a. Immediate halt of the bleeding
   b. Pain management, avoiding aspirin
   c. Early treatment to avoid crippling deformities (immobilize the affected joint and apply cold compresses)
   d. Surgical correction of musculoskeletal complications
   e. Genetic counseling
2. Nonpharmacologic interventions
   a. Careful planning for dental and surgical procedures. It may be necessary to give the patient a transfusion beforehand.
   b. Synovectomy, joint débridement, or arthroplasty to treat hemarthrosis complications

3. Pharmacologic interventions
   a. Transfusion of the deficient clotting factor is the mainstay of treatment. Two products of choice are cryoprecipitate, which is rich in factor VIII, and freeze-dried concentrates of factor VIII or IX. Genetically engineered synthetic factor VIII, or recombinant factor VIII, is also available.
   b. For persons with mild hemophilia, desmopressin, a synthetic analogue of human antidiuretic hormone, is the treatment of choice. It causes increased factor VIII release from storage sites within the body.
4. Special medical-surgical procedures
   a. Replacement of deficient factors before any invasive dental or surgical procedure
   b. The consultation of a hematologist to manage the care of the patient with hemophilia who requires surgery

Complications

1. **Hemarthrosis,** bleeding into a joint space (most commonly the knees, ankles, and elbows), is a hallmark of severe disease.
2. Repeated episodes of hemarthrosis lead to joint destruction and loss of motion. Joints become warm, edematous, and painful to touch. Cartilage is destroyed, and permanent bone deformities occur if the problem is left untreated.

Prognosis

1. Although blood screening and testing are not 100 percent exclusive for hepatitis and the human immunodeficiency virus, they have improved significantly since 1984. Therefore, with proper management the average life span of a person with hemophilia is relatively normal.
2. Before 1984, a significant number of persons with hemophilia became infected with the human immunodeficiency virus through transfusion, which shortened their life span dramatically.

Applying the Nursing Process

NURSING DIAGNOSIS: Altered tissue perfusion (vital organs) R/T hemorrhage

---

1. *Expected outcomes:* After intervention, the patient should be able to maintain hemodynamic stability and therefore tissue perfusion, as indicated by adequate cardiac output and avoidance of shocklike symptoms (decreased blood pressure, diaphoresis, and decreased urinary output).
2. *Nursing interventions*
   a. Monitor vital signs (blood pressure, pulse, etc.) frequently. Note changes.
   b. Transfuse clotting factors and blood products as necessary (Procedure 25–2).

P
Procedure 25–2
Transfusing Blood Products

Definition/Purpose	Transfusion of blood products is the delivery of a component of blood, such as packed red blood cells, plasma, or albumin, directly into the bloodstream. Transfusions of blood products are used to replace blood lost through surgery, disease, or trauma.
Contraindications/Cautions	Always verify the physician's order for blood product transfusion. Follow your institution's policies and procedures regarding the transfusion.

Preliminary Activities

Equipment	• Informed-consent form • 0.9 percent saline for infusion (normal saline)—Do not infuse the blood component with any solution other than normal saline. Neither should the intravenous (IV) line be primed or flushed with any solution other than normal saline. • 19-gauge or larger IV infusion device for adults • Y-tubing blood administration set with filter (or other tubing as specified in your institution's policies)—Do not transfuse the blood component without the appropriate filter.
Assessment/Planning	• Record the patient's vital signs before starting the infusion. If the temperature is elevated, notify the physician before transfusing the component. • Complete a full physical assessment of the patient, including auscultation of the lungs and bowels. • If the patient is receiving maintenance IV fluids, check with the physician to ensure that total IV fluids being infused do not exceed what the patient can tolerate.
Procedure	

Action	Rationale/Discussion
1. Obtain the physician's order for transfusion of blood product. Use only written orders, except in emergencies.	1. Transfusion of blood components requires a physician's order. Written orders help prevent errors. When you have to administer blood components with verbal orders during an emergency, obtain written order as soon as possible afterward.
2. Send the patient's blood sample to the laboratory for typing and crossmatching. Follow your institution's procedures for labeling and initialing the sample.	2. To avoid adverse reactions, the blood type and Rh factors of the donor and recipient must match.
3. Obtain informed consent for transfusion of the blood component. Teach the patient and family about the possibility of a transfusion reaction.	3. Informed consent is necessary except in emergency situations. Be sure the patient and family understand the importance of telling health care professionals about the 1st signs of a reaction: a rash, low-grade fever, or headache.
4. When the blood component arrives on the nursing unit, check for compatibility of ABO groups and Rh factor between the patient and the blood to be transfused.	4. This is one step in ensuring that the laboratory or blood bank sent the correct blood component.
5. With another nurse, check to be certain that the patient's name, blood type, Rh factor, and identification number are the same as those on the blood component bag. Document on appropriate forms that this check was completed. Document that the patient's identification band has the same name and number as shown on the label on the blood component.	5. This is a critical step in ensuring the patient's safety. Many institutions require that both nurses' signatures be recorded.
6. If you are unable to initiate the infusion of the blood component within a half hour of its arrival on the nursing unit, return the blood component to the transfusion service.	6. Some institutions allow 1 hour to pass before the blood component must be returned to the transfusion service. Know your institution's policy. Blood is kept refrigerated in the transfusion service. To prevent bacterial growth and hemolysis, it must be administered within the time allowed by institutional policy. *Never* refrigerate the blood component on the nursing unit.
7. Before starting the infusion, inspect the blood component container for any unusual appearance (bubbles, purplish color, or clots) or leakage.	7. If any of these changes are present, return the bag to the transfusion service.

(continued)

P

Procedure 25–2

(continued)

Action	Rationale/Discussion
8. Do not warm the blood component in the microwave or in hot water. If it must be warmed, use a blood warmer.	8. If a blood warmer is necessary because of the need to infuse multiple units of blood rapidly, follow the manufacturer's instructions and your institution's policy.
9. Take a new set of vital signs just before starting the infusion of the blood component. Stay with the patient during the first 15 to 20 minutes of the infusion. Allow only 25 to 30 ml of the component to infuse over that period.	9. Although complications can occur during the following 48 hours (or even 180 days), the most likely time for severe reactions to occur is the first 15 to 20 minutes of the transfusion.
10. The rate of infusion of the remainder of the blood component depends on the patient's medical condition. Generally, the blood component is infused as quickly as the patient's condition allows. No blood component should be allowed to infuse for longer than a total of 4 hours.	10. Some institutional policies allow for the component of blood to infuse over a total of 4 hours.
11. Do not remove identification information from the infusion bag until the transfusion is completed.	11. Some institutions require that the blood container be returned to the transfusion service when the transfusion is completed. Other institutions require other verification and paperwork. Be sure to know your institution's policy and follow it.
12. During the administration of blood products, follow body fluid precautions at all times. Maintain aseptic technique.	12. Protection of nursing professionals as well as the patient is essential.
13. If signs and symptoms of a negative reaction to the blood product transfusion occur, stop the transfusion. Change the tubing down to the infusion device and hang normal saline to keep the vein open or open it fully, depending on the patient's physical status. *Do not leave the patient alone.* Monitor vital signs and intake and output. Notify the physician. Follow orders from the medical team.	13. Signs and symptoms of a negative reaction include tachypnea, apnea, dyspnea, cough, wheezing, rales, elevated temperature, chills, chest pain, muscle aches, headache, diarrhea, bradycardia, tachycardia, change in blood pressure, cyanosis, decreased urine output, itching, diaphoresis, lumbar or low-back pain, tingling, numbness, nausea, a vague feeling of nervousness, confusion, anxiety, restlessness, sweating and pale cool extremities, decreased bowel sounds, and diminished peripheral pulses.
14. Recheck the blood component label, the patient's ABO and Rh group, and the crossmatch requisition.	14. Errors may have occurred despite the policy and procedures in place.
15. Expect to obtain blood samples to test for serum bilirubin, free hemoglobin, and prothrombin time and partial thromboplastin time. A repeat crossmatching will probably be ordered. A urine sample is needed to assess for free hemoglobin.	15. The blood sample is for rechecking the patient's type and crossmatch. A urine sample is used to assess for hemolysis.
16. Expect to administer injectable diphenhydramine (Benadryl) or a corticosteroid (hydrocortisone or prednisone).	16. These medications should be readily available when blood products are being administered.

c. Observe for signs and symptoms of acute hemorrhage, such as increased pain, swelling, fever, shock, pulse, or restlessness or decreased blood pressure.

d. Apply cold compresses and elevate the hemorrhagic area until the bleeding subsides. Immobilize the area.

e. Restrict strenuous activities for 48 hours after the bleeding episode.

NURSING DIAGNOSIS: Pain R/T ischemic and swollen tissues

1. *Expected outcomes:* After intervention, the patient should be able to do the following:
   a. Express relief of pain within 30 minutes after complaint
   b. Achieve satisfactory long-term management of pain
2. *Nursing interventions*
   a. Administer analgesics to manage pain but without IM

injections. Avoid medications that decrease platelet aggregation—aspirin, ibuprofen, dipyridamole, or any compounds containing these agents.

b. Assist the patient in performing range-of-motion exercises with the affected joints at least 48 hours after bleeding is controlled.

c. Teach relaxation, guided imagery, and therapeutic touch or massage to reduce the perception of pain (Learning/Teaching Guidelines for Self-Care of Hemophilia).

Discharge Planning and Teaching

1. Teach the patient precautions that he or she may take to avoid bleeding episodes.
2. Teach the patient techniques for management of acute bleeding episodes at home, including proper home administration of clotting factors.

LEARNING/TEACHING GUIDELINES
for Self-Care of Hemophilia

General Overview

1. Home management during the chronic state of hemophilia is vitally important, because of the disease's progressive course. Both quality and length of life may depend on the patient's ability to manage the disorder.
2. Most home care can be achieved with basic education of the affected individual and family.

Topics for Education

1. Patients should be referred to their local chapter of the Hemophilia National Foundation (see "Agencies") to obtain strategies for coping with this lifelong illness. A chapter can also serve as a source of referrals to support services.
2. Initial teaching focuses on recognizing disease-related problems that can be resolved at home and those that require hospitalization. Hospitalization is required for the following problems:
   - Severe pain or swelling of muscles and joints that restricts movements or inhibits sleep
   - Swelling that occurs in the neck or mouth
   - Any type of head injury
   - Hematuria
   - Melena or vomiting of blood
   - Abdominal pain
   - Large skin wounds in need of suturing
3. Patients should be taught to prevent injuries by taking the following actions:
   - Avoiding potential situations that could lead to trauma
   - Wearing work gloves when doing household tasks
   - Avoiding excessive use of sharp knives, awls, or heavy mechanical equipment
   - Asking for assistance when repair requires heavy supplies or equipment
   - Participating in noncontact sports only
4. Personal care includes the following:
   - Performing oral hygiene daily
   - Using very soft toothbrushes or tooth sponges
   - Applying lotions to keep the skin from drying and cracking
   - Wearing a medical alert bracelet or tag to identify the condition to health care providers
5. Medical self-care might involve the following:
   - Self-administration of antihemophilic factors
   - Care of long-term parenteral lines left in place

3. Assist patient and family members to understand the impact of a chronic illness on the growth and development of the person with hemophilia and on the family.
4. Address knowledge deficit and fear of multiple transfusions.
5. Introduce strategies for coping with lifelong illness.
6. Emphasize the need to wear a medical alert bracelet.
7. Identify organizations that provide information and support.

Public Health Considerations

1. Refer patient and family members to genetic counseling to identify carriers and discuss reproductive options.
2. Refer patients to a hemophiliac treatment center for comprehensive management.

◼ IMMUNE THROMBOCYTOPENIC PURPURA

Definition

1. Immune thrombocytopenic purpura (ITP) is a hemorrhagic disorder in which immunologic platelet destruction causes a marked decrease in the number of circulating platelets. It is also known as **idiopathic thrombocytopenic purpura.**

2. Immune thrombocytopenic purpura is the most common acquired thrombocytopenia.

Incidence and Socioeconomic Impact

1. Acute ITP usually affects children ages 2 to 9 and is postviral.
2. Chronic ITP mainly affects adults younger than 50, primarily women ages 20 to 40.

Risk Factors

1. Immune-related disorders
2. Exposure to viral infections
3. Pregnancy

Etiology

1. Immune-related disorders
2. Viral infections such as rubella, chicken pox, or a respiratory infection
3. Recent immunization with live vaccine for chickenpox, mumps, measles, or smallpox
4. Sensitivity to drugs, allergies (especially food allergies to beans and fruits), and blood transfusions
5. Exposure to insecticides and chemicals such as vinyl chloride

6. An immune response in which antibodies reduce platelets' life spans or an idiopathic autoimmune response

Pathophysiology

1. Platelets are manufactured and function in hemostasis. Surface antigens on the platelets cause them to be destroyed in the spleen.
2. A pronounced reduction in the circulating volume of platelets causes bleeding tendencies.

Clinical Manifestations

1. Insidious onset of bleeding from the mouth, nose, and skin upon slight injury
2. Spontaneous bleeding from the mucous membranes
3. Generalized weakness, fatigue, and lethargy; petechiae; and ecchymosis

Diagnostics

1. Document spontaneous bleeding episodes, a complete blood count with a severely low ($<20,000/mm^3$) platelet count, increased bleeding time, decreased platelet survival time, and possible platelet antibodies.
2. When taking the patient's history, include questions regarding exposure to toxic chemicals, recent immunization, and recent exposure to or contraction of a viral illness.
3. Assess for incidents of minor bleeding, epistaxis, or bruising tendencies.
4. Look for petechiae, hematomas, and superficial ecchymotic areas on the skin.
5. Note changes in level of consciousness, confusion, and lethargy, which might be signs of intracranial hemorrhage.
6. Palpate the abdomen for possible liver and spleen enlargement. Also look for lymphadenopathy.

Clinical Management

1. Goals of clinical management
   a. Acutely reduce and control the severity of the bleeding.
   b. Maintain hemodynamic stability.
   c. Identify the possible cause of the bleeding.
2. Nonpharmacologic interventions
   a. Plasmapheresis (a process that removes plasma from the blood and filters and possibly reinfuses it) for severe cases
   b. Splenectomy in chronic cases
3. Pharmacologic interventions
   a. Platelet transfusions
   b. High-dose gamma globulin to elevate the platelet count and reduce turnover
   c. Glucocorticoids, usually prednisone, to suppress the immune response in chronic ITP

d. Possible powerful immunosuppressives such as azathioprine (Immuran) and cyclophosphamide (Cyclosporin) or antithymocyte globulin

Complications

1. Uncontrolled bleeding and anemia
2. Acute hemorrhage that can lead to a fatal intracranial bleed

Prognosis

1. Recovery occurs within 1 to 2 months for most (up to 90%) patient with acute ITP.
2. About 10 to 20 percent of patient with chronic ITP recover without any treatment. After 6 months, ITP is considered chronic.
3. The risk of acute hemorrhage is greatest during the 1st 2 weeks of the disease. Intracranial bleeds can be fatal.

Applying the Nursing Process

NURSING DIAGNOSIS: Risk for injury R/T prolonged bleeding time

1. *Expected outcomes:* After intervention, the patient should remain free of hemorrhagic injury.
2. *Nursing interventions*
   a. Control localized bleeding.
   b. Transfuse as necessary.
   c. Prevent further injuries by limiting the patient's activities.
   d. Teach adequate oral hygiene, including the use of soft toothbrushes or tooth sponges and the need for frequent brushings.
   e. Prevent constipation through diet and fluids and stool softeners if necessary.
   f. Avoid drugs that decrease platelet aggregation, such as aspirin and other nonsteroidal anti-inflammatory drugs, and avoid IM injections.
   g. Caution the patient to avoid using razors with blades.
   h. Use normal saline nasal drops or sprays to decrease drying of mucous membranes, which can cause epistaxis.

Discharge Planning and Teaching

1. Teach the patient the early signs and symptoms of bleeding.
2. Teach the patient interventions to control bleeding.
3. Teach preventive oral hygiene measures.

Public Health Considerations

1. Teach people to avoid exposure to toxic chemicals.
2. Teach people to minimize their exposure to virus-infected individuals.

◻ *DISSEMINATED INTRAVASCULAR COAGULATION*

Definition

1. Disseminated intravascular coagulation (DIC) is a clinical syndrome of simultaneous clotting in the microvascular bed and profound bleeding due to consumption of clotting factors.
2. This disorder can be acute or chronic. The acute form of DIC produces the coagulation abnormalities and is symptomatic. This form is the medical emergency that usually warrants immediate attention. The chronic form (also known as **low-grade DIC** or **compensated DIC**) may or may not be symptomatic. It is managed by the patient.
3. A precipitating factor sets off the accelerated clotting cascade.

Incidence and Socioeconomic Impact

1. The impact of DIC is difficult to determine because of the varying degrees of clinical severity of this syndrome.
2. This syndrome is potentially fatal.

Risk Factors

1. Obstetric trauma (i.e., placental rupture or the syndrome of high blood pressure, elevated liver enzymes, and low platelets)
2. Neoplasms
3. Hematologic dysfunctions
4. Major tissue traumas (burns, crushing injuries, and trauma)
5. Severe infectious disease processes (especially gram-negative bacteremia and sepsis)
6. Systemic inflammatory response syndrome

Etiology

1. Disseminated intravascular coagulation occurs as a complication of various disease processes and conditions. It is not a disease in and of itself.
2. Three primary etiologic processes activate the clotting cascade: severe tissue injury, a vascular endothelial injury that triggers the intrinsic pathway of the clotting cascade, and a foreign body substance in the bloodstream.

Pathophysiology

1. A disease process or tissue injury overstimulates the pace of the clotting cascade to the point of exhaustion. Overproduction of thrombin rapidly converts fibrinogen to fibrin threads. These threads disseminate into the bloodstream, causing platelets to aggregate and develop into multiple, microscopic emboli. Microemboli form in the capillary beds, where they damage organ tissue. Peripheral ischemia also occurs.
2. A paradoxical syndrome of simultaneous bleeding and clotting occurs. Multiple clotting depletes clotting factors such as platelets and fibrinogen. Clot-dissolving mechanisms are triggered, and stable clots begin to break up before missing coagulation factors are replaced. This process is the body's attempt to restore microcirculation. Thus anticoagulant factors dominate and cause uncontrolled bleeding. Fibrin degradation products, which are the products of clot lysis, are released into the bloodstream. They contribute to the bleeding seen with DIC.

Clinical Manifestations

1. Thrombus formation and bleeding tendencies disseminated throughout the entire body are the basic clinical symptoms of DIC. Mild bleeding rapidly progresses to severe hemorrhage. Oozing for prolonged periods from minor trauma or invasive sites is usually a 1st symptom. Bleeding is seen from at least 3 unrelated sites. For example, ecchymosis, epistaxis, and hematuria may be seen simultaneously.
2. The systems most at risk for organ ischemia are the renal, cardiac, pulmonary, and central nervous systems. Infarcts result from clotting, and tissue damage results from bleeding.

Diagnostics

1. The diagnosis of DIC is difficult to confirm, because some laboratory tests are not abnormal until the DIC is in a severe stage.
2. Initial alterations in laboratory tests that lead to a preliminary diagnosis include the following:
   a. Prothrombin time is greater than 15 seconds (normal is 12–15 sec).
   b. Partial thromboplastin time is greater than 60 seconds (normal is 25–39 sec).
   c. Elevation of the prothrombin and partial thromboplastin times means that the enzymes responsible for converting fibrinogen into fibrin are in short supply.
   d. Fibrinogen level is below 195 mg per dl (normal value is 200–400 mg/dl).
   e. Platelet count is below 100,000 per mm^3 (normal is 150,000–400,000/mm^3).
   f. Fibrin degradation products are greater than 45 μg per ml or even 100 μg per ml (normal value is 10 μg/ml). The increase indicates that intravascular clots have formed and the body is attempting to dissolve them to restore microcirculation.
3. Other data might include the following:
   a. Tests to identify the underlying cause
   b. D dimer fibrin split-products test to confirm diagnosis (an increase may indicate DIC)
   c. Diminished factor V and VIII levels
   d. Positive fibrin monomers
   e. Decreased hemoglobin level
   f. Elevated blood urea nitrogen

g. Elevated serum creatinine level
h. Decreased urine output

4. The hallmark of DIC is abnormal bleeding without a history of a serious bleeding disorder. Note any signs of spontaneous bleeding to skin, mucous membranes, wounds, and invasive lines. Check for occult blood in emesis, urine, and stool.
5. Also assess skin for color changes—pallor, jaundice, or marked peripheral cyanosis—a key diagnostic symptom.
6. Ask about malaise and weakness. Note changes in level of consciousness.
7. Note other findings, such as nausea; vomiting; severe muscle, abdominal, and back pain; shocklike symptoms such as decreased blood pressure, tachycardia, and tachypnea; and petechiae, purpura, epistaxis, ecchymosis, and hematomas.

Clinical Management

1. Goals of clinical management
   a. Treat the underlying cause. If the cause is not eliminated or controlled, other treatment is futile.
   b. Replace deficient blood components and factors such as platelets, cryoprecipitate, fresh-frozen plasma, and RBCs.
   c. Control emboli formation.
   d. Administer anticoagulant therapy.
   e. Restore intravascular volume.
2. Nonpharmacologic interventions
   a. Supportive antishock care: fluid replacement, adequate oxygenation, and blood pressure support
   b. Evaluation of effectiveness of treatment through serial laboratory tests, including platelet counts, fibrinogen levels, prothrombin times, partial thromboplastin times, and fibrin degradation products
3. Pharmacologic interventions
   a. Heparin given IV or subcutaneously to treat the rampant microclotting and minimize tissue damage (be aware that it may also increase hemorrhage)
   b. Multiple transfusions of deficient clotting factors and blood components such as platelets, factors V and VII, packed cells, fresh-frozen plasma, and cryoprecipitate
   c. Antifibrinolytic therapy with epsilon-aminocaproic acid to disrupt fibrinolysis
   d. Specific drug treatment for the underlying cause
   e. Medications for pain control

Complications

1. Life-threatening uncontrolled hemorrhage leading to circulatory compromise
2. Multisystem organ failure due to infarcted vital organs
3. Hypoxia, cyanosis to peripheral tissues, adult respiratory distress syndrome, pulmonary embolism, and general pulmonary failure

Prognosis

1. Because of the varying degrees of severity of DIC, mortality rates vary. Mortality rates of 80 to 90 percent have

been reported. The rate is affected by the precipitating event.
2. Death is usually a result of multisystem organ failure, uncontrolled hemorrhage, or both.

Applying the Nursing Process

NURSING DIAGNOSIS: Altered tissue perfusion (vital organs) R/T hemorrhage due to altered coagulopathy

1. *Expected outcome* After intervention, the patient's risk of altered vital organ perfusion (i.e., shock) should be minimized through anticipatory and aggressive management of altered coagulopathy.
2. *Nursing interventions*
   a. Institute measures to control or prevent bleeding.
   b. Monitor serial laboratory work. Keep blood type and crossmatch current.
   c. Monitor for transfusion reactions from multiple transfusions.
   d. Accurately determine the patient's blood loss by weighing the dressing, recording amounts of drainage, and calculating blood loss from multiple blood draws.
   e. Observe for signs and symptoms of hypovolemic shock: decreased blood pressure, increased pulse, decreased urine output, and decreased skin turgor.
   f. Limit injections of any kind.
   g. Protect the patient from injuries. For example, use gentle patient positioning, padded side rails, and bed rest.
   h. Monitor the patient's neurologic status. Disseminated intravascular coagulation can affect cerebral circulation.

Discharge Planning and Teaching

1. Assist the family in coping with life-threatening illness.
2. Teach persons with chronic DIC the signs and symptoms of bleeding tendencies. Because of the poor prognosis in acute DIC, teaching and discharge planning are limited.

Public Health Considerations

1. Primary prevention of DIC is limited because of the vast array of etiologies and precipitating factors.
2. Onset is insidious after a catalytic cause.

◼ *VITAMIN K DEFICIENCY*

Definition

1. Vitamin K deficiency is an acquired coagulation disorder in which individuals are deficient in vitamin K.
2. Vitamin K is essential to liver synthesis of prothrombin and coagulation factors VII, IX, and X.

Incidence and Socioeconomic Impact

1. Vitamin K deficiency is common in neonates.
2. Bleeding problems occur in 25 percent of persons taking oral anticoagulants.

Risk Factors

1. Bowel resections
2. Ulcerative colitis
3. Cystic fibrosis with fat malabsorption
4. Chronic anticoagulation therapy

Etiology

1. Vitamin K deficiency is secondary to a disease process, such as bile obstruction, biliary fistula, malabsorption syndromes, bowel resection, chronic liver disease, or ulcerative colitis.
2. It is also secondary to the use of certain drugs, including prolonged use of anticoagulants and broad-spectrum antibiotics (penicillin and cephalosporins).

Pathophysiology

1. The body acquires vitamin K from the normal diet and as a by-product of intestinal bacteria.
2. Chronic liver disease leads to vitamin K deficiency by impairing synthesis of clotting factors. Vitamin K deficiency from liver disease is worsened by anorexia, poor food selection, and malabsorption. Liver synthesis of clotting factors is decreased by consumption of oral anticoagulants, salicylates, quinine, and barbiturates.

Clinical Manifestations

1. Bleeding of the mucous membranes and into the tissues
2. Decreased levels of prothrombin in the blood and prolonged prothrombin time

Diagnostics

1. Laboratory findings might include increased fibrinolysis; an elevated level of fibrin degradation products; a decreased platelet count; a decreased fibrinogen level; prolonged prothrombin time; and, in severe cases, prolonged partial thromboplastin time.
2. Thorough assessment of the patient's medical history involves looking for intestinal problems or long-term antibiotic therapy.
3. Skin assessment involves looking for petechiae, ecchymosis, and oozing of blood from orifices.
4. Palpation of the abdomen can identify liver and spleen enlargement.

Clinical Management

1. Replacement of deficient vitamin K, usually parenterally
2. Transfusion of fresh-frozen plasma, which contains vitamin K and vitamin K–dependent clotting factors
3. Temporary cessation of anticoagulant therapy

Complications

1. Potential for hemorrhage
2. Triggering of DIC

Prognosis

1. The prognosis is excellent if the deficiency is replaced. Vitamin K replacement takes up to 24 hours. Fresh-frozen plasma acts more rapidly but carries the risks of transfusion, such as transfusion reaction.
2. The underlying cause should also be identified.

Applying the Nursing Process

NURSING DIAGNOSIS: Risk for injury (bleeding tendencies) R/T nutritional deficiency and malabsorption of vitamin K

1. *Expected outcomes:* After intervention, the patient should remain free of injuries secondary to bleeding tendencies.
2. *Nursing interventions*
   a. Control the bleeding by applying localized pressure. Keep the head of the bed elevated.
   b. Avoid IV administration of vitamin K. Severe dysrhythmias can occur.
   c. Monitor the person's food consumption and elimination patterns.
   d. Provide foods rich in vitamin K, such as green leafy vegetables, fish meal, oats, wheat, rye, and alfalfa.

Discharge Planning and Teaching

1. Teach the patient about the disease process and its manifestations.
2. Teach the patient the signs and symptoms of early bleeding tendencies.
3. Stress the need to avoid contact with sharp objects until bleeding tendencies subside.

Public Health Considerations

1. Teach about malabsorption.
2. Teach about vitamin replacement therapy.

◼ OTHER HEMATOLOGIC DISORDERS

Multiple Myeloma

1. Definition: Multiple myeloma is a neoplastic disease in which bone and bone marrow are infiltrated by defective plasma cells that form multiple tumors.
2. Incidence and etiology
   a. Multiple myeloma is most common after age 50. It affects males twice as often as females and affects more Blacks than Whites by a 2:1 ratio.
   b. There are many theories about the cause of multiple myeloma, including viral influences, hypersensitivity reactions, and chronic inflammation. Genetic factors may play a role. The disease has been linked to chronic exposure to low-level radiation.
   c. The disease process involves excessive numbers of neoplastic plasma cells infiltrating bone marrow and developing into tumors. The plasma cells destroy bone and involve lymph nodes, the liver, the spleen, and the kidneys. An abnormal immunoglobulin formed by the plasma cells prevents further development of normal plasma cells and leads to immunocompromise.
3. Clinical manifestations
   a. Development is insidious and slow. The person complains of severe skeletal pain, usually in the pelvis, spine, and ribs, as a result of the excessive accumulation of abnormal plasma cells in the bone marrow. Osteoporotic lesions are seen in the skull, vertebrae, and ribs.
   b. Degeneration of bones leads to calcium loss into the serum and causes hypercalcemia. Hypercalcemia precipitates renal dysfunction, anorexia, confusion, and hyperuricemia.
   c. Thrombocytopenia, anemia, and granulocytosis may also be seen. Fatigue, weakness, and the degree of anemia are related to the percentage of plasma cells in the marrow.
   d. Assessment indicates anorexia, weight loss, and tingling or myalgias of extremities or paresthesias.
   e. Laboratory work indicates pancytopenia, an elevated serum protein level, hypercalcemia, hyperuricemia, and an elevated creatinine level. Bence Jones protein is present in urine. Skeletal radiographs and bone scans, including magnetic resonance imaging of the spine, determine osteoporosis, demineralization, tumors, and degree of skeletal involvement. Bone marrow aspiration and biopsy indicate significant number of plasma cells.
4. Clinical management
   a. Long-term (up to 10 years) management of symptoms of chronic disease involves pain control with medication or palliative radiation and the use of drugs to prevent complications, especially renal problems.
   b. The effects of hypercalcemia, hyperuricemia, and dehydration can be treated through ambulation, hydration, and the use of antigout agents. Calcium is reabsorbed through weight-bearing exercise. Serum protein and calcium can be diluted with fluids. Fluids should be administered to maintain an output of 1.5 to 2 liters per day.
   c. Orthopedic supports and localized radiation are used to manage skeletal pain. Assist the patient with mobility to prevent injury and implement weight-bearing exercises. Position the patient to prevent injury and provide maximum comfort.
   d. Plasmapheresis removes excessive M-protein from the blood and is used to treat patients with hyperviscosity syndrome.
   e. Chemotherapy treats the tumor lesions of bone marrow. Administration of alkylating agents solely or in combination with prednisone is the mainstay of treatment. Steroids are sometimes used for antitumor effects.
   f. Studies indicate that bone marrow transplant is the treatment of choice for younger patients.
   g. Diuretics, IV fluids, antigout agents, and other medications counteract hypercalcemic and hyperuremic conditions.
   h. Mild analgesics and nonsteroidal anti-inflammatory drugs to reduce bone pain may be more effective than narcotics. Radiotherapy to localized lesions may also be used. Good skin care should be given to those areas.
   i. Complications include renal failure; osteoporosis leading to orthopedic injury, such as pathologic fractures and compression fractures; and infection, especially pneumonia. Preventing complications is a goal of treatment.
   j. Symptoms may remit and return, causing multiple hospitalizations. Teach the patient about the disease process, including symptoms and recurrence. Support the patient and family in dealing with life-threatening illness.
   k. The long-term prognosis is poor. Final stages do not respond to treatment, and the disease becomes fatal quickly. Hospice care may be appropriate for the final stages of illness.

Hypersplenism

1. Definition: Hypersplenism is overactive destruction of circulating blood cells by the spleen. Splenomegaly often accompanies an overactive spleen.
2. Incidence and etiology: Hypersplenism can occur as a primary or secondary disorder. Its incidence varies with its etiology. It may accompany neoplastic disorders, infections, collagen disorders, anemias, thrombocytopenias, hypersensitivity reactions, or liver disease.
3. Clinical manifestations
   a. The spleen destroys circulating blood cells rapidly, decreasing the circulating blood volume of these components. The resulting splenomegaly often increases the spleen's filtration rate, further reducing blood components and inducing pancytopenia, anemia, or thrombocytopenia.

b. Complications include shock, hemorrhage, and infections.

c. Assessing for left-upper-quadrant tenderness and splenomegaly is important. Also assess the skin, noting bleeding tendencies. Ask questions regarding a recent history of any contributing disease.

d. Diagnosis obtained through laboratory values such as a complete blood count with differential indicates anemia, thrombocytopenia, or leukopenia. Ultrasonography, CT, or magnetic resonance imaging may indicate splenomegaly or splenic rupture.

4. Clinical management

a. Reverse pancytopenic conditions.

b. Eliminate the cause of the splenic disorder.

c. Prevent infection, shock, and hemorrhage.

d. Perform a respiratory assessment carefully, because splenomegaly may impede diaphragmatic expansion.

e. Splenectomy through surgical removal is the treatment of choice. Administer analgesia and provide postoperative pain management.

f. Radiation of the spleen is used in some circumstances.

g. Transfuse blood components.

h. Administer antibiotics to prevent infection. Patients who have undergone a splenectomy are especially vulnerable to infection, because of deficiencies in IgM antibodies. Young persons may be immunized against *Pneumococcus*, a common infection after splenectomy. Teach persons with hypersplenism to avoid exposure to those with respiratory infections.

Bibliography

Books

Ashwanden P, et al. (eds). *Oncology Nursing: Advances, Treatments, and Trends into the 21st Century.* Gaithersburg, MD: Aspen Publishers, 1990.

Brown BA: *Hematology Principles and Procedures.* Philadelphia: Lea & Febiger, 1988.

Burke MB, et al. *Chemotherapy Care Plans.* Boston: Jones & Bartlett, 1992.

Ewald GA, and McKenzie CR. *Manual of Medical Therapeutics—The Washington Manual.* Boston: Little, Brown & Co, 1995.

Fischbach F. *A Manual of Laboratory & Diagnostic Tests.* 4th ed. Philadelphia: JB Lippincott, 1992.

Gauntlett P, and Myers P. *Adult Health Nursing.* St. Louis: Mosby–Year Book, 1994.

Jandl JH. *Blood: Textbook of Hematology.* Boston: Little, Brown & Co, 1987.

Lewis JA (ed). *Illustrated Guide to Diagnostic Tests.* Springhouse, PA: Springhouse Corporation, 1992.

McNally JC, et al. *Guidelines for Oncology Nursing Practice.* 2nd ed. Philadelphia: WB Saunders, 1991.

Monahan FD, Drake T, and Neighbors M (eds). *Nursing Care of Adults.* Philadelphia: WB Saunders, 1994.

Powers LW. *Diagnostic Hematology.* St. Louis: CV Mosby, 1990.

Rapaport SI. *Introduction to Hematology.* Philadelphia: JB Lippincott, 1987.

Thomas CL (ed). *Taber's Cyclopedic Medical Dictionary.* 17th ed. Philadelphia: FA Davis, 1993.

Wyngaarden J, Smith L, and Bennett J (eds). *Cecil Textbook of Medicine.* 19th ed. Philadelphia: WB Saunders, 1992.

Chapters in Books and Journal Articles

Structure and Function

Haueber D, and Spross J. Alterations in protective mechanisms: Hematopoiesis and bone marrow depression. *In* Baird SB, McCorkle R, and Grant M (eds). *Cancer Nursing: A Comprehensive Textbook.* Philadelphia: WB Saunders, 1991, pp. 759–781.

Shannon-Bodnar RM. Patient assessment: History taking and physical examination. *In* Harold CE, et al. (eds). *Nurse Review.* Springhouse, PA: Springhouse Corporation, 1988.

Shaw CE. Diagnostic studies: Patient teaching preparation, and nursing care. *In* Harold CE, et al. (eds). *Nurse Review.* Springhouse, PA: Springhouse Corporation, 1988.

White Blood Cell Disorders

Armstrong TS. Stomatitis in the bone marrow transplant patient: An overview and proposed oral care protocol. *Cancer Nurs* 17:403–410, 1994.

Blake LS. "It's not in my head" . . . myalgic encephalomyelitis (ME), or chronic fatigue syndrome. *Can Nurse* 89(7):29–32, 1993.

Butler S, and Chalder T. Researching chronic fatigue. *Nurs Times* 86(47):40–43, 1990.

Carson C, and Callaghan ME: Hematopoietic and immunologic cancers. *In* Baird SB, McCorkle R, and Grant M (eds). *Cancer Nursing: A Comprehensive Textbook.* Philadelphia: WB Saunders, 1991, pp 536–566.

Cho WK, and Stollerman GH. Chronic fatigue syndrome. *Hosp Pract* 27:221–224, 227–230, 233–234, 1992.

Collins PM. Diagnosis and treatment of chronic leukemia. *Semin Oncol Nurs* 6:31–43, 1990.

King C, et al. Nurses' perceptions of the meaning of quality of life for bone marrow transplant survivors. *Cancer Nurs* 18:118–129, 1995.

Kumar L. Leukemia: Management of relapse after allogenic bone marrow transplantation. *J Clin Oncol* 12:1710–1717, 1994.

Lawrence J. Critical care issues in the patient with hematologic malignancy. *Semin Oncol Nurs* 10:198–207, 1994.

Maguire-Eisen M. Diagnosis and treatment of adult acute leukemia. *Semin Oncol Nurs* 6:17–24, 1990.

Meili L. Leukemia. *In* Otto S (ed). *Oncology Nursing.* 2nd ed. St. Louis: Mosby–Year Book, 1994, pp. 278–330.

Mitus AJ, and Rosenthal DS. Adult leukemis. *In* Holleb AI, Fink D, and Murphy G (eds). *American Cancer Society Textbook of Clinical Oncology.* Atlanta, GA: American Cancer Society, 1991, pp. 410–432.

Pavel JN. Leukocyte disorders: Acute and chronic leukemia. *In* Harold CE, et al. (eds). *Nurse Review.* Springhouse, PA: Springhouse Corporation, 1988.

Snyder AS, and McGlave PB. Treatment of chronic myelogenous leukemia with bone marrow transplant. *Hematol Oncol Clin North Am* 4(3):535–557, 1990.

Thompson KS, and Hogan RM. Hematologic problems. *In* Phipps WJ (ed). *Medical Surgical Nursing: Concepts and Clinical Practice.* 4th ed. St. Louis: Mosby–Year Book, 1991, pp. 775–811.

Verdonck L, and Rozenberg-Arska M. Infection prevention in autologous bone marrow transplantation and the role of protective isolation. *Bone Marrow Transplant* 14:89–93, 1994.

Volker DL. Research trends in bone marrow transplantation. *Nurs Acum* 3(3):2, 1991.

Whedon M, and Ferrell B. Quality of life in adult bone marrow transplant patients: Beyond the first year. *Semin Oncol Nurs* 10:42–57, 1994.

Yeager K, and Miaskowski C. Advances in understanding the mechanisms and management of acute myelogenous leukemia. *Oncol Nurs Forum* 21:541–548, 1994.

Disorders That Affect Coagulation

Acevedo M. Blood dyscrasias: Polycythemia, idiopathic thrombocytopenic purpura, and thrombotic thrombocytopenic purpura. *J Intravenous Nurs* 15:52–57, 1992.

Bussel JB, and Schreiber AD. Immune thrombocytopenic purpura, neonatal alloimmune thrombocytopenia, and post-transfusion purpura. *In* Hoffman R, et al. (eds). *Hematology: Basic Principles and Practice.* New York: Churchill Livingstone, 1991.

Esparaz B. Disseminated intravascular coagulation. *Crit Care Nurs Q* 13:7–13, 1990.

Lusher JM, and Warrier J. Hemophilia A. *Hematol Oncol Clin North Am* 6(5):1021–1033, 1992.

Moake JL. Thrombotic thrombocytopenic purpura and the hemolytic-uremic syndrome. *In* Hoffman R, et al. (eds). *Hema-tology: Basic Principles and Practice.* New York: Churchill Livingstone, 1991.

Omiboni AC. Infection in the neutropenic patient. *Semin Oncol Nurs* 6:50–60, 1990.

Schneiderman E. Thrombocytopenia in the critically ill patient. *Crit Care Nurs Q* 13:1–6, 1990.

Shelton BK. Acquired coagulation disorders: Thrombocytopenia, DIC, and other problems. *In* Harold CE, et al. (eds). *Nurse Review.* Springhouse, PA: Springhouse Corporation, 1988.

Shelton BK. Congenital coagulation disorders: Hemophila, Von Willebrand's dis-ease, and other problems. *In* Harold CE, et al. (eds). *Nurse Review.* Springhouse, PA: Springhouse Corporation, 1988.

Transcultural Considerations

Chrisman N. Cultural systems. *In* Baird SB, McCorkle R, and Grant M (eds). *Cancer Nursing: A Comprehensive Textbook.* Philadelphia: WB Saunders, 1991, pp 45–54.

Palos G. Cultural heritage: Cancer screening and early detection. *Semin Oncol Nurs* 10:104–113, 1994.

Agencies and Resources

American Cancer Society
National Headquarters
1599 Clifton Road NE
Atlanta, GA 30329
(404) 320–3333
(local chapters are nationwide)

Cancer Information Center
(800) 4–CANCER
(800) 638–6070 in Alaska
(808) 531–1662 in Hawaii

Choice in Dying
250 West 57th Street
New York, NY 10107
(212) 246–6962

Corporate Angel Network, Inc.
Building One
Westchester County Airport
White Plains, NY 10604
(914) 328–1313

Hemophilia National Foundation
Center for Dissemination of
    Information
Soho Building
212 Green Street Suite 406
New York, NY 10012
(212) 431–8541
(regional centers are also
    available)

Hospice Association of America
210 7th Street SE
Washington, DC 20003
(202) 547–5263

Leukemia Society of America
733 Third Avenue
New York, NY 10017
(212) 573–8484

U.S. Department of Labor
Occupational Safety and Health
    Administration
Directorate of Technical Support
200 Constitution Avenue NW
Washington DC 20210
(202) 523–7047

26
Caring for People with Urinary System Disorders

URINARY SYSTEM STRUCTURE AND FUNCTION

Structure of the Kidneys

1. Gross structure (Fig. 26–1 shows the renal anatomy and vasculature.)
   a. Lymphatic drainage arises from para-aortic chains and paravena caval chains.
   b. Innervation of autonomic motor and visceral sensory nerves arises from the celiac plexus, greater splanchnic nerve, intermesenteric plexus, and superior hypogastric nerve.
2. Microscopic structure (Fig. 26–2).

Functions of the Kidneys

1. Urine formation
   a. Renal blood flow determines the volume allocated for renal filtration and urine formation. Approximately 1200 ml per minute or 25 percent of cardiac output reaches the kidney. Blood is filtered at the level of glomerular capillary. Peritubular capillaries carry the reabsorbed portion of ultrafiltrate back to the circulation. Juxtamedullary nephrons contain complex vasculature (vasa recta) that enhance reabsorption of sodium and water.
   b. Urine forms through a series of processes in the nephron:
      (1) Filtration: The glomerulus filters blood, allowing only protein-free plasma to enter the nephron. Filtration efficiency is expressed as the glomerular filtration rate (GFR)—the amount filtered out by the glomerulus in a given period of time. The substance most commonly measured is creatinine, an intrinsic metabolic waste product.
      (2) Reabsorption: Tubules in the nephron (particularly the proximal tube) reabsorb salts, water, and other elements needed by the body and carry them to the kidney veins, which flow into the renal vein and then into general circulation (Fig. 26–3). Excess water and other waste materials (amino acids, urea, uric acid, and trace minerals) are poorly reabsorbed. They remain in the tubules as urine,

which moves from the tubules to a series of ducts, and then to the ureters.
      (3) Secretion: Tubules also secrete substances that facilitate transport of other substances from the blood into the tubules.
   c. The loop of Henle influences the reabsorption and excretion of water and sodium and accounts for approximately 25 percent of glomerular filtrate.
      (1) The descending loop is sodium impermeable and highly permeable to water.
      (2) The thin ascending limb is relatively impermeable to water with greater permeability to sodium and urea.
      (3) A stepwise concentration fluid shift (countercurrent multiplier system) allows concentration of urine with water conservation. The greatest concentration of sodium at the loop tip reaches 1400 mOsm per liter.
      (4) The length of the tube directly affects the ability to concentrate urine.
2. Homeostatic functions of the kidney
   a. Antidiuretic hormone, which promotes reabsorption from the collecting duct, is secreted by the pituitary gland when plasma osmolarity increases and blood volume decreases.
   b. Homeostasis of sodium and water is either intrinsic or extrinsic.
      (1) Intrinsic mechanisms: Kidneys reabsorb sodium in exchange for hydrogen ion excretion, a process that contributes to pH balance. When hypernatremia of the distal tube occurs, kidneys exchange sodium for hydrogen and potassium ions. The juxtaglomerular apparatus also influences sodium excretion or conservation.
      (2) Extrinsic mechanisms:
         • Antidiuretic hormone secretion stimulates reabsorption of water.
         • The renin-angiotensin system raises blood volume by regulating sodium (and water) reabsorption—sodium is reabsorbed, but potassium ion is lost in the exchange. The juxtaglomerular apparatus secretes renin enzyme when blood volume or pressure in the renal corpuscle decreases. Renin splits angiotensinogen to angiotensin I. Angiotensin I splits to angiotensin II in the lungs and liver. Metabolically active angiotensin II

GROSS STRUCTURE OF THE KIDNEYS

The kidneys are paired, bean-shaped organs located in the retroperitoneal space with the concave surface (the hilum) oriented toward the spine.

The upper pole is adjacent to the 12th thoracic vertebra, the lower pole to the 3rd lumbar vertebra. The right kidney is lower than the left because of the presence of the liver.

The adult kidney is approximately 11 cm long, 5–7.5 cm wide, and weighs approximately 115–155 gm.

Renal Vasculature

The renal artery, which is occasionally duplicated, exits the abdominal aorta at a 90-degree angle to enter the kidney hilum. The segmental, arcuate, and lobular arteries branch from the renal artery at near 90-degree angles.

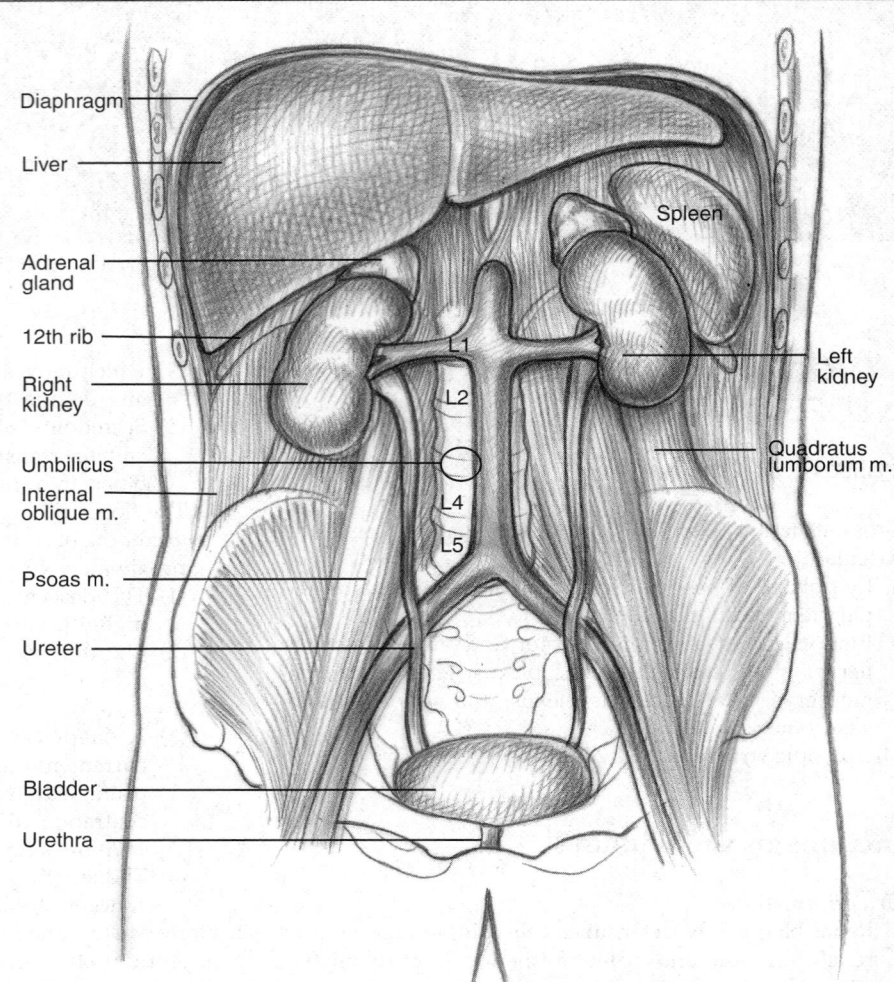

Coronal anatomy

Renal parenchyma *(renal medulla)*
• renal cortex
• pyramids

Renal hilum
• major calyx
• renal pelvis
• renal artery
• renal vein
• ureteropelvic junction

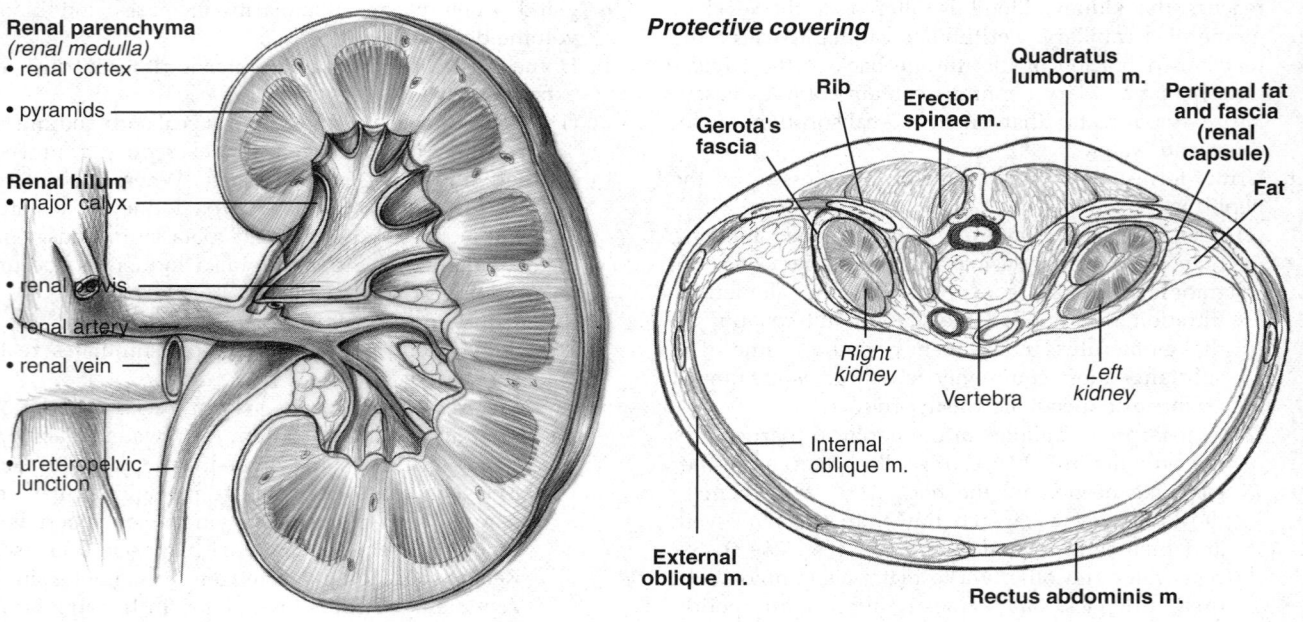

Protective covering

Gerota's fascia
Rib
Erector spinae m.
Quadratus lumborum m.
Perirenal fat and fascia (renal capsule)
Fat
Right kidney
Vertebra
Left kidney
Internal oblique m.
External oblique m.
Rectus abdominis m.

Figure 26–1.

MICROSCOPIC STRUCTURE OF THE NEPHRON

Nephron

The nephron consists of:

- Glomerulus and Bowman's capsule
- Proximal convoluted tubule
- Loop of Henle
- Distal convoluted tubule
- Collecting duct

Cortical nephrons, the short loop of Henle, constitute 85% of the approximately 1 million nephrons in the kidneys. Juxtamedullary nephrons, the longer loop of Henle, which dips deeply into the renal medulla, constitute 15% of nephrons.

Blood supply of the nephron:

The interlobular artery branches to the afferent arteriole, which is drained by the efferent arteriole after supplying the glomerulus. The peritubular capillaries branch from the efferent arteriole to follow the course of convoluted tubules, allowing reabsorption of fluids and other substances from ultrafiltrate or secretion into filtrate through the tubular cells.

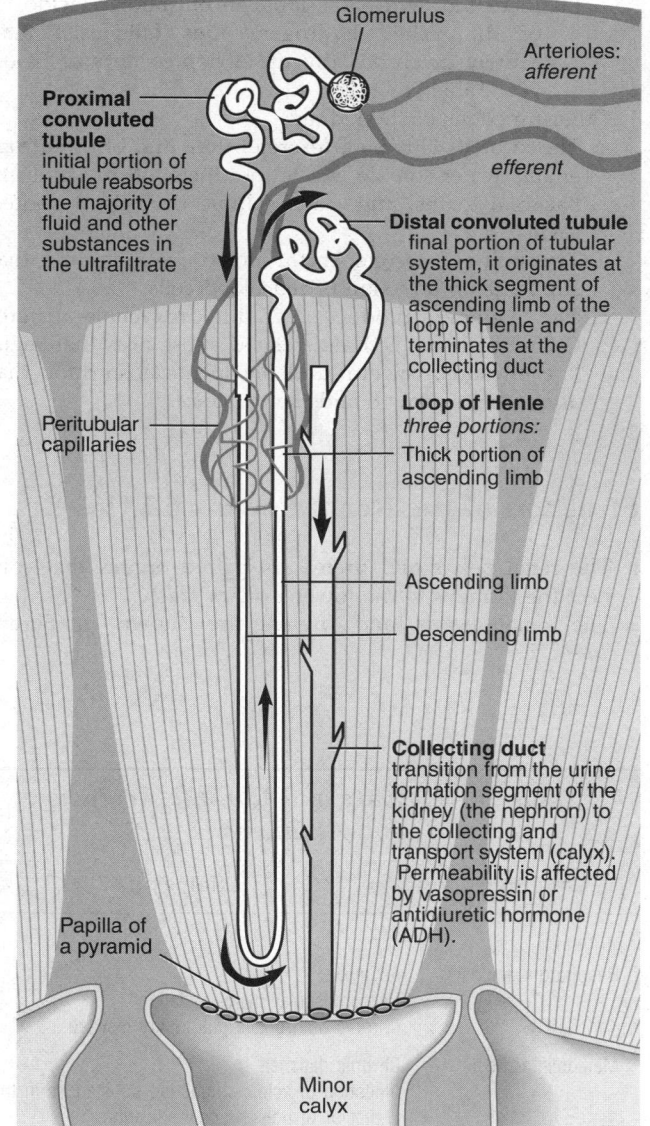

Glomerulus

Arterioles:
afferent

Proximal convoluted tubule
initial portion of tubule reabsorbs the majority of fluid and other substances in the ultrafiltrate

efferent

Distal convoluted tubule
final portion of tubular system, it originates at the thick segment of ascending limb of the loop of Henle and terminates at the collecting duct

Loop of Henle
three portions:

Thick portion of ascending limb

Peritubular capillaries

Ascending limb

Descending limb

Collecting duct
transition from the urine formation segment of the kidney (the nephron) to the collecting and transport system (calyx). Permeability is affected by vasopressin or antidiuretic hormone (ADH).

Papilla of a pyramid

Minor calyx

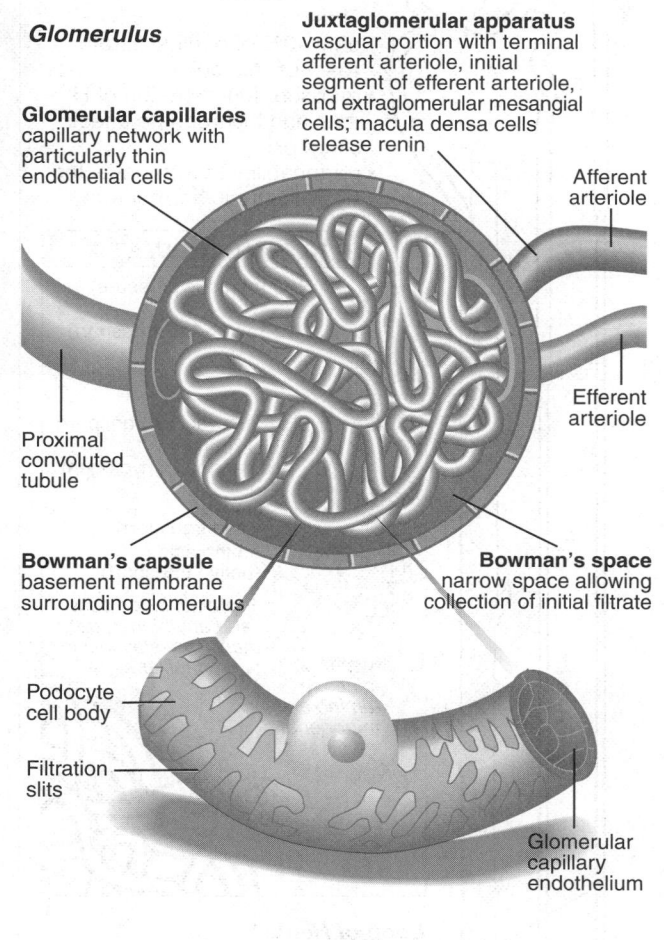

Glomerulus

Glomerular capillaries
capillary network with particularly thin endothelial cells

Juxtaglomerular apparatus
vascular portion with terminal afferent arteriole, initial segment of efferent arteriole, and extraglomerular mesangial cells; macula densa cells release renin

Afferent arteriole

Efferent arteriole

Proximal convoluted tubule

Bowman's capsule
basement membrane surrounding glomerulus

Bowman's space
narrow space allowing collection of initial filtrate

Podocyte cell body

Filtration slits

Glomerular capillary endothelium

Figure 26–2.

causes vasoconstriction, rapidly raising blood pressure. Angiotensin II also stimulates secretion of aldosterone, causing sodium and water reabsorption and increasing blood volume.

- Atrial natriuretic factor diminishes blood pressure, balancing the action of the renin angiotensin system. Atrial natriuretic factor is secreted by

the cardiac atrial wall when venous volume increases. It reduces renal reabsorption of sodium (and water) and inhibits antidiuretic hormone secretion.

c. Kidneys provide long-term pH balance for the body by excreting excess hydrogen ions and conserving bicarbonate ions, thus preserving the acid-alkaline balance.

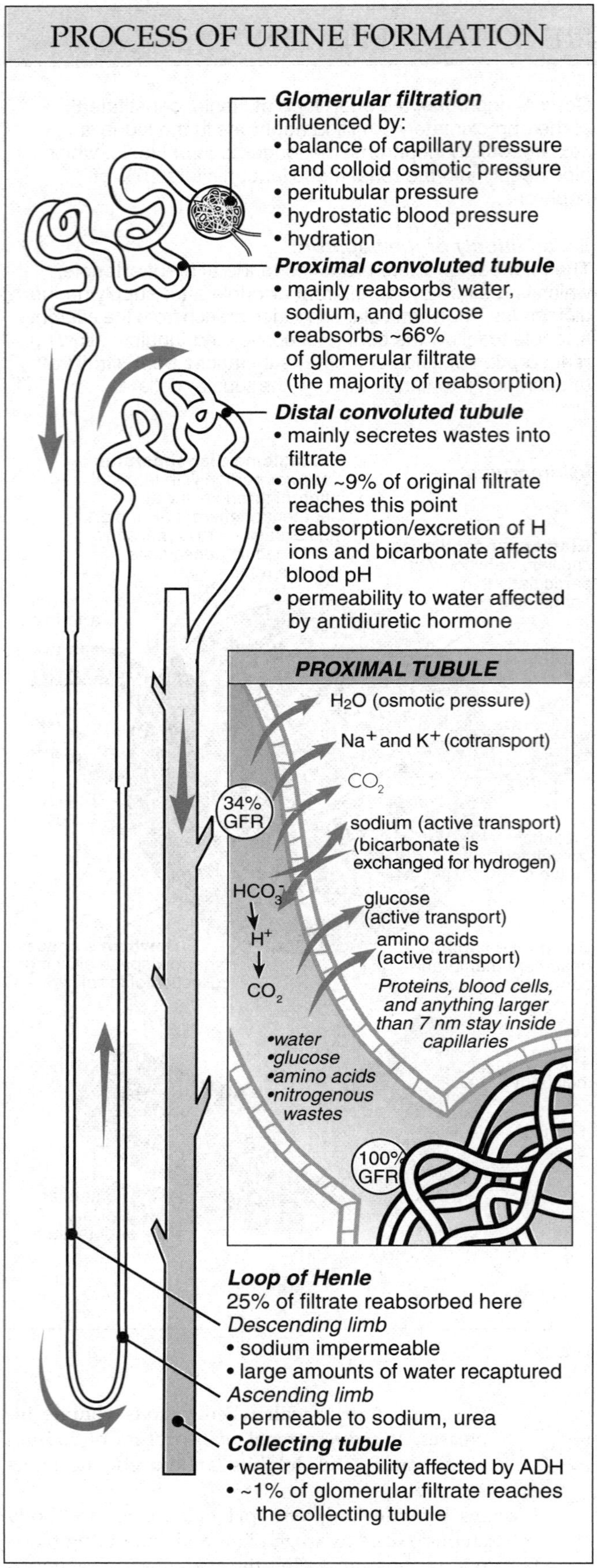

PROCESS OF URINE FORMATION

Glomerular filtration
influenced by:
• balance of capillary pressure and colloid osmotic pressure
• peritubular pressure
• hydrostatic blood pressure
• hydration

Proximal convoluted tubule
• mainly reabsorbs water, sodium, and glucose
• reabsorbs ~66% of glomerular filtrate (the majority of reabsorption)

Distal convoluted tubule
• mainly secretes wastes into filtrate
• only ~9% of original filtrate reaches this point
• reabsorption/excretion of H ions and bicarbonate affects blood pH
• permeability to water affected by antidiuretic hormone

PROXIMAL TUBULE

H_2O (osmotic pressure)

Na^+ and K^+ (cotransport)

CO_2

34% GFR

sodium (active transport) (bicarbonate is exchanged for hydrogen)

HCO_3^-
↓
H^+
↓
CO_2

glucose (active transport)
amino acids (active transport)

Proteins, blood cells, and anything larger than 7 nm stay inside capillaries

• water
• glucose
• amino acids
• nitrogenous wastes

100% GFR

Loop of Henle
25% of filtrate reabsorbed here
Descending limb
• sodium impermeable
• large amounts of water recaptured
Ascending limb
• permeable to sodium, urea
Collecting tubule
• water permeability affected by ADH
• ~1% of glomerular filtrate reaches the collecting tubule

Figure 26–3.

(1) Potent acids entering interstitial fluid space are neutralized by sodium bicarbonate produced in the kidney and lungs.
(2) Hydrogen ions are excreted in 1 of 2 ways. When release of a hydrogen ion depletes the body's store of bicarbonate, the hydrogen ion is excreted via the respiratory system. When a sodium-bound acid salt enters the nephron, the sodium ion is actively reabsorbed from the distal tubule in exchange for a hydrogen ion, which is excreted in the urine.
(3) Increased hydrogen ion concentrations (acidosis) or diminished hydrogens ions (alkalosis) may acutely or chronically upset homeostasis of blood pH (Table 26–1).
3. Other functions of the kidney
   a. The kidneys eliminate (excrete) urea and other nitrogenous water-soluble waste products of metabolism, bacterial toxins, and water-soluble drugs and related toxins.
   b. The kidneys secrete erythropoietin, a hormone that stimulates production of red blood cells.
   c. The kidneys produce 1,25-dihydroxycholecalciferol (1,25-dihydroxy D3) and related substances that regulate intestinal calcium and phosphate absorption that affects bone growth and maintenance.

Structure of the Renal Pelvis and Ureters

1. The renal pelvis and ureter are paired organs that connect the kidneys to the lower urinary tract.
2. The renal pelvis and ureters are shown in Figure 26–4.

Table 26–1. Acute and Chronic Acidosis and Alkalosis

Condition	Etiology
Acidosis	
Respiratory acidosis	Asphyxia
	Neuromuscular hypoventilation
	Chronic obstructive pulmonary disease
Metabolic acidosis	Chronic diarrhea
	Ingestion of acidic-containing substances in the diet or of poisons or medications
	Lactic acid buildup with atypical, severe exertion, resulting from shock
Alkalosis	
Respiratory alkalosis	Hyperventilation
	Altitude sickness causing hyperventilation
Metabolic alkalosis	Emesis of gastric contents
	Ingestion of alkaline substances via the diet or of toxic substances
	Diuretic ingestion causing acidic urine

URETERAL COURSE

Ureters are composed of a 24−30-cm tube that runs an inverted S-shaped course from the renal pelvis to the base of the bladder. The ureteral course travels medially from the ureteropelvic junction to pass over the psoas muscle, turns laterally toward the ischial spine of the bony pelvis, and curves back toward the base of the bladder to terminate at the ureterovesical junction.

Three areas of narrowing may become obstructed during passage of calculi from the kidneys to the bladder:
• ureteropelvic junction
• ureteral course near the iliac arteries
• ureterovesical junction, which consists of the lower portion of the ureter, the trigone muscle, and the adjacent wall of the bladder

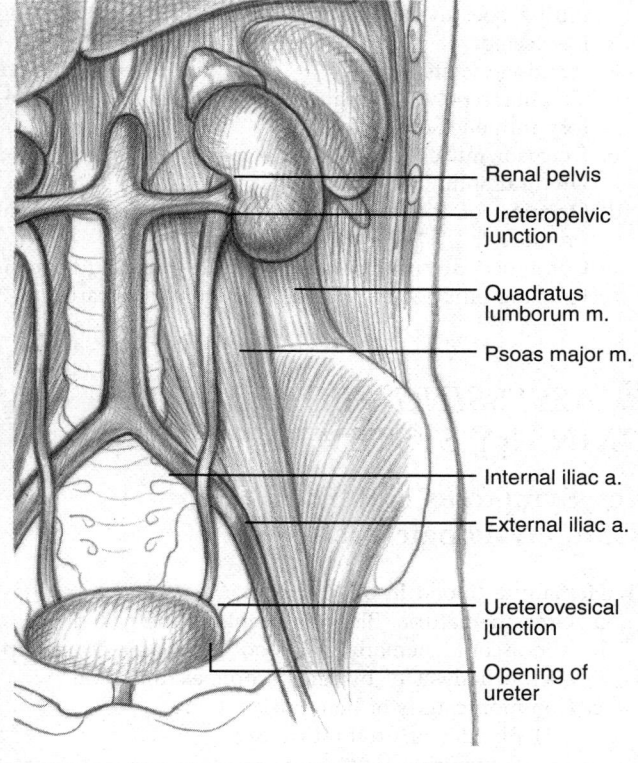

Renal pelvis

Ureteropelvic junction

Quadratus lumborum m.

Psoas major m.

Internal iliac a.

External iliac a.

Ureterovesical junction

Opening of ureter

Figure 26−4.

Functions of the Renal Pelvis and Ureters

1. The renal pelvis and ureters transport urine from the kidneys to the bladder.
   a. Efflux of urine is promoted (antegrade or forward movement of urine from upper to lower urinary tracts).
   b. Reflux of urine is prevented (retrograde or backward movement of urine from lower to upper urinary tracts).
2. Urine is transported via peristalsis—that is, propulsion of a bolus of urine via muscular contraction of the renal pelvis and ureteral wall.
3. Reflux of urine is prevented by mechanical and active components of the ureterovesical junction.

a. Bladder filling increases intramural pressure, mechanically closing the ureterovesical junction and intramural ureter during bladder filling.
b. Active contraction of ureteral smooth muscle and trigone prevents reflux during micturition.

Structure of the Bladder, Urethra, and Pelvic Muscles

1. Figure 26−5 shows the location of the urinary bladder.
   a. Blood is supplied through the inferior hypogastric or internal inial arteries in males and through the uterine, vaginal, or obturator arteries in females.
   b. Lymphatic drainage proceeds through the internal and common iliac chains and the hypogastric chains.
2. The male urethra and female urethra are shown in Figure 26−6.
3. Pelvic muscles and endopelvic fascia extend from the anterior to the posterior aspects of the bony pelvis, supporting its visceral contents.

STRUCTURE OF THE BLADDER

The urinary bladder is a hollow, muscle-lined organ located in the true pelvis of the adult. The base of the bladder is the lissosphincter and is fixed, but the body changes shape as it fills with urine. The muscle of the bladder is the detrusor. The empty bladder forms a tetrahedron, whereas the full bladder resembles an imperfect sphere. In cross-section, there are 2 ureteral inlets and a single outlet at the neck of the bladder.

Upper dome of bladder moves superiorly as bladder fills with urine

Detrusor muscle layer
Lissosphincter
Trigone m.
Interureteric fold

Orifice of ureter

Mucous membrane

Urethral outlet

Bladder neck
Urethral smooth m.

Periurethral m.

Rhabdosphincter m.

Ureter

Trigone m.

Ureterovesical junction

Figure 26−5.

MALE AND FEMALE URETHRAS: A COMPARISON

Male Urethra

The male urethra extends from the bladder neck to the meatus of the glans penis. The **bladder neck** is composed of circular, smooth muscle bundles, which form part of the urethral sphincter mechanism. The **prostatic urethra** extends approximately 3 cm along the vertical axis of the prostate. The **membranous urethra** pierces the pelvic floor muscles to form the terminal portion of the sphincter mechanism. The **pendulous urethra** is encased in corpus spongiosum, which extends from the **bulbous urethra** to the **fossa navicularis**. The fossa navicularis is the final urethral dilation in the posterior aspect of the flaccid penis. The urethral meatus is oval shaped near the end of the glans penis.

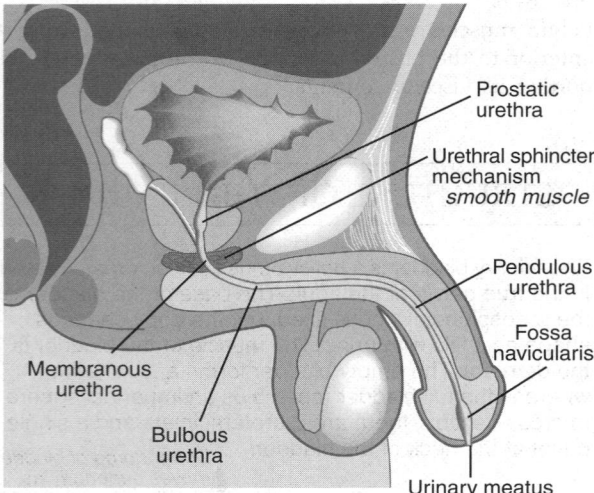

- Prostatic urethra
- Urethral sphincter mechanism *smooth muscle*
- Pendulous urethra
- Fossa navicularis
- Membranous urethra
- Bulbous urethra
- Urinary meatus

Female Urethra

The female urethra extends from the base of the bladder to the meatus immediately superior to the vaginal introitus. The bladder neck is composed of circular smooth muscle bundles, which make up part of the sphincter mechanism. The middle third of the urethra contains intrinsic **striated muscle**, which forms an aspect of the sphincter mechanism. The distal part of the urethra is fused to the anterior portion of the vaginal wall.

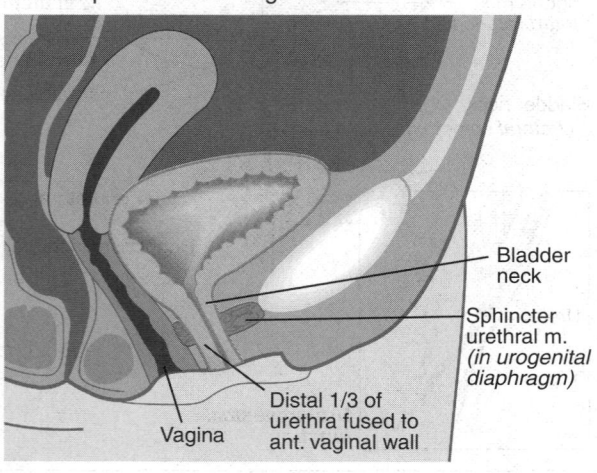

- Bladder neck
- Sphincter urethral m. *(in urogenital diaphragm)*
- Distal 1/3 of urethra fused to ant. vaginal wall
- Vagina

Figure 26–6.

Functions of the Bladder, Urethra and Pelvic Muscles

1. The bladder is the storage unit for urine. (The bladder in an adult holds 300–600 ml.)
2. Complete evacuation is achieved via micturition (emptying of the bladder) at regular intervals (normally more than every 2 hr) (Fig. 26–7). The urethral sphincter mechanism is shown in Figure 26–8.
3. Bladder filling and storage events occur as follows:
   a. Urine enters the bladder from the ureters, stimulating tension receptors in the bladder wall. The detrusor relaxes, and the urethral sphincter mechanism closes.
   b. Sufficient tension (usually filling of 90–200 ml) causes urgency (desire) to urinate, but the detrusor remains relaxed and the sphincter closed.
   c. Modulatory centers of the brain prevent micturition until a socially acceptable time and place for voiding is selected.
4. Micturition events
   a. Voluntary pelvic relaxation with release of the inhibitory influence of the brain
   b. Detrusor muscle contraction
   c. Urethral sphincter muscle relaxation
   d. Opening of the urethra under sufficient intravesical pressure
   e. Continued detrusor contraction until the bladder contents are emptied and filling and storage restarts

☐ ASSESSING PEOPLE WITH URINARY SYSTEM DISORDERS

Key Symptoms and Their Pathophysiologic Basis

1. Hematuria (blood in the urine)
   a. Gross hematuria: Blood is visible to the naked eye.
   b. Microscopic hematuria: Blood is observed on dipstick urinalysis or by microscopic examination.
   c. Common causes of hematuria
      (1) Bladder or urethral trauma
      (2) Penetrating renal trauma
      (3) Blunt renal trauma (contusion)
      (4) Injury to the vascular pedicle of the kidney
      (5) Iatrogenic bleeding following transurethral tissue resection; vigorous urethral instrumentation, including dilation; traumatic catheterization or endoscopic instrumentation; and open urologic surgery involving the kidneys, ureters, bladder, and urethra
      (6) Urinary tract infection
      (7) Urinary system tumors, including urethral tumors, bladder tumors (particularly transitional cell carcinoma), and renal tumors (including renal cell carcinoma)
      (8) Interstitial nephritis
      (9) Glomerulonephritis
      (10) Transient hematuria with vigorous exercise
      (11) Benign familial hematuria

NEURAL CONTROL OF THE BLADDER

Neural control of urinary bladder requires integration of central and peripheral nervous system and detrusor muscles.

The following brain centers act as a unit to provide stability (voluntary control) of urination. Dysfunction of any one brain center is likely to cause instability (loss of detrusor muscle control):

- Cerebral cortex
  (location of detrusor motor center)
- Thalamus
- Hypothalamus
- Basal ganglia
- Cerebellum

In the brain stem, the dorsal tegmentum of pons is the origin of the detrusor reflex and the coordination center between the detrusor and sphincter muscles.

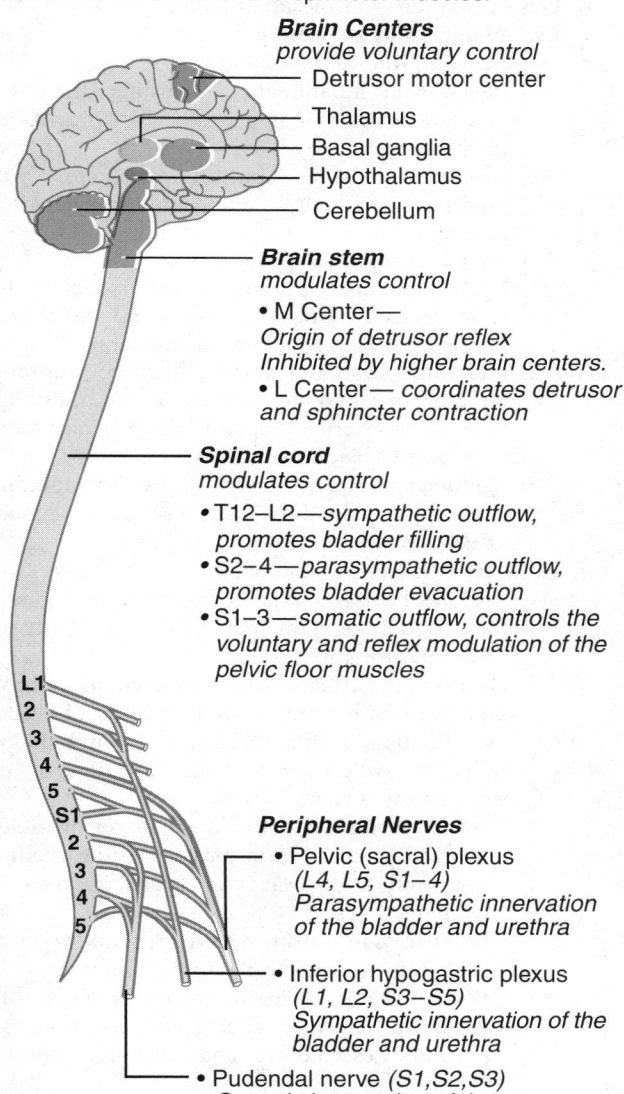

Brain Centers
provide voluntary control
— Detrusor motor center
— Thalamus
— Basal ganglia
— Hypothalamus
— Cerebellum

Brain stem
modulates control
- M Center—
  Origin of detrusor reflex
  Inhibited by higher brain centers.
- L Center— *coordinates detrusor and sphincter contraction*

Spinal cord
modulates control
- T12–L2—*sympathetic outflow, promotes bladder filling*
- S2–4—*parasympathetic outflow, promotes bladder evacuation*
- S1–3—*somatic outflow, controls the voluntary and reflex modulation of the pelvic floor muscles*

Peripheral Nerves
- Pelvic (sacral) plexus
  (L4, L5, S1–4)
  Parasympathetic innervation of the bladder and urethra
- Inferior hypogastric plexus
  (L1, L2, S3–S5)
  Sympathetic innervation of the bladder and urethra
- Pudendal nerve *(S1,S2,S3)*
  Somatic innervation of the periurethral muscles

Figure 26–7.

URETHRAL SPHINCTER MECHANISM

Elements of Compression:
The urethral wall softness provides a watertight seal between the bladder and the urethra. Mucosal secretions decrease surface tension and fill in the microscopic holes of the urethral mucosa. The submucosal vascular cushion changes shape and transmits pressure from the elements of tension, thus increasing the efficiency of the mucosal seal.

Elements of Tension:
Smooth muscle bundles at the bladder neck and proximal urethra sustain closure. The rhabdosphincter, a striated muscle contained entirely within the urethra, is specially designed to promote continence. The periurethral muscles contract rapidly during precipitous increases in abdominal pressure (e.g., from coughing, sneezing) to provide additional protection from urine loss.

Elements of Support:
Pelvic floor muscles provide support, maximizing efficiency of muscular components of the sphincter mechanism. The fascial reflections and pelvic ligaments provide additional support.

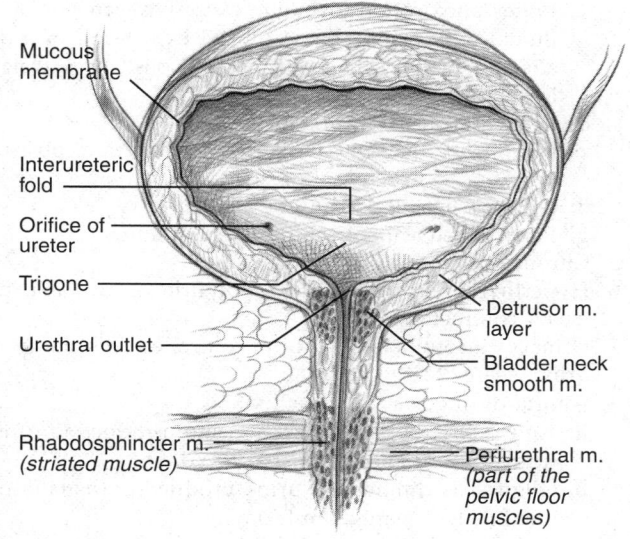

Mucous membrane
Interureteric fold
Orifice of ureter
Trigone
Urethral outlet
Rhabdosphincter m. *(striated muscle)*
Detrusor m. layer
Bladder neck smooth m.
Periurethral m. *(part of the pelvic floor muscles)*

Figure 26–8.

2. Proteinuria
   a. The presence of protein in the urine may indicate significant renal parenchyma damage and altered glomerular permeability.
   b. Transient or benign proteinuria is caused by the following:
      (1) Prolonged fever
      (2) Copious urinary sediment—red or white blood cells, bacterial or parasitic sediment
      (3) Pregnancy
      (4) Vigorous exercise
3. Irritative voiding symptoms: Causes of urgency to urinate, frequent urination (more than every 2 hr while awake), and nocturia (more than 1–2 times per night)
   a. Urinary tract infections (see p. 1207)

b. Radiotherapy (usually requires 6000–7000 rads over 6–7 weeks)

c. Chemotherapeutic agents (systemic and intravesical)

d. Interstitial or eosinophilic cystitis

e. Inflammatory lesions of the bladder (e.g., cystitis cystica or cystitis glandularis)

f. Urethritis

g. Pyelonephritis

h. Bladder malignancies, particularly carcinoma in situ

i. Bladder outlet obstruction

j. Detrusor instability

k. Dietary agents usually include the following:
   (1) Caffeine
   (2) Carbonated beverages
   (3) Alcohol (ethanol)-containing beverages
   (4) Chocolate
   (5) Spicy or greasy foods
   (6) Artificial sweeteners

l. Urethral syndrome (idiopathic irritative voiding symptoms)

4. Polyuria: Passage of a large volume of urine may result from the following:
   a. Diabetes mellitus
   b. Diabetes insipidus
   c. Water intoxication (drinking excessive water or other fluids), which may be a cultural expression of a desire to "purify" the body of "poisons" or a weight loss strategy
   d. Recovery phase of tubular necrosis
   e. Recovery after relief of acute urinary tract obstruction (postobstructive diuresis)
   f. Drugs, particularly diuretic agents
   g. Early phase acute or chronic renal failure

5. Chronic nephritis

6. Hyperthyroidism (may cause polyuria or unstable detrusor contractions)

7. Urinary incontinence—the uncontrolled discharge of urine (see p. 1218)

8. Anuria or oliguria
   a. Anuria is the absence of urine production (total urine output is less than 100 ml/day).
   b. Oliguria is diminished urine production (usually defined as less than 400 ml/day).
   c. Acute or chronic renal failure (insufficiency) is the cause.

9. Poor force of urinary stream: causes of intermittent or reduced force of urinary stream:
   a. Bladder outlet obstruction due to the following:
      (1) Prostatic enlargement
      (2) Bladder neck hypertrophy
      (3) Bladder neck contracture
      (4) Bladder neck dyssynergia
      (5) Urethral stricture
      (6) Vesicosphincter (detrusor–striated sphincter) dyssynergia
      (7) Severe pelvic descent in women
      (8) Pseudodyssynergia (functional obstruction produced by pelvic floor muscle contraction)
   b. Poor detrusor contraction strength due to the following:
      (1) Chronic overdistention caused by infrequent voiding habits

      (2) Sensory- or motor-impaired bladder as a result of diabetes mellitus, tabes dorsalis, sacral spinal lesions, or cauda equina syndrome
      (3) Drug-induced contraction strength deficiency from use of anticholinergics or antispasmodics, tricyclic antidepressants, antipsychotics, narcotics, recreational drugs (especially cannabis and hallucinogens), and calcium channel blockers
      (4) Fecal impaction or severe constipation

10. Acute urinary retention: The inability to urinate despite the presence of urine in the bladder is caused by the following:
    a. Complication of bladder outlet obstruction
    b. Drug-induced contraction strength deficiency (see p. 1226)
    c. Complication of deficient detrusor contraction strength

11. Urinary system pain. Areas of differences in urinary system pain include the following:
    a. Character and perceived intensity
    b. Onset, location, and radiation pattern
    c. Exacerbating and alleviating factors
    d. Urethral pain due to the following:
       (1) Infection or inflammation—burning discomfort of acute onset that is exacerbated by urination (dysuria)
       (2) Urethral syndrome—burning discomfort with gradual onset that is temporarily alleviated by urination
    e. Bladder pain due to the following:
       (1) Cystitis—acute, burning, suprapubic pain that is aggravated by urination (dysuria) and is temporarily relieved following micturition
       (2) Interstitial cystitis—chronic, burning, suprapubic pain that may be very intense, is transiently relieved with urination, and is often exacerbated by intake of bladder irritants
       (3) Bladder spasm (stranguria)—episodic, cramping suprapubic pain that is relieved by evacuation of urine from the bladder
    f. Flank pain due to the following:
       (1) Pyelonephritis—similar to bacterial cystitis with the addition of flank pain, it is transiently relieved by urination
       (2) Obstructing urinary calculi—cramping, throbbing pain with acute onset that is not alleviated by urination, position changes, or ambulation; radiation patterns reflect the location of the stone in the urinary system.
          • When calculi are in the lower ureter or ureterovesical junction, pain radiates to the groin in men and to the labia or broad ligament in women.
          • When calculi are in midureter, flank or lower back pain radiates to the lower abdomen.
          • When calculi are in the upper ureter or ureteropelvic junction, flank pain combines suprapubic discomfort and irritative voiding symptoms.

12. Edema: Excessive fluid in the interstitial space with swelling of dependent limbs or periorbital spaces is most often caused by the following:

a. Acute or chronic renal failure with compromised body water homeostasis
b. Pulmonary problems (see Chapter 22)
c. Cardiovascular problems (see Chapter 23)
d. Decreased plasma oncotic pressure with proteinuria
e. Chronic venous or arterial insufficiency

13. Hypertension: Persistent elevation of systemic diastolic and systolic blood pressures is caused by the following:
    a. Renal-related hypertension caused by ischemic-induced activation of renin-angiotension-aldosterone cascade
    b. Secondary hypertension—10 percent of all cases (approximately 80% of which are related to renal disease) are caused by chronic glomerulonephritis, reflux nephropathy, polycystic kidney disease, renal artery stenosis, and chronic pyelonephritis

Health History

1. The chief complaint and duration of symptoms
2. The impact of symptoms on self-image, activities of daily living, and social life
3. The patient's perception of symptoms and motivation to undergo specific treatments (such as organ transplantation or intermittent catheterization)
4. Current medications (prescribed, over-the-counter, and recreational)
5. The patient's usual voiding patterns can be characterized in a bladder diary (Fig. 26–9). The diary can document the following:
   a. Patterns of urinary elimination and leakage
   b. Functional capacity (the patient is given a graduated container to measure voided volume)
   c. Volume of fluid intake
   d. Intake of potential bladder irritants (patient must record types and amounts of beverages and food consumed)
   e. Diurnal urinary frequency (per hour)
   f. Nocturia (episodes per night)
   g. Urgency or hesitancy to urinate
6. Use of urinary containment devices
   a. Pads (type, number used per day)
   b. Adult briefs (type, number used per day)
   c. Condom catheter
7. Catheterization history
   a. Use of indwelling catheters
      (1) Urethral versus suprapubic
      (2) Catheter size
      (3) Material of construction (silicone, Teflon coated, Lubricous coated, polyurethrane)
      (4) Time since the catheter was originally inserted
   b. Use of intermittent catheterization
      (1) Actual frequency of catheterization (approximate times of days catheterization is performed)
      (2) Prescribed frequency of catheterization
8. Urinary incontinence (discussed on p. 1218)
9. History of urinary retention
10. Information on urinary system pain—location, character, severity, duration, and alleviating or aggravating factors
11. Change in urine appearance—color, visibility of blood or blood clots, and presence of sediment in the urine

12. Focused review of systems
    a. Urologic system
       (1) Urinary tract infections (febrile versus afebrile, frequency, association with incontinence)
       (2) Hematuria or urologic cancer
       (3) Passage of urinary calculi
       (4) Previous urologic surgery or endoscopic or extracorporeal procedures
    b. Neurologic system
       (1) Disorders of the brain, including tumor (benign or malignant), cerebrovascular accident, increased intracranial pressure, multiple sclerosis, Alzheimer's disease, parkinsonism, and traumatic brain injury
       (2) Disorders of the spinal cord, including traumatic injury, spinovascular disease, stenosis or disk disease, transverse myelitis, and spinal dysraphism
       (3) Disorders of the peripheral nervous system, including peripheral neuropathies related to diabetes mellitus, heavy metal toxicities, and chronic ethanol (alcohol) abuse; and infectious neuropathies, including herpes zoster infections, or shingles.
       (4) Surgery on the brain or spinal surgery
       (5) Orthopedic procedures on the spinal column
       (6) Orthopedic procedures requiring craniotomy
       (7) Benign or malignant tumors of the nervous system
       (8) Infections of the nervous system, including meningitis and encephalitis
    c. Gastrointestinal system
       (1) Frequency and consistency of bowel movements
       (2) Fecal incontinence, including frequency of incontinent episodes and volume (fecal soiling versus involuntary passage of formed stool)
    d. Male reproductive system
       (1) Erectile function and dysfunction and the frequency and timing of intercourse
       (2) Ejaculatory dysfunction
       (3) Infertility
       (4) Loss of libido
       (5) Prostate disorders, including infection or inflammation, benign prostatic hyperplasia (hypertrophy), and prostate cancer
       (6) Infection of the testis and epididymis
       (7) Malignancy of scrotal contents or the penis
       (8) Penile, scrotal, or prostate surgery
    e. Female reproductive system
       (1) Menses, including onset of menopause (if appropriate), onset of menarche, current menstrual frequency, and general characteristics of flow.
       (2) Reproduction, including pregnancies, deliveries (vaginal or cesarean section), use of forceps, and breech presentations
       (3) Signs and symptoms of pelvic descent, including suprapubic or vaginal pressure, lower back discomfort that is aggravated by exercise and prolonged periods of standing and is alleviated by resting in a supine position, and stress urinary incontinence
       (4) Malignancies of reproductive organs
       (5) Surgical procedures on the female reproductive system

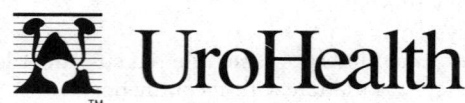

RECORD BOOK

(502) 893-3510
912A Dupont Road
Louisville, Kentucky 40207

Name: _____

Next Appointment Date: _____   Time: _____

Nurse's Name: _____

Instructions:

1. **In the 1st column, mark the time you urinated.**

2. **In the 2nd column, mark every time you leaked urine and indicate whether it was a large (L) or Small (S) amount.**

3. **In the 3rd column, place a check next to the time a wet pad was changed.**

4. **In the 4th column, enter the reason for incontinent episode, like sneezing, coughing, lifting, couldn't make it the bathroom, etc.**

Figure 26–9. Bladder record. (Courtesy of UroHealth, Louisville, KY.)

DAY 1   Date: _____

Time	Urinate in Toilet	Incontinent Episode L/S	Changed Wet Pad	Reason for Incontinent Episode
6 - 8 am				
8 - 10 am				
10 - 12 N.				
12 - 2 pm				
2 - 4 pm				
4 - 6 pm				
6 - 8 pm				
8 - 10 pm				
10 - 12M				
Overnight				
No. of pads used				
NOTES:				

Physical Examination

1. General assessment
   a. Mobility and manual dexterity (particularly the ability to perform self-care tasks)
   b. Cognition and the ability to store and recall information (compromised with central nervous system disease, including dementias and fluid and electrolyte imbalances related to renal insufficiency or functional urinary incontinence)
   c. Blood pressure in the supine and upright positions (elevated with renal failure or renovascular hypertension)

d. Inspection of skin
  (1) Pallor and yellow or sallow appearance (related to chronic anemia)
  (2) Pruritis and dry, thin brittle skin (protein deficiency related to renal failure)
  (3) Altered skin integrity and bruising (impaired wound healing related to renal failure or perineal, monilial, or ammonia contact dermatitis related to severe urinary incontinence)
2. Abdomen
  a. When the patient is supine following urination, check for contour and symmetry and presence of abdominal masses. A suprapubic mass may be related to urinary retention; an abdominal mass of the upper quadrant may be related to severe hydronephrosis or renal tumor.
  b. Before performing any palpation or percussion, auscultate the abdomen for the presence and frequency of bowel sounds; bruits in upper quadrants may be related to renal artery abnormality.
  c. Percuss the abdomen for the presence of a distended bladder (dull area at or above the umbilicus); costovertebral angle tenderness indicates pyelonephritis.
  d. Use light palpation to detect tenderness or muscle guarding.
  e. Use deep palpation to detect masses. Renal palpation is difficult except in very thin individuals.
3. Male genitalia (see Chapter 30): Assess for the following:
  a. Altered skin integrity with significant urinary leakage
  b. Altered sensations, absent bulbocavernosus reflex with localized neurologic deficit
  c. Urethral discharge with infection or inflammation
4. Female genitalia (see Chapter 31): Assess for the following:
  a. Altered skin integrity with significant urinary leakage
  b. Altered sensations, absent bulbocavernosus response with localized neurologic deficit
  c. Pelvic descent and cystocele: a bulging of the anterior vaginal wall with Valsalva maneuver
  d. Rectocele: A bulging of the posterior vaginal vault with exertion
  e. Enterocele: A gurgling near the vaginal vault with descent of the small bowel into the pouch of Douglas
  f. Uterine prolapse: A protrusion of the cervix and related vaginal wall with or without exertion (eversion of the vaginal wall in severe cases)

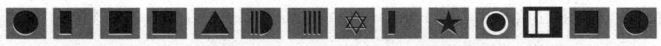

TRANSCULTURAL CONSIDERATIONS

Examination of the female genitalia is undertaken with extreme care for young women of the Islamic culture. The examination must be performed by a female clinician and extraordinary measures to ensure privacy must be observed. Failure to provide adequate privacy may significantly damage the woman's "prospects" for marriage to a man within her culture.

Table 26–2. Normal Findings in a Routine Urinalysis

Component	Normal Values
Color	Straw colored to darker yellow
Opacity	Clear
Specific gravity	1.002–1.035
Osmolality	275–295 mOsm/L
pH	4.5–8.0
Glucose	Negative
Ketones	Negative
Protein	Negative
Bilirubin	Negative
Red blood cells	0–3.5
White blood cells	0–5 high-power field
Bacteria	None
Casts	0–4 hyaline casts, low-power field
Crystals	None

From Black JM, and Matassarin-Jacobs E (eds). *Luckmann and Sorensen's Medical-Surgical Nursing: A Psychophysiologic Approach.* 4th ed. Philadelphia: WB Saunders, 1993, p 1427.

Special Diagnostic Studies

1. Urine studies (Tables 26–2 and 26–3 and Procedure 26–1): Normal findings in urinalysis:
  a. Color: Straw-colored to darker yellow
  b. pH: 4.5 to 8.0
  c. Specific gravity: 1.002 to 1.035
  d. Ketones: None
  e. Glucose: None

Table 26–3. Common Causes of Urine Discoloration

Color	Contributing Factors
Clear/colorless	High intake of water, clear liquids
Dark yellow	Dehydration
Bright yellow	Vitamins (B₂, A)
	Bilirubin (forms yellowish foam with agitation)
	Drugs (chloroquine phosphate, Gantrisin)
Red	Blood (fresh)
	Beets, blackberries
	Drugs (doxorubicin, ibuprofen, phenolphthalein, phenytoin, rifampin)
Brown	Hemoglobin (old blood)
	Melanin
	Hair coloring
	Drugs (chlorpromazine, levodopa, methyldopa, metronidazole, nitrofurantoin, Gantanol—specific ingredient in Septra, Bactrim)
Orange	Drugs (phenazopyridine, warfarin)
Blue or blue-green	Clorets (specific action of chlorophyll)
	Drugs (amitriptyline, cimetidine, indomethacin, Phenergan)
	Tryptophan

From Cohen M, and Thill J. What's the cause of abnormally colored urine? *Contemp Urol* 4(6):25–31, 1992.

Procedure 26–1
Urine Collection for Estimation of Serum Creatinine
Clearance: The 6-Hour Creatinine Clearance Test

Definition/Purpose	Glomerular filtration rate (GFR) is one of the major functions that decreases in the presence of renal disease. The driving principle for this test is that endogenous serum creatinine should remain constant throughout the day. Creatinine is readily excreted regardless of urinary flow. Efficient glomerular filtration also prevents reabsorption. In contrast, blood urea nitrogen (BUN) fluctuates in response to other disease processes and so is not an adequate measure of GFR.
Contraindications/Cautions	Many physicians order the creatinine clearance test as a 24-hour urine collection. The duration of collection is less important than the specimens being collected at precise intervals. When a patient is properly hydrated, the creatinine clearance test can be performed in a 4- to 6-hour period.
	Creatinine clearance values are generally not valid if voided specimens are obtained from patients with a postvoid residual volume of greater than 30 to 50 ml. If high postvoid residual volume is suspected, the specimens are collected by urethral catheterization.
	The patient must be able to understand and implement the procedure.
Learning/Teaching Activities	Explain the procedure thoroughly, answering any questions the patient has.
	Inform the patient of the duration of the test (6 hr).

Preliminary Activities

Equipment	• Three sterile urine collection containers, with labels
	• Pen or other implement for writing on container labels
	• 72 to 96 ounces of fluid for consumption by the patient
Assessment/Planning	• Ensure that the patient understands what to do.
	• Be prepared to monitor or assist the patient in carrying out urine collection.

Procedure

Action	Rationale/Discussion
1. The patient awakes and voids normally.	1. The first void is discarded.
2. After the 1st void, the patient drinks 12 to 16 ounces of fluid hourly during the ensuing 2 hours.	2. Necessary to ensure adequate urine output for samples.
3. The patient uses the 1st container to collect all urine voided in the 2-hour period after the initial void.	3. The patient should void as close as possible to the end of the 2-hour period.
4. The patient labels the container "Specimen 1" (or 2 for the 2nd collection or 3 for the 3rd collection).	4. Accurate labeling of specimens in the order they were taken is critical to the test.
5. The patient repeats steps 2 through 4 in the 2-hour period after the 1st collection and again in the 2-hour period after the 2nd collection.	5. Three samples is sufficient if timing of sample taking is accurate.

Final Activities

Measure each urine specimen to the nearest 5 ml. Pull 10 ml of urine from each container and place each sample in a separate vial, labeling each vial to match its original container. Prepare the vials of urine and blood test specimen for transport to the laboratory.

Review results: Normal values are 97 to 140 ml per minute in males and 85 to 125 ml per minute in females, with the exact clearance rate varying with the patient's body size and muscle mass.

Patients with mild renal insufficiency and a GFR of 50 to 75 ml per minute are at increased risk of postoperative renal failure.

f. Bilirubin: None
g. Red blood cells: 0 to 5 per high-power field
h. White blood cells: 0 to 5 per high-power field
i. Casts: 0 to 4 hyaline casts per low-power field

j. Urinalysis of red and white blood cells and casts requires microscopic examination.
2. Blood studies (see Chapter 25)
    a. Blood urea nitrogen (BUN) and serum creatinine

Table 26–4. Special Diagnostic Tests for Urinary Disorders

Name/Purpose	Preparation	Indications	Postprocedure Care
Kidney-ureters-bladder (KUB, plain abdominal film): a single antero-posterior view of urinary system and adjacent structures	None	Detect urinary calculi Preliminary to intravenous urography, voiding cystourethrogram, videourodynamic test	None
Intravenous pyelogram/intrave-nous urogram (IVP/IVU): serial radiographic views of kidney, ureters, and bladder following intravenous injection of contrast material	Screen for allergies to contrast materials, iodine-based solutions, shellfish. Clear liquids and a laxative maximize visualization of the kidneys; catharsis and dehydration procedures may be prescribed in special situations by consulting radiologist. Reassure patient that "warm flush" and foul taste in mouth are common.	Urinary calculi Recurrent or febrile urinary tract infection Hematuria of unclear etiology Abdominal or pelvic mass or tumor Congenital anomaly of urinary system	Determine severity of obstructive uropathy. Provide prompt hydration to prevent acute renal failure (uncommon).
Retrograde pyelogram (RPG): se-rial radiographs of the renal ure-ter, pelvis via retrograde injec-tion of contrast material during endoscopic examination	Ensure that urine is sterile before invasive cystoscopic instrumentation. Administration of local anesthesia or systemic sedation or anesthesia may be required.	Similar to IVP, but preferred for individuals allergic to contrast materials or with nonfunctioning kidneys or obstructed ureters	Monitor for signs and symptoms of febrile urinary infection. Extravasation may require transient ureteral stents.
Renal arteriogram: serial radio-graphic views of the renal vas-culature via intra-arterial injec-tion of contrast material	Screen for allergies to contrast material, iodine-bound solutions, shellfish. Systemic sedation is often required.	Intrarenal mass or tumor Renal trauma Renovascular hypertension	Monitor pressure dressing for signs of significant bleeding. Monitor peripheral pulses in affected extremity—diminished or absent pulses may indicate embolus or thrombus. Enforce strict bed rest and use a sandbag at insertion site 4–8 hr to diminish risk of bleeding or thromboembolic event.
Renal venogram: serial radio-graphs of renal venous system following intravenous injection of contrast material	Similar to arteriography, often follows renal arteriogram. Epinephrine injection 10 sec after arteriography enhances venographic images.	Renovascular hypertension Renal vein thrombosis Renal tumor (evaluate potential extension into vena cava) Congenital anomalies	Similar to arteriography.
Radionuclide renal studies: intrave-nous injection of radioisotope with serial, computer-generated image of kidneys, ureters, and bladder	Intravenous injection of radionu-clide minutes to hours before imaging. Urethral catheterization may be required.	Determined by specific isotope	Pregnant women should avoid contact with patient or urinary output for 24 hr.
Ultrasonography of the urinary system: serial ultrasonic images of the kidneys, ureters, bladder	None	Abdominal masses Urinary calculi Recurrent or febrile urinary infections	None
Magnetic resonance imaging (MRI) of the urinary tract: serial, com-puter-generated images of the kidneys, ureters, and bladder produced by radio waves and alteration of the magnetic field of human tissues	Careful instruction minimizes anxi-ety produced by limited space in imaging tube. Systemic sedation may be required. Remove all magnetic materials from the body before scanning. Contraindications: pacemaker, me-tallic implants.	Abdominal masses Urinary system tumors	None
Computerized tomography (CT): serial, computer-generated axial images of abdomen and pelvis, including urinary system	Intravenous or oral contrast mate-rials may be required as for IVP.	Abdominal or pelvic masses Staging malignancies	None
Bladder/urethral or ureteral biop-sies obtained during endoscopic examination (cystoscopy, ureter-oscopy required)	Same as for retrograde pyelogram.	Bladder or urethral mass Inflammatory lesions of the blad-der or urethra Ureteral masses	Mild hematuria typically resolves with time and adequate fluid intake. Potential for febrile or afebrile uri-

Table continued on following page

Table 26-4. Special Diagnostic Tests for Urinary Disorders (Continued)

Name/Purpose	Preparation	Indications	Postprocedure Care
			nary infection; may require antibiotic prophylaxis.
Renal biopsy: small section of renal parenchyma obtained during percutaneous or open surgical approach	General anesthesia may be indicated; local anesthesia, systemic sedation typically required. Contraindications: solitary kidney, irreversible hemorrhagic tendencies, sepsis.	Persistent proteinuria Nephrotic syndrome Unexplained hematuria with suspected renal origin	Serial urine samples may be kept to observe resolution of hematuria after procedure; persistent, significant hematuria may indicate significant intrarenal bleeding. Tight surgical dressing to prevent excessive bleeding. Monitor hematocrit and hemoglobin for 24–48 hr after biopsy. Apply direct pressure to site for at least 30 min or apply sandbag to pressure dressing to minimize bleeding. Bed rest for 8 hr or more. Adequate hydration (1500–2000 ml/day) to ensure adequate urinary flow.
Cystogram, voiding cystourethrogram (VCUG): serial radiographs of the lower urinary tract via retrograde, intravesical injection of contrast materials. Cystogram shows bladder filling; VCUG shows it emptying. Urodynamic testing: defines lower urinary tract function and dysfunction	Invasive catheterization required; eradicate bacteriuria before procedure. Ensure absence of urethral trauma (bleeding at meatus) when performing cystogram to evaluate pelvic trauma. See cystogram/VCUG. Patient to undergo uroflowmetry as part of urodynamics; should arrive with comfortably full bladder.	Recurrent afebrile or febrile urinary infections Vesicoureteral reflux Trauma of lower urinary tract or pelvis Congenital anomaly Urinary incontinence Voiding dysfunction (with or without urinary leakage) Neuropathic bladder dysfunction Urinary retention of unknown etiology	Monitor for signs of urinary tract infection. Ensure adequate hydration (1500–2000 ml/day) to minimize discomfort and risk of infection. Antibiotic prophylaxis indicated when reflux is present. See cystogram/VCUG.
Cystourethroscopy: direct visualization of the urethra, bladder and ureteral orifices using telescopic or fiberoptic technology; a form of endoscopy	Eradicate bacteriuria before procedure. Transurethral or percutaneous local anesthesia typically indicated. Systemic sedation or general anesthesia required for prolonged examination or adjunct procedures (e.g., biopsy, transurethral resection).	Urethral or bladder masses Bladder or urethral fistulas Vesicoureteral reflux (selected cases) Congenital anomalies of the lower urinary tract Urethral or bladder neck strictures or stenosis Neuropathic bladder (selected cases) Calculi in bladder or lower third of ureter	Adequate fluid intake and a warm sitz bath alleviate postprocedure discomfort. Monitor patient for signs of infection; serious, febrile infections may occur. Hematuria is expected when transurethral resection accompanies endoscopic examination; gross persistent hematuria with abdominal distention indicates possible bladder perforation. Microscopic hematuria (pink-tinged or clear urine) may occur with biopsy.
Ureteroscopy: direct visualization of the ureters using telescopic or fiberoptic technology; dilation of the orifice must be completed before examination; a form of endoscopy	Same as for cystourethroscopy.	Ureteral masses Ureteral strictures or obstructions (calculi, tumors, etc.)	See cystourethroscopy. Ureteral spasm may produce colic type pain similar to obstructing calculi. Loss of ureteral integrity may require temporary placement of stents.
Percutaneous nephroscopy: direct visualization of the pelvicaliceal system via a percutaneous route using telescopic or fiberoptic technology; a form of endoscopy	Spinal anesthesia with systemic sedation or general anesthesia required. Significant bleeding may occur; obtain blood for potential transfusion as indicated. Eradicate bacteriuria before invasive examination.	Calculi of renal pelvis or upper ureter Extrinsic compression or intrinsic obstruction from tumor	Assess for significant blood loss: passage of bright red blood or clots in urine. Monitor urine for presence of hematuria, bright red bleeding, or clots. Monitor percutaneous nephrostomy tube for output, presence of blood. Monitor hematocrit and hemoglobin for 48 hours or as directed.

b. Decreases in red blood cells, hemoglobin, and hematocrit as well as increased white blood cell count
3. Other tests (Table 26–4)

☐ *CARING FOR PEOPLE WITH ACUTE AND CHRONIC RENAL FAILURE*

Definitions

1. Renal failure is failure of the kidneys to maintain internal homeostasis.
2. Acute renal failure is the rapid loss of renal function over a period of days or weeks; it typically occurs in critically ill patients.
   a. In acute prerenal failure, renal blood flow is impaired, with decreased filtration pressure.
   b. Acute intrarenal failure occurs as a complication of prerenal failure or as a primary disorder (most often, as acute tubular necrosis).
   c. Acute postrenal failure is an obstruction of urinary outflow, with low bladder wall compliance.
3. Chronic renal failure is the slow, usually insidious loss of function occurring over a period of months or years. (It is often associated with a chronic disease.) It becomes irreversible at some unclear point.

Incidence and Socioeconomic Impact

1. The exact incidence of renal failure is unknown.
2. Approximately 90,000 people in the United States receive Medicare benefits for renal dialysis, with 8000 new cases being entered into the program annually.

Risk Factors

1. Acute renal failure
   a. Hypotensive episodes that produce renal ischemia precipitated by hypovolemia, hemorrhage, or septic shock
   b. Recent surgery (particularly cardiovascular or cardiac procedures)
   c. Multiple organ failure
   d. Preexisting renal disease
   e. Diabetes mellitus with other secondary complications
   f. Recent exposure to potentially nephrotoxic substance or pharmacologic agent
2. Chronic renal failure
   a. Chronic glomerulonephritis or pyelonephritis
   b. Diabetes mellitus
   c. Chronic misuse or abuse of analgesics
   d. Chronic intake of drugs with potential nephrotoxic side effects
   e. Autoimmune disorders
   f. Genetic disorders (polycystic kidney disease, among others)
   g. Prolonged urinary obstruction
   h. Recurrent obstructive urinary calculi

i. Multiple open surgical procedures requiring manipulation of 1 or both kidneys

TRANSCULTURAL CONSIDERATIONS

Those ethnic and racial groups that hold a cultural view that organs or bodies "wear out" due to overuse may interpret acute or chronic renal failure from that perspective. It is important to educate the patient regarding the physical causes of chronic or acute renal failure.

Etiology

1. Acute renal failure
   a. Prenal: Impaired renal perfusion due to the following:
      (1) Hemorrhage (gastrointestinal, trauma, postpartum)
      (2) Severe burns
      (3) Hypovolemia (increased sensible fluid losses or 3rd spacing of fluids)
      (4) Severe congestive heart failure
      (5) Renal hypoxia
   b. Intrarenal: Insult to the renal parenchyma due to the following:
      (1) Acute tubular necrosis (the most common cause occurring as postischemic sequelae or nephrotoxicity from antibiotics, including aminoglycosides, cephalosporins, tetracyclines, and sulfonamides; antineoplastics; anesthetics; analgesics; nonsteroidal anti-inflammatory agents; ethylene glycol; and radiographic contrast media)
      (2) Hypertensive sclerosis
      (3) Acute or chronic glomerulonephritis
      (4) Recurrent pyelonephritis
      (5) Diabetic nephrosclerosis (most commonly related to chronic renal failure)
   c. Postrenal: Obstruction of the urinary transport system due to the following:
      (1) Acute, bilateral ureteral obstruction
      (2) Acute obstruction of the bladder outlet or urethra
2. Chronic renal failure
   a. Diabetes mellitus
   b. Renal artery occlusion, stenosis, or thrombosis with coexisting hypertension
   c. Autoimmune disorders
   d. Metabolic disorders such as renal tubular acidosis, calcium phosphate disorders, and uric acid disorders
   e. Chronic urinary obstruction caused by the following:
      (1) Prostatic enlargement
      (2) Bladder neck contracture or hypertrophy
      (3) Vesicosphincter dyssynergia
   f. Low or poor bladder wall compliance
   g. Polycystic kidney disease
      (1) This hereditary disorder, which may strike during childhood or adulthood, is characterized by the

development of grapelike cysts that contain blood, serous fluid, or urine. These cysts eventually replace normal kidney tissue.

(2) Common manifestations include palpable kidney masses, dull aching lumbar or flank pain, proteinuria, pyuria, and calculi. Over a period of 15 to 30 years or more, the condition may progress to end-stage renal disease.

(3) As the disease process cannot be arrested, the goal of treatment is to preserve as much kidney function as possible, prevent urinary system infections, and control hypertension.

(4) Once a person is diagnosed, genetic counseling may help to prevent the transmission of this disorder to the next generation.

Pathophysiology

1. Acute renal failure
   a. Physical trauma, infection, inflammation, or exposure to toxic chemicals damages the renal tubules, causing tubular necrosis, or produces severe vasoconstriction of renal blood vessels, causing ischemia of kidney tissue.
   b. Excretion is impaired, allowing substances normally eliminated to accumulate in body fluids.
   c. Homeostatic, endocrine, and metabolic functions are disrupted.
   d. Acute renal failure proceeds through 3 phases
      (1) Oliguria-anuria: Urine volume declines to less than 400 ml per 24 hours. Serum concentrations of substances normally eliminated (e.g., magnesium, potassium, urea, uric acid) increase. Renal function may decrease as nitrogen retention increases. The GFR decreases. Duration is generally 8 to 15 days (the longer the duration, the less chance of recovery or survival).
      (2) Diuresis: BUN stops increasing and gradually begins to decrease. Urine volume gradually increases, and GFR begins to increase. Renal function remains abnormal.
      (3) Recovery: BUN is stable and normal. Urine volume is normal. Complete recovery may take 1 to 2 years. Some impairment of glomular filtration and concentrating ability may be permanent.
2. Chronic renal failure proceeds through the following stages:
   a. Decreased renal reserve
   b. Renal insufficiency
   c. Renal failure
   d. Uremia, which causes death in the absence of dialysis or kidney transplantation

Clinical Manifestations

1. General signs and symptoms
   a. Weight changes:
      (1) Weight gain with acute fluid retention

(2) Weight loss with altered nutritional status, nausea, and vomiting
   b. Electrocardiogram abnormalities:
      (1) Peaked T waves
      (2) Prolonged PR interval
      (3) Widened QRS complex
   c. Pulmonary signs:
      (1) Tachypnea—Kussmaul breathing or dyspnea; hypoxemia with fluid overload
      (2) Rales and rhonchi on auscultation
   d. Urinary signs:
      (1) Frequent urination of large volumes (early diuretic phase of acute failure or failure of ability to concentrate urine in chronic renal failure)
      (2) Infrequent urination of small volumes with advanced failure (oliguria)
      (3) Absent urination with advanced failure (anuria)
      (4) Suprapubic distention with urinary retention or obstruction
      (5) Dysuria, odor with infection
   e. Skeletal and integumentary signs:
      (1) Bone pain and fractures
      (2) Joint swelling and pain
      (3) Signs of demineralization
      (4) Calcium deposits in soft tissues
2. In acute renal failure, general signs and symptoms include the following:
   a. Confusion or altered mentation
   b. Pulmonary edema
   c. Gastrointestinal bleeding
   d. Congestive heart failure
   e. Altered serum chemistry levels including the following:
      (1) Increasing serum creatinine and BUN
      (2) Unexpectedly high serum levels of specific drugs
      (3) Low serum calcium
      (4) Increased serum phosphates
      (5) Increased serum osmolality
   f. Altered urine chemistry levels including the following:
      (1) High urine specific gravity with prerenal failure; low specific gravity with postrenal failure
      (2) Low urinary pH
      (3) Elevated urine creatinine with prerenal failure
3. Cause-specific signs and symptoms in acute renal failure:
   a. Decreased tissue turgor, diarrhea, dry mucous membranes, nausea and vomiting, and somnolence in prerenal failure
   b. Fever, skin rash, and edema in intrarenal failure
   c. Difficulty urinating and changes in urine flow in postrenal failure
4. Signs and symptoms in chronic renal failure (Fig. 26-10):
   a. Changes that become apparent when renal function decreases to below 25 percent of normal
   b. Urinary system changes including frequent, infrequent, or absent urination
   c. Oral changes
      (1) Cracked, bleeding gums
      (2) Foul breath (uremic fetor)
   d. Integumentary changes
      (1) Skin with a gray or bronzed appearance

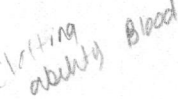

CHRONIC RENAL FAILURE

PATHOPHYSIOLOGY	CLINICAL MANIFESTATIONS	COMPLICATIONS
Metabolic Disorders–		
Metabolic acidosis	Confusion, apathy, stupor Shortened memory and attention span	Seizures, coma
Metabolic toxins build up	Nausea, vomiting	Pericarditis Peptic ulcers
Metabolic disorders	Restless leg syndrome • *peripheral neuropathies* • *lower extremity paresthesias*	
Abnormal calcium or phosphorus metabolism	Altered bone growth and replacement • *swollen, painful joints* • *soft tissue calcium deposits (brain, eyes, joints, heart, skin)* • *renal osteodystrophy*	
Hyperkalemia	Increased risk of cardiovascular disease • *compromised cardiac function*	Cardioarrhythmias Congestive heart failure Erectile dysfunction
Crystallization of calcium salts	Decreased oil and sweat production • *itching, excoriation* • *brittle nails and hair*	
Impaired secretion and prolonged increase in production of triglycerides		
Hyperlipidemia	Accelerated atherosclerosis	
Altered insulin production and metabolism	Carbohydrate intolerance	
Activated renin–angiotensin system	Fluid overload and retention of water and salt	Hypertension
	Edema	Pulmonary edema Pneumonia (uremic or viral)
Impaired coagulation, capillary fragility	• *contusions, bruises* • *bleeding gums* • *bleeding diathesis* • *pallor*	Anemia
Fragile GI mucosa	Susceptibility to peptic ulcers	
Pigment retention	Skin color gray or bronze	
Altered production of growth hormone	Altered growth in children	
Hyperprolactinemia • *diminished spermatogenesis, impaired testosterone function*	Subfertility in males Diminished libido	
• *impaired FSH, LH production*	Ovulatory disorders Amenorrhea	
Diminished immune response		
Excess salivary urea, stomatitis		

Figure 26–10.

Illustration continued on following page

ACUTE RENAL FAILURE

PATHOPHYSIOLOGY	CLINICAL MANIFESTATIONS
Metabolic acidosis • *retention of hydrogen ions* • *impaired ammonium ion production* • *buildup of metabolic toxins* • *impaired bicarbonate production*	Confusion, altered mentation *(drowsiness or coma)* Headache Kussmaul breathing Diminished RBC viability • *tachypnea, dyspnea* • *pulmonary edema*
Hyperkalemia	Compromised cardiac function • *cardiac arrhythmias* • *congestive heart failure* Hypotension • *diuretic phase* Hypertension • *fluid retention phase*
Impaired erythropoietin production	GI bleeding, anemia
Inability to concentrate urine	Azotemia *(altered serum and urine chemistry)* Polyuria • *dehydration* Anuria, oliguria • *weight gain*

Figure 26–10. *Continued*

(2) Pallor with anemia
(3) Itching and excoriation related to scratching
(4) Contusions or ecchymosis, even with minor trauma
(5) Brittle nails and dry, brittle hair
e. Fluid and electrolyte imbalances
 (1) Dehydration
 (2) Fluid overload in the oliguric-anuric stage
 (3) Metabolic acidosis
f. Cardiovascular system changes
 (1) Hypertension
 (2) Hyperkalemia
 (3) Pericarditis
 (4) Pleuritis
g. Pulmonary system changes (uremic pneumonia)
h. Gastrointestinal system changes
 (1) Nausea and vomiting, particularly in the morning because metabolic toxins accumulate during sleep
 (2) Fragility of gastrointestinal mucosa with susceptibility to ulceration and altered mucous secretions
 (3) Carbohydrate intolerance
 (4) Hyperlipidemia
 (5) Constipation

 (6) Anorexia
i. Endocrine system changes
 (1) Glucose intolerance
 (2) Disturbances of growth hormone (typically increased) and sex hormones
j. Reproductive system changes
 (1) Impaired fertility
 (2) Erectile dysfunction
k. Neurologic system changes
 (1) Cognitive changes (shortened memory and attention span, confusion)
 (2) Stupor, coma, or seizures
 (3) Peripheral polyneuropathies (lower extremity paresthesias, tingling, restless leg syndrome, burning feet)
 (4) Sleep disorders
 (5) Headache
 (6) Fatigue
l. Skeletal system changes
 (1) Renal osteodystrophy (demineralization of bone, pain, and pathologic fractures in advanced disease)
 (2) Hyperparathyroid bone disease
m. Personality changes
 (1) Apathy
 (2) Impatient, demanding behavior

Diagnostics

1. Assessment: Check for clinical manifestations
2. Medical diagnosis
 a. Acute prerenal failure
  (1) Serum creatinine is elevated and BUN levels increase with diminishing GFR.
  (2) Creatinine clearance decreases with diminishing GFR.
  (3) Urine sodium levels are low; specific gravity is high.
 b. Acute postrenal failure
  (1) Serum creatinine and BUN levels are elevated.
  (2) Creatinine clearance is decreased.
  (3) Urine sodium and specific gravity are normal.
 c. Chronic renal failure
  (1) Serum creatinine and BUN levels are elevated.
  (2) Urine is pH acidic; urinary volume is decreased (in advanced stages, diuretic phase with higher urinary volumes is noted in early stages).
  (3) Creatinine clearance and GFR are decreased.

Clinical Management

1. Goals of clinical management
 a. Remove or reverse predisposing factors
 b. Prevent or postpone advancement of renal insufficiency to acute or chronic renal failure
 c. Support or augment renal function
2. Nonpharmacologic interventions
 a. Controlling fluid and sodium intake

b. Providing nutritional support, including vitamin supplements as needed

c. Providing replacement fluids or blood as ordered to prevent renal ischemia from hypovolemic shock

d. Limiting protein intake to minimize progressive renal insufficiency (44 and 56 gm in women and men, respectively)

3. Pharmacologic interventions include antibiotics for urinary tract infection to reverse pyelonephritis.

4. Special medical-surgical procedures

a. Catheters are used to reverse obstructions

b. Dialysis supports or augments compromised or failed renal function (Fig. 26–11).

(1) Dialysis may take the form of peritoneal dialysis or hemodialysis. Schedule and type of dialysis should be determined by consultation among physician, patient, family.

(2) Both forms of dialysis remove toxins in the blood through ultrafiltration and diffusion. Ultrafiltration uses osmotic or hydrostatic pressure to remove excess fluid from the blood. Diffusion occurs when particles (ions) pass—or fail to pass (because of their size)—through the pores of a membrane (the peritoneal membrane in peritoneal dialysis, an artificial membrane in hemodialysis).

(3) The result of both peritoneal dialysis and hemodialysis is the removal from the blood of waste products such as urea and creatinine and excess fluid, the restoration of electrolytic balance, and elimination of acidosis.

c. In peritoneal dialysis, dialysate solution is instilled in the peritoneal cavity. Excess substances in the blood enter the dialysate and needed substances in the dialysate enter the blood, then the dialysate is removed. This cycle is repeated as needed.

(1) In intermittent peritoneal dialysis, an automated machine dialyzes for 8- to 12-hour periods 3 to 5 times per week.

(2) In chronic ambulatory peritoneal dialysis, nonautomated dialysis requires 3 to 5 passes every day (Fig. 26–12).

(3) In continuous cycling peritoneal dialysis, an auto-

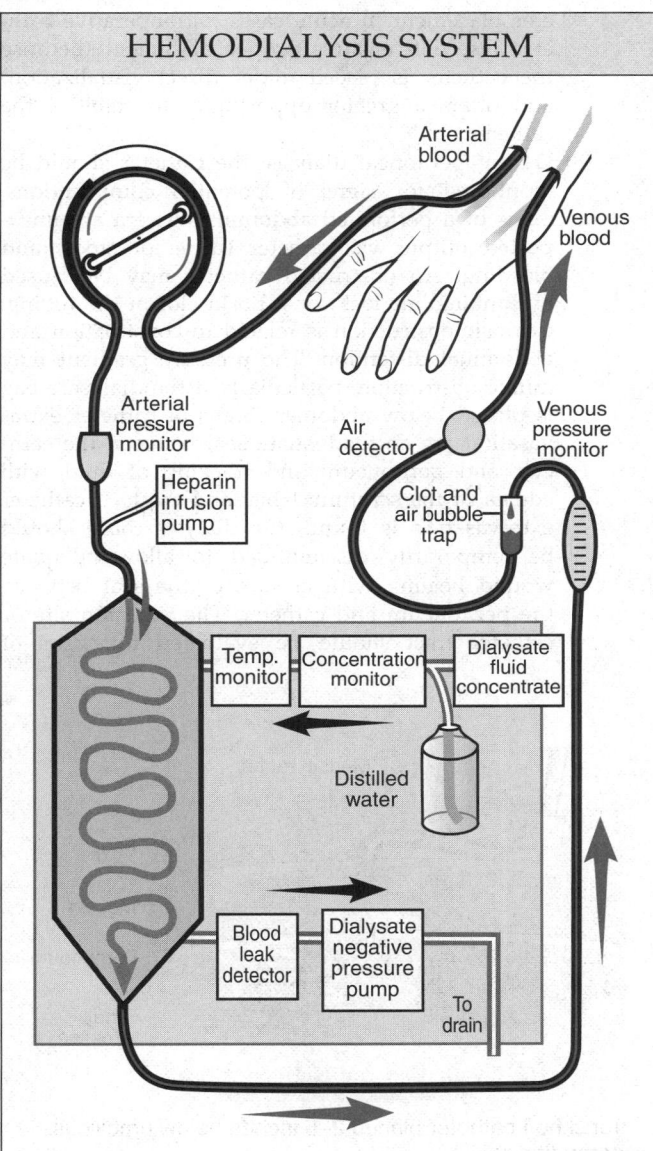

HEMODIALYSIS SYSTEM

Arterial blood

Venous blood

Arterial pressure monitor

Air detector

Venous pressure monitor

Heparin infusion pump

Clot and air bubble trap

Temp. monitor

Concentration monitor

Dialysate fluid concentrate

Distilled water

Blood leak detector

Dialysate negative pressure pump

To drain

Figure 26–11.

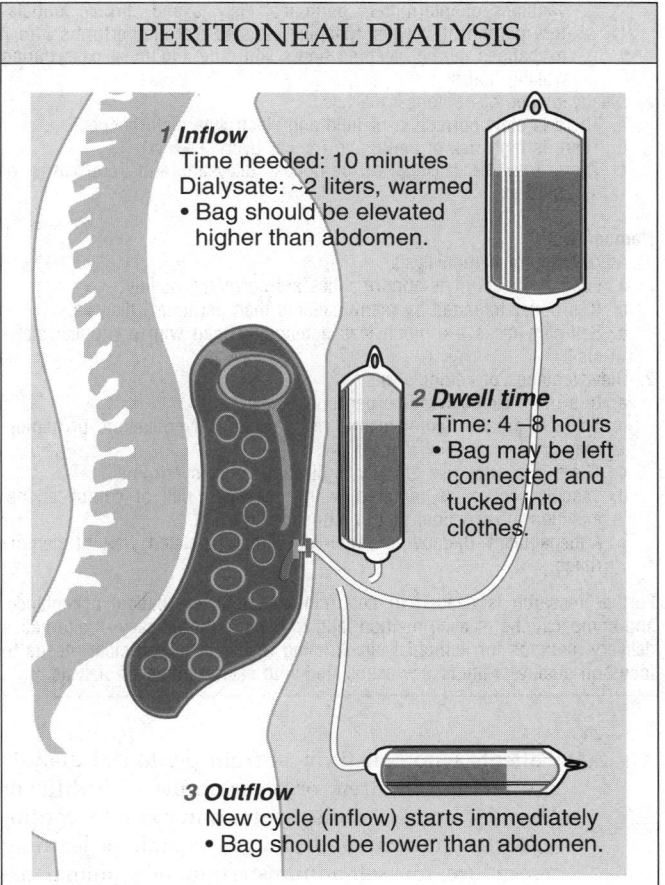

PERITONEAL DIALYSIS

1 Inflow
Time needed: 10 minutes
Dialysate: ~2 liters, warmed
• Bag should be elevated higher than abdomen.

2 Dwell time
Time: 4–8 hours
• Bag may be left connected and tucked into clothes.

3 Outflow
New cycle (inflow) starts immediately
• Bag should be lower than abdomen.

Figure 26–12. Components of long-term peritoneal dialysis system.

mated, closed system dialyzes 3 to 7 times during sleeping hours, with an additional nonautomated pass made during waking hours.

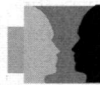

CLINICAL CONTROVERSIES

What's the best mode of dialysis? Ideally, dialysis should rapidly and effectively remove toxins and waste products at low cost and with minimal complications. It should be relatively easy for patients to self-administer and maximize their independence and mobility. There is no "ideal" system. Both peritoneal dialysis and hemodialysis have advantages and disadvantages.

Peritoneal Dialysis
1. Advantages of peritoneal dialysis
   a. It is inexpensive.
   b. It is hemodynamically well tolerated. There is low risk of hypotension, hypoxia, hemorrhage, or dialysis dysequilibrium syndrome (characterized by headache, seizure, and coma).
   c. No vascular access is required.
   d. No anticoagulant therapy is needed.
   e. Several forms of peritoneal dialysis are available.
      (1) Intermittent peritoneal dialysis requires dialysis passes only 3 to 5 times per week but a machine is required for dialysis. The procedure takes 8 to 12 hours but may be performed during sleeping hours. The risk of air embolus is avoided.
      (2) Chronic ambulatory peritoneal dialysis requires no machine. Physical mobility is maximized but dialysis must be done 3 to 5 times daily every day. The hazard of peritonitis is greater than with intermittent peritoneal dialysis.
      (3) Continuous cycling peritoneal dialysis attempts to combine advantages of intermittent peritoneal dialysis and chronic ambulatory peritoneal dialysis. Machine-assisted dialysis performs 3 to 7 exchanges during sleeping hours with one additional pass during waking hours.
2. Disadvantages of peritoneal dialysis
   a. There is slow correction of fluid and electrolyte disturbances
   b. There is high risk of peritonitis (recurs every 1–2 yr)
   c. There may be leakage of peritoneal dialysate and rare cases of hydrothorax.

Hemodialysis
1. Advantages of hemodialysis
   a. Fluid and electrolyte abnormalities are corrected rapidly.
   b. It is better tolerated by many patients than peritoneal dialysis.
   c. Self-care tasks are much less demanding than with peritoneal dialysis.
2. Disadvantages of hemodialysis
   a. It is more expensive than peritoneal dialysis.
   b. There is greater hemodynamic risk (hypoxia, hypotension, or hemorrhage).
   c. There is greater risk of dialysis disequilibrium syndrome.
   d. Vascular access is required, with associated risk of complications, infection, obstruction, or thromboembolic event.
   e. Anticoagulant therapy is required, with associated risk of hemorrhage.

Further research is needed to determine the efficacy, patient acceptance, and complications of each method, and to explore the efficacy of alternative delivery methods for hemodialysis. Nursing research, in particular, needs to focus on quality-of-life issues associated with each method of dialysis.

(4) Patients who benefit most from peritoneal dialysis are infants, children, or older adults with difficult vascular access; adults with compromised cardiovascular function; and patients capable of learning procedure for self-administration or minimal assistance administration of dialysis at home.

(5) Peritoneal dialysis requires insertion of a catheter for peritoneal access. Insertion may be done at the bedside for acute cases requiring immediate access or intraoperatively for chronic or prolonged dialysis.

(6) The procedure for catheter insertion is as follows. The abdomen is shaved and prepared at bedside. Local anesthesia is administered for pain control. The physician makes a midline incision 2 to 5 cm below the umbilicus. Incisional bleeding is controlled. The patient is asked to tighten abdominal muscles if feasible. A trocar is inserted through the incision into the peritoneum. The peritoneal cavity is often expanded using dialysate or dextrose in saline solution to ensure accurate placement of the trocar. The catheter is threaded via the trocar. The peritoneal cavity is flushed with antibiotic solution, and bleeding is evaluated.

(7) Intraoperative catheter insertion usually involves placement of a Tenckhoff catheter (Fig. 26–13). Although the procedure is similar to bedside catheter placement in acute cases, intraoperative catheter insertion ensures proper placement (because the catheter is placed under direct visualization) and offers a greater opportunity to stabilize the catheter.

(8) During peritoneal dialysis, the catheter should be monitored for signs of potential complications. Signs of a perforated abdominal viscera are unexpected output via catheter (urine or stool) and bleeding. An obstructed catheter may be caused by kinking, air lock, or a fibrin clot in the tubing; extrinsic obstruction is related to constipation and abdominal distention. The pressure gradient may mimic obstruction, particularly if the dialysate bag is placed below abdomen. Signs of catheter extravasation are an inadequate seal between the catheter and peritoneum and tracking of fluid with edema of the scrotum, labia, and thigh. If catheter extravasation is found, the dialysis route should be temporarily discontinued to allow adequate wound healing with closure of the seal between the peritoneum and catheter. The insertion site or catheter tract should be evaluated for signs of

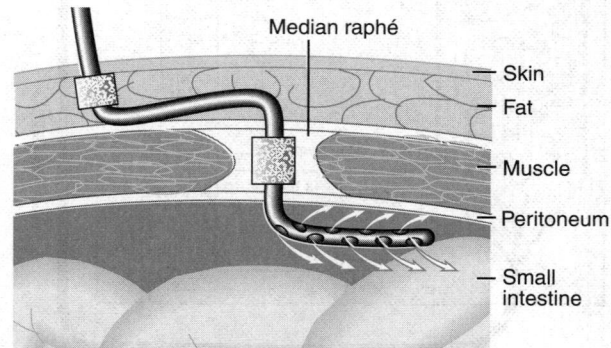

Tenckhoff catheter placed 2–5 inches below umbilicus, at median raphé

Figure 26–13. The Tenckhoff catheter is surgically implanted into the peritoneal space for long-term peritoneal dialysis.

LEARNING/TEACHING GUIDELINES
for Peritoneal Self-Dialysis

General Guidelines

1. Explain the schedule for dialysis and the time required to complete the procedure each time.
2. Describe factors that entered into selection of specific dialysate solution. Teach the patient to manipulate dialysate and dextrose solutions independently (higher concentrations of dextrose, up to 50 percent, are used to increase total dialyzed volume).
3. Teach the patient general guidelines and specific techniques for operating equipment based on the selected method and access route.
4. Stress the need for precision and sanitary measures.

Predialysis Self-Assessments

1. The patient should record vital signs daily. Measuring the apical pulse is particularly important, because it allows the patient to detect obvious dysrhythmias.
2. The patient should weigh self and take vital signs before and after each dialysis procedure.

Prevention and Self-Management of Complications

1. Infectious peritonitis: Signs and symptoms include fever, abdominal pain, and cloudy peritoneal outflow. The patient should contact a nurse or physician promptly so that trained medical personnel can do the following:
   a. Obtain a culture, institute continual peritoneal dialysis using dialysate solution with antibiotic solution, and heparinize the dialysate to prevent occlusion of the catheter.
   b. Provide sensitivity-driven antibiotics based on results of culture.
   c. Initiate treatment when a negative culture indicates aseptic or mechanical peritonitis. Initial treatment is similar to that for infectious peritonitis, but antibiotics are not given.

2. Loss of skin integrity may result from irritation caused by the presence of the catheter, tape, povidone–iodine cleansing solution, and excessive exposure to moisture. Self-management techniques include the following:
   a. Exposing the skin to dry air with a blow dryer at a low setting (soothes maceration).
   b. Application of a moisture barrier to prevent recurrence
   c. Changing the cleansing solution (Hibiclens or other substances) or type of tape to prevent hypersensitivity
3. To prevent or manage obstruction of dialysate solution outflow, patients should do the following:
   a. Empty their bowel before the procedure (aggressive program to prevent constipation may prevent obstruction)
   b. Check tubing for occlusion and kinking
   c. Ensure the correct, dependent position of the outflow bag
   d. Contact medical personnel to discuss the possible need for a radiograph of the catheter to exclude subcutaneous segment kinking or occlusion of the internal lumen
4. Pink-tinged effluent or the presence of small strings of blood in the outflow may or may not be cause for concern. The nurse should do the following:
   a. Assure the patient before the start of self-dialysis that some blood is normal for several days after catheter placement and that transient bloody effluent occurs for unclear reasons and is typically self-limiting.
   b. Instruct the patient to report larger quantities of bright, red blood in the effluent (rare).
5. If there is persistent ascites from a source other than the dialysis process, the patient should do the following:
   a. Substitute a lower concentration of dialysate whenever feasible
   b. Contact medical personnel who can provide aggressive intervention if respiratory compromise occurs (occasional)

local infection daily. The catheter is palpated weekly to detect infection. If rolling the subcutaneous catheter between thumb and index finger causes pain or swelling, the physician should be contacted and antibiotic agents administered promptly to prevent peritonitis.
(9) See Learning/Teaching Guidelines for Peritoneal Self-Dialysis.
d. In hemodialysis, toxin-filled (''dirty'') arterial blood flows into the dialyzer in a hemodialysis machine, where toxins and excess fluid pass through an artificial membrane into dialysate solution, and needed

electrolytes and other elements from the solution pass through the membrane and into the ''clean'' blood, which is then returned to the patient's venous system (Procedure 26–2).
(1) Access to the patient's blood depends on the patient's condition.
(2) For acute or temporary vascular access until renal function is reestablished or a chronic site is accessible, a subclavian catheter is inserted at bedside; patency requires heparinization between treatments. A femoral catheter is inserted at bedside before and removed after each treatment. An ex-

Procedure 26–2
Assisting with Hemodialysis

Definition/Purpose	Hemodialysis removes impurities from the blood such as in cases of acute or irreversible renal failure and fluid and electrolytic imbalances. It is also used to rapidly clear the body of toxins such as barbiturate overdoses.
Contraindications/Cautions	Hemodynamic instability, presence of other diseases, including coronary artery disease, hypertension, and diabetes, and advanced age of the patient are contraindications.
Learning/Teaching Activities	Explain the hemodialysis procedure. Review specific symptoms that occur during hemodialysis, including headache, nausea, vomiting, fever, dyspnea, and chest pain.

Preliminary Activities

Equipment	• Hemodialysis machine • Dialyzer • Dialysate solution • Vascular access route (external arteriovenous shunt, subclavian catheter, or internal arteriovenous fistula or graft) installed in or on a patient's forearm or lower leg before dialysis
Assessment/Planning	• Clear air from blood and dialysate channels to prevent vascular air embolus. Use 400 to 500 ml of saline solution to flush the blood channel; use the dialysate solution to flush the dialysis channel. • Determine the patient's weight. Calculate the ideal or "dry weight" based on previous trends or weight of the patient in an edema-free state and approximate the volume to be removed—typically 1.5 to 2.0 kg. • Assess the patient for abnormal vital signs, evidence of pulmonary edema, pericardial rub, or other potential complicating factors. • Draw a blood sample for clotting time determinations. Arrange for blood urea nitrogen, creatinine, and electrolyte analysis as indicated. • Make sure all equipment and supplies (especially correct dialysate fluid) are ready for use.
Procedure	

Action	Rationale/Discussion
1. Using meticulous technique, prepare the fistula site and dialysate solution as per institutional protocols.	1. Infection is a major potential complication of hemodialysis.
2. Administer the anticoagulant (typically heparin), as ordered.	2. This prevents formation of blood clot in the blood tubing and dialyzer membrane.
3. Connect the tube to the membrane compartment of the dialysis machine to the arterial connection in the patient's shunt-catheter-fistula-graft. Connect the tube, restoring clean blood to the venous connection in the patient's shunt-catheter-fistula-graft.	3. For dialysis to work, "dirty blood" must flow into the dialyzer and across the separating membrane to interact with the dialysate solution before returning to the patient.
4. Begin the flow of blood into the dialysis machine.	4. Begin the flow slowly (50 to 75 ml per minute). Gradually increase the flow to steady state (typically 250 to 300 ml per minute) over a 30-minute period. Total dialysis time normally ranges from 3 to 4 hours.
5. Assess the patient's vital signs at regular intervals during dialysis.	5. Indications of potential problems include changes in blood pressure, pulse rate, respirations, and temperature. Warning: Do not take blood pressure readings using the extremity connected to the machine.
6. Monitor the access device for bleeding, temperature, and signs of infection.	6. If signs of bleeding, infection, or poor extremity circulation appear, work with the physician to correct the problem.
7. Be alert for potential life-threatening complications if the dialysis machine alarm goes off.	7. The machine monitors for problems such as air in the blood tubing; changes in dialysate solution temperature; blood leakage in the dialysate compartment; changes in blood flow, pressure, or composition; and changes in the pressure or composition of the dialysate solution.
8. Prevent or promptly manage intradialysis complications such as hypotension, cardiac dysrhythmias, hemolysis, air embolus, and hyperthermia.	8. For hypotension, raise the patient's feet and legs to boost cardiac return, decrease blood flow into the dialyzer, lower the transmembrane hydrostatic pressure to diminish the volume of fluid removed from plasma, administer normal saline boluses (up to 500 ml) to increase the circulating plasma volume, and administer albumin (as ordered) to increase colloid oncotic pressure.

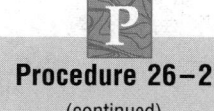

Procedure 26–2

(continued)

Action	Rationale/Discussion
	For cardiac dysrhythmias, monitor the electrocardiogram and administer antidysrhythmia medications as indicated.
	For hemolysis, immediately contact the physician, discontinue dialysis without clearing the fluid lines (see step 9), monitor vital signs, administer oxygen as indicated, and obtain hematocrit and hemoglobin immediately. For air embolus, contact the physician, discontinue dialysis immediately (see step 9), monitor vital signs, and administer oxygen as indicated.
	For hyperthermia, monitor vital signs (including temperature), observe temperature of dialysate in the dialyzer (verify with external monitor if necessary), discontinue dialysis (see step 9), evaluate for hemolysis, and contact the physician as indicated.
9. Terminate dialysis after prescribed treatment is completed or if complications occur.	9. For scheduled or routine termination, stop the blood pump, clamp the arterial and access lines, disconnect the arterial blood line from the access tubing, restart the blood pump with a slow infusion rate, return all blood to the patient using a saline chaser into the arterial blood line, and clamp and disconnect the venous and access lines.
	For emergency termination, stop the blood pump, clamp the access and blood lines, and disconnect patient from dialyzer.

Final Activities

Perform postdialysis evaluation by repeating vital signs to ensure continued stability, obtaining patient weight measurement and comparing it to the goal of "dry" weight, and assessing symptoms compared with predialysis evaluation. Assist the patient to arise slowly if hypotensive episodes have occurred during dialysis.

---

ternal arteriovenous (AV) shunt requires surgical placement; it is preferred for continuous AV hemofiltration.

(3) For prolonged or long-term dialysis, internal vascular access is achieved by
  • Internal AV fistula: A fistula is created that is not accessible for dialysis until weeks to months later, when wound healing occurs and edema subsides.
  • Internal graft AV fistula: Straight or looped natural or synthetic graft is placed in an arm or thigh; it is preferred for obese individuals.
  • Internal AV graft with external access device: An external access port is attached to an AV graft, bypassing the need for repeated needle insertions.

(4) Each access device poses risks of complications.
  • Thrombosis: The fistula is auscultated or gently palpated to ensure pulsations indicate patency. Blood pressure cuffs or constrictive tourniquets should not be used above the fistula or graft. The patient should be hydrated (within prescribed limits) to avoid hypovolemia and risk of clotting. Streptokinase prevents clotting.
  • Local infections: The site is assessed regularly for signs of infection. Antibiotics are administered. The patient should be taught to self-monitor for

infection, particularly when synthetic graft material is used (Learning/Teaching Guidelines for Hemodialysis Blood Access Devices: Self-Care and Self-Monitoring).
  • Aneurysms: The nurse should regularly observe the patient for aneurysm formation. The site of venipuncture should be rotated.
  • Steal syndrome (ischemic pain related to vascular insufficiency from fistula creation): The patient should be assessed for diminished pulses, pallor, and pain distal to the site. Surgical revision or additional procedures are indicated when steal syndrome occurs.

e. Renal transplantation reestablishes failed renal function (Procedure 26–3; Fig. 26–14).
  (1) The organ may be donated by a living person or removed from a cadaver.
  (2) Factors in selecting a donor of either kind include the following:
    • ABO compatibility: Incompatibility contraindicates transplantation.
    • Histocompatibility: The greatest reliability is with living, related donors.
    • White blood cell cross match: A positive response contraindicates transplant.

LEARNING/TEACHING GUIDELINES
for Hemodialysis Blood Access Devices: Self-Care and Self-Monitoring

General Guidelines

Because much of a hemodialysis patient's time is spent away from medical facilities, it is important for such patients to understand the need and procedures for dealing with their blood access devices when they are not on the dialysis machine.

Teach Patient Care of Insertion Site

1. Review potential complications and indications requiring the patient to contact a nurse or physician.
2. Address discomfort issues
   a. Discomfort at the incisional site lessens with maturation of the insertion wound, typically within days to several weeks; 2 to 4 weeks after insertion, all signs of inflammation should disappear.
   b. Discomfort is felt with distention of the abdomen and is alleviated by changing positions.
3. Stress the need for cleanliness of the insertion site to prevent infection.
   a. Teach aseptic technique; have the patient provide a return demonstration.
   b. Emphasize the need to maintain meticulous cleanliness at the catheter insertion (exit) site during wound healing, when opening the system, and when exchanging fluid.
      (1) Using sterile gauze, the patient should clean the site, catheter, and immediately adjacent skin with povidone–iodine solution daily.
      (2) The patient should rinse the site to minimize

irritation from the povidone–iodine solution and dry thoroughly.
      (3) The patient should place sterile gauze on either side of the catheter and curl the tube over this dressing. Additional sterile gauze is placed over the catheter and dressing; clear film or nonadhesive tape dressing is used to seal the gauze.
      (4) In some cases, a dressing may not be needed, but daily cleansing is always vital.
   c. After the wound heals, the patient may take showers but should be discouraged from bathtub bathing. After a shower, the patient should follow the routine cleansing procedure described previously, including dressing the insertion site (if appropriate).

Teach Patient to Protect Site from Inadvertent Trauma

1. Describe the need to use small dialysate volumes during the first 2 weeks after insertion to minimize the risk of leakage and to encourage wound healing.
2. Because the presence of leakage increases risk of infection, provide both verbal and written instructions on self-monitoring for signs of insertional site infection and peritoneal infection.
3. Explain that complications may necessitate replacement of the catheter; reassure and support the patient during transitional periods.

- Mixed lymphocyte culture and reaction: Five days are needed, which is not feasible for a cadaveric donor kidney.
(3) In addition to the risks of surgery, transplant patients face the prospect of organ rejection.
   - Hyperacute rejection occurs immediately after transplantation; it is a rare occurrence, given the increased sophistication in histopathologic compatibility screening. No effective treatment is available.
   - Acute rejection occurs 1 to 2 weeks after transplantation. Prompt management with intravenous Solu-Medrol or prednisolone or local irradiation usually reverses symptoms.
   - Chronic rejection occurs over months or years, gradually increasing creatinine and fluid retention. Immunosuppressive medications and diet slow—but rarely reverse—rejection.

Complications

1. Acute renal failure
   a. Metabolic acidosis

   b. Hypertension
   c. Severe anemia
   d. Infection
   e. Hyperkalemia with cardiac dysrhythmias
2. Chronic renal failure
   a. Hypertension
   b. Hyperkalemia with cardiac dysrhythmias
   c. Congestive heart failure
   d. Pulmonary edema
   e. Pericarditis
   f. Pneumonia
   g. Accelerated atherosclerosis
   h. Bleeding diathesis
   i. Peptic ulcers
   j. Seizures, stupor, and coma

Prognosis

1. Acute renal failure: The mortality rate exceeds 50 percent; 15 to 35 percent are inpatients in intensive care units. Risk increases as the number of related medical problems, including other organ failure, increases.
2. Chronic renal failure: The mortality rate without dialysis

Procedure 26-3
Assisting with Renal Transplantation

Definition/Purpose	Replacement of 1 kidney with a donor organ from a living or cadaverous donor sustains life in a patient with end-stage renal disease as an alternative to routine dialysis.
Contraindications/Cautions	Age younger than 4 or older than 70 years, advanced uncorrectable cardiac disease, malignant neoplasms, active vasculitis, extreme obesity, severe psychiatric disorders, and history of intravenous drug abuse are contraindications.
Learning/Teaching Activities	Assist the patient to feel "ready" to receive the transplanted organ by reviewing the cause of the original failure, including bilateral nephrectomy that removed native kidneys serving as a focus of persistent infection or systemic illness leading to failure such as systemic lupus erythematosus and Goodpasture's syndrome.
Teach the patient about the procedure and necessary posttransplant lifestyle changes.
Counsel the patient on the need to stop smoking before surgery to minimize the risk of posttransplant pulmonary infection.
Carefully evaluate patients with noncompliant behavior related to dialysis before surgery. Discuss the need for compliance with posttransplant procedures and routines.

Preliminary Activities

Equipment	See Chapter 13.
Assessment/Planning	• Assess for and plan nursing intervention for other conditions that increase risks of transplant or mitigate its success, including voiding dysfunction or bladder outlet obstruction that contribute to renal distress, severe vesicoureteral reflux, aggressive or nonactive tuberculosis (increases risk of pulmonary infection following transplant), peptic ulcers (posttransplant steroids increase risk of gastrointestinal distress from active ulcers), liver disease, including cirrhosis and hepatitis, and active infections.
• Assist with determining cardiovascular system readiness (patency of iliac vessels, overall cardiac function, and severity of atherosclerotic disease and coronary artery disease, which may be particularly severe in diabetic patients).
• Plan for nursing management of diabetes or other chronic illnesses, including careful neurologic monitoring for seizure disorders immediately after surgery. Remind patient that combined pancreatic-kidney transplant may be performed in diabetic persons, if indicated. Instruct the patient as appropriate. Monitor for hyperglycemia or accelerated atherosclerotic changes in diabetic patients.
• Review laboratory values to ensure acceptable levels before transplant surgery, including serum creatinine of more than 5 mg/dl, blood area nitrogen (BUN) of more than 70 mg/dl, and creatinine clearance of more than 15 ml per minute.
• Schedule assessment procedures several weeks ahead of the transplant operation if possible. Because the availability of the transplant organ cannot be predicted, the transplantation team must be flexible in its scheduling of evaluation procedures.

Procedure

Action	Rationale/Discussion
1. The kidney is removed from a living or cadaverous donor.	1. See text.
2. The transplanted kidney is placed in the anterior iliac fossa. The kidney is oriented to place the renal artery anterior and the vein posterior.	2. This placement allows for simpler reanastomosis of the kidney vasculature and ureter and minimizes manipulation of bowel, postoperative discomfort, and risk of peritonitis.
3. The renal artery and vein are anastomosed to the external iliac or hypogastric artery and veins. The ureter is implanted into the bladder (ureteroneocystostomy) in a nonrefluxing (or occasionally refluxing) manner; or, the ureter is anastomosed to the recipient's native ureter (ureteroureterostomy).	

Final Postoperative Activities

Activity	Rationale/Discussion
1. Evaluate renal function on a continuous basis.	1. Areas to monitor include BUN, serum creatinine, urine creatinine clearance, fluid status (blood pressure, edema, fluid intake, and urinary

(continued)

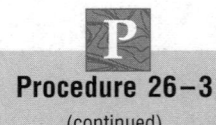

Procedure 26-3

(continued)

Final Postoperative Activities

Activity	Rationale/Discussion
	output), radionuclide renal scans (1st postoperative day and as indicated after this baseline study), and renal biopsy as indicated when other variables indicate possible rejection of the organ.
2. Provide adequate fluid intake.	2. This minimizes the risk of occlusion or infection and encourages spontaneous voiding after catheter removal.
3. Maintain catheter to bedside drainage only as long as needed.	3. The catheter allows monitoring of urinary output and prevents retention. When the risk of urinary retention has passed, discontinue the catheter in early morning (approximately 2:00 A.M.) to minimize the risk of retention. Reinsert the catheter or teach intermittent catheterization as directed if the patient cannot urinate.
4. Monitor urine characteristics.	4. Pink-tinged output is normal. Notify the physician of the presence of bright red bleeding or clots that may indicate loss of anastomotic integrity.
5. Limit the patient's sitting upright.	5. A 90-degree angle may kink the ureter and obstruct urinary outflow.
6. Observe the patient for fluid and electrolyte imbalances; manage any apparent imbalances.	6. For hypokalemia, hyponatremia, and hypovolemia resulting from osmotic diuresis, administer replacement fluids and electrolytes as indicated. For fluid overload, hypertension, congestive heart failure, or pulmonary edema related to rejection, acute tubular necrosis, or technical complications, monitor urinary output and administer diuretics as indicated; prepare the patient for surgery if necessary.
7. Discontinue intravenous fluids and restart oral fluids as bowel function return.	7. Administer stool softeners as needed; constipation is often exacerbated by surgical manipulation of the sigmoid colon.
8. Administer immunosuppressive drugs as indicated.	8. See Chapter 21.
9. Arrange for psychiatric evaluation, if indicated.	9. Steroids may exacerbate psychosis and paranoia.
10. Monitor for signs and symptoms of organ rejection: • Oliguria or anuria • Fever (may be masked by steroid effect) • Boggy, tender kidney on palpation • Fluid retention with weight gain and hypertension • Malaise • Changes in renal function measured by urine and serum studies • Changes noted on biopsy and radionuclide scans	10. Promptly manage rejection syndrome to prevent rejection of transplant organ.

or transplantation approaches 100 percent. With dialysis and ongoing care, prognosis is 25 years and more. Uncontrolled diabetes increases the risk of dangerous complications.

Applying the Nursing Process

NURSING DIAGNOSIS: Altered nutrition R/T chronic renal failure

1. *Expected outcomes:* Following intervention, the person should be able to do the following:
   a. Maintain adequate nutritional intake
   b. Prevent complications secondary to nutritional deficits
2. *Nursing interventions*
   a. In conjunction with the physician, nutritionist, and patient, design a diet to meet the following goals:

   (1) Prevent hypervolemia and hypertension
   (2) Prevent catabolism
   (3) Prevent dangerous electrolyte imbalances
   b. Diet, to be determined in consultation with the nutritionist and physician, should be defined by allowances of sodium, potassium, calories, and fluids. (The individual prescription for diet varies according to the specific conditions of the patient.)

NURSING DIAGNOSIS: Altered skin integrity R/T chronic renal failure

1. *Expected outcomes:* Following intervention and instruction, the person should be able to do the following:
   a. Prevent changes in skin integrity
   b. Avoid complications related to development of pressure ulcers

KIDNEY TRANSPLANT

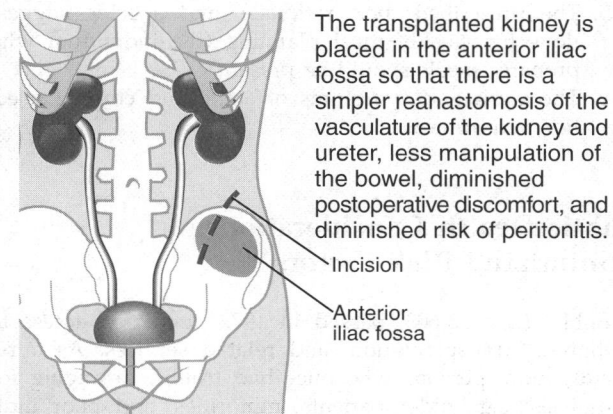

The transplanted kidney is placed in the anterior iliac fossa so that there is a simpler reanastomosis of the vasculature of the kidney and ureter, less manipulation of the bowel, diminished postoperative discomfort, and diminished risk of peritonitis.

Incision

Anterior iliac fossa

The kidney is oriented to place the renal artery anteriorly, the renal vein posteriorly. The renal artery and vein are anastomosed to the external iliac or hypogastric artery and veins. The ureter is implanted into the bladder (a ureteroneocystostomy) in a nonrefluxing or occasionally refluxing manner; or the ureter is anastomosed to the recipient's native ureter (a ureteroureterostomy).

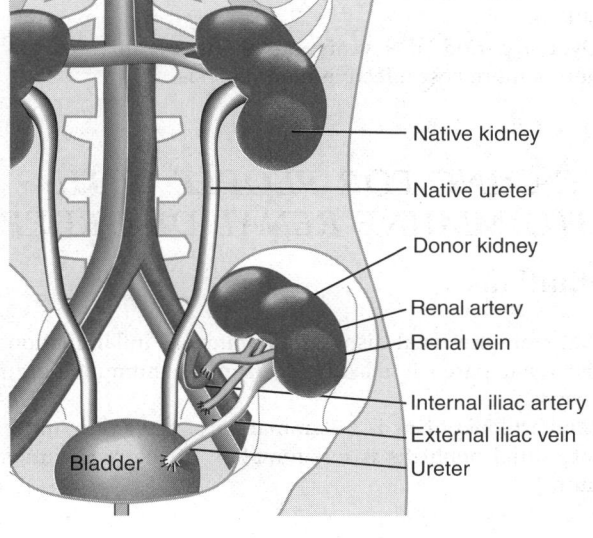

Native kidney

Native ureter

Donor kidney

Renal artery

Renal vein

Internal iliac artery

External iliac vein

Ureter

Bladder

Figure 26–14.

2. *Nursing interventions*
   a. Teach the patient proper skin care.
      (1) Regular bathing is essential, but soap should be used sparingly.
      (2) Encourage use of bath oils and lotions to prevent overdrying of skin.
      (3) Shampooing should be limited to minimize drying of hair.
   b. Turn and reposition bed-ridden patients frequently and use pressure relief or reduction devices (see Chapter 7).
   c. Control phosphate levels to reduce calcium deposition and itching.

d. Administer antipruritic medications as ordered.
e. Maintain short cuticles.

NURSING DIAGNOSIS: Fluid volume excess R/T chronic renal failure

1. *Expected outcomes:* Following intervention, the person should be able to do the following:
   a. Adhere to a fluid regimen
   b. Identify sources of excess fluid and electrolytes
   c. Prevent complications related to fluid volume excess
2. *Nursing interventions*
   a. Restrict fluids to total urine output plus 500 to 600 ml per day to account for insensible losses.
   b. Explain the importance of adherence to the prescribed diet to prevent intake of excessive fluids or electrolytes from food or beverages.
   c. Administer dialysis, as ordered, to remove excessive fluids and associated electrolytes.

NURSING DIAGNOSIS: Altered cardiovascular tissue perfusion R/T chronic renal failure

1. *Expected outcomes:* Following intervention, the person should be able to do the following:
   a. Identify symptoms and discuss treatment of hyperkalemia
   b. Self-administer antihypertensives
   c. Adhere to a dietary regimen
2. *Nursing interventions*
   a. Monitor vital signs, especially the pulse.
   b. Monitor serum potassium and electrocardiographic changes.
   c. If significant hyperkalemia occurs (>6.5 mEq/L), promptly administer medications, as ordered.
      (1) For severe hyperkalemia, administer hypertonic glucose and regular insulin to move potassium into the intracellular space, sodium bicarbonate to reduce metabolic acidosis, calcium gluconate to minimize cardiac effects, and sodium polystyrene sulfonate (Kayolexate) to reduce potassium levels.
      (2) For moderate hyperkalemia, administer sodium polystyrene to reduce potassium.
   d. Administer antihypertensive medications, as ordered. Explain the administration schedule.
   e. Alter antihypertensive medication dosages before dialysis, as ordered—fluid removal may reduce blood pressure significantly.
   f. In conjunction with the physician, nutritionist, and patient, develop a diet that restricts fluids, dietary sodium, and potassium intake. The diet should also be low in dietary fats and cholesterol to prevent accelerated atherosclerotic changes associated with renal failure.

NURSING DIAGNOSIS: Altered tissue perfusion, generalized R/T anemia

1. *Expected outcomes:* Following counseling and intervention, the person should be able to do the following:
   a. Discuss signs, symptoms, and treatment of anemia
   b. Use supplements to prevent anemia
2. *Nursing interventions*
   a. Explain the causes of anemia, its indications, and treatment.
   b. Take precautions to prevent anemia:
      (1) Avoid unnecessary venipuncture for diagnostic tests.
      (2) Rinse dialyzer thoroughly to avoid excessive hemolysis.
   c. Provide iron and folic acid supplements, as ordered.
   d. Give blood transfusions, as ordered, for severe anemia.
   e. Administer erythropoietin, as ordered, to encourage production of erythrocytes.

NURSING DIAGNOSIS: Altered gastrointestinal tissue perfusion R/T chronic renal failure

---

1. *Expected outcomes:* Following interventions, the person should be able to do the following:
   a. Discuss potential gastrointestinal symptoms
   b. Prevent gastrointestinal complications
   c. Design and adhere to a dietary regimen that reduces potential for nausea, vomiting, and constipation
2. *Nursing interventions*
   a. Administer antiemetics, as ordered, for severe nausea and vomiting.
   b. Alter oral hygiene as indicated. Use a soft-bristled toothbrush and oral rinses to minimize the risk of ulceration.
   c. Give small, bland meals and avoid giving early morning meals to reduce nausea and anorexia.
   d. Encourage adequate dietary fiber and fluid intake.
   e. Administer stool softeners, as ordered.
   f. Avoid using magnesium-containing enemas when removing impaction.

Discharge Planning and Teaching

1. After the initial diagnosis and institution of dialysis, instruct patient and family regarding the following:
   a. Prescribed medications and their actions, dosages, administration, and common side effects
   b. Prescribed diet, including rationale and specific suggestions for weekly meal planning (the individual who prepares meals should be present)
   c. Access site care for hemodialysis or peritoneal dialysis, including prevention and management of complications
   d. Principles of dialysis, with specific instruction for use of all home dialysis equipment (other persons who are likely to assist with the patient's care should be present)
2. After renal transplantation, teach the patient and family about the following:

   a. The action of immunosuppressive medications and their administration, dosages, and common side effects (see Chapter 21)
   b. The prescribed diet, rationale, and specific suggestions for weekly meal planning (the individual who prepares meals should be present)
   c. The signs and symptoms of acute and chronic rejection syndromes

Public Health Considerations: Minimizing Risk Factors

1. Public Law 92-603, passed in 1972, increased access to dialysis, transplantation, and related services. As a result, more persons who once had trouble arranging for dialysis (e.g., older patients, minorities, and poor individuals) make up a greater percentage of persons on dialysis.
2. Dialysis facilities and transplant services have grown proportionally with greater access to care, increasing from less than 200 dialysis centers in the United States before 1972 to more than 1000 in 1990.
3. Total costs incurred by the Medicare population with renal failure for 1996 are projected to be more than $4 billion.
4. Over a period of 9 years, successful organ transplantation is more cost effective than dialysis.

■ CARING FOR PEOPLE WITH AUTOIMMUNE RENAL DISORDERS

Definitions

1. Autoimmune renal disorders manifest as inflammation of the renal parenchyma arising from an immunologic response.
2. Glomerulonephritis is inflammation of the glomeruli.
3. Interstitial nephritis is inflammation of the renal interstitium.

Incidence and Socioeconomic Impact

1. Approximately 5 percent of all streptococcal infections produce acute poststreptococcal glomerulonephritis; 5 percent progress to irreversible renal failure.
2. Chronic glomerulonephritis is the most common cause of chronic renal failure in adults.
3. Interstitial nephritis is the 2nd leading cause of chronic renal failure in adults.
4. Immune complex glomerulonephritis accounts for approximately 90 percent of all cases of glomerulonephritis in adults.
5. Antiglomerular basement membrane glomerulonephritis accounts for approximately 5 percent of all cases of glomerulonephritis in adults.

Risk Factors

1. Systemic autoimmune disorders
   a. Systemic lupus erythematosus
   b. Goodpasture's syndrome (pulmonary-renal hypersensitivity disorder of unknown etiology), especially in antiglomerular basement membrane glomerulonephritis
2. Bacterial infections caused by the following:
   a. Group A β-hemolytic streptococci
   b. Staphylococci
   c. *Treponema pallidum*
3. Viral illnesses
   a. Mumps
   b. Measles
   c. Hepatitis β virus infection
   d. Epstein-Barr virus infection
   e. Coxsackie virus infection
4. Pharmacologic agents, including the following:
   a. Penicillins—ampicillin, methicillin
   b. Penicillamine
   c. Phenindione
   d. Sulfonamides
   e. Phenytoin
5. Parasitic illnesses
   a. Schistosomiasis
   b. Malaria

Etiology and Pathophysiology

1. Etiology is unknown.
2. In immune complex glomerulonephritis, endogenous or exogenous antigens in the bloodstream stimulate antibody synthesis, creating an antibody-antigen complex deposited in the glomerular capillary. Release of immunologic agents damages the glomerulus and increases permeability, with severity dependent on the number of glomeruli injured.
3. In antiglomerular basement membrane glomerulonephritis, antibodies act directly at the glomerular basement membrane.
4. In interstitial nephritis, autoimmune cascade causes inflammation of the renal interstitium; antibodies are commonly observed in the renal tubular basement membrane. During the acute phase, renal function declines precipitously. The disorder progresses with few clinical manifestations. The resolution of symptoms leaves a scarred, dysplastic kidney with poor ability to concentrate urine. Endocrine functions of the kidney are often affected as follows:
   a. Renin-mediated hypertension
   b. Erythopoietin-mediated anemia
   c. Insufficiency of cholecalciferol with abnormal calcium-phosphorous metabolism

Clinical Manifestations

1. Gross or microscopic hematuria
2. Hypertension

3. Renal failure (acute and chronic)
4. Proteinuria
5. Edema with hypoalbuminemia, hypercholesterolemia
6. Anemia

Diagnostics

1. Assess for signs of the following:
   a. Headache, malaise, fever, and chills
   b. Nausea and vomiting
   c. Flank pain
   d. Skin rash
2. Urinalysis
   a. Glomerulonephritis is characterized by the following:
      (1) Dark brown or rust colored urine
      (2) Gross or microscopic hematuria
      (3) Red blood cell casts
      (4) Proteinuria
   b. Interstitial nephritis is characterized by the following:
      (1) Sterile pyuria
      (2) Hematuria (gross or microscopic)
      (3) Eosinophilic casts
      (4) Low specific gravity
3. Serum studies
   a. In glomerulonephritis, studies show the following:
      (1) Low serum albumin
      (2) High serum lipids
      (3) Increased serum creatinine and BUN
      (4) Low hematocrit and hemoglobin
      (5) Diminished creatinine clearance
   b. In interstitial nephritis, eosinophilia is shown.
   c. Renal biopsy shows the following:
      (1) Pathologic changes on light and electron microscopic examination
      (2) Presence of complement C3, IgG, IgM, or other antibody deposits with immunofluorescent staining

Clinical Management

1. Goals of clinical management
   a. Prevent complications
   b. Promote kidney function
2. Nonpharmacologic interventions
   a. Restriction of dietary protein when BUN is elevated or oliguria is present
   b. Bed rest during acute illness
3. Pharmacologic interventions
   a. Corticosteroid or immunosuppressive therapy administered only in specific cases of glomerulonephritis associated with the following:
      (1) Systemic lupus erythematosus
      (2) Goodpasture's syndrome
   b. Antibiotic therapy for residual infection, acute post-streptococcal glomerulonephritis, or interstitial nephritis with bacterial infection
   c. Various medications to manage symptoms of associated systemic illness and complications
4. Special medical-surgical procedures include dialysis (see p. 1191) if fluid retention and uremia are not otherwise controlled.

Complications

1. Fluid overload may occur with pulmonary edema and congestive heart failure.
2. Seizures
3. Irreversible, chronic renal failure

Prognosis

1. In acute poststreptococcal glomerulonephritis, 95 percent of patients recover renal function that lasts for decades.
2. In glomerulonephritis of unknown cause, there is significant risk of acute or chronic renal failure; routine follow-up is required over the years.
3. In rapidly progressive glomerulonephritis, renal failure occurs within weeks to months.
4. In glomerulonephritis with Goodpasture's syndrome, irreversible renal failure occurs within months to years.
5. In interstitial nephritis, approximately 15 percent of cases progress to acute renal failure.

Applying the Nursing Process

NURSING DIAGNOSIS: Altered renal tissue perfusion R/T glomerulonephritis

1. *Expected outcomes:* Following interventions, the person should be able to do the following:
   a. Avoid complications associated with glomerular inflammation
   b. Maintain adequate fluid and electrolyte balance
2. *Nursing interventions*
   a. Teach the person to self-administer medications to reverse glomerular inflammation.
   b. Closely monitor urine function as follows:
      (1) Urine output versus intake
      (2) Serum creatinine and BUN
      (3) Urine creatinine clearance
      (4) Hematocrit, hemoglobin
      (5) Serum potassium, sodium
      (6) Serum calcium, serum phosphate
   c. Administer dialysis, as ordered.

NURSING DIAGNOSIS: Fluid volume excess R/T glomerulonephritis

1. *Expected outcomes:* Following intervention, the person should be able to do the following:
   a. Maintain adequate fluid and electrolyte balance
   b. Recognize and report signs and symptoms of fluid overload
   c. Self-administer medications
2. *Nursing interventions*
   a. Teach the patient to self-monitor for symptoms of fluid overload as follows:
      (1) Hypertension

(2) Peripheral edema, bulging of neck veins
(3) Weight gain
(4) Signs of congestive heart failure or pulmonary edema
(5) Central venous pressure
   b. Teach the patient to limit fluid, sodium, and potassium intake.
   c. Administer diuretic medications, as ordered.
   d. Administer cardiac glycosides, as ordered.

NURSING DIAGNOSIS: Fluid volume deficit R/T early-stage interstitial nephritis

1. *Expected outcomes:* Following intervention, the person should be able to do the following:
   a. Maintain adequate fluid and electrolyte balance
   b. Recognize and report signs and symptoms of fluid deficit
   c. Self-administer medications
2. *Nursing interventions*
   a. Teach the patient to self-assess for signs of dehydration.
   b. Instruct the patient in monitoring urinary output versus fluid intake.
   c. Administer oral or intravenous fluids, as ordered.

NURSING DIAGNOSIS: Altered nutrition, less than body requirements, R/T glomerulonephritis with proteinuria

1. *Expected outcomes:* Following interventions, the person should be able to do the following:
   a. Assess changes in body weight and maintain body requirements
   b. Discuss the importance of maintaining adequate nutritional supplementation
   c. Self-administer dietary supplements
2. *Nursing interventions*
   a. Assess for signs of protein-based nutritional deficit (e.g., weight loss, low total protein intake, or hypoalbuminemia).
   b. Encourage dietary protein intake of approximately 1 mg per kg of body weight plus the volume lost in 24-hour urine.
   c. Teach the patient to monitor fluid intake.
   d. Provide nutritional supplements or parenteral nutrition, as ordered, for severe deficits caused by nausea and vomiting.

NURSING DIAGNOSIS: Risk for infection R/T glomerulonephritis

1. *Expected outcomes:* Following intervention, the person should be able to do the following:
   a. Avoid complications associated with urinary tract infections
   b. Recognize signs and symptoms of infection
   c. Describe ways to prevent infection
   d. Self-administer medications

2. *Nursing interventions*
   a. Assess the patient for signs of urinary tract infection, and teach the patient the following signs:
      (1) Cloudy, odorous urine
      (2) Dysuria, suprapubic discomfort
      (3) Fever, nausea, flank pain with upper urinary tract involvement
   b. Administer prophylactic or therapeutic antibiotic agents, as ordered.
   c. Explain how to prevent urinary tract infections.

Discharge Planning and Teaching

1. Review renal function status.
2. Explain the need to monitor renal function on an ongoing basis. Emphasize the significance of follow-up blood, urine, and imaging studies.
3. Describe the need for ongoing monitoring of blood pressure following cases of interstitial nephritis.
4. Teach specific strategies to prevent further loss of renal function, including dietary alterations.
5. Encourage close follow-up and management of systemic autoimmune disorder to prevent recurrent glomerulonephritis.

Public Health Considerations: Minimizing Risk Factors

1. Pharyngitis and other streptococcal infections should be aggressively treated to reduce the risk of poststreptococcal glomerulonephritis.
2. Ongoing monitoring of renal function and dietary control may reduce the number of patients whose disease progresses to chronic renal failure or it may slow the rate of progression.

◼ CARING FOR PEOPLE WITH METABOLIC RENAL DISORDERS

Definitions

1. Metabolic renal disorders are abnormalities of renal function that disturb internal homeostasis.
2. Renal tubular acidosis (RTA) is a metabolic disorder of the renal tubule predisposing the person to metabolic acidosis excretion from a distal tubule defect; it is most common in children with predisposing factors.
3. Nephrotic syndrome is a cluster of symptoms primarily related to excessive loss of protein (particularly albumin) in the urine, with generalized edema, hyperlipidemia, and lipiduria.

Risk Factors and Etiology

1. Renal tubular acidosis is associated with the following:
   a. Autosomal dominant or recessive or sex-linked recessive genetic predisposition

   b. Biliary cirrhosis
   c. Active hepatitis
   d. Obstructive uropathy
   e. Vitamin D intoxication
   f. Hypergammaglobulinemia
   g. Hyperparathyroidism
2. Nephrotic syndrome is associated with the following:
   a. Glomerulonephritis
   b. Diabetic nephropathy
   c. Pharmacologic agents
   d. Allergic response to toxic or natural substances such as pollens, insect stings, and poison ivy

Pathophysiology

1. Type 1 RTA (most common form)
   a. A defect in the distal tubule causes the hydrogen secretion mechanism to fail. Kidney cannot acidify urine.
   b. Retained ions cause metabolic acidosis.
   c. Hydrogen-sodium ionic exchange decreases and sodium-potassium exchange increases, causing lowered serum pH, hypokalemia, and hypovolemia.
   d. The body pulls calcium from bones to neutralize excess endogenous acids, causing hypercalcemia and hypercalciuria with demineralization of bone.
2. Type 2 RTA
   a. Failure of hydrogen ion secretion in the proximal tubule causes failure of the bicarbonate exchange process. Excess is excreted in urine.
   b. Excess hydrogen ions produce metabolic acidosis, with metabolic consequences similar to those in Type 1 RTA.
3. Type 4 RTA (no type 3)
   a. Aldosterone deficiency (hypoaldosteronism) or target tissue (renal tubule) resistance to aldosterone causes diminished exchange of hydrogen ions for sodium and reduces potassium excretion.
   b. Hyperkalemia acidosis results.
4. Nephrotic syndrome
   a. Excessive protein loss in the kidney causes abnormal catabolism of albumin.
   b. Altered permeability of basement membrane allows greater filtration of smaller proteins (i.e., albumin).
   c. Reduction of net electrical charge within the glomerular capillary promotes protein losses and proteinuria.
   d. Resulting hypoalbuminemia causes edema.
      (1) Reduced oncontic pressure drives water from vascular to extracellular spaces.
      (2) Loss of water and sodium from vascular spaces stimulates the renin-angiotensin system. The resulting fluid retention exacerbates edema, because additional fluid is rapidly lost from the vascular space.

Clinical Manifestations

1. Renal tubular acidosis is characterized by the following:
   a. Weakness and lethargy
   b. Hyperventilation

c. Obstructive symptoms due to calculi formation (see p. 1210)
d. Incidental finding of nephrocalcinosis on radiographic studies
2. Nephrotic syndrome is characterized by the following:
   a. Generalized edema, with weight gain and pitting edema of the extremities and around the eyes
   b. Oliguria, frothy urine, or fat cells floating in urine
   c. Fatigue
   d. Nausea and vomiting

Diagnostics

1. Renal tubular acidosis
   a. Urinalysis reveals the following:
      (1) pH greater than 5.5 despite metabolic acidosis
      (2) First morning urine pH greater than 5.5
      (3) Hypercalciuria
   b. Serum studies confirm diagnosis of metabolic acidosis.
   c. An acid load test is performed when metabolic acidosis is not apparent with random serum tests.
   d. Kidney, ureter, and bladder (KUB) or intravenous pyelogram (IVP) is used to assess urinary calculi (nephrocalcinosis on KUB in type 1 RTA)
   e. Urinary citrate excretion test distinguishes RTA types 1 (low citrate levels) and 2 (high citrate levels)
   f. Serum aldosterone testing reveals hyperkalemia with hypoaldosteronism in type 4 RTA.
2. Nephrotic syndrome
   a. Urinalysis reveals proteinuria and lipiduria, with a total protein measurement of greater than 3 to 5 gm per day
   b. Serum studies measure albumin and vitamin D levels; serum albumin is less than 30 gm per liter

Clinical Management

1. The goal of clinical management is to control metabolic acidosis.
2. Nonpharmacologic interventions
   a. Potassium supplements for RTA
   b. In nephrotic syndrome
      (1) Increased dietary protein unless GFR is compromised
      (2) Limited sodium intake
      (3) Adequate caloric intake to offset accelerated protein catabolism
      (4) Protein diet supplements
      (5) Adequate fluid intake
      (6) Small, easily digested meals with oral hygiene before eating to reduce nausea
3. Pharmacologic interventions
   a. RTA
      (1) Control of metabolic acidosis by binding hydrogen ions in the vascular space with bicarbonate
      (2) Citrate solution to minimize gastrointestinal upset and distention
      (3) Potassium citrate solution as an alternative to bicarbonate or citrate solutions

      (4) Alkalinizing drugs as indicated
      (5) Thiazide diuretics to enhance proximal tubular reabsorption in type 2 RTA
   b. Nephrotic syndrome
      (1) Immunosuppressive agents for inflammation (e.g., prednisone, azathioprine, chlorambucil, and antineoplastic agents such as cyclophosphamide)
      (2) Suppressive or therapeutic antibiotics for bacterial infection
      (3) Diuretics to alleviate fluid overload
      (4) Albumin to increase plasma oncotic pressure and replace losses

Complications

1. Metabolic acidosis
2. Osteomalacia (with RTA)
3. Urinary calculi (particularly in type 1 RTA)
4. Infection
5. Atherosclerosis
6. Renal vein thrombosis (in nephrotic syndrome)
7. Sepsis
8. Acute or chronic renal failure
9. Venous thrombosis

Prognosis

1. Renal tubular acidosis is incurable, but the prognosis is good with proper management of acidosis and associated symptoms.
2. Nephrotic syndrome
   a. Minimal change syndrome responds to therapy with recovery of renal function.
   b. Severe change syndrome typically progresses to renal failure.
   c. Sepsis is a serious, potentially fatal complication of nephrotic syndrome.

Applying the Nursing Process

NURSING DIAGNOSIS: Excess fluid volume R/T RTA

1. *Expected outcomes:* Following intervention, the person should be able to do the following:
   a. Maintain adequate fluid and electrolyte balance
   b. Recognize and report signs and symptoms of fluid overload.
   c. Self-administer medications
2. *Nursing interventions*
   a. Teach the patient to self-monitor fluid volume homeostasis for evidence of fluid overload, including home monitoring for blood pressure, signs of peripheral edema, abdominal ascites, signs of pulmonary edema, and changes in daily weight, and to limit sodium and fluid intake.

b. Monitor urine protein, specific gravity and serum protein, albumin, and hematocrit for evidence of reduced plasma oncotic pressure.

c. Administer diuretics, albumin, or both, as ordered.

NURSING DIAGNOSIS: Altered nutrition, less than body requirements, R/T acidosis

---

1. *Expected outcomes:* Following intervention, the person should be able to do the following:
   a. Maintain adequate nutritional intake
   b. Adhere to dietary regimen
   c. Describe signs and symptoms of poor nutritional balance
2. *Nursing interventions*
   a. Working with the physician, nutritionist, and patient, develop a diet plan that includes adequate calories and protein.
   b. Monitor laboratory data (e.g., total protein) for adequacy of dietary plan.
   c. Provide protein dietary supplements, as ordered.

NURSING DIAGNOSIS: Altered renal tissue perfusion R/T acidosis

---

1. *Expected outcomes:* Following instruction, the person should be able to do the following:
   a. Describe signs and symptoms of urinary tract infection
   b. Identify signs of renal failure
   c. Maintain adequate urine output
   d. Prevent development of complications
2. *Nursing interventions*
   a. Monitor for signs of renal failure (see p. 1188).
   b. Administer immunosuppressive agents, as ordered. Monitor the patient for evidence of infection while on immunosuppressive therapy, including monitoring temperature and urine culture and watching for altered wound healing.
   c. Teach the patient to reduce the risk of infection by avoiding persons with communicable diseases (e.g., upper respiratory infections).

NURSING DIAGNOSIS: Altered peripheral tissue perfusion R/T to hypovolemia

---

1. *Expected outcomes:* Following intervention, the person should be able to do the following:
   a. Remain free of thrombosis
   b. Recognize signs of altered tissue perfusion
   c. Discuss the importance of anticoagulant therapy and preventing thrombosis
   d. Self-administer anticoagulants
2. *Nursing interventions*
   a. Monitor extremities for evidence of thrombosis related to fluid shift from the vascular space with "thickening" of blood.

b. Monitor hematocrit, hemoglobin, and blood clotting studies.

c. Provide maximal hydration.

d. Administer anticoagulants, as ordered. Demonstrate proper administration procedures and have the patient perform a return demonstration.

e. Explain the purpose and importance of anticoagulant therapy in preventing thrombosis.

NURSING DIAGNOSIS: Body image disturbance R/T to generalized edema

---

1. *Expected outcomes:* Following interventions, the person should be able to do the following:
   a. Identify changes in body image related to generalized edema
   b. Express concerns regarding body image
   c. Identify support groups and caregivers appropriate for psychologic assistance and advice
2. *Nursing interventions*
   a. Discuss body image changes caused by the edema with the patient and the patient's family.
   b. Encourage the patient to express feelings related to the change in body appearance.
   c. Emphasize reversibility of the changes with treatment and recovery of renal function.
   d. Provide information on support groups. Refer complex problems to a psychologist or psychiatrist.

Discharge Planning and Teaching

1. Explain the nature of metabolic renal disorder and its relationship to current symptoms.
2. Teach the patient to collect urine specimens and evaluate the urine for pH, calcium, and protein.
3. Make sure the patient understands medication dosages, administration methods and schedule, and side effects.
4. Describe complications of metabolic disorders and preventive and management strategies.
5. Emphasize the potential for relapse of symptoms and the necessity of prompt care.
6. Gently introduce the possibility of renal failure and the significance of ongoing evaluation of renal function.

Public Health Considerations: Minimizing Risks

Adequate control of diabetes may reduce the risk of nephrotic syndrome.

◼ CARING FOR PEOPLE WITH RENOVASCULAR DISORDERS

Definitions

1. Renovascular disorders involve compromised renal function related to vascular disorders.

2. Nephrosclerosis is damage to the renal vascular system related to prolonged elevations of blood pressure; changes may be rapid (occurring over months, rather than years) if hypertension is malignant, with precipitous changes in blood pressure.
3. Renal artery stenosis (and occlusion) or renal vein thrombosis is the narrowing of the renal artery or vein.

Incidence and Socioeconomic Impact

1. Primary hypertension of unknown cause accounts for approximately 90 percent of all affected individuals. Risk of nephrosclerosis increases with severity and duration.
2. Secondary hypertension accounts for approximately 10 percent of affected individuals; 80 percent is attributable to renal causes, but only a small portion is attributable to vascular stenosis or thrombosis.

Risk Factors

1. Nephrosclerosis
2. Risk factors for renal artery stenosis or renal vein thrombosis
   a. Arteriosclerotic disease
   b. Fibromuscular disease
   c. Nephrotic syndrome

Etiology

1. Nephrosclerosis is due to renal deterioration and hypertension.
2. Renal artery stenosis is due to congenital or acquired occlusion of unilateral or bilateral renal artery or fibromuscular vascular disease affecting the renal artery.
3. Renal artery occlusion is due to embolus from myocardial infarction, mitral valve stenosis, or subacute endocarditis. (It may result from congenital defect.)
4. Renal vein thrombosis is due to thrombus from dehydration, sepsis, or invasive tumor causing partial obstruction.

Pathophysiology

1. Nephrosclerotic changes occur over years of untreated or poorly controlled hypertension, which causes the following:
   a. Arterial spasms and thickening with subsequent hypertrophy
   b. Hyaline degeneration of the renal arterial system
2. In renal artery stenosis, ischemia to glomerulus stimulates secretion of renin, raising systemic blood pressure. The contralateral kidney is affected (nephrosclerosis) as is the entire body (secondary hypertension).
3. Renal artery occlusion causes cessation of blood flow with coagulation necrosis of the affected kidney; acute renal failure ensues in persons with a solitary kidney, single functioning kidney, or bilateral occlusion.

Clinical Manifestations

1. Nephrosclerosis is characterized by elevated blood pressure with headache, dizziness, fatigue, palpitations, and blurred vision.
2. Renal artery stenosis and renal vein thrombosis are characterized by the following:
   a. Severe flank pain
   b. Hypertension with associated findings

Diagnostics

1. Assessment
   a. Check blood pressure for presence of hypertension.
   b. Auscultate abdomen for bruits with renal artery stenosis.
   c. Intravenous pyelogram may show a small kidney, parenchymal thickening, and delayed excretion of contrast material.
   d. Rapid sequence pyelography detects unilateral renovascular disease.
   e. Diethylenetriamine pentaacetic acid (DTPA) radionuclide renal scan determines comparative perfusion.
   f. Special tests include renal arteriography for renal stenosis and renal venography for thrombus.
2. Medical diagnosis
   a. In nephrosclerosis, findings include hypertension with proteinuria, elevated BUN, serum creatinine, and positive renal biopsy.
   b. In renal artery stenosis, findings include narrowed segment on imaging study or unilateral perfusion reduction on radionuclide scan.
   c. In renal vein thrombosis, findings include filling defect on renal venography and perfusion anomalies on radionuclide scan.

Clinical Management

1. Goals of clinical management
   a. Control blood pressure to slow renal deterioration
   b. Delay renal failure
2. Management of nephrosclerosis
   a. Pharmacologic management of elevated blood pressure
   b. Behavioral management of hypertension by exercise and diet
3. Management of renal artery stenosis
   a. Pharmacologic management of hypertension, including use of angiotensin-converting enzyme inhibitors
   b. Anticoagulation therapy in some cases
   a. Transmural balloon dilation
   b. Vascular reconstruction in selected cases, including aortorenal bypass and autogenous renal artery bypass
   c. Nephrectomy for nonfunctioning, infection-prone kidney
4. Management of renal vein thrombosis includes anticoagulation therapy.

Complications

1. Chronic renal failure
2. Death

Prognosis

1. Rapid, appropriate intervention results in approximately 50 percent cure or improvement.
2. Progression of symptoms occurs when renal function is severely compromised before discovery of disease or when therapy for residual hypertension is not continued.

Applying the Nursing Process

NURSING DIAGNOSIS: Altered renal tissue perfusion R/T damage to nephrons

1. *Expected outcomes:* Following intervention, the person should be able to do the following:
   a. Reverse or improve hypertension
   b. Preserve renal function
   c. Prevent other complications of prolonged hypertension
2. *Nursing interventions*
   a. Determine and monitor renal function in consultation with the physician through the measurement of serum creatinine and BUN, and the use of radionuclide renal scan, intravenous pyelography, or nephrographic phase of contrast-enhanced arteriography.
   b. Administer anticoagulants, as ordered, to prevent or reduce thrombus or alleviate arterial occlusion.
   c. Administer antihypertensive medications to control hypertension and diminish the risk of nephrosclerosis.
   d. Teach the patient to manage fluid and sodium intake (consult the physician and nutritionist as needed).

NURSING DIAGNOSIS: Pain R/T renal vascular occlusion (see Chapter 11)

1. *Expected outcomes:* Following intervention, the person should be able to do the following:
   a. Control pain
   b. Institute alternative nonpharmacologic pain management techniques
   c. Self-administer pain medication
2. *Nursing interventions*
   a. Monitor location, character, duration, and intensity of pain.
      (1) Intense flank pain of long duration occurs in renal vascular occlusion.
      (2) Sudden exacerbation of pain occurs in acute occlusion in a partially compromised kidney.
   b. Administer narcotic or other analgesics, as ordered.

   c. Teach nonpharmacologic strategies to manage pain (see Chapter 11).

Discharge Planning and Teaching

1. Provide the patient with a detailed explanation of the relationship between renal function and chronically elevated blood pressure. Stress the need for ongoing administration of antihypertensives. Dispel the myth that resolution of symptoms of hypertension is a cure.
2. Emphasize the importance of ongoing health care follow-up and repeated evaluation of renal function to prevent or slow the progression of symptoms and the disorder.
3. Teach the administration, dosage, action, and potential side effects of all medications.
4. Explain the need for follow-up evaluation after transmural or surgical manipulation of renal artery stenosis or venous thrombosis.

Public Health Considerations: Minimizing Risk Factors

1. Nephrosclerosis, stroke, and other cardiovascular risk factors require aggressive public health programs to aggressively treat hypertension.
2. Careful screening for secondary causes of hypertension, including renovascular disorders, is vital, because 50 percent or more cases are cured or improved as a result.

◻ CARING FOR PEOPLE WITH URINARY SYSTEM INFECTIONS

Definitions and Classifications

1. Urinary system infection is any infection of the urinary tract that causes inflammation of that system.
2. Classification by location
   a. Urethritis is infection of the urethra.
   b. Cystitis is infection of the bladder.
   c. Pyelonephritis is infection of the upper urinary tract.
   d. Urosepsis is pyelonephritis with blood-borne infection.
3. Classification by symptoms
   a. Afebrile infection is confined to the lower urinary system (i.e., bladder, urethra).
   b. Febrile infection involves the upper urinary tract.
4. Classification by clinical course (particularly useful for recurrent urinary system infections in women)
   a. In first-time infection, the initial episode is of symptomatic bacteriuria.
   b. In recurrent infection, symptomatic bacteriuria recurs after successful resolution (as determined by culture) of a previous episode of infection.
   c. In persistent infection, bacteriuria persists despite appropriate antibiotic therapy.
   d. In unresolved infection, bacteriuria persists because of inappropriate or incomplete treatment.

Incidence and Socioeconomic Impact

1. Prevalence of urinary system infections is second only to respiratory infections.
2. Women have a 10 to 20 percent likelihood of experiencing at least 1 episode of symptomatic cystitis in their lifetime.
3. Incidence increases with institutionalization and repeated instrumentation of the urinary system.

Risk Factors

1. Urinary retention related to deficient detrusor contraction strength or bladder outlet obstruction or as neuropathic bladder dysfunction
2. Other risk factors
   • Hospitalization or institutionalization
   • Immobility
   • Indwelling catheter
   • Calculi or foreign body in bladder
   • Pregnancy
   • Dehydration
   • Sexual intercourse (more for women than for men)
   • Previous urinary infection

Etiology

1. Routes of infection include the ascending urethral route (most common) and the vascular route.
2. Pathogens
   • *Escherichia coli*
   • *Klebsiella pneumoniae*
   • *Pseudomonas aeruginosa*
   • *Proteus mirabilis*
3. Sources of pathogens
   a. Typically, pathogens originate from gastrointestinal (perianal) or vaginal flora.
   b. Iatrogenic sources are from urethral instrumentation and intravesical infusion and irrigation.

Pathophysiology

1. The pathogen enters the urinary system via the ascending urethral or vascular route.
2. Pathogenic reproduction overwhelms host defense mechanisms (see Chapter 8), including the following:
   a. Mechanical flushing of urine via micturition (bladder must completely evacuate urine and foreign objects, if any)
   b. Anti-infective properties of urine
   c. Polymorphonucleocyte response
3. The urinary system becomes inflamed.
   a. The bladder or urethral wall is invaded by polymorphonucleocytes.
   b. Polymorphonucleocytes occur in urine.
4. The severity of infection depends on the virulence of the pathogen and host immune response.

Clinical Manifestations

1. Urethritis
   a. Dysuria
   b. Urethral burning
   c. Discomfort between episodes of urination
2. Cystitis (afebrile infection)
   a. Irritative voiding symptoms
      (1) Diurnal frequency greater than 2 hours
      (2) Dysuria
      (3) Urgency to urinate
      (4) Urge incontinence in patients with such a predisposition
      (5) Suprapubic discomfort
   b. Hematuria (grossly visible or microscopic)
3. Pyelonephritis (febrile infection)
   a. Irritative voiding symptoms (see cystitis)
   b. Flank pain
   c. Fever (typically greater than 100 degrees Fahrenheit)
   d. Chills
   e. Nausea and vomiting

Diagnostics

1. Assessment
   a. History of current symptoms and predisposing factors
   b. Urethral swab culture and sensitivities
   c. Urine culture and sensitivities via
      (1) Clean-catch specimen (midstream preferred) (Procedure 26-4)
      (2) Catheterized specimen (sterile technique)
      (3) Suprapubic needle aspiration (most accurate)
   d. Blood specimen for culture and sensitivites
   e. Cystourethroscopy as indicated to detect the presence of foreign objects
   f. Imaging studies, including voiding cystourethroscopy and intravenous pyelography to determine the presence of calculi, diverticulae, or vesicoureteric reflux
   g. Urodynamic testing to determine the nature of associated voiding dysfunction
   h. Costovertebral angle tenderness with pyelonephritis
2. Medical diagnosis
   a. Urethritis
      (1) Purulent drainage from the urethra
      (2) Positive urethral swab culture
      (3) Coexistent bacteriuria
   b. Cystitis
      (1) Irritative voiding symptoms with or without hematuria
      (2) Detectable bacterial colony-forming units (CFU) in urine (some clinicians require greater than 100,000 CFU), or the presence of fungi or other pathogens in urine
   c. Pyelonephritis
      (1) Bacteriuria with irritative voiding symptoms
      (2) Fever greater than 100 degrees Fahrenheit
   d. Urosepsis
      (1) Bacteriuria with fever
      (2) Blood culture showing the same pathogen as in the urine culture

Procedure 26–4
Collection of a Midstream Clean
Catch Urine Specimen

Definition/Purpose	A midstream clean-catch urine specimen is routinely performed to rule out the presence of a urinary tract infection via Chemstrip urinalysis and microscopic analysis.
Contraindications/Cautions	The patient must be able to understand and follow directions precisely.
Learning/Teaching Activities	Remind the patient that the goal of the test is to determine whether bacteria are present in the urine. Thus, it is important that the test be performed as "clean" as possible so that other bacteria do not contaminate the specimen.
	Teach proper handwashing technique to be used before collection of urine.
	Explain the need for the patient to open the sterile container and place the lid of the container "upside down" on the counter. (Failure to do so will contaminate the specimen when the lid is replaced on the container.)
	Tell uncircumsized male patients to retract the foreskin before collecting the midstream urine.

Preliminary Activities

Equipment	• Sterile urine collection container
	• Antiseptic cleansing solution or soap
	• Antiseptic towelette
	• Label for collection container and pen or other implement with which to write on the label
Assessment/Planning	Ensure that the patient understands what do do.
Procedure	

Activities	Rationale/Discussion
1. Patients wash their hands thoroughly, remove the lid of the container and place it upside down on a counter, and use the towelette to clean the urethral meatus. Uncircumsized male patients retract the foreskin of the penis.	1. This reduces the risk of nonurinary bacteria contaminating the specimen.
2. The patient begins voiding normally into the toilet. After a small amount of urine has passed, the patient interrupts the stream and attempts to collect approximately 30 ml of urine in the container.	2. Not collecting the 1st portion of the urinary stream allows urine to flush out the urethra. It may be easier for females to sit facing the commode while collecting the specimen.
3. The patient replaces the lid on the container, taking care not to contaminate the specimen.	
4. Place the label on the specimen container with the patient's name, date of birth, and date and time that the specimen was obtained.	4. Proper labeling is needed to ensure accurate report by the laboratory.

Clinical Management

1. Goals of clinical management
   a. Eradication of infection
   b. Relief of symptoms
   c. Prevention of renewed infection
2. Nonpharmacologic interventions
   a. Maintain adequate hydration
   b. Encourage regular, complete bladder evacuation
      (1) Timed voiding
      (2) Double voiding in which the patient voids as completely as possible, then repeats the voiding effort after 3 to 5 minutes
   c. Intermittent catheterization (see p. 1222)
3. Pharmacologic interventions

   a. Anti-infective medications to eradicate bacterial, fungal, or parasitic infection (Table 26–5)
   b. Urinary analgesics to relieve discomfort

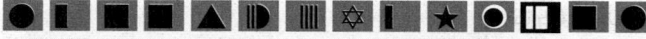

TRANSCULTURAL CONSIDERATIONS

Because the urinary system is located in proximity to sexual organs, many cultural views related to sex and reproduction carry over into attitudes toward the urinary system and its treatment. With their wide variety of signs and symptoms, urinary system infections lend themselves well to combinations of medical management and traditional home remedies that may offer patients both physical and psychologic comfort.

Table 26–5. Oral Anti-infective Medications for Urinary Tract Infections

Medication	Nursing Implications
Ampicillin	Provide adequate hydration. Observe for hypersensitive reactions. Observe for diarrhea. Observe for nausea and vomiting; consult physician for alternative agent (such as amoxicillin) if nausea persists.
Trimethoprim-sulfamethoxazole (Bactrim, Septra)	Administer with liquid. Maintain adequate hydration (crystalization may compromise urinary function). Observe for hypersensitivity reaction. Observe for nausea, vomiting; may administer following meal. Closely observe clotting times in patients receiving anticoagulant therapy.
Nitrofurantoin (Macrodantin, Macrobid)	Observe nausea and vomiting; administer with meals or snack. Observe for signs of pneumonitis in patient with compromised pulmonary function. Assess for tingling or burning discomfort of peripheral polyneuropathy with prolonged use.
Cephalosporins (Keflex, Keftab)	Observe for nausea, vomiting; administer with meal or snack. Observe for diarrhea; alter diet and fluid intake or administer Lactinex as directed for diarrhea.
Fluoroquinolones (Cipro, Maxaquin, Noroxin, Floxin)	Administer in consultation with physician or pharmacologist in younger patients. Observe for nausea and vomiting; may administer with meal or snack.

Complications

1. Urosepsis, shock, death
2. Persistent or recurrent infection
3. Epididymitis in males
4. Vaginitis in females
5. Infectious urinary calculi, particularly with urea-splitting pathogens

Prognosis

1. Prognosis is excellent unless urosepsis occurs.
2. The likelihood of renal failure is significantly increased when febrile urinary infections occur.

Applying the Nursing Process

NURSING DIAGNOSIS: Altered urinary elimination R/T urinary system infection

1. *Expected outcomes:* Following intervention, the person should be able to do the following:
   a. Remain infection-free
   b. Restore urinary elimination to premorbid patterns
   c. Alleviate or reverse predisposing factors
   d. Prevent or promptly manage recurrent infection or complications
   e. Discuss the importance of adequate fluid hydration
   f. Identify potential bladder irritants
2. *Nursing interventions*
   a. Encourage adequate fluid intake—15 ml per pound of body weight. Encourage intake of water and clear liquids.
   b. Caution the patient about behavior that is likely to exacerbate irritative voiding symptoms.
      (1) Dehydration causes concentration of urine, which exacerbates irritation.
      (2) Beverages with caffeine (coffee, tea, many carbonated beverages), alcoholic beverages, and artificial sweeteners should be limited or avoided.
      (3) Chocolates or other foods likely to irritate the bladder lining should be limited or avoided.
   c. Recommend ingestion of yogurt, buttermilk, or other dairy products with active cultures to restore and maintain normal flora.

NURSING DIAGNOSIS: Pain R/T urinary system infection

1. *Expected outcomes:* Following intervention, the person should be able to do the following:
   a. Control pain through a combination of medication and alternative nonpharmacologic pain management techniques
   b. Self-administer pain medicaton
2. *Nursing interventions*
   a. Provide warm sitz baths.
   b. Stress the importance of adequate fluid intake and avoidance of foods or beverages that irritate the bladder.
   c. Administer urinary system analgesics, as ordered, to relieve irritative voiding symptoms and lower urinary tract discomfort.
   d. Administer analgesics, as ordered.
   e. Administer anti-infective medications to eradicate infection, inflammation, and related pain.

NURSING DIAGNOSIS: Noncompliance with therapeutic regimen R/T lack of knowledge about the regimen

1. *Expected outcomes:* Following interventions, the person should be able to do the following:
   a. Explain the importance of compliance with antibiotic regimens
   b. Comply with pharmacologic therapy routines and recommendations
   c. Identify nonpharmacologic management techniques for preventing recurrence

2. *Nursing interventions*
   a. Explain that anti-infective therapy should be taken for the duration of the prescribed course (typically 3 to 5 days)—even if the patient feels better sooner—to prevent persistent bacteriuria or recurrence.
   b. Administer 1-time intramuscular therapy, as ordered, when compliance with ongoing oral therapy is not feasible.
   c. Instruct the patient to contact health care providers if side effects (e.g., nausea and diarrhea) render prescribed anti-infective medication intolerable.
   d. Teach strategies to minimize side effects of anti-infective medications (e.g., taking medication with meals).
   e. Advise the patient to avoid "saving" a portion of anti-infective medication for recurrence. Teach nonpharmacologic strategies to prevent reinfection.

Discharge Planning and Teaching

1. Explain the signs of infection and specific risk factors for recurrent urinary system infection.
2. Teach nonpharmacologic interventions to prevent recurrence of infection as follows:
   a. Maintain adequate hydration
   b. Evacuate bladder regularly and completely
   c. Use timed voiding, double voiding, or intermittent catheterization using clean technique as indicated (see p. 1209)
   d. Evacuate bladder before intercourse (women)
   e. Avoid bubble baths
   f. Use proper perineal hygiene for women (wipe from urethral meatus to anal area, not vice versa)
3. Review dosage, administration, potential side effects, and duration of therapy for current urinary infection. Teach dosage, administration, potential side effects, and duration for suppressive or prophylactic therapy.
4. Teach persons on suppressive or prophylactic therapy to administer their medication before sleeping to provide maximum anti-infective activity during the period of longest urinary retention.

Public Health Considerations: Minimizing Risks

1. Use of indwelling catheters to manage incontinence should be avoided unless absolutely necessary.
2. Education regarding risk factors and strategies to prevent nonfebrile urinary system infections should be aimed at women of childbearing age who are most at risk.

◼ CARING FOR PEOPLE WITH INTERSTITIAL CYSTITIS

Overview

1. Interstitial cystitis is chronic pancystitis of the bladder wall, causing pain and voiding dysfunction.

2. Incidence and socioeconomic impact
   a. Incidence is estimated at 1 in every 300 to 400 persons seeking care for persistent bladder pain. The ratio of affected women to affected men is 10 to 1.
      (1) The incidence is highest in middle-aged women.
      (2) There is a slightly higher incidence among Jewish women.
   b. Prevalence is approximately 20,000 to 90,000 in the United States known to have interstitial cystitis. Due to suspected underdiagnosis or misdiagnosis, the true prevalence may be up to 5 times this number.
3. There are no identified risk factors.

Etiology

1. The cause is unknown.
2. Several causes have been postulated:
   a. Occult infection (infection not readily diagnosed by urine culture)
   b. Vascular or lymphatic obstruction (unlikely cause)
   c. Altered glycosaminoglycan layer function, that is, pain caused by loss of the protective mucous lining of the bladder
   d. Psychologic (unlikely cause)
   e. Reflex sympathetic dystrophy in which the chronic hypertonicity of sympathetic receptors produce ischemia and chronic pain
   f. Toxic urinary agents in which an unidentified toxin or pathogen damaging the glycosaminoglycan protective layer causes chronic pain and discomfort
   g. Immune response in which a chronic inflammatory cascade occurs as a response to antigens in urine or as an autoimmune response

Pathophysiology

1. Inflammation causes chronic bladder pain over the suprapubic area, sometimes radiating to the labia.
2. Chronic bladder pain causes voiding dysfunction with reduced capacity (<400 ml), diurnal urinary frequency (>every 2 hr), and nocturia (>2 episodes per night).
3. Chronic pain and voiding dysfunction cause fatigue and loss of stamina, which, in turn, alter work and recreational patterns. Chronic pain with significant intensity contributes to sexual dysfunction.

Clinical Manifestations

1. Diurnal frequency is marked (urination occurring every 10–60 min is common).
2. Nocturia may exceed 4 to 12 episodes per night.
3. Pain is typically characterized as burning with moderate to severe intensity (often reported at 7 to 10 on objective pain assessment scales).
4. Pain lasts over a period of weeks to years and is unrelieved by antibiotics or antispasmodic therapy.
5. Urination offers transient relief, but, as the bladder refills, pain rapidly crescendos in intensity (unlike the urgency characteristic of urge incontinence).

6. Postponing urination and intake of bladder irritants exacerbate pain.
7. Pain and nocturia profoundly alter sleep patterns.
8. Vaginismus and dyspareunia are common in women.

> According to an Urban Health study of 1000 sufferers of interstitial cystitis, 63 percent had dyspareunia at the onset, with 65 percent indicating they had pain "usually" or "always." At least 57 percent indicated that the dyspareunia persisted. A Duke University study demonstrated that 90 percent of patients with interstitial cystitis had pain upon insertion of the penis or after coitus. Less than 35 percent had pain during foreplay or orgasm.

Diagnostics

1. Assessment
   a. The history of symptoms and their duration should be sought. The patient should rate pain on an objective pain scale to document its intensity.
   b. The patient should keep a bladder record to establish objective documentation of voiding dysfunction.
   c. Symptomatic history establishes a probable diagnosis of interstitial cystitis; definitive diagnosis is made by a combination of symptoms and physical findings.
2. Medical diagnosis
   a. Exclude other causative factors
      • Recurrent or chronic urinary tract infection
      • Inflammatory lesions of the bladder wall
      • Bladder cancer
      • Detrusor instability, hyperreflexia, or urge incontinence
      • Urethritis
      • Prostatitis in men
   b. Diagnostic studies
      (1) Urethral swab, urinalysis, and urine culture may exclude urinary tract infection. In interstitial cystitis, urinalysis shows an absence of bacteria and urine culture is negative.
      (2) Urine cytology may be completed to exclude cancer.
      (3) Cystoscopy can exclude inflammatory lesions of the bladder wall and cancer of the bladder wall; it can identify characteristics of interstitial cystitis including generalized inflammation (and resultant fragile bladder mucosa), petechiae, cracking and bleeding of the bladder wall with filling, and Hunner's ulcers (a rare occurrence, but considered the "classic cystoscopic finding").
      (4) Urodynamics studies can exclude detrusor instability; identify characteristic findings, that is, reduced bladder capacity (<400 ml) and pain induced by bladder filling; and identify low compliance of late-stage disease.

Clinical Management

1. The goal of clinical management is to control symptoms. (No interventions are considered curative.)

2. Nonpharmacologic interventions
   a. Transvaginal, transcutaneous, or transrectal electrical stimulation to reduce bladder pain
   b. Behavioral therapy and biofeedback to increase bladder capacity and alleviate voiding dysfunction
3. Pharmacologic interventions
   a. Analgesics (often narcotics) to relieve pain
   b. Antihistamines or steroids to reduce inflammation of the bladder wall and associated pain
   c. Urinary analgesics and antispasmodics to increase bladder capacity
   d. Intravesical chemotherapy to relieve pain and inflammation
      (1) Dimethyl sulfoxide to reduce inflammation
      (2) Heparin (sometimes combined with other agents) to relieve ischemic-related pain or discomfort from glycosaminoglycan layer damage
      (3) Steroids to reduce inflammation
      (4) Silver nitrate, a caustic antiseptic and astringent, to relieve inflammation
   e. Calcium channel blockers or amitriptyline to relieve chronic, burning-type discomfort
4. Special medical-surgical procedures
   a. Cystoscopy under anesthesia with hydrodistention: Transient mechanical distention of the bladder and local denervation are sometimes combined with intravesical silver nitrate instillation and transurethral fulguration of inflammatory regions.
   b. Laser fulguration of inflammatory areas.
   c. Surgical reconstruction of the urinary system (rare, even with severe symptoms, because of the risk of persistant suprapubic pain, or pain within the urinary diversion).
      (1) Augmentation enterocystoplasty: typically increases bladder capacity but rarely reduces associated pain.
      (2) Ileal conduit: Incontinent diversion may be combined with cystectomy, but pain may still occur at the site of the conduit or recur in the suprapubic area.
      (3) Continent urinary diversion: Pain may occur at the site of the diversion or the suprapubic area.

Complications

1. There may be poor (low) bladder wall compliance with pyelonephritis and ureterohydronephrosis in advanced disease.
2. Bacteriuria markedly exacerbates symptoms.
3. Secondary coping disorders are caused by chronic pain and fatigue.

Prognosis

1. Chronic condition persists for years; the condition is not considered fatal.
2. Poor bladder wall compliance is seen during later stages of disease and may predispose the patient to compromised renal function unless it is managed properly.

Applying the Nursing Process

NURSING DIAGNOSIS: Pain R/T bladder inflammation

1. *Expected outcomes:* Following intervention, the person should be able to do the following:
   a. Control pain
   b. Report improved levels of comfort
   c. Identify bladder irritants
2. *Nursing interventions*
   a. Teach the patient to self-administer analgesia, calcium channel blockers, amitriptyline, as ordered, to relieve bladder pain.
   b. In consultation with the physician, institute transvaginal or transrectal electrostimulation to relieve pain.
      (1) Assist the patient to obtain a "take home" stimulator unit set with short pulse width frequency and 10-to-20-Hz frequency.
      (2) Teach the patient to control current delivered by the unit and to adjust the current so that warm, tingling stimulation, not stinging pain, is perceived.
      (3) Instruct the patient to perform stimulation for 1 to 2 sessions per day for 10 to 15 minutes.
      (4) Evaluate progress using a combination of an objective pain scale and bladder record and voiding diary to assess changes in pain and voiding dysfunction.
   c. To identify bladder irritants that exacerbate interstitial cystitis–related pain, have the patient eliminate these substances 1 at a time, then reintroduce them in the diet to judge their effect on the bladder. Substances include the following:
      (1) Caffeinated beverages (decaffeinated brews may or may not irritate bladder)
      (2) Carbonated beverages, particularly those containing artificial sweeteners (particularly aspartame) and caffeine
      (3) Artificial sweeteners
      (4) Spicy or greasy foods
      (5) Dairy products
      (6) Acidic fruits
   d. Encourage the patient to stop smoking (nicotine is a bladder irritant).
   e. Assist with temporary comfort measures:
      (1) A warm sitz bath
      (2) A knee to chest position
      (3) Relaxation techniques such as visualization and deep breathing
   f. Reassure the patient that frequent voiding is a necessary pain reduction strategy.

NURSING DIAGNOSIS: Altered urinary elimination R/T bladder pain, inflammation

1. *Expected outcomes:* Following intervention, the person should be able to do the following:
   a. Improve voiding function (especially reduce diurnal frequency)
   b. Increase functional bladder capacity
2. *Nursing interventions*
   a. Encourage intake of an adequate volume of water and other nonirritating beverages to avoid chronic dehydration, concentration, or infection of urine.
   b. Warn the patient to avoid prolonged dehydration, which concentrates urine and increases the risk of urinary tract infection.
   c. Advise the patient to abstain temporarily from fluids when toilet facilities are not available.
   d. Assist the patient to anticipate the need to urinate frequently by doing the following:
      (1) Locating toilet facilities rapidly, before there is an immediate need to urinate
      (2) Maintaining a urinal for use in vehicles (disposable urinals designed for women are available)
      (3) Using results of the bladder record to determine typical voiding patterns and anticipate schedule accordingly

NURSING DIAGNOSIS: Fatigue R/T bladder pain

1. *Expected outcomes:* Following intervention, the patient should be able to do the following:
   a. Reduce nocturia and nighttime bladder pain, restoring normal sleep patterns and reducing fatigue
   b. Control pain (see Chapter 11)
2. *Nursing interventions*
   a. Administer analgesics and sleep aids, as ordered.
   b. Teach the patient to avoid consumption of bladder irritants within 2 hours of sleep and to consume only sips of beverages needed to take medications for 1 to 2 hours before bed time.
   c. Encourage the patient to take naps during day.

NURSING DIAGNOSIS: Ineffective individual coping R/T chronic pain and fatigue

1. *Expected outcomes:* Following interventions, the person should be able to do the following:
   a. Identify support groups for assistance
   b. Develop strategies to maximize social and recreational activities
   c. Express feelings and frustrations
2. *Nursing interventions*
   a. Provide names of support groups to patients and family. Assist the patient and family to identify educational resources in the health care community.
   b. Reassure the patient that frequent voiding is necessary and, with proper planning need not prohibit social activities.
   c. Encourage the patient to vent feelings about interstitial cystitis.
   d. Support the patient's efforts to try alternate means of pain control.

NURSING DIAGNOSIS: Sexual dysfunction R/T bladder pain

1. *Expected outcomes:* Following interventions, the person and the person's partner should be able to do the following:
   a. Express concerns about sexual dysfunction
   b. Understand that avoidance of pain is not the same as rejection of intimacy
   c. Identify alternate means of sexual expression that do not cause pain
2. *Nursing interventions*
   a. Provide opportunities for the patient and family to express concerns (separately, if necessary) and to meet with support groups.
   b. Reassure the patient that temporary withdrawal from sexual intercourse is entirely natural when pain is experienced. Advise the patient's partner that intolerance to intercourse is a response to pain, not a rejection of intimacy.
   c. Offer suggestions for alternate sexual expressions to provide mutual stimulation and satisfaction without intercourse.

Discharge Planning and Teaching

1. Teach medications, dosage, schedule, and side effects.
2. Reinforce instruction in alternate methods of pain control.
3. Teach the patient principles to identify dietary substances that may act as bladder irritants.
4. Teach principles of interstitial cystitis and its management to all family members.

◼ *CARING FOR PEOPLE WITH URINARY CALCULI (STONES)*

Definitions

1. Urinary calculi are stones formed in the kidneys from crystalline substances in the urine.
2. Nephrolithiasis is renal stone disease.
3. Urolithiasis is stones in the urinary system.

Incidence and Socioeconomic Impact

1. Each year, approximately 500,000 persons in the United States experience urinary calculi and between 1 and 5 percent of Americans experience stone disease at some time during their lives.
2. The incidence of upper urinary tract stones is greater in industrial countries, such as the United States and countries of Europe, than in developing nations.
3. The incidence of calculi is higher in Whites and Eurasians than in Blacks, Native Americans, and native Israelis.
4. Incidence of urinary calculi peaks between the 3rd and 5th decades of life.

5. Urinary calculi are more common in men than in women.
6. Between 70 and 80 percent of stones are made up primarily of calcium oxalate crystals; the rest contain calcium phosphate salts, struvite (magnesium, ammonium, and phosphate), uric acid, or cystine (an amino acid).

Risk Factors

1. Calcium-based stones: renal tubular acidosis, hypercalcemia, hypercalciuria
2. Oxalate stones: hyperoxaluria
3. Struvite stones (which account for most large "staghorn" stones occupying the majority of the pelvicaliceal system): urea-splitting pathogens of urinary tract infections
4. Uric acid stones: gouty arthritis
5. Cystine stones: cystinuria
6. Any foreign body in the bladder serves as a nidus for infection and calculi formation.
7. Urinary stasis is related to a neuropathic bladder and immobility.
8. Acute or chronic dehydration probably exacerbates associated risk factors.
9. Hyperuricosuria is related to leukemia and lymphoma treatment.
10. Dehydration and immobility exacerbate the risk of calculus formation.

Etiology and Pathophysiology

1. Etiology is unknown.
2. Pathophysiologic consequences of calculi arise from their potential to obstruct the urinary system.
   a. Obstruction causes pain, because pressure distends the urinary tract proximal to the blockage.
   b. Urinary stasis above the obstruction exacerbates the risk of infection, the risk of pyelonephritis, and urosepsis.
   c. Prolonged obstruction compromises the function of the affected kidney. Bilateral calculi may lead to acute or chronic renal failure.
3. The most common sites of urinary tract obstruction (Fig. 26–15)
   a. The ureteropelvic junction
   b. The ureteral curve at the iliac artery
   c. The ureterovesical junction

Clinical Manifestations

1. Clinical manifestations vary with the location and size of the calculus.
2. In renal colic, intense intermittent periods of pain are followed by periods of relief (dull ache) when the calculus obstructs the upper ureter and renal pelvis; renal colic persists with radiating pain to the umbilicus, posterior abdomen, or genitalia with midureteral calculus.
3. Nausea, vomiting, and ileus occur with severe renal colic.
4. Suprapubic pain occurs with irritative voiding symptoms and stranguria with calculus entrapped in the ureterovesical junction.

STONE ENTRAPMENT SITES AND ASSOCIATED PAIN

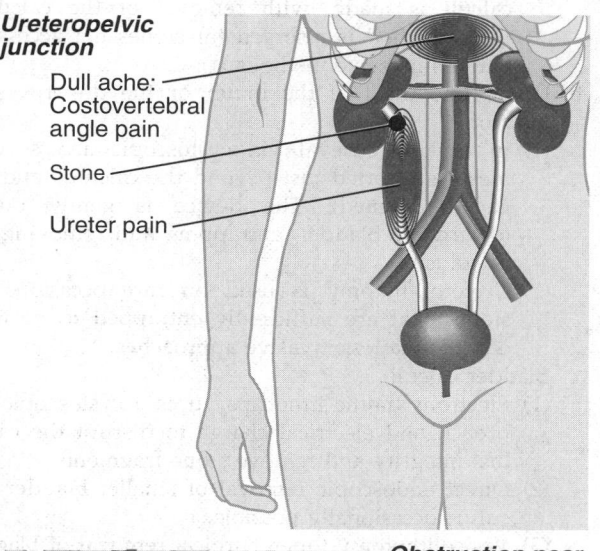

Ureteropelvic junction

Dull ache: Costovertebral angle pain

Stone

Ureter pain

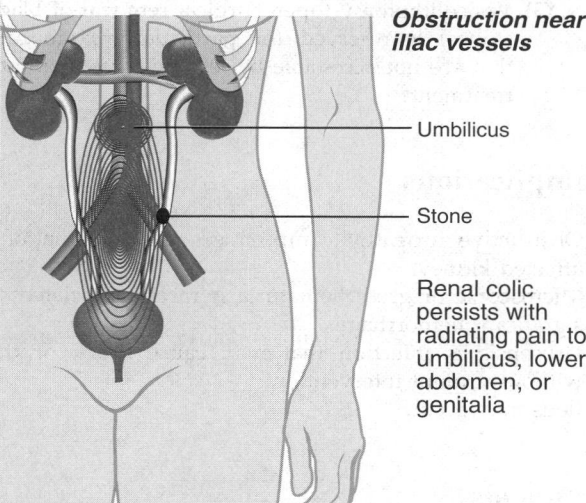

Obstruction near iliac vessels

Umbilicus

Stone

Renal colic persists with radiating pain to umbilicus, lower abdomen, or genitalia

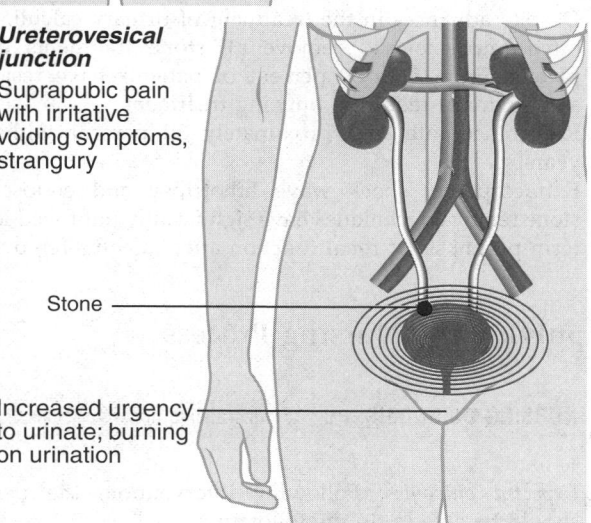

Ureterovesical junction

Suprapubic pain with irritative voiding symptoms, strangury

Stone

Increased urgency to urinate; burning on urination

Figure 26–15.

5. Restlessness occurs with increased pulse and blood pressure, and tachypnea as the patient seeks relief.
6. Microscopic or gross hematuria, pyuria, or bacteriuria are manifestations.
7. Fever accompanies signs of pyelonephritis and urosepsis (uncommon).

Diagnostics

1. Assessment
   a. History
      (1) Prior stone formation
      (2) Renal or bladder colic type pain without objective evidence of calculi formation
      (3) Risk factors
      (4) Location, character, and duration of current pain
      (5) Current and previous radiation patterns (indicates possible location and movement of calculus through the urinary system)
   b. Physical examination
      (1) Vital signs include increased pulse, respirations, and blood pressure associated with colicky pain; fever indicates serious infection.
      (2) Hyperactive bowel sounds occur with nausea and vomiting; hypoactive or absent bowel sounds occur with ileus.
2. Diagnostic studies
   a. Urinalysis, urine culture, and sensitivity testing determine the presence of urinary tract infection, hematuria, or urine crystals.
   b. Radiographic studies
      (1) Ninety percent of calculi are visible on radiographic images.
      (2) Calcium phosphate stones are brightest on radiograph; uric stones are least visible (radiolucent).
      (3) KUB using plain abdominal film detects larger, radiopaque stones.
      (4) IVP locates radiopaque stones, allowing evaluation of associated obstructive uropathy and crude evaluation of renal function (i.e., the ability to concentrate and excrete contrast material).
      (5) Tomograms locate stones in the pelvicaliceal system. They are performed in combination with IVP.
      (6) Renal and bladder ultrasound locates stone, creates hypoechogenic "shadow," and gives some indication of associated obstructive uropathy.
      (7) Computed tomography scan locates radiopaque stones.
      (8) Radionuclide study is an alternative technique for locating calculi among patients allergic to contrast materials or in a nonfunctioning kidney.
   c. Among endoscopic procedures, cystoscopy is performed for bladder stone, ureteroscopy for ureteral calculus, and nephroscopy for stone in the pelvicaliceal system.
   d. Laboratory studies
      (1) Serum chemistry tests identify calcium, phosphate, oxalate, cystine metabolism, and renal function (creatinine, BUN) abnormalities.
      (2) Complete blood count detects systemic infection.

(3) Twenty-four–hour urine collection measures excretion of phosphorous, calcium, uric acid, and creatinine levels.

(4) Stone analysis determines the composition of the calculus and assists in designing a preventive program.

e. Visualization of the stone on imaging study or via endoscopic visualization provides definitive diagnosis. Calculus is suspected when colic-type pain occurs and the stone is not visualized (the suspect calculi may be excreted before diagnostic evaluation).

Clinical Management

1. Goals of clinical management
   a. Locate and remove the obstructive calculi
   b. Prevent or eradicate infection
   c. Control pain
   d. Restore the best possible renal function
   e. Identify risk factors and prevent recurrence
2. Nonpharmacologic interventions
   a. Increasing fluid intake to maintain adequate urinary output for body weight and fluid loss
   b. "Watchful waiting" in which adequate fluid hydration and analgesia for pain control are maintained while waiting for spontaneous excretion of the calculus (approximately 50% "pass" spontaneously). Invasive treatments are reserved for stones that are entrapped, large, or produce complications.
3. Pharmacologic interventions
   a. Analgesia during the watchful waiting period
      (1) Narcotic analgesia is typically required.
      (2) Regular administration, rather than as needed dosage, is recommended to achieve adequate pain control.
   b. Medications to prevent or dissolve the calculi
      (1) D-penicillamine, captopril, and α-mercaptopropinoglycide prevent cystine calculi.
      (2) Allopurinol to prevent uric acid stones; sodium bicarbonate or citrate increases urinary pH and encourages dissolution of existing uric acid stones.
      (3) Pyridoxine or cholestyramine to prevent oxalate stones.
      (4) Hydrochlorthiazide, orthophosphate, cellulose phosphate, and potassium citrate to prevent calcium or calcium-oxalate calculi.
4. Special medical-surgical procedures
   a. Pelvicaliceal system or upper two thirds of the ureter
      (1) In extracorporeal shock wave lithotripsy, sound waves are passed through degassed water or other medium, disrupting the integrity of the calculi without harming surrounding tissue. (Calculi in the ureter may be pushed back into the renal pelvis for the procedure.)
      (2) In direct lithotripsy, sound waves are applied during endoscopy.
      (3) In percutaneous nephrolithotomy, calculi are removed using an endoscopic access tract created into the renal pelvis through the flank.
      (4) In open nephrolithotomy, the pelvicaliceal system

is opened by surgical incision and the stone is removed. (This method is reserved for stones not accessible via other methods.)

(5) In ureterolithotomy, open, surgical incision of the calculi is made, with removal of the calculus. (This method is reserved for stones not accessible via less invasive methods.)

b. Lower one third of the ureter or the ureterovesical junction
   (1) In basket retrieval via cystoscopic access, wire mesh is inserted just beyond the calculus and engaged (opened). The device is gently pulled toward the bladder, entrapping and removing the calculus.
   (2) Ureterolithotomy is used on rare occasions for stones that are sufficiently entrapped to be inaccessible via less invasive approaches.

c. Bladder calculi
   (1) Electrohydraulic lithotripsy uses a cystoscopic approach and electrical charge to disrupt the calculus' integrity and remove stone fragments.
   (2) Direct endoscopic removal of smaller bladder calculi is occasionally possible.
   (3) Vesicolithotomy (open surgical removal of bladder stones) is reserved for particularly large calculi that are not accessible by less invasive methods of treatment.

Complications

1. Obstructive uropathy compromises the function of the affected kidney.
2. Microscopic or gross hematuria is rarely associated with significant hemorrhage.
3. Urosepsis is infection that may cause shock or death without prompt intervention.
4. Ileus may occur.

Prognosis

1. Despite advances in the treatment of urinary calculi, it is often impossible to remove all stone fragments completely. From 5 to 30 percent of patients have residual stone burden requiring ongoing treatment.
2. Recurrence rate is approximately 30 percent within 6 years.
3. Extracorporeal shock wave lithotripsy and endoscopic stone removal techniques have significantly improved long-term prognosis of renal function after calculus removal.

Applying the Nursing Process

NURSING DIAGNOSIS: Pain R/T obstructing urinary calculus

1. *Expected outcomes:* Following intervention, the person should be able to do the following:

a. Control pain and discomfort of acute episode of stone excretion
b. Prevent urinary calculus formation
2. *Nursing interventions*
   a. Assess character, location, intensity, and duration of discomfort. Note particularly renal or bladder colic symptoms; location of pain may indicate the site for treatment.
   b. Administer analgesia during the period of watchful waiting.
   c. Limit environmental noise and lighting to promote comfort and rest.
   d. Apply warm, moist compresses to the affected flank or abdomen to relieve discomfort.
   e. Encourage and assist the patient to ambulate to "free" the stone from the site of obstruction and alleviate related pain via mechanical means.
   f. Supply fluid intake sufficient to provide urinary output of approximately 1500 ml per day to relieve the obstruction and associated pain.

NURSING DIAGNOSIS: Altered urinary elimination R/T presence of urinary calculi

1. *Expected outcomes:* Following interventions, the person should be able to do the following:
   a. Return to normal patterns of urinary elimination
   b. Recognize altered patterns of elimination as temporary changes while the obstruction passes through the urinary system
2. *Nursing interventions*
   a. Explain the changes that will occur as the stone moves through the patient's system.
      (1) Detrusor instability and urge incontinence may occur as the stone passes from the ureterovesical junction into the bladder.
      (2) Urinary frequency, urgency, and strangury abate with passage or removal of the calculus.
      (3) A brief period of increased diuresis with urinary frequency follows passage or removal of the calculus.
   b. Supply adequate fluids during postobstructive diuresis to flush toxins and stone debris from the urinary system.
   c. Encourage frequent voiding during the transient period of urge incontinence.

NURSING DIAGNOSIS: Risk for infection R/T obstructing urinary calculus

1. *Expected outcomes:* Following interventions, the person should be able to do the following:
   a. Identify signs and symptoms of urinary tract infection
   b. Practice adequate fluid hydration
   c. Prevent complications of stone disease such as renal damage and urinary infection
2. *Nursing interventions*

a. Evaluate the patient for signs of febrile urinary tract infection.
b. To prevent urosepsis, obtain a urine culture and begin broad-spectrum anti-infective medications, as ordered, before invasive procedures are undertaken.
c. Encourage adequate fluid intake to promote flushing of toxins from the body.
d. Provide intravenous fluid hydration in consultation with the physician if the patient is unable to tolerate oral intake.

NURSING DIAGNOSIS: Altered renal peripheral tissue perfusion R/T postrenal obstruction

1. *Expected outcomes:* Following interventions, the person should be able to do the following:
   a. Explain the importance of prevention
   b. Practice principles of prevention
   c. Maintain adequate fluid hydration
2. *Nursing interventions*
   a. Emphasize the importance of prevention as the key to reducing the risk of compromised renal function or acute or chronic renal failure related to recurring obstructive calculus formation.
   b. Strain all urine during the watchful waiting period to provide material for metabolic stone analysis and creation of a preventive program.
   c. Encourage routine fluid intake sufficient to create urine production equivalent to 15 ml per pound of body weight or approximately 1500 ml to 2000 ml per day.
   d. Describe the signs and symptoms of dehydration caused by bouts of vomiting and diarrhea. Warn the patient to promptly seek assistance if dehydration occurs.
   e. Advise the patient to avoid dehydration, such as that produced following heavy intake of alcohol.
   f. Describe the specific risk factors and preventive measures based on laboratory analysis of blood, urine, and stone fragments in consultation with the physician.
   g. Provide information and advice regarding dietary measures to reduce the risk of calculus formation based on analysis of specific risk factors for that patient.
      (1) Food sources rich in calcium are dairy products, sardines, canned salmon, and dark green leafy vegetables.
      (2) Foods rich in oxalates are worcestershire sauce, almonds, cashews, raspberries, cranberries, asparagus, plums, and beets.
      (3) Foods rich in uric acid are organ meats (liver, kidneys), whole grains, and lean meats.

Discharge Planning and Teaching

1. Describe general and specific risk factors in urinary calculus development.

2. Teach the early warning signs of urinary calculi and the importance of prompt intervention.
3. Explain the signs and symptoms of urinary tract infection and the risk of systemic infection when complicated by an obstructing calculus.
4. Instruct the patient to maintain adequate fluid hydration and avoid or promptly manage dehydration.
5. Teach administration, dosage, scheduling, and side effects of preventive medications.
6. Stress the importance of ongoing administration of preventive medications, despite the absence of symptoms.

Public Health Considerations

1. Because specific geographic regions (known as "stone belts") have particularly high numbers of individuals with calculi, public health resources and education should be concentrated in these areas.
2. Mobile lithotripters have proven more efficient and cost effective (despite costing more than $500,000) than stationary units.

■ CARING FOR PEOPLE WITH URINARY INCONTINENCE

Definitions

1. Urinary incontinence (UI) is an involuntary loss of urine sufficient to cause hygienic or social problems for the patient or family
   a. Acute (transient) urinary incontinence is the acute onset of urinary leakage, which is resolved when the underlying cause is corrected.
   b. Chronic (established) urinary incontinence is the persistent leakage of urine despite the absence or correction of acute or transient factors; it includes several subtypes.
      (1) Extraurethral (constant) incontinence: urine loss due to anatomic defects of the urinary system or surgical intervention. The North American Nursing Diagnosis Association (NANDA) diagnosis is total incontinence.
      (2) Instability incontinence: loss of urine with unstable (hyperactive) or hyperreflexic contractions of the detrusor. The NANDA diagnoses are urge or reflex incontinence.
      (3) Overflow (paradoxic) incontinence: leakage of urine related to significant urinary retention, caused by deficient detrusor contraction strength or obstruction. The NANDA diagnosis is urinary retention.
      (4) Stress urinary incontinence (SUI): loss of urine during physical exertion; the NANDA nursing diagnosis is "stress incontinence" or total incontinence if the volume of urine loss is significant. (Fig. 26–16).
   c. Functional incontinence: urine loss due to environmental, cognitive, mobility, or dexterity deficiencies
   d. Enuresis: involuntary urine loss during sleep, or bed-

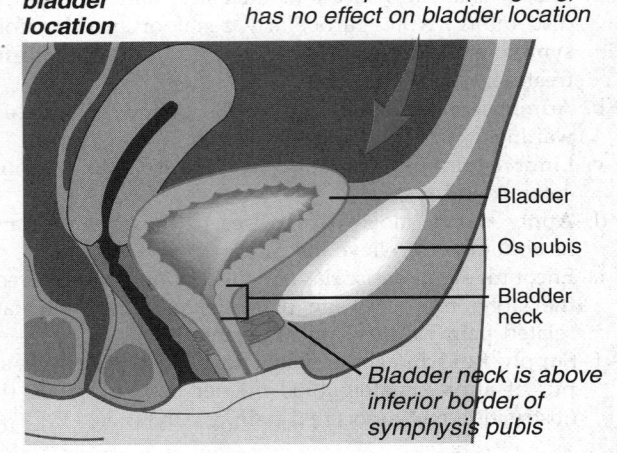

STRESS INCONTINENCE

Normal bladder location

Abdominal pressure (coughing) has no effect on bladder location

Bladder
Os pubis
Bladder neck

Bladder neck is above inferior border of symphysis pubis

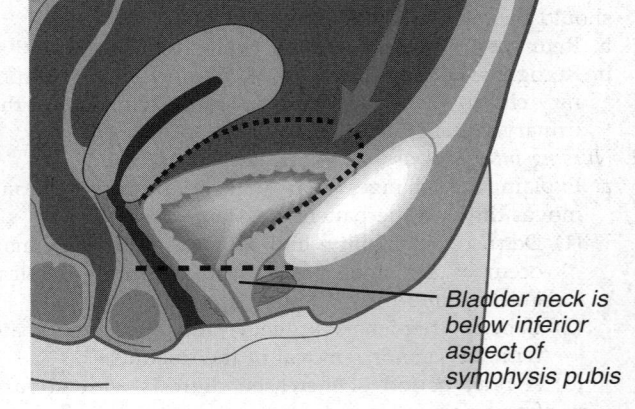

Stress urinary incontinence

Bladder and urethra demonstrate hypermobility

Abdominal pressure (coughing) causes bladder to displace downward

Bladder neck is below inferior aspect of symphysis pubis

Figure 26–16.

wetting after the age of bladder control (see Chapter 15)
   e. Total incontinence: unpredictable urine loss related to intrinsic sphincter deficiency or extraurethral causes.
2. Urinary incontinence is a symptom of an underlying problem rather than a disease.
3. At least 10 million adults in the United States have some form of urinary incontinence, including approximately 50 percent of institutionalized elderly persons and 35 percent of persons in acute care facilities.
4. Urinary incontinence is a significant economic burden, with estimated costs being $10.3 billion annually.

Risk Factors and Etiology

1. Because UI is a symptom, not a disease, its causes range from self-limiting mechanical disorders to life-threatening neurological or urologic conditions.

a. Pregnancy and number of vaginal deliveries increases the risk of pelvic floor descent (urethral hypermobility with or without rectocele or cystocele). Forceps-assisted delivery, breech birth, prolonged delivery, central episiotomy, and uncontrolled "tearing" are also risk factors.

b. In pelvic floor denervation, neurologic lesions predispose the patient to urinary retention or overflow incontinence.
  (1) Lumbosacral spinal lesions include trauma myelodysplasia, tethering of the spinal cord, and lesions of multiple sclerosis.
  (2) Cauda equina syndrome is injury to nerves exiting the lower spinal column.
  (3) Tabes dorsalis is a complication of tertiary syphilis.

c. Other risk factors
  (1) Extensive pelvic surgery
  (2) Repeated urethral suspension procedures
  (3) Trauma, particularly pelvic fracture
  (4) Hormonal changes from menopause and following hysterectomy or bilateral oophorectomy
  (5) Neurologic lesions (above S2, lesions produce detrusor hyperreflexia)
  (6) Stool impaction

2. Pharmaceuticals
  a. Antiparkinsonians, antidepressants, and psychotropic drugs create drowsiness and exert an antispasmodic effect that predisposes the patient to functional UI and urinary retention.
  b. Antihypertensives (diuretic agents) predispose the patient to polyuria; α blocking agents exacerbate SUI.
  c. Calcium channel blockers diminish detrusor contraction strength.
  d. Polyuria exacerbates urinary incontinence.
  e. Drugs especially predispose elderly persons to urinary incontinence.

3. Predisposers for and causes of extraurethral urinary incontinence are
  a. Ectopia of the ureter, bladder, and urethra
  b. Fistula between the bladder, proximal urethra and skin, and the vagina
  c. Surgical reconstruction (incontinent urinary diversion)

4. Predisposers for and causes of functional incontinence
  a. Narcotics in quantities that restrict mobility
  b. Other sedatives and hypnotics that restrict mobility or cause mental confusion
  c. Cognitive deficit (confusion, dementia) and lack of awareness of need to urinate
  d. Immobility or inability to move to the toilet
  e. Poor dexterity or inability to maneuver onto the toilet or remove clothing for toileting
  f. Environmental barriers to toilet
  g. Psychologic factors such as patient apathy (rare)

5. Predisposers for and causes of instability incontinence
  a. Frequent or chronic urinary tract infection and consequent bladder irritation
  b. Bladder cancer
  c. Radiation- or chemotherapy-induced cystitis
  d. Polyuria

e. Neurologic lesion or disorder
  (1) Cerebrovascular accident
  (2) Multiple sclerosis
  (3) Spinal injury
  (4) Central nervous system tumors
  (5) Hydrocephalus
  (6) Spinovascular diseases
  (7) Poliomyelitis and postpolio syndrome
  (8) Complications of acquired immunodeficiency syndrome

f. Obstruction

g. Inflammation of lower urinary tract

h. Idiopathic cause (may be maturational deficit or subtle neuropathy)

i. Associated with SUI, but the exact relationship is unclear

j. Atrophic vaginitis that irritates the urethra

k. Diuretics, which create polyuria

l. Instability incontinence (divided into reflex incontinence and urge incontinence, based on differing causes and resultant responses)
  (1) In reflex incontinence, unpredictable urine loss occurs with detrusor hyperreflexia due to spinal cord abnormalities.
  (2) In urge incontinence, urine loss is with a precipitous desire to void due to loss of volitional control over detrusor activity as a result of disease or trauma to the nervous system. Cardinal signs are urgency to urinate, frequency of urination ($>$ every 2 hr), and nocturia ($>$1 or 2 episodes/night).

6. Predisposers for and causes of overflow incontinence
  a. Infrequent voiding habits
  b. Obstruction, including an enlarged prostate, urethral stricture, or sphincter dyssynergia (also for urge incontinence)
  c. Dribbling urinary leakage from an overdistended bladder

7. Predisposers for and causes of SUI (Table 26–6)
  a. Estrogen deficiency, which thins the urethral vascular cushion
  b. Urethral hypermobility in which muscle weakness allows excessive movement of the urethra with loss of urine during physical exertion
  c. Intrinsic sphincter deficiency in which there is weakness of muscular elements of the urethral sphincter mechanism
  d. Exacerbation by polyuria

Table 26–6. DIAPPERS Mnemonic for Acute or Transient Urinary Incontinence

D	Delirium or confusion
I	Infection
A	Atrophic urethritis or vaginitis
P	Pharmaceuticals
P	Psychologic
E	Endocrine
R	Restricted
S	Stool impaction

Pathophysiology

1. In extraurethral incontinence, the urethral sphincter mechanism is bypassed, causing continuous, uncontrolled urine loss.
2. In instability incontinence, hyperactive detrusor contractions cause loss of bladder control, triggering contraction by volume or other provocation, which, in turn, causes precipitous micturition, regardless of proximity to a toilet.
3. In overflow incontinence, damage to the detrusor prevents the bladder from contracting and emptying completely, allowing dribbling of urine.
4. In stress urinary incontinence:
   a. Urethral hypermobility moves the urethra out of the abdominal pressure transmission zone and compromises the efficiency of the sphincter muscle to close the urethra during physical stress.
   b. An intrinsic sphincter deficiency prevents muscular elements of the sphincter from maintaining closure of the urethra during periods of physical exertion.

Diagnostics

1. Assessment
   a. History
      (1) Duration of symptoms
      (2) Patterns of urine elimination and incontinence, including fluid intake patterns and types of beverages typically consumed
      (3) Type of incontinence
      (4) Characteristics of urinary stream
      (5) History of urinary retention or feelings of incomplete bladder emptying
      (6) A focused urologic review, including urinary infections, congenital defects, inflammatory lesions of the lower urinary tract, and obstructive lesions
      (7) A focused neurologic review
      (8) Female reproductive and gynecologic status, including number of pregnancies and deliveries, forceps use, complicated or difficult deliveries, menstrual history, current status, and gynecologic disorders, particularly pelvic descent
      (9) Male reproductive system review, including prostate disorders
      (10) Patterns of bowel elimination, focusing on constipation or fecal incontinence
      (11) Previous surgeries, focusing on neurologic and abdominopelvic or surgeries for UI
      (12) Detailed review of medications, including over-the-counter and recreational drugs (legal and illegal)
   b. Physical assessment
      (1) Palpate abdomen to assess distention or masses. Lower abdominal distention or mass occurs with fecal impaction; suprapubic distention occurs with significant urinary retention.
      (2) Inspect the external genitalia and perineum for altered skin integrity related to urinary leakage.
      (3) Inspect vaginal tissue for evidence of hormonal insufficiency (e.g., loss of rugation, pale or dry appearance, or tenderness).
      (4) Assess for evidence of pelvic floor descent in females:
         • Cystocele: Bulging of anterior vaginal wall with straining
         • Rectocele: Bulging of posterior vaginal wall with straining
         • Uterine prolapse (hypermobility of the cervix, which may protrude from the vagina without provocation in severe cases)
      (5) In females, reproduce sign of SUI when feasible: Ask the patient to cough, and observe the urethral meatus for leakage while observing the urethra for signs of hypermobility.
      (6) Perform a complete examination of the female genitalia with digital assessment of the circumvaginal muscle strength and the presence of bulbocavernosus reflex by placing 1 or 2 gloved fingers in the central aspect of the vault. The clinician checks for bulbocavernosus reflex (contraction of circumvaginal and perirectal muscles with gentle tapping of the clitoris; absent reflex indicates denervation), profound weakness (the patient cannot exert any force against fingers), moderate weakness (the patient is able to exert perceptible force against the fingers but is unable to pull the fingers toward the posterior aspect of vault), minimal weakness (the patient is able to exert perceptible force against the fingers with slight movement toward the posterior aspect of the vault), and brisk force against the fingers that are gently pulled toward the cervix and posterior aspect of the vault.
      (7) A digital rectal examination in men determines the presence of a fecal mass or hardened impaction in the rectum. The bulbocavernosus reflex is assessed by gently squeezing the glans penis. Contraction of the sphincter indicates the presence of reflex; an absent reflex indicates denervation. The size and consistency of the prostate should be assessed. An enlarged prostate may obstruct the bladder outlet, predisposing the patient to urinary retention.
   c. Diagnostic tests
      (1) Urinalysis for cause of incontinence: Positive "blood" may indicate bladder cancer, inflammatory lesion, or infection. Positive glucose may indicate polyuria related to diabetes mellitus. Positive leukocytes may indicate infection.
      (2) Urine culture and sensitivity test: Performed when urinalysis or clinical symptoms raise suspicion of urinary tract infection as the cause of UI
      (3) Bladder record or voiding diary
      (4) Endoscopy: Performed when the suspected cause is bladder cancer or there are specific inflammatory lesions, fistulas, ectopia, or other anatomic abnormalities
      (5) Urodynamics tests: Performed to determine incontinence type when simpler methods fail to provide adequate information

(6) Videourodynamics: Performed for complex SUI in cases of failed surgical repair or suspicion of intrinsic sphincter deficiency, performed to evaluate bladder outlet obstruction (to locate obstruction, assess obstructive uropathy, and determine hostile potential of bladder), and, performed for complex UI that is not adequately evaluated by simpler means

(7) Voiding cystourethrogram: Performed to assess anatomic bladder defects and vesicoureteric reflux

2. Medical diagnosis

   a. In extraurethral incontinence, there is anatomic evidence of ectopia, fistula, or surgical ostomy.

   b. Functional incontinence is demonstrated by environmental assessment, functional evaluation, and mini mental status examination in combination with screening evaluation and bladder record; urodynamics tests are performed when coexisting chronic UI is suspected.

   c. Instability incontinence

      (1) In reflex incontinence urodynamics testing is recommended. Cystometrogram is used to diagnose hyperreflexic bladder contraction, and sphincter electromyogram is used to assess vesicosphincter dyssynergia. Videourodynamics tests are used when feasible.

      (2) In urge UI, a presumptive diagnosis is based on symptoms and bladder record unless the patient fails therapy or there is a complicating condition (urinary retention or infection).

   d. Overflow incontinence is demonstrated by ultrasonography of the bladder or kidneys or by cystoscopy with cystography to detect residual urine.

   e. Stress urinary incontinence is shown when it is reproduced on physical examination or by urodynamic or imaging study in selected cases.

Clinical Management

1. Goals of clinical management

   a. Restore normal patterns of urinary elimination (i.e., diurnal frequency of more than every 2 hours and nocturia 0 to 1 time per night in patients younger than 70 years of age and 0 to 2 times per night in patients older than 70 years).

   b. Correct urinary leakage or provide patient devices and education to adequately contain leakage

   c. Prevent complications

   d. Restore dignity and correct social isolation produced by UI

2. Extraurethral incontinence

   a. Nonpharmacologic interventions

      (1) Urinary containment devices (e.g., pads with 500 ml capacity to accommodate the continuous nature of urine leakage or adult containment briefs)

      (2) Skin care to prevent infection

   b. Pharmacologic interventions include sclerosing therapy.

      (1) Liquid tetracycline is infused into the fistulous tract to sclerose (scar) the extraurethral passage.

      (2) Treatment often requires repeated application to achieve permanent closure of the fistulous tract.

   c. Special medical-surgical procedures include surgical closure of the fistula or excision of ectopic ureter.

3. Instability incontinence

   a. Nonpharmacologic interventions

      (1) Timed voiding in which the patient is taught to void at timed intervals, using a graded program with voiding intervals increased 15 to 30 minutes each week

      (2) Control of fluid intake in which the patient avoids ingestion of large quantities of fluid during a brief period, limits intake with meals to 8 ounces, takes sips of water or clear liquids throughout day, and takes sips of fluid only for 1 to 2 hours before bedtime

      (3) Biofeedback

   b. Pharmacologic interventions

      (1) Anticholinergics or antispasmodics to inhibit unstable detrusor muscle contractions and reduce urgency

      (2) Calcium channel blockers to decrease contractility of the detrusor muscle by reducing the available calcium ions required for muscle contraction

      (3) Anticholinergic pharmacotherapy with intermittent catheterization to inhibit all bladder contractions in favor of regular catheterization schedule

      (4) Alpha-adrenergic blocking agents to reduce obstruction from vesicosphincter dyssynergia (application limited to reflex incontinence)

   c. Special medical-surgical procedures

      (1) Surgical management through augmentation enterocystoplasty (surgical enlargement of the bladder), autoaugmentation of the bladder, incontinent urinary diversion, or continent urinary diversion

      (2) Sphincterotomy with application of a condom device to contain urinary leakage in quadriplegic males

      (3) Intermittent catheterization performed by the patient (Learning/Teaching Guidelines for Intermittent Self-Catheterization)

4. Overflow incontinence

   a. Nonpharmacologic interventions include double voiding.

   b. There are no pharmacologic interventions.

   c. Special medical-surgical procedures

      (1) Intermittent catheterization

      (2) Temporary placement of an indwelling Foley catheter

      (3) Surgical resection of constricted tissue

5. Stress urinary incontinence

   a. Nonpharmacologic interventions include

      (1) Pelvic floor (Kegel) exercises to strengthen the sphincter mechanism (Fig. 26–17). The patient isolates and contracts periurethral (circumvaginal or perirectal) muscles, beginning with 10 repetitions and gradually building to 35 to 50 repetitions. For maximal strength and endurance exercise, the patient should contract as much as possible for 6 to 10 seconds followed by a 10-second relaxation period. Exercises should be performed every other day for 6 to 12 weeks.

LEARNING/TEACHING GUIDELINES
for Intermittent Self-Catheterization

General Guidelines

1. Intermittent self-catheterization is an important factor in managing many cases of urinary incontinence, because it can provide regular, complete bladder evacuation.
2. Be sure to teach patients sanitary measures to prevent infection.

Preparing for Self-Catheterization

1. Teach the patient to make sure all necessary equipment is gathered before beginning.
2. Patients must wash their hands thoroughly before commencing self-catheterization.
3. Explain the need to wash the catheter with warm soap and water and dry it thoroughly. An alternate cleaning method is to wash the catheter with soap and water, place it in a paper bag, and microwave (with 8 ounces of water in a glass next to the catheter bag) for 10 minutes.

Instructions to the Patient on Self-Catheterization

1. Clean the perineum with soap and water or with towelettes (impregnated, disposable cloth).
2. Lubricate the catheter with sufficient water-soluble lubricant.
3. Locate the catheter insertion point:
   a. Women can locate the urethral meatus by a combination of visualization and palpation; the goal is to self-catheterize by "feel" alone.
   b. Men catheterize by visualizing the penile meatus.
4. Insert the catheter slowly until urine return is attained.
5. Once the bladder is drained, gently remove the catheter.
6. Immediately rinse the catheter with cool tap water to remove residue. Dry thoroughly. *Never* store the catheter wet or in "antiseptic solution."

---

(2) Weighted vaginal cones that force circumvaginal muscles to contract to hold the cones in place
(3) Incontinence containment devices. Incontinence pads with Superabsorbents are recommended. (Feminine hygiene pads are not designed to contain urine.) Pads that absorb at least 300 to 500 ml are indicated when urine loss is significant. Adult briefs are required only for markedly severe cases. Condom catheter containment is a viable alternative for men, but is rarely viable for women.

b. Pharmacologic interventions
(1) Alpha-sympathomimetics (ephedrine, pseudoephedrine, phenylpropanolamine) to increase muscle tone
(2) Topical or oral estrogens to reverse atrophic vaginitis
(3) Imipramine for combined α-sympathomimetic and anticholinergic effects

c. Special medical-surgical procedures
(1) Insertion of a temporary indwelling catheter (Box 26–1)
(2) Intermittent self-catheterization
(3) Insertion of a pessary to support a cystocele and prevent urethral hypermobility
(4) Electrostimulation therapy: transcutaneous or transvaginal application of a non-painful, low-voltage (20 to 50 Hz) current to pelvic floor muscles to stimulate muscle contraction; may be performed by patient using home device
(5) Periurethral injection of glutaraldehyde cross-linked collagen
(6) Surgical repairs, including the following:
   • Retropubic urethropexy: The bladder neck and adjacent structures are elevated by anchoring

them to the periosteum of the symphysis pubis (Marshall-Marchetti-Krantz) or Cooper's ligament (Burch's procedure) through an abdominal incision.

BOX 26–1. Insertion of a Temporary Indwelling Catheter

1. Select a catheter designed for ongoing use: hydrogel-bonded, silicone catheters are preferred for prolonged use.
2. Select the appropriate size: typically, a 14 to 18 French catheter is used in adults. Larger catheters increase the risk of urethral erosion.
3. Select a special-feature catheter as indicated. A man with an enlarged prostate may require a coude-tipped catheter for atraumatic insertion.
4. Select an appropriate drainage system—a large drainage bag with an antireflux valve and adequate length tubing. An easy-to-use drainage mechanism is important.
5. Select a leg bag (indicated only in patients able to routinely open the system without recurrent, symptomatic infections) with a baffled design, cloth sleeve, Velcro leg straps, and easy-to-use drainage mechanism.
6. Insert the catheter using strict aseptic technique.
7. Ensure that there is adequate lighting and position of the patient before catheter insertion.
8. Wash the meatus with a povidone-iodine solution.
9. In women, coat the catheter with water-soluble lubricating jelly and insert gently with labial tissue pulled away from the meatus.
10. In men, inject 10 ml of lubricating jelly into the urethra before catheter insertion, coating the catheter as well.
11. Insert the catheter beyond the point of urine return.
12. Inflate the retention balloon, per the manufacturer's recommendation. Overinflation rarely prevents leakage around the catheter.
13. Anchor the catheter with a cloth strap to avoid traction or inadvertent removal.

MUSCLES OF THE PELVIC FLOOR –FEMALE

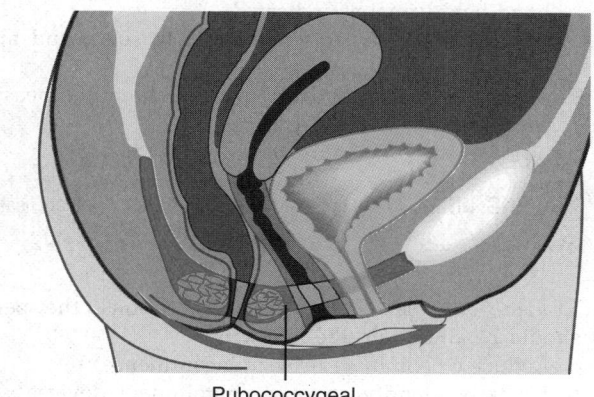

Pubococcygeal
muscle

Contraction of the pubococcygeal muscle causes muscle to move forward (anteriorly) toward the os pubis, closing all external openings.

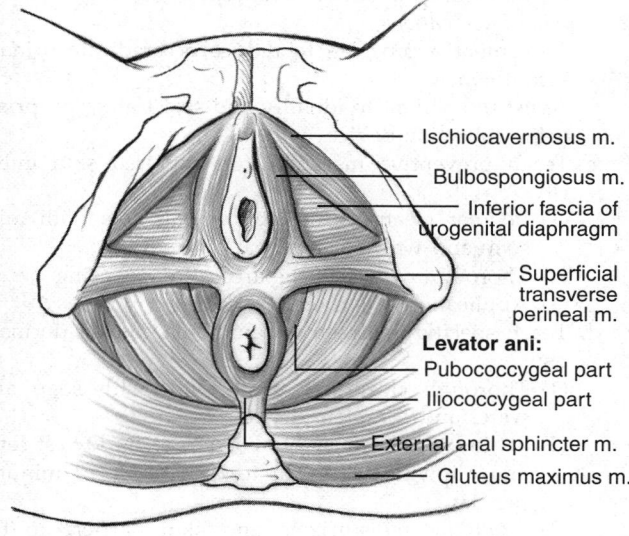

Ischiocavernosus m.

Bulbospongiosus m.

Inferior fascia of urogenital diaphragm

Superficial transverse perineal m.

Levator ani:
Pubococcygeal part

Iliococcygeal part

External anal sphincter m.

Gluteus maximus m.

Figure 26–17.

- Anterior repair: From a vaginal approach, silk mattress sutures are placed on either side of the urethra to restore more normal anatomic relations.
- Transvaginal needle bladder neck suspensions: The urethra and bladder neck are fixed in retropubic position via endopelvic fascia lateral to the bladder neck, typically through a vaginal incision and 2 small abdominal incisions (Raz procedure).
- Suburethral sling: The proximal urethra is supported with a sling of fascia or synthetic material (Marlex, Goretex) placed beneath the urethra through an abdominal incision. (An additional incision for harvesting the sling may be needed.)

- Artificial urinary sphincter: A synthetic device is implanted via an abdominal incision (Box 26–2).

Complications

1. Urinary tract infection
2. Altered skin integrity
3. Depression and social isolation
4. Odor
5. Compromised renal function (particularly in the presence of severe obstruction)
6. Urinary retention

Prognosis

1. Prognosis is excellent except when severe obstruction causes overwhelming infection or acute or chronic renal failure.
2. Associated and causative conditions may alter the prognosis.

Applying the Nursing Process

NURSING DIAGNOSIS: Total incontinence R/T fistula, ectopia, or surgical intervention

1. *Expected outcomes:* Following interventions, the person should be able to do the following:
   a. Properly identify and use containment devices when urinary leakage is not cured
   b. Prevent altered skin integrity
   c. Show signs of restored dignity, improved self-esteem, and reduced feelings of social isolation
   d. Describe corrective surgery
2. *Nursing interventions*
   a. Assist the patient to identify and apply adequate containment devices for continuous leakage.

BOX 26–2. Implanting an Artificial Urinary Sphincter

1. The surgeon places the cuff around the proximal urethra or bladder neck.
2. The surgeon places the pump device in the scrotum of males and under the labia majoris in females. (Use of artificial urinary sphincters has declined in women due to poor results.)
3. An abdominal reservoir is created to activate and deflate pump.
4. Activated pump: The periurethral cuff is filled with solution from the abdominal reservoirs, creating pressure on the urethral lumen, closing the urethra.
5. Deflation: Squeezing the pump baffling fluid from the cuff to the abdominal reservoir allows the bladder to empty by voiding or catheterization.
6. The cuff passively refills over a period of 1 to 2 minutes.
7. The pump device contains a deactivation device, allowing prolonged baffling of fluid from the cuff to the abdominal reservoir. (Incontinence recurs when the cuff is deactivated.)
8. Significant complications include infection, mechanical failures, and urethral erosion.

b. Teach the patient preventive measures for altered skin integrity.
c. Prepare the patient for sclerosing therapy.
   (1) Carefully shield surrounding skin using absorptive barriers and create a narrow window pane for introduction of the sclerosing agent
   (2) Cover all exposed skin adjacent to the fistula with an appropriate moisture barrier before treatment
d. Arrange for the patient to meet with the enterostomal therapy nurse to learn pouching techniques and peristomal skin care before creation of an incontinent urinary stoma.
e. In conjunction with other team members, answer the patient's questions about the surgical procedure.

NURSING DIAGNOSIS: Functional incontinence R/T impaired mobility, cognition, and environmental barriers

1. *Expected outcomes:* Following interventions, the patient (and caregivers, as appropriate) should be able to do the following:
  a. Initiate a prompted voiding program
  b. Recognize environmental barriers to toileting
  c. Properly identify and use containment devices when urinary leakage is not cured
  d. Prevent altered skin integrity
  e. Report restored dignity, improved self-esteem, and reduced feelings of social isolation
2. *Nursing interventions*
  a. Teach the patient a patterned urge response toileting program or a prompted voiding program.
    (1) Evaluate the frequency of bladder evacuation by regular monitoring via a specially designed bladder record.
    (2) Have the patient toilet on a schedule based on determined patterns of urinary elimination. (Patients with a voiding frequency of <2 hr are poor candidates for this program.)
    (3) Assist and encourage the patient to toilet.
    (4) Reward successful toileting and dry episodes with verbal praise.
    (5) Limit socialization during pad or containment device changes.
  b. Have caregivers remove environmental barriers to toileting.
    (1) Install grip bars and raised toilet seats.
    (2) Help the patient attain a portable or hand-held urinal.
    (3) Ensure adequate lighting in the toilet area; remove articles that impede access.
  c. Maximize the patient's mobility and dexterity.
    (1) Assist the patient to attain ordered assistive devices (e.g., cane, walker, or wheelchair).
    (2) Encourage elderly patients to select and wear shoes with nonskid soles.
    (3) Assist patients to alter their clothing to simplify removal for toileting (e.g., the patient may use Velcro rather than buttons or zippers, use stretch waist bands, and wear few undergarments).

    (4) Arrange for the patient to meet with a physical therapist or occupational therapist to assist with maximizing mobility and dexterity.
d. Assist the patient to obtain and use a bedside toilet or hand-held urinal as indicated.
e. Assist the patient and caregivers to select and apply containment devices.
f. Teach the patient and caregivers preventive measures for impaired skin integrity.

NURSING DIAGNOSIS: Impaired skin integrity R/T urinary leakage

1. *Expected outcomes:* Following interventions, the person should be able to do the following:
  a. Reduce or eliminate urinary incontinence
  b. Properly identify and use containment devices when urinary leakage is not cured
  c. Prevent altered skin integrity
  d. Report restored dignity, improved self-esteem, and reduced feelings of social isolation
2. *Nursing interventions*
  a. Implement a program to reduce or eradicate urinary incontinence.
  b. Assist the patient to identify and select an appropriate urine collection device.
  c. Teach preventive measures for impaired skin integrity:
    (1) Regular cleansing of the perineal area with mild soap and water or perineal cleanser
    (2) Thorough drying of the area after cleansing
    (3) Application of a moisture barrier
  d. Teach specific treatment of ammonia contact dermatitis:
    (1) Thorough cleansing of the skin with soap and water and complete drying
    (2) Setting a hand-held blow dryer at its lowest level and applying warm air to the area for 5 minutes per day
    (3) Applying moisturizers and skin barriers to the area as ordered
  e. Teach specific treatment of monilial skin rash:
    (1) Following the 1st 2 steps for ammonia contact dermatitis as discussed previously
    (2) Applying antimonilial powder, brushing over the area, and sweeping away all excess powder. The patient should avoid applying a thick layer that clumps and retains moisture.

NURSING DIAGNOSIS: Social isolation R/T stigma of urinary incontinence

1. *Expected outcomes:* Following interventions, the person should be able to do the following:
  a. Identify resources for education and support
  b. Report restored dignity, improved self-esteem, and reduced feelings of social isolation
2. *Nursing interventions*

a. Reassure the patient that incontinence is treatable and is not an inevitable consequence of aging.
b. Encourage the patient to seek out information and participate in support groups and informational advocacy groups.

Discharge Planning and Teaching

1. Teach the patient the importance of ongoing adherence to the prescribed bladder management program.
2. Inform the patient that successful programs often involve a combination of treatment modalities and that, if the current program does not meet expectations, alternative treatments should be explored.

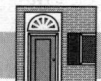 **HOME CARE STRATEGIES**

Indwelling Catheters

Maintenance of an indwelling urinary catheter can be overwhelming for the patient and family. Care of the catheter rests with the patient and caregiver, who are instructed by the nurse. Maintaining patency, preventing trauma, reducing the risk of infection, and changing the catheter are the objectives. Provide the caregiver with information (name and telephone number) about the medical supply company to obtain necessary supplies.

Maintaining Patency

- Instruct the patient and caregiver to have liquids within reach and offered hourly.
- Suggest the use of liquid-based foods.
- Instruct on assessing for and avoiding kinks in the tubing.
- Suggest the use of a bucket under the drainage bag at night in the event of leaks. Empty the drainage bag into a designated container on rising, at bedtime, and every 6 to 8 hours during the day.

Preventing Trauma

- Instruct the caregiver to secure the tubing so that it does not catch on the bed rails, walker, or wheelchair.
- Suggest that small children and pets be monitored so that unintentional pulling of the tubing does not occur.

Reducing the Risks of Infection

- Good hand washing with an antibacterial soap is a must.
- Gloves are not necessary for the patient and caregiver but may be used if preferred.
- The catheter and tube should be wiped with 70 percent alcohol before and after disconnection.
- The drainage bag should not rest on the floor.

Changing the Catheter

- Your equipment should include a flashlight or headlight.
- Chux, a clean towel, or a sheet is used to protect the linen and maintain a clean field.
- Two catheters are always on hand in case of malfunction or contamination.
- Leave a 30-ml syringe in the home to empty the balloon and remove the catheter.
- Use positioning techniques, pillows, and help from the caregiver to assist with insertion of the catheter.
- Dispose of catheter supplies in a leakproof plastic bag.

3. Describe the behavioral antecedents, provocative maneuvers, and bladder irritants associated with UI.
4. Explain dosage, administration, scheduling, and side effects of medications.
5. Teach ongoing care of indwelling catheters:
   a. In daily catheter care, the exposed tube and meatus are gently cleansed with mild soap and water or specific perineal cleanser.
   b. The catheter is anchored.
   c. The drainage bag is kept below the level of the bladder at all times.
   d. The drainage bag system is kept closed except during routine drainage.
   e. The drainage bag is emptied before it becomes completely full.
   f. The bag is cleaned by filling it with several ounces of cool tap water or water with 1 teaspoon per pint of household vinegar, agitating briskly for several minutes, and emptying it. The procedure is repeated.
   g. Several ounces of a solution of 15 percent Dakin's solution (household bleach) are poured over the drainage mechanism and the connection to the catheter.
   h. The solution is poured into the catheter bag and agitated for several minutes. It is emptied via the drainage mechanism.
   i. The bag is rinsed with cool tap water and allowed to air dry thoroughly before subsequent use.
6. Teach patients with indwelling cathethers to watch for signs and symptoms of urinary tract infection and to have adequate fluid intake—15 ml per pound of body weight—to prevent symptomatic infection.
7. Teach care of a vaginal pessary
   a. The patient should undergo regular follow-up with a health care provider.
   b. The patient should learn how to insert estrogen creams.
   c. The patient should learn self-monitoring for signs of erosion or infection—odorous vaginal discharge or new onset of vaginal discomfort when the pessary is in place.
8. Teach patients who have had augmentation enterocystoplasty to irrigate the augmented bladder pouch, to prevent infection by ingesting cranberry juice (which encourages formation in urine of hippuric acid, a natural mucolytic agent), and to ingest adequate fluid to reduce obstructing mucus formation.

Public Health Considerations

1. Less than 50 percent of all persons with incontinence report their condition to a health care provider. Many use absorbent products rather than seek treatment.
2. To educate clinicians on the evaluation and treatment of incontinence, the U.S. Department of Health and Human Services through the Agency for Health Care Policy and Research (AHCPR) has developed the *Clinical Practice Guideline for Urinary Incontinence in Adults*. This document contains treatment algorithms for UI.

◼ CARING FOR PEOPLE WITH URINARY RETENTION

Definitions

1. Urinary retention is the inability of the bladder to completely empty by micturition, despite continuing urine production.
2. Chronic urinary retention is the persistent inability to completely empty the bladder of urine.
3. Acute urinary retention is the inability to evacuate even part of the bladder's contents.

NURSE ADVISORY

Acute urinary retention is a medical emergency calling for immediate catheterization.

Incidence and Socioeconomic Impact

1. Bladder outlet obstruction, a common cause of urine retention, affects men much more frequently than women.
   a. Benign prostatic hypertrophy (BPH) is the most common cause of bladder outlet obstruction in males (see Chapter 30).
   b. One in 4 American males who lives to age 80 years will be treated for BPH.
   c. Annual costs related to BPH and its management are approximately $4.5 billion per year.
2. Deficient detrusor contraction strength (poor muscle strength of the detrusor), which can also cause urine retention, affects men and women.

Risk Factors

1. Urethral strictures
2. Urethral cancer
3. Congenital anomalies of the urinary tract or external genitalia
4. Infrequent voiding with overdistension of the bladder
5. Neuropathic lesions of the lower spine and pelvic nerves
6. Bladder dysfunction, neuropathy, or chronic overdistention associated with polyuria of diabetes mellitus or diabetes insipidus
7. Prolonged use or abuse of specific drugs
8. Fecal impaction or recurrent constipation
9. Prostate disorder
10. History of poliomyelitis
11. Recurrent or acute herpetic infection

Etiology

1. Obstruction may be due to the following:
   a. Urethral stricture

b. Detrusor striated sphincter dyssynergia, in which there is loss of coordination between the detrusor and striated muscles of the sphincter mechanism
   c. Bladder neck dyssynergia
   d. Bladder hypertrophy
   e. Bladder neck contracture
   f. Urethral distortion in women (uncommon)
   g. Benign prostatic hyperplasia (hypertrophy)
   h. Prostatitis and prostatodynia (symptoms of prostatitis without evidence of infection or inflammation)
   i. Levator ani syndrome (prostatodynia may represent one form of this syndrome)
2. Deficient detrusor contractility may be due to the following:
   a. Transient or reversible causes
      (1) Decongestants (α-sympathomimetics) and mixed agents (over-the-counter cold remedies), particularly among patients with prostatic enlargement
      (2) Anticholinergic, antispasmodic, and parasympatholytic drugs
      (3) Antidepressants such as tricyclics and structurally related agents
      (4) Psychotropic drugs
      (5) Hallucinogens, including cannabis
      (6) Narcotics
      (7) Alpha-adrenergic agonists
      (8) Fecal impaction
      (9) Acute immobility associated with serious illness
      (10) Acute phase following spinal injury (detrusor contractions may or may not return, based on the level of injury and vascular extension)
      (11) Hysterical response (uncommon)
      (12) Water intoxication (persistent overhydration with excess intake of water or other fluids)
   b. Chronic causes
      (1) Spinal injury to orthopedic level T12 or lower or neurologic outflow from levels S2 and below
      (2) Tabes dorsalis
      (3) Diabetes mellitus (combination of neuropathy and mechanical effect of chronic overdistention)
      (4) Diabetes insipidus (mechanical effect of chronic polyuria with overdistention)
      (5) Poliomyelitis
      (6) Postpolio syndrome
      (7) Herpes infection affecting the sacral dermatomes (simplex or zosteriform)
      (8) Multiple sclerosis with plaques affecting the lower spine
      (9) Lumbosacral myelodysplasia or meningocele
      (10) Spina bifida occulta associated with tethering of the spinal cord
      (11) Sacral agenesis

Pathophysiology

1. Retention may be due to obstruction (Fig. 26–18).
   a. Anatomic or functional disorder blocks urinary outflow. The bladder cannot evacuate contents despite adequate detrusor contraction strength.
      (1) Note in Figure 26–18 that hydronephrosis is the distention of the renal pelvis and calices with urine.

COMMON OBSTRUCTIONS OF THE URINARY SYSTEM

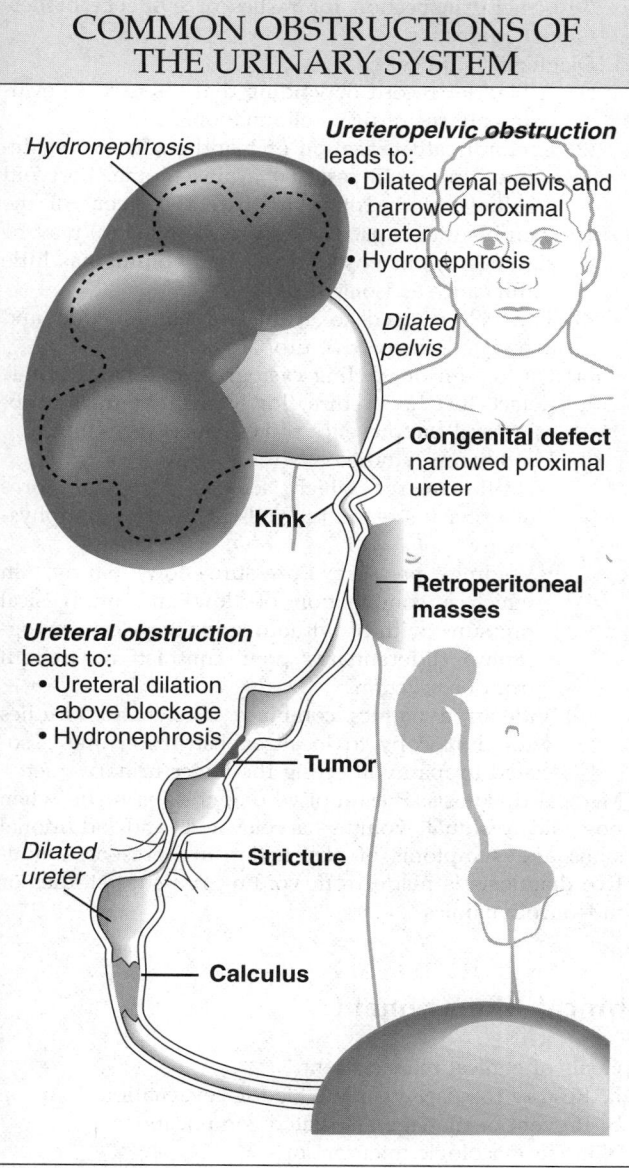

Hydronephrosis

Ureteropelvic obstruction
leads to:
- Dilated renal pelvis and narrowed proximal ureter
- Hydronephrosis

Dilated pelvis

Congenital defect
narrowed proximal ureter

Kink

Retroperitoneal masses

Ureteral obstruction
leads to:
- Ureteral dilation above blockage
- Hydronephrosis

Tumor

Dilated ureter

Stricture

Calculus

Figure 26–18.

(2) Hydronephrosis results from an obstruction of normal urine flow. The obstruction may be due to a congenital defect, calculus, tumor, scar tissue, or a kink in the ureter.

(3) Without intervention, the functioning units of the kidney will be destroyed by the sustained or intermittent pressure within the renal pelvis, calices, and nephrons.

   b. The severity of the obstruction correlates with the risk of complicating factors, including infection, vesicoureteric reflux, ureterohydronephrosis, and chronic or acute renal failure.

2. Retention may be due to deficient detrusor contraction strength.
   a. A weak detrusor cannot open the urethra long enough to completely evacuate urine from the bladder.
   b. Ureterohydronephrosis or other uropathy is uncommon. The bladder is enlarged but not trabeculated.

Clinical Manifestations

1. Chronic urinary retention
   a. Frequent urination (more than every 2 hr while awake)
   b. Frequent nocturia (2 or more episodes per night)
   c. Postvoid dribbling
   d. Possible overflow incontinence
   e. Frequent voiding accompanied by abdominal straining
   f. Diminished force of stream, prolonged or intermittent urinary stream
   g. Splaying or splitting of urinary stream with urethral stricture
2. Acute urinary retention
   a. Inability to urinate
   b. Marked suprapubic discomfort
   c. Lower abdominal (suprapubic) distention

Diagnostics

1. Assessment
   a. Acute and chronic retention should be differentiated (Table 26–7).
   b. History
     (1) Duration of symptoms
     (2) Patterns of urinary elimination and incontinence (if present)
     (3) Characteristics of urinary stream
     (4) Previous surgeries

Table 26–7. Differentiating Acute from Chronic Urinary Retention

Characteristic	Acute Retention	Chronic Retention
Onset	Sudden, occurring over days or hours	Gradual, occurring over weeks to years
Discomfort	Marked suprapubic discomfort	Little discomfort, often asymptomatic
Extent of retention	Complete inability to void	Voiding compromised but not absent
Accompanied by overflow urinary incontinence	Yes	Yes

(5) Detailed review of current medication, including use of over-the-counter medications and recreational drugs (both legal and illegal)

(6) Neurologic system review

(7) Review of female or male reproductive systems

(8) Gastrointestinal system review with emphasis on fecal constipation and impaction

(9) For suspected BPH, complete specific symptom score (no widely accepted tools are available for other forms of obstruction) (Fig. 26–19)

c. Physical examination

(1) Inspection and palpation of the abdomen for distention and tenderness

(2) Neurologic examination with emphasis on the perineal area

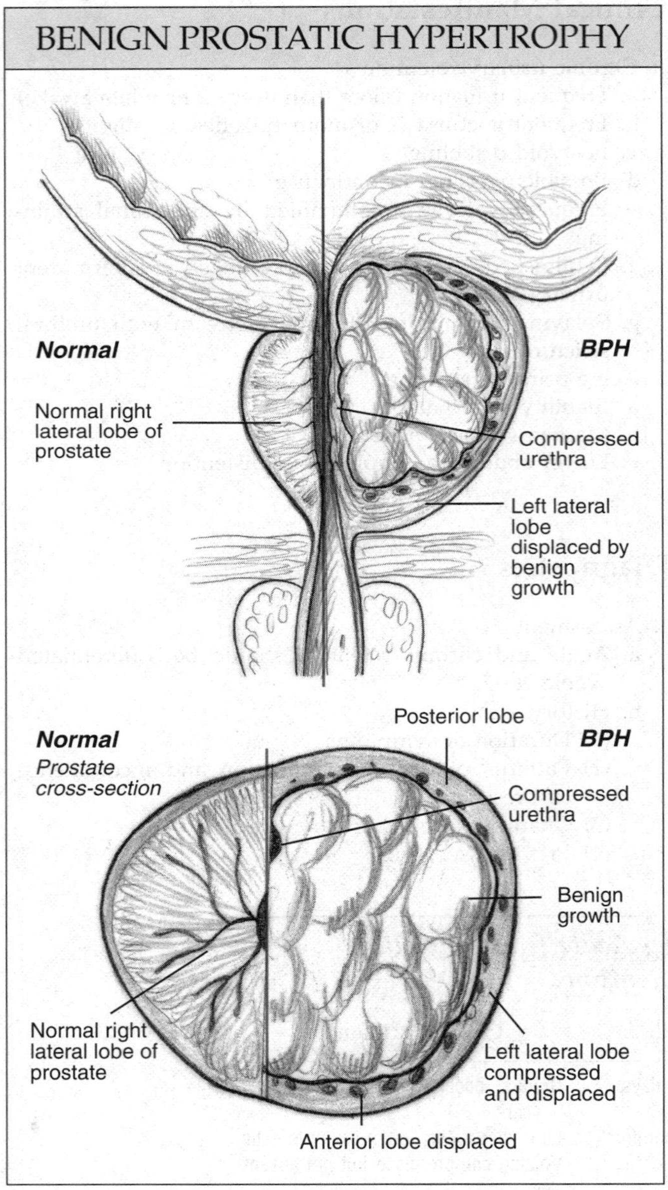

(3) General inspection for rashes or evidence of herpetic infection

d. Diagnostic studies

(1) A bladder record or voiding diary is used to evaluate patterns of urine elimination.

(2) Urethral catheterization or bladder ultrasound determine postvoid residual urine volume. Postvoid residual volume of more than 25 percent of the total bladder capacity or more than 200 ml may be significant, but postvoid residual volume has little significance as isolated datum.

(3) The IVP is used to evaluate renal function and associated obstructive uropathy.

(4) Cystogram or voiding cystogram detects anatomic defects of the urethra, lower urinary tract uropathy, and the presence of vesicoureteric reflux.

(5) Urodynamic studies

• Uroflowmetry, which screens for poor force of urinary stream, but fails to define pathophysiology

• Voiding pressure (pressure–flow) study, in which a combination of flow and intravesical pressure (with or without sphincter electromyography) differentiates poor contraction strength from obstruction.

(6) Videourodynamics combines urodynamic studies with fluroscopy to localize obstruction and associated uropathy affecting the lower urinary tract.

2. Medical diagnosis: Presumptive diagnosis is made when postvoid residual volume is elevated and additional signs and symptoms of obstruction are present; definitive diagnosis is made from voiding pressure studies or videourodynamics.

BENIGN PROSTATIC HYPERTROPHY

Normal

Normal right lateral lobe of prostate

BPH

Compressed urethra

Left lateral lobe displaced by benign growth

Posterior lobe

Normal

Prostate cross-section

BPH

Compressed urethra

Benign growth

Normal right lateral lobe of prostate

Left lateral lobe compressed and displaced

Anterior lobe displaced

Figure 26–19.

Clinical Management

1. Goals of clinical management
   a. Restore regular, complete bladder evacuation
   b. Prevent or manage associated complications
2. Nonpharmacologic interventions
   a. For acute urinary retention, immediate catheterization
   b. For chronic urinary retention,
      (1) Double voiding (see p. 1209)
      (2) Timed voiding
      (3) Indwelling catheterization (see p. 1222)
      (4) Intermittent catheterization (see p. 1222)
3. Pharmacologic interventions: See Table 26–8.
4. Special medical-surgical procedures
   a. Resection or removal of the lesion causing the obstruction
   b. Dilation of the obstructive stricture or stenosis
   c. Surgical repair of the urethral distortion
   d. Table 26–9 lists surgical treatments of BPH.

Complications

1. Urinary tract infections (the patient may be febrile)
2. Vesicoureteral reflux and possible hydronephrosis

Table 26–8. Pharmacologic Treatment of Urinary Retention

Drug Classification	Trade or Chemical Names	Potential Side Effects
Alpha-adrenergic blockers	Phenoxybenzamine Prazosin Terazosin Doxazosin	Orthostatic or postural hypotension, tachycardia, lethargy, fatigue, rhinitis
Cholinergic analog	Bethanecol chloride (Urecholine); Urecholine cannot be given intramuscularly or intravenously	Hypotension with reflex tachycardia, nausea, malaise, "hot flashes" Antidote: atropine
5 α-reductase inhibitors	Finasteride (Proscar); Proscar is not indicated for use in women or children.	Erectile dysfunction, decreased libido, decreased volume of ejaculate, headache

3. Compromised renal function, acute or chronic renal failure (uncommon)
4. Acute urinary retention
5. Low or poor bladder wall compliance (predisposing the patient to compromised renal function)
6. Instability (urge) incontinence with unstable detrusor contractions

Prognosis

1. Prognosis depends on location, duration, and severity of retention.
2. Severe obstruction of 7 days' duration can cause significant renal damage. If the obstructive lesion is corrected within 2 weeks or less, partial recovery is typical. If severe obstruction persists for more than 3 weeks, up to 50 percent of normal kidney function may be lost.
3. Prognosis is worsened when the obstruction is complicated by infection.
4. Generally, prognosis is excellent with ongoing treatment for urinary retention.

Applying the Nursing Process

NURSING DIAGNOSIS: Urinary retention (acute) R/T deficient detrusor contraction strength or obstruction

1. *Expected outcomes:* Following interventions, the person (with assistance) should be able to do the following:
   a. Regularly and completely empty the bladder
   b. Perform clean intermittent catheterization
   c. Ensure proper care for an indwelling catheter
   d. Prevent or properly manage symptomatic urinary tract infection
2. *Nursing interventions*
   a. Teach preventive measures to patients at risk for acute retention.
      (1) Patients should avoid medications containing α-adrenergic agonists. Advise the patient to consult a pharmacist, nurse, or physician before taking any over-the-counter or prescribed decongestants or dietary pills.

(2) Patients should avoid medications that reduce contractility of detrusor. Advise the patient to consult a physician, nurse, or pharmacist before beginning prescribed medications.
(3) Patients should avoid consumption of large volumes of fluid over short time periods because rapid diuresis predisposes the patient to retention.
(4) Patients should limit alcohol consumption because diuretic sedative effects may predispose the patient to acute retention.
(5) Patients should avoid prolonged exposure to cold environments. The body should be warmed before the first attempt to urinate when prolonged exposure to cold temperatures occurs.
   b. Teach strategies to promote urination.
      (1) Patients should drink warm tea or coffee to stimulate the desire to urinate.
      (2) Patients should assume the sitting position in a quiet, warm bathroom.
      (3) Patients should sit in the bathtub or shower with warm water to stimulate urination. Patients should urinate in the shower or bathtub or move immediately to a toilet and attempt to urinate.
   c. Instruct patients and their families to seek urgent medical assistance if acute retention persists more than 8 hours or if the patient is in acute discomfort and distress.

NURSING DIAGNOSIS: Urinary retention (chronic) R/T deficient detrusor contraction strength or obstruction

1. *Expected outcomes:* Following interventions, the person should be able to do the following:
   a. Regularly and completely empty the bladder
   b. Practice preventive measures
   c. Seek medical assistance for complete urinary retention
   d. Perform clean intermittent catheterization or manage an indwelling catheter (with assistance, if necessary)
2. *Nursing interventions*
   a. Teach the double-voiding technique.
   b. Institute a schedule of timed voiding—indicated for patients with poor sensation of bladder filling and poor muscle contractility.
   c. In consultation with the physician, teach self-intermittent catheterization.

Table 26–9. Surgical Treatment of Benign Prostatic Hypertrophy

Procedure	Description	Complications	Nursing Implications
Transurethral resection of prostate gland (TUR-P)	Surgical resection of tissue under endoscopic control. Commonly performed; the "gold standard" to which other procedures are compared. Indwelling catheter with 30-ml retention balloon under gentle traction used to tamponade prostatic vascular bed after surgery. Continuous bladder irrigation approximately 24 hours after procedure.	Hemorrhage TUR syndrome (potentially life-threatening electrolyte imbalance characterized by bradycardia, agitation) Vomiting during first postoperative day Acute urinary retention Stress urinary incontinence (uncommon) Erectile dysfunction Infertility	Brief hospitalization (1–3 days after procedure). Maintain catheter traction and inform surgeon immediately if catheter becomes dislodged. Monitor bladder irrigation system to avoid bladder overdistention or obstruction of catheter as clots or other debris drains from catheter. Monitor for signs of TUR syndrome, maintain adequate fluid hydration, and immediately inform surgeon if symptoms occur.
Transurethral incision of the prostate (TUIP)	Limited transurethral incision of prostatic capsule from bladder neck to edge of veromontanum. Often done on outpatient basis or with less than 24-hr observation period.	Similar to TUR-P	Complications are less likely with TUIP than TUR-P because of the limited area of incision. Teach patient and family to monitor for complications and call physician immediately if symptoms occur.
Balloon dilatation of prostate	Transurethral dilation of prostatic capsule using intraurethral balloon.	Hematuria	Frequency of this procedure is declining rapidly; it should no longer be considered viable treatment because it produces only transient therapeutic response.
Transurethral ultrasonic laser incision of the prostate (TULIP)	Ablation of prostate using ultrasonic imaging and laser energy from side-firing neodymium YAG laser in a transurethral sheath. Typically performed as outpatient procedure.	Bleeding Injury to adjacent tissue Prostatic edema with urinary retention that may persist for 1–2 wk	Manage bleeding complications (rare due to coagulation ability of laser). Teach patient and family to monitor for complications (particularly urinary retention) and call physician promptly if symptoms occur. Teach patient to care for suprapubic catheter and advise that the tube will remain in place for at least 2 wk, or until spontaneous voiding returns.
Visual laser ablation of the prostate (VLAP)	Laser energy from neodymium YAG laser under direct, endoscopic visualization.	Similar to TULIP Prostatic swelling and edema possibly producing transient urinary retention	Similar to TULIP
Vaporization of the prostate (Vaportrobe)	Vaporization of prostatic tissue using a Vaportrobe device; energy source identical to that used for resectoscope.	Prostatic swelling and edema possibly producing dysuria Transient urinary retention	Similar to VLAP
Interstitial laser therapy	Application of laser energy directly to prostate tissue using lower energy beam over a period of 5–10 min; may use transurethral, transrectal, or transperineal route.	Similar to TULIP and VLAP, but risk of injury to adjacent tissues may be lessened	Procedure remains "experimental;" clinical role in management of benign prostatic hypertrophy (BPH) remains unclear. May cause less postprocedural edema and urinary retention than VLAP or TULIP.
Transurethral needle ablation (TUNA)	Ablation of prostate tissue with transurethral application of radiofrequency energy (ultrasound used to image prostate and determine location of needle used to deliver energy).	Unclear	Undergoing clinical testing at 27 centers; clinical role in management of BPH remains unclear.

Table 26–9. Surgical Treatment of Benign Prostatic Hypertrophy (Continued)

Procedure	Description	Complications	Nursing Implications
Cryotherapy	Cooling of prostate tissue with subsequent slough.	Incontinence Injury to adjacent tissues Urinary retention	Rarely applied to BPH; role in clinical management remains unclear.
Hyperthermia of prostate	Transfer of heat to prostate tissue with subsequent tissue necrosis. Applied via transrectal or transurethral routes using microwave energy. Performed in outpatient settings.	Injury to adjacent tissues Urinary retention	May not provide dramatic improvement in symptoms noted with TUR-P. Transient urinary retention requires catheter drainage: teach catheter care to patient. Teach patient and family to monitor for complications and contact physician promptly if symptoms occur. Undergoing clinical testing; clinical role in BPH management remains unclear
Intraurethral stents	Stainless steel mesh or spiral stents that mechanically open prostatic urethra are inserted via transurethral route. Urethral mucosa overgrows mesh over period of time.	Infection Urinary retention Dysuria Incontinence Calculi possibly form when elements of stent extend into bladder	Temporary suprapubic catheter required. Provide patient medi-alert bracelet informing others that implant is present in urethra. Persistent pain and dysuria may indicate infection or failure of urethral epithelialization over device: teach patient to self-monitor for complications and promptly report symptoms to physician. Stent may be difficult to remove after epithelialization occurs.

d. Insert an indwelling catheter, as ordered.
e. Teach the patient and family to care for a chronic, indwelling catheter (see Box 26–1).
f. Begin a fluid management program to ensure adequate fluid intake and to avoid overhydration or dehydration.
  (1) Determine fluid needs (approximately 15 ml per pound of body weight).
  (2) Teach the patient to avoid consuming large volumes of fluid over brief periods of time.
  (3) Encourage the intake of clear liquids and water.
  (4) Limit the patient's fluid intake to sips 2 hours before sleep to minimize nocturia.
g. Prepare the patient for surgery or invasive procedures to resect or correct anatomic obstructions, as ordered.

NURSING DIAGNOSIS: Risk for infection R/T urinary retention

1. *Expected outcomes:* Following interventions, the person should be able to do the following:
  a. Describe the relationship between urinary tract infection and urinary retention
  b. Maintain adequate fluid hydration
  c. Prevent urinary tract infections

2. *Nursing interventions*
  a. Explain the association between urinary tract infection and urinary retention.
  b. Maintain adequate fluid hydration in the patient to flush toxins from the urinary system. Teach the patient the principles of hydration.
  c. Teach the patient about prophylactic anti-infective medications ordered by the physician.
    (1) Describe the need to take medications before sleeping unless otherwise directed.
    (2) Identify the side effects and emphasize that these may occur at any time while taking the drug.
    (3) Warn the patient of the potential for "breakthrough" infection that is resistant to suppressive anti-infective medication.

Discharge Planning and Teaching

1. Provide information about drugs and behaviors likely to aggravate urinary retention.
2. Teach care of catheters and related supplies.
3. Teach signs and symptoms of urinary tract infections.
4. Teach methods to access emergency care if acute urinary retention occurs.

■ *CARING FOR PEOPLE WITH URINARY SYSTEM CANCER*

Definitions

1. Cancer is uncontrolled cellular growth with potential for metastasis. Left untreated, local tumor growth and distant metastasis cause morbidity and premature death.
2. Classifications are according to site (location), extent of local invasion, presence of distant metastasis (staging system). Further classification is according to malignant potential (grade) (Fig. 26–20).

a. Renal tumors: Adenocarcinomas account for more than 90 percent of primary tumors of the renal parenchyma.
   (1) Stage I: Tumor is confined to renal capsule.
   (2) Stage II: Local invasion is into the perirenal fat and ipsilateral adrenal gland.
   (3) Stage IIIa: Metastasis is to the renal vein or the inferior vena cava.
   (4) Stage IIIb: Metastasis is to regional lymph nodes.
   (5) Stage IV: Local spread is beyond Gerota's fascia, and there is metastasis to distant organs.
b. Bladder and ureteral tumors: Transitional cell carcinomas account for more than 95 percent of primary bladder tumors and more than 90 percent of ureteral or upper urinary tract malignancies (Fig. 26–21).

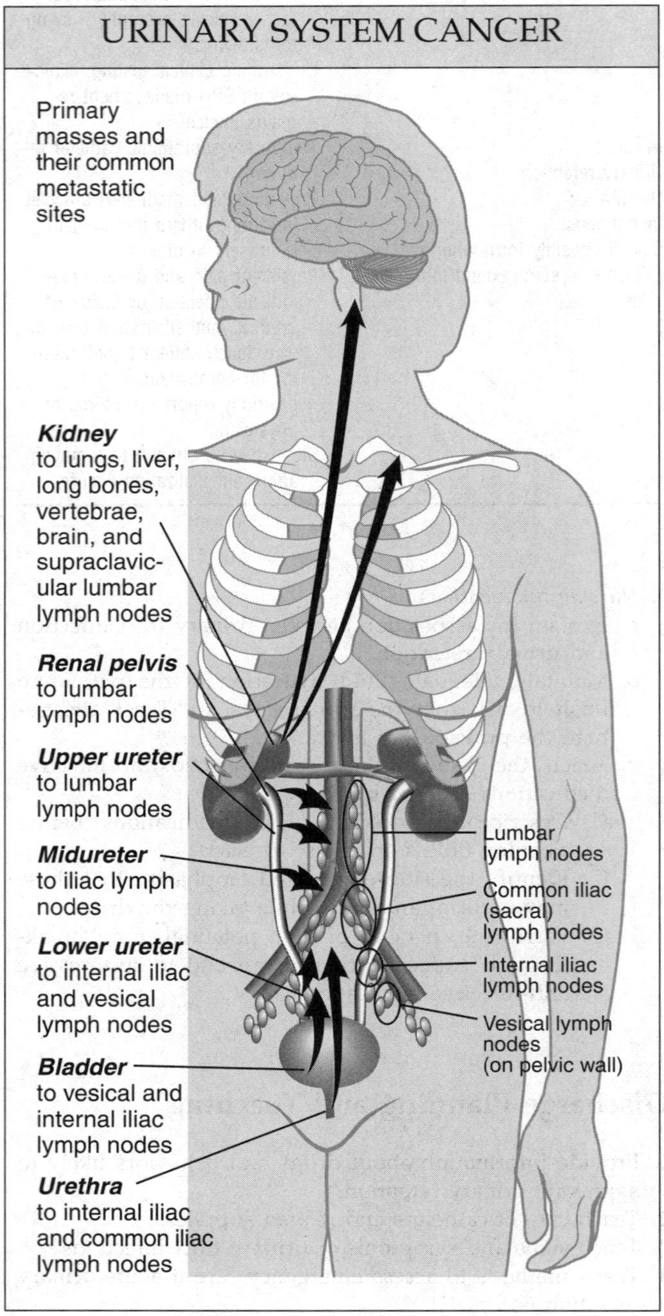

Incidence and Socioeconomic Impact

1. Renal adenocarcinoma appears predominantly between the ages of 50 to 60 years.
2. Approximately twice as many men are affected as women.
3. Bladder tumors are the 2nd most common form of genitourinary tumors and the 4th most common cause of

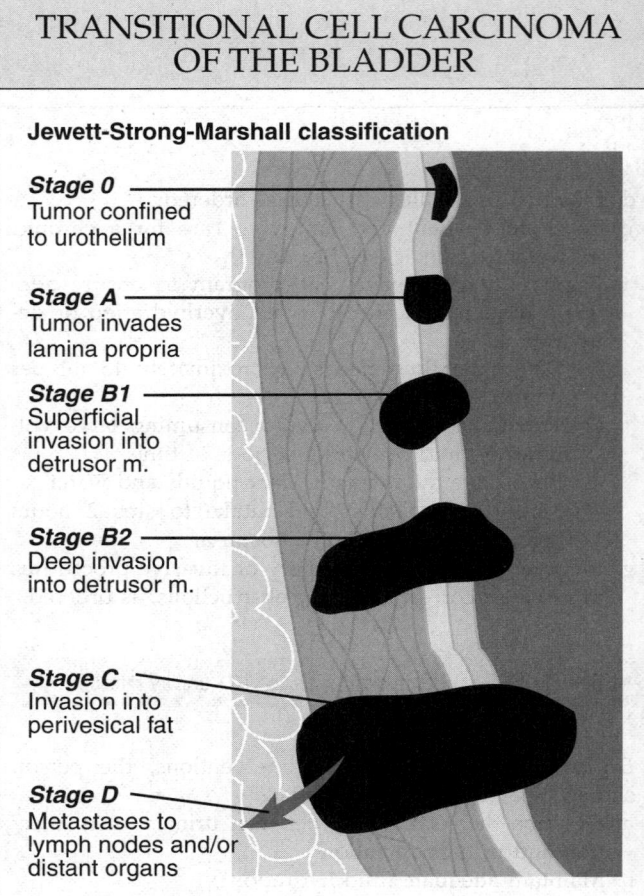

Figure 26–20.

Figure 26–21.

cancer deaths among 75-year-old men in the United States.
4. Bladder tumors occur predominantly in the 6th decade of life and are more common in men than women by a margin of 3.5 to 1.
5. Bladder cancer is more common among Whites than Blacks.
6. Approximately 85 percent of bladder cancers manifest as a low-grade superficial disease; 50 to 60 percent of ureteral tumors appear in the same manner. Thus, early detection is important.
7. Exposure to occupational carcinogens is linked to nearly 25 percent of all bladder cancers in the United States.

Risk Factors and Etiology

1. Risk factors for renal tumors
   a. Adult polycystic disease
   b. Von Hippel-Lindau disease
   c. Horseshoe renal anomalies
   d. Abuse of analgesics (phenacetin)
   e. Cigarette smoking and exposure to occupational carcinogens and toxins (unconfirmed but suspected)
2. Risk factors for bladder or ureteral tumors are similar to those of renal cancer, with the addition of the following:
   a. Cigarette smoking (up to 4 times the incidence in smokers)
   b. Chronic cystitis
   c. Familial patterns
   d. Excessive coffee ingestion
   e. Use of artificial sweeteners
3. Etiology is unknown.

Pathophysiology

1. Renal tumors
   a. Renal tumors arise from the proximal renal tubular epithelial cells (may be bilateral).
   b. Renal tumors have a high propensity for rapid metastatic spread with significant morbidity and death rates.
2. Bladder and ureteral tumors
   a. Activation of oncogenes with inhibition of suppressor mechanisms may contribute to the pathogenesis.
   b. Papillary tumors arise from the bladder epithelium and appear as a "cauliflower" configuration on a thin stalk attached to the bladder or ureteral lining.
   c. Ninety percent of bladder carcinomas exhibit transitional cell histology; approximately 11 percent of patients with superficial papillary tumors have carcinoma in situ (transitional cells confined to the epithelium).
   d. Seventy percent of transitional cell carcinomas appear as papillary lesions, with the remaining 30 percent appearing as nodular and mixed forms.

Clinical Manifestations

1. Renal tumors
   a. Hematuria, gross or microscopic

b. Fatigue, lethargy, pallor, and anemia
c. Palpable mass in upper abdominal quadrants
d. Flank pain with obstruction
e. Bone pain (typical of advanced-stage disease with metastasis)
2. Bladder or ureteral tumors
   a. Gross hematuria
   b. Irritative bladder symptoms such as urinary frequency and urgency
   c. Flank pain with ureteral obstruction
   d. Lymphadenopathy and hepatomegaly in advanced metastatic cases

Diagnostics

1. Assessment
   a. History should establish general symptoms, including change in urine elimination patterns, hematuria not associated with infection, and general symptoms of cancer, including weight loss.
   b. On physical examination, the abdomen should be inspected and palpated for masses.
   c. Diagnostic studies
      (1) Urinalysis for hematuria
      (2) Complete blood count for anemia with significant tumor-related blood loss (there are no known serum markers for renal, ureteral, or bladder cancer)
      (3) Urine cytologic study for atypical cells for bladder cancer (less sensitive for diagnosis of renal cell carcinoma)
      (4) Flow cytometry for analysis of DNA content of exfoliated cells obtained from cytologic study to grade the biologic aggressiveness of the tumor
      (5) An IVP for presence of a renal mass, distortion of the pelvicaliceal system due to the mass effect, hydronephrosis, or filling defect shown on cystogram with bladder tumor
      (6) Ultrasound for solid mass with echogenicity similar to that of renal parenchyma
      (7) Abdominal computed tomography scan to differentiate a fluid-filled from a solid renal mass and to stage the tumor before surgery
      (8) Magnetic resonance imaging study to detect the presence of a mass, and stage the tumor
      (9) Renal angiography to detect the presence of a tumor via vascular characteristics including neovascularity and arteriovenous fistulas
      (10) Endoscopy and tissue biopsy for direct inspection of the lower urinary tract and some ureteral masses, and to obtain tissue samples for grading of the tumor
2. Medical diagnosis
   a. For renal tumors, presumptive diagnosis is based on imaging study and clinical presentation; definitive diagnosis is by pathologic analysis of tissue obtained during surgical tumor resection.
   b. For bladder or ureteral tumors, presumptive diagnosis is based on imaging studies and cytology report; definitive diagnosis is by pathologic analysis of tumor by transurethral tissue resection, open surgical resection, or transurethral biopsy.

Clinical Management

1. Goals of clinical management
   a. Contain and eradicate the primary tumor
   b. Prevent local extension and distant metastases
   c. Establish normal patterns of urinary elimination
   d. Resolve hematuria
   e. Control pain
2. There are no nonpharmacologic interventions.
3. Pharmacologic interventions
   a. For renal adenocarcinoma:
      (1) Single (vinblastine) or combination agent chemotherapy, which is rarely successful
      (2) Hormone therapy: Medroxyprogesterone acetate (progesterone) to slow or retard tumor growth
      (3) Immunotherapy: Interferon-α, -β, or -γ and interleukin-2, which produce somewhat more favorable results than other agents
      (4) Radiotherapy, which is a palliative measure
      (5) Analgesia for pain produced by metastases (typically narcotics)
   b. For transitional tumors of the bladder and ureter:
      (1) Intravesical chemotherapeutic agents (Table 26–10): Treatment begins 10 to 14 days after bladder tumor resection
      (2) Systemic chemotherapy: Used to reduce tumor bulk before radical cystectomy and to treat advanced-stage cancer (significant side effects reduce the efficacy of prolonged treatment in advanced-stage disease)
      (3) Vitamin therapy: B_6 and vitamin C enhance the immune response
      (4) Hematoporphyrin derivative phototherapy: Binds with cancer cells, with porphyrin destroying cancer cells during subsequent exposure to krypton-ion laser light (efficacy is limited to superficial tumors)
4. Special medical-surgical procedures
   a. Renal cell carcinoma
      (1) Radical nephrectomy: removal of the kidney, surrounding fascia (including Gerota's fascia), ipsilateral adrenal gland, proximal half of the ureter, and regional lymph nodes. The procedure is the first-line surgery for unilateral tumors and is indicated for stages I, II, or IIIa renal cell carcinoma.
      (2) Palliative nephrectomy: removal of the kidney in the presence of advanced-stage tumor to retard metastasis and associated morbidity. However, this is done infrequently.
      (3) Subtotal nephrectomy: removal of the renal pole or local resection of small stage I tumors.
   b. Bladder and ureteral tumors
      (1) Transurethral resection of bladder tumors: removal of the tumor via the transurethral approach. Follow-up monitoring with or without adjunctive intravesical chemotherapy is essential.
      (2) Laser fulguration is therapy for small bladder tumors.
      (3) Radical cystectomy may be performed with continent or incontinent urinary diversion.

Complications

1. Complications of renal tumors
   a. Significant blood loss
   b. Hypertension due to poor renal function
   c. Flank pain with obstruction of the urinary system

Table 26–10. Intravesical Medications Used for the Treatment of Bladder Cancer

Medication and Dosage	Mechanism of Action	Potential Side Effects	Notes
BCG (Bacillus Calmette-Guérin) Reconstitute with nonbacteriostatic normal saline.	Considered as immunotherapy. Mechanism of action is unknown.	Irritative voiding symptoms Possible chemical cystitis Flu-like symptoms Prostatitis Sepsis or miliary tuberculosis Death	Most effective for treatment of carcinoma in situ. Cannot be given if patient is on antibiotic therapy or is immunosuppressed. Systemic reactions may require treatment with isoniazid, rifampin, or cycloserine.
Thiotepa Reconstituted with sterile water to obtain a 1 mg/ml dilution	Alkylating agent	Irritative voiding symptoms Myelosuppression Leukopenia	Complete blood count should be performed to evaluate possible decreases in white blood cell count and platelet count.
Adriamycin (doxorubicin) Reconstitute with normal saline to obtain a 1 mg/ml dilution	Antibiotic, antineoplastic, intercalating agent.	Irritative voiding symptoms Chemical cystitis Rare systemic myelosuppression Allergic reaction	Very expensive compared to other agents.
Mitomycin-C Reconstitute with sterile water to obtain a 1 mg/ml dilution	Antitumor, antibiotic, alkylating agent that inhibits DNA synthesis of growing tumor cells.	Irritative voiding symptoms Maculopapular rash, palmar or genital rash due to contact with the skin	Patient must be instructed to wash hands and genitals thoroughly after voiding to avoid skin contact. Significant cost.

d. Significant painless hematuria
e. Liver, bowel, central nervous system dysfunction with metastasis
f. Pathologic fracture with metastasis
g. Death
2. Complications of bladder and ureteral tumors
 a. Significant blood loss from hematuria
 b. Metastatic disease affecting the lungs, liver, and skeletal system
 c. Death

Prognosis

1. Prognosis for individuals with superficial (stage O, A) transitional cell carcinoma is very good; only 10 to 15 percent of these tumors progress to invasive malignancies that require radical cystectomy with urinary diversion.
2. Survival rates for persons with low-grade bladder tumors (stages B1, B2) are approximately 30 to 40 percent over 5 years.
3. Upper tract (ureteral or renal) tumors develop in approximately 2 percent of bladder cancer patients.
4. Prognosis is poor for advanced-stage renal tumors—5-year survival rates vary from 0 to 30 percent. Stage I tumors have a better prognosis, with 5-year survival rates of 60 to 82 percent.

Applying the Nursing Process

NURSING DIAGNOSIS: Altered protection R/T urinary system cancer with potential for local and metastatic invasion

1. *Expected outcomes:* Following interventions, the person should be able to do the following:
 a. Maintain physical protective defenses
 b. Prevent complications
2. *Nursing interventions*
 a. Administer systemic chemotherapy, as ordered. Advise the patient of dosage, schedule, and potential side effects. Administer antiemetics, as ordered, for associated nausea and vomiting.
 b. Provide frequent, small meals to minimize nausea related to chemotherapy. Assist the patient with oral hygiene before meals to maximize the appetite. Offer food preferences with maximally flexible scheduling.
 c. Monitor laboratory tests, particularly white blood cell count. Consult with the physician concerning scheduling of chemotherapy sessions if significant myelosuppression is noted.
 d. Administer immunotherapy, as ordered. Teach the patient dosage, administration, schedule, and side effects. (Prolonged fatigue is common.) Assist the patient to maintain adequate nutritional intake.
 e. Administer intravesical chemotherapy as ordered (see Chapter 17). Advise the patient of dosage, administra-

tion, scheduling, and side effects. Assess the patient for myelosuppression before each treatment.
 f. Prepare the patient for surgery to debulk or eradicate the tumor burden, as ordered.

NURSING DIAGNOSIS: Altered urinary elimination R/T urinary system tumor and associated treatments

1. *Expected outcomes:* Following interventions, the person should be able to do the following:
 a. Urinate normally
 b. Understand and comply with pain relief measures
 c. Recognize symptoms that require medical attention
2. *Nursing interventions*
 a. Assist the patient to minimize irritative voiding symptoms by fluid management and avoidance of bladder irritants.
 b. Administer urinary analgesics or antispasmodic medications, as ordered, to manage intense bladder irritation induced by intravesical chemotherapy.
 c. Advise the person to seek care from a urologist or continence nurse specialist if irritative voiding symptoms persist for more than 6 months after successful treatment of bladder or ureteral cancer.

NURSING DIAGNOSIS: Altered tissue perfusion (cardiovascular, peripheral vascular, renovascular) R/T urinary system cancer

1. *Expected outcomes:* Following interventions, the person should be able to do the following:
 a. Recognize signs and symptoms that indicate complications
 b. Recognize hematuria
 c. Describe signs and symptoms of altered tissue perfusion
2. *Nursing interventions*
 a. Monitor hematocrit, hemoglobin, and complete blood count for anemia with renal cell carcinoma or blood loss from tumor.
 b. Teach the patient to monitor urine for hematuria.
 c. Monitor vital signs for hypertension or compromised renal function. Administer antihypertensives, as ordered.
 d. Prepare the patient for palliative or therapeutic radical nephrectomy, as ordered.

NURSING DIAGNOSIS: Pain R/T metastasis of a urinary system tumor

1. *Expected outcomes:* Following interventions, the person should be able to do the following:
 a. Report control of pain
 b. Use pharmacologic agents for pain under supervision
 c. Use alternative techniques to increase comfort
2. *Nursing interventions*
 a. Administer analgesia as indicated for cancer-related pain (regular administration of narcotics is often nec-

essary for advanced-stage tumors with metastatic disease). Teach the patient to operate patient-controlled analgesia pump (see Chapter 13) as ordered.
   b. Use therapeutic touch and relaxation techniques.
   c. Apply warm, moist compresses to the flank.
   d. Assist the patient in positional changes to relieve local or generalized discomfort from bone metastasis.

Discharge Planning and Teaching

1. Teach signs and symptoms of recurrent urinary system tumor and the importance of ongoing monitoring for the presence of hematuria and other signs of recurrence.
2. Stress strict compliance with follow-up visits.

Public Health Considerations: Minimizing Risks

1. Avoidance of predisposing risk factors, such as smoking and exposure to occupational carcinogens, is essential in preventing bladder cancer.
2. Public education of warning signs of renal and bladder cancer is urgently needed; early detection and treatment profoundly affect prognosis.

■ CARING FOR PEOPLE WITH URINARY SYSTEM TRAUMA

Definitions

1. Urinary system trauma is an injury to any part of the urinary system (renal, ureteral, bladder, or urethral).
2. Injury may be of a blunt or penetrating nature.

Incidence and Socioeconomic Impact

1. A total of 4.6 percent of females suffering pelvic fractures have a coexisting urethral injury.
2. Eighty-five percent of bladder rupture is associated with pelvic fracture and other pelvic trauma.
3. Urinary system injuries may go undiagnosed as health care providers focus on other, more readily apparent, injuries.
4. Traumatic urinary system injuries often accompany blunt or penetrating trauma to the lower abdomen, pelvis, or perineum.
5. Blunt renal trauma is 8 to 9 times more frequent than penetrating renal injury.
6. The kidney is the most commonly injured organ within the urinary system.
7. Ureteral trauma is more likely to occur in association with surgical misadventure than is blunt or penetrating trauma.

Risk Factors

1. Driving while under the influence of drugs or alcohol
2. Engaging in contact sports without wearing adequate protective gear

Etiology

1. Blunt trauma of the abdomen is related to the following:
   a. Motor vehicle accidents
   b. Kidney deceleration injuries due to falls and impact of projectiles
   c. Risk of injury to the lower urinary tract is enhanced by pelvic fracture or having a full bladder.
2. Penetrating injuries are related to the following:
   a. Surgical misadventure
   b. Gunshot wounds
   c. Stab wounds

Pathophysiology

1. Blunt renal trauma
   a. A fall or the impact of a projectile causes sudden deceleration of the kidney.
   b. Protective mechanisms (perirenal fat, fascial coverings, adjacent organs, and bony structures) partially protect the kidney but are overwhelmed. The result is a tearing of the intima of intrarenal arteries and veins (renal contusion or more serious hemorrhage).
   c. Microscopic or grossly visible hematuria and delayed function ensue.
   d. In rare cases (usually involving spinal hyperextension injuries), the ureteropelvic junction is disrupted.
2. Penetrating renal trauma
   a. Gunshot or stab wounds penetrate the renal pedicle or parenchyma, causing hemorrhage and delayed function.
   b. Injury to the renal pedicle irreversibly impairs organ function. Parenchymal damage or polar avulsion usually results in less profound functional impairment.
3. Ureteral injuries: Disruption of urinary transport causes collection of urine in the retroperitoneum (urinoma) and increased risk of infection with penetrating trauma.
4. Bladder trauma
   a. Bladder rupture
      (1) Intraperitoneal rupture typically affects the dome of the bladder.
      (2) Extraperitoneal rupture (associated with pelvic fracture) causes tearing of the bladder wall. Urine may extravasate into the abdomen or upper thighs.
      (3) Interstitial rupture is the tearing of the bladder wall.
   b. Bladder contusion accounts for approximately one third of all vesicle injuries.
5. Urethral trauma
   a. Posterior urethra: After a severe blow to the abdomen or pelvis, the symphysis pubis shifts. Shearing force pulls bone and the urethra in different directions, causing disruption.
   b. Anterior urethra of the male: Significant straddle injuries to the perineum crush the bulbous urethra against the pelvic arch.

Clinical Manifestations

1. Renal trauma
   a. Gross or microscopic hematuria in 95 percent of cases

b. Contusion of the abdomen or flank in 85 to 90 percent of cases

c. Entry wound, exit wound, or both from a knife, bullet, or other projectile, typically in the abdomen or flank

d. Rib fracture on chest film or plain abdominal film, typically involving 10th, 11th, or 12th rib

e. Hemorrhagic shock with significant penetrating injury to the vascular system (systolic blood pressure of less than 90 mm Hg)

2. Ureteral trauma

a. Abdominal contusion or penetrating trauma: Ureteral trauma is suspected when fever of more than 100 degrees Fahrenheit develops and increasing flank pain occurs 4 to 9 days after injury. (Hematuria is not predictive of ureteral trauma.)

b. Hyperextension injury of the spine, particularly in young or thin patients

3. Bladder rupture

a. Pelvic fracture with abdominopelvic injury

b. Hematuria (gross hematuria in more than 95 percent of cases)

c. Nonspecific abdominal pain with inability to urinate

d. Intraperitoneal injury with abdominal distention and sanguineous fluid in the peritoneal cavity

e. Absent bowel sounds following abdominal injury

4. Urethral rupture

a. Vaginal bleeding with pelvic fracture in 80 percent of cases involving women

b. Gross hematuria (acute phase) following injury

c. Sanguineous discharge from the urethral meatus seen at the beginning or end of the urinary stream

d. Acute urinary retention

e. In men, anterior urethral damage (contusions and edema of the penile shaft and scrotum)

Diagnostics

1. Assessment

a. History

(1) The circumstances of trauma, including blunt trauma (location, type of object involved, body position during injury), penetrating injuries, hyperextension of spine, and fullness of bladder at the time of injury

(2) Preexisting hematuria or pain

b. Physical examination

(1) Prioritization of the patient's injuries. Life-threatening injuries receive priority.

(2) Measurement of vital signs to rule out hypovolemic shock and sepsis.

(3) Assessment of the flank or abdomen for signs of bruising, penetrating injury, or distention. The abdomen should be palpated to assess the location and quality of tenderness.

(4) Examination of the perineum for contusion of the penis or scrotum, vaginal bleeding, or butterfly contusion of the perianal area and scrotum with penile or urethral injury.

(5) Digital rectal examination of the male to detect upward displacement of the prostate toward the symphysis pubis ("high-riding prostate" with posterior urethral damage).

c. Diagnostic studies

(1) Urinalysis for hematuria (the severity of hematuria does not correlate with the severity of trauma)

(2) Serum studies: Complete blood count, hematocrit, and hemoglobin levels are measured to evaluate hemodynamic status.

(3) Plain film of the abdomen for fractured ribs

(4) Intravenous urogram for disruption of the kidneys, ureters, and bladder

(5) Nephrotomograms (similar to IVP) for anatomic integrity of kidneys

(6) Computed tomography scan for disruption of urinary structures

(7) Retrograde urethrogram to detect urethral rupture (performed before urethral catheterization)

(8) Cystogram to detect bladder rupture

(9) Radionuclide scan to determine differential renal function after injury

(10) Surgical exploration for direct visualization and assessment of trauma

(11) Intraoperative injection of methylene blue to detect ureteral trauma

(12) Exploratory laparotomy to detect intraperitoneal injury

2. Diagnosis

a. Renal trauma

(1) In blunt trauma, diagnosis is based on abdominal or flank trauma with or without trauma and hematuria persisting for days or weeks and anatomic distortion of kidney on imaging study.

(2) In penetrating trauma, diagnosis is based on distortion of anatomy on imaging study and direct visualization during surgical exploration or repair.

b. In ureteral trauma, diagnosis is based on the following:

(1) Disruption of the ureteral course on imaging study

(2) Direct visualization of the ureteral disruption during surgical procedure

c. In bladder trauma, diagnosis is based on the following:

(1) Extravasation of fluid on imaging study

(2) Direct visualization of disruption with exploratory laparotomy

d. In urethral trauma, diagnosis is based on the following:

(1) Extravasation on retrograde urethrogram

(2) Direct visualization of disruption on exploratory laparotomy or during endoscopic examination

Clinical Management

1. Goals of clinical management

a. Prevent life-threatening hemorrhage, sepsis, and related complications

b. Restore normal urinary function and prevent further damage to the urinary system

c. Prevent sepsis or formation of fistula or stricture
d. Reduce pain associated with trauma
2. Nonpharmacologic interventions
   a. For renal trauma, bed rest, serial urinalysis, and monitoring of vital signs (mild to moderate blunt trauma)
   b. For ureteral trauma, none
   c. For bladder trauma, bed rest (limited to contusion, minor injuries), indwelling catheterization (approximately 10 days for extraperitoneal ruptures)
   d. For urethral trauma, suprapubic catheterization and bed rest
3. Pharmacologic interventions
   a. Anti-infective agents to prevent or manage infection
   b. Analgesia for pain
   c. Intravenous hydration as indicated
   d. Transfusion of blood or blood components as indicated
4. Special medical-surgical interventions
   a. For renal trauma:
      (1) Partial nephrectomy for disruption of the renal pole
      (2) Nephrectomy for extensive renal injury
   b. For ureteral trauma:
      (1) Ureteral stents (under endoscopic control) for partial disruption
      (2) Primary reanastomosis
      (3) Ureteroneocystostomy for lower ureteral injury
      (4) Ureteroureterostomy (union of injured ureter with contralateral ureter for higher ureteral injuries)
   c. For bladder trauma:
      (1) Catheter diversion
      (2) Exploratory laparotomy with primary closure of the bladder wall and placement of a Jackson-Pratt drain

NURSE ADVISORY

It is vital to assess urethral trauma before inserting a catheter for bladder rupture.

      (3) Subsequent repair of fistulas, if required
   d. For urethral trauma (surgery delayed to allow initial healing and "strengthening" of tissues):
      (1) Suprapubic catheterization
      (2) Temporary diversion (rare)
      (3) Reanastomosis of the urethra

Complications

1. Complications of renal trauma (complications noted within the 1st month of injury):
   a. Hemorrhagic shock
   b. Retroperitoneal hematoma (develops in the 1st 2 weeks after injury)
   c. Abscess, sepsis, extravasation of urine, and fever
   d. Urinary fistula
   e. Hydronephrosis
   f. Pyelonephritis (febrile urinary tract infection)

g. Transient renin-mediated hypertension
2. Complications of ureteral injuries:
   a. Peritonitis
   b. Uroascites with respiratory distress
   c. Impaired renal function
3. Complications of bladder rupture:
   a. Urine extravasation into the peritoneum with uroascites and acute respiratory distress
   b. Sepsis
   c. Urinary incontinence
   d. Stricture or contracture of the bladder outlet
   e. Persistent fistula
4. Complications of urethral trauma:
   a. Strictures
   b. Incontinence
   c. Erectile dysfunction
   d. Increased risk of complications due to delayed diagnosis or inappropriate instrumentation of the urethra before specific evaluation for urethral trauma

Prognosis

1. Mortality directly related to urinary system trauma is rare.
2. Seriously compromised renal function is uncommon (less than 5%) with blunt trauma but more common (up to 50%) with penetrating injury

Applying the Nursing Process

NURSING DIAGNOSIS: Altered (renal) tissue perfusion R/T urinary system trauma

1. *Expected outcomes:* Following interventions, the person should be able to do the following:
   a. Be free of complications from urinary system trauma
   b. Experience optimal healing of the wound or contusion
2. *Nursing interventions*
   a. Continuously assess the patient for urinary system trauma, particularly after life-threatening injuries.
   b. Monitor vital signs and laboratory values for signs of significant bleeding due to blunt or penetrating renal trauma; serum and urine creatinine and serum BUN; and serial urinalyses for resolution of hematuria as renal trauma heals.
   c. Administer intravenous fluids, blood, or blood components, as ordered.
   d. Prepare the patient for diagnostic tests.
   e. Prepare the patient with significant trauma for surgery, as ordered.
   f. Provide adequate bed rest. Severely limit exertion, particularly during the acute phase after trauma.
   g. Insert an indwelling urethral catheter (after ensuring the absence of urethral rupture), as ordered. Teach the patient care of the catheter.
   h. Alert all staff to existing urethral trauma and instruct "no urethral instrumentation."

i. Monitor all wounds related to trauma, including surgical wounds, for signs of healing. Consult with the physician and the enterostomal therapy nurse regarding a poorly healing wound.

NURSING DIAGNOSIS: Risk for infection R/T urinary system trauma

1. *Expected outcomes:* Following interventions, the person should be able to do the following:
   a. Avoid complications of urinary system trauma
   b. Recognize signs and symptoms of infection
2. *Nursing interventions*
   a. Monitor vital signs for evidence of systemic infection or urosepsis.
   b. Monitor laboratory values, urine and blood cultures, and sensitivity reports for signs of specific infection. Consult the physician for sensitivity-driven antibiotic therapy.
   c. Administer anti-infective medications to prevent or treat infection, as ordered.
   d. Teach the patient to self-monitor for urinary tract infection.
   e. Encourage adequate fluid intake (15 ml/pound of body weight) to flush toxins and sediment from the urinary tract.

NURSING DIAGNOSIS: Pain R/T urinary system trauma

1. *Expected outcomes:* Following interventions, the person should be able to do the following:
   a. Report control of pain
   b. Maintain adequate hydration
2. *Nursing interventions*
   a. Assess pain for location, quality, duration, intensity, alleviating, or aggravating factors.
      (1) In renal trauma, assess for dull, boring, flank pain of prolonged duration; intensity may be severe with obstruction, mimicking obstructing calculus.
      (2) In ureteral trauma, assess for intense flank pain (steadily increasing) with ureteral rupture and formation of urinoma.
      (3) In bladder trauma, assess for burning suprapubic discomfort with episodes of sharp, cramping pain produced by unstable detrusor contractions ("bladder spasms").
      (4) In urethral trauma, assess for burning sensation in the urethra (penis or near vagina) that is aggravated by urination.
   b. Ensure adequate fluid intake (15 ml/pound of body weight). Emphasize intake of water and clear liquids.
   c. Teach the patient to avoid bladder irritants.
   d. Administer analgesics, as ordered.
   e. Teach positioning and relaxation techniques to promote comfort.
   f. Promote bed rest.

NURSING DIAGNOSIS: Altered nutrition, less than body requirement, R/T multiple system trauma

1. *Expected outcomes:* Following interventions, the person should be able to do the following:
   a. Identify nutrients essential to healing
   b. Maintain optimal levels of nutrition
2. *Nursing interventions*
   a. Discuss the need for increased intake of essential nutrients to promote wound healing.
   b. Administer supplemental nutrients (oral, enteral, or parenteral routes may be required depending on the nature or extent of injuries).
   c. Consult a nutritionist as indicated.
   d. Monitor laboratory values and status of wound healing in relation to nutritional status.

Discharge Planning and Teaching

1. Teach the patient and family to monitor for hematuria, either visually or via serial dipstick urinalyses, and signs and symptoms of urinary tract infection.
2. Reinforce the significance of follow-up care to remove the ureteral stint after trauma.
3. Teach urethral or suprapubic catheter care.
4. Discuss the potential for renovascular hypertension following renal trauma and advise the patient to routinely monitor blood pressure throughout life.

Public Health Considerations: Minimizing Risks

Penetrating renal trauma most commonly occurs as a result of a gunshot or stab wound; public policy designed to reduce violence and the access to weapons of human destruction is urgently needed.

Bibliography

Books

Benson JT (ed). *Female Pelvic Floor Disorders: Investigation and Management.* 1st ed. New York: WW Norton, 1992.

Brundage DJ. *Renal disorders.* St. Louis, Mosby–Year Book, 1992.

Gillenwater JY, et al (eds). *Adult and Pediatric Urology.* 3rd ed. Chicago: Mosby–Year Book, 1996.

Gray ML. *Genitourinary Disorders.* St. Louis: Mosby–Year Book, 1992.

Gray ML. *Urology Nursing Drug Reference.* St. Louis: Mosby–Year Book, 1996.

Krane R, and Siroky MB (eds). *Clinical Neuro-Urology.* 2nd ed. Boston: Little, Brown & Co, 1991.

Kunin CM. *Detection, Prevention, and Management of Urinary Tract Infections.* 4th ed. Philadelphia: Lea & Febiger, 1987.

Ostergard DR, and Bent AE (eds). *Urogynecology and Urodynamics.* Baltimore: Williams & Wilkins, 1991.

Tanagho EA, and McAninch JW (eds). *Smith's General Urology.* 12th ed. Englewood Cliffs, NJ: Prentice-Hall, 1988.

Torrens M, and Morrison JFB (eds). *The Physiology of the Lower Urinary Tract.* London: Springer-Verlag, 1987.

Walsh PC, et al (eds). *Campbell's Urology.* 6th ed. Philadelphia: WB Saunders, 1992.

Chapters in Books and Journal Articles

Colapinto V, and McCallum RW. The urethral injury in the fractured pelvis: A new understanding of the mechanism of injury. *In* Carlton CE Jr (ed). *Controversies in Urology.* Chicago: Year Book Medical Publishers, 1989.

Grasso M. Resecting upper-tract urothelial Ca by ureteroscopy. *Contemp Urol* 5:12, 1993.

Gray M. Electrostimulation in the management of voiding dysfunction. *Urol Nurs* 12:73–74, 1992.

Gray ML. Assessment and investigation of urinary incontinence. *In* Jeter KF, Faller NA, and Norton C (eds). *Nursing for Continence.* Philadelphia: WB Saunders, 1990.

Harrison LH. Differential diagnosis of uncomplicated versus complicated urinary tract infection. *In* Harrison LH (ed). *Management of Urinary Tract Infections. International Congress and Symposium Series.* London: Royal Society of Medical Services, 1990.

Herr HW. Transurethral resection and intravesical therapy of superficial bladder tumors. *Urol Clin North Am* 18:3, 1991.

Hudson ML. Toward a practical understanding of carcinoma in situ of the bladder. *Contemp Urol* 5:6, 1993.

Kelly M. Clinical snapshot: Chronic renal failure. *Am J Nurs* 96(1):36, 1996.

Labasky RC. Urodynamics. *In* Smith JA Jr (ed). *High Tech Urology; Technological Innovations and Their Clinical Applications.* Philadelphia: WB Saunders, 1992.

Lamm DL, et al. Prospective randomized comparison of intravesical with percutaneous bacillus Calmette-Guérin versus intravesical bacillus Calmette-Guérin in superficial bladder cancer. *In* Gillenwater JY, and Howards SS (eds). *Year Book of Urology 1992.* St. Louis: Mosby–Year Book, 1992.

Lee JY, and Cass AS. Evaluating lower urinary tract injuries. *Contemp Urol* 5:6, 1993.

Lynes WL, et al. The histology of interstitial cystitis. *In* Gillenwater JY, and Howards SS (eds). *Year Book of Urology 1991.* St. Louis: Mosby–Year Book, 1991.

Mostofi FK, Cavis CJ, Sesterhenn IA. Carcinoma of the male and female urethra. *In* Crawford ED, and Das S (eds). *Urol Clin North Am* 19:2, 1992.

Moul JW, et al. A range of genetic upsets may contribute to rcc. *Contemp Urol* 4:7, 1992.

Newman DK, and Smith DA. Pelvic muscle reeducation as a nursing treatment for incontinence. *Urol Nurs* 12:1, 1992.

Nurse DE, Parry JRW, and Muncy AR. Problems in surgical treatment of interstitial cystitis. *In* Gillenwater JY, Howards SS (eds). *Year Book of Urology 1992.* St. Louis: Mosby–Year Book, 1992.

Pearson BD. Liquidating a myth: Reducing liquid intake is not advisable for elderly with urine control problems. *Urol Nurs* 13:3, 1993.

Slade DKA. Interstitial cystitis: A challenge to urology. *Urol Nurs* 9:5, 1989.

Snyder JA, and Lipsitz DU. Evaluation of female urinary incontinence. *In* Leach GE (ed). *Urol Clin North Am* 18:2, 1991.

Stanton, SL. Stress incontinence: Why and how operations work. *Urol Clin North Am* 12, 279–284, 1985.

Stone AR. Treatment of voiding complaints and incontinence in painful bladder syndrome. *In* Leach GE (ed). *Urol Clin North Am* 18:2, 1991.

Switters DM, Soares SE, and de Vere White RW. Nursing care of the patient receiving intravesical chemotherapy. *Urol Nurs* 12:4, 1992.

Vapnek JM, Hricak H, and Carroll PR. Recent advances in imaging studies for staging of penile and urethral carcinoma. *In* Crawford ED, and Das S (eds). *Urol Clin North Am* 19:2, 1992.

Wein AJ. Pharmacologic management of non-BPH-induced voiding dysfunction: II. *In* Stamey TA (ed). *1993 Monographs in Urology* 14:6, 1993.

Resources and Agencies

Agency for Health Care Policy and Research
AHCPR Clearinghouse
P.O. Box 8547
Silver Spring, MD 20907
(800) 358–9295

American Cancer Society
1180 6th Avenue
New York, NY 10036
(800) ACS–1234

American Kidney Fund
6110 Executive Boulevard,
Suite 1010
Rockville, MD 20852
(800) 638–8299

American Nephrology Nurses' Association (ANNA)
ANNA National Office
East Holly Avenue—Box 56
Pitman, NJ 08071–0056
(609) 256–2320

National Association For Continence
P.O. Box 8310
Spartanburg, SC 29305
(800) BLADDER

The National Kidney Foundation
30 East 33rd Street
New York, NY 10016
(800) 622–9010

Sexuality Information and Education Council of the U.S. (SIECUS)
130 West 42nd Street, Suite 350
New York, NY 10036
(212) 819–9770

Simon Foundation For Continence (I Will Manage Programs)
P.O. Box 835
Wilmette, IL 60091
(800) 23–SIMON
(847) 864–3913
Information on setting up support groups and patient education on incontinence.

Society of Urologic Nurses and Associates
East Holly Avenue
Box 56
Pitman, NJ 08071–0056
(609) 256–2335

Wound, Ostomy, Continence Nurses' Society
2755 Bristol Street, Suite 110
Costa Mesa, CA 92626
(714) 476–0268

27
Caring for People with Gastrointestinal Disorders

■ GASTROINTESTINAL STRUCTURE AND FUNCTION

Structure of the Gastrointestinal System

The gastrointestinal (GI) system (Fig. 27–1) consists of the following:

1. Alimentary canal (GI tract): Essentially a long, hollow tube of muscle that includes the mouth, esophagus, stomach, small intestine, large intestine, rectum, and anus. It is made up of 4 layers: the mucosa, submucosa, muscularis, and serosa (adventitia).
2. Accessory organs: liver, pancreas, and gallbladder

Structure of the Gastrointestinal Tract

1. The mouth (buccal or oral cavity) consists of the teeth, tongue, hard and soft palates, cheeks, lips, pharynx, and 3 salivary glands (Fig. 27–2).
   a. Parotid glands produce serous secretions containing salivary amylase (ptyalin).
   b. Submandibular glands produce mucus and serous secretions through Wharton's ducts.
   c. Sublingual glands produce thick mucus.
2. The esophagus is a muscular tube 2.5 cm in diameter and about 25 cm long that extends from the pharynx to the stomach (Fig. 27–3).
   a. It lies posterior to the trachea and in front of the vertebral column.
   b. It contains 2 sphincters:
      (1) The upper pharyngoesophageal sphincter
      (2) The lower esophagogastric (cardiac) sphincter
3. The stomach is a distensible organ that can reach a size of 25 cm by 10 cm (Fig. 27–4).
   a. It is located in the left upper quadrant of the abdomen below the diaphragm.
   b. The stomach has 4 anatomic divisions:
      (1) Cardiac region
      (2) Fundus
      (3) Body
      (4) Pylorus (antrum)
   c. There are 2 sphincters at each end of the stomach.

(1) Esophagogastric (cardiac): Prevents reflux of acidic stomach contents back up into the esophagus
(2) Pyloric (at duodenum): Has protective and transport functions
4. The small intestine is a tubelike structure about 1 inch in diameter and 18 feet long (Fig. 27–5).
   a. It is divided into 3 regions:
      (1) Duodenum: 1st region, C-shaped
      (2) Jejunum: midportion
      (3) Ileum: last section
   b. It has cellular layers that are similar to the rest of the GI tract except that the mucosa and submucosa have circular folds known as plicae circulares, and the mucosal surface is covered with villi. These 2 structures greatly increase the absorptive surface of the small intestine.
5. The large intestine is a tubelike structure approximately 5 to 6 feet long and 2 inches in diameter that consists of the following:
   a. Cecum: First segment (at the junction of the ileum and colon), containing the ileocecal valve and the appendix
   b. Ascending colon: Extends from the cecum to the hepatic flexure
   c. Transverse colon: Crosses the abdominal cavity from right to left (hepatic flexure to splenic flexure)
   d. Descending colon: Runs down the left side of the abdomen from the splenic flexure to the iliac crest
   e. Sigmoid colon: The S-shaped last section of the colon that ends at the rectum
   f. Rectum: Last portion of the large intestine, about 5 inches long; it follows the sigmoid colon in the midsacral area and connects to the anal canal.
6. Innervation of the GI tract occurs in 2 ways:
   a. Neural transmission to the smooth muscle that stimulates movement of food through the GI tract; it results from distention of the myenteric plexus (found in longitudinal and circular smooth muscle) or the submucosal plexus (found in the submucosa).
   b. Autonomic nervous innervation results from the following:
      (1) Sympathetic stimulation: The thoracic and lumbar splanchnic nerves inhibit secretions and movement and contract sphincters.
      (2) Parasympathetic stimulation: The vagus nerve increases motor and secretory activity and relaxes sphincters.

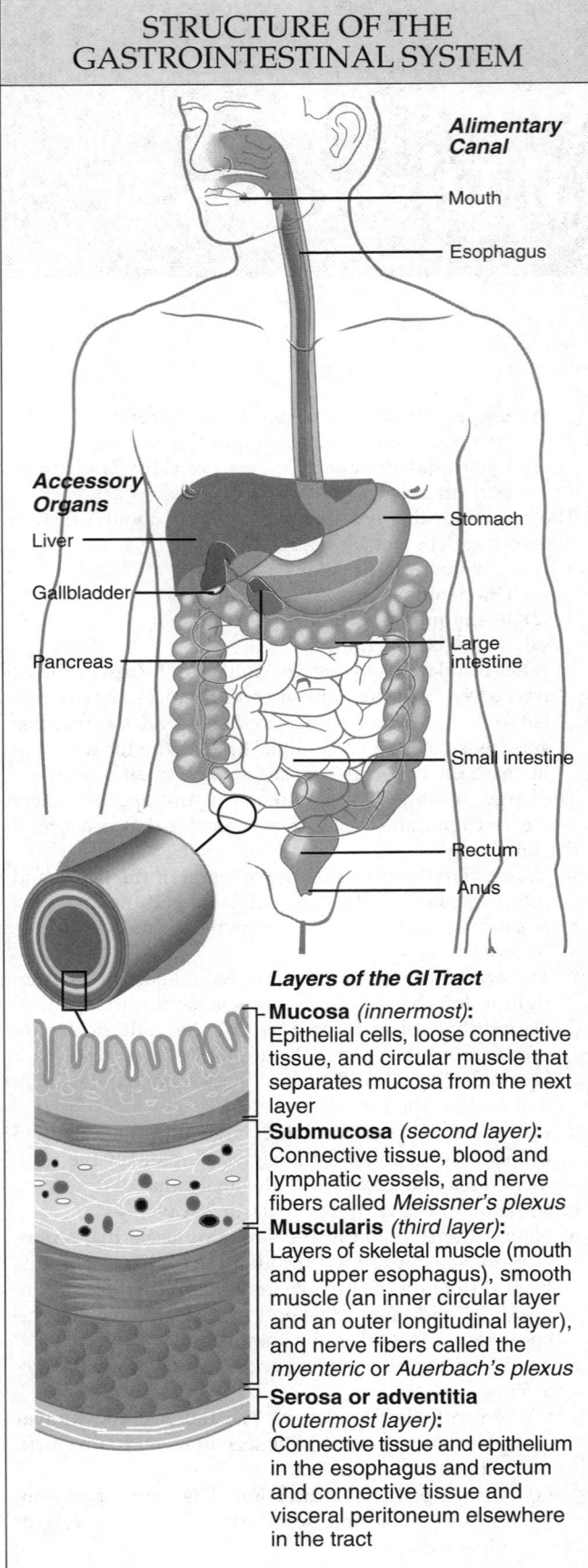

STRUCTURE OF THE GASTROINTESTINAL SYSTEM

Alimentary Canal

— Mouth

— Esophagus

Accessory Organs

Liver —

Gallbladder —

Pancreas —

— Stomach

— Large intestine

— Small intestine

— Rectum

— Anus

Layers of the GI Tract

Mucosa *(innermost)*:
Epithelial cells, loose connective tissue, and circular muscle that separates mucosa from the next layer

Submucosa *(second layer)*:
Connective tissue, blood and lymphatic vessels, and nerve fibers called *Meissner's plexus*

Muscularis *(third layer)*:
Layers of skeletal muscle (mouth and upper esophagus), smooth muscle (an inner circular layer and an outer longitudinal layer), and nerve fibers called the *myenteric* or *Auerbach's plexus*

Serosa or adventitia *(outermost layer)*:
Connective tissue and epithelium in the esophagus and rectum and connective tissue and visceral peritoneum elsewhere in the tract

Figure 27–1.

STRUCTURE OF THE MOUTH

— Teeth

— Hard palate

— Soft palate

— Uvula

— Tonsil

— Tongue

Parotid gland

Parotid duct

— Ducts of sublingual gland

— Sublingual gland

— Submandibular gland

Sublingual caruncle (opening of submandibular duct or Wharton's duct)

Figure 27–2.

Functions of the Gastrointestinal System

1. Functions of the GI tract are to ingest, transport, digest, absorb, and eventually eliminate nutrients from the body.
2. The process begins in the mouth.
   a. Teeth chew (masticate) the food. Mastication breaks large particles into small ones. It also stimulates the release of ptyalin (Table 27–1), which does the following:
      (1) Acts to break down polysaccharides
      (2) Provides the initial stimulus that starts the enzymatic digestion process
   b. The secretion of saliva softens food.
   c. The tongue forces the food bolus into the pharynx, and swallowing begins.
3. The bolus travels from the pharynx to the esophagus, where peristalsis propels food toward the stomach.
   a. Peristalsis is a wormlike movement that results from

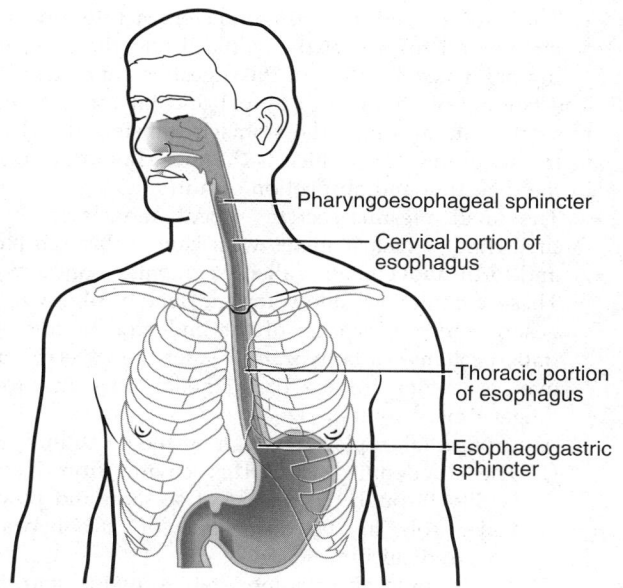

Figure 27-3. Structure of the esophagus.

STRUCTURE OF THE STOMACH

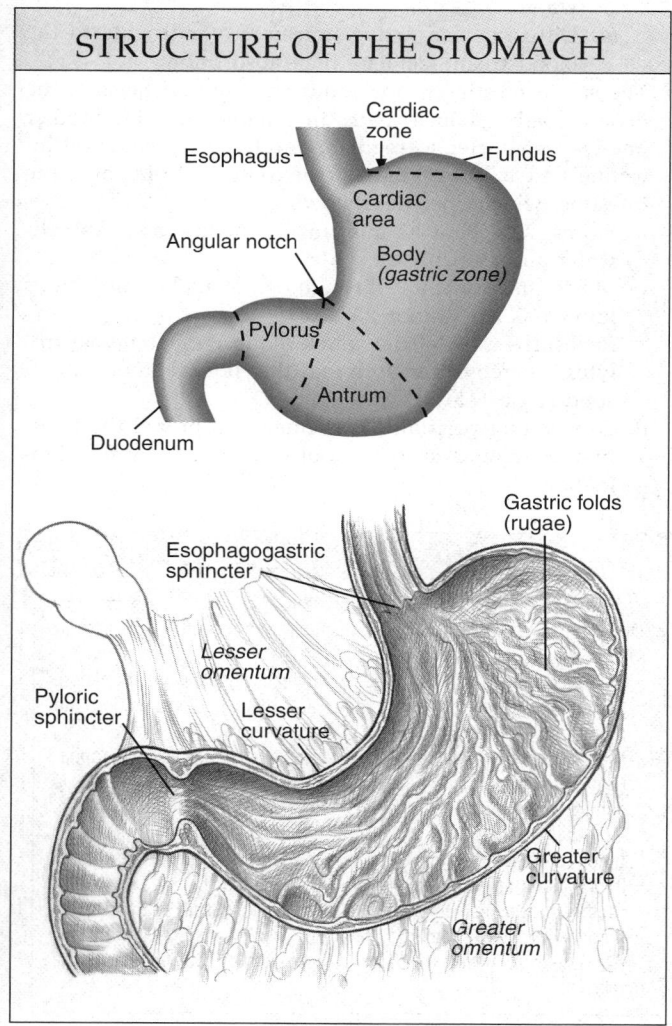

Figure 27-4.

STRUCTURE OF THE SMALL AND LARGE INTESTINES

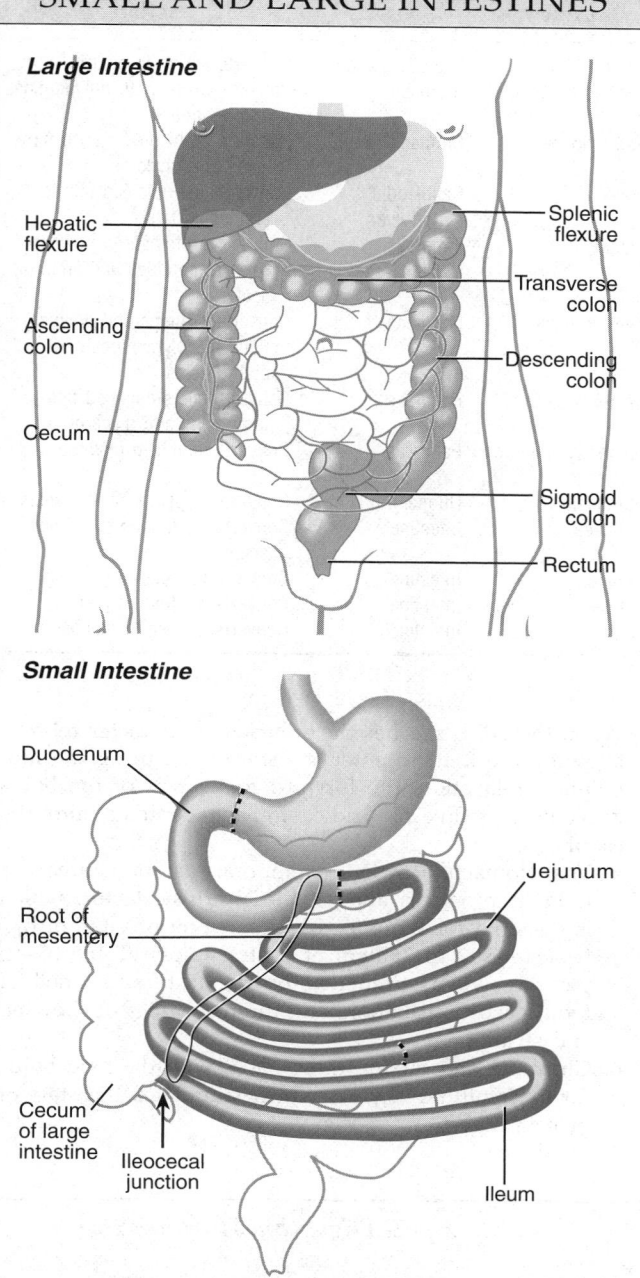

Figure 27-5.

relaxation and contraction of the longitudinal and circular fibers of the muscularis and sphincters throughout the GI tract.

(1) It moves small amounts of food into the stomach and also helps to mix the food with gastric juice.

(2) In combination with the secretion of hormones and enzymes, it promotes digestion throughout the tract.

b. The esophagus secretes mucus continually to lubricate and aid peristalsis.

Table 27–1. Digestive Enzymes

Enzyme	Source	Action
Ptyalin	Salivary glands	Converts starch to dextrin
Protease (pepsin)	Stomach	Converts proteins to polypeptides and peptides
Gastric lipase	Stomach	Converts emulsified fats to fatty acids and glycerol
Bile	Gallbladder and liver	Converts unemulsified fats to emulsified fats
Trypsin	Pancreas	Converts proteins and polypeptides to peptides and amino acids
Chymotrypsin	Pancreas	Converts proteins and polypeptides to polypeptides and amino acids
Pancreatic lipase	Pancreas	Converts bile-emulsified fats to fatty acids and glycerol
Pancreatic amylase	Pancreas	Converts starch to maltose
Enterokinase	Duodenum	Converts trypsinogen to trypsin
Peptidase	Intestine	Converts dipeptides to amino acids
Sucrase	Intestine	Converts sucrose to glucose
Maltase	Intestine	Converts maltose to glucose
Lactase	Intestine	Converts lactose to glucose

4. When the bolus reaches the stomach, a sphincter relaxes, allowing the food to enter the stomach. During the momentary relaxation, the forward movement of the bolus prevents a reflux of acidic stomach contents into the esophagus.
   a. The stomach acts as a temporary storage area for food. It produces and secretes intrinsic factor, which is essential for the effective absorption of vitamin B_{12}. It secretes 2 to 3 liters of gastric juices (Table 27–2) per day when stimulated by the taste and smell of food, gastric distention, and the mechanics of chewing and swallowing.
   b. Churning and mixing these juices with the food bolus forms semifluid chyme, which stimulates the start of protein digestion.

Table 27–2. Digestive Hormones

Hormone	Source	Action
Gastrin	Secreted by gastric mucosa	Stimulates motility and secretion of pepsin and HCl
Gastric inhibitory peptide (GIP)	Secreted by small intestine	Inhibits motility and decreases gastric secretion
Cholecystokinin	Secreted by duodenum	Stimulates gallbladder releases of, and increases, pancreatic enzymes
Secretin	Secreted by duodenum	Stimulates secretion of pancreatic juices and bile, inhibits stomach contractions
Pancreozymin	Secreted by duodenum	Stimulates secretion of pancreatic juices

c. The cardiac and pyloric sphincters act to transport chyme and to protect the stomach and the surrounding organs from reflux of the digestive contents.
5. The volume of chyme and its pH and fat content determine the rate at which the stomach transfers the chyme to the small intestine, which is the most important organ in the digestion and absorption of nutrients.
   a. The small intestine secretes mucus and watery intestinal fluid, which it mixes with chyme through back-and-forth movements called segmental contractions. These contractions allow for nutrient breakdown, digestion, and absorption of the end-product nutrients (fats, proteins, carbohydrates, water, and electrolytes) over a greater surface of epithelial cells and for a longer time.
   b. Absorption takes place throughout the small intestine.
      (1) The duodenum neutralizes chyme from gastric acidity through the release of secretin and plays a major role in the absorption of carbohydrates, iron, and calcium.
      (2) The jejunum absorbs most fats, proteins, and vitamins.
      (3) The ileum absorbs intrinsic factor–vitamin B compound and nutrients that are not absorbed elsewhere.
      (4) Diffusion and active transport of nutrients to the bloodstream facilitate their absorption.
6. The small intestine propels nutrients by peristalsis to the ileocecal valve, which works in conjunction with another one-way sphincter to regulate emptying of the small intestine and to prevent reflux of contents from the large intestine, which does the following:
   a. Stores and moves intestinal contents and absorbs water and electrolytes
   b. Mixes its contents through segmental contractions known as haustrations
   c. Reabsorbs most of the water, along with some electrolytes, thereby transforming the liquid stool into a solid stool (feces)
   d. Uses strong peristaltic movements to propel the intestinal contents and force stool into the rectum for elimination

ELDER ADVISORY

Over time, changes in the gastrointestinal tract occur that can result in problems for older people.
- In the mouth, gingivitis causes gum recession and inflammation. Salivary glands secrete less saliva and ptyalin. Dental caries and tooth loss are common.
- In the esophagus, peristaltic action increases. The lower esophageal sphincter may relax or become incompetent. Hiatal hernia is common. All of these changes result in swallowing difficulties, increases in heartburn, and complaints of reflux or regurgitation.
- In the stomach, gastric emptying decreases, as do secretions of hydrochloric acid and pepsin, as well as lipase activity.
- In the intestines, secretions of pepsin and lipase decrease. Absorption of many nutrients (fats, dextrose, xylose, calcium, iron, B_2, B_{12}) is reduced. The internal sphincter of the large intestine relaxes.

■ ASSESSING PEOPLE WITH GASTROINTESTINAL DISORDERS

Key Symptoms and Their Pathophysiologic Bases

1. Common major symptoms in gastrointestinal disorders include pain or discomfort, nausea or vomiting, and changes in bowel habits.
2. To determine the significance of these symptoms, ask the person these questions:
   a. How would you describe the symptom?
   b. How long have you experienced the symptom? Have you ever had it before?
   c. When did the symptom start?
   d. Did it start suddenly or gradually; has it been continuous or intermittent?
   e. Does anything relieve the symptom or make it worse?
   f. Has the symptom interfered with your ability to eat or otherwise carry on your daily routine?
   g. Do any specific activities seem to bring it on?
   h. Do you have any other symptoms that are associated with it?
   i. What do you think is causing the symptom?
3. Pain or discomfort
   a. Characteristics: Abdominal pain can be described as dull, aching, sharp, burning, stabbing, cramping, gnawing, or colicky. Anal discomfort is described as an itching, burning, or stinging pain.
   b. Location: Abdominal pain is identified by the quadrant involved. Pain may radiate or spread to other areas (Fig. 27–6).
   c. Duration: Abdominal pain can be intermittent or continuous: it can come on gradually or suddenly, or it can gradually intensify. The onset of pain from intes-

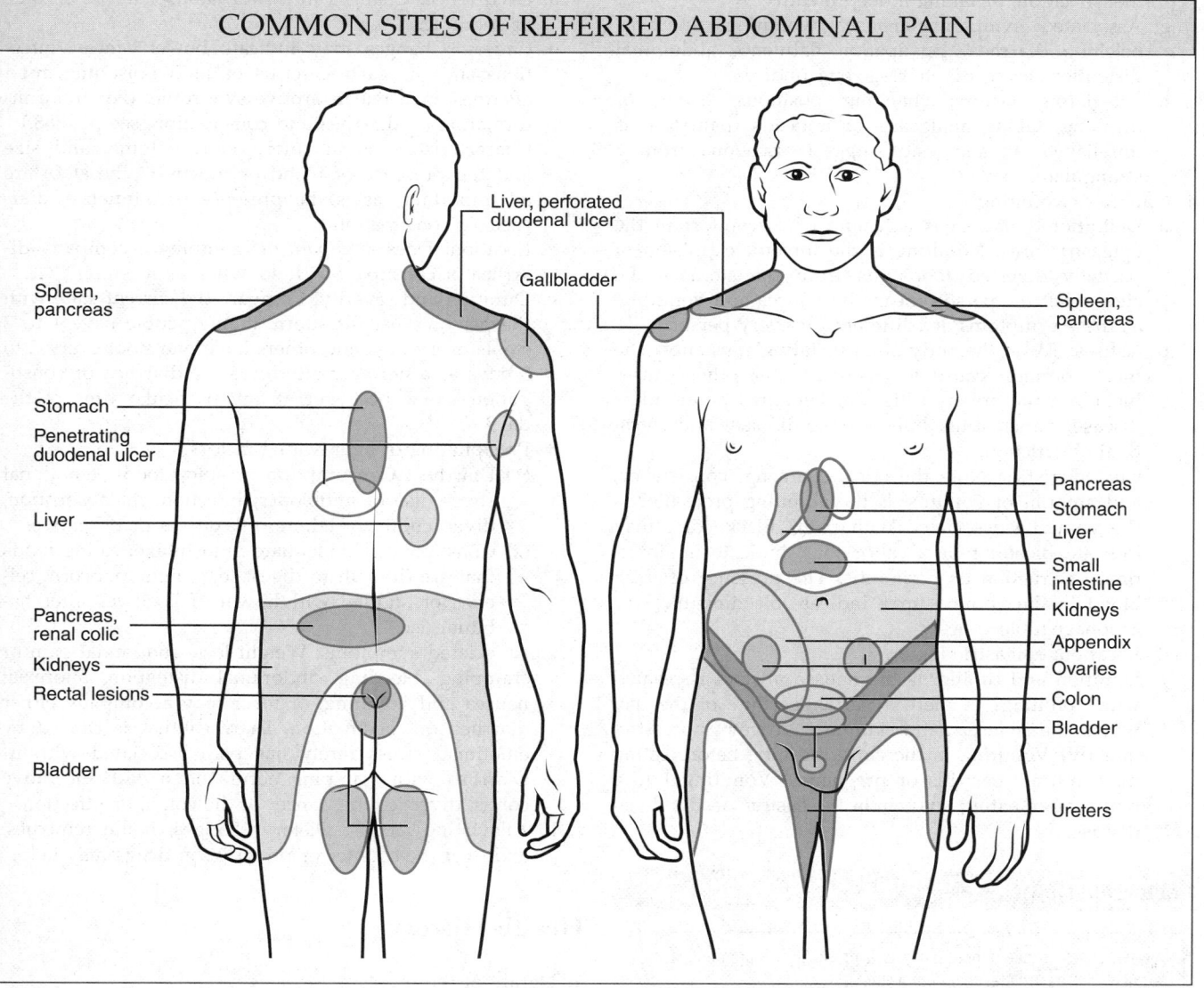

COMMON SITES OF REFERRED ABDOMINAL PAIN

Liver, perforated duodenal ulcer

Gallbladder

Spleen, pancreas

Stomach

Penetrating duodenal ulcer

Liver

Pancreas, renal colic

Kidneys

Rectal lesions

Bladder

Spleen, pancreas

Pancreas

Stomach

Liver

Small intestine

Kidneys

Appendix

Ovaries

Colon

Bladder

Ureters

Figure 27–6.

tinal obstruction or appendicitis is usually gradual, whereas pain from a perforated ulcer is sudden.

d. Severity: Quantify the pain on a scale of 1 (no pain) to 10 (most severe pain). Pain severity is usually a good indicator of the severity of the disease.

e. Types of abdominal pain
   (1) Visceral pain originates in the abdominal organs and is usually diffuse, poorly localized, and intermittent. It may be described as dull or aching, burning, or cramping.
   (2) Parietal (or somatic) pain develops after the visceral pain occurs and is caused by inflammation. It is more localized, steady, and severe than visceral pain.
   (3) Referred pain is felt at a site distant from, but of the same dermatome as, the spinal root of the affected organ and is usually localized at the site.

f. Precipitating or aggravating factors: eating, drinking, having a bowel movement, walking, changing positions, taking certain medications, emotional stress, menstruation, or taking a deep breath

g. Associated symptoms: nausea, vomiting, anorexia, belching, diarrhea, constipation, flatulence, abdominal distention, fever, diaphoresis, or jaundice

h. Alleviating factors: changing positions, eating or drinking, taking analgesics or antacids (pain that is unrelieved by analgesics suggests ischemia from a strangulated bowel).

4. Nausea or vomiting
   a. Definitions: Nausea is a feeling of discomfort in the epigastric area. Vomiting is the forceful expulsion of partially digested foodstuffs from the stomach. Be clear what the person means by nausea and vomiting, as these symptoms are different for every person.
   b. Causes: To rid the body of an irritating substance. The most common cause is gastroenteritis; other causes include acute appendicitis, flu, hepatitis, peptic ulcer disease, pancreatitis, biliary tract disease, and intestinal obstruction.
   c. Characteristics: Note the odor, character, consistency, and amount of vomitus. Is the vomiting projectile? Is the vomiting associated with pain? Black color may indicate bleeding; fecal odor may indicate an intestinal obstruction or peritonitis. The presence of fresh blood in the vomitus may indicate bleeding ulcer or esophageal bleeding.
   d. Location: epigastric region
   e. Duration and timing: Is the nausea always associated with vomiting? Is there a particular time of the day when the nausea and vomiting occur more frequently? Vomiting in the early morning before eating may indicate gastritis or pregnancy. Vomiting 1 to 4 hours after eating may indicate gastric or duodenal disease.

NURSE ADVISORY

Always check to see if pregnancy is a possibility in premenopausal women with gastrointestinal complaints.

f. Severity: Check to see if the person can keep down any foods or liquids. Severe nausea and vomiting can result in a fluid and electrolyte imbalance or a metabolic problem. In addition, severe or prolonged vomiting poses the threat of aspiration, especially in the elderly.

g. Precipitating or aggravating factors: Food, alcohol, drugs, odors, position, emotional upsets, or stress can trigger or worsen nausea and vomiting.

h. Associated symptoms: Anorexia, diarrhea, constipation, abdominal pain, fever, headache, or weight loss may accompany nausea and vomiting. Nausea and vomiting with generalized or localized right lower quadrant abdominal pain may indicate appendicitis. Explore any weight gain or loss.

i. Alleviating factors: What types of fluids and diet are being tolerated? Does it help to change positions? Do over-the-counter or prescription antiemetic medications help?

5. Changes in bowel habits
   a. Occurrence: Changes in bowel habits may be chronic or sporadic.
   b. Causes: Changes may indicate bowel cancer, infections such as gastroenteritis or food poisoning, food allergies, or a malabsorptive syndrome. (For more information on diarrhea and constipation, see p. 1288.)
   c. Characteristics: Fecal color, odor, volume, and size and the presence of blood or mucus in the stool are all important, as is the presence of flatulence, diarrhea, or constipation.
   d. Location: Does any pain or cramping accompany diarrhea or constipation? If so, where is it tender?
   e. Duration and severity: Compare the current state with the person's usual pattern. (Some people have 1 to 2 stools every day, and others have one stool every 2 to 3 days as a normal pattern.) Is the diarrhea or constipation worse or better at any particular time of the day?
   f. Precipitating or aggravating factors
      (1) Diarrhea: Consumption of spicy foods, emotional stress, use of antibiotics, infection, malabsorption, diverticulitis, or taking of laxatives or purgatives
      (2) Constipation: Inadequate fluid intake, eating foods that are difficult to digest (e.g., nuts, popcorn, celery), or sudden withdrawal of laxatives after habitual use
   g. Associated symptoms: Weight loss, abdominal pain or cramping, bleeding, abdominal distention, anorexia, nausea and vomiting, or fever may accompany either diarrhea or constipation. Diarrhea that is caused by emotional stress rarely has pain associated with it. Diarrhea with cramping occurs often with ulcerative colitis, diverticulitis, cancer of the colon, or infection.
   h. Alleviating factors: Dietary changes, home remedies, and over-the-counter or prescription drugs may help.

Health History

1. Nature of the problem
   a. Investigate all GI complaints carefully, even "vague"

complaints of indigestion or heartburn, loss of appetite, unexplained weight loss, passing a lot of gas, or feelings of fullness.
   b. Many of the complaints are difficult to describe, so listen and question fully.
   c. Many GI complaints are "private," and some people will not discuss them openly.
   d. Be careful to determine what is normal for this person and what is not right about the current state.
2. Major illnesses and hospitalizations: Conditions that have the greatest impact on current GI status are diabetes mellitus, heart disease, alcoholism, liver disease, pancreatic disease, gallbladder disease, jaundice, bleeding disorders, ulcer disease, colitis, hernia, hemorrhoids, cancer of the GI tract, and previous abdominal surgery.
3. Medications
   a. Medications often cause gastrointestinal disturbances. Note all medications that are being taken, with times, route, and dosage.
   b. Over-the-counter medications, such as aspirin, vitamin supplements, laxatives, antacids, or enemas, are particularly important. Aspirin can predispose the person to ulcer disease. Long-term use of laxatives can cause dependence.
   c. Gastrointestinal disease can interfere with the normal use and uptake of medications.
4. Nutritional status
   a. Assess for any special diet or dietary restrictions.
   b. Determine the usual foods eaten daily, and approximate amounts, times, and frequency of meals. Pay particular attention to consumption of caffeine and alcohol, as both contribute to GI tract disease.

TRANSCULTURAL CONSIDERATIONS

Assess for cultural and religious patterns. Spicy cooking styles precipitate or aggravate gastrointestinal complaints. Fasting and abstinence patterns are also important. Assess immigrants and refugees for dietary changes that result from the acculturation process —different daily eating patterns, unavailability of traditional foods, and incorporation of "fast food" into the diet.

---

   c. Determine whether there have been any changes in diet as a result of the recent illness.
5. Family history: Assess for family history of heart disease, diabetes mellitus, liver disease, pancreatic disease, bleeding disorders, alcoholism, ulcers, colitis, or cancers of the GI tract.
6. Social history
   a. Age, gender, race, religion, and occupation increase the likelihood of some GI disorders, such as cancers, hiatal hernia, ulcerative colitis, diverticulosis, and ulcers.
   b. Recent travel out of the country may cause GI problems, especially infections.
   c. Tobacco use predisposes to several oral cancers.
   d. Does the person have adequate financial means to obtain proper medical care and sound nutrition? Financial problems can also increase stress, which (regardless of its source) can lead to GI disorders.

Physical Examination

1. Height and weight (see Chapter 5 for details)
2. Anthropometric arm measurements (see Chapter 10 for details)
3. Mouth and pharynx
   a. Inspect the outer lips for color, symmetry, and presence of any abnormalities.
   b. Using a penlight and tongue depressor, inspect the inner surfaces of the lips and oral mucosa, noting the condition of the membranes.
   c. Assess the tongue, noting color, coating, ulcers, and any variations in size or shape.
   d. Inspect the teeth and gums for dental caries, absence of teeth, inflammation, or signs of bleeding.
   e. Note any significant mouth odors.
   f. Assess the pharynx for signs of inflammation and the presence of tonsils, exudate, swelling, or ulcerations.
   g. Ask the person to say "ah," and note the normal retraction of the uvula with an intact vagus nerve.
4. Abdomen
   a. General principles
      (1) Use the 4 techniques of examination but in a different sequence; perform auscultation before percussion and palpation so that you do not change intestinal activity, and hence the presence or character of bowel sounds.
      (2) Proceed systematically with the examination from the upper right quadrant, moving clockwise.
      (3) Examine any areas of pain or tenderness last. Approach these areas very cautiously; observe the person for signs of pain or distress to prevent inadvertent tensing of the patient's abdominal muscles.
   b. Preparing for the examination
      (1) Ask the patient to empty the bladder.
      (2) Have the patient lie supine with keens slightly bent and arms at the sides.
   c. Inspection—Inspect all quadrants or regions of the abdomen, noting abnormalities and visualizing the underlying structures and organs in order to better examine the person (Figure 27–7).
      (1) Skin: Inspect the skin of the neck, shoulders, and chest for the presence of spider telangiectases, small, red, vascular lesions that are indicative of liver cirrhosis. See Chapter 5 for more detail.
      (2) Architecture: Observe the contour and symmetry of the abdomen, noting the shape and position of the umbilicus.
      (3) Movement: Look for the normal rise and fall of inspiration and expiration; note any pulsations, particularly in the area of the abdominal aorta. Although they are only rarely seen on inspection, report any visible peristaltic movements, including the quadrant of origin and direction of flow, as these may indicate intestinal obstruction.

ABDOMINAL QUADRANTS AND REGIONS

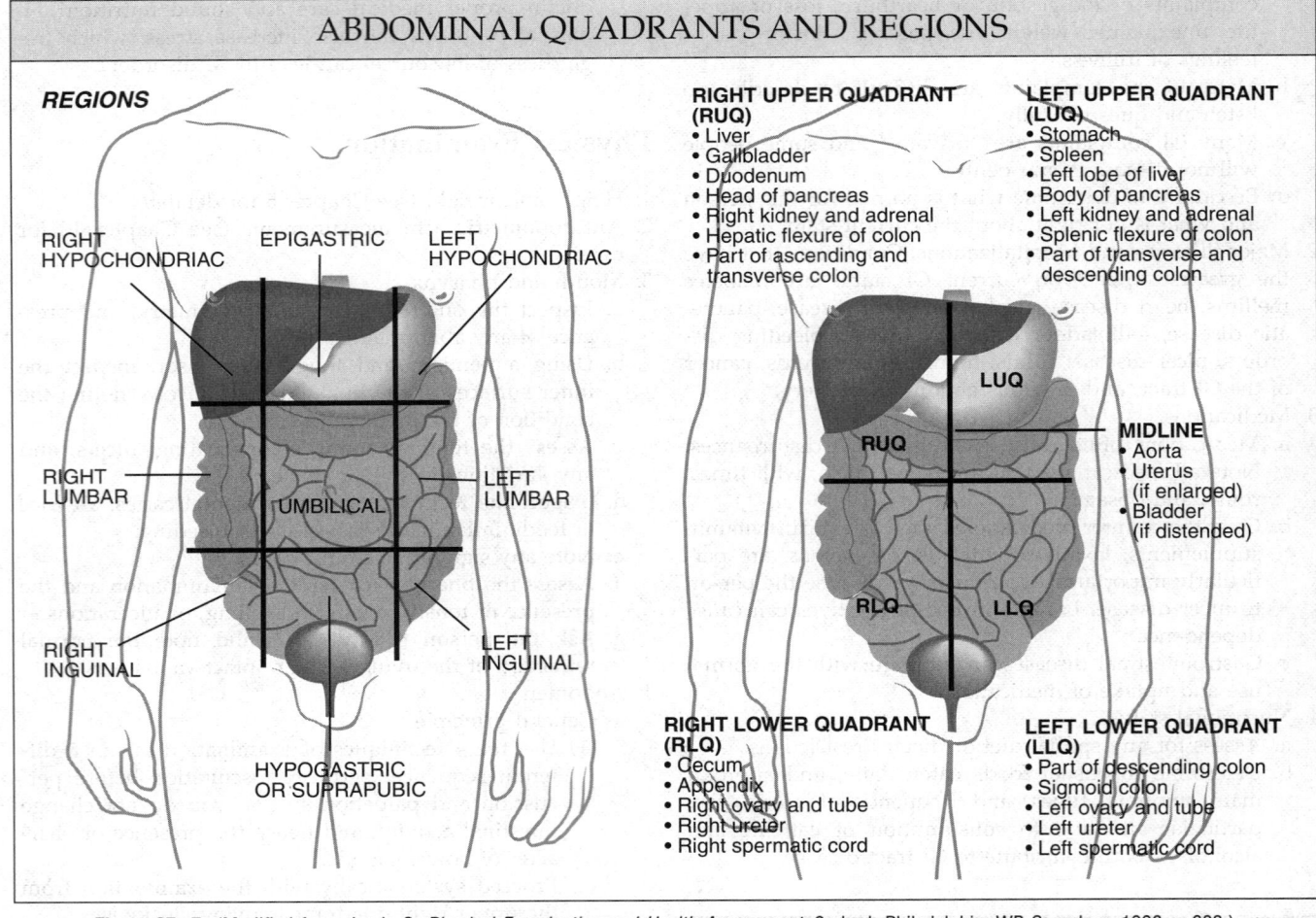

REGIONS

RIGHT HYPOCHONDRIAC

EPIGASTRIC

LEFT HYPOCHONDRIAC

RIGHT LUMBAR

UMBILICAL

LEFT LUMBAR

RIGHT INGUINAL

LEFT INGUINAL

HYPOGASTRIC OR SUPRAPUBIC

RIGHT UPPER QUADRANT (RUQ)
• Liver
• Gallbladder
• Duodenum
• Head of pancreas
• Right kidney and adrenal
• Hepatic flexure of colon
• Part of ascending and transverse colon

LEFT UPPER QUADRANT (LUQ)
• Stomach
• Spleen
• Left lobe of liver
• Body of pancreas
• Left kidney and adrenal
• Splenic flexure of colon
• Part of transverse and descending colon

MIDLINE
• Aorta
• Uterus (if enlarged)
• Bladder (if distended)

RIGHT LOWER QUADRANT (RLQ)
• Cecum
• Appendix
• Right ovary and tube
• Right ureter
• Right spermatic cord

LEFT LOWER QUADRANT (LLQ)
• Part of descending colon
• Sigmoid colon
• Left ovary and tube
• Left ureter
• Left spermatic cord

Figure 27–7. (Modified from Jarvis C. *Physical Examination and Health Assessment.* 2nd ed. Philadelphia: WB Saunders, 1996, p 603.)

d. Auscultation
   (1) Bowel sounds: Use the diaphragm of the stethoscope and listen in all 4 quadrants, noting the character and frequency of the sounds. Bowel sounds are normally heard as soft clicks and gurgles that occur every 5 to 15 seconds, with a normal frequency range of 5 to 34 per minute.
   (2) Circulatory sounds: Use the bell of the stethoscope and place lightly on the abdomen over the aorta, renal arteries, and iliac arteries. Listen for bruit, friction rub, and venous hum (see Chapter 28 for details).
e. Percussion
   (1) Percussing the abdomen determines the size and density of solid organs and the presence of masses, fluid, and air.
   (2) The percussion notes heard over the abdomen are tympanic (over air-filled intestine) or dull (over a solid organ such as the liver or a mass).
   (3) To percuss the size of the liver span, see Chapter 28.
   (4) Percussion can also be used to determine the size and position of the spleen (at the 10th intercostal space, midaxillary line), the presence of the gastric bubble (left of the midline at the left lower anterior rib cage border, indicating an air-filled stomach), or the height of a distended bladder.
f. Palpation
   (1) Light palpation, which may be used to detect large masses and areas of tenderness, is performed by placing the palm and fingers of the hand lightly on the abdomen, depressing only 1 to 2 cm in depth as you move your hand smoothly and systematically from quadrant to quadrant.
   (2) Deep palpation, which can be used to further determine the size and shape of abdominal organs and masses, is performed by using the palm and fingers of 1 or both hands to palpate to a maximum depth throughout the abdomen.
   (3) Rebound tenderness is elicited when you perform deep palpation. Press your hands into the abdomen slowly and firmly, then quickly withdraw them. Where did it hurt? Did it hurt more on pressing in or letting go? Pain on release of pressure is called "rebound tenderness" and is a reliable sign of peritoneal inflammation.
   (4) For the techniques of liver palpation, see Chapter 28.
5. Other findings
a. A protuberant abdomen with bulging flanks suggests fluid buildup known as ascites.

(1) Ascites produces a finding that is called a "shifting dullness." When percussion is performed outward from the umbilicus, the percussion tones normally go from tympany to dullness.

(2) When ascites is present, ask the person to turn onto 1 side, and these tones will change. The dullness shifts to the more dependent areas.

b. Assess the legs for thigh and leg edema. If present, note any decreases in circulation by checking the dorsalis pedis and posterior tibial pulses.

c. Assess for asterixis, also called liver flap. See Chapter 28.

Special Diagnostic Studies

1. Laboratory tests
   a. Blood level assessments
      (1) Calcium is measured to detect blood clotting deficiencies, GI tract malabsorption, or renal and endocrine disorders
      (2) Potassium is assessed to evaluate renal and endocrine disorders
      (3) Ammonia is utilized to rebuild amino acids, or for conversion to urea for excretion. Elevations are seen with cirrhosis of the liver, liver dysfunction, or hepatic failure.
      (4) Carcinoembryonic antigen (CEA) is a glycoprotein that is found on the surface cells of the GI tract during fetal life; it becomes elevated with heavy smoking, biliary obstruction, or alcoholic hepatitis. Because it may be secreted again in the presence of a neoplasm, CEA measurements are used to evaluate the effectiveness of cancer treatments, such as surgery and chemotherapy, and to determine the possibility of cancer recurrence.
      (5) Amylase is an enzyme formed by the pancreas for digestion of starches; it becomes elevated in pancreatic inflammation such as pancreatitis.
      (6) Lipase is an enzyme that is necessary for digestion of fats; it is elevated during pancreatic inflammation.
      (7) D-Xylose absorption: D-Xylose is a sugar that is absorbed in the small intestine; decreased levels of the sugar are seen when the integrity of the mucosa of the small bowel is compromised in malabsorptive syndromes such as celiac disease, steatorrhea, short bowel syndrome, starvation, and milk sensitivity. To measure D-xylose levels, maintain an overnight fast, give oral D-xylose, and measure both serum and urine xylose levels after 1 to 2 hours.
   b. Urine and stool analysis
      (1) The Schilling test is used to determine vitamin B_{12} absorption; decreased levels are seen with pernicious anemia and some malabsorptive syndromes. To prepare for the test, maintain an overnight fast, then give radioactive vitamin B_{12} capsules. Begin a 24-hour urine collection. After 2 hours, give an intramuscular injection of nonradioactive vitamin B_{12}. The urine is analyzed to compare relative absorption of the 2 isotopes.

      (2) Check the stool for occult blood. Measure the amount of blood in the stool, which possibly results from GI bleeding, colorectal cancer, or other GI disorder. Usually 3 stools are collected, and each must reach laboratory analysis within 6 hours.
      (3) Analyze the stool for fecal fat. Measure any abnormal levels of fat in the stool. The test may be performed on a random stool, or the person may adhere to a 3-day high-fat diet followed by a 72-hour collection of stool. Elevated levels of fat are seen in malabsorptive syndromes such as Crohn's disease.
      (4) Prepare stool for culture. Measure the presence of any bacteria or ova and parasites to determine the cause of intestinal infections. Collect a freshly passed stool specimen and transport immediately to the laboratory.
   c. Gastric analysis: Measures the stomach's secretion of hydrochloric acid and pepsin
      (1) To prepare, allow the person nothing by mouth (NPO) for at least 12 hours before the test. A nasogastric tube is inserted (see Procedure 27–1) and residual contents of the stomach are removed and discarded. During the analysis, the nasogastric tube is hooked to suction and the contents are collected at 15-minute intervals for 1 hour. This measures the level of basal gastric secretion.
      (2) This test can be followed up using a measurement of gastric acid stimulation by administering a stimulant for gastric acid secretion such as pentagastrin or histalog and again collecting specimens at 15-minute intervals for 1 hour.
      (3) Elevated gastric acid secretions are seen in Zollinger-Ellison syndrome and gastric and duodenal ulcers; decreased levels are suggestive of gastric carcinoma.
2. Radiologic tests
   a. Upper GI and small bowel series
      (1) Purpose: The upper GI series visualizes the lower esophagus, stomach, and duodenum. The small bowel series continues through the small intestines to, and including, the ileocecal junction. It is used to detect esophageal disorders, gastric ulcers, tumors, and small bowel disorders.
      (2) Preparation: Maintain the person on NPO status after midnight. If possible, the person may be placed on a low-residue diet for 48 hours before the test.
      (3) Procedure: The person drinks a mixture of barium sulfate. Fluoroscopy traces the barium through the esophagus and stomach for about 30 minutes. To include the small bowel series, the person must drink more barium. Then, additional radiographs are taken every 30 minutes for 2 to 6 hours.
      (4) Follow-up: A laxative is usually ordered for natural elimination.
   b. Barium swallow
      (1) Purpose: The barium swallow visualizes the pharynx and esophagus to detect tumors, strictures, hiatal hernia, varices, ulcers, or motility disorders.

(2) Preparation: Maintain the person on NPO status after midnight.

(3) Procedure: The person begins the procedure while in an upright position and drinks a barium mixture or Hypaque; fluoroscopy begins visualizing down the esophagus. It may be necessary to place the person in other positions (e.g., side to side or lying flat).

(4) Follow-up: A laxative may be ordered.

c. Barium enema

(1) Purpose: The barium enema visualizes the large intestine to detect polyps, masses, strictures, colorectal cancers, diverticulosis, and inflammatory bowel disease.

(2) Preparation: Maintain the person on a clear liquid diet for at least 24 hours before the examination and on NPO status after midnight before the procedure. Usually, a potent laxative or oral liquid bowel preparation and enemas are given to cleanse the bowel the evening before the test.

(3) Procedure: The barium mixture is inserted into the bowel through a rectal catheter, as with an enema. The person is placed in various positions and instructed to hold the barium, even if the urge to defecate is great, while the radiographs are being taken. The test usually takes 1 hour.

(4) Follow-up: A mild laxative or cleansing enemas may be ordered. Monitor the elimination of the barium carefully, because it can cause an obstruction if it is not eliminated completely.

d. Ultrasound

(1) Purpose: Ultrasound uses sound waves to image soft tissues and organs of the abdomen.

(2) Preparation: The person should maintain an NPO status for 8 to 12 hours before the examination.

(3) Procedure: A lubricated microphone transducer is placed on the abdomen and rubbed over the skin to image the structures below. There is no follow-up.

e. Computed tomography

(1) Purpose: This form of radiograph visualizes differences in tissue densities and thus detects tumors and masses.

(2) Preparation: Maintain the person on NPO status for 8 to 12 hours before the radiograph is taken. An oral contrast medium may be given 4 to 6 hours before the procedure to enhance visualizations.

(3) Procedure: The person is placed on a radiograph table and moved "inside" the scanning machine, which emits loud "clicking" sounds as it moves to different positions. An intravenous injection of contrast may also be given to further enhance the imaging. There is no follow-up.

f. Magnetic resonance imaging (MRI)

(1) Purpose: In MRI, a radiofrequency and magnetic field produce images of soft tissues, organs, and blood vessels to detect the presence of abnormal masses, abscesses, fistulas, tumors, bleeding, and metastases.

(2) Preparation: Maintain the person on NPO status for 4 to 6 hours before the scan. Patients who have metal implants such as heart valves, surgical clips, orthopedic clips, or pacemakers cannot have an MRI because the powerful magnet can move these implants within the body. All jewelry, metal hair clips, and clothing with metal fasteners must be removed as well.

(3) Procedure: The person is placed on a radiograph table and moved inside the narrow scanner tunnel, which emits "thumping" sounds as the machine scans. There is no follow-up care.

3. Special diagnostic procedures

a. Esophagogastroduodenoscopy (Fig. 27–8)

(1) Purpose: Esophagogastroduodenoscopy uses a flexible endoscope to provide direct visualization of the esophagus, stomach, and proximal duodenum and thus diagnose esophageal and gastric lesions, bleeding, and motility disorders.

(2) Preparation: Keep the person on NPO status for at least 4 to 6 hours before the examination to reduce the risk of vomiting and aspiration. Medications, such as atropine and intravenous sedation, may be given before the procedure to dry secretions and help the person to relax. A topical anesthetic is applied to the throat to block the gag reflex and to aid in the passage of the endoscope.

(3) Procedure: The flexible, lubricated endoscopic tube is passed down the GI tract in stages while each area is examined. Monitor vital signs and airway, with careful attention to the quantities of secretions and any signs of pain, bleeding, or perforation.

(4) Follow-up: The person must remain on NPO status until the gag reflex returns (usually 2–4 hours). Any remaining throat irritation is usually relieved with saline gargles or throat lozenges. Continue to monitor vital signs and secretions. Do not allow the patient to drive for 12 hours. Postprocedure complications can include perforation of the GI tract and aspiration pneumonia.

b. Colonoscopy

(1) Purpose: Colonoscopy is a direct visualization of the large intestine from the rectum to evaluate for malignancy, diverticulitis, inflammatory bowel disease, polyps, strictures, and bleeding.

(2) Preparation: Keep the patient on a liquid diet for 24 hours before the test. A laxative and an oral liquid preparation or tap water enemas are given for bowel cleansing the evening before. The person is usually given intravenous sedation just before the test to promote relaxation during the procedure.

(3) Procedure: The person is placed on the left side and a lubricated colonoscope is passed through the rectum while the person is instructed to take long, slow, deep breaths. Air may be used to help distend the walls of the colon for better visualization.

(4) Follow-up: Monitor vital signs carefully and observe for signs of perforation, pain, abdominal rigidity, distention, and bleeding.

ENDOSCOPY

Endoscopy is a direct visualization through the insertion of a hollow tube or endoscope into the lumen of the gastrointestinal (GI) tract.

General Preprocedure Instructions
1. Obtain informed consent for the procedure.
2. Explain the need for NPO (nothing by mouth) status for the specified period of time prior to the procedure.
3. Teach the person about the type of local anesthesia and sedation to be used. Explain what each test is, what will be visualized, and what the person can expect to happen during the procedure, including positioning and loss of reflex or function.

General Postprocedure Instructions
1. The person should not drive for 12 hours after the procedure because of sedation and should be accompanied by a responsible adult during and after the procedure if it is to be done on an outpatient basis.
2. Watch for signs of perforation:
- Upper GI tract: fever; difficulty or pain on swallowing; any other abnormal areas of pain including the shoulder, the epigastric or substernal areas, or the back; bleeding; vomiting; or shortness of breath.
- Lower GI tract: fever, rectal bleeding, abdominal pain, changes in bowel elimination or distention.
3. Other specific instructions:
- Upper GI tract: Withhold food and fluids until the gag reflex has returned completely and the person is able to swallow without difficulty.
- Lower GI tract: Instruct the person that there may be a lot of flatus due to the insufflation of air into the colon.

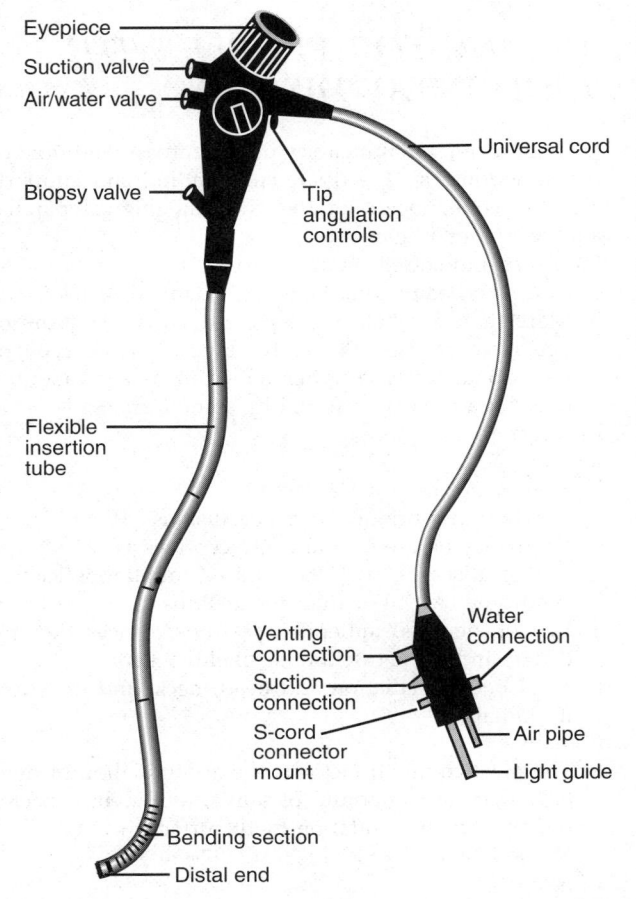

Figure 27–8.

c. Proctosigmoidoscopy
   (1) Purpose: By using either a rigid proctosigmoidoscope or a flexible sigmoidoscope or colonoscope, this procedure provides direct visualization of the rectum and the sigmoid colon. Flexible sigmoidoscopy seems to be better tolerated than rigid proctosigmoidoscopy, and it allows for examination of more of the colon than is possible with the proctoscope. This procedure is used to evaluate rectal bleeding, polyps, tumors, persistent diarrhea, and inflammatory bowel disease and as an initial colorectal cancer screen.
   (2) Preparation: A saline enema or low-volume preparation enema (e.g., Fleet) is given a few hours before the examination. Usually, no medication is necessary.
   (3) Procedure: The person is placed in a lateral knee-chest position and is asked to bear down while the scope is passed into the rectum. Instruct the person to breathe slowly and deeply as the scope continues to be inserted.
      After it reaches the desired depth, the scope is

withdrawn slowly while the mucosal wall of the bowel is examined carefully.
   (4) Follow-up: The person is instructed to watch for signs of perforation and rectal bleeding.
d. Anal manometry
   (1) Purpose: Anal manometry helps with assessment of anal and rectal muscle and sphincter problems associated with several disorders, especially fecal incontinence, and is also useful in evaluating chronic constipation.
   (2) Preparation: A low-volume enema is given the evening before the test to aid in bowel evacuation.
   (3) Procedure: Instruct the person to empty the bladder. Position the person in a left lateral decubitus position with knees flexed. Provide for the person's comfort and hygiene during this procedure. The manometry catheter is inserted and sterile water is infused through eight luminal openings in the catheter. Measurements of anal sphincter length and resting and squeeze pressures are performed as the tube is pulled out. The pressures are recorded on a graph in a computer. The entire

procedure takes about 30 minutes. There is no follow-up care.

◼ CARING FOR PEOPLE WITH PERIODONTAL DISEASE

1. Definition: an inflammatory degenerative condition of the periodontium (the tissue surrounding and supporting the teeth), including the gingiva, gingival papilla, and periodontal ligament
2. Incidence and socioeconomic impact
   a. Common health complaint in the United States
   b. More than one half of people older than 18 years of age have at least the early stage of some type of periodontal disease. After 35 years of age, about 3 out of 4 adults are affected by some form.
3. Risk factors
   a. Poor diet
   b. Smoking or chewing tobacco
   c. Poorly fitting bridges or malocclusions
   d. Pregnancy or use of oral contraceptives
   e. Certain diseases, such as acquired immunodeficiency syndrome (AIDS) or diabetes mellitus
   f. Use of steroids, antiepilepsy drugs, cancer therapy drugs, and some calcium channel blockers
   g. Total body irradiation and head, neck, and oral cavity radiation
4. Etiology
   a. The most common factor is the accumulation of dental plaque (a compound of saliva, food debris, bacteria, and organic acids) on tooth surfaces
   b. Malocclusion
   c. Stress
5. Pathophysiology
   a. Accumulation of plaque leads to formation of calculus on teeth.
   b. Plaque erodes enamel on teeth, which allows development of tooth decay and inflammation of the gingiva (gingivitis).
   c. Gingivitis causes the gum to separate from the surface of the tooth, thereby creating pockets wherein bacteria can accumulate, causing bleeding and pus from the gums.
   d. The disease eventually invades the periodontal ligament and the alveolar bone that supports the teeth. The teeth become loose and can be lost.
6. Clinical manifestations
   a. Early symptoms include bleeding, swelling, and inflammation of the gums.
   b. Buildup of plaque on the teeth
   c. Tooth pain
7. Diagnostics
   a. History
      (1) Determine normal daily oral hygiene patterns.
      (2) Assess for any complaints of pain, sensitivities to heat or cold, or bleeding.
   b. Examination
      (1) Assess the condition of the teeth and gums.
      (2) Examine teeth for dental caries and plaque buildup.
      (3) Observe gums for signs of inflammation, bleeding, swelling, and pus.
8. Clinical management
   a. Goals are to correct periodontal disease and to enhance proper oral hygiene.
   b. Nonpharmacologic interventions
      (1) Improve brushing technique: Instruct the patient to brush outside, inside, and chewing surfaces of the teeth with a soft, rounded toothbrush placed just at gum surface, and to brush back and forth with small strokes.
      (2) Include flossing at least daily to remove plaque and foodstuffs between teeth.
      (3) Assess the need for assistive equipment for brushing and flossing.
   c. Pharmacologic interventions
      (1) Fluoride rinses for 1 to 3 minutes daily after brushing either in the morning or the evening
      (2) Medication for pain, if severe
   d. Special medical-surgical procedures
      (1) Early treatment: Scaling of the teeth (removal of calculus)
      (2) Gingivectomy: Removal of gum tissue and diseased areas
      (3) Gingivoplasty: Repair and rebuilding of gum tissue
      (4) For advanced disease that cannot be treated, tooth extraction and dentures can be used.
9. Complications
   a. Loss of teeth
   b. Systemic infection
10. Prognosis: In severe cases that involve the periodontal ligament and alveolar bone, removal of teeth and dentures may be the only solution.
11. Applying the nursing process

NURSING DIAGNOSIS: Pain in gums and teeth R/T inflammation and swelling

   a. *Expected outcomes:* Following intervention, the person should be able to do the following:
      (1) Report relief from pain
      (2) Achieve proper oral hygiene
   b. *Nursing interventions*
      (1) Warm saline mouth rinses to soothe the pain of gum inflammation
      (2) During the acute period, analgesics to reduce pain

NURSING DIAGNOSIS: Risk for infection of the mouth R/T inflammation

   a. *Expected outcomes:* Following intervention, the person should be able to do the following:
      (1) Identify signs and symptoms of infection
      (2) Identify actions to prevent further dental caries or progression of the periodontal disease
   b. *Nursing interventions*

(1) Explain the need for water and hydrogen peroxide cleansing and rinsing of gums and teeth to reduce inflammation.

(2) Monitor the person's brushing and flossing techniques to ensure that they are being done properly. Encourage continued brushing and flossing per routine during acute phase

(3) Continue to assess the status of the teeth and gums for signs of developing infection.

(4) Provide information to the person regarding the signs of infection: swelling, redness, increased pain in the teeth or gums, or radiating pain to the jaw or ear.

12. Discharge planning and teaching
   a. Describe how to prevent dental caries and periodontal disease.
   b. Teach thorough brushing for 2 to 5 minutes after each meal with fluoride toothpaste and fluoride rinse, followed by flossing to decrease the plaque buildup between teeth.
   c. Explain the importance of a well-balanced diet, including decreased intake of sugar.
   d. Stress the need for regular dental examinations.

13. Public health considerations: Fluoridation of the public water supply is recommended for prevention of dental caries and periodontal disease, as is childhood fluoridation of the teeth.

■ *CARING FOR PEOPLE WITH STOMATITIS*

1. Definition: an inflammatory disorder of the lining of the mouth that is often characterized by ulcers on the gums and oral mucous membranes

2. Incidence and socioeconomic impact: The American Cancer Society estimates that 40 percent of chemotherapy patients experience stomatitis at some time during their treatment.

3. Risk factor: lowered immune resistance

4. Etiology
   a. Can be a primary lesion, such as with aphthous stomatitis (canker sores), with herpes simplex stomatitis, or following a mechanical trauma to the oral mucosa
   b. Can be a secondary infection caused by a viral or bacterial invasion (e.g., candidiasis or secondary herpes simplex) that is due to lowered resistance from another disease process (e.g., allergies, nutritional disorders, renal failure, diabetes, leukemia, AIDS) or treatment (e.g., drugs such as steroids and antibiotics, and immunosuppressive therapies such as radiation therapy and chemotherapy)

5. Pathophysiology
   a. Primary lesions develop as circular areas of erythema that ulcerate (usually in the center). These appear as areas of eroded mucosa.
   b. Candidiasis—also called moniliasis or "thrush"—is caused by *Candida albicans* (part of the normal oral flora) and develops as white, curdlike patches.

6. Clinical manifestations
   a. Sore mouth and throat
   b. Reddened, painful ulcerations on the mucosa
   c. White, dry patches on the tongue or mucosa that are accompanied by inflammation
   d. Foul breath odor
   e. Excessive salivation

7. Diagnostics
   a. History: Any history of weight loss? Complaints of burning or stinging mouth pain?
   b. Examination: Assess lips and mucous membranes for ulcers or vesicles, or reddened or whitish patches.
   c. Exfoliative cytology: A scraping of the lesion is taken and a culture or smear made for examination.

8. Clinical management
   a. Goals are to relieve discomfort, enhance or maintain the integrity of the mucous membranes, and assist in controlling infection.
   b. Nonpharmacologic interventions
      (1) Assess mucous membranes daily for any breaks in the tissue.
      (2) Give oral hygiene with soothing solution, and use a soft toothbrush or foamswabs.
      (3) Encourage a soft, bland diet and water or other fluid intake. Popsicles are a good source of calories and are cool and numbing to the mucous membranes.
      (4) Lubricate or moisten lips.
   c. Pharmacologic interventions: Give topical medications, such as viscous Xylocaine, to reduce discomfort, especially just before meals; give antifungals (oral, topical, or systemic) to treat candidal infection.

9. Complications
   a. Infection
   b. Decreased nutritional intake

10. Prognosis: Recurrence of primary lesions is common.

11. Applying the nursing process

NURSING DIAGNOSIS: Altered nutrition, less than body requirements R/T to discomfort of stomatitis

---

   a. *Expected outcomes:* After intervention, the person should be able to do the following:
      (1) Increase oral intake of identified nonirritating foods and fluids
      (2) Maintain stable weight and adequate nutrition
   b. *Nursing interventions*
      (1) Assess the person's general level of nutrition. Poor nutrition can impair healing and increase risk for infection.
      (2) Identify specific foods and fluids that are usually nonirritating, and discuss with the person their preferences.
      (3) Provide sufficient quantities of nonirritating foods and fluids to maintain adequate nutrition.
      (4) If discomfort becomes too great to allow oral intake, consider inserting a nasogastric tube to provide nutrition (see Procedure 27–1).

NURSING DIAGNOSIS: Pain R/T inflammation of oral mucous membranes

a. *Expected outcomes:* Following intervention, the person should be able to do the following:
   (1) Report relief from pain
   (2) Describe techniques to decrease the pain
b. *Nursing interventions*
   (1) Give warm normal saline or water and hydrogen peroxide rinses to soothe mild pain.
   (2) For severe pain, give prescribed analgesics or topical anesthetics to ease discomfort and to increase the person's ability to take adequate nutrition.

NURSING DIAGNOSIS: Risk for infection R/T alteration of oral mucous membrane

a. *Expected outcomes:* Following intervention, the person should be able to do the following:
   (1) Identify actions to reduce the risk of infection
   (2) Prevent the spread of infection through proper oral hygiene measures
b. *Nursing interventions*
   (1) Provide information regarding the signs of infection: swelling, redness, increased pain, or onset of or increase in exudate or drainage from the stomatitis.
   (2) Monitor the ability of the person to continue with proper oral hygiene (brushing teeth, rinsing and cleaning of mouth after eating).
12. Discharge planning and teaching: Teach the person about the importance of oral hygiene in preventing infection, the probable causes of stomatitis, the importance of proper nutrition and oral fluid intake, and measures to decrease pain.
13. Public health considerations: Proper infection control measures in families, daycare centers, workplaces, and hospitals are essential in preventing the spread of stomatitis.

■ CARING FOR PEOPLE WITH ESOPHAGITIS

1. Definition: an inflammation of the esophagus, also called heartburn (pyrosis)
2. Incidence: Occurs frequently
3. Risk factors
   a. Smoking
   b. Obesity
   c. Pregnancy
4. Etiology
   a. The most frequent cause is gastroesophageal reflux disease, but it can also be caused by *C. albicans*, herpes simplex, or cytomegalovirus.
   b. Associated with irritants such as alcohol, caffeine, spicy foods, dust, or ingestion of chemicals
   c. Cancer of esophagus

5. Pathophysiology
   a. Normally, reflux is prevented by pressures that exist between the cardiac sphincter of the stomach and the lower esophagus and the acute angle between the left part of the esophagus and where it enters into the stomach (angle of His).
   b. Inflammation of the gastric mucosa occurs when an incompetent lower esophageal sphincter (LES), with decreased pressure, allows gastric acid and pepsin from the fundus of the stomach to back up into the esophagus.
   c. Prolonged or frequent contact with gastric secretions inflames or damages the mucosa, eventually causing superficial erosions or deeper ulcerations.
6. Clinical manifestations
   a. Localized pain
   b. Belching
   c. Difficulty swallowing
7. Diagnostics
   a. History: Assess dietary patterns, alcohol intake, and nutritional status.
   b. Examination
      (1) Measure weight.
      (2) Observe person's swallowing.
   c. Esophagoscopy can detect erosions, inflammation, edema, or bleeding.
   d. Barium swallow can assess the shape of the esophagus and detect any structural abnormalities such as strictures that are seen in severe disease.
   e. Bernstein's acid perfusion test: Administration of an acid solution through a tube placed in the esophagus quickly produces pain and heartburn in people with esophagitis. This test distinguishes epigastric pain from pain of cardiac origin.
8. Clinical management
   a. Goals are to increase the pressure of the LES and to reduce the acidity of gastric secretions.
   b. Nonpharmacologic interventions
      (1) Give a bland, low-fat, nonirritating diet.
      (2) Keep the head of the bed elevated (at least equivalent to a 2-pillow elevation) after meals and during sleep.
      (3) Limit food and fluid intake 2 to 4 hours before bedtime.
   c. Pharmacologic interventions
      (1) The usual 1st approach is to administer antacids (Table 27–3) to reduce gastric acidity: they are

Table 27–3. Common Antacids

Antacid	Action
Mylanta or Maalox (aluminum hydroxide, magnesium hydroxide)	Reduces or neutralizes gastric acidity
Riopan (magaldrate)	Reduces or neutralizes gastric acidity in those with sodium restrictions
Amphogel (aluminum hydroxide)	Neutralizes gastric acidity
PeptoBismol (colloidal)	Protects the gastric mucosa

Table 27–4. Histamine H$_2$-Receptor Antagonists

Medication	Length of Action	Side Effects
Cimetidine (Tagamet)	6 hr	Diarrhea, headache, fatigue
Ranitidine (Zantac)	10 hr	Headache
Famotidine (Pepcid)	10 hr	Dizziness, headache
Nizatidine (Axid)	10 hr	Fatigue

most often given 1 hour before meals, 2 to 3 hours after meals, and at bedtime.

   (2) If this approach fails to control symptoms, histamine H$_2$-receptor antagonists (Table 27–4) may be prescribed. Histamine is believed to be the final activator of hydrochloric acid secretion; these drugs are antisecretion drugs. They should be taken with meals or at bedtime; at least 1 hour should elapse between the administration of an antacid and the taking of an H$_2$-receptor antagonist.

   d. Special medical-surgical procedures: Surgery may become necessary if medication treatment alone does not relieve symptoms.
9. Complications: Esophageal strictures
10. Prognosis: Control with medications is generally good if the person avoids other contributing factors, such as smoking, alcohol, and highly acidic foods.
11. Applying the nursing process

NURSING DIAGNOSIS: Pain R/T regurgitation and eructation

   a. *Expected outcomes:* Following intervention, the person should be able to do the following:
   (1) Report relieved or reduced discomfort in esophageal pain or heartburn
   (2) Identify actions to reduce or relieve the discomfort of esophageal pain
   b. *Nursing interventions*
   (1) Monitor the person for effective relief of pain while using the prescribed antacid and antisecretory medications.
   (2) Discuss with the person the importance of eating a diet of foods that are more easily tolerated. Develop a list of foods that do not cause heartburn and recommend that those foods be included regularly in the diet.
   (3) Teach the effect of maintaining the upright position before, during, and after eating. Explain that the recumbent position increases regurgitation and can exacerbate symptoms.

NURSING DIAGNOSIS: Risk for impaired tissue integrity R/T inflammation of the esophagus secondary to the presence of gastric acid

   a. *Expected outcomes:* After intervention, the person should be able to do the following:
   (1) Identify causes of risk for impairment of tissues
   (2) Participate in the medication regimen to prevent impaired tissue integrity
   b. *Nursing interventions*
   (1) Explain the causes of esophageal tissue impairment and associated risk behaviors.
   (2) Administer prescribed medications to decrease gastric acid production and neutralize any gastric acids already produced.
12. Discharge planning and teaching
   a. Teach the person to recognize and avoid causative agents.
   b. To prevent symptoms, explain the importance of drug therapy and of critical timing (the proper timing of medications, e.g., antacids given 1 hr before meals, 2–3 hr after meals, and at bedtime).
   c. Recommend bland, low-fat foods; advise the patient to avoid caffeine, chocolate, orange juice, and tomato products, which are known to increase reflux.
13. Public health considerations: Educate the public regarding the risk factors in esophagitis and how to minimize them.

■ CARING FOR PEOPLE WITH GASTROESOPHAGEAL REFLUX DISEASE (REFLUX ESOPHAGITIS)

1. Definition: a backflow of contents from the stomach or duodenum into the esophagus that occurs without vomiting
2. Incidence and socioeconomic impact: The most frequent problem that occurs in the esophagus and perhaps the most frequent problem that occurs in the GI tract
3. Risk factors
   a. Diet: A diet high in fatty foods, chocolate, xanthine-containing drinks (cola, tea, coffee), and alcohol
   b. Cigarette smoking
4. Etiology
   a. Occurs whenever there is inappropriate relaxation of the LES, decreased LES tone, increased intra-abdominal pressures, or increased volume of the stomach, as a result of the following:
   (1) Incompetent LES
   (2) Fatty meals
   (3) Cigarette smoking
   (4) Pregnancy
   (5) Pyloric stenosis
   (6) Motility disorders
5. Pathophysiology
   a. Reflux occurs if the highly acidic contents of the stomach flow back into the esophagus.
   b. The mucosal barrier in the esophagus breaks down and inflammation results from exposure of the esophagus to the gastric acid and pepsin, which occurs because of the following:
   (1) Transient LES relaxation
   (2) Free reflux due to decreased LES tone

(3) Increased intra-abdominal pressure due to muscular contraction

(4) Increased gastric volume

c. The degree of inflammation and extent of destruction of the mucosa depend on the number of reflux episodes, the length of exposure time, and the acidity of the contents.

6. Clinical manifestations
   a. Heartburn or pyrosis
   b. Intermittent chest pain (dyspepsia)
   c. Regurgitation
   d. Odynophagia
   e. Dysphagia (difficulty swallowing)
   f. Hypersalivation ("water brash") in response to the reflux

7. Diagnostics
   a. History
      (1) Assess "heartburn" pain and dysphagia to determine the cause and course of their development.
      (2) Determine usual dietary patterns, foods eaten and amounts, and timing of meals.
   b. Esophagoscopy with or without biopsy to detect erosions, inflammation, edema, or bleeding
   c. Barium swallow to detect the shape of the esophagus and any structural or sphincter abnormalities.
   d. Esophageal manometry to measure esophageal motility and the resting pressure of the lower esophageal sphincter. A water-infusion catheter that is connected to pressure transducers at each of its luminal openings is inserted into the nose or mouth and passed through the esophagus into the stomach. The catheter is then slowly withdrawn at intervals to measure the pressure in the esophagus at various sites, especially the LES.
   e. Monitoring of esophageal acidity (pH) every hour for 24 hours

8. Clinical management
   a. Goals are to minimize symptoms and to decrease reflux.
   b. Nonpharmacologic interventions
      (1) Maintaining upright positioning during and after meals facilitates downward flow of food.
      (2) Modify the diet to reduce intake of foods that aggravate symptoms. Consume small, frequent meals.
   c. Pharmacologic interventions
      (1) Administer antacids (see p. 1255) to provide symptomatic relief for heartburn.
      (2) Administer histamine H_2-blockers (see p. 1255) to reduce gastric acid secretion.
      (3) Administer bethanechol (Urecholine) or metoclopramide (Reglan) to persons who are experiencing severe esophagitis with reflux. Bethanechol, a cholinergic, causes an increase in LES pressure but also increases gastric acid secretions and must be administered along with a histamine H_2-antagonist. Metoclopramide, a dopamine antagonist, increases the rate of gastric emptying.
   d. Special medical-surgical procedures: Surgery is not the treatment of choice; however, there are several "anti-reflux" surgical procedures that involve wrapping the fundus of the stomach around the lower esophagus. For more on these procedures, see page 1257.

9. Complications
   a. Esophageal strictures
   b. Hemorrhage (upper GI bleed)
   c. Perforation
   d. Barrett's esophagus: Development of a premalignant type of columnar epithelium that replaces normal squamous epithelium in the esophagus in the body's attempt to protect esophageal mucosa from acid reflux episodes during healing
   e. Esophageal cancer
   f. Pulmonary aspiration

10. Prognosis: Medical treatment is generally effective; however, this tends to be a recurring problem.

11. Applying the nursing process

NURSING DIAGNOSIS: Pain R/T acid reflux

   a. *Expected outcomes:* After intervention, the person should be able to do the following:
      (1) Report relief from pain
      (2) Identify measures to reduce the incidence of reflux
   b. *Nursing interventions*
      (1) Assess and document the effectiveness of prescribed antacid and antisecretory medications in relieving pain and reducing the incidence of reflux.
      (2) Teach the person the causes of reflux and the importance of carefully following the medication regimen and dietary modifications to control the pain and the incidence of reflux.
      (3) Determine the person's understanding of the importance of timing medications with the intake of food.

12. Discharge planning and teaching
   a. Explain the relationship between positioning and onset of symptoms, and recommend that the person not eat before going to bed or lying down.
   b. Teach dietary modifications that include eating small frequent meals rather than large meals and avoiding high-fat foods, chocolate, caffeine, alcohol, and smoking, as they all delay gastric emptying and decrease LES pressure.
   c. Discuss weight loss, if appropriate.

13. Public health considerations: Educate the public about gastroesophageal reflux as a cause of epigastric pain and its association with cigarette smoking, obesity, and fatty foods.

◼ CARING FOR PEOPLE WITH HIATAL HERNIA

1. Definition: protrusion of the lower part of the esophagus or a portion of the stomach through an opening in

A hiatal hernia is a protrusion of the lower part of the esophagus or a portion of the stomach through an opening in the diaphragm into the thoracic cavity.
It is also called an esophageal or diaphragmatic hernia.

Types of Hiatal Hernias

Sliding:
Most common type of hernia. Results from the junction of the esophagus and the fundus of the stomach moving above the diaphragmatic opening in the thorax.

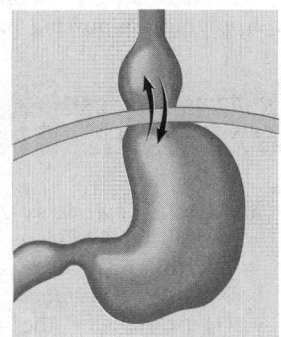

Rolling or paraesophageal:
Hernia that results from the greater curvature of the stomach and the fundus rolling through the diaphragmatic opening in the thorax. The junction of the esophagus and the stomach remains in place, and the herniated portion sits beside the esophagus in the thorax.

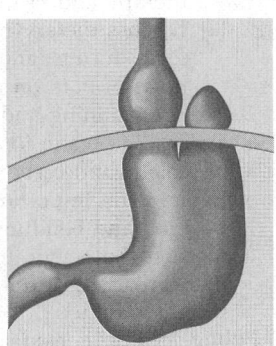

Surgical Repair

Surgical repair of the hernia involves "wrapping" the fundus of the stomach around the lower portion of the esophagus to reinforce the lower esophageal sphincter. The three types of this surgery are:

Nissen fundoplication:
Uses a transabdominal approach to the wrapping of the fundus of the stomach around the lower esophagus, reinforcing the sphincter and returning the esophageal junction to the normal position. Involves a 360-degree gastric wrap of the distal esophagus.

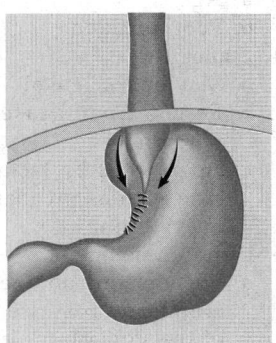

Hill gastroplexy: Involves a posterior approach, anchoring the stomach and the esophagus to a ligament. Consists of a 180-degree wrap of the stomach around the distal esophagus.

Belsey repair: Uses a transthoracic approach that attaches the anterior and lateral aspects of the stomach onto the esophagus. Involves a 270-degree wrap of the stomach and the distal esophagus.

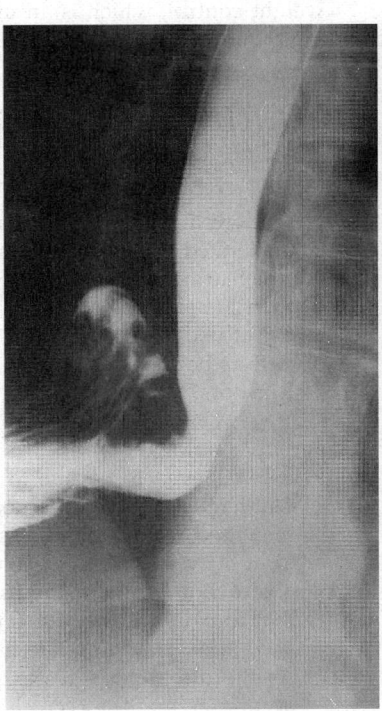

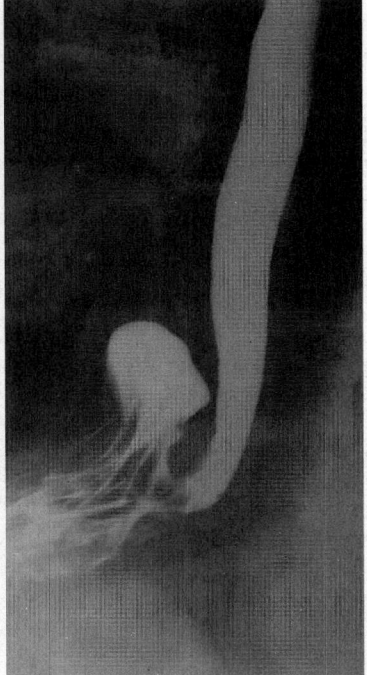

(Radiograph of paraesophageal hernia courtesy of the University of Maryland Medical Center.)

Figure 27–9.

the diaphragm into the thoracic cavity; also called esophageal or diaphragmatic hernia

2. Incidence and socioeconomic impact
   a. One of the most frequent GI problems
   b. Occurs more frequently in women than in men
3. Risk factors
   a. Age
   b. Poor nutrition
4. Etiology
   a. May be congenital
   b. Results from weakening of the muscles of the diaphragm
   c. Aggravated by factors that increase abdominal pressure such as pregnancy, ascites, obesity, tumors, and heavy lifting
5. Pathophysiology
   a. The opening in the diaphragm through which the esophagus passes enlarges, allowing the upper part of the stomach to pass into the thoracic area.
   b. There are 2 types of hiatal hernias (Fig. 27–9): sliding (the more common type) and rolling (paraesophageal).
6. Clinical manifestations
   a. May or may not be symptomatic
   b. Heartburn (pyrosis)
   c. Feeling of fullness
   d. Discomfort or pain
   e. Regurgitation
   f. Dysphagia (difficulty swallowing)
   g. Odynophagia
   h. Lump in the throat
   i. Bleeding
7. Diagnostics
   a. History: Any chest pain or difficulty breathing?
   b. Examination: Assess the person's ability to swallow and eat.
   c. Barium swallow is the main diagnostic test for visualizing the abnormality.
   d. Esophagoscopy may be done to determine the presence of gastric reflux or inflammation or to perform a biopsy.
8. Clinical management
   a. Goals are to relieve discomfort and to prevent gastroesophageal reflux.
   b. Nonpharmacologic interventions
      (1) Implement a high-protein, low-fat diet to maintain nutrition and to reduce weight, if necessary.
      (2) Introduce small, frequent quantities of food and minimize liquids to decrease the incidence of reflux.
      (3) Have the person sit upright while eating and for 30 minutes afterward to promote downward passage of food.
   c. Pharmacologic interventions
      (1) Antacids (see p. 1254) to relieve heartburn and increase lower esophageal sphincter pressure (thereby decreasing gastroesophageal reflux)
      (2) Histamine H_2-receptor blockers (see p. 1255) alternately with antacids
   d. Special medical-surgical procedures: Surgical removal of the hiatal hernia may be necessary if phar-

macologic treatment does not bring relief, or if complications arise.

9. Complications
   a. Hemorrhage
   b. Strangulation of the hernia
   c. Severe esophagitis
10. Prognosis: Surgery is often inevitable.
11. Applying the nursing process

NURSING DIAGNOSIS: Pain R/T gastroesophageal reflux of acid contents of stomach

   a. *Expected outcomes:* After intervention, the person should be able to report a reduction or an alleviation of pain and a decrease in reflux symptoms.
   b. *Nursing interventions*
      (1) Administer the prescribed regimen of antacid therapy and H_2-receptor antagonists.
      (2) Discuss dietary modifications and positioning before, during, and after eating (see nursing diagnosis of pain on p. 1256).
12. Discharge planning and teaching
   a. Teach the person to avoid alcohol, smoking, caffeine, chocolate, and carbonated beverages.
   b. Explain the importance of avoiding both a reclining position and bending-down motions after eating.
   c. Instruct the person to avoid tight, restrictive clothing that increases intra-abdominal pressure and hence increases reflux.
13. Public health considerations: Educate the public on weight control, which is an important factor in preventing the development of hiatal hernia.

◼ CARING FOR PEOPLE WITH ACHALASIA

1. Definition: a motility disorder of the esophagus that is characterized by a progressively worsening loss of esophageal peristalsis and defective LES function
2. Incidence and socioeconomic impact
   a. Onset usually occurs between 30 and 50 years of age
   b. Affects both sexes equally
3. Risk factors: None known
4. Etiology: Unknown
5. Pathophysiology
   a. It is believed to be due to a lack of peristalsis in the esophagus along with a poorly relaxing LES.
   b. Increased resting LES pressure and failure of the LES to fully relax when swallowing cause a functional obstruction between the esophagus and the stomach that impairs transit between the two and causes food and fluids to accumulate in the distal esophagus.
   c. As the disease progresses, dilation of the esophagus occurs.
6. Clinical manifestations
   a. Difficulty swallowing (dysphagia) both solids and liquids
   b. Regurgitation

c. Chest discomfort

d. Weight loss

7. Diagnostics

    a. History

        (1) When did the 1st episode of dysphagia occur? How has it progressed? Does anything make it worse? Ease it?

        (2) Assess history of weight carefully.

    b. Barium swallow to detect absence of peristalsis and any dilation of the esophagus

    c. Esophagogastroduodenoscopy to detect structural abnormalities

    d. Esophageal manometry (see p. 1256) to check motor function and to measure pressures of the LES and the esophagus at rest and during swallowing

    e. Routine chest radiograph to check for widened mediastinum with a dilated esophagus

8. Clinical management

    a. Goals are to reduce symptoms, relieve obstruction, and prevent the development of complications.

    b. Nonpharmacologic interventions

        (1) Diet of semisolid foods, which are tolerated best, with any changes in diet or introduction of new foods carefully monitored

        (2) Upright positioning during meals and for at least 2 hours after meals

    c. Pharmacologic interventions

        (1) Nitrates, such as sublingual isosorbide dinitrate (Isordil), a long-acting nitrate, may reduce LES pressure. They should be given 15 to 20 minutes before meals and at bedtime, with peak action occurring at between 15 and 90 minutes. Reducing LES pressure may relax the sphincter and relieve dysphagia.

        (2) Calcium channel blockers (nifedipine) interfere with calcium flux across the cell membrane and diminish contraction of both vascular and visceral smooth muscle. Capsules should be chewed and given 30 to 45 minutes before meals and at bedtime.

    d. Special medical-surgical procedures

        (1) Pneumatic dilation of the LES can be accomplished by passing an esophageal ''bougie'' with a pneumatic dilator under local anesthesia.

          • The person is put on clear liquids 1 to 2 days before dilation and must be on NPO status for 8 hours before the procedure.

          • A guidewire is passed by means of endoscopy, the endoscope is removed, and the dilator is passed over the wire.

          • The dilator is inflated for 30 to 60 seconds and then deflated for an equal time. It is reinflated and deflated once more.

          • The major complication is esophageal perforation.

        (2) Esophagomyotomy (modified Heller myotomy) enlarges the LES by cutting several of the muscle fibers around the sphincter. The major complication associated with this surgery is gastroesophageal reflux.

9. Complications

a. Pulmonary disorders caused by aspiration

b. Cancer of the esophagus

10. Prognosis: This is a chronic condition that can usually be treated, and the person can adapt to the symptoms.

11. Applying the nursing process

> **NURSING DIAGNOSIS:** Altered nutrition, less than body requirements R/T dysphagia

    a. *Expected outcomes:* After intervention, the person should be able to do the following:

        (1) Maintain stable weight and adequate nutritional status

        (2) Discuss measures for increasing ability to tolerate the intake of foods

    b. *Nursing interventions*

        (1) Monitor the effectiveness of medication therapy aimed at relaxing the pressures of the LES and increasing the person's ability to swallow without discomfort, regurgitation, and nausea.

        (2) Discuss dietary modifications that will increase tolerance for food and maintain the necessary daily dietary intake.

> **NURSING DIAGNOSIS:** Anxiety R/T difficulty or inability to swallow

    a. *Expected outcomes:* After intervention, the person should be able to describe effective measures for dealing with fears and anxieties regarding achalasia.

    b. *Nursing interventions*

        (1) Provide emotional support.

        (2) Supply information regarding the disease, normal esophageal functioning, and available treatment options.

12. Discharge planning and teaching

    a. Teach the person to eat slowly and to chew foods well. Attempts at introduction of new foods or changes in the diet should be made carefully to monitor pressure and reflux changes.

    b. Encourage the person to drink fluids with meals to ease swallowing.

◨ *CARING FOR PEOPLE WITH DIVERTICULA (ZENKER'S DIVERTICULUM)*

1. Definition: Outpouchings of 1 or more layers of the esophageal mucosa that are found in 3 areas:

    a. Above the esophageal sphincter (Zenker's)

    b. At the midpoint of the esophagus

    c. Just above the LES

2. Incidence and socioeconomic impact

    a. Esophageal diverticula are not common.

    b. The most frequent are Zenker's diverticula, which occur more often in men older than 50 years of age.

3. Risk factor: Previous esophageal trauma
4. Etiology: Unclear
5. Pathophysiology
   a. Diverticula may develop from a congenital weakness in the esophageal wall or from a previous trauma to the wall that has left it weakened.
   b. They are most often associated with a motor abnormality of the esophagus, usually in the upper esophageal sphincter.
6. Clinical manifestations
   a. Transient dysphagia (difficulty swallowing)
   b. Feelings of aspiration
   c. Gurgling in the throat
   d. Regurgitation
   e. Visible mass on the neck
7. Diagnostics
   a. History: Ask about prior trauma or surgery to the esophagus
   b. Administer barium swallow to detect any structural abnormalities, particularly within the sphincters.
8. Clinical management
   a. Goals are to relieve the discomfort associated with the diverticula and to maintain adequate nutritional status.
   b. Nonpharmacologic interventions
      (1) Keep the head of bed in an elevated position for sleeping.
      (2) Change the diet (e.g., eat smaller amounts) to increase the patient's ability to tolerate the intake of food. Evaluate foods carefully when an episode of intolerance occurs.
   c. Pharmacologic interventions: None
   d. Special medical-surgical procedures: Excision of diverticula may become necessary if the person begins to become malnourished because of poor food intake.
9. Complications
   a. Esophageal perforation
   b. Aspiration pneumonia
10. Prognosis: Surgery may be necessary.
11. Applying the nursing process

NURSING DIAGNOSIS: Altered nutrition, less than body requirements R/T dysphagia

   a. *Expected outcomes:* After intervention, the person should be able to do the following:
      (1) Maintain stable weight and adequate nutritional status
      (2) Identify measures to maintain intake of adequate nutrition
   b. *Nursing interventions*
      (1) Assess the person's ability to maintain nutritional status. (Surgery may be required if the person is at risk for malnutrition.)
      (2) Monitor food intake, carefully noting which foods the person is able to eat and which cause problems.
      (3) Monitor weight daily.

NURSING DIAGNOSIS: Pain R/T dysphagia and feeling of fullness and pressure in sternal region

   a. *Expected outcomes:* After intervention, the person should be able to do the following:
      (1) Report relief or reduction in pain
      (2) Describe measures that can be taken to reduce or eliminate pain
   b. *Nursing interventions*
      (1) Discuss position changes and dietary modifications that may be necessary to improve comfort.
      (2) Administer prescribed medications to promote comfort.
12. Discharge planning and teaching: Instruct the person to sleep with the head of the bed elevated, and not to eat food within 2 to 4 hours of going to bed.

◼ CARING FOR PEOPLE WITH GASTRITIS

1. Definition: generalized inflammation of the gastric mucosa as a result of some sort of irritant and an impairment of the gastric protective mechanisms; can be either acute or chronic
   a. In acute gastritis, varying degrees of inflammation, ulceration, and erosive damage to the mucosa result from ingestion of certain drugs, from excessive alcohol intake, or from consumption of spicy or contaminated foods.
   b. In chronic gastritis, progressive, diffuse inflammation of the mucosal lining results from the normal aging process or from the course of certain diseases (e.g., pernicious anemia, peptic ulcer disease, stomach cancer, chronic alcohol ingestion, or chronic nonsteroidal anti-inflammatory drug [NSAID] ingestion).
2. Incidence and socioeconomic impact
   a. A common problem of the stomach
   b. More frequent in men than women
   c. Most frequently seen in patients who are between 50 and 60 years of age
3. Risk factors
   a. Smoking
   b. Heavy alcohol intake
   c. Dietary indiscretions
   d. Acute systemic inflection
   e. Excessive use of aspirin or other NSAIDs
4. Etiology and Pathophysiology
   a. The normal mucosal barrier of the stomach breaks down and is inflamed by an organism such as *Helicobacter pylori*.

Helicobacter pylori (originally identified as *Campylobacter pylori*) are "curved bacilli" (S- or C-shaped) that are found in the gastric mucosa. These gram-negative bacteria, with their smooth outer coat and 2 to 4 imipolar flagellae, infect and irritate the stomach mucosa, most often causing gastritis of the antrum of the stomach. This organism also is directly associated with gastric ulcers, peptic ulcer disease, and gastric cancer. However, many people older than 65 years have this organism and remain asymptomatic. Although, fortunately, it is sensitive to antibiotics and bismuth compounds, researchers do not know its origin or how it is spread.

b. Inflammation of the gastric mucosa allows hydrogen ions to diffuse back into the epithelial cells of the gastric mucosa, causing erosion, ulceration, or bleeding.

c. In acute gastritis, the back-diffusion of hydrogen ions causes a release of histamine, which further stimulates increased secretion of hydrogen ions by the parietal cells of the mucosa. Bleeding can result.

d. In chronic gastritis, the protective mucosal lining thins (may atrophy), glandular activity decreases, and gastric functioning slows. There may even be bile reflux from the duodenum as the condition progresses.

5. Clinical manifestations
   a. Abdominal discomfort or pain
   b. Nausea and vomiting
   c. Increased saliva production
   d. Hiccuping
   e. Bleeding

6. Diagnostics
   a. History
      (1) Note pertinent risk factors and whether peptic ulcer disease has developed.
      (2) Question the person about symptoms of anorexia, nausea, vomiting, or food intolerance. Take a diet history to determine normal eating patterns and food choices.
   b. Examination: Assess for abdominal pain and signs of bleeding.
   c. Gastroscopy with gastric biopsy to culture the mucosa is the test of choice.
   d. Barium swallow may be done to rule out other esophageal and gastric problems.
   e. Serum gastrin levels may be determined to check functioning.
   f. Gastric analysis may be performed.

7. Clinical management
   a. Goal is to eliminate the cause of the gastritis.
   b. Nonpharmacologic interventions
      (1) Begin NPO status with intravenous fluids, if nausea and vomiting are severe. Replace fluids and electrolytes to balance losses from vomiting.
      (2) Use nastogastric decompression and suction, if gastritis is severe.
      (3) Resume clear liquids slowly and progress to bland diet.
   c. Pharmacologic interventions
      (1) Administer antacids (see p. 1254) for abdominal discomfort.
      (2) Give antiemetics for nausea and vomiting.
      (3) Use histamine H_2-receptor antagonists (see p. 1255) to reduce or inhibit gastric acid secretions.
      (4) Give combination therapy of bismuth compound (Pepto-Bismol) and an antimicrobial (amoxicillin or metronidazole) to treat *H. pylori* bacteria.
   d. Special medical-surgical procedures
      (1) Surgery may be necessary if pharmaceutic treatment alone does not work.
      (2) Gastrectomy: Partial gastrectomy involves removal of the distal $\frac{2}{3}$ to $\frac{3}{4}$ (the antrum and pylorus) of the stomach to eliminate the ulcer and to reduce gastric acid secretion. Total gastrec-

tomy (esophagojejunostomy) involves complete removal of the stomach at the LES with attachment of the esophagus to the jejeunum or duodenum.
      (3) Vagotomy: This surgical division of the vagus nerve is performed to eliminate the vagal impulses that stimulate hydrochloric acid secretion in the stomach. There are three main types of vagotomy:
   • Selective vagotomy severs only the branches of the vagus that innervate the stomach, thereby interrupting acid secretion.
   • Truncal vagotomy severs both the anterior and posterior trunks of the vagus nerve at the level of the esophagus before the stomach, thus decreasing acid secretion and gastric motility.
   • Parietal vagotomy (highly selective vagotomy) severs only the portion of the vagus that innervates the parietal acid-secreting cells of the stomach.
      (4) Pyloroplasty: This enlargement of the pyloric sphincter of the stomach prevents or decreases pyloric obstruction and enhances gastric emptying. However, it does not decrease the release of gastric acid secretions. Sometimes a vagotomy is done in conjunction with a pyloroplasty.
   e. Gastrointestinal intubation
      (1) Gastrointestinal tubes can be placed in different locations.
   • Nasogastric: Is inserted into the nares and ends in the stomach.
   • Orogastric: Is inserted into the mouth and ends in the stomach.
   • Intestinal (nasoenteric, nasoduodenal, or nasojejunal): Is usually inserted into the nares and ends in the intestines
   • Gastrostomic: Is inserted into the stomach through an incision in the abdominal wall
   • Jejunostomic: Is inserted into the jejunum through an incision in the abdominal wall
      (2) Gastric intubation is done for the following reasons:
   • Decompression: To manage distention, or to empty the stomach of contents, secretions, and gas
   • Compression: To stop bleeding
   • Feeding or gavage: To provide nutrition
   • Lavage: To irrigate and clear the stomach of blood or other secretions
   • Gastric analysis: To obtain a laboratory sample
      (3) The purpose of the gastric intubation determines the type of tube to be used.
      (4) Tubes used for decompression
   • Levin: A single-lumen stomach tube that is used to remove gastric contents or to provide tube feedings
   • Salem sump: A double-lumen stomach tube; it is the most frequently used tube for decompression with suction.
      (5) Tubes used for compression
   • Sengstaken-Blakemore: A triple-lumen gastric tube that has an inflatable esophageal balloon,

Procedure 27–1
Insertion, Discontinuance, Irrigation, and Care of
Nasogastric and Intestinal Tubes

Definition/Purpose	To insert, maintain, and discontinue a nasogastric tube—a tube inserted in the nose, through the esophagus into the stomach. The nasogastric tube is used for diagnostic, therapeutic, and nutritional purposes.
Contraindications/Cautions	1. Some tubes are inserted only by physicians. 2. During the procedure, if the person experiences difficulty breathing or any respiratory distress (gagging, coughing, dyspnea, or cyanosis), pull back on the tube and wait until the distress subsides. 3. When discontinuing an intestinal tube, dispose of the mercury in the appropriate manner per your facility's policy.
Learning/Teaching Activities	Provide the following information about the procedure: (1) Purpose of the tube, (2) How long the tube will be in place, and (3) any necessary restrictions while the tube is in place

Preliminary Activities

Equipment	• Nasogastric tube • Emesis basin • 1/2-inch tape • Glass of water with a straw • Gloves • Water-soluble lubricant • 35–50 ml catheter tip syringe • Normal saline • Stethoscope
Assessment/Planning	• Examine the mouth and nasal structures of the person for any structural abnormalities that may interfere or cause difficulties with the passage of the tube. • Ask the person if he or she has ever had previous nasal or oral surgeries.
Preparation of the Person	• Position the person upright in bed at about a 90-degree angle, if that position can be tolerated. • Otherwise, position the patient on their right side. • Check the patency of the nasogastric tube by running water through the tube before insertion. Also check for the presence of any holes or nicks in the tube.

Procedure

Action	Rationale/Discussion

Insertion of a Nasogastric Tube

1. Select the nares to be used for its patency.

2. Measure the length of tube needed— usually done by placing the tube at the tip of the nose and measuring by extending the tube to the ear lobe and then down to the xiphoid process. Mark the tube at that length.

3. Lubricate about 3 inches of the tube at the insertion end with a water-soluble jelly.

4. Insert the tip of the tube through 1 nostril and begin to advance the tube backward toward the ear and through the nasopharynx (down the nasal passage). *Do not force the tube.*

5. As you reach the nasopharynx, instruct the person to bend the head forward and take a sip of water. Continue to advance the tube as the person swallows.

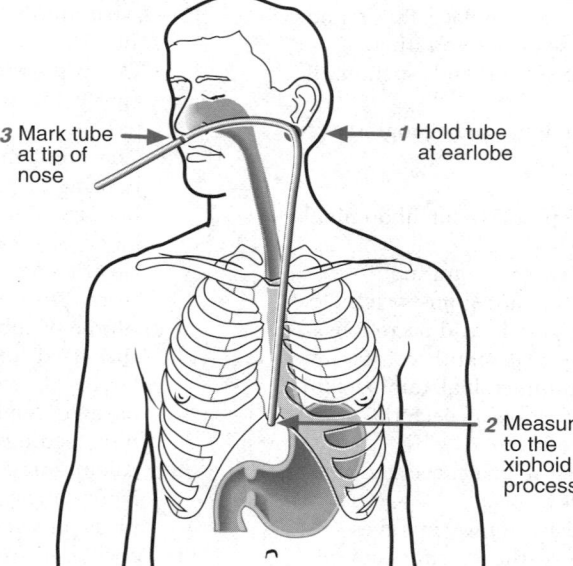

3 Mark tube at tip of nose

1 Hold tube at earlobe

2 Measure to the xiphoid process

1. The nostril with the better air flow is usually chosen.

2. The average length for an adult is about 22 to 26 inches.

3. The use of water-soluble lubricant prevents the development of pneumonia, a complication that can develop if the tube accidentally goes into the bronchus with an oil lubricant.

4. Insert slowly to avoid pressure on any structures, which might cause bleeding or pain.

5. Bending the head forward closes the epiglottis (closing the trachea) and opens the esophagus. Taking a sip of water helps with passage of the tube into the esophagus.

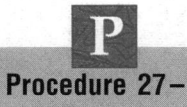

Procedure 27–1
(continued)

Action	Rationale/Discussion
6. Advance the tube until you reach the mark for the desired length of tube per your measurements.	6. Continue to advance slowly and carefully.
7. For intestinal tubes, allow the tube to advance over several hours until the correct length of tube has advanced. The tube is inserted through the nares and threaded into the stomach. Position the person on the right side to facilitate passage through the pylorus of the stomach and into the small intestine.	7. The mercury weights within the tube facilitate the movement of the tube through the stomach into the intestine.
8. To confirm placement, aspirate for gastric contents, or auscultate for swooshing sounds in the stomach while air is injected as you listen.	8. If no gastric contents are aspirated, the tube has not advanced into the stomach. A swooshing sound heard with the stethoscope means that the tube is in the stomach. A radiograph confirms the tube placement.
9. Secure the tube to the person's nose with an attachment device or with a piece of adhesive tape that is split to form a Y.	9. To maintain security of the tube and to prevent as little tugging on the tube as possible.

Discontinuance of Nasogastric Tube

Action	Rationale/Discussion
1. Discontinue the suction apparatus and clamp the tube to prevent escape of fluid during removal. Remove the tape around both the tube and the person's nose carefully.	1. Clamping the tube prevents the escape of any gastric contents that could be irritating or cause aspiration during removal.
2. Deflate the balloon or aspirate the mercury contents of an intestinal tube balloon.	2. To allow for easy removal.
3. Instruct the person to exhale and remove the tube with 1 very smooth, continuous pull.	3. This will close the epiglottis and allow for easy withdrawal through the esophagus into the nose.
4. Remove an intestinal tube about 6 inches every 10 minutes until it reaches the stomach, and then withdraw it as you would the nasogastric tube.	4. This avoids pulling on the intestines.
5. Dispose properly of the disposable materials.	5. Per facility policies.

Basic Care of the Nasogastric Tube

Action	Rationale/Discussion
1. Maintain and check patency of the tube every 4 hours.	1. To prevent vomiting and maintain decompression.
2. Note color of the drainage—dark brown, dark red, green, or "coffee-ground" material.	2. Normally gastric drainage is colorless or mucusy yellow. The color and consistency of the drainage are significant in determining the presence of different materials: Green suggests bile, "coffee-ground" material suggests the presence of old blood, and so forth.
3. Measure an accurate intake and output every 8 hours.	3. To maintain fluid balance.
4. Give routine mouth care.	4. The person with a nasogastric tube tends to mouth-breathe and will have extreme drying of the mouth.
5. Give routine nares care.	5. The person with a nasogastric tube will have increased nasal secretions, and crusting builds up easily in and around the nares.

Irrigation of a Nasogastric Tube

Action	Rationale/Discussion
1. Clamp the nasogastric tube and disconnect the tube from the feeding or suction apparatus. Determine the correct placement of the tube in the stomach before beginning the irrigation.	1. This is essential for the safe performance of the irrigation and for prevention of complications.
2. Insert a 30 to 50-ml syringe filled with water or normal saline into the tube. Unclamp the tube and inject the irrigating solution slowly.	2. Throughout the irrigation, evaluate the person's ability to tolerate this procedure.
3. If resistance is met, check the tubing to see if it is kinked or blocked anywhere, or have the person change positions. If neither of these techniques allows you to continue, call the physician.	3. Placement and patency of the tube are important for the performance of the procedure.
4. Pull back on the syringe plunger or bulb to withdraw the irrigating fluid.	4. Withdrawal of the instilled fluid allows the nurse to check the patency of the tube and the gastric contents.
5. Assess and measure the aspirated contents, document the character and amount of aspirate.	5. Accurate recording of the amount instilled and the amount withdrawn will prevent a fluid imbalance, which could result in abdominal distention, or vomiting at the very least.
6. Repeat the irrigation if the tube remains sluggish.	
7. Reclamp the tube, disconnect the syringe, and reconnect the tube to the suction or feeding apparatus. Then, unclamp.	

(continued)

P

Procedure 27–1

(continued)

Action	Rationale/Discussion
Basic Care of Intestinal Tubes	
1. Check hospital policy for the nurse's role in the care, advancement, and removal of intestinal tubes.	1. Facility policies vary with regard to the nurse's role in caring for intestinal tubes.
2. Do not secure the tube to the face until it has reached the final placement. It can be taped to the forehead with a setup that allows for continued advancement of the tube.	2. To allow for full advancement of the tube without restriction.
3. Intestinal tubes are not usually irrigated by the nurse for obstruction; if the tube is blocked, a small amount of air injected into the lumen can clear the tube. This should first be reported to the physician.	
4. Maintain and check patency of the tube every 4 hours. Check for evidence of mercury balloon rupture.	4. To ensure continued functioning of the tube.
5. Note color and consistency of the drainage—dark brown, dark red, green, "coffee-ground" material.	5. The color and consistency of the drainage are significant in determining the presence of different materials: Green suggests the presence of bile, "coffee-grounds" suggests the presence of old blood.
6. Measure an accurate intake and output every 8 hours.	6. To monitor fluid balance.
7. Give routine mouth care.	7. The person with a nasointestinal tube will tend to mouth-breathe with the presence of the tube and will have extreme drying of the mouth.
8. Give routine nares care.	8. The person with a nasointestinal tube will tend to have increased nasal secretions, and crusting builds up easily around and inside the nares.

Final Activities

1. Document the insertion or discontinuation of a nasogastric tube. Record the type and size of tube inserted, any difficulties encountered during the procedure, how well the person tolerated the procedure, and if any air, fluid, or other material was used to inflate the balloon portion of the tube.
2. Record the person's understanding of the purpose of the nasogastric tube and any restrictions that may have to be followed.
3. After discontinuation of the nasogastric tube, assist the person with mouth and nares care. Include assistance with the removal of any tape residue left on the nose.

an inflatable stomach balloon, and a gastric suction lumen; it is used for treatment of bleeding esophageal varices and is usually inserted along with another nasogastric tube to collect secretions above the esophageal balloon.
- Linton-Nachlas: A 4-lumen gastric tube that has an inflatable esophageal balloon, an inflatable stomach balloon, and 2 suction lumina, 1 in the stomach and the other in the esophagus; it is used to treat bleeding esophageal varices.

(6) For feeding, use the Keofeed, which is a special tube made of silicone rubber; it is soft and pliable, and it comes in small sizes for long-term feeding use.

(7) Tubes used for lavage
- Levacuator: A double-lumen vinyl tube that is used to evacuate gastric contents through 1 lumen and to irrigate through the other
- Ewald: A reusable, single-lumen large tube that is used for rapid, 1-time irrigation and evacuation

(8) Intestinal intubation is used to do the following:
- Decompress the bowel
- Remove intestinal contents
- Provide a feeding

These tubes are longer and usually have a balloon at the distal end to keep them in place. Types of intestinal tubes include the following:
- Cantor: A single-lumen tube with a mercury-filled balloon and a suction port
- Miller-Abbott: A double-lumen tube, 1 for the mercury balloon and the other for suction or drainage
- Harris: A single-lumen tube with a mercury-filled balloon and a suction port

(9) See Procedure 27–1 for information on inserting, caring for, and removing nasogastric and intestinal tubes.

8. Complications
   a. Hemorrhage
   b. Pernicious anemia
   c. Ulceration

9. Prognosis: Treatment with medication is often successful.
10. Applying the nursing process

NURSING DIAGNOSIS: Pain R/T increased gastric secretions and gastric inflammation

a. *Expected outcomes:* After intervention, the person should be able to do the following:
   (1) Report relief of or reduction in epigastric pain
   (2) Identify factors that aggravate the pain
   (3) Describe measures that decrease or alleviate epigastric pain
b. *Nursing interventions*
   (1) Assist the person to identify factors that aggravate the pain and that should be avoided. This may result in dietary modifications, such as reducing or eliminating spicy foods and foods with caffeine, or identification of a particular medication that is causing distress. Emphasize that only foods that aggravate the pain and inflammation must be eliminated or reduced.
   (2) Administer and evaluate prescribed medication therapy, including antacids and antisecretory drugs. Evaluate the effectiveness of medications so that the proper combination therapy can be reached.

NURSING DIAGNOSIS: Altered nutrition, less than body requirements R/T anorexia, nausea and vomiting, and distress

a. *Expected outcomes:* After intervention, the person should be able to do the following:
   (1) Maintain stable weight and adequate nutritional status
   (2) Identify dietary modifications that are necessary to decrease symptoms and to improve food intake.
b. *Nursing interventions*
   (1) Discuss dietary modifications with the person to achieve a well-balanced diet that is easily tolerated.
   (2) Administer prescribed medication therapy to reduce symptoms of nausea and vomiting.
11. Discharge planning and teaching
   a. Discuss the role of causative agents, such as aspirin, alcohol, caffeine, smoking, and emotional stress.
   b. Teach the person the importance of taking antacids and antisecretory drugs and following the prescribed schedule.
   c. Discuss dietary restrictions and the need for continual monitoring of foods that aggravate symptoms.
   d. Teach the person the signs of GI bleeding, such as dark tarry stools, fatigue, pain, and vomited blood.
12. Public health considerations: Prevention should focus on cessation of smoking, limiting intake of alcohol and caffeine, and the use of stress-reduction techniques.

■ CARING FOR PEOPLE WITH GASTRIC ULCER DISEASE

1. Definitions
   a. Peptic ulcer disease is a broad term that is used to classify any ulceration of the mucosa of the esophagus, stomach, or duodenum. The most common peptic ulcers are gastric ulcers and duodenal ulcers.
   b. Gastric ulcers involve ulceration of the mucosal lining that extends through the muscularis mucosae to the submucosal layer of the stomach. They are usually found in the central area of the stomach at the lesser curvature (see Color Fig. 27–2.)
2. Incidence and socioeconomic impact
   a. Usually occurs between 45 and 70 years of age
   b. Equal incidence among men and women
   c. Less common than duodenal ulcers
   d. Impact of stress and lifestyle on the development of peptic ulcer disease remains controversial.
3. Risk factors
   a. Chronic use of aspirin, other NSAIDs, corticosteroids
   b. Cigarette smoking
   c. Family history of ulcer disease
   d. Alcohol use
   e. Gastritis
4. Etiology and Pathophysiology
   a. Changes in the mucosa may occur as a result of the following:
      (1) Back-diffusion of hydrogen ions into the epithelium, which causes a release of histamine and stimulates the production of more acid
      (2) Dysfunction of the pyloric sphincter, which allows reflux of bile from the duodenum into the stomach
   b. The mucosa's increased permeability to back-diffusion of hydrogen ions impairs its ability to protect against damage from toxins.
   c. Gastric secretion levels are usually normal in patients with gastric ulcers, so there is controversy over whether these secretions damage the normal mucosa or cause the ulcerations once the damage to the mucosa occurs.
5. Clinical manifestations
   a. A gnawing, sharp pain that occurs in, or left of, the midepigastric region 1 to 2 hours after eating
   b. Nausea and vomiting
   c. Bleeding
6. Diagnostics
   a. History
      (1) Assess the person for abdominal pain. Determine the location, timing, and severity of pain, along with associated symptoms and precipitating factors.
      (2) Assess for recent weight loss.
   b. Examination: Palpate the abdomen carefully for pain, which is usually present in the upper epigastrium, left of the midline.
   c. Esophagogastroduodenoscopy (or gastroscopy alone) is the 1st choice for diagnosis and may be repeated at 4 to 6 week intervals to evaluate response to therapy.

d. Upper GI series are not precise at diagnosis, because many gastric ulcers are superficial and are difficult to detect with barium studies.

e. Exfoliative cytology (examination of secretions and cells that are scraped or brushed from the mucous membranes) helps to distinguish malignant from benign ulcers.

f. Gastric analysis has limited value because many of the gastric secretion levels are normal in ulcer disease.

7. Clinical management

a. Goals are to eliminate causative agents, to reduce or neutralize gastric acid secretions, and to enhance mucosal resistance.

b. Nonpharmacologic interventions

(1) During the active disease state, small, frequent bland feedings may help with food tolerance, but they can be foods of the person's own choosing.

CLINICAL CONTROVERSIES

Diet is a controversial issue in ulcer therapy. Current evidence does not suggest that diet contributes to healing. However, foods such as caffeine and chocolate are known to increase acid secretion.

(2) Maintain adequate hydration.

(3) Adequate rest and relaxation are important to the healing process.

c. Pharmacologic interventions

(1) Administer histamine H_2-receptor antagonists (see p. 1255) to decrease the secretion of gastric acids.

(2) Give antacids (see p. 1254) to neutralize gastric acid secretions and to decrease discomfort.

(3) Give anticholinergics such as Pro-Banthine to reduce gastric motility and to decrease acid secretions.

(4) Administer mucosal barrier protectants, such as sucralfate, which appear to bind with proteins at the ulcer site to form a protective coat and to prohibit the actions of gastric acids and pepsin on the mucosa. These medications should be taken 1 hour before each meal.

(5) Prostaglandins, such as Cytotec, are used for both cytoprotective and antisecretory purposes. These are newer drugs that are usually given in conjunction with one of the other drug therapies to increase the strength of the treatment (Table 27–5).

d. Special medical-surgical procedures

(1) Surgery may be necessary. The decision to do surgery is usually based on the severity and duration of the ulcer disease, compliance with the treatment regimen, and response to the medication and diet therapy. Several options for surgery exist (Box 27–1).

(2) Total gastrectomy or vagotomy (see p. 1261 for details on both procedures) may be necessary.

(3) Gastric resection (antrectomy) removes the

Table 27–5. Cytoprotective Agents and Other Gastrointestinal Drugs

Medication	Action
Sucralfate (Carafate)	A mucosal barrier fortifier that forms a protective coat over the ulcer, shielding it from gastric secretions
Misoprostol (Cytotec)	A synthetic prostaglandin that reduces the production of gastric acid and protects the mucosa
Omeprazole (Prilosec)	A proton pump inhibitor that stops the production of gastric acid by inhibiting gastric parietal cell secretion (H,K,ATPase inhibitor)
Metoclopramide (Reglan)	A cholinergic and dopamine antagonist that promotes gastric emptying and increases LES tone
Propantheline bromide (Pro-Banthine)	An anticholinergic that reduces acid secretion and decreases gastric motility

lower half of the stomach. This procedure usually includes a vagotomy.

(4) Billroth I (gastroduodenostomy) involves partial gastrectomy (see p. 1267) with anastomosis of the gastric stump to the duodenum (Fig. 27–10).

(5) Billroth II (gastrojejunostomy) involves partial

Box 27–1. Care of the Person Undergoing Gastric Surgery

Preoperative Management

1. Provide instructions regarding the specific surgery.
2. Discuss with the person the goals of the surgery and the expected outcomes.
3. Discuss the need for a nasogastric (NG) tube to remove secretions and empty the stomach.
4. Explain what to expect during the immediate postoperative period, such as NPO status (nothing by mouth), NG tube with suction apparatus, intravenous therapy, Foley catheter, coughing and deep breathing, ambulation schedules, wound care, pain medication.

Postoperative Management

1. Provide fluid and electrolyte replacements via intravenous therapy.
2. Maintain NPO status for 1 to 3 days until peristalsis returns.
3. Monitor NG tube for drainage and maintain connection to suction for postoperative decompression.
4. Strictly record intake and output.
5. Assess bowel sounds.
6. Provide wound care per specific surgery.
7. Provide drain care per specific surgery.
8. Encourage ambulation as soon as the surgery allows.
9. Observe for signs and symptoms of complications:
   - Nausea and vomiting
   - Diarrhea, constipation, or both
   - Paralytic ileus
   - Wound dehiscence or evisceration
   - Infection
   - Shock
   - Hemorrhage
   - Pulmonary complications
   - Thrombosis
   - Dumping syndrome

TYPES OF GASTRIC SURGERY

Gastric Resection
Also called antrectomy. Removes the lower half of the stomach. Usually includes a vagotomy.

Total Gastrectomy
Also called esophagojejunostomy. Removal of the entire stomach at the LES with attachment of the esophagus to the jejunum or duodenum.

Pyloroplasty
The enlargement of the pyloric sphincter of the stomach to prevent or decrease pyloric obstruction, enhancing gastric emptying. This does not decrease the release of gastric acid secretion. Sometimes a vagotomy is done in conjunction with a pyloroplasty.

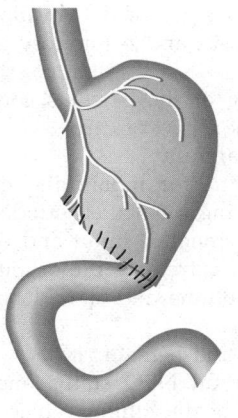

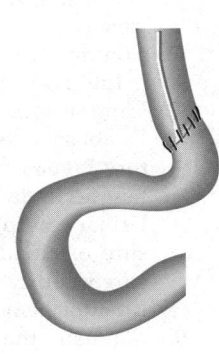

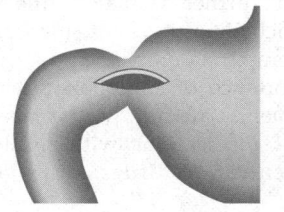 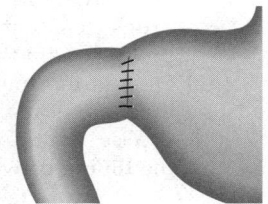

Vagotomy
The surgical division of the vagus nerve.
This is done to eliminate the vagal impulses that stimulate hydrochloric acid secretion in the stomach.
The 3 main types of vagotomy are:
- *selective vagotomy*, which severs only the branches of the vagus that innervate the stomach, interrupting acid secretion
- *truncal vagotomy*, which severs both the anterior and posterior trunks of the vagus nerve at the level of the esophagus prior to the stomach, which in turn decreases acid secretion and gastric motility
- *parietal vagotomy (highly selective vagotomy)*, which severs only the portion of the vagus that innervates the parietal acid-secreting cells of the stomach.

Billroth I
Also called gastroduodenostomy. Involves partial gastrectomy (removal of antrum and pylorus of stomach) with anastomosis of the gastric stump to the duodenum.

Billroth II
Also called gastrojejunostomy. Involves partial gastrectomy (removal of antrum and pylorus of stomach) with anastomosis of gastric stump to the jejunum.

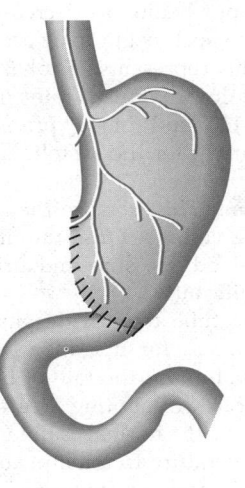

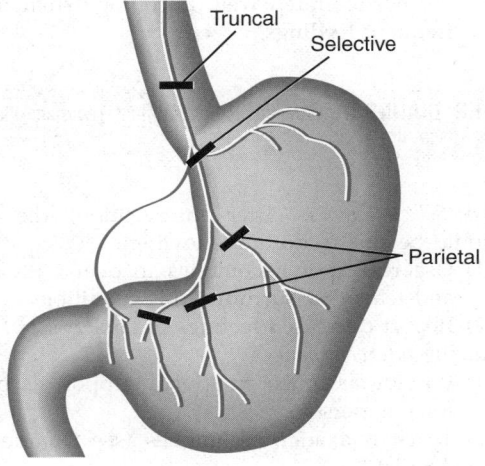

Figure 27–10. LES, Lower esophageal sphincter.

gastrectomy with anastomosis of the gastric stump to the jejunum (see Fig. 27–10).

(6) Pyloroplasty enlarges the pylorus to prevent or decrease pyloric obstruction, thereby enhancing gastric emptying. Sometimes a vagotomy is done in conjunction with the pyloroplasty.

(7) Postoperative complications include dumping syndrome, hypoglycemia, and diarrhea.

8. Complications

    a. Gastrointestinal bleeding
    b. Pyloric obstruction
    c. Perforation

9. Prognosis: Only about 8 percent of gastric ulcers are malignant.

10. Applying the nursing process

NURSING DIAGNOSIS: Pain R/T increased gastric secretions

a. *Expected outcomes:* After intervention, the person should be able to report reduction or elimination of gastric irritation and pain.

b. *Nursing interventions*

(1) Administer antacids and antisecretory drugs on an alternating basis (to neutralize the gastric acid secretions and to attempt to block the continued secretion of the hydrochloric acid), along with cytoprotective agents (to protect the mucosal barrier from further damage) and other drugs (e.g., anticholinergics, antiemetics, and prostaglandin therapy) as prescribed.

(2) Discuss the importance of compliance with the medication regimen, particularly the need for precise timing of medications with meals and the timing between various drugs.

NURSING DIAGNOSIS: Altered nutrition, less than body requirements, R/T pain, food intolerance, and nausea and vomiting

a. *Expected outcomes:* After intervention, the person should maintain stable weight and adequate nutritional status.

b. *Nursing interventions*

(1) Discuss the controversy surrounding dietary modifications in the treatment of gastric ulcer disease. Focus on identifying and avoiding foods that increase acid secretion and tend to aggravate the condition.

(2) In conjunction with the patient and a dietitian, develop a plan for a well-balanced diet that is easily tolerated, restricting only those foods that are not tolerated well. Encourage smaller, more frequent feedings.

NURSING DIAGNOSIS: Anxiety R/T treatment regimen, lifestyle changes, discomfort

a. *Expected outcomes:* After intervention, the person should be able to do the following:

(1) Use relaxation techniques to deal with anxiety and fears that surround this condition

(2) Report decreased feelings of anxiety

b. *Nursing interventions*

(1) Provide as much emotional support as possible for this person.

(2) Teach relaxation techniques (see Chapter 6 for details).

(3) Explore the person's use of cigarettes and alcohol for decreasing stress and anxiety, as they will contribute to or aggravate this condition.

(4) Explain thoroughly all treatments, medications, procedures, and restrictions. Allow the person to ask any questions that are of concern.

(5) Discuss the controversial role that stress plays in the development and exacerbation of the ulcer disease. Suggest that patients consider decreasing the emotional, physical, and psychologic stresses in their lives.

NURSING DIAGNOSIS: Risk for fluid volume deficit R/T upper GI hemorrhage

a. *Expected outcomes:* After intervention, the person should do the following:

(1) Have fluid homeostasis restored

(2) Experience no further hemorrhaging

b. *Nursing interventions*

(1) Assess the person for signs of dehydration, hypovolemic shock, sepsis, and respiratory insufficiency.

(2) Continual monitoring of the person's condition is the most important aspect of care.

(3) Monitor vital signs carefully.

(4) Establish a central line for monitoring circulatory homeostasis during the acute period. Maintain accurate measurement of input and output. Urinary output is an extremely important measure of circulatory volume and should be measured hourly.

(5) Monitor hemoglobin and hematocrit.

(6) Maintain the person on NPO status and give intravenous fluids to begin volume replacement. Give blood transfusion per physician order.

(7) Attempt to assess or estimate the amount of bleeding.

• Less than 500 ml: This is about 10 percent of circulating volume. Pulse rate is beginning to rise.

• 500–1000 ml: This is about 25 percent of circulating volume. Pulse rate increases to between 100 and 110, and blood pressure begins to decrease. Urine output begins to decrease. Signs and symptoms of shock begin to appear.

• 1000–2000 ml: This represents 25 to 40 percent of circulating volume. Pulse rate increases beyond 110 to 120 and blood pressure decreases by 20 mm Hg for the systolic measurement.

• More than 2000 ml: This is more than 40 percent of circulating volume. Pulse rate increases to beyond 120; blood pressure and urine output decrease significantly.

(8) Insert a nasogastric tube to provide gastric decompression and access for irrigation, to allow collection of information on the rate of bleeding, and to reduce the risk of vomiting. Begin lavage through the tube with normal saline or tap water at room temperature to attempt to reduce active bleeding and measure amounts of bleeding until other treatments are initiated.

(9) If saline lavage does not immediately stop the bleeding, institute other treatments per the physician's order:

• Intravenous vasopressin to reduce partial pressure and slow the bleeding

• Endoscopic variceal ligation or endoscopic sclerotherapy

• Balloon tamponade

(10) Once the acute episode is under control, diagnose and correct the underlying condition.

11. Discharge planning and teaching
    a. Teach the person the importance of diet and medications in the treatment of this conditon.
    b. Instruct the person to avoid aspirin and other NSAIDs, and not to smoke.
    c. Explain the need for lifestyle modifications: moderate activity, adequate rest, and decreased stress.
12. Public health considerations
    a. One method of preventing disease involves providing education about smoking cessation programs. Smoking has been shown to have a direct effect on the mucosa of the GI tract.
    b. The direct link between stress and the development of ulcer disease remains controversial; however, educating the public regarding stress reduction and relaxation techniques is a positive preventive measure.

◼ CARING FOR PEOPLE WITH DUODENAL ULCERS

1. Definition: a break in the mucosa of the duodenum—most often in the pyloric region—that can extend through the muscularis mucosa
2. Incidence and socioeconomic impact
   a. Eighty percent of all peptic ulcers
   b. Four times more common than gastric ulcers
   c. Usually occur between 40 and 60 years of age
   d. Three times more common in men than in women
3. Risk factors
   a. Associated with such diseases as chronic obstructive pulmonary disease, cirrhosis, chronic pancreatitis, chronic renal failure, and Zollinger-Ellison syndrome (pancreatic islet cell tumor)
   b. Dietary factors: alcohol and caffeine intake
   c. Smoking
   d. Use of corticosteroids, aspirin, and NSAIDs
   e. Stress
4. Etiology
   a. Primary cause: increased levels of gastric acid secretion by the parietal cells
   b. Alcohol intake
   c. Cigarette smoking
   d. Caffeine
   e. Stress
   f. Infection with *Helicobacter pylori*
5. Pathophysiology
   a. Duodenal ulcers may result either from high acid secretion by gastric parietal cells or from decreased mucosal resistance to injury or impaired mucosal defense mechanisms.
   b. Ulceration results when hydrogen ions successfully diffuse back into the gastric epithelium, either because of excessive acid or because of a weakened mucosa.
6. Clinical manifestations
   a. Burning pain in the midepigastric region, usually 2 to 4 hours after eating or during the night
   b. Pain that is often relieved by eating
7. Diagnostics
   a. History

(1) Assess for epigastric pain severity, timing, and duration. Often, the person has had this pain for weeks or even a year or more before seeking attention.
(2) Assess for occurrence of vomiting and diarrhea.
   b. Examination: Palpate the abdomen for areas of tenderness or pain, noting the location of pain and any presence of rigidity.
   c. Endoscopy: Use procedure to visualize ulcer location, size, and condition.
   d. Barium contrast studies: To check for delayed emptying
   e. Exfoliative cytology
   f. Elevated serum gastrin levels
   g. Gastric analysis is of limited benefit to show the presence of hyperacidity.
8. Clinical management
   a. Goals of clinical management are to eliminate the ulcer-causing agents, to decrease gastric acidity, and to prevent complications.
   b. Nonpharmacologic interventions
      (1) Provide for adequate physical and emotional rest.
      (2) Recommend a bland diet with small, frequent feedings.
      (3) Encourage the reduction or cessation of smoking because smoking delays ulcer healing.
   c. Pharmacologic interventions
      (1) Give antacids (see p. 1254) as necessary to neutralize acid secretions.
      (2) Administer histamine H_2-receptor antagonists (see p. 1255) to block continued secretion of acids.
      (3) Sucralfate (Carafate) has aluminum hydroxide that may bind with the ulcer base if it is taken 30 to 60 minutes before meals.
   d. Special medical-surgical procedures
      (1) Surgery is normally performed only in cases involving hemorrhage, obstruction, or perforation.
      (2) In severe cases of recurrent ulcer history, highly selective vagotomy may be offered as elective surgery.
9. Complications
   a. Bleeding or hemorrhage
   b. Perforation
   c. Gastric outlet obstruction
   d. Intractable disease
10. Prognosis
    a. Treatment begins with use of medications. Surgery is performed only if the ulcer is unresponsive to the medications.
    b. Usually remission is seen only with healing of the ulcer.
11. Applying the nursing process (see p. 1268)
12. Discharge planning and teaching
    a. Teach the person about the link between disease and causative and contributing factors.
    b. Educate the person about the importance of the medication schedule.
    c. Describe the signs of bleeding or hemorrhage.
13. Public health considerations
    a. Primary prevention should emphasize the link between smoking and ulcer disease and should support smoking cessation programs.

b. Controversy remains about the link between stress and ulcer disease; however, stress reduction and relaxation techniques are valuable tools to enhance a healthy lifestyle.

CARING FOR PEOPLE WITH CROHN'S DISEASE (REGIONAL ENTERITIS)

1. Definitions
   a. A chronic, recurrent inflammation of the mucosa and surrounding musculature of the GI tract; it can involve any segment of the bowel but usually affects the terminal ileum.
   b. Regional enteritis refers to Crohn's disease that is limited to the small bowel.
   c. Crohn's colitis is used to refer to disease that affects the colon (Fig. 27–11).
2. Incidence and socioeconomic impact
   a. Most common age of onset: 15 to 30 years of age
   b. Both sexes affected equally
   c. Most frequent among Whites of European Anglo-Saxon background
   d. Higher incidence among European and North American Jewish populations than non-Jewish populations.

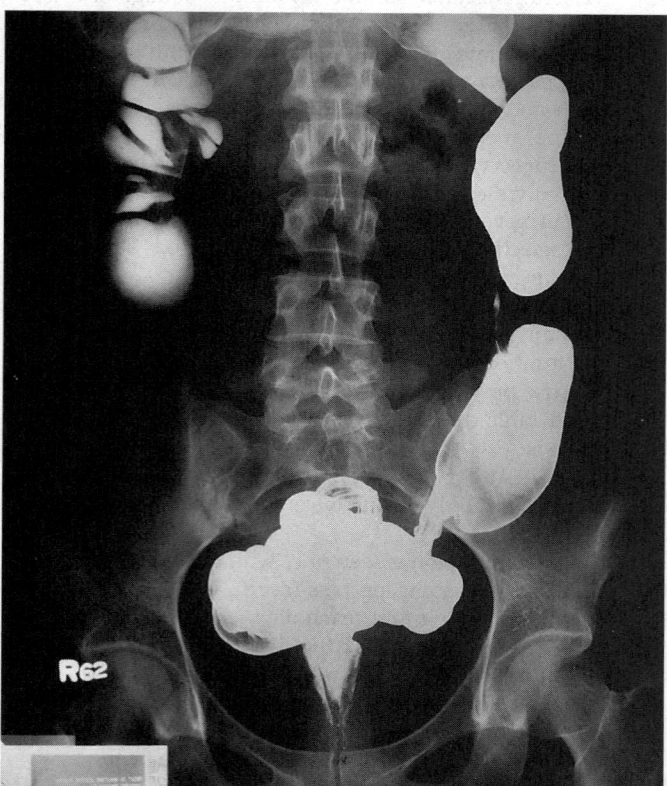

Figure 27–11. Barium enema radiograph showing multiple strictures of the descending colon in Crohn's disease. (Courtesy of the University of Maryland Medical Center.)

3. Risk factors: family predisposition
4. Etiology
   a. Exact etiology unknown
   b. Viral or bacterial
   c. Associated with some sort of altered immune response

CLINICAL CONTROVERSIES

Most theories of altered immune response—including altered autoimmune reactions, lymphocyte-mediated reaction (IgE), and host resistance—as a direct cause of Crohn's disease have been disproved. Indeed, a key question today is whether the immune responses involved are causes or effects.

   d. Dietary factors in Western cultures
   e. Psychosomatic factors—more involved in exacerbations than in the development of the condition
5. Pathophysiology
   a. The earliest lesions start as ulcers and develop into deep fissures in the bowel wall that penetrate into the submucosal layer or through the wall, creating fistulas and abscesses. The changes in the bowel wall involve the lymph nodes, as well as dilation of the lymphatic channels.
   b. As the disease worsens, the inflammation of the bowel wall increases and the wall becomes congested and thickened, which narrows the lumen. Normal tissue between the areas of involvement is called "skip" lesions.
6. Clinical manifestations
   a. Insidious onset
   b. Diarrheal stools
   c. Crampy abdominal pain
   d. Abdominal distention
   e. Fever
   f. Anorexia, nausea, and vomiting
   g. Weight loss
   h. As the disease worsens, there is increased abdominal discomfort, malnutrition, anemia, or dehydration with fluid and electrolyte imbalances.
   i. Extraintestinal symptoms affect the following:
      (1) Joints: colitic arthritis, ankylosing spondylitis, sacroiliitis, finger clubbing
      (2) Eye: conjunctivitis, uveitis, episcleritis
      (3) Skin: erythema nodosum, pyoderma gangrenosum
      (4) Vascular system: thromboembolic disease
      (5) Hepatobiliary system
7. Diagnostics
   a. History
      (1) Ask about perianal problems that cause discomfort or pain.
      (2) Assess for extraintestinal symptoms (see above).
   b. Examination
      (1) Examine the perianal area for breakdown.
      (2) Assess for extraintestinal symptoms.
   c. Barium enema detects the affected bowel segments, ulcers, fissures, and fistulas and can also show the

''string sign'' (visible areas of diseased bowel that are separated by segments of normal bowel).
   d. Colonoscopy or sigmoidoscopy provides direct visualization of the bowel.
   e. Complete blood count (CBC) detects anemia.
8. Clinical management
   a. Goals are to control diarrhea, achieve relief from abdominal pain and cramping, treat and control any infections or complications, provide emotional support to decrease stress, and correct any fluid and electrolyte imbalances.
   b. Nonpharmacologic interventions
     (1) Patient may need to be on NPO status; give fluids intravenously during the acute exacerbation.
     (2) Provide for adequate rest and comfort.
     (3) Give parenteral or enteral nutrition if the person does not respond and seems unable to tolerate added oral feedings, or for the malnourished or preoperative person, to allow the bowel to rest while supplying adequate nutrition. This can be done by an elemental tube feeding or by total parenteral nutrition.
     (4) Give elemental supplemental feedings during exacerbation to assist with nutrition.
     (5) After exacerbation is under control, begin a regular, balanced, high-calorie, high-nitrogen, no-fat, no-residue diet. Avoid milk or milk products if the patient is lactose intolerant.
   c. Pharmacologic interventions
     (1) Corticosteroids during exacerbation may decrease the inflammatory response within the intestine and also help with some extraintestinal symptoms.
     (2) Sulfasalazine may decrease inflammation if there is disease in the colon. Give it with adequate fluids to prevent crystalluria.
     (3) Administer antidiarrheals as necessary.
   d. Special medical-surgical procedures
     (1) Surgery is not a 1st choice and is reserved for intractable disease or repair of complications.
     (2) The extent of surgery depends on which part of the bowel is affected and the general condition of the person.
     (3) Possible surgeries include colostomy and ileostomy; procedural choice depends on the severity and extent of the disease.
9. Complications
   a. Fistulas are the most frequent complication; several different kinds can arise with Crohn's disease:
     (1) Cutaneous fistulas in the perianal area
     (2) Rectourinary fistulas
     (3) Rectovaginal fistulas
   b. Abscesses
   c. Perforation
   d. Obstruction
   e. Malabsorption
   f. Perianal complications including anal skin tags, fissures, abscesses, and excoriated skin.
10. Prognosis: Crohn's is a recurrent disease and the course of the disease varies significantly. Some people have acute exacerbations and long remissions, whereas others with Crohn's have more severe disease.
11. Applying the nursing process

NURSING DIAGNOSIS: Diarrhea R/T inflammation of the small intestine

   a. *Expected outcomes:* Following intervention, the person should be able to do the following:
     (1) Report a reduction in the frequency of stools and the return of stools to a more normal consistency
     (2) Identify factors that may aggravate the diarrhea
   b. *Nursing interventions*
     (1) Administer prescribed medication therapy.
     (2) Assess the severity of the diarrhea and the effectiveness of the medications.
     (3) Monitor for skin integrity problems as a complication of diarrhea. Discuss proper perianal hygiene and the possible development of fissures and skin breakdown with severe diarrhea. Teach the use of routine sitz baths during exacerbations.

NURSING DIAGNOSIS: Altered nutrition, less than body requirements, R/T anorexia, nausea and vomiting, or malabsorption

   a. *Expected outcomes:* Following intervention, the person should be able to do the following:
     (1) Maintain stable weight
     (2) Increase intake of tolerated foods and fluids to improve nutritional status
   b. *Nursing interventions*
     (1) Assist the person with the development of a well-balanced nutrition plan that includes foods that the person likes and can tolerate.
     (2) Suggest supplements to regular meals that can provide much-needed calories during periods of disease exacerbation. Encourage patients to eat whatever they want and to limit only those foods that worsen the disease.

NURSING DIAGNOSIS: Ineffective individual coping R/T chronic condition and anxiety regarding diagnosis and disease

   a. *Expected outcomes:* Following interventions, the person should be able to do the following:
     (1) Report decreased feelings of anxiety regarding this illness and its treatment
     (2) Identify successful personal coping mechanisms to use throughout the exacerbation period of the disease
   b. *Nursing interventions*
     (1) Provide adequate education and psychologic and emotional support. Help the person to identify successful coping mechanisms and to focus on personal strengths, rather than on the weaknesses of this chronic condition.
     (2) Provide for adequate rest and comfort to decrease stress and to make the person feel some control.

(3) Discuss the relationship between exacerbations of the disease and major life events or changes.

(4) Refer the person for additional counseling, if necessary.

12. Discharge planning and teaching
   a. Explain the disease process, the course and chronic nature of Crohn's disease, the need for follow-up care, and the symptoms of recurrence and how to respond to them, including signs and symptoms of complications.
   b. Teach the importance of a well-balanced diet and the need for rest and use of stress-reduction techniques.
   c. Instruct the person on proper hygiene and how to maintain the integrity of the perianal area during recurrent episodes of irritating diarrhea.
   d. Teach the importance of identifying life stresses or the approach of major life events or changes to plan how these events will be approached.

13. Public health considerations
   a. Identify those who are at risk for developing the disease and educate them concerning diet, rest, and low-stress lifestyle.
   b. Support groups for people with Crohn's can offer support and assistance to maintain a fairly normal life, despite chronic disease.

◼ CARING FOR PEOPLE WITH ULCERATIVE COLITIS

1. Definition: diffuse inflammation of the mucosal wall of the large intestine and rectum
2. Incidence and socioeconomic impact
   a. Familial tendency
   b. Occurs most often between 20 and 40 years of age
   c. Equal incidence among males and females
   d. More common in Whites than non-Whites
   e. More frequent in European and North American Jews
3. Risk factors
   a. There is a significant relationship between ulcerative colitis of longer than 10 years and cancer of the colon.
   b. Family history
4. Etiology
   a. Exact etiology is unknown—possibly viral or bacterial infection
   b. Autoimmune response
   c. Psychosomatic factors—more involved in exacerbations than in the development of the condition
5. Pathophysiology
   a. Inflammation begins in the rectum or lower rectum and spreads proximally to the cecum.
   b. The inflammation involves the mucosa and submucosa and causes the mucosa of the colon to become thick and edematous.
   c. Chronic inflammation of the wall causes bleeding.
   d. Abscesses can develop and become necrotic, leading to purulent exudate and bloody stools.
6. Clinical manifestations

a. Intermittent recurrence of disease is common.
b. Crampy abdominal pain
c. Bloody, mucousy diarrhea; may pass visible pus as disease progresses
d. Weight loss
e. Anorexia, nausea, and vomiting
f. Left lower quadrant abdominal pain
g. Abdominal distention
7. Diagnostics
   a. History
      (1) Assess the normal pattern of bowel habits for this person. Does anything increase or decrease the frequency of bowel irregularities?
      (2) Take a complete diet history.
   b. Examination
      (1) Listen to bowel sounds.
      (2) Assess for signs of dehydration, poor skin turgor, dry skin, thirst, dry mucous membranes, and sunken eyeballs from the diarrhea and malabsorption.
      (3) Assess for extra intestinal problems, such as liver disease, skin problems, inflammation of the eye, and joint problems to differentiate between Crohn's and ulcerative colitis (Table 27–6).
   c. Check stool specimens for blood, mucus, and pus.
   d. Perform a complete blood count and chemical panel to determine anemia and electrolyte imbalances.
   e. Colonoscopy or proctosigmoidoscopy with rectal biopsy determines the extent of disease and the condition of the mucosa.
   f. Barium enema may be done to identify abnormal mucosa.
8. Clinical management
   a. Goals are to decrease the inflammation, allow the bowel to rest, and correct nutritional deficiencies.
   b. Nonpharmacologic interventions
      (1) Provide bed rest to promote healing and decrease intestinal activity.
      (2) Assist with personal hygiene, focusing on the perianal area after each episode of diarrhea. Pay close attention to skin assessment and care because of the malnutrition and the debilitated condition of the person. Prevent skin breakdown (see also Chapter 7).
      (3) Rectal pouching for severe diarrhea may be helpful in the weakened person.
      (4) Maintain accurate input and output records, recording the number of bowel movements and the amount and character of the stool.
      (5) Initially, the person may be on NPO status with fluids and electrolyte replacements given intravenously. Total parenteral nutrition may also be necessary to correct nutritional and electrolyte deficiencies.
      (6) High-calorie, high-protein, low-fat, low-residue elemental feedings are used to begin oral intake. Small, frequent meals may be best tolerated. Any dietary restrictions should be based on tolerance of food; only foods that are found to be irritating should be eliminated. Supplemental feedings may enhance nutrition during acute exacerbations. A

Table 27–6. Major Differences Between Crohn's Disease and Ulcerative Colitis

	Crohn's Disease	Ulcerative Colitis
Age of Onset	Adolescent and young adult	Young and middle adult
Incidence	Uncommon	Frequent
Etiology	Familial	Unknown
Location of disease		
Small intestine	Yes	No
Rectum involved	Occasionally	Yes
Lymph nodes	Involved	Normal
Mesentery	Thick	Normal
Extent of Disease	Entire wall	Mucosa
Fistulas	Yes	Rare
Toxic Megacolon	Rare	Yes
Ulcerations	"Skip" areas, deep	Extensive, superficial
Obstruction	Yes	Rare
Perforation	Rare	Yes
Malabsorption	Yes	Rare
Rectal Lesions	Yes	Rare
Bleeding	Rare	Rectal
Weight Loss	Severe	Yes
Diarrhea	Nonbloody	Bloody
Abdominal Pain	Yes	Yes
Fever	Yes	Rare
Cure with Surgery	No; Recurrence	Yes
Predisposition to Malignancy	Rare	Yes

calorie count may be necessary to monitor intake. Necessary caloric intake varies by individual need, condition, amount of bowel affected, surgery, and the like (see also Chapter 10).

(7) Emotional support is also extremely important to assist the person in coping with stress, necessary lifestyle changes, and the chronic nature of the condition. Help focus thoughts and energies away from the bowel problems.

c. Pharmacologic interventions
 (1) Antidiarrheals for exacerbations—document the effectiveness of the medication
 (2) Sulfasalazine (Azulfidine), a sulfanimide, to decrease secondary infections
 (3) Corticosteroids, given orally, intravenously, or as an enema to decrease the inflammatory response
 (4) Anticholinergics to decrease peristalsis and to relieve cramping

d. Special medical-surgical procedures
 (1) Surgery is indicated when the person does not respond to medical treatment, or if the onset is abrupt and fulminant and results in complications (see below). Several types of surgeries can be done.
 (2) Colectomy (removal of the colon) may stop uncontrolled bleeding.
 (3) Proctocolectomy, removal of the rectum and colon that is needed for massive bleeding or

other severe complications, along with permanent ileostomy.
 (4) Continent ileostomy (Kock pouch) involves creation of an internal ileal pouch that is connected to the abdominal wall by a stoma that is continent through the intussusception of a piece of ileum between the stoma and the pouch.
 (5) Ileoanal anastomosis, with colectomy, removes the diseased colon, creates an ileal reservoir (Fig. 27–12) from the terminal ileum, and connects this to the anus. This procedure preserves the rectal neuromusculature and allows the person to maintain some continent control of feces and gas.

9. Complications
a. Hemorrhage and coagulation defects related to vitamin K deficiency
b. Perforation
c. Toxic megacolon: This is a life-threatening complication that results from the spread of severe inflammation through the mucosal layers of the colon. The smooth muscle of the wall relaxes and becomes paralyzed. The colon dilates and fails to move its contents along, with the bacteria and toxins found in the colon being absorbed by the dilated walls. Frequency of stools decreases with pain and distention. Surgery is needed.
d. Cancer of the colon

KOCK POUCH

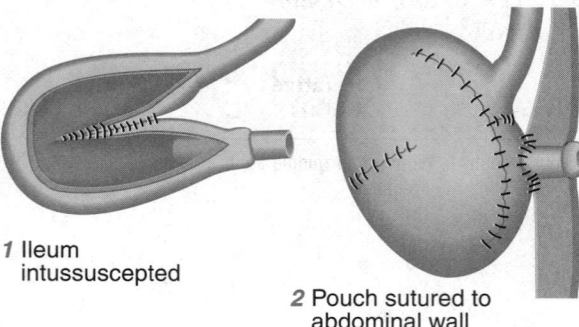

1 Ileum
intussuscepted

2 Pouch sutured to
abdominal wall

ILEAL "J" POUCH

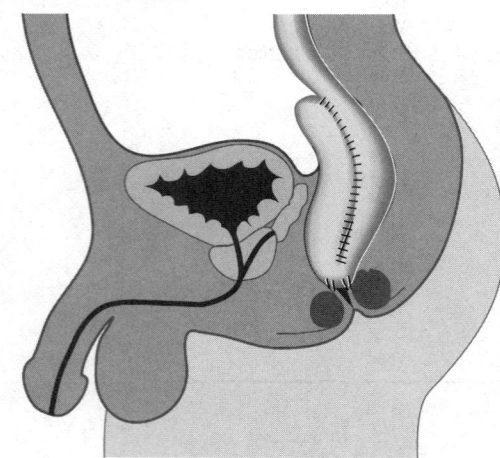

Figure 27–12. Kock pouch and ileal reservoir.

10. Prognosis: About 85 percent of persons with ulcerative colitis can be successfully treated pharmaceutically. The other 15 percent require surgical intervention.
11. Applying the nursing process

NURSING DIAGNOSIS: Pain R/T inflammation, cramping, frequent diarrhea

a. *Expected outcomes:* Following intervention, the person should be able to do the following:
    (1) Report relief from, reduction in, or control of the pain
    (2) Identify relaxation techniques
    (3) Describe the successful use of 1 form of relaxation or diversion
b. *Nursing interventions*
    (1) Assess the extent of the pain and attempt to provide relief through medications, positioning changes, and restrictions of certain foods that the person may indicate seem to increase the discomfort. Pain will vary greatly among different people.
    (2) Teach relaxation techniques (see Chapter 6) and diversions to cope with the discomfort.

NURSING DIAGNOSIS: Diarrhea R/T the inflammatory process

a. *Expected outcomes:* After intervention, the person should be able to do the following:
    (1) Report a reduction in the frequency of stools and the return of stools to normal consistency
    (2) Identify factors that aggravate the diarrhea
    (3) Establish a regular pattern of bowel elimination
b. *Nursing interventions*
    (1) Administer prescribed medications to treat diarrhea and cramping.
    (2) Record the amount, consistency, and frequency of stools, noting any observed relationships between the occurrence of diarrhea and the intake of medications, diet, and patient activities. Observe for signs and symptoms of possible complications related to continued uncontrolled diarrhea, and report these as soon as noted.
    (3) Assess the effectiveness of medication.

NURSING DIAGNOSIS: Altered nutrition, less than body requirements, R/T inadequate intake, diarrhea, dietary restrictions, malabsorption

a. *Expected outcomes:* After intervention, the person should be able to do the following:
    (1) Maintain stable weight through progression of diet
    (2) Maintain adequate intake of foods and fluids or nutritional supplements
    (3) List foods that are easily tolerated and identify foods that may aggravate symptoms
    (4) Describe nutritional requirements
b. *Nursing interventions*
    (1) Provide nutritional support (see Nonpharmaceutical Interventions, earlier), including parenteral nutrition, if necessary. Gradually move the person to liquids, then to a soft, bland diet, and finally to a normal dietary pattern. Add foods 1 at a time to test tolerance for each newly added food.
    (2) Discuss the impact of high-fiber and bulky foods on the GI tract. Have the person identify foods that produce gas and irritate the bowel.

NURSING DIAGNOSIS: Risk for fluid volume deficit R/T diarrhea or malabsorption

a. *Expected outcomes:* After intervention, the person should be able to do the following:
    (1) Maintain an adequate fluid volume
    (2) Be free of signs and symptoms of dehydration
b. *Nursing interventions*
    (1) Monitor input and output.
    (2) Provide for adequate fluid volume replacement.
    (3) Encourage adequate fluid intake (3000–4000 ml per day).
    (4) Observe for signs and symptoms of fluid and electrolyte imbalance, including skin turgor, mucous membranes, vital signs, urine specific gravity, and other serum electrolyte values.

a. *Expected outcomes:* After intervention, the person should be able to do the following:
   (1) Express feelings related to the disease process
   (2) Acknowledge personal strengths and past methods of coping
   (3) Identify successful coping mechanisms and the appropriate situations in which to use them
b. *Nursing interventions*
   (1) Assess the person's strengths and weaknesses and past methods of coping with life stress.
   (2) Encourage expression of feelings about living with a chronic illness and dealing with lifestyle adaptations.
   (3) Be sensitive and help patients identify ways to adapt their lifestyles to limitations and restrictions that may be necessary.
   (4) Involve family members in discussions of ways to support the person, to help identify coping mechanisms, and to implement necessary lifestyle changes for the family.
   (5) Arrange for volunteers from support groups to talk and share living experiences with patients and their families.
12. Discharge planning and teaching
    a. Discuss the treatment regimen and how the person can manage the medication, nutrition, and lifestyle adjustments.
    b. Instruct the person about the signs and symptoms of disease recurrence and when to seek medical attention.
    c. Teach signs of electrolyte imbalance and loss of sodium and potassium. Alert those with ostomies that during the summer months, supplemental fluid intake (e.g., Gatorade or other electrolyte solutions) may be necessary because of perspiration and loss of fluids.
    d. Explain the need to avoid smoking, as this increases intestinal motility.
13. Public health considerations: Educate the public about the need for surveillance for colon cancer, based on the strong relationship between long-standing ulcerative colitis and cancer of the colon.

◼ CARING FOR PEOPLE WITH DIVERTICULOSIS, DIVERTICULITIS, AND MECKEL'S DIVERTICULUM

1. Definitions
   a. A diverticulum is an outpouching of the bowel mucosa. It may be found anywhere along the gastrointestinal tract from the esophagus to the rectum but is seen most often in the sigmoid colon (see Color Fig. 27–3).
   b. Diverticulosis is a condition in which there are multiple diverticula found in the GI tract.
   c. Diverticulitis is a complication of diverticulosis in which an inflammation or perforation of the diverticulum results.
   d. Meckel's diverticulum is a congenital outpouching of the distal ileum near the cecum. Symptoms are similar to those of appendicitis. Clinical manifestations include abdominal pain and dark blood in the stools.
2. Incidence and socioeconomic impact
   a. About 50 percent of the population 40 years of age and older have diverticula; the incidence rises as age increases.
   b. Such problems are more frequent in Western countries than in Eastern or developing countries.
   c. They are seen more frequently in men than in women.
3. Risk factors
   a. Increasing age
   b. Lack of fiber and bran in the diet
   c. Stress
4. Etiology: Trapped undigested food particles and bacteria in the diverticula
5. Pathophysiology
   a. A diverticulum forms in the wall of the intestine as a herniation of the mucosa and submucosa between muscle fibers in response to increased pressures during segmentation. This herniation forms the diverticulum.
   b. Diverticulitis results when food particles and bacteria become trapped in a diverticulum, thereby creating a hardened mass called a fecolith.
   c. The inflammation that results spreads to the surrounding mucosa, and edema results.
   d. This edema occludes the area and causes more inflammation and decreased blood supply to the area, which can cause the diverticulum to perforate and bleed; also, with continued trapped fecal contents, an obstruction can result.
6. Clinical manifestations
   a. The presence of diverticula does not necessarily mean that symptoms will occur. Many patients are asymptomatic.
   b. If symptoms are present, they vary according to the extent of the inflammation; these symptoms include abdominal pain, alternating diarrhea and constipation, bleeding, gas formation, abdominal distention, and fever.
7. Diagnostics
   a. History
      (1) Assess for abdominal discomfort, especially in the left lower quadrant.
      (2) Question the person about changes in bowel patterns. Take a complete bowel history, noting complaints of, or increases in, constipation.
      (3) Take a diet history, noting the amounts of bran, fruits, and vegetables that are included in the regular diet.
   b. Examination
      (1) Assess abdominal pain and tenderness, guarding, rebound tenderness, and distention.

(2) Monitor vital signs for fever and tachycardia.

(3) Check stools for occult blood.

c. Ultrasonography may be used to check for the presence of diverticula during exacerbation.

d. Barium enema may be performed after the acute inflammation has decreased.

e. Rectal examination with sigmoidoscopy or colonoscopy provides direct visualization of the diverticula.

8. Clinical management

a. Goal is to decrease the inflammatory process.

b. Nonpharmacologic interventions

(1) During the acute phase, it is important to take measures to rest the bowel and decrease intestinal motility.

(2) Institute NPO status with intravenous fluids to maintain hydration.

(3) Provide bed rest to decrease activity and stress.

(4) Use a nasogastric tube with suction for decompression of the bowel.

(5) Provide a diet that begins with clear liquids and advances as tolerated; it should include high-fiber foods when solids are tolerated.

(6) Advance activity as tolerated.

c. Pharmacologic interventions

(1) Give broad-spectrum antibiotics—ampicillin for mild cases and cephalosporin for more severe cases.

(2) Use anticholinergics (such as propantheline or Pro-Banthine) to reduce colonic contractions or hypermotility.

(3) Provide pain medications, such as meperidine hydrochloride (Demerol), as necessary, for severe discomfort.

(4) Give bulk-forming laxatives and stool softeners, if needed to maintain bowel function.

d. Special medical-surgical procedures

(1) Surgery may be performed if any of the emergency complications results or with disease that is unresponsive to medical intervention.

(2) Excision or bowel resection of the involved segment of the colon with anastomosis is an option.

(3) A diverting temporary colostomy may be created if inflammation is too severe for anastomosis. The colostomy is usually reduced in 3 months.

9. Complications

a. Partial or complete obstruction

b. Perforation

c. Peritonitis

d. Hemorrhage

(1) Recognize the possibility of this complication if the person is experiencing lower GI bleeding.

(2) Measure amounts of bloody stool passage, monitor vital signs, and measure output (nasogastric and urinary) carefully. Increases or changes in any of these measures can be early signs of hypovolemia.

(3) Assess the person for abdominal distention and for increasing abdominal pain and rigidity; these are signs of perforation or peritonitis.

(4) Emergency surgery may be required if bleeding cannot be controlled.

e. Fistula formation

10. Prognosis: Approximately 75 percent of persons who are succcessfully treated for diverticulitis for the 1st time will have no or only minimal symptoms after treatment and may never require surgery.

11. Applying the nursing process

NURSING DIAGNOSIS: Constipation R/T lack of bran or fiber in the diet

a. *Expected outcomes:* After intervention, the person should be able to do the following:

(1) Establish a daily or regular pattern of bowel elimination

(2) Report reduction or alleviation of constipation

b. *Nursing interventions*

(1) Teach the person the relationship between constipation and the lack of adequate fluids, bran or fiber, and bulk in the daily diet. Fluid intake should measure at least 2500 ml per day, if the medical condition allows.

(2) Explain the development of diverticular disease and how it increases in the presence of constipation.

(3) In the person with diverticulosis, assess the effectiveness of medications to increase colonic activity; these include stool softeners and bulk-producing laxatives.

NURSING DIAGNOSIS: Pain R/T inflammation of the diverticula

a. *Expected outcomes:* After intervention, the person should be able to do the following:

(1) Report reduction or alleviation of pain

(2) Describe methods to reduce or alleviate painful episodes

b. *Nursing interventions*

(1) In the person with diverticulosis, assess the effectiveness of bulk-producing laxatives for decreasing the pain and discomfort of constipation and for increasing colonic activity.

(2) In the person with diverticulitis, assess the effectiveness of medications to relieve pain and decrease colonic activity.

NURSING DIAGNOSIS: Fear R/T medical diagnosis of chronic disease

a. *Expected outcomes:* After intervention, the person should be able to do the following:

(1) Openly discuss fears associated with the disease process and treatment

(2) Identify personal strengths and successful mechanisms to cope with fears

(3) Report reduction in or alleviation of fears

LEARNING/TEACHING GUIDELINES
for Ostomy Self-Care

General Overview

1. An *ostomy* is an opening from an internal organ through the abdominal wall by which a portion of the organ is brought to the surface of the skin. It provides an outlet for the organ for excretion or for feeding.
2. An intestinal ostomy, which is more often called a colostomy, ileostomy, or cecostomy, creates an opening from the bowel through the abdominal wall; it allows the person to evacuate feces through the opening or ostomy.
3. Ostomies are classified according to the type of diversion, their location, and whether they are temporary or permanent.

Preoperative Teaching

1. Discuss the particular disorder that may require the creation of an ostomy for treatment and alleviation of the disease: Crohn's disease, ulcerative colitis, diverticulitis, and colon and rectal cancer.
2. Describe what an ostomy is (see above).
3. Show the person pictures of the ostomy to be made (the size and shape) and discuss what it will feel like (mucous membrane feeling) and look like (a red beefy color).
4. Differentiate the particular ostomy to be created from others, such as a colostomy or an ileostomy, a gastrostomy, a jejunostomy, or a nephrostomy.
   a. *Colostomy* is a surgical opening created from the colon through the abdominal wall. The most frequent sites of this surgery are the descending and sigmoid colon. Discuss normal functioning of the colostomy.
   b. *Cecostomy* is an opening from the cecum through the abdominal wall. This type of colostomy is usually done to treat obstructions in the ascending colon.
   c. *Ileostomy* is an opening from the ileum through the abdominal wall. Discuss the normal functioning of the ileostomy.
5. Explain whether the person's ostomy will be permanent or temporary.
   a. A colostomy is considered permanent when the rectum, anus, or distal portion of the bowel has to be removed.
   b. A colostomy is considered temporary if reanastomosis is possible when the rectum and anus are left intact. Temporary colostomies are often done after the occurrence of trauma, bowel resection, or major abdominal surgery, or to provide decompression of the bowel with obstruction.
      (1) Loop colostomy is a temporary colostomy that is made when immediate relief is needed for the bowel, often because of an obstruction. A loop of bowel is brought to the skin surface and stabilized to the surface. Only the anterior wall of the loop is opened; the posterior wall remains intact. This opening allows for fecal elimination and decompression of the bowel.
      (2) Double-barrel colostomy is a temporary colostomy that is made after bowel resection, if anastomosis is not an option at the time of surgery, usually because of infection or ischemia. Two stomas are brought to the skin surface: the proximal stoma to drain feces, and the distal stoma to drain mucus from the distal bowel and rectum.
6. Arrange a visit from someone with an ostomy to discuss what life is like living with an ostomy.
7. Include basic abdominal preoperative teaching:
   a. What to expect in the immediate postoperative period: intravenous fluids, nastrogastric (NG) tube, Foley catheter, coughing and deep-breathing exercises, early ambulation
   b. How, after the surgery, the stoma is monitored (checking for color, size and shape, status of skin, and presence of any irritation, pain, redness, swelling, and bleeding) and bowel sounds are auscultated (noting the number, location, and quality of the sounds)
   c. How important it is for the person to communicate when he or she feels the need to pass gas or stool, as this is a sign of returning peristalsis, and that the feces will be monitored for amount, consistency, and color
   d. That to make assessment of the stoma and fecal contents easier, a transparent drainage bag will originally be used
   e. That the postsurgery diet will start out as clear liquids, advance first to full liquids, then to a bland diet, and finally on to a regular diet as tolerated

Postoperative Teaching

1. It is important to begin the discharge teaching of the person early in hospitalization. Include family members or significant others in this education as appropriate.
2. Drainage
   a. Discuss with the person the type of drainage bag or pouching system to be used. Factors that should be included in this discussion are the following:
      (1) Condition of the stoma. Some persons are able to simply wear a small patch over the stoma and do not require the use of a pouch at all.

(continued)

LEARNING/TEACHING GUIDELINES
(continued)

(2) The person's ability for self-care: Does the patient have any physical limitations? Can a friend or relative help with care after the return home?

(3) Will the person's insurance or private means be adequate to cover the costs of the surgery and proper postsurgical care?

b. Explain that the stoma will continue to change and get smaller over the 1st year and that the patient must continue to measure the stoma to ensure that the pouch fits properly.

c. Demonstrate the use of the pouch.

(1) Make sure that throughout the demonstration the person can see everything you do.

(2) Assemble all materials needed. Suggest that the person make a list of what is needed for a change—pouch, scissors, tissues, soap, towel, washcloth, and bag for disposal—and use it to be sure that all items are gathered before beginning the procedure.

(3) Remove the old pouch carefully and put it in the disposal bag.

(4) Clean around the stoma, first removing any fecal material with the tissues. Cleanse the stoma and skin around the stoma with non-irritating soap (optional) and water. Dry gently by patting the stoma and skin around it.

(5) Teach the person to assess the stoma and skin at this time. Assess the size, color, and shape of the stoma, looking for signs of bleeding, irritation, skin breakdown, swelling, redness, or anything unusual. Explain the other types of problems that can occur with an ostomy—diarrhea, constipation, and obstruction—and what to do about each.

(6) Prepare the skin around the stoma with an appropriate skin barrier. Discuss the choices of skin barriers: stomahesive, karaya gum, liquid skin sealant, or spray skin sealant. Explain which is best for this person's situation. After applying the skin barrier, place the pouch over the stoma and press it to the skin, holding it in place for 2 to 3 minutes.

(7) Explain that the pouch should be changed about every 5 days, depending on the type of pouch and how well it remains in place and sealed to the skin.

(8) Demonstrate the emptying of the pouch.

• Demonstrate the position used to empty the pouch—seated on the toilet with the legs spread.

• Assist the person to sit on the toilet in the position you just demonstrated.

• To empty the pouch, unclamp it at the end. Fold up the ends of the pouch like a cuff to prevent soiling and accumulation of feces on the end of the pouch and to limit odors. Holding the pouch in the middle, point it downward between the person's legs into the toilet to empty it.

• Have patients who cannot use the leg-spread-on-toilet position either sit on a chair next to the toilet and empty the pouch into the toilet or sit on the toilet and empty the pouch into something else.

• Once the pouch is empty, rinse the inside of the pouch with warm tap water to clean it out. Unfold the end of the pouch, clean off the end, and reclamp the pouch.

d. Ask the person to demonstrate the procedure to be sure he or she understands and can perform it.

e. Explain that the pouch should be emptied when it is no more than one-half full to prevent leakage, overfilling, or the possibility of its coming off.

f. Discuss with the person how to obtain the supplies that will be needed to care for the ostomy.

g. Address concerns about bowel control with use of a pouch. Note that the farther along in the intestine that the colostomy is created, the more formed the stool will be and the better the chances are of achieving some regularity in control and frequency of drainage from the ostomy.

h. Address any concerns about odor emanating from the pouch.

(1) Discuss odor-producing foods and gas-producing foods and the time interval between eating them and emission of gas and odors.

(2) Explain that, although most pouches are odor-proof, the person may wish to take the following precautions:

• Promptly drain and change the pouch if there is a leak.

• Use room deodorants when changing the pouch and draining the contents.

3. Irrigation

a. The decision to irrigate or not has to be made by each individual, depending on their ability and desire to control the daily output of the colostomy.

b. Explain that colostomy irrigation is similar to an enema and is used to regulate colostomy output.

c. Demonstrate the procedure

(1) Set out all supplies to be used: irrigation set, enema bag, lubricant, gloves.

(2) Fill the irrigation set with 500 to 1000 ml warm tap water and flush the tubing. Begin with only a 500-ml instillation for the 1st few irrigations, and gradually increase the amount to 1000 ml for each irrigation. *Never force the catheter tip into the stoma. If resistance is met,*

LEARNING/TEACHING GUIDELINES
(continued)

digitally remove any feces that may be blocking the stoma. If cramping occurs during instillation, slow the flow.

(3) Instill a lubricated, cone-shaped irrigation catheter tip or regular irrigation catheter tip (if a cone-shaped irrigation catheter tip is not available) into the stoma opening about 7.5 cm. The cone prevents the possibility of perforation.

(4) Unclamp the irrigation bag and allow the irrigation fluid to begin to flow. It should flow slowly over 10 to 15 minutes.

(5) After the irrigation has infused, remove the catheter tip. It will take about 15 to 30 minutes for the feces and irrigation to be expelled.

(6) Clean the stoma and the skin around the stoma, and dry the skin carefully. Replace the ostomy pouch or dressing.

(7) The next time irrigation is scheduled, have the person perform the procedure to ensure that it is understood and performed properly.

4. Diet modifications
   a. Explain to the person that, although there are no strict diet restrictions following surgery and the ostomy, not all foods are equally well tolerated by those with ostomies. Low-fiber and low-residue foods are best tolerated. Foods that are usually tolerated in *limited quantities* (although they need not be eliminated totally) include spicy foods, fruits such as prunes, and any food that produces gas, odor, diarrhea, or constipation. Foods with a cellulose base, such as nuts and seeds, tend to be undigestible and should be avoided.
   b. Recommend introducing new foods slowly, 1 at a time, to check for tolerance.
   c. Teach the person to chew all foods thoroughly

and thus eliminate the problems of undigestible large chunks of food.

5. Living with an ostomy
   a. Explain that there are no activity limitations associated with the ostomy. The person can go back to work, have a social life, travel, and go on with life as before. For example, the person can bathe and shower normally, with the pouch on or off, depending on control of the ostomy.
   b. The only limitations on those with ostomies involve the need to *plan* to care for the ostomy. For example, the person should be alert to tight or restrictive clothing that could interfere with drainage into the pouch.
   c. Provide information about local ostomy support groups for educational, emotional, and psychologic support as needed.

6. Psychologic concerns
   a. Patients undergoing ostomy procedures often need substantial psychologic support. Maintain open communication, and encourage the patient to discuss concerns not only with you, but also with other members of the medical team, with their families and significant others, and with members of ostomy support groups.
   b. Discuss the person's concerns about self-care abilities. Be supportive during the 1st return demonstrations of ostomy care, as some of the activities involved are very technical and threatening to the lay person.
   c. Encourage the patient to discuss the following:
      (1) Concerns about anticipated changes in lifestyle and family relationships
      (2) Concerns regarding body image changes, especially fears regarding loss of sexual attractiveness
      (3) Feelings of grief for their lost body part and for the diagnosis or prognosis they may be facing.

b. *Nursing interventions*
   (1) Provide complete explanations of the disease process, the treatment regimen, and any possible options.
   (2) If appropriate, discuss the person's responsibility in preventing further progression of this disease through compliance with major dietary modifications.
   (3) If surgery is prescribed, explain the procedure and the temporary or permanent nature of the surgical outcome.
   (4) Provide information about what the person can expect in the immediate postoperative period, such as a nasogastric tube, intravenous fluids, what and where the colostomy will be, and what it will look and feel like.

12. Discharge planning and teaching
    a. Provide preoperative and postoperative teaching as necessary. See Learning/Teaching Guidelines for Ostomy Self-Care.
    b. Teach the person to avoid very large meals, to avoid foods that are difficult to digest (e.g., nuts, popcorn, and celery), and to increase fiber and bran in the diet (i.e., to add wheat bran, whole grain breads and cereals, and fresh fruits and vegetables).

NURSE ADVISORY

Caution: Add fiber gradually to the diet, as it can increase flatulence.

c. Explain the need to avoid alcohol and smoking.
d. Provide information about stress-reduction and re-laxation techniques (see Chapter 6).
e. Provide information on the signs and symptoms of acute diverticulitis recurrence—pain, bloody stools, fever, gas, and abdominal distention.
f. Instruct the person to use only bulk-producing laxa-tives, such as Metamucil, if constipated.
13. Public health considerations: Prevention can be achieved with proper diet—increase amounts of whole grain breads and cereals; participate in the "Strive for Five" program for fresh fruits and vegetables in the daily diet.

◼ *CARING FOR PEOPLE WITH IRRITABLE BOWEL SYNDROME*

1. Definition: a functional disorder that affects the fre-quency or consistency of stool; a chronic spasticity of the colon
2. Incidence and socioeconomic impact
   a. A common disorder
   b. Most frequently found in those 20 to 40 years of age
   c. More frequent in women than men
3. Risk factors: Smoking
4. Etiology
   a. Unknown
   b. Emotional and psychologic stress
   c. Intake of certain foods that are spicy or high in fat
5. Pathophysiology
   a. It is called a syndrome because there is no patho-logic condition that explains the symptoms.
   b. It is a disorder of GI motility with progressive changes in bowel function from diarrhea to constipa-tion, or alternating diarrhea and constipation.
6. Clinical manifestations
   a. Episodic abdominal pain and cramping
   b. Alternating periods of diarrhea and constipation
   c. Bloating
   d. Flatulence
7. Diagnostics
   a. Must be distinguished from inflammatory bowel dis-ease (Crohn's disease and ulcerative colitis), from which it differs in location, distribution, and depth of mucosal involvement
   b. History
      (1) Ask the person about changes in bowel habits; most often complaints of constipation are reported.
      (2) Question the patient about the presence of pain, its location, and whether it is relieved by defeca-tion.
      (3) Assess dietary history; question about eating very rich foods and usual alcohol consumption.
      (4) Determine history of cigarette smoking.
      (5) Assess for high levels of anxiety with job or oc-cupation or at home, depression, or obsessive-compulsive and rigid behaviors.
   c. Examination
      (1) Inspect the abdomen for distention; palpate areas

of tenderness and pain, especially in the left lower quadrant.
      (2) Auscultate bowel sounds, noting frequency and location.
   d. Endoscopy: to visualize mucosa and to check for presence of spastic contractions
   e. Upper GI series and barium enema: to detect the presence of any structural abnormalities such as a narrowed lumen
   f. Stool for blood, cultures, and ova and parasites: to rule out other causes of diarrhea
8. Clinical management
   a. Goal is to restore regular bowel patterns.
   b. Nonpharmacologic interventions
      (1) Encourage a well-balanced, high-fiber diet for constipation; limit fiber and irritating foods with acute diarrhea.
      (2) Increase or maintain fluid intake at 8 glasses per day.
   c. Pharmacologic interventions
      (1) With complaints of constipation, administer pre-scribed bulk-forming laxatives, such as psyllium hydrophilic mucilloid (Hydrocil, Mucillium, or Metamucil), to prevent dry, hardened stools and to normalize stool consistency.
      (2) With complaints of diarrhea, administer pre-scribed antidiarrheal medications, such as atro-pine sulfate (Lomotil) or loperamide (Imodium), to decrease the frequency of stools, and anticho-linergics, such as propantheline bromide, to re-lieve cramping and spasm of the bowel.
      (3) May have to administer a mild tranquilizer.
   d. Special medical-surgical procedures: none
9. Complications: weight loss
10. Prognosis: This is a long-term, chronic problem.
11. Applying the nursing process

NURSING DIAGNOSIS: Diarrhea R/T increased bowel motility

   a. *Expected outcomes:* After intervention, the person should be able to do the following:
      (1) Report relief from, or reduction in, the diarrhea and the return of stools to normal consistency
      (2) Establish regular bowel elimination patterns
   b. *Nursing interventions*
      (1) Record the amount, consistency, and frequency of stools, noting any observed relationships be-tween the presence of the diarrhea and medica-tions given, diet, stress, and activities.
      (2) Assess the effectiveness of medications.
      (3) Observe for signs and symptoms of increased frequency of diarrhea, fatigue, or increased ab-dominal pain.

NURSING DIAGNOSIS: Constipation R/T decreased bowel activity

   a. *Expected outcomes:* After intervention, the person should be able to do the following:

(1) Report reduction or alleviation in constipation
(2) Establish a daily or regular pattern of bowel elimination
(3) Describe required daily actions to avoid a pattern of constipation
b. *Nursing interventions*
(1) Teach the person about the relationship between constipation and the lack of adequate fluids and bran or fiber and bulk in the daily diet. Explain the patient's responsibility in the success of therapy for this syndrome, that is, in increasing dietary fiber and ensuring adequate fluid intake.
(2) Record the amount, consistency, and frequency of stools, noting any relationships between bowel movement and foods or activities.
(3) Assess the effectiveness of medications.

NURSING DIAGNOSIS: Ineffective individual coping R/T anxiety over life stressors and irritable bowel syndrome

12. Discharge planning and teaching
a. Encourage the person to establish a regular time and habit for bowel elimination.
b. Provide diet counseling: Encourage brans, whole grain breads and cereals, and fresh fruits and vegetables as a routine part of the diet; discourage alcohol and caffeine; there is no need to limit or avoid any certain foods unless they can be identified as irritating or causing the diarrhea.
c. Teach the person about irritable bowel syndrome and the causative link with stress.
d. Provide information to assist in stress management (see Chapter 6).
e. Teach about the importance of the medication therapy.
13. Public health considerations
a. Primary preventive measures in young teens and adults aim at minimizing emotional and psychologic stress.
b. Educate the public about the importance of eating a well-balanced diet and avoiding very high-fat foods.

◼ CARING FOR PEOPLE WITH MALABSORPTIVE SYNDROME

1. Definition: a syndrome that results from impaired absorption of fats, carbohydrates, proteins, fat-soluble vitamins, minerals, and water.
2. Incidence: There are 25 different reported disorders.
3. Risk factors
a. Previous GI surgery
b. Travel to a developing country
4. Etiology: Anything that causes an interruption to the process of absorption in the intestine
a. Sprue syndrome
b. Lactase deficiency
c. Gastric resections
d. Crohn's disease
e. Ulcerative colitis
f. Liver and pancreatic abnormalities
5. Pathophysiology
a. Nutrients (fats, carbohydrates, proteins, vitamins, minerals, and water) are normally digested and absorbed in the intestine.
b. Three types of pathologic change are involved:
(1) The presence of a disorder that affects digestion and the preparation of nutrients—an enzyme deficiency
(2) The presence of a lesion in the mucosa—a disruption of the mucosa from disease, surgery, or other factors
(3) The presence of a lesion that affects lymph vessels that carry lipids, causing an obstruction to lymph flow
6. Clinical manifestations
a. Steatorrhea (fatty stools)
b. Diarrhea
c. Weight loss
d. Possible pain or cramping
e. Bloating and flatulence
f. Bone pain
7. Diagnostics
a. History
(1) Question the person about bowel symptoms, such as the presence and frequency of diarrhea, gas, and bloating.
(2) Determine the presence of any other symptoms, especially bone pain.
(3) Take a complete diet history.
(4) Determine recent travel history.
(5) Ask about any weight loss despite normal food intake.
b. Physical examination
(1) Inspect for distention and bloating.
(2) Listen to bowel sounds.
(3) Palpate the abdomen for tenderness or discomfort.
c. Blood studies: to reveal vitamin, mineral, and electrolyte deficiencies
d. Stool specimen for culture, fecal fat, ova, and parasites: to identify any causative agent
e. Abdominal radiographs, ultrasonography, or CT scan: to detect tumors
f. Barium enema: to detect mucosal changes
8. Clinical management
a. The goal is to treat the cause and alleviate symptoms.
b. Nonpharmacologic interventions: Modify the diet to avoid foods that aggravate symptoms—may have to limit fats; provide a gluten-free diet for celiac sprue; give a high-protein, high-calorie diet after gastric resection surgery.
c. Pharmacologic interventions
(1) Provide antibiotics, if necessary, to treat the causative agent.
(2) Give vitamin and mineral supplements to complement the diet.
(3) Administer antidiarrheal medications, such as atropine sulfate (Lomotil).

d. Special medical-surgical procedures: none
9. Complications: weight loss
10. Prognosis
    a. Prognosis varies depending on the cause of the malabsorption.
    b. Celiac sprue is a life-long condition that requires strict adherence to diet modifications.
11. Applying the nursing process

NURSING DIAGNOSIS: Diarrhea R/T malabsorptive syndrome

---

a. *Expected outcomes:* After intervention, the person should be able to do the following:
   (1) Report a decrease in the frequency and quantity of stools and a return to normal consistency of stools
   (2) Establish a regular bowel elimination pattern
b. *Nursing interventions*
   (1) Monitor frequency, amounts, and changing character of stools.
   (2) Evaluate the effectiveness of medication treatment to control diarrhea or steatorrhea.
   (3) Observe the person for signs and symptoms of fluid or electrolyte deficiencies, especially calcium, potassium, magnesium, and iron.

NURSING DIAGNOSIS: Altered nutrition, less than body requirements, R/T poor absorption, nutrient loss

---

a. *Expected outcomes:* After intervention, the person should be able to do the following:
   (1) Maintain stable weight throughout treatment
   (2) Maintain adequate intake of foods and fluids or nutritional supplements
   (3) Describe nutritional requirements
b. *Nursing interventions*
   (1) Discuss the importance of dietary modifications for the success of treatment of this syndrome.
   (2) If the cause of the malabsorption is known, discuss the types of foods that must be eliminated from the diet and how this can be accomplished, taking into account the likes and dislikes of the person. Involve both the patient and a dietitian in discussions of dietary restrictions and in the development of a proper diet plan.
   (3) If the cause is not known, involve the person in identifying foods that aggravate the diarrhea and in limiting or restricting those foods.
12. Discharge planning and teaching
    a. Provide information and rationale for diet modifications.
    b. Explain drug therapy and, if the patient is taking antibiotics, the need to take the entire course of treatment.
13. Public health considerations: Educate the public on the importance of nutrition to the overall health of the body.

◼ CARING FOR PEOPLE WITH PARASITIC DISEASES

1. Definition: infestation of the GI tract with protozoa and helminths, resulting in infections that vary in symptoms and severity (see also Chapter 8)
2. Incidence and socioeconomic impact (see Chapter 8)
3. Risk factors
   a. Travel
   b. Daycare centers
   c. Immunodeficiencies
   d. Oral-anal sexual practices
4. Etiology
   a. The protozoa found most frequently in the United States are *Giardia lamblia* (causing giardiasis) and *Entamoeba histolytica* (causing amebisasis or amebic dysentery). Protozoa exist as cysts (which are ingested and passed) and trophozoites (which adhere to the bowel wall).
   b. Common helminths include nematodes (roundworms), cestodes (tapeworms), trematodes (flukes), *Enterobius vermicularis* (a common roundworm), and pinworm.
   c. Contact with these parasites is usually from contaminated water, food, or feces.
5. Pathophysiology
   a. Parasites invade, inflame, and sometimes ulcerate the wall of the GI mucosa of both the small and the large intestines.
   b. Diarrhea and malabsorptive signs and symptoms usually result from the epithelial changes and abnormalities.
6. Clinical manifestations
   a. Diarrhea
   b. Flatulence
   c. Abdominal cramps
   d. Anorexia and nausea
7. Diagnostics
   a. History
      (1) Assess the person's living, working, and travel history.
      (2) Ask about oral-anal sexual practices.
   b. Examination
      (1) Inspect and palpate the abdomen.
      (2) Listen to bowel sounds for hyperactivity or changes in character.
   c. Collect at least 3 fresh stool specimens to assess for the presence of a parasite in the stool.
   d. Occasionally, a biopsy of the intestinal wall may be necessary. This is accomplished through endoscopy.
8. Clinical management
   a. Goals are to relieve symptoms and to eradicate the causative parasite.
   b. Nonpharmacologic interventions
      (1) Proper diet, rest, and hygiene
      (2) Use and teaching of universal precautions when handling stool
   c. Pharmacologic interventions
      (1) Oral antibiotics: see Chapter 8

(2) Antidiarrheal medications to control the frequency of diarrhea

(3) Antispasmodics to decrease colonic motility

d. Special medical-surgical procedures: Biopsy may be needed to determine the causative agent, if all diagnostic tests are negative.

9. Complications
   a. Weight loss
   b. Malabsorption

10. Prognosis: Serious or fatal disease may result if condition is not treated and eradicated.

11. Applying the nursing process

NURSING DIAGNOSIS: Diarrhea R/T inflammation of mucosa secondary to parasitic invasion

a. *Expected outcomes*
   (1) The patient should report a decrease in the frequency and quantity of stools and a return to normal consistency of stools
   (2) The patient should establish a regular bowel elimination pattern.

b. *Nursing interventions*
   (1) Monitor the frequency, amount, and character of stools, noting changes in elimination pattern.
   (2) Evaluate the effectiveness of medications.
   (3) Explain the use of universal precautions when handling stool. Discuss the modes of transmission of the parasites and their infectious nature.

NURSING DIAGNOSIS: Knowledge deficit R/T unknown disease process, treatment, and prognosis

a. *Expected outcomes:* After intervention, the person should be able to do the following:
   (1) Describe the disease process and the treatment plan
   (2) Identify necessary lifestyle changes and participate in the treatment regimen

b. *Nursing interventions*
   (1) Provide information regarding parasitic infections, modes of transmission, and methods of prevention.
   (2) Discuss possible necessary lifestyle changes and allow the person to ask questions and express concerns about the acquisition of this infection.

12. Discharge planning and teaching
   a. Explain the sources of parasitic infection and the modes of transmission.
   b. Teach universal precautions for handling feces.

13. Public health considerations
   a. Water purification and proper food handling methods are vital in preventing parasitic infections.
   b. Prepare traveler advisories for common parasites, their mode of transmission, and areas or countries in which they are found.
   c. Educate the public about fecal-oral transmission of infections or disease.

◨ CARING FOR PEOPLE WITH INGUINAL OR FEMORAL HERNIA

1. Definition: an abnormal protrusion of the intestine or other abdominal organ through a weakness or defect in the musculature into another cavity (Fig. 27–13).

2. Incidence and socioeconomic impact
   a. Hernias are a widely occurring problem.
   b. Indirect inguinal hernias are the most frequent type of hernia.

3. Risk factors
   a. Obesity
   b. Pregnancy
   c. Occupations that involve heavy lifting

4. Etiology and pathophysiology: A congenital or acquired muscle weakness in the abdominal musculature gives way under increased intra-abdominal pressure, as from lifting heavy objects.

5. Clinical manifestations
   a. Complaint of "bulging" abdomen
   b. Abdominal pain

6. Diagnostics
   a. History: Ask about any recent lifting of heavy objects, previous abdominal surgery, or previous herniation.
   b. Examination
      (1) Observe the abdomen for bulges.
      (2) Listen for the presence and character of bowel sounds—changes may be an early sign of obstruction, if hernia is strangulating.
      (3) Palpate carefully for abdominal masses.
      (4) Hernia examination: Insert a finger in the inguinal wing, instruct the person to cough, and note changes or palpable hernia.
   c. Abdominal radiograph: to visualize the presence of a hernia

7. Clinical management
   a. The goals are to relieve herniation and reduce discomfort.
   b. Nonpharmacologic interventions
      (1) Provide adequate rest.
      (2) Prepare the person for surgery.
      (3) Postoperatively, apply scrotal support or an ice bag to the inguinal-scrotal area to reduce postoperative swelling.
      (4) Encourage postoperative deep breathing and lung expansion. However, postoperative coughing should be avoided.
      (5) Check postoperative return of normal voiding within 6 to 8 hours after surgery.
   c. Pharmacologic interventions: pain medication, if necessary
   d. Special medical-surgical procedures
      (1) Herniorrhaphy: Surgical repair of the hernia through ligation and removal of the hernia defect
      (2) Hernioplasty: Surgical repair of the hernia with reinforcement of the weakened musculature with fascia or a Dacron mesh

8. Complications
   a. Incarceration

TYPES OF ABDOMINAL HERNIAS

Abdominal hernias occur as a result of a defect in the integrity of the muscular wall or an increased intra-abdominal pressure. The types of abdominal hernias are:

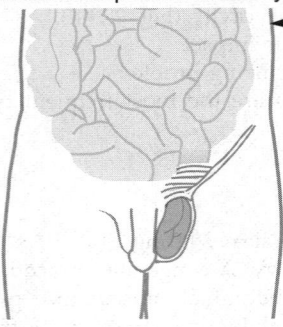

◄ Indirect Inguinal Hernia
The intestine or other abdominal structure protrudes along the inguinal ring (indirect protrusion), following the spermatic cord in males or the round ligament in females, to the inguinal canal and into the scrotum or labia.

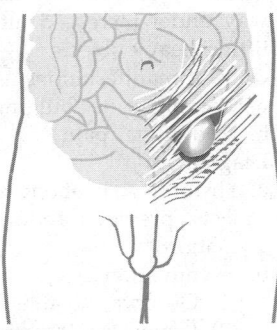

Direct Inguinal Hernia ►
The intestine or other abdominal structure protrudes directly through the posterior inguinal wall.

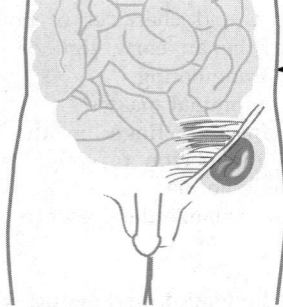

◄ Femoral Hernia
The intestine or other abdominal structure protrudes through the femoral ring in the groin.

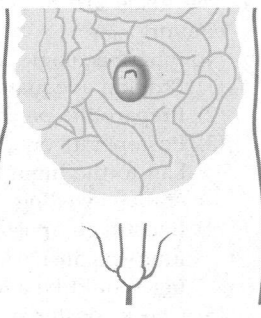

Umbilical Hernia ►
The abdominal structure protrudes through the abdominal musculature around the umbilicus.

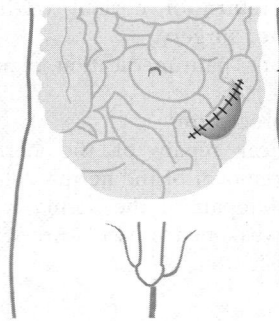

◄ Ventral or Incisional Hernia
An abdominal structure protrudes through a weakness in the abdominal wall, most often from a previous surgery site.

Figure 27–13.

b. Strangulation
c. Bowel perforation
d. Postoperative wound infection
e. Postoperative wound dehiscence or evisceration
f. Postoperative scrotal edema
9. Prognosis
  a. Normal activities are usually resumed in 2 weeks.
  b. Recurrence is common.
10. Applying the nursing process

NURSING DIAGNOSIS: Risk for injury R/T possible complications: strangulation, incarceration

a. *Expected outcomes:* After intervention, the person should be able to do the following:
  (1) Identify factors that increase the risk for injury or complication
  (2) Describe safety or prevention measures to use when hernia occurs
b. *Nursing interventions*
  (1) Assess the person for the development of any complication, such as strangulation or incarceration. Look for symptoms such as abdominal or groin pain, abdominal distention, nausea and vomiting, tachycardia, dyspnea, or any other signs of distress.
  (2) Notify the physician should any of these signs or symptoms appear.
  (3) Teach the person safety or prevention measures to be used to prevent the development of complications.

NURSING DIAGNOSIS: Anxiety R/T surgical procedure

a. *Expected outcomes:* After intervention, the person should be able to do the following:
  (1) Report decreased anxiety related to impending surgical procedure
  (2) Explain the reason for hernia repair, describe the surgical procedure, and identify ways to prevent wound infection and other postoperative complications
b. *Nursing interventions*
  (1) Explain the hernia repair procedure and what the immediate postoperative period will be like. This surgery is often done on an outpatient basis, so discussion of transportation home and the need for someone to assist the person immediately after surgery is important in the preoperative teaching.
  (2) The person should understand the physical limitations of the recovery period. Wound dehiscence, a frequent complication after hernia repair because of the site of surgery, often results from everyday activities that increase intra-abdominal pressure, such as coughing, sneezing, and straining during bowel movements.
  (3) Postoperative teaching should include providing information on the signs of wound infection and prevention of postoperative complications.

11. Discharge planning and teaching
    a. Teach proper wound care, techniques for dressing change, and signs and symptoms of wound infection.
    b. Caution the patient not to lift objects weighing more than 5 pounds for at least 2 weeks (longer, if necessary).
    c. Explain the need to avoid constipation (and, thus, straining on defecation) by drinking plenty of fluids and increasing fiber in the diet.
12. Public health considerations
    a. Educate the public regarding body mechanics and proper lifting techniques to prevent injuries.
    b. Weight-control programs are an important strategy in preventing hernias, as obesity increases the risk of herniation.

◼ CARING FOR PEOPLE WITH ANORECTAL ABSCESS

1. Definition: localized infection involving accumulation of pus in tissue spaces around the rectum and anus
2. Incidence and socioeconomic impact: Most frequent forms are perianal or ischiorectal.
3. Risk factors
    a. Trauma to rectal or anal tissue
    b. Presence of Crohn's disease
4. Etiology
    a. Possible complication of inflammatory bowel disease
    b. Infected anal hair follicles
    c. Trauma or abrasion from anal intercourse
5. Pathophysiology
    a. Result of an infection that develops from an accumulation of feces with toxic and purulent materials
    b. Materials collect in an anal crypt and form cysts in the crypts that can eventually extend into the submucosal wall.
    c. Anal glands are usually obstructed.
6. Clinical manifestations
    a. Throbbing anorectal pain that worsens with sitting or walking
    b. Swelling of the anal area
    c. Purulent drainage
7. Diagnostics
    a. History: Assess for changes in bowel habits, diarrhea, constipation, bleeding, or pain on defecation.
    b. Examination: Inspect the outside anal area for visible signs of purulent drainage or infection.
    c. Anoscopy or sigmoidoscopy can locate the source of the abscess.
8. Clinical management
    a. Goals are to relieve pain and treat infection.
    b. Nonpharmacologic interventions
       (1) The abscess usually must be incised and drained.
       (2) Postoperatively, give sitz baths to ease the discomfort.
    c. Pharmacologic interventions
       (1) Antibiotics, if ordered, for infection
       (2) Analgesics for pain
       (3) Stool softeners to ease painful defecation
    d. Special medical-surgical procedures: Surgical excision and drainage may be done with local anesthesia on an outpatient basis.

9. Complications
    a. Recurrent abscess formation
    b. Fistula
    c. Septicemia
10. Prognosis: Can recur
11. Applying the nursing process

NURSING DIAGNOSIS: Pain R/T inflammation and infection

---

   a. *Expected outcomes:* After intervention, the person should be able to do the following:
      (1) Report relief of pain
      (2) Describe measures to increase comfort
   b. *Nursing interventions*
      (1) Preoperatively, soothe the abscess pain with ice packs or witch hazel pads (Tucks).
      (2) Postoperatively, provide sitz baths to alleviate the discomfort and to cleanse the perianal area.
      (3) Evaluate the effectiveness of pain medication and the use of sitz baths.
12. Discharge planning and teaching
    a. Teach careful perianal cleansing after all bowel movements.
    b. Establish regular bowel elimination patterns by attempting to go the same time of the day and to be free of distractions. This is important in decreasing the incidence of constipation; failure to respond to the urge to defecate results in pain and difficulty on defecation.
13. Public health considerations: Stress the importance of a high-fiber diet with fluids to assist with regular soft stools.

◼ CARING FOR PEOPLE WITH ANAL FISTULA AND ANAL FISSURE

1. Definitions
    a. Anal fissure (fissure-in-ano): a longitudinal ulceration or thin crack in the skin of the anal canal
    b. Anal fistula: an abnormally formed tunnel from the rectum or anus to the vagina or outside skin
2. Incidence and socioeconomic impact: Do not occur often in the general population
3. Risk factors
    a. Fissures—Crohn's disease, trauma following childbirth
    b. Fistulas—Crohn's disease, ulcerative colitis
4. Etiology
    a. Fissures—trauma, constipation, or local infection
    b. Fistulas—Crohn's disease
5. Pathophysiology
    a. Fissures most often occur along the midline of the posterior anal canal and are ulcerations that arise from stretching or tearing.
    b. Fistulas are found between the anal canal and the outside or between the anal canal and the vagina; they are communicating tracts that are created from an infection or abscess.

6. Clinical manifestations
   a. Fissures
      (1) Sharp burning pain on defecation
      (2) Painful spasms
      (3) Anal itching
      (4) Severe tearing with discharge of bright red blood on defecation
   b. Fistulas
      (1) Purulent drainage of pus, blood, mucus, and stool
      (2) In women, passage of flatus and feces through the vagina
      (3) Pain
      (4) Pruritus
7. Diagnostics
   a. Fissures
      (1) History: Assess for pain on defecation.
      (2) Examination: Inspect for tearing or stretching of the skin and the occurrence of bleeding. Perform a rectal examination.
      (3) Anoscopy or sigmoidoscopy
   b. Fistulas
      (1) History: Assess for history of anorectal abscess or infection.
      (2) Examination: Inspect for visible signs of fistula to the outside or purulent drainage with stool.
      (3) Perform anoscopy or sigmoidoscopy to locate the source of the fistula.
   c. May need to rule out associated inflammatory bowel disease
   d. Give barium enema to detect structural abnormalities.
8. Clinical management
   a. Goals are to relieve discomfort and heal or repair fissures or fistulas.
   b. Nonpharmacologic interventions
      (1) Fissures: Use warm sitz baths for comfort and cleansing, and give careful attention to proper cleansing after bowel movements.
      (2) Fistulas: Provide wound care with packing to allow the fistula to granulate.
   c. Pharmacologic interventions
      (1) Fissures
         • Use analgesic ointments or suppositories, if ordered.
         • Take bulk-producing laxatives, such as psyllium hydrophilic mucilloid (Metamucil), to increase the consistency and soften the stool.
      (2) Fistulas: antibiotics for infection, if ordered
   d. Special medical-surgical procedures
      (1) Fissures
         • Surgical excision under local anesthesia
         • Sphincterotomy: surgical excision for chronic fissures
      (2) Fistulas
         • Fistulotomy: surgical excision to correct deep fistulas
         • Fistulectomy: surgical excision to repair straight, superficial fistulas
9. Complications
   a. Bleeding
   b. Infection

10. Prognosis: Recurrence is common.
11. Applying the nursing process

NURSING DIAGNOSIS: Pain R/T ulcerations, inflammation, infection, and need to defecate

a. *Expected outcomes:* After intervention, the person should be able to do the following:
   (1) Report relief from, or reduction in, pain
   (2) Describe actions that relieve or reduce pain or discomfort on defecation
b. *Nursing interventions*
   (1) Evaluate the effectiveness of pain medication and comfort measures used.
   (2) Discuss the use of bulk-producing laxatives as a mechanism for creating stools that are easier to pass; this would minimize some of the discomfort experienced before, during, and after defecation. The need for adequate fluid intake (8 glasses of fluid daily) is part of this regimen.

NURSING DIAGNOSIS: Risk for impaired skin intergrity R/T fissure or fistula disease process

a. *Expected outcomes:* After intervention, the person should be able to do the following:
   (1) Be free of signs and symptoms of infection
   (2) Describe proper perianal hygiene measures to prevent infection
b. *Nursing interventions*
   (1) Assess postoperative healing.
   (2) After excision of fissures or fistulas, the wound is often left open for drainage and granulation to occur naturally. Meticulous wound care with gauze packing can help the granulation process.
   (3) Teach proper hygiene techniques.
12. Discharge planning and teaching: Teach the importance of careful perianal cleansing after each stool.

◼ CARING FOR PEOPLE WITH HEMORRHOIDS

1. Definition: dilated (distended) veins in the anal and rectal areas that are located either internal (not visible on inspection or found above the pectinate line) or external (visible in the anal region or found below the pectinate line) to the anal sphincter (Fig. 27–14)
2. Incidence and socioeconomic impact: Usually appear in adults 20 to 50 years of age
3. Risk factors
   a. Pregnancy
   b. Prolonged constipation
   c. Straining during defecation
   d. Portal hypertension
4. Etiology

HEMORRHOIDS

Normal Anatomy of the Rectum

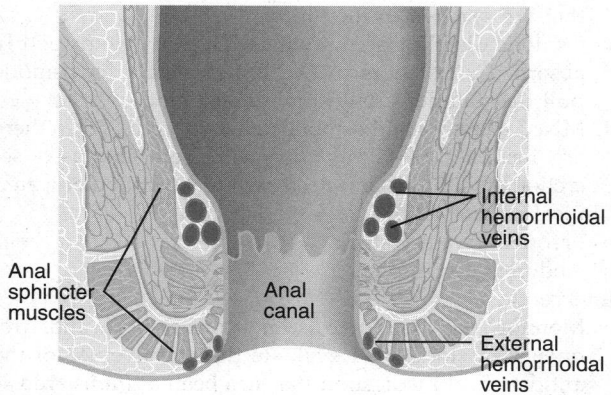

Hemorrhoidal Condition

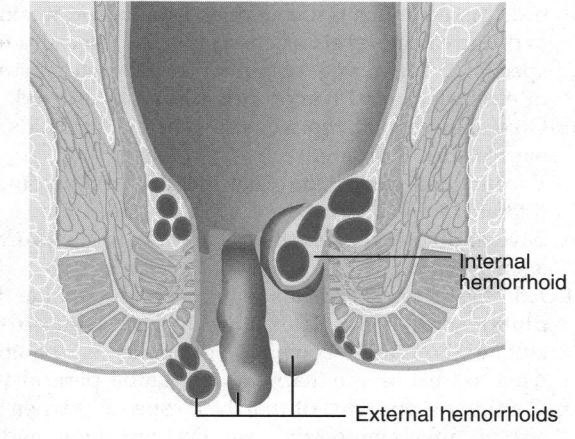

Figure 27–14.

a. Straining with constipation
b. Venous congestion with congestive heart failure or portal hypertension
5. Pathophysiology
  a. Dilated anorectal veins distend in response to increased intra-abdominal pressure and an engorgement of the blood supply to the veins of the anorectal region.
  b. These distended veins separate from the smooth muscle around them and prolapse. They can become thrombosed or inflamed, or they may bleed.
6. Clinical manifestations
  a. Internal or external bulge
  b. Pain
  c. Itching
  d. Mucous discharge
  e. Bleeding with bowel movements
7. Diagnostics
  a. History
    (1) Assess for pain, itching, or visible bleeding.

(2) Question the person about bowel habits: Any straining on defecation?
  b. Examination
    (1) Inspect for external hemorrhoids or prolapse of internal hemorrhoids.
    (2) Perform digital rectal examination.
  c. Proctosigmoidoscopy, if necessary, can locate and visualize the hemorrhoids.
8. Clinical management
  a. Goals are relief of discomfort and reduction of symptoms.
  b. Nonpharmacologic interventions
    (1) Maintain a recumbent position to relieve pressure, edema, and prolapse.
    (2) Consume a regular high-fiber diet to promote bowel movements without straining.
    (3) Increase fluid intake to ensure soft, formed stools.
    (4) Apply cold packs at the onset of pain, then local moist heat and sitz baths, to relieve continuing discomfort.
    (5) Use a flotation pad to increase comfort while sitting in bed or on chairs.
    (6) For thrombosed hemorrhoids: Apply cold packs initially, then heat.
  c. Pharmacologic interventions
    (1) Take stool softeners to aid in regular and easier defecation.
    (2) Use bulk-forming laxatives to reduce constipation.
    (3) Apply ointments, creams, and suppositories to relieve mild and moderate pain and itching.
  d. Special medical-surgical procedures
    (1) Hemorrhoidectomy: Surgical removal of hemorrhoids
    (2) Sclerosing of the hemorrhoid: Injection of the submucous tissue around the hemorrhoidal tissue, which causes shrinking of the tissues
    (3) "Rubber banding" (elastic band ligation): Application of several bands together at the base of moderate-sized hemorrhoids, causing interruption of the blood supply and infarction of the hemorrhoids before sloughing off
9. Complications
  a. Bleeding with resulting anemia
  b. Strangulation
  c. Thrombosis of the hemorrhoid
10. Prognosis: Recurrence rate is 50 percent after sclerosing treatment. There is a better prognosis with ligation and hemorrhoidectomy.
11. Applying the nursing process

NURSING DIAGNOSIS: Pain R/T inflammation of hemorrhoidal tissue

a. *Expected outcomes:* After intervention, the person should be able to do the following:
  (1) Report reduction in or alleviation of pain
  (2) Describe actions that reduce pain or discomfort

b. *Nursing interventions*
(1) Evaluate the effectiveness of measures used to promote comfort, such as oral and anal medications, sitz baths, a flotation pad, and positioning. Assist the person by making additional recommendations or corrections in positioning and use of comfort measures.
(2) Discuss the need for high-bran and high-fiber diets with adequate fluid intake to soften stool and relieve anal pressure.
12. Discharge planning and teaching
a. Teach the person self-care and proper hygiene for postoperative care to the anal area.
b. Instruct the person in ways to reestablish routine bowel habits with minimal discomfort.
c. Discuss dietary considerations (see earlier).
d. Teach methods to prevent constipation and avoid straining.
13. Public health considerations: Educate the public on the importance of a high-fiber diet and adequate fluid intake.

CARING FOR PEOPLE WITH PILONIDAL CYST

1. Definition: a hair-containing cyst that is usually located in the midline on the posterior surface of the sacrum
2. Incidence and etiology
a. A congenital disorder, it is usually diagnosed in adolescence or early adulthood.
b. The cyst is formed under the skin and at the gluteal cleft on the lower surface of the sacrum.
c. A tuft of hair is usually present, which communicates with the outside of the skin through a small sinus opening.
3. Clinical manifestations appear in adolescence
a. Presence of an abscess or irritating drainage
b. Pain
c. Hair follicle that protrudes from the cyst
4. Clinical management
a. Avoid constipation by consuming a diet that is high in bulk and fiber and drinking ample water.
b. Give antibiotics.
c. If infection and abscess have resulted, recommend surgical excision of the cyst and drainage of the abscess.
d. Promote postsurgical pain relief.
(1) Pain is usually relieved by positioning the patient on the side with a pillow between the legs.
(2) Medication may be necessary for extreme postoperative discomfort.

CARING FOR PEOPLE WITH DIARRHEA

1. Definition: an increase in frequency or fluidity of stool
2. Etiology
a. Any condition that increases secretion in the GI tract (*Escherichia coli* and *Vibrio cholerae*), interferes with reabsorption in the GI tract (malabsorption syndromes), or increases motility in the GI tract (inflammatory bowel disease, irritable bowel syndrome) can cause diarrhea.
b. Secretory diarrhea occurs when a significant increase in secretory stimuli causes overproduction of GI fluid, which increases the volume of water and electrolytes that are secreted in the lumen.
c. Osmotic diarrhea occurs when unabsorbable or poorly absorbed substances in the lumen create an osmotic pull that interferes with the reabsorption of water.
d. Mixed secretory and osmotic diarrhea occurs when there are increases in GI motility with both increased secretion of GI fluids and decreased reabsorption of water.
3. Clinical manifestations
a. Frequent, watery stools
b. Abdominal cramping
4. Interventions
a. Monitor the quantity, color, consistency, and frequency of stools, and evaluate the effectiveness of the antidiarrheal medication that has been administered.
b. Continually monitor for signs and symptoms of fluid volume deficit. Maintain accurate input and output records. Assess mucous membranes, skin turgor, weakness, and decreasing levels of consciousness. Measure urine specific gravity, and obtain other laboratory studies of electrolytes and hemoconcentration, if ordered.
c. Give intravenous replacement therapy of fluids and electrolytes, if ordered.
d. Encourage a clear liquid diet initially, and advance as tolerated.
e. Give antibiotic therapy that is specific to the causative agent.
f. Administer antidiarrheals as ordered: loperamide (Imodium) or diphenoxylate hydrochloride with atropine sulfate (Lomotil). Codeine, an opiate, is sometimes used to treat severe diarrhea and inhibit peristalsis.
g. Continuing episodes of diarrhea, especially when they are of unknown origin, can be frustrating and exhausting for the person. Providing physical and emotional support throughout the diagnostic and treatment process is very important.

CARING FOR PEOPLE WITH CONSTIPATION

1. Definition: the infrequent passage of stool, or difficulty in attempting to pass dry, hardened stool
2. Etiology
a. Reduced colonic motility due to decreased muscle tone of the intestinal smooth muscle and reduced neuromuscular reflex activity
b. Reduced dietary fiber and bulk
c. Inadequate fluid intake
d. Sedentary lifestyle or forced bed rest due to illness or incapacitation
e. Medications: aspirin, anticholinergics, aluminum hydroxide calcium carbonate antacids, tranquilizers, tricyclic antidepressants, iron, and diuretics
f. Types of constipation by etiology
• Rectal: often caused by a habit of delaying the elimination of stool

- Colonic: caused by delayed passage of feces through the colon, leading to hardened stool as a result of inadequate fluid intake or mechanical obstruction
- Hypertonic: caused by increased segmental contractions of the musculature that create dry, hard stools and abdominal cramping
- Hypotonic: caused by decreased segmental contractions that create soft, putty-type stool
- Dyzschezial: caused by overuse of laxatives

3. Clinical manifestations
   a. Abdominal discomfort
   b. Abdominal bloating
4. Interventions
   a. Remove impaction, if present (Procedure 27–2).
   b. Administer medications as ordered: bulk-producing laxatives or stool softeners; use stimulant laxatives, suppositories, and enemas only if necessary.

c. Assist the person in identifying a routine for bowel elimination: same time of the day, after a meal, and free of distractions. Stress the need to respond immediately to the urge to defecate.
d. Explain the reasons for constipation, and discuss ways of alleviating causative factors in the person's life.
e. Work with the person to develop a dietary program that promotes normal bowel movements. Teach the importance of bulk, fiber, and fruits and vegetables in the diet. Stress the need for increased fluids in the diet, at least 6 to 8 glasses of fluid per day. These should *not* include coffee, tea, or grapefruit juice, because these fluids are natural diuretics that decrease the body's fluids.
f. Recommend ways to increase exercise or activity level, if not contraindicated. Walking is an excellent choice.

P

Procedure 27–2
How to Remove a Fecal Impaction

Definition/Purpose	To remove fecal matter that is obstructing normal bowel function
Contraindications/Cautions	None
Learning/Teaching Activities	Explain the need for the procedure and what will occur.

Preliminary Activities

Equipment	• Bedpad • Disposable gloves • Lubricant jelly • Bedpan
Assessment/Planning	Throughout the process, observe for signs of pallor, diaphoresis, or change in pulse rate (the manual stimulation in the rectum can cause a vagal stimulation). Ask patients at frequent intervals how they are doing.

Procedure

Action	Rationale/Discussion
1. Protect bed linens with a bedpad, and place the person in a side-lying position with the knees flexed.	1. This position provides maximum access.
2. Put on the disposable glove, put lubricant jelly on your index finger, and insert it into the patient's rectum. Carefully move your finger along the rectal wall upward. Attempt to dislodge the hardened stool by moving your index finger into the stool and breaking it apart. Then gently move the stool down the rectum.	2. When moving your finger within the patient's rectum, be careful not to injure the mucosal wall.
3. Remove as much stool as possible.	3. If ordered, follow the removal with a cleansing enema or an oral laxative.

Final Activities

1. Assist the person to use the bedpan or commode to expel other bits of stool after completion of the procedure.
2. Assist the person with follow-up hygiene, if necessary.

◼ CARING FOR PEOPLE WITH FUNCTIONAL OBSTRUCTION OR PARALYTIC ILEUS

1. Definition: a functional or neurogenic obstruction of the intestines with failure of the intestinal contents to move through the GI tract because of decreased or lost peristalsis
2. Incidence and etiology
   a. More frequent in middle-aged or older adults
   b. Occurs after the bowel is handled during abdominal surgery
   c. Abdominal infection
   d. Electrolyte imbalance
   e. Peritonitis
3. Clinical manifestations
   a. Diminishing bowel sounds: Early in the developing obstruction, hyperactive bowel sounds are audible in the quadrants above the obstruction. Eventually, there is complete absence of bowel sounds.
   b. Nausea and vomiting
   c. Failure to pass stool
   d. Absence of flatus postoperatively
   e. Abdominal distention
4. Interventions
   a. Keep the person on NPO status with intravenous fluid and electrolyte replacements.
   b. Insert a nasogastric tube for decompression (see pp. 90–91). Provide gastric suction until bowel functioning returns. Ileus usually resolves as the bowel rests.
   c. Maintain accurate intake and output measurements that include amounts of vomitus and nasogastric suction fluids.
   d. Monitor the person for signs of impending hypovolemia: check vital signs, look for signs of dehydration (dry mucous membranes, poor skin turgor, sunken eyeballs, decreased urine output, weakness), assess level of consciousness, and note increasing abdominal distention, if it occurs.
   e. Administer pain medication for severe discomfort, as ordered.
   f. Evaluate the effectiveness of medications, positioning, and comfort measures to alleviate abdominal pain.
   g. Keep the head of the bed elevated to promote intestinal motility and prevent respiratory distress.
   h. Determine the effect of pain on breathing and lung expansion, and assist postoperative patients to continue coughing and deep-breathing exercises to prevent other complications.

◼ CARING FOR PEOPLE WITH MECHANICAL OBSTRUCTION

1. Definition: failure of contents to move through the GI tract due to an occlusion to the lumen
2. Etiology and pathophysiology
   a. Three possible etiologies
      • Related to changes in the bowel wall from inflammatory bowel disorders or tumors
      • Intraluminal, with fecal impaction (especially in the elderly), food that is difficult to digest, gallstones
      • Extraluminal, including volvulus, adhesions, intussusception, and strangulated hernia
   b. Pathophysiology: Occlusion of the bowel lumen with accumulation of intestinal contents proximal to the obstruction causes the distal end of the bowel to collapse. Initially, intestinal activity proximal to the obstruction may increase.
3. Clinical manifestations
   a. Abdominal distention
   b. Pain
   c. Possible vomiting
   d. Hyperactive tinkling bowel sounds: Peristalsis initially increases, then decreases.
   e. Failure to pass stool
4. Interventions
   a. Maintain hemodynamic status: Positive fluid balance is critical when patients return to surgery for correction of obstruction. Keep patients on NPO status with intravenous fluids and electrolytes for replacement.
   b. Monitor nastrogastric tube for decompression.
   c. Maintain accurate intake and output measurements that include amounts of vomitus and nasogastric suction fluids.
   d. Monitor the person for signs of impending hypovolemia.
   e. Prepare the person for impending surgery to correct the mechanical obstruction. Explain the reasons for surgery, what will be done, and what the immediate postoperative period will be like.
   f. Administer prescribed pain medications for severe discomfort.
   g. Evaluate the effectiveness of medications, positioning, and comfort measures to alleviate abdominal pain.
   h. Determine the effect of pain on breathing and lung expansion, and assist postoperative patients to continue coughing and deep-breathing exercises to prevent other complications.

◼ CARING FOR PEOPLE WITH APPENDICITIS

1. Definition and incidence
   a. An inflammation of the vermiform appendix
   b. Most frequent reason for emergency surgery
   c. Seen in men more often than in women
2. Etiology and pathophysiology
   a. An obstruction of the lumen of the appendix occurs from a fecalith, from fibrous disease in the bowel wall, or from adhesions.
   b. Obstruction causes inflammation of the appendix.
   c. Appendicitis results, the mucosa ulcerates, blood supply is decreased, and the lumen fills with pus.
   d. Gangrene and perforation can result.
3. Clinical manifestations
   a. Acute abdominal pain that begins in the epigastric region and spreads to the lower right quadrant
   b. Anorexia, nausea, and vomiting
   c. Low-grade fever
   d. Rovsing's sign is elicited by palpating the left lower quadrant; pain is felt in the right lower quadrant

4. Interventions
   a. Keep the patient on NPO status with intravenous replacement of fluids and electrolytes.
   b. Give preoperative teaching that provides information on appendicitis, appendectomy, and what to expect in the postoperative period, such as the need for intravenous fluids, NPO status, and the importance of coughing and deep breathing.
   c. Allow the person to express fears about the upcoming surgery. Answer all questions and concerns about the surgery. Involve family members in preoperative teaching and support.
   d. High anxiety levels increase the patient's pain and discomfort from appendicitis and appendectomy and can interfere with coping. Help the patient to identify successful relaxation techniques that have worked in the past (teach new ones, if necessary), and encourage use of these techniques as an adjuvant therapy to use of pain medications. Explain that relaxation can help to reduce both anxiety and pain.
   e. Administer prescribed antibiotics both preoperatively and postoperatively to prevent sepsis if the appendix has ruptured.
   f. Administer pain medications, as prescribed.
   g. Monitor the person for complications:
      • Perforation: Ruptured appendix is an emergency condition that results from perforation of the appendix with outflow of appendiceal contents into the peritoneal cavity. Symptoms include low-grade fever, vomiting, acute abdominal pain with rebound tenderness, and eventual development of ileus. White blood cell counts are highly elevated. Surgical intervention is necessary after the patient is stabilized with intravenous fluids, gastric suctioning, and antibiotics.
      • Abscess formation
      • Peritonitis
   h. Evaluate the effectiveness of pain medication, positioning, and comfort measures.
   i. Ambulation should begin on the day of surgery. Recovery is rapid, with many activities being resumed within 1 to 2 weeks.
   j. Advance diet as tolerated.

◼ CARING FOR PEOPLE WITH PERITONITIS

1. Definition: an inflammation of the peritoneum of the abdomen
2. Etiology and pathophysiology
   a. Inflammation results when toxins enter the abdominal cavity from a traumatized or ruptured organ.
   b. The peritoneum becomes edematous, secretes an exudate, and attempts to wall off the toxins and localize the infection.
   c. Fluids, proteins, and electrolytes are lost into the abdominal cavity, which causes decreased plasma volume that can result in hypovolemic shock.
   d. As the inflammation progresses, intestinal motility decreases and ileus results.

3. Clinical manifestations
   a. Pain that can be localized or general and that may increase with movement
   b. Rigidity of abdominal muscles
   c. Abdominal distention
   d. Anorexia, nausea, and vomiting
   e. Low-grade fever
   f. Absence of bowel sounds
4. Interventions
   a. Maintain hemodynamic status: Positive fluid balance is critical when the patient returns to surgery for correction of obstructions. Keep the patient on NPO status with intravenous fluids with proteins and electrolytes for replacement.
   b. Monitor vital signs and input and output carefully as measures of possible fluid deficits. Include amounts of vomitus and nasogastric suction fluids. Monitor serum electrolytes.
   c. Monitor the person for signs of impending hypovolemia.
   d. Provide a nasogastric tube for decompression of obstruction.
   e. Administer broad-spectrum antibiotics to treat infection.
   f. Give preoperative teaching on peritonitis—what it is, what surgery will be done, and what to expect in the postoperative period (e.g., the need for intravenous fluids and NPO status, and the importance of coughing and deep breathing).
   g. Encourage the person to express fears about surgery. Answer all questions and concerns about the surgery. Involve family members in preoperative teaching and support.
   h. A high anxiety level increases the patient's pain and discomfort and can interfere with coping. Help the patient to identify successful relaxation techniques that have worked in the past (teach new ones, if necessary), and encourage use of these techniques as an adjuvant therapy to use of pain medications. Explain that relaxation can help to reduce both anxiety and pain.
   i. Administer prescribed analgesics as needed, and evaluate the effectiveness of pain medication, positioning, and comfort measures.
   j. Postoperative care includes monitoring the surgical incision and the patency of abdominal drains. Note amount, color, and odor. Assess for return of bowel sounds.

◼ CARING FOR PEOPLE WITH GASTROENTERITIS

1. Definition and incidence
   a. An inflammation of the mucosa of the stomach and intestines
   b. More likely to occur in developing countries; also called "traveler's diarrhea"
   c. More frequent in the very young and in older adults
2. Etiology and pathophysiology
   a. Normal bacterial flora and gastric acidity usually protect the GI tract against invasion from pathogens,

such as *Campylobacter jejuni*, *E. coli*, and *Shigella*. Conditions that decrease the normal acidity or that alter the normal flora of the GI tract can cause this disorder.
   b. The resulting altered bacteria interfere with protective mechanisms such as the secretion of enterotoxin that causes inflammation and secretory diarrhea, the destruction of the intestinal wall by bacterial invasion, and the destruction of absorption cells.
3. Clinical manifestations
   a. Abdominal cramping
   b. Anorexia, nausea, and vomiting
   c. Diarrhea
   d. Fever
   e. Weakness and malaise
4. Interventions
   a. Keep the person on NPO status while vomiting is occurring. Administer fluid and electrolyte replacements intravenously as necessary. Give oral fluids as soon as they can be tolerated, and resume a diet with small amounts of clear liquids that are rich in electrolytes (e.g., ginger ale, Seven-Up, flavored gelatin, sherbet, and broth).
   b. Monitor weight, intake, and output, especially the amount of stool and vomitus and characteristics of both. Monitor hydration status carefully for signs of dehydration.
   c. Treat the patient with appropriate antibiotic therapy after the causative agent has been identified.
   d. Give antidiarrheal and antiemetic medications, if ordered

NURSE ADVISORY

Antidiarrheal medications, such as anticholinergics, and some antiemetic medications that slow intestinal motility are usually contraindicated in gastroenteritis because they interfere with the body's attempt to expel the cause of the diarrhea.

   e. Assist the person with meticulous perianal hygiene and comfort measures. Pay careful attention to the perianal skin to prevent breakdown from the irritation of frequent diarrhea.
   f. Note response of the patient to medications.
   g. Teach about the infectious nature of this disease, the fecal-oral route of transmission with these types of infections, and the need to use universal precautions when handling the infected stool. Instruct the person on proper handling, preparation, and storage of foods.
   h. Alert prospective travelers to the risks and high rate of traveler's diarrhea infection in particular travel areas or countries.

▣ CARING FOR PEOPLE WITH CANCER OF THE ESOPHAGUS

1. Definition: an abnormal malignant growth in the esophagus (Fig. 27–15)
2. Incidence and socioeconomic impact
   a. Usually occurs between 50 and 70 years of age

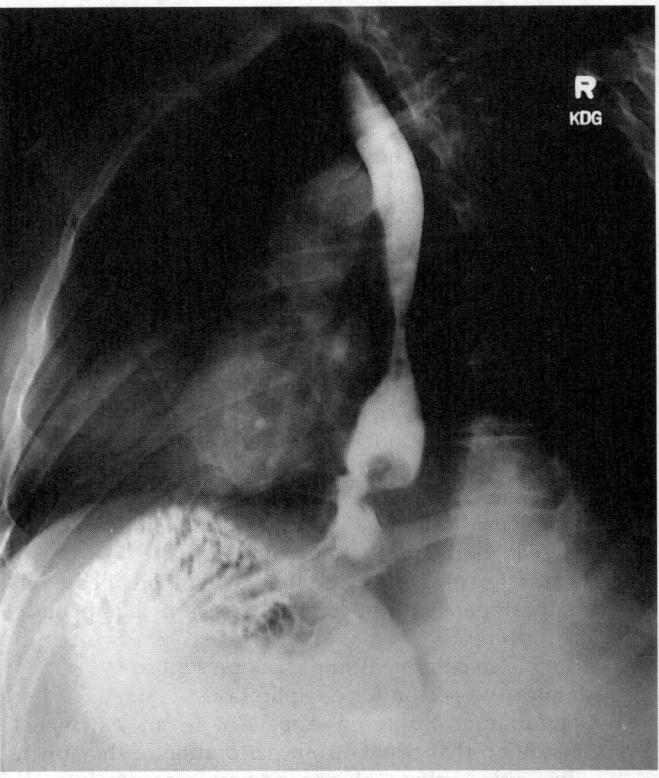

Figure 27–15. Barium enema radiograph showing cancer of the esophagus. (Courtesy of the University of Maryland Medical Center.)

   b. More frequent in men than in women
   c. In 1995, an estimated 10,200 people died from esophageal cancer, and another 11,300 cases were diagnosed.
   d. High incidence in China
3. Risk factors
   a. Dietary factors
   b. Smoking
   c. Heavy alcohol consumption
   d. Possible genetic link
4. Etiology
   a. Exact cause unknown
   b. Diet high in nitrosamines, intake of foods that are salt cured or smoked
   c. Diet that is deficient in riboflavin
   d. Presence of achalasia, hiatal hernia, and Barrett's esophagus
5. Pathophysiology
   a. Altered epithelial changes due to a variety of factors increase the susceptibility of the esophageal epithelium to malignant changes.
   b. Squamous cell carcinomas, the most frequent type, occur in the area between the pharynx and the gastroesophageal junction.
   c. Adenocarcinomas usually occur between the gastroesophageal junction and the stomach.
6. Clinical manifestations
   a. Vague initial symptoms
   b. Indigestion
   c. Abdominal pressure and feelings of GI fullness

d. Later symptoms (often appear after the disease is very advanced): dysphagia (difficulty swallowing), anorexia, and weight loss

e. Substernal or back pain due to metastasis into the mediastinum

7. Diagnostics

a. Esophageal cancer is difficult to diagnose in the early stages, because no routine screening techniques are used in the United States, and many signs and symptoms occur late in the disease. It has often metastasized before diagnosis.

b. History

• Assess for history of indigestion and feelings of fullness. How long have symptoms been noted?

• Determine how the onset of dysphagia began and when it finally bothered the person enough to seek medical attention.

c. Physical examination: It is very difficult to examine the esophagus unless a tumor is palpably evident.

d. Endoscopy visualizes the tumor, with tissue biopsy for diagnosis.

e. Exfoliative cytology is used to obtain cells and examine them for diagnosing and staging.

f. Barium swallow detects the presence of the mass or tumor.

8. Clinical management

a. Goals are to remove the tumor, establish adequate nutrition, and restore and maintain swallowing.

b. Nonpharmacologic interventions are limited to palliative measures that provide comfort and reassurance.

c. Pharmacologic interventions

(1) Provide pain medications, if ordered.

(2) Chemotherapy may be used in combination with cisplatin.

d. Special medical-surgical procedures: Esophagogastrectomy is the surgery of choice. The tumor is resectioned and the stomach is elevated to the remaining portion of the esophagus and anastomosed. Key interventions in the postoperative period involve maintaining the nasogastric tube carefully. Because placement of the tube is crucial after surgery, call a physician to do any manipulation that is called for by problems with nasogastric output.

(1) Occasionally, too much of the esophagus has to be removed for esophagogastrectomy. In such cases, surgeons perform a colon or jejunal interposition, using a segment of colon or jejunum to replace the esophagus that has been resected during the tumor removal, thus retaining peristalsis.

(2) Radiation therapy has been used as a preoperative, postoperative, or primary method of palliative treatment.

e. Palliative treatment for advanced esophageal cancer includes the following:

(1) Esophageal dilation and placement of a stent to maintain the esophageal lumen

(2) Use of laser photoablation therapy (yttrium-aluminum-garnet or YAG) to destroy the tumor and relieve the obstruction

(3) Photodynamic therapy, a newer laser technique that is more selective, in affecting only the abnormal cancer cells, than YAG: The person is given an injection of Photofrin II (dihematoporphyrin ethers), which is taken up by all cells but within 48 hours is minimal in normal cells.

NURSE ADVISORY

A note of caution regarding laser photoablation therapy: A side effect is increased sensitivity to light, especially sunlight. Advise patients to protect themselves from sunburn for 4 to 8 weeks; avoid windows: pull shades and draperies in daylight; and wear protective clothing, including sunglasses, gloves, hats, and long sleeves. After about 6 weeks, they can increase exposure to sunlight gradually.

9. Complications

a. Aspiration pneumonia

b. Vocal cord paralysis

10. Prognosis: poor, with a 5-year survival rate of 9 percent

11. Applying the nursing process

NURSING DIAGNOSIS: Knowledge deficit R/T diagnostic procedures, disease process, possible surgical procedures, and diagnosis of cancer

a. *Expected outcomes:* After intervention, the person should be able to describe the diagnosis, disease process, and treatments, including possible surgery.

b. *Nursing interventions*

(1) It is essential to provide information to patients and their families regarding diagnostic testing, such as the necessity of each test, what will occur, and why.

(2) Be open. Discuss and answer all questions the person may have regarding the diagnosis. Provide as much factual information as possible.

(3) Thoroughly explain surgery as the treatment of choice. Information should include what the surgery is, expected outcomes, and what the immediate postoperative period will be like.

NURSING DIAGNOSIS: Pain R/T pressure of the tumor

a. *Expected outcomes:* After intervention, the person should be able to report relief from, or reduction in, pain and describe actions to relieve or reduce pain.

b. *Nursing interventions*

(1) Teach the person how to optimize pain medication by taking it immediately when it is needed, and not waiting until the pain gets unbearable.

(2) Teach the person relaxation techniques to help control pain (see Chapter 6).

(3) Assess comfort level and response to, and effectiveness of, pain therapy.

NURSING DIAGNOSIS: Anxiety R/T difficulty swallowing, unknown problem, feelings of helplessness, and cancer diagnosis

a. *Expected outcomes:* After intervention, the person should be able to do the following:
   (1) Report decreased feelings of anxiety due to an unknown medical problem
   (2) Discuss openly the diagnosis of cancer and feelings about it
   (3) Demonstrate the use of appropriate coping mechanisms to participate in treatment
b. *Nursing interventions*
   (1) Provide an open environment in which the person and the family can share feelings about the condition. Encourage open discussion of the problems, the cancer diagnosis, and the feelings associated with each of those.
   (2) Supply continuing information regarding treatment, progress, and options so that patients feel they are informed and in control of the situation.
   (3) Identify the person's and the family's strengths and weaknesses and previous methods of dealing with a significant life stressor, such as the one they are currently facing.
   (4) Help the person to identify suitable coping mechanisms for use during treatment and recovery.

NURSING DIAGNOSIS: Anticipatory grieving R/T terminal prognosis

a. *Expected outcomes:* After intervention, the person should be able to do the following:
   (1) Openly express feelings of grief
   (2) Describe the dying process
   (3) Discuss feelings of grief with family and significant others
   (4) Continue to plan for the time remaining
b. *Nursing interventions*
   (1) Be aware that the diagnosis of cancer usually leads to feelings of powerlessness, fear, denial, anger, isolation, bargaining, sadness, and profound depression.
   (2) If culturally appropriate (see Chapters 2 and 43 for more on this issue), initiate frank and open discussions with the person that are aimed at encouraging expression of feelings and acceptance of the situation. Support and assist patients and their families through the grieving process and continue to identify positive coping mechanisms.
   (3) Identify coping strategies that were used successfully in the past, or teach new coping strategies to help patients accept their diagnosis and prepare and plan for the limited time that is left.
   (4) Assess the coping mechanisms of the individual and the family on an ongoing basis.
12. Discharge planning and teaching
    a. Teach the person about long-term problems that can accompany this type of surgery, including gastroesophageal reflux, esophagitis, early satiety, and dysphagia.

b. Instruct the person in ways to decrease the likelihood that these complications will interfere with lifestyle: Encourage small meals, low-fat foods, and maintenance of an upright position after eating.
    c. Explain the use of antacids and histamine H_2-antagonists, if necessary.
13. Public health considerations: China, a country with a high rate of esophageal cancer, performs mass screenings of high-risk populations by inserting a nasogastric tube with netting attached to obtain cells for cytologic study. This has been 90 percent successful in attaining earlier diagnosis for high-risk people.

■ CARING FOR PEOPLE WITH CANCER OF THE STOMACH

1. Definition: an abnormal malignant growth in the stomach (see Color Fig. 27–4).
2. Incidence and socioeconomic impact
   a. More frequent among those 50 to 80 years old
   b. Twice as frequent among men as women
   c. Incidence in the United States has been decreasing since 1930
   d. Very high incidence in Japan
   e. Adenocarcinomas are most frequent
   f. About one half are found in the pyloric region of the stomach.
3. Risk factors
   a. Diet that is high in complex carbohydrates, grains, and salt but low in animal fat and fresh, green leafy vegetables and fresh fruit
   b. Nitrites and nitrates
   c. Smoking
   d. Alcohol consumption
   e. Previous gastric ulcers
4. Etiology
   a. Unknown
   b. Strong environmental link
5. Pathophysiology
   a. Invasion by carcinoma occurs directly through the gastric mucosal layers into the peritoneum, peritoneal cavity, and lymphatic nodes.
   b. Pathologic effects are due to obstruction of stomach sphincters and bleeding from stomach vessels.
6. Clinical manifestations
   a. Often asymptomatic until later stages
   b. Weight loss
   c. Fatigue
   d. Anemia
   e. Anorexia, nausea, vomiting, indigestion
   f. Epigastric discomfort
   g. Difficulty swallowing (dysphagia)
   h. Palpable abdominal mass
7. Diagnostics
   a. History: Is the patient experiencing pain, heartburn or indigestion, nausea and vomiting, anorexia, belching, or bleeding? Take a complete diet history that includes information on intake of foods that are high in nitrates or in fats and alcohol.
   b. Examination: Inspect for visible signs of the mass or tumor. Palpate the abdomen for masses or tumors.

c. Barium swallow (upper GI series) is often done 1st to assess for the presence of obstruction.

d. Esophagogastroduodenoscopy or gastroscopy directly visualizes a suspected tumor and allows an epithelial scrape for cytologic study.

e. Exfoliative cytologic examination evaluates the presence of cancer cells.

f. Carcinoembryonic antigen: Radioimmunoassay uses a plasma tumor marker that is elevated in gastric carcinoma.

8. Clinical management
   a. Goals are to remove the tumor and establish a nutrition program.
   b. Nonpharmacologic interventions
      (1) Maintain on NPO status with intravenous fluids or total parenteral nutrition
      (2) Nasogastric tube for decompression to prevent complications postoperatively
      (3) Blood transfusions to correct anemia, if present
   c. Pharmacologic interventions
      (1) Administer pain medications, if ordered.
      (2) Chemotherapy is used as adjuvant therapy; in most cases, this is usually a combination of fluorouracil (5-FU) and other agents.
   d. Special medical-surgical procedures
      (1) Surgical resection of the tumor involves removing as much of the stomach as necessary to remove all of the tumor (see p. 1267).
      (2) Radiation therapy has limited use with gastric cancers because of the proximity of adjacent organs, although its use has increased with unresectable tumors.

9. Complications
   a. Hemorrhage
   b. Obstruction
   c. Metastases
   d. Postprandial dumping syndrome: This condition results from a loss in the stomach absorptive surface and in the function of the pylorus after surgery (especially Billroth I). Symptoms, which usually occur 30 minutes after eating, include nausea, vomiting, abdominal cramping, diarrhea, feelings of fullness, palpitations, diaphoresis, dizziness, and weakness. Treatment includes modifications to the diet, such as eating small meals, avoiding fluids with food, reducing carbohydrates and increasing protein intake, and taking antiperistaltic medications.

10. Prognosis
    a. Without lymph node involvement, about 5 to 15 percent of persons have a 5-year survival rate.
    b. Survival is decreased considerably if lymph nodes or adjacent organs are involved.

11. Applying the nursing process

NURSING DIAGNOSIS: Knowledge deficit R/T impending surgery, diagnosis, and disease process

NURSING DIAGNOSIS: Altered nutrition, less than body requirements, R/T anorexia, nausea and vomiting, and difficulty swallowing

a. *Expected outcomes:* After intervention, the person should be able to do the following:
   (1) Maintain stable weight throughout the treatment process
   (2) Maintain adequate intake of food and fluids or nutritional supplements
b. *Nursing interventions*
   (1) Supply proper nutrition and nourishment, including nutritional supplements if the person's condition has deteriorated, to prepare the person for surgery.
   (2) Small, frequent, bland, and easily digestible meals are better tolerated. In addition, vitamin and mineral supplements may be necessary.
   (3) Monitoring the person's nutritional state is extremely critical to this person's condition: input and output, calorie counts, and daily weights.

NURSING DIAGNOSIS: Anticipatory grieving R/T diagnosis and prognosis

12. Discharge planning and teaching
    a. Instruct the person about the possibility of long-term postoperative complications that may develop and interfere with their nutrition and lifestyle.
    b. Provide information regarding support groups for those who survive gastric carcinoma.
13. Public health considerations: Identify persons who are at high risk for stomach cancer.

◼ CARING FOR PEOPLE WITH CANCER OF THE COLON OR RECTUM

1. Definition: an abnormal malignant growth that involves the colon or rectum (Fig. 27–16 and Color Fig. 27–5)
2. Incidence and socioeconomic impact
   a. Highest incidence is in Western cultures and industrialized countries; decreased incidence in Asia and Africa
   b. Higher incidence for men than women
   c. Most often seen in those 50 to 60 years of age
   d. Most often adenocarcinomas
   e. Most frequent sites—the rectosigmoid, then the cecum
3. Risk factors
   a. Environmental factors
   b. Dietary factors
   c. Polyposis syndrome
   d. Ulcerative colitis of more than 10 years' duration
   e. Genetic factors
4. Etiology
   a. Exact cause unknown
   b. Familial polyposis
   c. Chronic ulcerative colitis
   d. High-fat diets
5. Pathophysiology
   a. The tumor originates in the mucosal and submucosal

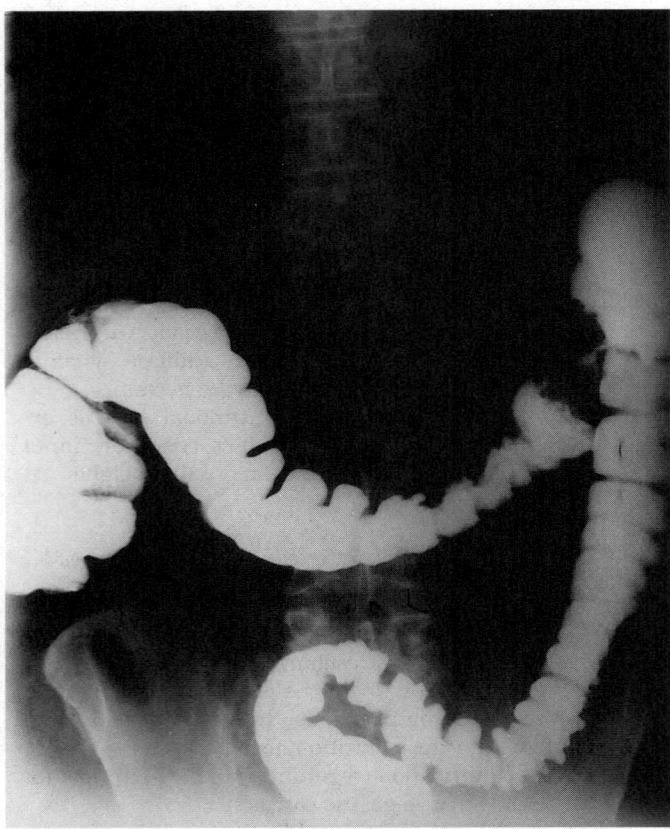

Figure 27–16. Barium enema radiograph showing cancer of the distal transverse colon. (Courtesy of the University of Maryland Medical Center.)

layers. Eventually, it invades deeper layers and may spread to the lymph system.

  b. Polyps can arise from the mucosal surface of the colon.

    (1) Adenomatous polyps are flat or pedunculated (on a stalk) premalignancies. Familial polyposis is a rare genetic disorder with multiple adenomatous polyps; it has an almost 100 percent cancer development rate.

    (2) Villous adenomatous polyps are soft and bleed easily. They have an increased malignancy potential.

  c. Metastasis to the liver is common.

6. Clinical manifestations

  a. Signs and symptoms are usually vague in early stages and later vary, depending on the side of the colon involved.

  b. Changes in bowel habits occur more frequently with cancers of the left side of the colon.

  c. Weakness, fatigue, and anemia may be the first signs of a right-sided colon cancer.

  d. Cancers on either side may show signs such as bloody stool, rectal bleeding, anemia, and abdominal pain.

7. Diagnostics

  a. History

    (1) Assess for changes in bowel habits, passing blood in the stool, or the presence of blood on the tissue wipe.

    (2) Assess for unexplained weight loss and signs of anemia.

    (3) Determine diet history and identify intake of high-risk foods.

  b. Physical examination

    (1) Auscultate bowel sounds.

    (2) Palpate the abdomen for masses and areas of tenderness or pain.

    (3) Perform digital rectal examination to detect any gross abnormalities.

  c. Assess the stool with guaiac to test for occult bleeding.

  d. Perform endoscopy or proctosigmoidoscopy to directly visualize the intestine and detect the presence of a tumor.

  e. Use a barium enema to detect abnormal masses and tumors in the intestine.

8. Clinical management

  a. Goals are to remove the tumor and establish a bowel regimen.

  b. Nonpharmacologic interventions

    (1) Maintain NPO status with intravenous fluid and electrolyte replacement

    (2) Nasogastric tube to suction for decompression until the bowel begins to function again

  c. Pharmacologic interventions

    (1) Administer pain medication, if ordered.

    (2) Chemotherapy (most often 5-FU, in combination with cisplatin, mitomycin, and others) is commonly used as an adjuvant therapy.

  d. Special medical-surgical procedures. Surgical removal of the tumor depends on the place and extent of the cancer.

    (1) Right hemicolectomy (removal of terminal ileum cecum and right portion of transverse colon) is the surgery of choice for tumors of the cecum and ascending colon.

    (2) Left hemicolectomy is used for tumors of the descending colon.

    (3) Abdominal-perineal resection is used for lesions of the middle and lower portions of the rectum or for familial multiple polyposis. It requires 3 incisions: an abdominal incision to remove the colon; a left abdominal stab wound to form the colostomy or ileostomy; and the perineal incision. The wounds are usually left open and packed with drains inserted. Monitor the amount and type of drainage, and any unusual odor or bleeding. Radiation is used primarily for those with unresectable tumors.

9. Complications

  a. Obstruction

  b. Anemia

10. Prognosis

  a. Five-year survival rate for localized disease is about 50 percent.

  b. Five-year survival rate for disease that is found in adjacent organs or nodes is also about 50 percent.

  c. Response rates for chemotherapy vary widely.

11. Applying the nursing process

NURSING DIAGNOSIS: Knowledge deficit R/T impending surgery, diagnosis and disease process, creation of ostomy

a. *Expected outcomes:* After intervention, the person should be able to describe the diagnosis, disease process, and treatments, including possible surgery.
b. *Nursing interventions*
   (1) It is essential to provide information to patients and their families regarding diagnostic testing: the necessity of each test, what will occur, and why.
   (2) Thoroughly explain surgery as the treatment of choice. Information should include what the surgery is, expected outcomes, and what the immediate postoperative period will be like.
   (3) Discuss the creation of an ostomy with the person *before* surgery. After surgery, explain procedures for care of the ostomy and begin to involve the person in the care of the stoma; attempt to establish a normal bowel regimen through care and regulation of the ostomy.

> **NURSING DIAGNOSIS:** Anticipatory grieving R/T cancer diagnosis

> **NURSING DIAGNOSIS:** Body image disturbance R/T surgery, creation of colostomy

a. *Expected outcomes:* After intervention, the person should be able to do the following:
   (1) Openly express feelings about the stoma or disease and its effect on self and lifestyle
   (2) Begin to report feelings of acceptance of changes in body appearance and functioning
   (3) Begin to participate in care of the stoma
b. *Nursing interventions*
   (1) Encourage the person to express feelings about the colostomy.
   (2) Teach the person care of the stoma, and be supportive through initial hesitancy to care for and touch the stoma. Allow the person to ask questions, and go slowly with the teaching.
   (3) Support the person in identifying things that might interfere with normal daily activities and possible compromises.
   (4) Support the person in discussions about the impact of the colostomy on sexual functioning and feelings of desirability and adequacy.
   (5) Encourage the person to include discussions of the impact of the colostomy on lifestyle among family and significant others.
12. Discharge planning and teaching
   a. Explain proper care of the stoma and signs of problems.
   b. Teach the importance of including fiber, betacarotene, calcium, and fresh fruits and vegetables in the diet.
13. Public health considerations

HOME CARE STRATEGIES

Ostomy Care

The patient with a new ostomy often experiences anger and grief because of loss of control and a dramatic change in body image. During the hospital stay, patients are physically ill and emotionally overwhelmed. The main focus and goal of teaching is to help them become self-sufficient in caring for their stomas and pouches and regain control of body functions, independence, and self-image.

Focus on 1 aspect of ostomy care at each visit. Increase patient participation each time. Be gentle, positive, and insistent.

Daily Care

- Store all ostomy equipment and supplies in an organized container in the bathroom.
- Empty the pouch directly into the toilet when it is one-third full and rinse with clear cool water.
- Use a biologic odor eliminator spray rather than air freshener.
- Knowledge of good hand-washing technique and proper waste disposal should never be assumed.

Pouch Change

- Change the pouch in the bathroom. Privacy, good lighting, water, and work space are essential.
- Prepare the new pouch before removing the old one.
- Inspect the stoma and peristomal skin for problems, and treat them promptly. Perform each step in sequence without taking shortcuts. Repetition and written guidelines promote success.

Ordering Supplies

Supplies are expensive, and insurance coverage is usually partial and limited. Be sure the supplier carries the correct type of pouch in stock.
- Instruct the patient in remeasuring the stoma size 3 to 4 times a year and modifying the size of the pouch.
- Provide a written supply list including the name and phone number of the supplier and the brand name and order number of all supplies.

Community Support

Evaluate community support if the patient is ready to participate in a support group.
- Supply the name and telephone number of the local ostomy association.
- Inform the patient if telephone advice is accessible from your agency.
- Provide the patient with the name of a hospital-affiliated enterostomal therapy nurse.

a. Persons who are at risk for cancer of the rectum or colon should pay close attention to annual screening examination recommendations and should be taught to recognize the need to seek medical attention for changes in bowel habits or any rectal bleeding.
b. Recommended annual screenings for the general population include a stool for guaiac test to be performed annually for everyone older than 50 years of age and a digital rectal examination to be given annually for everyone older than 40 years of age.

Bibliography

Books

American Dental Association. *Periodontal Disease*. Chicago: American Dental Association, 1992.

Bates B. *A Guide to Physical Examination and History Taking*. 5th ed. Philadelphia: JB Lippincott, 1990.

Doughty DB, and Jackson D. *Gastrointestinal Disorders*. St. Louis: Mosby–Year Book, 1993.

Drossman D. *Manual of Gastroenterologic Procedures*. 3rd ed. New York: Raven Press, 1993.

Guyton A. *Human Physiology and Mechanisms of Disease*. 5th ed. Philadelphia: WB Saunders, 1992.

Hamilton H, and Rose M (eds). *Gastrointestinal Disorders*. Springhouse, PA: Springhouse Corporation, 1985.

Hellemans J, and Vantrappen G. *Gastrointestinal Tract Disorders in the Elderly*. New York: Churchill Livingstone, 1984.

Jones R (ed). *Gastrointestinal Problems in General Practice*. Oxford: Oxford Medical Publications, 1993.

Malasanos, L, et al. *Health Assessment*. 4th ed. St. Louis: Mosby–Year Book, 1990.

Morton P. *Health Assessment in Nursing*. 2nd ed. Springhouse, PA: Springhouse Corporation, 1991.

Powell L, and Piper D (eds). *Fundamentals of Gastroenterology*. New York: McGraw-Hill, 1991.

Sleisenger M, and Fordtran J. *Gastrointestinal Disease*. Philadelphia: WB Saunders, 1993.

Society of Gastroenterology Nurses and Associates. *Gastroenterology Nursing: A Core Curriculum*. St. Louis: Mosby–Year Book, 1993.

Spiro H. *Clinical Gastroenterology*. New York: McGraw-Hill, 1993.

Yamada T, et al. *Atlas of Gastroenterology*. Philadelphia: JB Lippincott, 1992.

Chapters in Books and Journal Articles

Gastrointestinal Structure and Function

Esberger K. Guide to gastrointestinal problems of elders. *Geriatr Nurs.* 12(2):74–75, 1991.

Kain C, Reilly N, and Schultz E. The older adult: A comparative assessment. *Nurs Clin North Am* 25(4):833–848, 1990.

Assessing People with Gastrointestinal Disorders

Gruber M, et al. Palatability of colonic lavage solution is improved by the addition of artificially sweetened flavored drink mixes. *Gastroenterol Nurs* 14(3):135–137, 1991.

Holmgren C. Abdominal assessment. *RN* 55(3):28–34, 1992.

Massoni M. GI handbook. *Nursing 90* 20(11):65–80, 1990.

O'Toole M. Advanced assessment of the abdomen and gastrointestinal problems. *Nurs Clin North Am* 25(4):771–776, 1990.

Patras A, and Brozenec S. Gastrointestinal assessment. *AORN J* 40(5):726–731, 1984.

Spada I, Taylor G, and McWeeny K. Endoscopic ultrasonography. *Gastroenterol Nurs* 12(3):24–28, 1990.

Swartz M. Nulytely. *Gastroenterol Nurs* 14(4):200–203, 1992.

Sweeney J. Endoscopy assessment tool—A new approach. *Gastroenterol Nurs* 13(2):71–76, 1990.

Sweeney J. Assessing the patient undergoing GI endoscopy. *Gastroenterol Nurs* 14(5):266, 1992.

Whitney L. Acute abdominal pain. *Nursing 93*. 23(9):34–41, 1993.

Wilkinson M. Nursing implications after endoscopic retrograde cholangiopancreatography. *Gastroenterol Nurs* 13(4):105–107, 1991.

Caring for People with Disorders of the Mouth

Graham KM, Ventura M, and Meyer CC. Reducing the incidence of stomatitis using a health assessment and improvement program. *Cancer Nurs* 16(2):117–122, 1993.

Caring for People with Disorders of the Esophagus

Alibertai L. Managing esophageal achalasia: Medical and nursing implications. *Gastroenterol Nurs* 16(3):126, 1993.

Kirby D. Management of esophageal varices: A review of treatment options and the role of the gastroenterology nurse and associate. *Gastroenterol Nurs* 12(1):10–14, 1989.

Sauderlin G. Esophageal achalasia. *Gastroenterol Nurs* 15(3):191–196, 1993.

Wilkinson M. Nursing care and patient teaching with percutaneous transhepatic biliary catheter. *Gastroenterol Nurs* 13(4):227–236, 1991.

Winchester C. New approach to esophageal varices: Endoscopic variceal ligation. *Gastroenterol Nurs* 14(1):4–8, 1991.

Caring for People with Disorders of the Stomach

Bhattacharya I. Evaluation and management of dyspepsia. *Hosp Pract* 27(10A):93–96, 1992.

Liebler J, et al. Respiratory complications in critically ill medical patients with acute upper gastrointestinal bleeding. *Crit Care Med* 19(9):1152–1157, 1991.

Looguran E. Therapies for acid peptic disease. *Gastroenterol Nurs* 13(4):198–201, 1991.

Mamel J. Clinical pharmacology of commonly used drugs in GI practice, Part I. *Gastroenterol Nurs* 15(3):114, 1992.

Mamel J. Clinical pharmacology of commonly used drugs in GI practice, Part II. *Gastroenterol Nurs* 15(4):156–162, 1993

Wardell T. Assessing and managing a gastric ulcer. *Nursing 91* 21(3):34–41, 1991.

Young R, and Murray N. *Helicobacter pylori*: A cause of chronic abdominal pain in children. *Gastroenterol Nurs* 15(6):247–251, 1993.

Caring for People with Disorders of the Small Intestine

Bingham W. Nutritional consequences and therapy in Crohn's disease. *Gastroenterol Nurs* 12(3):189–192, 1990.

Kinash R, et al. Coping patterns and related characteristic in patients with IBD. *Gastroenterol Nurs* 16(1):9, 1993.

Swartz M. Beyond the scope: A nursing view of extraintestinal manifestations of IBD. *Gastroenterol Nurs* 12(1):3, 1989.

Caring for People with Disorders of the Large Intestine

Bayless T, Phillips S, and Rogers A. Malabsorption: Fine-tuning the workup. *Patient Care* 25(19):17–20,25–26,28, 1991.

Coellen D. Understanding diverticular disease. *Enterostom Ther* 16(4):176–180, 1989.

Hanauer S, Peppercorn M, and Present D. Current concepts, new therapies in IBD. *Patient Care* 26(13):79–84,86–90, 93–104, 1992.

Meissner J. Caring for patients with ulcerative colitis. *Nursing 94* 24(7):54–55, 1994.

Paulford-Lecher N. Teaching your patient stoma care. *Nursing 93* 23(9):47–49, 1993.

Trier J. Clinical clues to malabsorption. *Emerg Med* 24(6):122–124,127–130,135–136, 1992.

Zelosney C. Giardiasis. *Gastroenterol Nurs* 14(6):313, 1992.

Caring for People with Disorders of the Anorectal Area

Chiappone G. Endoscopic retrograde hemorrhoidal sclerotherapy. *Gastroenterol Nurs* 15(2):78–80, 1992.

Caring for People with Other Disorders of the Gastrointestinal System.

Camp D, and Otten N. How to insert and remove nasogastric tubes. *Nursing 90* 20(9):59–64, 1990.

Falconio M, Kokosyka J, and Prasad M. Anorectal manometry. *Gastroenterol Nurs* 15(3):110–113, 1992.

Hoebler L, and Irwin M. Gastrointestinal tract cancer: Current knowledge, medical treatment, nursing and management. *Oncol Nurs Forum* 19(9):1403–1404, 1992.

Rice P, and Phaasawasdi K. Understanding idiopathic chronic constipation: An understated problem. *Gastroenterol Nurs* 12(2):90–97, 1989.

Savas K, and Zeroske J. Nonresectable esophageal cancer. *Gastroenterol Nurs* 15(3):98–103, 1992.

Stalzer R. Three dimensional imaging of the anal sphincter: A new approach to anorectal manometry. *Gastroenterol Nurs* 14(1):14–17, 1991.

Williams S, and DiPalma J. Constipation in the longterm facility. *Gastroenterol Nurs* 12(3):179, 1990.

28

Caring for People with Hepatic, Biliary, and Pancreatic Disorders

◼ HEPATIC, BILIARY, AND PANCREATIC STRUCTURE AND FUNCTION

The Hepatic System

1. Structure
   a. The hepatic system consists of the liver and the hepatic circulation, which is composed of the hepatic artery, portal vein (formed at the junction of the superior and inferior mesenteric veins and the splenic vein), and hepatic vein.
   b. The liver, which is the largest internal organ in the body, weighs approximately 1.5 kg (3.3 lb) and is composed primarily of Kupffer's cells and hepatocytes (Fig. 28–1).
   c. The portal vein and the hepatic artery supply the liver with 75 percent and 25 percent of its blood, respectively. The liver receives approximately 30 percent of total cardiac output.
      (1) The hepatic artery carries oxygenated blood, and the portal vein carries unoxygenated blood.
      (2) The portal vein delivers nutrients, metabolites, and toxins from the digestive organs to the liver for processing, detoxification, and assimilation.
   d. The hepatic vein transports venous blood from the liver via the portal vein and returns it to the inferior vena cava and, ultimately, to the right side of the heart. Thus, any condition that impedes blood flow through the right side of the heart can cause liver enlargement.
2. Function
   a. In conjunction with the biliary system and exocrine functions of the pancreas, the hepatic system produces, detoxifies, and stores substances responsible for digestion, assimilation, and use of nutrients.
   b. Hepatocytes of the liver metabolize carbohydrates, proteins, and fats by
      (1) Converting glucose to glycogen, then storing it and breaking it down as needed
      (2) Synthesizing amino acids, albumin, globulins, prothrombin, fibrinogen, and other coagulation factors
      (3) Converting ammonia to urea

   (4) Forming lipoproteins, phospholipids, and cholesterol
   (5) Storing fat-soluble vitamins, vitamin B_{12}, copper, and iron
   (6) Producing 600 to 1000 ml of bile each day to facilitate the digestion of fat.
      • Bile consists of bile pigments (principally bilirubin and urobilinogen) and bile salts along with water, electrolytes, and other significant substances, including lecithin, fatty acids, and cholesterol.
      • Bilirubin helps give bile its greenish yellow color. It is metabolized by bacteria in the small intestine and results from the breakdown of hemoglobin.
      • Urobilinogen, a by-product of bilirubin, gives feces their characteristic brown color.
      • Bile salts help break down fat globules and absorb fatty acids, monoglycerides, cholesterol, and other lipids.
   c. Kupffer's cells of the liver
      (1) Perform phagocytosis by trapping foreign bodies
      (2) Detoxify toxic substances such as drugs and toxins

The Biliary System

1. Structure
   a. The biliary system consists of the gallbladder, biliary circulation, and the ductal system (see Fig. 28–1).
   b. The gallbladder is a saclike organ approximately 7 to 10 cm (2.8 to 4 inches) long.
2. Function
   a. The left and right hepatic ducts transport bile from the liver to the gallbladder.
   b. The gallbladder does the following:
      (1) Acts as a reservoir of bile that comes from the liver, holding a maximum volume of 40 to 70 ml
      (2) Concentrates bile by absorbing salts and water
      (3) Responds to ingestion of fats by releasing bile to the duodenum through the sphincter of Oddi
   c. If the gallbladder is removed surgically, biliary ducts enlarge and take over the bile storage function but are not able to respond consistently to ingestion of fatty foods.

STRUCTURE OF THE HEPATIC AND BILIARY SYSTEMS AND OF THE PANCREAS

Liver

The liver is located in the right upper quadrant of the abdomen and fits snugly against the right inferior diaphragm; it is attached to the anterior portion of the abdomen between the diaphragm and umbilicus by the falciform ligament. It is surrounded by connective tissue called Glisson's capsule, which is covered by serosa and which contains blood vessels and lymphatics. The liver's 4 major lobes are the right, left, caudate, and quadrate. Within them lie the functional units of the liver, the lobules or sinusoids. Located within the liver are receptacles for bile called canaliculi.

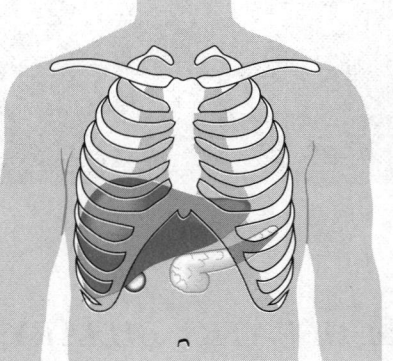

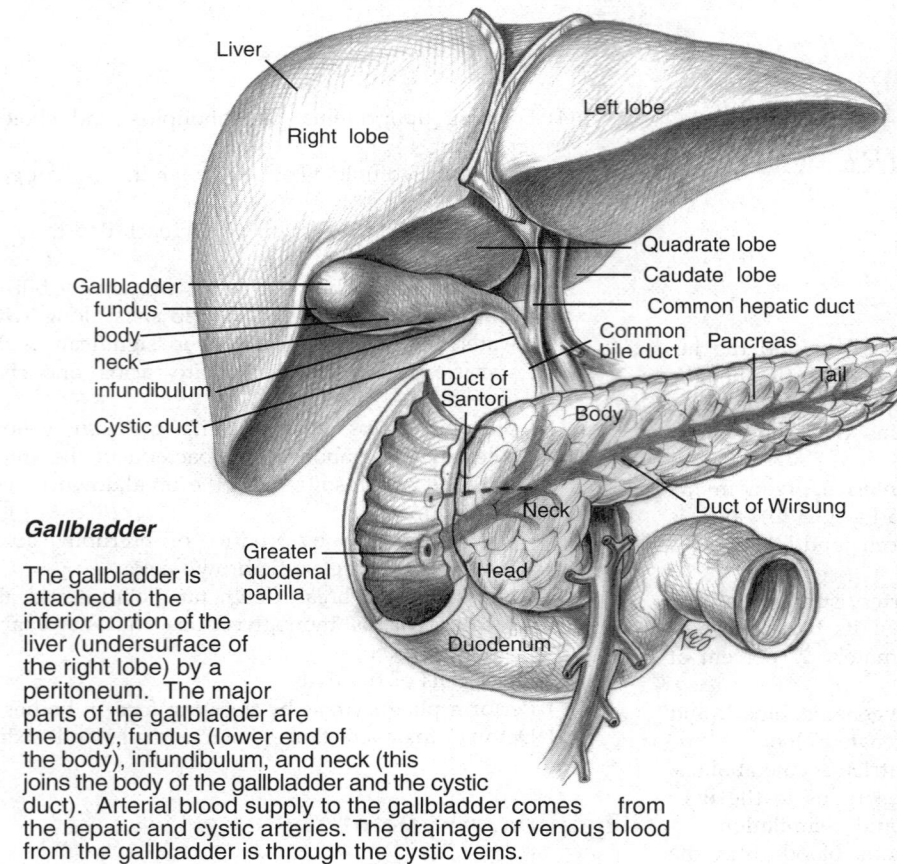

Pancreas

The pancreas is located retroperitoneally, in the space behind the duodenum and the spleen. The 3 major parts of the pancreas are the head and neck (constituting about 30% of the pancreas, lying within the duodenum), the body (largest part, lying behind the stomach), and the tail (thin, narrow part of the pancreas, extending to the spleen).

The 2 ducts of the pancreas are the duct of Wirsung and the duct of Santori. Duct of Wirsung: Main pancreatic duct, which traverses the entire length of the pancreas from left to right. It joins the common bile duct within the ampulla of Vater (short segment of the duct of Wirsung located near the duodenal opening) before it enters into the duodenum. Duct of Santori: An accessory pancreatic duct, present in approximately 15% of the population. When present, the duct of Santori enters the duodenum proximal to the duct of Wirsung.

Gallbladder

The gallbladder is attached to the inferior portion of the liver (undersurface of the right lobe) by a peritoneum. The major parts of the gallbladder are the body, fundus (lower end of the body), infundibulum, and neck (this joins the body of the gallbladder and the cystic duct). Arterial blood supply to the gallbladder comes from the hepatic and cystic arteries. The drainage of venous blood from the gallbladder is through the cystic veins.

Figure 28–1.

The Pancreatic System

1. Structure
   a. The pancreatic system consists of the pancreas and the pancreatic ducts (see Fig. 28–1).
   b. The pancreas is a large, elongated gland weighing approximately 70 to 120 gm (2.8 to 4.8 oz) and is between 12 and 20 cm (4.8 and 8 inches) long.
      (1) It is made up of 2 main cell types: exocrine cells (acinar cells) and endocrine cells (islet of Langerhans).
      (2) The islet of Langerhans has 4 cell subtypes: alpha, beta, delta, and pancreatic polypeptide.
   c. The pancreatic ducts are the duct of Wirsung and the duct of Santorini.
2. Functions
   a. Exocrine functions
      (1) The pancreas secretes bicarbonate ions, water, sodium, potassium, and digestive enzymes (trypsin, amylase, lipase, ribonuclease, and deoxyribonuclease) when chyme is present in the small intestine.
      (2) Trypsin breaks down amino acids.
      (3) Amylase breaks down complex carbohydrates into simple sugars.
      (4) Lipase breaks down triglycerides into fatty acids and glycerol.

Table 28–1. Functions of Various Cell Types in the Islet of Langerhans

Cell Type	Secretion	Action of Secretion
Alpha cells	Glucagon	Break down hepatic glycogen into glucose and adipose tissue into triglyceride
		Stimulate gluconeogenesis from amino acids
Beta cells	Insulin	Facilitate the use of glucose by the tissues
Delta cells	Somatostatin	Inhibit insulin, glucagon, and growth hormone secretion
		Exact function not fully understood
Pancreatic polypeptide	Polypeptide	Causes diarrhea and gastrointestinal hypermotility in animals
		Exact effects in humans are not clearly understood

(5) Ribonuclease and deoxyribonuclease break down nucleic acids into free mononucleotides.

(6) The amount of bicarbonate ion secreted by the pancreas is approximately equal to the amount of acid secreted by the stomach.

b. Endocrine functions: Various cells of the pancreas secrete insulin, glucagon, somatostatin, and other polypeptides (Table 28–1; see Chapter 29).

c. Pancreatic secretions are controlled by vagal and hormonal stimulation.

(1) Vagal stimulation causes the pancreas to secrete the enzymes trypsin and chymotrypsin. Parasympathetic stimulation is initiated by the sight, smell, and thought of food and by food entering the stomach.

(2) The hormones secretin and cholecystokinin (which are secreted in response to gastrin and the presence of chyme in the duodenum) stimulate secretion of the pancreatic enzymes trypsin, chymotrypsin, and carboxypolypeptidase. Entrance of food in the small intestine stimulates secretion of bicarbonate ions.

ASSESSING PEOPLE WITH HEPATIC, BILIARY, AND PANCREATIC DISORDERS

Key Symptoms and Their Pathophysiologic Bases

1. Abdominal pain or discomfort
   a. Location: The location of the pain, which often reflects the specific organ involved, can be determined using the four-quadrant landmark.
   b. Characteristics: Descriptions of the severity and duration of abdominal pain range from absent (as in most liver disorders) to dull and aching to sharp. Sharp pains may be intermittent (as in cholecystitis) or unrelenting (as in pancreatitis and pancreatic cancer).
      (1) Visceral pain arises from organic lesions or functional disturbance within the abdomen. The pain is usually dull and poorly localized.
      (2) Somatic pain arises from the pathways in the nervous system and is usually sharp and well localized.
      (3) Referred pain is experienced in an area other than where the organ is located.
   c. Precipitating and aggravating factors: For example, eating fatty foods may trigger abdominal pain in patients with cholecystitis.
2. Nausea and vomiting: These symptoms are part of the general response of the sympathetic nervous system to stress but require careful nursing attention. Excessive vomiting can lead to large losses of water, electrolytes, bile salts, and gastric acid, all of which can cause fluid and electrolyte imbalances and lower blood acidity.
3. Anorexia: Prolonged lack of desire for food—whether the result of nausea brought on by a disorder or a related problem (e.g., alcoholism in cirrhosis)—can lead to life-threatening problems associated with malnutrition and fluid and electrolyte imbalance.
4. Weight loss
   a. Loss of weight may stem from decreased food intake for reasons such as anorexia, dysphagia, vomiting, and insufficient supplies of food; defective absorption of nutrients through the gastrointestinal tract; increased metabolic requirements; and loss of nutrients through acute injury response.
   b. When weight loss is present, it should be determined whether the intake of food had diminished proportionately or whether it has remained the same or even increased.
5. Fluid and electrolyte imbalances: These may arise if the liver cells cannot synthesize sufficient albumin to maintain intravascular colloidal osmotic pressure and to metabolize aldosterone properly (see Chapter 9).
6. Jaundice (also called icterus): This symptom appears when the liver is unable to metabolize bilirubin. Elevated bilirubin levels in the blood cause the characteristic yellow discoloration of the skin, sclera, and mucous membranes.
   a. Discoloration varies from a slight yellow tint of the sclera to a deep bronze yellow overall color of the skin. Degree of yellowing depends on the severity of the disease and the patient's intrinsic skin color. For example, jaundice is pronounced in Whites with cirrhosis and liver failure.

b. In persons with severe jaundice, bile salts also accumulate on the skin.

7. Altered mental or neurologic status (encephalopathy)
   a. This symptom has been attributed to increased levels of ammonia and other protein by-products in the blood because of the inability of the liver to metabolize them into urea. Serum ammonia level is normal in 10 percent of patients with liver disease, however, and the degree of neurologic impairment does not completely correlate with ammonia level.
   b. It has been suggested that such encephalopathy may result from an amino acid imbalance. In patients with liver disease, the blood concentration of branched-chain amino acids (valine, leucine, and isoleucine) is usually decreased, whereas levels of aromatic amino acids (methionine, phenylalanine, and tyrosine) are increased, interfering with neurotransmitter synthesis.

8. Increased susceptibility to infection
   a. A decreased ability of the liver to perform phagocytosis may result in increased susceptibility to infection.
   b. Altered function of the mononuclear phagocytic system may be due to portal hypertension in those with hepatic disorders.

9. Altered bleeding tendencies: These arise if the liver becomes unable to manufacture clotting factors or clear fibrinolysins. Most often, these tendencies arise when the ability of the liver to absorb vitamin K interferes with hepatic synthesis of prothrombin and other clotting factors.

10. Fatty food intolerance: This symptom is manifested as pain on ingestion of fat when an inflamed gallbladder contracts to release bile, its normal function.

11. Dark, tea-colored urine or clay-colored stools: Excessive amounts of conjugated bilirubin in the bloodstream cause the kidneys to increase their excretion of bilirubin and other bile pigments so much that small amounts of urobilinogen (a dark pigment) are excreted in the urine instead of the feces.

12. Altered bowel habits: Changes in the venous blood flow of the gastrointestinal mucosa are thought to result from blood congestion in the hepatic vasculature.

Health History

1. Medical history
   a. Many prescription medications (e.g., steroids, birth control pills, sulfa drugs, thiazides) and over-the-counter drugs (e.g., antidiarrheal agents, stool softeners, antacids, acetaminophen) affect either the liver or the pancreas.
   b. Conditions such as diabetes mellitus, Reye's syndrome, gastrointestinal bleeding, protracted vomiting, and prolonged diarrhea can affect hepatic, biliary, and pancreatic performance. In the medical history, any exposure to hepatitis or receipt of hepatitis B vaccination should be particularly noted.
   c. Confirm whether the patient has previously undergone diagnostic studies such as upper gastrointestinal series, abdominal ultrasound, cholangiography, endoscopy, and liver biopsy.
   d. Explore reported recent changes in weight and elimination thoroughly.
      (1) Bowel habits should be discussed, including color of stool, and history and frequency of diarrhea or constipation.
      (2) The amount of unintentional weight loss and any associated symptoms (e.g., nausea, anorexia) should be discussed. The patient may have subtle signs of malnutrition such as weakness, easy fatigability, cold intolerance, and flaky dermatitis.

2. Nutritional history
   a. Eating habits
      (1) Intake, that is, the nutritional content of foods, including daily calories ingested, is a factor of nutritional history. Protein depletion is a risk factor for development of cirrhosis. Excessive intake of cholesterol and unsaturated fat increases the risk for development of cholelithiasis and pancreatic cancer.
      (2) The person's economic status, and cultural and religious beliefs with regard to food should be examined. Many cultures use spices or hot pepper in cooking, and these can aggravate or precipitate symptoms of indigestion. Religious patterns of fasting or abstinence can exacerbate hepatic, biliary, and pancreatic conditions. Cultural, religious, and related attitudes toward eating may require a careful series of compromises between medical personnel and a patient with a disorder that requires dietary changes.
   b. Chronic indigestion: Any distress associated with eating is chronic indigestion. Some patients use this term synonymously with heartburn, excessive gas, or feelings of abdominal fullness after meals. For any such symptoms, patients should be asked about what (especially foods) seems to cause it, what relieves it, and any associated symptoms.
      (1) Heartburn is a sense of burning or warmth felt retrosternally; it may radiate from the epigastrium to the neck.
      (2) Excessive gas is manifested by frequent belching, abdominal bloating or distention, or flatus.
      (3) Abdominal fullness after meals may be linked to medications that the patient is taking (especially anticholinergic drugs).

3. Social history and lifestyle
   a. Alcohol use: Investigation should be made regarding the type of alcohol consumed, how much and how often it is consumed, duration of the drinking habit, treatment for alcohol abuse, and history of withdrawal symptoms. Excessive alcohol consumption can damage the liver and the pancreas.
   b. Smoking: Investigation should be made regarding the type used (e.g., cigarettes, pipe, snuff), how often it is used (e.g., packs per day), at what age the habit began, and exposure to secondhand smoke. Cigarette smoking is a risk factor for development of liver and pancreatic cancers.

c. Living environment: Investigation should be made regarding the number of people in the household and its sanitation conditions. Hepatitis A is transmitted through unsanitary living conditions.

d. Sexual history: Investigation should be made regarding the frequency of sexual activity, the number of sexual partners, and the age at which sexual activity began. Sexual activity with many partners is a risk factor for development of hepatitis B and C.

e. Recent and remote travel: Investigation should be made regarding the location and duration of travel, sanitation conditions, native foods eaten, and inoculations received before travel. Diseases such as hepatitis A and E and schistosomiasis are common in Third World countries.

f. Intravenous drug use: The nurse should ask whether intravenous drugs are being used or have been used in the past. Investigation is made regarding the type and frequency of intravenous drug use as well as whether needles are shared.

g. Transfusion history: Investigation is made regarding whether the patient has received a transfusion of blood or blood products within the last 5 years. Many viral pathogens affecting the liver are blood borne.

Physical Examination

1. General observations include the following:
   a. Any signs of grimacing or obvious pain, or nonverbal cues regarding the presence of pain
   b. Abnormal skin color (either pallor or jaundice)
   c. Posture, that is, whether the person assumes a specific position other than upright or erect to be comfortable
   d. Any obvious enlargement or pulsations of the abdomen
2. Auscultation of the abdomen should be done before percussion and palpation.
   a. All 4 quadrants of the abdomen should be assessed for frequency and character of bowel sounds.
   b. The diaphragm of the stethoscope should be pressed lightly on the abdomen to avoid compressing the blood vessels when listening for bowel sounds.
   c. If bowel sounds are hypoactive, it may be necessary to listen for a full 2 to 5 minutes per quadrant.
   d. Normal bowel sounds are low pitched.
   e. Other relevant auscultatory findings include the following:
      • Presence of bruits in the region of the abdominal aorta (epigastric area), denoting blood vessel aneurysms or constrictions

PHYSICAL EXAMINATION OF THE LIVER
Palpation and Percussion

Percussion

With a quick, sharp, but relaxed motion, strike the pleximeter finger with the right middle finger (plexor) aiming at the distal interphalangeal joint. The plexor should be almost at right angles with the pleximeter. The tip of the plexor finger should be used and not the finger pad.

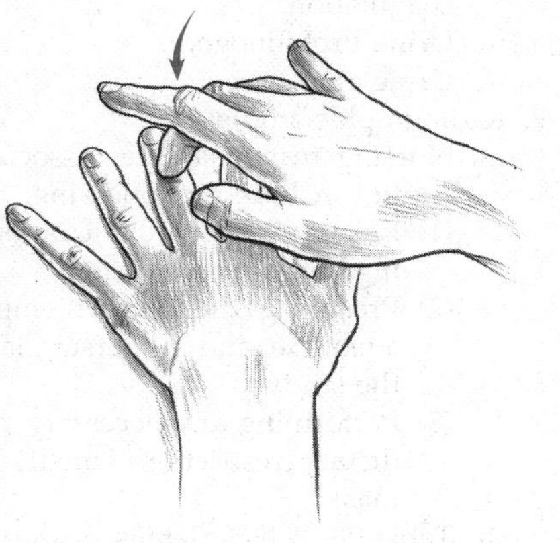

Palpation

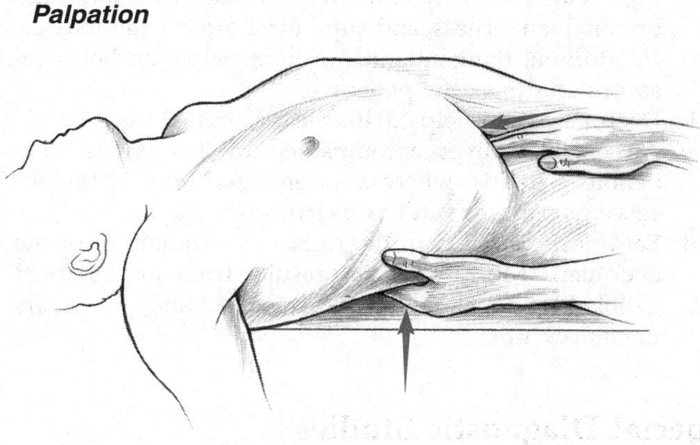

Ascertain the lower border of the liver by lightly percussing upward starting at a level below the umbilicus to the midclavicular line. The span of liver dullness is approximately 6–12 cm in the right midclavicular line.

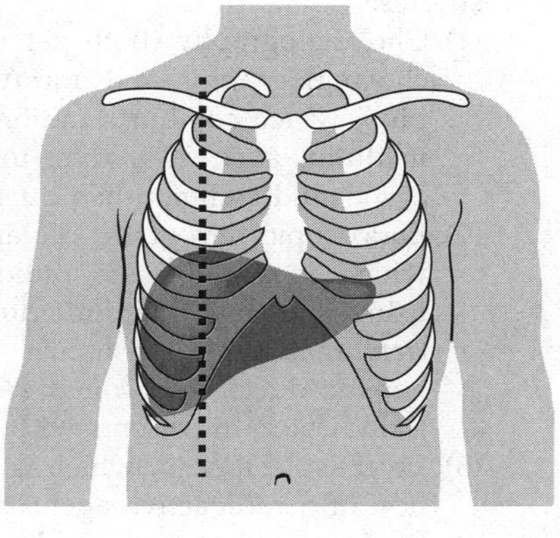

As the patient exhales, the examiner presses in and up at the midclavicular line to feel for the edge of the descending liver.

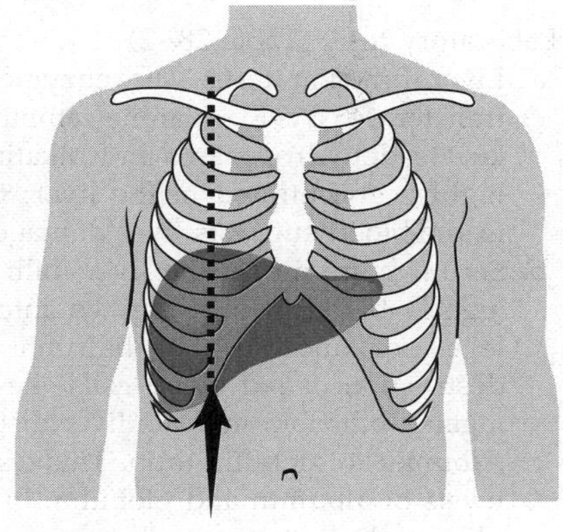

Figure 28–2.

- Venous hum in the area over the liver, denoting liver disease or thrombosis of the portal vein
- Friction rub over the area of the liver, denoting the presence of tumor
3. Percussion examination includes both upper and lower borders of the liver area (Fig. 28–2) to establish enlargement of the liver and presence of a tumor or fluid.
   a. The lower border of the liver is ascertained by lightly percussing upward, starting at a level below the umbilicus (in an area of tympany) to the midclavicular line.
   b. The upper border of the liver can be determined by lightly percussing from lung resonance down toward liver dullness.
   c. The span of liver dullness is approximately 6 to 12 cm (2.4 to 4.8 inches) on the right midclavicular line

NURSE ADVISORY

Some differences exist in normal liver spans. In general, normal liver span is greater in men than in women and in tall than in short people. Estimates of liver size generally vary from 2 to 3 cm, depending on the force of percussion.

4. Palpation is one of the most important parts of any abdominal examination. It is used to identify specific areas of pain or discomfort and to detect organ enlargement (see Fig. 28–2).
   a. Light palpation helps identify muscular resistance, abdominal tenderness, and superficial organs and masses. In addition, the gentleness of light palpation helps reassure and relax the patient.
   b. Deep palpation helps delineate abdominal masses.
   c. An enlarged liver accompanied by tenderness may denote hepatitis, whereas an enlarged liver in the absence of pain may indicate cirrhosis.
   d. Pain on inspiration in the right upper quadrant of the abdomen (Murphy's sign) results from an inflamed gallbladder touching the examiner's hand, as occurs in cholecystitis.

Special Diagnostic Studies

1. Laboratory tests (Table 28–2)
   a. Liver function tests: The enzymes aspartate aminotransferase (AST), alanine aminotransferase (ALT), lactate dehydrogenase, and alkaline phosphatase are highly concentrated in the liver; thus, their presence in the blood suggests liver damage.
   b. Serum bilirubin: In the liver, bilirubin normally conjugates before being excreted into the bile. Elevated levels of unconjugated bilirubin indicate increased destruction of red blood cells; elevated levels of conjugated bilirubin indicate liver disease.
   c. Albumin to globulin ratio: This test identifies shifts in levels of albumin and globulin. In liver disease, globulin levels increase as albumin levels decrease.
   d. Total protein level: Although this test sometimes helps determine the ability of the liver to carry out protein metabolism, the total protein level may remain normal in chronic liver disease despite altered liver function because globulin levels increase as albumin levels decrease.
   e. Serum α-fetoprotein: α-Fetoprotein is produced in large amounts only during the 1st year of life and in persons with liver cancer, in whom the rapidly multiplying liver cells resume α-fetoprotein production.
   f. Pancreatic function tests: Elevated levels of the pancreatic digestive enzymes (amylase and lipase) in the blood indicate pancreatic disease.
   g. Serum ammonia level: Ammonia, an end product of protein metabolism, is converted to urea in the liver and excreted by the kidneys. Although levels of serum ammonia do not directly correspond with the degree of hepatic encephalopathy, decreasing levels of ammonia do indicate improving liver function.
   h. Complete blood count: This test is usually used to determine baseline status of the patient's red blood cells, white blood cells, and platelets.
   i. Serum glucose and blood sugar level (see Chapter 29)
   j. Serum electrolyte profile, including sodium, potassium, chloride, and calcium measurements
   k. Prothrombin time: This test uses vitamin K–dependent factors II, V, VII, and X to assess the intrinsic and common pathways of coagulation.
   l. Partial (and activated partial) thromboplastin time: This test measures factors I, II, V, VIII, IX, X, XI, and XII to assess the intrinsic and common pathways of coagulation.
   m. Urine urobilinogen
   n. Urine amylase
2. Radiographic studies
   a. Nursing responsibilities associated with radiographic studies include the following:
      (1) Ensuring maximum comfort for the patient during and after the study
      (2) Preparing the patient emotionally by providing adequate and understandable information about the study
      (3) Performing any necessary prestudy activities (e.g., dietary restrictions, medication adjustments, enemas)
   b. Table 28–3 lists details of the following radiographic studies:
      (1) Cholangiography (both percutaneous transhepatic cholangiography and intravenous cholangiography), which combines radiography and a contrast medium, such as a dye, to outline the hepatic, cystic, and common bile ducts
      (2) Endoscopic retrograde cholangiopancreatography, which is an invasive radiographic examination using a flexible fiberoptic duodenoscope and contrast material to visualize the pancreatic ducts, hepatic ducts, and common bile ducts. It is contraindicated in patients with acute pancreatitis.
      (3) Liver–spleen scan, which is an intravenous injection of a radioactive agent taken up primarily by the liver and secondarily by the spleen that helps identify liver and spleen tumors and abscesses

Table 28-2. Laboratory Studies of Hepatic, Biliary, and Pancreatic Function

Tests	Normal Values*	Procedure/Nursing Considerations	Interpretation
Liver function tests		Blood for liver function tests is drawn without special preparation.	
Aspartate aminotransferase (AST)	Men: 8–46 U/L Women: 7–34 U/L	Draw 5 ml venous sample. Note on the laboratory slip any drugs being taken by the patient.	AST is found in many body organs; thus, its specificity is limited. However, extreme elevations of AST occur in acute pancreatitis and fulminant hepatic failure. Intramuscular injection and drugs such as salicylates and antibiotics interfere with test results.
Alanine aminotransferase (ALT)	10–30 IU/L	Draw 5 ml venous sample. Note on the laboratory slip drugs being taken by the patient.	The highest concentration of ALT is found in the liver. Elevations of 30 to 50 times the normal AST value occur in toxic hepatitis. Drugs such as meperidine, gentamicin, salicylates, indomethacin, and erythromycin cause decreased levels of ALT.
Lactate dehydrogenase LDH$_4$ LDH$_5$	70–250 U/L 5–15% of total 2–20% of total	Draw 5 ml venous sample.	High concentrations of isoenzymes LDH$_4$ and LDH$_5$ are found in the liver. Levels of both isoenzymes are elevated in cases of liver disease.
Alkaline phosphatase (ALP) 5′ Nucleotidase (5′N) Gamma glutamyl trans-peptidase (GGTP)	20–130 U/L 0–1.6 U 6–37 U/L	Draw 3 ml venous sample. Handle specimen gently to prevent hemolysis.	ALP isoenzymes 5′N and GGTP are primarily seen in the liver. Elevated levels of these isoenzymes indicate liver disease.
Total serum bilirubin Direct (conjugated) Indirect (unconjugated)	0.3–1.2 mg/dl 0.1–0.4 mg/dl 0.3–1.1 mg/dl	Have patient fast for 4 hours. Draw 5 ml venous sample. Protect sample from ultraviolet light.	Elevated levels of conjugated bilirubin indicate biliary obstruction. Elevated levels of unconjugated bilirubin indicate hepatocellular dysfunction.
Albumin to globulin ratio	1.5:1–2.5:1	Draw 5 ml venous sample. (No special preparation is needed.)	In the presence of acute liver disease, globulin increases whereas albumin decreases or remains unchanged.
Total serum protein	6.6–7.9 g/dl	Draw 5 ml venous sample. (No special preparation is needed.)	In the presence of liver disease, insufficient protein forms, thus decreasing serum levels.
Serum α-fetoprotein	<30 ng/dl	Draw 5 ml venous sample. (No special preparation is needed.)	This is a tumor marker in the liver. Elevated levels are seen in the presence of hepatic carcinoma.
Serum amylase	60–160 Somogyi units/dl	Draw 3 ml venous blood. (No special preparation is needed.)	Because amylase is released with the breakdown of acinar cells, elevated levels are seen in acute pancreatitis; however, elevated serum amylase levels appear only for 24 to 48 hr after the onset of pain.
Serum lipase	0–1.5 U	Have patient fast at least 4 hr. Draw 3 ml venous blood.	Because lipase is released with the breakdown of acinar cells, elevated levels of serum lipase may indicate acute pancreatitis.
Serum ammonia	40–100 μg/dl	Have patient fast at least 4 hr. Draw 3 ml venous sample.	Elevated levels indicate hepatic dysfunction—the inability of the liver to convert ammonia to urea for excretion in the kidneys.
Complete blood count		Blood for complete blood count analysis is drawn without special preparation. Total amount of blood drawn is approximately 10 ml.	
Red blood cell count Hemoglobin	Men: 4.2–5.5 million/mm³ Women: 3.6–5.0 million/mm³ Men: 14–16.5 g/dl Women: 12–15 g/dl		Decreased red blood cell count (including hemoglobin and hematocrit) indicates anemia, recent bleeding, or liver disease that causes premature de-

Table continued on following page

Table 28–2. Laboratory Studies of Hepatic, Biliary, and Pancreatic Function (Continued)

Tests	Normal Values*	Procedure/Nursing Considerations	Interpretation
Hematocrit	Men: 37–45% Women: 42–50%		struction of red blood cells. Elevated levels indicate hemoconcentration caused by dehydration.
White blood cell count	5000–10,000/mm³		Elevated levels of white blood cell counts reflect infections such as pancreatitis and cholecystitis.
Platelet count	150,000–400,000/mm³		Platelets primarily function to control bleeding. Decreased levels of platelets indicate liver disease.
Serum glucose–blood sugar	60–110 mg/dl	Have patient fast at least 4 to 6 hours. Draw 5 ml venous sample.	Decreased levels are seen in 50% of patients with acute viral hepatitis caused by depleted glycogen stores, decreased gluconeogenesis, and poor intake. Elevated levels are seen in chronic hepatitis and in pancreatic disease.
Serum electrolyte profile		Draw 10 ml venous sample. (No special preparation is needed.)	
Sodium	136–145 mEq/L		Serum sodium is usually elevated in dehydration. In patients with cirrhosis, serum sodium may be low because of water retention (dilutional hyponatremia).
Potassium	3.5–5.0 mEq/L		Low serum potassium is seen in patients with liver and pancreatic disease, in the presence of vomiting, and in those receiving diuretics. Elevated serum potassium is seen in renal failure.
Chloride	96–106 mEq/L		Because chloride preserves electroneutrality in the extracellular fluid, changes in serum chloride affect acid-base balance. Elevated serum chloride indicates acidemia. Low serum chloride reflects alkalemia.
Calcium	8.0–10.5 mg/dl		Low serum calcium (hypocalcemia) is seen in patients with pancreatic and liver disease and those receiving multiple blood transfusions. Elevated serum calcium is seen in renal failure.
Prothrombin time (PT)	12–15 sec	Draw 5 ml venous sample. (No special preparation is needed.)	Prolonged PT may indicate deficiencies in vitamin K or coagulation factors such as factors II, V, VII, and X (seen in liver disease). Anticoagulant therapy also causes prolonged PT. A prolonged PT reflects abnormal bleeding tendencies.
Partial thromboplastin time (PTT) or activated partial thromboplastin time (APTT)	25–38 sec	Draw 5 ml venous sample. (No special preparation is needed.)	Because some coagulation factors are synthesized in the liver and are vitamin K dependent, prolonged PTT or APTT is seen in patients with hepatic disease or biliary obstruction. Prolonged PTT or APTT indicates the presence of bleeding tendencies.
Urine urobilinogen	1–4 mg/24 hr	Perform 24-hour urine collection. Keep specimens refrigerated. (If patient is catheterized, keep catheter bag on ice.)	Urine urobilinogen level is increased in hepatobiliary disease and in other diseases that increase bilirubin and prevent removal of reabsorbed urobilinogen from the portal circulation.

| | | Procedure/Nursing | |
Tests	Normal Values*	Considerations	Interpretation
Urine amylase	1–17 U/hr	Perform urine collection for 2, 4, 6, 8 or 24 hr. Keep specimens refrigerated. (If the patient is catheterized, keep catheter bag on ice.) Elevated levels of urine amylase occur in pancreatitis and pancreatic obstruction. Urine amylase values usually increase together with serum amylase. However, decline in urine amylase values takes longer than in serum amylase.	

Table 28–2. Laboratory Studies of Hepatic, Biliary, and Pancreatic Function (Continued)

* Normal values may differ among institutions.

(4) Oral cholecystogram (gallbladder series), which allows radiographic visualization of the gallbladder and thus helps evaluate gallbladder function and diagnose gallbladder disease and gallstones

(5) Hepatobiliary scan (imaging), which detects hepatobiliary abnormalities more rapidly than oral cholecystography and which can be done even if serum bilirubin is more than 1.8 mg per dl: A dye such as technetium-labeled hepato-iminodiacetic acid (HIDA) is sometimes to enhance the image.

(6) Radionuclide scanning (scintigraphy), which uses an intravenous infusion of gamma-emitting isotopes such as gallium (to determine the presence or absence of inflammation of the liver, gallbladder, or pancreas), technetium (to evaluate liver and biliary tract function), or selenium (to identify pancreatic abnormalities)

(7) Magnetic resonance imaging, which produces cross-sectional images of tissues used to study blood flow as well as identify areas of malignancy

(8) Computed tomography scan, which creates 3-dimensional images to help identify tumors and other diseases, cysts, abscesses, and hematomas and to distinguish between obstructive and nonobstructive jaundice

(9) Angiography, which uses a contrast dye to allow visualization of the viscera for identification of abnormalities of vascular structure and function, presence of a mass, and sites of bleeding

3. Abdominal ultrasound
   a. This noninvasive procedure uses high-frequency, inaudible sound waves to form images of internal structures. Sound waves are directed toward the area to be studied. When they hit internal organs, they are reflected back and are converted to an image on a screen.
   b. Ultrasound is used to detect abscesses, gallstones, size of abdominal organs, hematomas, and metastasis and to assess vascular patency in the hepatic artery and portal vein.

4. Biopsy: Tissues removed from an organ either by needle aspiration or by peritoneoscopy are studied (Procedure 28–1).

5. Peritoneoscopy
   a. Structural changes in the liver that are reflective of cirrhosis and cancer are visualized by laparoscopy.
   b. Peritoneoscopy is contraindicated in patients with infections of the abdominal cavity, prolonged prothrombin time and partial thromboplastin time, or intestinal obstruction. Obesity and ascites interfere with test results.
   c. Nursing responsibilities are to validate informed consent, administer preprocedural medications, ensure adequate prothrombin time and partial thromboplastin time, check for allergies, direct the patient to hold breath while the needle is inserted, and monitor the patient for signs of pneumothorax, air embolism, bile leakage, or perforation of hollow organ after the procedure.

6. Portal pressure measurements
   a. A minor surgical procedure is performed in either the operating room or the special studies laboratory and often involves use of a contrast dye.
   b. Measurements of portal pressure and blood flow help diagnose portal hypertension and determine its severity. Common types of portal pressure measurements are the following:
      (1) Wedged hepatic vein pressure: Using the antecubital vein or the femoral vein, the physician catheterizes the hepatic vein and indirectly obtains portal pressure.
      (2) Umbilical vein catheterization: Percutaneous catheterization of the umbilical vein permits direct measurement of portal pressure.
      (3) Splenic pulp manometry: While the patient holds breath, the physician places a needle between 2 of the lower ribs and inserts a manometer into the spleen.
   c. Nursing responsibilities are to apply standard preoperative procedures, and, after the procedure, to assess for bleeding and hematoma formation at the needle

Table 28–3. Radiographic Studies of Hepatic, Biliary, and Pancreatic Function*

Radiographic Study	Patient Preparation	Procedural Care	Postprocedure Care
Cholangiography			
Percutaneous transhepatic cholangiography	No formal preparation is needed. Ask patients about allergies to iodine or seafood. Obtain informed consent.	A needle is inserted into the liver under fluoroscopic guidance while patient holds breath to help stabilize the liver. The dye is injected as the needle is removed. The outline of the biliary tree is visualized under fluoroscopy. Total time for the test is approximately 30 minutes.	Place the patient on bed rest for at least 8 hours. Inspect the injection site for bleeding, bile leakage, tenderness or abdominal distention. Monitor vital signs. Apply pressure on insertion site as ordered.
Intravenous cholangiography	Same as in percutaneous transhepatic cholangiography	A contrast material (dye) is given intravenously while the patient is in the radiology department. Radiographic films are obtained at 15- to 20-min intervals until the biliary ducts are visualized (usually within 1 to 2 hr). Total time for the test is approximately 2 to 4 hr.	No postprocedural care is needed.
Endoscopic retrograde cholangiopancreatography	The patient should take nothing by mouth for at least 6 to 8 hr before the procedure. Obtain informed consent. Obtain baseline vital signs. Administer ordered medications at least 30 min before the procedure. Valium may be ordered to calm the patient. Atropine may also be ordered to dry secretions. ERCP is contraindicated if the patient's bilirubin is greater than 3.5 mg/dl.	A local anesthetic is sprayed into the patient's throat to prevent gag reflex and make swallowing difficult. A flexible endoscope is passed down the esophagus and advanced to the duodenum and into the biliary tract. Contrast medium is injected through the endoscope. Radiographic films are obtained to evaluate the biliary tract. Total time for the test is approximately 1 hr.	Monitor vital signs. Keep patient NPO until gag reflex returns. Assess the patient for signs of cholangitis or perforation (e.g., fever, abdominal pain—especially on the right upper quadrant—hypotension, and tachycardia).
Liver-spleen scan	Instruct patient to lie still. Patient receives intravenous injection of radioactive colloid at least 15 min before the procedure to allow for uptake. Reassure patient that this injection only has an extremely small amount of radioactivity, and thus is not dangerous.	While on the scan table in the nuclear medicine department, the patient is placed in many different positions to allow for optimal visualization of the liver. Total time for the test is approximately 1 to 2 hr.	No postprocedural care is needed.
Oral cholecystography or gallbladder series	Do not perform this test if serum bilirubin level is greater than 1.8 mg/dl Have patient eat a fat-free meal the evening before the test. Keep patient NPO except for water at least 4 hr before the procedure. Obtain information regarding allergies to iodine, contrast dyes, or seafood. Administer six iopanoic acid tablets (one at a time at 5-min intervals) after the patient's evening meal. Observe patient for side effects of the tablets (e.g., abdominal cramping, diarrhea, and vomiting). If present, report to the physician immediately. If patient vomits after ingesting tablet, examine emesis for undigested tablets. If present, notify physician immediately so that the dye can be prescribed again or the test rescheduled.	While on the x-ray table, the patient assumes various positions and several radiographic films are taken. The test may take several hours.	No postprocedural care is needed.

Table 28–3. Radiographic Studies of Hepatic, Biliary, and Pancreatic Function (Continued)

Radiographic Study	Patient Preparation	Procedural Care	Postprocedure Care
Hepatobiliary scan	Keep patient NPO 4–6 hr before the procedure. Radioactive isotope dye is given at least 15 min before the procedure.	While in the nuclear medicine department on the scan table, the patient is placed in many different positions to allow for optimal visualization of the liver.	No postprocedural care is needed.
Radionuclide scanning or scintigraphy	Keep patient NPO except for giving clear liquids at least 3 to 4 hr before the procedure. Obtain informed consent. Administer pain medications as ordered before the test to facilitate patient positioning. Patient receives an intravenous injection of a small amount of radioactive isotope at least 15 min before the test.	While on the scan table in the nuclear medicine department, the patient is placed in different positions. Total time for the test is several hours. Occasionally, additional scanning may be done within 24 hr of the initial scan.	No postprocedural care is needed.
Magnetic resonance imaging Computed tomography of the abdomen	Keep patient NPO at least 4 hr before procedure.	While on the scan table, the patient is placed in many different positions to allow for optimal visualization. A water-soluble contrast dye may be used to clearly delineate pancreatic margins. Total time for this test is usually 30 min to 1 hr.	No postprocedural care is needed.
Angiography	Obtain informed consent. Ask patient about allergies to contrast dyes, iodine, or seafood.	A needle is inserted into the femoral artery and a contrast dye is injected. The needle is exchanged for a catheter, which is then passed into the celiac, superior mesenteric, or hepatic artery. A sequence of radiographic films are obtained. This test may take several hours.	Place patient on bed rest for 2 to 4 hr after the procedure. Monitor vital signs. Observe injection site for bleeding or hematoma formation.

* In all of these tests, the procedure should be explained to any individual who is awake and alert. If the patient is not awake and alert, the procedure must be explained to family or relevant friends.

insertion site and for signs of pneumothorax after splenic pulp manometry.
7. Analysis of biliary drainage
  a. This procedure is an alternative for patients who are allergic to contrast dye.
  b. Nursing responsibilities are to ensure the patient receives nothing by mouth for at least 6 to 8 hours before the study begins.
  c. The procedure is undertaken as follows:
    (1) The physician inserts a single-lumen nasogastric tube into the stomach and aspirates the stomach contents.
    (2) The physician slowly advances the tube to the duodenum. (The position of the tube in the duodenum is indicated by clear, yellow, alkaline aspirate.)
    (3) Magnesium sulfate is instilled into the tube to stimulate the flow of bile to the duodenum. Intravenous administration of secretin followed by

oral pancreatic enzyme (pancreozymin) may be used instead of magnesium sulfate.
    (4) Bile from the duodenum is aspirated and sent to the laboratory for analysis of enzyme, bile, and bicarbonate content.
    (5) Disproportions in the ratio between bile and pancreatic juice indicate biliary or pancreatic duct obstruction. Presence of cholesterol crystals in the collected drainage indicates cholelithiasis.

◼ CARING FOR PEOPLE WITH HEPATIC DISORDERS

Hepatitis

1. Definition: Hepatitis is inflammation of the liver caused by virus, bacteria, or exposure to hepatotoxins or drugs.

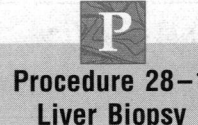

Procedure 28–1
Liver Biopsy

Definition/Purpose	Needle aspiration of a core of liver tissue for analysis and diagnosis of liver disease.
Contraindications/Cautions	Do not perform this procedure if the individual has a platelet count below 100,000 units. Other contraindications include the presence of local infection at the base of the right lung, peritonitis, massive ascites, or cholecystitis.
Learning/Teaching Activities	• Describe the procedure. • Identify the nature and risks of the biopsy and ascertain that the person understands them. • Discuss the importance of the person's cooperation throughout the procedure (especially of holding the breath on exhalation during the procedure to stabilize the liver).

Preliminary Activities

Equipment	• Biopsy needle (14 or 18 gauge) • Glass slides, specimen bottles containing fixative and test tubes • Local anesthetic • Syringes • Sterile gloves, sterile fenestrated towels • Betadine for local skin cleansing • 4 × 4 gauze for dressing the needle insertion site • Hypoallergenic adhesive tape • Pillows and pressure bags
Assessment/Planning	• Obtain informed consent before the procedure. • Know the latest series of vital sign readings for this person and be cognizant of the trend. • Know the latest prothrombin levels and platelet count; it may be necessary to postpone the biopsy if the prothrombin time is prolonged or if the platelet count is too low because of potential intractable bleeding.
Preparing the Patient	• Give patient nothing by mouth 4 to 8 hours before the procedure. • This restriction is necessary because complications of the procedure may require emergency surgery. • Administer prescribed sedation at least 30 minutes before the procedure to allow time for the medication to take effect. • Place the individual in supine or left lateral position with the right arm extended above the head to widen the intercostal spaces and fully expose the hepatic area.

Procedure

Action	Rationale/Discussion
1. Stay with the person throughout the procedure.	1. The nurse's presence provides emotional support to the patient.
2. Stand on the individual's left side and hold the left hand. At the same time, place one hand lightly on the individual's right arm.	2. Holding the right arm allows the nurse to quickly restrain the arm from movement during the procedure.
3. Before the biopsy needle is inserted, instruct the individual to inhale fully and hold the breath on exhalation while the specimen is obtained.	3. On exhalation, the diaphragm ascends and the risk of puncturing the lung is minimized. In addition, holding the breath stabilizes the liver, thus minimizing the incidence of liver laceration.
4. The physician inserts the liver biopsy needle through the sixth and seventh or eight and ninth ribs and removes a sample of liver tissue.	4. This is the liver span during exhalation.
5. Apply pressure dressing once the biopsy needle is withdrawn.	5. Dressing decreases the incidence of infection and hemorrhage from the biopsy site

Final Activities

1. Maintain the person on bed rest for 8 to 24 hours to decrease the incidence of bleeding.
2. Apply pressure on the site of biopsy for the first few hours by turning the person to the right side with pillows or sandbags. This position compresses the liver capsule against the chest wall, minimizing the leakage of blood or bile.
3. Monitor the person carefully for signs of hemorrhage, such as frank bleeding or tenderness around the biopsy site. Laceration of the liver or puncture of a blood vessel within or surrounding the liver can cause hemorrhage.

P

Procedure 28-1

(continued)

4. Check vital signs and inspect site at least every 15 minutes for the first hour, then every 30 minutes, and then hourly. Complications of liver biopsy are bleeding and bile peritonitis, which can cause changes in vital signs.
5. Observe for signs of pneumothorax (which can result from improper position of the biopsy needle that punctures the lung) such as increased respiratory rate, pleuritic chest pain, shoulder pain, shortness of breath, decreased breath sounds.
6. Administer vitamin K, if prescribed, to reduce the risk of bleeding by improving clotting time.
7. Provide pain medications as needed. Some pain in the right upper quadrant and right shoulder is common because of leakage of small amounts of bile, blood, or both from the biopsy site. However, if pain is severe and unrelenting, notify the physician immediately.

---

a. Viral hepatitis, which involves widespread inflammation of liver cells, is the most common form of hepatitis.
b. Researchers have clearly identified 5 hepatotrophic viruses that cause viral hepatitis: hepatitis A (HAV), B (HBV), C (HCV), D (delta hepatitis), and E (HEV) (Table 28-4). In addition, 1 or more as yet unnamed viruses appear to cause hepatitis.
2. Incidence and socioeconomic impact
   a. Hepatitis A infection
      (1) Is commonly seen in areas of poverty and overcrowding, poor hygiene, and inadequate sewage disposal
      (2) Has a seasonal incidence; is commonly seen during fall and winter
      (3) Has an incidence of 90 percent in developing areas of the world, and 40 to 90 percent in the United States
   b. Hepatitis B infection
      (1) Is common among drug abusers
      (2) Is nonseasonal
      (3) Has increased in incidence by 37 percent in the past decade in the United States
      (4) Causes 4000 to 5000 deaths annually, although

more than 50 percent of cases of hepatitis are subclinical and usually go unnoticed.
   c. Hepatitis C infection
      (1) Occurs year round
      (2) Leads to chronic liver disease in 10 to 40 percent of patients with infection
      (3) Has an incidence of as many as 170,000 new infections annually in the United States
   d. Hepatitis D infection
      (1) Is endemic in the Mediterranean and Middle Eastern areas but its occurrence is uncommon in the United States, accounting for less than 2 percent of all hepatitis cases
      (2) Is commonly seen among drug abusers
      (3) Leads to chronic liver disease in 80 percent of patients with infection
   e. Hepatitis E infection
      (1) Is endemic after a heavy rain in areas of the world where sewage disposal is inadequate or where communal bathing in contaminated rivers is practiced. Large outbreaks have been reported in Asia, Africa, the former Soviet Union, and Mexico.
      (2) Is the leading cause of acute viral hepatitis in

Table 28-4. Types of Viral Hepatitis

Type of Hepatitis	Mode of Transmission	Incubation Period
Hepatitis A	Fecal–oral route On rare occasions, may be airborne if body secretions are copious May be transmitted parenterally	2–6 wk
Hepatitis B	Parenteral Sexual contact Occasionally, fecal–oral route	6–24 wk
Hepatitis C (formerly known as non-A, non-B hepatitis)	Contact with blood and body fluids	5–10 wk
Hepatitis D (delta hepatitis)	Close personal contact Coinfects with hepatitis B	7–8 wk
Hepatitis E	Fecal–oral route	2–9 wk

young to middle-aged adults in developing countries

3. Risk factors
   a. Risk of infection with HAV is increased
      (1) By personal contact with infected materials
      (2) By handling contaminated feces
      (3) By consuming raw fish
   b. Risk of infection with HBV is increased
      (1) By receiving multiple blood transfusions
      (2) In health care providers in contact with blood and blood products
      (3) In hemodialysis patients
      (4) By sharing toothbrushes
      (5) During the perinatal period (especially during the 3rd trimester) when vertical transmission may occur from mother to child
      (6) In sexually active individuals, especially those with multiple partners
   c. Risk of infection with HCV is the same as for HBV.
   d. Risk of infection with delta hepatitis is the same as for HBV.
   e. Risk of infection with HEV is the same as for HAV.

4. Etiology
   a. Hepatitis A virus is transmitted via the following:
      (1) Poorly washed utensils
      (2) Infected water, milk, or food, especially raw shellfish
   b. Hepatitis B virus is transmitted via the following:
      (1) Infected blood and blood products
      (2) Infected saliva or semen
   c. Hepatitis C virus is transmitted as for HBV; it is the major cause of post-transfusion hepatitis.
   d. Delta hepatitis can only infect persons who have previously contracted hepatitis B. It is transmitted via contact with blood and blood products among persons already infected with HBV and is otherwise transmitted the same as for HBV.
   e. Hepatitis E virus is transmitted as for HAV.

5. Pathophysiology
   a. Virus, bacteria, or toxins invade the portal tracts, periportal space, and liver lobules.
   b. In the early stages of hepatitis, a widespread accumulation of inflammatory cells (e.g., Kupffer's cells, monocytes, and lymphocytes) and edema are present. Some localized necrosis may also be present.
   c. As the disease progresses, the simultaneous appearance of inflammation, necrosis, degeneration, and regeneration of liver cells distorts the normal lobular pattern. This distortion interferes with normal blood flow in the liver lobules, causing an increased pressure in the portal circulation. Liver function decreases.
   d. When phagocytic and enzymatic reactions eventually remove the damaged liver cells, the remaining cells cannot regenerate.

6. Clinical manifestations
   a. Symptoms of viral hepatitis vary greatly from no symptoms to hepatic failure or hepatic encephalopathy.
   b. Symptoms associated with viral hepatitis are usually divided into 3 stages:

   (1) Pre-icteric (prodromal) symptoms include fatigue, malaise, anorexia, nausea and vomiting, vague abdominal discomfort, progressive darkening of the urine, elevated levels of AST, ALT, and bilirubin, joint pain, weight loss, right upper quadrant abdominal pain, changes in taste, headache, and cold symptoms.
   (2) Icteric symptoms include jaundice, elevated levels of direct bilirubin, persistent anorexia, clay-colored stools, right upper quadrant abdominal pain, dark or tea-colored urine, enlarged and tender liver, pruritus (due to increased bile deposits on skin), and spider angiomas.
   (3) Post-icteric (convalescent) symptoms include fatigue, decreasing jaundice, return to normal of stool and urine color, and improved appetite.

7. Diagnostics (see pp. 1306–1309)
   a. Laboratory tests measure elevated serum levels of AST, ALT, lactate dehydrogenase, bilirubin, serum glucose; elevated alkaline phosphatase; and presence of bilirubin in the urine.
   b. Liver biopsy shows the extent of hepatocellular damage.
   c. Ultrasound shows enlargement of the liver.
   d. Specific diagnostic tests detect the following:
      (1) Hepatitis A infection
         • Presence of anti-HAV IgM confirms the diagnosis of hepatitis A in the acute phase.
         • Presence of anti-HAV IgG indicates previous hepatitis A infection and lifelong immunity to the virus.
      (2) Hepatitis B infection
         • Presence of hepatitis B surface antigen indicates recent acute infection (also positive in chronic carriers of the virus).
         • Presence of hepatitis B e antigen indicates high infectivity and a greater chance of development of chronic disease.
         • Presence of antibody to hepatitis B surface antigen indicates immunity to hepatitis B. It is also a marker of immune response to immune globulin or the hepatitis B vaccine.
         • Presence of antibody to hepatitis B core antigen indicates previous hepatitis B infection. It does not appear after hepatitis B vaccination.
      (3) Hepatitis C infection: Presence of antibody to HCV indicates previous hepatitis C infection.
      (4) Hepatitis D infection: Presence of antibody to delta hepatitis indicates past or present infection with the delta virus.
      (5) Hepatitis E infection: There is no test available.

8. Clinical management
   a. Goals of clinical management are to focus on supportive therapy for existing symptoms and to prevent transmission of the disease.
   b. Nonpharmacologic interventions
      (1) Bed rest is usually prescribed for 1 to 2 weeks, with activity gradually increased as the patient can tolerate.
      (2) A low-fat, low-sodium, high-protein, high-carbohydrate diet is recommended.

- For anorexia, small frequent meals with increased amounts of clear liquids should be ingested.
- Increased carbohydrates provide the calories needed for energy to help heal the damaged liver.
- A low-fat diet counterbalances reduced bile production from the liver.
- The patient should eat a diet high in protein. Serum ammonia and blood urea nitrogen levels should be closely monitored.
  (3) The patient should abstain from ingesting alcohol which is toxic to the liver.
  (4) Serum bilirubin should be monitored.
  (5) Increased fluid intake should be recommended.
  (6) Universal precautions should be taken at all times.

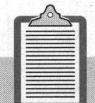

NURSING MANAGEMENT

Nurses and other health care personnel who are injured by contaminated needles (and have not received the hepatitis B vaccine) have a 6 to 30 percent chance of becoming infected with hepatitis B virus. Such personnel will benefit from post-accident vaccination against hepatitis B virus but should also receive hepatitis B hyperimmunoglobulin. With regard to other forms of hepatitis, the incidence of acquiring hepatitis C from a contaminated needle is only about 2 to 3 percent; accidental transmission of hepatitis D virus is only possible in persons who already have hepatitis B. The incidence of acquiring hepatitis A and E can be dramatically decreased if nurses observe enteric precautions.

c. Pharmacologic interventions include the following:
  (1) Dimenhydrinate (Dramamine) or trimethobenzamide (Tigan) for severe nausea
  (2) Intravenous fluids to prevent dehydration
  (3) Vitamin B complex to compensate for the inability of the liver to absorb water-soluble vitamins
  (4) Vitamin K, if prothrombin time is prolonged
  (5) Steroids, which are controversial, because they have not been proven effective in treating viral hepatitis, except for hepatitis C

DRUG ADVISORY

In patients with viral hepatitis, corticosteroids can further increase serum bilirubin levels, interfere with the action of birth control pills, increase sodium and water retention, and cause blood sugar elevation. Nurses should monitor blood sugar, blood pressure, and daily weights in such patients and continuously assess them for edema.

9. Complications
  a. Cirrhosis (see p. 1316)
  b. Portal hypertension (see pp. 1322–1323)
  c. Fulminant hepatic failure (see p. 1326)
  d. Hepatocellular carcinoma (see p. 1328)

e. Hepatic encephalopathy (see p. 1321)
10. Prognosis
  a. Recovery with only mild damage is common.
  b. Residual liver damage depends on severity of the illness.
11. Applying the nursing process

NURSING DIAGNOSIS: Altered nutrition, less than body requirements, R/T anorexia or nausea and vomiting

  a. *Expected outcomes:* Following intervention, the patient should be able to do the following:
    (1) Ingest prescribed daily caloric requirement
    (2) Verbally express and physically manifest decreased incidence of nausea and vomiting and presence of moist mucous membranes
  b. *Nursing interventions*
    (1) Provide a high-carbohydrate, low-fat diet. If moderate amounts of protein are added to the diet, monitor the patient for changes in mental status indicative of hepatic encephalopathy.
    (2) Provide small frequent feedings to avoid tiring the patient and to alleviate vomiting.
    (3) Administer antiemetics 30 minutes before meals if needed.
    (4) Implement strict calorie count.
    (5) Provide intravenous or enteral feeding for patients unable to ingest food orally.
    (6) Give daily vitamin supplements.

NURSING DIAGNOSIS: Activity intolerance R/T the infectious process

  c. *Expected outcomes:* Following interventions, the patient should be able to do the following:
    (1) Report absence of fatigue associated with normal activity
    (2) Achieve maximum activity level
    (3) Return to preillness activities of daily living
  d. *Nursing interventions*
    (1) Coordinate nursing care to provide planned periods of rest.
    (2) Provide bed rest in a quiet environment.
    (3) Assist the patient who is extremely fatigued to turn, cough, and perform passive range-of-motion exercises while on bed rest to avoid complications of immobility such as pneumonia and thrombophlebitis (see Chapter 7).
    (4) Gradually increase the patient's activity levels.

NURSING DIAGNOSIS: Risk for impaired skin integrity R/T pruritus (see p. 1322)

12. Discharge planning and teaching: See Learning/Teaching Guidelines for Self-Care of Patients with Viral Hepatitis

LEARNING/TEACHING GUIDELINES
for Self-Care of Patients with Viral Hepatitis

General Overview

1. Describe the disease process and the importance of good personal hygiene in decreasing the spread of hepatitis types A, B, and E.
2. Provide information on measures to prevent the transmission of hepatitis.
3. Refer the patient to a home-care agency as needed.

Diet

1. Stress the importance of eating a high-calorie, moderate-protein diet that is still low in fat. Hard candies are good source of carbohydrates.
2. To achieve a general decrease in dietary fat, instruct the person to:
   a. Avoid sauces, gravies, and fatty meats.
   b. Avoid using cream and eating rich desserts.
   c. Broil or grill foods instead of frying them.
3. Provide the person with an American Diabetes Association Fat Portion Exchange List.
4. Encourage the person to eat smaller, more frequent meals.
5. Emphasize the importance of abstaining from alcohol.

Measures to Prevent Transmission of Infection

1. Provide instructions on hygenic measures:
   a. The patient should not share bathroom facilities unless the patient adheres to strict personal hygiene measures.
   b. Individual washcloths, towels, and drinking and eating utensils must be clearly labeled and must not be shared.
   c. Toothbrushes and razors must be labeled and must not be shared.
   d. Frequent handwashing is essential.
2. Emphasize that the person should not prepare food for family members and should not be in the business of handling food.
3. Advise the person not to donate blood.
4. Explain to the person the importance of not taking any drug that is not prescribed by the physician.
5. Encourage the person to gradually return to normal activity, while preventing fatigue.
6. If the person has hepatitis A or B, advise family members to have immunoglobulin injections or vaccinations (Heptavax-B, Recombinant HB)
7. Explain that improvements in water purification and sewage treatment systems are extremely important.
8. Explain that close personal contact such as hugging and kissing are not advisable until hepatitis B surface antigen test results are negative.

Resources Available

1. Persons with hepatitis and their families may obtain more information on infection control from their local health department.
2. Assistance of a home aide may be necessary in the first few weeks after hospital discharge while the person is gradually recovering.
3. Stress the importance of keeping appointments for follow-up care.

13. Public health considerations
    a. During the 1st year after medical diagnosis, patients should carry a medical alert card noting the date of hepatitis onset.
    b. Patients requiring medical or dental care during the 1st year after medical diagnosis should inform health care professionals of the date of onset of hepatitis.
    c. Patients with hepatitis should not donate blood.
    d. High-risk groups such as health care professionals should be vaccinated with hepatitis B immune globulin.
    e. Individuals who have been in direct contact with persons with hepatitis should be given hepatitis B vaccine or gamma globulin as soon as possible.
14. Other types of viral hepatitis are listed in Table 28–5.

Cirrhosis

1. Definition
   a. This chronic liver disease is characterized by a grad-ual, insidious, and progressive degeneration of the liver parenchyma, with diffuse hepatocellular necrosis, widespread hepatic fibrosis, and nodular regeneration.
   b. There are 4 clinically distinct forms of cirrhosis: Laennec's, postnecrotic, biliary, and cardiac (Table 28–6).
2. Incidence and socioeconomic impact
   a. Cirrhosis accounts for more than 26,000 deaths in the United States annually.
   b. Approximately 80 percent of individuals with Laennec's cirrhosis have a history of chronic ingestion of alcohol.
   c. Primary biliary cirrhosis is more common in women than in men.
   d. Postnecrotic cirrhosis is the most common form of cirrhosis worldwide.
3. Risk factors
   • Malnutrition
   • Protein depletion
   • Metabolic disease
   • Drug toxicity

Table 28–5. Other Types of Hepatitis

Type of Hepatitis	Definition	Incidence/Etiology	Clinical Manifestations	Intervention
Alcoholic hepatitis	Either an acute or chronic inflammation of the liver accompanied by parenchymal necrosis as a result of alcohol intoxication	Heavy alcohol ingestion	Anorexia Nausea Abdominal pain Jaundice Hepatomegaly Splenomegaly Anemia Elevated serum bilirubin Ascites Hepatic encephalopathy (in the progressive stage)	Restricted alcohol ingestion High-calorie, high-carbohydrate diet Vitamin supplements, especially folic acid Same as in cirrhosis
Chronic hepatitis	Inflammation of the liver that continues longer than 3–6 months	Hepatitis B, C, or D virus Idiopathic cause Cytomegalovirus infection Common in males	Discomfort in the upper right quadrant of the abdomen Nausea Anorexia Hepatomegaly Elevated aspartate aminotransferase levels	Discontinuation of medications that may be causing the hepatitis Bed rest High-calorie, high-protein, low-fat diet with vitamin supplements Steroids as prescribed
Toxic nonviral hepatitis	Hepatitis following exposure to hepatotoxins	Exposure to drugs such as acetaminophen, chloroform, aspirin, isoniazid, tetracycline, and benzenes Ingestion of *Amanita* mushrooms Occurrence of toxic, nonviral hepatitis dependent on the toxicity of the substance or the genetic makeup of the individual	Fever Arthralgia (joint pains) Increased white blood cell count (especially eosinophils) Fever Elevated liver function tests	Elimination of the causative agent Bed rest High-calorie diet with fats (if not contraindicated) and proteins if hepatic encephalopathy is not present Steroids for hypersensitive reactions

4. Etiology
 • Chronic alcoholism—major cause
 • Hepatitis
 • Biliary obstruction
 • Chronic congestive heart failure
 • Repeated exposure to toxic chemicals

• Metabolic disorders (e.g., Wilson's disease, Budd-Chiari syndrome)
5. Pathophysiology
 a. There is diffuse destruction and regeneration of the liver parenchymal cells.

Table 28–6. Comparison of Different Forms of Cirrhosis

Criteria	Laennec's	Primary Biliary	Postnecrotic	Cardiac
Occurrence	Commonly seen in North America and Western Europe	No specific distribution	Most common form of cirrhosis seen worldwide	Common in individuals with chronic right-sided congestive heart failure
Etiology	Increased alcohol consumption (called alcoholic cirrhosis) Protein malnutrition	Autoimmune mechanism, cholelithiasis, or biliary tumor or atresia (secondary) causing destruction of bile ducts	Viral hepatitis B Ingestion of toxic drugs or chemicals Metabolic disorders	Prolonged constrictive pericarditis Decompensated cor pulmonale Atrioventricular valve disease
Gender differences	More common among males	More common in women between 35 and 65 yr	Males and females equally affected	Males and females equally affected
Major clinical features	Portal hypertension Muscle wasting Jaundice Ascites	Jaundice with pruritus Hepatomegaly Hypercholesterolemia Steatorrhea	Similar to Laennec's cirrhosis	Jaundice Hepatomegaly Ascites

b. The regeneration causes fibrous tissue formation, which causes irregularity in the liver lobules.

c. Eventually nodular formation occurs in the liver, causing compression of blood, lymph, and bile channels.

d. Increased resistance to portal blood flow occurs because of distortion and constriction of the liver lobules.

e. Degeneration and decreased liver functioning occur after prolonged periods of damage and scar tissue formation.

6. Clinical manifestations

a. Abdominal pain

b. Altered hair distribution due to the inability of the liver to detoxify estrogen

c. Altered bleeding tendencies

d. Anemia due to increased destruction of red blood cells as a result of elevated levels of unconjugated bilirubin or, in alcoholic cirrhosis, due to the inability of bone marrow to produce normal red blood cells because alcohol is toxic to the bone marrow

e. Anorexia

f. Ascites due to decreased albumin resulting in decreased vascular colloidal osmotic pressure (see p. 1303), and portal hypertension

g. Asterixis (liver flap or hepatic tremor) due to hepatic encephalopathy caused by formation of toxic products such as ammonia and mercaptans, which interfere with brain metabolism

(1) To identify asterixis, the patient is asked to extend an arm, dorsiflex the wrist, and extend the fingers.

(2) Asterixis is present if rapid nonrhythmic extensions and flexions of the wrist and fingers are present.

h. Caput medusa (dilated abdominal veins) due to the increased congestion in the superficial veins in the abdominal wall caused by the shunting of blood to the umbilical area

i. Chronic dyspepsia (indigestion) due to gas accumulation associated with impaired fat digestion and absorption

j. Constipation or diarrhea

k. Dark or tea-colored urine

l. Edema of extremities due to decreased serum albumin and decreased ability of the liver to metabolize aldosterone

m. Fatigue due to decreased energy reserve as a result of the inability of the liver to metabolize carbohydrate

n. Splenomegaly—enlargement of the spleen secondary to portal hypertension

o. Hepatomegaly due to fat-infiltrating liver cells, causing enlargement; however, the liver decreases in size with progression of hepatocellular necrosis

p. Hypercholesterolemia due to the inability of the liver to metabolize fats

q. Jaundice

r. Musty-sweet breath (fetor hepaticus), which is thought to arise from mercaptans that are absorbed from the gut and are inadequately metabolized

s. Palmar erythema (warm and bright red palms of the hands and soles of the feet) due to high circulating levels of estrogen

t. Portal hypertension due to obstruction in the portal venous system as a result of changes in the hepatic vasculature (see p. 1321)

u. Pruritus due to increased deposits of bile salts in the skin

v. Spider angiomas and telangiectasia due to the formation of collateral blood vessels resulting from obstruction in liver blood flow

w. Testicular atrophy and gynecomastia due to increased conversion of androgens to estrogen, resulting in increased estrogen levels in the blood

7. Diagnostics

a. Laboratory studies reveal bile in the stool; the presence of urobilinogen in the urine; elevated AST, ALT, alkaline phosphatase, serum bilirubin, blood urea nitrogen, serum globulin, serum ammonia; prolonged prothrombin time; decreased fibrinogen level, serum albumin, and platelets.

b. Radiographic studies

(1) Percutaneous transhepatic portography shows portal hypertension.

(2) Endoscopic retrograde cholangiopancreatography shows common bile duct obstruction.

(3) Liver scan shows hepatomegaly early in cirrhosis and hepatoatrophy and splenomegaly in the later stage of cirrhosis.

c. Liver biopsy confirms cirrhosis.

d. Ultrasound shows liver damage.

8. Clinical management

a. Goals of clinical management are to eliminate or relieve causative factors, treat problems that have occurred as a result of liver damage, prevent further liver damage, and provide supportive care.

b. Nonpharmacologic interventions

(1) Bed rest

(2) A high-carbohydrate, low-sodium, low-fat diet with vitamin supplements and with protein content adjusted according to blood urea nitrogen and serum ammonia levels

(3) Monitoring of serum ammonia levels (increasing levels are associated with encephalopathy), prothrombin time, and bilirubin

(4) Observation of bleeding precautions such as use of electric razor in shaving and using a soft-bristled toothbrush for dental care

c. Pharmacologic interventions

(1) Potassium-sparing diuretics such as spironolactone (Aldactone) if ascites is present

(2) Salt-poor albumin to restore plasma volume

(3) Vitamin K to bring prothrombin time close to normal

(4) Vitamin B complex (because the liver cannot synthesize fat-soluble vitamins)

(5) Cautious use of antiemetics, such as dimenhydrinate (Dramamine); these medications often require adequate liver function for detoxification

(6) Lactulose to decrease serum ammonia level and improve encephalopathy

(7) Propranolol (Inderal) to decrease portal pressure in cases of esophageal varices (see p. 1323)

Caution should be used when administering lactulose to older patients because lactulose induces diarrhea. Older people are more prone to fluid imbalances than are young and middle-aged adults because they have less body water and have an altered thirst mechanism that prevents adequate fluid intake. Older patients must be closely monitored for signs of dehydration.

d. Special medical-surgical procedures
  (1) Paracentesis (Procedure 28–2) may temporarily help patients with ascites when the large volume of ascitic fluid compromises breathing, but ascitic fluid tends to reaccumulate. Paracentesis is also a diagnostic tool.
  (2) Le Veen shunt is shown in Figure 28–3.
9. Complications: Table 28–7 describes diagnostics and nursing care for individuals with 1 or more of the common complications of cirrhosis: portal hypertension, ascites, hemorrhage, and hepatic encephalopathy.
10. Prognosis
  a. More than 50 percent of patients die within 5 years of onset, even without complications.
  b. Among patients in whom ascites develops, the mortality rate is 70 to 90 percent within 5 years of onset.
11. Applying the nursing process

NURSING DIAGNOSIS: Impaired gas exchange R/T increased pressure on the diaphragm from ascites

a. *Expected outcomes:* Following intervention, the person should have the following:
  (1) Clear lungs on auscultation
  (2) Adequate oxygenation (demonstrated by blood gases or pulse oximetry)
b. *Nursing interventions*
  (1) Monitor respiratory rate, depth, rhythm, and work of breathing.
  (2) Monitor blood gases or pulse oximetry.
  (3) Assist patient to a comfortable position that maximizes lung expansion.
  (4) Assist physician with paracentesis to relieve pressure on the diaphragm.
  (5) Encourage use of incentive spirometer to maximize lung expansion (see Chapter 22).

NURSING DIAGNOSIS: Altered nutrition, less than body requirements, R/T nausea, vomiting, anorexia, impaired metabolism of nutrients, and impaired storage of vitamins

a. *Expected outcomes:* Following intervention, the patient should be able to do the following:
  (1) Report decreased nausea and vomiting
  (2) Ingest and digest meals to meet prescribed daily caloric requirement

PLACEMENT OF THE LEVEEN SHUNT

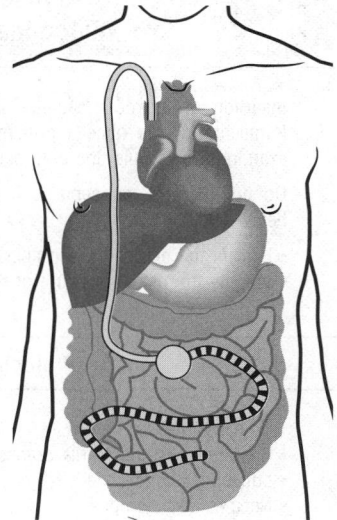

The LeVeen shunt allows for the continuous shunting of ascitic fluid from the abdominal cavity through a 1-way, pressure-sensitive valve into a silicone tube that empties into the superior vena cava.
The valve is implanted while the patient is under anesthesia.

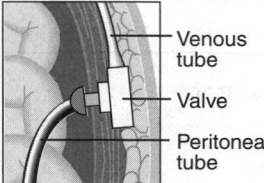

Venous tube
Valve
Peritoneal tube

The 1-way, pressure-sensitive valve opens when the pressure in the abdominal cavity increases to approximately 3 cm of water pressure such as when the diaphragm moves down during inhalation. While the abdominal cavity pressure increases, pressure in the superior vena cava decreases. Because of the decrease in pressure, ascitic fluid enters the venous system via the superior vena cava.

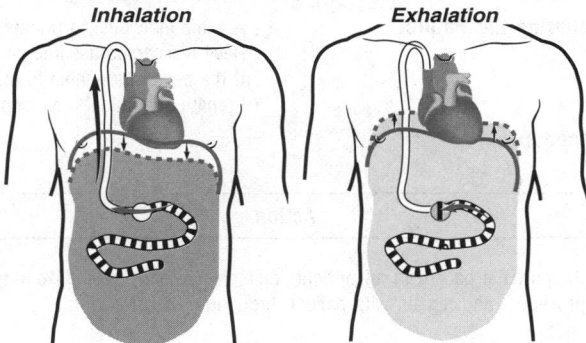

Inhalation   *Exhalation*

During exhalation, the pressure within the abdomen decreases while pressure in the superior vena cava increases, thus closing off the 1-way valve and stopping the flow of ascitic fluid.

Following the procedure, continue to measure abdominal girth, obtain accurate intake and output, administer diuretics as prescribed to facilitate fluid elimination, monitor for signs of congestive heart failure (see Chapter 23), peritonitis, and bleeding, and monitor daily weight to determine if there is any continuing fluid retention.

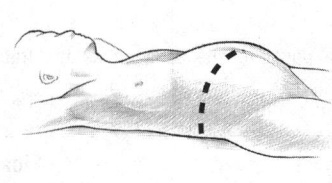

To measure abdominal girth
1 Place the patient supine.
2 Bring the tape measure around the patient.
3 Measure at the largest diameter of the abdomen.
4 Before removing the tape, mark the position of the tape on the patient's flanks and midline to ensure consistent measurement.

Figure 28–3.

Procedure 28–2
Abdominal Paracentesis

Definition/Purpose	Insertion of a trocar catheter into the abdomen to remove and drain ascitic fluid in the peritoneal cavity. Paracentesis was once a primary treatment modality for ascites, but is currently used as a diagnostic tool to examine ascitic fluid and as a palliative measure to relieve abdominal pressure that causes respiratory distress.
Contraindications/Cautions	Do not perform paracentesis if the person has peritonitis, the person is hypovolemic, or the platelet count is below 100,000 units.
Learning/Teaching Activities	• Explain the procedure and answer patient's questions. • Identify the risk and nature of the procedure and ascertain that the person understands them.

Preliminary Activities

Equipment	• Trocar catheter • Sterile gloves and sterile drapes • Local anesthetic • Needles and syringes • Betadine for local skin cleansing • Container for the collected fluid specimen if laboratory tests are ordered • Ascitic fluid collection bottle (regular or vacuum) • Paracentesis tray
Assessment/Planning	• Obtain informed consent. • Know the latest series of vital sign readings for this person. • Measure abdominal girth. • Obtain latest weight.
Preparing the Patient	• Ask the individual to urinate before the procedure to prevent puncturing the bladder. • Have the person assume an upright position at the side of the bed with the feet propped on a stool. • If the person is unable to tolerate sitting position, have the person assume a high Fowler's position. • Prepare abdominal area with Betadine to decrease surface organisms (and thus risk of infection).
Procedure	

Action	Rationale/Discussion
1. Support the patient in an upright (or high Fowler's) position during the procedure and remain with patient throughout the procedure.	1. This position allows the intestine to float posteriorly and helps prevent laceration during catheter insertion. The presence of the nurse provides emotional support to the person.
2. The physician inserts a trocar catheter with a metal guide through an incision made below the umbilicus.	2. The metal guide facilitates the insertion of the catheter into the peritoneal cavity.
3. When the catheter is in place, the physician removes the metal guide and connects the remaining plastic cannula from the trocar to the drainage tube.	3. The trocar allows the removal of the ascitic fluid either by gravity or vacuum.
4. Monitor vital signs at least every 15 minutes during the drainage procedure.	4. Excessive loss of abdominal ascites may cause hypovolemia and precipitate shock. (A drop in blood pressure seen during the initial volume loss is not cause for alarm.) Usually not more than 1000 ml is removed to avoid hypotension.
5. Observe ascitic fluid for color and consistency.	5. Ascitic fluid should be clear and straw-colored. The presence of blood may denote injury during catheter insertion. Cloudy fluid may indicate some pus. Presence of stool may indicate intestinal laceration.
6. Apply a sterile dressing on the puncture site as soon as the trocar catheter is removed.	6. This prevents or decreases the incidence of infection.

Final Activities

1. Measure and document amount of drainage obtained during the procedure on the intake and output sheet.
2. Send specimens for laboratory analysis if ordered. Otherwise, dispose of ascitic fluid properly.

P

Procedure 28-2
(continued)

3. Maintain the person on bed rest until vital signs are stable or have returned to baseline. Pay particular attention to occurrence of hypotension, which can occur as a result of fluid shift from the circulatory system to the peritoneum to replace aspirated ascitic fluid.
4. Monitor the person for electrolyte imbalances, including assessment of the abdominal dressing for excessive fluid leakage that can cause fluid and electrolyte imbalances.

b. *Nursing interventions*
(1) Observe food tolerances and aversions.
(2) Give small, frequent feedings of high-carbo-hydrate, low-sodium, low-protein, and low-fat foods.
(3) Record patient's caloric intake.
(4) Provide oral care frequently and before meals.
(5) Administer prescribed antiemetics before meals.
(6) Provide vitamin supplements as appropriate.

NURSING DIAGNOSIS: Fluid volume excess R/T changes in hydrostatic and oncotic pressures

a. *Expected outcomes:* Following intervention, the patient should exhibit the following:
(1) Balanced intake and output
(2) Decreased edema of the extremities
b. *Nursing interventions*

Table 28-7. *Complications of Cirrhosis and Associated Nursing Care*

Complication	Assessment	Nursing Care
Portal hypertension: Persistent increase in pressure within the portal vein. Develops as a result of increased resistance or obstruction to the flow of blood in the portal vein and its tributaries	Assess abdominal girth for presence of ascites. Assess for presence of caput medusae. Assess for presence of hemorrhoids. Assess for hepatomegaly and splenomegaly.	Monitor the patient for signs of bleeding. Administer propranolol (Inderal) as prescribed to help alleviate portal hypertension. Monitor patient's blood pressure and heart rate closely.
Ascites: Presence of excessive fluid in the peritoneal cavity	Same as in portal hypertension Assess for bleeding tendencies. Assess for fluid and electrolyte imbalance.	Administer sodium supplement (250 to 500 mg of sodium is usually prescribed). Limit fluid intake to 1000 to 1500 ml/day. Administer potassium-sparing diuretic therapy (e.g., spironolactone—Aldactone) as prescribed. If this does not produce adequate fluid loss, furosemide (Lasix) may be ordered. Administer albumin (e.g., salt-poor albumin) as ordered to increase plasma colloid osmotic pressure. Assist in paracentesis (see Procedure 28-2) to remove ascitic fluid. Provide postoperative care following shunt procedure (e.g., Le Veen shunt).
Hemorrhage	Assess patient for petechial hemorrhages in the eye, skin, or mucous membrane (caused by spontaneous rupture of small blood vessels). Assess for presence of ecchymosis. Observe patient for bleeding from the gums after brushing the teeth or from the nose after forceful blowing. Observe presence of blood in the stool and urine.	Administer aqueous solution of vitamin K parenterally as prescribed. Administer fresh-frozen plasma as prescribed to replace clotting factors. Administer blood replacement therapy as prescribed if hemoglobin and hematocrit are critically low.
Hepatic encephalopathy (also called hepatic coma)	Assess for presence of asterixis. Assess for presence of musty-sweet odor from the breath (fetor hepaticus). Observe for neurologic signs and symptoms such as decreased attention span, confusion, slowing of thought processes.	Restrict protein intake. Administer lactulose as prescribed to decrease absorption of ammonia. Administer neomycin as prescribed to decrease ammonia-forming bacteria in the intestine. Implement skin care protocol to prevent breakdown as a result of lactulose-induced diarrhea.

(1) Record the patient's intake and output; weigh the patient daily.
(2) Assess the patient for presence of edema; if present, document its degree and location.
(3) Monitor serum electrolytes (especially sodium and potassium), albumin, and ammonia levels.
(4) Measure abdominal girth to assess ascites and report any changes.
(5) Restrict fluid and sodium intake.
(6) Administer diuretics as prescribed to promote diuresis.
(7) See also Chapter 9.

NURSING DIAGNOSIS: Risk for injury R/T decreased clotting factors and inability to metabolize vitamin K

a. *Expected outcomes:* Following intervention, the patient should do the following:
(1) Be free from bleeding (e.g., hematoma formation or ecchymosis)
(2) Exhibit improved prothrombin time (as close to normal as possible)
(3) Be able to describe and use bleeding precautions
b. *Nursing interventions*
(1) Monitor prothrombin time.
(2) Observe and document the presence of bleeding, including melena and hematemesis.
(3) Monitor hemoglobin and hematocrit.
(4) Avoid use of razor blades and hard-bristled toothbrushes.
(5) Advise patients to avoid straining during bowel movement and to avoid forceful nose blowing.
(6) Avoid giving intramuscular injections.

NURSING DIAGNOSIS: Risk for impaired skin integrity R/T bile salts deposited in the skin, poor nutritional status, compromised immunologic status, and excessive ascites

a. *Expected outcomes:* Following interventions, the patient should be free from the following:
(1) Skin breakdown
(2) Excessive dryness of the skin
b. *Nursing interventions*
(1) Regularly assess skin for breaks and reddened areas.
(2) Reposition the patient frequently to minimize pressure on high-pressure areas.
(3) Keep the patient's fingernails short; consider having the patient wear cloth gloves to minimize scratching.
(4) Avoid use of soap and adhesive tape when possible.
(5) Use gentle rubbing or patting of the skin when pruritus is present.
(6) Administer antipruritic medications and lotions as prescribed.
(7) Use a mattress that allows for capillary–skin interface pressure of 32 mm Hg at most.

(8) Keep skin well lubricated and dry to avoid dermal injury.
12. Discharge planning and teaching
a. Emphasize the importance of adhering to treatment.
b. Provide the patient and family with information on symptoms and signs of impending complications.
c. Provide a list of common foods and their sodium and protein content.
d. If cirrhosis is alcohol related, provide names of support groups and detoxification programs to encourage withdrawal from alcohol.
e. Explain the importance of frequent medical checkups beyond the first year of medical diagnosis.
13. Public health considerations: Both local and national efforts focus on increasing awareness of problems associated with excessive alcohol consumption. Programs may be offered by organizations, businesses, or schools.

Esophageal Varices

1. Definition: Esophageal varices are dilated and tortuous vessels of the esophagus that are at high risk for rupture if portal circulation pressures rise.
2. Incidence and socioeconomic impact: Approximately one third to one half of patients with esophageal varices eventually bleed or hemorrhage.
3. Risk factors
a. Gastric acidity irritation
b. Spasmodic vomiting
c. Excessive alcohol intake
4. Etiology: Varices can be classified according to the point of origin of portal hypertension—prehepatic, intrahepatic, or posthepatic (Table 28–8).

Table 28–8. Etiology of Esophageal Varices

Point of Origin	Possible Cause
Prehepatic	Splenic vein thrombosis
	Portal vein thrombosis
Intrahepatic	Polycystic disease
	Alcoholic hepatitis
	Liver cirrhosis
	Amyloidosis
	Tuberculosis
	Sarcoidosis
	Acute fatty liver of pregnancy
	Schistosomiasis
	Portal hypertension
	Biliary cirrhosis
	Hepatocellular carcinoma
	Increased levels of vitamin A
	Arsenic and copper sulfate poisoning
Posthepatic	Budd-Chiari syndrome
	Constrictive pericarditis
	Congenital malformations and thrombosis of the inferior vena cava
Other	Arteriovenous fistulas in the aortomesenteric or aortoportal areas

5. Pathophysiology
   a. The portal vein delivers approximately 75 percent of the blood to the liver.
   b. Obstruction of blood flow through the liver increases pressure in the portal venous system.
   c. When the gradient between portal venous pressure and inferior vena cava pressure exceeds 10 mm Hg, portal venous blood is directed away from the liver into lower pressure venous beds.
   d. Collateral channels develop around high-pressure areas (e.g., the abdominal wall, rectum, and stomach) to decompress the portal system. Because these collateral channels are fragile and tortuous, they bleed easily.
   e. Increased vascular resistance to portal blood flow results in portal hypertension.
   f. Portal veins become hypertrophied, especially in the submucosa of the lower esophagus.
6. Clinical manifestations
   a. Hematemesis, melena, and tarry stools, all caused by bleeding esophageal varices
   b. Ascites (see p. 1318)
   c. Jaundice
   d. Hepatomegaly (see p. 1318)
   e. Dilated abdominal veins caused by shunting of blood to the umbilical area
   f. Hemorrhoids that result when backflow of blood from the portal system drains into the venous plexus formed by the superior hemorrhoidal veins
   g. Splenomegaly (see p. 1318)
7. Diagnostics
   a. Laboratory tests demonstrate guaiac-positive stools, an abnormal coagulation profile, decreased hemoglobin and hematocrit, and elevated liver function enzymes and serum ammonia.
   b. Angiographic studies, such as splenoportography, hepatoportography, or celiac angiography, show tortuous vessels in the portal venous system.
   c. Abdominal ultrasound identifies disturbance in blood flow in the portal venous system.
   d. Endoscopy confirms the presence of varices.
8. Clinical management
   a. Goals of clinical management are to control bleeding, prevent complications, and avert recurrence of bleeding.
   b. Nonpharmacologic interventions
      (1) The patient should be given nothing by mouth.
      (2) Hemoglobin and hematocrit should be monitored to estimate the amount of bleeding.
      (3) Coagulation factors should be assessed.
      (4) Vital signs and urine output should be monitored to assess fluid volume status. Orthostatic changes in vital signs should be assessed.
      (5) Level of consciousness should be monitored.
   c. Pharmacologic interventions
      (1) Vasopressin (Pitressin) may be given intravenously or by intra-arterial infusion to induce vasoconstriction and reduce bleeding from varices. Because of its potent vasoconstrictive effects, however, it is usually contraindicated in patients with coronary heart disease.
      (2) Nitroglycerine is usually administered in con-

junction with vasopressin because of its systemic vasodilator effect. Nitroglycerine causes vasodilation of the portosystemic collateral blood vessels and simultaneously reduces portal pressure and side effects associated with administration of vasopressin alone.
      (3) Beta-blockers such as propranolol (Inderal) may be used to prevent initial bleeding or recurrence of bleeding and to reduce portal hypertension, but these drugs are not effective during the acute bleeding phase.
      (4) Intravenous fluids are needed to restore fluid volume and electrolyte imbalances when patients are given nothing by mouth. Blood or blood products are given for bleeding varices.
      (5) Oxygen is usually given to prevent hypoxia and maintain adequate blood oxygenation.
   d. Special medical-surgical procedures
      (1) Endoscopic injection sclerotherapy: Through endoscopy, a sclerosing agent such as morrhuate sodium is injected into and around bleeding varices. Complications include chest pain, pleural effusion, perforation of the esophagus, aspiration pneumonia, and esophageal stricture.
      (2) Endoscopic variceal ligation: Through endoscopy, varices are ligated with an elastic rubber band. Sloughing, followed by superficial ulceration, usually occurs in the area of ligation within 3 to 7 days.
      (3) Balloon tamponade (Procedure 28–3): A variety of tubes may be used:
         • Sengstaken-Blakemore tube: a triple-lumen tube with ports for gastric aspiration, inflation of a gastric balloon, and inflation of an esophageal balloon
         • Minnesota tube: a modification of the Sengstaken-Blakemore tube that has 4 lumens, with the additional lumen used to aspirate esophagopharyngeal secretions (making the nasogastric tube unnecessary)
         • Linton tube: a single-lumen tube with 2 ports —esophageal and gastric—for suctioning, is used for gastric tamponade
      (4) Surgically implanted shunts are shown in Figure 28–4.
9. Complications
   a. Variceal bleeding
   b. Hepatic encephalopathy (see Table 28–7)
   c. Hemorrhagic shock
10. Prognosis
   a. The mortality rate with the 1st bleeding episode is 45 to 50 percent, making esophageal varices 1 of the major causes of death for patients with cirrhosis.
   b. Rebleeding occurs in one third of patients with esophageal varices.
   c. Prognosis depends on severity of the underlying liver disease and the course of the bleeding.
11. Applying the nursing process

NURSING DIAGNOSIS: Risk for aspiration R/T hematemesis

a. *Expected outcomes:* Following intervention, the patient should exhibit the following:
  (1) Clear lungs on auscultation
  (2) No signs of respiratory distress
b. *Nursing interventions*
  (1) Monitor vital signs every 5 to 10 minutes during episodes of bleeding.
  (2) Monitor lung sounds.
  (3) Assess for presence of respiratory distress symptoms (e.g., gasping, flaring of the nostrils, and use of accessory muscles of respiration).
  (4) Elevate the head of the patient's bed, if not contraindicated.
  (5) Apply a nasogastric tube (see Chapter 22).

NURSING DIAGNOSIS: Fluid volume deficit R/T bleeding

a. *Expected outcomes:* Following intervention, the patient should do the following:
  (1) Show no signs of active bleeding
  (2) Have approximately equal intake and output
b. *Nursing interventions*
  (1) Monitor hemoglobin, hematocrit, and coagulation profile.
  (2) Maintain an accurate recording of intake and output, and weigh the patient daily.
  (3) Monitor vital signs as often as necessary.

Procedure 28–3
Insertion of Esophagogastric Balloon Tamponade
(Sengstaken-Blakemore Tube, Minnesota Tube, or Linton Tube)

Definition/Purpose	Sengstaken-Blakemore, Minnesota, or Linton tubes are used to apply pressure against the esophageal veins and thus control bleeding in this area.
Contraindications/Cautions	Do not insert an esophagogastric tamponade tube if the person has ulceration or necrosis of the esophagus, with a Salem sump tube if the balloon tamponade used is the Sengstaken-Blakemore or Linton tube, or if the person has had previous esophageal surgery.
Learning/Teaching Activities	• Describe the procedure (regardless of the person's level of consciousness). • Explain that the person will not be able to swallow. • Explain the need for patient restraints to decrease the incidence of pulling out the tube.

Preliminary Activities

Equipment	• Esophagogastric balloon • Salem sump tube • Suction catheters • Sterile gloves • Sphygmomanometer • Football helmet or overbed traction apparatus and 1-pound traction weight • Suction set-up • 50-ml syringe (with catheter tip) • Soft wrist restraint • Hypoallergenic adhesive tape • Gauze • Large scissors • Water-soluble lubricant • Emesis basin • Clamps for the tubing
Assessment/Planning	• Check the patency and integrity of all balloons by inflating and deflating them before insertion. • Identify and label each lumen of a tube to prevent errors in adding or removing pressure and air volume. • Lubricate the entire tube before insertion. • Ensure that a chest radiographic film is immediately available on tube insertion. • Have suction readily available.
Preparing the Patient	• Anesthetize the nose and oropharynx of the patient using a spray anesthesia. • Suction the patient just before tube insertion to clear the oropharynx of secretions. • Place the person in left lateral or semi-Fowler's position. • Administer preinsertion medications ordered (e.g., morphine, Valium).

Procedure

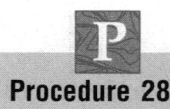

Procedure 28–3

(continued)

Action	Rationale/Discussion
1. The physician gently inserts the esophagogastric tube into the stomach. Inflate the gastric balloon with 50 ml of air upon insertion.	1. The tip of the tube must reach the stomach so that the balloon can be anchored appropriately. Inflating the gastric balloon at this time prevents air leakage.

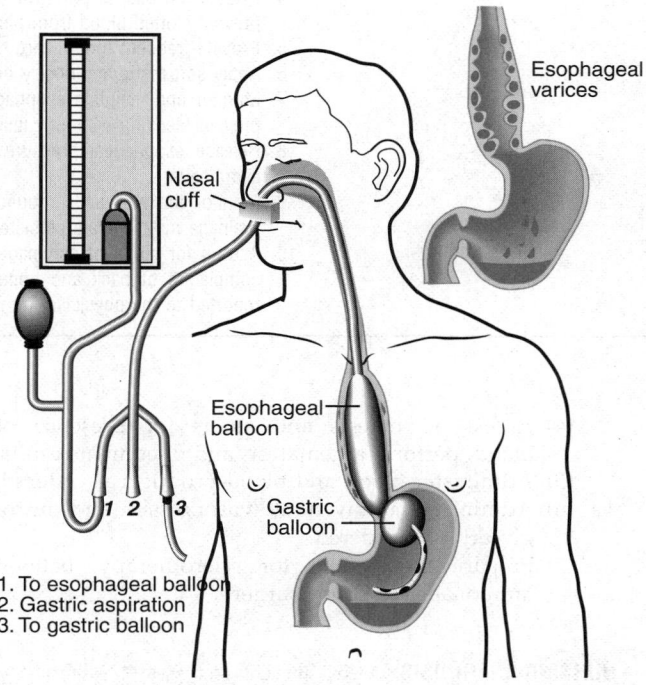

Nasal cuff

Esophageal varices

Esophageal balloon

Gastric balloon

1. To esophageal balloon
2. Gastric aspiration
3. To gastric balloon

Action	Rationale/Discussion
2. Obtain a chest radiographic film immediately upon tube insertion to verify tube placement.	2. Verification of tube placement is crucial before balloon inflation to ensure that the gastric balloon is located in the cardia of the stomach and not in the esophagus (see Figure).
3. After verifying tube position, the physician aspirates and irrigates the stomach.	3. This cleans the stomach and prevents aspiration, occluded airway, and respiratory compromise.
4. Inflate the gastric balloon with a minimum of 150 ml of air to a maximum of 300 ml.	4. This helps anchor the tube and creates tamponading pressure.
5. Assist the physician in securing the tube and applying traction either by taping the tube to the faceguard of a football helmet or by securing it to an overbed traction apparatus and applying a 1-pound traction weight.	5. This provides additional tamponading pressure.
6. Inflate the esophageal balloon to between 20 and 30 mm Hg pressure using a sphygmomanometer.	6. This pressure level prevents rupture of the esophagus from overinflation.
7. Apply a cut gauze sponge around the tube under the patient's nose.	7. This alleviates pressure on the nares and prevents pressure necrosis.
8. Keep the head of the bed elevated once the tube is in place.	8. This position enhances lung expansion and reduces portal blood flow, permitting effective compression of the varices.

Final Activities

1. Double clamp balloon parts to prevent air leaks (which, in turn, keeps the gastric balloon from riding up into the esophagus).
2. Keep scissors at the bedside at all times. Cut the tube and remove it immediatley if signs of respiratory distress occur, as may happen if the gastric tube migrates upward to the esophagus and laryngopharynx causing airway obstruction.

(continued)

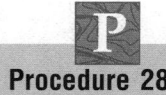

Procedure 28–3

(continued)

Final Activities

3. If a Sengstaken-Blakemore tube or Linton tube is used, insert a Salem sump tube in the esophagus above the inflated balloon to allow for suctioning of secretions that accumulate in the esophagus and oropharynx such as blood and saliva, thus, reducing the risk of aspiration. This is not necessary if a Minnesota tube is used; such a tube has an additional lumen (port) situated above the esophageal balloon to allow suctioning of esophageal secretions.
4. Irrigate the gastric port with room temperature water as frequently as prescribed and connect to suction to prevent clotted blood from plugging the gastric lumen.
5. Provide frequent mouth care to relieve halitosis and discomfort from inability to swallow and mouth breathing.
6. Apply soft restraints loosely on patient's hands if necessary to prevent patient pulling out the tube.
7. Monitor and maintain esophageal balloon pressure between 20 and 25 mm Hg to compress the varices and prevent bleeding without causing overinflation.
8. Release esophageal pressure at specified intervals to minimize incidence of ulceration or necrosis to the esophagus.
9. Monitor the type and amount of drainage coming from the gastric and esophageal ports. Increased bloody drainage may indicate persistent bleeding.
10. Assess for signs of esophageal rupture (e.g., drop in blood pressure, increased heart rate accompanied by complaints of back and upper abdominal pain). Esophageal rupture is a medical emergency and must be reported to the physician immediately.

---

(4) Assess all emesis and stools for presence of blood, perform a hematest, and document results.
(5) Administer blood and blood products as ordered.
(6) Administer intravenous vasopressin and nitroglycerine as ordered.
(7) Prepare the patient for sclerotherapy, balloon tamponade, or shunt surgery.

NURSING DIAGNOSIS: Altered thought processes R/T impairment of the detoxification function of the liver

a. *Expected outcomes:* Following intervention, the patient should exhibit the following:
   (1) Improved level of consciousness
   (2) Decreased serum ammonia level
b. *Nursing interventions*
   (1) Monitor serum ammonia levels.
   (2) Monitor serum electrolyte levels.
   (3) Monitor patient's level of consciousness.
   (4) Restrict the patient's protein intake.
   (5) Avoid giving narcotics, sedatives, and tranquilizers as much as possible.
   (6) Administer medications such as neomycin and lactulose as ordered to reduce intestinal bacterial flora, which is a rich source of nitrogen.
12. Discharge planning and teaching
a. Emphasize the importance of abstaining from alcohol.
b. Encourage wearing a medical alert bracelet.
c. Discuss options for altering lifestyle in the future to avoid further complications.
d. Refer to support groups in the community to help ease the transition of lifestyle.
e. Explain that follow-up endoscopy examinations are

recommended at 6-month intervals to monitor for recurrence of varices.
13. Public health considerations: Efforts focus on increasing the public's awareness of alcohol-related diseases and discouraging the drinking of alcohol.

Fulminant Hepatic Failure

1. Definition
a. Fulminant hepatic failure is a clinical syndrome characterized by sudden clinical and biochemical presence of liver disease or severe impairment of liver function due to massive hepatocellular necrosis in someone with previously normal liver function.
b. Hepatic encephalopathy (hepatic coma) generally develops in patients with fulminant hepatic failure within 8 weeks or less of onset of symptoms. The encephalopathy seen in fulminant hepatic failure is directly attributed to hepatocellular necrosis, unlike the encephalopathy seen in cirrhosis, which is due to increased levels of serum ammonia.
2. Incidence and socioeconomic impact
a. The risk of fulminant hepatic failure developing after acute hepatitis A infection is approximately 1 to 2 percent.
b. Hepatitis B infection, either alone or together with hepatitis D, accounts for more than 50 percent of all cases of fulminant hepatic failure.
c. Hepatitis D alone accounts for approximately 30 percent of all cases of fulminant hepatic failure.
3. Risk factors
a. Reye's syndrome

SURGICAL SHUNT PROCEDURES
used to reduce portal pressure

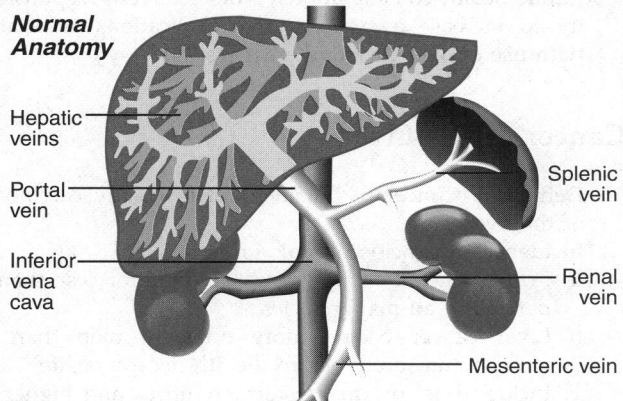

Normal Anatomy

Hepatic veins

Portal vein

Inferior vena cava

Splenic vein

Renal vein

Mesenteric vein

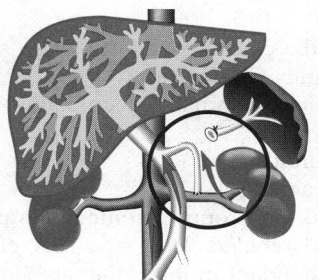

Splenorenal Shunt:
Surgical shunting that involves a splenectomy with anastomosis of the splenic vein to the left renal vein.

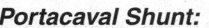

Portacaval Shunt:
Surgical shunting of the blood from the portal system (portal vein) to the venous system (inferior vena cava).

Mesocaval Shunt:
This shunt involves a side anastomosis of the superior mesenteric vein to the proximal end of the inferior vena cava.

Transjugular Intrahepatic Portosystemic Shunt:
A new interventional radiologic surgical procedure that uses the normal vascular anatomy of the liver to create a shunt with the use of a metallic stent. The shunt is between the portal and systemic venous system within the liver and is aimed at relieving portal hypertension. Patients are given intravenous sedation and should be monitored for vital signs and for the presence of arrhythmias.

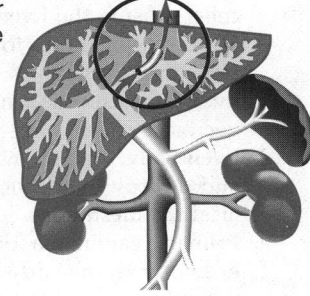

Figure 28–4.

b. Use of drugs such as acetaminophen, isoniazid, rifampin, and halothane
c. Hepatitis B contracted through unprotected sexual activity
d. Exposure to chemicals such as carbon tetrachloride
e. Budd-Chiari syndrome

4. Etiologic factors
   a. Excessive alcohol ingestion
   b. Ingestion of poisonous mushrooms (e.g., *Amanita* mushrooms)
   c. Acute fatty liver of pregnancy
   d. Amebic abscess of the liver
   e. Herpes simplex, cytomegalovirus, or Epstein-Barr virus in immunocompromised patients
   f. Wilson's disease
   g. Idiopathic conditions

5. Pathophysiology
   a. Precipitating factors cause hepatocellular necrosis, leading to loss of the synthetic and excretory functions of the liver.
   b. The inability of the liver to conjugate ammonia causes serum ammonia levels to increase.
   c. The liver also loses the ability to produce adequate quantities of clotting factors.

6. Clinical manifestations
   a. Jaundice
   b. Asterixis (see p. 1318)
   c. Palmar erythema (see p. 1318)
   d. Hepatomegaly during the acute stage (later, the progression of hepatocellular necrosis causes the liver to shrink and become smaller in size)
   e. Positive Babinski's sign due to meningeal irritation caused by hepatic encephalopathy
   f. Loss of mental clarity (ranging from mild confusion and decreased attention to stupor and coma) secondary to hepatic encephalopathy
   g. Hypotension (systolic blood pressure usually less than 90 mm Hg) due to fluid depletion in the intravascular space as a result of decreased colloidal osmotic pressure
   h. Altered bleeding tendencies
   i. Renal failure, probably due to decreased kidney perfusion, resulting in increased renal vascular resistance
   j. Electrolyte disturbances
   k. Hypoglycemia due to the altered metabolic function of the liver, including an inability to produce glucose as needed
   l. Increased susceptibility to infection

7. Diagnostics
   a. Electroencephalogram shows generalized abnormality and slowing.
   b. Laboratory findings are the same as in cirrhosis (see p. 1318)
   c. Radiologic findings are the same as in cirrhosis (see p. 1318)
   d. Spinal tap findings include elevated levels of the amino acid glutamine

8. Clinical management
   a. Goals of clinical management
      (1) Supportive care to deal with complex problems of associated multisystem organ dysfunction

(2) Preparing the patient for liver transplantation, if necessary

b. Nonpharmacologic interventions
   (1) Monitoring serum ammonia levels
   (2) Monitoring serum blood urea nitrogen levels and serum electrolyte levels (especially potassium, calcium, and magnesium)
   (3) Monitoring the patient's level of consciousness
   (4) Monitoring blood gases
   (5) Monitoring the patient for dysrhythmias. Most patients with liver failure exhibit a sinus tachycardia rhythm. Other dysrhythmias (e.g., nonspecific ST segment and T-wave abnormalities) are usually secondary to changes in acid-base balance.
   (6) Monitoring renal function

c. Pharmacologic interventions
   (1) Neomycin is used as an enema to cleanse the bowel and decrease enteric organisms that produce ammonia when they break down nitrogenous substances.
   (2) Lactulose, which is usually given orally or rectally, decreases absorption of bowel ammonia.
   (3) Intravenous fluids are given for fluid resuscitation in the presence of hypotension.
   (4) Electrolyte replacements (e.g., calcium, magnesium) and vitamin K to correct prothrombin time.
   (5) Sucralfate (Carafate) is given prophylactically to prevent gastrointestinal bleeding.

d. Special medical-surgical procedures
   (1) Detoxification of blood, using resins, charcoal, or plasma exchange
   (2) Use of bioartificial liver as a bridge to transplantation to provide missing synthetic and detoxifying liver functions
   (3) Liver transplant, which is the only "cure" for liver failure (see pp. 1330–1332)

9. Complications
   • Portal hypertension
   • Ascites
   • Renal failure
   • Cardiac dysrhythmias
   • Hypovolemic shock
   • Cerebral edema
   • Sepsis
   • Respiratory failure

10. Prognosis depends on the patient's ability to obtain a liver transplant. Moving patients to medical centers that perform such transplantations can increase their chances of a "match." Without a transplant, patients who have fulminant hepatic failure usually die in 1 to 5 weeks.

11. Applying the nursing process: Actions are similar to those for cirrhosis (see pp. 1319–1322)

12. Discharge planning and teaching
   a. Emphasize the importance of adhering to the treatment regimen.
   b. Encourage patient to have frequent medical follow-ups.
   c. Explain the need to avoid excessive use of over-the-counter drugs.
   d. Refer patients to social services, pastoral care, or psychotherapists to address psychologic complications.

13. Public health considerations: Nurses have a responsibility to increase awareness of complications associated with use of over-the-counter drugs.

Cancer of the Liver

1. Definition: Cancer of the liver refers to any carcinoma of the liver.
2. Incidence and socioeconomic impact
   a. Primary hepatic carcinomas account for less than 2 percent of all malignancies.
   b. Liver cancer occurs more often in men than in women and rarely before the 5th decade of life.
   c. Incidence is low in Western countries and higher in South Africa, Asia, and the Pacific Islands.
3. Risk factors
   a. Cirrhosis (especially the postnecrotic form)
   b. Hepatitis B and hepatitis C infection
   c. Hemochromatosis (the abnormal accumulation of iron in the tissues)
   d. Use of androgenic steroids
   e. Type II glycogen storage disease
   f. Ingestion of aflatoxins—a group of compounds produced by the mold *Aspergillus flavus* and *Aspergillus parasiticus*, 2 toxins abundant in foods that are stored under humid conditions, such as bean sprouts and unroasted peanuts
   h. Cigarette smoking (especially when combined with alcohol use)
   i. Exposure to chemicals such as vinyl chloride (used for processing various rubber and plastic products)
   j. Ingestion of nitrosamines (found in smoked meats)
4. Etiology: The exact cause of primary carcinoma of the liver is unknown.
5. Pathophysiology
   a. Primary carcinoma of the liver is rare. Most cancer of the liver occurs because of metastasis. Metastasis to the liver occurs because of the vast capillary circulation in the hepatic region. Malignant cells enter the bloodstream and migrate and lodge within the liver via the portal system, the lymphatic channels, or by direct extension from an abdominal trauma.
   b. As malignant cells grow (whether the original malignant cells in liver cancer are primary or secondary to another carcinoma), they compress the normal liver cells, causing the liver to enlarge.
   c. Cancer cells travel to the vascular bed of the liver, impeding receipt of oxygen and nutrients by the liver, thus, subsequently leading to hemorrhage and necrosis.
   d. Eventually, malignant cells outnumber normal cells and destroy liver function.
6. Clinical manifestations
   a. Primary carcinoma of the liver is difficult to diagnose during the early stages.
   b. Patients may exhibit no symptoms or be extremely ill.

c. Common symptoms of liver cancer include jaundice, weight loss, fatigue, abdominal pain, and presence of a mass on the right upper quadrant of the abdomen.
7. Diagnostics
   a. Serum α-fetoprotein is excreted in patients with carcinoma and serves as a tumor marker.
   b. Liver biopsy confirms the presence of carcinoma and identifies the type of cancer cell.
   c. Other methods of confirming the presence of a tumor in the liver include ultrasound, computed tomography, magnetic resonance imaging, and hepatic scintigraphy.
8. Clinical management
   a. Goals of clinical management are similar to those for cirrhosis (see p. 1318), but with more focus on supportive therapies.
   b. Nonpharmacologic interventions
      (1) Bed rest minimizes metabolic requirements and promotes comfort.
      (2) Diet should be high carbohydrate, high calorie, low fat, low sodium, and low protein.
   c. Pharmacologic interventions
      (1) Chemotherapeutic agents such as doxorubicin (Adriamycin) or 5-fluorouracil
      (2) Pain medications, which, although important, must be used judiciously because they are metabolized in the liver
      (3) Antiemetics for nausea or vomiting
   d. Special medical-surgical procedures
      (1) Liver resection may be done as a palliative measure (usually only when the tumor is confined to 1 lobe). Because the liver has excellent regenerative abilities, up to 90 percent of it can be removed. Survival after liver resection is up to 5 years. Standard postoperative care is necessary after resection of the liver.
      (2) Radiation therapy (see Chapter 17) may be used.
      (3) An intravenous pump may be implanted under the skin of the chest or abdominal wall. It supplies continuous chemotherapy infusion to the liver through the hepatic artery (see Chapter 17). Heparinized saline is used to maintain patency of the pump when chemotherapy is not being administered.
9. Complications
   a. Metastases, which occur primarily to the lung and may also involve the regional lymph nodes, adrenals, bone, kidneys, heart, pancreas, and stomach
   b. Hepatic encephalopathy
10. Prognosis
   a. Patients with carcinoma of the liver have a poor prognosis. Most die within 6 months of medical diagnosis.
   b. Even with surgical removal of the tumor or liver transplantation, the survival rate of patients with carcinoma of the liver remains poor because most patients have advanced cancer before medical diagnosis.
11. Applying the nursing process

NURSING DIAGNOSIS: Fatigue R/T increased metabolic demands

   a. *Expected outcomes:* Following intervention, the patient should do the following:
      (1) Report absence of fatigue
      (2) Describe realistic activities that can be carried out without incurring further increases in metabolic needs
   b. *Nursing interventions*
      (1) Maintain patient on bed rest.
      (2) Provide for a high-calorie, high-carbohydrate diet.
      (3) Coordinate activities to provide for planned periods of rest.
      (4) Encourage the patient to use relaxation tapes and exercises or guided imagery therapy.
      (5) Help the patient to identify priority activities and eliminate or delegate low-priority activities.
      (6) Teach energy conservation techniques such as encouraging small, frequent feedings and frequent rest periods.

NURSING DIAGNOSIS: Anticipatory grieving R/T poor prognosis

   c. *Expected outcomes:* Following intervention, the patient should be able to do the following:
      (1) Openly express feelings of grief (if it is acceptable within the patient's culture)
      (2) Share concerns with family and friends
   d. *Nursing interventions*
      (1) Provide for the patient's expression of grief.
      (2) Encourage the patient to share concerns with family or health care providers.
      (3) Promote family cohesiveness by allowing for increased family interactions.
      (4) Help the patient and family identify their strengths and weaknesses.
      (5) Encourage the patient and family to join support groups and seek emotional and religious support from various sources.
      (6) As appropriate, help the patient and family plan for death (see Chapter 43).

NURSING DIAGNOSIS: Risk for impaired skin integrity R/T bile deposits in the skin (see p. 1322)

12. Discharge planning and teaching
   a. Refer the patient and family to visiting nurses for continuous support.
   b. Provide information on support groups and local hospice organizations.
13. Public health considerations
   a. Coordinate efforts with industries to have high-risk

employees (e.g., those working in rubber and plastic companies) undergo a complete physical yearly.

b. Discourage smoking.

Other Hepatic Disorders

(Table 28–9)

Liver Transplantation

1. Liver transplantation is an accepted therapeutic option for patients with irreversible end-stage liver disease. Indications include the following:
   - Cirrhosis, both primary biliary and alcoholic
   - Sclerosing cholangitis
   - Chronic active hepatitis
   - Confined hepatic malignancy
   - Fulminant hepatic failure
   - Biliary atresia
   - Budd-Chiari syndrome

- Metabolic liver disease (Wilson's disease and Reye's syndrome)

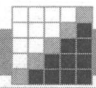
LEGAL AND ETHICAL CONSIDERATIONS

Should people with alcoholic cirrhosis receive liver transplants? This issue is a sensitive one in view of the chronic shortage of transplant organs. Some argue that because alcoholic cirrhosis is a self-induced problem, the relatively few transplantable livers available should not be "wasted" on these patients. Others say that everyone deserves a "second chance." At present, most transplant centers require a 6-month period of abstinence before a patient can become a transplant candidate, although some centers waive this requirement. This ethical dilemma will continue to exist unless the disparity between the number of organs donated for transplant and the number of patients with end-stage organ disease is resolved.

2. Contraindications
   - Metastatic tumors
   - Psychosis
   - Active suicidal thoughts

Table 28–9. *Other Hepatic Disorders*

Hepatic Disorder	Definition	Incidence/Etiology	Clinical Manifestations	Clinical Management
Liver abscess	Abscess formation in the liver secondary to infection	Bacterial infection in the portal vein (usually after bowel perforation) Amebiasis Bacterial cholangitis Diverticulitis Metastatic liver tumor Diabetes mellitus	Pain and tenderness on the right upper quadrant of the abdomen Shoulder pains Nausea and vomiting Hepatomegaly Weight loss Elevated temperature Right pleural effusion (complication of liver abscess because of proximity of liver to right lung) Elevated aspartate aminotransferase, bilirubin, and alkaline phosphatase Blood culture positive for bacterial infection	Drainage of the abscess either percutaneously or surgically Antimicrobial therapy Active pulmonary toilet to prevent complications Monitoring of vital signs (especially temperature and pulse rate) Fluid replacement therapy to prevent dehydration Emotional support for patient and family
Acute fatty liver	Infiltration of lipids in the liver resulting in hepatomegaly, increased firmness, and (eventually) decreased function	Obesity Chronic alcoholism Prolonged use of parenteral nutrition Diabetes mellitus Malnutrition Pregnancy Cushing's syndrome	Usually asymptomatic in mild cases Anorexia Jaundice Abdominal pain Elevated serum bilirubin and alkaline phosphatase	Providing adequate nutrition Counseling patient on proper diet Maintaining metabolic balance Emotional support for patient and family before, during, and after diagnostic procedures
Liver trauma	Blunt or penetrating injuries to the liver causing hemorrhage or laceration.	Knife wounds to the abdomen Gunshot wound to the abdomen Injuries from steering wheel or fall, or other crush injuries	Pain Hemorrhage Liver hematomas	Monitoring vital signs (especially blood pressure and heart rate Control of bleeding Débridement of hematoma Monitoring for postoperative complications such as peritonitis and liver abscess

• Active substance abuse or dependence
• History of serious noncompliance

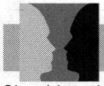

CLINICAL CONTROVERSIES

Should patients with active hepatitis receive transplants? Or are the associated increases in morbidity and mortality enough to justify such procedure? The main factors contributing to increased morbidity and mortality are recurrence of hepatitis associated with bacterial and fungal sepsis. In 1986, Demetris and colleagues reported 1- and 3-year survival rates of 57% and 40%, respectively, in patients with positive serology for hepatitis B surface antigen. In addition, reports of the use of hepatitis B hyperimmunoglobulin to prevent and control graft reinfection with hepatitis B virus are conflicting. Mora and colleagues reported that passive immunization with hepatitis B hyperimmunoglobulin did not affect the rate of recurrence of hepatitis.

3. Preoperative nursing care
   a. Ascertain medical necessity.
      (1) Liver function tests, quantitative assessment of liver metabolism and clearance, may be done to determine functional hepatocyte mass and, thus, hepatic reserve.
      (2) A useful test to assess liver metabolism and clearance is measurement of galactose elimination capacity (obtained by calculating the maximal removal rate of galactose by the liver).
   b. Determine psychologic suitability.
      (1) Personal and family life are important considerations. The patient should have a good support system so that recovery can be optimized.
      (2) Some psychiatric disturbances may be absolute contraindications to transplantation.
   c. Determine physiologic suitability.
      (1) Extrahepatic disease may contraindicate transplantation.
      (2) Blood and tissue must be typed for appropriate matching of donor and recipient.
   d. Patients approved to receive a transplant are placed on the United Network for Organ Sharing waiting list with information regarding blood type and organ size.
4. There are 2 types of operative approaches to liver transplantation: orthotopic and heterotopic.
   a. Orthotopic transplantation, which is the removal of the diseased liver before the new one is transplanted, is the most common.
   b. In heterotopic transplantation, the diseased liver is left in place and the new one is transplanted.
   c. The actual liver transplant procedure takes between 8 and 16 hours; total surgery time is up to 22 hours.
   d. During transplantation, surgeons complete five anastomoses between the recipient and donor organs: at the suprahepatic inferior vena cava, infrahepatic vena cava, portal vein, hepatic artery, and biliary tract (may involve end-to-end anastomosis between the donor and recipient common bile duct or anastomosis between the donor common bile duct and the recipient jejunum).
5. Postoperative nursing care (see pp. 1332–1333)
   a. In the immediate postoperative period, while the patient is in the critical care unit, the nurse should do the following:
      (1) Assess cardiovascular and hemodynamic status to ascertain early changes in cardiac and circulatory status
      (2) Assess the patient for signs of bleeding
      (3) Assess the patient for functional liver graft (bile characteristics, coagulation times, liver function tests, serum bilirubin)
      (4) Monitor the patient for respiratory compromise and wean the patient from mechanical ventilation (see Chapter 22). Patients are usually extubated after 24 hours if there are no complications.
      (5) Assess for patency of wound drains
      (6) Administer medications and otherwise assist the patient in pain management
   b. During the recovery period, the nurse should do the following:
      (1) Monitor liver function
      (2) Monitor the patient for respiratory complications
      (3) Continue pain management
      (4) Provide adequate nutrition
      (5) Initiate physical therapy as soon as possible
      (6) Continue monitoring wound drains
      (7) Follow immunosuppressive protocols (Table 28–10)

DRUG ADVISORY

Two of the most dangerous side effects of cyclosporine are renal failure and seizures. Because both of these side effects are dose related, drug levels must be monitored in the first week following transplantation and dosage adjusted according to these levels. After the first week, drug levels should still be monitored, but less frequently. Because the toxicity of cyclosporine is dose related, if patients develop seizures or extreme elevations in blood urea nitrogen and creatinine, the drug dose must be lowered.

6. Complications
   a. Infection, which is the primary threat to graft and patient survival
   b. Rejection, which is a T-cell–mediated response (Table 28–11) that usually occurs within the 4th to the 10th postoperative day. Liver biopsies are used to diagnose rejection. Symptoms of rejection:
      • Decreased flow of bile
      • Colorless instead of yellow bile
      • Jaundice
      • Increased prothrombin time
      • Fever
      • Tachycardia
      • Right lower quadrant or flank pain
      • Increased serum bilirubin
      • Increased in ALT, AST, and alkaline phosphatase
   c. Acute renal failure
   d. Hemorrhage
   e. Pancreatic complications (pancreatic pseudocysts and pancreatic fistulas)
   f. Common bile duct obstruction
7. Applying the nursing process

Table 28–10. Immunosuppressive Agents Commonly Used Following Liver Transplantation*

Agent†	Action	Side Effects	Nursing Care
Cyclosporine A (Sandimmune)	Suppresses helper and cytotoxic T cells with minimal effect on B lymphocyte	Hypertension Renal failure Hyperkalemia Seizures Increased susceptibilty to infection	Monitor blood pressure. Assess for complications of hypertension (e.g., headaches, dizziness, and vision changes). Monitor serum potassium level. Monitor urine output. Monitor serum blood urea nitrogen and creatinine. Monitor drug level (seizures are related to high drug levels).
Prednisone (corticosteroid)	Reduces accumulation of macrophages and leukocytes Inhibits phagocytosis and lysosomal enzyme release Reduces neutrophil and monocyte response Reduces T lymphocytes, monocytes, and eosinophils	Peptic ulcer Sodium and water retention Hyperglycemia Delayed wound healing Mood disturbances Increased susceptibilty to infections	Provide low-salt diet. Monitor serum glucose. Monitor wound sites and report any signs of infection. Monitor blood pressure. Monitor for signs of bleeding ulcer (e.g., hematemesis or tarry stools). Instruct patient to report epigastric pain. Monitor patient's weight.
Azathioprine (Imuran)	Blocks DNA synthesis, thus preventing the rapid cell division that accompanies the immune response. Other rapidly dividing cells are also affected, leading to bone marrow suppression.	Thrombocytopenia Increased susceptibilty to infection Nausea and vomiting Increased risk of neoplasms	Monitor for signs of bleeding due to decreased platelet count. Monitor white blood cell count (the basis for drug dosage). Same as for cyclosporine A.

* Immunosuppressant regimens following liver transplantation vary considerably with respect to specific drugs and dosages, and from one institution to another; however, the usual regimen consists of either the double- or triple-therapy approach. Double-therapy immunosuppression consists of loading and maintenance doses of cyclosporine and corticosteroid. Triple-therapy immunosuppression includes the addition of azathioprine.

† New transplant drugs in various stages of experimental and clinical trials are cyclosporine G, OKT4, FK-506 (Prograf).

NURSING DIAGNOSIS: Ineffective breathing pattern R/T postoperative pain (see Chapter 22)

a. *Expected outcomes:* Following intervention, the patient should exhibit the following:
(1) Respiratory rate and oxygenation within the patient's normal limits
(2) Clear lungs on auscultation

b. *Nursing interventions*
(1) Monitor oxygenation through pulse oximetry.
(2) Administer pain medications as often as needed so that pain does not become so severe that it interferes with normal breathing.
(3) Assist the patient with progressive ambulation and in assuming a position to maximize lung expansion.
(4) Encourage the use of incentive spirometry.
(5) Encourage deep breathing and coughing exercises as often as necessary while the patient is awake.

Table 28–11. Types of Rejection Seen Following Organ Transplantation

Type*	Occurrence	Treatment
Hyperacute	During surgery, immediately after donor organ is transplanted and while circulation is being established	Remove transplanted organ. Retransplant with new organ (if available) or return patient to United Network for Organ Sharing waiting list.
Accelerated	Within 1 to 5 days after transplantation	Same as for hyperacute.
Acute	Within 7 to 14 days after transplantation	Increase dosage of immunosuppressive agents. Continue to monitor for signs of rejection. Monitor for signs of renal failure (most immunosuppressive agents are nephrotoxic). Administer OKT3 (a monoclonal antibody preparation) for additional immunosuppression.
Chronic	Months to years after transplantation	Patient may require retransplantation.

* Both hyperacute and accelerated types of rejection are rare in patients receiving liver transplant.

NURSING DIAGNOSIS: Risk for infection R/T immunosuppressive therapy and surgical procedure

c. *Expected outcomes:* Following intervention, the patient should exhibit the following:
  (1) Absence of wound infection and signs of rejection
  (2) Normal wound healing
d. *Nursing interventions*
  (1) Assess the wound for signs of infection.
  (2) Assess skin for breakdown and institute skin care protocol.
  (3) Provide mouth care as often as possible to prevent bacterial growth.
  (4) Use aseptic technique when handling drains and in changing dressings.
  (5) Administer antibiotics as prescribed.

NURSING DIAGNOSIS: Fluid volume excess or deficit R/T perioperative or postoperative imbalance

e. *Expected outcomes:* Following intervention, the person should exhibit the following:
  (1) Intake that approximates output
  (2) Normal skin turgor
f. *Nursing interventions*
  (1) Monitor urine output and drainage tube output, and accurately record intake and output.
  (2) Monitor serum sodium and potassium.
  (3) Weigh the patient daily.
  (4) Administer diuretics as prescribed.
  (5) Assess hydration status such as examining the skin turgor and the presence of peripheral edema.

NURSING DIAGNOSIS: Pain R/T surgical procedure (see Chapter 11)

8. Discharge planning and teaching
  a. Keep the patient well informed. The patient's survival depends largely on an understanding of the illness and treatment regimen.
  b. Teach the patient the signs and symptoms of rejection, including subtle signs such as fever. Stress the need to notify a nurse or physician immediately if these occur.
  c. Discuss the medications the patient will need. Emphasize the importance of taking immunosuppressive medication without fail. Develop a schedule for taking these medications. Teach the patient to self-administer medications.
  d. Explain the need for the patient to limit activities until fully recovered and to avoid people with infections (including colds and flu) that can be life threatening to persons with immunocompromised systems.
  e. Advise the patient to wear a medical alert bracelet.

  f. Schedule clinic visits, and emphasize the importance of keeping follow-up appointments.

◨ CARING FOR PEOPLE WITH BILIARY DISORDERS

Cholecystitis

1. Definition: Cholecystitis is inflammation of the gallbladder wall, which can be acute or chronic.
2. Incidence and socioeconomic impact
  a. Approximately 90 percent of cases of cholecystitis are caused by gallstones.
  b. The acalculous type accounts for approximately 4 to 8 percent of all cases of acute cholecystitis.
  c. Acute cholecystitis can affect any age group.
  d. Chronic cholecystitis primarily affects middle-aged and obese older women.
  e. Incidence of chronic cholecystitis has a female to male ratio of 3:1.
  f. A higher incidence of cholecystitis is seen among individuals with a sedentary lifestyle.
  g. Italian, Jewish, and Chinese ethnic groups are predisposed to cholecystitis.
3. Risk factors
  a. In acute cholecystitis, risk factors are the following:
    • Gallstones
    • Sepsis due to invasion by bacteria (usually *Escherichia coli*, salmonella, or streptococcus) via the lymphatic or vascular route
    • Abdominal surgery for adhesions
    • Trauma
    • Multiple childbirth
    • Prolonged anesthesia
    • Prolonged dehydration
    • Long-term dietary fasting
    • Prolonged immobility
    • Excessive narcotic use
    • Familial tendency to biliary disease
    • Insulin-dependent diabetes
    • Cholelithiasis (calculous type)
  b. In chronic cholecystitis, risk factors are the following:
    • Cholelithiasis
    • Obesity
    • Acute cholecystitis
4. Etiology: The exact etiology of cholecystitis is unknown.
5. Pathophysiology
  a. Acute cholecystitis
    (1) Normal flow of bile from the gallbladder to the duodenum is obstructed by gallstones, trauma, or other factors. Venous return is also impeded, resulting in vascular congestion.
    (2) Edema occurs, causing further congestion and progression of the inflammatory process.
    (3) When the trapped bile is reabsorbed, it acts as a chemical irritant to the gallbladder wall, producing an inflammatory effect.
    (4) The presence of bile, in combination with im-

paired circulation, edema, and distention, causes ischemia of the gallbladder wall, resulting in tissue sloughing with necrosis and gangrene.

    (5) Perforation of the gallbladder wall may occur. If the perforation is small and localized, an abscess may form.

  b. Chronic cholecystitis

    (1) Persistent inflammation of the gallbladder wall results in a fibrotic and contracted gallbladder.

    (2) This fibrosis impairs the ability of the gallbladder to concentrate bile. Even more important, the fibrosis decreases gallbladder motility, which, in turn, leads to ineffective bile emptying.

6. Clinical manifestations

  a. In acute cholecystitis, manifestations are the following:

    • Abdominal pain, especially in the right upper quadrant and epigastric area

    • Nausea and vomiting

    • High-grade fever due to gallbladder inflammation

    • Positive Murphy's sign (see p. 1306)

    • Flatulence and eructation (belching) because of gas accumulation resulting from impaired fat digestion and absorption

  b. In chronic cholecystitis, manifestations are the following:

    • Vague and nonspecific abdominal pains

    • Low-grade fever

    • Jaundice

    • Clay-colored stools

    • Steatorrhea (presence of fat in the stool) resulting from the same causes as flatulence in acute cholecystitis

7. Diagnostics

  a. Laboratory tests demonstrate elevated AST, alkaline phosphatase, lactate dehydrogenase, white blood cell count, and serum bilirubin (both conjugated and unconjugated).

  b. Gallbladder ultrasound confirms presence of gallbladder inflammation.

  c. Hepatobiliary imaging shows gallbladder inflammation; oral cholecystogram images are poor.

8. Clinical management

  a. Goals of clinical management

    (1) Provide pain relief through dietary restrictions

    (2) Relieve biliary obstruction

    (3) Prevent gallstone formation

  b. Nonpharmacologic interventions

    (1) A low-fat diet to decrease stimulation of the gallbladder

    (2) Weight reduction, including a prescribed diet and exercise program

    (3) Intravenous fluids for patients given nothing by mouth

    (4) Monitoring of serum bilirubin

    (5) Assessment for abdominal guarding and rigidity, two reliable indicators of peritoneal irritation

  c. Pharmacologic interventions

    (1) Anticholinergics such as propantheline bromide (Pro-Banthine) to relax the smooth muscles and prevent biliary contraction

    (2) Narcotic analgesics such as meperidine to relieve pain and decrease incidence of spasms

    (3) Antiemetics such as prochlorperazine (Compazine) to provide relief from nausea and vomiting

    (4) Oral gallstone-dissolving drugs such as chenodeoxycholic acid for patients with cholelithiasis

  d. Special medical-surgical procedures

    (1) Nastrogastric intubation to decompress the stomach for severe nausea and vomiting

    (2) Cholecystectomy

    (3) Insertion of a T tube following cholecystectomy (Fig. 28–5)

9. Complications

  • Pancreatitis

  • Cholangitis

  • Peritonitis

10. Prognosis: Most patients with cholecystitis make a full recovery, but they should maintain dietary restrictions (low fat intake) for pain control.

11. Applying the nursing process

NURSING DIAGNOSIS: Fluid volume deficit R/T vomiting or nasogastric suction

  a. *Expected outcomes:* Following intervention, the patient should exhibit the following:

    (1) Moist mucous membranes

    (2) Normal skin turgor

    (3) Urine output greater than 30 ml per hour

  b. *Nursing interventions*

    (1) Carefully document intake and output and daily weights.

    (2) Monitor serum electrolyte levels.

    (3) Assess the patient for signs of dehydration.

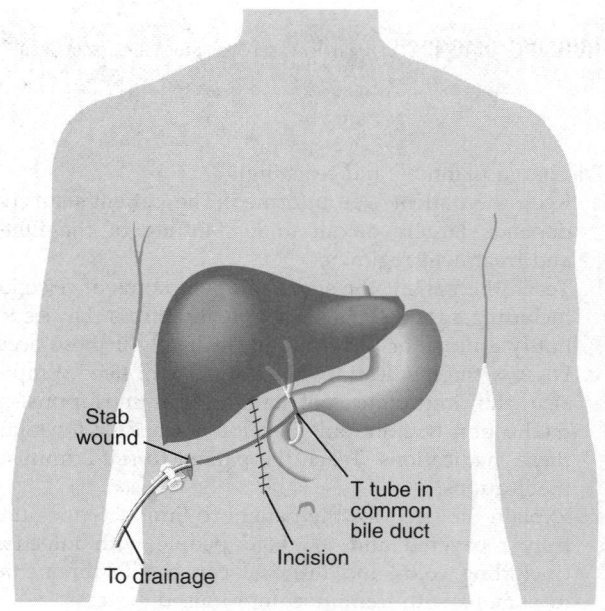

Figure 28–5. T-tube placement.

LEARNING/TEACHING GUIDELINES
for Self-Care Following Conventional Cholecystectomy

General Overview

1. Describe the disease process and the importance of leaving the T tube in place for a period of days.
2. Emphasize the importance of returning for a follow-up cholangiogram as instructed.
3. Refer the patient to a home-care agency as needed.

Diet

1. Stress the importance of limiting fat intake.
2. To achieve a general decrease in dietary fat, instruct the person to:
   a. Avoid sauces, gravies, and fatty meats.
   b. Avoid using cream and eating rich desserts.
   c. Broil or grill foods instead of frying.
3. Provide the person with an American Diabetes Association Fat Portion Exchange List.

Wound Care

1. Instruct the person to wear loose fitting clothing to prevent wound irritation.
2. Explain the importance of taking showers and avoiding baths to prevent bacterial infection of the open wound.
3. Emphasize the importance of reporting presence of redness, swelling, or pain in the wound area, because these are the early signs of infection.
4. Instruct the person to report wound drainage if it increases, becomes purulent or foul-smelling, because these are signs of infection.
5. Instruct the person to avoid lifting heavy objects to prevent straining the wound.
6. Instruct the person to avoid driving for at least 6 weeks after surgery to prevent unnecessary pressure or strain on the wound.

Care of T Tube

1. Emphasize the importance of keeping the T tube drainage bag below the level of the suture line to prevent the backflow of bile.
2. Demonstrate how to change the dressing around the T tube and instruct the person to change the dressing at least daily to prevent infection.
3. Have the person give a return demonstration.
4. Emphasize the importance of attaching the T tube to the abdomen or clothing using a tape or other fastener to prevent pull on the tube from the weight of the drainage.
5. Instruct the person to keep the T tube free of kinks to prevent reflux of bile.
6. Advise the person to expect possible bile leakage and select clothing that can easily be washed to remove any stains.
7. Demonstrate the correct procedure for opening and emptying the T-tube drainage bag.
8. Have the person give a return demonstration.
9. Advise the person to empty the T-tube drainage bag at the same time each day.

---

      (4) Administer intravenous fluids and antiemetics as ordered.
12. Other nursing diagnoses
   • Pain (see Chapter 11)
   • Ineffective breathing pattern related to pain (see p. 1332).
13. Discharge planning and teaching

NURSE ADVISORY

> Most biliary disorders are the consequence of lifestyle. Thus, nurses need to assess each patient's lifestyle before devising a discharge teaching plan. The best opportunity to explain the risks of detrimental lifestyles and their relationship to biliary disease (especially gallstone formation) is while providing discharge instructions.

   a. Assess the living environment regarding the patient's ability to procure and prepare foods.
   b. Meet with patient and family to discuss activity restrictions.
   c. Recommend a low-fat diet and continuation of a weight reduction regimen.
   d. Discuss care of the T tube, if appropriate (Learning / Teaching Guidelines for Self-Care Following Conventional Cholecystectomy).
   e. Discuss wound care and follow-up appointments with postoperative patients.
14. Public health considerations
   a. Screening programs that check blood cholesterol levels can detect cholecystitis.
   b. Primary prevention focuses on effects of fatty foods and the importance of dietary restrictions, especially for high-risk groups.
   c. Businesses should be encouraged to offer their employees health promotion programs that include diet and exercise regimens.

Cholelithiasis

1. Definition
   a. Cholelithiasis is the formation or presence of stones

or calculi in the gallbladder. Gallstone formation takes place in the gallbladder, the common bile duct, and the duodenum.

  b. Types of gallstones

    (1) Cholesterol gallstones contain at least 50 percent cholesterol by weight.

    (2) Pigment gallstones are made up of bile pigments and are caused by increased production and excretion of bilirubin or stasis of bile such as in cirrhosis, hemolysis, and infections of the biliary tree.

2. Incidence and socioeconomic impact

  a. Twenty to 25 million Americans have gallstones, with approximately 1 million new cases being diagnosed each year.

  b. Cholelithiasis is 3 to 4 times more common in women than in men until women reach menopause, then differences in occurrence decrease.

  c. Incidence of cholelithiasis is higher among Native Americans and Whites than among Asians and Blacks.

  d. Cholesterol gallstones represent 70 to 80 percent of stones found in Americans and are more common than pigment gallstones.

3. Risk factor

  a. Aging: Cholesterol gallstones are rare before the age of 20 years and increase in prevalence with each successive decade.

  b. Gender: Women are twice as likely as men to have gallstones. Use of birth control pills further increases the risk of cholesterol gallstone formation due to increased biliary cholesterol saturation.

  c. White race

  d. Factors that alter sterol metabolism—obesity, prolonged periods of weight loss (especially from fad diets), bile acid malabsorption, and ingestion of a combination of antihyperlipoproteinemic drugs such as clofibrate (Atromid-S)

4. Etiology: The exact etiology of gallstone formation is unknown, but it appears to arise secondary to alteration in lipid metabolism.

5. Pathophysiology (Fig. 28–6)

  a. Gallstones form when the bile in the gallbladder or common bile duct becomes supersaturated with cholesterol.

  b. Cholesterol monohydrate crystals nucleate and precipitate. These crystals then begin to increase in size, joining together to form macroscopic cholesterol gallstones.

  c. Less is known about the formation of pigment gallstones.

6. Clinical manifestations

  a. Intolerance to fatty foods

  b. Nausea with or without vomiting

  c. Pain or discomfort in the right upper quadrant of the abdomen, occasionally radiating to the chest

  d. Positive Murphy's sign (see p. 1306)

  e. Low-grade fever due to gallbladder inflammation

  f. Steatorrhea (see p. 1334)

  g. Clay-colored stools, dark-colored urine, or jaundice caused by obstructed bile ducts

7. Diagnostics

  a. Elevated serum levels of unconjugated bilirubin occur especially in patients with pigment gallstones.

  b. Computed tomography scan, abdominal ultrasound, cholecystogram, or cholangiography detects the presence of gallstones.

  c. Hepatobiliary imaging visualizes any pathologic condition in the bile ducts.

  d. Cholescintigraphy confirms the presence of gallstones.

8. Clinical management

  a. Goals of clinical management

    (1) Asymptomatic cases are treated conservatively with dietary restrictions.

    (2) Treatment of symptomatic cases focuses on relieving the symptoms, which usually requires removal of the gallstones.

  b. Nonpharmacologic interventions

    (1) Bed rest

    (2) Nothing by mouth and insertion of a nasogastric tube for symptomatic patients

    (3) Low-fat diet for patients who are able to eat

  c. Pharmacologic interventions

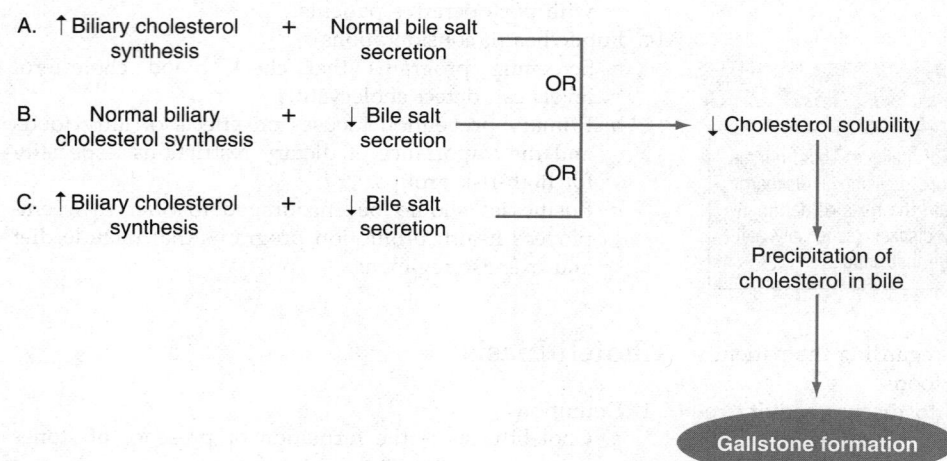

Figure 28–6. The exact mechanism of cholesterol gallstone formation is unknown. This illustration shows the possible abnormalities that would predispose a person to cholesterol gallstone formation. The common mechanisms identified here are (*A*) increased biliary synthesis, (*B*) decreased biliary salts, and (*C*) a combination of both. Bile salts are responsible for increasing the solubility of cholesterol. Thus, decreased level of bile salts available in the bile would increase the change of cholesterol precipitation.

(1) Intravenous fluids rehydrate patients who are vomiting and receive nothing by mouth.

(2) Antiemetics are given for persistent vomiting.

(3) Antispasmodics relieve colic.

(4) Analgesics relieve pain. (Demerol does not produce spasms of the sphincter of Oddi as opiates do.)

d. Special medical-surgical procedures (Table 28–12)

Table 28–12. Nursing Care of Patients Undergoing Medical-Surgical Procedures for Cholelithiasis

Procedure	Patient Preparation Nursing Care	Complications
Dissolution therapy	No preprocedural preparation is needed. To decrease the incidence of nausea, discontinue contact solvent infusion during meals. Provide bland diet to help relieve nausea. Administer antiemetics if gastric symptoms continue despite nonpharmacologic measures. Administer antidiarrheal medications if necessary.	Nausea and vomiting Diarrhea Anorexia Abdominal pain Gastritis Liver damage
Endoscopic sphincterotomy	Give patient nothing by mouth (NPO) at least 6 hr before the procedure. Administer prophylactic antibiotics as prescribed. Following the procedure, keep patient NPO until gag reflex returns. With return of gag reflex, start patient on liquid diet and progress to regular low-fat diet. Maintain patient on bed rest at least 6 hr after the procedure. Monitor for signs of bleeding (e.g., tarry stools, hematemesis). Administer pain medication as prescribed.	Pancreatitis Perforation of the duodenum Bleeding
Extracorporeal shock-wave lithotripsy	Administer medications the evening before the procedure as prescribed to decrease gas in the intestine (gas interferes with shock waves). Keep patient NPO at least 6 hr before the procedure to decrease risk of vomiting. Insert intravenous line before the procedure to facilitate medication administration. Monitor patient closely throughout the procedure. Instruct patient to expect transient gross hematuria after the procedure. Adminster pain medication as prescribed after the procedure (patients usually experience right upper quadrant pain). Provide instructions on adjuvant oral bile acid therapy as prescribed. Instruct patient to report signs of fever, persistent hematuria, abdominal pain, severe nausea, and vomiting. Schedule patient for return visit.	Damage to the gallbladder and surrounding tissues Acute cholecystitis Obstruction of bile duct by stone fragments Pancreatitis Recurrence of stone formation
Laparoscopic laser cholecystectomy	Provide standard preoperative preparation for procedures done under general anesthesia. After surgery, encourage patient to ambulate as soon as possible. When gag reflex returns, start patient on liquids and progress to regular low-fat diet. Assist patient in pain management. If diaphragmatic irritation occurs, place patient on left side with the right knee and thigh drawn up toward chest and left arm along the back. This position helps move the gas pocket away from the diaphragm. Check incision site for bleeding.	Bleeding Peritonitis Irritation of the diaphragm (due to incomplete release or absorption of carbon dioxie)
Abdominal cholecystectomy	Provide standard preoperative preparation for procedures done under general anesthesia. Provide aggressive pulmonary care following surgery (breathing tends to be shallow because of the effect of anesthesia and incisional pain). Secure T tube and collection drainage to avoid dislodgment. Monitor drainage from the T tube. Monitor for signs of bleeding (e.g., excessive sanguineous drainage on the dressing). Provide pain relief. Initiate progressive ambulation. When gag reflex returns, start patient on clear liquids and progress to regular low-fat diet. Perform progressive clamping of T tube as prescribed.	Recurrence of stone formation Peritonitis Bleeding Wound infection Respiratory problems
Percutaneous cholecystolithotomy	Same as in laparoscopic cholecystectomy. Start adjuvant oral bile acid therapy as prescribed.	Bleeding Recurrence of gallstones Peritonitis

(1) Dissolution therapy
  • One form of this therapy uses contact solvents (e.g., monooctanoin) that chemically react with cholesterol gallstones on contact, causing the gallstones to dissolve. Contact solvents are usually infused through a nasobiliary tube for 1 to 3 weeks. During the infusion, cholangiography is done every 3 days to monitor the dissolution of the stones.

 CLINICAL CONTROVERSIES

Research is being done on the direct instillation of methyl tertiary butyl ether (MTBE), a contact solvent, into the gallbladder, either through a transhepatic catheter or a nasobiliary catheter. Once the catheter is inserted, the bile is aspirated from the gallbladder and methyl tertiary butyl ether is instilled. After several minutes, methyl tertiary butyl ether is withdrawn and a fresh solvent is instilled. This procedure is done under flouroscopic guidance. Early reports show that stone dissolution is complete with this form of therapy. In comparing the transhepatic or nasobiliary catheter insertion approach, the nasobiliary method appears advantageous because it dissolves gallstones faster and requires less patient preparation.

  • Another type of dissolution therapy uses bile acids such as chenodeoxycholic acid or ursodeoxycholic acid. Oral bile acids facilitate the gradual dissolution of cholesterol gallstones by decreasing the amount of cholesterol in the bile and increasing cholesterol solubility. Oral bile acid therapy is used primarily for patients who are poor surgical risks or as prophylaxis against formation of new calculi in patients with recurrent cholecystitis. Oral bile acids interfere with the action of oral contraceptives.
(2) Extracorporeal shock-wave lithotripsy is a noninvasive procedure that uses high-energy or high-pressure sound waves to break gallstones into small fragments so that they can pass through the common bile duct into the duodenum. Stone fragments may also be removed by endoscopy or may be dissolved with oral bile acid or solvents.
(3) In laparoscopic laser cholecystectomy, a laparoscope is inserted, usually below the umbilicus after insufflation with carbon dioxide. Cholecystectomy is then performed through the laparoscope, guided by the image projected on the video monitor.
(4) In abdominal cholecystectomy, the surgeon works through a high right subcostal incision and excises the gallbladder and ligates the cystic duct. Drain options include a Penrose drain in the wound (see Chapter 22) and a T tube (see Fig. 28–6) inserted into the common bile duct to ensure its patency. Initial T-tube drainage is approximately 500 ml in the first 24 hours. The amount of drainage decreases as edema in the common bile duct subsides.
(5) Percutaneous cholecystolithotomy uses cystoscopes, stone baskets, and other instruments designed for nephrolithotomy to extract gallstones. If a stone is too large to be extracted percutaneously, a lithotriptor or laser fiber is used to break it down into fragments.
(6) Endoscopic sphincterotomy uses an incision in the sphincter of Oddi to remove gallstones in the common bile duct.
9. Complications
  • Cholecystitis
  • Infections
  • Abscess and fistula formation
10. Prognosis
  a. Patients with cholelithiasis usually have complete recovery after removal of the gallstones.
  b. A small percentage of patients have recurrent gallstones. Patients who are medically managed require continual dietary restrictions.
11. Applying the nursing process

NURSING DIAGNOSIS: Altered skin integrity R/T surgical incision, T-tube placement, or presence of drains

  a. *Expected outcomes:* Following intervention, the patient should exhibit no skin breakdown or sign of excoriation around the wound site.
  b. *Nursing interventions*
    (1) Change the dressing frequently if the drain is in place, because the drainage contains bile that is irritating to the skin (Procedure 28–4).
    (2) Use Montgomery straps to secure the dressing instead of plain tape so that skin irritation from tape removal is minimized.
    (3) Use aseptic technique during dressing changes.
    (4) Cleanse the suture line and around the T-tube site, and apply an antiseptic with each dressing change.
12. Discharge planning and teaching
  a. Emphasize the importance of eating a low-fat diet and avoiding fried foods and heavy cream.
  b. Make the patient aware that gallstones sometimes recur.
  c. Instruct postoperative patients on the care of suture lines and drains that remain in place.
  d. Stress the need for postoperative patients to resume normal activities gradually and to avoid lifting heavy objects for at least 6 weeks.
  e. Counsel obese patients on weight reduction.
13. Public health considerations are the same as those for cholecystitis

Other Biliary Disorders

1. Although less common than cholecystitis and cholelithiasis, choledocholithiasis, gallbladder carcinoma, and sclerosing colangitis are not obscure ailments.
2. Table 28–13 characterizes these disorders.

Procedure 28–4
Changing the Dressing Around the T Tube

Definition/Purpose	A T tube is usually inserted to ensure patency of the common bile duct. In cholecystitis and postoperative cholelithiasis, the common bile duct may be inflamed, which can impede bile flow and contribute to bile stasis.
Contraindications/Cautions	Because the T tube is inserted surgically, it is not recommended in persons who are poor surgical risks.
Learning/Teaching Activities	• Describe the procedure (regardless of the person's level of consciousness). • Explain that it is advisable to wear loose clothing to avoid irritation at the wound site. • Explain that the T tube must be below the level of the gallbladder to allow for free-flowing bile drainage.

Preliminary Activities

Equipment	• Clean, precut dressing • Adhesive tape • Antiseptic • 4 × 4 or 2 × 2 gauze • Sterile gloves • Karaya or any skin protective agent
Assessment/Planning	• Assemble materials necessary to change the dressing. • Wash hands thoroughly. • Empty bile bag carefully without contaminating the opening.
Preparing the Patient	Place person in semi-Fowler's position to ensure good visualization.
Procedure	

Action	Rationale/Discussion
1. Open the packet of gauze but do not remove it from the packet. Open the precut dressing packet but do not remove it from the packet. Open packet of antiseptic.	1. This ensures easy access to the equipment needed without contaminating them.
2. Put on clean gloves and remove old dressing while holding the T tube in place.	2. This prevents contaminating the clean surgical wound, thus decreasing risk of infection.
3. Inspect old dressing for pus or bloody drainage, and estimate the amount of drainage on this dressing. Inspect insertion site for swelling, inflammation, erythema, warmth, excessive drainage, or irritation.	3. These signs and symptoms of infection must be reported immediately to the physician.
4. Remove soiled gloves, wash hands, and put on sterile gloves.	4. Observing good aseptic technique decreases risk for iatrogenic infection.
5. If there is some leakage of bile around the area of the tube, wipe it with clean gauze.	5. Removing excess bile around the skin area prevents skin excoriation.
6. Cleanse the area around the insertion site with gauze moistened with sterile water or normal saline using a circular pattern and starting at the insertion site going outward. Then wipe the area of the tube close to the skin.	6. This prevents catheter infection.
7. Apply antimicrobial agent (e.g., Neosporin) around the insertion site and a protective agent (e.g., karaya) on the skin. Place clean, precut dressing around the T tube.	7. This prevents infection and protects the skin from irritation.
8. Secure the T tube and the dressing in place with hypoallergenic adhesive tape. Make sure that there is no kink or pull on the T tube.	8. This prevents strain on the T tube, thus decreasing incidence of dislodging the tube.

Final Activities

1. Dispose of all contaminated materials properly.
2. Wash hands thoroughly.
3. Observe the amount and color of drainage emptied from the bile bag. Changes in volume and character of drainage may indicate complications such as obstruction.

Table 28–13. Other Biliary Disorders

Biliary Disorder	Definition	Incidence/Etiology	Clinical Manifestations	Interventions
Choledocholithiasis	Presence of stones in the common bile duct	Occurs in approximately 8–15% of cholelithiasis cases Incidence increases with age Etiology is same as in cholelithiasis	Biliary colic Cholangitis (inflammation of the common bile duct) Pain in the right upper quadrant of the abdomen Jaundice (present if there is obstruction of the bile duct) Chills and fever Mild elevation of serum bilirubin level Asymptomatic elevation of alkaline phosphatase	Antibiotic therapy in the presence of cholangitis Removal of stones either by extracorporeal shock-wave lithotripsy, or endoscopic sphincterotomy (recommended in patients with previous cholecystectomy) Monitoring of drainage from T tube postoperatively Dietary restrictions of fat Prevention of pulmonary complications postoperatively
Gallbladder carcinoma	Cancer of the gallbladder	Most common malignant lesion of the biliary tract Accounts for 5% of all cancers Female to male ratio is 3:4 Increased incidence is seen over the age of 50 yr Hispanics, Native Americans, Northeastern Europeans, and Israelis are usually at high risk In the United States, 4000–6000 cases annually	Pain Weight loss Jaundice Anorexia Palpable mass in the right upper quadrant of the abdomen Other clinical manifestations depend on absence or presence of preexisting biliary symptoms	Radiation Chemotherapy Radical resection of the gallbladder Opening of the bile duct to relieve obstruction
Sclerosing cholangitis	A progressive autoimmune disease of the bile duct starting as an inflammation and progressing to fibrosis and strictures of extrahepatic and intrahepatic biliary ducts	Common in young males, with a male to female ratio of 3:2 Approximately two thirds of cases occur in persons younger than age 45 yr Usually caused by infectious agents Persons with altered immunity are at high risk Usually associated with chronic inflammatory bowel disease and risk of colon cancer	Anorexia Weight loss Jaundice Nonspecific upper quadrant abdominal pain Fatigue Pruritus	Long-term antibiotic therapy Use of corticosteroids Immunosuppressants Colchicine Surgical opening of the bile ducts (biliary reconstruction for extrahepatic strictures and percutaneous dilatation for intrahepatic strictures) Urodeoxycholic acid (experimental drug) may be helpful in preventing biliary cirrhosis.

◻ CARING FOR PEOPLE WITH PANCREATIC DISORDERS

Acute Pancreatitis

1. Definition: Pancreatitis is the acute or chronic inflammatory response in the pancreatic tissue secondary to premature activation of pancreatic digestive enzymes.
2. Incidence and socioeconomic impact
   a. Pancreatitis caused by alcoholism is more common in men than in women.
   b. A higher incidence of pancreatitis caused by biliary tract disorders is seen in women than in men.
3. Risk factors
   a. Undergoing operative procedures such as cardiopulmonary bypass or abdominal surgery
   b. Undergoing invasive procedures such as endoscopy
   c. Familial tendency
   d. Use of drugs such as thiazides, sulfas, estrogen, tetracycline, and oral contraceptives
4. Etiologic factors
   • Alcoholism (most common cause of chronic pancreatitis)
   • Hyperlipidemia
   • Hypercalcemia
   • Biliary tract disease (most common cause of acute pancreatitis)
   • Blunt or penetrating trauma to the pancreas
   • Hyperparathyroidism
   • Cholelithiasis

- Ischemic vascular disease
- Peptic ulcer disease
- Bacterial or viral infection, such as mumps

5. Pathophysiology
   a. Injuries to the pancreas cause an abnormal activation of the pancreatic proteolytic enzymes trypsin, chymotrypsin, and elastase.
   b. The increased release of pancreatic enzymes destroys tissues in and around the pancreas by autodigestion.
   c. The pancreatic inflammatory response causes increased concentration of phospholipase A, which damages the acinar cell membrane.

6. Clinical manifestations
   a. Pain
      (1) Pain may manifest as unrelenting abdominal pain or tenderness, usually localized in the epigastric area and periumbilical region.
      (2) Pain sometimes radiates to the chest and back.
      (3) Pain may be accompanied by abdominal distention, a poorly defined palpable abdominal mass, decreased peristalsis, and abdominal guarding.
   b. Jaundice
   c. Weight loss
   d. Low-grade fever due to pancreatic inflammation
   e. Anorexia due to severe abdominal pain
   f. Dehydration due to vomiting
   g. Dark amber or brown and foamy urine, which denotes the presence of bile
   h. Steatorrhea (see p. 1334)
   i. Grey Turner's sign—discoloration or bruising (blue, green, or brown) of the flank, usually secondary to bleeding
   j. Cullen's sign—discoloration as for Grey Turner's sign, but present around the umbilicus and usually present in hemorrhagic pancreatitis
   k. Pleural effusion due to the spread of inflammation created by the pancreatic enzymes as inflammation passes from the peritoneal cavity into the pleural cavity via the transdiaphragmatic lymph channels
   l. Signs of peritonitis—abdominal tenderness, rigidity, and guarding
   m. Persistent vomiting because pain stimulates the vomiting center

7. Diagnostics
   a. Laboratory studies demonstrate the following:
      (1) Elevated levels of AST, ALT, lactate dehydrogenase, alkaline phosphatase, serum amylase and lipase, bilirubin, triglycerides, urine amylase, and serum glucose (elevation transient) accompanied by glycosuria
      (2) Elevated white blood cell count
      (3) Decreased levels of serum protein, albumin, potassium (in cases of persistent vomiting), and calcium (due to calcium deposited in areas of fat necrosis and calcium trapped by undigested intestinal fat)
   b. Upper gastrointestinal series usually shows delayed gastric emptying and enlargement of the duodenum due to edema of the head of the pancreas.
   c. Abdominal film may show presence of dilated loops

of small bowel ("sentinal loop") adjacent to the pancreas. In chronic pancreatitis, abdominal film shows calcification of the pancreas.
   d. Endoscopic retrograde cholangiopancreatography can confirm the presence of pancreatitis.
   e. Computed tomography shows abscesses or tumors as well as pancreatic pseudocysts.

8. Clinical management
   a. Goals of clinical management center on controlling the cause of pancreatic inflammation and its symptoms and on preventing and treating its complications, because there is no known cure.
   b. Nonpharmacologic interventions
      (1) The patient should be given nothing by mouth to rest the pancreas.
      (2) A bland, low-fat, low-protein diet is given for patients able to eat. Caffeine and alcohol should be avoided.
      (3) Serum glucose and electrolytes are monitored closely.
   c. Pharmacologic interventions
      (1) Medications such as meperidine (Demerol) for pain (morphine and other opiates are usually avoided because they can cause spasms of the sphincter of Oddi)
      (2) Anticholinergic agents, given in combination with pain medications
      (3) Insulin, usually given as a continuous infusion if there is glucose intolerance
      (4) Prophylactic antibiotics
      (5) Histamine (H_2) antagonist to decrease hydrochloric acid, thus decreasing production of pancreatic enzymes
      (6) Intravenous fluids and plasma expanders to correct fluid imbalances
      (7) Aggressive pulmonary care
   d. Special medical-surgical procedures
      (1) Insertion of a central venous catheter or a pulmonary artery catheter to monitor for hypovolemic shock and guide fluid therapy
      (2) Intubation with a nasogastric tube to remove hydrochloric acid before it can enter the duodenum and stimulate secretion of pancreatic enzymes
      (3) Placement of external biliary drains and stents placed in the pancreatic duct via endoscopy to help decrease the production of pancreatic enzymes

9. Complications
   - Hemorrhage
   - Acute respiratory failure
   - Sepsis
   - Abscess formation
   - Pseudocyst
   - Acute renal failure
   - Myocardial depression
   - Electrolyte disturbance (e.g., hypocalcemia)
   - Metabolic disturbance (e.g., hyperglycemia)
   - Disseminated intravascular coagulation (due to the release of necrotic tissue and enzymes into the bloodstream as a result of the complex physiologic changes occurring in the pancreas)

10. Prognosis
    a. Mortality rate ranges from 5 percent in the mildest form of acute pancreatitis to greater than 50 percent in hemorrhagic pancreatitis.
    b. In 5 to 15 percent of patients with pancreatitis, the disease takes on a fulminant course, and 20 to 60 percent of these patients usually die.
    c. Overall mortality rates are reported at 10 to 20 percent.
11. Applying the nursing process

NURSING DIAGNOSIS: Impaired gas exchange R/T shallow, guarded respirations because of pain and pleural effusion

    a. *Expected outcomes:* Following interventions, the patient should be able to do the following:
        (1) Exhibit clear lungs on auscultation and oxygenation within the patient's normal limits
        (2) Cough and take a deep breath without pain
    b. *Nursing interventions*
        (1) Monitor lung sounds.
        (2) Monitor oxygen saturation by pulse oximetry.
        (3) Assist patient to a position that promotes maximum respiratory expansion.
        (4) Encourage the patient to cough and breathe deeply as frequently as possible while awake.
        (5) Encourage use of incentive spirometry.
        (6) See Chapter 22.

NURSING DIAGNOSIS: Fluid volume deficit R/T vomiting, gastric suctioning, and activation of pancreatic enzymes

    c. *Expected outcomes:* Following intervention, the patient should exhibit improved fluid volume, as evidenced by the following:
        (1) Normal skin turgor
        (2) Moist mucous membranes
        (3) Intake approximate to output
        (4) Central venous pressures within normal limits
        (5) Stable blood pressure
    d. *Nursing interventions*
        (1) Monitor vital signs as frequently as needed.
        (2) Monitor daily intake and output.
        (3) Assess mucous membranes for dryness.
        (4) Monitor serum electrolytes, especially sodium.
        (5) Administer intravenous fluids and antiemetics as ordered.

NURSING DIAGNOSIS: Altered nutrition, less than body requirement, R/T vomiting and anorexia

    e. *Expected outcomes:* Following intervention, the patient should do the following:
        (1) Have blood urea nitrogen within normal limits to confirm positive nitrogen balance
        (2) Express and exhibit signs of decreased nausea and vomiting

    f. *Nursing interventions*
        (1) Record caloric intake.
        (2) Provide oral care frequently and before meals.
        (3) Administer antiemetics as ordered before meals.
        (4) Note food tolerances and aversions, and prepare meals accordingly.
        (5) Give small, frequent feedings of high-carbohydrate, low-protein, low-fat foods, and eliminate spices, coffee, and tea.
        (6) Administer pancreatic enzyme replacement immediately after meals.

NURSE ADVISORY

Do not mix pancreatic enzyme preparations with foods containing protein. Enzymatic action dissolves such foods into watery substances. Rather, mix these supplements with fruit juices or applesauce to make them more palatable. After the patient has ingested the enzyme preparation, the patient's lips should be wiped with a wet towel because residual enzymes can cause irritation and skin breakdown.

        (7) If the patient is unable to eat, provide total parenteral nutrition.
12. Other nursing diagnosis: Pain related to pancreatic inflammation
13. Discharge planning and teaching
    a. Explain the importance of eating a bland, low-fat, high-calorie, high-carbohydrate diet while avoiding alcoholic and caffeinated beverages.
    b. Provide instructions regarding taking pancreatic enzyme replacement.
    c. Refer patients with a history of alcohol to rehabilitative treatment and support groups for both themselves and their families.
14. Public health considerations
    a. Prevention begins with educating patients of all ages and backgrounds on the dangers of excessive drinking and consumption of fatty foods.
    b. Persons in high-risk groups should be screened for key signs on a regular basis.
    c. The American Diabetes Association's Fat Portion Exchange List should be made easily available.

Chronic Pancreatitis

1. Definition: Chronic pancreatitis is a progressive, inflammatory disease, consisting of fibrosis and degeneration of the pancreas.
2. Incidence and socioeconomic impact
    a. In the United States, the incidence of chronic pancreatitis is 4 per 100,000 population.
    b. It is common among individuals who abuse alcohol.
    c. It is seen more in men than in women.
    d. The age of occurrence is variable, but is usually between 45 and 60 years.

3. Risk factors
   - Excessive alcohol ingestion
   - Biliary tract disease
   - Pancreatic pseudocysts
   - Postoperative ductal scarring
   - Cancer of the pancreas or duodenum
   - Prolonged starvation
4. Etiologic factors
   - Alcoholism (most common cause)
   - Hyperparathyroidism
   - Pancreatic trauma
   - Protein malnutrition
5. Pathophysiology
   a. Repeated attacks of acute pancreatitis cause irreversible scarring and calcification of pancreatic tissue.
   b. Scarring leads to histologic changes that, in turn, cause metaplasia (cell replacement) and fibrosis.
   c. Intraductal calcification and marked pancreatic parenchymal destruction develop in the late stages of disease.
   d. Acinar cell atrophy causes the pancreas to become hard and firm, leading to pancreatic insufficiency.
   e. This progressive destruction of the pancreas affects both endocrine and exocrine functions of the pancreas.
6. Clinical manifestations
   - Unrelenting abdominal pain described as burning or gnawing dullness
   - Vomiting
   - Fever
   - Jaundice
   - Weight loss
   - Hyperglycemia due to damage to the islet of Langerhans
   - Steatorrhea (see p. 1334)
   - Abdominal distention with flatus and cramps due to gas accumulation as a result of decreased fat absorption
7. Diagnostics
   a. Laboratory test results demonstrate mild elevation of white blood cell count and elevated serum amylase and bilirubin.
   b. Computed tomography shows degeneration of the pancreas.
   c. Ultrasound depicts fibrosis of the pancreas.
   d. Cholangiography shows alteration of the biliary structure.
8. Clinical management
   a. Goals of clinical management are to relieve pain and restore normal endocrine and exocrine functions of the pancreas as much as possible.
   b. Nonpharmacologic interventions
      (1) Providing nutritional support, that is, either total parenteral nutrition or enteral feeding of a low-fat diet for patients unable to take food orally, or a bland, low-fat, low-protein, high-carbohydrate diet for patients able to take food orally
      (2) Monitoring blood sugar and serum electrolytes
      (3) Providing bed rest and preventing skin breakdown
   c. Pharmacologic interventions

   (1) Analgesics, beginning with nonnarcotic analgesics such as pentazocine (Talwin) to avert possible narcotic dependency, then administering narcotic analgesics such as meperidine hydrochloride (Demerol) if nonnarcotics fail.
   (2) Exogenous insulin therapy to compensate for destruction of the islet of Langerhans (see Chapter 29)
   (3) Pancreatic enzyme replacement therapy such as pancreatin and pancrelipase
   (4) Vitamin supplements (especially fat-soluble vitamins)
   (5) Histamine-H_2 antagonists to decrease production of hydrochloric acid, and thus decrease stimulation of pancreatic activity
   d. Special medical-surgical procedures (Fig. 28–7)
      (1) Sphincteroplasty (incision of the sphincter and dilation of the pancreatic duct) may be done to enlarge the sphincter if it is fibrotic. The procedure has only limited application in pancreatitis, however.
      (2) In pancreaticojejunostomy (side-to-side), the surgeon opens the pancreatic duct and anastomoses it to the jejunum to relieve obstruction. The most successful surgical procedure for pancreatitis, pancreaticojejunostomy relieves pain and preserves pancreatic tissue and function. It is usually indicated when gross dilation of the pancreatic duct is due to calculi.
      (3) Caudal pancreaticojejunostomy is the procedure of choice if stenosis of the pancreatic duct is present but does not involve the ampulla of Vater.
      (4) Pancreaticoduodenal resection is indicated when pancreatic changes are confined to the head of the pancreas. This procedure usually preserves the pylorus.
      (5) Subtotal pancreatectomy (resection of the pancreas) is usually performed on patients with disabling pain.
      (6) Postoperative nursing responsibilities for all pancreatic surgeries involve awareness of the location and purpose of drains and stents, monitoring of proper functioning of these drains and stents, and monitoring for signs of peritonitis.
9. Complications
   - Those of acute pancreatitis (see p. 1341)
   - Peritonitis
   - Narcotic drug dependency
10. Prognosis
    a. The prognosis is good when the patient abstains from drinking alcohol and attacks of acute pancreatitis decrease.
    b. The prognosis is poor when the patient continues to drink alcohol.
11. Applying the nursing process is the same as for acute pancreatitis (see p. 1342)
12. Discharge planning and teaching
    a. Stress the need for the patient to abstain from alcohol.
    b. Elicit participation from the patient's family in planning a diet of bland, low-fat, low-protein, high-car-

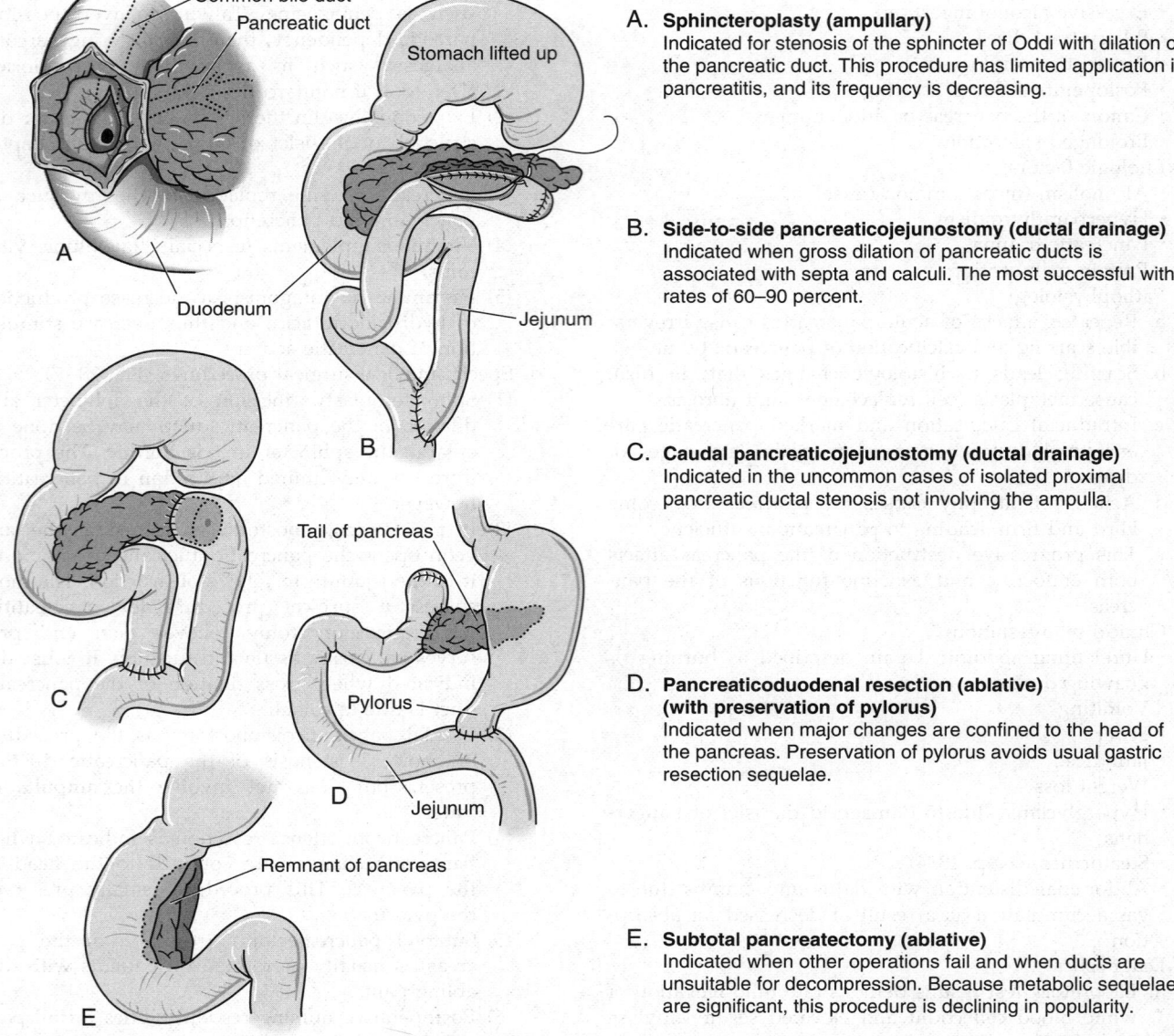

A. **Sphincteroplasty (ampullary)**
Indicated for stenosis of the sphincter of Oddi with dilation of the pancreatic duct. This procedure has limited application in pancreatitis, and its frequency is decreasing.

B. **Side-to-side pancreaticojejunostomy (ductal drainage)**
Indicated when gross dilation of pancreatic ducts is associated with septa and calculi. The most successful with rates of 60–90 percent.

C. **Caudal pancreaticojejunostomy (ductal drainage)**
Indicated in the uncommon cases of isolated proximal pancreatic ductal stenosis not involving the ampulla.

D. **Pancreaticoduodenal resection (ablative)**
(with preservation of pylorus)
Indicated when major changes are confined to the head of the pancreas. Preservation of pylorus avoids usual gastric resection sequelae.

E. **Subtotal pancreatectomy (ablative)**
Indicated when other operations fail and when ducts are unsuitable for decompression. Because metabolic sequelae are significant, this procedure is declining in popularity.

Figure 28–7. Different surgical procedures for chronic pancreatitis. (Redrawn from Black JM, and Matassarin-Jacobs E [eds]. *Luckmann and Sorensen's Medical-Surgical Nursing: A Psychophysiologic Approach.* 4th ed. Philadelphia: WB Saunders, 1993, p 1752.)

bohydrate foods. Caution the patient against ingesting caffeinated beverages or rich and spicy foods that are known to precipitate pancreatitis attacks.

c. Provide instructions and a written schedule on how and when to take prescribed medications.

d. Explain activity limitations.

e. Show a reliable friend or family member how to give intramuscular injections for pain medication. Observe a return demonstration.

g. Teach the patient to monitor blood sugar using glucose monitoring meters. Observe a return demonstration.

h. If applicable, teach the patient to self-administer subcutaneous insulin injections. Observe a return demonstration.

Pancreatic Cancer

1. Definition: Pancreatic cancer is carcinoma of the pancreas.
2. Incidence and socioeconomic impact
   a. Approximately 25,000 new cases of pancreatic cancer occur annually.
   b. Peak incidence of pancreatic carcinoma occurs in the 5th and 6th decades of life.
   c. Two thirds of pancreatic carcinomas occur at the head of the pancreas; the rest occur in the body or tail of the pancreas.
3. Risk factors
   • Cigarette smoking
   • Increased fat consumption

- Increased alcohol consumption
- Diabetes mellitus (especially in women)
4. Etiologic factors
   - Diseases of the gallbladder
   - Diseases of the extrahepatic bile duct
5. Pathophysiology
   a. Pancreatic cancers are usually adenocarcinomas that originate from the epithelial lining of the duct areas of the pancreas.
   b. As the tumor mass grows, it blocks the ducts.
   c. Pancreatic tumors usually grow rapidly and metastasize to nearby structures (e.g., liver, stomach, intestines, bones) as well as to lymph nodes.
6. Clinical manifestations
   a. Weight loss (usually rapid and progressive) in approximately 75 percent of patients with carcinoma of the head of the pancreas
   b. Vague abdominal pain
   c. Jaundice, indicative of metastasis to the liver or gallbladder
   d. Hepatomegaly, in approximately 50 percent of patients with carcinoma of the pancreas
   e. Palpable mass in the right upper quadrant of the abdomen in approximately 20 percent of patients with carcinoma of the pancreas, which nearly always signifies surgical incurability
   f. Nausea and vomiting
   g. Anorexia
7. Diagnostics
   a. Laboratory studies demonstrate elevated alkaline phosphatase and serum bilirubin and lipase as well as electrolyte imbalances.
   b. Percutaneous aspiration biopsy identifies the types of pancreatic cancer cells.
   c. Abdominal angiography shows either encasement of the major arteries and veins by the pancreatic tumor or increased vascularity of abnormal vessels in the area of the tumor.
   d. Endoscopic retrograde cholangiopancreatography detects metastasis in the walls of the duodenum.
   e. Computed tomography confirms the presence of pancreatic tumors.
8. Clinical management
   a. Goals of clinical management focus on palliation of symptoms in various ways.
   b. Nonpharmacologic interventions
      (1) Nutritional support is given as a high-calorie, low-fat diet for patients who can eat and total parenteral nutrition for those who cannot.
      (2) Blood sugar levels and serum electrolytes are monitored.
      (3) Blood transfusions are supplied to correct anemia.
   c. Pharmacologic interventions
      (1) Vitamin K is given to correct prothrombin deficiency.
      (2) Pain medications include meperidine (Demerol) or morphine as continuous infusions.
      (3) Chemotherapeutic agents are used.
   d. Special medical-surgical procedures
      (1) The Whipple procedure (radical pancreaticoduodenectomy) is done only if just the head of the pancreas is involved and there is no evidence of metastasis. The surgeon removes the proximal pancreas, duodenum, lower half of the stomach, and gallbladder and implants the pancreatic duct into the jejunum and the hepatic duct into the remaining stomach. The procedure allows gastric, hepatic, and pancreatic secretions to empty into the jejunum so that reasonably normal digestion may take place.
      (2) Cholecystojejunostomy (anastomosis of the gallbladder to the jejunum) allows bile to flow directly into the intestine, bypassing any obstruction caused by an inoperable tumor of the pancreas.
      (3) Central venous catheter or pulmonary artery catheters may be used to guide fluid therapy.
   e. Palliation of symptoms often requires a combination of simple surgical procedures (such as cholecystojejunostomy), radiation, and chemotherapy.
9. Complications include respiratory failure and sepsis.
10. Prognosis
   a. Most patients with pancreatic carcinomas die within a year of medical diagnosis.
   b. The five-year survival rate for carcinoma of the head of the pancreas is approximately 10 percent. The overall survival rate of patients with pancreatic carcinoma is less than 1 percent.
   c. Pancreatic carcinoma is the 3rd leading cause of death due to cancer in men aged 35 to 54 years.
11. Applying the nursing process

NURSING DIAGNOSIS: Altered nutrition, less than body requirement, R/T anorexia

   a. *Expected outcomes:* Following intervention, the patient should be able to do the following:
      (1) Maintain body weight
      (2) Take in at least 75 percent of prescribed caloric requirement
   b. *Nursing interventions*
      (1) Administer parenteral nutrition if necessary.
      (2) If the patient takes food orally, provide a high-carbohydrate, high-protein diet with vitamin and mineral supplements.
      (3) Maintain a record of the patient's caloric intake.
      (4) Maintain a consistent oral hygiene routine for the patient.

ELDER ADVISORY

Older patients are at high risk for the development of hepatic, biliary, and pancreatic disease because of normal aging changes that occur in body systems. When any of these diseases develops in an older patient, clinical manifestations may be atypical and symptoms more severe. For example, pruritus due to jaundice is intensified because of thinning of the epidermal skin layers. Anorexia is more problematic because of diminished salivary flow and changes in the sense of smell that may further decrease appetite.

Table 28–14. Other Pancreatic Disorders

Pancreatic Disorder	Definition	Incidence/Etiology	Clinical Manifestations	Interventions
Pancreatic pseudocysts	Localized collections of pancreatic enzymes in a cystic structure outside of the parenchyma of the pancreas	Accounts for up to 75% of all cystic lesions in the pancreas Commonly seen in alcoholic pancreatitis	Nausea and vomiting Abdominal pain Early satiety Jaundice	Follow-up monitoring of the patient with abdominal ultrasound to detect whether pseudocysts are resolving Percutaneous drainage Surgical removal if pseudocyst does not resolve
Pancreatic fistula	Formation of an abnormal tract connecting the abscess site in the pancreas with the abdominal wall	Pancreatic abscess secondary to acute pancreatitis Pancreatic pseudocysts	Elevated temperature Presence of a small, reddened area that is warm to the touch in the abdominal wall Presence of purulent, foul-smelling drainage in the abdominal wall	Antibiotic therapy Wound irrigation Packing of the wound with sterile wet gauze in between wound irrigation Culture drainage Monitoring of vital signs (especially temperature and heart rate) Monitoring of drainage from fistula Skin care
Pancreatic trauma	Injury to the pancreas associated with blunt or penetrating abdominal trauma	Majority of trauma to the pancreas caused by penetrating injuries Injury to the pancreas seen in 2% of abdominal traumas	Mild epigastric pain and tenderness especially in blunt trauma Hemorrhage (especially in penetrating injuries) Hypovolemia	Surgical intervention to control hemorrhage Débridement of nonviable pancreatic tissues and hematomas Insertion of pancreatic sump tube to drain pancreatic secretions
Pancreatic abscess	Presence of infected, necrotic pancreatic tissue occurring after severe acute pancreatitis, exacerbations of chronic pancreatitis, and biliary tract surgery	Development of a single abscess or multiloculated abscesses due to extensive inflammatory necrosis of the pancreas, which is readily invaded by infectious organisms Common causative organisms: *Escherichia coli, Klebsiella, Bacteroides, Staphylococcus,* and *Proteus* Recurrent abscesses in most patients Mortality rate associated with pancreatic abscess as high as 60%, even with surgical drainage; 100% mortality rate without surgical drainage	Similar to pancreatic pseudocysts; however, patients with pancreatic abscess may experience temperature as high as 104°F (40°C) Pleural effusions common in pancreatic abscesses	Surgical drainage of abscesses as soon as possible to prevent sepsis Antibiotic therapy in conjunction with surgical drainage Analgesics for pain Emotional support for patient and family Good handwashing technique Adequate nutrition

NURSING DIAGNOSIS: Powerlessness R/T rapid progression of pancreatic cancer

    c. *Expected outcomes:* Following intervention, the patient should be able to do the following:
      (1) Verbalize factors that he or she can control
      (2) Participate in decision making regarding treatment

    d. *Nursing interventions*
      (1) Avoid jargon in explaining procedures and treatments to the patient and family.
      (2) Insofar as is possible, let patients manipulate their own environment (e.g., lighting, sound, room temperature).
      (3) Allow patients to make decisions regarding visiting with family and friends.

(4) Encourage patients to participate in decisions regarding their care (e.g., when to have a bath).

(5) Develop a conference schedule for the patient, family, and health care providers to assess progression of the disease and long-term plans for therapy.

> **NURSING DIAGNOSIS:** Risk for infection R/T presence of invasive catheters

e. *Expected outcomes:* Following intervention, the patient should be free from infection, as exhibited by the following:

(1) White blood cell count within normal limits

(2) No fever

(3) No redness or abscess at catheter sites

f. *Nursing interventions*

(1) Use strict aseptic technique and follow dressing change protocols when handling catheters.

(2) Use universal precautions when handling drainage.

(3) Develop skin care protocol to prevent skin breakdown.

(4) Administer antibiotics as ordered.

12. Other nursing diagnoses
   - Pain related to tumor stimulating sensory nerves
   - Anticipatory grieving related to impending death (see Chapter 43)

13. Discharge planning and teaching
   a. The patient should be made as comfortable as possible for the remainder of his or her life.
   b. The patient and family should be referred to support groups and hospice centers.

14. Public health considerations
   a. The public should be made aware of correlations between pancreatic cancer and lifestyle choices such as cigarette smoking, alcoholism, and high-fat diet.
   b. Patients should be screened for pancreatic disorders, especially diabetic women who smoke.

Other Pancreatic Disorders

1. Table 28–14 details some less common pancreatic disorders.
2. These include pancreatic pseudocysts, pancreatic fistulas, pancreatic trauma, and pancreatic abscesses.

Bibliography

Books

Black JM, and Matassarin-Jacobs E (eds). *Luckmann and Sorensen's Medical-Surgical Nursing: A Psychophysiologic Approach.* 4th ed. Philadelphia: WB Saunders, 1993.

Bongiovanni G. *Clinical Gastroenterology.* New York: McGraw-Hill Book Co, 1988.

Guyton AC. *Textbook of Medical Physiology.* 9th ed. Philadelphia: WB Saunders, 1991.

Ignatavicius DD, Workman ML, and Mishler MA (eds). *Medical-Surgical Nursing: A Nursing Process Approach.* 2nd ed. Philadelphia: WB Saunders, 1995.

Payer L. *Medicine and Culture.* New York: Henry Holt, 1988.

Sherlock S, and Dooley J. *Disease of the Liver and Biliary System.* 9th ed. Oxford: Blackwell Scientific, 1993.

Vander AJ, Sherman JH, and Luciano DS. *Human Physiology.* 6th ed. New York: McGraw-Hill Book Co, 1994.

Chapters in Books and Journal Articles

Assessing People with Hepatic, Biliary, and Pancreatic Disorders

Briones TL. The gastrointestinal system. *In* Alspach JG (ed). *Core Curriculum for Critical Care Nursing.* 4th ed. Philadelphia: WB Saunders, 1991.

O'Toole MT. Advanced assessment of the abdomen and gastrointestinal problems. *Nurs Clin North Am* 25:771, 1990.

Caring for People with Hepatitic Disorders

Gurevich I. Hepatitis part I. Enterically transmitted viral hepatitis: etiology, epidemiology, and prevention. *Heart Lung* 22:370, 1993.

Gurevich I. Hepatitis part II. Viral hepatitis B, C and D. *Heart Lung* 22:450, 1993.

Kools AM. Hepatitis A, B, C, D and E. Update on testing and treatment. *Postgrad Med* 91:109, 1992.

Lisanti P, and Talotta D. Hepatitis update: the delta virus. *AORN J* 55:790, 1992.

Maddrey WC. Chronic viral hepatitis: diagnosis and management. *Hosp Pract* 29:117, 1994.

Marx JF. Viral hepatitis: Unscrambling the alphabet. *Nursing* 3:36, 1993.

O'Grady J. Management of acute and fulminant hepatitis A. *Vaccine* 10(suppl): S21, 1992.

Rosman AS, et al. Hepatitis C virus antibody in alcoholic patients. Association with the presence of portal and/or lobular hepatitis. *Arch Intern Med* 153:965, 1993.

Schiff ER. Hepatitis C among health care providers: Risk factors and possible prophylaxis. *Hepatology* 16:1300, 1992.

Cirrhosis

Briones TL. The gastrointestinal system. *In* Alspach JG (ed). *Core Curriculum for Critical Care Nursing.* 4th ed. Philadelphia: WB Saunders, 1991.

Butler RW. Managing the complications of cirrhosis. *Am J Nurs* 94:46, 1994.

Gines A, et al. Incidence, predictive factors, and prognosis of the hepatorenal syndrome in cirrhosis with ascites. *Gastroenterology* 105:229, 1993.

Henriksen JH, and Ring-Larsen H. Ascites formation in liver cirrhosis: the how and the why. *Dig Dis* 8:152, 1990.

Neuschwander-Tetri BA. Organ interactions in the hepatorenal syndrome. *New Horizons* 2:527, 1994.

Esophageal Varices

Adams L, and Soulen MC. TIPS, a new alternative for the variceal bleeder. *Am J Crit Care* 2:196, 1993.

Briones TL. The gastrointestinal system. *In* Alspach JG (ed). *Core Curriculum for Critical Care Nursing.* 4th ed. Philadelphia: WB Saunders, 1991.

Burns SM, and Martin MJ. VP/NTG therapy in the patient with variceal bleeding. *Crit Care Nurse* 10:42, 1990.

Burns SM, et al. Evaluation and revision of a vasopressin/nitroglycerine protocol for use in variceal bleeding. *Am J Crit Care* 2:202, 1993.

Kerber K. The adult with bleeding esophageal varices. *Crit Care Clin North Am* 5:153, 1993.

Mahl TC, and Grozzman RJ. Pathophysiology of portal hypertension and variceal bleeding. *Surg Clin North Am* 70:251, 1990.

Paquet KJ, et al. Surgical procedures for bleeding esophagogastric varices when sclerotherapy fails: A prospective study. *Am J Surg* 160:43, 1990.

Peck SN, and Griffith DJ. Reducing portal

hypertension and variceal bleeding. *Dimensions Crit Care Nurs* 7:269, 1988.

Fulminant Hepatic Failure

Chang TMS. Artificial liver support based on artificial cells with emphasis on encapsulated hepatocytes. *Artif Organs* 16:71, 1992.

Katelaris PH, and Jones DB. Fulminant hepatic failure. *Med Clin North Am* 73:955, 1989.

Kelso LA. Fluid and electrolyte disturbances in hepatic failure. *AACN Clin Issues* 3:681, 1992.

Kucharski SA. Fulminant hepatic failure. *Crit Care Nurs Clin North Am* 5:141, 1993.

LePage EL, et al. A bioartificial liver used as a bridge to liver transplantation in a 10-year-old boy. *Am J Crit Care* 3:224, 1994.

Cancer of the Liver

Harris CC. Hepatocellular carcinogenesis: Recent advances and speculations. *Cancer Cells* 2:146, 1990.

Keehn DM, and Frank-Stromborg M. A worldwide perspective on the epidemiology and primary prevention of liver cancer. *Cancer Nurs* 14:163, 1991.

Rustgi V. Epidemiology of hepatocellular carcinoma. *Gastroenterol Clin North Am* 16:545, 1987.

Vargas V, Castells L, and Esteban J. High frequency of antibodies to the hepatitis C virus among patients with hepatocellular carcinoma. *Ann Intern Med* 112:232, 1990.

Wogan G. Dietary risk factors for primary hepatocellular carcinoma. *Cancer Detect Prev* 14:209, 1989.

Other Hepatic Disorders

Bergman MM, and Ciak CS. A novel approach to an uncommon problem: liver abscess. *Hosp Pract* 24:37, 1989.

Liver Transplantation

Bass PS, Bindon-Perler PA, and Lewis RJ. Liver transplantation: the recovery phase. *Crit Care Nurs Q* 13:51, 1991.

Smith SL, and Ciferni M. Liver transplantation for acute hepatic failure: A review

of clinical experience and management. *Am J Crit Care* 2:137, 1993.

Tuel SM, Meythaler JM, and Cross LL. Inpatient comprehensive rehabilitation after liver transplantation. *Am J Phys Med Rehabil* 70:242, 1991.

United Network for Organ Sharing. *Scientific registry*. Richmond, VA: United Network for Organ Sharing, May 1993.

Caring for People with Biliary Disorders

Duane WC. Pathogenesis of gallstones: Implications for management. *Hosp Pract* 25:65, 1990.

Holland P, and Hussain I. Biliary lithotripsy: Nonsurgical treatment of gallstones. *Soc Gastrointest Assist J* 3:158, 1989.

Jackson DC, et al. Endoscopic laser cholecystectomy. *AORN J* 51:1546, 1990.

Johnston DE, and Kaplan MM. Pathogenesis and treatment of gallstones. *N Engl J Med* 328:412, 1993.

Kohn CL, Brozenec S, and Foster PF. Nutritional support for the patient with pancreatobiliary disease. *Crit Care Nurs Clin North Am* 5:37, 1993.

Ondrusek RS. Cholecystectomy: An update. *RN* 23:28, 1993.

Weltman DI, and Zeman RK. Acute diseases of the gallbladder and biliary ducts. *Radiol Clin North Am* 32:933, 1994.

Other Biliary Disorders

Babb RR. Acute acalculous cholecystitis: a review. *J Clin Gastroenterol* 15:238, 1992.

Boland G, Lee MJ, and Mueller PR. Acute cholecystitis in the intensive care unit. *New Horizons* 1:246, 1993.

Jones RS. Palliative operative procedures for carcinoma of the gallbladder. *World J Surg* 15:348, 1991.

Rattner DW, Fergusson C, and Warshaw AL. Factors associated with successful laparoscopic cholecystectomy for acute cholecystitis. *Ann Surg* 217:233, 1993.

Wanebo HJ, and Vezeridis MO. Carcinoma of the gallbladder. *J Surg Oncol* 3:134, 1993.

Weltman DI, and Zeman RK. Acute diseases of the gallbladder and biliary ducts. *Radiol Clin North Am* 32:933, 1994.

Caring for People with Pancreatic Disorders

Axon AT. Endoscopic retrograde cholangiopancreatography in chronic pancreatitis. *Radiol Clin North Am* 27:39, 1989.

Brodrick RL. Preventing complications in acute pancreatitis. *Dimens Crit Care Nurs* 10:262, 1991.

Brown A. Acute pancreatitis. Pathophysiology, nursing diagnoses, and collaborative problems. *Focus Crit Care* 18:121, 1991.

Kohn CL, Bronzenec S, and Foster PF. Nutritional support for the patient with pancreatobiliary disease. *Crit Care Nurs Clin North Am* 5:37, 1993.

Krumberger JM. Acute pancreatitis. *Crit Care Nurs Clin North Am* 5:185, 1993.

Levelle-Jones M, and Neoptolemos J. Recent advances in the treatment of acute pancreatitis. *Ann Surg* 22:235, 1990.

Pancreatic Cancer

Lygidakis NJ, et al. Resectional surgical procedures for carcinoma of the head of the pancreas. *Surg Gynecol Obstet* 168:157, 1989.

Morel P, et al. Pylorus-preserving duodenopancreatectomy: Long-term complications and comparison with Whipple procedure. *World J Surg* 14:642, 1990.

Reber HA. Pancreatic cancer: Presentation of the disease, diagnosis and surgical management. *J Pain Symptom Manage* 3:164, 1988.

Other Pancreatic Disorders

Ahearne PM, et al. An endoscopic retrograde cholangiopancreatography-based algorithm for the management of pancreatic pseudocysts. *Am J Surg* 163:111, 1992.

D'Egidio A, and Schein M. Pancreatic pseudocysts: A proposed classification and its management complication. *Br J Surg* 78:981, 1992.

Grace PA, and Williamson RCN. Modern management of pancreatic pseudocysts. *Br J Surg* 80:573, 1993.

Leppäniemi A, et al. Pancreatic trauma: Acute and late manifestations. *Br J Surg* 75:165, 1988.

Sukul K, Lont HE, and Johannes EJ. Management of pancreatic injuries. *Hepatogastroenterology* 39:447, 1992.

Agencies/Resources

Alcoholics Anonymous (AA)
468 Park Avenue South
New York, NY 10016
(212) 686–1100

American Cancer Society
1599 Clifton Road NE
Atlanta, GA 30329
(404) 320–3333

American Liver Foundation
30 Sunrise Terrace
Cedar Grove, NJ 07009
(201) 857–2626

American Society for Parenteral and
Enteral Nutrition (ASPEN)
8605 Cameron Street
Suite 500
Silver Spring, MD 20910
(301) 587–6315

National Digestive Diseases Education and
Information Clearinghouse
1255 23rd Street NW, No. 275
Washington, DC 20037
(202) 296–9610

29

Caring for People with Endocrine Disorders

◼ *ENDOCRINE SYSTEM STRUCTURE AND FUNCTION*

Overview of Structure and Function

1. The endocrine system is composed of many glands that release their secretions directly into the blood (Fig. 29–1). In contrast, the exocrine glands, such as the liver, release their secretions onto body surfaces or internal organs.
2. The endocrine glands produce hormones that may act locally or generally and contribute to the following:
   a. Growth and development
   b. Homeostasis
   c. Response to stress and injury
   d. Reproduction
   e. Energy metabolism
3. The need for hormonal secretion is triggered by the negative feedback system (Fig. 29–2).

Thyroid Structure and Function

1. The structure of the thyroid gland is shown in Figure 29–3.
   a. Thyroid hormones affect the following functions:
      (1) Carbohydrate metabolism
      (2) Fat metabolism
      (3) Basal metabolic rate
      (4) Body weight
      (5) Cardiovascular system—blood flow, cardiac output, and heart rate
      (6) Respiration
      (7) Gastrointestinal tract
      (8) Central nervous system
      (9) Muscle function
      (10) Sleep
      (11) Sexual function
      (12) Other endocrine functions, such as pancreas and glucose metabolism, bone formation and parathyroid hormone (PTH), and adrenal glucocorticoid inactivation
   b. Thyrocalcitonin lowers calcium levels. (For details, see the discussion of the parathyroid, below.)
2. Thyroid gland function is influenced by the secretion of thyroid-stimulating hormone (TSH, or thyrotropin) from the anterior pituitary gland.
   a. Thyroid-stimulating hormone works via the negative feedback system.
   b. It is controlled by thyrotropin-releasing hormone (TRH) from the hypothalamus.

Parathyroid Structure and Function

1. The parathyroid structure is shown in Figure 29–3.
2. The function of the parathyroid glands is to secrete parathyroid hormone (PTH).
   a. Parathyroid hormone controls calcium concentration in the extracellular fluid. It is released in response to the calcium level in the extracellular fluid, which depends on the following:
      (1) Calcium and phosphate absorption from the bone
      (2) Loss of phosphate in the urine
      (3) An increase in reabsorption of calcium in the kidneys
      (4) An indirect effect of calcium absorption in the gastrointestinal tract
   b. Vitamin D works in conjunction with PTH to promote absorption of calcium and bone deposition.
   c. High calcium concentrations trigger the C cells in the thyroid to secrete thyrocalcitonin, which inhibits bone resorption.

Adrenal Structure and Function

1. The structure of the adrenal glands is shown in Figure 29–4.
2. Adrenal hormone secretion
   a. Mineralocorticoid (aldosterone) secretion is influenced by the following:
      (1) Extracellular fluid volume
      (2) Blood volume
      (3) Extracellular fluid volume concentrations of sodium and potassium
      (4) Arterial pressure
      (5) Renin-angiotensin system
   b. Secretion of glucocorticoids is controlled by adrenocorticotropic hormone (ACTH) from the anterior pituitary gland.

STRUCTURE AND FUNCTION OF THE ENDOCRINE SYSTEM

The endocrine system is composed of the pituitary (*hypophysis*), hypothalamus, thyroid, parathyroids, thymus, adrenals, ovaries and testes, and pancreas (*islets of Langerhans*). The endocrine glands produce hormones that may act locally or generally. Hormonal secretion occurs in response to nerve stimuli and nerve and neuroendocrine activity in the hypothalamus.

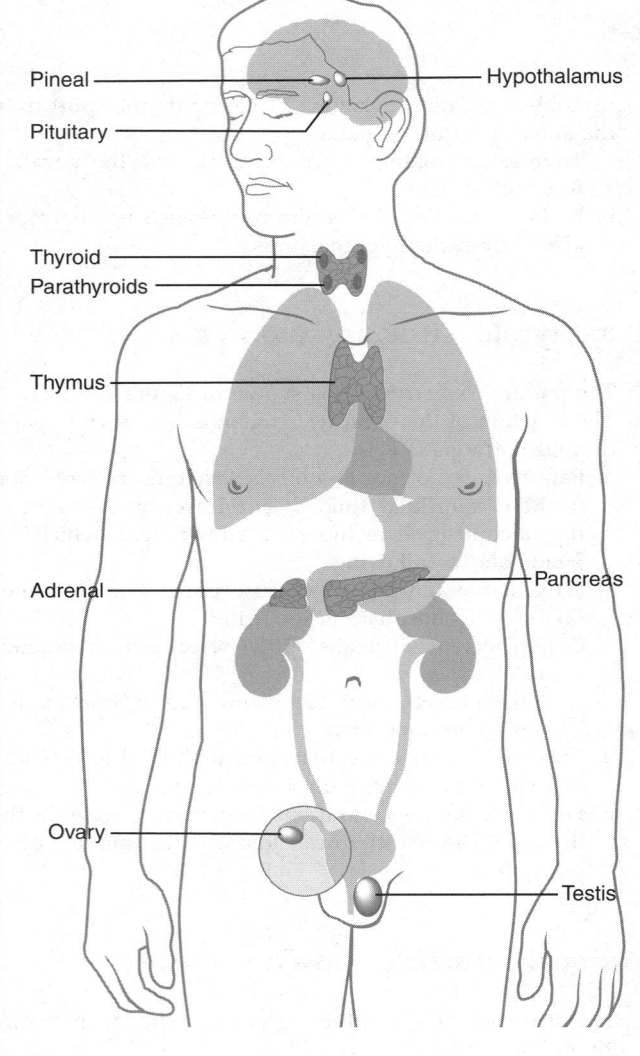

Figure 29-1.

(1) Adrenocorticotropic hormone is secreted within minutes in response to stressors such as trauma, extreme temperature variation, infection, surgery, injection of necrotizing substances beneath the skin, injection of norepinephrine or other sympathomimetic drugs, or psychologic distress.

(2) The secretory rates of ACTH and glucocorticoids follow a circadian rhythm: The levels are high early in the morning and low late in the evening.

3. Adrenal cortical function is necessary to maintain life.
   a. Effects of aldosterone: Influences potassium excretion and sodium retention and water balance.
   b. Effects of cortisol
      (1) Blocks early stages of inflammation or infection by

NEGATIVE FEEDBACK SYSTEM

Hormonal production and secretion is controlled primarily by the anterior pituitary and the hypothalamus. The anterior pituitary is controlled by hypothalamic-releasing hormones and inhibitory hormones, which are secreted from the hypothalamus.

The hypothalamus receives signals from the nervous system indicating which hormones are to be secreted. The releasing or inhibiting hormones are then absorbed into the hypothalamic-hypophysial portal capillaries and are transmitted to the anterior pituitary gland. The releasing or inhibiting hormones then reach the target glands (thyroid, adrenal cortex, ovaries, testicles).

Release of most hormones is controlled by a negative feedback system. Hormones are secreted in response to a stimulus. The increased level of the released hormone inhibits further secretion. This negative feedback loop keeps hormone levels within a narrow range.

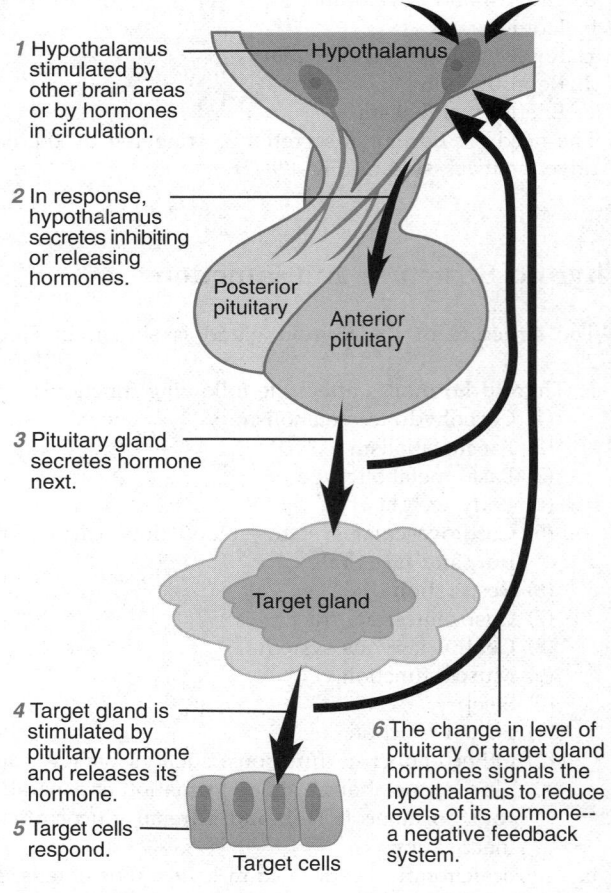

Figure 29-2.

STRUCTURE AND LOCATION OF THYROID AND PARATHYROIDS

Thyroid Gland

The thyroid is located below the cricoid cartilage in the neck. It has 2 lobes, 1 on each side of the trachea, joined by a thin isthmus. In the normal adult, each lobe measures 2-3 cm in vertical diameter and 1 cm in width. Each lobe is made of nodules, which are composed of tiny follicles filled with colloidal material called thyroglobulin. The thyroid hormones are synthesized and stored here. The thyroid gland is vascularized by the superior thyroid artery (a branch of the external carotid artery) and the inferior thyroid artery (a branch of the subclavian artery). Innervation by the adrenergic and cholinergic nervous systems arises from the cervical ganglia and vagus nerve, respectively.

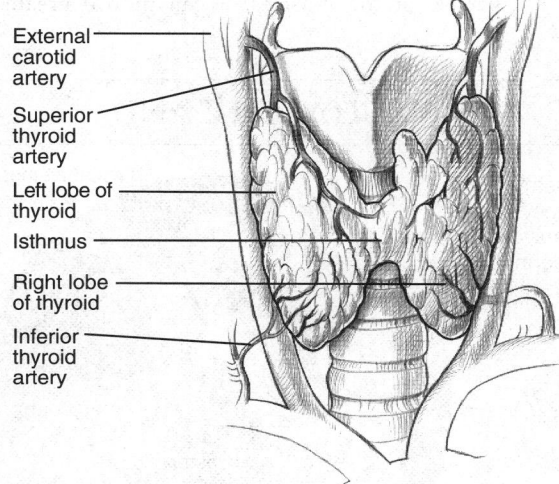

External carotid artery
Superior thyroid artery
Left lobe of thyroid
Isthmus
Right lobe of thyroid
Inferior thyroid artery

Parathyroid Glands

Four parathyroid glands are located in the posterior section of the thyroid. One parathyroid gland is located in each of the upper and lower lobes of the thyroid. Each parathyroid is approximately 6 mm long, 3 mm wide, and 2 mm thick. Each resembles a piece of dark brown fat embedded in the thyroid.

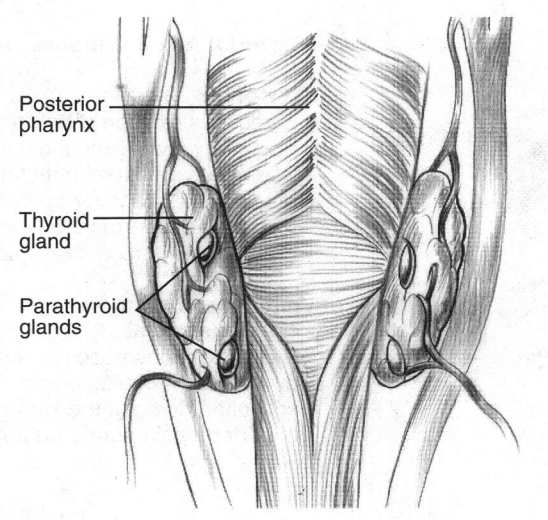

Posterior pharynx
Thyroid gland
Parathyroid glands

Figure 29-3.

STRUCTURE AND LOCATION OF THE ADRENAL GLANDS

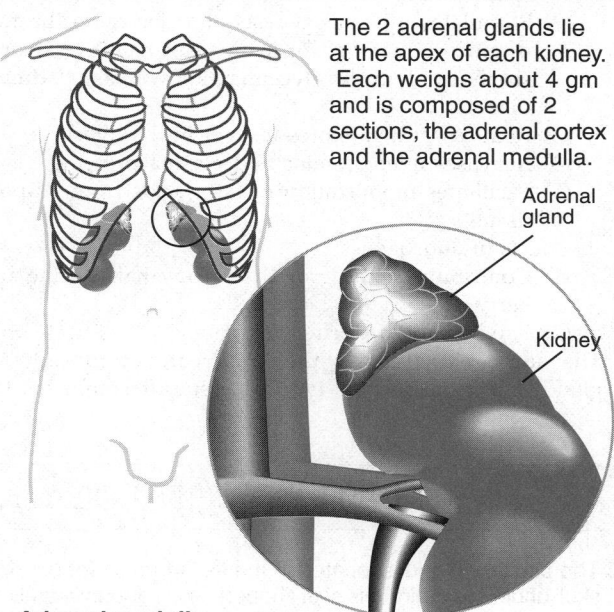

The 2 adrenal glands lie at the apex of each kidney. Each weighs about 4 gm and is composed of 2 sections, the adrenal cortex and the adrenal medulla.

Adrenal gland
Kidney

Adrenal medulla

The inner core of the adrenal gland, made of 1 type of tissue. It produces 80% epinephrine (adrenalin) and 20% norepinephrine. These elevate blood pressure, convert glycogen to glucose when needed by muscles for energy, increase the heart rate, increase cardiac contractility, and dilate the bronchioles.

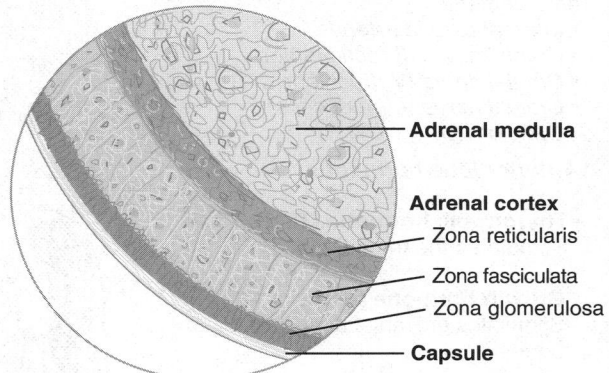

Adrenal medulla
Adrenal cortex
Zona reticularis
Zona fasciculata
Zona glomerulosa
Capsule

Adrenal cortex

Constitutes approximately 80% of the adrenal gland and is composed of 3 layers of adrenal tissue, each of which secretes a unique hormone. All corticoids are important for defense against stress or injury.

Aldosterone, a mineralocorticoid, is secreted by the zona glomerulosa (outermost layer). Tends to increase sodium retention and potassium excretion.

Cortisol (from the glucocorticoid group) is secreted by the zona reticularis, the most central layer of cortex, and the zona fasciculata (middle layer). Promotes carbohydrate, protein, and fat catabolism and increases tissue responsiveness to other hormones.

Androgens (male hormones) are secreted by the zona reticularis and the zona fasciculata. Govern certain secondary sex characteristics.

Figure 29-4.

interfering with an established inflammatory response

(2) Stimulates gluconeogenesis and decreases the rate of glucose metabolism, which can result in a cortisol-induced hyperglycemia known as "adrenal diabetes"

(3) Reduces protein stores (except in the liver)

(4) Increases liver proteins and plasma proteins

(5) Facilitates mobilization of fatty acids from adipose tissue

c. Effects of androgens

(1) Contribute to the growth of body hair during puberty

(2) Are important during pregnancy

4. The adrenal medulla is the inner core of the adrenal gland and is made of 1 type of tissue. It comprises the central 20 percent of the adrenal gland and is functionally related to the sympathetic nervous system.

a. It secretes epinephrine and norepinephrine in response to sympathetic stimulation. Epinephrine makes up about 80 percent and norepinephrine about 20 percent of the hormones secreted by the adrenal medulla. Both epinephrine and norepinephrine cause vasoconstriction of most blood vessels.

(1) Epinephrine increases the basal metabolic rate of the body and converts glycogen to glucose when the muscles need glucose for energy. It has a greater effect than norepinephrine on cardiac contraction, because it stimulates the β-receptors more effectively.

(2) Because norepinephrine particularly constricts the vessels of the muscles, it can induce greater pe-

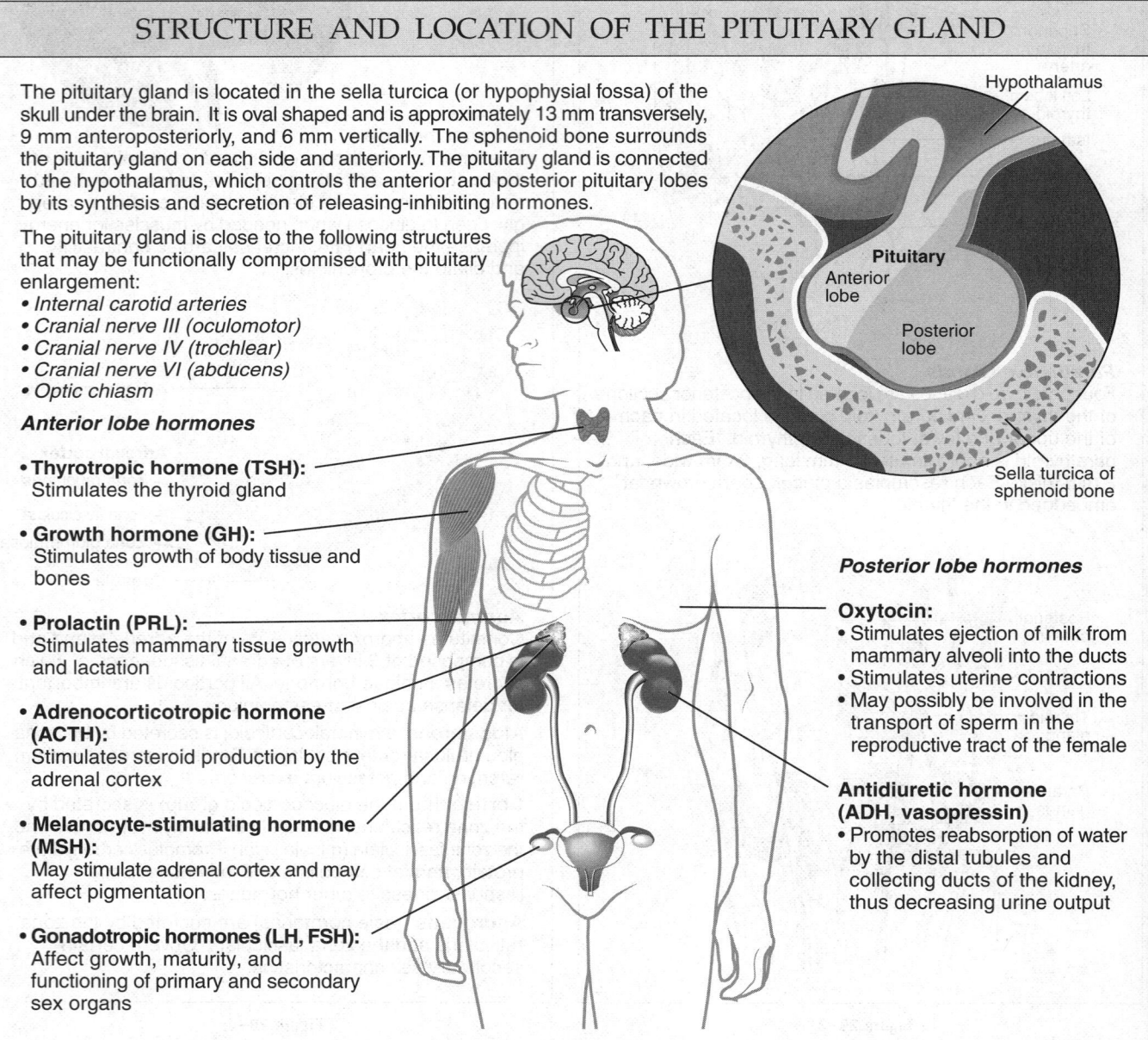

STRUCTURE AND LOCATION OF THE PITUITARY GLAND

The pituitary gland is located in the sella turcica (or hypophysial fossa) of the skull under the brain. It is oval shaped and is approximately 13 mm transversely, 9 mm anteroposteriorly, and 6 mm vertically. The sphenoid bone surrounds the pituitary gland on each side and anteriorly. The pituitary gland is connected to the hypothalamus, which controls the anterior and posterior pituitary lobes by its synthesis and secretion of releasing-inhibiting hormones.

The pituitary gland is close to the following structures that may be functionally compromised with pituitary enlargement:
• *Internal carotid arteries*
• *Cranial nerve III (oculomotor)*
• *Cranial nerve IV (trochlear)*
• *Cranial nerve VI (abducens)*
• *Optic chiasm*

Anterior lobe hormones

• **Thyrotropic hormone (TSH):**
Stimulates the thyroid gland

• **Growth hormone (GH):**
Stimulates growth of body tissue and bones

• **Prolactin (PRL):**
Stimulates mammary tissue growth and lactation

• **Adrenocorticotropic hormone (ACTH):**
Stimulates steroid production by the adrenal cortex

• **Melanocyte-stimulating hormone (MSH):**
May stimulate adrenal cortex and may affect pigmentation

• **Gonadotropic hormones (LH, FSH):**
Affect growth, maturity, and functioning of primary and secondary sex organs

Hypothalamus

Pituitary
Anterior lobe
Posterior lobe

Sella turcica of sphenoid bone

Posterior lobe hormones

Oxytocin:
• Stimulates ejection of milk from mammary alveoli into the ducts
• Stimulates uterine contractions
• May possibly be involved in the transport of sperm in the reproductive tract of the female

Antidiuretic hormone (ADH, vasopressin)
• Promotes reabsorption of water by the distal tubules and collecting ducts of the kidney, thus decreasing urine output

Figure 29–5.

ripheral vascular resistance than epinephrine and can therefore increase arterial blood pressure.

Pituitary Structure and Function

1. The pituitary structure is shown in Figure 29–5.
2. Anterior pituitary lobe (adenohypophysis)
   a. The anterior lobe is larger than the posterior lobe, making up about 80 percent of the gland. It is regulated by 6 releasing and inhibitory hormones secreted by the hypothalamus:

(1) Growth hormone–releasing hormone
(2) Growth hormone–inhibiting hormone (also called *somatostatin*)
(3) Thyrotropin-releasing hormone
(4) Corticotropin-releasing hormone
(5) Gonadotropin-releasing hormone
(6) Dopamine (prolactin-inhibiting hormone)

   b. The releasing or inhibiting hormones enter the hypothalamic-hypophyseal portal blood supply and then become part of the anterior pituitary gland.
   c. The anterior pituitary itself stores and releases 6 hormones (Table 29–1).

Table 29–1. *Pituitary Hormones, Target Organs, Functions, and Related Diseases*

Hormone	Target Organs	Functions	Diseases Related to Hypofunction	Diseases Related to Hyperfunction
Anterior Lobe				
Growth hormone (GH)	Entire body	Promotes growth of cells, bones, and tissues. Influences carbohydrate, fat, and protein metabolism. Increases blood glucose utilization. Is insulin antagonist. Increases lipolysis, free fatty acid levels, and ketone formation.	Primary pituitary failure GH deficiency secondary to hypothalamic dysfunction dwarfism Adults: no clinical manifestations Children: decreased body growth development	Somatotroph tumor Pre-epiphyseal closure Gigantism Acromegaly in adults
Prolactin	Breast Gonads	Is imperative for breast development and lactation. Controls reproductive function in males and females.	None	Prolactinoma
Thyroid-stimulating hormone (TSH)	Thyroid gland	Is imperative for growth and function of thyroid gland.	Hypothyroidism	Hyperthyroidism
Adrenocorticotropic hormone	Adrenal cortex	Is imperative for growth and size of adrenals. Controls release of glucocorticoids (cortisol) and adrenal androgens. Has a slight role in release of mineralocorticoids (aldosterone).	Cushing's disease or syndrome	Secondary adrenal cortical insufficiency Addison's disease
Gonadotropins (1) Follicle-stimulating hormone	Testes Ovaries	Stimulates the development of gametes (ovum and spermatozoan) in males and females.	None	Gonadotroph adenoma
(2) Luteinizing hormone	Testes and ovaries	Growth of follicles and increased secretion of estrogen and progesterone; increased testosterone secretion in males.	None	Amenorrhea
Posterior Lobe				
Antidiuretic hormone or vasopressin	Kidneys	Regulates osmolality and water volume. Increases permeability of collecting ducts in kidney to water, resulting in increased water reabsorption.	Diabetes insipidus	Syndrome of inappropriate antidiuretic hormone (SIADH)
Oxytocin	Breast tissue Uterus	Influences milk "letdown" in lactating breast. Causes uterine contractions in labor.	None	May contribute to SIADH-like manifestations

3. Posterior pituitary lobe (neurohypophysis)
   a. The posterior pituitary gland connects to the pituitary stalk and the hypothalamus via a rich nerve supply.
   b. The posterior lobe stores and releases 2 hormones that are actually synthesized in the hypothalamus and transported along nerve axons to the posterior pituitary.

STRUCTURE AND LOCATION OF THE PANCREAS

The pancreas is located behind the stomach. The head of the pancreas is found within the curve of the duodenum. The pancreas is a fish-shaped organ measuring 12–15 cm long, 3–5 cm wide, and a maximal thickness of 2–3 cm.

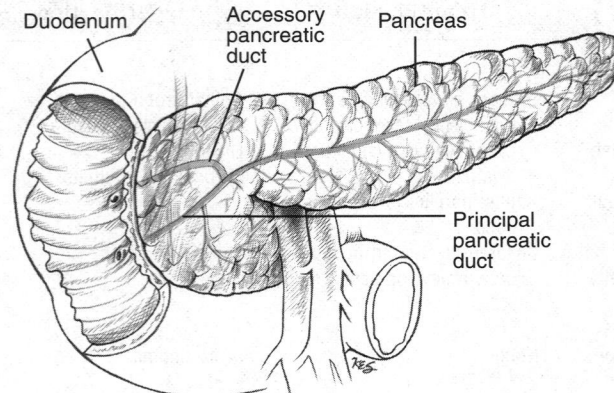

Duodenum *Accessory pancreatic duct* *Pancreas*

Principal pancreatic duct

Two major tissue types

Acini:
Secrete digestive juices into the duodenum (exocrine function)

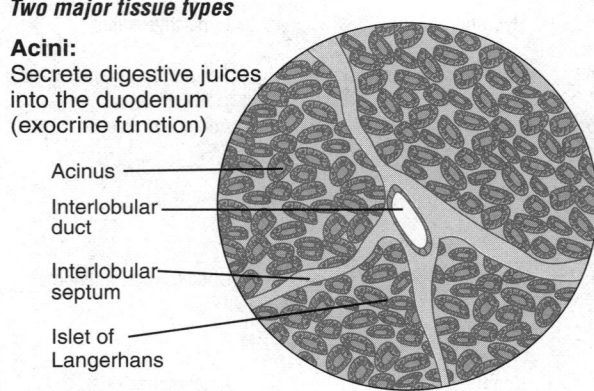

Acinus

Interlobular duct

Interlobular septum

Islet of Langerhans

Islets of Langerhans:
Secrete insulin and glucagon directly into the blood (endocrine function). The islet cells are composed of *alpha cells*, which make up about 25% of all cells and secrete glucagon; *beta cells*, which make up about 60% of all cells and secrete insulin; and *delta cells*, which make up about 10% of all cells and secrete somatostatin.
- Insulin: promotes metabolism of carbohydrates, protein, and fat, thus decreasing blood glucose levels
- Glucagon: mobilizes glycogen stores, thus raising blood glucose levels
- Somatostatin: decreases secretion of insulin, glucagon, growth hormone, and several gastrointestinal hormones (gastrin, secretin)

Figure 29–6.

Pancreatic Structure and Function

1. The structure and location of the pancreas are shown in Figure 29–6.
2. Secretion of glucagon and insulin
   a. Glucagon is released from the alpha cells in response to *decreasing* blood sugar. It increases the blood sugar level by promoting the conversion of glycogen to glucose within the liver.
   b. Insulin is released from the beta cells in response to *increasing* blood sugar. Its purpose is to enable blood sugar to enter a cell, where it can be used as an energy source. In conjunction with ACTH, corticosteroids, epinephrine, and thyroid hormones, insulin influences carbohydrate metabolism. Insulin's other functions include the following:
      (1) Assisting fat and protein metabolism
      (2) Promoting conversion of glucose to glycogen for storage
      (3) Inhibiting conversion of glycogen to glucose
      (4) Promoting conversion of fatty acids into fat and facilitating storage of fat as adipose tissue, mobilization of fat, and conversion of fat to ketone bodies
      (5) Stimulating protein synthesis within tissues
      (6) Inhibiting breakdown of protein into amino acids

◼ ASSESSMENT OF PEOPLE WITH ENDOCRINE DISORDERS

Key Symptoms and Their Pathophysiologic Bases

The key symptoms of endocrine disorders and their pathophysiologic bases are listed in Table 29–2.

Health History

1. History pertinent to all thyroid disorders
   a. History of head or neck radiation, surgery, or cancer
   b. Any neck pain, swelling, or fullness
2. See specific disorders for details on other relevant history issues.

Physical Examination

1. Check for key signs and symptoms (see Table 29–2).
2. See specific disorders for details on areas for especially close examination.

Diagnostic Studies

Diagnostic studies for the endocrine system are presented in Table 29–3.

Text continued on page 1361

Table 29–2. Key Symptoms of Endocrine Disorders and Their Pathophysiologic Bases

Key Symptom	Disorder	Pathophysiologic Basis
Mental Status Change		
Shortened attention span	Hyperthyroidism	Increased sympathetic nervous system activity
	Hypoglycemia	Insufficient glucose to the brain
Mental slowness or dullness	Hyperparathyroidism	Elevated serum calcium level
	Hypothyroidism	Decreased metabolism
	Hypoglycemia	Decreased glucose to brain
Irritability	Hypoparathyroidism	Hypocalcemia
	Hypocalcemia	Decreased glucose to brain
	Diabetes insipidus (DI)	Absence of antidiuretic hormone (ADH) results in excretion of polyuria and electrolyte imbalance
Delirium	Syndrome of inappropriate antidiuretic hormone (SIADH)	
	Hypoparathyroidism	Hypocalcemia
	Cushing's disease or syndrome	Hypercortisolemia
Vital Sign Alteration		
Hypothermia	Hypothyroidism	Decreased body metabolism and heat production
	Hypopituitarism	Head trauma or infiltrative disorders crowd sella, causing hypofunction of anterior pituitary hormones
Hyperthermia	Hyperparathyroidism	
	Hyperthyroidism	Increased metabolic rate
	Thyroiditis	Reaction to viral (subacute thyroiditis) or bacterial (acute thyroiditis) invasion
Tachycardia	Hyperthyroidism	Increased sympathetic nervous system rate
	Hypoglycemia	Compensatory mechanism influenced by epinephrine release
	Pheochromocytoma	Excess release of epinephrine
Bradycardia	Hypothyroidism	Decreased thyroid hormone
	Hyperparathyroidism	Hypercalcemia affects myocardial cells
Tachypnea	Diabetic ketoacidosis (DKA)	Compensatory mechanism for acidosis and volume depletion
Bradypnea	Hypothyroidism	Decreased circulating thyroid hormone
		Decreased body metabolism
Hypertension	Pheochromocytoma	Excess release of norepinephrine, epinephrine, and dopamine elevates blood pressure
	Hyperparathyroidism	Associated with chronic renal changes
		Hypercortisolemia
		Volume expansion, increased peripheral vascular resistance
Hypotension	DKA	Volume depletion secondary to polyuria
	Addison's disease (orthostatic hypotension)	Hypocortisolism contributes to volume depletion
	Hyperaldosteronism	Orthostatic hypotension without reflex tachycardia
	Hypopituitarism	Related to hyponatremia or adrenocorticotropin hormone deficiency
	DI	Absence of ADH and excessive polyuria
Weight Change		
Gain	Hypothyroidism	Decreased metabolic rate
	Cushing's disease	Redistribution of fat
	SIADH	Excess ADH retains large amounts of water (no edema)
		Related to degree of hyponatremia
Loss	Hyperthyroidism	Increased metabolic rate
	Addison's disease	Volume depletion secondary to hypoaldosteronism
	Hyperglycemia	Hyperglycemia's influences: osmotic diuresis and polyuria
	Hypoparathyroidism	Hypocalcemia's influences: gastrointestinal irritability, nausea, and vomiting
	Hyperparathyroidism	Hypercalcemia's influences: nausea and vomiting
	Pheochromocytoma	Related to prolonged paroxysm that includes nausea and vomiting
	DI	Absence of ADH causes polyuria
Change in Hair		
Fine hair	Hyperthyroidism	Increased metabolic rate and protein loss
Coarse hair	Hypothyroidism	Decreased metabolic rate
Eye Change		
	Diabetes mellitus (DM)	Hyperglycemia's influences: retinopathy, microangiopathy, and neuropathy

Table continued on following page

Table 29–2. Key Symptoms of Endocrine Disorders and Their Pathophysiologic Bases
(Continued)

Key Symptom	Disorder	Pathophysiologic Basis
	Hyperthyroidism (Graves' disease)	Exophthalmos related to excess periorbital fat, lid retraction, muscle swelling, and tissue edema
	Pituitary tumor	Tumor size contributing to exophthalmos or visual changes
Bone Change		
	Hyperparathyroidism	Bone resorption related to hypercalcemia
	Hyperpituitarism	Increase in growth hormone (acromegaly)
	Cushing's syndrome	Increased adrenal activity causes osteoporosis
Skin Change		
	Hypothyroidism	Dry skin related to decreased heat production
	Hyperthyroidism	Increased metabolic rate produces warm, moist skin
	Addison's disease	Hypocortisolism causes hyperpigmentation
	Hypoparathyroidism	Horizontal ridges of nails and dry, scaly skin related to hypocalcemia
	Cushing's disease	Acne, oily skin, abdominal striae, and easy bruising related to increased steroids
	Hypopituitarism	Multiple endocrine abnormality causes symptoms of Addison's disease (except for the skin changes) and hypopigmentation
	DI	Dry skin and mucous membranes secondary to polyuria
Neuromuscular Alteration		
Tremors	Hyperthyroidism	Increased sympathetic nervous system activity
	Hypoglycemia	Epinephrine release
	Pheochromocytoma	Hypersecretion of catecholamines
Weakness	Hyperthyroidism	Increased sympathetic nervous system activity causes excessive muscular activity with little rest
	Hyperparathyroidism	Myopathy influenced by neuropathic atrophy
	Cushing's disease	Proximal myopathy secondary to hypokalemia
		Protein tissue wasting
	SIADH	Related to degree of hyponatremia
Cramps	Hypoparathyroidism	Depressed parathyroid hormone (PTH) causes hypocalcemia
	Addison's disease	Hypoaldosteronism causes volume depletion and electrolyte imbalances
	SIADH	Electrolyte imbalances
Paresthesias	Hypoparathyroidism	Depressed PTH produces hypocalcemia and hypophosphatemia
	DM	Neuropathy and angiopathy
Hyperreflexia	Hyperthyroidism	Increased sympathetic system activity
	Hypoparathyroidism	Depressed PTH causes hypocalcemia
Hyporeflexia	Hyperparathyroidism	Hypercalcemia
	Hypothyroidism	Decreased body metabolism
	SIADH	Related to electrolyte imbalances
Fatigue	Hypoparathyroidism	Hypocalcemia causes neuromuscular symptoms that influence fatigue
	Hyperthyroidism	Increased metabolic rate
	Hypoglycemia	Decreased energy to muscles
	Pheochromocytoma	Paroxysms influenced by excess epinephrine release
	SIADH	Related to hyponatremia
Change in Sexual Function		
Decreased libido	Cushing's disease	Increased circulating sex hormones
	Hypopituitarism	Decreased sex hormones
Impotence	Hypothyroidism	Decreased sex hormones
	DM	Related to diabetic neuropathy and microvascular changes
	Cushing's disease	Increased estrogen and progesterone in males
	Hypopituitarism	Decreased sex hormones
Irregular menses	Hypoparathyroidism	Decreased sex hormones
	Hypothyroidism	Decreased sex hormones
	Addison's disease	Hypercortisolism

Table 29–3. Diagnostic Studies for the Endocrine System

Test	Description	Nursing Care	Significance of Findings
Pancreatic Function Studies			
Blood sugar, blood glucose	Evaluates current level of glucose in blood sample.	None	↑ : hyperglycemia, related to infection, stress, recent meal, steroid use, insulin underdose
Fasting blood sugar (FBS)	Evaluates glucose level in blood sample after fasting state.	Patient NPO at least 4 hr before phlebotomy. If known diabetic, hold A.M. food and insulin until blood drawn.	↓ : related to timing of hypoglycemic agent or insulin dose. Addison's disease, pituitary disorders, reactive hypoglycemia
Blood glucose finger-stick	Self-monitoring of blood sugar that is usually done to spot-check blood sugar when symptomatic or response to new treatment.	None	
Glycosylated hemoglobin, glycohemoglobin	Measures average of blood sugars in samples taken over 3 mo.	Sample may be obtained any time.	↑ : inadequate control or compliance
Glycosylated albumin (fructosamine)	Measures average of blood sugars in samples taken over previous 7–10 days.		↓ : inappropriate control or compliance
Ketones	May use urine or serum sample. Evaluates ketone presence as end product of fatty acid catabolism.	No preparation necessary.	↑ : lipolysis, hyperglycemia, acidosis, starvation
Glucose tolerance test (GTT) or oral glucose tolerance test	Evaluates pancreas's ability to tolerate an oral glucose load. FBS drawn prior to GTT. 100 gm concentrated glucose ingested by patient when NPO. Urine collected with phlebotomy at 30 min, 1 hr, 2 hr, and 3 hr after glucose ingestion.	Confirm NPO status with MD during test. Drugs that may interfere in nondiabetic patient: nicotine, aspirin, steroids, thiazide, oral contraceptives.	↑ : >200 mg/dl at 2 hr—diabetes, hyperglycemia in nondiabetic patient with hyperthyroidism, infection, or cancer
Thyroid Function Studies			
Blood tests			
Thyrotropin or thyroid-stimulating hormone (TSH)	TSH, which controls triiodothyronine (T_3) and thyroxine (T_4) production	None	↑ : hypofunction of thyroid gland or anterior pituitary; primary hypothyroidism ↓ : pituitary disorders; hyperthyroidism; high dosages of dopamine or corticosteroids
Thyroid antibodies	Measures presence of antibodies produced by body that may cause inflammation and destruction of thyroid gland.	Oral contraceptives may elevate titers.	↑ : thyroiditis
Free thyroxine index			↑ : hyperthyroidism ↓ : hypothyroidism
T_4	Provides a direct measurement of total amount of T_4 present in blood.	Fasting recommended. Note on lab slip if patient is taking thyroid supplements. Levels can be increased. Pregnancy or oral contraceptives may increase levels.	↑ : hyperthyroidism ↓ : hypothyroidism
T_3 by radioimmunoassay (RIA)	Measures small amount of potent thyroid hormones. T_3 is active form of thyroid hormone.	Same as T_4.	↑ : hyperthyroidism, pregnancy, oral contraceptives ↓ : hypothyroidism, hypoprotein conditions
T_3 resin uptake	Measures protein-bound T_3.	None	↑ : hyperthyroidism, low serum protein levels
Thyroid-binding globulins	Measures protein-bound T_4.	None	↓ : high serum protein hypothyroidism
Radioactive Tests			
Radioactive iodine uptake test (RAIU) ^{131}I uptake	24-hr urine collection begins after oral tracer dose has been given. Thyroid is scanned after 24 hr. Determines metabolic activity of thyroid gland by measuring absorption of ^{131}I by thyroid.	Patient education: radioactive dose is small and harmless. Contraindicated in pregnancy. Drugs that may elevate results: barbiturates, estrogen, lithium, phenothiazines.	↑ : hypothyroidism, thyroiditis, liver cirrhosis ↓ : hyperthyroidism

Table continued on the following page

Table 29–3. Diagnostic Studies for the Endocrine System (Continued)

Test	Description	Nursing Care	Significance of Findings
		Seafood may elevate results. Drugs that may decrease results: Lugol's solution, saturated solution of potassium iodide (SSKI), antithyroid, cortisone, aspirin, antihistamines.	
Parathyroid Function Studies			
Parathormone or parathyroid hormone (PTH)	Blood study that measures the amount of circulating PTH. Results usually correlated with serum calcium level drawn at same time.	No preparation	↑ : look for hypocalcemia and hyperphosphatemia, primary hyperparathyroid tumor ↓ : look for hypercalcemia, hyperphosphatemia, trauma, surgery, infection, and tumor
Serum calcium (total serum calcium)	Measures calcium in its free (ionized) calcium form and in its protein-bound form (albumin).	Thiazide diuretics and excessive ingestion of calcium-containing antacids may increase results.	↑ : check serum albumin, hyperparathyroidism, non–PTH-producing tumors ↓ : check serum albumin, hypoparathyroidism, renal failure
Ionized calcium	Sensitive measurement of serum calcium that is not influenced by serum albumin.	No preparation	↑ : hyperparathyroidism ↓ : hypoparathyroidism
Adrenal Cortex Function Studies			
Dexamethasone suppression test for cortisol levels	Dexamethasone given before phlebotomy to suppress diurnal formation of adrenocorticotropin hormone (ACTH). 1 mg of dexamethasone is given at 11:00 P.M. to suppress ACTH formation in time for 8:00 A.M. phlebotomy and later at 8:00 P.M.	None	↑ : pituitary tumor, Cushing's syndrome or disease, hyperplasia of adrenal cortex (benign or malignant) ↓ : Addison's disease
Fasting prephlebotomy for cortisol plasma level	Measures cortisol levels in the blood.	Plasma cortisol levels have diurnal effect: levels higher in A.M. than P.M. 2 hr of supine activity are necessary before test, because activity increases cortisol level. Estrogens increase level. Aldactone (spironolactone) can cause false-positive result.	↑ : pregnancy, activity, obesity, Cushing's disease or syndrome ↓ : Addison's disease
17-Hydroxysteroids (Porter-Silber test) 17-OCHS	Measure metabolites of glucocorticoids and aldosterone in urine.	24-hr urine collection to be kept on ice. Many drugs can invalidate results.	↑ : Cushing's disease or syndrome; ACTH administration; nonadrenal ACTH-producing tumor ↓ : Addison's disease or exogenous steroid suppression.
17-Ketosteroids	Measure steroid metabolites from adrenal cortex and testes (not including testosterone) in urine.	24-hr urine test; keep collection cold; may need preservative. Many drugs can invalidate results.	↑ : tumors of adrenal cortex or testes ↓ : hypofunction of adrenal or in patients who have had testes or ovaries removed
Aldosterone	Blood test measures mineralocorticoid production.	Patient to be supine 2 hr before phlebotomy. An increase in aldosterone can elevate extracellular fluid. Oral contraceptives, sodium restriction, and potassium may increase level.	↑ : primary or secondary hyperaldosteronism, severe liver dysfunction ↓ : Addison's disease
Urinary cortisol level	Measures cortisol, not metabolites, in urine.	None.	↑ : adrenal hyperfunction, Cushing's syndrome ↓ : not necessarily adrenal hypofunction
Renin level	Measures renin, an enzyme produced by juxtaglomerular apparatus in response to decreased blood flow to kidneys.	Patient in supine position. Results higher in A.M. Note sodium content in diet on lab slip.	↑ : hypertension, upright position with phlebotomy ↓ : high-sodium diet

Table 29–3. *Diagnostic Studies for the Endocrine System* (Continued)

Test	Description	Nursing Care	Significance of Findings
ACTH	Tests anterior pituitary function.	Drugs that interfere with results: diuretics, estrogens, oral contraceptives, antihypertensives. Fasting sample. Stress may artificially increase results.	↑: Cushing's syndrome due to bilateral adrenal hyperplasia or ectopic ACTH-producing tumors; Addison's disease due to adrenal gland failure, surgical removal of adrenals, or adrenal suppression with long-term exogenous steroid supply ↓: Addison's disease due to hypopituitarism; Cushing's syndrome when hyperfunction causes adrenal adenoma
Captopril test	Uses glomerular filtration rate (GFR) to rule out renal artery stenosis.	Nuclear medicine captopril renal scan done first to evaluate resting GFR. Captopril administered orally. GFR reevaluated after captopril.	↑: GFR: renal artery stenosis ↓: GFR after captopril: negative for renal artery stenosis

Adrenal Medulla Function Studies

Test	Description	Nursing Care	Significance of Findings
Epinephrine, norepinephrine levels	Measures catecholamines in blood.	NPO, resting serum sample.	↑: pheochromocytoma
Vanillylmandelic acid (VMA)	Urine test that measures catecholamine breakdown (epinephrine and norepinephrine).	24-hr iced or refrigerated urine collection. Patient to eliminate foods with VMA 3 days before collection: These are bananas, fruit juices, chocolate, tea, coffee, carbonated drinks, vanilla products, cheese, gelatins. Drugs that may increase results: salicylates, sulfonamides, penicillin, chlorpromazine isoproterenol, levodopa, lithium, nitroglycerin, methenamine, methocarbamol. No drugs 3 days before collection if possible.	↑: pheochromocytoma, neuroneoplasms, some foods and drugs ↓: uremia, drugs, some antihypertensives

Anterior Pituitary Gland Function Studies

Test	Description	Nursing Care	Significance of Findings
Testosterone	Measures circulating hormone produced by adrenal cortex, testes, and ovaries.	No preparation is necessary.	↑: androgenital syndrome (decreased cortisol and increased androgens) ↓: anterior pituitary insufficiency, testicular failure, alcoholism, hypopituitarism
Growth hormone (GH)	Blood drawn at intervals up to 120 min. Measures anterior pituitary gland release of GH.	GH is suppressed by hyperglycemia. GH is stimulated by hypoglycemia, levodopa, insulin, bromocriptine. Phlebotomy is drawn in A.M. because GH release is diurnal.	↑: in children, giantism; in adults, acromegaly, related to anterior pituitary tumors ↓: hypofunction of pituitary secondary to trauma, tumor, or unknown causes
Prolactin (PRL)	Measures anterior pituitary gland release of PRL.	Drug that may decrease level: levodopa. Many drugs may elevate level. Fasting specimen preferred.	↑: pregnancy, lactation, tumors of anterior pituitary, ectopic tumors of lung, hypothyroidism ↑: hypofunction of pituitary
Follicle-stimulating hormone (FSH)	May be serum or urine collection.	Note on lab slip if patient is taking oral contraceptives and phase in menstrual cycle.	↑: menopause, FSH-producing pituitary tumor, orchiectomy, hysterectomy, oophorectomy ↓: neoplasms of ovaries, testes, or adrenals; hypopituitarism; anorexia nervosa

Table continued on following page

Table 29–3. Diagnostic Studies for the Endocrine System (Continued)

Test	Description	Nursing Care	Significance of Findings
Luteinizing hormone (LH)	Blood test that measures anterior pituitary's release of LH.	Drugs that influence levels: oral contraceptives, estrogens, testosterone.	↑: amenorrhea, pituitary or testicular tumors ↓: primary hypogonadism, pituitary insufficiency (secondary hypogonadism)
Estradiol	Evaluates gonadal dysfunction.	Record phase of menstrual cycle on lab slip.	↑: primary amenorrhea, ovarian failure, hypopituitarism, menopause ↓: ovarian tumors, testicular tumors, adrenal hyperplasia
Estrogen	May reflect production from ovaries, adrenal cortex, or testes.	Oral contraceptives, estrogens, and steroids can increase level.	↑: ovarian tumors, adrenal hyperplasia, testicular tumor, cirrhosis of the liver ↓: postmenopausal, ovarian failure, primary hypogonadism, pituitary insufficiency
Progesterone	Measurement of progesterone from corpus luteum of ovaries.	Include last normal menstrual period or trimester of pregnancy on lab slip. Drugs that may influence results: ACTH, progesterone preparations.	↑: ovulation, third trimester of pregnancy, neoplasms of adrenal cortex and ovaries ↓: look for decreased LH during first part of menstrual cycle
Posterior Pituitary Gland Function Studies			
Water deprivation test	Evaluates ADH response to an artificially induced dehydrated state.	Patient NPO 4–18 hr during testing. Compare to urine output. Urine specific gravity is obtained and measured hourly while patient is NPO.	Absence of ADH: patient develops diabetes insipidus with increased urine output, decreased urine osmolarity. Presence of ADH: patient does not develop diabetes insipidus with decreased urine output, increased urine osmolarity.
Radiographic Studies			
Thyroid scan	Radioactive substances (injected isotopes or radioactive iodine taken orally) help visualize thyroid gland. Scanning done 24 hr later.	No preparation. Dose is harmless. Contraindications: SSKI, Lugol's solution, seafood intake, thyroid medications.	Cold nodules: cancer. Hot nodules: benign.
Ultrasonography	Identifies location and size of glands and nodules. Differentiates solid tumors from fluid-filled cysts.	No preparation is necessary. Provide patient education to alleviate anxiety (e.g., explain that patient will *not* be radioactive).	See specific disorders.
Magnetic resonance imaging	Reveals gland size and location and abnormalities.	Contraindicated for patients with pacemaker, arthroplasty, or metal skull plate. Assess patient for allergy to contrast media. Inquire about claustrophobia.	See specific disorders.
Computed tomography	Identifies location and structure of glands. Noninvasive. Contrast media may be used.	Provide patient education. Note allergy history.	See specific disorders.
Angiography of adrenals	Reveals neovascularization of gland for evaluation for neoplasms.	Contraindications: same as for any angiography. Note allergy to contrast media. Complications: hemorrhage, health crisis, extremity, ischemia or infarction from dislodgement of atherosclerotic plaque.	See "Caring for People with Adrenal Disorders."
X-rays	X-ray of sella turcica or pituitary to identify size, location, abnormalities.	No preparation necessary.	See specific disorders.
Other Procedures Used to Diagnose Endocrine Disorders			
Fine-needle aspiration	Provides sample of cells for histologic studies. Usually used as thyroid biopsy.	Patient education for short, relatively pain-free procedure. Observe site for swelling and bleeding.	Benign or malignant.

■ *CARING FOR PEOPLE WITH PANCREATIC DISORDERS*

Diabetes Mellitus

1. Definition and classification
   a. Diabetes mellitus (DM) is a chronic disorder involving impaired glucose tolerance. It is characterized by abnormal carbohydrate metabolism and altered fat and protein metabolism. A deficiency of insulin to meet the body's demands (as well as an increase in the counterregulatory hormones—cortisol, epinephrine, glucagon, and growth hormone) results in hyperglycemia, or elevated blood sugar.
   b. Two major types of DM are covered in this section: types I and II (Fig. 29–7).
   c. Type I DM is insulin-dependent diabetes mellitus (IDDM) and is usually characterized by the following:

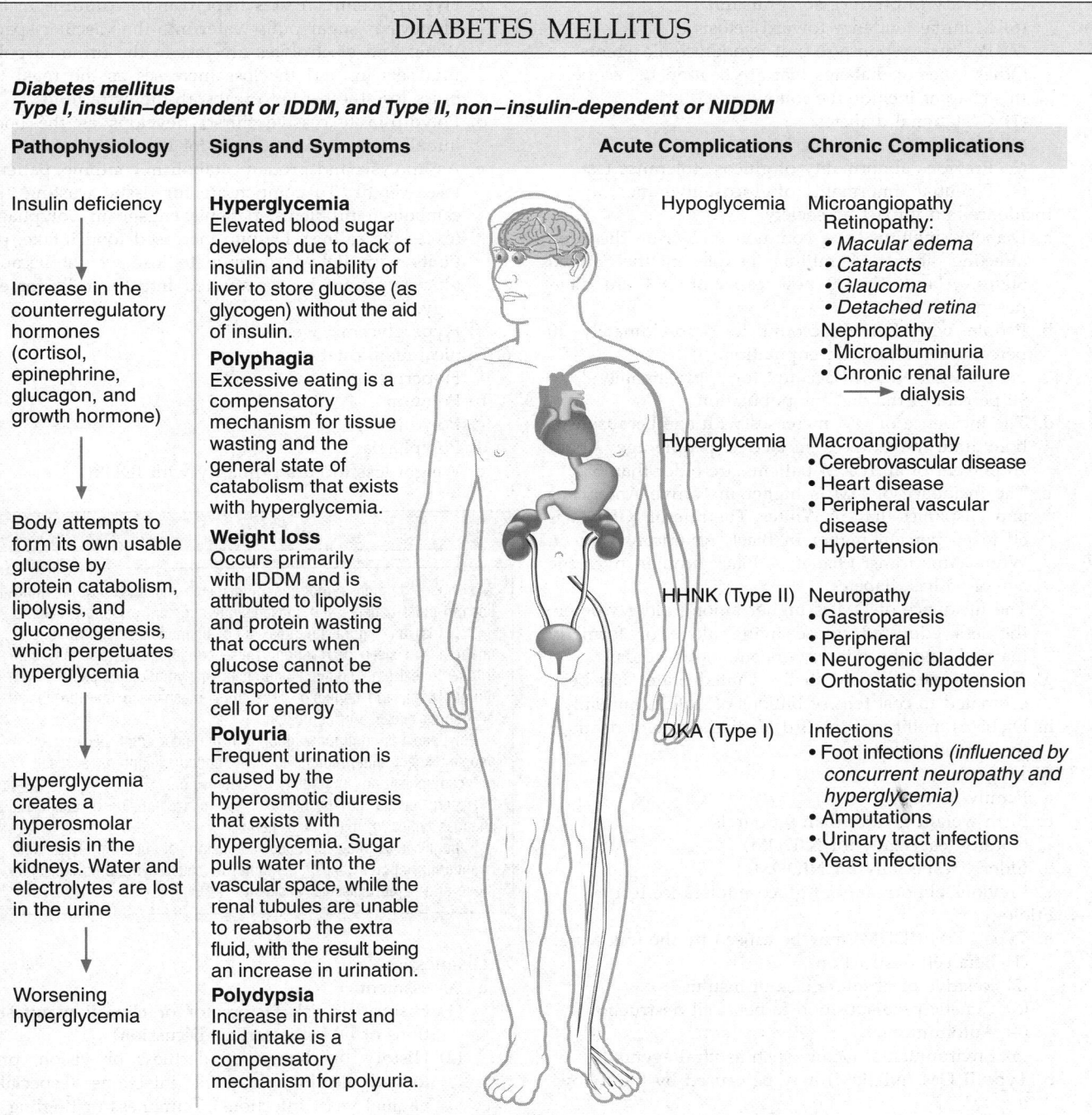

DIABETES MELLITUS

Diabetes mellitus
Type I, insulin–dependent or IDDM, and Type II, non–insulin-dependent or NIDDM

Pathophysiology	Signs and Symptoms	Acute Complications	Chronic Complications
Insulin deficiency ↓ Increase in the counterregulatory hormones (cortisol, epinephrine, glucagon, and growth hormone) ↓ Body attempts to form its own usable glucose by protein catabolism, lipolysis, and gluconeogenesis, which perpetuates hyperglycemia ↓ Hyperglycemia creates a hyperosmolar diuresis in the kidneys. Water and electrolytes are lost in the urine ↓ Worsening hyperglycemia	**Hyperglycemia** Elevated blood sugar develops due to lack of insulin and inability of liver to store glucose (as glycogen) without the aid of insulin. **Polyphagia** Excessive eating is a compensatory mechanism for tissue wasting and the general state of catabolism that exists with hyperglycemia. **Weight loss** Occurs primarily with IDDM and is attributed to lipolysis and protein wasting that occurs when glucose cannot be transported into the cell for energy **Polyuria** Frequent urination is caused by the hyperosmotic diuresis that exists with hyperglycemia. Sugar pulls water into the vascular space, while the renal tubules are unable to reabsorb the extra fluid, with the result being an increase in urination. **Polydypsia** Increase in thirst and fluid intake is a compensatory mechanism for polyuria.	Hypoglycemia Hyperglycemia HHNK (Type II) DKA (Type I)	Microangiopathy Retinopathy: • *Macular edema* • *Cataracts* • *Glaucoma* • *Detached retina* Nephropathy • Microalbuminuria • Chronic renal failure → dialysis Macroangiopathy • Cerebrovascular disease • Heart disease • Peripheral vascular disease • Hypertension Neuropathy • Gastroparesis • Peripheral • Neurogenic bladder • Orthostatic hypotension Infections • Foot infections *(influenced by concurrent neuropathy and hyperglycemia)* • Amputations • Urinary tract infections • Yeast infections

Figure 29–7. DKA, Diabetic ketoacidosis; HHNK, hyperglycemic, hyperosmolar, nonketotic.

(1) Onset before 30 years of age

(2) Rapid onset of hyperglycemia

(3) Failure to respond to oral hypoglycemic agents

(4) Tendency toward ketosis

(5) Need for exogenous insulin

d. Type II DM is non–insulin-dependent diabetes mellitus (NIDDM) and is usually characterized by the following:

(1) Onset after age 30

(2) Obesity

(3) Genetic predisposition (familial tendency)

(4) Insidious onset

(5) Ability to produce some insulin

(6) Minimal tendency toward ketosis

(7) Positive response to oral hypoglycemic agents

e. Other types of diabetes that are beyond the scope of this chapter include the following:

(1) Gestational diabetes

(2) Impaired glucose tolerance

(3) Previous abnormality of glucose tolerance test

(4) Potential abnormality of glucose tolerance

2. Incidence and impact on society

a. Diabetes mellitus is a common endocrine disorder, affecting about 14 million people in the United States. About 725,000 new cases of DM are diagnosed each year.

b. People with IDDM account for approximately 10 percent of the diabetic population.

c. People with NIDDM account for approximately 85 to 90 percent of the diabetic population.

d. The incidence of DM increases with age because carbohydrate intolerances surface as people age. About 70 percent of all IDDM patients are older than 55.

e. The incidence of DM is higher in Native Americans and Hispanics than in Whites. The rate of NIDDM is 50 to 60 percent higher in Black Americans than in White Americans. One in 4 Black women over the age of 55 has diabetes.

f. The incidence of DM is higher among older women, the less educated, those living alone or formerly married, and those in low-income households.

g. The treatment of DM in the United States has been estimated to cost tens of billions of dollars annually.

h. Diabetes mellitus is the 3rd leading cause of death in the United States.

3. Risk factors

a. Family history

b. Birth weight greater than 9 pounds

c. Obesity (especially for NIDDM)

d. Elderly (especially for NIDDM)

e. Previous abnormality of glucose tolerance test

4. Etiology

a. Type I DM (IDDM) may be caused by the following:

(1) Beta cell destruction

(2) Relative or absolute lack of insulin

(3) Genetic predisposition to beta cell destruction

(4) Autoimmunity

(5) Environmental factors such as viral agents

b. Type II DM (NIDDM) may be caused by the following:

(1) Impaired insulin secretion

(2) Insulin resistance or insensitivity

(3) Heredity

(4) Obesity

(5) Lack of exercise, which accentuates obesity

5. Pathophysiology

a. When insulin is deficient relative to blood sugar level, the blood sugar level rises. The lack of insulin also keeps the liver from storing glucose (as glycogen), exacerbating the problem.

b. The body attempts to form its own usable glucose by protein catabolism and gluconeogenesis. This process perpetuates the hyperglycemic state.

c. Hyperglycemia creates hyperosmolar diuresis in the kidneys as sugar pulls water into the vascular space. Water and electrolytes are lost in the urine as polyuria sets in, and the loss increases as the renal tubules lose the battle to reabsorb the extra fluid.

d. Polydipsia (excessive thirst) develops as the body initially tries to compensate for the fluid loss.

e. As lipolysis and protein catabolism continue, patients lose weight. To compensate for tissue wasting and catabolism problems, patients engage in polyphagia (excessive eating). Despite increased food intake, patients with IDDM continue to lose weight because glucose cannot be transported into the cells for energy.

f. Hyperglycemia worsens.

6. Clinical manifestations

a. Hyperglycemia

b. Polyuria

c. Polydipsia

d. Polyphagia

e. Weight loss (occurs primarily with IDDM)

ELDER ADVISORY

The most common symptoms of diabetes mellitus may go unnoticed in older patients and consequently augment existing problems.

Polyuria may aggravate preexisting incontinence, contributing to nocturia and sleep deprivation. These conditions in turn may contribute to extreme fatigue, night falls, dehydration (especially with diuretic use), and confusion. The thirst mechanism may be absent or ignored because of confusion.

Polyphagia is commonly ignored in the older adult, because many people expect older adults to have added weight as a result of reduced socializing, immobility, or depression.

Hyperglycemia may be mistaken for mild confusion or behavioral changes typical of many older people.

Hypoglycemia may produce confusion or behavioral changes (wandering, aggression, or paranoia) or cause symptoms similar to those of a cerebrovascular accident.

7. Diagnostics

a. Assessment

(1) History of risk factors for or clinical manifestations of DM (see earlier discussion)

(2) History of change in alertness or vision, prolonged healing, frequent infections (especially vaginal yeast infections), numbness or tingling of hands or feet, or fatigue

Table 29–4. Comparison of Therapies for Diabetes Mellitus

	Conventional Therapy	Intensive Therapy
Insulin administration	One or 2 daily injections, including mixtures of rapid- and intermediate-acting insulins. Daily adjustments are not made.	Administration of insulin 3 or more times daily by injection or insulin per an insulin pump. Dosage adjusted according to SMBG, dietary intake, and anticipated exercise.
Goals	Absence of symptoms R/T glycosuria or hypoglycemia. Absence of ketonuria. Maintenance of normal growth and development. Ideal body weight. Freedom from frequent or severe hypoglycemia.	Fasting blood sugar 70–120 mg/dl. Postmeal blood sugar <180 mg/dl. Weekly 0300 blood sugar >65 mg/dl. Monthly glycosylated hemoglobin <6%.
Monitoring	Daily monitoring of urine or blood glucose. Examination every 3 mo.	SMBG at least 4 times daily. Follow-up monthly and more frequently by telephone.
Education	Regarding diet and exercise.	Regarding diet, exercise, and how to adjust insulin dosages.

SMBG, Self-monitoring blood glucose.

(3) For established diabetics, history of dietary habits, nutritional status, weight; details of previous and current treatment modalities (including diabetic education); exercise history; frequency, severity, and cause of acute complications, prior or current infections, symptoms and treatment of chronic complications; medications that may affect blood glucose control; risk factors for atherosclerosis; gestational history, including hyperglycemia, birth weight greater than 9 pounds, toxemia, stillbirths, other complications

(4) Psychosocial and economic factors that might influence the management of DM

(5) Transcultural considerations (see Chapter 2)
  • Cultural dietary practices such as fasting and consumption of holiday foods
  • Long-term insulin treatment as it is affected by cultural concepts of time
  • Patient's explanatory model of disease

(6) Physical examination findings: Patients presenting with new onset of hyperglycemia may be asymptomatic. Patients with more advanced DM may demonstrate any of the following:
  • General findings: obesity or lethargy
  • Integumentary system: evidence of poor healing, lipodystrophy, or lipohypertrophy
  • Eyes: fundoscopic evidence of maculopathy, cataracts, microaneurysms, hypertensive retinopathy, dot hemorrhages, or hard exudates
  • Neuromuscular system: weakness or paresthesias of the extremities (may be asymmetric)
  • Cardiovascular system: evidence of atherosclerotic disease with poor circulation to the feet, hypertension, cool extremities, bruits or thrills, or orthostatic hypotension
  • Gastrointestinal system: hypoactive bowel sounds, pain, or rigidity

b. Medical diagnosis (see also Table 29–3) is based on the following:
  (1) Blood sugar greater than 150 mg per dl
  (2) Fasting blood sugar greater than 150 mg per dl × 3

(3) Glycosylated hemoglobin greater than 7.5 to 8.0 percent
(4) Elevated glycosylated albumin
(5) Ketones in urine or serum
(6) Glucose tolerance test: blood sugar greater than 200 mg per dl at 2 hours
(7) Fasting lipid profile: total cholesterol, high-density lipoproteins, low-density lipoproteins, and triglycerides

8. Clinical management
  a. Goals
    (1) Control glycemia. The Diabetes Control and Complications Trial demonstrated that intensive control of blood sugar in type I diabetes can prevent or delay complications of diabetes. Those with type II diabetes benefit similarly from tight glycemic control (Table 29–4 and Box 29–1).
    (2) Prevent or minimize complications.
    (3) Educate patients on their lifelong responsibilities regarding diabetic care (Box 29–2).
  b. Nonpharmacologic interventions
    (1) A diet prescribed according to the American Diabetic Association guidelines will reflect calories based on current or desired weight (Procedure 29–1), a diet high in complex carbohydrates and low in fat (Tables 29–5 and 29–6), and behavior

---

BOX 29–1. The Diabetes Control and Complications Trial

The Diabetes Control and Complications Trial (DCCT) was a multicenter, randomized, nearly 10-year (1983–1993) clinical trial designed to compare the results of intensive diabetes therapy with those of conventional diabetes therapy regarding their effects on the development and progression of the early vascular and neurologic complications of type I diabetes mellitus. Table 29–4 compares the conventional therapy and intensive therapy regimens.

Results of the study: Intensive therapy delays the onset and slows the progression of chronic complications of diabetes by 35 percent to more than 70 percent. On the basis of these results, the DCCT recommends that most patients with type I diabetes mellitus be treated with closely monitored intensive regimens.

BOX 29-2. Management of Diabetes

Staged Diabetes Management (SDM) was developed by the International Diabetes Center in Minneapolis, Minnesota, in an effort to understand the current state of diabetes care and develop a new approach consistent with national practice standards.

On the basis of 3000 cases of diabetes of several types, researchers developed a series of guidelines that lead to "Decision-Paths" that show the sequence of therapy options and tell patients and health care providers where therapy has been and where it is going in terms of phase and stage. Goals are clearly stated, as are stages of therapies and criteria for moving from one to another. Detailed manuals further explain the use of these devices.

In addition to clarifying therapeutic options and monitoring progress, a major advantage of SDM is team building. It includes the patient and family, in setting goals, deciding on treatments, and communicating the success or failure of those therapies.

Type II Diabetes Practice Guidelines

Diagnosis	Majority are over age 40 (with risk factors over age 30) and obese*
Plasma blood glucose:	*Random* ≥ 200 mg/dl plus symptoms or *Fasting* ≥ 140 mg/dl on 2 occasions
Symptoms:	*Often none* *Common (classic)*: Blurred vision, urinary tract infection, yeast infection, dry/itchy skin, numbness/tingling in extremities, fatigue *Occasional (subtle)*: Increased urination, thirst, and appetite; nocturia; weight loss
Urine ketones:	Negative (usually)
Risk factors:	• Obese (particularly increased waist-to-hip ratio) • Previous gestational diabetes (GDM) • Positive family history • Age >40 (risk increases with age) • Previous impaired glucose tolerance (IGT) • Ethnicity: American Indian, African American, Asian American, or Hispanic
Treatment Options	Food plan and exercise; oral agent; combination therapy; insulin stages 2, 3A, 4A
Targets	More than 50% of values should be within target range
Self-monitored blood glucose:	• 80–140 mg/dl (pre-meal) 100–160 mg/dl (pre-evening snack) • No severe (assisted) or nocturnal hypoglycemia Adjust target if decreased life expectancy; frail elderly; cognitive disorders; or other medical concerns (cardiac disease, stroke, hypoglycemia unawareness, end-stage renal disease); consider target of 100–160 mg/dl pre-meal
Hemoglobin A_{1c} (HbA_{1c}):	Within 1.5% of upper limit of normal (e.g., normal 6%; target <7.5%) and test 3–4 times per year. HbA_{1c} can be used to verify self-monitored blood glucose (SMBG) data or if no SMBG data available. If possible, obtain prior to clinic visit to assist in clinical decision-making. If HbA_{1c} does not correlate with SMBG, check meter accuracy, assess patient SMBG skills, monitor BG more frequently, and/or refer for diabetes education.
Monitoring	
Blood glucose:	2–4 times per day (before each meal and the evening snack) May be modified for other reasons (cost, technical ability)
Method:	Meter with memory recommended
Follow-up	
Monthly:	Office visit during adjust phase (weekly phone contact may be necessary)
Every 3–4 months:	Hypoglycemia, weight or BMI (kg/m² = weight/height²), medications, blood pressure, SMBG data (cleaning and checking meter), food plan, exercise, foot care, and HbA_{1c} (or fructosamine)
Yearly:	History and physical, fasting lipid profile, urinalysis, microalbumin, neurologic examination, eye examination with dilation, dental examination, diabetes and nutrition continuing education

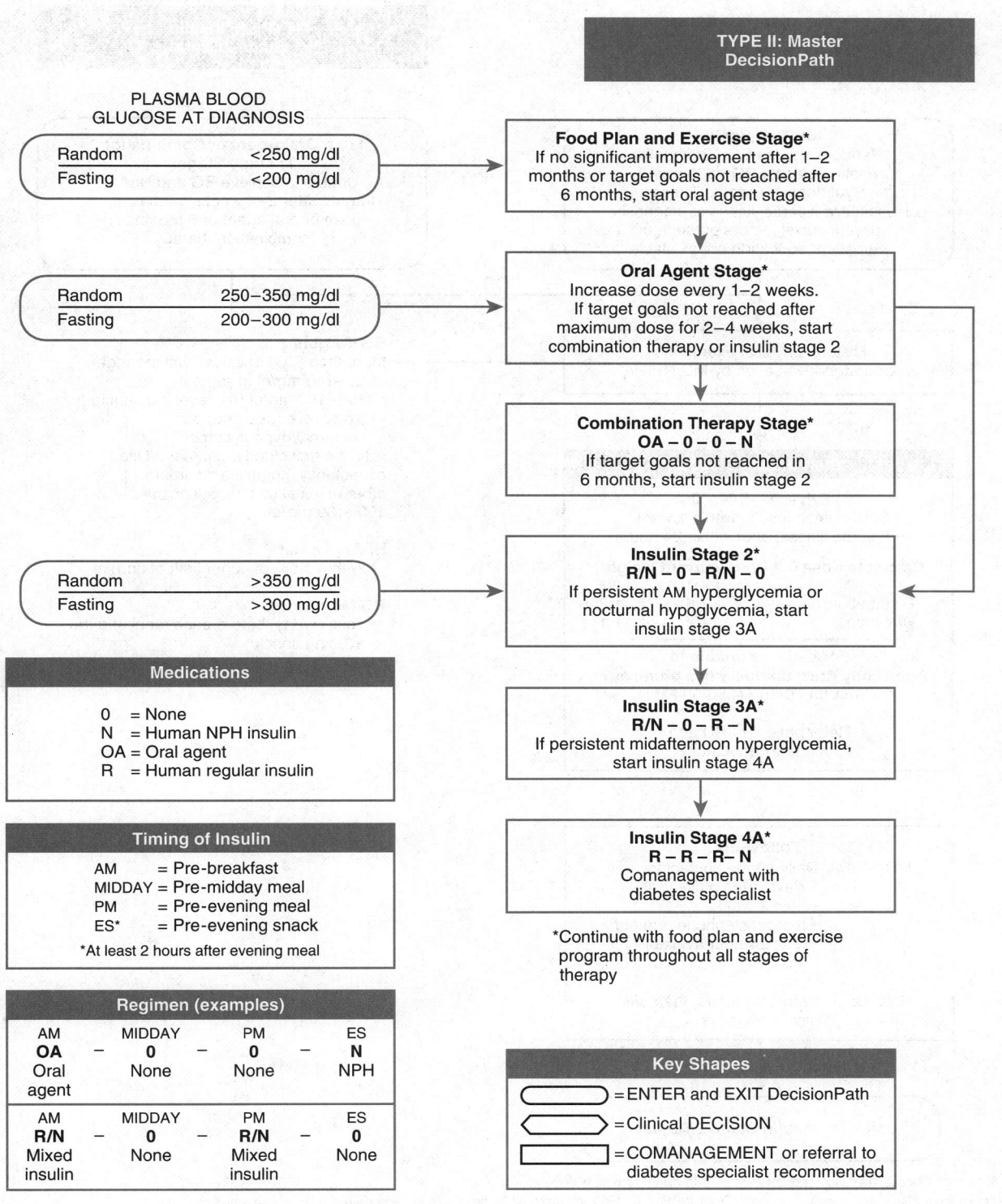

TYPE II: Master
DecisionPath

PLASMA BLOOD
GLUCOSE AT DIAGNOSIS

| Random | <250 mg/dl |
| Fasting | <200 mg/dl |

| Random | 250–350 mg/dl |
| Fasting | 200–300 mg/dl |

| Random | >350 mg/dl |
| Fasting | >300 mg/dl |

Food Plan and Exercise Stage*
If no significant improvement after 1–2
months or target goals not reached after
6 months, start oral agent stage

Oral Agent Stage*
Increase dose every 1–2 weeks.
If target goals not reached after
maximum dose for 2–4 weeks, start
combination therapy or insulin stage 2

Combination Therapy Stage*
OA – 0 – 0 – N
If target goals not reached in
6 months, start insulin stage 2

Insulin Stage 2*
R/N – 0 – R/N – 0
If persistent AM hyperglycemia or
nocturnal hypoglycemia, start
insulin stage 3A

Insulin Stage 3A*
R/N – 0 – R – N
If persistent midafternoon hyperglycemia,
start insulin stage 4A

Insulin Stage 4A*
R – R – R– N
Comanagement with
diabetes specialist

*Continue with food plan and exercise
program throughout all stages of
therapy

Medications

0	= None
N	= Human NPH insulin
OA	= Oral agent
R	= Human regular insulin

Timing of Insulin

AM	= Pre-breakfast
MIDDAY	= Pre-midday meal
PM	= Pre-evening meal
ES*	= Pre-evening snack

*At least 2 hours after evening meal

Regimen (examples)

AM	MIDDAY	PM	ES
OA	– **0**	– **0**	– **N**
Oral agent	None	None	NPH

AM	MIDDAY	PM	ES
R/N	– **0**	– **R/N**	– **0**
Mixed insulin	None	Mixed insulin	None

Key Shapes

= ENTER and EXIT DecisionPath
= Clinical DECISION
= COMANAGEMENT or referral to diabetes specialist recommended

Box continued on following page

BOX 29–2. Management of Diabetes *Continued*

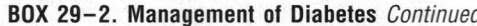

TYPE II: Insulin
Stage 2/Start

At Diagnosis
Random plasma BG >350 mg/dl
Fasting plasma BG >300 mg/dl
Symptoms, +/– acute illness
Hospitalize if acute illness at diagnosis,
psychosocial factors present, or
outpatient education not available

From **Oral Agent** or **Combination
Therapy Stages**
Unable to achieve BG and HbA₁c
targets after 2–4 weeks on maximum
dose of oral agent or 6 months on
combination therapy

OR

History, physical exam, and
laboratory evaluation by MD/NP/PA

BG Targets
More than 50% of values within range
• 80–140 mg/dl (pre-meal)
  100–160 mg/dl (pre-evening snack)
• No severe (assisted) or
  nocturnal hypoglycemia
Adjust if frail elderly, decreased life
expectancy, cognitive disorders,
other medical concerns, consider
100–160 mg/dl

HbA₁c Target
• Within 1.5% of upper limit of normal

BG Monitoring
• Test 4x/day, before each meal and the
  evening snack

Start Insulin Stage 2

R/N – 0 – R/N – 0
• Start human insulin within 1 week
• If acute illness, start within 24 hours

Calculate dose 0.3 U/kg (current weight)

	AM	PM
Distribution	2/3	1/3
R/N ratio	1:2	1:1

**For patients unable to
correctly draw up dose, use premixed
insulin 70/30 AM 50/50 PM**

Refer patient to RD and
diabetes educator

Follow-up
MD/NP/PA: Daily phone contact for
3 days, then office visit
within 2 weeks
Emergency phone number
within 24-hour availability
necessary

RN/RD: Within 24 hours, then office
visit in 2 weeks

Move to **Insulin Stage 2/Adjust**

* *Note:* Oral Glucose Tolerance Test is rarely used to diagnose type II diabetes.
Redrawn from Staged Diabetes Management *DecisionPaths,* © 1995 International Diabetes Center, Minneapolis, MN, with permission.

modification and evaluation of eating habits as factors in weight control.

(2) As an alternative to the traditional food exchange from the American Diabetic Association diet,

physicians may prescribe adherence to the dietary guidelines for Americans (Food Guide Pyramid) issued by the U.S. Departments of Agriculture and Health and Human Services in 1992 or

Text continued on page 1374

Procedure 29–1
How to Calculate Caloric Needs for the Patient with Diabetes Mellitus

Procedure	Example

Method 1†

For Women

1. Start by assuming 100 lb of body weight for the first 5 ft of height.

2. Add 5 lb for each inch above 5 ft, or subtract 5 lb for each inch below 5 ft.

3. To account for body frame, add 10% of the total in step 2 for a large frame, or subtract 10% for a small frame to arrive at *estimated body weight*.

4. To determine *basic caloric need,* multiply the estimated body weight from step 3 by 10.

5. To account for activity level
   a. Add 3 kcal/lb of estimated body weight to basic caloric need for an inactive woman.
   b. Add 5 kcal/lb of estimated body weight to basic caloric need for a normally active woman.
   c. Add 8–10 kcal/lb of estimated body weight to basic caloric need for a very active woman.

6. To account for menopausal status, subtract 25% from the total in step 5 for a postmenopausal woman.

In a normally active, small-framed, 5-ft 4-in postmenopausal woman, the calculation is as follows:

1. 100 lb
2. $+(4 \times 5) = 120$ lb
3. $-(120 - 10\%) = 108$ lb
4. $\times 10 = 1080$ kcal
5. $+(108 \times 5) = 1620$ kcal

6. $-(1620 \times 25\%) = 1215$ kcal

For Men

1. Start by assuming 106 lb of body weight for the first 5 ft of height.

2. Add 6 lb for each inch above 5 ft, or subtract 6 lb for each inch below 5 ft.

3. To account for body frame, add 10% of the total in step 2 for a large frame, or subtract 10% for a small frame to arrive at *estimated body weight*.

4. To determine *basic caloric need,* multiply the estimated body weight from step 3 by 10.

5. To account for activity level
   a. Add 3 kcal/lb of estimated body weight to basic caloric need for an inactive man.
   b. Add 5 kcal/lb of estimated body weight to basic caloric need for a normally active man.
   c. Add 8–10 kcal/lb of estimated body weight to basic caloric need for a very active man.

In a very active, large-framed, 5-ft 11-in man, the calculation is as follows:

1. 106 lb
2. $+(11 \times 6) = 172$ lb
3. $+(172 + 10\%) = 189.2$ lb

4. $\times 10 = 1892$ kcal

5. $+(9 \times 189.2) = 3594.8$ kcal

Method 2‡

1. Convert body weight from pounds to kilograms by multiplying by 0.45.

2. To determine *caloric need,* multiply weight in kilograms by 30 for a normally active person, by 35–40 for a very active person, or by 25 for an inactive person.

In a normally active, 120-lb adult, the calculation is as follows:

1. $120 \times 0.45 = 54$ kg

2. $\times 30 = 1620$ kcal

---

* These methods are a starting point. Caloric needs should be fine-tuned to account for individual variations.
† This method can be used when the patient's height is known, but weight is not.
‡ This less precise method can be used when the patient's weight is known.
From Ignatavicius DD, and Bayne MV. *Medical-Surgical Nursing: A Nursing Process Approach.* Philadelphia: WB Saunders, 1991, pp 1617–1618.

Table 29–5. Exchange Lists for Diabetes Nutrition Management

Starch/Bread List

Each item in this list contains approximately 15 gm carbohydrate, 3 gm protein, a trace of fat, and 80 kcal. Whole-grain products average about 2 gm fiber per serving. Some foods are higher in fiber.

Starch exchanges can be chosen from any of the items on this list. The general rule for starch foods not on this list is that:

½ cup of cereal, grain, or pasta is one serving.

1 oz of a bread product is one serving.

Cereals/Grains/Pasta

*Bran cereals, concentrated	⅓ cup
*Bran cereals, flaked	½ cup
(such as Bran Buds, All-Bran)	
Bulgur (cooked)	½ cup
Cooked cereals	½ cup
Cornmeal (dry)	2½ T
Grape-Nuts	3 T
Grits (cooked)	½ cup
Other ready-to-eat unsweetened cereals	¾ cup
Pasta (cooked)	½ cup
Puffed cereal	1½ cup
Rice, white or brown (cooked)	⅓ cup
Shredded Wheat	½ cup
*Wheat germ	3 T

Dried Beans/Peas/Lentils

*Beans and peas (cooked)	⅓ cup
(such as kidney, white, split, blackeye)	
*Lentils (cooked)	⅓ cup
*Baked beans	¼ cup

Starchy Vegetables

*Corn	½ cup
*Corn on cob, 6-in long	1
*Lima beans	½ cup
*Peas, green (canned or frozen)	½ cup
*Plantain	½ cup
Potato, baked	1 small (3 oz)
Potato, mashed	½ cup
Squash, winter (acorn, butternut)	¾ cup
Yam, sweet potato, plain	⅓ cup

Bread

Bagel	½ (1 oz)
Bread sticks, crisp, 4-in long × ½ in	2 (⅔ oz)
Croutons, low-fat	1 cup
English muffin	½
Frankfurter or hamburger bun	½ (1 oz)
Pita, 6-in across	½
Plain roll, small	1 (1 oz)
Raisin, unfrosted	1 slice (1 oz)
*Rye, pumpernickel	1 slice (1 oz)
Tortilla, 6-in across	1
White (including French, Italian)	1 slice (1 oz)
Whole wheat	1 slice (1 oz)
Taco shell, 6-in across	2
Waffle, 4½-in square	1
Whole wheat crackers, fat added (such as Triscuits)	4–6 (1 oz)

Crackers/Snacks

Animal crackers	8
Graham crackers, 2½-in square	3
Matzoth	¾ oz
Melba toast	5 slices
Oyster crackers	24
Popcorn (popped, no fat added)	3 cups
Pretzels	¾ oz
Rye Crisp, 2-in × 3½-in	4
Saltine-type crackers	6
Whole wheat crackers, no fat added (crisp breads, such as Finn, Kavli, Wasa)	2–4 slices (¾ oz)

Starch Foods Prepared with Fat
(Count as 1 starch/bread serving, plus 1 fat serving)

Biscuit, 2½-in across	1
Chow mein noodles	½ cup
Corn bread, 2-in cube	1 (2 oz)
Cracker, round butter type	6
French-fried potatoes, 2-in to 3½-in long	10 (1½ oz)
Muffin, plain, small	1
Pancake, 4-in across	2
Stuffing, bread (prepared)	¼ cup

* Foods with 3 or more gm of fiber per serving.

Meat List

Each serving of meat and substitutes on this list contains about 7 gm of protein. The amount of fat and number of calories vary, depending on the kind of meat or substitute chosen. The list is divided into three parts based on the amount of fat and calories: lean meat, medium-fat meat, and high-fat meat. One ounce (1 meat exchange) of each of these includes:

	Carbohydrate (gm)	Protein (gm)	Fat (gm)	Calories
Lean	0	7	3	55
Medium-fat	0	7	5	75
High-fat	0	7	8	100

Table 29–5. Exchange Lists for Diabetes Nutrition Management (Continued)

Lean Meat and Substitutes
(One exchange is equal to any 1 of the following items.)

Beef:	USDA Good or Choice grades of lean beef, such as round, sirloin, and flank steak; tenderloin; and chipped beef†	1 oz
Pork:	Lean pork, such as fresh ham; canned, cured, or boiled ham;† Canadian bacon,† tenderloin	1 oz
Veal:	All cuts are lean except for veal cutlets (ground or cubed). Examples of lean veal are chops and roasts.	1 oz
Poultry:	Chicken, turkey, Cornish hen (without skin)	1 oz
Fish:	All fresh and frozen fish	1 oz
	Crab, lobster, scallops, shrimp, clams (fresh or canned in water†)	2 oz
	Oysters	6 medium
	Tuna† (canned in water)	¼ cup
	Herring (uncreamed or smoked)	1 oz
	Sardines (canned)	2 medium
Wild Game:	Venison, rabbit, squirrel	1 oz
	Pheasant, duck, goose (without skin)	1 oz
Cheese:	Any cottage cheese	¼ cup
	Grated Parmesan	2 T
	Diet cheeses† (with less than 55 kcal/oz)	1 oz
Other:	95% fat-free luncheon meat	1 oz
	Egg whites	3 whites
	Egg substitutes with less than 55 kcal per ¼ cup	¼ cup

Medium-Fat Meat and Substitutes
(One exchange is equal to any 1 of the following items.)

Beef:	Most beef products fall into this category. Examples are: all ground beef, roast (rib, chuck, rump), steak (cubed, Porterhouse, T-bone), and meatloaf.	1 oz
Pork:	Most pork products fall into this category. Examples are: chops, loin roast, Boston butt, cutlets.	1 oz
Lamb:	Most lamb products fall into this category. Examples are: chops, leg, and roast.	1 oz
Veal:	Cutlet (ground or cubed, unbreaded)	1 oz
Poultry:	Chicken (with skin), domestic duck or goose (well-drained of fat), ground turkey	1 oz
Fish:	Tuna† (canned in oil and drained)	¼ cup
	Salmon† (canned)	¼ cup
Cheese:	Skim or part-skim milk cheeses, such as:	
	Ricotta	¼ cup
	Mozzarella	1 oz
	Diet cheeses† (with 56–80 kcal/oz)	1 oz
Other:	86% fat-free luncheon meat†	1 oz
	Egg (high in cholesterol, limit to 3/wk)	1
	Egg substitutes with 56–80 kcal per ¼ cup	¼ cup
	Tofu (2½ in × 2¾ in × 1 in)	4 oz
	Liver, heart, kidney, sweetbreads (high in cholesterol)	1 oz

High-Fat Meat and Substitutes

Remember, these items are high in saturated fat, cholesterol, and calories, and should be used only three (3) times per week. (One exchange is equal to any 1 of the following items.)

Beef:	Most USDA Prime cuts of beef, such as ribs, corned beef†	1 oz
Pork:	Spareribs, ground pork, pork sausage† (patty or link)	1 oz
Lamb:	Patties (ground lamb)	1 oz
Fish:	Any fried fish product	1 oz
Cheese:	All regular cheeses,† such as American, Blue, Cheddar, Monterey, Swiss	1 oz
Other:	Luncheon meats,† such as bologna, salami, pimento loaf	1 oz
	Sausage,† such as Polish, Italian	1 oz
	Knockwurst, smoked	1 oz
	Bratwurst†	1 oz
	Frankfurter (turkey or chicken)	1 frank (10/lb)
	Peanut butter (contains unsaturated fat)	1 T

Count as 1 high-fat meat plus 1 fat exchange:

	Frankfurter† (beef, pork, or combination)	1 frank (10/lb)

† Foods with 400 mg or more of sodium per exchange.

Vegetable List

Each vegetable serving on this list contains about 5 gm carbohydrate, 2 gm protein, and 25 kcal. Vegetables contain 2–3 gm of dietary fiber. Vegetables are a good source of vitamins and minerals. Fresh and frozen vegetables have more vitamins and less added salt.

Unless otherwise noted, the serving size for vegetables (1 vegetable exchange) is:

½ cup of cooked vegetables or vegetable juice.

1 cup of raw vegetables.

Artichoke (½ medium)	Cabbage, cooked	Mushrooms, cooked	Spinach, cooked
Asparagus	Carrots	Okra	Summer squash (crookneck)
Beans (green, wax, Italian)	Cauliflower	Onions	Tomato (one large)

Table continued on following page

Table 29–5. Exchange Lists for Diabetes Nutrition Management (Continued)

Bean sprouts	Eggplant	Pea pods	Tomato/vegetable juice†
Beets	Greens (collard, mustard, turnip)	Peppers (green)	Turnips
Broccoli	Kohlrabi	Rutabaga	Water chestnuts
Brussels sprouts	Leeks	Sauerkraut†	Zucchini, cooked

Starchy vegetables such as corn, peas, and potatoes are found on the Starch/Bread List.
† 400 mg or more sodium per exchange.

Fruit List

Each item on this list contains about 15 gm of carbohydrate and 60 kcal. Fresh, frozen, and dry fruits have about 2 gm fiber per serving. Fruit juices contain very little dietary fiber.

The carbohydrate and calorie content for a fruit serving are based on the usual serving of the most commonly eaten fruits. Use fresh fruits or fruits frozen or canned without sugar added. Whole fruit is more filling than fruit juice and may be a better choice for those who are trying to lose weight. Unless otherwise noted, the serving size for 1 fruit serving is:

½ cup of fresh fruit or fruit juice.
¼ cup of dried fruit.

Fresh, Frozen, and Unsweetened Canned Fruit

Apple (raw, 2-in across)	1 apple	Mango (small)	½ mango
Applesauce (unsweetened)	½ cup	*Nectarine (1½-in across)	1 nectarine
Apricots (medium, raw) or	4 apricots	Orange (2½-in across)	1 orange
Apricots (canned)	½ cup, or 4 halves	Papaya	1 cup
		Peach (2¾-in across)	1 peach, or ¾ cup
Banana (9-in long)	½ banana		
*Blackberries (raw)	¾ cup	Peaches (canned)	½ cup, or 2 halves
*Blueberries (raw)	¾ cup		
Cantaloupe (5-in across)	⅓ melon	Pear	½ large, or 1 small
(cubes)	1 cup		
Cherries (large, raw)	12 cherries	Pears (canned)	½ cup or 2 halves
Cherries (canned)	½ cup		
Figs (raw, 2-in across)	2 figs	Persimmon (medium, native)	2 persimmons
Fruit cocktail (canned)	½ cup	Pineapple (raw)	¾ cup
Grapefruit (medium)	½ grapefruit	Pineapple (canned)	⅓ cup
Grapefruit (segments)	¾ cup	Plum (raw, 2-in across)	2 plums
Grapes (small)	15 grapes	*Pomegranate	½ pomegranate
Honeydew melon (medium)	⅛ melon	*Raspberries (raw)	1 cup
(cubes)	1 cup	*Strawberries (raw, whole)	1¼ cup
Kiwi (large)	1 kiwi	Tangerine (2½-in across)	2 tangerines
Mandarin oranges	¾ cup	Watermelon (cubes)	1¼ cup

Dried Fruit

*Apples	4 rings
*Apricots	7 halves
Dates	2½ medium
*Figs	1½
*Prunes	3 medium
Raisins	2T

Fruit Juice

Apple juice/cider	½ cup
Cranberry juice cocktail	⅓ cup
Grapefruit juice	½ cup
Grape juice	⅓ cup
Orange juice	½ cup
Pineapple juice	½ cup
Prune juice	⅓ cup

* 3 or more gm of fiber per serving.

Milk List

Each serving of milk or milk products on this list contains about 12 gm of carbohydrate and 8 gm of protein. The amount of fat in milk is measured in percent (%) of butterfat. The calories vary, depending on the kind of milk chosen. The list is divided into 3 parts based on the amount of fat and calories: skim/very low fat milk, low-fat milk, and whole milk. One serving (1 milk exchange) of each of these includes:

	Carbohydrate (gm)	Protein (gm)	Fat (gm)	Calories
Skim/Very low fat	12	8	trace	90
Low fat	12	8	5	120
Whole	12	8	8	150

Table 29–5. Exchange Lists for Diabetes Nutrition Management (Continued)

Skim and Very Low Fat Milk

Skim milk	1 cup
½% milk	1 cup
1% milk	1 cup
Low-fat buttermilk	1 cup
Evaporated skim milk	½ cup
Dry nonfat milk	⅓ cup
Plain nonfat yogurt	8 oz

Low-Fat Milk

2% milk	1 cup fluid
Plain low-fat yogurt (with added nonfat milk solids)	8 oz

Whole Milk

The whole milk group has much more fat per serving than the skim and low-fat groups. Whole milk has more than 3¼% butterfat. Try to limit choices from the whole milk group as much as possible.

Whole milk	1 cup
Evaporated whole milk	½ cup
Whole plain yogurt	8 oz

Fat List

Each serving on the fat list contains about 5 gm fat and 45 kcal. The foods on the fat list contain mostly fat, although some items may also contain a small amount of protein. All fats are high in calories and should be carefully measured. Everyone should modify fat intake by eating unsaturated fats instead of saturated fats. The sodium content of these foods varies widely. Check the label for sodium information.

Unsaturated Fats

Avocado	⅛ medium
Margarine	1 tsp
‡Margarine, diet	1 T
Mayonnaise	1 tsp
‡Mayonnaise, reduced-calorie	1 T
Nuts and seeds:	
Almonds, dry roasted	6 whole
Cashews, dry roasted	1 T
Pecans	2 whole
Peanuts	20 small or 10 large
Walnuts	2 whole
Other nuts	1 T
Seeds, pine nuts, sunflower (without shells)	1 T
Pumpkin seeds	2 tsp
Oil (corn, cottonseed, safflower, soybean, sunflower, olive, peanut)	1 tsp
‡Olives	10 small or 5 large
Salad dressing, mayonnaise-type	2 tsp
Salad dressing, mayonnaise-type, reduced-calorie	1 T
‡Salad dressing (all varieties)	1 T
†Salad dressing, reduced-calorie	2 T

(Two tablespoons of low-calorie salad dressing is a free food.)

Saturated Fats

Butter	1 tsp
‡Bacon	1 slice
Chitterlings	½ oz
Coconut, shredded	2 T
Coffee whitener, liquid	2 T
Coffee whitener, powder	4 tsp
Cream (light, coffee, table)	2 T
Cream, sour	2 T
Cream (heavy, whipping)	1 T
Cream cheese	1 T
‡Salt pork	¼ oz

‡ If more than 2 servings eaten, these foods have 400 mg or more sodium.

Free Foods

A free food is any food or drink that contains less than 20 kcal/serving, and can be taken in unlimited amounts. Two or 3 servings per day of those items that have a specific serving size can be eaten.

Drinks
Bouillon† or broth without fat
Bouillon, low sodium
Carbonated drinks, sugar-free
Carbonated water
Club soda
Cocoa powder, unsweetened (1 T)
Coffee/tea
Drink mixes, sugar-free
Tonic water, sugar-free

Nonstick pan spray

Fruit
Cranberries, unsweetened (½ cup)
Rhubarb, unsweetened (½ cup)

Vegetables (raw, 1 cup)
Cabbage*
Celery*
Chinese cabbage*
Cucumber
Green onion
Hot peppers
Mushrooms
Radishes
Zucchini*

Salad greens
Endive
Escarole
Lettuce
Romaine*
Spinach*

Sweet substitutes
Candy, hard, sugar-free
Gelatin, sugar-free
Gum, sugar-free
Jam/jelly, sugar-free (2 tsp)
Pancake syrup, sugar-free (1–2 T)

Sugar substitutes (saccharin, aspartame)
Whipped topping (2 T)

Condiments
Catsup (1 T)
Horseradish
Mustard
Pickles†, dill, unsweetened
Salad dressing, low-calorie (2 T)
Taco sauce (1 T)
Vinegar

Table 29–5. Exchange Lists for Diabetes Nutrition Management (Continued)

Seasonings can be very helpful in making food taste better. Be careful of how much sodium is used. Read the label, and choose those seasonings that do not contain sodium or salt.

Basil (fresh)	Flavoring extracts (vanilla, almond,	Lemon juice	Pepper
Celery seeds	walnut, peppermint, butter,	Lemon pepper	Pimento
Cinnamon	lemon, etc.)	Lime	Spices
Chili powder	Garlic	Lime juice	Soy sauce†
Chives	Garlic powder	Mint	Soy sauce, low sodium ("lite")
Curry	Herbs	Onion powder	Wine, used in cooking (¼ cup)
Dill	Hot pepper sauce	Oregano	Worcestershire sauce
	Lemon	Paprika	

* 3 gm or more of fiber per serving.
† 400 mg or more of sodium per serving.

Combination Foods

These combination foods do not fit into only 1 exchange list. It can be quite hard to tell what is in a certain casserole dish or baked food item. This is a list of average values of some typical combination foods.

Food	*Amount*	*Exchanges*
Casseroles, homemade	1 cup (8 oz)	2 starch, 2 medium-fat meat, 1 fat
Cheese pizza,† thin crust	¼ of 15 oz or ¼ of 10 in	2 starch, 1 medium-fat meat, 1 fat
Chili with beans*† (commercial)	1 cup (8 oz)	2 starch, 2 medium-fat meat, 2 fat
Chow mein*† (without noodles or rice)	2 cups (16 oz)	1 starch, 2 vegetable, 2 lean meat
Macaroni and cheese†	1 cup (8 oz)	2 starch, 1 medium-fat meat, 2 fat
Soup		
Bean*†	1 cup (8 oz)	1 starch, 1 vegetable, 1 lean meat
Chunky, all varieties†	10¾ oz can	1 starch, 1 vegetable, 1 medium-fat meat
Cream† (made with water)	1 cup (8 oz)	1 starch, 1 fat
Vegetable† or broth†	1 cup (8 oz)	2 starch, 1 medium-fat meat, 1 fat
Spaghetti and meatballs† (canned)	1 cup (8 oz)	2 starch, 1 medium-fat meat, 1 fat
Sugar-free pudding (made with skim milk)	½ cup	1 starch
If beans are used as a meat substitute:		
Dried beans,* peas,* lentils*	1 cup (cooked)	2 starch, 1 lean meat

Foods for Occasional Use

Moderate amounts of some foods can be used in the meal plan, in spite of their sugar or fat content, as long as blood glucose control is maintained. The following list includes average exchange values for some of these foods. Because they are concentrated sources of carbohydrate, the portion sizes are very small.

Food	*Amount*	*Exchanges*
Angel food cake	1/12 cake	2 starch
Cake, no icing	1/12 cake, or a 3-in square	2 starch, 2 fat
Cookies	2 small (1¾-in across)	1 starch, 1 fat
Frozen fruit yogurt	⅓ cup	1 starch
Gingersnaps	3	1 starch
Granola	¼ cup	1 starch, 1 fat
Granola bars	1 small	1 starch, 1 fat
Ice cream, any flavor	½ cup	1 starch, 2 fat
Ice milk, any flavor	½ cup	1 starch, 1 fat
Sherbet, any flavor	¼ cup	1 starch
Snack chips,‡ all varieties	1 oz	1 starch, 2 fat
Vanilla wafers	6 small	1 starch, 1 fat

* 3 gm or more of fiber per serving.
† 400 mg or more of sodium per exchange.
‡ If more than 1 or 2 servings are eaten, these foods have 400 mg or more sodium.
From Mahan LK, and Arlin MT. *Krause's Food, Nutrition, & Diet Therapy*. 8th ed. Philadelphia: WB Saunders, 1992, pp 541–545.

Table 29–6. Sample Diabetic Food Exchanges

		Number of Food Exchanges												
Calories		800	1000	1200	1400	1500	1600	1800	2000	2200	2400	2500	3000	3400
Breakfast	Meat	1	1	1	1	1	1	1	1	1	1	1	2	2
	Bread/starch	1	1	1	1	2	2	2	2	2	2	2	3	3
	Fruit		1	1	1	1	1	1	2	2	2	2	2	2
	Fat	1	1	1	1	1	1	1	1	1	1	1	2	2
	Skim milk			1	1	1	1	1	1	1	1	1	1	1
A.M. snack	Bread/starch												2	2
	Fruit	1	1	1	1	1	1	1	1	1	1	1	1	2
	Skim milk													
Lunch	Meat	2	2	2	2	2	2	3	3	3	3	3	4	5
	Vegetable	1	1	1	1	1	1	1	1	1	1	1	1	1
	Bread/starch	1	1	1	2	2	2	2	2	3	3	3	3	3
	Fruit		1	1	1	1	1	1	1	1	1	2	2	2
	Fat	1	1	1	1	1	1	1	1	1	1	1	1	1
	Skim milk		1	1	1	1	1	1	1	1	1	1	1	1
P.M. snack	Bread/starch			1	1	1	1	1	1	1	1	1	2	2
	Fruit												2	2
	Skim milk						1	1	1	1	1	1	1	1
Dinner	Meat	2	2	2	2	2	2	2	3	3	3	3	4	5
	Vegetable	1	1	1	1	1	1	1	1	1	1	1	1	1
	Bread/starch	1	1	1	1	1	2	2	2	3	3	3	3	3
	Fruit		1	1	1	1	1	1	1	1	1	2	2	2
	Fat	1	1	1	1	1	1	1	1	1	1	1	1	1
	Skim milk		1	1	1	1	1	1	1	1	1	1	1	1
Bedtime snack	Meat										2	2	2	2
	Bread/starch		1	1	1	1	1	2	2	2	2	2	2	2
	Fruit										1			2
	Fat										1	1		
	Skim milk	½	½	1	1	1	1	1	1	1	1	1		1

From Black JM, and Matassarin-Jacobs E (eds). *Luckmann and Sorensen's Medical-Surgical Nursing: A Psychophysiologic Approach*. 4th ed. Philadelphia: WB Saunders, 1993, p 1782.

Table 29–7. Currently Recommended Nutritional Guidelines for the Individual with Diabetes Mellitus

Calories	Sufficient to achieve and maintain reasonable weight.
Protein	Adequate to ensure maintenance of body protein stores. Individuals with diabetes have the same protein requirements as nondiabetics. In general, 10–20% of total daily calories should come from protein (approximately 0.8 gm/kg/day).
Fats	Less than 30% of calories should be from fat, with less than 10% of that from saturated fat sources. If individualized risk factors indicate elevated very low density lipoproteins and low-density lipoproteins, total calories from saturated fat may be reduced to 7%. Cholesterol intake should be limited to 300 mg/day or less.
Carbohydrates	50–60% of total calories should be from carbohydrates. Simple and complex sugars do *not* differ appreciably in their ability to worsen hyperglycemia.
Fiber	20–35 gm/day (same as for nondiabetics)

to recent recommendations from the American Diabetic Association for diabetics; daily percentages of carbohydrate, protein, fat, and fiber intake from total calories consumed daily (Table 29–7).

- Advantages: Patients have more flexibility in their diet and attain a sense of personal control by taking more responsibility for their insulin needs and blood sugar limits.
- Disadvantages: Patients must be very knowledgeable about and responsible for food intake, frequent blood sugar monitoring, and adjusting insulin intake to meet their needs.

(3) Exercise is important because it decreases cholesterol and triglyceride levels; lowers blood pressure; helps the body burn excess sugar; encourages weight loss and increases insulin receptor sites, decreasing the amount of oral hypoglycemics or insulin needed; and improves circulation (Table 29–8).

(4) For close monitoring of blood glucose levels, finger-stick monitoring has largely replaced urine testing in self-monitoring of blood sugar. Although they are far more accurate than urine tests, finger-stick tests do require patients to prick themselves (usually several times a day), involve higher costs for equipment and supplies, and require that the patient pay close attention to proper procedures to obtain accurate results (Procedure 29–2).

c. Pharmacologic interventions

(1) Oral hypoglycemic agents (Table 29–9): these drugs are *not* insulin; rather, they stimulate the pancreas to produce insulin. The 2 major classes of such agents are sulfonylureas and biguanides.

- **Sulfonylureas** are the most commonly used, and there are many from which to choose. Duration of action is the most significant difference. Side effects that require physician attention include lethargy, weakness, easy bruising, unexplained bleeding, and mouth ulcers.
- A **biguanide** derivative, metformin (Glucophage), decreases blood glucose in patients with type II diabetes by increasing the body's use of glucose and may be used alone or in combination with sulfonylureas to control hyperglycemia. Metformin also decreases triglyceride, low-density lipoprotein, and cholesterol levels. Side effects include gastrointestinal

Table 29–8. Dietary Adjustments and the Exercising Diabetic

Type of Exercise and Examples	If Blood Glucose Is:	Increased Food Intake by:	Suggestions of Food to Use
Exercise of short duration and of low to moderate intensity (walking a half mile or leisurely bicycling for less than 30 min)	Less than 100 mg/dl 100 mg/dl or above	10–15 gm carbohydrate per hour Not necessary to increase food	1 fruit or 1 starch/bread exchange
Exercise of moderate intensity (1 hr of tennis, swimming, jogging, leisurely bicycling, golfing, etc.)	Less than 100 mg/dl 100–180 mg/dl 180–300 mg/dl 300 mg/dl or above	25–50 gm carbohydrate before exercise, then 10–15 gm/hour of exercise 10–15 gm carbohydrate Not necessary to increase food Don't begin exercise until blood glucose is under better control	1 fruit or 1 starch/bread exchange
Strenuous activity or exercise (about 1 to 2 hr of football, hockey, racquetball, or basketball games; strenuous bicycling or swimming; shoveling heavy snow)	Less than 100 mg/dl 100–180 mg/dl 180–300 mg/dl 300 mg/dl or above	50 gm carbohydrate, monitor blood glucose carefully 25–50 gm carbohydrate, depending on intensity and duration 10–15 gm carbohydrate Don't begin exercise until blood glucose is under better control	1 meat sandwich (2 slices of bread) with a milk and fruit exchange ½ meat sandwich with a milk or fruit exchange 1 fruit or 1 bread exchange

Procedure 29–2
How to Use a Blood Glucose Monitor

Definition/Purpose	To provide the patient with current blood glucose levels. Monitoring blood glucose allows the patient to alter diet, insulin, or activity to maintain good glycemic control.
Contraindications/Cautions	• A blood glucose monitor (BGM) must be used with caution by patients with neuropathy or retinopathy. Patients with significant retinopathy may need partial or total assistance. • The procedure must be done precisely to achieve reliable results. If results do not seem reasonable, the patient should reread the instructions for the BGM, reassess technique, check expiration date of test strips, and perform procedure again to verify original results.
Learning/Teaching Activities	• Stress the importance of following the manufacturer's instructions for the patient's specific BGM. • Calibrate the monitor as instructed by the manufacturer. • Check the expiration date for the test strips.

Preliminary Activities

Equipment	• BGM • Test strips
Assessment/Planning	• Know the desired range of blood glucose control. • Know the rationale for monitoring blood glucose—what will the patient do with the results? • Know the desired frequency of using the BGM on normal days; sick days; and days when diet, insulin or oral hypoglycemic agent (OHA), or activity changes. • Assess the patient's eyesight to determine whether he or she can read the instructions and results (for at-home use). • Assess the patient for learning readiness.
Preparation of Patient	• Provide a comfortable learning environment. • The patient should be instructed about factors that influence blood glucose results: accuracy of procedure, timing and dosage of recent insulin or OHA; activity, recent dietary intake, and test strip viability.

Procedure

Action	Rationale/Discussion
1. Wash hands in warm water.	1. Hands must be clean and warm to prevent infection and to facilitate getting a large drop of blood.
2. Select the side of the finger pad as puncture site.	2. It is usually less uncomfortable to pierce the side of the finger than the end of the finger.
3. Hold hand in a relaxed position to collect a drop of blood on the test strip.	3. It is easier to obtain a drop of blood if the finger is relaxed (this improves vasodilation).
4. Start timing procedure as soon as a drop of blood touches the test strip or as soon as the monitor beeps.	4. This achieves the most accurate chemical response of blood on test strip.
5. At the time indicated, blot or wipe the test strip exactly as specified by the instructions that come with the monitor.	5. Alteration of this procedure affects accuracy of results.
6. Insert the test strip into the monitor and note the blood glucose reading.	6. Note carefully whether the directions indicate a longer waiting period for higher blood glucose values. Variations in time affect the accuracy of results.
7. Clean the BGM as directed by the manufacturer.	7. An unclean "window" affects the accuracy of results.
8. Calibrate the BGM regularly as indicated by the manufacturer.	8. Regular calibration helps keep the BGM accurate.

symptoms (anorexia, nausea, abdominal discomfort, and diarrhea) and (rarely) lactic acidosis. Metformin should not be used in patients with kidney or liver disease or cardiorespiratory insufficiency, persons who abuse alcohol, or pregnant women.

(2) Insulin therapy: The key to successful insulin therapy is the rate of absorption from site of injection. Intramuscular injections are absorbed faster than subcutaneous injections, especially in thin patients when subcutaneous injection is at-

Table 29-9. Oral Hypoglycemic Agents

Agent	Duration of Action	Frequency	Metabolism
First-Generation			
Tolbutamide (Orinase)	6–12 hr	1–3/day	By liver to inactive product
Tolazamide (Tolinase)	12–24 hr	1–2/day	By liver to active and inactive products requiring renal route
Acetohexamide (Dymelor)	12–18 hr	1–2/day	Same as tolazamide
Chlorpropamide (Diabinase)	60 hr	1/day	Approximately 70% by liver to less active products but renal route imperative
Second-Generation			
Glyburide (Diabeta; Micronase)	16–24 hr	1–2/day	By liver to mostly inert products
Glipizide (Glucotrol)	12–24 hr	1–2/day	By liver to inert products
Metformin (Glucophage)	12–14 hr	1–2/day	By kidney, unchanged

Adapted from Black JM, and Matassarin-Jacobs E (eds). *Luckmann and Sorensen's Medical-Surgical Nursing: A Psychophysiologic Approach.* 4th. Philadelphia: WB Saunders, 1993, p 1783.

Procedure 29-3
Subcutaneous Insulin Administration

Definition/Purpose   To administer insulin safely in order to maintain glycemic control.

Contraindications/Cautions
- Alter the prescribed dose of insulin when the patient is hypoglycemic.
- Patients with retinopathy may need syringes designed specifically for the visually impaired or prefilled syringes.
- Administer the insulin in the same general area to predict absorption rate. Rotate the exact site within an area.

Learning/Teaching Activities
- It is strongly recommended that a family member or friend also learn to give subcutaneous insulin in the event that the patient cannot.
- Teaching may begin while the nurse prepares the insulin and administers it to the patient.
- Formal teaching begins when the patient prepares and self-administers insulin.
- Coordinate actual administration of insulin with information on insulin overdosage and underdosage. Relate this to blood glucose level.

Preliminary Activities

Equipment
- Correct type of insulin—check expiration date
- Two alcohol swabs
- Insulin syringe and needle
- Puncture-proof container for used syringes and needles

Assessment/Planning
- Know the patient's prescribed insulin dose.
- Know what the insulin is for and the effects of underdosage and overdosage.
- Know the patient's latest blood sugar level; be able to relate blood sugar to recent diet, activity, and previous insulin dose and time.
- Prepare the patient:
  - Provide a comfortable learning environment.
  - Assess the patient for learning readiness.

Procedure

Action	Rationale/Discussion
1. Wash hands.	1. Washing minimizes the spread of bacteria.
2. Inspect the bottle to determine the type of insulin and expiration date.	2. Administering insulin of the wrong type may cause underdosage, overdosage, or other complications. Expired insulin may cause underdosage.
3. Roll the bottle of insulin between palms of hands.	3. Insulin should be mixed and at room temperature.
4. Wipe the top of the bottle with an alcohol swab.	4. Swabbing prevents contamination of the needle and insulin.
5. Remove the needle cover and pull back the plunger to draw air into the syringe. The amount of air should equal the insulin dose. Put the needle in the bottle and inject air.	5. This makes it easier to withdraw insulin.

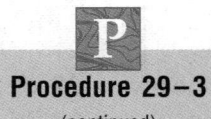

Procedure 29–3

(continued)

Action	Rationale/Discussion
6. Turn the bottle and syringe upside down in 1 hand and draw up the insulin dose into the syringe.	6. Inverting the bottle facilitates drawing insulin into the syringe.
7. Remove air bubbles in the syringe by tapping on the syringe or injecting the insulin back into bottle; redraw correct amount.	7. The presence of air bubbles prevents injection of full dose.
8. Remove the needle from the bottle and select a site for injection that has not been used in the past month.	8. Within an area, sites need to be rotated to ensure proper absorption of insulin.
9. Clean the site with an alcohol swab. Pinch up the area of skin and insert the needle at a 90-degree angle. Push the needle all the way in and inject the insulin.	9. The tip of the needle should reach fatty tissue.
10. Pull the needle straight out quickly.	10. Discomfort is minimized.
11. Dispose of the syringe and needle (without recapping) in a puncture-proof container (plastic, metal, or heavy cardboard).	11. Contamination from used needles is prevented.

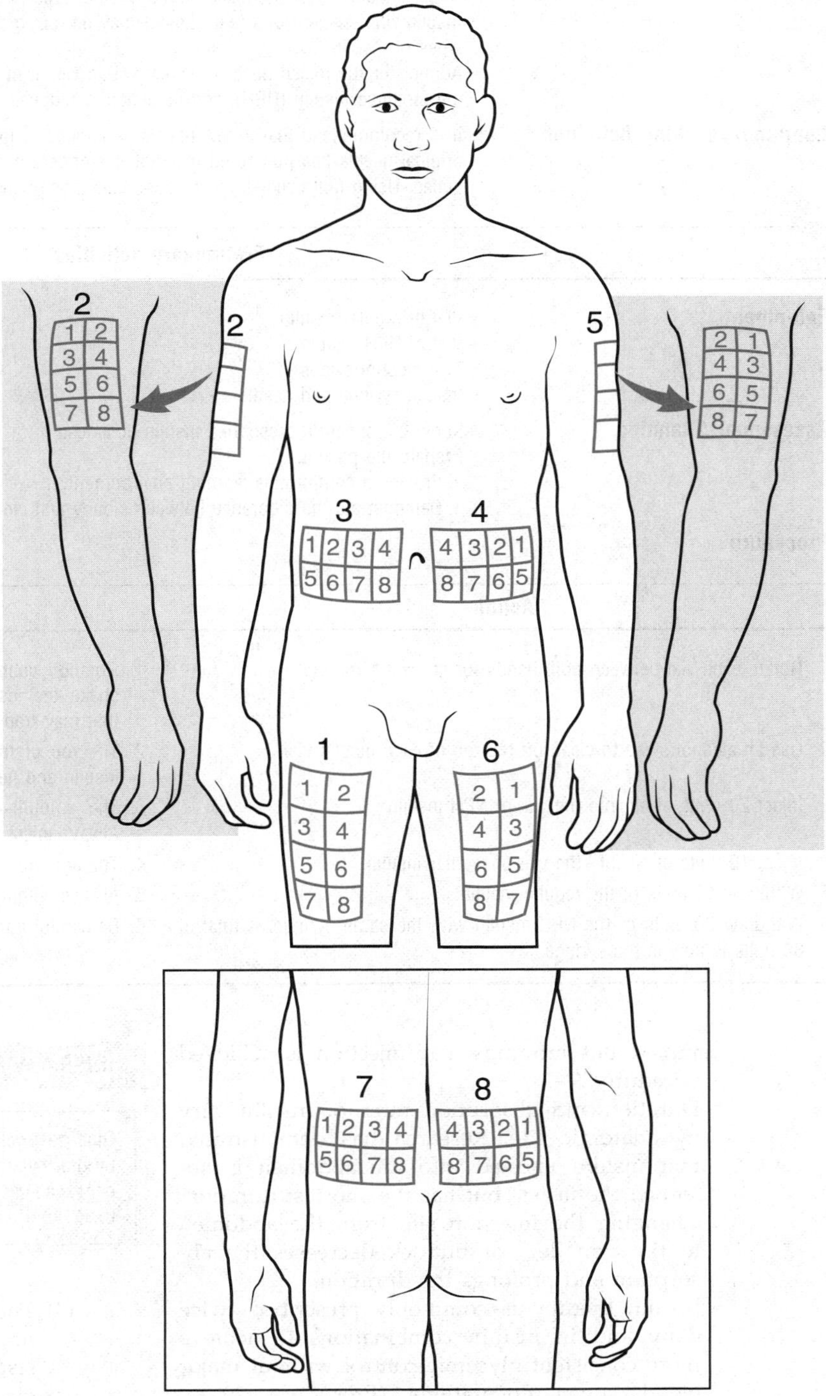

Adapted from Ignatavicius DD, and Bayne MV. *Medical-Surgical Nursing: A Nursing Process Approach.* Philadelphia: WB Saunders, 1991, p 1611.

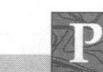

Procedure 29–4
Mixing Regular and NPH Insulin

Definition/Purpose	Mixing two insulins in one syringe allows the patient to inject only one time.
Contraindications/Cautions	• Be careful not to inject any regular insulin into NPH vial.
	• Regular insulin may be mixed with any other type of insulin.
	• Insulin zinc suspensions (e.g., Lente) may be mixed only with each other and regular insulin, not with other types of insulin.
	• Administer the mixed dose of insulin within 5 min of preparation. After this time, the regular insulin binds with the modified insulin (NPH), and its action is reduced.
Learning/Teaching Activities	• It is recommended that a new needle be applied to the syringe after insulin mixing is completed, because the original needle has punctured the rubber stoppers of 2 vials during the mixing procedure and is somewhat dulled. Using dull needles for injection can cause patients unnecessary discomfort.

Preliminary Activities

Equipment	• Vial of regular insulin
	• Vial of NPH insulin
	• Two alcohol swabs
	• Insulin syringe and needle
Assessment/Planning	• Know the patient's prescribed insulin dosages.
	• Prepare the patient:
	• Provide a comfortable learning environment.
	• Demonstrate the difference between cloudy and clear insulin.

Procedure

Action	Rationale/Discussion
1. Rotate each vial between both hands for at least 1 minute.	1. Rotation suspends the insulin and helps warm the medication. Do *not* shake the insulin vials, because shaking causes bubbles and foaming that may trap particles and alter insulin dosage.
2. Use an alcohol swab to clean off the top of each insulin vial.	2. The top of the bottle should be clean to prevent contamination of the insulin and needle.
3. Inject 20 units of air into the vial of NPH insulin.	3. The amount of air injected is equal to the dose of insulin desired. Always inject air into the longer-acting insulin first.
4. Inject 10 units of air into the vial of regular insulin.	4. The amount of air injected is equal to the dose of insulin desired.
5. Withdraw 10 units of the regular insulin.	5. Always withdraw the shorter-acting insulin first.
6. Withdraw 20 units of the NPH insulin with the same syringe. A total of 30 units is now in the syringe.	6. Be careful not to inject any short-acting insulin into the NPH bottle.

tempted but intramuscular injection is achieved (Procedure 29–3).

• Duration and absorption rates of insulin vary by anatomic site. Research has demonstrated that insulin injected into the abdomen is absorbed the fastest but has the shortest duration. Changing the injection site from the abdomen to the arm, leg, or buttock decreases the absorption and prolongs the duration.

• Insulin therapy is commonly prescribed twice daily and in insulin combinations to achieve more consistent glycemic control without major blood sugar fluctuations (Procedure 29–4). Most often, a short-acting insulin and an intermediate-acting insulin are combined (Table 29–10 and Fig. 29–8).

NURSE ADVISORY

Glucose levels controlled by insulin fall faster than those controlled by oral hypoglycemic agents. Therefore, patients with insulin-dependent diabetes mellitus are at greater risk for hypoglycemia than are those whose diabetes is not insulin dependent.

(3) The combined use of insulin and oral sulfonyl-ureas may be useful for patients exhibiting persistent fasting hyperglycemia despite maximal oral drug therapy. More studies are necessary to define the patient characteristics for which this combined therapy is most effective.

(4) Humulin insulin (rDNA biosynthetic human in-

Table 29–10. Types of Insulin

Type	Onset (hr)	Peak (hr)	Duration (hr)
Short Acting			
Humulin regular	½–1	1½–3	6–8
Humulin semilente	½–1	2–8	8–6
Intermediate Acting			
Humulin NPH (isophane insulin suspension)	2½–3	5–7	13–16
Humulin lente	1–3 (1–4)	6–12 (6–8)	(10–16)
Long Acting			
Protamine zinc insulin	4–6	18–24	28–36
Humulin ultralente insulin	4–6 (6–14)	14–24 (relatively peakless effect)	36 (18–36)
Premixed			
70% NPH and 30% regular	½	2–12	18–24

NPH, Neutral protamine Hagedorn.

sulin) offers so many advantages over the pork and beef insulins that it has totally replaced beef and pork insulins in the United States. These advantages are the following:

- Daily doses that are 10 to 25 percent lower
- No side effects or local reactions and few (<1%) allergic reactions
- Virtual elimination of the risk of lipoatrophy

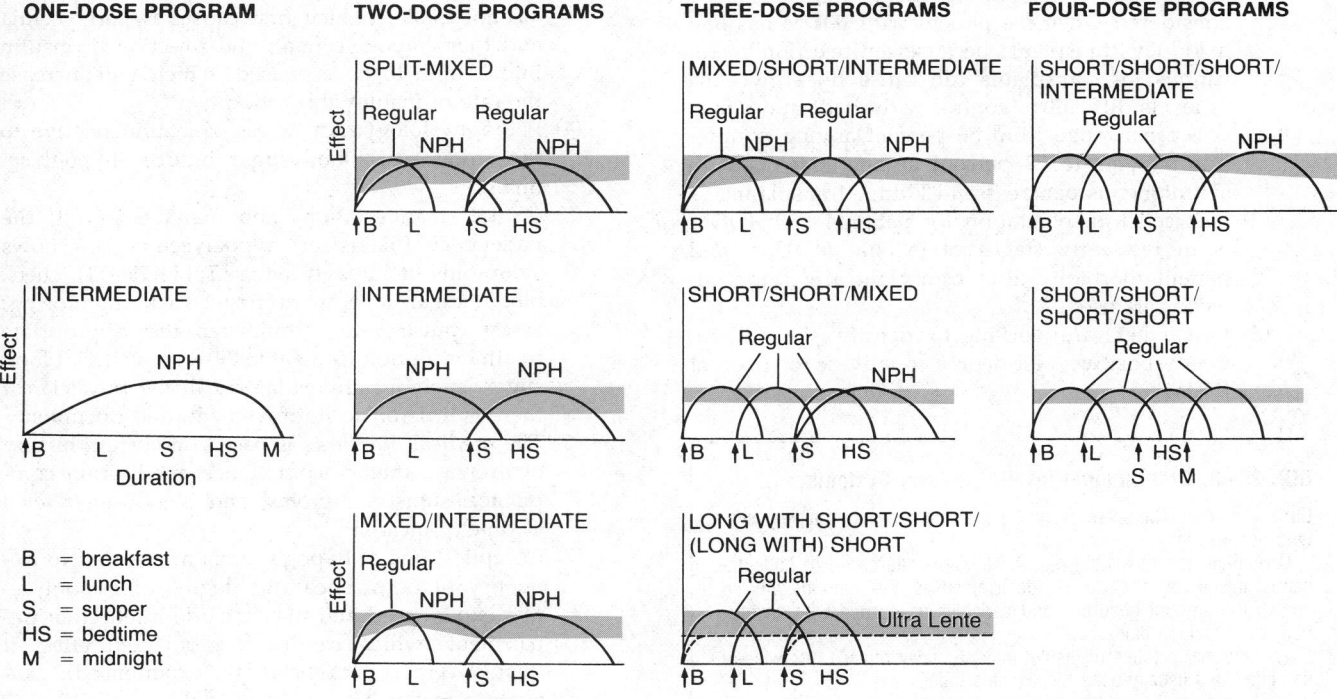

Figure 29–8. Insulin regimens. One injection a day of short-acting or intermediate-acting insulin may be enough to control blood glucose levels. However, split doses (2, 3, or 4 injections of the daily dose) or split mixed doses (a mixture of short- and longer-acting insulins) may give better control. *Note:* Screened areas represent range of glycemic control achieved with mixed insulins. (Modified from Ignatavicius DD, Workman ML, and Mishler MA. *Medical-Surgical Nursing: A Nursing Process Approach.* 2nd ed. Philadelphia: WB Saunders, 1995, p 1880.)

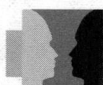

(5) The neutral protamine Hagedorn (NPH) insulin is more rapidly absorbed than the pork and beef insulins, but it is also of shorter duration, resulting in higher fasting blood sugars in the morning and raising the risk that injection before dinner instead of at bedtime might impair metabolic control during the night.

(6) The following are experimental insulin delivery systems (Box 29–3):

• Oral inhalation: Research continues into the amount inhaled versus the amount absorbed and variables associated with absorption, such as lung disease.

• Transdermal patches of insulin are currently under investigation.

• Implanted insulin delivery devices are being studied.

• An artificial pancreas: Efforts have focused on combining an implanted glucose administration device with a glucose sensor.

d. Special medical-surgical procedures

(1) A pancreas transplant (graft) is most seriously considered when the patient with IDDM has had a kidney transplant, because antirejection medications for transplants can cause hyperglycemia at levels difficult to control with medication. Success rates range from 56 percent among nonuremic patients to 77 percent among patients with simultaneous pancreas and kidney transplants.

(2) Islet cell transplantation for patients with IDDM is in the early stages of evaluation. Cost and patient morbidity after transplant are factors affecting its use.

(3) Researchers are working to identify islet cell, antibody-positive, 1st-degree relatives to prevent IDDM.

BOX 29–3. Experimental Insulin Delivery Systems

Currently, researchers are exploring a number of new delivery systems for insulin:

Oral inhalation of insulin may be a viable alternative to subcutaneous injections. Still to be determined is the amount inhaled versus the amount absorbed and variables associated with absorption, such as lung disease.

Transdermal patches of insulin may someday replace the twice-a-day injections usually used for diabetes today.

Implanted insulin delivery systems, possibly in combination with a glucose sensor to create an "artificial pancreas," offer yet another prospect for the future.

---

9. Complications: Approximately 75 percent of all patients with diabetes develop diabetes-specific complications. Factors that influence the development of complications and their morbidity include compliance with therapy, concurrent medical problems, age at diagnosis of diabetes, and genetic predisposition as part of the diabetes syndrome (a genetic hypothesis). Diabetic complications develop as a direct result of the hyperglycemia of diabetes (a metabolic hypothesis). *Acute* complications include hypoglycemia, diabetic ketoacidosis (DKA), and hyperglycemic hyperosmolar nonketotic coma (HHNK). Long-term complications include diabetic retinopathy, nephropathy, neuropathy, and macrovascular complications (macroangiopathy), as well as microangiopathy, hypertension, cardiovascular disease, stroke, peripheral vascular disease, and infection.

a. Hypoglycemia

(1) Definition: Blood sugar less than 50 mg per dl or a sudden large drop in blood sugar (e.g., from 180 to 90 mg/dl)

(2) Incidence and socioeconomic impact: The most common complication of DM, hypoglycemia occurs in approximately 90 percent of IDDM patients. The risk of hypoglycemia is greatest between dinner and breakfast, when insulin peaks, or before mealtime or snacktime.

(3) Etiology: overtreated hyperglycemia; vomiting, anorexia, or missed meals while still taking an oral hypoglycemic agent or insulin; increased exercise; medications that inadvertently block epinephrine activity (e.g., β-adrenergic blockers); erratic or altered insulin absorption; inadequate nutrient absorption secondary to gastric paresis; alcohol intake (which first causes hyperglycemia and then hypoglycemia); and injection of insulin into a limb to be exercised, which will increase the rate of insulin absorption.

(4) Pathophysiology: An excess of insulin relative to the amount of blood sugar induces hypoglycemia.

(5) Clinical manifestations and management: If the patient complains of hypoglycemia or shows symptoms of hypoglycemia (Table 29–11), check blood sugar level with finger-stick monitoring; assess pulse rate; administer the appropriate treatment option (see Table 29–11); recheck blood sugar level 15 minutes later; call the physician if there is little or no improvement; and document.

(6) The medical diagnosis is based on current history of exercise, dietary compliance, medication compliance, signs, symptoms, and blood sugar level at time of incident.

(7) Complications of hypoglycemia are related to frequency of occurrence and degree of hypoglycemia experienced and may include intellectual impairment (which can be a permanent effect if hypoglycemia is repeatedly experienced), seizures, and death.

(8) Discharge planning and teaching: Instruct the patient on the causes, signs, and symptoms of hypoglycemia; when to monitor blood sugar more

Table 29–11. Clinical Management for Hypoglycemia

Clinical Manifestations	Clinical Management
Mild Hypoglycemia Tremors Tachycardia Diaphoresis Paresthesias Excessive hunger Pallor Shakiness	10–15 gm carbohydrate = 4 oz orange juice 6 oz regular soda 6–8 oz 2% skim milk 6–8 Lifesavers 1 small (2 oz) tube of cake icing

Moderate Hypoglycemia
Above manifestations
  Headache
  Mood swings
  Irritability
  Inability to concentrate
  Drowsiness
  Impaired judgment
  Slurred speech
  Double or blurred vision
	20–30 gm carbohydrate
	Glucagon 1 mg subcutaneously or intramuscuarly (IM)

Severe Hypoglycemia Disorientation Seizures Unconsciousness	25 gm D-50 dextrose intravenously (IV) Glucagon 1 mg IM or IV

of DM; a history of medication, diet, and exercise compliance; identification of suspected cause of hyperglycemia (e.g., infection); clinical manifestations and vital signs; and results of diagnostic studies (blood glucose, glycosylated hemoglobin, arterial blood gases, presence of ketones in blood or urine, and serum electrolytes).

NURSE ADVISORY

To correct hyperglycemia, use an insulin drip made of regular insulin in intravenous (IV) solution of 0.90 normal saline (NS) or 0.45 NS, depending on the degree of dehydration. Prepare the least amount of insulin in the smallest bag available, depending on the patient's needs, for example, 100 units of regular insulin in 100 ml of 0.90 NS for a 1:1 ratio of regular insulin to IV fluid.

When preparing an insulin drip, remember that insulin adheres to IV tubing. Prime the tubing with IV solution before adding insulin. Place the insulin drip on an IV drip monitor (IMED or IVAC). Assess the IV drip monitor for correct working order throughout the procedure.

Always assess patients for hypoglycemia while they are on an insulin drip. Hypoglycemic symptoms may reflect a sudden decrease in blood sugar. If signs of hypoglycemia appear, take a finger-stick blood sugar test from the patient and decrease the amount of IV insulin as needed. Continue finger-stick glucose testing at least every 30 to 60 minutes until blood sugar reaches 250 to 300 mg per dl. Document the patient's blood sugar levels and correlate with vital signs, mentation, and other clinical manifestations of hypoglycemia.

The insulin drip is commonly discontinued when blood sugar reaches 250 mg per dl.

frequently; treatment options for mild to severe hypoglycemia; sources of fast-acting glucose; and not delaying meals for longer than 30 minutes after insulin has been administered (see also p. 1389).

b. Diabetic ketoacidosis

(1) Definition: DKA, a life-threatening emergency, is hyperglycemia that has progressed to include metabolic acidosis.

(2) Incidence and socioeconomic impact: DKA occurs most frequently in patients with IDDM. It accounts for 20 to 30 percent of patients with newly diagnosed DM and 2 to 14 percent of all hospitalizations of those with diabetes.

(3) Etiology: Insulin deficiency relative to glucose needed, dietary indiscretions, undiagnosed DM, and stress (infection, surgery, and emotional stress).

(4) Pathophysiology (Fig. 29–9): Insulin deficiency keeps glucose from entering cells. The body metabolizes fat for energy, converting free fatty acids to ketone bodies. Increased gluconeogenesis or glucose production in the liver occurs.

(5) Clinical manifestations: sunken eyeballs; dry mucous membranes; polyuria; muscle weakness; Kussmaul's respiration; acetone breath; warm, flushed skin; electrocardiographic (ECG) changes related to potassium imbalance; nausea and vomiting; abdominal pain and rigidity; oliguria and anuria (late signs); and hypotension (late sign)

(6) Medical diagnosis is based on previous diagnosis

(7) Clinical management: correct hyperglycemia with intravenous insulin drip. Correct dehydration with rapid infusion (varies somewhat, depending on coexisting medical problems) of intravenous (IV) fluids; 0.9 or 0.45 saline is recommended. Treat causes of hyperglycemia. Correct acidosis if pH is less than 7.10. Correct electrolyte imbalance. A patient with DKA may first demonstrate hypokalemia because of osmotic diuresis and dehydration. Later, the patient may exhibit hyperkalemia as acidosis occurs. When the patient receives insulin to lower the blood sugar level, expect the serum potassium to decrease as acidosis improves. Potassium replacement may then be indicated. Provide supplemental oxygen.

(8) Complications are related to the complex physiology from the hyperglycemia, metabolic acidosis, and osmotic diuresis and may include dehydration, electrolyte imbalance, cardiac dysrhythmia, shock, acute renal failure, respiratory acidosis, respiratory arrest, brain damage, coma, or death.

(9) Discharge planning and teaching: Instruct the patient on the causes of, signs and symptoms of, and ways to prevent DKA; when to call the physician; the consequences of late intervention for DKA; and monitoring urine for ketones (see also p. 1387).

CARBOHYDRATE METABOLISM   PROTEIN METABOLISM   FAT METABOLISM

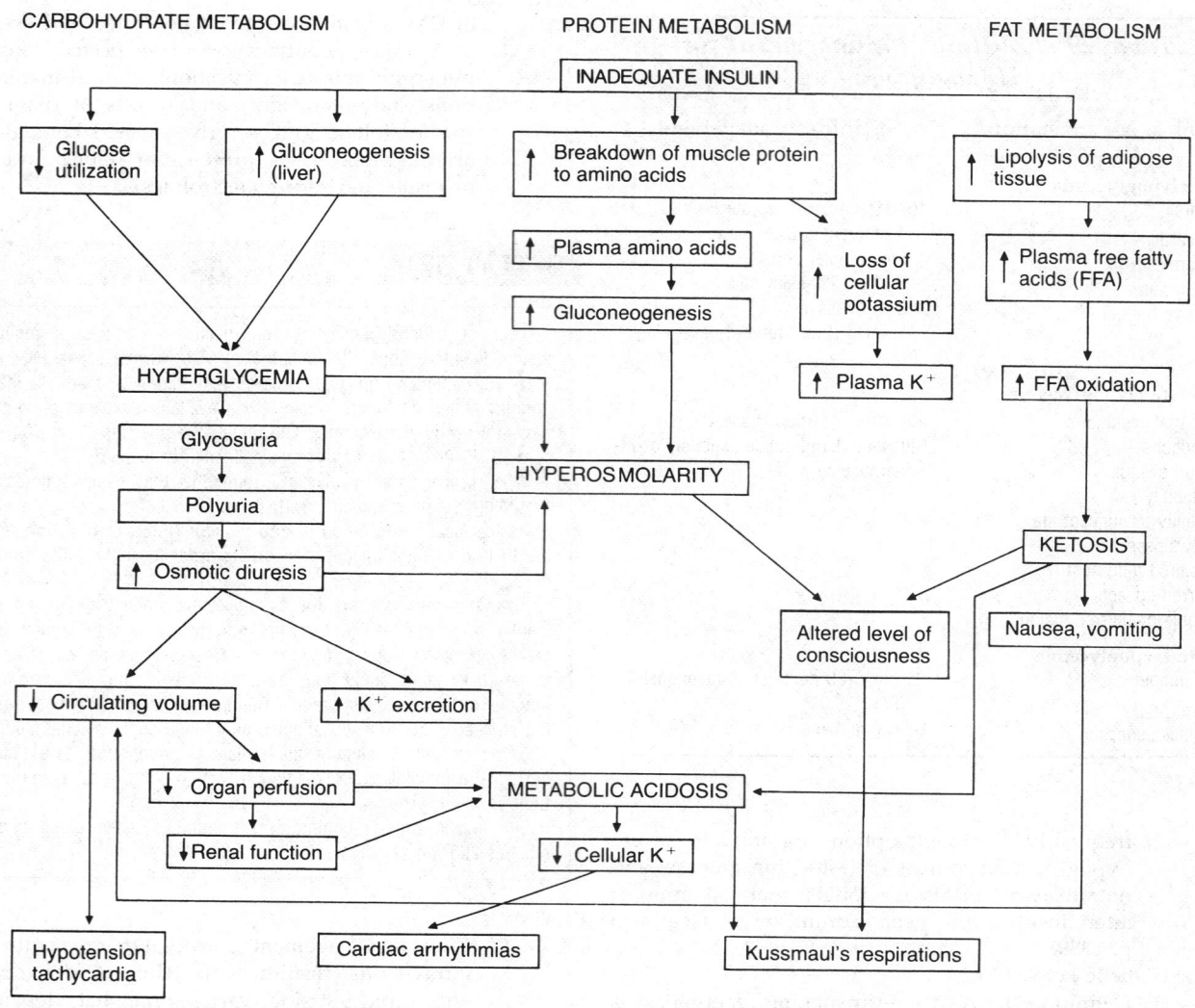

Figure 29–9. Pathophysiology of diabetic ketoacidosis. (From Black JM, and Matassarin-Jacobs E [eds]. *Luckmann and Sorensen's Medical-Surgical Nursing: A Psychophysiologic Approach.* 4th ed. Philadelphia: WB Saunders, 1993, p 1795.)

c. Hyperglycemic hyperosmolar nonketotic coma (HHNK)
  (1) Definition: Extreme hyperglycemia without acidosis
  (2) Incidence and socioeconomic impact: HHNK accounts for about 10 percent of hyperglycemic emergencies in people with type II DM. The mortality rate for HHNK is 10 to 70 percent, with mortality rising as osmolality increases.

  (3) Etiology and precipitating events: undiagnosed NIDDM presenting for the 1st time as HHNK, stress (e.g., infection, surgery, or trauma), medications (thiazides, steroids, or phenytoin), and hyperalimentation
  (4) Pathophysiology: A precipitating event causes hyperglycemia to develop. As hyperglycemia increases, hyperosmolar diuresis develops, causing polyuria. The patient initially responds to the polyuria with polydipsia, but as the polyuria progresses, dehydration worsens, electrolyte imbalance occurs, and the patient becomes obtunded and thus unable to respond to the thirst mechanism. (The degree of obtundedness depends in part on the precipitating factor; e.g., infection may cause fever, sepsis, dehydration, or hypotension.) While this cycle continues, ketosis does not develop, because patients with NIDDM have the ability to produce enough insulin to prevent metabolism of fats into energy.

(5) Clinical manifestations: polyphagia, polyuria, polydipsia, glucosuria, dehydration, abdominal discomfort, hyperventilation, alterations in level of consciousness, coma, hypotension, and shock

(6) The medical diagnosis is based on history of NIDDM, precipitating event, clinical manifestations, vital signs, absence of ketones in urine, serum osmolality, and electrolytes.

(7) Clinical management: Nonpharmacologic interventions include dietary education from a dietitian. Pharmacologic interventions include hydration with IV fluids (0.9 or 0.45 saline), with the rate and amount depending on the degree of dehydration, vital signs, and concurrent medical problems; potassium replacement, as indicated; and IV regular insulin via pump to correct hyperglycemia.

(8) Complications are related to progressive and untreated hyperglycemia, the precipitating event, and related physiology and may include dehydration, vascular collapse, shock, hypotension, electrolyte imbalance, cardiac dysrhythmias, coma, lactic acidosis, and death.

(9) Discharge planning and teaching: Instruct the patient on the causes of HHNK, the monitoring of blood sugar level with finger-stick testing, when to call the physician, and the consequences of prolonging treatment. Refer to a dietitian if needed (see also p. 1387).

d. Diabetic retinopathy
(1) Definition: a chronic and progressive noninflammatory disease of the retina that results from diabetes

(2) Incidence and socioeconomic impact: Although the onset is slow, diabetic retinopathy is the major cause of blindness among Americans with diabetes, with about 50 percent of all patients with IDDM showing some signs of it 7 to 10 years after the initial IDDM diagnosis.

(3) Risk factors and etiology: uncontrolled hypertension, atherosclerotic disease of the small vessels, poor glycemic control (especially hyperglycemia), duration of diabetes, and pregnancy in women with IDDM

(4) Pathophysiology: The diabetic disease process causes microvascular changes in the eyes, including thickening of the capillaries and damage to the basement membrane. Capillary destruction damages the microcirculation of the eye, depriving the eye tissue of oxygen. Tissue anoxia quickly develops. Not all diabetic retinopathy produces visual changes. What (if any) changes occur depend on the part of the eye circulation involved.

(5) Clinical manifestations: a change in vision (ruptured vessels), blurred vision (macular edema), sudden loss of vision (retinal detachments), and cataracts (lens opacity)

(6) The medical diagnosis is based on history of DM, hypertension, blood sugar control, and other known acute and chronic complications of dia-

betes. A physical examination with a fundoscope (ophthalmoscope) is vital for detecting diabetic retinopathy in asymptomatic patients because it reveals diabetes-influenced changes such as dot hemorrhages, hard exudates, ischemia, neovascularization, microaneurysms, cataracts, proliferative retinopathy, and retinal detachment. Fundus photography and fluorescein angiography are done as well.

(7) Clinical management: To minimize the potential for and degree of diabetic retinopathy, control of hypertension is strongly recommended. Tight glycemic control is also vital, delaying onset of retinopathy and decreasing microangiopathy-related morbidity in patients with IDDM. There are no treatments for early retinal change. Special medical procedures include laser therapy (photocoagulation) to remove hemorrhagic tissue to decrease scarring, vitrectomy to remove vitreous hemorrhages and thus decrease tension on the retina and prevent retinal detachment, and cataract removal with lens implant.

(8) Complications: permanent visual changes and blindness.

(9) Discharge planning and teaching: Instruct the patient on the need for eye examinations to be performed by an ophthalmologist every 6 to 12 months. Monitor the patient for failing visual acuity that impairs self-care (e.g., inability to read an insulin syringe or glucometer machine). Refer patients with such problems to appropriate agencies for syringe magnifiers or home care.

e. Diabetic nephropathy
(1) Definition: A progressive decrease in kidney function as a result of diabetes; it is associated with microalbuminuria.

(2) Incidence and socioeconomic impact: About 35 to 45 percent of people with IDDM and 20 percent of those with NIDDM have nephropathy. Symptoms appear within 5 to 10 years of diagnosis of diabetes in patients with NIDDM and 15 to 20 years for those with IDDM. Of persons with diabetic nephropathy, 30 to 40 percent of those with IDDM and 3 to 5 percent of those with NIDDM progress to erythrocyte sedimentation rate disorders.

(3) Etiology: unknown. Risk factors include poor glycemic control (probably), duration of disease, hypertension (family history or presence in the patient).

 DRUG ADVISORY

Procedures requiring radiocontrast materials may cause acute renal failure in 6 to 9 percent of diabetic patients. Make sure patients with diabetes are well hydrated and have normal creatinine levels before subjecting them to radiocontrast materials.

(4) Pathophysiology: Destruction of the diabetic kidney is probably influenced by hyperglycemia, hyperfiltration, increased blood viscosity, glomerular scarring and nodules, microalbuminuria with normal or elevated glomerular filtration rate, hypertension, glomerulosclerosis, and gross proteinuria.

(5) Clinical manifestations: Early stages of diabetic nephropathy are asymptomatic. Microalbuminuria, often the 1st indicator, precedes the development of the nephrotic syndrome and end-stage renal disease. Microalbuminuria is associated with hypertension and is twice as common in those with NIDDM as in IDDM. As the uremia develops, patients often manifest fatigue, anemia, dyslipidemia, weight loss, and (sometimes) malnutrition.

(6) The medical diagnosis is based on history of DM and its acute and chronic complications; and laboratory studies (urinalysis, 24-hour urine collection for protein creatinine clearance and glomerular filtration rate, serum creatinine level, and blood urea nitrogen).

(7) Clinical management: Minimize risk factors—control hypertension with angiotensin-converting enzyme inhibitors and calcium channel blockers; maintain acceptable blood sugar levels; monitor albuminuria; restrict dietary protein, sodium, and potassium; and facilitate weight management. Administer angiotensin-converting enzyme inhibitors to decrease microalbuminuria or protein excretion and slow decline in glomerular filtration rate in normotensive patients with IDDM. Special medical-surgical procedures are hemodialysis, continuous ambulatory peritoneal dialysis, and kidney transplants for patients with erythrocyte sedimentation rate disorders; pancreas or islet cell transplant to eliminate DM; and kidney and pancreas transplant.

(8) Complications: end-stage renal disease (which requires hemodialysis) and death from uremia (if untreated)

(9) Discharge planning and teaching: see page 1388.

f. Diabetic neuropathy

(1) Definition: damage to the somatic and autonomic nervous systems as a result of the diabetic disease process

(2) Incidence and socioeconomic impact: Neuropathy is the most common complication of diabetes, with about 60 percent of patients with diabetes showing signs of it and others suffering neuropathy but asymptomatic.

(3) Etiology: unknown. Poor glycemic control (probable; research is being done) and duration of diabetes are risk factors. Hyperglycemia is considered a major initiating factor.

(4) Pathophysiology: Hyperglycemia, glycosylation, and the polyol pathway damage the transportative abilities of the nerve axons and cause the protective myelin sheath to degenerate, possibly causing hypoxia. Vascular changes also occur.

Basement membranes thicken, allowing chemicals to gather near peripheral nerves, causing demyelination.

(5) Clinical manifestations diagnostics and management (Table 29–12 and Box 29–4).

(6) The medical diagnosis is based on history; physical examination; electrophysiologic studies; and autonomic testing (barium swallow to detect gastrointestinal problems, impotence testing, ECG to verify heart rate changes with respiration, and the Valsalva maneuver).

(7) Complications are foot injuries. Trauma and diabetic ulcers frequently involve amputation.

(8) Discharge planning and teaching: see page 1385.

g. Macrovascular complications (macroangiopathy)

(1) Definition: any of a number of macrovascular changes due to early atherosclerosis of the large arteries as a result of the diabetic disease process (may be cerebral vascular disease, heart disease, cardiomyopathy, peripheral vascular disease, hypertension, or infection).

(2) Incidence and socioeconomic impact: About 75 percent of people with diabetes (especially those with IDDM) experience macrovascular changes. Such changes are responsible for the majority of hospitalizations of persons with DM and roughly 40 to 60 percent of fatalities.

(3) Etiology and risk factors

• The exact etiology is unknown.

• Risk factors specific to diabetics include being female, having a history of hypertension (which may accelerate vascular complications), and having hyperinsulinemia caused by insulin resistance. It is thought that hyperinsulinemia causes hyperglycemia, hypertension, hypertriglyceridemia with low high-density lipoprotein cholesterol levels, and upper body obesity leading to atherosclerosis.

• People with DM are at greater risk of developing cardiovascular disease (especially those with NIDDM), cerebral vascular accidents and peripheral vascular diseases (2 to 5 times more likely than the general population), and hypertension (1.5 to 2.0 times more likely than nondiabetics).

• Risk factors for macrovascular changes shared by those with and without diabetes include angina, genetic predisposition, obesity, cigarette smoking, and hyperlipidemia.

BOX 29–4. Monofilament Tactile Testing

The monofilament is a soft fiber that the patient or health care professional can brush along the patient's extremity to assess for the absence of sensory perception or diminished sensory perception related to diabetic neuropathy. Monofilament tactile testing for blunt sensory perception can alert the patient to safety issues related to self-care, foot care, early infection detection and intervention, and injury prevention.

Table 29–12. Types, Clinical Manifestations, and Treatment of Diabetic Neuropathy

Type	Symptoms	Signs	Treatment
Sensorimotor	Paresthesia (numbness and tingling in stocking and, less commonly, glove distribution); progresses to hypoesthesia	Decreased or absent reflexes, and decreased sensation to vibration and light touch; wasting of interosseous muscles with flexion (claw toe) deformity	None, other than foot care to prevent trauma and ulcers
	Painful neuropathy (rare); dysesthesia with lancinating or burning pain; may be accompanied by anorexia and depression	Same as above	Tricyclic antidepressant drugs, phenytoin, carbamazepine, or topical capsaicin; avoid narcotics (high potential for addiction)
Focal Motor and Compression	Weakness or loss of sensation in distribution of nerve	Cranial- (III, IV, V, VI) or peripheral-nerve palsy; carpal tunnel syndrome, foot-drop	Improves spontaneously in 2–12 mo; surgical decompression for compression lesions
Autonomic			
Gastrointestinal	Gastroparesis (early satiety, nausea, vomiting)		Metoclopramide, erythromycin
	Diabetic diarrhea (nocturnal, with incontinence)		Clonidine, increase dietary fiber, abstinence from milk products
	Constipation (more common)		
Genitourinary	Impotence, retrograde ejaculation		Penile injections with papaverine, phentolamine, or prostaglandin (or a combination); vacuum or implantable devices
	Neurogenic bladder		
	Women: dyspareunia		Women: estrogen-containing lubricants
	Overflow incontinence		Teach signs and symptoms of URL, prn bladder training program
Cardiac	Dizziness	Postural hypotension, resting tachycardia	Fludrocortisone, salt
Adrenal Medulla	Hypoglycemic	No adrenergic symptoms	Monitor blood sugar qid
	Unawareness	Only mentation changes	Keep blood sugar slightly elevated
			Wear Medic-Alert band
			Liquid glucose or injection of glucose

Modified with permission from Nathan DM. Long-term complications of diabetes mellitus. *N Engl J Med* 328:1676–1685, 1993. Copyright © 1993, Massachusetts Medical Society. All rights reserved.

(4) Pathophysiology: The pathophysiology is the same as that of macrovascular changes not induced by diabetes, but changes are more diffuse and frequent and occur at an earlier age in people with diabetes.

(5) Clinical manifestations, medical diagnosis, and clinical management are presented in Table 29–13.

(6) Prognosis depends on degree of neuropathy, especially in lower extremities; glycemic control; compliance with weight reduction and diet regimes; and meticulous foot care (including performing daily inspections of and hygiene for the feet; clipping toenails so they are smooth and straight across; wearing clean, padded sport socks and well-fitting shoes; and obtaining prompt medical attention for foot deformities (calluses, hammer toes, and corns) and problems (ulcers, infections, and impaired circulation).

(7) Discharge planning and teaching: see page 1388.

10. The prognosis for DM depends highly on patient compliance, glycemic control, age at diagnosis, type of diabetes, age at onset of complications, weight, and coexisting medical problems.

11. Applying the nursing process

NURSING DIAGNOSIS: Knowledge deficit R/T new medical diagnosis or poor understanding from previous diabetic instruction regarding factors, manifestations, and prevention of complications from diabetes

a. *Expected outcomes:*
Following interventions, the person should be able to do the following:

(1) Demonstrate an understanding of the causes of DM and its complications and how to prevent complications

(2) Properly administer oral hypoglycemic agents or insulin as prescribed

(3) Describe how to shop and prepare meals for his or her prescribed diet

(4) Plan and relate the importance of a safe exercise program

(5) Demonstrate finger-stick glucose monitoring and recording

b. *Nursing interventions:* See Learning/Teaching Guidelines for the Diabetic Patient.

NURSING DIAGNOSIS: Anxiety R/T new disease and unknown impact on lifestyle

Table 29–13. Macroangiopathy: Clinical Manifestations, Medical Diagnosis, and Clinical Management

Clinical Manifestations	Medical Diagnosis	Clinical Management
Cerebral Vascular Disease		
Atherothromboembolic infarctions (transient ischemic attacks and cerebrovascular accidents) are more severe, have higher mortality rate, and have higher recurrence rate.	History Symptoms Physical exam Computed tomography Magnetic resonance imaging	Same as for nondiabetics, plus: Improved glycemic control Aspirin
Heart Disease (coronary heart disease and coronary artery disease [CAD])		
Diabetics have a higher incidence of coronary artery changes that influence decreased oxygen and nutrients to the myocardium. Patients have more angina and higher mortality with myocardial infarction. Patients with a history of diabetes mellitus (DM) and myocardial infarction have higher incidence of congestive heart failure, shock, and dysrhythmias. Cardiomyopathy may occur secondary to small vessel infarctions, causing myocardial fibrosis and hypertrophy.	History Symptoms Physical exam Electrocardiogram Cardiac enzymes Cardiac catheterization Stress test Autopsy	Same as for nondiabetics with CAD plus: Improved glycemic control Exercise Diet Use of diuretics may worsen NIDDM* hyperglycemia if hypokalemia exists and may adversely affect lipid levels. Additional CAD symptoms: Exertional weakness, peripheral edema, and orthopnea, fatigue
Infection		

Diabetics have a higher incidence of:
Pseudomonas external otitis, monilial skin infections. Common sites of infection in the diabetic include the urinary tract and skin.
Nephropathy
	History
	Symptoms
	Physical exam
	Lab data:
	  Increased WBC
	  Increased blood sugar
		Glycemic control
		Antibiotics and antifungals as required
		Follow-up with lab data
		Patient education

Peripheral Vascular Disease		
Carotid bruits, intermittent claudication, absent pedal pulses, and ischemic gangrene increase with DM. Peripheral vascular disease and neuropathy augment the morbidity associated with trauma and infection in the lower extremities.	History Symptoms Physical exam Doppler studies Angiogram Neuropathy identification	Patient education about meticulous foot care, padded sport socks, well-fitting shoes, and dangers of neuropathy Weight reduction Cessation of smoking Safe exercise programs
Hypertension		

	History
	Physical exam
	Orthostatic blood pressures (BPs) with pulse recordings
	BP lying, sitting, and standing
	Elevated BP readings at 2-3 recordings
	Urinalysis: 24-hr urine collection for protein, creatinine clearance, and glomerular filtration rate
		Eliminate risk factors
		Educate patient on this silent but deadly disease
		Diet education: low protein, low salt
		Pharmacologic interventions:
		  Diuretics
		  β-blockers
		  Angiotensin-converting enzyme inhibitors
		  Calcium channel blockers
		  α-blockers

a. *Expected outcomes:* Following interventions, the patient should be able to do the following:
   (1) Demonstrate understanding of the causes and complications of DM and the precautions necessary for dealing with it
   (2) Express lessened feelings of anxiety
b. *Nursing interventions*
   (1) Reassure the patient that control of diabetes is possible; stress the importance of good glycemic control for living safely with diabetes.
   (2) In combination with other team members, work with the patient to develop an individualized program that minimalizes upheavals in the patient's normal lifestyle.
   (3) Teach the patient about DM.

NURSING DIAGNOSIS: Altered nutrition, more than body requirements, R/T hyperglycemia

a. *Expected outcomes:* Following interventions, the person should attain an optimal blood sugar level.
b. *Nursing interventions*

LEARNING/TEACHING GUIDELINES
for the Diabetic Patient

1. Review the patient's knowldge about diabetes mellitus (DM).
2. Reteach or build on previously learned information to develop the patient's confidence.
3. General education
   a. Basic anatomy and physiology of the pancreas
   b. Definition of DM and its relationship to abnormal function of the pancreas
   c. Signs and symptoms of hyperglycemia
   d. Methods of controlling hyperglycemia
      (1) Diet: Refer the patient to a dietitian.
      (2) Exercise: The patient may need a complete physical examination before beginning an exercise program to assess cardiac status, neuropathy, retinopathy, and nutritional needs (weight loss is commonly indicated).
      (3) Oral hypoglycemic agents (see Table 29–9)
      (4) Insulin (see Table 29–10 and Fig. 29–8): Educate the patient on how, when, why, and where to give insulin combinations. Provide information on storage of insulin and needles and using, recycling, and disposing of needles.
      (5) What the patient should do when he or she is ill and when to call a physician
      (6) Daily blood sugar testing and recording and how to use a blood glucose monitor
      (7) Complications of DM: definition, cause, signs and symptoms, and treatment. Acute complications include hypoglycemia, diabetic ketoacidosis, and hyperglycemic hyperosmolar nonketotic coma. Chronic complications include microvascular problems, diabetic retinopathy, nephropathy, neuropathy, macrovascular problems, cardiovascular disease, hypertension, peripheral vascular disease, and infections.
      (8) Persons with DM need routine physician follow-up to provide early medical diagnosis and treatment for acute and chronic complications, evaluation of present means of care, and treatment of coexisting medical disorders.

---

(1) Assess blood sugar at insulin peaks as ordered or when the patient is symptomatic of hypoglycemia.
(2) Assess the patient for signs and symptoms of hypoglycemia.
(3) Treat hypoglycemia (see Table 29–11) and document accordingly.
(4) Arrange for a dietitian to teach the patient about his or her prescribed diet and weight reduction programs as indicated.

NURSING DIAGNOSIS: Altered nutrition, less than body requirements, R/T poor glucose utilization due to lack of insulin in a patient with diabetic ketoacidosis

a. *Expected outcomes:* After interventions, the patient should attain a blood sugar within normal range.
b. *Nursing interventions*
   (1) Administer IV fluids as ordered.
   (2) Administer IV insulin as ordered and monitor by finger-stick blood sugar test every 30 to 60 minutes.
   (3) Observe the patient for hypoglycemia.
   (4) Document the patient's blood sugar level, serum and urine ketones, and the patient's response and discuss them with the physician.
   (5) Treat the cause of DKA.
   (6) Refer the patient to a dietitian if dietary noncompliance contributed to hyperglycemia.

NURSING DIAGNOSIS: Fluid volume deficit R/T hyperglycemia and osmotic diuresis

a. *Expected outcomes:* Following interventions, the person should be able to do the following:
   (1) Decrease his or her blood sugar level while maintaining acceptable intake and output, vital signs, and electrolytes
   (2) Regain and maintain normal fluid volume, as evidenced by vital signs within acceptable parameters, urine output greater than 30 ml per hour, normal skin turgor, moist mucous membranes, and normal laboratory values
b. *Nursing interventions*
   (1) Monitor and record intake and output.
   (2) Obtain daily weights.
   (3) Assess skin turgor and mucous membranes for hydration.
   (4) Assess for signs of hypovolemic shock and electrolyte deficiency (especially hypokalemia).
   (5) Administer IV insulin and monitor the effectiveness of insulin through finger-stick glucose testing every 30 to 60 minutes until blood sugar is stable (250–300 mg/dl).
   (6) Monitor laboratory data: blood sugar, potassium, arterial blood gases, serum osmolality, serum and urine ketones, serum sodium, serum electrolytes, and urine-specific gravity.
   (7) Monitor vital signs and compare with previous

vital signs and laboratory data. Correlate vital signs with skin turgor and mental status.
 (8) Administer IV fluid replacement as ordered.

NURSING DIAGNOSIS: Ineffective breathing pattern R/T alteration in acid-base balance caused by increased production and decreased utilization of acetone bodies in a patient with diabetic ketoacidosis

  a. *Expected outcomes:* Following interventions, the person should be able to do the following:
   (1) Breathe normally
   (2) Exhibit signs of restored acid-base balance: normal pH, acceptable glucose level, and fewer or no acetones in serum and urine
  b. *Nursing interventions*
   (1) Monitor and record respirations.
   (2) Observe the patient for symptoms of Kussmaul's respiration and tachycardia.
   (3) Review arterial blood gases.
   (4) Monitor laboratory data for absence of ketones in urine and serum, hyperglycemia, and hypokalemia.
   (5) Provide oxygen therapy and monitor oxygen saturation as ordered.
   (6) Administer IV fluids as ordered.
12. Discharge planning and teaching
  a. Health teaching is directly related to quality of life for patients with diabetes.
  b. Teaching needs to begin as soon as the diagnosis of diabetes has been made and reinforced and updated at intervals thereafter.
  c. Begin by assessing the patient's individual needs and ability to learn.

 HOME CARE STRATEGIES

Diabetic Diet Instructions
When individuals with diabetes become aware of hidden sugar in their diets, they are more likely to decrease sugar intake, follow their diet, and maintain near normal blood glucose levels.
 As part of diabetic teaching:
 • Ask for your patient's permission to visit the kitchen area to discuss the contents of the refrigerator and cabinets. Bring attention to commonly overlooked potentially high sugar sources such as flavored instant drinks and cereals, sweetened canned or frozen fruit, baked beans, flavored yogurt, salad dressings, barbecue sauce, jellies, and glazed meats.
 • Show the patient how to interpret valuable information on the food labels including ingredients, serving size, and nutritional content.
 • Suggest the undesirable items be used by someone without diabetes or disposed of in a manner acceptable to the patient. Grocery stores will usually exchange nonperishable items without a receipt when informed their purchaser is diabetic.
 • Explain the benefits of consuming simple, basic foods such as lean meat, fresh or frozen vegetables, and whole grain breads. Processed or prepared foods should be avoided.
 • Have the patient keep a food diary for several days. It should include food eaten, portion size, and time of consumption so that together you can modify the diet as needed.

  d. Start with information already familiar to the patient to build confidence and a learning base.
13. Public health considerations
  a. Preventing diabetes through minimization of controllable risk factors
  b. Importance of early detection—stress the signs and symptoms of DM.

Reactive Hypoglycemia

1. Definition
  a. Reactive hypoglycemia exists when the homeostatic mechanism designed to regulate the blood sugar level fails to function, causing either over- or underproduction of insulin. It is usually measured as a blood glucose less than 50 mg per dl.
  b. Reactive hypoglycemia may develop spontaneously or after fasting.
  c. Reactive hypoglycemia is also known as *hypoglycemia in the fed state, functional hypoglycemia,* and *hyperinsulinism.*
2. Risk factors depend on etiology (see p. 1380)
3. Etiology and pathophysiology
  a. Hypoglycemia associated with fasting
   (1) Hypersecretion of insulin due to islet cell adenoma or carcinoma
   (2) Hepatic disease (ethanol hypoglycemia)
   (3) Sepsis
   (4) Endocrine deficiencies: anterior pituitary insufficiency, adrenocortical insufficiency, and hypothyroidism
   (5) Deficient carbohydrate stores or intake
  b. Reactive or stimulative hypoglycemia
   (1) Idiopathic functional hypoglycemia
   (2) Alimentary hyperinsulinism
   (3) Prediabetic functional hypoglycemia
   (4) Endocrine deficiencies
  c. Factitious and artificial hypoglycemia
   (1) Surreptitious insulin administration
   (2) Surreptitious ingestion of a sulfonylurea
   (3) Elevated leukocyte count—leukemia or polycythemia
4. Clinical manifestations are the same as in hypoglycemia with DM (see p. 1380). If left untreated or undetected, they may cause convulsive seizures and unconsciousness.
5. Diagnostic
  a. Assessment
   (1) History or current complaint of sudden hunger, irritability, anxiety, nervousness, tachycardia, or tremulousness after eating a large meal; history of gastric surgery; history of pancreatic tumors
   (2) Detailed dietary history—relate food intake and timing to onset of signs and symptoms
   (3) Physical examination for clinical manifestations and other signs and symptoms, such as cool or diaphoretic skin, hyperactive responses (common in early stages), or a sluggish reflex response (in later stages)
  b. Diagnostic tests

(1) Serum hypoglycemia: Blood sugar testing when symptoms develop may be helpful in diagnosing reactive hypoglycemia. However, the blood sugar level is not always low when the classic hypoglycemic symptoms develop, making this disorder difficult to diagnose.

(2) Measurement of plasma insulin in association with hypoglycemic glucose values: A mixed meal tolerance test may be administered. A standardized meal is eaten, and blood sugar level and symptoms are evaluated every 30 minutes for 5 hours.

(3) Oral glucose tolerance test extended to 6 hours.

(4) Tolbutamide tolerance test: Provides important information regarding the etiology of hypoglycemia. A rapid intravenous infusion of 1 gm of tolbutamide is given in the fasting state. Plasma samples for glucose are obtained at 2, 15, 30, 60, 90, and 120 minutes after the infusion. (Development of severe hypoglycemia often requires stopping the test before completion.) In normal patients, plasma glucose decreases significantly (may exceed 50% of fasting value) at 30 minutes; however, the value returns to normal at 2 hours. Patients with fasting hypoglycemia usually have a more profound decrease in plasma glucose that persists throughout the test.

(5) Calcium infusion test: Infusion of calcium over a 4-hour period may induce hyperinsulinemia and hypoglycemia in some patients with islet cell tumors.

6. Clinical management

a. Goals

(1) Control frequency of hypoglycemic reactions.

(2) Prevent the symptoms of hypoglycemia.

b. Nonpharmacologic interventions: Dietary intervention is the main treatment for reactive hypoglycemia.

(1) The treatment for severe reactive hypoglycemia is the same as for hypoglycemia in patients with DM (see p. 1381).

(2) Dietary modifications include small, frequent meals; meals that are relatively free of simple sugars; omission of refined sugar and white flour; a balanced intake of fats, protein, and the complex carbohydrates found in fruits, vegetables, and whole grains; no fasting.

c. Pharmacologic interventions

(1) Anticholinergic drugs to control intestinal motility associated with gastric surgery or intestinal bypass surgery: These surgeries can produce a "dumping syndrome"—delivery of a large bolus of food to the intestine, causing the pancreas eventually to react with a surplus of insulin.

(2) Dioxide therapy to suppress insulin secretion in patients with inoperable insulinomas

(3) Avoidance of drugs that may cause hypoglycemia: alcohol, salicylates, and propranolol

(4) Correction of any endocrine deficiency (e.g., hypopituitarism or adrenal insufficiency) that may be causing hypoglycemia

(5) Treatment of hepatic disease

7. Complications: Frequent or prolonged episodes may eventually cause progressive and irreversible neuropathy, retinal hemorrhages, cerebral vascular accidents, permanent personality changes, and intellectual damage (see p. 1380).

8. Prognosis is good if the patient complies with his or her medical prescription. Frequent episodes of hypoglycemia or severe hypoglycemia may affect the patient's quality of life.

9. Applying the nursing process: See nursing diagnoses "Fluid volume deficit" (p. 1387) and "Altered nutrition, more than body requirements" (pp. 1386–1387).

10. Discharge planning and teaching

a. Describe the diagnostic tests and procedures to the patient, and answer his or her questions.

b. As soon as reactive hypoglycemia is diagnosed, instruct the patient and family regarding the cause (if known) and treatment of this disorder, including dietary management and emergency treatment. Explain the consequences of frequent or prolonged hypoglycemia and how to avoid this state.

c. Prepare the patient for surgery (if indicated).

■ THYROID DISORDERS

Hypothyroidism

1. Definition

a. Hypothyroidism is underactivity of the thyroid, hyposecretion of thyroid hormone, and decreased body metabolism and heat production.

b. Myxedema, an extreme state of worsening hypothyroidism, is *not* the same as hypothyroidism; it is a *complication* of hypothyroidism (see p. 1392).

c. Hypothyroidism may be primary, secondary, or tertiary (see p. 1390).

2. Incidence and socioeconomic impact

a. Hypothyroidism affects women 4 times more often than it affects men.

b. The highest incidence of hypothyroidism is found among people older than 30.

c. About 95 percent of patients diagnosed with hypothyroidism have primary hypothyroidism (see p. 1390).

3. Risk factors

a. Patients living in areas with iodine-deficient water and soil are at risk for endemic goiter. In the United States, these areas include the Midwest, Northwest, and Great Lakes region. Food additives and the use of iodized salt have nearly eradicated this problem.

b. Ingestion of goitrogenic glycosides may cause sporadic goiter.

(1) Medicinal glycosides include thioureas (e.g., propylthiouracil), thiocarbamides (aminothiazole and tolbutamide), and large doses of iodine.

(2) If eaten in large quantities, nutritional glycosides in some foods (e.g., rutabagas, cabbage, soybeans, peanuts, peas, strawberries, and spinach) may inhibit thyroxine (T_4) production.

c. Genetic defects involving faulty iodine metabolism cause hypothyroidism.

4. Etiology
   a. Primary hypothyroidism (thyroid failure) may be caused by cretinism, defective hormone synthesis, iodine deficiency, antithyroid drugs, surgery, radiation therapy for hyperthyroidism, or the aftereffects of chronic inflammation of the thyroid. Hashimoto's thyroiditis is the most common cause of primary hypothyroidism.
   b. Secondary hypothyroidism occurs when TSH fails to stimulate the thyroid gland. Diseases of the pituitary or hypothalamus also may cause secondary hypothyroidism.
   c. Tertiary hypothyroidism (central hypothyroidism) may develop if tumors or lesions in the hypothalamic area interfere with normal hypothalamic function and cause it not to produce TRH. Lack of TRH, in turn, causes a decrease in TSH from the pituitary.

5. Pathophysiology
   a. Lack of iodine in the diet prevents the thyroid gland from producing the 3 thyroid hormones: T_4, triiodothyronine (T_3), and thyrocalcitonin (calcitonin) *or* some other factor suppresses production of these hormones. Decreased production of thyroid hormones slows the body's metabolic rate.
   b. In an attempt to restore thyroid hormone production to normal levels, the anterior pituitary vainly increases production of TSH, causing the thyroid gland to enlarge. Enlargement causes development of a goiter that may eventually grow large enough to compress structures in the neck and chest, resulting in respiratory problems and dysphagia.

6. Clinical manifestations are shown in Figure 29–10.

7. Diagnostics
   a. Assessment
      (1) History of neck or head radiation or surgery; neck pain or swelling; neck cancer; weight gain; anorexia; intolerance to cold; dry or thinning hair; mental slowness; unusual fatigue; decreased libido; impotence; irregular menses; constipation; lithium usage; iodine deficiency; or recent viral or bacterial infection with myalgia, arthralgia, or neck discomfort.
      (2) Physical examination: Check for clinical manifestations.
   b. Diagnostic studies
      (1) Blood tests for thyroid function show increased levels of TSH, decreased levels of thyroid hormones, presence of serum thyroid antibodies, and increased serum cholesterol levels. A complete blood count is needed to evaluate related anemia.
      (2) Additional laboratory tests may be indicated to confirm the effects of hypothyroidism on other body systems.
      (3) The ECG interpretation may reveal changes related to hypothyroidism (flat or inverted T waves, small ST segment depressions, or low-amplitude QRS complexes).
      (4) Radioactive iodine uptake test (RAIU) shows increased TRH levels in primary hypothyroidism

and decreased levels in secondary hypothyroidism. Subsequent scans of the thyroid can determine the size of the gland, the presence and number of nodules, and the degree of iodide uptake by any nodules. "Hot nodules" absorb more isotope than does normal tissue and are usually benign.
      (5) Needle biopsy may be used to check for malignancies.

ELDER ADVISORY

Approximately 5 percent of the older population has subclinical or asymptomatic hypothyroidism. Laboratory test results will include increased levels of thyroid-stimulating hormone and normal levels of thyroxine (T_4), free T_4, and triiodothyronine. Be alert for generic complaints of fatigue, weakness, slowed thinking, and feeling cold—all may indicate that a thyroid workup is in order. Also be sure to assess for tachycardia at rest; myopathy with proximal muscle loss; and unexplained congestive heart failure, palpitations, and atrial fibrillation.

8. Clinical management
   a. Goal: Restore and maintain the patient's euthyroid state for life.
   b. Nonpharmacologic interventions: For use in combination with pharmacologic interventions and while the patient is in a symptomatic hypothyroid state:
      (1) Sufficient physical and emotional rest and emotional support
      (2) Balanced diet with increased fiber
      (3) Adequate bowel elimination
      (4) Appropriate ambulatory aid to support weak muscles
      (5) Lotion for dry skin, as needed
   c. Pharmacologic interventions (dosages depend on the severity of the disease and the patient's general medical condition and response to treatment)
      (1) Thyroid hormone supplements: **Thyroid USP** (desiccated thyroid, thyroid extract), which contains T_4 and T_3, may cause side effects similar to hyperthyroidism and may exacerbate angina. **Synthetic T_4** (thyroxine, levothyroxine, or sodium L-thyroxine), a common form of Synthroid, has fewer side effects than thyroid USP and is the agent of choice.
      (2) Thyroid hormone replacement: Must be gradual and monitored by monthly measurements of TSH.
   d. Special medical-surgical procedures
      (1) Surgery may be performed to remove goiters endangering neck structures.

℞ **DRUG ADVISORY**

Although thyroxine treatment is beneficial in many cases, it does entail risks, such as the possibility of creating an adrenal crisis. In patients with positive cardiac histories, it can also cause angina or cardiac dysrhythmias and deterioration in the symptoms of ischemic heart disease and can even precipitate a myocardial infarction.

HYPOTHYROIDISM AND HYPERTHYROIDISM

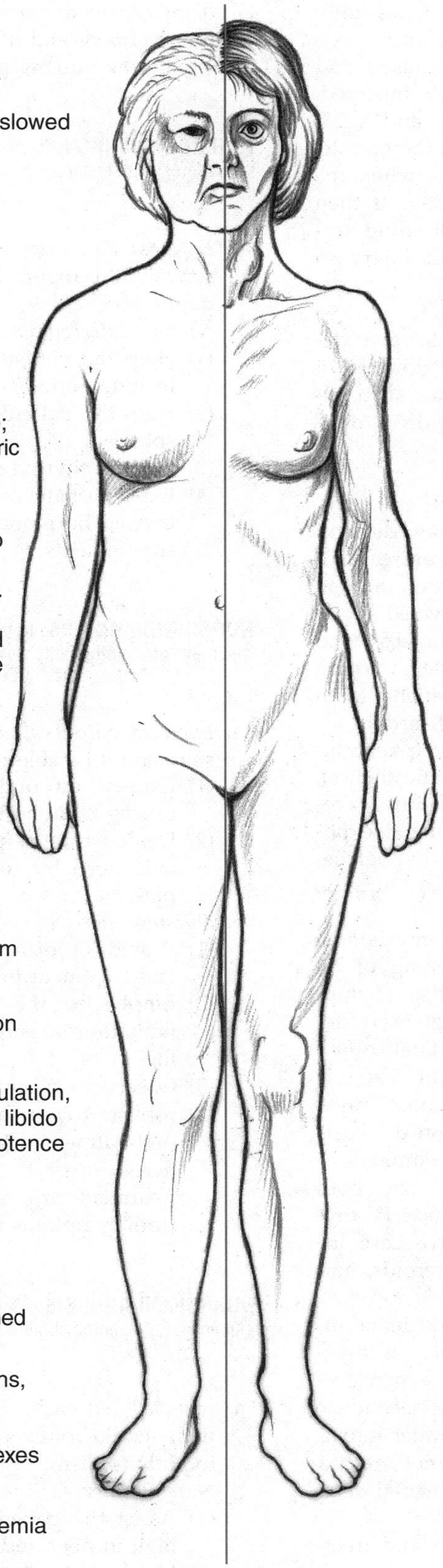

HYPOTHYROIDISM

Neurologic
- Apathy, depression, paranoia
- Impaired short-term memory
- Lethargy, thought processes slowed
- Slowed response

Eyes
- Periorbital puffiness

Facies
- Rounded face
- Dulled expression
- Relaxed features
- Indefineable puffiness

Neck
- No thyroid enlargement
- Diffuse enlargement possible; may be symmetric or asymmetric

Cardiovascular
- Heart rate: slow to normal. A slowed rate may contribute to a decreased cardiac output.
- Rhythm: dysrhythmias are rare.
- Blood pressure: normal to slight elevation of systolic and diastolic (causing an increase in peripheral vascular resistance).

Respiratory
- Dyspnea

Gastrointestinal
- Anorexia
- Increased weight gain
- Constipation
- Decreased bowel sounds
- Decreased protein metabolism
- Increased serum lipids
- Delayed glucose uptake
- Decreased glucose absorption

Reproductive
- Females: menorrhagia, anovulation, irregular menses, decreased libido
- Males: decreased libido, impotence

Integumentary
- Cold, dry, and thickened skin
- Nonpitting edema
- Occasional scaling
- Hair: Dry and coarse; lateral thirds of eyebrow may be thinned

Neuromuscular
- Slowed and deliberate motions, speech
- Generalized weakness
- Hypoactive deep tendon reflexes

Hematologic
- Normocytic or macrocytic anemia

HYPERTHYROIDISM

Neurologic
- Emotional instability, lability; anxiety, worry paranoia; irritability
- Depression or manic states may develop
- Easy to distract, unable to concentrate
- Quick responses to questions or stimuli

Eyes
- Lid lag, exophthalmos
- Often paresis of extraocular muscles

Facies
- Features thinned and sharp
- Frequent, fast facial movements

Neck
- Thyroid enlargement usual
- Tracheal displacement may occur
- Arterial thrill, arterial bruit may occur
- Nodules may be present

Cardiovascular
- Increased strength of myocardial contraction demonstrated by precordial thrust (palpitation)
- Tachycardia
- Rhythm: frequent atrial fibrillation or atrial flutter
- Blood pressure: usually systolic pressure elevated, diastolic decreased, giving a widened pulse pressure.

Respiratory
- Shortness of breath
- Increased rate and depth of respiration

Gastrointestinal
- Increased peristalsis
- Increased appetite
- Weight loss
- Diarrhea
- Increased use of adipose and protein stores
- Decreased serum lipids
- Increased gastrointestinal secretions
- Vomiting, abdominal pain

Reproductive
- Females: amenorrhea, irregular menses, decreased fertility, tendency for spontaneous abortion
- Males: impotence, decreased libido, decreased sexual development, prepuberty

Integumentary
- Nonpitting edema of the shins
- Soft, moist, diaphoretic, warm skin
- Hair: fine, oily, may have patchy alopecia

Neuromuscular
- Hyperkinesia
- Hyperactive deep tendon reflexes
- Fine tremor in fingers, tongue, and proximal muscle groups
- May be some generalized weakness in proximal muscle groups

Figure 29–10.

(2) Needle biopsy may be performed to rule out a malignancy. The procedure, which takes only about 10 minutes, may be performed on an outpatient basis. The thyroid area is cleansed and draped. Local anesthesia may be administered. The patient's neck is hyperextended, and a 23-gauge needle is used to aspirate from the nodule. Mild pressure is placed over the site when the needle is removed. An adhesive bandage is then applied. Complications such as a bleeding tracheal puncture, laryngoparalysis, and injury to the laryngeal nerve are rare.

9. Complications
   a. Because patients with hypothyroidism have a decreased ability to metabolize, the usual dosages of many drugs may produce toxicity. Monitor such patients closely for drug levels and signs of drug toxicity.
   b. Myxedema and myxedema coma
      (1) Definition: Myxedema is a rare but severe manifestation of hypothyroidism that may develop into myxedema coma or stupor if left untreated.
      (2) Incidence: Myxedema is most common among persons with undiagnosed or undertreated hypothyroidism (especially women in their 60s) who experience increased stress. Myxedema coma occurs most frequently in elderly patients with underlying pulmonary and vascular disorders.
      (3) Precipitating factors: infection, drugs (phenothiazines, barbiturates, narcotics, and anesthetics), respiratory failure, congestive heart failure, cerebral vascular accident, trauma, prolonged exposure to cold, metabolic disturbances (hypoglycemia, hyponatremia, and adrenal crisis), surgery, and seizures
      (4) Clinical manifestations: Symptoms of myxedema include hypothermia and the worsening of all signs and symptoms of hypothyroidism. Symptoms of myxedema coma reflect an intensely depressed metabolic rate progressing to fatal coma.
      (5) Medical diagnosis: Diagnosis is difficult. There is no specific laboratory test to diagnose myxedema. Laboratory tests are ordered on the basis of the patient's history and physical examination.
      (6) Clinical management: Interventions for both myxedema and myxedema coma include IV thyroid hormone replacement, supportive care for symptoms, stress dosages of corticosteroids, and correction of precipitating events.
      (7) Complications: Complications of myxedema include myxedema coma. Complications of myxedema coma include hyponatremia, hypercalcemia, respiratory or metabolic acidosis, secondary adrenal insufficiency, hypoglycemia, water intoxication, and severe hypothermia. If not treated promptly, it can result in permanent mental deterioration or death.
      (8) Prognosis: With appropriate diagnosis and treatment, the long-term prognosis for myxedema is excellent. The mortality rate for untreated myxedema coma is very high.

10. Prognosis for hypothyroidism: Patients with hypothyroidism can lead normal, productive lives with appropriate treatment and lifelong compliance.
11. Applying the nursing process

NURSING DIAGNOSIS: Activity intolerance R/T muscle fatigue and depression secondary to decreased metabolic state

---

a. *Expected outcomes:* Following interventions, the person should report increased energy and decreased depression.
b. *Nursing interventions*
   (1) Help the patient anticipate a daily schedule and include periods of rest alternating with activity.
   (2) Help the patient in establishing a relaxing atmosphere.
   (3) Provide thyroid supplements as ordered.
   (4) Explain that energy and interests will return as thyroid hormone levels rise as a result of thyroid supplements.

NURSING DIAGNOSIS: Knowledge deficit R/T new diagnosis and treatment of hypothyroidism

---

a. *Expected outcomes:* Following interventions, the person should be able to do the following:
   (1) Express an understanding of hypothyroidism's causes, complications, and treatments
   (2) Demonstrate a positive response to therapy, as evidenced by compliance with prescribed therapies
b. *Nursing interventions*
   (1) Provide information on hypothyroidism's causes and treatment to the patient and family.
   (2) Emphasize the necessity of lifelong treatment with thyroid supplements to enhance quality of life.
   (3) Observe for signs and symptoms of hyperthyroidism (overtreatment) and hypothyroidism (undertreatment). Monitor laboratory tests as ordered. Assist the patient in adjusting the treatment program to provide continuous relief from symptoms of hypothyroidism.

NURSING DIAGNOSIS: Constipation R/T decreased peristalsis influenced by hypometabolic state and activity intolerance

---

a. *Expected outcomes:* Following interventions, the patient should return to bowel habits established before hypothyroidism.
b. *Nursing interventions*
   (1) Assist the patient in developing a palatable diet high in fiber and high in liquids.
   (2) Monitor bowel patterns and bowel sounds.
   (3) Provide stool softeners and cathartics as ordered and needed.

a. *Expected outcomes:* Following interventions, the patient should report renewed self-esteem and self-confidence in the ability to cope with long-term hypothyroidism.

b. *Nursing interventions*

  (1) Repeatedly provide the patient small amounts of information about reasonable expectations for thyroid therapy.

  (2) Assist and encourage the patient to dress and maintain his or her activity level.

  (3) Allow and encourage the patient to choose menus or short-term activity ideas to promote thought initiation.

  (4) Include family and friends in effort to provide a positive, supportive environment for the patient.

12. Discharge planning and teaching

  a. Instruct the patient on the causes, complications, and treatment of hypothyroidism (including signs of under- or overtreatment).

  b. Emphasize the need to accept the chronicity of hypothyroidism.

  c. Inform the patient about thyroid supplements—how and when to take them and why they are necessary—and explain that physical manifestations of hypothyroidism will decrease over 3 to 12 weeks as TSH decreases.

  d. Stress the importance of thyroid hormone assessments and physician visits.

13. Public health considerations

  a. Focus is on primary prevention of hypothyroidism.

  b. Pregnancy, lactation, and growth spurts are times for increased thyroid hormones. Pregnant women, lactating mothers, and adolescents should be evaluated for adequate TSH and free (f)T_4 levels when symptoms of hypothyroidism surface.

Hyperthyroidism

1. Definition: Oversecretion of thyroid hormone, which accelerates many body functions, causing a hypermetabolic state

2. Incidence and socioeconomic impact: Hyperthyroidism occurs in women 4 times more often than in men. It is commonly diagnosed in the 20- to 40-year-old age group.

3. Risk factors

  a. Overtreatment for hypothyroidism

  b. Radioiodine therapy of partial thyroidectomy, causing a rebound effect that can produce hyperthyroid symptoms

  c. Pituitary disease

  d. Hypothalamic disease

4. Etiology

  a. Graves' disease, an autoimmune disorder, is the most common cause of hyperthyroidism. Thyroid-stimulating autoantibodies cause increased thyroid function and hyperplasia of the gland.

  b. Acute thyroiditis, a rare disorder that is bacterial in origin, produces fever and pain in the thyroid that radiates to the ears. Subacute thyroiditis, a more common condition that is viral in origin, produces pain from thyroid to the ears and local tenderness.

5. Pathophysiology

  a. Hyperthyroidism results when conditions such as autoimmune disorders and thyroiditis disrupt the normal regulatory controls (TSH from the anterior pituitary and TRH from the hypothalamus) over thyroid hormone secretion.

  b. Excess production of thyroid hormones overstimulates the body, causing hypermetabolism; increased sympathetic nervous system activity; and alteration of production and release of hormones produced in the gonads, hypothalamus, and pituitary.

6. Clinical manifestations are shown in Figure 29–10.

7. Diagnostics

  a. Assessment

  (1) History of neck or head radiation, surgery, or cancer; neck pain or swelling; dysphagia; hoarseness; tremors; palpitations; nervousness; muscle weakness; emotional lability; fatigue; heat intolerance; diphoresis; frequent bowel movements; and weight loss in spite of increased appetite

  (2) Physical examination: Check for clinical manifestations.

  b. Diagnostic studies

  (1) Typically decreased serum TSH and increased T_3, T_4, and fT_4

  (2) Elevated serum calcium level reflecting hypercalcemia secondary to alteration in calcium metabolism from hyperthyroidism

  (3) Increased red blood cell count secondary to increased formation of erythrocytes

  (4) Decreased white blood cell count due to a decline in neutrophils

  (5) 24-hour RAIU to distinguish Graves' disease from other causes of hyperthyroidism

  (6) Thyroid scan using radioactive tracers

8. Clinical management

  a. Goals

  (1) Restore and maintain the patient's euthyroid state for life

  (2) Control thyroid hormone secretion

  (3) Prevent complications

  b. Nonpharmacologic interventions: Prescribe a diet high in calories, fiber, and protein to compensate for hypermetabolism, with exact makeup dependent on concurrent medical problems such as kidney disease, heart disease, or DM.

  c. Pharmacologic interventions are listed in Table 29–14.

  (1) Antithyroid medications such as propylthiouracil (the drug of choice), methimazole, and carbimazole inhibit hormone synthesis and deplete hormone stores. Propylthiouracil and carbimazole also impair the conversion of T_4 to T_3 in the peripheral tissues. Medications may be needed

Table 29–14. Medications Used to Treat Thyroid Disorders

Medication	Use	Side Effects	Nursing Implications
Propythiouracil (PTU)	**Antithyroid medication** used to treat hyperthyroidism Inhibits thyroid hormone synthesis	Adverse responses are rare However, the following may occur: Nausea, vomiting, diarrhea, loss of taste, skin changes, headache, dizziness, drowsiness, lymphadenopathy, hypersensitivity, agranulocytosis, hypothyroidism	Use carefully in combination with any drug that causes agranulocytosis Monitor blood counts Should not be used in the last trimester of pregnancy or during lactation Report any symptoms of infection Give every 8 hr around the clock Urge continued compliance, because response is slow
Methimazole (Tapazole)	**Antithyroid medication** used to treat hyperthyroidism Inhibits thyroid hormone synthesis	Agranulocytosis, headache, drowsiness, diarrhea, nausea and vomiting, jaundice, urticaria, arthralgia, lymphadenopathy	Use carefully in pregnancy Monitor thyroid function closely Check CBC periodically Watch for signs of hypothyroidism, colds, and other infections Stop drug if rash or lymphadenopathy occurs Give with meals to decrease gastrointestinal effects Store in light-resistant containers
Saturated solution of potassium iodide	**Antithyroid medication** that blocks thyroid hormone production and release Used to treat hyperthyroidism	Diarrhea, nausea and vomiting, stomach pain, hypothyroidism, hypersensitivity, iodine poisoning, irregular heart beat, productive cough	Use with caution in patients with tuberculosis, hyperkalemia, acute bronchitis, impaired renal function, or cardiac disease Safety in pregnancy, lactation, or childhood has not been established Give after meals with fruit juice Monitor potassium level Avoid sudden withdrawal Keep in light-protected bottle Avoid use of over-the-counter drugs containing iodine Restrict iodine-rich foods and iodized salts Ensure preoperative compliance
Radioactive iodine (^{131}I)	**Antithyroid medication** that destroys thyroid tissue Used to treat hyperthyroidism May be used to treat thyroid cancer May produce remission without destroying entire thyroid gland	Feeling of fullness in neck, metallic taste, hypothyroidism, possible increased risk of leukemia later in life	Contraindicated in pregnancy and lactation for hyperthyroidism Stop all antithyroid medications 1 wk before ^{131}I administration Monitor thyroid function closely Give on empty stomach Institute radiation precautions on body secretions for 3 days after ingestion Teach patient to avoid close, prolonged contact with children for a week and to sleep alone for a week Patient should not resume antithyroid medications for 6 wk
Levothyroxine sodium (Synthroid)	**Thyroid replacement medication** T_4 used to treat hypothyroidism	Rare hyperthyroidism, tremors, hunger, palpitations, headache, nervousness, tachycardia, insomnia, heat intolerance, weight loss	Use with caution in patients with acute MI, hypertension, renal insufficiency, or diabetes and in elderly or pregnant patients Give a single dose in A.M. Watch for adverse effects early in treatment Do not use to treat depression or obesity Stress need for lifetime replacement Toxicity may last for weeks with overdosage Monitor for improvement of symptoms
Liothyronine sodium (Cytomel)	**Thyroid replacement medication** T_3 used to treat hypothyroidism	Signs of hyperthyroidism, diarrhea, abdominal cramps, vomiting, tachycardia, weight loss, heat intolerance	Use with caution in patients with acute MI, hypertension, renal insufficiency, or diabetes and in elderly or pregnant patients

Table 29–14. Medications Used to Treat Thyroid Disorders (Continued)

Medication	Use	Side Effects	Nursing Implications
			Give a single dose in A.M. Watch for adverse effects early in treatment Smaller doses required for older patients Monitor pulse, blood pressure, and thyroid function
Strong iodine solution (Lugol's solution)	Used in preparation for thyroid surgery Nonradioactive antithyroid medication Suppresses iodine uptake, inhibits thyroid hormone synthesis, and inhibits release of thyroid hormone	"Iodism" from chronic ingestion: brassy taste, burning sensation of mouth and throat, soreness of teeth and gums, frontal headache, coryza, salivation, and skin eruptions	Mix with juice or other beverage to disguise unpleasant taste Side effects will disappear when medication is discontinued
IV sodium iodide	Thyrotoxic crisis management Rapidly suppresses thyroid hormone release. Used with PTU and propranolol	Rare, although the following may occur: severe hypersensitivity reactions, immediate or delayed by several hours; angioedema; laryngeal edema (no antidote; supportive treatment is used)	Observe for side effects and hypothyroid signs and symptoms
Propranolol	Suppresses tachycardia and other symptoms of hyperthyroidism as β-adrenergic antagonist Does not reduce T_3 or T_4 level	Hypotension, headache, bradycardia, bronchoconstriction, central nervous system effects, congestive heart failure	Contraindicated in patients with known asthmatic or congestive heart failure

CBC, Complete blood count; IV, intravenously; MI, myocardial infarction; PO, orally; tid, 3 times daily.
Modified from Black JM, and Matassarin-Jacobs E (eds). *Luckmann and Sorensen's Medical-Surgical Nursing: A Psychophysiologic Approach.* 4th ed. Philadelphia: WB Saunders, 1993, p 1815

 DRUG ADVISORY

Roughly 10 to 14 days after administration of radioiodine, thyroiditis sets in and may cause the release of large quantities of stored thyroid hormone. This release can be hazardous to patients with underlying cardiac disease or systemic illnesses. It is recommended that patients be made euthyroid with antithyroid drugs before radioactive iodine is used.

A significant side effect of radioiodine and other antithyroid agents is the risk of inducing hypothyroidism. Those treated with radioiodine have a very high frequency (approximately 80%) of late hypothyroidism.

The most common side effect of antithyroid drugs (<1% of patients) is agranulocytosis, in which dramatic decreases in granulocyte production leave the patient defenseless against bacterial infection. Prompt withdrawal of the drug and treatment of the infection with antibiotics usually result in complete lymphocyte recovery.

for as little as 6 months or for the rest of the patient's life. Reduction of symptoms becomes apparent after about 2 weeks of therapy; full return to normal (normal TSH and T_4 levels and, in one half to two thirds of patients, reduction in size of the thyroid) takes about 6 weeks.

(2) Radioiodine decreases goiter size by destroying local thyroid tissue.

(3) Dexamethasone inhibits secretion of thyroid hormones and peripheral conversion of T_4 to T_3. It is used for rapid alleviation of hyperthyroidism and as an adjunct therapy.

(4) Beta-adrenergic antagonists help manage the cardiac side effects of hyperthyroidism. Propranolol controls tachycardia, hypertension, and atrial fibrillation.

d. Radiating the thyroid gland: oral ingestion of radioiodine

(1) The radioiodine is quickly absorbed and stored in the thyroid, acutely radiating the thyroid and causing thyroid atrophy. Symptoms gradually decrease after about 3 weeks; a euthyroid state returns after 3 months. Most (66%) patients need only 1 dose of radioiodine.

(2) To prepare the patient for radiation, explain the procedure and the expected results, inquire as to iodine or shellfish allergies, stop antithyroid medicine 4 to 7 days before administration of radioiodine begins, and instruct the patient to take nothing by mouth the night before the radioiodine is to be ingested.

(3) After the ingestion, increase oral fluids to promote excretion of the radioiodine. The patient's urine and saliva are very radioactive for 24 hours after ingestion, and vomitus is radioactive for 6 to 8 hours. Thus, the patient should void into a lead-lined urine container, use disposable utensils, and avoid close contact with children and pregnant women for 48 hours after ingestion. Fe-

male patients should use contraception and avoid pregnancy until advised by the physician. Symptoms related to radiation treatment—pain, swelling, and fever—should be reported to the physician.

(4) Routine follow-up with a physician to check thyroid levels is necessary to determine disease status.

e. Special medical-surgical procedures

(1) Thyroid biopsy may be performed to distinguish benign from malignant thyroid disease and to diagnose disorders such as subacute thyroiditis, Hashimoto's disease, and multinodular goiter.

(2) Surgery (subtotal or total thyroidectomy) may be performed when pharmacologic therapies fail or for thyroid cancer. To minimize the risk of thyroid storm (see "Complications"), the patient should be euthyroid, which may take 2 to 3 months. The patient is then prescribed a 10-day course of saturated solution of potassium iodide to decrease the vascularity and size of the thyroid before surgery. Common postoperative complications include bleeding into the operative site, laryngeal nerve damage, hypothyroidism, recurrent hyperthyroidism (less than 10% of patients), thyroid storm, hypoparathyroidism (transient or permanent) (Table 29–15).

9. Complications

a. Thyroid storm (also called *thyroid crisis* and *thyrotoxicosis*)

(1) Definition: an acute, potentially life-threatening exacerbation of all symptoms of hyperthyroidism

(2) Precipitating factors: untreated, progressive hyperthyroidism; any stressor that accelerates metabolic rate (e.g., infection); congestive heart failure; diabetic ketoacidosis; pregnancy; pulmonary embolism; and traumatic injury

(3) Symptoms: hyperthermia (38–41 degrees Celsius; 100–106 degrees Fahrenheit), tachycardia, atrial fibrillation, congestive heart failure; marked agi-

Table 29–15. Postoperative Care for the Patient with a Thyroidectomy

Postoperative Order	Rationale	Associated Nursing Interventions
Vital signs every 15 min until stable; then every 30 min for next 12 hr	After thyroidectomy, hemorrhage and respiratory obstruction may develop. Elevated pulse and hypotension indicate hemorrhage and shock. Dyspnea, stridulous respirations, and retraction of neck tissues indicate respiratory obstruction.	Check dressing after checking vital signs. Observe for bleeding at front, sides, and back of neck. Examine back of patient's neck and shoulders for bleeding, because blood tends to drain posteriorly. Check dressing for tightness; uncomfortable tautness may indicate bleeding into tissues. Loosen dressing and call surgeon immediately.
Semi-Fowler's position when conscious unless patient is hypotensive; support head and neck with pillows and sandbags; ambulate 2nd day as tolerated	Immobilization of head and neck is essential to prevent flexion and hyperextension of neck with resultant strain on suture line. Semi-Fowler's position is used for comfort.	Place sandbags on either side of patient's head for immobilization and maintenance of good alignment. Warn patient not to extend or hyperextend neck; reassure patient that sandbags will prevent moving head too much. Gently rub back of patient's neck to relieve tenson. Support patient's head and neck when moving or changing position.
Fluids by mouth as tolerated; if nauseated or vomiting, notify surgeon; soft diet on afternoon of 2nd day	Give intravenous fluids if nauseated or vomiting. Otherwise, start oral fluids as soon as patient is fully conscious.	Maintain intake and output record for 2 or 3 days. Assess for difficulty swallowing. Normally, this problem lasts for only 1 or 2 days postoperatively. Weigh patient once a full diet is started; weight lost during early postoperative period should be regained.
Meperidine (Demerol) or morphine sulfate, every 3–4 hr as needed for pain in throat area	Demerol and morphine sulfate are both used during early postoperative period to relieve pain and promote rest.	Do not give narcotics if respirations below 12/min or if respiratory congestion is present; consult physician for further orders.
Cough and deep-breathe every half hour; suction mouth and trachea if necessary	Pooling of mucous secretions in trachea, bronchi, and lungs will cause respiratory obstruction with resultant atelectasis and pneumonia. Secretions must be raised to prevent respiratory complications.	Instruct patient to cough and deep breathe as taught during preoperative period. If patient cannot raise secretions, gently suction mouth and trachea. Do not oversedate patient with profuse respiratory secretions; give narcotics judiciously.
Tracheostomy set, endotracheal tube, laryngoscope, and oxygen on hand in room.	Acute respiratory obstruction due to hemorrhage, edema of glottis, laryngeal nerve damage, or tetany is an emergency. Equipment for establishing an airway and administering oxygen must be available for immediate use.	Continuously assess for signs of airway obstruction, e.g., increasing restlessness, tachycardia, apprehension, cyanosis, stridulous respirations, and retraction of neck tissues. Report any of these signs to surgeon immediately.
Continuous mist inhalation until chest is clear	Humidification of air promotes easier breathing and helps to liquefy mucous secretions.	Keep doors closed so that moist air is retained in room.
Tympanic temperature every 4 hr for 24 hr; then oral temperature	One of the first signs of thyroid storm is an elevated temperature.	Carefully assess for signs of thyroid storm: elevated temperature, extreme restlessness, agitation, and tachycardia. Report any elevation over 37.2° C (99° F).

Modified from Black JM, and Matassarin-Jacobs E (eds). *Luckmann and Sorensen's Medical-Surgical Nursing: A Psychophysiologic Approach.* 4th ed. Philadelphia: WB Saunders, 1993, p 1823.

tation, restlessness, and tremor progressing to delirium; nausea, vomiting, and diarrhea

(4) Medical diagnosis is based on correlation of history, physical examination, and laboratory data.

(5) Clinical management: pharmacologic depression of TSH, symptomatic relief

DRUG ADVISORY

Tests of patients with thyrotoxicosis may reveal increased clotting factor III. Treating this situation with coumarin derivatives, a popular class of anticoagulants, can be problematic in people with hyperthyroidism. These individuals' increased metabolisms rapidly clear vitamin K–dependent clotting factors from their body. Because coumarin derivatives inhibit production of these factors, using them can result in a *shortage* of clotting factors over time.

b. Exophthalmos

(1) Definition: a rare eye condition marked by protrusion of the eyes

(2) Precipitating factors: prolonged hyperthyroidism's effects—proptosis, lid retraction, muscle swelling and tissue edema

(3) Symptoms: protruding eyes, gritty sensation in the eyes, photophobia, lacrimation, diplopia, and inflammatory changes

(4) Clinical management: Exophthalmos is generally lessened or resolved by treating hyperthyroidism. Surgical decompression is used in those rare cases in which eye function is jeopardized.

c. Heart disease

(1) The complication of heart disease in the hyperthyroid patient is influenced by the amount of cardiac reserve and the direct effects of the thyroid hormone on the heart.

(2) Disease states that might develop include atrial fibrillation, congestive heart failure, myocardial infarction, cardiomegaly, tachycardia, and angina.

(3) Propranolol is the drug of choice but is contraindicated if congestive heart failure or asthma is concurrently diagnosed.

10. Prognosis: Prompt (and, if necessary, lifelong) treatment of hyperthyroidism enables most patients to lead normal and productive lives without specific limitations.

11. Applying the nursing process

NURSING DIAGNOSIS: Hyperthermia R/T hypermetabolic state

a. *Expected outcomes:* Following interventions, the patient's body temperature should return to normal.

b. *Nursing interventions*

(1) Monitor temperature.

(2) Treat fever with nonaspirin antipyretics as ordered, cold packs, cool room, and hypothermia mattress.

NURSING DIAGNOSIS: Decreased cardiac output R/T compensatory response to hypermetabolic state or tachydysrhythmia

a. *Expected outcomes:* Following interventions, the patient's cardiac function should return to a normal heart rate, rhythm, and blood pressure.

b. *Nursing interventions*

(1) Create a quiet, nonstressful environment.

(2) Administer β-blockers as ordered.

(3) Administer sedatives as ordered.

(4) Monitor heart rate and rhythm and blood pressure frequently to assess response to complications from drug therapy, such as hypotension, congestive heart failure, or dysrhythmias.

(5) Auscultate heart sounds (S_1 gallop indicates cardiac failure).

(6) Explain the procedures to the patient to decrease anxiety and secondary increased heart rate (tachycardia).

NURSING DIAGNOSIS: Altered nutrition, less than body requirements, R/T catabolic state and increased energy expenditure

a. *Expected outcomes:* Following interventions, the person should be able to do the following:

(1) Describe the necessary components of a healthy diet

(2) Balance nutritional intake to match energy expenditures

b. *Nursing interventions*

(1) Monitor the patient's intake, output, daily weight, and electrolytes.

(2) Working with other team members and the patient, develop a diet plan that is high in fiber and calories.

(3) Encourage fluids.

(4) Administer antidiarrheal medication as ordered.

(5) Treat hyperthyroidism.

NURSING DIAGNOSIS: Anxiety R/T hypermetabolic state

a. *Expected outcomes:* Following interventions, the patient should express and demonstrate lowered anxiety.

b. *Nursing interventions*

(1) Reassure the patient that his or her anxiety is a symptom of hyperthyroidism and that nervousness will decline as medications become effective.

(2) Administer antithyroid drugs as ordered. Observe for desired and undesired effects. Be alert for the development of hypothyroidism.

(3) Administer medications to treat associated symptoms (e.g., β-blockers or sedatives). Observe for desired and undesired effects.

(4) Assess the patient's level of anxiety in relationship to declining thyroid hormone levels.

(5) Assess the patient for other causes of anxiety that may be augmenting this nervous state.

(6) Develop a schedule that provides the patient with short periods of activity alternating with rest. Provide emotional support.

12. Discharge planning and teaching
    a. Provide information about the causes, symptoms, and treatment of hyperthyroidism, especially the actions of, dosages for, and adverse reactions to medications (particularly hypothyroidism). Help the patient plan a medication schedule that enhances compliance.
    b. Explain that physician follow-ups are usually more frequent during the 1st year after diagnosis is made, so that T_4, T_3, fT_4, and TSH can be closely monitored. Visits may be yearly after the euthyroid state is reached and medication history is uneventful.
    c. If the patient has had a thyroidectomy, provide instruction on incision care to be performed at home.
13. Public health considerations: Hyperthyoidism is easily treated and its complications are very preventable if the disease is detected early.

Other Thyroid Disorders

1. Thyroiditis
    a. Definition, classification, and incidence
        (1) Thyroiditis is an inflammation of the thyroid gland. The thyroid gland may enlarge and become hypo- or hyperactive, depending on the etiology.
        (2) Forms of thyroiditis include acute, subacute, and chronic.
        (3) Thyroiditis is rare. Acute thyroiditis is most common in women aged 20 to 40; subacute thyroiditis occurs about twice as often in women as in men, usually in the 5th decade of life; chronic thyroiditis (Hashimoto's or lymphocytic thyroiditis) is found almost exclusively (95% of cases) in women, usually beginning between the 3rd and 5th decades of life. The incidence of chronic thyroiditis has increased as a result of improved diagnostics and growing recognition of the disorder.
    b. Etiology
        (1) Acute thyroiditis: a bacterial infection (most often *Streptococcus pyogenes*, *Staphylococcus aureus*, or *Streptococcus pneumoniae*) in the form of an abscess
        (2) Subacute thyroiditis: a viral syndrome of the thyroid, which usually develops after a respiratory illness
        (3) Chronic thyroiditis: Etiology is unknown, but there are several possible causes—familial tendency, autoimmune disease, surgery for hyperthyroidism, RAIU treatments for hyperthyroidism, amiodarone administration, and secondary hypothyroidism.
    c. Clinical manifestations
        (1) Common manifestations include signs of hyper- or hypothyroidism, possible thrill or bruit.
        (2) Acute thyroiditis usually is characterized by acute neck pain, unilateral tenderness in the thyroid area, fever, edema of the neck, and warmth over the infected area. Usually 1 lobe of the thyroid is more affected than the other.
        (3) Patients with subacute thyroiditis present with an enlarged and tender thyroid after a viral syn-

drome. Neck pain may radiate to the jaw or ear. Signs of hyperthyroidism—fever, malaise, myalgia, weight loss, or anorexia—may appear 3 to 4 weeks after the viral syndrome. Recovery phase may begin 2 to 4 months after onset.
        (4) Chronic thyroiditis is characterized by an enlarged thyroid gland. The patient may or may not have signs of hypothyroidism. Goiters may be asymmetrically enlarged and may impose on other neck structures, producing dyspnea or dysphagia. Chronic thyroiditis is rarely painful.
    d. Clinical management
        (1) Goal: restore the patient to a euthyroid state without complications
        (2) Nonpharmacologic interventions: comfort measures related to hypo- or hyperthyroidism
        (3) Pharmacologic interventions
            • Acute thyroiditis is usually treated with antibiotics.
            • Subacute thyroiditis usually benefits from analgesics. If pronounced, hyperthyroidism may need to be treated. Propranolol or steroids may be used. Hypothyroidism may be treated with supplements.
            • Chronic thyroiditis is commonly treated with supplements, such as levothyroxine sodium (Synthroid or Levothroid) to suppress goiter size and TSH release. Supplements are usually started at a low dose and titrated upward as tolerance rises, but full replacement dosages may be started immediately after a thyroidectomy. Therapy for chronic thyroiditis does not prevent progression of disease, but rather is aimed at symptomatic control.
        (4) Special medical-surgical procedures: For **acute thyroiditis,** incision and drainage may be performed. For **chronic thyroiditis,** a fine-needle biopsy may be done to rule out malignancy. Indications for surgery are localized cold nodule via ultrasound with negative serum thyroid antibodies, tracheal compression and airway obstruction, recurrent laryngeal nerve palsy, and localized suppuration after bacterial infection.
2. Thyroid cancer
    a. Definition: a rare group of malignancies ranging from low grade to very aggressive (Table 29–16).
    b. Incidence: Thyroid cancer is rare. It represents 90 percent of endocrine malignancies and 1 percent of all cancers. Women outnumber men 2.5:1.0. Most patients are aged 25 to 60.
    c. Risk factors, etiology, and pathophysiology: A family history of endocrine disorders, low-dose radiation to head or neck, or the presence of a goiter raises risks of thyroid cancer. The exact etiology of thyroid cancers is unknown, but risk factors must be considered carefully when trying to identify the disease. The pathophysiology of thyroid cancer is presented in Table 29–16.
    d. Clinical manifestations
        (1) A hard, painless nodule in an enlarged thyroid gland that shows as "cold" on an ultrasound

Table 29–16. Types of Thyroid Cancer: Incidence, Characteristics, and Clinical Management

Type	Incidence	Characteristics	Clinical Management
Papillary adenocarcinoma	Comprises 60% of thyroid cancers Mainly affects patients in their 40s	Slow-growing firm tumor Palpable nodule Spreads to regional nodes in approximately 50% of cases Radiation-related thyroid cancer with 10- to 20-yr latency period	Total or near-total thyroidectomy Others recommend lobectomy and isthmectomy
Follicular adenocarcinoma	Comprises 15% of thyroid cancers Mainly affects patients in their 50s	Slow-growing nodule with about 15% metastasis to regional nodes at diagnosis Associated with radiation, iodine deficiency, endemic goiter	Total thyroidectomy
Medullary carcinoma	Comprises 5–10% of thyroid cancers Mainly affects patients in their 40s and 50s	Tumor is hereditary and familial Tends to secrete adrenocorticotropic hormone, serotonin Metastases to surrounding structures at diagnosis in 50%	Total thyroidectomy Radical neck resection if metastasis
Anaplastic carcinoma	Comprises 5–15% of thyroid cancers Mainly affects patients in their 60s and 70s	Highly malignant Grows rapidly Local and widespread metastasis within 1 year	Combination of thyroidectomy, external radiation therapy, chemotherapy, and tracheostomy as needed

Modified from Black JM, and Matassarin-Jacobs E (eds). *Luckmann and Sorensen's Medical-Surgical Nursing: A Psychophysiologic Approach.* 4th ed. Philadelphia: WB Saunders, 1993, p 1827.

(2) Signs of hyper- or hypothyroidism
(3) Signs of compromised function related to metastasis (hoarseness or dysphagia)
(4) Palpable lymph nodes
(5) Sore neck or tenderness on palpation, with local or diffuse neck enlargement
(6) Enlargement of lymph nodes, thyroid nodules, or both (unilateral, bilateral, unifocal, or multifocal)
(7) Possible bruit or thrill
(8) Displaced trachea
e. Clinical management (see Table 29–16 for treatment of specific cancers)
  (1) Goals
    • Early recognition and medical diagnosis to delay or end metastasis
    • Improved prognosis (prognosis is excellent for papillary adenocarcinoma, good for follicular adenocarcinoma, poor for medullary carcinoma, and grave for anaplastic carcinoma)
  (2) Nonpharmacologic interventions: possible postoperative radiation therapy to the neck of the high-risk patients, to reduce the likelihood of recurring malignancy after modified neck mass dissection
  (3) Pharmacologic interventions: thyroid replacement therapy after a total thyroidectomy; thyroid supplement after an incomplete surgical resection; and palliative treatment for symptomatic relief with inoperable tumors
  (4) Special medical-surgical procedures
    • Total thyroidectomy with parathyroid autotransplantation, if possible
    • Subtotal thyroidectomy
    • Postoperative tracheostomy for airway management, if needed
    • Radioactive iodine ablation via radioiodine as supplemental therapy for high-risk patients
    • External radiation therapy for patients with residual recurrent regional metastatic disease that fails to trap radioiodine

■ PARATHYROID DISORDERS

Hypoparathyroidism

1. Definition: a condition of decreased secretion or peripheral action of PTH, with lessened PTH in bones and kidney contributing to hypocalcemia and hyperphosphatemia
2. Incidence and socioeconomic impact: More women than men are affected. Incidence is related to method of diagnosis, thyroidectomy surgery (temporary occurrence in 6.9–25.0% after total surgery and 1.6–9.0% after subtotal surgery).
3. Etiology and pathophysiology
  a. Hypoparathyroidism may arise from deficient PTH secretion secondary to the following:
    (1) Thyroidectomy (Postsurgical hypoparathyroidism, the most common form of hypoparathyroidism, occurs after a thyroidectomy and is usually, although not always, temporary.)
    (2) Radioactive iodine therapy for hyperthyroid disease (extremely rare)
    (3) Surgery for primary hyperparathyroidism
    (4) Suppressed PTH secretion
    (5) Metastasis of cancer (most commonly breast cancer) to parathyroids
    (6) Hypoalbuminemia

b. Pseudohypoparathyroidism, or Albright's hereditary osteodystrophy, is an unusual inherited disorder in which the target organ is unresponsive to PTH.

c. Idiopathic hypoparathyroidism occurs when a PTH deficiency exists without a defined cause.

4. Pathophysiology

a. Suppression of PTH or the inability of 1 or more organs to respond to it leads to a fall in serum calcium and an upset in the balance between serum calcium and serum phosphate.

b. Bone resorption slows, causing severe neuromuscular irritability and, if treatment is not prompt, permanent cataracts and brain calcifications.

5. Clinical manifestations

a. Neurologic manifestations (induced primarily by hypocalcemia): paresthesia of the lips, tongue, or fingers; tingling; tremor; hyperreflexia; positive Chvostek's or Trousseau's sign; muscle cramps; carpopedal spasm; irritability, delirium, tetany, or seizures; and hypocalcemia-induced convulsions

b. Respiratory: hoarseness and laryngeal stridor or edema

c. Gastrointestinal: nausea, vomiting, and abdominal pain

d. Cardiovascular: palpitations, cyanosis, ECG changes (prolonged QT interval, peaked or inverted T waves, or heart block)

e. Renal calculi formation with normal kidney function

f. Integumentary: vitiligo; thinning hair; dry, scaly skin and nails; horizontal ridges on nails; and brittle nails

g. Dental defects

h. Eyes: cataracts and papilledema

i. Signs of hypothyroidism in cases secondary to surgery for hypoparathyroidism

6. Diagnostics

a. Assessment

(1) History: head, neck, or thyroid surgery; muscle cramps; carpopedal spasms; convulsions; paresthesias; malnutrition; alcohol abuse

(2) Physical examination. Findings related to hypocalcemia (positive Chvostek's sign, positive Trousseau's sign, hyperactive deep tendon reflexes, and convulsions); see also p. 1356).

b. Diagnostic studies: See Table 29–3 and Table 29–17. Other useful tests include radiographs of the skull, computed tomographic (CT) scan of the head, and an ophthalmic examination (to reveal calcification of the lens that can lead to cataract formation).

7. Clinical management

a. Goals

(1) Maintain serum calcium concentrations high enough to prevent symptoms of hypocalcemia and progressive long-term complications.

(2) Increase intestinal calcium absorption by administering supplemental calcium and vitamin D.

b. Nonpharmacologic interventions: A low-sodium diet may be effective in some patients with mild hypoparathyroidism.

c. Pharmacologic interventions

(1) Vitamin D (calcitriol)

(2) Calcium supplements: oral calcium supplements for chronic management and calcium chloride or calcium gluconate for emergency use in life-threatening hypocalcemia

(3) Diuretics

(4) Oral phosphate binders (e.g., Amphojel)

8. Complications are related primarily to hypocalcemia.

a. Resistance to cardiac glycosides secondary to hypocalcemia

b. Poorly controlled hypoparathyroidism during pregnancy, leading to a form of secondary hyperparathyroidism (see p. 1401) in the fetus.

c. Complications from overtreatment (hypercalcemia or nephrolithiasis) or undertreatment (tetany or seizures)

d. Electrocardiogram

(1) Prolonged QT interval

(2) T-wave changes: peaking and inversion

e. Hyperresponse (in nearly all patients) to TRH

9. Prognosis: The prognosis is very good if the patient complies with prescribed treatment and has consistent physician follow-up.

10. Applying the nursing process

NURSING DIAGNOSIS: Ineffective airway clearance R/T diagnostic laryngeal studies of edema secondary to hypocalcemia

a. *Expected outcomes:* Following interventions, the patient's airway should remain open and effective respirations should occur.

Table 29–17. Diagnostic Laboratory Tests for Hyperparathyroidism and Hypoparathyroidism

	Hyperparathyroidism		Hypoparathyroidism
	Primary	*Secondary*	
Serum parathyroid hormone (RAI)	↑ in 80–90% of patients	↑	↓
Serum calcium	↑	↓	↓
Serum phosphorus	↓ in 50% of patients	↓	↑
Urine calcium	↑	↑	↓
Urine phosphorus	↑	↑	↓

RAI, Radioassay immune.

b. *Nursing interventions*
(1) Assess respiration rate and depth, skin color, and temperature.
(2) Auscultate lung sounds.
(3) Assess the patient for respiratory distress in response to activity.
(4) Administer calcium supplements, vitamin D, and phosphate binders as ordered.
(5) Monitor serum calcium levels.
(6) Use pulse oximeter as indicated.

NURSING DIAGNOSIS: Risk for injury R/T seizures or tetany secondary to hypocalcemia

a. *Expected outcomes:* Following interventions, the patient with hypocalcemia should be free of injury.
b. *Nursing interventions*
(1) Monitor vital signs and reflexes.
(2) Monitor serum calcium level.
(3) Assess the patient for signs and symptoms of hypocalcemia.
(4) Administer calcium supplements, vitamin D, and phosphate binders as ordered.
(5) Implement seizure precautions.
(6) Monitor for cardiac manifestations of hypocalcemia.

NURSING DIAGNOSIS: Knowledge deficit R/T hypocalcemic symptoms and self-administration of prescribed medications

a. *Expected outcomes:* Following interventions, the patient should be able to do the following:
(1) Demonstrate an understanding of parathyroid function
(2) Discuss hypoparathyroidism and the action and side effects of medications used to treat it
(3) Adhere to a daily medication schedule and make regular follow-up visits to a physician
(4) Describe the signs and symptoms of overtreatment and undertreatment of hypoparathyroidism
b. *Nursing interventions:* See next step.
11. Discharge planning and teaching
a. Provide the patient with information on normal parathyroid function and on hypoparathyroidism—its causes, signs and symptoms, diagnostics, treatment, and long-term care.
b. Explain the need for lifelong medication and the signs and symptoms of overtreatment, undertreatment, and side effects.
c. Assist the patient in planning a daily medication schedule (to enhance compliance) and follow-up care with physician.

Hyperparathyroidism

1. Definition and classification: overactivity of the parathyroid that may be classified as primary, secondary, or tertiary

2. Incidence and socioeconomic impact
a. Primary hyperparathyroidism is 2 to 4 times more common in women than in men. Most patients are diagnosed in the 6th decade of life.
b. Secondary hyperparathyroidism may be diagnosed at any age in the renal patient. Some degree of secondary hyperparathyroidism is present in nearly all patients with end-stage renal disease.
c. The incidence of tertiary hyperparathyroidism is unknown.
3. Risk factors
a. Chronic renal failure
b. Exposure to head and neck radiation and coexistence of Hashimoto's thyroiditis
c. History of neck exploration or thyroid surgery
4. Etiology
a. Primary hyperparathyroidism
(1) A single adenoma is the cause in 75 to 80 percent of cases.
(2) Hyperplasia (multiglandular) of the parathyroid gland accounts for 20 to 25 percent of patient diagnoses.
(3) A malignant gland is rare (less than 1% of cases).
b. Secondary hyperparathyroidism
(1) Glands that are hyperplastic as a result of malfunction of another organ system, such as the kidney, may cause secondary hyperparathyroidism.
(2) Paget's disease, multiple myeloma, and carcinoma with bone metastasis may also cause secondary hyperparathyroidism.
c. Tertiary hyperparathyroidism occurs when PTH production is irrepressible in patients with normal or low normal calcium levels.
5. Pathophysiology
a. Primary hyperparathyroidism
(1) Glands may be adenomatous (about 80% of cases), hyperplastic (about 20% of cases), or malignant (1% of cases).
(2) The severity of hypercalcemia depends on the quantity of hyperfunctioning tissue.
(3) Excessive PTH stimulates transport of calcium into the blood from the intestine, kidneys, and bone.
(4) Hypercalciuria develops to compensate for very elevated serum calcium levels.
(5) Nephrolithiasis (secondary to calcium phosphate kidney stones and the deposition of calcium in the soft tissues of the kidney) occurs in 20 to 30 percent of patients with hyperparathyroidism and may be complicated by pyelonephritis.
(6) Bone changes include bone resorption related to hypercalcemia.
b. Secondary hyperparathyroidism
(1) As the glomerular filtration rate decreases, a slight rise in serum phosphorus begins, causing the serum calcium level to fall, stimulating PTH secretion.
(2) Increased PTH levels decrease renal tubular reabsorption of phosphorus, causing serum phosphorus levels to return to normal.

(3) As the glomerular filtration rate continues to decrease, PTH is secreted in increased amounts to decrease tubular reabsorption of phosphorus and maintain serum phosphorus in, or close to, normal limits (the trade-off hypothesis).

6. Clinical manifestations
   a. Most patients show no physical signs of hyperparathyroidism.
   b. Those who do show signs may report the following:
      (1) Neurologic problems—fatigue, slowed mentation, depression, hyperactive reflexes, sensory losses, and emotional lability
      (2) Musculoskeletal problems—weakness (especially in proximal muscles), joint hyperextensibility, ataxic gait, bone deformities, shortened stature, arthralgias, and tenderness
      (3) Gastrointestinal problems—anorexia, nausea, weight loss, and constipation
      (4) Renal problems—polyuria, dysuria, and renal colic/stones

7. Diagnostics
   a. History: neck surgery, peptic ulcer disease, bone fractures with minimal trauma, polyuria, polyphagia, kidney stones, nausea, anorexia, constipation, dyspepsia, neuromuscular weakness, use of certain medications or supplements (thiazide, furosemide, vitamin D, vitamin A, calcium, and lithium)
   b. Physical examination: In addition to assessing for clinical manifestations, check for signs of hypertension and ECG changes (broad T waves, short or prolonged QT interval, and bradycardia).
   c. Diagnostic studies
      (1) See Table 29–18.
      (2) Radiographic examination is performed to determine bone resorption and to detect bone cysts with advanced disease, diffuse demineralization of bones (poor bones density), subperiosteal bone resorption ("salt and pepper erosion"), and loss of lamina dura surrounding the teeth.
      (3) Ultrasonography is the procedure of choice for preoperative localization of the parathyroid glands.
      (4) When ultrasonography fails to localize the parathyroid, CT scans can locate about 50 to 77 percent of parathyroid tumors (versus 25% for contrast dye enhancement of adenomas).
      (5) Magnetic resonance imaging (MRI) is used to detail parathyroid gland location on film.
      (6) Twenty-four-hour urine collection is used to determine creatinine clearance.
   d. Medical diagnosis can be difficult in the early stages.

8. Clinical management
   a. Goal: Eliminate signs and symptoms of hypercalcemia insofar as possible
   b. Nonpharmacologic interventions
      (1) Primary hyperparathyroidism: dietary management, including a diet low in calcium and vitamin D
      (2) Secondary hyperparathyroidism: dietary modifications, including calcium supplements and restriction of phosphorus
      (3) Kidney stones: an acidotic diet to help treat renal calculi
   c. Pharmacologic interventions are presented in Table 29–18 and Box 29–5.

 DRUG ADVISORY

The presence of other disorders complicates corticosteroid therapy. Use these drugs cautiously and monitor patients for potential problems:

Patients with diabetes mellitus may experience augmented hyperglycemia.

Patients with inflammatory bowel disorders may experience fluid retention that exacerbates peristalsis.

Patients with hypertension, congestive heart failure, and renal insufficiency may suffer increased fluid retention.

Corticosteroid are contraindicated for patients with viral, fungal, or tubercular infections.

Table 29–18. Pharmacologic Interventions for Hyperparathyroidism

Primary Hyperparathyroidism

- Hydration with saline solution to increase rapidly urinary excretion of calcium
- Diuretics (e.g., furosemide)
- Plicamycin (mithramycin), a toxic antibiotic that inhibits bone resorption and lowers serum calcium (delivery is intravenous; side effects are platelet suppression and renal failure)
- Didronel
- Glucocorticoids
- Phosphate as antihypercalcemic agent in patients not taking glucocorticoids (the combination may cause nephrolithiasis)
- Calcitonin in high doses without glucocorticoids (up to 3.5 glands removed)
- Estrogen to decrease bone resorption and serum calcium (if not contraindicated)
- Etidronate disodium

Secondary Hyperparathyroidism

- Phosphate-binding antacid (Alucaps or Basaljel) to enhance phosphorus excretion through the gastrointestinal tract
- Calcium supplement (calcium carbonate or calcitrol) to combat acidosis, act as a phosphate-binding agent, and serve as a nutritional supplement to the low-phosphate diet
- Vitamin D

BOX 29–5. Drugs That Affect Calcium Metabolism in Patients Treated with Calcium and Vitamin D Supplements

Thiazide diuretics: May enhance renal tubular reabsorption of calcium and precipitate hypercalcemia.
Loop diuretics: May increase calcium excretion and cause hypocalcemia.
Glucocorticoids: May antagonize the effects of vitamin D and decrease intestinal absorption.
Aluminum hydroxide and **magnesium hydroxide:** Precipitate calcium.
Cholestyramine: Prevents vitamin D absorption.
Anticonvulsant therapy (phenytoin or phenobarbital): Converts vitamin D to a less biologically active compound.
Oral contraceptives and **estrogen:** Decrease serum calcium levels by preventing bone resorption.
Citrate (an anticoagulant used in blood banking): Has a great affinity for calcium.

d. Special medical-surgical procedures
   (1) Surgery is indicated for most patients with complications related to hyperparathyroidism or adenoma, such as hypercalcemia, lithiasis, decreased renal function, or bone disease.
      • Subtotal parathyroidectomy is most often recommended and has a success rate of approximately 92 percent. Total parathyroidectomy with autotransplantation has limited success; the overall rate is lower for patients who have had previous exploration of the neck for hyperparathyroidism.
      • The key factors in success are the localization of glands and the surgeon's skill and knowledge.
      • Possible complications are hemorrhage (immediate or delayed by 2–3 days), hypocalcemia (12–72 hours after surgery in 20% of patients), tetany, recurrent hyperparathyroidism (in about 5% of patients with adenoma), hypercalcemia (when insufficient tissue is removed), respiratory obstruction, hematoma or edema of the wound, laryngeal nerve injury, and hypoparathyroidism (especially with total thyroidectomy).
   (2) Hemodialysis is used for end-stage renal failure with secondary hyperparathyroidism.
   (3) Renal transplant may reverse all complications related to secondary hyperparathyroidism. Success depends on the stage of renal hyperparathyroidism and osteodystrophy.
9. Complications
   a. Primary hyperparathyroidism
      (1) Chronic renal failure secondary to hyperparathyroidism
      (2) Arthritic changes secondary to soft tissue calcification
      (3) Bone tenderness, deformities, and fractures
      (4) Psychiatric manifestations
      (5) Pancreatitis
      (6) Severe hypertension
      (7) Peptic ulcer disease that resists treatment
   b. Secondary hyperparathyroidism
      (1) Chronic renal failure necessitating hemodialysis
      (2) Skeletal abnormalities associated with chronic renal failure (e.g., osteodystrophy and osteitis fibrosa cystica)
10. Prognosis
    a. Primary hyperparathyroidism: Prognosis is improved if the diagnosis is made before age 70 and before renal involvement has occurred.
    b. Secondary hyperparathyroidism presents an uncertain prognosis, because of the many variables that affect the quality of life of a patient on chronic hemodialysis or the renal transplant recipient. Early recognition and treatment may slow the disease course and improve quality of life.
11. Applying the nursing process

NURSING DIAGNOSIS: Risk for injury R/T demineralization of bones resulting in pathologic fractures

a. *Expected outcomes:* Following interventions, the person should be
   (1) Free of injury (especially pathologic fractures)
   (2) Free of hypercalcemia
b. *Nursing interventions*
   (1) Assess for pain—may indicate a pathologic fracture.
   (2) Keep patient's bed in the low position.
   (3) Assist the patient with ambulation as needed.
   (4) Maintain correct body alignment.

NURSING DIAGNOSIS: Altered urinary elimination R/T renal involvement secondary to hypercalcemia and hyperphosphaturia

a. *Expected outcomes:* Following interventions, the patient should return to normal urinary output, as evidenced by no development of stones and urine output of 30 to 60 ml per hour.
b. *Nursing interventions*
   (1) Encourage the patient to drink at least 3000 ml of fluid daily (if not contraindicated by other medical problems).
   (2) If a stone is suspected, strain urine.
   (3) Assess serum calcium levels.
   (4) Monitor intake and output as indicated.
12. Discharge planning and teaching
    a. Provide the patient with information on the normal function of the parathyroid glands and on hyperparathyroidism (cause; signs and symptoms; laboratory studies; and treatment, including specific medications, diet, and signs of overtreatment or undertreatment).
    b. Patients with secondary hyperparathyroidism are generally asymptomatic and reluctant to take medication early in the course of renal failure. Effective education about secondary parathyroidism and the role prescribed medications may have in control of complications is imperative.
    c. Stress the importance of long-term management of hyperparathyroidism, including medications; yearly follow-up, history, and physical examination; diagnostic tests; and the need for more aggressive management as signs or symptoms develop.

◨ ADRENAL DISORDERS

Cushing's Syndrome (Hypercortisolism)

1. Definition and classification: Cushing's syndrome is hypercortisolism caused by abnormalities of the pituitary or adrenal gland; it may also result from ACTH secretion by a nonpituitary tumor. Cushing's disease is a specific type of Cushing's syndrome that results from excessive pituitary ACTH secretion from a pituitary tumor.
2. Incidence and socioeconomic impact
   a. Cushing's syndrome occurs in women more than men in the 20- to 40-year-old age group. Ectopic

ACTH production and neoplasms account for 32 percent of all cases.

   b. Cushing's disease represents 68 percent of Cushing's syndrome.

3. Risk factors

   a. Administration of exogenous steroids

   b. Adrenal tumors

   c. Pituitary tumors (especially in Cushing's disease)

4. Etiology

   a. Cushing's syndrome may be either ACTH dependent, resulting from pituitary hyperplasia that causes excess pituitary ACTH; small cell (oat cell) carcinoma or carcinoid tumors that produce ectopic ACTH; or prolonged use of ACTH, or ACTH independent, resulting from adrenal neoplasm or prolonged use of steroids.

   b. Cushing's disease is ACTH dependent, the result of chronic ACTH hyperplasia of the adrenal glands.

5. Pathophysiology

   a. Cushing's syndrome

     (1) Primary adrenocortical disease increases cortisol secretion, which suppresses corticosteroid-releasing hormone release and action, which in turn suppresses ACTH secretion.

     (2) Reduced ACTH secretion causes the pituitary corticotrophs and the adrenal cortex to atrophy and adrenal carcinomas to produce large amounts of steroid hormones relative to size.

   b. Cushing's disease

     (1) The amplitude of ACTH secretory episodes increases, disturbing normal ACTH circadian rhythm.

     (2) Increased plasma levels of ACTH stimulate development of bilateral adrenocortical hyperplasia and hypersecretion of cortisol.

6. Clinical manifestations may be present 3 to 6 years before diagnosis (Fig. 29–11).

ELDER ADVISORY

Signs of Cushing's syndrome may be difficult to discern in the older adult because many older patients already have the characteristics of hypertension, diabetes, and osteoporosis.

7. Diagnostics

   a. Assessment

     (1) History: recent onset of weakness, increase in weight or abdominal girth, roundness of face or acne; impaired wound healing; more frequent infections; depression, mania, or psychosis; osteoporosis; clumsiness; easy bruising; polydipsia and polyuria; and impotence or decreased libido

     (2) Physical examination: Check for signs of clinical manifestations.

   b. Diagnostic study results

     (1) Increased serum cortisol

     (2) Decreased serum calcium

     (3) Increased plasma ACTH

     (4) Positive result on dexamethasone suppression test

     (5) Blood sugar increase in 25 percent of cases

     (6) Increased free cortisol and 17-hydroxycorticosteroid in 24-hour urine collection

   c. Other tests:

     (1) An MRI view of the pituitary to localize the tumor

     (2) A CT scan of the pituitary gland and adrenal glands to localize the tumor

     (3) Inferior petrosal sinus ACTH sampling for ACTH

     (4) Radiographs to detect osteoporosis (see Chapter 34)

CUSHING'S SYNDROME

Clinical Manifestations

Redistribution of fat
- Round "moon" face
- Dorsocervical fat pad (buffalo hump)
- Supraclavicular fullness
- Trunk obesity

Hypertension

Abdominal striae

Decreased libido, amenorrhea, oligomenorrhea, virilism in women, impotence or feminization in men

Neuropsychiatric dysfunction
- Emotional lability
- Agitated depression
- Panic attacks
- Mania or psychosis (hypercortisolemia)

Osteoporosis due to matrix wasting can cause pathologic fractures

Polyuria due to cortisol-induced suppression of ADH and hyperglycemia

Muscle weakness: proximal myopathy, secondary to hypokalemia and protein tissue wasting

Easy bruising

Poor wound healing, prolonged infections due to impaired immune system; lymphocytopenia

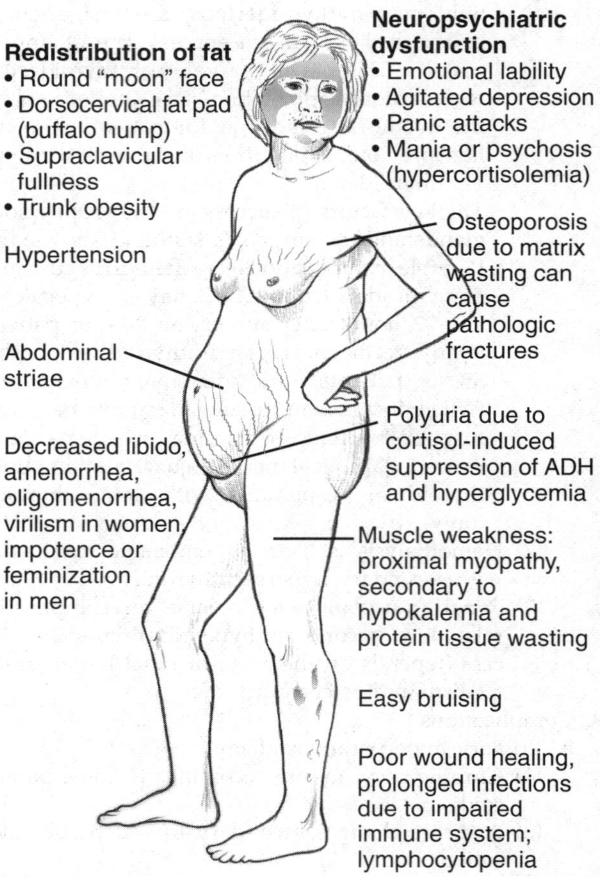

Complications
Cardiovascular complications are the major causes of morbidity and mortality. Other complications:
- Congestive heart failure
- Hypertension
- Dependent edema
- Left ventricular hypertrophy
- Pathologic fractures
- Masked infections

Figure 29–11.

8. Clinical management
   a. Goals
      (1) Restore normal cortisol levels as soon as possible, with few long-term effects.
      (2) Correct electrolyte imbalance.
      (3) Eradicate the tumor.
      (4) Avoid permanent dependence on synthetic steroids.
      (5) Avoid permanent hormone deficiency.
   b. Nonpharmacologic interventions
      (1) Diet with decreased calories and carbohydrates, low amounts of sodium, and high amounts of potassium
      (2) As a palliative measure to treat the tumor or residual tumor, radiation may be applied externally or internally to the pituitary gland.
   c. Pharmacologic interventions
      (1) Palliative treatment for hypercortisolism with nonlocated ACTH-secreting tumors includes cytoxic antihormonal agents to inhibit corticosteroid synthesis and cytoxic agents to block synthesis of glucocorticoids and adrenal steroids.
      (2) During and after elective surgeries, patients should be given higher than normal glucocorticoid replacement to avoid acute steroid withdrawal. Maintenance hydrocortisone should be given thereafter.
   d. Special medical-surgical procedures
      (1) Adrenalectomy and lifelong hydrocortisone replacement are indicated for all adrenal forms of Cushing's syndrome.
      (2) Transsphenoidal pituitary microsurgery (with or without pituitary radiation) is the treatment of choice for pituitary Cushing's disease. Prolonged high cortisol levels after surgery eventually suppress the hypothalamic-pituitary axis, causing the adrenal glands to atrophy within 6 weeks and adrenal insufficiency to develop (indications that all the pituitary tumor was removed). After successful surgery, the hypothalamic-pituitary-adrenal axis takes 12 to 24 months to recover, during which time replacement steroids are needed.
9. Complications
   a. Cardiovascular complications (the major cause of morbidity and mortality): congestive heart failure, hypertension, dependent edema, and left ventricular hypertrophy
   b. Pathologic fractures
   c. Masking of infections
10. Prognosis: The cure rate for transsphenoidal pituitary surgery is 85 to 90 percent, with success dependent on the surgeon's skills and the length of time the cortisol level has been elevated.
11. Applying the nursing process

NURSING DIAGNOSIS: Activity intolerance R/T muscle weakness and fatigue

a. *Expected outcomes:* Following interventions, the patient should exhibit a steady, safe gait and independent ambulation.
b. *Nursing interventions*
   (1) Provide planned periods of rest and activity.
   (2) Assess the patient and laboratory studies for hypokalemia, hypernatremia, and hypercortisolism that may contribute to weakness.
   (3) Treat electrolyte imbalance in collaboration with the physician.
   (4) Assess the patient for improved ambulation and increased tolerance for activity.

NURSING DIAGNOSIS: Body image disturbance R/T musculoskeletal changes (weakness or osteoporosis) and integumentary changes (thinning of skin, easy bruising, moon face, or Buffalo hump).

a. *Expected outcomes:* Following interventions, the patient should do the following:
   (1) Experience fewer or less intense bodily changes.
   (2) Demonstrate an understanding and acceptance of remaining body image changes.
b. *Nursing interventions*
   (1) Assess pressure points for skin integrity. Administer skin care to pressure points.
   (2) Change the patient's position every 2 hours.
   (3) Avoid tape or other skin irritants.
   (4) Provide a safe environment for the patient.
   (5) Provide ambulatory assistance as needed.
   (6) Plan for periods of rest.
   (7) Discuss the changes in the patient's body with him or her.
   (8) Inform the patient that fat accumulation will subside as treatment is implemented.
   (9) Assist the patient in identifying coping mechanisms for dealing with physical changes.

NURSING DIAGNOSIS: Risk for infection R/T impaired immune response

a. *Expected outcomes:* Following interventions, the patient should be free from infection.
b. *Nursing interventions*
   (1) Assess the patient for actual and potential infection sites.
   (2) Implement preventive measures for potential infection sites such as having the patient turn, cough, and take a deep breath; monitoring visitors for infections; and frequent hand washing.
   (3) Assess vital signs.
   (4) Use sterile technique when caring for areas of impaired skin integrity.
   (5) Provide antibiotic therapy as ordered.

NURSING DIAGNOSIS: Altered thought processes R/T elevated steroid levels

a. *Expected outcomes:* Following interventions, the patient should exhibit reduced signs of altered thought processes such as depression, mania, or psychosis.

b. *Nursing interventions*
   (1) Orient the patient as needed.
   (2) Provide an atmosphere that is calm, safe, and supportive.
   (3) Provide frequent contact with staff.
   (4) Explain medications and procedures clearly.
   (5) Encourage the patient to discuss his or her feelings.
   (6) Prevent emotionally upsetting scenarios.
   (7) Plan care with the patient and anticipate needs.
   (8) Discuss emotional reactions that are out of proportion for event and present a more realistic reaction or approaches for the future.

12. Discharge planning and teaching
   a. Provide the patient with information on normal adrenal function as well as the causes, signs, complications, and treatment of Cushing's syndrome. Make sure the patient understands the need for diagnostic tests and the consequences of unchecked disease.
   b. Assist the patient in arranging follow-up care.
      (1) Frequent follow-up with the physician to evaluate medication effectiveness and under- or overtreatment, laboratory tests, and additional medical problems.
      (2) Postoperative follow-up, including observation for return of the cortisol level to normal as the patient regains adrenal and anterior pituitary function
      (3) Physician visits every 3 to 4 months until normal cortisol levels are developed
      (4) Lifelong follow-up, even after surgery, to detect recurrences early

Hyperaldosteronism

1. Definition and classification
   a. Hyperaldosteronism is the overproduction of mineralocorticoids by the adrenal cortex.
   b. Depending on its etiology, hyperaldosteronism is usually classified as:
      (1) Primary aldosteronism, including adrenocortical adenoma (also known as *aldosterone-producing adenoma*) and bilateral adrenocortical hyperplasia (also known as *idiopathic hyperplasia*)
      (2) Secondary aldosteronism
   c. Bartter's syndrome, a rare syndrome of hyper-reninemia, hyperaldosteronism, hypokalemia, and alkalosis without hypertension or edema, is another form of hyperaldosteronism but is beyond the scope of this book.

2. Incidence and socioeconomic impact
   a. Estimates for the incidence of primary aldosteronism vary from 0.05 to 2.00 percent of the hypertensive population. Adrenocortical adenoma accounts for 60 percent of primary aldosteronism. Bilateral adrenocortical hyperplasia accounts for 20 percent.
   b. Women are diagnosed with primary aldosteronism twice as often as men.

c. Medical diagnosis is usually made between the ages of 30 and 60.

3. Risk factors
   a. Primary aldosteronism
      (1) Refractory hypertension without evidence of a secondary cause
      (2) History of difficulty maintaining a normal serum potassium level, despite treatment
   b. Secondary aldosteronism
      (1) Chronic heart failure
      (2) Cirrhosis of the liver with ascites
      (3) Nephrotic syndrome
      (4) Hypertension caused by renal artery disease

4. Etiology
   a. *Primary aldosteronism* is a generic term for disorders in which chronic aldosterone excess exists independently or semi-independently of the renin-angiotensin system, which results in hypertension and hypokalemia. It is caused by a unilateral or bilateral adrenal lesion.
   b. *Secondary aldosteronism* results from the formation of peripheral edema, as in cases of congestive heart failure, cirrhosis, or nephrotic syndrome.

5. Pathophysiology
   a. The pathogenesis of aldosterone-secreting adrenocortical tumors is unknown.
   b. All features of primary aldosteronism are related to the consequences of aldosterone excess:
      (1) Total body sodium content is elevated as a result of increased sodium reabsorption by the distal renal tubules. Because water is also retained, sodium concentration remains normal.
      (2) Hypertension arises from volume expansion and increased peripheral vascular resistance.
      (3) Hypokalemia results when aldosterone causes potassium loss in the distal renal tubule.
      (4) Metabolic alkalosis develops as the hypokalemia worsens.
      (5) Polyuria develops as renal concentrating ability decreases because of the hypokalemia.
   c. Secondary aldosteronism
      (1) Aldosterone secretion increases in response to a decrease in effective circulating blood volume caused by decreased output or transfer of intravascular volume into extravascular sites.
      (2) Decreased hepatic metabolism of aldosterone occurs in patients with hepatic disease.

6. Clinical manifestations: No distinct physical manifestations

7. Diagnostics
   a. Assessment
      (1) History: headaches, weakness, fatigue, tingling or paresthesias of lower extremities, dizziness with position change, increased thirst, swelling, and polyuria (especially at night)
      (2) Physical examination: fatigue, muscle weakness, paresthesias, positive Chvostek's sign, tetany, autonomic dysfunction, hypertension, postural hypotension without reflex tachycardia, and cardiomegaly
   b. Laboratory study results
      (1) Hypokalemia

(2) Metabolic alkalosis

(3) Kaliuresis

(4) Increased urinary excretion of aldosterone

(5) Low plasma renin activity

(6) Increased plasma aldosterone level

c. Other diagnostic studies

  (1) Electrocardiogram to reveal depressed ST segment and T wave, appearance of U wave, and premature ventricular contractions

  (2) Radiographs to visualize cardiac hypertrophy related to chronic hypertension

  (3) A CT scan or an MRI view of adrenal glands to identify hyperplasia or adenoma

  (4) Adrenal venous catheterization to sample aldosterone levels

8. Clinical management

a. Goals

  (1) Prevent morbidity and mortality associated with hypertension and hypokalemia.

  (2) Correct hypokalemia.

  (3) Prevent kidney damage.

  (4) Treat the cause of hyperaldosteronism.

b. Nonpharmacologic interventions: (These interventions are meant to contribute to the success of the pharmacologic treatment and are not to be used independently.)

  (1) Dietary management: low sodium (less than 2 gm/day)

  (2) Maintenance of ideal body weight

  (3) Avoidance of tobacco use

  (4) Regular aerobic exercise

c. Pharmacologic interventions

  (1) Spironolactone is the drug of choice because of its antihypertensive properties, its potassium-sparing qualities, and its ability to correct electrolytes unassisted. Preoperative blood pressure response to spironolactone is a predictor of blood pressure response to unilateral adrenalectomy.

DRUG ADVISORY

The administration of spironolactone is complicated because it has side effects of gastrointestinal discomfort, impotence, decreased libido, gynecomastia, and menstrual irregularities; increases the half-life of digoxin, thereby decreasing the patient's serum levels of prescribed digoxin; and interacts with salicylates, which increase renal tubular excretion of canrenone, the major active metabolite of spironolactone, thereby decreasing its effectiveness.

  (2) If hypertension persists despite dose titration, a 2nd agent may be added.

  (3) Hypertension may take 4 to 8 weeks to correct. Long-term dose titration after the patient is normokalemic is determined by blood pressure response and serum potassium level.

  (4) Amiloride is the drug of choice for patients intolerant to spironolactone.

d. Special medical-surgical procedures

  (1) Surgery is not indicated for a patient with idiopathic hyperplasia, because it is effective in controlling hypertension in only about one third of patients.

  (2) Unilateral or bilateral adrenalectomy is indicated for aldosterone-producing adenomas. Blood pressure control and correction of hypokalemia are attained preoperatively.

9. Complications

a. Chronic hypertension (hypertension usually exists 7 to 8 years before diagnosis)

b. Cerebral vascular accident

c. Prolonged and progressive hypokalemia (may be manifested by muscle weakness, ECG changes, dysrhythmias, heart failure, polyuria, dehydration, hypotension, polydipsia, metabolic alkalosis, tetany, or respiratory depression)

d. Prolonged and progressive hypernatremia (rarely develops into gross edema, because the kidneys are able to compensate for the hyperaldosteronism, allowing water excretion to balance with sodium intake)

e. Renal failure secondary to hypertension or renin angiotensin dependency (with idiopathic hyperplasia)

10. Prognosis

a. Hypertension related to aldosterone-producing adenoma typically resolves 3 to 6 months postoperatively.

b. The long-term cure rate for a unilateral adrenalectomy averages 69 percent.

11. Applying the nursing process

NURSING DIAGNOSIS: Fluid volume excess R/T hypernatremia

a. *Expected outcomes:* Following interventions, the patient should exhibit a lack of fluid volume symptoms.

b. *Nursing interventions*

  (1) Assess the patient's sodium level and signs of hypernatremia.

  (2) Auscultate lung sounds.

  (3) Assess for edema and manifestations of fluid volume overload.

  (4) Monitor daily weights.

  (5) Help the patient construct a satisfactory diet that is low in sodium.

NURSING DIAGNOSIS: Risk for injury R/T weakness, fatigue, paresthesia, or hypotension (orthostatic) caused by electrolyte imbalance

a. *Expected outcomes:* Following interventions, the patient should be free from injury.

b. *Nursing interventions*

  (1) Assess the patient's strength, balance, and gait for safety and reliability.

  (2) Keep the patient's bed in a low position, with side rails up and the call light within reach.

  (3) Provide ambulatory assistance as indicated.

  (4) Plan periods of activity alternating with rest.

  (5) Assess postural hypotension.

12. Discharge planning and teaching
    a. Provide information on the causes, complications, and treatment of hyperaldosteronism.
    b. Stress the importance of lifelong follow-up.

Addison's Disease

1. Definition and classification
   a. Addison's disease (also called chronic adrenal insufficiency, cortisol deficiency, and hypocortisolism) is a syndrome resulting from insufficient secretion of cortisol by the adrenal glands. In some cases, hypoaldosteronism coexists.
   b. Primary adrenal insufficiency is hypofunction of the adrenal gland that originates in the adrenal gland.
   c. Secondary adrenal insufficiency is hypofunction of the pituitary hypothalamic unit.
2. Incidence and socioeconomic impact
   a. Addison's disease affects about 1 in 100,000 people.
   b. It occurs in all age groups and afflicts men and women equally.
3. Risk factors
   a. Infectious processes (e.g., tuberculosis and histoplasmosis) that damage or destroy the adrenal glands
   b. Spread of a carcinoma (especially from the lungs or breast) that replaces the adrenal gland with tumor
   c. Large dosages of corticosteroids, which suppress the hypothalamic-pituitary-adrenal axis and cause atrophy of the adrenal glands
   d. Acquired immunodeficiency syndrome
4. Etiology
   a. Idiopathic Addison's disease is the most common cause of adrenal insufficiency.
   b. Primary adrenal insufficiency
      (1) Tuberculosis accounts for approximately 20 percent of cases.
      (2) Autoimmune-induced insufficiency (autoimmune adrenalitis with adrenal atrophy) may be idiopathic. It is associated with other clinical abnormalities, such as Hashimoto's thyroiditis, Graves' disease, simple goiter, pernicious anemia, DM, hypoparathyroidism, premature gonadal failure, chronic active hepatitis, alopecia, and lymphocytic hypophysitis.
   c. Secondary adrenal insufficiency
      (1) Chronic treatment with glucocorticoids for nonendocrine uses (the most common cause)
      (2) Bilateral adrenalectomy
      (3) Hemorrhagic infarction and necrosis of the adrenal glands
      (4) Hypopituitarism (possibly caused by a lesion in the pituitary or hypothalamus) resulting in decreased secretion of ACTH by the pituitary gland
      (5) Pituitary tumors
      (6) Pituitary infarction
      (7) Irradiation of the pituitary
5. Pathophysiology
   a. Idiopathic Addison's disease is usually caused by autoimmune destruction and shrinkage and atrophy of the adrenal glands. It is frequently accompanied by other immune disorders. Gradual destruction leads to chronic adrenocortical insufficiency.
   b. Lymphocytic infiltration of the adrenal cortex is the characteristic feature.
   c. Continued loss of cortical tissue accompanies a deficiency of mineralocorticoids as well as glucocorticoids, leading to the manifestations of chronic adrenocortical insufficiency.
   d. Rapid destruction of adrenal structure and function occurs in about 25 percent of the patients who are first diagnosed while they are having an adrenal crisis or when an adrenal crisis is impending.
6. Clinical manifestations
   a. More than 90 percent of the adrenal glands must be destroyed before the clinical picture of adrenal insufficiency emerges.
   b. Manifestations due to cortisol deficiency include weakness, fatigue, anorexia, nausea, vomiting, weight loss, hypotension, and hypoglycemia.
   c. Manifestations due to mineralocorticoid deficiency (all resulting from renal sodium wasting and potassium retention) include dehydration, hypotension, hyponatremia, hyperkalemia, and acidosis.
7. Diagnostics
   a. Assessment
      (1) History: weight loss, weakness, fatigue, dizziness with position change, darkening of skin, anorexia, nausea or vomiting, diarrhea, irritability, depression, craving for salty foods, hypoglycemia, and irregular or absent menses
      (2) Physical examination (in addition to clinical manifestations: hyperpigmentation of skin, decreased body hair, tachycardia, irritability, and depression
   b. Laboratory study results
      (1) Lowered serum cortisol
      (2) Elevated serum corticotrophin
      (3) Serum aldosterone undetectable; 17-hydroxysteroids decreased
      (4) Normal to low hyponatremia
      (5) Hyperkalemia
      (6) Anemia
      (7) Poor or no response on the ACTH stimulation test
   c. Other studies: radiographs, CT scans, or MRI views of the adrenal glands and pituitary gland to identify location and size of the glands and thus identify tuberculous changes
8. Clinical management
   a. Goals
      (1) Prevent morbidity and mortality associated with Addisonian crisis.
      (2) Correct hypotension.
      (3) Correct electrolyte imbalance.
   b. Nonpharmacologic interventions
      (1) Give high-sodium, low-potassium diet with increased fluids.
      (2) Prevent stressful events.
   c. Pharmacologic interventions are listed in Table 29–19.
   d. Special medical-surgical procedures: none

Table 29-19. Corticosteroids

Medication	Duration of Action	Indication	Mineralocorticoid or Glucocorticoid Activity	Side Effects (Relative to Dose and Duration)
Glucocorticoids				
Betamethasone (Celestone)	Short	Chronic adrenocortical insufficiency, inflammation	Mineralocorticoid high	Fluid and electrolyte disturbances: hypokalemic, hypocalcemia, congestive heart failure, hypertension
Cortisone (Cortone)	Long	Allergic disorders, Cushing's syndrome (suppression test)	Mineralocorticoid low–nil	Musculoskeletal: weakness, myopathy, aseptic necrosis femoral and humeral heads, spontaneous fractures, osteoporosis
Dexamethasone (Decadron)	Long	Adrenal hyperplasia	Mineralocorticoid nil	Cardiovascular: thromboembolism, cardiac dysrhythmias related to hypokalemia, hypertension, myocardial rupture following recent myocardial infarction
Hydrocortisone (Hydrocortone or Cortef)	Short	Chronic adrenal insufficiency, inflammatory disorders, allergic reactions, collagen disorders, nonsuppurative thyroiditis	Mineralocorticoid moderate	Gastrointestinal: pancreatitis, peptic ulcer, inflammatory bowel disease, ulcerative esophagitis
Methylprednisolone (Medrol)	Intermediate	Immunosuppressant for transplant patients, adrenogenital syndrome, rheumatoid arthritis	Mineralocorticoid nil	Integumentary: impaired wound healing, thin skin, petechiae, suppression of skin test reactions
Prednisolone (Delta-Cortef)	Intermediate	Inflammation, immunosuppression	Mineralocorticoid moderate	Neurologic: convulsions, steroid psychosis
Prednisone (Deltasone tablets, liquid prednisone syrup)	Intermediate	Inflammatory conditions	Mineralocorticoid moderate	Endocrine: amenorrhea, postmenopausal bleeding, development of Cushingoid state, growth suppression in children, secondary
Mineralocorticoids				
Desoxycorticosterone (Doca Percorten)	Long acting	Addison's disease, salt-losing adrenogenital syndrome	Glucocorticoid nil	Endocrine: drug-induced adrenal insufficiency Cardiovascular: hypertension fluid retention, weight gain, cardiomegaly
Fludrocortisone (Florinef)	Long acting	Chronic adrenocortical insufficiency, salt-losing adrenogenital syndrome	Glucocorticoid high	Immunosuppression Integumentary: bruising, diaphoresis Other: hypokalemia, allergic reaction

 DRUG ADVISORY

When administering diuretics to patients with the syndrome of inappropriate antidiuretic hormone, be sure to monitor for urinary losses of potassium, calcium, and magnesium and replace these elements as needed.

9. Complications
    a. Addisonian crisis (acute adrenal insufficiency)
       (1) Addisonian crisis develops in response to stress, infection, surgery, trauma, or dehydration.
       (2) Symptoms include sudden penetrating pain in lower back, abdomen, or legs; depressed mentation; severe vomiting and diarrhea; fever; dehydration and fluid volume depletion; hypotension and shock; and loss of consciousness. Death results if symptoms are untreated.
       (3) Interventions

- Administer dextrose in 5% normal saline intravenously at a rate of 500 ml per hour, or faster, to maintain blood pressure for 1st 4 hours and thus combat dehydration, salt depletion, and hypoglycemia. Provide plasma, oxygen, and vasopressor therapy as ordered and indicated. Initiate treatment for cause of crisis.
- Administer IV hydrocortisone immediately and as ordered thereafter (usually every 8 hr for 24 hr). If the patient improves, taper IV dosages; stop when the patient can tolerate oral hydrocortisone.
- Correct electrolyte imbalance if it has not been corrected by administration of cortisone and fluids.
- Treat coexisting disorders.

    b. Osteoporosis with excessive use of glucocorticoids
    c. Hyponatremia, hyperkalemia, lymphocytosis, eosinophilia, and hypoglycemia

10. Prognosis: Prognosis and quality of life are excellent for

patients who are motivated, comply with treatment, show up for appointments, and communicate concurrent medical problems (especially acute infections).

11. Applying the nursing process

NURSING DIAGNOSIS: Risk for injury R/T acute renal insufficiency secondary to stressor (infection, surgery, trauma, or emotional stress)

a. *Expected outcomes:* Following interventions, the patient should be free from injury.
b. *Nursing interventions*
  (1) Assess the patient for sources and signs of infection or other stressors.
  (2) Evaluate vital signs.
  (3) Assess laboratory values related to stressor.
  (4) Administer glucocorticoids or mineralocorticoids as ordered.
  (5) Evaluate serum cortisol level.
  (6) Monitor intake and output, daily weights, and skin turgor.
  (7) Administer IV fluids and vasopressors as ordered.
  (8) Monitor for signs of Addisonian crisis.
  (9) Evaluate for dysrhythmias secondary to hyperkalemia (hypokalemia with rehydration).

NURSING DIAGNOSIS: Fluid volume deficit R/T sodium wasting by kidneys

a. *Expected outcomes:* Following interventions, the patient should do the following:
  (1) Maintain acceptable intake and output
  (2) Exhibit good skin turgor and acceptable vital signs
b. *Nursing interventions*
  (1) Monitor intake and output, vital signs, and daily weights.
  (2) Assess skin turgor and mucous membranes.
  (3) Examine the patient for hypovolemia.
  (4) Evaluate the patient for signs and symptoms of hypercalcemia and hyponatremia.
  (5) Administer fluids as ordered.

NURSING DIAGNOSIS: Ineffective individual coping R/T irritability, depression, and possible hyponatremic state

a. *Expected outcomes:* Following interventions, the patient should do the following:
  (1) Experience increase of steroids to acceptable range
  (2) Demonstrate a positive outlook both verbally and nonverbally
b. *Nursing interventions*
  (1) Reassure the patient that irritability and depression will decline as steroid level improves.

  (2) Assess the patient for signs and symptoms of hyponatremia.
  (3) Correct hyponatremia with intravenous fluids.
  (4) Assess the patient for other sources of depression. Depending on the overall level of depression, the patient may need frequent or constant supervision. Consult with psychiatric therapists as needed.
  (5) Evaluate the patient's status relative to improving steroid level.

12. Discharge planning and teaching
  a. Provide the patient with information on normal adrenal functioning as well as the causes, signs, complications, and treatments (including the use, dangers, and side effects of medications) of Addison's disease.
  b. Help the patient identify stressors that may cause an increased need for steroid therapy: infections, viruses, temperature extremes, surgery, or psychologic stress.
  c. Give the patient guidelines for self-treatment for acute illness or stress.
    (1) Double the prescribed dose for up to 1 week.
    (2) Resume the normal dose when improvement occurs.
    (3) Contact the physician with questions or if symptoms persist.
    (4) Seek medical attention for severe infections, vomiting or diarrhea, dental surgery, profuse diaphoresis, fever, or emotionally charged situations.
    (5) Carry a needle, syringe, and injectable form of cortisol for emergencies when traveling.
  d. Encourage activity, if not contraindicated, to slow demineralization of bones (osteoporosis).
  e. Encourage frequent hand washing to decrease bacterial and viral infections.
  f. Stress to the patient the importance of always wearing a Medic Alert bracelet or carrying identification that specifies his or her name, medical problems, prescribed medications, and physician's name and phone number.
  g. Help the patient schedule the initial follow-up visit and explain the need for routine follow-ups every 6 months (more often for patients with complex medical histories or acute illness).

Pheochromocytoma

1. Definition
  a. A pheochromocytoma is a small chromaffin cell tumor that releases excess amounts of the catecholamines epinephrine and norepinephrine (and small amounts of another catecholamine, dopamine) and thus can bring on paroxysms (see "Pathophysiology").
  b. Pheochromocytomas may arise wherever there are chromaffin cells. The adrenal medulla contains the largest number of chromaffin cells.
2. Incidence and socioeconomic impact
  a. Pheochromocytomas are rare.

b. Approximately 0.1 to 0.2 percent of patients with diastolic hypertension have a pheochromocytoma.

c. Tumors are found in both sexes equally.

d. Although they occur in patients of any age, pheochromocytomas are most commonly diagnosed during the 4th decade of life.

e. About 95 percent of pheochromocytomas are found in the abdomen; 85 percent of these are found in the adrenal gland.

f. Fewer than 10 percent of pheochromocytomas are malignant.

3. Risk factors

a. Smoking

b. Micturition: In the case of pheochromocytoma of the urinary bladder, micturition can trigger the paroxysm of hypertension.

c. Drugs that may increase catecholamine release, such as histamines, some anesthetics (halothane, thiopental, cyclopropane, methoxylflurane, and Innovar), atropine, chlorpromazine, opiates, steroids, and glucagon.

d. The paroxysm of hypertension can be triggered by any activity that displaces abdominal organs, such as exercise, bending, straining, or vigorous palpation of the abdomen.

e. Pregnancy, especially the 3rd trimester, and labor.

4. Etiology: unknown

5. Pathophysiology

a. Pheochromocytomas hypersecrete catecholamines into the circulatory system, which trigger a paroxysm related to excesses of those hormones.

b. A paroxysm usually begins with a sensation of something deep in the chest.

c. Deep breathing begins.

d. The patient notes a pounding or forceful heartbeat from the β-receptor–mediated increase in cardiac output. Throbbing spreads to the trunk and head, causing a headache.

e. Intense α-receptor–mediated peripheral vasoconstriction causes cool, moist hands and feet and facial pallor.

f. The increase in cardiac output and vasoconstriction causes marked elevation of systolic and diastolic blood pressures when the catecholamines are released.

g. Tachycardia frequently results from epinephrine hypersecretion. Epinephrine also affects metabolism, causing carbohydrate intolerance (hyperglycemia) by inhibiting insulin.

h. The decreased heat loss and increased metabolism may cause a rise in temperature or flushing and diaphoresis.

i. When episodes are prolonged or intense, nausea, vomiting, visual disturbance, chest or abdominal pain, or seizures may develop.

6. Clinical manifestations

a. Symptoms vary in intensity and frequency and last minutes to hours, depending on the pheochromocytoma's paroxysmal release of catecholamines.

b. Hypertension is the major symptom.

c. Headache is reported in 80 to 90 percent of paroxysms.

d. Other commonly reported symptoms are diaphoresis, palpitations, anxiety, tremor, visual disturbances, nausea and vomiting, weight loss, fatigue and exhaustion, abdominal pain, chest pain, dizziness with position change, and irritability.

7. Diagnostics

a. Assessment

(1) History: uncontrolled hypertension and paroxysm alone or in concert with palpitations, chest pain, abdominal pain, constipation, feeling of fear or impending doom, headache, diaphoresis, nausea, tremor, weakness, pallor, or decreased urine output

(2) Physical examination (in addition to clinical manifestations): tachycardia, flushing, tachypnea, and feeling of apprehension or impending doom

b. Medical diagnosis

(1) Blood and urine test results (may not be helpful in diagnosing patients with brief or infrequent paroxysms)

- Elevated plasma levels of the catecholamines epinephrine and norepinephrine

- Increased vanillylmandelic acid found in 24-hour urine collection as a result of increased excretion of catecholamines

(2) A CT scan, an MRI view, and [I^{131}]m-iodobenzylguanidine scintigraphy to localize tumors

(3) Arteriography (usually reserved for cases in which the CT scan fails to reveal the adrenal gland adequately)

(4) Intravenous administration of glucagon to induce a paroxysm

---

NURSE ADVISORY

Intravenous administration of glucagon should *not* be used to induce paroxysms in patients who have angina, visual changes, or severe symptoms during an attack. In all such tests, be sure that phentolamine is available to terminate the induced paroxysm.

---

8. Clinical management

a. Goals

(1) Reduce blood pressure

(2) Reduce incidence of complications

(3) Prepare the patient for surgery

b. Nonpharmacologic interventions

(1) Dietary measures to help control catecholamine release (including no caffeine)

(2) Nonstressful environment

(3) Promotion of rest and sleep

c. Pharmacologic interventions

(1) Adrenergic antagonists prescribed for a few days to 2 weeks before surgery to decrease symptoms, reduce blood pressure, and eliminate paroxysms

(2) Agents include phenoxybenzamine, the drug of choice for frequent paroxysms or persistent hypertension; prazosin for blood pressure control; phentolamine, an α-blocker, as a competitive antagonist to norepinephrine; propranolol (adminis-

tered after α-receptor blockade is established; sedatives; and steroid replacement postoperatively.

(3) Patients who are not able to undergo surgery may be managed pharmacologically for prolonged periods.

(4) Successful treatment of malignant tumors involves chemotherapeutic agents and radiation therapy in addition to palliative treatment.

d. Special medical-surgical procedures

(1) Unilateral or bilateral adrenalectomy is indicated as soon as the blood pressure is decreased and paroxysms are eliminated.

(2) Highlights of postoperative care include monitoring blood pressure. It is common for the blood pressure to fall to 90/60 mm Hg. A total lack of a decline in blood pressure may indicate residual tumor tissue. Volume expanders or fluids may be indicated. Pressor therapy is usually not indicated. The patient should be regarded as having excessive catecholamine stores in sympathetic nerve endings for about 1 week postoperatively.

9. Complications
   a. Hypertensive retinopathy
   b. Hypertensive nephropathy
   c. Myocarditis
   d. Increased platelet aggregation
   e. Cerebral vascular accident
   f. Congestive heart failure
   g. Death due to myocardial infarction, cerebral vascular accident, dysrhythmias, irreversible shock, renal failure, and dissecting aortic aneurysm

10. Prognosis
    a. With early diagnosis and proper treatment, nearly all patients with benign pheochromocytomas recover completely.
    b. Surgical morbidity or mortality depends on whether the patient develops severe hypertension during anesthesia induction or develops hypotension postoperatively.
    c. The survival rate is 95 percent following the first 5 years after surgery.
    d. Recurrence of a pheochromocytoma after surgery is less than 10 percent.
    e. Early diagnosis is critical to survival in those with malignant pheochromocytomas.

11. Applying the nursing process

NURSING DIAGNOSIS: Risk for injury R/T altered cardiovascular, renal, or cerebral perfusion caused by hypertension

a. *Expected outcomes:* Following interventions, the patient should not experience any renal, cardiac, or neurologic complications from hypertension.
b. *Nursing interventions*
   (1) Assess the patient for signs and symptoms related to angina, congestive heart failure, and dysrhythmias.
   (2) Evaluate vital signs.

(3) Monitor cardiac functioning as needed.
(4) Assess the patient's renal function: Measure intake and output and daily weight, evaluate blood urea nitrogen, serum creatinine, and urine electrolytes as ordered, and perform urinalysis as indicated.
(5) Evaluate the patient's neurologic status.
(6) Administer antihypertensive drugs as ordered.
(7) Maintain a quiet environment

NURSING DIAGNOSIS: Pain R/T headache and surgery

a. *Expected outcomes:* Following interventions, the patient should express a decrease in or the absence of pain.
b. *Nursing interventions*
   (1) Assess the patient for pain.
   (2) Assess the patient for other symptoms if the pain is related to paroxysm.
   (3) Administer analgesics as ordered.
   (4) Assess vital signs, particularly blood pressure, after analgesics are given. Opiates can cause a hypertensive episode in a patient with pheochromocytoma. Narcotics and opiates can cause postoperative hypotension.

NURSING DIAGNOSIS: Anxiety R/T unfamiliarity with diagnosis of and treatment regimen for the disease and its clinical manifestation of hypertension

a. *Expected outcomes:* Following interventions, the patient should do the following:
   (1) Express reduced anxiety.
   (2) Demonstrate understanding of pheochromocytoma and its treatment.
   (3) Properly administer prescribed medications.
   (4) Acknowledge that medication administration will be a lifelong task and that a consistent administration schedule is the key to compliance.
b. *Nursing interventions*
   (1) When assessing for vital signs, paroxysms, or response to medications, inform patient of status or progress.
   (2) Depending on the patient's anxiety level, provide information on symptoms and medications when appropriate.
   (3) See next step.

12. Discharge planning and teaching
    a. Provide the patient with information on normal adrenal function as well as the causes, diagnosis, effects, and treatment options for pheochromocytoma.
    b. Describe the need for postoperative steroids (a lifetime prospect) and for consulting a physician before taking any prescribed or over-the-counter drugs.
    c. Help the patient arrange follow-up care to monitor blood pressure, steroid therapy, and clinical manifestations.

◼ *PITUITARY DISORDERS*

Hypopituitarism

1. Definition and classification
   a. Hypopituitarism, called *dwarfism* when it occurs in childhood, results from deficient hormonal secretion of one or more anterior pituitary hormones.
   b. Hypopituitarism results in retarded growth in children, sexual immaturity, and metabolic dysfunctions.
   c. Hypopituitarism may be primary or secondary, depending on its cause.
   d. Partial or total deficiency of all 6 pituitary hormones is called *panhypopituitarism*.
2. Incidence: All forms of hypopituitarism are rare.
3. Etiology
   a. Primary hypopituitarism results from damage to or destruction of the anterior pituitary as a result of the following:
      (1) Pituitary tumors (prolactinomas in 60% of cases) that compress or destroy the pituitary—the most common cause and may be linked to oral contraceptive use
      (2) Head trauma that produces injury to the pituitary
      (3) Postpartum hemorrhage that causes pituitary necrosis
      (4) Hypophysectomy (surgical removal of the pituitary), performed as a palliative measure in cases of breast cancer or diabetic retinopathy
      (5) Congenital defects of the anterior pituitary that cause growth hormone deficiencies
      (6) Radiation of the head and neck
      (7) Chemical agents
      (8) Rapid weight or fat loss or malnutrition (linked to anorexia nervosa, sickle cell anemia, and overtraining in sports)
      (9) Invasive neoplasms from primary or metastatic cancer of the breast, lung, or gastrointestinal tract
   b. Secondary hypopituitarism results from damage to the pituitary's ability to produce hormones needed to stimulate or inhibit hypothalamic activity (TSH and ACTH) as a result of the following:
      (1) Infection (e.g., tuberculosis and syphilis)
      (2) Head trauma that produces injury to the pituitary
      (3) Brain tumors (especially craniopharyngioma)
      (4) Infiltrative disorders (e.g., sarcoidosis and hemochromatosis) that compress or replace normal tissue in the hypothalamus or, less often, the pituitary
   c. The etiology of some hypopituitarism is unknown.
4. Clinical manifestations
   a. Because the pituitary has great functional reserves, signs and symptoms appear only when the disease has progressed to destroy 75 percent of the pituitary.
   b. Specific signs and symptoms of hypopituitarism depend on the age of onset and specific hormonal deficiencies. They include the following:
      (1) Deficiency of ACTH, causing secondary adrenal insufficiency: Manifestations include signs and symptoms of Addison's disease (see p. 1408), except for cardiovascular complications.
      (2) Deficiency of TSH, causing secondary hypothyroidism (usually less severe than primary thyroid failure)
      (3) Luteinizing hormone and follicle-stimulating hormone deficiencies, causing hypogonadism: Manifestations include amenorrhea, breast atrophy, and decreased vaginal secretions in women and decreased libido, impotence, reduced muscle strength, and testicular atrophy in men.
      (4) Growth hormone deficiency, causing dwarfism in children and hypoglycemia in all ages
      (5) Prolactin (PRL) deficiency, causing absence of lactation in postpartum women
   c. Other manifestations
      (1) Integumentary: hypothermia and wrinkled, waxy, smooth skin
      (2) Musculoskeletal: loss of muscle tone
      (3) Cardiovascular: brachycardia and hypotension
      (4) Neurologic: hypoactive reflexes
      (5) Reproductive: poorly developed secondary sexual characteristics, absence of lactation in postpartum women
      (6) Hematologic: anemia related to thyroid and androgen deficiencies
      (7) Signs of hypoglycemia, hypothyroidism, ACTH deficiency, and hyponatremia
5. Clinical management
   a. Goals
      (1) Correct hyposecretion of anterior pituitary hormones.
      (2) Preserve normal pituitary tissue.
      (3) Remove or suppress pituitary tumors.
   b. Nonpharmacologic interventions: none
   c. Pharmacologic interventions depend on the specific hormone deficiency and its extent.
      (1) Deficiency of ACTH: glucocorticoid support (be aware that attempting thyroid replacement before correcting a glucocorticoid deficiency may cause adrenal crisis)
      (2) Deficiency of TSH (secondary hypothyroidism): thyroxine supplement
      (3) Luteinizing hormone and follicle-stimulating hormone deficiencies that cause hypogonadism (only when patient is euthyroid)
         • Women: estrogens and progesterones to maintain secondary sexual characteristics, clomiphene citrate to promote ovulation, and small doses of long-acting androgens to improve diminished libido
         • Men: testosterone replacement to restore libido and potency and secondary sexual characteristics and chorionic gonadotropin, menotropins, or both to relieve aspermatogenesis (in some cases)
      (4) Growth hormone deficiency: exogenous hormone replacement for children
      (5) Deficiency of PRL: bromocriptine
   d. Special medical-surgical procedures
      (1) Transsphenoidal hypophysectomy for pituitary tumors that do not respond to suppressive drugs

(2) Radiation for patients with large pituitary tumors or an incomplete resection of such tumors

Hyperpituitarism

1. Definition
   a. Hyperpituitarism is the oversecretion of hormones from the anterior pituitary. Usually, a combination of hormones is hypersecreted, rather than single hormone.
   b. Syndromes that result from hormone hypersecretion include the following:
      (1) Prolactinoma from excessive PRL secretion
      (2) Acromegaly from excessive growth hormone secretion
      (3) Cushing's disease, a form of Cushing's syndrome (see pp. 1403–1404) from excessive ACTH secretion
2. Etiology
   a. Prolactinoma
      (1) Estrogen therapy or oral contraceptive use
      (2) Pregnancy (may increase tumor size and dysfunction)
      (3) Hypothyroidism
   b. Acromegaly (Fig. 29–12)

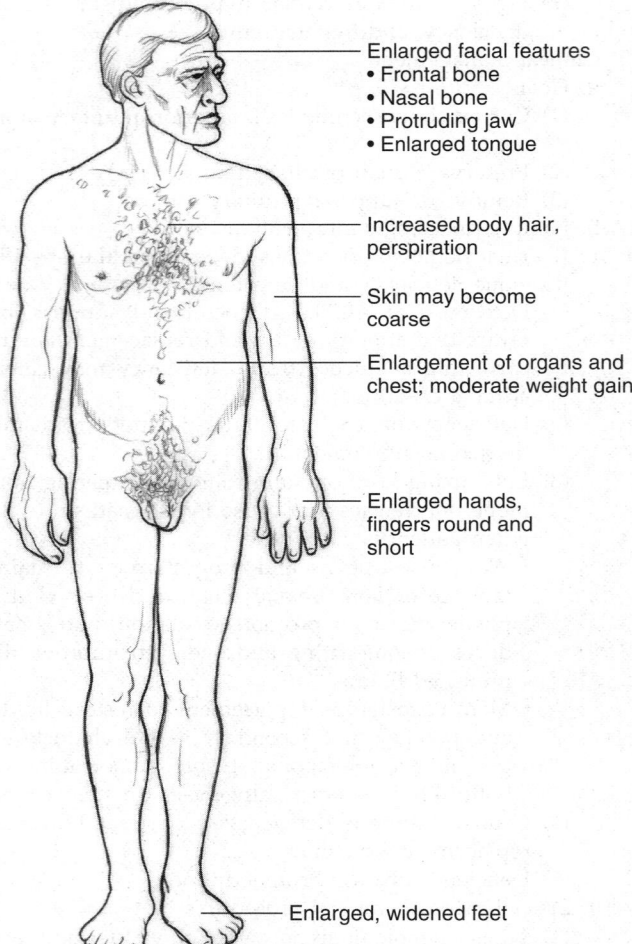

Enlarged facial features
• Frontal bone
• Nasal bone
• Protruding jaw
• Enlarged tongue

Increased body hair, perspiration

Skin may become coarse

Enlargement of organs and chest; moderate weight gain

Enlarged hands, fingers round and short

Enlarged, widened feet

Figure 29–12.

(1) Primary pituitary adenoma
(2) Abnormal hypothalamic function (rare)
3. Clinical manifestations depend on specific hormone oversecreted.
   a. Prolactinoma from oversecretion of PRL
      (1) Abnormal lactation secretion (galactorrhea) in nonlactating breast
      (2) Amenorrhea
      (3) Decreased vaginal lubrication
      (4) Decreased libido in men
      (5) Impotence
      (6) Depression
      (7) Anxiety
      (8) Headache
      (9) Visual loss
   b. Acromegaly from oversecretion of growth hormone
      (1) Local overgrowth of bone in skull and mandible
      (2) Soft tissue overgrowth
      (3) Lethargy
      (4) Weight gain
      (5) Paresthesias
      (6) Glucose intolerance
      (7) Coarse facial features
      (8) Irregular or absent menses
      (9) Enlargement of hands and feet over 1 to 10 years
      (10) Depression
      (11) Headache
      (12) Diaphoresis
      (13) Oily, thickening skin
      (14) Visual field defects
4. Clinical management
   a. Goals
      (1) Prolactinoma: Control PRL hypersecretion, eliminate galactorrhea, and restore normal gonadal function.
      (2) Acromegaly: Halt progression of disorder, prevent complications, remove or destroy the tumor, and reverse hypersecretion of growth hormone.
   b. Nonpharmacologic interventions: none
   c. Pharmacologic interventions
      (1) Prolactinoma: Bromocriptine can reduce PRL levels in approximately 90 percent of patients. However, adverse reactions, such as nausea, headaches, dizziness, nasal stuffiness, hypotension, and depression, may contribute to noncompliance.
      (2) Acromegaly: Bromocriptine can reduce growth hormone levels in 60 to 80 percent of patients. Somatostatin analogue octreotide, commonly used in conjunction with surgery for large tumors, is very effective in reducing growth hormone levels but may cause cholelithiasis.
   d. Special medical-surgical procedures
      (1) Transsphenoidal microsurgery may be used, although it can cause complications such as elevated hormone levels, visual loss, diabetes insipidus (DI), and postoperative infections.
      (2) Transfrontal craniotomy may be used for patients with large suprasellar extension of tumors not accessible by the transsphenoidal approach. Postoperative bromocriptine or radiation is required.

(3) Radiation therapy is used if pharmacologic and surgical interventions have failed. It may retard tumor growth or relieve its signs and symptoms. Complications include damage to the surrounding anatomy of the pituitary gland (may be minimized by using accelerated proton beam therapy that focuses on the pituitary); hypopituitarism (the most common side effect); and increased morbidity related to atherosclerotic disease, respiratory disease, hypertension, DM, and gastrointestinal cancer.

Diabetes Insipidus

1. Definition and incidence: a rare disorder of the posterior pituitary gland or hypothalamus in which hyposecretion of the antidiuretic hormone (ADH) vasopressin (or, in some cases, the kidney's inability to respond to ADH) results in failure of the kidney tubules to reabsorb water.
2. Etiology
   a. Central (neurogenic) DI: Neurosurgical interruption of anatomic integrity (cranial surgery for tumor or hypophysectomy) accounts for 20 percent of central DI. Localized or generalized edema secondary to head trauma or vascular lesions, central nervous system infections or inflammations, and vasopressin-inhibiting drugs (ethanol, glucocorticoids, adrenergic agents, phenytoin, and narcotic antagonists) account for 55 percent of central DI. Tumors of the hypothalamus or pituitary glands account for 25 percent of central DI.
   b. Complete DI: The complete absence of vasopressin disrupts the hypophysial tract, causing 80 percent degeneration of the supraoptic and paraventricular nuclei.
   c. Nephrogenic DI: Deficiency of vasopressin receptors in the renal collecting ducts results from a rare hereditary disorder or is acquired secondary to pyelonephritis, obstructive uropathy, or hypocalcemia.
   d. The etiology is idiopathic in about 30 percent of all patients with DI.
3. Clinical manifestations
   a. Genitourinary: polyuria (a few liters to 18 L/day), clear urine, frequent urination, and nocturia
   b. Gastrointestinal: weight loss and polydipsia (if thirst mechanism is intact)
   c. Integumentary: dry skin and mucous membranes
   d. Neurologic: changes in mentation as electrolyte imbalance and hypotension worsen
4. Clinical management
   a. Goals
      (1) Identify the cause (this can be difficult).
      (2) Prevent complications such as dehydration, electrolyte imbalance, and shock.
      (3) Correct the cause.
   b. Nonpharmacologic interventions: Increase oral fluids, especially water.
   c. Pharmacologic interventions
      (1) Intravenous fluids
      (2) Antidiuretic hormone replacement therapy

- Synthetic vasopressin (especially desmopressin nasal solution twice a day) may be given IV, subcutaneously, or intranasally. The onset of action is 1 hour, duration is 6 to 24 hours, and side effects are hyponatremia and water intoxication.
- Pitressin tannate in oil may be given intramuscularly daily.
- Lypressin nasal solution
- Aqueous pitressin
- Chlorpropamide may stimulate ADH release and help reduce symptoms.
- Thiazide diuretics may be used for overtreatment of synthetic vasopressin.

(3) Special medical-surgical procedures: hypophysectomy to remove posterior pituitary tumor

Syndrome of Inappropriate Antidiuretic Hormone

1. Definition: In syndrome of inappropriate antidiuretic hormone (SIADH, also called *Schwartz-Bartter syndrome*), the posterior pituitary and other ectopic sources continue to secrete vasopressin, despite the absence of either osmotic or nonosmotic stimuli.
2. Etiology
   a. Ectopic production of vasopressin by malignant tumors (e.g., bronchogenic, pancreatic, and prostatic carcinomas and lymphomas of the duodenum, brain, thymus, and bladder) is the most frequent cause of SIADH, and about 80 percent of patients with small cell carcinoma have SIADH.
   b. Other causes of SIADH
      (1) Vasopressin overuse (as in DI)
      (2) Increased intracranial pressure secondary to infectious processes or trauma to the brain
      (3) Infectious processes (e.g., viral and bacterial pneumonia) that produce ectopic vasopressin
      (4) Drugs that stimulate vasopressin release (e.g., vincristine, cyclophosphamide, thiazides, phenothiazides, carbamazepine, vinblastine, cisplatin, and oxytocin)
      (5) Endocrine diseases such as adrenal insufficiency, myxedema, and anterior pituitary insufficiency
      (6) Analgesics
      (7) Vomiting
3. Clinical manifestations
   a. Manifestations related to the degree of hyponatremia: confusion, lethargy, irritability, seizures, coma, and diminished gastrointestinal mobility (anorexia, nausea, and vomiting)
   b. Abrupt weight gain (without edema) of 5 to 10 percent
4. Clinical management
   a. Goals
      (1) Correct the cause, if possible.
      (2) Treat electrolyte imbalance.
      (3) Prevent complications.
      (4) Protect brain from insult secondary to hyponatremia.
   b. Nonpharmacologic interventions
      (1) Fluid restriction (it alone may control fluid excess)

(2) Sodium restriction
c. Pharmacologic interventions
  (1) Replacement of sodium with other hypertonic IV fluids.

DRUG ADVISORY

Demeclocycline may be nephrotoxic. Monitor renal function carefully (blood urea nitrogen, serum creatinine, and intake and output).

(2) Diuretics to correct low plasma osmolality.
(3) Demeclocycline to antagonize vasopressin.
(4) Hyperosmolar, low-volume enemas
(5) Metabolic emergencies: Administration of 3 percent hypertonic saline to quickly correct hyponatremia and increase serum osmolality (Use with caution: Fluid overload with this solution may cause congestive heart failure or circulatory collapse.)
(6) Vasopressin antagonists—still under investigation
d. Special medical-surgical procedures: none

Bibliography

Books

American Diabetes Association. *Intensive Diabetes Management* (Clinical Education Series). Alexandria, VA: Author, 1995.

Bardin CW (ed). *Current Therapy in Endocrinology and Metabolism.* 4th ed. Philadelphia: BC Decker, 1991.

Bates B. *A Guide to Physical Examination and History Taking.* 5th ed. Philadelphia: JB Lippincott, 1991.

Berne R, and Levy M. *Physiology.* 3rd ed. St. Louis, Mosby–Year Book, 1993.

Black J, and Matassarin-Jacobs E. (eds). *Luckmann and Sorenson's Medical-Surgical Nursing.* 4th ed. Philadelphia: WB Saunders, 1993.

Braverman L, and Higer R. (eds.). *Weiner and Ingbar's The Thyroid.* 6th ed. Philadelphia: JB Lippincott, 1991.

Cady B, and Rossi R. *Surgery of the Thyroid and Parathyroid Glands.* 3rd ed. Philadelphia: WB Saunders, 1991.

Corbett JV. *Laboratory Tests and Diagnostic Procedures with Nursing Diagnosis.* 3rd ed. Norwalk, CT: Appleton & Lange, 1992.

Falk S (ed). *Thyroid Disease—Endocrinology, Nuclear Medicine and Radiotherapy.* New York: Raven Press, 1994.

Felig P, et al. (eds). *Endocrinology and Metabolism.* 3rd ed. New York: McGraw-Hill, 1995.

Fitzgerald P. *Handbook of Clinical Endocrinology.* 2nd ed. Norwalk, CT: Appleton & Lange, 1992.

Guyton A: *Human Physiology and Mechanisms of Disease.* 5th ed. Philadelphia: WB Saunders, 1992.

Ignatavicius DD, Workman ML, and Mishler MA. *Medical-Surgical Nursing: A Nursing Process Approach.* 2nd ed. Philadelphia: WB Saunders, 1995.

Jarvis C. *Physical Examination and Health Assessment.* 2nd ed. Philadelphia: WB Saunders, 1996.

Kee JL. *Laboratory and Diagnostic Tests with Nursing Implications.* 3rd ed. Norwalk, CT: Appleton & Lange, 1991.

Lehne R. *Pharmacology for Nursing Care.* 2nd ed. Philadelphia: WB Saunders, 1994.

Malasanos L. *Health Assessment.* 4th ed. St. Louis, CV Mosby, 1990.

National Institutes of Health. *Diabetes in America.* 2nd ed. National Institute of Diabetes and Digestive and Kidney Diseases, NIH Publication No. 95-1468. Bethesda, MD: National Institutes of Health, 1995.

Olin BR (ed). *Drug Facts and Comparisons, 1994 edition.* St. Louis: Facts and Comparisons, 1994.

Pagana KD, and Pagana TJ. *Diagnostic Testing and Nursing Implications. A Case Study Approach.* 3rd ed. St. Louis: CV Mosby, 1990.

Phipps W, et al. (eds). *Medical-Surgical Nursing Concepts and Clinical Practice.* 4th ed. St. Louis: Mosby–Year Book, 1991.

Thompson J, et al. *Mosby's Clinical Nursing.* 3rd ed. St. Louis: CV Mosby–Year Book, 1993.

Tucker S, et al. *Patient Care Standards.* 5th ed. St. Louis: CV Mosby–Year Book, 1992.

Ulrich S, Canale S, and Wendell S. *Medical-Surgical Nursing Care Planning Guides.* 3rd ed. Philadelphia: WB Saunders, 1994.

Wilson J, and Foster D. (eds). *Williams Textbook of Endocrinology.* 8th ed. Philadelphia: WB Saunders, 1992.

Chapters in Books

Diabetes Mellitus

Franz M. Nutritional care in diabetes mellitus and reactive hypoglycemia. *In* Mahan LK, and Arlin MT (eds). *Krause's Food, Nutrition and Diet Therapy.* 8th ed. Philadelphia: WB Saunders, 1996, pp 681–716.

Guyton A. Insulin, glucagon and diabetes mellitus. *In* Guyton A. *Textbook of Medical Physiology.* 9th ed. Philadelphia: WB Saunders, 1995, pp 971–983.

Ward JD. Diabetic neuropathy. *In* Alberti KGMM, et al. (eds). *International Textbook of Diabetes Mellitus.* Vol. 2. New York: John Wiley & Sons, 1992, pp 1385–1414.

Reactive Hypoglycemia

Franz M. Nutritional care in diabetes mellitus and reactive hypoglycemia. *In* Mahan LK, and Arlin MT (eds). *Krause's Food, Nutrition and Diet Therapy.* 8th ed. Philadelphia: WB Saunders, 1996, pp 681–716.

Young C, and Karam J. Hypoglycemia disorders. *In* Greenspan F (ed). *Basic and Clinical Endocrinology.* 4th ed. Norwalk, CT: Appleton & Lange, 1994, pp 635–648.

Parathyroid Disorders

Alfrey A. Phosphate, aluminum and other elements in chronic renal disease. *In* Schrier R, and Gottschalk C (eds). *Diseases of the Kidney.* 5th ed. Boston: Little Brown & Co, 1992, pp 3153–3166.

Guyton A. Parathyroid hormone, calcitonin, calcium and phosphate metabolism, vitamin D, bone and teeth. *In* Guyton A. *Medical Physiology.* 9th ed. Philadelphia: WB Saunders, 1996, pp 985–1016.

Schteingart D. Disorders of calcium metabolism. *In* Price S, and Wilson L (eds). *Pathophysiology: Clinical Concepts of Disease Processes.* St. Louis: CV Mosby, 1992, pp 858–862.

Schteingart D. Pancreas: Glucose metabolism and diabetes mellitus. *In* Price S, and Wilson L (eds). *Pathophysiology: Clinical Concepts of Disease Processes.* St. Louis: Mosby–Year Book, 1992, pp 881–891.

Adrenal Disorders

Goldfien A. Adrenal medulla. *In* Greenspan F (ed). *Basic and Clinical Endocrinology.* 4th ed. Norwalk, CT: Appleton & Lange, 1991, pp. 370–391.

Keiser HR. Pheochromocytoma and related tumors. *In* DeGroot LJ (ed). *Endocrinology.* 3rd ed., vol. 2. Philadelphia: WB Saunders, 1995, pp 1861–1862.

Schteingart D. Adrenal cortex: Disorders of hypersecretion. *In* Price S, and Wilson L (eds). *Pathophysiology: Clinical Concepts of Disease Processes.* St. Louis: Mosby–Year Book, 1992, pp 877–880.

Pituitary Disorders

Findling J, and Tyrell B. Anterior pituitary gland. *In* Greenspan F (ed). *Basic and Clinical Endocrinology.* 4th ed. Norwalk, CT: Appleton & Lange, 1991.

Schteingart D. Disorders of the pituitary gland. *In* Price S, and Wilson L (eds). *Pathophysiology: Clinical Concepts of Disease Processes.* St. Louis: Mosby–Year Book, 1992, pp 840–848.

Articles

Diabetes Mellitus

American Diabetes Association. The pharmacological treatment of hyperglycemia in NIDDM. *Diabetes Care* 18(11):1510–1518, 1995.

American Diabetes Association. Standards of medical care for patients with diabetes mellitus (position statement). *Diabetes Care* 18(Suppl 1):8–15, 1995.

American Diabetes Association. Clinical practice recommendations for 1996. *Diabetes Care* 19(Suppl 1):S1–S113, 1996.

Anderson S. Seven tips for managing patients with diabetes. *Am J Nurs* 94(9):36–38, 1994.

Arbour R. Preventing hypoglycemic seizures. *Nursing* 24(1):33, 1994.

Bantle J, Neal L, and Frankamp L. Effects of the anatomical region used for insulin injections on glycemia in type I diabetes subjects. *Diabetic Care* 16(12):19, 1993. pp 1592–1597.

Caro J. Diabetes and hypertension: Not the final chapter. *Diabetes Care* 16(2):540–541, 1993.

Cirone N. Diabetes in the elderly. Part I: Unmasking a hidden disorder. *Nursing* 26(3):34–39, 1996.

Cirone N. Diabetes in the elderly. Part II: Finding the balance for drug therapy. *Nursing* 26(3):40–47, 1996.

David M. Diabetic retinopathy. *Diabetes Care* 15(12):1844–1874, 1992.

Diabetes Control and Complications Trial Research Group. The effect of intensive treatment of diabetes on the development and progression of long-term complications in insulin-dependent diabetes mellitus. *N Engl J Med* 329(14):977–986, 1993.

Diabetes Control and Complications Trial Research Group. Implementation of treatment protocols in the diabetes control and complications trial. *Diabetes Care* 18(3):361–376, 1995.

Diabetes Control and Complications Trial Research Group. Influence of intensive diabetes treatment on quality of life outcomes in the diabetes control and complications trial. *Diabetes Care* 19(3):195–203, 1996.

Donahue R, and Orchard T. Diabetes mellitus and macrovascular complications. *Diabetes Care* 15(9):1141–1155, 1992.

Dorgan MB, et al. Performing foot screening for diabetic patients. *Am J Nurs* 95(11):32–37, 1995.

Drass J. What you need to know about insulin injection. *Nursing* 22(11):40–45, 1992.

Eisenbarth G, et al. The design of trials for prevention of IDDM. *Diabetes* 42:941–947, 1993.

Engel S, et al. Diabetes care needs of Hispanic patients treated at inner-city neighborhood clinics in New York City. *Diabetes Educ* 21(2):124–128, 1995.

Fain J. National trends in diabetes: An epidemiologic perspective. *Nurs Clin North Am* 28(1):1–8, 1993.

Friedman E. Diabetic nephropathy. *Diabetes Spectrum* 2(2):86–95, 1989.

Goldschmid MG, et al. Diabetes in urban African Americans II. High prevalence of microalbuminuria and nephropathy in African Americans with diabetes. *Diabetes Care* 18(17):955–961, 1995.

Greene D, et al. Complications: Neuropathy, pathogenic considerations. *Diabetes Care* 15(12):1902–1925, 1992.

Haas L. Chronic complications of diabetes mellitus. *Nurs Clin North Am* 28(1):71–86, 1993.

Heinemann L, and Richter B. Clinical pharmacology of human insulin. *Diabetes Care* 16(Suppl 3):90–100, 1993.

Hoyson PM. Diabetes 2001: Oral medications. *RN* 58(5):34–40, 1995.

Johnson A, and Taylor R. Diabetes mellitus. *Postgrad Med J* 66:1010–1024, 1990.

Kannel WB, and McGee DL. Diabetes and cardiovascular disease: The Framingham Study. *JAMA* 241:2035–2038, 1979.

Kestel F. Using blood glucose meters. Part I. *Nursing* 23(5):34–41, 1993.

Kestel F. Using blood glucose meters. Part II. *Nursing* 23(5):50–53, 1993.

Kestel F. Using blood glucose meters. Part III. *Nursing* 23(5):51–54, 1993.

Knight-Macheca MK. Diabetic hypoglycemia: How to keep the threat at bay. *Am J Nursing* 93(4):26–30, 1993.

Lee ET, et al. Diabetes and impaired glucose tolerance in three American Indian populations aged 45–74 years: The Strong Heart Study. *Diabetes Care* 18(5):599–610, 1995.

LeMone P. Responses of the older adult to the effects and management of diabetes mellitus. *Med Surg Nurs* 3(2):122–127, 1994.

Mazze R, et al. (1994) Staged diabetes management: Toward an integrated model of diabetes care. *Diabetes Care* (Suppl 1):56–66, 1993.

McCance DR, et al. Long term glycaemic control and diabetic retinopathy. *Lancet* 2:824–827, 1989.

McNeely M, et al. The independent contributions of diabetic neuropathy and vasculopathy in foot ulceration. *Diabetes Care* 18(2):216–219, 1995.

Moser M, and Ross H. The treatment of hypertension in diabetic patients. *Diabetes Care,* 16(2):542–547, 1993.

Nathan D, et al. Glycemic control in diabetes mellitus. *Am J Med* 100(2):157–163, 1996.

Nathan DM. Medical progress: Long term complications of diabetes mellitus. *N Engl J Med* 28(23):1676–1685, 1993.

Peterson A, and Drass J. Managing acute complications of diabetes. *Nursing* 21(2):34–40, 1991.

Plummer ES, and Albert SG. Foot care assessment in patients with diabetes. A screening algorithm for patient education and referral. *Diabetes Educ* 21(1):47–51, 1995.

Ponte CD. The clinical use of oral sulfonylureas in the management of noninsulin dependent diabetes mellitus (NIDDM). *W V Med J* 86:455–458, 1990.

Reichard P, Nilsson B, and Rosenquist U. The effect of long term intensified insulin treatment on the development of microvascular complications of diabetes mellitus. *N Engl J Med* 329(5):304–313, 1993.

Reising DL. Acute hyperglycemia: Putting a lid on the crisis. *Nursing* 25(2):33–48, 49–50, 1995.

Reising DL. Acute hypoglycemia: Keeping the bottom from falling out. *Nursing* 25(2):41–48, 1995.

Robertson RP. Pancreatic and islet transplantation for diabetes—Curse or curiosities? *N Engl J Med* 327(26):1861–1868, 1992.

Ross M. Neuropathies associated with diabetes. *Med Clin North Am* 77(1):111–124, 1993.

Sabo C, and Michael S. Diabetic ketoacidosis: Pathophysiology, nursing diagnosis, and nursing interventions. *Focus Crit Care* 16(1):21–28, 1989.

Schernthaner G. Immunogenicity and allergenic potential of animal and human insulins. *Diabetes Care* 16(Suppl 3):155–165, 1993.

Selby JV, and Shang D. Risk factors for lower extremity amputation in persons with diabetes. *Diabetes Care* 18(4):509–516, 1995.

Spollett G. Intensive insulin therapy in insulin dependent diabetes and combination therapy. *Nurse Pract* 18(7):27–28, 33, 36–38, 1993.

Steil C, and Deakins DA. Oral hypoglycemics: What you and your patient need to know. *Nursing* 22(11):34–39, 1992.

Strowig S, and Raskin P. Glycemic control and diabetic complications. *Diabetes Care* 15(9):1126–1140, 1992.

Tanja JJ, and Langlass TM. Pharmacy update: Metformin: A biguanide. *Diabetes Educ* 21(6):509–510, 513–514, 1995.

Toyry LK, et al. Occurrence, predictors and clinical significance of autonomic neuropathy in NIDDM: Ten-year follow-up from diagnosis. *Diabetes* 45(3):308–315, 1996.

Weakland B. Administering insulin through an indwelling catheter. *Nursing* 23(11):58–61, 1993.

Reactive Hypoglycemia

Field J. Hypoglycemia—definition, clinical presentations, classification and laboratory tests. *Endocrinol Metab Clin North Am* 18(1):27–43, 1989.

Thyroid Disorders

Baher K, and Feldman J. Thyroid cancer. A review. *Oncol Nurs Forum* 20(1):95–104, 1993.

Block M. Surgical treatment of medullary carcinoma of the thyroid. *Otolaryngol Clin North Am* 23(3):453–473, 1990.

Corsetti A, and Buhl B. Managing thyroid storm. *Am J Nurs* 94(11):39, 1994.

Cummings C, Flint P, and Krause C. Neck cancer: What's optimal therapy? *Patient Care* 24(4):44–48, 53, 54, 57, 60, 61, 1990.

Eggo MC, et al. Expression of fibroblast growth factors in thyroid cancer. *J Clin Endocrinol Metab* 80(3):1006–1011, 1995.

Helfand M, and Crapo L. Screening for thyroid disease. *Ann Intern Med* 12(11):840–849, 1990.

Hershman J, Ladenson P, and Paulshock B. A savvy approach to thyroid testers. *Patient Care,* February 15, 1992.

Isley W. Thyroid disorders. *Crit Care Nurse* 13(3):39–49, 1990.

Johnson J, and Felicetta J. Hyperthyroidism: A comprehensive review. *J Am Acad Nurse Pract* 4(1):8–14, 1992.

Lammon CA, and Hart G. Action stat! Recognizing thyroid crisis. *Nursing* 23(4):33, 1993.

Lee K, and Loré J. The treatment of metastatic thyroid disease. *Otolaryngol Clin North Am* 23(3):475–493, 1990.

McMorrow ME. The elderly and thyrotoxicosis. *AACN Clin Issues Crit Care Nurs* 3(1):114–119, 1992.

Spittle L. Diagnoses in opposition: Thyroid storm and myxedema coma. *AACN Clin Issues Crit Care Nurs* 3(2):300–308, 1992.

Yoemans A. Assessment and management of hypothyroidism. *Nurse Pract* 15(11):8–16, 1990.

Parathyroid Disorders

Heath H. Primary hyperparathyroidism: Recent advances. *Adv Intern Med* 37:275–293, 1991.

Netterville J, Aly A, and Ossoff R. Evaluation and treatment of complications of thyroid and parathyroid surgery. *Otolaryngol Clin North Am* 23(3):529–552, 1990.

Petti G. Hyperparathyroidism. *Otolaryngol Clin North Am* 23(2):339–355, 1990.

Adrenal Disorders

Benowitz N. Diagnosis and management of pheochromocytoma. *Hosp Pract* 25(6):163, 1990.

Biglieri E. Spectrum of mineralocorticoid hypertension. *Hypertension* 17(2):251–261, 1991.

Brown CF, Renusch J, and Turner L. Addisonian crisis: Emergency presentation of primary adrenal insufficiency. *Ann Emerg Med* 20:802–806, 1991.

Cryer P. Pheochromocytoma. *West J Med* 156:399–407, 1992.

Davenport J, et al. Addison's disease. *Fam Physician* 43(5):1338–1342, 1991.

Findling J. Cushing syndrome—an etiologic work-up. *Hosp Pract* 27(10):107–122, 1992.

Ganguly A. Glucocorticoid-suppressible hyperaldosteronism: An update. *Am J Med* 88(4):321, 1988.

Grondel S, and Hamberger B. Primary aldosteronism. *Br J Surg* 79(6):484–485, 1992.

Handerhan B. Recognizing adrenal crisis. *Nursing* 22(4):33, 1992.

Klein I, and Ojamaa K. Cardiovascular manifestations of endocrine disease. *J Clin Endocrinol Metab* 75(2):339–342, 1992.

Melby J. Clinical review 1: Endocrine hypertension. *J Clin Endocrinol Metab* 69(4):697–703, 1989.

Norbiato G, et al. Cortisol resistance in acquired immunodeficiency syndrome. *J Clin Endocrinol Metab* 74(3):608–613, 1992.

Oldfield EH, et al. Petrosal sinus sampling with and without corticotropin-releasing hormone for the differential diagnosis of Cushing's syndrome. *N Engl J Med* 325:897–905, 1991.

Orth DN. Differential diagnosis of Cushing's syndrome. *N Engl J Med* 325(13):957–959, 1991.

Ringstad J, et al. Rapidly fatal Addison's disease: Three case reports. *J Intern Med* 230:465–467, 1991.

Shapiro B, and Gross M. Pheochromocytoma. *Crit Care Clin* 7(1):1–22, 1991.

Stoffer S. Addison's disease. *Postgrad Med* 93(4):265, 266, 271, 276, 1993.

Tahir A, and Sheeler LR. Recurrent Cushing's disease after transsphenoidal surgery. *Arch Intern Med* 152:977–981, 1992.

Winer N. Pheochromocytoma. *Crit Care Nurs Q* 13(3):14–22, 1990.

Wittert GA, et al. Acutely raised corticotropin levels in Addison's disease are not associated with increased plasma arginine vasopressin and corticotropin-releasing factor concentrations in peripheral plasma. *J Clin Endocrinol Metab* 76(1):192–196, 1993.

Young W, et al. Primary aldosteronism: Diagnosis and treatment. *Mayo Clin Proc* 65:96–110, 1990.

Yucha C, and Blakeman N. Pheochromocytoma—The great mimic. *Cancer Nurs* 14(3):136–140, 1991.

Pituitary Disorders

Blondell R. Hypopituitarism. *Am Fam Physician* 43(6):2029–2036, 1991.

Chipps E. Transsphenoidal surgery for pituitary tumors. *Crit Care Nurse* 12(1):30–39, 1992.

Constine L, et al. Hypothalamic-pituitary dysfunction after radiation for brain tumors. *N Engl J Med* 328(2):87–94, 1993.

Ezzat S. Hepatobiliary and gastrointestinal manifestations of acromegaly. *Dig Dis Sci* 10:173–180, 1992.

Giustina A, et al. Characterization of the paradoxical growth hormone inhibitory effect of Galanin in acromegaly. *J Clin Endocrin Metab* 80(4):1333–1340, 1995.

Greenman Y, et al. Relative sparing of anterior pituitary function in patients with growth hormone secreting macroadenomas. *J Clin Endocrinol Metab* 80(5):1577–1583, 1995.

Johnston D, et al. Metabolic changes and vascular risk factors in hypopituitarism. *Horm Res* 38(Suppl 1):68–72, 1991.

Katz E, and Adashi E. Hyperprolactinemic disorders. *Clin Obstet Gynecol* 33(3):621–639, 1990.

Melmed S. Acromegaly. *N Engl J Med* 322:966–977, 1990.

Molitch M. Clinical manifestations of acromegaly. *Endocrinol Metab Clin North Am* 21(3):597–613, 1992.

Nalbach D, and Carson M. Prolactinoma: A review and case study. *Crit Care Nurse* 11(9):48–49, 52–57, 1991.

Reasner C. Anterior pituitary disease. *Crit Care Nurs* 13(3):62–66, 1990.

Tordjman K, et al. The role of low dose adrenocorticotrophin test in the evaluation of patients with pituitary diseases. *J Clin Endocrinol Metab* 80(4):1301–1305, 1995.

Diabetes Insipidus

Cagno M. Nursing care plan: Diabetes insipidus. *Crit Care Nurse* 9(6):86–93, 1989.

Halloran T. Nursing responsibilities in endocrine emergencies. *Crit Care Nurs Q* 13(3):74–81, 1990.

Leahy N. Complications in the acute stages of stroke. *Nurs Clin North Am* 26(4):971–983, 1991.

Ober P. Diabetes insipidus. *Crit Care Clin* 7(1):109–126, 1991.

Shulman L, et al. Desmopressin for diabetes insipidus, hemostatic disorders and enuresis. *Am Fam Physician* 42(4):1051–1057, 1990.

Yucha C, and Suddaby P. David could have died of thirst. *Nursing* 21(7):42–45, 1991.

Syndrome of Inappropriate Antidiuretic Hormone

Brice J. S.I.A.D.H. *Nursing* 24(4):33, 1994.

Halloran T. Nursing responsibilities in endocrine emergencies. *Crit Care Nurs Q* 13(3):74–81, 1990.

Leahy N. Complications in the acute stages of stroke. *Nurs Clin North Am* 26(4):971–983, 1991.

Lindama C. SIADH—is your patient at risk? *Nursing* 22(6):60–63, 1992.

Segatore M. Hyponatremia after aneurysmal subarachnoid hemorrhage. *J Neurosci Nurs* 25(2):92–99, 1993.

Sterns R. The management of hyponatremic emergencies. *Crit Care Clin* 7(1):127–142, 1991.

Talmi Y, et al. Syndrome of inappropriate secretion of arginine vasopressin in patients with cancer of the head and neck. *Ann Otol Rhinol Laryngol* 101(11):946–949, 1992.

Agencies and Resources

American Diabetes Association National Center
1660 Duke Street
Alexandria, VA 22314
(800) 232–3472

American Dietetic Association
Suite 800
216 West Jackson Boulevard
Chicago, IL 60606
(312) 899–0040

International Diabetes Center
3800 Park Nicollet Boulevard
Minneapolis, MN 55416
(612) 993–3393

30

Caring for Men with Sexual and Reproductive System Disorders

☐ MALE REPRODUCTIVE STRUCTURE AND FUNCTION

Structure of the Male Reproductive Organs

1. The male reproductive organs consist of the penis, testicles, epididymis, and prostate gland (Fig. 30–1).
2. Structure of the penis
   a. The penis, a cylindric, pendulous structure, consists mainly of erectile tissue.
   b. The erectile tissue of the penis is arranged into 3 columns, which are contained within the body of the penis. The posterior ends of the columns extend into the root or base of the penis.
      (1) The corpus cavernosum is composed of 2 of the columns.
      (2) The corpus spongiosum is a 1-column structure that fills with blood during sexual excitement. This column also contains the urethra, which forms a pathway for the elimination of urine and semen.
   c. The penis is divided into 3 major parts.
      (1) The root, or base, is attached to the anterior pubic arch by fascia, a triangular suspensory ligament, and muscle tissue.
      (2) The body, corpus, or shaft is the pendulous, soft tissue portion that extends from the root to the distal end of the penis (glans penis).
      (3) The glans penis surrounds the slit-like opening of the urethral meatus.
   d. The penis is covered by skin that is dark, hairless, and loosely attached to the underlying fascia. This loose attachment allows the penis to enlarge during erections.
   e. The prepuce, or foreskin, is a continuation of the penile skin that covers the glans.
3. Structure of the testicles
   a. Each testis (testicle) is suspended in the scrotum by the spermatic cord, which provides the vascular, lymphatic, and nerve innervation to the testis.
      (1) Each testis has 600 to 12,000 seminiferous tubules, which consist of germinal epithelial cells and Sertoli's cells.
      (2) Leydig's cells, which secrete the major male hormone testosterone, are located in the interstitial tissue surrounding the seminiferous tubules.
   b. The epididymis is the 1st portion of the ductal system that transports spermatozoa from the testes to the urethra.

(1) The head of the epididymis is attached to the posterior aspect of the testis.
(2) The body of the epididymis descends along the lateral wall of the testis.
(3) The tail of the epididymis joins the vas deferens.
   c. The vas deferens transports spermatozoa from the epididymis to the ejaculatory ducts at the base of the prostatic urethra.
4. Structure of the prostate gland
   a. The prostate gland is a chestnut-shaped, fibromuscular, glandular organ.
   b. It is situated between the neck of the bladder and the urogenital diaphragm.
   c. It is separated from the anterior wall of the rectum by a thin fascial sheath that is part of the rectovesical septum.
   d. The urethra passes through the prostate gland from the internal urethral orifice at the neck of the bladder to the urethral sphincter in the urogenital diaphragm.
   e. The prostate is divided into 3 lobes, commonly referred to as a median lobe and 2 lateral lobes.
   f. Prostatic function is dependent on adequate levels of testosterone.

Function of the Male Reproductive Organs

1. The penis is the male organ for sexual intercourse and urination.
2. Function of the testes and epididymis
   a. The testes are a pair of ovoid organs that produce spermatozoa and testosterone.
   b. The seminiferous tubules are the functional unit of the testes and the site of spermatogenesis.
   c. Sertoli's cells develop spermatozoa in response to follicle-stimulating hormone (FSH).
   d. Leydig's cells secrete testosterone.
   e. The epididymis transports spermatozoa from the testes to the urethra.
3. Function of the prostate gland
   a. The prostate gland is the largest accessory gland of the male reproductive system.
   b. It secretes a milky alkaline fluid that adds bulk to the semen, neutralizes acidic vaginal secretions, and enhances spermatozoa motility.
   c. Fluid from the prostate gland comprises 20 to 30 percent of the total ejaculate.

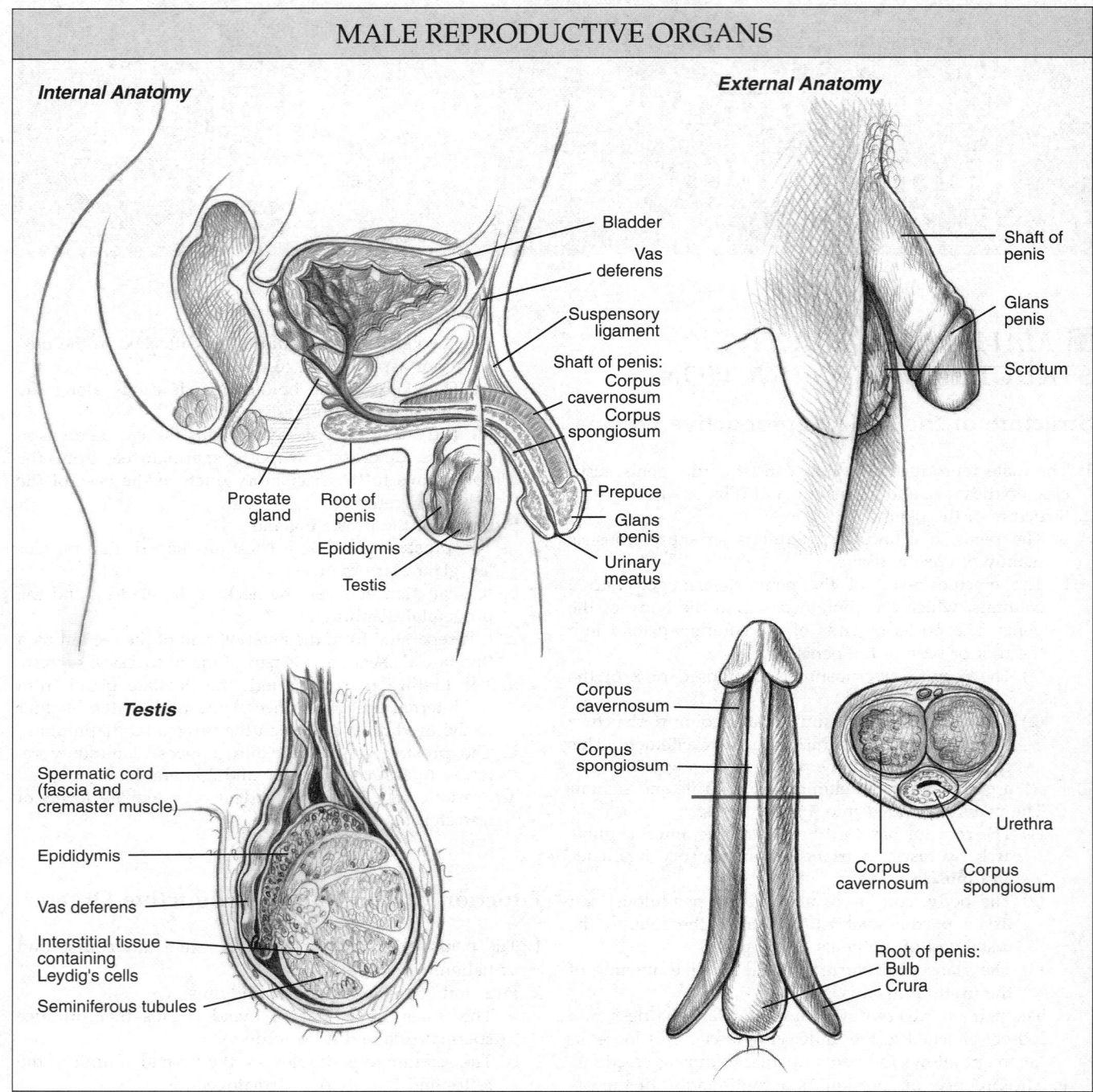

MALE REPRODUCTIVE ORGANS

Internal Anatomy

Bladder
Vas deferens
Suspensory ligament
Shaft of penis:
Corpus cavernosum
Corpus spongiosum
Prepuce
Glans penis
Urinary meatus

Prostate gland
Root of penis
Epididymis
Testis

External Anatomy

Shaft of penis
Glans penis
Scrotum

Testis

Spermatic cord (fascia and cremaster muscle)
Epididymis
Vas deferens
Interstitial tissue containing Leydig's cells
Seminiferous tubules

Corpus cavernosum
Corpus spongiosum

Urethra
Corpus cavernosum
Corpus spongiosum

Root of penis:
Bulb
Crura

Figure 30–1.

ASSESSING MEN WITH REPRODUCTIVE DISORDERS

Key Symptoms and Their Pathophysiologic Bases

1. Erectile dysfunction
   a. Characteristics include an inability to attain an erection, an inability to maintain an erection, or both.
   b. Erectile dysfunction is attributed to psychologic factors, physical factors, or a combination of both.
2. Urinary tract symptoms (see Chapter 26)
   a. Characteristics include urgency, frequency, inability to initiate a stream, postvoid dribbling, and burning sensation when urinating.
   b. Because of the proximity of the reproductive system to the urinary tract, a variety of reproductive disorders can cause problems with urinary elimination.
   (1) Disorders of the prostate gland obstruct the out-

flow of urine by encroaching on the bladder opening.
  (2) Invasive procedures or surgery on the urinary system may result in temporary or permanent changes in sexual function.
3. Lump or swelling in the testicle
  a. Problems or conditions that develop inside the scrotum usually occur as a mass or swelling.
  b. Inflammation or infection of the structures in the scrotum can also cause swelling or edema in the testicle.
4. Prostate pain
  a. Prostate pain is most often due to acute inflammation.
  b. There is usually discomfort in the lower back, rectum, and perineum.
5. Scrotal pain
  a. Scrotal pain generally arises from disorders of the testes or the epididymis.
  b. Acute scrotal pain is usually the result of trauma, torsion of a structure within the testicle, or inflammation, especially epididymitis.
  c. Persons with a hydrocele, varicocele, or testicular tumor are more apt to experience scrotal discomfort or a sense of fullness rather than pain.

Physical and Psychosocial Health History

1. Childhood and adolescent conditions
  a. The history of a cryptorchid, or undescended testicle, is one of the risk factors for the development of testicular cancer.
  b. The history of mumps orchitis may be a risk factor in the development of sterility.
2. Diseases and aging
  a. Disorders that have the greatest influence on the person's reproductive function are listed in Table 30–1.
  b. Other conditions that affect reproductive function are brain or spinal cord injury, pelvic irradiation, and surgical procedures on the prostate, bladder, or rectum.
  c. Normal changes of aging, such as loss of tissue elasticity or a decrease in testosterone levels, can also affect reproductive function.
  d. Age is an important consideration when evaluating a man for a reproductive disorder.
    (1) Testicular cancer is the 3rd leading cause of cancer deaths in young men.
    (2) Prostatic enlargement is nearly a universal condition in older men.
3. Medications
  a. Medications can have a significant impact on a person's reproductive or sexual ability.
  b. Medications that affect reproductive or sexual function include antihypertensive drugs, narcotics, antidepressants, estrogens, and antihistamines.
  c. Some cytotoxic chemotherapeutic agents, such as cyclophosphamide, may cause gonadal suppression, with resultant sterility. Other chemotherapeutic agents, such as vincristine and vinblastine cause neurotoxicities that lead to impotence.

Table 30–1. Effects of Specific Disorders on the Male Reproductive System

Disorder	Effect
Diabetes mellitus	Vascular changes
	Neuropathies
Cardiovascular disease	Decreased or occluded blood supply to
Arteriosclerosis	the penis
Hypertension	
Genitourinary diseases	
Peyronie's disease	Decreased blood flow to corporal bodies
Prolonged priapism	Tissue damage resulting from blood clotting in the tissue
Endocrine diseases	
Hypopituitarism	Decreased testosterone levels secondary to increased prolactin or decreased luteinizing hormone
Cushing's syndrome	Decreased testosterone
Addison's disease	
Neurologic diseases and injury	Decreased nerve innervation to either
Multiple sclerosis	sympathetic or parasympathetic nervous systems
Parkinson's disease	
Spina bifida	
Amyotrophic lateral sclerosis	
Myasthenia gravis	
Sympathectomy	
Trauma to spinal cord	

4. Social history and lifestyle
  a. Prostate cancer is the most common male cancer. It is more common after the age of 65, among African Americans, and among men who have large numbers of sexual partners.
  b. An assessment of the person's social history is important to ascertain his living situation, family structure, and employment status.
5. Sexual and reproductive history
  a. Although sexuality and reproductive function are closely linked, they are not the same thing.
  b. The importance of the ability to function sexually or to have children is unique to each man.
  c. Ask specific questions about sexual concerns especially if the man's chief complaint is related to a sexual problem.
  d. Questions should be objective and matter-of-fact. Homosexual or bisexual men need to feel acceptance to discuss their health concerns.
  e. The history should ascertain whether the man is in a relationship involving sexual intercourse.
  f. Determine the sexual preference of the man (i.e., heterosexual, homosexual, or bisexual).
  g. Find out whether the man has one or more sexual partners.
  h. Remember sexual behavior and preferences may change during a person's life.
  i. Determine the type of birth control method used, if any.
  j. Ascertain the number of children the man has fathered, if any.

6. Habits
   a. Intake of caffeine can irritate the prostate gland or impair erectile function.
   b. Alcohol can have an adverse effect on a person's sexual performance.
   c. Street drugs such as marijuana and cocaine can affect a person's sexual or reproductive abilities.
   d. Tight or restrictive clothing may raise scrotal temperature above optimum for spermatogenesis.

Physical Examination

1. General information
   a. The person's chief complaint or any problems identified while obtaining the history determine how extensive the physical examination should be.
   b. A complete physical examination is necessary for anyone undergoing a surgical procedure or for anyone who has symptoms that may have a cause outside of the genitourinary system.
   c. In most instances, a focused examination of the genitourinary tract is sufficient at the time of the initial examination.
2. General appearance
   a. Observe the person for evidence of any nutritional deficiencies, edema, pruritus, pallor, or ecchymoses. These conditions may indicate renal insufficiency from long-standing urinary obstruction.
   b. Assess the person for any signs and symptoms of depression. Observe his affect, mood, facial expressions, and body posture.
3. Abdomen
   a. The person should void before his physical examination.
   b. The abdominal and bladder examination are best carried out with the person in the supine position.
   c. Inspect, palpate, and percuss the person's abdomen for any evidence of a distended bladder.
      (1) With the person in the supine position, a full or overdistended bladder may be visible on inspection.
      (2) Percussion over the bladder may be particularly useful when obesity makes palpation difficult.
      (3) The bladder can usually be percussed if it contains more than 150 ml of urine.
      (4) Dullness occurs over a distended bladder, adipose tissue, fluid, or a mass.
4. Penis

NURSE ADVISORY

Always wear gloves during the examination of male genitalia.

---

   a. Inspection of the penis reveals any obvious lesions and whether the man is circumcised.
      (1) If the man has been circumcised, the glans and meatus can be inspected directly.
      (2) If the man has not been circumcised, foreskin is retracted to inspect the glandular surface of the foreskin as well as the glans and meatus.

   b. Palpation of the penile shaft is important to identify any areas of fibrous tissue.
   c. The urethra is examined for any evidence of urethral discharge.
5. Scrotum and scrotal contents (Fig. 30–2)

NURSE ADVISORY

It is always important to note the presence or absence of the testes.

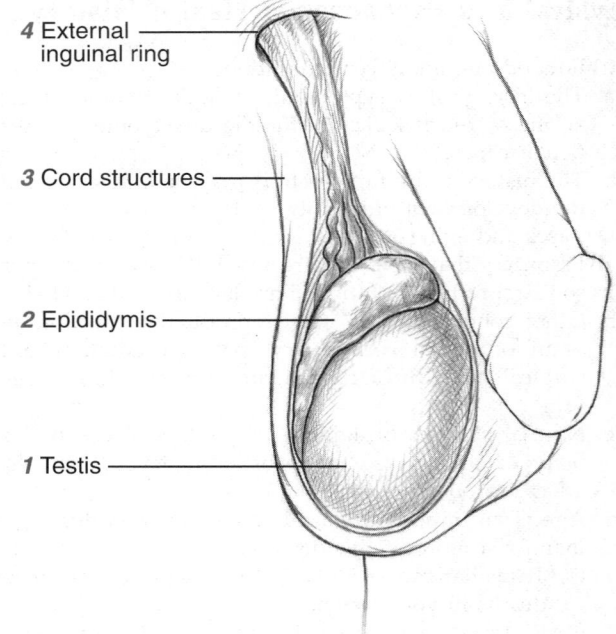

PHYSICAL EXAMINATION OF THE SCROTAL CONTENTS

Inspection of the scrotum is best carried out with the man in a standing position.

Palpate the scrotal contents in an orderly manner: first, the testes, then the epididymides, then the cord structures, and, last, the external inguinal ring to test for the presence of an inguinal hernia.

Examine in this order:

4 External inguinal ring

3 Cord structures

2 Epididymis

1 Testis

NURSE ADVISORY

Interventions that promote drainage of the scrotum are the following:
1. Bed rest
2. Elevation of the scrotum with a rolled towel
3. Ice pack, applied intermittently to the scrotum for the 1st 24 hours
4. Wearing of a scrotal support

Figure 30–2.

6. Prostate and rectum
   a. Because the prostate is close to the rectal wall, it is easily examined by a digital rectal examination.
   b. It is important not only to palpate the prostate gland but also to palpate the entire inside of the rectum to screen for other abnormalities.
   c. During the rectal examination, the posterior aspect of the prostate is palpated.
   d. Abnormalities of the prostate include an abnormal consistency, nodular abnormalities, areas of induration, and areas of bogginess or fluctuance.
   e. If necessary, the patient is prepared for a prostate massage by the physician or nurse practitioner to obtain prostate secretions for examination and culture (Fig. 30–3).

Special Diagnostic Studies

1. Special studies used to diagnose reproductive problems include the following:
   - Laboratory tests
   - Urodynamic tests
   - Radiology tests
   - Tumescence monitoring
2. Nursing interventions
   a. Educate the person about the purpose of the test and provide instructions about the actual procedure or test itself.
   b. Administer any preliminary procedures, such as enemas, that the person requires.
   c. Administer or adjust medication as needed.
   d. Provide physical and emotional support.
   e. Monitor the person after the procedure (vital signs, urine output).
3. Laboratory tests
   a. Blood tests
      (1) A complete blood count is a routine study that provides a red blood cell count, hematocrit, hemoglobin, corpuscular indices, white blood cell count, differential count, and platelet count.
      (2) Blood urea nitrogen and serum creatinine studies provide information about the person's renal function.
      (3) Prostate-specific antigen (PSA) test gives information about the activity of the person's prostate gland. The efficacy of this test as a screening tool for prostate cancer is a controversial issue.
      (4) Acid phosphatase and alkaline phosphatase studies are ordered as part of a metastatic workup when a prostate malignancy is suspected.
      (5) Beta subunit of human chorionic gonadotropin and α-fetoprotein are the primary tumor markers for testicular cancer, and tests are ordered for any young man with a testicular lump.
   b. Urine tests
      (1) Urinalysis includes tests for glucose, protein, blood, pus, and pH levels.
      (2) Urine culture and sensitivity is obtained based on the results of the urinalysis.
4. Urodynamic tests assess voiding and are important in the diagnosis of bladder neck obstruction.

PROSTATE MASSAGE AND DIGITAL RECTAL EXAMINATION

Prostate Massage

Starting from the side and superiorly and moving toward the midline of the prostate, roll the pad of your index finger across the prostate, which should feel rubbery, firm, movable, and nontender.

Possibly cancerous: firm area, not raised, with discernible borders

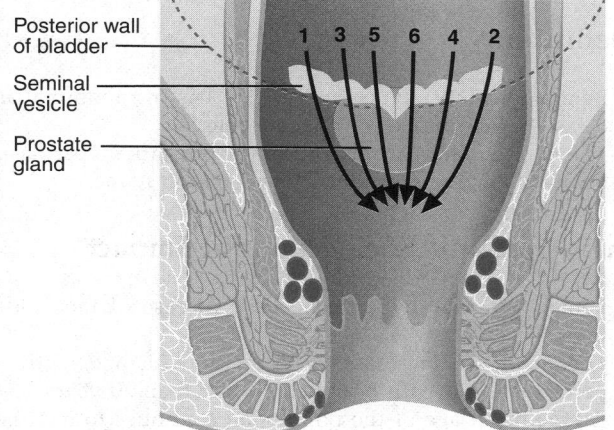

Posterior view of rectum

Use the same technique as that for the prostate massage, but extend your finger higher over the seminal vesicles.

Posterior wall of bladder

Seminal vesicle

Prostate gland

Digital Rectal Examination

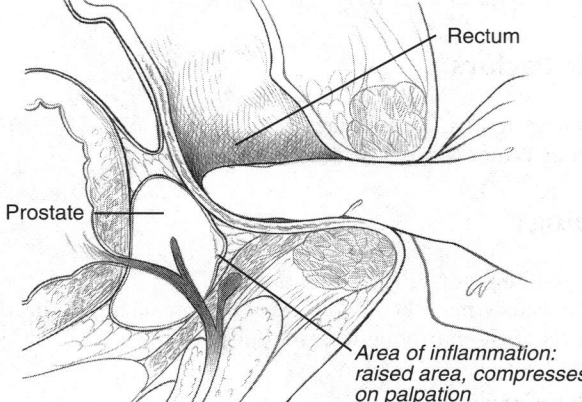

Rectum

Prostate

Area of inflammation: raised area, compresses on palpation

Put the pad of your index finger over the anus and ask the person to bear down. The anal sphincter will tighten, then relax. Slowly insert your finger into the anal canal while pointing your finger toward the umbilicus. Check for abnormalities such as tenderness, nodules, or masses.

Figure 30–3.

- Bladder capacity, pressure, and tone tests
- Urethral pressure
- Urinary flow
- Perineal muscle control and strength (see Chapter 26)
5. Common radiologic studies used in the workup of a man with symptoms involving his reproductive system include the following:
   a. Radiographs of the kidneys, ureters, and bladder together to demonstrate the placement of the urinary tract in the abdomen
   b. Intravenous pyelogram (IVP), which reveals the structure and function of the urinary tract
6. Penile tumescence monitoring
   a. Depending on his age, a man has approximately 3 to 5 erections, each lasting 10 to 25 minutes, during a night's sleep.
   b. The nocturnal penile tumescence test is used to measure and record nocturnal erections to help distinguish between psychologic and physiologic impotence.

▣ *BENIGN PROSTATIC HYPERTROPHY*

Definition

1. Benign prostatic hypertrophy (BPH) is an abnormal increase in the number of prostate cells.
2. The correct name of this process is prostatic hyperplasia, but prostatic hypertrophy is the common name.

Incidence and Socioeconomic Impact

1. Benign prostatic hypertrophy is a disease of men older than 40 years.
2. The incidence increases consistently with age, with 90 percent of men with BPH being older than 70 years.
3. As the mean age of the population continues to increase, the incidence of BPH will also increase, resulting in more procedures being performed and requiring more health care dollars to treat BPH.

Risk Factors

1. Increasing age is a risk factor.
2. Being White is a risk factor.

Etiology

1. The etiology of BPH is unknown.
2. The cause may be linked to systemic changes in the levels of the hormone testosterone.

Pathophysiology

1. The prostate gland enlarges and extends upward into the bladder.
2. The urethra becomes narrowed and obstructs the outflow of urine.

Clinical Manifestations

1. Usually, the person with BPH has a syndrome called prostatism, which includes the following symptoms:
   - Frequency
   - Nocturia
   - Decrease in stream
   - Postvoid dribbling
2. Prostatism refers to the obstruction of urinary flow due to an enlarged prostate (whether due to BPH, inflammation, or malignancy) (see Chapter 26).

Diagnostics

1. History
   a. The age of the person should be considered when obtaining a nursing history from someone who is suspected to have BPH.
   b. Question the person about his urinary pattern.
   c. Ask the person if he has experienced any hematuria.
2. Physical examination
   a. Refer to page 1423 for a description of the physical examination of the prostate.
   b. The prostate examination reveals a prostate that has a uniform, elastic, nontender enlargement.

Clinical Management

1. The goal of any intervention for BPH is to relieve the bladder neck obstruction.
2. There are 4 different approaches to prostate surgery: transurethral resection of the prostate, suprapubic prostatectomy, retropubic prostatectomy, and perineal prostatectomy (Fig. 30–4).
3. Factors influencing the choice of surgical procedures are the size of the prostate gland, the degree of urinary retention, and the age and medical condition of the person.
4. Preoperative evaluation and nursing interventions
   a. Evaluate thoroughly for any coexisting conditions such as cardiovascular disease, renal disease, diabetes, or pulmonary disease.
   b. Assess for any evidence of urinary tract infection and treat according to culture and sensitivity.
   c. Assess hemodynamic state, and type and crossmatch for possible blood transfusions. Blood loss is common during prostatectomies.
   d. Implement preoperative teaching plan to include discussion of anesthesia (general versus spinal) and urinary catheterization (with or without bladder irrigation). The person may have had a catheter placed preoperatively to relieve obstruction, facilitate bladder drainage, or improve renal function.
5. Postoperative management
   a. The postoperative care for prostate surgery is the same regardless of approach or anesthesia used.
   b. Urine output should be maintained.
      (1) Drainage should be observed for evidence of in-

SURGICAL APPROACHES TO PROSTATE SURGERY

1 *Transurethral Resection of the Prostate*
A small amount of prostate tissue is removed from around the urethra by an endoscope and related instruments.

2 *Suprapubic Prostatectomy*
This is performed when more prostate tissue needs to be removed than can be removed with a transurethral resection. An incision is made through the bladder to access the prostate; therefore, any coexisting bladder problems can also be corrected through this approach.

3 *Retropubic Prostatectomy*
Also performed when more prostate tissue needs to be removed than can be removed with a transurethral resection. An incision is made directly into the prostatic capsule, and the contents are removed.

4 *Perineal Prostatectomy*
This surgery removes the prostate tissue through an incision between the scrotum and the anus.

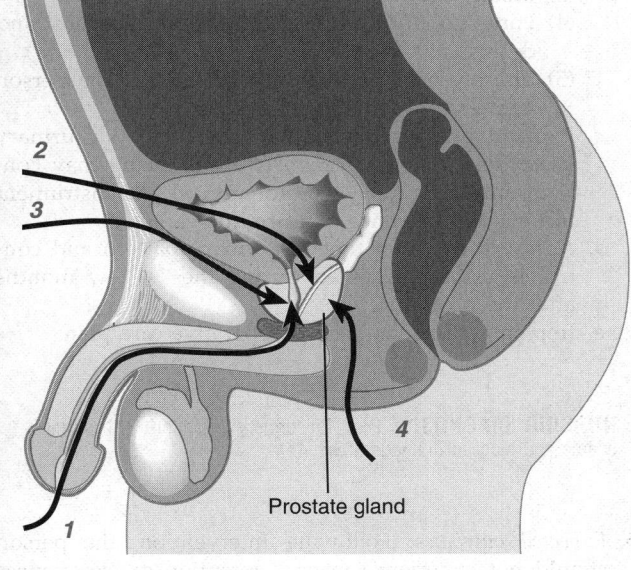

Prostate gland

Figure 30–4.

creased bleeding. Bright red suggests arterial bleeding; dark indicates venous bleeding. The presence or absence of clots is noted.

(2) The Foley catheter should be irrigated, or continuous bladder irrigation should be maintained as prescribed by the urologist.

(3) Bladder distention may increase bleeding.

(4) If the catheter is taped to the patient's thigh, he should keep his leg straight.

c. Nurses monitor and prevent complications by doing the following:

(1) Observe for signs and symptoms of hemorrhage.

(2) Assess vital signs based on clinical condition.

(3) Apply or maintain manual traction on the urethral catheter as directed.

(4) Prepare for blood component therapy or further surgery if bleeding persists.

(5) Monitor for hyponatremia, which occurs as a result of systemic absorption of bladder-irrigating fluid during surgery and the immediate postoperative period.

(6) Observe for vital sign changes (increased blood pressure, decreased pulse), confusion, and nausea.

(7) Monitor for other postoperative complications, such as infection, deep vein thrombosis, or pulmonary embolism.

6. Pharmacologic interventions

a. The presence of α-adrenergic receptors in the prostatic smooth muscle makes it treatable by α-blocking agents.

b. When α-blocking agents are given, the prostate gland constricts, thereby reducing urethral pressure, improving urine flow, and decreasing residual urine (Table 30–2).

7. Special medical-surgical procedures

a. The following measures help minimize obstructive symptoms by causing the release of prostatic fluid:
   - Prostatic massage
   - Frequent sexual activity leading to ejaculation
   - Masturbation

b. Measures aimed at preventing overdistention of the bladder
   - Avoiding drinking large amounts of fluid in a short time
   - Avoiding consumption of alcohol and caffeine
   - Voiding as soon as the urge is felt

c. The following medications cause urinary retention and should be avoided:
   - Anticholinergics
   - Antihistamines
   - Decongestants

Complications

1. In response to unrelieved outlet resistance, the bladder is affected in several ways.

2. First, the bladder becomes hyperirritable, which causes urgency and frequency.

3. As the bladder compensates for the increased workload, the muscles in the bladder wall hypertrophy (trabeculation).

4. Prolonged urine flow obstruction also results in a dilation of the ureters (hydroureter) and kidney (hydronephrosis).

5. Urinary retention or incomplete bladder emptying occurs.

Prognosis

1. The prognosis for the man undergoing treatment for benign prostate disease is excellent.

2. A wide variety of treatments and procedures are available to relieve urinary obstruction and prevent damage to the urinary system.

Table 30–2. Medications Used in the Treatment of Benign Prostatic Hypertrophy

Medication	Advantages	Disadvantages	Side Effects
α-Adrenergic–blocking agents Phenoxybenzamine Prazosin Terazosin Doxazosin	All medications are noninvasive.	Phenoxybenzamine has questionable carcinogenic effects. Prazosin may cause syncope and should be taken at night.	Tachycardia Palpitations Fatigue Nasal congestion Dry mouth Postural hypotension
Finasteride	Circulating testosterone levels are not affected, so there is no erectile dysfunction.		
Anti-androgen		All anti-androgens cause erectile dysfunction due to interruption of the androgen pathway.	Erectile dysfunction Diarrhea Gynecomastia

Applying the Nursing Process

> **NURSING DIAGNOSIS:** Anxiety R/T examinations (e.g., digital rectal examination, or DRE) and possible procedures (transrectal biopsy) or fear of cancer

1. *Expected outcomes:* Following instruction and explanation, the person should be able to do the following:
   a. Correctly state the causes, complications, and treatment options for men with BPH
   b. Review the diagnostic procedures related to prostate cancer
   c. Feel a decrease in anxiety related to DRE or biopsy
2. *Nursing interventions*
   a. Provide a supportive atmosphere for the person and his partner to discuss concerns. Involve the person's partner in the management of the condition.
   b. Explain all procedures and tests in easily understood terms.
   c. Provide diagrams to review anatomic structures and physiologic function to clarify the rationale for the test.
   d. Provide privacy for the person, both for discussion of fears and during the examination or procedures.

> **NURSING DIAGNOSIS:** Anxiety R/T transurethral resection of the prostate or prostatectomy

3. *Expected outcomes:* Following instruction, the person and family should not experience anxiety or fear, or experience minimal anxiety or fear, related to planned transurethral resection of the prostate or prostatectomy.
4. *Nursing interventions*
   a. Encourage the person and his family to talk about their concerns regarding the possible effect that the transurethral resection of the prostate or prostatectomy may have on bodily functioning, such as incontinence, erectile dysfunction, and discharge associated with the urethral catheter.
   b. Instruct the person and his family what to expect postoperatively so that they are not anxious when the following expected conditions occur:

   (1) Placement of a urethral catheter with possible continuous bladder irrigation
   (2) Bloody urine in drainage bag
   (3) Bloody drainage around the urinary meatus
   (4) Large amount of drainage from incisions and drains
   (5) The presence of a suprapubic tube if the person had a suprapubic prostatectomy
   c. Explain preoperatively that some of the urinary symptoms that the person is experiencing may continue postoperatively due to surgical and instrument trauma and presence of a urethral catheter.
   d. Assure the person that his urinary pattern and control is usually regained during the 1st few months after the procedure.
   e. Implement the standard preoperative care plan.

> **NURSING DIAGNOSIS:** Risk for urinary retention R/T surgical edema and blocked drainage tubes

5. *Expected outcomes:* Following intervention, the person should not experience urinary retention or experiences resolution of urinary retention if it occurs.
6. *Nursing interventions*
   a. Keep urethral drainage tubing free of kinks, and keep the collection bag below bladder level.
   b. Tape the catheter securely to the person's abdomen or thigh to prevent inadvertent trauma or removal.
   c. Maintain continuous bladder irrigation with normal saline or perform intermittent catheter irrigations as needed.
   d. Notify physician if urinary retention is not relieved.

> **NURSING DIAGNOSIS:** Fluid volume excess R/T absorption of irrigating solution during surgery

7. *Expected outcomes:* Following intervention, the person should not experience fluid volume excess or water intoxication.
8. *Nursing interventions*

LEARNING/TEACHING GUIDELINES
for Discharge Instructions for Transurethral Resection of the Prostate or Prostatectomy

The cut area inside the body takes approximately 8 to 12 weeks to heal completely. Stresses and strains that put tension on the area and cause damage should be avoided.

1. The person may eat and drink normally, but use alcohol, caffeine, soft drinks, and spicy food in moderation. These can irritate the resected prostate gland.
2. The person should keep urine output flowing freely by drinking lots of fluids during the day, that is, 3 quarts of fluid, or approximately 12 8-ounce glasses. It is best to space fluid consumption during the day and not to drink after 8 P.M. to decrease the number of times the person gets up during the night.
3. The person should not strain during bowel movements and should take a stool softener.
4. During the first 2 to 3 weeks, the person should not drive, ride in a car for more than 20 to 25 minutes, walk more than one-half mile, climb stairs fast, lift more than 8 pounds, engage in sexual intercourse, or play sports.
5. If there is some blood in the urine, the person should go to bed, rest quietly, and drink more fluids. If the bleeding continues, the doctor should be contacted.
6. People with desk-type jobs can go back to work in 2 to 3 weeks. People with physical jobs must wait 4 weeks.
7. The doctor should be contacted if there is a sensation of fullness in the person's bladder after voiding. This may signal urinary retention.
8. Kegel exercises help the person regain sphincter control.
9. When the person leaves the hospital, an appointment should be made to be seen by the doctor 3 weeks subsequently.
10. The person should write down any questions to ask at the next visit.

a. Use normal saline rather than hypotonic solutions for bladder irrigations to decrease the risk of additional fluid absorption and water intoxication.
b. Do not increase frequency of bladder irrigations or speed up the rate of the continuous irrigation.

NURSING DIAGNOSIS: Altered urinary elimination R/T incontinence

9. *Expected outcomes:* Following instruction, the person should experience minimal urinary retention or regain urinary control quickly after surgery. Most men experience dribbling or temporary loss of urinary sphincter control after urethral instrumentation or prostatectomy.
10. *Nursing interventions*
   a. Reinforce the fact that these symptoms are usually temporary.
   b. Instruct the person on exercises that increase urinary control, such as Kegel or pelvic floor exercises.
   c. Instruct the person to drink most of his fluids during the day to decrease the possibility of nighttime incontinence.

Discharge Planning and Teaching

1. Before discharge, the man should be instructed about possible complications of treatment such as infection, dysuria, dribbling of urine, temporary loss of urine control, and sexual dysfunction (if he underwent a prostatectomy) (see Learning/Teaching Guidelines for Discharge Instructions for Transurethral Resection of the Prostate or Prostatectomy).
2. Unless there is a complication of surgery, the man should be discharged without a dressing or indwelling catheter.

Public Health Considerations

1. Because BPH is a disease of aging, an increasing number of men will experience symptoms.
2. More procedures will result in more morbidity and more health care dollars spent.
3. More research in pharmacologic treatment and noninvasive or localized therapies is needed.

ADENOCARCINOMA OF THE PROSTATE

Classification

1. Ninety-five percent of cancers of the prostate are adenocarcinomas.
2. The remaining 5 percent are nonepithelial carcinomas, such as ductal carcinomas, transitional cell carcinomas, squamous cell carcinomas, and sarcomas.

Incidence and Socioeconomic Impact

1. Prostate cancer is the most common cancer affecting men.
2. It is the 2nd leading cause of cancer deaths among men.

3. The incidence increases with age, affecting 1 of 10 men during his lifetime.
4. As the mean age of society increases, the incidence of cancer of the prostate will increase, necessitating that more health care dollars be spent on treatment for prostate cancer.

Risk Factors

1. Black race is a significant risk factor.

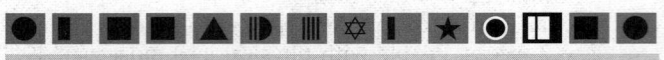

TRANSCULTURAL CONSIDERATIONS

Twice as many Black men as men of other races are diagnosed with prostate cancer.

2. Advanced age
   a. Prostate cancer is rare in men younger than 50 years of age.
   b. Eighty percent of cases are diagnosed in men older than 65.
   c. The average age at diagnosis is 73 years.
   d. Men with a positive family history for prostate cancer are at increased risk.

Etiology

1. The etiology is unknown.
2. Heredity and family history may play a role.

Pathophysiology

1. Prostate cancer occurs primarily in the periphery of the gland.
2. It is one of the slowest growing of all malignancies.
3. It metastasizes in a fairly predictable pattern. From the prostate gland it spreads to the following:
   a. The prostatic and perivesicular (surrounding the bladder) lymph nodes
   b. Regional pelvic lymph nodes
   c. Bone marrow
   d. Bones of the pelvis, sacrum, and lumbar spine
   e. Visceral organs (e.g., liver and lung) late in the course of the disease

Clinical Manifestations

1. Men with prostate cancer experience some of the same symptoms (prostatism) as men with BPH.
2. Painless hematuria is often found in persons with cancer of the prostate but is unusual in persons with BPH.

3. Prostate cancer can remain asymptomatic until metastasis occurs.
4. Bone pain in the lower back, pelvis, or upper thigh is usually a symptom of metastatic disease.

Diagnostics

1. Physical examination
   a. The DRE remains the standard screening examination for prostate cancer and is the most widely used. Findings that may indicate prostate cancer are a discrete hard nodule and a difference in consistency in 1 area of the gland.
   b. In the abdominal examination, the abdomen is palpated for the presence of any masses, and the liver is palpated for any evidence of enlargement.
   c. Inguinal, axillary, and cervical lymph nodes should be palpated for any evidence of swelling.
2. Laboratory studies
   a. Complete blood count
   b. Prostate-specific antigen levels, used in conjunction with DRE to diagnose prostate cancer. The PSA levels are also used as a tumor marker to monitor the progression of the disease or response to treatment.
   c. Serum alkaline phosphatase
   d. Serum acid phosphatase
3. Radiographic studies
   a. Chest radiograph
   b. Bone scan
   c. Transrectal ultrasound is used whenever the findings of the DRE or prostate-specific antigen tests are suspicious or abnormal.
4. Prostatic biopsies are done in an outpatient setting in conjunction with cystoscopy.
5. Transrectal ultrasound is used to isolate the area to be sampled.
6. Transrectal or transperineal biopsies are made using a coring type of needle.

Clinical Management

1. The goal of clinical management depends on the reason for the treatment. If the medical diagnosis is new and the cancer localized, the goal of treatment is cure. If the person has systemic disease, the goal of treatment may be to control the primary tumor or to relieve the person from symptoms of urinary retention or pain.
2. Factors that influence treatment selection
   a. The stage or extent of the cancer at the time of diagnosis
   b. The grade or aggressiveness of the tumor
   c. The person's age and medical condition
   d. The person's preference
3. Nonpharmacologic intervention
   a. Radical prostatectomy may be used with an abdominal or perineal approach. It involves complete removal of the prostate gland, seminal vesicles, and regional pelvic lymph nodes. Radical prostatectomy has a 50- to 90-percent chance of resulting in erectile dysfunction.

b. Transurethral resection of the prostate is used to remove tumor causing bladder neck obstruction. It does not remove the entire gland, only the tissue obstructing the urethra.

c. Bilateral orchiectomy is the surgical removal of the testicles (the major source of testosterone) and is used for management of metastatic disease.

d. The 2 types of radiation therapy used to treat localized tumors are external beam and interstitial implants. They are also used to treat bone metastasis. A possible result of radiation therapy is erectile dysfunction due to fibrosis of the pelvic arteries.

4. Pharmacologic intervention includes hormonal therapy. Because prostate cancer is dependent on testosterone for growth, blocking the binding of testosterone to its receptor sites can stop or slow the growth of the cancer. Endocrine therapy directly affects a person's sexuality by decreasing his libido or making an erection impossible. See Table 30–2 for a list of medications used for the treatment of prostate cancer.

Complications

1. Complications are the same as those for BPH, which also causes bladder neck obstruction.
2. The person may experience symptoms from the site of any metastatic disease.
3. Ten to 35 percent of affected persons have ureteral obstruction from local extension of the tumor.
4. The skeleton is the most common distant metastatic site.

Prognosis

1. Persons with localized prostate cancer, or cancer that has not spread outside of the gland, have a 91-percent 5-year survival rate.
2. The overall 5-year survival rate for prostate cancer is 76 percent.

Applying the Nursing Process

NURSING DIAGNOSIS: Ineffective individual or family coping R/T the diagnosis of cancer of the prostate

1. *Expected outcomes:* Following instruction and counseling, the person and family should demonstrate effective coping skills by verbalizing questions and concerns.
2. *Nursing interventions*
   a. Correct any knowledge deficits the person has about the cause of the disease, natural history of the disease, treatment options, and side effects.
   b. Involve the person's family in the management of the condition.
   c. Facilitate effective coping techniques by the person and his family. Some people equate the medical diagnosis of cancer with death.
   d. Establish a trusting relationship with the person.
   e. Encourage discussion of concerns and fears.
   f. Identify the person's own coping mechanisms and support systems.
   g. Provide the person with information about additional coping strategies.

NURSING DIAGNOSIS: Altered sexuality patterns or sexual dysfunction R/T prostate cancer and its treatment

3. *Expected outcomes:* Following instruction and counseling, the person and his partner should be able to adjust to the change in sexuality. Prostate cancer and its treatment can have definite impact on male sexuality potency. Even though this may have been explained and discussed in the pretreatment stage, experiencing a change in sexual ability can cause great anxiety. Table 30–3 lists hormonal therapy for metastatic prostate cancer.
4. *Nursing interventions*
   a. Investigate the meaning that sexuality has to the person before treatment.
   b. Plan with the person and his partner how to maintain sexual expression during and after treatment.
   c. Be aware of personal biases.
   d. Assist the person and his partner to investigate nontraditional expressions of sexuality.

Discharge Planning and Teaching

1. Before being discharged, the person and his family need to know the following:
   a. The natural history of prostate cancer
   b. The person's treatment plan
   c. The necessary surveillance follow-up studies
   d. Signs and symptoms of disease or treatment side effects that should be reported to the physician
2. The person should be given instructions on any self-care activities related to his treatment.

Public Health Considerations

1. Because the etiology of prostate cancer is unknown, the primary prevention is early detection.
2. American Cancer Society screening recommendations
   a. Every man should have annual DREs beginning at age 40 years.
   b. Men at high risk for prostate cancer (e.g., Black men or men with a first-degree relative with cancer of the prostate) should have a DRE and prostate specific antigen level drawn annually beginning at age 40 years.

Table 30–3. Hormonal Therapy for Metastatic Prostate Cancer

Medication	Advantages	Disadvantages	Side Effects
Estrogens (Diethylstilbestrol)	Agents may be orally administered. Side effects are reversible if treatment is discontinued within the first 2 years.	There is possible noncompliance due to side effects	Gynecomastia Edema Cardiovascular symptoms 　Myocardial infarction 　Hypertension 　Cerebrovascular accident Thrombophlebitis 　Pulmonary embolism Gastrointestinal symptoms 　Nausea/vomiting 　Abdominal cramping Erectile dysfunction Decreased libido
Luteinizing hormone–releasing agonists (leuprolide acetate, goserelin acetate)	Agents may be administered as a monthly injection.	Monthly office visits for injections.	Increased pain during the first 2 weeks of treatment Edema Hot flashes/sweats Anorexia Nausea/vomiting Erectile dysfunction
Anti-androgens (flutamide)	Agents may be orally administered. Agents may potentiate other hormonal therapies when used concomitantly.	Visits may not be covered by insurance.	Gynecomastia Diarrhea Erectile dysfunction

◼ PHYSIOLOGIC ERECTILE DYSFUNCTION

Definition

1. The term **erectile dysfunction** has replaced the term **impotence** to signify an inability to achieve an erection sufficient to permit intercourse, 25 percent of the time.
2. Erectile dysfunction is a component of the overall multifaceted process of male sexual function.

Incidence and Socioeconomic Impact

1. It is estimated that 10 to 20 million men in the United States have an erectile dysfunction.
2. Inclusion of men with partial erectile dysfunction increases the estimate to 30 million.
3. Erectile dysfunction is the leading complaint of men seeking help in sexual therapy clinics.
4. Fifty percent of men with erectile dysfunction have an underlying physical cause for their erectile disorder. Examples are the following:
   a. Vascular disease
   - Arteriosclerosis
   - Stroke
   - Hypertension
   - Decreased cardiac output
   - Abdominal aortic aneurysm
   b. Neurologic disease
   (1) Any disease affecting the brain, spinal cord, or peripheral nerves
   - Multiple sclerosis
   - Parkinson's disease
   - Amyotrophic lateral sclerosis
   - Alzheimer's disease
   (2) Any tumor, benign or malignant
   (3) Brain or spinal cord trauma
   c. Surgical procedures
   - Pelvic surgery
   - Prostate surgery
   - Perineal surgery
   - Vascular surgery
   d. Endocrine and metabolic disorders
   - Primary gonadal failure (hypergonadism and hypogonadism)
   - Thyroid disorders
   - Adrenal disorders
   - Diabetes mellitus
   e. Drug-induced effects
   - Antihypertensives
   - Psychotropic agents
   - Anticholinergic drugs
   - Commonly abused drugs, such as alcohol, cocaine, and marijuana
   - Sedatives and narcotics
   f. Other factors
   - Uremia
   - Dialysis
   - Pelvic radiation

Risk Factors

1. Age
   a. Five percent of men aged 40 years have an erectile dysfunction.
   b. Fifteen to 20 percent of men aged 65 years or older have an erectile dysfunction, but it is not necessarily a natural part of aging. It is usually the result of disease processes and pharmacotherapeutics that are more common in older persons.

ELDER ADVISORY

Erectile dysfunction is not an inevitable part of aging. It can be the symptom of many conditions, most of which can be treated. The patient should talk to his doctor if he is experiencing a problem with erections. The doctor may be able to help.

---

2. Approximately 50 percent of all men with diabetes mellitus also have an erectile dysfunction due to diabetic-associated neuropathies.

Etiology

1. Pathologic cause
   a. Because adequate arterial blood supply is needed for an erection, any disorder that impairs blood flow may play a role in causing an erectile dysfunction.
   b. Disorders that interfere with the corporal veno-occlusive mechanism result in a failure to trap blood in the penis. This causes an erection that cannot be maintained or is easily lost.
2. Iatrogenic cause
   a. Erectile dysfunction can be the result of treatment for another problem, such as the following:
      • Pelvic surgery
      • Prostatic surgery
      • Perineal surgery
      • Vascular surgery
   b. Drug-induced effects are caused by any agent that alters normal homeostasis through hormonal balance, somatic and autonomic neurotransmission, and vascular flow; or by medications such as antihypertensives, psychotropic agents, anticholinergic drugs, and substances of abuse, including alcohol.
3. Other causes
   • Uremia
   • Dialysis
   • Any chronic debilitating condition

Diagnostics

1. Sexual history
   a. The person's specific complaint distinguishes it from true erectile dysfunction, changes in sexual desire, and orgasmic or ejaculatory disturbances.
   b. The person should be specifically asked about the onset, frequency, quality, and duration of erections, the presence of nocturnal or morning erections, and the ability to achieve orgasm.
   c. Psychosocial factors, such as current sexual relationships, performance anxiety, and motivation for treatment, should be discussed.
   d. The man's partner should be included in discussion whenever possible.
2. Medical history
   a. The medical history is important in identifying specific organic causes that may contribute to or account for the person's erectile dysfunction.
   b. The review of systems includes
      (1) Vascular risk factors, such as hypertension, diabetes, smoking, and peripheral vascular disorders
      (2) Pelvic surgery or trauma
      (3) Neurologic causes, such as multiple sclerosis and alcoholism
      (4) Detailed medication and drug history, because approximately 25 percent of cases may be attributable to medications for other conditions
      (5) History of prior evaluation or treatment for erectile dysfunction
      (6) History of pelvic surgery, radiation therapy, pelvic or penile trauma, prostatitis, priapism, or any urinary problems
3. Physical examination
   a. An endocrine disorder may be indicated by changes in secondary male sex characteristics. Pubic, axillary, and facial hair should be assessed. Genital growth and development should be evaluated.
   b. Examination of the genitalia
      (1) Evaluate the size and consistency of the testes.
      (2) Palpate the shaft of the penis to determine the presence of fibrosis.
      (3) Perform a DRE of the prostate with assessment of anal sphincter tone.
      (4) Carry out sensation tests.
   c. The vascular examination
      (1) Note the presence of any bruits.
      (2) Take femoral and lower extremity pulses.
      (3) Note skin temperature, color, and hair distribution.
      (4) Perform an abdominal examination for possible abdominal aortic aneurysm.
   d. Neurologic examination focuses on deep tendon reflexes, perianal sensation, and bulbocavernosus reflex.
4. Laboratory studies
   a. Blood studies
      • Complete blood count
      • Fasting blood sugar
      • Creatinine
      • Testosterone
      • Prolactin
      • Luteinizing hormone
   b. Urinalysis
5. Other studies
   a. Doppler studies to assess blood flow in the penis
   b. Nocturnal penile tumescence
      (1) Men normally have 3 to 5 erections per night, each lasting 10 to 25 minutes.

(2) Various methods and devices are available to measure the presence of nocturnal erections.

Clinical Management

1. Goals of clinical management must be mutually set between the person and the health care provider.
   a. The person's partner must be included in the treatment plan.
   b. The goal of the treatment is to meet the person's need for sexual expression.
2. Nonpharmacologic management
   a. Through psychotherapy and counseling, attempts to decrease sexual anxieties are part of the treatment plan. Counseling alone is helpful to some men and their partners.
   b. The purpose of any medical treatment is to reverse any underlying conditions that contribute to erectile dysfunction. Adjustments may be made to the person's medication regimen, which may contribute to or cause the erectile dysfunction.
   c. Constrictive devices (e.g., vacuum devices, penile rings, Velcro bands) may be used to counteract the dysfunction.
   d. Surgical interventions
      (1) Vascular procedures, following which persons with erectile dysfunction secondary to arterial occlusion may have return of function after bypass surgery
      (2) Implantation of penile prostheses (i.e., semirigid, malleable, and inflatable). The complications and acceptability vary among the different types. Major complications are mechanical failure, infection, and erosion of penile skin (Fig. 30–5).
3. Pharmacologic management includes intracavernosal injection therapy, which is self-injection of medication, usually a combination of papaverine and phentolamine, directly into the corpora.

Applying the Nursing Process

NURSING DIAGNOSIS: Knowledge deficit R/T erectile dysfunction, its causes, and treatment options

1. *Expected outcomes:* Following instruction, the person and partner should be able to do the following:
   a. Demonstrate an understanding of erectile dysfunction by defining erectile dysfunction and explaining the difference between psychologic and physiologic impotence.
   b. Discuss the causes for the person's erectile dysfunction and select an appropriate treatment plan.
2. *Nursing interventions*
   a. Review the normal physiologic process responsible for erection.
   b. Discuss appropriate treatment options.
   c. Encourage the person and partner to ask questions so misconceptions can be addressed.

PENILE PROSTHESES

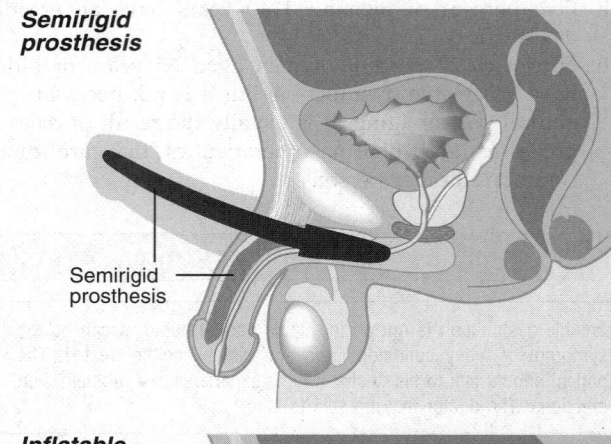

Semirigid prosthesis

Semirigid prosthesis

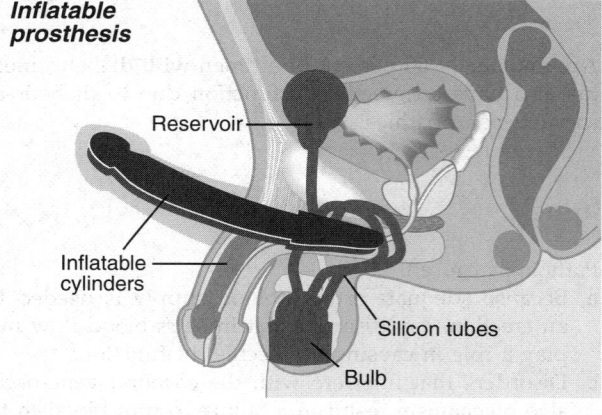

Inflatable prosthesis

Reservoir

Inflatable cylinders

Silicon tubes

Bulb

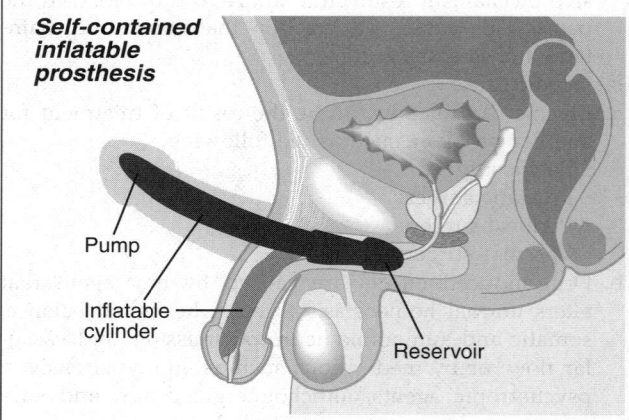

Self-contained inflatable prosthesis

Pump

Inflatable cylinder

Reservoir

Figure 30–5.

NURSING DIAGNOSIS: Altered sexuality patterns R/T erectile dysfunction

3. *Expected outcomes:* Following counseling, the person and partner should be able to do the following:
   a. Discuss the effects that erectile dysfunction has on the person's feelings of self-worth.

LEARNING/TEACHING GUIDELINES
for Discharge Instructions Following Penile Prosthesis Surgery

1. Stitches dissolve in approximately 2 weeks. The incision should heal completely in 3 to 4 weeks.
2. The person may shower or bathe the day after leaving the hospital.
3. There may be postoperative pain for several weeks after surgery. This is normal, and medication may be given to control the pain. There may also be pain temporarily as the prosthesis is inflated. This is also normal.
4. There is no need to wear a dressing, although it may be useful to keep the incision from rubbing on clothing and causing irritation.
5. Persons whose temperature exceeds 101 degrees Fahrenheit should contact their doctor or report to the closest emergency room.
6. Normal activity can be resumed, but without overdoing it. During the first 2 weeks, the person should avoid driving, car rides of longer than 30 minutes, climbing stairs more than once a day, lifting more than 8 pounds, or playing sports.
7. Persons should not have sexual intercourse until the doctor advises that it is safe to do so. Usually, intercourse is permitted 4 to 6 weeks after surgery.
8. After discharge, a follow-up visit should be scheduled. At that time, instruction on how to use the prosthesis is given.

b. Identify alternative expressions of sexuality besides intercourse.
c. Express feelings of comfort after experiencing different expressions of sexuality.
4. *Nursing interventions*
a. Support a positive self-image of the person regarding his male identity.
b. Provide privacy and opportunity for the person and his partner to discuss their feelings and concerns.
c. Assist the person and his partner to explore different means of expressing sexuality via oral stimulation, sexual devices, and manual stimulation.

Discharge Planning and Teaching

1. Unless the person undergoes surgery for the placement of a penile prosthesis, he will be managed in an ambulatory setting.
2. Provide appropriate instruction for the person's plan of care (i.e., instructions on devices or self-injections).
3. If the person has undergone a penile prosthesis placement, he will need to be given home care instruction regarding his specific prosthesis (Learning/Teaching Guidelines for Discharge Instruction Following Penile Prosthesis Surgery).

◼ *MALE FERTILITY AND INFERTILITY*

Male Fertility

1. Male fertility is defined as the ability to produce offspring within 1 year of unprotected sexual intercourse.
2. Male fertility is assessed through a semen analysis. This analysis is made on an ejaculated sample of semen and includes the following measures:
a. Spermatocyte count
b. Rating of the percent of sperm that are motile
c. Fluid volume
d. Fluid pH
3. Interventions
a. Nonsurgical interventions include a wide variety of birth control methods available for controlling male fertility. See Chapter 14.
b. Surgical interventions include vasectomy, which is an elective procedure for a man who wants a permanent method of contraception. A small incision is made in the scrotal skin, the vas is brought out through the incision and resected, the ends are ligated, and the incision is sutured. The person is instructed to resume intercourse when comfortable but to continue using contraception until a postprocedure spermatozoa analysis reveals azoospermia.

Male Infertility

1. Male infertility is defined as the inability to father a child after 1 year of unprotected sexual intercourse.
2. Incidence and socioeconomic impact
a. Approximately 15 to 20 percent of couples have difficulty achieving pregnancy by the end of 1 year of unprotected sexual intercourse.
b. A male infertility factor alone is found in approximately 30 percent of couples, and both a male and female factor is found in an additional 20 percent of infertility problems.
3. Risk factors
a. Cryptorchid or undescended testicle should be corrected before a child is 2 years old.
b. Infectious processes can destroy testicular tissue.
c. There is no known cause in 10 to 20 percent of infertility cases.
4. Etiology
a. Endocrine abnormalities include hypothalamic disease and pituitary disease.
b. Semen abnormalities
• Azoospermia (absence of spermatozoa)

- Oligospermia (decreased number of spermatozoa)
- Decreased spermatozoa motility
  c. Spermatozoa transport disorders
  - Congenital hypoplasia or absence of reproductive pathways
  - Congenital abnormalities in seminal vesicles or vas deferens
  - Ejaculatory duct obstruction (bilateral)
  - Scarring or obstruction of the vas from bacterial infections
  - Scrotal abnormalities (abnormal or arrested spermatogenesis in the testicle)
  - Other causes, including damage to the sympathetic nervous system from surgical trauma, diabetes, or spinal cord lesions; effects of pharmacologic agents; surgical procedures resulting in retrograde ejaculations; and infections
  d. Disorders of spermatozoa function or motility
  - Immotile cilia syndrome
  - Maturation defects
  - Immunologic defects
  - *Escherichia coli* semen infection
5. Diagnostics
  a. History should include questions regarding the following:
  - Childhood illnesses, specifically cryptorchidism, postpubertal mumps orchitis, and history of testicular pain or trauma
  - Puberty
  - Exposure to occupational or environmental chemicals or toxins, such as pesticides, heat from hot tubs or saunas, and exposure to radiation
  b. Drug and medication history should include use or receipt of the following:
  - Cancer chemotherapy
  - Anabolic steroids
  - Cimetidine
  - Spironolactone
  - Marijuana
  - Cocaine
  - Alcohol
  c. Surgical history should include details of the following:
  - Prostate surgery
  - Retroperitoneal surgery
  - Bladder neck surgery
  d. History of sexual habits should include details of the following:
  - Frequency of intercourse
  - Frequency of ejaculation
  - Use of lubricants
  - Knowledge of ovulation
  e. Physical examination
  (1) The person should be examined for signs and symptoms of hypogonadism and poorly developed secondary sex characteristics.
  (2) The scrotum and testes should be examined for symmetry, size, swellings, lumps, pain, or tenderness.
  (3) The person should be examined for any evidence of gynecomastia.

f. Laboratory studies include the following:
  - Fasting blood sugar
  - Serum testosterone levels
  - Semen analysis
6. Clinical management
  a. Nonpharmacologic interventions
  (1) Varicocelectomy is the most common urologic surgical procedure related to infertility. It improves semen quality in 70 percent of men.
  (2) Vasovasotomy is vasectomy reversal.
  (3) Orchidopexy is the surgical placement of a testicle into the scrotum.
  b. Pharmacologic interventions
  (1) Endocrine therapy replaces or adjusts hormone levels.
  (2) Immunologic therapy includes the use of corticosteroids to abort or modulate the production of antibodies.
  c. Special medical-surgical procedures are assisted reproductive techniques that include artificial insemination, semen processing, intrauterine insemination, and in vitro fertilization.
7. Complications related to the treatment of infertility are related to the method of treatment. Each method has its own rate of complication and success in achieving pregnancy.
8. In determining prognosis, the longer the period of infertility, the less likely the chance of successful treatment and pregnancy.
9. Applying the nursing process

NURSING DIAGNOSIS: Powerlessness R/T the diagnosis of infertility and the treatment

a. *Expected outcomes:* Following instruction and support, the person and his partner should be able to do the following:
  (1) Verbalize a sense of control over feelings associated with infertility
  (2) Discuss appropriate treatment options and select a treatment plan
b. *Nursing interventions*
  (1) Encourage the person and partner to talk about their feelings about infertility.
  (2) Maintain active communication with the person and partner during the diagnostic testing. This can be a stressful time for the couple.
  (3) Provide information concerning diagnostic testing and treatment options.

■ *TESTICULAR CANCER*

Classification

1. Most testicular tumors are malignant and are of germ cell origin (90–95%). They comprise the group of tumors called germinal tumors.

a. Seminoma is the most common type (occurring in 40% of cases).

b. Nonseminomatous tumors include embryonal tumors (20–25% of cases), teratomas (20–25% of cases), and choriocarcinomas (1% of cases).

c. Mixed tissue type tumors include teratocarcinomas (20–25% of cases).

Incidence and Socioeconomic Impact

1. There are 2 to 3 cases in 100,000 men, or approximately 7000 new cases per year in the United States.
2. Testicular cancer is the most common solid tumor found in young men aged 15 to 35 years.
3. It affects men most frequently during their early adult years, but it can occur at any time.

Risk Factors

1. History of cryptorchid or undescended testis increases risk by 40 times.
2. The disease is most common in White males.
3. The most common age at diagnosis is 15 to 35 years.

Etiology

1. The etiology is unknown.
2. In the case of a cryptorchid testicle, it is thought that the testicle involutes over time, giving rise to a malignant process.

Pathophysiology

1. Testicular cancer metastasizes mainly through the lymphatic system.
2. The lymph nodes of the retroperitoneum are the most common metastatic sites.
3. Visceral metastasis occurs late in the course of the disease.

Clinical Manifestations

1. The first sign of disease is the presence of a small, hard, painless lump in the testicle or a painless enlargement of the testis.
2. Other symptoms include a sensation of heaviness in the testicle or scrotum or sudden accumulation of fluid in the scrotum.
3. Approximately 10 percent of persons have symptoms of metastatic disease at the time of diagnosis.
   a. Testicular cancers are rapidly dividing cancers.
   b. The average time lapse from when the person finds the lump and evaluation by a health care professional is 2 to 5 months.
   c. The most common metastatic symptom is back pain.
   d. Other symptoms include cough or dyspnea and gas-

trointestinal symptoms such as anorexia, nausea, and vomiting.

Diagnostics

1. Physical assessment
   a. A testicular mass or diffuse enlargement that does not transluminate should be suspected as a malignancy.
   b. There may be gynecomastia or breast enlargement.
   c. Palpation of the abdomen may reveal retroperitoneal disease.
   d. Palpation may reveal scalene, supraclavicular, or inguinal lymph node enlargement.
   e. Epididymitis is the most common misdiagnosis in men with testicular cancer.
2. Laboratory studies
   a. Tumor markers
      (1) Serum tumor markers are useful in the cancer diagnosis and staging, and in the monitoring of the treatment response.
      (2) Human chorionic gonadotropin and α-fetoprotein are also useful markers.
   b. Radiographic and imaging studies
      (1) Ultrasound of the testis is done to evaluate the density of the testicle to determine whether it is filled with solid tissue or fluid.
      (2) A chest radiograph is obtained to evaluate for any evidence of metastatic disease in the lungs.
      (3) Computed tomography scans of the abdomen and chest are done to evaluate for any evidence of metastatic disease in the lungs.
   c. A radical orchiectomy through an inguinal incision is the biopsy procedure for testicular cancer.

Prognosis

1. The prognosis of testicular cancer is directly related to the stage or extent of disease at the time of diagnosis.
2. The cure rate of early stage testicular tumor is 90 percent.

Clinical Management

1. Nonpharmacologic management
   a. Surgery
      (1) **Radical orchiectomy** is performed on all persons at the time of diagnosis. It includes the removal of the testis, epididymis, a portion of the vas deferens, and the gonadal lymphatics.
      (2) **Retroperitoneal lymph node dissection** is the surgical removal of the lymph nodes deep in the retroperitoneum. All nodal tissue between the ureters from the renal vessels to the bifurcation of the common iliac vessels is removed.
   b. Radiation therapy
      (1) External beam radiation therapy to the retroperitoneal lymph nodes is the primary treatment for seminomatous testicular cancer.

(2) A lead cup is used to shield the remaining testicle.
2. Pharmacologic management
   a. Chemotherapy may be used before retroperitoneal lymph node dissection or after, depending on the findings of the surgery.
   b. The standard chemotherapy regimen is a combination of cisplatin, vinblastine, and bleomycin (PVB).

Applying the Nursing Process

> **NURSING DIAGNOSIS:** Knowledge deficit R/T testicular cancer and its treatment

1. *Expected outcomes:* Following instruction, the person and family should be able to do the following:
   a. Discuss testicular cancer, the cause, natural history, and treatment options based on correct information
   b. Identify the effects that testicular cancer and its treatment have on the person's sexuality
   c. Identify alternative methods of meeting reproductive needs
2. *Nursing interventions*
   a. Clarify any misconceptions that the person and family have regarding testicular cancer. Young men may believe that testicular cancer is related to sexual activity or is a punishment for sexual activity.
   b. Provide the person and his family with correct information about the cause of testicular cancer. Most men with testicular cancer are already oligospermic or aspermic at the time of diagnosis.
   c. Provide the person with information about the different interventions that are used to treat testicular cancer.
   d. Reinforce that, because the person has a remaining functioning testicle, he will be able to achieve an erection and orgasm.
   e. Encourage the person to verbalize his concerns related to his sexuality and reproductive capability.
   f. Explore options with the person and his family to meet his reproductive needs, such as sperm banking, donor insemination, and adoption.

Discharge Planning and Teaching

1. Discuss the ability of the remaining testis to compensate for loss of 1 testis.
2. Provide information about sperm banking.
3. Stress the importance of follow-up surveillance studies.
4. Discuss the pros and cons of a silicone testicular implant to restore normal appearance or body image.

Public Health Considerations

1. Primary prevention is by educating pediatric nurses and parents about the importance of correcting cryptorchid testicles as soon as possible (before age 2 years).
2. Early detection
   a. Testicular self-examination can detect cancer early (Box 30–1).

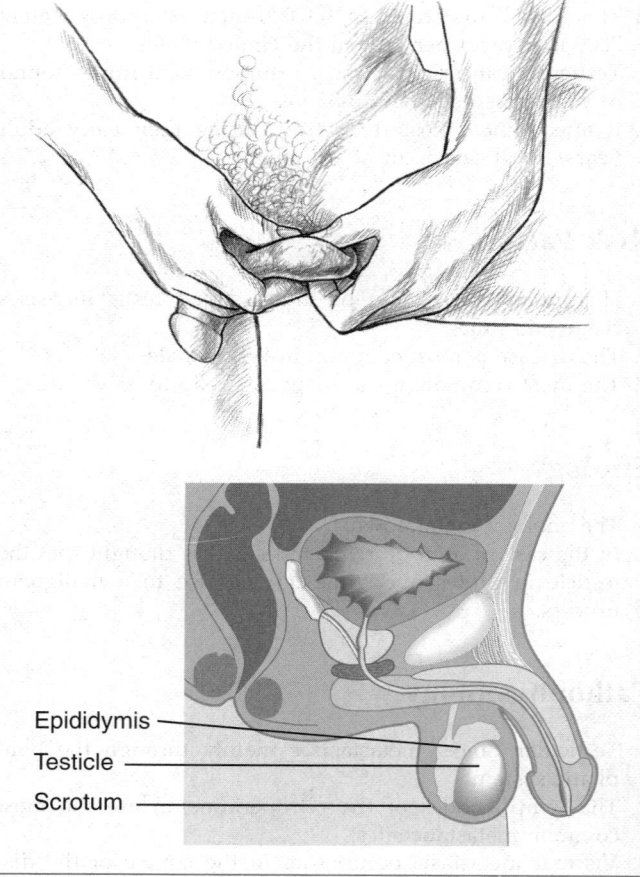

BOX 30–1. Testicular Self-Exam (TSE)

1. Every man should perform TSE monthly. The best time is right after a bath or shower. This is when the scrotal skin is most relaxed and the testicles are easy to feel.
2. Examine each testicle by gently rolling it between the thumbs and fingers. The index and middle fingers should be on the underside of each testicle and the thumbs on the top.
3. Report any lumps or swellings to your doctor. A normal testicle is shaped like an egg and is about 4 cm (1 5/8 inches) long. It feels firm but not hard and is smooth with no lumps.

Epididymis

Testicle

Scrotum

b. Emphasize during teaching that any abnormal lump, swelling, or mass should be evaluated as soon as possible by a health care provider to prevent any delays in treatment.

■ DISORDERS OF THE PENIS

Carcinoma of the Penis

1. Incidence is less than 1 percent of all malignancies in men in the United States and 12 percent in countries where circumcision is not practiced.
2. Clinical manifestations are a painless wartlike growth or ulcer on the glans under the prepuce (foreskin). The lesion may appear reddened with plaque.
3. Clinical management
   a. Surgical management

Table 30-4. Other Disorders of the Penis

Disorder	Etiology	Clinical Manifestations	Management
Phimosis	A constricted foreskin that cannot be retracted over the glans penis	May interfere with intercourse. Unable to clean under the foreskin.	Antibiotics, if infection is suspected. Warm soaks. Circumcision (surgical removal of the foreskin)
Paraphimosis	The foreskin is retracted behind the glans so that it cannot return to its normal position	Compression of dorsal veins and lymphatics of the distal penis, causing edema and pain in the glans	Manual reduction of the foreskin over the glans after pushing edematous fluid out of the glans. Circumcision may be done to prevent recurrence

    (1) Excisional biopsy
    (2) Penectomy (partial or total removal of the penis, depending on the extent of the tumor)
  b. Most penile cancers are squamous cell cancers and are treatable with radiation therapy.

Priapism

1. Priapism is defined as an uncontrolled and long-maintained erection without sexual desire.
2. Causes
  a. Neurologic causes include spinal cord injury that results in inappropriate stimulus of nerves, causing erections.
  b. Vascular causes include the following:
    • Thrombosis of the veins of the corpora cavernosa
    • Leukemia
    • Sickle cell anemia
  c. Pharmacologic causes include use of the following:
    • Psychotropic medications
    • Antidepressants
    • Antihypertensives
3. Clinical manifestations
  a. The penis becomes large, hard, and painful.
  b. The 2 corpora cavernosa are affected; the corpus spongiosum is not affected.
  c. Priapism is considered a urologic emergency because blood flow to the penis may be compromised.
  d. The person may be unable to void.
4. Clinical management
  a. Conservative measures include prostatic massage, sedation with meperidine, warm enemas, and urinary catheterization.
  b. Aspiration or irrigation of the corpora cavernosa with a large-bore needle is used to evacuate sludged blood.
  c. Blood can be surgically diverted from the corpora.

Other Disorders of the Penis

Refer to Table 30-4.

◼ INFECTIONS

Prostatitis

1. Prostatitis is an inflammation of the prostate gland. It may be the result of a variety of pathogens.
2. Abacterial prostatitis occurs after a viral illness or can occur after a decrease in sexual activity. It is also seen in men with occupations that involve long hours of sitting, delayed urination, and vibration such as in truck drivers or heavy equipment operators.
3. Bacterial prostatitis is associated with urethritis or urinary tract infections. Most common causative organisms are gram-negative such as *E. coli*, *Proteus*, and group D streptococci.
4. Chronic prostatitis is a long-term problem, sometimes necessitating up to 6 months of antibiotic therapy.
5. Clinical manifestations
  a. The prostate becomes edematous and tender.
  b. Abscesses may form.
  c. The person experiences perineal pain and irritation in voiding.
6. Clinical management
  a. The following are methods to facilitate drainage of the prostate:

Table 30–5. Disorders of the Testes

Disorder	Etiology	Clinical Manifestations	Management
Hydrocele	The result of a lymphatic disorder in the drainage of the scrotum	A cystic mass in the scrotum, usually filled with straw-colored fluid	1. Aspiration 2. Hydrocelectomy (surgical removal)
Spermatocele	A sperm-containing cyst	A cystic mass in the scrotum, which develops on the epididymis along the side of the testicle	Spermatocelectomy (surgical removal)
Varicocele	A cluster of dilated veins posterior to and above the testis	Scrotum feels like a "bag of worms" during palpation, usually on the left side. Have the person perform a Valsalva maneuver.	Varicocelectomy (surgical removal)
Torsion	Twisting of the spermatic cord. May occur after strenuous exercise or trauma, or may be spontaneous	Acute pain. Prolonged torsion of the spermatic cord results in tissue death in the testicle.	Unilateral orchlectomy (surgical removal of the testicle)

- Intercourse
- Masturbation
- Prostatic massage

b. The person should be instructed to use a condom when engaging in sexual activity with a partner.

Epididymitis

1. Definition
   a. Inflammation of the epididymis may be the result of a sexually transmitted disease such as gonorrhea or infection with *Chlamydia trachomatis.*
   b. The route of infection is usually along the vas deferens, from an infection in the urethra, prostate, or bladder.
   c. Inflammation may be the result of a long-term indwelling urinary catheter.
2. Epididymitis is the most common intrascrotal infection.
3. Clinical manifestations
   a. Early localized pain and edema
   b. Hemiscrotal erythema and pain

4. Clinical management
   a. Use of antibiotics
   b. Application of ice packs intermittently for the 1st 24 hours
   c. Bed rest with the scrotum elevated with a rolled towel
   d. Use of sitz baths
   e. Abstinence from sexual activity without a condom until the infection is resolved
   f. Use of a scrotal support
   g. If no improvement after 2 weeks of treatment (antibiotics and other measures), evaluation for testicular tumor
   h. Vasectomy for chronic infections secondary to long-term urinary catheter use

Orchitis

1. Definition
   a. Orchitis is testicular inflammation from either infection or trauma.
   b. Epididymis is usually involved (epididymo-orchitis).
2. Clinical manifestations
   a. There is direct spread of bacteria from other structures in the testicle.
   b. There is spread of bacteria from elsewhere in the body during pneumonia, tuberculosis, gonorrhea, syphilis, and mumps.

   c. There is scrotal edema and pain.
3. Interventions are the same as for epididymitis:
   • Bed rest with scrotal elevation
   • Application of ice
   • Use of antibiotics

Urethritis

1. Urethritis is inflammation of the urethra.
2. Clinical manifestations
   a. Urethritis causes frequency, nocturia, and burning on urination.
   b. Urethral discharge is usually present.
   c. A pathogen is usually involved.
      (1) Gonococcal urethritis is from infection with *Neisseria gonorrhoeae*.
      (2) Nongonococcal urethritis is from infection with *C. trachomatis*.
   d. Nonbacterial urethritis occurs with inflammation but no infection.
3. Clinical management includes administration of the proper antibiotic for the specific infection. (See Chapter 32.)

Other Disorders of the Testes

Refer to Table 30–5.

Bibliography

Books

American Cancer Society. *Cancer Facts and Figures—1994*. Atlanta: Author, 1994.
American Joint Committee on Cancer. *Manual for Staging of Cancer*. 4th ed. Philadelphia: JB Lippincott, 1992.
Belcher A. *Cancer Nursing*. St Louis: Mosby–Year Book, 1992.
Karlowitz KA (ed.) *Urologic Nursing Principles and Practice*. Philadelphia: WB Saunders, 1995.
Otto S. *Oncology Nursing*. St Louis: CV Mosby, 1995

Chapters in Books and Journal Articles

Cancers of the Male Reproductive Organs

Dixon D, and Moore RA. Tumors of the male sex organs. *In Atlas of Tumor Pathology* (fascicle 31b:32, series 1). Washington, DC: Armed Forces Institute of Pathology, 1952.
Flannery M. Reproductive cancers. *In* Clark JC, and McGee RF (eds). *Core Curriculum for Oncology Nursing*. 2nd ed. Philadelphia: WB Saunders, 1990.

Cancer Screening

Coyne CL. Early screening programs for prostate cancer. *Innovations Urol Nurs* 11(4):24–27, 1991.

Moore S, et al. Screening for prostate cancer: PSA, blood test, rectal examination, and ultrasound. *Urol Nurs* 12(3):106–107, 1992.

Early Detection

Friman PC, and Finney JW. Health education for testicular cancer. *Health Educ Q* 17(4):443–453, 1990.
Littrup J, Goodman AC, and Mettlin CJ. The benefit and cost of prostate cancer early detection. *CA Cancer J Clin* 44(3):134–149, 1993.
Murphy G. Report on the American Urologic Association/American Cancer Society Scientific Seminar on the Detection and Treatment of Early-Stage Prostate Cancer. *CA Cancer J Clin* 44(2):91–95, 1994.
Richie JP. Detection and treatment of testicular cancer. *CA Cancer J Clin* 43(3):151–175, 1993.
Willson P. Testicular, prostate and penile cancers in primary care settings: The importance of early detection. *Nurs Pract* 16(11):18–26, 1991.

Sexual Function

Costabile R. The effects of cancer and cancer therapy on male reproductive function. *J Urol* 149:1327–1330, 1993.
Jones K. Interventions for male clients

with reproductive problems. *In* Ignatavicius DD, Workman ML, and Mishler MA (eds). *Medical-Surgical Nursing: A Nursing Process Approach*. 2nd ed. Philadelphia: WB Saunders, 1995.
Kaiser F. Sexual function and the older cancer patient. *Oncology* 6(2):112–118, 1992.
Waxman E. Sexual dysfunction following treatment for prostate cancer: nursing assessment and interventions. *Oncol Nurs Forum* 20(10):1567–1571, 1993.

Benign Prostate Hyperplasia

Moore S, et al. Nerve-sparing prostatectomy. *Am J Nurs* 92(4):59–64, 1992.
Wozniak-Petrofsky J. BPH: Treating older men's most common problem. *RN* 54(7):31–37, 1991.

Erectile Dysfunction

Buczy B. Impotence in older men: A newly recognized problem. *J Gerontol Nurs* 18(5):25–30, 1992.

Other Problems Affecting Male Sex Organs

Kaker SR. Epididymitis in the young adult male. *Nurs Pract* 15(5):10–18, 1990.

Agencies and Resources

American Board of Urologic Allied Health
Professionals
407 Strawberry Hill Avenue
Stamford, CT 06902
(203) 323–1227

American Cancer Society
1599 Clifton Road NE
Atlanta, GA 30329
(404) 320–3333

American Fertility Society
1608 13th Avenue South
Suite 101
Birmingham, AL 35205
(205) 933–8494

Impotence Anonymous
P.O. Box 1257
Maryville, TN 37802
(615) 983–6064

OURS
(Organization for a United Response)
3148 Humbolt Avenue South
Minneapolis, MN 55408
(612) 827–5709

RESOLVE
P.O. Box 474
Belmont, MA 02178
(617) 484–2424

31
Caring for Women with Sexual and Reproductive System Disorders

◼ FEMALE REPRODUCTIVE STRUCTURE AND FUNCTION

Structure of the Female Reproductive System

1. The female reproductive system consists of external structures that extend from the pubis to the perineum and internal organs that are located in the pelvic cavity.
2. The external structures, or **vulva,** consist of the mons pubis, labia majora, labia minora, clitoris, vestibule, fourchette, perineum, and various glandular structures (Fig. 31–1).
   a. Mons pubis. The **mons pubis,** or **mons veneris,** is a fatty pad of tissue that covers the symphysis pubis. During puberty, the mons becomes prominent and covered with coarse, curly hair. The mons pubis protects the symphysis pubis and provides traction during coitus.
   b. Labia majora
      (1) The **labia majora** are 2 skin-covered vertical folds of fatty tissue that extend from the mons downward to the perineum. They protect the inner vulvar surfaces and enhance sexual arousal.
      (2) The labia majora become prominent during puberty. Hair develops on the outer surfaces of the labia, but the inner surfaces stay smooth. The labia contain sebaceous glands and are highly vascular.
   c. Labia minora
      (1) The **labia minora** are 2 thin vertical folds of reddish tissue located between the labia majora. They extend downward from beneath the clitoris to the fourchette. The labia minora have a rich nerve supply, are highly vascular, and contain many sebaceous glands, which lubricate the vaginal entrance. The tissues of the labia minora join above the clitoris, then branch to form the prepuce (a hoodlike covering over the clitoris) and the frenulum (a transverse fold of tissue beneath the clitoris).
      (2) The **fourchette** consists of thin, flat tissue and is formed by the joining of the labia minora in the midline below the vaginal opening.
   d. Clitoris
      (1) The **clitoris** is a short cylindric structure located beneath the arch of the pubis, between the prepuce and frenulum.
      (2) The clitoris consists of erectile tissue (comparable to that in the male penis) and many extremely sensitive sensory nerve endings. Clitoral stimulation is important in sexual arousal.
   e. Vestibule
      (1) The **vestibule** is an oval area located between the labia minora and clitoris and the fourchette. The vestibule contains openings to the urethra, Skene's glands, the vagina, and Bartholin's glands.
      (2) The **hymen** is a thin, elastic, membranous tissue that can partially or totally cover the vaginal opening in the vestibule.
      (3) **Skene's,** or **paraurethral, glands** are multiple tiny (0.5 cm diameter) organs located on each side of the urethral meatus. They are usually not visible.
      (4) **Bartholin's,** or **vestibular, glands** (0.5–1.0 cm diameter), are located on each side of the vaginal opening at the base of the labia majora. They are usually not visible.
      (5) **Skene's glands** and **Bartholin's glands** of the vestibule also lubricate the vaginal entrance during sexual arousal.
   f. Perineum
      (1) The **perineum** is the skin-covered muscular area between the fourchette and the anus that covers the pelvic structures.
      (2) Muscles, fascia, and ligaments that support the pelvic organs are anchored in the perineal body (see Fig. 31–1).
3. The internal reproductive structures are the uterus, fallopian tubes, ovaries, and vagina (see Fig. 31–1).
   a. Uterus
      (1) The **uterus** is a pear-shaped, flat, hollow organ approximately 7.5 × 5.0 × 2.5 cm in size. It is attached to the upper end of the vagina and is located in the true pelvis between the bladder and

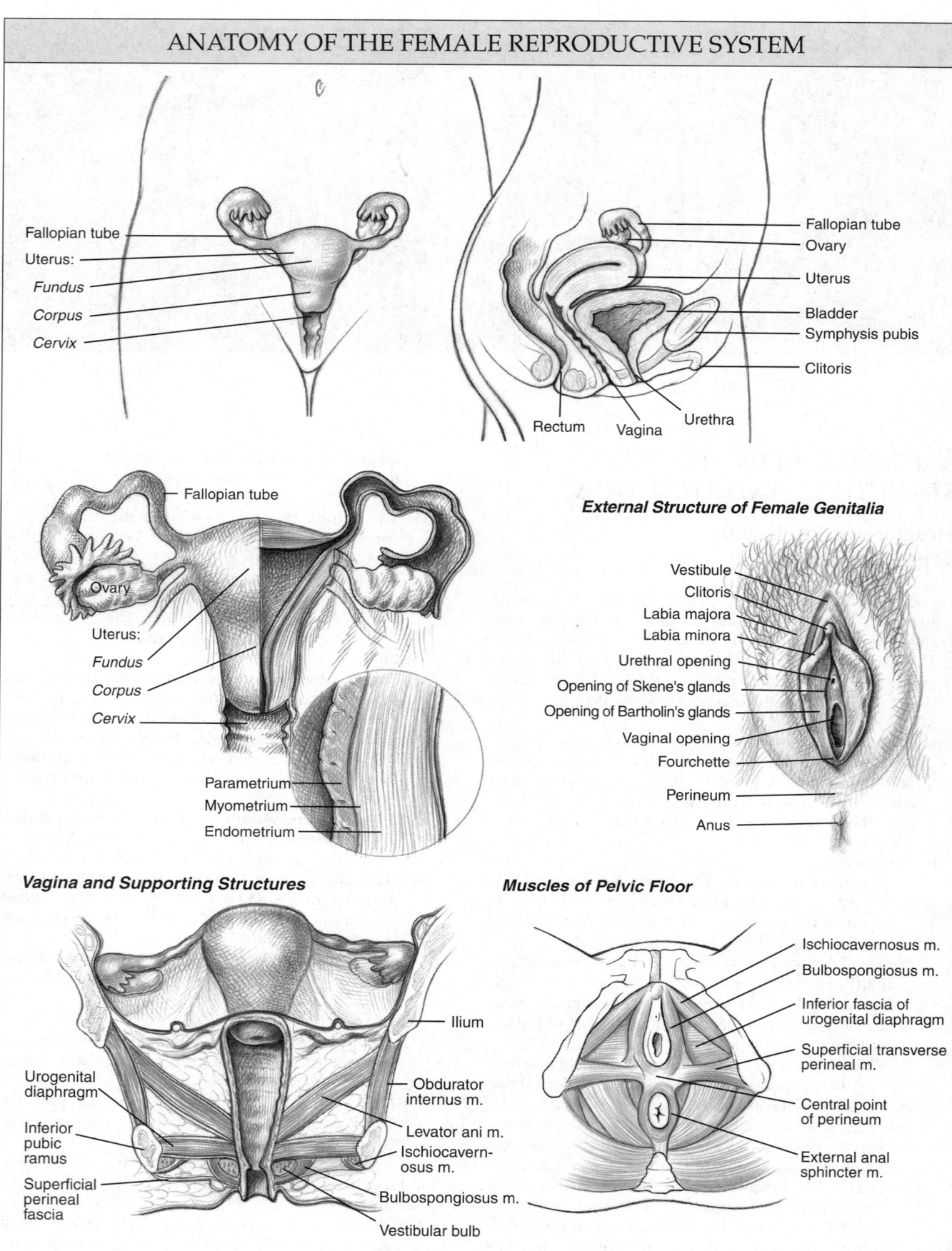

Figure 31–1.

rectum. The uterus is an organ of menstruation. It also receives, nurtures, and expels the products of conception.

(2) The uterus is a relatively mobile organ. Although normally it is anteverted (tipped forward) and slightly anteflexed (bent forward), it can also be retroverted or retroflexed (Fig. 31–2).

(3) The uterus has 2 main parts: the upper triangular portion, called the corpus, or body, and the lower cylindrical portion, called the cervix. The **fundus** is the upper portion of the corpus, into which the fallopian tubes insert. The **isthmus** (also called the **lower uterine segment**) is a constricted region that separates the corpus from the cervix. The uterus is supported by 4 pairs of ligaments: cardinal, uterosacral, round, and broad (see Fig. 31–1). The **rectouterine pouch,** or cul-de-sac of Douglas, is a deep recess posterior to the uterus.

(4) The **cervix** is approximately 2.5 cm long and is composed of fibrous connective and elastic tissue and muscles. It connects the uterine cavity to the vagina through the endocervical canal (canal inside the cervix). The **internal os** is the narrow opening between the uterine cavity and the endocervical canal. The external os is the opening that extends from the cervix to the vagina. Its shape ranges from oval in nulliparous women to an irregular transverse slit in women who have borne children. The **endocervical canal** is lined with columnar epithelium and covered with squamous epithelium. The site where the two types of epithelium meet is called the **squamocolumnar junction.** The recesses around the part of the cervix that protrudes into the vagina are called fornices.

(5) The uterine walls have three layers: the parametrium, or outer layer; the myometrium, or middle layer; and the endometrium, or inner layer (see Fig. 31–1). The **myometrium** is made up of 3

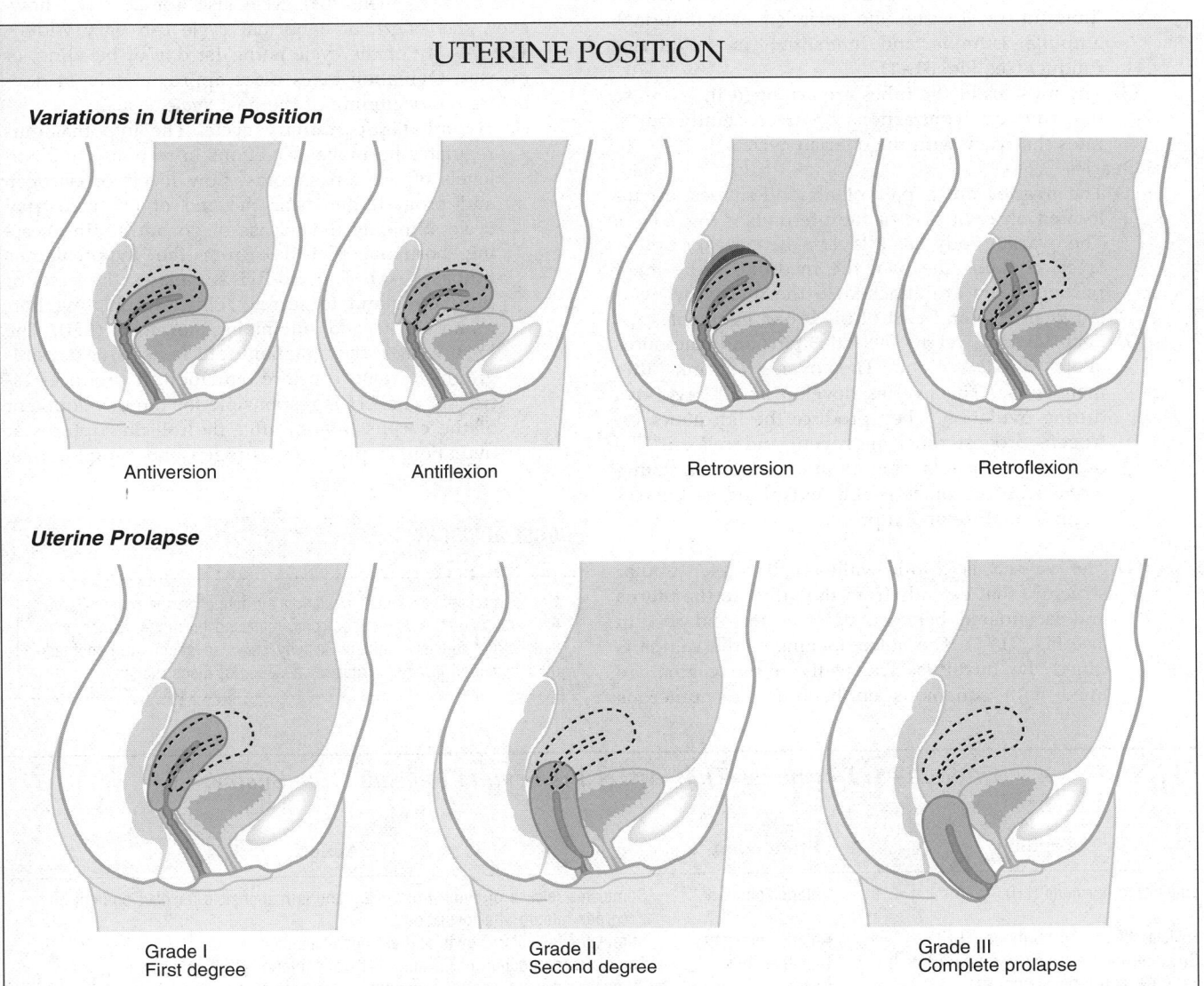

UTERINE POSITION

Variations in Uterine Position

Antiversion Antiflexion Retroversion Retroflexion

Uterine Prolapse

Grade I First degree Grade II Second degree Grade III Complete prolapse

Figure 31–2.

layers of muscle fibers arranged in opposing directions and interlaced with blood vessels. The **endometrium** also has 3 layers: a compact surface layer, a spongy middle layer, and a dense inner layer that connects the endometrium with the myometrium.

b. Fallopian tubes
   (1) The 2 **fallopian,** or **uterine, tubes** are attached to the uterine fundus and extend laterally to a site near the ovaries. Each tube is approximately 10 cm long and 0.6 cm in diameter. The opening has the same diameter as a pencil lead. Each tube is covered in peritoneum and lined with a mucous membrane of ciliated and secretory columnar cells that produce a current flowing toward the uterine cavity. The fallopian tubes serve as passageways between the ovaries and uterus for the ova. They are also the site of fertilization of an ovum by a sperm.
   (2) The fallopian tubes have 4 distinct sections: infundibulum (most distal and encircled with fimbriae), ampulla, isthmus, and interstitial (in the uterine fundus) (see Fig. 31–1).
   (3) The muscles of the tubes are arranged in layers so that rhythmic contractions occur constantly but at rates that vary with the ovarian cycle.

c. Ovaries
   (1) The **ovaries** are a pair of almond-shaped organs located on each side of the uterus (see Fig. 31–1). The ovarian body has 2 layers: the cortex, or outer layer, contains the ova; the medulla is the inner portion. They are attached to the uterus by ovarian ligaments and part of the broad ligament.
   (2) Each ovary weighs about 3 gm and measures about 3 × 2 × 1 cm. The ovaries shrink after menopause. The ovaries develop and release ova during ovulation. They produce the hormones estrogen, progesterone, androgen, and relaxin. The ovarian surface is smooth and white in young women but becomes rough and pitted as follicles begin to mature and rupture.

d. Vagina
   (1) The **vagina** is a thin-walled collapsible tubular structure that extends from the vulva to the uterus and is situated between the bladder and rectum (see Fig. 31–1). The outer opening of the vagina is called the **introitus.** The walls of the vagina are lined with squamous epithelium and numerous blood vessels. During the reproductive years, the walls are arranged in transverse folds called **rugae** that allow for expansion.
   (2) The vagina has minimal nerve supply and is relatively insensitive. It is a receptacle for the penis during intercourse. It also functions as the passageway for menstrual flow and the birth canal.

Functions of the Female Reproductive System

1. Menstruation and climacterium
   a. **Menarche** is the first menstrual period. It normally occurs between ages 10 and 16 years.
   b. **Menstruation** is the cyclic shedding of the endometrium by the uterus. It is controlled by a feedback system of 3 cycles: the hypothalamic-pituitary cycle, the ovarian cycle, and the uterine (endometrial) cycle. The average menstrual cycle lasts for 28 days; however, the length of a normal cycle can vary widely. The 1st day of the cycle is the 1st day of bleeding, or menses. Ovulation takes place approximately 14 days before the beginning of the next cycle.
      (1) **Hypothalamic-pituitary cycle.** The hypothalamus regulates hormonal secretions in response to blood levels of ovarian steroids. Low levels of estrogen and progesterone near the end of the menstrual cycle stimulate the release of gonadotropin-releasing hormone (Gn-RH) from the hypothalamus (Table 31–1). The Gn-RH stimulates the anterior pituitary gland to secrete follicle-stimulating hormone (FSH) and luteinizing hormone (LH). The FSH causes the graafian follicle (see next paragraph) to mature before ovulation. It produces estrogen. The LH is responsible for the development of the corpus luteum after the follicle ruptures at ovulation. It produces estrogen and progesterone.

NURSE ADVISORY

Oral contraceptives inhibit ovulation by acting on the hypothalamus to inhibit secretion of gonadotropin-releasing hormone. Stress, starvation, and intensive athletic activity can also affect the hypothalamus, resulting in amenorrhea, or absence of menstruation.

Table 31–1. Hormones That Affect the Female Reproductive System

Hormone	Site of Production	Action
Luteinizing hormone (LH)	Anterior pituitary	Stimulates release of ovum from ovary and is responsible for development of corpus luteum after ovulation
Follicle-stimulating hormone (FSH)	Anterior pituitary	Stimulates follicular growth and estrogen secretion
Gonadotropin-releasing hormone (GnRH)	Hypothalamus	Stimulates production of LH and FSH from anterior pituitary gland
Estrogen and progesterone	Ovary	Stimulates development of secondary sex characteristics; modulates cyclic changes of menstrual cycle

If fertilization and implantation do not occur, the levels of estrogen and progesterone decline. Menstruation occurs, and the cycle is repeated (see Fig. 31–2).

(2) **Ovarian cycle.** The 1st day of menses is the beginning of the follicular, or preovulatory, phase of the ovarian cycle. The variations in length of the follicular cycle are responsible for the variations in length of the menstrual cycle. One of the ovaries develops 20 or more estrogen-producing follicles in response to FSH stimulation. Usually, only 1 follicle matures to become the graafian follicle. The increased level of estrogen causes the pituitary gland to suppress FSH production and to increase LH production. A preovulatory surge of LH causes the graafian follicle to rupture. Ovulation occurs when the ovum is released about 24 hours after the LH surge. After ovulation, the luteal phase of the ovarian cycle begins. The ruptured follicle becomes the corpus luteum, which produces estrogen and progesterone for about 13 to 15 days. If pregnancy does not occur, the corpus luteum regresses and is reabsorbed. Estrogen and progesterone levels decline. The hypothalamus is stimulated to repeat the menstrual cycle (Fig. 31–3).

NURSE ADVISORY

Mittelschmerz is a pain felt by some women in the lower abdomen at the time of ovulation. It is thought to be caused by peritoneal irritation resulting from the release of follicular fluid from the ovulating ovary.

(3) Endometrial cycle. Menstruation is the 1st phase of the **endometrial, or uterine, cycle.** In response to decreased progesterone levels, the upper layers of the endometrial lining are shed over 1 to 5 days.

NURSE ADVISORY

The average length of the menstrual cycle is 5 days. The amount of blood loss is about 50 ml.

- The **proliferative phase** begins on about day 5 and extends to day 14, or ovulation. It corresponds with the follicular phase of the ovarian cycle. Estrogen promotes the thickening of the endometrial lining. It becomes more vascular and has increased glandular secretions.
- After ovulation, the **secretory phase** begins. Between days 15 and 25, the endometrium continues to become more vascular and rich in glycogen.
- If pregnancy does not occur, the **premenstrual phase** begins about day 25. As the corpus luteum regresses and levels of estrogen and progesterone decline, the endometrium begins to disintegrate. Constriction of blood vessels causes ischemia, and the endometrial tissue begins to slough off. The onset of bleeding begins the cycle again (see Fig. 31–3).

c. The **climacterium** is a transitional phase that begins with the initial decline of estrogen production and ends when all symptoms produced by this decline cease.

(1) **Menopause** is the last menstrual period. The average age at natural (nonsurgical) menopause is 51.4 years. Menopause is the biologic end of normal reproductive activity. Menopause can be diagnosed only in retrospect, after the woman has had no menstrual periods for 12 months. Surgical menopause occurs when the ovaries are removed in premenopausal women.

(2) Decreased estrogen resulting from declining ovarian function causes changes in the reproductive system. Atrophic tissue changes occur in the vagina, vulva, and urethra. Decreased estrogen also causes the symptoms of menopause, including vasomotor instability, or "hot flashes," and anovulatory cycles.

(3) Women are at higher risk for osteoporosis and heart disease after menopause.

2. Female sexual response cycle

a. The physiologic sexual response involves 2 processes: vasoconstriction and myotonia.

(1) With sexual stimulation, the circumvaginal blood vessels constrict, causing lubrication, engorgement, and distention of the genitals.

(2) Sexual arousal produces myotonia (increased muscular tension), which causes voluntary and involuntary rhythmic contractions.

b. The sexual response cycle has 4 phases: excitement, plateau, orgasmic, and resolution. Changes take place sequentially, but the duration and intensity of the phases vary among individuals.

(1) Excitement phase: In preparation for penetration, vaginal lubrication increases, the inner two thirds of the vagina lengthens and distends, the external genitalia darken with congested blood, the clitoris enlarges, and the uterus moves upward.

(2) Plateau phase: The outer vaginal walls and the labia become engorged and form an "orgasmic platform." The clitoris contracts under the hood. The labia minora become deeper in color.

ELDER ADVISORY

The older woman experiences changes in the sexual response cycle. In the excitement phase, there is a delay in vaginal lubrication. In the plateau phase, there is a decrease in expansion of the vagina; the labia majora remain flaccid; and the labia minora do not swell or darken. The clitoris decreases in size after age 60 years. The orgasmic phase is shorter, and resolution is more rapid.

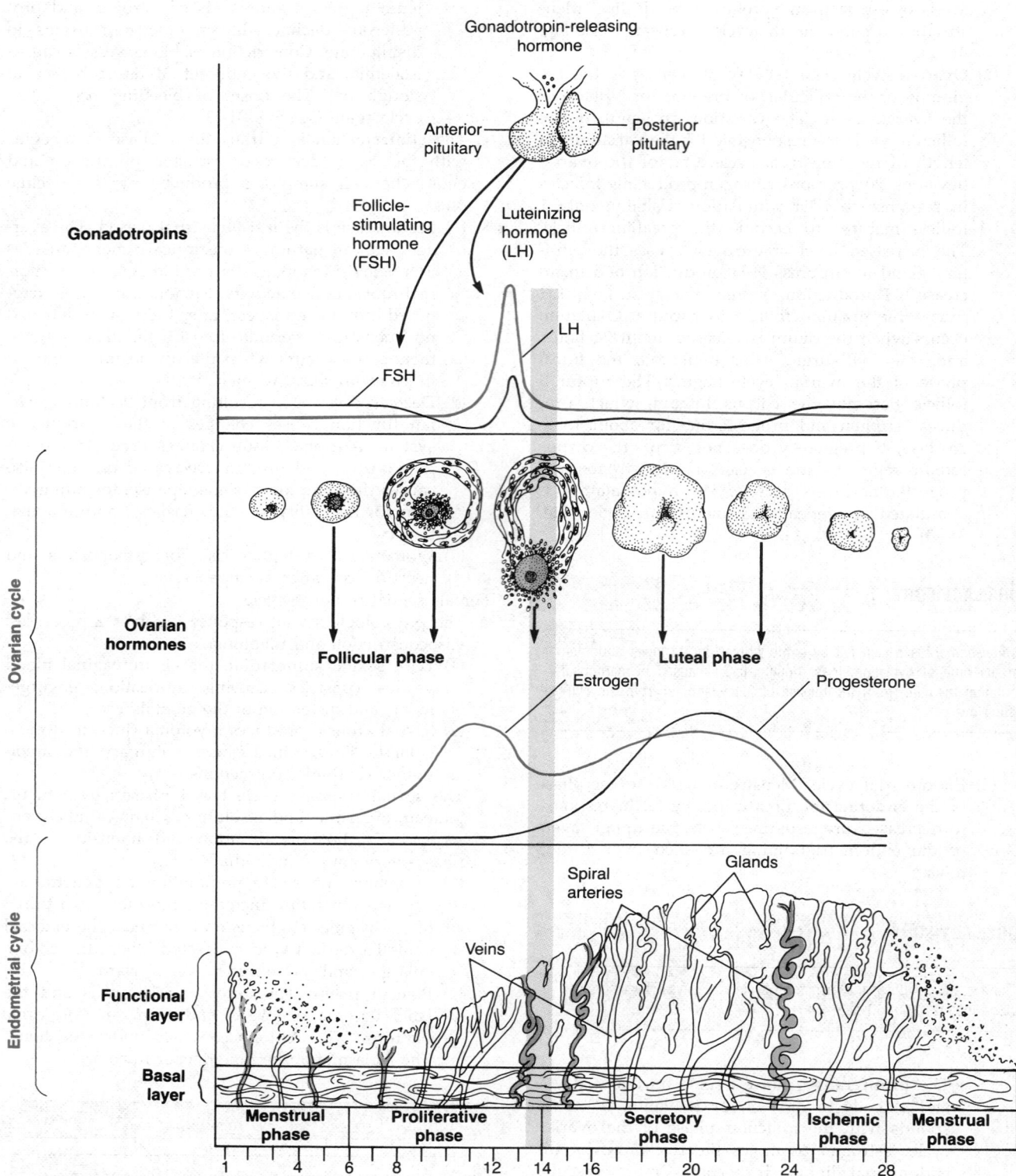

Figure 31–3. The menstrual cycle. (From Gorrie TM, McKinney ES, and Murray SS. *Foundations of Maternal Newborn Nursing.* Philadelphia: WB Saunders, 1994, p 61.)

(3) Orgasmic phase: Strong rhythmic contractions occur in the orgasmic platform. The uterus contracts rhythmically.

(4) Resolution: Vascular congestion decreases. The

organs rapidly return to a nonexcited state. The clitoris comes out from under its hood, and the uterus returns to its normal position.

c. Refractory period: This is the time required to repeat

the cycle. Because women physically never have a refractory period, multiple orgasms can occur.

ASSESSING WOMEN WITH SEXUAL AND REPRODUCTIVE DISORDERS

Key Symptoms and Their Pathophysiologic Bases

1. Bleeding or lack of bleeding
   a. Occurrence: Bleeding or lack of bleeding can occur at any time during the menstrual cycle, after menopause, with strenuous exercise, and during or after intercourse.
   b. Characteristics: Bleeding can be absent, spotty, light, heavy, and with or without clots.
   c. Location: Bleeding is usually vaginal.
   d. Duration: Bleeding can last for a few moments or for days or weeks.
   e. Severity: Severity is measured by the amount of bleeding—for example, the number and saturation of pads or tampons used in 24 hours.
   f. Precipitating or aggravating factors: Strenuous exercise, anxiety and stress, pregnancy, and poor nutrition (anorexia) can cause the absence of bleeding. Intercourse, trauma, hormonal imbalances, benign tumors, and cancer can cause bleeding.
   g. Associated symptoms: Pain, abdominal fullness, cramping, weight change, and bowel or urinary changes can accompany bleeding.
   h. Alleviating factors: Hormonal therapy or surgery may alleviate the bleeding.
2. Pain
   a. Occurrence: Pain can occur before or during menses, with voiding or defecation.
   b. Characteristics: Pain can be described as cramping, a dull ache, or sharp.
   c. Location: Pain may be in the lower abdomen, or it may be perineal or vaginal. It can also be in the lower back.
   d. Duration: Pain can occur several days before menses and cease at the start of menses. It can occur during the first 1 to 2 days of menses. The duration can vary greatly depending on the cause.
   e. Severity: The pain can be described as mild to severe. A pain scale can be used to quantify the amount of pain experienced.
   f. Precipitating or aggravating factors: Menses, endometriosis, tumors, premenstrual syndrome, intercourse, and exercise can trigger pain.
   g. Associated symptoms: Headaches, nausea and vomiting, bleeding, diarrhea, and bloating may accompany the onset of pain.
   h. Alleviating factors: Heat to the abdomen, exercise, massage, acupuncture, relaxation techniques, prostaglandin synthetase inhibitors, and analgesics have been used to relieve menstrual pain and other pain experienced in the female reproductive system.
3. Vaginal discharge
   a. Occurrence: Vaginal discharge can be acute or chronic.
   b. Characteristics: Discharge can be described as thick, heavy, watery, profuse, purulent, or odorless and can be further characterized by its color.
   c. Location: Discharge is vaginal or cervical.
   d. Duration: Duration of discharge may vary depending on the cause. Usually, discharge related to infection will persist until treatment is initiated.
   e. Precipitating or aggravating factors
      (1) Intercourse, wearing tight-fitting clothing, wearing noncotton underwear, using irritating douches or feminine hygiene products, and taking medications (antibiotics) can cause discharge.
      (2) Pregnancy and diabetes can increase the likelihood of vaginal infections.
      (3) Many sexually transmitted diseases (STDs) have a characteristic discharge.
   f. Associated symptoms: Vaginal discharge can be accompanied by pain, burning, dysuria, itching, fever, or rash.
   g. Alleviating factors: Sitz baths, warm soaks, topical creams (hydrocortisone), and treatment of infection can relieve the discomfort caused by vaginal discharge.
4. Sores or growths
   a. Occurrence: Sores can occur as a symptom of an STD. Masses can occur with benign and neoplastic changes in the reproductive system.
   b. Characteristics: Sores or masses can be described according to their texture (smooth, soft, firm, nodular, granular, fibrous), size (measured in centimeters), shape (e.g., angular, linear), mobility (fixed or freely moving), tenderness, heat, color, and induration.
   c. Location: Sores may be found on the external genitalia, in the vagina, and on the cervix. Masses may be found on the external genitalia or in the uterus, on the ovaries, or anywhere in the pelvic cavity.
   d. Duration: Sores caused by STDs are usually present when the infection is active. Masses such as uterine fibroids can be present for years and grow slowly.
   e. Precipitating or aggravating factors: Having intercourse with a partner who has an active STD can precipitate an occurrence of genital lesions. Benign tumors or cancer may be responsible for a mass.
   f. Associated symptoms: Bleeding and pain can accompany both benign and cancerous masses. Tissue or lymph node tenderness, dysuria, vaginal discharge, and dyspareunia can accompany sores caused by STDs.
   g. Alleviating factors: Using cool compresses, sitz baths, and heat lamps and keeping the area around the sore dry and clean can alleviate discomfort.

Health History

1. Menstrual history
   a. Age at menarche
   b. Date of last menstrual period (LMP)
   c. Number of days in cycle and regularity of cycles
   d. Characteristics of flow: amount (number and type of

pads or tampons), duration, presence and size of clots

e. Dysmenorrhea: frequency, onset, duration, relief measures

f. Spotting between periods

g. Premenstrual symptoms: headache, weight gain, edema, breast tenderness, mood swings

h. Menopausal symptoms: hot flashes, menstrual changes

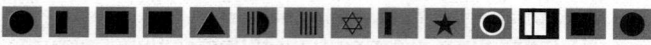

TRANSCULTURAL CONSIDERATIONS

In some cultures, menstruation is seen as a method of cleansing the body of impurities (bad blood). To some groups (e.g., Cubans, Haitians, Bahamians, Afghans, Appalachians), monthly menstruation literally means health. The interruption of menstruation signifies illness or impending illness. Excessive menstrual flow or bleeding between periods is regarded as abnormal because it weakens the body by decreasing the amount of blood or making it too thin, thereby causing bad blood. This makes the female vulnerable to illness, premature aging, or infertility.

2. Pregnancy history
   a. Gravidity: number of pregnancies
   b. Parity: number of term births, preterm births, abortions (spontaneous [miscarriages] and induced), and number of living children
   c. Complications of pregnancy, birth, and the postpartum period

3. Contraceptive history
   a. Current method: length of time used, effectiveness, consistency of use, satisfaction with method
   b. Previous methods: duration of use, reasons for discontinuing

4. Family history
   a. Reproductive history: history of multiple gestation, congenital anomalies, infertility
   b. Cancer of the reproductive system. Note whether woman's mother took diethylstilbestrol (DES) while pregnant.
   c. Menstrual problems, endometriosis
   d. Family history of diabetes

5. Medical history: Note that as many as half of all health problems are a result of lifestyle and behavior determined by cultural beliefs.
   a. Past gynecologic procedures or surgery: hysterectomy, tubal ligation, laparoscopy. Note when procedures were performed.
   b. Sexually transmitted diseases: Note type (gonorrhea, syphilis, genital herpes, hepatitis, human immunodeficiency virus [HIV], chlamydia, human papillomavirus [HPV], pelvic inflammatory disease [PID]) and when.
   c. Vaginal infections. Note type.
   d. Diabetes
   e. Cancer of the reproductive system

6. Current reproductive health status
   a. Medication use
      (1) Prescription or over-the-counter drugs: dosage
      (2) Drug allergies
   b. Sexually transmitted disease risk factors

c. Self-care behaviors
   (1) Last Papanicolaou (Pap) smear and results
   (2) Breast self-examination
   (3) Vulvar self-examination

7. Social history and lifestyle
   a. Age, race, ethnic group membership
   b. Support systems and marital status
   c. Occupational hazards, such as chemicals, radiation
   d. Use of alcohol, tobacco, illegal drugs
   e. Leisure activities: stress management strategies
   f. Nutritional status
      (1) Women who are anemic may complain of fatigue and decreased libido.
      (2) Obesity and high-fat diets may be risk factors for certain reproductive cancers (endometrial, breast, ovarian).
      (3) Calcium-deficient diets can result in osteoporosis.
      (4) Irregularities in ovulation can be caused by low body fat.

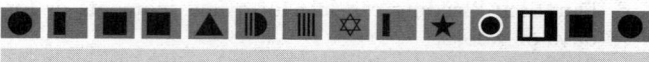

TRANSCULTURAL CONSIDERATIONS

To assess health beliefs from a cultural perspective, these questions might be helpful:
1. What is your religion?
2. Do you believe religious practices can influence your health?
3. What do you think causes you to be ill?
4. What do you do when you feel sick? Do you go to a doctor or someone else, or do you treat yourself?

8. Sexual relationships. A nondiscriminating attitude is essential in eliciting information. Lesbian issues are often not addressed by health care providers.
   a. Number of partners
   b. Age woman became sexually active
   c. Possible sexual abuse
   d. Sexual preference. Do not assume that the woman is in a heterosexual relationship.
   e. Satisfaction with sexual relationship
   f. Difficulties, concerns

NURSE ADVISORY

Some health history questions are for women of childbearing age and will not be applicable for young adolescent and postmenopausal women. Because some clients seeking health care may be lesbians, health history questions need to be phrased in nonsexist terms.

Physical Examination

1. General considerations
   a. Assess the woman's behavior for appropriateness. Ask yourself whether there are signs of obvious anxiety, fear, or embarrassment.

b. Ask the woman if this is her 1st pelvic examination. Explain the procedure. Maintain eye contact.

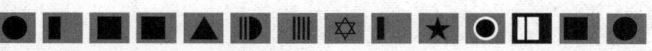

TRANSCULTURAL CONSIDERATIONS

Women from some cultures, such as Vietnamese, will not return eye contact, as a demonstration of respect to the care provider. Japanese women may prefer not to see the examiner and may request that a screen or sheet be held up. For some women (e.g., Islamic), female examiners are required. In cultures that require proof of virginity on the wedding night, problems are encountered when a pelvic examination is needed. Use of a pediatric speculum may be a solution.

c. Assist the woman to a lithotomy position, with her arms crossed over her chest, and her buttocks extending slightly over the edge of the examining table (Procedure 31–1).

d. Drape the woman if she desires, and offer her a mirror to watch the examination if she is interested in doing so.

2. External examination

a. Inspection and palpation are used to examine the external genitalia.

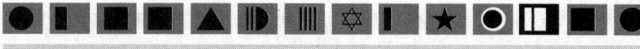

TRANSCULTURAL CONSIDERATIONS

Touching the genitals may be viewed as masturbation and deemed culturally inappropriate.

b. Teach the woman about vulvar self-examination (Learning/Teaching Guidelines for Vulvar Self-Examination).

c. Techniques for examining the external female genitalia are presented in Procedure 31–1.

Text continued on page 1454

Procedure 31–1
Pelvic Examination

Definition/Purposes	To inspect and palpate for symmetry, color, position, and size, as well as signs of inflammation, infection, trauma, tenderness, masses, nodules, enlargements, and changes in consistency
Contraindications/Cautions	Pelvic examination should not be deferred in older women. Privacy should be ensured. Have someone in the examining room to provide support for the woman and assistance to you if needed.

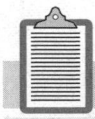

NURSING MANAGEMENT

Agency policy may require a male examiner to have a female assistant.

Learning/Teaching Activities	Provide the following information: (a) describe the procedure and (b) explain the use of equipment.

Preliminary Activities

Equipment	• Gloves • Water-soluble lubricant • Speculum • Light source • If indicated for Pap test or cultures: culture tubes, chlamydial enzyme immunoassay kit, glass slides, sterile cotton swabs, wooden or plastic spatulas, cytologic fixative
Assessment/Planning	• Make sure room is warm and private. • Consider age-related factors that might affect the examination. • Decide which hand will insert the speculum and which hand will be used for the vaginal examination. In general, it is best to use the dominant hand for vaginal palpation. • Become familiar with how the speculum operates before the examination.

(continued)

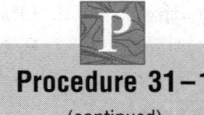

Procedure 31–1

(continued)

Patient Preparation

- The woman should empty her bladder before the examination.
- The woman should be in the lithotomy position with her feet in the stirrups and her arms across her chest or by her side. A Sims' position can also be used.

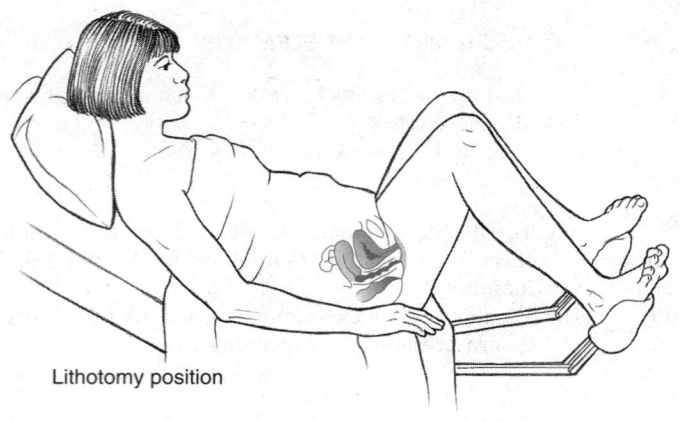

Lithotomy position

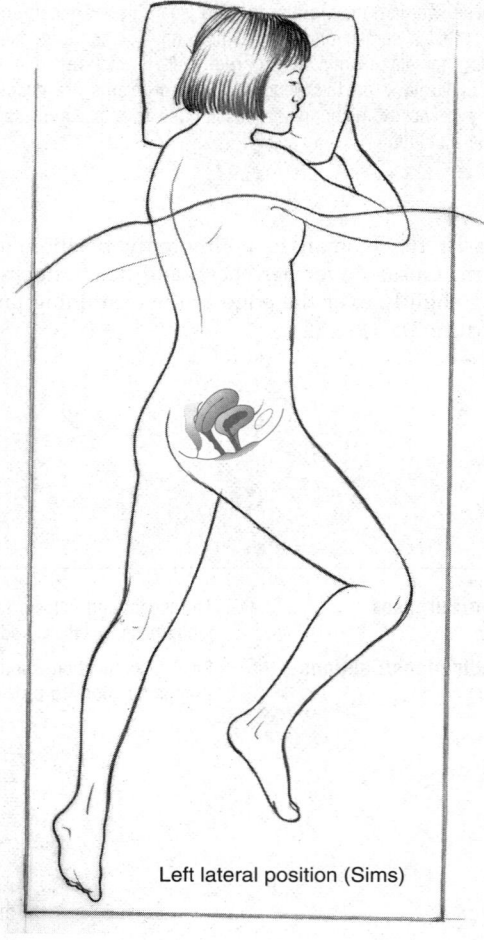

Left lateral position (Sims)

- Drape the woman if she desires.
- Offer to let her view the examination with a mirror if she desires.
- Encourage the woman to use relaxation techniques during the examination.
- Assure the woman that you will stop the examination if she feels discomfort.

Procedure

Actions	Rationale/Discussion
1. Wash hands before any examination.	1. Hand washing protects against possible cross-contamination from other women.
2. Wear gloves. Double glove if the woman is bleeding, if infection is suspected, or if you have cuts or lesions on your hands.	2. Gloves protect against possible infections.
3. Have the woman assume the lithotomy position with her feet stabilized in stirrups, her buttocks slightly over the edge of the table, and her arms across her chest.	3. This position facilitates examination. If the woman puts her arms behind her head, her abdomen will tense, which will hinder palpation.
4. Position yourself at the end of the examining table.	4. This position provides for ease of examination.
5. Begin the examination by telling the woman what you are going to do before you touch her.	5. Explanations decrease anxiety and promote a trusting relationship.

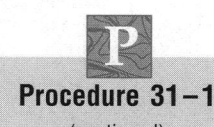

Procedure 31–1

(continued)

Actions	Rationale/Discussion
6. Ask the woman to spread her legs.	6. Because pelvic examination is an intrusive procedure, force should never be used.

External Genitalia Examination

1. Inspect the external genitalia, noting hair distribution and texture; general appearance; and symmetry of characteristics.
2. Palpate the external genitalia.
3. Separate the labia majora. Insert your fingers into the vagina to milk the urethra for discharge from Skene's glands. Palpate Bartholin's glands.

1. Look for lice, nits, lesions, edema, masses, hematomas, discharge, deviations from normal. Assess for age-appropriate development.
2. Assess for tenderness and consistency.
3. Assess for infection or inflammation, tenderness, swelling. Discharge should be cultured for *Neisseria gonorrhoeae* and/or *Streptococcus.*

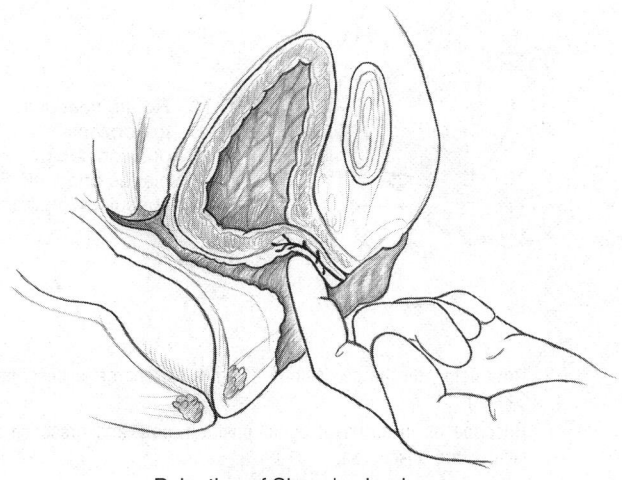

Palpation of Skene's gland

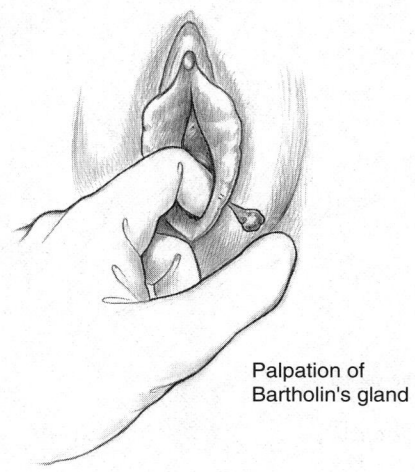

Palpation of
Bartholin's gland

Actions	Rationale/Discussion
4. Palpate the perineum.	4. Normally, the perineum feels smooth and thick in nulliparous and thin and rigid in multiparous women.
5. Ask the woman to squeeze the vaginal opening around your 2 fingers.	5. Test for muscle tone.
6. Place 2 fingers in the vagina and ask the woman to bear down on them	6. Assess for bulging or urinary incontinence. A bulging anterior wall indicates a cystocele; bulging of the posterior wall indicates a rectocele. Prolapse of the uterus is seen as a protrusion of the cervix or uterus.

Internal Examination

1. Begin the examination by selecting the speculum of appropriate size and lubricate it with warm water if needed.

2. Insert the speculum by placing two fingers of one hand into the vagina and press down gently. Ask the woman to breathe slowly and to bear down.
3. Hold the speculum in your other hand with the index finger over the blades and the other fingers around the handle.
4. Hold the closed speculum obliquely and insert it at a 45-degree angle down and posteriorly.
5. After the speculum is in the vagina, remove your fingers and rotate the speculum to a horizontal position.
6. Open the blades slowly to expose the cervix and lock the speculum in place.

1. Select the smallest size possible that allows examination of the internal genitalia. Lubricants other than water will interfere with the Pap test and culture results.
2. This procedure encourages pelvic relaxation and ease of insertion.

3. This maneuver prevents the speculum from opening during insertion.

4. The angle of the speculum matches the angle of the vagina and avoids trauma to the urethra and vaginal walls.
5. This step opens the speculum.

6. This step avoids pinching and stabilizes the speculum in open position.

(continued)

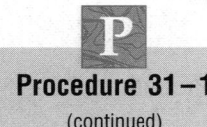

Procedure 31–1

(continued)

Actions	Rationale/Discussion

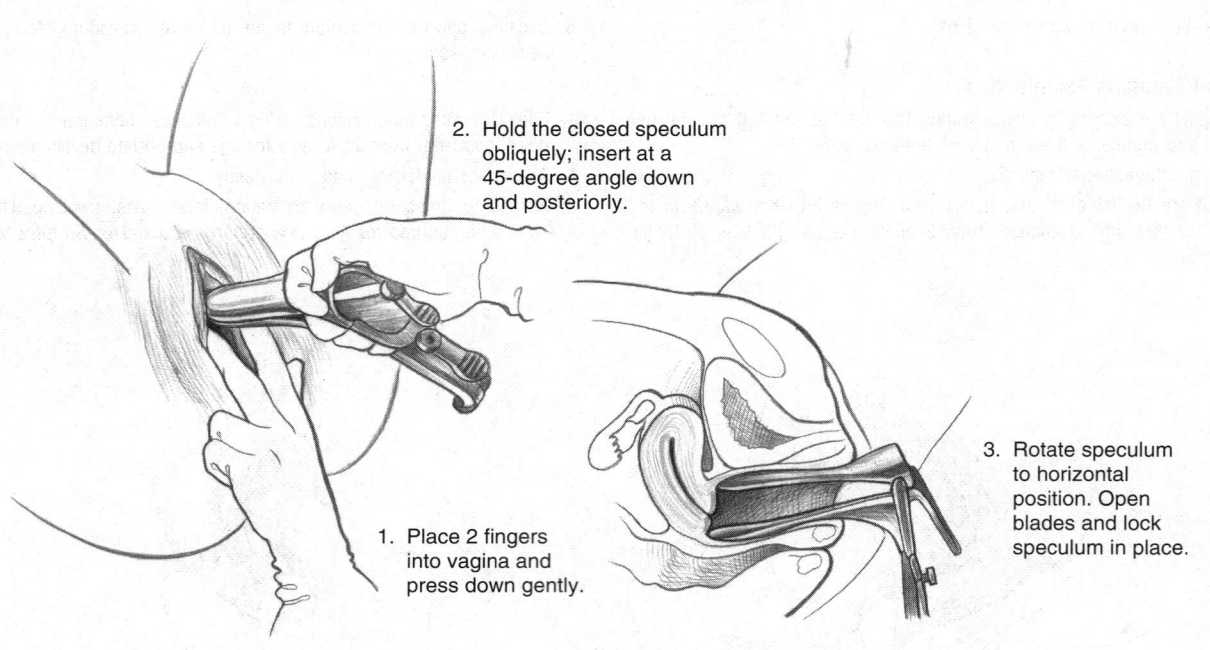

2. Hold the closed speculum obliquely; insert at a 45-degree angle down and posteriorly.

1. Place 2 fingers into vagina and press down gently.

3. Rotate speculum to horizontal position. Open blades and lock speculum in place.

7. Inspect the vagina.	7. Note color, discharge, lesions. (Vaginal discharge is described in Table 31–6.)
8. Inspect the cervix.	8. Describe os in terms of color, position, size, and presence of erosion, lacerations, discharge.

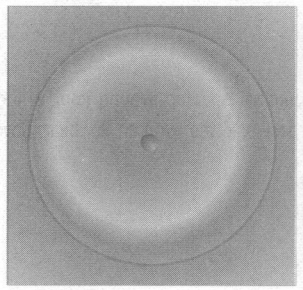

Nulliparous cervix

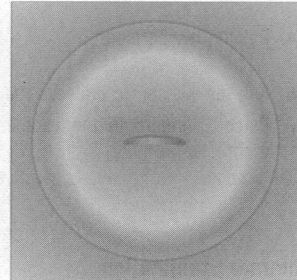

Parous cervix

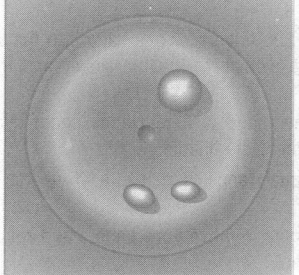

Nabothian cyst

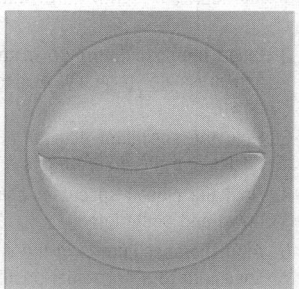

Bilateral transverse laceration

P

Procedure 31–1
(continued)

Actions	Rationale/Discussion

9. Obtain smears and cultures as needed.

9. Smears and cultures are taken in the following order: Pap test, gono-coccal culture, chlamydial culture, wet prep slides. (See Procedure 31–2 for collection methods.)

10. Unlock the blades and remove the speculum while rotating it to a vertical position.

10. This step avoids trauma and pinching of vaginal mucosa on removal.

Bimanual Examination

1. Stand up to do the bimanual examination. Insert lubricated gloved 1st 2 fingers of 1 hand into the vaginal opening. Wait until the vaginal walls relax; then insert your fingers fully into vagina.

1. Both hands are used. One hand is placed on the abdomen, and 2 fingers of the other hand are inserted into the vagina.

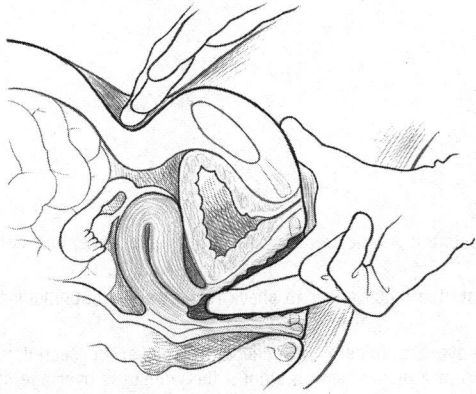

Bimanual examination

2. Palpate the vaginal wall.

2. Normally, it feels smooth, nontender, without nodules or bulging.

3. Locate the cervix, using the palmar surface of your fingers. Note consistency, contour, and mobility. Insert the tip of your finger into cervix to assess patency and fornices.

3. The cervix is usually smooth and firm in the midline. It can be moved from side to side without discomfort. The os should admit the fingertip 0.5 cm. The fornices should feel smooth.

4. Palpate the uterus by pressing downward on the abdominal wall with 1 hand while pushing up on either side of the cervix with 2 fingers of the other hand. Determine size, shape, and position of the uterus.

4. The abdominal hand should be placed halfway between the umbilicus and symphysis. Position, or version, compares the long axis of the body of the uterus with the long axis of the body. Usually, the uterus is anteverted and the fundus is palpated at the level of the pubis, with the cervix pointing posteriorly.

5. Palpate the uterine wall with fingers in fornices.

5. Normally it feels firm and smooth. The uterus is pear-shaped and 5.5 to 8 cm long.

6. Gently move the uterus between the abdominal and vaginal hands.

6. Assess mobility and tenderness. A fixed uterus indicates adhesions.

7. Palpate the ovaries and fallopian tubes by pressing downward on the abdominal wall while pressing upward with the fingers in the vagina on the left and right sides of the uterus. Note size, shape, mobility, and tenderness.

7. This should be a stroking motion with the fingers of both hands pushing together as the hands move downward. Often, the ovaries and fallopian tubes are not palpable. If palpable, the ovaries are firm, smooth, mobile ovoid, and about $3 \times 2 \times 1$ cm in size. Fallopian tubes are not usually palpable.

8. Withdraw the hand from the vagina and check secretions on the glove before discarding it.

8. Normal secretions are clear or creamy and odorless.

Rectovaginal Examination

1. Perform a rectovaginal examination. Change gloves and lubricate the middle and index fingers.

1. Gloves avoid spreading possible infection.

(continued)

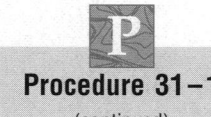

Procedure 31–1

(continued)

Actions	Rationale/Discussion
2. Insert the index finger into the vagina and the middle finger into the anus. Place the other hand on the abdomen.	2. Having the woman bear down will relax the anal sphincter and facilitate insertion.

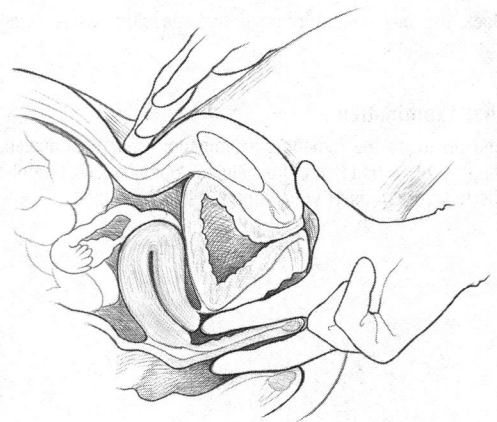

Rectovaginal examination

Actions	Rationale/Discussion
3. Palpate the anterior rectal wall for thickness, tone, and nodules.	3. The rectovaginal septum should feel smooth, thin, pliable. You may feel a retroflexed uterus.
4. Rotate the rectal finger to check rectal wall and sphincter tone.	4. The wall should be smooth; the sphincter should feel tight around your finger.
5. Remove the fingers and check the glove for secretions and stool. Perform a guaiac test on stool if the woman is over age 40 years.	5. The test identifies occult blood.
6. Give the woman tissues to wipe the perineum.	6. The woman should remove secretions, fecal material, and lubricant.
7. Assist the woman to slide back on the examining table and help her remove her feet from the stirrups if needed.	7. Prevents her from falling off the table and reduces strain on the perineal area and lumbosacral ligaments.
8. Remind the woman to sit up slowly.	8. Orthostatic hypotension may be experienced.
9. Provide a perineal pad if needed and provide privacy for dressing.	9. The pad protects clothing from secretions. Demonstrates respect and caring for woman.

Final Activities

Record findings on the chart. The description should include normal findings on external, internal, and rectovaginal examinations as well as deviations from normal.

---

3. Internal examination
   a. A speculum is inserted into the vagina to inspect the vagina and cervix.
   b. Specimens for Pap testing and gonococcal and chlamydial cultures may be obtained if indicated.
   c. Techniques for internal genitalia examination are presented in Procedure 31–1.
4. Bimanual vaginal examination
   a. Palpation of internal genitalia is done with 2 fingers of a lubricated, gloved hand inserted into the vagina and the other hand placed on the abdomen.
   b. Note location, size, and mobility of masses or areas of tenderness.

   c. Techniques for bimanual examination and normal and abnormal findings are presented in Procedure 31–1.
5. Rectovaginal examination: This technique is used to assess the rectovaginal septum, posterior uterine wall, cul de sac, and rectum.
   a. Change gloves and lubricate index and middle fingers. Insert index finger into vagina and middle finger into rectum.
   b. Explain that the examination may be uncomfortable and that she may feel as if she is moving her bowels.
   c. Techniques for the complete pelvic examination are presented in Procedure 31–1.

LEARNING/TEACHING GUIDELINES
for Vulvar Self-Examination

Overview

1. Explain why monthly examination of the vulvar area is important.
2. Teach the woman to perform the examination between menstrual periods.
3. Remind the woman that most signs and symptoms do not mean cancer but that early detection of vulvar cancer usually means cure if it is treated early.

Technique of Examination

1. Assist the woman to find a comfortable position—on the edge of her bed or bathtub or on the floor—in a well-lighted area (or use a flashlight).

2. Instruct her to use a hand mirror to examine the external genitalia.
3. Point out the genital organs that make up the vulvar area.
4. Assist the woman in examining the area around the vaginal opening from the mons pubis to the anus.
5. Instruct the woman to palpate as well as look at the vulvar area.
6. Instruct the woman to report any lumps, masses, growths, sores, changes in skin color, painful areas, or itching to her health care provider.

---

6. Pelvic examination after hysterectomy
   a. Assess the external genitalia in the same manner used for a woman who has not had a hysterectomy.
   b. During the internal examination, note whether a vaginal cuff (surgical scar) is present on the posterior fornix.
   c. A Pap test may be done on the cells at the vaginal cuff. Be sure to label the specimen as vaginal cells if sending it to a laboratory.
   d. Samples for gonococcal and chlamydial cultures may be taken from the vestibule.
   e. Examine for signs of rectocele, cystocele, and stress incontinence (see p. 1218, 1487).
   f. Perform a bimanual examination to assess for lumps or masses, adhesions, tenderness. Palpate ovaries and fallopian tubes if present.
7. Pelvic examination of the older woman
   a. The examination procedure is the same as for younger adult women.

ELDER ADVISORY

Physical changes with age found on pelvic examination include
- Thin, sparse pubic hair that may also be gray
- Flatter labia and smaller mons pubis due to decreased fatty deposits
- Smaller clitoris after age 60 years
- Urethral meatus appearing as a slit located more posteriorly because of relaxed perineal musculature
- Vaginal introitus that may be smaller
- Vagina shorter, pink with smaller rugae
- Smaller and paler cervix that protrudes less far into the vagina
- Smaller uterus that may not be palpable on bimanual examination
- Nonpalpable ovaries due to atrophy
- Nonpalpable fallopian tubes
- Smoother, thinner rectovaginal septum

Note: Palpable structures of the adnexa suggest abnormality and need further investigation.

b. After menopause, numerous physical changes take place.
c. Because pelvic relaxation can occur, assess for stress incontinence, uterine prolapse, or other structural changes.
d. The older woman may need more assistance in assuming the lithotomy position or in supporting her legs.
e. Disabled women may need to be examined in the Sims' position (see Procedure 31–1).
f. A smaller speculum may be needed, and more lubrication may be needed on instruments and hands.

Special Diagnostic Studies

1. Special studies used to diagnose female reproductive problems include laboratory tests, vaginal smears and cultures, radiographic examinations, endoscopic studies, biopsy studies, dilation and curettage (D & C), and ultrasound.
2. Nursing responsibilities include the following:
   a. Providing the woman with accurate and understandable information about the purposes of the tests
   b. Giving the woman information about preparation for specific tests
   c. Scheduling the test (in some settings)
   d. Promoting maximum physical and emotional comfort during the tests
   e. Providing information about follow-up after the tests are performed
3. Laboratory tests
   a. Serum hormone levels
      (1) Follicle-stimulating hormone and LH levels are measured to assess pituitary function.
      (2) Prolactin levels are measured to detect hyperprolactinemia.
      (3) Human chorionic gonadotropin (hCG) levels are measured to detect pregnancy.

Table 31–2. Classifications of Pap Smears

Numeric Class	Traditional	Dysplasia	Cervical Intraepithelial Neoplasia (CIN)	Bethesda*
Class I	Class I	Normal	Normal	Normal
Class II	Class II	Atypical squamous	No designation	Atypical squamous cells
Class III	Class III	Mild dysplasia	CIN I	Low-grade squamous lesion
	Moderate dysplasia	Moderate dysplasia	CIN II	High-grade squamous lesion
Class IV	Severe dysplasia	Severe dysplasia	CIN III	High-grade squamous lesion
	Carcinoma in situ	Carcinoma in situ		
Class V	Invasive cancer	Invasive cancer	Invasive cancer	Invasive cancer

* The Bethesda system is the preferred system. The class, traditional, and dysplasia systems are infrequently used.
Data from Herbst A, et al. *Comprehensive Gynecology*. 2nd ed. St. Louis: CV Mosby, 1992; Meissels A, and Morin C. *Cystopathology of the Uterine Cervix*. Chicago: ASCP Press, 1991; and National Cancer Institute Workshop. The 1988 Bethesda System for reporting cervical/vaginal cytological diagnoses. *JAMA* 262:931, 1989.

(4) Progesterone and estradiol are measured to assess ovarian function.
b. Serologic tests (i.e., VDRL and treponemal antibody absorption test) are done to detect syphilis.
c. Thyroid function tests are done to assess thyroid function.
4. Pap test or smear: The Pap test is used to detect precancerous and cancerous cells in the cervix and vagina. Procedure 31–2 describes how to perform a Pap test, and Table 31–2 explains the interpretation of the results.

NURSE ADVISORY

Recommendations for routine Pap screening vary. The American Cancer Society recommends yearly Pap tests for women over the age of 18 years who are sexually active. After 2 or more negative test results 1 year apart, less frequent testing may be performed on the advice of the health care provider. Most sources agree that high-risk women should have annual Pap tests. Women who have had hysterectomies but still have ovaries need annual pelvic examinations and vaginal cytology every 3 to 5 years. Women older than 65 years of age who have had normal results on Pap smears may not need annual screening.

5. Wet smears
a. Secretions from the vaginal pool are obtained during a speculum examination. A sterile cotton swab is used to collect the specimen, which is then placed on a glass slide and treated with 1 drop of normal saline or potassium hydroxide (KOH) and covered with a glass cover. The slide is examined under a microscope to detect pathogens.
b. Table 31–3 describes the wet preparations used in diagnosing common vaginal infections.
6. Cultures
a. Specimens for gonococcal and chlamydial culture analysis are obtained from discharge from the endocervix, vagina, and urethra. (See Chapter 32 for discussion of sexually transmitted diseases.)
b. Sterile swabs are used to collect specimens, which

are then placed in a culture tube or swabbed onto a culture plate to be sent to the laboratory for analysis.
7. Pelvic and abdominal ultrasound is used to assess such problems as uterine fibroids, ovarian cysts, and pelvic masses. Ultrasound uses high-frequency sound waves to produce a 3-dimensional image of the organs.
a. The woman should have a full bladder to enhance visualization of the uterus.
b. For an abdominal scan, the woman's abdomen is exposed, and oil or transmission gel is applied to the area being scanned.
c. For a transvaginal scan, the transducer is covered with a condom or vinyl glove that has been coated with transmission gel before insertion into the vagina.
d. The woman may be able to see the monitor during the examination. She may be curious about landmarks and structures, but she may also notice abnormal or negative findings.
8. Radiographic examinations
a. **Computed tomography (CT)** is a noninvasive scanning technique that produces 3-dimensional cross-sectional images. The CT scans can differentiate solid tissue masses from cystic masses and are useful in distinguishing benign and malignant tumors.
(1) No preparation is needed other than emptying the bladder and removing all metal objects from the body.
(2) The woman should be informed that she will hear a clicking sound as the scanner rotates around her. She must remain still during the test.

Table 31–3. Wet Preparations for Diagnosis of Vaginal Infections

Wet Preparation	Vaginal Infection
Normal saline	*Trichomonas* vaginitis
	Cervicitis
	Nonspecific vaginitis
Potassium hydroxide (KOH)	Moniliasis *(Candida albicans)*
	Gardnerella vaginitis

Procedure 31–2
Obtaining a Specimen for a Papanicolaou Test

Definition/Purpose	To detect precancerous and cancerous cells of the cervix and vagina.
Contraindications/Cautions	The woman should not be menstruating because blood can interfere with interpretation of the test. She should not douche, put any medication into her vagina, or have intercourse for at least 24 hours before the test.
Learning/Teaching Activities	Provide the following information: explain the procedure. Explain that she should not feel any discomfort except possibly when the speculum is inserted. Instruct her not to douche, insert vaginal medications, or have sexual intercourse for at least 24 hours before the test.

Preliminary Activities

Equipment	• Speculum • Sampling tools (e.g., cytobrush, cotton-tipped applicators, wooden or plastic spatulas, endocervical aspirator) • Glass slides • Fixative spray • Gloves • Lamp or other light source
Assessment/Planning	• Choose the appropriate size speculum. • Warm the speculum before inserting it. Use only water for lubrication. • Make labels for slides, indicating site of sample—endocervix or exocervix. • Schedule the test before ovulation for premenopausal woman to get the best-quality sample. • Schedule the test any time for the postmenopausal woman unless she is on hormone replacement therapy. In that case, the test should be scheduled for the first half of the cycle when she is not taking progesterone, which suppresses maturation of squamous epithelium and can affect the quality of the sample.
Patient Preparation	• Have the woman empty her bladder before the procedure. • Assist the woman to a lithotomy position. • Drape the woman if she desires. • Explain each step in the examination before it is performed. • Encourage the woman to use relaxation techniques, such as folding her arms across her chest or using breathing patterns or a visual focal point.

Procedure

Actions	Rationale/Discussion
1. Insert the speculum (see Procedure 31–1).	1. Examine the site of sample collection.
2. Wipe away excess mucus if present.	2. Mucus can interfere with interpretation of the sample.
3. Obtain the endocervical sample by inserting a premoistened cotton applicator into the os and rotating it 360 degrees on the surface of the squamocolumnar junction.	3. The mucus around the squamocolumnar junction will contain more carcinoma cells than mucus from other parts of the vagina. Saline prevents cells from being absorbed by the cotton.

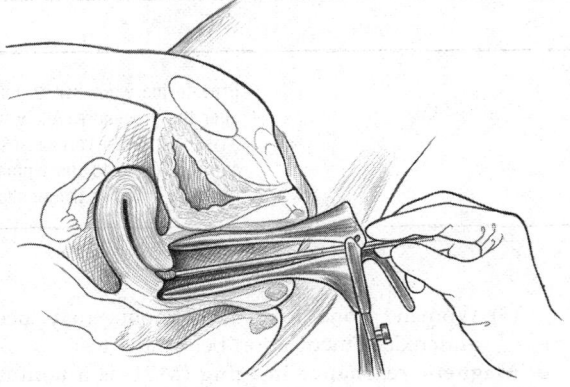

Cotton applicator
inserted into os

(continued)

P

Procedure 31–2

(continued)

Actions	Rationale/Discussion
4. Roll the swab on a glass slide to deposit the cells.	4. Spread thinly for easier examination of cells.
5. Spray the slide immediately with fixative.	5. Fixative prevents drying of cells.
6. Alternate collection methods for specimens. Use a cytobrush for endocervical cells and a spatula for ectocervical cells. Wooden, plastic, or metal spatulas can be used.	6. The cytobrush improves sample quality. The woman may experience spotting after this procedure. If spatulas are used, the longer end is inserted into the cervix.
7. To obtain a specimen from the vaginal pool, insert a cotton-tipped applicator or rounded end of the spatula into the posterior fornix and rotate it 360 degrees.	7. Cells from the endometrium, endocervix, ectocervix, and vagina are obtained for examination.

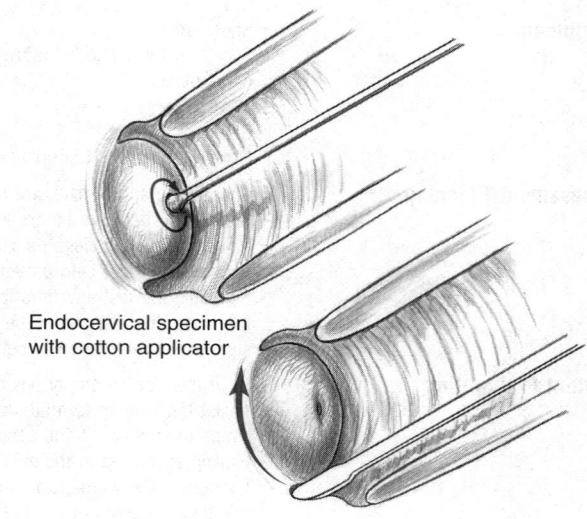

Endocervical specimen
with cotton applicator

8. Spread the sample gently onto the glass slide and immediately spray with fixative.	8. Fixative prevents cells from drying out.
9. Label specimens. Include name, age, date of last menstrual period, known infections, hormone ingestion, previous abnormal cytology.	9. This information is necessary for accurate interpretation and minimizes the chance of mismatched specimens.
10. If the woman's history indicates or you notice abnormal discharge, obtain a sample for microscopic study (see Table 31–3).	10. Cultures are done after the Pap specimens are obtained to prevent interference with adequate cell collection for interpretation.
11. Remove the speculum as described in Procedure 31–1.	
12. Assist the woman to sitting position.	12. She may experience orthostatic hypotension.

Final Activities

Provide the woman with tissues for wiping secretions; offer a perineal pad to protect clothing in case she bleeds after the procedure. Allow privacy for dressing. Send slides to the laboratory, where they will be interpreted. Table 31–2 lists the various classifications that may be used in reporting Pap test results. The results can be communicated to the woman in person, by letter, or by telephone. Abnormal results should be followed up with retesting or other diagnostic procedures as indicated.

    (3) Women prone to claustrophobia may need an antianxiety medication before the test.
b. **Magnetic resonance imaging (MRI)** is a noninvasive scanning technique that provides multiplane cross-sectional imaging using a magnetic field and radio-frequency energy to produce images. Magnetic resonance scanners may interfere with the programming of permanent pacemakers. Magnetic resonance imaging is used to detect pelvic tumors.
(1) Patient preparation is similar to that for CT.

(2) The woman should be informed that she will hear a thumping sound during the procedure and that she must remain still during the test.

(3) Women prone to claustrophobia may need an antianxiety medication before the test.

c. In **hysterosalpingography,** the uterus and fallopian tubes are radiographed following injection of a contrast dye. A hysterosalpingogram is useful in an infertility workup to evaluate tubal and uterine abnormalities.

(1) The test should be performed before ovulation to prevent fetal injury in an undiagnosed pregnancy.

(2) The woman should empty her bladder before the procedure.

(3) Premedications may include analgesics or nonsteroidal anti-inflammatory agents.

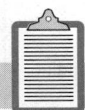

NURSING MANAGEMENT

Remind nursing and medical personnel about diagnostic procedures that require written informed consent from the woman. Instruct personnel to explain the reasons for the procedure; alternatives to the procedure; what to expect before, during, and after the procedure; risks; and benefits.

(4) During the procedure, the woman may be encouraged to use relaxation techniques to cope with any discomfort.

(5) After the procedure, the woman may experience referred shoulder pain due to irritation of nerves by the dye.

(6) Postprocedure instructions include reporting bleeding or discharge that lasts more than 4 days and any signs of infection.

9. Endoscopic examinations

a. **Colposcopy** is the direct visualization of the vagina and cervix with a binocular microscope. The procedure is used to locate the exact site of precancerous and malignant lesions for biopsy and for screening women at high risk for developing cervical and vaginal clear cell adenocarcinoma because of exposure to DES while in utero.

(1) The woman is placed in a lithotomy position.

(2) A speculum is inserted into the vagina.

(3) The cervix is cleaned with 3 percent acetic acid, which allows for better visualization of the squamocolumnar junction. A biopsy may be performed (see later discussion).

(4) After the procedure, the woman is given supplies to clean the perineal area and a perineal pad to absorb any secretions.

b. **Laparoscopy** is the use of a lighted, flexible instrument to visualize the pelvic cavity to diagnose causes of infertility, ectopic pregnancy, endometriosis, ovarian tumors and cysts, and pelvic masses.

(1) Preparation includes an explanation of the procedure, risks, and discomforts. Regional or general anesthesia may be used. Nothing by mouth (NPO) status is maintained for at least 8 hours before the procedure.

(2) During the procedure, the woman will be in a modified lithotomy position or Trendelenburg's position. A needle is inserted below the umbilicus to infuse CO_2 into the pelvic cavity to enhance visibility. A trocar and cannula are inserted into an incision. The trocar is removed, and the laparoscope is inserted (Fig. 31–4).

(3) After the procedure, the woman receives postoperative care until her condition is stable. Discomfort from referred shoulder pain caused by residual CO_2 in the peritoneal cavity usually disappears within 48 hours.

(4) Discharge teaching includes observation for and reporting of signs of infection and avoidance of strenuous activity for 1 week.

c. **Hysteroscopy** is the endoscopic examination of the uterine cavity to evaluate infertility and unexplained bleeding. The procedure should be performed before ovulation to prevent fetal injury in an undiagnosed pregnancy.

(1) The woman is placed in a lithotomy position and given regional anesthesia.

(2) During the procedure, an endoscope is inserted

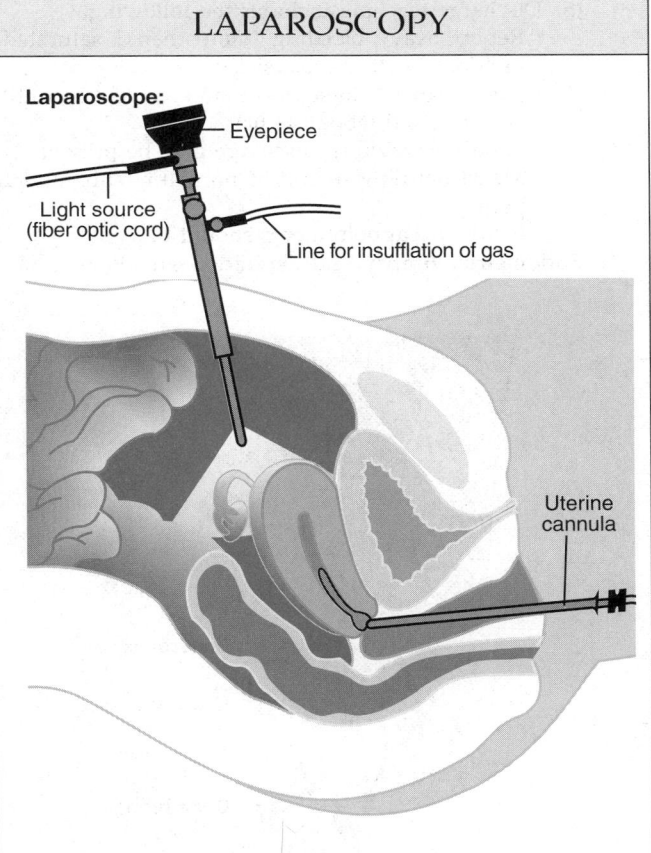

LAPAROSCOPY

Laparoscope:

Eyepiece

Light source (fiber optic cord)

Line for insufflation of gas

Uterine cannula

Figure 31–4.

through the cervix, and CO_2 is used to distend the uterus for better visibility.

   (3) After the procedure the woman may experience some cervical and uterine cramping that usually resolves within 24 hours. Instruct the woman to observe for signs of bleeding and infection.

10. Biopsies

  a. **Cervical biopsy** is the removal of cervical tissue for cytologic study to confirm a cancer diagnosis or to evaluate other cervical abnormalities.

    (1) A **punch biopsy,** in which tissue is removed with a needle punch device, is done when the lesion is visible with use of a colposcope.

    (2) A **cone biopsy,** or **conization,** is the removal of a cone-shaped portion of the cervix with a scalpel. This procedure is used when lesions are not visible or when malignancy is suspected (Fig. 31–5).

    (3) Preparation is similar to that for a pelvic examination. Punch biopsy is done without anesthesia; cone biopsy requires at least local anesthesia. The woman may be anxious because of the fear of malignancy. Relaxation techniques may be helpful. To minimize bleeding, the procedure should be done 1 week after menses.

    (4) During the procedure, the woman is in the lithotomy position. After the sample is taken, the biopsy site is cauterized, and a tampon or vaginal packing is inserted into the vagina and left in place for several hours.

    (5) Discharge teaching includes the following:
- Report heavy bleeding (more than 1 saturated pad in 1 hr) to the physician.
- Avoid sexual intercourse and douching until site is healed (about 72 hr).
- A heavy brownish discharge may be present.
- Menstrual flow should be normal in subsequent periods.
- Follow-up appointments should be kept.

  b. **Endometrial biopsy** and **aspiration** are done to ob-

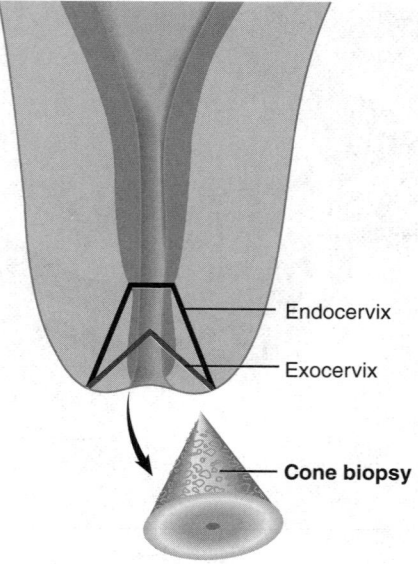

Figure 31–5. Cone biopsy.

BOX 31–1. Conscious Sedation

Intravenous (IV) conscious sedation can minimize discomfort or reduce anxiety when local anesthesia is used for operative procedures (e.g., dilation and curettage, ovarian cyst removal). The woman will have a reduced level of consciousness but will be able to maintain a patent airway independently and should be able to respond to verbal commands and physical stimulation.

Drugs commonly used for conscious sedation include midazolam (Versed), diazepam (Valium), morphine, meperidine (Demerol), and fentanyl (Sublimaze). The onset of action varies with the drug used but ranges from 1 to 5 minutes. The duration of effect also varies but ranges from 30 minutes to 2 hours or longer.

Nursing Actions:

1. If you administer conscious sedation, you are responsible for preoperative assessment and teaching.
2. Establish baseline data (cardiac rate, rhythm, blood pressure, respiration rate, oxygen saturation level, and level of consciousness).
3. Administer the drug according to physician order.
   - Give the drug over at least a 2-minute interval.
   - Wait at least 2 to 5 minutes to evaluate effectiveness.
   - Titrate doses to individual patient effect (e.g., sedative endpoint or slurring of speech).
   - Avoid excessive doses or rapid dosing that can lead to respiratory depression.
   - If there is significant change in physiologic status—for example, oxygen saturation level (SaO_2) drops below 94%—stop dosing and notify physician.
4. Monitor patient status every 5 minutes during the operative procedure.
5. Oxygen is usually not given without physician order unless the oxygen saturation level (SaO_2) drops below 94%. Oxygen is not given for respiratory depression as it can mask signs of oversedation.
6. Emergency equipment must be available (e.g., suction, positive pressure oxygen device, crash cart with defibrillator).
7. Document all assessments, interventions, and patient reactions.
8. After the operative procedure, the patient may be discharged to home or returned to the hospital unit. She may be sleepy but arousable for several hours.

Note: Registered nurses who wish to perform conscious sedation must be permitted to do so by state nurse practice laws and by institutional policies and procedures. They must also be able to document certain skills necessary for the procedure. These include ACLS certification or similar training, pulse oximetry, drug doses, and intravenous administration techniques.

Adapted from Batson VD. Conscious sedation: Implications for perioperative nursing practice. *Sem Periop Nurs* 2(1):45–57, 1993.

---

tain endometrial cells to evaluate infertility, precancerous changes, and anovulatory bleeding.

    (1) Preparation is similar to that for a pelvic examination and may be done with or without local anesthesia. Advise the woman that she may experience some cramping, and that relaxation techniques or premedication (nonsteroidal anti-inflammatory agents) may help.

    (2) The procedure is performed just before menses to assess ovulation and progesterone influences. Postmenopausal women can have the biopsy done at any time.

    (3) During the procedure, the uterus is measured with a metal sound and the cervix is dilated. A curette is inserted, and a tissue sample is re-

---

BOX 31-2. Discharge Instructions After Dilation and Curettage

- Take your temperature for at least 2 days. Call your doctor if it is more than 100 degrees Fahrenheit (38 degrees Celsius).
- Report any bleeding that is heavier than your normal menstrual period. The bleeding should not last more than 2 weeks.
- Use a heating pad or hot water bottle to relieve the discomfort from uterine cramping.
- Take a mild analgesic such as acetaminophen for abdominal pain.
- To prevent infection and allow healing, avoid sexual intercourse, douching, use of tampons, and tub baths for 2 weeks.
- Keep your follow-up appointment.

---

moved. The sample may also be obtained with a suction apparatus.

    (4) After the procedure, the woman is given a perineal pad to wear. Spotting may be present for 1 to 2 days. Postprocedure instructions are similar to those for cervical biopsy.

11. **Dilation and curettage** is a procedure in which the cervix is dilated and the uterine lining is surgically removed. A D & C is indicated for evaluation of suspected uterine malignancy, infertility, and dysfunctional uterine bleeding. There are also therapeutic indications for performing a D & C, including treatment of heavy bleeding, dysmenorrhea, incomplete abortion, and polyp removal.

    a. Preparation for a D & C may include maintenance of NPO status for 12 hours before the procedure and explanation of the procedure.

    b. During the procedure, the woman is placed in the lithotomy position. Local, regional, or general anesthesia or conscious sedation may be used (see Box 31-1 for nursing implications). A pelvic examination is performed, and a speculum is inserted into the vagina to examine the cervical os. The os is dilated, and a curette is inserted to scrape out the uterine lining.

    c. After the procedure, the woman's vital signs and vaginal bleeding are monitored until her condition is stable. Discharge instructions are summarized in Box 31-2.

◼ *AMENORRHEA*

Definition

1. **Amenorrhea** is absence of menstruation.
2. **Primary amenorrhea** is the failure to menstruate by about 16 years of age. **Secondary amenorrhea** is the absence of menstruation for at least 3 months after menarche.

Incidence and Socioeconomic Impact

1. Primary amenorrhea affects less than 0.1 percent of young women.
2. Secondary amenorrhea affects about 0.7 percent of young women.

Risk Factors

1. For primary amenorrhea, risk factors include congenital defects that cause an estrogen deficiency.
2. For secondary amenorrhea, risk factors are strenuous exercise, starvation, lactation, pregnancy, stress, discontinuing oral contraceptive pills, low thyroid level.

Etiology

1. Estrogen deficiency
2. Suppression of hypothalamic activity

Pathophysiology

1. Hypothalamic-pituitary dysfunction
2. Dysfunction in ovarian or endometrial cycles of menstruation, or both

Clinical Manifestations

1. Absence of menses
2. Lack of menstruation as a secondary effect

Diagnostics

1. History: note the following:
    a. Age-related factors: onset and cessation of menses, menopausal symptoms
    b. Diet: weight loss or gain
    c. Stress or anxiety
    d. Hormone or drug use (e.g., oral contraceptives, phenothiazines)
2. Physical assessment
    a. Note unusual distribution or amount of body hair (hirsutism).
    b. Note signs of pregnancy, such as breast tenderness, skin changes (see Chapter 14).
3. Diagnostic studies: pregnancy test, pelvic ultrasound, pelvic examination to assess for congenital abnormalities, ovarian biopsy, hormone withdrawal test, determination of serum FSH, LH, prolactin, and thyroid levels

Clinical Management

1. Goal of clinical management: to have the woman begin or resume menstrual cycles.
2. Nonpharmacologic interventions depend on the cause of amenorrhea and can include weight loss or weight gain counseling, counseling about effects of strenuous exercise, and stress reduction techniques.
3. Pharmacologic interventions depend on the cause of amenorrhea and can include drugs to stimulate ovulation and periodic progesterone withdrawal.

Progesterone is given to stimulate withdrawal bleeding. Onset of bleeding indicates normal functioning of the hypothalamus, pituitary gland, ovary, and uterus.

Complications

1. Altered sexual functioning
2. Infertility

Prognosis

1. Prognosis depends on the cause.
2. Menstruation often resumes after treatment for secondary amenorrhea.

Applying the Nursing Process

NURSING DIAGNOSIS: Anxiety R/T causes, treatment, and prognosis of amenorrhea

1. *Expected outcomes:* After intervention, the woman should be able to do the following:
   a. Verbalize fears and anxiety about condition
   b. Demonstrate knowledge about cause of amenorrhea and treatments
   c. Verbalize feelings regarding sexuality and fertility
2. *Nursing interventions*
   a. Identify and correct misconceptions about causes and effects of amenorrhea.
   b. Discuss the woman's past coping mechanisms.
   c. Explain tests and treatment options in easily understandable terms.
   d. Provide emotional support and encourage expression of feelings about sexuality and fertility.

Discharge Planning and Teaching

1. Explain to the woman the type of amenorrhea she has.
2. Describe its treatment and prognosis.

◙ *DYSMENORRHEA*

Definition

1. Painful menstruation
2. **Primary dysmenorrhea** is pain that has no known pathologic origin. **Secondary dysmenorrhea** is pain associated with a pathologic condition.

Incidence and Socioeconomic Impact

1. As many as 75 percent of all women experience dysmenorrhea.
2. Approximately 15 percent of women miss school or work each month because of dysmenorrhea.

Risk Factors

1. Risk factors for primary dysmenorrhea include obesity, never having had children, and age under 20 years.

2. Risk factors for secondary dysmenorrhea include endometriosis, ovarian neoplasms, leiomyomas, PID, and use of intrauterine devices (IUDs).

Etiology

1. Primary dysmenorrhea is thought to be caused by increased production and release of prostaglandins.
2. Secondary dysmenorrhea is caused by organic problems.

Pathophysiology

1. Increased levels of prostaglandins stimulate the uterine muscle, causing severe spasms. These spasms constrict blood flow to the muscle, resulting in ischemia and pain.
2. Dysmenorrhea may be related to such conditions as endometriosis and leiomyomas.

Clinical Manifestations

1. Pain begins with the onset of menstrual flow and lasts 12 to 48 hours.
2. Pain is located in the lower abdomen but can radiate to the lower back and thighs.
3. Nausea and vomiting may occur.
4. Less frequent manifestations include headaches, bloating, breast tenderness, diarrhea, nervousness, and fatigue.

Diagnostics

1. Question the woman about her menstrual history, obstetric history, contraceptive method, types of pain, and pain relief measures.
2. Ask about signs and symptoms suggestive of pelvic problems such as endometriosis.
3. Ask about attitudes toward menstruation and perceptions about the extent of disruption of her life.
4. A pelvic examination, including a Pap smear, cervical cultures, and vaginal cultures, should be done to determine if an underlying pathologic condition is present.
5. Ultrasound, endometrial biopsy, laparoscopy, D & C, and hysteroscopy may be used to visualize organs and determine cause.

Clinical Management

1. Goal of clinical management: to relieve the pain
2. Nonpharmacologic interventions include hot baths, aerobic exercise, yoga or meditation, massage, orgasm, and heat to the abdomen. Dietary changes include increased vitamin B_6, calcium, magnesium, and protein and decreased sodium.
3. Pharmacologic interventions are aimed at inhibiting ovulation and decreasing prostaglandin levels (see Table 31-4). Analgesics are given for pain relief.
4. Special medical-surgical procedures: Temporary relief may be obtained by surgical dilation of the cervix. In

Table 31-4. Drugs Used to Treat Dysmenorrhea

Medication	Action	Side Effects	Contraindications	Nursing Implications
Ibuprofen (Motrin, Advil, Nuprin); naproxen sodium (Anaprox, Naprosyn, Aleve); mefenamic acid (Ponstel, Ponstan)	Inhibits prostagladin release; analgesia	Gastrointestinal upset; nausea; rash; pruritus; drowsiness; edema. Mefenamic acid may cause tinnitus, increased bleeding time	Pregnancy	Take with milk or meals. Watch for rash or pruritus. Do not take with aspirin. May cause drowsiness. Avoid alcohol. Bruising or bleeding may occur with mefenamic acid.
Aspirin	Same as above			
Oral contraceptives	Inhibit ovulation; decrease menstrual cramps and bleeding	Breast tenderness; nausea, weight gain; breakthrough bleeding; spotting; mood changes; depression; chloasma	Thrombophlebitis; history of cerebrovascular accident; coronary artery disease; history of or known breast cancer; history of or known estrogen-dependent tumor; impaired liver function; pregnancy	Take at same time every day. Smoking increases risks associated with oral contraceptives. Warning signs include severe chest pain, severe headache, unusual swelling or pain in legs, vision problems

Data from Gant NF, and Cunningham FG. *Basic Gynecology and Obstetrics.* Norwalk, CT: Appleton & Lange, 1993; Bobak I, Lowdermilk D, and Benson M. *Maternity Nursing.* 4th ed. St. Louis: CV Mosby, 1995.

rare cases in which there is no underlying disorder and medical treatment has not been effective, a hysterectomy, presacral sympathectomy, or uterosacral nerve ablation may be performed.

Complications

1. Dysmenorrhea can cause disruption of activities of daily living.
2. Dysmenorrhea can cause infertility.

Prognosis

1. Primary dysmenorrhea may be alleviated after vaginal childbirth.
2. Secondary dysmenorrhea will end at menopause.

Applying the Nursing Process

NURSING DIAGNOSIS: Pain R/T dysmenorrhea

1. *Expected outcomes:* After teaching and intervention, the woman should be able to do the following:
   a. Demonstrate use of effective pain relief measures
   b. Verbalize relief of pain
2. *Nursing interventions*
   a. Evaluate character and severity of pain.
   b. Provide information about pain control; for example, heat, diet, exercise, drugs (prostaglandin inhibitors, analgesics, nonsteroidal anti-inflammatory drugs).

NURSING DIAGNOSIS: Ineffective individual coping R/T stressors that may aggravate pain

1. *Expected outcomes:* After counseling, the woman should be able to do the following:
   a. Demonstrate effective coping behaviors
   b. Verbalize that disruptions to her daily life are minimal
2. *Nursing interventions*
   a. Explore the woman's behavior during dysmenorrhea to identify effects on lifestyle.
   b. Encourage the use of past effective coping mechanisms or refer to other resources as needed.

Discharge Planning and Teaching

1. Educate the woman about therapeutic measures for pain relief.
2. Help the woman identify ways to decrease stress and get adequate rest and exercise.
3. Discuss ways to treat the underlying condition, including surgical options.

◼ *PREMENSTRUAL SYNDROME*

Definition

Premenstrual syndrome (PMS) is a constellation of symptoms that appear before the onset of menses.

Incidence and Socioeconomic Impact

1. About 50 percent of all women experience some degree of PMS.
2. It is estimated that 9 to 12 million American women are affected.

TRANSCULTURAL CONSIDERATIONS

In the United States, premenstrual syndrome is often considered a culture-bound illness.

Risk Factors

1. Major life stressor
2. Age over 30 years
3. Depression

Etiology

1. The etiology of PMS is not well understood.
2. There may be many causes.

Pathophysiology

1. Symptoms appear only in the luteal phase of the menstrual cycle and disappear with menses.
2. A fall in estrogen and progesterone levels increases aldosterone production, which can result in sodium retention and edema.
3. Depression may be related to decreased brain levels of monoamine oxidase.
4. Mood swings may be caused by decreased serotonin levels.

Clinical Manifestations

1. Symptoms begin 5 to 10 days before menstruation.
2. Symptoms are listed in Table 31–5.

Diagnostics

1. History
   a. Identify symptoms and their timing.
   b. Assess effects on activities of daily living.
2. Physical examination: Fluid retention, breast tenderness, abdominal bloating, acne, paresthesia may be revealed.
3. Medical diagnosis includes ruling out other problems that have similar symptoms.
4. Information about type and timing of symptoms is most important in diagnosing PMS.
5. Suppression of ovulation with a gonadotropin-releasing hormone agonist relieves symptoms

Table 31–5. Premenstrual Syndrome (PMS)

System	Indicators
Dermatologic	Acne
	Urticaria
	Herpes
Respiratory	Sinusitis
	Asthma
	Rhinitis
	Colds
Urologic	Oliguria
	Cystitis
	Enuresis
	Urethritis
Ophthalmologic	Conjunctivitis
	Styes
	Glaucoma
Neurologic	Headaches
	Migraine
	Syncope
	Vertigo
	Numbness of hands and feet
	Epilepsy (if susceptible)
Emotional or psychologic	Depression
	Irritability
	Tension
	Panic attacks
	Change in libido
	Mood swings
	Anxiety
Behavioral	Lowered work performance
	Food cravings
	Alcohol and drug overindulgence
	Confusion
	Sleeplessness
	Lack of coordination
	Suicidal ideation
	Lethargy
	Child abuse
	Assaultive behavior
Metabolic	Edema
	Breast tenderness
Other	Allergies
	Hypoglycemia
	Joint pain
	Palpitations
	Water retention

Adapted from Ignatavicius DD, Workman ML, and Mishler M (eds). *Medical-Surgical Nursing: A Nursing Process Approach.* 2nd ed. Philadelphia: WB Saunders, 1995, p 2218.

Clinical Management

1. Goal of intervention: to reduce or eliminate the symptoms of PMS
2. Nonpharmacologic interventions

a. Limit intake of salt, caffeine, animal fats, refined sugars, stimulants, alcohol
b. Increase intake of carbohydrates, protein, fiber
c. Increase exercise and use stress reduction techniques
d. Obtain psychologic therapy or support as needed

3. Pharmacologic interventions
   a. Suppression of ovulation with danazol, gonadotropin-releasing hormone agonists, oral contraceptives
   b. Progesterone
   c. Antiprostaglandin agents for cramping
   d. Bromocriptine for breast tenderness
   e. Diuretics, tranquilizers, antidepressants such as fluoxetine (Prozac)
   f. Vitamin E, magnesium
4. Special medical-surgical procedures: Endometrial ablation is performed if underlying condition warrants it (see p. 1466).

Complications

1. Complications may be due to an underlying pathologic condition.
2. Premenstrual syndrome may have psychogenic complications.

Prognosis

1. Premenstrual syndrome will resolve at menopause.
2. Reduction of symptoms depends on how the individual woman reacts to therapy.

Applying the Nursing Process

NURSING DIAGNOSIS: Activity intolerance R/T fatigue or other symptoms that interfere with usual activities

1. *Expected outcomes:* After instruction, the woman should be able to do the following:
   a. Comply with the therapeutic interventions
   b. Demonstrate understanding of PMS and how it affects activity tolerance
   c. Report being able to function optimally in usual activities
2. *Nursing interventions*
   a. Identify the woman's activities and determine when PMS affects them.
   b. Discuss ways to decrease cyclic changes.

NURSING DIAGNOSIS: Pain R/T symptoms caused by hormonal shifts

1. *Expected outcomes:* After intervention, the woman should report less pain.
2. *Nursing interventions*
   a. Determine the severity of symptoms and provide information on pain control.
   b. Collaborate with other health care providers to ensure effective pain control.

NURSING DIAGNOSIS: Self-esteem disturbance R/T PMS

1. *Expected outcomes:* Following counseling, the woman should report a positive self-image.
2. *Nursing interventions*
   a. Discuss the woman's feelings about herself.
   b. Encourage the woman and her partner to participate in a support group or counseling.
   c. Assist the woman to identify self-care activities that reduce symptoms.

Discharge Planning and Teaching

1. Teach the woman to keep a menstrual chart for several months and to plot occurrence of symptoms.

LEARNING/TEACHING GUIDELINES
for Premenstrual Syndrome

General Overview

1. Describe the possible causes of premenstrual syndrome (PMS).
2. Discuss dietary modifications that may alleviate symptoms.
3. Point out the importance of rest, stress reduction, and exercise in reducing the impact of PMS symptoms.
4. Help the woman explore treatment options—drug therapy, support groups or counseling, psychotherapy.

Dietary Modifications

1. Eat small, frequent meals to avoid glucose fluctuations. Include protein, complex carbohydrates, fruits, and vegetables.
2. Limit salt intake to avoid fluid retention.
3. Avoid coffee, tea, chocolate, and colas with caffeine, as they may cause breast pain and depression.

Exercise

1. Walks in daylight may improve behavioral symptoms, such as mood swings.
2. Adequate rest may decrease PMS symptoms.

2. Help the woman to identify foods and vitamins that may alleviate symptoms.
3. Teach stress reduction.
4. See Learning/Teaching Guidelines for Premenstrual Syndrome.

Public Health Considerations

1. Nurses can provide public education about PMS.
2. Nurses can organize support groups for women and their family members who are affected by PMS.

◼ DYSFUNCTIONAL UTERINE BLEEDING

Definition

1. **Dysfunctional uterine bleeding (DUB)** is abnormal uterine bleeding.
2. It has a variety of causes.

Incidence and Socioeconomic Impact

1. Dysfunctional uterine bleeding is the most frequently encountered female reproductive system disorder. As many as 75 percent of the cases of abnormal bleeding are classified as DUB.
2. Half of the cases of DUB occur in women older than 40 years of age; 20 percent occur in adolescents, and 30 percent affect women 20 to 40 years of age.

Risk Factors

1. Stress
2. Extreme weight changes
3. Oral contraceptive use
4. Postmenopausal status

Etiology

1. Hormonal imbalance
2. Pelvic pathologic conditions such as tumors

Pathophysiology

1. Endometrial hyperplasia caused by persistent unopposed estrogen stimulation (e.g., taking estrogen without progesterone). When the endometrial lining can no longer be maintained by estrogen, it sloughs off, and vaginal bleeding occurs.
2. Follicular-phase defects cause a shortened proliferative phase, which can result in spotting.
3. Luteal-phase defects can cause profuse or prolonged

bleeding, or both, because the corpus luteum fails to regress appropriately, causing a progesterone deficiency.

Clinical Manifestations

1. Painless bleeding that is abnormal in amount, duration, or timing
2. Midcycle spotting
3. Oligomenorrhea

Diagnostics

1. The history should include questions about the menstrual cycle, exercise habits, weight change, and use of drugs.
2. The physical examination includes inspection for obesity, malnutrition, and abnormal hair growth. The abdomen is palpated for pain or masses.
3. Pelvic examination
4. Diagnostic tests include pelvic ultrasound, hysteroscopy, and endometrial biopsy.
5. Laboratory data include complete blood count, thyroid function tests, endocrine profile, serum progesterone levels, Pap smear, serum hCG.

Clinical Management

1. Goals of intervention: The woman should maintain adequate tissue perfusion, and abnormal bleeding episodes should be resolved.
2. Nonpharmacologic interventions: Adequate rest and a diet rich in iron may be suggested in addition to pharmacologic therapy.
3. Pharmacologic interventions
   a. Hormonal manipulation for anovulatory DUB involves oral contraceptives for 3 to 6 months and progesterone or medroxyprogesterone during the last 10 to 13 days of the cycle, to regulate uterine bleeding.
   b. Hormonal manipulation for ovulatory DUB involves administration of progestins during the luteal phase.
   c. Iron preparations may be prescribed.
4. Special medical-surgical procedures
   a. Dilation and curettage for acute bleeding episodes (see p. 1461).
   b. Endometrial ablation for bleeding in women who do not respond to medical management
      (1) Endometrial laser ablation is performed under local or general anesthesia as an outpatient procedure.
      (2) The uterine cavity is distended and irrigated with a normal saline solution.
      (3) Laser energy is directed through a hysteroscope.
      (4) A dragging technique is used to ablate the endometrium under video monitor control.
      (5) Risks of laser ablation include uterine scarring and possible sterility. The procedure may not be completely effective. Hemorrhage can occur, and normal tissues can be destroyed.

(6) Nursing care after ablation includes teaching about the signs of infection, good perineal hygiene, and keeping the area dry. Explain that vaginal discharge may be present for up to 4 weeks. Analgesics or nonsteroidal anti-inflammatory drugs or both may be prescribed for postoperative pain. Normal activities can be resumed in 1 to 2 days.

c. Hysterectomy is done only if other treatments fail (see p. 1474).

Complications

1. Hemorrhage
2. Anemia, weight loss
3. Altered sexual functioning

Prognosis

1. The prognosis depends on the cause of abnormal bleeding.
2. The woman's response to treatment also affects the prognosis.

Applying the Nursing Process

NURSING DIAGNOSIS: Anxiety R/T cause of DUB and its treatment

1. *Expected outcomes:* Following counseling the woman should verbalize decreased anxiety about DUB and its treatment.
2. *Nursing interventions*
   a. Provide information about the causes, treatment, and prognosis of DUB.
   b. Provide an opportunity for the woman to discuss fears and feelings about her condition.
   c. Discuss the woman's past coping strategies and teach new strategies if needed.

NURSING DIAGNOSIS: Potential for altered tissue perfusion R/T excessive uterine bleeding

1. *Expected outcomes:* Following intervention, the woman should demonstrate adequate tissue perfusion as evidenced by normal vital signs, serum hematocrit, and blood loss that is not excessive.
2. *Nursing interventions*
   a. Monitor blood loss, measure vital signs, and review laboratory findings such as hematocrit.
   b. Encourage fluid intake and rest.
   c. Give iron medication and blood products if ordered.

Discharge Planning and Teaching

1. Discuss self-medication, including actions and side effects, dosage, and frequency.
2. Discuss postoperative self-care if surgery is performed.

Public Health Considerations

1. Explain the importance of reporting future abnormal bleeding episodes.
2. All postmenopausal women should report any uterine bleeding to their physician.

◻ *ENDOMETRIOSIS*

Definition

1. Abnormal development of endometrial tissue
2. Tissue growth outside the uterus

Incidence and Socioeconomic Impact

1. Endometriosis affects 1 to 3 percent of women of childbearing age.
2. It is associated with as much as 30 percent of all cases of infertility.

Risk Factors

1. Nulliparity
2. History of endometriosis in mothers, siblings, or 1st-degree relatives
3. Endometriosis is more frequent in White women.

Etiology

1. The cause of endometriosis is unknown.
2. Several causes have been proposed.

Pathophysiology

1. Metaplasia: endometrial tissue develops from coelomic epithelial cells as a result of hormonal or inflammatory influences.
2. Retrograde menstruation: endometrial tissue flows back through the fallopian tubes during menstruation. These fragments implant on pelvic structures.
3. Dissemination through vascular or lymphatic routes

Clinical Manifestations

1. Lower abdominal and pelvic pain that is described as deep, constant pressure and radiates to the back and down the legs
2. Rectal pressure, painful defecation
3. Dyspareunia (painful intercourse)
4. Pain usually occurs in the second half of the cycle
5. Abnormal uterine bleeding

Diagnostics

1. A menstrual and obstetric history should determine characteristics of bleeding and pain.

NURSE ADVISORY

> The degree of pain does not indicate the severity of the endometriosis. Minimal disease can cause severe pain, whereas extensive endometriosis can occur without symptoms.

2. A physical examination identifies nodules, masses, tenderness, scarring, or uterine retroflexion.
3. Pelvic ultrasound to rule out other causes
4. Laparoscopy and biopsy to identify endometrial tissue outside the uterus (Fig. 31–6).

Clinical Management

1. Goal of clinical management: to relieve symptoms and to retain or improve fertility
2. Nonpharmacologic interventions
   a. Application of heat to the sacrum or abdomen
   b. Relaxation techniques, yoga, biofeedback, exercise
3. Pharmacologic interventions
   a. Mild analgesics, prostaglandin synthetase inhibitors
   b. Hormonal therapy: oral contraceptives, progesterone, androgen (danazol), Gn-RH
4. Special medical-surgical procedures
   a. Electrocauterization or laser ablation of adhesions and endometrial implants (see p. 1477).
   b. Hysterectomy and bilateral salpingo-oophorectomy for endometriosis unresponsive to other treatment (see p. 1477).

Complications

1. Infertility
2. Ectopic pregnancy

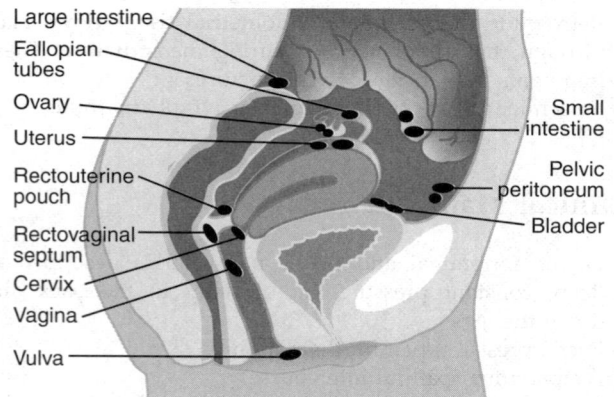

Large intestine
Fallopian tubes
Ovary
Uterus
Rectouterine pouch
Rectovaginal septum
Cervix
Vagina
Vulva
Small intestine
Pelvic peritoneum
Bladder

Figure 31–6. Common sites of endometriosis.

Prognosis

1. Prognosis depends on the treatment option.
2. Endometriosis may regress after pregnancy and at menopause.

Applying the Nursing Process

NURSING DIAGNOSIS: Self-esteem disturbance R/T the effects of endometriosis on sexual functioning, fertility

1. *Expected outcomes:* Following counseling the woman should verbalize a positive self-esteem.
2. *Nursing interventions*
   a. Encourage the woman to ventilate feelings about her self-image and sexual functioning.
   b. Involve significant others in discussions.
   c. Provide information about support groups or counseling as needed.

NURSING DIAGNOSIS: Pain R/T condition

1. *Expected outcomes:* Following teaching and intervention, the woman should do the following:
   a. Report an understanding of the various methods of pain relief
   b. Report decreased pain after implementing pain relief measures
2. *Nursing interventions*
   a. Determine severity of pain.
   b. Provide information about pain control measures, such as heat to the abdomen, relaxation techniques, and analgesics.

NURSING DIAGNOSIS: Knowledge deficit R/T the treatment options

1. *Expected outcomes:* Following counseling, the woman should verbalize understanding of the treatment options.
2. *Nursing interventions*
   a. Discuss hormonal and surgical treatment alternatives.
   b. Include significant others in discussions.

Discharge Planning and Teaching

1. If hormonal therapy is prescribed, the woman should be taught the dosages, frequency, actions, and side effects of the medication.
2. Information about support groups and counseling should be made available.
3. If surgery is to be done, postoperative instructions for self-care are needed.

Public Health Considerations

1. Nurses can organize support groups for women and their partners or families.
2. Nurses can provide information about endometriosis through community programs.

◼ *GYNECOLOGIC INFECTIONS*

Definition

1. Gynecologic infections can be local or systemic. They may or may not be sexually transmitted. Gynecologic infections that are sexually transmitted are discussed in Chapter 32.
2. Gynecologic infections include infection with *Candida albicans, Gardnerella vaginalis,* or *Trichomonas vaginalis;* bacterial vaginosis; PID; and toxic shock syndrome.

Incidence and Socioeconomic Impact

1. Bacterial vaginosis is the most common cause of vaginal symptoms in women of childbearing age.
2. The incidence is higher in women who use oral contraceptives.

Risk Factors

1. Use of oral contraceptives.
2. Obesity, diabetes, use of antibiotics, and pregnancy are risk factors for monilial infections.
3. Sexual activity and swimming in contaminated water are risk factors for trichomoniasis.

Etiology

1. Bacterial vaginosis is caused by a number of different bacteria.
2. Candidiasis (moniliasis) is a yeast infection caused by *C. albicans.*
3. Trichomoniasis is caused by *T. vaginalis.*

Pathophysiology

1. Microorganisms invade the vulva and vagina.
2. Altered pH, changes in normal flora, and low estrogen levels lower the woman's resistance to infection.
3. Menstrual blood provides a growth medium for pathogens.

Clinical Manifestations

1. Vaginal discharge
2. Itching
3. Vaginal burning or dysuria

Diagnostics

1. History includes questions about unprotected sexual activity, multiple partners, or known transmission of bacterial or other infection and description of symptoms.
2. Physical findings include vaginal discharge with or without odor, inflammation, edema, and scratch marks. Table 31–6 describes common vaginal discharges. Table 31–3 summarizes wet preparations for diagnosing vaginal infections.
   a. Bacterial vaginosis: culture of vaginal secretions for evidence of "clue cells," KOH wet preparation for whiff test (presence of fishy odor)
   b. Candidiasis: culture for yeast, KOH wet preparation to detect hyphae and *C. albicans* spores
   c. Trichomoniasis: normal saline wet preparation to detect protozoa

Clinical Management

1. Goal of intervention: to treat infections successfully and to prevent complications
2. Nonpharmacologic intervention
   a. Safer sex practices (e.g., condom use, monogamous relationship)
   b. Good genital hygiene
3. Pharmacologic intervention
   a. Bacterial vaginosis is treated with metronidazole. Both the woman and her partner are treated.
   b. Candidiasis is treated with antifungal agents. Both the woman and her partner receive treatment.

Table 31–6. Common Vaginal Discharges

Cause	Characteristics	Symptoms
Normal	Clear after menses; thicker, white, after ovulation; no odor	None
Monilia (*Candida albicans*)	Thick, white or yellow cheesy patches on cervix and vaginal walls; usually little odor	Itching, dysuria
Trichomonas vaginalis	Frothy, green discharge; strawberry spot on cervix; foul odor	Foul odor; profuse discharge; itching
Gardnerella vaginalis (bacterial vaginosis)	Thin, gray-white discharge; fishy odor	May be asymptomatic; fishy odor; itching
Atrophic vaginitis	Thin, whitish discharge; often blood-tinged; no odor; pale, thin, dry vaginal mucosa	Vaginal dryness; painful intercourse; itching

c. Trichomoniasis is treated with metronidazole for both the woman and her partner.

 DRUG ADVISORY

If a 1-time dose of metronidazole (Flagyl) is given, the patient should avoid alcohol for 48 hours. If a 7-day dose is given, alcohol should be avoided during this course and for 24 hours after the last dose.

Complications

1. Secondary infections
2. Neonatal exposure during childbirth
3. Congenital anomalies if infection occurs during pregnancy

Prognosis

Prognosis is good if treatment is completed.

Applying the Nursing Process

NURSING DIAGNOSIS: Knowledge deficit R/T causes, treatments, and prevention

1. *Expected outcomes:* Following counseling, the woman should verbalize understanding of the cause, treatment, and prevention of gynecologic infections.
2. *Nursing interventions*
   a. Discuss transmission, treatment, and prevention.
   b. Provide information on ways to practice safer sex.
   c. Explain why partners need to be treated as well.
   d. Advise sexual abstinence until follow-up visit after treatment.

NURSING DIAGNOSIS: Pain R/T infection

1. *Expected outcomes:* After counseling, the woman should do the following:
   a. Verbalize understanding of pain relief measures
   b. State that pain is lessened or relieved
2. *Nursing Interventions*
   a. Determine the severity of pain.
   b. Inform the woman that treatment decreases pain.
   c. Provide information about comfort measures, such as cool compresses and sitz baths.

Discharge Planning and Teaching

1. Teach good hygiene practices (Box 31–3).
2. Teach ways to minimize risk of reinfection.

BOX 31–3. Hygiene to Prevent Vaginal Infections
- Wash hands before and after genital contact.
- Wipe front to back after urinating or having a bowel movement.
- Wear all-cotton or cotton-crotch underpants.
- Avoid tight-fitting clothes, such as jeans, pantyhose.
- Do not douche or use feminine hygiene sprays.
- Use condoms during sexual intercourse.
- Avoid intercourse if you have a vaginal infection or if your partner has an infection of his sex organs.
- Remove damp exercise clothes (leotards, tights, swimsuits) promptly.

---

3. Describe treatment plan and need to take all the medication as prescribed and to return for follow-up appointment.

Public Health Considerations

1. All women need information about sexually transmitted diseases, ways to practice safer sex, and good perineal hygiene.
2. Information should be available in schools, health clinics, or offices. Public awareness programs should be available in communities.

■ UTERINE DISPLACEMENT AND PROLAPSE

Definition

1. **Uterine displacement** is a variation in placement of the uterus from the midline in the pelvis with the cervix posterior and body of uterus in slight anterior flexion (see Fig. 31–2).

Incidence and Socioeconomic Impact

1. Both uterine prolapse and uterine displacement are more common in older women.
2. Aging weakens the pelvic support structures.

Risk Factors

1. Prolapse of the uterus is seen less frequently in Black and Asian-American women than in White women.
2. Both uterine prolapse and uterine displacement are more common among elderly nulliparas and women who have experienced complicated childbirth.

Etiology

1. Displacement and prolapse of the uterus can be caused by congenital or acquired weakness of the pelvic support structures.

2. Pregnancy, birth, surgery, radiation, and aging are all causal factors.

Pathophysiology

1. Weakened pelvic supports allow the uterus to be displaced.
2. The uterus may become repositioned backward or prolapsed into the vaginal canal or outside the vaginal opening.

Clinical Manifestations

1. Pelvic pressure, pain
2. Backache
3. Visible uterine prolapse
4. Bowel or bladder prolapse (if rectocele, cystocele, or both are also present)

Diagnostics

1. The history should include information about infertility, backache, painful intercourse, sensations of pressure or heaviness in pelvis or the feeling that "something is in my vagina," history of pelvic trauma, pelvic surgery, or childbirth.
2. Pelvic examination may reveal structural disorders.

Clinical Management

1. Goal of intervention: to relieve pain and to treat the structural defect
2. Nonpharmacologic interventions
   a. Increasing muscle tone through Kegel exercises (Box 31–4)
   b. Use of pessaries to support the uterus (Fig. 31–7)

BOX 31–4. Kegel Exercises

Kegel exercises can strengthen the perineal muscles and improve muscle tone. To teach a woman to perform Kegel exercise correctly, have her start by trying to stop the flow of urine during urination. If she can do this, her pubococcygeal muscle tone is good.

The woman can practice Kegel exercises in 2 ways:
1. Slowly tighten the pubococcygeal muscle, hold for a count of 3 to 5, then relax it.
2. Quickly tighten the muscle and relax it as quickly as possible. Repeat with either method at least 10 to 24 times 4 times a day. Perform the exercise during urination as well as at other times.

---

3. Pharmacologic interventions
   a. Topical estrogen for regeneration of pelvic supports in older women
   b. Analgesic for discomfort
4. Special medical-surgical procedures
   a. Surgical repair of the prolapsed uterus
   b. Hysterectomy (see p. 1474)

Complications

1. Infertility
2. Bowel or bladder dysfunction
3. Infection

Prognosis

1. Surgical repairs are often successful.
2. Corrective procedures may shorten the vagina, which may cause painful intercourse.

Applying the Nursing Process

NURSING DIAGNOSIS: Knowledge deficit R/T causes of structural disorder and treatment options

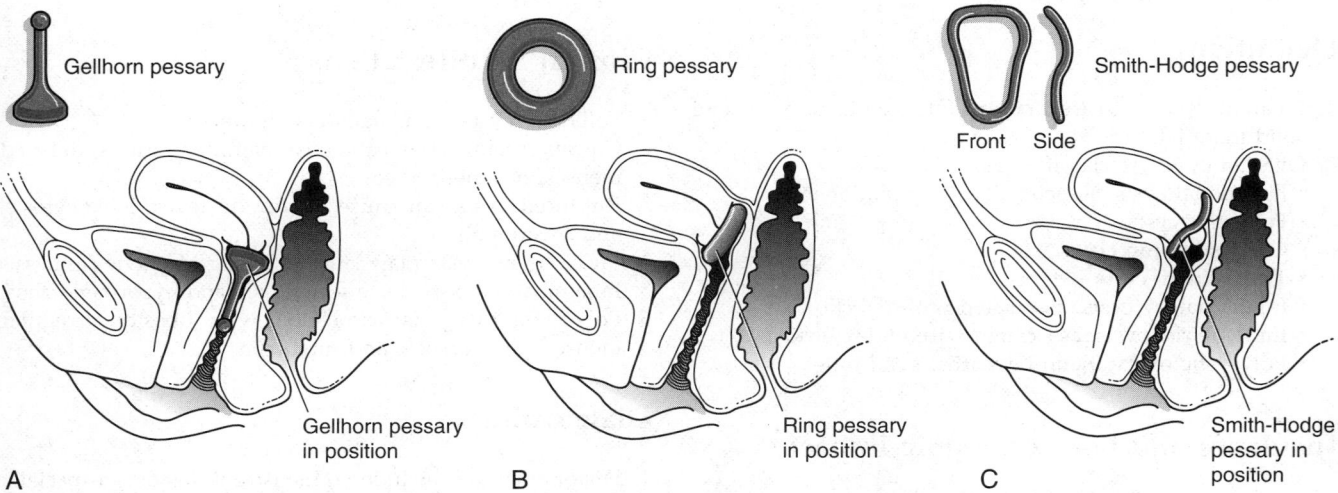

Gellhorn pessary

Gellhorn pessary in position

Ring pessary

Ring pessary in position

Smith-Hodge pessary

Front   Side

Smith-Hodge pessary in position

A   B   C

Figure 31–7. Types of vaginal pessaries. (From Monahan FD, Drake T, and Neighbors M. *Nursing Care of Adults.* Philadelphia: WB Saunders, 1994, p 1722.)

1. *Expected outcomes:* Following counseling, the woman should verbalize understanding about her diagnosis and treatment options.
2. *Nursing interventions*
   a. Encourage the woman to ask questions about her diagnosis and treatment.
   b. Provide information on the causes and treatment options, risks, and possible outcomes.
   c. Include partner in teaching process.

NURSING DIAGNOSIS: Anxiety R/T treatment and prognosis

---

1. *Expected outcomes:* Following teaching, the woman should verbalize decreased anxiety about treatment and her prognosis.
2. *Nursing interventions*
   a. Encourage the woman to discuss her feelings and concerns.
   b. Clarify misunderstandings about treatment and prognosis.
   c. Identify the woman's past coping mechanisms and encourage use.

Discharge Planning and Teaching

1. Explain nonsurgical treatment options such as Kegel exercises or use of a pessary.
2. Teach pre- and postoperative procedures as appropriate.

Public Health Considerations

1. Kegel exercises can strengthen the muscles of the perineum.
2. Avoiding closely spaced pregnancies may prevent this problem.

◼ *OVARIAN CYSTS*

Definition

1. **Ovarian cysts** are sacs that are filled with fluid or semisolid material.
2. Ovarian cysts are classified as
   • Functional cysts, associated with ovulation
   • Follicular cysts
   • Corpus luteum cysts
   • Theca lutein cysts
   • Inflammatory cysts, associated with infection
   • Endometrial cysts, associated with endometriosis
   • Polycystic ovary (Stein-Leventhal syndrome)

Incidence and Socioeconomic Impact

1. Ovarian cysts can develop at any age.
2. These cysts are uncommon after menopause.

NURSE ADVISORY

A woman who is perimenopausal or postmenopausal and has a palpable ovarian mass is more likely to have a malignancy than a cyst.

Risk Factors

1. Any ovulating female is at risk for functional ovarian cysts.
2. Prolonged Gn-RH therapy and hydatidiform mole are risk factors for theca lutein cysts.
3. Gonorrhea is a risk factor for inflammatory cysts.

Etiology

1. Polycystic ovary is caused by high levels of LH.
2. Corpus luteum cysts are caused by an unexplained increase of fluid in the corpus luteum.
3. Inflammatory cysts are caused by acute infection.
4. Endometrial cysts are caused by endometrial implants on the ovaries.

Pathophysiology

1. Follicular cysts develop as a result of the mature follicle's failure to rupture or an immature follicle's failure to reabsorb fluid after ovulation.
2. Corpus luteum cysts are enlargements caused by increased fluid secretion by the corpus luteum after ovulation.
3. Endometrial cysts are caused by endometrial implants and are often filled with old blood, in which case they are called **chocolate cysts.**
4. Inflammatory cysts develop as a result of infection of the ovary or fallopian tube.
5. Polycystic ovaries develop as a result of hyperstimulation of the ovaries caused by elevated levels of LH.

Clinical Manifestations

1. Follicular cysts are usually asymptomatic.
2. Corpus luteum cysts can cause pain, tenderness, delayed menses, or amenorrhea.
3. Ruptured cysts can cause low-grade fever, leukocytosis, and severe pain.
4. Theca lutein cysts may cause a feeling of pelvic fullness.
5. Inflammatory cysts cause severe pain and hypermenorrhea.
6. Polycystic ovary is associated with obesity, irregular menses, amenorrhea, and hirsutism.

Diagnostics

1. History should include a menstrual history, especially amount of bleeding; pain assessment; and a report of presenting symptoms.

2. Bimanual and rectovaginal palpation will reveal tenderness and presence of ovarian cyst.
3. Medical diagnosis
   a. Ultrasound to differentiate functional cysts from neoplastic (solid) cysts
   b. Laparoscopy to diagnose endometriosis and polycystic ovaries
   c. Abdominal radiograph to visualize functional cysts and differentiate them from neoplastic cysts
   d. Laboratory data:
      (1) The white blood cell count may be elevated with inflamed cysts.
      (2) Human chorionic gonadotropin levels may be elevated with theca lutein cysts.
      (3) Pregnancy test may be given, especially if theca lutein cyst is suspected.

Clinical Management

1. Goal of intervention: to reduce pain, treat the cause of the cyst, and prevent complications
2. Nonpharmacologic interventions include pelvic examinations at regular intervals to monitor ovarian cyst size. Follicular cysts may spontaneously disappear within 60 days.
3. Pharmacologic interventions include mild analgesics for pain, oral contraceptives to suppress ovulation and shrink functional cysts, and antibiotic therapy, either prophylactic or for infected cysts.
4. Special medical-surgical procedures: surgery to remove ovarian cysts
   a. Cystectomy, the removal of a cyst, is the preferred procedure.
   b. Oophorectomy, or removal of the ovary, is usually not recommended.

Complications

1. Infection
2. Rupture of cyst
3. Infertility
4. Hemorrhage
5. Recurrence of cyst

Prognosis

Most functional ovarian cysts disappear within 60 days with or without treatment.

Applying the Nursing Process

NURSING DIAGNOSIS: Pain R/T ovarian cysts

1. *Expected outcomes:* Following instruction, the woman should verbalize understanding of ways to manage pain.

2. *Nursing interventions:* Educate the woman about pain-relieving measures, including analgesics as ordered; comfort measures, such as moist heat to vulva or dry heat to the abdomen; and relaxation techniques.

NURSING DIAGNOSIS: Knowledge deficit R/T causes and treatment options of cysts

1. *Expected outcomes:* Following instruction, the woman should verbalize understanding of the causes and treatment options.
2. *Nursing interventions*
   a. Provide information on pre- and postoperative care if surgery is needed.
   b. Instruct the woman to take prescribed medications.

Discharge Planning and Teaching

1. Discuss the importance of keeping follow-up appointments for monitoring the cyst or for postoperative follow-up.
2. Teach signs of infection and postoperative incision care as needed.

Public Health Considerations

1. All women need to be educated about the importance of routine physical examinations throughout their lives.
2. Recommendations for intervals for screening should be available in clinics or physicians' offices.

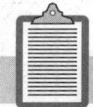

NURSING MANAGEMENT

Alert all personnel conducting admission interviews to ask the woman about her past use of the health care system. This information will provide a basis for discharge planning and health teaching.

◨ UTERINE LEIOMYOMAS

Definition

1. **Leiomyomas** are nonmalignant masses (nonencapsulated tumor) of the smooth muscle of the uterus.
2. Leiomyomas, or uterine fibroids, are classified as intramural (in the uterine wall), subserous (beneath the peritoneal cavity, projecting into the abdominal cavity), or submucus (beneath the endometrium, projecting into the uterine cavity) (Fig. 31–8).

Incidence and Socioeconomic Impact

1. About 20 percent of women older than 30 years of age have leiomyomas.

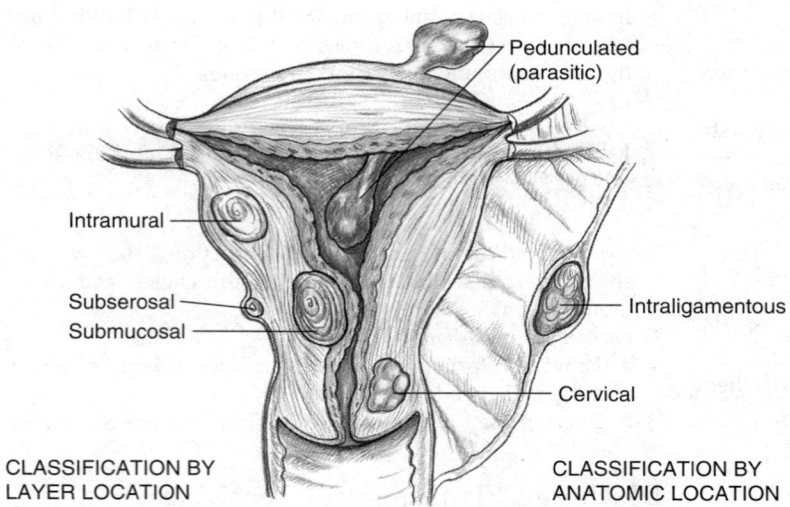

Figure 31–8. Classification of uterine leiomyomas.

2. Leiomyomas are more common in Black women than in White women in the United States.

Risk Factors

1. Age older than 50
2. Black women

Etiology

Unknown cause but may be related to estrogen stimulation

Pathophysiology

1. Leiomyomas are benign, slow-growing solid tumors that develop from uterine myometrium.
2. Leiomyomas are attached to the uterine wall by means of a pedicle, or stalk. They grow with use of oral contraceptives and usually regress after menopause.

Clinical Manifestations

1. Pain
2. Prolonged menses
3. Constipation, urinary frequency
4. Feelings of pelvic pressure
5. Bleeding
6. Most are asymptomatic

Diagnostics

1. History includes questions about bleeding, pain, pelvic pressure, and changes in the size or shape of the abdomen.
2. Physical examination may reveal uterine enlargement, irregularly shaped abdomen, and pain during bimanual palpation.
3. Medical diagnosis
   a. Pregnancy test to rule out pregnancy as cause for enlargement
   b. Laparotomy to visualize subserous leiomyomas
   c. Ultrasound to differentiate leiomyomas from endometriosis

Clinical Management

1. Goals of intervention: to monitor the status of the leiomyoma or remove it
2. Nonpharmacologic interventions: pelvic examinations at 4- to 6-month intervals to monitor status of leiomyoma. Monitoring is done for women who are asymptomatic or who desire childbearing.
3. Pharmacologic interventions include Gn-RH agonists, leuprolide acetate (Leupron) to reduce leiomyoma size in an effort to avoid surgery.
4. Special medical-surgical procedures
   a. In **myomectomy,** the leiomyoma is removed through an incision in the uterus; the uterus is not removed to preserve childbearing potential. Laser surgery can destroy fibroids through a laparoscopic approach. Fibroids can also be removed by surgical excision through an abdominal incision. Surgery is usually performed during the proliferative phase of the menstrual cycle to decrease blood loss.
   b. **Hysterectomy,** the removal of the uterus, is the usual treatment for symptomatic multiple fibroids. Abdominal hysterectomy is usually performed for fibroids that are larger than a 12-week fetus. Vaginal hysterectomy may be performed for removal of small fibroids. In both procedures, the uterus is removed from supporting ligaments (round, broad, and uterosacral), which are then attached to the vaginal cuff. Vaginal depth is maintained. In vaginal hysterectomy, the incision is internal, and the uterus is removed through

the vagina. In abdominal hysterectomy, the uterus is removed through an abdominal incision.

Complications

1. Infertility
2. Iron-deficiency anemia
3. Tissue necrosis

Prognosis

1. After menopause, leiomyomas often shrink without treatment.
2. Surgical removal by hysterectomy is successful.

Applying the Nursing Process

NURSING DIAGNOSIS: Anxiety R/T diagnosis and potential surgical treatment

1. *Expected outcomes:* Following consultation, the woman should verbalize decreased anxiety about medical diagnostic and surgical procedures.
2. *Nursing interventions*
   a. Encourage the woman to verbalize her concerns about her diagnosis and surgical treatment options.
   b. Assist the woman to identify and use coping mechanisms that have worked for her.
   c. Explore the significance of the loss of her uterus if appropriate.
   d. Provide information about support groups and counseling if needed.

NURSING DIAGNOSIS: Decisional conflict R/T treatment options

1. *Expected outcomes:* Following instruction, the woman should verbalize understanding of treatment options.
2. *Nursing interventions*
   a. Discuss procedures, risks, and advantages with the woman and her family.
   b. Describe pre- and postoperative procedures as applicable.
      (1) Preoperative care includes laboratory workup (complete blood count, hematocrit, blood type and crossmatch, urinalysis, electrocardiogram, chest radiograph), vaginal examination, abdominal-mons or perineal shave if ordered, NPO status past midnight, voiding before surgery, preoperative intravenous fluids and medications, identification band in place, and teaching about leg exercises, turning, coughing, and deep breathing.
      (2) Psychologic assessment includes significance of loss of uterus, concerns about sexual functioning, adequacy of support system, and too much or no anxiety concerning procedure.

(3) Postoperative care includes monitoring vital signs and condition until stable; turning, coughing, and deep breathing exercises (splinting incision); leg exercises, then ambulation; observing for infection, hemorrhage, and other complications (urinary tract infection, thrombophlebitis, pulmonary embolism, wound evisceration); auscultating lungs and bowel sounds; monitoring intake and output; observing for signs of depression and other psychologic reactions.
   c. Describe effects of surgery on childbearing potential if applicable.

NURSING DIAGNOSIS: Pain R/T surgical incision from hysterectomy

1. *Expected outcomes:* Following intervention, the patient should experience relief from pain as evidenced by the following:
   a. Stating that pain is relieved
   b. Vital signs within normal limits
   c. No diaphoresis
   d. Relaxed posture
2. *Nursing interventions*
   a. Assess for presence of pain.
   b. Administer prescribed analgesics before pain becomes severe. Discuss effectiveness of medication with the patient. Document effectiveness.
   c. Use nonpharmacologic methods of pain relief, such as position changes, heat to the abdominal incision, and massage.
   d. Encourage relaxation techniques such as slow breathing and guided imagery.
   e. Teach the patient how to splint the incision when coughing or getting out of bed.

NURSING DIAGNOSIS: Impaired skin integrity R/T surgery

1. *Expected outcomes:* Following intervention, the patient should demonstrate an intact incision as evidenced by the following:
   a. Normal temperature and other vital signs
   b. No redness, swelling, or drainage from incision
   c. Intact incision with well approximated edges
2. *Nursing interventions*
   a. Assess incision site for signs of infection on each shift.
   b. Maintain aseptic technique during wound care.
   c. Assess vital signs every 4 hours.
   d. Encourage patient to eat foods high in protein, iron, and vitamin C to promote wound healing.
   e. Administer antibiotics if ordered.

NURSING DIAGNOSIS: Risk for fluid volume deficit R/T decreased intake secondary to NPO status

1. *Expected outcomes:* Following intervention, the patient should demonstrate adequate fluid balance as evidenced by the following:

a. Oral intake of 3000 ml of fluid in 24 hours
b. Urine output of more than 1500 ml in 24 hours
c. Vital signs within normal limits
d. Urine specific gravity within normal limits
e. Good skin turgor
2. *Nursing interventions*
   a. Assess vital signs every 4 hours.
   b. Assess patient for signs of dehydration (e.g., poor skin turgor).
   c. Administer intravenous fluids as ordered.
   d. Encourage oral intake of fluids when the patient is allowed more than sips of clear liquids.
   e. Monitor intake and output with urine specific gravity every shift.

NURSING DIAGNOSIS: Body image disturbance R/T loss of uterus

1. *Expected outcomes:* Following counseling, the patient should accept the change in her body and incorporate the changes in her self-image as evidenced by the following:
   a. Taking an interest in her appearance
   b. Visiting with family and friends
   c. Verbalizing that she and her partner understand that sexual relations should be as satisfying as before surgery

Discharge Planning and Teaching

1. If observation only is recommended, discuss the importance of keeping follow-up appointments to monitor leiomyoma status.
2. If myomectomy or hysterectomy is performed, discharge instructions include the following:
   a. Limiting strenuous activities or lifting anything heavier than 20 pounds for 1 month
   b. Avoiding sexual intercourse for 3 to 6 weeks; use of water soluble lubricant may decrease discomfort of 1st intercourse
   c. Eating foods high in protein, iron, and vitamin C to aid in tissue healing; increasing fiber and fluids
   d. Tub baths should be avoided for the first 4 weeks. Showering and hair washing are not restricted.
   e. Douching should be done only on the advice of the health care provider.
   f. Keeping postoperative follow-up appointments
   g. Recognizing and reporting signs of complications, such as infection or hemorrhage
3. If a hysterectomy was performed, discuss expected physical changes such as cessation of menses, fatigue and weakness, and possible emotional reactions.
   a. Although menses will cease, the premenopausal woman will not experience surgical menopausal symptoms unless her ovaries are also removed.
   b. The most common emotional reaction to hysterectomy is depression. Women who have completed childbearing, work outside the home, have no misconceptions

about hysterectomy, and have family support usually adjust well. Women who become depressed or have other emotional reactions after hysterectomy may benefit from referral to a support group or individual counseling.
4. Myomectomy may be less successful than hysterectomy as leiomyomas can recur.

Public Health Considerations

Considerations are the same as those for ovarian cysts. See page 1473.

◻ CANCER OF THE ENDOMETRIUM

Definition

Endometrial cancer is a malignant neoplastic disease of the endometrium of the uterus.

Incidence and Socioeconomic Impact

1. Endometrial cancer is the most common cancer of the female reproductive system. It is more frequent in postmenopausal women.
2. Endometrial cancer is more common in White women in the United States.

Risk Factors

1. Obesity
2. Nulliparity
3. Late menopause (after age 52 years)
4. Family history of breast or uterine cancer
5. Diabetes mellitus
6. Estrogen stimulation, especially unopposed menopausal estrogen replacement therapy (no progestin therapy)

Etiology

1. Excessive exogenous estrogen has been implicated in the development of endometrial cancer.
2. The disease may be preceded by endometrial hyperplasia.

Pathophysiology

1. Most endometrial cancers are adenocarcinomas.
2. Endometrial cancer develops in the epithelial layer of the endometrial lining.
3. The tumor grows from the fundal portion of the uterine cavity, then spreads directly to the myometrium, cervix, fallopian tubes, and ovaries.
4. Metastatic spread

a. Lymphatic spread throughout the pelvis
b. Hematogenous spread to the lungs, liver, bones, and brain
c. Direct extension to adjacent structures.

5. Table 31–7 describes the clinical staging system for endometrial cancer developed by the International Federation of Gynecology and Obstetrics (FIGO).

Clinical Manifestations

Abnormal vaginal bleeding, postmenopausal bleeding

Diagnostics

1. History includes a reproductive history, the woman's report of abnormal bleeding, and identification of any risk factors.
2. Physical examination includes a pelvic examination that reveals the presence of a uterine mass or enlargement.
3. Diagnostic tests
   a. Pap tests are not reliable in detecting endometrial cancer.
   b. Endometrial biopsy or D & C are reliable diagnostic techniques for high-risk populations.
4. Laboratory procedures to determine spread of cancer include the following:
   • Complete blood count
   • Liver function tests
   • Renal function tests
5. Radiographic tests to determine spread may include the following:
   • Intravenous pyelogram (IVP) to assess ureter function
   • Cystoscopy to visualize the bladder
   • Computed tomography to identify the origin and spread of disease
   • Lymphangiogram to evaluate nodal involvement

Table 31–7. FIGO Staging of Endometrial Carcinoma

Stages and Characteristics

IA	Tumor limited to endometrium
IB	Invasion to < ½ myometrium
IC	Invasion to > ½ myometrium
IIA	Endocervical glandular involvement only
IIB	Cervical stromal invasion
IIIA	Tumor invades serosa or adnexa or positive peritoneal cytology
IIIB	Vaginal metastases
IIIC	Metastases to pelvic or paraaortic lymph nodes
IVA	Tumor invasion of bladder and/or bowel mucosa
IVB	Distant metastases including intraabdominal and/or inguinal lymph node

Group and Degree of Differentiation

G1	5% or less of a nonsquamous solid growth pattern
G2	6%–50% of a nonsquamous solid growth pattern
G3	More than 50% of a nonsquamous solid growth pattern

From McCorkle R, et al. *Cancer Nursing.* 2nd ed. Philadelphia: WB Saunders, 1996, p 711.

Clinical Management

1. Goal of intervention: to treat the cancer and prevent spread
2. Nonpharmacologic interventions
   a. Women may receive 6 weeks of external radiation therapy to destroy cancer cells in the pericervical lymphatics before surgery (see Chapter 17).
   b. Women may receive internal radiation therapy before surgery. Intracavitary radiation includes the placement of an applicator into the woman's uterus (through the vagina) under anesthesia. The correct placement of the applicator is confirmed by radiograph. The radioactive source is placed in the applicator (usually after the woman is returned to her room).
      (1) Preoperatively, the woman is given enemas, and an indwelling catheter is placed in her bladder.
      (2) During treatment, the woman is on isolation precautions. Radiation precautions (i.e., lead shielding) are practiced, and time at the bedside is limited.
      (3) The woman must remain on her back (head may be slightly elevated). Movement is restricted to prevent dislodgement of the radioactive source.
      (4) The woman is assessed for skin breakdown, given a low-residue diet, and encouraged to drink fluids.
      (5) Medications that may be ordered include broad-spectrum antibiotics, tranquilizers, analgesics, and antidiarrheals.
      (6) After the radioactive source is removed (24–72 hr), care includes a cleansing enema and vaginal douche (Procedure 31–3).
3. Pharmacologic interventions
   a. Chemotherapy may be used to treat advanced or recurrent disease. Chemotherapy is not as effective as progestin therapy. Chemotherapeutic agents used to treat endometrial cancer include cisplatin or carboplatin, doxorubicin (Adriamycin), cyclophosphamide (Cytoxin), 5-fluorouracil (5-FU), and vincristine (Oncovin) (see Chapter 17).
   b. Progestational therapy may be used to treat estrogen-dependent stage I and II cancers. Medroxyprogesterone acetate (Depo-Provera) and megestrol acetate (Megace) are the most commonly used progestin agents.
   c. Tamoxifen citrate (Tamofen), an antiestrogen, is also used, although it is still considered experimental for this type of cancer.
4. Special medical-surgical procedures: Surgical management is the usual treatment for endometrial cancer. A total abdominal hysterectomy and bilateral salpingo-oophorectomy (removal of fallopian tubes and ovaries) are recommended for stage I cancers. A radical hysterectomy with pelvic node dissection is usually performed for stage II cancers. Removal of the upper third of the vagina and parametrium is possible.

Complications

1. Recurrence
2. Metastasis
3. Death

Procedure 31–3
Vaginal Irrigation

Definition/Purpose	To irrigate the vagina for the purpose of cleansing or treating infection
Contraindications/Cautions	The procedure is not recommended during pregnancy. The solution should be introduced into the vagina under low pressure.
Learning/Teaching Activities	Provide the following information: describe the procedure and explain the use of equipment.

Preliminary Activities

Equipment	• Clean gloves • Vaginal irrigation set • Douche tip • Irrigation solution • Bedpan and underpads if the woman is unable to perform self-irrigation on toilet • Toilet tissue
Assessment/Planning	• Determine whether the woman can do self-irrigation or will need assistance. • Ensure privacy. • Be familiar with how the irrigation set operates. Check health care provider orders for type, temperature, and amount of irrigating solution (usually 1000 to 2000 ml at 105 degrees Fahrenheit or 40.5 degrees Celsius).
Patient Preparation	• The woman should empty her bladder before the procedure. • If the procedure is done in bed, the woman should be placed on the bedpan in the supine position with knees bent and feet flat on the bed. • Drape the woman if she desires. • Encourage the woman to relax. • Hang (hold) solution set 2 feet above the vaginal opening. • If the woman can perform the procedure, she may sit on the toilet to do so.

Procedure

Actions	Rationale/Discussion
1. Wash hands.	1. Hand washing protects against possible cross-contamination.
2. Wear gloves (optional for patient).	2. Gloves protect against possible infection.
3. With the woman in the supine position with knees bent in bed or while sitting on the toilet, spread the labia.	3. Position for ease of insertion.
4. Insert the douche tip about 3 to 4 inches.	4. Make sure solution flows into the vagina.
5. Open the clamp and allow the solution to flow in while rotating the douche tip.	5. Provide even flow of solution to all areas of the vagina.
6. Remove the douche tip from the vagina when the solution flow stops.	6. Prevent the solution from flowing outside the vagina.
7. Dry the perineum with toilet tissue.	7. Remove excess moisture.
8. Remove and clean equipment.	8. Irrigation sets and douche tips are reusable for the same patient.
9. Wash hands.	9. Prevent cross-contamination.

Final Activities

Record treatment on chart. Describe how well the woman tolerated the procedure.

Prognosis

1. The prognosis depends on the extent of the disease.
2. Five-year survival rates for stage I endometrial cancer are 76 percent; for stage II, 50 percent; for stage III, 30 percent; and for stage IV, 9 percent.

Applying the Nursing Process

NURSING DIAGNOSIS: Body image disturbance R/T diagnosis of cancer or the effects of treatment

1. *Expected outcomes:* After counseling, the woman should do the following:
   a. Verbalize understanding of the effects of cancer and its treatment on her body image
   b. State that her concerns about self-image are reduced
2. *Nursing interventions*
   a. Enable the woman to discuss her concerns about cancer or the effects of treatment.
   b. Provide emotional support.
   c. Include significant others in discussions when possible.

NURSING DIAGNOSIS: Fear R/T cancer and possible death

---

1. *Expected outcomes:* Following consultation, the woman should verbalize reduction of fear and anxiety about her diagnosis and treatment.
2. *Nursing interventions*
   a. Encourage the woman to express her feelings.
   b. Provide correct information about the diagnosis and treatment.
   c. Promote the use of effective coping strategies the woman has used in the past.
   d. Refer to a support group or other community resource as needed.

NURSING DIAGNOSIS: Pain R/T cancer or surgical procedures

---

1. *Expected outcomes:* Following instruction and intervention, the woman should verbalize a reduction in pain.
2. *Nursing interventions*
   a. Monitor type of pain.
   b. Encourage diversional activities.
   c. Teach the woman about nonpharmacologic pain relief measures, such as relaxation techniques and guided imagery.
   d. Encourage the woman to take pain medications as prescribed.
   e. Evaluate pain relief and the need for further interventions.

NURSING DIAGNOSIS: Sexual dysfunction R/T diagnosis of cancer or its treatment

---

1. *Expected outcomes:* Following consultation, the woman should report that she and her partner will be able to resume mutually satisfying sexual relations.
2. *Nursing interventions*
   a. Educate the woman and her partner about anatomic changes that result from surgery or radiation therapy.
   b. Encourage the woman and her partner to discuss their feelings and concerns. Clarify any misconceptions.
   c. Teach the woman and her partner specific techniques or positions to help them resume intercourse after cancer treatment (Box 31–5). Refer for sexual counseling if needed.

Box 31–5. Sexual Activity After Cancer Treatment

To assist the woman and her partner in resuming intercourse after treatment for gynecologic cancer, advise her to
• Use water-soluble lubricants for vaginal thinning or dryness.
• Use the rear-entry or woman on top position for intercourse rather than the traditional "missionary" position.
• Use vaginal dilators to decrease adhesions, prevent shortening of the vagina, and keep the vaginal orifice flexible. This is especially important for women who do not engage in sexual intercourse during and after radiation treatment.

NURSING DIAGNOSIS: Impaired skin integrity R/T surgery or radiation

---

1. *Expected outcomes:* Following instruction and intervention, the woman will not experience skin breakdown related to surgery or radiation therapy.
2. *Nursing interventions*
   a. Teach wound care for hysterectomy.
   b. Monitor incisional healing for signs of infection after surgical procedures.
   c. Teach the woman signs of skin breakdown during external radiation therapy. Teach her to avoid bathing and to avoid sun exposure to the markings for treatment.

Discharge Planning and Teaching

1. Before discharge, the woman needs to learn specific self-care activities related to the treatment of her cancer. Home care instructions after hysterectomy for endometrial cancer are the same as those for hysterectomy for leiomyoma. Because ovaries are removed, menopausal symptoms will occur in premenopausal women.
2. Women receiving external radiation or chemotherapy will likely be treated as outpatients and will need to plan for travel to the health care facility for the scheduled treatment.
3. After an internal radiation implant, the woman should be instructed to do the following:
   • Report side effects, such as vaginal bleeding, foul-smelling discharge, abdominal pain, or hematuria
   • Resume normal diet
   • Use a vaginal dilator with a water-soluble lubricant to prevent vaginal shrinkage
   • Take medications as prescribed
   • Keep follow-up appointments with her physician

Public Health Considerations

1. Women at high risk should have endometrial biopsies at least every 2 years to detect endometrial cancer in its earliest stages.
2. All women older than 40 years need to have annual physical and pelvic examinations.
3. Postmenopausal women should report any vaginal bleeding to their physicians promptly.

◼ OVARIAN CANCER

Definition

A malignant neoplasm of the ovary

Incidence and Socioeconomic Impact

1. Ovarian cancer is the leading cause of death from gynecologic cancer. It is estimated that 1 in 70 women will develop ovarian cancer. Survival rates are low because early diagnosis is difficult.
2. Ovarian cancer is the 2nd most frequent gynecologic cancer.
3. Japan is the only industrialized nation that does not have a high incidence of ovarian cancer. However, 2nd-generation Japanese-American women have rates almost as high as those of White women of northern European descent who are older than 50 years.

Risk Factors

1. Age older than 50 years
2. Family history of ovarian, breast, or colon cancer
3. Nulliparity or first pregnancy after age 30 years
4. Diet high in fat (a possible risk factor)
5. Use of talc (e.g., baby powder) (a possible risk factor)
6. Oral contraceptives may have a protective effect.

Etiology

1. The etiology of ovarian cancer is unknown.
2. Serous adenocarcinoma is the most common ovarian tumor.

Pathophysiology

1. Ovarian tumors are usually epithelial in origin
2. Spread of ovarian cancer
   a. Direct extension from the ovary to adjacent organs
   b. Peritoneal seeding of tumor cells
   c. Distal spread through lymphatic drainage to the liver and lungs

Clinical Manifestations

1. Early ovarian cancer often has no or only mild symptoms, such as indigestion or abdominal bloating or distention.
2. More advanced disease can manifest as an enlarged abdomen with ascites or abdominal or pelvic masses.

NURSE ADVISORY

Women may attribute symptoms related to ovarian cancer to midlife changes or stress. Women older than 40 years with persistent, vague gastrointestinal complaints should be evaluated for ovarian cancer.

Diagnostics

1. History includes a report of abdominal swelling or vague gastrointestinal symptoms, family history of cancer of the uterus or breast, and a reproductive history.
2. Physical examination may reveal an abdominal mass. A pelvic examination may not reveal any abnormality, but a palpable ovary in a postmenopausal woman needs further investigation.
3. Medical diagnosis
   a. A Pap test has limited diagnostic value because results are abnormal in only 20 to 30 percent of women with ovarian cancer.
   b. Computed tomography and ultrasound (vaginal and abdominal) are used to locate and evaluate masses.
   c. Diagnostic tests that are used to rule out other causes of a mass include barium enema, proctosigmoidoscopy, chest radiograph, and intravenous pyelogram.
   d. Cancer antigen (CA)-125 is an ovarian antibody that may be elevated if cancer is present.
   e. Staging of the tumor and precise diagnosis are done through exploratory surgery. Table 31–8 describes the clinical staging of ovarian cancer.

Clinical Management

1. Goals of intervention: to debulk (remove) or treat as much of the cancer as possible and to prevent complications
2. Nonpharmacologic interventions
   a. Nutritional support, such as supplements, enteral feeding, and parenteral hyperalimentation, may be needed as disease progresses.
   b. External radiation therapy (see Chapter 17) may be used after surgery if the cancer has spread to other organs, although its use is controversial.
   c. Referral to a cancer support group may be useful.
3. Pharmacologic interventions
   a. Intra-abdominal injection of chromic phosphate (^{32}P), a radioactive colloid, may improve survival in advanced ovarian cancer.
   b. Postoperative chemotherapy is given for stage II, III, and IV disease. Alkylating agents are useful but may increase the woman's risk of secondary leukemia. Combination drug therapy seems to be more effective than drugs used singly. (Combinations include cisplatin together with paclitaxel and cisplatin or carboplatin with cyclophosphamide.)

℞ DRUG ADVISORY

Paclitaxel (Taxol) has toxicities different than other chemotherapeutic agents, so that patients need special preparation and monitoring.
- Anaphylactic reactions can occur during administration. Premedication with dexamethasone, diphenhydramine, and cimetidine is common.
- Cardiac arrhythmias can occur.
- Emergency equipment—oxygen, ventilation equipment, electrocardiography machine, intravenous fluids, and medications (epinephrine, diphenhydramine, albuterol, steroids)—should be available.
Bone marrow depression and alopecia are experienced by almost all patients.

Table 31–8. FIGO Staging System for Ovarian Cancer*

Stage I	Growth limited to the ovaries.
Stage IA	Growth limited to one ovary; no ascites. No tumor on the external surface; capsule intact.
Stage IB	Growth limited to both ovaries; no ascites. No tumor on the external surfaces; capsules intact.
Stage IC†	Tumor either stage IA or IB but with tumor on surface of one or both ovaries; or with capsule ruptured; or with ascites present containing malignant cells or with positive peritoneal washings.
Stage II	Growth involving one or both ovaries with pelvic extension
Stage IIA	Extension or metastases, or both, to the uterus or tubes (or both).
Stage IIB	Extension to other pelvic tissues.
Stage IIC*	Tumor either stage IIA or IIB, but with tumor on surface of one or both ovaries; or with capsule(s) ruptured; or with ascites present containing malignant cells or with positive peritoneal washings.
Stage III	Tumor involving one or both ovaries with peritoneal implants outside the pelvis or positive retroperitoneal or inguinal nodes. Superficial liver metastasis equals stage III. Tumor is limited to the true pelvis but with histologically proved malignant extension to small bowel or omentum.
Stage IIIA	Tumor grossly limited to the true pelvis with negative nodes but with histologically confirmed microscopic seeding of abdominal peritoneal surfaces.
Stage IIIB	Tumor of one or both ovaries with histologically confirmed implants of abdominal peritoneal surfaces, none exceeding 2 cm in diameter. Nodes are negative.
Stage IIIC	Abdominal implants greater than 2 cm in diameter or positive retroperitoneal or inguinal nodes, or both.
Stage IV	Growth involving one or both ovaries with distant metastases. If pleural effusion is present, there must be positive cytology to allot a case to stage IV. Parenchymal liver metastasis equals stage IV.

* Based on findings at clinical examination or surgical exploration, or both. The histology is to be considered in the staging, as is cytology as far as effusions are concerned. It is desirable that a biopsy be taken from suspicious areas outside the pelvis.
† To evaluate the impact on prognosis of the different criteria for allotting cases to stage IC or IIC, it would be of value to know (1) if rupture of the cpasule was (a) spontaneous or (b) caused by the surgeon, or (2) if the source of malignant cells detected was (a) peritoneal washings or (b) ascites.
From McCorkle R, et al. *Cancer Nursing.* 2nd ed. Philadelphia: WB Saunders, 1996, p 715.

c. Six cycles of chemotherapy are the standard regimen, yielding a response rate of 60 to 70 percent and a 5-year survival rate of 10 to 20 percent.

d. Chemotherapeutic agents can be given intraperitoneally and may increase the cytologic effects.

4. Special medical-surgical procedures
   a. Surgery for ovarian cancer usually includes the removal of the ovaries and fallopian tubes (bilateral salpingo-oophorectomy) and hysterectomy and omentectomy (removal of peritoneal covering) with staging and debulking. Bilateral salpingo-oophorectomy is the surgical removal of both fallopian tubes and both ovaries. Preoperative and postoperative care for this procedure are similar to those for abdominal hysterectomy or tubal ligation.
   b. A laparoscopy or laparotomy may be performed after 6 months to 1 year of chemotherapy to confirm the presence or absence of tumor or to remove residual tumor.

Complications

1. Sepsis
2. Bowel obstruction
3. Cardiovascular collapse
4. Metastasis
5. Death

Prognosis

1. The overall survival rate for ovarian cancer is between 30 and 35 percent.

2. The prognosis is poor because most cases have progressed to stage III or IV by the time they are diagnosed.

Applying the Nursing Process

Nursing diagnoses, expected outcomes, and nursing interventions are similar to those for endometrial cancer (see earlier discussion). Because malignancy is usually in an advanced stage when diagnosed, the following nursing diagnosis is pertinent:

NURSING DIAGNOSIS: Anticipatory grieving R/T diagnosis, loss of uterus and ovaries, and prognosis

1. *Expected outcomes:* Following counseling the woman should express her feelings about loss and death.
2. *Nursing interventions*
   a. Encourage expression of feelings about the diagnosis, loss, or possible death.
   b. Provide accurate information about the treatment and prognosis.
   c. Encourage the woman to use her support system.
   d. Provide support and encouragement to the woman and her family and assist them to use effective coping strategies.
   e. Provide information about available community resources, such as cancer support groups and hospice, when indicated.

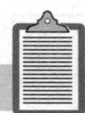

NURSING MANAGEMENT

A woman with ovarian cancer usually has ongoing needs for treatment and support. She and her family will be well known to the health team. Assignment of a primary caregiver for continuity of care may be useful in helping the woman and her family cope with the experience.

Discharge Planning and Teaching

1. Discharge planning after surgery is similar to that for a hysterectomy for leiomyoma (see p. 1476).
2. The woman who undergoes chemotherapy or radiation therapy will need information on management of side effects, such as nausea and vomiting, diarrhea, and alopecia (see Chapter 17).

Public Health Considerations

1. Screening techniques for ovarian cancer are limited. Women need to be educated to seek regular physical examinations, including a careful family history and pelvic examinations every 1 to 3 years before the age of 40 years and annually after age 40 years.
2. Women at high risk may have CA-125 determinations and transvaginal ultrasonic examinations annually.

◼ CANCER OF THE CERVIX

Definition

Neoplastic disease of the uterine cervix

Incidence and Socioeconomic Impact

1. Cancer of the cervix is the 3rd most common reproductive cancer.
2. Death rates have declined over the last 40 years, primarily because of widespread and effective screening techniques.

3. The incidence of invasive cancer has decreased 50 percent, but the incidence of cancer in situ has increased.
4. Cervical intraepithelial neoplasia most often occurs in women in their twenties; cancer in situ is more common in women in their thirties, and invasive cancer is more frequent in women older than 40 years.
5. Black women are twice as likely to have cervical cancer as White women in the United States. Hispanic and Native American women are also at increased risk.

Risk Factors

1. Low socioeconomic status
2. Cigarette smoking
3. Early age of onset of sexual intercourse
4. Multiple sex partners
5. Human papillomavirus infections

Etiology

1. Unknown for squamous cell carcinoma
2. Adenocarcinoma is thought to be related to in utero exposure to DES.

Pathophysiology

1. Cervical cancer begins as neoplastic changes in the cervical epithelium. Preinvasive lesions are limited to the cervix and usually originate in the squamocolumnar junction, or transformation zone (Fig. 31–9).
   a. A Pap test is the primary screening tool. It is repeated if atypical cells are found.
   b. Following a 2nd abnormal Pap test result, a colposcopic examination and biopsy of the transformation zone may be done.
   c. Magnetic resonance imaging or a CT scan may be done to identify the origin and spread of the tumor.

Clinical Manifestations

1. Preinvasive cancer is often asymptomatic.
2. Abnormal vaginal bleeding is the classic symptom of invasive cancer (e.g., postcoital bleeding).

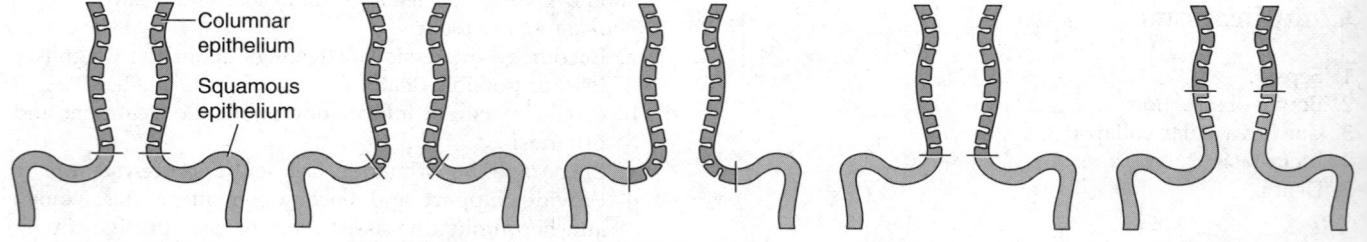

Figure 31–9. Location of the squamocolumnar junction (transformation zone) at various stages of adult development. (From Ignatavicius DD, Workman ML, and Mishler MA. *Medical-Surgical Nursing: A Nursing Process Approach.* 2nd ed. Philadelphia: WB Saunders, 1995, p 2251.)

3. Other late-stage symptoms include rectal bleeding, hematuria, anemia, and back or leg pain.

Diagnostics

1. History includes sexual activity, risk factors, presence of HPV infection, and bleeding episodes.
2. The pelvic examination results may be normal unless late-stage disease is present.
3. Table 31–9 describes the clinical staging for cancer of the cervix using the FIGO system.
4. Special medical-surgical procedures
   a. Laser surgery is useful when the limits of the lesion are visible under colposcopic examination and the endocervical biopsy is normal.
   b. Cryosurgery may be used to treat cervical intraepithelial neoplasia. In **cryosurgery,** a probe is used to freeze abnormal tissues with subsequent necrosis.
   c. Conization (see p. 1460) is the treatment of choice for microinvasive cervical cancer when the limits of the lesion cannot be seen on colposcopic examination
   d. Hysterectomy may be performed to remove the uterus. A radical hysterectomy and lymph node dissection may be done for cancers that have extended beyond the cervix but are still confined to the pelvis.
   e. A pelvic exenteration may be performed for recurrent cancer if no tumor is found outside the pelvis and there is no lymph node involvement.

   (1) An **anterior pelvic exenteration** is the removal of the uterus, ovaries, fallopian tubes, vagina, bladder, urethra, and pelvic lymph nodes. An ileal conduit is created for passage of urine (Fig. 31–10*A*). A neovagina may be constructed
   (2) A **posterior exenteration** is the removal of the uterus, ovaries, fallopian tubes, descending colon, rectum, and anal canal. A colostomy is created for the passage of feces (see Fig. 31–10*B*).
   (3) A **total exenteration** is a combination of anterior and posterior procedures (see Fig. 31–10*C*). A neovagina may be constructed.
   (4) Preoperative considerations include providing information about physical preparation, postoperative care, and recovery; assessing psychologic readiness for surgery, including sexual assessment; and discussing vaginal reconstruction if this is desired and is an option.
   (5) Preoperative preparation includes extensive bowel preparation and stoma site selection and referral to an enterostomal therapist for stoma placement and teaching.
   (6) Postoperative interventions include stabilization of physical status (often in an intensive care setting), monitoring for potential complications (e.g., shock, hemorrhage, pulmonary embolism, other pulmonary complications), management of ileal conduit or colostomy, and determination of psychologic status.

Table 31–9. FIGO Staging System for Cervical Cancer

Preinvasive Carcinoma

Stage 0	Carcinoma in situ, intraepithelial carcinoma (Cases of stage 0 should not be included in any therapeutic statistics)

Invasive Carcinoma

Stage I	The carcinoma is strictly confined to the cervix (extension to the corpus should be disregarded)
Stage IA	Preclinical carcinomas of the cervix, that is, those diagnosed only by microscopy
Stage IA^1	Minimal microscopically evident stromal invasion
Stage IA^2	Lesions detected microscopically that can be measured. The upper limit of the measurement should not show a depth of invasion of more than 5 mm taken from the base of the epithelium, either surface or glandular, from which it originates, and a second dimension, the horizontal spread, must not exceed 7 mm. Larger lesions should be staged as IB
Stage IB	Lesions of greater dimensions than stage IA2 whether seen clinically or not. Preformed space involvement should not alter the staging but should be specifically recorded so as to determine whether it should affect treatment decisions in the future
Stage II	The carcinoma extends beyond the cervix but has not extended onto the pelvic wall. The carcinoma involves the vagina, but not the lower third
Stage IIA	No obvious parametrial involvement
Stage IIB	Obvious parametrial involvement
Stage III	The carcinoma has extended onto the pelvic wall. On rectal examination, there is no cancer-free space between the tumor and the pelvic wall. The tumor involves the lower third of the vagina. All cases with hydronephrosis or nonfunctioning kidney
Stage IIIA	No extension onto the pelvic wall
Stage IIIB	Extension onto the pelvic wall or hydronephrosis (or both) or nonfunctioning kidney
Stage IV	The carcinoma has extended beyond the true pelvis or has clinically involved the mucosa of the bladder or rectum. A bullous edema as such does not permit a case to be allotted to stage IV
Stage IVA	Spread of growth to adjacent organs
Stage IVB	Spread to distant organs

From McCorkle R, et al. *Cancer Nursing.* 2nd ed. Philadelphia: WB Saunders, 1996, p 700.

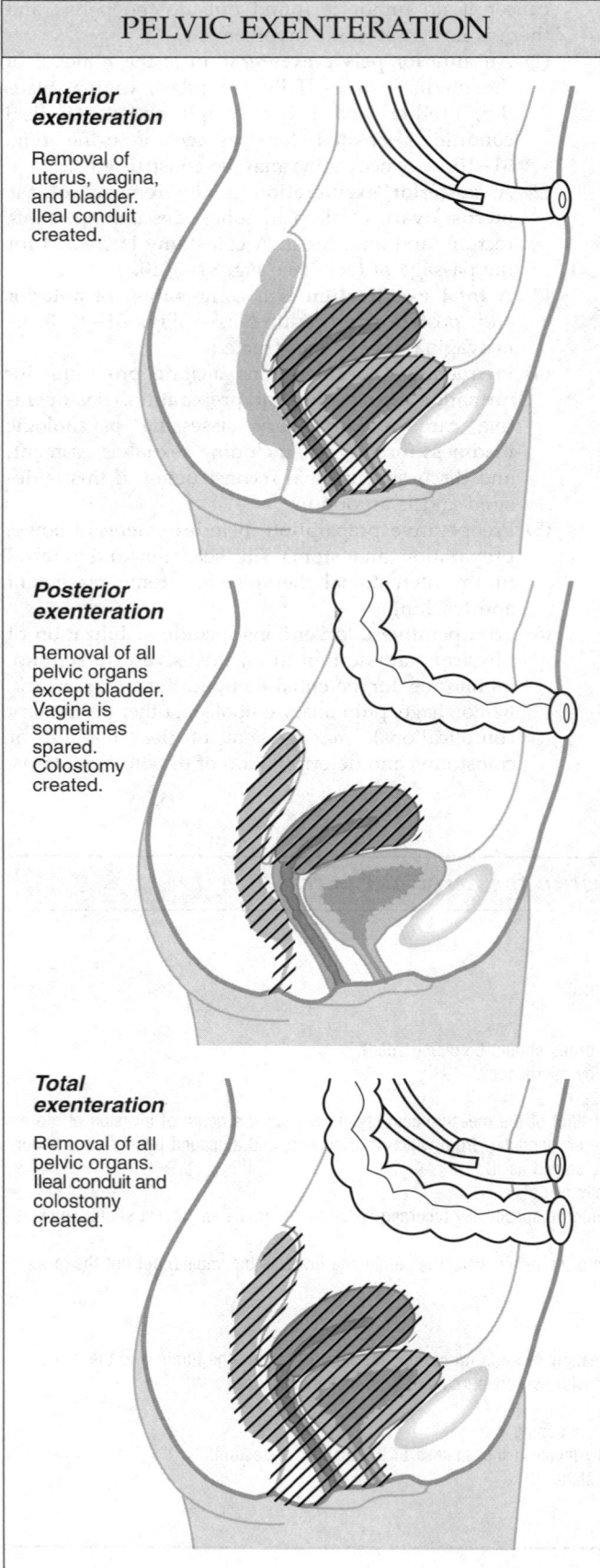

PELVIC EXENTERATION

Anterior exenteration

Removal of uterus, vagina, and bladder. Ileal conduit created.

Posterior exenteration

Removal of all pelvic organs except bladder. Vagina is sometimes spared. Colostomy created.

Total exenteration

Removal of all pelvic organs. Ileal conduit and colostomy created.

Figure 31–10.

Clinical Management

1. Goal of intervention: to treat the cancer and prevent recurrence
2. Nonpharmacologic interventions: Radiation therapy is used to treat invasive cancer of the cervix. Intracavitary radioactive implants (e.g., cesium) are used to treat tumors that have extended beyond the pelvic wall (see p. 1477). To shrink the tumor, external radiation is often administered before internal radiation (see Chapter 17).
3. Pharmacologic interventions: Chemotherapy may be used for recurrent tumors that cannot be removed or for disseminated metastasis. Cisplatin and 5-FU are 2 of the most common drugs used. Taxol may be given as a palliative measure (see Chapter 17). Squamous cell cancer spreads by direct extension to the vaginal mucosa, pelvic wall, bladder, and bowel. Metastasis is usually found only in the pelvis, but distant metastasis can occur through lymphatic spread (e.g., brain and lung metastases).

Complications

1. Metastasis
2. Recurrence
3. Death

Prognosis

1. Stage 0 and stage Ia squamous cell cancer of the cervix carry a 5-year survival rate of almost 100 percent.
2. Stage Ib disease has a 5-year survival rate of 90 percent.
3. The prognosis worsens as the stage increases.

Applying the Nursing Process

Nursing diagnoses, expected outcomes, and nursing interventions are the same as those for endometrial cancer. An additional nursing diagnosis is the following:

NURSING DIAGNOSIS: Impaired skin integrity R/T surgery

1. *Expected outcomes:* Following instruction, the patient should be able to perform necessary wound care.
2. *Nursing interventions*
   a. Perform and teach wound care for a pelvic exenteration, which includes perineal irrigation with a solution of one-half normal saline or other solution as ordered. Irrigation is followed by drying of the perineum with a hair dryer on cool setting or a heat lamp placed about 18 inches from the perineum (use with caution to prevent burns).
   b. Perform and teach care of the colostomy or ileal conduit (see Chapter 27).

Discharge Planning and Teaching

1. Before discharge, the woman needs to learn about self-care related to the specific treatment for cervical cancer.
2. Home care after cryosurgery or laser surgery includes the following:
   a. Avoiding intercourse and use of tampons as long as vaginal discharge is present
   b. Recognizing that a watery discharge will be present for several weeks after the procedure
   c. Recognizing early signs of infection and reporting these to the physician promptly
   d. Keeping follow-up appointments
3. Teaching and discharge planning for the woman who has had a hysterectomy, radiation therapy, or chemotherapy are the same as described for endometrial cancer (see p. 1479).
4. After pelvic exenteration, the woman will need the following information:
   a. Take all medications as prescribed.
   b. Care for your colostomy or ileal conduit as taught.
   c. Care for your neovagina as instructed.
   d. Wear perineal pads to protect clothing from discharge.
   e. Report signs of infection or bowel obstruction.
   f. Follow advice about resumption of sexual intercourse or alternative techniques and options for sexual experience. Twelve to 18 months may be needed for healing. Sexual counseling may be needed.
   g. Keep follow-up appointments.

Public Health Considerations

1. All sexually active women should know the risk factors for cervical cancer and should have annual physical examinations and Pap tests. Table 31–10 lists risk factors, warning signs, and screening frequencies for the major gynecologic cancers.
2. Information about cancer risk factors, warning signs, and screening guidelines should be readily available to the general public.

Table 31–10. Common Reproductive Cancers

Risk Factors	Cervical Cancer	Endometrial Cancer	Ovarian Cancer	Vulvar Cancer
Age	CIS 30–40 yr Invasive 40–60 yr	50–65 yr	>50 yr	60–70 yr
Family History		Increased risk	Increased risk	
Personal history	DES exposure	HX diabetes, HTN, breast cancer	HX breast, colon, endometrial cancer	HX vulvar disease, possibly diabetes
First sexual encounter	<18 yr			
Sexually transmitted diseases	HX HPV, genital warts, herpes			Genital warts, genital herpes
Parity	Multiparity	Nulliparity	Nulliparity	
Smoking	Increase ×2			
Estrogen use	Possible increase with OCP use	Possible increase with prolonged estrogen use	OCP use may have preventive effects	
Diet			High fat	
Body size		Obesity		Possible obesity
Race	African American	White		
Warning Signs	Abnormal bleeding between periods; bleeding after menopause or intercourse	Abnormal bleeding between periods; bleeding after menopause or intercourse	Enlarged abdomen without digestive disturbances; often no obvious symptoms	Sores that don't heal; ulcers; raised bumps; areas of itching; changes in skin color
Screening Procedure	Pap smear Pelvic examination	No practical screening for asymptomatic women; endometrial biopsy 80–90% reliable; Pap smear less than 50% reliable; pelvic examination	No practical screening for asymptomatic women; pelvic examination; physical examination	Vulvar self-examination; pelvic examination
Frequency	Yearly if at high risk or older than 40; every 1 to 3 years if three tests are negative and care provider agrees	Annual biopsy if at high risk, older than 40, or on unopposed estrogen therapy; every 1 to 3 years before age 40	Yearly examination after age 40; every 1 to 3 years before age 40	Monthly self-examination; yearly examination after age 40; every 1 to 3 years before age 40

CIS, Carcinoma in situ; DES, diethylstilbestrol; HX, history; HPV, human papillomavirus; OCP, oral contraceptive pills; HTN, hypertension.

◘ CANCER OF THE VULVA

Definition

Neoplastic disease of the vulva

Incidence and Socioeconomic Impact

1. Cancer of the vulva is the 4th leading cause of gynecologic cancer, constituting 3 to 4 percent of all gynecologic cancers.
2. The peak incidence of cancer of the vulva is in women older than 70 years.

Risk Factors

1. Age older than 60 years
2. Low socioeconomic status
3. History of benign vulvar disease, diabetes, HPV infection, herpes simplex virus type II infection, pruritus

Etiology

The etiology of vulvar cancer is unknown, although some relationship to sexually transmitted diseases has been suggested.

Pathophysiology

1. The primary site of vulvar cancer is usually the labia majora.
2. Vulvar cancer usually remains localized.
3. Most vulvar cancers are squamous cell carcinomas.
4. The 1st change is vulvar atypia, or vulvar intraepithelial neoplasia. These lesions can progress over time to carcinoma in situ and then to invasive cancer. Table 31–11 describes the clinical staging of vulvar cancer using the FIGO system.

Table 31–11. FIGO (1989) Staging of Vulvar Cancer

Stage 0	Carcinoma in situ; intraepithelial carcinoma
Stage I	Tumor confined to the vulva or perineum; 2 cm or less in greatest dimension; no nodal metastasis
Stage II	Tumor confined to the vulva or perineum; more than 2 cm in greatest dimension; no nodal metastasis
Stage III	Tumor of any size extending to the urethra, vagina, anus, or perineum but without grossly positive lymph nodes
Stage IVA	Lesions involving mucosa of the rectum, bladder, or urethra or involving the pelvic bone
Stage IVB	All cases with pelvic or distant metastases including pelvic lymph nodes

From McCorkle R, et al. *Cancer Nursing*. 2nd ed. Philadelphia: WB Saunders, 1996, p 723.

5. Metastasis is by direct extension and lymphatic spread; hematogenous spread to distal sites is rare.

Clinical Manifestations

1. Half of the women with vulvar intraepithelial neoplasia are asymptomatic.
2. There may be itching or a burning sensation in the vulva.
3. A mass or growth is present in the vulvar area.

Diagnostics

1. History includes an age assessment, reports of itching or burning in the vulvar area, complaints of a sore or growth on vulva, and risk factors.

> **ELDER ADVISORY**
>
> Many older women will treat themselves and delay seeking medical care or will be reluctant to tell the health care provider about their concerns because of embarrassment. The interview should be conducted in an unhurried, sensitive manner.

2. A pelvic examination will reveal a lesion or sore on the vulva. Palpation of the inguinal lymph nodes may reveal swelling.
3. Medical diagnosis
   a. Pelvic examination is the most important diagnostic test, revealing white or reddish multifocal lesions on the vulva.
   b. Vulvar cancer is diagnosed by local excisional biopsy of the lesion. Colposcopy may be used to select the biopsy site.
   c. Diagnostic tests to determine metastasis include chest radiograph, barium enema and proctosigmoidoscopy, cystoscopy with intravenous pyelogram, CT and MRI to identify retroperitoneal nodular areas.

Clinical Management

1. Goal of intervention: to treat the vulvar cancer and prevent its spread
2. Nonpharmacologic interventions: Radiation therapy may be used for palliative treatment in advanced disease (see Chapter 17).
3. Pharmacologic interventions: Chemotherapy may be used for palliative treatment in advanced cancer (see Chapter 17).
4. Special medical-surgical procedures: Surgery is the most common treatment for vulvar cancer.
   a. Laser surgery, cryosurgery, or electrocautery may be used to treat premalignant vulvar lesions.
   b. A simple vulvectomy—removal of the vulva, labia majora and minora, and possibly the clitoris—may be performed for carcinoma in situ, but it is uncommon.

c. A "skinning" vulvectomy—removal of the vulvar skin followed by split-thickness skin grafts—is more frequently performed for carcinoma in situ. Sexual functioning and appearance are better with this procedure (Fig. 31–11).

d. For invasive cancer, a modified radical vulvectomy (removal of the entire vulva, skin, labia majora and minora, clitoris, subcutaneous tissues, and possibly dissection of the inguinal and femoral lymph nodes) is performed.

e. Preoperative care includes thorough explanation of the procedure; exploration of fears and concerns related to physical changes and sexual functioning; and vaginal douche, enema, and perineal skin shave.

f. Postoperative interventions include care of the wound suction drains, indwelling bladder catheter care, incision care, and pain management.

Complications

1. Wound breakdown after surgery
2. Deep vein thrombosis, pulmonary embolism
3. Metastasis
4. Recurrence
5. Death

Prognosis

1. Prognosis is related to the stage of cancer and involvement of lymph nodes.
2. The 5-year survival rate for women with no lymph node involvement is 85 percent.

Applying the Nursing Process

The nursing diagnoses, expected outcomes, and nursing interventions are similar to those for endometrial cancer (pp. 1478–1479) and cervical cancer (p. 1484).

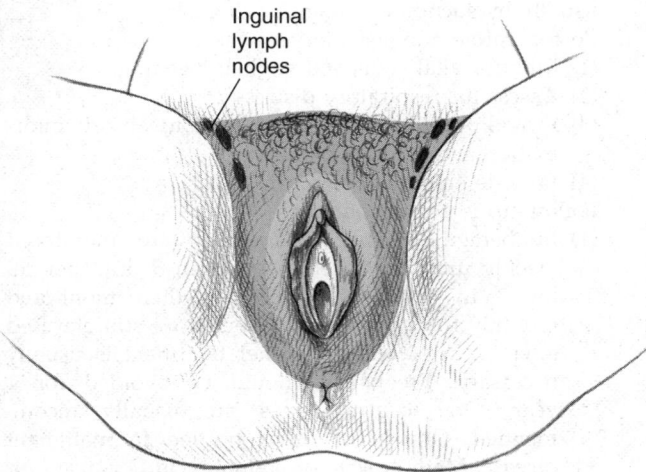

Figure 31–11. "Skinning" vulvectomy or radical vulvectomy.

Discharge Planning and Teaching

1. Inform the woman of possible complications after radical surgery, such as wound breakdown, chronic leg edema, and stress incontinence.
2. Teach the woman and family how to perform wound care after vulvectomy. Infection and wound breakdown occur in about 50 percent of women. A solution of one-half strength normal saline or other ordered solution is used to irrigate the wound. The wound is dried with a heat lamp set about 18 inches from the wound or a hair dryer on cool setting. Home health care may be needed.
3. Encourage the woman to eat foods high in protein, iron, and vitamin C to promote wound healing.
4. Discuss available pain management methods.
5. Teach the woman to control urine flow by using a funnel or standing while urinating.
6. Address the woman's concerns about sexual functioning.
   a. If the clitoris is removed, loss of orgasm usually occurs. Use of vaginal dilators and a water-soluble lubricant may relieve dyspareunia. Refer for sexual counseling if necessary.
7. Explore the need for counseling related to low self-esteem and negative body image.

Public Health Considerations

1. Teach women how to perform vulvar self-examination (see Learning/Teaching Guidelines for Vulvar Self-Examination).
2. Educate women to have annual pelvic examinations after the age of 40 years.
3. Provide information to all women about safe sex practices.

◨ OTHER GYNECOLOGIC CANCERS

Cancer of the Vagina

1. Definition: Neoplasm of the vagina, most often squamous cell in origin, usually occurring in the lower third of the vagina
2. Incidence and etiology
   a. Vaginal cancer is rare, accounting for less than 2 percent of all gynecologic cancers.
   b. Women older than 50 years are most frequently affected.
   c. Young women between the ages of 14 and 30 years may have clear cell adenocarcinoma of the vagina as a result of maternal ingestion of DES during pregnancy.
   d. Risk factors include DES exposure, Black race, low socioeconomic status, age older than 50 years, and history of vaginal trauma, HPV infection, or radiation therapy.
   e. Etiology is unknown, but the condition may be caused by genital viruses or chronic irritation.
3. Clinical manifestations

a. An abnormal Pap test result
b. Abnormal vaginal bleeding
c. Foul-smelling vaginal discharge
d. Dysuria
4. Clinical management
a. Goals of intervention: to treat the cancer and prevent its spread
b. Nonpharmacologic interventions: Radiation therapy is used in all stages of vaginal cancer (see Chapter 17). Intracavitary radiation therapy is administered for vaginal cancer limited to the vaginal walls. External radiation therapy and internal radiation therapy are used for vaginal cancers that extend beyond the vaginal walls.
c. Pharmacologic interventions: Chemotherapy is ineffective for most vaginal cancers. Topical 5-FU cream can be applied to lesions.
d. Special medical-surgical procedures
   (1) Laser surgery can be effective for vaginal intraepithelial neoplasia.
   (2) Local excision may be used for single or multiple lesions clustered together.
   (3) Vaginectomy, removal of all or part of the vagina, with reconstructive surgery may be used to treat stage I disease.
   (4) Radical hysterectomy with lymphadenectomy or pelvic exenteration is used to treat extensive or recurrent cancer.
e. Nursing diagnoses, expected outcomes, and nursing interventions are the same as for other gynecologic cancers.

Cancer of the Fallopian Tubes

1. Definition: Neoplasm of the fallopian (uterine) tubes, primarily occurring in the lumen of the tubes
2. Incidence and etiology
   a. Cancer of the fallopian tubes is the rarest of all gynecologic cancers, with an incidence of less than 1 percent.
   b. Adenocarcinoma of the fallopian tubes is associated with age older than 50 years, nulliparity, infertility, and pelvic inflammatory disease.
   c. Etiology is unknown for squamous cell carcinoma.
3. Clinical manifestations
   a. Usually asymptomatic in early stages
   b. Clear vaginal discharge
   c. Lower abdominal pain
   d. Abnormal vaginal bleeding
4. Clinical management
   a. Goals of intervention: to treat the cancer and prevent its spread
   b. Nonpharmacologic interventions: External radiation has been used postoperatively in late-stage disease (see Chapter 17).
   c. Pharmacologic interventions: Chemotherapy may be used after surgery (see Chapter 17). Alkylating agents have been effective, although the success rate is unclear because of the small number of cases.
   d. Special medical-surgical procedures: Surgery for fallo-

pian tube cancer consists of an abdominal hysterectomy and bilateral salpingo-oophorectomy with omentectomy (removal of connective tissue covering the organs).
   e. Nursing diagnoses, expected outcomes, and nursing interventions are similar to those for the woman with ovarian cancer (see p. 1481).

Gestational Trophoblastic Disease

1. Definition: Complex neoplastic disorders that arise from the placenta and trophoblast and include hydatidiform mole, invasive mole, and choriocarcinoma
2. Incidence and etiology
   a. Hydatidiform mole is benign, occurring in 1 of every 1500 live births in the United States.
   b. Incidence is higher in women older than 40 years of age.
   c. Fifteen to 30 percent of molar pregnancies progress to choriocarcinoma.
   d. Etiology is unknown, but theories include nutritional deficiencies (e.g., carotene) and an ovum that does not contain chromosomes.
3. Clinical manifestations
   a. Pregnancy is usually the first symptom.
   b. Vaginal bleeding occurs in the 1st trimester; the blood is bright red or dark.
   c. Fluid-filled vesicles of trophoblastic tissue are passed vaginally.
   d. Uterine size is larger than expected for dates in 50 percent of women
   e. No heart sounds or fetal activity is noted.
   f. Preeclampsia occurs in 25 percent of women before 24 weeks' gestation.
   g. Hyperemesis gravidarum affects 25 percent of women.
   h. Hyperthyroidism occurs in 10 percent of women; these women are at risk for thyroid storm.
4. Clinical management
   a. Assessment usually includes ultrasound examination.
   b. Chest films rule out metastasis to lungs (most common site of metastasis).
   c. Surgical management is by evacuation of the uterus, usually by suction curettage.
   d. Postoperative nursing interventions
      (1) Monitor vital signs and vaginal bleeding.
      (2) Assess for respiratory distress.
      (3) Provide family and patient time to absorb information and recommendations.
      (4) Provide emotional support.
   e. Follow-up is very important.
      (1) In benign disease hCG levels are monitored weekly until the level is less than 5 mIU per ml for 3 to 4 weeks; levels are then monitored monthly for 1 year. If hCG levels are still elevated after 12 to 14 weeks, further treatment is usually necessary. Pregnancy should be avoided for 1 year. Oral contraceptives are usually recommended. Chemotherapy is needed in malignant disease. Methotrexate or actinomycin D is used for nonmetastatic disease. Multiple-agent chemother-

apy is required in metastatic disease (e.g., methotrexate, actinomycin D, and chlorambucil or cyclophosphamide).

OTHER SEXUAL AND REPRODUCTIVE DISORDERS

Postmenopausal Bleeding

1. Definition: Bleeding that occurs at least 1 year after menopause
2. Incidence and etiology
   a. Postmenopausal bleeding is related to gynecologic cancer in 20 to 40 percent of women who experience it.
   b. Risk factors include estrogen replacement therapy.
   c. Etiologic factors include endometrial abnormalities, cervical polyps, and atrophic vaginitis.
3. Clinical manifestations
   a. Bleeding or spotting after intercourse
   b. Any bleeding or spotting after menopause
4. Clinical management: The goal of intervention is to treat the cause of bleeding.
   a. Pharmacologic interventions
      (1) For atrophic vaginitis, estrogen is administered orally, transdermally, or vaginally.
      (2) For hyperplasia, progestin is added during the last 10 days of estrogen replacement therapy.
      (3) Table 31–12 describes hormone replacement therapy.
   b. Special medical-surgical procedures
      (1) Dilation and curettage for an acute bleeding episode (see p. 1461)
      (2) Hysterectomy for atypical hyperplasia or cancer (see p. 1474)
      (3) Surgical removal of polyps
   c. Nursing interventions
      (1) Encourage the woman to discuss her fears and concerns.
      (2) Provide information about possible causes and treatment options.
      (3) Provide support during diagnosis and treatment procedures.

Toxic Shock Syndrome

1. Definition: **Toxic shock syndrome** is an acute multisystem illness that primarily affects menstruating women.
2. Incidence and etiology
   a. Toxic shock syndrome develops in 3 to 14 of every 100,000 menstruating women per year.
   b. Risk factors include tampon use, surgical wound infection, age between 15 and 24 years, postpartum period, and use of diaphragm or vaginal sponge contraceptive methods.
   c. Toxic shock syndrome is thought to be caused by certain strains of *Staphylococcus aureus* that produce toxins.

> **Box 31–6. Methods for Reducing Risk of Toxic Shock Syndrome**
>
> · Insert tampons carefully to avoid trauma.
> · Change tampons every 3 to 6 hours.
> · Use perineal pads instead of tampons at night.
> · Do not use superabsorbent tampons.
> · Avoid diaphragm use; if one is used, remove it within 6 to 8 hours after intercourse.
> · Wash hands before inserting anything into the vagina.

---

3. Clinical manifestations
   a. High fever
   b. Rash with peeling
   c. Myalgia
   d. Fatigue
   e. Nausea and vomiting
   f. Sore throat
   g. Diarrhea
4. Clinical management
   a. Teach the woman about causes of toxic shock syndrome and how to prevent further infection
      (1) Avoid tampons or limit use and change frequently.
      (2) Change method of contraception.
   b. Pharmacologic interventions
      (1) Antibiotic therapy, such as cefoxitin or cefazolin
      (2) Topical corticosteroids for skin rash
      (3) Fluid replacement for electrolyte imbalance
   c. Special medical-surgical procedures: Possible transfusions of blood products to treat thrombocytopenia (platelet deficiency)
   d. Nursing interventions
      (1) Discuss the causes, treatment, and prevention of toxic shock syndrome (Box 31–6).
      (2) Discuss the importance of following the treatment regimen and keeping follow-up appointments.
      (3) Teach warning signs of complications (e.g., high fever, vomiting, diarrhea).

Pelvic Inflammatory Disease

1. Definition: **Pelvic inflammatory disease** is an infectious process that can involve the fallopian tubes, uterus, ovaries, and peritoneal surface.
2. Incidence and etiology
   a. Incidence is difficult to determine because PID is not a reportable disease.
   b. Fifteen to 25 percent of women who are infected become infertile.
   c. Chronic PID is common.
   d. Risk factors include IUD use, STDs, multiple sex partners, and history of PID.
   e. Pelvic inflammatory disease is caused by infections, such as gonorrhea, chlamydial infection, and mycoplasma infection, that are transmitted through sexual intercourse.
3. Clinical manifestations
   a. Severe lower abdominal pain and tenderness

Table 31–12. Hormone Replacement Therapy

Medication	Action	Side Effects	Contraindications	Nursing Implications

Estrogen
Oral
  Conjugated estrogen (Premarin); esterified estrogen (Estratab, Menest); estradiol (Estrace); estropipate (Ogen)
Topical
  Ortho Dienestrol, Premarin, Estrace
Transdermal
  Estraderm
Intramuscular
  Estroject, Estrone-5, Delestrogen
	Relieves vasomotor symptoms of menopause and atrophic vaginitis; provides some protection against osteoporosis and cardiovascular disease (taking progestin reduces this protection)	Chest pain, severe headache, visual disturbances, breast tenderness, edema, bloating, cholasma (dark, spotting on skin)	Presence or history of thromboembolitis disorders, breast or estrogen-dependent cancer, pregnancy; use with caution if woman has hypertension, gallbladder disease, migraine headaches, diabetes, renal disease	*All methods of administration:* Report breast tenderness, vaginal bleeding, swelling of feet and hands, and other adverse signs. Have a yearly physical examination and perform monthly breast self-examination. Oral therapy is usually cyclical—3 weeks on and 1 week off. Vaginal creams may cause local irritation. Apply at bedtime to increase effectiveness. Remain flat for 30 minutes after applying. Avoid using tampons. Systemic reaction is possible. Patches are changed twice weekly. Sites are rotated on the abdomen and buttocks. Watch for skin reaction. Patches are worn 3 weeks on and 1 week off. Combining progestin with estrogen is recommended to decrease risk of endometrial hyperplasia. Read patient information insert that accompanies the prescription.

Progestin *Oral* Medroxyprogesterone acetate (Provera)	Prevention of endometrial hyperplasia in women taking estrogen for menopausal symptoms	Depression, headache, breast tenderness, edema, breakthrough bleeding, hypertension, decreased libido	Presence or history of thromboembolitic disorders, breast cancer, liver dysfunction, pregnancy, gynecologic cancer, undiagnosed uterine bleeding	Take progestin for 10 days beginning on day 16 of estrogen cycle or as prescribed. Withdrawal bleeding may occur. Report side effects to physician. See patient information insert that accompanies the prescription. Yearly physical examination is advised and monthly breast self-examination. Not usually recommended for women who do not have a uterus and who are on estrogen replacement therapy.

Data from *Nursing 94 Drug Handbook*. Springhouse, PA: Springhouse Corp., 1994; Corson SL. Physiology of menopause and update on hormonal replacement therapy. *NAACOGs Clin Issues Perinat Women's Health Nurs* 2(1):483–496, 1991; Gant NF, and Cunningham FG. *Basic Gynecology and Obstetrics.* Norwalk, CT: Appleton & Lange, 1994; Patient information insert for Provera. Kalamazoo, MI: The Upjohn Company, 1992; Estrace information for the patient. Princeton, NJ: Mead Johnson Laboratories, 1992.

b. Fever
c. Purulent vaginal discharge
d. Dysuria

4. Clinical management
   a. The history elicits information about unprotected sexual activity with infected partner, recent IUD use, recent abortion or childbirth, prior episodes of PID or STDs, and symptoms such as fever, nausea, and lower abdominal pain.
   b. Pelvic examination reveals purulent cervical discharge and pain and abdominal guarding when the cervix and adnexa (tubes and ovaries) are manipulated.
   c. Nonpharmacologic interventions
      (1) Sitz baths for comfort
      (2) Heat to abdomen
      (3) Bedrest in semi-Fowler's position to promote drainage of discharge
   d. Pharmacologic interventions: Combination antibiotic therapy for 10 to 14 days. Drug selection depends on causative organism.
   e. Special medical-surgical procedures: laparotomy with incision and drainage of abscesses and lysis of adhesions if possible
   f. Nursing interventions

(1) Provide information about causes, risk factors, treatment, and prevention of reinfection.
(2) Provide information about comfort measures and pain control with medications.
(3) Encourage verbalization of concerns and feelings.
(4) Include partner in discussions as indicated.
(5) Refer to support group or counseling as needed.

Cystocele and Rectocele

1. Definition
   a. A **cystocele** is the protrusion of the bladder through the vaginal walls (Fig. 31–12).
   b. A **rectocele** is the protrusion of the rectum through the weakened vaginal wall (Fig. 31–12).
2. Incidence and etiology
   a. The incidence is unknown, but most women who have experienced vaginal childbirth have some degree of defect.
   b. Risk factors include obesity, age older than 35 years, and difficult childbirth.
   c. Congenital defect of supporting tissues, childbearing, and loss of estrogen after menopause are causes.
3. Clinical manifestations
   a. Cystoceles and rectoceles are often asymptomatic.
   b. Symptoms of cystocele include urinary frequency, retention, and incontinence.
   c. Symptoms of rectocele include constipation, flatus, and fecal incontinence.
4. Clinical management
   a. The history will elicit information about difficulty in emptying the bladder, urinary frequency, urinary tract infections, urinary or fecal incontinence, constipation, fecal impaction, or feelings of rectal or vaginal fullness.
   b. Pelvic examination reveals a bulge in the anterior vaginal wall when the woman is asked to bear down. Rectovaginal examination reveals a bulge in the posterior vaginal wall when the woman is asked to bear down.
   c. Nonpharmacologic interventions
      (1) No treatment may be necessary if the woman is asymptomatic and the cystocele or rectocele is small.
      (2) A diet high in fiber may relieve symptoms caused by the rectocele.
      (3) A pessary (device worn in vagina) may provide some relief for cystocele.
   d. Pharmacologic interventions
      (1) Stool softeners or mild laxatives may be prescribed for symptoms related to a rectocele.
      (2) Topical estrogen cream or estrogen replacement therapy may prevent atrophy and weakening of vaginal walls in postmenopausal women.
   e. Special medical-surgical procedures
      (1) For severe symptoms related to cystocele, anterior colporrhaphy, or anterior repair, may be performed. In this procedure, the pelvic muscles are shortened to provide better support of the bladder.
      (2) For severe symptoms related to rectocele, a posterior colporrhaphy, or posterior repair, is done. In

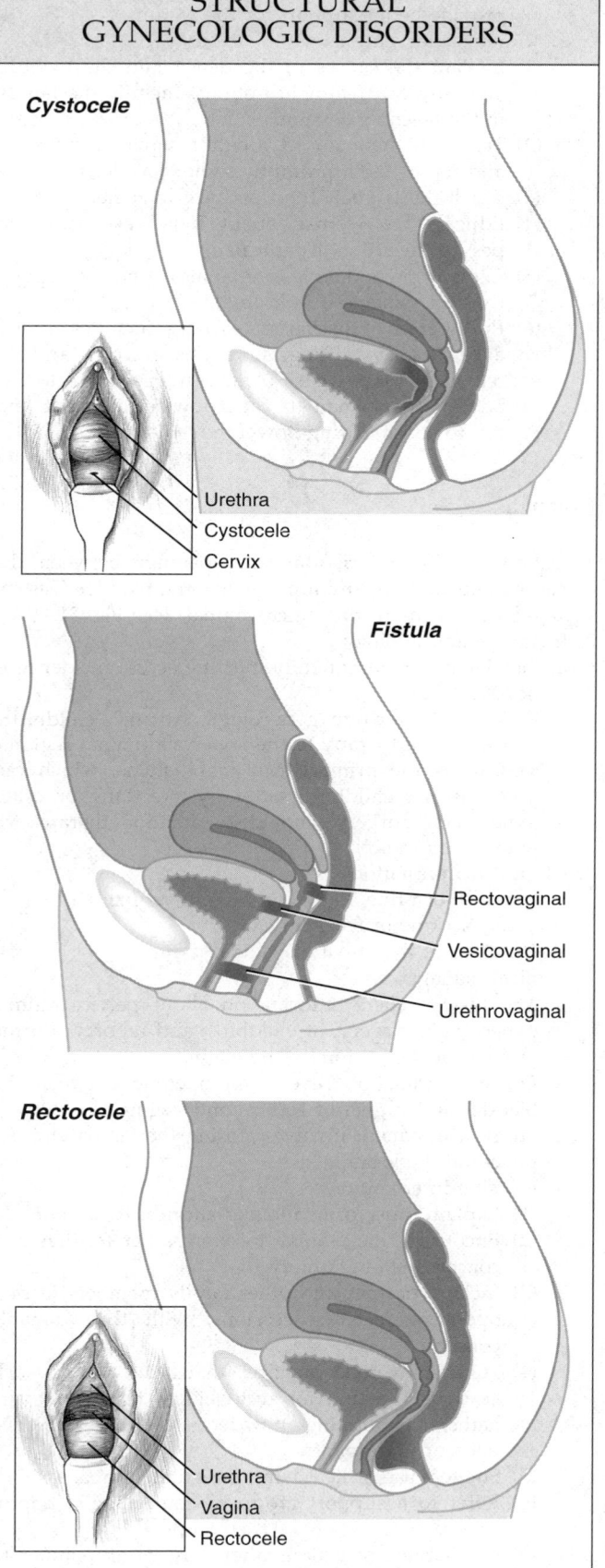

STRUCTURAL GYNECOLOGIC DISORDERS

Cystocele

Urethra
Cystocele
Cervix

Fistula

Rectovaginal
Vesicovaginal
Urethrovaginal

Rectocele

Urethra
Vagina
Rectocele

Figure 31–12.

this procedure, the pelvic muscles are shortened to provide better support for the rectum.

   f. Nursing interventions

     (1) Explain the causes of the defect and the medical and surgical treatment options. Include the family in the teaching session.

     (2) Teach the woman to identify signs of infection and report them promptly to her physician.

     (3) Teach the woman good perineal hygiene.

     (4) Educate the woman about Kegel exercises and pessary insertion, if indicated.

     (5) Explain preoperative preparation and postoperative assessments if indicated.

     (6) Postoperative discharge teaching includes avoidance of heavy lifting, strenuous exercise, and intercourse for 6 weeks. After surgery for rectocele, advise the woman to eat a low-residue diet and not to strain during bowel movements.

Fistulas

1. Definition: **Vaginal fistulas** are openings between the vagina and urethra (urethrovaginal), the bladder (vesicovaginal), and the rectum (rectovaginal) (see Fig. 31–12).
2. Incidence and etiology
   a. Fistulas occur infrequently, but the actual incidence is not available.
   b. Risk factors include gynecologic surgery, childbirth, and radiation therapy to the lower abdominal region.
   c. Trauma is the primary cause of fistulas, which can occur during childbirth, after hysterectomy or other gynecologic surgery, and after radiation therapy for gynecologic cancers.
3. Clinical manifestations
   a. Presence of urine, flatus, or feces in vagina
   b. Odor of urine or feces in vagina
   c. Irritation of the vulva or vaginal tissues
4. Clinical management
   a. The history elicits information about pelvic trauma, gynecologic surgery, or childbirth and reports of urine or feces or their odors in the vagina.
   b. Pelvic examination reveals an opening between the bladder and vagina or rectum and vagina.
   c. Surgical treatment involves closing the fistula and depends on the location.
   d. Nursing interventions
      (1) Explain cause of fistula and surgical treatment.
      (2) Encourage the woman to express her feelings and concerns about surgery.
      (3) Include partner and other family members in preoperative teaching sessions, with the woman's consent.
      (4) Suggest hygiene practices that reduce odor, such as douching (not for rectovaginal fistulas) or sitz baths, deodorizing powders, use of protective pads or underpants.
      (5) Suggest use of heat lamp on irritated area.
      (6) Refer to a support group or counseling if appropriate.
      (7) Discharge instructions after surgery are similar to those for cystocele and rectocele repair (see above).

Cervical Polyps

1. Definition: **Cervical polyps** are nonmalignant bulging growths that develop at the lower end of the endocervix. The surface is covered with columnar epithelium, with areas of metaplasia and ulceration. The polyp is usually filled with blood and is on a pedicle (stalk).
2. Incidence and etiology
   a. Polyps are the most common benign lesions of the cervix during the reproductive years.
   b. Risk factors include age over 40 years, use of oral contraceptives and multiparity.
   c. The cause is unknown, but polyps can result from hyperplasia of the endocervical epithelium or from inflammation.
3. Clinical manifestations
   a. Usually asymptomatic
   b. Bleeding after coitus
   c. Pre- or postmenstrual bleeding or spotting
4. Clinical management
   a. The goal of intervention is to treat the irregular bleeding by removal of the polyps.
   b. Special medical-surgical procedures: Usual removal is by grasping the polyp with a clamp and twisting to detach it. The specimen is then sent to the laboratory for evaluation. Electric or chemical cauterization will usually stop the bleeding at the operative site.
   c. Nursing interventions
      (1) Encourage the woman to discuss her feelings and concerns about the procedure.
      (2) Provide information on what to expect during the procedure.
      (3) Encourage use of relaxation techniques during the procedure.
      (4) Provide support during the procedure.
   d. Discharge instructions
      (1) Advise the woman to avoid tampon use, sexual intercourse, and douching for 4 to 7 days after the procedure.
      (2) Describe signs of complications such as heavy bleeding (more than 1 saturated pad in 1 hr) and signs of infection, which should be reported to the physician.
      (3) Encourage the woman to keep follow-up appointments.

Bartholin's Cysts

1. Definition: A cyst arising in the Bartholin's glands or ducts, filled with clear fluid
2. Incidence and etiology
   a. Bartholin's cysts are the most common vulvar disorder.
   b. Bartholin's cysts are caused by an obstruction of Bartholin's duct.
3. Clinical manifestations: Bartholin's cysts cause dyspareunia, vulvar pain, and a mass in the perineal area.
4. Clinical management
   a. Bed rest and application of moist heat to the vulva for infected Bartholin's cysts
   b. Mild analgesics for pain

c. Antibiotic therapy for infection

d. Marsupialization (the formation of a new duct opening for drainage) is sometimes needed for Bartholin's cysts. Bartholin's cysts tend to recur unless a new duct opening is established.

▣ *SEXUAL DYSFUNCTION*

Overview of Sexual Dysfunction

1. In **sexual dysfunction** pathophysiologic and psychogenic factors can interfere with the ability to have or enjoy the sexual experience.
2. Classifications include the following:
   a. General sexual dysfunction, in which a woman derives no sexual pleasure from sexual stimulation
   b. Orgasmic disorders, in which female orgasm is inhibited
   c. Sexual pain disorders, or vaginismus, in which recurrent, persistent involuntary spasms of the outer vaginal muscles interfere with coitus

Anorgasmia (Inhibited Female Orgasm)

1. Definition: The woman has a normal sexual response cycle through the excitement and plateau stages but cannot progress to orgasm or does not get adequate stimulation for the sexual response cycle to begin.
2. Incidence and etiology
   a. Inhibited female orgasm is the most prevalent sexual problem among women. Fewer than 20 percent of cases have a physiologic basis. Eight to 15 percent of American women have not experienced orgasm other than in their sleep.
   b. The incidence of situationally inhibited female orgasm is 50 percent.
   c. Risk factors include use of alcohol, barbiturates, or narcotics; inflammatory or infectious gynecologic conditions; ignorance of sexual techniques; stress; and fatigue.
   d. Etiology can be psychogenic, involving a woman's unconscious, unresolved conflicts about sexual activity, or organic, in which disease causes general debilitation or affects the sexual response cycle or drugs depress the central nervous system.
3. Clinical manifestations
   a. Complaints of not being able to have an orgasm
   b. History of the woman's presenting problem: onset, duration, frequency, situation (Box 31–7)
4. Clinical management
   a. Determine onset, duration, frequency of situation.
   b. Goals of intervention: to increase self-awareness and teach effective self-stimulation and achievement of orgasm
   c. Nonpharmacologic interventions
      (1) Masturbation training may be done for a woman who has never experienced orgasm.
      (2) Group therapy may be encouraged to help the woman discuss her problem and learn about sexual functioning. "Homework" assignments (e.g.,

---

Box 31–7. Sexual History

Privacy is essential when taking a sexual history. It is usually more effective to begin with less sensitive issues. Use language that the woman understands.
- Ask the woman about her sexual response with all partners, if applicable.
- Assess the sexual attitude of the woman and her partner.
- Assess use of sexual stimulation techniques, such as masturbation or vibrators.
- Assess history of depression and anxiety.
- Assess drug use (tranquilizers, oral contraceptives, narcotics).
- Determine whether the woman has a body image disturbance related to obesity, mastectomy, hysterectomy, rape, or any other factors.
- Assess cultural perspectives about sexual activities.

---

masturbation) are given to encourage practice at home.
      (3) Couple's therapy involves exercises in stimulation by the woman's partner to help her achieve orgasm.
   d. Pharmacologic interventions—for example, discontinuing use of tranquilizers or oral contraceptives—vary with the problem.
   e. Nursing interventions
      (1) Help the woman to express her feelings.
      (2) Offer understanding and support.
      (3) Provide accurate information to the woman and her partner, if indicated.
      (4) Teach what orgasm is like and what to expect.
      (5) Provide instructions for manual stimulation.
      (6) Refer to a sex therapist for counseling when appropriate.

Vaginismus

1. Definition: **Vaginismus** is a condition in which a woman develops an anxiety-fear-guilt cycle, so that negative thoughts become associated with the act of vaginal penetration and a conditioned reflex is established. The woman can experience sexual arousal and noncoital activity may be pleasurable, but vaginal penetration is not possible.
2. Incidence and etiology
   a. Vaginismus is relatively rare.
   b. Risk factors include fear of men; ignorance about sexual functioning and childbirth; and history of prior sexual trauma, rape, molestation.
   c. Etiology is related to an early traumatic event such as rape or sexual trauma. Ninety percent of cases are psychogenic.
3. Clinical manifestations: involuntary vaginal muscular spasms that prevent penetration or examination
4. Clinical management
   a. Review history of inability to insert tampons and pain on attempted intercourse.
   b. Goals of intervention: to assist the woman to understand what is occurring physiologically and to correct the condition
   c. Nonpharmacologic interventions

(1) Discuss physiologic responses

(2) Demonstrate vaginal spasm to show it is involuntary.

(3) Use graduated dilators to overcome the spasms and allow vaginal penetration.

(4) Recommend relaxation exercises and warm baths before sexual activities.

(5) Psychoanalysis, behavior therapy, and hypnosis may be useful to reduce a phobic avoidance of vaginal penetration.

d. Nursing interventions

(1) Encourage the woman to discuss her fears about intercourse, childbirth.

(2) Encourage open communication between the woman and her partner.

(3) Promote increased self-awareness.

(4) Provide information on use of dilators and manual exploration of the vagina.

(5) Encourage therapy at home.

(6) Refer for sexual counseling as needed.

Bibliography

Books

Agur AMR. *Grant's Atlas of Anatomy.* 9th ed. Baltimore: Williams & Wilkins, 1991.

American Cancer Society. *Cancer Facts and Figures 1996.* New York: Author, 1996.

Clarke-Pearson D, and Dawood MJ. *Green's Gynecology: Essential Clinical Practice.* 4th ed. Boston: Little, Brown, & Co, 1990.

Cunningham FG, et al. *William's Obstetrics.* 19th ed. Norwalk, CT: Appleton & Lange, 1993.

DiSaia PJ, and Creaseman WT. *Clinical Gynecological Oncology.* 4th ed. St. Louis: Mosby–Year Book, 1993.

Edge V, Miller M. *Woman's Health Care. Clinical Nursing Series.* St. Louis: Mosby–Year Book, 1994.

Gant NF, and Cunningham FG. *Basic Gynecology and Obstetrics.* Norwalk, CT: Appleton & Lange, 1993.

Guyton AC. *Textbook of Medical Physiology.* 8th ed. Philadelphia: WB Saunders, 1991.

Hatcher RA, et al. *Contraceptive Technology: 1994–96.* 16th ed. New York: Irvington Press, 1994.

Herbst A, et al. *Comprehensive Gynecology.* 2nd ed. St. Louis: Mosby–Year Book, 1992.

Horton JA. *The Women's Health Data Book.* 2nd ed. New York: Elsevier, 1995.

Lichtman R, and Papera S. *Gynecology: Well Woman Care.* Norwalk, CT: Appleton & Lange, 1990.

Lowdermilk D, Perry S, and Bobak I. *Maternity and Women's Health Care.* 6th ed. St. Louis: Mosby–Year Book, 1997.

McCorkle R, et al. *Cancer Nursing: A Comprehensive Textbook.* 2nd ed. Philadelphia: WB Saunders, 1996.

Nichols DH. *Gynecologic and Obstetric Surgery.* St. Louis: Mosby–Year Book, 1994.

Nichols DH, and Randall CL. *Vaginal Surgery.* 3rd ed. Baltimore: Williams & Wilkins, 1989.

Shephard BD, and Shephard CA. *The Complete Guide to Woman's Health.* New York: Plume, 1990.

Thibodeau GA, and Patton K. *Anatomy and Physiology.* 2nd ed. St. Louis: Mosby–Year Book, 1993.

Willson JR, and Carrington ER. *Obstetrics and Gynecology.* 9th ed. St. Louis: Mosby–Year Book, 1991.

Chapters in Books and Journal Articles

Anatomy and Physiology

Hamm T. Physiology of normal female bleeding. *NAACOGs Clin Issues Perinat Womens Health Nurs.* 2(3):289, 1991.

Lowdermilk DL. Assessment of the reproductive system. *In* Ignatavicius DD, Workman ML, and Mishler M (eds). *Medical-Surgical Nursing: A Nursing Process Approach.* 2nd ed. Philadelphia: WB Saunders, 1995.

Physical Assessment

Barkauskas VH, et al. Female genitalia. *In* Barkauskas VH (ed). *Health and Physical Assessment.* St. Louis: Mosby–Year Book, 1994.

Devy S. Lesbian health care. *In* Fogel C, and Woods N (eds). *Women's Health Care: A Comprehensive Handbook.* Thousand Oaks, CA: Sage, 1995.

Jarvis C. Female genitalia. *In* Jarvis C. *Physical Examination and Health Assessment.* 2nd ed. Philadelphia: WB Saunders, 1996, pp 803–846.

Kain CD, Reilly N, and Schultz ED. The older adult: A comparative assessment. *Nurs Clin North Am* 25(4):833–849, 1990.

Lawhead RA. Vulvar self-examination: What your patients should know. *Female Patient* 15:33–38, 1990.

Rudy EB, and Gray VR. Assessment of female genitalia and rectum. *In* Rudy E (ed). *Handbook of Health Assessment.* 3rd ed. Norwalk, CT: Appleton & Lange, 1991.

Seidel HM, et al. Female genitalia. *In* Seidel HM, et al. (eds). *Mosby's Guide to Physical Examination.* 3rd ed. St. Louis: Mosby–Year Book, 1995.

Stevens PE. Structural and interpersonal impact of heterosexual assumptions on lesbian health care clients. *Nurs Res* 44(10):25–30, 1995.

Special Diagnostic Studies

Barsevick A, and Lauver D. Womens' informational needs about colposcopy. *Image J Nurs Sch* 22:23–26, 1990.

Beal M. Cervical cytology. *NAACOGs Clin Issues Perinat Womens Health Nurs* 1(4):470–478, 1990.

Calle EE, et al. Demographic predictors of mammography and Pap smear screening in U.S. women. *Am J Public Health* 83:53–60, 1993.

Clay L. Midwifery assessment of the well woman: The Pap smear. *J Nurse Midwife* 35(6):341, 1990.

Germain M, et al. A comparison of the most common Papanicolaou smear collection techniques. *Obstet Gynecol* 84:168–173, 1994.

Ginsberg C. Exfoliative cytologic screening: The Papanicolaou test. *JOGNN* 20(1):39–46, 1991.

Harlan LC, Bernstein AB, and Lessler LG. Cervical cancer screening: Who is not screened and why? *Am J Public Health* 81(7):885, 1991.

Lauver D, and Rubin M. Women's concerns about abnormal Papanicolaou test results. *JOGNN* 20(2):154–159, 1991.

National Cancer Institute Workshop. The 1988 Bethesda System for reporting cervical/vaginal cytological diagnoses. *JAMA* 262:931–934, 1989.

Saigo P, et al. Understanding the Bethesda System. *Patient Care* April 30, 1993, pp 65–80.

Common Menstrual Disorders

Bernhard L, and Sheppard L. Health, symptoms, self-care, and dyadic adjustment in menopausal women. *JOGNN* 22(5):456–461, 1993.

Christian A. The relationship between women's symptoms of endometriosis and self-esteem. *JOGNN* 22(4):370–376, 1993.

Cook M. Perimenopause: An opportunity for health promotion. *JOGNN* 22(3):223, 1993.

Garry R, et al. Six hundred endometrial laser ablations. *Obstet Gynecol* 85:24–29, 1995.

Hsai LS, and Long MH. Premenstrual syndrome: Current concepts in diagnosis and management. *J Nurse Midwife* 35(6):351, 1990.

Lindow KB. Premenstrual syndrome: Family impact and nursing implications. *JOGNN* 20(2):135–138, 1991.

Mason E. Medical causes of abnormal vaginal bleeding. *NAACOGs Clin Issues Perinat Womens Health Nurs* 2(3):322, 1991.

Mitchell ES. The elusive premenstrual syndrome. *NAACOGs Clin Issues Perinat Womens Health Nurs* 2(3):294–303, 1991.

Murata, J. Abnormal genital bleeding and secondary amenorrhea in common gynecological problems. *JOGNN* 19(1):26–36, 1990.

Peck D. Premenstrual syndrome. *In* Lichtman R, and Papera S (eds). *Gynecology: Well-Woman Care.* Norwalk, CT: Appleton & Lange, 1990, pp 333–343.

Powell, L. Evaluation of abnormal genital bleeding. *NAACOGs Clin Issues Perinat Women's Health Nurs* 2(3):328, 1991.

Gynecologic Infections

Centers for Disease Control and Prevention. 1993 Sexually Transmitted Diseases Treatment Guidelines. *MMWR* 42(RR-14):1–102, 1993.

Eschenbach DA, and Mead PB. Vaginitis: Varying management approaches. *Contemp Obstet Gynecol* 37(1):25, 1992.

French JI. Abnormal bleeding associated with reproductive infections. *NAACOGs Clin Issues Perinat Womens Health Nurs* 2(3):313–321, 1991.

Jossens M, and Sweet R. Pelvic inflammatory disease: Risk factors and microbial etiologies. *JOGNN* 22(2):169–179, 1993.

McKeon VA: Hormone replacement therapy: Evaluating the risks and benefits. *JOGNN* 23(8):647–657, 1994.

Tuomala R. Gynecological infections. *In* Ryan K, Berkowitz J, and Babieri R (eds). *Kistner's Gynecology: Principles and Practices.* 5th ed. Chicago: Year Book Medical Publishers, 1990, pp 570–609.

Structural Disorders of the Uterus and Vagina

Ferguson K, et al. Stress urinary incontinence: Effect of pelvic muscle exercise. *Obstet Gynecol* 75:671, 1990.

Gynecologic Tumors

American College of Obstetricians and Gynecologists. *Laser Technology* (Technical Bulletin #146). Washington, DC: Author, 1990.

Bachmann GA. Psychosexual aspects of hysterectomy. *Women's Health Issues* 1(Suppl 1):41–49, 1990.

Boyle N, Bertin-Matson K, and Bratschi A. A patient's guide to Taxol. *Oncol Nurs Forum* 21(Suppl 9):1569–1572, 1994.

Dorsey JH. Endometrial ablation. *Obstet Gynecol Clin North Am* 18(3):475–489, 1991.

Huff BC. Gestational trophoblastic disease. *NAACOGs Clin Issues Perinat Womens Health Nurs* 1(4):453–458, 1990.

Lowdermilk DL. Nursing care update: Internal radiation therapy. *NAACOGs Clin Issues Perinat Womens Health Nurs* 1(4): 532–541, 1990.

Lowdermilk DL. Interventions for clients with gynecologic problems. *In* Ignatavicius DD, Workman ML, and Mishler M (eds). *Medical-Surgical Nursing: A Nursing Process Approach.* 2nd ed. Philadelphia: WB Saunders, 1995.

Lowdermilk DL. Reproductive surgery. *In* Fogel C, and Woods N (eds). *Women's Health Care: A Comprehensive Handbook.* Thousand Oaks, CA, Sage, 1995.

Martin LK, and Brally PS. Gynecologic cancer. *In* Baird SB, McCorkle R, and Grant M. *Cancer Nursing: A Comprehensive Textbook.* Philadelphia: WB Saunders, 1991, pp 502–535.

National Institutes of Health Consensus Conference. Ovarian cancer: Screening, treatment, and follow-up. *JAMA* 273(6):491–497, 1995.

Rostad ME. The radical vulvectomy patient: Preventing complications. *Dimens Crit Care Nurs* 7:289–294, 1988.

Rubin M, and Lauver D. Assessment and management of cervical intraepithelial neoplasia. *Nurse Pract* 15(10):23–31, 1990.

Shell JA. Sexuality for patients with gynecologic cancer. *NAACOGs Clin Issues Perinat Womens Health Nurs* 2(4):479–494, 1990.

Strohl RA. External radiation beam therapy in gynecologic cancers. *NAACOGs Clin Issues Perinat Womens Health Nurs* 2(4):525–531, 1990.

Wakczak J, and Klemm P: Gynecologic cancers. *In* Groenwald S, et al (eds). *Cancer Nursing: Principles and Practice.* 3rd ed. Boston: Jones & Bartlett, 1993.

Williamson ML. Sexual adjustment after hysterectomy. *JOGNN* 21(1):42–47, 1992.

Yoder L, and Rubin M. The epidemiology of cervical cancer and its precursors. *Oncol Nurs Forum* 19(3):84–90, 1992.

Sexual Dysfunction

Bernhard LA. Sexuality in women's lives. *In* Fogel C, and Woods N (eds). *Women's Health Care: A Comprehensive Handbook.* Thousand Oaks, CA: Sage, 1995.

Field ML. Psychomotor sexual dysfunction. *In* Fogel CI, and Lauver D. *Sexual Health Promotion.* Philadelphia: WB Saunders, 1990.

Fogel CI, Forker J, and Welch MB. Sexual health care. *In* Fogel CI, Lauver D. *Sexual Health Promotion.* Philadelphia: WB Saunders, 1990.

Rosenthal MB, Benson RC. Psychologic aspects of obstetrics and gynecology. *In* Pernoll ML. *Current Obstetric and Gynecologic Diagnosis and Treatment.* Norwalk, CT: Appleton & Lange, 1991.

Agencies

American Cancer Society
1599 Clifton Road
Atlanta, GA 30329
(800) ACS–2345

Association of Women's Health,
  Obstetrics, and Gynecologic
  Nursing
700 14th Street NW, Suite 600
Washington, DC 20005
(202) 662–1600

Endometriosis Association
8585 North 76th Place
Milwaukee, WI 53223
(414) 355–2200

National Gay and Lesbian Health
  Foundation
P.O. Box 65472
Washington, DC 20035
(202) 797–3708

National Women's Health Network
1325 G Street NW
Washington, DC 20004
(202) 347–1140

PMS Access
(800) 222–4PMS (4767)

Premenstrual Syndrome Action
P.O. Box 16292
Irving, CA 92713
(714) 854–4407

32

Caring for People with Sexually Transmitted Diseases

◼ *OVERVIEW OF SEXUALLY TRANSMITTED DISEASES*

Definition

1. **Sexually transmitted diseases** (STDs) are a group of diseases transmitted from 1 individual to another.
   a. Routes of transmission
      • Sexual intercourse
      • Intimate oral, genital, or anal contact
      • Blood
      • Transplacental
      • Transmembranous
      • Perinatal
      • Contact with bedding or clothing of infected person (lice and scabies)

Etiology

1. More than 20 diseases and syndromes are currently classified as STDs.
2. The rising incidence of STDs is due to the following:
   a. Increased identification of organisms
   b. Improved laboratory and diagnostic findings
   c. Increased number of sexually active people
   d. Increased number of people with multiple sex partners
3. Table 32–1 lists the most prevalent STDs and their causative pathogens.

Incidence

1. An estimated 10 to 13 million cases of STDs occur annually in the United States.
2. Table 32–2 shows the estimated incidence of common STDs.
3. The majority of STDs occur in people 15 to 30 years old.
4. State and local health officials are required to report each case of syphilis, gonorrhea, chancroid, hepatitis B, and human immunodeficiency virus (HIV) infection.
5. The true incidence of STDs is not known because of the following:
   a. The variability in state and local reporting requirements

   b. Absence of a national surveillance system
   c. Limited federal and state funds for screening programs
   d. Lack of money in local areas to collect and report information

Socioeconomic Impact

1. The person infected with STDs is at increased risk for the following:
   a. Infertility
   b. Life-threatening tubal pregnancy
   c. Congenital and perinatal infections
   d. Cervical, anal, and penile cancers
   e. Human immunodeficiency virus infection
2. The estimated direct and indirect costs of these infections exceed $6 billion.

Risk Factors

1. Lower socioeconomic status
2. Minority status
3. Drug abuse

BOX 32–1. U.S. Preventive Services Task Force Recommendations

These recommendations serve as a basis for forming health policy and preventive services throughout the United States.

Syphilis and Gonorrhea: Routine screening in asymptomatic people in high risk groups and pregnant women. Concentration of resources in the highest incidence areas.

Chlamydia: Improved diagnostic testing and treatment services. Routine screening for asymptomatic people and pregnant women at high risk.

Genital Herpes: Screening for genital herpes simplex virus infection is recommended for pregnant women with active lesions. Progress expected in the development of antiviral agents.

Genital Warts: Screening recommended for pregnant women. Increased research for diagnosis and treatment.

Hepatitis B: All pregnant women should be tested for hepatitis B surface antigen. Repeat the test in the third trimester for women at risk of exposure. Increased active cooperation from other agencies and private practioners to offer vaccination.

Adapted from Report of the U.S. Preventive Services Task Force *Guide to Clinical Preventive Services.* Baltimore: Williams & Wilkins, 1989.

Table 32–1. The Etiology of Sexually Transmitted Diseases

Disease	Etiology
Syphilis	*Treponema pallidum*
Gonorrhea	*Neisseria gonorrhoeae*
Chlamydia	*Chlamydia trachomatis*
Herpes genitalis	Herpes simplex virus type 1 or 2
Genital warts	Human papillomavirus
Bacterial vaginosis	*Gardnerella vaginalis*
Trichomoniasis	*Trichomonas vaginalis*
Candidiasis	*Candida albicans*
Hepatitis B	Hepatitis B virus
Chancroid	*Haemophilus ducreyi*
Lymphogranuloma venereum	L_1, L_2, L_3 *Chlamydia trachomatis*
Granuloma inguinale	*Calymmatobacterium granulomatis*
Pediculosis pubis	*Phthirus pubis*
Scabies	*Sarcoptes scabiei*

4. Multiple sexual partners
5. Young age (adolescents and young adults)
6. Limited access to medical care

Public Health Considerations: Primary Prevention

1. Identification and targeting of high-risk groups for education and treatment (Box 32–1)
2. Screening programs offered at STD, family planning, prenatal, and adolescent case clinics, emergency departments, physicians' offices, and college campuses
3. Dissemination of information on disease prevention and treatment
4. Presumptive treatment of sexual contacts of infected person irrespective of signs and symptoms for syphilis, gonorrhea, chancroid, lice, and scabies.
5. Goals of *Healthy People 2000,* a federal public health initiative
   a. Instruction in all middle and secondary schools on STD transmission, prevention, and treatment

Table 32–2. Common Sexually Transmitted Diseases in the United States

Disease	Estimated Incidence Per Year
Chlamydia	4 million cases
Pediculosis	3 million cases; not all sexually transmitted
Trichomoniasis	2.5–3 million cases
Gonorrhea	1.3 million cases
Genital warts	1–2 million cases
HIV infection	1 million people currently infected
Genital herpes	500,000 cases
Hepatitis B	300,000 cases; not all sexually transmitted
Syphilis	134,000 cases
Chancroid	3000–5000 cases

b. More primary care providers (e.g., physicians, nurses, nurse practitioners, and physician assistants) to provide age-appropriate counseling in high-incidence areas
c. Increased partner notification (contact tracing)
d. The advent of new antibiotics and the focus on behavioral interventions such as condom use to limit the spread of STDs have been only partly successful. Increased attention is being given to vaccine research.

■ ASSESSING PEOPLE WITH SEXUALLY TRANSMITTED DISEASES

Key Symptoms and Their Pathophysiologic Bases

See Table 32–3 for a clinical presentation of selected STDs.

Sexual Health History

1. The nurse should be aware of several personal and cultural factors that can influence the interview before obtaining a sexual health history.

Table 32–3. Clinical Presentation of Selected Sexually Transmitted Diseases

Syndrome	Potential Causes
Males	
Urethritis	Gonorrhea, chlamydia, genital mycoplasma infection
Epididymitis	Gonorrhea, chlamydia, and other bacterial infections
Prostatitis	Gonorrhea, chlamydia, staphylococcal/gram-negative infection
Proctitis or proctocolitis	Gonorrhea, herpes, enteric pathogens (e.g., amebiasis, syphilis, chlamydia)
Females	
Urethritis	Gonorrhea, nongonococcal urethritis
Vulvovaginitis	Trichomoniasis, vaginal candidiasis, bacterial vaginosis
Endocervicitis	Gonorrhea, chlamydia, genital herpes
Pelvic inflammatory disease	Gonorrhea, chlamydia, gram-negative/anaerobic infection
Males and Females	
Generalized rash	Hepatitis B, disseminated gonorrhea, syphilis, scabies, acute HIV infection
Genital ulcers	Syphilis, chancroid, genital herpes, granuloma inguinale, lymphogranuloma venereum
Arthritis	Disseminated gonococcal infection, Reiter's syndrome, hepatitis B

NURSE ADVISORY

1. To overcome barriers when dealing with sexual issues related to STD
   - Examine your attitudes and feelings through reflection and self-study.
   - Review current literature related to STDs and nursing practice, counseling skills, and sexual customs within cultures.
   - Set aside preconceived notions regarding sexuality of homosexuals, older people, and the disabled.
2. Do not ask questions merely to satisfy your curiosity.
3. As you take the history, start with general questions and progress to more specific questions.
4. Give positive verbal and nonverbal feedback.
5. Listen carefully to both spoken and unspoken patient concerns.
6. Avoid ambiguous terms.
7. Respect the person's identity.

2. Obtain a health history related to male and female genitourinary and sexual functioning. (See also Chapter 4.)
3. The purpose of the following questions is to assess the presence of common risk factors:
   - Have you ever been treated for an STD or for HIV?
   - Are you currently sexually active? For how long?
   - When was the last time you had sex?
   - Are you currently using birth control?

TRANSCULTURAL CONSIDERATIONS

Advise the use of barrier methods for safe sex. During the sexual assessment and interview, it is important to remember that there may be cultural or religious prohibitions against the use of barrier methods or any other method of birth control.

   - Are you currently sexually active with 1 or more partners?
   - Is your sexual preference for men, women, or both?

4. Ask the following questions to determine the significance of the patient's presenting symptoms:
   a. Where is the location of the symptom or symptoms?
   b. How long have you experienced the symptoms?
   c. Is the symptom related to a previous sexual activity?
   d. Have you been using over-the-counter medications or self-treatments for the symptoms you are currently experiencing?
   e. Is the symptom associated with other urinary tract infection symptoms such as painful urination, burning sensation while urinating, frequency, or urgency?

Physical Examination

1. General information
   a. A person may have more than 1 symptom.
   b. It is not unusual for an individual to harbor 1 or more organisms simultaneously.

NURSE ADVISORY

A person with a known STD should be advised to have periodic HIV screening. Informed consent should be obtained. The person should have adequate pre- and post-test counseling for both positive and negative results.

   c. Perform a focused examination on the following:
      (1) The oral cavity
      (2) The skin
      (3) The genitourinary tract
      (4) The anorectal area
      (5) The regional lymph nodes of the neck and pelvis
   d. See also Chapter 5.

Special Diagnostic Studies

1. Cultures can be obtained for the following (Procedure 32–1):

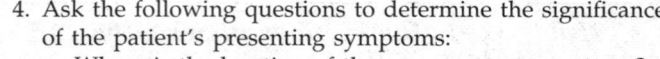

Procedure 32–1
Obtaining Culture for the Diagnosis of Bacterial Disease

Definition/Purposes	To obtain culture specimens for diagnosis of disease from the oropharynx, anal canal, male urethra, and cervix.
Learning/Teaching Activities	Provide the following information: (1) describe the procedure, (2) explain that the procedure will cause temporary discomfort, and (3) tell the patient that a chaperone is available to assist.

Preliminary Activities

Equipment	• Examination gloves • Vaginal speculum • Sterile cotton swabs

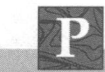

Procedure 32–1

(continued)

Preliminary Activities

- Sterile calcium alginate swabs
- Sterile wire loop
- Culture medium

Assessment/Planning
- Know which disease the culture is being done for.
- Know whether the person has had cultures done before.
- Make sure environment provides privacy and comfort.
- Schedule return visit as needed for results and possible follow-up culture.

Preparation of Person
- Individual should be undressed with adequate draping and lying down.
- Wash hands with soap and water before and after procedure.
- Don examination gloves.

Procedure

Actions	Rationale/Discussion

Male and Female Oropharynx Culture

1. Place the person in a sitting position.
2. Swab the pharynx and tonsil area bilaterally and posteriorly with a calcium alginate swab for 20 to 30 seconds.
3. Roll the swab in a large Z pattern on the selected medium.

1. For comfort and ease of obtaining specimen.
2. Specimen is obtained when there is a suspicion of disseminated gonococcal infection.
3. Provides exposure of the organisms on the medium.

Male and Female Rectal Culture

1. Place the person in a dorsal lithotomy position.
2. Insert sterile cotton swab 2.5 cm into the anal canal.
3. Insert the sterile calcium alginate swab approximately 2.5 cm into the anal canal moving it from side to side for 20 to 30 seconds.

1. For comfort and ease of specimen collection.
2. This swab clears feces from the anal canal.
3. Movement from side to side ensures that the specimen will be obtained and absorbed onto the swab.

Female Cervical Culture

1. This specimen is collected by using proper technique for inserting a vaginal speculum.
   a. Warm the speculum with water only.
   b. When separating the labia, depress the perineum and posterior vaginal wall with the finger while holding the speculum with the other hand.
   c. Have the woman take a deep breath and release it while you insert the speculum slowly and gently.
2. Clean the external cervical area with a large sterile cotton swab.
3. Insert the sterile calcium alginate swab into the endocervical canal, rotating it for 20 to 30 seconds.
4. Inoculate the selective culture medium with the specimen.
5. Instruct woman that procedure is completed.
6. Release the bivalve vaginal speculum slowly.
7. Dispose of equipment in the proper receptacle.

   a. Lubricants other than water interfere with specimen collection.
   b. Eases introduction of the speculum.

   c. Breathing out makes it difficult to tense the pelvic muscles, thereby allowing the speculum to slide in more easily.
2. Removes the excess cervical mucus normally present.
3. Ensures adequate sampling.

4. The Z pattern ensures isolated colonies of organisms.

Male Urethral Culture

1. Clean the external opening.
2. Insert sterile bacteriologic wire loop approximately 2 cm into the uretha, gently scraping the mucosa anterior to the urethra, or insert a sterile urethral calcium alginate swab until the tip is completely hidden. Rotate the swab for 20 to 30 seconds.
3. Remove the specimen from the urethra.
4. Inoculate the selective culture medium with the specimen.

1. Decreases the possibility of contamination from other organisms.
2. Ensures adequate sampling.

4. Culture is indicated if the Gram stain is negative or if the person is asymptomatic.

a. Gonorrhea
b. Chlamydial infection
c. Chancroid
d. Trichomoniasis
e. Bacterial vaginosis
2. See other diagnostic studies specific to each disease.

◼ SYPHILIS

Definition

Subacute to chronic infectious disease caused by the bacterium *Treponema pallidum*.

Incidence and Socioeconomic Impact

1. Syphilis is the 3rd most commonly reported communicable disease in the United States.
2. There are approximately 43,000 cases of reported primary and secondary syphilis and 22.3 per 100,000 cases of early latent and latent syphilis.
3. The southern United States has a higher proportion of the population living below the poverty line and a higher rate of syphilis.

Etiology

1. Syphilis is caused by *T. pallidum*.
2. Syphilis is acquired through sexual contact with an infected person.

Pathophysiology

1. The mechanism by which the bacterium, a spirochete, penetrates the mucocutaneous tissue is unknown, but it is capable of invading all tissue and persists within the cells.
2. The bacterium can move throughout the body, causing progressive damage to many organs over time.
3. The bacterium can be passed transplacentally from mother to fetus.

Clinical Manifestations

1. The incubation period for syphilis ranges from 10 to 90 days before the primary lesion (chancre) appears.
2. In the primary stage, a painless chancre appears, which is an ulcerated lesion with a raised border and an indurated base.
   a. In men the lesion is easily apparent.
   b. In women the lesion is most commonly found on the cervix or in the vagina.
   c. Extragenital sites may include the anus, mouth, oropharynx, and nipples.
   d. Painless inguinal lymphadenopathy is frequently present.

e. The primary chancre will disappear spontaneously in 2 to 6 weeks without treatment.
3. Secondary stage is the next phase of the disease if the person is not treated.
   a. This stage occurs 6 weeks to 6 months after the 1st chancre.
   b. A generalized rash occurs that includes the following:
      (1) Maculopapular lesions on the palms and soles
      (2) Moist patches with grey scaly lesions on the oral mucous membranes
      (3) Condylomata lata, which are flat papules, similar to genital warts, that develop in warm, moist areas
   c. Generalized lymphadenopathy
   d. Flulike symptoms, such as fever, malaise, anorexia, and joint and muscle pain. Symptoms spontaneously clear in 2 to 6 weeks.
4. The latent stage is divided into early and late phases.
   a. The early latent phase lasts less than 1 year and is associated with exacerbation of secondary syphilis.
   b. The late latent phase lasts longer than 1 year. In this phase, the disease cannot be transmitted sexually but can be passed transplacentally to the fetus.
5. Late (tertiary) stage
   a. One third of diagnosed cases progress to this stage, which involves the cardiovascular, central nervous, musculoskeletal, and organ systems.
   b. Cardiovascular manifestations include aortic aneurysm, aortic insufficiency, and damage to the heart valves and blood vessels.
   c. Central nervous system manifestations include general paresis, tabes dorsalis, optic atrophy, meningiovascular syphilis, dementia, and slurred speech.
   d. The musculoskeletal system and viscera are affected by inflammatory processes that can cause granulomatous lesions (gummas) in any part of the body.
   e. Ophthalmic complications include uveitis, neuroretinitis, optic neuritis, and blindness.
6. Congenital syphilis
   a. Result of maternal syphilis during pregnancy. It can cause fetal demise, stillbirth, or premature birth in 40 percent of infants born to women infected with primary or secondary stage syphilis.
   b. Most infants with early congenital syphilis are asymptomatic at birth but develop active disease within 10 days to 2 weeks.
   c. Symptoms include rhinitis, mucocutaneous eruptions, hepatosplenomegaly, and osteochondritis.
   d. Late congenital syphilis is rarely seen in the United States. It occurs when the disease persists beyond 2 years.

Diagnostics

1. See Sexual Health History, page 1497.
2. Physical Examination
   a. Focused examination
   b. Lymph node examination

(1) Cervical, axillary, and inguinal lymph nodes are palpated for swelling.
3. Laboratory tests
   a. Darkfield examination of the exudate from the lesions of primary or secondary syphilis
   b. A presumptive medical diagnosis is made using two types of serologic tests for latent and tertiary syphilis and screening of all women at the initial prenatal visit.
      (1) Examples of nonspecific non–treponemal antibody tests are the Venereal Disease Research Laboratory (VDRL) test and the rapid plasma reagin (RPR) test. False-positive results are more likely to occur with these tests because they are not specific for the treponemal antibody.
      (2) Conditions that warrant screening for syphilis include *mycoplasma pneumonia* infection, malaria, acute viral and bacterial infections, autoimmune diseases, and pregnancy.
      (3) A positive VDRL or RPR test result should be followed by a more specific treponemal antibody test, such as the fluorescent treponemal antibody absorption test (FTA-ABS).
      (4) Neurosyphilis is diagnosed by a combination of the following:
      • The VDRL-CSF test cerebrospinal fluid assay
      • High CSF cell and protein count
      • The FTA-ABS test for CSF (treponemal-specific test).
   c. Congenital syphilis and neurosyphilis are difficult to diagnose. However, the following new techniques have shown promise in clinical trials:
      (1) Direct antigen tests
      (2) Enzyme-linked immunosorbent assay (ELISA)
      (3) Polymerase chain reaction (PCR) techniques

Clinical Management

1. Goals
   a. The goal of intervention for syphilis is to cure the infection, stop further damage to organ systems, and treat sexual contacts of the infected individual.
2. Nonpharmacologic interventions
   a. Individuals infected with HIV should be monitored with VDRL testing at 1-, 2-, 3-, 6-, 9-, and 12-month intervals for evaluation of treatment effectiveness.
   b. Long-term sexual partners exposed to late latent syphilis and neurosyphilis should be evaluated clinically and serologically.
3. Pharmacologic interventions
   a. Centers for Disease Control and Prevention (CDC) treatment recommendations
      (1) The drug of choice for primary, secondary, and early latent syphilis (less than 1 year) is benzathine penicillin G.
      (2) If therapy is ineffective, CSF examination is appropriate and retreatment is necessary with benzathine penicillin G.
      (3) Sexual contacts exposed to primary, secondary, or early latent syphilis should be treated presumptively.
      (4) Alternate drugs for patients who are allergic to penicillin are doxycycline and tetracycline. These are contraindicated in pregnancy.
      (5) Late latent syphilis (more than 1 year's duration) gummas, and cardiovascular syphilis are treated with benzathine penicillin G.
   b. Neurosyphilis and syphilitic eye disease are treated with aqueous crystalline penicillin G. Compliant out-

---

LEARNING/TEACHING GUIDELINES
for Self-Administration of Antibiotics

Instruct people who are going to self-administer antibiotics to

A. Always take the medication on time and never skip doses.
B. Incorporate administration into daily routines (e.g., meal times, bedtime, and daily hygiene schedules).
C. Always report any side effects to the provider.
D. Watch for signs of allergic reaction. Have someone remain for 30 minutes after every injection.
E. Special considerations for the following medications:

1. Tetracycline
   a. Watch for rash, nausea, and diarrhea.
   b. Encourage increased fluid intake.
   c. Take medication on an empty stomach. Avoid dairy products and antacids.
2. Doxycycline
   a. Avoid iron and other mineral preparations.
   b. Avoid antacids.
3. Probenecid
   a. Take with food.
   b. Encourage increased fluid intake (8–10 glasses each day).

---

patients can take aqueous procaine penicillin with probenecid.
   (1) Additional benzathine penicillin is given after completion of the other medications.
4. Special medical-surgical procedures: Management of a person with a history of penicillin allergy should include a skin test, with monitoring for an anaphylactic reaction, and referral for desensitization if needed.

Complications

Long-term complications of syphilis are described on page 1500.

Prognosis

1. Cure is possible in all stages of syphilis except late (tertiary) syphilis. Cure is indicated by a 4-fold decrease in the VDRL or RPR titer.
2. Damage to organ systems due to tertiary syphilis is permanent.
3. Central nervous system involvement occurs much earlier in persons with HIV infection.

Applying the Nursing Process

NURSING DIAGNOSIS: Knowledge deficit R/T lack of information or misinformation about STDs, their modes of transmission, treatments, and self-care

1. *Expected outcomes:* Following instruction, the person should be able to do the following:
   a. Demonstrate ability to read and understand written materials
   b. Define the STD, or STDs, the person is being treated for

   c. List the myths and misinformation about STDs
   d. Discuss the significance of diagnostic test results
   e. Explain the treatment of STDs.
   f. List the protective measures to reduce risk of reinfection
2. *Nursing interventions*
   a. Have the person read sentences from the written information presented.
   b. Have the person discuss myths or misinformation they are aware of.
   c. Explain the steps in diagnostic test performed.
   d. Ask the person to review the prescribed treatment plan.
   e. List 3 protective measures to reduce the risk of reinfection.
   f. Encourage the person to call with any questions or concerns.
   g. Provide flexible hours for patient education and nursing services to fit the needs of the patient and community.

NURSING DIAGNOSIS: Altered health maintenance R/T repeated STD infections

1. *Expected outcomes:* Following interventions, the person should be free of reinfection.
2. *Nursing interventions*
   a. Establish a level of understanding of risk factors.
   b. Encourage abstinence as soon as symptoms occur and until treatment is completed and symptoms have completely resolved.
   c. Encourage monogomy on the part of patient and sexual partner.
   d. Encourage the use of a condom at all times even when another method of birth control is being used.
   e. Encourage screening and testing for STDs on a regular basis.
   f. Encourage treatment for the sexual partner or partners.

NURSING DIAGNOSIS: Anxiety R/T social stigma of contracting STDs

1. *Expected outcomes:* Patient should have decreased anxiety with increased knowledge about the disease and the necessity for completing treatment for cure or remission.
2. *Nursing interventions*
   a. Establish a trusting relationship.
   b. Provide calm relaxing surroundings.
   c. Provide both verbal and nonverbal openings to encourage the person to express feelings of guilt, shame, or anger.

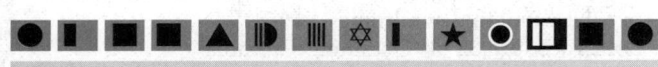

TRANSCULTURAL CONSIDERATIONS

Society sends a double message that women should be sexually appealing but are to blame for unwanted consequences of sex, such as STDs. Stigmatized by a self-caused illness, the woman is often considered unclean and sinful. This results in shame, low self-esteem, and self-blame. Women often use over-the-counter drugs and remedies, thereby delaying treatment.

   d. Provide privacy, confidentiality, support, and non-judgmental care.
   e. Be especially gentle in examining near open lesions and in areas that may be tender or painful.
   f. Offer factual information about STDs.
   g. Discuss the importance of completing treatment for cure or remission.

Discharge Planning and Teaching

1. Before discharge, instruct the patient about the disease process, the medications appropriate to the particular stage of disease, follow-up schedule, and prevention behaviors.
2. Discharge learning and teaching guidelines for all STDs are presented in Learning/Teaching Guidelines for Self-Care in Sexually Transmitted Diseases and for Self-Administration of Antibiotics.

Public Health Considerations

See the discussion of public health considerations in the overview of this chapter.

◨ *GONORRHEA*

Definition

Gonorrhea is a bacterial infection of the mucous membranes of the genitourinary tract, rectum, and pharynx (Figs. 32–1 and 32–2).

FEMALE UPPER REPRODUCTIVE TRACT INFECTIONS

Diseases, conditions, and organisms that can affect the female reproductive tract:
- Chlamydia
- Gonorrhea
- *Mycoplasma hominis*
- Bacterial vaginosis
- Streptococcus
- Staphylococcus
- *Escherichia coli*
- Other aerobic and anaerobic organisms

Routes of spread of upper reproductive tract infections:

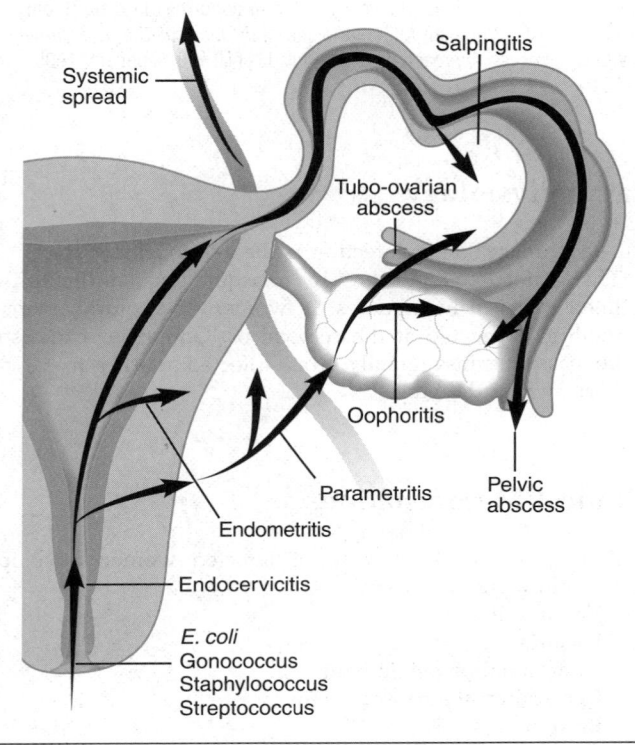

Figure 32–1.

Incidence and Socioeconomic Impact

1. Gonorrhea is the most commonly reported STD.
2. The incidence is highest among individuals 15 to 29 years old.
3. An increasing number of 10- to 14-year-olds are infected with gonorrhea.
4. The highest incidence is reported among non-Whites.

Etiology

Gonorrhea is caused by *Neisseria gonorrhoeae.*

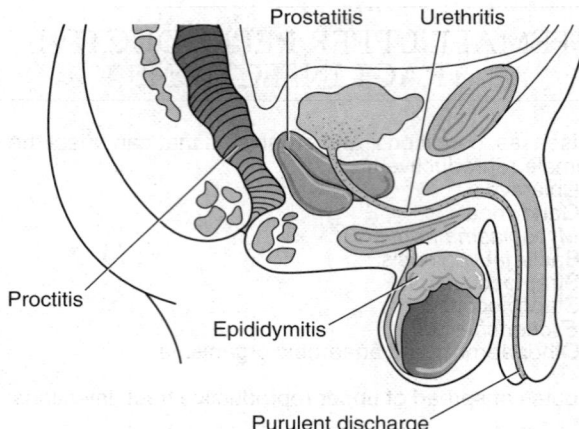

Figure 32–2. Some areas of involvement with gonorrhea in men. (From Ignatavicius DD, Workman ML, and Mishler MA. *Medical-Surgical Nursing: A Nursing Process Approach.* 2nd ed. Philadelphia: WB Saunders, 1995, p 2304.)

Pathophysiology

1. The primary site of infection is the genitourinary tract.
2. The gonococcus attaches to nonsquamous epithelium–lined mucosal membranes. In women, the columnar epithelium is located at the cervical os. Gonorrhea can also be passed transvaginally from infected mother to newborn during delivery.

Clinical Manifestations

1. Approximately 40 percent of infected women develop the following symptoms:
   - Vaginal discharge
   - Dysuria
   - Abdominal or pelvic pain
   - Cervical erythema and edema
   - Bartholinitis
   - Cervical-motion or adnexal tenderness
2. Nearly 100 percent of men develop the following symptoms:
   - Urethral discharge
   - Dysuria
   - Urinary frequency
   - Testicular or epididymal tenderness
3. Other clinical manifestations include the following:
   a. Anorectal
      - Itching or burning
      - Bleeding
      - Painful bowel movements
      - Mucopurulent discharge
   b. Pharyngeal
      - Sore throat
      - Redness and swelling
   c. Conjunctival
      - Redness and swelling
      - Mucopurulent discharge

Diagnostics

1. Refer to the earlier discussion of sexual health history and physical examinations in this chapter.
2. The presence of gram-negative diplococci, which supports an immediate presumptive diagnosis of gonorrhea.
3. Gram stain with culture remains the standard method of diagnosis for gonorrhea with results available in 48 to 72 hours.
4. A specimen is obtained with a sterile swab from the throat, male urethra, and female endocervical canal.
5. Differential medical diagnosis is made when gonorrhea is suspected, because the disease can be confused with chlamydial infection and the nongonoccocal, nonchlamydial exudative syndromes.
6. See Procedure 32–1, Obtaining Cultures

Clinical Management

1. Goals of clinical management
   a. Aggressive treatment with antibiotics
   b. Careful consideration of the anatomic site of infection
2. Pharmacologic interventions
   a. The CDC recommends cefixime, ceftriaxone, ciprofloxacin, and ofloxacin for treatment of gonorrhea.
   b. People identified as sexual contacts of an infected person are treated presumptively for gonorrhea irrespective of signs and symptoms for the following reasons:
      (1) Eliminates the need for additional office visit
      (2) Prevents complications, especially pelvic inflammatory disease (PID)
      (3) Breaks the transmission chain
   c. Special considerations are made for pregnant women (spectinomycin), and persons with gonococcal conjunctivitis (ceftriaxone), disseminated gonococcal infection (ceftriaxone), gonococcal meningitis and endocarditis (ceftriaxone), and pharyngeal gonococcal infection (ceftriaxone).
   d. Pharmacologic treatment for gonorrhea has changed over the years due to the development of resistant strains such as
      (1) Penicillinase-producing *N. gonorrhoeae* (PPNG)
      (2) Chromosomal-mediated resistant *N. gonorrhoeae* (CMRNG)
      (3) Tetracycline-resistant *N. gonorrhoeae*

Complications

1. Disseminated gonococcal infection has 2 stages.
   a. Early bacteremic stage is characterized by the following:
      - Chills
      - Fever
      - Skin lesions that resolve spontaneously
      - Bacterial endocarditis
      - Meningitis
   b. Septic arthritis stage: Purulent synovial effusion, most commonly affecting the knees, ankles, and wrists
2. Pelvic inflammatory disease. See Chapter 31.

Prognosis

1. Cure is possible for all types of gonorrhea.
2. Cure is indicated by resolution of symptoms.

Applying the Nursing Process

1. Nursing care is identical to that for syphilis (see pp. 1502–1503).

Discharge Planning and Teaching

1. See Learning/Teaching Guidelines for Self-Care in Sexually Transmitted Diseases and for Self-Administration of Antibiotics.
2. Follow-up is encouraged if symptoms persist. Persistent symptoms are most commonly due to reinfection rather than treatment failure or infection with *chlamydia trachomatis* or other organisms.

Public Health Considerations

1. See the discussion of public health considerations in the overview of this chapter.

■ *CHLAMYDIAL INFECTION*

Definition

Chlamydial infection is caused by *C. trachomatis*.

Incidence and Socioeconomic Impact

1. It is the most prevalent STD known.
   a. This disease is responsible for the large numbers of men who present with nongonococcal urethritis and women who present with mucopurulent cervicitis.
   b. Chlamydial infection is the STD that has the highest incidence among adolescents.

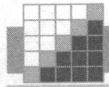

LEGAL AND ETHICAL CONSIDERATIONS

Teenagers often hesitate to get help for sexual problems because of concerns about confidentiality. Many young people fear their parents may have access to their medical records, and this concern is valid. It is a good idea to use abbreviations for the sexual health history. Codes are easy to devise and help to ensure confidentiality.

2. Although there has been a steady increase in the number of states mandating reporting of this disease, the exact number of cases is not known.
3. An estimated $1 billion is spent each year on chlamydial infection and its complications.

Etiology

1. *C. trachomatis* resembles a gram-negative bacterial pathogen and has RNA and DNA susceptibility to antibiotics.
2. Like a virus, it requires tissue culture for isolation.
3. *C. trachomatis* invades the same epithelial tissue as *N. gonorrhoeae*.

Pathophysiology

1. All chlamydiae share a common genus-specific antigen.
2. There are 2 stages in the life cycle of *C. trachomatis*
   a. Stage 1: In the infective stage, the elementary body attaches itself to a particular site on the cell and is capable of entering uninfected cells.
   b. Stage 2: The reticulate body multiplies by binary fission to produce the serotypes that are identified in the stained cells. Lysis occurs and release of a new elementary body begins the process again.
   c. The complete infectious cycle takes 2 to 3 days.
3. Currently there are 15 recognized serotypes of *C. trachomatis*.
4. Serotypes A, B, and C are associated with trachoma, a chronic conjunctivitis causing blindness.
5. Serotypes D through K are the oculogenital and sexually transmitted strains that cause inclusion conjunctivitis, newborn pneumonia, urethritis, cervicitis, epididymitis, salpingitis, acute urethra syndrome, and proctitis.
6. Serotypes L_1, and L_2, and L_3 cause lymphogranuloma venereum.

Clinical Manifestations

1. The incubation period for *C. trachomatis* infection is 6 to 14 days.
2. The longer the incubation period, the higher the rate of asymptomatic infection.
3. *C. trachomatis* is isolated in 72 percent of men found to have nongonococcal urethritis with the following symptoms:
   • Urinary frequency
   • Dysuria
   • Mucoid or mucopurulent discharge
   • Scrotal swelling
4. In women, chlamydial infection is usually asymptomatic. However, *C. trachomatis* is isolated in 90 percent of women found to have mucopurulent cervicitis with the following symptoms:
   • Yellow, mucopurulent vaginal discharge
   • Endocervicitis
   • Dysuria
   • Urinary frequency

Diagnostics

1. Refer to the earlier discussion of sexual health history and physical examination in this chapter.

2. Medical diagnosis is difficult and often missed because there are few or no symptoms.
3. A culture is obtained from the suspected site of infection (e.g., endocervix, urethra, rectum).
4. Two other types of tests for nonculture detection are the following:
   a. Direct fluorescent monoclonal antibody staining of chlamydial elementary bodies in smears obtained from specimens
   b. Enzyme-linked immunoassay for detection of chlamydial antigen in specimens
5. Presumptive medical diagnosis is made for men who have urethral discharge with greater than 4 polymorphonuclear leukocytes (PMNs) per high-power (oil immersion) field on microscopic examination of a smear.
6. Presumptive medical diagnosis can be made for women without mucopurulent discharge on the basis of the following criteria:
   a. Greater than 10 PMNs of a gram-stained specimen from the transitional zone of the cervix
   b. Friability of the cervix
   c. Erythema or edema of the cervix

Clinical Management

1. Goals of clinical management
   a. Treatment with a broad-spectrum antibiotic active against gram-positive cocci and *Escherichia coli*.
   b. Prevention of the spread of disease and further complications. If symptoms appeared within 30 days, treat regardless of culture results.
   c. Treat presumptively if person is being treated for gonorrhea.
2. Pharmacologic interventions
   a. The CDC recommends that chlamydial infection be treated with azithromycin and doxycycline.
   b. Nongonococcal urethritis and mucopurulent cervicitis are treated with doxycycline or erythromycin.
3. Special medical-surgical procedures. Obtain a good sample of epithelial cells (see Procedure 32–1).

Complications

1. Untreated chlamydial infection
   a. Men may experience the following:
      • Acute epididymitis
      • Prostatitis
      • Proctitis
      • Reiter's syndrome (an episode of arthritis associated with reactive urethritis in men or cervicitis in women)
      • Fitz-Hugh–Curtis syndrome (perihepatitis)
   b. Women may experience the following:
      • Bartholinitis
      • Salpingitis
      • Nonpuerpural endometritis
      • Reiter's syndrome
      • Fitz-Hugh–Curtis syndrome

• Pelvic inflammatory disease
• Infertility
• Spontaneous abortion or premature delivery during pregnancy

Prognosis

1. Disease is reversible and does not progress if individuals are screened and treated.
2. Cure is indicated by resolution of symptoms. If symptoms persist, retreatment is necessary.
3. In women, this disease can lead to long-term chronic PID and sterility if not treated.
4. In men, this disease can lead to sterility if not treated.

Applying the Nursing Process

See Applying the Nursing Process in the section on syphilis (pp. 1502–1503).

Discharge Planning and Teaching

1. See Learning/Teaching Guidelines for Self-Care in Sexually Transmitted Diseases and for Self-Administration of Antibiotics.
2. Take medication 1 to 2 hours after meals. Avoid iron, antacids, and dairy products.

Public Health Considerations

1. See the discussion of public health considerations in the overview of this chapter.

◼ *HERPES GENITALIS*

Definition

1. Herpes genitalis is a virus located in the genital area.
2. There are two types of herpes simplex virus (HSV).
   a. The first, HSV type 1 (HSV-1), generally causes lesions of the oral cavity, lips, and face, commonly called fever blisters or cold sores.
   b. The second, HSV type 2 (HSV-2), usually causes lesions in the perineal and rectal area.
   c. However, either type can cause lesions above or below the waist.
3. Approximately 15 percent of cases of primary genital herpes are caused by HSV type 1.

Incidence and Socioeconomic Impact

1. The HSV is endemic in the United States because approximately 1 to 2 percent of the population carry this virus.
2. Fifty to 80 percent of adults have antibodies to HSV type 1 or type 2.

Etiology

1. The HSV is a double-stranded DNA virus surrounded by a glycoprotein.
2. It forms 2 antigenically similar but distinct types.

Pathophysiology

1. Infection with HSV occurs by inoculation of mucous membranes or skin through close contact with an infected individual.
2. After infection occurs, the virus can become dormant, with HSV-1 residing in the trigeminal sensory nerve ganglia and HSV-2 residing in the dorsal sensory nerve ganglia.
3. Two hypotheses exist regarding recurrent episodes.
   a. In the "ganglion trigger" hypothesis, a stimulus affects the latent infected ganglion cells, producing viral replication. Flow of the virus down the peripheral nerve occurs.
   b. The "skin trigger" hypothesis posits that the virus is produced frequently by the ganglion, reaching the skin every few days. The body's immune defenses usually eliminate the virus. However, if local immunosuppression is present, there are enough viral products to cause a vesicular lesion.

Clinical Manifestations

1. The HSV may be either symptomatic or asymptomatic.
2. Primary genital herpes is considered the first episode, without circulating antibodies to HSV-1 or HSV-2.
3. The incubation period ranges from 2 to 20 days.
4. Localized genital symptoms include the following:
   - One or more painful lesions, which consist of vesicles progressing to ulcers
   - Edema
   - Secondary bacterial infection
   - Inguinal adenopathy
5. Systemic symptoms include the following:
   - Fever
   - Malaise
   - Headache
   - Nausea
6. Recurrent genital herpes
   a. The noticeable symptoms are local prodromal symptoms lasting about 2 days, including paresthesias, itching, and pain.
   b. Lesions appear in clusters, and vesicles rupture within 24 to 48 hours.
   c. Viral shedding lasts for about 4 to 5 days.
   d. Lesions are present for about 7 to 10 days.
7. Latency is the interval between clinical episodes.
8. Viral shedding can occur intermittently during this phase.

Diagnostics

1. Refer to the earlier discussion of sexual health history and physical examination in this chapter.

2. Perform a clinical examination of the oral, genital, and rectal areas for crops of vesicles and ulcers in various stages of progression.
3. Obtain a viral culture from the suspicious lesions, preferably within the first 4 days of the outbreak of disease.
4. Indirect immunoperoxidase and direct immunofluorescence tests may be useful.
5. Culture is still the standard method for medical diagnosis.

Clinical Management

1. Goals of clinical management
   a. Decrease the severity and duration of the lesions
   b. Provide supportive and symptomatic relief during outbreak
   c. Provide psychosocial support
2. Nonpharmacologic interventions
   a. Encourage frequent hand washing and bathing to avoid autoinoculation
   b. Increase fluid intake
   c. Decrease pain and discomfort
      (1) Using gloves, apply topical anesthetics to affected areas.
      (2) Apply heat or cold to lesions.
      (3) Encourage 3 to 4 warm baking soda sitz baths per day.
      (4) Spray water over genitalia while urinating to decrease burning.
      (5) Wear cotton underwear.
      (6) Discourage sexual activity during the prodromal phase and for approximately 10 days afterward when lesions are present.
      (7) Encourage condom use during all sexual contact.
3. Pharmacologic interventions
   a. Acyclovir is the drug of choice for both initial and recurrent attacks.
      (1) If there are more than 6 recurrent episodes per year, daily suppressive therapy with acyclovir is an option.
      (2) Severe HSV infection or its complications may necessitate hospitalization, and intravenous acyclovir administration.
   b. Vaccination for HSV is currently under study.
4. Special medical-surgical procedures: Viral culture with results in 48 to 72 hours

Complications

1. Increased possibility of spontaneous abortion
2. Transvaginal transmission to newborn
3. Greater risk of premature delivery
4. More severe and complicated course of HSV infection for those infected with HIV
5. Possible disseminated infection includes encephalitis, pneumonia, and hepatitis.

Prognosis

1. Infection with HSV is a chronic lifelong disease with recurrent episodes occurring at varying intervals.

Applying the Nursing Process

See Applying the Nursing Process in the section on syphilis (pp. 1502–1503).

Discharge Planning and Teaching

1. See Learning/Teaching Guidelines for Self-Care in Sexually Transmitted Diseases and for Self-Administration of Antibiotics.
2. See the previous discussion of nonpharmacologic interventions in the section on clinical management of this disease.

Public Health Considerations

1. See the discussion of public health considerations in the overview of this chapter.

◻ HUMAN PAPILLOMAVIRUS INFECTION (GENITAL WARTS)

Definition

1. Human papillomaviruses (HPVs) are members of the papovavirus family.
2. Approximately 60 types of HPV have been identified, and new ones are found each year.
3. Types of HPV vary as to both site of infection and biologic behavior.
4. Recurrence is a result of reactivation of a subclinical infection rather than reinfection from a partner.

Incidence and Socioeconomic Impact

Infection with HPV is the 2nd most common sexually transmitted viral infection.

Etiology

1. Genital warts have been associated with HPV types 6, 11, 16, 18, 31, 33, 35, and 39.
2. External genital warts and mild cervical intraepithelial neoplasia (CIN) have been associated with HPV types 6 and 11.
3. The HPV types 16, 18, 31, 33, and 35 are most frequently associated with severe CIN and premalignant and malignant lesions of the lower genital tract in both sexes.

Pathophysiology

1. This highly contagious virus is composed of double-stranded DNA. It infects the epithelial cells. DNA replication allows the infection to persist in a resting phase.
2. The transformation zone of the cervix is vulnerable to viral infections and neoplastic changes (Fig. 32–3).
3. Papillomavirus DNA can be found in adenocarcinoma, adenosquamous carcinoma, and squamous carcinoma of the cervix.

Clinical Manifestations

1. Genital warts can occur in the urogenital and anorectal regions.
2. The warts are pedunculated or broad based, pink to grey, soft, and fleshy and occur singularly or in clusters.
3. The exophytic lesions vary in size from pinhead to cauliflower and are often friable but without accompanying symptoms.
4. The endophytic lesions are generally seen on the cervix; however, they can also be found on the vulva, anus, and penis.

Diagnostics

1. Assessment is done by inspection of the anogenital region because the external warts are characteristic and easily identifiable.
2. Medical diagnosis of external warts is made on appearance alone.
3. If external warts are of questionable origin, the following diagnostic procedure can be done:
   a. Five percent acetic acid can be applied to the cervix, vulva, vagina, penis, scrotum, or anus.
   b. Lesions will whiten after 3 to 5 minutes, and examination can be made with a colposcope.
   c. Warts will be shiny white with irregular borders and accompanying satellite lesions.
4. If lesions are atypical, biopsy provides the definitive medical diagnosis.
5. Subclinical infection on and around the cervix can be made by a Papanicolaou (Pap) smear.
6. Differential medical diagnosis includes the following:
   • Cervical dysplasia
   • Squamous cell carcinoma

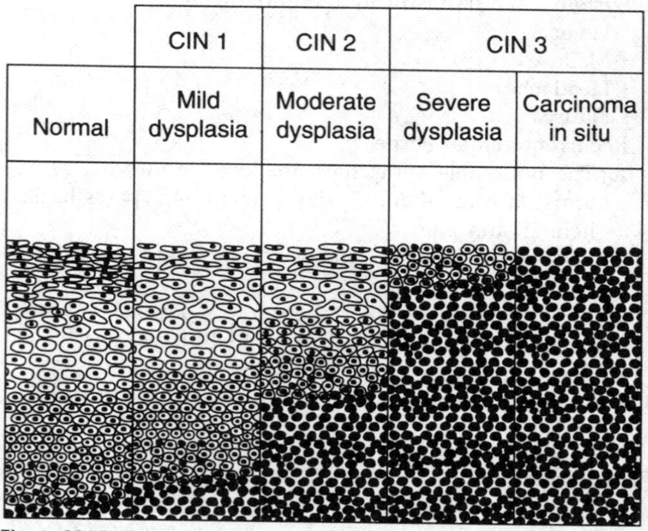

Normal	CIN 1	CIN 2	CIN 3	
	Mild dysplasia	Moderate dysplasia	Severe dysplasia	Carcinoma in situ

Figure 32–3. Schematic representation of CIN. (Reprinted with permission from Nolte S, and Hanjani P. Intraepithelial neoplasia of the lower genital tract. *Semin Oncol Nurs* 6[3], 181–189, 1990.)

- Secondary syphilis
- Benign neoplasia
- Hemorrhoids

Clinical Management

1. Goals of clinical management
   a. Remove the exophytic warts
   b. Control signs and symptoms of the disease
   c. Treatment is guided by the following factors:
      (1) Preference of the individual
      (2) Anatomic site and size
      (3) Number of warts present
      (4) Potential side effects
2. Pharmacologic interventions. The CDC recommends the following:
   a. For external genital or perianal warts:
      (1) Podofilox (Condylox) 0.5 percent solution. Apply with cotton swab to warts twice a day for 3 days. No application for 4 days. Repeat the cycle for 4 cycles. Contraindicated during pregnancy.
      (2) Podophyllin 10 to 25 percent in compound tincture of benzoin. Apply weekly; wash off 3 to 5 hours after application. May use up to 6 applications. If warts persist, other measures should be used. Contraindicated during pregnancy.
      (3) Trichloroacetic acid (TCA) 80 to 90 percent. Apply only to wart; powder with baking soda to remove unreacted acid. Repeat treatment weekly up to 6 applications. If warts persist, other measures should be used.
      (4) Cryotherapy with liquid nitrogen or cryoprobe.
   b. Treatment for the following locations:
      (1) Vagina: TCA, podophyllin, and cryotherapy with liquid nitrogen
      (2) Urethral meatus: podophyllin and cryotherapy with liquid nitrogen
      (3) Anal region: TCA, cryotherapy with liquid nitrogen, and surgical removal
      (4) Oral cavity: cryotherapy with liquid nitrogen and surgical removal
3. Special medical-surgical procedures. Patients with cervical and rectal mucosal warts should be referred to a specialist for surgical evaluation.

Complications

1. Strong association of HPV types, 16, 18, 31, 33, and 35 with cervical, vulvar, anal, and penile cancers.
2. Obstruction of the urethra, causing painful and difficult urination.
3. Decreased elasticity of the vagina, causing obstruction and bleeding during a vaginal delivery.
4. Laryngeal papillamatosis in children can be transmitted in utero and during delivery.

Prognosis

1. There is no curative treatment for HPV infection; it is a chronic lifelong disease.

2. Left untreated, genital warts have been known to resolve on their own, remain unchanged, or grow.

Applying the Nursing Process

1. See the section on Applying the Nursing Process under syphilis (pp. 1502–1503).

Discharge Planning and Teaching

1. Self-application of medication to warts
   a. Patient must be able to see and reach wart easily.
   b. Inform the patient who is using podophyllin that lesions may be painful for several days.
   c. The area around the wart should be coated with petroleum jelly.
   d. The patient should not leave the health care facility without demonstrating ability to apply medication.
2. Avoid sexual intercourse until treatment is completed because warts are highly contagious.
3. Follow-up should continue if warts persist, and an annual Pap smear is recommended even after warts have resolved.
4. See Learning/Teaching Guidelines for Self-Care in Sexually Transmitted Diseases.

Public Health Considerations

1. See the discussion of public health considerations in the overview of this chapter.

◼ *VULVOVAGINITIS*

Definition

1. Vulvovaginitis is an inflammation and infection of the vulva and vagina characterized by discharge, irritation, and itching.
2. Three types of infectious vulvovaginitis are bacterial vaginosis, trichomoniasis, and candidiasis (Table 32–4).

Incidence and Socioeconomic Impact

The most prevalent nonviral STD is trichomoniasis.

Classification

1. Bacterial vaginosis
   a. Definition
      (1) Bacterial vaginosis is a bacteria-caused infection of the vagina.
      (2) Bacterial vaginosis does not fall into a particular microbiologic category.
      (3) In the majority of cases, the organism identified is *Gardnerella vaginalis*, but others, such as *Mycoplasma hominis*, have been identified also.

Table 32–4. Characteristics of the Common Vaginal Infections

	Bacterial Vaginosis	Trichomoniasis	Vaginal Candidiasis
Etiology	*Gardnerella vaginalis* but may be unclear	*Trichomonas vaginalis*	*Candida albicans*
Vaginal discharge	Mildly increased, malodorous	Much increased, yellow	Increased with white curds
Other signs and symptoms	No erythema or pruritus	Vaginal erythema, vulvar pruritus	Vaginal erythema, vulvar pruritus
Microscopic findings	Clue cells, mixed flora	Trichomonads on wet prep white cells	White cells, yeast on KOH prep
Other findings	Fishy odor with KOH, pH > 4.5	Vaginal pH > 4.5	Vaginal pH > 4.7
Treatment of choice	Metronidazole	Metronidazole	Intravaginal clotrimazole
Treatment of partner	No, but examine for STDs	Yes, use same medication	Usually not; examine for STDs

b. Etiology
  (1) Bacterial vaginosis is characterized by a decrease in H_2O_2-producing aerobic lactobacilli and an increase in anaerobic lactobacilli.
  (2) Clue cells, free-floating bacteria, and absence of leukocytes are suggestive of bacterial vaginosis.
c. Pathophysiology
  (1) Bacterial vaginosis is caused by more than 1 bacterium.
  (2) The triggers for change in the vaginal flora have not been identified.
  (3) *G. vaginalis* ferments glycogen and produces substances that are metabolized by anaerobes, which release the malodorous amines that cause the distinctive fishy odor.
d. Clinical manifestations
  (1) Bacterial vaginosis can be detected in both symptomatic and asymptomatic women.
  (2) Symptoms include white vaginal discharge, fishy odor, and simultaneous urinary tract infection.
e. Complications
  (1) Upper genital tract infection (e.g., endometritis and salpingitis)
  (2) Pelvic inflammatory disease
  (3) Vaginal cuff cellulitis following invasive procedures, such as intrauterine device (IUD) placement, uterine curettage, hysterectomy, and cesarean section
  (4) Adverse outcomes of pregnancy including premature births and low–birth-weight infant
f. Diagnostics: Clinical medical diagnosis can be made if 3 of the following 4 symptoms are present:
  (1) White, uniformly distributed, and noninflammatory discharge from the vagina
  (2) Vaginal fluid with a pH of greater than 4.5
  (3) Vaginal discharge with a fishy odor or positive "whiff test" when 10 percent KOH is added
  (4) Presence of clue cells on microscopic examination
g. Clinical management
  (1) Pharmacologic interventions
    (a) Metronidazole is the mainstay of treatment.
    (b) Clindamycin is preferred by some physicians, especially for patients who are allergic to metronidazole and during the 1st trimester of pregnancy, when metronidazole is contraindicated.

 DRUG ADVISORY

Alcohol must be avoided while taking metronidazole and for 24 hours after treatment is completed. Otherwise, an Antabuse-like reaction can occur.

2. Trichomoniasis
  a. Definition
    (1) Trichomoniasis is primarily an infection of the urogenital tract.
    (2) Primary sites for infection are the urethra and prostate in men and the vagina in women. Up to 50 percent of males and females are asymptomatic.
  b. Etiology: Trichomoniasis is caused by *Trichomonas vaginalis*, an ovoid, flagellated, and motile anaerobic protozoan.
  c. Pathophysiology
    (1) The protozoan cytoplasm is rich in glycogen granules and ribosomes, which support optimal growth and reproduction under anaerobic conditions.
    (2) The organism engulfs and digests bacteria that assist with nutritional requirements. It then attaches to mucous membranes via a specific adhesion process, and produces phospholipases, which damage mucosal cells and fetal membranes.
    (3) Asymptomatic and symptomatic infections can persist for prolonged periods.
  d. Clinical manifestations
    (1) Symptoms appear within 4 to 25 days
    (2) In men symptoms include thin whitish discharge and painful and difficult urination.
    (3) In women symptoms include pruritus and inflammation of the labia, vulva, vaginal walls, and cervix; vaginal pH greater than 4.5; dyspareunia; painful urination; vaginal discharge with a mucopurulent foul odor; and small cervical and vaginal hemorrhages, commonly called "strawberry cervix."
  e. Complications
    (1) Adverse pregnancy outcomes such as preterm labor and premature rupture of membranes. Upper reproductive tract infections may occur after gynecologic surgical procedures.

f. Diagnostics
  (1) Medical diagnosis is made by microscopic "wet prep" evaluation in which a sample of vaginal fluid is placed in normal saline and viewed under the microscope for motile trichomonads and smaller white blood cells.
  (2) Pap smear
  (3) Culture with Diamond's media culture
g. Clinical management
  (1) Pharmacologic interventions: Metronidazole is currently the only effective drug. Treatment should include all sexual contacts, should continue through the woman's menstrual bleeding, and should be avoided during the 1st trimester of pregnancy.
3. Vulvovaginal candidiasis
  a. Definition
    (1) Candidiasis is an infection caused by a fungus of the genus *Candida*. Candidiasis may be present concurrently with other STDs.
    (2) Symptoms are caused by alteration of the vaginal environment rather than by sexually acquired or transmitted lesions.

NURSE ADVISORY

Recurrent and unresolved symptoms of candidiasis may be due to co-existing STDs or other medical conditions. Use of over-the-counter medications for vulvovaginitis may delay treatment of other STDs.

  b. Etiology: An overgrowth of *Candida* (usually *C. albicans*) colonizes the vaginal mucosa and adheres to the vaginal epithelial cells, causing an inflammatory response. The pH remains low.
  c. Pathophysiology: There are many different types of yeast, but *Candida* species are the most common.
  d. Clinical manifestations
    (1) In women, symptoms include vulvar pruritus and burning; vaginal soreness and irritation; vaginal discharge that is frequently minimal but varies from watery to homogeneously thick; entry dyspareunia; external dysuria; erythema and swelling of the labia, vulva, and vagina.
    (2) In male partners of women with vaginal candidiasis, symptoms include transient rash, erythema, and pruritus occurring minutes or hours after unprotected sex.
    (3) Risk factors for vaginal candidiasis include diabetes mellitus; corticosteroid therapy; pregnancy; antimicrobial therapy; estrogen therapy; use of diaphragm, IUD, sponge, and nonoxynol-9 for birth control; HIV infection; and tight-fitting synthetic undergarments.
    (4) Recurrent vulvovaginal candidiasis is defined as 3 or more episodes of symptomatic vulvovaginal candidiasis per year. The pathophysiology of recurrent vulvovaginal candidiasis is poorly understood. Management involves continuing treatment between episodes.

ELDER ADVISORY

Sexually active postmenopausal women can have the same risk factors for STDs as younger women (e.g., multiple sexual partners, new sexual partner, or a recent history of STDs). Older women should undergo the same routine diagnostic procedures (e.g., vaginal pH, wet mount, and KOH) and treatment regimens as younger women. Careful history taking, physical examination, and laboratory testing can rule out STDs.

  e. Diagnostics
    (1) Medical diagnosis is made when the vaginal pH is greater than 4.7, indicating bacterial vaginosis, trichomoniasis, or a mixed infection. (The normal pH is 4.0 to 4.5.)
    (2) Wet prep identifies yeast and mycelia and excludes the presence of clue cells and trichomonads.
    (3) Potassium hydroxide improves the visualization of yeast and mycelia.
    (4) Vaginal culture is done if microscopic results are negative.
  f. Clinical management
    (1) Pharmacologic interventions
      • Over-the-counter preparations include miconazole and clotrimazole.
      • Prescription preparations include butoconazole, teranazole, and terconazole.

 DRUG ADVISORY

Miconazole can cause vulvar burning. Self-medication with miconazole or clotrimazole should be adivsed only for those women who have been seen by a physician. The Centers for Disease Control and Prevention recommend that any woman whose symptoms persist after using an over-the-counter preparation or who experiences a recurrence of symptoms within two months should seek medical care.

    (2) Treatment of sex partners has not been demonstrated to reduce the frequency of recurrent vulvovaginal candidiasis.

Applying the Nursing Process

1. See Applying the Nursing Process under syphilis (pp. 1502–1503).

Discharge Planning and Teaching

1. See Discharge Planning and Teaching under Herpes Genitalis
2. See Learning/Teaching Guidelines for Self-Care in Sexually Transmitted Diseases

■ *HEPATITIS B VIRUS INFECTION*

Definition

1. Infection with hepatitis B virus (HBV) is referred to as serum hepatitis or long-incubation hepatitis. Viral hepatitis is a systemic infection that affects the liver.

Incidence and Socioeconomic Impact

1. More than 1.5 million people carry HBV in their blood, 6 to 10 percent of whom become chronic HBV carriers.
2. The HBV accounts for 5000 deaths from cirrhosis of the liver and hepatocellular cancer per year.

Risk Factors

1. Sex with infected person
2. Intravenous drug use
3. Occupational exposure (health care workers)
4. Hemodialysis
5. For infants, maternal HBV
6. Residence in developing country

Etiology

1. The HBV is transmitted through contact with body fluids containing the virus, such as blood, saliva, semen, or cervicovaginal secretions.
2. The corresponding antibody is hepatitis B surface antibody (anti-HBs).

Pathophysiology

1. A DNA virus is enveloped by surface antigen HBsAG.
2. Large amounts of HBV are produced and synthesized by the liver and then allowed to circulate freely.

Clinical Manifestations

1. Characterized by acute and insidious onset
2. The infection progresses through the incubation, preicteric, icteric, and convalescent phases.
   a. Incubation phase lasts 30 to 180 days.
   b. Preicteric phase usually lasts 3 to 10 days. Although many people remain asymptomatic up to this point, others will have some or all of the following symptoms:
   - Mild fever
   - Headache
   - Muscle aches
   - Fatigue
   - Loss of appetite
   - Nausea and vomiting
   - Diarrhea

   c. Icteric phase lasts 1 to 3 weeks and symptoms include the following:
   - Dark foaming urine
   - Pale feces
   - Abdominal pain
   - Jaundice
   d. Convalescence occurs after 3 weeks and may last up to 6 months. This period consists of resolution of symptoms.
3. Symptoms of fulminant viral hepatitis include the following:
   - Lethargy
   - Somnolence
   - Personality changes
   - Agitated behavior

Diagnostics

1. A full discussion can be found in Chapter 28.
2. The presence of HBsAg can be determined in the incubation and preicteric phases of the disease. If found 6 months after infection, HBsAg indicates development of chronic hepatitis or symptomatic carrier status.
3. Laboratory tests include
   a. Radioimmunoassay for HBsAG, HBcAg, anti-HBc, HBeAg, and anti-HBe
   b. Liver function tests, including prothrombin time (PT), international normalized ratio (INR), and assays for albumin, aspartate transferase (AST), and alanine transferase (ALT)

Clinical Management

1. Goals of clinical management
   a. Prevention, screening, and detection
   b. Universal vaccination

NURSE ADVISORY

A person known to be at high risk for acquiring hepatitis B virus (HBV) (e.g., persons with multiple sex partners or more than one sex partner in the preceding 6 months, sex partners of HBV carriers, intravenous drug users, homosexual and bisexual men) should be offered vaccination unless they are immune to HBV as a result of past infection or vaccination.

Adapted from Recommendations of the Advisory Committee on Immunization Practice (ACIP), Centers for Disease Control and Prevention.

2. Pharmacologic interventions
   a. Health care and laboratory workers are required to be vaccinated with 3 doses starting at 0-, 1- and 6-month intervals.
   b. The CDC recommends that infants be vaccinated at the same dosing intervals.
   c. Persons exposed to HBV through sexual contact should receive postexposure prophylaxis, followed by the standard three-dose immunization series.
3. Special medical-surgical procedures: see Chapter 28.

Complications

1. These range in severity and include the following:
   a. Acute hepatitis (life-threatening)
   b. Cirrhosis of the liver
   c. Hepatocellular carcinoma
   d. Immune system disorders

Prognosis

1. Hepatitis B is a life-long disease.
   a. Six to 10 percent of infected adults become carriers.
   b. Chronic hepatitis develops in 50 percent of carriers.

Applying the Nursing Process

See Chapter 28.

HOW TO USE A CONDOM

Because condoms protect against STDs, they should be used whenever you have sex. For added safety, a spermicide jelly containing nonoxynol 9 should also be used. Inspect the package for damage. Make sure the condom is not discolored or brittle.

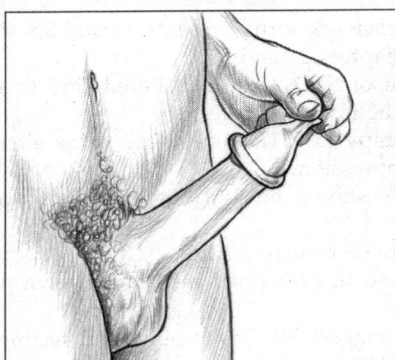

To use a condom, place the rolled-up condom over the tip of the penis.

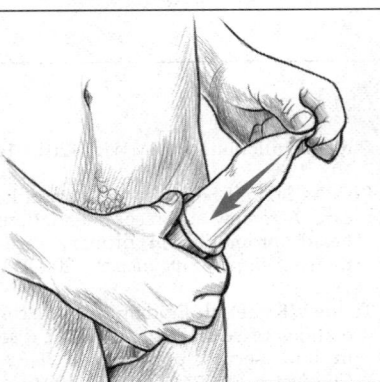

Hold the end of the condom to allow a little extra space at the tip, then unroll the condom over the penis.

Right after ejaculation, grasp the condom around the base of the penis before it is withdrawn.
The condom should be thrown away; never reuse condoms.
Wash hands and genitals.
Keep condoms in a cool, dry place out of direct sunlight.

Figure 32–4.

Discharge Planning and Teaching

1. Promote HBV vaccination.
2. Encourage sexually active persons to use condoms (Fig. 32–4) and to maintain a monogomous sexual relationship.
3. Warn against use of nonsterile drug injection equipment.
4. Discourage sharing of items that could infect others such as razors or toothbrushes.

Public Health Considerations

1. See the discussion of public health considerations in the overview of this chapter.
2. Universal vaccination as described by the Immunization Practices Advisory Committee of the Public Health Service and the American Academy of Pediatrics Committee on Infectious Diseases.
3. Pregnancy is not a contraindication to HBV vaccine administration; in fact, it is now considered part of routine prenatal care.

◙ *OTHER SEXUALLY TRANSMITTED DISEASES*

Chancroid

1. Incidence and etiology
   a. *Haemophilus ducreyi* is the causative organism.
   b. Ulcer appears 2 to 14 days after infection.
2. Clinical manifestations
   a. Painful genital ulcer and regional lymphadenopathy
   b. Bubo may develop after initial lesion, which ruptures and forms a large inguinal ulcer.
3. Diagnostics: Medical diagnosis is based on Gram-stained smears, culture, and lesion characteristics.
4. Clinical management
   a. Infected person and all infected sexual contacts require treatment.
   b. Azithromycin is the drug of choice for chancroid.
   c. Alternatives
      (1) Amoxicillin, plus clavulanic acid
      (2) Ciprofloxacin. This drug is contraindicated in pregnant and lactating women and children under 17 years of age.
   d. Follow-up to examine ulcers weekly until gone.

Lymphogranuloma Venereum

1. Incidence and etiology
   a. L_1, L_2, L_3 serotypes of *C. trachomatis* obtained through tissue culture isolation
   b. Ulcer appears 3 to 21 days after infection.
2. Clinical manifestations
   a. Primary state: Painless papule or vesicle appears in the anogenital area; lesion ulcerates, then heals within 3 to 5 days.

b. Secondary stage: Inguinal lymphadenopathy develops after 1 to 4 weeks. Fever, malaise, headache, myalgias may be present.
c. Tertiary stage: Fistula formation and scarring are seen.
3. Diagnostics: Medical diagnosis is based on clinical presentation and tissue culture isolation of *C. trachomatis.*
4. Clinical management
a. Pharmacologic therapy is with doxycycline, erythromycin, or sulfasoxazole. Erythromycin can be taken by pregnant and lactating women.

Pediculosis Pubis

1. Incidence and etiology
a. Causative agent is the crab louse, *Phthirus pubis.*
b. The incubation period is 30 days.
c. Infestation is caused by close sexual contact or contaminated bedding or clothing.
2. Clinical manifestations
a. Groin irritation pruritis secondary to bites
b. Louse found in the pubic, perineal, and perianal regions
3. Diagnostics: Crab louse can be seen with a magnifying glass.
4. Clinical management
a. The infected person, all sexual contacts within the last 30 days, and family members are treated.
b. Lindane 1% shampoo or permethrin 1% cream rinse as prescribed. Use a fine-tooth comb to remove nits from the hair shafts.
c. Bedding and clothing must be washed and dried using the heat cycle. Re-treat in 7 days if symptoms persist.
d. Pregnant and lactating women may use permethrin cream. Oral antihistamines may be indicated for itching.

Scabies

1. Incidence and etiology
a. An insect, *Sarcoptes scabiei,* is the cause.

b. Clinical infection occurs 4 to 6 weeks following contact.
2. Clinical manifestations
a. Nocturnal pruritus
b. Papular erythematous rash on the genitals, buttocks, wrists, elbows, ankles, feet, and skin folds
3. Diagnostics
a. Medical diagnosis is based on presenting symptoms alone.
b. Confirmation can be obtained through microscopic identification of the mite, eggs, or fecal pellets from the burrows.
4. Clinical management
a. Topical therapy involves one of the following: Permethrin, lindane, or crotamiton. Permethrin is the preferred treatment for pregnant and lactating women and infants.
b. Oral antihistamines may be indicated for itching.
c. Bedding and clothing must be washed and dried using the heat cycle. Re-treat in 7 days if symptoms persist.

◼ *HUMAN IMMUNODEFICIENCY VIRUS*

1. Human immunodeficiency virus presents a complex clinical picture. See Chapters 21 and 37.
2. The natural course of STDs may be altered due to the effects of HIV on the immune system.
3. Pharmacologic therapy for STDs may need to be altered due to immunosuppression.
4. A diagnosis of HIV should be considered in the following situations:
a. Unusually severe or recurrent STD
b. Failure to respond to prescribed medication for a particular STD
5. It is important to suggest HIV counseling and testing if there are multiple STD risk factors.

Bibliography

Books

Sweet RL, and Gibbs RS. *Infectious Diseases of the Female Genital Tract.* 2nd ed. Baltimore: Williams & Wilkins, 1990.
U.S. Department of Health and Human Services. *Healthy People 2000: National Health Promotion and Disease Prevention Objectives.* DHHS Publication No. (PHS) 91-50213, 1990.
U.S. Department of Health and Human Services. *Resource List for Informational Materials on Sexually Transmitted Diseases (STDs) and HIV/AIDS.* Publication No. (PHS) 734-643, 1992.
U.S. Preventive Services Task Force. *Guide to Clinical Preventive Services.* Baltimore: Williams & Wilkins, 1989.

Chapters in Books and Journal Articles

Overview of Sexually Transmitted Diseases

Adimora AA. Vaccines for classic sexually transmitted diseases. *Infect Dis Clin North Am* 8(4):859–876, 1994.
Alexander LL. Sexually transmitted diseases: Perspectives on this growing epidemic. *Nurse Practitioner* 17(10):31–42, 1992.
Nettina SL, and Kauffman FH. Diagnosis and management of sexually transmitted genital lesions. *Nurse Practitioner* 15(1):20–39, 1990.
1993 Sexually transmitted diseases treatment guidelines. *MMWR* 42(RR-14):1–102, 1993.
Roberts SJ, and Sorensen L. Lesbian health care: A review and recommendations for health promotion in primary care settings. *Nurse Practitioner* 20(6):42–47, 1995.
Toomey KE, et al. Epidemiological considerations of sexually transmitted diseases in underserved populations. *Infect Dis Clin North Am* 7(4):739–752, 1993.

Syphilis

Buckley HB. Syphilis: A review and update of this new infection of the '90s. *Nurse Practitioner* 17(8):25–32, 1992.

Larson SA, et al. Laboratory diagnosis and interpretation of tests for syphilis. *Clin Microbiol Rev* 8(1):1–21, 1995.

Sharts-Engel NC. Syphilis in pregnancy: Centers for disease control guidelines. *Matern Child Nurs J* 15(6):355, 1990.

Tillman J. Syphilis: An old disease, a contemporary perinatal problem. *JOGNN* 21(3):209–213, 1992.

Webster LA, Bergman SM, and Greenspan JR. Surveillance for gonorrhea and primary and secondary syphilis among adolescents, United States—1981–1991. *MMWR* 42(SS-3):1–11, 1993.

Webster LA, and Rolfs RT. Surveillance for primary and secondary syphilis, United States—1991. *MMWR* 42(SS-3):13–19, 1993.

Gonorrhea

Rice RJ, et al. Sociodemographic distribution of gonorrhea incidence: Implications for prevention and behavioral research. *Am J Public Health* 81(10):1252–1257, 1991.

Webster LA, Bergman SM, and Greenspan JR. Surveillance for gonorrhea and primary and secondary syphilis among adolescents, United States—1981–1991. *MMWR* 42(SS-3):1–11, 1993.

Zenilman JM. Gonorrhea: Clinical and public health issues. *Hosp Pract* 28(2A):29–50, 1993.

Zimmerman HL, et al. Epidemiologic differences between chlamydia and gonorrhea. *Am J Public Health* 80(11):1338–1342, 1990.

Chlamydial Infection

Keat A. Sexually transmitted arthritis syndromes. *Med Clin North Am* 74(6):1617–1631, 1990.

Stein AP. The chlamydia epidemic: Teenagers at risk. *Med Aspects Hum Sex* 25(2):26–33, 1991.

Webster LA, et al. An evaluation of surveillance for *Chlamydia trachomatis* infections in the United States, 1987–1991. *MMWR* 42(SS-3):21–40, 1993.

Zimmerman HL, et al. Epidemiologic differences between chlamydia and gonorrhea. *Am J Public Health* 80(11):1338–1342, 1990.

Herpes Genitalis

Apuzzio JJ, and Leo MV. Herpes in the pregnant woman. *Med Aspects Hum Sex* 25(6):54–58, 1991.

Davies K. Genital herpes: An overview. *JOGNN* 19(5):401–406, 1990.

Gurevich I. Counseling the patient with herpes. *RN* 53(2):22–28, 1990.

Holley HP, and Fowler SL. Update on herpes simplex infections. *Hosp Med* 29(5):28–46, 1993.

Human Papillomavirus Infection (Genital Warts)

Bergman A. HPV infection in men: Severing the link to cervical cancer. *Med Aspects Hum Sex* 25(12):20–26, 1991.

Carlson JW, Hill PS, and Robertson AW. Evaluation and treatment of human papillomavirus infection in men. *Med Aspects Hum Sex* 24(8):58–62, 1990.

Cohen PR. A quick diagnostic guide to genital warts in men. *Med Aspects Hum Sex* 25(6):40–41, 1991.

Lilley LL, and Schaffer S. Human papillomavirus: A sexually transmitted disease with carcinogenic potential. *Cancer Nurs* 13(6):366–372, 1990.

Tinkle MB. Genital human papillomavirus infection: A growing health risk. *JOGNN* 19(6):501–507, 1990.

Vulvovaginitis

Andrist LC, and Maillet A. Vulvovaginal conditions: Social, psychological, and sexual considerations. *Nurse Practitioner* 3(3):181–184, 1992.

Biswas MK. Bacterial vaginosis. *Clin Obstet Gynecol* 36(1):166–176, 1993.

Carcio HA, and Clarke-Secor RM. Vulvovaginal candidiasis: A current update. *Nurse Practitioner Forum* 3(3):135–144, 1992.

Heine P, and McGregor JA. *Trichomonas vaginalis:* A reemerging pathogen. *Clin Obstet Gynecol* 36(1):137–143, 1993.

Kent HL. Epidemiology of vaginitis. *Am J Obstet Gynecol* 165:1168–1176, 1991.

Peters NC. Vulvovaginitis in the postmenopausal woman. *Nurse Practitioner Forum* 3(3):152–154, 1992.

A rapid test for vaginosis. *Emerg Med Clin North Am* 25(5):109, 1993.

Sobel JD. Candidal vulvovaginitis. *Clin Obstet Gynecol* 36(1):153–165, 1993.

Hepatitis B Virus Infection

Heeg JM, and Coleman DA. Hepatitis kills. *RN* 55(4):60–68, 1992.

Margolis HS. Prevention of acute and chronic liver disease through immunization: Hepatitis B and beyond. *J Infect Dis* 168:9–14, 1993.

McClennen-Reece S. Immunization strategies for the elimination of hepatitis B. *Nurse Practitioner* 18(2):42–50, 1993.

Schiff ER. Viral hepatitis today. *Emer Med* 24(15):115–132, 1992.

Other Sexually Transmitted Diseases

Chirgwin K, et al. HIV infection, genital ulcer disease, and crack cocaine use among patients attending a clinic for sexually transmitted diseases. *Am J Public Health* 81(12):1576–1579, 1991.

Agencies and Resources

American Social Health Association
P. O. Box 13827
Research Triangle Park, NC 27709
(800) 227–8922 (National STD Hotline)
(800) 342–AIDS (National AIDS Hotline)

Centers for Disease Control and Prevention
National Center for Prevention Services (NCPS)
Information Services Office
1600 Clifton Road
Atlanta, GA 30333
(404) 639–3534

U.S. Department of Health and Human Services
Public Health Services and National Institute of Allergy and Infectious Diseases
Bethesda, MD 20892
(301) 496–4000

State Health Departments
STD Control Program
(Usually located in capital city of each state)

33

Caring for People with Breast Disorders

☐ BREAST STRUCTURE AND FUNCTION

Structure of the Breast

1. The breast consists of glandular, fibrous, and fatty tissue (Fig. 33–1).
   a. Glandular tissue is divided into 12 to 20 lobes.
      (1) Each lobe is divided into smaller lobules, each of which is composed of 10 to 100 acini (milk-producing glands).
      (2) Lobes empty into a system of collecting ducts, which join to form a single terminal collecting duct.
      (3) Each terminal duct exits on the nipple surface.
      (4) The largest amount of glandular tissue is located in the upper, outer quadrant of the breast.
   b. Fibrous tissue supports the glandular tissue.
      (1) Fibrous tissue is a layer of connective tissue under the skin that supports the breast.
      (2) Cooper's ligaments are fibrous bands that attach subcutaneous tissue to deep muscle fascia. They loosely connect the breast to the chest wall. Fat surrounds glandular tissue.
2. Lymphatic drainage is directed primarily toward the axilla (see Fig. 33–1).
   a. Pectoral nodes are located inside the anterior axillary fold.
   b. Subscapular nodes are located along the lateral border of the scapula.
   c. Lateral nodes are located along the upper humerus.
   d. Other lymphatic drainage goes to the subclavian, internal mammary, and subdiaphragmatic lymph nodes.
3. Breasts lie between the 2nd and 6th ribs, between the sternum and the midaxillary line.
4. Variation in size is common between sides.
5. Nervous innervation is provided by the 3rd and 4th branches of the cervical plexus to the upper breast, and by the thoracic intercostal nerves to the lower breast.
6. The major blood supply comes from the internal mammary artery.

Functions of the Breast

1. Lactation is a primary function of the breast.
   a. Hormonal changes during pregnancy cause proliferation of ducts and maturation of glandular tissue.
   b. Estrogen, progesterone, prolactin, and oxytocin interact to control lactation.
   c. In the 2nd trimester of pregnancy, acini produce colostrum, a thin yellowish fluid.
   d. Milk is produced 3 to 4 days after delivery.
2. Breasts are a source of sexual stimulation and may play an important role in sexual activity.
3. Large breast size as a source of sex appeal has been emphasized by the media.

☐ BREAST ASSESSMENT

Common Breast Symptoms

1. Tenderness, fullness, and nodularity (generalized lumpiness) are usually bilateral and in corresponding locations. Cyclic symptoms often occur 3 to 5 days before menstruation and resolve after menses.
2. Nipple inversion is normal if it is bilateral and present since puberty.

Symptoms of Possible Breast Problems

1. A breast mass may occur, with 50 percent located in the upper outer quadrant.
   a. Assess for number, size, shape, mobility, definition, consistency, and associated skin changes or adenopathy.
   b. Characteristics of malignant masses may include rough, irregular border; hard consistency; and fixation to the underlying tissue.
   c. Characteristics of benign masses may include smoothness, mobility, hard consistency, and a cystic quality.

NURSE ADVISORY

Any new breast lump or thickening needs full evaluation. Delayed or missed breast cancer diagnosis is the 2nd most common category of malpractice cases.

2. Skin dimpling or inflammation may result from lymphatic blockage by the breast cancer. Dimpling manifests

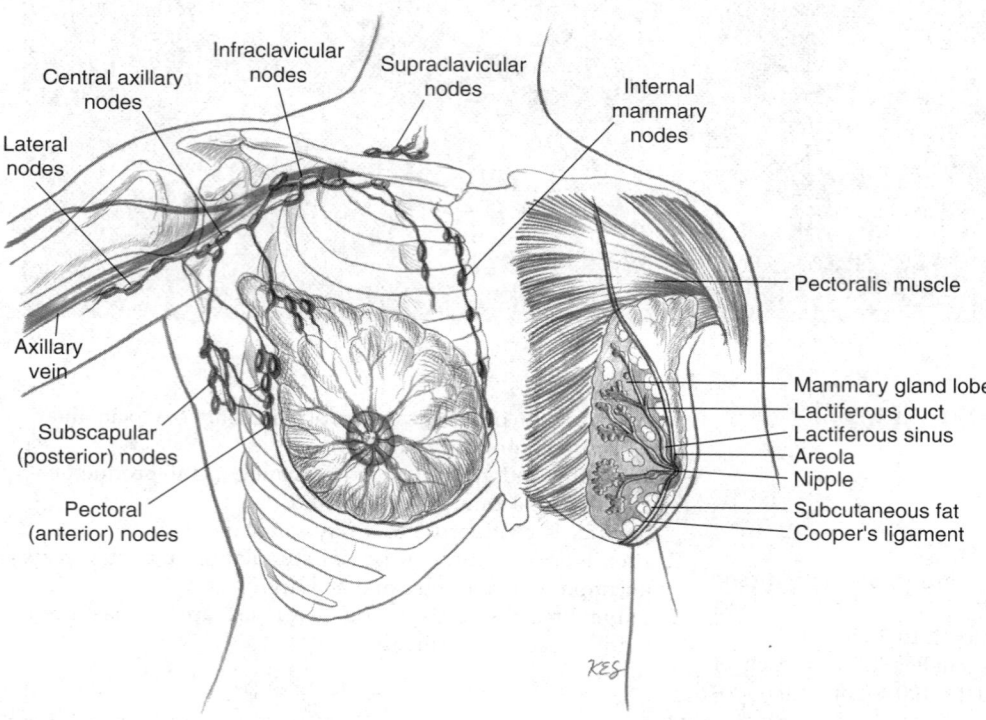

Figure 33–1. Structure and lymphatic drainage of the breast.

Labels (left): Central axillary nodes · Infraclavicular nodes · Supraclavicular nodes · Internal mammary nodes · Lateral nodes · Axillary vein · Subscapular (posterior) nodes · Pectoral (anterior) nodes

Labels (right): Pectoralis muscle · Mammary gland lobe · Lactiferous duct · Lactiferous sinus · Areola · Nipple · Subcutaneous fat · Cooper's ligament

as thickened, dimpled appearance of the skin termed "pig skin" or "peau d'orange" (orange peel–like skin).

3. Ulceration can occur from the growth of tumor through the skin.

4. Unilateral nipple inversion, deviation, edema, redness, erosion, and ulceration may be signs of underlying malignancy.

5. Nipple discharge may be seen, which is usually normal if it is present over many years and is bilateral.
   a. Certain medications, such as major tranquilizers, and elevated serum prolactin levels can cause bilateral discharge. A serum prolactin level is useful in evaluating bilateral nipple discharge.
   b. Discharges that are spontaneous, unilateral, of recent onset, dark, or bloody are ominous and require further evaluation.

6. Unilateral pain in an isolated area of the breast should be evaluated.

7. Adenopathy may be seen, which appears as enlarged axillary lymph nodes that manifest as a single, distinct node or as multiple, indistinct nodes (often called "shoddy").

Procedure 33–1
Physical Examination of the Female Breast

Definition/Purpose	A thorough, systematic examination of all breast tissue and regional lymph nodes performed by a health care provider to detect any signs of breast cancer.
Learning/Teaching Activities	Provide explanation and instructions on each step of the procedure as you are performing the examination to reinforce knowledge of breast self-examination. Assess for any concerns about ability to perform breast self-examination; some women find a breast "map," which outlines the different structures palpable on the breast examination, helpful in reinforcing what is felt during their own breast examination.

Preliminary Activities

Equipment	• Patient gown • Blanket or sheet • Lotion or powder

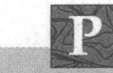

Procedure 33–1

(continued)

Preparation

- Ensure privacy and a warm room.
- Ask the woman to undress to the waist, leaving the gown open in the front.

Procedure

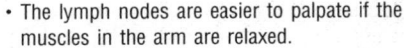

Action	Rationale/Discussion
1. Visual inspection is done with the woman sitting and moving her arms in four positions: • Arms at side, relaxed • Arms over her head • Arms pressed on her hips to flex the pectoral muscles • Leaning over at the waist and letting breast fall away from the chest wall.	1. The change in position allows the practitioner to observe for signs such as dimpling, skin retraction, or protrusions that may not be apparent with the breast relaxed against the chest wall.
2. Observe for the following: • Differences in size and symmetry between the breasts • Skin changes such as dimpling, edema, ulceration, prominent venous patterns, or masses • Nipple abnormalities, including retraction, rashes, or discharge	2. Any of these findings, especially if they are new for the woman, may represent signs of breast cancer and require further evaluation.
3. Tactile examination of lymph nodes • With the patient sitting, rest her forearm on your arm and palpate the axilla with the other hand. • Using a circular motion, reach high into the axilla, palpating behind the pectoral muscle, down over the ribs, inside the anterior and posterior axillary folds, and against the humerus. • Palpate the supraclavicular area above both of the clavicles.	• The lymph nodes are easier to palpate if the muscles in the arm are relaxed. • The lymph system from the breast drains to the axillary, mediastinal, and supraclavicular nodes. The axillary and supraclavicular nodes can be palpated if enlarged.

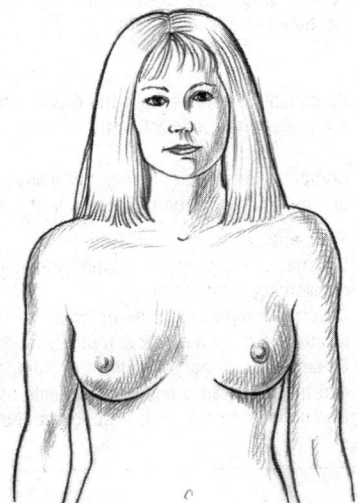

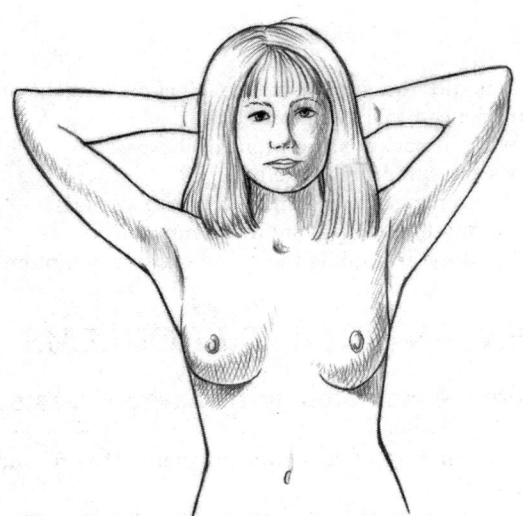

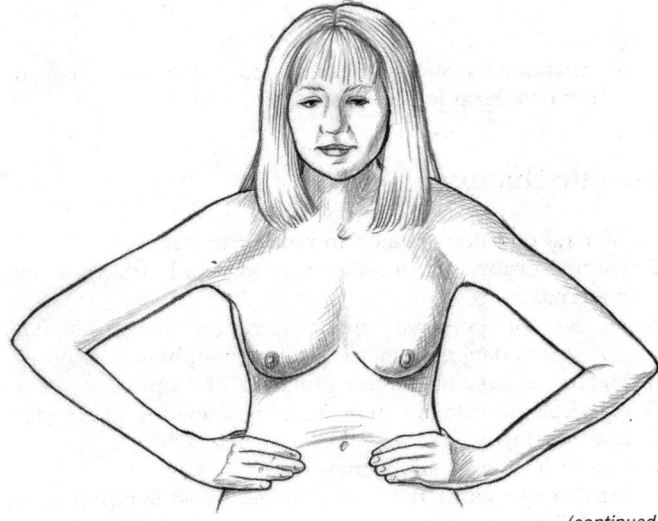

(continued)

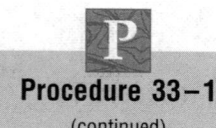

Procedure 33–1

(continued)

Action	Rationale/Discussion

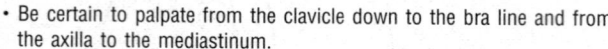

4. Tactile examination of the breast
   - Ask the patient to lay down and place her hands behind her neck. Put a small pad under the side to be examined.

   - Palpate in dime-sized circular motions, using light, medium, and deep pressure at each spot.

   - Palpate in a uniform pattern. Vertical strips have been shown to be the most effective method.

   - Be certain to palpate from the clavicle down to the bra line and from the axilla to the mediastinum.

   - Compress the nipple, noting any masses or discharge. Use a guaiac test on any discharge to determine the presence of occult blood.

5. Documentation
   - Describe adenopathy by location, number of involved nodes, size, consistency, and mobility.
   - Describe masses in terms of when the person first noticed them, the location, size, consistency, mobility, and associated skin changes.
   - Describe nipple abnormalities according to when they were noticed, and the appearance and characteristic of any discharge.
   - Document with narrative description and diagrams.

- Careful positioning helps flatten the breast tissue for a better examination.

- Using different pressures allows the practitioner to feel the different structures, especially deep in the thickest part of the breast.
- A uniform pattern helps minimize missed breast tissue. The vertical strip is the most efficient method to cover all the areas of the chest that need to be examined.
- Breast tissue is present up into the axilla (tail of Spence) and on the chest wall beyond the actual breast mound. The entire area needs to be examined for thoroughness.
- Bloody nipple discharge needs further evaluation to rule out pathology in the duct.

5. Careful documentation is vital for the evaluation of any breast abnormality, especially if the abnormality is going to be followed for changes rather than biopsied.

Final Activities

Ensure that the woman has full understanding of any abnormal findings in her breast and the follow-up plan, if needed. If the breast examination result was normal, emphasize the importance of following a full breast health screening program, including breast self-examination, clinical breast examination, and mammography.

---

a. Adenopathy should be assessed using the same criteria as those for a breast mass.

Health History

1. General questions related to risk for breast cancer
2. Family history of breast cancer on both paternal and maternal sides
3. History of personal previous cancer diagnosis (i.e., breast, ovarian, endometrial, colon, lymphoma)
4. History of previous breast problems or biopsies
5. Gynecologic history—menarche, menopause, pregnancy, and nursing
6. Use of hormonal supplements
7. Further questions that characterize breast symptoms are the following:

a. When did the symptom begin? How long have you experienced this symptom?
b. Have you had this symptom in the past?
c. Does the symptom come and go?
d. Does it change before and after your periods?
e. Does anything aggravate the symptom?
f. What do you think is the cause of your symptom?

■ BENIGN BREAST PROBLEMS

Problems Associated with Large Breasts

1. Difficulty finding clothes and brassieres that fit and are affordable.
2. Physical discomfort from back strain, shoulder pressure, and fungal rashes under the breasts.

3. Weight loss and well-fitting bras may provide some relief.
4. Breast reduction surgery is an option for discomfort that is not relieved by conservative measures.

Fibrocystic Breast Changes

1. Fibrocystic breast changes present as breast tenderness, increased nodularity (generalized lumpiness), and sometimes distinct cysts.
2. On palpation, multiple, indistinct smooth lumps may be felt, especially in the upper outer quadrants.
3. Symptoms are cyclic but may not resolve completely between periods.
4. Treatment may include caffeine restriction, increased intake of vitamins C and E, use of supportive bras, aspiration of distinct cysts, and hormonal therapy for severe symptoms.

Fibroadenomas

1. The most common cause of solid breast mass.
2. Occur most frequently in younger women.
3. Manifest as a solid, smooth, mobile singular mass.
4. Treatment involves local excision or the use of new core biopsy techniques. Fibroadenomas can be left in the breast unless they obscure mammograms or clinical breast examination.

Ductal Ectasia

1. Is caused by chronic inflammation of the terminal, subareolar ducts.
2. Commonly occurs in menopausal women.
3. Symptoms may include nipple discharge, subareolar tenderness, nipple retraction, and a mass.
4. Medical diagnosis is made by mammogram, galactogram, and biopsy.
5. Treatment may include antibiotics or excision of the involved ducts.

Intraductal Papilloma

1. Is caused by benign epithelial tumors in the ductal system.
2. May cause unilateral nipple discharge, tenderness, or an indistinct mass.
3. Microscopic evaluation of the nipple discharge, galactogram, and excision of the affected duct used to diagnose and plan treatment.

Mastitis

1. Breast infection that is usually associated with lactation. It occurs most often in mothers who are breast-feeding for the first time.

2. Bacteria may enter the breast through a cracked nipple and are usually carried by the mother, although the infant's mouth is another source of infection.
3. Clinical manifestations include a sore nipple and a reddened, edematous, hot, and tender breast. Progressive symptoms may include fever, chills, malaise, and headache.
4. Treatment: antibiotics, heat to promote comfort, emptying the affected breast to prevent stasis of milk, and meticulous hygiene. Lactation may have to be discontinued.

Breast Abscess

1. May occur during lactation, often as a result of mastitis. Subareolar abscess is a low-grade infection that can occur in nonlactating women.
2. Skin over the abscess is red and edematous. Pain, chills, and fever may occur. A mass may be palpable.
3. Treatment: antibiotics, analgesics, draining of the abscess, and application of warm, moist compresses. In lactating women, weaning may be necessary.

Fissure of the Nipple

1. A painful longitudinal ulcer that may occur in lactating women. The condition is aggravated by the infant's sucking.
2. Prenatal preparation of the nipple may prevent fissures.
3. Treatment: hand washing before breast-feeding, and washing and drying nipples after breast-feeding. Drying the nipples and exposing them to a heat lamp may also be helpful.
4. Avoiding astringent soaps and creams is important. Lanolin-based creams may relieve soreness.

◼ *THE MALE BREAST*

Physical Examination

1. Inspection and palpation can usually be performed while the man is sitting.
   a. Observe for skin changes, nipple swelling, or ulceration.
   b. Palpate the breast and areola for nodules, masses, and fatty or glandular enlargement.
   c. Document areas of abnormality.
2. Examination of the breast is important for men with gynecomastia.

Gynecomastia

1. Benign enlargement of 1 or both breasts in men.
2. Is caused by an increase in breast tissue.
3. Etiology idiopathic or caused by obesity, hormonal disorder, systemic disease, drugs (i.e., alcohol), or medications.

4. Treatment indicated if mass is present, breast is painful, or cosmetic changes cause psychologic distress.

Male Breast Cancer

1. Less than 1 percent of all breast cancer. In 1996, 1400 men were diagnosed with breast cancer; 260 men died from the disease.
2. Usually diagnosed at a later stage than that in women
3. Prognosis same as women of the same stage
4. All treatment options same as those for women, including adjuvant therapy and reconstructive surgery if desired to create new nipples

◼ *FEMALE BREAST CANCER*

Definition

1. Female breast cancer is a malignant neoplasm of breast tissue.
2. Cancer care is detailed in Chapter 17.

Incidence and Socioeconomic Impact

1. In 1995, 185,700 women were diagnosed with breast cancer.
2. Since 1970, the incidence of breast cancer has increased approximately 2 percent per year. This trend may be due to an aging population and improved diagnostic techniques.
3. One in 8 American women will develop breast cancer in her lifetime. The chance of developing breast cancer increases with age (Table 33–1).

ELDER ADVISORY

Many older women believe that the risk for breast cancer decreases with age, but it actually continues to rise. It is important that nurses continue to educate older women about the importance of early detection.

4. Only 1 percent of breast cancer occurs in men.
5. The incidence of breast cancer is highest in White women, who are followed by African Americans and then Hispanics. The lowest rate occurs in Asian Americans.

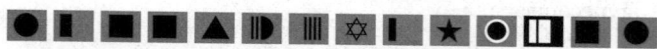

TRANSCULTURAL CONSIDERATIONS

African Americans are twice as likely to die of breast cancer as White Americans. It is not known whether this difference is related to the biology of the disease or to African Americans' limited access to medical care.

Table 33–1. Risk of Breast Cancer

Age	Related Risk
25	1 in 19,608
30	1 in 2,525
35	1 in 622
40	1 in 217
45	1 in 93
50	1 in 50
55	1 in 33
60	1 in 24
65	1 in 17
70	1 in 14
75	1 in 11
80	1 in 10
85	1 in 9
Ever	1 in 8

6. In 1996, 44,560 women died from breast cancer.
7. Ten-year survival rates range from 75 to 85 percent for stage I, 50 to 60 percent for stage II (depending on the number of nodes involved), and less than 30 percent for women with stages III and IV.

Risk Factors

1. Age and gender are the 2 main risk factors for breast cancer. Seventy percent of women have no major risk factors other than gender and age.
   a. Ninety-nine percent of breast cancer occurs in women.
   b. The rate of breast cancer increases with age.
2. Family history
   a. Genetic factors are rare, occurring in only 5 to 10 percent of women.
      (1) Genes may be inherited from the mother or father.
      (2) The BRCA1 gene is associated with breast and ovarian cancers and accounts for 45 percent of inherited breast cancers. Ashkenazic Jews have a greater risk of carrying a specific alteration of this gene.
      (3) The BRCA2 gene is associated with female and male breast cancers and accounts for 35 percent of inherited breast cancers.
      (4) The BRCA3 gene is associated with approximately 10 percent of inherited breast cancers.
      (5) The Li-Fraumeni syndrome, which is caused by a damaged P53 gene, increases a family's predisposition for a variety of cancers.
   b. A positive family history may be related to factors other than a specific gene. A greater risk is associated with afflicted 1st-degree relatives (mother, sister, daughter).
3. Personal history
   a. A prior history of breast cancer in 1 breast
   b. History of a benign breast biopsy that revealed breast tissue at risk for developing breast cancer (i.e., atypical hyperplasia or lobular carcinoma in situ)
4. Endogenous hormonal factors

a. Related to the length of time that the breast has been exposed to the woman's own estrogen
b. Factors that increase risk
   (1) Early age at menarche (younger than 12)
   (2) Late age of menopause (older than 52, or more than 40 years of menses)
   (3) Nulliparity
   (4) First full-term pregnancy after the age of 30 to 35 years
c. Factors that decrease risk
   (1) Early age of 1st pregnancy
   (2) Oophorectomy before the age of 30, without hormone replacement therapy
5. Obesity, especially after menopause. Currently, there is little evidence to support the correlation between obesity and breast cancer risk.
6. Diet
   a. A high-fat diet, especially at puberty, may increase risk. Further study is under way to explore this association.
   b. Excessive alcohol consumption appears to increase risk.
   c. Soy intake and foods high in antioxidant vitamins have been suggested as protectants against breast cancer. This association requires further study, as the present evidence is inconclusive.
7. Radiation exposure
   a. The risk of breast cancer development is greater for women who have been exposed to ionizing radiation at a young age.
   b. Women who have had repeated chest radiographs to screen for tuberculosis or who were treated with radiation for acne, mastitis, tonsillitis, or enlarged thymus gland have an increased risk of breast cancer.
8. Environmental causes: Pesticides and food additives are suspected risk factors for breast cancer, but results of studies are inconclusive.

Etiology

1. Growth factors may contribute to the development of breast cancer. These include the following:
   a. Insulin-like growth factor
   b. Transforming growth factor alpha
   c. Epidermal growth factor
   d. Ligands for erbB2 and erbB3
2. Molecular genetic events may contribute to the development of breast cancer. These include the following:
   a. Activation of certain oncogenes (e.g., erbB1, B2, B3)
   b. Inactivation of tumor suppression growth factors or genes (e.g., P53)
   c. Chromosomal locus for the loss of heterozygosity

Pathophysiology

1. Most human breast cancers are adenocarcinomas that are classified as ductal or lobular. Most ductal tumors appear to arise in the terminal sections of the ducts.
2. Most breast cancers may be further classified as in situ (within the duct or lobe) or invasive (broken through the duct or lobe into surrounding breast tissue) (Fig. 33–2).

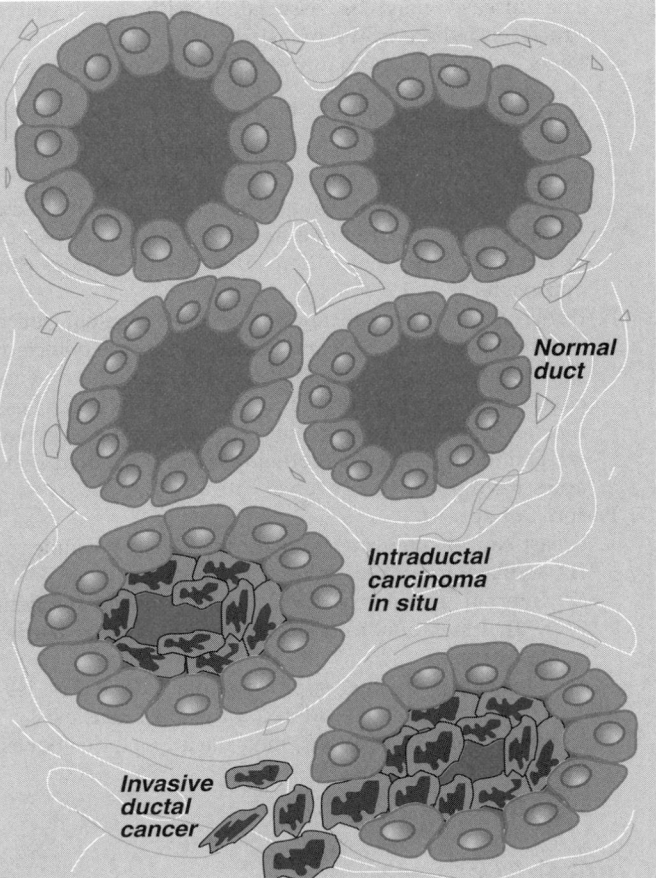

Figure 33–2. In situ versus invasive cancer.

a. In situ lobular carcinoma (LCIS) is considered a risk factor rather than a progression into invasive cancer. Women with LCIS have a 6 to 10 times greater risk of developing an invasive cancer (ductal or lobular) in either breast.
   (1) In situ lobular carcinoma is usually bilateral.
   (2) Treatment: close observation or bilateral prophylactic mastectomy. These women qualify for a chemopreventive trial with tamoxifen.
b. In situ ductal carcinoma is considered a "precancer" by many because it does not have the ability to metastasize without microinvasion. Subtypes include comedo, cribriform, and micropapillary. The comedo subtype is the most aggressive.
c. Invasive (infiltrating) ductal cancer is the most common and aggressive type.
d. Invasive lobular cancer has a greater chance of being bilateral. In pure form it is less aggressive, although a more aggressive variant occurs in some women.
3. Other, much less common, and often less aggressive types include medullary, mucinous, papillary, scirrhous, and tubular.
4. Inflammatory breast cancer involves the lymphatic channels of the skin. This form of cancer is considered very aggressive and is treated initially with chemotherapy.
5. Paget's disease is breast cancer of the nipple and is usually present unilaterally.

a. The disease may be associated with an invasive cancer elsewhere in the breast.
b. Paget's disease may manifest as itching and flaking of the nipple.

6. Theories of breast cancer
   a. Halstedian theory: Breast cancer spreads by direct extension from breasts through the lymph nodes out to the rest of the body. Thus, the rationale for radical mastectomies that remove as much of the disease as possible. It took more than 70 years to change this approach.
   b. Fisher theory: Breast cancer has been present for a minimum of 6 to 8 years before it can be detected. Therefore, systemic spread through lymphatic or vascular invasion has occurred before detection. Less radical surgeries have resulted in the same survival rates, and adjuvant chemotherapy and hormonal therapies have improved survival rates.

7. Patterns of spread
   a. Breast cancer often metastasizes to the lymph nodes.
      (1) Axillary metastasis is most common.
      (2) Internal mammary metastasis is more frequent with inner quadrant breast cancers and is harder to evaluate.
      (3) Metastasis to the supraclavicular nodes is less common and is considered a distant metastasis.
   b. Common organ sites of metastasis include bones, lungs, liver, and brain.

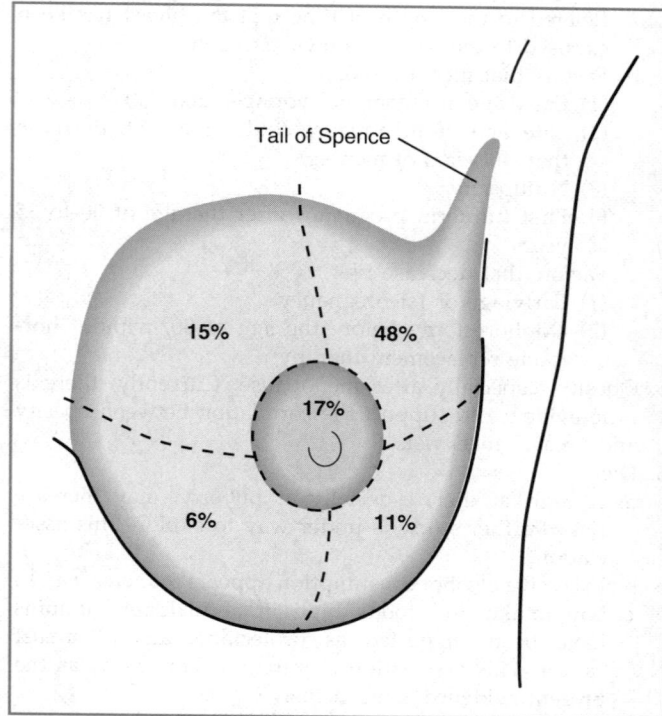

Figure 33–3. Frequency of occurrence of breast cancer according to location. Note the highest occurrence in the upper outer quadrant and tail of Spence. (Redrawn from Black JM, and Matassarin-Jacobs E [eds]. *Medical-Surgical Nursing: A Psychophysiologic Approach.* 4th ed. Philadelphia: WB Saunders, 1993, p 2178.)

Clinical Manifestations

1. Initially, breast cancer typically appears as a unilateral, single mass or thickening, usually in the breast's upper outer quadrant (Fig. 33–3).
2. The mass is usually painless, nontender, hard, irregular in shape, and immobile.

Diagnostics

1. Mammography: Diagnostic or tailored mammogram is used to evaluate women with current breast problems, a history of breast cancer, or breast implants in place.
2. Ultrasound
   a. Uses high-frequency sound waves to create a pattern or picture of breast structures
   b. Useful to help interpret a mammogram or to determine whether a lump is solid or cystic
   c. Useful in evaluating young women with a lump because no radiation is involved
   d. Useful to evaluate a breast symptom (e.g., a lump or pain) when mammogram results are normal
   e. Not useful for screening because it is difficult to interpret shadows created by all the contours of the breast.
3. Galactogram (ductogram)
   a. A radiopaque dye study to evaluate breast ducts in cases of spontaneous or bloody nipple discharge.
   b. Dye is injected into the draining ducts to search for abnormalities.
4. Magnetic resonance imaging (MRI)
   a. Uses a magnet to create an image of the breast
   b. Useful to identify leaks in silicone breast implants
   c. May be useful to search for an occult primary breast cancer when mammogram results are normal
   d. Will probably never be used for screening, because of cost
5. Radionucleotide studies (Sesta-MIBI)
   a. Experimental but may be useful to differentiate benign from malignant changes in the breast or to search for an occult primary breast cancer
   b. Current technology not compatible with use of this modality for wire localization or with biopsy-guided techniques, so that other procedures may be a problem when the abnormality is seen only with this type of imaging
6. Biopsy
   a. Fine-needle aspiration
      (1) Aspirates cells from the abnormal areas, which are evaluated by cytology
      (2) Can be done on palpable or nonpalpable lesions using ultrasound or stereotactic mammography to guide needle placement
   b. Core needle biopsy
      (1) Removes a core of tissue from abnormal areas, which is evaluated for pathologic changes
      (2) Maintains architecture so that diagnosis is easier and more accurate
      (3) Can be done on palpable or nonpalpable lesions using ultrasound or stereotactic mammography to guide needle placement

c. Incisional biopsy, which removes a portion of the abnormal area
d. Excisional biopsy
   (1) Removes entire abnormal area
   (2) May require placement of a wire, under mammography or ultrasound, to help localize nonpalpable lesion for the surgeon
7. Staging and prognostic factors
   a. Serve as a guide for therapy (Fig. 33–4)
   b. Help predict prognosis
   c. Serve as a basis to compare different treatment methods to achieve the best results
   d. The TNM system is accepted worldwide (Box 33–1).
      (1) T = tumor size
      (2) N = node involvement
      (3) M = metastasis
   e. Histologic grading as an important indicator of aggressiveness. Smith-Bloom-Richardson (SBR) is the standardized method of grading cancer.
      (1) Grade I—well differentiated, less aggressive
      (2) Grade II—moderately differentiated
      (3) Grade III—poorly differentiated, more aggressive
   f. Hormone receptor status is a significant indicator.
      (1) Some breast cancer cells have receptor sites on the cell wall for the female hormones estrogen and progesterone.
      (2) Receptor positivity is considered a good prognostic factor that does the following:
         • Allows more treatment options
         • Appears to be associated with a less aggressive cancer
         • Occurs more often in postmenopausal women
   g. Other prognostic factors have not been shown to be independently reliable in predicting prognosis. When used together, however, they may indicate the potential aggressiveness of a woman's breast cancer (Table 33–2).
   h. The staging workup varies with the clinical stage of the tumor.
      (1) Imaging studies may include bone scan, chest radiograph, and abdominal computed tomographic (CT) scan.
      (2) Laboratory tests may include calcium levels to evaluate for bone metastasis, alkaline phosphatase measurements to evaluate for bone and liver metastases, and liver function tests.

NURSE ADVISORY

Hypercalcemia, an elevated serum calcium over 11 mg per dl, is an oncologic emergency requiring immediate treatment. Treatment consists of vigorous hydration, diuresis, and, if needed, medications to inhibit bone resorption.

(3) Tumor markers are based on findings that tumor antigens can be measured in the blood of some patients. Tumor markers are sometimes used to monitor for recurrence or to evaluate efficacy of therapy. Specific markers include CA-15-3, CA-27-29, and CEA (carcinoembryonic antigen).

CLINICAL STAGING OF BREAST CANCER

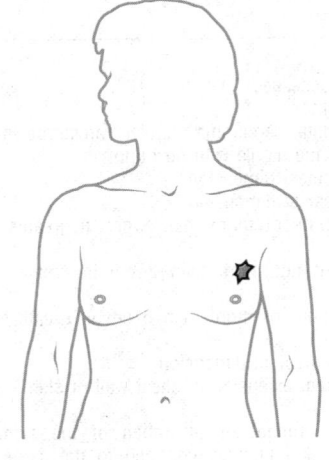

Stage I:
• Tumor less than 2 cm
• Confined to breast
• No positive lymph nodes
• No metastases present

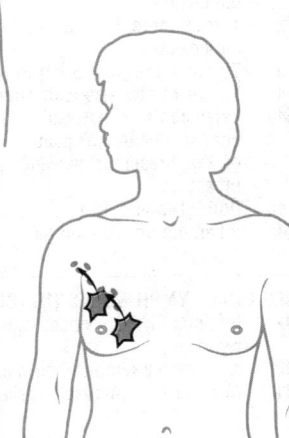

Stage II:
• Tumor less than 2 cm with positive lymph nodes; no metastases evident
• *Or* tumor 2–5 cm with or without positive lymph nodes; no metastases evident
• *Or* tumor greater than 5 cm with negative lymph nodes; no metastases evident

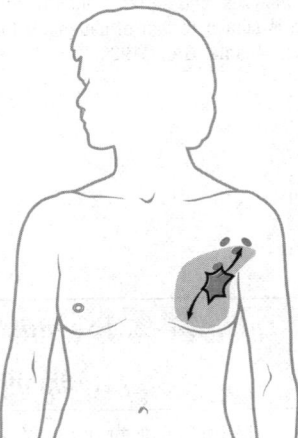

Stage III:
• Tumor larger than 5 cm with positive lymph nodes; no metastases present
• *Or* tumor extends to chest wall or skin
• *Or* positive internal mammary nodes are present; no metastases evident
• *Or* presence of positive lymph nodes fixed to one another

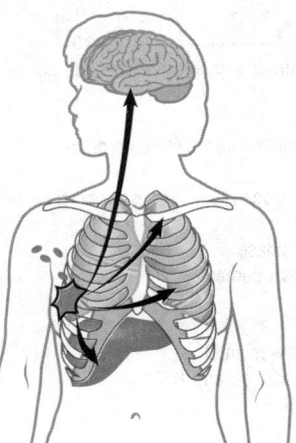

Stage IV:
• Any distant metastases to brain, lung, liver, or bone
• With or without positive lymph nodes

Figure 33–4.

BOX 33-1. Staging for Breast Carcinoma

T = Primary Tumor   N = Regional Lymph Nodes
M = Distant Metastasis

PRIMARY TUMOR (T)
TX Primary tumor cannot be assessed
T0 No evidence of primary tumor
Tis* Carcinoma in situ: Intraductal carcinoma, lobular carcinoma in situ, or Paget's disease of the nipple with no tumor
T1 Tumor 2 cm or less in greatest dimension
    T1a 0.5 cm or less in greatest dimension
    T1b More than 0.5 cm but not more than 1 cm in greatest dimension
    T1c More than 1 cm but not more than 2 cm in greatest dimension
T2 Tumor more than 2 cm but not more than 5 cm in greatest dimension
T3 Tumor more than 5 cm in greatest dimension
T4† Tumor of any size with direct extension to chest wall or skin
T4a Extension to chest wall
T4b Edema (including peau d'orange) or ulceration of the skin of the breast or satellite skin nodules confined to the same breast
T4c Both (T4a and T4b)
T4d Inflammatory carcinoma

REGIONAL LYMPH NODES (N) (CLINICAL)
NX Regional lymph nodes cannot be assessed (e.g., previously removed)
N0 No regional lymph node metastasis
N1 Metastasis to movable ipsilateral axillary lymph node(s)

N2 Metastasis to ipsilateral axillary lymph node(s) fixed to one another or to other structures
N3 Metastasis to ipsilateral internal mammary lymph node(s)

DISTANT METASTASIS (M)
MX Presence of distant metastasis cannot be assessed
M0 No distant metastasis
M1 Distant metastasis (includes metastasis to ipsilateral supraclavicular lymph node[s])

STAGE GROUPING

Stage	T	N	M
Stage 0	Tis	N0	M0
Stage I	T1	N0	M0
Stage IIA	T0	N1	M0
	T1	N1‡	M0
	T2	N0	M0
Stage IIB	T2	N1	M0
	T3	N0	M0
Stage IIIA	T0	N2	M0
	T1	N2	M0
	T2	N2	M0
	T3	N1, N2	M0
Stage IIIB	T4	Any N	M0
	Any T	N3	M0
Stage IV	Any T	Any N	M1

* Paget's disease associated with a tumor is classified according to the size of the tumor.
† Chest wall includes ribs, intercostal muscles, and serratus anterior muscle but not pectoral muscle.
‡ The prognosis of patients with pN1a is similar to that of patients with pN0.
From the American Cancer Society, Inc., Atlanta, GA. ©1989.

Clinical Management

1. Goals of clinical management
   a. Eliminate cancer
   b. Minimize trauma to the person
   c. Maintain a high quality of life
   d. Achieve long-term remission and cure
   e. Involve the patient in treatment decisions. In discuss-

Table 33-2. Prognostic Factors for Breast Cancer

Factor	Significance	Related Risk
Tumor size and lymph node status	The best predictor of risk of recurrence	Less than 1 cm tumor = low risk; greater than 3 cm = high risk Approximately 6% per node risk of recurrence
Nuclear and histologic grades	SBR scores based on mitosis, size and shape of nuclei, and tubule formation	SBR grade I = low risk SBR grade III = high risk
Estrogen and progesterone receptors	Receptors for female hormones present on breast cancer cells	Positive + lower risk and better response from hormone therapy
S phase	Measures cell proliferation. Reported as % cells in S phase	Low % = low risk
DNA content	Measures amount of DNA in tumor. Aneuploid = abnormal amount Diploid = normal amount	Diploid = low risk Aneuploid = high risk
Cathepsin D	Enzyme secreted by some breast cancers	Elevated cathepsin D = high risk
Her2/neu and P53	Oncogenes	Positive = high risk
EGFR	Epidermal growth factor receptors (EGFRs) may be present on some breast cancer cell walls	Positive = high risk

ing all treatment options with the person, review the following:

(1) Expected side effects and self-care measures to prevent or minimize them

(2) Amount of time anticipated for treatment

(3) Cost of treatment—financial, emotional, and long-term physical complications

(4) Cosmesis

(5) Rehabilitation options: Conserve the breast as much as possible. The trend is toward less surgery and more systemic therapy. Conservative breast surgery typically involves lumpectomy or quadrantectomy and radiation therapy. This approach is preferred to breast removal because the survival statistics are the same and the breast is preserved.

ELDER ADVISORY

Age discrimination and assumptions by professionals about body image among older women may lead to fewer treatment choices being offered to these women. All women should be given the opportunity to choose breast conservation, if it is medically indicated.

---

2. Nonpharmacologic interventions. Surgery and radiation therapy are used to treat local disease. Radiation therapy is both a primary treatment to the breast and a palliative treatment for metastasis to bone or brain. Local radiation is also used with mastectomy, for cancers with extension to skin or muscle or for recurrent breast lesions.

   a. Simulation

   (1) A treatment-planning session determines the treatment field.

   (2) Tattoos are used to outline the field for standardized positioning.

   b. Treatments take about 10 to 15 minutes and are usually given Monday through Friday over 5 to 6 weeks.

   c. Some women require an extra dose or a boost at the tumor site. This can be delivered by electron beam or by radioactive implants.

   d. Short-term side effects

   (1) Fatigue

   (2) Skin burn and, for some, blistering

   e. Long-term complications

   (1) Potential change in breast size, texture, and color

   (2) Secondary malignancies (sarcomas and lung cancer in smokers), although these are rare

   (3) Pneumonitis

3. Pharmacologic interventions. Breast cancer, even when diagnosed early, is often treated as a systemic disease because of the potential for micrometastasis. Use of chemotherapy and hormonal therapy is increasing.

   a. Adjuvant chemotherapy for localized disease

   (1) The effect on the disease-free interval has improved more than overall survival.

   (2) Combination chemotherapy is more effective than single-agent chemotherapy.

   (3) Adjuvant chemotherapy is more effective in premenopausal women.

(4) Combinations of drugs are used to maximize effectiveness while minimizing side effects. Protocols may be standard or experimental.

   • CMF—Cyclophosphamide (Cytoxan), methotrexate, and 5-FU (fluorouracil): the most common protocol, it is usually given for 6 months, and may be given as all intravenous, or as a combination of intravenous and pills.

   • CAF—Cytoxan, doxorubicin (Adriamycin), 5-FU: a more aggressive protocol that is used for some premenopausal women with positive nodes and is usually given as all intravenous therapy.

(5) Currently, research protocols are looking at the following:

   • More intense doses of chemotherapy over a shorter period of time (Adriamycin plus Cytoxan)

   • Different sequences of drugs (Adriamycin for 4 cycles followed by CMF)

   • Very high dose chemotherapy with stem cell rescue

   • Chemotherapy before primary surgery

   • Use of newer drugs in old combinations (paclitaxel [Taxol] with CMF or CAF)

(6) Possible short-term side effects

   • Standard CMF and CAF protocols are fairly well tolerated by most women.

   • Nausea and vomiting are usually minimized with new serotonin-related antiemetics.

   • Febrile neutropenia is uncommon with standard therapy but more common with newer dose-intensive therapy. Neutropenia can be treated with growth factors (granulocyte-colony stimulating factor [G-CSF] or granulocyte macrophage–colony stimulating factor [GM-CSF]), which stimulate the growth of neutrophils.

   • Alopecia (hair loss) is complete with Adriamycin but may occur only as thinning with CMF.

   • Fatigue is very common and may have the greatest effect on the quality of life.

   • Weight gain of 10 to 15 pounds is common. The etiology is unknown but may be minimized with a regimen of diet and exercise.

   • Bladder irritation and stomatitis also occasionally occur.

(7) Possible long-term complications

   • Premature menopause with increased risk for osteoporosis and cardiovascular disease

   • Infertility

   • Cardiomyopathy with anthracycline and related chemotherapy (Adriamycin, mitoxantrone)

   • Treatment-induced leukemia (0.1% risk)

   b. Adjuvant hormonal therapy for localized disease

   (1) The effect on the disease-free interval has improved more than overall survival.

   (2) Adjuvant hormonal therapy is more effective in postmenopausal women and more effective in women with positive estrogen and progesterone receptors.

   (3) Tamoxifen is both an estrogen agonist and antagonist and may prevent a breast cancer from devel-

oping in the contralateral breast. The agent is being used in prevention trials. Possible long-term complications include endometrial cancer and cataracts. Possible short-term side effects include the following:
- Hot flashes, vaginal discharge, or vaginal dryness
- Decrease in libido and increase in orgasmic threshold
- Depression, short-term memory loss
- Thromboembolic events

NURSE ADVISORY

All women on tamoxifen who have a uterus need to be informed of their risk for endometrial cancer and the need for yearly thorough gynecologic examinations.

(4) Oophorectomy is more effective in premenopausal women and may be used in addition to adjuvant chemotherapy for high-risk breast cancer.

c. Treatment for advanced or metastatic breast cancer
(1) Goals include long-term remission and palliation of symptoms.
(2) The treatment approach depends on the extent of disease, menopausal status, and hormone receptor status.
(3) A new approach for younger women with minimal disease is aggressive high-dose chemotherapy to attempt long-term remission.
(4) Women with hormone receptor–positive breast cancer may be able to control their cancer with hormone therapy for extended periods, thereby reserving chemotherapy for later.

d. Chemotherapy for advanced disease
(1) Adriamycin
- Single most effective agent against breast cancer
- Has a lifetime dose limit, but this may change with use of new cardioprotective drug (dexrazoxane [Zinecard])
- Usually used in combination with other drugs
(2) Taxol
- New antimicrotubule agent from the bark of a yew tree
- Approved by the U.S. Food and Drug Administration (FDA) for use in treatment of advanced breast cancer
- Peripheral neuropathy as dose-limiting toxicity
(3) Mitoxantrone
- Approved by the FDA for use in breast cancer
- Cardiomyopathy as dose-limiting toxicity

e. High-dose chemotherapy with stem cell rescue
(1) Trials are still under way to determine whether there is a long-term survival advantage over standard therapy. Early results indicate a survival advantage in women with newly diagnosed metastatic cancer and those with high-risk stage II or III disease.

(2) Because bone marrow suppression is a dose-limiting toxicity of chemotherapy, autologous stem cell rescue allows larger doses of chemotherapy to be given.
(3) Autologous stem cells are collected from the bone marrow in the iliac crest or from the peripheral circulation with plasmapheresis. Harvested stem cells are cryopreserved and then thawed and reinfused after completion of the chemotherapy regimen.
(4) The trend is toward having a larger portion of care given in ambulatory care settings to reduce cost.
(5) The intensive clinical course requires extensive physical, psychologic, and social support.
(6) There is a risk of long-term morbidity.

f. Hormonal therapy for advanced disease
(1) Tamoxifen (Nolvadex) is 1st-line hormonal therapy for women with metastatic breast cancer, unless the agent is already being used for adjuvant therapy.

NURSE ADVISORY

Women with bone metastasis are at risk for hypercalcemia whenever they start or change hormonal therapy. Monitor for signs and symptoms of hypercalcemia, including nausea, vomiting, constipation, polyuria, polydipsia, lethargy, and confusion. Monitor calcium levels carefully.

(2) Megestrol acetate (Megace)
- Second-line hormonal therapy
- Side effects, including significant weight gain and hot flashes
(3) Arimidex is a new aromatase inhibitor with fewer side effects. The chief side effect is transient nausea.
(4) Aminoglutethimide (Cytadren)
- Medical adrenalectomy—blocks the function of the adrenal gland
- Must be given with hydrocortisone
- Initial side effects of drowsiness and skin rash resolve with continuing therapy.

NURSE ADVISORY

Women need to be instructed not to discontinue medication because of rash or drowsiness, as these will resolve over 2 to 4 weeks. The woman should contact her physician if symptoms become severe.

(5) Other hormones that may be used include estrogen (diethylstilbestrol [DES]) and androgens (fluoxymesterone [Halotestin]).

4. Special medical-surgical procedures
a. Lumpectomy

(1) The tumor and a margin of healthy tissue around the tumor are removed.

(2) Moderate dose of radiation is used to eradicate any residual cancer in the breast.

(3) Axillary node dissection may also be performed.

(4) Complications may include hematoma, infection, pain, seroma, and emotional distress.

b. Quadrantectomy

(1) A quadrantectomy is the same as a lumpectomy but with a full quadrant of breast removed.

(2) The purpose is to ensure adequate removal of all tumor.

c. Mastectomy (Fig. 33–5)

(1) Mastectomy is still needed for some women, especially those with multifocal disease, a large tumor in relation to breast size, cancer in more than 1 quadrant of the breast, a history of collagen vascular disease, and a personal choice for this procedure.

(2) A simple, or total, mastectomy is removal of the entire breast, including the nipple, while preserving pectoral muscles.

(3) A modified radical mastectomy is removal of the entire breast, including the nipple, and an axillary node dissection.

(4) A radical mastectomy is removal of the entire breast, including the nipple, axillary nodes, and pectoral muscles. A radical mastectomy is rarely, if ever, necessary.

(5) Complications may include seroma, infection, skin necrosis, phantom breast sensation, and emotional distress.

d. Reconstruction after mastectomy

(1) Reconstruction can be immediate or delayed. Immediate reconstruction allows for immediate cosmetic results and fewer times for the patient to undergo general anesthesia. The disadvantage to immediate reconstruction is that it can be overwhelming to make 1 more decision at this time, and to weigh advantages and disadvantages of all the different types of reconstructive procedures.

(2) Reconstruction does not replace the need to grieve over a lost breast.

(3) Implants are placed below pectoral muscle to provide thicker covering and a more natural appearance and to allow for adequate clinical examination to check for recurrence. Types of implants include the following:

- Saline-filled in a silicone shell
- Silicone-filled: currently banned by the FDA because of possible association with autoimmune disorders but still available through research protocols for women with breast cancer
- Currently, clinical trials are under way with new substances (e.g., peanut oil).

(4) Tissue expanders are often used to stretch the skin and muscle to provide an adequate space for the implant and to allow a more natural droop.

(5) Complications related to implants include the following:

- Fibrous capsular contraction, which immobilizes the implant, creating asymmetry and discomfort. Implant massage has not been shown to be effective in preventing or treating contraction and is no longer routinely recommended because of the risk of leakage or rupture of the implant.
- Infection
- Leakage
- Erosion or extrusion of the implant

e. Autologous tissue reconstruction

(1) Myocutaneous flaps

- Tissue from the donor site is tunneled to the breast while maintaining the original blood supply.
- The latissimus dorsi flap uses the muscle from the back that moves the shoulder.
- The rectus abdominus muscle uses the large, vertical abdominal muscles.

(2) Free flaps

- Tissue from the donor site is completely removed and transferred to the breast, and the blood supply reanastomosed.
- The rectus abdominus muscle uses the large, vertical abdominal muscles.
- The superior gluteal muscle uses the muscle from buttocks.

Lumpectomy with lymph node dissection:
Only tumor and axillary lymph nodes removed.

Simple mastectomy:
Breast and usually nipple removed. Lymph nodes left intact.

Modified radical mastectomy:
Breast, nipple, and lymph nodes removed; muscle left intact.

Radical mastectomy:
Breast, nipple, muscles, and lymph nodes removed.

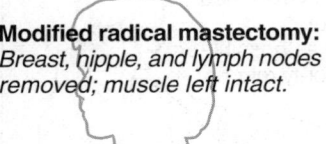
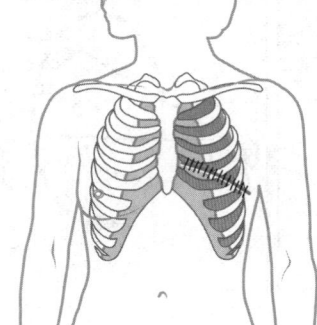

Figure 33–5. Types of surgery.

(3) Complications
- Flap necrosis, which is more common with smokers, diabetics, and those with peripheral vascular disease
- Decreased function of the donor muscle site (i.e., decreased shoulder motion and strength)
- Abdominal hernia

f. Nipple areolar reconstruction
(1) The procedure uses skin from the afflicted breast, groin, behind the ear, donor site, or other breast to create a new nipple areolar complex.
(2) The reconstructed nipple does not have sensation.
(3) The skin of the areola may be tattooed to match the contralateral breast.

g. Contralateral breast reconstruction

(1) An additional procedure may be needed to achieve symmetry. Mastoplexy raises the dropped breast. Reduction or augmentation may be needed to match the reconstructed breast.
(2) Most states mandate insurance coverage for breast reconstruction, but surgery on the contralateral breast may not be covered.

h. Axillary node dissections
(1) Useful to determine spread of breast cancer beyond the breast (Box 33–2)
(2) Complications (Fig. 33–6)
- Lymphedema
- Alteration in arm mobility
- Nerve damage with numbness
- Seroma

POSTAXILLARY DISSECTION EXERCISES

Arm Swings:
- Stand with feet 8 inches apart.
- Bend forward from waist, allowing arms to hang toward floor.
- Swing both arms up to sides to reach shoulder level.
- Swing back to center, then cross arms at center.
- Do not bend elbows.
- If possible, do this and other exercises in front of mirror to ensure even posture and correct motion.

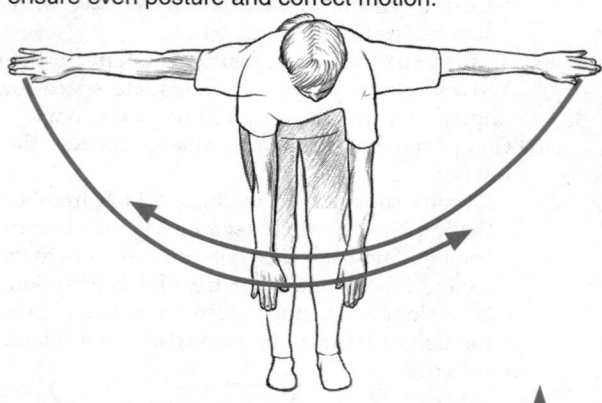

Pulley Motion:
- Using affected arm, toss a 6-foot rope over a shower rod or over the top of a door.
- Grasp 1 end of the rope in each hand.
- Slowly raise affected arm as far as comfortable by pulling down on the rope on opposite side
- Keep raised arm close to your head.
- Reverse to raise unaffected arm by lowering the affected arm.
- Repeat.

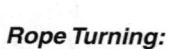

Hand Wall Climbing:
- Stand facing wall with toes 6–12 inches from wall.
- Bend elbows and place palms against wall at shoulder level.
- Gradually move both hands up the wall parallel to each other until incisional pulling or pain occurs. (Mark that spot on wall to measure progress.)
- Work hands down to shoulder level.
- Move closer to wall as height of reach improves.

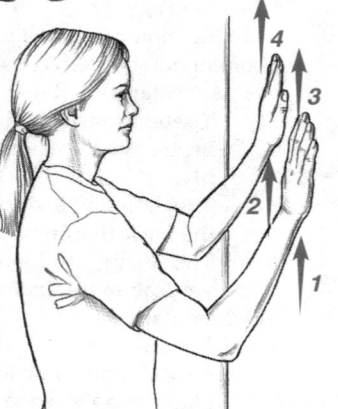

Rope Turning:
- Tie rope to door handle.
- Hold rope in hand of affected side.
- Back away from door until arm is extended away from body, parallel to floor.
- Swing rope in as wide a circle as possible
- Increase size of the circle as mobility returns.

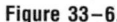

Figure 33–6.

BOX 33-2. Clinical Controversies Regarding Axillary Node Dissection

Axillary node dissection has been a standard of therapy for breast cancer for many years. Over the past few years, however, there has been increasing discussion on the value of node dissections compared to the morbidity from them.

In favor of dissection
- Node status, the *N* in the TNM staging system, is one of the key factors in the ability to predict prognosis and plan for adjuvant therapy.
- Better locoregional control is achieved by removing nodes that may contain micrometastasis.

Against dissection
- From 6 to 28 percent of women with axillary node dissections experience complications of lymphedema, arm numbness, or impaired shoulder mobility.
- Many women receive adjuvant therapy regardless of node status and therefore should be spared the morbidity of the surgery if the axilla is clinically negative.
- Some women, because of age or other medical conditions, will not receive adjuvant therapy regardless of node status and should therefore be spared the morbidity of surgery if the axilla is clinically negative.

NURSE ADVISORY

Place a sign over the hospital bed to remind all staff to avoid blood pressures, venipunctures, or injection in the arm that has undergone axillary node dissection.

Complications

1. Functional recovery depends on the woman's preexisting physical condition and other chronic illnesses that may be present. Recovery also depends on stage of breast cancer, extent of surgery, and extent of adjuvant therapy.
2. Long-term physical complications are not common.
   a. Frozen shoulder is due to alterations in mobility after axillary node dissection or radiation therapy.

ELDER ADVISORY

Older women with preexisting musculoskeletal conditions are at greater risk for complications. Assessment for risk factors should be done before or soon after surgery because early referral to physical therapy may prevent long-term complications.

   - Need to begin range-of-motion exercises as soon as drains are removed after surgery
   - Physical therapy referral if mobility does not return to normal by 4 to 6 weeks after surgery
   b. Lymphedema is blockage of lymph drainage in the arm due to scarring from surgery. Lymphedema can occur any time in the future (months, years) after axillary node dissection. Prevention (Box 33-3) is con-

troversial because there have been no studies to document a significant difference in lymphedema between women who follow the guidelines and those who do not. Goals of prevention are to avoid infection, constriction, or overuse of the arm. Treatment is aimed at control.
   - Compression stockings and gloves
   - Electrical gradient pumps
   - "Bandaging"—a technique of combining pressure with motion
   - Manual lymphatic drainage (MLD)—a specialized type of massage

Survivorship Issues

1. Every woman diagnosed with breast cancer is considered a cancer survivor from the day of diagnosis forward.
2. Emotional recovery may mean 1 to 2 years is required to establish emotional equilibrium after breast cancer diagnosis and treatment. Women describe the journey toward recovery as an "emotional roller coaster" that travels through many emotions of denial, anger, sadness, anxiety, and hope.
3. Many types of support are available.
   a. Studies have shown that women with metastatic breast cancer who actively participate in a support group live longer.
   b. One-on-one peer support, in which a breast cancer survivor acts as a guide through the initial phases of diagnosis and treatment, can be effective. One example of this is the American Cancer Society's Reach to Recovery Program.
   c. Professional counseling with a therapist may be beneficial.
4. Family and significant others must be involved in recovery.
   a. Daughters may feel especially vulnerable with mixed emotions of anger and guilt because of perceived increased risk for breast cancer.
   b. Adolescent daughters are at risk for developmental difficulties with the mother's diagnosis coming at a time when they are learning to adjust to their own developing breasts and sexuality.
5. Adapting a positive lifestyle includes the following:
   a. Eating healthy low-fat foods. Fruits and vegetables may provide a survival advantage. A new randomized study is under way at the University of California, Davis.
   b. Beginning an aerobic exercise routine. Exercise may minimize side effects of therapy, help maintain weight, and improve mental outlook.
   c. Controlling weight. Weight gain with therapy may make weight control especially important.
   d. Returning to work
      (1) Although job discrimination is illegal, some women report being passed over for jobs or promotions after a breast cancer diagnosis. The National Coalition for Cancer Survivors ([505] 764-9964) provides support for individuals who have concerns about work.

BOX 33-3. Eighteen Steps to Prevention for the Breast Cancer Patient Who Is at Risk of Lymphedema and for the Breast Cancer Patient Who Has Developed Lymphedema

WHO IS AT RISK?

At risk is anyone who has had a simple mastectomy, lumpectomy, or modified radical mastectomy in combination with axillary node dissection and, often, radiation therapy. Lymphedema can occur immediately postoperatively, or within a few months, a couple of years, or 20 years or more after cancer therapy. With proper education and care, lymphedema can be avoided or, if it develops, kept well under control. *The following instructions should be reviewed carefully preoperatively and discussed with your physician or therapist.*

1. Absolutely do not ignore any slight increase of swelling in the arm, hand, fingers, or chest wall *(consult with your doctor immediately).*
2. Never allow an injection or a blood drawing in the affected arm(s).
3. Have blood pressure checked in the unaffected arm.
4. Keep the edemic arm, or "at-risk" arm, spotlessly clean. Use lotion (Eucerin, Nivea) after bathing. When drying it, be gentle, but thorough. Make sure it is dry in any creases and between the fingers.
5. Avoid vigorous, repetitive movements against resistance with the affected arm (scrubbing, pushing, pulling).
6. Avoid heavy lifting with the affected arm. Never carry heavy handbags or bags with over-the-shoulder straps.
7. Do not wear tight jewelry or elastic bands around affected fingers or arm(s).
8. Avoid extreme temperature changes when bathing or washing dishes. Do not use a sauna or hot tub. Keep the arm protected from the sun.
9. Avoid any type of trauma (bruising, cuts, sunburn or other burns, sports injuries, insect bites, cat scratches).
10. Wear gloves while doing housework, gardening, or any type of work that could result in even a minor injury.
11. When manicuring your nails, avoid cutting your cuticles *(inform your manicurist).*
12. Exercise is important, but consult with your therapist. Do not overtire an arm at risk; if it starts to ache, lie down and elevate it. *Recommended exercises:* walking, swimming, light aerobics, bike riding, and specially designed ballet or yoga. *(Do not lift more than 15 lbs.)*
13. When traveling by air, patients with lymphedema must wear a compression sleeve. Additional bandages may be required on a long flight.
14. Patients with large breasts should wear light breast prostheses (heavy prostheses may put too much pressure on the lymph nodes above the collar bone). Soft pads may have to be worn under the bra strap. Wear a well-fitted bra: not too tight and with no wire support.
15. Use an electric razor to remove hair from axilla. Maintain electric razor properly, replacing heads as needed.
16. Patients who have lymphedema should wear a well-fitted compression sleeve during all waking hours. At least every 4 to 6 months, see your therapist for follow-up. If the sleeve is too loose, most likely the arm circumference has reduced or the sleeve is worn.
17. Warning: If you notice a rash, blistering, redness, increase of temperature, or fever, see your physician immediately. An inflammation or infection in the affected arm could be the beginning or a worsening of lymphedema.
18. Maintain your ideal weight through a well-balanced, low-sodium, high-fiber diet. Avoid smoking and alcoholic beverages. Lymphedema is a high-protein edema, but eating too little protein will not reduce the protein element in the lymph fluid—rather, this will weaken the connective tissue and worsen the condition. The diet should contain protein that is easily digested such as chicken, fish, or tofu.

Unfortunately, prevention is not a cure. But, as a breast cancer patient, you are in control of your ongoing cancer checkups and the continued maintenance of your lymphedema.

From National Lymphedema Network, San Francisco, CA.

---

(2) Some women are afraid to change jobs or venture into private practice because of fear of losing insurance.

(3) Some find it easier to reenter the work community by being straightforward and open with peers, to minimize miscommunication about illness and treatments.

6. It is important not to let insurance lapse at any time, because new insurance may not cover preexisting conditions. Many states now have high-risk insurance pools to cover people with histories of catastrophic illness.

7. Women may experience concerns regarding sex and sexuality.
   a. Changes in body image related to disease, surgery, chemotherapy, and hormonal therapy include alopecia of head and other body hair, loss of breast or breast scars, scars from reconstruction donor site, and weight gain.
   b. Hormonal changes may lead to decreased libido, vaginal dryness, or change in ability to have an orgasm.
   c. Communication breakdown and nonverbalized expectations may create tension between couples.

TRANSCULTURAL CONSIDERATIONS

Sexuality and sexual behavior may vary for different cultural groups. Members of some cultures are uncomfortable with open discussion of sexuality. The nurse needs to be sensitive to the issues that each woman may face and should find ways to provide support and needed information.

   d. Therapy is aimed at the cause of the sexual dysfunction.

(1) Provide information about prostheses, wigs, and makeup.

(2) Self-massage can help a woman accept physical changes that have occurred.

(3) Open communication with the woman's sexual partner is very important.

(4) Couples' counseling may be needed to improve communication, help couples face fears and disappointment, and attain healthy adjustment.

8. Pregnancy after breast cancer is still controversial, but most retrospective studies do not demonstrate any difference in survival. Many physicians advise a waiting period of 1 to 2 years to allow the body time to recover physically and emotionally.

NURSE ADVISORY

For women of childbearing age who are undergoing chemotherapy or hormonal therapy for breast cancer, the nurse needs to emphasize the importance of birth control. Oral contraceptives are not an option for women who are undergoing treatment for breast cancer, so information about other methods needs to be discussed.

9. Symptoms of menopause may include hot flashes, mood swings, vaginal dryness, and insomnia. Some women find that vitamins C and E help decrease some of these symptoms.

a. Risk for osteoporosis increases after menopause, and women should begin an exercise routine and calcium supplementation.

b. Risk for heart disease may be decreased with improvements in exercise and diet.

10. Traditionally, a woman was followed by her oncologist, surgeon, and primary physician at intervals over several years. There is an evolving trend to return the surveillance to the primary care physician when direct treatment is completed.

a. Clinical examinations and office visits are usually scheduled every 3 months for the first 1 to 2 years, every 6 months during years 3 to 5, and then yearly.

b. Laboratory studies may include complete blood count and blood chemistries. Some physicians follow tumor markers (CA 15-3 and CEA) on a regular basis.

c. The trend is to do less surveillance imaging (bone scan, CT scan) because these have not been shown to provide a survival advantage if metastasis is detected on scans before clinical manifestation.

d. It is common for women to experience anxiety and "mood swings" before routine checkups.

Applying the Nursing Process

NURSING DIAGNOSIS: Pain R/T biopsy and diagnostic tests

1. *Expected outcomes:* After intervention, the woman should be able to maintain a level of comfort throughout recovery.

2. *Nursing interventions*

a. Manage mild to moderate pain with extra strength Tylenol or a mild narcotic such as Vicodin or Percocet.

b. Instruct the woman about the use of pain medications, anticipating pain, and potential side effects.

c. Apply ice to the biopsy site for 4 to 6 hours to minimize hematoma and swelling.

d. Instruct the woman to wear a good, supportive bra for the 1st 48 hours after the tests.

e. Instruct the woman about nonpharmacologic pain interventions, including relaxation with imagery, music, and distraction.

NURSING DIAGNOSIS: Anxiety R/T potential cancer diagnosis

1. *Expected outcomes:* After intervention, the woman should be able to express anxiety and identify coping strategies to use during the wait.

2. *Nursing interventions*

a. Provide information as needed to minimize unrealistic fears.

b. Instruct the woman about anxiety-relieving techniques such as relaxation with imagery, "stop" talk, distraction, and exercise.

c. Acknowledge anxiety and *listen*. There is no such thing as "just a little biopsy." Even benign findings change a woman's approach to breast health forever.

NURSING DIAGNOSIS: Knowledge deficit R/T biopsy procedures

1. *Expected outcomes:* After intervention, the woman should be able to verbalize what to expect and understand preoperative instructions.

2. *Nursing interventions*

a. Provide preoperative instructions for a core biopsy.

(1) Eat a light breakfast.

(2) Do not use deodorant or powder.

(3) Wear 2-piece clothing, which is more comfortable.

(4) Take no anticoagulants, aspirin, or nonsteroidal analgesics for 48 to 72 hours before the biopsy. These agents increase bleeding time.

b. Provide preoperative instructions for an open biopsy.

(1) Take nothing by mouth after midnight because sedation or an anesthetic may be used.

(2) Use no deodorant or powder if wire localization will occur with the biopsy.

c. Provide postoperative instructions.

(1) Explain methods for managing pain.

(2) Instruct the woman about signs of infection. Explain that infection usually manifests 48 to 72 hours after the biopsy. Watch for skin that is hot to touch; redness; or an increase in level of pain, swelling, or purulent drainage.

(3) Inform the woman that ecchymosis may take 2 to 3 days to manifest completely and often appears in dependent positions in the breast.

(4) If a Penrose drain is in place, instruct the woman about dressing changes, if appropriate.

LEARNING/TEACHING GUIDELINES
for Self-Care After Mastectomy

General Overview

1. Describe the general course of recovery after mastectomy, including expected sensations, drains, incisions, dressings, and activities.
2. Individualize all instruction depending on the extent of surgery, reconstruction, and general health of the woman.
3. Provide detailed information for the immediate discharge period and general information with available resources needed for long-term recovery.
4. Provide as much information as possible in writing. With shortened hospital stays, many women are still under the effects of narcotics and anesthesia during instruction and need written material to reinforce teaching.
5. Provide surgeon-specific information, or instruct the woman when she can shower, shave her axilla, use deodorant, exercise, and use public swimming pools.

Drain Care

1. With shorter hospital stays, many women are discharged with surgical drains.
2. Discuss clean technique and the importance of hand washing before and after emptying drains.
3. Discuss the importance of keeping the drain secured to prevent it from being dislodged. The drain can be secured with a safety pin to clothing, or with new postsurgical belts or lingerie. If the surgeon allows showering with the drain in place, the woman can pin the drain to a cloth belt tied around the waist during the shower.
4. Demonstrate how to empty, reestablish vacuum, and close the drain.
5. Instruct on how to measure and record the amount of drainage.
6. If the drain is dislodged, instruct the woman to place a sterile gauze over the drain site and call her physician.

Incision Care

1. Inform the woman on dressing changes, if necessary. The dressings are rarely necessary for drainage (except possibly at the drain site) but may provide comfort to the chest during the immediate postoperative period.
2. Provide instructions on return appointments for suture or staple removal, if these are used to close the incision.
3. Inform the woman that the incision and surrounding area may have many different sensations, including phantom breast sensations, numbness, shooting pains, pruritus, and surgical pain. If an axillary node dissection was performed, the woman may experi-

ence numbness in the back of the arm extended down to the elbow, which usually resolves 1 to 2 weeks after surgery. Some women experience residual numbness.
4. If possible, show the woman the different options that are available in breast prostheses. During the immediate postoperative period, a woman may feel more comfortable wearing cotton T-shirts or specially designed camisoles with a pocket for a soft, lightweight cotton breast form. Over the first few weeks after surgery, a lightweight breast form is the most comfortable on the chest. Once the chest has completely healed, a weighted, properly fitted prosthesis will aid in restoring the woman's balance, posture, and self-esteem.

Exercise and Activity

1. Encourage the use of the arm after axillary node dissection for activities of personal hygiene like brushing teeth and eating. Instruct the woman to avoid stretching the arm away from the body or overhead until the drain has been removed.
2. Demonstrate exercises that help stretch the arm after drain removal. Tell the woman to inform her physician if full range of motion has not returned within a month after surgery.
3. Inform the woman to avoid heavy lifting, heavy housework, or strenuous sports activities (water skiing, weight lifting), generally for 6 to 8 weeks after mastectomy and 8 to 12 weeks after reconstructive surgery.
4. Emphasize the benefit of light aerobic activity, such as walking or riding a stationary bike, in reducing side effects of adjuvant therapy and improving a sense of well-being after surgery.
5. Encourage the return to normal sexual activities as soon as the woman is ready. Changes in positioning may be necessary if the chest wall is tender after the surgery.

Diet and Nutrition

1. Instruct the woman on the importance of maintaining a well-balanced diet during recovery and any follow-up therapy.
2. Inform the woman who is receiving adjuvant chemotherapy or postoperative radiation therapy that the average weight gain is 10 to 20 pounds. She should avoid increasing or decreasing caloric intake at this time.
3. Instruct the woman to talk with her physician about supplemental vitamins.
4. Provide information about the American Cancer Society and National Cancer Institute's Diet Recommendations:

(5) Explain that the woman usually can shower within 24 to 48 hours.

NURSING DIAGNOSIS: Knowledge deficit R/T breast cancer diagnosis and treatment options

1. *Expected outcomes:* After intervention, the woman should be able to verbalize the type of breast cancer she has and treatment options that are available (see Learning/Teaching Guidelines for Self-Care After Mastectomy).
2. *Nursing interventions*
   a. Help the woman focus on information gathering and decision making 1 phase of treatment at a time, to minimize information overload and feeling overwhelmed.
   b. Explain that the 1st decision is usually the type of local therapy—breast conservation versus mastectomy, with or without reconstruction.
   c. Explain that the many sources of information available include the following:
      (1) Books and videos
      (2) National Cancer Institute Cancer Information Hotline (1–800–4CANCER)
      (3) Y-me (1–800–221–2141) and the American Cancer Society (1–800–ACS–2345), both of which have early support programs from which women can receive support and guidance from breast cancer survivors.
      (4) A clinical nurse specialist or social worker, for whom a referral can be obtained, to help process information and identify resources

NURSING DIAGNOSIS: Pain R/T postoperative condition

1. *Expected outcomes:* After intervention, the woman should be able to maintain an acceptable level of comfort throughout recovery.
2. *Nursing interventions*

a. Monitor pain regularly and document the level of pain before and after the administration of medications.
b. Administer analgesics as needed.
   (1) Oral narcotics such as Vicodin or Percocet are usually all that is required for axillary node dissection, lumpectomy, or mastectomy without reconstruction.
   (2) Intravenous morphine, which is often delivered through a patient-controlled analgesic pump, is usually necessary for the first 24 to 48 hours after autologous tissue reconstruction.
c. Instruct the patient to anticipate pain medication needs before the pain becomes severe.
d. Position the patient with pillows to support the breast when on the side and to elevate the affected arm.
e. Nonpharmacologic management—including relaxation with imagery, focused breathing, music, and distraction—may be helpful.

NURSING DIAGNOSIS: Impaired physical mobility R/T axillary node dissection, drains, and pain from surgery

1. *Expected outcomes:* After recovery, the woman should achieve full mobility and strength in the affected arm.
2. *Nursing interventions*
   a. Position the affected arm on pillows above the level of the heart, to facilitate drainage.
   b. Avoid abduction and raising the arm above shoulder level. While the drain is in place, the arm may be used for some activities of daily living.
   c. Instruct the woman about doing isometric exercises by squeezing a ball, or opening and closing her fists, and also flexing and straightening her arm at the elbow several times a day for the first couple of days.
   d. Once the drain has been removed, begin exercises.
   e. If full mobility has not returned to normal in 4 to 6 weeks, refer to physical therapy. Women at risk for problems include those with the following:
      (1) History of shoulder injury

(2) Arthritis

(3) Latissimus dorsi reconstruction

NURSING DIAGNOSIS: Knowledge deficit R/T drain care

---

1. *Expected outcomes:* After intervention, the woman or an identified caregiver should be able to demonstrate skills in caring for the drain.
2. *Nursing interventions*
   a. Determine the woman's ability to care for the drain. If she is unable to care for it herself, help identify a caregiver or make a home health referral.
   b. Teaching about drains should begin soon after admission because many women are hospitalized for a day or less.
   c. Instruct the woman about the following:
      (1) Frequency of emptying the drain
      (2) Washing hands before and after procedures
      (3) Technique for emptying the drain and re-establishing vacuum
      (4) Securing the drain to clothing at all times
      (5) Documenting the amount of drainage

NURSING DIAGNOSIS: Altered tissue perfusion R/T potential or actual lymphedema secondary to scarring after axillary node dissection

---

NURSING DIAGNOSIS: Risk for infection R/T potential or actual lymphedema secondary to axillary node dissection

---

1. *Expected outcomes*: After intervention, the woman should exhibit no signs of lymphedema or related complications.
2. *Nursing interventions*
   a. Avoid blood pressure readings, venipunctures, and use of intravenous lines in the affected arm.
   b. Keep the arm elevated on a pillow while the patient is in bed.
   c. Instruct the woman about the steps to prevent lymphedema (Box 33–3).
   d. Instruct the woman about early signs of swelling and the importance of early interventions.
   e. For patients with lymphedema, refer early to a center or physical therapist experienced in treatment strategies. For the center nearest you, call the National Lymphedema Network ([800] 541–3259).

NURSING DIAGNOSIS: Body image disturbance R/T diagnosis and treatment of breast cancer

---

1. *Expected outcomes:* After intervention, the woman should be able to demonstrate coping skills in adapting to body image changes.
2. *Nursing interventions*
   a. Offer to be present when the woman initially looks at changes to her chest, although your presence may be impossible with shortened hospitalizations. Prepare her for what to expect of the physical appearance and possible emotional reactions. Many women find the 1st shower or bath a very emotional experience.
   b. For women who have undergone mastectomy without reconstruction, provide guidance about where to purchase a prosthesis. The American Cancer Society usually provides listings through the Reach to Recovery program.
      (1) Insurance coverage of prostheses varies, but insurance usually covers the basic prosthesis. Medicare pays for a new prosthesis every year as well as 2 specialty bras every 6 months.
      (2) It may take more than 6 weeks before the chest is healed enough to wear a heavy prosthesis. Many products are available for interim use.
      (3) It is important to go to a store with a full range of products and an experienced fitter. A proper fit improves comfort, self-esteem, and posture.
   c. For the woman who has undergone mastectomy and reconstruction, explain the following:
      (1) She will need to grieve over the lost breast and will need time to accept the new breast.
      (2) Reconstruction may take a period of several weeks to months to complete.
      (3) With the tissue expander type of reconstruction, she may need a temporary external prosthesis that can be changed in size as the breast is slowly inflated.
      (4) Artificial nipples are available for women who are waiting for, or choose not to have, nipple reconstruction.
   d. For the woman who has undergone breast conservation, explain the following:
      (1) She will need to grieve for the changes in her breast. The breast may be changed in size, shape, texture, sensation, or nipple position.
      (2) Occasionally, some women need a partial prosthesis to achieve symmetry in clothing.
      (3) Tattoos that mark the radiation field are very small but may be visible and distressing to some women. Makeup can be used to hide the tattoos that are not covered with clothing.
   e. Provide information about when hair loss may occur, how severe it may be, and when to expect regrowth.
   f. Provide information on where to shop for wigs, turbans, or other head coverings. A good resource is the Look Good, Feel Good program of specially trained cosmetologists who are experienced with persons who have cancer. They provide tips for wig care, makeup, and skin and nail care that are specific for women who are undergoing treatment for cancer. To find resources in your area, call 1–800–395–LOOK.
   g. Provide emotional support and encouragement regarding weight gain. A dietary consultation may be helpful. An aerobic exercise program can help with weight loss and can also improve the patient's sense of well-being.

NURSING DIAGNOSIS: Altered family process R/T hospitalization and prolonged therapy in some women (family unit may be traditional or any combination of significant others identified by the woman)

NURSING DIAGNOSIS: Risk for altered parenting R/T hospitalization and prolonged therapy in some women

1. *Expected outcomes:* After intervention, the woman should be able to adjust to changes while maintaining the integrity of the family.
2. *Nursing interventions*
   a. Monitor for risk factors, including young children, adolescent children, troubled relationships, families with a single parent, and lack of available extended family.
   b. Help the woman anticipate longer periods of recovery with larger reconstructive surgery or more intensive chemotherapy regimens.
   c. Help identify community resources.
      (1) Church groups that can help with providing meals, child care, or rides
      (2) American Cancer Society ride program
      (3) Flexible treatment schedules to accommodate family's work schedule, if possible
   d. Help the woman prioritize life chores: Which ones she can continue to do, which can be delegated to someone else, and which can be left undone.
   e. Promote honest, open communication within the family. Encourage family time away from chores and preoccupation with cancer, if possible.

NURSING DIAGNOSIS: Impaired home maintenance management R/T fatigue

NURSING DIAGNOSIS: Self-care deficit R/T fatigue

1. *Expected outcomes:* After intervention, the woman should be able to prioritize and perform activities of highest value.
2. *Nursing interventions*
   a. Provide tips on conserving energy.
   b. Assess sleep habits and diet.
   c. Encourage rest periods; however, naps do not always restore energy in people with cancer. Some studies demonstrate moderation of fatigue in women with breast cancer who engage in some form of exercise.
   d. Give permission to let go of low-priority activities or to ask for help if needed.

NURSING DIAGNOSIS: Fear R/T potential for recurrence or death

1. *Expected outcomes:* After intervention, the woman should be able to identify coping strategies for the fear.
2. *Nursing interventions*
   a. Provide meaningful information about risk of recurrence, if appropriate.
   b. Reassure the woman that fear is normal, especially before checkups and near anniversary dates of diagnosis.
   c. Provide ways to gain a sense of control over body:
      (1) Use of relaxation and imagery

      (2) Performing breast self-examination (BSE) regularly
      (3) Choosing a healthy lifestyle with improved diet and exercise
   d. Reassure the woman that many women place new significance on normal body symptoms like a backache or headache, fearing that they now represent metastasis.
   e. Instruct the woman to be concerned about any new symptom that persists longer than a week.
   f. Encourage the woman to consult her health care provider if she is concerned about a new symptom.
   g. Encourage expression of fears and explain the value of support groups. The American Cancer Society (1–800–ACS–2345) or the National Alliance of Breast Cancer Organizations (1–212–719–0154) can provide information about groups in your area.
   h. If fear becomes overwhelming, refer the woman to professional counseling, which may be beneficial.

NURSING DIAGNOSIS: Sexual dysfunction R/T altered body image, menopausal and hormonal changes, and side effects of therapy

1. *Expected outcomes:* After intervention, the woman and her sexual partner should be able to identify possible causes of sexual dysfunction, develop alternative methods of sexual expression if necessary, and maintain a healthy sexual relationship.
2. *Nursing interventions*
   a. Prepare the woman for body image changes.
   b. Follow the PLISSIT model for support.
      (1) *P*—Give the patient *P*ermission to talk about the subject and ask questions; provide an open door by including questions about sexual health in nursing assessment.
      (2) *LI*—Offer *L*imited *I*nformation about potential problems.
      (3) *SS*—Make *S*pecific *S*uggestions about how to overcome difficulties, if appropriate:
         • Pain in the breast or mastectomy site with pressure from traditional position during intercourse may require changing positions, placing a small soft pillow between partners, or positioning an arm over the chest to provide support.
         • Vaginal dryness and painful intercourse related to hormonal changes may indicate a need for lubrication. The best procedure is to use water-soluble lubricants on a routine basis, as well as at time of intercourse.
         • Fatigue may require that the couple schedule time for intimacy when energy levels are higher.
         • A decrease in libido may be temporary because of medications or prolonged hormonal changes. If the condition persists, instruct the woman to discuss this problem with her physician. Some women find relief with testosterone supplementation, if allowed.
      (4) *IT*—*I*ntensive *T*herapy may be needed for some couples who have persistent problems.
   c. Encourage continual open communication between partners about fears, expectations, and disappointments.

Discharge Planning and Teaching

1. Teaching needs
   a. Respect the patient's learning style and cultural diversity.
   b. Be aware of the limited amount of information that is absorbed during the crisis of new diagnosis and during the shorter hospital stays. Expect to repeat vital information several times and provide it in several types of media.
   c. Encourage the woman to tape-record teaching sessions and consultations.
   d. Provide written material in the patient's language and at the appropriate reading level, if available.
2. Discharge planning
   a. Hospital stays have become very short for women who are being treated for breast cancer. Home health referral may be necessary for drain and incision care as well as to reinforce teaching.

HOME CARE STRATEGIES

Caring for the Mastectomy Patient

Shorter hospital stays for patients undergoing mastectomy often necessitate home health care referrals for additional assessment and teaching. Physiologic and psychosocial management are paramount in achieving positive outcomes for these patients. Physiologic management consists of the following:

- Instruction regarding dressing changes and incisional care. Participation by the patient and family member will encourage visualization of the incision and facilitate body image adjustment.
- Instruction regarding milking, emptying, and compressing drainage tubes. Urinalysis or 1-ounce medication cups facilitate measurement. Patients can practice milking the drainage tube by using a rubber band.
- Securing the drainage tube to a blouse or robe with a safety pin to prevent tugging or kinking.
- Instruction to wash under both arms. Deodorant under the affected arm is often prohibited until authorized by the physician.
- Instruction on avoidance of venipuncture or blood pressure measurement in affected arm. Advise on wearing a medical alert bracelet.
- Instruction on arm and hand exercises. Examples include combing hair and finger crawling exercises.
- Referral to the physician for specific limitations on gardening, vacuuming, and bowling. Wearing a glove when gardening is recommended.
- Instruction about monthly breast self-examination. Augment teaching through brochures and breast models. A return demonstration is recommended.

Psychosocial management: Questions are often asked regarding reactions from spouse, family, friends, coworkers, sexuality, body image, prosthesis information, medical follow-up, and fear of future cancer diagnosis.

- Listen and provide emotional support. Be cognizant of verbal and nonverbal communication.
- Incorporate patient teaching materials. Excellent resources are the American Cancer Society and National Cancer Institute.
- Provide information about Reach to Recovery and breast cancer support groups.
- Provide a list of local suppliers of prosthetic devices. Wearing a brassiere with a soft cloth or pair of panties in the affected cup assists with cosmetic effect before prosthetic use.
- Assist in compiling a list of questions for the physician. Examples include prognosis, restrictions, and further therapy.
- Leave purchased or agency-prepared videotapes in the home between visits for reinforcement of teaching.

b. Nurses need to develop new ways to get information to women in a timely fashion. Issues such as sexuality and survivorship usually do not arise during the acute phase, and yet women may not have easy access to information at a later time.

Public Health Considerations

1. Prevention
   a. Diet: Low-fat diet, with less than 20 percent calories from fat, should be consumed.
   b. Exercise: Women of childbearing years who participate in 3 to 4 hours of aerobic exercise per week have a 30% to 40% reduced rate of breast cancer.
   c. Prophylactic mastectomy
      (1) Mastectomy never removes 100 percent of the breast tissue, so you can never completely remove the risk.
      (2) Subcutaneous mastectomy leaves even more breast tissue behind.
      (3) Should be considered for the following women:
         • Women who are at high risk because of strong family history
         • Women who have difficulty examining their breasts, both clinically and radiographically
         • Women who have persistent disabling fear that they will develop breast cancer
   d. Tamoxifen trial: A current chemoprevention study randomizing women at high risk for breast cancer to tamoxifen (an estrogen-like hormone) or a placebo for 5 years.
   e. Retinoids—vitamin A
      (1) Biologic regulators of orderly cell development
      (2) Powerful antioxidants that promote orderly cellular proliferation
2. Early detection
   a. Breast self-examination monthly, beginning by age 20 (Fig. 33–7)

ELDER ADVISORY

Arthritic changes and sensory loss may reduce a woman's ability to perform breast self-examination (BSE). Research on this population needs to determine the best method of BSE when impairment is present.

b. Clinical breast examination (CBE)

TRANSCULTURAL CONSIDERATIONS

Some cultural groups, such as Asian women, have taboos regarding touching their own breasts or having someone else touch their breasts for examination. A device (the Sensor Pad) that is currently under investigation by the FDA creates a physical barrier between the breast and fingers but does not inhibit tactile sensation. This may be useful in these situations. For now, nurses must be sensitive to the beliefs of all women.

Why do the breast self-exam?

There are many good reasons for doing a breast self-exam each month. One reason is that it is easy to do and the more you do it, the better you will get at it. When you get to know how your breasts normally feel, you will quickly be able to feel any change, and early detection is the key to successful treatment and cure.

When to do breast self-exam

The best time to do breast self-exam is right after your period, when your breasts are not tender or swollen. If you do not have regular periods or sometimes skip a month, do it on the same day every month.

Now, how to do breast self-exam

1. Lie down and put a pillow under your right shoulder. Place your right arm behind your head.

2. Use the finger pads of your three middle fingers on your left hand to feel for lumps or thickening. Your finger pads are the top third of each finger.

3. Press firmly enough to know how your breast feels. If you're not sure how hard to press, ask your health care provider. Or try to copy the way your health care provider uses the finger pads during a breast exam. Learn what your breast feels like most of the time. A firm ridge in the lower curve of each breast is normal.

4. Move around the breast in a set way. You can choose either the circle (A), the up and down line (B), or the wedge (C). Do it the same way every time. It will help you to make sure that you've gone over the entire breast area, and to remember how your breast feels.

5. Now examine your left breast using right hand finger pads.

6. If you find any changes, see your doctor right away.

For added safety:

You should also check your breasts while standing in front of a mirror right after you do your breast self-exam each month. See if there are any changes in the way your breasts look: dimpling of the skin, changes in the nipple, or redness or swelling.

You might also want to do a breast self-exam while you're in the shower. Your soapy hands will glide over the wet skin, making it easy to check how your breasts feel.

Remember: A breast self-exam could save your breast–and save your life. Most breast lumps are found by women themselves, but in fact, most lumps in the breast are not cancer. Be safe, be sure.

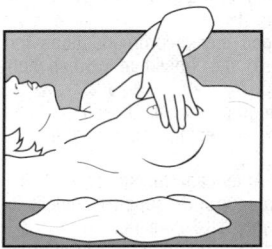 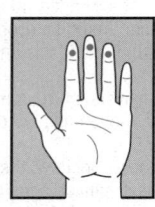

Finger pads

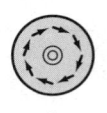 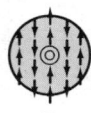 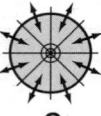

A **B** **C**

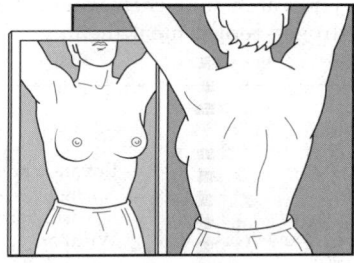

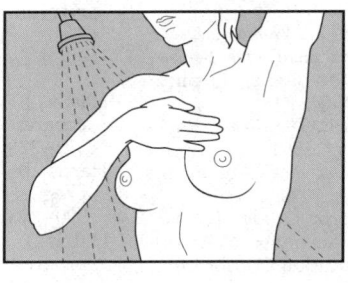

Figure 33–7. Technique for self-examination of the breast. (From American Cancer Society, "How to Do Breast Self-Examination," 1992.)

(1) Age 20 to 39, every 1 to 3 years
(2) Age 40 +, every year
c. Mammogram (Box 33–4)
  (1) Most effective tool for detecting a breast cancer up to 2 years before it could be detected clinically
  (2) Only 80 to 85 percent effective because some women's breast density obscures any occult malignancy. Therefore, it is important to use mammography in conjunction with BSE and CBE.
  (3) Guidelines:
    • Age 40 to 49, every 1 to 2 years
    • Age 50 +, every year

  (4) Controversy over stopping mammograms. Most agree that women should continue with annual mammograms until life expectancy is shortened because of other life-threatening illnesses.
  (5) Screening mammogram is used to find cancers in asymptomatic women.
  (6) Low-dose mammography is now the preferred method, with radiation dose .01 GY (1 rad) or less per 2 views of each breast. The risk of developing a cancer from this dose is equal to that associated with smoking 1.5 cigarettes.
3. Primary prevention

BOX 33–4. Clinical Controversies Concerning Mammography

The universal agreement is that women older than 50 years of age and younger women with a family history of breast cancer should have yearly mammograms.

Debate continues about the role of mammography for average-risk, asymptomatic women, aged 40 to 49.

The National Cancer Institute dropped any recommendations for this age group, leaving the decision to the individual woman and her physician.

Rationale: Meta-analysis of mammography trials does not demonstrate a survival advantage with screening mammogram in women ages 40 to 49.

The American Cancer Society, the American College of Radiologists, and many breast cancer consumer groups support guidelines for screening women ages 40 to 49 every 1 to 2 years.

Rationale: Breast cancer is the leading cause of death in women ages 40 to 44. One third of all breast cancer deaths occur in women ages 40 to 49.

---

   a. Need to educate the public about healthy lifestyles
   b. Need to support research investigating the influence of exercise and diet on women's health
   c. Need to support research into chemoprevention and the efficacy of estrogen replacement therapy

4. Empowering women to be active participants in their health and wellness
5. Secondary prevention or early detection
   a. Need to improve access to care
      • Minority women are less likely to have regular breast examinations and mammograms.
      • Nurses need to continue to advocate for insurance coverage for all people, even after a diagnosis of breast cancer
   b. Need to continue to regulate the quality of care
      • Support FDA requirements for ongoing certification of mammography centers
      • Support research to continue to explore the issue of screening mammograms for asymptomatic women between the ages of 40 and 49.
6. Stigma of breast cancer
   a. Advocate for improved media coverage of breast cancer, treatment, and the importance of early detection.
   b. Encourage the openness of celebrities who discuss their personal and family experiences with breast cancer.
7. Search for a cause and a cure
   a. Encourage participation of women in clinical trials, especially minority women who represent a very small portion of women traditionally enrolled in clinical trials.
   b. Lobby for continued funding for research.

Bibliography

Books

Baker N. *Relative Risk: Living with a Family History of Breast Cancer.* New York: Viking Penguin Books, 1991.

Bates B. *A Guide to Physical Examination and History Taking.* 5th ed. Philadelphia: JB Lippincott, 1991.

Berger K, and Bostwick J. *A Woman's Decision: Breast Care, Treatment and Reconstruction.* 2nd ed. St. Louis: Quality Medical Publishing, 1994.

Bland K, and Copeland E. *The Breast.* Philadelphia: WB Saunders, 1991.

Brack P. *Moms Don't Get Sick.* Aberdeen, SD: Melius Publishing, 1990.

Cederberg D, et al. *Breast Cancer: Let Me Check My Schedule.* Vancouver, WA: Innovative Medical Education Consortium, 1994.

Ham JR, et al. *Breast Disease.* 2nd ed. Philadelphia: JB Lippincott, 1991.

Kaye R. *Spinning Straw into Gold.* New York: Simon & Schuster, 1991.

Kelly P. *Understanding Breast Cancer Risk.* Philadelphia: Temple University Press, 1991.

Love S. *Dr. Susan Love's Breast Book.* 2nd ed. Reading, MA: Addison-Wesley, 1995.

McGinn K. *The Informed Woman's Guide to Breast Health.* Palo Alto, CA: Bull Publishing Co, 1992.

Murphy G, Lawrence W, and Lenhard R. *Textbook of Clinical Oncology.* 2nd ed. Atlanta: American Cancer Society, 1995.

Oktay J, and Walter C. *Breast Cancer in the Life Course.* New York: Springer Publishing Co, 1991.

Royak-Schaler R, and Benderly B. *Challenging the Breast Cancer Legacy.* New York: Harper Collins, 1992.

Wittman J. *Breast Cancer Journal.* Golden, CO: Fulcrum Publishing, 1993.

Articles

Breast Cancer—Overview

Harris J, et al. Breast cancer—Medical progress—Part 1. *N Engl J Med* 327(5):319–328, 1992.

Harris J, et al. Breast cancer—Medical progress—Part 2. *N Engl J Med* 327(6):390–398, 1992.

Harris J, et al. Breast cancer—Medical progress—Part 3. *N Engl J Med* 327(7):473–480, 1992.

Koshland D. Molecule of the year: An editorial. *Science* 262:1953, 1993.

Wingo P, Tong T, and Bolden S. Cancer statistics, 1995. *CA Cancer J Clin* 45(1):8–30, 1995.

Breast Cancer—Early Detection and Breast Evaluation

Campbell H, et al. Improving physicians' and nurses' clinical breast examination: A randomized controlled trial. *Am J Prev Med* 7:1–8, 1991.

Ellerhorst JM, et al. Evaluating benign breast disease. *Nurse Pract* 13:13–28, 1988.

Kelly P. Breast cancer risk: The role of the nurse practitioner. *Nurse Pract* 4:91–95, 1993.

Lerman C, et al. Mammography adherence and psychological distress among women at risk for breast cancer. *J Natl Cancer Inst* 85:1074–1080, 1993.

Metlin C, and Smart C. Breast cancer detection guidelines for women aged 40–49 years: Rationale for the American Cancer Society reaffirmation of recommendation. *CA Cancer J Clin* 44:248, 1994.

Pennypacker H. Achieving competence in clinical breast examination. *Nurse Pract* 4:85–90, 1993.

Breast Cancer—Prevention

Bernstein L, Herndenson B, Hanisch R, Sullivan-Halley J, and Ross R. Physical exercise activity and reduced risk of breast cancer in young women. *J Natl Cancer Inst* 86:1403, 1994.

Kritchevsky D. Nutrition and breast cancer. *Cancer* 66:1321–1325, 1990.

Breast Cancer—Treatment and Rehabilitation

Cooley M, Yeomans A, and Cobb S. Sexual and reproductive issues for women with Hodgkin's disease: Application of the PLISSIT model. *Cancer Nurs* 9:248, 1986.

Fisher B. The evolution of paradigms for management of breast cancer. *Cancer Res* 52:2371–2383, 1992.

Gelber R. Adjuvant therapy for breast cancer: Understanding the overview. *J Clin Oncol* 11:580–585, 1993.

Lerner L, and Jordan C. Development of antiestrogens and their use in breast cancer. *Cancer Res* 50:4177–4189, 1990.

Lippman M. Potential contributions of breast cancer biology to management of breast cancer. *Adv Oncol* 8:26–28, 1993.

Marchant D. Estrogen replacement therapy after breast cancer. *Cancer Suppl* 71:2169–2176, 1993.

Resources

American Cancer Society (ACS)
Call your local unit or state division office listed in the local telephone book. For more information, call (800) ACS–2345.
ACS professional and public resources (partial list of relevant pamphlets):

- "Special Touch: A personal plan of action for breast health." (1987)
- "Breast Self Examination: A New Approach." (1992)
- "Breast Cancer Dictionary." (1995)
- "After Diagnosis: Common Questions and Expectations of Cancer Patients and Their Families." (1993)
- "For Women Facing Breast Cancer." (1995)

National Cancer Institute (NCI) of the National Institutes of Health
For more information, call (800) 4–CANCER.
NCI resources available (partial list of relevant pamphlets):

- "Questions and Answers About Choosing a Mammography Facility." (1993)
- "Take Care of Your Breasts." (1993)
- "A Blueprint for Action: Establishing Workplace Cancer Screening Programs." (1991)

- "What You Need to Know About Breast Cancer." (1993)
- "Understanding Breast Changes: A Health Guide for All Women." (1993)
- "Taking Time: Support for People with Cancer and the People Who Care About Them." (1993)
- "Facing Forward: A Guide for Cancer Survivors." (1992)

Susan B. Komen Foundation
For more information, call the national office in Dallas, TX—214–450–1777.
Resources available (partial list of relevant pamphlets):

- "Breast Self Examination"
- "Mammography: A Picture That Can Save a Life"
- "Questions About Breast Cancer: What You Need to Know"
- "Caring for Your Breasts"

Y-Me
For more information, call the national office in Chicago—(800) 221–2141.
Resources available (partial list of relevant pamphlets):

- "Just for Teens." (1992)
- "When the Woman You Love Has Breast Cancer." (1994)
- "For the Single Woman with Breast Cancer." (1994)

Miscellaneous Publications and Resources on Breast Issues:

- American Association of Retired Persons: "Chances Are You Need a Mammogram: A Guide for Mid-life and Older Women."
- American College of Radiology: "Your Guide to Mammography."
- Bristol-Myers Squibb Oncology: "Sharing: A Woman's Guide to Breast Cancer." (1994)
- Bristol-Myers Squibb Oncology: "Sharing: A Family's Guide to Breast Cancer." (1994)
- National Alliance of Breast Cancer Organizations: "Breast Cancer Resource List."
- Rose Kushner Breast Cancer Advisory Center: "If You've Thought About Breast Cancer." (1994)
- The Mautner Project: "Lesbians and Cancer."

34

Caring for People with Musculoskeletal Disorders

◼ MUSCULOSKELETAL STRUCTURE AND FUNCTION

Structure of Bone

1. Classification of bones
   a. Bones are classified according to shape (Fig. 34–1).
      (1) Examples of long bones are the femur, humerus, radius.
      (2) Examples of short bones are the carpal, phalange, and tarsal.
      (3) Examples of flat bones are the sternum, rib, and skull.
      (4) Examples of irregular bones are the vertebrae and mandible.
      (5) An example of a sesamoid bone is the patella.
2. Gross structure of bones
   a. Long bones often bear weight and are made up of the following parts (Fig. 34–2):
      (1) The shaft, or diaphysis, and 2 knoblike ends called epiphyses
      (2) The metaphysis—the flared portion between the diaphysis and the epiphyses
      (3) The epiphyseal plate—the thin plate of cartilage between the metaphysis and the epiphysis
      (4) The periosteum—the connective tissue covering the bone
      (5) The medullary canal—the marrow in the center of the diaphysis
   b. Short bones bear little or no weight and are composed of the same structures as long bone.
   c. Flat bones protect vital organs and contain blood-forming cells.
   d. Irregular bones have unique shapes.
   e. Sesamoid bone is the least common type of bone and develops within a tendon.
   f. Bone has 2 layers.
      (1) The cortex, the outer layer also known as compact bone, is composed of dense, compact tissue.
      (2) The medulla, the inner layer also known as trabecular bone, is composed of spongy, cancellous tissue.
3. Microscopic structure of bone
   a. The haversian system, the structural unit of the cortex, contains blood vessels and lymphatics (see Fig. 34–2). It maintains and transports nutrients to compact bone tissue.

   b. Bone contains 3 types of cells.
      (1) Osteoblasts are formed in the periosteum and are essential for the formation of new bone.
      (2) Osteocytes are mature cells found embedded within lacunae, the little "lakes" of bone.
      (3) Osteoclasts are capable of resorption of either healthy or dead bone.
   c. Bone contains a matrix of organic and inorganic compounds.
      (1) Organic matrix, which constitutes 35 percent of bone weight, gives bone elasticity. It consists of collagen, protein, polysaccharide, and lipid.
      (2) Inorganic matrix constitutes 65 percent of bone weight and gives bone hardness. It consists of calcium and phosphorus.
4. Bone marrow
   a. Bone contains bone marrow, a blood-forming organ that produces most of the cellular elements of blood, including red blood cells, white blood cells, and platelets, and some immune reactive cells such as lymphocytes and macrophages.
5. Bone development
   a. Bone formation occurs in 2 phases: matrix formation, or the biosynthesis of collagen, and mineralization.
   b. Embryonic development occurs during uterine life.
   c. Endochondral ossification occurs when cartilage is replaced by bone in the embryo, during fracture healing, and in some bone tumors.
   d. Bone growth reaches maturity and maximal growth at puberty, is influenced by genetic and environmental factors, and is a continuous process of formation and resorption at equal rates until age 35 years. Bone resorption increases in later life, resulting in decreased bone mass and predisposition to injury.
   e. Bone modeling is the process that shapes bone.
      (1) It begins in embryonic life and lasts through adult life.
      (2) It serves a biomechanical purpose by producing bone structured to resist force.
      (3) Bone modeling may occur in response to abnormal influences, such as Paget's disease or vitamin deficiency.
   f. Remodeling is the process of fine-tuning bone modeling to maintain the physiologic and mechanical integrity of bone.
   g. Repair is the process that heals gross physical injury to restore bone function.

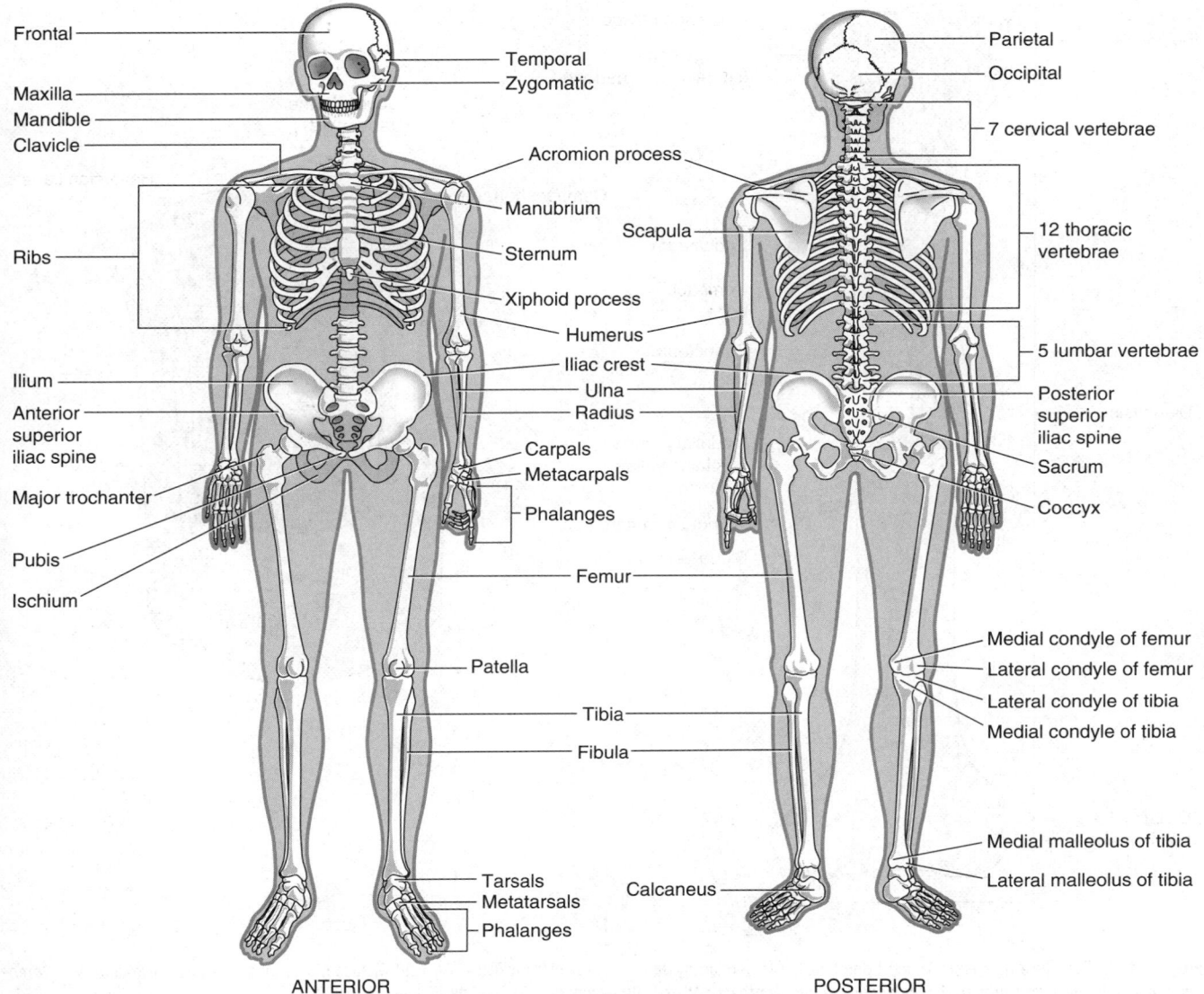

Figure 34—1. Human skeleton. (Redrawn from Black JM, and Matassarin-Jacobs E [eds]. *Luckmann and Sorensen's Medical-Surgical Nursing: A Psychophysiologic Approach.* 4th ed. Philadelphia: WB Saunders, 1993, p 1866.)

Structure of the Muscular System

1. Muscle types. The body has 3 types of muscle: smooth (see Chapter 18), cardiac (see Chapter 23), and skeletal (Fig. 34–3).
   a. Skeletal muscle is voluntarily controlled by the central and peripheral nervous systems.
      (1) It is composed of muscle and connective tissue.
      (2) Unique features include irritability, contractibility, extensibility, and elasticity.
   b. Skeletal muscles are named according to the following criteria:
      (1) Action—such as extensor (push) and flexor (pull)
      (2) Shape—such as quadrilateral (4 sided)
      (3) Origin—the stationary attachment of muscle to the skeleton

   (4) Insertion—the movable attachment of muscle to the skeleton
   (5) Number of divisions—such as triceps (3) and biceps (2)
   (6) Location
   (7) Direction of fibers—such as tranverse
2. Gross structure of muscle
   a. Muscle fibers are arranged in bundles, or fasciculi, and held together by connective tissue.
   b. Groups of bundles are similarly bound.
3. Connective tissue occurs throughout the musculoskeletal system. It makes up tendons, ligaments, and cartilage.
   a. Tendons are bands of strong, inelastic fibrous tissue that attach muscle to bone. They are an extension of the muscle sheath that attaches to the periosteum.

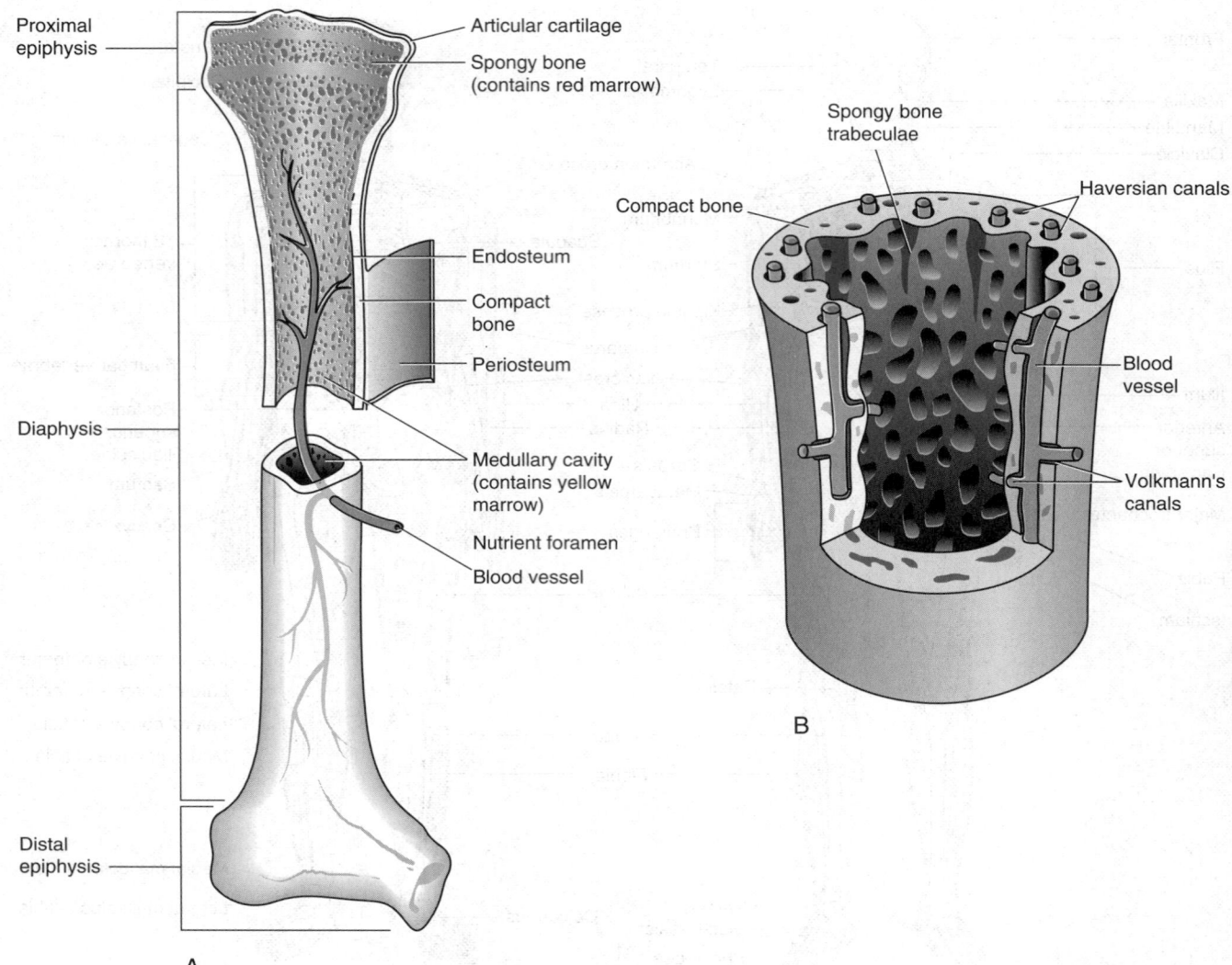

Figure 34–2. Structure of a typical long bone and the Haversian system. (Redrawn from Black JM, and Matassarin-Jacobs E [eds]. *Luckmann and Sorensen's Medical-Surgical Nursing: A Psychophysiologic Approach.* 4th ed. Philadelphia: WB Saunders, 1993, p. 1867.)

b. Ligaments connect bones at joints and provide stability during movement.
c. Cartilage is dense connective tissue that covers opposing ends of bones and is prevalent throughout the musculoskeletal system. It is highly resilient in resisting tension and compression. It has a limited supply of nerves and blood. Cartilage forms most of the embryo skeleton, slowly changing through ossification into bone. Cartilage has 3 forms:
  (1) Hyaline cartilage is the most common type and is capable of being calcified.
  (2) Fibrocartilage is found in certain ligaments, intervertebral disks, and articular disks.
  (3) Elastic or yellow cartilage is characterized by the presence of elastic fibers.
4. Joints
  a. Joints are commonly classified as 1 of the following:
    (1) Immovable or synarthroses
    (2) Slightly moveable or amphiarthroses
    (3) Freely movable or diarthroses
  b. Joints can also be classified as synovial or nonsynovial.

(1) Synovial or freely movable joints are lined with a membrane called synovium.
(2) Synovium secretes synovial fluid, a lubricant to minimize friction between adjoining bones.
(3) Immovable or nonsynovial joints have fibrous or cartilaginous tissue between adjoining bones.
(4) There are 6 types of synovial joints (Fig. 34–4): ball and socket (hip, shoulder), hinge (tibiofemoral joint), pivot (radioulnar joint), gliding (patellofemoral joint), saddle (carpometacarpal joint), and ellipsoid (radiocarpal joint).

Functions of the Skeletal System

1. The skeletal system provides shape and form to the body, protects organs and internal structures, supports the surrounding tissues, provides attachments for muscle to allow movement, manufactures blood cells in red bone marrow, and provides storage for mineral salts.

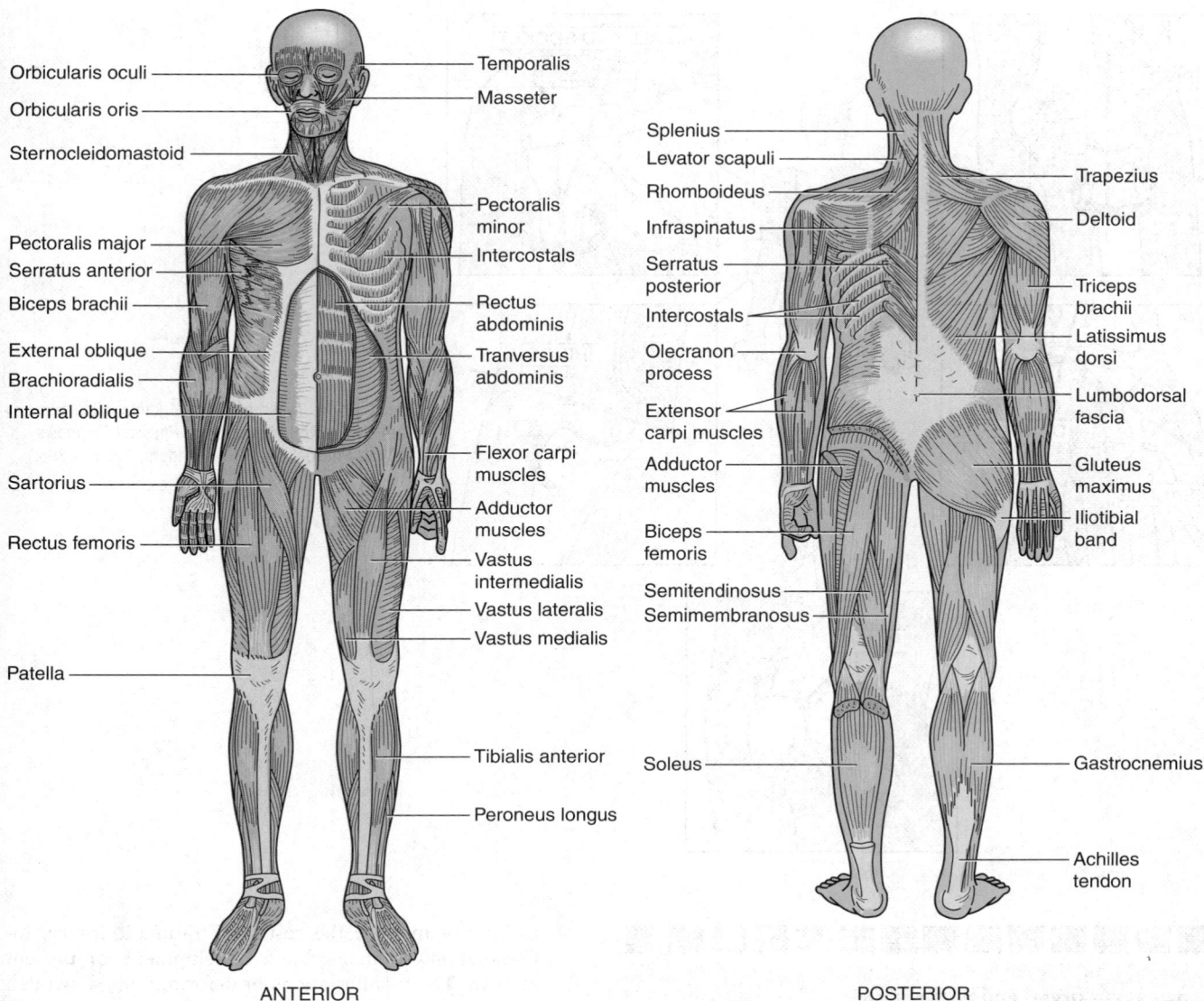

Figure 34–3. Principal muscle groups. (Redrawn from Black JM, and Matassarin-Jacobs E [eds]. *Luckmann and Sorensen's Medical-Surgical Nursing: A Psychophysiologic Approach.* 4th ed. Philadelphia: WB Saunders, 1993, p 1869.)

2. The primary function of the muscular system is movement of the body and its parts.
3. The primary function of joints is to allow movements of the body and its parts.

ASSESSING PEOPLE WITH MUSCULOSKELETAL DISORDERS

Key Symptoms and Their Pathophysiologic Bases

1. Pain (see Chapter 11)
   a. Pain is described as a personal and subjective experience with few or no objective measurements.
   b. Pain is more an experience than a symptom.
   c. Pain is elicited by threatened or actual tissue damage that stimulates nociceptive (pain sensitive) neural receptors.
   d. Acute pain may follow an acute injury or disease (e.g., fractured bone pain and postoperative pain).
   e. Chronic malignant pain is associated with cancer or other progressive disorder (e.g., malignant bone tumor and sickle cell crisis).
   f. Chronic nonmalignant pain is seen in persons whose tissue injury is nonprogressive or healed (e.g., low back pain and rheumatoid arthritis).
   g. Poorly localized pain is usually associated with blood vessels, joints, fascia, or periosteum.
   h. Throbbing pain is usually bone related.
   i. Aches are usually muscle related.
   j. Sharp pain is associated with fractures and bone infection.
   k. Pain associated with movement is typical of joint problems.

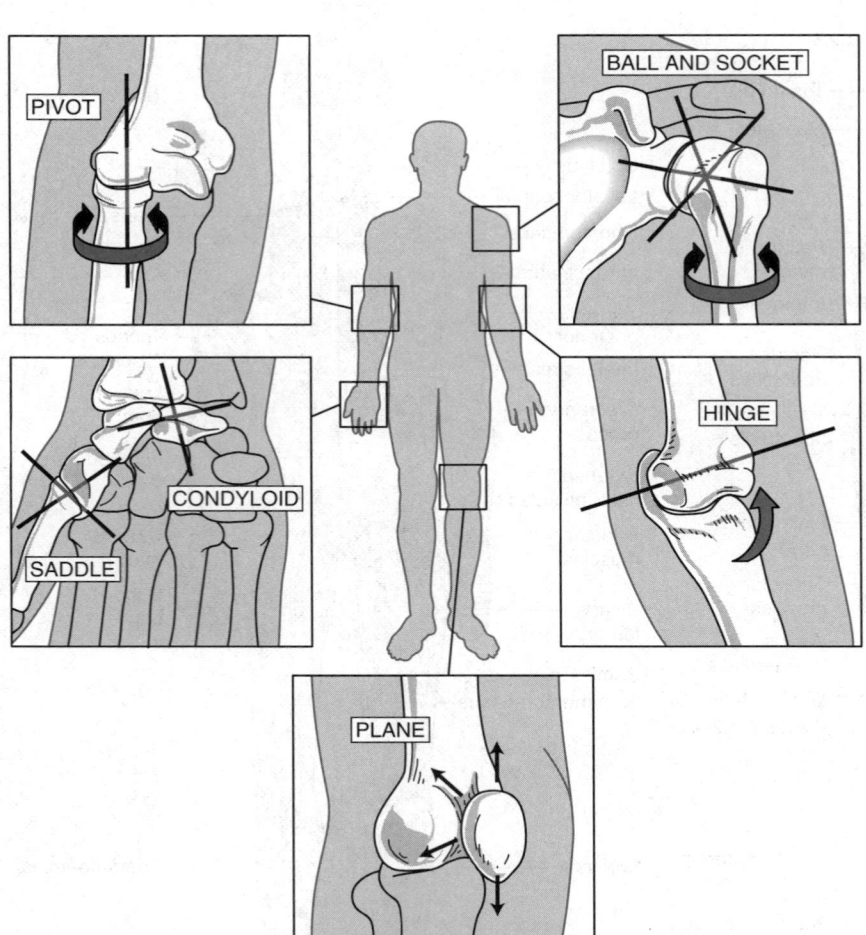

Figure 34-4. Types of synovial joints. (Redrawn from Swartz MH. *Textbook of Physical Diagnosis.* 2nd ed. Philadelphia: WB Saunders, 1994, p 396.)

TRANSCULTURAL CONSIDERATIONS

The biomedical explanation of osteoporosis as a softening or loss of bone density presents problems for Asians. Their cultural practices of digging up and reburying bones of dead ancestors belies the idea that bones degenerate. They point to the fact that the bones are there after years of burial so they must be strong to resist degeneration after death.

2. Swelling (edema) is an abnormal accumulation of fluid in the interstitial spaces between the cells.
   a. Trauma or injury to tissue increases capillary permeability.
   b. Histamine is released.
   c. There is increased blood flow to the area and decreased tissue perfusion.
   d. Swelling often accompanies bone and muscle injury.
   e. Elevation reduces swelling in acute injuries.
   f. If unchecked, edema may result in acute compartment syndrome, requiring immediate intervention.
3. Deformity is a disruption in the shape of a part of the body.

a. Deformity may be the result of traumatic injury, inflammation, edema, growth development, or present at birth. The manifestations of deformity are a swollen extremity, shortening of fractured extremity, and abnormal alignment of fractured bone.
   b. A gradually developing mass may indicate a tumor.
4. Immobility affects bones, muscles, and joints.
   a. Immobility results in the following: calcium resorption, osteoporosis, muscle atrophy, decreased strength, decreased endurance, shortened ligaments, shortened tendons, degenerated intra-articular surfaces, contracture development, and decreased range of motion.
   b. Immobility from degenerative joint disease varies with the severity of the condition.
5. Sensory changes alter the ability to perceive and respond to discomfort.
   a. Sensory changes specific to the person with musculoskeletal disorders include perception of light touch, pain versus pressure, vibration, position, object identification, and temperature.
   b. Manifestations of deficits include paresthesia (pins and needles), numbness, and tingling.
6. Muscle weakness is the inability of muscle to function at full potential over a period of time, allowing the forces of gravity to work against the individual. In the person

with musculoskeletal disorders, it manifests itself in wristdrop, footdrop, and lower back weakness.

7. Muscle spasms are muscle irritability causing the muscle to contract negatively, influencing function and producing pain.
   a. Myoclonus is sudden muscle contractions of varying intensity.
   b. In the person with musculoskeletal disorders, muscle spasms occur in response to a ruptured lumbar intervertebral disk, because of muscular dystrophy, and because of spinal cord injury.
   c. Application of heat may reduce muscle spasm.
8. Joint and muscle stiffness occurs in response to disuse or nonuse.
   a. In the person with musculoskeletal disorders, joint or muscle stiffness occurs with osteoarthritis of hands or knees and after participation in sports.
   b. Some conditions such as ankylosing spondylitis have remissions and exacerbations of muscle and joint stiffness.
   c. Application of heat may increase stiffness by increasing bleeding into and swelling of the joint.
9. Muscle cramps are a response of arms, legs, and occasionally, the abdomen related to sodium depletion from excessive perspiration. In the person with musculoskeletal disorders, muscle cramps occur during participation in sports and in response to a ruptured lumbar intervertebral disk.

Health History

1. Family history. Presence of the following conditions should be sought:
   • Muscular dystrophy
   • Arthritis: thirty percent of people with psoriatic arthritis have a family history of psoriasis.
   • Gout
   • Scoliosis
   • Ankylosing spondylitis
2. Past medical and surgical history
   a. A number of diseases can affect the musculoskeletal system.
   b. Childhood and adult-onset disorders may influence recovery from present illness.
   c. Previous trauma, accidents, or surgery involving the musculoskeletal system should be noted, including fractures, dislocations, strains, and sprains.
   d. Childhood and infectious diseases should be noted.
      (1) Hemophilia may cause bleeding in joints and produces pain, swelling, and deformity.
      (2) Psoriasis may precede psoriatic arthritis.
      (3) Possible sources of secondary infection should be identified.
   e. Previous treatments may include the following:
      (1) Traditional therapy, such as physical therapy, occupational therapy, hydrotherapy, and ice and heat applications
      (2) Complementary therapies, such as biofeedback, acupuncture, herbal remedies, chiropractic services, and transcultural therapies (e.g., herbal mixtures, copper bracelets, and the use of a talisman or good luck charms)

3. Diet history
   a. Dietary history may provide clues to musculoskeletal problems.
   b. Foods eaten by the patient on a typical day should be listed.
   c. The health care provider should assess adequate intake of vitamin A, vitamin D, calcium, and protein.
   d. Poor calcium intake can lead to bone demineralization and fractures.
   e. Excessive weight gain may place stress on the musculoskeletal system. Degenerative joint disease may be exacerbated by weight gain or obesity.
4. Medications
   a. Present prescription and over-the-counter medications taken by the patient should be identified.
   b. The health care provider should ask specifically about the following medications used for musculoskeletal problems:
      (1) Salicylates
      (2) Muscle relaxants
      (3) Nonsteroidal anti-inflammatory drugs (NSAIDs)
      (4) Corticosteroids, which may precipitate necrosis of the femoral head
   c. The following other medications may influence recovery:
      (1) Anticoagulants that may produce hemarthrosis (blood in joint)
      (2) Anticonvulsants that may cause osteomalacia
      (3) Hormone replacement therapy with estrogen in postmenopausal woman that modifies the effects of osteoporosis
5. Occupation
   a. Certain occupations require everyday activities that may predispose a person to musculoskeletal injuries. Examples are heavy lifting, strenuous activity, and repeated motions.
   b. Low back pain can arise in individuals who do a lot of driving.
   c. Habitually carrying heavy objects may place uneven pressure on the spinal column.
6. Lifestyle
   a. Habits and lifestyle can increase the risk of development of musculoskeletal disorders.
   b. Lack of exercise produces poor muscle tone that may lead to muscle strain.
   c. Contact sports such as football or hockey may lead to injury or fracture. Participants should do the following:
      (1) Use proper safety equipment
      (2) Warm up sufficiently before participating in exercises or sports
   d. There is a high incidence of accidental injury among people who pay little attention to safety practices.
   e. Abuse of alcohol and drugs influences judgment and may lead to motor vehicle or sport injury.

Physical Examination

1. The examination proceeds from head to toe, proximal to distal, assessing bones, muscles, and joints (see Chapter 5).
2. One side of the body is compared with the other.

In this section we are interested in learning how your illness affects your ability to function in daily life.

Name _____

Date _____

• Please check the one response which best describes your usual abilities OVER THE PAST WEEK:

	Without ANY Difficulty	With SOME Difficulty	With MUCH Difficulty	UNABLE To Do	FOR PHYSICIAN USE ONLY DO NOT WRITE IN THIS COLUMN
DRESSING & GROOMING					_____
Are you able to:					
Dress yourself including tying shoelaces and doing buttons?	_____	_____	_____	_____	
Shampoo your hair?	_____	_____	_____	_____	
ARISING					_____
Are you able to:					
Stand up from an armless straight chair?	_____	_____	_____	_____	
Get in and out of bed?	_____	_____	_____	_____	
EATING					_____
Are you able to:					
Cut your meat?	_____	_____	_____	_____	
Lift a full cup or glass to your mouth?	_____	_____	_____	_____	
Open a new milk carton?	_____	_____	_____	_____	
WALKING					_____
Are you able to:					
Walk outdoors on flat ground?	_____	_____	_____	_____	
Climb up five steps?	_____	_____	_____	_____	

• Please check any AIDS OR DEVICES that you usually use for any of these activities:

_____ Cane

_____ Walker

_____ Crutches

_____ Wheelchair

_____ Devices Used for Dressing (button hook, zipper pull, long-handled shoehorn, etc.)

_____ Built-Up or Special Utensils

_____ Special or Built-Up Chair

_____ Other (Specify: _____)

• Please check any categories for which you usually need HELP FROM ANOTHER PERSON:

_____ Dressing and Grooming

_____ Arising

_____ Eating

_____ Walking

Figure 34–5. Stanford Arthritis Center Disability and Discomfort Scale. (Reprinted with permission from James F Fries, MD, Department of Medicine, Stanford University, 1981.)

3. The examination should reflect the influence of musculoskeletal functioning on activities of daily living.
4. Figure 34–5 shows the Stanford Arthritis Center Disability and Discomfort Scale.

Diagnostic Studies

1. Special tests (Table 34–1)
2. Special laboratory studies (Table 34–2 and 34–3)

• Please check the one response which best describes your usual abilities OVER THE PAST WEEK:

	Without ANY Difficulty	With SOME Difficulty	With MUCH Difficulty	UNABLE To Do	FOR PHYSICIAN USE ONLY DO NOT WRITE IN THIS COLUMN
HYGIENE					————
Are you able to:					
Wash and dry your entire body?	————	————	————	————	
Take a tub bath?	————	————	————	————	
Get on and off the toilet?	————	————	————	————	
REACH					————
Are you able to:					
Reach and get down a 5-pound object (such as a bag of sugar) from just above your head?	————	————	————	————	
Bend down to pick up clothing from the floor?	————	————	————	————	
GRIP					
Are you able to:					
Open car doors?	————	————	————	————	
Open jars which have been previously opened?	————	————	————	————	
Turn faucets on and off?	————	————	————	————	
ACTIVITIES					————
Are you able to:					
Run errands and shop?	————	————	————	————	
Get in and out of car?	————	————	————	————	
Do chores such as vacuuming or yardwork?	————	————	————	————	

• Please check any AIDS OR DEVICES that you usually use for any of these activities:

———— Raised Toilet Seat   ———— Long-Handled Appliances for Reach

———— Bathtub Seat   ———— Long-Handled Appliances in Bathroom

———— Jar Opener (for jars   ———— Other (Specify: _____)
        previously opened)

———— Bathtub Bar

• Please check any categories for which you usually need HELP FROM ANOTHER PERSON:

———— Hygiene   ———— Gripping and Opening Things

———— Reach   ———— Errands and Chores

Disability Index   ————

We are also interested in learning whether or not you are affected by pain because of your illness.

• How much pain have you had because of your illness IN THE PAST WEEK?

Pain   ————

PLACE A MARK ON THE LINE TO INDICATE THE SEVERITY OF THE PAIN

NO PAIN   VERY SEVERE PAIN

├───┤
0   100

Figure 34–5. *Continued*

3. Bone marrow examination
   a. The primary function of bone marrow is to manufacture erythrocytes, leukocytes, and platelets.
   b. Examination includes aspiration, biopsy, and microscopic evaluation of red marrow.
   c. Results are used to confirm or rule out a suspected diagnosis, plan the course of treatment, and evaluate response to treatment.
   d. Musculoskeletal assessment indications include osteoporosis, metabolic bone disease, multiple myo-

Scoring

Each category (DRESSING AND GROOMING, ARISING, etc.) has two or more component questions.

Possible responses for the component questions are:

Without ANY difficulty = 0
With SOME difficulty = 1
With MUCH difficulty = 2
UNABLE to do   = 3

The highest score for any component question determines the score for that category. If a component question is left blank or the response is too ambiguous to assign a score, then the score for that category is determined by the remaining completed question(s). If all component questions are blank, then the category is left blank.

If the patient's mark is between the response columns, then move it to the closest one. If it's directly between the two, move it to the higher one.

If either devices and/or help from another person is checked for a category, the score = 2. This may determine the score unless the score on any other component question = 3. For example, the response to "Dress yourself…" is with SOME difficulty (score = 1). The patient has checked the use of a device for dressing, thereby increasing the score to 2. The response to "Shampoo your hair…" is UNABLE to do (score = 3). Therefore, the score for DRESSING category is 3.

Devices associated with each category:

DRESSING & GROOMING	Devices used for dressing (button hook, zipper pull, long-handled shoehorn, etc.)
ARISING	built-up or special chair
EATING	built-up or special utensils
WALKING	cane, walker, crutches
HYGIENE	Raised toilet seat bathtub seat bathtub bar long-handled appliances in bathroom
REACH	long-handled appliances for reach
GRIP	jar opener (for jars previously opened)

Devices written in the "Other" sections are considered only if they would be used for any of the stated categories.

Disability Index Calculation:

The index is calculated by adding the scores for each of the categories and dividing by the number of categories answered. This gives a score in the 0 to 3.0 range.

Pain Severity Coding

Pain is measured on a visual analog scale (a horizontal line where each end represents opposite ends of a continuum) 15 cm long, with "no pain" or 0 at one end and "very severe pain" or 100 at the other.

A score from 0 to 3.0 is determined based on the location of the respondent's mark. Some patients put more than one mark on the line. If that is the case, take the midpoint.

Using a metric rule, measure the distance from the left-hand side of the line to the mark (0 to 15.0 cm) and multiply by 0.2 to obtain a value from 0 to 3.0. Round to the even number of cm if the mark falls between two points. For example, if the mark is between 4.2 and 4.3 cm, use 4.2. There is a pain severity coding sheet (which follows) for your use. It converts the number of cm into the appropriate score.

PAIN SEVERITY CODING
(USING THE VISUAL ANALOG SCALE)

MEASUREMENT (CM) = SCORE	MEASUREMENT (CM) = SCORE
0 = 0	
.1 − .7 = .1	7.8 − 8.2 = 1.6
.8 − 1.2 = .2	8.3 − 8.7 = 1.7
1.3 − 1.7 = .3	8.8 − 9.2 = 1.8
1.8 − 2.2 = .4	9.3 − 9.7 = 1.9
2.3 − 2.7 = .5	9.8 − 10.2 = 2.0
2.8 − 3.2 = .6	10.3 − 10.7 = 2.1
3.3 − 3.7 = .7	10.8 − 11.2 = 2.2
3.8 − 4.2 = .8	11.3 − 11.7 = 2.3
4.3 − 4.7 = .9	11.8 − 12.2 = 2.4
4.8 − 5.2 = 1.0	12.3 − 12.7 = 2.5
5.3 − 5.7 = 1.1	12.8 − 13.2 = 2.6
5.8 − 6.2 = 1.2	13.3 − 13.7 = 2.7
6.3 − 6.7 = 1.3	13.8 − 14.2 = 2.8
6.8 − 7.2 = 1.4	14.3 − 14.7 = 2.9
7.3 − 7.7 = 1.5	14.8 − 15.0 = 3.0

Stanford Arthritis Center Disability and Discomfort Scale: Disability Index.
This is designed to assess the patient's functional ability over the past week; the patient is also asked to indicate the use of any aids or devices or if help is needed from another person for any of the activities. Responses for the component questions are

Without ANY difficulty = 0
With SOME difficulty = 1
With MUCH difficulty = 2
UNABLE to do   = 3

The highest score for any component question determines the score for that category.

Figure 34–5. *Continued*

clonia, and metastatic disease to bone (see Chapter 25).

4. Radiographic studies
   a. Radiographic studies offer a wide range of aids in the diagnosis of musculoskeletal disease (Table 34–4).

(1) Although fracture management is the primary indication, radiography can reveal bone deformity, joint congruity, bone density, and calcification.
(2) The texture, size, shape, localized destruction, and fracture of bone may be the result of hereditary,

Table 34–1. Special Tests Used to Assess for Musculoskeletal Disorders

Test	Description	Significance
Chvostek's test (hypocalcemia)	Tap the parotid gland lightly (in front of the ear).	Positive: Facial muscles twitch.
Adson's maneuver (thoracic outlet syndrome)	Palpate radial artery while abducting, extending, and externally rotating the arm. Have the person take a deep breath and turn head toward the arm being tested.	Positive: Marked decrease or loss of radial pulse during the test.
Apley's scratch test (shoulder range-of-motion)	Have the person reach up behind the head and touch the top of the opposite scapula.	Limited range of motion decreases ability to perform activities of daily living—hair combing, putting on brassiere, use of back pocket or zipper.
Drop arm test (rotator cuff tear)	Abduct person's shoulder to 90 degrees. Instruct the person to slowly lower the arms from a winglike position to the side.	Positive: Arm drops suddenly or sharp pain is felt as arm is lowered.
Finkelstein's test (tenosynovitis of the thumb)	The person makes a fist with the thumb inside the fingers. The examiner holds the forearm steady and deviates the wrist toward the ulnar side.	Positive: Experiences pain over thumb tendon.
Phalen's test (carpal tunnel syndrome)	Backs of hands are held together with wrists flexed to 90 degrees. Hold position for 60 seconds.	Positive: Tingling or burning in area of hand innervated by median nerve.
Hoover's test (lumbar spine disease; possible malingering)	The person lies supine on examination table. The examiner cups the patient's heels in hands. Ask the person to raise the weak leg.	Positive: When weak leg is raised, pressure is not felt in cupped hand supporting the other leg. Questionable attempt at leg raising.
Gaenslen's test (sacroiliac joint pathology)	The person lies on the side with the test leg as the upper leg, hyperextended at the hip. The patient holds the lower leg flexed against the chest. The examiner stabilizes the pelvis and extends the hip of the upper leg.	Positive: Can be caused by an ipsilateral sacroiliac joint lesion, hip pathology, or an L4 nerve root lesion.
Laségue's test (straight leg raising; herniated nucleus pulposus)	The person is supine. The examiner passively raises leg with knee extended until pain is felt. Leg is then extended slowly until there is no pain or tightness. The examiner dorsiflexes the person's foot.	Positive: Pain with dorsiflexion of foot.
Milgrim's test (herniated nucleus pulposus)	The person lies supine and raises leg approximately 2 inches off the examination table.	Positive: Unable to hold in raised position for 30 seconds.
Naffziger's test (increased intrathecal pressure)	The person lies supine. The examiner applies pressure to jugular veins for approximately 10 seconds. The face will flush. Ask the person to cough.	Positive: Pain experienced in lower back upon coughing.
Trendelenberg's sign (strength of gluteus medius muscle)	The person stands with back to the examiner. Observe the dimpled area over the posterior iliac spine. When the person stands with weight distributed evenly, the dimples appear at the same level. Have the person raise one foot off the ground.	Positive: Duck-like gait. The pelvis drops on the normal side when the person bears weight on the affected side.
True leg length (leg length discrepancy)	With the person supine, measure from the anterior iliac spine (fixed point) to medial malleolus (fixed point). Repeat for each leg, comparing measurements.	Normal: Should be equal or a minimum of 1 cm difference. Abnormal: Measurements greater than 1 cm difference either above or below the knee indicates leg length discrepancy.
Apparent leg length (leg length discrepancy)	With the person supine, measure from the umbilicus (nonfixed point) to the medial malleolus (fixed point). Repeat for each leg, comparing measurements.	Abnormal: When apparent leg length is unequal, evaluate for possible adduction, flexion hip deformity, or pelvic obliquity. Positive: True leg length is equal and apparent leg length is unequal.
Thomas test (hip flexion contracture)	With the person supine, flex one hip by bringing knee to chest. Instruct person to hold knee in place, and observe other leg.	Positive: Opposite leg raises off the table. Measure the area (angle) formed between the posterior thigh and the examining table to determine flexion contracture.
Anterior drawer test (ligament stability in knee)	The person lies on back with knee flexed to 90 degrees and hip flexed to 45 degrees. Secure foot of leg being tested by leaning against the examiner's hip. With thumbs on the medial and lateral joint lines, pull the tibia forward on femur with hands around the tibia.	There should be minimal movement—no more than 6 mm. Positive: More than 6 mm of movement indicates an unstable knee and a possible tear of the anterior cruciate ligament.

Table continued on following page

Table 34–1. Special Tests Used to Assess for Musculoskeletal Disorders (Continued)

Test	Description	Significance
Posterior drawer test (ligament stability in knee)	Position the person as above. Push the tibia back on the femur.	There should be minimal to no movement. Positive: Movement can be felt or observed, indicating injury to posterior cruciate ligament.
Lachman's test (injury to anterior cruciate ligament [ACL])	The person lies supine with knees between 30 degrees and full extension. The examiner holds the femur steady while using other hand to pull the tibia forward.	There should be minimal movement. Positive: When the tibia moves forward, the infrapatellar tendon slope disappears indicating anterior cruciate ligament injury.
McMurray's test (medial and lateral meniscus injury)	The person lies supine with injured leg fully flexed. The examiner cups heel with one hand and, using the other hand (fingers on medial joint line and thumb on lateral joint line), rotates the tibia medially, changing the degrees of flexion. Then, the examiner rotates the tibia laterally, continually changing the degrees of flexion.	Positive: A snap or click indicates a probable meniscus tear.

congenital, developmental, infectious, inflammatory, neoplastic, metabolic, vascular, neurologic, and degenerative disorders.

b. Preprocedure preparation
 (1) Persons requiring radiographic study need minimal preparation except when special techniques are used. Patients are instructed to sit, stand, or lie still in an appropriate position. Although taking radiographs is not painful, positioning may cause discomfort, especially with musculoskeletal disorders. Pain medication, analgesics, muscle relaxants, or sedatives may help lessen discomfort. Anxiety-reducing strategies such as relaxation techniques and imagery may facilitate compliance.

Table 34–2. Common Laboratory Studies Used in Diagnosing Musculoskeletal Conditions

Test/Normal Value	Significance of Results
Erythrocyte sedimentation rate (ESR) Normal: Westergren's method: Men, 0–15 mm/hr Women, 0–20 mm/hr Wintrobe's method: Men, 0–9 mm/hr Women, 0–15 mm/hr	Elevations common in arthritic conditions, infection, inflammation, cancer, cell or tissue destruction
Tests of Mineral Metabolism	
Calcium 8.0–10.5 mg/dl or 4.5–5.5 mEq/L	Decreased levels found in osteomalacia, osteoporosis Increased levels found in bone tumors, Paget's disease, healing fractures
Alkaline phosphatase 30–90 IU/L	Elevations found in bone cancer, osteoporosis, osteomalacia, Paget's disease
Phosphorus 2.5–4.0 mg/dl	Increased levels found in healing fractures, osteolytic metastatic tumor diseases
Muscle Enzymes	
Aldolase A 1.3–8.2 U/dl	Elevations in muscular dystrophy, dermatomyositis
Aspartate aminotransferase 10–50 mU/ml	Found in skeletal muscle, but primarily heart and renal cells
Creatine phosphokinase 15–150 IU/L	Increased levels found in traumatic injuries, progressive muscular dystrophy, polymyositis
Lactate dehydrogenase (LDH_4, LDH_5) 60–150 IU/L	Elevations in skeletal muscle necrosis, extensive cancer, progressive muscular dystrophy

From Black JM, and Matassarin-Jacobs E (eds). *Luckmann and Sorensen's Medical-Surgical Nursing: A Psychophysiologic Approach*. 4th ed. Philadelphia: WB Saunders, 1993, p 1880.

Text continued on page 1557

Table 34–3. Common Diagnostic Studies Used in Rheumatic Diseases

Test and Purpose	Normal Value	Significance
Antinuclear Antibody (ANA) ANA are gamma globulins that react to specific antigens. ANA titer indicates the presence of antibodies that are produced in response to the nuclear part of the white blood cell. If antibodies are present, further tests determine the type of ANA circulating in the blood.	Titer $\leq 1:32$	A small number of healthy adults have a positive ANA. ANA levels may increase with age, even in those without immune disease. Positive titers ($1:10-1:30$) are associated with SLE, SS, dermatomyositis, and Sjögren's syndrome. The higher the titer, the greater the degree of inflammation. A negative test for ANA is strong evidence against the diagnosis of SLE.
C4 Complement Method determines serum hemolytic complement activity. Complement is a protein that binds antigen–antibody complexes for purposes of lysis. Activation of the entire complement system leads to an inflammatory response that destroys or damages cells. When the number of antigen–antibody complexes increases markedly, complement is used for lysis, thus decreasing the amount available.	Men: 12–72 mg/dl Women: 13–75 mg/dl	Complement is increased in active inflammatory disease and in autoimmune disorders (rheumatoid spondylitis, JRA); it may be decreased in RA and SLE.
C-Reactive Protein (CRP) CRP indicates presence of abnormal plasma protein (glycoprotein) that appears as a nonspecific response to a variety of inflammatory stimuli.	Trace to 6 μg/ml	CRP is a nonspecific antigen–antibody reaction test to help determine the extent or severity of a disease process. Elevated measurements indicate active inflammation, both infectious and noninfectious. CRP is elevated in RA, bacterial and viral infections, disseminated lupus erythematosus. In RA, the test becomes negative with successful therapy, indicating that the inflammatory reaction has disappeared, although the ESR may continue to be elevated.

Erythrocyte Sedimentation Rate (ESR)
 	
ESR measures the rate at which RBCs settle out of unclotted blood in 1 hour.
	Wintrobe's method:
	  Men: 0–7 mm/hr
	  Women: 0–25 mm/hr
	Westergren's method:
	  Men: 0–20 mm/hr
	  Women: 0–30 mm/hr
	Higher elevations are seen in both men and women older than age 50 years.
		Increased rate is seen in inflammation and necrotic processes.
		Increase is often seen in any inflammatory connective tissue disease.
		An increase often indicates increased inflammation, resulting in clustering of RBCs, which makes them heavier than normal. The higher the sedimentation rate, the greater the inflammatory activity.
		ESR is particularly useful as a guide to the management of the patient with RA.
		ESR is decreased in salicylate toxicity.
		ESR is falsely elevated with excessive exercise, anxiety, pain, or dehydration.

HLA-B27 Antigen HLA-B27 antigen measures the presence of the human leukocyte antigen HLA-B27, which is used for tissue typing and tissue recognition Five series have been designated for HLA—A,B,C,D,DR —each with 10–20 distinct antigens.	Titer $\leq 1:32$	Primary use is to predict the compatibility of donor–recipient tissues and platelets. HLA-B27 is found in 80–90% of those with AS and Reiter's syndrome. It is also found in persons with the pauciarticular subgroup of JRA. Presence of HLA-B27 does not mean disease: HLA-B27 is also seen in 8% of the general population.

Table continued on following page

Table 34–3. *Common Diagnostic Studies Used in Rheumatic Diseases* (Continued)

Test and Purpose	Normal Value	Significance
Immunoglobulin Electrophoresis		

Values of immunoglobulins, serum antibodies produced by the plasma cells of the B lymphocytes, are measured.
5 classes:
  IgA—protects mucous membranes from viruses and bacteria
  IgM—first responder to appear after antigens enter body; produces antibody against rheumatoid factor
  IgG—produces antibodies against bacteria, viruses, toxins
  IgD—less active
  IgE—less active
	IgA: 85–385 mg/dl
	IgG: 565–1700 mg/dl
	IgM: 55–370 mg/dl
	IgD: trace
	IgE: trace
		Basic function of immunoglobulins is to neutralize toxic substances (antigens) to allow phagocytosis. They are unique because of their genetic coding: each immunoglobulin interacts with other molecules.
		The recognition mechanism of the immunoglobulin forms the basis of the immune response.
		Increased levels are found in autoimmune diseases, specifically IgM (SLE, RA) and IgG (RA)

LE Prep (Lupus Erythematosus Test)		
The number of LE cells, essentially a type of ANA, is measured. Repeat on 3 consecutive days to obtain the most accurate results.	Negative	Test is positive in 75–80% of patients with SLE. Positive results may also be associated with RA and SS.
Radioallergosorbent Test (RAST)		
Test measures the quantity and the increase of the antibody IgE present in the serum after exposure to a specific antigen.	0.01–0.04 mg/dl	Results are elevated with allergic reactions: asthma, hay fever, dermatitis RAST may be used to evaluate suspected allergic responses in patients on gold therapy.
Red Blood Cell Count (RBC)		
The number of circulating erythrocytes per cubic millimeter of blood is measured.	Men: 4.7–6.1 million/mm^3 Women: 4.2–5.4 million/mm^3	Normal values vary according to age. When the value is > 10% below the normal value, the patient is considered to be anemic. RBC is decreased in SLE, RA, chronic inflammation.
Rheumatoid Factor (RF)		
RF determines the measurement for RF, a macroglobulin (antibody) directed toward a gamma globulin (IgG).	≥ 1:160 considered significant in latex fixation	Positive RF present in 70–90% of persons with RA. Negative RF found in 10–30% of patients with clinical diagnosis of RA.
Two tests are used: latex fixation and sheep red cell agglutination	≥ 1:16 considered significant for agglutination titer	Positive RF may also suggest SLE or mixed connective tissue disease. The higher the titer (the number to the right of the colon), the greater the degree of inflammation. Titer is normally increased in older persons and those who have had multiple vaccinations or blood transfusions.
Salicylate Level		

Test determines whether salicylate (aspirin) level is within therapeutic range.
Test determines the severity of salicylate toxicity.
	No salicylates in blood	Different salicylate preparations are absorbed at varying rates by different persons, regardless of dose.
		Salicylate concentrations and toxicity levels are
		  Up to 50 mg/dl—no ill effects
		  50–80 mg/dl—mild toxicity
		  80–100 mg/dl—moderate toxicity
		  100–160 mg/dl—severe toxicity
		  > 160 mg/dl—lethal toxicity

SLE, Systemic lupus erythematosus; SS, system sclerosis; JRA, juvenile rheumatoid arthritis; RA, rheumatoid arthritis; RBCs, red blood cells; AS, ankylosing spondylitis.
From Maher AB, Salmond SW, and Pellino TA. *Orthopedic Nursing.* Philadelphia: WB Saunders, 1994, pp 378–379.

Table 34–4. Diagnostic Radiology for Musculoskeletal Procedures

Test	Indications	Preparation	Procedure	Aftercare
Bone scan	A nuclear medicine study that uses a radionuclide (99m Tc) to determine presence of various primary malignancies that metastasize to bone. Unable to determine whether tumor is benign or malignant. Other indications include: Fractures that may be difficult to see on radiograph alone Avascular necrosis Rheumatoid arthritis Metabolic disease (Paget's disease) Loosening or infected prosthesis Osteomyelitis	Instruct the patient that scan will take 10 min to 1 hr. Radionuclide is injected intravenously 3 hr before procedure. Unless contraindicated, increase fluid intake which increases voiding, facilitating decrease of radionuclide uptake in bladder. Patient empties bladder just before the scan. Answer all questions.	Skeletal imaging is done 2–3 hr after injection of radionuclide. Radionuclide localizes in bone and emits gamma radiation (x-rays). A normal scan is symmetric. Areas of increased uptake (hot spots) or decreased uptake (cold spots) activity are carefully reviewed.	Instruct patient to drink large quantities of fluid for next 24–48 hr. Urine is radioactive and safety procedures should be followed.
Magnetic resonance imaging (MRI)	Noninvasive examination that uses a magnetic field and radio waves to depict density of tissues in the body. More sensitive than computed tomography by identifying a change in tissue water content. Useful for examination of intraspinal contents, degenerative disk space, spinal stenosis, tumors. Differentiates among tendon, muscle and ligaments. Avascular necrosis.	Iron, nickel, cobalt, and other metals place the person at risk for displacement or dislocation of cardiac pacemakers, aneurysm clips, and electric neurostimulators. Persons requiring life support or oxygen may be excluded due to the potential of objects becoming airborne projectiles. Careful screening for any body metal. Any question warrants radiograph to verify. Remove all external metal devices or objects. Instruct the patient that examination will require 30–90 min, of which 20 will be in the magnet. The noise is significant from gradient coils. Some persons require a sedative to reduce anxiety while in the small inner chamber.	The person lies on imaging table with pillows beneath head and knees. Room is usually cool. Earplugs are needed for gradient noise. The patient must lie absolutely still.	The patient may resume diet and activity. Comfort measures taken are for any residual discomfort from lying still.
Computed tomography (CT)	CT scanner is a high-powered computer coupled with a special x-ray system. Spine CT for diagnosis of spinal cord and peripheral pathology. Fractures in areas difficult to assess.	Instruct the patient that scan will take between 30 to 90 min. Ascertain whether the patient is claustrophic. Verify any allergies to contrast medium or iodine. Contrast material may be injected or ingested.	The person lies supine on imaging table. Scanner is positioned and makes a 180-degree arc, 1 degree at a time. Loud clicking noises may be heard. In CT images, air is black, bone is white, and soft tissue is gray.	The patient may resume all activities. The patient may be sore from lying on table.

Table continued on following page

Table 34–4. Diagnostic Radiology for Musculoskeletal Procedures (Continued)

Test	Indications	Preparation	Procedure	Aftercare
Myelography	Evaluation of the spinal canal and contents by instilling contrast medium in subarachnoid space. Indicates an interruption in the flow of cerebrospinal fluid. Reveals distortion of the epidural, dural, and subarachnoid space. Often used in combination with CT scan. Provides a clear and detailed visualization of nerve roots.	Phenothiazines and neuroleptics should be discontinued 48 hours before the procedure because they lower the seizure threshold. Food and fluids may be held for 4 hours before test. Cleansing enema or colon lavage may be ordered to obviate possibility of gas shadows on radiograph. Instruct person to void before procedure.	The patient is positioned lying on side or prone for lumbar puncture. Metrizamide, a nonionic, water-soluble contrast medium, is instilled and does not need to be removed from subarachnoid space. Iophendylate is an oil-based contrast medium that tends to form globules in spinal canal and must be removed upon completion of procedure. Under fluoroscopy, the table is tilted to facilitate flow of medium. The person is secured by straps and with feet flat against an upright foot board to prevent slipping. Films are obtained as necessary.	Observe for meningeal irritation that may manifest in the following: Fever Headache Nausea Vomiting Convulsions Adverse reactions occur within 3–8 hr after injection. If oil-based dye is used, patient must lie supine 12–16 hr. If water-soluble contrast is used, patient must have head of bed elevated about 45 degrees for 6–8 hr. Because of the ability to lower the seizure threshold, phenothiazines and neuroleptics are held 24 hours after procedure.
Electromyography (EMG)	Examination of action potentials created during skeletal muscle contractions. Primary muscle disease and disruptions in transmission of electrical impulses at neural junctions. Degenerative disk disease.	No special preparation. Instruct patient of the need to insert a needle or wire electrodes to determine action potential of muscle.	The person may sit or lie down supine or prone. Skin is cleansed and electrodes applied. Normal muscles at rest have no action potentials. The patient alternately constricts and relaxes various muscles. Examination may last between 30 min and 2 hr.	Warm compresses or ice may be applied for any discomfort from pin pricks.
Thermography	Technique that measures and records heat from the body's surface. Variations in temperature are compared with the temperature of the opposite body part. Includes all forms of arthritis, carpal tunnel syndrome, reflex sympathetic dystrophy, bursitis, tendonitis, tumors, degenerative disk disease, and ankylosing spondylitis.	No physical therapy 1 day before examination. No injections 1 day before examination. No alcohol or caffeinated beverages. No topical ointments. No vasodilators 12 hr before examination. No smoking up to 8 hr before examination. No bathing is allowed within 30 min of the examination.	The person is placed in a draft-free room with constant temperature (usually 68 degrees Fahrenheit or 20 degrees Celsius) Patient sits or lies quietly in room for 10–20 min—allowing body temperature to adjust to the room temperature. A cooling spray may be used on the specific body area to be examined. Body part is scanned. Procedure takes less than 30 min.	Patient resumes diet and activity.
Gallium scan	Uses gallium citrate, a radioisotope that migrates to bone. Detects tumors, arthritis, osteomyelitis, osteoporosis, and compression fractures, and is used for unexplained bone pain. More specific and sensitive in detecting bone problems than bone scan.	Gallium is administered 1–3 days before scanning. Bone takes up gallium more slowly than technetium. Gallium is excreted through the intestines and serial enemas may be given before scan to prevent false reading on test. No other procedures requiring contrast media or	The scan takes 30–60 min, requiring that the person lie still. Mild sedation may be required to facilitate relaxation.	No special care is required after the test. Isotope is excreted through urine and stool. No special precaution with excreta need be taken.

Table 34–4. Diagnostic Radiology for Musculoskeletal Procedures (Continued)

Test	Indications	Preparation	Procedure	Aftercare
		other isotopes should be performed during this time.		
Indium imaging	Uses indium to tag leukocytes. Primarily detects bone infection.	None.	Leukocytes are separated from a blood sample, labeled or "tagged" with indium, and injected into the person intravenously. In acute bone infection, the leukocytes accumulate and are picked up by scanning.	None.

(2) All persons requiring radiographic study or enhanced imaging procedures should receive a thorough explanation of the procedure. The nurse should assess their levels of knowledge and gauge explanation toward their ability to understand. The explanation should include whether the procedure is painful, and available interventions should be offered.

5. Techniques for measuring bone density (Table 34–5) detect the amount of bone mass individuals have and their risk for fracture. The amount of bone mineral content and the bone mineral density, or how tightly packed the bone is, are measured.

6. Arthroscopy
   a. Arthroscopy is the examination of the interior of a joint with a small fiberoptic tube called an arthroscope.
   b. Arthroscopy allows for extensive, accurate visualization of the joint cavity and structures.
   c. Candidates for arthroscopy include the following:
      (1) Persons injured in an accident or by trauma, such as twisting or falling
      (2) Persons experiencing unexplained symptomatic joint complaints
      (3) Persons experiencing a disease process, such as exacerbation of degenerative or rheumatic disease
   d. In the knee, arthroscopic examination may reveal the following:
      (1) A tear in the meniscus
      (2) The condition of the articular cartilage
      (3) The condition of the anterior and posterior cruciate ligament
      (4) Synovial lesions
   e. Preprocedure care

Table 34–5. Techniques for Measuring Bone Density

Technique	Bones Measured	Examination Time
Dual energy x-ray absorptiometry (DXA) uses a double beam from a single x-ray source.	Spine, hip, total body	10–20 min
Dual photon absorptiometry (DPA) uses a double beam from a radioactive energy source.	Spine, hip, total body	20–40 min
Quantitative computed tomography (QCT) uses a conventional CT scanner with specialized software.	Spine	10–15 min
Peripheral QCT (pQCT) is a specialized version of the QCT that measures only the bone density of the wrist.	Wrist	10 min
Radiographs absorptiometry (RA) uses a radiograph of the hand and a small metal wedge to calculate bone density.	Hand	1–3 min
Single energy x-ray absorptiometry (SXA) uses an x-ray source to measure bone.	Wrist, heel	4 min
Single-photon absorptiometry (SPA) uses a single beam from an energy source passed through water.	Wrist	1–15 min

(1) Discontinue medications that may cause bleeding, such as aspirin and warfarin.

(2) Do not allow the patient to eat or drink before procedure, usually nothing after midnight the night before surgery.

f. The procedure may take from 15 minutes to several hours, usually 30 minutes.

(1) The joint is draped.

(2) A tourniquet may be applied.

(3) The irrigation system and wall suction are set up.

(4) A small stab wound is made.

(5) A small tube is inserted.

(6) Two more portals are made.

(7) The arthroscope is placed through the cannula of the tube.

(8) A light source is attached.

(9) Surgery is performed while the joint is continuously irrigated.

g. Postprocedure care

(1) The joint is elevated for the first 48 hours.

(2) Ice is applied for at least 24 hours after arthroscopy.

(3) Usually, the patient may partially bear weight with crutches.

(4) Mild analgesics are used.

(5) The physician should be contacted if there is increased swelling, elevated temperature, or increased joint pain.

(6) Follow-up appointment should be made within 7 days.

(7) The patient may shower 48 hours after surgery.

(8) The patient may return to sedentary work within 7 days.

7. Joint aspiration

a. Joint aspiration is a procedure to obtain synovial fluid for examination from any joint including the ankles, knees, hips, wrists, elbows, and shoulders.

b. Joint aspiration may be performed to evaluate inflammatory disorders, to relieve joint effusion, and to instill anti-inflammatory medications into the joint.

c. Preprocedure preparation includes assessment for allergies to antiseptic solutions and local anesthetics.

d. The procedure is performed with the physician using structural landmarks.

(1) Positioning varies depending on the joint to be aspirated.

(2) The skin is prepared.

(3) Local anesthetic is instilled.

(4) A large-bore needle is inserted and fluid aspirated.

(5) A steroid with or without local anesthetic may be instilled after aspiration.

e. In postprocedure care, the physician should be contacted if there is continued or additional joint swelling, elevated temperature, purulent drainage, redness, or increased pain or tenderness at site of aspiration.

◻ ORTHOPEDIC EQUIPMENT AND TREATMENT MODALITIES

Casts

1. Definition: Casting is the application of plaster of Paris or fiberglass to immobilize bones and surrounding tissues. This immobilization protects and supports realigned bone, prevents or corrects deformities, and supports unstable joints.

2. Types of casts include upper extremity, lower extremity, and body spica casts (Table 34–6).

Table 34–6. Cast Types and Common Uses

Type	Illustration	Body Part Covered	Common Uses
Short leg cast		Foot to below knee	Fracture of the foot, ankle, or distal tibia or fibula Severe sprain or strain Postoperative immobilization following open reduction and internal fixation Correction of deformity, such as talipes equinovarus
Leg cylinder cast		Ankle to upper thigh	Fracture or dislocation of the knee Soft tissue injury to the knee Postoperative immobilization following tibial valgus osteotomy Correction of varus or valgus deformity of the knee

Text continued on page 1561

Table 34–6. Cast Types and Common Uses (Continued)

Type	Illustration	Body Part Covered	Common Uses
Long leg cast		Foot to upper thigh	Fracture of the distal femur, knee, or lower leg Soft tissue injury to the knee or knee dislocation Postoperative immobilization following arthrodesis of the knee
Abduction boots		Feet to below knee or upper thigh	Postoperative immobilization following hip abductor release Maintain abduction
Unilateral hip spica cast		Entire leg and trunk to waist or nipple line	Fracture of the femur Postoperative immobilization following open reduction and internal fixation Correction of deformity, such as congenital soft tissue injury following dislocation of the hip
One and one-half hip spica cast	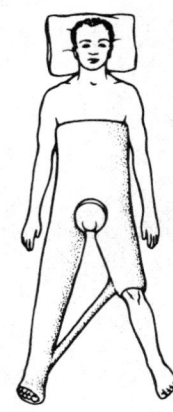	Entire leg, opposite leg to knee, and trunk to waist or nipple line	Fracture of the femur Postoperative immobilization following open reduction and internal fixation of the pelvis

Table continued on following page

Table 34–6. Cast Types and Common Uses (Continued)

Type	Illustration	Body Part Covered	Common Uses
Bilateral long-leg hip spica cast		Entire leg bilaterally to waist or nipple line	Fractures of femur, acetabulum, or pelvis Postoperative immobilization following open reduction and internal fixation
Short-leg hip spica cast		Knees or thighs bilaterally to waist or nipple line	Developmental dysplastic hip
Short arm cast		Hand to below elbow	Fracture of the hand or wrist Postoperative immobilization following open reduction and internal fixation
Long arm cast		Hand to upper arm	Fracture of the forearm, elbow, or humerus Postoperative immobilization following open reduction and internal fixation
Arm cylinder cast		Wrist to upper arm	Elbow dislocation Postoperative immobilization following open reduction and internal fixation

Table 34–6. Cast Types and Common Uses (Continued)

Type	Illustration	Body Part Covered	Common Uses
Shoulder spica cast		Trunk and shoulder, arm and hand	Shoulder dislocation Soft tissue injury to the shoulder, such as rotator cuff tear Postoperative immobilization following open reduction and internal fixation

From Maher AB, Salmond SW, and Pellino TA. *Orthopedic Nursing*. Philadelphia: WB Saunders, 1994, pp 279–281.

3. Assessment
   a. To assess the neurovascular status of casted extremity:
      (1) Palpate peripheral pulses if accessible, and compare to baseline assessment.
      (2) Compare fingers or toes of the casted extremity to fingers or toes of the opposite extremity to assess color, temperature, size, movement, and sensation.
   b. To assess skin integrity:
      (1) Look at the skin around the edges of the cast for signs of irritation.

LEARNING/TEACHING GUIDELINES
for Care of the Person in a Cast

General Overview

1. Describe the reason for the cast, and explain that it is a temporary method of immobilization, so that healing can occur.
2. Discuss the importance of watching for signs of potential complications including compartment syndrome, thrombophlebitis, infection, and cast syndrome.
3. Explain the measures required to prevent complications.
4. Discuss the importance of exercise and diet.

Potential Complications

1. Instruct persons with a cast to watch for the following signs and symptoms and to report them immediately to the physician:
   a. Numbness and tingling of the casted extremity
   b. Excessive edema of the extremity above or below the cast
   c. Decreased movement of the casted extremity
   d. Paleness or blueness of the casted extremity
   e. Increased pain or burning under the cast
   f. Foul odor from the cast
   g. Change in temperature of the extremity from warm to cold
   h. Chest pain or shortness of breath
   i. Nausea, vomiting, or abdominal pain if the person is in a body spica cast

Prevention of Complications

1. Instruct the person in the cast to:
   a. Inspect the skin around the cast edges daily. If a rough edge occurs, place adhesive tape over the edge.
   b. Notify the physician if the cast is rubbing and irritating the skin. Do not cut the cast.
   c. Do not put anything down the cast to scratch an itchy area. Articles dropped into a cast can cause infection and loss of skin.
   d. Avoid getting the cast wet. If the physician permits, a plastic bag or cast cover can be taped over the extremity so a shower can be taken.
   e. Notify the physician if the cast cracks or breaks.
   f. Elevate the casted extremity when sitting or lying.
   g. If in a body cast, turn every few hours to prevent respiratory congestion and skin pressure areas.

Exercise and Diet

Instruct the person in a cast to:

1. Exercise joints not in the cast to maintain strength and mobility.
2. Exercise casted extremity as directed by the physician.
3. Eat a balanced diet with emphasis on fiber to prevent constipation.
4. Drink extra water to prevent constipation.

Procedure 34-1
Care of the Person in a Cast: Applying a Cast

Definition/Purpose
The application of plaster of Paris or fiberglass to immobilize bones and surrounding tissues. This immobilization assists healing of fractures or assists with realignment of congenital deformities such as club foot.

Contraindications/Cautions
A cast should not be applied if there is a large amount of external tissue damage or swelling. After a cast is applied, it is important to watch for signs of compartment syndrome, cast syndrome, or excessive pressure on the skin under and surrounding the cast.

Learning/Teaching Activities
Provide the following information: (a) describe the procedure in terms that the person can understand; (b) explain that the skin under the cast will feel warm for a few minutes when the cast is applied; and (c) instruct the individual to keep the cast uncovered and to move the casted area carefully until it dries.

Preliminary Activities

Equipment
- Sheet wadding in appropriate size
- Plaster or fiberglass rolls (appropriate size)
- Stockinette (appropriate size)
- Container filled with warm water
- Gloves
- Scissors
- Covering to protect bed or floor
- Extremity holder or another person needed to hold body part in proper position

Assessment/Planning
- Check skin for open areas, rash, or other abnormalities.
- Cleanse skin gently if needed.
- Wounds should be closed and covered with sterile dressings.
- Assess need for pain medication before the procedure.

Preparation of Person
- The person should be in a comfortable position.
- Permit a child to handle cast material to reduce fears.
- If different colors of cast material are available, allow the person to choose the color.
- Allow family members to be present while the cast is applied.

Procedure

Actions	Rationale/Discussion
1. Open cast wadding, stockinette, and cast material and fill container with warm water.	1. Having all materials ready promotes a smoother procedure.
2. Position the area to be casted.	2. Proper body alignment is essential for healing.
3. Cover the skin that will be under the cast with sheet wadding and stockinette. Use additional padding if needed. Be sure to allow for extra stockinette at the ends so it can be pulled over to make a smooth edge for the cast.	3. Proper padding protects skin and bony prominences.
4. Dip the cast material 1 roll at a time into the warm water and squeeze excess water out gently.	4. Wetting 1 roll at a time eliminates waste of cast material, because it hardens quickly.
5. Apply the cast material smoothly and evenly, overlapping each turn of the roll by approximately one half of the preceding turn. Smooth the material to fit the contour of the area. If extra support is needed, longitudinal strips of cast material can be applied.	5. Using this technique helps prevent too tight a cast and does not put too much pressure over skin and bone.
6. Position the casted area on a smooth, firm surface. Place pillows without plastic covers under joints to maintain flexion if appropriate. Handle cast with palms of the hands and lift at 2 points of the extremity.	6. These measures prevent stress at the injury site and pressure areas on the cast.

Final Activities

Assess circulation and sensation of extremities. Watch for edema, keeping the casted area elevated above heart level. Document assessments and communicate any abnormalities to the physician. Give the patient cast care instructions.

(2) Smell the cast to check for foul odors.

(3) Feel the cast to check for areas of warmth.

c. To assess pain:

  (1) Assess the amount, character, location, and duration of pain.

  (2) Assess response to pain medication and other treatments for pain.

d. To assess mobility, the health care provider should observe the patient's ability to transfer and ambulate.

4. Clinical management (see Learning/Teaching Guidelines for Care of a Person in a Cast and Procedures 34–1 and 34–2.

Traction

1. Definition

a. Traction is the application of a pulling force to an injured or diseased part of the body.

b. Traction reduces fractures or dislocations; decreases muscle spasm and pain; corrects, lessens, or prevents deformities; promotes rest of an injured or diseased part; and promotes exercise.

2. Principles of traction

a. To be effective, traction requires countertraction, such as the weight of the person's body, elevation of the head or foot of bed, and use of weights pulling in the opposite direction. The person should not be allowed to slide down in bed.

b. To prevent friction:

  (1) Weights should move freely through pulleys.

  (2) The footplate should not rest on the end of the bed.

  (3) The person's body should be lifted rather than dragged when moving.

  (4) Weights should not rest on the floor.

c. A neutral line of pull should be maintained unless otherwise ordered by the physician.

d. Continuous or intermittent traction should be maintained as ordered.

Procedure 34–2
Care of the Person in a Cast: Removing a Cast

Definition/Purpose	Removal of a cast using a cast cutter.
Contraindication/Caution	Do not attempt to remove a cast on a restless or uncooperative patient unless sedation can be used.
Learning/Teaching Activities	Provide the following information: (a) Describe the procedure in terms that the person can understand; (b) explain that the cast cutter is noisy, but will not cut the skin; and (c) explain that the skin under the cast will be dry and tender.

Preliminary Activities

Equipment	• Cast cutter • Scissors with blunt ends • Cast spreader
Assessment/Planning	• Cast is to be removed only when the physician orders it.
Preparation of Person	• The individual should be in a comfortable position. • Permit the family to remain while the cast is removed, especially when being removed from children.
Procedure	

Actions	Rationale/Discussion
1. Depress the cutter blade into the cast and cut end to end along a lateral or anterior surface. For body casts, bivalve or cut both sides of the cast.	1. This method promotes smoother removal of the cast material.
2. Gently spread the cut area with the cast spreader.	2. This allows for easier cutting of underlying cast padding.
3. Gently cut the cast padding.	3. The area under the cast will be tender.
4. Lift the cast and paddings off the area while supporting the area.	4. The area under the cast will be weak and tender.

Final Activities

Document the condition of the area that was casted. Give the individual instructions for care of skin.

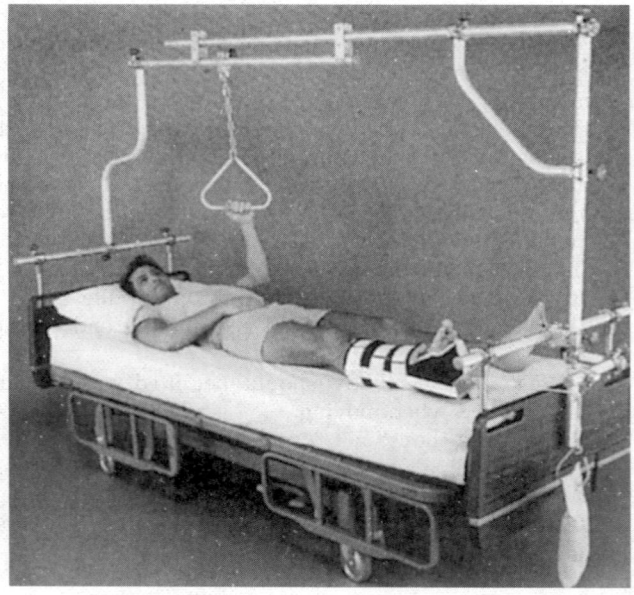

Figure 34–6. Buck's traction. (Courtesy of Zimmer, Inc.)

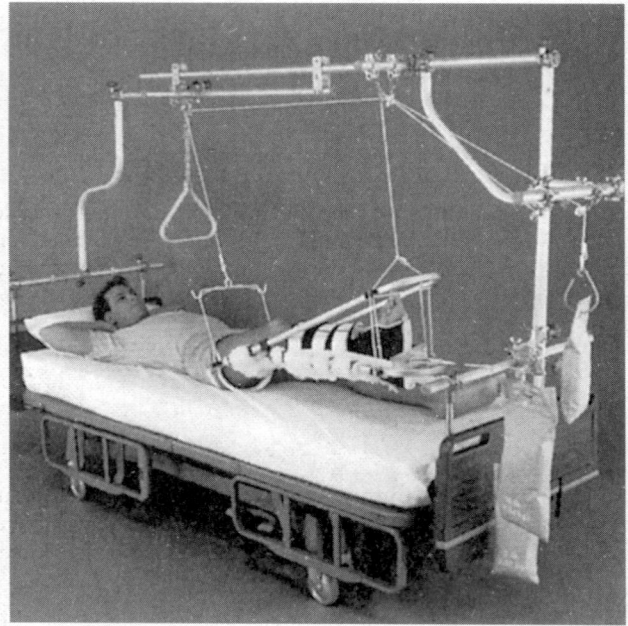

Figure 34–7. Skeletal traction. (Courtesy of Zimmer, Inc.)

3. Types of traction
   a. Skin traction
      (1) Traction attaches to skin and exerts a light pull (usually 5 to 8 pounds per extremity for adults).
      (2) More weight can be used for larger body areas such as the pelvis.
      (3) Traction is maintained for short periods of time.
      (4) Weight is applied by attachment of weight to a belt, boot, or Ace wrap that surrounds the body part (Procedure 34–3; Fig. 34–6).
   b. Skeletal traction (Procedure 34–4)
      (1) Traction attaches directly to bone, usually by means of a pin, and exerts a continuous pull.
      (2) A range of weights is used depending on injury, body size, and amount of muscle spasm.
      (3) A splint and balanced suspension may be used with the traction.
      (4) Weight is applied by attachment to pins or wires within the bone (Fig. 34–7).
   c. In manual traction, a steady pull is applied by the hands during casting, fracture reduction, and application of halo traction.

Splints and Braces

1. Definition
   a. Splints and braces are temporary immobilization devices that can be made from a variety and combination of materials, including plaster of Paris, fiberglass, plastic, Velcro, cloth, and metal.
   b. They may be individually designed or commercially prepared.
   c. They are external appliances that limit motion or weight bearing, protect weak and painful musculo-

skeletal areas, prevent and correct deformities, reduce axial load, and improve function.
2. Types of braces (orthoses)
   a. Ankle foot orthosis—short leg brace
   b. Knee, ankle, foot orthosis—long leg brace
   c. Hip, knee, ankle, foot orthosis—long leg brace with pelvic band
   d. Cervical thoracic lumbar sacral orthosis—Milwaukee brace
   e. Thoracic lumbar sacral orthosis—Boston brace (Fig. 34–8)
   f. Hip abduction orthosis—Scottish Rite brace.
3. Types of braces (splints)
   a. Static splints that hold the joint in a functional position: knee immobilizer, wrist immobilizer (Fig. 34–9) ankle immobilizer, and abduction pillow
   b. Dynamic splints that allow the joint to move, such as the metacarpal-phalanges (MP) arthroplasty splint

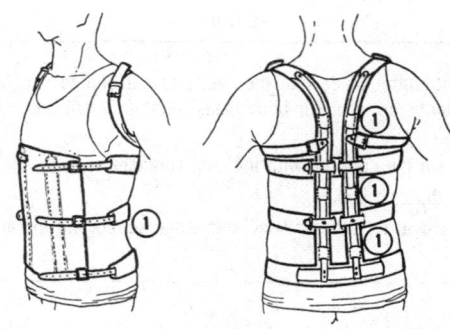

Figure 34–8. Thoracic lumbar sacral orthosis. (From Connolly JF. *Fractures and Dislocations.* Vol. 1. Philadelphia: WB Saunders, 1995, p 424.)

Procedure 34–3
Care of the Person in Traction: Skin Traction

Definition/Purposes	Skin traction is applied to relieve pain from muscle spasm or inflammation, to help lessen flexion contractures, or to treat overriding or shortening of fractures.
Contraindications/Cautions	Do not apply to skin that is damaged. Skin traction should not cause an increase in pain. Proper padding must be used to prevent nerve damage or skin damage.
Learning/Teaching Activities	Provide the following information: (a) Describe the procedure in terms that the person can understand; (b) explain that skin traction is for short-term use and it may be removed according to the physician's orders; and (c) reinforce that the individual must not remove the traction, but should call the nurse for assistance.

Preliminary Activities

Equipment	• Weights • Weight holder • Spreader bar • Nylon rope • Pulleys • Bed frame with traction bars • Traction devices: collar, boot, belt, sling or moleskin strips, and elastic (Ace) bandages
Assessment/Planning	• Know the physician's order for type of skin traction, amount of weight to be used, and length of time to be applied. • Assess the person's response to the traction: how long it was tolerated, any increase or decrease in pain.
Preparation of Person	• Individual should be placed comfortably in the proper position.
Procedure	

Actions	Rationale/Discussion
1. Check for proper size of the traction device.	1. Proper fit is needed for comfort and maximum effect.
2. Check for proper alignment of the traction device.	2. Proper alignment is needed for comfort and maximum effect.
3. Secure the traction device snugly, but not too tight.	3. Too loose or too tight a fit can decrease the effect or cause skin damage.
4. Tie the rope to the attachment on the end of the traction device and attach the weight holder to the other end of the rope.	4. This is for initial setup for skin traction. It will not be necessary to repeat this each time traction is applied.
5. Slowly add the weights to the weight holder.	5. Movement of the weights and rope should be careful so there is no discomfort for the person in traction.
6. Gently lower the weights until the rope is even within the pulley attached to the end of the bed.	6. Proper alignment is needed for comfort and maximum effect.
7. Check to see whether the position of the traction pull is direct and straight, and with no friction.	7. This position is the most effective.

Final Activities

Assess skin and bony prominences for signs of irritation and check extremity circulation and sensation for possible deficits. Document the individual's tolerance to skin traction and any other observations pertinent to use of the traction.

---

4. Assessment
   a. Skin: inspect for signs of irritation over bony prominences, around edges, and underneath the splint or brace.

   b. The nurse should check for proper fit by observing the following:
      (1) Correct position of the splint or brace on the body

Procedure 34–4
Care of the Person in Traction: Skeletal Traction

Definition/Purpose	To provide continuous traction for the treatment of fractures or other conditions.
Contraindication/Caution	Skeletal traction causes increased immobility due to prolonged bed rest.
Learning/Teaching Activities	Provide the following information: (a) describe the procedure in terms that the person can understand; (b) explain that the initial procedure may be uncomfortable, but the discomfort will decrease; and (c) instruct the individual in deep breathing, coughing, and ankle pumping exercises that will decrease chances for breathing or circulatory complications.

Preliminary Activities

Equipment	• Bed with traction set-up • Nylon rope • Pulleys • Weights • Weight holder • Sterile skeletal traction tray: towels, local anesthetic, skin prep, knife, blade, syringes, needles, skeletal pin • Balanced suspension materials: metal spreader bar, splint, leg attachment, foot support, support pads
Assessment/Planning	• Assess the person's peripheral pulses, color, temperature of injured extremity. Assess for edema, pain, and sensation. • Give pain medication or other sedation as ordered by the physician. • Obtain written consent of the individual before sedation, or, if the individual is unable to give consent, obtain it from the responsible person.
Preparation of Person	• Individual should be lying as comfortably as possible.

Procedure

Actions	Rationale/Discussion
1. Skin where pin is to be inserted is cleansed with antiseptic. Sterile drapes are applied around the pin site.	1. This action prevents infection.
2. Local anesthetic is injected around entrance and exit sites.	2. This action is for comfort of the person.
3. A small incision is made at the insertion site.	3. This action allows easier pin insertion.
4. The pin is drilled into the bone, through the bone and exit site.	4. Drilling is performed slowly to avoid increased loss of bone cells.
5. The spreader bar is attached to the pin and the rope is attached. The rope is guided over a pulley and attached to the weight holder at the end of the bed.	5. This equalizes the weight through the pin when the weights are applied.
6. The splint, leg attachment, and foot support are applied with ropes and another pulley to another weight holder.	6. This supports the leg and provides more comfort and better alignment. The foot support helps prevent foot drop.
7. Weights are slowly applied to the pin weight holder and the splint weight holder.	7. Weights are applied slowly for more comfort.
8. Countertraction is applied by adding weights equal to the weights of the pin to the splint portion of the traction.	8. Countertraction provides balance for the traction, so the person can move in bed without damaging the alignment.

Final Activities

Assess peripheral pulses, color, temperature, sensation, level of pain, and presence of edema. Document tolerance of skeletal traction and report any abnormalities to the physician. Watch for sign of pin tract infection. For persons in body spica casts, do not use the cross bar of the cast to move the person. The cross bar strengthens the cast and pulling on it could damage the cast.

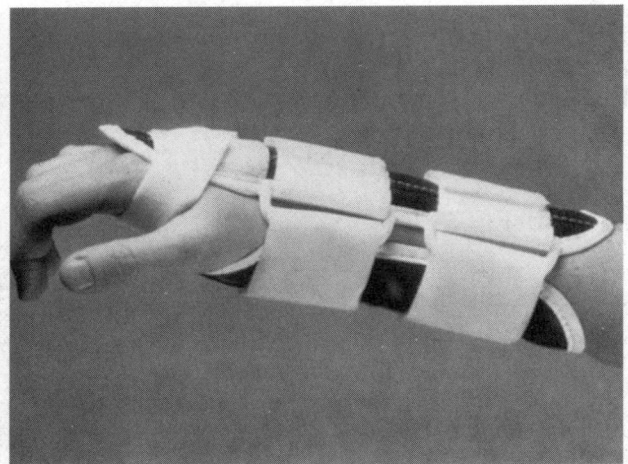

Figure 34–9. Wrist immobilizer. (Courtesy of Zimmer, Inc.)

(2) That straps are secure, but not too tight
(3) That the device does not slip down when the person moves

c. The patient should be taught when to wear the device, how to apply it, and how to care for it (i.e., keep it clean and dry; protect skin by wearing socks, tee shirt, or other appropriate cloth material under the device). The physician should be notified if the splint or brace begins to rub the skin or does not fit properly.

Continuous Passive Motion

1. Definition
   a. A machine applies gentle, continuous range of motion to a joint (Fig. 34–10).
   b. Continuous passive motion promotes early healing and assists in prevention of joint stiffness.
   c. Continuous passive motion is useful after total knee

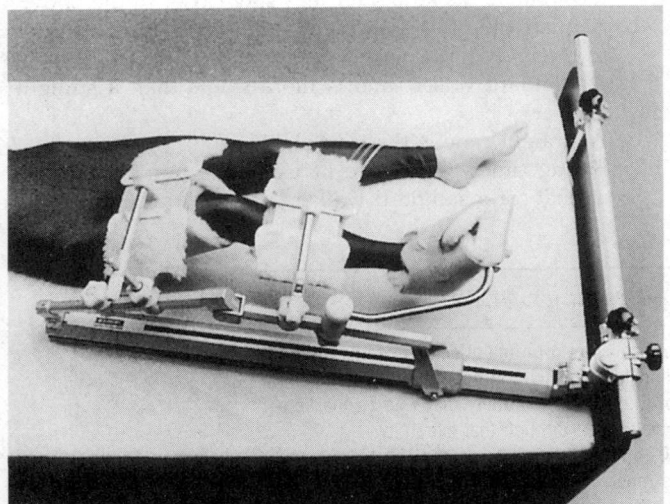

Figure 34–10. Sutter LiteLift Model 7000 continuous passive motion device. (Courtesy of Sutter Corporation.)

replacement, anterior cruciate ligament repair, and other orthopedic surgeries.
   d. Continuous passive motion can be used on other joints, such as the elbow, hand or wrist, and shoulder.
   e. Timing of application, amount of extension, and flexion, and increase of range of motion depends on physician order and patient tolerance.

2. Assessment
   a. To assess the skin, the nurse should inspect for signs of irritation wherever the continuous passive motion device is touching the body.
   b. To check for proper fit, the nurse should observe that the entire extremity is supported and that the extremity joint is in line with the continuous passive motion flexion-extension joint.
   c. To assess the patient's tolerance of flexion-extension therapy, the nurse should observe whether the person is able to tolerate increase in range of motion of the joint without increase in pain. If not, the physician should be notified.
   d. People using continuous passive motion devices at home should be instructed when to apply the device, how to apply it, and who to call with questions about its use.

Ambulation Techniques with Assistive Devices

1. Crutches
   a. Axillary crutches bear weight through the arms and hands (Table 34–7).
   b. Elbow crutches bear weight through the forearms.
   c. Loftstrand-Canadian crutches use bands that fit around the forearm and bear weight through the hands.

> **NURSE ADVISORY**
>
> It is important for the nurse to understand the different weight-bearing statuses for ambulation techniques so that further injury does not occur due to incorrect weight being applied to the extremity.

   d. Fitting crutches.
      (1) To fit axillary crutches, the person stands while being measured. Two to 3 fingers should fit between the crutch and the axilla, with crutches 2 inches lateral and 6 inches anterior to the foot. There should be 20 to 30 degrees of elbow flexion.
      (2) To fit platform crutches, the elbow should be positioned at 90 degrees of flexion with shoulders relaxed and in alignment (see Learning/Teaching Guidelines for Crutch Walking).

2. Walkers
   a. A standard walker provides a wider base of support than crutches or cane. A foldable type is convenient for traveling. It is used for non–weight-bearing or partial weight-bearing persons.

LEARNING/TEACHING GUIDELINES
for Crutch Walking

General Overview

1. Discuss the importance of safe ambulation.
2. Demonstrate the appropriate gait pattern.

Safe Ambulation

1. Instruct the person using crutches to:
   a. Wear shoes that will not slip (i.e., rubber-soled shoes).
   b. Watch the physical environment for possible hazards such as throw rugs, pets, small children, wet floors.
   c. Never walk with crutches if the individual feels dizzy or light-headed.
   d. Ask someone to walk with the person if the individual does not feel safe in any way.
   e. Not exceed the weight-bearing limitations given by the physician.
   f. Not attempt stairs unless the person has been given instruction and has demonstrated correct use of crutches on stairs.
   g. Use crutches that have been properly sized for the individual, have the axillary and hand grip pads in place, and have the rubber cups covering the tips of both crutches.
   h. Use both armrests of a chair when rising from a sitting position, so that the chair does not tip over.

Gait Patterns

Instruct the person in the appropriate gait pattern as indicated by the amount of weight bearing allowed.

1. Two-point gait: Advance the crutch with the opposite leg, then advance the other crutch with the other opposite leg. Used when partial weight bearing is allowed.
2. Three-point gait: Advance both crutches with the affected leg, bearing weight on the wrists and crutches instead of the leg. Used if no weight bearing to partial weight bearing is allowed.
3. Four-point gait: Advance 1 crutch, then the opposite foot, then the other crutch, then the other opposite foot. Used when weight bearing is allowed on both legs.
4. Walking up stairs: Advance the unaffected leg first, then advance the crutches together with the affected leg. If a banister is present and is secure, it may be used on 1 side in place of a crutch if the person feels comfortable doing so.
5. Walking down stairs: Advance the crutches and the affected leg first, then follow with the unaffected leg.

---

b. For platform walkers, arm support is applied for persons with upper extremity weakness, pain, or fracture. They are used for non–weight-bearing or partial weight-bearing persons.
c. Rolling walkers have wheels on the front legs of the walker. It is used for severe upper extremity weakness or for persons with balance problems.
d. Fitting walkers
   (1) To fit standard or rolling walkers, the person is measured while standing. With the person's arms at the sides, the handles of the device should be right at the bend of the wrist. There should be 20 to 30 degrees of elbow flexion.
   (2) To fit a platform walker use the technique same as that for platform crutches (see Learning/Teaching Guidelines for Use of a Walker).
3. Canes
   a. A pyramid cane, which resembles a step stool, is the most stable. Its straighter legs stay closer to the body.
   b. A quad cane has 4 legs. Its straighter legs stay closer to the body.
   c. A standard offset cane is more stable than a straight cane.
   d. A straight cane is the least stable.
   e. Fitting canes. Canes are fit using the same procedure as that for a standard walker.

Table 34–7. Weight-Bearing Status

Nonweight bearing	The patient does not bear weight on the affected extremity; the affected extremity should not touch the floor.
Touch-down weight bearing	The patient's foot of the affected extremity may rest on the floor, but no weight is distributed through that extremity.
Partial weight bearing	The patient bears 30–50% of his weight on the affected extremity.
Weight bearing as tolerated	The patient bears as much weight as he can tolerate on the affected extremity without undue strain or pain.
Full weight bearing	The patient bears weight fully on the affected extremity.

From Maher AB, Salmond SW, and Pellino TA. *Orthopedic Nursing*. Philadelphia: WB Saunders, 1994, p 324.

LEARNING/TEACHING GUIDELINES
for Use of a Walker

General Overview

Same as how to use crutches.

Safe Ambulation

Same as how to use crutches.

Gait Patterns

1. After rising from sitting to standing using the proper method, instruct the person to:

   a. Lift and move the walker forward 8 to 10 inches.
   b. Put body weight on the wrists and arms and step forward with the unaffected leg.
   c. Bring the affected leg forward, being careful to not put any more weight than is allowed on the affected leg.

---

  f. Gait
    (1) The person should be able to bear full or almost full weight on the affected extremity.
    (2) The cane is held in the hand opposite the affected extremity.
    (3) The cane is moved first, then the affected leg, then the unaffected leg. Or, the cane and affected leg are moved together, then the unaffected leg.

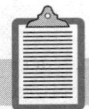

NURSING MANAGEMENT

The use of orthopedic equipment and procedures can overwhelm a nurse who does not routinely work in that area. Periodic in-service programs with opportunity for hands-on experience can assist in decreasing this anxiety.

☐ MUSCULOSKELETAL INJURIES AND OVERUSE SYNDROMES

Fractures

1. Definition: A fracture is a break in the continuity of a bone.
2. Types of fractures (Fig. 34–11)
  a. Classification by extent of damage
    (1) Open or compound fractures extend through the skin.
    (2) Closed or simple fractures do not extend through the skin.
    (3) Complete fractures extend from 1 side of bone to the other.
    (4) Incomplete fractures do not extend across the entire bone.
    (5) In displaced fractures, bone fragments are not aligned at the fracture site.
    (6) In undisplaced fractures, bone fragments are aligned at the fracture site.
    (7) In comminuted fractures, there are more than 1 fracture line and more than 2 fragments. The bone may be shattered or crushed.
    (8) In compression fractures, bone cracks are caused by unusual force.
    (9) Impacted fractures contain 1 bone fragment driven into another.
    (10) In avulsion fractures, bone fragment and tendons and ligaments are pulled away from the insertion site.
  b. Classification by fracture line
    (1) Transverse fracture lines are at a 90-degree angle to the bone.
    (2) Oblique fracture lines are at a 45-degree angle to the bone.
    (3) Spiral fractures twist around the bone.
  c. Fractures may also be classified by the following (Fig. 34–12):
    (1) Anatomic location, point of reference on a bone (e.g., femoral neck or intertrochanter)
    (2) The name of a person (e.g., Bennett's or Pott's)
    (3) The appearance of the fracture (e.g., burst or butterfly)
    (4) The method by which the fracture occurred (e.g., dashboard or bumper)
3. Incidence and socioeconomic impact
  a. Fractures occur in all age groups and affect any part of the skeletal system.
  b. Incidence of fracture peaks in males and females between the ages of 8 and 16 years, and in the older person.
  c. Approximately 90 percent of fractures cause restriction of activity or work disability.
  d. Approximately 26 percent of fractures require hospitalization.
  e. The most common sites of fractures are hand, foot, ribs, spine, and long bones of the extremities.
4. Risk factors
  a. Biologic risk factors
    • Osteoporosis
    • Neoplasms
    • Cushing's syndrome
    • Hormonal changes due to menopause
    • Cortisone therapy
    • Aging

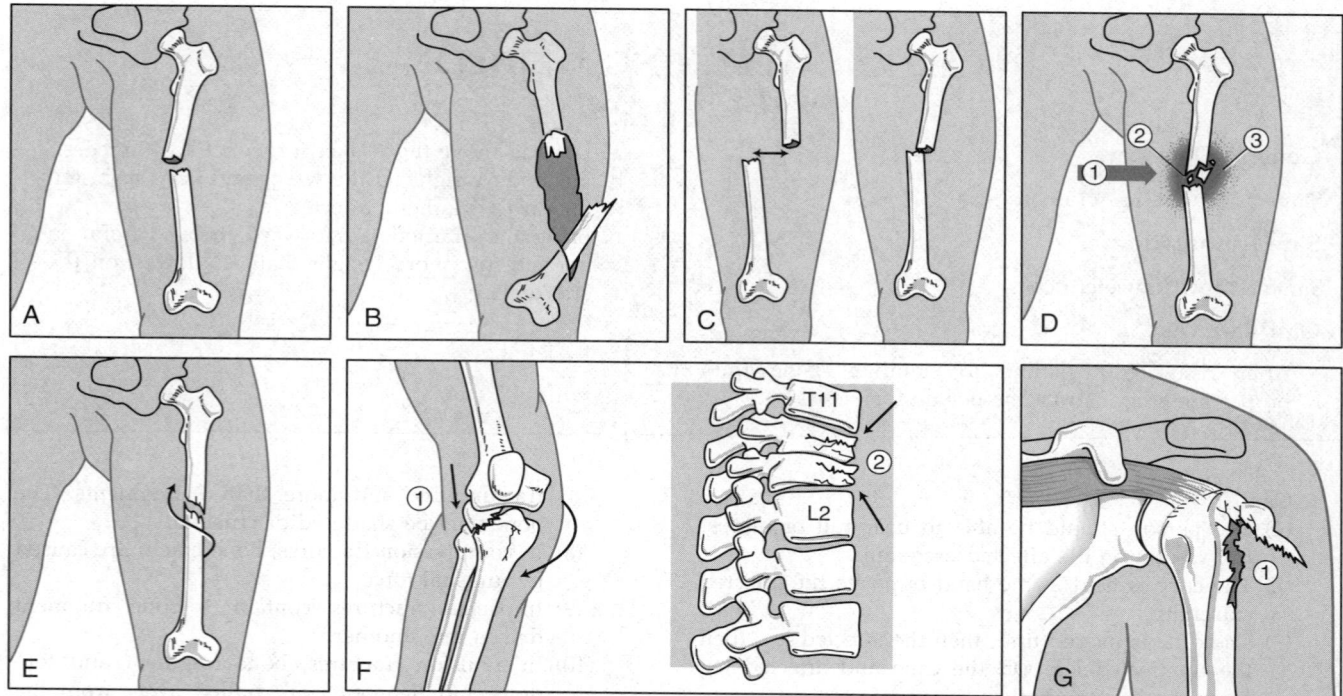

Figure 34–11. Classification of fractures by extent of damage and fracture line. *A*, Closed; *B*, open; *C*, displaced; *D*, comminuted; *E*, spiral; *F*, compression; *G*, avulsion. (Redrawn from Connolly JF. *Fractures and Dislocations*. Vol. 1. Philadelphia: WB Saunders, 1995, pp 5, 31, 29, 11, 6, 7, 8.)

- Malnutrition
- Osteogenesis imperfecta

  b. High-risk behavorial activities
- Skateboarding
- Skydiving
- Mountain climbing
- Rollerblading

  c. Child or elder abuse increases the incidence of fractures.

5. Etiology

  a. Fractures occur when a bone receives more stress than it can absorb.

  b. Fracture can occur from direct and indirect forces.

    (1) Direct force is when a moving object directly contacts the bone.

    (2) Indirect force is when a powerful force such as a muscle contraction pulls against the bone.

  c. Fractures are usually caused by motor vehicle accidents, falls, and other trauma. Pathologic fractures can also occur due to infection, bone tumors, metabolic disease, cystic bone disease, and developmental disorders.

  d. Common locations of fractures and their causes are as follows:

    (1) Sternum: automobile accidents

    (2) Ribs: direct or indirect cause

    (3) Upper extremity: direct blow or fall onto outstretched arm or hand

    (4) Pelvis: automobile accident, automobile-pedestrian accident, motorcycle accident, falls from great heights, and crush injuries

    (5) Proximal femur: osteoporosis, which may or may not be associated with a fall

    (6) Shaft of femur: automobile accident

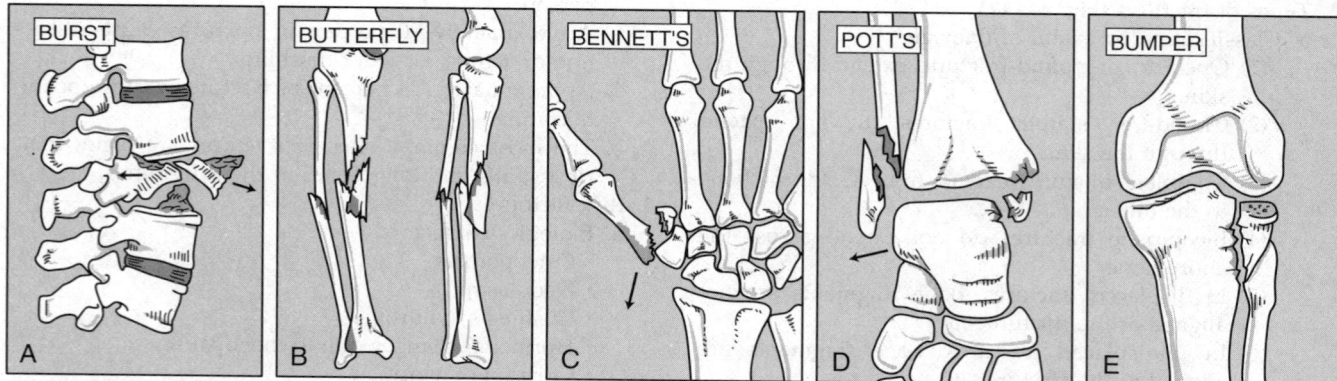

Figure 34–12. Classifications of fractures by anatomic location, person's name, method by which the fracture occurred. (Redrawn from Connolly J. *De Palma's The Management of Fractures and Dislocations*. 3rd ed. Philadelphia: WB Saunders, 1981.)

(7) Patella: automobile accident

(8) Tibia and ankle: sports injuries and falls

6. Pathophysiology

a. Small blood vessels of bone and surrounding tissues are torn and hemorrhage into the fracture site, forming a hematoma.

b. As the blood supply and bone cells begin to restore, the hematoma begins to break down and the newly formed tissue called callus begins to fill the fracture site.

c. The bone calcifies and models, and the fracture site heals completely.

d. The process of bone healing may take several weeks to a year, depending on the site of the fracture, the extent of the fracture, and the patient's general condition.

7. Clinical manifestations

a. Pain

b. Muscle spasms

c. Swelling

d. Ecchymosis

e. Change in length, stability, shape, alignment, and mobility of the bone

f. Numbness, tingling, or paralysis

8. Diagnostics

a. History should elicit careful questioning of the mechanism of the injury.

b. Physical examination

(1) Basic trauma care (airway, bleeding, circulation) should be followed.

(2) In the primary survey, life-threatening injuries should be evaluated and treated first.

- A cervical collar should be applied on all trauma cases at the scene if possible or on arrival at the emergency department.

- The collar remains in place until radiography rules out injury.

NURSE ADVISORY

Protect the cervical spine at all times until radiographic studies are complete and cervical injury is ruled out. When moving the patient, be sure to have someone support the patient's head and move the patient's body as one unit. The cervical collar may be loosened to inspect skin, but not until the cervical spine is cleared.

(3) In the secondary survey, clothing should be removed and the entire body inspected.

(4) Ecchymoses and lacerations should be sought. Neurovascular status should be evaluated frequently before and after fracture fixation, then at least every 4 hours afterward.

c. Radiographic studies

(1) Anteroposterior and lateral views are necessary.

(2) Oblique views may be needed to check for rotation or overriding fragments.

(3) Joints above and below the suspected fracture should be included.

d. Computed tomography scans, magnetic resonance imaging, or bone scans may be done to provide more in-depth views of the injury. Chest radiographs are used to assess fractured ribs and possible lung trauma.

e. Arthroscopy may be done to assess joint injuries.

f. Laboratory studies such as complete blood count, urinalysis, and cardiac enzyme studies may be done to detect blood loss and other injuries (see Chapter 12).

(1) Blood loss, which may cause hypovolemic shock, varies depending on fracture site.

- Tibia: 0.5 to 1.5 liters

- Femur: 1.0 to 2.5 liters

(2) Urinalysis shows evidence of myoglobinuria.

(3) Cardiac enzyme tests show evidence of cardiac contusion from a chest hitting a steering wheel.

9. Clinical management

a. Goals of clinical management are to manage pain (see Chapter 11), facilitate healing of fracture, and return the patient to preinjury mobility and function.

b. Nonpharmacologic interventions

(1) Application of cold

(2) Facilitate healing of fracture

(3) Prevent injury extension and loss of function

c. Pharmacologic interventions

(1) Narcotic analgesia

(2) Nonnarcotic analgesia

(3) NSAIDs

 DRUG ADVISORY

Nonsteroidal anti-inflammatory drugs (NSAIDs) are widely used in the care of persons with musculoskeletal disorders. It is important to take these medications with food to prevent gastrointestinal distress. Persons should also be alerted to watch for signs of gastrointestinal bleeding such as tarry stools, coffee ground or bright red emesis, abdominal pain, nausea, dizziness, or light-headedness. Edema from fluid retention caused by NSAIDs can also be serious, especially for older people with hypertension or congestive heart failure. Periodic monitoring of hemoglobin, hematocrit, blood urea nitrogen, creatinine, and potassium levels is recommended for persons older than 65 years of age who are on continuous NSAIDs therapy.

d. Special medical-surgical procedures

(1) Reduction and immobilization is the basis of treatment for most fractures.

(2) Fractures not requiring reduction include impacted fractures of the neck of the humerus, clavicle fractures, and in children, femoral or forearm fractures that are not angulated.

(3) Open fractures are considered an emergency requiring antibiotic therapy, débridement of dead tissue, and closure of the open wound, in addition to reduction of the fracture. The wound is considered infected and antibiotics should be started as soon as possible. Débridement of dead tissue and foreign material is essential for proper healing. Débridement may be repeated in 24 to 72 hours if needed. If the wound is not closed immediately, soft tissue reconstruction should occur within 5 to 7 days after injury, as

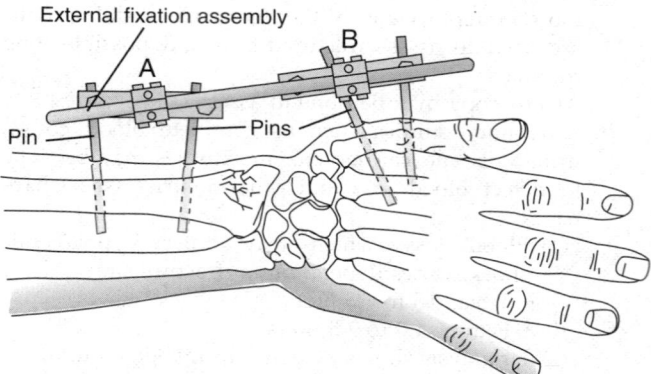

Figure 34–13. External fixator. In this example, pin set A is anchored in the ulna, and pin set B is anchored in the 5th metacarpal bone.

long as the wound is clean and stable. Skin grafts or muscle grafts may be required for soft tissue reconstruction.

(4) Closed fractures require alignment of fracture fragments using manual manipulation or traction. No internal fixation is required. External immobilization devices such as casts, splints, traction, braces, or external fixators hold fracture fragments in alignment while the fracture heals.

(5) External fixators are a series of pins connected to a metal frame and applied externally and directly to bone to hold reduction (Fig. 34–13).

- External fixators are used when there is extensive soft tissue damage or open wounds. They can be applied in a variety of positions and on various body parts such as the arms, legs, and pelvis. See Table 34–8 for a list of advantages and disadvantages of external fixation.
- A special type of external fixator, Ilizarov, was developed to allow limb lengthening by periodic distraction of the bone. The pins and wires from the device apply gentle traction to the bone that is surgically prepared to allow regeneration of new bone.

(6) Internal fixation by open reduction (Fig. 34–14) is used when closed treatment does not attain or maintain reduction, when disruption of major muscles or ligaments is present, or when closed reduction is known to be ineffective. Internal fixation allows early mobilization and promotes more rapid healing. It is used to hold bone fragments together, maintain bone length and alignment, prevent angulation and rotation, and apply compression if needed. The most common devices used for open reduction and internal fixation of fractures are the following:

- Wires and pins—used primarily for small bone fractures that do not need compression
- Bone screws and plates—generally used on the shaft of a bone
- Sliding screw or compression screw—used for femoral neck and intertrochanteric or subtrochanteric hip fractures
- Endoprosthesis—used for replacing the head of the femur when a femoral neck fracture disrupts the blood supply to the head of the femur
- Nails—intramedullary type

(7) Pin site reactions are characterized by redness, tenderness, swelling, and drainage, which may or may not be purulent. Loosening of the pin may also occur. Pin care, if ordered to prevent infection, consists of gently cleansing the skin around the pin with an antiseptic solution. Antibiotic ointment may or may not be applied. Some physicians think that it is better to not disrupt the crusting that occurs from the serous drainage that is present at the pin site.

e. Clinical management of different types of fractures (Table 34–9)

10. Complications

a. Acute compartment syndrome is a serious condition in which there is high pressure within 1 or more muscle compartments of an extremity, compromising circulation to the area.

Table 34–8. Advantages and Disadvantages of External Fixation

Advantages	Disadvantages or Potential Complications
Immediate fracture stabilization	Pin loosening and drainage
Rigid fixation with compression to ensure primary bone healing	Pin tract infection
Increased patient comfort	Loss of bone stabilization
Facilitates nursing care	Superficial and deep wound infection in patients with soft tissue injury
Ability to observe soft tissue injury	Skin excoriation and necrosis from the frame
Access to open wounds	Cutaneous nerve injury
Ability to maintain motion of adjacent joints	Muscle impingement
Decreased blood loss when used for pelvic fractures with compression of bleeding sites	Appearance of device may frighten patient and family
Decreased risk of sepsis	
Facilitation of vascular and soft tissue reconstruction	
Improved pulmonary function with improved mobility	
Fewer complications of immobility with early mobilization	

From Maher AB, Salmond SW, and Pellino TA. *Orthopedic Nursing.* Philadelphia: WB Saunders, 1994, p 301.

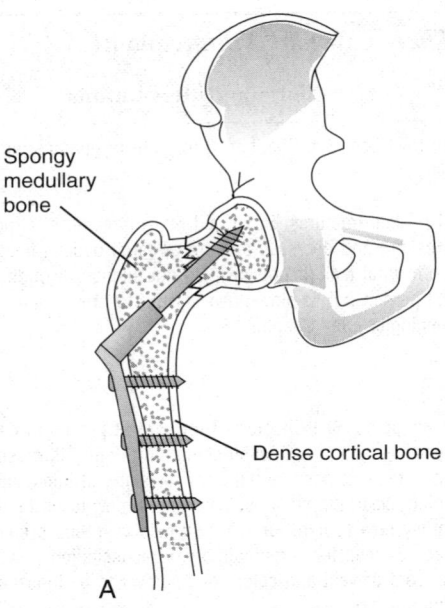

Spongy
medullary
bone

Dense cortical bone

A

COMPRESSION HIP SCREW FIXATION

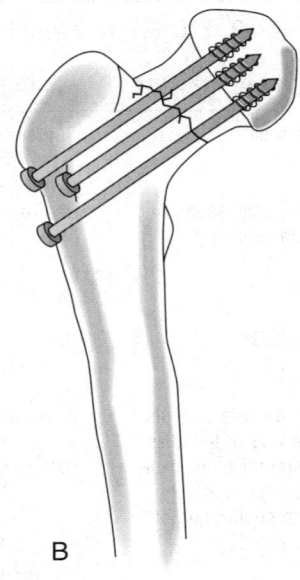

B

CANNULATED HIP SCREW FIXATION

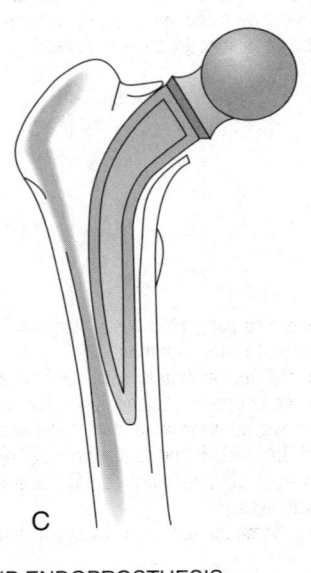

C

HIP ENDOPROSTHESIS

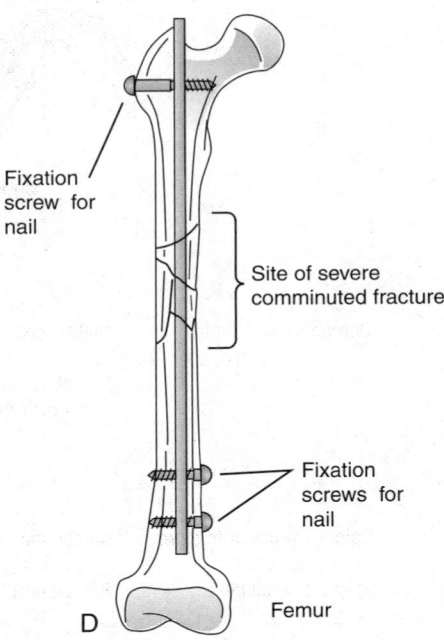

Fixation
screw for
nail

Site of severe
comminuted fracture

Fixation
screws for
nail

Femur

D

INTRAMEDULLARY NAIL FIXATION

Figure 34–14. Internal fixation devices.

(1) Distal portions of upper and lower extremities contain more compartments than the proximal portions, increasing the risk of incidence after injury (Fig. 34–15).

(2) The pressure source may be internal (e.g., with bleeding or fluid accumulation) or external (e.g., with casts or tight or bulky dressings).

(3) Compartment syndrome is seen not only in persons with musculoskeletal problems but also in those with severe burns, insect bites, or intravenous infiltration.

(4) Figure 34–16 shows the ischemia-edema cycle.

(5) If compartment syndrome is left untreated, irreversible neuromuscular damage occurs within 4 to 6 hours after onset.

(6) The affected limb can become useless within 24 to 48 hours.

(7) Compartment pressure may be monitored with

Table 34–9. Different Types of Fractures and Their Clinical Management

Fracture Site	Types of Fracture	Clinical Management	Nursing Interventions
Skull	Depressed	Surgery to elevate bone and remove bone fragments from tissue	Skull fractures: See Chapter 18 for care of persons with craniotomy.
Base of skull	Linear, depressed or comminuted	Bed rest with bed flat	Basilar skull fractures: Strict bed rest to decrease intracranial pressure and decrease amount of cerebrospinal fluid drainage from dural tear (if present). Do not suction through nares and tell person not to blow nose or sniff to prevent infection or meningitis. See Chapter 18.
Face	Mandibular	Open or closed reduction with wiring of mandible	
Cervical spine			Cervical spine: See Chapter 18 for care of person in cervical skeletal traction and when spinal cord injury is present. For halo traction, observe pin sites for signs of infection or loosening, clean pin sites per physician order, teach person and family how to care for skin and halo vest, and prepare vest in case of need for cardiopulmonary resuscitation (tape wrench to front of vest and color code screws to be loosened in emergency).
C1	Burst fracture disrupts the ring of the atlas	Halo traction	
C2	Bilateral posterior pedicle fracture of axis with subluxation of C2 and C3	Halo traction	Persons with halo traction need to be assisted with ambulation because of displaced center of gravity, loss of balance, and decreased peripheral vision. Teach the person to scan the area before moving by using eyes more and to get up slowly. A walker may be needed to provide stability.
Thoracic spine	Compression fracture	Stable: bed rest and brace Unstable: surgery with spinal instrumentation	Thoracic spine: See page 1611 for explanation of nursing care following spinal instrumentation. For bed rest, roll person side to side, keeping the body straight. When a brace is ordered, observe skin for signs of redness. The person should wear a tee shirt under the brace to protect skin. Teach the person and family how to apply the brace. Watch for signs of spinal cord compression (see Chapter 18) and paralytic ileus.
Lumbar spine	Spinous process fracture	Corset and brace	Lumbar spine: Same as nonsurgical care of thoracic fractures.
Ribs	Single or multiple	Rib support	Ribs: Observe for respiratory complications: pneumonia, pneumothorax, hemothorax. Encourage deep breathing and support fractured area with hands or rib belt. Monitor response to pain medication, intercostal nerve block, or administration of epidural analgesia.
Clavicle	Closed fracture	Clavicle strap or sling	Clavicle: Observe for tingling in hands if strap is too tight. Teach the person to exercise elbow, wrist, and fingers.
Shoulder	Fracture or dislocation	Closed reduction Sling and swathe Open reduction and internal fixation for recurrent dislocation	Shoulder, humerus fractures: Check sling and swathe or other immobilizer for correct fit. Observe circulation and sensation of arm and hand for deficits. Observe incisions for signs of infection. Teach the person and family how to gently wash axilla and apply a soft pad under axilla to prevent skin maceration. Teach shoulder and other exercises as ordered. Do not prop a hanging arm cast. It must hang free to provide the traction force needed for the fracture to heal. Check the cervical area for irritation and pad it if needed for comfort.
Head of humerus	Comminuted	Total shoulder arthroplasty	
Proximal humerus	Impact fracture	Sling and swathe	

Table 34–9. *Different Types of Fractures and Their Clinical Management* (Continued)

Fracture Site	Types of Fracture	Clinical Management	Nursing Interventions
Shaft of humerus	Fracture or dislocation	Closed reduction with hanging arm cast	
	Pathologic fracture	Open reduction and internal fixation with plate and screws or intramedullary rod	
Distal humerus	Supracondylar fracture	Closed reduction and posterior splint	
		Open reduction with pin if closed reduction is unsuccessful	
	Transcondylar fracture	Open reduction and internal fixation	
Olecranon	Articular fracture or dislocation	Open reduction and internal fixation	Olecranon, radius, ulna, wrist, hand, fingers and thumb: Observe circulation and sensation of upper extremity for deficits. Observe incision for signs of infection. Keep area elevated to prevent swelling. Check bandages, splints, and casts for signs of being too tight. Check pin sites of external fixators for signs of infection and provide or teach pin care as ordered. Encourage exercise of unaffected joints to prevent stiffness.
Radius head and neck	Nondisplaced fracture	Cast	
	Comminuted fracture	Open reduction and internal fixation; removal of loose fragments and excision of radial head	
Distal radius	Colles fracture with displacement of the radius	Cast	
		If severely comminuted, open reduction with wires and application of external fixator	
Ulna	Transverse or oblique	Open reduction with plate and screws or intramedullary rod; application of external fixator	
Wrist	Transverse or oblique	Cast	
Hand and fingers	Transverse or oblique	Closed reduction and cast or splint or open reduction and internal fixation	
Thumb	Intra-articular fracture of the base of the 1st metacarpal	Closed or open reduction with insertion of wire	
Pelvis acetabulum	Fracture with displacement of femoral head	Skeletal traction or open reduction and internal fixation or arthroplasty	Pelvis: Observe for signs of internal bleeding, thrombi, emboli, infection, bowel and bladder problems, circulation and sensation deficits, and paralytic ileus. For pelvic sling, observe for signs of skin redness and use preventive skin care. If able to turn person, use pillow between person's legs for support and comfort. When external fixator is present, provide or teach pin care as ordered. Encourage exercise of legs and feet. Ambulation training will be necessary if the person is able to walk. Maintain or teach weight-bearing precautions.
Pelvic wing	Fracture of ileum below anterior superior spine	Bed rest	
Pelvic ring	Comminuted or oblique and lateral	Open reduction and internal fixation or closed reduction and external fixation	
Pelvic rami	Bilateral fracture of superior and inferior pubic rami	Bed rest	

Table continued on following page

Table 34–9. *Different Types of Fractures and Their Clinical Management* (Continued)

Fracture Site	Types of Fracture	Clinical Management	Nursing Interventions
Proximal femur	Femoral neck or subcapital	Open reduction and internal fixation with compression screw, pins, or prosthesis	
	Intertrochanteric	Open reduction and internal fixation with compression screw, nails, or plate	
	Subtrochanteric	Open reduction and internal fixation with compression screw, intramedullary nail, or fixed-angle nail and plate	
Femoral shaft	Transverse or oblique	Closed reduction with intramedullary fixation or open reduction with intramedullary fixation	Femur fractures: Observe for circulation and sensation deficits in lower extremities. Observe incision for signs of infection. For skeletal traction, provide pin care as ordered and observe for signs of skin redness. For casts, splints, and other immobilizers, observe for proper fit and use preventive skin care. For hip fractures requiring replacement of the head of the femur with a prosthesis, maintain or teach abduction precautions (see page 1608). Teach ankle pumping and other exercises as ordered.
Distal femur	Condylar fractures	Open reduction with skeletal pins, screws, and plate and screws, or skeletal traction, cast brace, or spica cast	
Knee	Patella, nondisplaced	Knee immobilizer or cast	Knee, tibia, fibula fractures: Observe for circulation and sensation deficits in lower extremities. Observe incision for signs of infection. Maintain elevation of extremity to prevent excessive swelling. Observe for skin redness and use preventive skin care when casts, splints, or braces are used. Teach ankle pumping and other exercises as ordered. Teach ambulation techniques as ordered.
	Patella, comminuted	Open reduction and internal fixation with wires	
Tibia	Tibial plateau, displaced	Open reduction and internal fixation with plate and screws	
	Tibial plateau, nondisplaced	Posterior splint	
Shaft of tibia	Transverse	Cast or open reduction and internal fixation	
	Comminuted or open	Open reduction and internal fixation with plate and screws or external fixator	
Fibula	Single fracture of shaft	Cast	
Ankle	Lateral and medial malleoli	Open reduction and internal fixation with pins, screws, or plate and screws, and cast	Ankle, calcaneus, and foot: Observe for circulation and sensation deficits in lower extremities. Observe incision for signs of infection. Maintain elevation of area to prevent excessive swelling. Observe for skin redness and use preventive skin care when casts, splints, or braces are used. Teach ambulation techniques as ordered.
Calcaneus	Transverse or oblique	Open reduction and internal fixation with pins or staples, or closed reduction with pin	
Metatarsal bones	Transverse or oblique	Closed reduction or open reduction with wire or plate	

a. Fracture of femoral neck, or subcapital
b. Intertrochanteric fracture
c. Subtrochanteric fracture

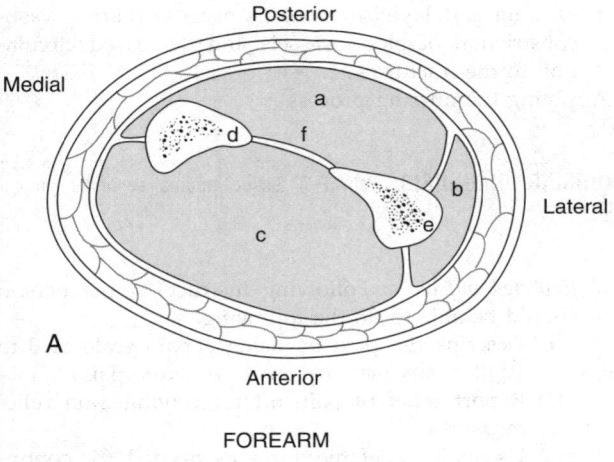

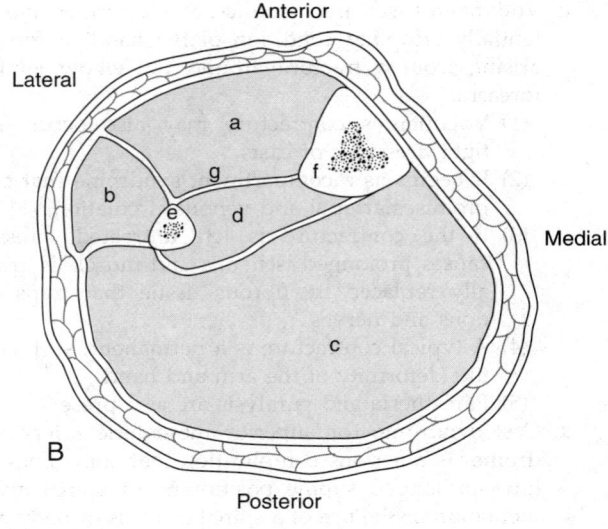

FOREARM

LOWER LEG

Figure 34–15. *A*, Compartments of the forearm. a, Posterior compartment; b, lateral compartment; c, anterior compartment; d, ulna; e, radius; f, interosseous septum. *B*, Compartments of the lower leg. a, Anterior compartment; b, lateral compartment; c, superficial posterior compartment; d, deep posterior compartment; e, fibula; f, tibia; g, interosseous septum.

a wick or slit catheter, usually in a critical care setting.

b. Delayed union, malunion, or nonunion of fracture
   (1) **Delayed union** is suspected when there occurs a continuation of or an increase in bone pain and tenderness beyond a reasonable healing period. Healing of the fracture is slowed but not completely halted. This may be caused by distraction of fracture fragments or infection. If the cause can be identified, healing usually occurs.
   (2) **Malunion** occurs when unequal biomechanical stresses at the fracture site result in an improper alignment of the fracture fragments. Malunion is associated with fractures treated with skeletal traction followed by plaster immobilization. It may develop when weight bearing occurs before medically indicated.
   (3) **Nonunion** occurs when fracture healing has not taken place 4 to 6 months after the fracture occurs and spontaneous healing is unlikely. It is caused by insufficient blood supply and uncontrolled repetitive stress on the fracture site. It

may be caused by interposed tissue between fracture fragments blocking the healing process. Other causes include prolonged or excessive traction, inadequate internal fixation, or infection. Treatment modalities include bone grafting, internal fixation, external fixation, electric bone stimulation, or combinations of these methods.

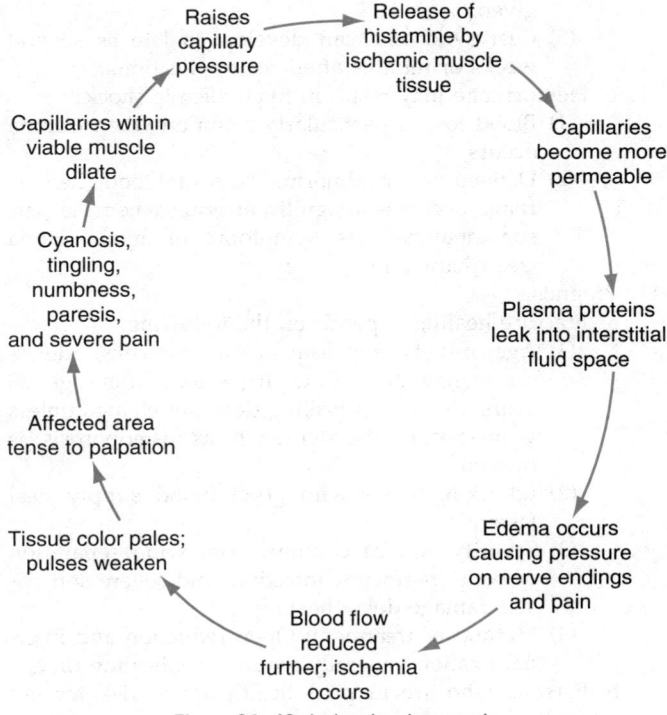

Figure 34–16. Ischemia-edema cycle.

c. Volkmann's ischemic contracture is a serious and potentially crippling condition of the hand or forearm arising from a fracture around the elbow joint or forearm.

   (1) Volkmann's contracture may also occur from tight dressings or casts.

   (2) It begins as a compartment syndrome that compromises arterial and venous circulation.

   (3) If the contracture is left untreated, pressure causes prolonged ischemia and muscle is gradually replaced by fibrous tissue that traps tendons and nerves.

   (4) A typical contracture is a permanent, stiff, claw-like deformity of the arm and hand.

   (5) Paresthesia and paralysis are also present.

d. Cast syndrome (or superior mesenteric artery syndrome) is a serious complication that sometimes follows prolonged supine positioning or spinal instrumentation or the use of a spinal orthosis or body cast.

   (1) Cast syndrome may also be associated with feelings of anxiety (claustrophobia) arising from any application of a cast, including one applied to an extremity.

   (2) Cast syndrome is characterized by nausea, abdominal pressure, and vague abdominal pain.

   (3) Cast syndrome may be caused by hyperextension of the spine, causing compression of the 3rd portion of the duodenum between the superior mesenteric artery anteriorly and the aorta and the vertebral column posteriorly.

   (4) Treatment for the person in a body cast is to cut or remove a large abdominal window, to bivalve, or to remove the cast. A nasogastric tube may be placed to remove gastric contents. Intravenous fluids and nothing by mouth may be given.

   (5) Cast syndrome can develop as late as several weeks or months after cast application.

e. Hemorrhage may result in hypovolemic shock.

   (1) Blood loss is particularly common when trauma occurs.

   (2) Defined as an abnormal loss of blood, hemorrhage becomes a significant issue when the person demonstrates symptoms of hypovolemia (see Chapter 12).

11. Prognosis

a. Fracture healing depends on the following:

   (1) Age: infants may heal in 4 to 6 weeks; adolescents may need 6 to 10 weeks; after age 20 years, the rate of healing does not change unless a metabolic disorder such as osteoporosis is present.

   (2) Location: bones with good blood supply heal faster.

   (3) Severity: severe comminution, wide separation of bone fragments, infection, and severe soft tissue damage delay healing.

   (4) Method of treatment: Open reduction and internal fixation generally require less healing time.

b. Persons who are in poor health are at risk for not healing properly.

c. Healing is delayed in smokers because there is vasoconstriction of blood vessels and decreased circulation to the fracture site.

12. Applying the nursing process

NURSING DIAGNOSIS: Pain R/T tissue trauma secondary to fracture

a. *Expected outcomes:* Following instruction, the person should be able to do the following:

   (1) Describe the pain by using a pain scale of 0 to 10 (0 = absence of pain; 10 = worst pain)

   (2) Report relief of pain after receiving pain relief measures

   (3) Use pain relief measures as needed for continued relief of pain

b. *Nursing interventions*

   (1) Assess the person's level of pain (see Chapter 11).

   (2) Teach the person techniques that help reduce pain.

    • Change position slowly and support the fractured area above and below the injury.

    • Elevate a fractured extremity unless contraindicated.

    • Apply ice if ordered.

    • Use relaxation techniques or imagery as described in Chapter 11.

    • Apply transcutaneous electrical nerve stimulation (see Chapter 11).

   (3) Assess the person's response to pain relief measures and investigate unrelieved pain. If the person is unable to verbalize pain relief, observe nonverbal responses such as facial grimacing or withdrawal.

NURSING DIAGNOSIS: Impaired physical mobility R/T activity restrictions and loss of muscle strength secondary to fracture

a. *Expected outcomes:* Following instruction, the person should be able to do the following:

   (1) Perform muscle strengthening (isometric) exercises

   (2) Perform range-of-motion exercises if indicated

   (3) Use assistive devices to increase mobility

b. *Nursing interventions*

   (1) Assess muscle strength daily.

   (2) Teach exercises as prescribed by the physician.

   (3) Instruct the patient on ambulation techniques.

NURSING DIAGNOSIS: Ineffective management of therapeutic regimen R/T insufficient knowledge of signs and symptoms of complications

a. *Expected outcomes:* Following instruction, the person should be able to do the following:

(1) State the signs and symptoms of complications that can occur following a fracture

(2) Recognize the importance of notifying the physician when the signs and symptoms of complications occur

b. *Nursing interventions*

(1) Teach the patient to recognize and report signs and symptoms of neurovascular compression of a fracture site
   - Severe pain
   - Numbness or tingling
   - Change in color of the skin
   - Excessive swelling
   - Change in the temperature of an extremity from warm to cool or cold

(2) Teach the patient to recognize and report signs and symptoms of infection
   - Chills, high fever
   - Pain or tenderness of the extremity
   - Increased drainage or change in appearance of drainage from an incision or wound
   - Foul-smelling drainage
   - Malaise

(3) Teach the patient to recognize and report signs and symptoms of respiratory complications
   - Shortness of breath
   - Chest pain
   - Coughing (check sputum to see whether it is a color other than clear white)

13. Discharge planning and teaching

a. Discharge planning begins as soon as the patient enters the hospital.

(1) Decisions must be made regarding whether the patient can be alone at home.

(2) If the family is unable to care for the patient and more therapy is required, a short-term stay in a nursing home with rehabilitation facilities or a skilled care unit within a hospital is needed.

(3) The social worker or discharge planner should be notified of a patient's admission so that home arrangements and equipment needs can be assessed.

b. Patients and families should be taught basic principles of wound care and symptom management, including signs and symptoms of infection and when to call the physician.

14. Public health considerations

a. Education is the focus of primary prevention. Teaching should stress the following:

(1) Avoiding high-risk activities such as high-impact sports, sky diving, and rollerblading

(2) Eating foods high in calcium and vitamin D

(3) Exercising regularly

(4) Avoiding safety hazards that lead to falls, particularly for older persons, such as throw rugs, pets running under foot, and loss of balance related to medications or visual problems

b. Home health nurses should assess the home environment for safety hazards and teach older persons with fractures how to prevent them.

ELDER ADVISORY

Inform older people to check for the following potential hazards in their homes or other places they may go: loose rugs or carpet, inadequate lighting, pets, electrical cords, slippery or wet floors, uneven floors, complex patterns on rugs or wallpaper, low or unstable furniture, lack of color discrimination between stairs and floor, and loose banisters. Also inform them that poorly adjusted eyewear, improper footwear, floor length skirts or slacks, inadequate nutrition, certain medications, alcohol consumption, and certain diseases can increase their risk of falling.

HOME CARE STRATEGIES

Modifying the Home Environment for Safety, Accessibility, and Convenience

Modifying the home environment is necessary to make the home accessible, safe, and convenient for the patient. Assess the patient's abilities to determine the modifications needed.

Range of Motion

This includes reaching, bending, squatting, and kneeling.
- Try to locate frequently used items within a patient's range of motion and reach.
- Evaluate items such as faucets, cabinets, shelves, electrical outlets, and personal items.
- Assistive devices such as a long-handled shoe horn or raised toilet seat can extend reach and reduce the need to squat.

Movement

- To get from one place to another, straight, smooth, flat, and wide pathways are best.
- Interior and exterior doorways must be wide enough to provide safe, easy passage.
- Lifts can replace stairs.

Dexterity

This will be demonstrated in fine finger movements, twisting, grasping, and turning.
- Select items that require less demand for fine movements.
- Consider lever-type faucets and a large-handled toothbrush.

Strength, Endurance, Stamina

Evaluate the ability to exert force and continue that force to perform tasks.
- Use light-weight objects.
- When possible, shorten distances.
- Position work stations at a height that allows a person to sit.

Safety

Safety risks are increased in patients who have musculoskeletal disorders. To help, do the following:
- Modify the environment to safeguard the patient against accidents and other risks.
- Help formulate an emergency escape plan in case of fire or other disasters.
- Make sure that the environment is clutter-free and has nonslip, smooth floor surfaces.
- Locate pet feeding centers outside of traffic areas.
- Remember that a room that is difficult to use, such as the bathroom, is a dangerous room.

Privacy and Community

- The environment should offer quality living, including opportunities for interaction and for being alone.
- Remove or provide barriers if necessary.

Sports Injuries

1. Knee injuries
   a. Definition: The knee is one of the joints most frequently injured during sports participation. Rupture or incomplete tears occur in the structures of the knee or in combinations: medial collateral ligament (MCL), lateral collateral ligament (LCL), anterior cruciate ligament (ACL), posterior crucial ligament (PCL), and menisci.
   b. Incidence and etiology
      (1) An MCL injury occurs when stress is applied on the lateral aspect of knee, forcing it to bend inward, stretching or tearing the MCL.
      (2) An LCL injury occurs when a blow is directed to the medial aspect of the knee, stressing the lateral aspect and causing injury to the LCL.
      (3) The ACL and PCL are main stabilizing ligaments of the knee that crisscross at the center of the knee. The ACL is the most frequently torn ligament, torn by excessive valgus force to the knee (e.g., clipping in football) and by hyperextension while the leg is externally rotated (e.g., while skiing, playing basketball, or performing gymnastics). Tear of the ACL occurs many times, along with torn menisci and collateral ligaments.
      (4) The menisci function as shock absorbers within the knee. Any injury to the knee may include a meniscal tear, and careful screening of these must be done.
   c. Clinical manifestations
      (1) At the time of injury to the MCL and the LCL, a tear may be felt or a "snap" may be heard. There is immediate pain, swelling, and instability. Ambulation is difficult without assistance.
      (2) At the time of injury to the ACL and the PCL, a tear may be felt or a "pop" may be heard. There is immediate pain, swelling, and instability. Ambulation is difficult. The Lachman test is positive.
      (3) In a meniscal tear, there is a popping or tearing sensation at the time of injury, with swelling of the knee over the next few hours. If the tear is significant, a piece may flip over and the knee may lock. Other manifestations include a clicking noise on ambulation, stiffness, giving way (buckling), and a positive McMurray's maneuver.
   d. Clinical management
      (1) For MCL and LCL, management includes the following:
         • Rest, ice, compression, and elevation (RICE) initially
         • Radiographic study to rule out avulsion fracture
         • Aspiration of blood from the knee joint
         • Nonsurgical treatment including a long leg limb brace or cast for 4 to 6 weeks with knee flexed at 45 degrees, quadriceps and hamstring strengthening exercise, ambulation with crutches with no weight bearing on the injured leg, active range of motion of the knee after the cast is removed, and an elastic brace if needed after the cast is removed. The person may return to sports activities when range of motion and strength are regained.
         • Surgical treatment that may include a long leg cast or long limb knee brace for 6 to 8 weeks with the knee flexed, quadriceps and hamstring strengthening exercises, ambulation with crutches with no weight bearing on the injured leg, and no weight bearing until there is 60 degrees of motion in the knee and the person can lift 15 pounds for 50 repetitions with the injured leg. Rehabilitation lasts 12 months or longer and a derotation brace may be required during sports activities. If surgical repair is delayed, physical therapy and bracing are used before surgery. If surgical repair is immediate, the person's own patellar tendon or semitendinosus ligament can be used or a synthetic ligament can be used. A long leg hinged brace is applied with knee flexion set at the desired flexion. Continuous passive motion is begun immediately or later per the physician's order. Isometric quadriceps setting, bent knee raises and ankle pump exercises are initiated. Ambulation is with crutches with no weight or partial weight (depending on type of ligament used in repair). As rehabilitation progresses, weights are added to the exercises, more progressive exercises are added, extension and flexion of the knee are adjusted per the physician's order, and weight bearing can increase. In 6 months, full range of motion, knee extension, and progressive resistive exercises are without limitation. A jogging program can be initiated if range of motion is normal and quadriceps strength is 75 percent of the nonoperative leg. Rehabilitation using artificial grafts produces faster rehabilitation time, that is, full range of motion.
      (2) For meniscal injuries, management includes the following:
         • Rest, ice, compression, and elevation
         • Quadriceps strengthening exercises
         • Arthroscopic removal or repair of injured meniscus if symptoms persist
         • Postoperative exercises, including quadriceps strengthening and range-of-motion
   e. Nursing interventions
      (1) Assess the neurovascular status of the injured extremity.
      (2) Observe for signs and symptoms of infection.
      (3) Evaluate the effectiveness of pain medications.
      (4) Teach cast care.
      (5) Teach quadriceps and hamstring strengthening exercises.
      (6) Teach non–weight-bearing ambulation with crutches.
      (7) Reinforce the importance of completion of the rehabilitation program.
2. Strains
   a. Definition: A strain is caused by a sudden traumatic forced motion that overstretches, misuses, or overextends the body of the muscle or attachment of a tendon beyond its normal range.

b. Incidence and etiology
  (1) Strains arise from twisting or wrenching movements.
  (2) The most common site of strains is the ankle.
  (3) Strains occur during athletic activity, including running, all ball sports, and unaccustomed vigorous exercise.
c. Clinical manifestations
  (1) A 1st-degree strain is the pulling of a musculotendinous unit with gradual onset muscle spasms, discomfort, and loss of range of motion.
  (2) 2nd-degree strain is the tearing of a musculotendinous unit with extreme muscle spasm, pain, immediate development of edema, and development of ecchymosis within a few hours.
  (3) A 3rd-degree strain is the complete rupture of a musculotendinous unit with severe muscle spasm, point tenderness, edema at the rim of injury, sensation of sudden tearing, snapping or burning sensation, and limited range of motion.
d. Clinical management
  (1) Radiographic examination rules out possible fracture.
  (2) Rest, ice, compression, and elevation is used for the first 24 to 48 hours after injury to reduce swelling.
  (3) Heat may then be prescribed for comfort, to reabsorb blood and fluid and to promote healing.
  (4) If there is rupture, surgical repair may be performed at the tendon–bone interface.
  (5) Movement is limited for 4 to 6 weeks.
e. Nursing interventions
  (1) Assess the neurovascular status of the injured extremity.
  (2) Evaluate the effectiveness of pain medication.
  (3) Teach use of crutches, sling, brace, elastic bandage, and ice, among other modalities.
3. Sprains
a. Definition: sprains are traumatic twisting injuries to joints in which an incomplete tear of the ligaments or their attachment and capsule occurs. The range-of-motion limits are exceeded, and there is forced hyperextension.
b. Incidence and etiology
  (1) Sprains may be mild, moderate, or severe as follows:
    • Grade 1—few fibers torn, minimal hematoma, no loss of function, ligament not weakened
    • Grade 2—up to half the ligaments torn, some loss of function, weakened ligament
    • Grade 3—ligament completely torn
  (2) The most common sites include the wrist, lateral ankle ligament, and knee.
  (3) High-risk athletic activities include football, skiing, basketball, and tennis.
  (4) Upper extremity sprains are caused by overstressing a joint, attempting to break a fall, and bracing during a motor vehicle accident.
  (5) Cervical sprains usually result from whiplash.
  (6) Ankle sprains result from missteps, motor vehicle accidents, and sports injury.

c. Clinical manifestations
  (1) The person may have a history of stepping on an uneven surface or of trauma.
  (2) The person may report that the joint feels like "something coming apart."
  (3) The person may report feeling a snap, pop, or tearing.
  (4) The amount of edema indicates severity of injury.
  (5) The site may be tender.
  (6) The person may have decreased motion and limited joint function.
  (7) Ecchymosis may not indicate the site or severity of injury.
d. Clinical management
  (1) Rest, ice, compression, and elevation
  (2) Immobilization by splinting, casting, or taping for 3 to 4 weeks
  (3) A planned exercise program after scar formation in 4 to 6 weeks
e. Nursing interventions
  (1) Assess the neurovascular status of the injured extremity.
  (2) Evaluate the effectiveness of pain medication.
  (3) Teach use of crutches, sling, brace, elastic bandage, and ice, among other modalities.
4. Dislocations and subluxations
a. Definition
  (1) Subluxation and dislocation are both displacements of the joint from its normal position.
  (2) Complete dislocation involves the complete separation of the articular surfaces of the joint.
  (3) Subluxation is a partial loss of contact between the articular surfaces of the joint.
  (4) Dislocations are described as anteroposterior or mediolateral.
  (5) Congenital dislocations are those that exist at birth, such as a congenital dislocated hip.
b. Incidence and etiology
  (1) Dislocations may be caused by direct or indirect forces including falls or weakening of a joint capsule secondary to surgery.
  (2) Subluxations may be caused by loose surrounding structures as a result of congenital problems, trauma, infection, and disuse, or atrophy.
  (3) The most commonly dislocated joints include the fingers, patella, and shoulder.
c. Clinical manifestations
  (1) Pain
  (2) Loss or change of normal contour of joint
  (3) Loss of length in an extremity (shortening)
  (4) Loss of normal mobility
  (5) Diagnosis confirmed by radiography
  (6) Often, associated fractures
d. Clinical management includes immobilization and reduction.
e. Nursing interventions
  (1) Assess the neurovascular status of the injured extremity.
  (2) Evaluate the effectiveness of pain medication.
  (3) Observe any incision for sign of infection.
  (4) Teach proper use of immobilization device.

LEARNING/TEACHING GUIDELINES
for Prevention of Sports Injuries

General Overview

1. Identify risk factors that can contribute to injury.
2. Recognize factors that need to be considered for a safe sports activity.

Risk Factors

1. Instruct the person to see a physician before participating in a sports activity if any of the following risk factors exists:
   a. Age older than 40 years
   b. Inactive lifestyle
   c. Twenty or more pounds overweight
   d. Medications being taken on a regular basis
   e. History of pain or pressure in the chest, arm, or throat
   f. Family history of cardiac disease
   g. Elevated cholesterol level
   h. Hypertension
   i. Smoker or history of pulmonary disease
   j. History of diabetes or other chronic disease
   k. History of joint disease

Factors for Safe Activity

1. Instruct the person to:
   a. Choose an activity that the person likes, can adapt to the person's routine, and that the person can physically manage.
   b. Choose equipment that fits properly and is appropriate for the activity.
      (1) Buy equipment that is fit for the individual. Do not borrow someone else's equipment.
      (2) Buy the appropriate equipment. Do not wear baseball shoes when playing football.
   c. Look for safety rather than cost or appearance when buying equipment.
   d. Learn the proper use of the equipment.
   e. Know the rules of play and follow them.
   f. Participate in preseason assessment and testing if in competitive sports. These programs help identify health problems and enable athletes to be matched according to size and weight rather than age.
   g. Prepare muscle groups before activity by developing strength, endurance, and flexibility.
   h. Maintain proper nutrition.
   i. Get proper rest and pace yourself.
   j. Always warm up before exercise and cool down afterward.
   k. Make sure the activity area is safe.

5. Contusions
   a. Definition: A contusion is blunt trauma to soft tissue that results in ecchymosis and edema.
   b. Incidence and etiology
      (1) Damage to the skin and soft tissue is a common occurrence.
      (2) A common contusion injury is the black eye caused by blunt trauma to the area from a fist, baseball, or racquetball.
   c. Clinical manifestations
      (1) Bleeding into soft tissue creates the characteristic purple ecchymosis.
      (2) The purple color fades to green and then yellow.
      (3) Discoloration disappears in approximately 10 days.
      (4) Other symptoms include pain and swelling.
   d. Clinical management
      (1) Rest, ice, compression, and elevation
      (2) Application of heat to the affected area after the initial 24 hours, 20 to 30 minutes at a time for 4 times a day
   e. Nursing interventions
      (1) Assess the neurovascular status of the affected area.
      (2) Evaluate the effectiveness of management modalities.
      (3) Encourage range of motion of joints.
      (4) Teach the person to avoid excessive exercise of the injured area.
      (5) Teach the person how to avoid reinjury (see Learning/Teaching Guidelines for Prevention of Sports Injuries).

Carpal Tunnel Syndrome

1. Definition: Carpal tunnel syndrome is the compression of the median nerve at the wrist, causing numbness and pain.
2. Incidence and socioeconomic impact
   a. Carpal tunnel syndrome can occur in adults of any age but peaks between ages 30 and 60 years.
   b. Women are 5 times more likely to experience the problem than men.
   c. Carpal tunnel syndrome affects the dominant hand more often.
   d. There is a higher incidence in postmenopausal women, persons with space-occupying lesions (e.g., rheumatoid arthritis, Colles' fracture of the wrist, ganglia of the wrist, or lipomas), and in persons with conditions causing an increase in fluid retention (e.g., diabetes, thyroid disease, and pregnancy).
3. Risk factors include repetitive hand activities involving pinch or grasp during wrist flexion or excessive hand

exercise for long periods of time, such as is done by factory workers, jackhammer operators, and computer programmers.

4. Etiology
   a. Compression of the median nerve by space-occupying lesions causes hemorrhage into the carpal tunnel.
   b. Increased fluid in tissue around the wrist compresses the median nerve.
   c. Repetitive hand activities stress the wrist.

5. Pathophysiology: The carpal tunnel is a rigid canal lying between carpal bone and fibrous tissue. Nine tendons enveloped by synovium share space with the median nerve, causing numbness and pain.

6. Clinical manifestations
   a. Burning pain and numbness of the hand
   b. Pain that is worse at night secondary to pressure and hand flexion
   c. Pain that may radiate to the arm, shoulder, neck, and chest
   d. Paresthesia or painful tingling and numbness of the thumb, index finger, middle finger, and radial aspect of the ring finger (median nerve distribution)
   e. Weak pinch, clumsiness, and difficulty with fine motor movements
   f. Muscle atrophy and wasting
   g. Skin discoloration
   h. Nail changes, including brittleness with increased or decreased palmar sweating

7. Diagnostics
   a. No specific laboratory tests detect carpal tunnel syndrome.
   b. Electromyography may be used to assist in providing a definitive diagnosis revealing nerve dysfunction before muscle wasting is observed.
   c. Phalen's wrist test produces paresthesia in median nerve distribution within 60 seconds.

8. Clinical management
   a. The goal of clinical management is to reduce or alleviate pain.
   b. Nonpharmacologic interventions include splinting the wrist and hand to prevent hyperextension and flexion. Approximately 70 percent of persons with carpal tunnel syndrome experience temporary relief.
   c. Pharmacologic interventions
      (1) Local injections of steroids to decrease inflammation
      (2) Short-term use of diuretics to reduce edema and oral vitamin B_6 for nerve tissue integrity and function
   d. Special medical-surgical procedures
      (1) Outpatient surgery to relieve pressure on the median nerve is necessary in approximately 40 percent of persons. Initially, the hand is kept immobile with a bulky dressing.
      (2) Postoperative care includes keeping the arm elevated for 1 to 2 days to reduce swelling. The patient should be instructed to exercise the fingers immediately to promote circulation and movement. Coolness or changes in color of the fingers should be reported to the physician. Check the pressure dressing for drainage and

tightness. The patient should be instructed to avoid hyperextension and flexion.

9. Complications: Decompression of the median nerve may be unsuccessful, especially in people with rheumatoid arthritis. Synovitis may recur, compressing the median nerve. Participation in the work environment may require the elimination of activities that promote flexion or hyperextension.

10. Applying the nursing process

> **NURSING DIAGNOSIS:** Pain R/T compression of the median nerve and activities that hyperextend and flex the wrist

   a. *Expected outcomes:* Following instruction and interventions, the person should be able to do the following:
      (1) Describe the pain by using a pain scale of 0 to 10 (0 = absence of pain; 10 = worst pain)
      (2) Report relief of pain after receiving pain relief measures
      (3) Use adaptive techniques or splints to maintain the wrist in neutral position
   b. *Nursing interventions*
      (1) Assess the person's level of pain (see Chapter 11).
      (2) Teach the person to use techniques that reduce pain, such as use of splints to maintain wrist in neutral position and use of pain medications as indicated.
      (3) Assess the person's response to pain relief measures and investigate unrelieved pain. Carpal tunnel syndrome may recur.

11. Discharge planning and teaching
   a. The patient should be taught proper application of adaptive equipment and wrist splint to maintain the wrist in neutral position.
   b. The person should be instructed and assisted with vocational retraining for persons working in occupations that require repetitive hand motion.
   c. Signs and symptoms of carpal tunnel syndrome should be taught so that the person knows what to expect if it recurs.
   d. Persons should be taught to avoid heavy lifting and repetitive motion for 3 to 4 weeks after surgery.

13. Public health considerations
   a. In some instances, carpal tunnel syndrome is preventable.
   b. Rotation of factory jobs among workers reduces the risk of carpal tunnel syndrome.

Low Back Pain, Sciatica, and Herniated Nucleus Pulposus

1. Definition
   a. Low back pain is pain in the lower back associated with or without radiating leg pain. (sciatica).
   b. Herniated nucleus pulposus, or "bulging disk," occurs laterally where the annulus fibrosus is weakest and the posterior longitudinal ligament is thinnest, resulting in spinal nerve root compression.

2. Incidence and socioeconomic impact
   a. Low back pain is one of the most common causes of disability and lost work time.
   b. Compensable low back pain is estimated to cost $11 billion annually.
   c. Low back pain is second only to headache as the most common complaint of individuals in the United States.
   d. Low back pain occurs most frequently in men between 30 and 50 years of age.
3. Risk factors
   • Poor posture
   • Wearing of high-heeled shoes
   • Poor physical conditioning
   • Repetitive overuse
   • Obesity
   • Pregnancy
4. Etiology
   a. Many disorders can produce low back pain, although most acute episodes are related to ligament and muscle injury and to degeneration of the spine.
   b. Ligament or muscle injury and, in the case of herniated nucleus pulposus, or ''bulging'' of the disk, commonly results from strenuous or improper lifting or bending
   c. Degeneration of the spine is part of normal aging, which may be accelerated by trauma, chronic overuse, chronic underactivity, or prolonged exposure to vibrating motion.
   d. If surrounding muscle or ligaments are weak, as in the case of herniated nucleus pulposus, the disk bulges.
   e. Painful muscle spasms may be related to stress.
   f. Some persons experience pain for which no physical basis can be found.
5. Pathophysiology
   a. Low back pain is more common than cervical pain.
   b. Lumbar herniation is more common than cervical herniation.
   c. Acute back pain is caused by the following:
      (1) Herniated nucleus pulposus (Fig. 34–17).
      (2) Ligament sprain
      (3) Disk injury from hyperflexion or muscle strain
      (4) Muscle spasm
      (5) Degenerative changes (osteoarthritis)
      (6) Osteoporosis
      (7) Spondylolysis or the breaking down of the vertebrae
      (8) Spondylolisthesis or the forward slipping of the vertebra, often resulting in stress fracture
      (9) Compression fractures due to minimal trauma, usually the result of cancer or osteoporosis
      (10) Scoliosis
   c. If pain continues for 3 months or if repeated episodes of pain occur, the back pain is diagnosed as being chronic.
   d. Pain may be aggravated by sneezing, coughing, or straining.
   e. Pain most often occurs at the L4–5 or L5–S1 level of spine.
   f. The sciatic spinal nerve root may be compressed.
6. Clinical manifestations
   a. Recent data indicate that most patients with acute low back pain recover within 4 weeks without specific treatment.
   b. The person with low back pain of less than 4 weeks' duration must be assessed to rule out serious disease.
   c. Persons in pain may walk in a stiff, flexed state or may be unable to bend.
   d. Sciatic nerve impairment may cause the person to walk with a limp.
   e. Heel-toe walking may cause severe pain in the affected leg or back.
   f. Low back pain is associated with frequent muscle spasm.
   g. Pain may radiate down the affected leg.
   h. The person may complain of the same type of pain in the middle of the buttock.
   i. The person may report complaints of sharp, burning, posterior thigh or calf pain.
   j. Sensory changes (paresthesia or numbness) may be evident in the involved limb.
   k. If the sciatic nerve is compressed, the person complains of severe pain when attempting to raise the leg straight.

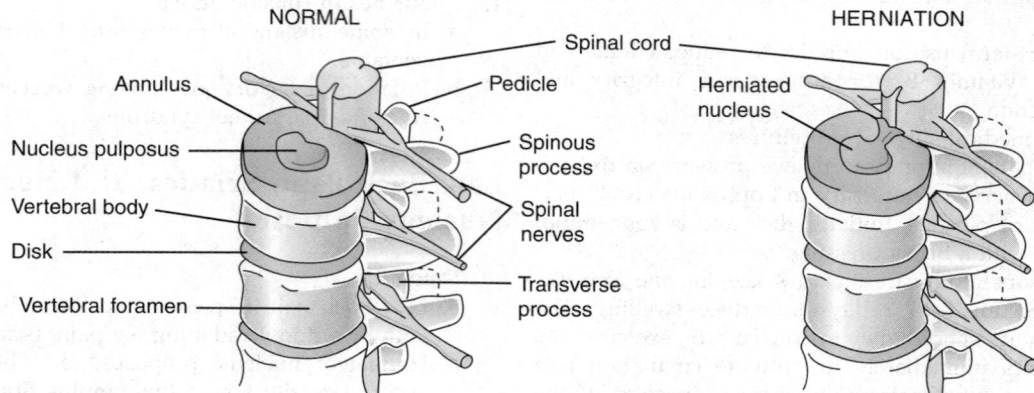

Figure 34–17. Herniated nucleus pulposus. (Redrawn from Ignatavicius DD, Workman ML, and Mishler MA [eds]. *Medical-Surgical Nursing: A Nursing Process Approach.* 2nd ed. Philadelphia: WB Saunders, 1996, p 1170.)

l. The following should be ruled out by medical history and physical examination:
  (1) Fracture, tumor, infection, or other serious conditions (red flags)
  (2) Nonspinal disorders that refer pain to the lower back
  (3) Sciatica or nerve root compromise
  (4) Nonspecific back pain or symptoms occuring primarily in the back

7. Diagnostics
  a. There are no special laboratory tests for back pain.
  b. Views for radiographic studies include anterior, posterior, and lateral spine.
  c. Computed tomography scan, with or without contrast of the spine, defines bony anatomy.
  d. Myelogram demonstrates neural encroachment.
  e. Magnetic resonance imaging defines soft tissue and is the procedure of choice in patients with previous back surgery. Magnetic resonance imaging can distinguish between disk herniation and scar tissue.
  f. Electromyelography may define subtle nerve root dysfunction.
  g. Sensory-evoked potentials may also be performed, especially in patients with suspected spinal stenosis.

8. Clinical management
  a. Goals of clinical management
    (1) The initial care of acute low back pain, with or without sciatica, is conservative.
    (2) Most patients recover within 4 weeks.
    (3) Patients who do not improve in 4 weeks require reassessment.
  b. Nonpharmacologic interventions
    (1) Symptom control includes use of manipulation such as chiropractic or osteopathic intervention, which is safe and effective during the 1st month of symptoms, application of heat or cold, and use of shoe insoles for persons who have to stand for long periods of time.
    (2) The following may be suggested but have not been proved effective for treating acute low back pain: corsets, traction, massage, diathermy, ultrasound, biofeedback, and transcutaneous electrical nerve stimulation (Fig. 34–18).
    (3) Activity may be restricted to avoid aggravation of symptoms. Restrictions are intended to allow the person to recover spontaneously and are prescribed for a limited period of time, usually not more than 3 months.
    (4) Exercise is undertaken to avoid debilitation due to inactivity and to increase activity tolerance. Aerobic exercise in the 1st few weeks decreases debility. Examples are walking, stationary bicycling, swimming, and light jogging. Exercises are used to strengthen the trunk muscles. Back stretching exercises have not been found to be helpful in acute low back pain.
    (5) Bed rest is reserved for persons with severe symptoms aggravated by any activity; usually a short period of 2 to 4 days is sufficient.
    (6) Sitting may aggravate symptoms in some individuals and these persons are advised to avoid

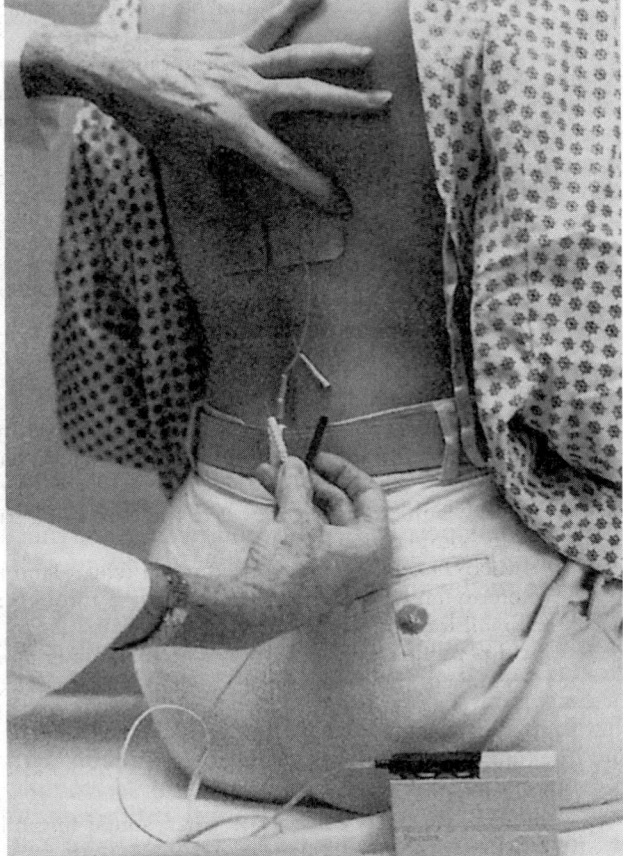

Figure 34–18. Transcutaneous electrical nerve stimulation. (From Ignatavicius DD, Workman ML, and Mishler MA [eds]. *Medical-Surgical Nursing: A Nursing Process Approach.* 2nd ed. Philadelphia: WB Saunders, 1996, p 137.)

prolonged sitting. They are advised to change position frequently. A chair with a lumbar support, arm rests, and a slightly reclining back may make sitting more comfortable.
  c. Pharmacologic interventions
    (1) Some persons respond well to over-the-counter analgesics.
    (2) Persons should be warned about the gastrointestinal irritation that may occur with NSAID use.
    (3) A short course of several days of a mild narcotic or muscle relaxant may be prescribed; however, there is no evidence that these are more effective than NSAIDs. Narcotics may cause drowsiness, and they have the potential for dependence and abuse.
    (4) Corticosteroids and antidepressants are not indicated for acute low back pain.
  d. Special medical-surgical procedures
    (1) Surgical intervention is indicated when all of the following criteria are present:
      • Sciatica is severe and disabling.
      • Sciatica is unimproved after 4 weeks of treatment.

- There is clear evidence of neurologic dysfunction.

    (2) Imaging is used to confirm the presence of neurologic compression. If imaging studies do not demonstrate a significant pathologic condition, the person is best treated conservatively.

    (3) To avoid surgery, epidural corticosteroid injection is an option.

    (4) The surgical goal is to decompress the nerve root by using the following:
    - Laminotomy, or incision of the lamina, part of the vertebral arch that forms the spinal canal
    - Laminectomy, or complete removal of one or more laminae
    - Diskectomy, or removal of disk fragments

    (5) Chemonucleolysis is a less invasive procedure and involves the injection of an enzyme that dissolves the disk. It is less effective than surgery or microdiskectomy and has rare but serious complications.

    (6) Microdiskectomy is a procedure in which laminotomy and diskectomy are performed through a small incision using a microscope.

    (7) In percutaneous diskectomy, the disk material is removed by means of a cannula inserted through skin.

    (8) Surgery for spinal stenosis usually requires complete laminectomy, followed by removal of osteophytes.

    (9) Spine fusion is considered when spinal instability is present.

9. Complications: Postlaminectomy syndrome occurs after unsuccessful surgery, exacerbating symptoms that may lead to repeated operations. Surgical complication rates are less than 1 percent for 1st-time surgery.

10. Prognosis
    a. In the absence of serious disease, approximately 90 percent of persons with low back pain or sciatica recover within 4 weeks.
    b. Persons with sciatica who have not recovered within 4 weeks and who have a clear evidence of neural compression are candidates for surgery. Surgery shortens the period of disability, but more than 80 percent of these persons eventually recover with or without surgery.

11. Applying the nursing process

NURSING DIAGNOSIS: Pain R/T spasms of the paraspinal muscles and/or compression of spinal nerves (in herniated nucleus pulposus)

a. *Expected outcomes:* Following instruction and treatment, the person should be able to do the following:
    (1) Describe the pain by using a pain scale of 0 to 10 (0 = absence of pain; 10 = worst pain)
    (2) Report relief of pain after receiving pain relief measures
    (3) Use pain relief measures as needed for continued relief of pain

b. *Nursing interventions*
    (1) Assess the person's level of pain (see Chapter 11).
    (2) Teach the person techniques that help to reduce pain.
    - Bed rest in a semi-Fowler's position with hips and knees flexed
    - Use of heat or ice on low back to relieve muscle spasm. Massage may also help to relieve muscle spasm.
    - Use of transcutaneous nerve stimulation (see Chapter 11)
    - Use of pain medications, muscle relaxants, and psychotropic medications
    (3) Assess the person's response to pain relief measures, and investigate unrelieved pain. If the person is unable to verbalize pain relief, note nonverbal responses such as facial grimace or withdrawal.

NURSING DIAGNOSIS: Ineffective management of therapeutic regimen R/T insufficient knowledge of condition and treatment

a. *Expected outcomes:* Following instruction, the person should be able to do the following:
    (1) Describe how low back pain affects lifestyle
    (2) Explain the proposed treatment plan
    (3) Demonstrate back exercises
    (4) Recognize methods to help prevent recurrence of low back pain

b. *Nursing interventions*
    (1) Help the person identify how the low back pain affects lifestyle.
    (2) Help the person identify how to cope with lifestyle changes that may continue, such as loss of work.
    (3) Discuss the proposed treatment plan with the person and answer questions about it. Encourage the person to also discuss the plan with the physician.
    (4) Teach the person back exercises that are designed to prevent recurrence of low back pain.
    (5) If surgery is required for herniated nucleus pulposus, see page 1611 for nursing care for laminectomy and spinal fusion.

12. Discharge planning and teaching
    a. Assure the patient that the condition usually improves within 4 weeks using conservative interventions.
    b. Instruct the patient in injury prevention strategies.
        (1) Proper lifting techniques
        (2) Proper posture when sitting or standing
        (3) Proper administration of medications, such as NSAIDs, muscle relaxants, and narcotics
    c. Instruct the patient in proper exercise techniques.
    d. Postoperative incision wound care after surgery for herniated nucleus pulposus
        (1) Instruct the person to notify the health care provider if any of the following occurs:

• Red and warm incision
• Drainage
• Elevated temperature
• Headache
• Recurrence or new onset of pain or numbness

   (2) The patient usually may shower the next day or when the dressing is removed. The patient should not sit in tub until the incision is completely healed.

13. Public health considerations
   a. Low back pain is one of the most common causes of disability and lost work time.
   b. With conservative treatment, most persons improve within 4 weeks.

◼ INFLAMMATORY MUSCULOSKELETAL DISORDERS

Gout

1. Definition: Gout is a hereditary metabolic disturbance of purine metabolism leading to excess urates that are deposited in body tissues and joints.
2. Incidence and etiology
   a. Gout predominantly affects middle-aged men.
   b. It can affect any joint but is predominant in the feet, legs, and great toe.
   c. The cause is unknown, but it is found to be linked with genetic defects in purine metabolism. Incomplete metabolism of purines builds up uric acid crystals in the body or leads to overproduction of uric acid.
   d. Overproduction of uric acid may also occur secondary to acquired disorders such as sickle cell anemia, malignant disease, and renal disease.
   e. Decreased renal function from prolonged use of certain medications (e.g., diuretics) can cause decreased excretion of uric acid from the kidneys.
3. Clinical manifestations
   a. Acute gout occurs in 3 stages:
      (1) Elevated serum uric acid
      (2) Painful, swollen joint with limited movement
      (3) Absence of symptoms for months or years
   b. Chronic gout occurs after several episodes of acute gout have occurred.
      (1) Persistent pain is present.
      (2) Hard, painless nodules called tophi are caused by collection of sodium urate crystals. These may be found in earlobes, fingers, hands, forearms, knees, feet, and on Achilles tendons.
   c. As gout progresses, degenerative arthritic changes such as destruction of cartilage and narrowing of joint space occurs.
4. Clinical management
   a. To achieve a low purine diet, the person should avoid red and organ meats, lunch meats, shellfish, sardines, anchovies, and meat gravies.
   b. Medication
      (1) During acute stages, the following medication may be given:

• Nonsteroidal anti-inflammatory drugs such as indomethacin, oxyphenbutazone, ibuprofen, naproxen, and sulindac.
• Colchicine, an anti-inflammatory drug specific for gout, which can be used with another anti-inflammatory drug
• Corticosteroids, if milder anti-inflammatory drugs are not effective

      (2) During chronic stages, the following medication may be given:
• Allopurinol, which suppresses uric acid production
• Probenecid and sulfinpyrazone, which increase excretion of uric acid

   c. The person should avoid excessive alcohol intake.
   d. The person should avoid starvation diets.
   e. The person should receive bed rest with immobilization of the affected area during acute attacks.
   f. Warm or ice packs may be applied.

5. Nursing interventions
   a. Keep covers off the affected area for comfort.
   b. Offer mild analgesics if needed to relieve discomfort.
   c. Instruct the person or family in how to prepare a low purine diet if ordered.
   d. Instruct the person or family in proper use of colchicine: Begin medication at the 1st sign of gout and follow the physician's orders for the schedule of medication.

Rx DRUG ADVISORY

During acute gout attacks, colchicine is administered every hour until symptoms subside, or until a total prescribed dose is given. If nausea, vomiting, abdominal cramping, or diarrhea occur, notify the physician because this is a sign of toxicity. These symptoms occur in approximately 80 percent of persons taking colchicine. Colchicine is also to be administered cautiously in elderly or debilitated persons and in those with renal, gastrointestinal, or heart disease.

   e. Instruct the person or family to avoid irritation of the inflamed area and to apply lotion to keep skin moist.
   f. Instruct the person or family that at least 2 liters of fluid should be consumed daily to avoid accumulation of uric acid crystals in the kidneys, which can lead to kidney stones. Ask the physician to verify that there are no contraindications to the person having this much fluid per day.

Paget's Disease (Osteitis Deformans)

1. Definition: Paget's disease is a disorder of the skeleton characterized by abnormally rapid bone turnover and resorption with excessive localized overgrowth of bone.
2. Incidence and etiology
   a. The etiology is unknown.
   b. Slow viral infection is contracted in young adulthood.
   c. Three million Americans older than age 40 years have Paget's disease.

d. Paget's disease occurs most frequently in persons between age 50 and 70 years.
e. There is a familial tendency.
f. The disease is slightly more common in men.

3. Clinical manifestations
   a. Ninety percent of persons with the disease are asymptomatic.
   b. Bone deformities include bone overgrowth and, in particular, bowed legs and an enlarged skull.
   c. Fatigue and intense skeletal pain may be experienced.
   d. Serum alkaline phosphatase is elevated.
   e. Radiograph of the skeleton is the primary means to confirm diagnosis of disease. A mosaic pattern in bone is seen on radiograph.

4. Clinical management
   a. Most affected persons are asymptomatic and require no treatment.
   b. Mildly symptomatic cases are treated with anti-inflammatory drugs and analgesics.
   c. Calcitonin may be given.
   d. Plicamycin (Mithracin) is an antibiotic used occasionally. It suppresses the action of osteoclasts.

5. Nursing interventions
   a. Assess which pain relief strategies the person is using and teach additional ones, if needed (see Chapter 11).
   b. Evaluate the effectiveness of pharmacologic and non-pharmacologic pain relief strategies.
   c. Assess mobility restrictions and ability to perform activities of daily living. The person may need a corset or brace, heel lifts, ambulation aids, or instruction in strengthening and weight-bearing exercises.
   d. Instruct the person on potential safety hazards.
   e. Discuss person's feelings regarding the disease and how it is affecting that person's life (Table 34–10).

Ankylosing Spondylitis

1. Definition: Ankylosing spondylitis is a systemic inflammatory condition of the vertebral column and the sacroiliac joints. Peripheral arthritis of the shoulders, knees, and hips occurs in 20 to 30 percent of affected persons.

2. Incidence and etiology
   a. There is possible autoimmune correlation.
   b. HLA-B27 antigen is present in 90 percent of affected people.
   c. Males are affected 8 to 1 over females.
   d. Peak incidence is in persons 20–40 years old.

3. Clinical manifestations
   a. There is a "bamboo spine" appearance on radiographic studies, and complete spinal fusion may be seen.
   b. There is excessive thoracic kyphosis and posterior rounding of the thoracic spine greater than 45 degrees.
   c. There is forward flexion of head and neck and low back pain.
   d. Sedimentation rate is elevated.
   e. Other systemic manifestations include pulmonary fibrosis, inflammatory bowel disease, and aortic insufficiency.

4. Clinical management
   a. Pain management includes the use of salicylates and NSAIDs, application of heat such as having a warm shower or bath, and phenylbutazone for severe cases, which should be limited due to the possibility of bone marrow depression.
   b. Education of the person and family should include managing activities of daily living.
      (1) Appropriate exercise includes swimming to promote spinal extension without increasing pain,

---

Table 34–10. Patient Education: Paget's Disease

Focus	Teaching Points
Pain related to bone deformities	Teach patient to take medications as prescribed and to position self with care in bed or chair. Instruct patient to move slowly and with measured steps; no abrupt movements.
Knowledge deficit related to disease process and drug therapy	Educate patient regarding the disease process and the drugs patient will be taking: Describe pagetic process to patient and provide information: Paget Foundation for Paget's Disease of Bone and Related Disorders (PFFPDBRD), 200 Varick Street, Suite 1004, New York, NY 10014–4810, (212) 229–1582, (800) 23–PAGET. When taking calcitonin: Teach self-injection and site rotation. Warn regarding side effects and that they are mild, infrequent, and usually diminish with continued use of calcitonin. When taking etidronate: Teach patient to take pills on empty stomach and not to eat for 90 min after dose. Divide daily dose to help minimize side effects. Tell patient to report any stomach cramps, diarrhea, new bone pain, or fractures. When taking plicamycin: Tell patient to watch for signs and symptoms of infection, temperature elevation, easy bruising, or bleeding. Tell patient to report any nausea, loss of appetite. Explain importance of completing regular follow-up laboratory tests.

From Maher AB, Salmond SW, and Pellino TA. *Orthopedic Nursing.* Philadelphia: WB Saunders, 1994, p 492.

range-of-motion exercises, and muscle strengthening exercises with a focus on spinal flexibility.

   (2) Maintenance of good posture includes use of furniture that does not keep the head, neck, and spine in constant flexion, sleeping flat in bed on one's back on a firm mattress. If a pillow is necessary, it should be as flat as possible. Sedentary persons should stretch or move around hourly.

   (3) Encourage good sleep habits.

   (4) Encourage maintenance of proper body weight.

5. Nursing interventions

  a. Discuss with the person how the disease affects that person's life.

  b. Evaluate the person's response to medications and other treatments.

  c. Assess the person's respiratory status. The person may have ineffective breathing patterns due to severe kyphosis.

Bursitis

1. Definition: Bursitis is a painful inflammation of a bursa, a closed, minimally fluid-filled sac that lubricates the space between tissue. Bursitis may be acute or chronic.

2. Incidence and etiology

  a. Activities requiring repetitive motion may aggravate or initiate the inflammation of joint.

  b. Bursitis may result from direct trauma to bursae or joint, infection, or rheumatoid arthritis or related conditions.

  c. The shoulder is the most commonly affected joint.

  d. Occurrence peaks in persons between 40 and 45 years of age.

  e. Slightly more women than men are affected.

3. Clinical manifestations

  a. Increased size of the bursa surrounding the joint as the sac fills with fluid

  b. Pain

  c. Erythema

  d. Localized increased skin warmth

  e. Increased discomfort upon motion

4. Clinical management

  a. Initially, ice and compression

  b. Rest of the affected area

  c. Aspiration of fluid from sac

  d. Nonsteroidal anti-inflammatory analgesics

  e. Cortisone injection into the joint–bursae space

5. Nursing interventions

  a. Evaluate the effectiveness of anti-inflammatory medication. The patient should take medication before activity.

  b. Teach use of heat and cold. Ice is applied for the first 24 to 48 hours to decrease swelling and inflammation. Moist heat is applied until pain subsides.

  c. Teach the person to rest, protect, and elevate the joint if appropriate. Instruct on the use of sling for subacromial bursitis, elastic bandage for olecranal bursitis, and felt pad or shoe with cut-out back for retrocalcaneol bursitis.

  d. Teach range-of-motion exercises to begin after pain subsides. For subacromial bursitis of the shoulder, instruct the person in the following techniques:

   (1) Passive pendulum: Tell the person to bend forward, allowing the affected arm to hang down. The person should slowly swing the arm in a small circle and gradually increase the size of the circle until full range of motion is achieved.

   (2) Wall walking: Tell the person to stand at arm's length from a wall and walk the fingers of the affected arm up the wall until the arm is elevated as far as possible.

  e. Encourage weight loss if needed for persons with trochanteric bursitis to decrease stress on the hip joint.

  f. Encourage the person to wear larger, easy-to-wear clothes to facilitate dressing during acute episodes.

Tendinitis (Tenosynovitis)

1. Definition: Tendinitis is inflammation of the sheath covering a tendon or group of tendons.

2. Incidence and etiology

  a. Tendinitis may be caused by repetitive motion or overuse, or inflammatory disease such as rheumatoid arthritis or gout.

  b. It may occur in persons with diabetes.

  c. Tendinitis may cause tears of the tendon sheath, bleeding in and around the tendon, loss of blood supply, and scar tissue or calcification at the tendon attachment.

  d. It occurs most commonly in the dominant extremity and can occur bilaterally.

  e. Tendinitis can affect the fingers, hands, wrists, elbows, shoulders, Achilles tendon, and patellar tendon.

  f. It frequently occurs with epicondylitis (inflammation of the tendons at the condyles) of the elbow.

  g. Tendinitis affects all age groups.

3. Clinical manifestations

  • Pain with motion

  • Edema

  • Point tenderness

  • Redness, warmth

  • Numbness or muscle weakness

4. Clinical management

  a. Rest

  b. Avoidance of motions that increase symptoms

  c. Application of ice for 24 to 48 hours, then of heat

  d. Range-of-motion exercises after inflammation subsides

  e. NSAIDs and nonnarcotic analgesics

  f. Cortisone injection

  g. Supports, such as forearm band for lateral epicondylitis, knee splint for patellar tendinitis, and heel pad or orthotic insert for Achilles tendinitis.

  h. If other measures do not help, surgery to remove calcified deposits and exostoses (bony outgrowths), repair tendon tears, and release and repair tendon sheath

5. Nursing interventions

a. Evaluate the effectiveness of medication.
b. Teach the rationale for the use of heat, cold, and rest.
c. Teach the proper application of forearm band, knee splint, or heel pads.

◼ MUSCULOSKELETAL INFECTIONS

Septic Arthritis

1. Definition: Septic arthritis is a bacterial invasion of a joint, originating in the joint or spreading from a nearby infection or through the bloodstream.
2. Incidence and etiology
   a. Septic arthritis is caused by various bacteria, viruses, or fungi.
   b. It can occur at any age.
   c. There is increased incidence in males and in children aged 2 years and younger.
   d. Untreated acute septic arthritis becomes chronic and causes joint destruction.
3. Clinical manifestations
   a. Fever and chills
   b. Pain and swelling of joint
   c. High serum and synovial fluid white blood cell count
   d. Elevated erythrocyte sedimentation rate and C-reactive protein
   e. Positive blood and joint cultures
   f. Bone destruction shown on radiographs
4. Clinical management
   a. Needle aspiration or open surgical drainage of infected joint fluid
   b. Pharmacologic interventions
      (1) Intravenous antibiotics
         • Type depends on age.
         • Children younger than 6 months receive gentamycin and nafcillin.
         • Children younger than 2 years receive chloramphenicol.
         • Adults receive penicillin G and other antibiotics as needed.
         • Therapy is for 2 to 3 weeks if there is no associated osteomyelitis.
      (2) Oral antibiotics initiated after clinical evidence of resolution of infection
5. Nursing interventions
   a. Monitor the wound site and report signs of increased purulent drainage.
   b. Evaluate the effects of nonnarcotic or narcotic analgesics.
   c. Teach the importance of taking antibiotics as ordered and informing the physician of any side effects.
   d. Teach the importance of maintaining a fluid intake of at least 3000 ml per day unless contraindicated.
   e. Teach the importance of the need for increase in protein and calorie intake to provide adequate nutrition during infection (see Chapter 8).
   f. Teach the importance of maintaining range of motion of joints. Have the patient demonstrate range-of-motion exercises.

g. Teach the proper use and care of splints needed for immobilization of affected joints. See pages 1565–1567.
h. Persons with chronic disease may need information regarding community resources that can assist with financial or emotional needs.
i. Instruct the patient on the principles of infection control: good handwashing, avoidance of people with colds and other infections, use of bleach to cleanse articles soiled with drainage, proper disposal of contaminated articles, and use of clean or sterile technique.

Infected Arthroplasty

1. Definition: Infected arthroplasty is infection of a total joint replacement. A superficial infection involves the suture line or drain site. An early deep infection is an infected hematoma with positive wound culture. A late deep infection involves the joint and prosthesis.
2. Incidence and etiology
   a. Causes include the following:
      (1) Infection elsewhere in the body
      (2) Contamination during surgery
      (3) Prior surgery in same area
      (4) Draining hematoma
      (5) Delayed wound healing
      (6) Joint aspiration
   b. Common organisms
      (1) Gram-negative organisms such as *Pseudomonas aeruginosa*, *Escherichia coli*, *Klebsiella*, and *Proteus vulgaris*
      (2) Gram-positive organisms such as *Staphylococcus aureus*, *Staphylococcus epidermidis*, and β-hemolytic streptococcus
   c. There is increased incidence in persons with the following:
      • Diabetes mellitus
      • Poor nutrition
      • Obesity
      • Autoimmune disease
      • Steroid dependency
      • Advanced age
   d. Infection rate is as follows:
      (1) Hips and knees: 1 to 2 percent
      (2) Shoulders: 1 to 2 percent
      (3) Elbows: 8 to 10 percent
3. Clinical manifestations
   a. Pain, swelling, and redness of joint
   b. Temperature spikes to 101 degrees Fahrenheit (38.3 degrees Celsius)
   c. Draining wound
   d. Decreased joint range of motion
   e. Elevated erythrocyte sedimentation rate
   f. Elevated white blood cell count
   g. Soft tissue swelling, periosteal new bone formation, and osteolysis shown on radiographs
   h. Limp
4. Clinical management
   a. The severity of infection determines its management.
   b. Intravenous antibiotics are given for 4 to 6 weeks. Type depends on the causative organism.

c. Irrigation and débridement of the wound may be undertaken.

d. The prosthesis may be removed and a cement spacer applied.

e. Skeletal traction may be used to preserve the joint space for reimplantation of prosthesis or to preserve leg length.

5. Nursing interventions
   a. Actions are the same as for septic arthritis, see page 1590.
   b. For care of persons in skeletal traction, see pages 1564–1566.

Tuberculosis of Bones and Joints

1. Definition: Tuberculosis of bones and joints is a secondary infection caused by *Mycobacterium* species that develops outside the pulmonary system.
2. Incidence and etiology
   a. Occurrence is most frequent in the spine (Pott's disease).
   b. Other common sites are the hip, knee, ankle, wrist, and elbow.
   c. Tuberculosis of bones and joints is the most common form of extrapulmonary tuberculosis.
   d. There is increased incidence in persons having compromised immune systems, diabetes mellitus, end-stage renal disease, positive results on tuberculosis skin test, and unsanitary living conditions.
   e. Destruction of bone is insidious.
3. Clinical manifestations
   a. Pain, swelling, stiffness, and reduced joint motion
   b. In the advanced stage:
      (1) Muscle atrophy and contractures
      (2) Abscess formation including sinus tracts that extend from bone to skin
      (3) Activation of pulmonary lesion causing low-grade fever, night sweats, anorexia, cough, and weakness
4. Diagnostics
   a. Synovial fluid analysis shows elevated white blood cell count, elevated protein, reduced or absent glucose, and poor mucin clot.
   b. Pure protein derivative test result is positive.
   c. Tubercle bacilli are isolated through biopsy of synovium, bony lesion, or lymph node.
   d. Radiographs may not show evidence of bone destruction for months or years.
   e. Chest radiograph may or may not show signs of tuberculosis.
5. Clinical management
   a. Pharmacologic interventions include strict therapy with antituberculosis drugs.
      (1) Combination therapy with isoniazid and rifampin for 12 to 24 months
      (2) Ethambutal to establish drug sensitivity or if there is history of previous drug therapy
   b. Special medical-surgical procedures
      (1) Synovectomy to remove infected tissue
      (2) Arthrodesis to fuse joint for stability and pain relief

(3) Spinal fusion, if the deformity progresses or if paraparesis or paraplegia occur

(4) After several years, total joint replacement

c. Splints are used to immobilize the affected joint, followed by physical therapy.

6. Nursing interventions
   a. See Chapter 8 for discussion of side effects of antituberculosis drugs.
   b. See page 1611 for nursing care related to spinal fusion and total joint replacement.
   c. The rehabilitative period may last as long as 1 to 2 years. Teach the need to continue medication, even when the person does not feel ill. Teach the use of splints, if needed, for immobilization of joints. See pages 1565–1567 for splint care. Reinforce the importance of continued follow-up to assess the success of treatment.
   d. Assess the person's home living conditions and teach principles of good hygiene if needed. Assess the availability of personal and community resources, nutritional status, and the presence of other health problems.

Osteomyelitis

1. Definition: Osteomyelitis is a pyogenic infection of the bone and surrounding tissue.
2. Incidence and etiology
   a. Osteomyelitis can be acute or chronic. Acute osteomyelitis can progress to chronic osteomyelitis if it is unidentified or not treated properly. Chronic osteomyelitis can lead to bone deformities, leg length discrepancies, or need for amputation.
   b. Organisms affecting adults include *E. coli, Neisseria gonorrhoeae,* staphylococci (*S. aureus* is the most common infecting organism, causing 90 percent of purulent osteomyelitis), and anaerobes.
   c. Occurrence is at any age (see Chapter 15).
   d. There is increased incidence in males, children younger than age 12 years, and adults older than age 50 years.
   e. In adults, risk factors include the following:
      (1) Genitourinary infection
      (2) Drug abuse
      (3) Vascular insufficiency related to diabetes or atherosclerosis
      (4) Unsanitary living conditions
      (5) Impaired immune response
      (6) Obesity
      (7) Malnutrition
      (8) Alcoholism
      (9) Smoking
      (10) Previous orthopedic surgery at the same site
      (11) Total joint surgery
      (12) Open trauma or fracture
3. Clinical manifestations
   a. For acute osteomyelitis, systemic symptoms include the following:
      • Temperature of 101 to 104 degrees Fahrenheit (38.3–40 degrees Celsius)

- Chills
- General malaise
- Elevated erythrocyte sedimentation rate
- Elevated white blood cell count

  b. For chronic osteomyelitis, localized symptoms include the following:

- Pain
- Swelling
- Redness
- Warmth
- Draining sinus tract

4. Clinical management

  a. Pharmacologic interventions

    (1) Parenteral antibiotics are started as soon as blood or wound cultures are obtained.

    (2) Penicillinase-resistant semisynthetic penicillin is given initially.

    (3) Other forms of antibiotics are added as needed, depending on the infective organism.

    (4) Intravenous antibiotics are given for 4 to 8 weeks.

    (5) Patients may go home with intravenous antibiotics if appropriate teaching is done and home health follow-up is in place.

    (6) Erythrocyte sedimentation rate studies are done to assess response to medications.

    (7) Oral antibiotics may be given for an additional 4 to 8 weeks after intravenous medication is completed. Oral antibiotics are started after there is evidence of resolution of the infection, that is, there is a decrease in erythrocyte sedimentation rate and no fever is noted.

    (8) To maintain proper levels of antibiotic in the blood, the minimum inhibitory concentration and the minimum bacterial concentration must be monitored.

    (9) There must be continuous irrigation of the antibiotic solution.

    (10) Antibiotic cement or beads may be inserted.

  b. Special medical-surgical procedures

    (1) For acute osteomyelitis, needle aspiration or percutaneous needle biopsy provides materials to determine causative organism. Irrigation and drainage of bone relieves pressure from purulent material inside bone. The endoprosthesis may be removed.

    (2) For chronic osteomyelitis, sequestrectomy removes dead bone. Saucerization removes all affected tissue, leaving a depression that looks like a saucer in the bone.

NURSE ADVISORY

Assess the patient every 8 hours for signs of superinfection, including continued fever or candidiasis of the mouth, throat, gastrointestinal tract, genitourinary tract, or vagina.

5. Nursing interventions. Actions are the same as for septic arthritis, see page 1590.

Osteoarthritis

1. Definition

  a. Osteoarthritis is a chronic, slowly progressive degenerative disease of movable joints.

  b. The cause of primary osteoarthritis is unknown, and it is more common in women.

  c. Secondary osteoarthritis is due to joint injury or disease, and it is more common in men.

  d. Localized osteoarthritis affects 1 or 2 joints.

  e. Generalized osteoarthritis affects 3 or more joints.

2. Incidence and socioeconomic impact

  a. Osteoarthritis is the most common form of arthritis, affecting more than 40 million Americans.

  b. It principally affects hips, knees, fingers, great toe, and spine.

  c. Occurrence peaks between the 5th and 6th decades of life.

  d. Five percent of people stop working each year due to disabling osteoarthritis.

  e. By age 70 years, more than 80 percent of people with osteoarthritis are symptomatic.

  f. Osteoarthritis is the number one cause of disability among older people.

3. Risk factors

  a. Obesity

  b. Family history

  c. Black race

  d. Hormonal factors

    (1) Hands are more affected in women.

    (2) Hips are more affected in men.

  e. Lifestyle and occupation. Repetitive motion activities affect shoulders, elbows, fingers, hips, knees, and ankles.

4. Etiology is unknown.

5. Pathophysiology: Cartilage covering the ends of bones within joints becomes soft, less elastic, and thinner. As cartilage wears away, the bones rub against each other and become rough, and bone tissue is damaged.

6. Clinical manifestations

  a. Loss of joint motion, causing joint stiffness

  b. Dull, aching pain in or around joint

    (1) Stiffness and pain is relieved by rest and worsened by activity.

    (2) As osteoarthritis progresses, pain occurs at night and during rest.

  c. Deformity of joints

    (1) Heberden nodes and Bouchard nodes develop in hands (Fig. 34–19).

    (2) Flexion contractures can develop in hips.

    (3) Knees may become bowed in appearance (varus), and flexion deformity may develop (Fig. 34–20).

    (4) In the spine, loss of joint space causes pain, numbness, and tingling as the spinal nerve is entrapped.

  d. When hips and knees are affected, a limp may occur due to pain, stiffness, and instability of the joint.

  e. Crepitation of the joint may be felt on movement.

7. Diagnostics

  a. Assessment

    (1) Health history. Note the following points when interviewing the person with osteoarthritis:

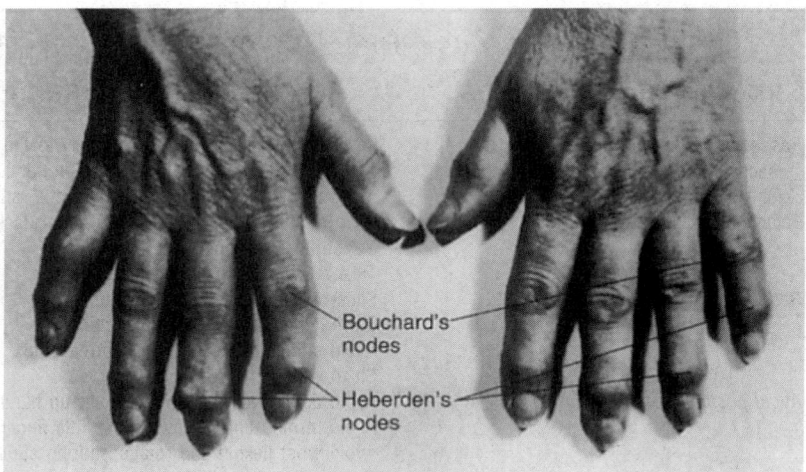

Figure 34–19. Heberden's and Bouchard's nodes. (From Polley HF, and Hunder GG. *Physical Examination of the Joints.* 2nd ed. Philadelphia: WB Saunders, 1978, p 120.)

- Presence of malaise, weakness, fatigue, and difficulty sleeping
- Character, location, and duration of pain and stiffness
- Level of activity; work and exercise history

(2) Physical examination
- Inspect and palpate joints for symmetry, size, shape, color, appearance, temperature, and pain.
- To assess the condition of joints, observe the ease of movement, presence of crepitus, and presence of squeaking, creaking, or grating with movement.
- Address how osteoarthritis affects the person's activities of daily living and role functions.
- Assessment tools such as the Stanford Arthritis Center Disability and Discomfort Scale can be useful (see Fig. 34–5). This scale assesses a per-

son's functional level for the past week and indicates what assistance the person needs to complete the listed activities.

b. Diagnostic studies
(1) In addition to the physical examination that identifies the clinical manifestations, diagnostic studies are useful in detection of the extent of the osteoarthritis and in differentiating it from rheumatoid arthritis. For a full explanation of rheumatoid arthritis, refer to Chapter 21.
(2) Radiographic studies show the following:
- Decreased joint space
- Subchondral sclerosis in which cartilage wears away and the bone under the cartilage touches the opposite side of the joint.
- Osteophyte formation (bone ridges or spurs)
(3) Bone scan determines which joints are affected.
(4) Magnetic resonance imaging determines the extent of joint destruction.
(5) There are no laboratory study abnormalities that characterize osteoarthritis.
(6) Synovial fluid analysis may be used to differentiate osteoarthritis from rheumatoid arthritis. In osteoarthritis, synovial fluid is clear yellow; in rheumatoid arthritis, it is milky, cloudy, or dark yellow.

8. Clinical management
a. Goals of clinical management
(1) Decrease pain
(2) Increase joint range-of-motion
(3) Maintain function
b. Nonpharmacologic interventions
(1) Application of heat and cold—cold during the acute inflammatory phase and heat after the acute flare-up
(2) Relaxation techniques, meditation, massage, biofeedback, and hypnosis
(3) Transcutaneous nerve stimulation
(4) Maintenance of optimal weight
(5) Use of assistive devices (e.g., crutches, cane)
(6) Joint protection techniques (Table 34–11)
(7) Range-of-motion and strengthening exercises
c. Pharmacologic interventions

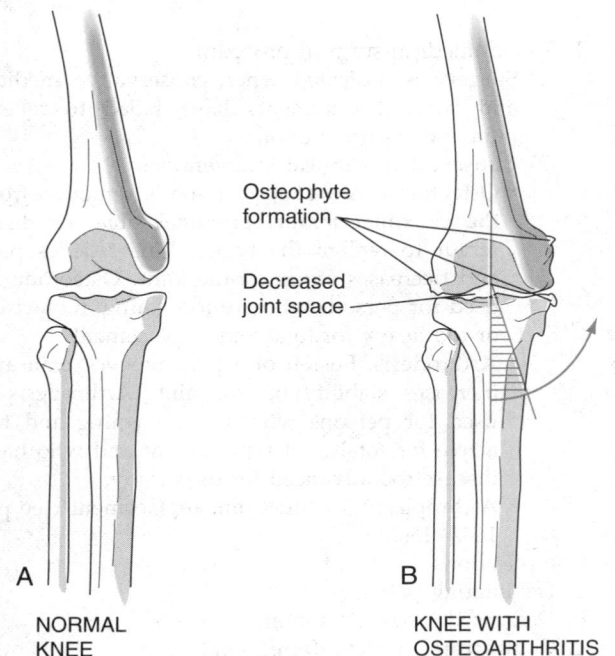

Figure 34–20. Comparison of a normal knee *(A)* with an arthritic knee *(B)*.

Table 34-11. Principles of Joint Protection and Associated Work Simplification Strategies

Joint Protection Principles	Strategies to Simplify Work
Respect pain (Fear of pain can lead to inactivity; ignoring pain can lead to joint damage)	Carry out activities and exercise only to the point of fatigue or discomfort. Reduce the time spent in doing painful activities. Avoid doing activities (other than gentle range of motion) when joints are inflamed.
Balance work and rest	Rest 5-10 min periodically when doing tasks that take more time. Get sufficient sleep. Take a 30-min rest during the afternoon.
Reduce effort to joints	Slide objects rather than lift them. Store items at appropriate heights. Avoid stooping, bending, or overreaching. Sit to work whenever possible.
Avoid positions of stress on joints	Avoid tight pinch or grip: use built-up handles and holders for objects such as toothbrushes and pens. Avoid turning fingers toward the little finger: turn fingers toward the thumb. Avoid wrist flexion and rotation during stirring. Example: use spoon like a dagger. Use two hands to lift or carry objects. Always consider adaptive devices (jar opener, reachers, built-up keys) to protect joints from deformities.
Use larger and stronger joints	Lift with palm and forearm instead of fingers. Use a backpack, waist pack, or shoulder bag instead of a handbag.
Use joints in most stable positions	Avoid or minimize excessive stretch of joint ligaments. Example: rise from chair symmetrically and avoid leaning to either side. Maintain good posture.
Avoid remaining in one position	Change position (or stretch) every 20 min. Balance sitting tasks with those that require moving around.
Avoid activities that cannot be stopped	Break activities into defined parts.

From Maher AB, Salmond SW, and Pellino TA. *Orthopedic Nursing*. Philadelphia: WB Saunders, 1994, p 384.

(1) Nonsteroidal anti-inflammatory drugs, which are indicated for mild to moderate pain relief. Therapeutic effects may not be noticed for 2 to 3 weeks. Because NSAIDs may irritate the gastrointestinal tract, give with food, antacids, or H_2-receptor antagonists such as Pepcid AC and 8 ounces of water. Watch for signs of abnormal bleeding. Use cautiously with persons older than 65 years of age or if hypertension, heart disease, or renal disease is present.

(2) Steroids, which are for intra-articular use only. They are given only once or twice a year for severe symptoms. A response usually takes 48 hours to occur.

(3) Analgesics
   • Aspirin that is enteric coated causes less gastrointestinal distress and has an anti-inflammatory effect.

DRUG ADVISORY

Persons taking high doses of aspirin need to be aware of side effects of salicylism: tinnitus, nausea, vomiting, drowsiness, and gastrointestinal bleeding (black tarry stools). They should also be instructed to check labels of other over-the-counter medications they are taking to avoid adding salicylates.

   • Acetaminophen causes no gastrointestinal distress and has no anti-inflammatory effect.

DRUG ADVISORY

Caution persons using acetaminophen in extra strength (500 mg per tablet) or regular doses (325 mg per tablet) not to take more than 2600 mg per day. Long-term uncontrolled use of acetaminophen or overdosage can cause liver damage.

d. Special medical-surgical procedures
   (1) Surgery is indicated when conservative medical and surgical treatments have failed to relieve pain and restore motion.
   (2) Conservative surgical interventions
      • Osteotomy. A wedge of bone is removed from the proximal femur, proximal tibia, or distal femur to realign the bones. This relieves pain and decreases stress on the joint. Osteotomy is used for persons who are too young, too active, or too heavy for total joint replacement.
      • Arthrodesis. Fusion of a joint relieves pain and increases stability of the joint. Arthrodesis is used for persons who are too young and too active for total joint replacement and who have disease too advanced for osteotomy.
      • Arthroplasty, or total joint replacement (see pp. 1607-1608).
9. Complications
   a. Debilitating pain
   b. Decreased range of motion
   c. Contractures of the affected joint

d. Loss of joint function

e. Loss of ability to independently care for self

10. Prognosis is improved quality of life with less pain and increased mobility.

11. Applying the Nursing Process

NURSING DIAGNOSIS: Pain R/T joint stiffness

---

a. *Expected outcomes:* Following instruction and treatment, the person should be able to do the following:

(1) Identify methods of pain management

(2) Participate in activities with decrease in pain

b. *Nursing interventions*

(1) Assess the person's pain, and identify present methods of pain management.

(2) Teach additional methods of pain management.

(3) Evaluate use of newly learned methods of pain management.

NURSING DIAGNOSIS: Impaired physical mobility R/T joint stiffness and destruction of joint

---

a. *Expected outcomes:* Following instruction and treatment, the person should be able to do the following:

(1) Identify techniques that will increase mobility

(2) Participate in activities that maintain increased mobility

b. *Nursing interventions*

(1) Assess range of motion of joints.

(2) Assess ambulation distance and endurance.

(3) Teach joint protection techniques (see Table 34–10).

(4) Teach strengthening and range-of-motion exercises.

- Passive range of motion is used during acute inflammation to stretch tightened muscles and prevent flexion contractures.

- Active stretching is used when pain and inflammation subside.

- Gradually progress to isometric exercises and gentle resistive exercises.

(5) Teach gait with assistive device if needed.

(6) Evaluate effectiveness of mobility techniques.

NURSING DIAGNOSIS: Impaired home maintenance management R/T pain, joint stiffness, or impaired activities of daily living

---

a. *Expected outcomes:* Following instruction and treatment, the person should be able to do the following:

(1) Identify methods that help increase participation in activities.

(2) Increase participation in activities.

b. *Nursing interventions*

(1) Assess the person's functional status using a standardized tool such as the Stanford Arthritis Center Disability and Discomfort Scale (see Fig. 34–5).

(2) Assist the person in identification of devices needed to help that person become more functional (e.g., gait devices, handrails, braces, elevated toilet seats and chairs, and shower stools).

(3) Assist the person in identifying needed changes in home environment such as having furniture rearranged and placing commonly used utensils within easier reach.

(4) Remind the person of joint protection principles and work simplification measures.

(5) Evaluate the effectiveness of changes and new techniques.

12. Discharge planning and teaching

a. Persons with osteoarthritis are usually not hospitalized unless surgery is required (see p. 1607–1608 for a discussion of total joint replacement).

b. Instruction can be given by nurses and physicians in the office regarding disease risk factors and aggravating factors (see p. 1592).

c. Referral to a self-help class can be helpful in teaching the person how to manage osteoarthritis.

NURSE ADVISORY

An arthritis self-help course sponsored by local Arthritis Foundation chapters teaches a multidisciplinary approach, pain management, disability management, and strategies for overcoming depression.

---

13. Public health considerations

a. At this time, there is no cure for osteoarthritis.

b. The following preventive measures are designed to maintain function and decrease pain through education:

(1) Light to moderate regular exercise

(2) Maintenance of normal weight

(3) Balancing rest with activity

(4) Stress management

(5) Joint protection

◼ *DEGENERATIVE MUSCULOSKELETAL DISORDERS*

Bunions (Hallux Valgus)

1. Definition: A bunion is a painful swelling of the bursae just above the lateral aspect of the great toe.

2. Incidence and etiology

a. Bunions may be acquired or congenital.

b. Bunions may be acquired from improperly fitting shoe apparel that is too narrow or pointed.

c. With congenital bunions, the great toe is angled at birth, displacing the other toes.

d. Bunions are the most common pain-inducing deformity of the great toe.

e. Bunions are 9 times more common in females than males.

3. Clinical manifestations

a. Valgus deformity of the great toe
b. Pain
c. Difficulty walking
d. Inflamed or ruptured bursae
4. Clinical management
   a. Conservative clinical management is to instruct the patient to change style of shoe apparel to sneakers or open-toed shoes (boxier-toed shoes).
   b. Pharmacologic interventions include administration of NSAIDs and antipyretics.
   c. Special medical-surgical procedures
      (1) Osteotomy
      (2) Soft tissue procedure to correct great toe deformity
5. Nursing interventions: After surgery, immediate postoperative care includes the following:
   a. Monitor circulation and sensation of toes of the affected extremity and compare with the toes of the other extremity. Report decreased circulation and sensation to the surgeon.
   b. Elevate the affected extremity to prevent excessive swelling and circulatory compromise.
   c. Evaluate the effectiveness of pain medication.
   d. Teach cast care if needed (see p. 1561).
   e. Teach ambulation with crutches if needed.

■ DEFICIENCY MUSCULOSKELETAL DISORDERS

Osteoporosis

1. Definition: Osteoporosis is an irreversible disease process in which there is a reduction of bone density, making bone more susceptible to fracture.
2. Incidence and socioeconomic impact
   a. Twenty-five million people suffer from osteoporosis in the United States: 20 million women and 5 million men.
   b. A total of 1.5 million fractures result from osteoporosis each year: 300,000 hip fractures, 500,000 vertebral fractures, and 200,000 wrist fractures.
      (1) White women 60 years of age or older have at least twice the incidence of fractures as Black women.
      (2) One of 5 Black women are at risk of developing osteoporosis. Black women have higher bone density.
      (3) A woman's risk of hip fracture development due to osteoporosis is equal to her combined risk for development of breast, uterine, and ovarian cancer.
      (4) Women can lose up to 20 percent of their total bone mass in the first 5 to 7 years after menopause.
3. Risk factors
   a. Genetic factors
      • Female
      • Asian or White, especially of northern European ancestry

• Small thin frame
• Family history of kyphosis or hip fracture
• Red or blonde hair
• Fair skin
• Mother who had osteoporosis
• Scoliosis
• Rheumatoid arthritis
   b. Nutritional factors
      • Lifelong low calcium diet
      • High sodium and protein diet
      • Strict vegetarian diet
      • Poor gastrointestinal absorption
   c. Lifestyle factors
      • Sedentary life
      • Tobacco use
      • Regular consumption of alcohol
      • High caffeine consumption
   d. Endocrinologic factors
      • Never being pregnant
      • Early menopause
      • Amenorrhea
      • Abnormally low weight or slimness
      • Hyperthyroidism
   e. Pharmacologic factors include consumption of the following:
      • Antacids containing aluminum
      • Seizure medications
      • Diuretics
      • Vitamin A
      • Corticosteroids
4. Etiology: The cause of osteoporosis is unknown.
5. Pathophysiology
   a. Bone resorption is more rapid than bone formation.
   b. Mineral and protein matrix is diminished, leading to decreased bone mass.
6. Clinical manifestations
   a. Osteoporosis is called the "silent disease" because bone loss occurs without symptoms.
   b. Collapsed vertebrae may be felt or seen in the form of severe back pain.
   c. Height may be lost.
   d. Spinal deformities may manifest as stooped posture or dowager's hump.
   e. Fractures are common.
7. Diagnostics
   a. Bone density testing
      (1) Detects osteoporosis before a fracture occurs
      (2) Predicts chances of future fractures
      (3) Determines rate of bone loss
      (4) Monitors the effect of treatment
   b. Techniques for measuring bone density
      (1) Quantitative computed tomography and dual photon absorptiometry (older methods)
      (2) Dual-energy x-ray absorptiometry (a newer method), giving more precise measurement, less radiation exposure, and shorter procedure time
   c. Laboratory tests
      (1) Urinary calcium may be elevated, but serum calcium is normal.
      (2) Serum bone Gla-protein (osteocalcin) is elevated.
   d. Special medical-surgical procedures: In a bone

LEARNING/TEACHING GUIDELINES
for Prevention of Osteoporosis

General Overview

1. Discuss the risk factors of osteoporosis.
2. Recognize the importance of preventing osteoporosis.
3. List steps required to prevent osteoporosis.

Risk Factors

1. Inform the person of risk factors
   a. Smoking
   b. Sedentary lifestyle
   c. Low calcium diet
   d. High intake of caffeine and alcohol
   e. Estrogen deficiency

Importance of Preventing Osteoporosis

1. Osteoporosis is irreversible.
2. Osteoporosis is a silent disease. You do not realize what is missing until it is gone.
3. Symptoms of osteoporosis include loss of height, dowager's hump (humpback), pain, and fractures.

Prevention

1. Prevention should start with children. Peak bone mass occurs at approximately 30 years of age.
2. Eat a balanced diet that includes the recommended amounts of calcium: 1200 mg for adolescents and adults and 1500 mg for postmenopausal women.
3. Avoid high protein intake, which causes increased loss of calcium from the kidneys.
4. Avoid high caffeine intake, which causes the body to lose fluid and calcium.
5. Avoid smoking: women who smoke experience menopause earlier than nonsmoking women.
6. Avoid high alcohol intake, which interferes with the intestinal absorption of calcium and interferes with the direct incorporation of calcium into the bone.
7. Treat estrogen deficiencies: amenorrhea due to excessive exercise, anorexia, bulimia, or surgical oophorectomy.
8. Exercise regularly: lack of regular exercise causes bone to demineralize. Thirty to 40 minutes of weight-bearing exercise 2 to 3 times a week is required.
9. Avoid stress, which causes loss of calcium from the body.

---

biopsy, a core of bone is taken from the anterior superior iliac spine to analyze structure and function of bone.

8. Clinical management
   a. Goals of clinical management
      (1) Preserve skeletal mass by inhibiting bone resorption
      (2) Prevent fractures
      (3) Relieve pain
   b. Nonpharmacologic interventions
      (1) Weight-bearing exercise as directed by a physician. High-impact or rotational type exercises of the spine must be avoided due to risk of fracture.
      (2) Increased calcium in the diet.
   c. Pharmacologic interventions
      (1) Estrogen replacement in postmenopausal women inhibits bone resorption. Side effects include headaches, bloating, increased vaginal bleeding, weight gain, tender breast, and mood swings.
      (2) Calcium supplements prevent bone resorption by stimulation of the parathyroid gland. Monitor for hypercalcemia (dehydration, lethargy, confusion, coma, abdominal pain, hypertension, muscle weakness, and fatigue).
      (3) Calcitonin slows bone breakdown and reduces pain associated with osteoporotic fractures. Side effects include nausea, vomiting, anorexia, urinary frequency, and mild, transient flushing of the hands and feet.

(4) Sodium fluoride, when taken with calcium, restores bone mass and is effective in spinal osteoporosis. Serum fluoride levels should be monitored.
(5) Etidronate (Didronel) inhibits resorption of bone. Side effects include transient elevation of creatinine and phosphate levels.

   d. Special medical-surgical procedures include surgical fixation of fractures if they occur. See page 1574 for a discussion of nursing care of fractures.

9. Complications
   a. Fractures: The most common sites are the hip, spine, and wrist (see p. 1570).
   b. Low back pain (see pp. 1583–1585).
10. Prognosis
   a. There is no cure for osteoporosis.
   b. Focus needs to be on prevention, starting with school-aged children (See Learning/Teaching Guidelines for Prevention of Osteoporosis).
   c. Goals for advanced osteoporosis are to maintain independence in activities of daily living and to prevent falls.
11. Applying the nursing process

NURSING DIAGNOSIS: Impaired physical mobility R/T the disease process

   a. *Expected outcomes:* Following instruction, the person should be able to do the following:

(1) Maintain or increase mobility
(2) Maintain or increase strength
b. *Nursing interventions*
(1) Teach strengthening exercises.
(2) Teach use of ambulatory devices (see pp. 1567–1568).
(3) Teach use of adaptive devices (see p. 1609).

NURSING DIAGNOSIS: Pain R/T disease process

---

a. *Expected outcomes:* Following treatment, the person should be able to do the following:
(1) Identify methods of pain relief
(2) Verbalize relief of pain
b. *Nursing interventions*
(1) Evaluate the effectiveness of medications given to relieve pain: narcotics, nonnarcotics, muscle relaxants, and NSAIDs.
(2) Teach nonpharmacologic methods to relieve pain: transcutaneous electric nerve stimulation, relaxation, and imagery (see Chapter 11).
(3) Teach use of brace if indicated (see pp. 1565–1567).
(4) Evaluate the effectiveness of use of heat to the affected area.

NURSING DIAGNOSIS: Altered nutrition, less than body requirements, R/T disease process

---

a. *Expected outcomes:* Following instruction, the person should be able to do the following:
(1) Recognize the importance of increased intake of calcium
(2) Include dietary sources of calcium in the daily diet
(3) Use calcium supplements if needed
b. *Nursing interventions*
(1) Teach that the body takes calcium from the bones if there is not enough in the daily diet. The recommended daily amounts are 1200 mg for adults and 1500 mg for postmenopausal women.
(2) Teach the makings of a balanced diet with emphasis on foods high in calcium: cheese, milk, dark green vegetables.
(3) Teach proper use of calcium supplements. Calcium carbonate (Tums) can be obtained over the counter.

NURSING DIAGNOSIS: Risk for injury R/T disease process

---

a. *Expected outcomes:* Following instruction, the person should be able to do the following:
(1) Recognize factors that can lead to falls and fractures
(2) Prevent falls and fractures
b. *Nursing interventions:* Teach factors that lead to falls.

12. Discharge planning and teaching. See Learning/Teaching Guidelines for Prevention of Osteoporosis.
13. Public health considerations. Public information programs about osteoporosis and its prevention and treatment are essential. The Osteoporosis Foundation is an excellent resource for information.

Osteomalacia

1. Definition: Osteomalacia is a condition of decalcification and softening of bones caused by vitamin D deficiency. Osteomalacia is called rickets in children.
2. Incidence and etiology
   a. Osteomalacia may be due to renal disease, with its increased losses of calcium or phosphorus.
   b. Osteomalacia may be caused by lack of exposure to sunlight, which is required to convert vitamin D into its absorbable form
   c. The combination of pregnancy and inadequate intake of vitamin D and calcium may cause osteomalacia.
   d. Gastrointestinal malabsorption may cause osteomalacia.
   e. Chronic diarrhea causes loss of calcium, leading to inadequate vitamin D absorption.
   f. Vitamin-D deficient rickets has almost completely disappeared due to vitamin D fortification of milk.
3. Clinical manifestations
   a. Fractured bones
   b. Progressive deformities of bones of extremities and the spine
   c. Persistent skeletal pain
   d. Progressive muscle weakness
   e. Presence of Looser's zones (decalcified areas in bone) on radiographs
   f. Elevated serum alkaline phosphatase
   g. Generalized bone demineralization and multiple bone deformities
   h. Decreased serum levels of calcium and phosphorus
4. Clinical management
   a. Increased dietary intake of vitamin D
   b. Calcium supplementation. Serial monitoring of serum calcium levels is important to detect hypercalcemia.
   c. Periods of sunlight exposure that is necessary for vitamin D metabolites to be converted to usable vitamin D in the body
5. Nursing interventions
   a. See nursing interventions for osteoporosis.
   b. Teach dietary sources of vitamin D: eggs, sardines, swordfish, mackerel, chicken liver, dairy products, and some cereals.
   c. Teach side effects of vitamin D toxicity: muscle weakness, fatigue, abdominal pain, confusion, lethargy, slow thinking, dehydration, hypertension, and coma.
   d. Reinforce the importance of follow-up care.

◻ *BONE TUMORS*

Primary Bone Tumors

1. Definition: Primary bone tumors are benign or malignant tumors that originate in bone. They may be chondro-

genic (from cartilage) or osteogenic (from bone) (Table 34–12).
2. Etiology: The cause of primary bone tumors is unknown.
3. Clinical manifestations (see Table 34–12)
4. Clinical management
   a. Nonpharmacologic and pharmacologic interventions: see Chapter 17.
   b. Surgery
      (1) Wide resection of the tumor removes the tumor along with a wide zone of normal tissue.
      (2) Amputation may be necessary.
   c. Chemotherapy or radiation therapy may also be indicated, especially with malignant tumors.
   d. See page 1604 for discussion of nursing care of amputations.

Metastatic Bone Lesions

1. Definition
   a. In metastatic bone lesions, malignant cells spread from the primary site to the bone via the following routes:
      (1) Direct route: spread from a local tumor
      (2) Hematogenous route: spread through the bloodstream
      (3) Lymphatic route: spread through the lymphatic system
   b. Two types of lesions are lytic lesions in which tumor cells cause destruction of bone, with greater chance for pathologic fracture, and blastic lesions in which tumor cells cause a reactive bone formation with less chance for pathologic fracture.

2. Incidence and etiology
   a. Metastatic bone disease occurs at any age.
   b. The most common sites of metastases:
      (1) Thorax and vertebrae, 50 percent
      (2) Extremities, 34 percent
      (3) Skull, 22 percent
   c. The most common primary sites:
      • Breast
      • Prostate
      • Lung
      • Kidney
      • Thyroid
      • Bladder
      • Lymph (Hodgkin's disease)
      • Pancreas
   d. Any malignant tumor can metastasize to bone.
3. Clinical manifestations
   a. Bone pain
   b. Paresthesia, paralysis, or radicular pain, indicating pressure on the spinal cord or vertebral collapse
   c. Hypercalcemia
   d. Elevated alkaline phosphatase
   e. Radiographs showing lytic or blastic lesions
   f. Bone scan showing areas of increased uptake
   g. Pathologic fracture
4. Clinical management
   a. Nonpharmacologic interventions
      (1) Radiation therapy, which promotes rapid destruction of tumor cells, followed by bone healing, recalcification, and relief from pain
      (2) Pain relief via imagery, relaxation, music therapy, and cutaneous stimulation

---

Table 34–12. Primary Bone Tumors

Classification/Name	Description
Benign chondrogenic	
Osteochondroma	Most common benign tumor. Commonly found in the femur and tibia; 10% develop into sarcoma.
Endochondroma	Common to mature hyaline cartilage in hands, feet, ribs, spine, sternum, or long bones. Frequently leads to pathologic fractures.
Benign osteogenic	
Osteoid, osteomas	Usually small tumors with clearly outlined area of reactive bone. Common to the proximal femur, tibia, scaphoid bone of the wrist, talus, or calcaneus of the foot. Causes pain at night.
Osteoblastoma	Evolves more rapidly and into a larger tumor than an osteoid osteoma. Found in vertebrae, distal femur, diaphysis of long bones, hands, and feet.
Giant cell tumor	Aggressive and extensive lesion. Has a tendency to recur and metastasize to the lung. Commonly found in the distal femur, tibia, distal radius, sacrum, proximal humerus, and proximal fibula. Produces pain, edema, and limitation in movement.
Malignant osteogenic	
Osteosarcoma	Most common malignant bone tumor. Occurs in the metaphysis of long bones, at the sites of the most rapid bone growth. Common to the distal femur, proximal tibia, and proximal humerus. Can be induced by ionizing radiation, and may follow therapeutic radiation. Causes pain, swelling, and pathologic fracture. Serum alkaline phosphatase is markedly elevated. Prognosis improving with combination therapies, reaching 65% survival.
Ewing's sarcoma	Common to young adults and found in the pelvis and lower extremities. Metastasizes quickly to the lungs and other bones. Clinical manifestations include pain, edema, low-grade fever, leukocytes, and anemia. Improving prognosis with aggressive therapy; 65% survival rate.
Chondrosarcoma	Common to the pelvis, ribs, proximal femur, and proximal humerus.
Fibrosarcoma	Common to the femur and tibia.

From Black JM, and Matassarin-Jacobs E (eds). *Luckmann and Sorensen's Medical-Surgical Nursing: A Psychophysiologic Approach.* 4th ed. Philadelphia: WB Saunders, 1993, p 1910.

(3) Assistive gait devices such as crutches, walkers, or canes
b. Pharmacologic interventions
(1) Chemotherapy that is appropriate to the primary site
(2) Pain relief via analgesics, NSAIDs, tricyclic antidepressants, and corticosteroids, which can be used alone or in combination as needed
5. Nursing interventions
a. See Chapter 17 for nursing care related to chemotherapy and radiation therapy.
b. See page 1574 for care of fractures.
c. See Chapter 11 for pain management.
d. See pages 1567–1569 for use of assistive gait devices.

Osteosarcoma

1. Definition: Osteosarcoma is a primary malignant bone tumor that most frequently affects the distal femur, proximal tibia, and proximal humerus.
2. Incidence and etiology
a. Osteosarcoma occurs in persons aged 10 to 30 years, with peak incidence between 10 and 20 years.
b. Osteosarcoma affects males slightly more than females.
c. Osteosarcoma is the most common sarcoma.
d. Children with familial retinoblastoma have approximately a 7 percent incidence of development of osteosarcoma.
e. Osteosarcoma is associated with Paget's disease in persons between age 50 and 60 years.
f. The cause is unknown.
3. Clinical manifestations
a. Progressive deep bony pain
b. Acute episode of pain or pathologic fracture, experienced as a dull, aching, constant pain, often worse at night
c. Elevated alkaline phosphatase
d. Radiographs showing destruction of bone cortex, bony expansion, calcifications, or "sunburst" appearance
e. Bone scan showing areas of increased uptake (hot spot)
f. Computed tomography scan and magnetic resonance imaging showing tumor invasion into bone, soft tissues, and neurovascular structures
g. Mass in the distal femur, proximal tibia, humerus, or mandible
h. Reluctance to use the affected part
4. Clinical management
a. Pharmacologic intervention is chemotherapy via a continuous intravenous infusion administered intraarterially.
b. Special medical-surgical procedures
(1) Limb salvage is the removal of the lesion along with a zone of normal surrounding tissue. An allograft, which is a cadaveric human bone graft, can be used to replace tumorous bone. Hemiarthroplasty, total arthroplasty, or joint fusion may be performed to stabilize the joint.

(2) Amputation is done if complete tumor eradication is not possible by other means. Amputation includes the joint above the tumor.
c. Nursing interventions. See Chapter 17 for nursing care related to chemotherapy, see page 1604 for nursing care related to amputation, and see page 1608 for nursing care related to total joint arthroplasty.

Multiple Myeloma—Bone Marrow Tumor

1. Definition: Plasma cell myeloma is also known as multiple myeloma, which is a malignant tumor of plasma cells in the bone marrow. Osteolytic lesions may form in the bones through the body (see Chapter 25).

◼ OTHER MUSCULOSKELETAL DISORDERS

Spondylolysis

1. Definition: Spondylolysis is a defect or break in the neural arch between the superior and inferior articulating surfaces of the vertebrae. It most commonly occurs at L4–5 or L5–S1.
2. Incidence and etiology
a. Hereditary defect or trauma due to repetitive stress to the low back may cause spondylolysis.
b. Defects occur in persons between the ages of 6 and 10 years, but they may be asymptomatic until adulthood.
c. Traumatic injury occurs at any age.
d. Spondylolysis occurs equally among males and females.
e. Five percent of people have spondylolysis.
3. Clinical manifestations
a. Acute muscle spasm
b. Leaning to 1 side
4. Clinical management includes use of orthosis.
5. Nursing interventions: See nursing interventions for low back pain.

Spondylolisthesis

1. Definition: Spondylolisthesis is a forward slip of 1 vertebra on another. It most commonly occurs at L4–5 or L5–S1 but can occur at any level of the spine.
2. Incidence and etiology
a. The cause is unknown.
b. Spondylolisthesis occurs in persons between the ages of 7 and 10 years.
c. Symptoms appear in late childhood or early adolescence.
d. The disease may go undetected until adulthood.
e. It is more frequent in males, gymnasts, weight lifters, and football linemen.
3. Clinical manifestations
a. Increased lumbar lordosis
b. Waddling gait

c. Difficulty touching toes and raising leg straight up while lying down
d. Bowel and bladder changes
e. Sensory and motor weakness in legs

4. Clinical management
    a. Orthosis
    b. NSAIDs (see Chapter 11)
    c. Physical therapy
    d. Epidural steroid injections (see Chapter 11)
    e. Spinal fusion (see pp. 1610–1611)

Spinal Stenosis

1. Definition: Spinal stenosis is a narrowing of the spinal canal.

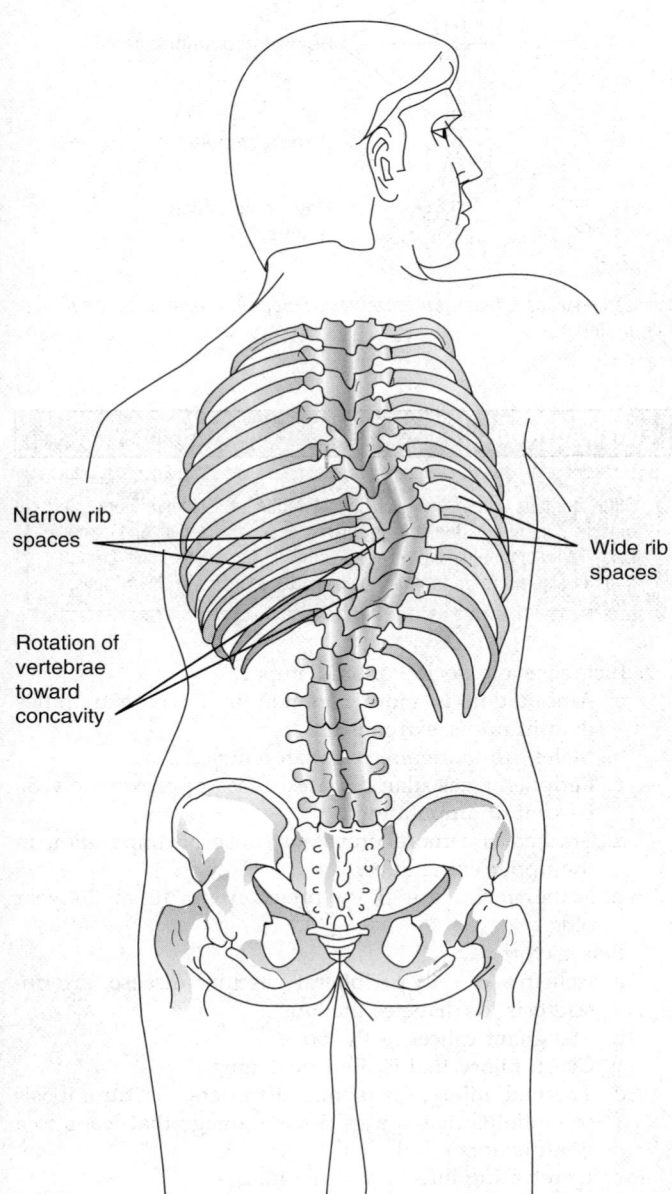

Narrow rib spaces

Wide rib spaces

Rotation of vertebrae toward concavity

Figure 34–21. Scoliosis.

2. Incidence and etiology
    a. Spinal stenosis occurs primarily in adults aged 60 and older.
    b. Degeneration of the disk is due to aging and arthritis.
    c. It can be congenital.
3. Clinical manifestations
    a. A flexed forward lumbar spine
    b. Crouched walk
4. Clinical management
    a. Use of NSAIDs (see Chapter 11).
    b. Use of transcutaneous electric nerve stimulation (see Chapter 11).
    c. Physical therapy
    d. Epidural steroid injections (see Chapter 11).
    e. Decompression laminectomy (see p. 1610).

Idiopathic Scoliosis

1. Definition: Idiopathic scoliosis is a lateral curvature of the spine with rotation of the vertebrae (Fig. 34–21). (See Chapter 15.)
2. Clinical management
    a. For adults, the curvature progresses slowly and should be monitored every 6 months to a year.
    b. Nonpharmacologic interventions: Bracing is with a thoracolumbosacral orthosis.
    c. Special medical-surgical procedures: Surgery is indicated if the curve is severe: 45 to 50 degrees, with subluxation of vertebra, pulmonary compromise, pain, or neurologic deficit. Spinal fusion is of the anterior, posterior, or anteroposterior approach (see p. 1610).

▣ *ORTHOPEDIC SURGERIES*

Amputation

1. Definition
    a. Amputation is the removal of a body part owing to disease or irreparable injury.
    b. It may be an open or closed procedure.
        (1) In an open procedure, the wound is left open and skin flaps are closed at a later time. It has a shorter operative time.
        (2) In a closed procedure, skin flaps are closed at the time of the amputation.
    c. The level of the amputation depends on the amount of affected tissue, the ability of the blood supply to promote healing, and the prognosis for fitting a functional prosthesis (Fig. 34–22).
    d. Different types of prostheses are available depending on the status of the residual limb.
        (1) A temporary prosthesis is usually applied after sutures are removed, in 2 to 6 weeks after surgery. Fitting of a temporary prosthesis requires application of a plaster of Paris bandage to form an impression of the stump. The temporary prosthesis is heavier and less cosmetic than a permanent prosthesis. It is held in place by a light belt or elastic sleeve. The usual wearing time for a

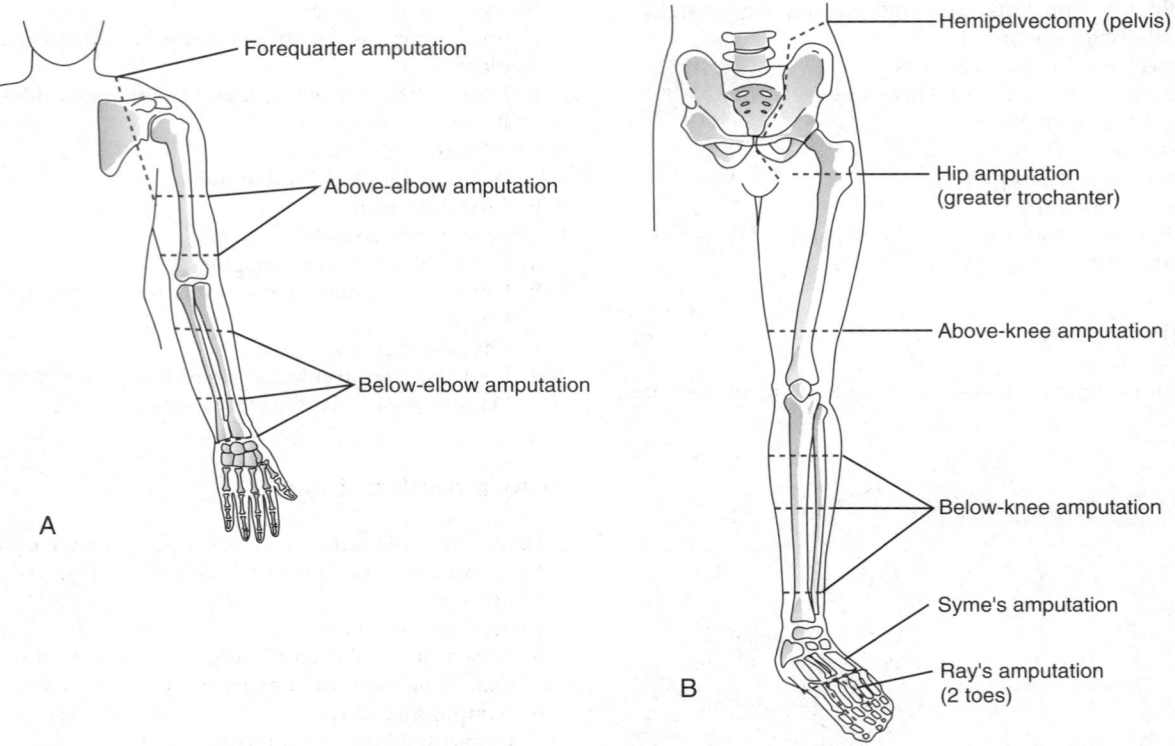

Figure 34–22. Common levels of amputation. (Redrawn from Black JM, and Matassarin-Jacobs E [eds]. *Luckmann and Sorensen's Medical-Surgical Nursing: A Psychophysiologic Approach.* 4th ed. Philadelphia: WB Saunders, 1993, p 1301.)

temporary prosthesis is 3 months. It may be necessary to have more than 1 temporary protheses due to changes in the size of the stump. Prosthetic socks are used to take up extra space in the socket of the prosthesis so it will fit better as the stump shrinks.

(2) A preparatory prosthesis may be used after a temporary prosthesis to provide a more accurate fit. Another casting is done and a transparent test socket is formed so that it can be seen through to determine proper fit. The preparatory prosthesis may be required for a few days or a few weeks.

(3) Permanent prostheses are custom made with plastic and foam. The design depends on age, location and length of stump, general medical condition, and desires of the person. Bone and muscle contouring is essential for flexible fitting. Stump measurements can be modified by a computer to produce the required shape which can then be shaped for fabrication by another computer. Cosmetic designs are soft, 1-piece materials and are not recommended for persons participating in athletics. Myoelectric arms and hands closely resemble human arms and hands and electronically move according to the person's muscle movements. Hydraulic knees offer smoother walking. The manual locking knee is better for persons who walk over uneven or rough surfaces.

ELDER ADVISORY

Older persons require special consideration of vascular, bone, and muscle contouring due to age-related changes in skin and circulation. The manual-locking knee prosthesis for above-knee amputations is also more appropriate because it reduces the risk of falls.

2. Incidence and socioeconomic impact
   a. Amputation is more common in lower extremities than in upper extremities.
   b. Males are more affected than females.
   c. Peripheral vascular disease causes approximately 80 percent of amputations.
   d. Trauma is a more prevalent cause of amputation in the upper extremities.
   e. Malignancies are more prevalent in 10 to 20 year olds.
3. Risk factors
   a. Ischemia due to peripheral vascular disease, arteriosclerosis, or diabetes mellitus
   b. Malignant cancer of the bone
   c. Crush injury that is life threatening
   d. Thermal injury, metabolic disorders, or thrombosis or embolus that causes tissue damage that leads to a nonfunctional limb
   e. Unrelenting infection of the limb
   f. Failed total knee arthroplasty with ischemia
4. Diagnostics: Preoperative assessment

a. History and physical examination to assess the following:
  - Mobility status, including use of assistive devices
  - Type, location, and severity of pain
  - Neurovascular status of affected and unaffected extremities. Note the presence of numbness or tingling. Note discoloration of skin due to circulatory problems, presence of ulcers, or presence of edema.
  - Condition of skin in the affected extremity

b. Laboratory work as determined by the physician; chest radiograph and electrocardiogram help evaluate general health condition and ability to tolerate surgery. Tests may be used to assess limb viability (Table 34–13).

c. Knowledge of the person and family regarding what the amputation will be and how it will affect the person after surgery: any cultural or religious beliefs or guidelines regarding amputation or handling the amputated parts; coping skills of the person and family.

5. Preoperative nursing interventions
  a. Teach the person and family about the surgical procedure and what will happen postoperatively (see p. 1604).
  b. Allow the person and family time to verbalize anxieties and fears regarding surgery and its outcomes.
  c. Report abnormal laboratory results and other tests to the physician.
  d. Discuss pain management strategies with the person and family. If chronic pain is present, the person may have strategies that have worked well in the past (see Chapter 11).
  e. Teach range-of-motion, flexibility, and strengthening exercises that will assist with mobility and prepare the person for rehabilitation after surgery (see p. 1605).
  f. Provide adequate nutrition for optimal healing.
    (1) Surgery, trauma, infection, and other systemic disease necessitate higher nutritional requirements.
    (2) Consult with the dietitian.
    (3) Provide a high-protein, high-calorie diet if not contraindicated by renal disease.
    (4) Provide oral supplements, tube feeding, or total parenteral nutrition, if indicated.

6. Intraoperative nursing interventions
  a. The prosthesis may be applied in the operating room for selected persons.
  b. A plaster cast is fitted over a closed stump and held in place by a harness or stockinette.
  c. Immediate-fit prostheses
    (1) Reduce edema
    (2) Prevent hematoma
    (3) Prevent injury to the affected extremity
    (4) Eliminate the need for rewrapping
    (5) Allow the stump to heal more rapidly
    (6) Allow earlier weight bearing

7. Postoperative nursing interventions
  a. Focus is on pain management, prevention of complications, mobilization, stump care, and assisting the person and family to cope with feelings.

Table 34–13. Tests for Assessment of Limb Viability

Invasive

Angiogram	Roentgenography following injection of radiopaque substance into blood vessel. Administer prophylaxis for allergic reaction. Monitor site for bleeding after procedure. (A pressure dressing is applied and sometimes augmented by a sandbag.) Monitor pulses distal to injection site for 4–6 hr.
Xenon 133	Radioactive isotope injected at the midpoint on the anterior portion of intended incision. Blood flow is recorded in milliliters per 100 g of tissue per minute. Flow rates greater than 2.4 ml/min/100 gm tissue predict the best results. Isotope not readily available.
Fluorescein fluorometry	Fluorescein (fluorescent) dye injected systemically and monitored by a fiberoptic fluorometer to determine nutritive blood flow to the affected area. Results measured in dye fluorescence index (DFI), which must average 79% to predict healing. Patient may experience nausea, urticaria, and pruritus on injection. Urine and sclera may be stained for 24 hr after injection.

Noninvasive

Doppler ultrasound	The most commonly used. Is a measure of systolic blood pressure. Cuff around affected extremity is inflated until the Doppler signal disappears. Cuff is slowly deflated until signal reappears. Pressure reading of 70 mm Hg is critical for healing.
Laser Doppler flowmetry	Laser beam reflected off of moving red blood cells. Can measure the difference in blood flow down to 1.5 mm from skin surface. May use same cuff technique as ultrasound, noting blood flow. Is comparable in accuracy and results to the xenon clearance technique. Can be used on all surfaces of lower extremity, including toes that are not testable by other methods, such as transcutaneous O_2 tension.
Transcutaneous O_2 pressure	The most promising and accurate test. Oxygen sensors are applied to the skin. Desirable oxygen tension is between 30 and 50 mm Hg. The sensor must be calibrated for temperature and atmospheric pressure, and the skin is warmed to 45 degrees Celsius. The surgeon can map out areas of greater and lesser perfusion in the involved extremity.
Thermography	Probe used to measure temperature in the ischemic limb at two sites from cutaneous tissue to center of bone. The lower the difference between the two readings, the greater the chance for healing.
Plethysmography	Segmental systolic blood pressure measurements to the lower extremity for evaluation of arterial flow to the area. Graph waveforms are dampened to flattened depending on amount of occlusion.

From Maher AB, Salmond SW, and Pellino TA. *Orthopedic Nursing*. Philadelphia: WB Saunders, 1994, pp 765. Adapted from Williamson VC. Amputation of the lower extremity: An overview. *Orthop Nurs* 11(2):57, 1992.

b. Most persons experience phantom limb sensation, that is, the perception of the amputated limb without pain, and many experience phantom pain, that is, the perception of pain in the limb that has been amputated.

c. Phantom limb sensation may be temporary or may last for years.

d. Phantom limb pain develops soon after surgery or may occur a few months after surgery.

(1) Phantom limb pain diminishes over time.

(2) It is more severe in above-the-knee amputations after gangrene and delay in amputating the extremity.

(3) The pain is described as "sharp," "burning," "electric," and "hot."

(4) The pain can be triggered by touching the stump or a "trigger point" on the trunk, opposite limb, or head; or by urination, defecation, sexual intercourse, angina, or cigarette smoking.

(5) Use of adequate postoperative analgesia for several days decreases the severity of phantom pain.

(6) Treatment of phantom pain depends on the type of pain.

- Beta-blockers increase serotonin levels for dull, aching, burning pain.
- Anticonvulsants ease stabbing pain.
- Baclofen controls spasms and cramps.
- Antidepressants increase serotonin levels to improve mood and alleviate insomnia.
- Narcotics do not help phantom pain because they do not alter the response of afferent nerve endings to painful stimuli.

e. Postoperative incisional pain is expected and should be treated with narcotic and nonnarcotic analgesics as needed.

f. For stump care, see Procedure 34-5.

8. Complications

a. Edema of the stump can occur due to decreased

P
Procedure 34-5
Stump Care

Definition/Purpose	To maintain skin integrity, decrease swelling, prevent adhesions, and decrease pain.
Contraindication/Caution	Continual assessment of the circulatory and skin status is essential to prevent complications that can occur from improper application or fitting of elastic bandages or shrinkers to stump.
Learning/Teaching Activities	Provide the following information: (a) instruct the person and family in proper incision care; (b) explain that improper wrapping of an elastic [Ace] bandage or a too tight stump shrinker will impair circulation; (c) instruct the person and family to notify the physician of any abnormal changes in the stump.

Preliminary Activities

Equipment	• Mild soap and water • Ace bandages or stump shrinker (appropriate size)
Assessment/Planning	• Obtain proper size of Ace bandage or shrinker. • The shrinker should not be used until sutures are removed and the incision is healed. • For below-knee amputation, use 2 4-inch Ace bandages. • For above-knee amputation, use 2 6-inch Ace bandages. • Check for history of allergy to soap. • Assess ability of the person and family to comprehend instructions.
Preparation of Person	• The individual should be relaxed and comfortable. • Answer questions and explain the procedure before beginning. • Explain the procedure in terms that the individual and family can understand. • Allow time for a return demonstration and repeat instructions as needed. • Provide the individual and family with written instructions and pictures for reference.
Procedure	

Actions	Rationale/Discussion
1. Wash the stump daily with mild soap and water.	1. Daily cleansing helps prevent infection.
2. Dry skin thoroughly and avoid use of creams or ointments.	2. Moisture may lead to skin breakdown and introduction of bacteria.
3. Keep incision clean and dry. Apply dry sterile dressing over sutures if drainage is present, and change dressing as needed.	3. Prevents irritation of skin and incision from drainage.
4. Inspect stump closely for signs of skin breakdown, redness, tenderness, increased warmth or coolness, numbness or tingling.	4. Signs of infection, circulatory compromise, or skin breakdown should be reported to the physician immediately.

P

Procedure 34–5
(continued)

Actions	Rationale/Discussion
5. Wrap the stump with Ace bandages using figure-of-8 turns.	5. The proper application of Ace bandages reduces edema and helps shape the stump.

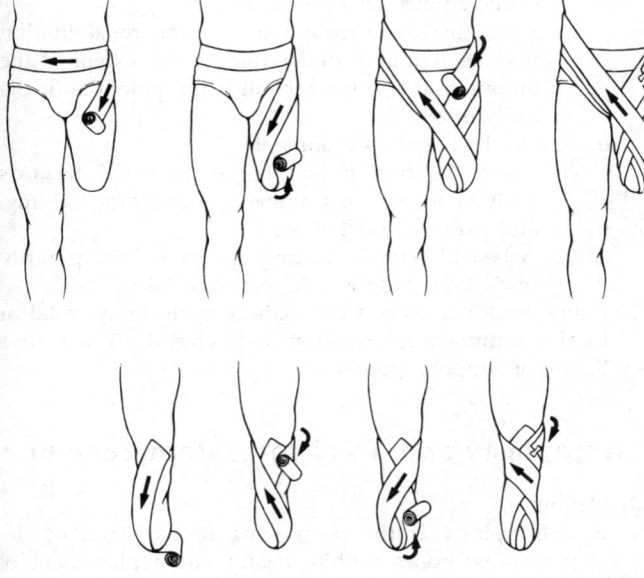

Actions	Rationale/Discussion
Do not wrap horizontally.	Horizontal wrap impedes circulation.
6. If shrinker is used, apply smoothly, making sure seams are in proper position. Apply nylon sock next to skin if skin irritation develops.	6. Proper application prevents skin irritation and circulatory complications.
7. Instruct individual to wear Ace bandages or shrinker until permanent prosthesis is ready or until pain and stump edema are well controlled.	7. Continual wearing of Ace bandages or shrinker will decrease edema and shape the stump for the prosthesis.
8. Massage the stump, and work up to patting it, rubbing it with a towel, and lightly slapping it to desensitize it.	8. Desensitization of the stump prevents adhesions and increases tolerance so that a prosthesis will not irritate it.
9. Wash Ace bandages, shrinkers, and the socket of the prosthesis daily and allow to dry thoroughly.	9. Thorough washing and drying prevent bacterial contamination and moisture that leads to skin breakdown.

Final Activities

Assessment of skin integrity, circulatory status, and tolerance of pain are ongoing activities. The physician, prosthetist, and physical therapist should be notified of any new or ongoing problems in these areas.

venous return. Elevation of the stump for the first 24 hours reduces edema and promotes venous return.

b. Hematoma may occur if bloody drainage collects within the spaces left when skin is pulled together to form the suture line. Monitor for oozing of blood and darkening of skin along the suture line, as well as for increased tenderness of the suture line.

c. Contractures can occur if the stump is elevated for longer than 24 hours or is left in a flexed position.
(1) Range-of-motion exercises should be performed regularly.

(2) Strengthening exercises also help prevent contractures. Quadriceps setting is done for above- or below-knee amputations. Straight leg raises are performed with the knee fully extended for below-knee amputations. Hip adduction is done for above-knee amputations. Biceps and triceps strengthening is done for below-elbow amputations.

(3) Instruct the person with above- or below-knee amputation to lie flat in bed in the prone position periodically to stretch muscles.

d. Monitor for signs of wound infection, wound dehiscence, hemorrhage, or shock. See Chapter 13 for a discussion of these complications.

9. Prognosis
   a. Rehabilitation potential depends on the general health of the person, the healing of the amputation site, the proper fitting of a prosthesis, and the coping skills of the person.
   b. A multidisciplinary team that includes the patient, family, physician, nurse, physical therapist, occupational therapist, social worker, prosthetist, psychologist, and vocational counselor can help ensure a successful transition.

10. Applying the nursing process

NURSING DIAGNOSIS: Impaired physical mobility R/T limited movement secondary to amputation

---

   a. *Expected outcomes:* Following instruction, the person should be able to do the following:
      (1) Demonstrate proper ambulation techniques
      (2) Increase activity level daily
   b. *Nursing interventions*
      (1) Instruct the person to perform exercises.
      (2) Instruct the person with lower extremity amputation in ambulation techniques. See pages 1567–1569. Persons with a lower extremity amputation, with or without a prosthesis, require special instruction on how to keep balanced when ambulating.
      (3) Instruct the person to take pain medication before activity, if needed.
      (4) Instruct the person to ask for assistance when ambulating until gait is steady and balance is good.
      (5) Instruct the person to gradually increase ambulation distance.

NURSING DIAGNOSIS: Grieving R/T loss of limb

---

   a. *Expected outcomes:* Following intervention, the person should be able to do the following:
      (1) Discuss feelings of grief
      (2) Recognize coping skills that can assist the person and family to deal with lifestyle changes
   b. *Nursing interventions*
      (1) Assess the person's and the family's perceptions of how the loss will affect them.
      (2) Provide opportunities for the person and family to discuss their feelings and the meaning of the loss.
      (3) Assist the person and family to recognize coping skills that have been successful in the past and that will be useful in this situation.
      (4) Use strategies for working through grief (see Chapter 39).

11. Discharge planning and teaching
    a. Assess equipment needs.
       (1) Assistive devices such as a walker or crutches may be needed.

    (2) Elastic (Ace) bandages and dressings may be needed temporarily until incision drainage stops.
    b. Assess financial support for purchase of prosthesis.
       (1) Inform the person and family to check with their insurance carrier for coverage of prosthesis.
       (2) The supplier of the prosthesis may have a financial counselor to assist persons in filing claims.
    c. Assess the need for follow-up.
       (1) Visiting nurses may need to be consulted to follow up on stump care teaching and preparation of the stump for a prosthesis.
       (2) After discharge from the hospital, rehabilitation may be required, depending on the extent of the amputation and the rehabilitation potential of the individual.
    d. Assess the home environment.
       (1) Teach the person and family to avoid hazards such as throw rugs, uneven floors, dim lighting, and cluttered walkways.
       (2) A bedside commode may be needed temporarily until the person is able to climb stairs.

12. Public health considerations. Check with the hospital or local community information and referral service for a listing of support groups.

Arthroplasty and Total Joint Replacement

1. Definition
   a. Arthroplasty is the resurfacing of damaged or degenerative bones within a joint and replacement of damaged bone and cartilage with metal and plastic components.
   b. The most commonly replaced joints are the following:
      (1) The hip, in which the head of the femur is removed and replaced; the acetabulum is resurfaced with a cup inserted (Fig. 34–23).

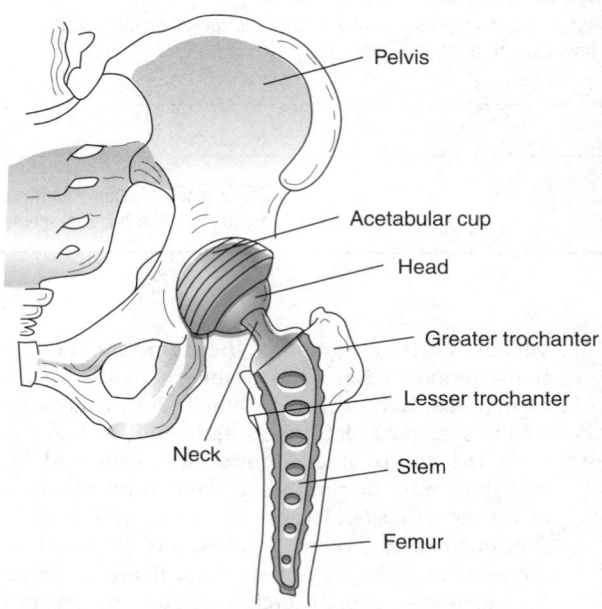

Figure 34–23. Total hip replacement.

(2) The knee, in which damaged bone from the proximal tibia and distal femur is removed and covered with the prosthesis (Fig. 34–24).

c. Other joints that can be replaced:
(1) Shoulder
(2) Elbow
(3) Ankle
(4) Joints of the hands and toes

d. Types of prostheses
(1) Cemented: Bone cement, methylmethacrylate, holds the prosthesis to the bone for immediate fixation. It is used primarily for older persons and those with poor bone strength due to osteoporosis and other conditions. It allows for immediate weight bearing on the operative leg.
(2) Uncemented: The porous texture of the prosthesis allows bone to grow into the prosthesis. It is used primarily for younger, more active, or heavier persons. It does not allow for immediate weight bearing. The person may need to wait 6 weeks before weight bearing is allowed.

3. Incidence and socioeconomic impact
a. Total hip arthroplasty is the most common major implant procedure in the world.

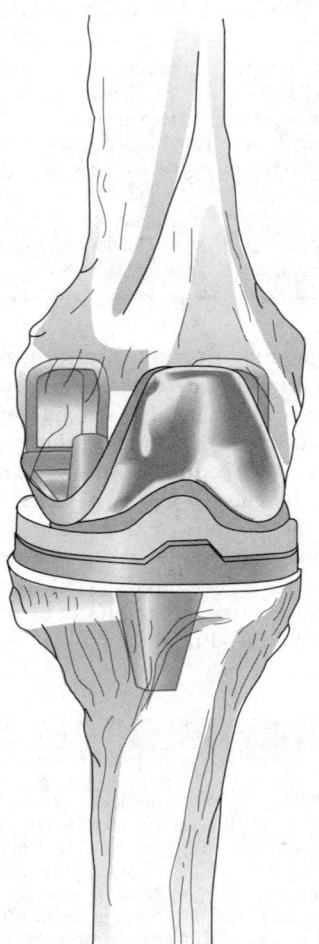

Figure 34–24. Total knee replacement.

b. More than 200,000 surgeries are performed yearly in the United States and more than 1 million are performed worldwide.

4. Risk factors
a. Severe pain in the joint
b. Extensive joint destruction
c. Severe limitation of joint motion
d. Infection in the joint, neurotropic joints, and inability to follow the postoperative treatment plan. Persons with such contraindications should not be considered for total joint replacement.

5. Diagnostics
a. Preoperative assessment
(1) History: Joint pain, loss of joint mobility, and difficulty with walking and other activities of daily living are revealed in the history. History of deep vein thrombosis or phlebitis increases the risk for developing these complications after total joint surgery.
(2) Physical examination
• Examine the joint requiring surgery, including range of motion and strength
• Assess muscle strength in the operative leg
• Assess the patient's ability to walk
• Dental examination detects problems that could lead to spread of infection through the bloodstream to the newly implanted joint.
• Assess tolerance to autologous blood donation. Most persons are able to donate their own blood before surgery, to be used for themselves during or after surgery. Usually, 2 to 3 units of blood are donated in anticipation of the blood loss during total joint replacement surgery. Assess whether the person is experiencing any dizziness, weakness, or other unusual symptom.
(3) Diagnostic tests: Preadmission laboratory testing should include studies required for any major surgery (see Chapter 13) (e.g., chest radiograph, electrocardiogram, and radiographs of the joint requiring surgery).

6. Clinical management
a. Preoperative nursing interventions
(1) In addition to preoperative assessment, preoperative teaching is essential. Instruction of preoperative and postoperative care, exercises, precautions, ambulation training, nutrition, and discharge planning should be included. This can be accomplished in the surgeon's office or at the hospital before surgery. The remainder of this discussion provides the content needed to instruct the person and family.
(2) Before entering the hospital, instruct the person to do the following:
• Inform the surgeon and family physician of any illness that occurs.
• Stop taking aspirin, anticoagulants, or NSAIDs as directed by the physician.
• Prepare the home for return after surgery. Have the bed moved downstairs temporarily if necessary. Remove throw rugs, electrical cords, and

any other article that could cause a fall. Prepare and freeze food ahead of time.
  - Eat a balanced diet with a concentration on foods high in iron, vitamin C, and protein.
  - Practice exercises that will be used postoperatively: quad sets, gluteal sets, ankle pumps, deep breathing, and relaxation.
  - Practice total joint precautions: No sitting in low chairs; no crossing of operative leg over the other leg (total hip); no bending over at the waist (total hip); no squatting; and no jumping, running, or playing high-impact sports.
  - Practice ambulation with a walker.
  - Determine discharge needs.
  (3) When the patient enters the hospital, the nurse should do the following:
  - Check any changes with health status and inform the physician of any abnormalities.
  - Check any laboratory studies ordered for the day of surgery and inform the physician of abnormalities.
  - Prepare the person for surgery (see Chapter 13).
b. Postoperative nursing interventions
  (1) In addition to the usual postoperative care for any surgical procedure, the person with total hip or knee replacement should be assessed for the following:
  - Circulation, sensation, and movement of the operative leg. All paramenters should be normal when compared with the preoperative assessment.
  - Blood loss in the wound drain, if one is used. If an autotransfusion device is used, reinfuse per hospital protocol. If a wound drain that cannot be reinfused is used or if no drain is present, notify the physician if more than 300 ml per 8 hours has drained.

NURSE ADVISORY

Blood from wound drainage can be collected intraoperatively or postoperatively and reinfused to the person undergoing certain types of orthopedic surgery.

During surgery, blood is aspirated from the surgical field, mixed with a heparin or citrated dextrose solution, filtered through a 140-micron filter, and placed in a centrifuge to separate red blood cells from waste products. The red blood cells are washed with normal saline, pumped into a blood bag, and transfused through a 20- to 40-micron filter.

When a postoperative drainage system is used, the wound drainage is collected in a closed container that has a filter inside. Within 6 hours of insertion of the drain, the blood must be collected and reinfused. A 40-micron filter is attached to the filtered blood tubing to further separate waste products. This blood is whole blood instead of red cells only.

  - Proper positioning of the operative extremity. After total hip replacement, the leg should be in the neutral position with the toes pointed upward. The legs are abducted with an abduction pillow or brace in place. Check with the

NURSE ADVISORY

It is important to position the abduction pillow correctly. The smaller end or top of the pillow should be just above the knees, and the wider end or bottom should be above or at the ankles. The straps should be secured when turning the person and when the person is sleeping to prevent dislocation of the hip; however, the straps should not be too tight. As the person learns how to properly hold and move the operative leg, the pillow may be removed and replaced with a regular pillow while the person is awake and lying on the back. The pillow is removed when walking, but may be needed when the person initially transfers to a chair.

surgeon regarding which side the person can turn toward. Avoid internal-external rotation of the operative leg and avoid flexion of the operative hip. After total knee replacement, the leg should be in the neutral position with the toes pointed upward. There may be a knee immobilizer on the leg to keep the knee straight or the leg may be on a continuous passive motion exerciser. Check with the surgeon regarding the parameters for their use (see Fig. 34–10).

NURSE ADVISORY

Continuous passive motion is used to increase motion of the knee joint, to help prevent deep vein thrombosis, and to help relieve pain due to joint stiffness. It is important to place the knee over the area where the machine bends. There may be straps that can be used to remind the person to not lift the leg up while the machine is in motion. Pad any areas in the groin that may be irritated from rubbing by the machine, if it extends into that area. The person should inform the nurse if there is an increase in knee pain while using the machine or if any other problem occurs.

  (2) Postoperative nursing care focuses on prevention of complications, pain management, and assisting the person in regaining strength and mobility.
  - Monitor use of anticoagulants and watch for signs of bleeding. Warfarin can be given by mouth. The dosage is determined by monitoring the protime or INR daily during the initial dosing. No daily laboratory studies are required for enoxaparin, but periodic complete blood counts are required to monitor possible internal bleeding.

 DRUG ADVISORY

Warfarin (Coumadin) or a low–molecular-weight heparin, enoxaparin, may be used in the hospital and at home after total joint replacement. It is essential that the person and family know the side effects of bleeding and when to notify the physician. Teach the person not to take any new prescribed or over-the-counter medications before checking with the physician who is monitoring the anticoagulant. Also, periodic laboratory work must be done after discharge from the hospital to monitor the effects of these medications and to determine what dosage of warfarin is needed.

- Monitor mechanical devices (e.g., sequential compressions devices that wrap around the legs or feet) used to prevent deep vein thrombosis, and watch for signs of skin irritation from these devices.
- Inspect the incision daily for signs of infection.
- Keep the operative leg in proper alignment to prevent dislocation of the prosthesis.
- Evaluate the pharmacologic and nonpharmacologic interventions used after total joint replacement
- During the first 2 to 3 days after surgery, epidural analgesia, patient-controlled analgesia, or intramuscular analgesia is used for management of the initial postoperative pain.
- Oral narcotic-nonnarcotic combinations such as hydrocodone with acetaminophen are used after discontinuation of the epidural, patient-controlled analgesia, or intramuscular analgesia. A decrease in amount of narcotic should be given when the person's level of pain has decreased. An NSAID such as Toradol may help in reducing the amount of narcotic needed.

- Nonpharmacologic methods such as transcutaneous electric nerve stimulation, relaxation, imagery, and ice pack application can decrease the amount of narcotic analgesia needed.
- Encourage the person to perform the exercises learned preoperatively and teach any new exercises ordered by the physician.
- Reinforce total joint precautions taught preoperatively.
- Reinforce ambulation techniques taught preoperatively.
- Reinforce the importance of eating foods high in iron, vitamin C, and protein.

7. Complications
   a. Complications can occur as with any surgical procedure (see Chapter 13).
   b. The following complications can occur with total joint replacement:
      (1) Deep vein thrombosis and pulmonary embolus
      (2) Infection
      (3) Dislocation of the prosthesis, with inward or outward rotation of the operative leg and increased pain and shortening of the leg (Fig. 34–25)
      (4) Loosening of the prosthesis (5–15 yr after surgery). Pain is a sign of a loosening prosthesis.
8. Prognosis
   a. Decrease in joint pain
   b. Increase in mobility
9. Applying the nursing process

NURSING DIAGNOSIS: Ineffective management of therapeutic regimen R/T insufficient knowledge of total joint precautions, use of adaptive equipment, and signs of complications

   a. *Expected outcomes:* Following instruction, the person should be able to do the following:
      (1) Demonstrate proper use of total joint precautions and adaptive equipment
      (2) Recognize signs and symptoms of complications
   b. *Nursing interventions*
      (1) Teach precautions
      (2) Teach proper use of adaptive devices:
         - A reacher to help pick up things so the person does not bend over
         - A sock donner that pulls on socks so the person does not bend over
         - A long-handled shoe horn, which assists with getting shoes on without bending forward
         - An elevated toilet seat or bedside commode to prevent the person from sitting on too low of a seat.
         - A shower chair to prevent the person from sitting in a bathtub or possibly falling while taking a shower.
         - A long-handled sponge, which helps the person avoid twisting to reach back while washing.
      (3) Teach signs and symptoms of complications:
         - Joint swelling, redness, or tenderness
         - Unusual pain

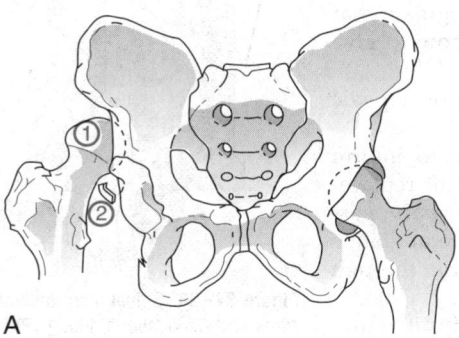
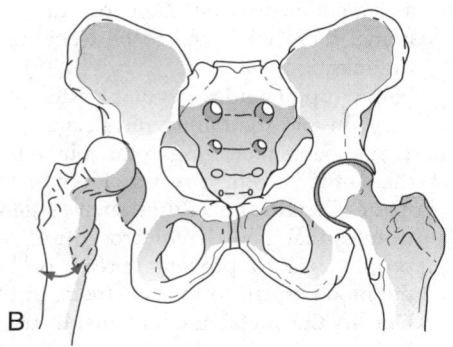

Figure 34–25. Hip dislocation. *A,* Posterial dislocation; *B,* anterior dislocation. (Redrawn from Connolly JF. *Fractures and Dislocations.* Vol. 1. Philadelphia: WB Saunders, 1995, pp 511, 528.)

A

B

- Reappearance of drainage that had previously stopped
- Elevated temperature
- Pain in calf, upper thigh, or chest
- Shortness of breath
- Burning with urination
- If after knee replacement, any change in the shape of the knee
- If after hip replacement, an inward or outward rotation of the leg with increased pain and shortening of the leg

NURSING DIAGNOSIS: Impaired physical mobility R/T postoperative pain and fatigue, and activity restriction

a. *Expected outcomes:* Following instruction, the person should be able to do the following:
  (1) Increase activity daily as tolerated
  (2) Recognize ways to become more independent while recovering from total joint replacement surgery
b. *Nursing interventions*
  (1) Reinforce exercise program as designed by physical therapy.
  (2) Reinforce use of ambulation techniques.
  (3) Offer pain medication before participation in therapy or exercise and ambulation on the nursing unit.
  (4) Schedule activities so that periods of rest alternate with the various activities.
  (5) Reinforce the importance of learning total joint precautions so that activities of daily living can be practiced safely and with less pain.
10. Discharge planning and teaching
  a. Discharge planning begins before hospitalization.
  b. Persons having total joint surgery must discuss their plans with their family.
  c. There may be need for equipment, visiting nurses, home or outpatient therapy, or continuing rehabilitation at a skilled nursing facility.
  d. Needs depend on family support and the person's general condition and ability to rehabilitate.
  e. Assessment of these areas needs to be done early to ensure a smooth transition from hospital to home or nursing facility.
  f. The person and family need to be taught how to use the equipment. If the person is to take enoxaparin—a subcutaneous injection of an anticoagulant—at home, there will need to be teaching of how to give the injection.
  g. Follow-up includes regular visits to the orthopedic surgeon and the family physician.
  h. Teach persons having total joint surgery to inform their other health care providers of the joint replacement. Certain procedures such as genitourinary, gastrointestinal, and dental procedures require antibiotic prophylaxis to prevent spread of bacteria through the bloodstream to the prosthetic implant.
  i. Due to the metal implant inside the body, it is im-

portant to inform technicians before a magnetic resonance imagery scan is obtained.
  j. The metal may also set off alarms found in security buildings and at airports. A card or note can be obtained from the surgeon stating that a person has a prosthesis.

Laminectomy and Spinal Fusion

1. Definition
  a. Laminectomy is excision of the lamina and the herniated disk. One level or multiple levels may be excised depending on the extent of the defect. It is usually done at the lumbar levels.
  b. Spinal fusion is fusion of 1 or more levels of vertebrae using bone graft with or without instrumentation.
    (1) Bone graft may be autologous (the person's own bone from the iliac crest or tibia) or allograft (bone from a bone bank).
    (2) Instrumentation consists of pedicle screws, plates, rods, hooks, or wires (Fig. 34–26).
    (3) Surgical approach can be anterior or posterior, depending on the diagnosis and location of the deformity. The anterior approach is used for lumbar scoliosis in an adolescent, lumbar scoliosis in an adult when it is the 1st of a 2-stage procedure, and with kyphosis. The posterior approach is used for fractures and spondylolisthesis. In some cases, anterior and posterior approaches may be done at the same time.
2. Incidence and socioeconomic impact. These procedures

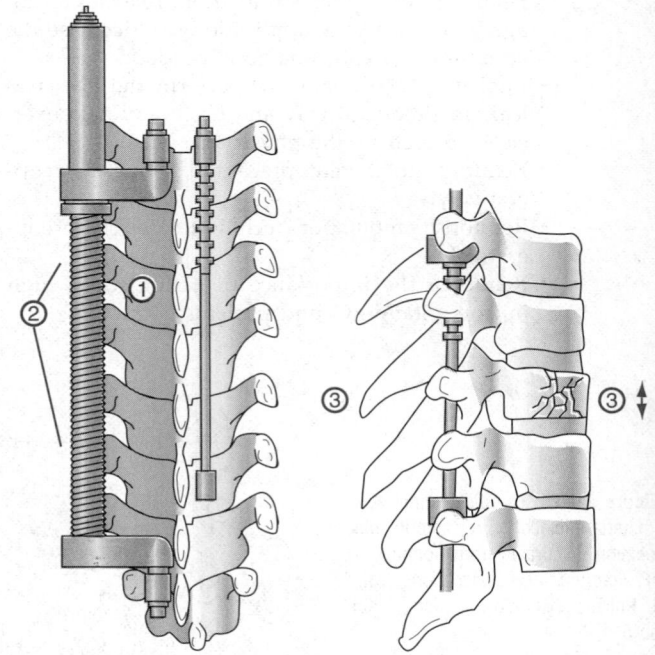

Figure 34–26. Spinal instrumentation. (Redrawn from Connolly JF. *Fractures and Dislocations.* Vol. 1. Philadelphia: WB Saunders, 1995, p 436.)

are done frequently for a variety of reasons. The exact numbers are unknown.

3. Risk factors
   a. For laminectomy, indications are herniated nucleus pulposus, spinal stenosis, and spinal tumors.
   b. For spinal fusion, indications are spinal fractures, spondylolisthesis, scoliosis, kyphosis, severe lordosis, and ankylosing spondylitis.

4. Diagnostics
   a. Preoperative assessment
      (1) Complete history and physical examination if possible
      (2) Assessment of the type, location, and severity of pain
      (3) Assessment of any neurologic deficits
      (4) Assessment of family support and resources
      (5) Psychosocial assessment, especially if an adolescent is undergoing spinal fusion for scoliosis
   b. Diagnostic tests: Laboratory tests are determined by the physician. Chest radiograph, spinal radiographs, and electrocardiogram may be indicated by age or condition.

5. Preoperative nursing interventions
   a. Teach the person and family about the surgical procedure and what will happen postoperatively.
   b. Allow the person and family time to verbalize anxieties and fears regarding the surgery and its outcomes.
   c. Report any abnormal laboratory results and other tests to the physician.
   d. Teach proper use of braces (e.g., thoracolumbosacral orthosis) that may be required after spinal fusion (see pp. 1565–1567).

6. Postoperative nursing interventions
   a. Focus is on pain management, prevention of complications, mobilization, and education of the person and family.
   b. Evaluate use of patient-controlled analgesia (PCA) or intramuscular narcotics for the first 48 to 72 hours.
   c. After patient-controlled analgesia or intramuscular narcotics are no longer needed, oral narcotic-non-narcotic combinations such as acetaminophen with codeine or hydrocodone can be given.
   d. Muscle relaxants such as diazepam may be used as adjunctive medication.
   e. Evaluate the incision for signs of dural leak (see Chapter 18).
   f. Monitor chest tube function and drainage if the anterior spinal approach is used.
   g. Watch for signs of infection in other areas such as the urinary tract or lungs.
   h. Monitor hemoglobin levels, hematocrit, and wound drainage and report abnormal findings per protocol.
   i. Reinfuse wound drainage if an autotransfusion unit was inserted or reinfuse autologous blood if predonation blood was used and such is ordered.
   j. Monitor neurovascular status every hour for 24 hours and every 4 to 8 hours thereafter until discharge.
   k. Monitor breath sounds every 4 hours and instruct the person to do deep breathing, coughing, and in-

centive spirometry every 1 to 2 hours until ambulatory.
   l. Monitor bladder and bowel function.
   m. Monitor the patient for deep vein thrombosis (see Chapter 24).
   n. Evaluate the person's ability to mobilize.
   o. Evaluate the person's educational needs.

7. Complications
   a. Neurologic impairment
   b. Respiratory problems: pneumonia, hemothorax or pneumothorax if a chest tube is inserted, and pulmonary embolus
   c. Infection in wound, lungs, or urinary tract
   d. Hemorrhage
   e. Spinal instrumentation failure and pseudarthrosis (later complication due to slippage of hooks or plates)

8. Prognosis: The operation is very successful in correction of scoliosis with a low incidence of complications (e.g., 1% incidence of neurologic deficits and 0.5% incidence of partial or complete paralysis).

9. Applying the nursing process

NURSING DIAGNOSIS: Impaired physical mobility R/T activity restrictions and fatigue

   a. *Expected outcomes:* Following instruction, the person should be able to do the following:
      (1) Demonstrate correct positioning and log-rolling techniques
      (2) Increase mobilization daily
   b. *Nursing interventions*
      (1) Teach correct body alignment while the patient is lying in bed, sitting, and standing:
         • When lying on their side, patients should keep the head of the bed flat with a pillow under their head and between their knees. Flexing knees slightly may be more comfortable.
         • When getting out of bed, patients roll to the edge, keeping their back straight.
         • When sitting on the side of the bed, patients raise their head and trunk at the same time as the legs are moving over the side of the bed. Instruct the person to ask for assistance when first doing this procedure to ensure smooth movements.
         • When standing, patients use 1 hand to support the stomach muscles and the other arm to push the body off the bed.
         • Patients apply the back brace, if ordered, before getting out of bed.
      (2) Instruct the person to take pain medication before activity, if needed.
      (3) Instruct the person to ask for assistance when ambulating, especially during the 1st few attempts and if dizziness or light-headedness occurs.
      (4) Instruct the person to alternate rest periods with periods of activity.

(5) Instruct the person to gradually increase ambulation distance and to not overdo it.
10. Discharge planning and teaching
    a. Discharge planning should begin before surgery if it is an elective procedure.
    b. Evaluate equipment needs and family supports.
    c. Reinforce education taught preoperatively (Table 34–14).

Surgical Complications

1. Deep vein thrombosis (see Chapter 24)
    a. Definition: A blood clot forms in the deep veins of the lower extremity.
    b. Incidence and socioeconomic impact
        (1) Deep vein thrombosis affects 45 to 70 percent of persons with total hip replacement, total knee replacement, total knee replacement, major knee reconstruction, or hip fracture.
        (2) Thromboembolism is responsible for 50 percent of postoperative mortalities in the 1st 3 months after total hip replacement.
        (3) Deep vein thrombosis affects 60 to 100 percent of persons having spinal trauma with neurologic involvement.
        (4) Incidence decreases with use of epidural anesthesia and analgesia, anticoagulants, sequential compression devices, and uncemented prostheses in total hip and total knee replacement.
2. Pulmonary embolus
    a. Definition: A clot travels from the systemic circulation to the pulmonary circulation and causes a partial or complete blockage in the pulmonary vasculature.
    b. Incidence and socioeconomic impact
        (1) Mortality ranges from 50,000 to 200,000 deaths per year.
        (2) Incidence can be as high as 20 percent in hip surgery patients.
        (3) Pulmonary embolism usually occurs 48 to 72 hours postoperatively or after injury.
        (4) See Chapter 22.
3. Fat embolus
    a. Definition: Fat embolus is the presence of fat globules in the bloodstream and lung tissue.
    b. Incidence
        (1) Fat embolus occurs in 0.5 to 2.0 percent of patients with long bone fracture.
        (2) Fat embolus occurs in 5 to 10 percent of patients with multiple fractures.
        (3) Fat embolus is more predominant in closed fractures than in open fractures.
        (4) Incidence is lower in children.
    c. Etiology
        (1) According to the mechanical theory, fat globules are released from the bone marrow into the blood.
        (2) According to the biochemical or metabolic theory, free fatty acids are released after trauma.
    d. Clinical manifestations
        • Dyspnea
        • Tachypnea
        • Tachycardia
        • Temperature greater than 103 degrees Fahrenheit
        • Subtle behavior changes, including irritability, confusion, restlessness, apprehension, and decreased level of consciousness
        • Chest pain
        • Petechiae on chest, axillae, and neck, only lasting a few hours
        • Arterial blood gases showing respiratory alkalosis

Table 34–14. Patient Education: Postoperative Home Management

Focus	Teaching Points
Mobility	To get in and out of bed, turn to side and use arms to push up from bed as you lower legs to floor.
	Increase walking gradually each day. Start with 100 ft and progress to several blocks.
	Have stand-by assistance for showering for the first week at home.
	Do not sit more than 30 min at a time if you have had lumbar spine surgery.
	Do not drive until your stamina has returned and you no longer require pain medication (except aspirin or acetaminophen) or muscle relaxants.
	Do not lift more than 5 to 10 pounds for 6 wk or until your physician advises an increase.
	Do not participate in strenuous activities.
	Swimming (without diving) and biking (in the erect position) are usually allowed after a few weeks. Ask your physician.
Wound care	Call the nurse or physician if the incision becomes reddened, if drainage develops, or if you have a fever.
	Wear a dressing on the incision if it is irritated by clothing, or if there is any drainage.
Nutrition	Eat a balanced diet.
	Consume approximately 1200 mg of calcium per day.
School/work activities	Have home tutor for 1 to 4 wk (depending on type of surgery).
	Anticipate 6 wk to 3 months off work (depending on type of surgery and type of employment).
	Discuss options for work retraining with rehabilitation counselor if you anticipate that you will not be able to return to your present occupation or profession.
Home maintenance	Have someone available to make meals, take care of household duties, and provide child care.
	Prepare and freeze meals before having surgery.
	Put commonly used household objects at level where you will not need to bend or reach for items.

From Maher AB, Salmond SW, and Pellino TA. *Orthopedic Nursing.* Philadelphia: WB Saunders, 1994, p 615.

- Thrombocytopenia
- Sudden decrease in hematocrit
- Chest radiograph showing snowstorm pattern
  e. Complications of fat embolus include adult respiratory distress syndrome and disseminated intravascular coagulation.
  f. Clinical management
    (1) Preventive measures
      - Early immobilization of fractures
      - Proper splinting and minimal manipulation of the fracture
      - Use of techniques in surgery to decrease pressure in medullary canal of bone and maintain intravascular volume
    (2) Supportive treatment
      - Oxygen therapy by mask or mechanical ventilation to maintain PO_2 at a minimum of 60 to 70 mm Hg
      - Fluid replacement to prevent or treat shock and hypotension
      - Medications (e.g., dopamine to improve urinary output, prevent edema, and increase cardiac output; nitroglycerin drip to improve arterial pressure and right ventricular afterload; digitalis if heart failure is present; and corticosteroids to decrease cerebral edema and to decrease inflammatory effects of fatty acids on alveolar membranes). Blood transfusion for low hemoglobin and hematocrit
    (3) For a comparison of pulmonary embolus and fat embolus, see Table 34–15.
  g. Nursing interventions
    (1) Move fractured extremities carefully and check immobilization devices for proper fit.
    (2) Monitor arterial blood gas results and report changes to the physician.
    (3) Monitor response to oxygen therapy and check for proper oxygen concentration delivery.
    (4) Keep the head of the bed elevated, if not contraindicated, and change the person's position frequently.
    (5) Assist the person with coughing and deep breathing exercises, and use of incentive spirometry.
    (6) Monitor fluid and blood replacement, and watch for signs and symptoms of congestive heart failure (see Chapter 23).
    (7) Monitor effects of medications and adjust or report as needed.
      - Dopamine increases blood pressure and must be watched closely. Also watch for sign of infiltration of the intravenous site because dopamine causes sloughing and necrosis of tissues.
      - Nitroglycerin can cause hypotension, so be cautious when getting the person out of bed. Elevate the head of the bed first, then dangle the person's feet before standing.
      - Digitalis lowers the heart rate. The pulse rate should be checked before giving the dose. Notify the physician if the pulse rate is below the range set for giving the medication.
      - Give corticosteroids slowly when giving intravenously.

    (8) Explain the treatment to the person and family, and reassure them that the person will be monitored closely.
    (9) Provide a means of communication for the person who is receiving mechanical ventilation.
4. Avascular necrosis (aseptic necrosis, osteonecrosis)
  a. Definition: Death of bone tissue is due to a lack of blood supply.
  b. Incidence and etiology
    (1) Avascular necrosis can occur at any age and in any bone.
    (2) The most common area affected is the femoral head.
    (3) Contributing conditions
      - Femoral neck fracture: 16 percent, which has a dramatically increased incidence if treatment is delayed 24 hours or more
      - Bone transplantation when new bone fails to develop adequate circulatory support
      - Long-term steroid therapy
      - Alcoholism
      - Exposure to x-rays, radioactive substances, or chemotherapeutic agents
  c. Clinical manifestations
    (1) Pain in the groin that radiates to the thigh or knee with any motion is a common complaint. Pain at rest is reported by 66 percent of patients, pain at night is reported by 33 percent of patients.
    (2) Decreased range of motion occurs in the affected area.
    (3) Computed tomography and magnetic resonance imaging are valuable in showing the staging of the disease
  d. Clinical management
    (1) Total hip arthroplasty or hemiarthroplasty for older patients provides relief of pain and restores joint motion.
    (2) Osteotomy or arthrodesis may be used for younger patients.
  e. Nursing interventions
    (1) See page 1608 for nursing care of persons requiring total hip arthroplasty.
    (2) Osteotomy requires use of a walker or crutches and arthrodesis may require use of a body cast (see pp. 1561–1564).
5. Myositis ossificans
  a. Definition: Myositis ossificans is the formation of heterotopic bone near bone and muscles in response to trauma
  b. Incidence and etiology
    (1) Occurrence is at any age.
    (2) Any part in the body can be affected.
    (3) Common sites are the arms, thighs, and hips.
    (4) Myositis ossificans circumscripta occurs in approximately two thirds of people undergoing acetabular open reduction and internal fixation.
  c. Clinical manifestations
    (1) History of injury or trauma, including surgery
    (2) Swelling
    (3) Inflammation of the area, indicating bleeding
    (4) Tenderness on palpation
    (5) Warm to the touch

Table 34–15. Comparison of Characteristics for Pulmonary Embolism and Fat Embolism Syndrome

Characteristic	Pulmonary Embolism	Fat Embolism Syndrome
Pathophysiology and etiology	Local venous trauma Venous stasis Hypercoagulability	Fat globule release from long bone or multiple fractures Stress-related release of catecholamines that mobilize lipids from adipose tissues
Risk factors	Immobility Age > 40 years History of heart disease, especially myocardial infarction or congestive heart failure Prior history of DVT or pulmonary embolus Surgery or trauma to hip, pelvis, or knee Obesity	Hypovolemia and shock Delayed immobilization or surgery Multiple traumatic injuries Joint replacement
Clinical manifestations*	Dyspnea Chest pain Apprehension or anxiety Cough or hemoptysis Tachypnea Localized rales Tachycardia Low-grade fever Thrombophlebitis	Dyspnea Restless, agitated, confused, stuporous Tachypnea > 30/min Diffuse rales (late) Tachycardia > 140/min Fever > 103 degrees Fahrenheit Petechial skin rash

Diagnostic assessment	ABGs ($PO_2 < 80$ mm Hg)
	Chest radiograph
	Electrocardiogram
	Lung scan
	Pulmonary angiography
		Hypoxemia ($PO_2 < 60$ mm Hg)
		Chest radiograph
		Electrocardiogram
		Laboratory
		   Thrombocytopenia
		   Decreased hemoglobin
		Fat in urine and blood
		Increased sedimentation rate
		Increased levels of fibrin split products

Prevention	Early ambulation
	Leg elevation
	Elastic stockings
	Leg exercises
	Intermittent pneumatic compression
	Medications
	   Anticoagulants
	   Antiplatelet agents
		Immobilize fractures
		Adequate hydration
		O_2
		Corticosteroids

Management	Anticoagulation
	Surgical intervention
	   IVC interruption
	   Embolectomy
	   O_2
		O_2
		Fluid replacement
		Mechanical ventilation with PEEP
		Corticosteroids
		Maintain adequate hemoglobin

* Occur within 48–72 hr in venous thromboembolism. Occur within 24–48 hr in fat embolism.
ABGs, Arterial blood gases; DVT, deep vein thrombosis; IVC, inferior vena cava; PEEP, positive end expiratory pressure.
From Black JM, and Matassarin-Jacobs E (eds). *Luckmann and Sorensen's Medical-Surgical Nursing: A Psychophysiologic Approach.* 4th ed. Philadelphia: WB Saunders, 1993, p 1922. Modified from Slye E. Orthopedic complications. *Nurs Clin North Am* 26(1):113–132, 1991.

    (6) Soft tissue mass shown on radiography
  d. Clinical management
    (1) Radiation therapy

    (2) Excision of heterotopic bone
  e. Nursing interventions. Routine incision care after excision of heterotopic bone.

Bibliography

Books

Agostini R. *Medical and Orthopaedic Issues of Active and Athletic Women.* Philadelphia: Hanley & Belfus, 1994.

Clark JC, and McGee RF. *Core Curriculum for Oncology Nursing.* 2nd ed. Philadelphia: WB Saunders, 1992.
Folcik MA, Carini-Garcia GK, and Birmingham JJ. *Traction: Assessment and Man-*

agement. St. Louis: Mosby–Year Book, 1994.
Kim MJ, McFarland GK, and McLane AM. *Pocket Guide to Nursing Diagnoses.* 5th ed. St. Louis: Mosby–Year Book, 1993.

Magee DJ. *Orthopaedic Physical Assessment.* 2nd ed. Philadelphia: WB Saunders, 1992.

Maher AB, Salmond SW, and Pellino TA. *Orthopaedic Nursing.* Philadelphia: WB Saunders, 1994.

McRae R. *Practical Fracture Treatment.* 3rd ed. New York: Churchill-Livingstone, 1994.

Mourad LA. *Orthopaedic Disorders.* St. Louis: Mosby–Year Book, 1991.

Mourad LA, and Droste MM. *The Nursing Process in the Care of Adults with Orthopaedic Conditions.* 3rd ed. Albany, NY: Delmar, 1993.

Petty W. *Total Joint Replacement.* Philadelphia: WB Saunders, 1991.

Salmond SW, Mooney NE, and Verdisco LA. *Core Curriculum for Orthopaedic Nursing.* 2nd ed. Pitman, NJ: National Association of Orthopaedic Nurses, 1991.

Chapters in Books

Follman DA. Assessment of clients with musculoskeletal disorders. *In* Black JM, and Matassarin-Jacobs E (eds). *Luckmann and Sorenson's Medical Surgical Nursing: A Psychophysiological Approach.* Philadelphia: WB Saunders, 1993.

Ignatavicius DD. Interventions for clients with musculoskeletal disorders. *In* Ignatavicius DD, and Bayne MV (eds). *Medical Surgical Nursing: A Nursing Process Approach.* Philadelphia: WB Saunders, 1991.

Rauscher NA. Nursing care. *In* Zuckerman JD (ed). *Orthopaedic Injuries in the Elderly.* Baltimore: Urban and Schwarzenberg, 1990.

Rauscher NA. Musculoskeletal assessment. *In* Salmond SW, Mooney NE, and Verdisco LA (eds). *Core Curriculum for Orthopaedic Nursing.* 2nd ed. Pitman, NJ: National Association of Orthopaedic Nurses, 1991.

Resnick D, and Niwayama G. Osteomyelitis, septic arthritis, and soft tissue infection: Mechanisms and situations. *In* Resnick D (ed). *Diagnosis of Bone and Joint Disorders.* 2nd ed. Philadelphia: WB Saunders, 1995.

Schmid FR. Principles of diagnosis and treatment of bone and joint infections. *In* McCarty DJ, and Koopman WJ (eds). *Arthritis and Allied Conditions.* 12th ed, vol. 2. Philadelphia: Lea & Febiger, 1993.

Whittington CF. Diagnostic studies. *In* Salmond SW, Mooney NE, and Verdisco LA (eds). *Core Curriculum for Orthopaedic Nursing.* 2nd ed. Pitman, NJ: National Association of Orthopaedic Nurses, 1991.

Journal Articles

Arlington RG, Costigan KA, and Aieroli CP. Postoperative orthopaedic blood salvage and reinfusion. *Orthop Nurs* 11(3):30–38, 1992.

Aspelin P, et al. Ultrasound examination of soft tissue injury of the lower limb in athletes. *Am J Sports Med* 20(5):601–603, 1992.

Barangan J. Factors that influence recovery from hip fracture during hospitalization. *Orthop Nurs* 9(5):19–29, 1990.

Barden RM, and Sinkora GL. Bone stimulators for fusions and fractures. *Nurs Clin North Am* 26(1):89–103, 1991.

Birge SJ. Osteoporosis and hip fractures in the care of the older woman. *Geriatr Med Clin* (9):69–86, 1993.

Boden SD, and Kaplan FS. Calcium homeostasis. *Orthop Clin North Am* 21(1):31–42, 1991.

Carroll P. Deep venous thrombosis: Implications for orthopaedic nursing. *Orthop Nurs* 12(3):33–42, 1993.

Chase JA. Spinal stenosis: When arthritis is more than arthritis! *Nurs Clin North Am* 26(1):53–64, 1991.

Chase JA. Outpatient management of low back pain. *Orthop Nurs* 11(1):11–20, 1992.

Childs S. Avascular necrosis of the bone: The causes and the cure. *Orthop Nurs* 12(4):29–34, 1993.

Commodore DI. Falls in the elderly population: A look at incidence, risks, healthcare costs, and preventive strategies. *Rehabil Nurs* 20:84–89, 1995.

Dowd SB. The radiographic appearance of gout. *Orthop Nurs* 12(1):53–55, 1993.

Eldridge J, and Bell D. Problems with substantial limb lengthening. *Orthop Clin North Am* 22(4):625–631, 1991.

Folcik M. Meniscal injuries. *Nurs Clin North Am* 26(1):181–198, 1991.

Freeman DA. Drug treatments for Paget's disease of bone. *Physician Assist* 16(30):125–126, 135–137, 162–164, 1992.

Fudman EJ, and Fox IH. When clinical clues point to gout. *J Musculoskeletal Med* 10(2):64–76, 1993.

Funk J, MacBrair B, and Peterson A. Tibial osteotomy. *Orthop Nurs* 9(2):29–36, 1990.

Galindo-Ciocon D, Ciocon JO, and Galindo D. Functional impairment among elderly women with osteoporotic vertebral fractures. *Rehabil Nurs* 20:79–83, 1995.

Hackfors AW. Orthopaedic manifestations of retroperitoneal infection. *Complications in Orthopaedics* 7(4):262–266, 1992.

Hay EK. That old hip: The osteoporosis process. *Nurs Clin North Am* 26(1):43–51, 1991.

Jenkins EA, and Cooper C. The epidemiology of osteoporosis: Who is at risk? *J Musculoskeletal Med* 10(3):18–33, 1993.

Johnson J, Anderson C, and Barrett A. Roller traction: Mobilizing patients with acetabular fractures. *Orthop Nurs* 14(1):21–24, 1995.

Lindly CA. Field assessment of the downed player. *J Am Acad Physician Assist* 7(6):394–402, 1994.

Lindsey B. Patient care guidelines—Cold and heat application in musculoskeletal injury. *J Emerg Nurs* 16(1):54–57, 1990.

Liscum B. Osteoporosis: The silent disease. *Orthop Nurs* 11(4):21–25, 1992.

McDowell JH, McFarland EG, and Nalli BJ. Use of cryotherapy for orthopaedic patients. *Orthop Nurs* 13(5):21–30, 1994.

Merkow RL, and Lane JM. Paget's disease of bone. *Orthop Clin North Am* 21(1):171–189, 1990.

Mooney NE. Pain management in the orthopaedic patient. *Nurs Clin North Am* 26(1):81–84, 1991.

Pavlik M. Measuring bone mineral content. *Orthop Nurs* 10(2):39–43, 1991.

Pellino TA. How to manage hip fractures. *Am J Nurs* 94(4):46–50, 1994.

Resnick B. Die from a broken hip? *RN* 57(7):22–27, 1994.

Ross D. Acute compartment syndrome. *Orthop Nurs* 10(2):33–38, 1991.

Santy J. Hip fractures: Can nursing make the difference? *Br J Nurs* 3(7; suppl): 335–339, 1994.

Slye DA. Orthopaedic complications: Compartment syndrome, fat embolism syndrome, and venous thromboembolism. *Nurs Clin North Am* 26(1):113–132, 1991.

Smith JE. Applying the continuous passive motion device. *Orthop Nurs* 9(3):54–56, 1990.

Smrcina C. Stress fractures in athletes. *Clin North Am* 26(1):1159–1166, 1991.

Strycula L. Traction basics, 3; Types of traction. *Orthop Nurs* 13(4):34, 38–44, 1994.

Strycula L. Traction basics, 4: Traction for lower extremities. *Orthop Nurs* 13(5):59–68, 1994.

Stulginsky MM. Nurse's home health experience. *Nurs Health Care* 14(8):402–407, 1993.

Thoren B, and Wigren A. Erythrocyte sedimentation rate in infection of total hip replacements. *Orthopedics* 14(4):495–497, 1991.

Weinerman SA, and Bockman RS. Medical therapy of osteoporosis. *Orthop Clin North Am* 21(1):109–119, 1990.

Williamson VC. Amputation of the lower extremity: An overview. *Orthop Nurs* 11(2):55–65, 1992.

35

Caring for People with Integumentary Disorders

◼ INTEGUMENTARY STRUCTURE AND FUNCTION

Structure of the Integument

1. The integument, or skin, consists of 3 major components: the epidermis, dermis, and epidermal appendages. It is supported by an underlying layer of subcutaneous tissue.
   a. The integument is the largest body system and accounts for approximately 15 percent of body weight.
   b. The structure of the skin varies from one part of the body to another.
2. The structure of the epidermis is shown in Figure 35–1.
3. Epidermal appendages consist of the hair, nails, apocrine sweat glands, eccrine sweat glands, and sebaceous glands (Fig. 35–2).
4. The structure of the dermis is shown in Figure 35–2.

Functions of the Integument

1. Regulation of body temperature
   a. Vasoconstriction conserves body heat.
   b. Vasodilation promotes body cooling.
   c. Eccrine glands promote cooling by increasing sweat production.
2. Protection
   a. The skin is a physical barrier to minor trauma; bacterial, chemical, and viral invasions; and excess loss of body fluid.
   b. The skin filters ultraviolet light (UVL) by producing melanin.
   c. Specialized Langerhans' cells in the skin initiate an immune response against invading antigens in the epidermis.
3. Regulation of excretion
   a. The skin minimizes loss of internal fluids.
   b. It excretes urea, lactic acid, sweat, and sodium chloride.
4. Regulation of blood pressure through vasoconstriction during hemorrhage, strenuous exercise, or emotional stress
5. Sensory perception of temperature, itching, pain, pressure, and touch

6. Synthesis of vitamin D precursors during exposure to ultraviolet irradiation (sunlight)
7. Repair of surface wounds through the escalation of replacement of cells.

◼ ASSESSING PEOPLE WITH INTEGUMENTARY DISORDERS

Key Symptoms and Their Pathophysiologic Bases (Box 35–1)

1. Erythema
   a. Occurrence: Erythema is a common symptom in many integumentary disorders, including erythema multiforme, eczema, many forms of dermatitis, cellulitis, infestations and insect bites, lupus erythematosus, drug eruptions, urticaria, erythroderma, and exfoliative erythroderma.
   b. Characteristics
      (1) Erythema is redness of the skin caused by superficial vasodilation and increased blood flow.
      (2) Erythematous lesions blanch if pressure is applied (in contrast to purpuric lesions, which do not blanch).
      (3) Erythematous skin feels warm to the touch.
      (4) Generalized erythematous conditions create intolerance to warm or cold temperatures.
   c. Location: The distribution of lesions is extremely important in diagnosis. Lesions may be generalized or localized.
   d. Duration: Erythema may be transient or prolonged, depending on its causative factor or factors.
   e. Severity: Erythematous lesions range from slightly pink to deep purple.
   f. Precipitating or aggravating factors: Exposure to sunlight, extremes of temperature, exercise, position changes, or emotional stress may change the degree of erythema experienced.
   g. Associated symptoms: Xerosis (dry skin), pruritus, intolerance to temperature variations, and emotional distress caused by a change in physical appearance may occur with varying degrees of erythema.
   h. Alleviating factors: Erythema is often decreased or relieved by topical steroids, a change in body position, antihistamines, or cool compresses.

STRUCTURE OF THE SKIN

Epidermis:

The epidermis is composed of 5 histologically distinct layers of avascular, stratified squamous epithelium.

The **stratum corneum** is the outermost layer of keratinized, dead squamous cells. It is constantly discarded and replaced with new cells produced in the basal layer. This renewal process requires 28 days from the initial cell division to the final stage of desquamation on the skin's surface. Keratin, a protein produced by keratinocytes in the epidermis, is an essential element of the barrier function of the skin.

The keratinocytes differentiate as they travel up through the **stratum spinosum**, **stratum granulosum**, and **stratum lucidum** layers into the stratum corneum.

The **basal layer** (stratum germinativum), or basement membrane, is the deepest layer of the epidermis. It produces new keratinocytes (squamous cells) to constantly renew the stratum corneum. The basal layer also contains melanocytes, the pigment-producing cells.

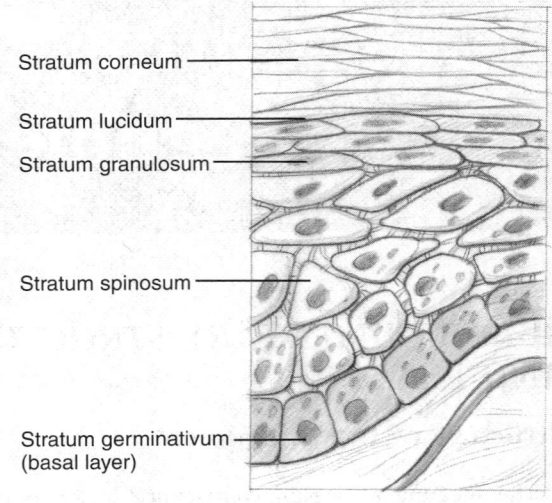

Stratum corneum
Stratum lucidum
Stratum granulosum
Stratum spinosum
Stratum germinativum (basal layer)

Dermis:

The dermis, composed of papillary and reticular layers, is a layer of highly vascular, connective tissue that supports and nourishes the epidermis. The vasculature controls body temperature and blood pressure.

The **papillary layer** contains papillae, finger-like projections that nourish the epidermal cells and provide a strong bond between the dermis and the epidermis.

The **reticular layer** contains connective tissue, blood vessels, lymphatics, and sensory and autonomic motor nerves and provides strength, stability, and elasticity.

The dermis is supported by the **hypodermis** (subcutaneous tissue), which is composed mainly of loose connective tissue and fat cells. The functions of the hypodermis are warmth, insulation, shock absorption, and caloric reserve.

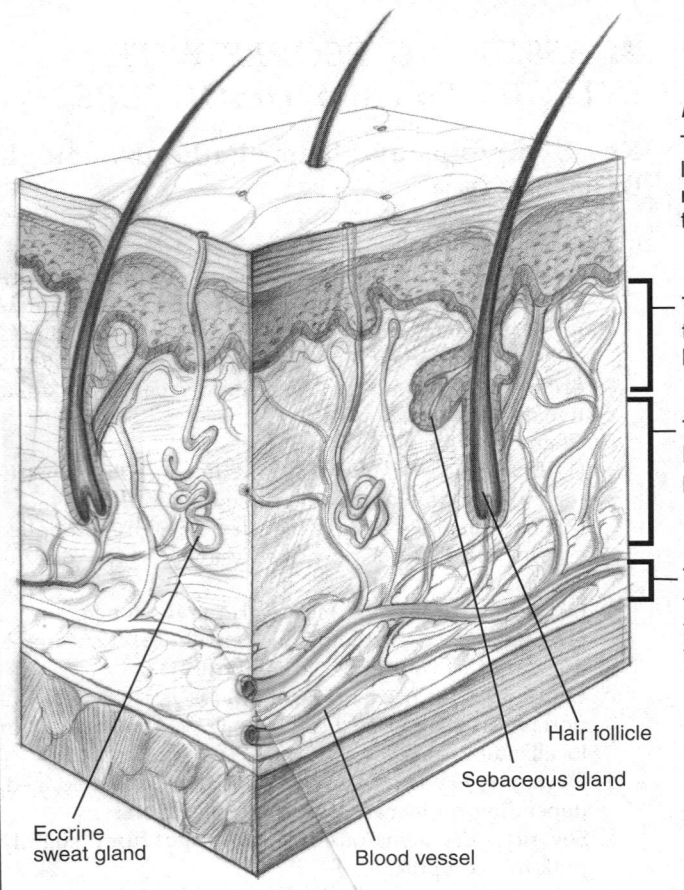

Hair follicle
Sebaceous gland
Eccrine sweat gland
Blood vessel

Figure 35–1.

2. Pruritus
   a. Occurrence: Pruritus is the most common symptom in many dermatologic disorders.
      (1) Pruritus is the major symptom in xerosis, eczema, allergic contact dermatitis, infestations, dermatitis herpetiformis, and insect-bite reactions.
      (2) It is often an underlying symptom of a systemic illness, such as renal or hepatic disease, hyperthyroidism, hypothyroidism, Hodgkin's disease, lymphoma, polycythemia vera, or iron deficiency anemia.
   b. Characteristics: Pruritus is often described as a tingling or crawling sensation. It may be intermittent or unrelenting and often becomes more pronounced at bedtime.

ANATOMY OF THE NAIL

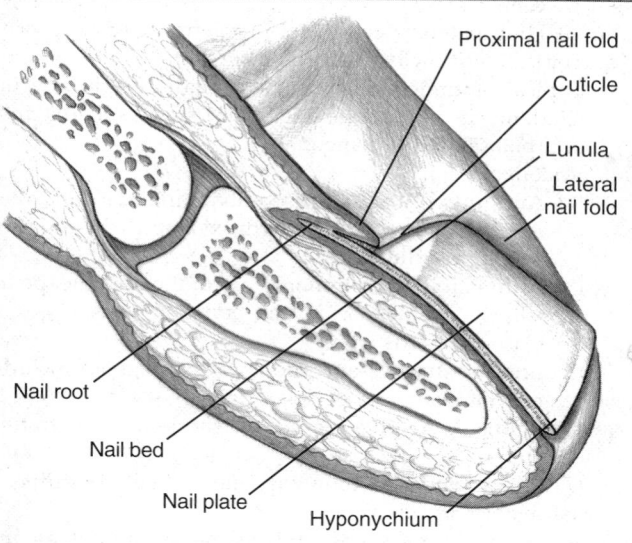

Proximal nail fold

Cuticle

Lunula

Lateral nail fold

Nail root

Nail bed

Nail plate

Hyponychium

Figure 35–2.

c. Location: Pruritus may be localized or generalized. When it is generalized, it is often intensified on the lower extremities (especially the anterior tibial area) and the back.

d. Duration: Pruritus may be self-limiting or protracted, depending on the underlying disorder. It may be episodic, paroxysmal, or continuous.

e. Severity: Pruritus ranges from mild to severe, according to the causative agent or disorder.

f. Precipitating or aggravating factors: Xerosis may be a causative factor, but it is also a major aggravating factor.

   (1) Environmental factors

     • Exposure to temperature extremes, especially hot weather

     • Low humidity (winter weather or air conditioning)

     • Extensive bathing or showering in hot water

     • Tight-fitting, woolen, or coarse synthetic clothing

     • Harsh soaps or chemicals

BOX 35–1. Key Symptoms of Integumentary Disorders

The major symptoms of people with integumentary disorders are (1) erythema, (2) pruritus, and (3) xerosis (dry skin). To determine the significance of these symptoms, ask the person the following questions:

• How long have you been experiencing the symptom(s)?
• Have you ever had this symptom or similar symptoms before? If the person answers yes, ask,
• Under what conditions did you experience the symptoms?
• Does the weather or seasons affect your symptoms?
• How did you alleviate the symptoms?
• What do you think is causing the symptoms?
• Are you having any other symptoms?
• Would it substantially improve your quality of life if we could relieve or alleviate this symptom?

---

   (2) Physical factors including sweating, emotional stress, and the habit of scratching.

g. Associated symptoms: Linear excoriation, lichenification (induration and thickening of the skin caused by chronic scratching behavior), and xerosis may accompany pruritus.

h. Alleviating factors: Pruritus is often relieved by the frequent use of emollients (ointments or creams); hydration of the stratum corneum followed by an emollient; less frequent bathing; cool compresses; antihistamines; and distraction techniques such as engaging in hobbies, recreation, or work.

3. Xerosis (dry skin)

a. Occurrence: Xerosis occurs as a primary disorder or as a secondary symptom in many integumentary disorders, such as atopic or contact dermatitis, ichthyosis vulgaris, and cutaneous T-cell lymphoma.

b. Characteristics: A superficial, fine scale appears, often accompanied by pruritus. Severe cases may cause cracking, fissuring, and erythema.

c. Location: Xerosis may occur anywhere, but the most common locations are the anterior legs, the dorsal surfaces of the hands, and the forearms.

d. Duration: The duration varies, depending on the causative factors and environmental conditions (it is exacerbated during winter months).

e. Severity: Dry skin is more severe during periods of low humidity.

f. Precipitating or aggravating factors: Excessive bathing or showering with hot water, low humidity (e.g., from using the furnace or air conditioner), and the use of harsh soaps or chemicals may trigger, or intensify, dry skin.

g. Associated symptoms: Pruritus is the most common associated symptom.

h. Alleviating factors: The use of emollients, less frequent bathing, the use of tepid water and mild soap and detergent, increased relative humidity, and hydration of the stratum corneum may alleviate dry skin.

ELDER ADVISORY

Older people are at increased risk for xerosis, especially during the winter months. They may not be aware of the significance of very dry skin and may not seek health care even if it becomes extremely symptomatic. Be sure to instruct the older person about xerosis. Xerosis most commonly affects the lower extremities. When bathing the older patient, use a mild, nondrying soap instead of the antibacterial, deodorant soap routinely found in institutional and acute care settings. Judiciously bathe the lower extremities and apply emollients at least 2 times a day to prevent xerosis and pruritus.

Physical and Psychosocial Health History

1. Family, childhood, and infectious diseases

a. Atopic dermatitis during childhood may resolve but recur in adulthood.

b. Hereditary angioedema, psoriasis, atopic dermatitis, acne, and neurofibromatosis are examples of familial disorders.

c. Infestations with lice or scabies are infectious and are transmittable to family members, daycare and school participants, and institutionalized populations.

2. Allergies

a. Allergic responses precipitate many skin reactions.

b. Identify food, environmental, drug, and family allergy history and determine exposure to any potential allergens.

c. Cosmetics, metal, chemicals, and leather are common culprits of contact dermatitis.

3. Major illnesses and hospitalizations

a. Major illnesses such as diabetes mellitus, hepatitis, immunodeficiency disorders, vascular insufficiency, and lymphomas commonly exhibit cutaneous manifestations.

b. Previous trauma or surgical sites provide clues to specific lesions.

4. Medications

a. Drug reactions may precipitate, imitate, exacerbate, or change a skin eruption or reaction.

(1) Low potency: hydrocortisone 1 percent

(2) Medium potency: triamcinolone acetonide 0.1 percent

(3) High potency: clobetasol propionate 0.05 percent

d. Topical antifungals (ketoconazole 2%)

e. Topical antimicrobial agents include erythromycin, clindamycin phosphate, bacitracin, silver sulfadiazine, and potassium permanganate.

f. Systemic therapy

(1) Antifungals include griseofulvin and ketoconazole.

(2) Antihistamines include hydroxyzine hydrochloride and terfenadines.

(3) Antimicrobials commonly used include the penicillins, cephalosporins, and erythromycins.

(4) Corticosteroids

(5) Immunosuppressant and cytotoxic agents include methotrexate and cyclosporine.

(6) Retinoids involve the use of isotretinoin or etretinate.

(7) Sulfonamides include dapsone and sulfapyridine.

5. Social history and lifestyle

a. Age, gender, race, and cultural background may increase the predilection for specific integumentary disorders.

TRANSCULTURAL CONSIDERATIONS

The use of home remedies for skin care is present among all cultures. The skin is a completely accessible organ and, as such, is susceptible to a multitude of home remedy concoctions.

- Ointments such as Tiger Balm, Vaporub, or arthritis pain relief formulas are commonly used for many ailments.
- Moxibustion, a Chinese American folk practice, involves placing ignited moxa plants near the ailing body part. This remedy can produce up to 1-cm depressed areas in the skin.
- Skin scraping, pinching, or cup suction practices are used by some Asian Americans for a variety of ailments. Bruising is commonly seen after these treatments.
- Hot or cold poultices are made from a variety of materials (herbs, roots, or animal or vegetable matter) and are applied directly to the skin in a number of cultures (Native Americans, European Americans, Appalachians, Mexican Americans, and Haitian Americans).

Assess patients for the use of home remedies and their potential to interfere with the prescribed treatment, induce an allergic reaction, or produce existing or additional skin lesions. To provide culturally appropriate nursing care, consider whether the home remedy is in direct conflict with the prescribed treatment plan. If it is not, and it is culturally important, incorporate it into the plan of care.

TRANSCULTURAL CONSIDERATIONS

Differences in age, gender, race, and cultural background may predispose some individuals to skin changes or skin disorders.

- Light-skinned races are at increased risk for developing skin cancers.
- Older persons are at increased risk for developing skin cancers, dry skin, and viral illnesses such as herpes zoster.
- Dark-skinned individuals more commonly develop keloids (hypertrophic scar formation) and dermatosis papulosa nigra (darker-colored, benign papules that usually appear in quantity around the face and neck). Mongolian spots (bluish discoloration of the lower back) are common among African Americans, Asian Americans, Mexican Americans, and Native Americans.
- Culturally related skin and hair changes may be seen as hair loss due to chronic trauma (the practice of cornrowing) or scars and mutilations related to custom or religious rituals (Aborigine tribes).
- Some skin disorders are associated with specific cultures. Hereditary polymorphic light eruption is limited to Native Americans in North America. Pemphigus vulgaris is more common among Ashkenazi Jews.

---

b. Common topical therapy involves the use of a specific pharmacologic agent (a corticosteroid or an antibiotic) delivered to the skin via the appropriate vehicle. The choice of the vehicle, in most cases, depends on the type of lesion, for example, wet versus dry (Table 35–1).

c. Topical corticosteroids are prescribed in a variety of strengths.

b. Cultural, ethnic, and religious beliefs provide valuable health assessment information. Determine the person's perception of health, illness, and current symptoms and illness. (See Chapter 2.)

c. A high level of daily stress increases the chances of incurring or exacerbating some illnesses, such as erythema or psoriasis.

d. Occupation and exposure to chemicals are important clues to a skin eruption.

Table 35–1. Vehicles for Topical Preparations

Vehicle	Action	Example of Use	Nursing Considerations
Gels	Cool and dry the skin.	Pruritic, weeping rash	May cause burning in open lesions. Watch for excess dryness. Are greaseless, nonstaining, and cosmetically acceptable.
Lotions, solutions	Dry the skin; are alcohol or water based.	Pruritic or moist lesions	Watch for excess dryness. Shake well before use.
Powders	Absorb fluid and moisture.	Intertriginous, moist areas	Apply to dry surface to prevent caking.
Pastes	Protect the skin.	Inflammatory lesions	Adhere best to the skin. Remove with mineral oil.
Aerosols	Dry and cool the skin.	Painful lesions, pruritus	Shake well before use. Avoid inhaling.
Creams	Moisturize and lubricate the skin.	Slightly to moderately dry lesions	Apply in direction of hair growth to prevent folliculitis. Apply in thin layer. Reapply as needed or as prescribed. Are usually the most cosmetically acceptable.
Ointments	Provide the best lubricating and emollient action. Decrease water loss. Protect the skin.	Severely dry and pruritic lesions	Promote absorption of topical medication. Feel greasy. Are easily removed with mineral oil. (See also creams.)

e. Certain habits, such as rubbing or picking the skin, squeezing facial acne, or tanning, may alter or exacerbate a skin eruption or disorder.

f. A travel history may furnish clues to an unusual infection or skin eruption.

6. A sexual history may reveal a sexually transmitted disorder that is producing cutaneous manifestations.

Physical Examination

1. First, assess the general appearance of the skin.
   a. When performing a skin examination, it is helpful to have adequate lighting, a magnifying lens, a penlight, tongue depressors, a centimeter ruler, and a glass slide.
   b. Examine the entire skin surface, not just the lesion or area in question. This is important so that a potentially problematic lesion, such as a skin cancer, is not missed. Maintain patient comfort and privacy during the examination.
   c. Assess the skin's dryness, color, temperature, mobility, turgor, and texture. Variations in color are best assessed by comparing the area with an area of unaffected skin. It is often more difficult to assess color variations in dark or pigmented skin.
      (1) Hyperpigmentation is excess pigmentation and may range from a very light tan to a deep brown.
      (2) Hypopigmentation is less or absent pigmentation, as seen in vitiligo.
      (3) Erythema may range from slight pink to deep red or purple.
      (4) Pallor is a paleness in normal skin tones or vasculature. It is most easily observed in the conjunctivae.
      (5) Cyanosis is a bluish or purplish discoloration of the skin or mucous membranes related to a deficiency in blood oxygenation. It is best assessed in the mucous membranes and nail beds.

      (6) Jaundice (icterus) is a yellowish discoloration best observed in the sclerae.
      (7) Vascular lesions vary from bright red to deep purple. If the vascular lesion is caused by dilated blood vessels, it will blanch or lose its color when compressed with a glass slide. This technique is called **diascopy**.
   d. Note any common, benign skin lesions (Table 35–2).
   e. Assess the general condition of the complexion, hair, nails, and mucous membranes.
2. Accurate observation and description of the lesion morphology, distribution, and configuration are essential in making a diagnosis.
   a. The **morphology** of a lesion is related to its size and structure.
   b. More than 1 type of skin lesion may be present.
   c. Assess for color, odor, texture, size, and presence of exudate as well as for pus, fluid-filled, elevated, and depressed lesions.
   d. Primary skin lesions are the skin's initial response to the underlying disease process (Fig. 35–3).
   e. Secondary skin lesions are modifications of a primary lesion caused by the natural evolution of the lesion. For example, a plaque may evolve into an ulceration. A secondary lesion may also result from trauma, such as scratching, or the application of medication to a primary lesion.
   f. The **distribution** of skin lesions refers to whether the lesions are generalized, localized, or specific to 1 body region.
      (1) Generalized skin lesions may be related to a systemic disorder, such as cutaneous T-cell lymphoma.
      (2) A localized red rash, such as on the left wrist, often indicates a contact dermatitis to jewelry or a wristwatch.
      (3) Lesions in body regions, such as erythema and maceration of the intertriginous areas, may indicate a fungal infection.

Table 35–2. Common Benign Skin Lesions

Skin Change	Description	Etiology/Pathophysiology	Management	Other
Corns (clavus)	A corn is a hyperkeratotic, painful, circumscribed area.	Repeated external pressure creates a localized accumulation of keratin. An elongated, hard plug forms in the horny layer of the epidermis.	The superficial layer of corn and hard plug in horny layer are excised.	Corns are found over bony prominences such as the interphalangeal joints of toes.
Calluses	A callus is a superficial, hyperkeratotic area.	Repeated friction or pressure stimulates the epidermis to increase cellular division, causing the stratum corneum to thicken.	Topical keratolytics are administered. Properly fitting shoes help prevent formation of calluses on the feet.	Calluses are commonly found on the palmar surfaces of the hands and the weight-bearing surfaces of the feet.
Papillomas (skin tags, acrochordons)	Papillomas are small, pedunculated, flesh-colored, tan, or pigmented growths, commonly seen on the neck, axillae, inguinal folds, eyelids, and upper chest.	Etiology is unknown. Lesions outpouch at skin surface with connective tissue and dilated capillaries.	Papillomas are removed by scalpel, electrodesiccation, or cryosurgery.	Most papillomas are asymptomatic, but some are easily irritated. They are associated with middle age and older adulthood, pregnancy, acromegaly, and family history.
Keratinous cysts: epidermal and sebaceous or pilar	Keratinous cysts are usually noninflammatory dermal cysts lined with epidermis and containing keratin. They are most often seen on face, neck, and upper trunk.	Keratinous cysts frequently occur after trauma, inflammation, or rupture of closed comedones. There is an increased tendency with a family history. Cystic rupture releases keratin, causing an inflammatory, foreign body response.	Complete wall-to-wall excision is curative. Intralesional corticosteroid injections reduce lesion size. Incision and drainage are performed if cyst is highly inflamed.	Self-manipulation leads to scarring and infection. Cysts are asymptomatic unless infected or inflamed. They frequently occur at sites of previous acne lesions.
Warts: common sessile, filiform, plantar, and flat	Warts are benign tumors of the skin common to the hands and feet. They occur singly or in groups and range in color from flesh to tan or gray-brown. Lesions are firm, flat, or slightly elevated.	Etiology is infection with human DNA papillomavirus. Autoinoculation is common. Course is unpredictable but may resolve spontaneously.	Keratolytics containing salicylic or lactic acid, cryosurgery, electrodesiccation and curettage, tape occlusion, and laser therapy are used. Surgical excision is used for plantar warts. Tretinoin cream .05–0.1% is used to induce inflammation for flat warts.	Warts are most common in children and young adults. They are often asymptomatic but create cosmetic concerns. They are diagnosed by their clinical appearance. No single treatment is effective for all warts.
Keloids	Keloids are areas of excessive hypertrophic scarring that enlarge to extend outside the area of injury. They are often erythematous or hyperpigmented and may be pruritic and painful. Purulent drainage may develop.	Keloids are the result of altered tissue response to skin injury in the fibroblastic phase of wound healing.	Intralesional corticosteroids, surgical excision or cryosurgery in combination with intralesional corticosteroids, and carbon dioxide laser excision are used.	Resolution is difficult, but size or progression can be decreased. There is an increased incidence of keloids in Blacks, burn patients, people with surgical wounds, and people ages 10–30. They are more common on the upper chest, ears, chin, shoulders, neck, back, abdomen, and legs.
Seborrheic keratoses	Seborrheic keratoses are benign, wartlike lesions, ranging up to several cm in diameter and light tan to black in color. They are common on the face, chest, shoulders, and back.	Etiology is unknown. A strong family history and sunlight exposure history predispose to development.	Excision, electrodesiccation and curettage, and cryosurgery are used.	A skin biopsy may be needed to confirm the diagnosis. Seborrheic keratoses are the most common skin tumor in older persons. They are generally asymptomatic but may be pruritic.
Actinic keratoses (solar and senile)	Actinic keratoses are the most common skin tumor. They occur in sun-exposed areas and	Etiology is premalignant transformation of keratinocytes caused by exposure to ultraviolet light.	Cryosurgery, curettage, chemical peel, dermabrasion, and topical fluorouracil are used.	Treatment is recommended owing to premalignant changes.

Table 35-2. Common Benign Skin Lesions (Continued)

Skin Change	Description	Etiology/ Pathophysiology	Management	Other
	are 1- to 5-mm, poorly circumscribed, erythematous papules. They are covered with white, rough scale.			
Moles (common acquired nevus)	Moles are the benign proliferation of melanocytes. They are well circumscribed, symmetric, and uniformly colored (tan to brown). The color is smooth and borders are regular. They are common on sun-exposed areas and are usually diagnosed by appearance.	Most moles are acquired and related to sun exposure.	No treatment is needed, but excision is done for cosmetic purposes or diagnostic concern. A biopsy is usually done on questionable moles.	New moles can appear throughout the life span. They are asymptomatic.

Table 35-3. Common Diagnostic Procedures

Diagnostic Procedure	Purpose	Procedure	Nursing Considerations
Wood's light	Detects fungal infections and disorders of hyper- and hypopigmentation.	Low-intensity ultraviolet light (blacklight) detects areas of fluorescence, pigment changes, and skin lesions. Painless.	Examination is done on clean hair/skin. Remove all creams, lotions, exudates from the skin and darken the room for the examination.
Potassium hydroxide (KOH) examination	Detects fungal and yeast infections of skin; is less reliable for detecting hair and nail fungal infections.	KOH-prepped microscopic slide examination of skin, hair, or nail scrapings is done. Procedure is painless.	Repeated scrapings may be necessary to rule out a fungal infection.
Tzank procedure	Is useful in blistering disorders such as herpes simplex, herpes zoster, varicella, and pemphigus vulgaris.	Microscopic slide examination is done. An examination of the blister roof often gives the best diagnostic results. Procedure is painless.	Results are available immediately.
Gram stain and culture	Determine gram positivity or negativity of bacteria. May help determine the type of infecting organism.	Microscopic examination of slide and culture prepared from lesion tissue or exudate is done. Procedure is painless.	Cultures require 48 hr for final results.
Skin biopsy	Determines histopathology of many skin lesions and disorders. Is a common diagnostic procedure.	This office or bedside procedure is done under local anesthetic. A shave, punch, or excisional biopsy is done, depending on lesion characteristics.	Results are usually available within 7 days. Results may be nondiagnostic, and the biopsy may need to be repeated. A punch or excisional biopsy may leave a small scar.
Phototesting	Detects photosensitivity to ultraviolet A or B light.	An artificial light source administers a controlled light dose to a small area of skin. Slight erythema often occurs to the area of exposure. Duplication of presenting symptom is a positive test reaction.	Procedure is usually done over several office visits. A positive reaction may generalize, producing total body redness, fever, anorexia, and nausea.
Patch testing (see also Chapter 21)	Detects contact sensitivities/allergies.	Small areas of skin are exposed to potential allergens for 48 hr with impregnated patches.	The exposed areas are measured for extent of erythema and induration to determine an allergic response.

PRIMARY SKIN LESIONS

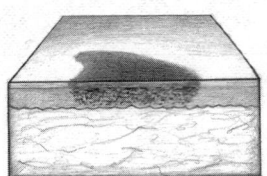

Macule: flat, less than 1 cm, various colors, nonpalpable, irregular, well circumscribed

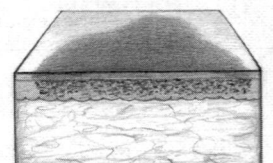

Patch: flat, greater than 1 cm, various colors, nonpalpable, irregular, well circumscribed

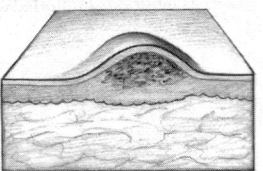

Papule: elevated, less than 1 cm, various colors, palpable, firm, well circumscribed

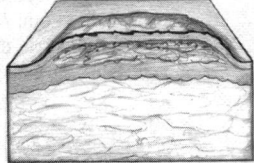

Plaque: elevated, greater than 1 cm, various colors, palpable, firm, flat topped

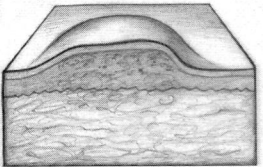

Wheal: elevated, variable size, pink to red in color, palpable edema, irregular shape

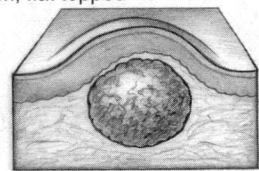

Nodule: elevated, 1-2 cm, flesh colored to red, palpable deeper into dermis, firm, well circumscribed; overlying skin is movable

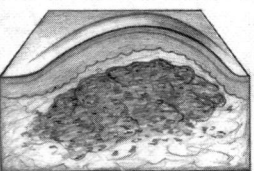

Tumor: elevated, greater than 2 cm, firm, various colors, palpable, variable demarcation

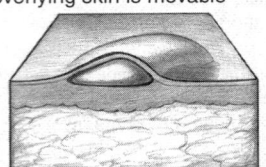

Vesicle: elevated, less than 1 cm, fluid filled, palpable, superficial, well circumscribed

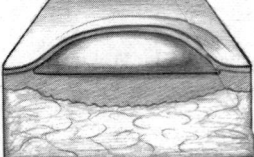

Bulla: elevated, a vesicle greater than 1 cm

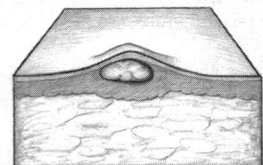

Pustule: elevated, less than 1 cm, contains purulent fluid, palpable, superficial, well circumscribed

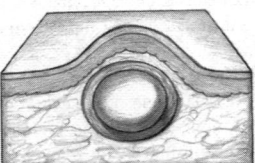

Cyst: elevated, variable size, contains liquid or semisolid material, encapsulated, palpable, and often compressible

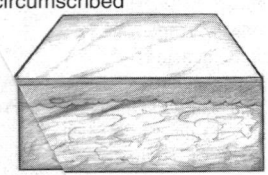

Telangiectasia: visible red small blood vessels caused by dilation of superficial capillaries

SECONDARY SKIN LESIONS

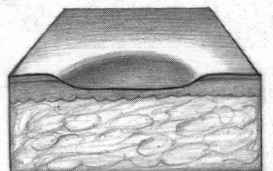

Erosion: areas of denudation of the epidermis with redness, weeping, and inflammation; following rupture of a blister

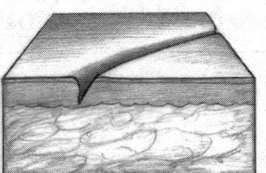

Excoriation: linear abrasion of the epidermis, usually self-induced

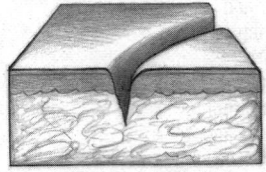

Fissure: linear crack from epidermis into dermis

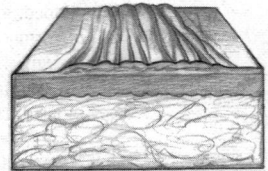

Lichenification: thick, rough epidermis caused by repeated scratching or rubbing

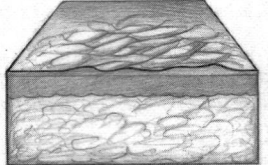

Scale: thin plates of dry, desquamating skin of various colors

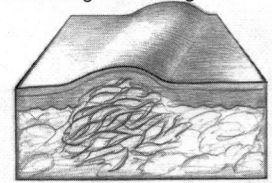

Scar: thick (hypertrophic) or thin (atrophic) fibrous tissue caused by dermal injury

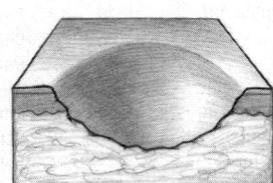

Ulcer: concave defect with epidermal and dermal tissue loss; may extend into subcutaneous tissue

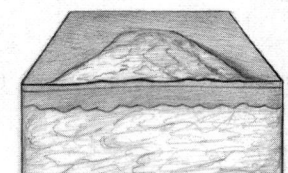

Crust: collection of dried serum, blood, or purulent material found on top of wound or weeping, eczematous lesions

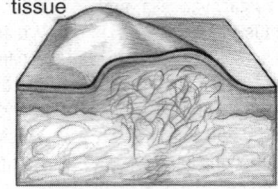

Keloid: hypertrophic scar extending beyond area of original injury

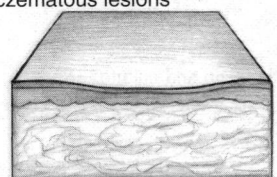

Atrophy: thinning of the epidermis, dermis, or subcutaneous tissue; loss of skin markings; skin is transparent

Figure 35–3.

g. **Arrangement** refers to single lesion configuration and grouping in relation to other skin lesions (Fig. 35–4 and Color Fig. 35–1).

Diagnostic Studies

See Table 35–3.

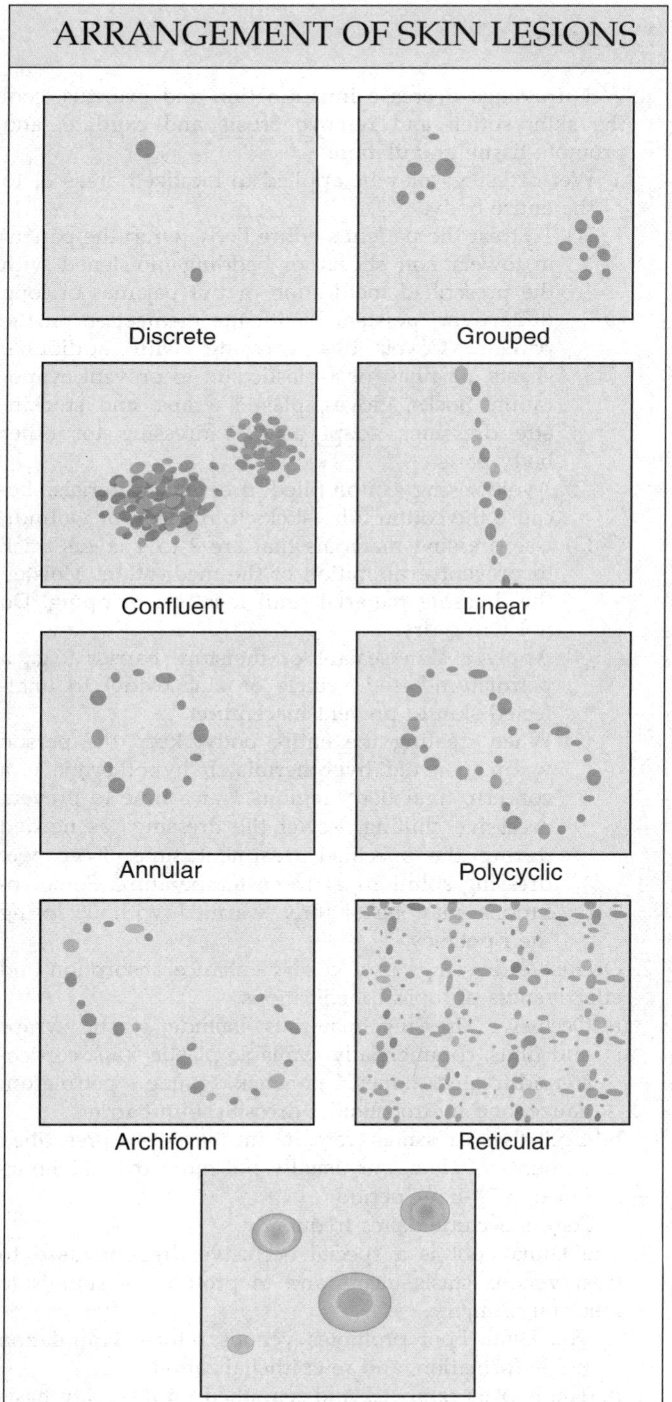

ARRANGEMENT OF SKIN LESIONS

Discrete

Grouped

Confluent

Linear

Annular

Polycyclic

Archiform

Reticular

Nummular

Figure 35–4.

TRANSCULTURAL CONSIDERATIONS

Consider the following guidelines when assessing the person with dark or pigmented skin:

1. Baseline skin color
   - The undertone of healthy black skin is a reddish color.
   - The oral mucosa and nail beds are pink; however, areas of oral hyperpigmentation occur in as many as 90 percent of dark-skinned individuals.
   - The sclera may have "freckles" that are additional deposits of melanin and may have a slightly yellow cast as a result of subconjunctival, fatty deposits.
2. Hyper- and hypopigmentation
   - Disorders that produce pigment loss (vitiligo) are more noticeable and distressful to the person with dark skin than the person with light skin.
   - Hyperpigmented scarring and keloid formation are more likely after an injury or inflammatory process.
3. Erythema
   - Redness is more difficult to detect. For an inflammatory process, inspect dark skin for a purple-gray cast.
   - Palpate for increased body temperature as a sign of inflammation.
   - Detect edema or infection by palpating for smooth or hard areas.
4. Cyanosis and pallor
   - Cyanotic, pigmented skin often appears gray.
   - Look for cyanotic changes around the mouth, over the cheekbones, and on the earlobes.
   - An absence of red undertones may indicate pallor. Check the areas with the least amount of pigment to detect pallor.
   - Assess for pallor by exerting pressure on the nail beds. Despite deeper pigment and perhaps thicker nails, a slow return of baseline color to the nail bed may indicate pallor or cyanosis.
5. Skin lesions
   - In dark skin, lesions are black, purple, or gray.
   - A rash may not be clearly visible. Ask the person whether there is a particularly itchy area.
   - Use light palpation to detect elevated borders and temperature differences in the skin.
   - Shine a penlight obliquely on the area to help detect papular lesions.
   - Gently stretch the skin over the area of the suspected rash. This technique decreases the reddish undertones and increases the visibility of the rash.

■ SPECIAL MEDICAL-SURGICAL TREATMENT MODALITIES

Baths (Balneotherapy)

1. Baths are a useful way to treat the entire body surface quickly and effectively.
2. The indications for therapeutic baths include the following:
   a. Treatment of widespread lesions
   b. Removal of crusts, scales, exudates, and previously applied topical medications
   c. Lubrication and hydration

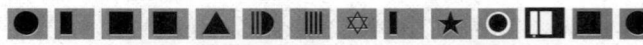

d. Anti-inflammatory and antipruritic effects.
3. The therapeutic agent used in the bath depends on the effect desired. A whirlpool bath and routine tub bath are effective means of delivering the treatment.
   a. Water and saline baths cool, soothe, and cleanse.
   b. Colloidal baths, such as oatmeal or starch, soothe and reduce itching.
   c. Bicarbonate of soda baths cool the skin.
   d. Tar preparations are useful in treating psoriasis and eczematous disorders. They have keratolytic and anti-inflammatory effects, in addition to increasing skin sensitivity to UVL.
   e. Potassium permanganate and aluminum acetate solutions (Burow's solution) have antibacterial as well as drying effects.
   f. Emollients (bath oils) lubricate and reduce itching.
4. Nursing interventions during a bath should follow several basic principles.
   a. The water is best at a warm, not hot, temperature; 96 degrees Fahrenheit is a good standard. Hot water dries the skin and causes more itching. Keep the room at a warm, comfortable temperature to avoid the temptation to use hot water in the bath.
   b. Discourage the use of washcloths during bathing. There is a tendency to use them for rubbing and scratching the skin. This only serves to stimulate the skin into an "itch-scratch-itch" cycle and causes lichenification of the skin from the repeated, vigorous rubbing motion.
   c. Bath medications may make the bathtub and floor slippery. Prevent any slips or falls with a bath mat and supervision, as appropriate. Elders are at in-

creased risk of falling and must be assisted to prevent injury. Emollients are especially slippery and should be used with discretion and caution.
   d. Slightly moist skin enhances absorption of topical preparations. To obtain the optimal absorption, hydration, and lubricating effects of the bath and any topical medications applied to the skin, pat the skin nearly dry and immediately apply the prescribed topical agent.

Dressings

1. Wet dressings decrease inflammation and pruritus, cool the skin, soften and remove crusts and exudate, and promote tissue granulation.
   a. Wet dressings may be applied to localized areas or to the entire body.
      (1) To treat the patient's entire body, wrap the patient in towels, soft sheets, or bedding moistened with the prescribed medication or put pajamas or long underwear moistened with the medication on the patient. Cover this dressing with additional sheets, pajamas, or a plastic suit to prevent evaporation. Socks, gloves, plastic wraps, and stockinette dressings adapt as wet dressing for other body parts.
      (2) Avoid using cotton-filled dressing materials, because the cotton filler sticks to the skin or wound.
      (3) Use dressing materials that are 2 to 4 layers thick to prevent evaporation of the medication. Moisten the dressing material until it is just dripping. Do not wring dry.
      (4) Apply a skin sealant or moisture barrier (e.g., a petrolatum-based vehicle or zinc oxide) to unaffected skin to prevent maceration.
      (5) When treating the entire body, keep the person warm to avoid hypothermia. If hypothermia is a concern, treat body regions 1 at a time to prevent excessive chilling. Rewet the dressings as needed during the specified treatment time. Keep wet dressing solutions at room temperature. Some solutions may be slightly warmed without losing their potency.
2. Occlusive dressings protect and enhance absorption and effectiveness of topical medications.
   a. Occlusive dressing materials include plastic wraps and films, commercially available plastic suits, corticosteroid-treated tapes, nonstick gauze, petrolatum gauze, and hydrocolloidal dressing film barriers.
   b. Occlusive dressings remain in place for prescribed amounts of time, but usually not more than 12 hours out of a 24-hour period.
   c. Assess occluded sites frequently.
3. The Unna boot is a special occlusive dressing used to treat venous stasis ulcers and to protect the skin from mechanical injury.
   a. The Unna boot promotes venous return, granulation tissue formation, and re-epithelialization.
   b. The boot is removed and reapplied on a weekly basis until the desired healing effect occurs. It is necessary

to assess the treated area for injury and infection on a routine basis.

Débridement

1. Débridement is a process to remove necrotic tissue.
2. In mechanical débridement, surgical technique is used to selectively remove dead tissue. It is more precise and spares more tissue than the wet-to-dry dressing technique. Wet-to-dry dressings débride wounds of both necrotic and new granulation tissue.
3. In chemical débridement, proteolytic enzymes (sutilains [Travase]) are used to liquefy necrotic tissue.
4. In autolytic débridement, the body's own defense mechanisms are allowed to destroy necrotic tissue. This process works best under occlusive dressings and is slower than mechanical or chemical débridement.

Phototherapy

1. Phototherapy is the use of artificially reproduced UVL in combination with oral or topical photosensitizing medications.
   a. The mechanism of action in phototherapy is not well understood. It inhibits cellular division caused by damage to the DNA in the cell. In psoriasis, this mechanism slows epidermal proliferation.
   b. The long-term risks of phototherapy include skin cancer, premature aging, and cataracts.
   c. Short-term side effects of phototherapy include dryness; pruritus; burns similar to a sunburn; exacerbation of herpes simplex; and delayed phototoxic reactions causing discomfort, redness, and blistering.
2. Short-wave ultraviolet B (UVB) light is helpful in treating psoriasis. Other disorders, such as atopic dermatitis, pruritus, pityriasis rosea, parapsoriasis, and cutaneous T-cell lymphoma, may respond to ultraviolet B light therapy.
   a. In the Goeckerman regimen, UVB and topical applications of crude coal tar are used in daily treatments for 2 to 3 weeks. The coal tar produces therapeutic pho-

tosensitivity and is also helpful in removing scale and thick plaques.
   b. Remissions of up to 1 year are possible with the Goeckerman regimen.
3. In long-wave UVL therapy, ultraviolet A light plus psoralen, a photosensitizing agent, are used.
   a. The acronym for psoralen plus ultraviolet A light is **PUVA.**
   b. The use of PUVA is therapeutic for psoriasis, cutaneous T-cell lymphoma, vitiligo, atopic dermatitis, lichen planus, pruritus, mastocytosis, graft-versus-host disease, and some cases of alopecia areata.
4. Before starting phototherapy, obtain the following data:
   a. Is the person taking any photosensitizing medications? If so, consider stopping them during therapy (Table 35–4).
   b. Is there a history of cataracts? A history of cataract formation may prevent the person from receiving phototherapy.

Table 35–4. Photosensitizing Drugs

Acne Preparations	Sulfonamides	Fluphenazine
Topical tretinoin	Sulfasalazine	Promethazine
Oral isotretinoin	Doxycycline	Thioridazine
Hexachlorophene	Griseofulvin	Trimeprazine
Antiarrythmics	Tetracycline	Haloperidol
Quinidine	**Antineoplastics**	Mesoridazine
Disopyramide	5-Fluorouracil	Methotrimeprazine
Amiodarone	Vinblastine sulfate	Perphenazine
Anticonvulsants	Procarbazine	Prochlorperazine
Carbamazepine	Dacarbazine	Promazine
Antidepressants	Methotrexate	Thiothixene
	Doxorubicin	Trifluoperazine
Imipramine	**Antiparasitics**	**Nonsteroidal Anti-Inflammatory Drugs**
Isocarboxazid	Bithionol	
Maprotiline	Quinine	Ketoprofen
Nortriptyline	Pyrvinium pamoate	Sulindac
Trimipramine	**Diuretics**	Piroxicam
Amitriptyline		Naproxen
Amoxapine	Chlorthalidone	**Oral Hypoglycemic Agents**
Desipramine	Furosemide	
Doxepin	Metolazone	Acetohexamide
Antihistamines	Hydrochlorothiazides	Chlorpropamide
	Thiazides	Glipizide
Cyproheptadine	Ethacrynic acid	Glyburide
Chlorpheniramine	**Estrogens**	Tolbutamide
Diphenhydramine hydrochloride	Conjugated estrogens	Tolazamide
Hydroxyzine	Diethylstilbestrol	**Others**
Promethazine	Esterified estrogens	
Antimalarials	Estradiol	Bergamot oils
	Estrone	Benzocaine
Chloroquine hydrochloride	Ethinyl estradiol	Cedar oils
Hydroxychloroquine	Quinestrol	Carbamazepine
Antimicrobials	**Furocoumarins**	Cyclamates
	Psoralens	Gold salts
Demeclocycline	**Neuroleptics**	Lime of citron
Hexachlorophene		Sodium aurothiomalate
Chlortetracycline	Chlordiazepoxide	Lavender
Minocycline	Chlorprothixene	Coal tar
Oxytetracycline	Chlorpromazine	

Table 35–5. Common Dermatologic Surgeries

Procedure	Description	Indications	Nursing Considerations
General Procedures			
Cryosurgery	Destruction of tissue by application of a frozen liquid such as liquid nitrogen or carbon dioxide. Cell damage occurs during thawing phase.	Benign lesions: actinic and seborrheic keratoses, lentigo, warts, cherry angiomas, and molluscum contagiosum. Malignant lesions: well-defined, superficial basal and squamous cell cancers less than 2 cm in diameter.	Patient needs to be taught the following: 1. The procedure may cause discomfort. 2. Scarring and hypo- or hyperpigmentation may occur. 3. Blisters may form at the treated site. 4. The signs/symptoms of infection. 5. Prevent infection by keeping the site clean and dry and not puncturing the blister. 6. Malignant lesions require 6–12 wk to heal.
Mohs' surgery	Microscopically controlled, staged excision of layers of tissue followed by frozen section review before further excision of tissue.	Interconnected tumors. Basal and squamous cell cancers greater than 2 cm and tumors located where tissue preservation is cosmetically and functionally crucial (eyes, ears, and nose). Selected cases of malignant melanoma.	Surgery is done under local anesthesia. This procedure often requires periods of waiting between removal of repeated layers of tissue. Prepare the person for an extended treatment time. Acetaminophen is usually adequate for pain control. Instruct the patient to avoid aspirin for 3–5 days to prevent bleeding and to cleanse the wound and apply antibiotic ointment twice daily to prevent infection.
Electrodesiccation and curettage	Under local anesthesia, tissue is destroyed by the application of electrical current (electrodesiccation) and removal of tissue with a loop-shaped cutting instrument (curet). Procedures are used separately or together.	Small benign lesions: skin tags, seborrheic keratoses, warts, and cherry and spider angiomas. Premalignant and malignant lesions: basal and squamous cell cancer, Bowen's disease, actinic keratoses. Not recommended for areas where scarring is a concern (e.g., the face).	Prepare the surgical area with an antibacterial cleansing agent. Prevent infection by applying topical antibacterial ointment; keep area clean and dry. A light dressing is optional.
Plastic Reconstructive Surgery			
Skin graft (free graft)	Detachment of a skin section from its blood supply and transfer of it to a recipient site. Skin for grafting is obtained from the affected individual (autograft), from another person (allograft), or from another species (xenograft).	Wound repair to cover defects from excision of tumors, to provide cover for denuded skin, and to allow closure of wounds.	Skin graft survival depends on an adequate blood supply at recipient site, firm contact of the graft with recipient site, immobilization of the graft, and an infection-free site. A vascularized graft usually appears pink. Instruct the person on the importance of recipient site immobilization, immediate reporting of signs/symptoms of infection, and infection prevention strategies.
Skin flaps (pedicle graft)	Grafting a portion of tissue (skin, muscle, mucosa, fat, bone, or omentum) with its blood supply still intact by a piece of pedicle tissue. Used to cover or close wounds or defects.	Used in areas with poor blood supply to repair defects from tumor ablation, congenital deformity, and trauma.	Assess psychologic preparation for surgery, nutritional status, and hematologic status. Teach the person and family members about the surgical procedure, postoperative recovery, and potential complications.
Free flap	Flap is detached from a donor site. Its blood supply is reattached at the recipient site by microvascular surgical techniques.	As above.	Grafted skin may be erythematous for several months; fading occurs gradually. Once healing occurs, treat donor sites with an emollient (mineral oil, lanolin) to lubricate and remove scales or crusts. Grafted skin is more vulnerable to sun exposure and should be protected with sunscreen.
Cosmetic Surgery			
Rhinoplasty	Removal of excess tissue and cartilage from the nose.	Septal defects; cosmetic appearance.	General considerations include preoperative teaching, postoperative care, potential complications, and expected cosmetic outcomes. Bruising and swelling are common after the procedures.
Rhytidectomy	Face lift.	Cosmetic repair of wrinkling or sagging of facial skin and tissue.	Healing times vary from 1 to 2 wk.
Blepharoplasty	Removal of excess fat and sagging tissue around the eyes.	Drooping eyelids and bagging skin under the eyes.	Postoperative activity is generally limited for 1 wk to decrease edema and promote healing.

Table 35–5. Common Dermatologic Surgeries (Continued)

Procedure	Description	Indications	Nursing Considerations
Chemical peels	Chemical solution applied to face causes superficial epidermal and dermal destruction. Type of chemical used determines depth of peel.	Fine wrinkles; superficial blemishes.	Complications include infection, hyperpigmentation, and scarring. Postoperatively, patient needs to be taught the following: 1. Keep head elevated to decrease edema and promote drainage. 2. Keep face immobile for 1–2 days to decrease discomfort. 3. Crusts form in several days and must not be removed until they fall off to prevent scarring. 4. Protect face from sun exposure for several days (exposure may cause pigment change).
Dermabrasion	Mechanical abrasion (sanding) of epidermis and part of dermis to promote tissue destruction followed by uniform and complete healing.	Deep acne, scars, aging, sun damage, hyperpigmentation.	Dressings are removed by the physician after 24 hr. Erythema may last weeks to months. Keep abraded areas soft and flexible with ointments and facial soaks when prescribed by the physician. (See also chemical peels.)
Collagen injection	Superficial injection of collagen material.	Fill in defects from small wrinkles and blemishes.	Contraindicated in persons with autoimmune disorders. Induration and swelling may occur at injection site.
Liposuction	Aspiration of fatty tissue.	Cosmetic body contouring, contour flaps, and removal of lipomas.	Complications include infection, hematoma, dimpling, and scarring. Final cosmetic results require 6 mo.

c. Is there a history of skin cancer? Therapy using UVL increases the risk of basal or squamous cell skin cancer.

d. Is there a history of lupus erythematosus? Exacerbations of lupus may occur with UVL exposure.

5. Assess the person on phototherapy routinely for signs of skin damage such as premature wrinkling, intense erythema, and skin cancers.

Dermatologic Surgery

Common dermatologic surgeries are listed in Table 35–5.

◼ PRIMARY BACTERIAL INFECTIONS (PYODERMAS): FOLLICULITIS, FURUNCLES, AND CARBUNCLES

Definitions

1. Folliculitis is a superficial or deep bacterial infection of the hair follicle that commonly occurs in the hair-bearing areas of the body subjected to friction or maceration. It may infect the surrounding dermis (see Color Fig. 35–2).

2. Furuncles (boils) may develop as a follicular infection spreads out from the hair follicle.

3. Carbuncles (abscesses) are more extensive and inflammatory lesions that develop from a follicular infection. They

are commonly found on thicker, less elastic skin, such as the back, neck, and thighs.

Incidence and Socioeconomic Impact

1. Folliculitis is a common skin disorder of adults and children. The incidence is increased in hospital environments, where there is a higher concentration of the causative organism.

2. People who are chronic carriers of nose and throat staphylococcus have an increased incidence of repeated follicular infections.

Risk Factors

1. Current skin lesions (e.g., an infected wound)
2. Obesity
3. Poor personal hygiene
4. Topical steroid therapy
5. Systemic steroid therapy or chemotherapy
6. Chronic hematologic disease (leukemia)
7. Immunodeficiency
8. Diabetes
9. Stiffened hairs
10. Hot climate

Etiology

1. The most common causative factor is *Staphylococcus aureus.*

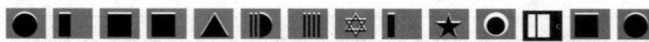

TRANSCULTURAL CONSIDERATIONS

Visible skin disorders, especially those of an infectious nature, stigmatize people in many cultures. Unfortunately, skin lesions are often readily visible and may enter into other people's judgment of a person's worth. Skin lesions may be attributed to excessive heat, bad blood, bad humors, vapors, wrongdoing, and evil spirits. Skin disease may be blamed on personal error or shortcomings rather than on a biomedical condition. For example,

• In Nigeria, skin disease is categorized with mental illness.
• In India, a diagnosis of leprosy constitutes legal grounds for divorce. Persons with vitiligo may be barred from using public transportation.

  Because of the important relationship between skin and one's culture, it is important to ask patients with skin disorders several questions regarding the impact of their disorder. On the basis of their response, it may be necessary to give them additional instructions or use alternative therapies.

• What do you think caused this illness?
• What effect has this disorder had on your family and social life?
• Should any home remedies or folk medicine be used to treat this illness?

2. Streptococcal infections are rare.

Pathophysiology

1. Folliculitis is a superficial inflammation of a hair follicle that results in papule or pustule formation.
2. More extensive inflammation produces an attempt by the host to wall off the infection. This produces inflammatory nodules or cysts (furuncles).
3. Carbuncles are more extensive furuncles, resulting in abscesses extending into and connecting within the fatty tissue.

Clinical Manifestations

1. Folliculitis manifests as tender, often pruritic papules and pustules.
2. Furuncles and carbuncles are very painful nodules, cysts, and abscesses and contain purulent, foul-smelling drainage. These lesions are often edematous and erythematous. They may cause systemic symptoms such as malaise and fever.

Diagnostics

1. Assessment
   a. History
      (1) Identify predisposing factors and determine whether the folliculitis is a recurring problem.
      (2) Determine hygiene practices when shaving areas of body hair.
   b. Physical assessment
      (1) Examine all hair-bearing areas for erythema, papules, pustules, nodules, cysts, and abscesses. Note their arrangement and distribution.
      (2) Palpate lesions for tenderness, firmness, and fluctuation (fluid-filled).
2. Diagnosis
   a. Diagnosis is often based on the clinical presentation.
   b. A Gram stain and culture identify the exact causative organism. These are often done to determine the appropriate antibiotic therapy.

Clinical Management

1. The goals of clinical management are to eliminate the infection and prevent recurrence.
2. Nonpharmacologic interventions
   a. Folliculitis may be treated with warm compresses and gentle cleansing with an antiseptic soap.
   b. Improved personal hygiene, less frequent shaving, and improved hydration of the skin during shaving may prevent or decrease future infections.
3. Pharmacologic interventions
   a. Topical antibiotics, such as erythromycin solution, may be administered.
   b. Furuncles and carbuncles are treated with systemic antibiotics (oral cloxacillin or dicloxacillin).
   c. For chronic carriers of staphylococcus, the nares are treated with a topical antibiotic ointment.
4. Special medical-surgical procedures
   a. Incision and drainage of furuncles and carbuncles are commonly done when the pus is localized and fluctuant.
   b. To prevent spread of infection, use universal precautions when handling the drainage from the incision and drainage procedure and the subsequent dressing materials.

Complications

• Cellulitis
• Bacteremia
• Systemic symptoms (malaise, fever, and chills)

Prognosis

1. Folliculitis often resolves spontaneously.
2. Furuncles and carbuncles usually respond rapidly to treatment, but recurrent infections are probable. This is due to the many risk factors involved and chronic carriers of the causative bacteria.

Applying the Nursing Process

NURSING DIAGNOSIS: Impaired skin integrity R/T disruption of skin surface and infectious process of skin

1. *Expected outcomes:* After instruction, the person should be able to do the following:
   a. Protect involved areas from trauma, friction, and maceration.
   b. Properly self-administer systemic and topical antibiotics.
   c. Demonstrate self-care of lesions by being able to do the following:
      (1) Wash involved area twice daily with an antibacterial soap.
      (2) Apply warm, moist compresses 3 to 4 times daily.
      (3) Avoid self-manipulation (picking and squeezing) of lesions.
   d. Demonstrate an understanding of the cause and treatment of folliculitis.
2. *Nursing interventions*
   a. Assess for risk factors and underlying disease process.
   b. Instruct the person on the cause and treatment of folliculitis, including the principles of administration of topical and systemic antibiotics.
   c. Help the person identify strategies to maintain personal hygiene and apply compresses or medications while preventing the spread of infection to family members. Instruct the person on proper hand-washing techniques.
   d. Caution the person about the detrimental effects of picking or squeezing lesions.

NURSE ADVISORY

Squeezing or manipulating facial furuncles and carbuncles greatly increases the risk of a fatal sinus thrombosis and pyemia, because these lesions drain directly into the cranial venous sinus. Educate persons with facial boils about this potentially fatal outcome of lesion manipulation.

Discharge Planning and Teaching

1. Provide information and materials (gloves and plastic bags) (e.g., on hand washing and isolation of contaminated articles) to prevent the spread of infection to self or others.
2. Advise the person to return for follow-up if the lesions do not resolve. This indicates that alternative antibiotic therapy is needed.

Public Health Considerations: Primary Prevention

1. Persons infected with furuncles and carbuncles should not work in food service or health care facilities until the lesions have healed.

2. Any contaminated items, such as linens and dressings, must be handled with universal precautions.

◼ OTHER PYODERMAS

Cellulitis and Erysipelas

1. Definitions
   a. Cellulitis is an acute, diffuse, primary skin infection that involves the dermis, lymphatics, and subcutaneous tissues.
   b. Erysipelas is a more superficial, acute form of cellulitis that affects the dermis, subcutaneous tissues, and lymphatics. It is also known as "St. Anthony's fire."
2. Incidence and etiology
   a. Cellulitis and erysipelas are fairly common. Erysipelas recurs more frequently
   b. The causative bacteria in most cases is group A β-hemolytic streptococci. Cellulitis may also be due to infection with *S. aureus*.
   c. Bacteria generally invade the tissue via a new or existing break in the skin surface. Cellulitis may occur in intact skin.
3. Clinical manifestations
   a. Cellulitis (see Color Fig. 35–3)
      (1) Cellulitis is brightly erythematous, edematous, inflamed, warm, and tender to the touch.
      (2) The lesions occur most commonly on the extremities and have ill-defined and generally nonpalpable borders.
      (3) Fever, chills, lymphangitis, and adenopathy are common.
      (4) Untreated cellulitis spreads easily to surrounding tissues and may result in septicemia, gangrene, or both.
   b. Erysipelas (see Color Fig. 35–4)
      (1) The affected area is similar in appearance to cellulitis, except that indurated, sharp borders are easily observed and palpated. Vesicles may or may not be present at the lesion borders.
      (2) The face is the most common site of infection. Lesions appear in a butterfly distribution.
      (3) Fever, chills, headache, and myalgias are common.
4. Intervention
   a. After tissue and blood cultures, penicillin is the drug of choice. For resistant organisms, penicillin derivatives (dicloxacillin) or cephalosporins may be used. Erythromycin is indicated for persons who are allergic to penicillin.
   b. Supportive care should be instituted to manage constitutional symptoms such as fatigue, fever, chills, headache, and myalgias.
   c. Warm compresses may be used to decrease discomfort, erythema, and edema.

Impetigo

See Chapter 15.

◪ FUNGAL INFECTIONS (TINEA)

Definition

1. Tinea is a dermatophyte fungal infection of the skin that involves overgrowths of plantlike organisms that consume organic matter.
2. Tinea infections involve multiple body sites.
   a. Tinea pedis (athlete's foot)
   b. Tinea cruris—groin (jock itch) (see Color Fig. 35–5)
   c. Tinea corporis—smooth body surfaces (ringworm) (see Color Fig. 35–6)
   d. Tinea capitis—scalp
   e. Tinea unguium (onychomycosis)—fingernails or, more commonly, toenails (see Color Fig. 35–7)

Incidence and Socioeconomic Impact

1. Tinea pedis is the most common of all fungal infections, occurring in the summertime and affecting up to 70 percent of the adult population at some time.
2. Concurrent fungal infections, such as tinea pedis and tinea cruris, are common.

Risk Factors

- Hot climate
- Poor nutrition and hygiene
- Immunosuppression or debilitating disease
- Exposure to organisms in other people, animals, or the soil
- Obesity

Etiology

1. Causative fungal organisms are human, animal, or soil related.
2. Poor host resistance increases the likelihood of infection.

Pathophysiology

1. Dermatophyte fungi survive in the dead layers of the epidermis.
2. There are many species of dermatophytes. *Trichophyton rubrum* is the most common cause of tinea pedis, tinea cruris, tinea unguium, and tinea corporis. *Trichophyton tonsurans* is the most common cause of tinea capitis.

Clinical Manifestations

See Table 35–6.

Diagnostics

1. History
   a. Inquire about exposure to other infected persons within the family, to family pets, or to soil as a potential source of infection.
   b. Determine whether risk factors are present.
   c. Does the person participate in athletics? This activity increases perspiration and opportunities for exposure to the fungi in gymnasiums.
   d. Determine the subjective symptoms experienced by the person. Ask whether there is itching, pain, or embarrassment associated with the tinea infection.
2. Physical assessment
   a. Examine all potential sites for a tinea infection. Look for evidence of scratching, vesicles, erythematous lesions, scaling, and maceration.
   b. Assess for signs and symptoms of secondary infection.
3. Diagnosis includes a potassium hydroxide preparation, fungal culture, and bacterial culture or Gram stain (if secondary bacterial infection is suspected).

Clinical Management

1. The goals of clinical management are to eliminate the infection and prevent reinfection.

Table 35–6. Clinical Manifestations of Tinea

Area Affected	Appearance	Distribution	Symptoms
Tinea corporis (body)	Ring-shaped, erythematous, and scaly, often with an area of central clearing; may be vesicular or papular	Anywhere on areas with no hair.	Pruritus
Tinea pedis (feet)	Scaling, maceration, and fissuring Dry, scaling hyperkeratosis Vesicular eruption	Between toes Moccasin distribution Sole or arch of foot.	Intense pruritus; acute lesions may be painful
Tinea cruris (jock itch) (groin)	Erythematous, scaly patches or plaques with elevated, marginated borders; may appear moist and weeping	Inguinal region; often extends into perineum and perianal areas	Moderate to severe pruritus and burning
Tinea capitis (scalp)	Erythematous, round patches with scales; may be patchy hair loss; hair is brittle and breaks off easily; pustules may be present	Single or multiple patches on scalp	Asymptomatic or mildly pruritic
Tinea unguium (nails)	Thickened nails that break and crumble easily; discoloration; nail plate may eventually separate from nail bed	Toenails most common; more than one nail may be involved, but rarely all 10	Asymptomatic

2. Nonpharmacologic interventions include measures to maintain a dry environment.
   a. Talcum or antifungal powders
   b. Cotton clothing to absorb perspiration
   c. Wearing shoes that allow air circulation and avoiding shoes that retain moisture (plastic or rubber).
3. Pharmacologic interventions
   a. Topical antifungal therapy (clotrimazole, miconazole, ketoconazole, or econazole) helps reduce symptoms and control the infection.
   b. Wet dressings with Burow's or Domeboro solution are necessary in more acute infections.
   c. If the infection does not respond to topical treatment, systemic antifungal therapy with agents such as griseofulvin and ketoconazole is used.

Complications

1. Superinfection of involved areas may occur.
2. Cellulitis and lymphangitis may result if secondary infection is present.

Prognosis

1. Most cases of tinea respond rapidly to treatment, but recurrence is a problem.
2. Immunocompromised individuals are at increased risk for recurrence, requiring continued treatment.
3. Chronic tinea pedis infections are common.

Applying the Nursing Process

> **NURSING DIAGNOSIS:** Knowledge deficit R/T tinea infections, including self-administration of antifungal medications and prevention of transmission and reinfection

1. *Expected outcomes:* After instruction, the person should be able to do the following:
   a. Discuss and identify risk factors for predisposition to tinea infections.
   b. Identify lifestyle changes to reduce identified risk factors.
   c. Properly self-administer topical or systemic antifungal therapy.
   d. Demonstrate no evidence of manipulation (scratching or picking) of involved areas.
2. *Nursing interventions*
   a. Provide information on required length of treatment and the importance of consistency for successful therapy.
   b. Provide encouragement and positive reinforcement for compliance with treatment, avoidance of self-manipulation, and lifestyle changes to reduce risk.
   c. Instruct the person on methods for application of topical antifungal creams and wet dressings or soaks.

Discharge Planning and Teaching

1. Encourage the person to seek follow-up care if the skin lesions do not respond to treatment.
2. Instruct the person on the use of appropriate clothing and shoes. Cotton underwear, undershirts, and socks help absorb perspiration. These items should be washed thoroughly with soap or detergent in hot water.
3. Advise the person to change socks and underwear frequently and to wear shoes that allow adequate airflow whenever possible. Shoes should be dry when worn.
4. Discuss the importance of properly drying the skin. All skin folds and spaces between the toes should be thoroughly dried. A clean cotton towel should be used daily. Talcum powder may help keep intertriginous areas dry.

Public Health Considerations

1. Public facilities such as swimming pools, gymnasiums, and locker rooms increase the likelihood of exposure to dermatophytes.
2. Persons who are susceptible to fungal infections should avoid such public facilities or take precautions to avoid exposure.

◼ *OTHER FUNGAL INFECTIONS*

Candidiasis

1. Definition—Candidiasis is a fungal infection of the skin or mucous membranes. Different terms are used depending on the area of infection.
   a. Paronychial candidiasis is involvement of the nail fold.
   b. Intertrigo is involvement in axillary, inframammary, groin, and perianal regions (see Color Fig. 35–8).
   c. Thrush is the involvement of oral mucosa.
   d. Vaginal candidiasis is involvement of the vaginal mucosa.
   e. Perlèche is involvement of the corners of the mouth.
2. Incidence and etiology
   a. Incidence
      (1) Hospitalized persons have an increased incidence of candidiasis.
      (2) Persons with identified risk factors demonstrate greater incidence than does the general population. Risk factors include diabetes; immunosuppression and immunosuppressive disorders; chronic illness and debilitation; use of corticosteroids, antibiotics, and oral contraceptives; obesity; an environment of warmth, moisture, maceration, and occlusion; pregnancy; and Cushing's disease.
   b. Etiology—Candidiasis is most commonly due to infection by *Candida albicans* in the presence of 1 or more risk factors.
3. Clinical manifestations
   a. Candidiasis that affects the skin is erythematous and surrounded by satellite pustules.

(1) The area may appear dry and scaly or moist and oozing.

(2) Pruritus and burning pain are common complaints; however, candidiasis may also be asymptomatic.

b. Thrush appears as a thick, white plaque on the mucous membranes of the mouth, throat, and tongue. Beneath the plaque, the mucosa is erythematous. The person may complain of pain while eating.

c. Vaginal candidiasis is characterized by intense pruritus; edema; erythema; and a thick, white, curdlike discharge.

d. Perlèche results in erythema, scaling, and fissuring of the corners of the mouth. These lesions are painful.

e. Paronychial candidiasis causes tenderness, erythema, and edema of the skin surrounding the nail. The posterior nail fold eventually lifts and rounds.

4. Intervention

a. The goals of intervention are to eliminate current infection, prevent future infections, and identify and eliminate or reduce risk factors.

b. Nonpharmacologic interventions

(1) The drying process is aided by cool, moist soaks for 10 to 15 minutes, followed by air drying of the affected intertriginous areas.

(2) Weight loss helps decrease excess skin folds.

(3) Talcum powder or corn starch produces a drying effect.

(4) Wearing protective gloves and avoiding exposure to moisture in the nail region is critical in the treatment of paronychial infections.

(5) Identify and eliminate or reduce risk factors.

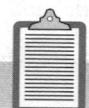

NURSING MANAGEMENT

People experiencing incontinence are at increased risk for developing perineal *Candida albicans* infections. These infections increase demand for nursing time, increase treatment costs and length of stay, delay healing, and produce discomfort for the individuals. Research demonstrates faster healing times when treatment for perineal candida infection adheres to the following regimen:
- Nursing intervention to keep skin clean and dry during episodes of incontinence.
- Consistent application of topical antifungals.
- Consistent application of a moisture barrier ointment, applied directly on top of the antifungal.

c. Pharmacologic interventions

(1) Topical antifungals, such as clotrimazole cream, are applied.

(2) Topical corticosteroids, such as hydrocortisone 1 percent, are useful for symptomatic relief.

(3) Systemic antifungals, such as ketoconazole, are useful for recurrent or resistant infections.

(4) Nystatin suspension or clotrimazole troches are helpful for thrush infections. For treatment to be successful, the antifungal mouthwash or troche must contact the oral mucosa sufficiently. Advise the person to cover all oral surfaces by thoroughly gargling and swishing the medication before swallowing it.

(5) Vaginal antifungals, such as nystatin or miconazole cream or suppositories, are administered nightly for 1 to 2 weeks.

Tinea Versicolor (Pityriasis Versicolor)

1. Definition—Tinea versicolor is a common, superficial fungal infection.

2. Incidence and etiology

a. Tinea versicolor affects approximately 5 percent of the U.S. population. All age groups can be affected, but the young adult age group predominates. Tinea versicolor occurs most commonly in the summer months.

b. The etiology of tinea versicolor is related to the overgrowth of the fungus *Pityrosporum furfur*. Risk factors attributable to its overgrowth include humidity, a warm climate, immunosuppression, heredity susceptibility, and pregnancy.

3. Clinical manifestations

a. Most commonly, tinea versicolor lesions are hypopigmented, scaling macules that are more prevalent in the summer and fall. The macular areas tend to enlarge, coalesce, or both, and they typically fail to tan with sun exposure (see Color Fig. 35–9).

b. The trunk is predominantly involved.

c. Itching is usually the only symptom, but the lesions may be entirely asymptomatic.

4. Intervention

a. Topical antifungal therapy is generally effective, but recurrence is common. Common topical agents include selenium sulfide (contraindicated in pregnancy), econazole, miconazole, and ketoconazole.

b. Systemic therapy with oral ketoconazole is also effective, but it is used only for very resistant cases because of its potential for hepatotoxicity. Liver enzymes must be monitored before initiation and after completion of treatment.

◼ HERPES ZOSTER

Definition

Herpes zoster (shingles) is an infection that is caused by a DNA virus and results in a vesicular eruption.

Incidence and Socioeconomic Impact

1. The incidence increases with age, with most reported cases occurring after the age of 40.

2. The incidence is much greater in immunocompromised individuals than in the general population.

Risk Factors

- Increasing age
- Physical trauma
- Debilitated or immunocompromised state
- Systemic illness
- Emotional stress
- Fatigue

Etiology

Herpes zoster is caused by a reactivation of the varicella-zoster virus, the causative virus for chickenpox.

Pathophysiology

1. After initial infection, the varicella-zoster virus remains dormant in the dorsal nerve root ganglia of the spinal and sensory cranial nerves.
2. Impaired immunologic function is implicated in the reactivation of the virus.

Clinical Manifestations

1. Classic lesions begin as papules or plaques, followed in 1 or 2 days by grouped, vesicular lesions. These primary vesicles later develop into pustules and crusted lesions.
2. The grouped vesicles of herpes zoster are distributed along a specific dermatome. The thoracic and cranial ophthalmic dermatomes are most commonly affected (see Color Fig. 35–10).
3. The outbreak of lesions is preceded by a prodromal period of 1 to 2 days. Prodromal symptoms are itching, burning, paresthesias, tingling, and pain over the dermatomal area.
4. Systemic symptoms during the prodromal period include headache, fever, pain, and fatigue.
5. Healing usually occurs within 2 to 3 weeks in the immunocompetent individual.

Diagnostics

1. Assessment
   a. A thorough history includes assessment for prodromal symptoms; current symptoms, especially pain level; identified risk factors; and psychosocial factors such as interference with activities of daily living.
   b. Physical assessment
      (1) Assess lesion characteristics and dermatomal distribution.
      (2) Assess for signs of secondary bacterial infection such as erythema, pus, and local edema.
2. Diagnosis
   a. With classic presentation, the clinical examination is diagnostic.

   b. A Tzanck preparation identifies the presence of multinucleated giant cells.
   c. Culture of the lesions provides the definitive diagnosis.

Clinical Management

1. The goals of intervention are to provide symptomatic relief of lesions, prevent secondary infection, speed healing of lesions, and reduce outbreak of new vesicles.
2. Nonpharmacologic interventions
   a. Cool compresses help decrease pruritus and inflammation.
   b. Biofeedback and transcutaneous nerve stimulation are alternative pain relief strategies for postherpetic neuralgia.
3. Pharmacologic interventions
   a. Uncomplicated cases
      (1) Antihistamines help reduce pruritus.
      (2) Analgesics help decrease lesional pain.
      (3) Topical soaks with Burow's solution keep the lesions clean, moist, and free of crusts.
      (4) Antiviral agents (e.g., oral acyclovir) may speed healing, decrease the number of new lesions, and decrease pain. Encourage fluids during oral acyclovir treatment to prevent nephrotoxicity.
   b. People who are immunocompromised or have disseminated infections may require intravenous acyclovir (vidarabine). Adequate hydration and monitoring of renal function are important in preventing nephrotoxicity from intravenous acyclovir.
   c. Persistent pain due to postherpetic neuralgia may respond to combination therapy of tricyclic antidepressants, narcotic analgesics, and intralesional injection of corticosteroids.

Complications

1. Complications include postherpetic neuralgia and disseminated herpes zoster.

> **ELDER ADVISORY**
>
> Herpetic neuralgia and disseminated herpes zoster are more common in the older person. The debilitated and frail older person is at even greater risk. Pain control and prevention of complications and disability are management priorities.

2. Trigeminal herpes zoster may lead to blindness with ophthalmic branch involvement. Facial and acoustic nerve involvement may lead to Bell's palsy, tinnitus, and hearing loss.

Prognosis

1. In immunocompetent persons, complete recovery is expected, but postherpetic neuralgia may affect persons older than 50.

2. Protracted infections or recurrent infections may occur in the immunocompromised person.

Applying the Nursing Process

> **NURSING DIAGNOSIS:** Pain R/T burning, pruritus, and paresthesias due to vesicular eruption and skin infection caused by herpes zoster

 HOME CARE STRATEGIES

Older Persons with Herpes Zoster (Shingles)

Herpes zoster is more commonly known as shingles. Focus care on managing symptoms and continuing daily activities.

Determine Cognitive Ability and Function

- Write key instruction points on index cards with a black marker and post in an obvious place (on refrigerator).
- Use a diary for the patient to log side effects, pain medication responses, and questions.

Determine Ability to Perform Activities of Daily Living

- Ask about a family member, friend, neighbor, or church member who can assist.
- Assess food supply.
- Refer to Meals on Wheels if needed.
- Utilize a social worker to assist with resources.
- Survey medicine cabinet for medications patient forgot to list. Encourage the patient to discard old medications.

Preventing Cellulitis

- Wash hands before and after caring for open areas.
- Use a gauze covering to keep open areas clean and protected.
- Double bag soiled dressings before placing in the trash.
- Wash soiled clothing in hot soapy water.
- Do not allow chickenpox-susceptible individuals or pregnant women to handle drainage.
- If eyes are affected, demonstrate proper eye hygiene.
- The cloth used to wipe the eyes should not be shared; launder it in hot soapy water.

Pruritus Management

- The affected areas are usually in places older people cannot reach. Discourage the use of objects to scratch. Keep nails clean and trimmed.
- If tub baths are unsafe, topical soaks can be used.
- If using antihistamines, observe for untoward effects, and teach precautions against falling.

Pain Management

- Observe for analgesic interactions and symptoms of toxicity from decreaesd liver or renal function.
- Assist in selecting loose fitting, cotton clothing (snap-front house dresses). Discourage the wearing of a bra or close-fitting clothes.
- Encourage participation in low-key activities or hobbies (puzzles, reading, knitting).

Maintain Socialization

- Encourage participation in social activities (church, bingo, shopping, social gatherings).
- Observe for symptoms of depression, and encourage the verbalization of feelings.

1. *Expected outcomes:* After treatment, the person should be able to do the following:
   a. Indicate a decrease in pain using a 10-point scale.
   b. Report adequate rest related to an increased comfort level and decreased pruritus.
   c. Demonstrate proper technique for application of compresses and soaks.
   d. Demonstrate lack of self-manipulation (scratching) and secondary infection.
2. *Nursing interventions*
   a. During the active lesion phase, assess for burning, paresthesias, pruritus, and pain using a 10-point scale.
   b. Use Burow's soaks or cool water compresses to prevent secondary infection and soothe burning and pruritus. Instruct the person on the correct use of these measures.
   c. Encourage consistent analgesia with acetaminophen or nonsteroidal anti-inflammatory drugs to alleviate discomfort and decrease the incidence of postherpetic neuralgia.
   d. Assess the level of pain on a 10-point scale if postherpetic neuralgia develops. Explore with the physician and the patient the use of additional analgesics and the use of alternative pain relief methods.
   e. Provide emotional support to the person with chronic pain.

Discharge Planning and Teaching

1. Discuss the treatment and expected course of uncomplicated herpes zoster.
2. Discuss methods to prevent secondary infection of lesions:
   a. Use of Burow's soaks
   b. Not scratching
   c. Cutting fingernails short to prevent excoriation of lesions
   d. Follow-up for nonhealing lesions or postherpetic neuralgia symptoms

Public Health Considerations

1. Individuals who have not been exposed to the varicella-zoster virus are susceptible to chickenpox.
2. Persons who had chickenpox are immune to herpes zoster infection from exposure to another infected individual.
3. Health care workers who are unsure of their immune status should have varicella titers done before exposure to a person with herpes zoster.

◼ OTHER VESICULOBULLOUS (BLISTERING) DISORDERS

Pemphigus Vulgaris

1. Definition—Pemphigus vulgaris is a chronic, progressive, potentially life-threatening, vesiculobullous skin

disorder that involves both the epidermis and mucous membranes.
2. Incidence and etiology
   a. Incidence
      (1) Pemphigus vulgaris is an uncommon disorder that affects both sexes and occurs primarily during the 4th through the 6th decades of life.
      (2) There is an increased incidence in people of Jewish, Mediterranean, and Indian descents.
   b. Etiology
      (1) The exact cause is unknown, but pemphigus vulgaris is considered an autoimmune disorder related to circulating IgG antibodies. These antibodies bind to the skin and cause a release of cellular inflammatory mediators.
      (2) Acantholysis (the dyshesion of epidermal cells) produces the characteristic intraepidermal vesicles and bullae.
3. Clinical manifestations
   a. The initial vesicles and bullae generally appear first on the mucous membranes, usually the mouth.
      (1) The bullae are flaccid or soft, arise from nonerythematous skin, rupture easily, and issue a malodorous drainage. Ruptured blisters result in erythematous, denuded, eroded areas. Blisters, especially those in the oral cavity, rarely remain intact, because of their extremely fragile nature (see Color Fig. 35–11).
      (2) The bullae enlarge readily at all peripheral edges. Minimal pressure on an intact blister produces involvement of surrounding skin. Lateral pressure or shear forces applied to normal skin cause easy detachment of the epidermis and newly eroded lesions (positive Nikolsky's sign).
   b. The spread of bullous lesions typically involves the scalp, face, trunk, umbilicus, and intertriginous areas. Lesions may also occur in the esophagus, larynx, and tracheobronchial tree.
   c. Eroded lesions often become secondarily infected, resulting in a typical clinical picture of crusting and a malodorous discharge.
   d. Lesions that heal spontaneously or with treatment generally do so without scarring.
   e. Pain is common at lesion sites, especially lesions on the mucous membranes. Eating is often painful, and maintaining oral nutrition is difficult.
   f. Systemic findings may include anemia, electrolyte imbalance, elevated sedimentation rate and leukocyte and eosinophil counts, and decreased serum protein.
4. Intervention
   a. Oral systemic corticosteroids are the mainstay of therapy. The corticosteroids are tapered over a period of months, according to the person's lesional response. Topical corticosteroids are appropriate for very mild outbreaks of pemphigus vulgaris.
   b. Concurrent immunosuppressive therapy with azathioprine or cyclophosphamide improves lesional response and allows a lower corticosteroid dose to be used. Coexisting infections must be controlled before initiating therapy. As the person's condition improves, these drugs are also tapered.

   c. Plasmapheresis may be used in life-threatening situations in which a great portion of skin is denuded and rapid clinical improvement is vital to survival.
   d. Supportive care includes hospitalization for severe cases, nutritional support, viscous lidocaine to painful oral lesions to promote an adequate nutritional intake, antibiotic therapy, blood transfusions for severe anemia, and topical care with colloidal oatmeal baths and cleansing or antibacterial compresses with Burow's solution and silver sulfadiazine.

Erythema Multiforme, Stevens-Johnson Syndrome, and Toxic Epidermal Necrolysis

1. Definition
   a. Erythema multiforme is an acute skin and mucous membrane reaction that results in erythematous macules, papules, and blistering lesions (see Color Fig. 35–12).
   b. Stevens-Johnson syndrome is a potentially life-threatening, clinical variant of erythema multiforme that results in severe blistering of the skin, eyes, and mouth.
   c. Toxic epidermal necrolysis is a life-threatening, severe form of erythema multiforme and Stevens-Johnson syndrome that produces large bullae and extensive skin sloughing.
2. Incidence and etiology
   a. These three disorders are uncommon to rare. Recurrent episodes are possible. Erythema multiforme is more prevalent in young adults, Stevens-Johnson syndrome is more common in young children, and toxic epidermal necrolysis occurs most often in older children.
   b. Etiology
      (1) The exact cause is unknown, but this complex of disorders is believed to be mediated by the immune system.
      (2) The onset may be idiopathic or due to a reaction to a known cause, such as a drug (penicillin, a sulfonamide, or a barbiturate), infection (herpes simplex, herpes zoster, mumps, influenza type A, syphilis, salmonellosis, or streptococcal), internal illness (graft-versus-host disease, lupus erythematosus, or cancer), chemicals, foods (shellfish), or physical agents (cold or sunlight).
      (3) Toxic epidermal necrolysis is almost always due to a drug reaction.
3. Clinical manifestations
   a. Erythema multiforme is characterized by "target" or "iris" plaques that have a bull's-eye appearance.
      (1) Plaques may be pink, red, white, or blue. Lesions enlarge slowly and clear centrally; new lesions typically form in the cleared center, giving the typical "target" appearance.
      (2) Vesiculobullous lesions may also be present.
      (3) Lesions are typically distributed over the extremities, palms, and soles, but they may appear elsewhere on the body.

(4) Erythema multiforme may be preceded by a pro-dromal period of fatigue, muscle pain, and fever. Skin lesions can be painful and pruritic.

b. Stevens-Johnson syndrome involves high fevers and severe blistering of the skin and mucous membranes. Eye involvement may result in photophobia and blindness. Tracheobronchial involvement may induce respiratory distress. This disorder is considered a dermatologic emergency.

c. Toxic epidermal necrolysis may be preceded by a sore throat, malaise, and then fever. It initially develops as erythematous blotches, but it quickly progresses to large bullae. These blistered areas slough, leaving large areas of denuded, sometimes necrotic, dermis. This disorder is considered a dermatologic emergency.

   (1) The entire body surface, eyes, and all mucous membranes may be involved and are painful.

   (2) Respiratory distress, bronchopneumonia, stomatitis, conjunctivitis, vulvitis, and balanitis (inflammation of the glans penis) are common.

   (3) Severe dehydration, electrolyte imbalances, and septicemia occur.

4. Intervention

   a. When possible, an identifiable cause should be eliminated.

   b. Mild cases of erythema multiforme often resolve without treatment and are typically managed with topical corticosteroids and antihistamines.

   c. Use of oral corticosteroids is controversial, but it is generally agreed that these drugs are most effective at the onset of the eruption. If they are given later in the illness, the chances that lesions will progress or a concurrent infection would contraindicate their use are greater.

   d. Discomfort is controlled with oral analgesics or narcotics for severe pain.

   e. Supportive care includes nutritional and electrolyte replacement and support, respiratory support, systemic antibiotic therapy specific to blood-cultured organisms, oral care with petrolatum for the lips, and viscous lidocaine for oral lesions.

   f. An ophthalmologic consult is needed to maintain eye health and prevent complications such as blindness, diminished vision, adhesions, and chronic dryness.

   g. Topical therapy must be used judiciously in severe cases, because of the skin's markedly decreased barrier function.

      (1) Warm water compresses are soothing for noninfected lesions.

      (2) Secondarily infected, eroded skin may be treated judiciously with Silvadene cream, dilute silver nitrate (0.25%), or acetic acid solution (0.1%).

      (3) Topical antibiotics should be avoided, because of the potential for increased systemic absorption and subsequent toxicity.

   h. Toxic epidermal necrolysis is most appropriately treated in an intensive care environment in a specialized burn unit.

Herpes Simplex

1. Definition—Herpes simplex is a common viral infection that results in clusters of vesicular lesions.

2. Incidence and etiology
   a. Incidence
      (1) Sixty to 70 percent of adults have antibodies to the herpes simplex virus.
      (2) Recurrent infections afflict approximately 20 to 45 percent of the U.S. population.
      (3) The incidence of recurrent infection is greatly increased in the debilitated or immunocompromised person.
   b. Etiology
      (1) Oral infection is caused by the herpes simplex virus type 1.
      (2) Genital infection is caused by the herpes simplex virus type 2.
      (3) Triggering factors for recurrent infections include emotional stress; the menstrual cycle; exposure to sunlight, cold, and wind; physical trauma; a debilitated or immunocompromised state; immunosuppression after a transplant; a high fever; viral illness; and systemic infection.

3. Clinical manifestations
   a. Classic lesions are grouped vesicles on an erythematous base (see Color Fig. 35-13). The vesicles eventually crust over before healing occurs. Lesions heal without scarring.
   b. Recurrent lesions are characterized by a prodromal state of burning, tingling, or itching. Active lesions are painful.
   c. Oral lesions generally appear on the lips, at the junction of the lips and skin, and in or around the nose. These lesions may interfere with eating and may be malodorous.
   d. Genital lesions may occur on any area of the genitalia or perianal region if anal intercourse is practiced.

4. Intervention
   a. The goals of intervention are to alleviate symptoms, prevent secondary infections, and reduce risk factors for recurrent infections.
   b. Nonpharmacologic interventions
      (1) Cool water compresses help decrease discomfort.
      (2) Frequent mouth care cleans and soothes affected mucous membranes.
      (3) Sitz baths for vulvar lesions may decrease discomfort and ease dysuria.
   c. Pharmacologic interventions
      (1) Acyclovir ointment may be beneficial in primary infections but is of little benefit in recurrent infections.
      (2) Systemic therapy with oral acyclovir may shorten the time of infection in primary infections and in immunocompromised persons.

◼ *PSORIASIS*

Definition

1. Psoriasis is a noninfectious, inflammatory skin disorder characterized by erythematous papules and plaques commonly covered by a silver-white scale.

2. Clinical presentations of psoriasis demonstrate multiple variants that include erythrodermic, pustular, and guttate forms.

Incidence and Socioeconomic Impact

1. Psoriasis is a common dermatologic disorder, affecting up to 2 percent of the U.S. population.
2. There is a familial tendency in 40 percent of cases.
3. Men and women are affected equally. The disorder may begin at any time throughout the life span, but it most commonly affects persons ages 10 to 40.

Risk Factors

1. A familial history predisposes a person to psoriasis.
2. Emotional distress, trauma, systemic illness, seasonal changes, and hormonal changes are linked to exacerbations.

Etiology

The etiology of psoriasis is unknown, but there may be a hereditary defect that overproduces keratin along with other immunologic and cellular abnormalities.

Pathophysiology

1. Psoriasis results from an abnormal, rapid proliferation of epidermal cells.
2. Normally, the length of time from cellular division in the basal layer to the shedding of cells in the stratum corneum is 28 days. In psoriasis, that process is accelerated to 3 to 4 days.

Clinical Manifestations

1. Psoriasis typically manifests as erythematous papules covered with silver-white scale. This papular appearance is known as **guttate psoriasis.** Over time, the papules tend to coalesce in sharply defined plaques (see Color Fig. 35–14).
2. Psoriatic lesions tend to be symmetric.
3. Affected areas include the scalp, elbows, knees, extensor surfaces of the arms and legs, lower back, sacrum, intergluteal fold, and genitalia.
4. Thickening, pitting, and discoloration of the nails occurs in approximately 50 percent of individuals with psoriasis.
5. Lesions are cosmetically troublesome and emotionally upsetting but are usually asymptomatic. Pruritus may be present.
6. Psoriasis is characterized by periods of remission and exacerbation.
7. New areas of traumatized skin may develop a psoriatic lesion during the healing process. For example, an area of newly scratched or newly sunburned skin may develop a psoriatic lesion. This is known as **Koebner's phenomenon.**

8. Psoriatic arthritis is associated with approximately 20 percent of persons with psoriasis.

Diagnostics

1. History
   a. Identify potential physical and emotional triggering factors. For example, psoriatic flare-ups typically follow a streptococcal pharyngitis infection by 7 to 10 days.
   b. Determine family history.
   c. Assess for local (lesional) and systemic complaints.
   d. Assess the person's psychosocial state. Try to determine whether an emotional upset or stressful event was associated with recent flare of psoriasis.
2. Physical examination
   a. Assess the distribution and severity of lesions.
   b. Identify areas of trauma.
3. Diagnosis
   a. Diagnosis is often based solely on the history and clinical presentation.
   b. A skin biopsy may be done if the diagnosis is difficult.
   c. Blood work may demonstrate an elevated uric acid, mild anemia, and elevated sedimentation rate.

Clinical Management

1. The goals of clinical management are to induce and maintain remission and alleviate symptoms.
2. Nonpharmacologic interventions
   a. Skin care using principles of hydration and lubrication
   b. Stress reduction strategies
   c. Careful exposure to sunlight (without burning), which may help control plaques
3. Pharmacologic interventions
   a. Topical corticosteroids inhibit epidermal cell mitosis and produce local anti-inflammatory and vasoconstrictive effects.
   b. Intralesional steroids (triamcinolone acetonide and triamcinolone hexacetonide) are used for specific lesions that do not respond to topical treatment.
   c. Coal tar preparations (Fototar cream, Estar gel, and PsoriGel), applied topically, inhibit DNA synthesis. They are often used in conjunction with ultraviolet B light therapy.
   d. Anthralin (Anthra-Derm and Drithocreme), a synthetic antipsoriatic agent, is effective for widespread, thickened plaques. Anthralin stains the skin and clothing and may cause skin irritation.
   e. Methotrexate, a cytotoxic agent, is effective, but it is reserved for severe psoriasis because of its potential for bone marrow suppression and liver toxicity.
   f. Etretinate (Tegison), a vitamin A derivative, is often used for more severe forms of psoriasis, such as erythrodermic or pustular psoriasis. Regular monthly follow-up is required, because of the potential for hematologic or liver toxicity.

LEARNING/TEACHING GUIDELINES
for Self-Care in Psoriasis

General Overview

1. Describe the disease process and overall treatment regimen.
2. Describe the proper administration of medications and their side effects. Discuss the name of each medication and its rationale for use, its dosage and frequency, and potential side effects and ways to reduce them.
3. Help the person and family members plan and carry out therapeutic skin care regimens.
4. Assist the person and family members in identifying potential stressors and ways to reduce or eliminate the stressors implicated in exacerbations of psoriasis.
5. Help the person and family members cope with a chronic illness.
6. Advise the person to avoid skin injury. Scratching, trauma, injury, and sunburn may elicit Koebner's phenomenon. Sunscreen should be used to prevent sunburn.
7. Emphasize the importance of lifelong medical follow-up in the care and control of psoriasis.

Psoriasis Therapies and Medications

1. For persons using topical steroid preparations, discuss the following points:
   a. Topical steroids reduce inflammation and inhibit cell growth.
   b. Occlusion of topical steroids enhances their effect and potency. Caution is required when occlusion is used. Watch the site(s) of occlusion for evidence of maceration and infection. Occlusion also increases the chance for systemic absorption of the steroid.
   c. Steroids with medium and high potency will irritate and macerate the face and intertriginous areas. They should not be used in these regions unless specifically prescribed and monitored by the physician.
   d. Topical gels and lotions are best suited for the scalp and other hairy areas. These preparations are best applied after the area has been washed. Shower caps are useful occlusive dressings for the scalp.
   e. Apply topical steroids in the direction the hair grows to prevent folliculitis.
2. For persons using topical tar preparations, discuss the following points:
   a. Topical tar preparations enhance the effects of ultraviolet light (UVL) therapy and inhibit cell division.
   b. Apply tar as prescribed in a thin layer in the direction the hair grows. This technique prevents the tar and its base from getting pushed into the hair follicles and causing folliculitis.
   c. Topical tar preparations have an unappealing

odor and are messy to apply. Encourage the use of the more aesthetically acceptable purified creams and gels.
   d. Tar preparations are often left on overnight, but the minimum effective exposure time on the skin is usually 2 hours.
3. For persons using topical anthralin preparations, discuss the following points:
   a. Anthralin inhibits cellular division, is a potent irritant, and helps flatten lesions.
   b. Anthralin is a potent medication and will irritate and burn unaffected skin. It must be carefully applied only to the involved areas. Open, oozing, and weeping lesions are not appropriate for anthralin application. It is available as a cream or an ointment.
   c. Anthralin stains the skin, clothing, and bathroom appliances. It is best applied when the person can limit his or her contact with items in the environment, and it should be wiped off with a previously stained towel or rag to prevent staining the sink, bathtub, and shower.
   d. Start with a low concentration of anthralin (0.1%) for 10 to 30 minutes and then wash off the medication. As tolerance to the anthralin builds, the concentration may be increased gradually up to 1 percent.
   e. Treatment with anthralin continues daily until the lesions flatten and clear. This often requires 8 weeks or longer.
4. For persons receiving UVL treatments, discuss the following points:
   a. Ultraviolet light therapy inhibits cellular division and promotes flattening of the psoriatic lesions.
   b. Most UVL treatments require the person to stand in a light treatment chamber for up to 15 minutes. This is demanding, both emotionally and physically.
   c. Safety precautions are required during UVL therapy. Protective wrap-around goggles prevent exposure of the eyes to UVL. Only those areas that require treatment should be exposed to UVL. For example, the face may be shielded with a loosely applied pillow case. Avoid direct contact with the light bulbs of the treatment unit to avoid burning the skin.
   d. Avoid photosensitizing medications to prevent burning during treatments.
   e. If an oral photosensitizing agent, such as psoralen, is used as part of the treatment, care must be taken to prevent skin burns and corneal damage for 24 hours after administration. Protective goggles, protective clothing, and sunscreens are necessary to prevent these complications. Nausea can occur with oral photosensitizing agents. This side effect is minimized if they are taken with food.

LEARNING/TEACHING GUIDELINES
(continued)

f. The side effects of UVL include severe skin burns. Symptoms such as swelling, pain, burning, and redness of the skin must be reported promptly.

5. For persons receiving systemic therapy with methotrexate, discuss the following points:
   a. Systemic medications inhibit cellular division, thereby flattening plaques and preventing new ones from forming.
   b. The side effects include damage to the bone marrow, liver, and gastrointestinal tract; nausea; fatigue, allergic reactions; and oral ulcerations.
   c. These side effects require close follow-up and frequent monitoring of affected body systems. The potential hepatotoxicity must be followed closely with liver enzyme testing and dose-related liver biopsies.
   d. Alcohol intake should be avoided at all costs to decrease the additive hepatotoxic effect. Acetaminophen and aspirin products should be avoided to prevent liver-related side effects. Adequate hydration is important to prevent kidney damage. Nausea is decreased if methotrexate is taken with food or used concurrently with an antiemetic.
   e. Pregnancy is to be avoided while this drug is being taken, because it will cause congenital defects.
   f. Side effects that must be reported immediately to the physician are jaundice, extreme fatigue, extensive mouth ulcerations, and increased bleeding tendencies.

Skin Care Principles

1. Instruct the person with psoriatic lesions about the following skin care principles to maintain skin wellness, alleviate dryness, and reduce pruritus:
   a. Keep the skin well lubricated at all times. Reapply lubricants and emollients as needed in between prescribed medications.
   b. Take baths in warm, not hot, water. Limit the time in the bath to 20 minutes. The bath is an appropriate time to try to loosen thickened scales and plaques. This must be done in a gentle fashion, rubbing the washcloth over the lesions in a circular manner. Discourage vigorous rubbing or pulling at scales, which will cause bleeding and may produce Koebner's phenomenon.
   c. Dry the skin by gently patting it. Apply any topical preparations immediately after taking a bath.

d. Avoid harsh soaps, chemicals, and cosmetics during skin care and personal hygiene routines.
2. Advise the person to make the following lifestyle and environmental changes to decrease skin irritation and dryness:
   a. Keep the humidity in the home at about 60 percent and avoid extremes of temperature.
   b. Wear loose-fitting, absorbent clothing made of a nonirritating cotton blend. Clothing made from wool is often irritating and itchy.
   c. Avoid contact with irritating chemicals in the home, at work, or during recreation.
3. Develop with the person a treatment schedule and plan that fits his or her lifestyle and treatment regimen needs.

Triggering Factors

1. Discuss the following factors related to psoriasis exacerbations:
   a. Although it is not scientifically proven, there seems to be a strong correlation between emotional or physical stressors and flare-ups of psoriasis. Physical illness should be treated promptly.
   b. Proper nutrition, exercise, and rest are general wellness-promoting strategies that may prevent recurrence of psoriasis.
   c. Stress reduction strategies include exercise, relaxation techniques, visual imagery, involvement in support groups, and recreation with friends and family members.
   d. Professional counseling is often helpful in identifying stressors and strategies for dealing with them.
   e. The National Psoriasis Foundation publishes a newsletter and offers local support groups and educational sessions that may help persons cope with this chronic illness.

Body Image Disturbance

1. Discuss with the person and family members the importance of sharing their feelings regarding the effect of psoriasis on body image and sexuality.
2. Advise the person and family members to talk with other persons affected by psoriasis at local support group meetings or during visits to the physician's office.
3. Discuss camouflage techniques with clothing that may be used as temporary measures while lesions are clearing.
4. Reinforce the disease course of psoriasis. It generally clears with treatment and does not produce scarring.

4. Special medical procedures include phototherapy with ultraviolet A or B light and the Goeckerman regimen. (See p. 1627 for a complete discussion of these phototherapy treatments.)

Complications

- Secondary infection of lesions
- Generalized exfoliative psoriasis

Prognosis

1. Psoriasis is an incurable, chronic illness characterized by periods of improvement and exacerbation.
2. Most cases of psoriasis can be treated and controlled with proper medical treatment.

Applying the Nursing Process

NURSING DIAGNOSIS: Impaired skin integrity R/T erythematous plaque with scale on knees, elbows, thighs, and hands

1. *Expected outcomes:* After instruction, the person should be able to do the following:
   a. Demonstrate an understanding of psoriasis by being able to:
      (1) Describe the basic pathophysiology of psoriasis.
      (2) State realistic expectations for prognosis and the understanding that long-term follow-up is required.
   b. Demonstrate appropriate daily skin care.
   c. Properly self-administer antipsoriatic medications.
   d. Develop a plan to eliminate or reduce identified triggering factors associated with flare-ups.
2. *Nursing interventions:* See Learning/Teaching Guidelines for Self-Care in Psoriasis.

NURSING DIAGNOSIS: Social isolation R/T emotional stress and treatment demands of psoriasis

1. *Expected outcomes:* After counseling, the person should be able to do the following:
   a. Develop a plan to reduce daily stress.
   b. Identify at least 2 coping skills that can be used to adapt to changes invoked by a chronic illness.
   c. Describe a plan to incorporate daily treatment schedule into routine of work, rest, and recreation.
   d. Use support systems to aid in effective coping with illness.
   e. Report an improved sense of well-being and socialization.
2. *Nursing interventions*
   a. Provide emotional support and encouragement for a physically and emotionally draining chronic illness.
   b. Discuss with the individual the triggering factors that may be involved in exacerbations and identify strategies to reduce or eliminate them.
   c. Help the person and family members identify strategies the person can use to maintain compliance with the prescribed medical regimen and manage this chronic illness.
   d. Teach the person and family members the rationale for each therapeutic regimen and correlate it with the disease course and expected response to treatment. Provide specific instructions on how to carry out each aspect of the medical treatment plan.
   e. Explore stress management and stress reduction strategies to enhance coping with a chronic illness and prevent exacerbations.
   f. Allow the person and family members to express their feelings concerning the impact of psoriasis on their lives. Facilitate discussion by asking open-ended questions.
   g. Provide information on local psoriasis support groups and encourage the involvement of all family members.
   h. Assess for signs and symptoms of depression.
   i. Involve family members in the treatment regimen whenever possible.
   j. Refer the person to social services or counseling services as needed.

Discharge Planning and Teaching

1. Provide information on the disease process, the treatment regimen, the use and side effects of medication, and the expected outcomes of therapy.
2. Give the person published information on support groups, newsletters, and the National Psoriasis Foundation.
3. Make a follow-up appointment for the person.
4. Encourage the person and family members to call with questions or concerns.

◼ ALLERGIC CONTACT DERMATITIS

Definition

Allergic contact dermatitis is an acute or chronic, noninfectious, inflammatory skin rash that results from a sensitivity to allergens or chemicals.

Incidence and Socioeconomic Impact

1. Allergic contact dermatitis is a commonly occurring dermatologic disorder that affects persons of all ages.
2. The incidence of contact dermatitis is directly related to exposure with the causative contact agent.

Risk Factors

1. Primary chemical irritants such as acid, alkalies, solvents, detergents, and oils are common causative agents.
2. In allergic contact dermatitis, sensitivity to a specific allergen occurs with exposure. Common allergens include poison ivy or oak, nickel, chromium, leather, epoxy resin, parabens, rubber, plants, cosmetics, and perfumes.
3. Persons with minimal skin pigment are more susceptible to irritant effects than those with heavier pigmentation.

Etiology

1. Contact with a primary irritant
2. Exposure to a substance to which there has been previous sensitization (delayed hypersensitivity reaction)

Pathophysiology

1. Mild irritants induce an inflammatory response over prolonged exposure. Strong irritants damage the skin on exposure. Contact with the irritant damages the stratum corneum and impairs its barrier function.
2. Cell-mediated immune responses induce the inflammatory reaction in allergic contact dermatitis. The response is a delayed hypersensitivity reaction.

Clinical Manifestations

1. Primary irritant dermatitis is characterized by dryness, erythema, fissures, blistering, or ulceration. Associated symptoms include pruritus and pain (see Color Fig. 35–15).
2. The distribution and location of lesions are indicative of the specific type of exposure.
3. The reaction may be acute, subacute, or chronic (Table 35–7).

Diagnostics

1. History
   a. Question the person about the home environment, work, hobbies, medications, clothing, laundry soap, cosmetics, and any other potential sources of irritants or allergens.
   b. Assess for symptoms such as pain, pruritus, fever, and malaise.
2. Physical examination
   a. Look for an unusual distribution and configuration of lesions. This is a classic indication of allergic contact dermatitis.
      (1) Airborne antigens have a photodistribution on all exposed areas.
      (2) Sharp angles, straight lines, and sharply margin-

ated plaques also suggest allergic contact dermatitis.
   b. Look for signs of secondary infection.
3. Diagnosis
   a. A clinical history and examination are usually sufficient to make a diagnosis of allergic contact dermatitis.
   b. Conduct patch testing for allergic contact dermatitis after the acute reaction subsides (see Chapter 21).

Clinical Management

1. The goals of intervention are to reduce inflammation, prevent secondary infection, and limit exposure to the causative agent.
2. The nonpharmacologic intervention is the application of cool compresses to reduce inflammation.
3. Pharmacologic interventions
   a. Burow's compresses (aluminum acetate in 1:20 dilution) may be used.
   b. Potassium permanganate compresses (1:16,000 to 1:4000 dilution) are both astringent and bactericidal.
   c. Systemic antihistamines (hydroxyzine and diphenhydramine) and topical antipruritics (calamine, camphor, and menthol) may be used for pruritus.
   d. Topical corticosteroids (e.g., triamcinolone acetonide 0.1%) may be used after oozing subsides.
   e. Systemic corticosteroids (e.g., prednisolone) may be needed for severe cases.

Complications

Secondary bacterial or yeast infections may develop.

Prognosis

1. The prognosis is good for localized reactions.
2. Dermal injury from caustic agents results in scarring.

Applying the Nursing Process

NURSING DIAGNOSIS: Impaired skin integrity R/T erythema, dryness, and vesicles of hands secondary to contact dermatitis

1. *Expected outcomes:* After instruction, the person should be able to do the following:
   a. Demonstrate consistent preventive measures essential to the promotion of healing by being able to
      (1) Reduce or eliminate exposure to any household or work irritants.
      (2) Keep the skin well lubricated.
      (3) Avoid abrasive soaps.
      (4) Eliminate exposure by wearing vinyl gloves with white cotton liners.

Table 35–7. Stages of Dermatitis

Stage	Clinical Features	Symptoms
Acute	Intense erythema, edema, erosions, papules, vesicles, crusting	Intensely pruritic
Subacute	Less intense erythema, fine diffuse scaling, scattered papules or plaques	Pruritic
Chronic	Lichenification (thick skin caused by chronic rubbing and scratching), dryness, scaling, postinflammatory hyper- and hypopigmentation	Pruritic

b. Guard against secondary infection by keeping the affected area clean and not scratching. It may be necessary for the person to cut the fingernails short.

2. *Nursing interventions*
   a. Help the person identify the causative agent and develop a plan to prevent reexposure.
   b. Help the person prevent secondary infection by providing instruction on antipruritic measures and demonstration of personal hygiene practices and handwashing techniques.

Discharge Planning and Teaching

1. Teach the person the use and side effects of medications and the signs and symptoms of a secondary infection.
2. Discuss ways to avoid the irritant or allergen, and help the person identify protective measures to promote healing.
3. Make an appointment for follow-up care.
4. Encourage the person and family members to call with questions or concerns.

Public Health Considerations

1. Provide education on ways to decrease exposure to household chemicals and occupational irritants.
2. Vesicle fluid is not contagious. For example, the exudate from poison ivy vesicles will not transfer the antigen to another person.
3. Allergic contact dermatitis that affects the hands significantly impairs the skin's barrier function in health care workers. Extreme caution must be used to prevent occupational exposure to pathogens.

◼ *ACNE VULGARIS AND ACNE ROSACEA*

Definition

1. Acne vulgaris is an inflammatory reaction of the sebaceous follicles (hair follicles with large, oil-producing glands). The reaction may result in papular, pustular, or nodular lesions.
2. Acne rosacea is a chronic erythematous eruption, located predominantly on the central area of the face. It is associated with a superimposed acneiform eruption (see Color Fig. 35–16).

Incidence and Socioeconomic Impact

1. Acne vulgaris is the most common skin disorder, occurring in more than 80 percent of the population.
   a. It most commonly appears in adolescence, but it may occur at any age. The most commonly affected age range is 12 to 35.

b. Adolescent males are more commonly affected than females.

2. Acne rosacea occurs during the 3rd to 5th decades of life and affects women more often than men. As many as 10 million Americans may be affected. The disorder worsens over time. Fair-skinned persons who blush easily are more likely to develop acne rosacea.

Precipitating Risk Factors

1. Precipitating factors for acne vulgaris include genetic predisposition; hormonal changes, such as those experienced in puberty or the menstrual cycle; emotional stress; a hot, humid climate; perspiration; use of cosmetics, steroids, or oral contraceptives; friction; and occlusive clothing.
2. Precipitating factors for acne rosacea are a fair complexion and conditions that promote vasodilation. These include exposure to sunlight, caffeine, alcohol, vasodilating drugs, hot liquids, temperature extremes, physical activity, infection, and emotional stress.

Etiology

The exact causes of acne vulgaris and acne rosacea are unknown.

Pathophysiology

1. In acne vulgaris, 3 major pathophysiologic processes are known (Fig. 35–5).
2. The pathophysiology of acne rosacea is similar to that of acne vulgaris in that there is an increase in sebum production and a proliferation of *Propionibacterium acnes*. However, there is no increase in epithelial cell shedding, and no comedones are formed.
   a. Vasomotor lability produces frequent vasodilation and may be responsible for persistent facial erythema and telangiectasia (dilated, small vessels) formation.
   b. The overgrowth of *P. acnes* results in papule and pustule formation.

Clinical Manifestations

See Table 35–8.

Diagnostics

1. History
   a. Acne vulgaris
      (1) Determine whether there is an endocrine-related pattern. Ask the following questions:
      • Are menstrual periods regular?
      • Is there any excessive hair growth?
      • Are oral contraceptives currently used, or have they been used within the past several months?

THE DEVELOPMENT OF ACNE

Three major pathophysiologic processes occur in the development of acne vulgaris.

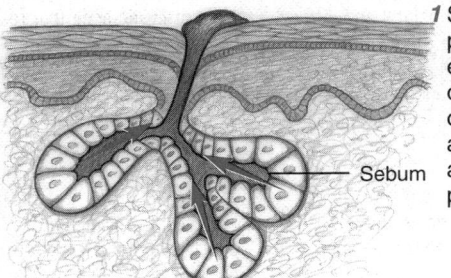

1 Sebum production is excessive and occurs with the onset of adrenal and gonadal androgen production.

Sebum

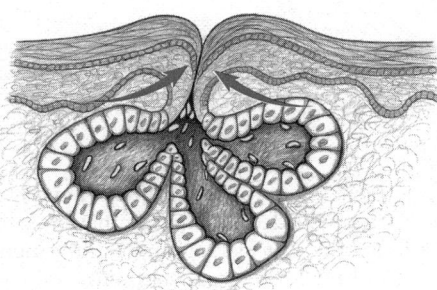

2 There is an increased shedding of epithelial cells lining the *sebaceous follicles* (hair follicles with oil-producing glands). This process expands and blocks the follicle.

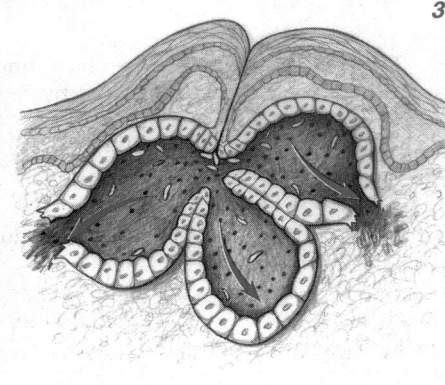

3 The cutaneous flora, *Propionibacterium acnes*, multiplies in this anaerobic environment and initiates an inflammatory response in the follicle. Open or closed comedones are then formed, and the follicle may rupture.

Figure 35–5.

- Does emotional stress have an effect on the lesions?
  (2) Determine whether there are environmental influences. Consider asking the following questions.
    - Do changes in the seasons affect the course of the disorder?
    - What cosmetics are used? There is often a desire to cover up lesions with heavy, oil-based makeup that clogs pores and aggravates lesions.

- Is there exposure to oils or greasy products in the work environment?
- What habits are aggravating the condition? Inquire about tight clothing; pressure; occlusion; and squeezing, picking, and rubbing of the affected area.
- How was the person's acne treated in the past, and what was the response? What over-the-counter preparations or home remedies have been used?
- Is the person taking corticosteroids, androgens, lithium, isoniazid, vitamin B_{12}, phenytoin (Dilantin), or hyperalimentation therapy? These medications may precipitate or aggravate acne vulgaris.
  (3) Explore concerns related to body image and self-esteem.
  b. Acne rosacea
    (1) Identify the onset of the disorder and its clinical characteristics to help distinguish it from acne vulgaris.
    (2) Carefully discuss known precipitating factors to identify individual pathophysiologic responses.
2. Physical examination—Focus on the clinical manifestations to arrive at the correct diagnosis.
3. The diagnosis for each disorder is based on the presenting history and clinical examination.

Clinical Management

1. The goals of clinical management are to reduce or eliminate lesions, prevent scarring and secondary infection, and reduce emotional distress.
2. Nonpharmacologic interventions
   a. Gentle, nonabrasive, routine cleansing of the skin
   b. Avoidance of precipitating factors
3. Pharmacologic interventions
   a. Acne vulgaris (Table 35–9).
   b. Acne rosacea
     (1) Systemic antibiotics such as tetracycline and erythromycin
     (2) Topical therapy with antibiotics such as metronidazole and sulfur-containing products such as Sulfacet-R
4. Special medical-surgical procedures
   a. Comedone extraction is done by applying gentle pressure over the lesion with a comedone extractor. It may be necessary to incise the opening of the follicle with a small-gauge needle to facilitate the expression of follicular contents. Repeated or forceful comedone extractions may lead to scarring.
   b. For acne rosacea, laser treatments may be helpful in removing telangiectasias. The associated rhinophyma may be surgically removed or laser treated.

Complications

- Secondary bacterial infection
- Emotional distress
- Ocular rosacea that may seriously damage vision
- Deep scarring

Table 35–8. Clinical Manifestations of Acne Vulgaris and Acne Rosacea

Type of Acne	Appearance	Distribution	Symptoms	Other Information
Acne vulgaris	Varying degrees of severity with multiple lesions possible, including open comedones (blackheads), closed comedones (whiteheads), inflamed papules, pustules, nodules, cysts. Scarring is common with more severe disease.	Face, chest, neck, and back. In extensive disease, the extremities, buttocks, and scalp are involved.	Nodular and cystic lesions are pruritic and painful and may rupture, draining purulent material. Lesions are emotionally distressing.	Acne conglobata is a severe form of cystic acne that results in ruptured cysts and nodules that coalesce under the skin to form very inflamed sinus tracts.
Acne rosacea	Lesions similar to acne vulgaris but without comedones. Flushing, erythema, and telangiectasias are common. Associated with rhinophyma, a thick, enlarged red nose with irregular skin	Predominantly on face, but may be seen on chest.	Burning or stinging during flushing episodes.	Sometimes associated with ocular symptoms of keratitis, blepharitis, and uveitis.

Prognosis

1. Neither disorder is curable, but both can be treated adequately to alleviate symptoms.
2. Untreated acne leads to lesional and emotional scarring.
3. Rosacea has a protracted course, extending over multiple decades of life.

Applying the Nursing Process

NURSING DIAGNOSIS: Impaired skin integrity R/T disruption of the epidermis and dermis secondary to nodulocystic lesions on face, neck, and back

1. *Expected outcomes:* After instruction, resolution of acne lesions should occur within 2 to 3 months, as evidenced by the following:
   a. The patient's verbalization of the importance of compliance with prescribed medical treatment
   b. Minimized scarring
   c. The absence of open or closed comedones
   d. The absence of acne nodules and cysts
   e. A return to nonerythematous skin tones
2. *Nursing interventions*
   a. Implement a teaching program on the cause of acne and strategies to prevent picking, squeezing, or manipulating of lesions.
   b. Review principles of skin care and topical treatments of acne.
   c. Apply warm compresses to promote suppuration of cysts.
   d. Help the patient develop a self-care regimen that facilitates compliance with the treatment plan.

   e. Help the patient recognize personal hygiene strategies that will decrease inflammation.
   f. Instruct the person and family members on the potential for long-term treatment.

NURSING DIAGNOSIS: Body image disturbance R/T nodulocystic acne and scarring on face

1. *Expected outcomes:* The person should experience improved body image and self-esteem, as evidenced by the following:
   a. Verbalization of improved psychologic well-being
   b. Improved social interactions with family and friends
   c. Improved eye contact
   d. Increased socialization as a result of treatment and use of camouflage techniques
   e. Positive body language (e.g., the person is smiling, hands and hair are away from the face, and the person holds his or her head up when talking and walking)
2. *Nursing interventions*
   a. Assess the person's self-perception and factors that influence it.
   b. Help the person focus on the realistic appearance of the disease and eliminate catastrophic or exaggerated perceptions of how others view the person.
   c. Encourage the person to discuss feelings of poor body image and validate those feelings. Approach all interactions in an accepting and positive manner. Maintain an honest but positive and caring perspective on treatment and expected outcomes.
   d. Demonstrate cosmetic camouflage techniques to decrease signs of erythema and scarring.
   e. Discuss available treatments and surgical procedures to minimize scarring.

Table 35–9. Pharmacologic Treatment of Acne Vulgaris

Medication	Uses	Action	Side Effects	Other Information
Topicals				
Tretinoin (vitamin A acid)	Drug of choice for noninflammatory lesions and comedones. Used in combination therapy in papular or pustular lesions.	Increases cellular turnover, clears out existing comedones, and prevents new ones.	Irritant reactions, especially in fair or sensitive skin. Increases susceptibility to sunburn, erythema, and peeling.	Symptoms of acne may worsen during first several weeks of treatment. Requires 3–5 months for resolution of lesions.
Benzoyl peroxide	Papular or pustular acne.	Antibacterial effect: Reduces proliferation of *Propionibacterium acnes*. Depresses sebum production.	Initial redness and scaling. Contact dermatitis may develop.	Often used in combination with tretinoin. Decrease irritant reaction by applying 10–15 min after washing the affected area.
Erythromycin, clindamycin, or tetracycline	Papular or pustular acne.	Suppresses growth of *P. acnes*; decreases free fatty acids on skin surface and inflammation.	Mild irritation. Rare side effect of clindamycin is pseudomembranous colitis. Discontinue use if diarrhea or intestinal symptoms occur.	Is applied 1–2 times daily. Treatment success is similar to that of benzoyl peroxide.
Systemic				
Tetracycline or erythromycin	Moderate to severe papular or pustular acne.	Suppresses *P. acnes*.	Tetracycline: photosensitivity and candida vaginitis. Contraindicated in pregnancy because of discoloration of fetal teeth. Erythromycin: gastrointestinal upset.	Tetracycline is the drug of choice. Successful treatment may require months to years.
Oral corticosteroids	Nodulocystic acne.	Potent anti-inflammatory and mild sebum-suppressing effects.	Chronic use has significant toxicity on multiple body systems, including the cardiovascular, central nervous, musculoskeletal, endocrine, and gastrointestinal systems.	Usually used only in a 2- to 3-wk treatment course.
Diaminodiphenylsulfane	Nodulocystic acne.	Sulfa-type antibiotic with antibacterial and anti-inflammatory effects.	Acute and long-term use may cause liver, bone marrow, and neurologic toxicity.	Requires careful follow-up during treatment.
Oral estrogens	Nodulocystic acne.	Suppresses sebum production.	Headaches and thrombosis.	Given to female patients only. Side effects are more severe in male patients.
Isotretinoin (synthetic vitamin A)	Nodulocystic acne.	Significantly suppresses sebum production and epidermal shedding. Prevents comedone formation.	Very dry lips and mouth, chapping of skin and mucous membranes. A significant and dangerous side effect is teratogenicity.	Used in nonresponsive cases. Female patients of childbearing potential *must* use contraceptives during treatment and for 8 wk afterwards.
Intralesional				
Corticosteroids	Papulopustular and nodulocystic acne.	Anti-inflammatory.	Temporary local atrophy of skin.	Produces rapid resolution of treated lesions within 2–3 days.

NURSING DIAGNOSIS: Risk for injury R/T side effects of oral isotretinoin

1. *Expected outcomes:* The risk of side effects should be minimized, as evidenced by the following:

a. No pregnancy during isotretinoin therapy and for 2 months after stopping the drug (in female patients)
b. No elevation of serum cholesterol, triglycerides, or liver function tests
c. Minimized skin scaling and lip and eye dryness
d. No muscle or joint pains
e. No headaches

2. *Nursing interventions*
   a. Instruct the person and family members on isotretinoin and its side effects.
   b. Obtain informed consent and a negative pregnancy test before starting treatment.
   c. Administer artificial tears, lip ointments, emollients, and moisturizers to decrease dryness.
   d. Administer analgesics for joint and muscle aches.
   e. Continually reassess patient's response and tolerance to treatment.
   f. Monitor laboratory values for elevated serum cholesterol, triglycerides, and liver function tests.

Discharge Planning and Teaching

1. Eliminate any myths the person may believe concerning the cause or treatment of acne vulgaris. Discuss the following points:
   a. Acne is not related to diet.
   b. Abrasive cleaning to "unblock pores" not only is ineffective, but also causes increased inflammation.
   c. Acne lesions are not caused by poor personal hygiene. (Review the known pathophysiology of acne vulgaris.)
   d. Acne is not a "stage of life" commonly experienced in the teenage years. It is a chronic disorder and may occur throughout the life span.
2. Make sure the patient thoroughly understands the course and treatment of the disorder so that compliance and positive therapeutic results are increased. The person needs to know when to seek care for potential side effects of medications.

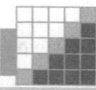

LEGAL AND ETHICAL CONSIDERATIONS

The risks for birth defects are so great during oral isotretinoin therapy that informed consent is required before therapy is instituted. Females of childbearing age who are taking oral isotretinoin must have a consistent and reliable form of birth control. In the consent process, some physicians require agreement to therapeutic abortion if a pregnancy does occur while oral isotretinoin is being taken. If compliance regarding the informed consent is in question, the physician may consider alternative treatments to avoid potential teratogenic complications and their potential legal ramifications.

◼ OTHER NONINFECTIOUS, INFLAMMATORY SKIN DISORDERS

Atopic Dermatitis

See Chapter 15.

Seborrheic Dermatitis

1. Definition
   a. Seborrheic dermatitis is a chronic, noninfectious, eczematous (inflammatory) reaction characterized by erythema and scaling. It is exacerbated by stress, infection, hormonal fluctuations, and poor nutrition.
2. Incidence and etiology
   a. Seborrheic dermatitis is a common dermatologic disorder with an increased incidence in the neonatal and postpubertal age groups.
   b. The etiology is unknown but involves a genetic predisposition. It is related to accelerated epidermal growth; however, despite its nomenclature, there is no associated increase in sebum production.
3. Clinical manifestations
   a. Typical lesions are pruritic, erythematous, greasy, and scaling and occur in areas well supplied with sebaceous glands, such as the scalp, face, and trunk. Skin folds, where bacterial counts are high, are also affected. Lesions are typically located in the scalp, face, trunk, and intertriginous areas (see Color Fig. 35–17).
   b. Erythema and fine, dry scale are present on the eyebrows, eyelids, nasolabial and postauricular folds, and facial hair areas.
   c. Secondary infection and impetiginization may occur.
   d. Periods of remission and exacerbation are common. Flare-ups commonly occur during cold weather.
4. Intervention
   a. The goals of intervention are to control the disorder and alleviate emotional distress.
   b. Pharmacologic interventions
      (1) Topical steroids may be used. The face and intertriginous areas require a mild, nonfluorinated cream such as hydrocortisone 1.0 percent. A midpotency steroid, such as betamethasone, is required for general body areas.
      (2) Topical antifungal therapy is often indicated for intertriginous areas.
      (3) Systemic antibiotic therapy with oral tetracycline is often indicated for resistant cases or coexisting acne rosacea.
      (4) Topical tar preparations, such as Doak tar lotion, may be used on a nightly basis. Because this is an aesthetically displeasing treatment, it is not routinely used.
      (5) Antiseborrheic shampoos, such as selenium sulfide and zinc pyrithione 1 to 2 percent, are necessary for scalp treatment. Steroid preparations for the scalp, such as Synalar, are often effective.

◼ MALIGNANT MELANOMA

Definition

1. Malignant melanoma is a skin cancer that results from the malignant transformation of epidermal melanocytes.
2. Melanoma skin cancers have a great proclivity for recurrence and local or systemic metastasis.

Incidence and Socioeconomic Impact

1. The incidence of melanoma is increasing rapidly worldwide, doubling over the past 2 decades. It accounts for 2

percent of all cancers, but its rate of incidence is increasing faster than any other cancer. Since 1950, the incidence of malignant melanoma has risen at a rate of 6 percent yearly.

2. Melanoma accounts for 5 percent of malignant skin tumors and is the primary cause of death from skin disorders. The incidence of deaths resulting from malignant melanoma is rising at a rate of 2 percent per year. At current rates of incidence and death, 1 person in 105 will develop malignant melanoma and 1 in 400 will die from it.

3. The incidence is higher in fair-skinned persons. Fair-skinned individuals are 10 times more likely than dark-skinned individuals to have melanoma.

Risk Factors

- Familial tendency
- Exposure to sunlight
- Being fair skinned and having blue or green eyes and blonde or red hair
- Dysplastic or congenital nevi
- Xeroderma pigmentosum

Etiology

The etiology of melanoma is unknown.

Pathophysiology

1. A neoplastic disorder of the melanocytes with a propensity for metastasis to other areas of the skin, brain, bone, liver, and lungs.
2. The propensity for metastasis is based on the thickness of the melanoma.

Clinical Manifestations

1. There are 4 types of melanoma.
   a. Superficial spreading melanoma, the most common type, occurs anywhere on the body (see Color Fig. 35–18).
   b. Lentigo maligna melanoma occurs on sun-exposed surfaces, commonly the face and neck.
   c. Acral-lentiginous melanoma occurs on the palms and soles and beneath the nails.
   d. Nodular melanoma, the 2nd most common melanoma, occurs anywhere on the body. It has a relatively smooth, well-defined border and surface and a uniform blue-black color. This melanoma has the poorest prognosis (see Color Fig. 35–19).
2. Except for nodular melanoma, the appearance of melanoma is characterized by the ABCDs of melanoma and its warning signs:
   a. *Asymmetry*
   b. *Border* irregularity
   c. *Color* variegation

(1) Brown
(2) Black
(3) Blue
(4) Red
(5) White
   d. *Diameter* (>5 mm)
   e. Warning signs are moles that change in size, color, shape, elevation, surrounding skin, surface, sensation, and consistency.

Diagnostics

1. History
   a. It is important to obtain a history of sun exposure.
   b. Information on family background is important to determine a genetic predisposition.
2. Physical examination
   a. Examine the entire body surface, including the nails and mucous membranes.
   b. Family members should also be checked for suspicious lesions.
   c. A penlight and oil aid the process of distinguishing border, color, and elevation irregularities.
3. Diagnosis
   a. A skin biopsy must be performed for any suspicious pigmented lesion. A punch or excisional biopsy is appropriate.
   b. Evaluation for possible metastatic disease should include a lymph node assessment, a complete blood count with differential, a liver profile, and chest radiographs.

Clinical Management

1. The goals of clinical management are early diagnosis and cure by complete excision.
2. Special medical-surgical procedures
   a. Surgical excision is the treatment of choice. The extent of resection is determined by the thickness of the tumor. A 1- to 3-cm margin of normal tissue is commonly practiced.
   b. Chemotherapy, radiation therapy, and immunotherapy may be indicated for metastatic disease.

Complications

Regional metastasis to the lymph nodes is most common. Distant metastasis occurs most commonly in the skin, followed by spread to the lungs, liver, bone, and brain.

Prognosis

1. With early diagnosis and treatment, 80 percent of melanomas are cured.
2. The person who has had a melanoma has an increased risk of developing a 2nd malignant melanoma.
3. The depth of the lesion is directly related to prognosis.

a. Breslow quantified prognosis via tumor thickness. People with tumors less than 0.76 mm thick experienced 100 percent survival 5 years after diagnosis. Persons with a tumor greater than 3.0 mm thick had a very poor prognosis.

b. Clark quantified prognosis on the basis of the degree of tumor invasion into the epidermis, papillary and reticular dermis, or subcutaneous tissue. Superficial invasion of less than 0.76 mm extends just into the papillary dermis and is associated with a favorable prognosis. Deep invasion into the reticular dermis and subcutaneous tissue has the poorest prognosis.

4. Melanoma that metastasizes to internal organs is almost universally fatal.

Applying the Nursing Process

NURSING DIAGNOSIS: Anxiety R/T fear of death or disfigurement caused by a diagnosis of malignant melanoma

1. *Expected outcomes:* After treatment and counseling, the person should be able to do the following:
   a. Express fears and anxiety concerning the diagnosis and treatment of melanoma.
   b. Identify at least 2 ways to gain more control over the situation.
   c. Express positive outcome of early diagnosis and treatment.
   d. Correctly demonstrate skin self-examination and verbalize a plan for incorporating this health practice into daily living.
   e. Demonstrate correct wound care to promote healing and prevent infection.
   f. State the importance of lifelong follow-up.

2. *Nursing interventions*
   a. Assist the person and family members in identifying coping strategies for dealing with the diagnosis and treatment of malignant melanoma.
   b. Provide the person with melanoma ample opportunity to express fears and anxiety concerning the diagnosis and treatment.
   c. Involve the person and family members in the assessment process.
   d. Teach the person and family members about the high cure rate associated with early diagnosis and treatment and the extreme importance of lifelong, twice-yearly, professional skin examinations by a dermatologist.
   e. Teach the person and family members about surgical techniques designed to preserve as much normal skin as possible. Show before and after pictures of positive surgical results.
   f. Instruct the person on postsurgical wound care and the signs and symptoms of infection.

Discharge Planning and Teaching

1. Make an appointment schedule for the postsurgical checkup and twice-yearly skin evaluations.
2. Provide instructions and a body diagram chart to facilitate monthly skin self-evaluations (Fig. 35–6).
3. Provide the person and family members information on support groups.
4. Encourage the person and family members to call with questions or concerns.

Public Health Considerations

1. Primary prevention depends on educating the public about the hazards of sun exposure and the ABCDs of

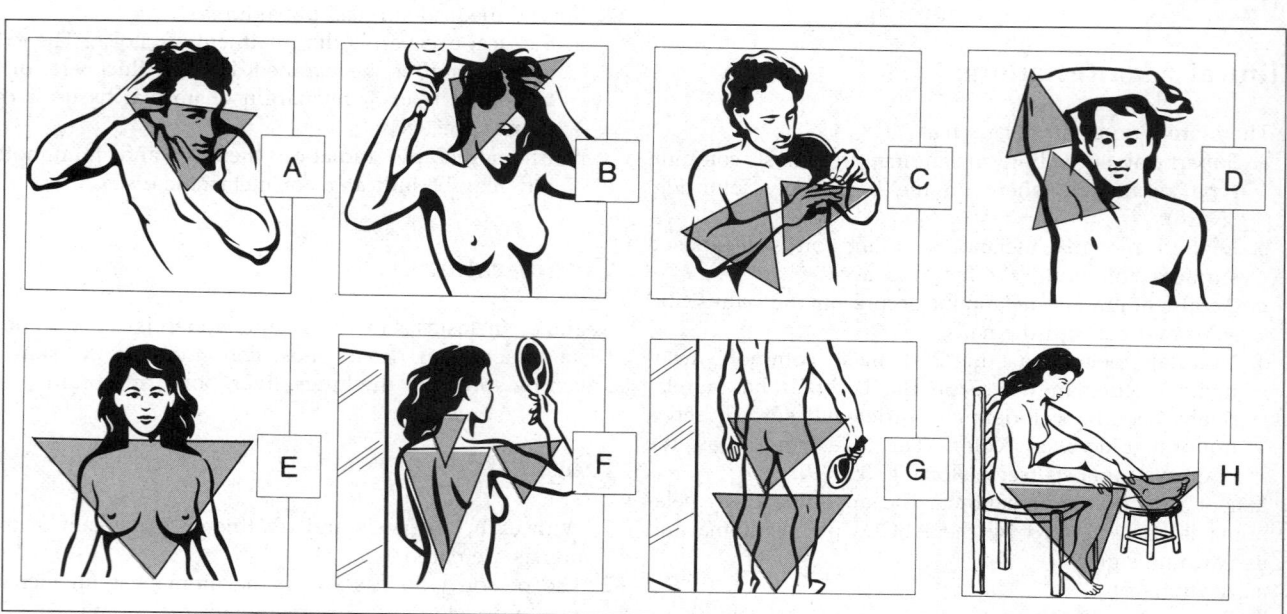

Figure 35–6. Skin self-examination. (Reproduced from the brochure *Skin Cancer: If You Can Spot It, You Can Stop It.* New York: The Skin Cancer Foundation, 1992. Copyright 1992, The Skin Cancer Foundation, New York. Published in cooperation with the Dermatology Nurses' Association.)

Table 35–10. Sun Protection Guidelines

Defining Skin Characteristics	Skin Type	Burn/Tanning History	Sun Protection Factor (SPF) Minimum Requirements	General Precautions for All Skin Types
Very fair skin with gray, green, or blue eyes and red, brown, or blonde hair	I and II	Burns easily with blistering, peeling, or minimal tanning.	SPF 15	Avoid exposure during peak times of 10 A.M.–3 P.M.
Medium fair skin and often brown hair and eyes	III	May burn but eventually tans.	SPF 15	Use caution on cloudy days. Sun damage still can occur. Wear protective, tightly knit clothing: Wide-brimmed hats, long sleeves, and long pants. Reapply sunscreens often, especially after exercising and swimming.
Light brown/olive skin with dark hair and eyes	IV	Rarely burns. Generally tans on first exposure.	SPF 15	Use SPF 15 lip protection. Use a broad-spectrum sunscreen that protects from
Medium brown skin and dark brown eyes	V	Rarely burns and easily tans.	SPF 15	ultraviolet A and B light. Cosmetics that induce an "indoor tan" do not provide added sun protection.
Dark brown or black skin	VI	Never burns.	SPF 15	Sand, water, and concrete can reflect up to 90% of the sun's rays and cause burning.

melanoma. Sun protection, using a broad-spectrum sunscreen, is necessary to prevent the hazards of sun exposure (Table 35–10).

2. Primary prevention also depends on educating physicians about the ABCDs of melanoma. With health care reform increasingly placing the focus of practice on general practitioners, their role in early detection and dermatologic referral for any suspicious lesion is vital.

◼ OTHER MALIGNANCIES INVOLVING THE INTEGUMENT

Basal Cell Carcinoma and Squamous Cell Carcinoma

See Table 35–11 and Color Figures 35–20 and 35–21.

Table 35–11. Comparison of Basal Cell and Squamous Cell Carcinomas

Cancer Type/Definition	Incidence/Etiology	Clinical Manifestations	Intervention
Basal cell cancer (BCC) is a slow-growing, malignant tumor of the epidermis. It rarely metastasizes, but it is locally destructive to tissue.	BCC is the most common skin cancer, accounting for 20% of cancers in men and 10% in women. It occurs most commonly on the head and neck in fair skinned or elderly persons or in persons with chronic sun damage. Incidence increases with previous lesions. The vast majority of cases are related to sun exposure. It is also linked to repeated low-dose x-ray exposure and arsenic ingestion. It may occur at the site of previous or repeated skin trauma.	BCC is usually asymptomatic; lesion is pruritic or tender if infected. BCC occurs anywhere, most commonly on sun-exposed areas. It may take multiple forms. A typical lesion is a pearl-colored plaque or nodule that ulcerates over time. External surface appears translucent. Size of lesion varies (see Fig. 35–25).	Surgical excision for well-defined lesions of 1–2 cm. Electrodesiccation and curettage for well-defined lesions less than 1 cm. Mohs' surgery for tumors that are recurrent, occur around nose and eyes, and are more than 2 cm. Cryosurgery if other methods are contraindicated. Cure rate is 95% with early diagnosis and treatment.
Squamous cell cancer (SCC) is a malignancy of the squamous epithelium. SCC is a faster growing skin cancer than BCC and has the potential to metastasize to lymph nodes.	SCC is the second most common skin cancer. It is a keratinocytic response to injury with an etiology similar to BCC. Other risk factors include tobacco use (oral lesions), chemical exposure (tars and oils), severe burn injury, and systemic disorders (lupus and xeroderma pigmentosum).	SCC is usually asymptomatic; lesion is pruritic or tender if infected. No classic clinical appearance. Distribution is similar to BCC. Typical lesion may be papular or nodular, with scaling and crusting, and tan, pink, red, or gray. SCC is locally destructive (see Fig. 35–26).	Surgical treatment is similar to that for BCC. In addition, radiation therapy is used for non-surgical lesions. Cure rate is 95–98% with early diagnosis and treatment.

Cutaneous T-Cell Lymphoma

1. Definition
   a. Cutaneous T-cell lymphoma (CTCL), also known as **mycosis fungoides,** is a chronic, progressive malignancy of T-helper lymphocytes that have an initial affinity for the skin. As the disease progresses, systemic involvement may occur in the lymph nodes, lungs, liver, and spleen.
   b. Sézary's syndrome, a leukemic variant of CTCL, results in malignant lymphocytes circulating in peripheral blood.
2. Incidence and etiology
   a. Cutaneous T-cell lymphoma is uncommon and affects mostly adults in middle age. Men are affected more than women by a 2:1 ratio.
   b. The exact etiology is unknown. Exposure to environmental toxins is one accepted causal theory.
3. Clinical manifestations
   a. Cutaneous T-cell lymphoma may present in 4 distinct stages or patterns or as a combination of stages.
      (1) Erythematous patches with scale
      (2) Indurated, potentially ulcerated, thickened plaques (see Color Fig. 35–22)
      (3) A tumor stage or tumor d'emble variant, in which the nodular or tumor lesions are the 1st presenting symptom
      (4) Erythrodermic or Sézary's syndrome, in which the skin has generalized erythema and scaling
   b. Clinical symptoms generally include intense pruritus; painful fissures of the palms and soles; hyperkeratosis; intolerance of temperature extremes; fever and chills; partial or total alopecia; and nail involvement (onycholysis), with pitting, ridging, thickening, and fissuring of the nails.
   c. Early-stage lesions typically appear on the buttocks, thighs, and trunk. As the disease progresses, lesions occur over the entire body.
4. Intervention
   a. Topical nitrogen mustard ointment, applied daily to the entire body except the face and intertriginous areas, is well tolerated. The most common side effect is allergic contact dermatitis.
   b. Local irradiation therapy is appropriate for localized lesions. More diffuse or thickened lesions are treated with total-body electron beam irradiation. Side effects include increased incidence of squamous cell carcinoma, alopecia, skin atrophy and aging, and transient loss of sweat gland function.
   c. Systemic therapy may include oral corticosteroids, multiagent chemotherapy, or high- or low-dose oral methotrexate therapy. These treatments have some palliative effect, but long-term survival is generally not affected.
   d. Topical photochemotherapy or PUVA (see p. 1627) is useful for early treatment of the patch or plaque stage.
   e. Topical corticosteroids are useful for symptom management. Some localized lesions respond therapeutically to more potent agents; however, high-potency topical steroids are not appropriate for total-body use.
   f. Extracorporeal photochemotherapy (photopheresis) is a U.S. Food and Drug Administration–approved therapy that exposes a photosensitized, leukocyte-enriched blood fraction, obtained through a 6-cycle centrifugation process, to ultraviolet A light within an extracorporeal (outside of the body) circuit (Fig. 35–7).
      (1) Photosensitization is accomplished 1 to 2 hours before initiating therapy with oral administration of 8-methoxypsoralen.
      (2) Exposure of the leukocyte-enriched fraction, composed of 300 ml of plasma and 240 ml of buffy coat, to ultraviolet A radiation inactivates the lymphocytes. Reinfusion of these inactivated cells modulates the immune system and may induce a therapeutic disease response (Fig. 35–8).
      (3) Treatments are administered on 2 consecutive days at monthly intervals. Six to 12 months of treatment may be required before a therapeutic response is seen. Photopheresis is well tolerated, and side effects are minimal.
      (4) Multicenter clinical trials of additional therapeutic applications of photopheresis are under way. These clinical investigations include treatment of organ transplant rejection, autoimmune disorders, and acquired immunodeficiency syndrome.

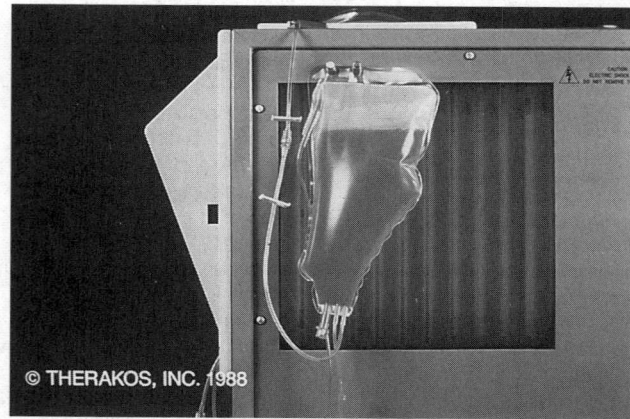

Figure 35–7. Photopheresis (UVAR) instrument with leukocyte-enriched blood component. (Copyright Therakos Inc., 1988.)

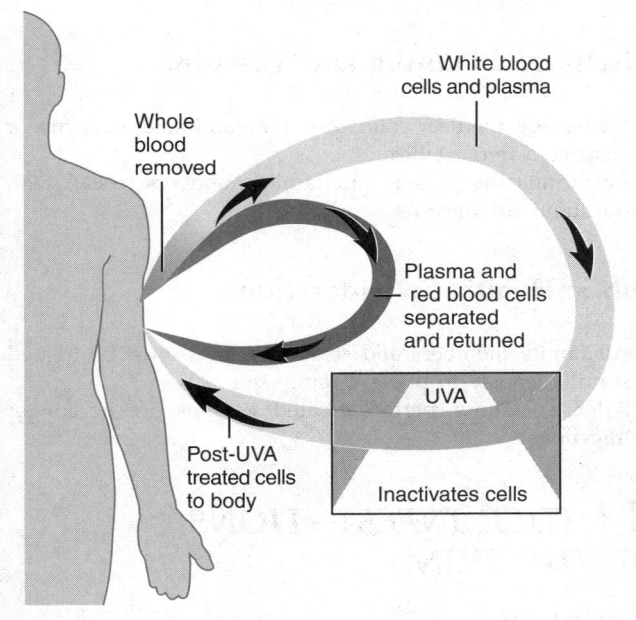

Figure 35–8.

Kaposi's Sarcoma

See Chapter 42.

☐ *SCABIES*

Definition

Scabies is a parasitic skin disorder caused by an infestation of the *Sarcoptes scabiei* (itch mite).

Incidence and Socioeconomic Impact

1. Scabies is endemic among schoolchildren and institutionalized populations, because of the close, personal contact experienced in those environments.
2. There is an increased incidence of scabies among persons of lower socioeconomic status.

Risk Factors

Close personal contact with an infected person or a contaminated article is a risk factor.

Etiology

The etiology of scabies is directly related to infestation with the itch mite.

Pathophysiology

1. The fertilized, adult female mite burrows and travels under the stratum corneum. Its life cycle of 1 to 2 months is completed on a human host.
2. There is a 1-month delay between the initial infestation and the onset of pruritus in the host. This phenomenon is related to a sensitivity that develops to the mite protein or its excrement.

Clinical Manifestations

1. Skin lesions are characteristically erythematous papules and pustules. A hallmark of a scabies infestation is threadlike, brownish, linear burrows up to 1 cm long. Excoriation or secondary infection may make the burrows invisible (see Color Fig. 35–23).
2. Secondary lesions consist of vesicles, crusts, reddish-brown nodules, and excoriations.
3. Common sites of infestation are the hands, feet, finger-webs, nipples, umbilicus, penis, intertriginous areas, soles, and palms.
4. Intense pruritus, which worsens at night, is a common symptom.

Diagnostics

1. History
   a. Ask the person about the itching. Where and when is itching the most bothersome?
   b. Assess for risk factors concerning exposure to the scabies mite. It is important to do this in a nonjudgmental manner.
2. Physical examination
   a. Burrows appear as brown or black, short, wavy, linear lesions. They are often difficult to see if the person has been scratching or rubbing the area.
   b. Check for papular, red lesions at the sites most likely to be infected.
3. Diagnosis
   a. Obtain skin scrapings for microscopic examination of an undisturbed papule or burrow. The specimen is best obtained with a no. 15 scalpel blade. Examine the specimen for eggs, feces, or the mite itself.
   b. Burrows are more easily identified by applying ink to suspected lesions. Once the ink is wiped away, a track is visible at the opening to the burrow.
   c. Multiple attempts to obtain a diagnostic scraping are commonly needed.

Clinical Management

1. The goals of clinical management are to prevent secondary infection and eradicate the infestation in the individual and any affected family members and close contacts.
2. Pharmacologic interventions
   a. Antihistamines or topical steroids help relieve itching.

b. Topical antiscabies creams or lotions, such as Kwell cream or Eurax, are necessary to kill the mites.
   (1) These preparations are applied to the entire body from the neck down for 6 to 24 hours, depending on the medication. Because the scabies mite rarely infects the head, it is generally not necessary to treat it.
   (2) The skin should be dry during application. Moist skin increases absorption and the potential for side effects.
   (3) The medication should be left on only for the specified amount of time; otherwise, skin irritation or side effects result. After treatment, remove the medication by washing with soap and water.

Complications

Secondary infection of lesions may occur, usually because of self-induced excoriation from scratching.

Prognosis

The prognosis is excellent once treatment is initiated. Reinfection will occur if all family members and close contacts are not treated simultaneously.

Applying the Nursing Process

> **NURSING DIAGNOSIS:** Knowledge deficit R/T lack of information about scabies infestation and treatment regimen

1. *Expected outcomes:* After treatment and instruction, the person should be able to do the following:
   a. Demonstrate an understanding of a scabies infestation, including its cause, treatment, and course.
   b. Demonstrate correct application of the topical therapy necessary for effective treatment.
   c. Describe the measures required to treat the environment and family members potentially affected by the scabies infestation.
   d. Identify a plan to prevent secondary infection and reinfestation of scabies.
2. *Nursing interventions*
   a. Instruct the person and family members on all aspects of treatment and prevention of reinfestation.
      (1) Bed linens and clothing can be disinfected by washing and drying using the hot cycle.
      (2) Dry clothing that is stored for longer than 48 hours is no longer infectious, because mites can live only 2 days apart from a host.
   b. Reinforce the need to treat all family members and help the person devise a plan to accomplish this task.
   c. Discuss the expected course of recovery.
      (1) Itching may persist for up to 4 weeks, because of a continued allergic reaction to mite proteins in the skin.
      (2) Instruct the person that he or she should not at-

tempt to alleviate continued pruritus by applying the topical medication beyond the prescribed length of time. Additional applications may produce toxicity.

Discharge Planning and Teaching

1. Encourage medical follow-up for continued pruritus or suspected reinfestation.
2. Encourage the person and family members to call with questions or concerns.

Public Health Considerations

1. All family members and sexual contacts must be treated simultaneously to prevent reinfection.
2. After a 24-hour period, treated persons are no longer infectious.

◼ OTHER INFESTATIONS OF THE SKIN

Pediculosis

See Chapter 15.

Lyme Disease

1. Definition—Lyme disease is a multisystem infection that results from a tick bite.
2. Incidence and etiology
   a. Lyme disease is the most common vector-borne illness in the United States. It is most prevalent during the summer months, because of increased outdoor exposure to the vector.
   b. The vectors responsible for the transmission of Lyme disease are the *Ixodes* ticks, which are carried by several species of deer. Persons bitten by the *Ixodes* ticks are infected with a newly identified spirochete, *Borrelia burgdorferi*.
3. Clinical manifestations
   a. The clinical manifestations of Lyme disease generally occur in 3 stages. Signs and symptoms may overlap among the defined stages (see Color Fig. 35–24).
   b. The hallmark of stage I is the development of erythema chronicum migrans. This skin rash develops within 2 to 30 days of infection, generally at the site of the tick bite.
      (1) The appearance of the rash may vary, but the classic appearance is an erythematous papule that develops into an annular lesion with a cleared center. Concentric rings may develop, giving it a bull's-eye appearance.
      (2) The lesion quickly enlarges up to 50 to 60 cm. Secondary, smaller lesions may develop farther away from the original tick bite.

Table 35–12. Characteristics of Alopecia

Classification	Pathophysiology	Clinical Manifestations	Management	Other Information
Nonscarring				
Androgenetic	Male-female pattern hair loss caused by androgens in genetically predisposed persons. Advancing age increases risk. Hair follicles decrease in size, with eventual loss of most hair follicles.	Diffuse hair loss on scalp. In men, frontal and temporal hair loss is most common. In women, vertex thinning and hair loss are most common.	Topical minoxidil (is expensive and requires long-term treatment), hair transplantation, or scalp reduction.	Androgenetic alopecia is the most common cause of diffuse hair loss in women. It is more severe in men, however.
Areata	Is associated with autoimmune disorders, family history, and immune dysfunction. Inflammatory.	Often occurs in patches but may affect entire scalp (alopecia totalis) or entire body (alopecia universalis). Asymptomatic. Exclamation mark hairs (distally thicker, broken-off hairs) located near margins of hair loss. Regrowth usually occurs in 6–12 mo, but hair loss may recur.	Localized disease: topical corticosteroids, anthralin, and minoxidil; intralesional corticosteroids; or immunotherapy with a topical contact allergen. Extensive disease: systemic corticosteroids; topical anthralin and immunotherapy; or topical/systemic psoralen and ultraviolet A light therapy.	Alopecia totalis and universalis have a poor prognosis for regrowth, especially if disease process occurs at an early age. The National Alopecia Areata Foundation is available for educational and emotional support.
Telogen effluvium	Increased shedding of hairs in resting phase (telogen phase) brought on by a triggering episode such as pregnancy, high fever, excessive stress, or physical illness.	Scalp hair loss exceeds the normal 50–100 strands lost daily. Hair loss occurs diffusely over the scalp and usually lasts 2–3 mo after triggering event. Is asymptomatic except for anxiety and emotional distress.	Spontaneous regrowth occurs without specific treatment.	An explanation of the disease process and prognosis allays fears of permanent hair loss. Regrowth takes about 6 mo.
Drug related	Hair in growth phase (anagen phase) is affected by antimitotic drugs, oral contraceptives, anticoagulants, anabolic steroids, β-blockers, and anticonvulsants.	Diffuse thinning and loss of hair in any hair-bearing area.	Hair loss is usually temporary; regrowth occurs after drug is discontinued.	Education and emotional support are helpful. Advise person to purchase a wig before total hair loss occurs.
Endocrine related	Hyperthyroidism—mechanism is unknown. Hypothyroidism causes early cessation of anagen phase and no start of new hair cycle.	Hyperthyroidism: Hair is fine and diffusely thinning. Hypothyroidism: Hair is dry, coarse, and brittle, with patchy or diffuse alopecia.	Correction of underlying metabolic disorder.	Successful treatment of thyroid disorder results in hair growth.
Trauma or chemical related	Related to physical trauma from tight ponytails or braiding or repeated use of hair dye, perm or straightener solution, or a hot curling iron.	Patchy alopecia with dry, brittle, and broken-off hair. Scalp may also be traumatized. Usually occurs around periphery of scalp.	Regrowth occurs after causative agent is discontinued. If follicle is destroyed, hair does not regrow.	Scarring may occur in some persons.

Table continued on following page

| | | Clinical | | |
Classification	Pathophysiology	Manifestations	Management	Other Information
Scarring				
Infectious process	Destruction of hair folli- cle related to tinea capitis and severe bacterial infections such as folliculitis de- calvans.	Patchy alopecia with scalp involvement.	Antifungals and antibiot- ics.	
Systemic or cutaneous disorders	Destruction of hair folli- cle related to discoid lupus erythematosus, scleroderma, lichen planus, or metastatic disease.	Patchy alopecia, usually of scalp.	Treatment of underlying disorder may halt or slow the process.	

Table 35–12. Characteristics of Alopecia (Continued)

(3) Most infected persons also develop flulike symp- toms that last 7 to 10 days and may recur later.
c. Stage II develops within 1 to 6 months in the majority of untreated persons. More serious sequelae include cardiac conduction defects and neurologic disorders such as Bell's palsy and paralysis that are usually not permanent.
d. The arthritic symptoms of stage III occur within a month to several months after initial infection. Arthralgias and enlarged or inflamed joints can per- sist for several years after the initial infection.
4. Intervention
a. Prevention, public education, and early diagnosis are vital to the control and treatment of Lyme disease.
b. A 3-week course of antibiotic therapy with oral doxy- cycline or amoxicillin is recommended during stage I. Later stages may require therapy with intravenous antibiotics such as penicillin G.

◼ ALOPECIA

Definition

1. Alopecia is the loss of hair caused by genetic factors, a disease process, or the aging process.
2. Hair loss is partial or total.

Incidence and Socioeconomic Impact

1. Alopecia areata (nonscarring, patchy hair loss) and an- drogenetic alopecia (common baldness) are very common disorders.
2. The incidence of alopecia in the absence of a genetic predisposition (trauma-induced, illness-related, or chemi- cal-induced alopecia) is commonly associated with the respective etiology (see Color Fig. 35–25).

Risk Factors

Risk factors vary with etiology. See Table 35–12 for a dis- cussion of risk factors, etiology, pathophysiology, clinical manifestations, and clinical management.

◼ VITILIGO

Definition

1. Vitiligo is a pigment disorder in which the degree of pigmentation or background color of the skin changes.
2. The skin in vitiligo is hypopigmented.

Incidence and Socioeconomic Impact

1. Vitiligo is fairly common and affects up to 1 percent of the population.
2. All races and both genders are affected.

Risk Factors

1. Vitiligo is associated with diabetes mellitus, Addison's disease, thyroiditis, and pernicious anemia.
2. There may be a family tendency in 25 percent of cases.

Etiology

The etiology of vitiligo is unknown, but autoimmune or endocrine disorders and exposure to toxins are potential factors.

Pathophysiology

1. The pathophysiology of vitiligo involves the destruction of existing melanocytes.
2. The destruction of melanocytes results in localized areas of depigmentation. These localized areas may progress to involve larger areas or the entire skin surface.

Clinical Manifestations

1. Localized lesions are macular, round, or oval in configuration and are white in color (see Color Fig. 35–26).
2. Affected areas of the scalp result in patches of white hair.
3. Commonly affected areas are the skin over bony prominences, around body orifices, in intertriginous areas, and in sun-exposed places.
4. Vitiligo is asymptomatic (except for the emotional distress related to appearance), but pigment loss is usually progressive. If repigmentation occurs, it affects small, centrally located, perifollicular sites.

Diagnostics

1. History
   a. Ask the person whether there is a family history of vitiligo or pigment changes.
   b. Assess for risk factors. Was the person exposed to toxins such as phenols, thiols, or quinones?
   c. On the basis of the history and physical examination, consider evaluating the person for vitiligo-associated disorders identified as potential risk factors.
2. Physical examination
   a. Assess for the classic configuration and distribution of vitiligo lesions.
   b. Examine the depigmented skin for any signs of solar damage. Look for lesions such as actinic keratoses or skin cancers.
   c. Check for areas of repigmentation. These occur around hair follicles and have a "salt and pepper" appearance.
3. Diagnosis is often based on the clinical examination. If necessary, it is confirmed with a skin biopsy demonstrating melanocyte absence in vitiligo-affected areas.

Clinical Management

1. The goals of clinical management are to stimulate repigmentation and protect depigmented skin from sun damage.
2. Pharmacologic interventions
   a. Clobetasol propionate (a potent topical corticosteroid), applied to localized areas of vitiligo, may stimulate repigmentation. Treating large areas with this regimen requires a 2-week limit on therapy to prevent systemic effects of the corticosteroid.

   b. Repigmentation of affected areas sometimes may be achieved with PUVA therapy. However, PUVA therapy increases the risk of photocarcinogenesis and photosensitivity reactions. For these reasons, it is important to administer PUVA therapy with extreme caution.
   c. If the vitiligo is extensive, depigmentation will lighten the surrounding areas of darker skin. Topical applications of hydroquinone or 20 percent monobenzyl ether will depigment darker skin. The cosmetic effect is a decrease in contrast between the pigmented and hypopigmented skin.

Complications

- Sun sensitivity
- An increased risk of developing skin cancer in areas of pigment loss

Prognosis

1. Spontaneous repigmentation occurs in only about 15 percent of affected individuals.
2. With treatment, repigmentation occurs in 30 to 40 percent of people.

Applying the Nursing Process

> **NURSING DIAGNOSIS:** Body image disturbance R/T embarrassment regarding patches of depigmented skin

1. *Expected outcomes:* After treatment and counseling, the person should be able to do the following:
   a. Demonstrate an understanding of the vitiligo disease and treatment process by being able to
      (1) Define vitiligo.
      (2) Discuss the various treatment regimens available for vitiligo.
      (3) Describe potential treatment outcomes and prognosis.
   b. Express feelings and emotions related to the diagnosis of vitiligo.
   c. Identify at least 2 strategies to cope positively with the body image changes related to vitiligo.
   d. Describe camouflage techniques, that is, ways that cosmetics, clothing, and hair can be worn to camouflage some areas of depigmentation.
2. *Nursing interventions*
   a. Encourage the person and significant others to express feelings concerning changes in physical appearance. Listen to them in an honest and nonjudgmental manner. Acknowledge feelings without agreeing with or minimizing them.
   b. Assist with the process of realistic self-evaluation. Examine catastrophic thoughts and feelings. Help the

person identify positive personal factors that help to define him or her. Reinforce these positive ideas and behaviors.

c. Discuss the disease process and its treatment honestly and completely. To enhance treatment compliance, make sure the person understands all the information.

d. Encourage the use of camouflage techniques involving cosmetics, clothing, hair, and accessories. Provide positive reinforcement to the person for using these techniques.

e. Initiate professional counseling if the person is unable to adjust to the long-term change in appearance.

Discharge Planning and Teaching

1. Make an appointment schedule for the person for the frequent return visits required for follow-up care.
2. Instruct the person on the importance of protecting the skin from damage caused by sun exposure. Protective clothing, hats, and sunscreens are necessary to prevent solar damage.

3. Teach the person and family members to examine their skin on a monthly basis for any signs of skin cancer.
4. Encourage the person and family members to call with questions or concerns.
5. Provide the person with information on support groups.

◼ SEXUALLY TRANSMITTED DISORDERS

See Chapters 30 through 32.

◼ BURNS

See Chapter 36.

◼ NAIL DISORDERS

See discussions of fungal infections and psoriasis on pages 1632 and 1637–1642.

Bibliography

Books

Basset A. *Dermatology of Black Skin*. Oxford: Oxford University Press, 1986.

Bondi EE, Jegasothy BV, and Lazarus GS (eds). *Dermatology: Diagnosis and Therapy*. Norwalk, CT: Appleton & Lange, 1991.

Burton JL. *Essentials of Dermatology*. 3rd ed. New York: Churchill Livingstone, 1990.

Carter R. *A Dictionary of Dermatologic Terms*. 4th ed. Baltimore: Williams & Wilkins, 1992.

Champion RH, Burton JL, and Ebling FJ. *Textbook of Dermatology*. 5th ed. Oxford: Blackwell Scientific Publications, 1992.

DuVivier A. *Dermatology in Practice*. Philadelphia: JB Lippincott, 1990.

Fitzpatrick TB. *Color Atlas and Synopsis of Clinical Dermatology*. 2nd ed. New York: McGraw-Hill, 1992.

Fitzpatrick TB, et al. (eds). *Dermatology in General Medicine*. 4th ed. New York: McGraw-Hill, 1993.

Glickman FS. *Fundamentals of Dermatology: A Study Guide*. New York: Marcel Dekker, 1990.

Habif TP. *Clinical Dermatology: A Color Guide to Diagnosis and Therapy*. 2nd ed. St. Louis: CV Mosby, 1990.

Lookingbill DP. *Principles of Dermatology*. 2nd ed. Philadelphia: WB Saunders, 1993.

Mackie RM. *Clinical Dermatology: An Illustrated Textbook*. 3rd ed. Oxford: Oxford University Press, 1991.

Moschella SL, and Hurley HJ (eds). *Dermatology*. 3rd ed. Philadelphia: WB Saunders, 1992.

Parish LC, and Lask GP. *Aesthetic Dermatology*. New York: McGraw-Hill, 1991.

Parish LC, and Millikan LE. *Global Dermatology: Diagnosis and Management According to Geography, Climate, and Culture*. New York: Springer-Verlag, 1994.

Rassner G. *Atlas of Dermatology*. 3rd ed. Philadelphia: Lea & Febiger, 1994.

Sams M, and Lynch P (eds). *Principles and Practice of Dermatology*. New York: Churchill Livingstone, 1990.

Sauer G. *Manual of Skin Diseases*. 6th ed. Philadelphia: JB Lippincott, 1991.

Scher R, and Daniel CR. *Nails: Therapy, Diagnosis, Surgery*. Philadelphia: WB Saunders, 1990.

Chapters in Books and Journal Articles

Integumentary Assessment

Cuzzell JZ. Clues: Pain, burning, and itching. *Am J Nurs* 90(7):15–16, 1990.

Erdos D. Redefining identity when appearance is altered. *Dermatol Nurs* 4(1):41–46, 1992.

Flory C. Perfecting the art: Skin assessment. *RN* 55(6):22–27, 1992.

Hill MJ. The skin: Anatomy and physiology. *Dermatol Nurs* 2(1):13–17, 1990.

Hunter L. Applying Orem to skin. *Nursing* 5(4):16–18, 1992.

Poorman SG. Sexuality and self-concept: Issues in skin disease. *Dermatol Nurs* 4(4):279–284, 1992.

Rudy SJ. From conception to birth: The development of skin and nursing implications. *Dermatol Nurs* 3(6):381–390, 1991.

Ruszkowski AM, Nicol NH, and Moore JA. Patch testing basics: Patient selection, application techniques, and guidelines for interpretation. *Dermatol Nurs* 7(suppl):11–19, 1995.

Dermatologic Surgery

Allen BJ. Moh's surgery: Nursing responsibilities, efficiency, and accountability. *Dermatol Nurs* 2(3):154–157, 1990.

Bergman KS, and Johannsen LL. Liposuction: A surgical intervention to improve body contour. *Dermatol Nurs* 6(4):239–245, 1994.

Hartwig PA. Lasers in dermatology. *Nurs Clin North Am* 25(3):657–666, 1990.

Meusch R, and Lillis PJ. Liposuction: The tumescent technique. *Dermatol Nurs* 3(4):255–260, 1991.

Norman MM. Painstaking Mohs' surgery conserves tissue, cures skin cancer. *Dermatol Patient Counseling Nurs* 2(3):11–13, 1994.

Ratner D, and Grande D. Moh's micrographic surgery: An overview. *Dermatol Nurs* 3(4):269–273, 1994.

Smalley PJ. Laser technology: A nursing perspective. *Dermatol Nurs* 3(4):241–245, 248–252, 1991.

Storck L. Deep peels: What the nurse does. *Dermatol Nurs* 3(3):164–171, 1991.

Whyte, A. Cryosurgery for the dermatology nurse. *Dermatol Nurs* 2(5):271–274, 1990.

Whyte A. Pre and postoperative evaluation of patients undergoing cutaneous surgery. *Dermatol Nurs* 6(4):248–250, 1994.

Special Treatment Modalities

Arndt KA, and Jorizzo JL. Which topical corticosteroid—and when. *Patient Care* 26(10):115–118, 121–123, 133–136, 1992.

Christensen I, and Heald P. Photopheresis in the 1990's. *J Clin Apheresis* 6:216–220, 1991.

Epstein JH. Phototherapy and photochemotherapy. *N Engl J Med* 322(16):1149–1151, 1990.

Habib K. A promising new use for UV light. *RN* 53:72–74, 1990.

Helm TN, and Dijkstra JW. PUVA therapy. *Am Fam Physician* 43(3):908–912, 1991.

Rolston KD, Gold MH, and Elson ML. Ultraviolet A treatment of pruritus secondary to hyperbilirubinemia: A case study. *Dermatol Nurs* 2(1):31–32, 1990.

Rook A, et al. Therapeutic applications of photopheresis. *Dermatol Clin* 11(2):339–347, 1993.

Shelk JL. Phototherapy: A nursing overview. *Dermatol Nurs* 3(6):401–407, 1991.

Folliculitis, Furuncles, and Carbuncles

Anastasi JK, and Rivera J. Identifying the skin manifestations of HIV. *Nursing* 22(11):58–61, 1992.

Raza A, et al. Bacterial infections. *In* Orkin M, Howard M, and Dahl M (eds). *Dermatology*. Norwalk, CT: Appleton & Lange, 1991.

Ritchie SR, et al. Primary bacterial skin infections. *Dermatol Nurs* 4(4):261–268, 1992.

VanNiel J. What's wrong with this peristomal skin? *Am J Nurs* 91(12):44–45, 1991.

Tinea and Candidiasis

Abramowicz M. Topical terbinafine for tinea infections. *Med Lett Drugs Ther* 35(903):76–78, 1993.

Bennett JE. Searching for the yeast connection. *N Engl J Med* 323(25):1766–1767, 1990.

Bergus GR, and Johnson JS. Superficial tinea infections. *Am Fam Physician* 48(2):259–268, 1993.

Bielan B. What's your assessment? *Dermatol Nurs* 5(3):207–208, 1993.

Bielan B. What's your assessment? *Dermatol Nurs* 6(5):334–335, 1994.

Bielan B. What's your assessment? *Dermatol Nurs* 6(6):408–409, 1994.

Buchholz MA. Prevention key to overcoming athlete's foot. *Dermatol Patient Counseling Nurs* 2(1):15, 1994.

Cuzzell J. Clues: Itching and burning skin folds. *Am J Nurs* 90(1):23–24, 1990.

Evans GV, and Dodman B. Comparison of terbinafine and clotrimazole in treating tinea pedis. *BMJ* 307(6905):645–647, 1993.

FDA Consumer. Recurring "yeast" infection may be early HIV sign. 27(1):5, 1993.

McMullen D. *Candida albicans* and incontinence. *Dermatol Nurs* 3(1):21–24, 1991.

Smith EB. Topical antifungal drugs in the treatment of tinea pedis, tinea cruris, and tinea corporis. *J Am Acad Dermatol* 28:S24–S28, 1993.

Tulumbas B. Onychomycosis explored. *Dermatol Patient Counseling Nurs* 2(1):12, 1994.

Vesiculobullous Disorders

Arbesfeld DM, and Thomas I. Cutaneous herpes simplex virus infection. *Am Fam Physician* 43(5):1655–1664, 1991.

Bielan B. What's your assessment? *Dermatol Nurs* 5(2):122–123, 1993.

Cuzzell JZ. Clues: Recurrent, punched-out lesions. *Am J Nurs* 90(5):21–22, 1990.

Engel JP, and Englund JA. Treatment of resistant herpes simplex virus with continuous infusion acyclovir. *JAMA* 263(12):1662–1664, 1990.

Gurevich I. Counseling the patient with herpes. *RN* 53(2):22–28, 1990.

Manek N. Herpes simplex virus. *Lancet* 335(8681):78, 1990.

Millikan LE. Vesiculobullous skin disease with prominent immunologic feature. *JAMA* 258(20):2910–2915, 1987.

Nahass G, and Goldstein BA. Comparison of Tzanck smear, viral culture, and DNA diagnostic methods in detection of herpes simplex and varicella-zoster infection. *JAMA* 268(18):2541–2544, 1992.

Parsons JM. Toxic epidermal necrolysis. *Int J Dermatol* 31:749–768, 1992.

Rasmussen JE. Erythema multiforme, Stevens-Johnson syndrome, and toxic epidermal necrolysis. *Dermatol Nurs* 7(1):37–43, 1995.

Rosen S, and Stanley JR. Pemphigus: Skin failure mediated by autoantibodies. *JAMA* 264(13):1714–1717, 1990.

Roujeau JC. The spectrum of Stevens-Johnson syndrome and toxic epidermal necrolysis: A clinical classification. *J Invest Dermatol* 102:285–305, 1994.

Rojeau JC. What's going on in erythema multiforme? *Dermatology* 188:249–250, 1994.

Schofield JK, Tatnal FM, and Leigh IM. Recurrent erythema multiforme: Clinical features and treatment in a large series of patients. *Br J Dermatol* 128:542–545, 1993.

Siegel D, and Golden E. Prevalence and correlates of herpes simplex infections. *JAMA* 268(13):1702–1708, 1992.

Simpson S, and Sadick S. HIV and associated cutaneous diseases. *Dermatol Nurs* 5(1):51–57, 1993.

Whitley RJ, and Gnann JW. Acyclovir: A decade later. *N Engl J Med* 327(11):782–789, 1992.

Psoriasis

Barker J. The pathophysiology of psoriasis. *Lancet* 338(8761):227–230, 1991.

Bielan B. What's your assessment? *Dermatol Nurs* 6(6):408–409, 1994.

Gilleaudeau P, and McClelland P. Cyclosporine: A new therapeutic option for severe, recalcitrant psoriasis. *Dermatol Nurs* 6(6):395–403, 1994.

Grizzard D. Understanding the pathophysiology of psoriasis: A nursing perspective. *Dermatol Nurs* 3(5):305–314, 1991.

Katz HI, et al. Waging war on psoriasis. *Care* 26(10):145–152, 157–158, 160–168, 171–175, 1992.

Lowe N. Systemic treatment of severe psoriasis: The role of cyclosporine. *N Engl J Med* 324(5):333–334, 1991.

McClelland P. The nursing challenge of psoriasis vulgaris. *Dermatol Patient Counseling Nurs* 1(2):7–8, 1991.

Mentor A, and Barker J. Psoriasis in practice. *Lancet* 338(8761):231–234, 1991.

Nicholson L. Get tough on psoriasis. *Prevention* 43(2):113–120, 1991.

Phillipps TJ, and Dover JS. Recent advances in dermatology. *N Engl J Med* 326(3):167–178, 1992.

Contact Dermatitis

Abel EA. Contact dermatitis: Recognition and management. *Hosp Med* 28(11):101–102, 105–108, 1992.

Beacham B. Common dermatoses in the elderly. *Am Fam Physician* 47(6):1445–1450, 1993.

Cameron J, et al. Contact dermatitis in leg ulcer patients. *Ostomy Wound Manage* 38(9):10–11, 1992.

Fisher AA. Allergic contact dermatitis. *Sportsmed* 21(3):65–72, 1993.

Hall AH, and Hogan DJ. Contact dermatitis from environmental exposures. *Am Fam Physician* 48(5):773–780, 1993.

Klaus MV, and Wieselthier JS. Contact dermatitis. *Am Fam Physician* 48(4):629–632, 1993.

Leritz N. Fragrances are chief causes of cosmetic-related dermatitis. *Dermatol Patient Counseling Nurs* 1(2):14–15, 1993.

Nicol NH, Ruszkowski AM, and Moore JA. Contact dermatitis and the role of patch testing in its diagnosis and management. *Dermatol Nurs* 7(suppl):5–10, 19, 1995.

Stewart LA, Engelken GJ, and Nicol NH. Essentials of occupational contact dermatitis. *Dermatol Nurs* 4(3):175–183, 1992.

Yotter M. Contact dermatitis: Nursing intervention. *Dermatol Nurs* 2(5):267–269, 1990.

Zamula E. Contact dermatitis: Solutions to rash mysteries. *FDA Consumer* 24(4):28–31, 1990.

Acne Vulgaris and Acne Rosacea

Dicken CH, et al. Retinoids: What role in your practice? *Patient Care* 26(10):18–21, 1992.

Drake LA, et al. Guidelines of care for acne vulgaris. *J Am Acad Dermatol* 4:676–680, 1990.

Duncanson C. A nurse's perspective on acne: Make the patient feel comfortable. *Dermatol Patient Counseling Nurs* 1(1):7, 1993.

Garver JH, et al. Flushing and rosacea: Overview and nursing interventions. *Dermatol Nurs* 4(4):271–277, 1992.

Henry SJ. Take control of rosacea. *Prevention* 44(12):107–111, 1992.

Jurzyk RS, and Spielvogel RL. Antiandrogens in the treatment of acne and hirsutism. *Am Fam Physician* 45(4):1803–1806, 1992.

Laudano JB, Leach EE, and Armstrong RB. Acne: Therapeutic perspectives with an emphasis on the role of isotretinoin. *Dermatol Nurs* 2(6):328–336, 1990.

Moritz DL. Surgical corrections of acne scars. *Dermatol Nurs* 4(4):291–299, 1992.

Phillips TJ, and Dover JS. Recent advances in dermatology. *N Engl J Med* 326(3):167–178, 1992.

Powell J. Adolescent skin problems: They're common and treatable. *Med Clin North Am* 4(27):3558–3565, 1992.

Rue NN. Acne alert. *Curr Health* 20(2):19–21, 1993.

Sharp K. Nurses can help ease the impact of rosacea. *Dermatol Patient Counseling Nurs* 2(5):12, 15, 1994.

Sober AJ. Management of rosacea. *Dermatol Nurs* 4(6):454–456, 1992.

Strauss J. Acne and rosacea. In Orkin M, Howard M, and Dahl M (eds). *Dermatology*. Norwalk, CT: Appleton & Lange, 1991.

Cutaneous Malignancies

Amonette RA, and Buker JL. Actinic keratosis: The most common precancer. *Skin Cancer Found J* 10:13, 77, 1992.

Anderson WK, and Silvers DN. Melanoma? It can't be melanoma! *JAMA* 266(24):3463–3465, 1991.

Bargoil SC, and Erdman LK. Safe tan: An oxymoron. *Cancer Nurs* 16(2):139, 1993.

Basler DE. Actinic keratosis and premalignant skin damage. *Dermatol Nurs* 3(1):37–40, 1991.

Bedell T. Missing some rays. *Men's Health* 6(3):20–21, 1991.

Bennett R. Cutaneous squamous cell carcinoma: Causes, recurrences, and metastases. *Skin Cancer Found J* 10:31, 95, 1992.

Bielan B. What's your assessment? *Dermatol Nurs* 6(4):254–255, 1994.

Birmingham DJ. Occupational risks for skin cancer. *Skin Cancer Found J* 10:11, 75, 1992.

Breslow A. Thickness, cross-sectioned areas and depth of invasion in the prognosis of cutaneous melanoma. *Ann Surg* 172(5):902–908, 1970.

Brozenza SJ, Waterman G, and Fenske NA. Malignant melanoma: Management guidelines. *Geriatrics* 45(6):55–58, 1990.

Canning S, and Kurban A. Laser treatment of cutaneous malignancies. *Dermatol Nurs* 5(6):447–451, 1993.

Clark WH. A classification of malignant melanoma in man correlated with histogenesis and biologic behavior. In Montagna WH (ed). *Advances in Biology of Skin*. London: Pergamon Press, 1966.

Crutcher WA, and Cohen PJ. Dysplastic nevi and malignant melanoma. *Am Fam Physician* 42(2):372–385, 1990.

Dean FA. Caring for CTCL patients undergoing photopheresis. *Dermatol Nurs* 2(1):26–28, 1990.

DeLaney TF. Radiation therapy for the treatment of skin cancers of the head and neck. *Dermatol Nurs* 6(2):104–109, 1994.

Dubois D, and Ledermann JA. Malignant melanoma. *Lancet* 340(8825):948–951, 1992.

Gantt G. Cutaneous squamous cell carcinoma characteristics. *Dermatol Nurs* 2(5):283–287, 1990.

Geller A. Valuable tools help nurses educate children on sun risks. *Dermatol Patient Counseling Nurs* 2(1):10–11, 1994.

Geller A, and Koh H. Effective early approaches make a difference in melanoma detection. *Dermatol Patient Counsel Nurs* 1(1):9–10, 1993.

Greeley A. No safe tan. *FDA Consumer* 25(4):16–21, 1991.

Halpern AC. Melanoma surveillance: The high-risk patient. *Skin Cancer Found J* 10:23, 89, 1992.

Harris JS, and Macey WH. Cutaneous T-cell lymphoma: A case study, treatment, and nursing implications. *Dermatol Nurs* 6(1):41–49, 1994.

Heald P, et al. Treatment of erythrodermic CTCL with extracorporeal photochemotherapy. *J Am Acad Dermatol* 27(3):427–433, 1992.

Ho VC, and Sober AJ. Therapy for cutaneous melanoma: An update. *J Am Acad Dermatol* 22:159–176, 1990.

Holloway K, Flowers F, and Ramos-Caro F. Therapeutic alternative in cutaneous T-cell lymphoma. *J Am Acad Dermatol* 27(3):367–378, 1992.

Kaminester LH. Skin cancer: Diagnosis and treatment. *Hosp Med* 26(3):99–116, 1990.

Karagas MR, and Stukel TA. Risk of subsequent basal cell carcinoma and squamous cell carcinoma of the skin among patients with prior skin cancer. *JAMA* 267(24):3305–3310, 1992.

Kopf AW, Vossaert KA, and Yadav S. Dermoscopy: A new technique to diagnose pigmented lesions. *Skin Cancer Found J* 10:29, 93, 1992.

Macey WH, and Harris JS. Photopheresis and the role of the nurse. *Dermatol Nurs* 7(1):13–21, 1995.

MacKie RM, and McHenry P. Accelerated detection with prospective surveillance for cutaneous malignant melanoma in high-risk groups. *Lancet* 341(8861):1618–1620, 1993.

Marks R. The public health approach to melanoma control. *Skin Cancer Found J* 10:9, 71, 1992.

Marks R. Skin cancer prevention activities around the world; Australia. *Skin Cancer Found J* 12:39, 95, 1994.

McFadden M. Cutaneous T-cell lymphoma. *Semin Oncol Nurs* 1:36–44, 1991.

Nicol NH. Early detection and prevention of skin cancer. *Dermatol Nurs* 1(1):11–20, 1989.

Pollack SV. Skin cancer and aging. *Skin Cancer Found J* 10:39, 101, 1992.

Preston DS, and Stern RS. Nonmelanoma cancers of the skin. *N Engl J Med* 327(23):1649–1662, 1992.

Rigel DS. Men versus women: Who gets melanoma? *Skin Cancer Found J* 10:7, 67, 1992.

Robins P, and Levine VJ. How to reduce the risk of recurrences: The value of follow-up for nonmelanoma skin cancers. *Skin Cancer Found J* 10:21, 83, 1992.

Sabatini MM. Skin cancer: The silent pandemic. *Dermatol Nurs* 7(1):45–50, 52, 1995.

Savage L, Myerly J, and Baynes N. Mycosis fungoides: Case study and nursing implications. *Dermatol Nurs* 2(4):215–220, 1990.

Schleper JR. Teaching skin self-examination. *Dermatol Nurs* 3(3):174–176, 1991.

Sober AJ. Melanoma in children. *Skin Cancer Found J* 10:15, 79, 1992.

Somma S, and Glassman D. Malignant melanoma. *Dermatol Nurs* 3(2):93–99, 1991.

Stoupa R. Understanding cutaneous T-cell lymphoma. *Dermatol Nurs* 2(1):19–25, 1990.

Stroll RA. The role of total skin electron beam radiation therapy in the management of mycosis fungoides. *Dermatol Nurs* 6(3):191–196, 220, 1994.

Toce J, and Strohl R. Radiation therapy in the management of skin cancers. *Dermatol Nurs* 3(1):31–35, 1991.

Vargo N. Basal cell carcinoma classifications and characteristics. *Dermatol Nurs* 2(4):209–214, 1990.

Infestations

Bielan B. What's your assessment? *Dermatol Nurs* 4(5):377–378, 1992.

Brodell RT, and Helms SE. Office dermatologic testing: The scabies preparation. *Am Fam Physician* 44(2):505–508, 1991.

Elgart ML. Scabies: Diagnosis and treatment. *Dermatol Nurs* 5(6):464–467, 1993.

Haag ML, and Brozena SJ. Attack of the scabies: What to do when an outbreak occurs. *Geriatrics* 48(10):45–53, 1993.

Harbit MD, and Willis D. Lyme disease: Implications for health educators. *Health Educ* 21:41–43, 1990.

Hart G. Risk profiles and epidemiologic interrelationships of sexually transmitted diseases. *Sex Transm Dis* 20(3):126–136, 1993.

Kaslow R. Current perspective on Lyme borreliosis. *JAMA* 267:1364–1367, 1992.

King MM. Lyme disease: A seasonal hazard. *Dermatol Nurs* 2(4):202–203, 1990.

Kolar KA, and Rapini RP. Crusted (Norwegian) scabies. *Am Fam Physician* 44(4):1317–1321, 1991.

Mocsny N. What's wrong with this patient? *RN* 52(5):61–63, 1989.

Sterling GB, and Fox MD. Scabies. *Am Fam Physician* 46(4):1237–1241, 1992.

Stroud S. Permethrin vs. lindane: Similar in efficacy, but not toxicity. *Am J Nurs* 90(8):50, 1990.

Taplin D, and Porcelain SL. Community control of scabies: A model based on use of permethrin cream. *Lancet* 337(8748):1016–1018, 1991.

Willis D. Lyme disease. *J Neurosci Nurs* 23:211–217, 1991.

Willis D. Early skin manifestations of Lyme disease. *Dermatol Patient Counseling Nurs* 1(1):8, 12, 1993.

Alopecia

Brandy DA. Fours solutions to balding. *Muscle Fitness* 54(7):50, 190, 1993.
Faliberte R. The great hair race. *Men's Health* 7(2):22–23, 1992.
Grimes PE. Hair and skin differences key to safe grooming for blacks. *Dermatol Patient Counseling Nurs* 1(4):6–7, 1993.
Spindler JR, and Data JL. Female androgenic alopecia: A review. *Dermatol Nurs* 4(2):93–99, 1992.
Warsen J. Hair-raising schemes. *Am Health* 12(3):12–17, 1993.
Weitzner JM. Alopecia areata. *Am Fam Physician* 41(4):1197–1201, 1990.

Vitiligo

Erdos D. Redefining identity when appearance is altered. *Dermatol Nurs* 4(1):41–46, 1992.
Moore S, and Lambert V. Vitiligo: Care and treatment. *Dermatol Nurs* 3(1):15–20, 1991.
Porter JR, and Beuf AH. Racial variation in reaction to physical stigma: A study of degree of disturbance of vitiligo among black and white patients. *J Health Soc Behav* 32(2):192–204, 1991.
Skolnick A. Undifferentiated cell transplant techniques appear effective in treating leg ulcers, vitiligo. *JAMA* 266(10):1331–1332, 1991.
Somma S. Vitiligo: Caring for patients. *Dermatol Patient Counseling Nurs* 11(2):6, 8, 1993.
Thompson F. Management of a vitiligo patient: A case study. *Dermatol Nurs* 5(2):139–144, 1993.

Agencies

Acne

Acne Research Institute
1236 Somerset Lane
Newport Beach, CA 92660
(714) 722–1805

Acquired Immunodeficiency Syndrome

American Foundation for AIDS
  Research
12th Floor
733 3rd Avenue
New York, NY 10017
(212) 682–7440

Gay Men's Health Crisis
129 West 20th Street
New York, NY 10011
(212) 807–6655

HIV Testing and Counseling—STD
  Clinic
Howard Brown Memorial Clinic
945 West George
Chicago, IL 60657
Contact: Social Services Department
(312) 871–5777

National AIDS Hotline:
800–342–AIDS

Pediatric AIDS Foundation
Suite 613
2407 Wilshire Boulevard
Santa Monica, CA 90403

San Francisco AIDS Foundation
P.O. Box 6182
San Francisco, CA 94101–6182
(415) 863–AIDS

Alopecia Areata

Help Alopecia International Research, Inc.
  (H.A.I.R., Inc.)
P.O. Box 1875
Thousand Oaks, CA 91358
(805) 494–4903

National Alopecia Areata Foundation
710 C Street, Suite 11
P.O. Box 150760
San Rafael, CA 94915–0760
(415) 456–4644

Anemia

Fanconi's Anemia International Registry
Laboratory for Investigative Dermatology
Rockefeller University
1230 York Avenue
New York, NY 10021–6399
(212) 327–8862

Arthritis (Rheumatoid)

Arthritis Foundation
1314 Spring Street, N.W.
Atlanta, GA 30309
(404) 872–7100

Ataxia

National Ataxia Foundation
15500 Wayata Boulevard
Wayzata, MN 55391–3750
Contact: Donna Gruetzmacher, Executive
  Director
(612) 473–7666

Behçet's Syndrome

American Behçet's Foundation, Inc.
421 21st Avenue, S.W.
Rochester, MN 55902
(507) 281–3059; (800) 723–4238

Bloom's Syndrome

Bloom's Syndrome Registry
% Laboratory of Human Genetics
New York Blood Center
310 East 67th Street
New York, NY 10021
(212) 570–3075

Cancer

American Cancer Society
1599 Clifton Road N.E.
Atlanta, GA 30329
(404) 329–7906

National Cancer Institute
National Institutes of Health
Building 31, Room 10A29
9000 Rockville Pike
Bethesda, MD 20892
(301) 496–6631

Dermatitis Herpetiformis

Celiac Sprue Association / USA
P.O. Box 31700
Omaha, NE 68131
(402) 558–0600

Gluten Intolerance Group of North
  America
(Dermatitis Herpetiformis)
P.O. Box 23053
Seattle, WA 98102–0353
(206) 325–6980

Dermatology

Dermatology Foundation
Suite 302
1560 Sherman Avenue
Evanston, IL 60201–4802
(708) 328–2256

International Foundation for Dermatology
Department of Medicine
University of British Columbia
855 West 10th
Vancouver, British Columbia, Canada
  V5Z1L7
(604) 874–6112

Dermatomyositis

Muscular Dystrophy Association
  (MDA)
810 7th Avenue
New York, NY 10019
(212) 586–0808

Dermatopathology

Dermatopathology Foundation
P.O. Box 377
Canton, MA 02021
(617) 821–0648

Ectodermal Dysplasia

National Foundation of Ectodermal
  Dysplasia
P.O. Box 114
219 East Main Street
Mascoutah, IL 62258
(618) 566–2020

Eczema

National Eczema Society
Travistock House North
London WC1 9SR United Kingdom
01–38804097

Eczema Association for Science and
  Education
Suite 303
1221 S.W. Yamhill
Portland, OR 97205
(503) 228–4430

Ehlers Danlos Syndrome

Ehlers Danlos National Foundation
P.O. Box 1212
Southgate, MI 48195
(313) 282–0180

Dystrophic Epidermolysis Bullosa
Research Association of America, Inc.
(D.E.B.R.A. of America, Inc.)
141 Fifth Avenue
New York, NY 10010
(212) 995–2220

Hemochromatosis

Hemochromatosis Research Foundation
P.O. Box 8569
Albany, NY 12208
(518) 489–0972

Ichthyosis

Ichthyosis Foundation of America
710 Laurel Avenue, B-8
San Mateo, CA 94401

Klippel-Trenaunay Syndrome

K-T Support Group
ST Syndrome
4509 Wood Dale Avenue
Edina, MN 55424

Leprosy

Damien Dutton Society for Leprosy Aid
616 Bedford Avenue
Bellmore, NY 11710
(516) 221–5929

Lupus

American Lupus Society
23571 Madison Street
Torrance, CA 90505
(310) 542–8891

Lupus Foundation of America, Inc.
Suite 203
1717 Massachusetts Avenue, N.W.
Washington, DC 20036
(800) 558–0121

National Lupus Erythematosus
  Foundation (NLEF)
Suite 206
2635 North First Street
San Jose, CA 95134
(408) 954–8600
In California: (800) 523–3363

Lymphomatoid Papulosis

Lymphomatoid Papulosis Central
  Registry
Department of Dermatology
Fargo Clinic
Fargo, ND 58123
(701) 237–2000

Melanoma

Melanoma Foundation
Suite 250
750 Menlo Avenue
Menlo Park, CA 94025

Muscular Dystrophy

Muscular Dystrophy Association
810 7th Avenue
New York, NY 10019
(212) 586–0808

Neurofibromatosis

National Neurofibromatosis Foundation
Suite 7-S
141 Fifth Avenue
New York, NY 10010
(212) 460–8980; (800) 323–7938

Ostomy

United Ostomy Association
Suite 120
36 Executive Park
Irvine, CA 92714
(714) 660–8624

Pediculosis

National Pediculosis Association
P.O. Box 149
Newton, MA 02161
(617) 449–6487

Plastic Surgery

Plastic Surgery Research Foundation
P.O. Box 2586
La Jolla, CA 92038
(619) 454–3212

Port Wine Stain

National Congenital Port Wine Stain
  Foundation
125 East 63rd Street
New York, NY 10021
(212) 755–3820

Pseudofolliculitis Barbae

PFB Project
Suite 400
4801 Massachusetts Avenue, N.W.
Washington, DC 20016–2087
(202) 364–8710

Pseudoxanthoma Elasticum

National Association for Pseudoxanthoma
  Elasticum
P.O. Box 6925
Albany, NY 12206–6925
(518) 485–8553

Psoriasis

Canadian Psoriasis Foundation
Suite 400
1565 Carling Avenue
Ottawa, Ontario Canada K1Z 8R1
(613) 728–4000

International Federation of Psoriasis
  Associations
Moneheia 80
4752 Hamresanden, Norway

National Psoriasis Foundation
Suite 210
6443 S.W. Beaverton Highway
Portland, OR 97221
(503) 297–1545

National Psoriasis Research Association
107 Vista del Grande
Dan Carlos, CA 94070
(415) 593–1394 (1 P.M.–10 P.M. western
  time)

Problem Psoriasis Clinic
909 Ridgeway Loop Road
Memphis, TN 38120
(901) 767–3612

Psoriasis Research Institute
600 Town & Country Village
Palo Alto, CA 94301
(415) 326–1848

Rare Disorders

National Organization for Rare Disorders
(NORD)
P.O. Box 8923
New Fairfield, CT 06812
(203) 745–6518

Scleroderma

Scleroderma Federation, Inc.
Suite 29 F
1725 York Avenue
New York, NY 10128
(212) 362–0077

Scleroderma Foundation of Greater
Chicago
Room 917
175 West Jackson
Chicago, IL 60604
(312) 922–3532

Scleroderma Research Foundation
Suite 307
2320 Bath Street
Santa Barbara, CA 93105
(805) 563–9133

Scleroderma Federation
1882 Teaneck Road
Teaneck, NJ 07666
(201) 837–9826
(508) 535–6600

United Scleroderma Foundation
P.O. Box 399
Watsonville, CA 95077
(408) 728–2202;
(800) 722–HOPE

Sjögren's Syndrome

National Sjögren Syndrome Association
21630 North 19th Avenue
Phoenix, AZ 85027
(602) 516–0787

Skin Cancer

Skin Cancer Foundation
Suite 2402
245 Fifth Avenue
New York, NY 10016
(212) 725–5176

Social Health

American Social Health Association
(ASHA)
P.O. Box 13827
Research Triangle Park, NC 27709
(919) 361–8400

Tuberous Sclerosis

National Tuberous Sclerosis Association
Suite 120
8000 Corporate Drive
Landover, MD 20785
(301) 459–9888; (800) CAL-NTSA

Vitiligo

National Vitiligo Foundation
P.O. Box 6337
Tyler, TX 75711
(903) 534–2925

Xeroderma Pigmentosum

Xeroderma Pigmentosum Registry
Department of Pathology
UMDNJ—New Jersey Medical School
185 South Orange Avenue
Newark, NJ 07103
(201) 982–4405

36

Caring for People with Burn Injuries

◼ OVERVIEW: TYPES AND INCIDENCE OF BURN INJURIES

Types of Injuries

1. Cutaneous burn injury results when the tissues of the body come into contact with or are exposed to a thermal, electric, chemical, or radioactive source.
2. Inhalation injury results from the inhalation of toxic fumes, gases, and particulate matter present in smoke. Vapors, such as hot steam, may also cause inhalation injury.

Incidence

1. Although the exact incidence of burn injury is unknown, estimates suggest that approximately 1.4 million people in the United States seek medical attention for burn injuries each year.
2. Approximately 54,000 people are hospitalized annually with severe burn injuries.
3. Approximately 5000 people die each year as a result of their burn injuries.
4. Nearly one third of all people admitted to burn centers in the United States have an associated inhalation injury.
5. Inhalation injury accounts for 60 to 70 percent of burn-patient fatalities.

◼ CUTANEOUS BURN INJURY

Types of Cutaneous Burn Injury

1. Thermal injury
   a. Thermal injury results from exposure to an explosive flash or flame or from contact with a hot object, liquid, semiliquid, or semisolid material. The severity of tissue damage from a thermal burn injury is directly related to the temperature of the burning agent and the duration of exposure.
   b. Thermal injuries include those sustained in a structure fire or explosive accident and those from contact with scalding water, steam, tar, or grease or a hot metal or glass object.

2. Electrical injury
   a. An electrical injury results from the heat that the electric current generates as it passes through the tissues of the body.
      (1) The duration of contact, type of current (direct or alternating), intensity of current (voltage), and resistance of the body determine the severity of tissue damage.
      (2) Alternating current is more dangerous than direct current because it may cause cardiopulmonary arrest and muscle tetany.
      (3) Current greater than 40 volts can cause injury. Current of more than 1000 volts is high voltage and is associated with greater tissue damage.
      (4) All body tissues conduct electricity. Different types of tissues, however, resist the electric current differently. For example, nerve tissue is less resistant to the electric current than bone or skin.
      (5) Electrical injuries are typically most severe at the contact sites and at sites of current arcing. Therefore, overall tissue damage may be much greater than what is evident owing to the internal tissue damage to muscle, nerves, and bone.
   b. Electrical injuries include those sustained when a person touches exposed or faulty electric wiring or high-voltage power lines and those sustained when a person is struck by lightning.

3. Chemical injury
   a. Chemical injury results from tissue or skin contact with strong acid, alkali, or organic compounds. The severity of injury is directly related to the type of offending chemical, the concentration and volume of the chemical, and duration of tissue contact.
   b. Chemical injuries include injuries resulting from contact with caustic chemicals found in industrial, agricultural, and military environments and injuries resulting from contact with common household chemicals and cleaning agents.

4. Radiation injury
   a. Radiation injury results from exposure to a radioactive source.
   b. Radiation injuries include those resulting from ionizing radiation used in industry, those from the medical use of therapeutic radiation, and those from nuclear accidents.

Table 36-1. Carbon Monoxide Poisoning

Carboxyhemoglobin Level (Percent)	Associated Physical Findings
<15	Asymptomatic or impairment of visual acuity
15-20	Flushing, headache
21-30	Nausea, impaired dexterity
31-40	Vomiting, dizziness, syncope
41-50	Obtundation, tachypnea, tachycardia
>50	Loss of consciousness, coma, death

From Carrougher GJ. Inhalation injury. *AACN Clin Issues Crit Care Nurs* 4(2):368, 1993.

◼ INHALATION INJURY

Types of Inhalation Injury

1. Carbon monoxide poisoning
   a. Carbon monoxide is a colorless, odorless, tasteless gas released when organic substances burn. It has an affinity for binding to hemoglobin that is 200 times greater than its affinity for binding to oxygen. When carbon monoxide is inhaled, oxygen molecules are displaced, and carbon monoxide binds reversibly to hemoglobin, forming carboxyhemoglobin.
   b. As carboxyhemoglobin levels increase, varying degrees of central nervous system dysfunction result (Table 36-1).
   c. Most fatalities occurring at a fire scene result from carbon monoxide poisoning and anoxia.
2. Direct injury to the respiratory tract
   a. Inhalation injuries often affect both the upper and lower airways.
   b. Injury above the glottis constitutes injury to the upper airways.

   (1) A thermal injury to the upper airways (nasal cavity, pharynx, larynx, and large bronchi) results from inhalation of heated air.
   (2) The airway mucosa appears erythematous with edema, blisters, or ulcerations. Mucosal edema is greatest in the first 24 to 48 hours after injury and may lead to upper airway obstruction.
   c. Injury below the glottis constitutes injury to the lower airways.
   (1) A thermal injury to the lower airways (small bronchi, bronchioles, and alveoli) is rare because heated air is rapidly cooled to body temperature as it passes through the upper airways.
   (2) A chemical injury to the lower airways is more common and results from inhalation of toxic fumes and particles of combustion (acroleins) produced in a fire.
   (3) Pathophysiologic changes resulting from chemical injury below the glottis include the following:
   · Impaired mucociliary activity
   · Tracheal membrane erythema
   · Hypersecretion of mucus by the cells lining the tracheobronchial tree
   · Edema
   · Ulcerations of the mucous membranes
   · Bronchospasm

◼ CLASSIFICATION OF BURN INJURY

Burn Severity

1. Burn depth
   a. The depth of injured tissue determines the type of wound care required (Fig. 36-1; Color Fig. 36-1; Table 36-2). Partial-thickness burn injuries are classi-

Table 36-2. Burn Wound Classification

	Injury Depth	Wound Appearance	Wound Sensation	Healing
1st Degree (partial thickness)	Epidermis	Bright red No blisters Blanches	Painful	Complete in 3-7 days
2nd Degree	Epidermis Part of dermis	Red, pink Blisters Wet, weepy Blanches	Painful Very sensitive	10-21 days for superficial burn More than 21 days for deeper burn
3rd Degree (full thickness)	Epidermis Dermis	Red, pearly white, brown, gray, or black Dry, leathery to touch Thrombosed vessels visible No blanching	Insensate (decreased pin-prick sensation)	Autografting required for healing
4th Degree	Epidermis Dermis Subcutaneous structures: nerves, fascia, muscle, bone	Similar in appearance to 3rd degree Charring in deepest areas	Insensate or no sensation	Autografting required for healing Amputation likely

BURN DEPTH COMPARISION

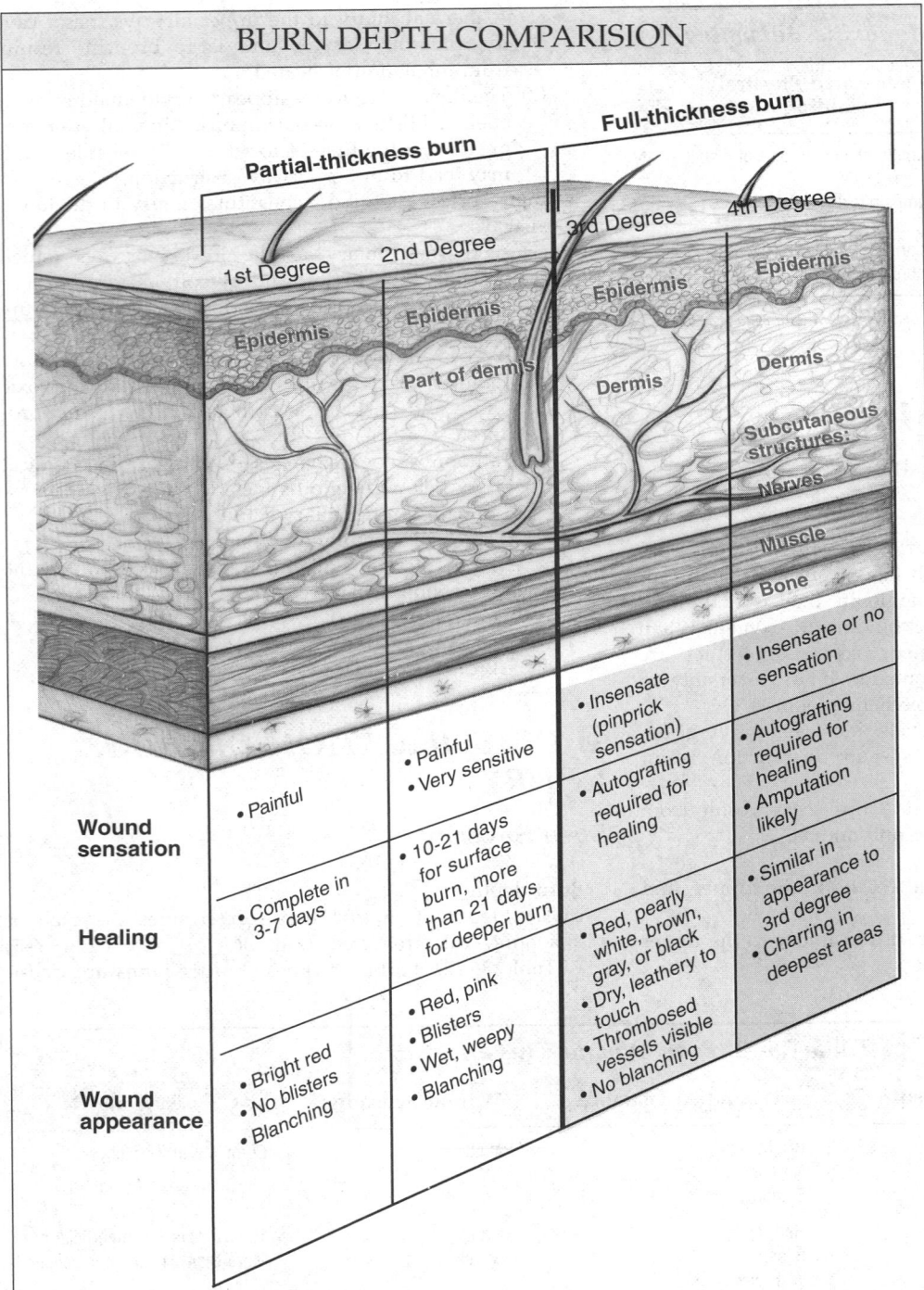

Figure 36–1. Depth of burn injury in skin and underlying tissue.

fied as 1st-degree burns and 2nd-degree burns (Color Fig. 36–2). Full-thickness burn injuries are classified as 3rd-degree burns (Color Fig. 36–3) and 4th-degree burns (Color Fig. 36–4).

   b. Burn injuries are usually a mixture of both partial-thickness and full-thickness injuries. As a rule, the greater the depth of tissue injury, the more severe the injury

2. Burn extent: The percentage of injured skin (excluding 1st-degree burns) determines the size or extent of the

burn injury. It is easiest to calculate the percentage of total body surface area (TBSA) burned by diagramming the burn injury and referring to 1 of several methods for determining burn extent.

   a. The rule of nines (Fig. 36–2)

   b. Burn diagram (Fig. 36–3)

3. Location of injury

   a. The location of the burn wound on the body is a key factor in determining the severity of injury.

   b. The face, hands, feet, genitalia, perineum, and major

MEASURING BURN EXTENT

The Rule of Nines

Often used in prehospital settings and emergency departments, the rule of nines is a quick, easy way to determine the percent of the total body surface area (TBSA) in burn patients.

Adult patient:

Body is divided into segments of 9 percent or multiples of 9 percent. The sum of percentages for all burned areas is an approximate total for the entire burn wound.

Estimate for small and/or scattered burns:

Use the person's palmar surface as a 1 percent estimate of TBSA.

Infant or child:

Trunk and arms are roughly the same as the adult's (9 percent for each upper extremity, 18 percent for the anterior trunk, and 18 percent for the posterior trunk). The infant's head and neck account for 18 percent, with each leg representing 14 percent. As the child grows, percentages are taken from the head and assigned to the legs.

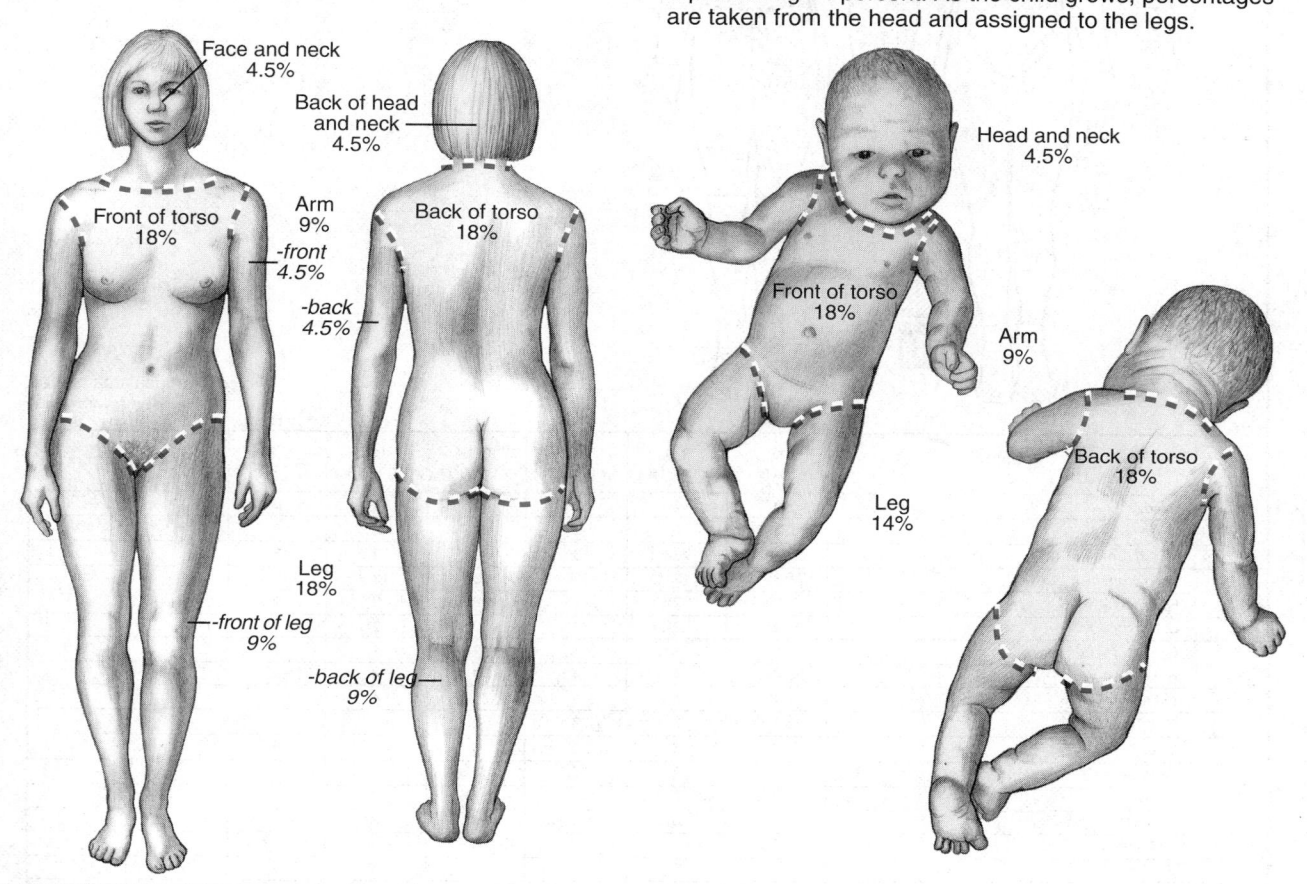

Figure 36–2.

---

joints are the body areas at greatest risk for functional or cosmetic impairment.

4. Age: Mortality rates are higher for burn patients younger than 4 and older than 65 years of age.
5. General health: Burn patients with preexisting cardiac, pulmonary, renal, or endocrine diseases have higher complication and mortality rates.
6. Mechanism of injury: The cause or mechanism of injury is an important determinant of injury severity.
   a. Although their injury may appear superficial, people who have sustained a high-voltage electrical injury may have suffered extensive damage to underlying organs, muscle, or soft tissue.
   b. People with chemical injuries may suffer from systemic toxicity from cutaneous absorption of the chemical in addition to their cutaneous injury.

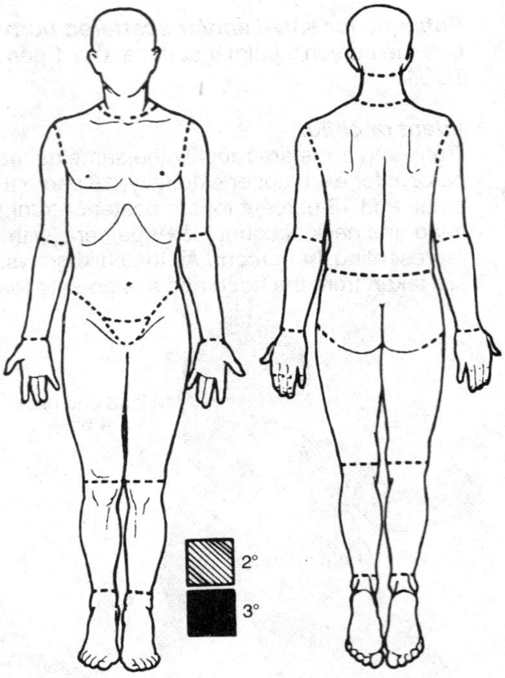

Date:______________________

Height:______________ Weight:__________

2° __________ + 3° __________ = __________%

Percent surface area burned (Berkow formula)

AREA	0-1 YEAR	1-4 YEARS	5-9 YEARS	10-14 YEARS	15 YEARS	ADULT	2°	3°
Head	19	17	13	11	9	7		
Neck	2	2	2	2	2	2		
Ant. Trunk	13	13	13	13	13	13		
Post. Trunk	13	13	13	13	13	13		
R. Buttock	2½	2½	2½	2½	2½	2½		
L. Buttock	2½	2½	2½	2½	2½	2½		
Genitalia	1	1	1	1	1	1		
R. U. Arm	4	4	4	4	4	4		
L. U. Arm	4	4	4	4	4	4		
R. L. Arm	3	3	3	3	3	3		
L. L. Arm	3	3	3	3	3	3		
R. Hand	2½	2½	2½	2½	2½	2½		
L. Hand	2½	2½	2½	2½	2½	2½		
R. Thigh	5½	6½	8	8½	9	9½		
L. Thigh	5½	6½	8	8½	9	9½		
R. Leg	5	5	5½	6	6½	7		
L. Leg	5	5	5½	6	6½	7		
R. Foot	3½	3½	3½	3½	3½	3½		
L. Foot	3½	3½	3½	3½	3½	3½		
TOTAL								

Figure 36–3. Burn diagram that outlines body percentages for body segment according to age. Used for all age groups to determine burn extent. Unlike the rule of nines, the Lund and Browder chart can be used reliably for infants and children with burn injuries. Acute care and burn centers regularly use burn diagrams because they provide the most accurate estimate of burn extent. (From Ignatavicius DD, Workman ML, and Mishler MA [eds]. *Medical-Surgical Nursing: A Nursing Process Approach.* 2nd ed. Philadelphia: WB Saunders, 1995, p 1985.)

The American Burn Association Severity Classification for Burn Injury

1. The American Burn Association (ABA) developed a classification schedule to assist clinicians in determining the severity of burn injury (Table 36–3).
2. The ABA classifies injuries as major, moderate, and minor according to extent and mechanism of injury, patient age, and location of injury.
3. After receiving emergency medical treatment at a local facility, people with major burn injuries usually require transfer to a special burn care facility.

Table 36–3. American Burn Association Burn Severity Classification Schedule

Degree of Burn	Criteria
Major burn injury	25% TBSA burn in adults <40 years old 20% TBSA burn in adults >40 years old 20% TBSA burn in children <10 years old
	Burn injury involving the face, eyes, ears, hands, feet, perineum likely to result in functional or cosmetic disability
	High-voltage electrical burn injury
	All burn injury with concomitant inhalation injury or major trauma
Moderate burn injury	15 to 25% TBSA burn in adults <40 years old 10 to 20% TBSA burn in adults >40 years old 10 to 20% TBSA burn in children <10 years old
	Less than 10% TBSA full-thickness burn without cosmetic or functional risk to burn involving the face, eyes, ears, hands, feet, perineum
Minor burn injury	<15% TBSA burn in adults <40 years old <10% TBSA burn in adults >40 years old <10% burn in children <10 years old
	No risk of cosmetic or functional impairment or disability

TBSA, total body surface area.
Adapted from American Burn Association. Guidelines for service standards and severity classification in the treatment of burn injury. *Am Coll Surg Bull* 69(10):2–28, 1984.

4. People with moderate, uncomplicated burn injuries can usually be treated at the receiving hospital as inpatients by medical personnel who have experience in the care of burn patients.
5. People with minor burn injuries usually require emergency care initially. They can then be discharged for follow-up outpatient care.

◼ PHASES OF A MAJOR BURN INJURY

Emergent Phase

1. The emergent (or resuscitative) phase begins at the time of injury and concludes with restoration of capillary permeability, typically 48 to 72 hours after a major burn injury.
2. The goals of medical and nursing care during the emergent phase of recovery are to do the following:
   • Stop the burning process
   • Stabilize the patient
   • Initiate prompt transport
   • Help the patient and family deal with the emergent aspect of the injury

Acute Phase

1. The acute phase begins when the person is hemodynamically stable, when capillary permeability has been re-

stored, and when diuresis has begun. This phase begins 48 to 72 hours after injury and concludes with discharge from the acute care setting.
2. The goals of medical and nursing care during the acute phase of recovery are to do the following:
   • Promote wound healing
   • Prevent infection
   • Promote physical therapy and recovery
   • Promote psychologic recovery

Rehabilitative Phase

1. The rehabilitative phase begins during the acute hospital stay, after the patient is stable, and continues until efforts to promote cosmesis, function, and adjustment are no longer required. The rehabilitative plan of care changes with time, reflecting the dynamic process of wound healing and patient independence and may last for several years after injury.
2. The goals of medical and nursing care during the rehabilitative phase of recovery are to do the following:
   • Attain quality function and cosmesis
   • Minimize hypertrophic scar development
   • Increase musculoskeletal strength
   • Overcome disabilities caused by related injuries, such as fractures, amputations, and nerve damage
   • Promote psychologic recovery

◼ LOCAL AND SYSTEMIC CHANGES AFTER A MAJOR BURN INJURY

Key Signs and Symptoms and Their Pathophysiologic Bases (Fig. 36–4)

> A burn injury affects all organ systems of the body. The physiologic changes that occur typically maximize during the first 2 weeks after burn injury and then slowly return to normal as the burn wound closes through either spontaneous healing or surgical closure (grafting).

1. Fluid shifts (see Chapter 9)
   a. The cellular injury caused by the burn results in the liberation of numerous vasoactive substances (serotonin, histamine, bradykinin, prostaglandins) that cause an increase in capillary permeability.
   b. With changes in capillary permeability, the intravascular fluid—composed of water, sodium, and plasma proteins—leaks into the extravascular space, resulting in tissue edema and hypovolemia.
      (1) Tissue edema is usually localized to the burn wound when the burn size is less than 25 to 30 percent TBSA.
      (2) Tissue edema becomes generalized to both burned and nonburned tissue when the burn size is greater than 25 to 30 percent TBSA.

KEY SIGNS AND SYMPTOMS OF BURN INJURIES AND THEIR PATHOPHYSIOLOGIC BASES

A burn injury affects all organ systems of the body. The physiologic changes that occur typically maximize during the first 2 weeks postburn and then slowly return to normal as the burn wound closes through either spontaneous healing or surgical closure (grafting).

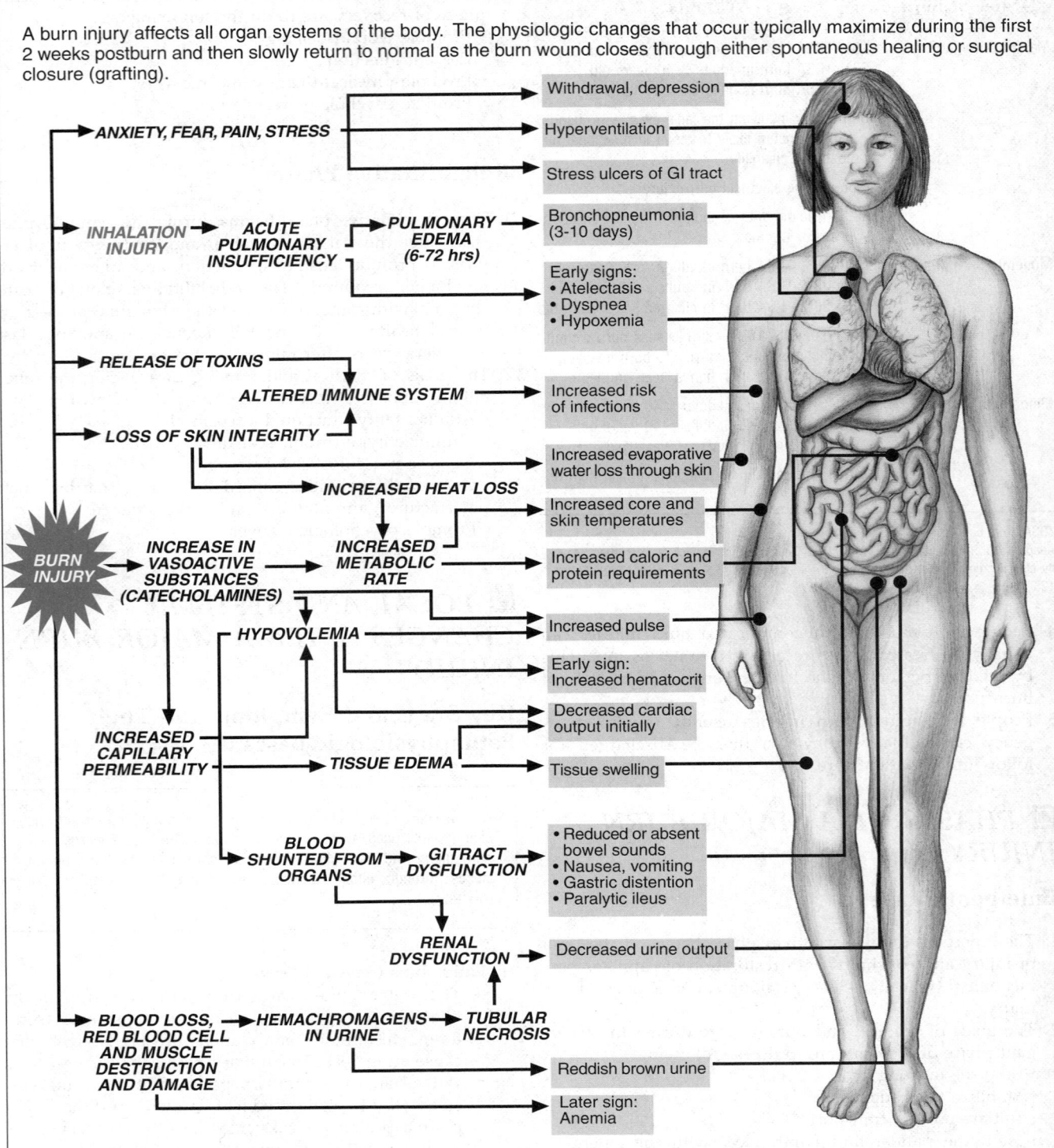

Figure 36-4.

(3) Maximum tissue edema typically occurs 18 to 24 hours after injury.

c. Capillary integrity returns to normal at approximately 18 to 36 hours after injury. Returning edema fluid, combined with intravenously replaced fluids, may lead to hypervolemia if the patient is not carefully monitored for fluid intake and output.

d. Evaporative water loss through burn tissue is higher than normal because of the loss of the epidermal skin layer.

(1) The amount of evaporative water loss is directly related to the percent of TBSA burn and can be estimated using the following formula:

Evaporative water loss (ml per hour)
= (25 + percentage of body surface burned)
× total body surface area in m².

(2) Evaporative water loss continues until the wound is closed.

2. Airway compromise: Inhalation injury often involves both upper and lower airways and may range from mild to severe.

a. Mild injury to the upper airway is associated with modest edema to the false cords but without compromise of the airway. Without signs of airway obstruction, a mild injury is treated with the administration of humidified air.

b. Moderate injury to the airways is associated with signs of airflow turbulence (hoarseness and stridor) and narrowing of the airway. Without signs of continued airway narrowing, treatment is aimed at decreasing further edema formation.

c. Severe injury to the airways is associated with edema to the false cords, mucosal erythema, and sloughing, leading to complete airway obstruction. Treatment is aimed at maintaining a patent airway, and patients should be intubated before the development of complete airway obstruction.

3. Pulmonary response (without inhalation injury)

a. Unless direct pulmonary injury occurs, initial clinical findings of pulmonary instability or insufficiency after a major burn injury are rare.

b. Minute ventilation typically remains normal during the emergent phase of recovery. After fluid resuscitation, minute ventilation increases (causing hyperventilation) according to burn size. This hyperventilation is thought to be caused by the postburn hypermetabolism and usually peaks at 2 weeks after injury. In addition, fear, ineffective pain management, and anxiety can cause the patient to hyperventilate further.

c. Immediately after injury, pulmonary vascular resistance increases slightly, and lung compliance decreases. The work of breathing increases proportionately with the decrease in lung compliance.

d. Immediately after a high-voltage electrical injury, respiratory arrest can occur.

4. Pulmonary response (with inhalation injury): In some patients with cutaneous burn and inhalation injuries, recovery can be complicated by the development of acute pulmonary insufficiency followed by pulmonary edema and pneumonia.

a. Acute pulmonary insufficiency is usually evident within the first 36 hours after injury. The following are manifestations:

• Hoarseness and stridor (indicative of damage or swelling to laryngeal structures with potential for upper airway obstruction)
• Atelectasis
• Dyspnea and wheezing (indicative of small-airway injury)
• Increased work of breathing
• Hypoxemia
• Respiratory acidosis

b. Pulmonary edema develops in 5 to 30 percent of patients with inhalation injury, typically within 6 to 72 hours after the injury. Treatment is aimed at judicious intravenous fluid administration.

c. Three to 10 days after injury, pneumonia develops in 15 to 60 percent of people with cutaneous burn and inhalation injuries. Treatment is aimed at identifying the causative organism and administering an appropriate antibiotic.

5. Cardiovascular response

a. Cardiac output: The fluid shifts and hypovolemia that are characteristic of a major burn injury lead to an initial depression in cardiac output with a marked increase in peripheral vascular resistance.

(1) In persons receiving adequate fluid resuscitation, cardiac output usually returns to normal 24 hours after burn injury and then to supranormal levels (2 to 2½ times normal) by 48 hours after injury. Cardiac output remains elevated until the burn wounds are closed.

(2) With inadequate fluid resuscitation, cardiac output continues to decrease, resulting in diminished blood flow to all body organs and continued maintenance of a high peripheral vascular resistance.

b. Pulse: Pulse rates are typically higher than normal because of hypovolemia and high amounts of circulating catecholamines.

c. Arterial blood pressure: Blood pressure is normal or slightly elevated unless hypovolemia is severe.

6. Electrolyte disturbances

a. Hyponatremia

(1) A mild, asymptomatic hyponatremia (serum sodium levels of 130 to 135 mEq/L) is common at the completion of fluid resuscitation.

(2) A symptomatic hyponatremia (serum sodium levels of less than 120 mEq/L) occurs with large volumes of hypotonic solution administration (e.g., 5% dextrose in water).

(3) Hyponatremia may also occur in burn patients with sepsis or prolonged use of dressings with 0.5 percent silver nitrate solution (sodium ions are leached from the eschar by the solution).

b. Hypernatremia

(1) Hypernatremia (serum sodium levels greater than 146 mEq/L) is the most common electrolyte imbalance that occurs during the acute phase of recovery.

(2) The primary cause of hypernatremia is inadequate replacement of evaporative water losses through the burn wound.

c. Hyperkalemia

(1) A mild to moderate hyperkalemia (serum potassium levels of 5.0–6.5 mEq/L) occurs after a burn injury because of release of potassium ions from damaged red blood cells and injured tissues.

(2) Hyperkalemia is further accentuated when lactic acidosis develops from impaired tissue perfusion.

7. Central nervous system response: No direct neurologic sequelae result from a cutaneous burn injury, unless the circumstances of the injury are associated with the following:

a. Neurologic trauma from a fall, motor vehicle accident, or explosion

b. Impaired perfusion to the brain during hypovolemic burn shock

c. Hypoxemia, if the person was trapped in a closed-space fire (the fire consumes available oxygen)

d. Inhalation injury with carbon monoxide poisoning or other asphyxiants (see Table 36–1)

e. Damage to central nervous system (spinal cord and peripheral nerves), especially with electrical injury.

8. Gastrointestinal response

a. Gastrointestinal function is often impaired after major burn injury because the body shunts blood away from the splanchnic vascular bed that supplies the stomach and intestines in response to hypovolemia. Symptoms that indicate decreased gastrointestinal motility include the following:
   • Hypoactive or absent bowel sounds
   • Gastric distention
   • Nausea
   • Vomiting
   • Paralytic ileus

b. With adequate fluid resuscitation, normal gastrointestinal function returns by 72 to 96 hours after injury.

c. Because of the stress of injury, burn patients are at risk for development of stress (Curling's) ulcers of the gastrointestinal tract.

(1) With decrease in gastric mucosal blood flow, superficial erosions in the stomach and duodenum occur.

(2) Prophylactic use of antacids or H$_2$ histamine receptor antagonists is commonly prescribed to prevent these focal lesions from developing into ulcerations of the gastrointestinal tract.

9. Renal response

a. Changes in renal function are frequently the result of hypovolemia.

(1) Initially, blood is shunted away from the kidneys as part of the normal neurohormonal stress response (see Chapter 26).

(2) Renal perfusion and glomerular filtration are decreased, resulting in low urine output.

(3) With adequate fluid resuscitation, renal blood flow returns to normal, signaled by an increase in urine output.

(4) This transient decrease in renal blood flow does not usually result in permanent renal dysfunction.

(5) With inadequate fluid resuscitation, renal blood flow continues to decrease and eventually leads to acute renal failure.

b. Hemachromagens found in the urine may adversely affect renal function.

(1) Hemachromagens (hemoglobin and myoglobin) are the byproducts of red blood cell and muscle tissue damage. They may cause acute renal failure.

(2) People with extensive burns or electrical injuries are at greatest risk for development of acute renal failure.

10. Immune alterations

a. Because the skin is the body's primary barrier to infection, people with major burn injuries are at serious risk for infection. A major burn injury minimizes the skin's defense.

b. A major burn injury alters normal immune function (see Chapter 21). For reasons not fully known, various compounds are released after a burn injury.

(1) These circulating toxins and hormones overstimulate suppressor T-cell function and the complement cascade system.

(2) At the same time, the toxins and hormones suppress other immune components: T-helper and T-killer cell activity and polymorphonuclear cell function.

11. Hematologic changes

a. Major burn injuries cause hematologic changes. A full-thickness burn destroys red blood cells in the immediate burn area. Red blood cell loss continues during the 1st week after injury.

b. During the emergent phase, the hematocrit increases to above normal because of hemoconcentration from the large fluid shifts. Hematocrit levels of 50 to 55 percent are expected during the first 24 hours after injury, with return to normal by 36 hours after injury.

c. During the acute phase, anemia typically develops as a result of the following:

(1) Red blood cell damage

(2) Reduced lifespan of the red blood cell

(3) Chronic blood loss from wounds

(4) Acute blood loss from burn-wound excision

(5) Blood sampling

12. Metabolic response

a. Increased basal metabolic rates (hypermetabolism) occur with burn injuries of about 30 percent TBSA or greater.

(1) Hypermetabolism in burn patients is related to burn size. For burns of less than 50 percent TBSA, the relationship is linear. For burns that cover more than 50 percent TBSA, this relationship plateaus, without further increase in metabolic rate.

(2) With burn wound closure, hypermetabolism diminishes, approaching normal metabolic rates by 1 year after injury.

b. The cause of the hypermetabolic response is related to the following:
  (1) Increases in circulating catecholamines (epinephrine and norepinephrine), leading to a hormonal stimulation of heat production.
  (2) Increases in evaporative and radiational heat losses.
  (3) An upward resetting of the hypothalamic thermoregulatory set point, causing an increase in heat production. Core and skin temperatures in burn patients are increased by 1 to 2 degrees Celsius above normal.
c. People with a burn that covers more than a 30 percent TBSA have increased caloric and protein requirements.
  (1) Various formulas are used to determine the increased energy needs of the burn patient. Calculations are based on the patient's age, gender, weight, extent of burn injury, and various activity factors. Table 36–4 outlines formulas used to calculate energy needs for burn patients. Protein requirements are closely tied to energy needs; 20 to 25 percent of the calories required should be of protein origin.
  (2) Methods for delivering nutritional support include oral diet, enteral tube feedings, peripheral parenteral nutrition, total parenteral nutrition, and a combination of these modalities. The preferred route for providing nutrition is the gastrointestinal tract (oral diet and enteral tube feedings). Parenteral nutrition is reserved for people who fail to meet their nutritional needs by the enteral route.
  (3) Failure to meet these elevated demands for nutritional repletion results in loss of muscle mass, delay in wound healing, further immunoincompetence, and infection.

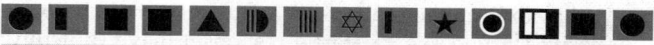

TRANSCULTURAL CONSIDERATIONS

Some Haitian, Cuban, Mediterranean, Latin American, and other Hispanic groups believe that solid-food intake and weight gain are signs of good or improving health. Members of these groups may become anxious at the need for liquid enteral feedings. In such cases, you should do the following:
- Obtain a diet history, including preferences, so you can determine whether ethnic foods brought to the patient are biomedically safe.
- Carefully explain the purpose and content of enteral feedings.
- Negotiate compromises when necessary. For example, blenderizing safe ethnic foods would reassure the family that the patient is getting culturally essential food.
- Carefully explain the purpose and content of intravenous fluids.

Psychologic Responses to a Major Burn Injury

1. Anxiety and fear
  a. A person commonly feels anxious and afraid after a traumatic injury.
  b. Family members are also often anxious and afraid. They may feel guilty for escaping injury while their loved one did not.
  c. Anxiety and fear (even fear of dying) may lead to

Table 36–4. Estimated Energy Calculation Formulas Used for Burn-Injured People

Author/Reference	Age Group (Years)	Caloric Needs/Day
Curreri 1990	0–1	BMR + (15 kcal × percent TBSA burn)
Curreri 1990	1–3	BMR + (25 kcal × percent TBSA burn)
Curreri 1990	4–15	BMR + (40 kcal × percent TBSA burn)
Curreri 1990	16–59	(25 kcal/kg body weight) + (40 kcal × percent TBSA burn)
Curreri 1990	>60	(20 kcal/kg body weight) + (65 kcal × percent TBSA burn)
Modified Harris-Benedict 1989	Adult	RMR × activity factor × injury factor
Hildreth 1990	Child (<12)	(1800 kcal/m² BSA) + (1300 kcal/m² TBSA burn)
Hildreth 1990	Adolescent	(1500 kcal/m² BSA) + (1500 kcal/m² TBSA burn)
USAISR 1995	Adult	Age- and sex-specific BMR × [0.89142 + (0.01335 × percent TBSA burn)] × m² × 24 × activity factor)

BMR, Basal metabolic rate; TBSA, total body surface area; RMR, resting metabolic rate.
Adapted from Rieg LS. Metabolic alterations and nutritional management. *AACN Clin Issues Crit Care Nurs* 4(2):390, 1993.

behavioral manifestations. The patient may become easily startled (i.e., a startle response), have difficulty concentrating and following instructions, withdraw, or not adhere to the treatment regimen.

2. Shock: Immediately after the injury, the person may be in shock, expressing disbelief and feelings of being overwhelmed.

3. Retreat: Shock often gives way to a need to retreat. The person may suppress feelings and try to withdraw from the nurse, visitors, other caregivers, and the environment.

4. Anger: The person may become angry for allowing the accident to occur or may be angry with those who caused the injury or escaped harm.

5. Depression: The person may become depressed at any time during recovery. The patient should be observed for apathy, tearfulness, insomnia, and loss of appetite.

TRANSCULTURAL CONSIDERATIONS

Some cultures consider anger and depression normal responses to upsetting situations. Use caution when interpreting psychosocial signs and symptoms.

6. Psychosis: While staying in the intensive care unit, the person may become psychotic as a result of the effects of medications, electrolyte and metabolic imbalances, drug withdrawal, sleep deprivation, or sensory overstimulation.

7. Grief: Patients may grieve for actual or perceived losses, such as limb amputations, death of loved ones, and their own functional limitations.

8. Acceptance: With time, recovery, and acceptance, the person can begin to plan for the future.

9. Post-traumatic stress disorder
   a. Post-traumatic stress disorder is characterized by the following symptoms:
      (1) Recurrent and intrusive recollections of the traumatic event
      (2) Avoidance of any circumstances or stimuli associated with the event
      (3) A numbing of general responsiveness (e.g., loss of interest in daily activities, feelings of isolation, memory impairment)
      (4) Hyperalertness
   b. The diagnosis of post-traumatic stress disorder is not made if the disturbance lasts less than 1 month.
   c. The most common precipitating events for post-traumatic stress disorder include the following:
      (1) A serious threat to one's life or physical integrity
      (2) A serious threat or harm to one's children, spouse, or other close relatives or friends
      (3) The sudden destruction of one's home or community
      (4) Seeing another person seriously injured or killed as a result of an accident or physical violence

Pain Response to a Major Burn Injury

1. Pain is the most severe recurrent experience endured by the burn-injured patient.

2. The pain experience depends on several factors:
   • Extent and depth of injury
   • Stage of wound healing
   • Age and stage of patient's emotional development
   • Patient's cognitive state
   • Responsiveness to pain medication
   • Pain threshold
   • Interpersonal and cultural factors

3. Burn patients typically describe 2 types of pain resulting from their burn injury.
   a. Background pain is continuous and low in intensity. Patients experience this pain during simple body movements (e.g., when shifting position in bed or with chest wall movements during a deep breath or cough).
   b. Procedural pain is acute and high in intensity. It is caused by recovery-process procedures: wound cleansing, wound débridement, dressing changes, and exercises.

◻ INITIAL CARE OF THE BURN-INJURED PERSON

Prehospital and Emergency Care

Prehospital and emergency care begins at the accident scene and continues until institutional emergency care takes over (see Chapter 35).

1. Remove the injured person from the source of the burn by performing the following:
   a. Extinguish burning clothes.
   b. Remove saturated clothing (in chemical or scald burns).
   c. Cool a tar burn.
      (1) Cold water soaks should be applied to the tar within 10 to 15 minutes from the time of injury. The soaking cools the tar and may limit the depth of injury. Cooling should be limited to avoid inducing hypothermia.
      (2) Do not attempt to remove the tar.
   d. Copiously irrigate a chemical burn. Burn patients with a chemical injury to the skin require prompt treatment initiated in the prehospital setting (field) and continued by emergency department personnel. The following should be performed:
      (1) Brush off any dry chemical promptly.
      (2) Remove all clothing immediately. It may retain the chemical and continue the burning process.
      (3) Remove all jewelry. It may restrict circulation to distal extremities.
      (4) Use continuous irrigation with water to dilute and remove the chemical. Acids can usually be removed with 30 to 60 minutes of continuous water irrigation. Alkali chemicals tend to bind more avidly to tissues and are more difficult to remove; they require hours of continuous water irrigation.
      (5) Do not use neutralizing agents. These create heat, further causing tissue damage.
   e. Remove the patient from contact with the electrical source.
      (1) Turn off electricity or use a dry, nonconductive object to remove the electrical source.

Date and time of call _____

Referring MD _____ Telephone _____

Hospital _____ City _____ State _____

PATIENT INFORMATION

Name _____ SSAN _____ Status: Active Duty _____
Retired _____
Age _____ Sex _____ Pre-Burn Weight _____ Dependent _____
VAB/BEC _____
Date of burn _____ Cause _____ PHS _____
Civilian _____
Extent of burn _____ 3rd Degree _____

Areas burned _____

Inhalation injury _____ Allergies _____

Associated injuries _____

Preexisting diseases _____

TREATMENT CHECK-LIST

Resuscitation: Calculated need (2 ml/kg/% TBS) _____

Fluid in _____ Urine Output _____

Airway_____ Blood gases _____ E−T Tube _____

Medications: Analgesics or sedatives _____ Tetanus _____

Antibiotics _____ Other Meds _____

Escharotomies: Arms _____ Legs _____ Chest _____

Wound Care: Wash and débride _____ Topical Agent _____

Lab tests: HCT _____ Electrolytes _____ BS _____ BUN _____

Request: Insert NG tube—Avoid general anesthesia or IM meds—Keep I & O

INFORMATION FOR FLIGHT PLAN

Burn Team _____ Family to accompany patient _____

Location of nearest airport with jet traffic _____

Transportation for team at destination _____

Figure 36–5. Patient transfer sheet. (Courtesy of U.S. Army Institute of Surgical Research.)

(2) To avoid becoming part of the electrical circuit, take all precautions when trying to remove the electrical source.
2. Assess the ABCs—establish the airway and ensure adequate breathing and circulation.
   a. Cardiopulmonary resuscitation may be required for patients who have sustained a high-voltage electrical injury.
   b. If the patient was burned in an enclosed-space fire, carbon monoxide poisoning should be suspected and 100 percent oxygen should be administered.

NURSE ADVISORY

Assess the ABCs:
- Establish the airway.
- Ensure adequate breathing—provide 100 percent oxygen through a nonrebreather face mask (conscious victim) or by endotracheal intubation and manual ventilation (unconscious victim) for suspected inhalation injury.
- Assess circulation.

3. Conserve the patient's body heat.
   a. The burn wound is covered with a clean sheet to prevent further wound contamination and to decrease pain.
   b. The patient is then covered with a clean blanket to conserve body heat.

NURSE ADVISORY

To reduce the depth of burn injury, cold water soaks may be applied to the burn:
- If the soaks are provided within 10 to 15 minutes of the time of injury.
- If the purpose is to cool scalding liquid and semiliquid materials (e.g., tar).
- If the soaks are limited to avoid inducing hypothermia.

---

4. Administer intravenous fluids if ordered.
   a. If the patient has only a burn injury (i.e., no other trauma) and transport to a medical facility can be achieved in less than 45 minutes, intravenous fluids do not need to be initiated in the field.
   b. If the patient suffers from multiple injuries or has experienced some blood loss or if transportation will require more than 45 minutes, a physiologic salt solution (e.g., normal saline or lactated Ringer's solution) should be administered through a peripheral vein and initiated in the field.
5. Transport should be to the closest medical facility for continued emergency care.

Transfer to a Burn Center

1. Before transfer to a burn center, the nurse should do the following:
   a. Ensure that the person has been initially stabilized.
   b. Contact the receiving facility. Transfer should be coordinated between the referring physician and the receiving physician at the burn center.
   c. Complete a patient transfer sheet to send with the patient (Fig. 36–5; see Table 36–3).

■ ASSESSING PEOPLE WITH MAJOR BODY INJURIES

Health History

1. Demographic information—patient's address, telephone number, language, religion, and occupation
2. Admission data—date and time of admission, next of kin, and reason for admission
3. Description of the burn injury, noting the following:
   - Causative agent
   - Duration of exposure
   - Circumstances of injury
   - Initial first aid given

4. The explanatory model, that is, the person's understanding of the injury (see Chapter 2)
5. Information regarding previous hospitalizations
6. Information regarding any health problems or patient concerns
7. The person's height and preinjury weight
8. Medication information—what medications the person is taking, how often, the reason for the medication, and when the last dose was administered
9. Data on the patient's use or abuse of drugs and alcohol, including the kinds and amounts consumed and the frequency of use
10. Smoking history and number of cigarettes smoked per day
11. Types of allergies or other sensitivities
12. Tetanus immunization status

NURSE ADVISORY

Before giving any medications, determine whether the patient has any allergies or sensitivities. If *yes*, ask about signs, symptoms, and actions taken for the allergic reaction. Document these findings so that all other health care professionals are aware of the patient's allergies.

---

13. Information regarding the person's eating patterns—number of meals per day, kind and frequency of snacks, and dietary restrictions
14. Information regarding whether the person has difficulty sleeping or uses sleeping aids
15. Information regarding gastrointestinal problems and use of any aids
16. Information regarding urinary frequency, burning, urgency, or other problems
17. Information regarding difficulty hearing, speaking, or seeing, and whether any aids are used for such difficulties
18. Information regarding how the person reacts to stressful situations
19. The person's special requests or concerns
20. Information regarding the availability of someone to assist the person at discharge

Physical Examination

Conduct a complete physical examination.

1. Note the date and time of the examination.
2. Describe the person's general appearance and emotional state.
3. Record the person's height and weight.
4. Describe the extent and depth of the burn injury. The extent and depth of burn injury are determined during the initial physical examination and such information is used to determine fluid resuscitation needs.
5. Review of each body system. A thorough review is necessary to identify any concomitant injuries or preexisting illnesses that may affect treatment choices and recovery.

INHALATION INJURIES

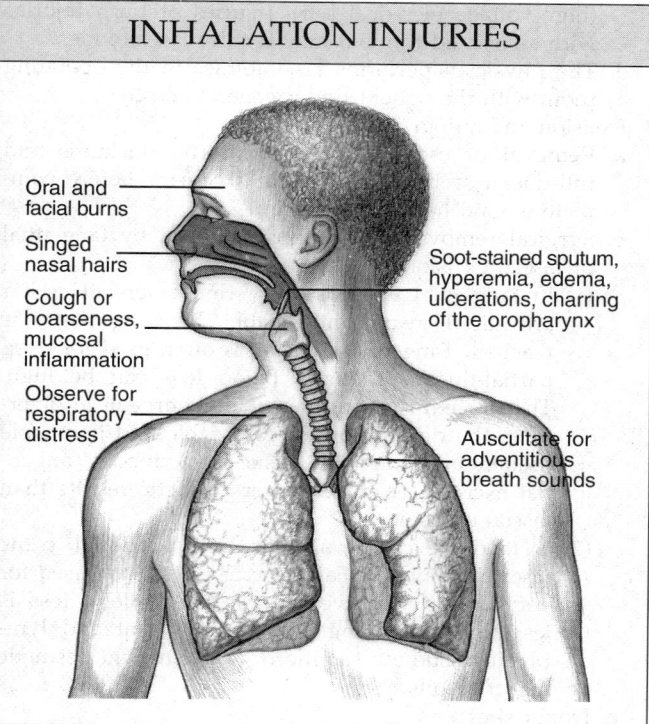

Oral and facial burns

Singed nasal hairs

Cough or hoarseness, mucosal inflammation

Observe for respiratory distress

Soot-stained sputum, hyperemia, edema, ulcerations, charring of the oropharynx

Auscultate for adventitious breath sounds

Figure 36–6. Examining for inhalation injury.

6. Assess associated trauma. Associated inhalation injury is also identified during the initial examination (Fig. 36–6).

Special Diagnostic Studies

1. Cutaneous burn or inhalation injury
   a. Baseline studies
      (1) Initial laboratory analyses of the following:
         • Complete blood count
         • Hemoglobin and hematocrit
         • Serum electrolytes
         • Blood glucose
         • Blood urea nitrogen
         • Arterial blood gas
         • Carboxyhemoglobin level—if carbon monoxide poisoning is suspected
         • Toxicology screen for opiates, anticonvulsants, and alcohol (if indicated)
      (2) A 12-lead electrocardiogram (for electrical injuries or preexisting cardiac disease)
      (3) A chest radiograph
      (4) Spine and long-bone radiographs to rule out concomitant trauma (if indicated)
      (5) Surveillance microbial cultures of the urine, wound, nares, and sputum
   b. Baseline studies are obtained to determine the patient's condition at the time of injury and to assist in the identification of any preexisting illnesses.
2. Inhalation injury
   a. Flexible fiberoptic bronchoscopy (see Chapter 22)
      (1) Flexible bronchoscopy allows direct examination of the upper airways and is used for early medical diagnosis of inhalation injury.
      (2) Common bronchoscopic criteria for diagnosing inhalation injury are laryngeal or tracheobronchial mucosal inflammation, hyperemia, edema, ulcerations, necrosis, presence of soot, and charring.
   b. ^{133}Xenon ventilation-perfusion scan: A positive scan indicates lower airway injury. It is best performed within 48 hours after the injury.
      (1) ^{133}Xenon isotope is injected intravenously. Serial scintiphotograms are then obtained to identify the pulmonary clearance of the xenon isotope.
      (2) A delay in pulmonary clearance (>90 seconds) or trapping of the isotope is considered a positive scan, indicative of injury.

◼ MANAGING BURN INJURIES

Special Burn Care Procedures

1. Escharotomy (Fig. 36–7)
   a. An **escharotomy** is an incision made through constricting eschar (nonviable burn tissue) to alleviate circulatory or ventilatory compromise.
      (1) Circulatory compromise: The incision lines are made in the midlateral or midmedial line, or both, of the compromised extremity and should extend from the distal to the proximal margin of the circumferential burn (Fig. 36–8).
      (2) Ventilatory compromise: The incision lines for chest wall escharotomies begin at the anterior axillary line and extend from the clavicle to the costal margin. They are performed bilaterally (see Fig. 36–8).
   b. Physicians generally perform escharotomies at the patient's bedside without local or general anesthesia. Escharotomy incision lines are placed only through insensate full-thickness burn wounds.
2. Fasciotomy

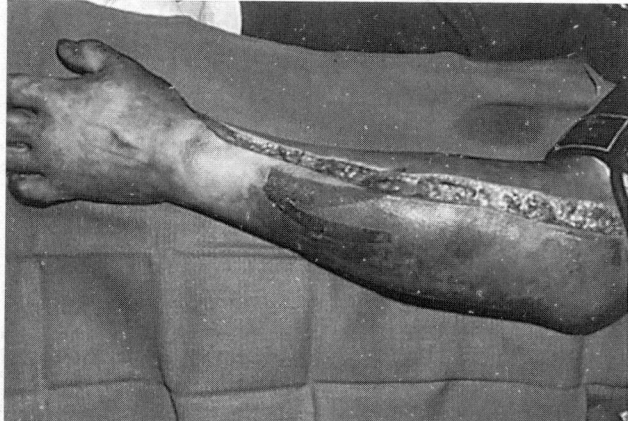

Figure 36–7. Escharotomy incision of full-thickness forearm burn. (Courtesy of the University of Washington Burn Center at Harborview Medical Center, Seattle, Washington.)

ESCHAROTOMY SITES

Circles denote joint areas
especially important
to relieve

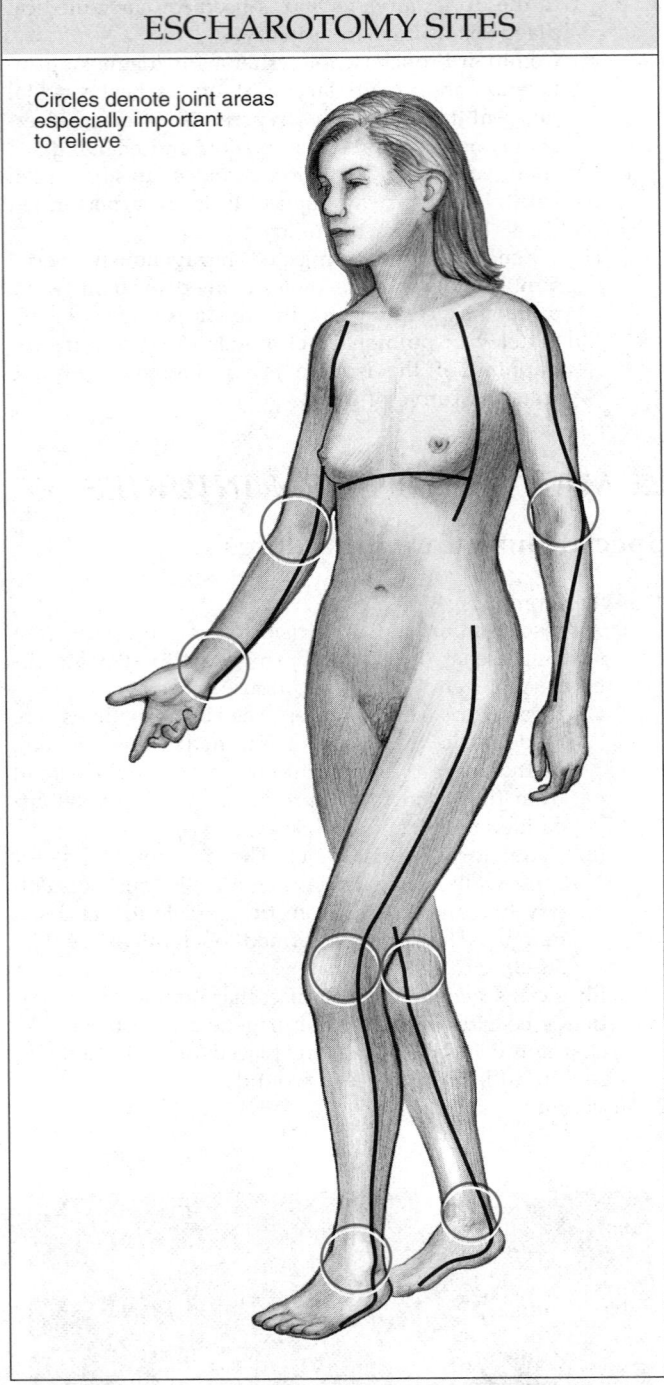

Figure 36–8. Preferred escharotomy incision lines of the thorax and extremities. The circles denote areas where the skin is more firmly attached to underlying tissue and constriction is likely to develop with circumferential burns.

A **fasciotomy** is an incision through constricting fascia.

b. If the peripheral pulses of injured extremities do not return after escharotomy, a fasciotomy should be considered.

c. Patients with full-thickness burns involving muscle (high-voltage electrical burn injuries or burn injuries with associated trauma) may require fasciotomies.

   d. The physician performs fasciotomies in the operating room with the patient under general anesthesia.

3. Excision and autografting procedures

   a. Removal of eschar from deep partial-thickness and full-thickness burn wounds is necessary before complete wound healing can occur.

   b. Surgical removal of eschar is achieved by tangential or fascial excision.

     (1) In tangential excision, very thin layers of eschar are sliced away until viable, bleeding tissue is reached. Tangential excision is often used for deep partial-thickness burns. Blood loss can be high. The procedure requires a skilled surgeon to determine the difference between viable and nonviable tissue. Only nonviable tissue is sacrificed. Tangential excision produces better cosmetic results than fascial excision.

     (2) In **fascial excision,** all injured tissue down to the fascia is removed. Fascial excision is often used for very deep, extensive burn injuries. Blood loss is less than with tangential excision. Fat and lymphatic tissue are sacrificed. A permanent cosmetic defect results.

   c. Donor sites

     (1) A donor site is created when a thin layer of unburned skin is surgically removed and placed (grafted) over excised burn wounds.

     (2) The size and location of the donor site and the condition of adjacent skin determine the selection of dressing material (see Table 36–8).

     (3) Nursing care depends on the type of dressing used.

   d. Autografting

     (1) **Autografting** is the surgical removal of the patient's own ("auto") unburned skin with application to the excised burn wound. Autografts can be applied as split-thickness skin grafts or as cultured epithelial autografts.

     (2) Split-thickness autografts can be applied in either a sheet form (sheet graft) or a meshed form (meshed graft). A sheet graft is applied to the excised wound bed without alteration in its integrity. Sheet grafts are often used to graft facial burns and small burns. A meshed graft has many small slits that allow for expansion of the graft. Meshing permits coverage of larger areas, coverage of irregular-shaped wounds, and drainage from a bleeding wound bed. When healed, the meshed pattern of the skin graft remains visible.

     (3) **Cultured epithelial autografts** are used in some burn centers in the treatment of patients with extensive burn injuries. Cultured epithelial autografts are produced in a laboratory by growing the patient's own keratinocytes into a thin, confluent sheet of epithelial cells. This process requires an initial biopsy of the patient's unburned skin and 3 to 4 weeks for cell growth before the graft can be applied to an excised wound bed. Successful use of cultured epithelial autograft to

treat extensive and deep burn injuries has been limited.

(4) Autografts are typically immobilized for 3 to 7 days after surgery, enabling the graft to adhere to the wound bed. Autograft immobilization is accomplished through positioning of the patient with splints, traction, or limb restraints. Nursing care should focus on preventing the hazards of immobility during this period.

Applying the Nursing Process

> **NURSING DIAGNOSIS:** Ineffective airway clearance R/T laryngeal and tracheal edema, airway epidermal sloughing, and depressed pulmonary ciliary action (inhalation injury)

1. *Expected outcomes:* Following interventions, the patient should be able to maintain an adequate airway.
2. *Nursing interventions*
   a. Elevate the head of the bed to reduce head and neck edema formation.
   b. Turn the patient and have the patient cough and take deep breaths every 1 to 2 hours for the first 24 hours, then every 2 to 4 hours while awake, as indicated.
   c. Place an oral suction device within the patient's reach for independent use.
   d. Monitor the patient for signs of impending airway obstruction and report the findings to the physician immediately. The nurse should watch for stridor, hoarseness, increased work of breathing, and respiratory distress.
   e. Assist with endotracheal intubation as needed. An endotracheal tube of at least 7.5 mm in diameter is recommended for use in the adult patient to facilitate pulmonary toilet.
   f. Perform endotracheal or nasotracheal suction as required. Document the volume and character of sputum

> **NURSING DIAGNOSIS:** Impaired gas exchange R/T inhalation of carbon monoxide and smoke toxins from inhalation injury or restrictive full-thickness chest wall burns

1. *Expected outcomes:* Following interventions, the patient should be able to maintain adequate gas exchange.
2. *Nursing interventions*
   a. Monitor for signs of respiratory distress as evidenced by the following:
      • Restlessness
      • Change in mental status
      • Labored breathing
      • Tachypnea
      • Dyspnea
      • Diminished or adventitious breath sounds
      • Tachycardia
      • Decrease in PaO_2 or SaO_2
      • Cyanosis (late finding)

   b. Monitor respiratory rate and rhythm, chest wall expansion, breath sounds, cough, and sputum production. Patients with restrictive chest wall burns may require chest wall escharotomies to allow adequate thoracic expansion and ventilation (see Fig. 36–8).
   c. Monitor arterial blood gas and continuous oxygen saturation levels (pulse oximeter) as needed.
   d. Administer humidified oxygen therapy as prescribed. For victims of carbon monoxide poisoning or inhalation injury, 100-percent oxygen should be administered through a nonrebreather face mask if the patient is conscious or with endotracheal intubation and mechanical ventilation if the patient is unconscious. Oxygen should be continued until the carboxyhemoglobin level is less than 15 percent.
   e. Turn the patient, and have the patient cough and take deep breaths every 1 to 2 hours for the first 24 hours, then every 2 to 4 hours while awake, as indicated.
   f. Teach the patient to use incentive spirometry.
   g. Place an oral suction device within easy reach so the patient can use it independently.
   h. Perform endotracheal or nasotracheal suction as required to assist with airway clearance.
   i. Elevate the head of the bed to facilitate the patient's lung expansion and gas exchange.
   j. Monitor the need for ventilatory support, and immediately report significant findings, such as hoarseness or stridor, to the physician.
   k. Assist with endotracheal intubation as needed. An endotracheal tube of at least 7.5 mm in diameter is recommended for use in the adult patient to facilitate pulmonary toilet.

> **NURSING DIAGNOSIS:** Fluid volume deficit R/T large fluid shifts from intravascular to extravascular space

1. *Expected outcomes:* Following fluid resuscitation, the patient should be able to maintain appropriate fluid volumes, maintain perfusion to vital organs, and avoid shock.
2. *Nursing interventions*
   a. Initiate fluid resuscitation in the emergency department (Box 36–1). Fluid administration requires placement of a central venous catheter or 2 large-bore peripheral intravenous catheters, preferably through nonburned skin. Table 36–5 lists formulas that have been used for fluid resuscitation of the burn-injured patient. The Parkland and modified Brooke formulas are commonly used for fluid resuscitation in burn-injured adults. Based on these formulas, a crystalloid-containing solution should be administered intravenously during the first 24 hours after the burn injury. Colloid-containing fluids (an albumin solution) are not used during this period because the increase in capillary permeability would allow leakage of the protein-rich fluids into the extravascular space, thus augmenting edema.
   (1) Administer one half of the calculated fluids within the 1st 8 hours after the burn injury.

BOX 36–1. Calculating Fluid Resuscitation Needs

To illustrate 1 approach to fluid resuscitation, consider the following patient scenario. D. Smith, a 42-year-old man, weighing 78 kg, was involved in a brush fire at 10:00 A.M. today. He sustained a 40-percent TBSA burn. Mr. Smith was immediately taken to a nearby hospital, where fluid resuscitation using the modified Brooke formula proceeded as follows:

Calculation of total 24-hour fluid requirements: 2 ml lactated Ringer's solution × 40 percent TBSA burned × 78 kg = 6240 ml lactated Ringer's

Calculation of 1st 8-hour fluid requirements: One half the total calculated fluid needs (3120 ml or 390 ml/hr) to be delivered intravenously over the 1st 8 hours after injury (10:00 A.M. to 6:00 P.M.)

Calculation of subsequent 16-hour fluid requirements: One half the total calculated fluid needs (3120 ml or 195 ml/hr) to be delivered intravenously over the subsequent 16-hour period (6:00 P.M. to 10:00 A.M.)

Note: The total fluid volume calculated by the resuscitation formula should be administered over the 1st 24 hours after injury and not after initiation of treatment. For example, if Mr. Smith's admission to the hospital had been delayed for 2 hours and he had not received any fluid resuscitation, the 1st one half of the 24-hour fluid needs (3120 ml) should be administered over the ensuing 6-hour period (12:00 P.M. to 6:00 P.M.).

---

(2) Administer one fourth of the calculated fluids during the 2nd 8-hour period (9 to 16 hours after injury).

(3) Administer one fourth of the calculated fluids during the 3rd 8-hour period (16 to 24 hours after injury).

(4) In the 2nd 24-hour period (24 to 48 hours after injury), a combination of crystalloid- and colloid-containing solutions is administered.

(5) The following information is necessary for successful fluid resuscitation:
- The patient's weight
- An accurate estimate of the percentage of TBSA (see Figs. 36–2 and 36–3)
- The time of injury (not the beginning of treat-

ment), as a base for calculating fluids to be administered in the first 24 hours
- Previous fluid administration

b. Monitor the following clinical signs during fluid resuscitation:

(1) Mentation: Unless the injury is complicated by a head injury or carbon monoxide poisoning, the patient should maintain a clear sensorium. Obtundation, lethargy, confusion, and agitation may be early signs of poor perfusion to the brain (secondary to hypovolemia), oxygenation and ventilation disturbances, undiagnosed head injury, or carbon monoxide poisoning.

(2) Urine output: Urine output is one of the most sensitive and reliable parameters of fluid resuscitation. An indwelling urinary catheter connected to a closed drainage system should be placed in the emergency department for all patients with major burn injuries. Monitor and record urine output for volume and hemachromagens at least every hour during the emergent period. Hemachromagens change the color of urine to a dark brown-red. For an adult (without urine hemachromagens), the hourly volume should be 30 to 50 ml. The hourly volume for children weighing less than 30 kg should be 1 ml per kg (see Chapter 15). For an adult (with urine hemachromagens or an electric injury, or both), the hourly volume should be 75 to 100 ml. The hourly volume for children weighing less than 30 kg should be 2 ml per kg.

(3) Pulse: Monitor the heart rate and rhythm continuously. A pulse rate of less than 120 beats per minute (<160 beats per minute in children) usually indicates adequate intravascular volume.

(4) Arterial blood pressure: Monitor blood pressure in an unburned extremity whenever possible. For the critically ill patient, an indwelling arterial catheter for continuous blood pressure monitoring may be placed. Maintain mean arterial blood pressure at 65 mm Hg or greater (40 mm Hg for children).

Table 36–5. Common Formulas for Fluid Resuscitation of Adult Burn Patients

Formula Name	First 24 Hours			Second 24 Hours		
	Electrolyte-Containing Solution	Colloid-Containing Solution	Dextrose in Water	Electrolyte-Containing Solution	Colloid-Containing Solution	Dextrose in Water
Evans	Normal saline 1 ml/kg/% burn	1 ml/kg/% burn	2000 ml	$\frac{1}{2}$ of 1st 24-hr requirement	$\frac{1}{2}$ of 1st 24-hr requirement	2000 ml
Brooke	Lactated Ringer's 1.5 ml/kg/% burn	0.5 ml/kg/% burn	2000 ml	$\frac{1}{2}$–$\frac{3}{4}$ of 1st 24-hr requirement	$\frac{1}{2}$–$\frac{3}{4}$ of 1st 24-hr requirement	2000 ml
Modified Brooke	Lactated Ringer's 2 ml/kg/% burn	None	None	None	0.3–0.5 ml/kg/% burn	Titrate to maintain urine output
Parkland	Lactated Ringer's 4 ml/kg/% burn	None	None	None	0.3–0.5 ml/kg/% burn	Titrate to maintain urine output

Adapted from Rue LW, and Cioffi WG. Resuscitation of thermally injured patients. *Crit Care Nurs Clin North Am* 3(2):185, 1991.

Blood pressure is usually maintained unless severe hypovolemia exists.

(5) Cardiac filling pressures and cardiac index: With a hemodynamically unstable patient (older individuals, patients with preexisting cardiac disease or dysrhythmias, or patients with extensive burn injuries complicated by a severe inhalation injury), a pulmonary artery catheter may be required to monitor cardiac filling pressures and cardiac index.

(6) Bowel sounds: For burn patients with 25 percent TBSA or greater, a nasogastric tube should be placed in the emergency department and connected to suction to decompress the stomach and prevent gastric distention. Monitor bowel sounds for indications that the gastrointestinal system is functioning.

(7) Serum electrolyte and hematologic studies: Continue to monitor baseline studies. Monitor serum electrolytes and hematocrit at least once daily during the early postburn period or more frequently as indicated. Compare test results to determine whether the patient's fluid status has changed.

NURSE ADVISORY

Fluid resuscitation formulas serve only as guides. To evaluate the adequacy of fluid resuscitation, you must monitor the following clinical signs:
- Mentation
- Urine output
- Pulse
- Arterial blood pressure
- Cardiac filling pressures and cardiac index (when indicated)
- Bowel sounds

It is also important to monitor any deviations from baseline laboratory studies.

c. Follow weight trends. Weigh patients daily without dressings at a consistent time of day using the same weight scale. For patients with extensive burns, a 15 to 20 percent increase in body weight after fluid resuscitation is not uncommon.

d. Monitor intake and output every hour during the initial 72 hours after injury and evaluate trends. Titrate intravenous fluid administration as prescribed according to the desired volume of urine output.

NURSING DIAGNOSIS: Altered tissue perfusion (peripheral) R/T constricting circumferential burns of extremities

1. *Expected outcomes:* Following interventions, the patient should have adequate tissue perfusion to burned extremities.
2. *Nursing interventions*
   a. Remove all constricting clothing and jewelry in the emergency department.
   b. Limit use of constricting blood pressure cuffs in affected extremities.

c. Monitor perfusion to all extremities. Clinical signs and symptoms of impaired circulation in a burned extremity include cyanosis of unburned skin, delayed capillary refill of unburned skin, progressive paresthesia, deep tissue pain, and loss of pulse by Doppler flowmeter.

(1) Loss of pulse is the most sensitive indicator of impaired circulation to an injured extremity.

(2) Pulses diminish or become absent with circulation impairment.

(3) Perform pulse checks every hour during the first 72 hours after injury in extremities at risk for circulatory compromise.

(4) Monitor pulses in the distal palmar arch vessels in the upper extremities or the posterior tibial artery in the lower extremities.

d. Encourage active range-of-motion exercises of affected extremities to promote venous return.

e. If the patient is hemodynamically stable, elevate the affected extremities to reduce dependent edema formation.

f. If circulation is impaired, prepare patient and family for escharotomy. Postescharotomy care includes the following:

(1) Monitoring the adequacy of circulation after escharotomy. The presence of arterial pulses should be documented, noting color, movement, and sensation of the affected extremity.

(2) Controlling bleeding with pressure, electrocautery, or suturing of bleeding vessels.

NURSING DIAGNOSIS: Risk for injury R/T the neurohormonal stress response of the burn injury

1. *Expected outcomes:* After implementation of the following interventions, the patient should remain free of stress (Curling's) ulcers.
2. *Nursing interventions*
   a. Monitor stomach aspirate for blood and pH.
   b. Administer antacid therapy or H_2 blockers to keep the gastric pH between 3.5 and 4.5, as prescribed.
   c. Notify the physician of any signs of blood in the gastric output.

NURSING DIAGNOSIS: Altered nutrition, less than body requirements, R/T increased metabolic needs for wound healing

1. *Expected outcomes:* Following interventions, the patient should be able to maintain lean body mass and prevent a weight loss of greater than 10 to 15 percent of the patient's preburn weight.
2. *Nursing interventions*
   a. Obtain accurate preburn weight.
   b. Consult a dietitian.
   c. Identify the patient's food preferences, eating habits and patterns, and food allergies.
   d. Monitor gastrointestinal function.

e. Weigh patient daily (except when operative procedure limits mobility).

f. Record enteral and parenteral intake and output.

g. Schedule patient care procedures to maximize nutritional intake.

h. Educate the patient and family about nutritional needs.

i. Encourage the family to bring favorite foods from home and to stay with the patient at mealtimes. A family might bring a specially prepared soup, for example, that would increase the patient's nutritional intake.

j. Consult with an occupational therapist about providing eating utensil aids to help the patient eat independently (Fig. 36–9).

k. Provide positive reinforcement for eating.

l. Provide oral hygiene.

> **NURSING DIAGNOSIS:** Infection, risk for, R/T loss of skin barrier, impaired immune response, presence of invasive catheters (indwelling urinary catheter and intravenous catheters), and invasive procedures (venous and arterial blood sampling and bronchoscopy)

1. *Expected outcomes:* After implementation of the following interventions, the patient should be able to avoid infection and sepsis.

2. *Nursing interventions*

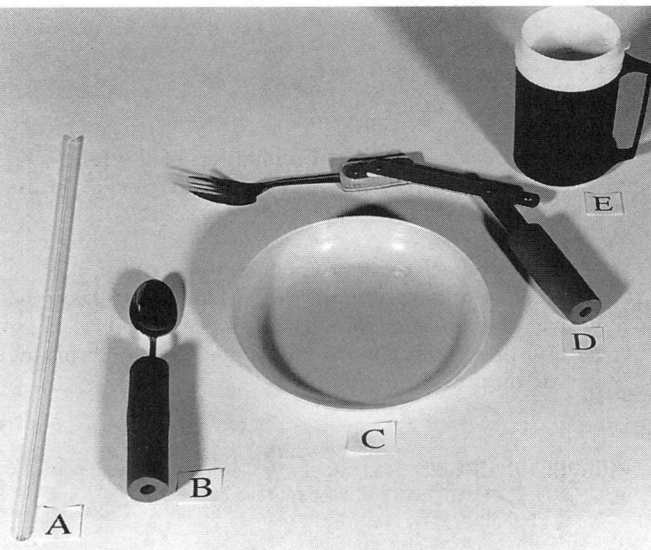

Figure 36–9. Assistive devices used during mealtime to increase the patient's independence. These devices are carefully selected by nurses and occupational therapists for use by patients during periods of immobility (e.g., after skin grafts to hands), when hand, wrist, or arm range of motion is limited. *A,* Long straw (pictured at 46 cm), which should be cut to required length. The straw enables a patient to drink from a cup when hands are immobilized. *B,* Spoon with built-up foam handle. The handle can also be used with a fork or knife. *C,* Plate with lip and skid pad, which facilitates placing food on a spoon or fork. The person can push against the lip while the pad holds the plate in place. *D,* Fork with extended, adjustable handle, used by patients with decreased elbow range of motion. *E,* Easy-grasp cup.

a. Determine tetanus immunization status in the emergency department (see Chapter 21). Tetanus prophylaxis for burn patients is guided by their previous immunization status.

(1) Patients from immigrant and refugee groups often have no record, and sometimes no knowledge, of whether they have been given tetanus immunization or boosters.

(2) Patients who have been immunized against tetanus, but not within the past 5 years, should receive a tetanus toxoid booster.

(3) Patients not previously immunized against tetanus should receive the tetanus human-immune globulin and the 1st of a series of active immunizations with tetanus toxoid.

(4) The only contraindication to tetanus immunization for the burn patient is a neurologic or severe hypersensitivity reaction to a previous dose. If a contraindication exists, the physician should consider passive immunization against tetanus.

b. Maintain infection control practices.

(1) The burn patient is at high risk for infection from autocontamination with microorganisms normally found in the oropharynx, in fecal flora, and on the unburned skin; cross-contamination from staff and visitors; airborne contaminants; and contaminants encountered at the scene of injury (e.g., jumping in polluted water, rolling in soil).

(2) Infection control practices differ throughout the United States. Most burn centers use caps, masks, eye protection, gloves, and impermeable aprons during wound care, when contamination is most likely to occur.

(3) Strict hand washing practices (before and after all patient contacts) are the most effective measures in reducing infection from cross-contamination.

(4) Staff and visitors with skin, gastrointestinal, or respiratory tract infections should not have contact with the patient.

c. Watch for clinical signs of infection including the following:

(1) Signs of wound infection and cellulitis:

Table 36–6. Types of Débridement

Method	Procedure
Mechanical débridement	Dressing materials (usually coarse mesh gauze) and a wetting solution (normal saline or antimicrobial agent) are applied to the wound. With wet-to-dry or wet-to-moist dressing, wound exudate and necrotic tissue become entrapped in the gauze and are débrided with gauze removal.
Sharp débridement	With careful use of forceps and scissors, blisters and loose eschar are lifted and trimmed away.
Enzymatic débridement	Commercially prepared ointments containing proteolytic enzymes digest necrotic tissue, facilitating eschar removal.

- Discoloration of wounds or drainage
- Odor
- Delayed wound healing

(2) Signs of pneumonia:
- Increase or change in character, color, or odor of sputum
- Adventitious breath sounds
- Fever
- Change in vital signs

(3) Signs of sepsis:
- Headache

- Chills
- Anorexia and nausea
- Change in vital signs
- Glucose intolerance (hyperglycemia and glycosuria)
- Paralytic ileus
- Confusion and restlessness

d. Monitor for signs of infection at catheter insertion sites twice daily.

e. Identify pathogenic organisms early to treat infections successfully. Obtain routine surface wound cultures to

---

Table 36–7. Topical Antimicrobial Agents Commonly Used in Burn Care

Agent	Description/Application	Side Effects
Creams and Ointments		
1% silver sulfadiazine cream	Broad-spectrum antimicrobial activity effective against both gram-positive and gram-negative organisms and fungi. Moderate eschar penetration. Apply 1 to 2 times/day in a thin layer (1 to 2 mm) directly to the burn wound. Antimicrobial activity lasts for 12 to 24 hr, depending on the amount of agent applied and wound characteristics. Pus and wound exudate can lessen or inhibit the antimicrobial activity. The open or closed method of wound dressing may be used.	Transient leukopenia possibly due to bone marrow suppression or eschar sequestration of leukocytes. Macular rash (uncommon). Local wound healing slowed.
Mafenide acetate (Sulfamylon) cream	Broad-spectrum antimicrobial activity similar to that of silver sulfadiazine, but with better coverage against *Pseudomonas aeruginosa* and anaerobes. Good eschar penetration. Apply every 12 to 18 hr in a thin layer (1 mm) directly to the burn wound. Pus and wound exudate do not inhibit the antimicrobial activity. The open or closed method of wound dressing may be used.	Pain and burning sensation upon application, especially when applied to partial-thickness burn wounds. Hyperchloremic metabolic acidosis due to carbonic anhydrase inhibition. The degree of metabolic acidosis is proportional to the body surface area treated. Maculopapular rash. Local wound healing impaired.
Povidone-iodine 1% ointment	Broad-spectrum antimicrobial activity effective against most gram-positive and gram-negative organisms and fungi. Moderate eschar penetration. Apply 2 to 3 times/day in a thin layer (1 mm) directly to the burn wound. The closed method of wound dressing is typically used.	Pain and burning on application. Iodine toxicity is uncommon unless renal dysfunction exists. Local wound healing impaired.
Nitrofurazone (Furacin) ointment or cream	Limited antimicrobial activity against *Staphylococcus aureus* and some gram-negative organisms. Ineffective against fungi and yeast. Limited eschar penetration. Apply 2 times/day to wound surface. The open or closed method of wound dressing may be used.	Pain and burning upon application. May be nephrotoxic if used in large quantities.
Polymyxin-based ointments	Antimicrobial activity against both gram-positive and gram-negative organisms. Limited eschar penetration. Apply directly to wound in a thin layer (1 mm). Reapply as necessary to keep agent in contact with wound. Typically used to treat small partial-thickness burn wounds. Dressings are unnecessary unless clothing must be protected.	Local wound healing slowed (less than with 1% silver sulfadiazine).
Solutions		
5% Mafenide acetate (Sulfamylon)	Broad antimicrobial activity. Moisten gauze dressing and apply directly to the burn wound or skin graft. Remove and reapply solution-moist dressings every 4 to 8 hr as prescribed. More frequent dressing changes (e.g., every 4 hr) facilitate wound débridement.	Pain and burning upon application (less than with mafenide acetate cream). Pruritus. Macular rash. Fungal colonization.
0.5% Silver nitrate	Antimicrobial activity against *S. aureus, Escherichia coli,* and *P. aeruginosa.* Poor eschar penetration. Moisten gauze dressing and apply directly to the burn wound. Ensure that dressings remain moist by wetting them every 2 hr with the silver nitrate solution. Remove and reapply solution-moist dressings every 8 to 12 hr as prescribed. Preserve solution in a light-resistant container. Protect environment (floors, walls, bed frame) with plastic to prevent staining.	Electrolyte abnormalities: hyponatremia, hypochloremia, hypokalemia, hypocalcemia.

identify potential pathogens. When hyperthermia or hypothermia develops, obtain cultures of the wound, blood, urine, and sputum.

  f. Administer systemic antibiotics for known infections, as prescribed. If the causative organism is unknown, the physician may initially order broad-spectrum antibiotics. Once Gram stain or culture results identify the causative organism, the physician makes the appropriate change in antibiotic coverage.

  g. Provide wound care.

    (1) Cleanse the wound using aseptic technique at the bedside or in a special tub, table, or shower (i.e., hydrotherapy). Use a mild surgical soap to wash the wound and remove any previously applied cream. Shave hair to within 1 inch of the burn wound periphery (except for the eyebrows). Rinse the wound thoroughly with water.

    (2) Débride the wound of all loose, nonviable skin and blisters (greater than 2 cm in diameter). Wound débridement may be accomplished by mechanical, sharp, or enzymatic means (Table 36–6).

    (3) Examine the wound after cleansing and débridement. Document the following wound characteristics: size, color, drainage (odor, color, amount), and presence of pain.

    (4) Apply the topical wound treatment as prescribed. Either the exposure method or closed method of

NURSE ADVISORY

Mechanical débridement—Mechanical débridement can be painful. Be careful to avoid injuring new granulation or epithelial tissues. Wetting the dressing with saline before its removal may help prevent injury and decrease pain.

Sharp débridement—Be careful not to cause bleeding. Bleeding may indicate injury to healthy tissue.

Enzymatic débridement—Contraindications for use of enzymatic débridement include wounds communicating with major body cavities, exposed nerves, and fungating neoplastic ulcers.

wound care should be used to apply topical antimicrobial creams. Table 36–7 describes the most commonly used antimicrobial creams. Table 36–8 describes temporary wound coverings, and Table 36–9 describes wound care to specialty areas. With the exposure method, apply the antimicrobial cream directly to the wound without dressings. Figure 36–10 illustrates the closed method.

NURSING DIAGNOSIS: Pain R/T burn injury, exposed nerve endings, treatments, and anxiety

Table 36–8. Temporary Wound Coverings Used in Burn Care

Name	Description	Indications and Use
Biologic		
Amnion	Amniotic membranes collected from human placenta under sterile conditions	To protect and facilitate healing of clean, partial thickness burn wounds
Allograft (homograft)	Human cadaver skin donated and harvested within 24 hr of death	To débride exudative wounds To protect excised wounds and test for receptivity before autograft application
Xenograft (heterograft)	Porcine skin harvested after slaughter, cryopreserved or lyophilized for storage	To protect and facilitate healing of clean, partial-thickness burn wounds To débride exudative wounds To protect excised wounds and test for receptivity before autograft application
Biosynthetic		
Biobrane (Winthrop Pharmaceuticals, New York City, NY)	Nylon fabric bonded to a silicone rubber membrane containing collagenous porcine peptides	Donor site dressing To protect and facilitate healing of clean, partial-thickness burn wounds
Synthetic		
Op-Site (3M Medical-Surgical Division, St. Paul, MN)	Semipermeable adherent polyurethane film	Donor site dressing (requires 2-inch margin of intact skin around donor site) To protect and facilitate healing of partial-thickness burn wounds
N-Terface Interpositional Surfacing Material (Winfield Laboratories, Inc., Richardson, TX)	Translucent netting material permeable to air and fluid	To protect newly applied meshed autografts or cultured epithelial autografts
Fine mesh gauze	Gauze dressing with or without impregnated petroleum	Donor site dressing To protect autografts before complete healing of interstices

Table 36–9. Burn Care for Special Areas

Body Area	Considerations for Care
Scalp	Shave hair in and around the wound margins (to within 1 inch).
Ears (auricles)	Protect burned ears from pressure; they are at risk for chondritis. Ensure there is no pillow beneath the patient's head. Use the exposure method to apply a topical antimicrobial agent to this area. Mafenide acetate (Sulfamylon) cream is commonly used to treat burned auricles. Inspect the ear canals daily for debris buildup and carefully remove debris.
Lips	Use a lubricant to keep the lips clean and moist.
Perineum	In male patients, the scrotum may become edematous and require protection from pressure and excoriation. Inspect the urinary catheter insertion site for drainage and erosion. Shave perineal hair in and around the wound margin (to within 1 inch). Cleanse perineal wound immediately after urine or stool incontinence and reapply the topical antimicrobial agent.

1. *Expected outcomes:* Following interventions, the patient should be able to state that pain is alleviated or reduced.
2. *Nursing interventions*
   a. During the emergent phase, give intravenous narcotics to manage pain. Morphine sulfate administered in small, frequent doses is the most commonly used pain medication during the emergent phase.

NURSE ADVISORY

Do not use the oral or intramuscular routes to administer pain medication for the patient with a major burn injury during the emergent phase of recovery. During this phase, gastrointestinal dysfunction, hypovolemia, and large intravascular fluid shifts make absorption of the medication unreliable.

   b. During the acute phase, use both pharmacologic and nonpharmacologic interventions for pain management.
      (1) Pharmacologic interventions include narcotics, hypnotics, sedatives, nonnarcotic analgesics, antianxiety medications, and subanesthetic doses of anesthetic agents.
         • Narcotics commonly used are morphine sulfate, meperidine, and hydromorphone.
         • Moderate to high doses are given for procedural pain.
         • Continuous intravenous infusions using morphine sulfate are used to treat background pain.
         • Patient-controlled analgesia, typically using morphine sulfate, provides the patient more pain control through self-administration of the prescribed analgesic (see Chapter 13).
         • Hypnotics, sedatives, nonnarcotic analgesics, and antianxiety medications are used in combination with narcotics. These medications help treat the psychologic component of pain.
         • Subanesthetic doses of anesthetic agents (e.g., ketamine, nitrous oxide) produce short-acting analgesia that relieves procedural pain during major dressing changes.
      (2) Nonpharmacologic interventions include hypnosis, relaxation techniques, music therapy, therapeutic touch, behavior modification, desensitization, and imagery. These interventions are used in conjunction with pharmacologic treatment.

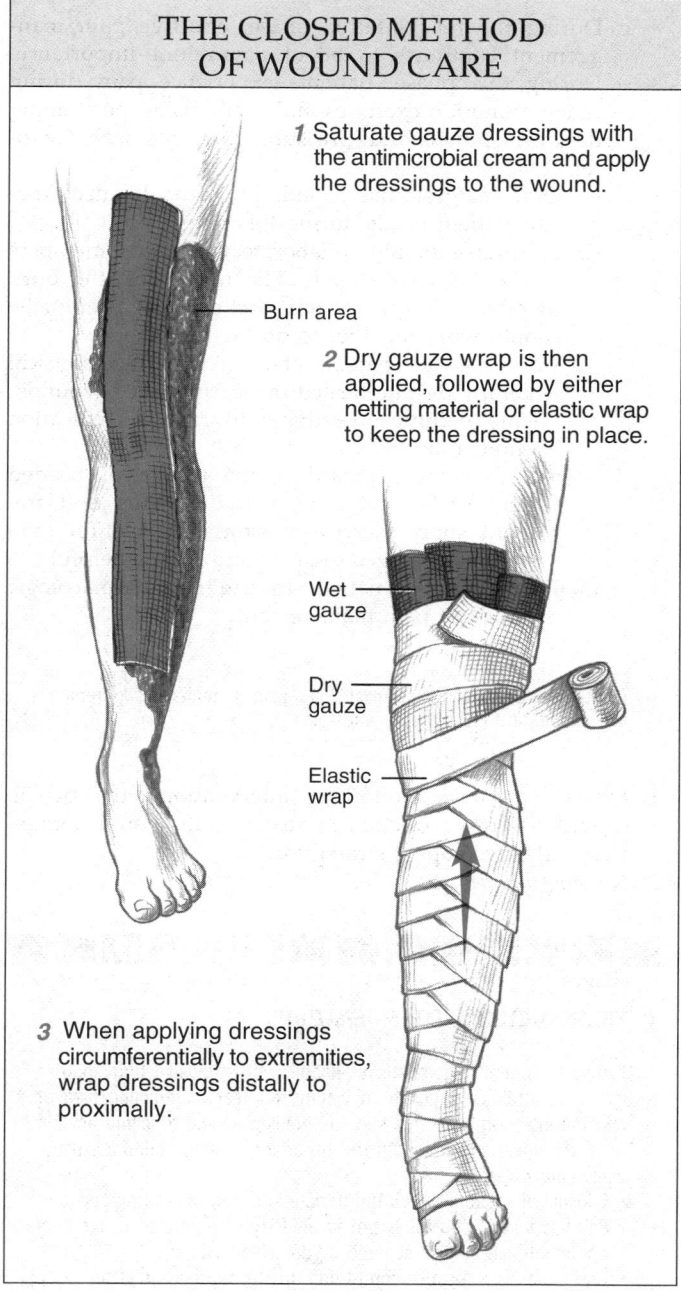

THE CLOSED METHOD OF WOUND CARE

1 Saturate gauze dressings with the antimicrobial cream and apply the dressings to the wound.

— Burn area

2 Dry gauze wrap is then applied, followed by either netting material or elastic wrap to keep the dressing in place.

Wet gauze —

Dry gauze —

Elastic wrap —

3 When applying dressings circumferentially to extremities, wrap dressings distally to proximally.

Figure 36–10.

(3) Both pharmacologic and nonpharmacologic treatments are individualized for each patient and are assessed daily for continued effectiveness.

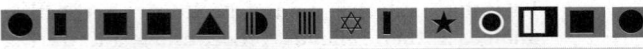

TRANSCULTURAL CONSIDERATIONS

With procedures that involve the genitals or other sexual organs, it is often important that the health care provider be the same gender as the patient. Same gender is especially important for cultures that believe in a strict division of labor between the sexes.

c. During the rehabilitative phase, effective pain management continues to be of paramount importance. During this phase, patients experience pain during range-of-motion exercises and while using positioning devices, splints, and pressure garments (see Chapter 7).
(1) Oral analgesic use is individualized to meet specific patient needs during this phase.
(2) The nurse should collaborate with other members of the burn care team. The nurse and the burn therapists (physical and occupational therapists) should work together to do the following:
 • Educate the patient about continuing physical therapy despite healed or nearly healed wounds
 • Time painful procedures to follow medication administration
 • Offer choices regarding the timing of needed therapy. For example, many patients find frequent short exercise sessions less painful than infrequent longer sessions and just as helpful.
(3) Encourage the patient to use nonpharmacologic methods of pain management.

NURSING DIAGNOSIS: Anxiety R/T pain, potential disfigurement, and change in future identity and role

1. *Expected outcomes:* Following interventions, the person should report a reduction in anxiety and should demonstrate effective coping strategies.
2. *Nursing interventions*

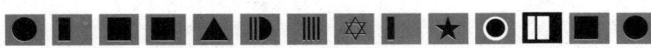

TRANSCULTURAL CONSIDERATIONS

Family members and friends of people with extensive burn injuries are often afraid to touch burn victims for fear of inflicting pain or causing infection. Gestures such as holding hands, touching an arm or a shoulder, and hugging are important in many cultures, especially Latin ones.
• Educate all visitors about appropriate infection control practices.
• Emphasize that contact is not forbidden but is limited to areas of unburned skin or skin covered by dressing materials.
• Use touch as a form of comforting in your nursing practice.

a. Determine how the patient has coped with stressful situations in the past. Assess patient and family coping abilities and strategies throughout hospitalization.
b. To reduce anxiety, explain the rationale for all treatments, procedures, and unfamiliar equipment to both the patient and the patient's family. The explanation should be brief, simple, and easy to understand.
c. Arrange for an interpreter for patients or family members with limited English proficiency.
d. Provide emotional support as needed.
e. Provide adequate pain medication (pain and discomfort magnify anxiety).

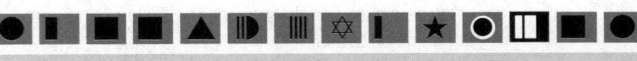

TRANSCULTURAL CONSIDERATIONS

In some cultures—Asian, Hispanic, and Native American among them—the family, not the individual, is the decision maker.

f. Give family members information regarding lodging, parking, area cafeterias and restaurants, visitation rules, and the burn center phone number.
g. Help the patient deal with stress by providing examples of coping strategies used by other people (e.g., diversion, music therapy, relaxation techniques).
h. Promote the patient's self-confidence and reduce the patient's anxiety by doing the following: Maintaining continuity in care providers, involving the patient and family members in care and treatment planning, and adhering to a consistent treatment schedule.
i. Provide an atmosphere of acceptance.
j. Consult with the psychiatric clinical nurse specialist, transcultural clinical nurse specialist, or psychologist when needed.

NURSING DIAGNOSIS: Fear R/T possibility of dying, pain, potential disfigurement, and change in future identity and role

1. *Expected outcomes:* Following interventions, the patient should be able to demonstrate effective coping strategies.
2. *Nursing interventions*
Refer to the interventions listed for anxiety.

NURSING DIAGNOSIS: Self-esteem disturbance R/T threatened or actual change in body image, physical loss, and loss of role responsibilities

1. *Expected outcomes:* Following interventions, the patient should be able to verbalize positive and realistic perception of the self.
2. *Nursing interventions*
a. Explore the patient's value system, expectations of hospitalization, and prior means of coping.
b. Assess the patient's support system. Work with the family to increase the patient's self-esteem.

c. Explain and reinforce the expected appearance of burns and grafts during the different phases of wound maturation.

d. Encourage a realistic perception of the changes in the patient's body image.

e. If current dependency is due to short-term limitations, reassure the person, without providing false hope, that independence will be regained.

f. Help the patient and family accept cosmetic and functional impairments. Encourage contact with others outside the patient's immediate family. Many burn centers make it possible for patients and family members to speak with other people who are injured or who have recovered from injury. Some centers offer both group support meetings and one-to-one sessions.

g. When medically appropriate, provide passes for brief excursions outside the hospital.

h. Discuss how to deal with potential social situations to help the person prepare for life after discharge.

i. Consult with the psychiatric clinical nurse specialist, transcultural clinical nurse specialist, or psychologist when needed.

NURSING DIAGNOSIS: Ineffective individual coping R/T emergency and critical nature of injury, and separation from family and friends

1. *Expected outcomes:* Following interventions, the patient should be able to verbalize feelings and to identify effective coping strategies.
2. *Nursing interventions*
   a. Provide an atmosphere of acceptance, trust, and caring. Communicate your accessibility to the patient.
   b. Encourage the patient to verbalize feelings, perceptions, and fears.
   c. Explore the patient's prior means of coping.
   d. Help the patient to identify new coping strategies.
   e. Provide positive reinforcement when effective coping strategies are utilized.
   f. Encourage the involvement of the patient's family in the coping process. Encourage visitation from family and close friends.
   g. Explain all procedures, diagnostic studies, and treatments. Ensure that the patient and family remain informed of the patient's physical condition and progress.
   h. Consult with pastoral care and social services as needed.

NURSING DIAGNOSIS: Impaired physical mobility R/T wound edema, pain, dressings, splints, enforced immobility due to surgical procedures, hypertrophic scarring, and wound contractures

1. *Expected outcomes:* Following interventions, the patient should be able to achieve maximum physical mobility.
2. *Nursing interventions*
   a. Perform a comprehensive assessment of the patient's range of motion, muscle strength, gait, general coordination and movement, and preinjury activity level.
   b. Assess pain level before and after activity. Administer analgesics before activity as needed.
   c. Provide physical therapy (see Chapter 7). Explain rationale for activities and positioning to the patient and family.
   d. Work closely with occupational and physical therapists to identify the physical therapy needs of burn patients. Physical therapy consists of active and passive range-of-motion exercises, stretching exercises, ambulation, splinting, and therapeutic positioning.
   e. Encourage active range-of-motion exercises every 2 to 4 hours while the patient is awake, unless such activity is contraindicated because of a recent surgical procedure. Active range-of-motion exercises help reduce edema and maintain strength and joint function.
   f. Provide passive range-of-motion and stretching exercises for patients who cannot perform active exercises (e.g., a comatose or chemically paralyzed patient). Passive range-of-motion exercises help to prevent tightening of muscles and ligaments that may form contractures.
   g. Encourage ambulation to maintain strength and range of motion in the lower extremities. Before placing a leg in any dependent position, wrap the burned legs and unburned legs with donor sites in elastic wraps using the figure-of-8 technique (see Fig. 36–10). As healing progresses, other elasticized support bandages or garments can be worn.
   h. Splint joints to maintain proper joint positioning and help prevent or correct wound contractures.
   i. Provide therapeutic positioning to help prevent or correct wound contractures (Table 36–10). Allowing the patient to assume a position of comfort often contributes to contractures. It is therefore important to position burned areas opposite to the anticipated contracture.
   j. Educate the patient and family regarding the need to continue physical therapy until the wounds have fully matured. This process may take many years from the time of injury.
   k. Plan rehabilitative care. The rehabilitative challenges facing the burn care team arise from the development of hypertrophic scarring and wound contractures.
      (1) Hypertrophic burn scar initially appears red and inflamed. The color of the scar typically changes from deep red or purple to pink during maturation. In the early stages of recovery, the scar is often fragile, lacks extensibility, and is raised above the normal skin level. The burn scar commonly matures in 6 to 18 months.
      (2) The severity of hypertrophic scarring depends on burn depth and extent, the type of graft, and the patient's age and race. Children tend to have more severe hypertrophic scarring and wound contractures than adults with similar burn injuries. For genetic reasons, some people scar worse than others, especially fair-skinned, Asian, and Black people.
   l. The burn scar is managed through both surgical and nonsurgical means.

Table 36–10. Therapeutic Techniques for the Adult Burn Patient

Burned Area	Therapeutic Position	Positioning Techniques
Neck		
Anterior	Extension	No pillow Small towel roll beneath cervical spine to promote neck extension (*A*)
Circumferential	Neutral toward extension	No pillow
Posterior or asymmetric	Neutral	No pillow
Shoulder/axilla	Arm abduction to 90-110°	Splinting Arms positioned away from body and supported on arm troughs (*B*)
Elbow	Arm extension	Elbow splint Elbows positioned in extension with slight bend at elbow (no greater than 10° elbow flexion) (*B*) Arms supported on arm troughs, forearm in slight pronation
Hand		
Wrist	Wrist extension	Hand splint
Metacarpal interphalangeal joints (MCP)	MCP flexion at 90°	Hand splint
Proximal and distal interphalangeal joints (PIP/DIP)	PIP/DIP extension	Hand splint
Thumb	Thumb abduction	Hand splint with thumb abduction
Web spaces	Finger abduction	Web spacers of gauze, foam, or thermoplastics to decrease webbing formation
Hip	Hip extension	Supine with head of bed flat, legs extended (*C*) Trochanter roll to maintain neutral hip rotation (toes should point toward ceiling) Prone positioning
Knee	Knee extension	Supine, knees extended (toes should point toward ceiling) Prone position, feet extended over end of mattress (*D*) Sitting in chair, legs extended and elevated Knee splint
Ankle	Neutral	Padded footboard Ankle positioning devices (avoid ankle inversion and eversion positions) (*E,F*)

A

B 90° 90°

C 15°

D 90°

E *F* 90°

From Carrougher GJ. Nursing care of the client with burn injury. *In* Black JM, and Matassarin-Jacobs E (eds). *Luckmann and Sorensen's Medical-Surgical Nursing: A Psychophysiologic Approach.* 4th ed. Philadelphia: WB Saunders, 1993.

(1) Surgical procedures depend on the anatomic area involved and the preferences of the surgeon. Procedures for the release of hypertrophic scar include split-thickness and full-thickness skin grafts, skin flaps (free flaps and pedicle flaps), Z-plasties, and tissue expansion.

(2) Pressure therapy is the primary nonsurgical approach to the prevention and control of a burn scar. Pressure dressings are used in the early stages of care, before complete wound closure. After tissue edema is reduced and the wounds are nearly closed, the patient should wear custom-fit pressure garments 23 hours per day until the scar has matured (Fig. 36–11). Garments are taken off for bathing, and patients should be fitted with at least 2 pairs of pressure garments to allow for cleaning of the garments between use.

NURSING DIAGNOSIS: Self-care deficit (grooming, bathing, eating, elimination) R/T functional deficits resulting from the burn injury, pain, dressings, splints, and enforced immobility due to surgical procedures and wound contractures

1. *Expected outcomes:* Following interventions, the patient should be able to achieve maximum independence in self-care activities.
2. *Nursing interventions*
   a. Perform a comprehensive assessment of the patient's ability to perform self-care activities.
   b. Consult with an occupational therapist regarding aids to assist the patient with feeding, bathing, and grooming. Provide assistive devices as needed.
   c. Develop an individualized teaching program for the patient. Specify a step-by-step plan of what the pa-

tient needs to know to overcome the deficit. Include time for teaching, return demonstration, and evaluation.
   d. Encourage the patient to participate in self-care tasks. This will help the patient to assume responsibility for care and provide information for continued assessment.
   e. Ensure that the patient has adequate time to accomplish the task.
   f. Provide positive reinforcement when tasks are accomplished.
   g. Consult with community health agency before discharge for evaluation of the home environment as needed.

NURSING DIAGNOSIS: Injury, risk for, R/T corneal abrasions or chemical injury to the eyes

1. *Expected outcomes:* Following interventions, the patient should incur no further injury from known complications of burn injury.
2. *Nursing interventions*
   a. For burn patients injured in a fire, flash, or explosion, evaluate the eyes for corneal injury in the emergency department.
      (1) Fluorescein staining is used to evaluate the condition of the cornea.
      (2) If a corneal abrasion is present, the nurse should ensure that the eyelashes are not turning in and scratching the cornea. The nurse should verify that the patient's eyes can close completely and should check for exudate buildup that may indicate infection. Apply appropriate agents to keep eyes moist and free from infection as prescribed.

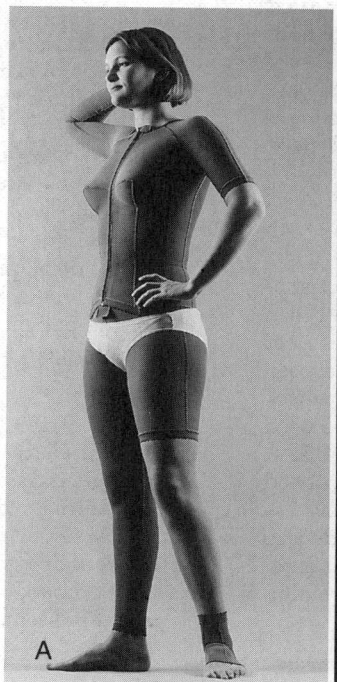
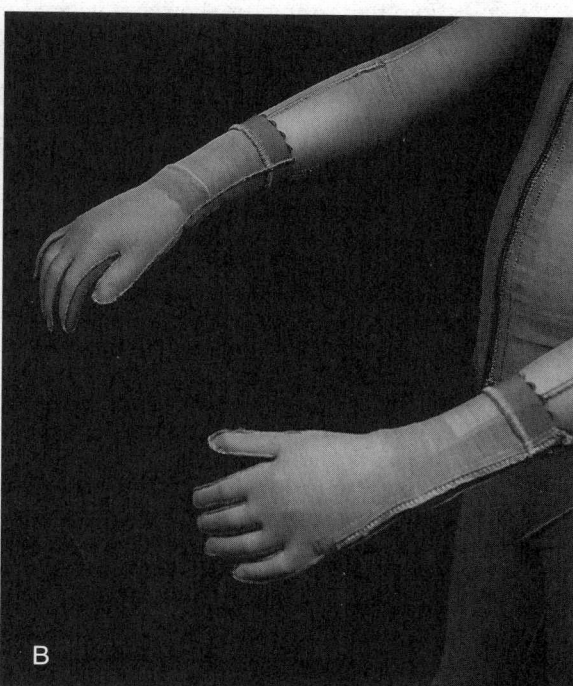

Figure 36–11. Custom-fit pressure therapy support garments. (Courtesy of Medical Z. Corp., San Antonio, TX.)

LEARNING/TEACHING GUIDELINES
for Skin Care After Hospitalization

General Overview

1. Describe the process of wound healing after a burn injury, emphasizing that newly healed skin requires special care after hospitalization.
2. Discuss bathing, care of dry skin and blisters, sun and cold exposure, and itching.
3. Discuss the importance of nutrition and diet to aid healing and skin maturation.
4. Discuss the importance of continuing with an exercise program at home to prevent contractures.

Skin Care

1. Educate your patient on the following skin care issues:
   a. Dry skin
      (1) Burn injuries can damage or destroy the glands that provide lubricating oils to the skin, leading to dry skin.
      (2) To prevent dryness, a thin layer of a moisturizer should be applied so that no oily film can be felt on the skin.
      (3) Natural lubricants such as vitamin E or cocoa butter are commonly used. Products that contain perfumes, alcohol, or lanolin should be avoided, because these products may tend to irritate and create blisters in newly healed skin.
   b. Bathing
      (1) Bathing should be in the patient's usual manner.
      (2) The water temperature should be tested before the bathtub or shower is entered. Healed burned skin is more sensitive to extreme temperatures and can be injured easily.
      (3) Washing should be gentle with a mild soap. All creams and loose particles of skin should be removed. The patient should rinse thoroughly and pat dry with a clean towel.
   c. Sun and cold exposure
      (1) Newly healed skin is more sensitive to both sun and cold exposure.
      (2) New skin tends to sunburn easily. Direct sunlight should be avoided at all times. When exposed to the sun, the patient should wear light clothing over body areas that have been burned and a large hat when the face or neck has been burned. A sunscreen should be used to block the sun's harmful ultraviolet rays. A light layer of sunscreen should be rubbed gently into the skin until it is completely absorbed. It should be reapplied as needed to keep the skin protected. Sunscreen is especially important when the person is swimming or sweating.
      (3) New skin is more sensitive to the cold because it is thinner than uninjured skin. Prolonged exposures to the cold should be avoided. Warm clothing should be worn. Some slight tingling is normal in hands and feet when the weather is cold but this sensation should diminish as the skin toughens.
      (4) Newly healed skin remains sun and cold sensitive for at least 1 year after injury.
   d. Blisters
      (1) Blisters often occur in newly healed skin because of friction (rubbing against bed linens), bumping against an object, or standing for prolonged periods without adequate support from pressure garments.
      (2) The tendency to form blisters decreases as the skin matures and thickens.
      (3) Before discharge, the patient should discuss how to care for blisters with the physician.
   e. Itching
      (1) Itching is usually associated with dry skin. Scratching may cause the skin to break open and should be avoided. The patient should soak in a tepid bath for short periods, then lightly apply a moisturizer to decrease itching. For severe itching, the physician may prescribe a medication to help relieve the itching.

Nutrition and Diet

1. Educate your patient about the importance of maintaining a healthy diet after discharge from the hospital.
   a. Nutrition and diet continue to be important for complete healing of skin and general health.
   b. A diet rich in protein is recommended. Protein may be obtained from beans, nuts, cheese, fish, eggs, meat, poultry, and milk.
   c. Vitamins and minerals are also important for healing and normal body functioning. They are found in whole-grain cereals, fruits and vegetables, dairy products, and protein-rich foods.
2. If the patient requires a special diet at home, ensure that the patient and dietitian meet before the patient is discharged.

Exercise

1. After discharge from the hospital, a home exercise program is necessary so that skin contractures and joint stiffness do not develop and muscle strength increases.
2. Ensure that a physical therapist has discussed a specific home exercise plan with the patient before the patient's discharge.

b. For the person with a chemical eye injury, immediately and continuously flush the injury with water or normal saline solution until the pH of the cul-de-sacs returns to normal (pH of 7.0). Irrigation systems using a small cannula sutured to the conjunctival sulcus or a scleral contact lens with an irrigating side arm have been used for extended eye irrigation.

(1) This treatment should begin in the field and be continued until an ophthalmologist has evaluated the patient.

(2) Neutralizing agents are generally not recommended because they generate heat (exothermic reaction) that could cause further ocular damage.

NURSE ADVISORY

To reduce the risk of hypothermia, avoid excessive patient exposure.

NURSING DIAGNOSIS: Ineffective thermoregulation R/T epithelial tissue loss

1. *Expected outcomes:* Following interventions, the patient should be normothermic to slightly hyperthermic.
2. *Nursing interventions*
   a. Minimize exposure by covering the patient with a clean, dry cloth while in the emergency department. Ice should not be applied to extensive burn injuries.
   b. Monitor rectal or core temperatures hourly during the emergent and early acute phases of recovery.
   c. Minimize exposure to heat loss during wound care.
      (1) Limit the amount of body surface area exposed.
      (2) Limit hydrotherapy treatment to less than 30 minutes using water temperatures of 37 to 39 degrees Celsius (98.6 to 102.2 degrees Fahrenheit).

TRANSCULTURAL CONSIDERATIONS

Some Hispanic, Asian, Mediterranean, and Middle Eastern groups have strong beliefs about heat and cold as causes and treatments of illness. People from these groups may have trouble understanding why burn patients should be immersed in warm water (hydrotherapy) as a treatment modality and may require further explanations.

(3) Maintain appropriate environmental temperatures for patient rooms, procedure rooms, and operative suites.

(4) Heat shields or heat lamps should be used as needed, with caution, to maintain body temperature.

NURSE ADVISORY

To prevent further injury when using external heat shields or radiant heat lamps, refer to the manufacturers' recommendation for the minimum distance between the patient and the heat source.

Discharge Planning and Teaching

1. Patient and family teaching needs
   a. Teaching should focus on specific needs related to wound care and maturation, infection, nutritional needs and diet, physical therapy and exercise, and emotional readjustment.
   b. Identify specific deficits in knowledge early and address them throughout the hospitalization (see Learning/Teaching Guidelines for Skin Care After Hospitalization).
   c. Specific written guides and handouts facilitate understanding and learning.
2. Discharge planning
   a. Discharge planning begins at the time of admission.
   b. To smooth the transition from hospital to home or rehabilitation facility, consult with the social worker and family to identify the patient's discharge needs in advance.
   c. Patients and their families may need help with insurance, housing, and long-term placement options in preparation for discharge.

HOME CARE STRATEGIES

Burn Care

The goal of care focuses on prevention of infection while promoting healing until a protective skin surface is restored. Patients and caregivers can be instructed in the following:

- The importance of good hand washing before and after dressing changes. Good personal and household cleanliness is important and should be encouraged.
- Dressing change technique. Often patients want to leave burns open to the air owing to discomfort from the dressing, or they believe air will help the site heal. Some patients apply petroleum jelly, thinking it will provide protection. Caution patients that only the prescribed treatment is to be applied to the burn site, and it should be covered with a protective dressing. Emollient lotion can be applied to healed skin.
- Proper storage and maintenance of supplies. Sterilize instruments by boiling or by soaking in an alcohol solution. Signs and symptoms of infection such as fever, redness, or foul odor should be reported.
- Use pain medications with dressing changes and at bedtime to provide maximum comfort.
- Importance of adequate nutrition. Encourage protein intake with each meal. Eggs, dried beans, and peanut butter are inexpensive sources of protein. Eat vitamin C–rich food, such as orange juice or tomatoes, daily to improve the rate of healing. Drink fluids liberally.
- Use basic safety measures to prevent repeat burn accidents. Use hot pads for lifting hot pots and pans as needed when hand grip and strength are a problem. Avoid smoking in bed. Double-check the bath water temperature on the inside of the arm before bathing. Use heating pads cautiously; never sleep on them.

◫ PUBLIC HEALTH CONSIDERATIONS: PREVENTION OF BURNS

Burn Prevention Education

1. Public burn prevention educational programs are provided throughout the United States. They play a critical role in reducing preventable burn injuries.
2. In areas with large populations of people with limited English proficiency, burn prevention programs and signs should be written in native languages.
3. Educational programs focus on the following:
   a. Reducing the likelihood of clothing ignition during routine meal preparation. For example:
      (1) Pot handles should be turned toward the back of the stove.
      (2) Heat controls should be on the front or side of the stove.
      (3) Clothing should be flame-retardant. Flame retard-

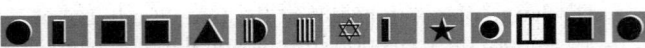

TRANSCULTURAL CONSIDERATIONS

Many Asian, Moslem, Hindu, North African, and Middle Eastern populations require women and female children to wear robes and other garments that are especially vulnerable to cooking fires. The risk is even greater for members of such groups who prefer charcoal fires and for those with little money who are cooking on unsafe stoves.

ant clothing for children has reduced the incidence of burn injuries caused by clothing ignition.

b. Reducing the likelihood of scald injuries.
   (1) The thermostat setting on hot water heaters should be set to produce a temperature of 54.5 degrees Celsius (130 degrees Fahrenheit) or lower. The Consumer Products Safety Commission and Underwriters Laboratory have encouraged manufacturers of hot water heaters to adjust thermostats to the lowest setting before shipping hot water heaters from the factory and to affix caution labels to all hot water heaters warning of the potential for injury.
   (2) A screen should be placed across the front of the stove to reduce the likelihood of children pulling pots off the stove.
   (3) Antiscald devices should be applied to faucets or shower heads. These automatically shut off water flow when the water temperature exceeds a predetermined temperature.
c. Reducing the incidence of residential fires.
   (1) Heating units and chimneys should be routinely checked and cleaned.
   (2) Wood-shingled roofs should be treated with a fire-retardant material.
   (3) A residential sprinkler system should be installed.
   (4) Smoke detectors should work correctly. When they are properly installed and well maintained, smoke and heat detectors provide residents with early warning of home fires, thus allowing time for escape.
   (5) A fire extinguisher should be available for home use.

Bibliography

Books and Manuals

Advanced Burn Life Support Manual. Lincoln, NE: Nebraska Burn Institute, 1990.

Boswick JA (ed). *The Art and Science of Burn Care.* Rockville, MD: Aspen Publishers, 1987.

Herndon DN (ed). *Total Burn Care.* London: WB Saunders Co, 1996.

Martyn JAJ (ed). *Acute Management of the Burned Patient.* Philadelphia: WB Saunders, 1990.

Wachtel TL, Kahn V, and Frank HA (eds). *Current Topics in Burn Care.* Rockville, MD: Aspen Systems Corp, 1983.

Chapters in Books and Journal Articles

American Burn Association. Guidelines for service standards and severity classification in the treatment of burn injury. *Am Coll Surg Bull* 69(10):24–28, 1984.

Ashburn MA. Burn pain: The management of procedure-related pain. *J Burn Care Rehabil* 16(3, part II):365–371, 1995.

Bayley EW. Wound healing in the patient with burns. *Nurs Clin North Am* 25(1):205–222, 1990.

Burgess MC. Initial management of a patient with extensive burn injury. *Crit Care Nurs Clin North Am* 3(2):165–179, 1991.

Calistro AM. Burn care basics and beyond. *RN* 56(3):26–31, 1993.

Carlson DE, and Jordan BS. Implementing nutritional therapy in the thermally injured patient. *Crit Care Nurs Clin North Am* 3(2):221–235, 1991.

Carrougher GJ. Inhalation injury. *AACN Clin Issues Crit Care Nurs* 4(2):367–377, 1993.

Carrougher GJ. Nursing care of the client with burn injury. *In* Black JM and Matassarin-Jacobs E (eds). *Luckmann and Sorensen's Medical-Surgical Nursing: A Psychophysiologic Approach.* 4th ed. Philadelphia: WB Saunders, 1993, pp 1985–2012.

Cioffi WG, and Rue LW. Diagnosis and treatment of inhalation injuries. *Crit Care Nursing Clin North Am* 3(2):191–198, 1991.

Cunningham JJ, Hegarty MT, and Burke JF. Measured and predicted calorie re-

quirements of adults during recovery from severe burn trauma. *Am J Clin Nutr* 49:404–408, 1989.

Curreri PW. Assessing nutritional needs for the burned patient. *J Trauma* 30(suppl):S20–S23, 1990.

Duncan DJ, and Driscoll DM. Burn wound management. *Crit Care Nurs Clin North Am* 3(2):199–219, 1991.

Dyer C, and Roberts D. Thermal trauma. *Nurs Clin North Am* 25(1):85–117, 1990.

Herndon DN, et al. Pulmonary injury in burned patients. *Surg Clin North Am* 67(1):31–45, 1987.

Hildreth MA, et al. Current treatment reduces calories required to maintain weight in pediatric patients with burns. *J Burn Care Rehabil* 11:405–409, 1990.

Kealey GP. Pharmacologic management of background pain in burn victims. *J Burn Care Rehabil* 16(3, part II):358–362, 1995.

Marvin JA. Pain assessment versus measurement. *J Burn Care Rehabil* 16(3, part II):348–357, 1995.

Molter NC. When is the burn injury healed?: Psychosocial implications of care. *AACN Clin Issues Crit Care Nurs* 4(2):424–432, 1993.

Pruitt BA, and Goodwin CW. Burn injury. *In* Moore EE, Ducker TB, and Edlick RF (eds). *Early Care of the Injured Patient.* 4th ed. Philadelphia: Dekker, 1990.

Pruitt BA, Goodwin CW, and Cioffi WG. Thermal injury. *In* Davis JH, and Sheldon GF (eds). *Clinical Surgery.* St. Louis: Mosby–Year Book, 1995, pp 643–720.

Rieg LS. Metabolic alterations and nutritional management. *AACN Clin Issues Crit Care Nurs* 4(2):388–398, 1993.

Rue LW, and Cioffi WG. Resuscitation of thermally injured patients. *Crit Care Nurs Clin North Am* 3(2):181–189, 1991.

Silverstein P, and Lack B. Fire prevention in the United States. *Surg Clin North Am* 67(1):1–14, 1987.

Summers TM. Psychosocial support of the burned patient. *Crit Care Nurs Clin North Am* 3(2):237–244, 1991.

Ward RS. The rehabilitation of burn patients. *CRC Rev Phys Rehabil Med* 2(3):121–138, 1991.

Watkins PN, et al. Psychological stages in adaptation following burn injury: A method for facilitating psychological recovery of burn victims. *J Burn Care Rehabil* 9(4):376–385, 1988.

Watkins PN, et al. Postburn psychologic adaptation of family members of patients with burns. *J Burn Care Rehabil* 17(1):78–92, 1996.

Williamson J. Actual burn nutrition care practices—A national survey (part II). *J Burn Care Rehabil* 10(2):185–194, 1989.

Wilmore DW. Nutrition and metabolism following thermal injury. *Clin Plas Surg* 1(4):603–619, 1974.

Agencies

American Burn Association
(800) 548–BURN

International Society for Burn Injuries
National Burn Institute (Advanced Burn Life Support)
(402) 464–7577

37

Caring for People Experiencing Emergencies

☐ OVERVIEW

Emergency Medical Services

1. Use and overuse of emergency care facilities
   a. The primary mission of an emergency department (ED) is to resuscitate, stabilize, diagnose, treat, and dispose of (admit, discharge, or transfer) individuals with actual or potential life-, limb-, or vision-threatening problems.
   b. Most patients present with a chief complaint or symptoms, rather than a specific diagnosis.
      (1) The emergency care team then function as "detectives" to identify the most likely problem.
      (2) Subtle symptoms may mask life-threatening problems.
   c. Despite the ED's mission, most problems treated in an ED are not life threatening.
   d. People with non–life-threatening problems seek ED care because of the following:
      (1) They lack access to care elsewhere because of time of day, physician unavailability, location, inconvenience, or insurance coverage.
      (2) They do not know where else to go.
      (3) They perceive the need for treatment to be immediate.
      (4) They are directed there by private physicians or office staff.
      (5) They can have a fairly thorough diagnostic workup done in a relatively short period of time.
   e. The consumer, not the staff, defines the emergency.
   f. Federal law requires EDs to assess every person who presents for care, regardless of how minor a problem appears; laws governing ED assessment are discussed in the legal section.
   g. Factors that impede emergency care include the following:
      (1) A large number of people with nonurgent problems
      (2) Limited impatient bed availability so patients are held in the ED for long periods
      (3) Space constraints that affect ability of staff to provide care to new patients
      (4) Diversion of ambulances to other facilities because of ED saturation or lack of critical care beds

   h. Time required for treatment is the most frequent reason for dissatisfaction among emergency patients.
      (1) Legal requirements, consumer perceptions of the urgency of health care need, and limited alternatives contribute to the problem.
      (2) Long waits for problems that are not emergencies are frustrating to both consumers and care providers.
   i. Major emergency nursing roles are to do the following:
      (1) Triage, assess, and set priorities for a wide spectrum of clinical situations of varying urgency, from life-threatening to chronic
      (2) Assess and provide care for individuals of all ages and conditions
      (3) Initiate timely care with limited information
      (4) Provide emotional support to the patient and family members
      (5) Facilitate spiritual support
      (6) Coordinate multiple diagnostic tests and care by multiple disciplines
      (7) Succinctly document and communicate information regarding care delivered and that needed for ongoing treatment
      (8) Facilitate referral for resolution of problems that cannot be addressed during the emergency care period
      (9) Assist the individual in the adaptations that are necessary to perform activities of daily living
      (10) Facilitate continuity of care through the use of community resources
      (11) Promote safe discharge and ongoing care through teaching and discharge planning
      (12) Comply with laws and procedures related to public health or welfare; for example, the emergency nurse must report communicable diseases, animal bites, potential criminal acts, and evidence collection
      (13) Communicate with, and provide on-line medical direction to emergency medical services (EMS) personnel
      (14) Facilitate institutional and community disaster response
2. Rural emergency care
   a. Providing emergency care in rural areas is a special challenge because of the following:

(1) Limited number of facilities and practitioners

(2) Hospital and ED closures for financial reasons, including low hospital occupancy rates and expensive regulatory requirements

(3) Limited continuing education opportunities

(4) Inadequate health care insurance coverage

(5) Vast geographic areas with disproportionate numbers of residents

(6) Prehospital emergency care constraints

- Heavy reliance on volunteer emergency medical technicians who may not be able to respond immediately to an emergency call
- Long travel times for volunteers to get to the station where the emergency vehicle is located
- Infrequent calls so that skill maintenance is impeded, creating significant training needs
- Geographic and topographic features such as mountains and wilderness create long scene response times and long transport times to an emergency facility.
- Limited advanced life support capabilities (e.g., intravenous therapy, medication administration, and invasive airway management [endotracheal intubation]) because the population density may not support such a level of care.

b. Transfer from a rural facility to an urban one may require ground or air medical transport teams.

(1) Team availability may be limited.

(2) Weather conditions may affect feasibility.

(3) Cost may be viewed as prohibitive.

3. Emergency medical services systems (EMSS)

a. Emergency medical services systems development in the United States is fairly recent.

(1) Research in the late 1960s indicated unnecessary death and disability were occurring due to the lack of a comprehensive system of care for the seriously ill or injured.

(2) The EMS Systems Act of 1973 was passed to address these needs.

b. The EMS Systems Act and state efforts identified and provided limited funding for essentials of an EMS system, including the following:

(1) Universal access (e.g., telephoning 911)

(2) Training of prehospital providers at the basic (emergency medical technician) and advanced (paramedic) life support level

(3) Facility designation for high-risk problems (trauma, cardiac incidents, and burns; neonatal, psychiatric, and pediatric emergencies)

(4) Radio communications between EMS providers and hospitals (Hospital emergency administrative radio [HEAR system])

(5) Prehospital and hospital equipment (e.g., ambulances, cardiac monitors, defibrillators)

(6) Disaster preparedness

(7) Public information and education on illness and injury prevention and proper use of EMS systems

c. The star of life, the symbol of EMS, illustrates key components: detection, reporting, response, on-scene care, care in transit, and transfer to definitive care.

d. Despite significant strides, many areas of the United States have inadequate EMS systems:

(1) Lack of 911 or centralized dispatch

(2) Long response times

(3) Limited access to EMS

(4) Lack of designated trauma facilities

(5) Inadequate funding for EMS

- Controversy over whether EMS is a right and must be provided by the local government or a privilege for which user fees should be charged.
- Concern that charging users for EMS may deter those who need it most
- Concern that a failure to charge fees results in abuse of the EMS system, with people using it as a taxi system, and tying up EMS personnel and vehicles; this adversely affects those who have real need for the service

e. With health care reform, there is concern that

(1) The EMS personnel will be expected to triage the sick and injured and deny transport to all but the most seriously ill or injured.

(2) Insurance plans may contract with selected ambulance services to provide EMS, thus significantly affecting the systems that have developed.

(3) Hospital contracts may require that patients be taken to a specific facility rather than to the most appropriate facility.

4. EMS communications

a. Adequate communication systems among the citizen who needs the service, dispatch centers, prehospital providers, and receiving facilities are essential.

b. The HEAR system was implemented as part of the EMS Systems Act; many other systems are now used.

c. Fire service frequencies if EMS is provided by a fire service.

d. Dedicated medical communication system, known as MEDCOM, is used.

e. Cellular phones may be used.

f. Satellites may enhance communication in rural or wilderness areas.

g. Radio or telephone lines are used to transmit cardiac rhythm strips or 12-lead electrocardiograms to ED medical control.

h. An ED may have a number of dedicated EMS radios and telephones that are answered only by specially educated medical or nursing personnel qualified to provide medical direction to EMS personnel.

i. Radio frequencies

(1) Frequencies are licensed by the Federal Communications Commission.

(2) Specific radio procedures must be used.

(3) Radio frequencies and cellular phone lines can be (and often are) monitored by the general public or the media.

(4) Patient name and sensitive information (e.g., human immunodeficiency virus [HIV] status) are not transmitted.

j. Well-educated dispatchers obtain information necessary to activate the appropriate response vehicle, reassure callers, and instruct them on measures to perform while EMS is en route, for example, care for a choking victim, cardiopulmonary resuscitation (CPR), and emergency childbirth.

5. Trauma care elements
   a. Trauma care requires a specific organized system of care, training of pre- and inhospital care providers, and facilities with immediately available personnel who are qualified to resuscitate, stabilize, perform prompt surgical intervention, and provide critical care services and rehabilitation.
   b. Trauma facilities that treat 500 or more cases per year have the best outcomes.
   c. Trauma center designation is required so that injured individuals are taken to the most appropriate trauma facility rather than simply the closest facility.
   d. Trauma centers are designated as levels 1 to 5, based on the American College of Surgeons criteria.
      (1) Level 1 center is the highest designation. It provides the most complex care, with a commitment to training, outreach services, and research.
      (2) Level 5 facility resuscitates, stabilizes, and transfers.
   e. Designation requires the following:
      (1) Written institutional commitment by the board of directors and medical staff levels
      (2) Necessary equipment, supplies, personnel, and support systems
      (3) Trauma registry
      (4) Ongoing evaluation of clinical outcomes
      (5) On-site visitation by a survey team composed of trauma surgeon, emergency physician, and trauma nurse coordinator
      (6) Periodic renewal by resurvey
   f. Trauma registry
      (1) Collects data on major trauma frequency and outcomes
      (2) Prehospital providers and trauma facilities collect and submit registry data to the state EMS office on a routine basis.
      (3) Calculates probability of survival or nonsurvival using physiologic parameters (e.g., trauma score and trauma injury severity score), mechanism of injury, and patient age
      (4) Targets injury prevention education and legislation

Medical, Legal, and Ethical Considerations

1. General concepts
   a. Emergency care providers often must initiate care in the absence of detailed information, are required to act quickly, and must make decisions that seem to be in the best interest of the individual when his or her wishes cannot be determined.
   b. Consent is assumed in persons who communicate their wishes.
   c. Emergency care providers are also required to consider the public health and safety, which may supersede the individual's right to privacy or confidentiality.

   d. Basic demographic and condition information about individuals who are cared for by public agencies (e.g., publically funded EMS or fire services) may be considered public information, and thus is not subject to the rules of confidentiality that generally apply to hospitalized individuals, especially if it is transmitted over radio frequencies.

2. Consent for care
   a. Consent to provide care is either expressed or implied.
      (1) Verbal or written consent to treat is expressed consent.
      (2) When a person is unable to give consent, by virtue of physical or mental impairment, consent to treat is implied.
   b. Although there may be state variation, in general, parental consent to treat is required for individuals younger than age 18, with the following exceptions:
      (1) Children age 14 or older may give consent for their own treatment of suspected sexually transmitted diseases, for pregnancy-related issues, and for treatment for alcohol or drug problems.
      (2) Children age 14 or older who are living independently and assuming responsibility for their own financial affairs may be considered "emancipated minors" and thus able to provide consent.
      (3) Children age 14 or older who are parents may give consent for the care of their children.
   c. In cases of suspected child abuse, contacting the parent for consent may endanger the child; administrative approval is usually obtained until court-authorized consent is obtained.
   d. Treatment is initiated on children who present with life-threatening conditions while efforts are made to contact parents or legal guardians.
      (1) Some facilities maintain preauthorized consent for care on file.
      (2) Consents provided by sitters or caregivers are generally accepted.
      (3) Consent is generally limited to emergency care and does not include surgery.
   e. Special consent may be required for certain procedures, depending on state law or hospital policy:
      (1) Testing for HIV
      (2) Blood or blood product administration
      (3) Drug testing for legal purposes
      (4) Alcohol testing for legal purposes
      (5) Evidence collection, such as in sexual assault cases
      (6) Photographs
      (7) Release of medical records to public safety agencies, for example, police, in probable or actual criminal cases
      (8) High-risk procedures

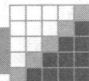

LEGAL AND ETHICAL CONSIDERATIONS

When immediate surgery is necessary and consent cannot be obtained from the patient or legal representative, the surgeon and the hospital administration assume responsibility for proceeding without consent.

f. A patient with a written "durable power of attorney for health care" has a representative who is authorized to make treatment decisions on behalf of the patient.

g. Only *written* advanced directives (e.g., "Do not resuscitate" orders) can be honored by emergency care personnel; this, unfortunately, causes much ill will at times when EMS personnel must refuse verbal instructions.

h. Most organ procurement agencies require consent of next of kin for organ or tissue donation, even though the patient may have a properly executed donor card.

3. Regulations related to providing emergency care
a. The Emergency Medical Treatment and Active Labor Act (EMTALA), part of the Consolidated Omnibus Budget Reconciliation Act (COBRA)
   (1) Originally called an antidumping law to prevent transfer of indigent people to another facility without assessment and stabilization; most people refer to it as COBRA
   (2) Requires medical screening for everyone who seeks emergency care or is in labor to determine whether an emergency exists
   (3) Does not require that screening be done by a physician
   (4) Prohibits transfer of a person to another facility without his or her permission
   (5) Authorizes fines and sanctions against the facility or practitioner for noncompliance
   (6) Mandates posting of informational signage in registration and treatment areas that outlines the requirement
   (7) Requires written evidence of compliance, usually through a transfer form signed by the patient and by the health care practitioner, attesting to reason for transfer, patient acceptance, and names of receiving facility agent and accepting physician
   (8) Requires appropriate care during transport
   (9) Includes "whistle blower" protection to prevent punishment of people who report potential COBRA violations
b. State and other federal laws require that charity care be provided.
c. Accrediting agencies' standards also address patient access to emergency care.

4. Good Samaritan laws
a. Provide protection from liability to individuals who voluntarily and without compensation provide assistance to ill or injured persons in a medical emergency
b. Health care professionals will most likely be held to a standard that is consistent with their education and experience.
c. Protection does not apply in cases of gross negligence.
d. Despite health care professionals' fears of liability, such claims have not been reported.

5. Evidence collection, preservation, and chain of custody
a. Emergency care personnel
   (1) Frequently encounter evidence associated with potential criminal acts (e.g., bullets, knives, tissue, blood, and clothing)
   (2) Are required to retrieve, handle, and secure evidence using well-defined procedures that protect the quality and integrity of the evidence
b. Basic concepts of evidence handling are discussed on page 1790.

◼ ESTABLISHING EMERGENCY CARE PRIORITIES

Ensuring Personal Safety

1. Evaluate the emergency scene to determine immediate threats to your welfare, such as the following:
   a. Oncoming traffic at the accident scene
   b. A disturbed person wielding a weapon
   c. Hazardous chemicals
   d. Blood-borne and airborne diseases such as acquired immunodeficiency syndrome (AIDS), hepatitis, tuberculosis, and meningitis
2. Wait for police to clear the scene if violence has been reported.
3. Ask someone to direct traffic if the emergency occurs on a roadway.
4. Recognize someone who is potentially violent, and try to defuse the situation.
5. If you must restrain someone, be sure help is available.
6. Use safety devices, protective garb, and appropriate equipment to prevent transmission of disease.

NURSE ADVISORY

Protective glasses or face shields, gowns, and thick gloves, such as chemotherapy gloves, are recommended when exposure to blood or other body fluids is likely.

---

7. Be very careful when checking clothing for identification or weapons. There may be broken glass, uncapped needles, or open knives.
8. Report exposures and get medical evaluation promptly.

Establishing Control and Rapport

1. People who are experiencing emergencies appreciate someone who takes control of the situation and directs others in the performance of meaningful activities.
2. Taking charge enables you to gain cooperation and provide direction to the ill or injured person and others.
3. Establish eye contact with the ill or injured person. Calmly and clearly state your name and role, and outline the steps you will be taking to address the emergency.
4. Clearly state what you expect from the ill or injured person.

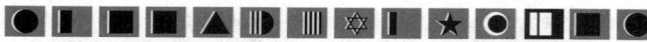

TRANSCULTURAL CONSIDERATIONS

Establishing or maintaining eye contact may be uncomfortable for certain cultural groups.

5. Ask the person's name while placing your hand on the person's hand or arm. This action accomplishes several things at once.

NURSE ADVISORY

The use of touch may be considered threatening in individuals with acute behavioral disturbances and in certain ethnic groups.

    a. It establishes connection with the person.
    b. It provides key assessment data:
       (1) Level of consciousness
       (2) Ability to follow commands
       (3) Orientation
       (4) Skin temperature
       (5) Skin moisture
       (6) Skin turgor
    c. It decreases the amount of stress, allowing the ill or injured person to focus on maintaining homeostasis, instead of using vital energy to deal with stress.

Triage and Setting Priorities

1. In an emergency, triage is the process of determining the nature and urgency of each person's health problem and further prioritizing the conditions that demand attention.
2. The triage category to which a person is assigned is based on the chief complaint or presenting problem, problem-focused historical data, mechanism of injury, preexisting health conditions, and primary and secondary surveys or assessments.
3. Emergency facilities and agencies generally use 1 of 3 kinds of triage systems:
    a. Numbers: category 1, 2, or 3, with 1 being the most critical and 3 being the least critical, although the opposite may be true. The number of categories may be greater as well (e.g., 1–6).
    b. Terms: emergent, urgent, nonurgent or immediate, delayed, minimal
    c. Colors: red, yellow, or green, with red being most critical and green being least critical
4. Triage categories used in day-to-day emergencies may differ from those used in disasters (see "Disaster Operations").

Performing the Primary Survey

1. The primary survey is a rapid, systematic assessment to identify and treat immediately life-threatening situations.

It involves the ABCs: *Airway, breathing, circulation;* consciousness and stability of the cervical spine are also assessed.

NURSE ADVISORY

In a multiply injured person, the most visible and dramatic injuries may be the least significant ones. Rapid systematic assessment of the ABCs and cervical spine protection are essential.

    a. Evaluate airway patency and effectiveness by looking for chest wall expansion and listening for and feeling airway exchange against your hand or face.
       (1) The airway is patent if the person can speak.
       (2) The number of words the person speaks before taking a breath indicates the degree of respiratory distress.
       (3) The respiratory rate indicates the amount of effort required to maintain oxygenation.
       (4) The amount of expired air indicates the degree of airway resistance or obstruction.
       (5) If there is insufficient or no air movement in a conscious person, consider the possibility of an airway obstruction due to foreign body (e.g., food) and perform the Heimlich maneuver (see Chapter 20).
       (6) An inadequate airway in an unconscious person may result from obstruction of the airway by the tongue; if there is no suspicion of cervical spine injury, the chin lift–head tilt maneuver may be used. If there is a potential cervical spine injury, use the jaw thrust maneuver to open the airway. Insert an oral or nasal airway to maintain a patent airway. If these measures are not adequate to establish or maintain the airway, endotracheal or nasotracheal intubation may be required.
    b. Evaluate *skin color* to check the degree of oxygenation. Skin color may also indicate other conditions such as blood loss, inadequate tissue perfusion, liver disease, and exposure to toxic materials (e.g., carbon monoxide, cyanide).
    c. Evaluate the effectiveness of *chest wall movement*, especially in chest trauma or in possible airway obstruction.
    d. Cover sucking chest wounds with air-tight dressing and mark the dressing with words "sucking chest wound" to prevent inadvertent removal.

NURSE ADVISORY

A tension pneumothorax may develop when a sucking chest wound has been completely sealed. Frequently reassess breath sounds and respiratory effort to detect this, and release a portion of the dressing if it occurs. The protocol in some EMS agencies is to cover these wounds with cellophane and seal only 3 sides; this allows excess air in the pleural space to escape, but prevents outside air from moving into the pleural space with inspiration.

e. If respiratory effort is inadequate:
   (1) Begin rescue breathing, using a pocket facemask, bag-valve mask, or mouth-to-mouth ventilation. The wisdom and efficacy of mouth-to-mouth ventilation are currently being debated.
   (2) Prepare for, or perform, endotracheal intubation (see Chapter 22 for general procedure). Intubation that occurs in a crisis situation may necessitate a procedure called "rapid sequence intubation or induction." The following medications and maneuvers are administered in sequence:
      • Atropine (vagolytic)
      • Lidocaine (antidysrhythmic and local anesthetic)
      • D-Tubocurarine or pancuronium (prevents fasciculations that occur with paralyzers)
      • Cricoid pressure to close off esophagus and minimize likelihood of vomiting and aspiration
      • Sodium thiopental or other sedating agent
      • Succinylcholine (muscle paralyzer) followed by insertion of the intubation tube when the muscles or the airway are completely relaxed
   (3) Because the person is completely paralyzed and unconscious, mechanical ventilation is required (with cricoid pressure sustained) if the 1st intubation attempt is not successful.
   (4) Mechanical ventilation is continued until the agents wear off and spontaneous breathing occurs.
   (5) An alternative to the standard endotracheal tube is the Combi-tube, a combination tracheal and esophageal intubation device that is used when endotracheal intubation cannot be accomplished.
   (6) A surgical airway via tracheotomy (see Chapter 20) or cricothyroidotomy may be necessary (Fig. 37–1). Cricothyroidotomy is a temporary procedure that is performed to establish an emergency airway, when tracheal intubation or tracheotomy cannot be performed immediately. It involves making an incision into the trachea and then inserting a small plastic tube or needle into the trachea to maintain the opening.
   (7) A chest radiograph is obtained as soon as possible to assess tube placement.

f. Assess breath sounds bilaterally, particularly in the asthmatic person or in trauma situations.
   (1) The absence of breath sounds unilaterally in a person with extreme respiratory distress and shock may be due to a *tension pneumothorax* (see p. 1780), a life-threatening condition requiring immediate insertion of a chest tube, a needle, or a catheter with a flutter valve to evacuate air that is compressing the heart and great vessels, thereby impeding both ventilation and venous return.

g. Evaluate circulation by palpating the radial pulse for approximate rate, rhythm, and volume (Table 37–1).
   (1) If there is no radial pulse, check for a carotid pulse. If the carotid pulse is absent, call for help and initiate CPR.
   (2) Determine *skin vital signs:* skin color, warmth, moisture, and capillary refill, which should be less than 2 seconds.
   (3) Observe for and treat life-threatening external bleeding (see p. 1723).
   (4) In the pregnant person, assess fetal heart tones and ask about fetal movement.

Table 37–1. Relationship of Pulse Location and Systolic Blood Pressure (BP)

Pulse Location	Estimated Minimal Systolic BP
Radial	80 mm Hg
Femoral	70 mm Hg
Carotid	60 mm Hg

NURSE ADVISORY

Even minimal trauma or minor medical conditions may cause fetal distress. Early and repeated assessment of fetal heart tones and fetal activity is a priority. Concurrent continuous fetal monitoring by a qualified obstetric clinician may be appropriate during the initial evaluation of the primary problem. Although the sudden decline in fetal activity is of concern, the presence of fetal activity does not rule out fetal distress. In high-risk situations, the mother may be transferred to Obstetrics for several hours of fetal monitoring before discharge.

(5) Start a large-bore (16–18 gauge) intravenous (IV) line if there is evidence of, or potential for, inadequate perfusion. Obtain necessary blood samples while starting the IV. Hang normal saline.

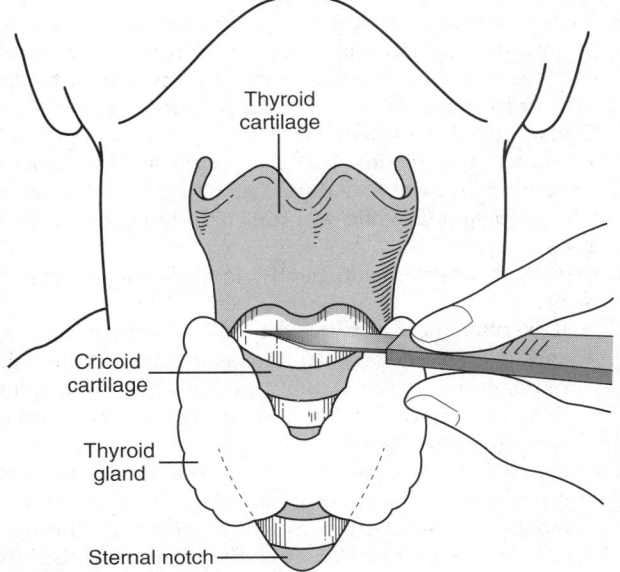

Figure 37–1. Cricothyroidotomy creates a temporary airway by making an opening into the trachea. The opening is maintained with a small plastic tube. (From Black JM, and Matassarin-Jacobs E [eds]. *Luckmann and Sorensen's Medical-Surgical Nursing: A Psychophysiologic Approach.* 4th ed. Philadelphia: WB Saunders, 1993, p 2223.)

CLINICAL CONTROVERSIES

There is ongoing controversy about both the type and amount of IV fluid to use for resuscitation. Although normal saline or Ringer's lactate remains the standard, there is much research regarding the use of hypertonic salt solutions and colloids such as albumin. In addition, the practice of vigorous fluid resuscitation is being questioned, with some researchers recommending that fluid resuscitation be delayed in persons with traumatic conditions.

    (6) If IV access cannot be achieved, an intraosseous fluid administration may be used, especially in children.

    (7) The "MAST" or "shock suit" or pneumatic anti-shock garment (PASG) may be applied if there is hypotension due to volume loss, or to temporarily tamponade bleeding in the abdomen or pelvis (see Chapter 12).

  h. Assess consciousness to evaluate cerebral perfusion and to identify the potential for ineffective airway management.

    (1) Determine the Glasgow Coma Scale Score.

    (2) Common causes of impaired consciousness include hypoglycemia and drugs, especially narcotics.

    (3) A "coma cocktail" of thiamine, 50% dextrose, and naloxone (Narcan) is commonly administered IV sequentially after blood is obtained for glucose.

NURSE ADVISORY

The sequence of administering the "coma cocktail" is important. Thiamine is administered 1st because a glucose load may precipitate acute Wernicke's encephalopathy in a person who is thiamine deficient, such as in malnutrition or alcoholism. Glucose is administered 2nd because hypoglycemia is one of the most common causes of altered consciousness. Narcan may not be needed if the person responds to intravenous glucose.

The routine use of this cocktail is being questioned at this time. A new, longer-acting narcotic antagonist, nalmefene (Revex), has become available in the United States; it is unclear if it will replace naloxone in the "coma cocktail." If benzodiazepine overdose is suspected, flumazenil may be administered.

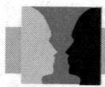

CLINICAL CONTROVERSIES

Although the components of the "coma cocktail" have been perceived for many years as innocuous, research suggests that 1 or more of the components may be hazardous in persons who have not used narcotics or are not hypoglycemic.

    (4) When toxic exposure is suspected, specific antidotes (e.g., atropine and 2-PAM chloride for organophosphate insecticide exposure, or cyanide antidote) may be administered (see "Poisoning, Overdose, or Intoxication").

  i. Establish or maintain stability of the cervical spine if there is history consistent with, or evidence of, neck trauma.

    (1) This is accomplished by doing the following:
- Applying a hard cervical collar while a 2nd person maintains the neck in a neutral position
- Several people placing the person on a spine board
- Securing the head, neck, torso, and extremities to the spine board

    (2) Secure the person in such a way that the entire board can be turned if the person is nauseated or vomits. A wedge is placed under the spine board of a pregnant patient to prevent or treat hypotension due to the gravid uterus compressing the aorta or vena cava.

Performing the Secondary Survey

1. Once the stability of the ABCs has been ensured, the secondary survey is performed. This is a systematic, head-to-toe, front-and-back assessment of the person to identify abnormalities.

2. The secondary survey is particularly important in a person with trauma or altered consciousness. These individuals, especially those with multisystem trauma, such as occurs in an automobile accident, may not be able to sense all of the areas that are painful for quite some time after the accident; therefore, a complete assessment is performed.

3. Once the secondary survey is completed, priorities for further diagnostic testing or intervention are determined.

4. Each practitioner establishes his or her own system for performing the secondary survey. Consistency in one's own assessment pattern is more important than having each practitioner perform the survey identically.

5. Explain what you will be doing, solicit the person's assistance, and request that the person let you know if something is painful. Additional historical information may be obtained while you are performing the secondary survey.

6. Expose the person sufficiently to perform the assessment.

  a. It is often necessary to cut off or remove clothing and jewelry to perform the assessment or to take radiographs. If the stability of the spine is in question, cut off the clothing so as not to risk further damage by movement.

  b. If possible, cut along seam lines so that garments can be salvaged. This is especially true with down garments; otherwise, feathers will be dispersed throughout the environment and may be inhaled by both the ill or injured person and caregivers.

  c. If there is a hole in a garment due to a bullet or a knife, avoid cutting through or near the hole. This is critical for police and forensic authorities (see p. 1790–1791).

d. Cover the person to maintain normal body temperature and dignity during the evaluation.

NURSE ADVISORY

Preventing hypothermia is a priority in persons who undergo resuscitation, children, and the elderly. This can be accomplished by limiting exposure during examination and procedures, warming the treatment room, using heat lamps or a heat shield, administering warmed intravenous fluids and blood, and using warmed blankets or external warming devices.

7. Obtain vital signs and apply monitoring devices (e.g., cardiac monitor, pulse oximeter).
8. Evaluate the head.
   a. Palpate and visualize the head and face for depressions, lacerations, ecchymosis (especially of the mastoid process and around the eyes—known as Battle's sign, associated with basilar skull fracture), and drainage from the nose or ears, especially cerebrospinal fluid. Remove earrings or necklaces that may interfere with taking a radiograph.
   b. Observe pupil size and reactivity; note eye movement and presence of contact lenses. Apply lens lubricant if the person's blink reflex is impaired. Assess visual acuity if relevant.
   c. Evaluate mouth and jaw occlusion, approximation of teeth, presence of loose or missing teeth, dentures, lacerations, deviation of the tongue, foreign materials. Remove loose dentures in the obtunded person to prevent airway impairment.
9. Assess the neck.
   a. Observe the anterior neck for trauma, position of the trachea, distended neck veins, medical alert devices. Remove jewelry that may interfere with taking radiographs.

NURSE ADVISORY

Necklaces and earrings interfere with the accuracy of cervical spine radiographs and CT scans, and may not be readily apparent when a cervical collar and immobilization device are in use. Ask the person about jewelry or check under the collar and head blocks; remove and secure it.

   b. Palpate the posterior neck for deformity and tenderness.
   c. Palpate the clavicle bilaterally from the sternal notch to the shoulder. Fractures that involve the inner 3rd of the clavicle are often associated with lacerations of major vessels, so palpate gently.
10. Evaluate the upper extremities.
    a. Palpate the anterior and posterior shoulder and put it through range of motion.
    b. Palpate the arm from shoulder to fingers.
    c. Palpate radial pulses bilaterally.

d. Perform range of motion of the elbow unless there is an obvious deformity of the elbow.
e. Have the person grip your hands and release.

NURSE ADVISORY

Injuries around the elbow require special caution because of the potential for lacerating nerves or arteries. If the person complains of elbow pain, do not move the joint. Immobilize the joint using a pillow splint.

11. Assess the chest.
    a. Observe for symmetry of chest wall movement, presence of deficits (e.g., flail chest), sucking chest wounds (which may be axillary wounds not identified earlier).
    b. Auscultate breath sounds bilaterally.
    c. Listen to heart sounds.
    d. Gently compress the chest wall anterior to posterior and laterally to midline to evaluate for rib or sternum fractures. Palpate ribs if this procedure elicits pain.
    e. Ask about the presence of shoulder pain.

NURSE ADVISORY

Nontraumatic shoulder pain (Kehr's sign) may be caused by irritation of the diaphragm from intra-abdominal bleeding. It is seen in trauma-induced bleeding and ruptured ectopic pregnancy.

12. Assess the abdomen.
    a. Observe for distention, injury, and ecchymosis, especially of the periumbilical area (known as Grey Turner sign), which suggests intra-abdominal bleeding.
    b. Auscultate bowel sounds.
    c. Palpate gently for pulsatile masses (associated with aortic aneurysm), direct or rebound tenderness, rigidity, and guarding.
    d. In a pregnant person, assess fetal movement and reassess fetal heart tones.
13. Assess the pelvis and hips.
    a. Observe for obvious deformity or ecchymosis.
    b. Palpate suprapubic area to determine bladder distention.
    c. Evaluate for pelvic fracture by gently pressing on the symphysis pubis anteriorly and compressing the hips laterally toward the midline.
    d. Place the hips through range of motion unless there is obvious deformity or pain.
    e. Palpate femoral pulses bilaterally.
14. Evaluate the external genitalia.
    a. Observe for external bleeding, evidence of incontinence, altered skin integrity, foreign material.
    b. Ask about desire to void, presence of tampons.

NURSE ADVISORY

The presence of blood at the urinary meatus suggests urethral injury, which may be worsened by insertion of a urinary catheter. Catheterization is generally deferred to a urologist; bladder catheterization via a suprapubic tube may be preferred.

15. Evaluate the lower extremities.
    a. Observe for injury, deformity, external or internal rotation of the leg, joint effusion, and ecchymosis.
    b. Palpate and mark pedal pulses.
    c. Perform range of motion of joints unless there is obvious dislocation, especially of the knee. Such action may impinge on and damage major blood vessels or nerves.
    d. Evaluate motor function.
    e. Test for Babinski's sign in persons over 2 years of age.
16. Evaluate the back.
    a. While maintaining stability of the spine, inspect and palpate the back, paying particular attention to the spinal column and the costovertebral angle (pain here may suggest renal trauma or pyelonephritis). This may be deferred until a radiograph indicates the cervical spine is cleared.
    b. Separate the buttock fold to observe for exit wounds in the person with a gunshot wound.
    c. Observe for skin discoloration (e.g., dark areas that may appear to be bruising), lesions, or redness suggestive of pressure areas, which may be due to laying on a spine board or in the same spot for prolonged periods of time.

TRANSCULTURAL CONSIDERATIONS

Mongolian spots, which are normal hyperpigmented areas found in dark-skinned people, may be incorrectly identified as bruises. Certain ethnic groups, especially southeastern Asians, may use remedies such as "cupping" or "coining," which may result in ecchymotic or hyperemic areas that can be misinterpreted as injuries. Ethnic and cultural practices need to be considered when skin variations cause concern about abuse or neglect.

17. Evaluate associated elements, including information provided by EMS providers, family, or others.
    a. Does the environment in which the person was found provide information that may assist in evaluation or management?
       (1) Are there pill bottles, medications, other containers?
       (2) Were there strange sights or smells?
       (3) Was the room temperature extremely cool or warm?
       (4) Were other persons present and ill or injured as well?

(5) Was a health warning alarm system present and is there someone who needs to be notified?

NURSE ADVISORY

Many people who live alone, especially those with physical disability, subscribe to health alert systems. They wear devices (usually necklaces) that, when activated, notify the system operator of the need for medical assistance. Subscribers are required to "check in" with the system operator at predetermined times each day. Failure to confirm well-being results in automatic activation of either EMS or other emergency response people. Health care providers who care for individuals using these systems should determine when the call needs to be made and notify the system operator so that the system is not activated.

       (6) Was the ill or injured person a caregiver for another who will now need assistance?
    b. What is the general appearance and hygiene of the person?
    c. Where was the person found (e.g., lying on the floor, thrown from a vehicle, in a bathtub or shower)?
    d. Determine the following in trauma situations:
       (1) What is the mechanism of injury (i.e., what happened)?
       (2) Why did the accident happen?
       (3) Were there antecedent events (e.g., did the person with a head laceration and a broken hip simply trip on a rug, or was the fall due to syncope from a cardiac dysrhythmia?)?
       (4) In gunshot or shotgun wounds, identify type of weapon, caliber and type of bullet, proximity to weapon, and location of entrance and exit wounds.
       (5) In vehicular accidents, what was the nature of the incident (e.g., head on, T-bone, rear ended); at what speed were the vehicles traveling; what is the condition of the vehicle (e.g., massive front end damage, broken steering wheel, airbag deployment, engine protrusion into compartment); were there deaths involving others in the vehicle; was there prolonged extrication; were restraining devices used (e.g., seat and shoulder belts, car seats)?
       (6) Was the incident witnessed, and if so, is the witness available for questioning?
18. Assess health history.
    a. Historical information is usually obtained concurrently in critical situations and includes history of the present problem and general health status information.
    b. Perform a symptom analysis of the current problem, using a PQRST format.
       (1) P = What precipitates or worsens the problem? What eases the problem?
       (2) Q = Quality and nature of the symptoms to include a numeric ranking of severity on a 1 to 10 scale, with 10 being the most intense.
       (3) R = Does pain radiate to any other area?

    (4) S = Associated symptoms (e.g., nausea, headache).

    (5) T = Timing. How long since the symptoms developed? How long do they last?

  c. Obtain general health history information, including the following:

    (1) General health status: major health problems such as diabetes, hypertension, heart disease, and pulmonary disease; significant surgeries; use of alcohol or tobacco

    (2) Medications used routinely or recently, including oral contraceptives

    (3) Allergies

    (4) Immunization status on children routinely and in adults in the presence of surface trauma

    (5) Treatments or medications used before arrival for treatment, including over-the-counter and home remedies and street drugs

    (6) Date of last *normal* menstrual period and occurrence of actual or potential pregnancy in females of childbearing age (important if radiographs or medications are ordered)

Providing Interventions Based on the Secondary Survey

1. Interventions that result from the secondary survey may be divided into 4 categories:
   a. Medical or nursing treatments to address defined problems; these include use of oxygen, positioning, splinting, application of ice or warmth, administration of pain medication, and so forth
   b. Diagnostic studies, such as laboratory tests, radiographs, or electrocardiogram (ECG), to define the problem and to establish a baseline
   c. Interventions that have previously been defined via guidelines, protocols, or care maps; these have been shown to be necessary to further diagnose problems, prevent complications, or monitor treatment effectiveness. An example is urinary catheter insertion to detect the presence of blood, prevent bladder distention, prevent bladder trauma during diagnostic peritoneal lavage, and monitor renal perfusion in the individual with multisystem trauma.
   d. Ongoing monitoring to evaluate the progress and effectiveness of interventions
2. Interventions are performed in order of priority (i.e., starting with whatever system disorder poses the greatest threat to the individual). In the multisystem-injured person, bleeding or injury is managed in the following order:
   a. Chest: because ineffective airway or impaired gas exchange is immediately life threatening. This may involve oxygen administration, insertion of a chest tube to remove air or blood, evacuation of a pericardial tamponade, or pulmonary treatments such as medication administration or assisted ventilation. Also, bleeding in the chest may be vigorous, causing impaired cardiac output and impaired tissue perfusion.

   b. Abdomen: Bleeding in the abdomen may also be vigorous, resulting in hypovolemic shock. Injuries that involve the bowel also predispose the person to sepsis.
   c. Head: Assuming adequate ventilation and perfusion, managing increased intracranial pressure is the next priority to prevent irreversible damage to central nervous system structures. This usually involves evacuation of epidural or subdural hematomas or prevention or management of cerebral edema. Once the cervical spine is cleared, either by physical examination or radiograph, the head is placed in a raised, neutral position; hyperventilation with oxygen to decrease carbon dioxide and administration of diuretics such as mannitol or furosemide are frequently used measures.
   d. Spine: Injuries to the spine are generally managed by immobilization and, in the case of cervical spine injuries, traction devices. High-dose steroids may be administered to decrease edema of the cord.
   e. Treatment of non–life-threatening vascular injuries
   f. Splinting or treatment of fractures
   g. Cleansing and repair of surface trauma (e.g., lacerations, abrasions)
   h. Administration of medications such as tetanus prophylaxis and antibiotics

Psychosocial Assessment

1. The emergency experience itself is frightening to most people; calm reassurance is required on the part of the caregiver to solicit the person's assistance in problem identification and resolution.
2. General elements to be assessed in the psychosocial assessment:
   a. The person's affect or behavior
   b. The person's understanding of what is happening, the plan of care, and timelines for accomplishing it
   c. The person's degree of coping with this situation
   d. The extent to which the person poses a threat to himself or others
   e. The presence or absence of developmental delay
   f. Orientation to person, place, and time
   g. Presence or use of mind-altering substances, including medications, street drugs, and alcohol
   h. The person's normal coping strategies
   i. The person's self-concept
   j. Support resources—human and financial
3. Accident and assault victims feel particularly vulnerable; they express a variety of emotions, ranging from a blunted affect to rage, hysteria, crying, and physical attacks on caregivers; there may be preoccupation with things that do not seem to be a high priority in light of the person's medical problems at the time, such as the condition and location of the car.
4. Because visits to the ED are often unplanned, notification of family or job; arrangements for child, elder, or pet care; and financial concerns may require attention.
5. Assessment of how the person is feeling or handling concerns needs to be validated with the individual.

6. Because the ED is the only resource for many individuals, issues such as shelter, clothing, and food may be the major priorities for nursing intervention.
7. Individuals who live alone, especially the elderly, may have concerns about their ability to perform activities of daily living, once discharged from the ED, and they may expect hospital admission, even if it is not clinically indicated. Temporary arrangements may be necessary.
8. Abused children and victims of domestic violence who are being evaluated for injuries may fear that the secret will be found out and that they will face repeated injury when they return home.
9. If the person feels responsible for the injury or death of another person, there may be significant guilt.
10. For some, the injury or illness may represent a major threat to their life plans or hopes for the future (e.g., the childless couple that has tried for many years to have a child and spent many thousands of dollars and is now experiencing a spontaneous abortion, or the person who is now a quadriplegic because of a spinal cord injury).
11. Psychosocial assessment also includes family dynamics and the extent to which family and friends are a support to the ill or injured person.

Communicating with Family Members

1. Timely notification of family or significant others who are unaware of the situation is a high priority in the emergency care setting, especially if the prognosis is poor or if death has already occurred.
2. Providing family members with the opportunity to see and speak to a loved one who is seriously ill or injured is critical in promoting normal grieving in the event of a bad outcome.
3. The family or significant others may be able to provide critical information regarding health status, allergies, current medications, and wishes regarding resuscitation.
4. Contacting family members gives them the opportunity to be present during resuscitative measures and to participate in decision making regarding continuance or termination of these efforts.
5. If telephone notification is required, a clear and organized plan is needed to ensure that key information is heard and understood and to promote the safety of the recipient while en route to the hospital.
   a. If possible, have the ill or injured person speak with loved ones; this is reassuring in itself, because it indicates that the person's condition is stable enough to allow this. The caregiver may need to clarify information with the significant others at the completion of the call.
   b. If a caregiver must make the call, he or she should have all the facts readily available before initiating the call:
      (1) What happened
      (2) Where it happened
      (3) The sequence of events, including use of EMS or police resources

(4) The person's condition on arrival at the hospital
(5) The nature and extent of the illness or injury
(6) The key parameters (e.g., level of consciousness, vital signs, respiratory effort, cardiac effort)
(7) The person's condition now (e.g., satisfactory, serious, critical, deceased) (Notification of a death by phone is controversial and should be avoided, if reasonable.)
(8) If possible, find out what the response of the significant other will be after receiving the information. Is that person physically or emotionally frail, requiring on-site support before receiving the notification?
(9) Is there someone other than the family member who should receive the information and be physically present when the person is advised of the situation?
c. The staff member who makes the call should do the following:
   (1) Introduce self by name, title, department, and institution.
   (2) Validate the person's relationship to the ill or injured person.
   (3) Establish whether another person is present if you are calling to advise that a person has died; this individual may be needed to evaluate the family member's ability to handle devastating news, to provide transportation, or to make arrangements for notification of other significant persons.
   (4) Give the information in a sequential manner with background information so that the recipient has a frame of reference for the event rather than stating the worst news 1st. For example, instead of saying "Your husband has had a massive heart attack, had a cardiac arrest, and we are doing CPR," say "Your husband developed chest pain while at work. He collapsed to the ground, and a coworker determined that he was not breathing and did not have a pulse. She started CPR right away and the paramedics were called. They continued CPR, put a tube into his trachea so that they could breathe for him, and gave him medications to try and get his heart to beat normally. This was continued during transport to the hospital, and we are continuing to do this now. He is unconscious and not feeling any pain. We are concerned that he has not responded to the treatment, but we are continuing our efforts. His condition is extremely critical, and we think that you should come to the hospital if you can."
   (5) Providing the information in a sequential way enables the recipient to process information gradually to the point that it is understood and helps to minimize the shock phase of grief and loss.
   (6) When a death has occurred, and information is given in a sequential manner, the recipient will often acknowledge the death before the caller states it.
   (7) To the extent possible, provide the family member with both the reality of the situation and a sense of hope, if resuscitation is continued.

(8) In situations in which death or brain death is likely, ask if the ill or injured person had any wishes regarding resuscitation or organ or tissue donation. Although this may seem insensitive, decisions to continue or terminate resuscitation are time sensitive.

(9) Ask whether the recipient is planning on coming to the hospital, and confirm the hospital name, the location of the loved one in the hospital, and directions to it.

(10) Reinforce safe driving and attentiveness and the value of having someone drive the person to the hospital.

Transcultural Considerations

1. Ethnicity and cultural norms and values may significantly affect the provision of emergency care in a variety of ways, including the following:

   a. Some diseases or injuries are predominant in a given group (e.g., thalassemia or sickle cell anemia, Kawasaki's syndrome).

   b. Physiologic differences such as skin and mucous membrane coloration may make assessment more complex (e.g., mongolian spots on dark-skinned children may be misidentified as bruises, with the potential for suspicion of child abuse).

   c. Hygiene differences can occur, such as use of depilatories versus shaving of the face in dark-skinned males, use of hair products, or not shaving facial hair for religious or cultural reasons.

   d. Language barriers may be noted, more in the use of certain words than as simple language differences.

   e. Culturally dictated surgical anatomic alterations render physical assessment difficult (e.g., female circumcision).

   f. Home remedies used to manage the problem, especially those that may appear as injuries or evidence of illness (e.g., skin cupping by Asian cultures), may result in petechial lesions that appear as bruising, causing one to question child abuse, clotting disorders, meningitis, or drug reactions.

   g. Alternative healers or spiritual leaders may be involved in the plan of care.

   h. Alternative therapies may be used.

   i. Rites and rituals may be used in the care of the ill or dying.

   j. Expectations can exist regarding presence of family members in the treatment area.

   k. Behavioral responses to illness or injury may be culturally mediated.

   l. Prohibitions may exist regarding certain treatments (e.g., blood product administration).

   m. There may be beliefs regarding contraception, pregnancy, childbirth, and childrearing.

   n. There can be prohibitions regarding male caregivers examining or providing care to female patients.

   o. Special considerations may apply regarding handling or internment of a deceased person.

   p. Restrictions can be imposed regarding removal of clothes or adornments.

   q. Past experience with health care providers in the home country can shape expectations regarding pain management, visitors, involvement in care decisions, and such; this is especially apparent in individuals from formerly Communist countries.

   r. Immigration status may cause individuals to be reluctant to seek regular care with the same provider or to provide correct addresses because of fear of being reported and deported.

   s. Recommendations regarding special diets may require evaluation for inclusion of foods or preparation techniques unique to a given group.

   t. Touching another person, sustained eye contact, and personal space considerations may affect the degree of ease the person feels.

2. In some cultures (e.g., Native Americans), illness or injury may be perceived as resulting from unacceptable behavior.

   a. Assessment of the individual, especially with regard to severity of symptoms, may be difficult, as persons often are somewhat stoic.

   b. There may be reluctance to verbalize the amount of pain being experienced, because of the belief that pain is punishment for inappropriate behavior.

   c. Pain management may be inadequate as a result of cultural norms.

   d. Offers to notify family members may be denied because of embarrassment.

3. In other cultures (e.g., Hispanic, Italian, and Jewish), vocalization of discomfort is normal.

4. Gypsy or Southeast Asian families may expect to remain in the treatment room with a loved one.

5. Mid-Eastern men often expect to remain in the examination rooms with their wives during examination and treatment.

6. Individuals providing care to persons from different ethnic and cultural backgrounds must learn what the norms and values are for a given group and tailor assessments, interventions, and teaching materials accordingly.

7. Interpreter services, either via an interpreter who is physically present or through a telephone interpreter service, are often important in obtaining health information and discharge teaching.

Performing and Assisting with Diagnostic Tests

1. Complete vital signs are needed to correctly determine triage category in all but the most obvious emergency situations.

   a. For adults and children older than 5 years of age, vital sign measurement includes blood pressure (BP), pulse, respiratory rate, and temperature.

      (1) Oral temperatures are preferred.

      (2) Tympanic or rectal temperature measurement is obtained in persons who have altered consciousness or in children younger than 1 year of age.

      (3) The use of electronic BP and pulse measurement has become commonplace and can improve efficiency; however, the pulse should also be as-

sessed manually to evaluate rate, rhythm, and character of the pulse, especially in older persons (see Chapter 23).

(4) The use of automatic BP machines can cause significant petechiae and hematomas both in normal persons and in those on anticoagulants.

(5) Blood pressure measurements are performed in both arms in people with chest pain to assess for dissecting thoracic aortic aneurysm.

(6) Postural vital signs, which include BP and pulse measurement with the person in supine, sitting, and standing positions, are routinely performed in individuals with actual or potential fluid loss (e.g., protracted diarrhea or vomiting), in those with abdominal pain, and in persons presenting with dizziness.

(7) When an automatic BP machine is used for postural vital signs, it is recommended that the machine be turned off between each position change, because the machine automatically cycles 20 to 40 mm Hg higher with each subsequent reading; this may cause considerable pain to the person and takes longer for cycling.

(8) Assessment of postural vital signs includes assessment of the person's response to position changes, such as lightheadedness or syncope.

(9) The definition of a postural change may be institution specific, but often includes a 20 mm Hg or greater fall in the BP, an increase of 20 or more in the pulse rate, or subjective reports of dizziness with position change, or a combination of these.

(10) Postural vital signs are not obtained in the person who is already hypotensive or in individuals in whom movement may worsen a condition.

(11) Although postural vital signs have had a long-standing and important role in evaluating hypotension in the emergency care setting, the value of this assessment is controversial because the presence of orthostasis does not reveal the pathophysiologic cause.

(12) The precise technique for performing postural vital signs is institution specific, with some agencies requiring a wait of 1 to 3 minutes between each position change and subsequent measurement and others requiring immediate measurement with each position change.

(13) Postural vital signs are generally not performed in children younger than 5 years of age.

(14) Routine vital sign measurement in children younger than 5 years of age is usually limited to temperature, pulse, and respiration, unless there has been trauma or significant volume loss.

2. Pulse oximetry is used (see Chapter 23).

a. Pulse oximetry is routinely used in the emergency care setting for persons who have respiratory symptoms and those who have evidence of poor perfusion.

b. Pulse oximetry is used to evaluate initial and ongoing tissue oxygenation, to guide the use of oxygen, and to assist in decision making regarding additional therapies.

c. Pulse oximetry is particularly helpful in evaluating oxygen saturation in a person with pulmonary disease during exertion, and may influence the perceived need for oxygen at home.

d. In most instances, the probe is placed on a finger or toe; however, devices for ear lobe and facial measurement are used in people with hypotension and poor peripheral perfusion.

e. The probe that is used must be tailored for size; an adult finger probe may give inaccurate readings when used on a small child.

f. When the probe is used on a digit, the accuracy of the reading may be affected by the presence of nail polish or artificial nails.

3. Electrocardiogram and cardiac monitoring are performed (see Chapter 23).

a. A 12-lead ECG is routinely performed in persons with chest pain suggestive of cardiac origin, individuals with chest trauma, those who have cardiac dysrhythmias detected during the physical assessment, and individuals presenting with weakness, dizziness, or a chief complaint related to cardiac rhythm (e.g., heart beating fast, fluttering sensation in the chest).

b. Cardiac monitoring is routinely used in the emergency care setting for individuals with chest pain, trauma, or respiratory distress; those who are or have the potential to become physiologically unstable; those with cardiac dysrhythmias; and individuals who have been exposed to or have ingested agents that affect the heart.

c. In most instances, a lead II configuration is used, with lead placement on the left and right shoulders and the left lower chest.

d. ST-segment monitoring is being used in some emergency care settings to evaluate individuals with chest pain after the initial ECG is done to detect ST-segment changes that may reflect a myocardial infarction.

4. Capnometry is measurement of the amount of carbon dioxide in expired air to ensure that the endotracheal tube is in correct position; it is measured by a disposable device that changes color in the presence of carbon dioxide or by attachment to a machine that measures end-tidal carbon dioxide of expired air.

5. The Doppler device detects wave motion via the use of a probe and special gel.

a. It is often used to measure BP when a pulse cannot be palpated or heard with a stethoscope.

b. It is used to diagnose arterial or venous occlusion by detecting the presence or absence of blood flow in arteries or veins.

c. It is also used to diagnose testicular torsion.

d. The Doppler is also helpful in detecting fetal heart tones, particularly in early pregnancy.

6. The Breathalyzer is a rapid way to measure approximate blood alcohol level and may be used by both clinicians and law enforcement officials.

a. A baseline Breathalyzer reading is helpful in differentiating whether altered consciousness is due to alcohol or other causes.

b. Repeated Breathalyzer measurements are used to monitor alcohol metabolism; there should be a direct correlation between the alcohol level and level of consciousness, if alcohol ingestion is the sole cause of altered consciousness.

c. In many states, a blood alcohol level must be less than 0.10 mg per dl before an intoxicated person can be evaluated by a mental health professional for involuntary commitment; the Breathalyzer is a quick way to evaluate this in persons who may not tolerate a venipuncture for blood alcohol measurement.

7. Laboratory studies play a critical role in the assessment and management of individuals in the emergency care setting.

a. Rapid turnaround of laboratory studies is key in diagnosing and treating problems quickly.

b. The tests routinely performed are those for which results can be attained quickly, usually within 1 hour.

c. Technologic advances now allow for multiple-study blood testing at the bedside, with results available in 1 to 2 minutes.

   (1) Although the cost of this technology is significant, its immediate value in timely management of the critically ill or injured justifies the expense.

   (2) The small amount of blood required to produce a large quantity of results makes it especially attractive for persons in whom venipuncture is difficult and for neonates who do not tolerate large-volume blood draws.

d. The most frequently ordered laboratory tests are the following:

   (1) Complete blood count, including differential

   (2) Glucose, electrolytes, blood urea nitrogen (BUN), creatinine

   (3) Cardiac enzymes

   (4) Coagulation studies: prothrombin time (PT), partial thromboplastin time (PTT)

   (5) Pregnancy test—human chorionic gonadotropin in blood is preferred; may be urine pregnancy test

   (6) Type and crossmatch, Rh

   (7) Liver function studies: amylase, lipase

   (8) Urinalysis, urine culture, and sensitivity

   (9) Strep screen or culture

   (10) Gonorrheal, chlamydial, and herpes cultures

   (11) Hepatitis screen

   (12) Calcium, phosphorus, magnesium levels

   (13) Thyroid function studies

   (14) Medication, street drug, and alcohol levels

8. Special studies performed in the emergency care setting include the following:

a. Culdocentesis: involves the insertion of a large spinal needle through the posterior wall of the vagina into the cul de sac and aspiration of fluid.

   (1) If blood is aspirated, and it does not clot, the test is determined as positive for either ruptured ectopic pregnancy or intra-abdominal bleeding due to trauma.

   (2) The presence of purulent material suggests pelvic inflammatory disease.

   (3) The procedure is quite painful, albeit short lived, but preprocedure medication with a sedative or narcotic may be appropriate.

   (4) The need for this procedure has decreased significantly because of rapid availability of ultrasound; however, it may be performed at times when ultrasound is not available.

b. Peritoneal lavage, also known as diagnostic peritoneal lavage, may be performed.

   (1) Peritoneal lavage is performed in individuals with abdominal or multisystem trauma to detect the presence of intra-abdominal blood.

   (2) It is usually performed when the person's condition is very unstable and using abdominal computed tomographic (CT) scan will result in too long a delay in diagnosis; in an unconscious multisystem trauma victim; or in a trauma situation in a person with spinal cord injury and impaired ability to communicate abdominal pain.

   (3) To prevent injury to the urinary bladder during the procedures, a Foley catheter is inserted and the bladder emptied. The procedure involves the insertion of a peritoneal dialysis catheter into the abdominal cavity through a small incision made in the abdominal wall, usually below the umbilicus; the skin is anesthetized with a local anesthetic containing epinephrine to achieve a bloodless field.

   (4) Once the catheter is in place, a syringe is attached to the catheter and an attempt is made to aspirate blood.

   (5) If there is no aspirate, warm saline or Ringer's lactate is infused through the catheter into the peritoneal cavity.

   (6) Once the solution is instilled, the bag is lowered and the fluid is allowed to drain back into the IV bag.

   (7) The fluid is visualized to determine if blood is present; this is done by attempting to read newsprint through the fluid.

   (8) Unless the solution is clearly bloody, the bag is sent to the laboratory for stat cell count, amylase, and bacteria.

   (9) The abdominal incision may be left open and covered with sterile gauze, or it may be sutured closed, pending laboratory analysis.

   (10) If the results are positive, exploratory laparotomy is scheduled promptly.

c. Lumbar puncture is used in the emergency care setting to diagnose meningitis, especially in young children, or to evaluate intractable headache in the presence of a normal result on head CT scan (see Chapter 18).

■ CARING FOR PEOPLE EXPERIENCING RESPIRATORY EMERGENCIES

Common or Serious Respiratory Emergencies

1. Anaphylaxis
2. Asthma

3. Acute exacerbation of chronic obstructive pulmonary disease (COPD)
4. Bronchitis
5. Pneumonia: bacterial, viral, aspiration
6. Pulmonary embolism
7. Toxic fume inhalation
8. Near drowning
9. Spontaneous pneumothorax
10. Congestive heart failure or pulmonary edema

Anaphylaxis or Anaphylactic Shock

1. Definition: Systemic antigen-antibody reaction due to exposure to an allergen, potentially resulting in the release of vasoactive substances that increase capillary permeability (see Chapter 21). Common allergens:
   a. Medications (e.g., antibiotics, immunizations, and desensitizing therapy)
   b. Bee or other insect stings
   c. Foods such as nuts, chocolate, strawberries, and seafood
   d. In some instances, the allergen may be unknown.
2. Clinical manifestations
   a. Localized or generalized tissue swelling
   b. Urticaria (hives)
   c. Laryngeal edema
   d. Bronchospasm
   e. Gastrointestinal symptoms: Nausea, vomiting, diarrhea
   f. Massive vasodilation and shock
   g. Cardiac arrest
3. Triage priority
   a. Immediate priority is given to a person with allergic reaction or a history of severe allergic or anaphylactic reaction.
   b. Severity of symptoms may not be readily apparent.
   c. Progression to profound shock, complete airway obstruction, or cardiac arrest can be rapid, occurring within minutes.
4. Diagnostics
   a. Relevant data
      (1) Method of exposure: ingestion, injection, insect sting, inhalation
      (2) Time since exposure
      (3) Treatment before arrival
   b. Physical examination findings
      (1) Respiratory symptoms: dyspnea, wheezing, shortness of breath, hoarseness
      (2) Central nervous system symptoms: syncope, headache, poor mentation, dizziness
      (3) Mucocutaneous symptoms: urticaria (hives), generalized swelling, or angioedema involving orbits, mouth, and upper airway; pruritus (itching), sensation of perineal burning
      (4) Gastrointestinal symptoms: nausea, vomiting, diarrhea
      (5) Behavioral response (e.g., sense of impending doom and intense fear) is common and understandable, given the life-threatening nature of this condition.
      (6) Central nervous system: level of consciousness and mentation
      (7) Respiratory assessment:
         • Airway patency
         • Ability to speak
         • Hoarseness
         • Wheezing
         • Stridor
         • Respiratory rate
         • Flaring of nostrils
         • Use of accessory muscles
         • Oximetry readings
      (8) Peripheral perfusion
         • Blood pressure
         • Pulse
         • Capillary refill
         • Skin vitals—skin warm and flushed
      (9) Location, nature, and magnitude of mucocutaneous symptoms
      (10) Gastrointestinal symptoms: bowel sounds, abdominal cramps, diarrhea
   c. Diagnostic studies: pulse oximetry, arterial blood gases if severe respiratory impairment; other studies as for shock management
5. Clinical management
   a. Goals of clinical management are to reverse the antigen-antibody reaction while maintaining adequate oxygenation and circulating volume and to prevent recurrence of anaphylactic reaction.
   b. Ensuring adequate oxygenation may include a variety of measures, depending on the severity of the symptoms: high-flow oxygen administration via nonrebreathing mask or nasal prongs, endotracheal intubation, cricothyroidotomy, and mechanical ventilation.
   c. Secure an IV line and hang a balanced salt solution; run at a rapid rate if hypotension is present.
   d. Stop the antigen-antibody reaction by doing the following:
      (1) Administer epinephrine.
      (2) In critical situations, epinephrine may be given IV in a diluted concentration.
      (3) If IV access is not feasible, epinephrine may be given via an endotracheal tube or injected sublingually.
      (4) In an insect sting or an injection in an extremity, a tourniquet may be applied between the site and the heart to prevent absorption of the antigen; a portion of the epinephrine may be injected around the site (distal to a tourniquet) and the remainder given subcutaneously or intramuscularly (IM) in another extremity.
   e. Reverse the histamine-induced increased capillary permeability, urticaria (hives), and itching. Administer diphenhydramine (Benadryl) IM or IV.
   f. Correct systemic vasodilation and hypotension with IV drip dopamine or other vasoconstrictor agents, titrated for effect.
   g. Decrease the inflammatory response and promote the stability of cell membranes by administering steroids (e.g., IV methylprednisolone [Solu-Medrol] or oral prednisone).

h. Treat bronchospasm.
 (1) Inhaled bronchodilators such as albuterol, using either a small-volume nebulizer or a metered-dose inhaler
 (2) Intravenous aminophylline
i. Minimize absorption of the antigen.
 (1) In insect stings, scrape away stinger if present; apply meat tenderizer (papain) paste and an ice pack to the site.
 (2) Use gastric lavage or emesis with syrup of ipecac to remove ingested allergen.
j. Provide care in a calm and reassuring manner, even if it appears that the person is unconscious and the prognosis is grave. Many individuals who have experienced anaphylactic shock and were clinically near death have, after recovering, reported in much detail specific conversations by clinicians about their condition and treatment.
6. Applying the nursing process

NURSING DIAGNOSIS: Impaired gas exchange R/T tissue edema, decreased tissue perfusion, and bronchospasm

a. *Expected outcomes:* Following interventions, the person should be able to demonstrate adequate gas exchange and tissue perfusion by having the following:
 (1) Normal pulse oximetry (oxygen saturation ≥ 90%)
 (2) Normal respiratory rate and effort
 (3) Normal skin color
b. *Nursing interventions*
 (1) Position person appropriately, given vital signs (e.g., sitting unless hypotensive).
 (2) Loosen constrictive clothing.
 (3) Initiate high-flow oxygen via nonrebreather mask or nasal prongs.
 (4) Initiate pulse oximetry monitoring.
 (5) Administer medications as indicated.
 (6) Be prepared to initiate or assist with endotracheal intubation, cricothyroidotomy, or other airway management strategies.

NURSING DIAGNOSIS: Decreased cardiac output R/T profound vasodilation, decreased venous return, and altered cell membrane permeability

a. *Expected outcomes:* Following intervention, the person should have normal BP, pulse, and respiration.
b. *Nursing interventions*
 (1) Maintain adequate tissue oxygenation by administering oxygen, using airway management devices or techniques, monitoring oximetry, evaluating arterial blood gases, and adjusting therapy.
 (2) Administer reversal agents and bronchodilators.
 (3) Establish and maintain IV access and administer IV fluids as needed to maintain adequate circulating volume.

 (4) Monitor BP, pulse, and urine output. For actual or potential impaired cardiac output, ensure adequate IV access, administer IV fluids, position person supine if hypotensive, administer medications as above, provide ongoing cardiac and BP monitoring.

NURSING DIAGNOSIS: Fear R/T loss of control and threat to life

a. *Expected outcomes:* Following intervention, the person should be able to do the following:
 (1) Verbalize the ability to cope with fear and anxiety
 (2) Identify support systems
b. *Nursing interventions*
 (1) Communicate with the person and colleagues in a calm and reassuring manner.
 (2) Allow family members to be in the room to serve as a source of comfort to the individual.
 (3) Explain all procedures, even when it seems that the person is unable to hear you.
 (4) Remain with the person until major symptoms are resolved; provide a call light when it is necessary to leave the room.

NURSING DIAGNOSIS: Knowledge deficit R/T avoidance of allergen and use of medications to treat anaphylaxis

a. *Expected outcomes:* Following intervention the person should be able to do the following:
 (1) Identify allergen and strategies to avoid it
 (2) State the proper use of medications
 (3) Describe the home-going treatment plan
b. *Nursing interventions*
 (1) Correct knowledge deficits regarding the cause and complications of the disorder, use of medications, and prevention strategies.
 (2) If the reaction is effectively reversed in the ED and discharge is deemed safe, the person must demonstrate knowledge regarding the following:
  • Home management of remaining symptoms, avoidance of allergens, and treatment of allergic reactions, if there is repeated exposure to the allergen.
  • Specific discharge teaching is included under "Discharge planning and teaching."
7. Criteria for discharge
a. Normal vital signs
b. Lung sounds clear; normal oximetry
c. Mucocutaneous symptoms resolved
d. Proximity to emergency treatment if symptoms return (e.g., if this is a 2nd or 3rd visit for the same exposure, the potential for treatment failure and return of symptoms is great; thus, individuals who live or work in remote areas where access to EMS is limited may require admission for observation rather than discharge)

e. Affected individual and family members articulate understanding of the life-threatening nature of this condition, treatment and follow-up plan, actions to take in event of return of symptoms, and avoidance measures.

8. Discharge planning and teaching
   a. Teach the patient what an allergic or anaphylactic reaction is, including probable sources of exposure, early signs and symptoms, and consequences of nontreatment.
   b. Explain medications, usually steroids and antihistamines, to be used after discharge, including tapering of steroids and safety considerations related to use of antihistamines.
   c. Stress the need for follow-up if the source of the allergen has not been identified; this may require skin testing.
   d. Demonstrate how and when to use an anaphylaxis treatment device called an EpiPen or an anaphylaxis kit containing epinephrine and Benadryl. Teaching pens without medication are available, and the person and family members must demonstrate how to use them. Make sure the patient or family member has the medication-filled EpiPen or anaphylaxis kit in hand before leaving the facility.
   e. Discuss the possibility of delayed reactions after the diphenhydramine has worn off, and how and why to get help quickly (e.g., call 911).
   f. Discuss strategies for avoiding allergens before discharge.

Asthma

1. Definition
   a. An obstructive pulmonary condition characterized by bronchial and bronchiolar smooth muscle spasm, mucosal swelling from increased capillary permeability, and hypertrophy of the mucous glands, producing excessive viscous mucus that can obstruct airways (see Chapter 20).
   b. Term **reactive airway disease** may be used.
   c. Individuals may have acute attacks that are short-lived or may progress to develop chronic asthma and COPD.
   d. *Status asthmaticus* is a life-threatening condition in which attack is unresponsive to standard therapy.
2. Incidence and socioeconomic impact
   a. Asthma deaths are on the increase, especially in children and young adults.
   b. Asthma may be intrinsic, with no apparent allergen source, or extrinsic, due to a wide range of allergens (see Chapter 22).
3. Clinical manifestations
   a. Swelling and increased mucus production impede both inspiratory and expiratory air flow, causing cough; wheezing; chest tightness; air hunger; hypoxemia; use of accessory muscles to breathe; fatigue; fear; and if severe, altered consciousness, respiratory arrest, and death.
4. Triage priority: Immediate priority is given because of

the impaired oxygenation and potential for sudden death.

5. Diagnostics
   a. Assessment: history of asthma; exposure to known allergens, including cigarette smoking; recent upper respiratory infection
      (1) Physical examination findings
         (a) Respiratory symptoms: shortness of breath, wheezing, exertional dyspnea, chest tightness, cough, increased sputum production
         (b) Central nervous system symptoms: anxiety, restlessness, fatigue, syncope, coma
         (c) Physical or emotional stress
         (d) Medications used, especially last dose of inhaled medications, use of steroids, and compliance with medication regimen; use of over-the-counter medications
         (e) Peak flow measurements, if being used to guide self-medication
         (f) Asthma history, including treatments that have been successful in the past, previous hospitalizations, and need for intubation and mechanical ventilation

> **NURSE ADVISORY**
>
> Obtain detailed information regarding the use and timing of asthma medications, including both prescriptive and over-the-counter medications. Individuals having an attack may have used inhalers more frequently than recommended and are at risk for cardiac dysrhythmias, especially if epinephrine is subsequently administered.

         (g) Level of consciousness: Individuals with an acute asthma attack are usually alert and quite anxious; the asthmatic patient with exhaustion or a decreased level of consciousness is of grave concern because of the likelihood of rapid progression to respiratory arrest.
         (h) Respiratory parameters, including breath sounds, especially inspiratory or expiratory wheezing

> **NURSE ADVISORY**
>
> The absence of wheezing in an asthmatic patient having an attack is an ominous sign. It may indicate that the airways are so constricted that air exchange is minimal.

- Air hunger
- Cough and sputum production
- Prolonged expiratory phase
- Hyperresonance to percussion
- Use of accessory muscles to breathe (e.g., sternomastoid and intercostal muscle retraction)
- Nasal flaring, especially in children
- Dyspnea, tachypnea, or both

- Pursed lip breathing
- Inability to speak more than a few words without taking a breath
  - (i) Peripheral perfusion
    - Skin vitals: pale, cool, and moist; cyanosis of ear lobe or perioral area is a very late sign of distress.
    - Capillary refill may be delayed.
    - Slight hypertension is common; hypotension is ominous.
    - Paradoxical pulse, if present, may indicate a severe attack, but is not always present.
    - Tachycardia is common, due both to the effect of medications and the stress of the physical work involved.
    - The oral temperature may be normal or low when the patient is evaluated initially; however, the reliability of an oral temperature is questionable, especially if the person is mouth breathing. Tympanic membrane temperatures are sometimes obtained but are of questionable validity as well. The temperature measurement may be deferred until treatment has been initiated and the person is less dyspneic and has been rehydrated. A subsequent temperature reading often shows a mild to moderate elevation, suggestive of an infectious etiology.
  - (j) Posture: The individual who is having an asthma attack usually prefers to sit straight up, often with the legs dangling over the side of the stretcher.
  - b. Diagnostic studies
    - (1) Pulse oximetry
    - (2) Peak flow measurement or spirometry
    - (3) Chest radiograph
    - (4) Arterial blood gases if oximetry is poor
    - (5) Sputum studies
    - (6) Complete blood count to determine leukocytosis (associated with infection), eosinophilia (associated with allergic responses), or elevated hematocrit (associated with increased red blood cell production in response to hypoxemia or dehydration)
    - (7) Theophylline level, if person is taking theophylline preparations
    - (8) Electrolytes, if the person is obtunded or not responding to therapy
6. Clinical management
  - a. Goals of clinical management are to improve air exchange and tissue oxygenation by relieving bronchospasm and to identify and treat etiology (e.g., infection).
  - b. Place the person in a sitting position, unless obtunded.
  - c. Administer humidified oxygen via nasal prongs.
    - (1) Alert individuals with air hunger usually tolerate nasal prongs better than oxygen masks.
    - (2) The liter flow is dependent on both the oximetry and arterial blood gas results and the presence or absence of COPD.
    - (3) High-flow oxygen administered to the person with

COPD may eliminate the respiratory drive completely and cause respiratory arrest because that person's stimulus to breathe is the oxygen level, not carbon dioxide as in normal individuals.
  - (4) A Venturi mask that delivers 24 or 28 percent oxygen may be used in the person with COPD, once the acute dyspnea is resolved.
  - (5) Humidification assists in loosening secretions, thereby facilitating removal and preventing mucus plugs.
  - d. Administer bronchodilators via a small-volume nebulizer or metered-dose inhaler.
    - (1) Medications frequently used include albuterol, isoetharine, terbutaline, and atropine.
    - (2) Carefully observe the person while he or she is using the metered-dose inhaler; many "treatment failures" are due to incorrect use of inhalers.
  - e. Administer bronchodilators such as subcutaneous epinephrine or terbutaline as an alternative or adjunct to inhaled agents.
    - (1) Epinephrine may be contraindicated in individuals with hypertension or those older than 40 years of age because of the cardiovascular effects.
    - (2) Subcutaneously administered epinephrine may result in significant systemic and localized vasoconstriction, as evidenced by elevation of the BP, headache, and a ring of pallor around the injection site. This will usually resolve within 20 minutes.

NURSE ADVISORY

Because of concern about carbon dioxide retention in persons with chronic obstructive pulmonary disease, medical air rather than oxygen may be used to deliver nebulizer treatments. It is critical that medical air flowmeters be removed from the wall at the completion of a treatment, lest someone inadvertently connect oxygen tubing to the device, causing hypoxemia to worsen.

  - f. Assess medication effectiveness immediately after completion of small-volume nebulizer, and within 20 minutes of metered-dose inhaler or injection therapy.
    - (1) Repeated doses, if needed, must be given in rapid sequence for maximal effectiveness; continuous therapy is now used in some facilities.
    - (2) Assessment parameters include breath sounds, vital signs, and peak flow measurements.
  - g. Establish an IV line for medication administration: Establishing IV access is usually done early in the course of treatment if IV medications are to be given; however, not all asthmatics require IV medications. If blood tests are ordered, it is prudent to start an IV and draw the blood from the IV; this decreases the number of venipunctures.
  - h. Administer IV steroids, usually methylprednisolone (Solu-Medrol); oral steroids may be given as well. Although this is uncommon, some individuals are allergic to certain steroid preparations, and their symptoms may worsen.

i. Aminophylline, IV bolus and maintenance drip, is sometimes used, but it is no longer part of the routine management. Obtain theophylline level (if on theophylline) before administering additional theophylline.
   (1) There is a very fine line between therapeutic and toxic levels of aminophylline.
   (2) Physical findings may not adequately forewarn of toxicity, but persons should be observed for tremulousness, tachycardia, nausea, vomiting, and central nervous system symptoms, including seizures.
j. Continuously monitor ECG for hypoxia or drug-induced dysrhythmias.
k. Administer antibiotics if there is evidence of bronchitis or pneumonia.

7. Applying the nursing process

NURSING DIAGNOSIS: Ineffective airway clearance R/T bronchospasm, edema of airways, and mucus production

a. *Expected outcomes:* Following interventions, the patient should be able to demonstrate effective airway clearance by
   (1) Absence of shortness of breath
   (2) Clear breath sounds
   (3) Ability to manage secretions
b. *Nursing interventions*
   (1) Minimize energy expenditure and oxygen need by transporting the person by wheelchair or stretcher. Restrict history taking, or phrase questions so that they may be answered with a "yes" or "no."
   (2) Promote maximal lung expansion by placing the patient in a sitting position and by loosening or removing restrictive clothing.
   (3) Administer oxygen, bronchodilators, and steroids.
   (4) Offer oral hydration to thin secretions and facilitate expectoration.
   (5) Obtain sputum specimen.
   (6) Provide an environment that is free from emotional or chemical irritants, including medical or nursing staff who may be wearing perfumes or colognes that worsen bronchospasm.

NURSING DIAGNOSIS: Impaired gas exchange R/T airflow obstruction

a. *Expected outcomes:* Following intervention, the patient should experience optimal tissue oxygenation as evidenced by an oxygen saturation of 90% or greater.
b. *Nursing interventions*
   (1) See nursing interventions for ineffective airway clearance.
   (2) Provide ongoing cardiac and oximetry monitoring, and frequently reassess respiratory status and level of consciousness (at least every 30 minutes); be prepared for endotracheal intubation and mechanical ventilation.

NURSING DIAGNOSIS: Fear or anxiety R/T inadequate airflow and possibly to previous hospitalizations for asthma

a. *Expected outcomes:* Following interventions, the patient should verbalize a decrease in anxiety and fear.
b. *Nursing interventions*
   (1) Involve the individual in plan of care.
   (2) Explain all procedures, and gain the person's assistance.
   (3) Ensure that call light is given and explained.
   (4) Accommodate request that curtains or doors be left open to decrease feeling of isolation.

NURSING DIAGNOSIS: Knowledge deficit R/T asthma management

a. *Expected outcomes:* Following interventions, the patient should do the following:
   (1) State the causes of the attack and the treatment after discharge, including avoidance of allergens and use of medications
   (2) Develop strategies to foster optimal health
b. *Nursing interventions*
   (1) Involve the person in his or her care; many asthmatics are used to managing their disease with a high degree of independence. Explain all therapies.
   (2) Provide discharge instructions as outlined below.
   (3) Consider referral to a community health nurse for evaluation of home or work environment, to determine whether either is a potential source of allergens.

8. Criteria for discharge
   a. Breath sounds are clear bilaterally.
   b. Peak flow is improved from baseline.
   c. Oximetry is within normal limits.
   d. Respiratory rate and effort are normal.
   e. Mentation and behavior are normal.
   f. Vital signs and skin vital signs are normal.
   g. The individual verbalizes that status has improved.
   h. The individual has the knowledge and capacity to care for self after discharge, including acquisition and use of medications.
   i. The individual demonstrates correct use of metered-dose inhaler. Teaching devices are available and should be used to ensure that the individual is able to perform a return demonstration correctly. Many treatment failures result from incorrect use of inhalers.
   j. The individual demonstrates the correct use of a peak flow meter and is able to articulate actions to take when peak flow decreases.
   k. The individual verbalizes the use and purpose of each medication prescribed.

9. Discharge planning and teaching
   a. Teach the basic pathophysiology of asthma, and precipitating causes.
   b. Review measures to be taken to prevent recurrence, including information on smoking cessation, if relevant.

c. Discuss medications to be used, especially how to use metered-dose inhalers and spacers, steroid tapering, and so forth.

d. Explain where and when to obtain follow-up care.

e. Review what to do in the event of recurrence of attack.

f. Stress the importance of hydration to facilitate expectoration of secretions.

Bronchitis

1. Definition: an inflammation of the bronchi that results from bronchial tissue irritation by agents such as tobacco smoke, pollen, and chemicals

2. Incidence, socioeconomic impact, and risk factors

 a. Acute bronchitis often follows an upper respiratory infection. Chronic bronchitis due to long-standing irritant exposure is a form of COPD and is characterized by persistent productive cough (see Chapter 22).

 b. Acute bronchitis is seen in all age groups. Chronic bronchitis is seen in middle-aged and older adults and occurs most often in winter and early spring.

 c. Men have a higher incidence of chronic bronchitis, but that may change as female smokers age.

3. Triage priority: usually not urgent unless hypoxemic

4. Diagnostics

 a. History of upper respiratory infection, chemical exposure, allergies, frequent respiratory infections, and smoking; occupational exposures; medications used; exposure to low-humidity air (e.g., airplane travel, arid climate)

 b. Physical examination findings

 (1) Cough: productive or nonproductive

 (2) Chest or back pain

 (3) Fever

 (4) Shortness of breath

 (5) Vital signs: tachypnea, fever, mild tachycardia, possible elevated BP

 (6) Use of accessory muscles, retraction, flaring of nostrils in children

 (7) Neck vein distention

 (8) Prolonged expiratory phase

 (9) Lung sounds: wheezes or rhonchi

 (10) Hyperresonance to percussion in those with chronic bronchitis

 (11) Sputum: ranging from thin and clear to thick and yellow or white

 (12) Anxiety and agitation, if severe dyspnea

 c. Diagnostic studies

 (1) Pulse oximetry may be normal in acute bronchitis and significantly lowered in chronic bronchitis.

 (2) Pulmonary function: peak flow

 (3) Arterial blood gases if oximetry poor

 (4) Complete blood count; leukocytosis, polycythemia, eosinophilia

 (5) Chest radiograph

 (6) Sputum evaluation

 (7) Theophylline levels, if appropriate

5. Clinical management

 a. Assist individual in assuming a position that maxi-

mizes ventilatory effort, usually sitting up; loosen belts, ties, and other restrictive clothing.

 b. Apply humidified oxygen, using a rate and device appropriate for oximetry levels and history of COPD (e.g., low-flow oxygen using a Venturi mask for individuals with COPD), remembering that high-flow oxygen may inhibit respiratory drive in these individuals.

 c. Administer medications as prescribed (e.g., bronchodilators [albuterol, metaproterenol] via small-volume nebulizer or metered-dose inhaler; steroids, theophylline preparations. Cough suppressants may be ordered for the person with acute bronchitis.

 d. Provide oral fluids for hydration and to thin secretions.

 e. Remove allergens from environment.

6. Applying the nursing process

NURSING DIAGNOSIS: Ineffective airway clearance R/T inflamed bronchial tissue

 a. *Expected outcomes:* Following interventions, the person should experience improved breathing and resolution of dyspnea.

 b. *Nursing interventions*

 (1) Administer medications as indicated.

 (2) Assist person to achieve a position that promotes maximal lung expansion.

NURSING DIAGNOSIS: Impaired gas exchange R/T increased mucus production

 a. *Expected outcomes:* Following interventions, the person should experience improved gas exchange as evidenced by an oxygen saturation of 90% or greater.

 b. *Nursing interventions*

 (1) Administer medications as prescribed.

 (2) Assist patient to a position that promotes maximal lung expansion.

 (3) Provide oral fluids to thin secretions.

 (4) Provide humidified oxygen, if appropriate.

 (5) Monitor oxygen saturation via pulse oximetry.

Additional Nursing Diagnosis

NURSING DIAGNOSIS: Knowledge deficit R/T bronchitis, factors that worsen symptoms and treatment plan, including use of medications

1. Discharge criteria

 a. Improvement of respiratory symptoms if small-volume nebulizer administered

 b. Room air pulse oximetry within normal limits for the individual

2. Discharge planning and teaching

a. Cigarette smoking or exposure to cigarette smoke is a major cause of bronchitis; hence information on strategies for smoking cessation (e.g., nicotine replacement therapy, smoking cessation classes) or smoke avoidance should be offered. Children of smokers have a higher incidence of bronchitis as well as otitis media.

b. Smoke from wood stoves may also be a factor in the development of bronchitis in both adults and children.

c. Bronchitis in the nonsmoker is often associated with upper respiratory infections; thus, prevention of these infections should be discussed.

d. Medications used in the treatment of bronchitis may include cough preparations containing narcotics (usually codeine), which may impair judgment and cause safety concerns.

  • Teaching includes alcohol avoidance and not operating a motor vehicle or machinery while taking the medication.

  • Codeine-containing medications may cause nausea if taken on an empty stomach; recommend taking them with meals.

  • Codeine preparations may cause constipation; advise the person to increase roughage and fluids in the diet to prevent this.

  • Cough-suppressing medications may interfere with activity, impede expectoration of mucus, and predispose the person to pneumonia; caution about overuse and the need to take deep breaths periodically.

e. Antibiotics may also be prescribed, and it is important that specific instructions be given about how to take them (e.g., with food or on an empty stomach), as well as the need to complete all medications, even though symptoms usually improve within 24 hours. Individuals with chronic bronchitis may have a routine standing order for antibiotics that is filled at the onset of symptoms; reinforce appropriate use of the antibiotics.

f. Plan for follow-up care: Include actions to take if symptoms worsen or do not improve within several days.

Acute Exacerbation of Chronic Obstructive Pulmonary Disease

1. Definition: a term given to chronic bronchitis, asthma, and emphysema (see Chapter 22)

2. Incidence and socioeconomic impact: Individuals seeking emergency care usually have varying degrees of hypoxemia and respiratory distress that often is exacerbated by pulmonary infection or exposure to pulmonary irritants. See Chapter 22 for discussion of pathophysiology.

3. Triage priority: immediate, due to hypoxemia

4. Diagnostics

a. Assessment: History of dyspnea at rest or with exertion; chronic productive cough; fatigue; weight loss or loss of appetite; anxiety; frequent pulmonary infections; exposure to irritants: cigarette smoke, pollution, occupational exposure; current and recent medications; include last dosages, especially of inhalers, theophylline preparations, and steroids. Medical history: heart disease, hypertension, diabetes, cigarette smoking, pulmonary disease. The person's wishes regarding endotracheal intubation and resuscitative measures. Individuals with end-stage COPD are extremely difficult to wean from a ventilator and may wish to limit their care to comfort and pharmacologic measures, but not intubation and mechanical ventilation.

b. Physical examination findings
   (1) Cyanosis
   (2) Altered mental status: restlessness, confusion, lethargy, or obtundation
   (3) Speaks in short sentences (3–4 words) because of dyspnea
   (4) Pursed-lip breathing
   (5) Cardiac dysrhythmias: premature ventricular contractions, tachycardia
   (6) Paradoxical pulse
   (7) Blood pressure may be elevated or low
   (8) Chest examination: rales, rhonchi, or wheezes; prolonged expiratory phase; increased anteroposterior diameter of chest (barrel chest); use of accessory muscles for breathing; diaphragmatic breathing

NURSE ADVISORY

Individuals with chronic obstructive pulmonary disease are at risk for spontaneous pneumothorax due to bleb rupture. Sudden worsening in respiratory status warrants attention to this possibility.

   (9) Requires sitting position; may dramatically worsen when placed supine

c. Diagnostic studies
   (1) Pulse oximetry
   (2) Peak flow meter or spirometry
   (3) Arterial blood gases: hypoxemia and hypercarbia
   (4) Chest radiograph
   (5) Sputum examination
   (6) Complete blood count to detect infection

5. Clinical management

a. Assist the person in assuming a position that optimizes air exchange, usually sitting up.

b. Apply humidified oxygen, usually low flow via a Venturi mask; observe carefully for evidence of decreased level of consciousness because oxygen administration may inhibit respiratory drive.

c. Prepare for the possibility of endotracheal intubation if the person is exhausted and profoundly hypoxemic.

d. Administer bronchodilators via small-volume nebulizer.

e. Steroids given IV or orally may be used.

f. Reassess efficacy of the small-volume nebulizer every 15 to 20 minutes using spirometry or peak flow measurements; small-volume nebulizers usually administered 3 times every 20 minutes, although a continuous small-volume nebulizer may also be used.

g. Provide oral fluids to facilitate thinning and expectoration of secretions.

h. Administer theophylline preparations. (See "Asthma.")

i. Individuals who are so profoundly hypoxemic that they require intubation and those who do not respond after 3 small-volume nebulizers generally require hospitalization.

6. Applying the nursing process (see "Asthma" and "Bronchitis" and Chapter 22)

7. Discharge planning and teaching

a. Once the acute crisis has resolved, explore strategies that will allow the person to carry out activities of daily living without becoming dyspneic, and determine treatments that the individual can use to avoid an acute crisis.

b. Review medications to be taken.

c. Discuss safety and dietary considerations related to the use of narcotic analgesics.

d. Describe the expected recovery course and the reasons to seek care again.

e. Explain the importance of coughing and deep breathing.

f. Stress increasing oral fluid intake to promote thinning and expectoration and to manage fluid loss associated with fever.

g. Explain how to increase caloric intake.

Pneumonia

1. Definition: Inflammation of pulmonary parenchyma caused by bacteria, viruses, fungi, mycoplasma, rickettsiae, or parasites (see Chapter 22). Chemical pneumonitis occurs from aspiration or toxic fume inhalation.

2. Triage priority

a. Variable depending on severity of symptoms.

b. Children and older patients may have less well-defined symptoms, and older people are at greater risk for developing complications such as empyema and meningitis.

c. Patients who are infected with the human immunodeficiency virus (HIV) are at risk for *Pneumocystis carinii* pneumonia, as well as for pulmonary tuberculosis.

d. Key is that many individuals seeking emergency care present with generalized malaise and fever without specific symptoms.

3. Assessment, clinical management, and nursing diagnoses. See Chapter 22.

4. Criteria for discharge

a. Normal vital signs

b. Oximetry within normal limits

c. Able to perform activities of daily living

d. Resources and ability to obtain medications (antibiotics and analgesics) and to take as prescribed

e. Ability to return if symptoms worsen

f. Consider community health nurse visitation for older patients, especially those who live alone.

5. Discharge planning and teaching

a. Review medications to be taken.

b. Explain safety and dietary considerations related to use of narcotic analgesics.

c. Describe expected recovery course and reasons to seek care again.

d. Stress the importance of coughing and deep breathing.

e. Explain increasing oral fluid intake to promote thinning and expectoration of secretions and to manage fluid loss associated with fever.

Pulmonary Embolism

1. Definition

a. Partial or complete obstruction of a branch of the pulmonary artery by a thrombus from elsewhere in the venous system, which may consist of clotted blood, amnionic fluid, fat, or bone (see Chapter 22).

b. Pulmonary embolism is most often seen in older patients, postoperatively, post–long bone fracture, in people who have been immobile, in dehydrated individuals, and in women using oral contraceptives, especially if they also use cigarettes.

2. Triage priority: High because of hypoxemia and potential for cardiac arrest; however, many individuals present with vague symptoms, and the nature of the problem is unclear. People with pulmonary embolism are hospitalized.

3. Diagnostics

a. Assessment (see Chapter 22)

b. Diagnostic studies

(1) Pulse oximetry may be only slightly abnormal.

(2) Chest radiograph is often normal.

(3) Cardiac rhythm indicates tachycardia.

(4) Petechiae are noted in those with fat embolism.

(5) Ventilation-perfusion lung scan is diagnostic.

4. Clinical management, complications, and nursing diagnoses (see Chapter 22)

Epiglottitis

1. Definition

a. Life-threatening inflammation of the epiglottis and supraglottic tissues that may rapidly result in complete airway obstruction (see Chapter 15)

b. Organism most often responsible is *Haemophilus influenzae*

c. Occurs most often in children (especially males), but may affect adults as well

d. Characterized by sudden onset of symptoms

2. Triage priority: immediate because of high potential for complete airway obstruction

3. Diagnostics

a. Assessment

(1) History of rapid development of high fever (above 101 degrees Fahrenheit); sore throat; drooling or inability to swallow secretions; lethargy; decreased appetite; and recent upper respiratory infection

(2) Physical examination is limited initially to whatever can be observed; do not attempt to visualize the throat or perform procedures or activities that may cause the patient to cry or change position.

This may result in airway obstruction. Findings are as follows:
- Vital signs, including temperature measurement, are often deferred until emergency airway management equipment and personnel are available.
- Characteristic posture in children, known as the tripod or sniffing position, which facilitates airway patency
- Patient appears ill or very pale and may have shadows beneath eyes
- Dysphagia
- Muffled voice—described as sounding as though the patient has mashed potatoes in his or her mouth
- Drooling
- Inspiratory stridor, expiratory snore
- Retractions
- High fever

NURSE ADVISORY

When epiglottitis is suspected, the priorities are to maintain a patent airway by minimizing activities that may obstruct the airway (such as crying), to obtain rapid radiographic evaluation to confirm the diagnosis, and to secure the airway through tracheal intubation. Because of the potential for sudden loss of the airway, the patient is continuously accompanied by personnel and equipment for surgical airway management. Typically, a soft tissue radiograph of the neck is taken immediately. If epiglottitis is present, the child is taken promptly to the operating room for tracheal intubation or immediate surgical airway, if intubation is not feasible. Other procedures and medications are deferred until the airway is secured.

  b. Diagnostic studies
   (1) Lateral neck radiograph is done very gently to minimize potential for airway obstruction; airway management resources must remain with patient during radiography. In many institutions, the patient is taken directly to the operating room for endotracheal intubation by direct or indirect laryngoscopy, with a set-up for tracheotomy immediately available.
   (2) Chest radiograph
   (3) Complete blood count
   (4) Arterial blood gases
   (5) Pulse oximetry
  4. Clinical management
   a. Establish and maintain airway; administer high-flow oxygen.
   b. Establish an IV line.
   c. Administer antibiotics.
   d. Once the airway is secured, sedation may be necessary for procedures and maximal ventilatory effort.
   e. Encourage family member to remain with the patient to allay fear, which may worsen the airway obstruction, or to facilitate patient cooperation with procedures.
   f. Provide a call light or other nonverbal means of communication.
  5. Applying the nursing process

NURSING DIAGNOSIS: Ineffective airway clearance R/T laryngospasm and edema of epiglottis

  a. *Expected outcomes:* Following interventions, the person should experience the following:
   (1) Breath sounds are equal bilaterally.
   (2) Oximetry is within normal limits.
   (3) Individual has improved respiratory rate, rhythm, effort, and tidal volume.
   (4) Intercostal, supraclavicular, and substernal retractions are decreased or absent.
   (5) There is minimal or no use of accessory muscles for breathing.
   (6) Color of skin and mucous membranes is improved.
   (7) Arterial blood gases are improved.
   (8) Secretions are expectorated.
  b. *Nursing interventions*
   (1) Secure airway. Endotracheal intubation may be necessary.
   (2) Monitor oxygen saturation via pulse oximetry.
   (3) Position person for optimal lung expansion.
   (4) Assist patient to expectorate secretions or suction as needed.

NURSING DIAGNOSIS: Anxiety R/T difficulty breathing, invasive procedures, separation from loved ones, and hospitalization

  a. *Expected outcomes:* Following interventions, the patient should be able to do the following:
   (1) Communicate decreased anxiety nonverbally or verbally
   (2) Be able to cooperate with procedures
  b. *Nursing interventions*
   (1) Stay with the person.
   (2) Allow person access to significant others.
   (3) Explain all procedures.
   (4) Approach person and family in a calm reassuring manner.
   (5) Administer anxiolytic medications as indicated.

Inhalation Injury Due to Smoke or Toxic Fumes

1. Definition: damage to the pulmonary system or the whole body due to inhalation of injurious material; bronchospasm, pneumonia, tracheitis, mediastinitis, pulmonary edema, and adult respiratory distress syndrome are not uncommon (see Chapters 36 and 38)
2. Risk factors and etiology
  a. Classic smoke inhalation from a house fire, with exposure to carbon monoxide, cyanide, and acrolein
  b. New smoke inhalation—injuries resulting from burning of synthetic products (e.g., plastics) in an enclosed space, with exposure to myriad toxins such as hydrogen chloride, toluene, chlorine gas, ammonia, and styrene (Table 37–2)

Table 37-2. Common Toxic Substances in Smoke Inhalation

Agent	Source	Toxic Substance	Site Affected
Polyvinyl chloride	Rubberized wall and floor coverings, pipes, cable insulation	Hydrogen chloride	Lungs
		Phosgene	Lungs
		Carbon monoxide	Systemic
Polyurethane	Upholstery	Isocyanates	Lungs
		Hydrogen cyanide	Systemic
Polystyrene	Foam products (e.g., cushions, pillows)	Styrene	Systemic
		Carbon monoxide	Systemic
Acrilan	Carpeting	Hydrogen cyanide	Systemic
Wall paper		Acid aldehyde	Lungs
Lacquered wood		Formaldehyde	Lungs
		Nitrogen oxides	Lungs
		Acetic acid	Systemic

c. Carbon monoxide from automobile exhaust fumes coming through the floor of car into passenger compartment, inadequate ventilation when oxygen-consuming engines are being used, faulty furnaces and heating systems, and fire in a closed space (see Chapter 38)

d. Industrial exposure both in the course of work and with a hazardous materials spill

3. Triage priority: immediate
4. Diagnostics
  a. Assessment
   (1) History of exposure often present, but may be obscure, such as carbon monoxide in a car or home, in which case altered consciousness may be the presenting symptom. Other data include the following: difficulty breathing; cough, which may or may not be productive; carbonaceous sputum with smoke inhalation; headache; and malaise; if work-related exposure, obtain information about likely substances (e.g., metal cleaning or glass etching).
   (2) Physical examination
     • Tachypnea, which worsens with minimal exertion
     • Soot on face, around and in nose and mouth
     • Singed facial hair and eyebrows
     • Facial, airway, or other burns
     • Respiratory symptoms: hoarseness, stridor, rales, rhonchi, wheezes
     • Carbonaceous or blood-tinged sputum; sputum may also be frothy, suggesting pulmonary edema
     • Skin color may be red because of carbon monoxide, cyanosis, or normal appearance
     • Pulse oximetry variable
     • Altered level of consciousness
     • Hypotension
     • Cardiac dysrhythmias may be present.
  b. Diagnostic studies
   (1) Arterial blood gases
   (2) Chest radiograph / lung scan
   (3) Electrocardiogram
   (4) Carboxyhemoglobin level—symptoms associated with various levels are listed in Table 37-3.
   (5) Cyanide levels
   (6) Toxicology screen, if there is fire involving a drug laboratory or job-related incident
5. Clinical management (see Chapter 36 for a detailed discussion)
  a. Airway management, which may include emergency laryngoscopy or bronchoscopy to remove soot from

Table 37-3. Signs and Symptoms Associated with Carbon Monoxide

Carboxyhemoglobin Level	Significance	Signs and Symptoms
0.3–10%	Normal	Increased blood flow to organs secondary to vasodilation; increased visual acuity
10–20%	Mild poisoning	Slight dyspnea, headache, flulike symptoms, decreased mental and visual acuity
20–40%	Moderate poisoning	Headache, feeling of constricting band around forehead, tinnitus, dizziness, weakness, yawning, dilated pupils, hypotension, tachycardia, ST-segment depression, atrial and ventricular dysrhythmias, pale or red-purple skin color
40–60%	Severe poisoning	Coma, seizures, cardiovascular collapse, death

airways, or endotracheal intubation and mechanical ventilation

b. High-flow humidified oxygen via tight-fitting mask; continuous positive airway pressure (CPAP) may be indicated

c. Hyperbaric oxygenation therapy

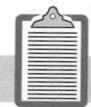

NURSING MANAGEMENT

The phone number of the closest medical hyperbaric chamber should be posted and immediately available. In addition, policies and procedures for preparing for and transporting a person to a hyperbaric chamber should be available.

d. Cyanide antidote, commercially available as Cyanide Antidote Package, includes amyl nitrite vaporettes, and sodium nitrite and sodium thiosulfate for IV use may be administered; fire departments now stock the antidote on EMS and fire rescue rigs for field administration.

e. Intravenous access and IV fluid restriction

f. Cardiac monitoring to detect ischemia and hypoxia-induced dysrhythmias

g. In smoke inhalation, absolute bed rest is recommended, even if there are minimal symptoms, because of the high potential for pulmonary edema with exertion.

h. Hospitalization is suggested for even minor smoke inhalation, especially that associated with plastics combustion.

i. Individuals with minor carbon monoxide exposures may be discharged; however, it is important to determine the cause, and to recommend community resources if residence cannot be reoccupied immediately.

6. Applying the nursing process (see Chapter 36). Common nursing diagnoses used are the following:
   • Ineffective airway clearance
   • Activity intolerance
   • Fear
   • Altered tissue perfusion

Near Drowning

1. Definition: also known as submersion injury or submersion incident; initial survival of person who has experienced water submersion

2. Incidence, socioeconomic impact, and risk factors
   a. Highest risk groups are children younger than 5 years of age and young adults between 15 and 24 years of age; people of all ages with seizure disorders are also at great risk during routine bathing.
   b. Submersion locations include bathtubs, swimming pools, oceans, lakes, quarries, canals, and buckets of water. Home swimming pools account for more than 50 percent of the drownings in young children.

Ocean drownings are less frequent than those in other locations due to lifeguard presence on public beaches.
   c. More than 50 percent of the victims are males.
   d. Black children have a 3 times greater incidence of drowning, and the location is more often a quarry or canal where lifeguards are not available.
   e. Alcohol, drug use, and medical conditions such as hypoglycemia or cardiac disorders are also associated with drowning.
   f. Drowning or near drowning may indicate child abuse or neglect; legal investigation is indicated.
   g. Drowning as a result of spinal cord injury sustained by diving into shallow water is very common among teenage and young adult males.
   h. Prevention strategies such as legislation requiring locked gates around pools have not been found to be particularly effective; research has demonstrated that although the barriers are in place, often the gate lock is unfastened or broken.
   i. Raising pool water level may also be a prevention measure; the average distance between the top of the water and the pool ledge is 12 to 14 inches—too great a height for a young child to pull him- or herself out of the pool. Raising the water level might decrease the incidence of drowning.
   j. Hypothermia often occurs in near drowning victims; depending on the degree of hypothermia, advanced cardiac life support (ACLS) measures (e.g., cardiotonic medications or defibrillation) may be ineffective until the person has been rewarmed. Resuscitation measures cannot be stopped until there has been adequate rewarming. (See Chapter 23 for discussion of ACLS protocols.)
   k. Despite differences in the tonicity of fresh water versus salt water, the major pathophysiologic changes that occur in a near drowning are essentially the same: hypoxemia (due to washout of pulmonary surfactant in most cases) and respiratory and metabolic acidosis.
   l. Although most near drowning victims aspirate a large amount of water ("wet drowning"), approximately 10 percent are "dry drownings" because of laryngospasm in response to the cold water. Although there may be no water aspiration, the airway closure still results in profound hypoxia, and the treatment for both groups is the same.
   m. Individuals who appear to have minimal submersion injury may develop delayed adult respiratory distress syndrome hours to days after the incident; hospitalization and careful monitoring are recommended.

3. Triage priority: Immediate, regardless of the initial presentation

4. Diagnostics
   a. Assessment
      (1) History of the event: fresh water versus salt water, cold versus warm water; length of submersion; witnessed or unwitnessed; risk for spinal cord or other injury; health status, especially conditions such as diabetes, seizures, cardiac problems, medication, alcohol or drug use

(2) Physical examination
- Many individuals are unconscious; thus information is obtained from bystanders or EMS personnel.
- Awake patients may minimize the degree of submersion and have few or no symptoms.
- Mild dyspnea, especially with activity, may be noted.
- Wheezing
- Cough
- Nausea or vomiting, or both, due to swallowing water
- Shaking chills or feeling cold
- ABCs—many individuals are in cardiac arrest and arrive while undergoing resuscitation efforts.
- Respiratory status: oximetry, breath sounds, secretions
- Cardiac rhythm, vital signs, with attention to temperature
- Evidence of, or potential for, injury
- Vomiting

b. Diagnostic studies
(1) Chest radiograph; cervical spine radiograph, if indicated
(2) Arterial blood gases
(3) Electrocardiogram
(4) Routine laboratory tests: complete blood count with platelets, electrolytes, BUN, serum osmolality, and clotting studies; urinalysis

5. Clinical management
   a. Establish and maintain airway; endotracheal intubation may be required. Administer oxygen as discussed later.
   b. Initiate cardiac monitoring.
   c. Follow ACLS protocols, if cardiac arrest.
   d. Establish IV access and draw blood for laboratory tests from site (if possible).
   e. Provide positive end-expiratory pressure (PEEP); CPAP; supplemental oxygen via non-rebreather mask or nasal prongs, depending on the severity of hypoxemia.
   f. Administer IV sodium bicarbonate for metabolic acidosis, depending on arterial blood gas results.
   g. Use rewarming procedures if hypothermic; prevent hypothermia, especially in children.
   h. Give antibiotics for pulmonary infection due to aspirated foreign material.
   i. Diuretics may be used to support both pulmonary and cerebral perfusion.
   j. Intravenous steroids may be used to stabilize surfactant-producing cells and decrease cerebral edema, but are controversial.
   k. Insert a nasogastric tube to remove swallowed water, allowing for maximal lung expansion and minimizing vomiting and aspiration.
   l. Use a Foley catheter, if consciousness is altered.
   m. Identify and treat other injuries.
   n. Provide supportive care.

6. Applying the nursing process

NURSING DIAGNOSIS: Impaired gas exchange R/T pulmonary edema and adult respiratory distress syndrome

a. *Expected outcomes:* Following interventions, the person should experience improved gas exchange as evidenced by the following:
(1) Oxygen saturation of 90% or greater
(2) Clear breath sounds
(3) Normal respiratory rate and effort
b. *Nursing interventions*
(1) Administer oxygen as ordered; monitor cardiovascular response to PEEP or CPAP.
(2) Set the patient in a position that maximizes oxygenation without compromising circulation.
(3) Monitor oximetry.
(4) Administer medications and respiratory treatments as indicated.
(5) Administer sedation and paralyzing agents as indicated for mechanical ventilation.

NURSING DIAGNOSIS: Fluid volume excess R/T aspiration of water

a. *Expected outcomes:* Following interventions, the person should experience a reduction in fluid volume as evidenced by the following:
(1) Clear breath sounds
(2) Absence of edema
(3) Normal serum osmolality
b. *Nursing interventions*
(1) Carefully monitor urine output and serum osmolality.
(2) Follow IV fluid restriction unless otherwise contraindicated.
(3) Administer diuretics as indicated.

NURSING DIAGNOSIS: Risk for infection R/T aspiration of contaminated water

a. *Expected outcomes:* Following interventions, the person should not develop an infection.
b. *Nursing interventions*
(1) Monitor temperature.
(2) Perform pulmonary toilet as indicated.
(3) Administer antibiotics as indicated.
(4) Encourage awake person to cough and deep breathe.

NURSING DIAGNOSIS: Hypothermia R/T cold water immersion and resuscitation efforts

a. *Expected outcomes:* Following interventions, the person should experience a return to normal body temperature.

b. *Nursing interventions*
(1) Monitor core temperature, cardiac rate and rhythm, and BP; be prepared for rewarming shock.
(2) Perform rewarming procedures.
(3) Increase room temperature, especially when person is uncovered for procedures.
(4) Use heat shield or heat lamps to prevent hypothermia.

NURSING DIAGNOSIS: Risk for injury R/T pulmonary aspiration, altered consciousness, invasive and noninvasive monitoring devices, altered immunity due to hemolysis

a. *Expected outcomes:* Following intervention, the person should be injury free while in a state of altered consciousness.
b. *Nursing interventions*
(1) Ensure that environment is free from devices that may cause pressure to the tissues.
(2) Reposition the unconscious person periodically, as cardiovascular status allows.

NURSING DIAGNOSIS: Post-trauma response R/T near drowning event

a. *Expected outcomes:* Following interventions, the person should experience a decrease in post-traumatic fears and concerns.
b. *Nursing interventions*
(1) Provide opportunity for expression of fears or concerns related to event.
(2) Provide support, reassurance, and factual information if there is guilt over injury or death of another person.
(3) Reinforce that feelings are normal after such a traumatic event.
(4) Offer prompt crisis intervention with a mental health professional or spiritual counselor.

NURSING DIAGNOSIS: Altered tissue perfusion (cerebral, cardiopulmonary, peripheral, and renal) R/T cardiopulmonary arrest or hypotension, hypothermia, and water aspiration

a. *Expected outcomes:* Following intervention, the person should have adequate tissue perfusion.
b. *Nursing interventions:* Administer medications and treatments to support adequate tissue perfusion.

NURSING DIAGNOSIS: Knowledge deficit R/T treatment plan for near drowning, potential complications in asymptomatic individual, or potential for future events in person with seizures or other medical conditions associated with altered consciousness

a. *Expected outcomes:* Following interventions, the person should understand the treatment being implemented.

b. *Nursing interventions*
(1) Explain all procedures.
(2) Explain the potential for delayed complications; asymptomatic individuals may have difficulty understanding the need for hospitalization.
(3) Propose that person with seizures use a "buddy system" so that someone is close at hand during bathing or other water activities, and that flotation devices be considered.
(4) Investigate if further evaluation or medication adjustment is needed to decrease likelihood of seizures or other medical conditions during water activities.

NURSING DIAGNOSIS: Fear R/T respiratory distress or mechanical ventilation

a. *Expected outcomes:* Following interventions, the person should experience a decrease in fear.
b. *Nursing interventions*
(1) Provide psychologic support and explain interventions.
(2) Provide sedation, if needed, when mechanical ventilation is used.
(3) Encourage family and significant others to remain with the person during treatment.
(4) Ensure that a call light is available.
(5) Explain that cardiac and other monitoring systems allow the nurse to continuously assess the person from afar.

NURSING DIAGNOSIS: Anticipatory grieving R/T near drowning of family member

a. *Expected outcomes:* Following counseling, the family should be able to do the following:
(1) Relate information given regarding the person's status and prognosis for survival
(2) Express grief in a manner consistent with their culture
(3) Identify available support systems
b. *Nursing interventions*
(1) The prognosis in an unconscious near drowning victim is extremely grave; although one does not want to present a picture of hopelessness, the family deserves to receive honest information about the likelihood of survival and return to normal function.
(2) Support the family's desire to remain with their loved one to the fullest extent possible; this allows them the opportunity to process the magnitude of the situation and perhaps to reconcile outstanding issues. At the very least, it provides them an opportunity to say to their loved one anything that they wish, so there are fewer regrets if the person does die.
(3) Offer spiritual support and consider needs for religious rites (e.g., Sacraments of the Sick).

(4) Because of their youth and the absence of multisystem organ failure, drowning victims are often ideal organ and tissue donors. If possible, determine wishes regarding organ and tissue donation and advanced directives.

(5) If the person does not survive, the death falls under the jurisdiction of the medical examiner or coroner; provide information regarding administrative processes.

(6) Provide the family or significant others with reference material on grief and loss, if appropriate.

NURSING DIAGNOSIS: Risk for altered parenting R/T inadequate supervision or child abuse or neglect

---

a. *Expected outcomes:* Following interventions, the parent should be able to do the following:
  (1) Identify parental behavior that may have contributed to the near drowning incident
  (2) State an understanding of the administrative policies concerned with protection of minors
b. *Nursing interventions*
  (1) The potential for child abuse or neglect is always considered when the near drowning victim is a young child.
  (2) Refer to agency policies and procedures regarding reporting of potential abuse or neglect to ensure protection of all concerned.
  (3) Consider referral for community health nurse assistance regarding parenting skills and child safety; parenting classes may also be beneficial.

Spontaneous Pneumothorax

1. Definition: partial or complete lung collapse for reasons other than trauma (see Chapter 22)
2. Incidence, socioeconomic impact, and risk factors
   a. Most commonly occurs from rupture of a bleb in individuals with COPD; however, it is also found in tall, thin males for unknown reasons.
   b. There is speculation that there is an increased incidence in individuals who use marijuana because of intense breath holding after inhalation.
3. Clinical manifestations
   a. Symptoms range from mild to severe respiratory distress.
   b. Tension pneumothorax (see p. 1780) can occur if the pneumothorax is large.
4. Diagnostics
   a. Assessment
     (1) History of shortness of breath; chest pain that is usually unilateral; COPD
     (2) Physical examination
       • Varying degrees of dyspnea, tachypnea, air hunger
       • Distended neck veins and hypotension if tension developing
       • Breath sounds diminished or absent

• Tympany to percussion, if entire side of lung affected
• Oximetry may be abnormal.
   b. Diagnostic study: Chest radiograph
5. Clinical management
   a. May be none if less than 20 percent involvement
   b. Removal of air using a needle or insertion of a catheter or chest tube
   c. Small catheters designed specifically for small pneumothorax may also have a flutter valve attached to the tube on 1 side and a drainage bag on the other; this allows the person to ambulate without regular chest drainage apparatus.
   d. A small pneumothorax may be treated on an outpatient basis with either observation or small chest tubes, as described above; a larger pneumothorax usually requires admission and observation for reexpansion.
6. Applying the nursing process: See Chapter 22.
7. Discharge criteria
   a. Small pneumothorax
   b. Person reliable enough to observe for worsening of symptoms and to return for treatment
   c. Normal oximetry results after tube placement and air removal
8. Discharge planning and instructions
   a. Provide explanation of what the problem is and how it will be managed.
   b. Supply the cause of the pneumothorax, if known.
   c. Discuss tube care, if relevant, including what to do if system becomes disconnected.
   d. Discuss pain management, if needed.
   e. Explain follow-up care.

■ *CARING FOR PEOPLE EXPERIENCING CARDIOVASCULAR EMERGENCIES*

Overview

1. Most frequent cardiovascular emergencies (see Chapter 23):
   a. Abnormal heart beat
   b. Myocardial infarction
   c. Angina pectoris, either newly diagnosed or unstable angina
   d. Dissecting aortic aneurysm
   e. Hypertensive crisis
   f. Pericarditis
2. Discussion in this section is limited to abnormal heart beat and care of the person with chest pain and probable myocardial infarction

Abnormal Heart Beat

1. Individuals of all ages present with abnormal heart beat. In some, the abnormality is due to noncardiac conditions (e.g., tachycardia due to fever, drug use, or

stress response); careful evaluation of likely causes of the abnormality is important in determining the priority for treatment. Even so, if the cardiac output is impaired, the etiology is of little importance in the initial triage.

2. This section focuses on either the most frequent or the most serious cardiac dysrhythmias. See Chapter 23 for more details.
3. The most common dysrhythmias
   a. Premature ventricular contractions (PVCs) or ventricular ectopic beats
   b. Ventricular tachycardia
   c. Supraventricular tachycardia (SVT)
   d. Frequent firing of an automatic implanted cardiac defibrillator
   e. Bradycardia
   f. Pacemaker malfunction
4. The primary concerns are the following:
   a. Effect of rhythm disturbance on cardiac output
   b. Potential for deterioration to a more life-threatening dysrhythmia
5. Premature ventricular contractions
   a. Definition: contraction of the ventricle early in the cardiac cycle and from an aberrant conduction pathway
   b. Incidence, socioeconomic impact, and risk factors
      (1) Occasional PVCs are not uncommon, may not be significant, and may not require treatment.
      (2) The presence of PVCs suggests myocardial irritability with potential to cause ventricular fibrillation.
   c. Triage priority: immediate or delayed, depending on the frequency and on other health problems
   d. Diagnostics, clinical management, and applying the nursing process (see Chapter 23)
6. Ventricular tachycardia
   a. Definition: Ventricular rate above 240 beats per minute; wide complexes. Rate interferes with adequate cardiac output. If untreated, usually progresses to ventricular fibrillation. In the awake person, it may be difficult to differentiate from supraventricular tachycardia with aberrant conduction.
   b. Triage priority: immediate
   c. Diagnostics: Usually limited to recognizing the rhythm; further detail deferred until after treatment because of life-threatening nature of the condition. See Chapter 23.
   d. Clinical management and applying the nursing process (see Chapter 23 for ACLS protocols)
7. Ventricular fibrillation
   a. Definition: disorganized and chaotic ventricular activity with no effective cardiac output; a form of cardiac arrest
   b. Triage priority: immediate
   c. Diagnostics: limited to recognizing dysrhythmia
   d. Clinical management: defibrillation; use ACLS protocol (see Chapter 23)
8. Supraventricular tachycardia
   a. Definition
      (1) Heart rate above 140 of supraventricular origin
      (2) May occur in the absence of cardiac disease

(3) Has a variety of etiologies and may be idiopathic
(4) May revert spontaneously
(5) Is of concern if cardiac output falls
   b. Triage priority: immediate
   c. Assessment
      (1) Historical or subjective
         • Patient reports that heart is racing or feels like it is pounding out of the chest or throat.
         • Patient may feel faint or have syncope.
         • Anxiety is not uncommon.
         • Patient may have a past medical history of same.
         • The feeling may be associated with eating a large meal accompanied by alcohol or with the use of medications, caffeine, or street drugs such as cocaine or amphetamines.
         • The condition may be associated with hyperthyroidism.
      (2) Objective: rapid radial pulse rate palpated; may be thready due to rapid rate; possible hypotension
      (3) Diagnostic studies: Cardiac monitor shows supraventricular tachycardia; 12-lead ECG.
      (4) Clinical management: done concurrently with assessment
         • Initiate oxygen by nasal prongs.
         • Establish IV access.
         • Maintain cardiac monitoring.
         • Perform Valsalva maneuver—The person may be instructed to bear down such as when having a bowel movement.
         • Provide stimulation of mammalian diving reflex by submerging nose and mouth in ice water; a cold wash cloth applied to the nose and mouth may accomplish the same result.
         • Perform carotid sinus massage on only 1 side at a time; performed by the physician in most settings.
         • Medications: adenosine (Adenocard) IV, diltiazem (Cardizem), verapamil IV, sedation IV or IM.
         • Use synchronized cardioversion (with prior sedation), if hemodynamically unstable and above therapies are not effective.
         • Some individuals convert spontaneously before treatment.
9. Automatic implantable cardiac defibrillator (AICD) frequent firing
   a. A permanent, surgically implanted device that is programmed to automatically deliver electrical current to the ventricle when the myocardium fibrillates; this creates a sensation of a small electrical shock that the patient can feel. (See Chapter 23.)
   b. Frequent firing occurs because of the following:
      (1) The person is actually having repeated episodes of ventricular fibrillation.
      (2) The AICD is malfunctioning.
   c. In both cases, additional treatment is needed.
   d. Diagnostics
      (1) Assessment: History of person reporting frequent firing. Caregiver can feel the AICD firing. Cardiac monitoring confirms frequent firing.

(2) Clinical management
- Under continuous cardiac monitoring, AICD is turned off using a special magnet, and the person is observed for ventricular fibrillation.
- If repeated ventricular fibrillation is noted, AICD is turned back on and antidysrhythmic drugs are administered.
- If repeated ventricular fibrillation is not documented, it is presumed that there is AICD misfiring, and reprogramming or replacement of the device is done.

10. Bradycardia
 a. Definition: ventricular rate of less than 60 beats per minute
 b. Incidence and socioeconomic impact: Many people, especially athletes, normally have a heart rate of less than 60 beats per minute and are asymptomatic. Bradycardia causes concern when it results in symptoms of inadequate cardiac output and hypoperfusion, such as weakness, syncope, or unconsciousness.
 c. Etiology: Bradycardia occurs for a variety of reasons:
 - Incomplete or complete heart block, which may be due to myocardial infarction or injury, or a primary conduction system defect
 - Drugs or toxic substances
 - Pain or psychic stress, causing vasovagal syncope
 - Increased intracranial pressure
 d. Diagnostics
 (1) Assessment: history of weakness, dizziness; altered level of consciousness; injury due to loss of consciousness (e.g., fractured hip, hypothermia, surface trauma); self-reported bradycardia; possible permanent pacemaker. Physical examination results include the following:
 - Pulse less than 60 beats per minute
 - Hypotension or postural hypotension
 (2) Diagnostic studies include cardiac monitoring, ECG, drug levels, and pacemaker function assessed with magnet.
 e. Clinical management
 (1) Atropine to increase heart rate
 (2) Use of CPR, an external pacemaker, or both if rate causes central nervous system symptoms
 (3) Temporary transvenous pacemaker
 (4) Admission for observation or permanent pacemaker
 (5) Complete primary and secondary survey, if person is unconscious
 f. Discharge criteria
 (1) Heart rate returns to normal and remains normal after a period of observation, usually 30 to 60 minutes.
 (2) Vital signs are within normal limits.
 (3) Once the rate has converted, there is no evidence of ischemia or other condition requiring admission.
 (4) Individual verbalizes understanding of problem and what to do if it returns.
 g. Discharge planning and teaching
 (1) Stress the avoidance of stimulants or causes of supraventricular tachycardia.

(2) Review the plan for follow-up.
(3) Explain what to do if supraventricular tachycardia returns.

■ CARING FOR PEOPLE EXPERIENCING OTHER EMERGENCY CONDITIONS

Bleeding or Shock

1. Bleeding may be obvious or occult; the most frequent sites or causes of bleeding seen in the emergency care setting are the following:
 a. Bleeding from a wound or surface trauma, which may be bright red, vigorous, arterial bleeding or darker red, oozing, venous bleeding.
 b. Vaginal bleeding, which may be bright red and profuse or scanty and dark.
 c. Epistaxis, which may be bright red and in copious amounts or may be occult as swallowed blood.
 d. Upper gastrointestinal bleeding, which is either bright red or coffee ground–colored.
 e. Lower gastrointestinal bleeding, which manifests as dark, tarry stools or, less often, as bright red bleeding.
 f. Abdominal or thoracic aneurysm rupture.
 g. Hematuria.
2. Although shock-producing bleeding is often visible, there are some conditions in which the major symptoms are syncope, hypotension, and pain such as the following:
 a. Aortic aneurysm leak or rupture
 b. Retroperitoneal bleeding due to pelvic fracture
 c. Intra-abdominal bleeding due to blunt or penetrating trauma (e.g., ruptured spleen)
 d. Pelvic or intrauterine bleeding such as from a ruptured ectopic pregnancy or abruptio placentae
3. Diagnostics
 a. Assessment
 (1) Bleeding was spontaneous or due to trauma. Amount of bleeding: Use household measures to elicit information (e.g., tablespoon or cup); ask about pad or tampon count in vaginal bleeding; duration of bleeding; associated symptoms (e.g., pain, dizziness, fatigue); measures to stop the bleeding; conditions that are associated with impaired coagulation (e.g., hemophilia, von Willebrand's disease)
 (2) Physical examination
 - ABCs, skin vital signs, orthostatic (postural) vital signs, if large amount of bleeding is suspected
 - Vigor of bleeding
 - Effects of direct pressure, if a wound or epistaxis
 - In hidden bleeding, assess girth of area.
4. Triage category: Priority depends on the likely source, magnitude of bleeding, and effectiveness of first aid measures to stop the bleeding (e.g., bleeding due to a wound that can be controlled with direct pressure is not an urgent priority unless other symptoms are present).
5. Clinical management
 a. Stop external bleeding.

(1) Epistaxis: Have person pinch nostrils or apply a nose clip. If external pressure does not stop posterior bleeding, posterior packing or a nasal balloon is needed.

(2) Bleeding due to a wound: Apply direct pressure (unless due to a penetrating foreign body) continuously for at least 5 minutes; elevate the part; apply an ice pack to the area; apply a pressure dressing: 4 × 4s or abdominal pads, Kling or Coban (a flexible adhesive wrap), applied with some tension; reassess to ensure that distal circulation is impaired. The use of an elastic bandage requires frequent reassessment. Apply pressure at pressure points (Fig. 37–2). In rare instances, apply a tourniquet, if other measures do not stop the bleeding.

6. Hemorrhagic shock—see Chapter 12.

Altered Consciousness

1. Common causes of altered consciousness are found in Table 37–4.
2. Nursing diagnoses related to care of the unconscious person are the following:
   a. Altered cerebral perfusion
   b. Ineffective airway clearance
   c. Impaired gas exchange
   d. Risk for injury
   e. Anticipatory grieving
3. Nursing interventions
   a. Ensure adequate airway and ventilation; keep neck in a neutral position to ensure adequate airway, promote venous outflow, and minimize development or worsening of cerebral edema.
   b. Administer oxygen.
   c. Position on side and elevate head of bed, if safe to do so.
   d. Cautiously administer IV fluid.
   e. Ensure adequate circulating volume.
   f. Provide continuous cardiac, BP, and oximetry monitoring; monitor neurologic status and Glasgow Coma Scale.
   g. Administer medications to decrease cerebral edema or treat etiology (e.g., anticonvulsants).

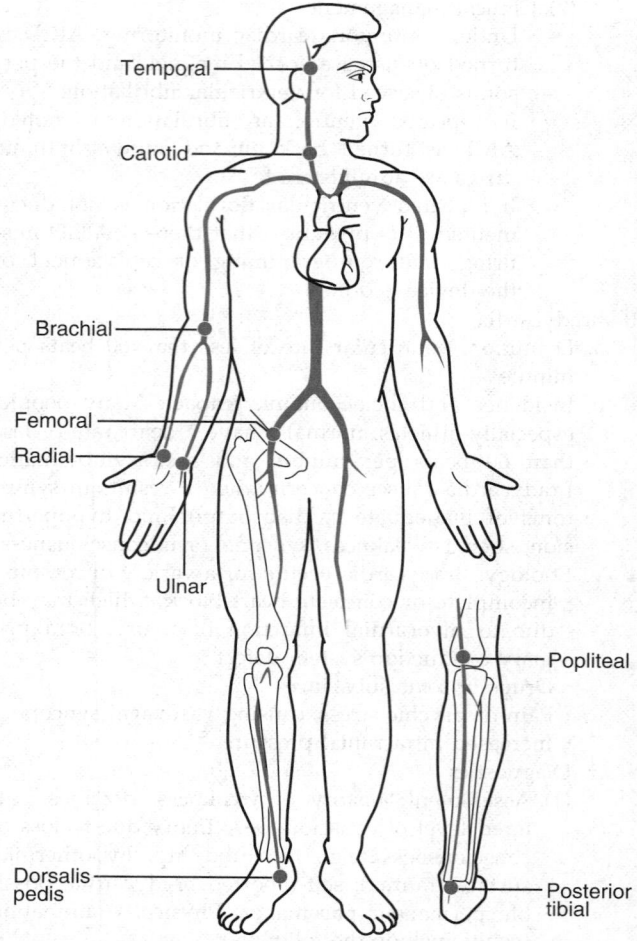

Figure 37–2. Pressure points for control of hemorrhaging by direct pressure.

   h. Monitor urine output; usually a Foley catheter is indicated.
   i. Explain what you are doing, even if it appears that the person cannot hear you; research has demonstrated that some seemingly unconscious people can hear.
   j. Prevent hypothermia, unless otherwise ordered for

Table 37–4. Common Causes of Altered Consciousness			
Metabolic	**Structural**	**Intoxication-Related**	**Functional**
Hyperglycemia	Central nervous system (CNS) hemorrhages	Alcohol	Hysteria
Hypoglycemia	CNS hematomas	Drugs	Catatonic reaction
Hypocalcemia	Nonvascular mass lesions (e.g., tumors, abscesses)	Poisons	
Hypotension		Toxins	
Hypoxemia	Seizures		
Hypothermia	Degenerative CNS disorders		

therapeutic reasons to decrease central nervous system metabolic needs.
k. Provide support to the family or significant others; sustained unconsciousness is a frightening and ominous sign.
l. Promote family presence at the bedside and encourage them to verbalize whatever they wish to say.
m. Facilitate diagnostic testing.
n. Address safety needs.
o. Inquire about desires for clergy attendance.
p. Inquire about advanced directives and consider organ or tissue wishes and potential, even though decisions that a person is brain dead are not usually made in the ED.
4. Clinical management of the unconscious person from unknown etiology:
   a. Provide airway or oxygen.
   b. Use cardiac monitoring.
   c. Obtain IV access; obtain blood for blood sugar and other routine laboratory tests; check blood sugar at bedside.
   d. Treat common causes of unconsciousness by administering "coma cocktail": IV naloxone (Narcan), flumazenil (Romazicon), thiamine, and 50 percent dextrose, as discussed earlier.
   e. Perform other diagnostic studies, if no response (e.g., CT scan, lumbar puncture).
5. Clinical management of seizures
   a. Provide oxygen, suction, protection from injury; nasal airway is helpful in maintaining a patent airway.
   b. Establish IV access; intraosseous access may be required in a small child.
   c. Stop seizures with diazepam or lorazepam; phenobarbital may be used in children. Rectal administration of anticonvulsants or sedatives may be necessary if IV or intraosseous access is not feasible.
   d. Continuously monitor respiration and oximetry.
   e. Draw blood for routine laboratory tests and anticonvulsant levels, if appropriate.
   f. If levels are subtherapeutic, administer anticonvulsants as ordered.
   g. Identify cause of seizures, if not previously diagnosed or not apparent (e.g., febrile seizure in child); administer antipyretics and initiate cooling measures in febrile seizures.
   h. Assess for injuries that may have occurred during the seizure.
   i. Monitor for return to normal level of consciousness; most people who have had a seizure sleep for a period of time after the seizure (post-ictal). Be prepared for the person to be confused or combative on wakening.
   j. Monitor urine output and observe for myoglobinuria, if there has been sustained seizure activity.
   k. Address hygiene needs: Incontinence or profuse sweating is normal during a seizure.
   l. Position person on side once the seizure has ceased.
   m. Initiate and maintain cardiac, BP, and oximetry monitoring until person is awake.
6. Discharge criteria
   a. Individuals with new-onset seizures, for which the

DRUG ADVISORY

Dilantin has the potential for causing significant hypotension, is highly irritating to veins, and may precipitate. Check institutional policy regarding administering through central lines. Dilantin is incompatible with many medications and intravenous solutions; it should be mixed with normal saline. Because of its propensity to precipitate, it is generally recommended that the intravenous drip be mixed immediately before administration.

etiology has not yet been determined, are usually admitted for diagnosis and seizure control; only those previously diagnosed with a seizure disorder or individuals for whom the cause of seizures can be identified (e.g., child with febrile seizures) are discharged from the ED.
   b. Fully awake, alert, and oriented.
   c. Neurologically intact.
   d. Reason for seizure is identified and controlled.
   e. A mature adult agrees to assume responsibility for observing the person; an individual who has had a seizure is not permitted to operate a motor vehicle until seizure-free for a period of 6 to 12 months, depending on state law.

NURSING MANAGEMENT

Out of interest for public safety, some states require treatment facilities or health care providers to notify the driver motor vehicle licensing agency when a licensed driver has a seizure. The agency then determines whether revocation of the driver's license is indicated. States may require a seizure-free period of 6 to 12 months before reissuing the driver's license. Policies and procedures to assist staff in making this notification are recommended.

Pain (see Chapter 11)

1. General considerations in assessment and management of pain in the emergency care setting:
   a. Acute or chronic pain is perhaps the most common reason why people seek emergency care and is an extremely important symptom.
   b. Timely pain relief is a priority for the person seeking care; this sometimes conflicts with caregiver needs to identify the cause of pain before treating it.
   c. Relieving pain before determining its cause is a concern because the character and progression of pain are often key to the diagnosis (e.g., in appendicitis, the pain is often periumbilical before it localizes to the right lower quadrant) and because certain types of pain respond best to certain medications or treatments.
   d. Spontaneous resolution of pain may indicate that a structure has ruptured (e.g., in a ruptured ectopic

pregnancy); thus, surgical intervention may become a higher priority.

e. Individuals who may require emergency surgery need to sign written informed consent; yet, many institutions have policies that prohibit a person who has been medicated with narcotics or mind-altering drugs from signing an operative permit within 4 hours of being medicated. Having the person sign an operative permit when it is not clear what surgical procedure will be needed is not an option, because it is not informed consent.

f. If narcotics must be used in the person who is a likely surgical candidate, the narcotic can be reversed with naloxone (Narcan); however, the pain that returns may be quite severe, necessitating remediation as soon as the permit is signed.

g. Narcotic analgesics are best given IV (titrated to effect), especially in the presence of hypotension; IM administration takes too long to be effective, the medication may accumulate in the muscles because of poor perfusion, and profound hypotension may result when resuscitative efforts improve the circulating volume to the point that the muscles are perfused and the medication moves into the systemic circulation.

h. Intravenous pain medication is used in persons with suspected myocardial infarction for several reasons:
   (1) The coronary vessel dilation caused by the medication improves myocardial perfusion, and this effect is desired immediately.
   (2) The medication decreases heart work, further decreasing myocardial oxygen consumption.
   (3) Skeletal muscle damage from IM injections may result in false-positive results on cardiac enzyme studies.
   (4) Thrombolytic therapy, often used in the treatment of acute myocardial infarction, may cause bleeding into and from IM injection sites.

i. Hypotension due to vasovagal stimulation and bradycardia from pain may be relieved with timely pain management.

j. Individuals who seek drugs frequent the ED, usually complaining of dental, back, or head pain.
   (1) Many clinicians are skeptical of persons whose pain is difficult to substantiate and who use the ED for their care on a routine basis, rather than establishing a relationship with a regular care provider.
   (2) Some communities have "drug alert" systems in which EDs check to see if a person who is complaining of pain has been seen or treated in another ED recently; the individual is then confronted if there is strong evidence of drug-seeking behavior.

k. There is some evidence that pain management may be less aggressive in certain ethnic groups; this suggests that caregivers should critically examine their own prescribing and administration practices to ensure that biases do not exist in the treatment of acute pain.

l. Pain scales that enable the patient to rank the pain severity on a 1 to 10 scale are useful and should be included in the initial and ongoing assessments to determine the progression of pain and the effectiveness of interventions. Visual pain scales may be used for children, developmentally delayed individuals, and persons with impaired verbal skills.

m. Pain management in the emergency care setting often requires immediate relief; thus, narcotics or nonsteroidal anti-inflammatory agents are often administered using IV push; this may amount to IV conscious sedation, requiring careful monitoring of vital signs and pulse oximetry.

n. Small doses of IV narcotics coupled with IM or IV nonsteroidal anti-inflammatory agents often produce longer analgesia than either one used alone.

o. The potential for serious allergic reactions always exists when narcotics or nonsteroidal anti-inflammatory agents are given IV; careful monitoring for at least 30 minutes is suggested.

p. In addition to pharmacologic strategies for pain relief, there are a number of other modalities that you may initiate to assist in relieving pain (see Chapter 11).

q. Safety concerns after discharge are important in determining agent, route, timing, and reassessment.
   (1) Be sure that the person has a way home with a responsible adult.
   (2) Reinforce no drinking alcohol, driving a motor vehicle, working at heights, or operating machinery for at least 4 hours after receiving narcotic analgesics or other central nervous system depressants.
   (3) Oral narcotics are administered immediately before discharge (assuming a short ride of less than 20 min) or nonsteroidal anti-inflammatory agents may be preferred if the person must drive.

2. Chest pain
   a. Common causes of chest pain include cardiovascular, pulmonary, gastrointestinal, musculoskeletal, systemic, and psychogenic causes (Table 37–5).
   b. Applying the nursing process (see Chapter 23 and Table 37–6)

3. Abdominal and flank pain (see Chapter 27)
   a. Abdominal and flank pain is also a common reason for seeking emergency care in all age groups; causes of pain include obstructive, inflammatory with or without perforation, hemorrhagic, cardiac, and systemic conditions (Table 37–7).
   b. Initial priorities in evaluating the person with abdominal pain are cardiovascular stabilization and determining whether the problem is an "acute abdomen"—one that requires prompt surgical intervention.
   c. Pain patterns may be visceral or referred, intermittent or constant, and of gradual or sudden onset; eliciting information about the nature of the pain is critical in determining triage priority and likely causes.
   d. History
      (1) When did the pain start and what was the severity at time of onset? Ruptured aortic aneu-

Table 37–5. Common Causes of Chest Pain

Cardiovascular	Pulmonary	Musculoskeletal	Gastrointestinal	Other
Myocardial infarction	Pneumonia	Rib fracture	Esophagitis	Herpes zoster
Angina pectoris	Pleuritis	Costochondritis	Hiatal hernia	Ketoacidosis
Pericarditis	Bronchitis	Tietze's syndrome	Esophageal reflux	Panic attack
Mitral valve prolapse	Pulmonary embolism	Muscle strain	Esophageal spasm	
Cardiomyopathy	Pneumothorax	Cervical disk disease	Mallory-Weiss tear	
Coronary artery disease	Pleural effusion	Arthritis	Cholecystitis	
Pericardial tamponade	Mediastinitis		Pancreatitis	
Cocaine use			Peptic ulcer	
			Gastritis	

rysm or perforation is associated with severe pain, but pain due to inflammation gradually worsens over time. Does the pain worsen with eating or several hours after eating?

(2) What is the nature of the pain? Is it constant or intermittent, penetrating or crampy, sharp, dull, or aching?

(3) What is the severity of the pain on a 1 to 10 scale, and has this changed from the onset?

(4) Where is the pain located and does it radiate? Have person point with 1 finger to location of the pain.

(5) Is there any history of trauma?

(6) Determine bowel movement pattern and use of laxatives, enemas, or suppositories.

(7) Are there associated symptoms: nausea, vomiting, diarrhea, gastrointestinal bleeding, increased flatus or abdominal bloating, change in skin color?

(8) Are there urinary tract or gynecologic symptoms, such as frequency, hematuria, dark urine, cloudy urine, or vaginal discharge?

(9) In females of childbearing age, when was the last normal menstrual period and is person sexually active?

(10) Is person exposed to heavy metals or fumes?

e. Physical examination
   (1) Activity (e.g., pacing versus lying quietly)
   (2) Observation, auscultation of bowel sounds, gentle palpation, starting with least painful areas 1st. Do not palpate the abdomen if a pulsatile mass is observed or an aortic aneurysm is suspected.
   (3) Postural vital signs, temperature, respirations

f. Diagnostic studies
   (1) Laboratory studies: complete blood count, chemistries, amylase and lipase if upper abdominal pain, PT and PTT, and hepatitis screen, if hepatic involvement suspected; pregnancy test, if in childbearing age; type and crossmatch, if intra-abdominal hemorrhage or gastrointestinal bleeding is suspected, or if surgery is anticipated; urinalysis
   (2) Radiographs of abdomen, CT scan, abdominal or pelvic ultrasound, intravenous pyelogram if hematuria or high likelihood of ureteral calculi

   (3) Peritoneal lavage may be done in blunt trauma to determine whether there is bleeding or bowel damage.
   (4) Use nasogastric tube, if gastrointestinal bleeding or pancreatitis is suspected; test gastric aspirate for blood.
   (5) Stool hemoccult

g. Clinical management
   (1) Cardiovascular stabilization
   (2) Definitive treatment based on diagnosis
   (3) Cautious and condition-specific pain management

h. Applying the nursing process (see Chapter 27)

i. Discharge criteria: The cause of abdominal pain may not be clear at the time of the initial visit; if the cause cannot be identified, the person must understand the rationale behind discharge and the need for follow-up.
   (1) Hemodynamically stable
   (2) Pain relieved or tolerable
   (3) Life-threatening conditions ruled out
   (4) Person reliable enough to return if symptoms worsen or do not resolve

j. Discharge planning and teaching
   (1) Discuss diagnosis or possible diagnoses.
   (2) Review dietary, activity, and work restrictions (e.g., a food handler who may have hepatitis A should not return to work until results of the hepatitis screen have been obtained).
   (3) Explain infection control considerations (e.g., dishwashing and food preparation or food sharing precautions in hepatitis, or abstinence from sexual activity in hepatitis or pelvic inflammatory disease).
   (4) Counsel those with hepatitis to avoid alcohol and acetaminophen.
   (5) Review the medications or treatments required.
   (6) List the symptoms to observe for and what to do if they occur.
   (7) Review the follow-up plan.

4. Head pain or headache (see Chapter 18)
   a. Headache is frequently encountered in the emergency care setting; an estimated 2 to 6 percent of patients who seek emergency care have a chief complaint of headache, with about 25 percent having migraine headache.

Text continued on page 1732

Table 37–6. Assessment of Chest Pain

Condition	Location	Quality	Severity	Course	Aggravating or Relieving Factors	Symptoms or Signs
Angina	Retrosternal region; radiates to neck, jaw, epigastrium, shoulders, or arms—left side common	Pressure, burning, squeezing, heaviness, indigestion	Moderate to severe	<10 min	Aggravated by exercise, cold weather, emotional stress, or after meals; relieved by rest or nitroglycerin; atypical (Prinzmetal's) angina may be unrelated to activity and caused by coronary artery spasm	S$_4$, paradoxical split S$_2$ during pain
Intermediate syndrome or coronary insufficiency	Same as angina	Same as angina	Increasingly severe	<10 min	Same as angina, with gradually decreasing tolerance for exertion	Same as angina
Myocardial infarction	Substernal, and may radiate like angina	Heaviness, pressure, burning, constriction	Severe, sometimes mild (in 25% of patients)	Sudden onset, 30 minutes or longer but variable; usually goes away in hours	Unrelieved	Shortness of breath, sweating, weakness, nausea, vomiting, severe anxiety
Pericarditis	Usually begins over sternum and may radiate to neck and down left upper extremity	Sharp, stabbing, knifelike	Moderate to severe	Lasts many hours to days	Aggravated by deep breathing, rotating chest, or supine position; relieved by sitting up and leaning forward	Pericardial friction rub, syncope, cardiac tamponade, pulsus paradoxus (Kussmaul's sign)
Dissecting aortic aneurysm	Anterior chest; radiates to thoracic area of back; may be abdominal; pain shifts in chest	Tearing	Excruciating, tearing, knifelike	Sudden onset, lasts for hours	Unrelated to anything	Lower blood pressure in one arm, absent pulses, paralysis, murmur of aortic insufficiency, pulsus paradoxus, stridor; myocardial infarction can occur
Mitral valve prolapse syndrome	Substernal; sometimes radiates to the left arm, back, jaw	Stabbing, sharp	Variable, generally mild, can become severe	Episodes are paroxysmal, may be prolonged	Not related to exertion, not relieved by nitroglycerin or rest	Variable palpitations, dizziness, syncope, dyspnea

Condition	Location	Quality	Severity	Duration	Aggravating factors	Associated features
Pulmonary embolism (most pulmonary emboli do not produce chest pain)	Substernal anginal	Not pleuritic unless infarction exists	Can be severe	Sudden onset; minutes to <hour	May be aggravated by breathing	Fever, tachypnea, tachycardia, hypotension, elevated jugular venous pressure, right ventricular lift, accentuated P_2, occasional murmur of tricuspid insufficiency and right ventricular S_4; with infarction usually in the presence of congestive heart failure, rales, pleural rub, hemoptysis, clinical phlebitis present in minority of cases
Pulmonary hypertension	Substernal	Pressure; oppressive	Variable		Aggravated by effort	Pain usually associated with dyspnea; right ventricular lift, accentuated P_2
Spontaneous pneumothorax	Unilateral	Sharp, well localized		Sudden onset, lasts many hours	Painful breathing	Dyspnea, hyperresonance, and decreased breath and voice sounds over involved lung
Pneumonia with pleurisy	Localized over area of consolidation	Pleuritic, well localized	Moderate		Painful breathing	Dyspnea, cough, fever, dull to flat percussion, bronchial breathing, rales, occasional pleural rub
Gastrointestinal disorders	Lower substernal area, epigastric, right or left upper quadrant	Burning, colic-like aching			Precipitated by recumbency or meals	Nausea, regurgitation, food intolerance, melena, hematemesis, jaundice
Musculoskeletal disorders	Variable	Aching		Short or long duration Prolonged period of time	Aggravated by movement, history of muscle exertion	Tender to pressure or movement
Neurologic disorders (herpes zoster)	Dermatomal in distribution			Unassociated with external events		Rash appears in area of discomfort with herpes
Anxiety states	Usually localized to a point	Sharp burning, commonly location of pain moves from place to place	Mild to moderate	Varies; usually very brief	Situational anger	Sighing respirations, often chest wall tenderness

1729

Table 37–7. Differential Diagnosis of Abdominal Pain

Condition	History Pattern	Pain Symptoms	Associated Findings	Clinical	White Blood Cell Count	Radiographs	Concerns
Gastroenteritis	Sudden onset; often occurs in epidemics	Diffuse, comes in waves	Vomiting, diarrhea, weakness	Fever, diffuse abdominal tenderness, dehydration	Normal or elevated	Normal	Severe volume deficits
Appendicitis	All age groups	Mild to severe epigastric or periumbilical; then localizes to right lower quadrant; pain decreases if rupture occurs until peritonitis results	Nausea, vomiting, anorexia	Fever, rebound tenderness	Elevated	Normal or distended bowel in right lower quadrant; fecolith may indicate gangrenous appendicitis	Diagnosis may be missed, especially ages <10 yr or >60 yr, and women. May have normal laboratory results and physical examination initially
Perforated or ruptured viscus	Causes: Perforated peptic ulcer, ruptured appendix, diverticulitis, vascular occlusion of bowel	Sudden, severe, worse with movement; diffuse	Variable, may be related to volume loss	Hypotension, shock, rigid abdomen, rebound pain, abdominal distention	Usually elevated	Upright film may show air under diaphragm; paralytic ileus	Urgent surgery required
Leaking abdominal aortic aneurysm	Hypertension, arteriosclerosis	Sudden or gradually worsening; severe midabdominal radiating to back; ripping sensation	Leg weakness, shock, diaphoresis, mottling below level of aneurysm, hematuria, sense of impending doom	Appears critically ill, pulsatile mass may be felt	Normal or elevated secondary to stress response	Plain films may show calcification of aorta, aneurysm; abdominal CT or ultrasound may show aneurysm	Surgical emergency, immediate surgery needed; MAST suit may tamponade bleeding as temporizing measure

Condition	History	Pain	GI Symptoms	Signs	WBC	X-ray/Diagnostic	Comments
Acute cholecystitis	Most common in females, ages 30–70. History of fatty food intolerance	Moderate to severe upper abdominal pain, worse after fatty meal. Pain may radiate to shoulder	Anorexia, nausea, vomiting	Fever, right upper quadrant tenderness, jaundice may be present; gallbladder may be palpable	Elevated	Plain films may show stones; gallbladder ultrasound usually diagnostic	Elevated bilirubin, amylase, lipase are common. Patient may be diaphoretic and appear like person with a myocardial infarction
Acute pancreatitis	May have history of cholecystitis or pancreatitis; alcoholism	Sudden, severe, continuous; bores through to back or flank. Worse with food	Nausea, vomiting, diaphoresis	May have hypovolemic shock, if hemorrhagic pancreatitis; fever, diffuse abdominal pain	Elevated	Normal or pancreatic calcification, if chronic	Elevated amylase diagnostic; electrolyte abnormalities common; may have elevated bilirubin; hypocalcemia not uncommon
Small bowel obstruction	Previous abdominal surgery and adhesions; constipation or obstipation × several days	Initially intermittent and colic-like, then continuous, severe. Usually midline and midabdomen	Vomiting, may be fecal smelling; anorexia	Hypovolemia, distended abdomen, visible peristalsis in thin person	Elevated	Plain films show distended loops of bowel, air-fluid levels, abnormal gas patterns	Significant fluid shifts and third spacing, creating serious fluid/electrolyte abnormalities
Mesenteric infarction	Middle-aged to elderly adults; often with cardiovascular disease, especially atrial fibrillation	Mild to severe central abdominal pain	Hematemesis, bloody stools, weakness	Shock, diffuse abdominal pain, Hematest positive stool	Elevated, but nonspecific	Ileus will develop	Difficult to diagnose, may mimic gastroenteritis or viral syndromes; significant findings may not occur until large amount of bowel necrosed. Surgery needed. May have massive fluid replacement needs
Mesenteric adenitis	May occur in epidemics	Moderate to severe, constant right lower quadrant	Vomiting; occasional diarrhea	Fever, right lower quadrant pain with rebound	Elevated	Abnormalities of terminal ileum	Difficult to diagnose; mimics appendicitis. Yersinia is a common cause

b. Headache is difficult to triage and evaluate; the severity of pain is not helpful in differentiating a non–life-threatening migraine or cluster headache from a truly life-threatening subarachnoid hemorrhage or epidural hematoma.

c. The presence of abnormal neurologic findings associated with headache is also not diagnostic; individuals with migraine headache may have focal neurologic signs.

d. Common types and causes of headache include the following:
   (1) Migraine
   (2) Cluster headache
   (3) Tension headache
   (4) Spinal headache, following lumbar puncture or spinal anesthesia
   (5) Headache associated with intracranial event:
       • Traumatic: subdural hematoma, epidural hematoma, intracerebral hematoma, subarachnoid hemorrhage associated with cervical neck strain or sprain, cerebral contusion, cerebral concussion
       • Nontraumatic: stroke, subarachnoid hemorrhage, mass lesion, meningitis, encephalitis, brain abscess, hypertensive crisis
   (6) Temporal arteritis
   (7) Medications or toxic substances: carbon monoxide, nitrates, atenolol, nifedipine, cimetidine, ranitidine, estrogens, monosodium glutamate, ethanol ingestion or withdrawal
   (8) Miscellaneous causes: sinusitis, exertion, cough, sexual activity, cold stimulus (ice cream headache)
   (9) Acute glaucoma

e. Assessment (history)
   (1) Severity of pain on 1 to 10 scale; be very concerned about the person who says that this headache "is the worst one I've ever had," as this may suggest that the problem is a subarachnoid hemorrhage. Massive and usually lethal subarachnoid hemorrhage is sometimes preceded by a smaller bleed that is manifested by headache.
   (2) Character of pain (e.g., stabbing, dull, constant, or throbbing)
   (3) Location
   (4) Onset and duration
   (5) Precipitating factors
   (6) Headache history
   (7) Medication or treatments used
   (8) Associated symptoms: nausea; vomiting; impaired mentation, cognition, motor function, or sensation; altered vision; fever; recent infection or upper respiratory infection

f. Physical examination
   (1) Complete vital signs
   (2) Neurologic function, gait
   (3) Visual acuity
   (4) Pain on palpation of head, neck, or face

g. Diagnostic studies
   (1) If history of migraine headache or source of headache is apparent, no studies may be ordered.
   (2) Complete blood count, chemistries, erythrocyte sedimentation rate, if temporal arteritis is suspected; blood cultures, if infectious process is suspected; toxicologic studies
   (3) Tonometry, if glaucoma is suspected
   (4) Head CT
   (5) Lumbar puncture
   (6) Sinus films, if facial tenderness

h. Clinical management of migraine headache: pharmacologic interventions
   (1) Phenothiazines (e.g., chlorpromazine), alone or in combination with dihydroergotamine, possibly preceded by a normal saline solution
   (2) Dihydroergotamine is a cranial vasoconstrictor.
   (3) Sumatriptan (Imitrex) given subcutaneously constricts edematous cranial arteries and decreases release of vasoactive peptides; does not cross blood-brain barrier, so no central nervous system depressant effect occurs.
   (4) Ketorolac, IM or IV
   (5) Narcotics

i. Nursing interventions
   (1) Provide a darkened, quiet environment to minimize painful stimulus.
   (2) Administer pain medications as ordered.
   (3) Consider nonpharmacologic strategies.
   (4) Elevate head of bed unless patient desires otherwise.
   (5) Follow safety considerations attendant to use of narcotics.
   (6) Have emesis basin, suction, or both immediately available.
   (7) Initiate automatic BP and other parameter monitoring so that the person is not disturbed during these measurements.
   (8) Reassess vital signs and effectiveness of pain medications at 15- to 30-minute intervals, depending on medications used, route, and probable diagnoses.
   (9) Reassess neurologic status at frequent intervals.

j. Criteria for discharge
   (1) Cause of pain identified
   (2) Pain significantly decreased or eliminated
   (3) Normal neurologic function
   (4) Responsible adult available to drive if central nervous system–altering medications given

k. Discharge planning and teaching
   (1) Review cause of headache.
   (2) Discuss common precipitating factors, if migraine headache (e.g., dietary).
   (3) Explain use of medications, especially ergotamine preparations or sumatriptan.
   (4) Recommend prevention strategies.
   (5) Remind the person about follow-up for further evaluation.
   (6) Review reasons to seek emergency care.

5. Back pain
   a. Back pain may herald a variety of conditions, some of which are life threatening. Most individuals who

present with back pain have acute mechanical low back pain without neurologic deficit of musculoskeletal origin associated with a defined incident, which resolves in a few days with anti-inflammatory analgesics and gradually increased activity. Other causes of back pain include the following:

   (1) Dissecting or rupturing abdominal aortic aneurysm

   (2) Ruptured ectopic pregnancy

   (3) Ureteral calculi producing renal colic

   (4) Compression fractures

   (5) Spinal stenosis

   (6) Osteoarthritis

   (7) Herniated disk, with or without cauda equina syndrome; sciatica

   (8) Spondylolysis or spondylolisthesis

   (9) Ankylosing spondylitis

   (10) Avascular necrosis of vertebrae (Scheuermann's disease)

   (11) Pyelonephritis

   (12) Infectious processes of the spine

    • Vertebral osteomyelitis

    • Epidural abscess

    • Diskitis, often postlumbar puncture

    • Reiter's syndrome

   (13) Herpes zoster (shingles)

   (14) Malignancy

b. Triage category: usually not urgent unless pain is severe

c. Assessment (history)

   (1) History of physical action that precipitated the event; such an event can be very minor (e.g., sneezing, turning, coughing)

   (2) Relationship of pain to activity (e.g., worsens with movement)

   (3) Motor and sensory function, including bowel or bladder laxity

   (4) Medications used

   (5) Chronic health problems (e.g., hypertension, diabetes)

   (6) Other associated symptoms (e.g., fever, hematuria, abdominal pain, groin pain)

d. Physical examination

   (1) Posturing (e.g., hyperextension of the back, which occurs with muscle spasm), preference for positioning (e.g., persons with muscle-related low back pain usually prefer to stand or lie flat, rather than sit)

   (2) Gait, movement, and flexibility; observe for evidence of foot drop; observe if person can bend over to remove shoes or clothing—assistance may be needed

   (3) Inspection and palpation of painful area

   (4) Leg raising tests are usually deferred to the treating practitioner

   (5) In an older person or one with hypertension, assess color of legs; back pain and leg numbness may be the presenting symptoms in the person with a dissecting abdominal aortic aneurysm; in this case, cyanosis of extremities and mid to lower abdomen are indicative of this condition.

e. Diagnostic studies

   (1) None, if muscle sprain or strain is suspected

   (2) Plain radiographs of the spine

   (3) A CT scan or a magnetic resonance imaging (MRI) view

   (4) Laboratory studies: complete blood count, urinalysis, erythrocyte sedimentation rate, others, depending on possible etiologies

f. Clinical management of muscle strain or sprain

   (1) Pain management: nonsteroidal anti-inflammatory agents such as ketorolac IM or IV, narcotics

   (2) Muscle relaxants (e.g., diazepam, Robaxin)

   (3) Ice pack to area

g. Criteria for discharge

   (1) Likely cause of pain identified and serious conditions ruled out

   (2) No neurologic abnormalities

   (3) Pain less severe or alleviated

   (4) Able to walk and perform activities of daily living

   (5) Able to void

h. Discharge planning and teaching

   (1) Discuss cause of back pain.

   (2) Review use of medications and prevention of constipation.

   (3) Review activity guidelines. Some practitioners recommend several days of bed rest; however, research suggests that early movement and return to work result in better outcomes.

   (4) Explain about ice massage, using an ice cube rubbed directly with pressure on the affected area for 15 to 20 minutes every few hours, which helps to decrease spasm initially; moist heat is usually recommended 3 days later.

   (5) Recommend back exercises after the acute period is over; many EDs have back care booklets that address back exercises as well as injury prevention.

   (6) Physical therapy referral may be ordered.

   (7) Explain how to perform activities of daily living during the acute phase (e.g., roll to the side of the bed and slide feet on the floor 1st, then push up with hands to get off the bed, rather than trying to sit up; a bedpan or urinal may be useful for persons with severe pain).

   (8) Recommend a bed board or firm mattress if appropriate; a sheet of plywood can be placed under the mattress.

   (9) A back support belt may be useful, although its value is not clearly established.

   (10) Recommend back supports on chairs for the person who sits a great deal.

   (11) Recommend smoking cessation, if disk disease is suspected; nicotine contributes to disk degeneration.

   (12) Weight loss (if appropriate) and measures to improve abdominal muscle tone assist in decreasing the recurrence of back muscle strain or sprain.

6. Leg pain

a. The most common causes of nontraumatic leg pain are the following:

   (1) Arterial occlusion

   (2) Deep vein thrombophlebitis (see Chapter 24)

(3) Disk disease with nerve root involvement (see Chapter 34)

b. Assessment, clinical management, and nursing interventions (see Chapter 11)

7. Joint pain
   a. Frequent causes of nontraumatic joint pain include the following:
      (1) Hemarthrosis in person with hemophilia or sickle cell disease
      (2) Septic joint, which may be nonspecific or associated with gonococcus
      (3) Arthritis
      (4) Tendonitis
      (5) Gout
   b. Assessment (history)
      (1) Painful joint in absence of trauma
      (2) History of hemophilia, sickle cell disease, or von Willebrand's disease
      (3) Redness and swelling of affected area
      (4) In septic joint, there may be history of gonococcal infection or of IV drug use.
   c. Physical examination
      (1) Reddened, swollen joint that is tender to touch
      (2) Fever may be present.
      (3) Restricted movement
      (4) In tendonitis, point tenderness may be elicited.
   d. Diagnostic studies
      (1) Laboratory studies: complete blood count, sickle cell preparation (if not previously diagnosed), erythrocyte sedimentation rate, uric acid, blood cultures, and Gram stain and culture of aspirate
      (2) Radiograph of joint
   e. Clinical management
      (1) Management is variable, depending on the presumed cause.
      (2) In sickle cell crisis, pain management and other systemic strategies are used to treat the crisis.
      (3) If pain is due to clotting factor deficiencies, replacement of factors, ice pack, and possible pressure bandage may help decrease bleeding.
      (4) A joint tap (aspiration) may be both diagnostic and therapeutic.
      (5) If septic joint is suspected, IV antibiotics are given, and the person is often hospitalized.
      (6) A splint or other immobilizing device may be used.
   f. Discharge criteria
      (1) Likely cause of joint pain identified
      (2) Condition amenable to outpatient treatment
      (3) Absence of systemic symptoms
   g. Discharge planning and teaching
      (1) Discuss the cause of the pain.
      (2) Review the medications.
      (3) Mention activity restrictions, if any.
      (4) Remind the patient about follow-up care.

Altered Body Temperature: Ineffective Thermoregulation

1. Hyperthermia
   a. Elevation of the body temperature above normal; may be caused by a variety of circumstances, both endogenous and exogenous.
   b. Endogenous causes include infection, central nervous system damage to temperature-regulating center of the brain, metabolic and endocrine disorders such as hyperthyroidism, and use of medications (e.g., malignant hyperthermia associated with succinylcholine, atropine and haloperidol, aspirin ingestion, cocaine, or amphetamines).
   c. Exogenous causes are environmental (e.g., hot environment, intense physical activity in a warm climate, or overdressing seen with children).
   d. Heat illnesses occur most often in the very young and in older people; obese individuals are at greatest risk.
   e. Heat stroke is the 3rd leading cause of death in athletes.
   f. Heat-related conditions include the following:
      (1) Heat edema
         (a) Swelling of the feet and ankles is due to vasodilation and prolonged standing or sitting, especially in persons new to a warm climate.
         (b) Elevation of the legs or feet and use of support hose are useful; diuretics are not helpful.
         (c) The condition should be recognized so that one does not associate it with heart failure or thrombophlebitis.
      (2) Heat syncope
         (a) Occurs from standing for long periods of time, especially with leg muscles tensed.
         (b) Results from blood pooling in the lower extremities.
         (c) Warning signs include vision changes, dizziness, and nausea.
         (d) Prevention includes flexing knees and leg muscles periodically.
         (e) Treatment involves removing person from hot environment, rest, and oral fluids.
      (3) Heat cramps
         (a) Characterized by severe muscle cramping of the thighs, calves, and abdomen.
         (b) Often occur after vigorous physical activity in a hot environment.
         (c) Result from sodium and fluid loss due to perspiration.
         (d) Treatment includes removing person to a cooler environment, rest, and drinking balanced salt solution.
      (4) Heat exhaustion
         (a) Results from sustained physical work in hot environment, resulting in salt and water loss.
         (b) Symptoms include temperature between 39 and 41 degrees Celsius; altered mental status such as confusion, giddiness, argumentativeness; dizziness; headache; nausea; vomiting; fatigue; and muscle cramping.
         (c) Treatment: cool environment, IV fluids such as normal saline solution or Ringer's lactate, observation.
      (5) Heat stroke
         (a) A life-threatening emergency, with signs and

symptoms of other heat injuries, but complicated by delirium, coma, and cardiovascular collapse

(b) Temperature 42 degrees Celsius or higher

(c) Categorized as either exertional or classic. Exertional occurs most often in young people because of intense physical activity; classic heat stroke occurs in older individuals and those with preexisting conditions such as heart or respiratory disease, diabetes, alcoholism, and the use of diuretics or medications that impair the ability to sweat, such as tricyclic antidepressants and phenothiazines. Heat stroke is often found in a hot environment.

(d) The person with heat stroke has profound vasodilation with peripheral pooling of blood and may have actual hypovolemia, resulting in inadequate organ and tissue perfusion.

(e) Localized or disseminated intravascular coagulation may occur.

(f) The elevated temperature causes cell damage and damage to autoregulatory mechanisms.

(g) Sweating may occur, but it is ineffective in reducing temperature.

(h) Assessment history includes a history of strenuous activity, chronic health problems, or use of above medications; and a history of change in behavior or consciousness.

(i) Physical examination findings
  • Central nervous system symptoms: confusion, coma, seizures
  • Vital signs: significantly elevated temperature, tachycardia, hypotension, cardiac dysrhythmias
  • Respiratory symptoms: pulmonary edema
  • Gastrointestinal symptoms: diarrhea, vomiting, bleeding
  • Renal function: may be impaired because of hypoperfusion or rhabdomyolysis; ketones, protein, red blood cells (RBCs), white blood cells (WBCs), and casts may be present.

(j) Diagnostic studies: arterial blood gases, complete blood count, electrolytes, BUN, creatinine, phosphate, calcium, serum glutamic-oxaloacetic transaminase, serum glutamic-pyruvic transaminase, lactate dehydrogenase, bilirubin, alkaline phosphatase, amylase, creatine phosphokinase including myocardial band isoenzymes of creatinine kinase, PT, PTT, platelets, fibrinogen, blood for type and screen, urinalysis, gastric and stool guaiac, chest radiograph, ECG

(k) Clinical management
  • ABCs; initiate continuous temperature monitoring via flexible rectal probe or esophageal probe.
  • Reduce body temperature as quickly as possible using a variety of modalities: external cooling with cool sponging (with evaporation enhanced with fans); cool packs to groin, axilla, base of neck, head; cool oxygen; gastric, peritoneal, or urinary bladder lavage with cool fluids; cool environment; hypothermia blanket; cool shower, if awake; cardiopulmonary bypass (rarely).
  • Insert a nasogastric tube to check for gastric bleeding and to perform lavage.
  • Other measures are done as for person with shock.
  • Administer antipyretics. Avoid using aspirin; acetaminophen may be given.
  • Avoid producing shivering because it will increase the body temperature; stop cooling measures if it occurs, or administer phenothiazines to stop shivering.
  • Avoid producing hypothermia or frostbite; protect hands, feet, breasts, and genitalia, if cooling blanket is used.

(l) Discharge criteria: Individuals with heat edema, heat cramps, and heat exhaustion may be discharged; persons with heat stroke are admitted to critical care for observation of delayed complications. Criteria for discharge:
  • Normal temperature and other vital signs
  • Normal mentation
  • Adequate urinary output
  • Environment to which person is returning can be cooled

(m) Discharge teaching
  • Teach prevention of heat-related disorders.
  • Remind the person to increase oral intake for next 24 hours.
  • Tell the patient to monitor voiding.
  • Stress the importance of staying in a cool environment.
  • Remind the person to rest.

2. Cold injuries
  a. Cold injuries include trench foot or immersion foot, frostnip, frostbite, hypothermia, cold urticaria, and snow blindness; only frostbite and hypothermia are addressed in detail in this section.
  b. Frostnip is ice crystal formation associated with vasoconstriction; it is superficial and reversible.
  c. Frostbite is tissue damage due to freezing of water in skin and subcutaneous tissues.
    (1) The pathophysiology of frostbite includes vasospasm, leakage of plasma, and crystal formation in the tissue; after thawing there is arterial spasm, venous dilation, and stasis of cold hypercoagulable blood with small emboli, leading to tissue hypoxia and, eventually, ischemia and gangrene.
    (2) The degree of damage is either mild, with no tissue loss, or severe, with tissue loss; some researchers cite a categorization of 1st through 4th degrees, with the latter representing significant tissue loss.
    (3) Frostbite occurs because of either the cold and associated external factors (e.g., wet clothing, wind chill), or internal factors, such as restricted clothing, inability to generate heat, and impaired circulation.

(4) Areas most often affected are the feet, hands, nose, and ears.

(5) Assessment (history)
- History of cold exposure
- Numbness of affected part
- Pain or burning sensation after rewarming
- Symptoms that occur days to weeks after the initial injury include paresthesias, electrical current–like sensation, resumption of burning sensation when normal weight-bearing activities occur, cold feet, excessive sweating of area, color changes, and joint pain.

(6) Physical examination
- Affected part may appear frozen: white or blue color, hard, cold, and not sensitive to touch.
- As thawing occurs, flushing of the skin, development of blisters or blebs, or tissue edema appears; gangrene develops in 9 to 15 days.

(7) Diagnostic studies
- None initially to specifically identify degree of tissue damage
- Routine laboratory studies

(8) Clinical management
- Primary and secondary survey; assess for hypothermia.
- Cardiac monitoring, if extensive involvement; potassium released during rewarming may affect cardiac activity.
- Establish IV access; prepare for, or administer, pain medication.
- Avoid handling injured part.
- Submerge part in warm water bath (104–110 degrees Fahrenheit or 40.0–43.3 degrees Celsius); do not allow injured part to touch the sides or bottom of the basin; a whirlpool can be used if immediately available.
- Monitor water temperature and add hot water to maintain desired temperature; do not put hot water on the injured part.
- Thaw for 20 to 45 minutes until color and sensation return and area is pliable.
- After thawing is complete, apply dry sterile dressing with cotton balls between digits.
- Do not allow person to walk on affected feet; use of hands is usually permitted unless there is extensive damage.

(9) Discharge criteria
- Hospitalization for observation, pain control, and treatment is generally recommended.
- If discharged, the person should understand that affected area is at great risk for repeated episodes of frostbite, so extra precautions must be taken.

d. Accidental hypothermia is defined as a core temperature of 35 degrees Celsius (95 degrees Fahrenheit) or less.

(1) Categorization
- Minor—temperature 32 to 35 degrees Celsius (89.8–95 degrees Fahrenheit)
- Moderate—temperature 30 to 32 degrees Celsius (86.6–89.8 degrees Fahrenheit)

- Severe—temperature less than 30 degrees Celsius (86.8 degrees Fahrenheit)

(2) Onset may be acute, as in immersion hypothermia, or chronic, from sustained exposure to cold or conditions that impede normal heat production.
- Older people, newborns, those who have chronic diseases or alcohol intoxication, persons who are on medications, and persons who are homeless are predisposed to hypothermia.
- In vulnerable individuals, hypothermia may occur in a normal environment.

(3) Effects of hypothermia on various organ systems:
(a) Central nervous system: apathy, lethargy, inappropriate behavior, argumentativeness, and slurred speech and vision changes, followed by stupor and coma, absence of reflexes, fixed and dilated pupils.
(b) Vascular effects: Decreased circulating volume, sludging of blood, fluid shifts causing elevated hematocrit, shifting of oxygen hemoglobin dissociation curve, hypotension, cold diuresis, metabolic acidosis.
(c) Cardiac events: Multiple cardiac dysrhythmias due to cold blood, altered pH, electrolyte abnormalities, and hypoxemia; characteristic "J" or Osborne wave may be seen; atrial fibrillation or bradycardia; asystole that converts to ventricular fibrillation during warming or manipulation.
(d) Respiratory symptoms: In sudden cold exposure, there is an increased respiratory rate, but a gradual decrease as metabolic need decreases; pulmonary edema occurs.
(e) Renal manifestations: Cold diuresis occurs with low specific gravity, but low urine output may occur.
(f) Glucose metabolism: Either hypo- or hyperglycemia may be noted; hypoglycemia is most prevalent in sudden hypothermia, because of use of glucose stores by shivering.
(g) Integument: Frostbite or pressure necrosis may occur.
(h) The symptoms associated with different body temperatures are outlined in Table 37–8.

NURSE ADVISORY

Hypothermia may significantly shift the oxygen-hemoglobin dissociation curve, necessitating arterial blood gas (ABG) analysis to guide therapy. Machines used for analyzing ABGs are calibrated for normal body temperature, and must be recalibrated when the person's blood is profoundly hypothermic. The nurse should ensure that the laboratory is advised of the patient's temperature.

(4) Clinical management
(a) The speed and magnitude of rewarming procedures are affected by the rate at which the hypothermia occurred and the initial temperature; the more quickly the hypothermia oc-

Parameter	Mild	Moderate	Severe
Temperature	95–98° F	90–94° F	Less than 90° F
Level of consciousness	Oriented, apathetic	Confused to stuporous	Coma
Blood pressure	Normal	Low or absent	Low or absent
Pulse	Elevated	Low	Low or absent
Respirations	Elevated	Variable, irregular	Low or absent
Skeletal muscle action	Shivering	Rigid, stiff distal movement	Absent
Electrocardiogram	Normal	Bradycardia	Osborn wave; V-tach, V-fib

Table 37–8. Symptoms of Hypothermia

curred, the more rapid the rewarming measures.

(b) Rewarming modalities include heated oxygen; external warming; warmed IV fluids; warm gastric, bladder, and peritoneal lavage; warmed pleural lavage; femoral-femoral bypass; open thoracotomy to rewarm.

(c) With mild hypothermia, external warming may be the only treatment needed; in severe hypothermia, however, external warming is not appropriate as it may precipitate rewarming shock due to cold blood moving to core organs.

(d) Key points in rewarming
- Consider electrical safety for staff when large amounts of warm water are used in the treatment area; rubber boots may be prudent.
- Handle the person very gently—manipulation can cause intractable ventricular fibrillation.
- Effectiveness of medications and electricity (defibrillation or external pacing) is impaired in a cold person.
- Treatment of metabolic acidosis with sodium bicarbonate during rewarming is not recommended, but adequate respiratory management may minimize the acidosis; acidosis will most likely correct itself when rewarming has been accomplished.
- Treatment of dysrhythmias that occur during rewarming is deferred until the person has been rewarmed.
- The person must be rewarmed before resuscitation efforts are stopped and death pronouncement made; there are numerous accounts of hypothermic persons who have been pronounced dead who later revived spontaneously after rewarming.

(5) Discharge criteria
- Mild hypothermia
- No evidence of frostbite
- Normal temperature and vital signs
- Normal mentation and cognitive function
- Has a warm environment to return to; social services assistance may be necessary

(6) Discharge planning and teaching

- Provide explanation of causes of hypothermia and prevention strategies.
- Make medication adjustment, if needed.
- Explain follow-up plan, if necessary.

Weakness, Dizziness, Fatigue, and Syncope

1. Complaint of weakness, dizziness, fatigue, or syncope is very common and presents a significant challenge to the emergency care practitioner.
2. The spectrum of problems associated with these complaints is quite large; the goal here is to identify the most common causes and the care priorities until the diagnosis is established.
3. Careful assessment provides clues to the areas that should be explored 1st; do not discount anything the patient tells you.
4. Major causes of weakness, dizziness, fatigue, or syncope
   a. Cardiovascular events
      (1) Cardiac dysrhythmia (e.g., bradycardia, Stokes-Adams attack, tachycardia, ventricular ectopy)
      (2) Myocardial infarction
      (3) Mitral valve prolapse
      (4) Heart failure
      (5) Hypovolemia
         - Loss of fluid due to use of diuretics, diarrhea, vomiting, diaphoresis
         - Blood loss (e.g., gastrointestinal bleeding, anemia, leukemia)
      (6) Hypo- or hypertension
      (7) Medication-related events
   b. Respiratory symptoms
      (1) Pneumonia
      (2) Chronic obstructive pulmonary disease with exacerbation
      (3) Pulmonary embolism
   c. Electrolyte abnormalities
      (1) Medication-related
      (2) Loss through excessive sweating, diarrhea, vomiting
   d. Neurologic events
      (1) Transient ischemic attack
      (2) Cerebrovascular accident
      (3) Subarachnoid hemorrhage
      (4) Central nervous system tumor
      (5) Meningitis or encephalitis
      (6) Intracranial hematoma

e. Ear, nose, and throat conditions
  (1) Acute labyrinthitis (Meniere's syndrome)
  (2) Sinusitis
  (3) Otitis media
f. Eye disorders: acute glaucoma
g. Genitourinary or gynecologic events
  (1) Cystitis, pyelonephritis
  (2) Ruptured ectopic pregnancy
  (3) Estrogen deficiency
h. Gastrointestinal abnormalities
  (1) Third spacing with bowel obstruction; mesenteric thrombosis
  (2) Gastrointestinal bleeding
  (3) Delayed rupture of the spleen
  (4) Hepatitis
i. Endocrine disorders
  (1) Hypoglycemia
  (2) Hyperglycemia—undiagnosed or uncontrolled diabetes mellitus
  (3) Hypocalcemia
  (4) Adrenal insufficiency
  (5) Hypothyroidism
j. Drug overdose or toxic substance exposure
  (1) Carbon monoxide
  (2) Heavy metals
k. Infectious disease
  (1) Flu
  (2) Rubella or rubeola
  (3) Varicella
  (4) Mononucleosis
  (5) Strep pharyngitis
  (6) Lyme disease
l. Autoimmune disorders
m. Behavioral disturbances (e.g., depression, Münchausen's syndrome)
5. History: based on likely causes
6. Physical examination
  a. Vital signs, including postural measurements
  b. Complete physical assessment
  c. Cardiac monitor
7. Diagnostic studies
  a. Oximetry
  b. Electrocardiogram
  c. Laboratory studies: complete blood count, electrolytes, BUN, sugar, calcium, phosphorus, thyroid function, drug levels, urinalysis, test of stool and gastric contents for blood, IgM heterophile antibodies (HA), strep screen, toxicology
  d. Head CT
8. Nursing interventions
  a. Provide safety during evaluation; do not allow unassisted ambulation.
  b. Initiate life-saving measures, if appropriate.
  c. Assist in identifying cause of symptoms.
  d. Monitor person during evaluation.
9. Criteria for discharge
  a. Normal vital signs, including posturals
  b. Able to ambulate without assistance
  c. Able to perform activities of daily living
  d. Capacity and resources to carry out plan of care

Surface Trauma

1. Definition
  a. Surface trauma is the term applied to injury to the skin and soft tissues.
  b. Included in this section are contusion, abrasion, avulsion, laceration, amputation, human and animal bites, puncture wounds, high-pressure injection injuries, burns, and common wound infections; tetanus and rabies prophylaxis is also addressed.
2. Goals of emergency care
  a. Minimize further tissue damage
  b. Prevent wound infection
  c. Promote optimal wound healing
  d. Promote optimal return of function
  e. Assist individual in coping with alterations in body function or image
  f. Prevent injury or illness involving other organ systems
3. General concepts of wound healing
  a. Wounds heal by either *regeneration* or *repair* of tissues. Regeneration is the replication of original cells; repair results from replacement of tissues with collagen that is deposited between the tissues.
    (1) Regeneration is noted in healing of nerves, epithelium, bone, liver, endothelium of blood vessels, and surfaces of joints, pleura, and peritoneum.
    (2) Repair is seen in the dermis, fat, tendons, fascia, cartilage, and all other internal organs.
  b. Wounds heal by 1 of 3 methods: primary, secondary, or tertiary intent.
    (1) Primary intent involves primary closure of a wound and epithelialization and scar repair. It is used in clean incised wounds, including most simple lacerations.
    (2) Secondary intent involves leaving the wound open and subsequent granulation, wound contraction, and epithelialization. It is used in grossly contaminated or infected wounds and avulsions and in those that have a high likelihood of becoming infected, such as human bites.
    (3) Tertiary (or 3rd) intent is also known as delayed primary closure and involves leaving the wound open for several days to allow for granulation and wound contraction, followed by surgical closure. It is used for potentially contaminated wounds that are likely to become infected if closed primarily (e.g., combat wounds, old wounds, and human or animal bites).
  c. Timing for wound closure is important; with the exception of the face, wounds more than 12 hours old are generally not sutured.
  d. Some of the interventions used to repair wounds may interfere with the phases of wound healing (e.g., topical and injected anesthetics containing vasoconstrictors may interfere with circulation to the area and with the movement of cells that fight infection; strong chemicals may also kill healthy cells).

e. Wounds normally swell, reaching the maximal size about 12 hours after the injury; this swelling may cause cross-hatching when sutures are in place, resulting in increased scarring. Pressure dressings are often applied to minimize tissue swelling; however, dressings that are too tight can interfere with circulation to the area.

4. Factors affecting wound healing
   a. Age of client and wound: Older clients heal less well; older wounds are likely to become infected.
   b. Race: Darker-skinned individuals are at greater risk for developing keloids.
   c. Health status: Poor nutrition and chronic health problems predispose a person to less effective wound healing.
   d. Medications such as steroids may delay wound healing.
   e. Location of injury: Injuries of the arms, neck, chest, and upper back are more likely to scar than those in other areas of the body.
   f. Blood supply to area: The more vascular the area, the more readily a wound heals; this affects suture removal time.
   g. Wound size, tidiness, degree of contamination: Larger wounds, those with ragged edges, and grossly contaminated wounds heal less quickly.

5. Assessment: Assess the total person. Surface trauma is often visually impressive; avoid being distracted by the obvious and failing to identify hidden, but more important, alterations in the ABCs.
   a. History
      (1) Nature and etiology of the injury; does the story fit the injury? Inconsistencies may indicate systemic problem (e.g., a cardiac event triggered the fall that caused the head laceration), domestic violence, child or vulnerable adult abuse or neglect, or a criminal act.
      (2) Mechanism of injury
      (3) Time injury occurred
      (4) Health status, allergies, medications
      (5) Immunization status
      (6) Tendency to scar
      (7) Treatments before arrival
      (8) If avulsion or amputation, location and condition of the missing tissue
   b. Physical examination
      (1) Type of surface trauma (e.g., avulsion, laceration, contused laceration)
      (2) Size and degree of involvement
      (3) Amount of bleeding, and whether controlled
      (4) Degree of contamination; presence of foreign body
      (5) Nerve, tendon, bone, or other vital structure involvement
      (6) Motor, sensory, and circulatory function

6. General concepts of wound cleansing and care
   a. Cover the wound with a saline-moistened dressing to prevent the dressing from sticking to the wound.
   b. The area around the wound may be shaved; do not shave eyebrows.
   c. Hair can be plastered down with water-soluble lubricant or hair gel, rather than shaved.
   d. Clean the area around the wound with a soap or antiseptic solution; place sterile gauze in the wound to prevent irritating chemicals from entering the wound.
   e. Irrigate the wound itself with either normal saline or special wound cleaners such as Shur-Clens—a nonirritating, noncaustic solution; a wound can never be irrigated too much. If disinfectants must be used, they should be well diluted; with the exception of human or animal bites, soap-free solutions are used.
      (1) One recommendation is to use 50 ml of irrigation fluid per inch length and depth for each hour since the wound was sustained, especially in grossly contaminated wounds.
      (2) Irrigate with a small stream of pressure; this is accomplished with an 18-gauge blunt-tipped needle or IV catheter attached to a 30- to 50-ml syringe; Asepto syringes or IV tubing does not produce adequate pressure to irrigate out foreign matter.
   f. Optimal wound cleansing is best accomplished with the area anesthetized; a variety of anesthetic agents are used for either wound cleaning or suturing:
      (1) Topical preparations
         • TAC—tetracaine, adrenalin, and cocaine—is used on intact skin, not on mucous membranes; it is applied by saturating a 2 × 2 pad with the agent and applying it to the wound with some pressure for at least 10 minutes. Adequate anesthesia becomes apparent by pallor of the tissues and patient report of no sensation.
         • A cocaine-free preparation known as LAT (lidocaine, adrenalin, and tetracaine) has been introduced in both liquid and gel forms and may very well replace TAC because of improved safety and reduced cost. These agents are not used on persons with hypertension or peripheral vascular disease, or on digits.
         • Lidocaine as jelly, ointment, or solution
      (2) Injectable agents
         • Lidocaine and a variety of other injectable anesthetics are available, plain or with epinephrine.
         • These agents can be painful during administration; adjusting the pH with sodium bicarbonate or warming the solution results in less painful infiltrations.
         • Anesthetics with epinephrine are not used on the fingers, toes, ears, nose, or penis, or for people with thin skin, or persons with hypertension.
         • Although it is rare, lidocaine can cause central nervous system stimulation and seizures or central nervous system depression; thus, the quantity used should be monitored.
      (3) Other anesthesia options
         • Diphenhydramine or saline infiltration

- Digital or regional nerve blocks
- Self-administered, inhaled anesthetics (e.g., Nitronox—a combination of nitrous oxide and oxygen)
- Dissociative anesthesia with ketamine
- Sedation
- Hypnosis
- Music

7. Dressings and immobilization
   a. Excellent outcomes require that attention be paid to applying the initial dressing and protecting the part during healing.
   b. A layered dressing, composed of a contact layer, an absorbent layer, and an outer wrap, is ideal for wounds such as lacerations and avulsions.
      (1) In sutured wounds, a small amount of petroleum-based ointment is applied to the suture line; this prevents crusting, which increases scarring.
      (2) The contact layer may contain a petroleum-based product (e.g., Vaseline gauze, Adaptic) or may be fine mesh gauze; this layer promotes drainage away from the wound and prevents it from drying out.
      (3) The middle layer is composed of absorbent material such as gauze sponges.
      (4) The outer layer keeps the layers of dressing in contact with one another, eliminating pockets where fluid can accumulate; it also serves to secure the dressing to the person. Common outer wraps are Kling, Kerlix, and tubular gauze.
      (5) If more pressure is desired, a material known as Coban, a combination of an adhesive and an elastic bandage, may be used.
      (6) Surgical net may be used to secure dressings, particularly in areas that are difficult to bandage or where adhesive tape is not desired.
      (7) If adhesive tape is used, avoid placing it over the wound itself; moisture can accumulate, increasing the likelihood of infection.
   c. Alternatives to a layered bandage include transparent dressings, adherent gel dressings, and liquid or spray sealants; the latter are used primarily on the scalp.
   d. Sutured areas that involve a joint should be immobilized to minimize motion that will place tension on sutures, thereby increasing the likelihood of scarring.
      (1) The bandage itself may be firm enough to splint the part.
      (2) Splints can be incorporated into the bandage.
      (3) For areas such as the knee, a premade immobilizer or plaster splint may be applied.

8. Tetanus prophylaxis
   a. The need for tetanus prophylaxis is assessed in all individuals with surface trauma, regardless of severity.
   b. Two different guidelines exist regarding the interval for tetanus prophylaxis, so be familiar with institutional guidelines.
   c. Tetanus prophylaxis is recommended if the person has not been immunized within 5 to 10 years.

   d. Adult or pediatric diphtheria tetanus toxoid is used in many areas of the United States.
   e. If the person has not had a complete series, and it is a tetanus-prone wound, tetanus immune globulin (Hyper-Tet) is administered.
   f. Discharge instructions should include the need for, and timing of completion of, series and frequent side effects of diphtheria tetanus booster (e.g., swelling and pain at the site, fever in some individuals) as well as comfort measures (e.g., analgesics and warm soaks).
   g. Although complications are exceedingly rare with diphtheria-tetanus boosters, federal law requires that the person (or parent) receive written information about immunizations and sign consent; in addition, the lot number must be recorded in either a log or the clinical record.

9. Discharge criteria
   a. Bleeding controlled
   b. Pain controlled
   c. No other organ systems involved
   d. Able to carry out activities of daily living
   e. If a burn, it meets the criteria for a minor burn (discussed later).
   f. Injury is not in an area in which contamination with stool is likely.
   g. Injury will not interfere with elimination.

10. Discharge planning and teaching
    a. Stress the importance of elevation and cold application.
    b. Keep clean and dry; people with head wounds may shower and wash their hair as long as the hair is dried well with a hair dryer or patting; change dressings that become wet.
    c. Teach the patient how to perform activities of daily living (e.g., wear gloves when performing activities that may soil or dampen the dressing).
    d. Describe wound care and dressing changes.
    e. Tell the patient where to obtain supplies for dressing changes.
    f. Explain what to watch for: signs of wound infection, dressing too tight.
    g. Describe normal wound healing: A wound often looks worse when sutures are removed than it did when the injury occurred; advise the patient that this is normal and that it takes about 6 months for the wound to mature; plastic surgery to revise a scar is generally not undertaken before this time.
    h. Discuss the reactions to tetanus and the need for an additional booster.
    i. Discuss follow-up care, including suture removal time.

11. Specific injuries
    a. Contusion
       (1) Definition: bruising of skin and possible hematoma formation; seen in crush injuries
       (2) Generally of no major consequence unless it affects a large area, leading to compartment syndrome (see Chapter 34), or occurs in a person with clotting disorders (e.g., hemophilia or von Willebrand's disease).

(3) May cause subungual hematoma (blood under finger- or toenail), which is evacuated by putting a hole in the nail; tetanus prophylaxis is given if this is done.

(4) Teaching includes monitoring extent of bruising and signs of compartment syndrome, if large area involved.

(5) Treatment includes ice, elevation, and possibly compression.

b. Abrasion

(1) Definition: loss of epidermis and portions of the dermis due to friction; also called rug or road burn

(2) Can be quite painful, especially if a large area is affected.

(3) Often grossly contaminated with dirt embedded in the wound; high risk for infection and tattooing if not cleaned very well.

(4) Cleaning may require use of a toothbrush or other brush, or manually removing all visible dirt with a needle.

(5) Once the wound is cleaned and irrigated, apply a thin layer of ointment or burn cream to prevent crusting; accumulation of bacteria under a thick eschar may cause infection.

(6) Instruct the patient to clean the area several times a day and to apply a thin layer of ointment.

(7) Transparent dressings may also be used and left on until wound healing lifts the dressing edges.

c. Avulsion

(1) Definition: loss of a portion of the skin through shear force; may be combined with a laceration

(2) Wound closure is difficult because of loss of skin.

(3) Skin grafting may be necessary if the avulsion is large or in a vulnerable area (e.g., tip of nose, finger).

(4) It may be necessary to allow wound to heal by 2nd intention; if so, the contact layer is left in place for 10 to 14 days to allow for granulation because premature removal of contact layer may remove granulation tissue.

d. Laceration

(1) Traumatically incised wound with straight, stellate (starlike from burst force), or irregular wound edges; often involves dermis and subcutaneous layers.

(2) Usually closed by suturing, use of adhesive skin closures (small wounds not over joints), or small staples (large, cosmetically unimportant areas) (Table 37–9).

(3) If layered closure is necessary, deeper layers are sutured with nonabsorbable material, and skin is sutured with monofilament nonabsorbable material (e.g., nylon), or closed with adhesive skin closures (most often used on the face).

• In facial injuries, the skin sutures may be removed after 3 days and replaced with adhesive skin closures to minimize scarring from sutures.

• See Learning/Teaching Guidelines for Self-Care of Sutured Lacerations.

e. Puncture wound

(1) Definition: Wound created by a thin, sharp object, such as a nail, ice pick, needle, splinter, or fish hook. Damage to deeper structures is not visible.

(2) Risk for wound infection and tetanus because of foreign material that is forced into wound at the time of injury, drainage inhibition by wound edges sealed by skin flaps, and inability to clean and irrigate the wound well; this is especially true in a nail wound of the foot in a person wearing rubber-soled tennis shoes, because there is a rubber plug deep in the wound.

(3) May cause damage to deeper structures, especially bone, causing osteomyelitis; this is especially true in nail wounds of the ball of the foot.

(4) Effective wound cleansing may require that the wound be incised and probed, then irrigated.

(5) A medication-impregnated wick (e.g., iodoform gauze) may be inserted into the wound to promote drainage.

(6) Discharge instructions include soaking the area 4 times a day in hot water, and carefully observing for infection.

(7) In needle puncture wounds, the needle may still be present and embedded in tissue; exploration and removal under fluoroscopy, or in surgery, may be needed.

(8) Wood splinters swell and break apart when wet, rendering removal very difficult; thus, these wounds are not cleaned before splinter removal.

(9) In removing a fish hook, it may be necessary to force the barbed end of the hook through the skin and cut off the barb; then, remove the rest of the hook through the same pathway as it most likely went into the skin. The area over the barb may be anesthetized first.

(10) Puncture wounds due to human or animal bite are discussed later.

f. High-pressure injection injury

(1) Definition: damage to deeper structures by foreign material that is injected under pressure through a small hole in the skin

Table 37–9. Suture Removal Times

Area	Time
Face*	3–5 days
Eyelids	3 days
Scalp	7–10 days
Trunk	7–10 days
Upper extremities	7–14 days
Lower extremities	14–21 days

* Adhesive skin closures are often placed over the wound if sutures are removed in 3 days.

LEARNING/TEACHING GUIDELINES
for Self-Care of Sutured Lacerations

General Overview

1. Describe the process of wound healing, and explain that complete tissue healing takes several months; although the wound often looks worse when the sutures are removed than it did when the injury occurred, the wound edges will gradually smooth out, and the redness will fade over the next several months. Plastic surgery for wound revision is generally not considered for at least 6 months.

2. Discuss steps the patient can take during the next several days to optimize wound healing and minimize scarring, such as limiting movement of the area, elevating the injured part, and applying cool packs to minimize tissue edema and decrease tension on the suture line.

3. Demonstrate how to clean the wound and apply prescribed ointments or creams and dressings.

4. Describe how to care for the wound and dressings, including keeping dressings clean and dry, daily gentle wound cleansing with mild soap and water to remove crusts, and the application of petroleum-based ointments to minimize crusting; in most instances, bathing, showering, or gentle shampooing is allowed, but the wound should be blotted dry as soon as possible.

5. Explain the use of adhesive skin closures (if applied), how to reinforce the ends if they curl up, and how to reapply the strips if they come off.

6. Describe how and where to obtain wound care materials, such as dressings and ointments.

7. Review the signs of infections (e.g., swelling, pain, redness or red streak extending from the wound), drainage, fever, and what do to if it occurs.

8. Provide information regarding follow-up care for wound check and suture removal, including specific number of days and where to have sutures removed. Suggest that the person call the next day for the appointment.

9. Discuss how to perform activities of daily living to protect the wound and dressings, such as wearing gloves, taping a piece of plastic over the area during bathing, and use of splints, slings, or other protective devices.

10. Investigate if the person needs written documentation for work or school to restrict activities.

11. Discuss pain management, including techniques for minimizing pain, use of medications, and concerns related to medications.

12. Discuss the common normal reactions to the diphtheria tetanus booster, including redness and swelling at the injection site and methods of minimizing discomfort (e.g., applying a heat pack to the site, oral Benadryl, or topical hydrocortisone cream); emphasize that these are not allergic reactions. If the person requires additional tetanus prophylaxis, explain when it is due and where to obtain it.

13. Discuss strategies for preventing future injuries, if appropriate.

Pain Management

1. Instruct the person regarding the use of pain medications.
   a. The anesthesia used during wound repair will wear off over the next few hours, and the area may become painful.
   b. Pain can be minimized by taking an over-the-counter analgesic, such as ibuprofen or acetaminophen, or a prescribed pain medication before the anesthesia wears off.
   c. Anti-inflammatory analgesics, such as ibuprofen, also help to decrease swelling and inflammation at the wound site itself.
   d. Pain medications should be taken with food to decrease gastric irritation.
   e. Discuss the appropriate dosage for over-the-counter medications, such as acetaminophen, aspirin, or ibuprofen; the manufacturer's dosing instructions are often more conservative than those recommended by health care professionals.
   f. Pain medications that contain narcotics may affect level of consciousness, blood pressure, dexterity, and judgment; do not use alcohol, drive a motor vehicle, operate dangerous machinery, or work at heights while taking narcotic analgesics.
   g. Because narcotic analgesics may cloud one's memory, write down the time that you take a medication to avoid accidental overdose.
   h. If there is significant pain, do not try to avoid the use of pain medication; once the pain becomes severe, it takes longer for pain medication to be effective.
   i. Alternating narcotic and nonnarcotic analgesics may enhance pain management.
   j. Do not take more medication than prescribed without consulting a health care practitioner; pain that is not relieved with the prescribed dose may suggest that there is a more serious problem that requires reevaluation.
   k. Narcotic analgesics may cause constipation; increase fiber, bulk, and fluids to minimize this.
   l. Pain from a sutured wound usually abates within 48 hours; the need for continued pain medication, especially narcotics, suggests a need for reevaluation.

2. Discuss nonpharmacologic pain management strategies:
   a. Minimize movement of the injured area for the 1st 24 to 48 hours; immobilizing devices, such as elastic bandages, slings, or splints, may be used.

LEARNING/TEACHING GUIDELINES
(continued)

b. Elevate the injured area above the heart to decrease swelling and promote drainage.

c. Apply cool packs to the area for 20 minutes every hour while awake for the first 48 hours; secure the cool pack with an elastic bandage and slight pressure so that there is good contact with the site. Ice packs should be covered with an absorbent material to prevent the dressing from becoming wet.

d. After 48 hours, use a warm pack to increase circulation to the area, and begin using the affected area, unless otherwise directed.

---

(2) Commonly caused by paint guns, grease guns, or medication guns injected into a small space (e.g., the finger or hand).

(3) Pressure causes material to dissect tissue, resulting in cellulitis and necrosis.

(4) Because the hole in the skin is minute (and may not be visible), the degree of damage and seriousness of the injury are often not appreciated by the novice practitioner or the patient; however, this can be a devastating injury, requiring prompt surgery to decompress tissue and remove foreign material. Even with prompt surgery, amputation of the part may eventually be necessary.

g. Human bite

(1) Human bites are of concern because of the high incidence of infection, especially in hand wounds; the rate of infection, excluding hand wounds, depends on the lapsed time from injury to treatment.

(2) A dental abrasion or clenched fist injury is a particularly dangerous form of human bite injury to the knuckle, which occurs when a person punches another in the mouth, causing the teeth to lacerate the area; the motion of unclenching the fist causes bacteria to travel into the dorsum of the hand, often involving the joint capsule or tendon sheath and setting up serious infection.

- The wound created usually does not appear significant; people often seek care several days later because of swelling and pain.

- The mechanism of injury increases the likelihood that there is a fracture as well, and the possibility of osteomyelitis.

- These wounds are difficult to treat, and it is not uncommon for significant infection to occur, requiring hospitalization, IV antibiotics, and surgery to facilitate drainage or amputation.

- Diabetics with hand bites have a higher incidence of infection and require special care.

(3) Human bites require scrupulous cleaning and irrigation; the use of disinfectants in these wounds is justified.

(4) Because of the potential for infection, the wound may be left open to heal by 2nd or 3rd intention, may be loosely sutured, or may be closed with adhesive skin strips, depending on the area injured and the size of the wound; the wisdom of suturing a human bite is controversial.

(5) Antibiotic therapy can be used.

- *Eikenella corrodens* and *Staphylococcus aureus* are common organisms in human bites.

- Antibiotics are usually prescribed for hand bites.

- Antibiotic options include the following: penicillin, dicloxacillin, amoxicillin, clavulanate, and cefuroxime; adults allergic to penicillin may be given tetracycline; children who have penicillin allergies may be given erythromycin.

(6) Criteria for discharge

- A completely reliable person who understands the seriousness of the injury and commits to compliance with antibiotic therapy and follow-up, which is usually daily until there is evidence of effective wound healing

- No fracture or involvement of joint capsule or tendon sheath

- No significant tissue loss

- Normal immune status

h. Animal scratches and bites

(1) Major concerns in the person with animal scratch or bite include infection, significant scarring due to large tissue loss, and complications such as cat-scratch disease and rabies.

(2) Thirty to 40 percent of cat scratches and puncture bites easily become infected; *Pasteurella multocida* is often the offending organism.

- Puncture wounds made by a cat's tooth are quite small but deep, and they seal off quickly; significant cellulitis can result rapidly, often within 24 hours.

- Cat scratches may result in permanent dermal dents, a form of scarring.

- Cat bites are generally not sutured.

- Antibiotic options include amoxicillin with clavulanate, oxacillin, penicillin, dicloxacillin, cefuroxime, and ceftriaxone; erythromycin and ciprofloxacin may be used in the person who is allergic to penicillin.

- Cat-scratch disease may occur from dog, cat, or monkey scratches or bites and is characterized by the development of a pustule or papule at the site several days after injury, followed by lymphadenitis within 2 weeks;

fatigue, fever, headache, and loss of appetite may also occur. Symptoms usually resolve spontaneously within 2 months, but tetracycline may be used.

(3) In dog bites, there is often an instinctual tearing motion that can result in a large amount of tissue loss and damage to deeper structures, including bone, especially in bites of the head, face, and hand.

- Suturing of dog bites is controversial, although the tendency now is to suture them unless they are high risk: The wound is more than 8 to 12 hours old, it involves the hand, it has obvious evidence of infection, or it involves deep fang wounds.
- Prophylactic antibiotics are also controversial, and there is a shift away from routine antibiotic therapy unless it is a high-risk wound, as discussed earlier.

(4) Although rabies can occur in domestic animals, most cases result from bites or exposure to the saliva of raccoons, skunks, and bats.

(5) The need for rabies prophylaxis usually requires consultation with public health officials regarding the prevalence of rabies in the area. It is customary for the rabies vaccination series to be given following public health agency approval. Also, in some areas, the cost of rabies prophylaxis is borne by the public health agency, and their permission is required.

(6) Key data that may assist in determining whether rabies prophylaxis is needed include the following:

- Does it involve a domestic or wild animal?
- If domestic, has the animal been immunized against rabies?
- What is the health status of the animal?
- Is the animal available for quarantine?
- Was the incident provoked or unprovoked? A unprovoked attack suggests that the animal is ill and may be carrying rabies; however, when the bite involves a small child, it is often difficult to determine whether it was unprovoked because children often unknowingly do things that would provoke a healthy dog or cat.

(7) Rabies prophylaxis involves the use of both rabies immune globulin and human diploid cell rabies vaccine.

- Half of the dose of rabies immune globulin is administered IM in the deltoid and the remaining half is injected subcutaneously around the site, unless the bite area is too small (e.g., finger); common reactions include fever and pain at the injection site.
- Human diploid cell vaccine is administered in 5 doses on days 0, 3, 7, 14, and 28; local reactions include redness and swelling at the injection site, and malaise, fever, muscle ache, headache, and abdominal pain. Administration is discontinued if tests of the animal are negative.

(8) Reporting of animal bites to health authorities or law enforcement is mandatory in many areas; in some cases the responsibility rests with the patient, and in other areas the hospital or practitioner must make the report. Document whether the report is made by the hospital or instructions are given to the patient regarding reporting responsibility.

(9) Animal bites, especially a dog bite to a child by a loving and loyal family pet, can be emotionally devastating, to both the patient and parents; in the parents' agitated state they often make hasty decisions and kill the animal or remove it from the home environment, creating long-lasting parent-child conflicts. Encourage parents to consider carefully the reason why the bite injury occurred and options for preventing future injuries. In general, children younger than 6 years of age should not be left unsupervised around a cat or dog, and all children should be educated about safe behavior around an animal.

i. Amputations (see Chapter 34)

(1) Traumatic amputation or avulsion of distal portions of fingertips, the nose, or larger areas requires attention to both the amputated part and the proximal site.

(2) The priority in care of the amputated part is to keep it viable in case reattachment efforts are made.

- Gently rinse the amputated part with saline; roll it so that skin is on the outside and subcutaneous tissue is on the inside to protect it from drying.
- Place the part in lightly moistened sterile gauze.
- Put the part in an airtight container, such as a plastic bag.
- Keep the bag in a cool area or on ice.
- Label the bag with the patient's name and tissue part.
- Check institutional protocols because local preferences may vary.

(3) Care of proximal end

- Control bleeding, if significant; a tourniquet may be needed on an arm or leg; pressure and elevation are usually adequate for smaller areas.
- Gently clean area.
- Apply a moist dressing, according to local preference; may be saline, povidone-iodine, or antibiotic solution.
- Repair of small amputations of the fingertip often does not include reattachment of the part, but rather bone ends are trimmed away and the area is covered with a nonadherent dressing (e.g., Owen's silk, fine mesh gauze, Adaptic) and allowed to heal by granulation.
- Radiograph of both parts may be ordered.
- Amputation of even small areas can be distressing; thus, psychologic support is important.

- Intravenous antibiotics may be ordered.
- Reattachment often requires care by a specialist using microsurgical instruments; anticipate the necessity for transfer if such facilities are not available at your institution so that care can be rendered as quickly as possible.
j. Burns (see Chapter 36)
    (1) Key elements in the care of any burned person are to do the following:
        (a) Stop the burning process by cooling and removing sources of heat (e.g., smoldering clothes or chemicals that may continue to burn).
        (b) Assess and monitor ABCs.
            - Consider smoke inhalation or carbon monoxide poisoning, especially if the fire was in an enclosed space (see p. 1716, "Inhalation Injury Due to Smoke or Toxic Fumes").
            - If circumferential burns of the chest are present, tissue swelling may compromise breathing and an escharotomy may be necessary.
            - Initiate cardiac, BP, and oximetry monitoring.
            - Obtain routine laboratory studies; consider carboxyhemoglobin level and arterial blood gases.
        (c) Estimate the percentage of the total body surface area (TBSA) affected, using the rule of nines for adults or special formulas for children, such as Lund and Browder or Berkow diagrams (see Chapter 36). This estimate is used to calculate necessary fluid volume replacement and to determine whether care at a burn center is indicated. For smaller burns, a rule of thumb is that the area the size of the patient's palm is equal to 1 percent TBSA.
        (d) Establish IV access for burns greater than 14 percent TBSA. For 15 to 40 percent TBSA, use 1 IV line. For over 40 percent TBSA, 2 IV lines. Local protocol may call for 2 lines in all people with greater than 15 percent TBSA. Avoid placing IV lines through or near the burn (if possible) and in lower extremities.
        (e) Initiate fluid resuscitation with Ringer's lactate, according to local protocol, for 24 hours, with half the total administered in the first 8 hours after the injury. Children may require additional maintenance fluids that contain dextrose, but glucose solutions are generally not administered to adults. Electrical burns may require additional fluids both because it is difficult to estimate the amount of tissue damaged and because of high risk for renal failure due to myoglobinuria; administer IV fluids to achieve a urine output of 100 ml per hour in electrical burns.

NURSE ADVISORY

The rate and volume of intravenous fluid administration are determined from the time the burn occurred, not the time of initiation of the fluid. Thus, the 1st 8 hours of intravenous fluid may need to be administered in less than 8 hours.

        (f) Insert a Foley catheter in a person with greater than 25 percent TBSA to monitor treatment effectiveness and guide fluid administration. Observe for red wine–colored urine, which suggests myoglobinuria, and increase IV fluids to clear the pigment.
        (g) Insert nasogastric tube if person has greater than 30 percent TBSA, is unconscious, or will be transported by air.
        (h) Assess circulation in burned extremities and adequacy of ventilation in chest burns—escharotomy may be needed.
        (i) Provide pain management with IV morphine in small doses, titrated for effect after fluid resuscitation has been initiated; monitor vital signs.
        (j) Wound care may be deferred if transfer to a burn center will be accomplished within 12 hours; cover person with a clean sheet and blanket. If transfer is delayed, burns are gently débrided, irrigated, and covered with a thin layer of Silvadene; ensure adequate pain management during the procedure.
        (k) Prevent hypothermia by keeping the person covered, increasing room temperature, and using a heat shield, as necessary.
        (l) Provide tetanus prophylaxis.
        (m) Criteria for referral to a burn center
            - Second- and 3rd-degree burns of greater than 10 percent TBSA in person younger than 10 years of age or older than 50 years of age
            - Third degree burns greater than 5 percent
            - Circumferential burns of extremities or chest
            - Second- and 3rd-degree burns involving hands, feet, face, perineum, or joints
            - Electrical burns, including lightning injuries
            - Associated with inhalation injury
            - Significant chemical burns
            - Burns in persons with significant preexisting disease (e.g., diabetes, heart disease, immunocompromise)
            - Burns in the presence of multisystem trauma
        (n) Wound management for minor burns
            - Provide adequate pain management, preferably with IV narcotics, before wound care.
            - In small burns, apply wet saline gauze sponges or immerse the burned area in

cool saline to provide immediate relief of pain. Periodically rewet the dressing by squirting more saline on the dressing, rather than removing and reapplying new dressings, which is painful.

- Gently clean area with soap and water or dilute povidone-iodine–saline solution.
- Gently débride nonviable tissue using iris scissors and forceps; do not pull off tissue; skin on the palms and soles may be left intact.
- Irrigate area well with normal saline solution.
- Apply Silvadene or other topical agents per protocol to fine mesh gauze, then apply to the burn area; applying topical agents directly to the burn is painful; cover with gauze sponges and wrap with flexible outer wrap.
- Surgical net can be used to secure dressings and is economical because multiple dressing changes will most likely be needed and it can be laundered and reused.
- Small burns may be covered with transparent dressings or colloidal dressings.
- Facial burns may be left unbandaged.

(o) Discharge instructions
- Explain how to perform wound care.
- Discuss where to obtain supplies.
- Describe signs of infection or reasons to return.
- Review when and where follow-up is to be done.
- Discuss pain management, including elevation.

k. Wound infections (see Chapters 8 and 13)
(1) Rate of infection in sutured lacerations is quite low, ranging from 3 to 6 percent. The infection rate in human bites is dependent on the location and ranges from 1 (face) to 40 percent (hand), with an average of approximately 18 percent for all sites. The incidence of infection in animal bites is species specific, ranging from 4.3 percent in dog bites to 50 percent in cat bites.
(2) Causative organisms
(a) *S. aureus* is the causative organism in the majority of nonbite wounds, followed by *Staphylococcus epidermidis, Streptococcus, Escherichia coli, Proteus, Enterobacter,* and *Klebsiella.*
(b) *P. multocida* is the predominant organism in dog and cat bites and is particularly virulent.
(c) *E. corrodens* is frequently noted in human bite wound infections, as are the organisms listed earlier.
(d) Less common, but potentially lethal, infections may include wound botulism from *Clostridium botulinum;* gas gangrene from *Clostridium perfringens* or anaerobic *Streptococcus;* tetanus from *Clostridium tetani;* and necrotizing fasciitis from *Streptococcus pyog-*

enes (so-called flesh-eating bacteria), which can be categorized as part of severe streptococcal invasive syndrome (SSIS).
- Gas gangrene creates massive local tissue damage characterized by tissue crepitation (due to gas in tissues) and gray, watery drainage; it may be treated with hyperbaric oxygenation as well as antitoxin.
- Tetanus is characterized by systemic symptoms, most commonly trismus and opisthotonus, and is treated with tetanus immune globulin (Hyper-Tet).
- Wound botulism also creates systemic rather than local symptoms and is treated with botulism antitoxin.
- Although hyperbaric oxygenation may be used in SSIS, its effectiveness may be limited because the organism is aerobic.
- Tetanus is clearly preventable with immunization, yet an average of 50 people die each year in the United States from this disease; the majority of them are women older than 50 years of age who have not had a diphtheria-tetanus booster every 10 years as recommended.
- Parental concern about complications of childhood immunizations, coupled with limited access to immunizations, has resulted in a decrease in the number of people who are immunized adequately; it is feared that there will be an increase in tetanus as well as in other previously rare, immunization-preventable diseases.
- Wounds that may cause these serious infections are not necessarily large or grossly contaminated; tetanus after a rose thorn puncture has been reported; thus, tetanus prophylaxis and discharge teaching are important for even the smallest wounds.

(3) Factors that increase the risk for infection are the same as those that influence wound healing:
- The nature of the wound: size and amount of tissue damage, mechanism of injury, age of the wound, degree of contamination or presence of a foreign body, and the body area involved. Wounds of the face and scalp heal well; wounds below the knee have the highest rate of infection.
- High-risk hosts: diabetics; immunocompromised individuals, by disease or corticosteroids; malnourished persons; older persons; those with liver or kidney disease; patients who are noncompliant with treatment or follow-up plan.
- Treatment-related factors: wound-cleansing agents (e.g., soaps); inadequate irrigation; rough handling of tissues; inadequate hemostasis and hematoma formation; use of anesthetics, especially those containing epinephrine; undesirable suture technique, with failure to close dead space; sutures that are too tight

or too loose; suture material used (some materials cause more tissue reactivity than others); and inadequate dressing.

    (4) Preventive measures (see Chapter 8)

    (5) Clinical management (see Chapter 13)

Visual Disturbances

1. Timely assessment of the person with an eye problem is a high priority because of the vital role of vision, and the limited time frame for intervention (see Chapter 19).
2. With few exceptions, basic nursing assessment of the person with an eye problem includes the following:
   a. Pupil size, shape, and response
   b. Visual acuity using a Snellen or similar eye chart (*Note:* In persons with excessive pain or tearing, it is often necessary to anesthetize the eye using short-acting topical anesthetic drops to obtain an accurate visual acuity; the use of this medication is by unit protocol.)
   c. Observation of the eye structures and surrounding tissues
   d. Everting eyelids to observe for foreign body
   e. In trauma situations, extraocular movement is also assessed.
3. More complex assessment includes the following:
   a. Funduscopic examination
   b. Fluorescein staining and visualization with a Wood's lamp (blue light)
   c. Use of the slit lamp
   d. Intraocular pressure measurement using a pneumotonometer or Schiøtz tonometer
4. Common or significant emergency eye problems
   a. Vitreous hemorrhage
       (1) Definition: Bleeding into the vitreous humor, which may be partial or complete, occurring spontaneously or as a result of trauma. Etiology may be spontaneous such as in diabetic retinopathy, retinal detachments, and retinal tears, or traumatic, resulting from blunt or penetrating trauma.
       (2) Triage category: Immediate
       (3) History
         • History of trauma
         • Associated with diabetes or primary eye problem such as retinal detachment
         • Varying degrees of vision loss
       (4) Physical examination
         • Funduscopic examination in partial hemorrhage reveals dark spots, which overlie the red reflex; a complete vitreous hemorrhage presents as a black uniform coloration with total loss of normal retinal red reflex.
         • Evidence of eye trauma may be noted.
       (5) Clinical management
         • Keep at rest with head of bed elevated.
         • If hemorrhage is due to protruding foreign body, immobilize the object and do not attempt to remove it.
         • Prepare for surgical intervention.
   b. Central retinal artery occlusion
       (1) Definition and etiology
         • Partial or complete loss of vision due to incomplete or complete occlusion of the retinal artery from embolized arteriosclerotic plaques from the carotid or heart valves, or due to inflammatory processes such as temporal arteritis.
         • Predisposing factors are vascular disease, diabetes, and hypertension.
         • Most often seen in older people, primarily men, occurring at night or early morning.
         • Permanent damage may occur if the condition persists for more than 2 hours.
       (2) Triage category: immediate
       (3) History: Sudden, painless loss of vision; some individuals may have transient episodes of decreased visual acuity lasting seconds to minutes before complete loss of vision occurs.
       (4) Clinical management
         • Apply intermittent digital pressure to the globe in an effort to dislodge the embolus performed by a physician or an advanced practitioner.
         • Promote vasodilation of retinal artery by elevating the level of carbon dioxide; this is accomplished by having the person breathe into a paper bag for 15 to 20 minutes.
         • Patient should inhale Carbogen (95 percent oxygen and 5 percent carbon dioxide) to dilate the vessels.
         • Remove fluid from the anterior chamber to decompress the globe and dislodge the embolus.
   c. Detached retina
       (1) Definition: A separation of the 2 layers of the retina resulting in varying degrees of unilateral or bilateral vision loss; may be due to a disruption in the inner layer as a result of trauma or traction, which permits fluid to separate the layers, or simply due to a buildup of fluid from a variety of causes such as tumors or vascular, inflammatory, or metabolic conditions.
       (2) History
         • Alteration in visual acuity may include "floaters" in the vitreous, blurred or foggy vision, flashes of light or sparks, or a sensation of a curtain moving across the eye.
         • More often noted in men, older people, those with severe myopia (nearsightedness), and persons with previous eye surgery.
       (3) Triage priority: immediate
       (4) Clinical management
         • Minimize further detachment by limiting head movement
         • Prepare for surgical management: scleral buckling, photocoagulation, air or silicon oil injections, cryotherapy
   d. Acute closed-angle (narrow-angle) glaucoma
       (1) Definition: Sudden onset of increased intraocular pressure due to impedance of outflow of aqueous humor from the anterior chamber, causing damage to the optic nerve, retina, iris, lens, and cornea; sustained pressure elevations may cause permanent blindness.
       (2) Triage priority: immediate. This is a true ophthalmologic emergency that can be reversed with immediate treatment.

(3) History
- Eye pain and blurred vision; however, some patients have no pain
- Halos around objects
- May occur as a result of pupillary dilation for any reason (e.g., clinician dilating pupils for examination, dark room, use of anticholinergic or sympathomimetic medications)
- Associated symptoms of nausea, vomiting, and headache

(4) Physical examination
- Bulging eye
- Sclera reddened and muddy
- Dilated pupil
- Cloudy cornea

(5) Diagnostic studies include measurement of intraocular pressure.

(6) Clinical management. Treatment is directed at urgently lowering intraocular pressure to below 40 mm Hg by doing the following:
- Interfering with production of aqueous humor through topical administration of β-adrenergic antagonists such as timolol, betaxolol, apraclonidine, or acetazolamide (Diamox) by oral, IM, or IV route
- Decreasing vitreous humor volume with systemic hyperosmolar medications such as IV mannitol or oral glycerol with lemon juice or oral isosorbide
- Increasing outflow of aqueous humor by constricting the pupil with 2 to 4 percent pilocarpine eye drops every 10 to 15 minutes for 1 to 2 hours (blue-eyed persons may respond to 2 percent pilocarpine; brown-eyed people may require a 4 percent concentration)
- Administering antiemetics if nausea or vomiting is present
- Surgical intervention by iridotomy is done after the acute crisis is managed.

℞ DRUG ADVISORY

Medications used to treat acute narrow-angle glaucoma may cause hyper- or hypotension. Blood pressure monitoring every 15 minutes, or more frequently, may be necessary in the initial treatment phase.

e. Chemical burn of the eye
(1) Definition
- Eye exposure to chemicals is a serious concern because of the potential for permanent vision loss.
- Alkaline burns are considered more serious than acid burns because alkali causes liquefaction, allowing for continued penetration of tissue long after initial exposure.
- Acids, however, precipitate eye protein on initial contact, which limits their penetrating ability; one exception to this is hydrofluoric acid, which has significant penetrating ability.
- Common alkaline substances that cause eye injury are drain and oven cleaners containing lye, plaster, or mortar; lime products; and fertilizers.
- Common acids that cause eye burns include car battery acid, bleach, hydrofluoric acid (used in glass etching, computer chip production, and gasoline processing), hydrochloric acid, and high concentrations of acetic acid.

(2) Triage: Irrigate the eye immediately; assessment is deferred until irrigation is under way.

(3) History
- Initially limited to history of exposure and treatment before arrival.
- Contact poison center for guidance regarding chemicals; have someone bring in the container if the chemical is unknown.

(4) Physical examination
- Depending on the chemical, the cornea may be opacified and the sclera and surrounding tissues reddened.
- Particulate matter may be trapped under the upper lids; the eyelid must be everted or a lid retractor used to identify and flush out the foreign material.
- Eyelid and facial burns may be present.
- Complete primary and secondary survey if the incident was an explosion or blast event; an intracranial or intraocular foreign body may be present.

(5) Clinical management
- If eye irrigation has already been done before arrival, use pH paper touched to lower conjunctiva to determine eye pH; the goal is a pH of 7.4 30 minutes after eye irrigation is complete.
- If eye irrigation was not done before arrival, irrigate the eye with a liter of normal saline and check the pH (Procedure 37–1).
- Because copious eye irrigation is usually required, the use of an eye irrigation lens is helpful.
- Most individuals undergoing eye irrigation experience blepharospasm, which can be relieved by anesthetic drops; these must be repeated frequently during the irrigation as the effect wears off quickly. A regional nerve block may also be needed to facilitate adequate irrigation.
- Medications used may include topical antibiotics, steroids, and cycloplegics as well as oral N-acetylcysteine (Mucomyst) to decrease collagenase synthesis and ascorbic acid to promote collagen synthesis.
- Pain management is accomplished with IV or oral narcotics, especially if facial burns are also present.
- Tetanus prophylaxis may also be ordered.
- Provide topical treatment of facial burns, according to unit protocol.
- Use unilateral or bilateral eye patching.
- Give reassurance that everything possible is being done, but honesty about the prognosis, especially with alkaline burns.

(6) Criteria for discharge
- Individuals with alkaline burns are usually admitted for continued irrigation.

Procedure 37–1
Ocular Irrigation

Definition/Purpose	To neutralize caustic chemical reaction after accidental exposure
Contraindication/Cautions	Immediate irrigation is imperative when a chemical is introduced into the eyes. *Do not* take the time to assemble ideal equipment if it is not readily available.
Learning/Teaching Activities	Provide the following information: (a) explain the procedure while you are starting it; (b) explain the imperative nature of neutralizing the chemical to prevent damage to the eye tissues.

Preliminary Activities

Equipment	• 1000-ml bag of normal saline • Macrodrip IV tubing • IV pole • Eyelid speculum • Nonsterile gloves • Towels • pH testing paper
Assessment/Planning	• Obtain a brief history of the accident while helping the person onto a stretcher or treatment table: (a) nature of injury, (b) irritant or chemical if known, (c) first aid given at scene, (d) allergies.

Procedure

Actions	Rationale/Discussion	
1. Use gloves.	1. Universal precautions	
2. Quickly place a strip of pH paper in the eyelid.	2. To determine whether substance is alkaline or acid	
3. With the person lying down or over a sink, direct the flow of saline into the eye or eyes.		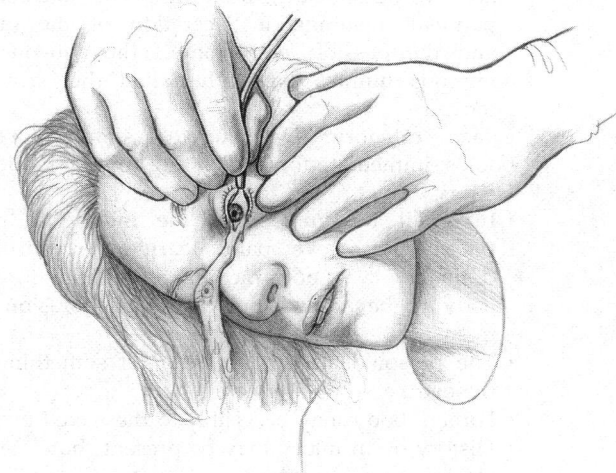
4. Continue the irrigation for 10–15 minutes without interruption.	4. Some chemicals adhere to the tissues and continue to cause damage.	
5. Assess the comfort of the person.		

Final Activities

Gently pat eye dry with soft towel. Apply eye patch or dressing, if indicated. Document person's response to procedure.

• Individuals with acid or other chemical burns may be discharged if they meet the following criteria: Normal eye pH; visual acuity returns to normal; no evidence of ulceration; assistance with activities of daily living is available if bilateral patches applied.

(7) Discharge planning and teaching
  • Discuss the use of medications and how to apply

or instill them; repeat cautions about topical anesthetics.
- Demonstrate the correct technique for applying eye patches.
- Review the follow-up plan.
- Discuss the expected outcome and time frames and complications.
- Review the safety considerations including impaired peripheral vision, the need to keep some distance from dangerous edges, and laws regarding wearing a temporary eye patch; some states prohibit driving a motor vehicle while wearing a temporary patch.
- Discuss prevention strategies.

f. Foreign body
   (1) Definition
      - Ocular foreign bodies range from barely visible tiny specks to impressive, large-diameter metal rods or pieces of wood, weeds, and grasses. Depending on the mechanism, they may affect only the cornea or sclera, or they may be intraocular or intracranial.
      - Superficial foreign bodies often include dirt or metal particles that blow into the eye and displaced contact lenses.
      - Intraocular foreign bodies are usually associated with metal-working or use of drills; there may be little external evidence of injury.
      - Penetrating foreign bodies occur from a variety of mechanisms, both domestic and occupational, resulting in laceration of the globe and the possible extrusion of the aqueous or vitreous humor, especially when they are removed.
   (2) Triage category: Delayed for simple foreign bodies; immediate for penetrating foreign bodies
   (3) History
      - In small foreign bodies, the individual may present with eye pain, tearing, or purulent drainage; it is not uncommon for the foreign body to be absent, but a corneal abrasion remains.
      - The person feels the sensation of something in the eye.
      - Foreign body may be visible to the naked eye.
      - History of an injury may be present, but often is elusive.
      - Visual acuity may be impaired because of pain and tearing, but may also be normal.
      - Photophobia may be present.
   (4) Physical examination
      - Foreign body visible
      - Corneal abrasion
      - Rust ring if the foreign body was metal
      - If there is a penetrating foreign body, there may be lacerations of the eyelid as well as globe, with extrusion of aqueous and vitreous humor.
   (5) Diagnostic studies
      - Tonometry
      - Fluorescein staining and visualization under blue light

- Head radiographs or CT, if possibility of intracranial foreign body

DRUG ADVISORY

Sterile fluorescein–impregnated paper strips are preferred over a fluorescein solution; solutions have been found to have bacterial contamination. To prevent corneal abrasion, it is suggested that the strip be moistened with a drop of saline or eye anesthetic, and that the fluorescein be allowed to drip into the lower conjunctival sac. Briefly irrigate the eye after fluorescein has been used, to prevent chemical conjunctivitis. Fluorescein is not to be used when there is a contact lens in place; it may cause permanent staining of soft and gas-permeable lenses.

   (6) Clinical management—simple foreign body
      - Topical anesthetics for comfort and initial evaluation
      - Eye irrigation with normal saline solution
      - Removal of foreign body using an eye spud, eye drill, or 27-gauge needle
      - Cycloplegics to decrease pupillary spasm, which causes pain
      - Topical antibiotic drops or ointment
      - The use of eye patching is controversial; some practitioners reserve the use of eye patching for only extensive abrasions.
      - If a patch is prescribed, it is removed after 24 hours and the abrasion reevaluated by a practitioner; alternatively, a reliable patient can determine if the patch should be continued, depending on the amount of discomfort when the patch is removed; simple corneal abrasions usually heal within 24 hours.
      - Tetanus prophylaxis
      - Oral pain medications, if severe abrasion
   (7) Clinical management—penetrating foreign body
      - Stabilize the object by building up the base with moistened gauze sponges, covered with an eye shield or cup, and secured to the face; do not attempt to remove the foreign body.
      - Immobilize the head with sandbags or sponge blocks (1000-ml IV bags can also be used if the other devices are not available); reinforce with the patient the need to keep the head still.
      - Establish IV access.
      - Administer IV antibiotics.
      - Provide pain relief; however, be cautious in person who may have an intracranial injury as well.
      - Give tetanus prophylaxis.
      - Monitor as for a head-injured person.
      - Prepare for immediate surgery.
   (8) Criteria for discharge—simple foreign body
      - No evidence of globe perforation
      - Able to perform activities of daily living or has assistance to do so
      - Able to carry out medication and patching regimen
   (9) Discharge planning and teaching—simple foreign body

- Same as for chemical burn of the eye.
- Caution person not to use anesthetic drops because they impede corneal healing; although these drops are never prescribed for use after discharge, some persons with chronic abrasions or arc welder burns have access to these agents.
- Infection may result in perforation of the globe or the development of herpetic keratitis with globe perforation; make sure the person knows the signs of infection.

g. Hyphema

(1) Definition: Accumulation of blood in the anterior chamber of the eye due to blunt or penetrating trauma, which damages small blood vessels of the ciliary body or iris; complications include glaucoma and corneal staining.

(2) Triage category: delayed

(3) History
- History of trauma: Common causes include racket or squash balls or rackets, baseballs, or punches to the eye.
- Vision impairment, if hyphema is large
- Headache
- Eye pain
- Photophobia
- Nausea or vomiting

(4) Physical examination
- Blood level is usually apparent with person sitting upright, although a small hyphema may be detected only with slit-lamp examination.
- Dilated pupil.
- Possibility of a blow-out fracture of the orbit, evidenced by asymmetry of the orbital bones and impaired extraocular movement due to entrapment of the eye muscle in the fracture.
- A small percentage of people develop signs of increased intracranial pressure, with decreased level of consciousness.

(5) Diagnostic studies
- Tonometry
- Orbital radiographs
- Computed tomography scan, if neurologic abnormalities are present
- Sickle cell prep for Black persons, if not previously tested (acetazolamide, which is used to decrease intraocular pressure, is contraindicated in persons with sickle cell disease or trait)

(6) Clinical management
- Limited activity or bed rest with head of bed elevated 45 degrees
- Eye rest
- Eye patch or shield
- Antiemetics
- Pain management with avoidance of aspirin or nonsteroidal anti-inflammatory agents, which may increase bleeding
- Beta-blocker drops (e.g., timolol)
- Mydriatics to decrease pain
- Steroids may be used
- Amicar to decrease clot lysis and prevent rebleeding

- Admission for observation, and possible surgery if large amount of bleeding

(7) Criteria for discharge
- Small hyphema (less than one third of the anterior chamber)
- Able and willing to decrease activity and rest eye
- Able and willing to return for daily reevaluation

(8) Discharge planning and teaching
- Discuss use of medications, including pain medications.
- Demonstrate how to apply eye patch or shield.
- Review how, when, and where to obtain follow-up.
- Explain complications and what to watch for.
- Stress safety considerations related to patching.

Gastrointestinal Disturbances

1. Disturbances involving the gastrointestinal tract may be primary gastrointestinal disorders or may reflect systemic conditions (e.g., diarrhea in the person with anaphylaxis) (see Chapter 27 for a detailed discussion).

2. Primary triage considerations
   a. Is the condition creating life-threatening hypovolemia (e.g., volume loss from gastrointestinal bleeding or profound diarrhea)? Children may deteriorate very quickly because of diarrhea.
   b. Is the problem one that requires surgical management (e.g., constipation due to a bowel obstruction)?
   c. If pain is present, does it require immediate intervention?
   d. Is the symptom characteristic of food-borne contamination that may affect a large number of people and may have significant public health implications (e.g., *E. coli*, botulism)? The recent outbreaks of *E. coli* with several deaths and a large number of people affected have caused health care providers to be anxious about a person with diarrhea.
   e. Is the symptom characteristic of a disorder that requires immediate isolation and special infection control precautions?

3. Some of the symptoms addressed here are associated with abdominal pain and are discussed in that section.

4. Diarrhea
   a. Causes of diarrhea
      (1) Infection:
         - Gastrointestinal: staphylococci, *Shigella*, *Salmonella*, *E. coli*, viral, amoebae, *Giardia*, parasites
         - Nongastrointestinal: otitis media, urinary tract infection, pneumonia
      (2) Obstruction
         - Small or large bowel obstruction
         - Intussusception, volvulus, foreign body, appendicitis
      (3) Medication, hyperosmotic or toxic substance ingestion
         - Antibiotics
         - Overuse of laxatives, cathartics, enemas
         - Lactose intolerance

- Candy, sugar substitutes in diet foods (e.g., sorbitol, mannitol, hexitol), chewing gum
- Wild mushrooms and other plants
- Paralytic shellfish poisoning—"red tide"
  (4) Enterotoxins
- Staphylococcal food poisoning
- *E. coli*
- Cholera
- Botulism
  (5) Inflammation or ischemia
- Colitis
- Mesenteric adenitis
- Diverticulitis or diverticulosis
- Hepatitis
  (6) Allergy
- Food
- Anaphylaxis
  (7) Malabsorption
- After surgery (e.g., gastrectomy)
- Pancreatitis
- Cystic fibrosis
- Hepatitis or hepatic failure
- Alcoholism
- Celiac disease
- Sprue
- Crohn's disease
  b. History
  (1) General health status; medication use
  (2) Nature, frequency, duration, character of diarrhea
  (3) Associated symptoms (e.g., nausea, pain)
  (4) Weight loss
  (5) In children, ask about activity, last voiding, appetite.
  (6) Other people in family or residence ill as well
  c. Physical examination
  (1) General assessment examination, with special attention to abdomen and neurologic status
  (2) Assessment of volume status: skin vital signs, tugor, softness of eyeballs, depressed fontanel, postural BP, pulse
  (3) Weight
  (4) Character, color of stool; Hematest
  d. Diagnostic studies
  (1) Complete blood count, chemistries, liver function studies, toxicologic studies, if appropriate
  (2) Stool analysis for Gram stain, culture and sensitivity, amoebae, parasites
  (3) Radiographic studies may be done, depending on likely causes.
  e. Clinical management
  (1) Provide IV volume replacement with saline solution if volume depletion; adults may require 1 to 3 liters of fluid before vital signs are normal.
  (2) Give oral hydration, if surgical problem ruled out, using an electrolyte solution (e.g., Pedialyte or Gatorade).
  (3) Administer medications.
- Antidiarrheals, depending on cause. Many clinicians avoid using these on the premise that they delay elimination of causative organism.
- Antibiotics
  (4) Assist with dietary adjustment, depending on probable cause and age.

- Adults: clear liquids for 12 to 24 hours, gradually advancing to solid food such as sugar-free rice or corn cereals, white bread, pasta, potatoes, rice, yellow vegetables, light-colored fruits, and meats; no dairy products for 3 to 6 days
- Children: clear fluids, electrolyte solution for infants; once diarrhea has stopped, advance to soy formula diluted with twice amount of water normally called for and advance to full strength over 24 hours; if not on formula, advance diet as for adult; avoid dairy products for 3 to 6 days.
  f. Discharge criteria
  (1) Able to retain oral fluids
  (2) Normal vital signs without postural hypotension
  (3) Frequency of diarrhea decreased
  (4) Normal mental status
  (5) Voiding normally
  g. Discharge planning and teaching
  (1) Review the cause of the diarrhea, if known or suspected.
  (2) Discuss the dietary plan.
  (3) Review the use of medications.
  (4) Remind the person of infection control procedures, especially if a child is involved, and of the need to ensure that caregivers exercise special precautions, if in a day care.
  (5) Discuss the complications of sustained diarrhea.
  (6) Explain the plan for follow-up care.
5. Constipation
  a. The major concern related to a complaint of sudden onset of constipation is the possibility of bowel obstruction or paralytic ileus.
  b. Other common causes of constipation include inadequate food or fluid intake, physical inactivity, and use of medications (e.g., codeine or other narcotics).
  c. History
  (1) Health status, medications
  (2) Associated symptoms (e.g., pain, nausea)
  (3) Last normal bowel movement
  (4) Recent surgery or trauma
  d. Physical examination
  (1) General assessment with attention to abdomen and bowel sounds
  (2) Evidence of volume depletion
  (3) Evidence of generalized conditions that may precipitate condition (e.g., neurologic disorders)
  e. Diagnostic studies
  (1) Complete blood count, routine chemistries
  (2) Abdominal radiographs (e.g., obstructive series, ultrasound, or CT scan)
  f. Clinical management
  (1) If stable and no gastrointestinal disorder identified, the person is usually discharged with prescriptions for enemas, cathartics, laxatives, bulking agents, dietary recommendations, medication adjustment.
  (2) Use other measures, if bowel obstruction or ileus suspected.
  g. Discharge criteria
  (1) No evidence of potential surgical problem
  (2) Person reliable enough to carry out plan

h. Discharge planning and teaching
  (1) Depends on cause, but usually involves discussion of dietary strategies to relieve problem.
  (2) Review how to use medications or treatments (e.g., enema).
  (3) Discuss the hazards of relying on long-term use of cathartics, purgatives, and the like.
  (4) Review the plan for follow-up care, especially the need for more complete diagnostic workup if problem is, or becomes, chronic; gastrointestinal tumors may be the cause.
6. Gastrointestinal bleeding
  a. Gastrointestinal bleeding includes hematemesis, melena, grossly bloody stools, and rectal bleeding, all of which can be life threatening.
  b. Gastrointestinal bleeding results from local trauma that causes erosion of the gastrointestinal mucosa (see Chapter 27).
  c. Certain medications such as iron and activated charcoal may produce black stools and cause concern that gastrointestinal bleeding is occurring.
  d. Triage category depends on the nature of bleeding and hemodynamic state.
  e. History
    (1) Nature and duration of problem
      • History of peptic ulcer, long-term use of antacids, and epigastric pain suggest a bleeding ulcer.
      • Long-term alcohol use, associated with other symptoms of cirrhosis, and a sudden welling up of blood in the throat indicate esophageal varices.
      • Acute alcohol use or significant use of aspirin or nonsteroidal anti-inflammatory agents suggests gastritis.
      • Hematemesis after protracted vomiting is characteristic of a Mallory-Weiss tear of the distal esophagus.
      • Bright red, blood-tinged stool, especially in the presence of rectal pain, is associated with bleeding hemorrhoids.
    (2) Health status and medication use
    (3) Associated symptoms (e.g., fatigue, syncope, weakness, shortness of breath)
  f. Physical examination
    (1) ABCs, including postural vital signs, if not hypotensive initially
    (2) General assessment with attention to evidence of liver disease and abdominal examination
    (3) Observe rectal area for hemorrhoids, if appropriate.
  g. Diagnostic studies vary, depending on likely cause, and are done concurrently with intervention in unstable person.
    (1) Complete blood count, electrolytes, BUN, creatinine, type, and crossmatch, if large amount of bleeding; clotting studies and liver function studies
    (2) Unless esophageal varices are suspected, a nasogastric tube may be inserted to assess for bleeding and for iced lavage if bleeding is present.
    (3) Stool Hematest
    (4) Fiberoptic endoscopic examination, if bleeding ulcer is suspected
    (5) Proctoscopic or anoscopic examination for rectal bleeding

NURSE ADVISORY

> Insertion of a nasogastric tube in a person with esophageal varices may cause massive bleeding because of damage to the varices.

    (6) Radiology: plain abdominal films, CT, or ultrasound
  h. Clinical management
    (1) Treat for shock (see Chapter 12).
    (2) Attempt to stem bleeding.
      • Blakemore-Sengstaken tube for esophageal varices
      • Gastric lavage with iced saline for peptic ulcer
      • Other endoscopic procedures to stop gastric bleeding
      • Silver nitrate cautery for bleeding hemorrhoids, or no treatment
      • Antacids, Donnatal, and viscous lidocaine (gastrointestinal cocktail), if gastritis or esophagitis is suspected
      • Intravenous antacids (e.g., Pepcid, cimetidine) for bleeding ulcer
  i. Criteria for discharge
    (1) Hemodynamically stable
    (2) Source of bleeding identified; normally upper and lower gastrointestinal bleeding and Mallory-Weiss syndrome warrant hospitalization, whereas gastritis and bleeding hemorrhoids do not.
  j. Discharge planning and teaching
    (1) Stress the avoidance of alcohol, spicy foods, and gastric irritants if gastritis is suspected.
    (2) Review medication usage.
    (3) In bleeding hemorrhoids, give information regarding stool softeners, adding fluid and bulk to diet, sitz baths, or other local treatments.
    (4) Discuss follow-up care.
7. Jaundice and hepatitis
  a. The most common causes of jaundice in adults are hepatitis, cirrhosis, and acute obstructive cholecystitis.
  b. See Chapter 28 for the assessment, diagnosis, and clinical management.
  c. Major emergency interventions are cardiovascular stabilization in acute obstructive cholecystitis with potential for sepsis and 3rd spacing, and infection control considerations related to hepatitis (e.g., hepatitis A in a food handler requires notification of public health officials so that exposed persons can be treated with gamma globulin), or to potential for exposure to intimate contacts in hepatitis B.
  d. Discharge criteria
    (1) Individuals with liver failure or obstructive cholecystitis are usually hospitalized.
    (2) Persons with hepatitis are usually discharged, if hemodynamically stable and adequate social support exists for care and nutrition.
  e. Discharge planning and teaching
    (1) Review the normal course of disease.
    (2) Test results indicating the type of hepatitis take several days; the plan for obtaining results needs to be clear.
    (3) Arrange for nutritional and medication counseling.

(4) Stress alcohol and acetaminophen avoidance.
(5) Discuss infection control issues (e.g., boiling dinnerware, avoiding intimate contact, handling of excretions).
(6) Plan follow-up, often with public health officials.
(7) Review reasons for return (e.g., intractable vomiting, gastrointestinal bleeding, worsening of symptoms).

Rash or Itching

1. Skin alteration, with or without itching (pruritus), is observed in a variety of practice settings and may be a diagnostic challenge to even the most expert practitioner (see Chapter 35).
2. The emergency nursing concerns are to determine whether the abnormality
   a. Reflects a serious or life-threatening problem (e.g., anaphylaxis, meningococcal meningitis, Kawasaki disease)
   b. Poses an infection control threat to staff, other patients, or visitors, such as rubella, rubeola, varicella, lice, scabies
3. History
   a. Time of onset and duration
   b. Associated symptoms (e.g., wheezing, malaise)
   c. Medications, including over-the-counter remedies used to treat the problem
   d. Location or distribution
   e. Illness in other family members
   f. History of recent bacterial or viral illness
   g. History of insect bite
   h. History of activity with exposure to ticks, fleas, spiders, or scabies
4. Physical examination
   a. General appearance and level of distress; routine assessment, including vital signs, with attention to temperature
   b. Breath sounds, if concern about an allergic reaction
   c. Is person scratching affected area or protecting it from clothing or touch?
   d. Evaluation of the rash itself
      (1) Location and distribution (e.g., extremities, torso, pressure areas from clothing)
      (2) Lesions flat or raised (macular, papular, vesicular, bullous)
      (3) Color—petechiae or purpura
      (4) Discrete borders or diffuse
      (5) Evidence of infection
      (6) Moist, dry, or scaling
5. The most important or most common rashes, and the reasons why they are important, are summarized in Table 37–10.

Poisoning, Overdose, or Intoxication

1. Individuals who ingest, inhale, or are exposed to health-threatening substances are encountered almost daily in the emergency care setting (see also Chapter 40).

2. The mechanisms may be accidental or intentional and may occur anywhere.
3. Although mortality and morbidity in children have decreased dramatically because of child safety caps, death due to intentional overdose has increased significantly in recent years, from both licit and illicit drugs.
4. Although every effort has been made to provide accurate treatment information, a poison center can be consulted as a matter of routine. Many EDs also have access to online computerized information regarding management of overdoses, poisonings, and exposures, as well as product identification. In addition, toxicology books are usually available.
5. Emergency departments frequently receive telephone requests for information on this topic.
   a. For both quality of care and liability reasons, it is strongly recommended that these calls be referred immediately to either a poison center or a pharmacy.
   b. Poison centers are well equipped not only to handle the calls but also to conduct follow-up, provide poison prevention information, and track and trend poisoning incidences and drug problems.
6. The spectrum of poisoning or overdose agents is massive; only the most frequent or most serious are addressed in this section.
7. Triage priority: variable, depending on agent and mechanism; usually given priority if delay will worsen the situation
8. Assessment
   a. History

NURSE ADVISORY

Unless an ingestion has been witnessed, the accuracy of the history is often suspect. Individuals with serious suicide intent may minimize the magnitude of the ingestion in the hope that treatment will be minimal and their goal will be achieved. Some people are embarrassed by their own ingestion or that of a child under their care. Others may exaggerate the ingestion as an attention-getting strategy. History is considered along with the clinical presentation and toxicology studies.

      (1) What substance is known or likely, and how much (i.e., is this a toxic amount)?
      (2) When did the incident occur?
      (3) Mechanism: ingestion, inhalation, IV, or contact
      (4) Location, especially in exposures or plant ingestions
      (5) Why did this occur—accidental, intentional, or unknown; is this possibly a suicide attempt, child neglect, due to memory lapse?
      (6) Is the container available?
      (7) Past medical history, allergies, and medication and alcohol use
      (8) Symptoms
      (9) Recent behavior, particularly if intentional overdose suspected
      (10) Is there a history or possibility of trauma?
   b. Physical examination
      (1) Are there strange smells or materials that sug-

Table 37–10. Common or Serious Rashes

Characteristics	Body Area	Possible Condition
Urticaria, hive, wheal, welt, may be diffuse swelling (giant hives), angioedema	Generalized	Anaphylaxis; viral illness; drug reaction; insect bite
Petechiae or purpura	May start on feet and spread rapidly	Meningococcal meningitis
	Generalized	Clotting disorder; mononucleosis
	Conjunctiva	Fat embolism
	Variable, but often palms and soles	Disseminated GC*
	Wrist, ankle, palm, sole initially, then to trunk	Rocky Mountain spotted fever†
Maculopapular	Face, then trunk	Rubella
		Rubeola
	Trunk, then face and legs	Varicella
		Roseola
Desquamation	Palms, soles	Toxic shock syndrome; Kawasaki syndrome‡; Stevens-Johnson syndrome
Pustules	Variable	Impetigo; candidiasis
Scales	Variable; may be along contact lines with clothing or diaper	Dermatitis (e.g., contact dermatitis, atopic dermatitis)
Vesicles or bullae	Variable	Contact dermatitis; poison oak, ivy, or sumac; Stevens-Johnson syndrome
Bullae and crepitus	Variable	Necrotizing fasciitis; gas gangrene *(Clostridium perfringens)*
	Genitalia	Herpes simplex—II
	Lip, mouth	Herpes simplex—I
	Dermatome	Herpes zoster
Scratch marks, wavy dark lines, and intense itching	Web spaces, body folds, hands, wrists, belt line	Scabies
Scratch marks and itching; possibly blue spots on skin; white nits in hair	Variable	Pediculosis—head, body, pubis
Scratch marks, itching with papule	Variable	Flea or insect bites
Erythematous, target-like lesion	Variable	Lyme disease
Red lesion with necrotic center	Variable	Brown recluse spider bite

* There may be macules, papules, vesicles, pustules, or purpura in disseminated gonococcus (GC).
† Rash initially papular, progressing to hemorrhagic lesions in about four days.
‡ Intense redness of sclera and conjunctiva and cracking of the lips are also noted in this condition.

gest a risk to the caregiver (e.g., organophosphate insecticide powders, chemicals)? If so, don appropriate protective garb before proceeding any further.

(2) Primary and secondary survey, with attention to the following:
  • ABCs, neurologic status
  • Presence of gag reflex
  • Pupils: dilated or pinpoint; pinpoint pupils are seen in narcotic overdoses; dilated pupils are seen in hypoxia, atropinics, amphetamines.
  • Skin: color, evidence of fresh or old needle marks or tracks, cellulitis, blisters (barbiturate), pressure injuries (from lying in one place for a long time)
  • Necrosis of nasal septum (associated with cocaine use)
  • Injury

NURSE ADVISORY

Single- or multisystem injury, a catastrophic central nervous system event, or systemic illness may be present in the person who is perceived as overdosed. These events can occur as a consequence of an ingestion, or simply be misinterpreted; thus, careful physical assessment and diagnostic studies may be warranted. Individuals who have been unconscious for a prolonged period of time may have injury or illness from immobility, such as rhabdomyolysis-induced renal failure due to sustained pressure on body parts, or aspiration pneumonia.

9. Clinical management—The acronym SIRES may be helpful in prioritizing care: *S*tabilize, *I*dentify, *R*everse, *E*liminate, *S*upport.
  a. Stabilize the person.

(1) Check ABCs.

(2) Establish IV line; draw routine laboratory tests and toxicology or drug levels, if appropriate.

(3) Initiate ongoing monitoring (cardiac, BP, and oximetry) to recognize changing status, which occurs often with some drug overdoses.

b. Identify the agent.

(1) Determining the agent or agents in the unconscious or uncooperative person with no history or other clues is challenging at best; clinical findings must be relied on because laboratory studies take time and many agents are not easily detected.

(2) Key clinical parameters

- Central nervous system
- Seizure activity
- Pupils
- Blood pressure
- Heart rate
- Respirations
- Temperature
- Skin and tissue appearance

(3) Symptoms associated with selected poisons, drugs, or toxic substances are summarized in Table 37–11.

c. Reverse the effects of the agent.

(1) Table 37–12 contains commonly used antidotes.

(2) With the exception of glucose, naloxone, thiamine, and flumazenil, antidotes or reversal agents are not often administered; it is prudent to review the available literature and consult with the poison center before administering less commonly used antidotes.

d. Eliminate the agent by decontamination, emesis, gastric lavage, or, less commonly, by hemodialysis or peritoneal dialysis, plasmapheresis, charcoal hemoperfusion, or gut lavage; only the 1st 2 are done in the ED.

e. Decontamination involves removing the agent from the skin and mucous membranes by washing the area, showering, or using more complex decontamination procedures.

f. Syrup of ipecac is used to induce vomiting to remove the agent from the stomach; home remedies (which often appear on containers) or mechanical methods of inducing vomiting are not recommended.

(1) Although its use was once widespread, the value of inducing emesis is being questioned, and there is a trend toward adsorbing the agent with activated charcoal.

(2) Emesis is contraindicated under the following circumstances:

- Decreased level of consciousness
- Seizures
- Decreased or absent gag reflex
- Ingestion of a known short-acting central nervous system depressant. The person's level of consciousness may be decreased by the time ipecac begins to work (usually 20–30 min after administration), resulting in the possibil-

ity of pulmonary aspiration of gastric contents.

- Hydrocarbon ingestion (e.g., petroleum distillates such as kerosene or gasoline); this area is controversial, and poison center guidance is recommended.
- Ingestion of strong acids or alkalis or a foreign agent that may do more damage during emesis

Table 37–11. Symptoms Associated with Various Overdoses or Poisonings

Pupils

Pinpoint (meiosis)—Opiates, cholinergics, antihypertensives, β-blockers, phenothiazines, barbiturates, chloral hydrate

Dilated (mydriasis)—Anticholinergics, sympathomimetics, phencyclidine, cocaine, cyanide, carbon monoxide

Note: Pupil size may be unpredictable in mixed overdose.

Breath odor

Garlic–Arsenic, organophosphates

Almond—Cyanide

Plastic—Placidyl

Pear—Chloral hydrate

Violets—Turpentine

Sweet—Chloroform

Shoe polish—Nitrobenzene

Fermented—Ethanol

Fruity—Ketosis (alcoholic ketoacidosis, diabetic ketoacidosis [DKA], etc.)

Skin

Flushed—Anticholinergics, phenothiazines, sympathomimetics, ethanol, carbon monoxide, insulin

Hyperventilation

Primary (aspirin)

Secondary

Anoxia (carbon monoxide, cyanide)

Acidosis

Extrapyramidal signs

Phenothiazines

Butyrophenones

Sympathomimetics (tachycardia, tachypnea, pyrexia, tremors, sweating)

Amphetamines

Cocaine

Phencyclidine

LSD

Alcohol, sedative, and/or hypnotic withdrawal

Anticholinergics (tachycardia, agitation, flushed, dry skin, urinary retention)

Polycyclic antidepressants

Antihistamines

Belladonna alkaloids

A mnemonic useful in determining anticholinergics is:

Mad as a hatter

Red as a beet

Dry as a bone

Hot as a hare

Blind as a bat

Cholinergics (bradycardia, hypersecretions, urinary and fecal incontinence; may see tachycardia, mydriasis, or hypertension if sympathetic ganglia are involved)

Organophosphates

Carbamates

Overtreated myasthenics

Modified from Rogers JH, Osborne HH, and Pousada L. *Emergency Nursing. A Practice Guide.* Baltimore: Williams & Wilkins, 1989, pp 176–177.

Table 37–12. Antidotes or Treatment Agents for Common Poisonings or Overdoses

Antidote	Use or Poisoning or Overdose Agent
Activated charcoal (plain and with sorbitol)	General use; adsorbent
Ammonium chloride	Acidifies urine to increase renal secretion of toxic substances; phencyclidine (PCP), amphetamines (speed), strychnine
Antitoxins:	
Botulinal antitoxin	Botulism
Antivenins:	
Latrodectus mactans	Black widow spider bite
Centruroides sculpturatus	U.S. scorpion
Crotalidae polyvalent	Pit vipers
Micrurus fulvius	Eastern coral snake
Atropine	Cholinesterase inhibitors (e.g., organophosphate insecticides, cholinergic agents, and mushrooms)
Bentonite (Fuller's earth)	Paraquat (herbicide)
Calcium chloride	Oxylates, ethylene glycol, calcium channel blockers
Calcium gluconate	Hydrofluoric acid burns, black widow spider bites
Cyanide Antidote Package (amyl nitrite, sodium nitrite, sodium thiosulfate)	Cyanide, sodium nitroprusside (Nipride)
Deferoxamine (Desferal)	Iron
Dextrose 50%	Hypoglycemia
Diazepam (Valium)	General sedation, treat seizures
Digoxin-specific antibody (Digibind, FAB)	Digitalis preparations
Dimercaprol (BAL—British Antilewisite)	Lead, arsenic, mercury, gold
Diphenhydramine (Benadryl)	Extrapyramidal (dystonic) reactions (e.g., phenothiazines)
Diuresis—acid	Phencyclidine, amphetamines, strychnine, quinine
Diuresis—alkaline	Salicylates, barbiturates, isoniazid
Edrophonium Cl (Tensilon)	Anticholinergics
Ethyl alcohol (ethanol)	Methanol, ethylene glycol
Ethylenediaminetetraacetic acid (calcium EDTA)	Heavy metals (e.g., lead, zinc)
Flumazenil (Romazicon)	Benzodiazepines
Folic acid	Methyl alcohol, methotrexate
Glucagon	Beta-blockers, calcium channel blockers, oral hypoglycemic agents, in hypoglycemia where intravenous access not available
Ipecac, syrup of	General—emetic
Lorazepam (Ativan)	Seizures
Magnesium sulfate citrate	General—cathartic
Methylene blue	Methemoglobinemia
N-acetylcysteine (NAC) (Mucomyst)	Acetaminophen
Naloxone (Narcan)	Narcotics, synthetic
Oxygen	Carbon monoxide, cyanide, general
Physostigmine (Antilirium)	Atropine, tricyclic antidepressants, anticholinergic agents
Pralidoxime chloride (2-PAM chloride)	Cholinesterase inhibitors
Protamine sulfate	Heparin
Pyridoxine hydrochloride	Isoniazid, ethylene glycol, certain mushrooms
Sodium bicarbonate	General alkalinizing agent, iron
Vitamin K	Coumadin, oral anticoagulants

- Children younger than 6 months of age
- When person has already vomited

(3) The appropriateness of promoting gastric emptying requires an analysis of the agent's characteristics and when it was ingested. Although many hours may have elapsed between ingestion and treatment, and presumably the agent has already passed out of the stomach, many drugs themselves by their effect on the sympathetic nervous system delay gastric emptying or are resecreted back into the stomach; gastric emptying via emesis or lavage may still be indicated.

(4) Syrup of ipecac is administered orally in age-

appropriate doses and is followed by several glasses of water.

- The use of carbonated beverages instead of water is controversial; although the patient may drink it more readily, there is concern that the carbonation may lead to gastric rupture.
- Some practitioners recommend having the person walk around to increase the effectiveness of syrup of ipecac, but this has not been well substantiated; the person should be observed, lest the level of consciousness decrease.
- The dose may be repeated after 20 to 30 min-

utes, if the initial dose does not produce results.

- Treatment failures occur when insufficient liquids are taken or the drug is an antiemetic.
- If adequate fluids have been given, a large amount of emesis will result; be prepared with a large basin.
- Observe the emesis for pill fragments, color, or other evidence of drug ingested; save the specimen for laboratory analysis.
- The effects of ipecac may last for an hour or longer; wait before administering charcoal.
- Protracted dry heaves without emesis can cause Mallory-Weiss tears of the distal esophagus; give additional fluids.

(5) Activated charcoal, with or without sorbitol (laxative), is given orally initially or after emetic therapy; it adsorbs the ingested agent.

- Activated charcoal is a fine, black powder that must be made into a slurry to administer it. It can be mixed with water or other liquid; however, milk is not recommended. Flavorings such as cherry syrup can be added to increase its palatability. Because it is a black liquid, some children and adults may be reluctant to drink it; using a straw and placing it in a covered container may be helpful. It is available commercially as a slurry in a specially designed bottle that allows for shaking or administration through a nasogastric or an Ewald tube.
- The 1st dose of activated charcoal administered usually contains sorbitol; however, subsequent doses should be plain activated charcoal only; profound diarrhea and fluid loss can occur with repeated doses of sorbitol.
- Plain activated charcoal may be ordered for small children; those who will be receiving an oral antidote (e.g., acetaminophen overdoses); those who require endoscopic procedures (e.g., acid or alkali ingestion), or those who have evidence of adynamic ileus or bowel obstruction.
- Charcoal pulsing, or hourly repeat dosing, is ordered for some ingestions.
- Activated charcoal may be given through a nasogastric or an Ewald tube if the person refuses it orally, or after gastric lavage.
- Activated charcoal is messy and may stain clothing; both the recipient and caregiver should wear protective garb.

(6) Gastric lavage

- This procedure involves inserting a large-bore (32–36 French) Ewald tube (adults) orally or a nasogastric tube and rinsing the stomach until the contents return clear.
- It is used under the following circumstances: The person has an altered level of consciousness, seizures, or an inadequate gag reflex; syrup of ipecac has been ineffective; or the person refuses to drink the syrup of ipecac.
- It is contraindicated in a person who has ingested a strong acid or alkali substance.
- Endotracheal intubation before lavage is indicated when there is a decreased level of consciousness or the gag reflex is decreased or absent.
- The procedure for gastric lavage is summarized in Procedure 37–2.

(7) Cathartics are used to hasten the elimination of the ingested agent through the system; a variety of options are available and may include the following:

- Adults: sorbitol, which comes mixed with charcoal; magnesium sulfate, which is contraindicated in persons with renal disease or in those whose ingestion may cause renal failure; magnesium citrate; sodium sulfate; or sodium phosphate.
- Children: sorbitol or magnesium sulfate.
- Oil-based cathartics are generally not used.

(8) Other strategies for enhancing elimination include the following:

- Diuresis with IV fluids and diuretics
- Alkalinization of the urine by administering sodium bicarbonate to prevent reabsorption by the kidney; this is used for barbiturates, salicylates, lithium, and isoniazid
- Acidifying the urine with oral or IV ascorbic acid, or ammonium chloride
- Hemodialysis or peritoneal dialysis
- Charcoal or resin hemoperfusion
- Exchange transfusion or plasmapheresis
- Immunotherapy, such as using hyperimmune sera for snake or insect bites, or Digibind for digoxin ingestion

g. Support

(1) Support includes physiologic and psychologic dimensions for the patient and significant others. Physiologic support involves frequent reassessment and ongoing monitoring to determine if there are additional symptoms and to evaluate therapy effectiveness. Hospitalization for at least 24 hours is the norm in many significant overdoses.

(2) Psychologic support is critical in any intentional overdose and in accidental ingestion in children; there is often a great deal of guilt on the part of parents or caretakers.

(a) Any person with an intentional overdose should be evaluated before leaving the ED by a mental health practitioner, to determine whether there is suicidal ideation; appropriate measures should be taken to protect the person from harm.

(b) Individuals who overdose experience significantly low self-esteem; this is worsened by insensitive caregivers who verbalize their anger at the patient for having overdosed; a better approach is to acknowledge that the person must have been feeling pretty badly to have resorted to overdose.

Procedure 37–2
Gastric Lavage for Toxic Substance Ingestion

Definition/Purpose
Irrigating the stomach to remove ingested toxic substances to minimize further absorption of the material. Also known as stomach pumping.

Contraindications/Cautions
Not performed if (a) stomach emptying can be achieved by emesis induced by syrup of Ipecac; (b) ingestion of corrosive or strychnine (may cause seizures); or (c) there has been a significant time lapse from ingestion to treatment. The value of gastric lavage is currently under debate. Because vomiting and aspiration may occur, the procedure is done only if the airway is secure by (a) intact gag reflex, or (b) tracheal intubation with a cuffed tube. Excessive fluid (e.g., more than 300 ml in an adult) may push gastric contents into the duodenum and increase absorption. Continuous blood pressure and cardiac monitoring is recommended because (a) vagal stimulation from the tube or gastric distention may cause bradycardia; and (b) many ingested substances affect the blood pressure and heart rate. Epistaxis may occur if the tube is placed nasally, rather than orally.

Learning/Teaching Activities
Provide the following information: (a) purpose of procedure, (b) what the procedure entails, (c) preparatory procedures (e.g., cardiac and blood pressure monitoring, use of restraints), (d) associated activities (e.g., oral suction, bite block or oral airway), (e) how the person can assist to get the procedure done in a timely manner, (f) how the person will communicate during the procedure (usually not able to talk because of tube size), and (g) reinforce that procedure is not being done for punitive reasons.

Preliminary Activities

Equipment
- Cardiac and blood pressure monitors
- Restraints (may not be necessary, but should be immediately available)
- Bite block or oral airway
- Tracheal intubation equipment
- Adhesive tape to secure tube and bite block
- Oxygen administration equipment
- Suction equipment—Yankauer
- Lavage tube (Ewald), 30–36 French for adults
- Lavage fluid—normal saline, water, tap water; 3000-ml bags of normal saline solution are available
- Tubing, Y connector, and straight connector
- Drainage collection receptacle
- Catheter tip syringe
- Unsterile gloves, face protector, impervious gown
- Bed protector
- Pillows to support person in sidelying position
- Specimen container (1000 ml)
- Stethoscope
- Medications: atropine, activated charcoal—plain or with sorbitol

Assessment/Planning
- Know the reason for lavage and the substance(s) most likely ingested.
- Assess vital signs, cardiac rhythm, oximetry.
- Secure intravenous access.
- Determine whether serum electrolytes have been obtained and reported (large-volume gastric lavage may cause hypokalemia).
- Assess gag reflex and level of consciousness (secure airway if diminished or absent gag reflex or decreased level of consciousness).
- Assess the degree of cooperation likely to determine if restraints and/or assistance will be needed.
- Assess body size to determine maximal amount of fluid to be instilled each time.
- Choose a stretcher or bed that permits Trendelenburg position.
- Ensure proximity of all equipment.
- Choose an appropriately sized lavage tube.
- Determine if urinary bladder catheterization is needed.

Preparation of Person
- Apply monitoring devices.
- Position individual on the left side of the bed in a Trendelenburg position; place pillows behind back to maintain sidelying position.
- Apply restraints; secure all straps on the same side so that the person can be turned to the side quickly if vomiting occurs.
- Secure small child on "mummy" board.
- Place protective pad under head.

(continued)

Procedure 37-2

(continued)

Preparation of Staff

- Don protective gown.
- Apply face shield or goggles.
- Don gloves.

Procedure

Actions	Rationale/Discussion
1. Connect tubing to fluid and drainage container.	1. System is ready to use.
2. Measure tube, from mouth to ear and xiphoid; mark tube at location of mouth.	2. Assists in determining amount of tube needed to reach stomach.
3. Flex person's neck and insert tube through the mouth.	3. Neck flexion minimizes inadvertent tracheal placement.
4. Ask the person to swallow during insertion.	4. Facilitates passage of tube.
5. Assess cardiac rate during tube insertion; interrupt procedure if bradycardia occurs, and resume procedure when it resolves. Consult with physician regarding administration of atropine to treat symptomatic bradycardia.	5. Stimulation of posterior pharynx can stimulate the vagus nerve, causing bradycardia. Atropine increases the heart rate.
6. Assess respiratory effort; remove tube if person is choking or unable to breathe.	6. Choking or impaired breathing indicates tube is in the airway.
7. Insert tube to predetermined mark; attach catheter-tip syringe, aspirate gastric contents, and place in specimen container.	7. Presence of gastric contents suggests correct tube placement. Gastric contents may be sent for analysis.
8. Inject 30 to 50 ml of air through the tube, while listening for air over the stomach.	8. Auscultating air over the stomach suggests correct tube placement.
9. Secure tube with adhesive tape.	9. Prevents inadvertent tube displacement.
10. Insert bite block, if necessary.	10. Prevents biting and occluding tube.
11. Connect tube to lavage fluid tubing and instill 100 ml of fluid, observing cardiac rate and patient response; suspend instillation if tachycardia, tachypnea, or other distress is noted.	11. A large amount of fluid can cause gastric distention, impaired respiration, or cardiac dysrhythmias.
12. Clamp inflow tubing, unclamp outflow tubing, note the quantity and character of return (e.g., color, pill fragments).	12. Allows fluid to drain into collection system; may validate ingestion.
13. Once outflow drainage has stopped, clamp outflow tubing; instill 300 ml of irrigation fluid, and repeat procedure until return fluid is clear.	13. Fluid washes gastric mucosa, removing gastric contents. Volumes as great as 40 liters may be required.
14. Periodically suction oral pharynx.	14. Secretions often accumulate here; the patient may feel a choking sensation.
15. Massage the area over the stomach or tilt person side to side.	15. Promotes freeing of material trapped in gastric folds.
16. Remove unreturned fluid using a catheter-tip syringe.	16. Tube position may impede fluid return; excessive fluid may cause gastric emptying into the duodenum and absorption of ingested material. Retention of large amounts of fluid may cause fluid or electrolyte abnormalities.
17. Instill activated charcoal per order.	17. Activated charcoal adsorbs remaining ingested material; sorbitol combined with charcoal is a cathartic that speeds gastrointestinal tract decontamination.
18. Instill 50 ml of fluid through tube after administering charcoal.	18. Promotes maximal dosing of charcoal and patency of tube.
19. Determine whether tube is to be removed or left in place.	19. Repeated doses of activated charcoal may be ordered over the next 24 hours, particularly in ingestion associated with enterohepatic recirculation.
20. Apply suction while withdrawing tube.	20. Minimizes aspiration of fluid in tube during removal.

Final Activities

Remove bite block and restraints, reposition in position of comfort, or as appropriate for level of consciousness. Document characteristics of gastric contents, type and volume of fluid instilled and removed, vital signs and other observations during the procedure, how procedure was tolerated, and restraint application and removal. Assess the need for repeat serum electrolyte measurements, if large-volume lavage was used. Arrange toxicologic evaluation of gastric contents, if indicated.

(c) Induction of emesis or gastric lavage should never be undertaken solely as a punitive measure or in an effort to prevent subsequent ingestions; research has demonstrated that this does not deter future attempts.

(d) The death of a person who has intentionally overdosed is often difficult for the staff and EMS personnel; critical incident stress debriefing may be in order.

10. Common or significant ingestions
    a. Narcotics and synthetic narcotics include heroin, morphine, meperidine (Demerol), hydromorphone (Dilaudid), hydrocodone (Hycodan, Vicodin), oxycodone (Percocet, Percodan), methadone, butorphanol (Stadol), fentanyl (Sublimaze), nalbuphine (Nubain), propoxyphene (Darvon), and pentazocine (Talwin).
       (1) Effects: Central nervous system depression, respiratory depression, pulmonary edema, pinpoint pupils, hypothermia, bradycardia, hypotension; hallucinations and dysphoria are seen with some agents (e.g., propoxyphene and pentazocine).
       (2) Treatment with narcotic antagonists such as naloxone (Narcan) or nalmefene (Revex)
          • Large doses of naloxone may be needed initially for some ingestions (e.g., propoxyphene).
          • The ingested drug may outlast the reversal agent, and redosing may be needed, although this may not be true with nalmefene.
          • Persons who have overdosed through recreational use may, on awakening, decide to leave the ED without further treatment; a decision may need to be made in advance about the use of restraints.
          • Some practitioners give IV heroin users a tetanus booster as a matter of routine.
    b. Benzodiazepines (e.g., Valium, Librium)
       (1) Effects: Central nervous system depression, drowsiness, ataxia, difficulty speaking, coma; paradoxical excitation may be noted. When even therapeutic doses are combined with alcohol, profound respiratory depression and death may occur.
       (2) Clinical management
          • Flumazenil (Romazicon) IV
          • Abrupt withdrawal from benzodiazepines in long-term user may result in seizures many days later; hospitalization for safe drug withdrawal may be indicated.
          • Gastric lavage is preferred to emesis because of the short onset of action.
          • Other routine poisoning management
    c. Tricyclic antidepressants (e.g., Elavil, Tofranil, Triavil); these are serious ingestions, resulting in a significant number of deaths.
       (1) Effects
          • Central nervous system: Confusion, excitability, hallucinations, abnormal muscle movement, hyperactive deep tendon reflexes, seizures, coma; the time frame from ingestion to onset of symptoms may be quite short.

• Cardiac: Initially tachycardia, possibly with prolonged QT interval, followed by bradycardia, delayed conduction, especially prolongation of all intervals, wide QRS, hypotension, ventricular ectopy, fibrillation, and death.
       (2) Clinical management
          • Gastric lavage
          • Charcoal pulsing due to enterohepatic recirculation
          • Alkalinization with sodium bicarbonate to achieve an arterial pH of 7.5 to 7.6
          • Phenytoin for cardiac dysrhythmias and seizures; reversal of QRS widening may be noted with phenytoin
          • Isoproterenol and pacemaker to treat symptomatic bradycardia; atropine is not used
          • Norepinephrine (Levophed) to treat hypotension
          • Continuous cardiac monitoring
          • Prolonged hospitalization with cardiac monitoring may be necessary; death from cardiac dysrhythmias several days after the ingestion has been reported.
    d. Amphetamines may be sniffed, ingested, or injected.
       (1) Effects
          • Central nervous system stimulation: restlessness, tremor, dilated pupils, confusion, agitation, delirium, violent behavior directed at self or others, seizures, coma
          • Cardiovascular: hypertension, tachycardia, intracranial hemorrhage due to hypertension
          • Extreme elevation of body temperature, which may cause coagulopathy
       (2) Clinical management
          • Gastric lavage
          • Sedation, if needed to perform procedures
          • Aggressive measures to manage hyperthermia
          • Antihypertensives (e.g., sodium nitroprusside)
          • Acid diuresis with mannitol, furosemide, or ammonium chloride, unless seizures or severe hyperthermia is present
    e. Cocaine may be snorted or injected IV, although significant overdose may be seen in a "body packer," a person smuggling cocaine by ingesting packets of cocaine that are usually wrapped in condoms.
       (1) Effects: Cocaine has a short half-life, usually within minutes after injection and 1 hour after mucous membrane exposure; the effects are similar to those of amphetamines with the following additional concerns:
          • Central nervous system: cardiovascular accident, subarachnoid or intracerebral bleed due to hypertension
          • Cardiovascular: acute myocardial infarction, hypertensive crisis, ventricular tachycardia, and fibrillation
          • Obstetric: may induce spontaneous abortion or labor in a full-term pregnancy
       (2) Clinical management: supportive; body packers may require surgery to remove the packets of cocaine.

f. Phencyclidine (PCP) may be inhaled or ingested; it is a common illicit street drug that may be taken alone or used to cut heroin or other drugs.
  (1) Effects
      • Central nervous system: psychotic state; delusions; bizarre behavior; altered perception of time, space, and sensations; behavior is totally unpredictable. One minute the person may seem logical and rational, and he or she may become totally psychotic the next minute. Nystagmus, ataxia, muscle twitching, and seizures may be noted.
      • Cardiovascular: hypertension and tachycardia
      • Temperature may be elevated.
      • Respiratory: initially tachypneic, followed by hypoventilation and apnea
      • Laboratory findings: hypoglycemia, elevated creatine phosphokinase, SGOT, and SGPT
  (2) Clinical management
      • Provide calm reassurance in a place with minimal stimulus.
      • Sedation may be appropriate.
      • Protective environment or restraints may be indicated.
      • Comatose person should be lavaged.
      • Use activated charcoal initially and cisapride (Propulsid) to speed drug's passage through gastrointestinal tract and decrease enterohepatic recirculation.
      • Employ forced diuresis with furosemide and ascorbic acid.
      • Treat seizures with diazepam and phenytoin.
g. With acetaminophen, also called paracetamol in European countries, toxicity may result from an intentional overdose or from use of drug in persons with alcohol use or abuse, or in those with liver disease. It is widely available over the counter alone or in combination with pain or cold relievers.
  (1) Effects
      • The major serious effect is liver failure. Symptoms are noted in phases: Phase 1—Nausea, vomiting, anorexia; symptoms may be so mild that person does not seek care; phase 2—Person may feel quite normal, or have mild right upper quadrant abdominal pain that may last up to 4 days; phase 3—Occurs 3 to 5 days after ingestion, and is characterized by symptoms of liver failure: Anorexia, abdominal pain, icterus, coma, and death.
      • Elevated liver enzymes become apparent during phase 2.
      • Acetaminophen level drawn 4 hours or more after ingestion is used to determine degree of injury and need for treatment; a special nomogram is used to evaluate risk.
  (2) Clinical management
      • Gastric emptying using syrup of ipecac if condition manifests shortly after ingestion
      • The use of activated charcoal is controversial; although there is concern that it will interfere with *N*-acetylcysteine (NAC), some research

suggests that activated charcoal is an adjunct to *N*-acetylcysteine.
      • If laboratory results indicate a toxic level, or if there will be a delay in obtaining results, *N*-acetylcysteine (Mucomyst) is administered orally, diluted 1:3 in juice or soft drink (to make it more palatable), or through a nasogastric tube if the person vomits the initial dose; repeated doses are given every 4 hours for 17 doses. Mucomyst may also be administered intramuscularly.
      • *N*-acetylcysteine is most effective if given within 16 hours of ingestion and is usually not given in ingestions older than 24 hours.
      • Daily liver function studies are performed to evaluate liver damage; if there are no elevations within 96 hours after the ingestion, it is presumed that the dose was not toxic.
h. Salicylates
  (1) Salicylate ingestion is primarily in the form of aspirin, although it may occur with oil of wintergreen.
  (2) Effects
      • Central nervous system stimulation, which may include tinnitus (ringing in the ears), hallucinations, and irritability, eventually leading to cerebral edema, seizures, and coma
      • Tachypnea, resulting in respiratory alkalosis; pulmonary edema
      • Hyperglycemia, but may vary widely
      • Evidence of impaired clotting
      • Nausea, vomiting, chest pain
      • Skin may be hot and dry; evidence of dehydration may be present
  (3) Clinical management
      • Emesis or lavage, followed by charcoal and cathartics; magnesium cathartics avoided
      • Vigorous IV fluid resuscitation
      • Cooling measures
      • Alkaline diuresis or hemodialysis
i. Alcohol
  (1) Ethyl alcohol (ethanol) is the most common overdose seen in the emergency care setting, either alone or in combination with other substances.
  (2) Effects
      • Variable, depending on the degree of tolerance; in nonalcoholic persons, blood alcohol levels above 100 mg per dl are associated with evidence of intoxication and those above 400 mg per dl, with death
      • Central nervous system: ataxia, dysarthria, nystagmus, seizures, coma, hypothermia, and death
      • Cardiovascular: hypotension, bradycardia until withdrawal
      • Respiratory: bradypnea or apnea, aspiration pneumonia
      • Gastrointestinal: nausea, vomiting, gastric or other gastrointestinal bleeding
      • Hypoglycemia may be present; vitamin defi-

ciency is often present in chronic alcoholics, so thiamine is routinely administered IV before glucose is given, to prevent the development of Wernicke's encephalopathy
- Renal impairment due to myoglobinuria from rhabdomyolysis, which results from lying in the same place for long periods of time
(3) Clinical management
- Supportive; there is no antidote or agent to increase the metabolism.
- Gastric lavage may be ordered if there is concern about coingestion.
- Airway management and mechanical ventilation may be necessary.
- Treat hypothermia, usually with external warming.
- Monitor blood alcohol level or Breathalyzer; there should be a correlation between level of consciousness and value; if not, other conditions (e.g., trauma, overdose) should be considered.

j. Methanol or methyl alcohol
(1) Methanol is widely available and is used in a variety of ways (e.g., paint thinners, to fuel fondue pots [Sterno]).
(2) Because it looks and smells similar to ethanol, ingestion may be accidental.
(3) Methanol ingestion is very serious, with symptoms occurring after ingestion of as little as 5 ml; its metabolism yields formaldehyde and formate.
(4) Effects
- Initial effects are similar to those of ethanol, but there may be greater drowsiness, euphoria, and muscle weakness; significant symptoms develop between 6 and 36 hours after ingestion.
- Central nervous system: headache, delirium, coma, fixed and dilated pupils, seizures, opisthotonus, cerebral edema
- Vision: Photophobia, blurred vision followed by irreversible blindness
- Respiratory: Dyspnea
- Gastrointestinal: Abdominal pain, which may be due to pancreatitis, diarrhea
- Significant metabolic acidosis
- Hyperglycemia and hyperosmolality
(5) Clinical management
- Check ABCs
- Gastric lavage and charcoal, if seen early
- Sodium bicarbonate to treat acidosis
- Intravenous alcohol bolus and drip to maintain blood alcohol level at 100 to 150 mg/dl; the alcohol competes with methanol for metabolism, preventing development of serious metabolites.
- Hemodialysis

k. Ethylene glycol
(1) Ethylene glycol is found in antifreeze and a variety of other substances; it may be accidentally or intentionally ingested, the latter most often by alcoholics who cannot get access to ethanol; symptoms are due to metabolites, including crystal formation in tissues.
(2) Effects occur over 72 hours.
- Central nervous system: Intoxication without smell of alcohol on breath, decreased tendon reflexes that progress to tetany and seizures, coma.
- Cardiovascular: hypertension, tachycardia
- Respiratory: tachypnea, pulmonary edema, cyanosis, pneumonitis
- Nausea, vomiting
- Genitourinary: Flank pain and costovertebral angle (CVA) tenderness, calcium oxalate crystals in urine, hematuria, renal failure
- Severe metabolic acidosis, hypocalcemia
(3) Clinical management
- Same as for methanol ingestion (e.g., IV alcohol, sodium bicarbonate)
- Calcium gluconate to treat hypocalcemia

l. Iron
(1) Ingestion occurs most often in children from over-the-counter or prescription iron preparations (e.g., multivitamins with iron); these medications often look like candy and are appealing to children.
(2) Death or serious injury can result from ingestion of just a few pills.
(3) Effects: The effects are in 3 phases:
- Phase 1: immediately after ingestion up to 6 hours—the irritating and corrosive effect of iron on the gastrointestinal tract may result in nausea, bloody vomiting and diarrhea, and hypovolemic shock.
- Phase 2: 6 to 24 hours after ingestion—clinical improvement may be noted.
- Phase 3: 24 hours after ingestion—there may be profound metabolic acidosis, liver and renal necrosis and failure, sepsis, and pulmonary edema.
(4) Clinical management
- Gastric emptying with emesis or lavage; the pills are often enteric coated and may form a solid ball that is radiolucent.
- Careful fluid resuscitation to prevent pulmonary edema, pressors, sodium bicarbonate.
- Deferoxamine lM or IV; a test dose may be given if special laboratory studies are not available. The urine turns a "vin-rosé" color if iron is present.

m. Insecticides—organophosphates and carbamates
(1) Insecticides, in powder or liquid form, are widely available in the home and in industry.
- They are readily absorbed through the skin, lungs, and mucous membranes, thus creating hazard for staff as well.
- Major action is interference with cholinesterase at the synaptic membrane and in cells.
(2) Effects over time: The acronym SLUD has been coined to remember the symptoms: *Salivation, Lacrimation, Urination, Diarrhea.*

- Central nervous system: inattentive, giddy, headache, confusion, delirium, tremors, slurred speech, weakness, twitching, muscle fasciculation, paralysis, seizures, coma, dilated pupils
- Cardiovascular: initially bradycardia, then tachycardia, hypertension, chest pain
- Respiratory: dyspnea, wheezing, increased pulmonary secretions
- Gastrointestinal: increased salivation, nausea, vomiting, diarrhea
- Other: diaphoresis, increased urination

(3) Clinical management
- Decontamination, if external
- Emesis or gastric lavage and charcoal and cathartics, if ingested
- Atropine: Atropine dosing is guided by resolution of symptoms—massive doses may be required.
- Pralidoxime (2-PAM) IV
- Benzodiazepines for seizures

n. Cyanide
(1) Cyanide exposure or ingestion may occur in a number of ways: Fire in an enclosed space, industry, fruit and seed pits, and during administration of IV sodium nitroprusside (antihypertensive); it interferes with cellular respiration, and death may occur rapidly.
(2) Effects
- Characteristic bitter almond odor
- Central nervous system: headache, giddiness, ataxia, seizures, coma
- Respiratory: dyspnea
- Gastrointestinal: possible nausea and vomiting
(3) Clinical management
- Airway management
- Amyl nitrite vaporettes crushed and held under nose or near endotracheal tube
- Establish IV line and administer IV sodium nitrite, followed by IV sodium thiosulfate.
- Hypotension may occur from these medications and is treated with pressors and change of position.
- The treatment objective is to cause methemoglobinemia (which competes for receptor sites), which may cause the person's skin to develop a bluish tinge; overtreatment can be reversed with IV methylene blue, although this may retoxify the person.

o. Mushroom poisoning
(1) Poisoning from mushroom ingestions can be quite complex to evaluate, because different mushrooms have different toxins, the intensity of which varies according to the age of the mushroom. Poisoning may be accidental or intentional. Most instances result from uninformed people picking mushrooms for food, but some are seeking hallucinogenic mushrooms.
(2) Two species cause the majority of mushroom poisonings: *Amanita muscaria* and *Amanita phalloides*.
(3) *Amanita muscaria*
- Symptoms develop within a few minutes to 2 hours after ingestion.
- Symptoms include SLUD as well as diaphoresis, pinpoint pupils, abdominal cramping, confusion, coma, and seizures (rare).
- Most people recover within 24 hours, but death has been reported.
- Treatment includes gastrointestinal decontamination, support, and IV atropine.
(4) *Amanita phalloides*
- Ingestion of 1 mushroom cap can be fatal.
- Symptoms develop 6 to 24 hours after ingestion.
- Common initial symptoms include severe abdominal pain, vomiting, and diarrhea, which may contain blood and mucus.
- Following these symptoms is a period of apparent recovery that occurs 12 to 24 hours after ingestion.
- After 24 to 72 hours, there is organ necrosis affecting the liver, heart, kidneys, and central nervous system, which is evidenced by coagulopathies, seizures, coma, and death.
- Hemodialysis may be useful.
- There is no antidote, and treatment is supportive.
(5) Hallucinogenic mushrooms that contain psilocin and psilocybin have been used for many years by Native Americans in religious ceremonies, and have attracted the attention of other groups.
- Symptoms include euphoria, hallucinations, tachycardia, dilated pupils, and paresthesias.
- Treatment includes reassurance and possible oral sedation.

p. Botulism
(1) Definition
- Food-borne botulism results from ingestion of food that contains *Clostridium botulinum* toxins; it results primarily from improperly home-canned or smoked foods but may result from commercially prepared foods and seafood.
- Infant botulism results from the ingestion of spores, subsequent gastrointestinal colonization, and release of toxins; it may occur from honey, vacuum cleaner dust, and dirt.
- Wound botulism results when the spore enters a break in the skin, and toxin is subsequently released.
(2) Effects
- The organism releases 7 toxins (A through G); toxins A, B, E, and F are responsible for most human poisonings.
- Symptoms may develop as early as 18 to 36 hours after ingestion, but the incubation period is 4 to 8 days.
- Bilateral neurologic abnormalities are charac-

teristic: There is descending weakness, starting with the cranial nerves.
- Symptoms include visual disturbances: Diplopia, ptosis of the eyelids, inability to accommodate to light, loss of pupillary reflex.
- Dry mouth, nausea, vomiting, diarrhea
- Weakness or paralysis of swallowing mechanisms: dysarthria and dysphagia, which may lead to aspiration
- Progressive muscle weakness involving the arms and legs
- Sensation, sensorium, vital signs, and laboratory study results remain normal.
- Constipation is common once the paresis descends.
- Respiratory failure and pneumonia are major concerns.
  (3) Clinical management of food-borne botulism
- Airway management and monitoring; there may be progressive respiratory failure.
- Gastrointestinal decontamination
- Intravenous fluids
- Nothing by mouth, if swallowing affected
- Botulism antitoxin—Obtain from the Centers for Disease Control and Prevention; may be beneficial even though many days may have elapsed from ingestion.
- Psychologic support
11. Criteria for discharge
    a. Fully awake, alert, and oriented
    b. Normal gait, motor and sensory function
    c. Ingestion or exposure not considered significant
    d. Person must be reliable regarding follow-up. Repeated laboratory studies may be necessary.
    e. No evidence of toxicity; symptoms controlled
    f. Not suicidal
12. Discharge planning and teaching in the poisoned or overdosed person
    a. Explain the effect of activated charcoal—It may cause stool to be black; this should not be confused with gastrointestinal bleeding.
    b. Describe symptoms to observe for and what to do if they occur.
    c. Remind the patient about follow-up studies, if indicated.
    d. Discuss prevention strategies.
    e. Give individuals with alcohol or drug problems information on referrals to alcohol or drug treatment programs.

Hazardous Materials Exposure

1. Definition
   a. A hazardous material (HAZ MAT), quite simply, is anything that may cause a person harm; it may be chemical, biologic, or radiologic.
   b. The term is most often applied to large quantities of chemicals found in industry, although a HAZ MAT incident can occur anywhere (e.g., explosion from

stored chlorine used for a private swimming pool, radioisotope accident in nuclear medicine).
   c. Although HAZ MAT incidents occur daily in most large cities, very few necessitate emergency medical care; each industry dealing with HAZ MATs is required to have a written plan and trained teams to manage incidents; thus, decontamination is often completed before a person reaches the hospital.
   d. Fire departments also have specially trained HAZ MAT teams and equipment for decontamination and cleanup; many fire departments require that industries handling or transporting HAZ MATs notify them in writing of the existence, risk, and location of the materials and further limit transport to times during which there is low risk to citizens in the event of a spill.
   e. Most HAZ MAT incidents occur in industry or are due to transportation accidents; individuals who transport HAZ MATs are required to register the shipment with the U.S. Department of Transportation and to display signs (placards) on the vehicle describing the nature of the HAZ MAT and the type of risk it entails. This enables law enforcement, fire, and EMS personnel to better know how to handle the incident.
   f. Placard and bill of lading information (detailing what chemical or material is being transported) is communicated to a central information source known as CHEM TREK (call 800 operator for correct phone number), who will advise rescue and health care personnel about the substance, its effects, and how to treat exposures.
   g. Raids of illegal methamphetamine laboratories have created HAZ MAT incidents; most law enforcement agencies are well versed in the types of chemical exposures that may result.
   h. Radiation-related accidents in hospitals are the responsibility of the radiation safety officer, who is usually affiliated with the radiology department.
2. Common or serious HAZ MAT exposures
   a. HAZ MATs can be divided into 2 categories:
      (1) Those that pose an immediate threat to life (e.g., chlorine, cyanide, ammonia, phosgene, hydrogen sulfide, organophosphate insecticides, nitrogen dioxide)
      (2) Those with cancer-causing potential (e.g., polychlorinated biphenyls)
   b. Persons with immediately life-threatening exposures are treated 1st and decontaminated during or after treatment; decontamination is done 1st in other exposures.
3. Triage category
   a. Hazardous materials that pose an immediate threat are an immediate priority.
   b. Evaluation of the person who is exposed to carcinogenic or teratogenic (fetal hazard) substances may be delayed if decontamination has been completed, but is immediate for decontamination procedures.
4. Effects
   a. Although the effects are agent specific, many HAZ MATs cause irritation of the lungs, skin, or eyes.
   b. Organophosphate and carbamate insecticides can

cause paralysis and death; the agents are absorbed through the skin.

5. Clinical management
   a. Before initiating treatment, it is important to assess the following:
      (1) Does the chemical pose a threat to caregivers?
      (2) If so, has person been decontaminated?
      (3) If the chemical poses no threat or decontamination has been done, treatment can proceed normally.
      (4) If the chemical poses a threat, the person has not been decontaminated, and the person has an immediately life-threatening condition, caregivers must don protective garb and provide necessary stabilization; the environment must be sealed off to prevent spread of contamination elsewhere.
      (5) If no immediate threat, and still contaminated, the person should be decontaminated 1st, preferably outside the facility to prevent contamination of treatment areas.
   b. Treatment is agent specific.
6. Decontamination
   a. Each hospital is required to have a chemical or radiologic decontamination plan and to practice it periodically; the following are general guidelines, and the reader is referred to specific institutional or community plans.
   b. Basic concerns
      (1) Decontamination of individual
      (2) Prevention of spread of contamination
      (3) Cleanup and removal of contaminated waste water and refuse
      (4) Monitoring and follow-up of personnel exposed, including caregivers
   c. Preparation
      (1) If there is a known community HAZ MAT incident, EMS or fire personnel usually notify the hospital so that it can set up a decontamination area or team.
      (2) It is not uncommon, however, for a single exposed worker to present to the triage desk with complaint of an exposure; this person may or may not have performed decontamination.
      (3) Assuming previous warning, the floor in the decontamination area is covered with an impervious material; this covering may extend through doorways and into the ambulance bay.
      (4) Air vents are sealed off (to prevent contamination of the whole facility).
      (5) The designated area is roped or taped off, and security staff are alerted; they will assist in keeping nonessential people away from the contaminated area.
      (6) Necessary equipment is placed in the room; equipment that may be needed is placed near the room but outside the contamination areas.
      (7) Supplies or equipment normally kept in the room may be removed or the closets and drawers sealed off.
   d. Decontamination procedures
      (1) A clean litter, preferably covered in plastic, is taken to the ambulance bay, and the person is moved onto the clean stretcher, covered with the plastic, and transported over the covered floor to the decontamination or treatment room by personnel in protective garb; the ambulance personnel then decontaminate themselves, their equipment, and their vehicle.
      (2) If appropriate, the person walks or is wheeled over the floor covering to the decontamination shower by a person wearing protective garb, which may include a respirator.
      (3) Clothing is removed and secured in a hazard bag; about 95 percent of the contamination is eliminated when clothing is removed.
      (4) Valuables are placed in a separate bag for later decontamination.
      (5) The person washes well with soap and water with attention paid to body orifices (especially nostrils) and hairy areas; the hair is shampooed well; wounds may require irrigation.
      (6) The waste water may be collected into a pool (e.g., a baby swimming pool) if there is no containment unit for the shower.
      (7) If there has been radiologic contamination, the body is scanned with a radiation detector meter, again with special attention to hairy areas and wounds; there is no detector available for chemical contamination.
      (8) While the person is showering, the floor cover may be removed and placed in a hazard bag; caregivers may remove and dispose of protective garb.
      (9) On completion of the decontamination shower, the person puts on a clean gown or clothes and steps onto the clean floor; medical evaluation can then proceed.
      (10) The principles are the same for decontamination of a stretcher-bound person; a hose and a slotted basket that allow the water to drain away from the person are ideal; special decontamination stretchers are available.
      (11) The plan should include responsibility for decontamination of the valuables and shower and removal of waste water and materials.
      (12) If care must proceed before the person is decontaminated, the treatment room itself is considered contaminated (may be called a hot zone or red zone); personnel may not enter and leave the room without using appropriate procedures. It is prudent to have a noncontaminated person stand at the door to serve as a scribe (medical records should not be taken into a contaminated room) and to get necessary equipment.
      (13) It is ideal if there are 2 doors to a decontamination shower so that the person exits into a different clean area, but this is not common.
      (14) Regulatory and institutional occupational health policies and procedures regarding recording exposure and follow-up should be implemented.
      (15) If large numbers of people are exposed and require decontamination, fire department, emer-

gency preparedness, and military resources may be called on.

(16) A significant HAZ MAT incident inevitably generates media attention; early involvement of hospital media relations, security, and local law enforcement helps prevent violation of contaminated areas and facilitates care of exposed persons.

(17) Decontamination procedures may be performed outside the department to prevent hospital contamination.

Sexual Assault

1. Definition
   a. Sexual assault, or rape (which is a legal, not medical, term), may be defined as sexual penetration of any body orifice without consent.
   b. It may be acute or chronic as in child sexual abuse.
   c. Adult women are sexually assaulted more often than adult men.
   d. Among children, more girls than boys seek treatment, but the actual incidence in both groups is probably greatly underreported.
   e. Rape includes sexual assault by a known or unknown assailant, date rape, and spousal rape (commonly seen in domestic violence).
   f. Although some sexual assault survivors may have serious injury requiring medical care, the care priorities for most are the following:
      (1) Psychologic support
      (2) Evidence collection and safeguarding
      (3) Pregnancy prevention
      (4) Sexually transmitted disease prevention
      (5) Referral for medical and emotional follow-up
      (6) Providing information regarding the legal processes that follow
2. Applying the nursing process
   a. In addition to those associated with physical injury, the following nursing diagnoses may apply to the sexual assault survivor:
      (1) Fear R/T rape itself, assailant harming again, possibility of pregnancy or of sexually transmitted diseases
      (2) Altered family processes R/T spouse or significant other blaming patient for causing the rape, or having difficulty understanding survivor's response to event
      (3) Rape trauma syndrome, compound reaction or silent reaction
      (4) Situational low self-esteem
      (5) Sexual dysfunction
      (6) Sleep pattern disturbance
      (7) Knowledge deficit R/T normal responses after rape, judicial system processes, follow-up care, coping
   b. The ED nurse cannot address most of the nursing diagnoses directly but can assist the patient by doing the following:
      (1) Ensuring privacy and consistency; have the same nurse provide all of the care, even though procedures may take 3 to 4 hours; providing a same-gender caregiver, unless specifically requested otherwise (e.g., a male patient may prefer a female caregiver, because the assaults are usually by males).
      (2) Providing care in a timely, compassionate, non-judgmental manner; this includes being knowledgeable about the fact that patients demonstrate a wide spectrum of responses, from crying to yelling to silence, and that a calm demeanor is no indicator of the degree of emotional stress the person is experiencing.
      (3) Providing the patient with the opportunity to make choices and take control whenever possible; this may include acknowledging the person's decision not to notify law enforcement and not to proceed with evidence collection.

> **NURSE ADVISORY**
>
> Some patients who have experienced sexual assault may initially decline to press charges, and refuse evidence collection at the time of initial evaluation. Although the choice is clearly the patient's, it is recommended that the evidence be collected and processed or stored in case the person decides at a later time to proceed with criminal investigation.

      (4) Respecting the person's need to express his or her emotions in whatever way he or she wishes, unless it poses a danger to self or others.
      (5) Respecting that the person may need time to gain emotional control before proceeding with procedures.
      (6) Obtaining the assistance of a rape crisis counselor who will come to the hospital, remain with the patient throughout the examination and police proceedings, provide support and information about procedures, facilitate discharge to a safe place, and provide follow-up information.
      (7) Explaining all procedures or actions beforehand and obtaining the patient's permission before doing any procedure.
      (8) Fastidiously collecting, labeling, securing, and transferring evidence.
      (9) Providing written and verbal discharge instructions.
3. Triage priority: Immediate, to move person to a quiet, private area; evidence collection can be deferred for a while, but evidence degrades or may be lost in the interim.
4. Assessment
   a. Assessment of the sexual assault survivor is guided by legal protocols and institutional policy, which should be used each time without fail; recording data on a special sexual assault form is recommended.
   b. Historical data should be obtained only once; survivors relate that repeating the story is like being raped a 2nd time.

c. The role of the triage nurse is to identify the complaint of sexual assault and identify life-threatening injuries, and defer to the primary nurse for all further assessment; in pediatric sexual abuse, the chief complaint may be of vaginal drainage or odor, perineal or groin area bruising, or unusual behavior or responses during bathing of the perineal area.

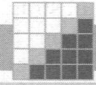
LEGAL AND ETHICAL CONSIDERATIONS

Sexual Assault Nurse Examiners are registered nurses who have received special education in the care of sexual assault survivors, including evidence collection, follow-up, and testifying in legal proceedings. These individuals may be the sole providers of care to the patient unless other physical injury necessitates physician involvement.

Nurses functioning in this role may also be called forensic nurses and may participate with law enforcement or the medical examiner or coroner in crime scene or death investigations. Forensic nurses are actively involved in educating law enforcement and participants in the judicial system about sexual assault and treatment of its survivors.

Certification in forensic nursing is available; contact the International Association of Forensic Nursing.

5. Sexual assault protocol
   a. Obtain written consent to collect evidence, including pictures, and to release information to law enforcement officials.
   b. Assess relevant health history, allergies, current medications.
   c. Evaluate injuries.
   d. Collect gynecologic history: last normal menstrual period and duration, use of contraception, gravity and parity, last voluntary coitus.
   e. Assault history: date and time (evidence examination may not be performed in assaults that occur more than 48 hours before arrival); number of assailants; type of assault: penis, finger, object; area: vagina, rectum, mouth; other: condom usage; whether assailant ejaculated; weapon used, and injuries from weapon.
   f. Postassault activities: bathed, douched, wiped genitals or other areas, voided, defecated, brushed teeth, ate, gargled, changed clothes, colored hair.
   g. Place paper on floor and have patient stand on paper while removing clothes; this allows any debris to be captured.
   h. Place clothing in paper bags or wrap in floor paper.
   i. Obtain head and pubic hair combings and controls, using a comb with cotton between the teeth, and plucking control hairs using tweezers; allow the patient to do this. Combings are placed in separate paper envelopes, sealed, and labeled with names of both the patient and the examiner.
   j. Collect fingernail scrapings and clippings, especially if patient has scratched assailant; these are also placed in paper envelopes and labeled.
   k. Photograph, or have forensic photographer take photographs of, injured areas, especially bite marks.
   l. Examine affected areas under a blue light (Wood's lamp); semen shows as yellow-white fluorescent color; swab areas to test for acid phosphatase, which is evidence of semen, even in vasectomized male.
   m. Swab the perineum with toluidine blue to detect fourchette lacerations, which are evidence of forced penetration; note that this may be the only evidence that an assault has occurred, especially if the assailant used a condom or did not ejaculate.
   n. Some institutions use a colposcope with a special camera to detect and document fourchette and other lacerations that may not be apparent to the naked eye.
   o. Pelvic, rectal, and oral examinations are performed; swabs (using cotton-tipped applicators) are obtained from each orifice. *Note:* Use water as a lubricant because lubricating jelly can alter the results.
   p. Specimens for wet mount to examine for presence of sperm are obtained from each orifice.
   q. Specimens are obtained for chlamydia and gonorrhea from each orifice.
   r. Gram stain and Papanicolaou (Pap) smear may be done but are of questionable value.
   s. Obtain blood for a baseline Venereal Disease Research Laboratories (VDRL) or rapid plasma reagin test and possibly for a pregnancy test; human immunodeficiency virus testing during the visit is generally not recommended because the records will be used in court; rather, it is recommended that the patient have the test done through the health department, by which confidentiality will be ensured.
   t. Evidence or specimen handling
      (1) Sent to hospital laboratory. Wet mounts, using chain of custody; swab or aspirate for acid phosphatase under chain of custody; VDRL, Gram stain, Pap smear, serum pregnancy test—no chain of custody.
      (2) Retained in medical record or hospital; released with subpoena
         • Consent for evidence collection
         • Sexual assault history and evidence collection form
         • Photographs taken by hospital staff
      (3) Taken by law enforcement under chain of custody
         • Swabs from each orifice and fluorescent areas after air-dried in a locked swab dryer
         • Clothing
         • Hair samples
         • Fingernail clippings
   u. Pregnancy prevention
      (1) Medication (Postcoital contraception includes oral agents such as Ovral and Danazol) to prevent pregnancy is usually ordered unless prohibited by institutional religious beliefs; if this is so, the patient should be referred to a provider who can assist in this regard.
      (2) These medications may cause nausea, so antiemetics are prescribed.
      (3) The patient must understand that the medication may be dangerous if she does become pregnant; institutions or practitioners often require written

informed consent indicating that the patient understands the risk and agrees to obtain voluntary termination of pregnancy before prescribing the medication.

    (4) Depo-Provera may also be used for pregnancy prevention.

  v. Sexually transmitted disease prophylaxis

    (1) Ceftriaxone IM or Suprax orally for gonococcus

    (2) Doxycycline (unless pregnant) orally for 7 days

  w. Other medications: Tetanus booster may be given if there are lacerations or abrasions; antibiotics may be given if there are bite wounds.

6. Discharge planning and teaching

  a. Discuss normal behavioral responses and rape trauma syndrome.

  b. Mention resources for counseling.

  c. Review follow-up for culture results and retesting.

  d. Provide information regarding human immunodeficiency virus testing.

  e. Provide information regarding pregnancy prevention medication, including warnings about nausea and abnormal bleeding.

Domestic Violence

1. Definition and magnitude of the problem

  a. Domestic violence may be defined as the physical, sexual, or psychologic abuse of an intimate or family member by another; this may include child, elder, or spouse abuse. However, the term "domestic violence" is most often used to describe an adult woman who has been physically or emotionally battered; this section focuses only on women who are battered.

  b. Domestic violence is a serious health and societal concern.

    (1) An estimated 1 out of 4 women are victims of domestic violence. Each year, 2 to 6 million women are beaten by their spouses, partners, or dates.

    (2) Two thousand to 4000 women are beaten to death annually; 40 percent of women and 10 percent of men are murdered by their partners.

    (3) Battering is the single major cause of injury to women, greater than auto accidents, rapes, or muggings.

    (4) Domestic violence affects all family members. It is believed that the abuser also abuses the children in one half of the cases, and the victim abuses children in another third. Even if children are not physically abused, witnessing abuse of a parent is a form of psychologic child abuse.

    (5) More than 1 million women seek emergency care for injuries due to battering each year; 35 percent of all visits by women to EDs are due to domestic violence; however, it is estimated that health care providers recognize it in only 1 out of 25 cases.

    (6) Domestic violence affects people of all ethnic and socioeconomic backgrounds but may be a special

problem in cultures new to the United States because of changing roles and norms.

    (7) Accurate statistics on the incidence of domestic violence are difficult to obtain because many victims do not report it to law enforcement for a variety of reasons; in most states, health care providers may not report it as a crime unless the patient agrees.

  c. A domestic violence victim leaves an abusive relationship an average of 7 times before finally terminating the relationship; an estimated 34 percent are battered after they leave the abusive relationship.

  d. Domestic violence should be considered in women who are injured, or in those with stress-related problems, or mental health concerns.

    (1) An estimated one third have anxiety or depression.

    (2) Twenty-six percent of all women who attempt suicide have experienced domestic violence.

    (3) More than 50 percent of Black women who attempt suicide are battered.

    (4) Sixty-six percent of women who are hospitalized for psychiatric reasons have been physically abused as an adult.

2. Characteristics

  a. Abusive men are manipulative and persistent, fostering a sense of low self-esteem and no worth, isolation, no rights, and no opinions.

  b. As part of their desire to control, as well as fear of being found out, abusers often demand to be present during the evaluation or repeatedly call the treating facility to inquire about the victim's status.

    (1) Abusers are often solicitous; they answer questions and do not allow the patient to express herself.

    (2) Extreme or inappropriate concern and demanding behavior may be clues that the person is an abuser.

  c. There is a pattern of control and constant vigilance regarding the patient's activities, finances, and social relationships.

  d. Victims often engage in self-blaming behavior, rationalizing that it was something they did or did not do that provoked the abuse.

  e. There are a number of reasons why victims do not leave an abusive relationship:

    (1) They love the abuser, and there are parts of the relationship that are rewarding.

    (2) Lack of resources (e.g., financial, housing, social support).

    (3) Fear that the abusive person will harm them, their children, or family pets; unfortunately, this is a legitimate fear because many of the murders of abused women occur after the victim leaves the abuser.

    (4) Social impact and embarrassment.

    (5) A belief that if they can avoid the behavior that causes the violence, it will stop.

3. Recognition

  a. Given evidence that health care providers often fail to recognize domestic violence and victims fail to report it, it is important for health care providers to ask specifically if the injury was caused by another person; some experts suggest that all women who seek health care for any reason should be asked if battering is occurring.

(1) Even when the question is asked, victims may deny that abuse is occurring.

(2) Victims indicate that they are both fearful that someone will ask about their injuries and fearful that they will not ask.

(3) It is often the questioning that helps the person realize that she does not need to put up with the abuse, and that there are alternatives and resources available.

b. Demeanor: Be concerned when the patient is hesitant or evasive with answers regarding mechanism of injury or has poor eye contact, or when the response to injury seems to be excessive for the injury.

c. The injury may be inconsistent with explanation or mechanism.

d. There may be multiple bruises in various stages of healing.

e. A delay may have occurred in obtaining treatment.

f. Injury in a pregnant person: An estimated 25 percent of all pregnant women are battered, often with injuries to the abdomen, face, and breasts; significant force (e.g., kicking to the abdomen in an attempt to terminate the pregnancy) is not uncommon.

g. The person may be injury prone or make frequent visits to the ED.

h. The person may have psychosomatic complaints.

i. The person may display fear or anxiety in the presence of her partner.

j. Sexual assault by the partner may have occurred (e.g., marital or date rape); up to 50 percent of abused women are raped by their husbands or boyfriends.

k. There may be evidence of drug or alcohol use or abuse, which may precipitate the event or be used as a means of coping with the violence.

l. Injury patterns: Injuries most often involve the face, chest, breasts, and abdomen; however, arm and leg injury may also occur.

m. Transport may be requested via EMS ambulance for even minor problems because that is the only way the person can get out of the house safely.

4. Assessment

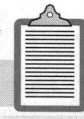

NURSING MANAGEMENT

Policies and procedures specifically designed to ensure safety of the domestic violence victim may be necessary. These include the ability to create an alias so the person's presence cannot be discovered, a chart or room flagging system to alert clinical staff and security that visitor access must be restricted, restrictions on computerized patient locater information, and a defined security or law enforcement response in the event that the abuser attempts to interfere with clinical care.

a. Provide a safe environment: Obtain the history and perform the assessment in a private, safe place without the partner present; if the partner objects to not being allowed to remain with the patient, advise that hospital regulations require this (batterers usually are not willing to allow the woman to be alone). Obtain assistance from security staff if necessary.

b. Confront the issue.

(1) Ask if someone caused the injury.

(2) Use phrasing such as, "Sometimes injuries like this are caused by someone hitting a person; did this happen to you?"

c. Document carefully what the patient says, using her own words, about how the injury was sustained or the reasons for her visit if not an injury.

d. If the patient verbalizes that she has been beaten, ask if she is willing to press charges; if yes, notify the police.

e. Identify, document, and photograph (if the patient allows) the injuries.

5. Nursing diagnoses

a. Fear R/T potential for injury and abuse from domestic violence

b. Risk for trauma R/T battering by abusive partner

c. Decisional conflict R/T perceived threat of injury from abusive spouse and lack of a support system

d. Situational low self-esteem R/T unwillingness to leave an abusive partner

e. Pain R/T injuries from battering by abusive partner

f. Hopelessness R/T lack of sufficient resources to leave an abusive relationship

g. Post-traumatic response R/T previous traumatic experiences perpetuated by abusive partner

h. Rape-trauma syndrome R/T forced nonconsensual sex with abusive partner

i. Powerlessness R/T battering relationship

j. Social isolation R/T constant vigilance and control of finances and social relationships by abusive partner

k. Altered family processes R/T battering by abusive partner

6. Clinical management, discharge planning, and teaching

a. Treat physical problems; hospitalization may be indicated for safety reasons, even if the injuries are not serious.

b. Provide counseling regarding options (this may also be done by social services).

(1) In many states, a restraining order can be obtained even without pressing charges.

(2) Some states have legislation requiring immediate jailing for domestic violence offenders as a cooling-off strategy whenever police encounter a domestic violence situation, even if the victim does not press charges.

(3) Some states offer relocation and new identity programs, similar to the federal witness protection programs.

(4) Determine natural support system (e.g., family, friends, or neighbors).

c. Provide information regarding making a safety plan.

(1) Make and secure copies of birth (own and children's) and marriage certificates, social security

card, bank account numbers, and medical insurance card.

(2) Obtain a spare credit card.

(3) Make an extra set of car and house keys.

(4) Obtain sufficient cash to last several days.

(5) Arrange for a place to go to (e.g., natural supports, a shelter).

(6) Have these items, as well as some clothing and a few children's toys, packed in a bag that is secured in a safe place (e.g., at a neighbor's house).

d. Provide information regarding resources.

(1) For safety reasons, it is suggested that any written resource information be generic without identifying that it is for victims of domestic violence because batterers often go through the victim's personal belongings; finding this information can provoke another beating.

(2) Numbers for domestic violence support groups; hot lines; and other community resources, such as food banks, shelters, and legal aid, are helpful.

e. If children are at risk, advise the patient of your obligation to notify the appropriate child protective agency; this action alone may cause the patient to realize the gravity of the situation and rethink the decision not to leave or press charges.

f. Couple counseling or batterer counseling has not proved to be effective and should not be recommended as a 1st step.

g. Recent public attention to both the frequency and often life-threatening nature of domestic violence has sparked much-needed discussion regarding the need for change in the way that society prevents and responds to domestic violence; the nurse should keep informed about changes in legislation that affect the management of this problem.

h. Health care providers often become frustrated when victims refuse to admit that injuries are due to domestic violence or are unwilling to leave an abusive relationship; this may affect their willingness to address the issue with future patients. Although this frustration can be appreciated, experts in the field are quick to point out that health care provider efforts in addressing the issue often provide the stimulus to the victims to take action, even if it is not apparent during the visit.

◻ CARING FOR PEOPLE WHO ARE INJURED

Major Injuries

1. Injury is the leading cause of death for all individuals between 12 and 44 years of age and the 5th leading cause of death for persons age 65 and over.

2. Priority setting

a. One of the axioms of trauma care is the "golden hour," which is a goal of resuscitation, stabilization, and definitive care (usually surgery) within 1 hour of injury.

b. Research has demonstrated that selected mechanisms and circumstances of injury are likely to produce certain injuries or potential lethality, and thus the person should be referred to a trauma center.

c. The decision by prehospital providers on where to transport a trauma victim (e.g., level 1 or 2 trauma center versus a regular ED) is dependent on this information as well as on the condition of the individual.

3. Assessment

a. Diagnostic and therapeutic measures are often based on the history of mechanism of injury rather than simply on the presenting findings. To the novice, initiating a variety of invasive and noninvasive measures before the diagnoses are made may seem a bit premature; however, injury research tells us of the likelihood that certain injuries are present more often than not.

b. Several important tools used to predict either the nature or severity of injury are the following:

(1) Mechanism of injury (e.g., fall from several stories, frontal impact at high velocity)

(2) History of incident and death of another person from the accident

(3) Trauma score

(4) Number of body systems involved

(5) Age of the individual

c. Mechanism of injury is the way an injury occurred; it may be categorized in several ways:

(1) Blunt or penetrating

(2) Low velocity or high velocity

(3) Blast or compression

(4) Area of impact (e.g., front-end or T-bone [in a motor vehicle accident], axial loading [something falling on the person's head or striking the top of the head on something])

d. The types of injuries associated with specific mechanisms are summarized in Table 37–13.

e. History of the accident and death at the scene in motor vehicle accidents:

(1) High-velocity motor vehicle accidents in which the vehicle strikes a stationary object (e.g., tree or guardrail), or those in which a person is ejected from a vehicle are more likely to result in serious injury than low-velocity ones or ones in which the person remains inside the vehicle.

(2) Research has demonstrated that the death of 1 person involved in an accident is often associated with more serious injury to other individuals involved in the same incident, thus necessitating transport to a trauma center.

f. Trauma score is also used to assess severity of injury and to guide transport decisions.

(1) The trauma score (Table 37–14) is based on several parameters including the following:

• Vital signs

• Glasgow Coma Scale

g. The number of body systems involved increases the likelihood of serious injury or of significant complications, necessitating a higher level of trauma care.

(1) In general, involvement of 2 or more body sys-

Table 37–13. Mechanisms of Injury

Mechanism	Resulting Injuries
Adult pedestrian struck by auto	Tibia, fibula, and femur fractures on side of impact
Child pedestrian struck by auto	Head, chest, and abdominal trauma
Pedestrian struck by large vehicle or dragged by vehicle	Above plus pelvic fracture
Front impact—unrestrained driver	Head, neck, chest, abdomen, and pelvis
Front impact—unrestrained passenger	Posterior hip dislocation, femur or patella fracture
Back seat passenger without safety belt	Cervical cord injury secondary to hyperextension of neck
Back seat passenger with only lap belt—rear impact	Lumbar spine fracture or dislocation
Fall on outstretched hand	Fractures of navicula (hand), wrist (Colles), or humerus
Blunt force to eye	Hyphema, blowout fracture of orbit
Blunt force to midface	Le Forte III fracture
Blunt force to neck	Laryngeal fracture
Diving into shallow water	Cervical spine fracture
Lifting child up with arms extended	Radius dislocation at elbow (nursemaid's elbow)
Blunt trauma to side of knee (e.g., "clipping" foul in football)	Knee dislocation
Fall from heights, landing on feet	Compression fracture of lumbosacral spine, calcaneus
Fall from standing position (elderly)	Hip fracture
Bicycle handlebars striking abdomen in child	Lacerated spleen
Fist versus blunt object	Fracture of head of 5th metacarpal (Boxer's fracture)
Eversion injury of ankle	Ligamentous injury of ankle, fracture of head of 5th metatarsal, possibly tibia-fibula fracture
Air bag deployment	Minor facial injuries; minor chemical irritation of face, eyes, or both

tems suggests a need for level 1 or 2 trauma center treatment.

(2) Isolated significant head or spinal cord injury may be referred directly to a trauma center, even though it is a single-system injury, because of the difficulty of evaluating the potential for internal injuries.

Table 37–14. Trauma Score

Parameter	Value	Score
A. Respiratory rate	10–24	4
	25–35	3
	>35	2
	<10	1
	0	0
B. Respiratory effort	Normal	1
	Shallow or retractive	0
C. Systolic blood pressure	>90	4
	70–90	3
	50–69	2
	<50	1
	0	0
D. Glasgow Coma Scale score	14–15	5
	11–13	4
	8–10	3
	5–7	2
	3–4	1

Trauma score = Sum of A + B + C + D.

h. Age: The likelihood of higher mortality and morbidity is, to some extent, age dependent.

(1) Even in the presence of the same trauma score and injury severity score, older persons have a higher risk for poor outcomes than do middle-aged people.

(2) Likewise, young children with smaller circulating volumes and impaired thermoregulation are less able to handle blood loss and hypothermia that may occur during trauma resuscitation. (Specific issues related to children are discussed later.)

i. Physical assessment of the trauma victim follows the assessment outlined at the beginning of the chapter—completing the primary and secondary survey, and intervening when life-threatening findings are noted.

(1) A key element of the secondary survey is assessing the back for injury, while maintaining cervical spine immobilization.

• Many individuals with blunt trauma have spinal immobilization composed of a hard cervical collar and foam blocks on either side of the head; the apparatus is secured to a long spine board, and the person is secured to the board as well.

• A cross-table lateral radiograph of the cervical spine is taken as soon as possible; once the cervical spine is "cleared," the person can be rolled gently to assess the back. If the spine cannot be cleared, cervical immobilization is maintained while the person is turned.

• Failure to assess the back is a major pitfall in trauma care; important injuries can be missed.

j. Diagnostic studies are dependent on the mechanism of injury and presenting problems.

(1) Laboratory studies: complete blood count, electrolytes, BUN, glucose, creatinine, amylase if abdominal trauma, type and crossmatch for 4 units packed RBCs, clotting studies if massive transfusion may be required or if the person is on anticoagulants, arterial blood gases if the person is hypotensive or if there is significant chest injury, urinalysis; clotting studies and fresh frozen plasma may be indicated after each 10 units of transfused blood, per institution's "massive transfusion policy." Toxicology, blood alcohol, and pregnancy tests may also be ordered.

(2) Radiology studies may include cervical spine and other spine films, chest, abdomen, extremity, CT of head or abdomen, ultrasound, dye studies (e.g., IV pyelogram, arteriogram).

- The registered nurse should accompany the patient to CT scan or radiography if the patient is actually or potentially hemodynamically unstable.
- Accomplish radiographs and other diagnostic studies quickly, and remove spine board as soon as possible.

NURSE ADVISORY

Spine boards, although important in immobilization and transport of injured or ill individuals, are extremely uncomfortable and may cause injury. Pressure necrosis can occur in less than 60 minutes, especially in persons who are, or have been, hypotensive. Every effort should be made to expedite diagnosis so that the spine board can be removed. Comfort measures, such as padding the board or massage, and support to the neck and lumbosacral area, are indicated if the person must remain on the board for safety reasons. Assess the skin after removal of the board to identify pressure areas, and provide measures to maximize circulation to these areas.

---

k. Although resuscitation is personalized, general standing orders include the following:

(1) High-flow oxygen via nonrebreather mask

(2) Two or more large-bore IV catheters (or intraosseous needles if a child) with Ringer's lactate or normal saline solution (do not use glucose-containing solutions that clog IV lines when blood is administered); the rate of IV fluid administration depends on the vital signs and other indicators of perfusion.

- Foley catheter, if no blood at urinary meatus (blood at meatus suggests a urethral laceration, necessitating urologist consultation, suprapubic catheter, or both); check for blood and send for analysis; check output every 15 to 30 minutes.
- Nasogastric tube (16 or 18 French for adults) for blood checking, for emptying the stomach and minimizing vomiting and aspiration, and for diagnostic purposes (air may be injected into the nasogastric tube to assess for free air under the diaphragm in stomach injuries).

NURSE ADVISORY

Insertion of a nasogastric tube may be contraindicated in a person with head injury and possible basilar skull fracture, because of the potential for inadvertent intracranial placement, brain injury, and death. If gastric tube insertion is considered essential, it may be placed orally or inserted through a nasal airway, with physician approval.

- Vital signs every 5 to 15 minutes until stable
- Continuous cardiac and oximetry monitoring in major trauma, hypotension, or chest injury
- Pain management, possibly in consultation with anesthesia staff
- Keep person warm using warmed environment, warming lights, blankets, and warmed IV fluids and blood.
- Tetanus prophylaxis, if indicated
- Reassess and mark pulses in injured areas; ice and splint possible fractures.
- Intravenous or IM antibiotics, if open wounds, shock, or possibility of bowel injury
- Provide wound care; irrigate and dress if closure will be delayed.

Trauma in Special Populations

1. The pregnant trauma victim
   a. The pregnant trauma victim requires special mention because of a variety of physiologic changes that may confuse the clinical picture, predispose the person to different injuries, or cause risk to the fetus.
   b. The change in center of gravity may predispose the pregnant person to falls.
   c. The dramatic increase in domestic violence in pregnancy may cause abdominal and intrauterine bleeding.
   d. The increased circulating volume in the latter part of pregnancy may result in delayed development of classic signs of hypovolemia, despite significant blood loss.
   e. Even very minor trauma may cause premature labor, delivery, or fetal distress; fetal monitoring, performed by an appropriately credentialed nurse, may be a part of the initial evaluation; simply obtaining 1 set of fetal heart sounds may not be sufficient to identify fetal distress. It is common practice to admit the person for several hours of fetal monitoring after emergency care has been completed.
   f. When the pregnant person is supine (e.g., on a spine board), the gravid uterus may compress the vena cava, causing hypotension or "vena cava syndrome"; the treatment is to tilt the spine board to the left side to relieve the compression, while still maintaining spinal immobilization.
   g. Incorrect placement of a lap belt, or not wearing a lap belt, may predispose the pregnant person to injury in even a minor motor vehicle accident.

h. The gravid uterus may impede lung expansion, and a minor pulmonary contusion or hemothorax may be life threatening.

i. The use of radiographs in a person in early pregnancy may warrant special consideration to minimize the amount of radiation exposure.

j. Some medications (e.g., antibiotics and analgesics) may be contraindicated in pregnancy.

k. The pregnant person in cardiac arrest due to trauma may be a candidate for postmortem cesarean section; although this procedure is exceedingly rare, and often not successful, emergency care providers should be prepared for the possibility.

l. Provide the obstetric, neonatal, and operating room staff with timely notice about the pregnancy status of a trauma victim so that appropriate resources can be mobilized.

2. The injured child (see Chapter 15)

a. The majority of injuries in children are due to blunt trauma, although the increase in handguns has been associated with an increase in gunshot wounds in children of all ages.

b. Normal anatomic differences predispose children to certain types of injuries.

(1) Spinal cord injury without radiographic abnormality: The radiographs are normal but there is neurologic deficit.

• Spinal cord injury without radiographic abnormality is seen in infants and young children and is due to the laxity of the ligaments and cartilage in cervical spine vertebrae, coupled with greater head size and weight relative to the rest of the body.

• Neurologic impairment is often progressive rather than being present at the time of initial evaluation; thus, careful monitoring is indicated.

• The cervical spine must be kept immobilized during initial evaluation and observation because radiographs may not be helpful.

(2) Splenic and renal injuries because of less protective tissue and normal childhood activities (e.g., bicycle riding and injuring abdomen on the handle bars).

c. Normal growth and development characterize both certain injuries and general treatment considerations.

(1) Children learning to walk or in play often fall, hitting their faces on objects such as furniture, resulting in facial lacerations.

(2) Sports injuries occur, such as femur, radius, ulna, or elbow fractures.

(3) Transient dislocation of the radial head, known as "nursemaid's elbow," occurs when a child is lifted up a step when the elbow is in extension.

(4) Initial and ongoing evaluation of pain in a non-verbal child is sometimes difficult, and is compounded by normal fears of childhood (e.g., parental separation).

(5) Sedation may be necessary for procedures that require the child to keep very still (e.g., CT scan), thus creating a new set of monitoring requirements.

3. The injured older person (see Chapter 16)

a. Injuries associated with physiologic changes in aging

(1) Hip, humerus, and radius or ulna fractures due to falls complicated by decreasing bone mass such as osteoporosis.

(2) Intracranial hemorrhages from minor head trauma due to either increased vessel fragility or medications that affect clotting; often, these hemorrhages may produce memory or behavior changes that are misidentified as normal aging or Alzheimer's disease.

(3) Motor vehicle accidents and household accidents due to impaired vision, hearing, or mobility; this may include the person either as a driver or as a pedestrian.

(4) Hypothermia because of altered thermoregulation.

b. Injuries caused by medications

(1) Postural hypotension, often associated with anti-hypertensive medications, may cause falls.

(2) Accidental drug overdose because of memory loss may cause falls due to hypotension or cardiac dysrhythmias.

(3) Persons on anticoagulants are at greater risk for significant bleeding in only minor trauma.

(4) Hypovolemia due to diuretic therapy may cause syncope, falls, and injury.

(5) Sedative or hypnotic medications may result in falls, injury, and hypothermia.

c. Injuries due to alcohol use

(1) An often unidentified problem among older people is alcohol use or abuse.

(2) The use of even small amounts of alcohol in combination with medications that affect the blood pressure or the sensorium may result in preventable injury.

Head Injury

1. Head injury can be classified as primary or secondary damage (see Chapter 18).

a. Primary impact damage is that which occurs at the time of impact (e.g., subdural hematoma).

(1) Direct (coup) injury is that done to tissues at the location of the impact.

(2) Indirect (contrecoup) injury results from the shifting of the brain within the cranial vault.

b. Secondary damage results from brain swelling and impaired circulation.

2. Head injuries may be blunt or penetrating and open or closed.

3. The most common types of head injuries seen in the ED are the following:

a. Skull fracture

(1) Linear

(2) Stellate

(3) Depressed

(4) Comminuted

(5) Basilar

b. Contusion: cerebral, cerebellar, and brain stem, in

which there is actual visible tissue damage and varying levels of altered neurologic status

c. Concussion: disruption of neuronal activity that causes immediate, but transient, alterations in mental status, ranging from confusion to unconsciousness and possible antegrade and retrograde memory loss

(1) Concussions are graded I to IV.

(2) Some individuals develop ''postconcussion syndrome,'' which may last weeks, months, or forever; it is characterized by inattentiveness, memory deficits, inability to perform complex tasks, and possibly headache.

d. Hematomas

(1) Epidural hematoma, usually associated with linear skull fracture, most often involving the temporal bone

(2) Subdural hematoma: may be acute, subacute, or chronic

(3) Intracerebral hematoma

e. Hemorrhage

(1) Subarachnoid

(2) Intracerebral

(3) Cerebellar

(4) Brain stem

4. A person with a head injury is assumed to have a cervical spine injury until proved otherwise.

5. General principles in the care of the head-injured person with altered consciousness (see Chapter 18 for more detail)

a. Ensure adequate airway and ventilation; administer high-flow oxygen and hyperventilate to decrease CO_2; maintain neck in neutral position.

b. Ensure circulating volume and cerebral perfusion—establish 1 to 2 large-bore IVs; draw blood for routine laboratory and toxicology; treat hypotension, but do not overresuscitate with IV fluids; use normal saline or Ringer's lactate.

c. Rule out cervical spine injury.

d. Once the cervical spine is cleared, elevate the head of the bed 45 degrees, keeping the neck neutral.

e. Monitor vital signs, oximetry, level of consciousness, Glascow Coma Scale score, and pupil response every 15 minutes until stable.

f. Evaluate carefully for other injuries; diagnostic peritoneal lavage or abdominal CT scan may be done because person is unable to communicate painful areas.

g. Use a Foley catheter to assess for injuries and to monitor the effectiveness of therapy.

h. Although controversial, diuretics such as furosemide or mannitol, or steroids such as dexamethasone or methylprednisolone sodium succinate may be ordered.

i. Insert a nasogastric tube to decrease gastric distention, check for bleeding, or administer antacids; no nasal placement of the tube in possible basilar skull fractures.

j. Registered nurse should accompany the patient for radiology studies (e.g., CT scan).

k. Provide emotional and spiritual support to patient and family.

l. In lethal head injury, introduction of the idea of organ or tissue donation may be considered.

m. In emergency situations, burr holes may be done in the ED to relieve an epidural hematoma; in some facilities, intracranial pressure monitoring may be initiated in the ED when the patient needs lengthy diagnostic testing or immediate surgery for other conditions.

6. Criteria for discharge

a. Diagnostic studies and neurologic evaluation normal

b. Alert and oriented

c. Normal vital signs

d. Responsible adult assumes accountability for observing person for next 24 hours

7. Discharge planning and teaching

a. Complications of head injury may not be present during the initial evaluation and may evolve over hours to weeks; it is critical that the adult patient and caregivers understand this and that there be a responsible adult who commits to careful observation of the patient during the next 24 hours, at a minimum.

b. Decrease activity or rest for the next 24 hours.

c. Have someone awaken the person every 2 hours to ascertain level of consciousness, orientation, motor function.

d. Eat light foods, preferably liquids for 24 hours.

e. Use only aspirin, acetaminophen, or ibuprofen for pain; do not use narcotics unless specifically prescribed.

f. Abstain from alcohol for 24 hours.

g. Mention the possibility of postconcussion syndrome and need for follow-up if symptoms occur or remain.

h. Return to the ED if any of the following symptoms appear:

(1) Headache unrelieved by nonnarcotic analgesics

(2) Altered level of consciousness or behavior

(3) Protracted vomiting (*Note:* Children often have 1 episode of vomiting after an injury, but continued vomiting is a concern.)

(4) Unequal pupils

(5) Weakness or inability to use an arm or leg

(6) Bleeding or clear drainage from the nose or ear

Spinal Column or Cord Injuries
(see Chapter 7 for long-term care)

1. The most common cause of spinal cord injury is trauma due to automobile or motorcycle accidents, falls, gunshot wounds, knife wounds, diving, and sporting accidents.

2. Disorders that may produce spinal cord injury include the following:

a. Tumors of the spinal cord and spinal column (see Chapter 18)

b. Vertebral metastases

c. Osteoporosis, which can result in compression fracture of the vertebrae (see Chapter 34)

d. Vascular disease

3. The most common types of spinal column or cord inju-

ries encountered in the emergency care setting are the following:

   a. Fracture, dislocation, or subluxation of the vertebral body with complete or incomplete transection of the spinal cord, most often in the cervical area

   b. Fracture, dislocation, or subluxation of the vertebral body, pedicles, or lamina without spinal cord injury

   c. Compression fractures of the thoracic or lumbar spine, often without spinal cord injury

4. The mechanisms of injury are the following (Fig. 37–3):

   a. Hyperflexion, such as in a motor vehicle accident

   b. Flexion rotation

   c. Hyperextension, due to a fall on the chin, or during endotracheal intubation in people with cervical spondylolisthesis or arthritis

   d. Axial loading, impact to the top of the head

   e. Compression, most often due to a fall from a height, landing on feet or buttocks but also seen spontaneously in older people, those with osteoporosis or spondylitis, or those with malignancy

   f. Penetrating wound (e.g., gunshot or stab wound)

   g. Cervical and lumbar fractures are considered unstable because of flexibility in those areas; thoracic fractures are considered more stable.

   h. The absence of motion or sensation in a person with an apparent spinal cord injury does not necessarily mean there is permanent cord damage; the potential exists for reversible injury such as cord impingement or spinal shock, which is causing the symptoms; thus, all persons with an apparent spinal cord

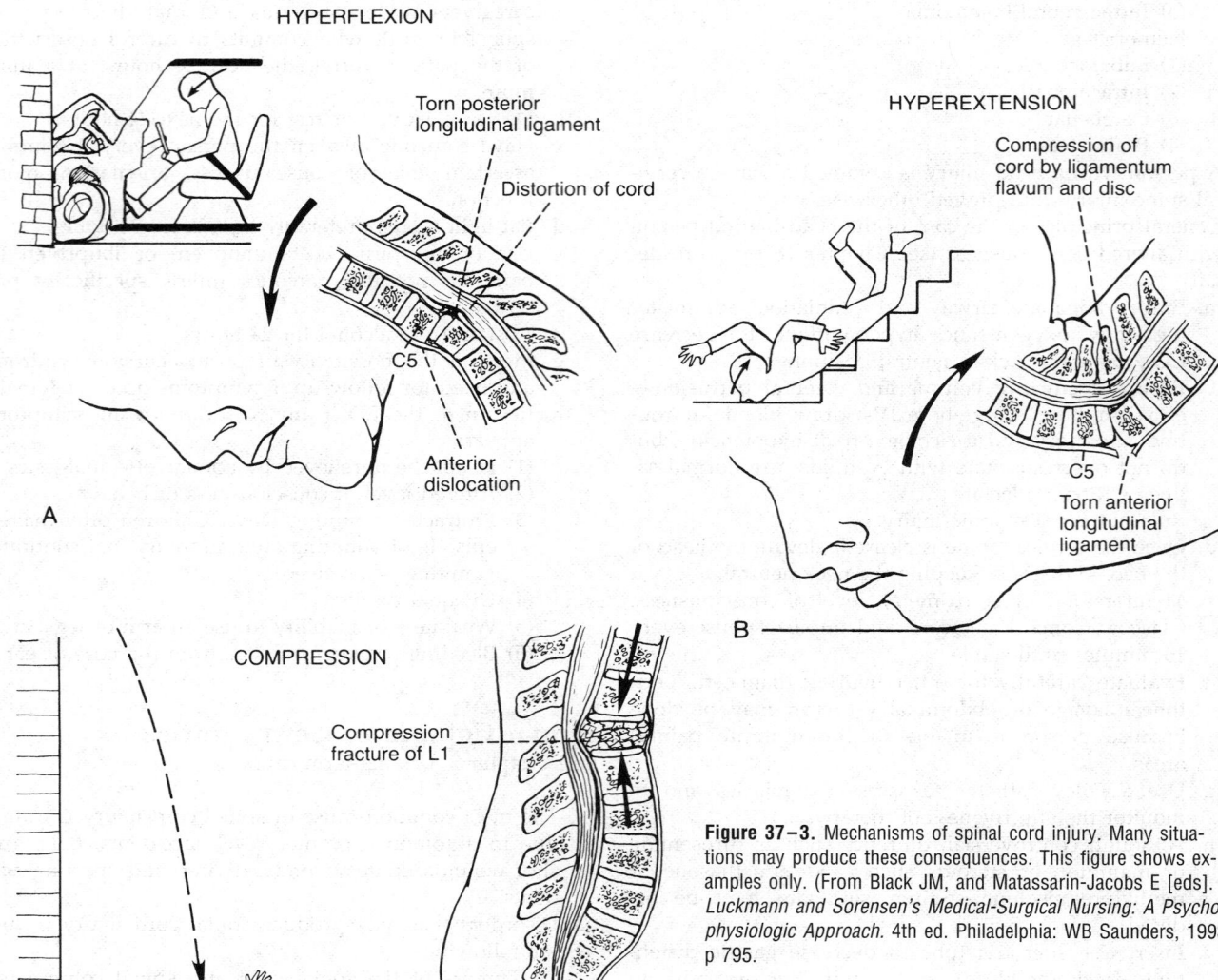

Figure 37–3. Mechanisms of spinal cord injury. Many situations may produce these consequences. This figure shows examples only. (From Black JM, and Matassarin-Jacobs E [eds]. *Luckmann and Sorensen's Medical-Surgical Nursing: A Psychophysiologic Approach.* 4th ed. Philadelphia: WB Saunders, 1993, p 795.

injury should be handled as if the condition were reversible.

5. Level of injury
    a. Injury to the spinal cord occurs when the vertebral column is displaced mechanically owing to trauma or tumors and the spinal cord tissues and nerve roots are compressed, pulled, or torn.
    b. Cervical spine and cord injuries produce quadriplegia.
    c. Thoracic and lumbar spinal injuries produce paraplegia.
    d. Injuries above the 4th cervical vertebra may cause death because of loss of innervation to the diaphragm and intercostal muscles.
    e. Ischemia, edema, and hemorrhage resulting from trauma also contribute to loss of spinal cord function.

6. Clinical manifestations
    a. Clinical manifestations depend on the level and severity of cord injury.
    b. Complete transection of the cord produces 2 stages: spinal shock and spasticity.
        (1) Spinal shock (which lasts from 7 days to 3 months) results in immediate loss of all sensation and function below the level of transection. Shock resolves when reflexes return.
        (2) Spasticity is a sign that recovery is progressing. On movement, the patient's limbs spasm into extension. Muscle spasms may be mild or violent. Cold weather and emotional upsets may trigger muscle spasms.
    c. Incomplete cord damage causes a variety of impairments, depending on the level of injury (Table 37–15).

7. Diagnostics
    a. Radiograph of the spinal column
    b. An MRI scan

8. Clinical management
    a. Immobilization
        (1) Cervical spine: Hard cervical collar, neck secured in immobilization device, spine board
        (2) Other fractures: Spine board
    b. ABCs—Spinal neural tissue is just as sensitive to hypoxemia as intracranial neural tissue, and the goal is to minimize tissue swelling; thus oxygen may be administered, and mechanical ventilation provided if respiratory effort is inadequate. Carefully monitor oxygen saturation, especially in thoracic and cervical cord injuries; respiratory failure may be insidious. Spinal shock, characterized by hypotension and bradycardia, may require IV fluids, vasoconstrictor agents, or both.
    c. High-dose steroids, although controversial, may be administered IV.
    d. Foley catheter
    e. Nasogastric tube, although this may be deferred if it poses a risk of movement or aspiration.
    f. Cervical traction through the use of Gardner-Wells spring-loaded tongs, inserted into the outer table of the skull just above the ears, and the attachment of weights (see Procedure 37–3).
    g. Cervical immobilization through the use of a halo device (see Chapter 18)
    h. If MRI scanning is anticipated, nonferrous tongs made out of carbon are used.
    i. When tongs are used, or when no traction is anticipated, the patient is placed on a special bed that allows for immobilization yet permits rotation of the

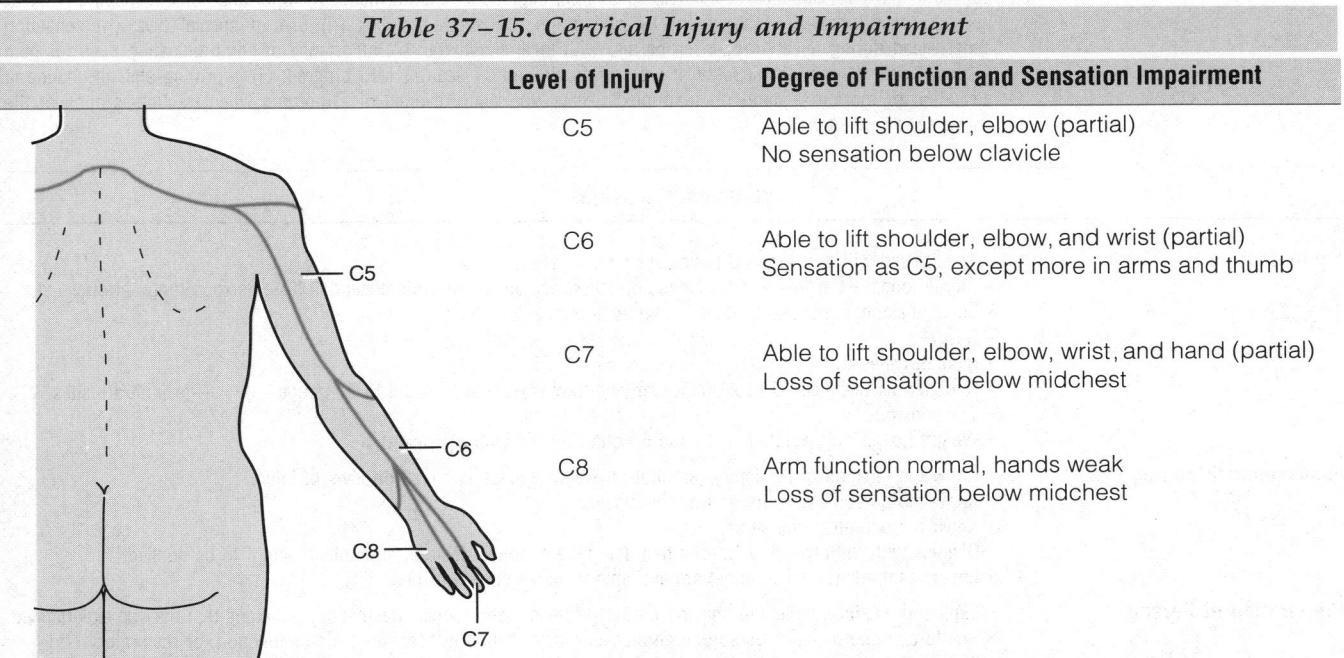

Table 37–15. *Cervical Injury and Impairment*

	Level of Injury	Degree of Function and Sensation Impairment
	C5	Able to lift shoulder, elbow (partial) No sensation below clavicle
	C6	Able to lift shoulder, elbow, and wrist (partial) Sensation as C5, except more in arms and thumb
	C7	Able to lift shoulder, elbow, wrist, and hand (partial) Loss of sensation below midchest
	C8	Arm function normal, hands weak Loss of sensation below midchest

From Black JM, and Matassarin-Jacobs E (eds). *Luckmann and Sorensen's Medical-Surgical Nursing: A Psychophysiologic Approach.* 5th ed. Philadelphia: WB Saunders, 1997.

bed from side to side or front to back to prevent pneumonia and other hazards of immobility. Note that if the patient must be transported by ambulance or helicopter, a Stryker frame or similar-size device is necessary; larger beds will not fit into these vehicles. Special spring traction devices are available to avoid the use of free-swinging weights in a moving vehicle.

j. Raise the head end of the bed to prevent weights from resting on the floor.

Procedure 37–3
Tong Insertion for Cervical Spine Traction

Definition/Purpose

Insertion of Gardner-Wells or Heifetz tongs into the scalp and application of cervical spine traction. Gardner-Wells are two-pronged; Heifetz are three-pronged; the third prong minimizes flexion or extension. Purpose is to reduce or realign cervical spine fracture or dislocation to prevent or minimize damage to spinal nerves or cord.

Contraindications/Cautions

Tong insertion is performed by a physician, usually a neurosurgeon. Tongs are generally not used in stable vertebral body compression fractures or fractures of the cervical spinous processes, unless there is ligamentous disruption. Maintain cervical spine immobilization via hard cervical collar until traction is achieved. Weights are applied and removed gradually under the supervision of a physician. Avoid sudden increase or decrease of traction or sudden movement of the bed or patient. Most stretchers are not designed to accommodate cervical tong traction; obtain the patient's hospital bed to avoid moving the person once the traction has been applied. A special therapy bed is often used. If transfer to another facility is required, a Stryker frame may be used, because it will fit into most ambulances and helicopters. A Collins spring-loaded traction device can be attached to a Stryker frame to prevent the hazard of swinging weights during air transport. Tongs are not inserted over skull fracture sites because of the creation of an open skull fracture and the possibility of intracranial infection. Radiographic confirmation of alignment is recommended each time weights are added or removed. If MRI is planned, special nonferrous tongs are used.

Complete seating of tongs may take 24 or more hours; they may slip out at any time. Hourly assessment of traction status is recommended. The traction may gradually pull the person to the head of the bed, with the weights resting on the floor, negating the traction. This can be minimized by elevating the head *end* (not the head) of the bed so that the body weight provides countertraction. Weights must hang free at all times.

The actual insertion of tongs is usually not painful because local anesthesia is injected over the insertion site; however, narcotic analgesia may be indicated for neck pain from the realignment and muscle spasm.

Learning/Teaching Activities

Provide the following information: (a) description of procedure, regardless of person's level of consciousness; (b) preparatory procedures (e.g., shaving small area of head, sensation of local anesthetic); (c) precautions that will be taken during movement to a special bed, especially if this will occur before tong insertion and traction application; (d) continuance of cervical collar until alignment is confirmed; (e) importance of not moving head or neck; (f) confirmation of alignment by radiograph, CT scan, or MRI; (g) use of special bed; (h) sensation experienced during injection of insertion site with local anesthetic; (i) importance of communicating need for pain management; (j) need for sedation if claustrophobic and CT scan or MRI ordered; (j) informing staff of change in sensation or motion (a para- or quadriplegic may experience reversal of symptoms when traction is applied; the converse is true as well).

Preliminary Activities

Equipment

- Special bed with traction and pulley system
- Sterile tongs—Gardner-Wells, Heifetz, or other, per physician preference; ask if nonferrous tongs are needed
- Local anesthetic, usually Lidocaine with epinephrine
- Razor
- Alcohol wipes
- Hypodermic needles: 18 to 20 gauge to withdraw anesthetic, and 25 to 27 gauge—1½"—to infiltrate sites
- Traction rope
- Weight holder and weights: 1, 2, and 5 pound (check with physician)

Assessment/Planning

- Know the location of the injury (amount of weight applied is based on level of injury).
- Know the person's sensory and motor function.
- Know the person's vital signs.
- Discuss with the physician: special bed use, type of tongs desired, amount of weight to be applied.
- Ensure that adequate personnel are available to move person to bed.

Preparation of Person

- Explain procedure, including shaving portion of head, use of local anesthetic, sensations that may be experienced.
- Reinforce importance of person communicating any change in sensation, motor function, or respiratory effort.
- Explain the use of special bed, including asking for antiemetic if nausea develops with rotation.
- Explain need for repeat radiographs or special procedures after insertion (e.g., CT scan, MRI).

P

Procedure 37–3
(continued)

Procedure—Gardner-Wells Tongs

Actions (* = physician activity)	Rationale/Discussion
1. Shave a 5-cm area 2 cm above each ear.	1. Promotes cleansing of insertion area.
2. Cleanse area with antiseptic solution.	2. Minimizes potential for infection.
3. *Infiltrate insertion sites with local anesthetic.	3. Minimizes pain from tong insertion.
4. *Place Gardner-Wells tong points on scalp below temporal ridge in line with the external ear canal, and tighten each pin until the spring-loaded portion of each pin extends approximately 1 mm.	4. Placement promotes proper alignment for traction; turning screw seats pins into scalp.
5. *Gently rock tongs back and forth.	5. Assists in seating tongs in skull.
6. Apply S-ring (if not already in place) and attach rope through pulley.	6. S-ring holds the rope to which the weightholder is attached; pulley height determines degree of cervical extension or flexion.
7. *Gradually add desired weights based on location of fracture/dislocation, usually 5 pounds for each cervical vertebra (e.g., C-3 fracture = 15 pounds of weight).	7. Weights are added gradually to avoid sudden movement of the cervical spine.
8. Assess motor and sensory function.	8. Traction may reverse or cause cord impingement.
9. Obtain cervical spine radiograph.	9. Used to assess alignment and traction effectiveness.
10. Apply antiseptic-soaked dressing around each pin insertion site.	10. Decreases potential for infection.
11. Place a small towel under person's neck; do not hyperextend the neck.	11. Provides comfort and support.
12. Place rolled towels, sponge blocks, or sand bags on either side of the head.	12. Minimizes side motion of head.

Final Activities

Document procedure, amount of weight applied, how procedure was tolerated, and sensory and motor status. Transport person slowly and gently, avoiding bumps and sudden stops or starts. Prevent weights from swinging. A registered nurse should accompany the person to continuously observe traction and patient response during transport.

---

k. Pain management: Although the person may have no sensation below the level of damage, there is often pain at the fracture site that should be treated; small doses of IV narcotics that can be titrated are preferred, especially because of the potential for spinal shock and impaired vasoconstriction, which might be exacerbated with large doses of narcotics.

l. Surgical exploration and decompression may be used in selected individuals, especially in the case of penetrating wound of the cord or column.

m. Psychologic support and social service referral: Spinal cord injury with permanent loss of function is a devastating condition that requires prompt and sustained psychologic support for the patient and family; crisis intervention and referral for assistance should be made early in the course of treatment. In the initial period after the injury, it is difficult to predict what the long-term outcome will be; hopefulness and honesty are paramount.

n. The long-term care of patients with spinal cord in-

jury is discussed in Chapter 7. The care of patients with spinal cord injury due to tumors of the spinal cord and spinal column is discussed in Chapter 18.

9. Complications

a. Autonomic dysreflexia (hyperreflexia) is a true emergency that may occur at any time: during the acute phase of spinal cord injury, during the rehabilitation period, during the 1st 1 or 2 years following injury, and up to 6 years following injury.

(1) This condition is defined as an uninhibited and exaggerated reflex response to noxious stimuli, such as pain, a distended bladder or rectum, or pressure on the patient's skin. It affects 85 percent of all patients with spinal cord injury above the level of the 6th thoracic vertebra.

(2) Clinical manifestations include immediate severe hypertension, a pounding headache, sweating, flushing of the skin above the level of injury, profuse diaphoresis, blurred vision, bradycardia, and nausea.

(3) Emergency care involves careful monitoring of the patient's blood pressure, elevation of the head of the bed to sitting level, administration of antihypertensives as prescribed (see Chapter 23), and checking the patient for the causative condition (e.g., bladder distention, bowel distention, a kinked catheter, or pain).

(4) Long-term measures include the prevention of constipation and impaction (see Chapters 7 and 27), urinary retention and urinary tract infections (see Chapters 7 and 26), skin ulcerations, and pressure sores (see Chapter 7).

b. Respiratory insufficiency

(1) Depending on the level of injury, the patient's intercostal and abdominal muscles may be paralyzed and the diaphragmatic muscle impaired. As a result, the patient may have an ineffective or weak cough. Also, vital capacity and inspiratory reserve volume may greatly diminish.

(2) To enhance vital capacity, teach the patient to use incentive spirometry and to perform diaphragmatic breathing (see Chapter 22).

(3) To maintain the airway, suction the person as needed and provide adequate fluids. Some patients may require mechanical ventilation (see Chapter 22).

(4) To promote effective coughing by the quadriplegic patient, do the following:

· Place the patient in a supine or low semi-Fowler's position.

· Place your hands on either side of the patient's rib cage or upper abdomen below the diaphragm.

· As the patient takes a deep breath, push upward to help the patient expand the lungs and cough.

· As the patient exhales and coughs, push your hands forward and down. This technique is sometimes called "assisted coughing," "cough assist," or the "quad cough."

c. Neurogenic bladder (see Chapters 7 and 26)

d. Respiratory and urinary infections (see Chapters 22 and 26)

e. Thromboembolitic disorders due to immobility (see Chapter 24)

f. Depression due to a loss of hope and a sense of powerlessness (see Chapter 7)

10. Applying the nursing process: The following nursing diagnoses may apply in the immediate and long-term care of the person with a spinal cord injury.

a. Ineffective airway clearance R/T weak cough reflex secondary to paralysis or impairment of respiratory muscles

b. Urinary retention R/T neuromuscular and sensory motor impairment

c. Constipation R/T neuromuscular impairment

d. Bowel incontinence R/T damage to sacral nerves that control anal sphincter

e. Thrombophlebitis R/T loss of muscle contraction in lower extremities and loss of venous return

f. Risk for injury R/T sensory deficit

g. Risk for impaired skin integrity R/T sensory deficits

h. Risk for autonomic dysreflexia R/T spinal cord injury

i. Pain R/T spinal cord injury

j. Impaired mobility R/T paralysis

k. Self-care deficit R/T loss of function secondary to spinal cord injury

l. Body image disturbance R/T paralysis and change in body functioning

m. Powerlessness R/T loss of independence and control over self-care

n. Anticipatory grieving R/T sudden change in body image and loss of independence

o. Sexual dysfunction R/T spinal cord injury

11. Discharge planning and teaching

a. The spectrum of problems associated with spinal cord injury is significant; care is best accomplished at a center that specializes in spinal cord injury management.

b. Transportation of such an individual requires a well-coordinated effort; consultation with the referral center regarding timing and mode of transport is important.

Chest Injury

1. The most common chest injuries

a. Hemothorax

b. Pneumothorax—simple or tension

c. Pulmonary contusion

d. Cardiac contusion

e. Aortic laceration or dissection

f. Rib fractures, with and without a flail segment

g. Sternum fracture

h. Pericardial tamponade

2. Mechanisms of injury

a. The majority of blunt chest injuries are seen in drivers involved in front impact motor vehicle accidents and in persons ejected or thrown from a vehicle.

b. Drivers are particularly at risk because the chest is thrust against the steering wheel, causing rib fractures, hemothorax, pulmonary and cardiac contusion, pericardial tamponade, and deceleration laceration of the thoracic aorta; the use of air bags may decrease these types of injuries dramatically.

c. Gunshot wounds most often create hemopneumothorax with massive bleeding; gunshot or stab wounds of the heart may cause pericardial tamponade or cardiac arrest due to laceration of coronary arteries.

d. Rib fractures can result from either blunt or penetrating trauma and may produce hemopneumothorax; fractures of the 1st or 2nd rib are particularly dangerous because of potential for lacerating major vessels such as the subclavian artery or vein.

e. Severe chest injuries that crush the chest and push the fractured rib segments into the lung tissue produce a flail chest (Fig. 37–4). This critical problem may be further complicated by hemopneumothorax. Pulmonary edema and atelectasis may also develop rapidly (see Chapter 22).

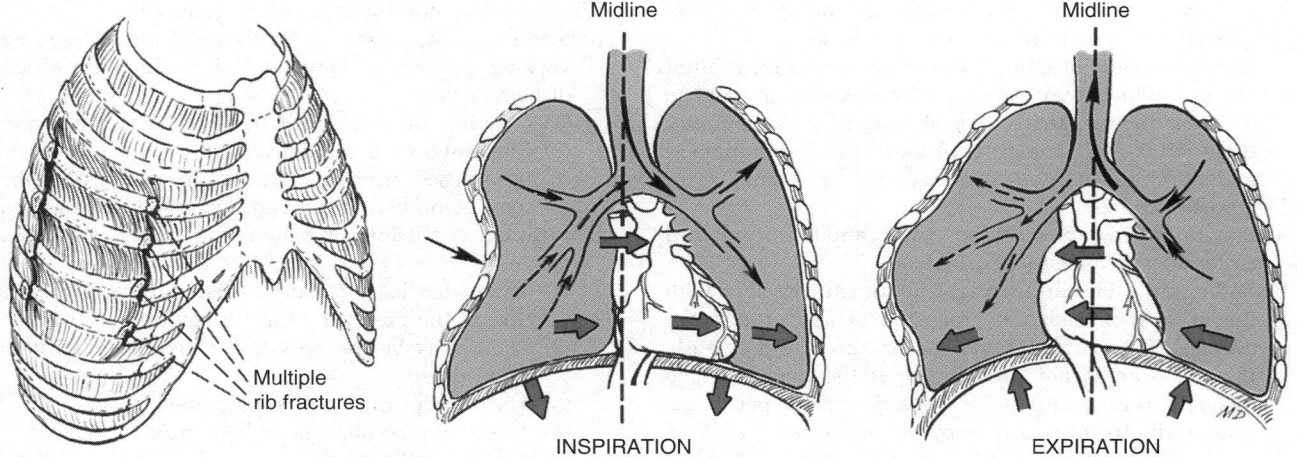

Midline   Midline

INSPIRATION   EXPIRATION

Figure 37–4. Flail chest. Thin solid arrows indicate air movement; thick arrows, structural movement. *A,* A flail chest consists of fractured rib segments that are unattached (free-floating) from the rest of the chest wall. *B,* On inspiration, the flail segment of ribs is "sucked" inward. The affected lung and mediastinal structures shift to the unaffected side. This compromises the amount of inspired air in the unaffected lung. *C,* On expiration, the flail segment of ribs "bellows" outward. The affected lung and mediastinal structures shift to the affected side. Some air within the lungs is shunted back and forth between the lungs instead of passing through the upper airway. (From Black JM, and Matassarin-Jacobs E [eds]. *Luckmann and Sorensen's Medical-Surgical Nursing: A Psychophysiologic Approach.* 4th ed. Philadelphia: WB Saunders, 1993, p 2237.)

3. History and physical examination
   a. Use of shoulder and lap restraint.
   b. The condition of the steering wheel: A deformed steering wheel suggests a high likelihood of pulmonary contusion, cardiac contusion, and aortic injury.
   c. The condition of the windshield: If the windshield shows a star pattern from the impact of the driver's head, there is a strong likelihood of chest injury.
   d. Chest and abdominal assessment
4. Diagnostic studies
   a. Chest radiograph
   b. Oxygen saturation
   c. Arterial blood gases
   d. A 12-lead ECG
   e. Chest CT or ultrasound
   f. Aortogram
   g. Cardiac enzymes
5. Clinical management of these conditions is focused on maintaining an adequate airway and ventilation; maintaining adequate cardiac output and perfusion; treating hemo- or pneumothorax.
   a. Chest tube or tubes for evacuation of air or blood
   b. Autotransfusion: have equipment ready to be attached to the chest drainage system
   c. Pericardiocentesis
   d. In rare instances, an open thoracotomy may be done to stop bleeding by cross-clamping the aorta or to repair holes in the heart.
   e. Pain management: If person is normotensive, medicate with IV narcotics before insertion of the chest tube, which is a painful procedure.
6. Criteria for discharge
   a. Chest radiograph, arterial blood gases, and oxygen saturation normal; note that a small pneumothorax of less than 20 percent may be treated on an outpatient basis, with either the insertion of a small catheter to remove air or observation only.

b. ECG and cardiac enzymes normal
   c. Vital signs within normal limits
   d. Pain controlled
7. Discharge planning and teaching
   a. Return if increasing chest pain, difficulty breathing, fatigue (may be due to blood loss from a small leaking thoracic aortic injury), hemoptysis.
   b. Discuss follow-up care, especially if catheter for relief of pneumothorax is inserted.
   c. Review pain management.

Abdominal Injury

1. Abdominal injury may result from either blunt or penetrating trauma and may result from even minor trauma.
2. The structures most often affected in blunt trauma are the following:
   a. Liver
   b. Spleen
   c. Pancreas
   d. Abdominal aorta, primarily in a motor vehicle accident when the person is wearing a lap belt without shoulder belt; flexion injury to the lumbar vertebrae also occurs from this mechanism.
   e. Normally hollow organs that are fluid-filled are at greater risk (e.g., full urinary bladder).
3. All abdominal structures and the spinal cord are at risk in penetrating trauma, especially that due to high-velocity gunshot wound; the structures that are damaged cannot be predicted by the wound of entry or exit, as bullets ricochet, turn, and twist along their path.
   a. Even when the bullet does not penetrate the peritoneum, the shock wave created by the bullet can damage deeper structures.
   b. Because of uncertainty about the location of the diaphragm when the bullet or knife wound is sustained,

penetrating wounds at or below the nipple are considered both chest and abdominal injuries.

   c. Retroperitoneal bleeding most often results from blunt trauma, which may cause pelvic fracture or damage to the kidneys, pancreas, or abdominal aorta; because these structures are retroperitoneal, the abdominal examination and peritoneal lavage may be normal.

4. Diagnostic studies
   a. Laboratory: complete blood count, amylase, type and crossmatch, chemistries, urinalysis
   b. Radiograph: Flat and upright abdomen, possibly with the upright preceded by injection of air through the nasogastric tube; abdominal CT or ultrasound or both.
   c. If a CT scan is not possible, or if the person is too unstable to undergo a CT scan, a diagnostic peritoneal lavage (discussed earlier) may be performed.

5. Clinical management of the person with abdominal trauma centers primarily around assessment and treatment of intra-abdominal bleeding and surgical repair of injured structures.
   a. Vigorous volume resuscitation may be needed.
   b. The shock suit may be used to tamponade intra-abdominal or retroperitoneal bleeding as a temporizing measure.
   c. A nasogastric tube for diagnostic and therapeutic purposes.
   d. A Foley catheter: Observe for blood at the urinary meatus that may suggest urethral injury and pelvic fracture.
   e. Intravenous antibiotics, if penetrating trauma or probable bowel injury.
   f. Small splenic injuries may be treated conservatively by observation rather than removing the spleen.
   g. Pain management: small doses of IV narcotics titrated for relief.
   h. If the results of diagnostic studies are negative, the person may be discharged with careful discharge teaching.
   i. Wounds that are not felt to penetrate the peritoneum may be explored, irrigated well, and sutured.
   j. Provide tetanus prophylaxis, if wounds are present.

6. Criteria for discharge
   a. Normal vital signs, including postural vital signs
   b. Pain controlled
   c. Adequate hemostasis of wounds
   d. Reliable patient or responsible adult to observe for complications

7. Discharge planning and teaching
   a. Blunt trauma to the abdomen may result in delayed rupture of the spleen or injuries not readily apparent at the time of visit; return to the ED if there is increasing abdominal pain, fatigue, or weakness.
   b. Return for reevaluation if hematuria, fever, or blood in stools occurs.
   c. Return for wound care follow-up, if appropriate.

Common Injuries: Genitourinary Trauma

1. Includes renal, urinary bladder, urethral, and penile injury (see Chapter 26 for a detailed discussion)

2. The most common injuries are the following:
   a. Contusion, laceration, or avulsion of the kidney, with varying degrees of hematuria, including the absence of hematuria
     (1) May be due to blunt or penetrating trauma
     (2) May involve the kidney itself, or the ureter may be avulsed from the kidney, in which case there may be no hematuria and decreased urine output
   b. Rupture, contusion, or penetrating injury of the bladder
     (1) These injuries most often result from pelvic fracture in the presence of a full bladder.
     (2) There may be the sensation to void but an inability to do so.
     (3) The bladder may not be palpable.
     (4) There may be oliguria or hematuria.
   c. Contused, lacerated, or transected urethra, with varying degrees of urinary retention
   d. Contused or lacerated penis, scrotum, or perineum; lacerations may produce significant blood loss
   e. Fractured or deformed penis with urethral obstruction
   f. Foreign bodies of the urethra or bladder, which may be asymptomatic or may cause hematuria or obstruction
   g. Testicular torsion, which is most often spontaneous, but may be due to trauma

3. Triage priority depends on condition and impact on hemodynamic status and reproductive potential; the following are usually a high priority:
   a. Lacerations that cause significant blood loss
   b. Obstructive injuries
   c. Testicular torsion, which requires urgent correction to prevent loss of blood supply to the area

4. Assessment: Nonspecific, but ability to void and hematuria are key elements.
   a. Doppler study may be used to assess blood supply in testicular torsion.
   b. A CT scan is used to evaluate renal trauma.
   c. Intravenous pyelogram and cystourethrogram may be used to assess hematuria.

5. Clinical management
   a. Cardiovascular stabilization
   b. Access for elimination, either urethral or via suprapubic tube
   c. Most significant injuries are treated surgically.
   d. Contusions that may impede voiding may be treated with a Foley catheter until the swelling subsides.
   e. Penile fracture may be treated with a catheter and splinting after realignment.
   f. Psychologic support and reassurance
     (1) Injuries involving the genitalia are often embarrassing; provide privacy and respect.
     (2) Male patients are often particularly concerned about the impact of the injury on their sexual function and reproductive potential; provide factual information about prognosis.

6. Criteria for discharge
   a. Able to void normally or urinary catheter in place
   b. Hematuria resolving
   c. Pain controlled
   d. Hemodynamically stable

7. Discharge planning and teaching
   a. Instructions depend on condition.
   b. Apply ice to injured tissue.
   c. Return if urinary retention, increasing bleeding, or evidence of infection.
   d. Remind the patient to pay careful attention to keeping wounds clean and dry.
   e. Provide information about when person can resume normal sexual activity, if appropriate.
   f. Discuss follow-up care, if needed.

Maxillofacial; Ear, Nose, and Throat; and Dental Injuries

1. Most common injuries include the following:
   a. Facial lacerations
   b. Fractures
      (1) Nasal bones
      (2) Maxilla
      (3) Mandible
      (4) Combinations of fractures known as Le Forte I, II, and III
         • Le Forte III are the most serious, involving the maxilla, zygoma, and nasal bones.
         • Fractures result from direct blow that creates a dishlike depression of the midface.
         • These fractures are serious because of the potential for airway obstruction.
   c. Epistaxis
   d. Hematoma, especially of the ear, creating a cauliflower ear
   e. Ruptured tympanic membrane, with bleeding, impaired hearing, and potential for infection
   f. Dental injury: avulsion, intrusion into socket, or fracture of the tooth
   g. Esophageal injury due to foreign body (e.g., bolus of food, bone [such as a fish bone], or small battery [in children]), or ingestion of caustic substance such as lye
   h. Laryngeal fracture
   i. Penetrating wounds of the neck
   j. Facial injuries may also be associated with significant central nervous system or eye injury.
2. Triage priority
   a. Injuries that cause actual or potential airway obstruction, ingestions, significant blood loss, and avulsed teeth are considered high priority.
   b. Injuries that cause disfigurement (e.g., nasal fracture) may be delayed if other concerns are absent.
3. Assessment
   a. ABCs
   b. Provide the patient with a mirror to help identify if there is injury present.
   c. Ask if dental alignment is normal for the patient.
   d. Be alert to hoarseness, which may suggest a laryngeal fracture.
   e. Assess hearing, if there is an ear injury.
   f. Palpation can often identify fractures.
4. Diagnostic studies
   a. Face, mandible, or neck radiographs
   b. Special dental radiographs (e.g., panograph), which are usually not available in a hospital
   c. Special swallowing studies for possible foreign body
   d. Endoscopic studies for foreign body or ingestions
5. Clinical management is condition specific.
   a. Nasal fractures may be left alone initially until the swelling subsides or may be realigned and splinted.
   b. Epistaxis is controlled with hemostasis agents (e.g., silver nitrate stick, collagen products), or with anterior or posterior packing.
   c. Avulsed or extruded teeth require immediate care to prevent permanent loss.
      (1) If completely out of the socket, gently rinse the tooth with saline.
      (2) Do not clean the tooth with sponges or a brush; this may damage the periodontal ligaments necessary for reattachment.
      (3) Return the tooth to the socket.
      (4) If this cannot be accomplished, put the tooth in a special tooth-saving solution (e.g., Save a Tooth), in milk, or under the person's tongue (if alert, oriented, and able to comply).
      (5) Reimplantation should be done immediately; after 15 to 30 minutes the likelihood of long-term success is minimal.
   d. Fractured teeth can be stabilized with a wax bridge.
   e. Control oral cavity bleeding with a dental roll and firm continuous pressure for 5 to 10 minutes.
   f. Significant facial fractures may be managed surgically.
   g. Penetrating neck wounds are evaluated in the operating room because of potential for damage to major structures.
   h. Hematomas of the ear may be evacuated and a pressure dressing applied.
   i. A ruptured tympanic membrane generally heals spontaneously, although antibiotic eardrops are often used.
   j. Larynx fracture.
      (1) Managed by hospitalization and observation because of the potential for airway obstruction
      (2) Endotracheal intubation or surgical airway (e.g., cricothyroidotomy or tracheotomy may be necessary)
   k. Esophageal foreign bodies
      (1) Food obstruction may be treated with the use of IV glucagon to relax the esophageal smooth muscle, allowing the foreign body to be swallowed.
      (2) Bones, batteries, and immovable food are removed by esophagoscopy.
      (3) There is the potential for serious infection involving the mediastinum, if esophageal perforation has occurred.
   l. Caustic substance ingestion
      (1) Usually requires endoscopy and hospitalization to observe for perforation of the esophagus or stomach
      (2) Antacids may be administered initially.
      (3) Nasogastric tube insertion is deferred to ear, nose, and throat specialist.
6. Discharge criteria. See specific conditions in Chapter 20.
7. Discharge planning and teaching. See specific conditions in Chapter 20.

Orthopedic Emergencies

1. Detailed assessment and management of orthopedic problems are discussed in Chapter 34. The focus in this section is on common problems and special considerations in emergency care. Common or significant orthopedic problems are the following:
   a. Sprains
      (1) Ankle
      (2) Knee
      (3) Wrist
   b. Strains
      (1) Lumbosacral
      (2) Cervical
      (3) Ankle
   c. Fractures
      (1) Humerus
      (2) Radius or ulna
      (3) Navicular of hand
      (4) Fifth metacarpal (boxer's fracture)
      (5) Pelvis
      (6) Femur
      (7) Patella
      (8) Tibia or fibula
      (9) Calcaneus
      (10) Fifth metatarsal
   d. Dislocation—either alone or in combination with a fracture
      (1) Shoulder
      (2) Elbow
      (3) Wrist
      (4) Fingers or toes
      (5) Hip or hip prosthesis
      (6) Knee
      (7) Patella
      (8) Ankle
   e. Tendon injuries
      (1) Flexor and extensor tendons of the fingers or hand due to blunt or penetrating trauma
      (2) Ruptured Achilles tendon
   f. Compartment syndrome—discussed in Chapter 34
2. Most significant concerns in the initial assessment and management
   a. Prevention and treatment of hemorrhagic shock, most often associated with pelvic and femoral fractures
   b. Arterial entrapment or rupture seen in hip and knee dislocation
   c. Nerve damage, most often seen in humeral fractures, and elbow and knee dislocations
   d. Pain management, especially with shoulder, hip, knee, and ankle dislocations and femoral fractures (the powerful contraction of the thigh muscles causes bone ends to override, increasing the pain)
   e. Infection, especially in open fractures, and in tendon injuries of the hand due to human bites
   f. Injuries that are difficult to diagnose, most often the navicular fracture and partial tendon injuries due to penetrating trauma
   g. Potential for, or presence of, compartment syndrome, primarily in fractures of the radius, ulna, or tibia and fibula

3. Triage priority
   a. Highest priority: injuries that have potential for significant blood loss, are very painful, and have impaired distal circulation, severely angulated fractures, and dislocations of major joints
   b. Intermediate priority: Digit dislocations, long bone fractures that can be splinted, potential tendon lacerations
   c. Lowest priority: sprains, strains, probable small bone fractures
4. Routine orthopedic assessment includes the following:
   a. History
      (1) Chief complaint—usually reported pain or observation of child's reluctance to use extremity
      (2) Mechanism of injury (e.g., inversion or eversion injury of the ankle)
      (3) When did injury occur?
      (4) Sensations or sounds (e.g., popping, cracking, ripping) at the time of injury
      (5) Ability to use area after the injury
      (6) Treatments initiated before arrival
         • Despite first aid teaching to apply ice to an injured area, many people persist in applying heat or soaking the part in hot epsom salt solutions immediately after the injury, thereby increasing swelling and rendering physical evaluation quite difficult.
         • Use of analgesics may cloud the pain assessment.
      (7) Pinpoint location of pain with 1 finger; radiation or other painful areas (e.g., inversion injuries of the ankle) are often associated with fracture of the 5th metatarsal or avulsion fracture of the fibula at the knee.
      (8) Occupation may influence who, where, and how injury is treated, and degree of contamination if open injury.
   b. Physical examination
      (1) Evidence of deformity, swelling, wounds, bleeding, poor skin color
      (2) Guarding or nonuse of injured part
      (3) Pulses, capillary refill, sensation, range of motion (ask the person to perform the activity, but do not attempt movement of elbow or knee joints that appear dislocated)
         • Mark pulses on feet with an X so that subsequent examiners can easily locate the pulse.
      (4) Gently palpate the area to determine location of pain, and presence of crepitus, or deformity.
      (5) Compare injured extremity with uninjured extremity.
      (6) Perform other standard assessment parameters.
   c. Diagnostic studies
      (1) Plain radiographs: Comparison views are often performed in children because of the difficulty of identifying fractures when the epiphyses are not calcified.
      (2) Compartment pressure monitoring may be performed in persons with radius, ulna, or tibia and fibula fractures.
      (3) Perform arteriogram or venogram, if vascular injury suspected.

(4) Arterial blood gases may be performed in the person with a femoral fracture because of the potential for fat emboli.

(5) Obtain a complete blood count and other routine laboratory tests if major blood loss suspected, or if operative management is required.

(6) A 12-lead ECG is routinely performed in older patients with a fractured hip because a cardiac event may have precipitated the fall, or because surgery will be required.

5. Clinical management

a. Hemodynamic stabilization

(1) Pelvic and femoral fractures may be associated with significant blood loss; patients may deteriorate during radiographic studies.

(2) Establish at least 1 large-bore IV line before movement to radiography.

b. Immobilization of fractures or dislocations is an early priority.

(1) Immobilization decreases pain significantly.

(2) It prevents vascular or nerve injuries from moving bone fragments.

(3) Many injuries can be immobilized with a standard padded splint.

(4) Femoral fracture often requires ankle hitch traction, along with Hare, Sager, or Thomas immobilization splint.

(5) Immobilize shoulder dislocations with the person sitting upright, the elbow bent, and the forearm resting on a pillow or in a sling; some patients prefer to lie face down on the stretcher, with the shoulder hanging over the side. This maneuver sometimes results in spontaneous relocation.

(6) Immobilize humeral fractures with elbow in flexion and a sling and swathe applied to keep the humerus against the lateral chest wall.

(7) Elbow or knee dislocation usually manifests with the joint in flexion, and it should remain in that position until radiographs are done; manipulation of the joint may cause vascular or nerve damage. Place pillows under joint for support.

(8) Splint severely angulated injuries with a moldable device such as a pillow, rather than a straight splint; do not attempt to straighten the extremity.

(9) Assess extremity pulse and sensation after splint application and after manipulation in radiography.

(10) Cover open fractures with a sterile moist saline or antiseptic solution dressing.

c. Apply ice pack with compression around the entire area, not just on the dorsum, to minimize swelling.

d. Pain management

(1) Some fractures or dislocations are extremely painful, warranting IV narcotics as soon as possible after arrival; IM narcotics are of little value in acute management.

(2) Relocation of dislocations or closed reduction of fractures other than the digits is often accomplished under IV conscious sedation; facility monitoring protocols should be carried out.

(3) In most instances, reduction or realignment and stabilization with plaster or fiberglass splinting result in dramatic reduction in pain; pain after these are accomplished necessitates reevaluation.

e. Definitive management

(1) Most fractures are splinted, rather than casted, because the postinjury swelling usually continues for 12 to 24 hours, and the cast could become too tight.

· Once the swelling goes down, the cast becomes too loose and its effectiveness is minimal.

· Splints are not designed for heavy activity or weight bearing; include this information in patient teaching.

· Once a fracture or dislocation has been reduced, postreduction radiographs are taken to confirm alignment.

(2) The types of splints or immobilization used for various injuries are summarized in Table 37–16.

6. Discharge planning and teaching

a. The acronym for musculoskeletal injury care is RICE— *rest*, *ice*, *compression*, and *elevation*.

(1) Resting the injured part allows bone ends to remain in alignment and decreases swelling.

(2) Ice is applied for 20 minutes every hour while the patient is awake; some experts believe that continuous cold application is not effective. Heat may be applied after 3 days.

(3) Compression, through the use of compression bandages (e.g., elastic bandage), is used for injuries that affect the joint; ice pack can be incorporated into the compression dressing.

(4) Elevation means keeping the injured part above the heart.

b. Teach individuals who are discharged with a splint, cast, or compression bandage to assess for adequacy of distal circulation: Capillary refill in nail beds, color, sensation, and what to do if symptoms occur.

c. Pain management: Discuss the use of prescribed or over-the-counter medications; return if pain not relieved with prescribed medications, and possibility of compartment syndrome.

d. Provide specific crutch-walking instructions for any person being discharged with crutches who has never used them before.

(1) Return demonstration is important in ensuring that the person has the physical agility and cognitive ability to use them correctly.

(2) Written teaching materials covering how to use crutches in activities of daily living are particularly helpful (see *Crutches on the Go* in the bibliography).

(3) The use of crutches by an individual who has received narcotics or who is under the influence of alcohol is generally contraindicated; a prescription for the crutches and information on where to get them at a later time can be provided.

(4) Crutches are expensive to buy, but they can be rented from most pharmacies.

(5) Individuals with chronic lack of stability while

Table 37–16. Splints or Immobilization Devices

Body Area or Injury	Device
Shoulder post relocation of dislocation; Acromioclavicular joint separation	Arm and shoulder immobilizer; sling, or sling and swathe (also called a Velpeau)
Humerus fracture	Arm and shoulder immobilizer, sling and swathe
Clavicle fracture	Clavicle strap; figure of 8
Elbow fracture	Long arm posterior splint or sugar tong splint; sling
Distal forearm fracture	Anterior posterior short or long arm splint; sugar tong
Wrist fracture	Colles splint; cockup splint; Mason Allen splint
Hand navicular (scaphoid) fracture	Volar splint with thumb immobilized (thumb spica or wrist gauntlet)
Finger and metacarpal fracture	Radial or ulnar gutter splint; buddy taping for fingers
Distal finger tendon avulsion with or without fracture (boutonniere injury)	Finger splint with metacarpophalangeal joint in extension or hyperextension
Femur fracture	Hare, Sager, or Thomas splint with ankle hitch traction; skeletal pin/wire with Thomas splint and traction
Knee sprain, strain, dislocation	Knee immobilizer or posterior long leg splint
Tibia-fibula fracture	Posterior splint, Jones compression splint
Ankle sprains, strains	Air cast, posterior splint, Jones compression splint
Calcaneus fracture	Hard-soled shoe
Metatarsal fracture	Posterior splint, Jones compression splint
Toe fracture	Buddy taping to next toe

walking may benefit from another device such as a cane or walker.

 e. Assess the person's ability to perform activities of daily living with the immobilization device, and consider a community health nursing referral if assistance is indicated, especially in humeral or wrist fractures, which usually involve the dominant hand and often occur in older people during a fall.

 f. Review when and where to obtain follow-up care; instruct patient to bring radiographs along when receiving follow-up care.

Behavioral Disturbances

1. A wide spectrum of behavioral problems is often encountered in the emergency care setting, ranging from anxiety to suicidal or homicidal attempts (see Chapter 41).

2. The goals of emergency care for behavioral disturbances are to do the following:

 a. Identify the individual at risk for harming self or others

 b. Provide a safe environment and protect the person from harming self or others while undergoing evaluation

 c. Conduct medical screening to determine whether the behavior is a result of, or associated with, organic problems (e.g., meningitis, brain tumor, drug overdose, dehydration)

 d. Treat or coordinate further diagnosis and treatment of organic problems

 e. Coordinate psychiatric evaluation and referral for treatment

 f. Ensure safe transport to a psychiatric treatment facility if inpatient care is required

 g. Ensure that the person's legal rights are protected

3. Priority for care

 a. Identifying a person who is at significant risk for harming self or others is a high priority.

 b. Even if the person is not a threat to self or others, bizarre behavior is frightening to others and embarrassing for the patient; for both confidentiality and safety reasons, the behaviorally disturbed person should be triaged quickly and placed in a safe treatment area where close observation can occur.

 c. For safety reasons, the person, clothing, and belongings should be checked for weapons, medications, or other items that may be dangerous.

4. Assessment

 a. Historical and subjective

  (1) Person's reason for seeking treatment

  (2) Suicidal or homicidal thoughts

   • Does the person admit to wanting to harm self or others?

   • If so, what does the plan involve and how well has it been thought out?

   • Does the person have the means to carry out the plan (e.g., a person who threatens to shoot himself and has a gun is considered at high risk)?

  (3) Past medical and psychiatric history

  (4) Use of medications, drugs, alcohol; recent or current drug overdose

  (5) Recent head injury or illness

  (6) Auditory or visual hallucinations

  (7) Delusions, delirium, disorientation

  (8) Social and support system

  (9) History from family or significant others, law enforcement

 b. Objective data

  (1) Mental status, orientation, memory, speech pattern, relevance of communication

  (2) Affect: depressed, anxious, angry, fearful, confused or disorganized, paranoid, visual or auditory hallucinations, withdrawal, nonresponsive

  (3) Appearance: disheveled, poor hygiene, evidence of injury or skin infection

(4) Vital signs
- Abnormal vital signs may suggest primary or associated systemic disease.
- Perform postural vital signs if person appears malnourished or dehydrated, or has abnormal gait.

(5) Evidence of alcohol ingestion or IV drug use
(6) Physical assessment

NURSE ADVISORY

Indicators that a person poses a serious risk to self or others may include: History of harming self or others, command hallucinations telling the person to do harm, psychotic state, verbalizations of desire to harm self or others, refusal to commit to verbal or written contract that she or he will not harm self or others, well-defined and feasible plan to harm self or others, hyperactive state as reflected by continuous pacing or motion, and profound depression, as well as alcohol or drug use or intoxication associated with the above.

c. Diagnostic studies
(1) Often none, unless there are historical or physical assessment data that suggest drug or alcohol use or systemic disease.
(2) Head CT may be done if there is a history of trauma or a history of sudden change in mental status.

d. After the person is medically cleared, a mental health assessment is carried out by a psychologist, a psychiatric nurse, or a mental health social worker to determine risk and interventions needed.
(1) For both clinical and legal reasons, psychiatric evaluation for possible involuntary commitment cannot be carried out when the person is intoxicated with alcohol or drugs; thus, it may be necessary to hold the person in the ED or admit to a medical service until detoxified.

5. Clinical management
a. Safety
(1) The individual who is a danger to self or others is placed in a safe treatment area under observation while undergoing medical screening and psychiatric evaluation; this may be a locked area or an area in which direct observation can occur.
- Maintain a calm demeanor and consistent approach.
- Provide a quiet, stimulus-free environment for the person who is hallucinating.
(2) De-escalation of potentially violent behavior is an important skill required of emergency care personnel; verbal de-escalation skill is preferred to restraint.
(3) If de-escalation strategies are unsuccessful, physical takedown and restraint may be needed.
(4) Restraint use requires a written physician order, documented as soon as possible; institutional

guidelines dictate the form and substance of the order.
(5) Individuals who are placed in restraints are at the mercy of the staff for all activities; most institutions require every-15-minute observation and periodic attention to hydration, nutrition, toileting, activity, and skin care while the patient is under the restraints.

b. Crisis intervention and referral for outpatient counseling may be all that is needed for those with acute anxiety or situational depression.

c. Hospitalization
(1) If the hospital psychiatric staff determine that psychiatric hospitalization is indicated, and the patient agrees, voluntary admission is accomplished.
(2) If the patient does not agree to voluntary hospitalization, involuntary commitment is requested by the county mental health professional who is legally empowered to order involuntary commitment. In most instances, the county commitment officer must reevaluate the person before authorizing involuntary commitment.
- The process of involuntary commitment may take many hours.
- During the intervening period, the use of psychotropic medication is generally not permitted because it affects the final evaluation by the commitment officer and is perceived to be a violation of the patient's rights.
- The net effect is that verbal de-escalation, seclusion, or restraints are the only options available to the ED staff until the commitment officer makes a decision.
- Individual states have specific regulations guiding the process of commitment and patient rights.

d. Medications
(1) Medications administered in the ED are generally limited to those needed to control acute anxiety, such as the following:
- Haloperidol (Haldol)
- Diazepam (Valium)
- Chlordiazepoxide (Librium)
- Lorazepam (Ativan)
- Clorazepate (Tranxene)
- Fluphenazine (Prolixin)
(2) Longer-term antipsychotic, psychotropic, or antidepressant medications are usually prescribed by a psychiatrist.

6. Criteria for discharge
a. No evidence of suicidal or homicidal behavior
b. Normal physical assessment and vital signs
c. No evidence of grave disability
(1) Although a person may be significantly impaired, hospitalization may be denied and discharge required.
- The closure of state psychiatric hospitals coupled with well-intentioned, but largely ineffective, policies and regulations ostensibly designed to protect the rights of the mentally ill have resulted in commitment denials of many seriously

impaired individuals who are then discharged back into communities that are ill-prepared to provide adequate outpatient mental health treatment or support.

(2) Many chronically mentally ill individuals are not suicidal, homicidal, or violent but rather pose a threat to themselves in less dramatic ways, such as the following:

- Inability to care for themselves in regard to daily living activities of nutrition, clothing, hygiene, housing, socialization, finances, and awareness of safety risks predisposes them to develop hypothermia or frostbite and to have malnourishment-related health problems.
- Because of their disoriented state, they are at risk for accidents or victimization, such as pedestrian victims of motor vehicle accidents or street crimes.

(3) If commitment is denied, staff may need to involve community agencies to provide immediate assistance in regard to food, clothing, shelter, finances, and general welfare.

- In cold weather, special arrangements may be necessary for homeless individuals to prevent the possibility of injury or death due to hypothermia.

(4) Discharge planning and follow-up care for the chronically mentally ill requires a coordinated effort with hospital and community resources.

◨ DISCHARGE PLANNING AND TEACHING

Most people seen in an ED are diagnosed, treated, and discharged. Because conditions vary, there can be no strict criteria for discharge; however, the following generally apply:

1. The condition for which treatment was sought has been identified, or serious conditions have been ruled out.
2. Symptoms are resolved or improved.
3. The person is alert and oriented or neurologically stable.
4. The person is able to ambulate and perform activities of daily living as before onset of condition, or arrangements have been made for assistance in that regard.
5. The vital signs and other physiologic parameters are normal for that person or are improved significantly.
6. There is a plan for follow-up care, if necessary.
7. The person has a means of transportation and a place to go.
   a. The nurse may need to assist the individual in obtaining transportation, which may include the hospital providing bus fare or taxi vouchers.
   b. If the person is homeless, check area shelters or missions for assistance.

Discharge Instructions

1. It is standard practice that every person who is discharged from the ED is provided with written and verbal discharge instructions that address the following:

   a. The probable diagnosis or diagnoses
   b. Activities that the person is to perform or avoid as part of the plan of care (e.g., bed rest, elevation of an extremity)
   c. Medications or treatments required or recommended
   d. Temporary readings of studies such as radiographs and ECG, and the fact that they will be read by a 2nd person; notification if subsequent reading differs from initial reading
   e. How test results not immediately available will be handled (e.g., culture results)
   f. Follow-up care that is required or recommended, including name and phone number of practitioner and timing of follow-up

2. Discharge instructions are generally written at the 4th grade level.
3. Written discharge instructions should be provided in the language of the patient.
   a. If it is impossible to obtain an interpreter locally, a language service, such as the AT&T language service, may be used; the appropriate operator can give the instructions in the native tongue over the phone and may be willing to fax instructions in the native language.
   b. Many discharge instruction software programs can produce printed instructions for the more common foreign languages.
4. Verbal and written instructions can be augmented with videotapes or booklets with pictures that reinforce the material; *Crutches on the Go* is one such example.
5. Discharge instruction software programs can be adjusted to print in larger type for those with impaired vision.
6. Instructions that include use of a psychomotor skill should involve a return demonstration.
7. The patient should be able to verbalize his or her understanding of the instructions.
8. Normally, a patient is requested to sign a copy of the instructions, indicating that they have been received and are understood.
9. Instructions for an individual who is returning to an extended care facility, congregate care facility, or correctional institution are given to the persons accompanying him or her and are also called in to the institution. For security reasons, an incarcerated person is not told the timing of follow-up visits (lest he or she plan an escape).
10. Intoxicated persons, or those who have received mind- or judgment-altering medications, should not be permitted to drive a motor vehicle or given crutches.
11. Discharging people in the middle of the night who have no one with them may be unwise; it may be safer to allow the person to wait until daylight hours.

COBRA and EMTALA

1. COBRA is the federal Consolidated Omnibus Budget Reconciliation Act, which includes an "antidumping" provision, and EMTALA is the Emergency Medical Treatment and Active Labor Act.

a. This legislation is designed to ensure access to emergency care to individuals with life-threatening health problems by preventing health care facilities and practitioners from doing the following:
   (1) Refusing to provide emergency care to ill or injured persons or to women in active labor
   (2) Transferring unstable individuals to another facility, unless the facility accepts the individual in transfer
   (3) Transferring a person without consent
b. The law, as amended, requires that a medical screening examination be conducted to determine if an emergency exists before any questions about health care insurance are asked.
c. Institutions must identify in writing who can perform a medical screening examination; the law does not specify that it must be a physician, and the screener is a registered nurse (usually the triage nurse) in some institutions.

2. Transfer to another facility has special requirements:
   a. The person must be stabilized to the greatest extent possible.
   b. The person or his or her physician must request the transfer.
   c. The specific risks (e.g., motor vehicle accident, deterioration en route) and the benefits of transfer must be explained to the patient and documented in writing; the patient or designee signs a statement that the risks and benefits have been explained and that the patient requests transfer.
   d. The names of both the physician who has agreed to assume care and the agent of the receiving facility must be documented.
   e. Copies of the clinical record and results of diagnostic tests must accompany the patient.
   f. Unless otherwise negotiated, the sending facility assumes responsibility until the patient is received at the accepting facility, including ensuring that appropriate staff and equipment are available during transport.
   g. Most institutions document all the requirements and signatures on a special transfer form; 1 copy becomes part of the original medical record, 1 copy goes with the patient, and there is often a 3rd copy that is used by the originating facility for quality improvement purposes.

3. Liability
   a. Failure to comply with COBRA regulations can result in a $25,000 to $50,000 fine per offense; both the institution and a practitioner can be fined.
   b. An allegation of a COBRA violation results in a lengthy investigation by both state and federal officials; the investigation is unannounced and involves review of many procedures and records, not just those related to the case.
   c. Although the original intent of the law was to ensure that unstable persons were not denied care for financial reasons, some individuals have attempted to use it in alleged malpractice (e.g., failure to diagnose a problem that was not life threatening); most courts have ruled this inappropriate.

d. Also, COBRA requires that institutions have a written "whistle blower" policy, prohibiting penalizing an individual who reports a suspected COBRA violation.
e. The COBRA regulations conflict with the widespread use of managed care plans that try to restrict use of the ED to those who have true emergencies; COBRA requires that every person be evaluated before information about insurance is obtained, although many managed care plans prohibit evaluation and will not reimburse the institution without prior permission to treat, except in life-threatening emergencies.
f. Legislative efforts are under way regarding "access to emergency care" that would require insurers to pay for evaluation of a problem that a reasonably prudent person would consider to be an emergency, even if it is later determined that the problem was not an emergency.

Transfer or Transport to Another Facility

1. Transfer is usually considered under the following conditions:
   a. The facility lacks the capability to provide services the patient requires (e.g., trauma, burns, reimplantation).
   b. The patient or designee requests it.
   c. The attending physician requests it.
   d. The health care insurer requests it and the patient agrees.
2. The mode of transport selected depends on the following:
   a. The urgency of the situation.
   b. The distance to the receiving facility.
   c. Care, equipment, and personnel required during transport. Some equipment may not fit in a helicopter.
   d. Weather conditions: Helicopters and some fixed-wing aircraft may not be able to fly in bad weather.
   e. Patient characteristics that may make flying a poor choice include claustrophobia, fear of flying, and violent behavior.
   f. Cost: Air medical transport is more expensive than ground transport.
3. Preparation for transport
   a. It is difficult to perform complex interventions in a moving vehicle; therefore, stabilization and insertion of devices are done before movement.
      (1) Airway is secured, which may require endotracheal intubation or surgical airway.
      (2) Two or more IV lines are established.
   b. Air expands at altitude and air-containing structures are at risk for rupture because of expanding gas; if a high-altitude, long trip is anticipated, tubes are placed into those structures.
      (1) Chest tubes are placed if there is pneumothorax present.
      (2) A nasogastric tube is inserted.
      (3) A urinary catheter is inserted; saline or water may be used to inflate the balloon.
      (4) Air splints may be replaced with regular splints.
   c. Safety considerations
      (1) Glass bottles are replaced with flexible ones or are wrapped with padded material.

(2) Free-swinging weights are replaced with spring-loaded devices.

(3) Agitated persons are sedated and possibly restrained in advance.

(4) Antiemetics are administered to the person who is prone to motion sickness, possibly including staff.

(5) A person who is unable to clear air from the eustachian canal may be given decongestants.

(6) Casts are bivalved so that there is an immediate method of removing the device if the circulation becomes impaired.

(7) Intravenous tubing that has 3-way stopcocks or needleless systems is used to prevent needle stick injury when giving medications en route.

d. Equipment that will be needed for transport is procured and must be vehicle adaptable.

(1) Some electrical equipment may interfere with aircraft operations; compatibilities must be established in advance if facility equipment is to be used.

(2) Back-up batteries may be necessary for battery-operated equipment.

(3) Special notice may be necessary for oxygen or compressed air–powered equipment.

(4) Hearing ability is impaired in most vehicles; take noninvasive BP monitoring equipment with you.

e. Supplies, medications, and additional IV fluids should accompany the person.

(1) Administer pain medication before transport; have additional doses available.

(2) Administer antibiotics before transport, and provide additional doses as required during transport.

(3) Other medications that may be needed during transport should be premixed in syringes that will fit into a syringe pump.

f. Temperature considerations for patient and staff: Ground and air ambulances can get very cold; provide extra blankets for the patient and ensure that staff have appropriate coats.

4. Helicopter safety

a. The moving blades of a helicopter can cause injury to an unknowledgeable person during both descent and ascent and when on the ground.

b. Approach only after cleared by the pilot.

c. Always approach and leave the aircraft in view of the pilot.

d. Stay away from the rear of the aircraft.

e. Keep your head down.

f. If the blades are moving, stoop down when you approach.

g. Do not hold IV bottles or devices above your head.

h. Walk, do not run, to and from the aircraft.

i. Allow the crew to load or unload the cot; they know best how it is to be placed.

j. The wind from moving blades can dislodge linen and devices; make sure blankets and sheets are tied down and that other devices are well secured.

k. Debris thrown by the aircraft can cause eye injury; wear protective goggles and keep your head down.

5. Medical orders and documentation

a. On-line medical direction may not be an option in some aircraft; therefore, obtain orders in advance for interventions that could be needed en route.

b. If a situation arises for which you have no orders or if you need physician guidance, the pilot may be able to contact a tower operator who can patch you through to a medical control physician.

c. Unscheduled landing of an aircraft on a nonapproved surface is discouraged for safety reasons; however, it may be necessary if the patient's condition deteriorates to the point that additional resources are needed.

d. Document assessments and interventions en route, providing a full verbal and written report to the receiving facility.

◼ PUBLIC HEALTH AND WELFARE CONCERNS AND DISASTER OPERATIONS

The emergency nurse plays a pivotal role in the recognition, management, reporting, and prevention of a number of public health and welfare issues.

1. Reportable diseases, potential epidemics, criminal or civil acts
2. Evidence collection, safeguarding, processing, and chain of evidence
3. Disaster operations
4. Injury prevention

Reportable Conditions

1. Although each state and local jurisdiction identifies what is reportable, to whom, and when, the most common reportable conditions are summarized in Table 37–17.
2. In some instances, there is immunity from reporting, liability, or both for failure to report.
3. Each institution has specific policies that describe the reporting process.
4. In matters related to the public health and welfare, the common good of all citizens may supersede individual rights to privacy and confidentiality.
5. The nurse may recognize trends that are potentially associated with an epidemic or serious health problem (e.g., a significant number of children with diarrhea that may be food-borne, many elderly stricken with influenza and pneumonia). It is often reporting by health care professionals, rather than laboratory data, that warns public health officials of a potentially serious condition (see Table 37–16).

Evidence Handling

1. Evidence is that which law enforcement determines is necessary to investigate or prosecute an actual or potential crime.
2. Evidence frequently encountered in the emergency care setting includes the following:

Table 37–17. Reportable Conditions

Agency	Condition or Situation
Law enforcement	Gunshot wounds Stab wounds Assault Motor vehicle accident Sexual assault* Domestic violence*
Medical examiner or coroner†	Deaths unattended by a physician‡ Accidental or traumatic deaths Deaths that are suspicious Deaths at work Deaths associated with a clinical procedure Suicides Homicides Deaths of public health interest† Stillborn (greater than 20 weeks) Death of unidentified person
Child protective services	Child abuse, neglect
Adult protective services	Elder abuse, neglect
Institutionalized elderly§	Suspected abuse, neglect of nursing home residents
Public health†	Infectious diseases Sexually transmitted diseases Potential outbreaks Food-related disorders (e.g., salmonella, shigella, *Escherichia coli*)
Law enforcement, public health, or other agency†	Animal bites

* Requires patient consent.
† Requirements vary according to local regulations.
‡ Patient's own physician; does not include emergency physician.
§ Not all states have this requirement.

   a. Clothing, linen, or valuables that may show evidence of a penetrating wound, such as a gunshot wound or stab wound, blood or other stains, and particulate matter
   b. Bullets, firearms, knives, other weapons, syringes, and needles
   c. Tissue found on the person that may belong to another person (e.g., tissue under the nails from scratching that belongs to another person)
   d. Body fluids (e.g., semen belonging to another)
   e. Blood or urine obtained for drug or alcohol testing; Breathalyzer results
   f. Drugs or other chemicals
   g. Photographs or videotapes taken of injured persons
   h. Injuries on the victim or assailant
   i. Clinical records that document findings and procedures
   j. Audio tapes or documentation of telephone or radio conversations (e.g., with EMS personnel)
3. Basic rules or evidence handling
   a. Limit the number of people who have access to the evidence to prevent contamination or tampering.
     (1) When it is clear that it is evidence that is being handled (e.g., specimens in a sexual assault case),

it is fairly easy to limit access; however, when it is a major trauma with multiple gunshot wounds, 1 of the 1st things to happen is that the clothes are cut off and usually end up in a pile with the evidence contaminated.
     (2) In critical situations, a number of clinicians may be involved; this takes precedence over protection of the evidence.
     (3) Evidence should be stored in a locked cabinet or closet with the key maintained on the person who placed it there.
     (4) A *chain of custody* log should be maintained, which clearly identifies the name and role of every person who has access to the evidence.
     (5) Every time evidence is transferred (e.g., specimens turned over to the laboratory or law enforcement), an entry should be made in the log.
     (6) Limiting access to the evidence may include limiting access of family or friends to the patient; this may need to be addressed on a case-by-case basis, especially when there is a death.
   b. Allow wet articles to air dry before they are packaged, if possible.
     (1) Hang clothing on a hanger to allow it to dry.
     (2) Bag evidence in paper, not plastic bags; wet articles mildew and degrade in plastic bags.
     (3) Advise law enforcement officials that materials are wet so they can make arrangements to dry them.
   c. When cutting off clothes, avoid areas where there are obvious holes or tears, lest you cut through the bullet hole and destroy key evidence.
   d. Handle bullets gently; the soft casing can be deformed with the use of regular surgical instruments, making it difficult to perform accurate ballistic studies.
     (1) The person who is removing or finding the bullet may write his or her initials on the end of the bullet, not on the side; this marking may be used later in court.
     (2) A bullet can be protected by placing it in a gauze sponge, and then placing it in an evidence envelope; it should not be simply tossed into a metal container.
   e. Label evidence bags or envelopes with the patient's identifying information, as well as the staff member's, and list the contents. Write across the envelope seal so that it is obvious if the seal was opened later.
   f. Complete an inventory form or document on the clinical record what evidence was obtained and transmitted and to whom, including name, agency, and badge number.
   g. Copies of clinical records are not given to law enforcement without written patient permission or subpoena, unless previously agreed on, such as in medical examiner cases.

Disaster Operations

1. A medical disaster is one in which the health needs of the ill or injured exceed normal capabilities.
   a. Disasters may be internal or external.
     (1) Internal disasters are limited to the facility, and

usually only a part of the facility (e.g., fire, flood); most agencies can handle internal disasters by modifying daily procedures and generally do not need external assistance.

(2) External disasters are those in which the facility is spared but there is a need to mobilize resources for the care of a large number of people.

(3) In some instances (e.g., earthquake), the disaster may be external and internal.

2. The general concepts of disaster operations are the following:

a. The overriding goal is to do the greatest good for the greatest number of people.

(1) This principle means that resources are directed at those with the strongest likelihood of survival and not at the massively injured person whose probability of survival is slim even under normal circumstances.

(2) Nurses may be called on to make triage decisions in a disaster, as they have in wartime mass casualty situations; making an active decision to withhold care to a massively injured person so that those who are salvageable can survive is perhaps the most difficult decision that any health care provider will ever make. It requires that the person have both superior assessment skills and solid clinical knowledge about the probabilities of survival with selected injuries.

b. Casualties are triaged and dispatched to separate treatment areas, according to previously determined categories; many agencies use colors that are linked to disaster tags to indicate categories:

(1) Immediate (red): require immediate intervention to save life (e.g., airway obstruction, arterial bleeding)

(2) Delayed (yellow): Require intervention, but are stable and can wait 30 to 60 minutes; examples may include penetrating abdominal injury, open head injury, eye injury, and moderate burns

(3) Minimal (green): require intervention, but are usually able to provide self-care; usually, the walking wounded with stable fractures or lacerations, or minor burns

(4) Expectant (black): injury so massive that probability of survival is minimal (e.g., massive burns, cardiac arrest, coma in open head injury)

• If a head-injured person who was responsive suddenly becomes unconscious, emergency burr holes may be done as a temporizing measure and the person would be placed in the immediate category; if the head injury is open, the person is already decompressing, and the use of burr holes would not make a difference.

• To estimate survivability in major burns, 1 guideline is that if the person's combined age and percent body surface area burned exceeds 100, the probability of survival is minimal.

• Placing a person in the expectant category does not mean that no care will be rendered; it simply means that the person is the last priority but that supportive and comfort measures are provided (e.g., pain management).

(5) Deceased

c. Care is standardized rather than individualized; standing orders are often used for IV fluids, laboratory studies, diagnostic and therapeutic measures, antibiotics, tetanus prophylaxis, and pain management.

d. Specialists become generalists (e.g., specialty surgeons all have general surgery as a part of their training, and can be tapped to provide general surgical care; a urologist or obstetrician can put in a chest tube if necessary).

e. Nurses may perform activities in a disaster that they do not normally perform (e.g., suturing, chest tube placement, surgical airway, tracheal intubation).

f. Diagnostic studies are limited, for both time and resource reasons (e.g., the routine practice of performing CT scans on people with trauma may need to be curtailed, both because there is a more urgent need to perform life-saving surgery and because of the high demand for the limited resource).

g. The use of resources may be determined by the disaster medical officer (e.g., what conditions get priority for operating rooms, how blood products will be dispensed).

h. Different areas of the hospital may need to be used for casualty care (e.g., an operating room in a labor and delivery suite may need to be used for general surgical procedures).

i. Media and traffic control become a priority.

j. Resources are needed to provide emotional and spiritual support to both casualties and family members.

k. Staff and others are at risk for critical incident stress; individual ability to function effectively needs to be assessed on a routine basis, and individuals may need to be removed from duty for rest.

l. Normal radio communications with EMS personnel may be affected, and casualties may arrive with no notice; in many disasters, casualties arrive separate from the normal EMS system, after finding their own transportation.

m. Ill or injured individuals who are not a part of the disaster are at risk for being overlooked; procedures need to be in place to either care for them or place the hospital on divert for all except disaster casualties.

n. Identification and tracking of casualties is difficult, especially because the normal way of processing is altered; the American Red Cross, as a part of its charter, is responsible for assisting and facilitating notification of next of kin.

(1) There is potential for a large number of unidentified people; procedures need to be established to preassign different "Doe" names so that errors are not made.

(2) In some disasters, nurses have played an important role in morgue duty, by assisting families to locate and identify loved ones.

o. In disasters such as a plane or train accident, industry or regulatory agency investigators may also be involved; evidence handling procedures may be necessary.

p. In a large-scale, protracted disaster, there is a need to have a preestablished staff rotation plan to ensure that personnel needs for rest, nourishment, and hygiene are addressed.

q. In large natural disasters, such as earthquake, infectious diseases also become a concern; mass immunization may be necessary.

r. Research in large natural disasters has demonstrated that many uninjured people, especially those rendered homeless, gravitate to the hospital as a logical source of support; separating them from the ill or injured is important.

3. Hospitals are required to exercise their disaster plans several times a year; knowledge of the plan and one's role in disaster operations is essential.

Injury and Illness Prevention

1. Preventable injury and illness is the leading cause of death and disability in this country; emergency nurses witness the senseless carnage on a daily basis, and are in an excellent position to do something about it.

2. Emergency and trauma nurses have formed groups to provide public education and information about injury prevention.

   a. Emergency Nurses Cancel Alcohol Related Emergencies—ENCARE—is a national organization that focuses its attention primarily on teaching teenagers to make smart decisions regarding drinking and driving; it has recently expanded its scope to include injury prevention among older persons.

   b. Trauma Nurses Talk Tough is another group that focuses on injury prevention, primarily related to drinking alcohol and driving.

3. A number of private and public organizations have programs on illness and injury prevention:

   a. The American Trauma Society, dedicated to injury prevention and trauma research, is composed of both health care professionals and the lay public; it has a number of publications, materials, and programs on injury prevention.

   b. The Emergency Nurses Association, EMS agencies, and the American Red Cross have injury and illness prevention as part of their programs; common topics include the following:

   (1) How and when to call 911

   (2) Driver safety

   (3) Use of automobile restraint devices

   (4) Signs of a heart attack

   (5) Basic first aid courses

   (6) Cardiopulmonary resuscitation

   (7) Child safety seats

4. Individual hospitals often have speaker bureaus in which medical and nursing staff provide information on both illness and injury prevention.

5. Opportunities for discussing prevention activities often surface during the routine nursing assessment or emergency care.

   a. Use of safety restraints and child safety seats is a part of the injury assessment.

   b. Safety considerations related to growth and develop-

ment can be included in the normal course of care of children.

   c. Immunization status should be included in the assessment of all individuals, and those who need updating can be either immunized or referred appropriately.

   • Many children are underimmunized or unimmunized; preventable illnesses are emerging that were once controlled.

   • The majority of the cases of tetanus in the United States occur in persons older than 50 years of age; many have never been immunized or have not had boosters for many years.

   • Immigrants are also at risk for being unimmunized.

   • Pertussis (whooping cough), once a rarity, and highly contagious, is re-emerging in both children and adults.

   d. Opportunities to address pregnancy and sexually transmitted disease prevention also surface during the assessment of female patients.

   e. Many EDs have a pamphlet rack that contains information on a variety of health and injury issues; written teaching materials often open up discussion of prevention issues.

6. One of the most serious preventable problems that is not being adequately addressed is that of suicide, particularly among teenagers and young adults.

   a. Information regarding the magnitude of the problem has not gained the attention it deserves.

   (1) The actual incidence of suicide is not known because the deaths may be incorrectly diagnosed or intentionally misreported.

   (2) In 1 study of all accidental deaths, more than 50 percent of the deaths were suicides; this did not include intentional drug overdose, which is a common means of suicide.

   (3) In a review of all gun-related deaths in the United States during 1 week, the majority of the deaths were suicides; many were by elderly people or those with terminal diseases.

   (4) Discussion of suicide is taboo in our society; although discussion of cause of death in accidents, cancers, or heart disease is commonplace, the same is not true for suicide.

   (5) Some people feel that discussing a suicide may cause vulnerable people to commit suicide.

   b. Many teenagers and young adults inadvertently commit suicide when all they wanted was to get someone's attention.

   (1) Ingestion of a seemingly safe medication such as acetaminophen may result in death because the lack of initial symptoms enables the person to hide the fact that they tried until several days later when the liver damage is irreversible.

   c. With most other deaths, a reason for the death can be determined; in suicide, the survivors are left to agonize over it.

   d. Accidents are understandable; taking one's own life is incomprehensible to most people.

   e. The spectrum of reasons why a person chooses to take his or her own life is so great that there is no simple prevention strategy.

   f. Prevention strategies that may make a difference

(1) Increased education about the magnitude of the problem

(2) Increased efforts to foster self-esteem, worth, and hopefulness among at-risk age groups

(3) Education of high-risk groups regarding signs to watch for and how to intervene if they observe these signs; teenagers especially seem to have a code that one does not report on a friend, and it will take some effort to get them to realize that this should be an exception.

(4) The incidence of suicide among older people or those with terminal diseases requires different strategies, such as more effective pain management, use of antidepressant medications, socialization, and improved quality of life.

7. Although voluntary efforts in injury or illness prevention are laudable, legislative efforts may have more immediate and profound impact.

a. Safety seats for children

b. Automatic restraint devices in automobiles

c. Helmets for bicyclists and motorcyclists

d. Lowering the legal blood alcohol level and creating stiffer penalties for driving while impaired

e. Handgun control: Mandating special triggers and locks that a child cannot release

f. Speed limit reduction

g. Providing safe areas for activities such as skateboarding and roller blading

h. Aggressive penalties for domestic violence, abuse, and sexual assault

i. Automatic smoke and carbon monoxide detector systems

j. Universal 911 access

k. Funding for illness and injury prevention research

8. Health care reform has made it clear to providers, insurers, and the public that the most effective way to reduce health care expenditures is to shift our energy and focus from injury and illness care to wellness care and prevention. Emergency nurses are in an ideal position to actively participate in this effort, and there is reason to be optimistic.

◼ DEATH AND DYING IN THE EMERGENCY CARE SETTING

1. Nursing considerations regarding death and dying are discussed in detail in Chapter 43. However, death in the emergency care setting has some unique characteristics that warrant special attention.

a. The death is usually unexpected, may be a result of injury or violence, and often occurs in young people.

b. As it is unexpected, there may be no time for the patient or family to prepare or to say good bye.

c. The patient's condition may be so unstable that resuscitation efforts and personnel may supersede the presence of loved ones, thus cutting off the opportunity for closure.

d. Many deaths are senseless and unnatural; there is often significant guilt on the part of loved ones, especially in suicides or home accidents.

e. There is often insufficient time to learn and process the facts and gain a clear understanding of what happened.

f. In suspicious or criminal acts, the involvement of law enforcement personnel and criminal investigation may limit the rights of loved ones.

(1) In most instances, securing the scene and preservation of evidence may preclude presence of the family.

(2) The person cannot be cleaned or devices removed before visitation by the family, and the hands may need to be covered with paper bags to preserve evidence; the sight of blood, devices, and the paper bags and the inability to hold a loved one's hands can be very difficult.

(3) Suspicious deaths fall under the jurisdiction of the medical examiner or coroner and usually require an autopsy; this may be counter to personal, religious, or cultural wishes.

(4) In some instances, the medical examiner's determination regarding the manner and cause of death may take some time because of the need for special laboratory and forensic studies.

g. In criminal acts, there may be no resolution until the perpetrator is tried and sentenced; in some cases there is no resolution.

h. Normal support systems used in times of crisis are often not immediately available.

i. The safety and welfare of family and friends who are not physically present, especially those who are in poor health or must travel, is a concern; the stress of death notification may create serious physical problems, distract a person so much that accidents occur, or cause a loved one to take his or her own life.

j. It is difficult for emergency care personnel to anticipate the way in which loved ones will respond to the news; responses vary from rage and verbal or physical attacks on caregivers to psychic blunting or quiet acceptance.

k. Cultural or religious norms and rites, not ordinarily encountered in the emergency care setting, may be important to some individuals.

2. Notification of loved ones of a seriously ill or injured person can be done in such a way that they can more effectively process the information and move through the grieving process.

a. If at all possible, notification should be made in person; however, this is often not possible in the ED.

b. If the physical or emotional stability of the recipient is of concern, determine whether there is another person present who can support the individual.

c. Identify yourself, your title, and your agency.

d. Confirm the name and relationship of the person with whom you are speaking.

e. Provide information in a sequential manner, starting from the beginning (e.g., "Mary collapsed at work about 3 o'clock this afternoon after having chest pain. Her coworkers determined that she wasn't breathing and did not have a pulse, so they started CPR and called 911. When the paramedics arrived, they determined that her heart wasn't beating effectively; they inserted a breathing tube, gave her medications, continued CPR, and brought her here to the emergency department. We are continuing to do CPR and give her medications. Her condition is critical at this time. She is not awake and she is not in pain.'').

   f. Ask whether there is any significant health history or medications, and ask whether there are any questions.

   g. Ask whether family members will be coming to the ED, and, if so, explain how to get there. Repeat the name of your facility and where in the facility the patient will be; emphasize driving safely.

3. When loved ones arrive, escort them to a quiet, private place with seating, clarify what they understand, and update them regarding the current situation. Provide something to drink, tissues, and access to a telephone. Explain the gravity of the situation, ask whether they would like a member of the clergy or a crisis worker called, and offer them the opportunity to be with their loved one.

   a. If family or significant others wish to be present in the resuscitation room, briefly explain in advance the various devices and activities that they will see; forewarn resuscitation staff, provide staff member accompaniment, and make sure there is a chair available.

     (1) To the greatest extent possible, allow the person closest to the patient access to the person, preferably at the head so they can say what they need to say.

     (2) If this is not possible, allow hand holding or touching the feet—some contact with the loved one.

     (3) Encourage them to say whatever they need or want to say, even though staff are present.

NURSE ADVISORY

> Family or significant other presence during resuscitation is a fairly recent advance in emergency care, and should be offered as a routine practice. For the welfare of all concerned, it may be desirable to bring in family or significant others after immediate interventions are completed (e.g., airway, intravenous lines, nasogastric tube, and Foley in place) and the situation is more controlled, but their wishes should be respected. Their need is to be with their loved one while she or he is technically still alive. Do not delay visitation to clean up the room; family and significant others tend to have tunnel vision and focus on their loved one rather than on the appearance of the room. Provide access so that they may touch or kiss their loved one. Observation often provides reassurance that everything possible was done, facilitates grieving, and often assists them in decision making to terminate resuscitation efforts.

   b. If the family does not wish to be present, keep them updated about how things are going; this allows anticipatory grieving and better prepares them if death occurs.

   c. If at all possible, ask about the patient's wishes regarding advance directives and organ or tissue donation.

4. If death has already occurred, the question of whether to give this information over the telephone becomes a con-

cern. Some institutions have guidelines to assist staff; however, the decision is usually the judgment of the staff.

   a. If the next of kin is located some distance away, it is probably best to tell them over the phone.

   b. If the next of kin is close by, the decision is based on conversation with the person. Some family members may be upset to learn that the person had already expired when they were 1st contacted and that the staff had not been honest with them.

5. Grief and loss research indicates that family visitation is important in the grief process; encourage the family to see their loved one, but respect their wishes if they decline.

   a. Although the resuscitation efforts or the nature of the injury may result in a messy treatment room, it is probably more important to allow family to see their deceased loved one as soon as possible than it is to clean up the room 1st; research has demonstrated that family focus on their loved one and are generally oblivious to the environment.

   b. If there are no concerns related to evidence, clean the person's face and hands, bandage wounds, and cover soiled linen.

   c. Use heat lamps to keep the person warm; family members sometimes comment on how cold their loved one is, raising a question about how long ago the person expired.

   d. Raise the deceased person's head slightly.

   e. Subdue lights so that contrasts and discoloration are not so stark.

   f. Put a child's gown on children, and wrap an infant in a clean blanket.

   g. Offer parents the opportunity to hold their child; provide a rocking chair and privacy.

   h. Leave wedding bands on until after visitation; give jewelry to family before they leave, unless the medical examiner requires that it be left on.

   i. Family may wish to have a lock of hair or a photograph.

   j. Have someone be with the family to support them during visitation; make chairs and tissues available.

   k. Offer to contact a member of the clergy.

   l. Families who have had some warning generally respond normally to the loss and do not remain long; assistance from crisis staff may be needed if the family seems totally irrational, suicidal, or refuses to leave.

6. Before leaving the hospital, the family should be provided with information regarding the following:

   a. Suspected cause of death, if determined

   b. Whether an autopsy will be done by the medical examiner or coroner; their right to have an autopsy done if the medical examiner does not assume jurisdiction

   c. Where valuables and clothing are located and when they can be returned (may be retained by law enforcement as evidence); explain if clothing was discarded because it was cut off.

   d. When the body will be released for burial. Ask if they know which funeral home will make the arrangements.

e. Procedures that will occur if the person was an organ or tissue donor, including communication with the organ procurement agency. Obtain phone numbers where the next of kin can be contacted regarding organ or tissue donation, if not already obtained.

f. The normal grieving process and strategies to deal with the coming days. Emphasize the need to take care of oneself, including adequate nutrition and safety.

(1) Provide booklets containing grief and loss information; the following references are especially helpful in unexpected death: *Healing Grief, Miscarriage, Grief by Homicide,* and *No Time for Goodbye.*

(2) Information on local support groups is also valuable.

g. How to tell children of the death of a parent, grandparent, or close family member.

h. Use of sedatives or hypnotics is generally not recommended.

i. Financial information: In some states, the assets of the deceased are frozen as soon as the death becomes a matter of public record; spouses may need to access some funds before this occurs so they have enough money for basic necessities.

j. The name and phone number of the ED and contact person if they have questions about the emergency care or about procedures; families often have questions or concerns that surface hours to days later.

7. Critical incident stress management techniques such as peer defusing or debriefing may be indicated for the personnel involved in the resuscitation, particularly in the death of a young person, or when the person was awake and alert on arrival and dies in the ED or shortly thereafter.

8. In some institutions, it is customary to send a bereavement card to the next of kin or for personnel to attend the funeral or memorial service.

Bibliography

Books

Auerbach PS, and Geehr EC (eds). *Management of Wilderness and Environmental Emergencies.* 3rd ed. St. Louis: CV Mosby, 1995.

Borg S, and Lasker J. *When Pregnancy Fails. Families Coping with Miscarriage, Stillbirth, and Infant Death.* Boston: Beacon Press, 1981.

Bourg P, Sherer C, and Rosen P. *Standardized Nursing Care Plans for Emergency Departments.* St. Louis: CV Mosby, 1986.

Bowen TE, and Bellamy RF (eds). *Emergency War Surgery. Second Revision of the Emergency War Surgery NATO Handbook.* U.S. Department of Defense. Washington, DC: U.S. Government Printing Office, 1988.

Buchsbaum HJ. *Trauma in Pregnancy.* Philadelphia: WB Saunders, 1979.

Burkel FM, Sanner PH, and Wolcott BW. *Disaster Medicine. Application for the Immediate Management and Triage of Civilian and Military Disaster Victims.* New York: Medical Examination Publishing Co, 1984.

Committee on Trauma Research, Commission of Life Sciences, National Research Council, and the Institute of Medicine. *Injury in America. A Continuing Public Health Problem.* Washington, DC: National Academy Press, 1985.

Elliott H, and Bailey B. *Ripples of Suicide.* Waco, TX: WRS Publishing, 1993.

Fassler J. *My Grandpa Died Today.* New York: Human Sciences Press, 1983.

Garcia LM. *Disaster Nursing. Planning, Assessment, and Intervention.* Rockville, MD: Aspen, 1985.

Giger JN, and Davidhizar RH. *Transcultural Nursing: Assessment and Intervention.* St. Louis: CV Mosby, 1991.

Hyman SE (ed). *Manual of Psychiatric Emergencies.* 2nd ed. Boston: Little, Brown & Co, 1988.

Judd RL, Warner CG, and Schaffer MA. *Geriatric Emergencies.* Rockville, MD: Aspen, 1986.

Kaplan EN, and Hentz VR. *Emergency Management of Skin and Soft Tissue Wounds. An Illustrated Guide.* Boston: Little, Brown & Co, 1984.

Kitt S, et al. *Emergency Nursing. A Physiologic and Clinical Perspective.* 2nd ed. Philadelphia: WB Saunders, 1994.

Klein AR, et al (eds). *Emergency Nursing Core Curriculum.* 4th ed. Philadelphia: WB Saunders, 1994.

Lord JH. *No Time for Goodbyes. Coping with Sorrow, Anger, and Injustice After a Tragic Death.* Ventura, CA: Pathfinder Publishing, 1987.

Mancini ME. *Decision Making in Emergency Nursing.* Philadelphia: BC Decker, 1987.

National Institutes of Health, National Asthma Education Program Expert Panel Report. *Guidelines for the Diagnosis and Management of Asthma.* NIH Publication No. 91-3042. Bethesda, MD, 1994.

Proehl J. *Adult Emergency Nursing Procedures.* Boston: Jones & Bartlett, 1993.

Qureshi B. *Transcultural Medicine: Dealing with Patients from Different Cultures.* 2nd ed. Boston: Kluwer Academic Press, 1994.

Raimond J, and Taylor JW. *Neurological Emergencies. Effective Nursing Care.* Rockville, MD: Aspen, 1986.

Rogers JH, Osborn HH, and Pousada L. *Emergency Nursing. A Practice Guide.* Baltimore: Williams & Wilkins, 1989.

Rund DA, and Rausch TA. *Triage.* St. Louis: CV Mosby, 1981.

Schaefer D, and Lyons C. *How Do We Tell the Children? Helping Children Understand and Cope When Someone Dies.* New York: Newmarket Press, 1986.

Trott A. *Wounds and Lacerations. Emergency Care and Closure.* St. Louis: CV Mosby, 1991.

Zuidema GD, Rutherford RB, and Ballinger WF. *The Management of Trauma.* 4th ed. Philadelphia: WB Saunders, 1985.

Chapters in Books and Journal Articles

Assessment and Stabilization

American Health Consultants. Code response team organization can help save time and lives. *ED Management* 7(5):49–55, 1995.

Bickell W, et al. Immediate vs delayed fluid resuscitation for hypotensive patients with penetrating torso injuries. *N Engl J Med* 331(17):1105–1109, 1994.

Childs SG. Syncope: Categories and considerations for practice. *J Emerg Nurs* 21(2):125–134, 1995.

Huston CJ. Emergency! Ruptured esophageal varices. *Am J Nurs* 96(4):43, 1996.

O'Hanlon-Nichols T. Clinical snapshot: Hyperglycemic hyperosmolar nonketotic syndrome. *Am J Nurs* 96(3):38–39, 1996.

Powell L, and Holt P. Rapid sequence induction in the emergency department. *J Emerg Nurs* 21(4):305–309, 1995.

Stapczynski JS. Fluid resuscitation in traumatic hemorrhagic shock: Challenges, controversies, and current clinical guidelines. *Emerg Med Rep* 15(25), 1994.

Thomas DO. How to deal with children in the emergency department. *J Emerg Nurs* 17(1):49–50, 1991.

Behavioral Emergencies

Meade D, Lynch T, and Fuller R. Adolescent suicide. *Emerg Med Serv* 24(3):27–35, 1995.

Meade D, and Riccio J. Signs of impending violence: Recognizing trouble before it begins. *Top Emerg Med* 16(3):18–29, 1994.

Cardiovascular Events

Fessmire FM, Wharton DR, and Calhoun FB. Instability of ST segment in the early stages of acute myocardial infarction in patients undergoing continuous 12-lead ECG monitoring. *Am J Emerg Med* 13:158–163, 1995.

Finefrock SC. Continuous 12 lead ST segment monitoring: An adjunct to identifying silent ischemia and infarct in the emergency department. *J Emerg Nurs* 21(5):413–416, 1995.

Ghosh RJ. Introducing the cardiac rhythm interpretation tree. *J Emerg Nurs* 21(3):226–227, 1995.

Jackson RR. Effect of patient's sex on the timing of thrombolytic therapy. *Ann Emerg Med* 27(1):8–15, 1996.

Meischke H, et al. Reasons patients with chest pain delay or do not call 911. *Ann Emerg Med* 25(2):193–197, 1995.

Page J, and Hubble MW. Recognizing infective endocarditis: Case study of a 28-year-old. *J Emerg Nurs* 22(1):24–28, 1996.

Pittman D, and Kirkpatrick M. Women's health and the acute myocardial infarction. *Nurs Outlook* 42(3):207–209, 1994.

Tsunoda D. Clinical snapshot: Acute myocardial infarction. *Am J Nurs* 96(5):38–39, 1996.

Wellford LA, and Young GP. Advances and updates in cardiovascular emergencies. *Emerg Med Clin North Am* 13(4), 1995.

Death and Dying

Oliver RC, and Fallat ME. Traumatic childhood death: How well do parents cope? *J Trauma* 39(2):303–308, 1995.

Snyder J. Bereavement protocols. *J Emerg Nurs* 22:39–42, 1996.

Yoder L. Comfort and consolation: A nursing perspective on parental bereavement. *Pediatr Nurs* 20(5):473–477, 1994.

Disaster Preparedness

Aghababian R, et al. Disasters within hospitals. *Ann Emerg Med* 23(4):771–777, 1994.

Amundson SR, and Burkle AM. Golden minutes: The Oklahoma City bombing—two ED nurses' stories. *J Emerg Nurs* 21(5):401–407, 1995.

Discharge Planning and Teaching

Jones JS, et al. Metered-dose inhalers: Do emergency health care providers know what to teach? *Ann Emerg Med* 26(3):3008–3011, 1995.

Spandorfer J, et al. Comprehension of discharge instructions by patients in an urban emergency department. *Ann Emerg Med* 25(1):71–74, 1995.

Thomas EJ, et al. Patient noncompliance with medical advice after the emergency department visit. *Ann Emerg Med* 27(1):49–55, 1996.

Domestic Violence

Hadley SM. Working with battered women in the emergency department: A model program. *J Emerg Nurs* 18(1):18–23, 1992.

Jezierski M. Abuse of women by male partners: Basic knowledge for emergency nurses. *J Emerg Nurs* 20(5):361–371, 1994.

McFarlane J, et al. Identification of abuse in the emergency department: Effectiveness of a two question screening tool. *J Emerg Nurs* 21(5):391–394, 1995.

EMS Systems and Access to Care

Bindman AB, et al. Preventable hospitalizations and access to health care. *JAMA* 274(4):305–311, 1995.

Campbell A, et al. Trauma centers in a managed care environment. *J Trauma* 29(2):246–253, 1995.

Derlet R, et al. Prospective identification and triage of nonemergency patients out of an emergency department: A 5-year study. *Ann Emerg Med* 25(2):215–223, 1995.

Meischke H, et al. Reasons patients with chest pain delay or do not call 911. *Ann Emerg Med* 25(2):193–197, 1995.

Ear, Nose, Throat, Dental, and Facial Emergencies

Camp JH. Dental trauma: Diagnostic considerations, emergency procedures and definitive management. *Emerg Med Rep* 16(9):79–116, 1995.

Colucciello SL. The treacherous and complex spectrum of maxillofacial trauma: Etiologies, evaluation, and emergency stabilization. *Emerg Med Rep* 16(7):59–70, 1995.

Neilson IR: Ingestion of coins and batteries. *Pediatr Rev* 16(1):35–36, 1995.

Singer JI, and McCabe JB: Epiglottitis at the extremes of age. *J Emerg Med* 6(3):228–231, 1988.

Eye Emergencies

Scott JL, and Ghezzi KT (eds). Emergency treatment of the eye. *Emerg Med Clin North Am* 13(3), 1995.

Genitourinary Disorders

Ruth-Sahd LA. Emergency! Renal calculi. *Am J Nurs* 95(11):50, 1995.

Stewart C. Sexually related trauma: A comprehensive review of diagnosis and management. *Emerg Med Rep* 15(4):31–40, 1994.

Geriatric Emergency Care

Foreman MD, and Zane D. Nursing strategies for acute confusion in elders. *Am J Nurs* 96(4):44–51, 1996.

O'Donnell ME. Assessing fluid with electrolyte balance in elders. *Am J Nurs* 95(11):41–46, 1995.

Oreskovich M, et al. Geriatric trauma: Injury patterns and outcome. *J Trauma* 24(7):565–572, 1984.

Shabot KK, and Johnson CL. Outcome from critical care in the "oldest old" trauma patients. *J Trauma* 39(2):254–260, 1995.

Stomatos CA, et al. Meeting the challenge of the older trauma patient. *Am J Nurs* 96(5):40–48, 1996.

Heat and Cold Injuries

Centers for Disease Control and Prevention. Heat-related mortality—Chicago, July 1995. *MMWR* 44:577–579, 1995.

Parks FB, and Calabro JJ. Hyperthermia. Performing when the heat is on. *JEMS* 15(8):24–32, 1990.

Stewart C. The destructive and unpredictable spectrum of chemical injuries to the skin. *Emerg Med Rep* 15(24):233–240, 1994.

White JD, et al. Evaporation versus iced peritoneal lavage treatment of heatstroke. *Am J Emerg Med* 11(1):1–3, 1993.

Legal Issues

Standing Bear ZG. Forensic nursing and death investigation: Will the vision be co-opted? *J Psychosoc Nurs Ment Health Serv* 33(9):59–64, 1995.

Neurologic Emergencies

Abramowicz M (ed). Drugs for migraine. *Med Lett Drugs Ther* 37(943):17–20, 1995.

Caesar R, and Gavin LJ. Acute headache management: The challenge of deciphering etiologies to guide assessment and treatment. *Emerg Med Rep* 16(13), 1995.

Chiocca EM. Emergency! Meningococcal meningitis. *Am J Nurs* 95(12):25, 1995.

Criss E. Back to back. Assessment of spinal trauma. *J Emerg Med Serv* 20(1):46–57, 1995.

Doynton S, and Roberts JR. Reappraisal of the "coma cocktail" dextrose, flumazenil, naloxone, and thiamine. *In Concepts and Controversies in Toxicology. Emerg Med Clin North Am* 12(2):301–313, 1994.

Hoffman RS, and Goldfrank LR. The poisoned patient with altered consciousness. Controversies in the use of a "coma cocktail." *JAMA* 274(7):562–569, 1995.

Huston CJ, and Boelman R. Emergency! Autonomic dysreflexia. *Am J Nurs* 95(6):55, 1995.

Kelly M. Emergency! Status epilepticus. *Am J Nurs* 95(6):50, 1995.

Lehman LH. The neurological causes of weakness. *Emerg Med* 28(8):22–40, 1995.

Starkman S, Barron D, and Kramer D. Stroke: Emergency evaluation and management. *Emerg Med Rep* 15(8):77–82, 1994.

Obstetric and Gynecologic Emergencies

Centers for Disease Control and Prevention. Ectopic pregnancy—United States, 1990–1992. *MMWR* 43(3):46–48, 1995.

Colucciello SA. The challenge of trauma in pregnancy: Guidelines for targeted assessment, fetal monitoring, and definitive management. *Emerg Med Rep* 16(4):171–182, 1995.

Mitchell L. Cardiac arrest during pregnancy: Maternal-fetal physiology and advanced cardiac life support for the obstetric patient. *Crit Care Nurse* 15(1): 56–60, 1995.

Pain

Abramowicz M (ed). Drugs for migraine. *Med Lett Drugs Ther* 37(943):17–20, 1995.

Caesar R, and Gavin LJ. Acute headache management: The challenge of deciphering etiologies to guide assessment and treatment. *Emerg Med Rep* 16(13):June 26, 1995.

Duda J. Drug update. The good, bad, and ugly: Using ketamine for pediatric patients. *J Emerg Nurs* 22(1):49–51, 1996.

Maikler V, et al. The child in pain. *Emerg Off Pediatr* 7(6):148–151, 1994.

Pasero CL. Pain control. Why withhold analgesia in the emergency department? *Am J Nurs* 95(12):15, 1995.

Tanabe P. Recognizing pain as a component of the primary assessment: Adding D for discomfort to the ABC's. *J Emerg Nurs* 21(4):299–304, 1995.

Wiens DA. Acute low back pain: Differential diagnosis, targeted assessment, and therapeutic controversies. *Emerg Med Rep* 16(14):129–140, 1995.

Poisoning, Overdose, and Hazardous Materials

Brent JA. Drugs of abuse: An update. *Emerg Med* 27(7):56–70, 1995.

Doynton S, and Roberts JR. Reappraisal of the "coma cocktail" dextrose, flumazenil, naloxone, and thiamine. *In Concepts and Controversies in Toxicology.* *Emerg Med Clin North Am* 12(2):301–313, 1994.

Hoffman RS, and Goldfrank LR. The poisoned patient with altered consciousness. Controversies in the use of a "coma cocktail." *JAMA* 274(7):562–569, 1995.

Huston CJ. Emergency! Carbon monoxide poisoning. *Am J Nurs* 96(1):45, 1996.

Neilson IR. Ingestion of coins and batteries. *Pediatr Rev* 16(1):35–36, 1995.

Prevention

Grossman DC, Mang K, Rivara FP. Firearm injury prevention counseling by pediatricians and family physicians. *Arch Pediatr Adolesc Med* 149:973–977, 1995.

Madden C, and Cole TB. Emergency intervention to break the cycle of drunken driving and recurrent injury. *Ann Emerg Med* 26(2):177–179, 1995.

McMahon MM. Managing accidents and injuries. *In* Luckmann J. *Your Health!* Englewood Cliffs, NJ: Prentice-Hall, 1990.

Rachuba L, Stanton B, and Howard D. Violent crime in the United States. An epidemiologic profile. *Arch Pediatr Adolesc Med* 149:953–960, 1995.

Respiratory Emergencies

Armstrong P. Inhalation injury. *Top Emerg Med* 17(1):25–34, 1995.

Graf WD, et al. Predicting outcome in pediatric submersion victims. *Ann Emerg Med* 26(3):312–319, 1995.

Halpern K. The treacherous clinical spectrum of allergic emergencies: Diagnosis, treatment, and prevention. *Emerg Med Rep* 15(22):211–222, 1994.

Harrigan R. Smoke inhalation injury and fire toxicology: Evaluation and management. *Emerg Med Rep* 15(21):203–210, 1994.

Jones JS, et al. Metered-dose inhalers: Do emergency health care providers know what to teach? *Ann Emerg Med* 26(3):3008–3011, 1995.

Levitt MA, Gambrioli EF, and Fink JB. Comparative trial of continuous nebulization versus metered dose inhaler in the treatment of acute bronchospasm. *Ann Emerg Med* 26(3):273–277, 1995.

Moran GJ, et al. Delayed recognition and infection control for tuberculosis patients in the emergency department. *Ann Emerg Med* 26(3):290–295, 1995.

Singer JI, McCabe JB. Epiglottitis at the extremes of age. *J Emerg Med* 6(3):228–231, 1988.

Somerson S, et al. Mastering emergency airway management. *Am J Nurs* 96(5): 24–31, 1996.

Sexual Assault

Burgess AW, Fehder WP, and Hartman CR. Delayed reporting of the rape victim. *J Psychosoc Nurs Ment Health Serv* 33(9):21–29, 1995.

Dwyer BJ. Rape: Psychological, medical, and forensic aspects of emergency management. *Emerg Med Rep* 16(12):106–116, 1995.

Ledray LE. Sexual assault: Clinical issues. Sexual assault evidentiary exam and treatment protocol. *J Emerg Nurs* 21(4):355–359, 1995.

Skin Disorders

Todd JK. Severe invasive streptococcal syndrome. *Hosp Med* 31(7):28–34, 1994.

Surface Trauma

Brogan GX Jr, et al. Comparison of plain, warmed, and buffered lidocaine for anesthesia of traumatic wounds. *Ann Emerg Med* 26(2):121–125, 1995.

Edlich RF, and Drake DB. Repair of lacerations. Technical considerations in wound closure. *Hosp Med* 31(7):35–39, 1995.

Ernst AA, et al. LAT (lidocaine-adrenalin-tetracaine) versus TAC (tetracaine-adrenaline-cocaine) for topical anesthesia in face and scalp lacerations. *Am J Emerg Med* 13(2):151–154, 1995.

Lewis KT, and Stiles M. Management of cat and dog bites. *Am Fam Phys* 52(2):479–485, 1995.

Stiles N. High-pressure injection injury of the hand: A surgical emergency. *J Emerg Nurs* 20(5):351–354, 1994.

Transcultural

Autotte PA. Folk medicine. *Arch Pediatr Adolesc Med* 149(9):949–950, 1995.

Blackhall LJ, et al. Ethnicity and attitudes toward patient autonomy. *JAMA* 272(10): 820–825, 1995.

Pachter LM, Cloutier MM, and Bernstein BA. Ethnomedical (folk) remedies for childhood asthma in a mainland Puerto Rican community. *Arch Pediatr Adolesc Med* 149:982–988, 1995.

Risse AL, and Mazur LJ. Use of folk remedies in a Hispanic population. *Arch Pediatr Adolesc Med* 149:978–981, 1995.

Todd KH, Samaroo N, and Hoffman JR. Ethnicity as a risk factor for inadequate emergency department analgesia. *JAMA* 269(12):1537–1539, 1993.

Trauma

Cheney P. Early management and physiologic changes in crush syndrome. *Crit Care Nurs Q* 17(2):62–73, 1994.

Colucciello SA. The challenge of trauma in pregnancy: Guidelines for targeted assessment, fetal monitoring, and definitive management. *Emerg Med Rep* 16(4): 171–182, 1995.

Criss E. Back to back. Assessment of spinal trauma. *J Emerg Med Serv* 20(1):46–57, 1995.

Laskowski-Jones L. Meeting the challenge of chest trauma. *Am J Nurs* 95(9):22–31, 1995.

Line RL, and Rust GS. Acute exertional rhabdomyolysis. *Am Fam Phys* 52(2): 502–506, 1995.

Pediatric emergencies. *Emerg Med Clin North Am* 13(2):267–268, 1995.

Polhgeers A, and Ruddy RM. An update on pediatric trauma. *In Pediatric Emergencies. Emerg Med Clin North Am* 13(2):267–268, 1995.

Quebec Task Force on Whiplash-Associated Disorders. Scientific monograph of the Quebec Task Force on whiplash-associated disorders: Redefining "whiplash" and its management. *Spine* 20(suppl), 1995.

Rogers FB, Shackford SR, and Keller MS. Early fixation reduces mortality and morbidity in elderly patients with hip fractures from low-impact falls. *J Trauma* 39(2):261–265, 1995.

Sampalas JS, et al. Trauma center designation: Initial impact on trauma-related mortality. *J Trauma* 39(2):232–239, 1995.

Shabot KK, and Johnson CL. Outcome from critical care in the "oldest old" trauma patients. *J Trauma* 39(2):254–260, 1995.

Stomatos CA, et al. Managing the challenge of the older trauma patient. *Am J Nurs* 96(5):40–48, 1996.

Swierzewski M, et al. Deaths from motor vehicle crashes: Patterns of injury in restrained and unrestrained victims. *J Trauma* 37(3):404–407, 1994.

Resources

Organizations

American Heart Association
Chapters in each state.
Focuses on research and education related to cardiovascular disease. Produces Basic Life Support and Advanced Life Support course materials and credentials participants.

American Red Cross
National Office
8111 Gatehouse Road
Falls Church, VA 22042
(703) 206–6000
Education in CPR, first aid, disaster preparedness, and shelter care. Identification and notification of family members.

American Trauma Society
8903 Presidential Parkway, Suite 512
Upper Marlboro, MD 20772–2656
(800) 556–7890
Focuses on injury prevention and research.

Emergency Nurses Association
216 Higgins Road
Park Ridge, IL 60068–5736
(800) 243–8362
Courses and materials on emergency nursing, trauma nursing core course, and emergency pediatric and advanced trauma course.

ENCARE—Emergency Nurses Cancel Alcohol Related Emergencies
c/o Emergency Nurses Association
(800) 243–8362
Classes on drinking and driving, directed at teenagers; also injury prevention for older adults.

International Association of Forensic Nursing
c/o SLACK, Inc.
6900 Grove Road
Thorofare, NJ 08086
(609) 848–8356
Sexual Assault Nurse Examiners, death investigation, and medicolegal issues.

International Critical Incident Stress Foundation
P.O. Box 204
Ellicott City, MD 21043
Hot Line: (410) 313–CISD (2473)
Education in stress prevention and management.

Medic-Alert Foundation
2323 Colonda Avenue
Turlock, CA 95382
(800) 344–3226
Produces identification devices that list significant medical information (e.g., allergies, diabetes, heart disease, and epilepsy); maintains a database that health care providers can call to obtain clinical information on persons who have registered with the organization.

38
Caring for People with Environmentally and Occupationally Induced Disorders

◧ ENVIRONMENTAL AND OCCUPATIONAL HEALTH NURSING: OVERVIEW

Definitions

1. **Occupational health nursing** is a specialty practice in community health nursing that provides for and delivers health care services to workers and worker populations. It is focused on the promotion, protection, and restoration of workers' health within the context of a safe and healthy work environment (Box 38–1).
2. **Environmental health** is that portion of community health nursing that analyzes those environmental factors (contaminated air, food, water, soil) that affect the health status of individuals and communities. Water and air quality are critical environmental health issues, as are toxic exposures caused by industrial accidents or by hazardous waste sites.
3. **Toxicity** refers to the capacity of a substance to cause harm.
4. **Hazard** is the probability that injury or illness will occur based on the use and handling of a toxic substance. For example, asbestos has the capacity to cause harm; therefore, it has inherent toxicity. It is not a hazard if it is sealed and undisturbed. It is a hazard, however, during demolition when it has the potential of being released in the breathing zone of a worker.
5. **Exposure** refers to the presence of a hazardous substance in the environment. Exposure is measured by environmental surveillance, for example, an air sample measurement of the airborne concentration of carbon monoxide.
   a. Federal Occupational Safety and Health Administration (OSHA) standards mandate a permissible exposure level for many chemicals, which is the legal limit an employer must not exceed.
   b. The American Conference of Governmental Industrial Hygienists publishes threshold limit values for chemicals, which are recommended exposure limits to protect against adverse health effects. Threshold limit values are often less than permissible exposure levels.

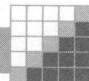

LEGAL AND ETHICAL CONSIDERATIONS

Employers must legally comply with the permissible exposure level in the OSHA standard, but this may not necessarily protect health. OSHA standards are consensus documents, wherein industry, labor, and scientific experts reach consensus on the acceptable risks and evaluate the economic impact of compliance with the standard.

In contrast, airborne concentrations of chemicals at or below the threshold limit values prevent adverse health effects. According to the ethical principle of **nonmaleficence,** or "do no harm," employers should strive to limit environmental airborne concentrations of hazardous chemicals to below the threshold limit value.

6. **Dose** refers to the amount of a substance delivered by inhalation, ingestion, or dermal or ocular absorption; it is measured by biologic measurements, for example, a blood level of lead.
7. **Ergonomics** is the study of the interface between the human body and the use of mechanical and electronic machines and tools. For example, an ergonomic evaluation determines whether there is a need for equipment redesign so that a 5-foot-tall woman can safely use a machine designed for a man who is 10 inches taller.

Basic Types of Hazards

1. **Physical hazards** include exposures to noise, heat, radiation, and vibration.
2. **Chemical hazards** include exposures to dusts, gases, fumes, and mists. Methylene chloride, a common solvent in many furniture stripping products, is an example of a potential chemical hazard.
3. **Psychophysiologic hazards** encompass the stressors associated with an imbalance between job demands and employee resources, including work stress, rotating shift work, and overtime. Violence is an increasingly prevalent example of a psychophysiologic hazard.
4. **Biologic hazards** include exposures to infectious agents, such as bacteria (tuberculosis) and viruses (hepatitis B). Exposures occur not only in patient care settings but also in research laboratories and animal care facilities.

BOX 38–1. Occupational and Environmental Health Team

Critical to occupational and environmental health program development, workers and their employers consult with the following team members:

- Occupational health nurse or nurse practitioner
- Occupational medicine physician
- Industrial hygienist
- Safety professional
- Workers' compensation carrier
- Rehabilitation counselor
- Employee assistance professional
- Ergonomic specialist
- Other resources: epidemiologist, toxicologist
- Other community health professionals, for example, sanitation experts

These team members may be employed by the industry and practice on site or they may be available through a workers' compensation insurance program. They may be employees of a local public health department or a freestanding clinic, or they may be employed by the employer through contractual agreements.

---

5. **Ergonomic hazards** include the mismatch or imbalance between a person and a machine or tool. Awkward posture, repetition, amount of weight, and degree of force are critical work variables, which, if not corrected, could lead to repetitive strain injuries, including tendonitis, carpal tunnel syndrome, strains, and sprains.

6. **Safety hazards** are associated with machine guarding, confined spaces, electrical systems, fire safety, vehicle safety, and emergency response.

Standards of Occupational and Environmental Health Nursing

1. The clinical standards of practice as set forth by the American Association of Occupational Health Nurses (AAOHN) are modeled after steps in the nursing process: assessment, nursing diagnosis, outcome identification, planning, implementation, and evaluation. The standards also include the following professional standards of practice: professional development and evaluation, quality improvement and assurance, collaboration, research, ethics, and resource management. A copy of the standards is available through the AAOHN.

2. There are no specific standards of practice for environmental health practice in nursing.

Transcultural Considerations

1. Environmental justice, or environmental equity, refers to the distribution of environmental risks across population groups and the recognition that there is disparity concerning these risks.

2. Frequently, low-income minority populations are subjected to multiple environmental risks and therefore have a greater environmental risk burden. For example, a child living in substandard housing may be exposed to both pesticides (from structural pest control applications)

and lead-based paint. Minorities continue to work disproportionately in higher risk jobs; non-White workers are concentrated in many of the most hazardous industries in the manufacturing sector.

3. It is estimated that 13 million preschoolers live in homes with lead-based paint. Poor non-Hispanic Black children who reside in urban areas are at increased risk for lead exposure.

Hazard Communication

1. The "right to know" about hazardous exposures at work and in the community is provided for by federal regulation; however, there are ethical considerations with right to know hazard communication programs.

2. Two key OSHA standards—the "Hazard Communication Standard" (Code of Federal Regulation [CFR] Title 29, Section 1910.1200) and "Access to Employee Exposure and Medical Records" (CFR 29, Section 1910.20)—require employers to provide certain hazard information to workers.

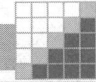 **LEGAL AND ETHICAL CONSIDERATIONS**

The right to know about hazardous chemicals and materials in the workplace or community involves the right to information so that appropriate action can be taken by the individual or group. This is the ethical principle of **autonomy.**

Employers who, knowingly or not, withhold toxics information from workers are legally out of compliance with the Hazard Communication Standard. Ethically, employers need to believe that workers have a right to this critical health and safety information. This information must be presented in a way that is tailored to the language and literacy skills of the work force. Likewise, involvement of worker groups in planning the hazard communication training and in the design of written hazard awareness educational materials integrates adult learning theory and risk communication principles. This illustrates the ethical principle of **beneficence,** or "doing good."

---

3. An important key provision of the Hazard Communication Standard is the Material Safety Data Sheet. The Material Safety Data Sheet is a summary of hazards for a chemical and outlines what to do for an emergency spill of that chemical. Workers must receive training in using the Material Safety Data Sheet, and they must be informed of hazardous chemicals that they may come in contact with in their workplace.

4. The OSHA Standard on Access to Employee Exposure and Medical Records provides access to aggregate exposure data of employees with similar work conditions, as well as giving employees access to their individual medical records.

5. Environmental regulation is by the Toxic Substances Control Act and by the Superfund Authorization Reconciliation Act III. Both require employers to report a certain level of toxic substance emissions into the environment.

6. The Environmental Protection Agency (EPA) monitors air and water quality. Federal regulation, such as the Clean Air Act, is implemented through state and local community agencies. For example, Air Quality Manage-

ment Districts monitor air for criteria pollutants (e.g., ozone) and toxic substances (e.g., benzene).

ASSESSING PEOPLE WITH OCCUPATIONALLY AND ENVIRONMENTALLY INDUCED DISORDERS

Key Symptoms and Their Pathophysiologic Basis

1. Symptoms of an occupational or environmental exposure may mimic other acute and chronic injury and illness. A careful history is needed to diagnose occupational and environmental conditions correctly.
2. Disease latency complicates accurate recognition of an occupational or environmental cause, for example, lung cancer that develops after a previous occupational exposure to a lung carcinogen such as asbestos or after an environmental exposure to radon.
3. Individuals may have multiple exposures at work, at home, and in the environment. For example, asthma caused by a work exposure to formaldehyde is exacerbated by passive smoking in the home and by ozone in air pollution.
4. Box 38–2 summarizes the occupational health objectives from *Healthy People 2000*.

BOX 38–2. Occupational Health Objectives for the Year 2000

1. **Work-related injury reduction:** reduce deaths, reduce lost time from work-related injuries.
2. **Cumulative trauma disorders:** reduce incidence rates; increase back injury prevention and rehabilitation programs.
3. **Occupational skin disorders:** reduce incidence rates of work-related skin disorders.
4. **Hepatitis B infection:** reduce incidence of hepatitis B cases; increase hepatitis B immunization for those at risk of work-related exposure.
5. **Vehicle safety:** increase use of seatbelts during all work-related travel.
6. **Noise-induced hearing loss:** decrease work-related exposure to below 85 dbA (decibel A).
7. **Lead exposure:** eliminate work-related exposure that results in blood levels greater than 25 μg/dl.
8. **Occupational health and safety programs:** implement state plans for the identification, management, and prevention of leading work-related injury and illness; increase employer-based programs on work health and safety; provide occupational health and safety consultation and assistance to small businesses.
9. **Occupational lung disease:** reduce the incidence of major occupational lung disorders: byssinosis (cotton), asbestosis, coal workers' pneumoconiosis, and silicosis.
10. **Occupational health history:** increase the proportion of primary care providers who routinely elicit occupational exposure data and provide relevant counseling.

From U.S. Department of Health and Human Services. *Healthy People 2000: National Health Promotion and Disease Prevention Objectives.* Washington, DC: U.S. Government Printing Office, 1991.

BOX 38–3. Environmental Health Objectives for the Year 2000

1. **Air quality:** reduce asthma morbidity; reduce human exposure to criteria air pollutants.
2. **Lead exposure:** reduce mental retardation; reduce lead in paint; lower blood lead levels in children; inform buyers of the presence of lead-based paint in property offered for sale.
3. **Water quality:** reduce outbreaks in waterborne disease from infectious agents and chemical poisonings; increase the supply of safe drinking water; improve the quality of surface water.
4. **Hazardous waste:** reduce human exposure to toxic pollutants and solid waste–related water, air, and soil contamination; eliminate significant health risks from hazardous waste sites on the National Priority List.
5. **Radon:** test for radon exposure in homes; adopt construction practices that minimize indoor concentrations of radon; inform buyers of radon concentrations in property offered for sale.
6. **Recycling:** establish recycling programs for households.
7. **Reporting:** establish a reporting system of sentinel environmental events.

From U.S. Department of Health and Human Services. *Healthy People 2000: National Health Promotion and Disease Prevention Objectives.* Washington, DC: U.S. Government Printing Office, 1991.

a. According to 1993 statistics from the Bureau of Labor Statistics, there were 6.7 million nonfatal work-related injury and illness cases reported in the private sector.
b. Of these, 6.3 million were injuries, mostly involving work-related musculoskeletal disorders. Manufacturing job injuries accounted for more than 50 percent of all newly reported illnesses, with injuries from repeated trauma, such as carpal tunnel syndrome, accounting for three fifths of the illness reports.

Reports of assaults and violent acts in the workplace have also increased across the United States (Box 38–3).

Health History

1. For a general screening of occupational and environmental risk factors, the following information should be obtained:
   a. The type and duration of all past and present work positions and associated job duties
   b. Whether there were any injuries or exposures to potentially hazardous toxins (e.g., exposure to asbestos or other dusts, solvents or other chemicals, lead or other metals, or radiation)
   c. Whether protective equipment (e.g., respirator, ear plugs, gloves) was used
   d. Whether there were any nonwork environmental exposures (e.g., associated with hobbies at home, passive smoking)
2. If pregnancy is desired, preconception counseling for both partners is of critical importance in assessing reproductive hazards (Tables 38–1 and 38–2). A list of telephone numbers for teratogen information is provided in *Case Studies in Environmental Medicine: Reproductive and Developmental Hazards.* (See Chapters 30 and 31.)

Table 38-1. Agents Associated with Adverse Female Reproductive Capacity or Developmental Effects in Human and Animal Studies*

Agent	Human Outcomes	Strength of Association in Humans†	Animal Outcomes	Strength of Association in Animals†
Anesthetic gases‡	Reduced fertility, spontaneous abortion	1, 3	Birth defects	1, 3
Arsenic	Spontaneous abortion, low birth weight	1	Birth defects, fetal loss	2
Benzo[a]pyrene	None	NA§	Birth defects	1
Cadmium	None	NA	Fetal loss, birth defects	2
Carbon disulfide	Menstrual disorders, spontaneous abortion	1	Birth defects	1
Carbon monoxide	Low birth weight, fetal death (high doses)	1	Birth defects, neonatal mortality	2
Chlordecone	None	NA	Fetal loss	2, 3
Chloroform	None	NA	Fetal loss	1
Chloroprene	None	NA	Birth defects	2, 3
Ethylene glycol ethers	Spontaneous abortion	1	Birth defects	2
Ethylene oxide	Spontaneous abortion	1	Fetal loss	1
Formamides	None	NA	Fetal loss, birth defects	2
Inorganic mercury‡	Menstrual disorders, spontaneous abortion	1	Fetal loss, birth defects	1
Lead‡	Spontaneous abortion, prematurity, neurologic dysfunction in child	2	Birth defects, fetal loss	2
Organic mercury	Central nervous system (CNS) malformation, cerebral palsy	2	Birth defects, fetal loss	2
Physical stress	Prematurity	2	None	NA
Polybrominated biphenyls	None	NA	Fetal loss	2
Polychlorinated biphenyls (PCBs)	Neonatal PCB syndrome (low birth weight, hyperpigmentation, eye abnormalities)	2	Low birth weight, fetal loss	2
Radiation, ionizing	Menstrual disorders, CNS defects, skeletal and eye anomalies, mental retardation, childhood cancer	2	Fetal loss, birth defects	2
Selenium	Spontaneous abortion	3	Low birth weight, birth defects	2
Tellurium	None	NA	Birth defects	2
2,4-Dichlorophenoxyacetic acid	Skeletal defects	4	Birth defects	1
2,4,5-Trichlorophenoxyacetic acid	Skeletal defects	4	Birth defects	1
Video display terminals	Spontaneous abortion	4	Birth defects	1
Vinyl chloride‡	CNS defects	1	Birth defects	1, 4
Xylene	Menstrual disorders, fetal loss	1	Fetal loss, birth defects	1

* Major studies of the reproductive health effects of exposure to dioxin are ongoing.
† 1 = limited positive data.
  2 = strong positive data.
  3 = limited negative data.
  4 = strong negative data.
‡ Agents may have male-mediated effects.
§ Not applicable because no adverse outcomes were observed.
From U.S. Department of Health and Human Services. *Case Studies in Environmental Medicine: Reproductive and Developmental Hazards.* Atlanta: Public Health Service, Agency for Toxic Substances and Disease Registry, 1993.

3. If a patient exhibits a specific symptom (e.g., a cough or skin rash), the following information should be sought:
   a. Potential work or home exposure that could cause the complaint
   b. Whether there has been a recent change in the work process or home situation that could account for the symptom
   c. Whether coworkers, other home residents, or neighbors have complained of similar symptoms
   d. Whether there is a temporal relationship to the symptom, for example, whether it is better on weekends, vacations, or during 1 season rather than another

NURSE ADVISORY

One exposed individual usually signifies more exposed individuals at the home, neighborhood, or workplace. Most occupational and environmental health conditions are preventable.

4. There are many sample formats for collecting an occupational and environmental health history. See Figure 38-1 for 1 suggested format for an exposure survey, work history, and environmental history.

Table 38–2. Exposures Associated with Male Reproductive Dysfunction

Agent	Human Outcomes	Strength of Association in Humans*	Animal Outcomes	Strength of Association in Animals*
Boron	Decreased spermatozoa count	1	Testicular damage	2
Benzene	None	NA†	Decreased spermatozoa motility, testicular damage	1
Benzo[a]pyrene	None	NA	Testicular damage	1
Cadmium	Reduced fertility	1	Testicular damage	2
Carbon disulfide	Decreased spermatozoa count, decreased spermatozoa motility	2, 3	Testicular damage	1
Carbon monoxide	None	NA	Testicular damage	1
Carbon tetrachloride	None	NA	Testicular damage	1
Carbaryl	Abnormal spermatozoa morphology	1	Testicular damage	1
Chlordecone	Decreased spermatozoa count, decreased spermatozoa motility	2	Testicular damage	2
Chloroprene	Decreased spermatozoa motility, abnormal morphology, decreased libido	2	Testicular damage	1
Dibromochloropropane	Decreased spermatozoa count, azoospermia, hormonal changes	2	Testicular damage	2
Dimethyl dichlorovinyl phosphate	None	NA	Decreased spermatozoa count	2
Epichlorohydrin	None	NA	Testicular damage	2, 3
Estrogens	Decreased spermatozoa count	2	Decreased spermatozoa count	2
Ethylene oxide	None	NA	Testicular damage	1
Ethylene dibromide	Abnormal spermatozoa motility	1	Testicular damage	2, 3
Ethylene glycol ethers	Decreased spermatozoa count	1	Testicular damage	2
Heat	Decreased spermatozoa count	2	Decreased spermatozoa count	2
Lead	Decreased spermatozoa count	2	Testicular damage, decreased spermatozoa count, decreased spermatozoa motility, abnormal morphology	2
Manganese	Decreased libido, impotence	1	Testicular damage	1, 3
Polybrominated biphenyls	None	NA	Testicular damage	1
Polychlorinated biphenyls	None	NA	Testicular damage	1
Radiation, ionizing	Decreased spermatozoa count	2	Testicular damage	2

* 1 = limited positive data.
  2 = strong positive data.
  3 = limited negative data.
  4 = strong negative data.
† Not applicable because no adverse outcomes were observed.
From U.S. Department of Health and Human Services. *Case Studies in Environmental Medicine: Reproductive and Developmental Hazards.* Atlanta: Public Health Service, Agency for Toxic Substances and Disease Registry, 1993.

5. For people at risk for an occupational or environmental exposure and for those who have sustained an occupational injury or illness, the following should be assessed:

  a. Cultural beliefs about health and preventive measures. Many occupational and environmental health conditions that occur in a specific region of the country or in a specific industry may be regarded as normal. For example, black lung in the coal miners in Appalachia, back pain in truck drivers, and hearing loss in rock and roll musicians may be viewed as anticipated and accepted risks of the job. Assessment of these health beliefs is critical when designing a teaching program for hazard reduction.

  b. Previous illness and course of recovery

  c. The meaning and expression of pain

  d. Work and functionality

  e. Disability and associated role change

  f. Healing practices

Physical Examination

1. Systems along the route of exposure (inhalation, ingestion, dermal) should be the focus of attention.
2. The examination should focus on any organ at potentially high risk of damage based on duration, dose, and nature of the substance or situation to which the patient has been exposed.

Selected Diagnostic Tests

- Pulmonary function tests (see Chapter 22)
- Audiograms (see Chapter 20)
- Patch testing (see Chapter 35)
- Nerve conduction studies (see Chapter 18)
- Radiographs or magnetic resonance imaging (see Chapter 34)
- Electrocardiograms and stress testing (see Chapter 23)

Text continued on page 1810

Exposure History Form

Part 1. Exposure Survey
Please circle the appropriate answer.

Name: _____ Date: _____

Birthdate: _____ Sex: M   F

1. Are you currently exposed to any of the following?

    metals

        no   *yes*

    dust or fibers

        no   *yes*

    chemicals

        no   *yes*

    fumes

        no   *yes*

    radiation

        no   *yes*

        loud noise, vibration, extreme heat or cold

        no   *yes*

        biologic agents

        no   *yes*

2. Have you been exposed to any of the above *in the past?*

        no   *yes*

3. Do any household members have contact with metals, dust, fibers, chemicals, fumes, radiation, or biologic agents?

        no   *yes*

If you answered *yes* to any of the items above, describe your exposure in detail—how you were exposed; to what you were exposed. If you need more space, please use a separate sheet of paper.

4. Do you know the names of the metals, dusts, fibers, chemicals, fumes, or radiation that you are/were exposed to?

        no   *yes* ■ ▬ ▬▬▬▬➤   If *yes*, list them below.

5. Do you get the material on your skin or clothing?

        no   *yes*

6. Are your work clothes laundered at home?

        no   *yes*

7. Do you shower at work?

        no   *yes*

8. Can you smell the chemical or material you are working with?

        no   *yes*

9. Do you use protective equipment such as gloves, masks, respirator, hearing protectors?

        no   *yes* ■ ▬ ▬▬▬▬➤   If *yes*, list the protective equipment used.

10. Have you been advised to use protective equipment?

        no   *yes*

11. Have you been instructed in the use of protective equipment?

        no   *yes*

12. Do you wash your hands with solvents?

        no   *yes*

13. Do you smoke at the workplace?   At home?

        no   *yes*   *no*   *yes*

14. Do you eat at the workplace?

        no   *yes*

Figure 38–1. Exposure history form. (From the U.S. Department of Health and Human Services. Case Studies in Environmental Medicine, October 1992. Originally developed by the Agency for Toxic Substances and Disease Registry, Atlanta, GA, in cooperation with the National Institute for Occupational Safety and Health.)

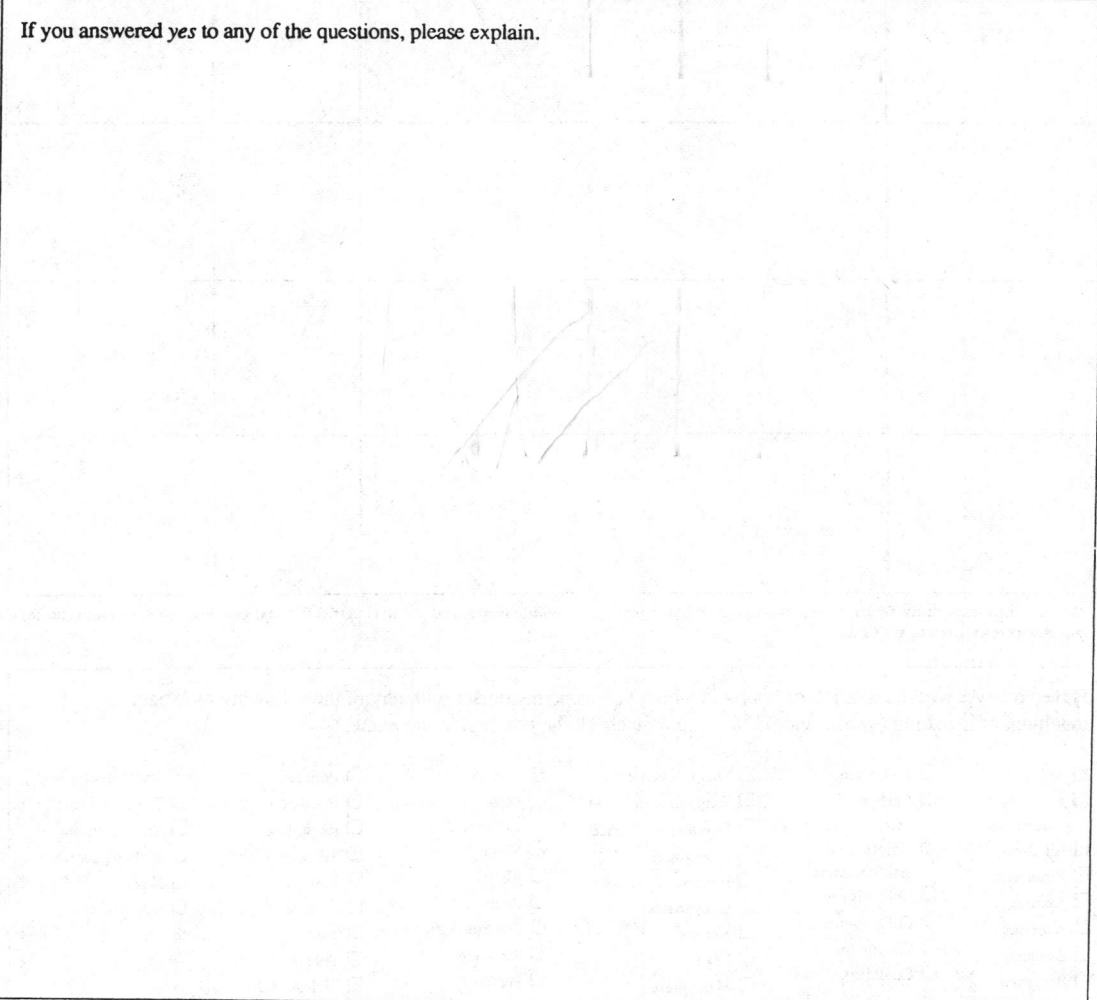

15. Do you know of any coworkers experiencing similar or unusual symptoms?
      no   *yes*

16. Are family members experiencing similar or unusual symptoms?
      no   *yes*

17. Has there been a change in the health or behavior of family pets?
      no   *yes*

18. Do your symptoms seem to be aggravated by a specific activity?
      no   *yes*

19. Do your symptoms get either worse or better at work?
      no   *yes*

   at home?
      no   *yes*

   on weekends?
      no   *yes*

   on vacation?
      no   *yes*

20. Has anything about your job changed in recent months (such as duties, procedures, overtime)?
      no   *yes*

If you answered *yes* to any of the questions, please explain.

Figure 38–1. *Continued*

Illustration continued on following page

Part 2. Work History
A. Occupational Profile

Name: _____

Birthdate: _____ Sex: M F

The following questions refer to your current or most recent job:

Job title: _____

Type of industry: _____

Name of employer: _____

Date job began: _____

Are you still working in this job?

     Yes   No

If no, when did this job end? _____

Describe this job:

_____

_____

_____

_____

_____

_____

Fill in the table below listing all jobs you have worked including short-term, seasonal, part-time employment, and military service. Begin with your most recent job. Use additional paper if necessary.

Dates of Employment	Job Title and Description of Work	Exposures*	Protective Equipment

*List the chemicals, dusts, fibers, fumes, radiation, biologic agents (i.e., molds, viruses) and physical agents (i.e., extreme heat, cold, vibration, noise) that you were exposed to at this job.

Have you ever worked at a job or hobby in which you came in contact with any of the following by breathing, touching, or ingesting (swallowing)? If yes, please check the box beside the name.

❑ Acids	❑ Cadmium	❑ Dichlorobenzene	❑ Mercury	❑ Phosgene	❑ Trichloroethylene
❑ Alcohols (industrial)	❑ Carbon tetrachloride	❑ Ethylene dibromide	❑ Methylene chloride	❑ Radiation	❑ Trinitrotoluene
❑ Alkalies	❑ Chlorinated naphthalenes	❑ Ethylene dichloride	❑ Nickel	❑ Rock dust	❑ Vinyl chloride
❑ Ammonia	❑ Chloroform	❑ Fiberglass	❑ PBBs	❑ Silica powder	❑ Welding fumes
❑ Arsenic	❑ Chloroprene	❑ Halothane	❑ PCBs	❑ Solvents	❑ X rays
❑ Asbestos	❑ Chromates	❑ Isocyanates	❑ Perchloroethylene	❑ Styrene	❑ Other (specify)
❑ Benzene	❑ Coal dust	❑ Ketones	❑ Pesticides	❑ Talc	
❑ Beryllium		❑ Lead	❑ Phenol	❑ Toluene	
		❑ Manganese		❑ TDI or MDI	

Figure 38–1. *Continued*

B. Occupational Exposure Inventory *Please circle the appropriate answer.*

1. Have you ever been off work for more than one day because of an illness related to work?   *no*   *yes*

2. Have you ever been advised to change jobs or work assignments because of any health problems or injuries?   *no*   *yes*

3. Has your work routine changed recently?   *no*   *yes*

4. Is there poor ventilation in your workplace?   *no*   *yes*

Part 3. Environmental History   *Please circle the appropriate answer.*

1. Do you live next to or near an industrial plant, commercial business, dump site, or nonresidential property?   *no*   *yes*

2. Which of the following do you have in your home?
   Please circle those that apply.

Air conditioner	Air purifier	Central heating (gas or oil?)
Gas stove	Electric stove	Fireplace
Wood stove	Humidifier	

3. Have you recently acquired new furniture or carpet, refinished furniture, or remodeled your home?   *no*   *yes*

4. Have you weatherized your home recently?   *no*   *yes*

5. Are pesticides or herbicides (bug or weed killers; flea and tick sprays, collars, powders, or shampoos) used in your home or garden, or on pets?   *no*   *yes*

6. Do you (or any household member) have a hobby or craft?   *no*   *yes*

7. Do you work on your car?   *no*   *yes*

8. Have you ever changed your residence because of a health problem?   *no*   *yes*

9. Does your drinking water come from a private well, city water supply, or grocery store?
   _____

10. Approximately what year was your home built?_____

If you answered *yes* to any of the questions, please explain.

Figure 38–1. *Continued*

Laboratory Work

- Liver function tests (see Chapter 28)
- Complete blood count (see Chapter 25)
- Blood lead levels
- Cholinesterase levels
- Carboxyhemoglobin levels

◪ *OCCUPATIONAL AND ENVIRONMENTAL DISORDERS*

Occupational Pulmonary Disorders

1. Pneumoconiosis: Pulmonary fibrotic conditions are a direct result of chronic pulmonary exposure to small particles of dust. Silica, asbestos, cotton dust, and coal dust are a few of the offending agents, in addition to hard metals, such as cobalt contained in dust. See Chapter 22 for a discussion on respiratory disorders.
2. Asbestosis
   a. Definition
      (1) Asbestosis is a pneumoconiosis caused by exposure to asbestos dust. Asbestos is a known carcinogen, causing cancers of the lung and gastrointestinal tract as well as mesotheliomas of the pleura and peritoneum.
      (2) Asbestosis can be caused from short exposures over a long period of time or from heavy exposures over a short period of time. Asbestosis cases have been recorded from an intense exposure over a 1-day period.
   b. Incidence and socioeconomic impact
      (1) Asbestos is the most widespread of the pneumoconioses, with use of asbestos being widespread from 1940 to 1970. Asbestos causes more lung inflammation, tissue injury, and fibrotic changes than silica or coal.
      (2) It is difficult to estimate the number of persons exposed to asbestos. Asbestos is ubiquitous in the environment. There is a long latency period of up to 15 to 40 years between exposure and onset of symptoms or radiologic changes.
   c. Risk factors
      (1) The construction, shipyard, and insulation industries used asbestos extensively between 1940 and 1970. Widespread application includes the use of asbestos in asbestos cement products (tiles, roofing, drain pipes); floor tile, insulation, and fireproofing materials (shipbuilding and construction); textiles; asbestos paper; and friction materials (brake and clutch linings in cars and trucks).
      (2) The EPA ordered a phased elimination of all new mining, importation, and application of asbestos in the early 1970s, but asbestos is still used in cement products.
      (3) Demolition, home remodeling, and auto repair work activities continue to expose workers to asbestos. Friability of the material containing asbestos is a critical consideration. If the material is friable, then there is a greater likelihood that breathable fibers of asbestos will be emitted.
      (4) Families can be exposed through asbestos dust on the skin and clothes of workers.
      (5) Water for drinking can contain asbestos through the natural erosion of asbestos rock, the contamination of water supplies through discarded mine tailings, and the passage of water through asbestos cement pipes.
      (6) Cigarette smoking greatly increases the risk of asbestos-associated lung cancer.
   d. Etiology
      (1) Asbestos is a fibrous, heat resistant, naturally occurring mineral silicate. There are several types of asbestos fibers. The type of asbestos used most is chrysotile of the serpentine class.
      (2) The primary route of exposure is through inhalation. Ingestion of asbestos fibers in mucus (coughed up in sputum) and water is an additional route of exposure.
      (3) The size and shape of the fibers determine whether the lung can effectively remove them. Only particles between 0.5 and 5.0 microns in diameter, with a length to width ratio of 3:1, are deposited in the alveoli and terminal bronchioles.
   e. Pathophysiology
      (1) Fibrotic lung changes result from the persistent release of inflammatory mediators such as interleukins and enzymes at the site of fiber penetration and deposition.
      (2) Unlike other pneumoconioses, asbestos affects the pleura of the lung, causing pleural thickening.
      (3) Asbestos fibers can persist in the lung many years after exposure. Asbestosis can progress even after exposure has ended.
   f. Clinical manifestations
      (1) Dyspnea is usually the 1st symptom of asbestosis, as shown by a decreased exercise tolerance.
      (2) A nonproductive cough is common.
      (3) Pleuritic pain and chest tightness may occur.
   g. Diagnostics (Some of the following diagnostics are mandated by the OSHA "Standard on Asbestos," CFR Title 29, Section 1910.1101.)
      (1) Health history includes the following:
         - Assessment for current and past sources of asbestos exposure at work and at home, including hobbies
         - An attempt to quantify moderate to severe exposure to asbestos by assessing how often the person worked in a white cloud of dust without appropriate respiratory protection
         - Assessment for history of shipyard work during World War II, which is usually significant for asbestos exposure
         - Assessment for other dust exposures, including silica dust, coal dust, cotton dust, and hard-metal–containing dusts
         - Assessment for a history of or current pattern of smoking
         - Use of a standardized respiratory questionnaire

for asbestos, which is included in the OSHA Standard Appendix

(2) Physical examination includes the following:
- Examination of the oronasopharynx to assess suspicious lesions
- Examination of the skin for cyanosis and the presence of skin nodules from asbestos fibers
- Examination of the nails for clubbing
- Examination of the pulmonary system for respiratory rate, nasal flaring, respiratory effort, and the presence of end-inspiratory rales
- Examination of the cardiovascular system
- Examination of the gastrointestinal system, including rectal examination

(3) Diagnostic studies include the following:
- Pulmonary function tests (see Chapter 22)
- Oblique and posteroanterior chest radiographs, specifically for fibrotic changes and pleural plaques and thickening. A "B" reader is recommended for interpretation and classification of chest radiographs of persons exposed to asbestos.
- Stool Hemoccult
- Computed tomography scan for evaluation of pleural plaques

h. Clinical management

(1) Goals of clinical management
- Because there is no medical or surgical treatment to reverse asbestosis, clinical management should focus on protecting the remaining lung function, with the goal to prevent future exposure to asbestos or other dusts.
- Smoking cessation is a critical consideration in a person with a prior or current exposure to asbestos.

(2) Nonpharmacologic interventions
- Education and counseling on managing the symptoms of dyspnea should be available to the patient and family (see Chapter 22).
- Smoking cessation group strategies should be instituted (see Chapter 40).
- The patient should be educated to observe for signs and symptoms of carcinoma.
- The patient should be given diet education to improve nutritional status and prevent protein-calorie malnutrition.

(3) Pharmacologic interventions include the following:
- Oxygen support at home, if needed
- Nicotine patches or gum for smoking cessation, if it is not contraindicated
- Aggressive treatment of any pulmonary infection
- Pneumococcal vaccine, with annual influenza vaccines

i. Complications

(1) Asbestosis can be a mild, nonprogressive disease, or it can advance to respiratory failure.

(2) Mesotheliomas of the pleura and the peritoneum are rare tumors exclusively caused by asbestos exposure. Mesothelioma is a separate entity, not viewed as a complication to asbestosis. There is no effective treatment.

(3) Lung cancer from asbestos exposure can occur after a latency period of 10 to 30 years. A synergistic risk for asbestos-associated lung cancer is noted in persons who smoke.

j. Prognosis

(1) Progression of asbestosis varies and can range from mild to severe pulmonary impairment.

(2) The prognosis for mesothelioma is poor.

(3) The treatment and prognosis of asbestos-associated lung cancer is similar to those of other lung cancers. Appropriate surgical and chemotherapeutic regimens are indicated.

k. Applying the nursing process

NURSING DIAGNOSIS: Impaired gas exchange R/T asbestos exposure

---

(1) *Expected outcomes:* Following instruction, the person should be able to do the following:
- Demonstrate an understanding of asbestos exposure by identifying that asbestos is a carcinogen and that there is a synergistic effect between smoking and the development of asbestos-associated lung cancer; identifying sources of potential asbestos exposure in the workplace, home, and with hobbies; listing ways to limit asbestos exposure, including ventilation, containment, personal protection controls (respirators and protective clothing), safe handling, and appropriate waste disposal; describing early symptoms and signs of pulmonary infection or carcinoma that need medical attention; and identifying diet considerations for improving nutritional status and preventing malnutrition
- Demonstrate the correct use of respiratory protection, if indicated
- If symptomatic, outline physiologic and psychosocial measures to manage dyspnea

(2) *Nursing interventions*
- Diaphragmatic breathing exercises
- Chest percussion
- Oxygen therapy
- Case management, with psychosocial support, is needed for patients with progressive pulmonary impairment.
- For patients currently exposed to asbestos, periodic surveillance is mandated by OSHA.

l. Discharge planning and teaching

(1) Reinforcement of the protection of pulmonary status with aggressive treatment of any pulmonary infection. Reinforcement of the need for annual influenza vaccine and smoking cessation.

(2) Protection from future exposure to asbestos and other pulmonary irritants.

m. Public health considerations
   (1) Work site visits by occupational health and safety specialists are recommended to evaluate for asbestos exposure.
   (2) Home remodeling is a potential source of asbestos exposure. Homeowners should determine whether their home has asbestos ceiling tile, insulation, or floor tiles before doing repairs. Professional consultation and removal by those certified in asbestos removal are required in many states.
   (3) The EPA monitors asbestos levels in water sources. The Asbestos in Schools Identification and Notification Act of 1982 outlines measures for the control of asbestos in school environments.
   (4) One occupational health objective in *Healthy People 2000* aims to reduce occupationally induced pulmonary disorders.
3. Occupational asthma
   a. Definition
      (1) Occupational asthma is airway obstruction that follows a workplace exposure to inhaled gases, dusts, fumes, or vapors.
      (2) It is a preventable condition, with the medical diagnosis made by eliciting a complete occupational and environmental health history.
   b. Incidence and etiology
      (1) At least 200 agents in the workplace have been shown to cause asthma (Table 38–3).
      (2) The prevalence of occupationally induced asthma is unknown. In 1991, however, an estimated 6.4 million (63%) of the 10.3 million persons with asthma in the United States resided in areas where at least one National Ambient Air Quality Standard was exceeded.
   c. Clinical manifestations
      (1) In allergic bronchospasm, IgE or IgG antibodies develop in susceptible persons after exposure to workplace antigens, such as animal and plant proteins. There may be a latency period between the 1st exposure and the onset of allergic bronchospasm.
      (2) After a workplace exposure, there can be an early or late onset of symptoms. After removal from exposure, some workers improve rapidly and recover to pre-exposure lung function within 24 hours. Others show progressive decrements in pulmonary function, not recovering to pre-exposure lung function until several days after removal from exposure.
      (3) Shortness of breath, wheezing, and cough are the usual symptoms of asthma. Occupational asthma, however, can usually be temporally linked to specific work practices wherein there is exposure to known respiratory allergens.
      (4) A progressive decline in forced expiratory volume in 1 second (FEV_1) while the person is at work, for example, a decline of 10 percent or more over the work shift as documented by a peak flowmeter, is a useful measurement in the diagnosis of occupational asthma.
   d. Intervention
      (1) Removal from exposure is the key intervention.
      (2) Protection of other workers from similar exposure is a public health consideration. The workplace

Table 38–3. Selected Causes of Occupational Asthma*

Agents	Occupation
High–molecular-weight compounds	
Animal products: dander, excreta, serum, secretions	Animal handlers, laboratory workers, veterinarians
Plants: grain, dust, flour, tobacco, tea, hops	Grain handlers, tea workers, bakers, and workers in natural oil manufacturing and in tobacco and food processing
Enzymes: *Bacillus subtilis,* pancreatic extracts, papain, trypsin, fungal amylase	Bakers and workers in the detergent, pharmaceutical, and plastic industries
Vegetable: gum acacia, gum tragacanth	Printers and gum-manufacturing workers
Other: crab, prawn	Crab and prawn processors
Low–molecular-weight compounds	
Diisocyanates: toluene diisocyanate, methylene-diphenyldiisocyanate	Polyurethane industry workers, plastics workers, workers using varnish, and foundry workers
Anhydrides: phthallic and trimellitic anhydrides	Epoxy resin and plastics workers
Wood dust: oak, mahogany, California redwood, Western red cedar	Carpenters, sawmill workers, and furniture makers
Metals: platinum, nickel, chromium, cobalt, vanadium, tungsten carbide	Platinum and nickel-refining workers and hard-metal workers
Soldering fluxes	Solderers
Drugs: penicillin, methyldopa, tetracyclines, cephalosporins, psyllium	Pharmaceutical and health care industry workers
Other organic chemicals: urea formaldehyde, dyes, formalin, azodicarbonamide, hexachlorophene, ethylene diamine, dimethyl ethanolamine, polyvinyl chloride pyrolysates	Workers in chemical, plastic, and rubber industries; hospitals; laboratories; foam insulation manufacture; food wrapping; and spray painting

* Mechanism believed to be immunoglobulin E–mediated for high–molecular-weight compounds and some low–molecular-weight compounds. The immunologic mechanism for asthma from many low–molecular-weight substances remains undefined.

From Levy BS, and Wegman DH (eds). *Occupational Health: Recognizing and Preventing Work-Related Disease.* 3rd ed. Boston: Little, Brown & Co, 1995, p 436.

environment should be evaluated to determine unsafe work processes or practices and relevant exposure levels. Controls (e.g., ventilation and enclosing of open systems) should be recommended to prevent exposure to specific chemical hazards. A respiratory protection program, as determined by the OSHA Respiratory Protection Standard (CFR Title 29, Section 1910.134), should be implemented.

Musculoskeletal Disorders

1. Musculoskeletal work-related disorders
   a. Definition
      (1) Soft tissue injuries of the back, cervical spine, and upper extremity are the most common work-related musculoskeletal disorders, involving strains (tendons) and sprains (ligaments). Fractures of the bones are an additional work-related injury.
      (2) Nerves, muscles, joints, skin, and vascular systems may be involved with work-related musculoskeletal disorders, in addition to the original injury to bones, tendons, and ligaments.
      (3) Work-related musculoskeletal disorders are of 2 types: acute injury and cumulative trauma. Low back pain is almost always classified as an injury, as are injuries from slips and falls. Cumulative trauma disorders are caused by overuse, with microtears to the soft tissue structures. Tendonitis is 1 example.
      (4) Repetitive strain injuries are directly related to the following work variables: repetitions (defined as a cycle time less than 30 sec), duration, forceful exertions, awkward postures, contact stresses (e.g., a hard edge of a desk), vibration, and cold temperature.
   b. Incidence and socioeconomic impact
      (1) The incidence of cumulative trauma disorders reported to the Bureau of Labor Statistics has increased. In 1993, 302,000 cases of cumulative trauma disorders were reported in the private sector, up from 281,000 cases in 1992.
      (2) *Healthy People 2000* notes that the 1987 baseline incidence rate of cumulative trauma disorders was 100 cases per 100,000 full-time workers; the goal is to reduce this rate to 60 cases per 100,000 full-time workers by the year 2000.
      (3) Many industries are reporting increased recognition of soft tissue injuries related to repetitive work, with associated increased workers' compensation costs. These costs are in diagnostics, medical treatment, lost time from work, and rehabilitation, in addition to lost productivity.
      (4) Draft ergonomic protection guidelines have been published by OSHA to help employers correct work stations and work processes to help prevent cumulative trauma disorders (see Learning/Teaching Guidelines for Assessment of and Solutions to Risks Associated with Manual Handling).

   (5) The National Institute for Occupational Safety and Health has established manual lifting guidelines, to prevent back and other injuries. These guidelines are integrated into the draft ergonomic guidelines published by OSHA.
   (6) The Agency for Health Care Policy and Research has published treatment guidelines in *Acute Low Back Problems in Adults: Assessment and Treatment,* outlining its research-based recommendations for low back pain assessment and management.
   (7) Many medical councils of state workers' compensation boards are detailing practice parameters for common work-related injury and illness management, including work-related musculoskeletal disorders.
   c. See Chapter 34 for the clinical management of these conditions.
2. Carpal tunnel syndrome
   a. Definition
      (1) Carpal tunnel syndrome is the compression of the median nerve at the wrist, under the transverse carpal ligament.
      (2) Carpal tunnel syndrome is associated with many conditions: diabetes, thyroid disorders, rheumatoid arthritis, amyloidosis, and in those persons with repetitious flexion-extension of the wrist.
      (3) Although not an inflammatory process, carpal tunnel syndrome is thought to be caused by venous congestion at the wrist and resultant scarring of the nerve sheaths or the nearby flexor tendon sheaths, which impinges on the median nerve.
      (4) Classic symptoms of carpal tunnel syndrome are the following:
         • Paresthesias in the median nerve distribution (thumb, 2nd and 3rd digits)
         • Nighttime wakening with these paresthesias
         • Motor loss of the thenar muscle, which is a late finding, signifying advanced carpal tunnel syndrome
   b. Incidence and socioeconomic impact
      (1) The incidence of carpal tunnel syndrome is difficult to quantify because of variable case definitions.
      (2) A Sentinel Event Notification System for Occupational Risks (SENSOR) project to document the true incidence of carpal tunnel syndrome related to work is under way in several states.
   c. See Chapter 34 for the management of carpal tunnel syndrome.

Occupational Cancers

1. Definition
   a. A number of occupational agents or exposures have been found to cause a variety of tumors (Table 38–4).
   b. Other nonchemical work-related exposures are linked to occupational cancers:
      • Radiation exposure and leukemia
      • Sun exposure and basal, squamous, and melanoma skin cancers

LEARNING/TEACHING GUIDELINES
for Assessment of and Solutions to Risks Associated with Manual Handling

Assessment of Risks Associated with Manual Handling

Manual Handling Checklist

Yes	No	
___	___	1. Are materials moved over a minimum distance?
___	___	2. Is the horizontal distance between the middle knuckle and the body less than 4 inches?
___	___	3. Are obstacles removed to minimize reaches?
___	___	4. Are walking surfaces level and well lit?
		5. Are objects
___	___	Able to be grasped by good handholds?
___	___	Stable?
___	___	Able to be held without slipping?
___	___	6. When required, do gloves improve the grasp without bunching up or resisting movement of the hands?
___	___	7. Is there enough room to access and move objects?
___	___	8. Are mechanical aids easily available and used whenever possible?
___	___	9. Are working surfaces adjustable to the best handling heights?
		10. Does material handling avoid
___	___	Movements below knuckle height and above shoulder height?

Yes	No	
___	___	Static awkward postures?
___	___	Sudden movements during handling?
___	___	Twisting of the trunk?
___	___	Excessive reaching while holding or moving the load?
___	___	11. Is help available for heavy or awkward lifts?
		12. Are high rates of repetition avoided by
___	___	Job rotation?
___	___	Self pacing?
___	___	Sufficient rest pauses?
		13. Are pushing and pulling forces reduced or eliminated by
___	___	Casters that are sized correctly and roll freely?
___	___	Handles for pushing and pulling?
___	___	Availability of mechanical assists?
___	___	14. Are objects rarely carried more than 10 feet?
___	___	15. Is there a preventive maintenance program for manual handling equipment?

If you answered no to any question in this section on manual material handling, please refer to Questions 1–7.

Possible Solutions to Risks Associated with Manual Handling

Area of Concern	Possible Solutions	Explanation
1. Do workers need to bend to handle items?	Awkward postures of the back include bending forward and backward or to either side. Activities include lifting, lowering, and stooping over workstations.	Bending occurs when the item is beyond reach. Use lifting tables to raise the work to an appropriate height. Design the material flow so that the work is at waist height and within reach.
2. Do workers twist while lifting?	Twisting usually occurs if 1. The lift and set-down positions are at an angle to one another. 2. The lifting motion is across the body. 3. The lift is done with the feet constrained (such as on a foot pedal). 4. The lift is done while the worker maintains balance on rough or uneven surface. Provide all materials and tools in front of the employee. Use equipment to change the direction. Eliminate or reduce the number of lifts performed in confined spaces.	Provide all materials and tools in front of the employee. Use equipment to change the direction. Eliminate or reduce the number of lifts performed in confined spaces.

LEARNING/TEACHING GUIDELINES
(continued)

Area of Concern	Possible Solutions	Explanation
3. Do workers reach too far?	Reaches beyond 20 inches (toes to middle knuckles) need to be reviewed. Excessive reaches stress the shoulders and back. Bending more than 20 degrees at the waist stretches the muscles and tendons in the back, legs, and knees. Bending at the waist can also create contact stress between the torso or legs and the edge of furniture or equipment in the workplace.	Provide a place for tools and materials within 15 inches of a seated workplace and 20 inches of a standing workplace. Reduce the size of materials or rotate the materials (pallet). Eliminate unnecessary obstructions.
4. Does the job require lifting too much weight?	The amount of weight that a person should lift depends on several factors. A few are the characteristics of the objects lifted, the posture of the worker during the lift, the frequency of the lift, and the muscle groups needed to perform the lift.	If the worker is lifting loads that are too heavy for the conditions, then either reduce the weight or increase the weight so that mechanical equipment is needed to perform the lift. The National Institute for Occupational Safety and Health lifting equation is useful for evaluating work conditions to determine whether too much weight is handled for the task conditions.
5. Does the work require excessive pushing, pulling, or carrying?	Items should not be carried more than 30 feet on a repetitive basis. Carrying requires a lift and sustained arm, shoulder, back, and leg muscle activity (often forearm and wrist too). Pushing is preferred to pulling. Both pushing and pulling involve an initial effort to start the object in motion, followed by a smaller effort to sustain the motion. Reducing the weight reduces the initial effort, while attention to surfaces and wheel condition reduces the sustained effort.	Eliminate the need to carry by using a material handling device, such as a cart. Eliminate the need to pull objects, and eliminate or reduce the force needed to push objects. Use powered materials handling equipment or better casters.
6. Does the job require handling patients or animals?	Unstable loads can create sudden high muscle forces that may result in musculoskeletal damage.	Unstable lifts should be performed by a 2 (or more) person team that has been trained in lifting. Other alternatives include lifting and transfer devices. For patient handling, modifications to the bathroom, toilet, and bed can reduce the effort needed to lift a person.
7. Are gloves needed?	Gloves may need to be worn when handling materials with sharp (rough) edges, in cold environments, or for chemical protection. Loose gloves require more grip than when no gloves are worn. Gloves that fit too tightly or are bulky also cause a person to grip harder.	When possible, it is better to eliminate the sharp edge or pad the edge of the material rather than to use gloves. Handles can eliminate the need for gloves. Good handles or handholds can reduce the effort needed to lift and eliminate contact stress. When gloves are needed for personal protection (e.g., against chemicals or cold), use gloves that combine protection and fit.

Adapted from Special Supplement, Appendix B. *Control of Risk Factor Exposures in the OSHA Draft Proposed Ergonomic Protection Standard: Summaries, Explanations, gulatory Text, Appendices A and B.* Washington, DC: Occupational Safety and Health Reporter, The Bureau of National Affairs, 1995.

- Chronic active surface antigen hepatitis B carrier status and liver hepatoma
c. An OSHA standard identifies, classifies, and regulates potential occupational carcinogens (CFR Title 29, Section 1990). The agency also publishes standards regulating known carcinogens (e.g., asbestos, benzene, and ethylene oxide).
Incidence and socioeconomic impact

a. An estimated 8 to 20 percent of all cancers are directly related to occupational exposures.
b. It is difficult to quantify the exact contribution of workplace exposures to cancer prevalence in the United States because of the following:
  - Multiple occupational and environmental exposures
  - Lack of accurate past exposure data on workers
  - Long latency of most cancers

Table 38–4. Some Occupational Carcinogens

Carcinogen	Human Cancer Site	Industry Setting
Acrylonitrile	Lung*, colon*, brain*, stomach*, prostate*	Used in acrylic fiber, chemical, and pesticide production
4-aminobiphenyl	Bladder	Formerly used as rubber antioxidant and dye intermediate
Arsenic and arsenic compounds	Lung, skin	Used in smelting, metallurgy, pigment and glass production, and pesticide manufacture and use
Asbestos	Lung, pleura, peritoneum, larynx, gastrointestinal tract	Used in insulation: e.g., ships, buildings, pipes, brake shoes
Benzene	Leukemia	Multiple uses in chemical products: e.g., adhesives, rubber, petrochemicals
Benzidine and salts	Bladder	Used in plastic, rubber, dye, chemical industries
Beryllium and certain beryllium compounds	Lung	Used in mining, electronics, chemical, electric, ceramics industries
Bis(chloromethyl) ether	Lung	Contaminant of CMME
Chloromethyl methyl ether (CMME)	Lung	Ion exchange resin; used in organic chemical manufacturing
Chromium	Lung, nasal cavity	Used in welding, etching, plating; steel and metal industries
Coal tars and coal tar pitches; soot	Lung, skin, kidney*, prostate*	Used in petrochemical and steel industries; fossil fuel combustion byproduc
Coke oven emissions	Lung, bladder, skin	Used in steel industry
1,2-dibromo-3-chloropropane	A	Used as former nematocide
1,2-dibromoethane, ethylene dibromide	A	Used as gasoline additive, solvent, pesticide
3,3'-dichlorobenzidine and salts	A	Used in polyurethane and pigment industries
1,4-dioxane	A	Used as solvent, degreaser
Epichlorohydrin	A	Used in chemical production
Ethylene oxide	A	Used as sterilizing agent
Formaldehyde	A	Used in manufacture of woods, resins, leather, rubber, metals
4,4'-methylene-bis-2-chloroaniline	A	Used in polyurethane, epoxy resin, elastomer manufacturing
Mineral oils (certain ones)	Skin, scrotum	Used as lubricant in metal-working; solvents in printing
Alpha-naphthylamine	Bladder	Used in chemical, textile, dye, rubber industries
Beta-naphthylamine	Bladder	No longer in commercial use
Nickel compounds	Lung, nasal cavity	Used in nickel refining and smelting
Polychlorinated and polybrominated biphenyls (PCBs and PBBs)	A	Used as flame retardants (PBBs); transformer and capacitor fluid solvents (PCBs)
Beta-propiolactone	A	Used in production and use of plastics, resins, and viricides
Vinyl chloride	Liver	Used in polyvinyl plastic production

* Possible human cancer sites.
A, Only animal evidence of carcinogenicity is currently satisfactory.
From Levy BS, and Wegman DH (eds). *Occupational Health: Recognizing and Preventing Work-Related Disease.* 3rd ed. Boston: Little, Brown & Co, 1995, p 291.

- The addition of family history and other personal risk factors
  c. Those cancers caused by occupational exposures are preventable; therefore, primary prevention measures to end these exposures should be the priority public health focus.
3. *Healthy People 2000* lists several cancer reduction objectives related to occupational and environmental exposure, specifically targeting lung cancer originating from radon and asbestos exposure (see Chapter 17).

Noise-Induced Hearing Loss

1. Definition
   a. Noise-induced hearing loss occurs when chronic exposure to noise causes direct damage to the hair cells in the cochlea, producing a sensorineural hearing loss.
   b. Noise-induced hearing loss involves loss of the high-frequency range.
   c. Comprehending speech is difficult, especially when

there is background noise. Vowel sounds are hear better than consonant sounds.
   d. Hearing loss may occur in 1 ear but is commonl bilateral, with gradual deterioration in hearing.
   e. The hearing loss may be partial or total, temporar or permanent.
   f. Hearing loss is directly related to duration and in tensity of noise exposure, with potential injury fro prolonged exposure to sounds higher than 85 dec bels.
2. Incidence and socioeconomic impact
   a. *Healthy People 2000* notes an estimated 8 millic workers in U.S. manufacturing industries are e: posed to noise of 80 decibels or greater for an 8-ho· day.
   b. More than 3 million workers in other occupations a exposed to noise of 85 decibels or greater for a 8-hour day.
   c. Public awareness of noise-induced hearing loss low. Children, parents, and hobby groups should t educated about the need for noise control.
3. Risk factors

a. A noisy home or work environment, without appropriate ear protection, is the major risk factor for noise-induced hearing loss (Table 38–5).

Etiology

a. Susceptibility to the effects of noise on hearing is highly variable.

b. Any prolonged noise higher than 85 decibels is potentially injurious.

Pathophysiology

a. An acoustic reflex partially protects the cochlea from the effects of continuous noise. This reflex is delayed with sudden impulse noise. An explosion, for example, is therefore particularly injurious.

b. The amount of progressive damage to the hair cells in the cochlea is based on duration and intensity of the noise.

c. Presbycusis is a sensorineural hearing loss associated with aging, with deterioration of hair cells in the cochlea, representing a loss in the higher frequencies (3000, 4000, and 8000 Hz).

Clinical manifestations

a. Noise-induced hearing loss occurs as difficulty in comprehending speech, especially when background noise is present.

b. Tinnitus may be associated with the hearing loss.

c. Other physiologic effects of noise are increased heart rate and increased blood pressure.

Diagnostics (Some of the following diagnostics are mandated by the OSHA "Occupational Noise Exposure Standard" CFR Title 29, Section 1900.95, if the individual has a work-related noise exposure that is over the OSHA limit.)

a. Health history

(1) Assessment for current sources of noise at home and at work, including hobbies

(2) Assessment for past history of military service, which is often significant in noise-induced hearing loss

(3) Assessment for other causes of sensorineural hearing loss, including the following:
- Ototoxic medications
- Other ototoxic exposures, for example, exposure to lead, solvents, arsenic, cyanide, or benzene
- A family history of early hearing loss
- Metabolic disorders (e.g., diabetes, autoimmune disorders)
- Meniere's disease
- Central nervous system disease (e.g., acoustic neuroma)

b. Physical examination

(1) Examination of the ear for excessive cerumen, abnormal color of tympanic membrane, obscure bony landmarks, fluid line, or an immobile tympanic membrane

(2) Examination of the nervous system to rule out central nervous system causes of the hearing loss

(3) Tuning fork tests (Weber and Rinne) to distinguish between a conductive and sensorineural hearing loss

(4) Testing of each ear with whisper or watch tick

c. Diagnostic studies

(1) Pure tone audiometry is the screening test most commonly used. Before testing, there should be no noise exposure for 14 hours (see Chapter 20).

(2) A complete audiogram includes pure tone audiometry in addition to speech reception, speech discrimination, tympanometry, and acoustic reflex testing. This testing is done by a certified audiologist.

(3) Sound level meters and dosimeter studies quantify the duration and intensity of noise exposure in the environment. Sound level meters take a one-time reading of noise levels. Dosimeters are worn by 1 worker during a typical work day to average the amount of noise exposure over an 8-hour work shift.

8. Clinical management

a. Goals of clinical management

(1) No medical or surgical treatment can reverse the effects of noise-induced hearing loss.

(2) Management should focus on protecting the remaining hearing ability, with the goal to prevent further noise exposure or future exposure to ototoxic medications.

b. Nonpharmacologic interventions

(1) Hearing amplification with hearing aids is most effective when speech reception threshold is below 25 decibels or with a speech discrimination score of less than 80 percent. Cosmetic concerns and the ability to use fine motion to set and adjust the hearing aid are patient selection criteria.

(2) Assistive listening devices may be helpful as may be aural rehabilitation classes.

c. Pharmacologic interventions

Table 38–5. Relative Intensity of Common Noises

Noise Level (dB)	Environmental Source	Human Speech
140	Air raid siren	. . .
120	Jet takeoff	. . .
110	Riveting machine	. . .
100	Pneumatic hammer	Shouting in ear
90	Subway train	Shouting at a distance of 2 feet
80	Vacuum cleaner	. . .
70	Freeway traffic	Loud conversation
50	Road traffic	Normal conversation
30	Library	Soft whisper
20	Broadcasting studio	. . .
0	Threshold of hearing	. . .

om LaDou J (ed). *Occupational Medicine.* Norwalk, CT: Appleton & Lange, 1990,).

(1) There are no pharmacologic interventions for noise-induced hearing loss.

(2) The use of ototoxic medications (e.g., aminoglycoside antibiotics, loop diuretics, certain antineoplastics, and salicylates) should be avoided.

DRUG ADVISORY

Preexisting noise-induced hearing loss can cause patients to be more susceptible to the ototoxic effects of aminoglycoside antibiotics (e.g., gentamycin), salicylates (e.g., aspirin), loop diuretics (e.g., furosemide), or antineoplastic agents (e.g., cisplatin).

9. Complications
   a. Total deafness can occur if the individual with noise-induced hearing loss is not removed from the noise stimuli.
   b. Tinnitus, which often accompanies noise-induced hearing loss, can be psychologically challenging, with the patient needing support groups and psychologic counseling to address the associated depression.
10. Prognosis
    a. Once the noise stimuli are removed, the hearing loss should stabilize; however, presbycusis may occur and potentiate the hearing loss.
11. Applying the nursing process

NURSING DIAGNOSIS: Auditory sensory-perceptual alterations R/T noise in work and/or home environments

   a. *Expected outcomes:* Following instruction, the person should be able to do the following:
      (1) Demonstrate the effects of noise on hearing.
         • Define noise-induced hearing loss.
         • Identify sources of noise exposure at home and at work.
         • Explain the results of pure tone audiometry.
      (2) Select hearing protection devices based on individual noise assessment.
      (3) Demonstrate correct placement and use of hearing protection devices.
   b. *Nursing interventions* (see Learning/Teaching Guidelines for Hearing Conservation Programs)
12. Discharge planning and teaching
    a. Reinforce the need for protection from future noise exposure, both at home and at work.
    b. Observe the correct use of hearing protection, and provide the person with sources of supply for the chosen method of hearing protection.
    c. Reinforce the need for an annual audiogram if the person is potentially exposed to a noisy environment.
    d. If a hearing aid is indicated, reinforce the importance of its use with the person and family members.
    e. If tinnitus is a primary associated symptom, refer the person to a tinnitus support group.
    f. Encourage the person or family members to call if they have questions or concerns.

13. Public health considerations
    a. Noise-induced hearing loss can be prevented. Education begins with school-aged children, teaching them to avoid prolonged exposure to loud noise.
    b. There is an OSHA occupational noise exposure standard that mandates a comprehensive hearing protection program for workplaces when there is noise exposure equal to or greater than 85 decibels for an 8-hour day.
    c. *Healthy People 2000* includes an objective to reduce the percentage of workers exposed to average daily noise levels that exceed 85 decibels.
    d. In the workplace, the following are ways to reduce noise exposure from specific work processes:
       (1) By replacing older machinery with newer, quieter machinery
       (2) By conducting maintenance of machinery frequently, for example, oiling parts often
       (3) By enclosing noisy machinery, using acoustic muffling if possible
    e. The amount of individual noise exposure can be reduced by limiting work time in noisy environments, for example, limiting noise exposure to 4 hours per shift.
    f. Hearing protection includes ear plugs or over-the-ear muffs, with varying noise reducing rates.
       (1) Most ear plugs have a noise reducing rate of 18 to 28 decibels, with ear muffs in the 20-25-decibel range.
       (2) Actual reduction is much lower if the devices are not worn properly.
       (3) When muffs and plugs are used together, an additional reduction of 5 to 10 decibels can be obtained, which is then added to the noise reducing rate of one of the devices.

Lead Poisoning

1. Definition
   a. Lead is a naturally occurring heavy metal with high density and corrosion resistance. Lead occurs in many ores in concentrations of 1 to 11 percent.
   b. Lead poisoning occurs when lead is absorbed through inhalation or ingestion.
   c. Lead poisoning is classified as mild, moderate, or severe according to blood lead levels.
      (1) Recent data indicate that there are adverse neurologic effects in children with lead levels more than 10 μg per 100 ml (dl) of blood. Therefore, the action level for children has been reduced to 10 μg per dl. Class I refers to a blood lead level less than 9 μg per dl in children. Class IIA and IIB refers to blood lead levels less than 19 μg per dl.
      (2) Moderate lead poisoning is indicated by blood lead levels between 20 and 44 μg per dl in children (Class III) and 40 and 60 μg per dl in adults.
      (3) Severe lead poisoning is indicated by blood lead levels between 45 and 69 μg per dl in children (Class IV) and 100 μg per dl or more in adults.

LEARNING/TEACHING GUIDELINES
for Hearing Conservation Programs

General Overview

1. Describe the prevalence and seriousness of noise-induced hearing loss at the national, state, local, and industry levels.
2. Explain that noise-induced hearing loss is a progressive loss of hearing over time due to cumulative noise exposure from work, home, and hobbies.
3. If the participants have noise exposure from a similar work process, identify those noisy areas in the workplace to help create a cue for learning.
4. Identify what the industry is currently doing to lower noise levels. Share some tangible examples of how management is supportive of safe noise levels.
5. Discuss briefly the noise standard, if participants have noise-induced hearing loss from their work sites.

Noise and Health Effects

1. Briefly discuss the normal anatomy of the ear and the physiology of hearing.
2. Brainstorm the health effects of noise to include hearing loss, increased heart rate, increased blood pressure, and increased stress levels.
3. Visually document the effects of noise on the hair cells of the cochlea.
4. Brainstorm those symptoms associated with hearing loss to include diminished speech discrimination and tinnitus.
5. Discuss other causes of hearing loss to include aging, ototoxic drugs, cerumen impaction, otosclerosis, and middle ear disease.
6. Compare temporary noise-induced hearing loss (called a temporary threshold shift) with a permanent threshold shift.
7. List the possible treatments (such as hearing aids, aural rehabilitation) for noise-induced hearing loss to demonstrate that once permanent, hearing loss is not reversible.

Evaluation of Noise Levels

1. Demonstrate sampling of various noise levels with a sound level meter. Collect noise levels at a whisper (30 decibels), a normal conversation (70 decibels), an alarm clock (80 decibels), a punch press (100 decibels), and a rock and roll band (110 decibels).
2. Demonstrate a dosimeter reading. It is helpful to have placed a dosimeter on one of the participants earlier in the day, if possible. Together, the group can calculate the average noise exposure over an 8-hour period.

Audiometry Interpretation

1. Review an example of pure tone audiometry results with the following findings:

a. Normal hearing
b. Noise-induced hearing loss
c. A conductive hearing loss associated with impacted cerumen
d. A hearing loss associated with aging
2. Graph collective audiometry results by department, if participants are from one industry.

If You Have a Noise-Induced Hearing Loss

1. Encourage discussion about protection of remaining hearing ability by avoiding loud noise at home, at work, and with hobbies.
2. Include education about avoidance of ototoxic medications and other exposures that may cause hearing loss (e.g., lead and solvents).
3. Discuss indications for hearing aids, aural rehabilitation, and need for referral to an ear, nose, and throat physician.
4. Discuss tinnitus support groups, if indicated.

Noise Control

1. Discuss feasible approaches to engineer out the noise, with keeping doors closed, sound shields, muffling, and acoustic barriers, in addition to oiling of machines.
2. Discuss goals to decrease overall exposure to noise and suggest splitting shifts to work in noisy areas only 4 hours per shift if possible.
3. Demonstrate various hearing protective devices, including disposable ear plugs, over-the-ear muffs, and designer ear plugs.
4. Include time to practice inserting different styles of hearing protection. It is important to have several different styles available for individual use.
5. There is varying compliance with using hearing protection, mainly because of altered social conversations. Therefore, recommend hearing protection only in the amount of noise-reducing capacity needed. For example, if the noise level is 100 decibels, the individual only needs a noise reducing capacity of 15 to 20 decibels. You do not need to recommend ear muffs, which have a noise-reducing capacity of 30 to 35 decibels, for this noise level.

Program Evaluation

1. If participants are in a work site, include direct observation of employees' use of hearing protection to evaluate whether the teaching program has been successful.
2. Labor union and management support of the program is important for overall program success.
3. Employees' safe work practices are a necessary component of job performance, and supervisors should reward consistent use of hearing protection, if indicated.

(continued)

LEARNING/TEACHING GUIDELINES
(continued)

4. Annual education for populations exposed to greater than 85 decibels of noise in an 8-hour average is required by OSHA. Involving your target population in the revision of program content and delivery is a strategy supported by adult teaching-learning theory.

A train the trainer model may be effective, depending on the size and needs of your target population.
5. Tailoring the guidelines for the educational and language background of your population is critical for program success.

---

blood lead level higher than 70 μg per dl (Class V) is a medical emergency in children.
  d. Lead affects several organ systems, with nervous, gastrointestinal, hemopoietic, reproductive, and renal systems being the most sensitive.
2. Incidence and socioeconomic impact
  a. Lead poisoning from environmental sources is one of the most common, preventable pediatric health problems in the United States.
  b. Lead is released into the environment from automobile emissions with the use of leaded gasoline and from the burning of coal.
  c. More than 30 states are mandated to report adult blood lead levels of more than 25 μg per dl.
  d. Large numbers of children continue to have blood lead levels in the toxic range. Approximately 1.7 million children aged 1 to 5 years have blood lead levels greater than 10 μg per dl.
  e. Work-related lead exposure continues to be a problem.
    (1) A total of 12,137 adult cases of blood lead levels exceeding 25 μg per dl were reported by 23 states in 1994.
    (2) Blood lead levels in the lower ranges (less than 39 μg per dl) have increased, but there has been a decrease in elevated blood lead levels of more than 40 μg per dl.
3. Risk factors
  a. Children ingest lead dust from environmental sources, including lead-painted walls, lead deposits in playground dirt, and lead in drinking water from lead-soldered plumbing. Children can be exposed from lead dust on the clothes of parents with an occupational exposure.
  b. Types of industries in which lead exposure is prevalent:
    • Battery manufacturing
    • Brass, copper, or lead foundries
    • Lead production or smelting
    • Radiator repairing
    • Recycling and scrap handling
    • Demolition of ships and bridges
    • Welding of old, painted metal
    • Ceramic glaze mixing
    • Working at a rifle firing range
    • Machining or grinding lead alloys
    • Lead soldering
    • Cable stripping

  c. Other risk factors include the following:
    (1) Folk remedies containing lead, such as azarcon, greta, pay-loo-ah, ghasard, bala goli, kandu, and kohl (alkohl).
    (2) Hobbies that use leaded solder for stained glass, artist's paints containing lead, molten lead to make fishing weights, or lead glazes in ceramics
4. Etiology
  a. Children are particularly sensitive to the adverse health effects of lead because they absorb and retain more lead in proportion to their weight than do adults.
  b. Lead readily passes through the placenta in pregnant women, placing the fetus at risk.
  c. Inhalation of lead fumes or dust and ingestion of lead dust are the major sources of exposure.
5. Pathophysiology
  a. Absorbed lead is bound to erythrocytes in the bloodstream.
  b. Bone constitutes the major site of deposition of absorbed lead. Lead is incorporated into the bone matrix much as is calcium.
  c. Lead interferes with numerous cellular enzymes, including those involved in heme synthesis. Lead also binds to mitochondrial structures and interferes with protein and nucleic acid synthesis.
  d. Excretion of lead is slow and is primarily through the kidneys. The half-life of lead is long, estimated to be from 5 to 10 years. Lead in dense bone is slowly mobilized and released over time, with increased lead levels being observed after bone fractures or osteoporosis.
  e. Iron and calcium deficiency can enhance lead absorption and aggravate pica; therefore, nutritional assessment is particularly important in children.
6. Clinical manifestations
  a. Lead poisoning may occur without symptoms.
  b. Mild lead poisoning
    (1) Occasional abdominal discomfort
    (2) Mild fatigue
    (3) Myalgias
  c. Moderate lead poisoning
    (1) Diffuse abdominal pain
    (2) Constipation
    (3) Nausea
    (4) Weight loss
    (5) Headache
    (6) Fatigue

    (7) Tremor
    (8) Difficulty concentrating
    (9) Emotional lability
  d. Severe lead poisoning
    (1) Colicky, severe abdominal pain
    (2) Diffuse abdominal pain
    (3) Paralysis
    (4) Encephalopathy

Diagnostics (Some of the following diagnostics are mandated by the OSHA ''Lead Standard'' CFR Title 29, Section 1910.1025, if the person has a work-related exposure over the OSHA limit.)
  a. Health history
    (1) When interviewing persons with lead exposure, a thorough occupational and environmental history should be obtained.
    (2) In children, the child's mouthing activities should be assessed, as should the existence of pica and the child's nutritional intake (especially the intake of calcium and iron).
    (3) Patient complaints of problems involving the gastrointestinal, neurologic, hematopoietic, and reproductive systems should be focused on.
  b. Physical examination
    (1) Blood pressure may be elevated if there is kidney involvement.
    (2) Lead deposition in the mouth can cause a blue-gray line in the buccal mucosa, called a lead line.
    (3) Examination of the target organs includes examination of the abdomen for tenderness; of the neurologic system for mental status changes, motor or sensory deficits, or tremor; and of the skin for signs of pallor.
    (4) In children, psychosocial and language development should be assessed.
  c. Diagnostic studies
    • Complete blood count with peripheral smear
    • Blood urea nitrogen and serum creatinine
    • Blood lead level
    • Erythrocyte protoporphyrin level
    • Urinalysis
    • Serum iron, iron-binding, and ferritin levels
    • Sperm analysis in adults if there is evidence of altered reproductive function

Clinical management
  a. Removal from exposure is the 1st goal of treatment.
  b. Chelation treatment using Calcium Disodium Versenate (CaNa$_2$EDTA) is usually reserved for adults with acute, brief exposures who have severe manifestations (e.g., hemolysis, encephalopathy, or renal injury) and a blood lead level more than 60 μg per dl. Chelation with the oral agent, dimercaptosuccinic acid (succimer) can be effective in adults and is the primary chelation agent for lead-exposed children.
  c. Chelation treatment in adults is not effective in chronic overexposure to lead; treatment with Calcium Disodium Versenate may cause acute tubular necrosis.
  d. Children with elevated blood lead levels greater than 45 μg per dl should receive chelation therapy. Succimer is an oral chelating agent approved by the U.S.

Food and Drug Administration for children with blood lead levels over 45 μg per dl. Protocols vary for children whose blood lead levels are between 25 and 40 μg per dl and for children who are symptomatic or asymptomatic.

DRUG ADVISORY

DMSA (meso 2,3-dimercaptosuccinic acid, or succimer), a chelating agent used in the treatment of lead toxicity, can be used in both adults and children. Administration of DMSA should never be a substitute for removal of lead exposure in the home or workplace.

  e. Dietary recommendations include ingestion of foods high in iron and calcium.
  f. Prompt treatment of iron deficiency anemia is recommended.
9. Complications
  a. Adverse reproductive outcomes include altered spermatogenesis and decreased libido in men and menstrual disturbances and spontaneous abortion in women.
  b. Mental retardation may occur in children exposed to high lead levels in utero.
  c. Normochromic anemia is found more frequently in children.
  d. Neurologic complications
    (1) Distal motor neuropathy (e.g., foot drop) occurs with long-term exposure to lead.
    (2) Lead encephalopathy, which occurs with acute exposure, is rare but is a medical emergency.
  e. Children with blood lead levels greater than 70 μg per dl (with or without symptoms) represent an acute medical emergency.
10. Prognosis
  a. Early diagnosis and treatment usually results in complete recovery.
  b. If there is neurologic or renal impairment, a complete recovery is not expected.
  c. Cognitive impairments in children are lifelong.
11. Applying the nursing process

NURSING DIAGNOSIS: Poisoning R/T lead exposure in the home or workplace

  a. *Expected outcomes:* Following instruction, the person should be able to do the following:
    (1) Demonstrate an understanding of lead poisoning by defining lead poisoning and identifying sources of lead exposure at home and at work
    (2) Remove all environmental sources of lead in the home
    (3) Demonstrate the appropriate use of a respirator for protection from lead dust and fumes
    (4) Explain the importance of laundering work clothes to prevent lead dust from entering the home environment

    (5) Describe the side effects of chelation
  b. *Nursing interventions*
    (1) In lead-exposed children, an aggressive case management approach is needed to ensure that the home environment becomes lead free.
    (2) Home or worksite visits to evaluate potential sources of lead exposure are recommended.
    (3) Using teaching materials that are culture and language relevant is highly recommended (Fig. 38–2).
12. Discharge planning and teaching
  a. Follow-up evaluation of an elevated blood lead level is important. The importance of such follow-up care should be stressed.
  b. If chelation was used, the blood lead level should be tested again after 7 to 10 days to determine the need for further treatment.
  c. Determining the source of lead exposure is critical for the prevention of continued exposure. Children, if hospitalized, should be discharged only to a lead-free environment.
  d. The person and family members should be encouraged to call with any questions or concerns.
13. Public health considerations
  a. Reduction and prevention of lead exposure in the environment
    (1) Since leaded gasoline was banned in most states, the EPA has reported a steady decline of lead levels in ambient air.

    (2) Since 1977, the Consumer Product Safety Commission has limited the use of lead in paints for residential use. The use of lead-containing solder in household plumbing was banned by the EPA in 1988.
    (3) Buildings built before 1950 are presumed to have paint containing lead pigment. Scraping and burning off of old paint may cause lead exposure. Appropriate ventilation during paint removal is highly effective at reducing this exposure.
    (4) Education about lead in selected folk remedies should be done by public health professionals.
    (5) Inexpensive lead testing kits can be purchased to test for the presence of lead pigment in ceramics.
    (6) Lead content in home water sources can be measured. Local public health departments are a resource for the names of toxicology laboratories that analyze water for a small fee. The EPA monitors lead levels in drinking water.
    (7) Playground soil may be contaminated with lead either from automobile emissions or paint chips. Soil samples can be sent to a recommended toxicology laboratory for a determination of lead level. Hand washing after outdoor play is recommended.
  b. *Healthy People 2000* lists several environmental and occupational objectives for the reduction of lead exposure for both children and adults.

Reducing Lead in Your Home

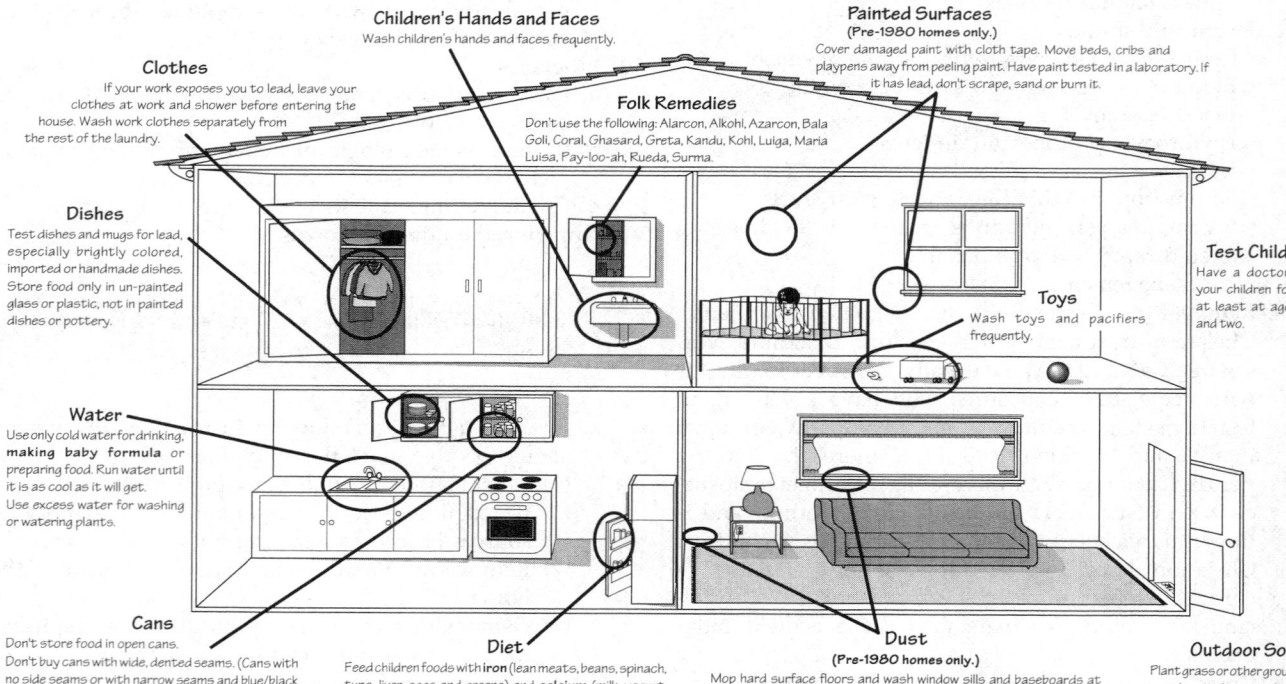

Children's Hands and Faces
Wash children's hands and faces frequently.

Painted Surfaces
(Pre-1980 homes only.)
Cover damaged paint with cloth tape. Move beds, cribs and playpens away from peeling paint. Have paint tested in a laboratory. If it has lead, don't scrape, sand or burn it.

Clothes
If your work exposes you to lead, leave your clothes at work and shower before entering the house. Wash work clothes separately from the rest of the laundry.

Folk Remedies
Don't use the following: Alarcon, Alkohl, Azarcon, Bala Goli, Coral, Ghasard, Greta, Kandu, Kohl, Luiga, Maria Luisa, Pay-loo-ah, Rueda, Surma.

Dishes
Test dishes and mugs for lead, especially brightly colored, imported or handmade dishes. Store food only in un-painted glass or plastic, not in painted dishes or pottery.

Test Children
Have a doctor test your children for lead at least at ages one and two.

Toys
Wash toys and pacifiers frequently.

Water
Use only cold water for drinking, **making baby formula** or preparing food. Run water until it is as cool as it will get. Use excess water for washing or watering plants.

Cans
Don't store food in open cans. Don't buy cans with wide, dented seams. (Cans with no side seams or with narrow seams and blue/black paint lines are lead-free.)

Diet
Feed children foods with **iron** (lean meats, beans, spinach, tuna, liver, eggs and greens) and **calcium** (milk, yogurt, cheese, tofu and cooked greens).

Dust
(Pre-1980 homes only.)
Mop hard surface floors and wash window sills and baseboards at least once a week with a string mop and a pail with a ringer. Don't use mops or rags for anything else.

Outdoor Soil
Plant grass or other ground cover as a barrier between lead in soil and your children.

Figure 38–2. Reducing lead in your home. (Used with permission of Consumer Action's Lead Poisoning Prevention Project, San Francisco.)

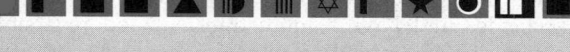

(1) The key focus is on screening and early medical diagnosis of lead-exposed children.

(2) The goal is to prevent any lead exposures over a blood lead level of 15 μg per dl in children and of 25 μg per dl in adults.

c. The OSHA "Lead Standard" outlines the components of a medical surveillance program for occupational lead exposure, and the steps for medical removal and reentry of the patient into a workplace when there is a lead exposure.

d. If blood lead levels are elevated or if air sampling reveals elevated lead levels in certain work areas, the goal is to reduce the exposure. The following workplace interventions are recommended:

(1) Substitution with a less hazardous lead-free material

(2) Installation of local ventilation systems to remove lead dusts and fumes

(3) Relocation of the employee to an area where lead is not being used

(4) Provision of an appropriate respirator, based on the type of lead exposure, for all potentially exposed employees if the other recommendations cannot be achieved

e. Lead is a known reproductive hazard for both men and women. Companies cannot discriminate against employees based on reproductive status, but they must strive to provide a safe workplace for both men and women employees and inform employees of hazards associated with lead exposure.

f. More than 30 states have mandatory reporting of blood lead levels of more than 25 μg per dl.

Pesticide Poisoning

1. Definition
   a. A pesticide is a substance used to prevent, destroy, repel, or mitigate any insects, rodents, nematodes, fungi, weeds, or other pest. A pesticide is any substance used to regulate, defoliate, or desiccate plants. Therefore, pesticide is a broad term that includes insecticides, rodenticides, nematocides, fungicides, herbicides, and fumigants.
   b. Pesticide poisoning occurs mainly from dermal absorption during mixing and application of pesticides, with eyes being a route of exposure for splashes and spills. Inhalation during pesticide manufacturing or through fumigation is a less common route of exposure.
   c. Pesticide exposure may also occur from eating foods containing pesticide residue. Breast milk and placental transfer are other routes of environmental exposure.
   d. Pesticide toxicity is mainly due to exposure to organophosphates and carbamates.
   e. Pesticides used in home and work settings affect mainly the dermatologic and neurologic systems in humans; many pesticides are known to cause cancer in animals and have reproductive toxicity in female animals. The major health concern for pesticide residues in food is their carcinogenic potential.
   f. U.S. military personnel who served in Vietnam between 1962 and 1969 were exposed to the herbicide Agent Orange, an equal parts mixture of 2,4-dichlorophenoxyacetic acid and 2,4,5-trichlorophenoxyacetic acid.

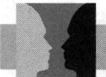

CLINICAL CONTROVERSIES

Herbicides were used in Vietnam to defoliate inland forests. Defoliation improved the ability to detect enemy forces and to destroy enemy crops. Aerial spraying began in 1962, peaked in 1967 to 1969, and was halted by 1971. Agent Orange was 1 of many herbicides used in Vietnam.

Dioxin (2,3,7,8-tetrachlorodibenzo-P-dioxin, or 2,3,7,8-TCDD) is an unavoidable byproduct of the manufacture of 2,4,5-trichlorophenoxyacetic acid, 1 of 2 herbicides used to manufacture Agent Orange. Dioxin is the focus of health concerns.

Little data on exposure were recorded during the Vietnam war, but it is presumed that any veteran who served in Vietnam between 1964 and 1975 was exposed to a herbicide containing dioxin.

Five conditions are service-connected as having an association with herbicide exposure: soft tissue sarcoma, non-Hodgkin's lymphoma, Hodgkin's disease, chloracne, and porphyria cutanea tarda (in genetically susceptible individuals).

The Veterans Administration has maintained an Agent Orange registry since 1978. In 1994, the Institute of Medicine recommended reconstruction of Agent Orange exposure models with further epidemiologic study of this population.

2. Incidence and socioeconomic impact
   a. In 1989, there were 729 active ingredient pesticide chemicals mixed with other ingredients and formulated into more than 22,000 products. In the United States, 1.5 billion pounds of pesticides are used annually.
   b. The greatest increase is in the use of herbicides for weed control. Of the 1 billion pounds of pesticides

used in agriculture, 750 million pounds are used on corn, soybeans, and cotton.

c. Consumers have expressed concerns about pesticide residues in food.

d. It is difficult to estimate the extent of pesticide-related injury and illness because of inaccurate medical diagnosis of mild toxicity and underreporting of pesticide-related illness. The EPA estimates a wide range of 20,000 to 300,000 acute poisonings annually in agricultural workers in the United States.

e. One third of all reported pesticide-related complaints are skin conditions, either irritant or allergic contact dermatitis.

3. Risk factors
   a. Pesticides can be used at home and at work.
   b. A total of 80 to 90 percent of all pesticides are used in commercial agricultural operations; 10 to 20 percent of all pesticides are used in structural pest control (e.g., for termites), horticulture, and home and garden use (Table 38–6).
   c. The highest exposure in an occupational setting is from the mixing and application of pesticides in agricultural pest control operations.

4. Etiology
   a. Organophosphate pesticides are the principal insecticides used in agriculture. They act by inhibiting acetylcholinesterase at nerve endings.

Table 38–6. Occupational and Environmental Pesticide Exposure Situations

Occupational Exposures

Research and development
Manufacturing: Technical grade material production
Formulation: Technical grade material mixed with "inert" ingredients such as solvents, adjuvants
Transportation
Pest control
Mixing: Commercial material diluted with water or other material
Loading: Into tanks in planes, ground rigs, backpacks, or hand-held sprayers
Application
Flagging: Standing at the end of fields to mark the rows to be sprayed by crop-dusting aircraft
Farm work: Contact with pesticide residues on leaves and fruit
Emergency and medical work: Personnel exposed to contaminated persons and equipment in the process of responding to spills, accidents, and poisonings

Environmental and Consumer Exposures

Accidents and spills: Especially ingestion by children
Suicide and homicide
Home use: House and garden
Structural use: Residents and occupants of buildings
Bystanders
Contamination: Food, water, air

From LaDou J (ed). *Occupational Medicine.* Norwalk, CT: Appleton & Lange, 1990, p 402.

b. The cholinesterase-inhibiting carbamates are all insecticides and have a more transient and reversible cholinesterase inhibition when compared with the organophosphates.

c. Both organophosphates and carbamates are applied either by hand or by aerial application, with most worker exposure by the dermal route.

5. Pathophysiology
   a. After human exposure to an organophosphate or carbamate pesticide, there is acetylcholine buildup at the nerve transmitter sites of specific organs (Table 38–7).
   b. Organophosphates can cause a delayed neuropathy. This finding is unrelated to its cholinesterase inhibition but rather is related to the inhibition of the neurotoxic esterase enzyme. Carbamates do not cause this delayed neuropathy.
   c. Most organophosphates and carbamates are primary skin irritants. A few pesticides (malathion, parathion, dichlorvos) are skin sensitizers that cause allergic contact dermatitis.
   d. Many pesticides have not been adequately tested for reproductive toxicity or carcinogenic effects in humans.

6. Clinical manifestations
   a. Table 38–7 details symptoms related to acute organophosphate poisoning. Cholinesterase-inhibiting carbamate poisoning incurs similar symptoms.
   b. Mild poisoning includes mild muscarinic signs and symptoms such as pupil constriction, increased salivation, and increased lacrimation.
   c. Moderate toxicity involves more than 1 system but does not require assistive breathing.
   d. Severe toxicity requires ventilatory assistance. Respiratory compromise is a result of combined muscarinic, nicotinic, and central nervous system effects.
   e. Skin exposure over a specific organ may reveal local findings such as fasciculations over a specific skeletal muscle or miosis in 1 exposed eye.
   f. Dermatitis symptoms include pruritic rash over affected skin areas.

7. Diagnostics
   a. Health history
      (1) Assessment for unprotected skin contact to organophosphates and carbamates, for example, reentry into a recently sprayed field
      (2) Assessment of temporal relationships or symptoms in other family members or coworkers to help make the diagnosis
   b. Physical examination
      (1) Examination of skin for dermatitis
      (2) Examination of neurologic systems for evidence of acetylcholine excess
   c. Diagnostic studies
      (1) Red blood cell cholinesterase level
      (2) Plasma cholinesterase level
          • Red blood cell and plasma cholinesterase levels measure 2 different enzymes; therefore, the results cannot be used interchangeably.
          • Cholinesterase levels are most valuable in assessing exposure to organophosphates. Expo-

Table 38–7. Signs and Symptoms of Acute Organophosphate Poisoning by Site of Acetylcholine Neurotransmitter Activity

System	Receptor Type	Organ	Action	Sign or Symptom
Parasympathetic	Muscarinic	Eye		
		Iris muscle	Contraction	Miosis
		Ciliary muscle	Contraction	Blurred vision
		Glands	Secretion	
		Lacrimal		Tearing
		Salivary		Salivation
		Respiratory		Bronchorrhea, pulmonary edema
		Gastrointestinal		Nausea, vomiting, diarrhea
		Urinary		Urination
		Sweat		Perspiration
(Sympathetic)		Heart		
		Sinus node	Slowing	Bradycardia
		Atrioventricular node	Refractory period increased	Arrhythmias, heart block
		Smooth muscle		
		Bronchial	Contraction	Bronchoconstriction
		Gastrointestinal wall	Contraction	Vomiting, cramps, diarrhea
		Sphincter	Relaxation	
		Bladder		
		Fundus	Contraction	Urination, incontinence
		Sphincter	Relaxation	
Neuromuscular	Nicotinic	Skeletal	Excitation	Fasciculations, cramps, followed by weakness, loss of reflexes, paralysis
Central nervous		Brain	Excitation (early)	Headache, dizziness, malaise, apprehension, confusion, hallucinations, manic or bizarre behavior, convulsions
			Depression (late)	Depression of, then loss of consciousness; respiratory depression

From LaDou J (ed). *Occupational Medicine*. Norwalk, CT: Appleton & Lange, 1990, p 412.

sure to carbamates has only a transient effect on cholinesterase levels.

- Certain organophosphates inhibit only 1 enzyme, thereby having a depressed plasma cholinesterase but a normal red blood cell cholinesterase level.
- Comparison of periodic cholinesterase levels to a baseline, pre-exposure level is the ideal method for biologic monitoring over time. Red blood cell cholinesterase is more reflective of cumulative absorption of organophosphate over time and, therefore, is the preferred blood test for biologic monitoring.
- A total of 25 to 30 percent of inhibition (70–75% of baseline) during periodic monitoring is a warning signal for overexposure to organophosphates. If this degree of inhibition is from chronic exposure, the person may be asymptomatic. However, if this inhibition occurred acutely, the person is symptomatic.

Clinical management

a. Goals of clinical management are to remove the patient from exposure and to provide respiratory support.

b. Nonpharmacologic interventions include decontamination techniques, which vary and must be in compliance with OSHA and EPA regulations. In general, decontamination includes flushing of the skin, including under the fingernails and exposed skin folds, shampooing of hair, and burning of contaminated clothing.

c. Pharmacologic interventions

(1) Atropine sulfate, which acts only on the muscarinic effects, should not be used if the patient has nicotinic or central nervous system signs and symptoms (e.g., muscle weakness or convulsions). Atropine does not affect the cholinesterase levels.

(2) Pralidoxime chloride. Serum cholinesterase levels should be measured before pralidoxime administration. Pralidoxime acts by breaking the bond between the acetylcholinesterase and the organophosphate, reactivating the enzyme and restoring the acetylcholine activity to normal. Pralidoxime can only be used in organophosphate poisoning and not carbamate poisoning.

9. Complications

a. Hypoxia may result from respiratory failure.

b. Delayed neuropathy may occur, and administration of atropine or pralidoxime does not influence the development of this condition.

10. Prognosis

a. Complete recovery is expected if tissue hypoxia does not occur.

b. If symptoms persist beyond 24 hours, then the person should be reassessed for a reservoir of continued exposure.

c. Sudden death occurs in a small percentage of recovered persons, most likely from ventricular arrhythmias.

d. A small percentage of persons, after recovery from acute exposure to organophosphates, report a persistent change in mood, lethargy, difficulty concentrating, and short-term memory loss. These reports need further investigation.

e. Delayed neuropathy may progressively improve over time with aggressive physical therapy, or it may worsen with development of paralysis.

11. Applying the nursing process

NURSING DIAGNOSIS: Risk for poisoning R/T organophosphate exposure from home or work environments

---

a. *Expected outcomes:* Following instruction, the person should be able to do the following:
   (1) Demonstrate an understanding of pesticide poisoning by defining pesticide poisoning and identifying sources of pesticide exposure at work and at home
   (2) Demonstrate safe handling and application of pesticides
   (3) Demonstrate appropriate use of respiratory protection
   (4) Explain the interval of time between spraying and field reentry with appropriate field posting
   (5) Maintain good hygiene when handling pesticides
b. *Nursing interventions*
   (1) Nurses should recognize that children may be exposed to pesticides, especially during the summer harvest season. A family and systems approach to nursing interventions should be used.
   (2) Aggressive case management is indicated to prevent pesticide exposure or re-exposure.
   (3) Language- and cultural-relevant teaching strategies are highly recommended.

12. Discharge planning and teaching
   a. Baseline cholinesterase levels obtained before pesticide exposure are very important.
   b. The person should be encouraged to have cholinesterase levels checked periodically.
   c. Children may also be exposed to pesticides, especially in migrant farm worker families and on family farms. Families should be educated about the safe handling of pesticides, including the need for good hygiene.
   d. The person and family members should be encouraged to call with any questions or concerns.

13. Public health considerations
   a. To reduce the amount of pesticides in use in the United States, the following integrated pest management techniques can be encouraged at the poli[cy] level:
      (1) Careful monitoring of pest populations
      (2) Exploitation of natural predators and processes
      (3) Judicious use of selective pesticides
      (4) Artificial disruption of pest populations
      (5) Mechanical methods of pest control (e.g., soil ae[r]ation, crop rotation, use of pest barriers)
   b. Culturally relevant teaching materials should be [de]veloped to meet the educational needs of a diver[se] group of workers who are potentially exposed [to] pesticides.
   c. The EPA, in conjunction with the Food and Dr[ug] Administration and the U.S. Department of Agric[ul]ture, monitors pesticide residues in food.
   d. Levels of pesticides in drinking water are monitor[ed] by the EPA, with information available from the [Of]fice of Pesticide Programs.
   e. Reporting of suspected and actual pesticide exposu[re] is required in many states.
   f. The EPA registers all pesticides and certifies sta[te] programs for licensing pesticide applicators.
   g. *Healthy People 2000* addresses not only a reduction [in] occupational skin disorders but also safe surfa[ce] drinking water.

Other Occupational and Environmental Disorders

1. Carbon monoxide exposure
   a. Definition
      (1) Carbon monoxide is an odorless, nonirritating g[as] that is produced by incomplete combustion [of] substances containing carbon.
      (2) Carbon monoxide acts as a chemical asphyxia[nt,] competing with oxygen at the oxygen-bindi[ng] sites on hemoglobin. The affinity of hemoglob[in] for carbon monoxide is 200 times greater than it [is] for oxygen.
   b. Incidence and etiology
      (1) Environmental sources of carbon monoxide i[n]clude automobile emissions, cigarette smokin[g,] home cooking, or heating with charcoal. Methy[l]ene chloride, a common solvent, is converted [to] carbon monoxide in the body.
      (2) Firefighters and parking lot attendants in enclose[d,] poorly ventilated garages are 2 high-risk occupatio[ns] for carbon monoxide exposure. Poor ventilation [is] a key risk factor for carbon monoxide poisoning.
      (3) Smokers have a baseline carboxyhemoglobin lev[el] of approximately 5 percent.
   c. Clinical manifestations
      (1) Acute symptoms include headache (at 10% ca[r]boxyhemoglobin levels); dizziness and dyspne[a] (at 20% carboxyhemoglobin levels); visual distu[r]bances and impaired judgment (at 30% carboxyh[e]moglobin levels); syncope, coma, and convulsio[ns] (at more than 40–50% carboxyhemoglobin level[s]) and angina, which can be precipitated with elev[ated]

tion in the carboxyhemoglobin levels (as low as 2.5% carboxyhemoglobin levels). With carbon monoxide exposure, there can be a decrease in exercise tolerance for persons with preexisting cardiovascular conditions.

(2) Chronic effects include neurologic deficits, cerebral infarction, myocardial infarction, and fetal damage.

(3) In severe cases, the blood is a cherry-red color.

d. Clinical management

(1) The person should be removed from exposure.

(2) Oxygen support should be given.

(3) There should be environmental evaluation with air sample measurements of carbon monoxide levels and evaluation of work processes and practices to locate sources of carbon monoxide exposure (including sources of methylene chloride).

(4) There should be assessment of ventilation, with location of clean air intake ducts.

(5) Respiratory protection should be given as outlined by the OSHA "Standard for Respiratory Protection" CFR Title 29, Section 1910.134.

(6) Cessation of smoking is important (see Chapter 40).

2. Building-associated illness

a. Definition

(1) Building-associated illnesses are health problems related to indoor air quality.

(2) Contaminants of indoor air may be from contents in the building or foundation, such as formaldehyde, asbestos, and radon; indoor human activities, such as cooking activities, smoking, heating, and cleaning; and infiltrated contaminants from outside air.

b. Incidence and etiology

(1) Conservation of energy has created "tight" buildings, with decreased fresh air exchange.

(2) Most indoor air quality problems are caused by inadequate ventilation, such as inadequate fresh air intake, poor air distribution and mixing, draftiness, poor temperature and humidity control, pressure differences between offices, and air filtration problems.

(3) Inside contamination can also cause poor indoor air quality from activities such as improper application of pesticides, use of various types of wet copiers, improper use of cleaning agents, tobacco smoking, and combustion byproducts from on-site cafeterias.

(4) Outside contamination sources include air intake vents near parking garages, with intake of nearby vehicle exhaust fumes, and air conditioning systems containing infectious agents, such as bacterial growth (e.g., *Legionella*).

c. Clinical manifestations

(1) Headache and mucous membrane irritation are the key symptoms of building-associated illness.

(2) Persons may report chest tightness or burning, dizziness, and fatigue.

(3) There is a temporal relationship to onset of symptoms upon entering the building and resolution of symptoms upon leaving the building.

(4) Physical examination findings are usually minimal, and, at times, a psychophysiologic somatoform diagnosis is made.

d. Clinical management

(1) A worksite evaluation by an industrial hygienist is indicated to assess the building for maintenance and upkeep of heating, air conditioning, and ventilation systems; any obvious sources of contamination; temperature and humidity control, with goals for a comfort zone at 73 to 77 degrees Fahrenheit, with relative humidity between 20 and 60 percent; number of air changes per hour, with percentage of recirculated air; measurement of carbon dioxide to determine adequacy of fresh air.

(2) Increasing the percentage of circulating fresh air may be effective at decreasing symptoms of building-associated illness. Regular maintenance of the heating, air conditioning, and ventilation systems is a usual recommendation.

(3) No-smoking policies at work sites should be enforced, with group smoking cessation strategies offered at the work site.

(4) Workers should be reassured that symptoms are usually self-limiting and should improve with time.

3. Occupational contact dermatitis

a. Definition

(1) Occupational contact dermatitis may be produced by either irritant or allergic sensitizers.

(2) The dermatitis occurs at the site of exposure, and the hands are usually involved (Tables 38–8 and 38–9).

b. Incidence and etiology

(1) Contact dermatitis accounts for almost 90 percent of all work-related skin disorders.

(2) *Healthy People 2000* notes an occupational skin disorder baseline rate of 64 cases per 100,000 full-time workers from 1983 to 1987 and recommends as a goal to reduce the incidence rate to no more than 55 cases per 100,000 full-time workers by 2000.

(3) Irritant contact dermatitis can range from mild to severe, with skin inflammation directly resulting from the irritant substance. Chemicals, such as hydrofluoric acid, can cause severe irritant contact dermatitis.

(4) Allergic contact dermatitis is a delayed hypersensitivity response to an allergen. Common work-related allergens that cause allergic contact dermatitis are poison oak, nickel, and latex.

c. Clinical manifestations

(1) A thorough occupational and environmental health history is key in the successful medical diagnosis of an occupational skin disorder.

(2) Occupational skin disorders often improve while the worker is away from the work site.

(3) A history of atopy is significant. Atopic individuals have a greater likelihood that allergic contact dermatitis will develop.

(4) Itching, redness, blisters, and edema are the primary skin symptoms and findings for both irritant

Table 38–8. Common Irritants in the Home and Workplace

Home	Epoxy resins
Bleaches	Foams (e.g., insulation foams)
Copper and metal brighteners	Noncarbon-required paper
Detergents	Powders
Drain cleaners	Aluminum
Fertilizers	Calcium silicate
Furniture polishes and waxes	Cement
Oven cleaners	Cleaning agents
Pesticides	Metallic oxides
Pet shampoos	Particles
Rug shampoos	Ore particles in mining
Scouring pads and powders	Plant particles
Soaps	Plastics, dry
Toilet bowl cleaners	Sawdust
Window cleaners	Wool
	Volatile substances
Workplace	Ammonia
Acid and alkalies	Formaldehyde
Cleaning products	Organic solvents

From U.S. Department of Health and Human Services. *Case Studies in Environmental Medicine: Skin Lesions and Environmental Exposures: Rash Decisions.* Atlanta: Public Health Service, Agency for Toxic Substances and Disease Registry, 1993.

and allergic contact dermatitis. Work-related skin disorders usually affect the hands, wrists, and forearms.

  (5) Patch testing with the suspected agent may be useful in determining the allergen. Caution is needed so that further sensitization does not occur.

  d. Clinical management

    (1) Removal of the person from the offending agent is the 1st step.

    (2) Topical or systemic corticosteroid therapy may be indicated, based on the severity of the symptoms.

    (3) For extensive weeping, a drying agent such as Burow's solution is indicated.

    (4) Signs of secondary infection should be investigated.

    (5) Worksite control strategies include the following:
      • Substitution of a less offensive agent
      • Enclosure of the work process
      • Good housekeeping so that exposure is limited
      • Use of appropriate gloves, determined by the type of exposure (cotton liners worn under the glove may be helpful in absorbing excess moisture)
      • Use of barrier creams if gloves cannot be worn

4. Gulf War illness
5. Violence in the workplace

  a. Definition

    (1) Work-related violence is defined as a fatality; an assault; an aggressive act of hitting, kicking, pushing, or scratching; a sexual act or attempted act, with or without a weapon; or any other such physical or verbal attack directed to the worker by a patient, client, relative, coworker, customer, or work-associated individual that arises during or as

Table 38–9. Common Causes of Allergic Contact Dermatitis

Germicides and biocides	Balsam of Peru
Formaldehyde-releasing compounds	Benzyl alcohol
Parabens	Cinnamic acid derivatives
Quaternary ammonium compounds	Citronella derivatives
Grains	**Metals**
Barley	Chromium
Oat	Cobalt
Rye	Nickel
Wheat	
Foods/spices	**Organic dyes**
Cardamom	*p*-Aminoazobenzene
Carrot	*p*-Phenylenediamine
Chicory	
Coconut	**Plastic resins**
Coffee	Epoxies
Endive	Formaldehyde-based acrylics
Lettuce	Phenolics
Potato	
Radish	*Rhus* plants*
Tamarind	Poison ivy
Turmeric	Poison oak
Vanilla	Poison sumac
Medication/product ingredients	**Rubber products**
Preservatives	Antioxidants
Lanolin	Polymerization accelerators
Thimerosal	**Topical medications**
Fragrances and perfumes	Benzocaine
	Neomycin

* For a more complete listing of plants that cause dermatitis, see Adams RM. *Occupational Skin Disease.* 2nd ed. Philadelphia: WB Saunders, 1990, pp 507–509.

From U.S. Department of Health and Human Services. *Case Studies in Environmental Medicine: Skin Lesions and Environmental Exposures: Rash Decisions.* Atlanta: Public Health Service, Agency for Toxic Substances and Disease Registry, 1993.

 CLINICAL CONTROVERSIES

A total of 700,000 U.S. troops were deployed to the Persian Gulf during operations Desert Shield and Desert Storm from 1990 to 1991. After returning from serving in the Persian Gulf War during that time, some veterans have reported persistent and chronic symptoms of fatigue, diarrhea, and rash.

The Veterans Administration and the Department of Defense established a health registry, and, through March 1995, approximately 59,000 veterans had registered health concerns related to service in the Persian Gulf region.

Efforts by the Veterans Administration and the Department of Defense have not identified a specific cause or biologic explanation for these illnesses, nor have specific diseases or syndromes been identified. However, in August 1996 the Department of Defense revealed possible troop exposure to low levels of chemical weapons during the Gulf War and therefore has resumed efforts to identify the possible effects of such low-level chemical exposure.

Research into this syndrome is ongoing. Veterans having continuing health problems are encouraged to register and obtain a health evaluation through the Veterans Administration or the Department of Defense.

Clinical manifestations include chronic, persistent symptoms of fatigue, diarrhea, other gastrointestinal complaints (gas, bloating, cramps, or abdominal pain), difficulty remembering or concentrating, and "trouble finding words," all lasting longer than 6 months. Standardized physical examination and laboratory results have not revealed consistent findings, as compared to exposed versus the nonexposed groups.

Treatment focuses on symptom management, psychosocial support, and referral of those symptomatic veterans to the health registries established by the Veterans Administration or Department of Defense.

a result of the performance of duties and that results in death, physical injury, or mental harm.

b. Incidence and etiology

  (1) Violent acts are underreported.

  (2) Homicide rates are highest for taxicab drivers, with a reported rate of 26.9 per 100,000 full-time workers per year. Other high-risk occupations include liquor store clerk, gas station attendant, convenience or grocery store clerk, and health care worker (emergency department personnel, community health workers, psychiatric personnel).

  (3) California OSHA has taken the lead in developing guidelines for workplace security, defining 3 types of violent workplace events:

    • Type I, although uncommon, includes work-related violent acts that are most likely to result in a fatality. Type I events include unknown assailants, who have no legitimate relationship to the work setting. They enter a work establishment and commit a violent act, usually during the course of a robbery. High-risk activities include having face-to-face contact with the public, exchanging money or goods with the public, having access to drugs, working alone, and working at night.

    • Type II events are the most prevalent work-related violent acts that most often result in nonfatal assaults. The assailant is someone who is a recipient of a service provided by the victim of violence, and, therefore, has a legitimate relationship with the work setting. A patient care situation is a good example of a setting for this type of violent act. Risk factors include being in any service-oriented profession, having open access to the work site, working in isolation with clients, performing night work, and making home visits by oneself.

    • Type III events are assaults perpetrated by someone who has some employment-related involvement with the workplace. The assailant may be a coworker, a supervisor, or an ac-

---

BOX 38–4. Hazard Correction: Workplace Security

Hazards that threaten the security of employees shall be corrected in a timely manner based on severity when they are first observed or discovered.

Corrective measures for type I workplace security hazards can include the following:

1. Making the workplace unattractive to robbers.
2. Utilizing surveillance measures, such as cameras or mirrors, to provide information as to what is going on outside and inside the workplace.
3. Procedures for reporting suspicious persons or activities.
4. Posting of emergency telephone numbers for law enforcement, fire and medical services where employees have access to a telephone with an outside line.
5. Posting of signs notifying the public that limited cash is kept on the premises.
6. Limiting the amount of cash on hand and using time access safes for large bills.
7. Employee, supervisor, and management training on emergency action procedures.
8. Other: _____

Corrective measures for type II workplace security hazards include

1. Controlling access to the workplace and freedom of movement within it, consistent with business necessity.
2. Ensuring the adequacy of workplace security systems, such as door locks, security windows, physical barriers, and restraint systems.
3. Providing employee training in recognizing and handling threatening or hostile situations that may lead to violent acts by persons who are service recipients of our establishment.

4. Placing effective systems to warn others of a security danger or to summon assistance (e.g., alarms or panic buttons).
5. Providing procedures for a "buddy" system for specified emergency events.
6. Ensuring adequate employee escape routes.
7. Other: _____
_____

Corrective measures for type III workplace security hazards include

1. Effectively communicating our establishment's antiviolence policy to all employees, supervisors, or managers.
2. Improving how well our establishment's management and employees communicate with each other.
3. Increasing awareness by employees, supervisors, and managers of the warning signs of potential workplace violence.
4. Controlling access to, and freedom of movement within, the workplace by nonemployees, including recently discharged employees or persons with whom one of our employees is having a dispute.
5. Providing counseling to employees, supervisors, or managers who exhibit behavior that represents strain or pressure that may lead to physical or verbal abuse of coworkers.
6. Ensuring that all reports of violent acts, threats of physical violence, verbal abuse, property damage, or other sign of strain or pressure in the workplace are handled effectively by management and that the person making the report is not subject to retaliation by the person making the threat.
7. Ensuring that employee disciplinary and discharge procedures address the potential for workplace violence.
8. Other: _____
_____

From Department of Industrial Relations. *Injury and Illness Prevention Program for Workplace Security.* San Francisco, CA: Cal–OSHA Consultation Service, 995.

quaintance or a spouse of an employee. Revenge is usually the precipitating variable, with the assailants perceiving themselves to be unfairly treated or to have unsatisfactory relationships. An example of type III violence is when a former employee enters a workplace and assaults a supervisor in revenge for termination.

c. Clinical manifestations
  (1) The risk for violence by a person is difficult to predict.
  (2) Agitation, making verbal threats, excessive alcohol or other drug use, having access to a gun, and having a history of violent behavior are all risk factors for a violent action (see Chapters 40 and 41).

d. Clinical management
  (1) Assessment of work site and community rates of violence is the 1st step.
  (2) The work site should be inspected to assess existing security measures and potential sites of violence, for example, places with poor visibility or unlocked windows and doors, or isolated work areas.
  (3) Control measures should be designed (Box 38–4).
  (4) There should be a management commitment to a zero tolerance of verbal or sexual threats or harassment in the workplace.

(5) All workers should be trained in workplace security policies and procedures.

■ SUMMARY

Poor occupational and environmental health conditions are almost 100 percent preventable. Recognition of these conditions is accomplished by obtaining a complete history of work, home, and community exposures.

Work-related musculoskeletal disorders continue to claim the most lost work days. The associated medical treatment, rehabilitation, and lost productivity contribute to escalating costs in both the health care and workers' compensation systems.

Violence in the workplace has become a more recognized problem, reflecting the overall societal concern about violence. This critical problem requires active involvement of employers and employees in implementing a workplace security program.

A community health focus, addressing primary prevention at the work site, is the only way to prevent work-related injury and illness. Preventing work-to-home exposure and industry-to-community transmission is a priority, especially with the persistence of lead exposure seen in children and adults. Correcting hazards close to the source is of paramount importance and requires a team approach of persons with occupational health and safety expertise.

Environmental health and safety continue to require grassroots community action for appropriate legislation and regulation to protect water, air, and soil quality.

Bibliography

Books and Reports

Association of Schools of Public Health. *Proposed National Strategies for the Prevention of Leading Work-Related Diseases and Injuries, Part 1*. Cincinnati: National Institute for Occupational Safety and Health, 1986.

Association of Schools of Public Health. *Proposed National Strategies for the Prevention of Leading Work-Related Diseases and Injuries, Part 2*. Cincinnati: National Institute for Occupational Safety and Health, 1988.

Burgel B. *Innovation at the Worksite: Delivery of Nurse Managed Primary Care Services*. Washington, DC: American Nurses Publishing Co, 1993.

LaDou J (ed). *Occupational Medicine*. Norwalk, CT, Appleton & Lange, 1990.

Levy BS, and Wegman DH. *Occupational Health: Recognizing and Preventing Work-Related Disease*. 3rd ed. Boston: Little, Brown & Co, 1995.

Rogers B. *Occupational Health Nursing: Concepts and Practice*. Philadelphia: WB Saunders, 1994.

U.S. Department of Health and Human Services. *Case Studies in Environmental Medicine: Exposure History*. Atlanta, GA: Agency for Toxic Substances and Disease Registry, October 1992.

U.S. Department of Health and Human Services. *Case Studies in Environmental Medicine: Reproductive and Developmental Hazards*. Atlanta, GA: Agency for Toxic Substances and Disease Registry, September 1993.

U.S. Department of Health and Human Services. *Healthy People 2000: National Health Promotion and Disease Prevention Objectives*. DHHS Publication No. (PHS) 91-50212. Washington, DC: U.S. Government Printing Office, 1991.

U.S. Department of Labor. *Occupational Injuries and Illnesses in the United States by Industry, 1993*. Washington, DC: Bureau of Labor Statistics, 1994.

Journal Articles

Burgel B, and Quinlan P. Control of occupational and environmental hazards. *Nurse Practitioner Forum* 6(2):72–78, 1995.

Neufer L, and Narkunas D. Hazardous substance releases at the community level. *AAOHN J* 42(7):329–335, 1994.

Rogers B. Linkages in environmental and occupational health: Assessing, detecting, and containing exposure sources. *AAOHN J* 42(7):336–343, 1994.

Salazar MK, and Primomo J. Taking the lead in environmental health: Defining a model for practice. *AAOHN J* 42(7):317–324, 1994.

Snyder M, et al. Environmental and occupational health education: A survey of community health nurses' need for educational programs. *AAOHN J* 42(7):325–328, 1994.

Twining S. The occupational and environmental health history: Guidelines for the primary care nurse practitioner. *Nurse Practitioner Forum* 6(2):64–71, 1995.

Wallerstein N. Health and safety education for workers with low-literacy or limited English skills. *Am J Ind Med* 22:751–765, 1992.

Regulations

Code of Federal Regulations:
CFR 29, Section 1910.1200. Hazard Communication.
CFR 29, Section 1920.20. Access to Employee Exposure and Medical Records.

Occupational Pulmonary Disorders

Books and Reports

U.S. Department of Health and Human Services. *Case Studies in Environmental Medicine: Asbestos Toxicity.* Atlanta, GA: Agency for Toxic Substances and Disease Registry, June 1990.

Journal Articles

Centers for Disease Control and Prevention. Asthma—United States, 1982–1992. *MMWR* 43(51/52):952–955, 1995.

Regulations

Code of Federal Regulations (OSHA Standards):
9 CFR 1910.134. Respiratory Protection.
9 CFR 1910.1000. Air Contaminants.
9 CFR 1910.1101. Asbestos.

Musculoskeletal Disorders

Books and Reports

U.S. Department of Health and Human Services. *Acute Low Back Problems in Adults: Assessment and Treatment.* Publication No. 95-0643. Washington, DC: Agency for Health Care Policy and Research, 1994.
U.S. Department of Health and Human Services. *Application Manual for the Revised NIOSH Lifting Equation.* Publication No. 94-176930. Cincinnati: National Institute for Occupational Safety and Health, 1994.

Journal Articles

Bureau of National Affairs. OSHA draft proposed ergonomic protection standard: Summaries, explanations, regulatory text, appendices A and B, March 20, 1995. *Occup Safety Health Rep* 24(42):S-1–S-248, 1995.
Childre F, and Winzeler A. Cumulative trauma disorder: A primary care provider's guide to upper extremity diagnosis and treatment. *Nurse Practitioner Forum* 6(2):106–119, 1995.
Moore JS. Carpal tunnel syndrome. *Occup Med* 7(4):741–763, 1992.

Occupational Cancers

Regulations

Code of Federal Regulations (OSHA Standards):
CFR 29 1990. Identification, Classification, and Regulation of Potential Occupational Carcinogens.

Other relevant standards for carcinogens:
CFR 29 1910.1001. Asbestos.
CFR 29 1910.1028. Benzene.

Noise-Induced Hearing Loss

Reports

National Institutes of Health. *Noise and Hearing Loss: NIH Development Conference Consensus Statement.* Washington, DC: Author, 8(1):1–24, January 22–24, 1990.

Journal Articles

Adera T, et al. Assessment of the proposed draft American National Standard Method for evaluating the effectiveness of hearing conservation programs. *J Occup Med* 5(6):568–573, 1993.
Miller MH, Crane MA, and Fox J. When air conduction is not enough and related issues: A critique of the OSHA Occupational Hearing Conservation Standard. *J Occup Med* 34(3):293–296, 1992.

Regulations

Code of Federal Regulations (OSHA Standards):
CFR 29 1910.95. Occupational Noise Exposure.

Lead Exposure

Books, Reports, and Pamphlets

California Occupational Lead Poisoning Prevention Program. *Lead in the Workplace.* Berkeley, CA: California Department of Health and Human Services, 1994.
Coalition to Prevent Lead Poisoning. *Reducing Lead in Your Home.* San Francisco: Consumer Action, 1992.
Olson K (ed). *Poisoning and Drug Overdose.* 2nd ed. Norwalk, CT, Appleton & Lange, 1994.
U.S. Department of Health and Human Services. *Case Studies in Environmental Medicine: Lead Toxicity.* Atlanta, GA: Agency for Toxic Substances and Disease Registry, 1990.
U.S. Department of Health and Human Services. *Preventing Lead Poisoning in Young Children.* Washington, DC: U.S. Government Printing Office, 1991.

Journal Articles

Centers for Disease Control and Prevention. Adult blood lead epidemiology and surveillance—United States, 1994 and First Quarter 1995. *MMWR* 44(27):515–517, 1995.
Centers for Disease Control and Prevention. Blood lead levels—United States, 1988–1991. *MMWR* 43(30):545–548, 1994.
Centers for Disease Control. Lead poisoning associated with use of traditional

ethnic remedies—California, 1991–1992. *MMWR* 42(27):521–524, 1993.

Regulations

CFR 29, Section 1910.1025. Lead Exposure.

Pesticides

Books and Reports

Institutes of Medicine. *Veterans and Agent Orange: Health Effects of Herbicides Used in Vietnam.* Washington, DC: National Academy Press, 1994.
U.S. Department of Health and Human Services. *Case Studies in Environmental Medicine: Cholinesterase-Inhibiting Pesticide Toxicity.* Atlanta, GA: Agency for Toxic Substances and Disease Registry, 1993.
U.S. Department of Health and Human Services. *Case Studies in Environmental Medicine: Dioxin Toxicity.* Atlanta, GA: Agency for Toxic Substances and Disease Registry, 1990.

Journal Articles

Henry T. Pesticide exposure seen in primary care. *Nurse Practitioner Forum* 6(2):90–98, 1995.
Lang L. Are pesticides a problem? *Environ Health Perspect* 101(7):578–583, 1993.
Moses M, et al. Environmental equity and pesticide exposure. *Toxicol Ind Health* 9(5):913–959, 1993.

Other Occupational and Environmental Disorders

Books and Reports

Department of Industrial Relations: *California OSHA Guidelines for Workplace Security.* San Francisco: Division of Occupational Safety and Health, 1994.
Department of Industrial Relations. *Model: Injury and Illness Prevention Program for Workplace Security.* San Francisco: Division of Occupational Safety and Health, 1995.
U.S. Department of Health and Human Services. *Case Studies in Environmental Medicine: Skin Lesions and Environmental Exposures: Rash Decisions.* Atlanta, GA: Agency for Toxic Substances and Disease Registry, 1993.

Journal Articles

Centers for Disease Control and Prevention. Unexplained illness among Persian Gulf War veterans in an air national guard unit: Preliminary report. *MMWR* 44(23):443–447, 1995.
NIH Technology Assessment Workshop Panel. The Persian Gulf experience and health. *JAMA* 272(5):391–395, 1994.
Simonowitz JA. Violence in health care: A strategic approach. *Nurse Practitioner Forum* 6(2):120–129, 1995.

Agencies and Resources

Agency for Toxic Substances and Disease
  Registry
1600 Clifton Road, NE
Atlanta, GA 30333
(404) 639–6206

American Association of Occupational
  Health Nurses
50 Lenox Pointe
Atlanta, GA 30324
(800) 241–8014

American Board for Occupational Health
  Nurses, Inc.
201 East Ogden Ave. #114
Hinsdale, IL 60521–3652
(708) 789–5799

County Poison Control Centers
Local and state health departments

Environmental Protection Agency (10 regions throughout the United States—see the federal government telephone listings)
Internet Website: http://www.dtic.mil/gulflink/dmdcz.htm/

National Institute for Occupational Safety
  and Health
Technical Information Branch
4676 Columbia Parkway
Cincinnati, OH 45226
(513) 533–8326, (800) 35–NIOSH

Occupational Safety and Health
  Administration
U.S. Department of Labor (10 regions across the United States—see the federal government telephone listings)

Caring for People with Special Psychosocial Needs and Problems

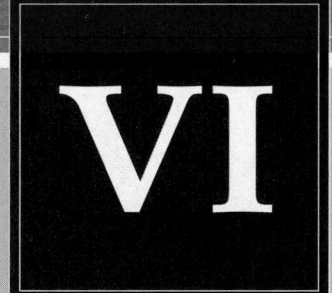

VI

39

Caring for People
Experiencing Life Crises

◀ OVERVIEW OF CRISIS AND STRESS

Stress

Stress is a condition that drains resources, endangers well-being, or is perceived as taxing.

Stress can come from the person, the environment, or more commonly, from a combination of both.

Stressors

Stressors are the events and situations that affect individuals, cause a perception of stress, and require a coping response.

Serious illness, death of a friend, marriage, hurricanes, or a final examination—although very different experiences—could all be stressors.

Stress Response

The person's mental and physical reactions to a stressor constitute a **stress response.**

See Chapter 6 for further information on the stress response.

Coping

Coping is the way people try to reduce or manage stress. People cope with stress in many different emotional and physical ways (Box 39–1).

Successful coping results in resolution or acceptance of the stressor. It can also lead to positive adaptation and personal growth. Unsuccessful coping can lead to crisis. It also contributes to poor adaptation.

Adaptation

Adaptation comprises the adjustments, accommodations, and assimilations that occur in work, social life, morale, and health as a result of coping with the crisis event.

2. Adaptation can be positive or negative. Signs of successful adaptation:
   - Improved morale
   - Improved physical health
   - Increased social functioning
   - Ability to cope in new and effective ways
   - Perception of the crisis event in a positive light
   - Ability to focus on aspects of life other than the crisis event

   Signs of poor adaptation:
   - Continued anxiety
   - Feelings of vulnerability and inadequacy
   - Symptoms of poor mental health, such as anxiety, psychosis, or depression
   - Continued signs of physical distress

Life Events

1. A **life event** is a measurable environmental stressor of importance to the individual. Major life events include childbirth, divorce, accidents, and start of a new job.
2. The number and quality of life events experienced in a given period are often measured to give a sense of the level of stress experienced. Stress cannot be predicted by numbers of life events alone, however, nor is the magnitude of the event predictive of a person's response. Sometimes an accumulation of the little annoyances of life can be just as stressful as a major event.
   a. Factors that increase the risk that a life event will become a crisis:
      - An event that is unexpected, overwhelming, and extraordinary
      - Inadequate social support, information, and resources
      - Unrealistic perception of the life event
      - Poor or inadequate coping strategies
   b. Factors that decrease the risk that a life event will become a crisis:
      - An event that is anticipated and commonly experienced
      - Adequate social support, information, and resources
      - Realistic perception of the life event
      - Good coping ability

1835

BOX 39–1. Common Coping Strategies Used by People in Crisis

Distancing themselves from the problem
Denying that the problem exists
Fantasizing or using wishful thinking
Isolating themselves from the problem or from other people
Blaming themselves for causing the problem
Accepting responsibility for the problem
Emphasizing the positive aspects of the problem
Drawing strength from adversity and seeing themselves as stronger people
Becoming hostile and angry
Becoming fatalistic
Using prayer and other practices of faith
Reviewing the event alone or with others
Trying to maintain self-control
Using tension-reducing strategies such as eating certain foods, exercising, and engaging in hobbies
Making use of available social support

Crisis Event

1. A **crisis** is a sudden, intense stressor that causes disequilibrium and sometimes acute emotional upset and physical distress. Crises often occur abruptly, allowing no time for adequate preparation and leaving the person struggling to adapt.
2. Life crises have identifiable characteristics:
   a. Universal experience: Crises affect almost everyone but are experienced in different ways by different people. They need not be associated with psychopathology.
   b. Short duration: Crises are acute and self limited, usually lasting 4 to 6 weeks.
   c. Identifiable beginning: Crises are precipitated by an identifiable event.
   d. Predictable development: Crises follow a predictable pattern from start to finish.

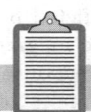

NURSING MANAGEMENT

Remind personnel that health problems can precipitate crisis in anyone. Crisis is not limited to those who have had psychologic difficulties in the past.

■ TYPES OF LIFE CRISIS

Situational Crises

1. **Situational crises** are unexpected occurrences that threaten self-esteem or physical safety. People will often say, "I never thought such a thing could happen to me."
2. Many different types of events can result in situational crises. Examples include crimes such as muggings, burglaries, and rapes; loss of a job; health problems; family problems; and death of a close friend or family membe[r]. Not every person who experiences such events exper[i]ences a crisis. Common characteristics of events that ca[n] precipitate situational crises include the following:
   - Accidental nature
   - Sudden or unexpected onset
   - Emergency quality

Maturational and Developmental Crises

1. **Maturational crises** occur during transitions from [one] phase of life to the next, such as from childhood t[o] adolescence and from adolescence to adulthood.
2. **Developmental crises** occur during transitional li[fe] changes, such as marriage and parenthood.
3. Precipitating factors in maturational and developmenta[l] crises
   a. A transition that is disrupted. For example, a youn[g] adult might not find a job after graduation. In nor[n] Western cultures, a disrupted transition might be th[e] failure of the community to provide formal rites [of] passage.
   b. Lack of necessary skills, knowledge, or resources t[o] effect a transition. For example, a teenaged mother [of] a newborn might be unable to meet her new respo[n]sibilities.
   c. Not accepting the time or the activities of transitio[n.] For example, a woman forced into early retirement [or] a woman who does not accept menopause may b[e] demonstrating lack of acceptance.
   d. Unexpected timing of the transition. For example, [a] young person who is widowed must make an une[x]pected transition.

Adventitious Crises

1. **Adventitious crises** are situational crises that affe[ct] many people at the same time. They include natur[al] disasters such as earthquakes, hurricanes, tornadoes, an[d] floods and human-made disasters such as fire and n[u]clear and chemical accidents.
2. Disasters caused by people cause long-term coping diff[i]culties more often than natural disasters because huma[n] errors are seen as preventable (see Chapter 37).

Stages of Life Crisis

1. A life crisis can be divided into stages.
2. The most common classification system includes [five] stages: precrisis, impact of event, crisis, resolution, an[d] postcrisis. (Fig. 39–1).
3. The end of crisis often means the resolution of th[e] stressor or acceptance of the situation. The cessation [of] the crisis can itself be a crisis for some indivic[d]uals. Not all crises are resolved, however; some lead t[o] long-term problems, such as post-traumatic stre[ss] disorder.

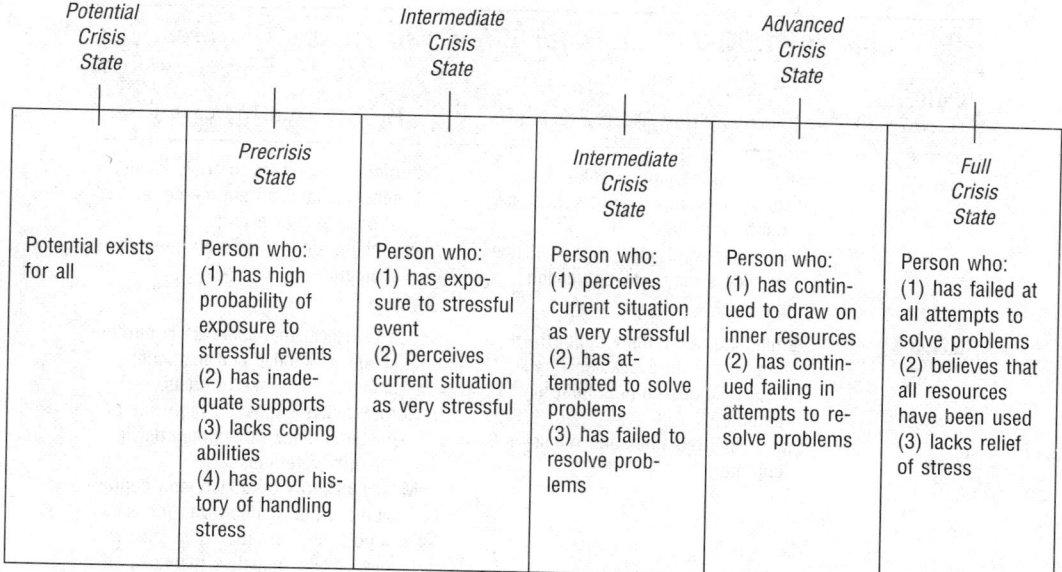

Figure 39–1. Crisis continuum. (From Brownell JM. The concept of crisis: Its utility for nursing. *Advances in Nursing Science: Crisis Intervention* 6 [4]:17, 1984. Copyright © 1984, Aspen Publishers, Inc.)

☐ TRANSCULTURAL FACTORS IN LIFE CRISES

Western versus Non-Western Perspectives

1. The Western focus is on mind-body split, emphasizing biomedical approaches, whereas the non-Western approach relies less on modern medicine and surgery. In non-Western cultures, symptoms of crisis are seen holistically, not as separate physical and psychologic manifestations.

2. What Western medicine views as an abnormal reaction to stress may be normal in some cultures. For example, loud vocalizations of distress or fainting are common expressions among some peoples. The nurse must avoid imposing personal values and thereby misinterpreting the reaction.

3. The family is more important than the individual in some non-Western cultures. To achieve effective care, people from such cultures must be treated within the context of the family.

4. Traditional healers are used for crisis prevention in some non-Western cultures (e.g., in renewal ceremonies and rites of passage).

5. In some refugee and immigrant groups, acute stress may be blamed on outside evil forces, such as magic, hexes, and witchcraft. Practitioners may do best to treat the physical signs and symptoms and use traditional healers to treat the believed cause.

Cultural Groups

All cultures provide support in times of crisis—for example, the large extended families of Italian Americans, the acceptance of family members with mental illness by people of Indian origin, and the religious faith of the Irish. All people deserve culturally sensitive care that takes these factors into consideration (Table 39–1).

2. Conversely, all cultural groups have characteristics that increase the risk of crisis. The high rate of alcoholism among Native Americans and the reticence of some American men to seek or accept psychologic help are two such factors. Be aware of what cultural factors hinder as well as help in crisis care.

☐ ASSESSING PEOPLE EXPERIENCING LIFE CRISES

Obtaining a Description of the Crisis

1. Onset: Crisis events have an identifiable beginning. Ask specific questions about when the crisis started. For people from non-Western cultures, ask when the physical signs and symptoms first appeared.

2. Precipitating event or events: Find out what precipitated the crisis. Allow the person to sort out the who, what, when, where, and hows.

3. Threats, loss, and challenges: Determine whether the crisis is a threat, loss, or challenge to social, physical, psychologic, or spiritual integrity.

4. Characteristics of the crisis event
   a. Predictability: The more predictable an event, the less stressful it will be.
   b. Timing: The timing of an event influences its psychologic impact. People and the societies in which they live have timelines for events such as marriage, death, and childbirth. When an event occurs at an unexpected time, there is increased stress. For example, young widows may experience more stress than older widows because widowhood is unexpected at an early

Table 39–1. Risk Factors for Life Crisis Across Cultures

Cultural Group	Factors That Decrease Risk	Factors That Increase Risk
Asians	Family loyalty is important. Balance (yinyang) is important in all matters of life. Folk healers and alternative medicine providers may provide needed support.	Common responses to crisis include a sense of fatalism and perceived lack of control over events. Psychiatric difficulties may be seen as shameful.
Blacks	Family and community support are important and available. Strong religious commitment is common. Use of folk remedies and medicine is common.	Use of dialect may increase communication difficulties and misunderstandings in times of crisis. Some studies suggest a high rate of post-traumatic stress disorder in minority veterans. Most measures of anxiety and depression are not standardized for black populations and may give false-positive or false-negative results.
Hispanics	Culture favors close, consistent relationships. Strong family ties and values are common. Coping strategies may include folk medicine and spiritualism. Seeking out faith healers is common.	Lack of fluency in English may impede getting help during crisis. Although folk beliefs are not necessarily problematic, they can be crisis producing. For example, the "evil eye" can be anticipated if a nurse admires but does not touch a child while giving care. Some have a fatalistic attitude toward crisis.
Native Americans	Family is very important. Wisdom and knowledge of older members are sought. Harmony with the environment is sought.	Talking about self is discouraged as bragging, making some mental health interventions difficult. Rates of alcohol abuse are high. Rates of suicide are high.

age. The young widows experience more stress in part because they have few peers with similar problems, and there has been little time to prepare for a new role.

c. Duration: The longer the duration of the event, the harder it is to cope with the crisis. The internal and external resources needed to cope with the event may become exhausted.

d. Sequencing: People expect events to occur in a certain order. For example, parents expect that they will die before their children. Events that occur out of the expected order are more stressful.

Exploring the Patient's History and Available Resources

1. A thorough history will help in planning the care. The history should include physical, psychologic, social, and spiritual health experiences, coping strategies used, and resolution of prior problems.

   a. Strength of feeling: The more strongly a person feels about an event or situation, the stronger the threat crisis.

   b. Commitment: The greater the commitment to a event or situation, the greater the chance for crisis the event is altered or threatened. Be aware of ea individual's level of commitment before planni care.

   c. Cultural belief systems: Culture influences reactions life events. To be effective, all care plans must culturally sensitive.

   d. Spiritual beliefs: Spirituality influences how a cris event is viewed as well as how it is dealt with by t person.

   e. Prior experience: Experience with an event can help person understand what to expect and how to pr pare for the event.

      (1) Positive experiences, knowledge, and preparatio can help a person react in a more effective way crisis.

      (2) Prior negative experiences can hinder reactio and ability to deal with the present similar crisis.

   f. Locus of control: The perceived locus, or source,

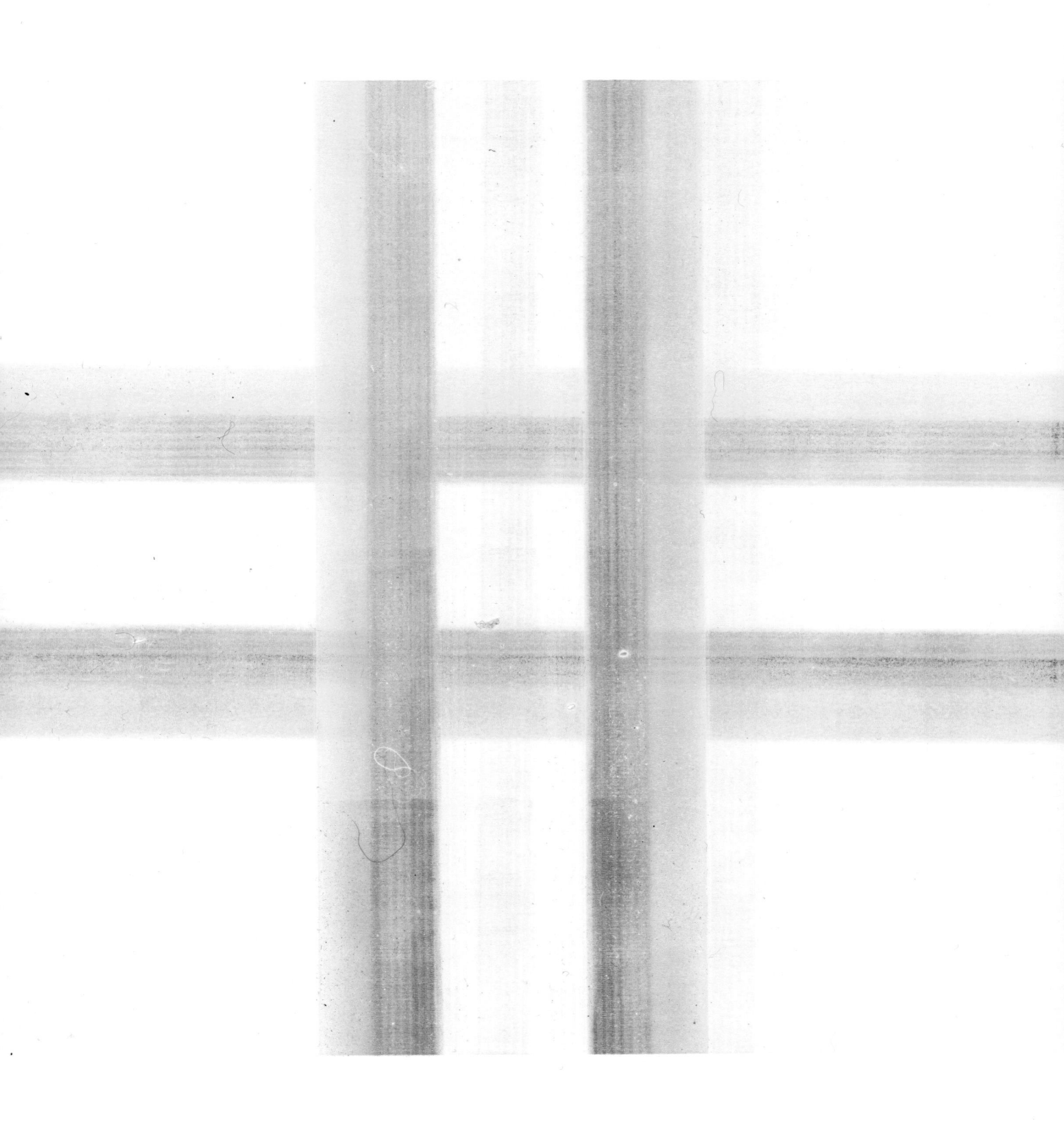

control for life events can be internal, external, or situational.

g. Prior use of coping strategies: Find out how the person coped in the past and what coping strategies are being used now. Experience with similar situations may aid coping. People use a variety of coping strategies to deal with crisis events. Cultural beliefs and mores influence coping strategies. The person in crisis might confront the problem and try to solve it with available coping skills or might confront the emotions involved and try to master feelings by using coping strategies (see Box 39–1).

Reviewing the person's current resources will determine what help is available. Ask whether the person has friends or family, community resources, or other sources of support.

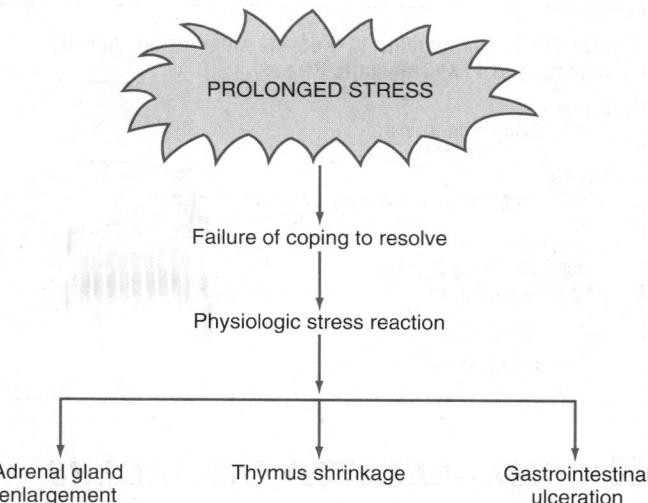

Figure 39–2. Selye's classic physiologic stress reaction. Adrenal enlargement, shrinkage of the thymus, and gastrointestinal ulceration comprise the classic stress reaction first identified by Selye.

DER ADVISORY

Factors that can augment the development of crisis in older people include the following:

Inaccurate perception of life events related to acute and chronic illness
Reduced social support and other coping resources
Problems in performing activities of daily living
Changes in the environment that disturb mental and physical equilibrium

ysical and Psychosocial Assessment

Keep in mind that not all people view the mind as separate from the body, so that questions about psychosocial issues may be inappropriate. The health care provider should consider that the balance between psychosocial and physical assessment may vary for people from different cultures. For many non-Western populations, the physical signs and symptoms are considered to be the only presenting problems (see Chapter 6).

Psychosocial assessment: To provide effective nursing care, perform an in-depth psychosocial assessment. Although everyone reacts differently, a crisis often results in 1 or more of the following key signs and symptoms:

a. Anger, loss of temper
b. Resentment toward health care workers or others who provide help
c. Resistance to treatments or diagnostic tests
d. Withdrawal from normal activities, friendships, or family relationships
e. Overuse of medications, drugs, alcohol, or food
f. Excessive excitement
g. Confusion and forgetfulness
h. Nervousness, irritability, and anxiety

Physical assessment: All people in crisis should have a physical examination to rule out physical causes of signs and symptoms and to provide a baseline for assessing future change. Although some people can tolerate the prolonged stress of unresolved crisis, others develop classic physiologic stress reactions (Fig. 39–2). Ask about physical signs and symptoms that are associated with crisis:

a. Headaches
b. Shaking or tremors
c. Restlessness
d. Muscle tension
e. Rapid speech, stuttering, stammering
f. Fatigue
g. Rapid pulse and elevated blood pressure
h. Digestive troubles, such as diarrhea, constipation, stomach upset
i. Menstrual cycle changes
j. Frequent urination
k. Heart palpitations
l. Hot flashes, chills, dry mouth
m. Crying

Assessment of Present Dangers

1. Carefully consider the likelihood of suicidal or violent behavior.
2. It is especially important to assess the threat of danger or harm with situational crises. Ask specific questions about safety. People who appear suicidal or dangerous to others should always be referred immediately for help (see Chapter 41).

Special Diagnostic Studies

1. Many different tests exist for measuring aspects of the crisis response (e.g., depression, coping, anxiety, and post-traumatic stress disorder).
2. Box 39–2 lists some commonly used tests.

◼ CRISIS-RELATED DISORDERS

Post-Traumatic Stress Disorder

1. Definition: **Post-traumatic stress disorder** (PTSD) is a common sequela of unresolved crisis.
2. This disorder is characterized by recurrent episodes in which the person relives the trauma. Symptoms include nightmares, sleep disturbances, guilt over surviving, psychic numbing, difficulty in concentrating, flashbacks, aggressive behavior, impulsiveness, panic attacks, phobic responses, and hyperalert states.
3. Among refugees, PTSD is common.

Adjustment Disorders

1. Definition: An **adjustment disorder** is a maladaptive response to a known event that results in social, physical, or psychologic problems.
    a. There is a clear change in the person's personality and behavior that is not attributable to a known mental illness.
    b. Most adjustment disorders start within 3 months of the onset of stress and resolve within 6 months.
    c. Treatment includes short-term supportive psychotherapy and occasionally pharmacotherapy.
    d. Adjustment disorders are differentiated by their symptoms. Examples include adjustment disorder with depressed mood and adjustment disorder with anxiety. See Box 39–3 for a list of the *Diagnostic and Statistical Manual of Mental Disorders* (DSM-IV)– accepted adjustment disorders.

2. Those influenced by non-Western cultures may exhibit crisis through "culture bound syndromes."
    a. "Falling out" is seen in African-American and Caribbean Blacks. Signs and symptoms include a sudden collapse without signs of seizure. The person can hear but cannot respond; the eyes are open, but the person does not appear to see. It is treated through religious rituals such as Catholic exorcism or voodoo ceremonies.
    b. "Susto" is seen in Mexicans and Central and Latin Americans. It is thought to occur when a frightening experience leads to a loss of one's spirit. Symptoms include crying, insomnia, anorexia, diarrhea, and fever. It is treated by a native healer with herbs, potioning, and prayer.
    c. "Lattah," manifested by trancelike behavior, is seen among Malaysians, Indonesians, Filipinos, and Japanese.
    d. "Amok," or wildman behavior, is seen in Indonesians, Malaysians, and others. "Nerves" are a common complaint among Appalachians, Chinese, and others.

◼ CRISIS MANAGEMENT

Goals of Crisis Management

1. Reduce debilitating effects of stress and inadequate coping.
2. Reestablish the ability to cope or help the patient improve coping skills.

Crisis Intervention

1. **Crisis intervention** is the help provided to people during or immediately after a crisis-producing event (see Chapter 41). Crisis intervention is classified as 1st- or 2nd-level assistance.
    a. First-level help is sometimes called psychologic first aid. It occurs directly after the event, is given in a community setting, and is provided by many different first-line caregivers, including police, clergy, social workers, nurses, and doctors. The goal of psychologic first aid is to reestablish the ability to cope.
    b. Second-level help is called crisis intervention. It is directed toward resolving the problems caused by the crisis when the problem is too complex or coping abilities are inadequate for 1st-level care.
        (1) It requires more time and more specialized therapeutic skills than 1st-level care. Crisis intervention is most effective immediately after the crisis.
        (2) There are 4 major goals of 2nd-level crisis intervention therapy.
            • Restore or maintain physical health and preserve life
            • Express feelings about the crisis
            • Understand the crisis and come to terms with it
            • Make necessary behavioral changes
2. Psychologic interventions: In the 6 weeks or so after

crisis, most people remain in a state of disequilibrium. Help is most effective during this period and can promote positive growth.

a. First-level help strategies
   (1) Allow the person to talk through the situation.
   (2) Communicate acceptance, concern, empathy, and a willingness to help.
   (3) Listen for both facts and feelings. Accept both as important to the person.
   (4) Give as much information as possible.
   (5) Establish physical contact: hold the person's hand or touch an arm. The use and amount of appropriate physical contact varies depending on the person involved and the circumstances of the crisis.
   (6) Determine specific needs. Help may include making telephone calls, locating a bed, finding transportation, and so forth. Take into account the safety of the person and any legal concerns.
   (7) Make use of community resources, such as rape support groups, the Red Cross, the Salvation Army, Parents without Partners, and Mothers Against Drunk Driving, as well as therapists and native healers.

b. Second-level help strategies: Many different therapeutic strategies can be used to help the person in crisis (see Chapter 41). Issues specific to the crisis should be addressed in therapy.
   • Reduce anxiety to increase the sense of control and mastery often lost in crisis.
   • Provide help in exploring and understanding what happened and why. Reflecting back the person's words often helps to foster understanding of the event. Help the person identify missing pieces of information, areas of distortion, and misinterpretations.
   • Explore the relationship among crisis and beliefs, life goals, and dreams for the future. Crisis events often radically change views about the world and the person's place in it. Work with the person to make the necessary adjustments and to build new dreams, goals, and aspirations.
   • Establish health care routines that promote physical well-being. Adequate nutrition, sleep, relaxation, and exercise facilitate crisis resolution.
   • Teach relaxation techniques, such as progressive muscle relaxation, yoga, and massage.
   • Identify and refer those for whom suicide or physical harm to others appears to be a real possibility. See Chapter 41 for further information about suicide prevention intervention.

Table 39–2. Pharmacologic Agents Used in Crisis Intervention

Drug Classification	Medications
Antianxiety Drugs	
Short acting	Oxazepam, alprazolam, lorazepam
Moderately long acting	Chlordiazepoxide
Long acting	Halazepam, diazepam, prazepam, clorazepate
Antidepressants	
Tricyclics	Amitriptyline, imipramine, amoxapine, doxepin
Monoamine inhibitors	Phenebizine, tranylcypromine, isocarboxazid
Atypical agents	Trazodone, fluoxetine, bupropion

(1) Individual therapy: Individual counseling can help the person in crisis reduce anxiety, learn new coping strategies, and understand the crisis event. Remember that family and friends may need to be involved if therapy is to be effective. For persons of non-Western cultures it may be more appropriate to address the presenting physical signs and symptoms, without emphasizing the Western view of underlying psychologic crisis.

(2) Family therapy: The individual in crisis is usually part of a family that may also experience either primary or secondary effects of the same crisis. The family should be assessed and help provided as warranted. Most family crisis counseling is problem focused and involves a limited number of sessions.

(3) Group therapy: Many individuals in crisis benefit from joining groups that meet on a short-term basis to focus on problem solving. Members who have experienced the same crisis can help each other work through feelings and seek solutions. Resource groups are of tremendous help in facilitating behavioral changes.

(4) Pharmacologic interventions: Medications may sometimes be prescribed during the crisis period. Commonly, medications are given to help decrease anxiety and depression (Table 39–2).

c. Health promotion: Health care routines that promote physical well-being facilitate crisis resolution. Stress the importance of adequate nutrition, sleep, relaxation, and exercise. People should be encouraged to avoid inappropriate or excessive use of drugs or alcohol. Relaxation techniques (e.g., progressive muscle relaxation, yoga, or massage) can be useful.

d. Models of crisis intervention: Available programs include mobile crisis intervention, rape crisis intervention, and telephone crisis centers or hotlines.

Applying the Nursing Process (Box 39–4)

NURSING DIAGNOSIS: Disabling ineffective family coping R/T destruction of home by fire

1. *Expected outcomes:* Following intervention, the family members should be able to do the following:
   a. Realistically describe the crisis situation of losing one's home to a fire.
   b. State that emotional stress levels are decreased.
   c. Report feeling protected from additional stressors.
   d. Mobilize resources necessary to obtain needed clothing, housing, and other necessities.
   e. Return to precrisis or higher level of coping ability.
2. *Nursing interventions*
   a. Ask about living and housing arrangements. If assistance is needed, help family contact appropriate social service agency.
   b. Provide family counseling sessions in immediate post-fire period.
      (1) Facilitate discussion about feelings of loss.
      (2) Encourage grief response as appropriate.
      (3) Review family coping strategies for effectiveness. Suggest alternatives when appropriate.
   c. Work with family to mobilize support from friends, family, and community.

NURSING DIAGNOSIS: Anxiety R/T prolonged hospitalization for recovery from injuries from automobile accident

---

1. *Expected outcomes:* Following intervention, the person should be able to do the following:
   a. State that anxiety about prolonged hospitalization is reduced.
   b. Realistically describe losses brought on by prolonged hospitalization.
   c. Implement plans to solve problems related to prolonged hospitalization.
2. *Nursing interventions*
   a. Encourage individual to ventilate feelings of anxiety.
   b. Obtain consultation regarding need for professional counseling.

BOX 39–4. Nursing Diagnoses for People Experiencing Crises

Many nursing diagnoses may be appropriate for an individual or family in crisis, although not all are relevant for all cultures. Examples of nursing diagnoses appropriate to crisis situations are

Anxiety
Decisional conflict
Defensive coping
Ineffective denial
Compromised, ineffective family coping
Disabling, ineffective family coping
Family coping: potential for growth
Ineffective community coping
Impaired adjustment
Post-trauma response
Rape-trauma syndrome: compound reaction
Rape-trauma syndrome: silent reaction
Situational low self-esteem

---

c. Identify problems brought on by prolonged hospitalization (e.g., work, financial, family).
d. Work with the person to develop a plan to address problems of prolonged hospitalization. Facilitate person's obtaining resources necessary to address problems. Make use of available community resources specific to individual problems (e.g., Salvation Army, religious organizations, social service agencies).

NURSING DIAGNOSIS: Post-trauma response R/T being victim of serious crime

---

1. *Expected outcomes:* After intervention the person should be able to do the following:
   a. Experience a decrease in disturbing symptoms.
   b. Demonstrate new coping strategies.
2. *Nursing interventions*
   a. Document signs of trauma exposure.
   b. Monitor the person for symptoms that focus on re-experiencing the trauma, avoiding the trauma, and altered lifestyle.
      • Re-experiencing: nightmares, daydreams, excessive talk about event, anger, anxiety, hyperalert state, and abnormal startle reactions
      • Avoidance: impaired memory, confusion, amnesia, feelings of numbness, and reduced function
      • Altered lifestyle: lack of impulse control, sleep disturbances, self-destructive behaviors, chronic depression, and difficulty with interpersonal relationships
   c. Assist the person in working through the event.
      (1) Help the client reconstruct the event.
      (2) Validate the person's perception of reality and feelings about the event.
      (3) Help the person find meaning in experience.
   d. Help the client learn new coping strategies (e.g., relaxation techniques, mental imagery, new hobbies).

■ HEALTH TEACHING AND CRISIS PREVENTION

Individual Activities to Prevent Crisis

1. Eliminate hazardous situations that can produce crisis. For example, ensure that work safety guidelines are followed to prevent situational or adventitious crises.
2. Identify vulnerable groups (e.g., police, members of the military) before exposure to hazardous or stressful situations. Provide anticipatory education about stress reduction and coping strategies.
3. Advise those exposed to crisis-producing situations about coping alternatives and available resources.
4. Increase repertoire and effectiveness of coping strategies through health education.

Provide additional physical, social, and informational resources to individuals under stress.

ommunity Crisis Prevention

Primary prevention: social action aimed at increasing the community's ability to react to crisis

2. Secondary prevention: community programs aimed at decreasing the number and seriousness of crisis situations by providing access to early diagnosis and effective treatments

3. Tertiary prevention: the establishment of rehabilitation programs aimed at increasing functioning of those individuals who have experienced crisis

bliography

oks

uilera DC. *Crisis Intervention: Theory and Methodology.* 6th ed. St. Louis: Mosby– ear Book, 1989.

stin LS. *Responding to Disaster: A Guide r Mental Health Professionals.* Washington, DC: American Psychological Society, 1992.

le JS, and Andrews MM. *Transcultural oncepts in Nursing Care.* Glenview, IL: cott Foresman & Co, 1989.

olan G. *Principles of Preventive Psychiary.* New York: Basic Books, 1964.

anti GA. *Caring for Patients from Different Cultures: Case Studies from American ospitals.* Philadelphia: University of ennsylvania Press, 1991.

y F, and Kavanaugh CK. *Psychiatric Mental Health Nursing.* Philadelphia: JB ippincott, 1991.

er JC, and Davidhizer RE. *Transcultural ursing: Assessment and Intervention.* St. ouis: Mosby–Year Book, 1991.

ff LA. *People in Crisis: Understanding and elping.* 3rd ed. Menlo Park, CA: Adison-Wesley, 1989.

arus RS, and Folkman S. *Stress, Apraisal, and Coping.* New York: Springer, 984.

Farland GK, and Thomas MD (eds).

Psychiatric Mental Health Nursing: Application of the Nursing Process. Philadelphia: JB Lippincott, 1991.

Pruett H, and Brown VB (eds). *Crisis Intervention and Prevention.* San Francisco: Jossey-Bass, 1990.

Qureshi B. *Transcultural Medicine: Dealing with Patients from Different Cultures.* Boston: Klewer Academic Press, 1989.

Roberts J. *Crisis Intervention Handbook: Assessment, Treatment, and Research.* Belmont, CA: Wadsworth Press, 1990.

Spielberger CD, Gorsuch RC, and Lushene RE. *Manual for the Stat-Trait Anxiety Inventory.* Palo Alto, CA: Consulting Psychologists Press, 1970.

Stuart GW, and Sundeen SJ. *Principles and Practice of Psychiatric Nursing.* 4th ed. St. Louis: Mosby–Year Book, 1990.

Townsend MC. *Psychiatric/Mental Health Nursing.* Philadelphia: FA Davis, 1992.

Wilson HS, and Kneisel CR. *Psychiatric Nursing.* Menlo Park, CA: Addison-Wesley, 1992.

Journal Articles

Bamber M. Victims of violence. *Occup Health* 44(4):115–117, 1992.

Beck AT, et al. An inventory for measuring depression. *Arch Gen Psychiatry* 52:53–63, 1961.

Castledine G. First-aid management of psychological emergencies. *Br J Nurs* 2(21):1079–1080+, 1993.

Cumbie B. Treating a PTSD flashback. *Nursing* 24(2):33, 1994.

Heiney SP, et al. The aftermath of bone marrow transplant for parents of pediatric patients: A post-traumatic stress disorder. *Oncol Nurs Forum* 21(5):843–847, 1993.

Keane TM, Caddell JM, and Taylor KL. Mississippi scale for combat-related post-traumatic stress disorder: Three studies in reliability and validity. *J Consult Clin Psychol* 56:85–90, 1988.

McCubbin HI, Larson A, and Olson DH. *Family Crisis Oriented Personal Evaluation Scales (F-Copes).* St Paul, MN: Family Social Science, 1981.

Morrison RA. Early identification of post-traumatic stress disorder by nurses. *Orthop Nurs* 13(4):22–24, 1994.

Steefl L. The World Trade disaster: Healing the wounds. *J Psychosoc Nurs Ment Health Serv* 31(6):5–7, 1993.

Tyra P. Older women: Victims of rape. *J Gerontol Nurs* 19(5):7–12, 1993.

Woods ST, and Campbell JC. Post-traumatic stress in battered women: Does the diagnosis fit. *Issues Ment Health Nurs* 14(2):173–186, 1993.

esources

h community has social service ncies that assist people in cri-
 The following are examples of ncies with national as well as al branches. Please refer to your al directories for addresses and

telephone numbers of other agencies.

Alzheimers Disease National
 Headquarters
(800) 621–0379

American Cancer Society
(800) 562–2623

American Red Cross
(800) 922–5986

Samaritan International
(800) 532–1737

40

Caring for People with Tobacco, Alcohol, and Other Drug Addictions

◼ OVERVIEW

Key Definitions and Concepts

1. A psychoactive substance distorts the operations of the central nervous system. Substances of abuse can create a rapidly obtained pleasurable effect or relief from discomfort, which reinforces their use. Substance use can be viewed as a progression from experimental use to addiction.
2. Experimental use of psychoactive substances has become a part of our culture and is almost expected among the young. "Gateway" or easily obtained drugs that introduce individuals to substance use include tobacco, alcohol, and inhalants.
3. Social or recreational use of psychoactive substances is use that is infrequent and sporadic, with little impact on the person's life. Habituation is a definite pattern of use such as a cup of coffee in the morning; the user will use that drug no matter what happens that day.
4. Psychoactive substance abuse is a pattern of heavy use despite social, psychologic, or medical problems, or a combination of these, that are directly related to use. There is no physiologic dependence.
5. Psychologic dependence
   a. Increased reliance on the substance for "medicinal" purposes, such as stress management and ability to socialize. Sometimes called "self-medicating."
   b. Substance use takes on a larger role in the coping mechanisms of the person, and increased use may create physical changes in the nervous system.
6. Psychoactive substance dependence (addiction)
   a. Physical dependency, which can be characterized by increased amount needed for desired effect or decreased effect when taking the same amount of the substance (tolerance)
   b. Characteristic withdrawal pattern with certain substances
   c. Continued use despite adverse consequences
   d. Compulsive use such that the person spends most of the time getting, using, or thinking about the substance
   e. World Health Organization definition: "a behavioral

pattern in which the use of a given psychoactive dr is given a sharply higher priority over other behav that once had a significantly higher value"
7. Tolerance
   a. Long-term exposure of brain cells to certain su stances induces changes that alter the sensitivity the cell at the synaptic site to communication fr other cells (neuroadaptation). This translates i needing more of the substance to get the same le of effect.
   b. Alcohol and some of the other central nervous syst depressants initiate the microsomal enzyme oxidizi system (MEOS/enzyme induction) in the liver.
      (1) This can increase the breakdown not only of al hol, but of any drug that is metabolized in liver.
      (2) Metabolism transforms the drugs through the p cess of oxidation into water-soluble compou more easily eliminated by the kidneys. Damage the liver or kidneys can result in toxic levels chemicals in the body.
   c. The individual with tolerance to a substance may able to consume amounts that would have produc symptoms of toxicity at the time of initial use.
8. Physical dependence
   a. The body comes to require the presence of a su stance to maintain normal levels of functioning.
   b. On interruption of use, a characteristic withdraw syndrome appears that is relieved by more drug the same group.
   c. The discomfort of abstinence (or fear of discomfo can lead to relapse. Initial stages of abstinence wi drawal may produce a powerful desire to resume u of the substance (cravings).
      (1) Reduced levels of neurotransmitters (norepinep rine, dopamine, serotonin, and endorphins) m create the biochemical basis of craving.
      (2) Repeated experience of alcohol withdrawal a associated limbic-neuronal discharge may induc permanent state of limbic hyperexcitability know as "kindling." Subsequent episodes of limbic d charge may be precipitated during abstinence alcohol-related cues or may occur spontaneously

Alcohol abuse is used here as the primary example because (a) more research has been done on the nature and impact of alcoholism and (b) alcohol has the most all-encompassing physiologic effects of any addictive substance.

Impact of Drug Addictions

Impact on the individual
a. Physiologic impact
   (1) Approximately 18 to 20 percent of all patients seen in ambulatory settings have substance abuse problems.
   (2) Thirty to 50 percent of all hospital admissions are related to the effects of substance abuse.
b. Psychologic impact
   (1) An estimated 20 to 36 percent of suicide victims have a history of alcohol abuse or were drinking shortly before their suicides. Alcohol use is particularly common in impulsive (as opposed to premeditated) suicides.
   (2) Low self-esteem; problems with problem solving; diminished work performance; and increased risk of legal, financial, and spiritual problems are common in alcohol abusers.

Impact on family members
a. Untreated alcoholics and their families have higher general health care costs than nonalcoholics and their families.
b. Parental substance abuse or dependence increases rates of child abuse and neglect, independent of social and environmental factors.
c. Alcohol use increases the chance of spousal abuse.

Socioeconomic
a. The Office of Substance Abuse Prevention reports 15 to 18 percent of Americans (36–43 million people) will develop a disorder of dependence on alcohol or other drugs in their lifetime.
b. Alcohol has been implicated in the leading causes of accidental death in the United States, including motor vehicle accidents, pedestrian accidents, airplane accidents, falls, fires, and burns.
c. Alcohol has been a factor in from 25 to 85 percent of homicides and 50 to 81 percent of rape cases.
d. Fetal alcohol syndrome (FAS) resulting from maternal alcohol consumption during pregnancy is the leading known cause of preventable mental retardation in newborns.

Impact on the American economy
a. The National Institute on Alcoholism and Alcohol Abuse estimates the loss to the nation's gross national product from alcohol problems and alcoholism at $142 billion in 1986, citing such causes as absenteeism, accidents, emergency agency involvement, and health care utilization.
b. In 1990, the Substance Abuse and Mental Health Services Administration (SAMSA) estimated a loss to the economy of $99 billion from alcohol abuse and $67 billion from illegal drug use.

Theories of Substance Use and Addiction

1. Biologic theories
   a. Genetic predisposition: Twin and adoption studies show that biologic children of alcoholics are more likely to have problems with alcohol than biologic children of nonalcoholics, even when raised in nonalcoholic environments; the genetic factor does not guarantee that an individual will become addicted; it only indicates increased susceptibility.
   b. Biochemical mechanisms: Excessive alcohol use is associated with concurrent opiate use in some persons, suggesting the lack of sufficient neurotransmitters such as endorphins or serotonin, which relate to pain and mood regulation (substance use is an attempt to make up for this deficit so the individual can feel "normal").
   c. Compulsion curve
      (1) People are born with sensitivities to specific drugs.
      (2) Stress or use of a drug increases sensitivity, but people with low sensitivity have to use a lot of a drug to become addicted.
      (3) Sensitivity may or may not return to normal if substance use stops; complete abstinence may be needed to avoid readdiction.
   d. Substance abuse is secondary to biologically based affective disorders such as depression or anxiety; treatment of the underlying disorder could result in an end to substance abuse (the individual would no longer need to self-medicate).
2. Psychosocial theories
   a. Personality traits such as low self-esteem, emotional immaturity, low frustration tolerance, difficulty dealing with tension, and genetic factors may create an individual in need of external coping mechanisms such as substances.
   b. Family phenomena such as lack of emotional warmth, parental rejection or overprotection, inconsistent and unclear behavioral limits, lack of role clarity for individuals, low parental aspirations for their children, and a high level of conflict and violence create an environment supporting the use of substances to cope.
      (1) Family patterns of self-medication model substance use.
      (2) Negative communication patterns (criticism, blaming, lack of praise) characterize families of adolescent substance abusers.
   c. Addiction as coping: societal support for "quick fixes" versus anxiety tolerance or delayed gratification.
      (1) The individual expects the substance to perform to reduce pain or anxiety; when it succeeds, the behavior is reinforced and will be repeated, even when consequences are periodically negative.
      (2) Type A occupational stresses: pressure to perform or to succeed may cause people to feel that they "can't measure up," so they turn to substance use.
   d. General psychosocial reasons why people use psychoactive substances
      (1) Pleasure, leisure, and euphoria
      (2) Curiosity, experimentation, decrease boredom, and sensation seeking

(3) Enhance social interaction by boosting self-confidence and performance, allowing relaxation and disinhibition, reducing anxiety, encouraging celebration, and responding to feelings of rebellion and peer pressure and the desire to appear more adult or sophisticated and to emulate admired figures.

3. Environmental theories
   a. Urban slums create an atmosphere of hopelessness and defeat for the poor; substances provide needed, although temporary, relief.
      (1) The social environment of the city emphasizes noninvolvement with others, diminished social responsibility, and anonymity.
      (2) Reactivity versus proactivity is common in the urban setting; one way to adapt is to become ill or addicted.
   b. Academic and social pressures are high in some middle-class families, so children in these families use substances to alleviate the pressure.
   c. Adolescents feel impotent and alienated; substance use becomes both a way to feel more adult and also a way to numb the negative feelings.
      (1) Role models related to a person's reference group and self-concept are lacking.
      (2) Identification with and responsibility for "family" processes—with things greater than self, with how what one does affects others, with shared investment in outcomes, with accountability to others for behavior—is lacking.
      (3) People face the choice of using the skills and attitudes necessary to work through problems and believing that they can be solved through the application of personal resources versus using the "miracle" solution of substance use.
      (4) Many people lack the intrapersonal and interpersonal skills of communication and the ability to share feelings, to trust, to empathize, and to give feedback.
   d. Peer group pressure encourages young people to use addictive substances despite the admonitions of adults and may determine which drug type has status and which route of administration is preferred (e.g., injection).
   e. Media messages raise expectations of solutions to problems from substance use such as tension relief, increased social skills, and sexual desirability. These messages suggest that problem resolution should be fast and easy.

Transcultural Attitudes Toward Drug Use and Abuse

1. Basic principles
   a. Culture defines acceptable and unacceptable alcohol and drug use in the community. Appropriate use of substances will be modeled by the adults, and alcohol or drugs may be employed as part of social gatherings, meals, celebrations, and religious ceremonies.
   b. Culture influences what behaviors are seen as problems. In some cultures any alcohol or drug use is forbidden, so any use is a problem (Mormon, Islam, some Christian).
   c. Different cultures have differing attitudes towards intoxication.
      (1) Groups (such as most northern European and some Native American cultures) that have few proscriptions against public intoxication have high rates of alcoholism.
      (2) Groups with proscriptions against public intoxication (such as the Jewish and Italian cultures) have low rates of alcoholism.
   d. Traditional beliefs explaining the cause of addiction (from stress to hexes and spells) can differ from culture to culture; the treatment prescribed arises from the explanatory model.
      (1) For groups using traditional methods, Western medical practitioners may be seen as nontraditional healers and therefore as less likely to diagnose and treat the problem correctly.
      (2) Having a practitioner of the same ethnic background as the person seeking care has been shown to increase the use of clinic facilities. In communities with small numbers of a group there may be reluctance to use an ethnically matched program or counselor because of concerns about confidentiality.
   e. Note that individuals of different cultures vary in the degree to which they identify with their particular cultural group and the degree to which they have acclimated and adapted to the majority culture.

2. Major cultural groups
   a. Asian American
      (1) Little is known about substance use and abuse among Asians, as no national alcohol survey has ever been done and no drug use pattern surveys were done before 1983. This group is typically included in an "other" category (along with Native Americans and Alaskan Eskimos); the sample size becomes especially small when Hawaii is excluded from studies.
         (a) The "model minority" stereotype maintains the idea that this group has a low incidence of substance use, and research has neglected those who have become heavy or problem drinkers. Community groups note the increase of alcohol and drug misuse, particularly among the youth and immigrant populations. Immigrants may have difficulty acculturating socially because of inadequate housing and crowdedness, socioeconomic hardships, difficulties with language and development of social and vocational survival skills, and loss of supportive networks.
         (b) Low alcohol abuse rates have been attributed to the response to alcohol known as the "flushing reaction" (face flushing when the person drinks alcohol; caused by genetic lack of enzyme ADLH-1 needed for alcohol metabolism), but cultural norms may have a stronger influence than genetics.

(c) Some areas of drug abuse have been missed owing to flaws in research methodology. Heavy methaqualone use by Asian youth in the 1980s was not recorded on major databases because studies relied on data from established heroin, cocaine, and amphetamine treatment programs.

(d) Use patterns may reflect generational differences between native-born and foreign-born Asians, geographic region, socioeconomic status, and gender and sexual orientation. In a driving while intoxicated survey, Japanese respondents reported consuming alcohol 3 times as often as Pacific Islanders, yet Pacific Islanders reported drinking twice as much as the Japanese at each occurrence of alcohol use.

(e) In 1989 a study found that Asians constitute 0.6 percent of the total population in substance abuse treatment while being 2.9 percent of the general population.

(2) Asian cultural norms include moderate drinking as a social event in prescribed situations. It is usually accompanied by food and is used to enhance social interaction. Women are expected to drink little or not at all.

(a) Aggressive, disorderly, and noisy behaviors that are observed when people are intoxicated are particularly condemned. Because these would ordinarily signal substance abuse problems in the larger community, problems may be hidden.

(b) Children are introduced to alcohol in the context of formal events such as wedding and funeral ceremonies and Shinto rituals, which reinforces the connection between alcohol use and social propriety.

(3) Substance abuse is a taboo issue and considered to be a serious breach of behavior leading to loss of face for the individual and the family. This fact may lead to underdocumentation of need for treatment, as the family attempts to cure the addict itself.

(a) The family may try traditional methods such as shaming, castigating, or scolding to resolve the issue.

(b) In extreme cases, the family may disown the person.

(c) Intervention is likely to begin with the family, later the extended family, and finally friends, elders, and the extended network. Only when all traditional avenues have been exhausted will nontraditional treatment resources be tried.

(d) Families may be looking for a quick-fix solution, failing to understand the role of the family in contributing to the continuation of drug abuse. The Asian value of familial interdependence versus individual independence may result in codependency and enabling the abuser to continue in the addicted lifestyle.

(4) An educative and supportive approach works better than confrontation to allow family members to begin shifting their behaviors of interdependency and possibly codependency toward better understanding and communication. Family approaches emphasizing respect and achieving alliances with the parents establish stronger therapeutic bonds between the counselor and the family.

b. Blacks

(1) Each group within the designation "Black" (e.g., African Americans and Caribbean Blacks) has a different history and so will have different specific cultural attitudes and norms about chemical use and abuse.

(2) Differences in attitudes toward alcohol and drug use may be seen in those growing up in rural versus urban settings.

(3) Social injustice, societal inconsistency, and personal impotence characterize the African-American experience, creating stress that may be medicated by alcohol and drugs.

(4) Despite similar use patterns with Whites, Black men experience a higher rate of problems associated with alcohol use, including higher cirrhosis and esophageal cancer death rates.

(a) White men tend to drink most heavily between 18 to 29 years old, so heavy drinking is associated with youthful behavior. Black men have a later onset of heavy drinking, so heavy drinking becomes associated with ongoing adult coping behavior.

(b) Blacks are often more vulnerable to substance-related disease than Whites who use the same amount of alcohol or drugs.

(5) The number 1 cause of death among young Black men aged 15 to 34 is homicide; alcohol and drugs are implicated in at least 70 percent of Black homicide incidents.

c. Hispanics

(1) There is a great cultural diversity within the Hispanic community, with associated diversity in patterns of substance use.

(2) The degree of behavioral acculturation of the individual and the differences in acculturation among family members both relate significantly to substance involvement.

(a) During the process of cultural adaptation, the family becomes a source of intergenerational conflicts and interpersonal dysfunctions between parents and children rather than a protection or buffer against a hostile new world. The children learn to speak the language of the new country and are immersed in the new culture, whereas the parents tend to hold onto familiar patterns from the "old country."

(b) Acculturation increases the likelihood of acquiring drug-using friends and when combined with low education and low income greatly enhances the likelihood of drug use. When acculturation is accompanied by inclusion in the mainstream economy, the probability of use decreases. Hispanic narcotic addicts are more likely to be involved in drug dealing and violent crime than White or Black addicts. Methadone treatment has not been very effective in changing this. There is an overrepresentation of Hispanics among acquired immunodeficiency syndrome (AIDS) cases. Hispanics constitute 8.4 percent of the total U.S. population but make up 16 percent of reported AIDS cases (more than half of which are associated with intravenous drug use).

(c) More highly acculturated men and women are more likely to be drinkers and to drink heavily with patterns similar to those of the mainstream culture than those less acculturated. Hispanic women drink less than Hispanic men. Drinking decreases with age although at a slower rate than within the White or Black community. Drinking appears to increase with income and education. Norms and restrictions on consumption become more permissive with acculturation. Mexican-American men hold more permissive norms towards drunkenness than Cubans and Puerto Ricans.

(3) Patterns of drug use do not differ greatly among Whites, Blacks, and Hispanics. Whites use all drugs at greater levels than Hispanics except the youngest Hispanics (12–17 years old), whose cocaine use exceeds that of their White and Black counterparts. Except for inhalants, drug use is most prevalent among the Puerto Rican community and least prevalent among the Cuban community.

(4) Stress plays a part in the etiology of drug use. This group has the following stressors: low English-speaking skills, lack of job skills, residence in poor neighborhoods with high crime rates, and concerns over liberal family beliefs of the larger Anglo society.

(5) The ability to communicate in one's preferred language is important in recovery and personal integration. Alcoholics Anonymous, Al-Anon, and Narcotics Anonymous have literature in Spanish, and some communities have meetings conducted in Spanish.

(6) Treatment with a *curandero* (healer) may be indicated for those with strong ties to traditional beliefs.

d. Native Americans

(1) Seventy-five percent of all traumatic deaths and suicides are alcohol related, particularly for those 25 to 44 years old.

(2) Binge drinking is characteristic of many tribes, especially on the reservation. Bloods levels of alcohol greater than 0.2 are associated with the onset of serious organ damage, so this behavior increases the likelihood of physiologic damage.

(3) Women may be more susceptible to alcohol-related health problems; despite relatively low consumption levels, women account for nearly half of cirrhosis deaths of all Native Americans.

(4) Fetal alcohol syndrome is a major health problem in this community.

(5) Native American philosophies of healing that may affect substance abuse treatment

(a) Nature is structured and follows rules of cause and effect but not necessarily in a manner understandable to humans. A person may be reluctant to actively work at solving problems, as in making relapse prevention plans.

(b) Living in harmony with nature is accomplished by following the traditions of the tribe. Breaking a taboo or ignoring a tradition can result in a state of disharmony, which can be manifested in an individual as disability, disease, or distress.

(c) All of life is seen as a spiritual process; individuals are considered relatively insignificant compared with the tribe, and an individual's problems are considered a problem of the group.

(d) The extended family, friends, and neighbors are mobilized to support the individual and integrate him or her into the social life of the group.

(e) Typically the healing ceremonies occur in the person's usual surroundings rather than in an unfamiliar place such as a hospital or clinic.

(f) When seeing a traditional healer, the person simply presents with a problem and it is up to the healer to diagnose the cause of the problem. Insight into the problem and curative powers are assumed to lie with the healer, not the person. In addition, the healer makes a diagnosis without asking the person personal questions or expecting intimate self-disclosure.

■ PRINCIPLES OF ASSESSMENT AND INTERVENTION FOR SUBSTANCE ADDICTION

Substance Assessment Overview

1. Preassessment (Box 40–1)
2. Assessing for characteristics of the drug

BOX 40–1. Nurse Self-Questioning Before Performing an Assessment

1. Do I drink (or use other substances)? If so, when, where, how much, how often, and for what reasons?
2. If not, what causes me to abstain?
3. What did I learn about alcohol and drugs when I was growing up?
4. What are my attitudes now about alcohol and drug use?
5. What do I experience when I see an intoxicated person?
6. Can I distinguish between social use and problem use?
7. Can I talk rationally with others about their use, especially when their patterns of use differ greatly from mine?
8. What is my belief about the prognosis for a substance use disorder?
9. Do I know what to do once I have determined a possible substance use disorder?

a. Dose, potency, and frequency relate to how much of a substance is taken, how strong the substance is, and how frequently the person repeats doses.

b. Route of administration affects the length of time it takes the substance to get to the brain as well as the onset of effects, the peak effects, and the duration of effects. The routes most frequently used for psychoactive substances are smoking (fastest onset, high peak, short duration of effect), oral (slower onset, longer duration), insufflation (snorting), and injection.

c. Pharmacokinetics: absorption, distribution, metabolism (biotransformation); excretion: what the body does to a substance, how the body brings the substance to the site of action (such as the brain), how and where the substance is broken down, and how it is removed.

d. Legal status of a drug: The legal status of a drug can create unique problems in use and in getting an accurate picture of use patterns.
  (1) The person may be reluctant to discuss concerns about use if afraid of being reported to authorities.
  (2) The underage person frequently "chugs" alcohol to avoid detection of use by authorities, which can create a life-threatening condition of overdose. This group is also often unskilled in driving, which makes mixing alcohol and driving particularly dangerous.

e. Environment of use: The setting itself, the lighting, and other factors may enhance certain aspects of a substance. For example, a cocktail lounge has subdued lighting and music, which encourages the relaxing aspects of alcohol.

f. Substance interactions (when the person takes more than 1 substance at a time)
  (1) Independent: no effect on each other
  (2) Antagonistic: "2 + 2 = 0" or "2 + 2 = 3." Effects of 1 or the other or both are blocked or reduced.
  (3) Additive: "2 + 2 = 4." Taking 2 different drugs is like doubling the dose of either of the substances.
  (4) Synergistic or potentiating: "2 + 2 = 5." The effect of 2 substances is greater than the additive effect. One substance may alter the distribution of the other or intensify or prolong the effects by changing the patterns of metabolism or elimination. **Potentiation** occurs when 1 substance intensifies the action of another. **Synergism** is a cooperative, facilitative, superadditive effect of 2 or more substances having the same drug action. Often results in overdose and death.
  (5) Cumulative effects develop when a 2nd dose is given before the 1st dose is fully metabolized. With alcohol, this could mean a rise in the blood alcohol level. The greater the amount of the substance in the bloodstream, the more likely it will affect parts of the brain such as the breathing centers.

g. Cross-tolerance is a type of substance interaction. Tolerance to any 1 of the sedative-hypnotic drugs, antianxiety drugs, or alcohol results in tolerance to any other of these general central nervous system depressants.

  (1) Use of 1 drug stops the withdrawal syndrome of another, so can be used in detoxification.
  (2) These can combine to work in an additive fashion. A dose that would not lead to drug dependency by itself will contribute to drug dependency when added to a 2nd drug of the general depressant type.

3. Assessing for characteristics of the person
  a. Age
    (1) Newborns have undeveloped enzyme systems. Their liver and kidneys are not fully formed, so they have trouble metabolizing drugs.
    (2) Older adults may have decreased kidney and liver functions and experience difficulty with homeostatic adjustments.
  b. Gender
    (1) Women differ from men in fat to water to muscle mass ratios. With their higher proportions of body fat, women achieve a higher blood alcohol concentration than men of comparable weight.
    (2) Rate of absorption of alcohol varies during the menstrual cycle (the highest absorption is premenstrually).
    (3) Men have a greater amount of alcohol dehydrogenase (ADH) produced by the gastric lining. For nonalcoholic men, up to 20 percent of alcohol consumed may be metabolized in the stomach, rather than waiting to be passed through the liver.
  c. Weight (related to blood volume): The greater the blood volume, the more diluted the drug will be in the system.
  d. Presence of medical or surgical disorders
    (1) Diseases of the liver and kidneys affect the ability of the body to metabolize and eliminate substances. Drug levels in the body may rise to a toxic, even lethal, level.
    (2) A poor nutritional state affects the enzyme production needed for substance metabolism, leading to higher drug levels.
  e. Idiosyncrasies: Some people do not respond to substances in a predictable fashion. A person might experience sedation taking a stimulant drug or stimulation taking a sedating drug.
  f. User expectation
    (1) This is derived from experience with the substance, friends' accounts, mass media, education, and training.
    (2) A person learns to compensate for the effects on the body, such as walking without staggering.
    (3) For some drugs, the user must learn to recognize the desired effects (e.g., marijuana users learning to identify the high of the drug).
    (4) Placebo studies show the impact of expectation on substance reactions: when a person expects to experience a certain response from ingesting a substance, that response can be produced even when no active ingredient is present. Research subjects expected and experienced sedation when given a substance they were told was a sedative (it was a stimulant). In the 1960s reported "highs" were achieved by smoking dried banana peels or mix-

ing cola with aspirins (none of which have mood-altering ingredients, except the caffeine in the cola).
g. User mood can enhance substance effects. A depressed person may become more depressed after ingesting a sedating drug; an excited person may become more excited when taking a stimulant.
h. The user's history of drug use
4. Development of defense mechanisms
a. Pathologic patterns begin to appear with increased reliance on a substance to modulate internal psychologic distress. These patterns intensify as reliance increases.
(1) These mechanisms often develop out of ignorance of the signs and symptoms of addiction (due to lack of information, lack of clear social norms about use and abuse, and the person's drug-affected brain) and a desire to use substances as others appear to.
(2) Denial: inability to perceive the deterioration and lack of acknowledgment of the problem with substance use
(3) Minimization: failing to perceive the degree of deterioration or failing to admit the seriousness of the problem
(4) Rationalization: giving excuses for the deterioration other than substance use and giving reasons for continuing to use
(5) Avoidance: avoiding situations or people (including health care practitioners) who might point out deterioration
(6) Projection of blame: finding others to blame for the deterioration and problems caused by substance use, again protecting the substance use pattern
b. Adolescent developmental task completion is often affected, and the user may demonstrate regressive coping mechanisms. Ability to socialize, to learn employment skills, to solve problems, to be assertive, and to delay gratification may be affected.
c. Development of despair with deterioration
(1) The person loses hope for positive change and doubts an ability to return to a prepathologic state.
(2) The person experiences feelings of loneliness, alienation, and futility and a sense of meaninglessness. This may come from the loss of everything holding meaning for the person: home, job, and family. For some this is identified as a spiritual crisis and can result in "hitting bottom."
(3) Self-esteem declines as deterioration progresses, and the self is blamed for the deterioration rather than recognizing the effect of substance-using behavior. The substance-using behavior becomes increasingly more protected. The addict frequently isolates himself or herself, cutting off possible information about the degree to which problems stem directly from continued use of the substance.
5. Substance use history
a. Find out how often, in what form, how much of each substance, and each form of substance a person consumes. Ask when the substance use started, the route of administration, the period of heaviest use, the last use, whether attempts were made to stop the use, and the consequences of use.

(1) Begin with the most benign substances 1st such coffee and tobacco and lead up to alcohol a other substances.
(2) Equivalent doses in taking an alcohol history: T alcohol content in 12 ounces of beer equals ounces of wine, which equals 1.5 ounces of distil spirits. Higher alcohol amounts are found in mix drinks and fortified wines (e.g., sherry). Have t person define a "drink." (One drink might be t whole martini shaker or a quart of beer).
(3) Given the reluctance of talking about substa use, the phrasing and intonation of questions important. Examples of questions for the drinki history: "How much alcohol do you drink day?" "Do you take more than 6 drinks a day "Do you have more than 12 beers on a Saturd night?" (People are more likely to go down th up in estimates, so aim high.) Pay attention to amount of time it takes to answer, as there may discomfort in answering honestly. Other dr amounts are often quoted in dollar amounts.
(4) Ask explicitly about each type of beverage co sumed on a specific recent day.
(5) Remind the person to think of alcohol consum between, as well as with, meals.
(6) Ask "Does it take more or less alcohol or drugs get you high than it used to?"
(7) Ask the person whether he or she ever thoug about cutting down on substance use. If the a swer is affirmative, ask why (consequences). L ten for references to worry, remorse, fruitless forts at control.
(8) If the person states that no substances are bei used, ask whether they were in the past, whi ones, and how often, and why they are not us now. Ask about past periods of abstinence, cons quences of substance use when they were bei used (especially with alcohol), especially bla outs, fights, legal charges, job losses, and relatic ship difficulties.
(9) Provide information and ask "What do y think?", being sure to provide the information i nonjudgmental, low-key manner. For example, all pregnant women know that smoking a drinking affect the health of the fetus, so give formation that promotes a discussion and may timately result in a plan for change of behavior.
6. Screening tools
a. Used to supplement the history taking from the pers
(1) Approach: asking where use fits into the perso general lifestyle and stresses (e.g., "Where d your use of alcohol or other drugs fit into this?"
(2) Asking about substance use in reference to a sp cific health problem. (Box 40–2)
(3) Questions can be embedded in a self-administer health questionnaire. Response rates seem to better when mailed to the patients, rather th administered by office receptionists.
b. Formalized tests such as Michigan Alcoholism Scree ing Test (MAST) (Box 40–3) and the Drug Abu Screening Tool (DAST): self-reports that indicate t presence and severity of substance use–related pr

BOX 40-2. CAGE: Quick Alcohol Abuse Assessment Tool

Have you ever felt you ought to **C**ut down on your drinking?
Have people **A**nnoyed you by criticizing your drinking?
Have you ever felt bad or **G**uilty about your drinking?
Have you ever had a drink 1st thing in the morning, to steady your nerves or get rid of a hangover? **E**ye-opener

Score: 1 for each positive answer; 2 to 3 points is suggestive of alcohol dependence (especially if cutting down is included), and 4 points is diagnostic.

From Ewing J. Detecting alcoholism: The CAGE questionnaire. *JAMA* 252(14):1905–1907, 1984. Copyright 1984, American Medical Association.

BOX 40-3. Brief Michigan Alcoholism Screening Test (B-MAST)

Answer the following to the best of your ability:

1. Do you feel you are a normal drinker? (A normal drinker is a person who drinks less than or as much as most other people). Yes _____ No _____
2. Do friends or relatives think you are a normal drinker? Yes _____ No _____
3. Have you ever attended a meeting of Alcoholics Anonymous or Narcotics Anonymous for your personal concerns about your own drinking or drugging? Yes _____ No _____
4. Have you ever lost friends or girlfriends or boyfriends because of drinking? Yes _____ No _____
5. Have you ever gotten into trouble at work because of drinking or drugging? Yes _____ No _____
6. Have you ever neglected your obligations, your family, or your work for 2 or more days in a row because you were drinking or drugging? Yes _____ No _____
7. Have you ever had delirium tremens (DTs), severe shaking, heard voices, or seen things that weren't there after heavy drinking? Yes _____ No _____
8. Have you ever gone to anyone for help about your drinking or drugging? Yes _____ No _____
9. Have you ever been in a hospital because of your drinking or drugging? Yes _____ No _____
10. Have you ever been arrested for drunken driving, driving while intoxicated, or driving under the influence of alcoholic beverages or drugs? Yes _____ No _____

Scoring: Substance abusing indication responses: *yes* to all but numbers 1 and 2. 2 points for each except numbers 3, 8, and 9, which each count as 5 points.

Interpretation: Less than 3 points: nonalcoholic or addict
4 points: suggests alcoholic or addict
5 or more points: indicates alcoholic or addict

From Selzer ML. The Michigan Alcoholism Screening Test: The quest for a new diagnostic instrument. *Am J Psychiatry* 127(12):1653–1658, 1971; and Pokorny AS, et al. The brief MAST: A shortened version of the Michigan Alcoholism Screening Test. *Am J Psychiatry* 129(3):342–345, 1972. Copyright 1971, 1972, the American Psychiatric Association. Reprinted by permission.

lems. When a person screens positive for drug consequences, ask for clarification. "You indicated your spouse criticizes your use. Can you tell me more about this?"

c. *Diagnostic and Statistical Manual of Mental Disorders* (4th ed.) (DSM IV) criteria (Box 40–4): The DSM IV interview has been shown to be more reliable as an assessment tool for identifying substance abuse than physiologic tests, particularly urine tests.

BOX 40-4. DSM-IV Criteria for Psychoactive Substance Abuse and Substance Dependence

Criteria for Substance Abuse

A. A maladaptive pattern of substance use leading to clinically significant impairment or distress, as manifested by one (or more) of the following, occurring within a 12-month period:
   (1) Recurrent substance use resulting in a failure to fulfill major role obligations at work, school, or home (e.g., repeated absences or poor work performance related to substance use; substance-related absences, suspensions, or expulsions from school; neglect of children or household).
   (2) Recurrent substance use in situations in which it is physically hazardous (e.g., driving an automobile or operating a machine when impaired by substance use).
   (3) Recurrent substance-related legal problems (e.g., arrests for substance-related disorderly conduct).
   (4) Continued substance use despite having persistent or recurrent social or interpersonal problems caused or exacerbated by the effects of the substance (e.g., arguments with spouse about consequences of intoxication, physical fights).
B. The symptoms have never met the criteria for Substance Dependence for this class of substance.

Criteria for Substance Dependence

A. A maladaptive pattern of substance use, leading to clinically significant impairment or distress, as manifested by three (or more) of the following, occurring at any time in the same 12-month period.
   (1) Tolerance, as defined by either of the following:
      (a) A need for markedly increased amounts of the substance to achieve intoxication or desired effect.
      (b) Markedly diminished effect with continued use of the same amount of the substance.
   (2) Withdrawal as manifested by either of the following:
      (a) The characteristic withdrawal of syndrome for the substance.
      (b) The same (or a closely related) substance is taken to relieve or avoid withdrawal symptoms.
   (3) The substance is taken in larger amounts or over a longer period than was intended.
   (4) There is a persistent desire or unsuccessful efforts to cut down or control substance use.
   (5) A great deal of time is spent in activities necessary to obtain the substance (e.g., visiting multiple doctors or driving long distances), use the substance (e.g., chain smoking), or recover from its effects.
   (6) Important social, occupational, or recreational activities are given up or reduced because of substance use.
   (7) The substance use is continued despite knowledge of having a persistent or recurrent physical or psychological problem that is likely to have been caused or exacerbated by the substance (e.g., current cocaine use despite recognition of cocaine-induced depression, or continued drinking despite recognition that an ulcer was made worse by alcohol consumption).

Specifiers: with or without physiological dependence.

Reprinted with permission from American Psychiatric Association. *Diagnostic and Statistical Manual of Mental Disorders.* 4th ed. Washington, DC: Author, 1994, pp 182–272. Copyright 1994, American Psychiatric Association.

Substance Abuse Intervention Overview

1. Sources of help for those addicted to substances
   a. The family practitioner: the first line of treatment. Advice about the need for behavior change can be a strong motivator, especially for users who are just beginning to get into trouble.
   b. Drug and alcohol counseling: professionals specially trained in assessing and treating addictions. Many communities have a continuum of treatment, from assessment to intensive inpatient treatment. The nurse may want to establish a relationship with individuals or agencies in the community to facilitate referrals.
   c. Self-help groups
      (1) Twelve-step–based groups (e.g., Alcoholics Anonymous) offer free ongoing support and behavior change guidance for individuals who feel comfortable with a spiritually based program.
      (2) Other groups such as Rational Recovery and Women in Sobriety are available in some communities.
   d. Workplace programs
      (1) Deterioration in work performance may be the 1st problem spotted. Desire to keep employment provides a strong reinforcer for problem identification and behavior change.
      (2) Employee assistance programs may be available to provide services to employees facing various physical and mental health problems, problems with family or other relationships, or problems in their environment that cause personal difficulties. Some provide treatment on site; others evaluate and refer out. Many companies have policies developed regarding drug or alcohol-affected workers. Transportation workers are 1 group that now have regular, mandatory (random) drug screens. Issues of right to privacy have been brought to court, but the legality of testing thus far has been upheld.
      (3) Be aware that the work environment itself has risk factors for substance misuse.
         (a) Internal risk factors: alienation and powerlessness, work stress, structural features of the workplace that weaken social controls over work behavior (e.g., shift work, forced retirement, unemployment, and work roles with little or no supervision), administrative subcultures whose norms tolerate or encourage substance use or even abuse, poorly implemented intervention policies
         (b) External risk factors: higher rates associated with socioeconomic class and certain ethnic groups (see Chapter 2), widespread availability of substances, importation into workplace of occupational cultures characterized by heavy drinking norms and high occupational autonomy (such as in traveling sales), societal support for substance use
2. The referral process
   a. General considerations
      (1) The person may need to be referred to other health professionals such as chemical depende[nce] counselors for further evaluation.
      (2) Considerations in referring to a specific progra[m]: types of substances; substance use history, [in]cluding extent of use; need for detoxificati[on]; past attempts at sobriety and treatment, incl[ud]ing Alcoholics Anonymous, Narcotics Ano[ny]mous, Cocaine Anonymous, and the like; a[ge]; gender; psychologic and cognitive functioni[ng]; cultural concerns, including language; sexual [ori]entation; veteran status; financial resources ([pri]vate vs. public insurance); availability of app[ro]priate facility; willingness to go into treatment
3. Principles of intervention
   a. Soft intervention: Advice about the need for behav[ior] change from a primary health care provider can m[oti]vate change.
   b. Formal intervention (Johnson Institute model)
      (1) An intervention by those important to him [or] her, forces the person to recognize the negat[ive] consequences of substance abuse, allowing [the] person to change before health, finances, and [re]lationships are totally lost.
      (2) An intervention generally relies on the element [of] surprise.
      (3) A professional trained in conducting interv[en]tions is contacted, and he or she plans and str[uc]tures the intervention. This person can co[me] from a variety of disciplines but should hav[e] background education in substance abuse tr[eat]ment and experience in using this model of or[ga]nized confrontation of the addict.
      (4) First, the interventionist provides substa[nce] abuse and addiction education to the fam[ily,] friends, employers, and others representing s[ig]nificant areas of the person's life who will [be] participating in the intervention.
      (5) Education about addiction helps these people [to] clarify how the addiction has affected them p[er]sonally and to begin to work together as a te[am.] Education about treatment options is also [dis]cussed.
      (6) The interventionist discusses any issues or r[ea]sons for the intervention and may need to cla[rify] any hidden agendas on the part of those seek[ing] the intervention (e.g., punishment of the addic[t]).
      (7) Participants in the intervention write letters [to] the person, outlining specific incidents when [the] person exhibited out-of-control behavior owing [to] substance use, and should be willing to re[ad] them aloud at the time of the intervention. Fo[cus] is on the feelings the person had at the time [of] the incident, not on blaming the addict.
      (8) A treatment center will have been contacted a[nd] an assessment arranged for immediately follo[w]ing the intervention (if the person is willing to g[o]).
      (9) The person is confronted by the participants [of] the intervention, who are supported by the int[er]ventionist. The person is asked to listen and [not] respond and is told by those intervening of [the] care and concern they have for the person.

(10) Consequences for lack of change or failure to go to treatment can be outlined. Care must be taken to say only those things family members and other participants are willing to do (e.g., sleep in another room, not tell untruths about absences from work).

(11) The participants will debrief with the interventionist, whether the person follows through with treatment or not. More than 1 intervention can be done.

c. If the person refuses to go to treatment the nurse can do the following:

(1) Negotiate an agreement with the person about the steps to be taken if future problems arise

(2) Inform and involve community health workers or other human service workers with the person, family, or both

(3) Provide necessary, ongoing medical care whether related or unrelated to alcohol or substance abuse or dependence

(4) Make the primary problem clear to the person and the family and others involved in general care

(5) Remain ready to arrange and facilitate treatment

(6) Teach significant others to avoid enabling the person to continue alcohol or substance abuse.

For example, do not authorize "sick time" for hangovers; be alert to the next crisis.

4. The rehabilitation or recovery process. The nurse may be able to use the following barriers and incentives to identify problems and issues that will hinder full recovery and help the person form a strategy about what to do to stay motivated (Fig. 40–1).

a. Barriers to recovery

(1) Denial: The person refuses to accept that problems are substance-use related.

(2) Poverty: Life may not get a lot better in recovery, so hope is lacking.

(3) Fear of withdrawal: Fear of pain and suffering from withdrawal symptoms keeps a person using.

(4) Lack of alternative methods of coping: Use of the substance or substances has become the primary method of dealing with stress and anxiety.

(5) Lack of clean and sober leisure activities: Substance use (and the socialization that may accompany it) provides the only fun in the person's life.

(6) Grief or loss: The substance has become the person's best friend; there is a fear of change and the unfamiliar (e.g., a substance-free lifestyle).

(7) An underlying or coexisting problem may be

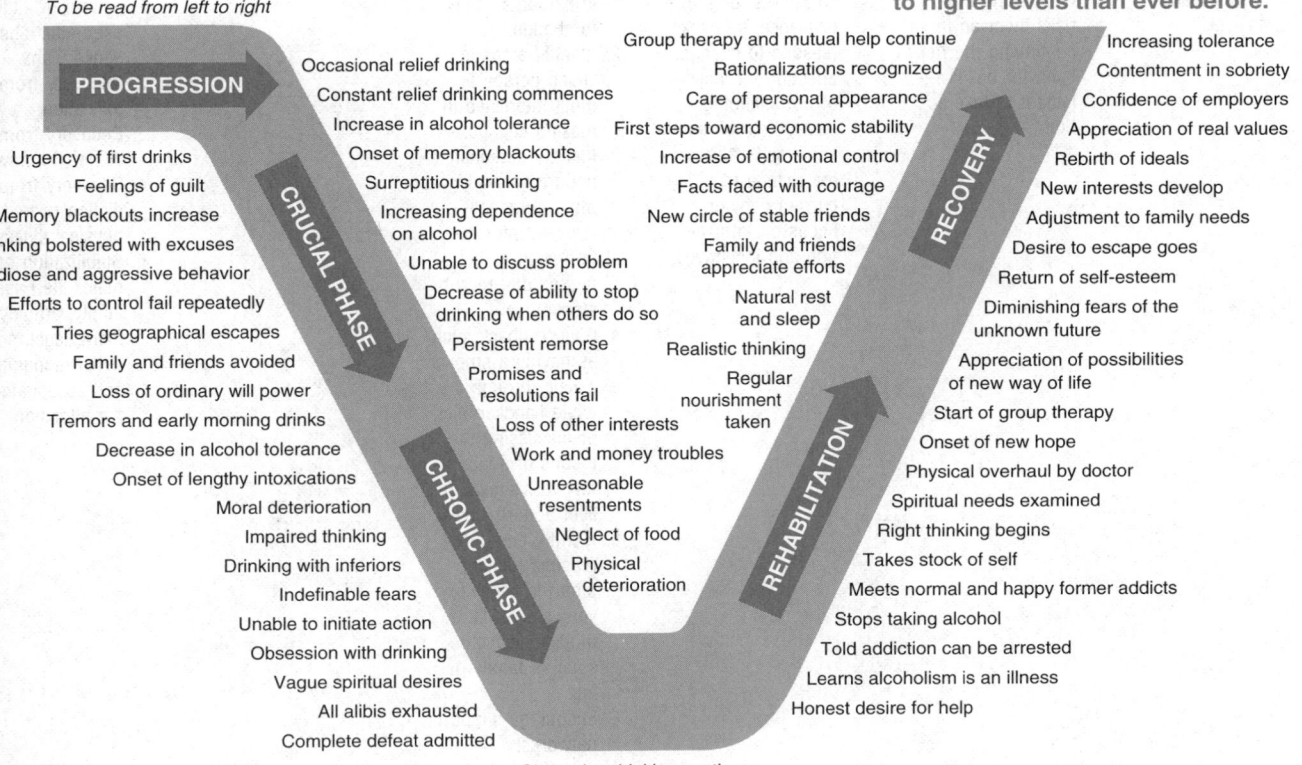

Figure 40–1. The progression and recovery of the alcoholic in the disease of alcholism. (From Glatt M. *The Alcoholic and the Help He Needs.* 2nd ed. York: Taplinger Publishing Co., Inc., 1974. ©1969 by Max Glatt. Reprinted by permission.)

Table 40–1. The Recovery Process: Transtheoretical and Relapse Prevention Models

Change Stage	Identifying Behavior	Nursing Interventions	Therapeutic Tasks	Developmental Model/Relapse Prevention	Tasks
Precontemplation	Person does not see a problem and therefore has no motivation to change, no reason to attempt to change; may have rationalizations and blame projection regarding continued use.	Raise doubt. Increase the person's perception of risk and problems with current behavior. A sensitive, empathic manner is important at this stage to aid in forming a working therapeutic alliance.	1. May prescribe attempting controlled use (such as 2 drinks per day, not to be saved up for the weekend), delayed use. 2. Other tasks to increase intellectual understanding: keeping a log, talking with a recovering person, learning about the effect of drugs, identifying own personal reasons for continued use. 3. Encourage verbalization of emotions regarding change. 4. Indicate readiness to help when ready to make change.	Transitional	1. Develop a histo of problems rel to the addiction
Contemplation: "risk-reward analysis"	Person has begun to understand the risks involved in continuing the risky behavior but is reluctant to take action.	Tip the balance. Person has strong ambivalence, so evoke reasons to change, question the risks of not changing, strengthen the person's self-efficacy for change of current behvior. Focus on information and incentives.	1. Increase confidence in person's ability to change. 2. Identify areas in which person is most interested in making change. 3. Identify personal use triggers and other personally relevant information such as illnesses due to substance use. 4. Give feedback such as having a smoker exhale through a white handkerchief, or discussing the results of a laboratory test showing liver abnormalities. 5. Identify personal reasons for stopping the behavior versus external motivating factors such as family or job. 6. Encourage support networks.	Stabilization	1. Interruption of pattern of addic use: initial absti nence plan. 2. Recovery from toxication. 3. Recovery from acute withdrawa 4. Recovery from diction-related physical illness. 5. Stabilization of major life crises family, employ- ment, legal, soc 6. Initial recognitio and acceptance the addiction.
Determination/ Preparation: commitment to action, making a plan	Person is still making the decision whether to stop throughout this stage.	Assess the strength and levels of commitment. Help the person to determine the best course of	1. Help resolve ambivalence. 2. Assess levels of physical and emotional dependency.	Early recovery	1. Establish an ext nally regulated r covery program (treatment). 2. Personal and fa

Table 40–1. *The Recovery Process: Transtheoretical and Relapse Prevention Models* (Continued)

Change Stage	Identifying Behavior	Nursing Interventions	Therapeutic Tasks	Developmental Model/Relapse Prevention	Tasks
		action to take in seeking change (engage problem-solving skills).	3. Assess situations (people, places, and things) which might sabotage recovery. 4. Identify coping mechanism and strengths of the person to offset triggers. 5. Help make written, comprehensive, individualized treatment plan. Focus on manageable steps; reward small changes made.		education about addiction and recovery. 3. Self-assessment aimed at recognition and acceptance of disease. 4. Learning to be honest with self. 5. Learning to talk and listen to others. 6. HALT: not too *H*ungry, *A*ngry, *L*onely, *T*ired. 7. Managing cravings. 8. Avoid places, people, events where substances are used.
Implementing the plan	Change has begun.	Help the person to take steps toward change, providing external confirmation of the plan, giving support, increasing self-efficacy, working as an external monitor of activity.	1. Set short-term goals. 2. Identify (social) support needed. 3. Problem-solve barriers. 4. Use self-help materials. 5. Establish follow-up. 6. Identify nonchemical means for comfort and leisure. 7. Usually takes 3–6 months to complete.	Middle and late recovery: Maintaining responsibility	1. Learns nonchemical coping skills. 2. Developing sobriety-centered value system; values clarification. 3. Sobriety-based social support. 4. Development of a nonsubstance user identity: sober self-esteem. 5. Examination of realistic responsibility for addiction. 6. Resolution of shame, guilt, and remorse. 7. Acceptance of loss of old lifestyle: grief work plan. 8. Overcoming addictive obstacles to self-esteem. 9. Establishing a self-regulated recovery program. 10. Learning to recognize personal health preferences. *Late Recovery Tasks:* 1. Cognitive restructuring: changing self-talk via affirmations and injunctions. 2. Affective restructuring: changing feelings through

Table continued on following page

Table 40–1. The Recovery Process: Transtheoretical and Relapse Prevention Models (Continued)

Change Stage	Identifying Behavior	Nursing Interventions	Therapeutic Tasks	Developmental Model/Relapse Prevention	Tasks
					conscious reex[perience]. 3. Behavior restru[c]turing: changin[g] what is done a[nd] maintain chang[e] until habitual. 4. Developing hea[lthy] intimacy.
Maintenance	New behavior is becoming firmly established.	Help the person to identify and use strategies to prevent relapse; provide help during crises. Provide reassurance, including feedback about change process.	1. Problem-solve difficulties. 2. Identify local resources and support. 3. Identify relapse strategy. 4. Problem-solving skills, social and environmental support. 5. Anticipation for potential difficulties (e.g., vacations).	Stability or Maintenance: establishing a balanced lifestyle.	1. Improved prob[lem] solving abilities 2. Management o[f] change withou[t] substance use. 3. Ongoing growt[h] and developme[nt] often related t[o] dealing with ot[her] long-standing [emo]tional or behav[ioral] problems begin[n]ing in childho[od].
Relapse	Person has been overwhelmed and unable to maintain the new behavior. This may be actual return to use or may be a return of patterns that could indicate risk of use (e.g., negativity, increased fighting, cravings).	Help the person to renew the processes of contemplation, determination, and action, without becoming stuck or demoralized because of relapse.	1. Support in reexamination. 2. Development of refined plan.	Lapse or relapse	1. Encourage a re[turn] to sobriety, exp[lore] what was lackin[g] in the old plan. 2. Write out a very [spe]cific new plan a[nd] have the perso[n] carry the plan a[t all] times. Identify [early] warning signals[,in]cluding what cr[e]ated the relaps[e] this time; what [was] learned; what n[eeds] to be done diff[er]ently; what resources can be called on that w[ere] not used durin[g the] relapse; and rea[sons] for not usi[ng] these resources

present, such as mental illness, head injuries, or developmental disabilities, such that the person may have greater than usual trouble with problem solving and impulse control.

b. Incentives for recovery
   (1) A return to normal functioning in the family; to maintain or regain lost relationships with the family
   (2) To keep a job or maintain a societal role
   (3) Personal discomfort at being controlled by the substance

   (4) Court requirements
   (5) Medical necessity
   (6) Financial instability
   (7) To normalize relationships with friends and [de]crease social isolation

5. The use of the transcultural model of change and developmental or relapse-prevention models can give [the] nurse a framework to use in developing a plan of in[ter]vention with the substance user (Table 40–1).

6. Significant others and the recovery process

a. Significant others can help provide a more accurate history of substance use.

b. The threatened loss of important relationships often provides motivation for change.

c. Social support aids in managing stress.

d. Changes for the addict also mean changes for significant others.

   (1) Lack of understanding the rationale for these changes may result in sabotage of the recovery process, such as undermining regular support group attendance.

   (2) The family needs support during the changes to reduce relationship stress and anxiety.

e. Significant others have been affected by the addiction.

   (1) Significant others need to focus on their own issues, including feelings of helplessness, hopelessness, anger, resentment, and fear of relapse, to actively heal; the addict's becoming sober does not solve these problems for significant others. Refer them to family support groups (Al-Anon, Nar-Anon, Alateen, Alatot).

   (2) Children need age-appropriate information about addiction and recovery, especially the fact that they did not create the family crisis and are not responsible for the substance use. Refer children to Alateen or Alatot.

f. Codependency: This dysfunctional and progressive life pattern focuses on the addictive behavior of another person and is characterized by denial of the basis of the problem, obsessive-compulsive behavior regarding attempts to change the substance abuser's behavior, and emotional repression.

   (1) Could be seen to be a normal response to an abnormal situation (the substance abuse). The significant other tries to handle a crisis, usually by attempting to be more controlling.

   (2) Often means doing for adults what they could do for themselves, thereby protecting substance abusers from the consequences of their actions.

   (3) How the substance abuser is doing becomes the measure for how the codependent is doing (external locus of control).

   (4) Codependency is not the same as caring for someone or helping someone when they need it. It involves rescuing and taking over the problem from the person who needs to learn how to handle the problem.

   (5) Nurses may use codependent behavior with those they care for unless they confront personal issues.

   (6) The concept has been criticized because of the lack of a workable definition (static personality traits versus behaviors), lack of research, feminist objections to labeling codependence as a stereotypic experience for women, and characteristics that are a result of socialization rather than personal inadequacy or dysfunction.

3. Resources for significant others

   (1) Treatment programs often provide counseling for the family or significant others.

   (2) Al-Anon is for those in relationships with alcoholics. Nar-Anon is for those in relationship with

drug abusers. These 12-step groups focus on how the significant others were affected by the addiction and what to do about it, not on how to fix the addict.

   (3) Adult Children Anonymous (ACA): also known as Adult Children of Alcoholics (ACOA). For adults who have grown up in dysfunctional families.

   (4) Alateen: for teenagers growing up with an alcoholic in their lives. Some groups also talk about the teen's substance use.

   (5) Alatot: usually associated with an Al-Anon group. For younger-aged children growing up with an alcoholic.

   (6) Codependents Anonymous (CoDA): For those who recognize codependency patterns.

7. Follow-up care: Planning for aftercare once a person has completed treatment.

   a. Schedule a posttreatment meeting to assess continuing treatment needs.

   b. Identify stressors on the person and the significant others, including any medical limitations.

   c. Identify resources in the community care network to involve in planning, to participate in management, and to assist in monitoring the person's status.

■ CARING FOR PEOPLE WHO ABUSE TOBACCO

Tobacco Addiction

1. Nicotine use is the largest single preventable cause of illness and premature death in the United States.
2. Smoking costs business $26 billion a year in lost productivity and $8 billion in smoking-related medical costs.
3. Most smokers begin smoking during childhood or adolescence (89% of daily smokers tried their first cigarette by or at age 18, and 71% of those who have ever smoked daily began smoking daily by age 18).

Tar and Nicotine

1. Can be taken by any method of administration but is usually inhaled or absorbed buccally.
2. It is poorly absorbed from the stomach but is absorbed from the small intestines. It is widely distributed, easily crosses the blood-brain and placental barriers, and is found in breast milk.
3. Nicotine releases dopamine, norepinephrine, acetylcholine, vasopressin, serotonin, and β-endorphins. These neurotransmitters enhance mood and performance.
4. Tobacco stimulates the same areas of the brain as cocaine and amphetamines. A few hours of smoking develops tolerance—faster than with heroin or cocaine.
5. Cigarette smoke contains more than 80 toxic substances; carbon monoxide is 1 of the most hazardous.
6. Tar is composed of 2 parts: neutral and basic. The neutral part contains benzopyrene, making it the most carcinogenic. The basic part contains the nicotine and other irritating chemicals.

7. Causes direct stimulation of the cells of the cerebral cortex, leading to feelings of increased alertness and causing the muscles to relax. It also stimulates the gastrointestinal tract and causes the adrenal gland to release catecholamines, which accelerate the heart rate.
8. It is metabolized mainly by liver enzymes but also by enzymes in the lung and kidney.
9. Smoking causes oxygen deprivation by impairing the blood's capacity to carry oxygen.

Assessing People with Tobacco Addiction

1. Key signs and symptoms
   a. Nicotine addiction differs from other drug addictions only in the lack of certain social consequences; this is changing with stricter laws limiting smoking and information about the effects of side-stream or second-hand smoke.
   b. Coughing, wheezing, trouble catching breath, smells like tobacco smoke.
2. Taking a tobacco use history
   a. Age of 1st use
   b. Age of 1st regular use (how many years smoking?)
   c. On the average, number of cigarettes currently smoking per day
   d. Number over the past 6 months
   e. Time of day of 1st cigarette (within 30 min of wakening is a reliable index of nicotine dependency).
   f. When is smoking the heaviest?
   g. Do you inhale?
   h. Use of other methods: pipes, cigars, chew or snuff tobacco; do you smoke other nontobacco products?
   i. Time of day of heaviest use.
   j. Have you tried to cut down or quit? Number of times (including number of times stopping smoking for at least a day).
   k. What methods have you tried to stop smoking?
   l. Which would be the hardest cigarette to give up?
   m. Do you have trouble not smoking in places where it is forbidden?
   n. In what situations do you not smoke?
   o. Currently or in the past have you had symptoms, a disease, or illness you believe was caused or made worse by your smoking?
   p. Does your desire for a cigarette ever disrupt the activities you are involved in?
   q. Do you lose time from work or other planned activities because of smoking?
   r. Do you smoke when you are so ill that you are not able to carry on your normal activities?
   s. Do you ever smoke more than you intended?
   t. Has a health practitioner ever told you to stop smoking?
   u. Have you ever experienced uncomfortable symptoms when you stopped smoking? What were they?
   v. Do others around you (friends, coworkers, family) smoke?
   w. Are there people close to you who want you to stop smoking?
   x. Do you have a quit date?
   y. Cost of smoking.

3. Physical examination
   a. History: Ask about trouble breathing or shortness breath, frequent coughing, getting tired in a sh time, pain or tightness in the chest.
   b. Auscultate heart and lungs.
   c. Perform oral examination.
   d. Check for associated cancers.
4. Special diagnostic tests
   a. Pulmonary function tests
   b. Carboxyhemoglobin tests
   c. Measures of alveolar carbon monoxide

Routes of Administration

1. Smoking: Reaches the brain in 7 seconds; the effects 30 minutes to 1 hour. Plasma half-life is about 2 hou which is decreased by caffeine.
2. Chewing: Placed between the teeth and cheek, tobacco absorbed more gradually through the mucous me branes of the mouth.

Risk Factors

1. The risk for smoking increases 3-fold if a 1st-degree logic relative smokes.
2. Currently young women are the fastest growing gro of new smokers despite information about the risks. Sm ing is associated with attempts at weight management

Pathophysiology

1. Mechanism of action: Nicotine causes ganglionic stim tion by depolarization in low doses but ganglionic blo ade at high doses. Nicotine receptors also exist in central nervous system, where nicotine freely penetra and stimulates and then depresses the vital medull and respiratory centers.
   a. Immediate effects of tobacco: raised arousal level, creased attention to extraneous stimuli, fine trem shortness of breath, decreased appetite, antidiur effect, decreased aggressiveness, sedation
   b. Acute effects or short-term adverse effects: increa heart rate, and blood pressure; cardiac contractility; sodilation; irritability; tremors; intestinal cramps; d rhea; nausea; vomiting; and water retention. Chew tobacco can produce toxic nicotine levels in the bloo
   c. Long-term effects due to nicotine, carbon dioxide, tars
      (1) Smoking is the primary cause of cancers, incl ing lung, esophageal (especially when combi with alcohol), kidney, and pancreatic cancers.
      (2) Smoking increases the risk of cancers of the cavity, larynx, and urinary bladder. It also creases the risk of leukemia.
      (3) Smoking increases the risk of heart attack, ath sclerosis, stomach ulcers, chronic bronchitis, physema, and decreases the high-density lipo tein levels in the blood.

Text continued on page 1

LEARNING/TEACHING GUIDELINES
for Counseling Substance-Using Pregnant Women

General Overview

1. Keep messages clear, simple, and realistic.
   a. Sensationalism and humor are not effective approaches.
   b. Stay abreast of myths and dangerous practices by pregnant women in your community.
2. Stress the positive. See example below.
3. Do not predict the outcome of a particular pregnancy.
   a. Statistics are not cases.
   b. Exaggerated warning about risks may reduce credibility and thus your role as a health resource if a drug-abusing women gives birth to an apparently healthy baby; emphasize the hope that the mother may be lucky and escape the odds this time.
4. Deliver personal, individually tailored messages.
   a. Even brief comments, delivered in person, are more effective than written information or audiovisual presentations without follow-up or discussion.
   b. Sensitivity to the communication styles of different groups can also enhance their receptiveness and understanding.
   c. Remember that some women are socialized not to ask questions, even when they do not understand the information given.
5. Be sensitive to the legal implications. In some states continuing substance use by a pregnant woman constitutes child abuse or neglect, which may mean suspension of parental rights once the child is born.

Help Women Assess Their Risk

1. Observation: You notice the pattern suggestive of substance use.
2. Direct questioning: Ask specifically about substance use.
3. Informed testing, with follow-up counseling and support. Use of self-report tests, such as MAST and DAST, and blood or urine screens to determine use.
4. When the person identifies a problem or possible risk there will be a better chance for cooperation and compliance with the needed treatment regimen.

5. Evaluate the risk of exposure to the human immunodeficiency virus.
6. Assess phase of change readiness in Table 40–1: The Recovery Process.

Motivate Risk Reduction and Provide Ongoing Hope

1. Help the woman to set realistic goals for possible change.
   a. Awareness of substance use antecedents and behavioral cues: reasons for use.
   b. Increase self-efficacy by finding alternatives to use.
2. Support change by relevant suggestions and attainable interim steps. Identify network from which person can draw support.
3. Consistently praise monitored behavior; a one-shot effort is not sufficient to keep the person working on behavior change.
4. Emphasize the benefits of quitting as soon as possible, as the developing fetus may have a chance to catch up in growth and to recuperate from some types of drug-related damage if the mother's use is reduced or halted after pregnancy begins.
5. Recommend substance abuse treatment when goals for abstention are not easily achieved.

Provide Special Help with Parenting

1. A mother's anxiety and guilt about giving birth to a drug-affected baby are likely to interrupt mother-infant attachment processes.
2. The baby's prolonged stay in the hospital, as well as the infant irritability and adjustment difficulties, can frustrate the mother and increase her stress and anxiety.
3. Some developmental outcomes can be helped with proper infant stimulation and play therapy. Referral to parenting training may be appropriate, as some of these parents may have lacked adequate role models of healthy parenting.

Sample Counseling Approaches

Positive Approach	Negative Approach
If you stop drinking now, you have a better chance of having a healthy baby.	Your drinking has already damaged your baby.
Your concern for your baby will help you be a good mother.	If you really love your baby, you would not drink so much.
You will feel better when you are sober and so will your child.	Continued drinking will ruin your health and prevent your child from developing normally.

ted from Cook PS, Petersen RC, and Moore DT. *Alcohol, Tobacco, and Other Drugs May Harm the Unborn.* Rockville, MD: U.S. Department of Health and Human Services,

Table 40–2. Reference Guide to Commonly Abused Substances

Drug	Route and Duration	Physical Findings in Intoxication	Behavioral Cues
Central Nervous System (CNS) Stimulants			
Nicotine	Smoking Absorption through oral mucosa Reaches brain in 7 sec, lasts 30 min to 1 h Plasma half-life 2 hr, decreased by caffeine	Raised arousal level Increases in heart rate, blood pressure, cardiac contractility, vasodilation Decreased attention to extraneous stimuli Fine tremor Shortness of breath Decreased appetite or intestinal cramps Antidiuretic effect Can decrease aggressiveness May increase irritability Sedation	Chronic cough Smells like tobacco Stained teeth Excessive skin wrinkling Chain smoking History of smoking when ill, 1st thing in the morning
Central Nervous System Depressants			
Alcohol	Oral; metabolized and excreted in 12 hr	CNS depression Decreased cognition and inhibitions Relaxation Impaired neuromuscular coordination Shortened rapid eye movement sleep with restlessness and early wakening Tremors, fatigue, and irritability Headache and gastrointestinal upset Tolerance shown by increased intake without visible signs of intoxication	Alcohol on breath Gait problems Cigarette burns, especially on hands and chest Bruises on lower extremities, arms, chest History of accidents Euphoria Mood swings Belligerence Intense use of mouthwashes, breath mints, or scents Depression in combination with unreasonable resentments and jealousy Social discomfort Poor judgment may result in financial losses, fights, accidents, child neglect, domestic violence Tardiness and absenteeism at work Decreased productivity Family disruption Social isolation Arrests

Adverse Effects	Overdose Symptoms	Withdrawal Symptoms	Detoxification Protocol
oking linked to pulmonary dis-ase; cancer of mouth, throat, nd lungs; cardiovascular dis-ase wing linked to oral cancer idental death due to fire result-ng from careless habits eased incidence of peptic lcers and cirrhosis luced effectiveness of medica-ions eased risk of hemorrhage, es-ecially cerebral hemorrhage in vomen older than 35 who moke and take birth control ills regnancy, increased risk of low irth weight babies, sudden in-ant death syndrome, spontane-us abortion reted in breast milk; may in-ibit milk production ond-hand smoke: cancers, pper respiratory infections in thers including children	At low and medium doses: in-creased blood pressure At high doses: fall in blood pres-sure Nausea Dizziness	Maximal intensity 24–48 hr after last use, decreasing over several weeks Reduced heart rate and blood pressure Craving Anxiety Restlessness Difficulty concentrating Disruption in sleep Excessive eating, especially sweets Irritability, frustration, anger Headaches Gastrointestinal disturbance	Transdermal patch (4–8 wk) Nicotine gum up to 6 months Clonidine up to 6 wk Antidepressants
sea, vomiting, diarrhea versible brain damage r damage tritis, ulceration, hemorrhage th from respiratory arrest with rge doses regnant women, crosses pla-ental barrier, affecting infant abolic disorders eased incidence of oral cancer ohagitis and varices liomyopathy eased incidence of lung infec-ons nutrition ers seizure threshold kouts eased accidents reased fertility r judgment eased fights chosocial deterioration r clotting, anemia e disorders	Highest risk with young drinkers (chugging contests) Decreased neuromuscular control leading to gait and speech dis-turbance, stupor, coma Occasionally violent outbursts and combative behavior Respiratory distress and failure	*First phase: symptoms begin within 6–8 hr of last use, last-ing a few hours to days (usually begin to abate within 48 hr):* Insomnia Increased blood pressure, pulse and body temperature Tremors Muscle weakness Profuse perspiration Headache Nystagmus Gait problems Anorexia Nausea Vomiting Abdominal cramps Flushed face Disorientation Intense craving for alcohol *After 8–12 hr:* Hallucinations *After 24–48 hr:* Seizures *Second-phase withdrawal or delir-ium tremens, beginning 72 hr after last drink:* Fever Tachycardia Profuse sweating Severe tremor Profound disorientation	Thiamine. In malnourished alcohol-ics, thiamine should be given before providing glucose calo-ries. Vitamin B-100 complex orally may be given additionally **Chlordiazepoxide** This long-acting benzodiazepine is used in the acute phase of alco-hol withdrawal and has both sedative and anticonvulsant ef-fects. **Beta-blockers** Reduce symptoms of autonomic nervous system dysfunction, de-crease the total dose of sedative hypnotics needed to control withdrawal symptoms These do not prevent withdrawal seizures or delirium tremors so should not be used as the sole pharmacologic intervention for moderate to severe alcohol ab-stinence syndrome.

Table continued on following page

Table 40–2. Reference Guide to Commonly Abused Substances (Continued)

Drug	Route and Duration	Physical Findings in Intoxication	Behavioral Cues
Central Nervous System Depressants (Continued)			
Alcohol (Continued)			
Central Nervous System Depressants			
Opiates and synthetic: Butorphanol (Stadol) Codeine Opiate designer drugs: fentanyl analogues Heroin Hydromorphone (Dilaudid) Methadone (Dolophine) Morphine sulfate Opium Opiates combined with nonsteroidal anti-inflammatory drugs (NSAIDs)	Oral, IV, IM, intranasal, smoked Lasts 4–12 hr	Pupillary constriction Depressed respiration Needle marks with IV use Scarred veins Inflammation of nasal mucosa with edema Drowsiness ("nodding") Lowered blood pressure Slurred speech Psychomotor retardation Cough suppression Itching Lowered temperature	Lethargy Euphoric mood Social withdrawal Episodes of stupor Wearing of covering clothing ev in hot weather Use of sunglasses indoors Uninterested in hygiene and ap pearance Preoccupied with obtaining and using drugs Prostitution, theft, selling drugs support habit

Adverse Effects	Overdose Symptoms	Withdrawal Symptoms	Detoxification Protocol
		Intense and frightening hallucinations Agitated delirium with possible violent behavior	**Lorazepam** Useful in elderly patients and those with hepatic dysfunction Shorter half-life and low accumulation of drug: more frequent administration and longer dosage taper Discontinue drug if person becomes obtunded Mental status should clear more rapidly than with chlordiazepoxide Not appropriate in those with a high tolerance for sedative-hypnotics and normal liver metabolism *Characteristics of candidates for lorazepam protocol:* Documented cirrhosis Symptoms of active alcoholic hepatitis (jaundice, fever, right upper quadrant abdominal pain) Massively enlarged liver Ascites Previous history of variceal bleeding Previous history of hepatic encephalopathy Older age Available intramuscularly (IM) or intravenously (IV) **Phenytoin** Sometimes given to persons with history of alcohol abstinence seizures. Monitor therapeutic doses of other medications such as phenytoin and coumadin, whose metabolism may be altered with the absence of alcohol.
ma spiratory depression or failure reased risk for hepatitis, acquired immunodeficiency syndrome (AIDS), tuberculosis terial endocarditis nal failure diac arrest zures rmatitis monary emboli anus lulitis, abscesses	Loss of consciousness Pale, cool, clammy skin with cyanotic tinge Respiratory depression or arrest Coma Shock Convulsions Death	**Adult** *Grade 0:* (4 hr after last dose) Anxiety Craving for drugs *Grade 1:* (8 hr) Yawning Lacrimation Rhinorrhea Perspiration	**Clonidine** Establish opiate abstinence syndrome; dose before symptoms become severe. A patient on doses of methadone higher than 30 mg/day may not tolerate abrupt abstinence even with the use of clonidine.

Table continued on following page

Table 40–2. Reference Guide to Commonly Abused Substances (Continued)

Drug	Route and Duration	Physical Findings in Intoxication	Behavioral Cues
Central Nervous System Depressants *(Continued)*			
Opiates and synthetic (Continued)			
Oxycodone (Percodan)		Lack of secretions (dry nose and mouth)	Look of contentment with loss of worry, sexual desire, appetite
Pentazocine (Talwin)		Slowed gastrointestinal activity	Impaired memory, concentration judgment
Propoxyphene (Darvon)			
Central Nervous System Depressants (Sedative Hypnotics)			
Barbiturates			
Amobarbital (Amytal)	Oral: capsules or pills	Slurred speech	Disinhibition of sexual or aggressive drives
Butabarbital (HMB, Quibron Plus)	IV	Lack of coordination	sive drives
Phenobarbital (Luminal, Antrocol, Bronkolixir, Quadrinal)	May last from 3–8 hr	Unsteady gait	Impaired judgment
		Drowsiness	Impaired social or occupational functioning
Secobarbital (Seconal, Tuinal)		Decreased blood pressure	functioning
Pentobarbital sodium (Nembutal)		Decreased pulmonary function	Impaired attention or memory
		Nystagmus	Irritability
Benzodiazepines and the like		Additive effects of alcohol may lead to coma sooner	Lethargy
Alprazolam (Xanax)			Neglect of activities of daily living
Chloral hydrate			Accidents
Chlordiazepoxide (Librium)			Acute confusion state
Diazepam (Valium)			
Glutethimide (Doriden)			

Adverse Effects	Overdose Symptoms	Withdrawal Symptoms	Detoxification Protocol
Circular-appearing scars from healed skin lesions Malnutrition Constipation Hypoglycemia Neurologic disorders Perforation of nasal septum Erectile dysfunction Irregular menses		*Grade 2:* (12 hr) All of the above plus the following: Mydriasis Piloerection Tremors Hot and cold flashes Aching bones and muscles Anorexia *Grade 3:* (18–24 hr) Increased intensity of the above plus the following: Insomnia Restlessness Nausea Increase in blood pressure, temperature, respiratory rate and depth, and pulse rate *Grade 4:* (24–36 hr) Increased intensity of the above plus the following: Curled-up position Vomiting Diarrhea Weight loss (up to 5 lb daily) Spontaneous ejaculation or orgasm Decreased concentration Leukocytosis Eosinophilia Hyperglycemia **Infant** Hyperactivity Tremors Frantic sucking Regurgitation and poor weight gain Irritability Diarrhea Fever High-pitched cry Seizures	Discontinue as soon as possible. Doxepin may help insomnia and depression. NSAIDs for muscle cramps Encourage participation in decision making about doses with person, especially tapers Failure to progress: reevaluate drug history for additional drugs of addiction or suspect drug use in treatment Random, supervised drug screens indicated If also withdrawing from benzodiazepines or alcohol, diazepam or chlordiazepoxide may be used instead of phenobarbital. Pain medication and sedation should not be ordered on demand after stabilization.
Cardiovascular or respiratory depression or arrest Coma Shock Convulsions Death Weight loss and malnutrition Cellulitis or vascular complications after IV use	Slurred speech Staggering gait Sustained nystagmus Slowed reactions Lethargy Progressive respiratory depression, evidenced by shallow and irregular breathing Stupor or coma Death, if untreated	Time of onset depends on half-life of the drug and dose. May be within 24 hr on cessation or may be delayed for several days **Adult** *High dose, minor syndrome* Anxiety Insomnia Nightmares Tremors Weakness Sweating	Stabilization on a dose of benzodiazepine or phenobarbital sufficient to control symptoms.

Table continued on following page

Table 40–2. *Reference Guide to Commonly Abused Substances* (Continued)

Drug	Route and Duration	Physical Findings in Intoxication	Behavioral Cues
Central Nervous System Depressants (Sedative Hypnotics) *(Continued)*			
Benzodiazepines and the like (Continued)			
Lorazepam (Ativan)			
Meprobamate (Equanil, Miltown)			
Oxazepam (Serax)			
Methaqualone (Quaalude)			
Inhalants			
Glue	Inhaled	Vertigo	Telltale chemical odors
Gasoline	Effects are brief, from a few minutes to 1 hr	Incoordination	Unexplained listlessness
Solvents		Slurred speech	Confusion
Aromatics		Nystagmus	Poor judgment
Spray can propellants		Unsteady gait	Accidents
Spray paint		Depressed reflexes	Drunken gait and behavior
Paint thinner		Psychomotor retardation	Impulsive behavior
Hair spray		Tremor	Destructive behavior
Amyl nitrite		Generalized muscle weakness	Euphoric
Butyl nitrite		Blurred vision or diplopia	
		Excess nasal secretions	
		Watering of eyes	

Adverse Effects	Overdose Symptoms	Withdrawal Symptoms	Detoxification Protocol
		Restlessness Reflexes may be hyperactive Elevated pulse, blood pressure, or both Loss of appetite Nausea Vomiting Weight loss *Major syndrome* Grand mal seizures High body temperature Psychosis Thought disorder (agitation, confusion, hallucinations, amnesia) *Low-dose benzodiazepine* Wax and wane separated by 2–10-day cycles Anxiety Panic Tachycardia Pupillary dilation Increased blood pressure Impairment of memory and concentration Parasthesias ("pins and needles") Feelings of unreality Altered sensations Insomnia Muscle spasm Overt psychosis Sometimes is anxiety symptom re-emergence Infant High-pitched cry Tremors Restlessness Sleep disturbances Hyperreflexia Hyperphagia Diarrhea or vomiting Seizures	
rdiopulmonary arrest (death rom asphyxiation, freezing the ungs, coating the lungs) in damage er damage e marrow depression ght loss nory and concentration impairment al damage	Loss of consciousness Hypoxia Respiratory failure	None identified	General

Table continued on following page

Table 40–2. Reference Guide to Commonly Abused Substances (Continued)

Drug	Route and Duration	Physical Findings in Intoxication	Behavioral Cues
Inhalants *(Continued)*			
Central Nervous System Stimulants			
Amphetamines Dextroamphetamine (Dexedrine) Methamphetamine (Methedrine, Desoxyn, "Ice") Racemic amphetamine (Benzedrine)	Orally: pill, capsule Subcutaneously IV Smoke Lasts 1–14 hr	Tachycardia or bradycardia Cardiac arrhythmias Dilated pupils Elevated blood pressure Nausea or vomiting Twitching Muscle weakness Respiratory depression Increased temperature Perspiration or chills Evidence of weight loss Local anesthesia	Constantly runny nose (snorting) Increased confidence, elation Psychomotor agitation Hypervigilance Talkativeness Irritability Euphoric mood Grandiosity or "specialness" Impaired judgment Impaired social and occupational functioning Stereotypic and repetitive behavior Mood swings
Cocaine and crack (free base)	High obtained in 3 min by snorting, 20 sec by IV, 4–6 sec by smoking Duration of average high: cocaine: 15–60 min; crack: 5–7 min	Tachycardia or bradycardia Dilated pupils Elevated blood pressure Insomnia Anorexia Perspiration or chills Nausea or vomiting Psychomotor agitation or retardation Muscular weakness Respiratory depression	Elation Grandiosity Resistance to fatigue Impaired judgment Paranoid thinking Disturbed concentration Psychosis Violent temper outbursts Hallucinations involving animals bugs crawling under skin
Caffeine	Orally through liquids, foods, pills, capsules Reaches peak blood plasma level within 30 min after ingestion, lasts 6–16 hr	Restlessness Excitement Insomnia Flushed face Diuresis	Periods of inexhaustibility Nervousness Rambling flow of thought and speech

Adverse Effects	Overdose Symptoms	Withdrawal Symptoms	Detoxification Protocol
...usea or vomiting ...creased myocardial contractility, ...rrhythmias ...scular and joint pain ...scle weakness ...ual or auditory hallucinations ...s of consciousness ...soning ...dden death ...orientation			
...ression and fatigue ...glect of nutrition and appear- ...nce ...ulsive, assaultive behavior ...y use sedative to induce sleep ...ight loss ...diac irregularities, hypertension ...anoid delusions ...ual, auditory, and tactile halluci- ...ations ...ere or panic level of anxiety ...nted affect ...ial withdrawal ...th worn down from bruxism ...vered seizure threshold	Respiratory distress Chest pain or cardiac arrhythmias Confusion Dyskinesias Dystonias Ataxia Hyperpyrexia Convulsions Coma Death associated with hyperpy- rexia, convulsions, cardiovascu- lar shock	"Crash" with lethargy and in- creased desire for sleep Severe depression lasting for months Agitation Apathy Disorientation Suicidal ideation Vivid, unpleasant dreams Increased appetite Psychomotor retardation or agita- tion	Focus on keeping person comfort- able. Decrease drug cravings. Provide adequate calories for re- pletion of body weight. Anxiety and agitation: low-dose benzodiazepine, e.g., chlordiaze- poxide every 4–6 hr. Taper and discontinue after symptoms have stabilized. Insomnia: First try diphenhydra- mine hydrochloride at hour of sleep, which may be repeated once during the night. Severe insomnia: increase benzo- diazepine or use chloral hydrate. Depression, continued insomnia, or severe cravings: evaluate for antidepressants.
...ydrug or alcohol abuse ...anoid delusions and hallucina- ...ons ...rs and abscesses ...ression or suicide ideation ...forated nasal septum ...onic insomnia ...ere headaches ...r or decreased sexual perform- ...nce ...eased risk for AIDS ...kinesias, dystonias ...diac arrhythmias	Seizures Chest pain Cardiac arrest Respiratory depression or arrest Convulsions Hyperpyrexia Stroke Confusion	"Crash" with lethargy and in- creased sleeping initially Vivid, unpleasant dreams Increased appetite Dysphoria, depression Agitation Anxiety Psychomotor retardation or agita- tion Insomnia Muscle cramps Stomach pain Intense craving for drug	Keep patient comfortable. Evaluate for medical problems and addiction to other drugs. Provide adequate calories for re- pletion of body weight. Anxiety and agitation may require sedation with chlordiazepoxide. Larger dose may be given every hour of sleep for insomnia. Taper and discontinue after symptoms have stabilized. May benefit from antidepressant therapy. In cases of severe prolonged drug cravings, a trial of bromocrip- tine, with gradually increasing doses over a 10-day period, can be used.
...d indigestion ...tic ulcer ...eased intraocular pressure in ...nregulated glaucoma	Diuresis Marked hypotension and circula- tory failure Agitation	Headache Restlessness Lethargy Inability to work productively	General

Table continued on following page

Table 40–2. Reference Guide to Commonly Abused Substances (Continued)

Drug	Route and Duration	Physical Findings in Intoxication	Behavioral Cues
Central Nervous System Stimulants (*Continued*)			
		Gastrointestinal complaints	
		Cardiac arrhythmias	
		Psychomotor agitation	
		Muscle twitching	
Psychotomimetics			
Cannabinoids	Smoking	Dry mouth	Can act as stimulant or depressant
Marijuana	Oral	Reddened eyes	Use of sunglasses to hide redness
Hashish	May accumulate in fatty tissues for	Increased heart rate	of eyes
Delta-9-tetrahydrocannabinol (THC)	up to 1 month	Impaired coordination and reaction	Increased use of eyedrops
	Effects generally last 3–4 hr, can	time	Impaired learning and retention
	last 12–24 hr	Increased appetite	Distorted sensory perceptions
		Sensory distortion in higher doses	Time distortion
		Exaggeration of emotions	Grandiosity
			Hazardous driving from poor coordination and judgment
			Occasional flashbacks
			Euphoria
			Inappropriate laughter, silliness
			Heightened sensitivity to external stimuli
			Talkative
			Increased appetite
			Sedation, lethargy
Hallucinogenics	Oral	Dilated pupils	Intense distorted perceptions
Lysergic acid diethylamide (LSD)	IV	Hyperreflexia	Impaired judgment and suggestibility
Mescaline	Lasts 2–24 hr (depends on substance)	Increased blood pressure	Flight of ideas
Psilocybin		Increased body temperature	Social isolation
3-4 methylenedioxyamphetamine (MDA)		Piloerection	Self-absorption
		Tachycardia	Paranoia, fear
		Senses intensified	Memory impairment
Phencyclidine (PCP, angel dust)	Smoking	Numbness or diminished responsiveness to pain	Accidents
	Oral		Ataxia
	Snorting	Excitement	Loss of concentration and memory
	Injection	Confusion	Assaultiveness
		Visual disturbances	Belligerence
		Distorted body perceptions	Impulsiveness
		Delirium	Unpredictability
		Panic	Impaired judgment and social and occupational functioning
		Vertical or horizontal nystagmus	Confused wandering
		Increased blood pressure, pulse, temperature	

Adverse Effects	Overdose Symptoms	Withdrawal Symptoms	Detoxification Protocol
achycardia ncreased plasma glucose and lipid levels ncreased incidence of angina and myocardial infarction xacerbation of anxiety	Sensory disturbances: ringing in ears, flashes of light Tachycardia Psychomotor agitation Arrhythmias Insomnia Grand mal seizures (more than 10 g) Respiratory failure	Irritability	
ethargy nhedonia ear of insanity eglect of appearance nage distortion nxiety ausea emors allucinations fficulty carrying out complex mental processes apired short-term memory owed speech and thought patterns itation of lung tissue, smoker's cough ss of motivation oodiness, irritability paired judgment esity ales: decreased sperm count, decreased testosterone levels with gynecomastia males: Menstrual irregularities that may persist for months gal problems	Feelings of loss of control, depression, nausea or vomiting Fatigue Paranoia	*Within hours of last dose:* Fat stores depleted in 10–12 days Irritatilibity Restlessness Nausea Loss of appetite, possible weight loss Sleep disturbance Diaphoresis Tremors	Symptoms may begin within hours after the last does of THC, but abstinence does not begin until fat stores are depleted, which may take 10–12 days. Mild sedation may be helpful initially if symptoms of anxiety, irritability, and sweating predominate, even in the 2nd week of withdrawal. Chlordiazepoxide is usually adequate. An alternative is use of a β-blocker in low dose or tricyclic antidepressant.
nic with impulsive behavior shbacks ychosis xiety usea, chills, tremors pid mood swings oression ual hallucinations	Psychosis Brain damage	Cravings to return to use	General
anoid psychosis arre, volent behavior ss of pain sensation oression oherent, aggressive acts toward self or others otional lability ggressive behavior (e.g., public masturbation) reased risk for AIDS, hepatitis diovascular toxicity	Psychosis Possible hypertensive crisis, cardiovascular accident Respiratory arrest Hyperthermia Seizures Coma, with aspiration Renal impairment Catatonic mutism with posturing	Craving to return to use of drug	General

Table continued on following page

Table 40–2. Reference Guide to Commonly Abused Substances (Continued)

Drug	Route and Duration	Physical Findings in Intoxication	Behavioral Cues
Psychotomimetics *(Continued)*			
Phencyclidine (PCP, angel dust) *(Continued)*		Ataxia Muscle rigidity Seizures Blank stare Chronic jerking Agitated, repetitive movements Needle tracks	

Drug	Route and Duration	Desired Effects	Findings in Intoxication	Behavioral Cues
Anabolic-Androgenic Steroids (AAS)	Oral Injectable "Stacking": alternating oral and IM over 4–18 wk	Increased weight Increased lean muscle mass and strength Increased confidence	Euphoria Diminished fatigue Increased aggressiveness Dizziness Nausea Muscle spasms	"Rhoid rage" Impaired social relationships due to mood swings

Modified with permission from Appendix A, *The Core Curriculum of Addictions Nursing NNSA*, Midwest Education Association, Inc., 1990. Data from Kraus ML, et al. Randomized and clinical trial of atenolol in patients with alcohol withdrawal. *N Engl J Med* 313:905–909, 1985; Clarke HW, and Longmuir. Northern California Society for Treatment Alcohol and Other Drug Dependencies News 13(1), 1986; Gawin FH, and Kleber HD. Cocaine abuse treatment. *Arch Gen Psychiatry* 41:903–909, 1984; Dackis CA, and Gold MS. Pharmacologic approaches to cocaine addiction. *J Subst Abuse Treatment* 2:139–145, 1985; Giannini, AJ, Baumgartel P, and DiMarzio L. Bromocriptine therapy in coca withdrawal. *J Clin Pharmacol* 27:267–270, 1987; Busto U, et al. Withdrawal reaction after long-term therapeutic use of benzodiazepines. *N Engl J Med* 315(4):854–859, 198; Smith DE, and Wesson DR. Benzodiazepine dependence potential: Current studies and trends. *J Psychoactive Drugs* 1:163–167, 1984.

(4) Smokeless tobacco damages the soft and hard oral tissue, increases heart rate and blood pressure, increases the risk of cancers, and is associated with the development of leukoplakia, a disease manifested by thick, white irregular patches inside the mouth (and often evolves into squamous cell carcinomas).

(5) Smokeless tobacco use has been linked to su pressed immunologic responses, increased den caries, gingival inflammation, and cancers of t pharynx, esophagus, urinary bladder, and pancre

(6) Risk of cerebral hemorrhage increases in wom older than 35 who smoke and take birth cont pills.

Adverse Effects	Overdose Symptoms	Withdrawal Symptoms	Detoxification Protocol
Respiratory problems including apnea, bronchospasm			

Adverse Effects	Overdose Symptoms	Withdrawal Symptoms	Detoxification Protocol	General Detoxification Protocol
endonitis isruption of reproductive system oscesses oody cysts in the liver hange in blood lipids creased blood pressure dema ypercalcemia enal calculi cne with permanent scarring uffy face roke creased risk of AIDS *en* ldness rophy of testes creased sperm count creased sex drive necomastia *omen* creased breast size toral enlargement creased facial hair epening of voice enstrual irregularities *uth* emature closing of growth plates	Priapism Gastrointestinal distress Diarrhea Jaundice	Depression Fatigue Restlessness Anorexia Insomnia	Follow procedures for corticosteroid taper.	1. Take regular vital signs every 2–4 hr; encourage fluids and nutritious diet; use medications such as acetaminophen, antacids, and milk of magnesia for general symptomatic relief. 2. Mild exercise, stretching or walking, relaxation classes, warm baths, or massage may aid in relief of withdrawal symptoms. Distraction rather than reliance on medication is advised, particularly once physical stabilization has been achieved.

Smoking and pregnancy
a. Decreased oxygen to the fetus leads to decreased birth weight
  (1) Increased risk of mortality due to increased risk of spontaneous abortion, fetal death, bleeding early and late in pregnancy, and premature and prolonged rupture of the amniotic membranes
  (2) Long-term effects on the baby's growth, intellectual development, and behavior
b. Associated with increased risk of sudden infant death syndrome
3. Smoking and breast-feeding: Nicotine is secreted in breast milk, seems to inhibit milk production, and reduces the level of vitamin C in the milk (see Learning/

Teaching Guidelines for Counseling Substance-Using Pregnant Women).

Withdrawal

1. Symptoms: Cravings for nicotine, anxiety, restlessness, difficulty concentrating, disruption in sleep, excessive eating, irritability, constipation, headaches, gastrointestinal disturbance (nausea, constipation or diarrhea), decrease in heart rate and blood pressure, decrease in level of adrenal hormones, and decrease in general arousal level (Table 40-2).
2. Most withdrawal symptoms reach maximal intensity 24 to 48 hours after cessation of tobacco use and gradually diminish in intensity over several weeks. Some behaviors such as eating more than usual, weight gain, and craving cigarettes (particularly in stressful situations) may persist for months or even years.

Drug Interactions

Smoking reduces the effectiveness of medications, including oral contraceptives, insulin, bronchodilators, and antidepressants.

Interventions

1. Nonpharmacologic interventions: identify minimal-contact strategies to stop smoking (e.g., National Cancer Institute, self-help programs)
   a. Ask about smoking at every opportunity, advise all smokers to stop, assist the person in stopping, and arrange for follow-up support.
   b. Refer to minimal-contact or self-help stop smoking or chewing tobacco programs such as those of the National Cancer Institute.
   c. Refer to specialized programs along with minimal-contact programs.
   d. Create a smoke-free office, including elimination of all tobacco advertising from the waiting room.
   e. Identify all smoking patients; use a permanent progress card for each smoking person and develop a patient's smoking cessation plan.
2. Pharmacologic interventions
   a. Transdermal nicotine patches (4–8 wk)
   b. Nicotine polacrilex (gum; up to 6 months)
   c. Clonidine (up to 6 wk)
   d. Antidepressants

Complications

1. Second-hand smoke is associated with more than 3000 cases of lung cancer among nonsmokers each year.
2. Children in smoking homes have greater risk of upper respiratory infections and asthma than those in non-smoking homes.
3. Risk for fires and burn injuries.

Prognosis

Relapse rates after abstinence appear to be similar those for heroin and alcohol; about 60 percent of quitte relapse within 3 months and 75 percent within 6 months.

Public Health Considerations

Nurses can advocate for smoke-free environments a prevention programs to reduce the numbers of new users

◾ CARING FOR PEOPLE WHO ABUSE ALCOHOL

Assessing People Who Abuse Alcohol

1. Key signs and symptoms
   a. Observe current behavior and physical base line: sess patterns to determine problems.
      • Does the person appear intoxicated?
      • Alcohol on breath?
      • Eyes dilated? Nystagmus?
      • Gait problems not explained by other causes?
      • Cigarette and other burns on hands or chest?
      • Bruises on the lower extremities, arms, or chest?
      • History of accidents?
      • Puffy eyes unaccounted for by uremia or allergy?
      • Red, puffy face?
      • Reddened conjunctivae?
      • Tremulousness of hands?
      • Diaphoresis?
   b. Note any physical problems possibly related to ac (intoxication, overdose, withdrawal) or chronic s stance use. See complications list below.
   c. Mental or psychologic indicators: mood or men functioning changes that might indicate substance u euphoria, mood swings, depression, paranoia (unr sonable fears or suspicions), belligerence. The indiv ual is not likely to be aware of these, so discuss with family members may be advised.
   d. Central nervous system depressants (alcohol, opiat sedatives): depression in combination with unreas able resentments and jealousy, paranoid attitudes, cial discomfort
   e. Alcohol: reports of blackouts or impaired memory what happens during drinking episodes; intense of mouthwash or scents. The consequences of dri ing are a better guide to assessing problem drink than simply the amounts consumed.
2. Alcohol use history (see p. 1850)
3. Physical examination
   a. History of major operations, seizures (describe), cers, cirrhosis or hepatitis, pancreatitis, tuberculo emphysema, bronchitis, asthma, hypertension, c betes, heart disease, venereal disease, recent injur pregnancy, and fractures; ask about psychiatric tory.
   b. Check the head, eyes, ears, nose, and throat; palp

the head, check for "battlesign" (thumbprint bruise behind ear); check the size of the head to rule out swelling. Check the eyes, ears, and throat for signs of inflammation, infection, drainage, bleeding, trauma, or deformity.

c. Auscultate the lungs for sounds of wheezes; percuss the back; ask regarding changes in respiratory status, congestion, or shortness of breath; ask whether pain increases with inspiration and about any recent trauma.

d. Auscultate the heart, checking for irregular beats and physiologic splitting, and ask about a history of chest pain. Ask about a previous history of myocardial infarctions and changes in electrocardiogram results.

e. Abdomen
   (1) Perform deep palpations of the 4 quadrants, looking especially for tenderness over the liver; look for contour symmetry and spider lesions.
   (2) Ask about changes in appetite, bowel habits, onset of nausea or vomiting, abdominal pain, and epigastric pain.
   (3) The liver is normally at the right costal margin, but a diseased liver can extend below the costal margin and is measured by finger widths; the spleen is normally above the left costal margin but when enlarged can be palpated on inspiration.

f. Neurologic: Check for extraocular movements and nystagmus; mental status and speech, cranial nerves, motor system, sensory system, and reflexes. Observe gait. Check for muscle tremors; strength in extremities; brief comparison of light touch over arms and legs; reflexes of biceps, triceps, brachioradiali, and abdominal muscles; knee; ankle; plantar, and peripheral neuropathy.

g. Skin: Check for diaphoresis, lesions, rashes, abnormal color (jaundice, redness of infections), and needle tracks.

Special diagnostic tests: These lack specificity in diagnosing alcoholism but are helpful in breaking through denial and increasing motivation for change.

a. Blood alcohol level (blood, urine, Breathalyzer)

b. Liver function tests
   (1) Gamma-glutamyltransferase (GGT)
   (2) Glutamate dehydrogenase (GDH)
   (3) Serum γ-glutamyltranspeptidase (SGGTP) shows some promise as a screening test for alcoholism but is not specific only to alcoholism. It is more predictive when the following are also elevated:
   (4) Serum glutamate pyruvate transaminase (SGPT)
   (5) Serum glutamic-oxaloacetic transaminase (SGOT)
   (6) Lactate dehydrogenase (LDH)
   (7) Alkaline phosphatase (AP)
   (8) Prothrombin (PT)
   (9) Bilirubin levels

c. Other tests to screen for physical damage from substance abuse
   (1) Serum carbohydrate-deficient transferrin has a higher correlation with ethanol consumption than does GGT, aspartate aminotransferase (AST), alanine aminotransferase (ALT), or mean corpuscular volume but may have limited sensitivity in patients with liver damage or in those with early-stage alcohol problems.
   (2) Low fasting blood sugar
   (3) Low blood urea nitrogen (BUN)
   (4) Electrolytes
   (5) Stool for occult blood
   (6) Electrocardiogram
   (7) Chest radiograph
   (8) Check for abnormal findings in macrocytosis; elevated mean corpuscular volume: less sensitive but more specific than GGT as a biologic marker of alcohol abuse; low hemoglobin and low hematocrit levels (common except in dehydrated persons, who would have elevated levels; low magnesium, phosphate, and potassium levels; elevated high-density lipoprotein levels; and uric acid levels.

Route and Duration

Alcohol is ingested orally; is metabolized in the liver; and is excreted by the kidneys, lungs, and sweat in 12 hours.

Risk Factors

1. Gender
   a. Men are 3 to 4 times more likely to develop alcohol problems than are women.
   b. Women typically begin drinking at an older age than men. They tend to develop higher blood alcohol concentrations than men because of lower percentage of body water and higher percentage of body fat, and they metabolize alcohol more slowly because of a lack of alcohol dehydrogenase in the mucosal lining of the stomach, so they have the same range of health and other problems as men by middle age.
2. Age
   a. The 1st episode of alcohol intoxication is likely to occur in midteens.
   b. There is a risk of concurrence of antisocial and conduct disorders in youth who begin to use alcohol before age 16.
3. Family history: Men with 2 or more alcoholic relatives are about 3 times more likely to become alcohol dependent than those without.
4. Culture: Northern European and some Native American groups are at increased risk of developing drinking problems.

Pathophysiology

1. Mechanism of action: Ethanol (ETOH) is a central nervous system depressant that produces sedation and, ultimately, hypnosis with increasing dosage. Alcohol synergizes many sedative agents and can result in life-threatening central nervous system depression when used with antihistamines or barbiturates.
2. Immediate effects of alcohol use:
   a. Intoxication: see Table 40–3

Table 40–3. Acute Effects of Alcohol (Related to Blood-Alcohol Level)*

Drinks per Hour	Blood Alcohol Level	Effects
2 drinks	.05	Reduced alertness; release of inhibitions; impaired judgment; vision may already start to double; there is some trouble distinguishing sounds, a decreased sensitivity to touch, an increase in reaction time, and probably some deficits in taste and smell.
5 drinks	.10	Slowed reaction time, impaired vision, impaired motor function, and less caution shown. Constitutes legal intoxication in most states.
	.15	Large, consistent increase in reaction time; impaired gait, standing, or talking.
10 drinks	.20	Marked decrease in sensorimotor capabilities, trouble staying awake; serious tissue damage may begin at this blood alcohol level.
15 drinks	.30	Stuporous but conscious.
20 drinks	.40	Depressed reflexes; state of unconsciousness or coma likely; LD 1 (minimum level for death).
25 drinks	.50	Complete unconsciousness, deep coma if not death.
	.60	Death most likely due to depression of nerve centers controlling heart rate and breathing.

* For a 150-lb man.

b. Blackouts: Transient episodes of amnesia that occur during a period of intoxication may be caused by a decrease in the transmission of certain nerve signals carried by serotonin and by disruptions at excitatory neurotransmitter synapses
3. Acute effects of alcohol use: overdose
   a. The threshold toxic dose depends on physical factors such as amount consumed, size of drinker, and the like. Usually, a blood alcohol level of greater than 400 mg per dl in nontolerant individuals constitutes a toxic dose.
   b. Overdose symptoms include irregular behavior, decreased neuromuscular control leading to gait and speech disturbance, stupor, coma, respiratory distress, and failure.
   c. The most common alcohol overdose victim is the young, inexperienced drinker who drinks a large amount of alcohol (e.g., a bottle of bourbon) quickly, usually on a dare. A person drinking at a normal rate would lose consciousness before the blood alcohol level could rise to lethal levels.
4. Adverse effects of short-term use: impaired coordination, poor judgment, possible increase in fights, accidents (driving impaired), shortened rapid eye movement sleep
5. Effects of long-term alcohol use
   a. Alcohol is carried in the water of the body, so it affects more systems than any other mind-altering substance.
   b. Malnutrition plays a major role in the physical harm done by alcohol to the body. Alcohol appears to block vitamin absorption, so damage is done even when vitamins are present in meals or taken as supplements.

c. Deterioration of functioning in all life roles.
6. Alcohol and pregnancy: FAS and fetal alcohol effect
   a. Ongoing use of alcohol during pregnancy may cau characteristic damage to the fetus, including FAS. A cohol does cross the placenta.
   b. No safe use level has been established for pregna women, so advise the patient to abstain. If she h already used, advise her to stop (see Learning/Teac ing Guidelines for Counseling Substance-Using Pre nant Women).
   c. Symptoms of FAS include growth deficiencies befc delivery and postbirth and characteristic facies (sm head, flat midface, indistinct philtrum); many childr have eye and ear problems.
   d. The most serious impact is on the central nervo system—low IQ, trouble retaining information, tro ble learning from mistakes.
   e. Recognition of the syndrome permits entry into habilitation and respite programs for the child a family.
   f. Fetal alcohol effects: Children are not so clearly fected as those with FAS but have difficulties such limited attention span (poor problem solving), lack appropriate social interaction, and apparent inabil to learn from mistakes. Currently these children not qualify for special programs.
7. Alcohol and breast-feeding
   a. Alcohol may reach the same concentration in mother's breast milk as in her blood and is rapi transmitted to the nursing infant. Chronic exposure the nursing infant to high doses of alcohol is pote tially dangerous as the infant oxidizes alcohol m slowly than an adult.
   b. Heavy drinking can decrease milk supply as well inhibit the milk-ejection reflex. Be aware that "c wives' tales" said to drink a beer before nursing, new mothers in particular may have been told this well-meaning but ill-informed family members other health practitioners.

NURSE ADVISORY

Clues for revealing substance abuse in the hospitalized patient or the person in rehabilitation
- Failure to respond to standard doses of tranquilizers or sedatives (suggests increased tolerance)
- Mood changes especially around visiting times: family or friends may be bringing in alcohol or drugs
- Overabundance of mouthwashes or toiletries, which could be a source of alcohol
- Frequent references to drinking or being intoxicated
- Multiple bruises, burns, abrasions at different stages of healing (especially at table-top height or on hands and face) caused by falls and accidents when intoxicated
- Scars from self-mutilation or suicide attempts
- Appearing older than one's stated age
- High rate of recidivism in rehabilitation
- Slow healing, requiring more clinic visits
- More frequent crises than others with a comparable diagnosis
- Emergence of signs of alcohol withdrawal

Withdrawal

General overview
a. The major concern is safety.
b. Aim of care: relieve symptoms, prevent seizures and delirium tremens (DTs), prepare for long-term rehabilitation

Principles
a. The more of the substance the person has used and the longer the time they have used it, the more serious the potential problems in detoxification.
b. The human and physical environment may need to be regulated during withdrawal (need for reduced stimulation).
c. The progression of withdrawal symptoms in some drugs such as alcohol can be stopped by replacing the short-acting drug by longer-acting drugs.
d. The need for pharmacologic support is indicated by vital signs (blood pressure, pulse, respirations) and other symptoms such as state of alertness and sweating.
e. Evaluate for other conditions and symptoms (head trauma, diabetes, fever).
f. Give support and encouragement

Assessment
a. Is there a history of withdrawal seizures or DTs?
b. What is the amount, duration of use, form of alcohol, and time of last use? (You may need to ask "How often do you go to the liquor store?" "How much do you purchase?" "How long does this amount last?")
c. Are other drugs used (polydrug abusers have 3 times the likelihood of seizures)?
d. General health status
e. Current signs of withdrawal (diaphoresis, tremulousness, rapid pulse, elevated blood pressure, sleeping a lot)?
f. Any changes in tolerance (may indicate liver problems). Ask "What is the amount of alcohol you need to drink to feel the effects or feel comfortable?"

Alcohol detoxification symptoms
a. Initial stage of minor withdrawal: tremors, weakness, profuse perspiration, headache, anorexia, nausea, abdominal cramps, vomiting, flushed face, disorientation, convulsions
 (1) Tremors occur within 6 to 8 hours after the last drink.
 (2) Auditory hallucinations in a person with otherwise clear senses (occasionally visual or other sensory hallucinations) occur 8 to 12 hours after last drink. Symptoms usually last a few hours to a few days.
 (3) Seizures may begin 7 to 38 hours after the last drink, typically peaking after 24 hours. They occur in series of 2 to 6 episodes, will progress to repeated or prolonged seizures or status epilepticus. Thirty percent will go on to develop DTs.
b. May progress on to major withdrawal (DTs), which is life threatening: fever, tachycardia, profuse sweating, severe tremor, profound disorientation, intense and frightening hallucinations, or agitated delirium with possible violent behavior. Occurs 72 hours after the last drink.

5. Indications for 24-hour care
 a. Previous withdrawal seizures or DTs
 b. Coexisting health problems, especially head injuries, bleeding, or fever
 c. Pregnancy
 d. Hallucinations
 e. Worsening of symptoms of withdrawal (increased symptoms over time, climbing blood pressure or pulse rate)
 f. Extreme anxiety or agitation, irritability, restlessness, hyperreflexia
 g. Changing mental status, mental confusion, fluctuating orientation

Drug Interactions

Alcohol is preferentially metabolized over substances including food, so it can affect blood levels of a wide variety of medications and other drugs, including the creation of lethal levels in the blood (usually respiratory arrest with other central nervous system depressants) (Table 40–4).

Clinical Management

1. Detoxification
 a. Nonpharmacologic approaches: rehydrate, keep in calm environment with minimal noise and soft lights when possible, as the nervous system will be in hyperarousal.
 b. Pharmacologic approaches: Drugs used in detoxification are the longer-acting benzodiazepines, phenobarbital, and antihistamines. Doses are related to the detoxification symptoms. See Table 40–2.
2. The rehabilitation process: see Table 40–1
 a. Stabilize the addicted individual
 b. Establish the need for long-term sobriety
 c. Establish a balanced lifestyle
 d. Self-help programs

Complications

1. Central nervous system complications include altered brain waves; perceptual difficulties; changes in the brain anatomy (atrophy, enlarged ventricles, widening sulci); autoimmune response (attacking own tissue); and disturbed blood flow to the brain, including increased clumping (agglutination) as blood alcohol levels rise. This clumping cuts off circulation in smaller vessels to the point of rupture and bleeding and results in edema and may occur in social drinkers as well as in alcoholics.
 a. Wernicke-Korsakoff syndrome
 (1) Caused by vitamin B_1 deficiency, which results in small hemorrhages and bleeding in the brain stem, patchy cell death, and alterations in nerve fibers
 (2) Symptoms: motor incoordination, hypothermia, trouble learning new or retaining old information, confabulation (making up facts to hide the lack of memory)

Table 40-4. Selected Alcohol-Medication Interactions

Medication	Effect When Combined with Alcohol
Anesthetics	Need for increased dose of anesthesia in newly sober alcoholics, but once asleep, sleep is deeper and longer
Anticonvulsants	
Phenytoin (Dilantin)	Diminished anticonvulsant effect with chronic alcohol abuse
	Enhanced anticonvulsant effect with acute intoxication
Antihistamines	Drowsiness due to additive effect
Anti-infectives	
Antibiotics	Higher blood levels (kanamycin) or lower blood level (penicillin)
Chloramphenicol	Minor disulfiram-like symptoms
Isoniazid	Diminished effect with chronic alcohol abuse
Metronidazole (Flagyl)	Minor disulfiram-like symptoms
Quinacrine (Atabrine)	Minor disulfiram-like symptoms
Antidepressant	
Tricyclics (Elavil)	Magnified motor impairment, increased elimination
Monoamine oxidase inhibitors (Parnate)	Hypertensive crisis
Antipsychotics	
Chlorpromazine (Thorazine)	Reduced elimination so increased anticholinergic side effects
Antisecretory	
Ranitidine (Zantac)	Increased blood alcohol level
Cimetidine (Tagamet)	
Cardiac medications	
Anticoagulants, oral	Reduced anticoagulant effect, enhanced central nervous system (CNS) depression
Digitalis	Arrythmias, digitoxicity
Hydrochlorothiazide	Enhances blood pressure lowering effects; can precipitate postural hypotension
Nitroglycerin	
Reserpine	
Propranolol	Dysrhythmias, angina
Disulfiram (Antabuse)	Abdominal cramps, flushing, vomiting, psychotic episodes, confusion, headaches, convulsions, unconsciousness, death
Hypoglycemics	
Chlorpropamide (Diabinese)	Minor disulfiram-like symptoms
Phenformin (DBI; Meltrol)	Lactic acidosis
Tolbutamide (Orinase)	Diminished hypoglycemic effect with chronic alcohol abuse
Insulin	Enhanced hypoglycemic effect with ingestion of alcohol, particularly in fasting people; minor disulfiram-like symptoms.
NSAIDs	
Salicylates	Increased risk of gastrointestinal bleeding
Acetaminophen	Increased risk of liver toxicity
Ibuprofen	Higher or prolonged blood alcohol levels
Opiates	Serious CNS depression due to synergism
Sedatives and tranquilizers	
Barbiturates	Diminished sedative effect with long-term alcohol abuse
	Enhanced CNS depression with acute intoxication
Chloral hydrate (Notec)	Prolonged hypnotic effect
Benzodiazepines (Valium)	Enhanced CNS depression; risk of overdose

Modified from Black JM, and Matassarin-Jacobs E (eds). *Luckmann and Sorensen's Medical-Surgical Nursing: A Psychophysiologic Approach.* 4th ed. Philadelphia: WB Saunders, 1993, p 2212.

b. Peripheral neuropathies
  (1) Caused by degeneration of myelin (protective sheath around the nerves) due to vitamin B_1 and other B vitamin deficiencies
  (2) Symptoms: slow onset pain, tingling, numbne[ss] starting in the farthest out nerves as axons [die] and moving toward the center; "stocking-glo[ve] effect," which is usually bilateral and symmetr[ical]

reflexes are absent; progression to muscle wasting and paralysis is possible; drop foot or wide-based gait may be seen.

c. Alcoholic cerebral atrophy
  (1) Autoimmune response due to antigens in the blood causes destruction and atrophy of the frontal lobes.
  (2) Symptoms: fatigue, listlessness, depression, irritability, confusion, and memory deficits

d. Alcoholic pellagra
  (1) Due to vitamin B_3 (niacin) deficiencies
  (2) Symptoms: clouding consciousness, cogwheel rigidity and emergence of primitive sucking and grasping reflexes. Depression, diarrhea, dermatitis. Good prognosis in milder cases; poor prognosis once severe mental symptoms show up; sudden death can occur despite apparent satisfactory progress in treatment.

e. Sleep disorder
  (1) Destruction of serotonergic and other neurons, causing sleep fragmentation
  (2) Symptoms: Alcohol produces decreased rapid eye movement with sedation; in detoxification rapid eye movement increases (rebound) as sedation level drops.

f. Mental or emotional disorders or psychosocial deterioration: increased depression, suicidal ideation; high risk of suicide completion when intoxicated, particularly when means are readily available

g. Secondary factors causing brain damage
  (1) Coma with hypoventilation due to high blood alcohol level
  (2) Vomiting with aspiration of gastric contents, causing hypoxia
  (3) Head injury due to accidents or trauma
  (4) Alcoholic hypoglycemia (inadequate glucose available for brain function)
  (5) Hepatic encephalopathy occurs with elevated serum ammonia levels.

Cardiac complications: alcoholic cardiomyopathy
a. The number 1 cause of death in alcoholics. Alcoholism doubles men's and quadruples women's chances of myocardial infarction.
b. Myocardial infarction occurs frequently when large amounts of alcohol are used for more than 5 years. Even though the person is usually well nourished, it is due to the direct toxic effect of alcohol on the heart muscle plus vitamin deficiencies.
c. Symptoms: fatigue, dyspnea (trouble breathing on exertion), cardiac murmur, edema (swelling), increased blood pressure, changes in electrocardiogram results, and arrythmias. The heart increases in size; it may become flabby and have fat deposits. The condition progresses to congestive heart failure.

Pulmonary complications: related to impaired immune system
a. Tuberculosis
b. Pneumonia

Hematologic complications
a. Due to malnutrition, especially vitamin C deficiency
b. Anemia: Immature red blood cells are released. Decreased energy due to decreased oxygen-carrying capacity of the blood.
c. Poor clotting: Platelet numbers are decreased along with the ability to aggregate, resulting in increased bleeding time (in a population with a high rate of accidents).

5. Gastrointestinal complications
a. Malnutrition even in the presence of an adequate diet. Vitamin metabolism in particular is severely affected.
b. Esophagitis due to increased gastric acid secretion and increased vomiting and the direct toxic effect of the alcohol.
c. Eophageal varices: Cirrhosis of the liver causes portal hypertension. As the pressure in the blood vessels increases, the blood backs up, creating varicose veins of the esophagus. With rupture of the veins, the person can bleed to death (the rupture can be caused by eating rough food).
d. Gastric ulcer: impaired mucosal cell layer barrier.
e. Increased risk of cancers of the mouth, tongue, and esophagus.
f. Pancreatitis: acute and chronic due to the toxic effects of the alcohol.
g. Liver (fatty liver, alcoholic hepatitis, cirrhosis)
  (1) Fatty liver: Decreased glycogen and increased lipid formation causes an increase in size, which is reversible with abstinence.
  (2) Alcoholic hepatitis: inflammation (not related to an infectious organism).
  (3) Cirrhosis: Cells die due to alcohol's toxic effects. This condition is not reversible. One in 4 alcoholics are affected, and the risk increases with a family history.

6. Muscle wasting
a. Skeletal muscles: Muscle wasting with pain or tenderness is caused by injury to the cell membranes and alteration of active transport system.
b. Muscle wasting can be caused by a negative nitrogen balance due to poor nutrition, impaired carbohydrate metabolism, and, in the case of those with liver disease, an increased requirement for amino acids.
c. The symptom is weakness.

7. Endocrine complications
a. Men: impotence that is partially reversible, decreased libido (desire), decreased testosterone, increased estrogen (secondary sex characteristics may be lost, which may lead to breast development or loss of facial hair), testicular atrophy, and decreased sperm count
b. Women: increased painful menstruation or no menstruation, increased risk of spontaneous abortions, and decreased fertility

8. Fluid and electrolyte imbalances often appear in the detoxification process, because alcohol is a diuretic.

9. Skin disorders: Vitamin deficiencies increase the fragility of the skin and interfere with healing.

10. Bone disorders
a. Osteoporosis: Loss of bone mass occurs due to protein and calcium deficiencies. Alcohol appears to have a direct toxic effect on the osteoblasts (which deposit new bone).
b. Osteomalacia (rickets): Newly formed bone fails to mineralize (resulting in soft bones) when the liver is

too damaged to convert vitamin D into its active form. Vitamin D stimulates calcium absorption in the intestine.

   c. Secondary hyperparathyroidism related to chronic osteomalacia or long-standing protein deficiency leads to further loss of bone mineral content. Alcohol intoxication causes a transitory elevation in parathyroid levels with resultant high levels of calcium in the blood (taken from the bones).

   d. Fractures: The risk of fractures increases owing to accidents.

   e. Avascular necrosis due to poor blood supply. Experienced as joint pain, mainly on motion. As the condition progresses, the pain is experienced in motion and at rest, as is restriction of movement in the affected joint.

Issues in Rehabilitation

1. The importance of sobriety and the need for ongoing support
2. Disulfiram (Antabuse)
   a. Action: Prevents full oxidation of alcohol (increased acetaldehyde), creating unpleasant flulike symptoms and chest pain that mimicks a heart attack in the presence of alcohol. It is useful in early recovery to help the person stop and think before consuming alcohol.
     (1) Disulfiram is highly lipid soluble, rapidly absorbed when taken orally, and quickly converted to active metabolite by serum enzymes.
     (2) It is further metabolized in the liver and excreted in the urine; its short half-life is due to metabolism by serum enzymes.
     (3) It has a long duration of action owing to the permanent inactivation of the enzyme aldehyde dehydrogenase.
   b. Nursing teaching: Some people are sensitive to alcohol in cosmetics or hand creams, mouthwashes, cough syrups, and other over-the-counter medications, so there is a need to be attentive to labels. Only give disulfiram to persons who have adequate impulse control and the ability to make informed decisions. It can be given on an outpatient basis after the person is alcohol free for 4 to 5 days. Disulfiram is contraindicated in pregnancy and in decompensated cardiac patients.
3. Naltrexone (ReVia) has been approved by the U.S. Food and Drug Administration for use with alcoholics in recognized treatment programs to reduce the incidence of cravings, particularly to curb further alcohol intake after a slip. For more information on naltrexone, see the section on opiate treatment.

Public Health Considerations

1. Know the resources in the community for appropriate referrals for evaluation and treatment.
2. Alcohol education, including the importance of responsible drinking, should be increased.

3. Early case finding of mothers at risk for having FA children.

CARING FOR PEOPLE WHO ABUSE CONTROLLED DRUGS

Statistics on Abuse of Controlled Drugs

1. Increases in the use of illicit drugs, including alcohol and tobacco, were reported by high school seniors in the class of 1994, marking the 2nd year in a row such trends have been reported and reversing a trend toward decreased drug use.
2. Current use rates are below 1981 levels, but both young and older students saw less risk involved in taking drugs than did previous graduating classes.
3. Emergency department records from 1991 to 1993 chronicle increases in drug abuse involving cocaine, heroin, marijuana, hashish, phencyclidine (PCP), and amphetamines. The only reduction was in lysergic acid diethylamide (LSD) (down 4%). However, LSD use has increased in some communities.

Legal Implications of Controlled Drug Abuse

The majority of funds designated for the "war on drugs" was spent on law enforcement.

1. Interdiction of supply received 60 percent of the money appropriated by Congress; however, this approach has not controlled drug availability.
2. Antidrug laws have not provided a sufficient deterrent to stop the use of drugs.
   a. The laws do not address the reasons people use illicit drugs, including escapes from poverty and feelings of hopelessness.
   b. Problems of insufficient number of law enforcement personnel, inadequate detention facilities, and backlogged court calendars mean that much drug traffic goes unchecked.
   c. Large amounts of money are involved, so corruption has been documented at all levels of law enforcement.
3. The level of violence around drug dealing and use has increased as rival gangs fight to control territory. Innocent bystanders have often become victims during turf wars.
4. Given the close association between drug use and crime, there has been confusion and ambivalence about treating the addict as a sick person or a criminal.
   a. Some addicts charged with crimes, particularly victimless crimes or those related to their own drug procurement, are given the opportunity to receive deferred prosecutions or deferred sentences for successfully completing drug treatment. This approach should reduce the likelihood of repeated offenses.
   b. When the addict is involved in serious crimes (especially against persons), treatment may be available while the person is incarcerated.

c. Dealers without addiction problems should be considered the same as anyone else involved in criminal activity; punishment is more appropriate than treatment.

Assessing People Who Abuse Controlled Drugs

Key signs and symptoms

a. Behavioral: Signs and symptoms are often tied to the progression of dysfunction. Note if the person refers often to substance use (being "bombed" or "stoned"), especially in idealizing the substance or the feeling. This may give a better indication of the importance of substances in his or her life than that obtained by direct questioning.

b. In users of central nervous system depressants (alcohol, opiates, sedatives): depression in combination with unreasonable resentments and jealousy, paranoid attitudes, social discomfort

c. In users of opiates: wearing long sleeves even in hot weather, being uninterested in hygiene and appearance, being preoccupied with obtaining and using drugs

d. In users of stimulants: paranoia along with the biochemical effects; feeling "special" because of the nature of the drug

e. In users of nasal cocaine: constantly runny nose, "sniffing," agitation, restlessness

f. In users of hallucinogenics and marijuana: withdrawal, self-absorption, paranoia, fear

g. In users of marijuana, hallucinogenics, and opiates: wearing sunglasses indoors owing to the effect of drugs on the pupils or to hide the eyes or the frequent use of eyedrops

h. In users of inhalants: telltale chemical odors; slurred speech; lack of coordination; unexplained listlessness, anorexia, and moodiness, especially in children and adolescents

Taking a controlled drug history (see the earlier section on taking a substance use history; Table 40–5)

Physical examination

a. Assess for drug injection, especially for the presence of abcesses.

NURSE ADVISORY

A pattern of the following behaviors indicates possible abuse of medications:

1. Vague complaints of psychologic distress, especially tied to drug seeking from the practitioner
2. History of lost prescriptions or stolen medications
3. Failure to follow up on referrals for testing or consultation
4. Pressuring for drugs
5. Sense of self-prescription through professional:
   • "I'm allergic to _____" (shifts away from suggested medication to drug with abuse potential):
   • "My former doctor always gave me _____"
   • "My neighbor takes _____"

b. Evaluate for possible endocarditis, a common complication of intravenous drug use (see Chapter 23).

4. Special diagnostic tests
   a. Blood or urine tests, or both, for the presence of substances. Some of these are expensive, and the nurse will have to specify which drugs are being looked for.
   b. Blood culture to rule out endocarditis. Echocardiography may aid in confirming the diagnosis.
   c. Complete blood count and serum electrolyte and enzyme levels to assess for possible disease states
   d. Test for the human immunodeficiency virus (HIV) as needed
   e. Weight changes (stimulant abusers)

Central Nervous System Depressants Other Than Alcohol

1. **Opiates** provide relief from anxiety, induce sleep, diminish the response to pain, quiet the cough center, and provide a rush of intense pleasure following injection.
   a. Mechanism of action: Opiates bind with specific protein receptors in the central nervous system and gastrointestinal tract. Opioid receptors are most dense in the brain stem, medial thalamus, spinal cord, hypothalamus, and limbic system.
   b. Classes of opiates are natural (opium); semisynthetic (heroin), synthetic (Demerol), and designer drugs. These are structural analogues, which are chemically identical to substances identified as illegal under the Controlled Substances Act except for a minor, insignificant difference. This allows manufacture and distribution to be legal. Fentanyl analogues have pharmacologic properties similar to heroin and morphine. They are known as "synthetic heroin," "China white," and "new heroin."
   c. Route and duration of action: oral, intravenous, intramuscular, or intranasal. The effects last 4 to 12 hours.
   d. Findings in intoxication: central nervous system depression, pupillary constriction ("pinpoint pupils"), depressed respiration, needle marks with intravenous drug use, scarred veins, inflammation of nasal mucosa with edema, drowsiness ("nodding"), lowered blood pressure or bradycardia, slurred speech, psychomotor retardation, and decreased body temperature
   e. Adverse effects of short-term use: Tolerance and physical dependence develop rapidly; therapeutic doses taken regularly over a 2- to 3-day period can lead to some tolerance and dependence (showing symptoms of withdrawal when the drug is discontinued). Many complications are related to unsanitary administration of the drugs or what the drug has mixed in it.
   f. Effects of long-term use (also due to the administration of adulterated substances versus the long-term effect of the drug on the system): increased risk for AIDS, increased risk for infections, hepatitis A and B, bacterial endocarditis, cardiac arrest, seizures, dermatitis, pulmonary emboli, tetanus, abscesses, constipation, hypoglycemia, neurologic disorders related to coma, and cerebral anoxia

Table 40–5. Controlled Substances—Uses and Effects

Drugs/CSA Schedules		Trade or Other Names	Medical Uses	Dependence	
				Physical	*Psychologic*
Opium	II III V	Dover's Powder, Paregoric, Parapectolin	Analgesic, antidiarrheal	High	High
Morphine	II III	Morphine, MS Contin, Roxanol, Roxanol-SR	Analgesic, antitussive	High	High
Codeine	II III V	Tylenol w/Codeine, Empirin w/Codeine, Robitussin A-C, Fiorinal w/Codeine	Analgesic, antitussive	Moderate	Moderate
Heroin	I	Diacetylmorphine, Horse, Smack	None	High	High
Hydromorphone	II	Dilaudid	Analgesic	High	High
Meperidine (pethidine)	II	Demerol, Mepergan	Analgesic	High	High
Methadone	II	Dolophine, Methadone, Methadose	Analgesic	High	High to low
Other narcotics	I II III IV V	Numorphan, Percodan, Percocet, Tylox, Tussionex, Fentanyl, Darvon, Lomotil, Talwin[2]	Analgesic, antidiarrheal, antitussive	High to low	High to low

Depressants

Chloral hydrate	IV	Noctec	Hypnotic	Moderate	Moderate
Barbiturates	II III IV	Amytal, Butisol, Fiorinal, Lotusate, Nembutal, Seconal, Tuinal, Phenobarbital	Anesthetic, anticonvulsant, sedative, hypnotic, veterinary euthanasia agent	High to moderate	High to moderate
Benzodiazepines	IV	Ativan, Dalmane, Diazepam, Librium, Xanax, Serax, Valium, Tranxene, Verstran, Versed, Halcion, Paxipam, Restoril	Antianxiety, anticonvulsant, sedative, hypnotic	Low	Low
Methaqualone	I	Quaalude	Sedative, hypnotic	High	High
Glutethimide	III	Doriden	Sedative, hypnotic	High	Moderate
Other depressants	III IV	Equanil, Miltown, Noludar, Placidyl, Valmid	Antianxiety, sedative, hypnotic	Moderate	Moderate

Stimulants

Cocaine[1]	II	Coke, flake, snow, crack	Local anesthetic	Possible	High
Amphetamines	II	Biphetamine, Delcobese, Desoxyn, Dexedrine, Obetrol	Attention deficit disorders, narcolepsy, weight control	Possible	High
Phenmetrazine	II	Preludin	Weight control	Possible	High
Methylphenidate	II	Ritalin	Attention deficit disorders, narcolepsy	Possible	Moderate
Other stimulants	III IV	Adipex, Cylert, Didrex, Ionamin, Melfiat, Plegine, Sanorex, Tenuate, Tepanil, Prelu-2	Weight control	Possible	High

Hallucinogens

LSD	I	Acid, microdot	None	None	Unknown
Mescaline and peyote	I	Mexc, buttons, cactus	None	None	Unknown
Amphetamine variants	I	2.5-DMA, PMA, STP, MDA, MDMA, TMA, DOM, DOB	None	Unknown	Unknown
Phencyclidine	II	PCP, angel dust, hog	None	Unknown	High
Phencyclidine analogues	I	PCE, PCPy, TCP	None	Unknown	High
Other hallucinogens	I	Bufotenine, Ibogaine, DMT, DET, Psilocybin, Psilocyn	None	None	Unknown

Cannabis

Marijuana	I	Pot, Acapulco gold, grass, reefer, sinsemilla, Thai sticks	None	Unknown	Moderate
Tetrahydrocannabinol	I II	THC, Marinol	Cancer chemotherapy antinauseant	Unknown	Moderate
Hashish	I	Hash	None	Unknown	Moderate
Hashish oil	I	Hash oil	None	Unknown	Moderate

CSA, Controlled Substance Act.
[1] Designated a narcotic under the CSA.
[2] Not designated a narcotic under the CSA.
From Black JM, and Matassarin-Jacobs E (eds). *Luckmann and Sorensen's Medical-Surgical Nursing: A Psychophysiologic Approach.* 4th ed. Philadelphia: WB Saunders, 1993, pp 2200–2201. Originally in *Drugs of Abuse.* U.S. Department of Justice Drug Enforcement Administration, 1989.

Tolerance	Duration (hours)	Usual Methods of Administration	Possible Effects	Effects of Overdose	Withdrawal Syndrome
Yes	3–6	Oral, smoked	Euphoria, drowsiness, respiratory depression, constricted pupils, nausea	Slow and shallow breathing, clammy skin, convulsions, coma, possible death	Watery eyes, runny nose, yawning, loss of appetite, irritability, tremors, panic, cramps, nausea, chills and sweating
Yes	3–6	Oral, smoked, injected			
Yes	3–6	Oral, injected			
Yes	3–6	Injected, sniffed, smoked			
Yes	3–6	Oral, injected			
Yes	3–6	Oral, injected			
Yes	12–24	Oral, injected			
Yes	Variable	Oral, injected			
Yes	5–8	Oral	Slurred speech, disorientation, drunken behavior without odor of alcohol	Shallow respiration, clammy skin, dilated pupils, weak and rapid pulse, coma, possible death	Anxiety, insomnia, tremors, delirium, convulsions, possible death
Yes	1–16	Oral			
Yes	4–8	Oral			
Yes	4–8	Oral			
Yes	4–8	Oral			
Yes	4–8	Oral			
Yes	1–2	Sniffed, smoked, injected	Increased alertness, excitation, euphoria, increased pulse rate and blood pressure, insomnia, loss of appetite	Agitation, increase in body temperature, hallucinations, convulsions, possible death	Apathy, long periods of sleep, irritability, depression, disorientation
Yes	2–4	Oral, injected			
Yes	2–4	Oral, injected			
Yes	2–4	Oral, injected			
Yes	2–4	Oral, injected			
Yes	8–12	Oral	Illusions and hallucinations, poor perception of time and distance	Longer, more intense "trip" episodes, psychosis, possible death	Withdrawal syndrome not reported
Yes	8–12	Oral			
Yes	Variable	Oral, injected			
Yes	Days	Smoked, oral, injected			
Yes	Days	Smoked, oral, injected			
Possible	Variable	Smoked, oral, injected, sniffed			
Yes	2–4	Smoked, oral	Euphoria, relaxed inhibitions, increased appetite, disoriented behavior	Fatigue, paranoia, possible psychosis	Insomnia, hyperactivity, and decreased appetite occasionally reported
Yes	2–4	Smoked, oral			
Yes	2–4	Smoked, oral			
Yes	2–4	Smoked, oral			

/ are schedules of various drugs.
hese drugs have no legal use (category includes investigative drugs).
Drugs with a high potential for abuse; known to be addictive.
Drugs with lower abuse potential than those of schedule II.
Same as schedule III, except they have different penalties for possession. Falsely considered by many people not to be addictive drugs.
Drugs with low abuse potential, may be purchased over the counter.

g. Overdose: Symptoms: loss of consciousness, pale, cool, clammy skin with cyanotic tinge, respiratory depression/arrest, coma, shock, convulsions. Management of overdose includes the use of narcotic antagonists such as naloxone administered intravenously. This will cause a dramatic reversal, but the person should be monitored closely because the action of the antagonist is shorter than that of the opiate on the breathing centers.

h. Withdrawal occurs when someone stops using opiates after 2 to 3 weeks of continuous use. See Table 40–4 for symptoms and detoxification protocols. Adult symptoms are yawning, gastrointestinal upset, restlessness, chills, dilated pupils, insomnia, aches, pains, upper respiratory symptoms (runny nose and sneezing), and profuse diaphoresis. Usually not life threatening. Infant withdrawal includes hyperactivity, tremors, frantic sucking, regurgitation, poor weight gain, irritability, diarrhea, fever, high-pitched cry, and seizures.

i. Drugs used in detoxification:

(1) **Methadone** can be used as an inpatient or an outpatient treatment to taper a person off opiates. Dosed according to severity of withdrawal symptoms, it is a replacement of euphoric opioid with a noneuphoric opioid.

(2) **Clonidine** (Catapres) transdermal patches are used to reduce the symptoms of withdrawal. Oral doses may also be necessary during the 1st 2 days because the patch takes time to deliver effective blood levels. There is currently no Food and Drug Administration approval for the use of clonidine for opiate withdrawal. A norepinephrine autoreceptor agonist, rapidly absorbed when taken orally, it blocks the symptoms of withdrawal, which are thought to be due to hyperactivity of norepinephrine neurons. It reaches peak plasma concentration at 1 to 3 hours, is lipid soluble, has a plasma half-life of 9 hours, is metabolized by liver enzymes, has no active metabolites, and is one-half of patent compound found in urine.

(3) **Naltrexone** (Trexan) is an opioid receptor antgonist that is used to block the opiate receptor sites to speed the person through withdrawal, usually in conjunction with clonidine to reduce the symptoms of the withdrawal. It is also in long-term treatment to assist in motivation for staying clean (see later discussion).

j. Effects of drugs used in detoxification

(1) Methadone maintenance (long-acting orally effective synthetic opiate administered once a day) may be used to stabilize the person by providing a long-acting opiate under strict supervision and connected with treatment. Levomethadyl acetate (LAAM) is being investigated as an even longer-acting replacement. The person must meet criteria such as a proven history of opiate addiction and a current level of addiction (demonstrate withdrawal sickness) before qualifying. The rationale for allowing a person to become addicted to the methadone is that there is a demonstrated reduction in criminal behavior, a reduction in or cessation of other drug abuse, a significant reduction of exposure to and infection with diseases transmitted by use of unsterile injection equipment and an increased psychosocial stabilization due to mandated treatment.

Researchers hypothesize that some individuals may be born with low endogenous endorphin levels or dysfunction in the endorphin system such that replacement narcotics permit normal functioning. For this reason, encouragement toward getting off methadone or reducing the dose may not be appropriate. Patient retention in treatment is high when the dose is high enough to cover withdrawal symptoms. Research finds that outcome (socialization and productivity) is improved with longer retention in the program. Owing to social stigmas (including in 12-step associations) against methadone use, the person who is stabilized on the medication may need special encouragement.

Levomethadyl acetate is a longer-acting (48–72 hr) opiate replacement drug currently available at approved narcotic treatment programs (methadone programs). It is not available to pregnant women.

(2) Buprenorphine is an opiate agonist-antagonist which at low doses acts like an opiate but at high doses blocks the opiate receptors and is used as a transitionary drug between methadone and naltrexone.

(3) Naltrexone (Trexan) is a long-acting opiate receptor antagonist that binds to the opiate receptor site so the euphoric feeling of opiates is blocked giving people less reinforcement to continue using because they cannot get "high". It is lipid soluble, effective orally, and rapidly absorbed with peak blood levels after 1 to 2 hours. Naltrexone is metabolized by liver enzymes and excreted in urine and has a half-life of 10 hours but converts to an active metabolite with a longer half-life. Its duration of action is 24 hours. Side effects include stomach irritation and mild elevation in blood pressure. There is less treatment compliance because, unlike methadone, naltrexone does not have mood-altering effects, and missed doses do not result in withdrawal. Many people have difficulty complying with a medication regimen designed to prevent, rather than cure, an illness.

Naltrexone may be appropriate and useful for health care providers recovering from narcotic dependency; it is the only narcotic-dependency medication acceptable to most licensing boards.

(4) Pregnancy: Heroin and methadone freely cross the placental barrier so the fetus readily becomes drug dependent. Methadone maintenance is often preferred over the risk of continued heroin use. Participation in a monitoring program and improved prenatal care are encouraged. There is a reduced risk

infection associated with unsanitary drug administration problems. The alternating toxic and withdrawal effects experienced by a substance-using mother results in an unstable uterine environment; withdrawal late in the 3rd trimester may precipitate labor.

(5) Breast-feeding: Heroin, methadone, and other narcotics are secreted in breast milk. A breast-fed baby could become opioid dependent from the mother through nursing. This does not preclude a methadone-maintained mother from breast-feeding, but nursing beyond 3 to 6 months may be inadvisable.

k. Pain management: An addict's physiology is changed in ways that necessitate higher narcotic doses for pain relief. When persons with addiction histories need pain medication, such as at times of surgery, they will need to be assisted in using narcotics appropriately, as well as in finding nonchemical ways of managing pain (e.g., medication, imagery, diversion, ice or heat, self hypnosis).

Barbiturates were formerly the treatment of choice for sedation and sleep induction. They are classified according to their duration of action.

a. Mechanism of action: Barbiturates are thought to inhibit the mesencephalic reticular activating system by interfering with sodium and potassium transport across cell membranes. Polysynaptic transmission within the central nervous system is also inhibited.

b. The chance of abuse rises with the rapidity of the onset.
   (1) Short- and intermediate-acting: Secobarbital (Seconal) "reds" can cause sleep or euphoria. Other barbiturates in this category are pentobarbital (Nembutal) and amobarbital (Tuinal).
   (2) Long-acting: Phenobarbital is used in the treatment of epilepsy; this form has even less protein binding, so it is less lipid soluble than short-acting barbiturates. Thirty to 50 percent of a dose of phenobarbital will be excreted unchanged in the urine.

c. It is believed that the persistence of low concentrations of barbiturates in the body may account for the "hangovers" after the therapeutic effect has worn off.

d. Care must be taken to avoid abrupt termination of these medications, because withdrawal can be life threatening.

e. The same drug may have different effects depending on the dose.
   (1) Sedatives reduce arousal and anxiety.
   (2) Hypnotics initiate sleep.
   (3) Anesthetics remove sensation.

f. Route of administration: oral or injected

g. Findings in intoxication: slurred speech, incoordination, unsteady gait, drowsiness, decreased blood pressure, and decreased pulmonary function. The additive effects of alcohol may lead to coma sooner than the use of barbiturates or alcohol alone.

h. Adverse effects of short-term use: disinhibition of sexual or aggressive drives, impaired judgment, impaired social or occupational functioning, impaired attention, irritability, lethargy, neglect of activities of daily living, accidents, and acute confusion.

i. Overdose
   (1) The toxic dose depends on the drug. An average would be 2 to 5 grams of barbiturate.
   (2) Symptoms: Slurred speech, staggering gait, sustained nystagmus, slowed reactions, lethargy, progressive respiratory depression evidenced by shallow and irregular breathing, and coma.

j. Drug interactions: The sedative effect is increased by the use of alcohol, tricyclic antidepressants, opiates, antipsychotics, and antihistamines.

k. Withdrawal: Barbiturate withdrawal is life threatening.
   (1) Assess the risk by asking how much the person has been taking ("How long does a prescription last? How many sources for the prescription?")
   (2) Symptoms of withdrawal are similar to those for alcohol: seizures (rare unless high doses are taken, usually shows up at the end of the 1st 7 days), anxiety, sleep disturbance, irritability, postural hypotension, hyperpyrexia, tachycardia, altered perceptions, depression, nausea and vomiting, sweating, muscular cramps, and nightmares; psychologic distress can persist for 6 weeks. Withdrawal severity varies with the half-life of the drug.
   (3) Infant withdrawal: high-pitched cry, tremors, restlessness, sleep disturbances, hyperreflexia, hyperphagia, diarrhea, vomiting, and seizures
   (4) Drugs used to stabilize withdrawal are similar to those used in alcohol withdrawal: longer-acting benzodiazepines.

l. Effects of long-term use: cellulitis or vascular complications after intravenous use

m. Pregnancy: Other than addiction, barbiturates do not appear to injure the fetus.

n. Breast-feeding: Barbiturates do cross into breast milk.

3. **Benzodiazepines** (e.g., diazepam [Valium], chlordiazepoxide hydrochloride [Librium], alprazolam [Xanax], clonazepam [Klonopin], triazolam [Halcion]) are the most widely used anxiolytic drugs and have largely replaced barbiturates in the treatment of anxiety.

a. Mechanism of action: Benzodiazepines reduce neural excitability by inhibiting the action of γ-aminobutyric acid (GABA).

b. Tolerance to sedation and ataxia develop rapidly, whereas tolerance for the antianxiety (anxiolytic) effect appears to develop slowly.

c. Overdose: drowsiness, loss of consciousness, depressed breathing, and coma; benzodiazepines are a lower risk in overdose than barbiturates unless mixed with alcohol.

d. Withdrawal: Symptoms are present if dependence has developed (if 10–20 times normal dosage is taken for several months).

e. Detoxification: Taper off slowly, usually using a longer-acting benzodiazepine.

f. Pregnancy: There is an increased incidence of cleft palate in mothers who take diazepam during early pregnancy.

4. Other sedative-hypnotics:
- **Quaaludes** have been withdrawn from the legitimate market, although counterfeit versions are on the street.
- **Ethchlorvynol (Placidyl)** is an older sedative hypnotic.
- **Zolpidem** (Ambien): benzodiazepine-like mechanism of action.
- **Meprobamate** (Miltown) was an anti anxiety medication widely prescribed in the 1950's with a high risk of tolerance/addiction.
- **Buspirone** (BuSpar) is a nonaddicting, nonsedating medication used to treat anxiety, and in higher doses is being used to treat depression. It is rarely abused.

Inhalants or Volatile Substances

1. Types
   a. Volatile solvents (e.g., glue, lighter fuel, paint thinners, degreasing compounds, gasoline)
   b. Aerosols (e.g., hair sprays, deodorants, vegetable frying pan lubricants, spray paints)
   c. Anesthetics (chloroform, nitrous oxide)
   d. Volatile nitrites (amyl nitrite, butyl nitrite)
2. Routes of administration: sniffed or snorted (inhaled by nose), "huffed" (inhaled by mouth; soaking in a rag and inhaling from it), bagging (inhaling the substance from an enclosed bag), and spraying (spraying the inhalant into the nose or mouth). This and direct ingestion of volatile substances are the most toxic methods because of pulmonary membrane damage and high dosage. Effects can last from minutes to hours depending on substance and dose.
3. Findings in intoxication
   a. At low dose the user is giddy and euphoric and experiences altered perceptions.
   b. At high dose there is numbing and hallucinations, unconsciousness, vertigo, incoordination, confusion, mood change, slurred speech, and impulsive and destructive behavior.
4. Adverse effects of short-term use: respiratory depression including suffocation, coma, lung tissue damage, brain injury, and poisoning
5. Withdrawal: The psychologic symptoms and physical symptoms are not well established.
6. Effects of long-term use: physical tolerance, impaired judgment; "sudden sniffing death" (may occur when the abuser exerts himself physically or emotionally such as in anger), possible long-term central nervous system damage, depression of myocardial contractility, cardiac arrhythmias, lack of coordination, weakness, inability to concentrate, and disorientation
7. Special concerns: These substances are used primarily by young people owing to low cost, easy availability, convenient packaging, and legality. They are responsible for up to 1200 deaths per year.

Central Nervous System Stimulants

1. Types
   a. Cocaine: refined coca leaves made into cocaine (salt form of the drug).
   b. Crack (freebase cocaine): An alteration in cocaine using ether or baking soda and heat, which gives a lower melting point so it can be smoked and therefore delivered to the brain faster and with greater intensity than any other method. Its popularity is due in part to smoking being a more socially acceptable route of administration than injection; to the reduced risk of acquiring HIV-AIDS by avoiding possibly contaminated needles; to its sale in smaller, more affordable units; and to the fact that in most communities there are more dealers (smaller amount of money needed to capitalize a "business").
   c. Amphetamines (amphetamine sulfate, Dexedrine, methedrine [crank]): artificial stimulants
   d. Ice: smokable form of methamphetamines
2. Mechanism of action: Cocaine and amphetamines block the presynaptic reuptake of norepinephrine and dopamine, leaving more neurotransmitter available at postsynaptic sites to keep up activation. The neurotransmitters at the synapse are eventually depleted; stimulation begins at the cortical level but ultimately migrates to the medullary centers.
3. Route and duration of action
   a. Insufflation or "snorting": 3 minutes until reaching the brain
   b. Smoking: 4 to 6 seconds to brain
   c. Intravenous injection: 20 seconds to brain
   d. Duration of action: 20 minutes (insufflation), 60 minutes (ingested); 5 to 7 minutes (injected or smoked)
4. Findings in intoxication: a "rush" (burst of energy accompanied by a physical sensation in the head and neck), tachycardia, dilated pupils, elevated blood pressure, insomnia, anorexia, and increased temperature. These are due to agonist action leading to central nervous system stimulation, agonist action on organs stimulated by neurons of the sympathetic nervous system, agonist action on receptors on heart muscle, and local anesthetic action, particularly on the heart muscle.
5. Effects of short-term use: increased confidence, elation, grandiosity, impaired judgment, paranoid thinking, disturbed concentration, psychosis, violent temper outbursts, hallucinations involving animals or bugs crawling under skin ("formication"), hyperarousal, hypervigilance, hostility, loquacity, and emotional lability
6. Overdose: seizures, cardiac arrest, respiratory depression or arrest, convulsions, hyperpyrexia, strokes, and death. Physical tolerance is experienced to the euphoria and self-rewarding aspects of stimulants but not to the effects on blood pressure.
7. Withdrawal: Fatigue, depression, apathy, anxiety or agitation, sleepiness, disorientation, and suicidal ideation may occur. Cardiac arrest has been reported following cocaine withdrawal.
   a. Little more than observation with hydration, rest, and nutrition may be necessary to physically stabilize the person.
   b. Antidepressants may be prescribed long-term during withdrawal and recovery. Amino acid replacement Tryptophan, especially for sleep, may be given in the first 3 days of withdrawal. Precursor amino acid treatment has not proved to be as useful in neurotransmitter rebalancing as had first appeared.

c. Carbamazepine (Tegretol) is 1 of several drugs being tried to reduce the cravings for cocaine.

8. Effects of long-term use: malnutrition, teeth worn down from bruxism, exacerbated hypertension, paranoid delusions and hallucinations (depletion of monoamine neurotransmitters and reduced sensitivity to receptor stimulation), scars and abscesses, depression or suicidal ideation, perforated nasal septum, chronic insomnia, chronic fatigue, severe headaches, poor or decreased sexual performance, and increased risk for AIDS.

9. Pregnancy
   a. Actions on the cardiovascular system of the mother and fetus result in constriction of blood vessels and decreased blood flow to the placenta. This diminishes oxygen and nutrient delivery to the fetus.
   b. Potential consequences: abruptio placentae, amonionitis, breech presentation, chorioamnionitis, eclampsia, gestational diabetes, intrauterine death, intrauterine growth retardation, placental insufficiency, postpartum hemorrhage, preeclampsia, preterm labor, premature rupture of membranes, and septic thrombophlebitis. Birth defects may affect the genitourinary tract, cardiovascular system, central nervous system, and extremities.
   c. Some studies have found no association between stimulant use and physical development defects when associated factors (prenatal care, lifestyle, multiple drug use) are controlled for.
   d. After heavy stimulant exposure, the infant at birth may demonstrate jitteriness, poor muscle tone, and poor feeding.

0. Breast-feeding: stimulants pass through the milk, creating tremulousness, irritability, startle responses, neurologic abnormalities, and even convulsions in the infant.

Psychomimetics

. Cannabinoids
   a. Mechanism of action: Tetrahydrocannabinol (THC) is the main alkaloid contained in marijuana. Its mechanism of action is uncertain.
   b. Route and duration of action: smoking, oral. Accumulation in fatty tissue permits cannabinoids to remain in circulation for up to 1 month after the last ingestion. Contains 400 to 500 different chemicals, 30 of which have psychoactive effects. Delta-9-tetrahydrocannabinol, which may act on benzodiazepine receptors, is recognized as the most psychoactive. When smoked, the dose depends on the speed of smoking, the puff duration, the volume inhaled, and the amount of time the user withholds expiration.
   c. Findings in intoxication: giddiness, dry mouth, reddened eyes, increased heart rate, impaired coordination and reaction time, increased appetite, and sensory distortion in higher doses. Cannabinoids tend to exaggerate emotions; they can act as a stimulant or a depressant.
   d. Adverse effects of short-term use: cough, motor impairment, and short-term memory impairment
   e. Overdose: feelings of loss of control, depression, nausea or vomiting, fatigue, and paranoia

f. Withdrawal: tolerance increases rapidly. Symptoms of withdrawal after long-term use include irritability, restlessness, decreased appetite, sleep disturbance, diaphoresis, tremors, nausea or vomiting, and diarrhea. Symptoms are fairly mild and not life threatening.

g. Effects of long-term used: lethargy, anhedonia, impaired learning and retention, personality changes, impaired driving ability, occasional flashbacks, anxiety, tremors, hallucinations, slowed speech and thought patterns, lung tissue irritation, moodiness, irritability, possible hormone disruption, delayed emotional development and "amotivational syndrome" (see later discussion).
   (1) Males: decreased sperm count and decreased testosterone levels with gynecomastia
   (2) Females: menstrual irregularities that may persist for months

g. Rehabilitation
   (1) Amotivational syndrome: occurs with prolonged use and is characterized by difficulty in planning and following through with plans.
   (2) The illegal nature of use may make it difficult to get accurate information to assess and treat the problem.
   (3) Recreational use: The drug was originally seen as benign; the lack of severe consequences compared with those of other drugs makes it difficult to motivate the person to change. With increased potency and compulsive use patterns, and addictive potential is being reevaluated.
   (4) Some individuals are reluctant to give up the drug because their high baseline level of irritability and ineffective anger management will return.

h. Pregnancy: Placental transfer of the drug is higher early in pregnancy; increased carbon monoxide level in the mother's blood creates lower fetal oxygen levels.

i. Newborns show increased tremulousness, altered visual response to light stimulus, and an increased startle reflex.
   (1) Disturbances of sleep and of intellectual development and behavior (inattention and hyperactivity) have been identified in prenatally exposed infants and children.
   (2) There are few or no effects on growth or physical development.

j. Breast-feeding: Cannabinoids pass into breast milk; no specific effects are noted.

2. Hallucinogens induce altered perceptions similar to dream states. These states are often characterized by bright colors and fluid changing shapes in the environment.
   a. Mechanism of action: Increased action of dopamine, seretonin (5-HT), and norepinephrine either by direct agonist activity or inhibition of reuptake.
   b. Types
      (1) Indole psychedelics: LSD, psilocybin and psilocin (magic mushrooms), morning glory seeds, dimethyltryptamine, ibogaine, yage
      (2) Phenylalkylamine psychedelics: mescaline (peyote), designer psychedelics (MDA [3,4-methylene-

dioxyamphetamine], MDMA [methyldioxymeth-amphetamine], ["Ecstasy," a combination of synthetic mescaline and an amphetamine], MMDA [3-methyoxy-4,5-MDA], STP/DOM [25-dimethoxy-4-methylamphetamine])

   (3) Anticholinergic psychedelics: belladonna, henbane, mandrake, datura, nutmeg, mace, and amanita mushrooms
   (4) Phencyclidine (PCP, or "angel dust"): This drug can act as a stimulant, depressant, or hallucinogen.

c. Route and duration of action: oral; lasts 2 to 24 hours, depending on the drug
d. Findings in intoxication: intense, distorted perceptions; impaired judgment and suggestibility; flight of ideas; intensification of the senses, dilated pupils, and increased blood pressure
e. Adverse effects of short-term use: extreme fright and nausea and vomiting from natural substances
f. Threshold toxic dose or overdose: depends on substance; can lead to psychosis, brain damage, and death
g. Withdrawal: generally believed not to occur
h. Effects of long-term use: panic with impulsive behavior, flashbacks, psychosis, anxiety, nausea, chills, tremors, rapid mood swings, depression, and visual hallucinations.
i. Pregnancy: Newborns of mothers who use PCP have increased emotional lability with a decreased ability to be consoled and poor visual coordination. Damage may not show up until months after birth.
j. Breast-feeding: These drugs do transfer into breast milk.

Anabolic-Androgenic Steroids

1. Anabolic-androgenic steroids ("rhoids") are used by athletes to enhance muscle building and strength, appearance, aggressiveness, and confidence despite negative consequences; they mimic the anabolic actions of testosterone with minimal androgenic effects: there is a shift to positive nitrogen balance as a result of increased nitrogen retention through improved utilization of ingested protein, but the effects may be short-lived.
2. Route of administration: oral and injectable
   a. "Stacking": alternating oral and intramuscular administration over several weeks to minimize the side effects and decrease the risk of detection
   b. "Cycling": taking the drugs for a 4- to 18-week period, then stopping, then restarting the cycle
3. Intoxication produces a stimulant-like high including euphoria, diminished fatigue, and increased aggressiveness
4. Effects of short-term use: tendonitis, disruption of the reproductive system, and infection from contaminated needles or poor injection technique
5. Effects of long-term use
   a. Impaired social relationships due to mood swings, psychologic dependence, "rhoid rage" (manic rage with possible violence)
   b. Increased risk of HIV-AIDS

   c. Bloody cysts in the liver (peliosis hepatitis), change in blood lipids leading to atherosclerosis (increases total serum cholesterol and lowers high-density lipoproteins), raised blood pressure, increased edema (due to retention of water and salt), and severe acne
   d. Males: baldness, atrophy of testes and decreased sperm count, and development of feminine breasts
   e. Females: decreased breast size, fluid retention, clitoral enlargement, increased facial hair, and deepening of the voice
   f. Pediatric: may cause premature closing of growth plates
6. Withdrawal: depression, fatigue, restlessness, anorexia, and insomnia
7. Rehabilitation
   a. To bypass denial, take a urinalysis of the person with a history of intensive weight lifting and athletic involvement when 2 or more symptoms not otherwise explained arise: dizziness, nausea, muscle spasms, urinary frequency, or menstrual irregularity.
   b. Human chorionic gonadotropin may be used to restart the body's hormone production after steroid abuse, but toxic effects have been reported.

Intervention

See Table 40–4 for treatment and Table 40–5 for the rehabilitation process.

◼ PREVENTION OF SUBSTANCE ABUSE

Health Promotion

1. Decrease or eliminate abuse and addiction by promoting health-oriented lifestyles.
   a. Institute wellness counseling, including monitoring of people in the community to prevent relapse/gain overall health improvement, substance use assessment, nutritional counseling, smoking cessation, weight loss, physical exercise, and stress management
   b. Reduce health risks in drug-using patients by providing information and strategies regarding more healthy ways to deal with life issues. Use the harm reduction approach (gradual modification of behavior to reduce risks).
   c. Education about alcohol and drug use
      (1) Include ways to modify behaviors (e.g., how to modify blood alcohol levels by eating food with alcohol, alternating alcoholic with nonalcoholic drinks, drinking slowly).
      (2) Educate the community and high-risk populations concerning the properties and dangers of substance abuse (e.g., FAS).
      (3) Employ stress management, values clarification, communication techniques, goal-setting skills, problem-solving techniques, time management, and assertiveness training to influence drug use decisions positively.

(4) Role model to demonstrate alternatives to substance abuse.

2. Early case finding: Include brief substance use and consequences tool such as CAGE as part of community wellness screening along with blood pressure, cholesterol, smoking, obesity, physical fitness, and stress.

3. Follow up: Reach out to those at risk; ensure successful referrals and prescribed treatment, and assist with reentry after treatment.

4. Support public policies and legislation to minimize social problems due to abuse and addiction.

◼ CARING FOR PEOPLE WHO ABUSE OTHER DRUGS

Caffeine

1. Oral, reaches blood plasma level within 30 minutes after ingestion, reaches peak blood levels about 60 minutes after consumption, and then fades in about 3.5 hours

2. Findings in intoxication: restlessness, excitement, insomnia, flushed face, diuresis, gastrointestinal complaints, cardiac arrhythmias, and psychomotor agitation

3. Effects of short-term use: nervousness and rambling flow of thought

4. Toxic or overdose: 5 to 10 gm (50–100 cups of coffee). Symptoms include diuresis, marked hypotension and circulatory failure, agitation, sensory disturbances, arrythmias, and insomnia

5. Caffeinism (chronic toxicity or poisoning): mood change, anxiety, suspiciousness, sleep disturbance, body complaints, muscle twitching, tremors, headache, ringing ears, dry mouth, lethargy, depression, palpitations, change in heart rate, change in blood pressure, nausea and vomiting, stomach pain, diuresis, and diarrhea

6. Withdrawal: headache, restlessness, lethargy, inability to work productively, and irritability

7. Effects of long-term use: gastric irritation, peptic ulcer, increased intraocular pressure in unregulated glaucoma, tachycardia, increased plasma glucose and lipid levels, and increased incidence of angina and myocardial infarction

8. Pregnancy and breast-feeding: Although no clear connection has been found between caffeine use and birth defects, women are advised to drink no more than 3 caffeinated drinks per day. Caffeine does pass into breast milk, and the child may show the effects of the stimulant.

Prescribed Medications

1. Consumers tend to ignore potential dangers because the drugs are prescribed by a health professional.

2. The dangerous practice of prescription drug sharing is common especially when resources are limited.

3. Prescription drugs are more likely to be used by women than men.
   a. More than half of the more than 121 million prescriptions for psychotropic drugs are written for women.
   b. Women are more likely than men to use pills to self-medicate and to determine their own dosage and frequency of use without medical consultation.

4. Prescribers are often pressured to increase or continue (or both) mind-altering medications.

5. Prescription drug use often starts with sleep problems, anxiety, or somatic complaints.
   a. Social biases against mental health diagnoses and counseling encourage the focus on somatic complaints, and a person may find it more acceptable to take medications than to deal with the root causes of the physical complaint or to identify the need for psychologic attention.
   b. The person may rationalize continued use on the basis of the original complaint, but with tolerance and addiction he or she will seek out multiple providers to obtain sufficient supplies of the medication.

Over-the-Counter Drugs

1. Patterns of misuse and abuse have been poorly studied.
2. Use patterns need to be documented as part of the medical record.
   a. Many people do not consider their use of medications such as cold medications (many of which contain alcohol) as drug use.
   b. Explore actual use patterns of medications. Package directions are sometimes ignored, causing rebound problems (e.g., with nasal decongestants) or complications when mixed with prescription medications.
3. Long-term use of laxatives, diuretics, or diet pills is connected with eating disorders and can cause life-threatening electrolyte disturbances (especially when combined with self-induced vomiting).

The Impaired Professional

1. Definition: A professional whose practice is or has a strong likelihood of becoming below the standard of care owing to chemical dependence or physical or psychologic illness.
   a. The American Nurses' Association defines "impaired practice" rather than "impaired professional."
   b. Drug diversion is often the 1st indicator of a problem rather than deteriorating performance.
2. Scope of the problem
   a. Six to 8 percent of nurses have alcohol or drug-related problems; 7 to 11 percent have psychiatric disorders.
   b. Two thirds of cases before state boards of nursing are the result of substance abuse.
   c. Physicians and nurses appear to have substance abuse prevalency rates on a par with the population as a whole.
3. Risk factors
   a. Family background: heavy drinking, death of 1 or both parents from alcoholism or drug addiction, alcoholic family member, or depression in a family member
   b. History of sexual dysfunction

c. Current life circumstances: divorce, or an alcohol-dependent spouse
4. Symptoms of impairment (patterns)
   a. Family background: family history of addiction, history of frequent change of workplace, prior health history requiring pain control, and reputation as conscientious and responsible
   b. Behavioral patterns
      (1) Increasing isolation from colleagues, friends, and family
      (2) Frequent complaints about family problems
      (3) Frequent reports of illness, accidents, and emergencies
      (4) Complaints from others about work performance, cooperation, and even use
      (5) Mood swings, irritability, depression, or suicide threats or attempts; may go from being irritable and tense to seeming calm or euphoric
      (6) Unusual interest in patient's pain control and medications, especially when an as needed medication is available
      (7) Frequent trips to bathroom or other abscences from the work site, especially after being in the narcotics cabinet (may be accompanied by elaborate excuses)
      (8) Requests for assignments that involve fewer people and less supervision, perhaps transferring to the night shift
      (9) Decreased work performance (e.g., sloppy or illogical charting, missing deadlines)
      (10) Being absent or late to work, especially after several days off
      (11) Sleeping or dozing while on duty
      (12) Increased errors in patient care and charting
      (13) Being on the unit when off duty
      (14) Eager to administer medications for others when they are busy
      (15) Manipulating possession of the narcotic keys for a particular shift (excuse may be inventory control)
   c. Physical symptoms
      (1) Odor of alcohol on breath or strong odor of mouthwash or mints
      (2) Tremulousness of hands
      (3) Watery eyes; pupils either dilated or constricted
      (4) Diaphoresis
      (5) Unsteady gait
      (6) Runny nose
      (7) Flulike symptoms
      (8) Weight gain or loss
      (9) Deterioration in personal appearance
      (10) Lapses in memory or periods of confusion
      (11) Frequent injuries to self
      (12) Clothing inappropriate to the climate and environment (covering injection sites)
   d. Discrepancies in controlled substances
      (1) Incorrect narcotic counts
      (2) Alteration of drug packaging
      (3) Patient reports of ineffective pain relief
      (4) Discrepancy among records of drug use (patients' charts, narcotic records, order sheets)
      (5) Patient reports of medication use that conflict with charted medication

(6) Records of large amounts of wasted narcotics
(7) More narcotic use on 1 unit than others
(8) Numerous corrections on narcotic record
(9) Use of maximum as needed doses when other nurses administer less
(10) Emergency department supplies missing
(11) Entire stock of a drug from the pharmacy missing, as well as the sign-out sheet (sometimes written off as an accounting error)

5. Clinical management
   a. Most frequently involves supervisor and representative of peer assistance program
   b. May include family
   c. Relies on the element of surprise and accurate recording of lapses of work performance, which are required to break through the person's defense system
   d. Need for structure and a plan for expected outcome
   e. Specifics of treatment (much the same as those for other persons)
      (1) There may be difficulty in assuming the patient' role.
      (2) Nurse self-help groups and peer assistance programs or medical professional groups can address issues unique to health care professional such as feelings of guilt and shame for violating professional standards of practice, anger with the profession, and work-related issues, especially about handling controlled substances.
6. Monitoring recovery: Need for clear return-to-work contracts
   a. May have limited or no access to narcotics cabinet
   b. Urinalysis (care about over-reliance on results; behavioral signs are more likely to be reliable in the long run
   c. Willingness to follow through with recommended treatment plan, including attendance at recovery based support groups such as Alcoholics Anonymous or impaired nurses group (may want to have verification) and work with a therapist, sponsor, or advocate
   d. Clearly spelled out consequences for failure to comply with the agreement
   e. Need for managers and coworkers to assess their own biases about recovery and allow for coworker's acceptance back in the workplace

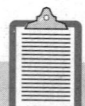

NURSING MANAGEMENT

When a problem is suspected, documentation of day, time, and behaviors will be valuable if you need to confront the employee, especially for an intervention.

▣ APPLYING THE NURSING PROCESS

NURSING DIAGNOSIS: Sensory-perceptual alteration R/T withdrawal from psychoactive substances

1. *Expected outcomes:* Following intervention, the person should be able to do the following:
   a. Achieve detoxification in a safe environment in 5 to 7 days
   b. Maintain homeostasis, including stable vital signs
   c. Not harm self or others during hospitalization and experience no seizures or hallucinations
   d. Be oriented to time, place, person, and circumstance
   e. Develop a trusting relationship with the staff, identify signs and symptoms of withdrawal, and request medication as needed
   f. Proceed with a recovery plan by the end of detoxification
   g. Begin to do own activities of daily living
   h. Become substance free and fully oriented to the unit by the end of detoxification.
2. *Nursing interventions*
   a. Assess degree of intoxication and determine withdrawal stage.
   b. Monitor withdrawal signs, especially pulse and blood pressure at least every 4 hours in early detoxification, to help determine the need for medication.
   c. Administer medication to minimize withdrawal progression or complications and to facilitate sleep.
   d. Offer food and nourishing fluids as soon as they can be tolerated, avoiding caffeine.
   e. Reorient the person to person, time, place, and situation as needed. Reassure that any hallucinations that occur are not real.
   f. Keep language clear and direct; avoid discussing feelings or lifestyle changes while the person is intoxicated or in withdrawal.
   g. Enhance homeostatic balance of the nervous system by promoting rest and sleep. Decrease environmental stimuli (e.g., bright lights, television, loud conversation) when possible.
   h. Assess risk of suicide.
   i. Teach about the process of detoxification, including signs and symptoms.
   j. Assess fetal development in the case of the pregnant substance user, and continue to assess even after birth; refer if indicated.
   k. Provide emotional support, maintaining a nonjudgmental attitude.

NURSING DIAGNOSIS: Sleep pattern disturbance R/T stimulant use as evidenced by verbal complaints of sleeping inability, nightmares, or interrupted sleep

. *Expected outcomes:* Following intervention, the person should be able to do the following:
   a. Have periods of undisturbed sleep
   b. Carry out measures to promote sleep within 1 week
      (1) Identify activities that promoted sleep in the past
      (2) Identify factors that currently interfere with sleep routine
      (3) Make a plan for regulating sleep, including diet management, daily activities, exercise, relaxation techniques, and environmental alterations
      (4) Identify and receive help in dealing with emotions that may be interfering with sleep

   c. Report feeling rested on awakening
   d. Identify how substance use affects sleep
2. *Nursing interventions*
   a. Determine the extent of sleep pattern disturbance, and monitor actual sleeping pattern.
   b. Provide exercise opportunities and a quiet, dark room for sleep.
   c. Establish which activities must be attended, and allow for rest in early treatment.
   d. Observe for anxiety; help with resolution of problems.
   e. Collaborate with physician to give non–mood-altering sleep medication.
   f. Teach sleep-promoting measures to promote normal sleep patterns (see Learning-Teaching Guidelines for Self-Care with Sleep Disorders).

NURSING DIAGNOSIS: Knowledge deficit regarding health risks involving substance abuse

1. *Expected outcomes:* Following instruction, the person should be able to do the following:
   a. Verbalize an understanding of the addictive process
   b. Verbalize knowledge of the effects of drug or alcohol use on the body; identify own consequences of use
   c. Define characteristics of the addiction, such as tolerance and compulsion and interference in social or occupational functioning, especially as related to own behavior
   d. Recognize the link between drug-using behavior and possible risks to health and identify own pattern of substance abuse as a chronic illness
   e. Verbalize the importance of abstaining from substance use
   f. Recognize and state (in simple terms) the physiologic basis for cravings
   g. Communicate the need for continued support outside the treatment setting
   h. Define the philosophy of self-help and support groups
2. *Nursing interventions*
   a. Encourage the person to identify the problem, and assess current knowledge about substance abuse and addiction.
   b. Dispel myths about chemical abuse by providing factual information about addiction patterns.
      (1) Provide a nonthreatening, nonjudgmental learning environment, allow an opportunity for patient feedback, including questions and reflections.
      (2) The teaching plan should include disease states associated with addictions; feelings associated with addiction; nutritional considerations; family interaction in addictive environments; and positive coping mechanisms, including improved communication skills, support and self-help group philosophy, and safe sexual practices and HIV-AIDS information.
      (3) Supplement information with movies, tapes, and printed materials.
   c. Direct the person's focus to his or her present situation. Focus on problems of substance abuse. Avoid distractions (e.g., outside problems, blaming others for

LEARNING/TEACHING GUIDELINES
for Self-Care with Sleep Disorders

General Overview

1. Insomnia can be the difficulty in getting to sleep or waking up and being unable to go back to sleep. It is not a disease.
2. Hypnotic drugs are taken to fall asleep faster or to sleep longer; most hypnotic drugs suppress rapid eye movement sleep, and when the drug is discontinued even after a single dose there is a rebound in rapid eye movement sleep with vivid dreams and increasing awakening.
3. After 3 weeks of continuous therapy, most drugs are no longer effective.
4. Rule out depression or other disease states.
5. The following symptoms indicate need for a referral to a sleep disorders center: Insomnia persisting 6 months or more that seriously affects daytime functioning; great difficulty staying awake during the day (especially if daytime sleepiness has caused an accident); sleep disturbed by breathing difficulties, including snoring with long pauses, chest pain, leg twitching, excessive pain, or other medical conditions.

Sleep Hygiene

1. Assess how much time you are actually asleep and awake.
2. Avoid lying in bed; get up and do a quiet activity for 30 minutes.
3. Assess how much food intake before bed helps or hinders sleep (carbohydrate snacks may help sleep onset, protein may inhibit).
4. Engage in quiet activities for a period of time before bed.
5. Avoid caffeine and alcohol: both can cause insomnia.
6. Participate in sufficient activity during the day to need sleep.
7. Increase your ability to deal with problems more effectively (e.g., get support).
8. Keep your bedroom just for sleeping.
9. Keep the temperature of the bedroom a comfortable one for sleeping.
10. Participate in nightly rituals before bed.
11. Keep the same bedtime; maintain a daily schedule for waking, sleeping, and resting.
12. Do not nap during the day.
13. Use "white noise" such as a fan for a noisy environment.
14. Try nonchemical sleep aids: warm bath, soft music, relaxation, and breathing exercises.

---

problems) by exploring underlying feelings, and then return to the task.

d. Identify problems in the person's life and their relation to substance abuse. Obtain history to demonstrate compulsion, interference in family, and social and occupational roles.

e. Identify potential relapse situations, and create opportunities for the person to rehearse alternative behavior.

f. Identify cravings as predictable occurrences. Explain in clear, basic terms how cravings occur physiologically. Have the person record triggers to be able to view their frequency and type (Box 40–5).

g. Include sources for family support in teaching about tools of recovery.

NURSING DIAGNOSIS: Self-esteem disturbance R/T unmet expectations, coping difficulties, guilt and shame about substance abuse

1. *Expected Outcomes:* Following treatment, the person should be able to do the following:
   a. Make positive statements regarding self-concept and report improved self-esteem, a sense of hope about the future, and faith in his or her ability to make positive changes
   b. Demonstrate increased confidence through sharing feelings within a group and in individual settings and through the ability to communicate assertively with others
   c. Recognize dependency needs and fulfill them using methods that are not self-destructive
   d. Realistically identify own strengths and weaknesses

BOX 40–5. Symptoms of Post–Acute Withdrawal Syndrome

The nurse can decrease anxiety in early recovery by teaching that the following are normal symptoms, which may last up to 2 years. Plans can be developed in advance to deal with them.

1. Increased desire for sugar
2. Periods of increased energy
3. Food binges, increased appetite, weight fluctuations
4. Jumping due to sudden noise
5. Fatigue during the day
6. Irritability and angry outbursts
7. Feelings of sadness, depression, tearfulness
8. Feeling keyed up and jittery
9. Marked mood fluctuations
10. Difficulty sleeping
11. Desire or cravings for substance
12. Dreaming about the substance

e. Identify emotions and experiences linked with cravings that occur during treatment

f. Replace feelings of isolation and self-defeat with active participation in treatment

g. Develop alternative methods of dealing with stress or conflict

Nursing interventions

a. Establish a trusting realtionship.

b. Assess for the risk of suicide.

c. Be accepting of the person and any evident negativism. Spend time with the person to convey acceptance and contribute toward feelings of self-worth.

d. Help the person to recognize and focus on strengths and accomplishments and how to build on them.

e. Discuss past (real or perceived) failures, but modulate amount of attention devoted to them to prevent feelings of hopelessness.

f. Identify choices to increase a sense of personal empowerment.

g. Provide positive feedback and support for life changes.

h. Help the person respect the strength of emotional links to substance use, and determine specific situations that the person must avoid during early recovery.

i. Monitor for grandiosity, excessive guilt, shame, or remorse.

j. Encourage participation in group activities from which the person may receive positive feedback and support from peers.

k. Help the person identify areas of change in self and assist with problem solving toward this effort.

l. Teach effective communication techniques such as the use of "I" messages and placing emphasis on ways to avoid making judgmental statements (assertiveness training).

m. Promote ongoing participation in support groups; encourage the person and family members to get sponsors if attending 12-step recovery-based support groups.

NURSING DIAGNOSIS: Ineffective individual coping R/T maladaptive reliance on alcohol and other drugs

Expected outcomes: Following intervention, the person should be able to do the following:

a. Complete a biography of substance use and consequences and demonstrate knowledge of the connection between substance use and coping strategy deficits resulting in negative consequences; accept personal responsibility for substance using behavior

b. Address issues related to family addictions, pain and stresses, or both that influence behavior during the active addictive disease process, recognize the negative effects of one's behavior on others

c. Communicate how life may be more manageable and less fearful without the addictive substance or behavior

d. Verbalize adaptive coping mechanisms other than substances in response to stress; develop acceptable alternative methods of dealing with feelings and situations

e. Accurately identify and appropriately express feelings

f. Exhibit increased feelings of self-worth as evidenced by verbal expression of positive aspects about self, past accomplishments, and future prospects

g. Identify coping mechanisms to be used to deal with emotions and experiences linked with substance use

h. Maintain abstinence from chemical substances

i. Demonstrate awareness of the role of various drugs in chemical use pattern and their potential to act as trigger mechanisms in relapse

j. Verbalize events that lead to increase of substance intake

k. Identify coping mechanisms and behavior strategies to use when confronted with the opportunity to return to the addictive behavior and demonstrate the ability to use these strategies while still on the unit

l. Identify actions to be taken in case of a slip; develop a relapse prevention plan

m. Participate in recovery-based support groups and report talking in the meetings.

n. Handle emotional situations appropriately and verbalize feelings; decrease risk-taking and impulsive behavior

2. *Nursing interventions*

a. Establish a therapeutic relationship, including appropriate limit setting and honest feedback.

b. Instruct the person in making a "biography," focusing on the way substance use has affected life areas such as relationships, health, occupation, socialization, and the like to see more clearly how substances have functioned as a stress modifier.

c. Identify key areas of coping deficits (e.g., lack of assertion, poor relaxation skills).

d. Identify ways to make up the deficits: list those groups or classes available in the treatment center, and encourage participation.

e. Give the person community resources for those specific skills training classes not available in the center.

f. Provide positive feedback for demonstration of new behaviors by the person while on the unit.

g. Promote involvement in recovery-based support groups, including a sponsor when involved in 12-step groups.

h. Encourage open exploration of feelings, particularly about the effects of addiction on the person's life, to promote motivation for positive change.

i. Help the person recognize and use strengths.

j. Help with a plan (alternative behaviors) for dealing with times, places, activities, and feelings associated with using that might be high risk for relapse.

k. Encourage expression of feelings about grief and loss related to loss of alcohol or drugs from life.

NURSING DIAGNOSIS: Altered family processes R/T role disruptions caused by substance abuse

1. *Expected outcomes:* Following treatment, the family should be able to do the following:

a. Regularly attend support groups or family programs (if available)
b. Acknowledge that the addiction has been destructive to the whole family
c. Identify the specific ways the addiction has affected the family system and each member individually (e.g., trust broken, feelings of shame and guilt)
d. Improve communication: recognize unhealthy patterns of communication, reduce blaming, avoidance, placating, and covering up; increase open expression of feelings
e. Develop a plan to support each member's recovery
f. Experience positive growth in social and family relationships
g. Identify strategies to enhance sexual functioning and satisfaction (sober sex) with partner
h. Participate in codependency treatment

2. *Nursing interventions*
   a. Provide education about the progression of addiction to the family.
   b. Assist family members to understand the nature of substance abuse, including the natural responses to deterioration of the relationship owing to substance use; identify specific patterns and behaviors of enabling, controlling, anger, and frustration.
   c. Help family members to find new patterns of communication; reinforce strengths.
   d. Assist the family in developing problem-solving and decision-making skills.
   e. Identify stressors that decrease family functioning.
   f. Provide family counseling or refer to an outside counselor for work on codependency issues.
   g. Provide written and oral information about self-help groups such as Al-Anon, Nar-Anon, Codependents Anonymous, Adult Children Anonymous, and other community resources.

h. Suggest a plan for each member of the family t identify needed behavioral and communication styl changes.
i. Support attendance at family support groups to fos ter greater understanding and healing.
j. Teach about addictions to children in an age-appro priate way.
k. Assist the family in doing a genogram to examin ways addictions are transmitted from 1 generation t the next.
l. Identify family members who may also have sub stance abuse disorders and refer for an evaluation.
m. Encourage exploration of sexual intimacy issues i the relationship with spouse or partner.

◼ DISCHARGE PLANNING AND TEACHING

1. If referred, collaborate with the treatment agency abou the person and the plan for the person's return.
2. Collaborate with other health care providers for follow up care of medical problems; set up an appointmen following discharge.
3. Have the person identify the support group meeting h or she will attend as part of the relapse preventio plan.
4. Identify community resources for the person and th family.
5. If medications such as disulfiram (Antabuse), naltrexon (Trexan), methadone, or antidepressants have been pre scribed, be sure the person has a supply at discharg and knows how to self-administer them (except whe dispensed by a treatment agency). See specific informa tion presented earlier.

Bibliography

Overview on Addiction and Drug Effects

Books and Reports

Ianaba DS, and Cohen WE. *Uppers, Downers, All Arounders: Physical and Mental Effects of Psychoactive Drugs.* 2nd ed. Ashland, OR: CNS Productions, 1993.
Julien RM. *A Primer of Drug Action.* 6th ed. New York: WH Freeman & Co, 1992.
Leccese, AP. *Drugs and Society: Behavioral Medicines and Abusable Drugs.* Englewood Cliffs, NJ: Prentice-Hall, Inc, 1991.
Ray O, and Ksir C. *Drugs, Society and Human Behavior.* St. Louis: Times Mirror / Mosby, 1990.
U.S. Department of Health and Human Services. *Sixth Special Report to the U.S. Congress on Alcohol and Health,* 1987.
U.S. Department of Health and Human Services. *Seventh Special Report to the U.S. Congress on Alcohol and Health,* 1990.

Chapters in Books and Journal Articles

Drugs and Drug Abuse Education Newsletter 25 (11 & 12), 1994.
Glover LV. The addictions liaison nurse and substance abuse issues in medical surgical nursing. *Addic Nurs* 6(1):13–18, 1994.
Gorman M, and Morris A. Developing clinical expertise in the care of addicted patients in acute care settings. *Addic Nurs Net* 4(4):106–121, 1992.
Hands M, and Dear G. Co-dependency: A critical review. *Drug Alcohol Rev* 13:437–445, 1994.
Kneisl, C. Nursing care of clients with substance abuse. *In* Black JM, and Matassarin-Jacobs E (eds). *Luckmann and Sorensen's Medical-Surgical Nursing: A Psychophysiologic Approach.* 4th ed. Philadelphia. WB Saunders, 1993.
Neiss R. The role of psychobiological states in chemical dependency: Who be-

comes addicted? *Addiction* 88(6):745–75 1993.
Salaspuro M. Biological state markers o alcohol abuse. *Alcohol Health Res Worl* 18(2):131–135, 1994.
Sands BF, Knapp CM, and Ciraulo DA Medical consequences of alcohol-dru interactions. *Addict Nurs* 6(2):56–61, 199
Santomier JP, and Hogan PI. Health impli cations of alcohol and other drug use: teaching module. *Addict Nurs* 6(2):46 53, 1994.
Solari-Twadell PA. Recreational drugs: So cietal and professional issues. *Addic Nurs Netw* 4(1):2–7, 1992.
Stammer ME. Cultural path effects o chemical dependency and recovery i professional nurses. *Addict Nurs Net* 1(4):17–19, 1989.
Sullivan EJ, Handley SM, and Connors H The role of nurses in primary car Managing alcohol-abusing patients. *A cohol Health Res World* 18(2):158–16 1994.

akoff B, et al. Advances in neurochemstry. *Alcohol Health Res World* 14(2), 38–143, 1990.

otta D, and Iisanti P. Nursing care of endocarditis: A common complication of ntravenous drug use. *Addict Nurs Netw* 5(3), 1993.

sessment

oks

nerican Psychiatric Association. *Diagnosic and Statistical Manual of Mental Disorders*. 4th ed. Washington, DC: Author, 1994.

es N, and Heinemann E. *Alcoholism: Development, Consequences, and Interventions*. 3rd ed. St. Louis: CV Mosby, 1986.

nney J. *Clinical Manual of Substance Abuse*. St. Louis: CV Mosby, 1991.

ssetti LM (ed). *Developmental Problems of Drug Exposed Infants*. San Diego: Singular Publishing Group, 1992.

th P (ed). *Alcohol and Drugs Are Women's Issues. Vol. 1: A Review of the ssues*. Metuchen, NJ: Women's Action Alliance and the Scarecrow Press, 1991.

urnal Articles

inemann AS, et al. Prescription medication misuse among persons with spinal cord injuries. *Int J Addict* 27(3):301–316, 1992.

nders JB, et al. Alcohol consumption, and related problems among primary health care patients: WHO collaborative project on early detection of persons with harmful alcohol consumption. *Addiction* 88(3):349–362, 1993.

derson CA. Detecting alcohol-related problems in trauma center patients. *Alcohol Health Res World* 18(2):127–130, 1994.

anscultural Considerations

oks and Reports

landi MA (ed). *Cultural Competence for Evaluators: A Guide for Alcohol and Other Drug Abuse Prevention Practitioners Working with Ethnic/Racial Communities*. OSAP Cultural Competence Series 1. Rockville, MD: U.S. Department of Health and Human Services, Public Health Service, ADAMHA (ADM) 92-1884, 1992.

5. Department of Health and Human Services. *NIDA Second National Conference on Drug Abuse Research and Practice: An Alliance for the 21st Century. Addressing Special Population Needs: Hispanics*. Rockville, MD: Author, 1993, pp 185–89.

hapters in Books and Journal rticles

lding JM, et al. Alcohol use, depressive symptoms and cultural characteristics in

two Mexican-American samples. *Int J Addict* 28(5):451–456, 1993.

Hallowell RA. Native American alcoholics. *Focus* Oct.–Nov., 30–44, 1991.

Ja DY, and Aoki B. Substance abuse treatment: Cultural barriers in the Asian-American community. *J Psychoactive Drugs* 25(1):61–71, 1993.

Johnson RC, and Nagoshi CT. Asians, Asian-Americans and alcohol. *J Psychoactive Drugs* 22(1):45–52, 1990.

Meyers RS, and Kail BL. Hispanic substance abuse: An overview. *In* Mayers RS, Kail BL, and Watts TD. *Hispanic substance Abuse*. Springfield, IL: Charles C Thomas, 1993.

Neft JA. Life stressors, drinking patterns and depressive symptomatology, ethnicity and stress-buffer effects of alcohol. *Addict Behav* 18(4):373–387, 1993.

Santisteban D, and Szapocznic J: Substance abuse disorders among Hispanics: A focus on prevention. *In* Becerra RM, et al (eds). *Mental Health and Hispanic Americans: Clinical Perspectives*. New York: Grune & Stratton, 1994.

Shai D. Mortality associated with drug misuse among blacks in New York City, 1979–1981. *Int J Addict* 27(12):1433–1443, 1992.

Szalay LB, et al. Vulnerabilities and cultural change: Drug use among Puerto Rican adolescents in the United States. *Int J Addict* 28(4):327–354, 1993.

Thomason TC. Counseling Native Americans: An introduction for non-native American counselors. *J Counseling Devel* 69:321–327, 1991.

Weatherspoon AJ, Danko GP, and Johnson RC. Alcohol consumption and use norms among Chinese Americans and Korean Americans. *J Stud Alcohol* 55(2):March: 203–206, 1994.

Tobacco

Books

Lynch BS, and Bonnie RJ (eds). *Growing Up Tobacco Free*. Washington, DC: National Academy Press, 1994.

Journal Articles

Leech TB. The stages of change in the treatment of nicotine dependence. *Addict Nurs* 6(3):86–89, 1994.

Alcohol

Books

Royce JE. *Alcohol Problems and Alcoholism: A Comprehensive Survey*. Rev. ed. New York: Free Press, 1989.

Journal Articles

The Alcoholism Report. 23(2), 1995.

Bradley K. The primary care practitioner's role in the prevention and management

of alcohol problems. *Alcohol Health Res World* 18(2):97–104, 1994.

Caetano R. The association between severity of DSM III-R alcohol dependence and medical and social consequences. *Addiction* 88 (5):631–642, 1993.

Day NL, Richardson GA. Comparative teratogenicity of alcohol and other drugs. *Alcohol Health Res World* 18(1):42–48, 1994.

de Boer MC, et al. Alcohol and social anxiety in women and men: Pharmacological and expectancy effects. *Addict Behav* 18:117–126, 1993.

Fromme K, and Dunn ME. Alcohol expectancies, social and environmental cues as determinants of drinking and perceived reinforcement. *Addict Behav* 17(2):167–177, 1992.

Klein H, et al. The relationship between emotional states and alcohol consumption. *Int J Addict* 28(1):47–61, 1993.

Smith MJ, et al. Reasons for drinking alcohol: Their relationship to psychosocial variables and alcohol consumption. *Int J Addict* 28(9):881–908, 1993.

Trice HM. Work-related risk factors associated with alcohol abuse. *Alcohol Health Res World* 16(2):106–110, 1992.

Amphetamines, Crack, and Cocaine

Books

Smith DE, et al. *Treating the Cocaine Abuser*. Center City, MN: Hazelden, 1985.

Journal Articles

Gawin F, and Klever H. Pharmacologic treatments of cocaine abuse. *Psychiatr Clin North Am* 9(3):573–583, 1986.

Nuckols CC, and Greeson J. Cocaine addiction: Assessment and intervention. *In* I. Nursing Interventions for Addicted Patients. *Nurs Clin North Am* 24(1):33–43, 1989.

Zacny JP, et al. Effects of setting on the subjective and behavioral effects of d-amphetamine in humans. *Addict Behav* 17:27–33, 1992.

Psychotomimetics

Gold MS. *Marijuana*. New York: Plenum Medical Book Co, 1989.

Inhalants

Crider RA, and Rouse BA (eds). *Epidemiology of Inhalant Abuse: An Update*. NIDA Research Monograph Series 85. Rockville, MD: U.S. Department of Health and Human Services, 1988.

Flanagan RJ, and Ives RJ. Volatile substance abuse. UN International Drug Control Programme. *Bull Narc* 46(2):49–73, 1994.

Sharp CW, and Carroll LT. Voluntary inhalation of industrial solvents. Rockville, MD: U.S. Department of Health, Education, and Welfare, Public Health Service, November 1978.

Recovery

Books and Reports

Gorski TT. *Passages Through Recovery.* New York: Harper Collins, 1989.

Jack L (ed). *National Nurses Society on Addictions. Nursing Care Planning with the Addicted Client.* Vols I and II. Skokie, IL: Midwest Education Association, Inc, 1989.

Marlatt GA, and Gordon JR (eds). *Relapse Prevention: Maintenance Strategies in the Treatment of Addictive Behaviors.* New York: Guilford Press, 1990.

Miller WR, and Rollnick S. *Motivational Interviewing: Preparing People to Change Addictive Behavior.* New York: Guilford Press, 1991.

National Institute on Alcohol Abuse and Alcoholism. *Motivational Enhancement Therapy Manual, Twelve Step Facilitation Therapy Manual, Cognitive Behavioral Coping Skills Therapy Manual.* Project Match Monograph Series. DHHS Publication No. (ADM) 92-1895, Rockville, MD: U.S. Department of Health and Human Services, 1992.

Smith DE, and Wesson DR, et al. *Treating Opiate Dependency.* Center City, MN: Hazelden, 1989.

Chapters in Books and Journal Articles

Massman JE. Normal recovery symptoms frequently experienced by the recovering alcoholic. *In* Galanter M (ed). *Currents in Alcoholism,* vol. VI. New York: Grune & Stratton, 1979.

Hoffman AL, and Estes NJ. Body and behavioral experiences in recovery from alcoholism. *Rehab Nursing* 12(4):188–192, 1987.

I. Nursing Interventions for Addicted Patients. *Nurs Clin North Am* 24(1), 1989.

Spear SF, and Mason M. Impact of chemical dependency on family health status. *Int J Addict* 26(2):179–187, 1991.

Prevention

Books and Reports

Cook PS, et al. *Alcohol, Tobacco and Other Drugs May Harm the Unborn.* DHHS Publication No. (ADM) 90-171. Rockville, MD: U.S. Department of Health and Human Services, Public Health Service, 1990.

A Manual on Adolescents and Adults with Fetal Alcohol Syndrome with Special Reference to American Indians. Rockville, MD: U.S. Department of Health and Human Services, Public Health Service; Indian Health Service, 1988.

Journal Articles

Barr HM, et al. Prenatal exposure to alcohol, caffeine, tobacco, and aspirin: Effects on fine and gross motor performance in 4-year-old children. *Dev Psych* 26(3):339–348, 1990.

Fitzpatric JL, and Gerard K. Community attitudes toward drug use: The need to assess community norms. *Int J Addict* 28(10):947–957, 1993.

O'Connor J, et al. Drug education: An appraisal of a popular preventive. *Int J Addict* 27(2):165–185, 1992.

Peterson PL, and Lowe JB. Preventing fetal alcohol exposure: A cognitive behavioral approach. *Int J Addict* 27(5):613–626, 1992.

Sexson WR. Cocaine: A neonatal perspective. *Int J Addict* 28(7):585–598, 1993.

Streissguth AP, et al. Fetal alcohol syndrome in adolescents and adults. *JAMA* 265(15):1961–1967, 1991.

Agencies and Resources

Addiction Research Foundation (ARF)
33 Russell Street
Toronto, Ontario, Canada M5S 2S1
(416) 595–6059
Education and research

Adult Children of Alcoholics
Interim World Service Organization
P.O. Box 3216,
2522 West Sepulveda Boulevard
Torrance, CA 90505
(213) 534–1815

Alcoholics Anonymous (AA) General Services Office
Box 459 Grand Central Station
New York, NY 10163
(212) 686–1100
Literature, audiovisual materials, information

American Academy of Health Care Providers in the Addictive Disorders
260 Beacon Street
Somerville, MA 02143
(617) 661–6248

American Council for Drug Education (ACDE)
204 Monroe Street
Rockville, MD
(301) 294–0600
Education, focus on high-risk groups

American Public Health Association (APHA)
Section on Alcohol and Drugs
1015 Fifteenth Street N.W.
Washington, DC 20005
(202) 789–5600
Policy formation

Children Are People Too
493 Selby Avenue
St. Paul, MN 55102
(612) 227–4031
Produces materials for and trains adults in prevention work with 5–12 year olds

Children of Alcoholics Foundation, Inc.
200 Park Avenue, 31st Floor
New York, NY 10166
(212) 351–2680
Program development, research

Drug and Alcohol Nursing Association, Inc. (DANA)
113 West Franklin Street
Baltimore, MD 21201
(410) 752–3318
Organization of nurses working in the field of substance abuse

Hazelden Foundation
Box 11
Center City, MN 55012
(800) 822–0800 (training and education)
(800) 328–9000 (educational materials)
(800) 257–7800 (Hazelden-Cork Sports Center)
Training and treatment.

International Nurses Anonymous (INA)
1020 Sunset Drive
Lawrence, KS 66044
(913) 842–3893
Provides a mechanism for networking and mutual support among recovering nurses

Narcotics Anonymous
PO Box 9999
Van Nuys, CA 91409
(818) 780–3951

National Consortium of Chemical Dependency Nurses, Inc. (NCCDN)
975 Oak, Suite 675
Eugene, OR 97401
(800) 87–NCCDN; (503) 485–4421
Professional organization, advocates for recovery and reinstatement of impaired professionals, certification

National Institute on Alcohol Abuse and Alcoholism (NIAAA)
Parklawn Building
5600 Fishers Lane
Rockville, MD 20857
(301) 443–3885
Sponsors research and information, some free

National Institute on Drugs (NIDA)
Parklawn Building
5600 Fishers Lane
Rockville, MD 20857
(301) 443–6480
Research, education

National Nurses' Society on Addiction
5700 Old Orchard Road, First Floor
Skokie, IL 60077–1024
(708) 966–5010
Professional organization; certification

National Self-Help Clearinghouse
25 West 43rd Street
New York, NY 10036
(212) 642–2944
Training, research, information and
  referral

Office for Substance Abuse Prevention
  (OSAP)
ADAMHA
5600 Fishers Lane, Room 9A54
Rockville, MD 20857
(301) 443–0365
Operates demonstration grant proposals,
  manages National Clearinghouse for
  Alcohol and Drug Information

Smokers Anonymous (SA) World Services
2118 Greenwich Street
San Francisco, CA 94123
(415) 922–8575

☐ OVERVIEW OF MENTAL HEALTH AND MENTAL ILLNESS

Mental Health–Mental Illness Continuum

Mental health is a lifelong process of successful adaptation to a changing internal and external environment. This successful adaptation is characterized by the ability to love, work, and create and to resolve conflicts within a framework of reasonability for one's group, age, background, and life experience.

Mentally healthy adults function comfortably within their society in contact with reality and in harmony with their environment.

Mental health is a relative, dynamic state. During the process of adapting to certain stressors, a person's usual level of functioning may temporarily diminish, such as during a crisis (see Chapters 37 and 39).

A particular individual's capacity to adapt to stressors is influenced by many factors, including genetic predisposition, childhood influences, previous related experience, physiologic health, and energy reserves.

Persons who lose the ability to respond to their environment in ways that are in accord with their own or society's expectation may be considered to be mentally ill or to have a mental disorder.

Mental disorders are characterized by thought or behavioral patterns that cause the person distress, impaired functioning, or the significant risk for these, again measured within the context of what society considers the norm. In a multicultural society, behavioral norms differ among cultures as well as from those of the society at large. Grief, or bereavement, is an example of a behavioral pattern with culturally defined norms. (See Transcultural Considerations.)

A person's mental state, or mental status, reflects how well that person is processing and interacting within the environment at that particular time (see p. 1902). An altered mental status does not necessarily imply the presence of a mental disorder, which involves a pattern of maladaptive behaviors persisting over time.

Incidence of Mental Illness

1. Approximately 22 percent of the population suffers from a mental or substance-related disorder (see Chapter 40) at some time in their lives.
2. As many as 50 million Americans are affected each year.
3. Up to 75 percent never receive treatment.
4. Anxiety disorders, substance-related disorders, and depressive disorders are the most prevalent medically diagnosed mental disorders.
5. Schizophrenia and depression are the most frequently cited reasons for mental health treatment.

Impact of Mental Illness

1. Impact on the individual
   a. An episode of mental illness interferes with how a person perceives and relates to others and the world.
   b. Persons with chronic mental disorders may have residual impairments in social skills and functioning, even between episodes of acute illness.
   c. Societal misunderstanding of some of the behaviors of mental illness has resulted in the "stigmatization," or marking, of persons with mental disorders as different, inferior, and to be feared or avoided.
      (1) Only 25 percent of surveyed Americans described themselves as well informed about mental illness, yet 33 percent reported having sought mental health assistance for themselves or a loved one.
      (2) Mental health facilities remain unwelcome in many neighborhoods and communities.
      (3) Depression is still viewed by many as personal weakness.
      (4) Movies and other media continue to portray both mentally ill persons and some treatments as dangerous and horrific.
   d. This societal stigma, in turn, produces a number of harmful effects on the already vulnerable mentally ill person:
      (1) Decreased self-esteem
      (2) Difficulty in making friends
      (3) Difficulty in finding employment
      (4) Reluctance to acknowledge (or receive treatment for) a mental disorder

2. Impact on family
   a. Family and friends bear much of the burden of care for the chronically mentally ill. To prevent acute episodes, loved ones try to protect the affected person from potential stressors, thereby increasing their own economic, social, and emotional strain.
   b. Feelings most often reported by family and friends are the following:
      (1) Shame and guilt surrounding possible family origins of the illness, be they genetic or environmental
      (2) Fear that siblings and children may be at increased risk for development of mental illness
      (3) Embarrassment, if bizarre behaviors are present
      (4) Powerlessness to influence behaviors or to plan future events
      (5) Prolonged, unresolved grief when the illness is chronic and debilitating.
   c. Services that family and friends request most often
      (1) Education
      (2) Support
      (3) Respite
      (4) Crisis services
   d. Economic costs to family have been estimated at $2.5 billion; the average family with a chronically mentally ill member pays $11,500 annually in unreimbursable expenses.
3. Socioeconomic impact
   a. Direct costs for treating mental disorders were $67 billion in 1990, $148 billion when indirect costs are included.
   b. Most persons with mental disorders do not receive care, including up to 5 million children with problems severe enough to require treatment.
   c. The "deinstitutionalization" movement of the past 25 years has reduced the number of resident inpatients by more than half. However, community resources have not kept up with the needs of these persons. Without sufficient support networks, the following trends have emerged:
      (1) Repeated, brief inpatient hospitalizations have generally replaced long-term hospitalization for the chronically ill. This practice is known as the "revolving door" phenomenon.
      (2) As many as half of the severely mentally ill complicate their situations with substance-related disorders.
      (3) There is an increase in urban homelessness—one third to one half of the homeless have a mental or substance-related disorder (see p. 1928).
      (4) There is an increase in the number of mentally ill persons who are in jails or prisons (see p. 1928).

Transcultural Considerations

1. Culture and mental health
   a. Culture determines what is considered appropriate or acceptable behavior. Eye contact, personal space, dress, and somatic expression are examples of norms determined by culture.
   b. What 1 culture calls mental illness, another may ca demonic possession, channeling, having visions, being under a spell.
   c. How to respond to patterns of abnormal behavio when to seek treatment, and from whom to seek (e.g., physician, spiritual healer, homeopathic herba ist, elder, exorcist) are also culturally determined. Fa tors that influence these decisions include the follow ing:
      • Religious beliefs and world-view
      • Relationships and support systems
      • Culturally approved healing practices
      • Stigma of behaviors and of seeking help
2. Culture-bound syndromes
   a. The Diagnostic and Statistical Manual of Mental Di orders (DSM-IV) describes certain syndromes, or clu ters of symptoms, that seem to be culture specific.
   b. These syndromes may be geographically localize and the behaviors may be quite specific (see Chapt 39).
   c. Less specific syndromes
      (1) Nervous or ataque de nervios
      (2) Mal de ojo or "evil eye"
   d. Industrialized nations also have culture-specific sy dromes: Anorexia nervosa and dissociative identi disorder are almost never seen in less developed n tions.
3. Attitudes of specific cultural groups: Many persons ethnic origin have become increasingly acculturated the dominant culture. The traditional attitudes may seen in varying degrees.
   a. Native Americans
      (1) Traditional healers, or shamans, combine spiritu and herbal healing practices. They take pride tradition and heritage, which include these pra tices.
      (2) Persons may appear reserved; they do not u touch casually as in the dominant culture, ar they do not express emotions demonstrativel Persons may have real difficulty discussing pro lems with strangers.
      (3) Many hold strong beliefs about the spirit of a d ceased person. Occasionally this develops in "ghost sickness," a preoccupation with death th may cause many symptoms of depression physical illness.
      (4) There is a high incidence of alcohol abuse in th culture.
   b. Blacks
      (1) Extended kinship ties have great importance; i creasingly, the head of the family is a matriarch.
      (2) There is considerable belief in the healing pow of religion.
      (3) Traditional remedies have included certain food or soul food.
      (4) The locus of control may be considered to be e ternal to self, especially in less educated person In these persons, there may be little future orie tation.
   c. Asians
      (1) Persons share a belief in a harmonious interactio

with the family as the social unit, deserving loyalty and not to be shamed. Elders are revered, and multigenerational families live together.

   (2) Eye contact may not be considered appropriate.

   (3) Health and illness are attributed to the presence or absence of harmony and balance; psychiatric illness may be considered as a shame to the family.

   (4) Views on suicide may differ from those of the dominant culture.

d. Hispanics

   (1) Family, religion (Catholicism), and culture are very important.

   (2) Family is male dominated.

   (3) Psychologic distress is often manifested somatically.

   (4) Substances abused are usually alcohol or marijuana.

   (5) Folk healers may be used; symptoms of mental illness may be believed to be caused by spirits; hearing voices or seeing visions may be culturally acceptable.

e. European Americans

   (1) Persons may have accepted the dominant culture; views on family are diverse.

   (2) Religious beliefs influence future or present orientation; they may also influence views on alcohol consumption.

   (3) Persons may ascribe more to the biologic model.

4. Nursing implications

a. Assessment and intervention require a trusting relationship and understanding of behaviors. This may require the following:

   (1) A skilled interpreter, one who can explain cultural nuances as well as translate language.

   (2) Increased self-awareness, particularly of nonverbal behaviors, such as touch, eye contact, and personal space.

   (3) Recognizing that cultural diversity may also mean a diversity in socioeconomic and educational levels and value systems.

b. A nonjudgmental attitude coupled with genuine advocacy for the patient may result in the examination of some long-held beliefs and values on the part of the practitioner.

   (1) Traditional healing practices, including herbs, foods, and incantations, should be supported unless they are considered poisonous.

   (2) Physical complaints may be the only acceptable outlet for great emotional pain and anxiety, including that of separation and acculturation (see p. 1916).

Legal and Ethical Considerations

1. Involuntary admission

a. Except in the case of a minor, only the potential patient may sign the consent for admission for psychiatric treatment. When inpatient treatment is necessary to prevent imminent harm to the affected person or others, that person may be involuntarily hospitalized through a legal process of committal. This judicial process requires "clear and convincing" evidence and after the evaluation of 2 clinicians.

b. Before the formal judicial process takes places, states incur an emergency detention process, and there is a finite period of protective custody to provide for the safety and thorough evaluation of the possibly mentally ill person who is at risk for harm to self or others. After this evaluation, the person may be committed, admitted voluntarily, or released.

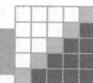

LEGAL AND ETHICAL CONSIDERATIONS

In most states, "competency," which is the legal right to make decisions, execute contracts, and manage financial affairs, is not compromised by admission to a psychiatric unit, even if it is via the committal process. Mentally ill people are considered competent unless there has been a separate competency adjudication.

   This competency affords clients protection to exercise their civil rights as well as the additional rights afforded to mental health unit patients. Involuntary admission (i.e., committal) only suspends the right to leave.

2. After admission to a unit, a person may request discharge at any time. State regulations, depending on the nature of the unit, may allow the care team several hours to consider the request. If it is denied, committal processes must begin.

3. Persons on mental health units retain their constitutional and statutory rights. The Mental Health Systems Act of 1980 included a recommended patient's bill of rights. It is the individual state's domain to enact such laws, and most have. Many require that the patient's bill of rights be posted clearly on mental health units, and some require the patients to receive or sign a copy.

LEGAL AND ETHICAL CONSIDERATIONS

Beyond constitutional and statutory rights, the patient's bill of rights often includes

1. The right to a clean, humane environment, free from abuse.
2. The right to appropriate treatment, in the least restrictive setting, with an individualized treatment plan and with the patient participating in the planning.
3. The right to refuse treatment, which is only rescinded in emergency situations or when incompetency is adjudicated.
4. The right to optimal freedom, that is, to have visitors, to go outside, to wear own clothing, and to use the telephone, unless restriction is specifically part of the treatment plan.
5. The right to confidentiality and to access of own records.
6. The right to information about rights and treatment, in language understandable by the person.

Data from Laben J, and MacLean CP. *Legal Issues and Guidelines for Nurses Who Care for the Mentally Ill.* 2nd ed. Owings Mills, MD: National Health Publications, 1989; Wilson H, and Kniesel C. *Psychiatric Nursing.* 4th ed. Redwood City, CA: Addison-Wesley, 1992; and the *Patients Bill of Rights,* Texas Department of Mental Health and Mental Retardation.

4. The right to be treated within the "least restrictive environment" is the basis for strict policy and procedures governing the use of seclusion and restraint. This right has been upheld in the courts, along with the right to refuse treatment.

◼ ASSESSING PEOPLE WITH MENTAL DISORDERS

Signs and Symptoms

1. Terms such as **psychotic, manic,** and **schizophrenic** describe specific clusters of symptoms of mental disorders but are often misused in the lay media. Box 41–1 defines frequently used terms.
2. Although delusions and hallucinations are classic symptoms of mental disturbance, they can be secondary to an organic medical process. Conversely, persons may be extremely mentally ill without psychosis.
3. Extremes on either side of the bell-shaped curve of "normal behavior" may signal a mental disorder, especially when these behaviors interfere with a person's functioning.
   a. Substance abuse, eating disorders, and phobias are examples of behavior excesses that interfere with daily living.
   b. Personality traits, such as suspiciousness or dependence, may also be carried to an extreme, signaling mental illness when they interfere with a person's daily functioning.
4. A professional examination is warranted whenever a person's thinking, judgment, or behavior veers significantly from a "baseline" personality. Examples are the following:
   a. A reasonably cautious adult who begins to spend vast sums of money
   b. A usually outgoing, positive person who becomes withdrawn and secluded
5. Mental disorders may interfere with physical functioning. Symptoms include changes in appetite, libido, sleep pattern, or general energy level. Signs may include weight changes, changes in hygiene, or changes in general appearance.
6. The severity of a specific mental disorder is related to the following:
   a. The degree to which symptoms interfere with a person's daily functioning
   b. Whether reality testing is impaired
   c. Whether the illness is a single episode or recurrent
   d. The person's level of functioning before and subsequent to the acute illness

Major Risk Factors

The lifetime risk for development of a mental health problem that meets the criteria for a specific diagnosis is approximately 1 in 5. Certain diagnoses have specific predis-

BOX 41–1. Terms Frequently Used in Mental Health

Affect—Observable, objective behavior that expresses a subjective mood or emotion. Affect is described as flat, blunted, appropriate, labile, or inappropriate.

Autism—Focused inward, sometimes to the exclusion of the external environment. May involve self-stimulation or highly individualized behaviors.

Compulsion—A repetitive behavior, often performed in a stereotyped ritualistic way. Carrying out the behavior is not pleasurable, rather it is intended to diminish the discomfort of not doing it.

Delusion—A fixed false belief, which is not congruent with a person's cultural beliefs. A psychotic disorder of thought content. Delusions may be categorized as grandiose, persecutory, religious, sexual, somatic, or nihilistic.

Derailment—See Loose Associations.

Hallucination—A sensory perception or experience that does not have an identifiable external stimulus. Hallucinations are often present in psychosis, although they may be the result of an organic disorder as well. One may have hallucinations of any of the 5 senses.

Illusion—A misperception of an external stimulus.

Loose associations—A pattern of thinking characterized by speech that shifts from 1 topic to another, with each successive topic only obliquely related to the preceding one, if at all. Also called *derailment*, because thoughts seem to gently slip off track, with little linkage. The rate of speech is normal to slow.

Mania—A syndrome characterized by an elevated, expansive, or irritable mood. Behaviors include hyperactivity, impulsiveness, inability to attend or to respect external limits. Inflated self-esteem, increased talking or writing, decreased eating and sleeping are seen. Thoughts are often described as "racing." Mania may escalate until psychosis results.

Milieu—The external environment of a person. This term often denotes the surroundings that may or may not be conducive to treatment. A **therapeutic milieu** is one that has been manipulated to produce a treatment effect.

Mood—Subjective experience of emotion; mood is relatively sustained and is generally expressed verbally. Mood may be inferred by *affect*.

Obsession—A persistent, recurrent thought that is difficult to dismiss or control.

Psychosis—A state of gross impairment of reality testing. Distorted thoughts, perceptions, or both are present. Judgment is therefore impaired when based on these thoughts or perceptions.

Schizophrenia—A mental disorder, usually chronic, which is characterized by periods of psychosis. There is also disorganization of thinking and disintegration of aspects of the personality. Not a "split (or multiple) personality."

Data from American Psychiatric Association. *Diagnostic and Statistical Manual of Mental Disorders.* 4th ed. Washington, DC: Author, 1994; Andreasen N, and Black D. *Introductory Textbook of Psychiatry.* Washington, DC: American Psychiatric Press, 1991; Carson R, and Butcher J. *Abnormal Psychology and Modern Life.* 9th ed. New York: Harper Collins, 1992; and Townsend M. *Psychiatric Mental Health Nursing: Concepts of Care: Community Health Supplement.* Philadelphia: FA Davis, 1995.

posing factors. Predisposing factors may be grouped into categories.

1. Biologic risk factors
   a. Genetic predisposition, anatomic abnormalities, and results of head trauma or brain insults all contribute to the risk of development of abnormal brain functioning that may manifest as a mental disorder. Schizophrenia and bipolar disorder are both widely recognized as being disorders of brain chemistry and having a strong biologic component.

b. Chronologic age: There seem to be "critical periods" for the appearance of the major mental illnesses.
   (1) Some disorders manifest in childhood by definition. These include autism, attention deficit and hyperactivity disorder, developmental disorders, and mental retardation. Some anxiety disorders manifest in early childhood.
   (2) Young adulthood is when schizophrenia and bipolar illness usually manifest, as do eating disorders and personality disorders.
   (3) Cognitive disorders are associated with increased age.
c. Gender
   (1) Female gender appears to be a risk factor for certain anxiety disorders, unipolar depressive disorders, eating disorders, dissociative disorders, and certain personality disorders. More females seek treatment for mental or emotional problems. (See Sociocultural Risk Factors.)
   (2) Male gender is associated with higher rates of antisocial personality disorder, attention deficit and hyperactivity disorder, and childhood disorders involving aggression (i.e., conduct and oppositional defiant disorders).
d. Physical illness: The presence of physical illness, acute or chronic, increases the risk for adjustment and depressive disorders. Seizure disorders, cerebrovascular illness, and endocrine disorders all have an increased concordance rate for mood or cognitive disorders.
2. Psychologic risk factors
   a. Coping skills, temperament, interpersonal relationships, and even genetics appear to be involved in the formation of a person's psychologic makeup.
   b. Different theories attach varying degrees of importance to the effect of early childhood experiences in the formation of character traits.
   c. Particular traits associated with mental health include positive self-regard, psychobiologic resilience, autonomy, and integrity.
3. Sociocultural risk factors
   a. Environmental stressors are associated with both psychotic and nonpsychotic disorders.
   b. Poverty and its deprivation are stressors that are concentrated in lower socioeconomic groups. Exposure to violence, trauma, and abuse is not limited to any group.
   c. Role overload, with its accompanying lack of leisure time and decrease in average night's sleep, is a current sociologic trend that increases vulnerability to mental health problems. Women in American society may be more prone to role overload, especially during the childbearing years.
   d. Relocation and the fragmentation of the family is a common stressor in American society. Members of cultural minorities and recent immigrants are vulnerable to a kind of "cultural overload" as well as to the stress of relocation (see Chapter 39).

Health History

1. Mental disorders may have physical symptoms. Physiologic disorders may manifest with an altered mental status. A complete history and physical examination, including laboratory testing, is warranted to rule out the presence of treatable physical illness.
2. For a patient with a mental disorder, the history includes additional information:
   a. Any previous history of psychiatric illness, substance abuse, or suicide attempts in either the person or the blood relatives
   b. A history of current and previous role and social functioning
   c. A corroborative history from a friend or family member describing behaviors and timeframe

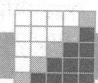

LEGAL AND ETHICAL CONSIDERATIONS

The person's right to confidentiality carries special significance in the area of mental health. Communication about a patient is limited to persons who have been specifically designated by the patient. The presence of the patient in treatment may not be acknowledged to anyone without a release from the patient. This may complicate history taking or validation.

The current third-party system compromises these rights in some areas when unknown insurance clerks have access to such personal information. Professionals must be cognizant of confidentiality issues, whether they involve not posting names on the unit or refraining from conversation about work, even when names are not used.

Physical Examination

1. Many states require that a physical examination be completed within the first 24 hours of psychiatric hospitalization; others allow several days.
2. Persons with chronic mental illness should have a complete physical examination with each exacerbation. These persons may have new concurrent medical problems, which they may have neglected or misinterpreted.
3. The physical examination includes a comprehensive neurologic assessment.

Diagnostics

1. Laboratory testing
   a. There are no specific laboratory tests for diagnosing a specific mental illness.
   b. Laboratory tests commonly ordered to rule out many physiologic causes of altered mental status include the following:
      • Complete blood count with differential
      • Chemistry panel
      • Thyroid profile
      • Blood and urine levels for intoxicating substances
      • Serologic tests for syphilis and human immunodeficiency virus tests
      • Arterial blood gas
      • Urinalysis
      • Urine culture and sensitivity
   c. Therapeutic drug levels may be ordered throughout a person's course of treatment.

d. The dexamethasone suppression test, once used in the diagnosis of depressive disorders, is currently rarely ordered.

2. Brain imaging
   a. Acute onset of symptoms, advanced age, or a history of head trauma increases the likelihood that a brain lesion is present. Imaging diagnostics are used to rule out the presence of such a lesion (see Chapter 18).
   b. Computed tomography or magnetic resonance imaging scans may reveal the presence of a structural abnormality (e.g., infarct, neoplasm, and hematoma) in the brain.
   c. Single-photon emission computed tomography and positron emission tomography provide graphic images of the metabolic activity (functioning) of specific areas of the brain.
      (1) Decreased activity in the temporal lobes has been correlated with depression.
      (2) Decreased prefrontal activity is seen in some types of schizophrenia.
   d. Electroencephalograms may detect focal areas of abnormal electrical activity, which may affect thinking processes, mood, or personality.

Mental Status Examination

1. More than a simple test for orientation, the mental status examination (MSE) is a comprehensive examination of the person's appearance, behavior, and patterns of thinking and communication.
2. Although direct questioning is involved, much information is acquired by quiet observation of behaviors (e.g., how the client communicates), the "process" as well as the content.
3. The MSE, which is usually administered by an advanced practitioner, and the admitting nurse's assessment data overlap in some areas.

Psychologic Testing

1. The physician may order psychologic tests to assist in the diagnostic process. A neuropsychologic battery is specified if an organic disorder is suspected.
2. Testing may be administered only by a licensed examiner and interpreted by a doctorally prepared psychologist.

3. Various psychiatric symptom rating scales may be administered by other professionals, including nurses. Table 41–1 includes some of the more frequently ordered psychologic tests and Table 41–2, the common psychiatric rating scales.

Nursing Assessment

Nursing assessment of the client with a mental disorder is a holistic one. Although the psychosocial aspects are emphasized, attention should be given to physical, emotional, and spiritual needs. Language difficulties or culture-specific practices that influence the person's adaptation should be addressed as early as possible. (See the chapters in Unit II.)

1. The nurse's ongoing assessment mirrors the MSE, but on a continuous basis. The nursing assessment includes the following:
   a. Observations of a person's affect, appearance, orientation, speech, and activity patterns
   b. Documentation of even subtle behavioral changes that can be instrumental in the diagnostic process
2. Assessment of potential safety issues for these patients is ongoing, including the following:
   a. Their ability to care for themselves safely
   b. The risk of harm they present to themselves or others
      (1) Most clients are not dangerous; however, risk must be continuously assessed throughout treatment
      (2) Suicidal risk may change dramatically throughout treatment; direct verbal as well as nonverbal assessment is required (see Chapter 37 and p. 1925)
      (3) A history of aggressive or assaultive behavior is the best predictor of future aggressive behavior.

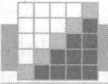

LEGAL AND ETHICAL CONSIDERATIONS

If a person needs to be restricted while on the unit, documentation must support that the person was a danger to self or others and that lesser steps were not effective.

Restrictive means might be the use of a quiet, seclusion room or physical restraints. Policy and procedure for the use of these means (e.g., regarding frequency of checks and release and duration of a physician's order for restraints) must be adhered to scrupulously.

Continual explanation to the person and reassessment of the need for the intervention are both legally (in provision of the "least restrictive environment") and ethically mandated.

Table 41–1. Psychologic Tests Frequently Administered

Information Sought	Test	Specifics
Intellectual functioning (IQ test)	Wechsler Adult Intelligence Survey, Revised (WAIS-R)	Scored on verbal and nonverbal performance. Mean = 100
Personality traits	Minnesota Multiphasic Personality Inventory (MMPI-2)	A true–false test of 290 items; scores are on different aspects or traits (depression, paranoia) with established norms.
Perceptions	Rorschach and Thematic Apperception Tests (TATs)	Client's subjective interpretation of pictures is analyzed.

Compiled with the assistance of Dora Winsorova, PhD, RN, and data from Andreasen N, and Black D. *Introductory Textbook of Psychiatry*. Washington, DC: American Psychiatric Press, 1991; and Batzer E, and Laraia M. Psychiatric evaluation. *In* Stuart G, and Sundeen S (eds). *Principles and Practice of Psychiatric Nursing*. 4th ed. St. Louis: CV Mosby, 1991.

Axis I—Clinical disorders and major mental disorders and other conditions that may be a focus of clinical attention
Axis II—Personality disorders, mental retardation. Includes mental retardation and specific developmental delays. May also list frequently used defense mechanisms. (See example.)
Axis III—General medical conditions
Axis IV—Psychosocial and environmental problems. Includes problems with support system, educational or occupational problems, and housing, economic, or legal problems.
Axis V—Global assessment of functioning (GAF). The rater assesses the individual's overall level of functioning. This is expressed as a number, using the GAF scale of 0 to 100, based on psychologic, social, and emotional functioning. The score is meant to reflect a point on the mental health–mental illness continuum. Problems that are derived from physical illness are not included. Comparison scores are useful and are often stated, comparing current level and past year or ratings at admission and discharge.

Example of a Multiaxial DSM-IV Diagnosis
(Axes I and II also have numeric codes, and all diagnoses that apply are recorded.)

Axis I:	296.23	Major depressive disorder, single episode, severe without psychotic features
	305.00	Alcohol abuse
Axis II:	301.6	Dependent personality disorder, frequent use of denial
Axis III:	History of peptic ulcer disease	
Axis IV:	Threat of job loss, marital problems, pending charge of driving while under the influence	
Axis V:	GAF = 35, current	

Data from American Psychiatric Association. *Diagnostic and Statistical Manual of Mental Disorders.* 4th ed. Washington, DC: Author, 1994.

DIAGNOSING PEOPLE WITH MENTAL DISORDERS

The Diagnostic and Statistical Manual of Mental Disorders, 4th edition, or DSM-IV

Published by the American Psychiatric Association, the DSM-IV provides the common language used by mental health professionals in the United States. It lists specific criteria necessary for the assignment of a specific mental disorder diagnosis.

2. The DSM-IV uses a multiaxial system of evaluation to give a comprehensive picture of a person's situation (See Box 41–2).
   a. Each of the 5 axes refers to a specific aspect of a comprehensive evaluation.
   b. Axes I and II diagnoses carry numeric codes that correspond to the International Classification of Diseases coding for worldwide statistical purposes.

Major Categories of Mental Disorders

1. In dividing specific disorders, each disorder must meet certain minimal criteria for its assignment.
2. Table 41–3 lists the major categories in the DSM-IV, as well as the central concept that distinguishes each major category.

CARING FOR PEOPLE WITH SCHIZOPHRENIA AND OTHER PSYCHOTIC DISORDERS

Definition and Key Criteria

1. Psychotic disorders are characterized by a loss of contact with or a distorted perception of reality. Perception, af-

TRANSCULTURAL CONSIDERATIONS

The diagnostic criteria for these mental disorders were revised in the early 1990s, and the difficulty of ascribing a unified set of norms to a multicultural society was acknowledged. In establishing criteria for most disorders, a fundamental principle is whether the behaviors are accepted within a given culture or whether the behaviors cause distress or interfere with functioning.

Areas such as sexual disorders and gender identity are value-laden for patients, their families, and health care professionals. Cultures and subcultures have differing views on these issues. It is the affected person's culture that must be considered, and it is that person's ability to function confidently within that culture that is the focus in psychiatry.

Table 41-2. Psychiatric Rating Scales

Information Sought	Scale	Specifics
Mood/depressive symptoms	Beck Hamilton Zung	All give numeric scores that are meant to reflect degree of depressive symptoms.
Thought disorders	Brief Psychiatric Rating Scale (BPRS)	Items measure psychosis and related behaviors.
Orientation, cognition	Mini-Mental State (Folstein) Short Portable Mental Status Questionnaire (Pfeifer)	5–10 min assessment of recall, orientation, concentration.

Compiled with the assistance of Dora Winsorova, PhD, RN, and data from Andreasen N, and Black D. *Introductory Textbook of Psychiatry.* Washington, DC: American Psychiatric Press, 1991; and Batzer E, and Laraia M. Psychiatric evaluation. *In* Stuart G, and Sundeen S (eds). *Principles and Practice of Psychiatric Nursing.* 4th ed. St. Louis: CV Mosby, 1991.

Table 41–3. DSM-IV Classification of Mental Disorders

Category Included	Core Concept	Major Diagnoses
Disorders first diagnosed in infancy, childhood, or adolescence (see Chapter 15)	The inability to attain certain developmental milestones and the functions, capabilities, and behaviors associated with those levels	Mental retardation Learning disorders Communication disorders Attention-deficit, hyperactivity disorders Autism Pervasive developmental disorders Feeding and eating disorders of infancy and childhood Motor skills disorders Tic disorders Elimination disorders Separation anxiety
Delirium, dementia, and amnestic and other cognitive disorders (formerly known as "organic disorders") (see Chapters 16, 18, and 40)	The presence of an impairment in thinking (cognition) or memory that is clinically significant and is a significant change from a previous level of functioning. The etiology is a general medical condition, as compared with a psychologic origin.	Delirium Dementias (e.g., Alzheimer's disease) Amnestic syndrome
Mental disorders due to a general medical condition	Occurrence of a mental disorder that is judged to be directly caused by a concurrent medical condition.	Behavioral change related to a general medical condition. The condition is named if known (e.g., catatonia related to frontal lobe lesion, or depression related to hepatoencephalopathy)
Substance-related disorders* (see Chapter 40)	Occurrence of behavioral, psychologic, and physiologic effects related to the taking of a drug of abuse, side effects of a medication, or to toxin exposure	Disorders of intoxication, dependence, abuse, and withdrawal from alcohol, amphetamines, caffeine, cannabis, cocaine, heroin, hallucinogens, and the like
Schizophrenia and other psychotic disorders (see p. 1905)	Characterized by distorted reality testing, an impairment in logical thought or communication, bizarre or disorganized behavior	Schizophrenia and its subtypes, schizophreniform disorder, schizoaffective disorder, delusional disorder
Mood disorders (see p. 1911)	Characterized by a disturbance of mood, persisting from 2 weeks to 2 years, which may be sufficient to impair functioning	Major depressive disorder Bipolar disorders Mood disorders due to a general medical condition Substance-induced mood disorders
Anxiety disorders (see p. 1914)	Characterized by the experience of anxiety that is more frequent, intense, or of longer duration than that experienced by the average person in everyday life. This abnormal degree of anxiety may result in the development of behaviors of avoidance, rituals, physiologic or psychologic responses.	Panic disorder Phobias Generalized anxiety disorder Obsessive-compulsive disorder Post-traumatic stress disorder Anxiety disorder due to a general medical condition Substance-related anxiety disorder
Somatoform disorders (see p. 1916)	Characterized by the presence of physical symptoms or complaints that suggest a general medical condition, but are not supported by or fully explained by the effects of a medical or other mental disorder. The complaints or preoccupation with them cause significant distress or functional impairment.† These disorders are often seen in medical settings.	Somatization disorder Conversion disorder Hypochondriasis Body dysmorphic disorder Pain disorder Undifferentiated somatoform disorder
Factitious disorders	An attempt to feign physical or emotional illness to assume the sick role	Factitious disorder, with predominantly psychologic, physical, or combined symptoms
Dissociative disorders (see p. 1916)	The essential feature is a disruption in the normally integrated functions of consciousness, memory, identity, or perception. It may be sudden or gradual, transient or chronic.	Dissociative amnesia Dissociative fugue Dissociative identity disorder Depersonalization disorder

Table 41–3. DSM-IV Classification of Mental Disorders (Continued)

Category Included	Core Concept	Major Diagnoses
...exual and gender identity disorders (see Chapters 30 and 31)	Disturbances in the processes that characterize the sexual response cycle, as well as sexual acts or fantasies that involve inhuman objects or produce suffering or humiliation in nonconsenting persons	Sexual dysfunctions of desire, arousal, or orgasm Sexual pain disorders (not due to a general medical condition) Exhibitionism Fetishism Frotteurism Pedophilia Sexual masochism Sexual sadism Transvestic fetishism Voyeurism
...ating disorders (see Chapter 10)	Characterized by severe disturbances in eating behaviors, not related to a general medical condition. A disturbance in the perception of body shape and weight is an essential feature.	Anorexia nervosa Bulimia nervosa
...eep disorders	A disturbance in the normal process of sleep—its initiation and maintenance—or its occurrence at the appropriate time	Insomnia Hypersomnia Circadian rhythm sleep disorder Breathing-related sleep disorder Nightmare disorder Sleepwalking disorder Sleep disorder due to a general medical disorder Sleep terror disorder Substance-induced sleep disorder
...pulse control disorders (not otherwise classified)	Characterized by the failure to resist an impulse or by the drive to perform an act that is harmful to the person or others	Intermittent explosive disorder Kleptomania Pyromania Trichotillomania Pathologic gambling

...djustment disorders (see Chapter 39)	The development of emotional or behavioral symptoms in response to an identifiable stressor. The symptoms must develop within 3 months after the onset of the stressor, and must be in excess of what might be expected.	Adjustment disorder
		    with depressed mood
		    with anxiety
		    with disturbance of conduct
		    with mixed anxiety and depressed mood

...rsonality disorders (PDs) (see p. 1917)	An enduring pattern of inner experience and behavior that deviates markedly from the individual's culture, is pervasive and stable over time, and leads to distress or impairment	Paranoid PD Schizoid PD Schizotypal PD Antisocial PD Borderline PD Histrionic PD Narcissistic PD Avoidant PD Dependent PD Obsessive–compulsive PD

Major DSM-IV diagnostic classes each include a category with a substance usage or a medical condition as the etiology (e.g., Substance-Induced Mood Disorder or Anxiety ...order due to a Medical Condition).
Note the important intentional difference in the next grouping.
...ta from American Psychiatric Association. *Diagnostic and Statistical Manual of Mental Disorders*. 4th ed. Washington, DC: Author, 1994. Copyright 1994, American Psychiatric ...sociation.

...fect, and thought processes are disturbed. This is evidenced by problems with logical thought and with communication and sometimes by disorganized or bizarre behavior.

Disorders in this group by definition involve a period of psychosis.

Table 41–3 lists the DSM-IV diagnoses that involve psychotic processes.

Incidence and Socioeconomic Impact

1. Schizophrenia afflicts approximately 1 percent of the population worldwide, crossing all cultures. This rate has remained relatively stable since statistics have been collected.

2. At least two thirds of persons with schizophrenia have

recurrent acute episodes of psychosis, with residual impairment to some degree.

3. Schizophrenia is the most frequent diagnosis for inpatients in county or state facilities and is the 2nd most frequent in every other type of inpatient psychiatric facility.

4. The cost of care for patients with schizophrenia exceeds $33 billion, with twice that amount being incurred in lost productivity.

Risk Factors

1. The most significant risk factor for schizophrenia is the presence of the illness in a 1st-degree relative.
   a. Siblings of a person with schizophrenia have a 10 percent risk, and children with 1 parent with the illness have a 5 to 10 percent risk of disease development.
   b. Twin studies show a concordance rate of 46 to 50 percent for monozygotic twins and 14 percent for fraternal twins (roughly the same as for any sibling).
   c. The diagnosis of schizophrenia is more common among lower socioeconomic groups; however, this may be a result of the effects of the illness or of the associated high stress of poverty.

Etiology

1. Although there are psychologic, sociocultural, and environmental theories for the cause of schizophrenia, biologic theories are the focus of most schizophrenia research.

2. The biologic theories include the following, either alone or in combination:
   • Genetic abnormality
   • Dopamine dysregulation
   • Viral effect (delayed)
   • Neuroanatomic defects

3. Most experts agree that genetics seem only to predispose a person (as evidenced by the twin studies). This predisposed individual must also be subjected to some other environmental stressors, in utero or afterward (e.g., a maternal virus in the latter half of pregnancy), to effect the anatomic and physiologic changes in the developing brain of the fetus (see below).

4. Maturational factors play a role in the manifestation of schizophrenia. Age of onset is between 18 and 30 years old in the majority of cases.

5. A precipitating stressor usually precedes the 1st and subsequent acute psychotic episodes.

6. The other diagnoses in this category have not been so closely tied to a biologic cause, although dopamine appears to be involved in the syndrome of psychosis.

Pathophysiology

1. The brains of persons with schizophrenia may differ both structurally and functionally from those of normal control subjects. The frontal cortex and the limbic system have been most studied.
   a. Computed tomography and magnetic resonance imaging studies show increased ventricle size, implying lack of brain development or a loss of tissue. Some limbic system structures, the thalamus in particular, also show decreased size.
   b. Positron emission tomography scans of persons with chronic schizophrenia show a below-normal activity level in the prefrontal cortex area when compared with control subjects performing the same task. This "hypofrontality" was present whether or not the persons with schizophrenia had ever taken antipsychotic medication.

2. Dopamine, as well as other neurotransmitters, appears to be out of balance.
   a. An excessive amount of dopamine in certain areas produces the delusions and hallucinations.
   b. A deficit of dopamine in other areas may account for the withdrawn symptoms, such as anergy and flattened affect.

Clinical Manifestations

1. Delusions, hallucinations, disorganized thoughts, and bizarre behaviors are the hallmark of schizophrenia and other psychotic disorders.

2. These "positive symptoms" of schizophrenia are obvious by their presence; "negative symptoms" refer to the absence or diminution of normal characteristics. Table 41-4 lists both the positive and negative symptoms. There is no one symptom specific to this illness.

3. Positive symptoms are more prominent during acute psychotic exacerbations; the negative symptoms tend to be more chronic and are less responsive to medication.

Table 41–4. Positive and Negative Symptoms of Schizophrenia

Positive Symptoms	Negative Symptoms
Delusions	Apathy Poor hygiene Lack of persistence
Hallucinations	Inattentiveness
Bizarre behaviors Inappropriate acts (social, sexual, aggressive) Bizarre clothing, appearance	Affective flattening Decreased facial expression or spontaneous movements Lack of vocal inflection
Formal thought disorder Marked by tangentiality, looseness of associations, incoherence or illogicality	Associality Impaired intimacy, few activities
	Alogia Poverty of speech, blocking

Adapted from Andreasen NC. The diagnosis of schizophrenia. *Schizophr Bull* 13:9, 1987.

4. A generalized decline in social functioning and self-care accompanies whatever other symptoms are present when the diagnosis is schizophrenia.

5. Other mental disorders that include psychosis (cognitive, mood, delusions, and substance-related disorders) share some of these positive symptoms, without the generalized decline, disorganization, and negative symptoms more specific to schizophrenia. Other psychotic disorders do not involve the disintegration of the personality. Persons with delusional disorders, for example, often continue to function quite well in society. (Refer to DSM-IV.)

Diagnostics

1. As with any mental disorder, physiologic causes must be ruled out (see pp. 1902–1903).
2. The history and MSE remain the primary assessment tools. The diagnosis of schizophrenia requires that several DSM-IV criteria be met.
   a. Disordered thinking is evidenced in both the thought content and form (how it is communicated). The MSE is challenging when communication is tangential, loose, or does not follow generally accepted usage.
   b. Perceptual disturbances may need to be inferred by observing a patient's behavior. For example, a person may appear to be listening or responding to some stimulus, yet may verbally deny hallucinations. Auditory hallucinations are the most prevalent in schizophrenia.
   c. Affect, behavior, cognition, sense of self, and relationship to the world are disintegrated in schizophrenia, sometimes seeming incongruent and disconnected. The person may behave bizarrely.
3. Nursing assessment includes observing the person for evidence of physical illness and deficits in self-care as well as the person's interaction with the environment and other people.

Complications

1. Persons with schizophrenia report a rate of alcohol disorders 10 times greater than their peers; drug use disorders are 7 times greater.
2. Approximately 1 in 10 persons with schizophrenia eventually commits suicide; clinical depression develops in 6 in 10.
3. Physical illnesses may go unnoticed or untreated in these persons. Life expectancy is shortened by these illnesses, accidents, vulnerability to violent crime, and increased rate of suicide.
4. With typical onset in young adulthood, schizophrenia can prevent the achievement of life potential. Declining social and occupational functioning may contribute to permanent disability.

Clinical Management (see p. 1919)

1. Treatment goals
   a. Maintenance of safety for the person experiencing psychosis
   b. Relief of psychotic symptoms

   c. A return to the highest possible level of functioning
2. Nonpharmacologic interventions
   a. Provision of a safe, structured environment
      (1) This may be in the hospital, day treatment center, boarding home, or person's own home.
      (2) Extreme situations may require the use of a quiet room or restraints if the client is in imminent danger to self or others.
      (3) The "least restrictive environment" must always be used to achieve safety and security goals (see Special Medical–Surgical Procedures).
   b. Psychotherapy
      (1) For the chronic schizophrenic patient, psychotherapy is more reality focused and practical, offering support and encouraging specific problem-solving and coping strategies.
      (2) Family therapy is also focused on coping and adapting to the challenges of having a member of the family with chronic mental illness.
   c. Psychoeducation, which is the current term used for the process of teaching the patient and family members about the illness, symptom recognition, and management
   d. Activity and recreational therapies
      (1) Occupational and recreational therapists assess current functioning and assist the client to learn and improve skills for living.
      (2) Vocational rehabilitation may help those with severe illness learn job skills and find employment.
   e. Milieu therapy
      (1) For persons with psychotic disorders, a safe environment is provided as previously described.
      (2) Stimuli may need to be decreased or increased (as distraction) for persons who are bothered by auditory or visual hallucinations.
3. Pharmacologic interventions
   a. Antipsychotic medications are used during psychotic episodes; maintenance doses may be necessary for life (see p. 1919).
   b. The short-term extrapyramidal side effects of antipsychotic medications are alleviated by anticholinergic, antihistaminic, gabaergic, and dopaminergic medications (see p. 1919).
   c. Lorazepam, lithium, propranolol, and carbamazepine have each been used to augment the efficacy of the antipsychotic drugs in selected cases (see p. 1919).
4. Special procedures
   a. When patients are unable to control aggressive impulses, the use of a quiet room or seclusion or restraints may be ordered by the physician.
   b. The nurse's early assessment of escalating behavior and prompt intervention, with talk or pharmacotherapy, often eliminate the need for these more restrictive means.

Applying the Nursing Process

NURSING DIAGNOSIS: Social isolation R/T altered sensory perceptions—auditory hallucinations and autistic withdrawal as evidenced by remaining in room, verbally responding to unseen stimuli, and attempting to plug ear canals

LEARNING/TEACHING GUIDELINES
for Persons with Chronic Mental Illness

General Overview

1. Chronic mental illness is thought to be the result of a combination of biologic and situational factors.
2. As with other chronic illnesses, there are periods of stability and periods when symptoms worsen. Medication may be required for long periods, perhaps throughout life, and their effects may be unpleasant.
3. People can help themselves or family members by learning about the illness, what factors they can control, how to manage medication, and where and when to get more help.
4. Teaching should be kept simple. Even with sufficient education and no language barrier, some illnesses affect the thought processes, and people lose the ability to abstract, or concentrate.
5. If there have been problems with trust, the educator should be a person familiar to the person, not someone new.
6. Denial of one's illness—or one's control over it—may go on for years. This is complicated by the fact that it is the organ of thinking and reasoning itself that is affected.

Medication Education

1. Antipsychotic drugs (all psychotropic medications) affect chemical systems in the brain. This results in improvement in symptoms as well as other effects that may be frustrating.
2. It is important for the patient to stay on the medication, even when he or she is feeling better. This reduces the chances of another flare-up of the illness.
3. These medications do not cause a high feeling, are not addicting, and have no street value.
4. Some side effects (dry mouth, blurred vision) diminish as tolerance develops. Occasionally, a new side effect can develop over time. Persons should be encouraged to write down questions and ask a health care professional. Written material given to the persons should have clear, concrete examples.

5. If blood samples are to be drawn, the person should take evening medication, but not the morning dose.
6. If a sore throat or fever develops, it could be serious. Specific medications (clozapine, lithium, monoamine oxidase inhibitors) have potentially lethal adverse effects. Persons should be able to recite their warning signs and carry information about the drugs with them.
7. Restlessness (akathisia), weight gain, and mental dullness are side effects that contribute significantly to noncompliance. Medication can help the restless feelings; each person needs to learn individual dietary limits. Diabetes and cultural dietary habits must be considered. A dietitian may be able to help, depending on the person's receptiveness.
8. Frustrations with symptoms or side effects contribute to the high rate of substance abuse in persons with mental disorders.
9. Other substances—cultural remedies, over-the-counter medications, street drugs, alcohol—can interfere with thinking, symptoms, or medication. The health care professional must ask specific questions, but in a nonjudgmental way. A tone should be set for the person to feel comfortable in discussing any and all substances being used. Concrete thinking and lack of trust often lead to communication breakdowns.
10. Mentally ill persons are unable to tolerate many of the stressors that are considered routine. Family and friends' expectations of these persons should be examined. Nonpharmacologic interventions may include long-term participation in psychoeducational sessions and support groups by all concerned.
11. The gradual acceptance of responsibility for some aspects of the illness and recognition of the limits of control may never be achieved. A spiritual belief system may be helpful. Cultural views may help or contribute to stigma. These aspects are important to consider in planning an individual's education and discharge.

---

1. *Expected outcomes:* After interventions the person should be able to do the following:
   a. Spend 50 percent of the day shift out of the room by time of discharge
   b. Interact with other persons at least minimally in 2 activities a day, with improved attention to outside stimuli
   c. Verbally report absence or minimal interference from voices
2. *Nursing interventions*
   a. Make brief one-to-one contact with the patient, frequently but without demands. Allow much personal space.
   b. Observe the patient for evidence of listening behav-

iors or of talking to unseen stimuli. Observe the patient for changes in affect or behavior, which suggest that voices are more menacing. If changes are noted ask the person about thoughts or plans to harm sel (see pp. 1913 and 1925).
   c. As the relationship builds, explain about illness and the voices; teach the patient to use distraction to interrupt or decrease the interference.
   d. Explain in concrete terms how medication will help with the voices (Learning/Teaching Guidelines for Persons with Chronic Mental Illness).
   e. Initially take medication to the person; gradually request that the person come to the station to receive it

f. Accompany the person out of the room for brief interaction; gradually increase time out of room, praise each effort and allow the person to retreat if feeling threatened.

Expected outcomes: Following interventions the person (and family) should be able to do the following:
a. Explain that the illness affects some brain processes, causing certain symptoms
b. Recognize behaviors and symptoms that are a result of the illness
c. Recite several nonpharmacologic methods of dealing with symptoms
d. Recite medication regimen, how to deal with side effects, and when to call or return to see the mental health professional
e. Demonstrate more than 95 percent compliance with medications at first follow-up appointment
Nursing interventions: see Learning/Teaching Guidelines for Persons with Chronic Mental Illness

Prognosis

Brief psychotic disorder lasts less than 1 month with no residual impairment.
Schizophreniform disorders and mood disorders with psychotic features are likely to be chronic illnesses, with varied levels of residual impairment.
The prognosis for a psychotic disorder due to a medical condition depends on the nature of the organic illness.

Discharge Planning and Teaching

Medication education is paramount; approximately 50 percent of clients with schizophrenia are noncompliant with medication.
Education about the disorder as well as sources for aftercare support is essential for both patients and their families. First appointments should be made before discharge. Increased stress in the environment may precipitate a relapse. Professionals in other disciplines should be consulted to foster a predictable, structured lifestyle and case management in the aftercare plan.

CARING FOR PEOPLE WITH MOOD DISORDERS

Definition and Key Criteria

This group is characterized by the development of an abnormal mood, which may last from 2 weeks to 2 years. Mood disorders occur as clusters of recurrent symptoms in the patient. They are categorized as bipolar (periods of high and depressed mood) or depressive (unipolar) disorders.
3. Symptoms may be insufficient to interfere with functioning or they may be severe enough to cause impaired judgment or psychosis.
4. Mood disorders may be primary or related to substance usage or a general medical condition.
5. Diagnoses of mood disorders as defined by the DSM-IV
   • Major depressive disorder
   • Dysthymic disorder
   • Depressive disorder, not otherwise specified
   • Bipolar I disorder
   • Bipolar II disorders
   • Cyclothymic disorder
   • Bipolar disorder, not otherwise specified
   • Substance-induced mood disorder
   • Mood disorder due to a general medical condition
   • Mood disorder, not otherwise specified

Incidence and Socioeconomic Impact

1. Unipolar depressive disorders (major depressive disorder, or MDD, and dysthymic disorder) are 2 to 3 times more likely to affect females than males. Lifetime risk for MDD is 7 to 12 percent in men and 20 to 30 percent in women. At any point in time, 5 to 9 percent of adult women and 2 to 3 percent of adult men suffer from an MDD. In the United States, 11.5 million persons are affected each year.
2. Clinical depression rates peak in the 22 to 44-year-old age group, although persons in younger age groups are increasingly given the diagnosis.
3. Costs to society include suicides and lost productivity exceeding every other disorder except cardiovascular disease. The total cost of clinical depression is nearly $44 billion per year.
4. Bipolar disorders affect males and females more equally than do MDDs.

Risk Factors

1. Female gender carries a 2:1 prevalence ratio worldwide.
2. First-degree relatives of persons with bipolar disorders have an increased risk for bipolar illness; MDD has an increased familial risk but to a lesser degree.
3. Medical conditions including cerebrovascular accident, myocardial infarction, cancer, and diabetes are associated with rates of MDD of 25 percent or more (see also Chapter 42).
4. Loss, low self-esteem, and situational stressors that involve relationships or esteem (e.g., rape, abuse) play a significant role in the onset of depressive disorders.

Etiology and Pathophysiology

1. In the biologic model, mood disorders involve chemical changes in the brain. Whether these changes are cause or effect of mood changes is unclear.

a. Depressed states may involve at least 3 neurotransmitters (norepinephrine, serotonin, and dopamine) as well as several hormonal systems, including the pituitary, thyroid, and adrenal systems.

b. Manic states seem to include excess amounts of catecholamines.

c. Disruptions in circadian rhythms, diet, and exposure to light have been associated with mood dysregulation, but the connections are not wholly understood.

2. Psychologic models for the etiology of depressive states include the following:

a. The analytic model of "aggression turned inward"

b. The cognitive model of negative thoughts preceding negative feelings

c. The behavioral and social learning model—positive interactions provide positive reinforcement and positive mood, whereas few or nonrewarding interactions worsen the mood.

d. Other theories involve aspects of loss, lack of attachment, and lack of esteem, agency, and hope.

e. Mania is seen as a denial of what is basically a depressive state.

3. The biopsychosocial or integrated model recognizes the importance of both biologic and psychologic influences in both the etiology and treatment of mood disorders.

Clinical Manifestations

1. The cardinal symptom of depressive disorders is the presence of a depressed mood or loss of interest or pleasure—anhedonia—which may be reported by the person or concerned others. This change lasts at least 2 weeks, outside the normal bereavement process.

2. Other signs and symptoms

a. Changes in sleep, appetite, and weight, and loss of libido

b. Generalized slowing in thinking and psychomotor activities or increased agitation and irritability

c. Reported feelings of guilt, dread, worthlessness, and hopelessness

d. Fatigue and loss of energy

e. Recurrent thoughts of death, dying, or suicide

3. The cardinal symptom of a manic or hypomanic episode is an abnormally, persistently elated, elevated, expansive, or irritable mood, for at least 4 days (hypomania) to a week.

4. Additional symptoms

a. Inflated self-esteem, grandiosity

b. Decreased need for sleep

c. Increased rate of thinking or talking, with increased distractibility

d. Increased activity, often in pleasurable activities, without heed to possibly dangerous consequences

5. The person who is manic may be engaging or hostile. The dress may be outlandish; the behaviors are impulsive. Persons do not realize that they are ill; they may see themselves as invincible or may disregard their own behavioral code.

Diagnostics

1. Mood disorders must be differentiated from physiolog illness, substance disorders, and schizophrenia. A histor of a head injury or substance usage must be explored.

2. Family history is assessed for the presence of mood di orders or suicide (see pp. 1902–1903).

3. Symptoms must meet DSM-IV criteria before the diagno sis is made. Modifiers are attached, depending c whether psychosis is involved, and whether the episod is singular or a recurrence.

Clinical Management

1. Treatment goals

a. Maintenance of safety while the person's mood is a tered

b. The return of a level, normal (euthymic) mood state

c. The return to optimal level of functioning

2. Nonpharmacologic interventions

a. A safe environment should be provided (see p. 1909 The acutely depressed or manic person is at risk fc harm to self, intentionally or accidentally. Suicida tendencies must be continually assessed. Suicide pre cautions or high-risk status may be required at inte vals throughout treatment (see p. 1925).

b. Assistance with activities of daily living is necessar when persons are too depressed or too distracted b mania to care for themselves. In outpatient setting this may involve family or home health personnel.

c. Psychotherapy may be individual, group, family, c marital. It may be primary treatment or adjunct t pharmacologic treatment. Cognitive therapy is specif for depressive disorders (see p. 1924).

d. Psychoeducation is as previously described.

e. Community support services are available.

(1) Local affiliates of national groups sponsor educa tional and support groups (see p. 1930).

(2) Community crisis lines are instrumental in suicid prevention.

f. Biologic treatment

(1) Light therapy has proved useful for seasonal kind of depression. Exposure to full spectrum light, vi a special light box or visor, may be prescribed b a physician. Exposure time is titrated to achiev therapeutic effect.

(2) Restructuring of the sleep cycle and circadia rhythm is also being used to break depression.

3. Pharmacologic interventions (see p. 1919)

a. Antipsychotic medications are used if delusions c hallucinations (psychosis) are present, or for rapi control of mania.

b. Antidepressant medications are used.

c. Mood stabilizing medications

(1) Lithium (carbonate or citrate) has been used fo mania and bipolar disorders since the 1970s.

(2) Carbamazepine and valproic acid–sodium va proate are anticonvulsants being used to manag bipolar disorders that are refractory to lithium c when lithium cannot be tolerated.

. Special medical-surgical procedures

a. Electroconvulsive therapy (ECT) has been shown to have a greater than 80 percent success rate in treating persons with acutely psychotic, suicidal depressions or severely depressed persons who are refractory to or cannot tolerate medications. This therapy has a lower morbidity and mortality rate than antidepressant medications and is equal to that of any minor surgery requiring general anesthesia.

   (1) Electroconvulsive therapy is performed as an inpatient or outpatient procedure. Six to 12 treatments may be required. The preparation and recovery are similar to any procedure involving general anesthesia (see p. 1925 and Chapter 13).

   (2) The procedure lasts less than 30 minutes, and persons are reoriented during recovery.

   (3) Short-term memory can be affected during treatment with ECT. Although recall problems are generally transitory, memory storage during the treatment period is affected.

Applying the Nursing Process

(See p. 1925 for care of suicidal persons.)

NURSING DIAGNOSIS: Hopelessness and self-care deficit RIT feelings of guilt, ambivalence, low energy, and decreased self-esteem, as evidenced by weight loss, lack of hygiene, slowed thinking, sad affect, and insomnia

Expected outcomes: After interventions the person should be able to do the following:

a. Demonstrate improved mood and outlook by

   (1) Being up and dressed every morning without assistance.

   (2) Consuming sufficient calories to maintain weight, with gradual regain of loss if desired

   (3) Sleeping 7 hours per night without awakening

   (4) Having a brighter affect; initiating activity; laughing

b. Prevent relapse by verbalizing

   (1) Knowledge of the illness of depression

   (2) Signs of relapse

   (3) The importance of following the treatment regimen

Nursing interventions

a. Actively assist with activities of daily living, gradually transferring responsibility to the patient as mood lifts

b. Allow time for the person to think and speak; spend time with the person, even without conversation

c. Assess for suicidal ideation as energy level increases

d. Monitor intake; offer snacks frequently; weigh the patient twice a week

e. Administer and teach the patient about antidepressant medications

f. Teach the patient about the various nonpharmacologic

interventions of exercise, cognitive restructuring, and decreasing isolation (see pp. 1910–1911).

NURSING DIAGNOSIS: High risk for injury R/T excessive energy, poor impulse control of mania as evidenced by no sleep or food in 2 days, garish makeup, and pressured speech

1. *Expected outcomes:* Following interventions, the person should be able to do the following:

   a. Be free of injury (to self or by others)

   b. Sleep at least 4 hours a night

   c. Maintain adequate intake of food and fluids

   d. Be able to apply internal controls to impulsive acts

2. *Nursing interventions*

   a. Maintain a safe, subdued environment; remove hazardous objects

   b. Monitor the person closely (every 15 minutes) while allowing the person some space.

   c. Administer scheduled medications and calming medications at the first sign of escalation or to encourage sleep.

   d. Offer frequent high-calorie finger foods and fluids to meet increased nutritional needs during mania.

   e. Encourage safe physical activity and exercise to redirect energy.

Prognosis

1. Depression is a treatable illness—65 percent of patients respond to antidepressant medications; 85 percent respond when they receive both pharmacologic and psychotherapeutic interventions.

2. Bipolar disorders have a 75 to 80 percent successful treatment rate with lithium or anticonvulsant medication.

3. An untreated episode of depression may last from 6 months to 2 years, with some or all of the symptoms persisting.

4. An MDD is associated with high mortality; up to 15 percent of persons with severe MDD die by suicide.

5. Persons diagnosed with MDD have a 50 percent chance of having a 2nd episode; the recurrence rate for a manic episode is 75 to 90 percent.

Discharge Planning and Teaching

1. The person and family should have a knowledge of the disorder and early signs of relapse and recurrence.

2. Understanding the medication regimen, its timetable, and its side effects contributes to adherence to the treatment plan. Written materials should accompany the person. The person should verbalize understanding of the regimen as well.

3. The person and family should have aftercare plans and know how to access community resources, including crisis lines and the support services of national and local mental health advocacy groups (see Agencies and Resources).

CARING FOR PEOPLE WITH ANXIETY DISORDERS

Definition and Key Criteria

1. Anxiety is a fear, the object of which is unknown. From a Greek root meaning "to strangle" or "press tight," anxiety is a diffuse apprehension, vague in nature, and associated with feelings of uncertainty and helplessness.
2. Anxiety is the following:
   a. A subjective experience, not directly observable, but only inferred through observing behaviors
   b. The result of any perceived threat to a person's self-concept
   c. Communicated interpersonally, or it may be considered "contagious," easily transmitted from 1 person to another
   d. A universal human experience
3. Anxiety exists along a continuum—mild, moderate, severe, or panic. Although mild anxiety is beneficial, increased anxiety levels lead to decreased effectiveness as focus narrows.
4. Anxiety prompts physiologic responses, which are deleterious when sustained over a prolonged period.

5. A panic level of anxiety can be associated with psychos or loss of accurate reality testing.
6. These disorders are characterized by anxiety that beyond the norm in intensity, duration, or the behavio that the anxiety precipitates.

DSM-IV Diagnoses for Anxiety-Related Disorders (Table 41–5)

Incidence and Socioeconomic Impact

1. The lifetime prevalence rate for anxiety disorders is a proximately 15 percent, with women affected twice often as men.
2. Simple phobias, obsessive-compulsive disorder, an agoraphobia have the highest prevalence.

Risk Factors

1. A family history of problems with anxiety; up to percent of cases have a familial component.
2. A personal history of separation anxiety or other chil hood anxiety disorder

Table 41–5. Anxiety Disorders

Disorder	DSM-IV Diagnosis	Description
Panic attack	A discrete period of intense fear or discomfort, which has a sudden onset and builds rapidly to a peak	Often accompanied by a sense of imminent doom and nee to escape. These attacks are often physiologic in manife tation (dizziness, palpitations, chest pain, choking) and are not traceable to a particular precipitating stimulus
Panic disorder	Characterized by recurrent panic attacks	Persons with panic disorder may develop agoraphobia, a fear of being in places where escape might be difficult. is considered to be the result of fear of having a panic attack away from home.
Phobia-specific	An excessive fear of a particular stimulus, resulting in extreme avoidance of the stimulus. Social phobia is the extreme fear of exposure to certain social settings. Some variants include "stage fright" or fear of speaking in public.	When exposed directly to the feared stimulus, extreme an ety results.
Obsessive-compulsive disorder	The presence of recurrent thoughts (obsessions) or repetitive, ritualized behaviors (compulsions), or both.	Affected persons recognize the thoughts and behaviors as excessive, irrational, and interfering with functioning. E amples of obsessions are recurring ideas of blasphemy or aggression that cause a person distress. Compulsior often involve ritualized washing, checking, or counting.
Post-traumatic stress disorder	As a result of exposure to unusually traumatic events (war, torture, rape, murder) with an accompanying feeling of intense horror or hopelessness, a person develops a syndrome of behaviors.	Syndrome of behaviors includes reexperiencing the event dreams or flashback), emotional numbing, and increase arousal (that is, irritability or startle response). Acute stre disorder is similar but lasts 4 weeks or less, whereas post-traumatic stress disorder has a longer duration.
Generalized anxiety disorder	Chronic, unrealistic, generalized worry, without a particular stimulus or response	Symptoms include physical as well as intrapsychic compo nents and must be present for at least 6 months. Orga illness (including premenstrual syndrome, caffeine addi tion or withdrawal) must be ruled out.

3. A personal history of having experienced a trauma, especially one that threatened a person's own life

Etiology and Pathophysiology

1. Severe anxiety, or its avoidance, results in physiologic or behavioral symptoms sufficient to interfere with daily functioning.
2. These responses are often not conscious, occurring without awareness.
3. Onset is often subsequent to the loss of an important relationship or to other highly stressful life circumstances.
4. Psychologic theories focus on anxiety as a learned response, resulting from childhood or adult situations that were perceived as threatening.
5. Biologic models
   a. Neurologic pathways in several areas of the brain regulate response to fear, and this response may not be conscious. Panic attacks have been the most studied, with the hippocampus and amygdala being implicated as factors.
   b. Several neurotransmitters may be involved including norepineprine, γ-aminobutyric acid and serotonin. The autonomic system mediates some somatic responses.

Clinical Manifestations

1. Individual anxiety disorders are characterized by specific clusters of responses.
2. The physical symptoms of certain anxiety disorders lend themselves to extensive physical workups and consultations with multiple medical specialists (see below).
3. The sequelae of anxiety disorders may mask or complicate the underlying primary diagnosis. Persons may present with the following:
   a. Stress-related physiologic illness, such as peptic ulcers or hypertension
   b. Chemical dependence or abuse
   c. Major depression

Diagnostics

Organic causes to be ruled out include the following:
a. Mitral valve prolapse
b. Endocrine disorders such as hyperthyroidism or hypoglycemia
c. Substance intoxication (including caffeine)
   (1) Withdrawal may precipitate panic attacks or mimic anxiety.
   (2) A substance usage history and drug screen is recommended.
Other psychiatric disorders to be ruled out include depression, somatoform disorder, and personality disorder. Nursing assessment includes observing for triggering situations as well as the person's strengths and coping skills. A specific anxiety disorder must meet the DSM-IV criteria (e.g., duration of symptoms).

Clinical Management

1. Goals of intervention are the resolution or diminution of symptoms or decreasing the distress surrounding them.
2. Nonpharmacologic interventions
   a. Behavioral therapies—desensitization and flooding techniques; thought stopping for obsessive thoughts
   b. Relaxation therapies—relaxation response, imagery, biofeedback for somatic responses
   c. Psychotherapy—individual; group psychotherapy, especially effective for post-traumatic stress disorder
3. Pharmacologic interventions
   - Benzodiazepines
   - Tricyclic antidepressants
   - Monoamine oxidase inhibitors
   - Nonbenzodiazepine anxiolytics (buspirone)
   - Carbamazepine, propranolol, and hydroxyzine
4. Special procedures such as hypnosis and sodium amobarbital (Amytal) interview are used infrequently. They may facilitate psychologic release of a traumatic event (see p. 1919).

Applying and Nursing Process

NURSING DIAGNOSIS: Panic level of anxiety R/T perceived threat (internal or external) as evidenced by tachycardia, sense of doom, diaphoresis

1. *Expected outcomes:* After interventions, the person should be able to do the following:
   a. Have a heart rate lower than 100 beats per minute
   b. Verbalize feeling safe in the environment
   c. Recognize symptoms of escalating anxiety and intervene before they reaching severe or panic level
2. *Nursing interventions*
   a. Stay with the person to promote security during acute or severe panic.
   b. Communicate with simple, brief, 1-step directions; reassure that the person is safe physically.
   c. Decrease external stimuli; explain any surrounding events that may be misperceived as threatening.
   d. Offer an anxiolytic agent.
   e. After the acute stage has passed, help the person reconstruct antecedent events, identifying possible triggering stimuli.
   f. Teach relaxation and thought-stopping techniques.

NURSING DIAGNOSIS: Powerlessness R/T ritualistic, compulsive behaviors, such as taking excessively long (e.g., 4 hr) to bathe and dress

1. *Expected outcomes:* Following interventions the person should be able to bathe and dress in less than 2 hours without an increase in anxiety or development of new rituals.
2. *Nursing interventions*
   a. Do not interfere with compulsive behaviors initially.

b. Help the person establish goals for gradual decrease of total time spent on compulsive behaviors.

c. Stay with the person during these targeted minutes initially, providing diversional activity and giving positive feedback throughout.

d. Teach the person about the use of antidepressants or behavioral therapies to decrease symptoms (see Learning/Teaching Guidelines for Persons with Chronic Mental Illness).

Prognosis

1. Approximately 25 percent of persons with anxiety disorders seek treatment. Prognosis is good for those who seek help before the effects become disabling.
2. Major depression, substance abuse, or a personality disorder may be concurrent diagnoses and would need treatment as well.

Health Teaching and Discharge Planning

1. Supportive, relaxation, and behavioral therapies are integral to the long-term success of treatment. Medication is only 1 of the tools.
2. Family may need to adjust old patterns of responses to the patient's symptoms. If there is a behavioral plan, family must be included and be ready to consistently follow it.
3. Medication teaching for anxiolytics includes the following:
   a. Warning against the use of other central nervous system depressants, such as alcohol
   b. Cautioning that benzodiazepines should not be discontinued abruptly
   c. Warning that stimulants (e.g., caffeine) may be contraindicated in certain disorders

◼ CARING FOR PEOPLE WITH SOMATOFORM DISORDERS

Definition

1. Somatoform disorders are characterized by persistent worry or complaints about physical illness or symptoms for which there are no supporting physical findings. These disorders are related to the anxiety disorders, but the anxiety is redirected into a somatic concern
2. Table 41–3 describes the specific disorders. Pain disorders, although grouped as somatoform disorders, may have a physical basis (see Chapter 11).

Incidence and Etiology

1. According to the DSM-IV, all somatoform disorders are more prevalent in women, except the body dysmorphic disorder, which occurs equally in males and females.

Somatization disorder has an increased incidence in 1s degree female relatives of women with the disorder.

2. Certain culture-bound syndromes may be related to th somatoform disorders. Cultural norms regarding somati expression vary, and symptoms must be evaluate within a cultural context.
3. The precipitating factors may or may not be identifiabl Persons do *not intend* to feign illness; their complaint are not under conscious control. (To intend so is calle "malingering" or a factitious disorder.)

Clinical Manifestations

1. Persons with somatoform disorders are often seen i general medical and surgical areas, and may have ha many procedures performed. Their distress is real, yet may be unrelieved when no organic problem is found.
2. The person with a conversion disorder may be an excep tion, showing inordinately little concern in response t an acute loss of function.

Clinical Management

1. The primary care practitioner's relationship with the per son may be the most important aspect of intervention.
2. Research has shown that conservative care with minim psychotropic medication can have good results whe trust is developed in the patient and the patient does n see multiple practitioners.
3. Attempting to convince these persons that it is "all i your head" is counterproductive.
4. Antidepressants or anxiolytics may be helpful, but ben zodiazepines should be used sparingly.
5. Pain disorders have responded well to multidisciplinar treatment, which includes supportive group therapy an the use of antidepressant medications.

◼ CARING FOR PEOPLE WITH DISSOCIATIVE DISORDERS

Definition

1. Dissociative disorders are characterized by periods disruption in the functions that tie people to their env

ronment. These functions involve consciousness, memory, identity, and perception of the environment.
The DSM-IV diagnoses include the following:
- Dissociative amnesia
- Dissociative fugue
- Depersonalization disorder
- Dissociative identity disorder formerly known as multiple personality disorder

ncidence and Etiology

Brief depersonalization may be experienced by almost anyone during a highly stressful situation. Depersonalization disorder has recurrent episodes that interfere with functioning. Dissociative fugue disorder is rare. Dissociative amnesia and dissociative identity disorder, once considered rare, are being increasingly reported.
The repression of unbearable memories is part of the etiology of all these disorders. The dissociative response is a defense against the overwhelming anxiety surrounding these events. War and disasters were once considered the primary cause, but severe abuse sustained during childhood has become the primary cause of dissociative identity disorder.

linical Manifestations

The inability to account for periods of time or to recall specific events is the hallmark of these disorders. This must not be a result of physiologic effects of a substance or physical condition. In fugue, the person suddenly travels to a new place, with no recall of life before the flight. In persons with dissociative identity disorder, at least 2 distinct identities emerge periodically; patients also have problems with recall.

CLINICAL CONTROVERSIES

the early 1990s, there was a proliferation of treatments to recover ressed memories. Some of the methods used, as well as the numbers persons believed to have experienced this repression, have come under ious scrutiny. Some persons needed this help, but others may have en convinced of a need or scenario that was exaggerated or did not st.

linical Management

Psychotherapy helps the person to reintegrate the repressed material and deal with the emotional responses to the memories.
Medications, specifically anxiolytics and antidepressants, are used periodically.
Hospitalization may be required if persons become suicidal; however, most treatment occurs on an outpatient basis.
Hypnosis and sodium amobarbital (Amytal) interviews are sometimes used to elicit repressed material.
Persons with dissociative disorders are among those who may be prone to self-mutilating behaviors.

◼ CARING FOR PEOPLE WITH PERSONALITY DISORDERS

Definition and Key Criteria

1. Personality disorders (PDs) are characterized by enduring patterns of inner experience and behavior that are maladaptive, are not culturally appropriate, and cause distress or functional impairment. The pattern is stable, inflexible, and persists over time and different aspects of life. Every person has traits that may be maladaptive, but a PD permeates the way a person sees and acts in life.
2. This history of a pattern may require several interviews, often requiring more than the patient as informant.

DSM-IV Subcategories

1. Personality disorders are recorded on axis II of the multiaxial diagnostic system. Major depression or other axis I disorders may be experienced by persons with certain PDs, and both diagnoses would be recorded.
2. DSM-IV includes 10 PDs, which are grouped into 3 "clusters." The clusters differ greatly in presentation; diagnoses within a cluster share some styles of response. Table 41–6 describes the disorders by cluster and specific diagnosis.
3. A PD is not an "illness" but rather the manner in which a person relates to the world.

Clinical Manifestations

1. Persons with PDs are seen in all settings. The patterns described in Table 41–6 manifest in problems in self-esteem, relating, and trusting.
2. Maladaptive psychologic defense mechanisms are used frequently—projection, regression, and splitting are frequently evident. Attempts to control may be overt or covert (manipulative), or there may be no acceptance of responsibility. These behaviors often trigger a visceral response in the professional.
   a. Persons with borderline PD may engage in self-mutilation as well as other self-destructive impulses, such as binge eating and shopping. Instability and rapid shifts of mood present many challenges to safety.

NURSE ADVISORY

Persons with antisocial, borderline, and paranoid personality disorders (PDs) are at high risk for dangerous, aggressive behaviors. The aggression may be toward self, others, or both, and escalation may be rapid.
Persons with borderline PD (and occasionally persons diagnosed with a dissociative disorder) may engage in self-mutilating behavior (e.g., cutting or burning oneself). Usually, these acts are not intended as a suicide attempt; however, they are a safety risk that must be addressed. A no-harm contract is not always sufficient, and one-to-one monitoring may be required.

Table 41–6. Personality Disorders—DSM-IV Diagnoses

Disorder	Brief Description	Prevalence/Etiology
Cluster A*		
Paranoid	Pervasive pattern of distrust, to the extent that others' motives are considered malevolent	0.5–2.5% in the general population
Schizoid	Pervasive pattern of social detachment and restricted range of emotions; seems cold, indifferent to praise or criticism	Uncommon; diagnosed slightly more in males
Schizotypal	Schizoid pattern plus cognitive or perceptual distortions; eccentricities; magical thinking	Approximately 3% of the population; may be slightly more prevalent in males.
Cluster B†		
Antisocial	Pervasive pattern of disregard for the rights of others; deceit, manipulation, lack of remorse	Not diagnosed in those under 18 years old (in younger persons, it may be a conduct disorder) 3% of males, 1% of females May be associated with substance-related disorders
Borderline	Pervasive pattern of instability of interpersonal relationships, self-image, and affects. Impulsivity, self-destructive behaviors and instability of mood. Many behaviors are attempts to avoid perceived abandonment	Approximately 2% of the population; 5 times more common in 1st-degree relatives of those with this disorder Physical and sexual abuse, neglect, or loss is common in the childhood histories
Histrionic	A pervasive pattern of excessive emotionality and attention seeking Desire to be the center of attention in speech, dress, or behavior.	Approximately 2–3% of the population
Narcissistic	Pervasive pattern of grandiosity, entitlement, and need for admiration and a lack of empathy	1–2% of the population; 50–75% of whom are male
Cluster C‡		
Avoidant	Pervasive pattern of social inhibition, feelings of inadequacy, fear of criticism	0.5–1.0%
Dependent	Pervasive pattern of need to be cared for; clinging, unable to function alone	Structured assessment tools report similar rate in males and females.
Obsessive-compulsive personality disorder	Pervasive pattern of preoccupation with orderliness and control, at the expense of flexibility and efficiency	Approximately 1%

* Cluster A disorders are characterized by odd, eccentric, isolative or suspicious behaviors. These persons are often loners, and the patterns often develop early in life.
† Cluster B disorders are characterized by behaviors that are either very dramatic, erratic and impulsive, or lacking in empathy.
‡ Cluster C personality disorders are characterized by anxious or fearful behaviors.
Data from American Psychiatric Association. *Diagnostic and Statistical Manual of Mental Disorders.* 4th ed. Washington, DC: Author, 1994. Copyright 1994, American Psychiatric Association.

  b. Persons with dependent PD are needy, whiny, fearful, yet demanding. Many persons regress during medical illness, but only a long-standing behavioral pattern is a PD.
3. Cultural differences must be kept in mind. Persons whom 1 culture may label as passive or obsessive-compulsive may be fulfilling role expectations of another culture. Or, persons who have lived under conditions of war, hostility, or deprivation may demonstrate a suspiciousness that was necessary to survive in that setting, not paranoia.

Clinical Management

1. Kind firmness and consistency of approach are necessary in dealing with most of the maladaptive behaviors.
2. Staff must be open and honest with persons who are suspicious or fearful. Explaining all procedures, routines, and medication changes helps fearful and withdrawn

persons. Whispering or talking in groups, or changing rules for certain persons is thought of as malevolent when a person has a paranoid PD.
3. Consistency among staff is necessary to prevent the manipulation and splitting seen in cluster B disorders. Setting limits that are swift, nonjudgmental, and predictable is most important. Limit-setting includes keeping relationships with these persons strictly professional.
4. Modeling assertiveness is important in both the passive and aggressive disorders. Positive reinforcement and praise for patients who demonstrate assertiveness is needed.
5. Psychodynamic individual psychotherapy and group therapies are the treatments of choice when persons wish to change pervasive maladaptive patterns. Families and friends may also need counseling in dealing with both old and new behaviors.
6. Pharmacologic interventions are of limited value. Antipsychotics help during the brief periods of psychosis that a person with a borderline PD may have; antidepressants and mood stabilizers help with mood shifts, rage, and

excessive behaviors. Depression, anxiety, or substance abuse may also be treated.

THERAPEUTIC OPTIONS FOR PEOPLE WITH MENTAL DISORDERS

Pharmacologic Approaches

Medications have made it possible for persons with major mental illness to live relatively normal lives, yet medication compliance is often 50 percent or less. Noncompliance is the primary reason for rehospitalization for many persons with mental disorders. Uncomfortable side effects, denial of illness, and misunderstanding of the medications are the major factors—and challenges for the nurse (see Learning/Teaching Guidelines for Persons with Chronic Mental Illness).

2. Antipsychotic medications
   a. Antipsychotic medications are the mainstay in treating psychosis, whether it is from schizophrenia, a psychotic mood disorder, or acute psychosis from medical condition.
   b. The primary mechanism of action is the blocking of dopamine at the (D_2) receptor site.
   c. Dopaminergic blockade also results in the extrapyramidal side effects that trouble patients in differing degrees and contribute to the 50 percent noncompliance rate for these medications. Table 41–7 lists

Table 41–7. Antipsychotic Medication Therapy

Generic Name	Actions	Comments	Side Effects	Nursing Considerations
Chlorpromazine Thioridazine Mesoridazine Haloperidol Loxapine Molindone Perphenazine Trifluoperazine Thiothixene Fluphenazine Risperidone Clozapine†	The exact mechanism of the antipsychotics is unknown. Most are believed to block dopamine at D_2 receptor sites. Clozapine and risperidone are believed to also affect serotonin receptors, possibly more so with clozapine.	These medications are not lethal and have no upper limit, except thioridazine.† Side effects are generally dose related and are similar for all except clozapine.‡ Tolerance to some side effects develops over weeks; other side effects emerge over time. Once a day dosing is usually at night, owing to likelihood of drowsiness.	Neurologic* Extrapyramidal Cardiovascular Postural changes Dizziness Tachycardia Endocrine Weight gain Photosensitivity— sun and heat intolerance Gynecomastia Impotence Anticholinergic Blurry vision Drowsiness Dry mouth Constipation Urinary retention	• Dry mouth is bothersome; offer hard candy and fluids. • Constipation may be moderate to severe. If diet, fluids, and exercise are not effective, medication may be needed. Withdrawn persons will not ask for help; nursing must be proactive in monitoring elimination. • Protect the skin from sunburn with hats and clothing. There is also increased risk for heat stroke with some medications. • Blurred vision as a side effect should resolve after several weeks of medication. • Urinary retention can be especially problematic in males with prostatic hypertrophy. Monitor intake and output. • The extrapyramidal side effects (EPS) of these medications are generally short term, except for tardive dyskinesia, which may be later onset and may be irreversible. (See Table 41–8.) Many states require signed informed consent for antipsychotic agents because of the risk of tardive dyskinesia. • Medications that alleviate short-term EPS may be prescribed prophylactically or as needed if signs occur. These medications are benztropine, trihexyphenidyl, biperiden, procyclidine, diazepam, lorazepam, diphenhydramine, orphenadrine, and amantadine. • Assess for short-term EPS by observation and checking for stiffness in the elbow and wrist or in ambulation. The Simpson-Angus Scale is used to measure short-term EPS. The Abnormal Involuntary Movement Scale is used to assess for long-term movement disorder effects. It should be administered periodically to all persons on these medications for more than several weeks.

*All antipsychotics lower the seizure threshold.
†Thioridazine may cause retinopathy at doses > 800 mg/day.
‡The side effect profile of clozapine is unique. Some usual anticholinergic symptoms (e.g., dry mouth) are not seen; hypersalivation and urinary incontinence are common during titration. Sedation, tachycardia, constipation, and orthostatic hypotension are seen, as is weight gain. Seizures may occur in higher dosages. See Nurse Advisory box regarding agranulocytosis. Extrapyramidal symptoms are not a problem with clozapine. Research has shown a reversal of tardive dyskinesia with use of clozapine.

Data from Crismon M, and Dorson P. Schizophrenia. *In* DiPiro J, et al (eds). *Pharmacotherapy: A Pathophysiologic Approach*. Norwalk, CT: Appleton & Lange, 1993, and Laraia and Stuart G. *Quick Psychopharmacology Reference*. 2nd ed. St. Louis: CV Mosby, 1995.

these medications and describes the side effects; Table 41–8 describes extrapyramidal side effects in detail.

d. Clozapine is atypical in its side effect profile.

e. Route of administration is usually oral but may be via intramuscular injection. Haloperidol and fluphenazine are also available for intramuscular injection in a long-acting (2 to 3 week) depot-type formulation.

f. Antipsychotic medications are similarly effective at therapeutic-equivalent doses. Relative potency correlates with the side effect profile of a particular agent and the side effect profile is usually how a particular agent is chosen.

g. Antipsychotic agents have low abuse potential and low lethality. Higher doses may be necessary in acute psychosis; lower doses for maintenance. In acute situations, a short-acting benzodiazepine may be added.

3. Antidepressant medications

ELDER ADVISORY

Several side effects of antipsychotic agents and tricyclic antidepressants may be extremely problematic for the older patient.

- The anticholinergic effect may be contraindicated for patients with glaucoma.
- The urinary retention effect may be complicated by preexisting prostatic hypertrophy.
- If anticholinergics are used to control extrapyramidal side effects, the effect may cause some cognitive changes in susceptible older persons. Anticholinergic crisis or delirium may result if several anticholinergic medications (including over-the-counter medications) are taken concurrently.
- Orthostatic hypotension is the most common cardiovascular side effect of antipsychotic and tricyclic drugs. Older patients may have preexisting postural changes, and a baseline blood pressure obtained while the patient is lying, sitting, and standing should be established before these medications are initiated as well as during treatment. Patients should be instructed to change position slowly, especially when getting out of bed at night to use the bathroom. The rapid change from lying to standing could lead to syncope or a fall, which is so dangerous in older persons.
- Research shows that older women have the highest risk for acquiring tardive dyskinesia.

NURSE ADVISORY

Agranulocytosis is a rare, potentially life-threatening side effect of several antipsychotic medications. Clozapine carries a 1 to 2 percent risk of agranulocytosis. To minimize the risk, the U.S. Food and Drug Administration has mandated weekly complete blood counts be obtained for any person who takes clozapine for as long as it is taken. A national registration bank is maintained to prevent a person from ever restarting the medication if it has been discontinued previously for this reason. Persons receiving this medication should be instructed to report any symptoms of infection to the health care provider.

Neuroleptic malignancy syndrome (NMS) is an idiosyncratic response to psychotropic medications that is rare and life threatening. Any person may become ill with NMS, regardless of the length of time that the person has been taking the medication. All antipsychotic drugs, lithium, and some antidepressants have been implicated in the development of NMS. Fever, profuse sweating, muscle rigidity, unstable pulse and blood pressure, and delirium are the signs of NMS. An elevated creatinine phosphokinase level is evidence of muscle breakdown and is considered diagnostic for NMS. Supportive treatment, including a medical ICU, may be required during the acute stage. This syndrome is considered a medical emergency, with a 20 percent mortality rate.

Table 41–8. Extrapyramidal Side Effects of Antipsychotic Medications*

Effect	Signs and Symptoms	Time of Onset	Factors
Acute dystonic reaction	Prolonged tonic muscle contractions of the neck and mouth, tongue protrusion, oculogyration, blepharospasm, laryngopharyngospasm	Within 96 hours of initiating or increasing antipsychotic medication Also seen with phenothiazine antiemetics	May be life threatening Administer anticholinergic intramuscularly High risk in young males and patients with high-potency medications
Akathisia	Motor restlessness; difficulty sitting still; tapping feet; inner tension	Anytime within the 1st few days to the 1st few weeks of therapy	May be mistaken for anxiety Common with high-potency medication
Pseudoparkinsonism	Any symptoms of Parkinson's disease: decreased movement, masklike facies, rigidity (with or without cogwheeling), shuffling gait, hypersalivation	1–2 wk after initiation or increase of dose	Risk slightly greater for older patients and patients with high-potency medications
Tardive dyskinesia	Abnormal involuntary movements, including blinking, oral or tongue movements, involuntary swallowing, limb or trunkal movements	Slow, later developing and may be irreversible Movements are rhythmic, increase with anxiety and cease during sleep	Risk increases with each year of antipsychotic usage Risk has become a medicolegal issue

* The extrapyramidal tracks of the brain arise in the basal ganglia and are responsible for the unconscious stability of movements and balance, posture, and gait. This system is affected by the imbalance of neurotransmitters that results from the dopamine blockade of the antipsychotics.
Data from Crismon M, and Dorson P. Schizophrenia. In DiPiro J, et al (eds). *Pharmacotherapy: A Pathophysiologic Approach.* 2nd ed. Norwalk, CT: Appleton & Lange, 1993.

a. There are 3 major classes of antidepressant medications: tricyclics, monoamine oxidase inhibitors, and selective serotonin reuptake inhibitors, plus "others."

b. Classes differ in mechanism of action. Within each class the differences are primarily in the degree of specific side effects (Table 41–9).

c. The selective serotonin reuptake inhibitors are currently the drug of choice, with a shorter onset of action, fewer side effects, and little danger from overdose or abrupt withdrawal.

d. The tricyclics and monoamine oxidase inhibitors carry different risks, but either can be lethal in the hands of a suicidal person.

 DRUG ADVISORY

Dietary restrictions should be initiated at least 1 day before, throughout treatment, until 2 weeks after cessation of therapy with any monoamine oxidase inhibitor. Persons should be thoroughly instructed in its use, given a wallet card, and given a medical alert–type bracelet.

Foods to be eliminated
- Aged cheeses
- Aged meats
- Aged red wine
- Fermented drinks and foods
- Overripe fruit, banana peels

Medications* to avoid
- Stimulants
- Ephedrine or pseudoephedrine
- Decongestants and inhalers, including over-the-counter cold medicines
- Narcotics
- Meperidine
- Methyldopa

Acceptable in moderation are
- Chocolate and caffeinated drinks
- White wine
- Sour cream and yogurt

*Persons should call the prescribing professional before taking any new prescription nonprescription drug, due to the multiple agents involved.

e. Antidepressant medications are also used for the following:
- Pain management
- Panic disorders
- Obsessive-compulsive disorder
- Sleep disorders
- Bulimia
- Social phobia

Mood-stabilizing medications

a. Lithium carbonate has been the drug of choice for bipolar disorder since the 1970s. The exact mechanism is still unknown.

b. The anticonvulsants of carbamazepine and valproic acid are used as 2nd-line or adjuvant therapies.

c. Mood stabilizers are also used to decrease the aggression and impulsivity of some other disorders.

d. Therapeutic blood levels must be maintained to stabilize the mood. None of these medications works im-

mediately to lower a manic high. All are administered orally only.

e. Compliance during nonacute periods is essential in preventing relapse. Intermittent noncompliance with lithium may also decrease its long-term effectiveness.

f. Lithium toxicity can be a life-threatening situation; some signs of neurotoxicity may also be seen with the anticonvulsants. (See Chapter 18 for additional information on carbamazepines and valproic acid.)

5. Antianxiety medications

a. The benzodiazepines are the primary class of currently used antianxiety drugs. Of the drugs listed in Table 41–9, only buspirone is a nonbenzodiazepine and has different properties.

 DRUG ADVISORY

Increasing lithium levels should be recognized early, when holding or lowering dose is sufficient treatment.

1. The earliest signs of toxicity (1.5 mEq/L or less) include nausea, vomiting, diarrhea, muscle weakness, and coordination problems.
2. Generalized muscle and central nervous system problems manifest at 2.0 mEq/L. Signs include dysarthria, coarse tremor, twitching, hyperreflexia, fasciculation, myoclonus, incontinence, ataxia, agitation, giddiness, and vertigo.
3. Vascular and cardiac symptoms, seizures, and coma occur at 2 to 3 mEq/L. This is a medical emergency.

b. Similar in action, benzodiazepines differ by half-life. Lorazepam is used parenterally for rapid onset and clearance, but oral administration is the usual route for benzodiazepines.

c. Addictive properties depend on the half-life as well as the individual. Physiologic withdrawal occurs if the usage exceeds several weeks; longer half-life agents may be used to decrease symptoms.

d. The danger from overdose is small when the agent is not combined with other agents.

6. Other drugs

a. Beta-blockers (e.g., propranolol and pindolol) are sometimes used to decrease impulsivity and aggressive outbursts.

b. Stimulants (e.g., methylphenidate, dexamphetamine, and pemoline) are used in the treatment of attention deficit–hyperactivity disorder in children. Stimulants are also used for depressive symptoms in some older and medically ill persons.

c. Thyroid hormone replacement (or lithium) may be used to potentiate the effect of an antidepressant.

d. Medications used to reverse the short-term extrapyramidal side effects of the antipsychotics include the following (Table 41–10):
- Anticholinergics (benztropine, trihexyphenidyl)
- Antihistamines (diphenhydramine)
- Benzodiazepines (lorazepam, diazepam)
- Beta blockers (propranolol)
- Dopaminergics (amantadine)

Table 41–9. Antidepressant and Mood Stabilizing Medications

Medication	Actions	Comments	Side Effects	Nursing Considerations
Antidepressants				• Safe use during pregnancy has not been established for any of these classes.
Serotonergic Agents Fluoxetine Paroxetine Sertraline	Agents inhibit the reuptake of serotonin at the neuronal receptor site.	Onset of action is 5–7 days. Fluoxetine is also used for treating obsessive–compulsive disorder and problems with behavior excess (e.g., binge eating). Side effect profile may be used (e.g., to aid in treating premature ejaculation).	Nausea Diarrhea Insomnia Headache Sweating Drowsiness Dizziness Muscle twitching Nervousness Sexual dysfunction (delayed climax or ejaculation)	• For anticholinergic side effects, see Table 41–7. • Weight gain may occur with the tricyclics and may require reduced caloric intake. Moderate exercise has a primary depression–alleviating effect and helps with the side effects of weight gain and constipation. • The risk of suicide by overdose or hoarding of medication may be greatest as depression starts to lift. • Patients should be told that these medications do not immediately lift the mood. Effects take several weeks. • Patient education must include the importance of continuing the medication, even after certain symptoms have lifted. • Time of administration should correlate with side effects (e.g., give sedating types at bedtime, stimulatory types early in the day).
Nonselective reuptake-inhibitor: venlafaxine	Agent inhibits uptake of both serotonin and norepinephrine.	Onset of action may be more rapid (3 days).	May contribute to hypertension in high doses.	
Nontricyclic/Nonserotonergic Maprotiline Bupropion Trazodone Nefazodone	Mechanism of action is not clear but probably works on serotonin and norepinephrine (also dopamine for bupropion).	Agents are contraindicated in persons with seizure disorders. Bupropion requires twice daily dosing. Agents are more sedating than serotonergic agents and cause less postural hypotension than tricyclics or monoamine oxidase inhibitors (MAOIs).	Seizures occur at higher dosages. Maprotiline side effects are more like those of tricyclics. Bupropion side effects include seizures (at higher doses), headaches, weight loss, agitation. Trazodone side effects are like those of tricyclics with less orthostasis; Priapism is rare.	
Tricyclic Antidepressants Amitriptyline Amoxapine Clomipramine Doxepin Desipramine Trimipramine Nortriptyline Protriptyline	Agents prevent the reuptake of norepinephrine and serotonin by the presynaptic neuron. Increased amounts are available at the synapse.	Clomipramine is the drug specific for obsessive–compulsive disorder. Tricyclics can be lethal when overdosed. Beneficial effects occur after 2–3 weeks. Agents are contraindicated for persons with angle-closure glaucoma and acute recovery from myocardial in-	Anticholinergic (Table 41–7) Orthostasis Weight gain Cardiac dysrhythmias Seizures at high-doses Drug interactions with central nervous system and antihypertensive agents	

Drug	Action	Side Effects	Nursing Considerations
Monoamine Oxidase Inhibitors Phenelzine Isocarboxazid Tranylcypromine	Agents inhibit production of the enzyme monoamine oxidase. This enzyme breaks down norepinephrine and serotonin. Without breakdown, norepinephrine and serotonin availability is increased.	Hypotension and postural changes Drowsiness or insomnia Edema Weight gain	Without this enzyme, the amino acid tyramine cannot be broken down. Dietary tyramine must be restricted, or hypertensive crisis can result.* Strict dietary compliance is necessary. Many medications are also contraindicated.
Mood Stabilizers Lithium carbonate or citrate	Exact mechanism of action is unknown. Na$^+$ and K$^+$ cell membrane transport is affected.	Thirst Polydipsia Weight gain Fine hand tremor Fatigue, lethargy Gastrointestinal distress Polyuria Metallic taste As blood levels increase >1.5 mEq/L: Coarse tremor Nausea, vomiting Diarrhea Slurred speech Long-term side effects: Hypothyroidism Renal changes	• Education must include the effects of dehydration, changed sodium intake, and exercise on the blood lithium levels. • Fluid balance should include 2–3 L/day if not contraindicated. • Diuretic therapy or dietary sodium should not be changed without increased monitoring of lithium levels. • The loss of fluid and electrolytes through vomiting or diarrhea increases lithium level and could contribute to escalation of an already high level (See Drug Advisory). • Weight gain is common, and diet may need modification. • Long-term effects include renal and thyroid changes. • Blood levels are drawn frequently during titration; blood should be drawn before the morning dose is given.
	Lithium is a naturally occurring substance, but it becomes toxic at certain blood levels. Lithium is used for long-term treatment of bipolar disorder or as adjunct to antidepressants. Lithium has a therapeutic blood level of 0.6–1.4 mEq/L (lower in geriatric populations).		
Anticonvulsants as Mood Stabilizers Carbamazepine Valproic acid Clonazepam	Agents diminish the "kindling effect" phenomenon. Clonazepam is a long-lasting benzodiazepine.	Carbamazepine: Agranulocytosis Rash Carbamazepine and valproate: Nausea Gastrointestinal upset Neurotoxicity: Ataxia Slurred speech Clumsiness Drowsiness Tremor Hepatotoxicity See Table 41–10.	**Anticonvulsants** • Frequent complete blood counts as well as drug levels are recommended with carbamazepine. • Because of the combined risk for agranulocytosis, carbamazepine use with clozapine is contraindicated. • Symptoms of neurotoxicity and hepatotoxicity are dose related and are similar for carbamazepine and valproic acid.
	Agents are used alone to prevent mania in patients refractory to or intolerant of lithium. Carbamazepine is therapeutic at blood levels of 8–12 µg, not as precise as for anticonvulsant uses. It may be used adjunctively or as sole mood stabilizer. Clonazepam also has been used as a mood stabilizer.		

* Hypertensive crisis may be treated with intravenous chlorpromazine or phentolamine.

Data from Laraia M, and Stuart G. *Quick Psychopharmacology Reference*. 2nd ed. St. Louis: CV Mosby, 1995; Andreasen N, and Black D. *Introductory Textbook of Psychiatry*. Washington, DC: American Psychiatric Press, 1991; and Spratto G, and Woods A. *RN's NDR 1993: Nurses' Drug Reference*. Albany, NY: Delmar, 1993.

Table 41–10. Anxiolytic Medication Therapy

Medication	Actions	Comments	Side Effects	Nursing Considerations
Benzodiazepines Alprazolam Chlordiazepoxide Clorazepate Diazepam Halazepam Lorazepam Oxazepam Prazepam	Agents are thought to work in parts of the limbic system and reticular formation, facilitating GABA, a neurotransmitter. Also used for ethyl alcohol detoxification and as a muscle relaxant.	Agents are safe in high doses. Main difference is in duration of action. Psychologic and physical dependence occur. Tapering decreases withdrawal symptoms.	Drowsiness Ataxia Increased irritability Memory problems Rebound insomnia	• Older persons are at higher risk for ataxia, falls, and paradoxical excitement. • Withdrawal symptoms may continue for weeks. Symptoms range from agitation and insomnia to psychosis and seizures. Tapering is necessary if anxiolytics have been used for more than several weeks.
Buspirone	Mechanism is not the same as for benzodiazepines. Agent binds with dopamine and serotonin receptors.	Agent is not addictive. It may not be used to detoxify or decrease withdrawal syndrome. Agent may require 2 wk of treatment before effects are seen.	Nausea Dizziness Extrapyramidal symptoms (see Table 41–7) Central nervous system effects	• May cause drowsiness, should not be combined with alcohol or central nervous system depressants. • Antacids interfere with absorption. • Buspirone should be given with food to decrease nausea.

Data from Laraia M, and Stuart G. *Quick Psychopharmacology Reference*. 2nd ed. St. Louis: CV Mosby, 1995; and Spratto G, and Woods A. *RN's NDR 1993: Nurses' Drug Reference*. Albany, NY: Delmar, 1993.

Psychotherapeutic Approaches

1. Individual psychotherapy
   a. Psychoanalysis, based on Freud's technique, involves years of almost daily sessions. Focusing primarily on early experiences, the therapist remains relatively neutral, allowing the patient to "transfer" to the therapist all old feelings and experiences, bringing to consciousness feelings that have been unconscious. It is for nonpsychotic people with good resources, both psychologic and financial. Analysts must have received several years of specialized analytic training.
   b. Psychodynamic therapy is another relatively long-term therapy, with a goal of restructuring some basic components of the personality. The focus may be on early experiences as well as the present. This is also called "long-term" psychotherapy in the current health care environment. It is helpful in the treatment of PDs and is primarily used for nonpsychotic disorders.
   c. Short-term therapy or brief problem-oriented therapy may be for individuals, couples, or family and is for 1 to 6 sessions usually. Several therapeutic techniques are used, but this format is geared to helping persons work on a particular problem. The therapist may act as a coach or active participant in the process. The therapy uses problem-solving methods, with the patient defining the problem. Therapy focuses on the person's strengths and on the present.
   d. Behavioral–social learning therapies are aimed at changing responses to stimuli, not gaining insight or restructuring personality. Usually geared to the individual, these therapies may be very structured and are excellent for treatment of phobias and compulsive disorders. Specific techniques include the following:
      • Flooding
      • Desensitization
      • Aversion
      • Thought stopping
      • Imagery
      • Behavioral modification
      • Relaxation techniques
   e. Cognitive-behavioral therapy is used primarily as a treatment for depression. This structured therapy is aimed at replacing negative thoughts that precede negative feelings. After the thoughts are identified, there is a process of restructuring the thoughts by recognizing their errors and replacing them. Therapy may be geared to individuals or groups. The person must be motivated, literate, and nonpsychotic.
2. Participatory therapies are those in which the patient physically carries out an activity, expressing or "acting out" inner conflicts in a safe environment and in a nondestructive way.
   a. Play therapy for children may be for individuals or groups. While the children engage in play, the therapist may identify conflicts and children may work them out.
   b. Psychodrama is a group experience used for adolescents and adults, involving a therapist with special training. A dramatization of personal events is carried out by participants, and insights are shared. Persons must be able to abstract and have some insight.
3. Group therapies
   a. Group psychotherapy may take place in an inpatient or outpatient setting and is facilitated by a profes

sional therapist. Members with different backgrounds come together, and the interactions within the group bring about changes in the insight and behavior of individual members. Groups may be open or closed (e.g., not open to new members once started).

b. Support groups and therapeutic or self-help groups focus on a shared problem, whether it be an addiction, grief, or physical illness. Members support and draw strength from one another. Support groups may have a permanent leader with professional training; self-help groups have a fellow member as a leader.

c. Marital and family therapies focus on the communication problems and process within the system. There are several schools of technique.

Milieu therapy uses the environment as a therapy. Related to behavioralism, this therapy involves shaping the person's environment to maximize the possibility of appropriate behaviors taking place. Also called "therapeutic environment" or "therapeutic community," the surroundings and atmosphere are used to teach lessons of responsibility and dealing with situations. From rules of governing to the use of color, the milieu is anything external to the person.

Activities therapies

a. Occupational and recreational therapies teach the use of exercise, crafts, and leisure activities to promote health and self-esteem. Occupational therapy may assess the person's ability to live independently after discharge.

b. Music and art therapies encourage creative expression as an outlet. Drawing has recently been used extensively for those children and adults who have experienced trauma.

c. Life skills therapy is the learning or relearning of social skills and day-to-day tasks and is often a group therapy for very regressed or withdrawn persons. Nurses or activity therapists may lead these groups.

Reminiscence or life review therapies benefit older adults. The intentional calling up of old memories and experiences may be helpful when dealing with aging and its losses. These 2 therapies are related but not identical.

a. Reminiscence therapy (group or individual) is primarily positive, suppressing conflicts and shoring up strengths and self-esteem.

b. Life review therapy uses the recall of past experiences, but it is more analytic of a person's life, often including unresolved past issues. Thus, it requires a trained psychotherapist.

pecial Procedures

In ECT (see p. 1913), a very small amount of electric current is delivered to the temporal area to stimulate a seizure. The seizure is the treatment; the current merely stimulates the seizure. A tonic-clonic seizure of 30 to 60 seconds' duration is preferred.

a. The psychiatrist performs this procedure with an anesthesiologist; the entire process, including recovery, takes as little as 30 minutes.

b. Anesthetized with a short-acting agent, the person then receives a muscle relaxant, so that the seizure may only be seen in the electroencephalogram and the 1 extremity that received minimal muscle relaxant.

c. Electroconvulsive therapy requires a signed informed consent.

d. The nurse is responsible for care of the patient before, during, and after treatment (Procedure 41–1).

e. Education, advocacy, and support is nursing's role throughout the course of treatment.

CLINICAL CONTROVERSIES

The use of electroconvulsive therapy (ECT) remains controversial in some areas, despite research supporting its safety and efficacy. Patients, families, and professionals are still influenced by the presentation of ECT in movies. Videotapes are now used so health care professionals and consumers may view the current procedures.

Research on attitudes of health care professionals (medical doctors, nurses, psychologists, and social workers) showed a correlation of knowledge and clinical experience with positive attitudes toward ECT as an effective modality. Nurses must be aware of their own feelings and educate themselves so that they can educate and support persons making decisions about treatment.

2. Psychosurgery
   a. Only a few neurosurgeons are skilled in the newer forms of psychosurgery, which have replaced the old frontal lobotomies of the 1940s and 1950s. It is considered the treatment of last resort.
   b. Currently, surgery is reserved for patients who have devastating symptoms of obsessive-compulsive disorder and depressive disorders or who have not been helped by any other treatments.
   c. The surgery itself involves removal or ablation of very small, discrete sections of the brain, often involving the gyrus cinguli (cingulotomy) or disconnection of the limbic system from the frontal lobes (capsulotomy).

◼ CARING FOR PEOPLE WITH PSYCHIATRIC EMERGENCIES

The Suicidal Person

1. Incidence and etiology
   a. Whereas psychiatric illnesses increase the risk for suicidal behavior, certain demographic and situational factors also increase risk.
   b. Most persons who attempt suicide have spoken to someone about it within the previous week.
   c. When suicide is an impulsive act, it is often as a result of the use of alcohol or other substances that alter judgment.
   d. Gunshot wounds account for the majority of the completed suicides in the United States.
2. Risk factors for completed suicide
   - White race
   - Male gender
   - Advanced age
   - Living alone

P

Procedure 41–1
Electroconvulsive Therapy

Preliminary Activities

Preparation of Person

Night Before Treatment
- Instruct or assist patient in shampooing hair to remove hair products that may interfere with conduction.
- Check chart to verify orders and signed consent. Check for changes to oral medications. Medications that raise the seizure threshold (e.g., benzodiazepines) may be contraindicated.
- Give nothing by mouth after midnight to decrease the risk of aspiration during the procedure.
- Check the treatment suite for supplies, emergency cart, and medications. Some additional supplies may need to be accessible during treatment.

Morning of Treatment
- Remind patient of the scheduled ECT and of the nothing-by-mouth status. Address any questions or concerns. The patient may have forgotten due to anxiety or memory difficulties from the ECT itself, or the patient may just need reassurance.

Procedure

Action	Rationale

Pretreatment

1. Assist the patient with gown or comfortable front-opening clothing.
2. Remove prostheses—hearing aids, dentures, glasses.
3. Remove hairpins, hair nets, barrettes.
4. Encourage the patient to void immediately before treatment.
5. Check vital signs.
6. Administer intramuscular anticholinergic agent 30 minutes before treatment.

7. Administer oral analgesic if ordered.
8. Accompany patient to the treatment room, via wheelchair or stretcher if the patient is unsteady.

1. Access is necessary for placement of electrocardiographic leads.
2. Items could be damaged or misplaced during treatment.
3. Items interfere with conduction of electricity.
4. Early voiding prevents incontinence during the induced seizure.
5. Establishes a preprocedure baseline.
6. Such administration decreases the risk of
   - Bradycardia during treatment
   - Aspiration of secretions
7. Analgesic is prophylaxis for a post-ECT headache.
8. Such accompaniment promotes safety and provides opportunity for offering support.

In the Treatment Room

1. Introduce the patient to all team members, explaining their roles.
2. Assist the patient to the stretcher; remove the patient's shoes and socks.
3. Cleanse placement areas and assist with placement of electroencephalographic and electrocardiographic electrodes.
4. Apply pulse oximeter and sphygmomanometer cuff.
5. Apply a 2nd blood pressure cuff to 1 ankle. (After administration of the anesthetic and muscle relaxant by the physician, anesthesia staff ventilate the patient with pure oxygen and monitor vital signs [VS].)
6. Insert a bite block just before delivery of the stimulus. Position it to separate upper and lower teeth, with the rim separating the lips and teeth.
7. Support the block and chin during the seizure. (The physician administers the electric pulse via a special machine. The current precipitates the seizure of 30 to 60 seconds, ideally.)
8. Monitor VS either continuously or every 1 minute during the procedure.

1. This decreases anxiety; many persons participate in the treatment.
2. Ankles must be bare to apply electrocardiographic leads and to obser the foot for tonic–clonic activity.
3. A clean area improves contact.

4. Equipment provides continuous monitoring during the procedure.
5. The cuff occludes blood flow to the extremity, limiting the flow muscle relaxant to the area. Thus, that foot still provides evidence seizure activity to validate electroencephalographic tracing.
6. Despite use of the relaxant, the position of the electrodes causes dire stimulation to the jaw. Clenching occurs, and tongue or teeth could damaged.
7. This assists in maintaining a patent airway and lowers the risk of inju to tongue and teeth.

8. Some patients experience a spike in blood pressure or a brief period asystole during and immediately after the procedure.

After Treatment

1. Remove the bite block and ankle cuff.
2. Monitor VS before and after the patient is cleared to transfer to a recovery area (every 2 to 5 minutes).
3. Decrease stimuli in the recovery area.
4. Monitor VS and oxygenation.

1. These are no longer necessary.
2. The responsibility for monitoring is transferred to the nurse from th anesthesiologist.
3. The patient is post-ictal and sensitive to stimuli.
4. Medications given during the procedure may still be affecting bloc pressure, cardiac, and respiratory functions.

P

Procedure 41–1

(continued)

5. Protect the patient from falls, frequently check mental status, and reorient the patient during arousal.

6. When the patient is stable, assist the patient to a room, via a wheelchair if the patient is unsteady.

7. The patient may nap or activities may be resumed.

8. Check for return of gag reflex before offering oral medications or nutrition. If the patient is awake and talking, offer breakfast.

9. Offer analgesia for headache or muscle soreness.

10. Gently reorient the patient as needed, verbally and through resumption of daily routine.

5. There is restlessness during this period, and the patient is at risk for falls and aspiration. Post-ictal and postanesthesia states cause confusion.

6. Patients often remain drowsy for a time after treatment.

7. Resuming activities helps with reorienting.

8. The gag reflex prevents aspiration. Breakfast stabilizes blood glucose level and helps the patient with orientation.

9. These are the most frequent physical complaints after ECT.

10. Retrograde amnesia is expected after ECT.

ata from Stuart G. Somatic therapies. *In* Stuart G, and Sundeen S (eds). *Principles and Practice of Psychiatric Nursing.* 5th ed. St. Louis: CV Mosby, 1995; Duffy and Conradt, ectroconvulsive therapy: The perioperative process. *AORN J* 50(4):806–809, 811–812, 1989. The assistance of L. Jeanette Weston, RN, in the preparation of this procedure is reatly appreciated.

- Feelings of hopelessness
- Medical illness
- Substance abuse
- Psychosis
- History of suicide attempts by person or family members

. Verbal and nonverbal interventional behavior of the professional must be swift, direct, and life affirming.

   a. Persons should be asked directly whether suicide is being considered and whether they have a plan and the means.

   b. Regardless of the setting, one-to-one continuous observation is the treatment of choice for the acutely suicidal person until the immediate crisis has lessened.

   c. Verbal contracts should be specific—not to harm self, to talk to someone if tempted. Contracts may be written or oral and should be for a specific time frame with frequent renewals.

   d. Maintenance of a safe environment includes removal of all potential weapons, even low lethality items such as shoelaces. Medication monitoring is necessary. A desperate person may break a lightbulb or save a plastic fork to fashion a weapon; 24-hour vigilance is the primary safety intervention

   e. Outpatient status may be maintained if verbal contracts are agreed to and persons have family members capable of monitoring them.

   f. The attitude of health care professionals toward the person must be one of confidence that the person has value and that together they will successfully resolve the crisis.

. The underlying illness or situational stressor should be addressed during and after the immediate crisis.

   a. Substance abuse, chronic mental illness, and physical illness may need treatment.

   b. Psychiatric illness, if previously diagnosed, may have been undertreated, or there may be noncompliance.

   c. Psychotherapy is helpful for issues of loss, low self-esteem, and depression.

   d. Persons should have available the telephone numbers for crisis lines if the problem recurs.

3. If a suicide has been completed, family or staff need to address the issues and feelings surrounding the event, as well as whether clues were missed or procedures were inadequate.

The Assaultive Person

1. Incidence and etiology

   a. Violence in the workplace has become a universal concern, regardless of the setting.

   b. Psychiatric inpatient units have been surpassed by emergency areas and medical-surgical units as the most dangerous units for nursing staff.

   c. Most psychiatric patients are not dangerous; the presence of certain conditions are better indicators of potential for aggression.

   d. Variables that increase the possibility for violence
   - A history of violent behavior
   - Organic brain insult—be it from substance abuse, injury, or disease process
   - Escalating hostility or paranoia
   - Poor impulse control
   - Impaired reality or sensorium

   e. Early cues and gradual escalation may be absent when there is organicity.

2. Clinical management

   a. Prevention techniques

      (1) There should be continuous monitoring of the safety of a person's environment. Institutions may

want to install metal detectors, and caregivers should be aware of how to exit a patient's area. Vigilance is important.

(2) Preparedness is maintained by periodic drills or rehearsals of simulated situations; in some states, annual training is mandatory for maintaining licensure of psychiatric units.

(3) The assaultive potential of each patient, including criteria previously listed, must be assessed early and often, with changes noted in status, such as increased motor activity, loudness, making of verbal threats, or clenching of fists.

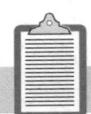

NURSING MANAGEMENT

Psychiatric unit staff are often more prepared for assaultive situations than staff working on other units. Medical-surgical and long-term care units also need periodic training in dealing with these issues.

(4) Persons should be aware of their own verbal and nonverbal behavior. Body language, tone, or prolonged eye contact may be threatening to a person.

b. Early intervention

(1) A person's own verbal and nonverbal behavior can be used to deescalate a situation. Calm, matter-of-fact instruction should be used in calm, brief interactions.

(2) Pharmacologic (anxiolytics or antipsychotics) or nonpharmacologic (a time out or quiet room use) means may be used to regain control.

c. Crisis techniques are implemented when the safety of the patient or others is jeopardized. Staff should implement the procedures of their unit or facility, including the following:

(1) The use of sufficient staff, who have made a plan of intervention before implementing it

(2) Designating a leader who directs the procedure and explains to the person what is transpiring and why

(3) Chemical restraint, if required, with the use of injection of a short-acting anxiolytic agent alone or an antipsychotic drug. An emergency situation can supercede the need for consent to medicate assaultive patients.

(4) If seclusion or restraints are used, the policies and procedures of the facility must be followed. (See pp. 1901 and 1909 regarding the least restrictive environment.)

d. Postincident procedures

(1) A debriefing-type session should be held for both the patient and the staff as soon as possible after the incident. A nonblaming attitude is necessary. Legal, ethical, and emotional issues may warrant a consultation with another health care professional.

(2) Implementation of the procedures should be evaluated for effectiveness or need for revision.

(3) If a staff person is assaulted, that person will need additional help to work through the post-trauma feelings. Professional or peer counseling are options. Some states allow charges to be filed against assaultive patients.

■ PUBLIC HEALTH CONSIDERATIONS AND PRIMARY PREVENTION

Caring for the Mentally Ill Homeless

1. Two hundred thousand mentally ill persons are among the homeless. Causes include deinstitutionalization, poverty and lack of low-income housing, substance abuse and the release of mentally ill persons from prison.

2. Schizophrenia, substance-related disorders, and mood disorders (bipolar, manic) are the most prevalent disorders in this population. Many use substances as well.

3. Inadequate sleep and nutrition, a head injury, or substance abuse can cause psychosis in persons who do not have a mental illness.

4. Local resources differ. Storefront clinics, outreach mobile teams, and screening facilities in shelters are the most common. Follow-up is nearly impossible for the homeless who are transient.

5. Caring for these persons requires compassion, coordination, and advocacy. Innovative programs must include simple housing and daily case management. Such programs are few.

6. Some states use the "outpatient committal" or "mandatory outpatient treatment" judicial process as a means to compel the chronically mentally ill to comply with pharmacologic and outpatient treatment. The long-acting intramuscular formulations of haloperidol and fluphenazine are helpful for some.

Caring for the Mentally Ill in Jails and Prisons

1. A total of 1.5 million persons are in US prisons and jails. At least 15 percent of them have major mental illness. The penal system and nursing homes are the 2 largest residential "treatment centers" for the mentally ill.

2. Three of 4 prisoners have problems with substance; only 1 in 3 receives treatment.

3. Prisons provide acute mental health services, rendered either at state mental hospitals or prison hospital psychiatric wards, but follow-up is lacking for many patients.

4. Local jails, however, may have no detoxification facilities or psychiatric treatment programs.

5. The lack of reentry programs for released prisoners is considered a contributing factor to the number of homeless and homeless mentally ill.

Trends in Mental Health Care

1. The 1990s were declared the "Decade of the Brain" by Congress. As a result

a. A total of $2 billion per year was allocated for brain research.

b. The physiologic bases for mental disorders are being more clearly delineated.

. Health care reform and managed care have decreased the length of stay for inpatients. Traditional inpatient treatments (e.g., ECT and treatment for substance abuse) are becoming outpatient modalities. Partial hospitalization and psychiatric home health services are being increasingly used.

. Cost-contained mental health care focuses on outcomes. In the future, these outcomes should attempt to measure improved quality of life (e.g., continued employment), not merely time between hospitalizations.

. To be truly cost effective, mental health care will require more funds dedicated to prevention, promotion, and rehabilitation outside the acute facilities.

a. Prevention and promotion efforts will focus on children and "at-risk" populations, with care provided in diverse settings (see below).

b. The aging of the baby boomers (born between 1947 and 1961) will be reflected in an increased emphasis on the cognitive mental disorders, such as community programs for cognitively impaired older adults, allowing affected persons to remain in the community.

. Nonpharmacologic, more holistic interventions (e.g., sleep reordering and light therapy) will be pursued for cost effectiveness and safety, especially in older adults.

. Increasing cultural diversity will influence societal attitudes about the holistic nature of humans, strengthening trends toward alternative or complementary treatments.

. Emerging knowledge of psychoneuroimmunology will add impetus to holistic models of health and disease, with mental health being viewed as integral to physical health.

Primary Prevention Measures

1. Biologic models are the focus currently; prevention in that mode involves identifying genetic markers and persons who are biologically at risk.
2. Psychologic and sociologic vulnerabilities have been identified for years (see also Chapter 39).
3. *Healthy People 2000,* a project of the U.S. Public Health Service, has identified prevention and promotion objectives for mental health and mental disorders. These include the following:
   a. Reducing suicides and suicide attempts by children and adolescents
   b. Targeting stress—decreasing it at work, reducing its health effects, and reducing its violent sequelae
   c. Increasing access to and use of mental health systems already in place—community support systems and treatment for depressive disorders and other emotional disorders
   d. Increasing primary care providers' attention to mental and emotional functioning of their patients
4. Schools are beginning to teach conflict resolution and coping strategies to young people, but fiscal constraints and "downsizing" are limiting the availability of programs, adding stress to the workplace and decreasing the time health care professionals can spend with their patients
5. Informing the public and raising the collective consciousness to value prevention are roles that nurses can play. Volunteer and grass roots organizations will play an increasing role. Promoting mental health in children is the primary prevention.

Bibliography

Books

American Psychiatric Association. *A Psychiatric Glossary.* 6th ed. Washington, DC: Author, 1988.

American Psychiatric Association. *Diagnostic and Statistical Manual of Mental Disorders.* 4th ed. Washington, DC: Author, 1994.

Andreasen N, and Black D. *Introductory Textbook of Psychiatry.* Washington, DC: American Psychiatric Press, 1991.

Baldessarini R. *Chemotherapy in Psychiatry: Principles and Practice, Revised.* Cambridge: Harvard University Press, 1985.

Carson R, and Butcher J. *Abnormal Psychology and Modern Life.* 9th ed. New York: Harper Collins, 1992.

Giger J, and Davidhizar R. *Transcultural Nursing: Assessment and Intervention.* St. Louis: CV Mosby, 1991.

Kaplan H, and Sadock B. *Comprehensive Textbook of Psychiatry.* 6th ed. Baltimore: Williams & Wilkins, 1995.

Laraia M, and Stuart G. *Quick Psychopharmacology Reference.* 2nd ed. St. Louis: CV Mosby, 1995.

McFarland G, and Thomas M. *Psychiatric Mental Health Nursing: Application of the Nursing Process.* Philadelphia: JB Lippincott, 1991.

Spratto G, and Woods A. *RN's NDR 1993: Nurses' Drug Reference.* Albany, NY: Delmar, 1993.

Stuart S, and Sundeen S. *Principles and Practice of Psychiatric Nursing.* 5th ed. St. Louis: CV Mosby, 1995.

Townsend M. *Psychiatric Mental Health Nursing: Concepts of Care.* Philadelphia: FA Davis, 1993.

Townsend M. *Psychiatric Mental Health Nursing: Concepts of Care: Community Health Supplement.* Philadelphia: FA Davis, 1995.

Wilson H, and Kniesl C. *Psychiatric Nursing.* 4th ed. Redwood City, CA: Addison-Wesley, 1992.

Chapters in Books and Journal Articles

The Mental Health–Mental Illness Continuum

Drake R, Alterman A, and Rosenberg S, Detection of substance abuse disorders in severely mentally ill patients. *Community Ment Health J* 29(2):175–192, 1993.

National Advisory Mental Health Council. Health care reform for Americans with severe mental illnesses. *Am J Psychiatry* 150:1447–1457, 1993.

News and notes: Mental illness remains a source of stigma. *Hosp Community Psychiatry* 41(7):819, 1990.

Regier DA, et al. The de facto U.S. mental and addictive disorders system. *Arch Gen Psychiatry* 50(2):85–94, 1993.

Assessment and Diagnostics

Batzer E, and Laraia M. Psychiatric evaluation. *In* Stuart G, and Sundeen S (eds). *Principles and Practice of Psychiatric Nursing.* 4th ed. St. Louis: CV Mosby, 1991.

Ribeiro CM, et al. The DST as a predictor of outcome in depression: A meta-analysis. *Am Psychiatry* 150(11):1618–1629, 1993.

Schizophrenic Disorders

Books

Torrey F. Causes of schizophrenia. *Surviving Schizophrenia: A family manual.* New York: Harper & Row, 1989.

Chapters in Books and Journal Articles

Andreasen NC, et al. Thallamic abnormalities in schizophrenia visualized through magnetic resonance image averaging. *Science* (266):294–298, 1994.

Black D, Yates W, and Andreasen N. Schizophrenia, schizophreniform and delusional (paranoid) disorders. *In* Talbot J, Hales R, and Yudofsky S (eds). *The American Psychiatric Press Textbook of Psychiatry*. Washington, DC: American Psychiatric Press, 1988.

Crismon M, and Dorson P. Schizophrenia. *In* DiPiro J, et al. (eds). *Pharmacotherapy: A Pathophysiologic Approach*. 2nd. ed. Norwalk, CT: Appleton & Lange, 1993.

Rosenthal T, and McGuiness T. Dealing with delusional patients: Discovering the distorted truth. *Issues Ment Health Nurs* 8(2):143–154, 1986.

Mood Disorders

Depression Guideline Panel. *Depression in Primary Care: Detection, Diagnosis and Treatment: Quick Reference Guide for Clinicians, Number 5*. Rockville, MD: U.S. Department of Health and Human Services, Public Health Service, Agency for Health Care Policy and Research, 1993.

Greenberg P, et. al. The economic burden of depression in 1990. *J Clin Psychiatry* 54(11):405–418, 1993.

Anxiety Disorders

Hayes P, and Kirkwood C. Anxiety disorders. *In* DiPiro J, et al. (eds). *Pharmacotherapy: A Pathophysiologic Approach*. 2nd ed. Norwalk, CT: Appleton & Lange, 1993.

May R. *The Meaning of Anxiety*. New York: Ronald Press Co, 1950.

Peplau H. A working definition of anxiety. *In* Burd S, and Marshall M (eds). *Some Clinical Approaches to Psychiatric Nursing*. New York: Macmillan, 1963.

Regier D, Burke J, and Burke K. Comorbidity of affective and anxiety disorders in the NIMH epidemiologic catchment area program. *In* Maser J, and Cloninger C (eds). *Comorbidity of Anxiety and Mood Disorders*. Washington, DC: American Psychiatric Press, 1990.

Stuart G, and Sundeen S. Anxiety. *In* Stuart G, and Sundeen S (eds). *Principles and Practice of Psychiatric Nursing*. 4th ed. St. Louis: CV Mosby, 1991.

Dissociative Disorders

Pawlilcki C, and Gaumer C. Nursing care of the self-mutilating patient. *Bull Menninger Clin* 57(3):380–389, 1993.

Stafford L. Dissociation and multiple personality disorder: A challenge for psychosocial nurses. *J Psychosoc Nurs Ment Health Serv* 31(1):15–20, 30–31, 1993.

Therapeutics

Books

American Psychiatric Association: *The Practice of Electroconvulsive Therapy: Recommendations for treatment, training, and privileging*. Washington DC: Author, 1990.

Chapters in Books and Journal Articles

Blair D, and Dauner A. Extrapyramidal symptoms are serious side-effects of antipsychotic and other drugs. *Nurse Practitioner* 17(11):61–66, 1992.

Blair D, and Dauner A. Neuroleptic malignancy syndrome: Liability in nursing practice. *J Psychosoc Nurs Ment Health Serv* 31(2):5–13, 1993.

Burns C, and Stuart G. Nursing care in electroconvulsive therapy. *Psychiatr Clin North Am* 14:971–984, 1991. [Entire volume is devoted to ECT.]

Crismon M, and Dorson P. Schizophrenia. *In* DiPiro J, et al. (eds). *Pharmacotherapy: A Pathophysiologic Approach*. 2nd. ed. Norwalk, CT: Appleton & Lange, 1993.

Dauner A, and Blair D. Akathesia: When treatment creates a problem. *J Psychosoc Nurs Ment Health Serv* 28:13–16, 1990.

Duffy WJ, and Conradt H. Electroconvulsive therapy. The perioperative process. *AORN J* 50(4):806–809, 811–812, 1989.

Forman L. Medications: Reasons for interventions for noncompliance. *J Psychosoc Nurs Ment Health Serv* 31(10):23–26, 1993.

Glod C, and Mathieu J. Expanding uses of anticonvulsants in the treatment of bipolar disorder. *J Psychosoc Nurs Ment Health Serv* 31(5):37–39, 1993.

Jaritz N, Flowers E, and Millsap L. Clozapine: Nursing care considerations. *Perspect Psychiatr Care* 28:19–25, 1992.

Littrell K, and Magill A. The effect of clozapine on preexisting tardive dyskinesia. *J Psychosoc Nurs Ment Health Serv* 31(9):14–18, 1993.

Rappaport Z. Psychosurgery in the modern era: Therapeutic and ethical aspects. *Med Law* 11(5–6):449–453, 1992.

Valenti S. Electroconvulsive therapy. *Arch Psychiatr Nurs* 4:223–230, 1991.

Wengel S, et al. Use of benzodiazepines in the elderly. *Psychiatr Ann* 23:325, 1993.

Psychiatric Emergencies

Cahill C, et al. Inpatient management of violent behavior: Nursing prevention and intervention. *Issues Ment Health Nurs* 12(3):239–252, 1991.

Fauman B, Terranova G, and Phillips R. The psychiatric emergency: Heading off trouble. *Patient Care* 28(18):130–2, 135–8, 141–142, 1994.

Kanak F. Interventions related to patient safety. *Nurs Clin North Am* 27(2):371–395, 1992.

Trends and Prevention

Mandersheid R, Sonnernshein M, eds. *Mental Health U.S., 1992*. Washington DC: U.S. Department of Health and Human Services, Center for Mental Health Services, 1994.

U.S. Department of Health and Human Services. *Healthy People 2000*. Washington, DC: Public Health Service, 1990.

U.S. Government Accounting Office. *Mentally ill inmates: Better data would help determine protection and advocacy needs*. Publication GAO-GDD 91-35. Washington, DC: U.S. Government Printing Office, 1991.

Agencies and Resources

National Institute of Mental Health (NIMH)
5600 Fishers Lane
Room 15C-05
Rockville, MD 20857
http://www.nimh.nih.gov

National Mental Health Association
1021 Prince Street
Alexandria, VA 22314–2971
http://www.worldcorp.com/dc-online/nmha

National Alliance for the Mentally Ill (NAMI)
2101 Wilson Boulevard
Suite 302
Arlington, VA 22009–1604
http://www.cais.net/vikings/nami

National Depressive and Manic Depressive Association
730 North Franklin Street
Suite 501
Chicago, IL 60610

The Obsessive–Compulsive Disorder Foundation
P.O. Box 70
Milford, CT 06460

42

Caring for People with Human Immunodeficiency Virus Disease

☐ OVERVIEW OF HUMAN IMMUNODEFICIENCY VIRUS DISEASE

Definitions

1. The first stage after exposure to human immunodeficiency virus (HIV) is HIV infection, manifested by the appearance of HIV antibodies in the blood, usually within 6 to 12 weeks after infection.
2. The entire continuum from initial, asymptomatic HIV infection to diagnosis of acquired immunodeficiency syndrome (AIDS) is referred to as **HIV/AIDS** or HIV disease.
3. The final clinical stage of HIV infection is **AIDS.** Results include progressive damage to the immune system and organ systems, especially the central nervous system.
4. **HIV-1** is the retrovirus that causes HIV infection. It has appeared in North America, South America, Europe, sub-Saharan Africa, and most other countries.
5. **HIV-2** causes similar pathology but is serologically and geographically distinct from HIV-1. HIV-2 is found primarily in West Africa.
6. **AIDS-related complex** is a term that was formerly used to refer to pre-AIDS conditions such as persistent generalized lymphadenopathy.
7. The Centers for Disease Control and Prevention (CDC) has continually refined definitions and diagnostic criteria since HIV was identified in 1983 (Table 42–1).

Classifications and Stages

1. The CDC clinical classification system
   a. Category A includes 1 or more of the following in an adolescent or adult with documented HIV infection:
      (1) Asymptomatic HIV infection
      (2) Persistent generalized lymphadenopathy
      (3) Acute HIV infection with accompanying illness or a history of acute HIV infection
   b. Category B includes symptomatic conditions in an

HIV-infected adolescent or adult that are not listed in Category C and meet 1 or more of the following criteria:
   (1) The conditions are due to HIV infection, indicate a defect in cell-mediated immunity, or both.
   (2) Physicians consider the conditions to have a clinical course or management complicated by HIV infection.
   (3) The person manifests such conditions as oral or vaginal candidiasis, fever or diarrhea for more than 1 month, and idiopathic thrombocytopenia purpura.
   c. Category C includes the 25 clinical conditions listed in the AIDS surveillance case definition presented in Box 42–1.
2. The CDC laboratory categories
   a. Category 1: 500 or more CD4 cells per mm^3
   b. Category 2: 200 to 499 CD4 cells per mm^3
   c. Category 3: fewer than 200 CD4 cells per mm^3
3. Progression of HIV/AIDS
   a. Initial infection
      (1) A person usually develops HIV antibodies 6 to 12 weeks after exposure to HIV. Some people take up to 12 months to develop antibodies, however.
      (2) Some persons experience flulike symptoms 2 to 6 weeks after infection, but others remain asymptomatic.
   b. Asymptomatic HIV infection
      (1) People experience no clinical symptoms.
      (2) During this stage, which can last 10 years or longer, many people are unaware that they are HIV infected.
   c. Development of symptoms (Table 42–2)
      (1) Persistent generalized lymphadenopathy may precede an AIDS diagnosis.
      (2) The person may also experience weight loss, weakness, fevers, and diarrhea.
   d. AIDS, the final clinical stage of disease
      (1) The CD4 count drops to 200 or below, which increases the likelihood of developing AIDS-defining opportunistic infections or neoplasms. Refer to Box 42–1 for a list of the clinical conditions that are considered AIDS defining or "indicator dis-

Table 42–1. The Development of the Definition of Human Immunodeficiency Virus Disease

Year	Development
1983	Human immunodeficiency virus (HIV) is identified as the causative agent for HIV disease.
1986	The Centers for Disease Control and Prevention (CDC) publishes a classification system for HIV disease.
1987	The CDC adds acquired immunodeficiency syndrome (AIDS) dementia and wasting syndrome to the list of 23 AIDS-defining conditions.
1993	The CDC revises the definition of AIDS surveillance to include recurrent bacterial pneumonias, pulmonary tuberculosis, and invasive cervical cancer. CD4 cell counts of 200 mm^3 or lower are also considered AIDS defining.

eases.'' One or more of these indicator conditions must be present for a patient to receive a diagnosis of AIDS.

(2) After a diagnosis of AIDS, life expectancy is 3 to 5 years. Improved therapies continue to lengthen and maintain quality of life.

Incidence and Mortality Rates

1. U.S. data
   a. Overall statistics: There are 1 million HIV-infected people in the United States. More than 513,000 Americans have been diagnosed with AIDS since 1981. The fatality rate is 62 percent.

BOX 42–1. Conditions That Indicate Acquired Immunodeficiency Syndrome

Recurrent bacterial pneumonia
Invasive cervical carcinoma, confirmed by biopsy
Candidiasis of bronchi, trachea, or lungs
Esophageal candidiasis
Cryptococcosis, extrapulmonary
Coccidioidomycosis, disseminated or extrapulmonary
Cryptosporidiosis, chronic intestinal for more than 1 month
Cytomegalovirus disease (other than liver, spleen, or nodes)
Cytomegalovirus retinitis (with vision loss)
Human immunodeficiency virus encephalopathy
Herpes simplex (chronic ulcers for more than 1 month) or bronchitis, pneumonitis, or esophagitis
Histoplasmosis, disseminated or extrapulmonary
Isosporiasis, chronic intestinal for more than 1 month
Kaposi's sarcoma
Lymphoma, Burkitt's (or equivalent term)
Lymphoma, immunoblastic (or equivalent term)
Lymphoma, primary, of brain
Mycobacterium avium-intracellulare complex, disseminated or extrapulmonary
Mycobacterium tuberculosis, any site (pulmonary or extrapulmonary)
Pneumocystis carinii pneumonia
Pneumonia, recurrent
Progressive multifocal leukoencephalopathy
Salmonella septicemia, recurrent
Toxoplasmosis of brain
Wasting syndrome (loss of more than 10% of baseline body weight, with chronic diarrhea or fever)

---

b. Geography: New York, the District of Columbia, Puerto Rico, California, Florida, and Texas rank among the highest states in number of diagnosed cases. In New York and a growing number of other states, AIDS has become the leading cause of death for women of childbearing age.

c. Racial and ethnic groups: The racial composition of the United States is 80 percent White, 12 percent Black, 6 percent Hispanic, and 2 percent other. In many communities, Blacks and Hispanics are disproportionately represented among those with AIDS. These 2 groups represent more than 50 percent of cases in New York and Chicago.

2. World data: The World Health Organization has estimated that 20 million people have been infected with HIV. An estimated 4.5 million of these people have developed AIDS. Four million became infected with HIV in 1993 alone.

3. Trends
   a. In the United States, the HIV infection rate is increasing substantially among adolescents and women, with African-American women in the South one of the fastest-growing affected populations.
   b. The epidemic is exploding in Asia, which is expected to become the new center of the epidemic.
   c. Prevention is the most effective approach, but current strategies—including sex education, condom distribution, and protection of the blood supply—have been inadequate.
   d. A small percentage of people with HIV infection do not experience disease progression, even after 12 years. Researchers studying this population are seeking medical clues to explain their longevity.

4. Projections for the future
   a. In the United States by the year 2000, 125,000 children and adolescents will have become orphans as a result of AIDS.
   b. Indicators suggest that AIDS may have peaked among gay men, but numbers continue to increase among gay teens and young adults.
   c. Acquired immunodeficiency syndrome is expected to be the 3rd most common cause of death in the United States by the turn of the century.
   d. The increasing rate of heterosexual transmission will result in more women and children in need of care.

Table 42–2. Effects of Human Immunodeficiency Virus and Acquired Immunodeficiency Syndrome–Defining Conditions on Organ Systems

System	Manifestations	Related to
Central nervous system	Encephalopathy → dementia, peripheral neuropathy, and vacuolar myelopathy	Direct results of human immunodeficiency virus (HIV) infection
	Toxoplasmosis encephalitis, cytomegalovirus encephalitis, and cryptococcal meningitis	Opportunistic infections (OIs)
	Primary central nervous system lymphoma and other metastatic lymphomas	Neoplasms
Respiratory	*Pneumocystis carinii* pneumonia and pulmonary tuberculosis	OIs
Genitourinary	HIV-associated nephropathy	Renal invasion by opportunistic pathogens; also use of nephrotoxic drugs to treat OIs
	Vaginal candidiasis	Often first sign in women with HIV infection
	Invasive cervical cancer	Neoplasm that became an acquired immunodeficiency syndrome (AIDS)–defining condition in 1993
Ocular	Cytomegalovirus (CMV) retinitis	OI caused by CMV
	Retinal vasculitis manifested by cotton wool spots on retina	May be direct effect of HIV
Cardiac	Myocarditis → congestive heart failure or dysrhythmia	May be direct effect of HIV
Gastrointestinal	HIV wasting syndrome without enteric OI	AIDS-defining condition as of 1987
	Anorexia, weight loss, and diarrhea	*Candida, Cryptosporidium,* and CMV
	Obstruction	Kaposi's sarcoma (KS)
	Hepatic disease	CMV, KS, and *Cryptosporidium*
Skin	Reddish brown nodules and patches	KS
	Warts	Papilloma
	Petechiae and ecchymoses	Thrombocytopenia
	Dry skin	Nutritional losses

e. The World Health Organization has estimated that 30 to 40 million men, women, and children will be HIV infected by 2000.

Socioeconomic Impact

1. Financial impact
   a. A 1991 study showed that among people in all stages of HIV disease, 28 percent had private insurance, 53 percent were covered by public entitlements like Medicaid, and 19 percent had no coverage at all. Estimates suggest that it costs $119,000 to care for a person from initial infection until death.
   b. Shorter and less frequent hospital stays and better home supports have reduced the total amount spent on care. If progress continues, in the future HIV disease will become a moderately expensive chronic illness.
2. Social impact

   a. Acquired immunodeficiency syndrome kills people in their most productive years—almost three fourths of deaths occur between the ages of 25 and 44.
   b. Discrimination and denial have slowed the national response to this epidemic, which demands strong, positive leadership for care and prevention.
   c. HIV disease inevitably becomes connected with other societal crises—homelessness, substance abuse, and domestic violence.

Transcultural Considerations

1. Providing culturally sensitive health care means encouraging early diagnosis and treatment and recognizing barriers to care, including financial difficulties, lack of transportation, and child care duties. Discrimination and isolation affect not only the persons with HIV infection or AIDS but also their families and friends.

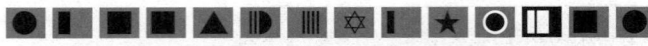

TRANSCULTURAL CONSIDERATIONS

When working with Hispanic people, remember that the family is a particularly important source of support in Hispanic culture. Smooth, positive relationships are valued, and respect and deference in a relationship are very important.

2. Opportunities to enroll in clinical trials have not been readily available for women, adolescents, and people of color because of inadequate support and education in existing primary care programs.
3. The World Health Organization's Global Programme on AIDS defines the family in its broadest sense, as any group of people united by feelings of trust, mutual support, and a common destiny. A blood relationship, marriage, sexual partnership, or adoption is not essential to this definition of family.
4. Cultural beliefs may adversely affect the use of safer sexual practices. For example, some cultures consider condom use an indicator of promiscuity. Women in many cultures defer to men regarding sexual practices (e.g., it is considered inappropriate for Hispanic women to suggest using condoms). Sexual practices that affect the integrity of the vaginal or anal mucosa (e.g., the use of irritants to increase sexual pleasure) may increase the likelihood of HIV infection by allowing HIV easier entry into the circulatory system.
5. Many communities of color manifest a pervasive denial that HIV is transmitted through sexual activity and a persistent belief that HIV affects only Whites. Bisexual men of color who are HIV infected may not identify themselves as gay and consequently do not use services targeted to gay men. Native Americans describe gay or bisexual persons as "two-spirited." Racial inequality in the delivery of health care must be forcefully addressed by all levels of government.
6. HIV-infected people who use injectable drugs need ready access to drug treatment programs as well as primary care for HIV infection.
7. Cultural restrictions and conflicting opinions about the appropriate sex education of adolescents have a negative impact on adolescent HIV prevention. The care of adolescents with HIV infection demands attention to specific issues:
   a. Geographic differences in the prevalence of HIV infection among teens, from a low rate in the north central states to a high rate in urban areas in the east and Texas
   b. A variety of laws that affect consent and confidentiality for minors (teens younger than 18)
   c. Inadequate clinical services to treat adolescents
   d. The lack of models of care that succeed in keeping youth in care throughout the course of the disease
8. The care of gay men infected with HIV is often hampered by stereotypic thinking, stigmatization, and homophobia.

Risk Factors

1. Sexual transmission
   a. Male-to-female transmission and female-to-male transmission have been established, but the relative efficiency of these routes has not been established.
   b. Male-to-male transmission has been established, as has (though rarely) female-to-female transmission.
   c. Transmission by oral sex has been reported.
   d. The presence of other sexually transmitted diseases that result in ulcerations in the genital mucosa may increase susceptibility to infection with HIV.
2. Blood-borne transmission
   a. The use of injectable drugs transmits HIV through the sharing of needles, syringes, and other equipment.
   b. Recipients of HIV-contaminated blood and blood products may become infected. Testing of the U.S. blood supply began in 1985. Before this time, more than half of all persons with hemophilia and people diagnosed with other clotting disorders acquired HIV infection through transfusions of factor concentrates.
3. Perinatal transmission
   a. Women become infected with HIV primarily by using injectable drugs and by having unprotected intercourse with an HIV-infected man. Blood transfusions and other exposures account for 15 percent of cases of transmission.
   b. In the United States, a pregnant women who is HIV positive has a 16 to 30 percent chance of transmitting the virus to her infant either during the pregnancy or at the time of delivery.
4. It is at-risk behaviors, rather than membership in a specific group, that contribute to the spread of HIV. At-risk behaviors include the following:
   a. Having unprotected sex with multiple partners
   b. Sharing needles with HIV-infected persons
   c. Receiving HIV-infected blood or blood products
   d. Being the sexual partner of an HIV-infected person and engaging in unprotected sex, including anal intercourse by both homosexual and heterosexual couples

Reducing the Risk of Human Immunodeficiency Virus Transmission

1. Universal precautions (see Box 8–3), including hand washing (see Procedure 8–1)

NURSE ADVISORY

It is possible to develop human immunodeficiency virus (HIV) infection through work-related exposure. Needlestick injuries pose the greatest threat. After a needlestick injury the risk of becoming HIV positive is 0.4 percent. This risk can be reduced significantly by the use of universal precautions. The likelihood that HIV-infected health care workers will infect a person receiving care is remote. The Centers for Disease Control and Prevention has conducted exhaustive studies and found no evidence to support prohibiting HIV-infected health care workers from providing patient care.

Precautions in the hospital environment

a. Room cleaning: Recommend standard procedures for cleaning the room of a person with HIV, both when the person occupies the room and on discharge. Germicide (e.g., 1 part bleach and 10 parts water) is used when any surface is contaminated visibly with body fluids.

b. Waste disposal: Follow institutional procedures for handling infective waste, which often requires double-bagging and marking the outer bag as infective or hazardous waste.

c. Linen: Use the same careful handling used with all soiled linen. No special procedures are necessary.

d. Sterilization: Recommend standard procedures for sterilizing. Common germicides are very effective against HIV.

Body substance isolation, an alternative to universal precautions (see Box 8–2): All body substances are considered potentially infective. Instead of placing signs requesting specific types of barrier protection only on some rooms, place signs describing appropriate barrier protection on *all* rooms.

Precautions in nonhospital settings

a. Home: Use universal precautions (see Box 8–3).

b. Nursing homes and long-term care facilities: No additional precautions beyond those described previously are needed.

c. Psychiatric facilities: No special restrictions are placed on persons with HIV infection, unless they are demonstrating unacceptable behaviors such as aggressive actions or lack of control of secretions and excretions.

d. Schools: Maintain the HIV-infected child's confidentiality, telling only those with a valid "need to know"; use universal precautions for any child who sustains an injury.

e. Occupational health settings: Use the usual universal precautions when handling a work-related emergency. A worker infected with HIV is protected from on-the-job discrimination through the Americans with Disabilities Act of 1990.

Etiology

In June 1985, the CDC announced that HIV is the etiologic agent for AIDS.

A retrovirus belonging to the subfamily of lentiviruses, HIV causes lifelong infection in a person.

Infection with HIV results in the following:

a. Gradual destruction of the body's immune system

b. Infection of the central nervous system

c. Progressive susceptibility to opportunistic infections

d. An increased likelihood of developing neoplasias

New research indicates that HIV causes cancer through some specific but as yet unknown mechanism, rather than indirectly through immunosuppression. This finding could lead to a better understanding of the role of viruses in other cancers.

Pathophysiology

1. When a person becomes infected with HIV, the body mounts an impressive immune response. (See Chapter 21.)

2. Although in most cases, the body responds within 6 months after infection by manufacturing HIV antibodies, the virus eventually prevails and begins to cause progressive immune system damage.

3. Currently, how low the CD4 cell level drops is thought to predict the extent of immunosuppression.

4. Normal CD4 cell levels range from 600 to 1200 mm^3. In the person with HIV infection, a CD4 level of 200 or lower indicates a diagnosis of AIDS.

5. The presence of p24 antigen, a protein found in the viral core of HIV, can sometimes serve as a marker for HIV infection. Persistent p24 antigenemia may indicate an increased risk of progression to AIDS for an HIV-infected person.

6. New tests to measure viral load, that is, the amount of HIV in the body, may prove helpful in predicting disease progression and measuring the efficacy of antiviral drugs.

◼ ASSESSING PEOPLE WITH HUMAN IMMUNODEFICIENCY VIRUS DISEASE

Key Symptoms and Their Pathophysiologic Bases

1. Symptomatic HIV infection

a. Persistent generalized lymphadenopathy: Diffuse, chronic lymph node enlargement is present for 3 months or longer. Affected nodes include cervical, axillary, inguinal, supraclavicular, infraclavicular, and popliteal. Paradoxically, shrinkage of nodes may predict disease progression.

b. Weight loss: The most important objective measure of disease progression is weight loss caused by reduced food intake, poor absorption of nutrients, and altered metabolism.

c. Oral candidiasis (also called thrush): These discrete or confluent white patches on the mucous membranes of the mouth or throat are caused by *Candida albicans* and may be the only early indicator of HIV infection.

d. Oral hairy leukoplakia: These painless, white, corrugated lesions, which are caused by Epstein-Barr virus, appear on the lateral surfaces of the tongue but may spread across the entire dorsal surface of the tongue. Like oral candidiasis, oral leukoplakia is significant as an early indicator of HIV infection (see Color Fig. 42–1).

e. Vaginal candidiasis (commonly called yeast infection): This severe itching of the labia and vulva, accompanied by thick white or yellow vaginal discharge and dysuria, is caused by several types of *Candida*. Association with HIV infection should be suspected if more than 2 episodes occur in 6 months or if the candidiasis persists after 2 courses of treatment. Vaginal candidiasis may be the only clinical indicator of HIV infection in women.

f. Fever: Low-grade, intermittent fever often accompanies persistent generalized lymphadenopathy. The person may also experience drenching night sweats. Persistent fever or the new onset of a fever higher than 103 degrees Fahrenheit requires a search for the focus of infection.

g. Diarrhea: More than 2 unformed stools per day for 30 days or longer is symptomatic of HIV infection. Causes of diarrhea may be multifactorial, or there may be no identifiable etiologic agent.

2. AIDS-defining conditions

a. *Pneumocystis carinii* pneumonia is the most common life-threatening infection in both genders. *P. carinii* is the causative organism. Symptoms may be nonspecific and include fever, nonproductive cough, tachypnea, and shortness of breath. Diagnosis requires finding *P. carinii* in sputum or lung tissue.

b. Cryptosporidiosis was first identified in humans in 1976. *Cryptosporidium* is the causative organism. Symptoms include profuse, watery diarrhea, abdominal cramping, fever, nausea, and vomiting. Diagnosis involves fecal smear or intestinal biopsy.

c. Toxoplasmosis is a major cause of encephalitis when a person has AIDS. *Toxoplasma gondii*, the causative agent, produces infection in approximately 50 percent of American adults. Symptoms may be vague and include headache, changes in mental status, fever, hemiparesis, seizures, aphasia, ataxia, and visual changes. To avoid brain biopsy, diagnosis is presumptive in the presence of symptoms and laboratory confirmation of HIV infection; computed tomography or magnetic resonance imaging may assist with diagnosis.

d. Esophageal candidiasis marks the progression of HIV infection and is AIDS defining when it occurs with candidiasis of the bronchi, trachea, or lungs. The causative organism is *C. albicans*, which does not respond to topical treatment when it has invaded the esophagus. Symptoms include painful swallowing and substernal pain. HIV infection is diagnosed presumptively with the preceding symptoms, especially in the presence of oral candidiasis.

e. Cytomegalovirus (CMV) retinitis is the most clinically important type of infection in the presence of HIV infection. Cytomegalovirus produces lifelong infection and may facilitate the development of neoplasms. Symptoms include floaters, decreased vision, progression to both eyes, and blindness unless treated promptly. Cytomegalovirus retinitis is diagnosed with clinical evidence and an eye examination.

f. Tuberculosis in the presence of HIV infection has great potential to progress from latent to active. *Mycobacterium tuberculosis*, the causative agent, is spread through the respiratory route by coughing, singing, or talking. Multidrug-resistant strains of tuberculosis

result from inadequate treatment and pose life-threatening risks for both the source patients and those who acquire active disease from them, including health care workers. Nonspecific symptoms include persistent fever, night sweats, weight loss, fatigue, anorexia, a productive cough, and dyspnea. Diagnostics include screening for infection with purified protein derivative as well as anergy screening, chest radiographs, and sputum cultures.

NURSE ADVISORY

Because of the increasing incidence of tuberculosis associated with human immunodeficiency virus infection, a hospitalized person with a cough should be kept in respiratory isolation until tuberculosis is ruled out with two successive negative sputum examinations.

g. Disseminated *Mycobacterium avium-intracellulare* complex infection affects 15 to 25 percent of persons with AIDS in the United States. *M. avium-intracellulare* is found in soil, water, animals, birds, and foodstuffs. Nonspecific symptoms include fever, night sweats, weight loss, anorexia, chronic diarrhea, weakness, and abdominal pain. Infection with this complex is diagnosed with blood cultures and biopsy of the lymph node, liver, or bone marrow.

h. Histoplasmosis, endemic in the central and south central states, is caused by *Histoplasma capsulatum*. This condition initially manifests as a pulmonary infection, but it can disseminate quickly in the person with AIDS. Symptoms include fever, night sweats, anorexia, weight loss, shortness of breath, abdominal pain, diarrhea, cough, central nervous system changes, and skin lesions. Diagnosis involves culture of blood and bone marrow and lymph node, liver, or lung biopsy.

i. Cryptococcosis, estimated to affect 6 to 12 percent of persons with AIDS in the United States, is caused by *Cryptococcus neoformans*, a pervasive yeastlike fungus found worldwide. It can result in pulmonary, central nervous system, and disseminated forms of infection. Symptoms may be subtle and include headaches, stiff neck, photophobia, nausea, vomiting, malaise, altered mental status, and seizures. Diagnosis is based on the serum antigen test, identification of the fungus in cerebrospinal fluid, and culturing of the fungus.

j. Coccidioidomycosis, seen most commonly in the southwestern United States, Mexico, and Central America, is caused by *Coccidioides immitis*. The lungs are usually the primary site of infection. Symptoms include fever, weight loss, cough, and fatigue. Diagnosis is confirmed with tissue cultures.

k. Kaposi's sarcoma (KS) is a neoplasm that affects the skin, mucous membranes, internal organs, or all of these. Although KS is on the decline, it is still a common AIDS-indicator malignancy, seen most frequently in men with a history of same-sex partners. The cause of KS is unknown; some researchers sus pect an infectious agent, and others believe HIV itself may influence the development of KS. Symptoms include reddish-blue lesions on the skin or in the oral cavity early in the disease (Color Figs. 42–2 and 42–3). Late disease results in swelling and pain in the lower extremities, penis, scrotum, or face (Color Fig. 42–4). If KS is disseminated, it affects the skin, lymphatic system, lungs, and gastrointestinal tract. Diagnosis involves punch biopsy of cutaneous lesions and biopsy of pulmonary and gastrointestinal lesions.

l. Lymphomas—cancers of the immune system—have been AIDS-indicator conditions since the onset of the epidemic; 25 percent of lymphomas affect the central nervous system. The cause is unknown, although there are reports of lymphomas in men after long-term antiviral therapy. Presenting symptoms include fever, night sweats, and weight loss. Other symptoms depend on the site of the lymphoma. Diagnosis is difficult because of the possibility of other AIDS-defining conditions. With gastrointestinal involvement, biopsy of enlarged lymph nodes and computed tomography may prove helpful.

m. Invasive cervical cancer became an AIDS-indicator condition in January 1993. Infection with HIV predisposes the woman to neoplastic changes in cervical lesions caused by the human papillomavirus. Early symptoms include painless intermenstrual bleeding. Late symptoms include leg and flank pain, dysuria, hematuria, rectal bleeding, and obstipation. Diagnosis involves Papanicolaou (Pap) smears and colposcopy.

n. HIV encephalopathy is also referred to as AIDS dementia complex (ADC) and became an AIDS-indicator disease in 1987. AIDS dementia complex is caused by neurotropic changes created by HIV. Symptoms include cognitive dysfunction, leg weakness, ataxia, apathy, reduced spontaneity, and withdrawal. Diagnosis of ADC is based on the presence of neurologic deficits, computed tomographic and magnetic resonance imaging scans, and analysis of cerebrospinal fluid.

Health History

Obtain a history of the present illness: Inquire about HIV testing, and assess current symptoms.

Review current medications, both prescription and over-the-counter medications.

Obtain a past medical history.

a. Chronic diseases and major illnesses: Ask about hepatitis and tuberculosis.

b. Surgical history: Include instances of receiving blood or blood products.

c. Childhood illnesses: Inquire about varicella and other childhood diseases and immunization history.

d. Obstetric and gynecologic history: Elicit the number of pregnancies, children, complications of labor, and incidence of pelvic inflammatory disease.

e. Sexually transmitted diseases: Conditions that produce genital lesions increase the risk of HIV infection. Note the dates, locations, and treatments for STDs.

f. Significant family history: Ask if the patient has a family history of tuberculosis or diabetes. Also inquire if there is a family history of depression or suicide.

g. Other care: Note whether the patient is currently receiving care from another physician or clinic and mental health counseling.

4. Obtain a social history.

a. Sexual orientation, modes of sexual expression, and sexual practices: Ask about the use of condoms, spermicides, and birth control methods.

b. Drug use
   (1) Noninjectable drugs such as alcohol and volatile nitrites (poppers) may act as cofactors in HIV disease, because of their immunosuppressive effect.
   (2) For injectable drugs, the greatest risk is in sharing dirty drug-injecting equipment.

c. Occupation: Ask about the person's occupational history and the likelihood of work-related exposure to blood.

d. Travel: Inquire about frequency and locations.

e. Living situation: Ask about the adequacy of the person's housing and finances and the HIV status of others in the household.

f. Support systems: Ask about significant others, children, parents, siblings, friends, and participation in support groups.

Physical Examination

1. General appearance: The initial impression of the person's appearance, demeanor, and affect can be important as the disease progresses.

2. Vital signs
   a. Weight should be recorded at each visit.
   b. Height should be measured once and is needed to determine the body surface area for medication dosage calculations.
   c. Hypertension is a common finding and requires blood pressure evaluation.
   d. Temperature should be recorded at each visit, because high or persistent fever is an indication of opportunistic infection.

3. Lymph nodes: Palpation and measurement of nodes are important to accurate disease staging. Note the location, size, consistency, tenderness, and mobility of affected nodes. New, rapid enlargement of lymph nodes may dictate fine-needle aspiration.

4. Skin: All skin areas require examination. Include the scalp, axillae, palms, pubic and perianal regions, and soles of the feet. Completely describe all noted skin lesions.

5. Eyes: Note the presence of white retinal spots, infiltrates, or hemorrhages. To rule out intracranial lesions, test for extraocular movements and size and reaction of pupils. Refer the person to an ophthalmologist for semiannual examinations when the CD4 level falls below 100 per mm^3.

6. Ears and nose: The ears and nose are common sites for KS lesions. Sinusitis is frequently seen in HIV-positive persons.

7. Oral cavity: Clinicians should wear gloves, use gauze pads to draw out the tongue, and examine the mouth thoroughly. Assess the status of the gums and teeth. Look for warts, ulcers, white plaques, macules, or papules.

8. Lungs: Auscultate and percuss the lungs. The presence of rales or rhonchi may indicate a bacterial infection.

9. Heart: Note the presence of murmurs, especially if there is a history of injectable drug use. Note sounds that may indicate cardiomyopathy.

10. Breasts: Palpate for masses. In men taking ketoconazole, breast enlargement may occur.

11. Abdomen: An enlarged liver or spleen may indicate mycobacterial or fungal infection and lymphoma. Hepatitis B and C are common findings. Infection with HIV may increase liver enzymes.

12. Extremities and musculature: Assess for muscle bulk, tenderness, and weakness. Note changes in the fingernails and toenails, such as clubbing, cyanosis, and fungal infections.

13. Genitals and rectum: Carefully inspect external regions for lesions, which may require culturing. Women must have a pelvic examination with a Pap smear, a swab for gonococcal and chlamydial infection, and a posterior swab for vaginitis. The presence of genital warts demands careful studies for cervical cytopathology. Prostate tenderness and enlargement require evaluation. In persons with a history of anal intercourse, note rectal tone, tenderness, and discharge.

14. Neurologic system: The mental status examination includes orientation, judgment, recent and remote memory ability, and capacity to calculate. Assess extremity strength and gait, which are often abnormal in early HIV dementia and in HIV with neuropathies. Fine motor skills may show abnormalities in the presence of HIV dementia.

Diagnostic Tests

1. Serologic tests: The enzyme-linked immunosorbent assay is used as a screening test to detect HIV antibodies. The Western blot is used to confirm the presence of HIV antibodies after 2 reactive enzyme-linked immunosorbent assays.

2. CD4 lymphocyte counts: CD4 counts are considered a primary test for measuring immune function. The normal range is 600 to 1200 cells per mm^3. CD4 counts should be made every 6 months when the count is greater than 600 and at least every 3 months when the count is between 200 and 600. In advanced disease, the CD4 count may drop to 10 or even be undetectable.

3. Complete blood cell count with differential and platelets: Assess for anemia, thrombocytopenia, and leukopenia. When the test result is normal, repeat it every 6 to 12 months.

4. Sequential Multiple Analyzer (SMA)-20: Monitor renal and liver function, electrolyte imbalances, and drug toxicities. When the test result is normal, repeat it yearly.

5. Urinalysis: Urinalysis detects proteinuria and pyuria and rules out HIV-associated nephropathy and heroin-asso-

ciated nephropathy. When the test result is normal, repeat it yearly.

6. Purified protein derivative: With an anergy panel, the purified protein derivative test screens for latent tuberculosis. Repeat the test annually after negative findings and no sign of anergy. If the person is living in an area with a high prevalence of tuberculosis, test every 6 months.

7. Venereal Disease Research Laboratories or rapid plasma reagin test: Screen for syphilis. When the test result is normal, repeat it yearly.

8. Hepatitis B serology: This test screens for hepatitis B. When results are normal, consider use of vaccine.

9. Pap smear: The Pap smear detects cell changes of the cervix. When the test result is normal, repeat it every 6 months.

Medical Diagnoses

1. A medical diagnosis of HIV infection indicates that HIV serology testing (enzyme-linked immunosorbent assay and Western blot) has revealed HIV antibodies.

2. A medical diagnosis of acute HIV infection refers to a primary HIV infection characterized by a flulike illness, which usually occurs within 6 weeks of initial exposure to HIV.

3. A medical diagnosis of persistent generalized lymphadenopathy is considered a pre-AIDS condition.

4. An AIDS diagnosis is confirmed with laboratory evidence of HIV infection and 1 or more of the following:
   a. A CD4 cell count below 200 per mm^3
   b. A CD4 cell percentage below 14 percent
   c. The presence of or a history of 1 of the 25 AIDS-indicator conditions (see Box 42–1)

◨ MANAGEMENT OF HUMAN IMMUNODEFICIENCY VIRUS DISEASE

Clinical Management

1. Goals of intervention
   a. Help persons living with HIV/AIDS achieve optimal symptom management to maintain or improve quality of life.
   b. Initiate actions to minimize disabilities caused by progressive HIV infection.
   c. Ensure that all nursing interventions are planned within the framework of the person's support systems and community.

2. Nutrition and diet: People with HIV/AIDS require 16 to 18 calories per pound of body weight each day to *maintain* weight. Adequate caloric intake is imperative to fighting infections, supporting the immune system, and maintaining energy levels.
   a. Calorie distribution should be as follows:
      (1) Fifty to 55 percent from carbohydrates

(2) Fifteen to 20 percent from protein

(3) Thirty percent or less from fat

b. Modify the diet in the presence of common nutrition-related problems that affect food intake.

  (1) Nonirritating foods in the presence of thrush and herpes

  (2) A low-residue diet to control diarrhea

  (3) Nutritional supplements for maintaining or gaining weight when calorie intake declines

  (4) Smaller, more frequent meals to improve digestion and increase calories

c. Consider referral to a registered dietitian.

d. Food safety is essential to preventing food-borne illnesses. Avoid unpasteurized dairy products and undercooked poultry, fish, shellfish, or meat. Exercise caution with organically grown fruits or vegetables.

. Psychosocial needs

a. Control issues: Many people living with HIV/AIDS feel strongly about staying in charge of their lives; nurses must provide the necessary information to enable people to make informed decisions regarding their treatment plans.

b. Maintaining independence: Independent functioning for as long as possible is facilitated through good discharge planning and case management.

c. Acknowledging stigmatization: No other life-threatening disease in recent memory has generated the extent of discrimination that ultimately will confront the person with a diagnosis of AIDS.

d. Establishing support systems: New sources of social support are often necessary to prevent the negative effects of isolation and loneliness.

e. Coping with stress: Lifestyle changes, rejection, financial concerns, and deteriorating health contribute to feelings of anxiety, insecurity, and alienation.

CLINICAL CONTROVERSIES

*though research indicates that there is an association between psychologic *ress* and changes in the immune system, a clear relationship between *ress*-related immune suppression and illness has not been documented.

. Symptom management

a. Fatigue: Identify fatigue-contributing factors—shortness of breath, inadequate nutrition, anemia, and diarrhea. Develop a schedule that will allow the person to pace activities of daily living over 24 hours. Include adequate rest periods.

b. Pain: Identify activities that aggravate or precipitate pain. Control pain with prescribed medication and comfort measures such as massage, applications of heat and cold, positioning, and air mattresses.

c. Fever: Use prescribed antipyretics, tepid sponge baths, and bed rest. Ensure adequate fluid and calorie intake.

d. Respiratory distress: Promote good pulmonary hygiene with position changes, coughing and deep-breathing exercises, and a fluid intake of 2.5 to 3 liters per day.

e. Gastrointestinal symptoms

  (1) Anorexia: Encourage small, frequent feedings. Use nutritional supplements and antiemetics as needed.

  (2) Dysphagia: After determining the cause of dysphagia (thrush, herpes, or neurologic disorder), promote good oral hygiene. Explain to the person that soft, nonirritating foods and cold foods may be swallowed more easily.

  (3) Nausea and vomiting: When the person is vomiting, withhold food and fluids for 2 hours; then introduce ice chips or clear liquids at 30 ml per hour. Provide good oral hygiene and prescribed antiemetics.

  (4) Diarrhea: Increase fluid intake, limit fiber intake, and use antidiarrheal medications as ordered.

  (5) Constipation: Ensure adequate fluid intake, including 2 liters of water each day in addition to other fluids. Promote regular exercise, regularly scheduled meals, and adequate fiber intake.

f. Weight loss

  (1) Identify the person's food preferences and ability to prepare meals.

  (2) Instruct the person about high-protein, high-carbohydrate foods. Encourage the use of prepared foods.

  (3) Refer the person to a dietitian if necessary.

  (4) Consider a home-delivered meal program, if one is available in the community.

g. Skin or mucous membrane lesions

  (1) Dry or broken lesions are left open to air.

  (2) Draining lesions require cleansing and normal saline dressings for comfort or a topical antibiotic.

  (3) Encourage the use of prescribed medications for specific conditions such as herpes, *C. albicans* infection, and KS.

NURSE ADVISORY

> Occlusive dressings such as Op-site, Stomahesive, and Duoderm are contraindicated, because their use may have a shearing effect on the skin of a person with a compromised immune system.

h. Dementia

  (1) Determine the onset, precursors, and duration of confusion.

  (2) Communicate with the person in simple terms.

  (3) Educate caregivers about memory cues and other strategies to keep the person oriented. Provide a calm, safe environment.

5. Pharmacologic interventions

a. Antiretrovirals: Drugs with antiviral effects interfere with the replication of HIV and are thought to slow disease progression. The 4 most common antiretrovirals are zidovudine (formerly called AZT), didanosine (ddI), dideoxycytidine (ddC), and deoxythymidine (d4T)

 DRUG ADVISORY

> A reported side effect of both didanosine and dideoxycytidine is life-threatening pancreatitis; peripheral neuropathy is a common side effect of all 4 antiretrovirals.

b. Antifungals: Antifungal agents are used primarily to treat candidiasis. Topical lesions require nystatin or clotrimazole. For disseminated candidiasis, ketoconazole or fluconazole is used, and in severe cases amphotericin B is prescribed.

DRUG ADVISORY

Amphotericin B must be used with extreme caution when the person is receiving other nephrotoxic drugs such as pentamidine and aminoglycosides. Amphotericin B is a very toxic drug, and may cause seizures, anaphylaxis, headache, or decreased renal function when infused.

c. Prophylaxis: Used in conjunction with antiretrovirals, prophylactic agents are generally initiated when CD4 cells are under 200. Co-trimoxazole (Septra) and pentamidine prevent *P. carinii* pneumonia. Acyclovir prevents recurrence of herpes infections. Foscarnet is used for acyclovir-resistant herpes infections.
d. Protease inhibitors
  (1) Protease inhibitors are used in combination with other antiretroviral drugs, for example, zidovudine and ddI.
  (2) Protease inhibitors produce the most potent antiviral effects of any group of drugs to date. Saquinavir, ritonavir, and indinavir have all been approved by the U.S. Food and Drug Administration.
  (3) The effectiveness of these drugs is based on their ability to lower a person's viral load significantly, in some cases to undetectable levels. Small research studies have indicated reduced death rates.
  (4) Health care providers must use these multidrug regimens correctly or infected individuals will develop resistance to protease inhibitors.
  (5) Protease inhibitors are very expensive. A multidrug regimen may cost between $12,000 and $70,000 annually.
e. Antibiotics: A wide range of antibiotics help control the many bacterial infections to which a person with HIV infection is susceptible.
f. Antineoplastics: Drugs such as doxorubicin (Adriamycin), cyclophosphamide (Cytoxan), and methotrexate (Folex) are used to treat KS and non-Hodgkin's lymphoma.
g. Antianxiety agents: Commonly used antianxiety agents are lorazepam (Ativan) and haloperidol (Haldol) for more severe mental changes.
6. Special medical-surgical procedures
a. Aerosolized pentamidine for *P. carinii* pneumonia prophylaxis: For the safety of patient and health care workers, treatments should be administered in well-ventilated treatment rooms with room air exhausted directly to the outside of the building.
b. Enteral-parenteral devices: Enteral nutrition is used for persons unable to take food by mouth, and peripheral and central lines are used primarily for administration of intravenous medications or nutritional support and frequent blood draws or transfusions.
7. Alternative therapies: Alternative treatment often causes a person to feel more in control of the disease process and should be viewed nonjudgmentally.
a. Alternative nutrition: Macrobiotic diets are gaining in acceptance; foods include steamed grains and vegetables. The diet requires balancing yin (acid-forming) and yang (alkaline-forming) foods.
b. Vitamin therapy: Vitamins play an important role in immune function. Deficiencies in vitamins A, B_6, and E reportedly decrease cellular immunity and antibody responses. Megadoses of vitamins may be used in conjunction with special diets to enhance immune function.
c. Minerals: Copper, iron, magnesium, and zinc are all considered major nutrients that affect the immune system.
d. Chinese herbs: Plants possess unique chemicals that can be extracted and used as medicines in both tea and powder form. Compound Q is an example of an herbal extract that has shown some promise in destroying HIV-infected cells.
e. Mind work
  (1) Relaxation: Stress management can have a positive effect on immune function.
  (2) Laughter and humor: Norman Cousins in *Anatomy of an Illness* spelled out the mind-body connection and the importance of humor in the healing process.
  (3) Meditation: Focusing on 1 thing at a time results in both physical and psychologic symptom reduction.
  (4) Visualization: Introduced by Dr. O. Carl Simonton in the mid-1970s as a complementary therapy for cancer treatment, visualization entails mental imaging of the body to martial its defenses against the invading organism.
f. Body work
  (1) Massage: Stimulation of muscle groups heightens a person's awareness of the body in a positive way.
  (2) Therapeutic touch: Delores Krieger, a nurse, proposes that therapeutic touch by the practitioner interacts with a person's energy system.
  (3) Yoga: Body positions and stretching contribute to a sense of balance and stamina.

Complications

1. Neurologic complications: A wide variety of conditions affects both the central nervous system and the peripheral nervous system. Progressive depletion of immune function increases the risk of opportunistic neurologic diseases.
a. Focal central nervous system disorders: The clinical presentation is affected by the location of brain lesions. Manifestations include the following:
  (1) Cerebral toxoplasmosis
  (2) Primary central nervous system lymphoma

(3) Progressive multifocal leukoencephalopathy
b. Peripheral nervous system disease
   (1) Peripheral neuropathy is thought to be related to HIV infection, but its etiology and pathology are not clearly understood. The disease is characterized by burning or painful sensations in the feet that may interfere with ambulation.
   (2) Drug-related peripheral neuropathies are caused by didanosine, dideoxycytidine, and deoxythymidine, with characteristic aching of feet, with or without other foot dysthesias.
c. AIDS dementia complex is a clinical syndrome that results in both cognitive and motor impairments as well as changes in behavior. Staging of ADC is based on the person's ability to manage job responsibilities and activities of daily living:
   (1) Mild—There is clinical evidence of motor or cognitive dysfunction, but the person is able to work and perform all activities of daily living.
   (2) Moderate—The person is unable to manage job responsibilities but continues to be independent with self-care. The person may need a cane for walking.
   (3) Severe—Serious cognitive deficits are present, such as the inability to follow complicated conversations or motor dysfunction (e.g., impaired ambulation that requires the use of a walker).
   (4) End stage—Cognitive and social skills at the most basic levels are lost (e.g., the person is paraplegic or incontinent of bowel and bladder).
2. Ocular complications: Many people develop ophthalmic diseases during the course of HIV disease, and 20 percent experience severe loss of vision from infections of the eye. Holland describes 4 categories of ocular changes in AIDS:
   a. Infection with HIV may cause direct infection of structures of the eye or may serve as a cofactor with cytomegalovirus, resulting in more severe pathology.
   b. Microvasculopathy affects the retina, conjunctiva, and optic nerve and is caused by a variety of pathogens. Cotton wool spots, the most common ocular lesions, are discrete, opaque patches on the retina near the optic nerve.
   c. Neoplasms of the eye include KS, which involves the conjunctiva, and intraocular lymphomas, which may be symptomatic of disseminated lymphoma.
   d. Ophthalmic signs as indicators of neurologic disease include abnormal eye movement, cranial nerve palsies, visual field deficits, papilledema, pupil changes, and atrophy of the optic nerve.
3. Gastrointestinal complications
   a. The entire gastrointestinal system, from mouth to anus, is a major target for AIDS-related diseases; 50 to 90 percent of people with AIDS develop gastrointestinal problems.
   b. As the life spans of people with AIDS lengthen, more gastrointestinal infections and primary lymphomas of the gastrointestinal tract will be seen.
   c. Causes of gastrointestinal problems are usually multifactorial and include the following:
      (1) Opportunistic pathogens

(2) Neoplasms—KS and lymphomas
(3) Medications
(4) Unknown etiologies
d. Gastrointestinal symptoms, which affect nutritional status, include dysphagia, anorexia, weight loss, nausea and vomiting, and diarrhea.
e. Affected structures
   (1) Esophagus: Opportunistic infections of the esophagus reflect a severely compromised immune function and a poor chance of survival.
   (2) Stomach: The same disease processes that affect the esophagus affect the stomach.
   (3) Large and small intestines: Inflammation results in diarrhea, which leads to malnutrition and wasting.
   (4) Hepatobiliary system: Primary opportunistic infections, HIV, drugs used in treatment, and hepatitis viruses affect the hepatobiliary system. Complications are related to risk factors of anal intercourse and injectable drug use.

CLINICAL CONTROVERSIES

It is unclear at this time whether diarrhea is caused by human immunodeficiency virus itself or by one of the opportunistic pathogens.

   (5) Pancreas: Inflammation and endocrine or exocrine failure are caused by drugs, opportunistic infections, neoplasms, and possibly HIV itself.
f. Gastrointestinal disease has enormous clinical significance and can contribute to the progression of the HIV infection, exacerbate immune dysfunction, and result in morbidity and death.

Prognosis

1. Disease progression and CD4 counts
   a. Early disease (CD4 count $\geq 500/mm^3$) is generally asymptomatic. The risk of developing an AIDS-defining condition that progresses to death in 18 to 24 months is less than 5 percent.
   b. Midstage disease (CD4 count $200-499/mm^3$) continues to be asymptomatic. Many clinicians initiate antiretroviral therapy, but even without treatment there is only a 20 to 30 percent chance of developing an AIDS-defining condition that progresses to death within 18 to 24 months.
   c. Late disease (CD4 count $50-199/mm^3$) results in a high risk for developing opportunistic infections. Without treatment, there is a 50 to 70 percent likelihood of developing more than one AIDS-related condition that will lead to death within 18 to 24 months.
   d. Advanced disease (CD4 count $<50/mm^3$) is marked by development of additional AIDS-defining illnesses associated with severe immunosuppression, such as CMV retinitis and disseminated *M. aviumintracellulare* complex. Death is likely within 2 years.
2. Indicators of disease progress

a. Time frame: Within a median time frame of 10 to 12 years from initial HIV infection to first AIDS-defining illness, a few people progress to AIDS in only a year and a half, while a few other HIV-infected people may not develop AIDS for 18 years.

b. Laboratory findings: The CD4 cell count is currently the best predictor of disease status. Measures of viral burden, which is known to increase with disease progression, may eventually prove to be a better laboratory predictor than the CD4 cell count.

3. Variability in course and rate of HIV disease: As is the case with many other life-threatening diseases, it is difficult to predict individual outcomes accurately. People should be encouraged and helped to live the fullest and most satisfying lives possible.

Applying the Nursing Process

> **NURSING DIAGNOSIS:** Knowledge deficit R/T transmission, treatment, and course of disease

1. *Expected outcomes:* After instructions, the person should be able to do the following:
   a. Describe the routes of HIV transmission.
   b. Use appropriate prevention measures, including sexual abstinence, correct use of condoms and spermicides, and appropriate methods of cleaning needles and syringes if unable to stop injecting drugs.
   c. Encourage sexual partners to seek HIV testing.
   d. Verbalize an understanding of the time frame and stages of HIV infection and differentiate between HIV infection and AIDS.
   e. Safely and consistently self-administer medications.
   f. Adhere to good health practices, including following a diet that meets nutritional needs and maintains weight, exercising as tolerated, obtaining adequate rest, and using safer sexual practices.
   g. Understand and appropriately use universal precautions.

2. *Nursing interventions*
   a. Describe basic HIV/AIDS terminology, routes of HIV transmission, personal behaviors to prevent transmission, and the importance of routine health supervision.
   b. Reinforce the preceding information with printed materials available from local health departments.
   c. Review prescribed medications and their potential side effects. Ensure that a payment source for prescriptions is established.
   d. Review the person's current dietary intake and its ability to supply necessary nutrients and adequate calories.
   e. Explain the urgency of HIV testing for sexual partners and provide information on counseling and testing resources in the community.
   f. Emphasize the following food safety procedures:
      (1) Avoid raw eggs; unpasteurized milk; and undercooked meat, poultry, and seafood.

(2) Peel and cook organically grown fruits and vegetables; careful washing before preparation is essential.
(3) Avoid soft, ripened cheeses such as brie or feta. Also avoid aged cheeses.
(4) Clean the refrigerator frequently to avoid the growth of molds.
(5) Wash dishes in the usual manner—using hot, soapy water and rinsing thoroughly in hot water.
(6) When eating in restaurants, inquire about methods of food preparation and request thoroughly cooked foods.

g. Discuss an appropriate exercise program.
   (1) Regular aerobic exercise (e.g., cycling, swimming, running, or walking) begun early in HIV disease can help avoid the wasting that sometimes characterizes this illness.
   (2) Even after the onset of wasting or weakness, a low-impact aerobic exercise program can delay further wasting.
   (3) Exercise helps relieve stress and augments a person's sense of body control.
   (4) Yoga and tai chi are other exercise programs that can benefit both mind and body.

h. Discuss the importance of rest and relaxation.
   (1) The person needs to know how to determine his or her energy levels and avoid overdoing.
   (2) Help the person plan for an adequate night's sleep and rest periods during the day if needed.
   (3) Help the person identify strategies for conserving energy, such as sitting to prepare food, shave, or dress.
   (4) Encourage the person to use assistive devices—such as a cane, walker, wheelchair, or trapeze—as necessary.
   (5) In a 24-hour schedule, plan periods of activity alternating with rest periods.

> **NURSING DIAGNOSIS:** Altered sexuality patterns R/T risk of transmitting HIV during intercourse

1. *Expected outcomes:* After instructions, the person should be able to do the following:
   a. Verbalize an understanding that HIV infection is lifelong and he or she can transmit the virus even though asymptomatic.
   b. Understand the dangers of reinfection with HIV through unprotected anal or vaginal intercourse with a partner who is HIV positive.
   c. Discuss feelings and concerns about sexual behaviors.
   d. Identify safer sexual practices that are satisfying and prevent the transmission of body fluids during sex.
   e. Use barrier protection and a spermicide to prevent the transmission of infectious semen, blood, or vaginal secretions.

2. *Nursing interventions*
   a. Establish a comfortable relationship that allows for open discussion of sexual concerns.

b. Reinforce the person's understanding of safer sexual behaviors and the correct use of barrier protection by supplying printed materials from a local health department.

c. Discuss safer sexual alternatives, such as masturbation, massage, hugging, sex toys, or dildoes.

d. Refer the person for counseling or to a support group for people living with HIV, if appropriate.

NURSING DIAGNOSIS: Decisional conflict R/T childbearing

1. *Expected outcomes:* After instructions, the person should be able to do the following:
   a. Understand the likelihood (16–30%) of delivering a baby who will develop AIDS.
   b. Know that using zidovudine during pregnancy may prevent transmission of HIV to the fetus.
   c. Use the double protection method of oral contraceptives and condoms with spermicide to prevent pregnancy.
   d. Receive support from health care providers to make an informed decision regarding future pregnancies.
2. *Nursing interventions*
   a. Review the benefits and risks of becoming pregnant when HIV infected.
   b. Discuss methods of contraception and protection against sexually transmitted diseases.
   c. Advise women who are HIV infected or at risk of infection to avoid using intrauterine devices, which increase the likelihood of developing pelvic inflammatory disease.
   d. Support the woman in her reproductive choices and help her obtain necessary gynecologic or obstetric services.

NURSING DIAGNOSIS: Anxiety R/T changes in health status, loss of control, and threat of death

1. *Expected outcomes:* After instructions, the person should be able to do the following:
   a. Identify issues that are of greatest concern.
   b. Decide which concerns demand immediate attention and develop a plan to address them.
   c. Actively seek appropriate community resources to meet identified needs.
   d. Value autonomy and the right to make personal decisions.
   e. Demonstrate an understanding of the disease process sufficient to make informed choices.
2. *Nursing interventions*
   a. Establish a communication pattern that allays fears and facilitates problem solving.
   b. Encourage independent decision making based on an adequate understanding of the demands of the situation.

c. Refer to accessible community resources that are most likely to provide needed assistance; help the person to avoid unnecessary red tape.

d. Use strategies that foster the person's autonomy and conserve the person's energy.

NURSING DIAGNOSIS: Body image disturbances R/T wasting, disfiguring skin conditions, and loss of function

1. *Expected outcomes:* After instructions, the person should be able to do the following:
   a. Identify the body changes that are the most distressing.
   b. Use techniques to minimize or disguise the changes in appearance.
   c. Safely maintain mobility by using a cane, walker, or wheelchair to the extent necessary.
2. *Nursing interventions*
   a. Help the person verbalize feelings and concerns about changes in appearance.
   b. Suggest ways to cope with the changes:
      (1) Wearing makeup to cover KS lesions
      (2) Wearing scarves or hairpieces to conceal hair loss
      (3) Wearing loose-fitting clothing to conceal wasting
   c. Instruct the person on the safe use of assistive devices to ensure continued mobility.

NURSING DIAGNOSIS: Knowledge deficit R/T use of universal precautions

1. *Expected outcomes:* After instructions, the person should be able to do the following:
   a. Use universal precautions appropriately to prevent exposure to blood-borne pathogens.
   b. Verbalize an understanding of universal precautions.
   c. Ensure that others in his or her household also use universal precautions.
   d. Wash hands at appropriate times and for 15 seconds each time.
2. *Nursing interventions*
   a. Explain the need for caregivers to follow the universal blood and body fluid precautions, which prevent parenteral, mucous membrane, and nonintact skin exposure to blood-borne pathogens (see Box 8–3).
   b. Demonstrate the correct use of protective barriers such as gowns, gloves, masks, and protective eyewear. Ensure that the household has an adequate supply of these items.
   c. Stress the importance of hand washing as the first line of defense for both the person with AIDS and the caregiver (see Procedure 8–1).

NURSING DIAGNOSIS: Risk for altered body temperature R/T infection or dehydration

HOME CARE STRATEGIES

Infection Control Guidelines

Infection control in the home setting is based on universal precautions that are familiar to all health care providers. In the home, you will have to adapt the guidelines to the equipment and supplies available and provide training to the patient and caregiver.

Equipment

- Instruct the household on selecting and using protective equipment.
- List activities that require the use of gloves, and identify the proper gloves to use.
- Use an apron if clothing is likely to become contaminated.

Hand Washing

- Demonstrate good hand-washing technique to all household members.
- Instruct the family on when hand washing is appropriate.

Sharps Disposal

- If a sharps container is not available, use a puncture-resistant, opaque container such as a detergent bottle or coffee can with the lid securely taped.
- Be familiar with your agency policy and local ordinances regarding sharps disposal.

Bandages and Linens

- Soiled dressings should be sealed tightly in a plastic bag and disposed of in the patient's trash bag.
- Clothing and linens soiled with body fluids should be stored in a plastic bag until laundered and then washed in water as hot as the fabric will tolerate. Add 1 cup of bleach or Lysol to the detergent in each load.
- If no washer or dryer is available, use the bathtub to wash linens and allow them to air dry, preferably in the sun.

Spills

- Contaminated surfaces should be washed with detergent and water. The surface should then be washed with a freshly made solution of 1:10 household bleach.
- Disposable toweling should be used.
- Blood and body wastes can be poured down a drain connected to a sanitary sewage system.

Dishes

- Leftover portions of uneaten food should not be saved.
- Soiled dishes should be washed in detergent and hot water immediately after use.

1. *Expected outcomes:* After instructions, the person should be able to do the following:
   a. Take and record his or her temperature.
   b. Know what to do to control fever.
   c. Identify the signs and symptoms of incipient infections and dehydration.
   d. Seek additional help if a fever does not respond to fever-control measures.
2. *Nursing interventions*
   a. Review the procedure for taking a temperature and obtain a return demonstration.
   b. Carry out measures to reduce fever: Give prescribed antipyretics and tepid sponge baths, push fluids, and maintain bed rest.

c. Increase the person's caloric intake with more frequent feedings and nutritional supplements.
d. Maintain the person's comfort by changing linen as needed and providing good skin care.
e. Promote safety by monitoring the person's mental status and ensuring that the person can ambulate independently.

NURSING DIAGNOSIS: Risk for infection R/T immunosuppression

1. *Expected outcomes:* After instructions, the person should be able to do the following:
   a. Identify potential infectious agents, such as people with respiratory infections, pets, and molds.
   b. Explain the signs and symptoms of incipient infections.
   c. Seek medical help appropriately and promptly.
   d. Discuss behaviors that may depress immune function, such as alcohol consumption and use of injectable drugs.
2. *Nursing interventions*
   a. Review good personal hygiene practices and housekeeping strategies to minimize the person's exposure to pathogens.
   b. If pets are in the household, remind the person of the following:
      (1) Animals may carry pathogens that can be dangerous to a person with HIV/AIDS.
      (2) Cleaning out fish tanks, cat or dog feces, or bird droppings should be avoided if at all possible.
      (3) If the person must clean up after a pet, a mask and gloves should be used, and hands should be washed thoroughly afterward.
      (4) Pets kept inside pose much less danger to their owners than do pets that are allowed to go outside.
      (5) Hands should be washed after playing with pets.
      (6) Care should be taken to avoid animal scratches and bites.

NURSING DIAGNOSIS: Diarrhea R/T infections, chemotherapy, or radiation

1. *Expected outcomes:* After instructions, the person should be able to do the following:
   a. List factors that contribute to diarrhea.
   b. Adhere to a low-residue, high-protein, high-calorie diet with a fluid intake of 2.5 to 3 liters per day.
   c. Use scrupulous skin care in the perianal area.
   d. Self-administer antidiarrheal medications as prescribed.

2. *Nursing interventions*
   a. Observe the person for signs of orthostatic hypotension, dehydration, and electrolyte imbalance.
   b. Advise the person that antidiarrheal drugs should be taken on a regularly scheduled basis rather than as needed.
   c. Instruct the person on the cleansing of the perianal region and the use of creams to maintain skin integrity.
   d. Encourage the use of adult diapers if incontinence is occurring.
   e. Advise the person to eat small frequent meals; take dietary supplements; avoid very hot, cold, or spicy foods; and use lactose-free dairy products (if the person is intolerant to lactose).

NURSING DIAGNOSIS: Impaired gas exchange R/T respiratory infections

1. *Expected outcomes:* After instructions, the person should be able to do the following:
   a. Identify factors that exacerbate respiratory distress.
   b. Promptly report symptoms such as worsening dyspnea on exertion.
   c. Use breathing exercises such as pursed-lip breathing to improve respiratory status.
   d. Avoid hyperventilating as a response to anxiety by using relaxation techniques.
   e. Pace activities of daily living to maximize energy conservation and decrease respiratory effort.
2. *Nursing interventions*
   a. If the person is a smoker, suggest strategies that will at least ameliorate the effects of smoking. For example, counsel against smoking before meals and before, during, and right after performing activities of daily living.
   b. Promote good pulmonary hygiene.
      (1) Have the person change position frequently and do coughing and deep-breathing exercises.
      (2) Ensure adequate hydration by providing 2.5 to 3 liters of fluid per day.
      (3) Initiate the use of a spirometer and chest physiotherapy, if not contraindicated.

NURSE ADVISORY

> Because of the possibility of pneumothorax or hemorrhage, coughing, deep breathing, and chest physiotherapy are contraindicated in the presence of *Pneumocystis carinii* pneumonia or Kaposi's sarcoma of the lung.

      (4) Plan care in such a way that the person's energy is conserved and fewer demands are placed on respiratory function.

NURSING DIAGNOSIS: Altered nutrition: less than body requirements R/T stomatitis, impaired absorption, loss of appetite, and fatigue

1. *Expected outcomes:* After instructions, the person should be able to do the following:
   a. Maintain or gain weight.
   b. Develop strategies for coping with loss of appetite, chewing difficulties, and dysphagia or odynophagia.
   c. Consume a well-balanced diet that provides adequate protein and caloric intake.
   d. Access community resources, such as home-delivered meals, food stamps, and public assistance.
2. *Nursing interventions*
   a. Monitor the person's nutritional status, including height and weight, intake of calories, skin integrity, and laboratory values.
   b. Ensure good oral hygiene.
   c. Encourage use of antiemetics 1 hour before mealtime to decrease nausea and increase tolerance for food.
   d. Provide nutritional supplements and small, frequent feedings to increase the person's caloric intake.
   e. Refer the person to a nutritionist if necessary.

NURSING DIAGNOSIS: Pain R/T tumors, opportunistic infections, neuropathies, and generalized joint and muscle pain

1. *Expected outcomes:* After instructions, the person should be able to do the following:
   a. Identify factors that precipitate or worsen pain.
   b. Know and use measures to control pain.
   c. Achieve good pain management.
2. *Nursing interventions*
   a. Instruct the person to use analgesics on a regularly scheduled basis rather than as needed.
   b. The daily plan of care should be scheduled according to the analgesic routine (i.e., administer the analgesic prior to bathing, ambulating, etc.).
   c. Initiate comfort measures such as massage, the use of a foam mattress, applications of heat and cold, and the proper support of limbs when the person is sitting or lying down.
   d. Consider nonpharmacologic pain management techniques, such as relaxation and imaging.

NURSING DIAGNOSIS: Altered thought processes R/T memory loss, impaired judgment, drug side effects, or depression

1. *Expected outcomes:* After instructions, the person should be able to do the following:
   a. Participate in decision making to the extent possible.
   b. Express concerns, anxieties, and fears.
   c. Remain free from injury.
   d. Participate in diversional activities as tolerated.
2. *Nursing interventions*
   a. Involve the primary caregiver in developing a plan of care.
   b. Encourage the person to keep a written schedule of activities to be followed by all those responsible for the person's care.
   c. Promote orientation by calling the person by name, identifying yourself, and using a calendar and watch to keep the person oriented to time.

d. Maintain a safe home environment.

e. Ensure that caregivers understand what the person can manage independently and with which activities the person needs assistance.

f. Encourage friends to spend time with the person and engage in activities such as reading, watching television, and taking walks with him or her.

NURSING DIAGNOSIS: Risk for caregiver role strain R/T demands of caregiving, poor prognosis, and impending loss

---

1. *Expected outcomes:* After counseling, the caregiver should be able to do the following:
   a. Verbalize concerns regarding the prognosis, decision making, and care.
   b. Identify and accept the need for respite from caregiving responsibilities.

c. Understand the unpredictability of the course of the disease and understand that death can come either swiftly or slowly.

2. *Nursing interventions*
   a. Determine the caregiver's health status.
   b. Identify the caregiver's need for respite from caregiving tasks.
   c. Encourage the caregiver to use home support services and volunteers.

NURSING DIAGNOSIS: Spiritual distress R/T feelings of hopelessness, loss of control, and self-blame

---

1. *Expected outcomes:* After counseling, the person should be able to do the following:
   a. Verbalize concern about life and death issues and possible conflicts about beliefs.

Table 42–3. Options for Long-Term Care for Persons with Acquired Immunodeficiency Syndrome

	Advantages	Disadvantages
Home care	Enhances quality of life by allowing the person to remain in familiar surroundings. Promotes autonomy. Allows family members and friends to assist with care. Allows for case finding and health teaching in the community.	Home care is not always less expensive than institutional care. Care may be compromised through the caregivers' failure to diagnose drug dependence or severe cognitive impairment. Family members and friends may experience caregiving burnout. Housing may lack convenient bathroom facilities, provide no refrigerated storage for food and drug supplies, or threaten the safety of the person with acquired immunodeficiency syndrome (AIDS) and the home care staff.
Nursing home	May be an alternative when home care is not possible. Is less expensive than continued hospitalization, although levels of Medicaid reimbursement vary from state to state. May be used on a short-term basis to provide respite for fatigued caregivers. Ensures that physical needs, such as meals and medication, are addressed. May provide special programs for persons with AIDS.	Both the person with AIDS and family members and friends may be reluctant to consider a nursing home. A lack of willingness to accept persons with AIDS is sometimes evident in the provision of marginal care. The institutional environment may increase dependence and have a negative impact on the return to normal functioning.
Hospice (See also Chapter 43.)	Is an ideal model of care incorporating interdisciplinary holistic health care. Emphasizes quality of life over quantity of life. Provides expert symptom management during end-stage disease for common problems such as pain, diarrhea, nausea and vomiting, dehydration, urinary incontinence, fever, respiratory distress, pressure ulcers, dementia, and fear.	Medicare-established rates for hospice care fail to cover the costs associated with the clinical needs of AIDS patients. Palliative care issues, such as continuing intravenous drug therapy to prevent the onset of blindness from cytomegalovirus retinitis and using blood transfusion to counteract anemia, need redefinition.

b. Request pastoral counseling or a visit from a member of the clergy.

c. Achieve a sense of peace, contentment, and resolution of concerns regarding treatment options.

. *Nursing interventions*

a. Communicate with the person in a way that encourages the person to share concerns, ensures confidentiality, and is nonjudgmental.

b. Provide a referral to appropriate pastoral counseling, if requested by the person.

c. Ask the person about usual spiritual practices and whether he or she desires assistance in pursuing them.

Discharge Planning and Teaching

. The goals of clinical management of HIV disease are to provide good care, coordinate services and avoid fragmented care, enhance or maintain the person's quality of life, and contain costs. Options for care are summarized in Table 42–3.

. Needs assessment includes personal and family information, names of people involved in care, the person's functional status, clinical needs, legal issues, social data, financial information, and names of providers and agencies involved in the case. The needs assessment process involves the following:

a. Developing a written plan of care in cooperation with the person and family members and friends involved in providing care

b. Implementing the plan through referral, coordination, counseling, and advocacy

c. Monitoring activities to ensure that necessary services are being provided

d. Evaluating the person on a regularly scheduled basis and modifying the written plan as needed

e. Identifying closure when mutually agreed-on criteria have been achieved

Preparation for death means validating individual treatment goals. Some people wish to pursue all available treatment options; others choose palliative care.

a. If treatment shifts from cure to care, maximize the person's comfort, optimize the person's function in spite of disease progression, and minimize suffering.

b. Reassess the adequacy of home support services.

c. Assist family and friends with anticipatory grieving. Prepare them for the downward spiral of the disease process, and caution them about the unpredictability of its course.

Public Health Considerations

Policy formation is ongoing and requires that health care providers know AIDS-related laws as they apply in their states. Relevant federal legislation includes the Americans with Disabilities Act of 1990, which covers HIV-infected people and prohibits discrimination and the Ryan White CARE Act of 1990, which provides comprehensive services for people living with HIV/AIDS.

2. Fair policymaking seeks a balance between the rights of the infected and the rights of those not infected.

3. Populations that should be tested for HIV include the following.

a. In 1993 the CDC recommended that hospitals with a seroprevalence rate of 1.0 per 1000 discharges consider routine HIV counseling and testing to all admissions ages 15 to 54.

b. Health care workers with identifiable risks for HIV infection should consider anonymous HIV testing. It is unlikely that an HIV-infected worker could infect a patient (Box 42–2).

c. At-risk populations and mandatory testing pose a dilemma. Enforced testing may deter those who otherwise would seek testing.

4. There are several types of HIV testing.

a. Mandatory testing is used for blood donors and recruits for Job Corps or the military. Large-scale mandatory testing such as premarital testing has proved to be ineffective.

b. Confidential testing links test results to the person but protects the person's identity.

c. Anonymous testing, available from many health departments, uses an identification number rather than a name.

5. Counseling is offered both before and after the test.

a. Pretest counseling describes the test itself, what the test results will mean, how the virus is transmitted, risk reduction activities (e.g., safer sex), available resources, and the value of knowing one's antibody status.

b. Posttest counseling

(1) If results are negative, retest in 3 months if the person is involved in high-risk behaviors. Review prevention strategies and make necessary referrals such as health care and drug rehabilitation.

BOX 42–2. Rights and Responsibilities of the Health Care Worker Infected with Human Immunodeficiency Virus

For the Worker

- Seek anonymous testing if you are at risk.
- If you are involved in "exposure-prone invasive procedures," accept the recommendations of an expert panel.
- Restrict practice only in case of invasive procedures.
- Know that licensure should not be linked to human immunodeficiency virus (HIV) or hepatitis B virus status.
- Expect your confidentiality to be protected and discrimination to be prohibited.
- Expect reasonable accommodations in your schedule and job responsibilities as your physical condition warrants them.

For the Employer

- Recognize your obligation to offer employment to an applicant with acquired immunodeficiency syndrome (AIDS) unless the person is incapable of performing the duties of the job.
- Do not require HIV testing for pre-employment or as part of the general workplace physical examination.
- Enforce universal precautions.
- Protect the confidentiality of the employee's medical record.
- Endorse nondiscriminatory employment policies and AIDS education programs at all levels of management.
- Do not force an employee with AIDS to take a medical leave unless the person is unable to perform the job.

(2) If results are positive, provide crisis intervention counseling. Discuss follow-up testing and care for partners and children. Review ways to prevent transmission. Refer the person for medical care and other services as required.

6. At-risk populations and the general public need basic information about HIV infection and ways to reduce risks and make behaviors safer.

a. Reducing risk from sexual transmission: Partners should be notified either by the HIV-infected person or by the health department to ensure early diagnosis and prompt treatment for exposed individuals. Correct condom use requires the use of latex condoms with spermicides and the proper application of the condom. Specific guidelines are available from the CDC and local health departments.

b. Reducing risk from blood-borne transmission: Administration of blood and blood products is regulated by the U.S. Food and Drug Administration. These products have been tested for HIV since 1985. Persons at risk for HIV should not donate plasma; blood; organs; tissue; or cells, including semen. People who use needles to inject drugs need to be instructed to flush equipment with bleach followed by water.

c. Reducing risk from perinatal transmission: Voluntary HIV testing before and during pregnancy should be routinely available, according to U.S. Public Health Service recommendations.

Bibliography

Books

Agency for Health Care Policy and Research. *Evaluation and Management of Early HIV Infection*. Rockville, MD: Agency for Health Care Policy and Research, 1994.

Andrews J, Novick B, and Associates. *HIV Care: A Comprehensive Handbook for Providers*. Thousand Oaks, CA: Sage Publications, 1995.

Benenson A (ed). *Control of Communicable Diseases in Man*. 15th ed. Washington, DC: American Public Health Association, 1990.

Broder S, Merigan T, and Bolognesi D (ed): *Textbook of AIDS Medicine*. Baltimore: Williams & Wilkins, 1994.

Cousins N. *Anatomy of an Illness*. New York: WW Norton & Co, 1979.

Ferri J. *There Is Hope: Learning to Live with HIV*. North Suburban Cook County, IL: HIV Coalition for North Suburban Cook County, 1993.

Ferri J, Roose R, and Schwendeman J. *There Is Hope: Learning to Live with HIV*. 2nd ed. North Suburban Cook County, IL: HIV Coalition for North Suburban Cook County, 1994.

Miller H, et al. (eds). *AIDS: The Second Decade*. Washington, DC: National Academy Press, 1990.

Miller S, et al. (eds). *Handbook for Assisted Living*. Chicago: Bonaventure House Inc, 1993.

Moyers B. *Healing and the Mind*. New York: Doubleday, 1993.

The National Commission on Acquired Immune Deficiency Syndrome: *America Living with AIDS*. Washington, DC: National Commission on AIDS, 1991.

Smith JW. *AIDS and Society*. Upper Saddle River, NJ: Prentice-Hall, 1996.

Swift R (ed). *Clinical Management of the HIV-Infected Adult: A Manual for Mid-Level Clinicians*. 2nd ed. Chicago: Midwest AIDS Training and Education Center at the University of Illinois, 1993.

The United States Conference of Mayors & The United States Conference of Local Health Officers. *Assessing the HIV-Prevention Needs of Gay and Bisexual Men of Color*. Washington, DC: The U.S. Conference of Mayors & The U.S. Conference of Local Health Officers, 1993.

Chapters in Books and Journal Articles

Transcultural Issues Involving HIV Disease

Anderson S, and Kaleeba N. AIDS Care in the family. *World AIDS Day Newsletter*, No. 3, 1994.

Kelly P, and Holman S. The New Face of AIDS. *Am J Nurs* 93(3):26–34, 1993.

Rose M. Health concerns of women with HIV/AIDS. *J Assoc Nurs AIDS Care* 4(3):39–45, 1993.

Responses to the Challenge of HIV Disease

Douard J, and Durham J. HIV-Infected women and children: Social and ethical perspectives. *In* Cohen F, and Durham J (eds). *Women, Children, and HIV/AIDS*. New York: Springer Publishing Co, 1993.

Flaskerud J. Overview: HIV disease and nursing. *In* Flaskerud J, and Ungvarski P (eds). *HIV/AIDS: A Guide to Nursing Care*. 2nd ed. Philadelphia: WB Saunders, 1992.

Epidemiology

AIDS Conference News: Ten million HIV babies by 2000. IXth International AIDS Conference, Berlin, June 10, 1993.

Altman L. At AIDS talks, science faces a daunting maze. *New York Times*, June 6, 1993.

Cohen F. The etiology and epidemiology of HIV infection and AIDS. *In* Durham J, and Cohen F (eds). *The Person with*

AIDS. 2nd ed. New York: Springer Publishing Co, 1991.

Global AIDS News. UN chief urges global mobilization against AIDS. Geneva Switzerland: World Health Organization's Global Programme on AIDS 93(1):1, 1993.

Hein K. "Getting real" about HIV in adolescents. *Am J Public Health* 83(4):492–494, 1993.

Pathophysiology

Grady C. HIV disease: Pathogenesis and treatment. *In* Flaskerud J, and Ungvarski P (eds). *HIV/AIDS: A Guide to Nursing Care*. 2nd ed. Philadelphia: WB Saunders, 1992.

Assessing People with HIV Disease

Agency for Health Care Policy and Research. Primary care physicians often fail to recognize important signs of HIV infection. *Res Activities* 190:10, 1996.

Cohen F. HIV infection and AIDS: An overview. *In* Cohen F, and Durham J (eds). *Women, Children, and HIV/AIDS*. New York: Springer Publishing Co, 1993.

Flaskerud J. Cofactors of HIV and public health education. *In* Flaskerud J, and Ungvarski P (eds). *HIV/AIDS: A Guide to Nursing Care*. 2nd ed. Philadelphia: WB Saunders, 1992.

Ungvarski P. Nursing management of the adult client. *In* Flaskerud J, and Ungvarski P (eds). *HIV/AIDS: A Guide to Nursing Care*. 2nd ed. Philadelphia: WB Saunders, 1992.

Clinical Picture of HIV Disease

Chavez C. Clinical update from Berlin. *Monthly Journal of Test Positive Aware Network*. Chicago: Test Positive Aware Network, July 1993.

Cohen F. The clinical spectrum of HIV infection and its treatment. *In* Durham J and Cohen F (eds). *The Person with*

AIDS. 2nd ed. New York: Springer Publishing Co, 1991.

Cohen F. HIV infection and AIDS: An overview. *In* Cohen F, and Durham J (eds). *Women, Children, and HIV/AIDS.* New York: Springer Publishing Co, 1993.

Grady C, Bechtel-Boenning C, & Boland, M (eds): HIV Infection/Perinatally Transmitted HIV Infection. *Nurs Clin North Am* 31(1), 1996.

Holland G. Ocular sequelae. *In* Broder S, Merigan T, and Bolognesi D (eds). *Textbook of AIDS Medicine.* Baltimore: Williams & Wilkins, 1994.

McKusick L. The end of life in HIV disease. *HIV Frontline Newsletter.* San Francisco, Professional Healthcare Communications, May/June 1993.

McKusick L. Riding the HIV roller coaster: Counseling and care in later-stage illness. *HIV Frontline Newsletter.* San Francisco, Professional Healthcare Communications, January/February 1993.

Whipple B, and Scura KW. The overlooked epidemic: HIV in older adults. *Am J Nurs* 96(2):23–29, 1996.

Williams A. The epidemiology, clinical manifestation and health maintenance needs of women infected with HIV. *Nurs Pract* 17(5):27–44, 1992.

Interventions Used to Treat HIV/AIDS

Altman L. New AIDS therapies arise, but who can afford the bill? *New York Times,* February 6, 1996.

Dickhens K. What you don't see can hurt you. *Monthly Journal of Test Positive Aware Network.* Chicago: Test Positive Aware Network, March 1993.

Hultz B. Protect your lungs. *Monthly Journal of Test Positive Aware Network.* Chicago: Test Positive Aware Network, July 1992.

Lein B. Rebuilding the immune system. *Monthly Journal of Test Positive Aware Network.* Chicago: Test Positive Aware Network, Aug/Sept 1993.

Martin J. Sustaining care of persons with AIDS. *In* Durham J, and Cohen F (eds). *The Person with AIDS.* 2nd ed. New York: Springer Publishing Co, 1991.

National Association of People with AIDS: Viral load and disease progression. *Med Alert* 3(7):6, 1996.

Physicians Association for AIDS Care. *HIV Disease Nutrition Guidelines.* Chicago: Physicians Association for AIDS Care, February 1993.

Project Inform. The new era in AIDS treatment: Protease inhibitors. *PI Perspective* 18:1, 1996.

Ungvarski P. Nursing management of the adult client. *In* Flaskerud J, and Ungvarski P (eds). *HIV/AIDS: A Guide to Nursing Care.* 2nd ed. Philadelphia: WB Saunders, 1992.

Alternative Therapies

Brodsky M. Paying lip service to calories: Oral nutrition supplements. *Monthly Journal of Test Positive Aware Network.* Chicago: Test Positive Aware Network, March 1993.

Flaskerud J. Psychosocial aspects. *In* Flaskerud J, and Ungvarski P. *HIV/AIDS: A Guide to Nursing Care.* 2nd ed. Philadelphia: WB Saunders, 1992.

Physicians Association for AIDS Care. *HIV Disease Nutrition Guidelines.* Chicago: Physicians Association for AIDS Care. February 1993.

Strawn J. Complementary therapies: Maximizing the mind-body connection. *In* Meisenhelder J, and LaCharite C. *Comfort in Caring.* Glenview, IL: Scott Foresman & Company, 1989.

Helping People Live with HIV Disease

Berk R, et al. Healthcare needs scale for patients with HIV/AIDS: Content validation. *J Assoc Nurs AIDS Care* 3(3):10–18, 1992.

Kelly P, and Holman S. The new face of AIDS. *Am J Nurs* 93(3):26–34, 1993.

McKusick L. Riding the HIV roller coaster: Counseling and care in later-stage illness. *HIV Frontline Newsletter.* San Francisco: Professional Healthcare Communications, January/February 1993.

van Servellen G, et al. The relationship of stressful life events, health status, and stress resistance resources in persons with AIDS. *J Assoc Nurs AIDS Care* 4(1):11–22, 1993.

Helping Family Members Cope with HIV Disease

Brown M, and Powell-Cope G. AIDS family caregiving: Transitions through uncertainty. *Nurs Res* 40(6):338–345, 1991.

Strawn J. The psychosocial consequences of HIV infection. *In* Durham J, and Cohen F (eds). *The Person with AIDS.* 2nd ed. New York: Springer Publishing Co, 1991.

Precautions to Prevent Transmission of HIV

Midwest AIDS Training and Education Center. *Taking Care: A Manual for AIDS Caregivers.* Minneapolis: School of Public Health, University of Minnesota, 1990.

Parris N. Infection control. *In* Flaskerud J, and Ungvarski P (eds): *HIV/AIDS: A Guide to Nursing Care.* 2nd ed. Philadelphia: WB Saunders, 1992.

Zelewsky M, and Birchfield M. Common ground: The nurse's role in caring for terminally ill patients with cancer or human immunodeficiency virus disease. *Home Healthc Nurse* 10(4):12–17, 1992.

Nursing Goals, Diagnoses, and Management

Nelson W. Nursing care of acutely ill persons with AIDS. *In* Durham J, and Cohen F (eds). *The Person with AIDS.* 2nd ed. New York: Springer Publishing Co, 1991.

Zelewsky M. Communicable diseases. *In* Matassarin-Jacobs E. *Saunders Review for NCLEX-RN.* 2nd ed. Philadelphia: WB Saunders, 1994.

Health Teaching and Prevention of HIV Disease

Dickhens K. What you don't see can hurt you: Tips for home food safety. *Monthly Journal of Test Positive Aware Network.* Chicago: Test Positive Aware Network, March 1993.

Ferri J. Learning to live with HIV. *In* Ferri J. *There Is Hope: Learning to Live with HIV.* North Suburban Cook County, IL: HIV Coalition for North Suburban Cook County, 1993.

Harris M. Preventing HIV infection. *In* Durham J, and Cohen F (eds). *The Person with AIDS.* 2nd ed. New York: Springer Publishing Co, 1991.

Kurth A. Reproductive issues, pregnancy, and childbearing in HIV-infected women. *In* Cohen F, and Durham J (eds). *Women, Children, and HIV/AIDS.* New York: Springer Publishing Co, 1993.

Physicians Association for AIDS Care. *HIV Disease Nutrition Guidelines.* Chicago: Physicians Association for AIDS Care, February 1993.

HIV and Public Policy

Centers for Disease Control. Recommendations for HIV testing services for inpatients and outpatients in acute-care hospital settings and technical guidance on HIV counseling. *MMWR* 42(RR–2):1–17, 1993.

Centers for Disease Control. Update: Investigations of persons treated by HIV-infected health-care workers—United States. *MMWR* 42(17):329–331, 1993.

Durham J, and Douard J. The challenge of AIDS for health care workers. *In* Cohen F, and Durham J (eds). *Women, Children, and HIV/AIDS.* New York: Springer Publishing Co, 1993.

Pearsaul S. Nurses with HIV: Should they tell? "Nursing News," *Chicago Tribune,* July 14, 1993.

Nursing Process Care Plan

Cohen F. The clinical spectrum of HIV infection and its treatment. *In* Durham J, and Cohen F (eds). *The Person with HIV/AIDS.* 2nd ed. New York: Springer Publishing Co, 1991.

Ungvarski P. Nursing management of the adult client. *In* Flaskerud J, and Ungvarski P (eds). *HIV/AIDS: A Guide to Nursing Care.* 2nd ed. Philadelphia: WB Saunders, 1992.

Zelewsky M. Communicable diseases. *In* Matassarin-Jacobs E. *Saunders Review for NCLEX-RN.* 2nd ed. Philadelphia: WB Saunders, 1994.

Agencies

National AIDS Education and Training Centers

The AIDS Education and Training Centers (AETCs) are federally funded programs under the auspices of the U.S. Public Health Service. The goal of these training centers is to provide education and training for health care providers who care for persons with HIV/AIDS. The 15 regional centers are listed below.

Midwest AIDS Training and Education Center
University of Illinois at Chicago
808 South Wood Street (M/C 779)
Chicago, IL 60612–7303
(312) 996–1373
Fax (312) 413–4184
Serves Illinois, Indiana, Iowa, Minnesota, Missouri, Wisconsin

Mid-Atlantic AIDS Training and Education Center
Virginia Commonwealth University
P.O. Box 980159
Richmond, VA 23298–0159
(804) 828–2447
Fax (804) 828–1795
Serves Delaware, Maryland, Virginia, West Virginia, Washington, D.C.

New England AIDS Training and Education Center
320 Washington Street, Third Floor
Brookline, MA 02146
(617) 566–2283
Fax (617) 566–2994
Serves Connecticut, Maine, Massachusetts, New Hampshire, Rhode Island, Vermont

AIDS Training and Education Center for Texas and Oklahoma
The University of Texas
1200 Herman Pressler Street
P.O. Box 20186
Houston, TX 77225
(713) 794–4075
Fax (713) 792–5292
Serves Texas and Oklahoma

Pennsylvania AIDS Training and Education Center
University of Pittsburgh
Graduate School of Public Health
130 DeSoto Street, Room A427
Pittsburgh, PA 15261
(412) 624–1895
Fax (412) 624–4767
Serves Pennsylvania

New Jersey AIDS Training and Education Center
University of Medicine and Dentistry of New Jersey Center for Continuing Education
30 Bergen Street, ADMC #710
Newark, NJ 07107–3000
(201) 982–3690
Fax (201) 982–7128
Serves New Jersey

Florida AIDS Training and Education Center
University of Miami
Department of Family Medicine
South Shore Hospital
600 Alton Road, Suite 502
Miami, FL 33139
(305) 531–1224 x3549
Fax (305) 532–9604
Serves Florida

Puerto Rico AIDS Training and Education Center
University of Puerto Rico
Medical Sciences Campus
GPO 36-5067, Room A-956
San Juan, PR 00936–5067
(809) 759–6528
Fax (809) 764–2470
Serves Puerto Rico

New York/Virgin Islands AIDS Training and Education Center
Columbia University School of Public Health
600 West 168th Street, 7th Floor
New York, NY 10032
(212) 305–3616
Fax (212) 305–6832
Serves New York and the Virgin Islands

Northwest AIDS Training and Education Center
University of Washington
1001 Broadway, Suite 217
Box 359932
Seattle, WA 98122
(206) 720–4250
Fax (206) 720–4218
Serves Washington, Alaska, Montana, Idaho, Oregon

Great Lakes to Tennessee Valley AIDS Training and Education Center
Wayne State University
2727 Second Avenue, Room 142
Detroit, MI 48201
(313) 962–2000
Fax (313) 962–4444
Serves Ohio, Michigan, Kentucky, Tennessee

Pacific AIDS Training and Education Center
University of California, San Francisco
5110 East Clinton Way, Suite 115
Fresno, CA 93727–2098
Western Division
(209) 252–2851
Fax (209) 454–8012
Southern Division
(213) 342–1846
Fax (213) 342–2051
Serves Nevada, Arizona, Hawaii, California

Southeast AIDS Training and Education Center
Emory University
735 Gateswood Road, N.E.
Atlanta, GA 30322–4950
(404) 727–2929
(404) 727–4562
Serves Alabama, Georgia, North Carolina, South Carolina

Delta Region AIDS Training and Education Center
LSU Medical Center
136 South Roman Street, 3rd Floor
New Orleans, LA 70112
(504) 568–3855
(504) 568–7893
Serves Arkansas, Louisiana, Mississippi

Mountain Plains Regional AIDS Training and Education Center
University of Colorado
4200 East Ninth Avenue, Box A-096
Denver, CO 80262
(303) 355–1301
Fax (303) 355–1448
Serves North Dakota, South Dakota, Utah, Colorado, New Mexico, Nebraska, Kansas, Wyoming

National AIDS Information Hotlines

Centers for Disease Control and Prevention National AIDS Information Clearinghouse
(800) 458–5231 (English, Spanish, and French)
(800) 243–7012 (hearing-impaired TTY/TDD)
Operators answer questions and mail publications. Free database searches are available. Referrals on all aspects of HIV infection are offered.

Centers for Disease Control and Prevention National AIDS Hotlines
(800) 342–2437 (English)
(800) 344–7432 (Spanish)
(800) 243–7889 (hearing-impaired TTY/TDD)
These 24-hour toll-free hotlines provide confidential information, referrals, and educational materials to callers.

National Native American AIDS
  Hotline
(800) 283–2437
Provides information addressed
  specifically to Native Americans.

Teens AIDS Hotline
(800) 234–8336
This hotline is operated by teens for teens
  and provides information, education,
  and referrals.

National Organizations

AIDS Clinical Trials Information
  Service
P.O. Box 6421
Rockville, MD 20849
(800) 874–2572
(800) 243–7012 (hearing impaired TTY/
  TDD)
Supplies telephone or printed information
  on ongoing private and federally
  funded clinical trials throughout the
  United States.

American Foundation for AIDS Research
733 Third Avenue
New York, NY 10017
(212) 682–7440
Supports research, including community-
  based clinical trials, and public policy
  development.

American Red Cross
430 17th Street, N.W.
Washington, DC 20006
(202) 737–8300
Many Red Cross chapters offer HIV/AIDS
  education for the community, and they
  are good resources for printed and
  audiovisual materials.

Association of Nurses in AIDS Care
1555 Connecticut Avenue, N.W.
Suite 200
Washington, DC 20036
(202) 462–1038
This specialty organization for nurses has
  local groups throughout the United
  States and publishes the *Journal of the
  Association of Nurses in AIDS Care*
  quarterly.

The NAMES Project
AIDS Memorial Quilt
2362 Market Street
San Francisco, CA 94114
(415) 882–5500

National Association of Persons with
  AIDS
1413 K Street, NW
Washington, DC 20005
(202) 898–0414
Offers information and education
  resources and advocacy for people
  living with HIV/AIDS.

National Hemophilia Foundation
The Soho Building
110 Greene Street
New York, NY 10012
(212) 219–8180
(800) 42–HANDI (424–2634)
Operates the Hemophilia and AIDS/HIV
  Network for the Dissemination of
  Information to provide information on
  hemophilia and HIV/AIDS as it relates
  to hemophilia.

National Minority AIDS Council
300 I Street, NE
Washington, DC 20002-4390
(800) 669–5052
Assists minority organizations with HIV/
  AIDS resources.

National Pediatric HIV Resource Center
15 South Ninth Street
Newark, NJ 07107
(201) 268–8251
(800) 362–0091 (resource center)
Provides consultation and training for
  professionals caring for children, youth,
  and families affected by HIV infection.

Project Inform
1965 Market Street
San Francisco, CA 94103
(800) 822–7422 (hotline operates 10 A.M. to
  4 P.M., Pacific time, Monday through
  Saturday)
Offers HIV/AIDS treatment information
  and advocacy.

◼ OVERVIEW

Definitions

1. **Terminal illness** refers to a health condition that is certain to result in the patient's physical decline and death. Treatment options may be available to slow the progression of the disease, but the person has no possibility for complete cure.
2. **Anticipatory grief** refers to the anticipation of a future loss and includes many of the symptoms and processes of grief after a loss. Anticipatory grief may be experienced by the dying person as well as his or her family and friends.
3. **Palliative care** is the care that professionals from many disciplines offer the dying person to improve the quality of his or her life by reducing pain and other distressing symptoms. The World Health Organization has developed a set of palliative care principles to guide clinical practice (Box 43–1).
4. **Palliative treatments** are often used to reduce distressing symptoms, but no cure is expected to result from them.
   a. **Palliative surgery** is often used to manage malignant obstructions related to cancer of the gastrointestinal tract, genitourinary tract, bile ducts, and blood vessels. Surgical procedures may be necessary to relieve discomfort associated with extensive local disease, pathologic fractures, and ulcers that result from tumor growth. Surgical placement of shunts or catheters for drainage of accumulated fluid in body cavities usually relieves distressing symptoms. Surgical placement of catheters may be necessary to deliver specific analgesic intervention (see Chapter 11).
   b. **Palliative radiotherapy** is very effective in providing pain relief related to bone metastases in cancer patients. Radiotherapy is the treatment of choice in preventing tumor-related spinal cord compression, which can lead to paralysis. Rapid relief from obstructive symptoms of superior vena cava syndrome is usually obtained from high-dose radiotherapy. Patients with brain and skin metastases are treated with radiotherapy, resulting in neurologic and integumentary improvements.
   c. **Palliative chemotherapy** may be used to reduce a cancer tumor mass or symptoms resulting from pleural effusion or superior vena cava obstruction. No cure is expected to result from palliative chemotherapy.
5. **Dying** is a continuous process in which the body and brain are unable to cope with hypoxia, electrolyte imbalance, and toxins that are not cleared from the body.
   a. Emotion, cognition, behavior, and autonomic function all deteriorate, and, in most cases, coma ensues before death.
   b. The duration of the process of dying may last a few hours to days, depending on the precipitating cause. Dying may be rapid after sudden serious traumatic injury. Chronic illnesses such as cancer or acquired immunodeficiency syndrome may initiate a slower process of dying.
6. **Death** may be defined across 4 dimensions of life: social, psychologic, biologic, and physiologic.
   a. **Social death** is the symbolic death of the patient that occurs because of lifestyle changes brought about by illness. Decreased functional capacity related to illness may interfere with usual patterns of work and recreation, limiting opportunities for social contact. Premature social death may be prevented by discussing ways to enable the patient to engage in the social life of family and friends.
   b. **Psychologic death** is the withdrawal of certain aspects of the dying person's personality. Causes of psychologic death include loss of autonomy, biochemical changes precipitated by disease and medication, grief reactions to anticipated future losses, and change in relationships related to decline in functional or cognitive abilities.
   c. **Biologic death** occurs when the human traits of consciousness and awareness no longer exist. Artificial life support systems may sustain organ function, but the self-sustaining mind and body of the person are no longer present.
   d. **Physiologic death** occurs when all vital organs stop functioning.

Theoretical Perspectives on Dying

1. Pattison conceptualized a terminally ill person's awareness of dying as a trajectory from an acute crisis to a terminal phase (Fig. 43–1). Many people assume that they will have a life span of 70 years or more. People

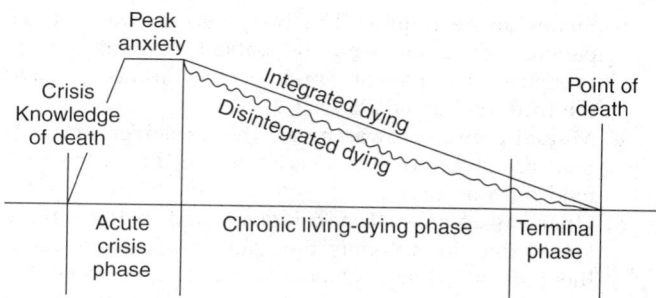

Figure 43-1. Pattison's trajectory of personal awareness of dying. (From Pattison EM. *The Experience of Dying.* Englewood Cliffs, NJ: Prentice-Hall, 1977. Used by permission of the publisher, Prentice-Hall, a division of Simon & Schuster.)

diagnosed with a terminal illness become aware of their shortened life spans.

a. The "acute crisis phase" occurs when the person receives the prognosis of a terminal illness. The person and his or her family members usually experience high levels of anxiety and are faced with altering their expectations about the future.

b. The "chronic living-dying phase" is initiated when the patient and family receive a poor prognosis. This living-dying interval may extend over several years and may include long-term disruption as a result of increased social, financial, physical, and emotional stressors. Patients and families may need assistance from professional and nonprofessional resources to adapt to the chronic living-dying phase.

(1) "Disintegrated dying" results when patients do not integrate knowledge of their dying into their lifestyles. Consultations with social service and mental health professionals may be helpful for some patients and families. Also, support groups provide a forum where they can obtain valuable information and social support.

(2) Remissions and relapses during terminal illness are difficult intervals for patients, family members, and staff. Decision making about treatment options is difficult for patients and families, because they fear side effects and are uncertain of the potential benefits.

c. The "terminal phase" is usually signaled by the patient's physical decline. Patient-family assessment at this time usually indicates a need for support services. Not all patients and families accept support from community-level services, however.

2. Kübler-Ross' stages of response to awareness of terminal illness provide insight into potential psychologic reactions (Table 43-1). Patients may not experience all 5 reactions, however, and there has been no research to show that these reactions occur in a progression of predictable stages.

Transcultural Variations in Dying

1. Variations in truth telling: Glaser and Strauss identified 4 types of communication patterns between dying patients and professional caregivers. Similar interactions may exist between patients and family members. Despite the lack of systematic cross-cultural studies, these patterns are also thought to be reflected within American subcultures.

a. **Closed awareness:** The caregiver is aware of the patient's condition but keeps this information from the patient.

Stage	Patient Responses
Denial	Denial allows the patient to mobilize coping defenses.
	The patient experiences temporary numbness or shock.
	Social withdrawal is possible.
	Discussion about the prognosis is avoided.
	Denial is usually replaced with other coping methods.
Anger	Anger is frequently directed at family and staff.
	Expression of anger may provide some relief.
Bargaining	The patient negotiates with the Supreme Being in an attempt to extend life.
Depression	Depression allows the patient to mourn for past and future losses.
	Expressions of sorrow may occur.
Acceptance or resignation	Hope is maintained and quality of living enhanced.

Table 43-1. Kübler-Ross' Reactions to Awareness of Terminal Illness

Adapted with the permission of Macmillan Publishing Company from Kübler-Ross E. *On Death and Dying.* New York: Macmillan, 1969. Copyright © 1969 by Elizabeth Kübler-Ross, MD.

b. **Suspicion awareness:** The caregiver is aware of the patient's condition, and the patient suspects a poor prognosis. The patient simultaneously wants to know the truth and avoids it.

c. **Mutual-pretense awareness:** The caregiver and patient are aware of the severity of the illness but pretend they are not.

d. **Open awareness:** The caregiver and patient share knowledge, information, thoughts, and feelings about the patient's dying. Open communication about the illness among family members has the potential to promote growth and cohesiveness. The advantage of open awareness is that the patient can make important end-of-life decisions.

2. Variations in response to dying: Every culture provides beliefs, values, and behaviors that guide thinking and practices associated with death for members of the group. Practices and beliefs may vary widely among members of a group. Religious traditions may guide beliefs about dying.

a. Hindus believe that the quality of one's life is shaped by one's deeds in a previous life and that the quality of one's death is shaped by how well one has behaved in this life. In Hindu culture, dying and death are acceptable topics and are openly discussed among family members.

b. According to Islamic beliefs, the dying person should be surrounded by friends and relatives. Islam directs persons who are aware of their imminent death to ask forgiveness of God and others, to pay off their debts, and to make a will. The dying person is also obligated to recite the Koran and perform specific cleansing rituals.

c. Native Americans are divided into 511 federally recognized entities. At present, much of the Native American population is located in 3 western states: Oklahoma, Arizona, and California. The great diversity among Native Americans, who speak more than 2000 native languages, makes generalizations impossible. Most Native Americans, however, prize self-reliance and are reluctant to ask for and receive assistance.

(1) Many Native American tribes also have a tradition of shared decision making among extended family members.

(2) Many Native Americans are accepting of death and view life and death as circular. Children are taught through ceremonies and stories that death is a part of life.

(3) Dying and death are usually accepted in a stoic manner. Yet Navajos are fearful of death, so that terminally ill Navajos may prefer to spend their last days in a setting apart from their families.

d. Many Blacks believe in immortality, and funeral rites are characterized as celebrations of life. For many, death is perceived to be a reunification with those who have died in the past. Strong multigenerational ties connect members of the extended family.

(1) Research has identified that nonverbal patterns of communication are emphasized within Black culture. Actions in response to immediate situations

are often more highly valued than discussions o the future. Open expression of feelings is valued.

(2) Blacks may perceive that they have little contro over their lives. This perception has developed a a result of being oppressed for many years by th dominant culture.

(3) Death has been more visible to Americans of Afri can descent than to Americans of European o Anglo descent. Violent deaths among young Blac men, for example, are common in urban centers.

(4) Extended family, friends, and church member may gather at the bedside to offer support an pray with the dying person.

e. Americans of European and Anglo descent form th dominant culture in the United States and consist o many subgroups.

(1) Expressions of sadness and grief are learne within the family and demonstration of emotio varies widely among White Americans. Stoicisr rather than open expression of grief may be dis played by family members of dying patients.

(2) Western culture has become characterized a death denying. Because of decline in multigenera tional living, death is less visible. For most peopl death has been removed from everyday famil life.

(3) Many Americans of European or Anglo heritag believe in immortality and place high value o family closeness. Spiritual beliefs and traditior vary across the subgroups.

f. Hispanic Americans are represented by diverse cu tures, such as Latino, Spanish American, and Chican Each of these subgroups may differ in its traditiona beliefs about death and dying and its practices in th care of the dying.

(1) Death is a family event, and children are full pa ticipants in the rituals and customs surroundin death. Some Hispanic Americans have a long tr dition of death acceptance that can be traced t Spain and Mexico.

(2) Many Hispanic Americans' religiosity is non institutional—that is, it tends to be home centere rather than church centered. Symbols and ritua are very important to many Hispanic American and provide comfort to the dying person and fam ily members.

(3) Often, major decisions about surgery and hospita ization are made by a group of the dying person family members.

(4) Open expression of grief is expected among Hi panic women but may be denied to Hispanic me

g. Asian Americans are represented by many subgroup including Chinese, Japanese, Koreans, Filipinos, Cam bodians, Hmong, Laotians, and Vietnamese. Belie and values vary across these groups.

(1) Most Asian Americans have a holistic conceptio of health and illness, seeing physical and ment functioning as intimately linked.

(2) Many Asian Americans believe in both Easter and Western medicine. Supporting traditional ap proaches is important when possible.

(3) Asians have strong reverence for their ancestors. Ritual ceremonies that honor dead ancestors may be incorporated into the care of the dying.

(4) In traditional Asian families, family members play a key role in decision making about the patient's medical care. Those who follow traditional Asian cultural patterns give up their right to autonomous decision making.

. Cultural assessment

a. Do not make assumptions about patients and their families solely on the basis of their cultural heritage.

b. To plan appropriate interventions, assess families' cultural backgrounds during the terminal phase of illness.

c. To identify strengths and needs in the family system, assess family roles, usual lifestyle, developmental level, authority patterns, and resources.

• What roles is the dying person relinquishing?
• Who will be affected by the illness situation?
• What are the expectations of family members?
• What are the family members' occupational patterns?
• What adaptations need to be made?
• Who are close friends and family?
• What are the economic resources?
• Are there any other concurrent stressors?
• What childrearing activities are present?
• Are there other caregiving responsibilities?
• Who will participate in decision making?
• What is the patient's and family's level of participation in religion?
• Does the spiritual tradition provide hope?

Variations in care after death: Recognize that the United States is composed of a variety of ethnic groups. All groups experience the phenomenon of dying, and many may have rituals that give meaning to the events of illness, dying, and death. Yet members of ethnic groups differ with respect to the need and desire for ritual after the death of a loved one.

a. Many cultures that specify rituals and specific time frames for mourning offer group members a means to express their grief within the community.

b. Be aware and respectful of culturally determined attitudes, beliefs, and values about death, dying, and bereavement.

c. Understand your own values and perspectives on death and dying. Be careful not to impose your own values on others and respect cultural divergence from mainstream American views.

egal and Ethical Considerations in Death nd Dying

Patients' right to information

a. All patients have the right to accurate information about their health status and prognosis. Medical professionals have an ethical and a legal obligation to provide honest answers to patients' questions.

b. Patients' constitutional right to engage in decision making regarding medical interventions at the end of their life is now protected through federal legislation. The Patient Self-Determination Act of 1990 requires all Medicare- and Medicaid-funded health care facilities to advise patients of their legal right to refuse or accept medical treatment.

2. Wills

a. People are free to distribute their property to anyone they wish according to the terms they state in a will. Wills are guided by statutes that vary from state to state. A will must be signed by at least 2 witnesses who stand to gain nothing as a result of the will. A will that does not comply with the statutes of the state in which the person resides will have no legal effect, and the property will pass under the laws of intestacy.

b. A person dying without a valid will is regarded as having "died intestate." Intestacy statutes are drafted and enacted by a state's legislators. The details of these statutes vary across states, but a surviving spouse and children are the preferred heirs.

c. Business affairs must be concluded after a person's death. All debts, taxes, funeral, and administrative expenses must be paid and the property owned at the time of death distributed to others. The management, administration, and transfer functions are accomplished through the probate process under the supervision of a court.

3. Will substitutes: To avoid the expense and time of probate, people may choose to transfer their property to their heirs while they are still alive. State regulations guide this transfer process.

4. Advance directives and living wills

a. Advance directives are prospective statements made by competent individuals that specify their medical choices in the event that they are unable to participate in decision making (Box 43–2). Advance directives give patients the opportunity to communicate their unique preferences about end-of-life care before they are unable to make their wishes known. Living wills and durable power of attorney are 2 forms of advance directives that are currently available in most states.

(1) Living wills document individuals' choices regarding life-sustaining procedures if for any reason they become unable to participate in decisions regarding their medical care. Information about withholding or withdrawing procedures such as surgery, administration of antibiotics, cardiac resuscitation, respiratory support, and artificial administration of nutrition and fluids may be stated in living wills.

(2) The patient's delegation of the power of attorney to another person authorizes the person (known as the proxy) to make decisions about withholding or withdrawing medical interventions. The proxy makes decisions regarding medical care only when the patient becomes unable to participate in decision making.

b. The Joint Commission on Hospital Accreditation requires all member hospitals to have policies related to Do Not Resuscitate (DNR) decision making, resolu-

BOX 43-2. Advance Directive

Living Will and Health Care Proxy

Death is a part of life. It is a reality like birth, growth and aging. I am using this advance directive to convey my wishes about medical care to my doctors and other people looking after me at the end of my life. It is called an advance directive because it gives instructions in advance about what I want to happen to me in the future. It expresses my wishes about medical treatment that might keep me alive. I want this to be legally binding.

If I cannot make or communicate decisions about my medical care, those around me should rely on this document for instructions about measures that could keep me alive.

I do not want medical treatment (including feeding and water by tube) that will keep me alive if:
• I am unconscious and there is no reasonable prospect that I will ever be conscious again (even if I am not going to die soon in my medical condition), *or*
• I am near death from an illness or injury with no reasonable prospect of recovery.

I do want medicine and other care to make me more comfortable and to take care of pain and suffering. I want this even if the pain medicine makes me die sooner.

I want to give some extra instructions: [*Here list any special instructions, e.g., some people fear being kept alive after a debilitating stroke. If you have wishes about this, or any other conditions, please write them here.*]

The legal language in the box that follows is a health care proxy.
It gives another person the power to make medical decisions for me.

I name _____ , _____ , who lives at _____

_____ , phone number _____ ,

to make medical decisions for me if I cannot make them myself. This person is called a health care "surrogate," "agent," "proxy," or "attorney in fact." This power of attorney shall become effective when I become incapable of making or communicating decisions about my medical care. This means that this document stays legal when and if I lose the power to speak for myself, for instance, if I am in a coma or have Alzheimer's disease.

My health care proxy has power to tell others what my advance directive means. This person also has power to make decisions for me, based either on what I would have wanted, or, if this is not known, on what he or she thinks is best for me.

If my first choice health care proxy cannot or decides not to act for me, I name _____ ,

address _____ ,

phone number _____ , as my second choice.

I have discussed my wishes with my health care proxy, and with my second choice if I have chosen to appoint a second person. My proxy(ies) has (have) agreed to act for me.

I have thought about this advance directive carefully. I know what it means and want to sign it. I have chosen two witnesses, neither of whom is a member of my family, nor will inherit from me when I die. My witnesses are not the same people as those I named as my health care proxies. I understand that this form should be notarized if I use the box to name (a) health care proxy(ies).

Signature _____

Date _____

Address _____

Witness' signature _____

Witness' printed name _____

Address _____

BOX 43–2. Advance Directive *(Continued)*

Witness' signature _____

Witness' printed name _____

Address _____

Notary [to be used if proxy is appointed] _____

Drafted and distributed by Choice In Dying, Inc.—the national council for the right to die. Choice In Dying is a national not-for-profit organization which works for the rights of patients at the end of life. In addition to this generic advance directive, Choice In Dying distributes advance directives that conform to each state's specific legal requirements and maintains a national Living Will Registry for completed documents. (5/92)

CHOICE IN DYING, INC.—
the national council for the right to die
(formerly Concern for Dying/Society for the Right to Die)
200 Varick Street, New York, NY 10014   (212) 366-5540

tion of disputes, and protection of patients' rights. It is important that each patient's wishes are clearly documented in his or her medical record. If a patient has not put forth advance directives or a living will and is incompetent, a Do Not Resuscitate decision may be made jointly by the health care team and family members.

End-of-Life Decisions

Completing personal business
a. Patients may engage in activities that help keep memories of them alive for family and friends. Writing journals and letters, recording shared times on videotape, recording personal messages, taking photos, and giving personal possessions to loved ones are all meaningful ways to complete personal business.
b. Patients may convey their preferences about types of care and procedures and make decisions related to estate planning, funeral arrangements, and preferred location for dying.
Deciding where to die: Patients and families need information and support as they make choices about where the patient will live during the last phase of his or her life. Many people experience difficulty in making this important decision. Patients may say that they do not want to be a burden on family and friends. Family and friends may say that they do not want to abandon the patient at the end of life. Hospital discharge planners and social work professionals are available in most settings to provide the necessary assistance for this important decision.

a. Nursing homes: Patients and families choose a nursing home as the setting for the phase of final physical decline for many reasons. This setting offers 24-hour nursing care. Arrangements may also be available through community-based hospice agencies to provide hospice services to the dying patient and his or her family.
b. Hospitals: Patients die in hospitals when they have sustained sudden serious changes in health status (e.g., myocardial infarction or a traumatic injury). Also, terminally ill patients may die while being hospitalized for symptom management.
c. Home: Many patients prefer to live the last days of life in their home. Services provided by home health care agencies make this choice possible.
d. Hospice: Hospice is a form of health care designed to meet the needs of patients and their families during the last 6 months of life. A physician-directed multidisciplinary team composed of nurses, social workers, chaplains, bereavement counselors, and volunteers provides a wide range of services. Physical and occupational therapists; pharmacologists; and psychiatric, pediatric, medical, and radiation oncology specialists may be available for consultation and intervention. Hospice services may be delivered in free-standing hospice facilities, hospitals, nursing homes, or the patient's home. In the United States there are few free-standing hospice facilities that deliver 24-hour inpatient care. Hospice care is frequently delivered in the home.
(1) The goals of hospice care are to support the physical, emotional, social, and spiritual aspects of life until the end of life; preserve human dignity,

maintain comfort, and provide autonomy and power of decision making for the dying person; and help family and friends cope with the reality of terminal illness.

(2) The availability of hospice services varies across the country. Although few inpatient hospice settings are available, community hospitals and nursing homes are making "respite care" available. Respite care includes 24-hour nursing care for a very limited time, usually less than 2 weeks. Respite care offers a break to primary caregivers of hospice patients.

(3) Most hospice services are community based. Services are available 24 hours a day on an on-call basis in many communities. Visits from skilled nurses and home health aides are regularly scheduled. Nurses teach family members specific patient care activities. For a limited time, around-the-clock respite care may be carried out at home or in an inpatient hospice facility if one is available.

(4) Admission to hospice and provision of services are based on need, rather than ability to pay. Third-party reimbursement and hospice Medicare benefits are available to people who qualify.

(5) Specially trained hospice volunteers provide companionship to patients and scheduled respite to caregivers in the home. Hospice volunteers may assist with transportation and errands.

(6) Coordination of durable medical equipment and supplies as well as assistance with funeral arrangements may also be provided.

(7) Hospice admission criteria include the following: a statement from the patient's primary physician certifying that the patient's life expectancy is not likely to exceed 6 months, the patient's and primary caregiver's awareness of the terminal prognosis, and the availability of a primary caregiver in the home with the hospice patient.

3. Deciding on organ donation
   a. Before death, anatomic organs can be removed only in the interests of the dying person or with the consent of the person or legal guardian.
   b. The Uniform Anatomical Gift Act of 1968 provides for organ donation procedures in all 50 states of the United States. Most states provide short, simple organ donation forms on driver's licenses. If a person has documented his or her intent to donate organs, the organs may be removed according to the terms of the donation, although the family's wishes are usually considered. If a person has not documented the intent to donate organs and has not expressed opposition to donation, the next of kin or other legitimate guardian assumes both the right and the responsibility for disposal of remains.
   c. Knowing that donated organs are providing new life to another person may provide some comfort to family survivors. This decision is difficult for many family members to make, however. Many regions have transplant coordinators who have special skills in discussing organ donation with family members. Some people are reluctant to sign an organ donation docu-

ment because they fear that medical professionals w[ill] not give them all possible life-sustaining assistance [if] they are in need of an organ for transplant. Vario[us] statutory definitions of death have been adopted [to] safeguard against this possibility. Generally, death [is] declared when the brain has undergone irrevocab[le] damage with no evidence of recovery, as demonstrate[d] by cessation of cardiac, respiratory, and neural activit[y].
   d. Many vital organs, such as the liver, heart, and kidney[s] must be transplanted immediately to avoid tissue det[e]rioration that leads to harm or death of the recipien[t]. Many types of organs, such as corneas, pituitary gland[s], and skin, can be stored in organ banks until needed.

4. Involving others in end-of-life decisions
   a. Family members and significant others may have [to] make difficult decisions about the use of life-sustai[n]ing interventions on the patient's behalf. In such [a] stressful situation, many emotions, such as fear, anx[i]ety, and sadness, are common. Family members w[ill] be called on to refuse or accept treatment for th[e] person who has become unable to participate in dec[i]sion making and has not documented his or h[er] choices in an advance directive or living will.
   b. The American Nurses' Association (ANA) has form[u]lated position statements on the nurse's role in en[d] of-life decisions (Box 43–3).

BOX 43–3. American Nurses' Association Position Statements on End-of-Life Decisions

1. Nursing and the Patient Self-Determination Act

   The American Nurses' Association (ANA) believes that nurses should play a primary role in implementation of the Patient Self-Determination Act (PSDA). It is the responsibility of nurses to facilitate informed decision making for patients making choices about end-of-life care. The nurse's role in education, research, patient care, and advocacy is critical to implementation of the PSDA within all health care settings.

   The ANA supports the patient's right to self-determination and believes that nurses will and must play a primary role in the implementation of the law.

2. Promotion of Comfort and Relief of Pain in Dying Patients

   Nurses should not hesitate to use full and effective doses of pain medication for the proper management of pain in the dying patient. The increasing titration of medication to achieve adequate symptom control, even at the expense of life, thus hastening death secondarily is ethically justified.

   The patient should have whatever medication, in whatever dosage, and by whatever route is needed to control the level of pain as perceived by the patient. The proper dose is the dose that is sufficient to reduce pain and suffering.

3. Foregoing Artificial Nutrition and Hydration

   The ANA believes that the decision to withhold artificial nutrition and hydration should be made by the patient or surrogate with the health care team. The nurse continues to provide expert care to patients who are no longer receiving artificial nutrition and hydration.

   It is morally, as well as legally, permissible for nurses to honor the refusal of food and fluid by competent patients in their care. Efforts to ensure "food nutrition" are unnecessary and can be inappropriate.

For a copy of the full text of these position statements, call the ANA at (8[00]) 637–0323 and request the *Compendium of Position Statements on the Nurse's R[ole] in End-of-Life Decisions*, catalog number PR-9. This summary is reprinted with p[er]mission of the American Nurses' Association. Washington, DC, 1992.

ASSESSING THE DYING PATIENT

Assessing Physical Comfort

Assessing pain
a. People usually learn ways of interpreting, expressing, and responding to pain within their social group. For example, a person may deny pain because of a fear that pain signals the progression of disease.
b. People with similar social learning experiences are likely to have similar patterns of pain perception, verbal and behavioral expressions of pain. Pain reporting varies widely with age, gender, and culture. (See Chapter 11.)
c. Attitudes, coping patterns, and reporting styles related to pain are influenced by ethnocultural background. People often define pain symptoms after consultation with their family members. (See Chapter 11.) Patient and family beliefs about pain remedies or the possibility of addiction may be a potent factor in the effectiveness of a pain management plan.
d. Patients who are depressed or anxious are more likely to have elevated levels of pain. Pain is also associated with sleep disturbance. Adjunctive interventions aimed at relief of depression, anxiety, and insomnia are helpful in a pain management plan.

Assessing other symptoms: Chart reviews and patient interviews indicate that pain, nausea, dyspnea, delirium, and drowsiness are the most common physical symptoms experienced by cancer patients with advanced disease. Other symptoms frequently mentioned include dysphagia, urinary retention or incontinence, fatigue, weakness, fever, constipation, anorexia, xerostomia, and sleep disturbance.

Assessing Psychosocial Needs

Feelings of uncertainty, anxiety, sadness, loneliness, anticipatory grief, spiritual distress, diminished hope, and loss of control have been reported by seriously ill persons.

A dying patient who is experiencing unrelieved symptoms or depression may verbalize a desire to commit suicide. Do not avoid discussion of suicide. Immediately refer the person to an appropriate source of support, while providing improved symptom control.

Assessing Spiritual Needs

Spirituality encompasses the significant meanings and values of an individual's life. The practice of spiritual beliefs or philosophy is not limited to participation in formal, institutional religions; attendance at churches or temples; or adherence to theologies or doctrines.

Nurses have an obligation to respect belief systems and to have a nonjudgmental perspective on spiritual philosophies different from their own. A spiritual assessment interview can guide nurses' actions in support of a patient's or family's beliefs. Such an assessment might include the following questions:
- What gives meaning to your life?
- Is religion or God significant to you?
- What is your source of strength or hope?
- What helps you the most when you feel afraid or need special help?
- Are there any spiritual practices, such as prayer or meditation, that help you?
- Is there someone, such as a member of your clergy or church, whom I could contact to assist you with your spiritual practices?

SUPPORTIVE CARE FOR THE DYING

Goals of Supportive Care

1. The following are the goals of supportive care for patients who are dying:
   a. To increase the quality of life by controlling pain and distressing symptoms.
   b. To offer strategies to patients and families dealing with debilitating and protracted illness.
   c. To provide psychologic support to patients and families facing multiple stressors associated with the end of life.
2. *Supportive care* describes a wide array of services for patients and their families.

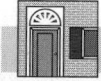

HOME CARE STRATEGIES

Palliative Care for the Dying

The goal of palliative care is to treat symptoms, optimize comfort, and improve the quality of life for the patient and loved ones. An in-depth interdisciplinary assessment and care plan that includes physical, psychosocial, and spiritual aspects of care is most important. When physical symptoms are present, the patient will have difficulty dealing with other care needs. It is important to assess and treat physical symptoms. In addition to physical symptoms, there are 2 main areas of concern that the patient and family usually wish to address:

How the Patient Will Die

- Patients are often worried that they will die in pain, that they will lose dignity or become a burden to their family. All health care disciplines need to listen carefully to what the patient is saying. Answer questions openly and honestly, and be ready to provide emotional support when needed.
- Both written and oral instructions need to be provided when appropriate.

How the Patient's Death Will Affect Family Members

- Identify fears and concerns related to patient care, financial issues, dying and funeral planning, and life after death.
- An evaluation of previous coping skills allows the family to identify what has been of value to them in the past and how to utilize those skills in dealing with caregiving, death, and the future.
- Help the family identify current supports, and refer to additional community resources.

Providing Supportive Care

1. Control pain. The following are the key principles of pain management:
   - Trust the validity of the patient's report of pain.
   - Evaluate concurrent psychosocial factors.
   - Evaluate the effect of pain medication using a simple valid measure of pain intensity (see Chapter 11).
   - Assess the impact of pain and pain management on the patient's mood and functional status, the patient's and family's acceptance of the pain management plan, and the patient's overall quality of life.
   - Anticipate and treat the side effects of the analgesic regimen.
2. Provide pain medications. The total absence of pain is not always achievable, but an effort to alleviate all causes of pain should be made (Box 43–4).
   a. Efficacy: Drug combinations should provide additive analgesia and reduce side effects. For example, non-steroidal anti-inflammatory drugs used in conjunction with opioids provide better pain relief than opioids alone in the treatment of bone metastases.
   b. Route: Use the simplest administration route, and adjust it according to the changing needs of the patient. Opioid medication may need to be administered by alternative routes (Table 43–2).
   c. Dosage: Analgesic medication should be titrated to maintain plasma drug concentrations associated with maximal pain control and minimal side effects.
   d. Frequency: Analgesic medication should be scheduled

BOX 43–4. Widespread Undertreatment of Pain by Professional Caregivers

The goal of pain management is to prevent or completely control pain. Although not all pain and associated symptoms can be completely eliminated, research shows that the major impediment to pain control is the health care team's lack of responsiveness to patients' reports of pain. Pain is related to physical, behavioral, and psychosocial factors. The cause(s) of pain and factors contributing to it need to be identified so that appropriate interventions can be implemented.

Many patients experience more than one type of pain simultaneously, and it is imperative that a pain control strategy be planned to manage diverse types of pain and associated symptoms (e.g. fatigue, functional disability, and affective depression). Somatic, visceral, and neuropathic pain, for example, require specific management strategies.

Unrelieved pain affects the physical, psychologic, social, and spiritual well-being of patients and their families. Failure to control pain with analgesic therapy believed to be adequate may lead to the false assumption that the patient is psychologically addicted to the drug. Addiction should never be an issue with palliative care of dying patients.

Barriers to adequate pain management are frequently related to inadequate assessment of pain. Factors that have been cited for inadequate control of pain include incomplete assessment of all factors contributing to pain; fear of respiratory depression, addiction, and drug abuse; and lack of a pain control plan that includes drug and nondrug approaches to physical and psychosocial aspects of the patient's experience of pain.

The World Health Organization and the Agency for Health Care Policy and Research are developing clinical standards and guidelines for available medications and other methods to address the problem of unrelieved pain.

Table 43–2. Possible Routes of Administration for Opioids

Route	Comment
Oral	Oral administration is preferred. Morphine is available in slow-release and immediate-acting tablet and liquid preparations.
Transmucosal	Molded lactose-based tablets of morphine or other opioids can be placed under the tongue or in the buccal pouch in patients who are unable to swallow liquids.
Rectal	Morphine, oxymorphone, and hydromorphone are available and are generally believed to be as effective when administered rectally as when given orally.
Transdermal	Fentanyl is formulated as a topical patch.
Subcutaneous 　Continuous infusion 　Repetitive bolus	Ambulatory pumps make outpatient infusion possible; morphine and hydromorphone have been used the most successfully.
Intramuscular	Intramuscular administration has a limited role in the delivery of opioids to patients in chronic pain.
Intravenous 　Repetitive bolus 　Continuous infusion	Patient-controlled analgesia pumps may be used.
Spinal 　Epidural 　　Repetitive bolus 　　Continuous infusion 　Intrathecal	The spinal route is a well-accepted route for which a variety of protocols are available.

Adapted from Portenoy RK. Practical aspects of pain control in the patient with cancer. *CA Cancer J Clin* 38:327–352, 1988.

around the clock to provide adequate pain relief. Sustained-release medications decrease the need for frequent medications and provide longer periods of uninterrupted sleep for the patient. Breakthrough pain may indicate that the medication regimen needs to include an additional agent to ameliorate these episodes. Increased sedation and confusion also indicate the need to evaluate the pain regimen.

e. Resistance: The fear of addiction related to administration of narcotic medications is prevalent among professional and family caregivers. The use of opioid medications in medical patients is very rarely associated with the development of addiction. Only 4 patients out of a sample of 11,882 with no history of addiction were identified as at risk for addiction. In addition, individuals who have a history of drug addiction require higher than normal doses of narcotics for adequate pain relief. To overcome fears related to administration of narcotics, education about the value of providing adequate pain relief is necessary.

TRANSCULTURAL CONSIDERATIONS

Cultural affiliation is an important influence on pain perception and response. A recent cross-ethnocultural study demonstrated that the best predictors of pain intensity in a sample of patients with chronic pain were ethnic group affiliation and locus of control style.

f. Tolerance: Tolerance is the need to increase a dosage over time to maintain the same level of pain relief. Usually the 1st indication of tolerance is a decrease in the duration of analgesia for a given dosage. Opioid tolerance and physical dependence are expected with long-term treatment and should not be confused with psychologic dependence (addiction). Patients are often reluctant to take opioid medication because they fear that if they start it too soon, it will not effectively relieve their pain in the future. However, this is not true, and nurses need to dispel this myth.

g. Patient-controlled analgesia: Patient-controlled analgesia allows patients to control the amount of analgesia they receive. Oral, subcutaneous, epidural, and parenteral routes are available for administration. Most pain relief medication is delivered on a regularly scheduled basis. Patient-administered boluses may be used when the patient experiences breakthrough pain. Patient-controlled analgesia accommodates transient changes in patients' analgesic requirements (e.g., increased activity, repositioning, dressing change).

Provide adjunctive pain relief: Adjunctive pain relief strategies are useful for patients early in the dying trajectory. (See Chapter 11.) Many of the pain relief strategies that rely on cognitive or distraction techniques are not well suited for patients close to death, because of these patients' diminished cognitive abilities. Most dying patients, who are in physical decline, do not have the

energy to practice relaxation strategies (Box 43–5 and Learning/Teaching Guidelines for Relaxation Imagery).

4. Control other symptoms.
   a. Activity limitation: Anticipate a progressive decline in functional abilities in patients who are experiencing terminal illness.
   b. Self-care deficits and problems with mobility increase the patient's reliance on others and may be a stressful transition for both the family and the patient. Suggest adaptive approaches and assist both the patient and the family through the transition. Consultation with physical or occupational therapists may provide solutions to mobility problems that the patient encounters during physical decline.
   c. Fatigue: Exhaustion that is unrelieved by rest or sleep may be a serious problem for dying patients. Patients may need assistance with setting priorities for activities and planning rest periods. Patients should do important activities first; nonessential activities should be eliminated. Distraction and relaxation techniques may be helpful. Patients may need to verbalize feel-

---

BOX 43–5. Adjunctive Pain Relief Techniques

Cognitive-Behavioral Interventions

Cognitive-behavioral interventions can help patients increase their control over symptoms and side effects of therapy and decrease their sense of helplessness and hopelessness. The mechanisms by which cognitive-behavioral techniques relieve pain are not known, but patients report altered perceptions of pain. Distraction helps reduce the awareness of pain by redirecting attention. Relaxation techniques reduce muscle tension and sympathetic arousal. These techniques are *not* a substitute for adequate analgesic control of pain, but they are adjunctive. Confusion and delirium limit the ability to use cognitive-behavioral techniques.

Certain factors influence whether successful outcomes result from cognitive-behavioral techniques. The patient must
- Be highly motivated to learn the new strategy.
- Have incentive to practice the technique.
- Be interested in participating actively in self-care.
- Have the energy to learn the technique, usually achieved by introducing it early in the illness.
- Have clear mentation.
- Have mild to moderate pain.

Relaxation-Imagery

Relaxation-imagery uses mental images in combination with relaxation. The patient is encouraged to assume a comfortable position, breathe slowly and deeply, and visualize a peaceful scene, such as clouds floating in the sky, or waves rolling onto a beach (see Learning/Teaching Guidelines for Relaxation-Imagery).

Music-Assisted Relaxation

Music-assisted relaxation redirects attention away from pain, negative emotions, and boredom to an instrumental audiotape selected by the patient. Clinical research shows that the use of music results in decreased pain.

Cutaneous Stimulation

Massage, pressure, and vibration help patients relax or provide distraction from pain. Common forms of massage are stroking, kneading, and rubbing using rhythmic, circular distal-to-proximal motions. An alcohol-free lotion used during massage decreases friction.

LEARNING/TEACHING GUIDELINES
for Relaxation-Imagery

General Overview

In a quiet environment, review the goal of the technique and instructions with the patient, taking time to answer questions about the expected benefits. Help the patient assume a comfortable position and provide instructions in a calm tone of voice. Provide positive feedback and elicit an evaluation. A copy of the instructions (a typed pamphlet or audiotape) should be given to the patient at the end of the session. Encourage the patient to practice this technique every day and to increase practice time to 20 minutes over the next week.

Instructions for Relaxation-Imagery

1. Breathe in slowly and deeply during this time (pause).
2. As you breathe out (pause), feel the tension leave your body (pause), feel yourself begin to relax (pause).
3. Breathe in and out slowly (pause) and rhythmically (pause).
4. Counting will help you to breathe slowly (pause).
5. Breathe in and count silently to yourself (pause) "one (pause), two (pause), three" (pause).
6. Breathe out and count silently to yourself (pause): "one (pause), two (pause), three" (pause).
7. Each time you breathe out (pause), you may say "peace" (pause) or "relax" (pause) or another word that you would like.
8. Now picture a place where you have felt peaceful or relaxed (pause).
9. You can imagine white clouds moving slowly across a blue sky (pause) or waves gently rolling onto the shore (pause) or some other favorite place where you felt relaxed (pause).
10. Continue to breathe slowly in and out (pause) and picture the peaceful place where you felt relaxed (pause).
11. End this session with a slow deep breath (pause). As you breathe out, say to yourself, "I feel alert and relaxed."

---

ings of frustration and disappointment related to increased fatigue. Extremes in environmental temperature may increase fatigue. Temperatures greater than 75 degrees Fahrenheit and humidity levels greater than 60 percent may increase the sense of fatigue.

   d. Sedation: Sedation may be an effect of the pain medication regimen and interfere with patients' daily activities and social interactions. Adjustments in the pain medication regimen may be needed. The use of caffeine or cerebral stimulants decreases sedation.

   e. Mood changes: Psychosocial reactions to physical decline may result in anger, hostility, depression, isolation, hopelessness, and loss of self-esteem. Patients and families need to know that mood changes may occur and that a variety of approaches to dealing with emotions are available (e.g., support groups and cognitive and behavioral therapy). Psychosocial support should be planned for the family as well as the patient.

   f. Side effects from treatments: Patients may experience distressing side effects from palliative therapies such as radiation therapy or surgery. Patients with progressive cancer may require palliative treatments to decrease the effects of the tumor.

   g. Nausea (see Chapter 27)

   h. Vomiting (see Chapter 27)

   i. Constipation (see Chapter 27)

   j. Anorexia (see Chapter 27)

   k. Dyspnea (see Chapter 22)

5. Manage unrelieved symptoms. Patients may present symptoms that cannot be managed with conventional treatments. The burden of dealing with these symptoms places increased stress on the patient, the family, and the professional staff.

6. Help the family live with protracted illness. A lo[ng] period of serious illness places great demands on [the] physical, emotional, social, and financial resources o[f the] family.

   a. Family caregivers, as well as the patient, may expe[ri]ence guilt and uncertainty over the disruption in fa[m]ily life related to the illness.

   b. Family members may have conflicting goals. The [pa]tient may be ready to die, but the family and phy[si]cian may continue efforts to sustain life. Convers[ely,] the patient may be holding onto life, and the fam[ily] may be ready to discontinue life-sustaining efforts.

7. Provide psychologic support. Family and friends m[ay] experience some of the same feelings that the dying [pa]tient experiences, such as uncertainty, anxiety, sadn[ess,] loneliness, anticipatory grief, spiritual distress, dim[in]ished hope, and loss of control. The timing of these fe[el]ings, however, may not be identical to the patien[t's,] presenting a complex situation for nursing interventi[on.] The patient and individual family members may ne[ed] different types of support at different times:

   • Consider family members' needs when planning care.

   • Evaluate the primary caregiver's ability to prov[ide] care.

   • Evaluate the primary caregiver's need for respite.

   • Determine the family's ability to adopt new ideas.

   • Assess the family's reactions to stress.

   • Assess the family's acceptance of support from sour[ces] outside the family.

   • Be accessible. Spend time with the patient and famil[y.]

   • Ask the patient what is needed.

   • Allow the patient to talk about him- or herself.

   • Introduce life review for patient self-expression.

   • Encourage family communication.

- Facilitate diminished guilt within relationships.
- Encourage conflict resolution.
- Help the patient maintain control by offering choices.
- Provide continuity through consistent staffing.
- Demonstrate a supportive presence.

Facilitate the experience of spirituality. Being aware of your own spiritual beliefs helps assist patients and families with this aspect of human life. Each person is the "expert" in a personal life journey. Nurses can assist patients through receptive listening. The following points, based on Burkhardt and Nagai-Jacobson's work, are helpful in facilitating the spiritual dimension of care:

- Know yourself as a spiritual being.
- Recognize that spirituality does not depend on the ability to define or describe God or the Ultimate Being.
- Encourage and share in reminiscing.
- Experience the present moment and whatever joy, pain, or grief it may hold.
- Recognize the importance of "being present with" patients as they describe the meaning or pain in their lives.
- Recognize that ambiguities, struggles, and searching are aspects of spirituality.

Assisting with the Dying Process

1. Making special arrangements
   a. Contacting clergy: Patients and family members may be comforted by the presence of clergy from their religious tradition. Provide information about available pastoral services in the care setting and determine whether the patient and family would like to contact clergy of their choice.
   b. Contacting and comforting family: Family members often want to be notified immediately about a decline in the patient's status. Many family members wish to be present with the dying patient as death approaches. Family members should decide among themselves who should be contacted at the patient's decline or death. The names and phone numbers of the family member(s) should be clearly documented so that all nursing staff will be able to contact the family.
   c. Providing time and privacy: Facilitate the practice of rituals (e.g., prayers) during the terminal phase.
   d. Mortuary services: Hospice home care agencies provide prior notification to mortuaries that death is expected in the home setting. This communication facilitates transfer of the body to the mortuary and prevents police involvement at the time of death.
   e. Contacting a counselor or social worker: The presence of a professional to support the patient and family members during the last phase of life may be beneficial for some families. Patients and family members may benefit from the psychosocial support provided by a professional who is experienced in assisting people through stressful times.
   f. Arranging for a bedside vigil: Patients may identify a person or persons whom they would like to be present near the time of death. Arrangements for this are usually made by the nurse and may entail providing a roll-away cot, comfortable chairs, fruit juice, and coffee and calling the person when it is time to be at the patient's bedside.

2. Providing life support for patients with end-stage disease. You may initiate life-saving measures in accordance with the patient's wishes about resuscitative measures. To guide life-saving interventions, written documentation should be evident in the patient's medical chart.

3. Identifying Do Not Resuscitate status. Patients' living wills should specify Do Not Resuscitate directives (see Box 43–2).

4. Withholding or withdrawing life support systems. The Patient Self-Determination Act was passed in 1990 as part of the Medicare Omnibus Reconciliation Act (Box 43–6). The patient has the right to refuse life-sustaining treatment. The patient should be encouraged to formulate an advance directive.

5. Withholding or withdrawing nutrition and fluids:
   - Support the patient's choices.
   - Help the family and patient clarify values.
   - Provide comfort measures.

6. Noting signs of imminent death:
   - Fluid intake becomes diminished or impossible.
   - Urine output is decreased or absent.
   - Responsiveness is altered, and the patient eventually becomes unconscious.
   - Blood pressure decreases.
   - Peripheral cyanosis increases.
   - Breathing diminishes, and apnea lengthens.
   - Pulmonary and pharyngeal secretions may accumulate.

7. Providing care at the time of death.
   - Provide time for the family to remain at the bedside for last good-byes after death.
   - Determine whether family members want to assist with postmortem care. Family members who have provided physical care during the patient's illness may find meaningful closure in assisting with postmortem care.

BOX 43–6. Withdrawing and Withholding Life-Sustaining Support

All institutions that receive Medicare or Medicaid funding must provide all adult patients with written information about choices regarding life support. Documentation in the patient record should note whether the patient has written advance directives. The American Nurses' Association has formulated a position statement entitled "Nursing Care and Do Not Resuscitate Decisions":

Nurses bear a large responsibility at the time a patient experiences cardiac arrest for either initiating resuscitation or ensuring that unwanted attempts to resuscitate do not occur. The choices and values of the competent patient should always be given highest priority, even when these wishes conflict with those of health care providers and families.

Nurses have the duty to educate patients and their families about all types of termination of treatment decisions and should encourage patients and their families to think about these decisions before admission to health care facilities. Nurses have a responsibility to educate patients and their families about various forms of advance directives such as living wills and durable power of attorney. If it is the nurse's personal belief that her/his moral integrity is compromised by her/his professional responsibility to carry out a particular Do Not Resuscitate (DNR) order, then the responsibility for the patient's care should be transferred to another nurse.

Reprinted with permission from *Compendium of Positions Statements on the Nurse's Role in End-of-Life Decisions*, © 1992, American Nurses Association, Washington, DC.

- Provide privacy and time for rituals and prayers in keeping with the traditions of the family.
- Provide support and comfort measures to the grieving family.

Care of the Body After Death

1. The care of the body after death is a nursing responsibility. Create an uncluttered environment in the patient's room by removing supplies and equipment, and make space to accommodate family members comfortably if they wish to view the body and grieve at the bedside.
   a. Remove blood, secretions, and intravenous tubing from the body. Place absorbent pads under the body to absorb urine or feces, because the sphincter muscles relax after death.
   b. Place the body in a supine position, with the arms comfortably resting at the side or folded on the chest. Gently close the eyelids and place dentures in the mouth to give the face a more familiar appearance.
   c. If the lower jaw is drooping, place a small rolled towel under the chin to close the mouth. The body needs to be positioned before rigor mortis (stiffening of the dead muscles as a result of chemical changes) makes it impossible. Rigor mortis begins with the jaw and progresses downward. It usually begins 2 to 3 hours after death and is completed in 6 to 8 hours. Purple blotches, known as livor mortis, appear on the dependent areas of the body about 20 to 30 minutes after death. Livor mortis is caused by gravity's pull on noncirculating blood. Placing a pillow under the head and the body in a supine position will prevent livor mortis from affecting the face.
2. Family members may wish to practice traditional rituals or religious practices at the bedside of the deceased. Give them the time and privacy for these practices.
3. Respectful handling of the body is an important component of postmortem care. Create a respectful atmosphere in the room through the tone of your voice and choice of conversation. It is most distressing for family members to hear laughing or loud discussions coming from the professional caregivers who are providing final care to their deceased loved one.
4. Family members may be invited to help bathe the body. Some family members who participated in care while their loved one was dying find this to be a natural part of the separation process.

◼ HELPING THE BEREAVED SURVIVORS

Definitions

1. **Loss** is a universal experience repeatedly encountered throughout life. Any loss results in a deprivation of some kind, either tangible or symbolic. The death of a loved one is usually experienced as a significant loss. Many losses, such as the loss of a loved one as a result of illness, are clearly recognized as negative. The importance of a loss varies according to the meaning the individual attaches to it.
2. **Grief** may be described as the process of psychological, social, and somatic reactions to loss. Grief is the normal reaction to loss. Grief reactions or symptoms might include anger, guilt, physical complaints and illness, despair, and sadness. The intensity of the symptoms varies across individuals and is influenced by the type of loss, the situation surrounding the loss, the personality of the bereaved, concurrent stressors, the availability of social support, and the strength of the attachment to the deceased.
3. **Bereavement** is the state of loss of a significant other through death. For most survivors, bereavement is experienced as a process. Each bereaved person is unique, and the course of bereavement is influenced by many variables. Be compassionate and aware of the differences among the bereaved, so that interventions are appropriate.
4. **Mourning** refers to the rituals and behaviors, usually culturally defined, that may be performed after a death. Mourners often have a visitation period before the funeral and a graveside service before the burial.

Theoretical Perspectives on Bereavement

1. Sanders's integrative theory of bereavement for survivors: Sanders' perspective includes both biologic and psychologic factors. Nurses need to be aware of the different factors surrounding each bereaved person (Fig 43-2). The integrative theory of bereavement includes the following:
   a. Assessment of personality factors: A person's psychologic health and successful use of coping strategies in the past influence his or her ability to cope with the loss of the loved one.
   b. Assessment of external and internal moderator factors: External mediators that influence bereavement patterns include the availability of social support systems, the circumstances surrounding the death, the bereaved person's relationship to the deceased, socioeconomic status, and concurrent stressors. Internal mediators include age, gender, personality, health, and feelings about the relationship with the deceased loved one.
   c. Phases of bereavement: People vary in the ways they grieve and the amount of time they need to go through the phases of the grief process. According to Sanders, the phases of bereavement are shock, awareness of loss, conservation-withdrawal, healing, and renewal. The bereavement process does not progress in a linear fashion but entails periods of overlapping phases and regression.
   d. Bereavement may result in the following outcomes: psychologic growth, no substantial change, or an adverse change in health or functioning.
2. Martocchio's theory of grieving: According to Martocchio, grief is the process of moving through the pain of loss. It is characterized by complex thoughts and emotions and is a time for healing, adaptation, and growth.

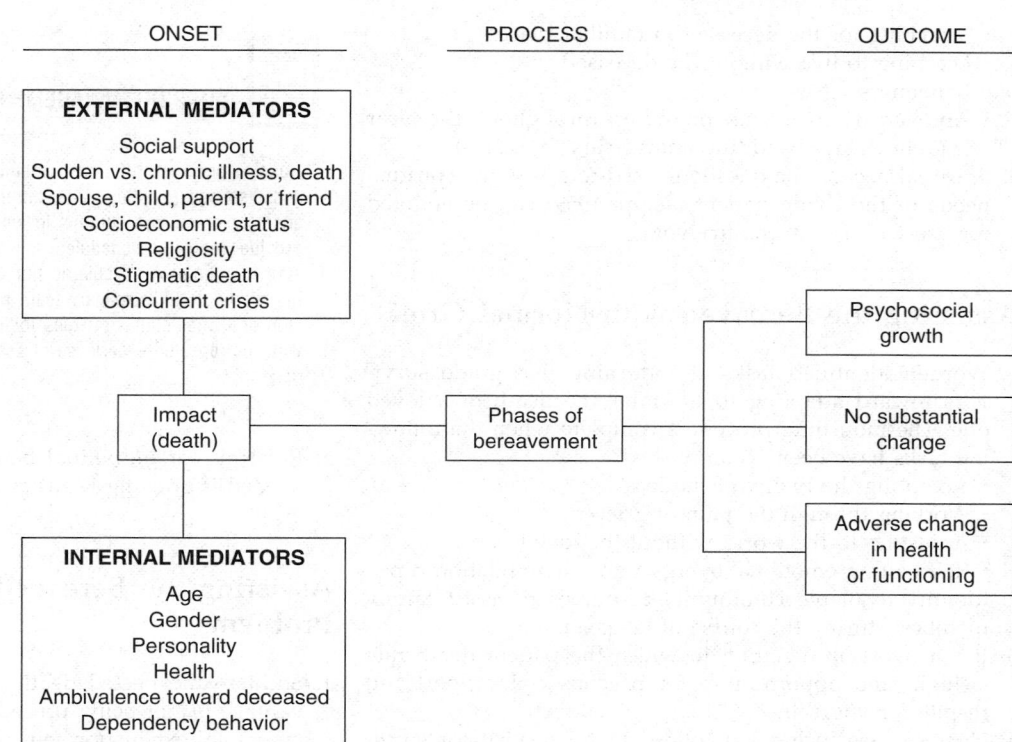

| ONSET | PROCESS | OUTCOME |

EXTERNAL MEDIATORS
Social support
Sudden vs. chronic illness, death
Spouse, child, parent, or friend
Socioeconomic status
Religiosity
Stigmatic death
Concurrent crises

Impact
(death)

Phases of
bereavement

Psychosocial
growth

No substantial
change

Adverse change
in health
or functioning

INTERNAL MEDIATORS
Age
Gender
Personality
Health
Ambivalence toward deceased
Dependency behavior

Figure 43–2. Integrative theory of bereavement for survivors. (Reprinted by permission from Sanders C. *Grief: The Mourning After.* New York: John Wiley & Sons, 1989. Copyright ©1989, John Wiley & Sons, Inc.)

a. Martocchio, a nurse researcher, described clusters of reactions that are not bound in time and may overlap. The clusters that form the framework include shock and disbelief; yearning and protest; anguish, disorganization, and despair; identification in bereavement; and reorganization and restitution.

b. According to Martocchio, the time line for grief resolution is variable. It may be shorter than a year or much longer than a year. Moreover, reactions to loss may last a lifetime. Anniversaries and holidays may be particularly difficult for survivors, bringing to mind memories of the deceased loved one.

d. The goal of successful grief work, according to Martocchio, is to be able to remember the loved one without major emotional pain and to reinvest emotional energy in living.

Transcultural Considerations

Cultural patterns of mourning vary widely. Members of a culture may have certain expectations of the newly bereaved with respect to participation in festivities and formation of new attachments.

Mourning traditions may restrict the style and color of clothing that mourners can wear for a defined period after the death of a loved one. For example, widows in some Mediterranean cultures wear conservative black clothing for anywhere from a full year to the rest of their lives.

Religious traditions may require mourners to perform memorial rituals or prayers for the deceased on designated days of the year. For example, some Chinese religious traditions that honor deceased ancestors include prayers and ritual offerings at an altar in the home.

Assessing the Bereaved

1. Physiologic effects of normal grief: Bereaved individuals experience any combination of the following somatic reactions:
   · Anorexia or other gastrointestinal disturbances
   · Weight loss
   · Inability to sleep
   · Crying
   · Tendency to sigh
   · Lack of strength
   · Physical exhaustion
   · Feelings of emptiness and heaviness
   · Feelings of "something caught in the throat"
   · Heart palpitations
   · Nervousness and tension
   · Loss of sexuality or hypersexuality
   · Lack of energy and psychomotor retardation
   · Restlessness and searching for something to do
   · Shortness of breath

2. Psychosocial effects of normal grief: Bereaved individuals experience any combination of the following psychosocial reactions:
   · Restlessness and inability to sit still
   · Inability to initiate and maintain organized patterns of activity
   · Withdrawal from social interaction
   · Preoccupation with thoughts of the deceased
   · Dreaming about the deceased

- Searching for the deceased in familiar places
- Learning to live without the deceased
- Loneliness
- Anniversary reactions on dates throughout the year (e.g., birthdays, wedding anniversary, holidays)

3. Spiritual needs: The questions used to assess the spiritual needs of the dying patient (see p. 1959) can be adapted for use with bereaved survivors.

Assisting the Bereaved with Normal Grief

1. Worden identified tasks of mourning that guide survivors toward adapting to life after the death of a loved one. The mourning process is complete when the following tasks have been accomplished:
   - Accepting the reality of the loss
   - Working through the pain of grief
   - Adjusting to the world without the loved one
   - Reinvesting emotional energy into a new relationship
2. Identify available community resources to assist family members during the course of bereavement.
3. If you work in a setting in which the patient death rate is high, find opportunities for psychosocial support and respite for yourself.
4. Hospice care includes a follow-up home visit for survivors. During this visit, give survivors information about bereavement support groups available in their community. Survivor support groups are offered through community- and hospital-based hospices, mental health agencies, and religious affiliations. Such support provides survivors an opportunity for reality checking, allows them to validate their feelings, and decreases their social isolation (Table 43–3).

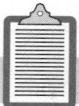

NURSING MANAGEMENT

Hospice agencies offer staff members weekly opportunities to discuss feelings resulting from caring for dying patients. Nurse managers in other care settings in which patients are terminally ill can provide regularly scheduled meetings to decrease stress among staff members. A psychiatric nurse liaison or another skilled member of the multidisciplinary team may facilitate a supportive discussion and offer staff strategies for coping with the stress associated with the repeated experience of death.

5. Referrals for individual bereavement counseling may be needed if grieving is sustained.

Assisting the Bereaved with Special Problems

1. Sudden unexpected death: A sudden death has the advantage of not being preceded by a time of financial and emotional exhaustion, but the disadvantage is that survivors have no warning and no time to prepare for the shock of loss. Myocardial infarction and an automobile accident are events that may result in sudden death.
   a. Interactions after an unexpected death event have significant impact on the survivors' grief process.
   b. Dubin and Sarnoff outlined interventions to facilitate the grief process for survivors of unexpected sudden loss (Table 43–4).

Table 43–3. Resources for Assisting the Bereaved

Organization	Form of Assistance
American Association of Suicidology	Provides information and referrals about local support groups for people who have lost a loved one through suicide.
Candlelighters Child Cancer Foundation	Provides group support and education for parents of seriously ill children.
Compassionate Friends	Offers support meetings for anyone who has lost a child. Has more than 600 local chapters.
National Organization for Victim Assistance	Supplies information and support to all victims of violent crime, including victims of domestic violence.
National Victim Center	Provides information through a national clearinghouse.
Parents of Murdered Children	Offers information and support to parents whose child has been murdered.
Resolve Through Sharing Bereavement Services	Provides information and supportive services to parents who have experienced miscarriage, stillbirth, or infant death. Offers support groups for bereaved parents and grief training sessions for professionals who interact with them.
The Sudden Infant Death Syndrome Alliance	Educates and supports parents who have lost an infant through sudden infant death syndrome.
Unite Grief Support	Supports parents who have experienced miscarriage, stillbirth, or infant death through telephone contact, educational programs, and parent-to-parent discussions.

Note: For the addresses and telephone numbers of these organizations, see "Agencies."

Table 43–4. Interventions for Survivors After Sudden Unexpected Death

Phase	Nursing Responsibilities
1. Contacting the survivors	Identify yourself and the hospital. Establish the identity of the survivor. Make sure to communicate with an adult. Determine whether someone else is present to provide emotional or physical support to the survivor. Generally, do not tell of the death over the telephone; instead, say that the relative is seriously ill or injured. Encourage the survivor to travel with another person who can provide emotional support. Encourage survivors to allow friends to drive them to the hospital.
2. Arrival of the survivors	Have staff available to meet the survivors. Verify the identity of the survivors. Escort the family to a private area. If the patient is alive, have a staff member contact the family every 15 min. Remember that informing the family about the death is the physician's responsibility. The physician has the most authority and can answer family members' questions about the patient's medical status and treatments.
3. Notifying the survivors about the death	Allow supportive persons to remain in the room with the family members if the family members wish it. Present events factually and in chronologic order. Tell the family about problems, actions taken, and the patient's response. Avoid jargon and be specific. Reassure the family that everything possible was done.
4. The grief response	Recognize that cultural norms influence expression of grief. Initial response may include numbness, disbelief, and shock. Demonstration of feelings will begin in a few minutes. Symptoms of normal grief include fatigue, shortness of breath, dizziness, palpitations, feelings of numbness, irritability, restlessness, headache, diarrhea, appetite loss, insomnia, inability to organize daily activities, self-blame, preoccupation with the image of the deceased, guilt, and hostility toward staff who attended the deceased. Encourage the expression of emotional reactions. Discourage use of tranquilizers, which only delay the grief reaction. Maintain a patient, understanding, and quiet presence. Be sure that staff respond to survivors without defensiveness or guilt and in an unhurried manner, even though anger about the death is often displaced onto them. Discourage survivor guilt.
5. Viewing the body	Do not refer to the deceased as "the body" or "it." Recognize that viewing the body facilitates grief because it forces survivors to confront the reality of the loved one's death. Remove blood and prepare the body for the survivors' visit, to preserve the deceased person's dignity. Move extra medical equipment away from the bedside. Leaving some medical equipment in the room, however, conveys a subliminal message to the survivors that efforts were made to save the person's life. Keep staff outside the room but available for support while the survivors view the body. Do not hurry the survivors through the viewing. Generally, survivors leave within 15 min.
6. Concluding the process	Offer the survivors information about their responsibilities in the transfer of the body to the medical examiner's office or funeral home. The family may be required to sign papers. Explain how to obtain copies of the autopsy or medical examiner's report. Give the survivors the opportunity to ask any remaining questions.

Table continued on following page

Table 43–4. Interventions for Survivors After Sudden Unexpected Death (Continued)

Phase	Nursing Responsibilities
	Explain symptoms of the grief response. Giving the survivors written material to take home is helpful.
	Obtain assurance that a friend or family member is available to stay with the survivor for the next 24–48 hr.
	Have a staff member accompany the survivors to the door.
	Make follow-up telephone calls to the survivors.

Adapted from Dubin WR, and Sarnoff JR. Sudden unexpected death: Interventions with the survivors. *Ann Emerg Nurse* 15(1):54–57, 1986.

2. Death of a spouse: The death of a spouse is considered one of the greatest loss events of a lifetime. Adjustment to living without a spouse is very difficult, and mutual-assistance groups have demonstrated effectiveness in helping widowed persons in a social setting. Support to widowed persons is offered through a variety of community- and church-affiliated groups.
3. Death of a child: Parents whose child has died demonstrate the range of grief reactions and may experience intense survivor guilt. Parents' grief symptoms are usually severe and long lasting. They may believe they failed to protect the child. Many parents require assistance with identifying and changing irrational beliefs and expectations that intensify their feelings of guilt. Individual counseling or group support may be beneficial.
4. Death of a parent with dependent children:
   a. Identify the information needs of all family members, including children. Alert the surviving parent to the differences between children's and adults' grief reactions.
   b. Children's questions and reactions related to the loss of a loved one may seem insensitive, but responses are usually consistent with their social, emotional, and cognitive development.
   c. Encourage honest discussion of terminal illness among adults and children within the family. Chil-

dren's fantasies about death will decrease if informa-tion is presented at the appropriate cognitive lev (Table 43–5).
   d. Encourage family members to discuss their hone feelings openly with children if such discussion is cultural norm. Do not lie or distort the truth abou death. In certain cultures, open expression of gri establishes a model for children that may be fostere within the family.
   e. Encourage families to share values, beliefs, and ritua related to death with children.
   f. Encourage family members to reassure children th family integrity, home, and love will continue despi the sadness related to illness and death.
5. Death by suicide: Suicide makes grief resolution difficu for many survivors. Western culture has traditional perceived suicide as sinful, criminal, or indicative of weak character. In contrast, other cultures view suicic as a rational choice or an honorable act. Offer survivo of suicide information about available grief counseling.
   a. Survivors may blame themselves for failing to preve the suicide.
   b. Survivors may also need to work through feelings anger and abandonment.
   c. If suicide was consciously chosen as a way to en

Table 43–5. Children's Cognitive Development of the Concept of Death

Predominant Death Concepts	Piaget's Period/Stage of Cognitive Development	Life Period
There is no concept of death.	Sensorimotor period	Infancy
Death is seen as reversible; a temporary departure or sleep.	Preoperational thought	Late infancy Early childhood
Death is seen as irreversible but capricious with external-internal physiologic explanations.	Concrete operations	Middle childhood Late childhood Preadolescence
Death is perceived as irreversible, universal, and personal but distant and having natural, physiologic, and theologic explanations	Formal operations	Preadolescence Adolescence Adulthood

From Wass H, and Corr CA. *Childhood and Death.* New York: Hemisphere Publishing, 1984. Reproduced with permission. All rights reserved.

debilitating illness, this fact may offer survivors an explanation that can help them deal with it.

d. Survivors may experience a social stigmatization that could slow the recovery process.

Death by murder: When someone dies suddenly and violently, survivors may experience not only intense grief reactions, but also anger and rage. Information and support resource networks have been established across the United States to meet the needs of family and friends of murder victims. Referrals to local and national agencies that provide information and guidance about criminal justice, crime victims' compensation, court accompaniment, and bereavement services are important to establish ongoing support for the grieving survivors of violent death.

Complicated grief and loss reactions

a. Persons who experience the deaths of more than 1 person in a relatively short time have an increased risk of complicated grief. For example, people who have witnessed illness and death from acquired immunodeficiency syndrome often experience complex reactions over a long period.

b. Parkes and Weiss identified a profile of families at risk for problems after death. The risk of problems increases when
- The family's socioeconomic status is low.
- The family's health status is poor.
- The death was sudden or followed a short period of illness.
- The family perceives a lack of social support.
- A religious belief system is absent.
- Family members are not supportive of one another.
- There is a history of psychiatric illness in the family.
- Multiple concurrent losses have occurred.
- Family relationships are dysfunctional.
- The family is geographically distant from the extended family.
- Guilt exists within family relationships.
- There is a high level of dependency among survivors.
- Family relationships are ambivalent.

Bibliography

Books, Reports, and Pamphlets

Agency for Health Care Policy and Research. *Depression in Primary Care: Clinical Practice Guideline.* No. 5. AHCPR Publication No. 93-0550. Rockville, MD: U.S. Department of Health and Human Services, Public Health Service, 1993.

Amenta MO, and Bohnet NL (eds). *Nursing Care of the Terminally Ill.* Boston: Little, Brown & Co, 1986.

American Nurses Association. *Compendium of Position Statements on the Nurse's Role in End of Life Decisions.* Washington, DC: Author, 1992.

American Nurses Association. *Position Statements on Nursing and the PDSA.* Washington, DC: Author, 1991.

American Pain Society. *Principles of Analgesic Use in the Treatment of Acute Pain and Cancer Pain.* 3rd. ed. Skokie, IL: Author, 1992.

Armstrong-Daily A, and Goltzer S (eds). *Hospice Care for Children.* New York: Oxford University Press, 1993.

Barlett J (ed). *Care and Management of Patients with HIV Infection.* East Islip, NY: Program Management Services, 1993.

Berger A, et al. (eds). *Perspectives on Death and Dying: Cross-cultural and Multidisciplinary Views.* Philadelphia: The Charles Press, 1989.

Blues A, and Zerwekh J. *Hospice and Palliative Nursing Care.* Orlando, FL: Grune & Stratton, 1984.

Bonica JJ. *The Management of Pain.* 2nd ed. Philadelphia: Lea & Febiger, 1990.

Carson V (ed). *Spiritual Dimensions of Nursing Practice.* Philadelphia: WB Saunders, 1989.

Choice in Dying. *Advance Directive: Living Will and Health Care Proxy.* New York: Author, 1992.

Doyle D, Hanks G, and MacDonald N (eds). *Oxford Textbook of Palliative Medicine.* New York: Oxford University Press, 1993.

Enck RE. *The Medical Care of Terminally Patients.* Baltimore: The Johns Hopkins University Press, 1994.

Flaskerud J, and Ungvarski P. *HIV/AIDS: A Guide to Nursing Care.* 2nd ed. Philadelphia: WB Saunders, 1992.

Foley KM, Bonica JJ, and Ventaffidda V (eds). *Advances in Pain Research and Therapy.* New York: Raven Press, 1990.

Gallagher-Allred C, and Amenta M (eds). *Nutrition and Hydration in Hospice Care: Needs, Strategies, and Ethics.* Binghamton, NY: The Haworth Press, 1993.

Giger J, and Davidhizar R. *Transcultural Nursing Assessment and Intervention.* St. Louis: Mosby–Year Book, 1991.

Glaser BG, and Strauss AL. *Awareness of Dying.* Chicago: Aldine, 1965.

Jacox A, Carr DB, and Payne R. *Management of Cancer Pain.* Clinical Practice Guideline No. 9. AHCPR Publication No. 94-0592. Washington, DC: U.S. Department of Health and Human Services, Public Health Service, Agency for Health Policy and Research, 1994.

Johanson G. *Physician Handbook of Symptom Relief in Terminal Care.* 4th ed. Santa Rosa, CA: Sonoma County Academic Foundation for Excellence in Medicine, 1993.

Johnson C, and McGee M. *How Different Religions View Death and Afterlife.* Philadelphia: The Charles Press, 1991.

Kalish RA. *Death, Grief, and Caring.* Monterey, CA: Brooks/Cole Publishing, 1985.

Kalish RA (ed). *Death and Dying: Views from Many Cultures.* Amityville, NY: Baywood, 1980.

Kübler-Ross E. *On Death and Dying.* New York: Macmillan, 1969.

Markides KS, and Mindel CH. *Aging and Ethnicity.* Newbury Park, CA: Sage, 1987.

McCaffery M, and Beebe A. *Pain: Clinical Manual for Nursing Practice.* Philadelphia: CV Mosby, 1989.

McFarland GK, Wasli EL, and Gerety EK. *Nursing Diagnoses and Process in Psychiatric Mental Health Nursing.* Philadelphia: JB Lippincott, 1992.

National Hospice Organization. *Standards of a Hospice Program of Care.* Arlington, VA: Author, 1993.

Osterweis M, Solomon F, and Green M (eds). Committee for the Study of Health Consequences of the Stress of Bereavement, Institute of Medicine. *Bereavement Reactions, Consequences, and Care.* Washington, DC: National Academy Press, 1984.

Parkes CM, and Weiss RS. *Recovery from Bereavement.* New York: Basic Books, 1983.

Parry JK (ed). *Social Work Practice with the Terminally Ill: The Transcultural Perspective.* Springfield, IL: Charles C Thomas, 1990.

Pattison EM. *The Experience of Dying.* Englewood Cliffs, NJ: Prentice-Hall, 1977.

Rando T. *Grief, Dying, and Death: Clinical Interventions for Caregivers.* Champaign, IL: Research Press Co, 1984.

Rosen E. *Families Facing Death: Family Dynamics of Terminal Illness.* New York: Lexington Books (Simon and Schuster), 1990.

Sanders CM. *Grief: The Mourning After.* New York: John Wiley & Sons, 1989.

Saunders C, and Sykes N. *The Management of Terminal Malignant Disease.* Boston: Edward Arnold, Division of Hodder & Stoughton, 1993.

Sudnow D. *Passing On: The Social Organization of Dying.* Englewood Cliffs, NJ: Prentice-Hall, 1967.

Turk D, and Feldman C. (eds). *Noninvasive Approaches to Pain Management in the Terminally Ill.* New York: The Haworth Press, 1993.

U.S. Bureau of the Census. *A Statistical Profile of the American Indian Population: 1980 Census (Census Fact Sheet).* Washington, DC: U.S. Government Printing Office, 1984.

Wass H, and Corr CA. *Childhood and Death.* New York: Hemisphere Publishing, 1984.

Worden JW. *Grief Counseling and Grief Therapy.* 2nd ed. New York: Springer Publishing Co, 1991.

World Health Organization. *Cancer Pain Relief and Palliative Care.* Report of WHO Expert Committee, Geneva: Author, 1990

Zimmerman JM. *Hospice: Complete Care for the Terminally Ill.* 2nd ed. Baltimore: Urban & Schwarzenberg, 1986.

Chapters in Books and Journal Articles

Anderson BL. Psychological interventions for cancer patients to enhance the quality of life. *J Consult Clin Psychol* 60(4): 552–568, 1992.

Bates MS, Edwards WT, and Anderson KO. Ethnocultural influences on variation in chronic pain perception. *Pain* 52:101–112, 1993.

Beck SL. The therapeutic use of music for cancer-related pain. *Oncol Nurs Forum* 18(8):1327–1337, 1991.

Benoliel JQ. Loss and terminal illness. *Nurs Clin North Am* 20(2):439–448, 1985.

Benoliel JQ. Health care providers and dying patients: Critical issues in terminal care. *Omega* 18(4):341–363, 1987–88.

Bourne V, and Meier J. What is happening? A booklet to be read to young children experiencing the terminal illness of a loved one. *Oncol Nurs Forum* 15(4): 489–493, 1988.

Brown MA, and Powell-Cope G. Themes of loss and dying in caring for a family member with AIDS. *Res Nurs Health* 16:179–191, 1993.

Bruera E, and MacDonald RN. Nutrition in cancer patients: An update and review of our experience. *J Pain Symptom Manage* 3(3):133–140, 1988.

Bruera E, Macmillan K, Pither J, and MacDonald RN. Effects of morphine on dyspnea of terminal cancer patients. *J Pain Symptom Manage.* 5(6):341–344, 1990.

Bruera E, et al. Estimate of survival of patients admitted to a palliative care unit: A prospective study. *J Pain Symptom Manage* 7(2):82–86, 1992.

Bruera E, et al. Cognitive failure in patients with terminal cancer: A prospective study. *J Pain Symptom Manage* 7(4):192–195, 1992.

Burkhardt M, and Nagai-Jacobson MG. Dealing with spiritual concerns of clients in the community. *J Community Health Nurs* 2(4):191–198, 1985.

Bushkin E. Principles of oncology nursing. *In* Holland JF, et al. (eds). *Cancer Medicine.* 3rd ed. Philadelphia: Lea & Febiger, 1993.

Canty SL. Constipation as a side effect of opioids. *Oncol Nurs Forum* 21(4):739–745, 1994.

Carrieri VK, et al. Desensitization and guided mastery: Treatment approaches for the management of dyspnea. *Heart Lung* 22(3):226–232, 1993.

Carroll R. Mourning: A concern for medical-surgical nurses. *MedSurg Nurs* 2(4): 301–303, 338, 1993.

Chrisman N. Cultural systems. *In* Baird S, McCorkle R, and Grant M (eds). *Cancer Nursing: A Comprehensive Textbook.* Philadelphia: WB Saunders, 1991.

Christ GH, et al. Impact of parental terminal cancer on latency-age children. *Am J Orthopsychiatry* 63(3):417–425, 1993.

Cleeland CS. Nonpharmacologic management of cancer pain. *J Pain Symptom Manage* 2(2):523–528, 1987.

Cohen SR, and Mount BM. Quality of life in terminal illness: Defining and measuring subjective well-being in the dying. *J Palliat Care* 8(3):40–45, 1992.

Coyle N, et al. Character of terminal illness in the advanced cancer patient: Pain and other symptoms during the last four weeks of life. *J Pain Symptom Manage* 5(2):83–93, 1990.

Creighton H. Decisions on food and fluid in life-sustaining measures. *Nurs Manage* 15(6):47–49, 1984.

Decker S, and Young E. Self-perceived needs of primary caregivers of home-hospice clients. *J Community Health Nurs* 8(3):147–154, 1991.

Degner LF, Gow CM, and Thompson LA. Critical nursing behaviors in care for the dying. *Cancer Nurs* 14(5):246–253, 1991.

Demi AS, and Miles MS. Suicide bereaved parents: Emotional distress and physical health problems. *Death Stud* 12:297–307, 1988.

Dimond EP. The oncology nurse's role in patient advance directives. *Oncol Nurs Forum* 19(6):891–896, 1992.

Dimond EP. Two years of the patient self-determination act. *Oncol Nurs Patient Treatment Support* 1(2):1–14, 1994.

Dobratz MC. Hospice nursing: Present perspectives and future directives. *Cancer Nurs* 13(2):116–122, 1990.

Dubin WR, and Sarnoff JR. Sudden unexpected death: Intervention with the survivors. *Ann Emerg Nurs* 15(1):54–57, 1986.

Ekberg J, Griffith N, and Foxall M. Spouse burnout syndrome. *J Adv Nurs* 11:161–165, 1986.

Fainsinger R, et al. Symptom control during the last week of life on a palliative care unit. *J Palliat Care* 7(1):5–11, 1991.

Ferrell BR, McCaffery M, and Rhiner M. Pain and addiction: An urgent need for change in nursing education. *J Pain Symptom Manage* 7(2):117–124, 1992.

Foley KM. Management of cancer pain. *In* Holland JF, et al. (eds). *Cancer Medicine.* Philadelphia: Lea & Febiger, 1993.

Fulton R. Anticipatory grief, stress, and the surrogate griever. *In* Tache J, Se H, and Day S (eds). *Cancer, Stress Death.* New York: Plenum, 1979.

Fulton R, and Fulton JA. A psychoso aspect of terminal care: Anticipate grief. *Omega* 2:91–99, 1971.

Gift A. Therapies for dyspnea relief. *Ho tic Nurs Pract* 7(2):57–63, 1993.

Gift A, and Pugh L. Dyspnea and fatig *Nurs Clin North Am* 28(2):226–232, 19

Grant M. Nutritional intervention: Incre ing oral intake. *Semin Oncol Nurs* 2: 43, 1986.

Horne BK. Hospice care for the termina ill. *Case Manage* 4(3):80–89, 1993.

LaFromboise T. American Indian men health policy. *Am Psychol* 43(5):388–3 1988.

Lindsey A. Cancer cachexia: Effects of t disease and its treatment. *Semin On Nurs* 2:19–29, 1986.

Loscalzo M, and Jacobsen PB. Practical b havioral approaches to the effecti management of pain and distress. *J Ps chosoc Oncol* 8:(2/3):139–169, 1990.

Martocchio B. Grief and bereavemer Healing through hurt. *Nurs Clin Nor Am* 20:327–341, 1985.

Melzack R. The tragedy of needless pai A call for social action. *In* Dubner Gebhart GF, and Bond MR (eds). *Pr ceedings for the 5th World Congress Pain.* New York: Elsevier Science Pu lishers, 1988, pp 1–11.

Pickett M. Cultural awareness in the co text of terminal illness. *Cancer Nu* 16:102–106, 1993.

Piper BF, Lindsey AM, and Doff MJ. Fa tigue mechanisms in cancer patient Developing nursing theory. *Oncol Nu Forum* 14(6):17–23, 1987.

Portenoy RK. Cancer pain: Epidemiolog and syndromes. *Cancer* 63:2298–230 1989.

Saunders JM, and McCorkle R. Models care for persons with progressive cance *Nurs Clin North Am* 20(2):365–377, 1985

Tripp-Reimer T, and Brink P. Culture bro kerage. *In* Bulechek G, and McCloskey (eds). *Nursing Interventions: Treatment for Nursing Diagnoses.* Philadelphia: W Saunders, 1985.

Turk D, Flor H, and Rudy T. Pain and families. Etiology, maintenance, and psychological impact. *Pain* 30:3–27, 1987

Wachtel T, et al. The end stage cancer pa tient: Terminal common pathway. *Hos pice J* 4(4):43–80, 1988.

Wimberly E. Minorities. *In* Wicks R, Par sons R, and Capps D (eds). *Clinica Handbook of Pastoral Counseling.* New York: Integration Books, Paulist Press 1985.

Winningham ML, Nail LM, and Burke MB. Fatigue and the cancer experience The state of the knowledge. *Oncol Nurs Forum* 21(1):23–36, 1994.

Wurzbach ME. The dilemma of withhold ing or withdrawing nutrition. *Image* 22(4):226–230, 1990.

Zimmerman L, et al. Effects of music in patients who had chronic cancer pain. *West J Nurs Res* 11(3):298–309, 1989.

gencies

erican Association of Suicidology
e 310
1 Connecticut Avenue, N.W.
shington, DC 20008

ıdlelighters Child Cancer Foundation
te 460
0 Woodmont Avenue
hesda, MD 20814
)) 366–2223

npassionate Friends, Inc.
). Box 3696
k Brook, IL 60522–3696
3) 990–0010

tional Organization for Victim
Assistance
7 Park Road, N.W.
shington, DC 20010
2) 232–6682

National Victim Center
Suite 300
2111 Wilson Boulevard
Arlington, VA 22201
(703) 276–2880

Parents of Murdered Children, Inc.
100 East 8th Street, B41
Cincinnati, OH 45202
(513) 721–5683

Resolve Through Sharing Bereavement
Services
1910 South Avenue
LaCrosse, WI 54601
(800) 362–9567 ext. 4747
(608) 791–4747

The Sudden Infant Death Syndrome
Alliance
Suite 210
1314 Bedford Avenue
Baltimore, MD 21208
(800) 221–SIDS

Unite Grief Support, Inc.
c/o Jeanes Hospital
7600 Central Avenue
Philadelphia, PA 19111–2499
(215) 728–3777
(215) 728–2082

APPENDIX A:
Traditional Health Beliefs and Practices of Selected Cultures

Illness	Causation	Prevention/Treatment
ack (African American)*†		
tural Illnesses	Failure to follow God's plan to maintain harmony in the world	Follow natural laws and fulfill social and religious obligations.
ly wears out	Failure to get enough rest	Lead moderate lifestyle.
	Failure to lead a moderate lifestyle	Consume adequate diet.
	Aging process	Do not overeat.
	Overuse of a body part, as in physical labor or sports	Get adequate rest.
		Take self-care measures and get help from family and friends.
		Seek biomedical treatment for sign or symptom relief.
		Use over-the-counter drugs.
od irregularities	Improper diet produces too much or too little blood	Seek biomedical treatment for signs or symptoms.
	Allowing impurities to build up in body	Use appropriate over-the-counter drugs.
	Failure to correlate medical treatment of a body part with zodiac signs to affect blood flow	Take self-care measures and get help from family and friends.
		Check diet and use herbs, tonics, iron pills and a variety of home remedies.
		Read zodiac signs and avoid treatment on or surgery to body part when one's zodiac sign is in ascendancy.
ld	Cold air entering body slows circulation and "thins" the blood. Thin blood lessens natural protection against colds, respiratory infections, and arthritis.	Avoid cold air.
spiratory disease		Dress adequately for the elements.
eumatism		Get biomedical treatment for signs or symptoms.
		Use appropriate over-the-counter drugs.
		Take self-care measures and get help from family and friends.
ivine Punishment	Retribution from God for failure to live life as God intended	Go to church, pray, and live one's life according to the word of God.
ental retardation	Improper behavior toward other persons	Make contact with God directly and repent for one's sin.
roke		Acknowledge the sin, feel remorse over the sin, and vow to take action to improve.
nvulsions		Avoid gossip; speak well of others; share whatever one possesses with others; never see self as better than others.
nnatural Illnesses	God withdraws divine protection from "grave" sinners, leaving them vulnerable to unnatural phenomena such as magic, witchcraft, or sorcery.	Get treatment from traditional healer, who is able to manipulate the supernatural world (see Table 2–8).
ness due to sorcery and witchcraft (magical illnesses)	Personal attack by an enemy or manipulation by kin	Get treatment from traditional healer to remove hex, spell, voodoo, conjure, roots, poison, and counteract black magic.
astrointestinal signs or symptoms:	Magical potion put in food or drink	Prevent through wearing amulets, drinking special potions, being careful not to offend or create envy in other persons and to dispose carefully of one's personal items and body substances (hair, fluid, fecal matter, nail clippings).
Weight loss	Natural illness signs or symptoms may convert to unnatural illness signs or symptoms if the person has a guilty conscience or has been told he or she will have the sign or symptom.	
Nausea		
Vomiting		
Foul taste in mouth		
Abdominal pain		
Diarrhea		

Table continued on following page

APPENDIX A:

Traditional Health Beliefs and Practices of Selected Cultures
(Continued)

Illness	Causation	Prevention/Treatment
Behavioral signs or symptoms: 　Inability to do everyday tasks 　Acting crazy 　Depression	Change in usual behavior Expressing fear of being unable to control own behavior.	Treatment by traditional healer
Unusual symptoms	Presence of animals in the body Symptoms never seen before Symptoms unresponsive to biomedical treatment	Treatment by traditional healer

Black (Haitian)*†

Supernatural Illnesses

Illness	Causation	Prevention/Treatment
Signs or symptoms that are internal and that persist over time 　Earache 　Toothache 　Abdominal pain 　Back pain 　Nausea 　Loss of energy	Failure to honor and serve one's spirit protector Failure to honor deceased kinsmen	*Prevention* Perform the appropriate rituals to honor s▮ protectors *(loa)* and deceased ancesto▮ *Treatment* Arrange for a divination ceremony by vood▮ priest *(houngan)* or priestess *(mambo* to ascertain causation and determine treatment.
Sudden onset of life-threatening illness or sudden death	Witchcraft and sorcery done by one's enemies	*Prevention* Avoid social conflict with family, kin, and others in one's interpersonal network. *Treatment* Arrange for a divination ceremony to deter▮ mine cause. Seek a more powerful sorcerer to countera▮ the magic or spirits sent by the sorce▮ hired by one's enemies.
Illness affecting a newborn or young child	Failure of parents or other kin to honor spirit protectors or fulfill obligations to ancestors	As above for spirit protector or dead ance▮
Congenital abnormalities, stillbirth, or death of a young child	Death of a child or fetus is always thought to be caused by one's enemies.	As above for witchcraft or sorcery

Natural Illnesses

Illness	Causation	Prevention/Treatment
Pain 　Head 　Stomach 　Legs 　Back 　Shoulders Rheumatism Anemia	Gas *(gaz)* enters the body through its natural orifices (mouth, ears, nose, vagina). It travels throughout the body causing pain. Enters via ears = Headache Enters via mouth = Abdominal pain Enters via vagina postpartum = Postpartum pain Gas travels from the stomach to: 　Legs = Rheumatism 　Back = Back pain 　Shoulder = Shoulder pain 　Intestine = Appendicitis	*Prevention* Avoid eating leftover food Drink tea made from garlic, mint, and clov▮ Eat solid foods capable of expelling gas (e▮ corn or plantain). Wear tight belt or linen around waist post-partum. Consult secular healers: 　*Fam saj* 　*Dokte fey* 　*Droquist*
Bone displacement 　Sprain 　Stiff or twisted neck 　Displaced vertebrae	Injury or physical exertion	Physically manipulate affected part by mas▮ sage or chiropractor. Warm poultices Oil massage

APPENDIX A:

Traditional Health Beliefs and Practices of Selected Cultures
(Continued)

Illness	Causation	Prevention/Treatment
esses caused by movement and consistency of milk in lactating mother	Milk of lactating mother is stored in breast and can cause problems for mother and breast-feeding newborn.	Avoid frightening or angering breast-feeding woman.
mpetigo in newborn	Milk is too thick.	Home remedies
Diarrhea, headache, postpartum depression, or violent behavior in mother	Milk becomes too "thin" if mother experiences sudden fright or anger. It rises to the brain, causing violent behavior, headache, or postpartum depression in the mother.	Consult *fam saj* or *dokte fey.*
wborn poisoning	Milk becomes mixed with mother's blood and is spoiled and can result in death of newborn.	*Prevention* Give mother rest and special care and diet for 12–18 months postpartum *Treatment* Wean child immediately Consult *fam saj* or *dokte fey* Home remedies
t or cold disequilibrium	Imbalance of hot and cold elements in the body, generally related to gender and reproduction Females are warmer than males. Pregnant women who have just given birth are warmer than other women.	*Prevention* Home remedies, diet, and herbs *Treatment* Consult *dokte fey, fam saj,* and family members. Home remedies, diet, and herbs
andering womb Postpartum weakness, dizziness, confusion, and pain	Type of organ displacement Result of sudden disruption at birth of the physical and emotional attachment between womb and fetus Womb moves frantically throughout body in search of fetus	Massage by *fam saj* to locate and reposition womb. Family and spouse must provide diet of rich and plentiful food to fill empty womb.
erdition Arrested fetal development Fetus trapped in womb	*Natural* Fetal development stops and is reversed until fetus becomes a speck in the womb. Causation may be walking barefoot on cold wet ground carrying a heavy load. When causation of arrested development is determined and alleviated, fetal development begins anew, ending with delivery 9 months later. The woman is considered pregnant the entire time in perdition and will menstruate. Perdition is not a miscarriage or an indication of psychosis. It is a culturally acceptable explanation for infertility.	Consult *fam saj.* Consult *dokte fey.* Consult *houngan* or *mambo* to divine causation. Self-care measures Home remedies Consult family. Obtain biomedical evaluation.
	Supernatural Spell cast by enemy on pregnant woman or her family or kin	Divination by *houngan* or *mambo* with appropriate action to remove spell.
Blood irregularities Quantity Color Viscosity Temperature Purity	Central dynamic of Afro-Caribbean health-culture beliefs and practices related to health maintenance, illness treatment, and body functions.	Dependent on status of blood. Generally regulated by diet, activity level, herbs, and home remedies. Consult family and friends and take self-care measures. Consult all types of traditional healers as determined by cause.

Table continued on following page

APPENDIX A:
Traditional Health Beliefs and Practice of Selected Cultures
(Continued)

Illness	Causation	Prevention/Treatment
		Use over-the-counter drugs. Seek biomedical evaluation and treatment.
Movement of disease Expansion or relocation of disease	Migration of disease from primary site to secondary site. Cultural explanation for radiating pain or need to seek care	Take self-care measures. Seek biomedical and ethnomedical evaluatio and treatment as indicated by causatio attributed to signs or symptoms.
Fright	Sudden shock or violent emotion disrupts body function. Extreme indignation after victimization or suffering injustice. Blood rises to head, causing partial loss of vision, headaches, temporary mental disturbance, and thinning of milk of lactating mother. In extreme cases, insanity may result if the blood is not returned to its normal position.	Use home remedies, self-care measures, or an appropriate traditional healer as dete mined by the attributed cause. The goa is to return blood to its normal positio and prevent spoilage. In violent episodes of emotion, home remedies may include tying a band around the victim's head or pouring coffee on the head.

Asian American (Chinese)*†

Natural Illnesses

Loss of ch'i or loss of blood

Illness	Causation	Prevention/Treatment
Anemia Fatigue Weakness Lack of energy Impatience or infertility Psychosomatic illnesses Loss of consciousness Excessive sleepiness	Depletion of *ch'i* (life energy) via loss of blood Obstruction or blockage of flow of *ch'i* along meridian pathways Aging process Overwork and overexertion Giving blood for laboratory tests Sudden fright during pregnancy	Use acupuncture or acupressure to remove blockage along meridian pathways. Take vitamin B_{12} injections Refuse to donate blood Avoid overexertion. Restore body balance of yin and yang.

Excessive ch'i

Illness	Causation	Prevention/Treatment
Anger Excessive talking and singing Restlessness and running about Scolding people incessantly Auditory and visual hallucinations Self-aggrandization	Abnormal or excessive food intake Obstruction of flow of *ch'i* Adolescence and young adulthood Experiencing sudden emotional distress	Use acupuncture or acupressure to restore flow of *ch'i* on meridian pathways. Take medications. Reduce food intake. Restore body balance of yin and yang.

Disturbances of hot and cold

Hot Conditions

Illness	Causation	Prevention/Treatment
Acne Dry mouth, throat, and nostrils Poor digestion Tiredness Sleeplessness Pregnancy	Improper food intake leading to excessive heat in the body Excessive intake of fried, spicy, and "rich" foods Dominance of yang Overexertion Excessive exposure to heat	Modify food intake. Take herbs and medications. Restore balance of yin and yang. Avoid exposure to heat.

Cold Conditions

Illness	Causation	Prevention/Treatment
Respiratory symptoms Dizziness Blurred vision Arthritic pain Postpartum	Exposure to cold temperature, wind, and rain Improper food intake Excessive intake of green, leafy vegetables Infancy, young childhood, and older people are prone to be in a "cold" body state Dominance of yin	Modify food intake. Take herbs and medications. Restore balance of yin and yang. Avoid exposure to cold and wind.

APPENDIX A:
Traditional Health Beliefs and Practices of Selected Cultures
(Continued)

Illness	Causation	Prevention/Treatment
nd Illnesses		
d conditions	Wind entering body via orifices and causing illness	Avoid exposure to cold and wind.
atedness	Exposure to cold and wind	Protect body orifices.
thy sputum		Use coining, burning, pinching, or cupping of the affected area.
ulence		Take herbs and medications.
bles in stool		Modify food intake.
stoperative distention		
stpartum conditions		
n		
ritic or joint pain		
adache		
ache		
sea or vomiting		
son Illnesses		
ignant tumors	Ingestion of poisons, chemicals, and other elements in food	Take herbs and medications to rid the body of poisonous substances.
ctions	Tumors and other internal growths give off poisons	Use coining, burning, pinching, or cupping of the affected area.
rgic conditions	Chemicals, air pollutants, and other pollutants that enter the body	
ayed healing of wounds		
ernatural Illnesses		
fortune		
onic illnesses	Unresolved family and social conflicts	Consult with fortune teller or shaman.
den, acute illnesses	Failure to fulfill obligations to parents, elders, and dead ancestors	Complete proper burial rituals for dead ancestors.
genital abnormalities	Interpersonal arguments	Worship gods regularly.
	Immoral behavior	Consult with gods and dead ancestors before important undertakings.
	Failure to worship or propitiate gods	Wear amulets.
	Violation of social taboos	
I loss		
ss fails to respond to treatment	Capture of one of a person's multiple souls by unhappy or unfulfilled ghost or spirit	Consult with shaman or medium.
onic illness exacerbates	Children are susceptible because their souls are loosely attached	Appease offended supernatural being.
fortune and bad luck	Dead ancestors are unhappy with final burial site or are angered or shamed by behavior of survivors	Make atonement for one's failures.
		Rectify improper or offending behavior.
panic Americans (Puerto Rican)*†		
ernatural Illnesses		
de ojo (evil eye; bad eye)		
(See Table 2–14)		
r	Envy of others	*Prevention*
iting	Admiring a child	Wear amulets.
rhea	Eyeing a child	Touch a child while saying "God bless you."
rexia	Causes blood to heat up or boil in the body causing signs and symptoms	*Treatment*
ng		Consult family.
ght loss		Consult *espiritista*
essness		Consult *curanderos* or *curanderas*.
		Pray.
		Massage with oil.
		Pass unbroken egg over body to draw out heat.

Table continued on following page

APPENDIX A:
Traditional Health Beliefs and
Practices of Selected Cultures
(Continued)

Illness	Causation	Prevention/Treatment
Mal puesto (bad deed) Paranoia Restlessness Anorexia	Spell cast on victim by an enemy	Consult *espiritista*.
Natural Illnesses *Imbalance of hot and cold*	Form of the humoral theory of health and illness. Illnesses and conditions are classified as hot or cold.	Neutralize the illness state by adding or subtracting foods, medicines, herbs, or fluids classified as hot or cold. Use self-care, family, *yerberos, partera,* and *curanderos* or *curanderas*.
Hot illnesses or conditions Constipation Diarrhea Pregnancy Rashes Sore throat Ulcers Warts	Body in a hot state	Use self-care, family, *yerberos, partera,* or *curanderos* or *curanderas*. Take cold or cool foods, medicines, herbs, and fluids. Avoid becoming overheated.
Cold illnesses or conditions Arthritis or joint pains Chest pain Colds Colic Earache Headache Menstrual period Postpartum Rheumatic fever Teething pain Tuberculosis	Body in a cold state	Use self-care, family, *yerberos, parteras,* and *curanderos* or *curanderas*. Take hot or warm foods, medicines, herbs, and fluids. Avoid drafts and becoming cold.
Susto (fright or soul loss) Diarrhea Restless sleep Lethargy Anorexia Paleness Weight loss Withdrawal or depression Loss of interest in personal appearance or hygiene Motor disability Decreased libido	The body is composed of a corporeal (physical) being and 1 or more souls (immaterial essences). The soul(s) are capable of leaving the body and wandering freely during dreams or after experiencing or witnessing a frightening event.	Use family, *curandero,* or *curandera* to lure soul back into body. Use massage. Take herbs to relax person.
Empacho (upset or obstructed stomach) Anorexia Diarrhea Fever Nausea Stomach cramps Vomiting	Witchcraft Ball of undigested food in stomach or other part of gastrointestinal tract Overeating and lying about amount of food eaten	Employ *espiritista* or spiritualist to perform countermagic. Use family, *yerberos, sobadores, cuandero,* or *cuandera*. Use prayer, herbs, and vigorous massage over back or stomach until loud crack is heard.

APPENDIX A:

Traditional Health Beliefs and Practices of Selected Cultures
(Continued)

Illness	Causation	Prevention/Treatment
ernal organ dislocation *da de la mollerea* (fallen fontanel)		Use family, *curandero* or *curandera*.

ing	Rapid removal of nipple from the infant's
	    mouth causing soft palate to become de-
	    pressed
		Press upward on soft palate.

hydration		Stimulate sucking reflex.
pressed anterior fontanel	Falling on the head	Spoon feed water.
rrhea	Not placing cap or cover on baby's head	Hold infant upside down over a pail of hot or

ficulty sucking	Doctor or nurse touching the baby's head
	    during physical examination or measuring
	    head circumference
		warm water.

ver		
nken eyes		
miting		
smo (paralysis)		

ralysis-like symptoms or spasm of vol-
    untary muscles, usually of the face or
    limbs
	Imbalance of hot and cold elements
	Body overheats and becomes chilled
		Consult family, *yerberos,* or *sabadores.*
		Consult *curandero* or *curandera.*
		Prevent exposure to extremes of hot and cold.
		Massage affected part.
		Consume herbs, food, and fluids of appropri-
		    ate temperature.

ld condition that becomes chronic	Body in a cold state	Consume herbs, food, and fluids of appropri- ate temperature.
al aire (bad air)	Imbalance of hot and cold elements	*Prevention*
quent explanation for:	Cold air entering body through various orifices	Take self-care measures.
Backache	and causing pain in affected body part	Consult family.
Chest cramps	Exposure of overheated body to cold wind,	Consult *curandero* or *curandera.*
Earache	air, or water	Consult *espiritista.*
Headache	May also have supernatural causation when	Use foods, herbs, and fluids of appropriate
Muscle spasms	essences or emanations from certain	temperature.
Pain from sprains	things affect the person. Emanations may	Wear amulets or religious medals.
Paralysis	be from persons, animals, the dead,	
Rheumatism	places, and heavenly bodies, for example,	
Stomach cramps	going near a cat that has just given birth,	
Temporary stiffness	menstruating or pregnant women step-	
Cessation or decrease of menstrual flow	ping over a child, contact with a dead	
Painful menstruation	corpse, or passing by a cold, damp place.	

Postpartum pain or distention	Postpartum: Air enters body through vagina
	    and causes abdominal distention or pain-
	    ful menstruation. May cause cessation
	    of menstrual period or decrease in nor-
	    mal flow. Interference with menstrual
	    flow may result in impurities building up
	    in blood.
		Take self-care measures.
		Consult family, *partera,* or *espiritista.*

aque de nervios (Nervous attack or
    Puerto Rican syndrome)
	Cultural response to acute stress, tension, and
	    anxiety
		Consult family.
		Protect self or others if aggressive behavior
		    occurs.

lling to ground		Consult *espiritista.*
yperkinetic episode		
creaming		
eizure pattern		
rashing		
ostepisode stupor		

Table continued on following page

APPENDIX A:

Traditional Health Beliefs and Practices of Selected Cultures
(Continued)

Illness	Causation	Prevention/Treatment
Mental Illnesses *Locura* (insanity; craziness) Homicidal behavior Suicidal behavior Unpredictable behavior	May have natural or supernatural causation *Natural causation due to biologic factors:* Drug abuse Alcohol abuse Heredity Head trauma Malnutrition *Natural causation due to social and psychological factors:* Excessive worry Family problems Obsessing Poor working conditions Poverty Sexual excess *Supernatural causation due to the following:* Spiritism Witchcraft *(dano)* Fate Bad luck Envy of others	Consult family, *curandero* or *curandera*, espiritista, or *yerbero*. Consult family. Consult *espiritista* for countermagic.
Enfermedad de los nervious (sickness of the nerves) Brooding Continued agitation Excessive crying Inability to concentrate	*Natural causation:* Excessive worry Family problems Poor working conditions Poverty *Supernatural causation:* Bad luck Envy of others Fate Spiritism Witchcraft *(dano)*	Consult family, *curandero* or *curandera*, or *yerbero*. Use talk, rest, herbs and medications for relaxation and calming. Consult family. Consult *espiritista*.

Illness	Causation	Other Causation
White Americans*† *Germ theory* (contact or contagion)	Illness caught from "other" persons through the air or direct contact with lesions or secretions	The specific microorganism may not be known. All microorganisms may be referred to as a "bug."
Colds Measles Chickenpox Tuberculosis	Virus or bacteria transmitted from 1 person to another Breathing in something from the air Bacteria and not taking care of oneself	Environmental changes Inherited predisposition Breathing in outside irritants like dust
Shingles	Virus and direct contact with lesions of another person	Nerves
Ringworm	Direct contact with lesions of another person	

APPENDIX A:
Traditional Health Beliefs and Practices of Selected Cultures
(Continued)

Illness	Causation	Other Causation
vironmental conditions		
anges in climate	Related to changes in temperature or exposure to the elements	
ds	Exposure to drafts and cold air: cold air enters the body, getting overheated and cooling off too rapidly	Viruses
eumonia		Contact with others who have the condition
urisy		Letting oneself get "run down"
nchitis	Failure to adequately protect oneself against the elements with proper clothing, blankets and adequate shelter	
ughs		
hritis	Changes in the weather	Body wears out
ckache		Normal part of the aging process
neral aches and pains		
estyle	Failure to lead a moderate lifestyle	
pertension	Stresses of everyday life	Obesity or heredity
ves	Emotional upset	
esity	Overeating	Diet
betes	Overeating sweets or sugar	Diet or heredity
nstipation	Becoming tense and upset	Diet
adaches		
igestion	Not letting the stress out	Failure to take laxatives on a regular basis
mach ulcer		
erculosis	Not taking care of oneself	Germs
		Heredity
icer	Smoking, diet, hormone pills	Hereditary

Illness	Causation	Prevention/Treatment
od irregularities	Allowing impurities (poisons or toxins) to build up in the blood	
s	Impurities in the blood trying to come out	Contact with lesions of others
hes	Impurities accumulate owing to the following:	Dirty skin
ples	Diet of rich foods	Microorganisms
etigo	Eating processed foods	
gworm	Failure to take laxatives	
	Failure to drink fluids	
erculosis	Germs entering the blood and making it impure	Heredity
		Breathing in dust
betes	Build up of impurities in the kidneys and blood	Lifestyle
		Heredity
	Chemical impurities in food	
creatitis	Chemical impurities in food	
mia (weak blood)	Impurities destroy blood	Loss of blood
		Diet
edity (runs in the family)	Weakness inherited for a certain illness or the illness inherited directly	
cer	Weakness for illness inherited	
betes		
erculosis		
defects	Direct inheritance	
rgies	Sensitivity to food and chemicals	

Table continued on following page

APPENDIX A:

Traditional Health Beliefs and Practices of Selected Cultures
(Continued)

---

* Represents the modal traditional beliefs and practices often attributed to Blacks, Asians, Hispanics, and Whites as groups. Cannot be generalized.

† The section on Blacks (African Americans) is based on data from Jackson J. Urban black americans. In Harwood A (ed). *Ethnicity and Medical Care*. London: Harvard University Press, 1981; Snow LF. *Walk' Over Medicine*. Boulder, CO: Westview, 1993; Snow LF. Sorcerers, saints and charlatans: Black folk healers in urban America. *Culture, Medicine and Psychiatry* 2:69–106, 1978; Snow LF. Popular medicine in a black neighborhood. *In* Spicer EH (ed). *Ethnic Medicine in the Southwest*. Tucson, AZ: University of Arizona Press, 1977. The section on Black (Haitian) is based on data from DeSantis L. Cultural factors affecting newborn and infant diarrhea. *J Pediatr Nurs* 3(6):391–398, 19 Farmer P. Sending sickness: Sorcery, politics, and changing concepts of AIDS in rural Haiti. *Med Anthropol Q* 4(1):6–12, 1990; Farmer P. Bad blood, spoiled milk: Bodily fluid as moral barometers in rural Haiti. *Am Ethnol* 15(1):62–83, 1988; Laguerre M. *Afro-Caribbean Folk Medicine*. South Hadley, MA: Bergin & Garvey, 1987; Laguerre M. Haitian Americans. *In* Harwood A (ed). *Ethnicity and Medical Care*. Cambridge, MA: Harvard University Press, 1981. The section on Asian American (Chinese) is based on data from Ahern EM. The power and pollution of Chinese Women. *In* Wolf AP (ed). *Studies in Chinese Society*. Stanford, CA: Stanford University Press, 1978; Chen-Louie T. Nursing care of Chinese American patients. *In* Orque MS, Bloch B, and Monrroy LSM (eds). *Ethnic Nursing Care: A Multicultural Approach*. St. Louis: Mosby, 1983; Gaw A. Chinese Americans. *In* Gaw A (ed). *Cross-Cultural Psychiatry*. Boston: Wright, 1982; Pachuta DM. Chinese medicine: The law of five elements. *In* Sheikh AA, and Sheikh KS (eds). *Eastern a Western Approaches to Healing: Ancient Wisdom and Modern Knowledge*. New York: Wiley, 1989; Wolf AP. Gods, ghosts, and ancestors. In Wolf AP (ed). *Studies in Chinese Society*. Stanford, CA: Stanford University Press, 1978; Wu DYH. Psychotherapy and emotion in traditional Chinese Medicine. *In* Marsella AJ, and White GM (eds). *Cultural Conceptions of Mental Health and Therapy*. New York: MacMillan, 1977. The section on Hispanic Americans (Puerto Rican) is based on data from Harwood A. The hot-cold theory of disease: Implications for treatment of Puerto-Rican patients. *JAMA* 216(7):1153–1158, 1971; Goldwater C. Traditional medicine in Latin America. *In* Bannerman RH, Burton S, and Wen-Chieh C (ed). *Traditional Medicine and Health Care Coverage*. Geneva: The World Health Organization, 1983; Maduro R. Curanderismo and Latino views of disease and caring. *West J Med* 139:868–874, 1983; Martinez RA. *Hispanic Culture and Health Care*. St. Louis: Mosby, 1978. The section on White Americans is based on data from Bauwens E. Medical beliefs and practices among lower-income Anglos. *In* Spicer EH (ed). *Ethnic Medicine in the Southwest*. Tuscon, AZ: University of Arizona Press, 1979; Hautman MA, and Harrison JK. Health beliefs and practices in a middle-income Anglo-American neighborhood. *Adv Nurs Sci* 4(1):49–64, 1982; Spector RE. *Cultural Diversity Health and Illness*. Norwalk, CT: Appleton & Lange, 1991.

APPENDIX B:

Guidelines for Obtaining Specific Laboratory Cultures

	Patient Preparation	Procedure	Results
...od culture	Cleanse the area over the venipuncture with alcohol and then with an iodine solution. Allow the iodine solution to remain on the skin for 1 minute before removal with an alcohol swab. Wear sterile gloves if palpating the venipuncture site after it is cleansed.	Perform a venipuncture and withdraw at least 10 ml of blood. Place half the blood into a culture tube for aerobic organisms and half into a tube for anaerobic organisms. Blood cultures are usually drawn on at least 2 consecutive days.	Normally, blood is sterile. If pathogens are present, most can be detected in blood after 72 hours of culture. Bacteria found in blood culture include *Streptococcus* sp., *Escherichia coli*, *Staphylococcus aureus*, *Bacterioides*, and *Neisseria meningitidis*. Viruses and fungi can also be detected.
...sopharyngeal culture	Explain that a specimen will be obtained from the back of the throat and that the procedure may cause some discomfort or trigger a gag reflex.	To collect the specimen, use a cotton swab attached to a flexible tube. Tilt the patient's head back and gently pass the swab through the nose and into the nasopharynx. Rotate the swab before removing it. Either streak the swab onto a culture plate immediately or send the swab, in a tube with transport medium, to the laboratory.	Pathogens may include *Bordetella pertussis*, *Haemophilus influenzae*, *Neisseria meningitidis*, *Corynebacterium diphtheriae*, group A β-hemolytic *Streptococcus*, and *Candida albicans*.
...utum culture	Teach the patient to expectorate sputum by 1st taking a few deep breaths and then coughing deeply. Be sure to obtain a sputum and not a saliva sample. The patient may require increased fluid intake, tracheal suctioning, or postural drainage to obtain sputum.	Wear a mask during the procedure. Use a sterile sputum cup or sputum trap if tracheal suctioning is used. Send the specimen to the laboratory immediately.	Sputum culture results are often difficult to interpret because the specimen is contaminated with flora in the oral cavity and trachea. Pathogens may include *Streptococcus pneumoniae*, *Mycobacterium tuberculosis*, *Enterobacteriae*, *H. influenzae*, *Pseudomonas aeruginosa*, and *S. aureus*.
...ol culture	If the patient is to collect the specimen at home, provide instructions about the proper collection technique.	Collect the stool specimen directly into a plastic-coated container or a clean, dry bedpan and transfer the specimen to the container with a tongue blade. Do not allow stool to contact urine. If blood or mucus is present, include it with the specimen. One gm of solid stool or 15 ml of liquid stool are enough. If using a sterile swab to obtain the specimen, insert it past the anal sphincter and rotate it several times before removal. Either innoculate a culture plate with the swab immediately or place the swab into a tube with buffered transport medium. If protozoa are suspected, collect specimens over several days, to increase the chance of sampling protozoa with cyclic life cycles. Use cellophane tape pressed over the perineal area to collect pinworms. Send to the laboratory immediately because some fecal organisms die with a fall in temperature.	Pathogenic organisms may include *Clostridium difficile*, *Clostridium botulinum*, *Clostridium perfringens*, *Salmonella*, *Shigella*, *S. aureus*, *Campylobacter jejuni*, *Vibrio cholerae*, helminths, and protozoa.

APPENDIX B:

Guidelines for Obtaining Specific Laboratory Cultures *(Continued)*

	Patient Preparation	Procedure	Results
Throat culture	Inform the patient that swabbing of the throat may cause a gag reflex.	Use a tongue depressor to avoid contact with structures in the oral cavity. Examine the throat with a flashlight. With a sterile swab, wipe the posterior pharynx, including areas of suspected infection (inflammation, ulceration, vesicles). Place the swab in a sterile collection tube and send to the laboratory immediately.	Pathogens may include group A β-hemolytic streptococcus, *S. pneumoniae*, *C. diphtheriae*, *B. pertussis*, *H. influenzae*, and *C. albicans*.
Urine culture	Instruct the patient about collection of a clean-voided midstream specimen to avoid contamination of the specimen with flora in the perineal area. If catheterization or suprapubic aspiration will be used to obtain the specimen, explain the procedure.	Collect the specimen as ordered. Collect at least 1 ml, but do not fill the container more than halfway. If collecting the specimen from an indwelling catheter, withdraw urine from a port in the tubing after wiping it with alcohol, using a sterile syringe. Do not take urine from the drainage bag. Send the specimen to the laboratory immediately. If transport to the laboratory is delayed longer than 30 min, refrigerate the specimen at 4°C. If the patient is undergoing diuresis, note this on the laboratory requisition because dilute urine can lower bacterial counts.	Bacterial counts of 100,000/ml of urine or more are a definite indication of urinary tract infection. Bacterial counts of 10,000–100,000/ml indicate probable infection, especially if the specimen was obtained by catheterization. Bacterial counts less than 10,000/ml usually indicate a contaminated specimen but could indicate infection in a symptomatic patient. The most common organism causing urinary tract infection is *E. coli*. A acid-fast stain can be requested to detect *M. tuberculosis* in the urinary tract.
Wound culture	Cleanse the skin around the wound to avoid contamination of the specimen with skin flora.	Collect specimens using a sterile swab, gently rotating it before removal. A minimum of 0.5 ml is required. Collect samples from several wound sites, including superficial and deep areas. Use a different swab or syringe for each site. Place 1 sample into a culture tube for aerobic organisms and another into a culture tube for anaerobic organisms. Be careful not to allow contact with air, which can kill anaerobic organisms. Send specimens to the laboratory immediately.	Organisms most frequently causing a wound infection include *S. aureus*, *E. coli*, *Pseudomonas*, *Proteus*, *Streptococcus*, *Bacterioides*, *Clostridium*, and fungi.

APPENDIX C:
Clinical Laboratory Values

Symbols and Units of Measurement

α	alpha
AU	arbitrary units
cc	cubic centimeter
cm	centimeter
dl	deciliter
fL	femtoliter
γ	gamma
g	gram
gm	gram
IU	international unit
kg	kilogram
L	liter
μg	microgram
mEq	milliequivalent
mg	milligram
mIU	milliinternational unit
ml	milliliter
mm	millimeter
mm Hg	millimeters of mercury
mmol	millimole
mOsm	milliosmole
mu	micro (μ)
ng	nanogram
%	percentage
pg	picogram
SI	Système International (international system)
U	unit
μ	micro

Normal Values: Whole Blood, Serum, and Plasma Tests

Name of Test	Conventional Values	SI Units
tivated partial thromboplastin time		
Average value	25–35 seconds	Same
Newborn	< 90 seconds	Same
renocorticotropic hormone		
In A.M.	25–100 pg/ml	25–100 ng/L
In P.M.	0–50 pg/ml	0–50 ng/L
renocorticotropic hormone stimulation test: a rise of plasma cortisol level within 30–60 minutes	≥ 18 μg/dl	≥ 497 nmol/L
anine aminotransferase		
Average adult range	10–35 IU/L at 37° C	Same
Newborn–1 year	13–45 IU/L at 37° C	Same
bumin		
Adult > 60 years	3.4–4.8 g/dl	34–48 g/L
Adult < 60 years	3.5–5 g/dl	35–50 g/L
Child	3.2–5.4 g/dl	32–54 g/L
Newborn	2.8–4.4 g/dl	28–44 g/L
bumin : globulin ratio	> 1	Same
dosterone		
Adult—Average sodium diet		
Supine	3–10 ng/dl	0.08–0.27 nmol/L
Upright	5–30 ng/dl	0.14–0.83 nmol/L
After fluorocortisone suppression or intravenous infusion	< 4 ng/dl	< 0.11 nmol/L
Adrenal vein	200–800 ng/dl	5.54–22.16 nmol/L

Table continued on following page

APPENDIX C:
Clinical Laboratory Values
(Continued)

Normal Values: Whole Blood, Serum, and Plasma Tests

Name of Test	Conventional Values	SI Units
Child		
11–15 years	<5–50 ng/dl	<0.14–1.39 nmol/L
3–5 years	<5–80 ng/dl	<0.14–2.22 nmol/L
1 week–1 year	1–160 ng/dl	0.03–4.43 nmol/L
Alkaline phosphatase		
Adult	4.5–13 King-Armstrong units/dl	32–92 U/L
	1.4–4.4 Bodansky units	
Infant	10–30 King-Armstrong units/dl	71–213 U/L
Alkaline phosphatase isoenzymes	*Percent Inactivation*	*Fractional Inactivation*
	16 Minutes at 55° C	*16 Minutes at 55° C*
Liver	50–70	0.5–0.7
Bone	90–100	0.9–1
Intestine	50–60	0.5–0.6
Placenta	0	0
Regan	0	0
Alpha$_1$-fetoprotein		
Adult	2–16 ng/ml	2–16 μg/L
Normal pregnancy	550 ng/ml	550 μg/L
Ammonia		
Adult	15–45 μg/dl	11–22 μmol/L
Neonate	90–150 μg/dl	64–107 μmol/L
Amylase		
Adult	60–180 Somogyi units	25–125 U/L
Neonate	5–65 U/L	Same
Androstenedione		
Adult male	75–205 ng/dl	2.6–7.2 nmol/L
Adult female	85–275 ng/dl	3–9.6 nmol/L
Child 10–17 years	8–240 ng/dl	0.3–8.4 nmol/L
Newborn	20–290 ng/dl	0.7–10.1 nmol/L
Angiotensin-converting enzyme		
Male	12–36 IU/L	Same
Female	10–30 IU/L	Same
Anion gap	10–15 mEq/L	10–15 mmol/L
Anti-DNA antibody	Negative	Same
Radioimmunoassay method	<10% binding	<0.1 binding fraction
Enzyme immunoassay method	<250 U/L	Same
Indirect immunofluorescent method	<1:10	Same
Antiglobulin test, direct	Negative	Same
Antiglobulin test, indirect	Negative	Same
Antinuclear antibody	Negative at a 1:20 dilution	Same
Antithrombin III	21–30 mg/dl	210–300 mg/L
	86–113%	86–113 AU
Aspartate aminotransferase		
Adult	8–20 U/L	Same
Newborn	16–72 U/L	Same
Bilirubin, direct		
Adult	0–0.4 mg/dl	<5 μmol/L
Bilirubin, indirect		
Adult	0.2–0.8 mg/dl	3.4–13.6 μmol/L
Bilirubin, total		
Adult	0.3–1 mg/dl	5–17 μmol/L
Child	0.2–0.8 mg/dl	3.4–13.6 μmol/L
Full-term neonate	6–10 mg/dl	103–171 μmol/L
Premature neonate*	<12 mg/dl	<205 μmol/L
Blood gases, arterial		
pH	7.35–7.45	7.35–7.45

APPENDIX C:
Clinical Laboratory Values
(Continued)

Normal Values: Whole Blood, Serum, and Plasma Tests

Name of Test	Conventional Values	SI Units
Pco₂	35–40 mm Hg	4.7–5.3 kPa
HCO₃⁻	21–28 mEq/L	21–28 mmol/L
Po₂		
Adult	80–100 mm Hg	10.6–13.3 kPa
Newborn	60–70 mm Hg	8–10.33 kPa
Oxygen saturation		
Adult	>95%	Fraction saturated: >0.95
Newborn	40–90%	Fraction saturated: 0.4–0.9
Base excess	± 2 mEq/L	± 2 mmol/L
ood gases, mixed venous		
pH	7.33–7.43	7.35 ± 0.05
Pco₂	40–45 mm Hg	5.3–6 kPa
HCO₃⁻	24–28 mm Hg	24–28 mmol/L
ood volume, total	60–80 ml/kg	Same
lcitonin, serum		
Adult	150 pg/ml	150 ng/L
Infant (cord blood)	25–150 pg/ml	25–150 ng/L
Infant (7 days old)	70–350 pg/ml	70–350 ng/ml
lcitonin, plasma		
Male	≤19 pg/ml	≤19 ng/L
Female	≤14 pg/ml	≤14 pg/L
lcium, total		
Adult	8.2–10.2 mg/dl	2.05–2.54 mmol/L
Child, 1 month–1 year	8.6–11.2 mg/dl	2.15–2.79 mmol/L
Newborn–1 month	7–11.5 mg/dl	1.75–2.87 mmol/L
lcium, ionized	44–55% of total serum calcium	0.45–0.55 fraction of serum calcium
Adult, serum	4.65–5.28 mg/dl	1.16–1.32 mmol/L
Child, serum	4.8–5.52 mg/dl	1.2–1.38 mmol/L
ancer antigen 125	<35 U/ml	<35 kU/L
arbohydrate antigen 19-9		
Adult	<37 U/ml	<37 kU/L
arbon dioxide, total		
Adult, venous	22–26 mEq/L	22–26 mmol/L
Adult, arterial	19–24 mEq/L	19–24 mmol/L
Infant, capillary	20–28 mEq/L	20–28 mmol/L
arcinoembryonic antigen		
Adult, nonsmoker	<2.5 ng/ml	2.5 μg/L
Adult, smoker	Up to 5 ng/ml	Up to 5 μg/L
arotene		
Adult	40–200 μg/dl	0.7–3.7 μmol/L
Infants	<60 μg/dl	<1.52 μmol/L
atecholamines (standing)†		
Epinephrine	<900 pg/ml	<4914 pmol/L
Norepinephrine	125–700 pg/ml	739–4137 nmol/L
Dopamine	<87 pg/ml	<475 pmol/L
eruloplasmin		
Adult	20–40 mg/dl	200–350 mg/L
Neonate–3 months	5–18 mg/dl	50–180 mg/L
hloride		
Adult	98–107 mEq/L	98–107 mmol/L
Newborn	98–113 mEq/L	98–113 mmol/L
Premature infant	95–110 mEq/L	95–110 mmol/L
holesterol, total	120–200 mg/dl	3.11–5.18 mmol/L
lot retraction time	1–24 hours	Same
Average time	4 hours	Same
lotting time	8–15 minutes	Same

Table continued on following page

APPENDIX C:
Clinical Laboratory Values
(Continued)

Normal Values: Whole Blood, Serum, and Plasma Tests		
Name of Test	*Conventional Values*	*SI Units*
Coagulation factor assay (general values)	50–150%	50–150 AU
Complement, total	75–160 U/ml	75–160 kU/L
Complete blood count		
Hematocrit		
Male	40–54%	0.4–0.59 (volume fraction)
Female	38–47%	0.38–0.47 (volume fraction)
Hemoglobin		
Male	13.5–18 g/dl	135–180 g/L
Female	12–16 g/dl	120–160 g/L
Red cell count		
Male	$4.6–6.2 \times 10^6/\mu l$	$4.6–6.2 \times 10^{12}/L$
Female	$4.2–5.4 \times 10^6/\mu l$	$4.2–5.4 \times 10^{12}/L$
Red cell indices		
Mean corpuscular volume	$80–96\ \mu m^3$	80–96 fL
Mean corpuscular hemoglobin	27–31 pg	27–31 pg
Mean corpuscular hemoglobin concentration	32–36%	0.32–0.36 (mean concentration fraction)
Red cell distribution width	13.1%	—
White cell count	$4.5–11 \times 10^3/\mu l$	$4.5–11 \times 10^9/L$
Platelets		
Adult	150,000–450,000 cells/L	$150–450 \times 10^9/L$
Newborn	84,000–478,000 cells/L	$84–478 \times 10^9/L$
Cortisol		
8 A.M.–10 A.M.	5–23 μg/dl	138–635 nmol/L
4 P.M.–6 P.M.	3–13 μg/dl	83–359 nmol/L
C-reactive protein	<1 mg/dl	<10 mg/L
Creatinine		
Adult male	0.7–1.3 mg/dl	62–115 μmol/L
Adult female	0.6–1.1 mg/dl	53–97 μmol/L
Newborn	0.3–1 mg/dl	27–88 μmol/L
Creatine phosphokinase		
Adult male	38–175 U/L	Same
Adult female	25–135 U/L	Same
Child, male	35–185 U/L	Same
Child, female	50–100 U/L	Same
Newborn	10–200 U/L	Same
Isoenzymes		
Creatine phosphokinase–MM	5–70 U/L	Same
	90–97% (of total CPK)	0.9–0.97 (fraction of total creatine phosphokinase)
Creatine phosphokinase–MB	0–7 U/L	Same
	0–6% of total creatine phosphokinase	0–0.06 (fraction of total creatine phosphokinase)
Creatine phosphokinase–BB	0.3 U/L	Same
	0–3%	0–0.03 (fraction of total creatine phosphokinase)
D-Dimer	<250 ng/ml	<250 μg/L
	No D-dimer fragments are present	Same
Dexamethasone overnight, single dose suppression test		
Plasma cortisol	Suppression to <5 μg/dl	Suppression to <138 nmol/L
D-Xylose absorption test		
Child–1 hour	>30 mg/dl	>2 mmol/L
Adult (2 hours, 5-g dose)	>20 mg/dl	>1.33 mmol/L
Adult (2 hours, 25-g dose)	>25 mg/dl	>1.67 mmol/L

APPENDIX C:
Clinical Laboratory Values
(Continued)

Normal Values: Whole Blood, Serum, and Plasma Tests

Name of Test	*Conventional Values*	*SI Units*
stein-Barr titer		
Viral capsid antigen—IgM	<1:10	Same
Viral capsid antigen—IgG	<1:10	Same
Epstein-Barr antinuclear antibody	<1:5	Same
Early antigen	<1:10	Same
rthrocyte sedimentation rate		
Adult		
<50-year-old male	0–15 mm/hour	Same
<50-year-old female	0–20 mm/hour	Same
Adult		
>50-year-old male	0–20 mm/hour	Same
>50-year-old female	0–30 mm/hour	Same
Child	0–10 mm/hour	Same
rythropoietin	5–36 μU/ml	5–35 IU/L
stradiol		
Premenopausal female	30–400 pg/ml	110–1468 pmol/L
Postmenopausal female	0–30 pg/ml	0–110 pmol/L
Male	10–50 pg/ml	37–184 pmol/L
striol, pregnancy		
28–30 weeks	38–140 ng/ml	132–486 nmol/L
32–34 weeks	35–260 ng/ml	121–902 nmol/L
36–38 weeks	48–570 ng/ml	167–1978 nmol/L
40 weeks	95–460 ng/ml	330–1596 nmol/L
globin clot lysis	1.5–4 hours	Same
ctor II	0.5–1.5 U/ml	0.5–1.5 kU/L
	60–150%	60–150 AU
ctor V	0.5–2 U/ml	0.5–2 kU/L
	60–150%	60–150 AU
ctor VII	65–135%	65–135 AU
ctor VIII	60–145%	60–145 AU
ctor IX	60–140%	60–140 AU
ctor X	60–130%	60–130 AU
ctor XI	60–135%	60–135 AU
ctor XII	60–150%	60–150 AU
ctor XIII	Clot is stable in 5 mol of urea for 24 hours	Same
rritin		
Adult male	20–250 ng/ml	20–250 μg/L
Adult female	10–120 ng/ml	10–120 μg/L
Newborn	25–200 ng/ml	25–200 μg/L
brinogen		
Adult	200–400 mg/dl	2–4 g/L
Newborn	125–300 mg/dl	1.25–3 g/L
brin split products	<10 μg/ml	<10 mg/L
'-Nucleotidase (adult)	2–17 IU/L	Same
ollicle-stimulating hormone		
Adult male	1–7 mU/ml	1–7 U/L
Adult female		
Follicular phase	1–9 mU/ml	1–9 U/L
Midcycle peak	6–26 mU/ml	6–26 U/L
Luteal phase	1–9 mU/ml	1–9 U/L
amma-glutamyl transferase		
Average adult range	5–40 IU/L	Same
Male adult	22.1 ± 11.7 IU/L	Same
Female adult	15.4 ± 6.58 IU/L	Same

Table continued on following page

APPENDIX C:
Clinical Laboratory Values
(Continued)

Normal Values: Whole Blood, Serum, and Plasma Tests		
Name of Test	*Conventional Values*	*SI Units*
Gastrin		
Adult male	< 100 pg/ml	< 100 ng/L
Adult female	< 75 pg/ml	< 75 ng/L
Newborn	120–183 pg/ml	120–183 ng/L
Globulin	2.8–4.4 g/dl	28–44 g/L
Glucagon, fasting	50–100 pg/ml	25 ng/L
Glucose, fasting		
Adult		
Whole blood	60–110 mg/dl	3.3–6.1 mmol/L
Serum, plasma	70–120 mg/dl	3.9–6.7 mmol/L
Elderly	80–150 mg/dl	4.4–8.3 mmol/L
Child, < 2 years old	60–100 mg/dl	3.3–5.6 mmol/L
Infant	40–90 mg/dl	2.2–5 mmol/L
Newborn	30–60 mg/dl	1.7–3.3 mmol/L
Glucose monitoring (capillary blood)	60–110 mg/dl	3.3–6.1 mmol/L
Glucose-6-phosphate dehydrogenase screen	Enzyme activity is present	Same
Glucose tolerance test, oral (adult fasting)		
Baseline fasting blood glucose	70–105 mg/dl	3.9–5.8 mmol/L
30-minute fasting blood glucose	110–170 mg/dl	6.1–9.4 mmol/L
60-minute fasting blood glucose	120–170 mg/dl	6.7–9.4 mmol/L
90-minute fasting blood glucose	100–140 mg/dl	5.6–7.8 mmol/L
120-minute fasting blood glucose	70–120 mg/dl	3.9–6.7 mmol/L
Glucose, 2-hour postprandial	< 140 mg/dl	< 7.78 mmol/L
Glycosylated hemoglobin assay	5–8% of total hemoglobin	0.05–0.08 fraction of total hemoglobin
Growth hormone		
Adult		
Male	0–5 ng/ml	0–5 µg/L
Female	0–10 ng/ml	0–10 µg/L
Child	0–16 ng/ml	0–16 µg/L
Growth hormone stimulation test		
With arginine	> 7 ng/ml	> 7 µg/L
With insulin	> 20 ng/ml	> 20 µg/L
Growth hormone suppression test	< 3 ng/ml	< 3 µg/L
Hematocrit		
Male	40–54%	0.4–0.59 (volume fraction)
Female	38–47%	0.38–0.47 (volume fraction)
Hemoglobin		
Male	13.5–18 g/dl	135–180 g/L
Female	12–16 g/dl	120–160 g/L
Hemoglobin electrophoresis		
Hb A	95–98%	0.95–0.98 Hb fraction
Hb A_2	1.5–3.5%	0.015–0.035 Hb fraction
Hb F	0–2%	0–0.02 Hb fraction
Hb C	Absent	Same
Hb S	Absent	Same
Hemoglobin, fetal		
Adult	< 2% Hb F	< 0.02 mass fraction Hb F
Newborn	77 ± 7.3% Hb F	0.77 ± 0.073 mass fraction Hb F
Hepatitis A antibody	Negative	Same
Hepatitis B core antibody	Negative	Same
Hepatitis Be antibody	Negative	Same
Hepatitis Be antigen	Negative	Same
Hepatitis B surface antigen	Negative	Same
Hepatitis C antibody	Negative	Same
Hepatitis delta antibody	Negative	Same

APPENDIX C:
Clinical Laboratory Values
(Continued)

Normal Values: Whole Blood, Serum, and Plasma Tests		
Name of Test	*Conventional Values*	*SI Units*
gh-density lipoprotein cholesterol		
Male	44–45 mg/dl	1.24–1.27 mmol/L
Female	55 mg/dl	1.425 mmol/L
stoplasmosis serologic study		
Complement fixation titer	<1:4	Same
Immunodiffusion test	Negative	Same
uman immunodeficiency virus serologic study	Negative	Same
uman chorionic gonadotrophin		
Male and nonpregnant female	<5 mU/ml	<5 U/L
Pregnant female		
1 week gestation	5–50 mU/ml	5050 U/L
4 weeks' gestation	1000–30,000 mU/ml	1000–30,000 U/L
6–8 weeks' gestation	12,000–270,000 mU/ml	12,000–270,000 U/L
12 weeks' gestation	15,000–270,000 mU/ml	15,000–270,000 U/L
uman leukocyte antigen	No destruction of lymphocytes	Same
sulin (fasting)		
Adult	5–25 µU/ml	34–172 pmol/L
Newborn	3–20 µU/ml	21–138 pmol/L
1 hour after eating	50–130 µU/ml	347.3–902.8 pmol/L
2 hours after eating	<30 µU/ml	<208.4 pmol/L
trinsic factor antibodies	Negative	Same
on		
Adult male	65–175 µg/dl	11.6–31.3 µmol/L
Adult female	50–170 µg/dl	9–30.4 µmol/L
Newborn	100–250 µg/dl	17.9–44.8 µmol/L
on-binding capacity, total	218–385 µg/dl	39–69 µmol/L
etones	Negative	Same
actate dehydrogenase	70–200 IU/L	Same
actate dehydrogenase isoenzymes		
LDH$_1$	14–26%	0.14–0.26 (fraction of total LDH)
LDH$_2$	29–39%	0.29–0.39 (fraction of total LDH)
LDH$_3$	20–26%	0.2–0.26 (fraction of total LDH)
LDH$_4$	8–16%	0.08–0.16 (fraction of total LDH)
LDH$_5$	6–16%	0.06–0.16 (fraction of total LDH)
actic acid	1–2 mEq/L	1–2 mmol/L
actose tolerance test, blood glucose	>20–30 mg/dl	1.1–1.7 mmol/L
ow-density lipoprotein : high-density lipoprotein	<3	Same
E cell test	Negative	Same
eucine aminopeptidase		
Adult male	80–200 U/ml (Goldberg-Rutenberg units)	19.2–48.0 U/L
Adult female	75–185 U/ml (Goldberg-Rutenberg units)	18–44 U/L
pase (adult)	<200 U/L	Same
pids, total	400–800 mg/dl	4–8 g/L
ong-acting thyroid stimulation	None; no long-acting thyroid stimulator present	Same
ow-density lipoprotein cholesterol	<130 mg/dl	<3.37 mmol/L
iteinizing hormone		
Adult male	1–8 mU/ml	1–8 U/L
Adult female		
Follicular phase	1–12 mU/ml	1–12 U/L
Midcycle peak	16–104 mU/ml	16–104 U/L
Luteal phase	1–12 mU/ml	1–12 U/L
Postmenopausal	16–66 mU/ml	16–66 U/L
Child, 6 months–10 years	1–5 mU/ml	1–5 U/L

Table continued on following page

APPENDIX C:
Clinical Laboratory Values
(*Continued*)

Normal Values: Whole Blood, Serum, and Plasma Tests		
Name of Test	*Conventional Values*	*SI Units*
Magnesium		
Adult	1.3–2.1 mEq/L	0.65–1.05 mmol/L
Child		
12–20 years	1.56 ± 0.21 mEq/L	0.78 ± 0.11 mmol/L
6–12 years	1.56 ± 0.18 mEq/L	0.78 ± 0.09 mmol/L
5 months–6 years	1.65 ± 0.23 mEq/L	0.83 ± 0.12 mmol/L
Newborn–4 days	1.2–1.8 mEq/L	0.6–0.9 mmol/L
Malaria smear	No organisms identified	Same
Metyrapone stimulation test (11-deoxycortisol)	>7 µg/dl	>200 nmol/L
Microfilariae smear	No parasites visualized	Same
Mononucleosis tests		
Monotest	Negative; nonreactive	Same
Heterophil titer	<1:56	Same
Neutrophil alkaline phosphatase	Score: 40–130	Same
Osmolarity		
Adult	285–319 mOsm/kg H_2O	285–319 mmol/kg H_2O
Child	270–290 mOsm/kg H_2O	270–290 mmol/kg H_2O
Osmotic fragility		
Initial hemolysis of erythrocytes	0.45% NaCl	4.5 g/L NaCl
Complete hemolysis of erythrocytes	0.3% NaCl	3 g/L NaCl
Parathyroid hormone		
Intact parathyroid hormone	210–310 pg/ml	210–310 ng/L
N-terminal	230–630 pg/ml	230–630 ng/L
C-terminal	410–1760 pg/ml	410–1760 ng/L
Parietal cell antibody	Negative	Same
pH (fetal scalp)	7.25–7.35	Same
Phenylalanine		
Guthrie test	<2 mg/dl	121 µmol/L
Fluorometry method		
Adult	0.8–1.8 mg/dl	48–109 µmol/L
Normal newborn	1.2–3.4 mg/dl	73–206 µmol/L
Premature newborn	2–7.5 mg/dl	121–454 µmol/L
Phosphorus, serum		
Adult		
12–60 years	2.7–4.5 mg/dl	0.87–1.45 mmol/L
>60 years	2.3–3.7 mg/dl	0.74–1.2 mmol/L
Child		
2–12 years	4.5–5.5 mg/dl	1.45–1.78 mmol/L
10 days–2 years	4.5–6.7 mg/dl	1.45–2.16 mmol/L
Infant 0–10 days	4.5–9 mg/dl	1.45–2.91 mmol/L
Premature infant	5.4–10.9 mg/dl	1.74–3.52 mmol/L
Cord blood	3.7–8.1 mg/dl	0.85–1.5 mmol/L
Phosphate, plasma (adult)	8.2–14.5 mg/dl	0.85–1.5 mmol/L
Plasma cell volume	40–50 ml/kg	Same
Platelet aggregation	3–5 minutes	Same
Platelet count		
Adult	150,000–450,000 cells/µl	150–450 × 10^9/L
Newborn	84,000–478,000 cells/µl	84–478 × 10^9/L
Potassium		
Adult	3.5–5.1 mEq/L	3.5–5.1 mmol/L
Newborn	3.7–5.9 mEq/L	3.7–5.9 mmol/L
Progesterone		
Adult male	13–97 ng/dl	0.4–3.1 nmol/L
Menstruating female		
Follicular phase	15–70 ng/dl	0.5–2.2 nmol/L
Luteal phase	200–2500 ng/dl	6.4–79.5 nmol/L

APPENDIX C:
Clinical Laboratory Values
(Continued)

Normal Values: Whole Blood, Serum, and Plasma Tests		
Name of Test	*Conventional Values*	*SI Units*
Pregnant female		
7–13 weeks' gestation	1025–4400 ng/dl	32.6–139.9 nmol/L
30–42 weeks' gestation	6500–22,900 ng/dl	206.7–728.2 nmol/L
Prolactin		
Adult	0–20 ng/ml	0–20 μg/L
Pregnancy		
Third trimester	34–306 ng/ml	34–306 μg/L
Lactating mother	<40 ng/ml	<40 μg/L
Newborn	<300 ng/ml	<300 μg/L
Prostate-specific antigen (male >15 years)	0.81 ± 0.89 ng/mL	0.81 ± 0.89 g/L
Prostatic acid phosphatase 4-Nitrophenylphosphate method (male)	0.13–0.63 U/L	2.2–10.5 U/L
Protein C	71–142%	0.71–1.42 fraction of whole
	2.82–5.65 μg/ml	2.82–5.65 mg/L
Protein electrophoresis		
Adult		
Albumin	3.5–5 g/dl	35–50 g/L
Alpha$_1$-globulin	0.1–0.3 g/dl	1–3 g/L
Alpha$_2$-globulin	0.6–1 g/dl	6–10 g/L
Beta globulin	0.7–1.1 g/dl	7–11 g/L
Gamma globulin	0.8–1.6 g/dl	8–16 g/L
Child		
Albumin	3.6–5.2 g/dl	36–52 g/L
Alpha$_1$-globulin	0.1–0.4 g/dl	1–4 g/L
Alpha$_2$-globulin	0.5–1.2 g/dl	5–12 g/L
Beta globulin	0.5–1.2 g/dl	5–11 g/L
Gamma globulin	0.5–1.7 g/dl	5–17 g/L
Protein S	61–130%	0.61–1.3 fraction of whole
Protein, total		
Adult, ambulatory	6.4–8.3 g/dl	64–83 g/L
Adult, recumbent	6–7.8 g/dl	60–78 g/L
Newborn	4–7 g/dl	40–70 g/L
Prothrombin time		
Average	10–13 seconds	Same
Newborn–6 months	13–18 seconds	Same
Red cell volume		
Male	25–35 ml/kg	Same
Female	20–30 ml/kg	Same
Renin, plasma		
Supine	12–79 mU/L	Same
Upright	13–114 mU/L	Same
Reticulocyte count		
Adult	0.5–1.5%	0.005–0.015 number fraction
	25,000–75,000/μl	25–75 × 10^9/L
Newborn	1.1–4.5%	0.011–0.045 number fraction
Rheumatoid factor	Negative	Same
Serotonin	50–175 ng/ml	0.28–0.99 μmol/L
Sickle cell tests	Negative	Same
Sodium		
Adult	136–145 mEq/L	136–145 mmol/L
Newborn	133–146 mEq/L	133–146 mmol/L
Syphilis serologic studies		
Venereal Disease Research Laboratory	Negative; nonreactive	Same
Rapid plasma reagin	Negative; nonreactive	Same
Fluorescent treponemal antibody absorption test	Negative; nonreactive	Same

Table continued on following page

APPENDIX C:
Clinical Laboratory Values
(Continued)

Normal Values: Whole Blood, Serum, and Plasma Tests		
Name of Test	*Conventional Values*	*SI Units*
Microhemagglutination assay – *Treponema pallidum*	Negative; nonreactive	Same
Testosterone, free		
Adult male	52–280 pg/ml	180.4–971.6 pmol/L
Adult female	1.6–6.3 pg/ml	5.6–21.9 pmol/L
Child 1–10 years	0.15–0.66 pg/ml	0.5–2.1 pmol/L
Testosterone, total		
Adult male	300–1000 ng/dl	10.4–34.7 nmol/L
Adult female	20–75 ng/dl	0.69–2.6 nmol/L
Child 1–10 years	<3–10 ng/dl	<0.1–0.35 nmol/L
Thyroid microsomal autoantibodies	Titer <1:1000; negative	Same
Thyroglobulin autoantibodies	Titer <1:1000; negative	Same
Thyrotropin		
Adult	0.4–8.9 μU/ml	0.4–8.9 mU/L
Newborn, whole blood	<20 μU/ml	<20 mU/L
Thyrotropin-releasing hormone test		
Throid-stimulating hormone value		
Male	14–24 μIU/ml	14–24 mIU/L
Female	16–26 μIU/ml	16–26 mIU/L
Thyroxine		
Adult	5–12 μg/dl	64.4–154.4 nmol/L
Child 1–10 years	6.4–15 μg/dl	82.4–193.1 nmol/L
Newborn	6.4–23.2 μg/ml	82.4–298.6 nmol/L
Thyroxine-binding globulin	16–34 μg/ml	16–34 mg/L
Thyroxine, free	0.9–1.7 ng/dl	11.5–21.8 pmol/L
Tolbutamide stimulation, serum insulin level	<195 μU/ml	1354 pmol/L
Toxoplasmosis serologic study	IgM antibody titer: <1:8	Same
Transferrin		
Adult <60 years	200–400 mg/dl	2–4 g/L
Newborn	130–275 mg/dl	1.3–2.75 g/L
Transferrin saturate	20–50%	Same
Triglycerides		
Male <40 years	46–316 mg/dl	0.52–3.57 mmol/L
Female <40 years	37–174 mg/dl	0.42–1.97 mmol/L
Male >50 years	75–313 mg/dl	0.85–3.54 mmol/L
Female >50 years	52–200 mg/dl	0.59–2.26 mmol/L
Triiodothyronine		
Adult	95–190 ng/dl	1.5–2 nmol/L
Child 1–10 years	94–269 ng/ml	1.4–4.1 nmol/L
Newborn	32–250 ng/ml	0.49–3.8 nmol/L
Triiodothyronine, free	0.2–0.52 ng/dl	3–8 pmol/L
Triiodothyronine resin uptake		
Adult	25–35% of total	0.25–0.35 fraction of total
Free thyroxine index	1.3–4.2	Same
Free triiodothyronine index	24–67	Same
Urea nitrogen		
Adult	5–20 mg/dl	1.8–7.1 mmol/L
Newborn–infant	4–16 mg/dl	1.4–5.7 mmol/L
Uric acid		
Adult <60 years		
Adult male	4.5–8 ng/dl	0.27–0.47 mmol/L
Adult female	2.5–6.2 ng/dl	0.15–0.37 mmol/L
Adult >60 years		
Male	4.2–8 ng/dl	0.25–0.47 mmol/L
Female	2.7–6.8 ng/dl	0.16–0.4 mmol/L
Child <12 years	2–5.5 ng/dl	0.12–0.32 mmol/L

APPENDIX C:
Clinical Laboratory Values
(Continued)

Normal Values: Whole Blood, Serum, and Plasma Tests

Name of Test	Conventional Values	SI Units
asopressin		
With osmolarity of >290 mOsm/kg	2–12 pg/ml	1.85–11.1 pmol/L
With osmolarity of <290 mOsm/kg	<2 pg/ml	<1.85 pmol/L
itamin D, activated	25–45 pg/ml	60–180 nmol/L
hite blood cell differential (adult),		
Segmented neutrophils	56%	0.56 (mean number fraction)
	1800–7800/μl	1.8–7.8 × 10⁹/L
Bands	3%	0.03 (mean number fraction)
	0–700/μl	0–0.07 × 10⁹/L
Eosinophils	2.7%	0.027 (mean number fraction)
	0–450/μl	0–0.45 × 10⁹/L
Basophils	0.3%	0.003 (mean number fraction)
	0–200/μl	0–0.2 × 10⁹/L
Lymphocytes	34%	0.34 (mean number fraction)
	1000–4800/μl	1.0–4.8 × 10⁹/L
Monocytes	4%	0.04 (mean number fraction)
	0–800/μl	0–0.8 × 10⁹/L

Normal Values: Urine Tests

Name of Test	Conventional Values	SI Units
ldosterone	2–26 μg/24 hours	6–72 nmol/24 hours
alcium (adult)		
Normal calcium intake	100–300 mg/day	2.5–7.5 mmol/day
Infant and child	<6 mg/kg/day	<0.15 mmol/kg/day
atecholamines		
Norepinephrine	15–56 μg/24 hours	88.6–331 nmol/24 hours
Epinephrine	<15 pg/ml	<82 nmol/24 hours
Dopamine	100–400 pg/ml	625–2750 nmol/24 hours
Vanillylmandelic acid	2–7 mg/24 hours	10–35 μmol/24 hours
Metanephrine	24–96 μg/24 hours	131–524 nmol/24 hours
Normetanephrine	75–375 μg/24 hours	409–2047 nmol/24 hours
hloride		
Adult	110–250 mEq/24 hours	110–250 mmol/24 hours
Adult >60 years	95–195 mEq/24 hours	95–195 mmol/24 hours
Child 10–14 years		
Male	64–176 mEq/24 hours	64–176 mmol/24 hours
Female	36–173 mEq/24 hours	36–173 mmol/24 hours
Child 6–10 years		
Male	36–110 mEq/24 hours	36–110 mmol/24 hours
Female	18–74 mEq/24 hours	18–74 mmol/24 hours
Child <6 years	15–40 mEq/24 hours	15–40 mmol/24 hours
Infant	2–10 mEq/24 hours	2–10 mmol/24 hours
ortisol, free (adult)	0–110 μg/24 hours	0–303.6 nmol/24 hours
reatinine clearance		
Adult male	1–2 g/day	8.8–17.7 mmol/L
Adult female	0.8–1.8 g/day	7.1–15.9 mmol/L
Child	70–140 ml/minute/1.73 m²	1.17–2.33 ml/second/m²
examethasone suppression test, low dose		
(adult)		
17-hydroxycorticosteroid	<4 ng/24 hours	<138 nmol/L
Free cortisol	<4 ng/ml	<11.04 nmol/24 hours
-Xylose absorption test		
Child	16–33% of ingested dose/5 hours	0.16–0.33 fraction of ingested dose/5 hours
Adult, 5-g dose	>1.2 g/5 hours	>8 mmol/L/5 hours
Adult, 25-g dose	>4 g/5 hours	>26.64 mmol/L/5 hours
Adult >65 years	3.5 g/5 hours	>23.31 mmol/L/5 hours

Table continued on following page

APPENDIX C:
Clinical Laboratory Values
(Continued)

Normal Values: Whole Blood, Serum, and Plasma Tests		
Name of Test	*Conventional Values*	*SI Units*
Estriol, pregnancy		
28–30 weeks	5–18 mg/24 hours	17–62 μmol/L
32–34 weeks	2–26 mg/24 hours	24–90 μmol/L
36–38 weeks	10–36 mg/24 hours	35–125 μmol/L
40 weeks	13–42 mg/24 hours	45–146 μmol/L
Estrogens		
Postmenopausal female	<20 μg/24 hours	69 μmol/24 hours
Premenopausal female	15–80 μg/24 hours	52–277 μmol/24 hours
Male	15–40 μg/24 hours	52–139 μmol/24 hours
Child	<10 μg/24 hours	<35 μmol/24 hours
5-Hydroxyindoleacetic acid, quantitative, adult	1–7 mg/24 hours	5–37 μmol/24 hours
Glucose	Negative	Same
Fibrin split products	<0.25 μg/ml	<0.25 mg/L
Follicle-stimulating hormone		
Adult male	4–18 U/24 hours	Same
Female		
Follicular phase	3–12 U/24 hours	Same
Midcycle peak	8–60 U/24 hours	Same
Hemosiderin	Negative	Same
Human chorionic gonadotropin		
Male, nonpregnant female	Negative	Same
Pregnant female	Positive	Same
17-Hydroxycorticosteroids		
Adult male	4.5–12 mg/24 hours	12.4–33.1 μmol/24 hours
Adult female	2.5–10 mg/24 hours	6.9–27.6 μmol/24 hours
Child		
8–12 years	<4.5 mg/24 hours	<12.4 μmol/24 hours
<8 years	<1.5 mg/24 hours	<4.14 μmol/24 hours
17-Ketogenic steroids		
Male	4–14 mg/24 hours	13–49 μmol/24 hours
Female	2–12 mg/24 hours	7–42 μmol/24 hours
Child		
11–14 years	2–9 mg/24 hours	7–31 μmol/24 hours
<11 years	0.1–4 mg/24 hours	0.3–14 μmol/24 hours
Ketones	Negative	Same
17-Ketosteroids		
Male	10–25 mg/24 hours	37–87 μmol/24 hours
Female	6–14 mg/24 hours	21–49 μmol/24 hours
Child		
10–14 years	1–6 mg/24 hours	3–21 μmol/24 hours
<10 years	<3 mg/24 hours	<10 μmol/24 hours
Lactose tolerance test		
Urine lactose		
Adult	12–40 mg/dl/24 hours	0.7–2.2 mmol/L
Child	<1.5 mg/100 dl	—
Leukocyte esterase	Negative	Same
Casts	0–4 hyaline casts/low-power field	Same
Crystals	Few	Same
Luteinizing hormone		
Adult male	9–23 U/24 hours	Same
Female	4–30 U/24 hours	Same
Male 1–10 years	<1–5.6 U/24 hours	Same
Female 1–10 years	1.4–4.9 U/24 hours	Same
Magnesium	7.3–12.2 mg/dl/day	3–5 mmol/day

APPENDIX C:
Clinical Laboratory Values
(Continued)

Normal Values: Whole Blood, Serum, and Plasma Tests		
Name of Test	*Conventional Values*	*SI Units*
smolarity		
Normal diet and fluid intake	500–800 mOsm/kg H_2O	500–800 mmol/kg H_2O
Range	50–1400 mOsm/kg H_2O	50–1400 mmol/kg H_2O
va and parasites	Negative	Same
henylalanine	Negative	Same
otassium		
Adult	25–125 mEq/24 hours	25–125 mmol/24 hours
Child 10–14 years		
Male	22–57 mEq/24 hours	22–57 mmol/24 hours
Female	18–58 mEq/24 hours	18–58 mmol/24 hours
Child 6–10 years		
Male	17–54 mEq/24 hours	17–54 mmol/24 hours
Female	8–37 mEq/24 hours	8–37 mmol/24 hours
Infant	4.1–5.3 mEq/24 hours	4.1–5.3 mmol/24 hours
regnanetriol		
Adult	<2 mg/day	<5.9 μmol/day
Child		
0–6 years	<0.2 mg/day	<0.6 μmol/day
7–16 years	<0.3–1.1 mg/day	<0.9–3.3 μmol/day
rotein	40–150 mg/24 hours	Same
rotein electrophoresis	40–150 ng/24 hours	40–150 mg/24 hours
chilling test		
Stage 1	10–40% cobalt-58, vitamin B_{12} excretion/24 hours	0.1–0.4 fraction of dose excreted
Stage 2	0–42% cobalt-57, vitamin B_{12}, and intrinsic factor excretion/24 hours	0–0.42 fraction of dose excreted
Cobalt-57 : cobalt 58 ratio	0.7–1.3	Same
odium		
Adult	40–220 mEq/24 hours	40–220 mmol/24 hours
Child 10–14 years		
Male	63–117 mEq/24 hours	63–117 mmol/24 hours
Female	48–168 mEq/24 hours	48–168 mmol/24 hours
Child 6–10 years		
Male	41–115 mEq/24 hours	41–115 mmol/24 hours
Female	20–69 mEq/24 hours	20–69 mmol/24 hours
ric acid (adult, average diet)	250–750 mg/24 hours	1.48–4.43 mmol/24 hours
rinalysis		
Specific gravity	1.003–1.029	Same
pH	4.5–7.8	Same
Protein	Negative	Same
Bilirubin	Negative	Same
Urobilinogen	Normal	Same
Glucose	Negative	Same
Ketone	Negative	Same
Occult blood	Negative	Same
Red blood cells (male)	0–3/high-power field	Same
Red blood cells (female)	0–5/high-power field	Same
White blood cells	0–5/high-power field	Same
Bacteria	Negative	Same
robilinogen		
Male	0.3–2.1 mg/2 hours	0.5–3.6 μmol/2 hours
Female	0.1–1.1 mg/2 hours	0.2–1.9 μmol/2 hours
ater deprivation		
Specific gravity	1.025–1.032	Same
Urine osmolarity	>800 mOsm/kg	>800 mmol/kg

Table continued on following page

APPENDIX C:
Clinical Laboratory Values
(Continued)

Normal Values: Body Fluids			
Body Fluid	**Name of Test**	**Conventional Values**	**SI Units**
Amniotic fluid	Amniotic fluid analysis		
	Chromosome analysis	Normal karyotype	Same
	Alpha$_1$-fetoprotein	0.5–3 Multiples of median (MoM)	Same
	Acetylcholinesterase	Negative	Same
	Rh incompatibility	Negative/1+	Same
	Bilirubin	0.01–0.03 mg/dl	0.02–0.06 μmol/L
	Creatinine		
	36 weeks' gestation	1.6–1.8 mg/dl	141–159 μmol/L
	37–38 weeks' gestation	>2 mg/dl	>177 μmol/L
	Lecithin to sphingomyelin ratio	>2	Same
	37–38 weeks' gestation		
	Phosphatidylglycerol	Present	Same
	Pulmonary surfactant	Positive; foam stability index, >0.48	Same
	Meconium	Absent	Same
Cerebrospinal fluid	Cerebrospinal fluid analysis		
	Pressure	90–180 mm H$_2$O	Same
	Appearance	Clear, colorless	Same
	Leukocyte count		
	Adult	0–5 cells/μl	0–5 $\times$ 10^6/L
	Child 5–18 years	0–10 cells/μl	0–10 $\times$ 10^6/L
	Neonate–1 year	0–30 cells/μl	0–30 $\times$ 10^6/L
	Lymphocytes (adult)	40–80%	0.4–0.8 fraction
	Monocytes	15–45%	0.15–0.45 fraction
	Neutrophils	0–6%	0–0.06 fraction
	Lymphocytes (neonate)	5–35%	0.05–0.35 fraction
	Monocytes	50–90%	0.5–0.9 fraction
	Neutrophils	0–8%	0–0.08 fraction
	Lactate	10–22 mg/dl	1.1–2.4 mmol/L
	Glucose	50–80 mg/dl	2.75–4.4 mmol/L
	Total protein	15–45 mg/dl	150–450 mg/L
	Albumin	10–30 mg/dl	100–300 mg/L
	IgG	1–4 mg/dl	10–40 mg/L
	Protein electrophoresis		
	Prealbumin	2–7%	0.02–0.07 fraction
	Albumin	56–76%	0.56–0.76 fraction
	Alpha$_1$-globulin	2–7%	0.02–0.07 fraction
	Alpha$_2$-globulin	4–12%	0.04–0.12 fraction
	Beta globulin	8–18%	0.08–0.18 fraction
	Gamma globulin	3–12%	0.03–0.12 fraction
	Myelin-basic protein	0–5% μg/L	Same
Effusion fluid	Carcinoembryonic antigen		
	Adult, nonsmoker	<2.5 ng/ml	2.5 g/L
	Adult, smoker	Up to 5 ng/ml	Up to 5 g/L
Gastric secretion	Gastric analysis		
	pH	<2	<2
	Basal acid output		
	Male	4.2 mEq/hour	4.2 mmol/hour
	Female	1.8 mEq/hour	1.8 mmol/hour
	Maximal acid output		
	Male	22.6 mEq/hour	22.6 mmol/hour
	Female	15.2 mEq/hour	15.2 mmol/hour
	Peak acid output		
	Male	35 mEq/hour	35 mmol/hour
	Female	25 mEq/hour	25 mmol/hour
	Basal acid output : maximal acid output	<0.4 (40%)	<0.4 (40%)

APPENDIX C:
Clinical Laboratory Values
(*Continued*)

Normal Values: Body Fluids			
Body Fluid	*Name of Test*	*Conventional Values*	*SI Units*
Peritoneal fluid	Peritoneal fluid analysis		
	Appearance	Clear, odorless, pale, yellow, scanty	Same
	Ammonia	<50 μg/dl	—
	Amylase	138–404 amylase units/L	Same
	Bacteria, fungi	None present	Same
	Cells	No malignant cells present	Same
	Glucose	70–90 mg/dl	3.89–4.99 mmol/L
	Protein	0.3–4.1 g/dl	3–41 g/L
	Red blood cells	None	None
	White blood cells	<300/μl	<300 × 10^6/L
Perspiration	Sweat test	5–40 mEq/L	5–40 mmol/L
Semen	Semen analysis		
	Appearance	Opalescent gray-white color	Same
	Volume	2–5 ml	0.002–0.005 L
	Liquefaction	10–60 minutes	Same
	pH	7.2–7.8	Same
	Acid phosphatase	>200 U/ejaculate	Same
	Citric acid	>52 μmol/ejaculate	Same
	Fructose	>13 μmol/ejaculate	Same
	Zinc	>2.4 μmol/ejaculate	Same
	Motility	>50%	>0.5 number fraction
	Concentration	20–250 × 10^6/ml	20–250 × 10^9/L
	Morphologic characteristics	>50% normal, mature spermatozoa	>0.5 number fraction
	Viability	>50% live spermatozoa	>0.5 number fraction
	Leukocytes	<1 × 10^6/ml	<1 × 10^9/L
Synovial fluid	Synovial fluid analysis		
	Appearance	Crystal clear, transparent, pale yellow	Same
	Viscosity	High	Same
	Volume	<3.5 ml	Same
	Red blood cells	Absent	Same
	White blood cells	0–200/mm³	0–200 × 10^6/L
	Nucleated cell count	<200 cells/μl	<200 × 10^6 cells/L
	Granulocytes	<25% of nucleated cells	<0.25 of nucleated cells; number fraction of granulocytes
	Protein	3 g/dl	30 g/L
	Uric acid	<8 mg/dl	476 mol/L
	Glucose (fasting)	70–110 mg/dl	3.9–6.1 mmol/L
	Blood-synovial fluid glucose difference	<10 mg/dl	<0.56 mmol/L
	Fibrin clot	Negative or absent	Same
	Mucin clot	Positive or abundant	Same
	String test	Formation of a long string	Same
	Culture	No growth	Same
	Rheumatoid factor	Negative	Same
Vaginal secretions	Prostatic acid phosphatase	<2 U/L	Same

* The values for premature neonates vary according to the degree of prematurity.
† Values are lower when the patient is in a supine position.
Modified from Malarkey LM, and McMorrow ME. *Nurse's Manual of Laboratory Tests and Diagnostic Procedures*. Philadelphia: WB Saunders, 1996, pp 942–969.

APPENDIX D:

Guideline for Isolation Precautions in Hospitals

◼ INTRODUCTION

To assist hospitals in maintaining up-to-date isolation practices, the Centers for Disease Control and Prevention (CDC) and the Hospital Infection Control Practices Advisory Committee (HICPAC) have revised the "CDC Guideline for Isolation Precautions in Hospitals."

The revised guideline contains 2 parts. Part I, "Evolution of Isolation Practices," reviews the evolution of isolation practices in U.S. hospitals, including their advantages, disadvantages, and controversial aspects, and provides the background for the HICPAC-consensus recommendations contained in Part II, "Recommendations for Isolation Precautions in Hospitals." The guideline supersedes previous CDC recommendations for isolation precautions in hospitals.

The guideline recommendations are based on the latest epidemiologic information on transmission of infection in hospitals. The recommendations are intended primarily for use in the care of patients in acute-care hospitals, although some of the recommendations may be applicable for some patients receiving care in subacute-care or extended-care facilities. The recommendations are not intended for use in daycare, well care, or domiciliary care programs. Because there have been few studies to test the efficacy of isolation precautions and gaps still exist in the knowledge of the epidemiology and modes of transmission of some diseases, disagreement with some of the recommendations is expected. A working draft of the guideline was reviewed by experts in infection control and published in the *Federal Register* for public comment. However, all recommendations in the guideline may not reflect the opinions of all reviewers.

◼ TYPES OF ISOLATION PRECAUTIONS

The "Guideline for Isolation Precautions in Hospitals" was revised to meet the following objectives: (1) to be epidemiologically sound; (2) to recognize the importance of all body fluids, secretions, and excretions in the transmission of nosocomial pathogens; (3) to contain adequate precautions for infections transmitted by the airborne, droplet, and contact routes of transmission; (4) to be as simple and user friendly as possible; and, (5) to use new terms to avoid confusion with existing infection control and isolation systems.

The revised guideline contains two tiers of precautions. In the first, and most important, tier are those precautions designed for the care of all patients in hospitals regardless of their diagnosis or presumed infection status. Implementation of these "Standard Precautions" is the primary strategy for successful nosocomial infection control. In the second tier are precautions designed only for the care of specified patients. These additional "Transmission-Based Precautions" are used for patients known or suspected to be infected or colonized with epidemiologically important pathogens that can be transmitted by airborne or droplet transmission or by contact with dry skin or contaminated surfaces.

Standard Precautions synthesize the major features of Universal (Blood and Body Fluid) Precautions (designed to reduce the risk of transmission of bloodborne pathogens) and Body Substance Isolation (designed to reduce the risk of transmission of pathogens from moist body substances). Standard Precautions apply to (1) blood; (2) all body fluids, secretions, and excretions *except sweat*, regardless of whether or not they contain visible blood; (3) nonintact skin; and, (4) mucous membranes. Standard Precautions are designed to reduce the risk of transmission of microorganisms from both recognized and unrecognized sources of infection in hospitals.

Transmission-Based Precautions are designed for patients documented or suspected to be infected or colonized with highly transmissble or epidemiologically important pathogens for which additional precautions beyond Standard Precautions are needed to interrupt transmission in hospitals. There are three types of Transmission-Based Precautions: Airborne Precautions, Droplet Precautions, and Contact Precautions. They may be combined for diseases that have multiple routes of transmission. When used either singularly or in combination, they are to be used in addition to Standard Precautions.

The revised guideline also lists specific clinical syndromes or conditions in both adult and pediatric patients that are highly suspicious for infection and identifies appropriate Transmission-Based Precautions to use on an empiric, temporary basis until a diagnosis can be made; these empiric, temporary precautions are also to be used in addition to Standard Precautions.

◼ RECOMMENDATIONS

The recommendations presented below are categorized as follows:

- *Category IA.* Strongly recommended for all hospitals and strongly supported by well-designed experimental or epidemiologic studies.
- *Category IB.* Strongly recommended for all hospitals and reviewed as effective by experts in the field and a con

sensus of HICPAC based on strong rationale and suggestive evidence, even though definitive scientific studies have not been done.

- *Category II.* Suggested for implementation in many hospitals. Recommendations may be supported by suggestive clinical or epidemiologic studies, a strong theoretical rationale, or definitive studies applicable to some, but not all, hospitals.
- *No recommendation; unresolved issue.* Practices for which insufficient evidence or consensus regarding efficacy exists.

The recommendations are limited to the topic of isolation precautions. Therefore, they must be supplemented by hospital policies and procedures for other aspects of infection and environmental control, occupational health, administrative and legal issues, and other issues beyond the scope of this guideline.

Administrative Controls

A. Education
   Develop a system to ensure that hospital patients, personnel, and visitors are educated about use of precautions and their responsibility for adherence to them. *Category IB*
B. Adherence to Precautions
   Periodically evaluate adherence to precautions, and use findings to direct improvements. *Category IB*

Standard Precautions

Use Standard Precautions, or the equivalent, for the care of all patients. *Category IB*

A. Hand washing
   (1) Wash hands after touching blood, body fluids, secretions, excretions, and contaminated items, whether or not gloves are worn. Wash hands immediately after gloves are removed, between patient contacts, and when otherwise indicated to avoid transfer of microorganisms to other patients or environments. It may be necessary to wash hands between tasks and procedures on the same patient to prevent cross-contamination of different body sites. *Category IB*
   (2) Use a plain (nonantimicrobial) soap for routine handwashing. *Category IB*
   (3) Use an antimicrobial agent or a waterless antiseptic agent for specific circumstances (e.g., control of outbreaks or hyperendemic infections), as defined by the infection control program. *Category IB* (See Contact Precautions for additional recommendations on using antimicrobial and antiseptic agents.)
B. Gloves
   Wear gloves (clean, nonsterile gloves are adequate) when touching blood, body fluids, secretions, excretions, and contaminated items. Put on clean gloves just before touching mucous membranes and nonintact skin. Change gloves between tasks and procedures on the same patient after contact with material that may contain a high concentration of microorganisms. Remove

gloves promptly after use, before touching noncontaminated items and environmental surfaces, and before going to another patient, and wash hands immediately to avoid transfer to microorganisms to other patients or environments. *Category IB*
C. Mask, Eye Protection, Face Shield
   Wear a mask and eye protection or a face shield to protect mucous membranes of the eyes, nose, and mouth during procedures and patient-care activities that are likely to generate splashes or sprays of blood, body fluids, secretions, and excretions. *Category IB*
D. Gown
   Wear a gown (a clean, nonsterile gown is adequate) to protect skin and to prevent soiling of clothing during procedures and patient-care activities that are likely to generate splashes or sprays of blood, body fluids, secretions, or excretions. Select a gown that is appropriate for the activity and amount of fluid likely to be encountered. Remove a soiled gown as promptly as possible, and wash hands to avoid transfer of microorganisms to other patients or environments. *Category IB*
E. Patient-Care Equipment
   Handle used patient-care equipment soiled with blood, body fluids, secretions, and excretions in a manner that prevents skin and mucous membrane exposures, contamination of clothing, and transfer of microorganisms to other patients and environments. Ensure that reusable equipment is not used for the care of another patient until it has been cleaned and reprocessed appropriately. Ensure that single-use items are discarded properly. *Category IB*
F. Environmental Control
   Ensure that the hospital has adequate procedures for the routine care, cleaning, and disinfection of environmental surfaces, beds, bedrails, bedside equipment, and other frequently touched surfaces, and ensure that these procedures are being followed. *Category IB*
G. Linen
   Handle, transport, and process used linen soiled with blood, body fluids, secretions, and excretions in a manner that prevents skin and mucous membrane exposures and contamination of clothing, and that avoids transfer of microorganisms to other patients and environments. *Category IB*
H. Occupational Health and Bloodborne Pathogens
   (1) Take care to prevent injuries when using needles, scalpels, and other sharp instruments or devices; when handling sharp instruments after procedures; when cleaning used instruments; and when disposing of used needles. Never recap used needles, or otherwise manipulate them using both hands, or use any other technique that involves directing the point of a needle toward any part of the body; rather, use either a one-handed "scoop" technique or a mechanical device designed for holding the needle sheath. Do not remove used needles from disposable syringes by hand, and do not bend, break, or otherwise manipulate used needles by hand. Place used disposable syringes and needles, scalpel blades, and other sharp items in appropriate puncture-resistant containers, which are located as close as practical to

the area in which the items were used, and place reusable syringes and needles in a puncture-resistant container for transport to the reprocessing area. *Category IB*

(2) Use mouthpieces, resuscitation bags, or other ventilation devices as an alternative to mouth-to-mouth resuscitation methods in areas where the need for resuscitation is predictable. *Category IB*

I. Patient Placement

Place a patient who comtaminates the environment or who does not (or cannot be expected to) assist in maintaining appropriate hygiene or environmental control in a private room. If a private room is not available, consult with infection control professionals regarding patient placement or other alternatives. *Category IB*

Airborne Precautions

In addition to Standard Precautions, use Airborne Precautions, or the equivalent, for patients known or suspected to be infected with microorganisms transmitted by airborne droplet nuclei (small-particle residue [5 μm or smaller in size] of evaporated droplets containing microorganisms that remain suspended in air and that can be dispersed widely by air currents within a room or over a long distance). *Category IB*

A. Patient Placement

Place the patient in a private room that has (1) monitored negative air pressure in relation to the surrounding areas, (2) 6 to 12 air changes per hour, and (3) appropriate discharge of air outdoors or monitored high-efficiency filtration of room air before the air is circulated to other areas in the hospital. Keep the room door closed and the patient in the room. When a private room is not available, place the patient in a room with a patient who has active infection with the same microorganism, unless otherwise recommended, but with no other infection. When a private room is not available and cohorting is not desirable, consultation with infection control professionals is advised before patient placement. *Category IB*

B. Respiratory Protection

Wear respiratory protection when entering the room of a patient with known or suspected infectious pulmonary tuberculosis. Susceptible persons should not enter the room of patients known or suspected to have measles (rubeola) or varicella (chickenpox) if other immune caregivers are available. If susceptible persons must enter the room of a patient known or suspected to have measles (rubeola) or varicella, they should wear respiratory protection. Persons immune to measles (rubeola) or varicella need not wear respiratory protection. *Category IB*

C. Patient Transport

Limit the movement and transport of the patient from the room to essential purposes only. If transport or movement is necessary, minimze patient dispersal of droplet nuclei by placing a surgical mask on the patient, if possible. *Category IB*

D. Additional Precautions for Preventing Transmission of Tuberculosis

Consult CDC "Guidelines for Preventing the Transmission of Tuberculosis in Health-Care Facilities" for additional prevention strategies.

Droplet Precautions

In addition to Standard Precautions, use Droplet Precautions, or the equivalent, for a patient known or suspected to be infected with microorganisms transmitted by droplets (large-particle droplets [larger than 5 μm in size] that can be generated by the patient during coughing, sneezing talking, or the performance of procedures). *Category IB*

A. Patient Placement

Place the patient in a private room. When a private room is not available, place the patient in a room with a patient(s) who has active infection with the same microorganism but with no other infection (cohorting). When a private room is not available and cohorting is not achievable, maintain spatial separation of at least 3 ft between the infected patient and other patients and visitors. Special air handling and ventilation are not necessary, and the door may remain open. *Category IB*

B. Mask

In addition to standard precautions, wear a mask when working within 3 ft of the patient. (Logistically, some hospitals may want to implement the wearing of a mask to enter the room.) *Category IB*

C. Patient Transport

Limit the movement and transport of the patient from the room to essential purposes only. If transport or movement is necessary, minimize patient dispersal of droplets by masking the patient, if possible. *Category IB*

Contact Precautions

In addition to Standard Precautions, use Contact Precautions, or the equivalent, for specified patients known or suspected to be infected or colonized with epidemiologically important microorganisms that can be transmitted by direct contact with the patient (hand or skin-to-skin contact that occurs when performing patient-care activities that require touching the patient's dry skin) or indirect contact (touching) with environmental surfaces or patient-care items in the patient's environment. *Category IB*

A. Patient Placement

Place the patient in a private room. When a private room is not available, place the patient in a room with a patient(s) who has active infection with the same microorganism but with no other infection (cohorting). When a private room is not available and cohorting is not achievable, consider the epidemiology of the microorganism and the patient population when determining patient placement. Consultation with infection control professionals is advised before patient placement. *Category IB*

B. Gloves and Handwashing

In addition to wearing gloves as outlined under Standard Precautions, wear gloves (clean, nonsterile gloves are adequate) when entering the room. During the course of providing care for a patient, change gloves after having contact with infective material that may contain high concentrations of microorganisms (fecal material and wound drainage). Remove gloves before leaving the patient's environment and wash hands immediately with an antimicrobial agent or a waterless antiseptic agent. After glove removal and handwashing, ensure that hands do not touch potentially contaminated environmental surfaces or items in the patient's room to avoid transfer of microorganisms to other patients or environments. *Category IB*

C. Gown

In addition to wearing a gown as outlined under Standard Precautions, wear a gown (a clean, nonsterile gown is adequate) when entering the room if you anticipate that your clothing will have substantial contact with the patient, environmental surfaces, or items in the patient's room, or if the patient is incontinent or has diarrhea, an ileostomy, a colostomy, or wound drainage not contained by a dressing. Remove the gown before leaving the patient's environment. After gown removal, ensure that clothing does not contact potentially contaminated environmental surfaces to avoid transfer of microorganisms to other patients or environments. *Category IB*

D. Patient Transport

Limit the movement and transport of the patient from the room to essential purposes only. If the patient is transported out of the room, ensure that precautions are maintained to minimize the risk of transmission of microorganisms to other patients and contamination of environmental surfaces or equipment. *Category IB*

E. Patient-Care Equipment

When possible, dedicate the use of noncritical patient-care equipment to a single patient (or cohort of patients infected or colonized with the pathogen requiring precautions) to avoid sharing between patients. If use of common equipment or items is unavoidable, then adequately clean and disinfect them before use for another patient. *Category IB*

F. Additional Precautions for Preventing the Spread of Vancomycin Resistance

Consult the HICPAC report on preventing the spread of vancomycin resistance for additional prevention strategies.

From Garner JS, Hospital Infection Control Practices Advisory Committee. *Guideline for Isolation Precautions in Hospitals.* Public Health Service, US Dept. of Health and Human Services, Centers for Disease Control and Prevention, Atlanta, GA, 1996.

Index

ISBN 0-7216-5017-1

PROCEDURES